ICD-10-CM Mappings

Linking ICD-9-CM to All Valid ICD-10-CM Alternatives

2016

Publisher's Notice

The *ICD-10-CM Mappings* is designed to be an accurate and authoritative source regarding coding and every reasonable effort has been made to ensure accuracy and completeness of the content. However, Optum360 makes no guarantee, warranty, or representation that this publication is accurate, complete or without errors. It is understood that Optum360 is not rendering any legal or other professional services or advice in this publication and that Optum360 bears no liability for any results or consequences that may arise from the use of this book.

Our Commitment to Accuracy

Optum360 is committed to producing accurate and reliable materials.

To report corrections, please visit www.optumcoding.com/accuracy or email accuracy@optum.com. You can also reach customer service by calling 1.800.464.3649, option 1.

Acknowledgments

Lauri Gray, RHIT, CPC, AHIMA-Approved ICD-10-CM/PCS Trainer, *Product Manager*
Karen Schmidt, BSN, *Technical Director*
Stacy Perry, *Manager, Desktop Publishing*
Lisa Singley, *Project Manager*
Karen Krawzik, RHIT, CCS, AHIMA-Approved ICD-10-CM/PCS Trainer, *Clinical/Technical Editor*
Peggy Willard, CCS, AHIMA-Approved ICD-10-CM/PCS Trainer, *Clinical/Technical Editor*
Tracy Betzler, *Senior Desktop Publishing Specialist*
Hope M. Dunn, *Senior Desktop Publishing Specialist*
Katie Russell, *Desktop Publishing Specialist*
Kate Holden, *Editor*

Copyright

Made in the USA
ISBN 978-1-62254-026-6

Technical Editors

Karen Krawzik, RHIT, CCS, AHIMA-Approved ICD-10-CM/PCS Trainer
Clinical/Technical Editor

Ms. Krawzik has expertise in ICD-10-CM, ICD-9-CM, and CPT/HCPCS coding. Her coding experience includes inpatient, ambulatory surgery, and ancillary and emergency room records. She has served as a DRG analyst and auditor of commercial and government payer claims, and as a contract administrator. Most recently she was responsible for the conversion of the ICD-9-CM code set to ICD-10 and for analyzing audit results, identifying issues and trends, and developing remediation plans. Ms. Krawzik is credentialed by the American Health Information Management Association (AHIMA) as a Certified Coding Specialist (CCS) and is an AHIMA-approved ICD-10-CM/PCS trainer. She is an active member of AHIMA and the Missouri Health Information Management Association.

Peggy Willard, CCS, AHIMA-Approved ICD-10-CM/PCS Trainer
Clinical/Technical Editor

Ms. Willard has several years of experience in Level I Adult and Pediatric Trauma hospital coding, specializing in ICD-9-CM, DRG, and CPT coding. She has been extensively trained in ICD-10-CM and PCS. Her recent experience includes in-depth analysis of medical record documentation, ICD-10-CM code assignment, and DRG shifts based on ICD-10-CM code assignment. Ms. Willard's expertise includes conducting coding audits, conducting coding training for coding staff and clinical documentation specialists, and creating internal ICD-10-CM coding guidelines/tips. Ms. Willard is an active member of the American Health Information Management Association (AHIMA) and the Minnesota Health Information Management Association (MHIMA).

Summary of Changes

ICD-10 GEMs FY2016 Version Update

Update Summary

Examples of the official updated GEMs entries are provided in the following pages.

ICD-10-CM to ICD-9-CM GEM entry for "Persistent atrial fibrillation"

2015 entry		Updated 2016 entry	
I48.1	Persistent atrial fibrillation	I48.1	Persistent atrial fibrillation
To		To	
427.32	Atrial flutter	427.31	Atrial fibrillation

Comment: Typographical error. The ICD-10-CM code specifies atrial fibrillation.

ICD-10-CM to ICD-9-CM GEM entry for "thoracic disc disorder with radiculopathy"

2015 entry		Updated 2016 entry	
Example		Example	
M51.14	Intervertebral disc disorders with radiculopathy, thoracic region	M51.14	Intervertebral disc disorders with radiculopathy, thoracic region
M51.15	Intervertebral disc disorders with radiculopathy, thoracolumbar region	M51.15	Intervertebral disc disorders with radiculopathy, thoracolumbar region
To		To	
724.4	Thoracic or lumbosacral neuritis or radiculitis, unspecified	722.92	Other and unspecified disc disorder, thoracic region

Comment: The updated entry is a closer match. The ICD-9-CM tabular instruction for 724.4 excludes radiculitis due to intervertebral disc disorder.

ICD-10-CM to ICD-9-CM GEM entry for "lumbar disc disorder with radiculopathy"

2015 entry		Updated 2016 entry	
Example		Example	
M51.16	Intervertebral disc disorders with radiculopathy, lumbar region	M51.16	Intervertebral disc disorders with radiculopathy, lumbar region
M51.17	Intervertebral disc disorders with radiculopathy, lumbosacral region	M51.17	Intervertebral disc disorders with radiculopathy, lumbosacral region
To		To	
724.4	Thoracic or lumbosacral neuritis or radiculitis, unspecified	722.93	Other and unspecified disc disorder, lumbar region

Comment: The updated entry is a closer match. The ICD-9-CM tabular instruction for 724.4 excludes radiculitis due to intervertebral disc disorder.

ICD-10-CM to ICD-9-CM GEM entry for "Hydronephrosis with ureteral stricture"

2015 entry	Updated 2016 entry
N13.1 Hydronephrosis with ureteral stricture, not elsewhere classified To 591 Hydronephrosis	N13.1 Hydronephrosis with ureteral stricture, not elsewhere classified To *Choice List 1* 591 Hydronephrosis AND *Choice List 2* 593.3 Stricture or kinking of ureter

Comment: The updated entry is a more complete translation of the condition specified in the ICD-10-CM code. N13.1 is a combination code, and requires an ICD-9-CM translation cluster specifying both the hydronephrosis and the ureteral stricture.

ICD-10-CM to ICD-9-CM GEM entry for "Hydronephrosis with renal/ureteral calculous"

2015 entry	Updated 2016 entry
N13.2 Hydronephrosis with renal and ureteral calculous obstruction To 591 Hydronephrosis	N13.2 Hydronephrosis with renal and ureteral calculous obstruction To *Choice List 1* 591 Hydronephrosis AND *Choice List 2* 592.Ø Calculus of kidney OR 592.1 Calculus of ureter OR 592.9 Urinary calculus, unspecified

Comment: The updated entry is a more complete translation of the condition specified in the ICD-10-CM code. N13.2 is a combination code, and requires an ICD-9-CM translation cluster specifying both the hydronephrosis and the urinary calculus.

ICD-9-CM to ICD-10-CM GEM entries for "Open skull fracture with concussion"

2015 entry	Updated 2016 entry
Example 8ØØ.99 Open fracture of vault of skull with intracranial injury of other and unspecified nature, unspecified concussion 8Ø1.99 Open fracture of base of skull with intracranial injury of other and unspecified nature, unspecified concussion 8Ø3.99 Other open skull fracture with intracranial injury of other and unspecified nature, unspecified concussion To *Choice List 1* SØ2.ØXXA Fracture of vault of skull, initial encounter for closed fracture AND *Choice List 2* SØ6.89ØA Other specified intracranial injury without loss of consciousness, initial encounter OR SØ6.9X9A Unspecified intracranial injury with loss of consciousness of unspecified duration, initial encounter	Example 8ØØ.99 Open fracture of vault of skull with intracranial injury of other and unspecified nature, unspecified concussion 8Ø1.99 Open fracture of base of skull with intracranial injury of other and unspecified nature, unspecified concussion 8Ø3.99 Other open skull fracture with intracranial injury of other and unspecified nature, unspecified concussion To *Choice List 1* SØ2.ØXXA Fracture of vault of skull, initial encounter for closed fracture AND *Choice List 2* SØ6.89ØA Other specified intracranial injury without loss of consciousness, initial encounter OR SØ6.9XØA Unspecified intracranial injury without loss of consciousness, initial encounter

Comment: Typographical error. 800.99, 801.99 and 803.99 are translated to S06.9X9A in choice list 2 of the cluster. This has been changed to S06.9X0A.

Contents

Preface

The *International Classification of Diseases, 10th Revision, Clinical Modification* (ICD-10-CM) is an advanced coding and classification system which has been developed to accommodate the ever-changing needs of the health care industry, incorporating changes in medical science, clinical terminology, and technology. As a result, the ICD-10-CM classification system includes exponentially more specific data granularity than does ICD-9-CM, such as extensive, updated clinical concepts, patient encounter information, different classification axes, and anatomic designations not included in ICD-9-CM. Therefore, making correlations between codes in the two classification systems requires some decision making because there may be more than one code alternative in the other code set. *ICD-10-CM Mappings: Linking ICD-9-CM to All Valid ICD-10-CM Alternatives* is a translation tool providing all valid alternative code choices designated in the official Diagnosis Code Set General Equivalence Mappings (GEM), 2016 Version, released by the National Centers for Health Statistics (NCHS).

ICD-10-CM Mappings serves as a companion to the ICD-9-CM and ICD-10-CM code sets and is designed to assist in training and preparation processes for the transition to the new coding classification system. It is an essential tool in the transition process for any health care entity. This manual presents the official general equivalence mapping results in an easy-to-use table format. The organization of the tables assumes the user is more familiar with reporting and collecting coded data using ICD-9-CM. Therefore, the information is arranged numerically by ICD-9-CM code and then by ICD-9-CM chapters. Each ICD-9-CM code will be presented with all valid ICD-10-CM code alternatives that reflect the clinical meaning of the ICD-9-CM code. *ICD-10-CM Mappings* is the first step in the process of determining the best alternatives for ICD-9-CM codes. In order to attain reasonable mapping results, code set tabular instructions, index entries, guidelines, and coding advice must also be considered when selecting the most appropriate translations. Using *ICD-10-CM Mappings* in concert with the ICD-10-CM code book will help the user determine the best translation results.

The key benefits of *ICD-10-CM Mappings* are to:

- Provide a quick reference to validate ICD-10-CM coding accuracy and the decision logic for encoder or other software applications
- Serve as a cost-effective alternative to the purchase of certain software applications
- Help focus internal coding training on those sections of the code set most important to the facility or practice to assist in focusing the efforts of the hospital, facility or physician practice on the critical coding and documentation issues which pose significant challenges to the reimbursement process and maintaining data integrity
- Verify code selections on updated forms, reports, and all other data systems

Mapping is not a straightforward correlation between codes of the two classification systems, and caution must be exercised when using the information provided. The user of the mapping data must determine the best decision-making process when selecting the best code alternatives based upon the documentation available and the ultimate use of the data. Also, each health care entity has unique documentation and treatment profiles that impact code alternative selections. It is the responsibility of the user of the mapping data to evaluate those factors, review all code choices provided, and reference the ICD-10-CM classification system to verify code selection.

Official Classification Systems

ICD-10-CM Mappings references two classification systems, both of which are maintained and updated by the federal committee, the ICD-10-CM Coordination and Maintenance Committee. The following information below specifies the version of each system included in this manual.

ICD-9-CM

The *International Classification of Diseases, 9th Revision, Clinical Modification* (ICD-9-CM) codes in this manual are consistent with the government's version of ICD-9-CM effective October 1, 2014, through September 30, 2015. **Note:** The codes provided in the official GEMs released in May 2015 include the code updates to ICD-9-CM effective October 1, 2014.

ICD-10-CM

The *International Classification of Diseases, 10th Revision, Clinical Modification* (ICD-10-CM) is the United States' clinical modification of the World Health Organization's ICD-10, the *International Statistical Classification of Diseases and Related Health Problems, 10th Revision*. ICD-10 is also the classification used in cause-of-death coding in the United States. The WHO Collaborating Center for the Family of International Classifications (FIC) in North America, housed at the National Center for Health Statistics (NCHS), has responsibility for the implementation of ICD and other WHO-FIC classifications and serves as a liaison with WHO, fulfilling international obligations for comparable classifications and the national health data needs of the U.S.

The ICD-10-CM classification system conforms to the conventions of ICD-10. The term clinical is used to emphasize the modification's intent: to serve as a useful tool in the area of classification of morbidity data for indexing of medical records, medical care review, and ambulatory and other medical care programs, as well as for basic health statistics. To describe the clinical picture of the patient, codes must be more precise than those needed only for statistical groupings and trend analysis.

ICD-10-CM far exceeds its predecessor ICD-9-CM in the number of clinical concepts, body part specificity, patient encounter information, and classification axes. To include health-related conditions and to provide greater specificity, ICD-10-CM has been expanded to the sixth-digit level with a seventh character extension. The sixth and seventh characters are not optional; when provided, they are required for recording the information documented in the clinical record.

General Equivalence Mappings (GEM)

The National Center for Health Statistics (NCHS) is the U.S. government agency that, jointly with the Centers for Medicare and Medicaid Services (CMS), refines the diagnostic portion of ICD-9-CM and is responsible for the modification of ICD-10-CM. The current official 2016 release of ICD-10-CM, including guidelines and General Equivalency Mapping (GEM) files, may be downloaded from the NCHS website at: http://www.cdc.gov/nchs/icd/icd10cm.htm or CMS' website at: http://www.cms.gov/Medicare/Coding/ICD10/2016-ICD-10-CM-and-GEMs.html.

Note: The GEM files do not include code titles and are source files that include the code pairs and the attribute codes, or computer logic flags, that define the relationship between the code pairs. These are raw files intended to be used by healthcare entities to design and create mapping applications.

Introduction

On January 16, 2009, the Department of Health and Human Services (HHS) published a final rule in the *Federal Register,* 45 CFR part 162, "HIPAA Administrative Simplification: Modifications to Medical Data Code Set Standards to Adopt ICD-10-CM and ICD-10-PCS." This final rule adopts modifications to standard medical data code sets for coding diagnoses and inpatient hospital procedures by adopting ICD-10-CM for diagnosis coding, including the Official ICD-10-CM Guidelines for Coding and Reporting, and ICD-10-PCS for inpatient hospital procedure coding, effective October 1, 2013. This rule may be downloaded at: http://edocket.access.gpo.gov/2009/pdf/E9-743.pdf.

On April 17, 2012, HHS released notice to postpone the date by which certain health care entities have to comply with International Classification of Diseases, 10th Edition diagnosis and procedure codes (ICD-10). The compliance date for implementation of ICD-10-CM and ICD-10-PCS as a replacement for ICD-9-CM was postponed to October 1, 2014.

The ICD-9-CM Coordination and Maintenance Committee implemented a partial code set freeze of the ICD-10-CM codes prior to the initial implementation date of October 1, 2013. As a result, on October 1, 2013, there were only limited code updates to the ICD-10-CM code sets to capture new technologies and diseases as required by section 503(a) of Pub. L. 108-173.

The ICD-10 Coordination and Maintenance Committee (formerly the ICD-9-CM Coordination and Maintenance Committee) implemented a partial freeze of the ICD-9-CM and ICD-10 (ICD-10-CM and ICD-10-PCS) codes prior to the implementation of ICD-10 which would end one year after the implementation of ICD-10.

On April 1, 2014, the Protecting Access to Medicare Act of 2014 (PAMA) (Pub. L. No. 113-93) was enacted with a provision that stated that the Secretary of Health and Human Services may not adopt ICD-10 prior to October 1, 2015.

The U.S. Department of Health and Human Services issued an interim final rule on August 4, 2014 finalizing October 1, 2015 as the new ICD-10 compliance date. This rule will also require HIPAA covered entities to continue to use ICD-9-CM through September 30, 2015. This interim final rule may be viewed at http://www.gpo.gov/fdsys/pkg/FR-2014-08-04/pdf/2014-18347.pdf

The partial freeze will be implemented as follows:

- The last regular, annual updates to both ICD-9-CM and ICD-10 code sets were made on October 1, 2011.
- On October 1, 2012, October 1, 2013, October 1, 2014, and October 1, 2015 there will be only limited code updates to to ICD-10 code sets to capture new technologies and diseases as required by section 503(a) of Pub. L. 108-173.

ICD-10-CM is an advanced coding and classification system, and as such, the inherent classification and terminology revisions, coupled with the increased detail, have resulted in code classifications that are exponentially more specific. To facilitate the conversion from ICD-9-CM to ICD-10-CM and to establish a common translation baseline, the general equivalence mappings (GEMs) were developed by the government as official tools that serve as general purpose translations for all types of health care entities. The GEM files were developed to be used in varied coded data use applications, but not as a quick reference or as a general resource. Therefore, *ICD-10-CM Mappings* was developed to translate the mappings for general use in an easy-to-use format. All mappings contained in this manual are based on the official GEM files.

General equivalence mappings are relationships established between corresponding code sets in which the most likely code linkages are provided for the user. In certain circumstances, the relationships and linkages between the code sets are fairly close—at times a one-to-one correlation. However, in many cases, this direct linkage is not possible. Mappings can result in multiple translation alternatives in ICD-10-CM to represent the complete meaning of the code in ICD-9-CM.

The version GEM files represented in this manual are between ICD-10-CM and ICD-9-CM (volumes 1 and 2). These mappings are differentiated from "crosswalks" in that their purpose is to help the user navigate between systems, translate code meanings, and compare and analyze data. From these mappings, users may develop customized mappings suited to their individual needs.

Because both systems are revisions of the International Classification of Diseases, they have much in common. The organization, formatting, and conventions of the two systems are similar, and as a result, many mappings are straightforward. However, due to the increased data granularity (specificity) of the 10th revision, a series of possible code choices are often presented as linkages between certain codes. For example, ICD-10-CM contains certain severity and anatomic specificity data elements that ICD-9-CM does not provide. In such cases, a seamless linkage is not possible.

The mappings included in this manual are bi-directional, meaning that the alternative code translations in both the ICD-9-CM to ICD-10-CM (forward) mapping and the ICD-10-CM to ICD-9-CM (backward) mapping are provided. It is important to recognize that differences in mapping results generally are due to the differences in clinical concepts, classification axes, and specific conventions between the two systems. It is the responsibility of the user of the mapping data to evaluate those factors, review all code choices provided, and reference the ICD-10-CM classification system to verify code selections.

Reconciliation methods between the two systems may vary according to the intended use of the data. For example, data needs for claims adjudication may not be the same as those for research or statistical analysis. Following are a few mapping characteristics to consider when deciding on a reconciliation method:

- One-to-one mapping: Provides a direct code-to-code linkage, which offers the most likely code choice or "best compromise" between codes (e.g., claims analysis)
- One-to-many mapping: Provides a comparison of all possible code linkages (e.g., statistical analysis, data trending, epidemiology)
- Forward mapping: Translation of existing ICD-9-CM coding data into ICD-10-CM equivalents
- Backward mapping: Translation of ICD-10-CM information back to ICD-9-CM for comparison

Each of these characteristics of mapping is discussed in the following sections and presented with examples and cautions.

One-to-One Mapping

Because ICD-9-CM and ICD-10-CM share a common heritage as classification systems, many of the clinical concepts and conventions have been continued. In these cases, the mapping is considered "equivalent" in both forward and backward mappings.

Example

ICD-9-CM

ØØ1.9 Unspecified cholera

ICD-1Ø-CM

AØØ.9 Cholera unspecified

One-to-one mappings exist where certain variables such as severity indicators, axis refinements, and anatomic specificity have been built into the ICD-10-CM system and the mapping is considered "approximate." Certain clinical concepts and code axes in ICD-9-CM have been deemed nonessential, no longer clinically accurate, or pertinent. In these cases, code descriptions or classifications have been either eliminated or reassigned in ICD-10-CM. For example, state of control is no longer a factor in code assignment for diabetes mellitus. ICD-10-CM diabetes mellitus codes are combination codes that indicate the type (I or II), the body system affected, and the presence and nature of certain complications.

Example

Type 1 diabetes mellitus, without mention of complication

ICD-9-CM

25Ø.Ø1 Diabetes, without mention of complication, type I [juvenile type], not stated as uncontrolled

ICD-1Ø-CM

E1Ø.9 Type 1 diabetes mellitus without complication

In ICD-10-CM, code classifications for diabetes mellitus no longer include the clinical concept of "controlled" or "uncontrolled" disease. Therefore, the one-to-one mapping is considered 'approximate' rather than 'equivalent' since the two classification systems do not contain exactly the same clinical concepts.

The complete meaning of a code must include consideration of the coding instructions and guidelines of the code sets. Use of the *ICD-10-CM Mappings* in concert with the ICD-10-CM code book ensures the best translation results.

One-to-Many Mapping

ICD-10-CM contains a greater number of codes with a higher level of specificity than ICD-9-CM. Therefore, in most cases, one ICD-9-CM code is mapped to multiple ICD-10-CM codes.

Example

Carpal tunnel syndrome

ICD-9-CM

354.Ø	Carpal tunnel syndrome

ICD-1Ø-CM

G56.ØØ	Carpal tunnel syndrome, unspecified upper limb
G56.Ø1	Carpal tunnel syndrome, right upper limb
G56.Ø2	Carpal tunnel syndrome, left upper limb

In the example above, the inclusion of laterality in ICD-10-CM for classifying carpal tunnel syndrome creates a one-to-many code linkage from ICD-9-CM to ICD-10-CM.

There are cases in which one ICD-10-CM code maps to multiple ICD-9-CM codes. This occurs when a classification axis that provided greater detail in ICD-9-CM no longer exists in ICD-10-CM.

Example

ICD-9-CM

Ø1Ø.ØØ	Primary tuberculous infection, unspecified
Ø1Ø.Ø1	Primary tuberculous infection, bacteriologic or histological examination not done
Ø1Ø.Ø2	Primary tuberculous infection, bacteriologic or histological examination unknown (at present)
Ø1Ø.Ø3	Primary tuberculous infection, tubercle bacilli found (in sputum) by microscopy
Ø1Ø.Ø4	Primary tuberculous infection, tubercle bacilli not found (in sputum) by microscopy, but found by bacterial culture
Ø1Ø.Ø5	Primary tuberculous infection, tubercle bacilli not found by bacteriological examination, but tuberculosis confirmed histologically
Ø1Ø.Ø6	Primary tuberculous infection, not found by bacteriological or histological examination but tuberculosis confirmed by other methods [inoculation of animals]

ICD-1Ø-CM

A15.7	Primary respiratory tuberculosis

The fifth-digit assignment choices for ICD-9-CM subcategory 010.0 describe the method of diagnosis confirmation, but this axis of classification is not included in ICD-10-CM. Therefore, each code in the 010.00–010.06 range maps to the single ICD-10-CM code A15.7. This is a many-to-one scenario in the forward mapping.

Review of all the alternatives provided by the mappings is critical for selecting the best translation according to the documentation available and the use of the coded data.

Introduction

Combination Codes

ICD-10-CM uses combination code conventions similar to those in ICD-9-CM. A combination code is a single code used to describe both the diagnosis and the associated manifestation, complication, or cause. Codes in either system may be linked to more than one code, depending on the nature of the classification changes. For example, two ICD-9-CM codes are required to describe diabetes with gangrene. In ICD-10-CM one code describes both the underlying condition (type I diabetes mellitus with peripheral circulatory disorders) as well as the manifestation (gangrene).

Example

ICD-9-CM

250.71	Diabetes with peripheral circulatory disorders, type I [juvenile type], not stated as uncontrolled
443.81	Peripheral angiopathy in diseases classified elsewhere
785.4	Gangrene

ICD-10-CM

E10.52	Type 1 diabetes with diabetic peripheral angiopathy w gangrene

Mapping Caution: In the example above, type I diabetes mellitus with peripheral circulatory disorders, is linked to E10.51 Type 1 diabetes with diabetic peripheral angiopathy without gangrene in the forward (ICD-9-CM to ICD-10-CM) mapping and is indicated as "approximate." In the backward mapping (ICD-10-CM to ICD-9-CM) type I diabetes mellitus with peripheral circulatory disorders is linked to three ICD-10-CM code alternatives.

E10.51	Type 1 diabetes with diabetic peripheral angiopathy w/o gangrene
E10.52	Type 1 diabetes with diabetic peripheral angiopathy w gangrene
E10.59	Type 1 diabetes mellitus with other circulatory complications

Since the combination of DM with gangrene is not absolute and either 250.71or 785.4 may be assigned in combination or separately depending upon the circumstances, there are several alternative code choices provided by the mappings for code 250.71. The proper mapping selection must be made from a list of alternatives. It is critical to consider both the ICD-9-CM and the ICD-10-CM coding guidelines and instructions when selecting the most appropriate alternative for a given coding issue.

In the following example, changes to the ICD-10-CM structure result in one-to-many linkages in the backward mapping.

Example

ICD-9-CM

555.0	Regional enteritis of small intestine
560.9	Unspecified intestinal obstruction

ICD-10-CM

K50.012	Crohn's disease of small intestine with intestinal obstruction

Scenarios

The GEMs include combinations, or groups, of codes that are necessary to satisfy the complete meaning of an ICD-9-CM code. There are also instances when there could be several combinations, any of which might satisfy the meaning of an ICD-9-CM code. When there are several groups of combinations, they are referred to as "scenarios."

Example

ICD-9-CM

806.00	Closed cervical fracture C1-C4 level with unspecified spinal cord injury

ICD-10-CM

Scenario 1: Closed fracture at **C1** cervical spine level

S14.101A	Unspecified injury at C1 level of cervical spinal cord, initial encounter
S12.000A	Unspecified displaced fracture of 1st cervical vertebra, initial encounter for closed fracture
S12.001A	Unspecified nondisplaced fracture of 1st cervical vertebra, initial encounter for closed fracture

Scenario 2: Closed fracture at **C2** cervical spine level

S14.1Ø2A Unspecified injury at C2 level of cervical spinal cord, initial encounter

S12.1ØØA Unspecified displaced fracture of 2nd cervical vertebra, initial encounter for closed fracture

S12.1Ø1A Unspecified nondisplaced fracture of 2nd cervical vertebra, initial encounter for closed fracture

Scenario 3: Closed fracture at **C3** cervical spine level

S14.1Ø3A Unspecified injury at C3 level of cervical spinal cord, initial encounter

S12.2ØØA Unspecified displaced fracture of 3rd cervical vertebra, initial encounter for closed fracture

S12.2Ø1A Unspecified nondisplaced fracture of 3rd cervical vertebra, initial encounter for closed fracture

Scenario 4: Closed fracture at **C4** cervical spine level

S14.1Ø4A Unspecified injury at C4 level of cervical spinal cord, initial encounter

S12.3ØØA Unspecified displaced fracture of 4th cervical vertebra, initial encounter for closed fracture

S12.3Ø1A Unspecified nondisplaced fracture of 4th cervical vertebra, initial encounter for closed fracture

The ICD-9-CM code describes a closed fracture of the vertebral column with spinal cord injury at C1-C4. ICD-10-CM has separate codes for each of the cervical levels. As a result, there are four coding scenarios that describe the vertebral fracture with spinal cord injury at each cervical level.

Conventions Used in *ICD-10-CM Mappings*

To use this mapping manual appropriately, the user must first understand the format, organization, and symbols in the guide. The codes and mapping relationships are based on the most recently updated GEM mapping file released in May 2015. All codes and code titles are based on the ICD-9-CM codes effective October 1, 2014, through September 30, 2015, and the ICD-10-CM version 2016.

- **Format:** The manual is formatted in two columns. The first column contains the ICD-9-CM diagnosis codes in numerical order with an abbreviated code title. The second column contains the ICD-10-CM diagnosis code(s) with abbreviated code titles that map to the ICD-9-CM codes using both forward and backward mapping. Every other row is shaded to make it easier to track across the row.
- **Organization:** The manual is organized into the same chapters as the ICD-9-CM code book. Dictionary headings at the top and outside edge of each page provide the name of the chapter and the range of ICD-9-CM codes contained on that page.
- **Code Titles:** Both ICD-9-CM and ICD-10-CM codes are provided with abbreviated code titles, which are necessary to accommodate the format of the manual. An abbreviation key is provided as Appendix B.

  Note: The ICD-10-CM code titles are the official sixty character abbreviation released by the Centers for Medicare and Medicaid Services (CMS).
- **Symbols:** The following symbols are used in the manual:

  European zero: Because ICD-10-CM uses the letter O, which could be confused with the number zero (0), this mapping guide uses a European zero, which contains a slanted vertical line through the character. This differentiates all zeroes from those ICD-10-CM codes that begin with the letter O.

Example

ICD-9-CM		ICD-10-CM	
63Ø	HYDATIDIFORM MOLE	**OØ1.Ø** **OØ1.1** **OØ1.9**	CLASSICAL HYDATIDIFORM MOLE INCOMPLETE AND PARTIAL HYDATIDIFORM MOLE HYDATIDIFORM MOLE UNSPECIFIED

Equivalent Mapping: The arrow symbol ➡ designates a mapping relationship that is considered an "Equivalent Mapping." The clinical concept between the two codes in ICD-9-CM and ICD-10-CM are considered completely equivalent.

Example

ICD-9-CM		ICD-10-CM		
593.1	HYPERTROPHY OF KIDNEY	➡	**N28.81**	HYPERTROPHY OF KIDNEY

Users should be aware that just because a target ICD-10-CM code does not have an arrow, it does not mean that the clinical concepts are completely dissimilar. There may be additional clinical concepts that add specificity in ICD-10-CM that should be considered. For example, ICD-9-CM code 595.0 represents acute cystitis. In the ICD-9-CM to ICD-10-CM forward mapping, the code is mapped to two ICD-10-CM codes, N30.00 and N30.01.

Example

ICD-9-CM		ICD-10-CM	
595.Ø	ACUTE CYSTITIS	**N3Ø.ØØ**	ACUTE CYSTITIS WITHOUT HEMATURIA
		N3Ø.Ø1	ACUTE CYSTITIS WITH HEMATURIA

ICD-10-CM combines the clinical concepts of cystitis and hematuria, which ICD-9-CM does not. Therefore, although both N30.0- codes are mapped to 595.0, it is not considered an equivalent mapping because an additional code for the hematuria would be required in ICD-9-CM coding for the clinical concepts to match. Both of the examples above are considered one-to-one mapping relationships, yet one is equivalent and the other approximate. One code from the source system is mapped to one code option in the target system

See Appendix A: The flag symbol ◘ designates those code mapping relationships that require multiple ICD-9-CM codes to satisfy the clinical concepts described in one ICD-10-CM code in the backward mapping:

Example

ICD-9-CM		ICD-10-CM		
Ø15.ØØ	TUBERCULOSIS VERTEBRAL COLUMN CONF UNSPEC	◘	**A18.Ø1**	TUBERCULOSIS OF SPINE

Appendix A provides all the ICD-9-CM code combinations required to complete the meaning of A18.01 tuberculosis of the spine.

A18.Ø1 Ø15.ØØ and 711.48; Ø15.ØØ and 72Ø.81; Ø15.ØØ and 73Ø.88; Ø15.ØØ and 737.4Ø

There are four coding scenarios for this particular example: tuberculosis of the spine maps back to arthropathy associated with tuberculosis, inflammatory spondylopathy due to tuberculosis, other infections (tuberculosis) involving bone, and curvature of the spine due to tuberculosis.

- **Scenarios: Use of "and" and "or" Operators:**
  GEM scenarios are the combinations of ICD-10-CM codes that are required to satisfy the meaning of an ICD-9-CM code. The user must take special note of the "and" and "or" operators found throughout the mapping guide. Whenever these operators appear, they are shaded in red as an alert that additional selection logic must be applied.

Example

ICD-9-CM		ICD-10-CM		
Ø73.Ø	ORNITHOSIS WITH PNEUMONIA	**A7Ø**	CHLAMYDIA PSITTACI INFECTIONS	*and*
		J17	PNEUMONIA IN DISEASES CLASSIFIED ELSEWHERE	

The equivalent clinical concept of the ICD-9-CM code for ornithosis with pneumonia requires both ICD-10-CM codes A7Ø and J17 to be assigned.

In the following example, the ICD-9-CM code specifies that the traumatic amputation is bilateral but does not specify whether it is partial or complete. Because both pieces of information — left or right foot and partial or complete amputation — are specified in separate codes in ICD-10-CM, the entry in the ICD-9-CM to ICD-10-CM GEM is a "scenario" entry. Because two ICD-10-CM codes are required to satisfy the equivalent meaning in the ICD-9-CM combination code, and because the injury can be partial on one side and complete on the other, both sides partial, or both sides complete, there are four different scenarios from which to select based upon available documentation.

Example

ICD-9-CM		ICD-10-CM		
896.2	TRAUMATIC AMP FT BILATERAL WITHOUT MENTION COMP	**S98.911A**	COMPLETE TRAUMAT AMP RT FT LEVEL UNS INITIAL ENC	*or*
		S98.921A	PART TRAUMAT AMP RT FT LEVEL UNS INITIAL ENC	*and*
		S98.912A	COMPLETE TRAUMAT AMP LT FT LEVEL UNS INITIAL ENC	*or*
		S98.922A	PART TRAUMATIC AMP LT FT LEVEL UNS INITIAL ENC	

Example

ICD-9-CM		ICD-10-CM		
912.7	SHLDR & UPPER ARM SUP FB NO MAJ OPN WOUND INFECTED	**S4Ø.259A**	SUPERFICIAL FB UNS SHOULDER INITIAL ENC	*or*
		S4Ø.859A	SUPERFICIAL FB UNS UPPER ARM INITIAL ENC	*and*
		LØ8.89	OTH SPEC LOCAL INFECTIONS THE SKIN & SUBQ TISSUE	

Because the ICD-9-CM coding system combines superficial foreign body codes for shoulder and upper arm into a single code and ICD-10-CM does not, the user must make a selection between the separate ICD-10-CM codes related to body site. Regardless of that choice, the secondary code (LØ8.89) indicating the infection must be assigned in addition to the primary code for the foreign body.

- **Brackets:** Some ICD-10-CM codes appear in this manual with brackets as a space-saving convention. The character values in the brackets correspond to the valid values for the character position where the brackets appear. For example:

Original ICD-10-CM Codes:

MØ5.441 Rheumatoid myopathy with rheumatoid arthritis of right hand

MØ5.442 Rheumatoid myopathy with rheumatoid arthritis of left hand

MØ5.449 Rheumatoid myopathy with rheumatoid arthritis of unspecified hand

Bracketed ICD-10-CM Codes:

MØ5.44**[1,2,9]** Rheumatoid myopathy with rheumatoid arthritis of hand

6th character meanings for codes as indicated
1 RIGHT 2 LEFT 9 UNSPECIFIED

Example

ICD-9-CM		ICD-10-CM	
714.Ø	RHEUMATOID ARTHRITIS	**MØ5.4Ø**	RHEUMATOID MYOPATHY WITH RA, UNSPECIFIED SITE
		MØ5.41[1,2,9]	RHEUMATOID MYOPATHY WITH RA, SHOULDER
		MØ5.42[1,2,9]	RHEUMATOID MYOPATHY WITH RA,ELBOW
		MØ5.43[1,2,9]	RHEUMATOID MYOPATHY WITH RA,WRIST
		MØ5.44[1,2,9]	RHEUMATOID MYOPATHY WITH RA,HAND
		MØ5.45[1,2,9]	RHEUMATOID MYOPATHY WITH RA, HIP
		MØ5.46[1,2,9]	RHEUMATOID MYOPATHY WITH RA, KNEE
		MØ5.47[1,2,9]	RHEUMATOID MYOPATHY WITH RA, ANKLE AND FOOT
		MØ5.49	RHEUMATOID MYOPATHY WITH RA, MULTIPLE SITES
		MØ5.5Ø	RHEUMATOID POLYNEUROPATHY W/ RA, UNSPECIFIED SITE
		MØ5.51[1,2,9]	RHEUMATOID POLYNEUROPATHY WITH RA, SHOULDER
		MØ5.52[1,2,9]	RHEUMATOID POLYNEUROPATHY WITH RA, ELBOW
		MØ5.53[1,2,9]	RHEUMATOID POLYNEUROPATHY WITH RA,WRIST
		MØ5.54[1,2,9]	RHEUMATOID POLYNEUROPATHY WITH RA, HAND
		MØ5.55[1,2,9]	RHEUMATOID POLYNEUROPATHY WITH RA, HIP
		MØ5.56[1,2,9]	RHEUMATOID POLYNEUROPATHY WITH RA, KNEE
		MØ5.57[1,2,9]	RHEUMATOID POLYNEUROPATHY W/RA,ANKLE & FOOT
		MØ5.59	RHEUMATOID POLYNEUROPATHY WITH RA, MULTIPLE SITES
		MØ5.7Ø	RA W/RHEUMATOID FCT W/O ORGN OR SYS INVLV
			6th Character meanings for codes as indicated ***1 RIGHT 2 LEFT 9 UNSPECIFIED***

The sixth character 1, 2, or 9 may be assigned to code MØ5.44 to represent laterality. Each page with bracketed codes has a key near the bottom of that table entry that provides the meanings for the characters within the brackets. Most bracketed characters involve those in either the sixth or seventh character position. Bracketed characters, along with their corresponding key, appear in blue type.

- **"Continued" and "Continued on next page":** Users should be aware that some mapping tables contain many code alternatives. If all the information cannot be displayed on one page, the words "Continued on the next page" in red type appear at the end of the table. The code is continued on the next page with a designation "Continued" in red type underneath the ICD-9-CM code in the table. For instance, code 733.81 Malunion of fracture, does not contain site-specific information in ICD-9-CM, but the ICD-10-CM codes do. As a result, the ICD-10-CM codes that map to 733.81 encompass more than 19 pages.
- **No Diagnosis:** There are ICD-9-CM codes for which ICD-10-CM does not have an equivalent code(s) and no mapping can be made. These codes will have "NO DIAGNOSIS' in the ICD-10-CM column.

Example

ICD-9-CM	ICD-10-CM
E85Ø.8 ACCIDENTAL POISN OTH SPEC ANALGES & ANTIPYRETICS	NO DIAGNOSIS

How to Use the *ICD-10-CM Mappings: Linking ICD-9-CM to All Valid ICD-10-CM Alternatives*

It is recommended that the following steps be followed when using this manual:

1. Locate the ICD-9-CM code, keeping in mind that the book is organized in numeric ICD-9-CM chapters, just as the ICD-9-CM code book is. Ensure that the code is valid and contains the full number of digits required for that category or subcategory. The ICD-9-CM codes are always located in the left column of the manual. Remember this version of the mappings includes the code changes effective October 1, 2014.
2. Review the ICD-10-CM codes that appear in the same row on the right side of the page that are considered alternatives to the source ICD-9-CM code.
3. Note whether any "arrow" symbol appears, designating that ICD-10-CM code as an equivalent match, meaning that the clinical concepts represented by each code are considered equal or equivalent.
4. Note whether any "flag" symbol appears, indicating that there is a complex combination mapping relationship between the coding systems in the backward mapping of ICD-10-CM to ICD-9-CM. If a flag appears next to an ICD-10-CM code, proceed to step 5. If no flag appears proceed to step 6.
5. Refer to Appendix A to review combinations of ICD-9-CM codes that satisfy the complete meaning of the listed ICD-10-CM codes. There may be more than one combination of codes or more than one scenario. Appendix A is arranged in ICD-10-CM alpha-numeric order and contains several different types of coding combinations. In some cases the user will be required to select a code from several different pick lists and assign the codes in combination with other codes. In this way, the clinical concept represented by the target ICD-10-CM code will be satisfied and a more equivalent coding scenario will be represented.
6. Note whether the right-hand column is shaded in red or blue and displays the operators "and" and "or." These operators indicate that a combination of codes must be selected. If there is more than one set of combinations or scenarios, the user must read the code descriptors carefully and then choose the best scenario that completes the meaning of the ICD-9-CM code based upon documentation or information available.
7. Refer to the tabular lists in the official ICD-9-CM and ICD-10-CM code books to review the codes, their inclusion terms, and other instructional notes that may affect code assignment. When reviewing the ICD-10-CM code book, the user will also note that separate codes are represented by the bracketed convention used in this manual, whereby all valid characters are "rolled up" and included in brackets in place of individual codes.
8. Once the ICD-10-CM code selections are made that satisfy the complete meaning of ICD-9-CM code meaning based on the documentation available and the coding practices of the facility or practice, the mapping exercise is complete.

Infectious and Parasitic Diseases

ICD-9-CM			ICD-10-CM	
001.0	CHOLERA DUE TO VIBRIO CHOLERAE	➡	A00.0	Cholera due to Vibrio cholerae 01, biovar cholerae
001.1	CHOLERA DUE TO VIBRIO CHOLERAE EL TOR	➡	A00.1	Cholera due to Vibrio cholerae 01, biovar eltor
001.9	UNSPECIFIED CHOLERA	➡	A00.9	Cholera, unspecified
002.0	TYPHOID FEVER		A01.00 A01.01 A01.02 A01.03 A01.04 A01.05 A01.09	Typhoid fever, unspecified Typhoid meningitis Typhoid fever with heart involvement Typhoid pneumonia Typhoid arthritis Typhoid osteomyelitis Typhoid fever with other complications
002.1	PARATYPHOID FEVER A	➡	A01.1	Paratyphoid fever A
002.2	PARATYPHOID FEVER B	➡	A01.2	Paratyphoid fever B
002.3	PARATYPHOID FEVER C	➡	A01.3	Paratyphoid fever C
002.9	UNSPECIFIED PARATYPHOID FEVER	➡	A01.4	Paratyphoid fever, unspecified
003.0	SALMONELLA GASTROENTERITIS	➡	A02.0	Salmonella enteritis
003.1	SALMONELLA SEPTICEMIA	◪	A02.1	Salmonella sepsis
003.20	UNSPECIFIED LOCALIZED SALMONELLA INFECTION	➡	A02.20	Localized salmonella infection, unspecified
003.21	SALMONELLA MENINGITIS	➡	A02.21	Salmonella meningitis
003.22	SALMONELLA PNEUMONIA	➡	A02.22	Salmonella pneumonia
003.23	SALMONELLA ARTHRITIS	➡	A02.23	Salmonella arthritis
003.24	SALMONELLA OSTEOMYELITIS	➡	A02.24	Salmonella osteomyelitis
003.29	OTHER LOCALIZED SALMONELLA INFECTIONS		A02.25 A02.29	Salmonella pyelonephritis Salmonella with other localized infection
003.8	OTHER SPECIFIED SALMONELLA INFECTIONS	➡	A02.8	Other specified salmonella infections
003.9	UNSPECIFIED SALMONELLA INFECTION	➡	A02.9	Salmonella infection, unspecified
004.0	SHIGELLA DYSENTERIAE	➡	A03.0	Shigellosis due to Shigella dysenteriae
004.1	SHIGELLA FLEXNERI	➡	A03.1	Shigellosis due to Shigella flexneri
004.2	SHIGELLA BOYDII	➡	A03.2	Shigellosis due to Shigella boydii
004.3	SHIGELLA SONNEI	➡	A03.3	Shigellosis due to Shigella sonnei
004.8	OTHER SPECIFIED SHIGELLA INFECTIONS	➡	A03.8	Other shigellosis
004.9	UNSPECIFIED SHIGELLOSIS	➡	A03.9	Shigellosis, unspecified
005.0	STAPHYLOCOCCAL FOOD POISONING	➡	A05.0	Foodborne staphylococcal intoxication
005.1	BOTULISM FOOD POISONING	➡	A05.1	Botulism food poisoning
005.2	FOOD POISONING DUE TO CLOSTRIDIUM PERFRINGENS	➡	A05.2	Foodborne Clostridium perfringens intoxication
005.3	FOOD POISONING DUE TO OTHER CLOSTRIDIA		A05.8	Other specified bacterial foodborne intoxications
005.4	FOOD POISONING DUE TO VIBRIO PARAHAEMOLYTICUS	➡	A05.3	Foodborne Vibrio parahaemolyticus intoxication
005.81	FOOD POISONING DUE TO VIBRIO VULNIFICUS	➡	A05.5	Foodborne Vibrio vulnificus intoxication
005.89	OTHER BACTERIAL FOOD POISONING		A05.4 A05.8	Foodborne Bacillus cereus intoxication Other specified bacterial foodborne intoxications
005.9	UNSPECIFIED FOOD POISONING	➡	A05.9	Bacterial foodborne intoxication, unspecified
006.0	ACUTE AMEBIC DYSENTERY WITHOUT MENTION ABSCESS	➡	A06.0	Acute amebic dysentery
006.1	CHRONIC INTEST AMEBIASIS WITHOUT MENTION ABSC	➡	A06.1	Chronic intestinal amebiasis
006.2	AMEBIC NONDYSENTERIC COLITIS	➡	A06.2	Amebic nondysenteric colitis
006.3	AMEBIC LIVER ABSCESS	➡	A06.4	Amebic liver abscess
006.4	AMEBIC LUNG ABSCESS	➡	A06.5	Amebic lung abscess
006.5	AMEBIC BRAIN ABSCESS	➡	A06.6	Amebic brain abscess
006.6	AMEBIC SKIN ULCERATION	➡	A06.7	Cutaneous amebiasis
006.8	AMEBIC INFECTION OF OTHER SITES		A06.3 A06.81 A06.82 A06.89	Ameboma of intestine Amebic cystitis Other amebic genitourinary infections Other amebic infections
006.9	UNSPECIFIED AMEBIASIS	➡	A06.9	Amebiasis, unspecified
007.0	BALANTIDIASIS	➡	A07.0	Balantidiasis
007.1	GIARDIASIS	➡	A07.1	Giardiasis [lambliasis]
007.2	COCCIDIOSIS	➡	A07.3	Isosporiasis
007.3	INTESTINAL TRICHOMONIASIS		A07.8	Other specified protozoal intestinal diseases
007.4	CRYPTOSPORIDIOSIS	➡	A07.2	Cryptosporidiosis
007.5	CYCLOSPORIASIS	➡	A07.4	Cyclosporiasis
007.8	OTHER SPECIFIED PROTOZOAL INTESTINAL DISEASES		A07.8	Other specified protozoal intestinal diseases
007.9	UNSPECIFIED PROTOZOAL INTESTINAL DISEASE	➡	A07.9	Protozoal intestinal disease, unspecified
008.00	INTESTINAL INFECTION DUE TO UNSPECIFIED E COLI		A04.4	Other intestinal Escherichia coli infections
008.01	INTESTINAL INFECTION DUE ENTEROPATHOGENIC E COLI	➡	A04.0	Enteropathogenic Escherichia coli infection
008.02	INTESTINAL INFECTION DUE ENTEROTOXIGENIC E COLI	➡	A04.1	Enterotoxigenic Escherichia coli infection
008.03	INTESTINAL INFECTION DUE ENTEROINVASIVE E COLI	➡	A04.2	Enteroinvasive Escherichia coli infection
008.04	INTESTINAL INF DUE ENTEROHEMORRHAGIC E COLI	➡	A04.3	Enterohemorrhagic Escherichia coli infection
008.09	INTESTINAL INF DUE OTH INTESTINAL E COLI INFS		A04.4	Other intestinal Escherichia coli infections
008.1	INTEST INF DUE ARIZONA GROUP PARACOLON BACILLI		A04.8	Other specified bacterial intestinal infections
008.2	INTESTINAL INFECTION DUE TO AEROBACTER AEROGENES		A04.8	Other specified bacterial intestinal infections
008.3	INTESTINAL INFECTIONS DUE TO PROTEUS		A04.8	Other specified bacterial intestinal infections

ICD-9-CM		ICD-10-CM	
ØØ8.41	INTESTINAL INFECTIONS DUE TO STAPHYLOCOCCUS	**AØ4.8**	Other specified bacterial intestinal infections
ØØ8.42	INTESTINAL INFECTIONS DUE TO PSEUDOMONAS	**AØ4.8**	Other specified bacterial intestinal infections
ØØ8.43	INTESTINAL INFECTIONS DUE TO CAMPYLOBACTER	➡ **AØ4.5**	Campylobacter enteritis
ØØ8.44	INTESTINAL INFS DUE YERSINIA ENTEROCOLITICA	➡ **AØ4.6**	Enteritis due to Yersinia enterocolitica
ØØ8.45	INTESTINAL INFECTIONS DUE CLOSTRIDIUM DIFFICILE	➡ **AØ4.7**	Enterocolitis due to Clostridium difficile
ØØ8.46	INTESTINAL INFECTIONS DUE TO OTHER ANEROBES	**AØ4.8**	Other specified bacterial intestinal infections
ØØ8.47	INTESTINAL INFECTIONS DUE OTH GM-NEGATIVE BACTER	**AØ4.8**	Other specified bacterial intestinal infections
ØØ8.49	INTESTINAL INFECTION DUE TO OTHER ORGANISMS	**AØ4.8**	Other specified bacterial intestinal infections
ØØ8.5	INTESTINAL INF DUE UNSPEC BACTERL ENTERITIS	➡ **AØ4.9**	Bacterial intestinal infection, unspecified
ØØ8.61	INTESTINAL INFECTION ENTERITIS DUE TO ROTAVIRUS	➡ **AØ8.Ø**	Rotaviral enteritis
ØØ8.62	INTESTINAL INFECTION ENTERITIS DUE TO ADENOVIRUS	➡ **AØ8.2**	Adenoviral enteritis
ØØ8.63	INTESTINAL INFECTION ENTERITIS DUE NORWALK VIRUS	**AØ8.11**	Acute gastroenteropathy due to Norwalk agent
ØØ8.64	INTEST INF ENTERITIS DUE OTH SMALL ROUND VIRUSES	**AØ8.19**	Acute gastroenteropathy due to other small round viruses
ØØ8.65	ENTERITIS DUE TO CALICIVIRUS	➡ **AØ8.31**	Calicivirus enteritis
ØØ8.66	INTESTINAL INFECTION ENTERITIS DUE TO ASTROVIRUS	➡ **AØ8.32**	Astrovirus enteritis
ØØ8.67	INTESTINAL INFECTION ENTERITIS DUE ENTRVRUS NEC	**AØ8.39**	Other viral enteritis
ØØ8.69	INTESTINAL INF ENTERITIS DUE OTH VIRAL ENTERITIS	**AØ8.39**	Other viral enteritis
ØØ8.8	INTESTINAL INFECTION DUE TO OTHER ORGANISM NEC	**AØ8.4** **AØ8.8**	Viral intestinal infection, unspecified Other specified intestinal infections
ØØ9.Ø	INFECTIOUS COLITIS ENTERITIS AND GASTROENTERITIS	**AØ9**	Infectious gastroenteritis and colitis, unspecified
ØØ9.1	COLITIS ENTERIT&GASTROENTERIT INF ORIGIN	**AØ9**	Infectious gastroenteritis and colitis, unspecified
ØØ9.2	INFECTIOUS DIARRHEA	**AØ9**	Infectious gastroenteritis and colitis, unspecified
ØØ9.3	DIARRHEA OF PRESUMED INFECTIOUS ORIGIN	**AØ9**	Infectious gastroenteritis and colitis, unspecified
Ø1Ø.ØØ	PRIMARY TUBERCULOUS COMPLEX CONFIRMATION UNSPEC	**A15.7**	Primary respiratory tuberculosis
Ø1Ø.Ø1	PRIM TB CMPLX EX NOT DONE	**A15.7**	Primary respiratory tuberculosis
Ø1Ø.Ø2	PRIM TB CMPLX EX UNKN	**A15.7**	Primary respiratory tuberculosis
Ø1Ø.Ø3	PRIM TB COMPLEX TUBERCLE BACILLI FOUND MIC	**A15.7**	Primary respiratory tuberculosis
Ø1Ø.Ø4	PRIMARY TB COMPLEX-CULT DX	**A15.7**	Primary respiratory tuberculosis
Ø1Ø.Ø5	PRIMARY TB COMPLEX-HISTO DX	**A15.7**	Primary respiratory tuberculosis
Ø1Ø.Ø6	PRIMARY TB COMPLEX-OTH TEST	**A15.7**	Primary respiratory tuberculosis
Ø1Ø.1Ø	TUBERCULOUS PLEURISY PRIM PROGS TB CONF UNSPEC	**A15.6**	Tuberculous pleurisy
Ø1Ø.11	TB PLEURISY PRIM PROGS TB EX NOT DONE	**A15.6**	Tuberculous pleurisy
Ø1Ø.12	TB PLEURISY PRIM PROGS TB EX RSLTS UNKN	**A15.6**	Tuberculous pleurisy
Ø1Ø.13	TB PLEURISY IN PRIMARY PROGRESSIVE TB-MICRO DX	**A15.6**	Tuberculous pleurisy
Ø1Ø.14	TB PLEURISY IN PRIMARY PROGRESSIVE TB-CULT DX	**A15.6**	Tuberculous pleurisy
Ø1Ø.15	TB PLEURISY IN PRIMARY PROGRESSIVE TB-HISTO DX	**A15.6**	Tuberculous pleurisy
Ø1Ø.16	TB PLEURISY IN PRIMARY PROGRESSIVE TB-OTH TEST	**A15.6**	Tuberculous pleurisy
Ø1Ø.8Ø	OTH PRIM PROGS TUBERCULOSIS INF CONF UNSPEC	**A15.7**	Primary respiratory tuberculosis
Ø1Ø.81	OTH PRIM PROGS TB INF EX NOT DONE	**A15.7**	Primary respiratory tuberculosis
Ø1Ø.82	OTH PRIM PROGS TB INF EX UNKN	**A15.7**	Primary respiratory tuberculosis
Ø1Ø.83	OTH PRIM PROGS TB INF TUBERCLE BACILLI FOUND MIC	**A15.7**	Primary respiratory tuberculosis
Ø1Ø.84	OTH PRIMARY PROGRESSIVE TB-CULT DX	**A15.7**	Primary respiratory tuberculosis
Ø1Ø.85	OTH PRIMARY PROGRESSIVE TB-HISTO DX	**A15.7**	Primary respiratory tuberculosis
Ø1Ø.86	OTH PRIMARY PROGRESSIVE TB-OTH TEST	**A15.7**	Primary respiratory tuberculosis
Ø1Ø.9Ø	PRIMARY TUBERCULOUS INFECTION UNSPEC CONF UNSPEC	**A15.7**	Primary respiratory tuberculosis
Ø1Ø.91	PRIM TB INF UNS EX NOT DONE	**A15.7**	Primary respiratory tuberculosis
Ø1Ø.92	PRIM TB INF UNS EX UNKN	**A15.7**	Primary respiratory tuberculosis
Ø1Ø.93	PRIM TB INF UNSPEC TUBERCLE BACILLI FOUND MIC	**A15.7**	Primary respiratory tuberculosis
Ø1Ø.94	UNS PRIMARY TB INFECTION-CULT DX	**A15.7**	Primary respiratory tuberculosis
Ø1Ø.95	PRIM TB INFECTION UNS-HISTO DX	**A15.7**	Primary respiratory tuberculosis
Ø1Ø.96	UNS PRIMARY TB INFECTION-OTH TEST	**A15.7**	Primary respiratory tuberculosis
Ø11.ØØ	TUBERCULOSIS LUNG INFILTRATIVE CONF UNSPEC	**A15.Ø**	Tuberculosis of lung
Ø11.Ø1	TB LUNG INFILTRAT EX NOT DONE	**A15.Ø**	Tuberculosis of lung
Ø11.Ø2	TB LUNG INFILTRAT EX UNKN	**A15.Ø**	Tuberculosis of lung
Ø11.Ø3	TB LUNG INFILTRAT TUBERCLE BACILLI FOUND MIC	**A15.Ø**	Tuberculosis of lung
Ø11.Ø4	TB OF LUNG-INFILTRATIVE-CULT DX	**A15.Ø**	Tuberculosis of lung
Ø11.Ø5	TB OF LUNG-INFILTRATIVE-HISTO DX	**A15.Ø**	Tuberculosis of lung
Ø11.Ø6	TB OF LUNG-INFILTRATIVE-OTH TEST	**A15.Ø**	Tuberculosis of lung
Ø11.1Ø	TUBERCULOSIS LUNG NODULAR CONFIRMATION UNSPEC	**A15.Ø**	Tuberculosis of lung
Ø11.11	TB LUNG NODULR EX NOT DONE	**A15.Ø**	Tuberculosis of lung
Ø11.12	TB LUNG NODULR EX UNKN	**A15.Ø**	Tuberculosis of lung
Ø11.13	TB LUNG NODULAR TUBERCLE BACILLI FOUND MIC	**A15.Ø**	Tuberculosis of lung
Ø11.14	TB OF LUNG-NODULAR-CULT DX	**A15.Ø**	Tuberculosis of lung
Ø11.15	TB OF LUNG-NODULAR-HISTO DX	**A15.Ø**	Tuberculosis of lung
Ø11.16	TB OF LUNG-NODULAR-OTH TEST	**A15.Ø**	Tuberculosis of lung
Ø11.2Ø	TUBERCULOSIS LUNG W/CAVITATION CONF UNSPEC	**A15.Ø**	Tuberculosis of lung
Ø11.21	TB LUNG W/CAVITATION EX NOT DONE	**A15.Ø**	Tuberculosis of lung

ICD-9-CM		ICD-10-CM	
Ø11.22	TB LUNG W/CAVITATION EX UNKN	**A15.Ø**	Tuberculosis of lung
Ø11.23	TB LUNG W/CAVITATION TUBERCLE BACILLI FOUND MIC	**A15.Ø**	Tuberculosis of lung
Ø11.24	TB OF LUNG WITH CAVITATION-CULT DX	**A15.Ø**	Tuberculosis of lung
Ø11.25	TB OF LUNG WITH CAVITATION-HISTO DX	**A15.Ø**	Tuberculosis of lung
Ø11.26	TB OF LUNG WITH CAVITATION-OTH TEST	**A15.Ø**	Tuberculosis of lung
Ø11.3Ø	TUBERCULOSIS BRONCHUS CONFIRMATION UNSPECIFIED	**A15.5**	Tuberculosis of larynx, trachea and bronchus
Ø11.31	TB BRONCHUS EX NOT DONE	**A15.5**	Tuberculosis of larynx, trachea and bronchus
Ø11.32	TB BRONCHUS BACTERIOLOGICAL/HISTOLOGICAL EX UNKN	**A15.5**	Tuberculosis of larynx, trachea and bronchus
Ø11.33	TUBERCULOSIS BRONCHUS TUBERCLE BACILLI FOUND MIC	**A15.5**	Tuberculosis of larynx, trachea and bronchus
Ø11.34	TB OF BRONCHUS-CULT DX	**A15.5**	Tuberculosis of larynx, trachea and bronchus
Ø11.35	TB OF BRONCHUS-HISTO DX	**A15.5**	Tuberculosis of larynx, trachea and bronchus
Ø11.36	TB OF BRONCHUS-OTH TEST	**A15.5**	Tuberculosis of larynx, trachea and bronchus
Ø11.4Ø	TUBERCULOUS FIBROSIS LUNG CONFIRMATION UNSPEC	**A15.Ø**	Tuberculosis of lung
Ø11.41	TB FIBROF LUNG EX NOT DONE	**A15.Ø**	Tuberculosis of lung
Ø11.42	TB FIBROF LUNG EX UNKN	**A15.Ø**	Tuberculosis of lung
Ø11.43	TB FIBROSIS LUNG TUBERCLE BACILLI FOUND MIC	**A15.Ø**	Tuberculosis of lung
Ø11.44	TB FIBROSIS OF LUNG-CULT DX	**A15.Ø**	Tuberculosis of lung
Ø11.45	TB FIBROSIS OF LUNG-HISTO DX	**A15.Ø**	Tuberculosis of lung
Ø11.46	TB FIBROSIS OF LUNG-OTH TEST	**A15.Ø**	Tuberculosis of lung
Ø11.5Ø	TUBERCULOUS BRONCHIECTASIS CONFIRMATION UNSPEC	**A15.Ø**	Tuberculosis of lung
Ø11.51	TB BRONCHIECTASIS EX NOT DONE	**A15.Ø**	Tuberculosis of lung
Ø11.52	TB BRONCHIECTASIS EX UNKN	**A15.Ø**	Tuberculosis of lung
Ø11.53	TB BRONCHIECTASIS TUBERCLE BACILLI FOUND MIC	**A15.Ø**	Tuberculosis of lung
Ø11.54	TB BRONCHIECTASIS-CULT DX	**A15.Ø**	Tuberculosis of lung
Ø11.55	TB BRONCHIECTASIS-HISTO DX	**A15.Ø**	Tuberculosis of lung
Ø11.56	TB BRONCHIECTASIS-OTH TEST	**A15.Ø**	Tuberculosis of lung
Ø11.6Ø	TUBERCULOUS PNEUMONIA CONFIRMATION UNSPECIFIED	**A15.Ø**	Tuberculosis of lung
Ø11.61	TB PNEUMON EX NOT DONE	**A15.Ø**	Tuberculosis of lung
Ø11.62	TB PNEUMON BACTERIOLOGICAL/HISTOLOGICAL EX UNKN	**A15.Ø**	Tuberculosis of lung
Ø11.63	TUBERCULOUS PNEUMONIA TUBERCLE BACILLI FOUND MIC	**A15.Ø**	Tuberculosis of lung
Ø11.64	TB PNEUMONIA [ANY FORM]-CULT DX	**A15.Ø**	Tuberculosis of lung
Ø11.65	TB PNEUMONIA [ANY FORM]-HISTO DX	**A15.Ø**	Tuberculosis of lung
Ø11.66	TB PNEUMONIA [ANY FORM]-OTH TEST	**A15.Ø**	Tuberculosis of lung
Ø11.7Ø	TUBERCULOUS PNEUMOTHORAX CONFIRMATION UNSPEC	**A15.Ø**	Tuberculosis of lung
Ø11.71	TB PNEUMO EX NOT DONE	**A15.Ø**	Tuberculosis of lung
Ø11.72	TB PNEUMO BACTERIOLOGICAL/HISTOLOGICAL EX UNKN	**A15.Ø**	Tuberculosis of lung
Ø11.73	TB PNEUMO TUBERCLE BACILLI NOT FOUND MIC	**A15.Ø**	Tuberculosis of lung
Ø11.74	TB PNEUMOTHORAX-CULT DX	**A15.Ø**	Tuberculosis of lung
Ø11.75	TB PNEUMOTHORAX-HISTO DX	**A15.Ø**	Tuberculosis of lung
Ø11.76	TB PNEUMOTHORAX-OTH TEST	**A15.Ø**	Tuberculosis of lung
Ø11.8Ø	OTH SPEC PULMONARY TUBERCULOSIS CONF UNSPEC	**A15.Ø**	Tuberculosis of lung
Ø11.81	OTH SPEC PULM TB EX NOT DONE	**A15.Ø**	Tuberculosis of lung
Ø11.82	OTH SPEC PULM TB EX UNKN	**A15.Ø**	Tuberculosis of lung
Ø11.83	OTH SPEC PULM TB TUBERCLE BACILLI FOUND MIC	**A15.Ø**	Tuberculosis of lung
Ø11.84	OTH SPEC PULMONARY TB-CULT DX	**A15.Ø**	Tuberculosis of lung
Ø11.85	OTH SPEC PULMONARY TB-HISTO DX	**A15.Ø**	Tuberculosis of lung
Ø11.86	OTH SPEC PULMONARY TB-OTH TEST	**A15.Ø**	Tuberculosis of lung
Ø11.9Ø	UNSPEC PULMONARY TUBERCULOSIS CONF UNSPEC	**A15.Ø**	Tuberculosis of lung
Ø11.91	UNS PULM TB EX NOT DONE	**A15.Ø**	Tuberculosis of lung
Ø11.92	UNS PULM TB BACTERIOLOGICAL/HISTOLOGICAL EX UNKN	**A15.Ø**	Tuberculosis of lung
Ø11.93	UNSPEC PULM TB TUBERCLE BACILLI FOUND MIC	**A15.Ø**	Tuberculosis of lung
Ø11.94	UNS PULMONARY TB-CULT DX	**A15.Ø**	Tuberculosis of lung
Ø11.95	UNS PULMONARY TB-HISTO DX	**A15.Ø**	Tuberculosis of lung
Ø11.96	UNS PULMONARY TB-OTH TEST	**A15.Ø**	Tuberculosis of lung
Ø12.ØØ	TUBERCULOUS PLEURISY CONFIRMATION UNSPECIFIED	**A15.6**	Tuberculous pleurisy
Ø12.Ø1	TB PLEURISY EX NOT DONE	**A15.6**	Tuberculous pleurisy
Ø12.Ø2	TB PLEURISY BACTERIOLOGICAL/HISTOLOGICAL EX UNKN	**A15.6**	Tuberculous pleurisy
Ø12.Ø3	TUBERCULOUS PLEURISY TUBERCLE BACILLI FOUND MIC	**A15.6**	Tuberculous pleurisy
Ø12.Ø4	TB PLEURISY-CULT DX	**A15.6**	Tuberculous pleurisy
Ø12.Ø5	TB PLEURISY-HISTO DX	**A15.6**	Tuberculous pleurisy
Ø12.Ø6	TB PLEURISY-OTH TEST	**A15.6**	Tuberculous pleurisy
Ø12.1Ø	TUBERCULOSIS INTRATHORACIC NODES CONF UNSPEC	**A15.4**	Tuberculosis of intrathoracic lymph nodes
Ø12.11	TB INTRATHOR NODES EX NOT DONE	**A15.4**	Tuberculosis of intrathoracic lymph nodes
Ø12.12	TB INTRATHOR NODES EX UNKN	**A15.4**	Tuberculosis of intrathoracic lymph nodes
Ø12.13	TB INTRATHOR NODES TUBERCLE BACILLI FOUND MIC	**A15.4**	Tuberculosis of intrathoracic lymph nodes
Ø12.14	TB OF INTRATHORACIC LYMPH NODES-CULT DX	**A15.4**	Tuberculosis of intrathoracic lymph nodes

ICD-9-CM		ICD-10-CM	
Ø12.15	TB OF INTRATHORACIC LYMPH NODES-HISTO DX	**A15.4**	Tuberculosis of intrathoracic lymph nodes
Ø12.16	TB OF INTRATHORACIC LYMPH NODES-OTH TEST	**A15.4**	Tuberculosis of intrathoracic lymph nodes
Ø12.2Ø	ISOLATED TRACHEAL/BRONCHIAL TUBERCULOSIS UNSPEC	**A15.5**	Tuberculosis of larynx, trachea and bronchus
Ø12.21	ISOLATED TRACHEAL/BRONCH TB EX NOT DONE	**A15.5**	Tuberculosis of larynx, trachea and bronchus
Ø12.22	ISOLATED TRACHEAL/BRONCH TB EX UNKN	**A15.5**	Tuberculosis of larynx, trachea and bronchus
Ø12.23	ISOLATED TRACHEAL/BRONCHIAL TB-MICRO DX	**A15.5**	Tuberculosis of larynx, trachea and bronchus
Ø12.24	ISOLATED TRACHEAL/BRONCHIAL TB-CULT DX	**A15.5**	Tuberculosis of larynx, trachea and bronchus
Ø12.25	ISOLATED TRACHEAL/BRONCHIAL TB-HISTO DX	**A15.5**	Tuberculosis of larynx, trachea and bronchus
Ø12.26	ISOLATED TRACHEAL/BRONCHIAL TB-OTH TEST	**A15.5**	Tuberculosis of larynx, trachea and bronchus
Ø12.3Ø	TUBERCULOUS LARYNGITIS CONFIRMATION UNSPECIFIED	**A15.5**	Tuberculosis of larynx, trachea and bronchus
Ø12.31	TB LARYNGITIS EX NOT DONE	**A15.5**	Tuberculosis of larynx, trachea and bronchus
Ø12.32	TB LARYNGITIS EX UNKN	**A15.5**	Tuberculosis of larynx, trachea and bronchus
Ø12.33	TB LARYNGITIS TUBERCLE BACILLI FOUND MIC	**A15.5**	Tuberculosis of larynx, trachea and bronchus
Ø12.34	TB LARYNGITIS-CULT DX	**A15.5**	Tuberculosis of larynx, trachea and bronchus
Ø12.35	TB LARYNGITIS-HISTO DX	**A15.5**	Tuberculosis of larynx, trachea and bronchus
Ø12.36	TB LARYNGITIS-OTH TEST	**A15.5**	Tuberculosis of larynx, trachea and bronchus
Ø12.8Ø	OTH SPEC RESPIRATORY TUBERCULOSIS CONF UNSPEC	**A15.8** **A15.9**	Other respiratory tuberculosis Respiratory tuberculosis unspecified
Ø12.81	OTH SPEC RESP TB EX NOT DONE	**A15.8**	Other respiratory tuberculosis
Ø12.82	OTH SPEC RESP TB EX UNKN	**A15.8**	Other respiratory tuberculosis
Ø12.83	OTH SPEC RESP TB TUBERCLE BACILLI FOUND MIC	**A15.8**	Other respiratory tuberculosis
Ø12.84	OTH SPEC RESPIRATORY TB-CULT DX	**A15.8**	Other respiratory tuberculosis
Ø12.85	OTH SPEC RESPIRATORY TB-HISTO DX	**A15.8**	Other respiratory tuberculosis
Ø12.86	OTH SPEC RESPIRATORY TB-OTH TEST	**A15.8**	Other respiratory tuberculosis
Ø13.ØØ	TUBERCULOUS MENINGITIS CONFIRMATION UNSPECIFIED	**A17.Ø**	Tuberculous meningitis
Ø13.Ø1	TB MENINGITIS EX NOT DONE	**A17.Ø**	Tuberculous meningitis
Ø13.Ø2	TB MENINGITIS EX UNKN	**A17.Ø**	Tuberculous meningitis
Ø13.Ø3	TB MENINGITIS TUBERCLE BACILLI FOUND MIC	**A17.Ø**	Tuberculous meningitis
Ø13.Ø4	TB MENINGITIS-CULT DX	**A17.Ø**	Tuberculous meningitis
Ø13.Ø5	TB MENINGITIS-HISTO DX	**A17.Ø**	Tuberculous meningitis
Ø13.Ø6	TB MENINGITIS-OTH TEST	**A17.Ø**	Tuberculous meningitis
Ø13.1Ø	TUBERCULOMA OF MENINGES CONFIRMATION UNSPECIFIED	**A17.1**	Meningeal tuberculoma
Ø13.11	TUBERCULOMA MENINGES EX NOT DONE	**A17.1**	Meningeal tuberculoma
Ø13.12	TUBERCULOMA MENINGES EX UNKN	**A17.1**	Meningeal tuberculoma
Ø13.13	TUBERCULOMA MENINGES TUBERCLE BACILLI FOUND MIC	**A17.1**	Meningeal tuberculoma
Ø13.14	TUBERCULOMA OF MENINGES-CULT DX	**A17.1**	Meningeal tuberculoma
Ø13.15	TUBERCULOMA OF MENINGES-HISTO DX	**A17.1**	Meningeal tuberculoma
Ø13.16	TUBERCULOMA OF MENINGES-OTH TEST	**A17.1**	Meningeal tuberculoma
Ø13.2Ø	TUBERCULOMA OF BRAIN CONFIRMATION UNSPECIFIED	**A17.81**	Tuberculoma of brain and spinal cord
Ø13.21	TUBERCULOMA BRAIN EX NOT DONE	**A17.81**	Tuberculoma of brain and spinal cord
Ø13.22	TUBERCULOMA BRAIN EX UNKN	**A17.81**	Tuberculoma of brain and spinal cord
Ø13.23	TUBERCULOMA BRAIN TUBERCLE BACILLI FOUND MIC	**A17.81**	Tuberculoma of brain and spinal cord
Ø13.24	TUBERCULOMA OF BRAIN-CULT DX	**A17.81**	Tuberculoma of brain and spinal cord
Ø13.25	TUBERCULOMA OF BRAIN-HISTO DX	**A17.81**	Tuberculoma of brain and spinal cord
Ø13.26	TUBERCULOMA OF BRAIN-OTH TEST	**A17.81**	Tuberculoma of brain and spinal cord
Ø13.3Ø	TUBERCULOUS ABSCESS BRAIN CONFIRMATION UNSPEC	**A17.81**	Tuberculoma of brain and spinal cord
Ø13.31	TB ABSC BRAIN EX NOT DONE	**A17.81**	Tuberculoma of brain and spinal cord
Ø13.32	TB ABSC BRAIN EX UNKN	**A17.81**	Tuberculoma of brain and spinal cord
Ø13.33	TB ABSC BRAIN TUBERCLE BACILLI FOUND MIC	**A17.81**	Tuberculoma of brain and spinal cord
Ø13.34	TB ABSCESS OF BRAIN-CULT DX	**A17.81**	Tuberculoma of brain and spinal cord
Ø13.35	TB ABSCESS OF BRAIN-HISTO DX	**A17.81**	Tuberculoma of brain and spinal cord
Ø13.36	TB ABSCESS OF BRAIN-OTH TEST	**A17.81**	Tuberculoma of brain and spinal cord
Ø13.4Ø	TUBERCULOMA SPINAL CORD CONFIRMATION UNSPECIFIED	**A17.81**	Tuberculoma of brain and spinal cord
Ø13.41	TUBERCULOMA SP CORD EX NOT DONE	**A17.81**	Tuberculoma of brain and spinal cord
Ø13.42	TUBERCULOMA SP CORD EX UNKN	**A17.81**	Tuberculoma of brain and spinal cord
Ø13.43	TUBERCULOMA SP CORD TUBERCLE BACILLI FOUND MIC	**A17.81**	Tuberculoma of brain and spinal cord
Ø13.44	TUBERCULOMA OF SPINAL CORD-CULT DX	**A17.81**	Tuberculoma of brain and spinal cord
Ø13.45	TUBERCULOMA OF SPINAL CORD-HISTO DX	**A17.81**	Tuberculoma of brain and spinal cord
Ø13.46	TUBERCULOMA OF SPINAL CORD-OTH TEST	**A17.81**	Tuberculoma of brain and spinal cord
Ø13.5Ø	TUBERCULOUS ABSC SPINAL CORD CONFIRMATION UNSPEC	**A17.81**	Tuberculoma of brain and spinal cord
Ø13.51	TB ABSC SP CORD EX NOT DONE	**A17.81**	Tuberculoma of brain and spinal cord
Ø13.52	TB ABSC SP CORD EX UNKN	**A17.81**	Tuberculoma of brain and spinal cord
Ø13.53	TB ABSC SPINAL CORD TUBERCLE BACILLI FOUND MIC	**A17.81**	Tuberculoma of brain and spinal cord
Ø13.54	TB ABSCESS OF SPINAL CORD-CULT DX	**A17.81**	Tuberculoma of brain and spinal cord
Ø13.55	TB ABSCESS OF SPINAL CORD-HISTO DX	**A17.81**	Tuberculoma of brain and spinal cord
Ø13.56	TB ABSCESS OF SPINAL CORD-OTH TEST	**A17.81**	Tuberculoma of brain and spinal cord
Ø13.6Ø	TUBERCULOUS ENCEPHALITIS/MYELITIS CONF UNSPEC	**A17.82**	Tuberculous meningoencephalitis

ICD-9-CM		ICD-10-CM	
Ø13.61	TB ENCEPHALIT/MYELITIS EX NOT DONE	**A17.82**	Tuberculous meningoencephalitis
Ø13.62	TB ENCEPHALIT/MYELITIS EX UNKN	**A17.82** **A17.83**	Tuberculous meningoencephalitis Tuberculous neuritis
Ø13.63	TB ENCEPHALIT/MYELITIS TUBERCL BACILLI FOUND MIC	**A17.82**	Tuberculous meningoencephalitis
Ø13.64	TB ENCEPHALITIS OR MYELITIS-CULT DX	**A17.82**	Tuberculous meningoencephalitis
Ø13.65	TB ENCEPHALITIS OR MYELITIS-HISTO DX	**A17.82**	Tuberculous meningoencephalitis
Ø13.66	TB ENCEPHALITIS OR MYELITIS-OTH TEST	**A17.82**	Tuberculous meningoencephalitis
Ø13.8Ø	OTH SPEC TUBERCULOSIS CNTRL NERV SYS CONF UNSPEC	**A17.89**	Other tuberculosis of nervous system
Ø13.81	OTH SPEC TB CNTRL NERV SYS EX NOT DONE	**A17.89**	Other tuberculosis of nervous system
Ø13.82	OTH SPEC TB CNTRL NERV SYS EX UNKN	**A17.89**	Other tuberculosis of nervous system
Ø13.83	OTH TB CNTRL NRV SYS TUBERCL BACILLI FOUND MIC	**A17.89**	Other tuberculosis of nervous system
Ø13.84	OTH SPEC TB OF CENTRAL NERVOUS SYSTEM-CULT DX	**A17.89**	Other tuberculosis of nervous system
Ø13.85	OTH SPEC TB OF CENTRAL NERVOUS SYSTEM-HISTO DX	**A17.89**	Other tuberculosis of nervous system
Ø13.86	OTH SPEC TB OF CENTRAL NERVOUS SYSTEM-OTH TEST	**A17.89**	Other tuberculosis of nervous system
Ø13.9Ø	UNSPEC TUBERCULOSIS CNTRL NERV SYS CONF UNSPEC	**A17.9**	Tuberculosis of nervous system, unspecified
Ø13.91	UNS TB CNTRL NERV SYS EX NOT DONE	**A17.9**	Tuberculosis of nervous system, unspecified
Ø13.92	UNS TB CNTRL NERV SYS EX UNKN	**A17.9**	Tuberculosis of nervous system, unspecified
Ø13.93	UNS TB CNTRL NERV SYS TUBERCL BACILLI FOUND MIC	**A17.9**	Tuberculosis of nervous system, unspecified
Ø13.94	UNS TB OF CENTRAL NERVOUS SYSTEM-CULT DX	**A17.9**	Tuberculosis of nervous system, unspecified
Ø13.95	UNS TB OF CENTRAL NERVOUS SYSTEM-HISTO DX	**A17.9**	Tuberculosis of nervous system, unspecified
Ø13.96	UNS TB OF CENTRAL NERVOUS SYSTEM-OTH TEST	**A17.9**	Tuberculosis of nervous system, unspecified
Ø14.ØØ	TUBERCULOUS PERTONITIS, UNSPECIFIED	**A18.31**	Tuberculous peritonitis
Ø14.Ø1	TB PERTONITIS EX NOT DONE	**A18.31**	Tuberculous peritonitis
Ø14.Ø2	TB PERITONITIS EX UNKN	**A18.31**	Tuberculous peritonitis
Ø14.Ø3	TB PERITONITIS TUBERCLE BACILLI FOUND MIC	**A18.31**	Tuberculous peritonitis
Ø14.Ø4	TB PERITONITIS-CULT DX	**A18.31**	Tuberculous peritonitis
Ø14.Ø5	TB PERITONITIS-HISTO DX	**A18.31**	Tuberculous peritonitis
Ø14.Ø6	TB PERITONITIS-OTH TEST	**A18.31**	Tuberculous peritonitis
Ø14.8Ø	TB INTST PERITON&MESENTERIC GLND OTH CONF UNSPEC	**A18.32** **A18.39** **A18.83**	Tuberculous enteritis Retroperitoneal tuberculosis Tuberculosis of digestive tract organs, NEC
Ø14.81	TB INTST PERITON&MESENTERIC GLND OTH EX NOT DONE	**A18.32** **A18.39**	Tuberculous enteritis Retroperitoneal tuberculosis
Ø14.82	TB INTST PERITON&MESENTERIC GLND OTH EX UNKN	**A18.32** **A18.39**	Tuberculous enteritis Retroperitoneal tuberculosis
Ø14.83	OTH TB INTEST-PERITONEUM-MESENTER GLAND-MICRO DX	**A18.32** **A18.39**	Tuberculous enteritis Retroperitoneal tuberculosis
Ø14.84	OTH TB INTEST-PERITONEUM-MESENTER GLAND-CULT DX	**A18.32** **A18.39**	Tuberculous enteritis Retroperitoneal tuberculosis
Ø14.85	OTH TB INTEST-PERITONEUM-MESENTER GLAND-HISTO DX	**A18.32** **A18.39**	Tuberculous enteritis Retroperitoneal tuberculosis
Ø14.86	OTH TB INTEST-PERITONEUM-MESENTER GLAND-OTH TEST	**A18.32** **A18.39**	Tuberculous enteritis Retroperitoneal tuberculosis
Ø15.ØØ	TUBERCULOSIS VERTEBRAL COLUMN CONF UNSPEC	**A18.Ø1**	Tuberculosis of spine
Ø15.Ø1	TB VERT COLUMN EX NOT DONE	**A18.Ø1**	Tuberculosis of spine
Ø15.Ø2	TB VERT COLUMN EX UNKN	**A18.Ø1**	Tuberculosis of spine
Ø15.Ø3	TB VERTEBRAL COLUMN TUBERCLE BACILLI FOUND MIC	**A18.Ø1**	Tuberculosis of spine
Ø15.Ø4	TB OF VERTEBRAL COLUMN-CULT DX	**A18.Ø1**	Tuberculosis of spine
Ø15.Ø5	TB OF VERTEBRAL COLUMN-HISTO DX	**A18.Ø1**	Tuberculosis of spine
Ø15.Ø6	TB OF VERTEBRAL COLUMN-OTH TEST	**A18.Ø1**	Tuberculosis of spine
Ø15.1Ø	TUBERCULOSIS OF HIP CONFIRMATION UNSPECIFIED	**A18.Ø2**	Tuberculous arthritis of other joints
Ø15.11	TB HIP BACTERIOLOGICAL/HISTOLOGICAL EX NOT DONE	**A18.Ø2**	Tuberculous arthritis of other joints
Ø15.12	TB HIP BACTERIOLOGICAL/HISTOLOGICAL EXAM UNKNOWN	**A18.Ø2**	Tuberculous arthritis of other joints
Ø15.13	TUBERCULOSIS HIP TUBERCLE BACILLI FOUND MIC	**A18.Ø2**	Tuberculous arthritis of other joints
Ø15.14	TB OF HIP-CULT DX	**A18.Ø2**	Tuberculous arthritis of other joints
Ø15.15	TB OF HIP-HISTO DX	**A18.Ø2**	Tuberculous arthritis of other joints
Ø15.16	TB OF HIP-OTH TEST	**A18.Ø2**	Tuberculous arthritis of other joints
Ø15.2Ø	TUBERCULOSIS OF KNEE CONFIRMATION UNSPECIFIED	**A18.Ø2**	Tuberculous arthritis of other joints
Ø15.21	TB KNEE BACTERIOLOGICAL/HISTOLOGICAL EX NOT DONE	**A18.Ø2**	Tuberculous arthritis of other joints
Ø15.22	TB KNEE BACTERIOLOGICAL/HISTOLOGICAL EX UNKNOWN	**A18.Ø2**	Tuberculous arthritis of other joints
Ø15.23	TUBERCULOSIS KNEE TUBERCLE BACILLI FOUND MIC	**A18.Ø2**	Tuberculous arthritis of other joints
Ø15.24	TB OF KNEE-CULT DX	**A18.Ø2**	Tuberculous arthritis of other joints
Ø15.25	TB OF KNEE-HISTO DX	**A18.Ø2**	Tuberculous arthritis of other joints
Ø15.26	TB OF KNEE-OTH TEST	**A18.Ø2**	Tuberculous arthritis of other joints
Ø15.5Ø	TUBERCULOSIS LIMB BONES CONFIRMATION UNSPECIFIED	**A18.Ø3**	Tuberculosis of other bones
Ø15.51	TB LIMB BNS EX NOT DONE	**A18.Ø3**	Tuberculosis of other bones
Ø15.52	TB LIMB BNS BACTERIOLOGICAL/HISTOLOGICAL EX UNKN	**A18.Ø3**	Tuberculosis of other bones
Ø15.53	TUBERCULOSIS LIMB BNS TUBERCLE BACILLI FOUND MIC	**A18.Ø3**	Tuberculosis of other bones

ICD-9-CM		ICD-10-CM	
Ø15.54	TB OF LIMB BONES-CULT DX	**A18.Ø3**	Tuberculosis of other bones
Ø15.55	TB OF LIMB BONES-HISTO DX	**A18.Ø3**	Tuberculosis of other bones
Ø15.56	TB OF LIMB BONES-OTH TEST	**A18.Ø3**	Tuberculosis of other bones
Ø15.6Ø	TUBERCULOSIS OF MASTOID CONFIRMATION UNSPECIFIED	**A18.Ø3**	Tuberculosis of other bones
Ø15.61	TB MASTOID EX NOT DONE	**A18.Ø3**	Tuberculosis of other bones
Ø15.62	TB MASTOID BACTERIOLOGICAL/HISTOLOGICAL EX UNKN	**A18.Ø3**	Tuberculosis of other bones
Ø15.63	TUBERCULOSIS MASTOID TUBERCLE BACILLI FOUND MIC	**A18.Ø3**	Tuberculosis of other bones
Ø15.64	TB OF MASTOID-CULT DX	**A18.Ø3**	Tuberculosis of other bones
Ø15.65	TB OF MASTOID-HISTO DX	**A18.Ø3**	Tuberculosis of other bones
Ø15.66	TB OF MASTOID-OTH TEST	**A18.Ø3**	Tuberculosis of other bones
Ø15.7Ø	TUBERCULOSIS OF OTHER SPECIFIED BONE UNSPECIFIED	**A18.Ø3**	Tuberculosis of other bones
Ø15.71	TB OTH SPEC BN EX NOT DONE	**A18.Ø3**	Tuberculosis of other bones
Ø15.72	TB OTH SPEC BN EX UNKN	**A18.Ø3**	Tuberculosis of other bones
Ø15.73	TB OTH SPEC BONE TUBERCLE BACILLI FOUND MIC	**A18.Ø3**	Tuberculosis of other bones
Ø15.74	TB OF OTH SPEC BONE-CULT DX	**A18.Ø3**	Tuberculosis of other bones
Ø15.75	TB OF OTH SPEC BONE-HISTO DX	**A18.Ø3**	Tuberculosis of other bones
Ø15.76	TB OF OTH SPEC BONE-OTH TEST	**A18.Ø3**	Tuberculosis of other bones
Ø15.8Ø	TUBERCULOSIS OTH SPEC JOINT CONFIRMATION UNSPEC	**A18.Ø2**	Tuberculous arthritis of other joints
Ø15.81	TB OTH SPEC JNT EX NOT DONE	**A18.Ø2**	Tuberculous arthritis of other joints
Ø15.82	TB OTH SPEC JNT EX UNKN	**A18.Ø2**	Tuberculous arthritis of other joints
Ø15.83	TB OTH SPEC JOINT TUBERCLE BACILLI FOUND MIC	**A18.Ø2**	Tuberculous arthritis of other joints
Ø15.84	TB OF OTH SPEC JOINT-CULT DX	**A18.Ø2**	Tuberculous arthritis of other joints
Ø15.85	TB OF OTH SPEC JOINT-HISTO DX	**A18.Ø2**	Tuberculous arthritis of other joints
Ø15.86	TB OF OTH SPEC JOINT-OTH TEST	**A18.Ø2**	Tuberculous arthritis of other joints
Ø15.9Ø	TUBERCULOSIS UNSPEC BNS&JOINTS CONF UNSPEC	**A18.Ø2** **A18.Ø3** **A18.Ø9**	Tuberculous arthritis of other joints Tuberculosis of other bones Other musculoskeletal tuberculosis
Ø15.91	TB UNS BNS&JNT EX NOT DONE	**A18.Ø2** **A18.Ø3**	Tuberculous arthritis of other joints Tuberculosis of other bones
Ø15.92	TB UNS BNS&JNT EX UNKN	**A18.Ø2** **A18.Ø3**	Tuberculous arthritis of other joints Tuberculosis of other bones
Ø15.93	TB UNSPEC BNS&JNT TUBERCLE BACILLI FOUND MIC	**A18.Ø2** **A18.Ø3**	Tuberculous arthritis of other joints Tuberculosis of other bones
Ø15.94	TB OF UNS BONES & JOINTS-CULT DX	**A18.Ø2** **A18.Ø3**	Tuberculous arthritis of other joints Tuberculosis of other bones
Ø15.95	TB OF UNS BONES & JOINTS-HISTO DX	**A18.Ø2** **A18.Ø3**	Tuberculous arthritis of other joints Tuberculosis of other bones
Ø15.96	TB OF UNS BONES & JOINTS-OTH TEST	**A18.Ø2** **A18.Ø3**	Tuberculous arthritis of other joints Tuberculosis of other bones
Ø16.ØØ	TUBERCULOSIS OF KIDNEY CONFIRMATION UNSPECIFIED	**A18.11**	Tuberculosis of kidney and ureter
Ø16.Ø1	TB KIDNEY EX NOT DONE	**A18.11**	Tuberculosis of kidney and ureter
Ø16.Ø2	TB KIDNEY BACTERIOLOGICAL/HISTOLOGICAL EX UNKN	**A18.11**	Tuberculosis of kidney and ureter
Ø16.Ø3	TUBERCULOSIS KIDNEY TUBERCLE BACILLI FOUND MIC	**A18.11**	Tuberculosis of kidney and ureter
Ø16.Ø4	TB OF KIDNEY-CULT DX	**A18.11**	Tuberculosis of kidney and ureter
Ø16.Ø5	TB OF KIDNEY-HISTO DX	**A18.11**	Tuberculosis of kidney and ureter
Ø16.Ø6	TB OF KIDNEY-OTH TEST	**A18.11**	Tuberculosis of kidney and ureter
Ø16.1Ø	TUBERCULOSIS OF BLADDER CONFIRMATION UNSPECIFIED	**A18.12**	Tuberculosis of bladder
Ø16.11	TB BLADD EX NOT DONE	**A18.12**	Tuberculosis of bladder
Ø16.12	TB BLADD BACTERIOLOGICAL/HISTOLOGICAL EX UNKNOWN	**A18.12**	Tuberculosis of bladder
Ø16.13	TUBERCULOSIS BLADD TUBERCLE BACILLI FOUND MIC	**A18.12**	Tuberculosis of bladder
Ø16.14	TB OF BLADDER-CULT DX	**A18.12**	Tuberculosis of bladder
Ø16.15	TB OF BLADDER-HISTO DX	**A18.12**	Tuberculosis of bladder
Ø16.16	TB OF BLADDER-OTH TEST	**A18.12**	Tuberculosis of bladder
Ø16.2Ø	TUBERCULOSIS OF URETER CONFIRMATION UNSPECIFIED	**A18.11**	Tuberculosis of kidney and ureter
Ø16.21	TB URETER EX NOT DONE	**A18.11**	Tuberculosis of kidney and ureter
Ø16.22	TB URETER BACTERIOLOGICAL/HISTOLOGICAL EX UNKN	**A18.11**	Tuberculosis of kidney and ureter
Ø16.23	TUBERCULOSIS URETER TUBERCLE BACILLI FOUND MIC	**A18.11**	Tuberculosis of kidney and ureter
Ø16.24	TB OF URETER-CULT DX	**A18.11**	Tuberculosis of kidney and ureter
Ø16.25	TB OF URETER-HISTO DX	**A18.11**	Tuberculosis of kidney and ureter
Ø16.26	TB OF URETER-OTH TEST	**A18.11**	Tuberculosis of kidney and ureter
Ø16.3Ø	TUBERCULOSIS OTH URINARY ORGANS CONF UNSPEC	**A18.13**	Tuberculosis of other urinary organs
Ø16.31	TB OTH URIN ORGN EX NOT DONE	**A18.13**	Tuberculosis of other urinary organs
Ø16.32	TB OTH URIN ORGN EX UNKN	**A18.13**	Tuberculosis of other urinary organs
Ø16.33	TB OTH URINARY ORGN TUBERCLE BACILLI FOUND MIC	**A18.13**	Tuberculosis of other urinary organs
Ø16.34	TB OF OTH URINARY ORGANS-CULT DX	**A18.13**	Tuberculosis of other urinary organs
Ø16.35	TB OF OTH URINARY ORGANS-HISTO DX	**A18.13**	Tuberculosis of other urinary organs
Ø16.36	TB OF OTH URINARY ORGANS-OTH TEST	**A18.13**	Tuberculosis of other urinary organs
Ø16.4Ø	TUBERCULOSIS EPIDIDYMIS CONFIRMATION UNSPECIFIED	**A18.15**	Tuberculosis of other male genital organs

ICD-9-CM		ICD-10-CM	
Ø16.41	TB EPIDIDYMIS EX NOT DONE	**A18.15**	Tuberculosis of other male genital organs
Ø16.42	TB EPIDIDYMIS EX UNKN	**A18.15**	Tuberculosis of other male genital organs
Ø16.43	TB EPIDIDYMIS TUBERCLE BACILLI FOUND MIC	**A18.15**	Tuberculosis of other male genital organs
Ø16.44	TB OF EPIDIDYMIS-CULT DX	**A18.15**	Tuberculosis of other male genital organs
Ø16.45	TB OF EPIDIDYMIS-HISTO DX	**A18.15**	Tuberculosis of other male genital organs
Ø16.46	TB OF EPIDIDYMIS-OTH TEST	**A18.15**	Tuberculosis of other male genital organs
Ø16.5Ø	TUBERCULOSIS OTH MALE GENITAL ORGANS CONF UNSPEC	**A18.14** **A18.15**	Tuberculosis of prostate Tuberculosis of other male genital organs
Ø16.51	TB OTH MALE GENIT ORGN EX NOT DONE	**A18.14** **A18.15**	Tuberculosis of prostate Tuberculosis of other male genital organs
Ø16.52	TB OTH MALE GENIT ORGN EX UNKN	**A18.14** **A18.15**	Tuberculosis of prostate Tuberculosis of other male genital organs
Ø16.53	TB OTH MALE GENIT ORGN TUBERCL BACILLI FOUND MIC	**A18.14** **A18.15**	Tuberculosis of prostate Tuberculosis of other male genital organs
Ø16.54	TB OF OTH MALE GENITAL ORGANS-CULT DX	**A18.14** **A18.15**	Tuberculosis of prostate Tuberculosis of other male genital organs
Ø16.55	TB OF OTH MALE GENITAL ORGANS-HISTO DX	**A18.14** **A18.15**	Tuberculosis of prostate Tuberculosis of other male genital organs
Ø16.56	TB OF OTH MALE GENITAL ORGANS-OTH TEST	**A18.14** **A18.15**	Tuberculosis of prostate Tuberculosis of other male genital organs
Ø16.6Ø	TUBERCULOUS OOPHORITIS&SALPINGITIS CONF UNSPEC	**A18.17**	Tuberculous female pelvic inflammatory disease
Ø16.61	TB OOPHORITIS&SALPINGITIS EX NOT DONE	**A18.17**	Tuberculous female pelvic inflammatory disease
Ø16.62	TB OOPHORITIS&SALPINGITIS EX UNKN	**A18.17**	Tuberculous female pelvic inflammatory disease
Ø16.63	TB OOPHORITIS & SALPINGITIS-MICRO DX	**A18.17**	Tuberculous female pelvic inflammatory disease
Ø16.64	TB OOPHORITIS & SALPINGITIS-CULT DX	**A18.17**	Tuberculous female pelvic inflammatory disease
Ø16.65	TB OOPHORITIS & SALPINGITIS-HISTO DX	**A18.17**	Tuberculous female pelvic inflammatory disease
Ø16.66	TB OOPHORITIS & SALPINGITIS-OTH TEST	**A18.17**	Tuberculous female pelvic inflammatory disease
Ø16.7Ø	TUBERCULOSIS OTH FE GENITAL ORGANS CONF UNSPEC	**A18.16** **A18.17** **A18.18**	Tuberculosis of cervix Tuberculous female pelvic inflammatory disease Tuberculosis of other female genital organs
Ø16.71	TB OTH FE GENIT ORGN EX NOT DONE	**A18.16** **A18.17** **A18.18**	Tuberculosis of cervix Tuberculous female pelvic inflammatory disease Tuberculosis of other female genital organs
Ø16.72	TB OTH FE GENIT ORGN EX UNKN	**A18.16** **A18.17** **A18.18**	Tuberculosis of cervix Tuberculous female pelvic inflammatory disease Tuberculosis of other female genital organs
Ø16.73	TB OTH FE GENIT ORGN TUBERCLE BACILLI FOUND MIC	**A18.16** **A18.17** **A18.18**	Tuberculosis of cervix Tuberculous female pelvic inflammatory disease Tuberculosis of other female genital organs
Ø16.74	TB OF OTH FEMALE GENITAL ORGANS-CULT DX	**A18.16** **A18.17** **A18.18**	Tuberculosis of cervix Tuberculous female pelvic inflammatory disease Tuberculosis of other female genital organs
Ø16.75	TB OF OTH FEMALE GENITAL ORGANS-HISTO DX	**A18.16** **A18.17** **A18.18**	Tuberculosis of cervix Tuberculous female pelvic inflammatory disease Tuberculosis of other female genital organs
Ø16.76	TB OF OTH FEMALE GENITAL ORGANS-OTH TEST	**A18.16** **A18.17** **A18.18**	Tuberculosis of cervix Tuberculous female pelvic inflammatory disease Tuberculosis of other female genital organs
Ø16.9Ø	UNSPEC GENITOURINARY TUBERCULOSIS CONF UNSPEC	**A18.1Ø**	Tuberculosis of genitourinary system, unspecified
Ø16.91	UNS GU TB BACTERIOLOGICAL/HISOTOLOGICAL NO EX	**A18.1Ø**	Tuberculosis of genitourinary system, unspecified
Ø16.92	UNS GU TB BACTERIOLOGICAL/HISTOLOGICAL EX UNKN	**A18.1Ø**	Tuberculosis of genitourinary system, unspecified
Ø16.93	UNSPEC GU TB TUBERCLE BACILLI FOUND MIC	**A18.1Ø**	Tuberculosis of genitourinary system, unspecified
Ø16.94	UNS GENITOURINARY TB-CULT DX	**A18.1Ø**	Tuberculosis of genitourinary system, unspecified
Ø16.95	UNS GENITOURINARY TB-HISTO DX	**A18.1Ø**	Tuberculosis of genitourinary system, unspecified
Ø16.96	UNS GENITOURINARY TB-OTH TEST	**A18.1Ø**	Tuberculosis of genitourinary system, unspecified
Ø17.ØØ	TB SKIN&SUBCUT CELLULAR TISSUE CONF UNSPEC	**A18.4**	Tuberculosis of skin and subcutaneous tissue
Ø17.Ø1	TB SKN&SUBQ CELLR TISS EX NOT DONE	**A18.4**	Tuberculosis of skin and subcutaneous tissue
Ø17.Ø2	TB SKN&SUBQ CELLR TISS EX UNKN	**A18.4**	Tuberculosis of skin and subcutaneous tissue
Ø17.Ø3	TB SKN&SUBQ CELLR TISS TUBERCL BACILLI FOUND MIC	**A18.4**	Tuberculosis of skin and subcutaneous tissue
Ø17.Ø4	TB OF SKIN&SUBCUTANEOUS CELLULAR TISSUE-CULT DX	**A18.4**	Tuberculosis of skin and subcutaneous tissue
Ø17.Ø5	TB OF SKIN&SUBCUTANEOUS CELLULAR TISSUE-HISTO DX	**A18.4**	Tuberculosis of skin and subcutaneous tissue
Ø17.Ø6	TB OF SKIN&SUBCUTANEOUS CELLULAR TISSUE-OTH TEST	**A18.4**	Tuberculosis of skin and subcutaneous tissue
Ø17.1Ø	ERYTHMA NODOSUM W/HYPERSENS REACT TB CONF UNSPEC	**A18.4**	Tuberculosis of skin and subcutaneous tissue
Ø17.11	ERYTHMA NODOSUM W/HYPERSENS REACT TB EX NOT DONE	**A18.4**	Tuberculosis of skin and subcutaneous tissue
Ø17.12	ERYTHMA NODOSUM W/HYPERSENS REACT TB EX UNKN	**A18.4**	Tuberculosis of skin and subcutaneous tissue
Ø17.13	ERYTHEMA NODOSUM W/HYPERSENS REACT TB-MICRO DX	**A18.4**	Tuberculosis of skin and subcutaneous tissue
Ø17.14	ERYTHEMA NODOSUM W/HYPERSENS REACTION TB-CULT DX	**A18.4**	Tuberculosis of skin and subcutaneous tissue
Ø17.15	ERYTHEMA NODOSUM W/HYPERSENS REACT TB-HISTO DX	**A18.4**	Tuberculosis of skin and subcutaneous tissue
Ø17.16	ERYTHEMA NODOSUM W/HYPERSENS REACT TB-OTH TEST	**A18.4**	Tuberculosis of skin and subcutaneous tissue
Ø17.2Ø	TUBERCULOSIS PERIPHERAL LYMPH NODES CONF UNSPEC	**A18.2**	Tuberculous peripheral lymphadenopathy
Ø17.21	TB PERIPH NODES EX NOT DONE	**A18.2**	Tuberculous peripheral lymphadenopathy

ICD-9-CM		ICD-10-CM	
Ø17.22	TB PERIPH NODES EX UNKN	**A18.2**	Tuberculous peripheral lymphadenopathy
Ø17.23	TB PERIPH NODES TUBERCLE BACILLI FOUND MIC	**A18.2**	Tuberculous peripheral lymphadenopathy
Ø17.24	TB OF PERIPHERAL LYMPH NODES-CULT DX	**A18.2**	Tuberculous peripheral lymphadenopathy
Ø17.25	TB OF PERIPHERAL LYMPH NODES-HISTO DX	**A18.2**	Tuberculous peripheral lymphadenopathy
Ø17.26	TB OF PERIPHERAL LYMPH NODES-OTH TEST	**A18.2**	Tuberculous peripheral lymphadenopathy
Ø17.3Ø	TUBERCULOSIS OF EYE CONFIRMATION UNSPECIFIED	**A18.5Ø**	Tuberculosis of eye, unspecified
		A18.51	Tuberculous episcleritis
		A18.52	Tuberculous keratitis
		A18.53	Tuberculous chorioretinitis
		A18.54	Tuberculous iridocyclitis
		A18.59	Other tuberculosis of eye
Ø17.31	TB EYE BACTERIOLOGICAL/HISTOLOGICAL EX NOT DONE	**A18.5Ø**	Tuberculosis of eye, unspecified
		A18.51	Tuberculous episcleritis
		A18.52	Tuberculous keratitis
		A18.54	Tuberculous iridocyclitis
		A18.59	Other tuberculosis of eye
Ø17.32	TB EYE BACTERIOLOGICAL/HISTOLOGICAL EXAM UNKNOWN	**A18.5Ø**	Tuberculosis of eye, unspecified
		A18.51	Tuberculous episcleritis
		A18.52	Tuberculous keratitis
		A18.54	Tuberculous iridocyclitis
		A18.59	Other tuberculosis of eye
Ø17.33	TUBERCULOSIS EYE TUBERCLE BACILLI FOUND MIC	**A18.5Ø**	Tuberculosis of eye, unspecified
		A18.51	Tuberculous episcleritis
		A18.52	Tuberculous keratitis
		A18.54	Tuberculous iridocyclitis
		A18.59	Other tuberculosis of eye
Ø17.34	TB OF EYE-CULT DX	**A18.5Ø**	Tuberculosis of eye, unspecified
		A18.51	Tuberculous episcleritis
		A18.52	Tuberculous keratitis
		A18.54	Tuberculous iridocyclitis
		A18.59	Other tuberculosis of eye
Ø17.35	TB OF EYE-HISTO DX	**A18.5Ø**	Tuberculosis of eye, unspecified
		A18.51	Tuberculous episcleritis
		A18.52	Tuberculous keratitis
		A18.54	Tuberculous iridocyclitis
		A18.59	Other tuberculosis of eye
Ø17.36	TB OF EYE-OTH TEST	**A18.5Ø**	Tuberculosis of eye, unspecified
		A18.51	Tuberculous episcleritis
		A18.52	Tuberculous keratitis
		A18.54	Tuberculous iridocyclitis
		A18.59	Other tuberculosis of eye
Ø17.4Ø	TUBERCULOSIS OF EAR CONFIRMATION UNSPECIFIED	**A18.6**	Tuberculosis of (inner) (middle) ear
Ø17.41	TB EAR BACTERIOLOGICAL/HISTOLOGICAL EX NOT DONE	**A18.6**	Tuberculosis of (inner) (middle) ear
Ø17.42	TB EAR BACTERIOLOGICAL/HISTOLOGICAL EXAM UNKNOWN	**A18.6**	Tuberculosis of (inner) (middle) ear
Ø17.43	TUBERCULOSIS EAR TUBERCLE BACILLI FOUND MIC	**A18.6**	Tuberculosis of (inner) (middle) ear
Ø17.44	TB OF EAR-CULT DX	**A18.6**	Tuberculosis of (inner) (middle) ear
Ø17.45	TB OF EAR-HISTO DX	**A18.6**	Tuberculosis of (inner) (middle) ear
Ø17.46	TB OF EAR-OTH TEST	**A18.6**	Tuberculosis of (inner) (middle) ear
Ø17.5Ø	TUBERCULOSIS THYROID GLAND CONFIRMATION UNSPEC	**A18.81**	Tuberculosis of thyroid gland
Ø17.51	TB THYROID GLAND EX NOT DONE	**A18.81**	Tuberculosis of thyroid gland
Ø17.52	TB THYROID GLAND EX UNKN	**A18.81**	Tuberculosis of thyroid gland
Ø17.53	TB THYROID GLAND TUBERCLE BACILLI FOUND MIC	**A18.81**	Tuberculosis of thyroid gland
Ø17.54	TB OF THYROID GLAND-CULT DX	**A18.81**	Tuberculosis of thyroid gland
Ø17.55	TB OF THYROID GLAND-HISTO DX	**A18.81**	Tuberculosis of thyroid gland
Ø17.56	TB OF THYROID GLAND-OTH TEST	**A18.81**	Tuberculosis of thyroid gland
Ø17.6Ø	TUBERCULOSIS ADRENAL GLANDS CONFIRMATION UNSPEC	**A18.7**	Tuberculosis of adrenal glands
Ø17.61	TB ADRENL GLND EX NOT DONE	**A18.7**	Tuberculosis of adrenal glands
Ø17.62	TB ADRENL GLND EX UNKN	**A18.7**	Tuberculosis of adrenal glands
Ø17.63	TB ADRENAL GLANDS TUBERCLE BACILLI FOUND MIC	**A18.7**	Tuberculosis of adrenal glands
Ø17.64	TB OF ADRENAL GLANDS-CULT DX	**A18.7**	Tuberculosis of adrenal glands
Ø17.65	TB OF ADRENAL GLANDS-HISTO DX	**A18.7**	Tuberculosis of adrenal glands
Ø17.66	TB OF ADRENAL GLANDS-OTH TEST	**A18.7**	Tuberculosis of adrenal glands
Ø17.7Ø	TUBERCULOSIS OF SPLEEN CONFIRMATION UNSPECIFIED	**A18.85**	Tuberculosis of spleen
Ø17.71	TB SPLEEN EX NOT DONE	**A18.85**	Tuberculosis of spleen
Ø17.72	TB SPLEEN BACTERIOLOGICAL/HISTOLOGICAL EX UNKN	**A18.85**	Tuberculosis of spleen
Ø17.73	TUBERCULOSIS SPLEEN TUBERCLE BACILLI FOUND MIC	**A18.85**	Tuberculosis of spleen
Ø17.74	TB OF SPLEEN-CULT DX	**A18.85**	Tuberculosis of spleen
Ø17.75	TB OF SPLEEN-HISTO DX	**A18.85**	Tuberculosis of spleen
Ø17.76	TB OF SPLEEN-OTH TEST	**A18.85**	Tuberculosis of spleen
Ø17.8Ø	TUBERCULOSIS ESOPHAGUS CONFIRMATION UNSPECIFIED	**A18.89**	Tuberculosis of other sites
Ø17.81	TB ESOPH EX NOT DONE	**A18.89**	Tuberculosis of other sites
Ø17.82	TB ESOPH BACTERIOLOGICAL/HISTOLOGICAL EX UNKNOWN	**A18.89**	Tuberculosis of other sites

ICD-9-CM			ICD-10-CM	
Ø17.83	TUBERCULOSIS ESOPH TUBERCLE BACILLI FOUND MIC		**A18.89**	Tuberculosis of other sites
Ø17.84	TB OF ESOPHAGUS-CULT DX		**A18.89**	Tuberculosis of other sites
Ø17.85	TB OF ESOPHAGUS-HISTO DX		**A18.89**	Tuberculosis of other sites
Ø17.86	TB OF ESOPHAGUS-OTH TEST		**A18.89**	Tuberculosis of other sites
Ø17.9Ø	TUBERCULOSIS OTH SPEC ORGANS CONFIRMATION UNSPEC		**A17.83**	Tuberculous neuritis
			A17.9	Tuberculosis of nervous system, unspecified
			A18.82	Tuberculosis of other endocrine glands
		▣	**A18.84**	Tuberculosis of heart
			A18.89	Tuberculosis of other sites
Ø17.91	TB OTH SPEC ORGN EX NOT DONE		**A18.84**	Tuberculosis of heart
			A18.89	Tuberculosis of other sites
Ø17.92	TB OTH SPEC ORGN EX UNKN		**A18.84**	Tuberculosis of heart
			A18.89	Tuberculosis of other sites
Ø17.93	TB OTH SPEC ORGN TUBERCLE BACILLI FOUND MIC		**A18.84**	Tuberculosis of heart
			A18.89	Tuberculosis of other sites
Ø17.94	TB OF OTH SPEC ORGANS-CULT DX		**A18.84**	Tuberculosis of heart
			A18.89	Tuberculosis of other sites
Ø17.95	TB OF OTH SPEC ORGANS-HISTO DX		**A18.84**	Tuberculosis of heart
			A18.89	Tuberculosis of other sites
Ø17.96	TB OF OTH SPEC ORGANS-OTH TEST		**A18.84**	Tuberculosis of heart
			A18.89	Tuberculosis of other sites
Ø18.ØØ	ACUTE MILIARY TUBERCULOSIS UNSPECIFIED		**A19.Ø**	Acute miliary tuberculosis of a single specified site
			A19.1	Acute miliary tuberculosis of multiple sites
			A19.2	Acute miliary tuberculosis, unspecified
Ø18.Ø1	ACUT MILIARY TB EX NOT DONE		**A19.2**	Acute miliary tuberculosis, unspecified
Ø18.Ø2	ACUT MILIARY TB EX UNKN		**A19.2**	Acute miliary tuberculosis, unspecified
Ø18.Ø3	ACUTE MILIARY TB TUBERCLE BACILLI FOUND MIC		**A19.2**	Acute miliary tuberculosis, unspecified
Ø18.Ø4	ACUTE MILIARY TB-CULT DX		**A19.2**	Acute miliary tuberculosis, unspecified
Ø18.Ø5	ACUTE MILIARY TB-HISTO DX		**A19.2**	Acute miliary tuberculosis, unspecified
Ø18.Ø6	ACUTE MILIARY TB-OTH TEST		**A19.2**	Acute miliary tuberculosis, unspecified
Ø18.8Ø	OTH SPEC MILIARY TUBERCULOSIS CONF UNSPEC		**A19.8**	Other miliary tuberculosis
Ø18.81	OTH SPEC MILIARY TB EX NOT DONE		**A19.8**	Other miliary tuberculosis
Ø18.82	OTH SPEC MILIARY TB EX UNKN		**A19.8**	Other miliary tuberculosis
Ø18.83	OTH SPEC MILIARY TB TUBERCLE BACILLI FOUND MIC		**A19.8**	Other miliary tuberculosis
Ø18.84	OTH SPEC MILIARY TB-CULT DX		**A19.8**	Other miliary tuberculosis
Ø18.85	OTH SPEC MILIARY TB-HISTO DX		**A19.8**	Other miliary tuberculosis
Ø18.86	OTH SPEC MILIARY TB-OTH TEST		**A19.8**	Other miliary tuberculosis
Ø18.9Ø	UNSPECIFIED MILIARY TUBERCULOSIS UNSPECIFIED		**A19.9**	Miliary tuberculosis, unspecified
Ø18.91	UNS MILIARY TB EX NOT DONE		**A19.9**	Miliary tuberculosis, unspecified
Ø18.92	UNS MILIARY TB EX UNKN		**A19.9**	Miliary tuberculosis, unspecified
Ø18.93	UNSPEC MILIARY TB TUBERCLE BACILLI FOUND MIC		**A19.9**	Miliary tuberculosis, unspecified
Ø18.94	UNS MILIARY TB-CULT DX		**A19.9**	Miliary tuberculosis, unspecified
Ø18.95	UNS MILIARY TB-HISTO DX		**A19.9**	Miliary tuberculosis, unspecified
Ø18.96	UNS MILIARY TB-OTH TEST		**A19.9**	Miliary tuberculosis, unspecified
Ø2Ø.Ø	BUBONIC PLAGUE	➡	**A2Ø.Ø**	Bubonic plague
Ø2Ø.1	CELLULOCUTANEOUS PLAGUE	➡	**A2Ø.1**	Cellulocutaneous plague
Ø2Ø.2	SEPTICEMIC PLAGUE	➡	**A2Ø.7**	Septicemic plague
Ø2Ø.3	PRIMARY PNEUMONIC PLAGUE		**A2Ø.2**	Pneumonic plague
Ø2Ø.4	SECONDARY PNEUMONIC PLAGUE		**A2Ø.2**	Pneumonic plague
Ø2Ø.5	PNEUMONIC PLAGUE, UNSPECIFIED		**A2Ø.2**	Pneumonic plague
Ø2Ø.8	OTHER SPECIFIED TYPES OF PLAGUE		**A2Ø.3**	Plague meningitis
			A2Ø.8	Other forms of plague
Ø2Ø.9	UNSPECIFIED PLAGUE	➡	**A2Ø.9**	Plague, unspecified
Ø21.Ø	ULCEROGLANDULAR TULAREMIA	➡	**A21.Ø**	Ulceroglandular tularemia
Ø21.1	ENTERIC TULAREMIA		**A21.3**	Gastrointestinal tularemia
Ø21.2	PULMONARY TULAREMIA	➡	**A21.2**	Pulmonary tularemia
Ø21.3	OCULOGLANDULAR TULAREMIA	➡	**A21.1**	Oculoglandular tularemia
Ø21.8	OTHER SPECIFIED TULAREMIA		**A21.7**	Generalized tularemia
			A21.8	Other forms of tularemia
Ø21.9	UNSPECIFIED TULAREMIA	➡	**A21.9**	Tularemia, unspecified
Ø22.Ø	CUTANEOUS ANTHRAX	➡	**A22.Ø**	Cutaneous anthrax
Ø22.1	PULMONARY ANTHRAX	▣	**A22.1**	Pulmonary anthrax
Ø22.2	GASTROINTESTINAL ANTHRAX	➡	**A22.2**	Gastrointestinal anthrax
Ø22.3	ANTHRAX SEPTICEMIA	▣	**A22.7**	Anthrax sepsis
Ø22.8	OTHER SPECIFIED MANIFESTATIONS OF ANTHRAX	➡	**A22.8**	Other forms of anthrax
Ø22.9	UNSPECIFIED ANTHRAX	➡	**A22.9**	Anthrax, unspecified
Ø23.Ø	BRUCELLA MELITENSIS	➡	**A23.Ø**	Brucellosis due to Brucella melitensis
Ø23.1	BRUCELLA ABORTUS	➡	**A23.1**	Brucellosis due to Brucella abortus
Ø23.2	BRUCELLA SUIS	➡	**A23.2**	Brucellosis due to Brucella suis

ICD-9-CM			ICD-10-CM	
Ø23.3	BRUCELLA CANIS	➡	A23.3	Brucellosis due to Brucella canis
Ø23.8	OTHER BRUCELLOSIS	➡	A23.8	Other brucellosis
Ø23.9	BURCELLOSIS, UNSPECIFIED	➡	A23.9	Brucellosis, unspecified
Ø24	GLANDERS	➡	A24.Ø	Glanders
Ø25	MELIOIDOSIS		A24.1	Acute and fulminating melioidosis
			A24.2	Subacute and chronic melioidosis
			A24.3	Other melioidosis
			A24.9	Melioidosis, unspecified
Ø26.Ø	SPIRILLARY FEVER	➡	A25.Ø	Spirillosis
Ø26.1	STREPTOBACILLARY FEVER	➡	A25.1	Streptobacillosis
Ø26.9	UNSPECIFIED RAT-BITE FEVER	➡	A25.9	Rat-bite fever, unspecified
Ø27.Ø	LISTERIOSIS		A32.Ø	Cutaneous listeriosis
			A32.11	Listerial meningitis
			A32.12	Listerial meningoencephalitis
			A32.7	Listerial sepsis
			A32.81	Oculoglandular listeriosis
			A32.82	Listerial endocarditis
			A32.89	Other forms of listeriosis
			A32.9	Listeriosis, unspecified
Ø27.1	ERYSIPELOTHRIX INFECTION		A26.Ø	Cutaneous erysipeloid
			A26.7	Erysipelothrix sepsis
			A26.8	Other forms of erysipeloid
			A26.9	Erysipeloid, unspecified
Ø27.2	PASTEURELLOSIS	➡	A28.Ø	Pasteurellosis
Ø27.8	OTHER SPECIFIED ZOONOTIC BACTERIAL DISEASES		A28.2	Extraintestinal yersiniosis
			A28.8	Oth zoonotic bacterial diseases, not elsewhere classified
Ø27.9	UNSPECIFIED ZOONOTIC BACTERIAL DISEASE	➡	A28.9	Zoonotic bacterial disease, unspecified
Ø3Ø.Ø	LEPROMATOUS LEPROSY	➡	A3Ø.5	Lepromatous leprosy
Ø3Ø.1	TUBERCULOID LEPROSY	➡	A3Ø.1	Tuberculoid leprosy
Ø3Ø.2	INDETERMINATE LEPROSY	➡	A3Ø.Ø	Indeterminate leprosy
Ø3Ø.3	BORDERLINE LEPROSY		A3Ø.2	Borderline tuberculoid leprosy
			A3Ø.3	Borderline leprosy
			A3Ø.4	Borderline lepromatous leprosy
Ø3Ø.8	OTHER SPECIFIED LEPROSY	➡	A3Ø.8	Other forms of leprosy
Ø3Ø.9	UNSPECIFIED LEPROSY	➡	A3Ø.9	Leprosy, unspecified
Ø31.Ø	PULMONARY DISEASES DUE TO OTHER MYCOBACTERIA	➡	A31.Ø	Pulmonary mycobacterial infection
Ø31.1	CUTANEOUS DISEASES DUE TO OTHER MYCOBACTERIA	➡	A31.1	Cutaneous mycobacterial infection
Ø31.2	DISSEMINATED DISEASES DUE TO OTHER MYCOBACTERIA	➡	A31.2	Dissem mycobacterium avium-intracellulare complex (DMAC)
Ø31.8	OTHER SPECIFIED DISEASES DUE OTHER MYCOBACTERIA	➡	A31.8	Other mycobacterial infections
Ø31.9	UNSPECIFIED DISEASES DUE TO MYCOBACTERIA	➡	A31.9	Mycobacterial infection, unspecified
Ø32.Ø	FAUCIAL DIPHTHERIA	➡	A36.Ø	Pharyngeal diphtheria
Ø32.1	NASOPHARYNGEAL DIPHTHERIA	➡	A36.1	Nasopharyngeal diphtheria
Ø32.2	ANTERIOR NASAL DIPHTHERIA		A36.89	Other diphtheritic complications
Ø32.3	LARYNGEAL DIPHTHERIA	➡	A36.2	Laryngeal diphtheria
Ø32.81	CONJUNCTIVAL DIPHTHERIA	➡	A36.86	Diphtheritic conjunctivitis
Ø32.82	DIPHTHERITIC MYOCARDITIS	➡	A36.81	Diphtheritic cardiomyopathy
Ø32.83	DIPHTHERITIC PERITONITIS		A36.89	Other diphtheritic complications
Ø32.84	DIPHTHERITIC CYSTITIS	➡	A36.85	Diphtheritic cystitis
Ø32.85	CUTANEOUS DIPHTHERIA	➡	A36.3	Cutaneous diphtheria
Ø32.89	OTHER SPECIFIED DIPHTHERIA		A36.82	Diphtheritic radiculomyelitis
			A36.83	Diphtheritic polyneuritis
			A36.84	Diphtheritic tubulo-interstitial nephropathy
			A36.89	Other diphtheritic complications
Ø32.9	UNSPECIFIED DIPHTHERIA	➡	A36.9	Diphtheria, unspecified
Ø33.Ø	WHOOPING COUGH DUE TO BORDETELLA PERTUSSIS		A37.ØØ	Whooping cough due to Bordetella pertussis without pneumonia
			A37.Ø1	Whooping cough due to Bordetella pertussis with pneumonia
Ø33.1	WHOOPING COUGH DUE TO BORDETELLA PARAPERTUSSIS		A37.1Ø	Whooping cough due to Bordetella parapertussis w/o pneumonia
			A37.11	Whooping cough due to Bordetella parapertussis w pneumonia
Ø33.8	WHOOPING COUGH DUE TO OTHER SPECIFIED ORGANISM		A37.8Ø	Whooping cough due to other Bordetella species w/o pneumonia
			A37.81	Whooping cough due to oth Bordetella species with pneumonia
Ø33.9	WHOOPING COUGH UNSPECIFIED ORGANISM		A37.9Ø	Whooping cough, unspecified species without pneumonia
			A37.91	Whooping cough, unspecified species with pneumonia
Ø34.Ø	STREPTOCOCCAL SORE THROAT		JØ2.Ø	Streptococcal pharyngitis
			JØ3.ØØ	Acute streptococcal tonsillitis, unspecified
			JØ3.Ø1	Acute recurrent streptococcal tonsillitis
Ø34.1	SCARLET FEVER		A38.Ø	Scarlet fever with otitis media
			A38.1	Scarlet fever with myocarditis
			A38.8	Scarlet fever with other complications
			A38.9	Scarlet fever, uncomplicated
Ø35	ERYSIPELAS	➡	A46	Erysipelas
Ø36.Ø	MENINGOCOCCAL MENINGITIS	➡	A39.Ø	Meningococcal meningitis
Ø36.1	MENINGOCOCCAL ENCEPHALITIS	➡	A39.81	Meningococcal encephalitis

[Brackets] indicate valid character values for each code. Character value meanings provided for each code grouping.

ICD-9-CM			ICD-10-CM	
036.2	MENINGOCOCCEMIA		A39.2	Acute meningococcemia
			A39.3	Chronic meningococcemia
			A39.4	Meningococcemia, unspecified
036.3	WATERHOUSE-FRIDERICHSEN SYNDROME MENINGOCOCCAL	➡	A39.1	Waterhouse-Friderichsen syndrome
036.40	MENINGOCOCCAL CARDITIS, UNSPECIFIED	➡	A39.50	Meningococcal carditis, unspecified
036.41	MENINGOCOCCAL PERICARDITIS	➡	A39.53	Meningococcal pericarditis
036.42	MENINGOCOCCAL ENDOCARDITIS	➡	A39.51	Meningococcal endocarditis
036.43	MENINGOCOCCAL MYOCARDITIS	➡	A39.52	Meningococcal myocarditis
036.81	MENINGOCOCCAL OPTIC NEURITIS		A39.82	Meningococcal retrobulbar neuritis
036.82	MENINGOCOCCAL ARTHROPATHY		A39.83	Meningococcal arthritis
			A39.84	Postmeningococcal arthritis
036.89	OTHER SPECIFIED MENINGOCOCCAL INFECTIONS	➡	A39.89	Other meningococcal infections
036.9	UNSPECIFIED MENINGOCOCCAL INFECTION	➡	A39.9	Meningococcal infection, unspecified
037	TETANUS	➡	A35	Other tetanus
038.0	STREPTOCOCCAL SEPTICEMIA	▣	A40.0	Sepsis due to streptococcus, group A
		▣	A40.1	Sepsis due to streptococcus, group B
		▣	A40.3	Sepsis due to Streptococcus pneumoniae
		▣	A40.8	Other streptococcal sepsis
		▣	A40.9	Streptococcal sepsis, unspecified
038.10	UNSPECIFIED STAPHYLOCOCCAL SEPTICEMIA	▣	A41.2	Sepsis due to unspecified staphylococcus
038.11	METHICILLIN SUSCEPTIBLE STAPH AUREUS SEPTICEMIA	▣	A41.01	Sepsis due to Methicillin susceptible Staphylococcus aureus
038.12	METHICILLIN RESISTANT STAPH AUREUS SEPTICEMIA	▣	A41.02	Sepsis due to Methicillin resistant Staphylococcus aureus
038.19	OTHER STAPHYLOCOCCAL SEPTICEMIA	▣	A41.1	Sepsis due to other specified staphylococcus
038.2	PNEUMOCOCCAL SEPTICEMIA	▣	A40.3	Sepsis due to Streptococcus pneumoniae
038.3	SEPTICEMIA DUE TO ANAEROBES	▣	A41.4	Sepsis due to anaerobes
038.40	SEPTICEMIA DUE UNSPEC GRAM-NEGATIVE ORGANISM	▣	A41.50	Gram-negative sepsis, unspecified
038.41	SEPTICEMIA DUE TO HEMOPHILUS INFLUENZAE	▣	A41.3	Sepsis due to Hemophilus influenzae
038.42	SEPTICEMIA DUE TO ESCHERICHIA COLI	▣	A41.51	Sepsis due to Escherichia coli [E. coli]
038.43	SEPTICEMIA DUE TO PSEUDOMONAS	▣	A41.52	Sepsis due to Pseudomonas
038.44	SEPTICEMIA DUE TO SERRATIA	▣	A41.53	Sepsis due to Serratia
038.49	OTHER SEPTICEMIA DUE TO GRAM-NEGATIVE ORGANISM	▣	A41.59	Other Gram-negative sepsis
038.8	OTHER SPECIFIED SEPTICEMIA	▣	A41.81	Sepsis due to Enterococcus
		▣	A41.89	Other specified sepsis
		▣	A42.7	Actinomycotic sepsis
038.9	UNSPECIFIED SEPTICEMIA	▣	A41.9	Sepsis, unspecified organism
039.0	CUTANEOUS ACTINOMYCOTIC INFECTION		A43.1	Cutaneous nocardiosis
			L08.1	Erythrasma
039.1	PULMONARY ACTINOMYCOTIC INFECTION		A42.0	Pulmonary actinomycosis
			A43.0	Pulmonary nocardiosis
039.2	ABDOMINAL ACTINOMYCOTIC INFECTION	➡	A42.1	Abdominal actinomycosis
039.3	CERVICOFACIAL ACTINOMYCOTIC INFECTION	➡	A42.2	Cervicofacial actinomycosis
039.4	MADURA FOOT		B47.9	Mycetoma, unspecified
039.8	ACTINOMYCOTIC INFECTION OF OTHER SPECIFIED SITES		A42.81	Actinomycotic meningitis
			A42.82	Actinomycotic encephalitis
			A42.89	Other forms of actinomycosis
			A43.8	Other forms of nocardiosis
039.9	ACTINOMYCOTIC INFECTION OF UNSPECIFIED SITE		A42.9	Actinomycosis, unspecified
			A43.9	Nocardiosis, unspecified
			B47.1	Actinomycetoma
040.0	GAS GANGRENE	➡	A48.0	Gas gangrene
040.1	RHINOSCLEROMA		A48.8	Other specified bacterial diseases
040.2	WHIPPLES DISEASE	➡	K90.81	Whipple's disease
040.3	NECROBACILLOSIS		A48.8	Other specified bacterial diseases
040.41	INFANT BOTULISM	➡	A48.51	Infant botulism
040.42	WOUND BOTULISM	➡	A48.52	Wound botulism
040.81	TROPICAL PYOMYOSITIS		M60.009	Infective myositis, unspecified site
040.82	TOXIC SHOCK SYNDROME	➡	A48.3	Toxic shock syndrome
040.89	OTHER SPECIFIED BACTERIAL DISEASES		A48.2	Nonpneumonic Legionnaires' disease [Pontiac fever]
			A48.4	Brazilian purpuric fever
			A48.8	Other specified bacterial diseases
041.00	UNSPEC STREPTOCOCCUS INFECTION CCE & UNS SITE		A49.1	Streptococcal infection, unspecified site
			B95.5	Unsp streptococcus as the cause of diseases classd elswhr
		▣	J20.2	Acute bronchitis due to streptococcus
041.01	STREPTOCOCCUS INFECTION CCE & UNS SITE GROUP A	➡	B95.0	Streptococcus, group A, causing diseases classd elswhr
041.02	STREPTOCOCCUS INFECTION CCE & UNS SITE GROUP B	➡	B95.1	Streptococcus, group B, causing diseases classd elswhr
041.03	STREPTOCOCCUS INFECTION CCE & UNS SITE GROUP C		B95.4	Oth streptococcus as the cause of diseases classd elswhr
041.04	STREP INF CCE & UNS SITE GROUP D ENTEROCOCCUS	➡	B95.2	Enterococcus as the cause of diseases classified elsewhere
041.05	STREPTOCOCCUS INFECTION CCE & UNS SITE GROUP G		B95.4	Oth streptococcus as the cause of diseases classd elswhr

ICD-9-CM		ICD-10-CM	
Ø41.Ø9	OTHER STREPTOCOCCUS INFECTION IN CCE & UNS SITE	**B95.3**	Streptococcus pneumoniae causing diseases classd elswhr
		B95.4	Oth streptococcus as the cause of diseases classd elswhr
		MØØ.2Ø	Other streptococcal arthritis, unspecified joint
		MØØ.211	Other streptococcal arthritis, right shoulder
		MØØ.212	Other streptococcal arthritis, left shoulder
		MØØ.219	Other streptococcal arthritis, unspecified shoulder
		MØØ.221	Other streptococcal arthritis, right elbow
		MØØ.222	Other streptococcal arthritis, left elbow
		MØØ.229	Other streptococcal arthritis, unspecified elbow
		MØØ.231	Other streptococcal arthritis, right wrist
		MØØ.232	Other streptococcal arthritis, left wrist
		MØØ.239	Other streptococcal arthritis, unspecified wrist
		MØØ.241	Other streptococcal arthritis, right hand
		MØØ.242	Other streptococcal arthritis, left hand
		MØØ.249	Other streptococcal arthritis, unspecified hand
		MØØ.251	Other streptococcal arthritis, right hip
		MØØ.252	Other streptococcal arthritis, left hip
		MØØ.259	Other streptococcal arthritis, unspecified hip
		MØØ.261	Other streptococcal arthritis, right knee
		MØØ.262	Other streptococcal arthritis, left knee
		MØØ.269	Other streptococcal arthritis, unspecified knee
		MØØ.271	Other streptococcal arthritis, right ankle and foot
		MØØ.272	Other streptococcal arthritis, left ankle and foot
		MØØ.279	Other streptococcal arthritis, unspecified ankle and foot
		MØØ.28	Other streptococcal arthritis, vertebrae
		MØØ.29	Other streptococcal polyarthritis
Ø41.1Ø	UNSPEC STAPHYLOCOCCUS INFECTION CCE & UNS SITE	**B95.8**	Unsp staphylococcus as the cause of diseases classd elswhr
		MØØ.ØØ	Staphylococcal arthritis, unspecified joint
		MØØ.Ø11	Staphylococcal arthritis, right shoulder
		MØØ.Ø12	Staphylococcal arthritis, left shoulder
		MØØ.Ø19	Staphylococcal arthritis, unspecified shoulder
		MØØ.Ø21	Staphylococcal arthritis, right elbow
		MØØ.Ø22	Staphylococcal arthritis, left elbow
		MØØ.Ø29	Staphylococcal arthritis, unspecified elbow
		MØØ.Ø31	Staphylococcal arthritis, right wrist
		MØØ.Ø32	Staphylococcal arthritis, left wrist
		MØØ.Ø39	Staphylococcal arthritis, unspecified wrist
		MØØ.Ø41	Staphylococcal arthritis, right hand
		MØØ.Ø42	Staphylococcal arthritis, left hand
		MØØ.Ø49	Staphylococcal arthritis, unspecified hand
		MØØ.Ø51	Staphylococcal arthritis, right hip
		MØØ.Ø52	Staphylococcal arthritis, left hip
		MØØ.Ø59	Staphylococcal arthritis, unspecified hip
		MØØ.Ø61	Staphylococcal arthritis, right knee
		MØØ.Ø62	Staphylococcal arthritis, left knee
		MØØ.Ø69	Staphylococcal arthritis, unspecified knee
		MØØ.Ø71	Staphylococcal arthritis, right ankle and foot
		MØØ.Ø72	Staphylococcal arthritis, left ankle and foot
		MØØ.Ø79	Staphylococcal arthritis, unspecified ankle and foot
		MØØ.Ø8	Staphylococcal arthritis, vertebrae
		MØØ.Ø9	Staphylococcal polyarthritis
Ø41.11	METHICILLIN SUSCEPTIBLE STAPH INF CCE & UNS SITE	**A49.Ø1**	Methicillin suscep staph infection, unsp site
		B95.61	Methicillin suscep staph infct causing dis classd elswhr
Ø41.12	METHICILLIN RESISTANT STAPHYLOCOCCUS AUREUS	**A49.Ø2**	Methicillin resis staph infection, unsp site
		B95.62	Methicillin resis staph infct causing diseases classd elswhr
Ø41.19	OTHER STAPHYLOCOCCUS INFECTION IN CCE & UNS SITE	**B95.7**	Oth staphylococcus as the cause of diseases classd elswhr

 [Brackets] indicate valid character values for each code. Character value meanings provided for each code grouping.

ICD-9-CM			ICD-10-CM	
Ø41.2	PNEUMOCOCCUS INFECTION IN CCE & UNS SITE		B95.3	Streptococcus pneumoniae causing diseases classd elswhr
		■	MØØ.1Ø	Pneumococcal arthritis, unspecified joint
		■	MØØ.111	Pneumococcal arthritis, right shoulder
		■	MØØ.112	Pneumococcal arthritis, left shoulder
		■	MØØ.119	Pneumococcal arthritis, unspecified shoulder
		■	MØØ.121	Pneumococcal arthritis, right elbow
		■	MØØ.122	Pneumococcal arthritis, left elbow
		■	MØØ.129	Pneumococcal arthritis, unspecified elbow
		■	MØØ.131	Pneumococcal arthritis, right wrist
		■	MØØ.132	Pneumococcal arthritis, left wrist
		■	MØØ.139	Pneumococcal arthritis, unspecified wrist
		■	MØØ.141	Pneumococcal arthritis, right hand
		■	MØØ.142	Pneumococcal arthritis, left hand
		■	MØØ.149	Pneumococcal arthritis, unspecified hand
		■	MØØ.151	Pneumococcal arthritis, right hip
		■	MØØ.152	Pneumococcal arthritis, left hip
		■	MØØ.159	Pneumococcal arthritis, unspecified hip
		■	MØØ.161	Pneumococcal arthritis, right knee
		■	MØØ.162	Pneumococcal arthritis, left knee
		■	MØØ.169	Pneumococcal arthritis, unspecified knee
		■	MØØ.171	Pneumococcal arthritis, right ankle and foot
		■	MØØ.172	Pneumococcal arthritis, left ankle and foot
		■	MØØ.179	Pneumococcal arthritis, unspecified ankle and foot
		■	MØØ.18	Pneumococcal arthritis, vertebrae
		■	MØØ.19	Pneumococcal polyarthritis
Ø41.3	KLEBSIELLA PNEUMONIAE INFECTION	➡	B96.1	Klebsiella pneumoniae as the cause of diseases classd elswhr
Ø41.41	SHIGA TOXIN-PRODUCING ESCHERICHIA COLI		B96.21	Shiga toxin E coli (STEC) O157 causing dis classd elswhr
Ø41.42	OTH SHIGA TOXIN-PRODUCING E COLI INF CLASS ELSW		B96.22	Oth shiga toxin E coli (STEC) causing diseases classd elswhr
Ø41.43	UNS SHIGA TOXIN-PRODUCING E COLI INF CLASS ELSW		B96.23	Unsp shiga toxin E coli (STEC) causing dis classd elswhr
Ø41.49	OTH & UNS E COLI INFECTION CLASS ELSW UNS SITE		B96.2Ø	Unsp Escherichia coli as the cause of diseases classd elswhr
			B96.29	Oth Escherichia coli as the cause of diseases classd elswhr
Ø41.5	HEMOPHILUS INFLUENZAE INFECTION CCE & UNS SITE		A49.2	Hemophilus influenzae infection, unspecified site
			B96.3	Hemophilus influenzae as the cause of diseases classd elswhr
		■	J2Ø.1	Acute bronchitis due to Hemophilus influenzae
Ø41.6	PROTEUS INFECTION IN CCE & UNS SITE	➡	B96.4	Proteus (mirabilis) (morganii) causing dis classd elswhr
Ø41.7	PSEUDOMONAS INFECTION IN CCE & UNS SITE	➡	B96.5	Pseudomonas (mallei) causing diseases classd elswhr
Ø41.81	MYCOPLASMA INFECTION IN CCE & UNS SITE		A49.3	Mycoplasma infection, unspecified site
			B96.Ø	Mycoplasma pneumoniae as the cause of diseases classd elswhr
		■	J2Ø.Ø	Acute bronchitis due to Mycoplasma pneumoniae
Ø41.82	BACT INF COND CLASS ELSW BACTEROIDES FRAGILIS	➡	B96.6	Bacteroides fragilis as the cause of diseases classd elswhr
Ø41.83	CLOSTRIDIUM PERFRINGENS INFECTION CCE & UNS SITE		B96.7	Clostridium perfringens causing diseases classd elswhr
Ø41.84	INFECTION DUE TO OTHER ANAEROBES CCE & UNS SITE		B96.82	Vibrio vulnificus as the cause of diseases classd elswhr
			B96.89	Oth bacterial agents as the cause of diseases classd elswhr
Ø41.85	INF DUE OTH GM-NEGATIVE ORGANISMS CCE & UNS SITE		B96.89	Oth bacterial agents as the cause of diseases classd elswhr
Ø41.86	HELICOBACTER PYLORI INFECTION	➡	B96.81	Helicobacter pylori as the cause of diseases classd elswhr
Ø41.89	INFECTION DUE OTHER SPEC BACTERIA CCE & UNS SITE		A49.8	Other bacterial infections of unspecified site
			B96.89	Oth bacterial agents as the cause of diseases classd elswhr
		■	MØØ.8Ø	Arthritis due to other bacteria, unspecified joint
		■	MØØ.811	Arthritis due to other bacteria, right shoulder
		■	MØØ.812	Arthritis due to other bacteria, left shoulder
		■	MØØ.819	Arthritis due to other bacteria, unspecified shoulder
		■	MØØ.821	Arthritis due to other bacteria, right elbow
		■	MØØ.822	Arthritis due to other bacteria, left elbow
		■	MØØ.829	Arthritis due to other bacteria, unspecified elbow
		■	MØØ.831	Arthritis due to other bacteria, right wrist
		■	MØØ.832	Arthritis due to other bacteria, left wrist
		■	MØØ.839	Arthritis due to other bacteria, unspecified wrist
		■	MØØ.841	Arthritis due to other bacteria, right hand
		■	MØØ.842	Arthritis due to other bacteria, left hand
		■	MØØ.849	Arthritis due to other bacteria, unspecified hand
		■	MØØ.851	Arthritis due to other bacteria, right hip
		■	MØØ.852	Arthritis due to other bacteria, left hip
		■	MØØ.859	Arthritis due to other bacteria, unspecified hip
		■	MØØ.861	Arthritis due to other bacteria, right knee
		■	MØØ.862	Arthritis due to other bacteria, left knee
		■	MØØ.869	Arthritis due to other bacteria, unspecified knee
		■	MØØ.871	Arthritis due to other bacteria, right ankle and foot
		■	MØØ.872	Arthritis due to other bacteria, left ankle and foot
		■	MØØ.879	Arthritis due to other bacteria, unspecified ankle and foot
		■	MØØ.88	Arthritis due to other bacteria, vertebrae
		■	MØØ.89	Polyarthritis due to other bacteria
Ø41.9	BACTERIAL INFECTION UNSPECIFIED CCE & UNS SITE		A49.9	Bacterial infection, unspecified
			B96.89	Oth bacterial agents as the cause of diseases classd elswhr
Ø42	HUMAN IMMUNODEFICIENCY VIRUS [HIV]	➡	B2Ø	Human immunodeficiency virus [HIV] disease
Ø45.ØØ	ACUT PARALYT POLIOMYEL SPEC BULBR UNS POLIOVIRUS		A8Ø.39	Other acute paralytic poliomyelitis
Ø45.Ø1	ACUT PARALYT POLIOMYEL BULBR POLIOVIRUS TYPE I		A8Ø.39	Other acute paralytic poliomyelitis

ICD-9-CM		ICD-10-CM	
Ø45.Ø2	ACUT PARALYT POLIOMYEL BULBR POLIOVIRUS TYPE II	**A8Ø.39**	Other acute paralytic poliomyelitis
Ø45.Ø3	ACUT PARALYT POLIOMYEL BULBR POLIOVIRUS TYPE III	**A8Ø.39**	Other acute paralytic poliomyelitis
Ø45.1Ø	ACUT POLIOMYEL W/OTH PARALYSIS UNSPEC POLIOVIRUS	**A8Ø.Ø** **A8Ø.1** **A8Ø.2** **A8Ø.3Ø** **A8Ø.39**	Acute paralytic poliomyelitis, vaccine-associated Acute paralytic poliomyelitis, wild virus, imported Acute paralytic poliomyelitis, wild virus, indigenous Acute paralytic poliomyelitis, unspecified Other acute paralytic poliomyelitis
Ø45.11	ACUT POLIOMYEL W/OTH PARALYSIS POLIOVIRUS TYPE I	**A8Ø.39**	Other acute paralytic poliomyelitis
Ø45.12	ACUT POLIOMYEL W/OTH PARALYSIS TYPE II	**A8Ø.39**	Other acute paralytic poliomyelitis
Ø45.13	ACUT POLIOMYEL W/OTH PARALYSIS TYPE III	**A8Ø.39**	Other acute paralytic poliomyelitis
Ø45.2Ø	ACUTE NONPARALYTIC POLIOMYEL UNSPEC POLIOVIRUS	**A8Ø.4**	Acute nonparalytic poliomyelitis
Ø45.21	ACUTE NONPARALYTIC POLIOMYEL POLIOVIRUS TYPE I	**A8Ø.4**	Acute nonparalytic poliomyelitis
Ø45.22	ACUTE NONPARALYTIC POLIOMYEL POLIOVIRUS TYPE II	**A8Ø.4**	Acute nonparalytic poliomyelitis
Ø45.23	ACUTE NONPARALYTIC POLIOMYEL POLIOVIRUS TYPE III	**A8Ø.4**	Acute nonparalytic poliomyelitis
Ø45.9Ø	ACUTE UNSPEC POLIOMYELITIS UNSPEC POLIOVIRUS	**A8Ø.9**	Acute poliomyelitis, unspecified
Ø45.91	ACUTE UNSPEC POLIOMYELITIS POLIOVIRUS TYPE I	**A8Ø.9**	Acute poliomyelitis, unspecified
Ø45.92	ACUTE UNSPEC POLIOMYELITIS POLIOVIRUS TYPE II	**A8Ø.9**	Acute poliomyelitis, unspecified
Ø45.93	ACUTE UNSPEC POLIOMYELITIS POLIOVIRUS TYPE III	**A8Ø.9**	Acute poliomyelitis, unspecified
Ø46.Ø	KURU	➡ **A81.81**	Kuru
Ø46.11	VARIANT CREUTZFELDT-JAKOB DISEASE	➡ **A81.Ø1**	Variant Creutzfeldt-Jakob disease
Ø46.19	OTHER AND UNSPECIFIED CREUTZFELDT-JAKOB DISEASE	**A81.ØØ** **A81.Ø9**	Creutzfeldt-Jakob disease, unspecified Other Creutzfeldt-Jakob disease
Ø46.2	SUBACUTE SCLEROSING PANENCEPHALITIS	➡ **A81.1**	Subacute sclerosing panencephalitis
Ø46.3	PROGRESSIVE MULTIFOCAL LEUKOENCEPHALOPATHY	**A81.2** **I67.3**	Progressive multifocal leukoencephalopathy Progressive vascular leukoencephalopathy
Ø46.71	GERSTMANN-STRAUSSLER-SCHEINKER SYNDROME	➡ **A81.82**	Gerstmann-Straussler-Scheinker syndrome
Ø46.72	FATAL FAMILIAL INSOMNIA	➡ **A81.83**	Fatal familial insomnia
Ø46.79	OTH & UNS PRION DISEASES CENTRAL NERVOUS SYSTEM	**A81.89**	Other atypical virus infections of central nervous system
Ø46.8	OTHER SPEC SLOW VIRUS INFECTION CNTRL NERV SYS	**A81.89**	Other atypical virus infections of central nervous system
Ø46.9	UNSPECIFIED SLOW VIRUS INFECTION CNTRL NERV SYS	➡ **A81.9**	Atypical virus infection of central nervous system, unsp
Ø47.Ø	MENINGITIS DUE TO COXSACKIE VIRUS	**A87.Ø**	Enteroviral meningitis
Ø47.1	MENINGITIS DUE TO ECHO VIRUS	**A87.Ø**	Enteroviral meningitis
Ø47.8	OTHER SPECIFIED VIRAL MENINGITIS	**A87.Ø** **A87.8**	Enteroviral meningitis Other viral meningitis
Ø47.9	UNSPECIFIED VIRAL MENINGITIS	**A87.9** **GØ3.2**	Viral meningitis, unspecified Benign recurrent meningitis [Mollaret]
Ø48	OTHER ENTEROVIRUS DISEASES OF CNTRL NERV SYS	**A88.Ø**	Enteroviral exanthematous fever [Boston exanthem]
Ø49.Ø	LYMPHOCYTIC CHORIOMENINGITIS	➡ **A87.2**	Lymphocytic choriomeningitis
Ø49.1	MENINGITIS DUE TO ADENOVIRUS	➡ **A87.1**	Adenoviral meningitis
Ø49.8	OTH NON-ARTHROPOD-BORN VIRL DZ CNTRL NRV SYS	**A85.Ø** **A85.1** **A85.8** **A88.8**	Enteroviral encephalitis Adenoviral encephalitis Other specified viral encephalitis Other specified viral infections of central nervous system
Ø49.9	UNS NON-ARTHROPOD-BORN VIRAL DZ CNTRL NERV SYS	**A86** **A89**	Unspecified viral encephalitis Unspecified viral infection of central nervous system
Ø5Ø.Ø	VARIOLA MAJOR	**BØ3**	Smallpox
Ø5Ø.1	ALASTRIM	**BØ3**	Smallpox
Ø5Ø.2	MODIFIED SMALLPOX	**BØ3**	Smallpox
Ø5Ø.9	UNSPECIFIED SMALLPOX	**BØ3**	Smallpox
Ø51.Ø1	COWPOX	➡ **BØ8.Ø1Ø**	Cowpox
Ø51.Ø2	VACCINIA NOT FROM VACCINATION	➡ **BØ8.Ø11**	Vaccinia not from vaccine
Ø51.1	PSEUDOCOWPOX	➡ **BØ8.Ø3**	Pseudocowpox [milker's node]
Ø51.2	CONTAGIOUS PUSTULAR DERMATITIS	**BØ8.Ø2**	Orf virus disease
Ø51.9	UNSPECIFIED PARAVACCINIA	**BØ8.Ø4**	Paravaccinia, unspecified
Ø52.Ø	POSTVARICELLA ENCEPHALITIS	**BØ1.11**	Varicella encephalitis and encephalomyelitis
Ø52.1	VARICELLA PNEUMONITIS	➡ **BØ1.2**	Varicella pneumonia
Ø52.2	POSTVARICELLA MYELITIS	➡ **BØ1.12**	Varicella myelitis
Ø52.7	CHICKENPOX WITH OTHER SPECIFIED COMPLICATIONS	**BØ1.Ø** **BØ1.81** **BØ1.89**	Varicella meningitis Varicella keratitis Other varicella complications
Ø52.8	CHICKENPOX WITH UNSPECIFIED COMPLICATION	**BØ1.89**	Other varicella complications
Ø52.9	VARICELLA WITHOUT MENTION OF COMPLICATION	➡ **BØ1.9**	Varicella without complication
Ø53.Ø	HERPES ZOSTER WITH MENINGITIS	➡ **BØ2.1**	Zoster meningitis
Ø53.1Ø	HERPES ZOSTER W/UNSPEC NERVOUS SYSTEM COMP	**BØ2.29**	Other postherpetic nervous system involvement
Ø53.11	GENICULATE HERPES ZOSTER	➡ **BØ2.21**	Postherpetic geniculate ganglionitis
Ø53.12	POSTHERPETIC TRIGEMINAL NEURALGIA	➡ **BØ2.22**	Postherpetic trigeminal neuralgia
Ø53.13	POSTHERPETIC POLYNEUROPATHY	➡ **BØ2.23**	Postherpetic polyneuropathy
Ø53.14	HERPES ZOSTER MYELITIS	➡ **BØ2.24**	Postherpetic myelitis

ICD-9-CM			ICD-10-CM	
Ø53.19	OTH HERPES ZOSTER W/NERVOUS SYSTEM COMPLICATIONS		BØ2.Ø	Zoster encephalitis
			BØ2.29	Other postherpetic nervous system involvement
Ø53.2Ø	HERPES ZOSTER DERMATITIS OF EYELID		BØ2.39	Other herpes zoster eye disease
Ø53.21	HERPES ZOSTER KERATOCONJUNCTIVITIS	➡	BØ2.33	Zoster keratitis
Ø53.22	HERPES ZOSTER IRIDOCYCLITIS	➡	BØ2.32	Zoster iridocyclitis
Ø53.29	OTHER OPHTHALMIC HERPES ZOSTER COMPLICATIONS		BØ2.3Ø	Zoster ocular disease, unspecified
			BØ2.31	Zoster conjunctivitis
			BØ2.34	Zoster scleritis
			BØ2.39	Other herpes zoster eye disease
Ø53.71	OTITIS EXTERNA DUE TO HERPES ZOSTER		BØ2.8	Zoster with other complications
Ø53.79	OTHER SPECIFIED HERPES ZOSTER COMPLICATIONS		BØ2.8	Zoster with other complications
Ø53.8	UNSPECIFIED HERPES ZOSTER COMPLICATION		BØ2.7	Disseminated zoster
			BØ2.8	Zoster with other complications
Ø53.9	HERPES ZOSTER WITHOUT MENTION OF COMPLICATION	➡	BØ2.9	Zoster without complications
Ø54.Ø	ECZEMA HERPETICUM	➡	BØØ.Ø	Eczema herpeticum
Ø54.1Ø	UNSPECIFIED GENITAL HERPES		A6Ø.ØØ	Herpesviral infection of urogenital system, unspecified
			A6Ø.9	Anogenital herpesviral infection, unspecified
Ø54.11	HERPETIC VULVOVAGINITIS		A6Ø.Ø4	Herpesviral vulvovaginitis
Ø54.12	HERPETIC ULCERATION OF VULVA		A6Ø.Ø4	Herpesviral vulvovaginitis
Ø54.13	HERPETIC INFECTION OF PENIS	➡	A6Ø.Ø1	Herpesviral infection of penis
Ø54.19	OTHER GENITAL HERPES		A6Ø.Ø2	Herpesviral infection of other male genital organs
			A6Ø.Ø3	Herpesviral cervicitis
			A6Ø.Ø9	Herpesviral infection of other urogenital tract
			A6Ø.1	Herpesviral infection of perianal skin and rectum
Ø54.2	HERPETIC GINGIVOSTOMATITIS	➡	BØØ.2	Herpesviral gingivostomatitis and pharyngotonsillitis
Ø54.3	HERPETIC MENINGOENCEPHALITIS		BØØ.4	Herpesviral encephalitis
Ø54.4Ø	UNSPEC OPHTHALMIC COMPLICATION HERPES SIMPLEX	➡	BØØ.5Ø	Herpesviral ocular disease, unspecified
Ø54.41	HERPES SIMPLEX DERMATITIS OF EYELID		BØØ.59	Other herpesviral disease of eye
Ø54.42	DENDRITIC KERATITIS		BØØ.52	Herpesviral keratitis
Ø54.43	HERPES SIMPLEX DISCIFORM KERATITIS		BØØ.52	Herpesviral keratitis
Ø54.44	HERPES SIMPLEX IRIDOCYCLITIS	➡	BØØ.51	Herpesviral iridocyclitis
Ø54.49	HERPES SIMPLEX W/OTHER OPHTHALMIC COMPLICATIONS		BØØ.53	Herpesviral conjunctivitis
			BØØ.59	Other herpesviral disease of eye
Ø54.5	HERPETIC SEPTICEMIA	➡	BØØ.7	Disseminated herpesviral disease
Ø54.6	HERPETIC WHITLOW		BØØ.89	Other herpesviral infection
Ø54.71	VISCERAL HERPES SIMPLEX		BØØ.81	Herpesviral hepatitis
Ø54.72	HERPES SIMPLEX MENINGITIS	➡	BØØ.3	Herpesviral meningitis
Ø54.73	HERPES SIMPLEX OTITIS EXTERNA		BØØ.1	Herpesviral vesicular dermatitis
Ø54.74	HERPES SIMPLEX MYELITIS	➡	BØØ.82	Herpes simplex myelitis
Ø54.79	OTHER SPECIFIED HERPES SIMPLEX COMPLICATIONS		BØØ.89	Other herpesviral infection
Ø54.8	UNSPECIFIED HERPES SIMPLEX COMPLICATION		BØØ.9	Herpesviral infection, unspecified
Ø54.9	HERPES SIMPLEX WITHOUT MENTION OF COMPLICATION		BØØ.9	Herpesviral infection, unspecified
Ø55.Ø	POSTMEASLES ENCEPHALITIS	➡	BØ5.Ø	Measles complicated by encephalitis
Ø55.1	POSTMEASLES PNEUMONIA	➡	BØ5.2	Measles complicated by pneumonia
Ø55.2	POSTMEASLES OTITIS MEDIA	➡	BØ5.3	Measles complicated by otitis media
Ø55.71	MEASLES KERATOCONJUNCTIVITIS	➡	BØ5.81	Measles keratitis and keratoconjunctivitis
Ø55.79	OTHER SPECIFIED MEASLES COMPLICATIONS		BØ5.1	Measles complicated by meningitis
			BØ5.4	Measles with intestinal complications
			BØ5.89	Other measles complications
Ø55.8	UNSPECIFIED MEASLES COMPLICATION		BØ5.89	Other measles complications
Ø55.9	MEASLES WITHOUT MENTION OF COMPLICATION	➡	BØ5.9	Measles without complication
Ø56.ØØ	UNSPECIFIED RUBELLA NEUROLOGICAL COMPLICATION	➡	BØ6.ØØ	Rubella with neurological complication, unspecified
Ø56.Ø1	ENCEPHALOMYELITIS DUE TO RUBELLA	➡	BØ6.Ø1	Rubella encephalitis
Ø56.Ø9	OTHER NEUROLOGICAL RUBELLA COMPLICATIONS		BØ6.Ø2	Rubella meningitis
			BØ6.Ø9	Other neurological complications of rubella
Ø56.71	ARTHRITIS DUE TO RUBELLA	➡	BØ6.82	Rubella arthritis
Ø56.79	RUBELLA WITH OTHER SPECIFIED COMPLICATIONS		BØ6.81	Rubella pneumonia
			BØ6.89	Other rubella complications
Ø56.8	UNSPECIFIED RUBELLA COMPLICATIONS		BØ6.89	Other rubella complications
Ø56.9	RUBELLA WITHOUT MENTION OF COMPLICATION	➡	BØ6.9	Rubella without complication
Ø57.Ø	ERYTHEMA INFECTIOSUM	➡	BØ8.3	Erythema infectiosum [fifth disease]
Ø57.8	OTHER SPECIFIED VIRAL EXANTHEMATA		BØ9	Unsp viral infection with skin and mucous membrane lesions
			L44.4	Infantile papular acrodermatitis [Gianotti-Crosti]
Ø57.9	UNSPECIFIED VIRAL EXANTHEM		BØ9	Unsp viral infection with skin and mucous membrane lesions
Ø58.1Ø	ROSEOLA INFANTUM UNSPECIFIED	➡	BØ8.2Ø	Exanthema subitum [sixth disease], unspecified
Ø58.11	ROSEOLA INFANTUM DUE TO HUMAN HERPESVIRUS 6	➡	BØ8.21	Exanthema subitum [sixth disease] due to human herpesvirus 6
Ø58.12	ROSEOLA INFANTUM DUE TO HUMAN HERPESVIRUS 7	➡	BØ8.22	Exanthema subitum [sixth disease] due to human herpesvirus 7
Ø58.21	HUMAN HERPESVIRUS 6 ENCEPHALITIS	➡	B1Ø.Ø1	Human herpesvirus 6 encephalitis
Ø58.29	OTHER HUMAN HERPESVIRUS ENCEPHALITIS	➡	B1Ø.Ø9	Other human herpesvirus encephalitis

ICD-9-CM			ICD-10-CM	
Ø58.81	HUMAN HERPESVIRUS 6 INFECTION		**B1Ø.81**	Human herpesvirus 6 infection
Ø58.82	HUMAN HERPESVIRUS 7 INFECTION		**B1Ø.82**	Human herpesvirus 7 infection
Ø58.89	OTHER HUMAN HERPESVIRUS INFECTION		**B1Ø.89**	Other human herpesvirus infection
Ø59.ØØ	ORTHOPOXVIRUS INFECTION UNSPECIFIED		**BØ8.Ø9**	Other orthopoxvirus infections
Ø59.Ø1	MONKEYPOX	➡	**BØ4**	Monkeypox
Ø59.Ø9	OTHER ORTHOPOXVIRUS INFECTION		**BØ8.Ø9**	Other orthopoxvirus infections
Ø59.1Ø	PARAPOXVIRUS INFECTION UNSPECIFIED	➡	**BØ8.6Ø**	Parapoxvirus infection, unspecified
Ø59.11	BOVINE STOMATITIS	➡	**BØ8.61**	Bovine stomatitis
Ø59.12	SEALPOX	➡	**BØ8.62**	Sealpox
Ø59.19	OTHER PARAPOXVIRUS INFECTIONS	➡	**BØ8.69**	Other parapoxvirus infections
Ø59.2Ø	YATAPOXVIRUS INFECTION UNSPECIFIED		**BØ8.7Ø** **BØ8.79**	Yatapoxvirus infection, unspecified Other yatapoxvirus infections
Ø59.21	TANAPOX	➡	**BØ8.71**	Tanapox virus disease
Ø59.22	YABA MONKEY TUMOR VIRUS	➡	**BØ8.72**	Yaba pox virus disease
Ø59.8	OTHER POXVIRUS INFECTIONS		**BØ8.8**	Oth viral infections with skin and mucous membrane lesions
Ø59.9	POXVIRUS INFECTIONS UNSPECIFIED		**BØ8.8**	Oth viral infections with skin and mucous membrane lesions
Ø6Ø.Ø	SYLVATIC YELLOW FEVER	➡	**A95.Ø**	Sylvatic yellow fever
Ø6Ø.1	URBAN YELLOW FEVER	➡	**A95.1**	Urban yellow fever
Ø6Ø.9	UNSPECIFIED YELLOW FEVER	➡	**A95.9**	Yellow fever, unspecified
Ø61	DENGUE	➡	**A9Ø**	Dengue fever [classical dengue]
Ø62.Ø	JAPANESE ENCEPHALITIS	➡	**A83.Ø**	Japanese encephalitis
Ø62.1	WESTERN EQUINE ENCEPHALITIS	➡	**A83.1**	Western equine encephalitis
Ø62.2	EASTERN EQUINE ENCEPHALITIS	➡	**A83.2**	Eastern equine encephalitis
Ø62.3	ST. LOUIS ENCEPHALITIS	➡	**A83.3**	St Louis encephalitis
Ø62.4	AUSTRALIAN ENCEPHALITIS	➡	**A83.4**	Australian encephalitis
Ø62.5	CALIFORNIA VIRUS ENCEPHALITIS	➡	**A83.5**	California encephalitis
Ø62.8	OTHER SPEC MOSQUITO-BORNE VIRAL ENCEPHALITIS		**A83.6** **A83.8**	Rocio virus disease Other mosquito-borne viral encephalitis
Ø62.9	UNSPECIFIED MOSQUITO-BORNE VIRAL ENCEPHALITIS	➡	**A83.9**	Mosquito-borne viral encephalitis, unspecified
Ø63.Ø	RUSSIAN SPRING-SUMMER ENCEPHALITIS	➡	**A84.Ø**	Far Eastern tick-borne encephalitis
Ø63.1	LOUPING ILL		**A84.8**	Other tick-borne viral encephalitis
Ø63.2	CENTRAL EUROPEAN ENCEPHALITIS	➡	**A84.1**	Central European tick-borne encephalitis
Ø63.8	OTHER SPECIFIED TICK-BORNE VIRAL ENCEPHALITIS		**A84.8**	Other tick-borne viral encephalitis
Ø63.9	UNSPECIFIED TICK-BORNE VIRAL ENCEPHALITIS	➡	**A84.9**	Tick-borne viral encephalitis, unspecified
Ø64	VIRAL ENCEPHALIT TRNSMTTED OTH&UNSPEC ARTHROPODS	➡	**A85.2**	Arthropod-borne viral encephalitis, unspecified
Ø65.Ø	CRIMEAN HEMORRHAGIC FEVER	➡	**A98.Ø**	Crimean-Congo hemorrhagic fever
Ø65.1	OMSK HEMORRHAGIC FEVER	➡	**A98.1**	Omsk hemorrhagic fever
Ø65.2	KYASANUR FOREST DISEASE	➡	**A98.2**	Kyasanur Forest disease
Ø65.3	OTHER TICK-BORNE HEMORRHAGIC FEVER		**A98.8**	Other specified viral hemorrhagic fevers
Ø65.4	MOSQUITO-BORNE HEMORRHAGIC FEVER		**A91** **A92.Ø**	Dengue hemorrhagic fever Chikungunya virus disease
Ø65.8	OTHER SPEC ARTHROPOD-BORNE HEMORRHAGIC FEVER		**A98.8**	Other specified viral hemorrhagic fevers
Ø65.9	UNSPECIFIED ARTHROPOD-BORNE HEMORRHAGIC FEVER		**A99**	Unspecified viral hemorrhagic fever
Ø66.Ø	PHLEBOTOMUS FEVER	➡	**A93.1**	Sandfly fever
Ø66.1	TICK-BORNE FEVER		**A93.2**	Colorado tick fever
Ø66.2	VENEZUELAN EQUINE FEVER	➡	**A92.2**	Venezuelan equine fever
Ø66.3	OTHER MOSQUITO-BORNE FEVER		**A92.Ø** **A92.1** **A92.4** **A92.8** **A93.Ø** **B33.1**	Chikungunya virus disease O'nyong-nyong fever Rift Valley fever Other specified mosquito-borne viral fevers Oropouche virus disease Ross River disease
Ø66.4Ø	WEST NILE FEVER UNSPECIFIED	➡	**A92.3Ø**	West Nile virus infection, unspecified
Ø66.41	WEST NILE FEVER WITH ENCEPHALITIS	➡	**A92.31**	West Nile virus infection with encephalitis
Ø66.42	WEST NILE FEVER W/OTHER NEUROLOGIC MANIFESTATION	➡	**A92.32**	West Nile virus infection with oth neurologic manifestation
Ø66.49	WEST NILE FEVER WITH OTHER COMPLICATIONS	➡	**A92.39**	West Nile virus infection with other complications
Ø66.8	OTHER SPECIFIED ARTHROPOD-BORNE VIRAL DISEASES	➡	**A93.8**	Other specified arthropod-borne viral fevers
Ø66.9	UNSPECIFIED ARTHROPOD-BORNE VIRAL DISEASE		**A92.9** **A94**	Mosquito-borne viral fever, unspecified Unspecified arthropod-borne viral fever
Ø7Ø.Ø	VIRAL HEPATITIS A WITH HEPATIC COMA	➡	**B15.Ø**	Hepatitis A with hepatic coma
Ø7Ø.1	VIRAL HEPATITIS WITHOUT MENTION OF HEPATIC COMA	➡	**B15.9**	Hepatitis A without hepatic coma
Ø7Ø.2Ø	VIRL HEP B W/HEP COMA ACUT/UNS W/O HEP DELTA		**B16.2** **B19.11**	Acute hepatitis B without delta-agent with hepatic coma Unspecified viral hepatitis B with hepatic coma
Ø7Ø.21	VIRAL HEP B W/HEP COMA ACUTE/UNSPEC W/HEP DELTA		**B16.Ø**	Acute hepatitis B with delta-agent with hepatic coma
Ø7Ø.22	VIRL HEP B W/HEP COMA CHRN W/O MENTION HEP DELTA		**B18.1**	Chronic viral hepatitis B without delta-agent
Ø7Ø.23	VIRAL HEP B W/HEP COMA CHRONIC W/HEP DELTA		**B18.Ø**	Chronic viral hepatitis B with delta-agent
Ø7Ø.3Ø	VIRL HEP B W/O HEP COMA ACUT/UNS W/O HEP DELTA		**B16.9** **B19.1Ø**	Acute hepatitis B w/o delta-agent and without hepatic coma Unspecified viral hepatitis B without hepatic coma
Ø7Ø.31	VIRL HEP B W/O HEP COMA ACUT/UNS W/HEP DELTA		**B16.1**	Acute hepatitis B with delta-agent without hepatic coma

[Brackets] indicate valid character values for each code. Character value meanings provided for each code grouping.

ICD-9-CM			ICD-10-CM	
Ø7Ø.32	VIRL HEP B W/O HEP COMA CHRN W/O HEP DELTA		**B18.1**	Chronic viral hepatitis B without delta-agent
Ø7Ø.33	VIRL HEP B W/O MENTION HEP COMA CHRN W/HEP DELTA		**B18.Ø**	Chronic viral hepatitis B with delta-agent
Ø7Ø.41	ACUTE HEPATITIS C WITH HEPATIC COMA	➡	**B17.11**	Acute hepatitis C with hepatic coma
Ø7Ø.42	HEP DELTA W/O MENTION ACTV HEP B DZ W/HEP COMA		**B17.Ø**	Acute delta-(super) infection of hepatitis B carrier
Ø7Ø.43	HEPATITIS E WITH HEPATIC COMA		**B17.2**	Acute hepatitis E
Ø7Ø.44	CHRONIC HEPATITIS C WITH HEPATIC COMA		**B18.2**	Chronic viral hepatitis C
Ø7Ø.49	OTHER SPECIFIED VIRAL HEPATITIS W/HEPATIC COMA		**B17.8**	Other specified acute viral hepatitis
Ø7Ø.51	ACUTE HEPATITIS C WITHOUT MENTION HEPATIC COMA	➡	**B17.1Ø**	Acute hepatitis C without hepatic coma
Ø7Ø.52	HEP DELTA W/O MENTION ACTV HEP B DZ/HEP COMA		**B17.Ø**	Acute delta-(super) infection of hepatitis B carrier
Ø7Ø.53	HEPATITIS E WITHOUT MENTION OF HEPATIC COMA		**B17.2**	Acute hepatitis E
Ø7Ø.54	CHRONIC HEPATITIS C WITHOUT MENTION HEPATIC COMA		**B18.2**	Chronic viral hepatitis C
Ø7Ø.59	OTH SPEC VIRAL HEP WITHOUT MENTION HEP COMA		**B17.8** **B18.8** **B18.9**	Other specified acute viral hepatitis Other chronic viral hepatitis Chronic viral hepatitis, unspecified
Ø7Ø.6	UNSPECIFIED VIRAL HEPATITIS WITH HEPATIC COMA	➡	**B19.Ø**	Unspecified viral hepatitis with hepatic coma
Ø7Ø.7Ø	UNSPECIFIED VIRAL HEPATITIS C W/O HEPATIC COMA	➡	**B19.2Ø**	Unspecified viral hepatitis C without hepatic coma
Ø7Ø.71	UNSPECIFIED VIRAL HEPATITIS C WITH HEPATIC COMA	➡	**B19.21**	Unspecified viral hepatitis C with hepatic coma
Ø7Ø.9	UNSPEC VIRAL HEPATITIS WITHOUT MENTION HEP COMA		**B17.9** **B19.9**	Acute viral hepatitis, unspecified Unspecified viral hepatitis without hepatic coma
Ø71	RABIES		**A82.Ø** **A82.1** **A82.9**	Sylvatic rabies Urban rabies Rabies, unspecified
Ø72.Ø	MUMPS ORCHITIS	➡	**B26.Ø**	Mumps orchitis
Ø72.1	MUMPS MENINGITIS	➡	**B26.1**	Mumps meningitis
Ø72.2	MUMPS ENCEPHALITIS	➡	**B26.2**	Mumps encephalitis
Ø72.3	MUMPS PANCREATITIS	➡	**B26.3**	Mumps pancreatitis
Ø72.71	MUMPS HEPATITIS	➡	**B26.81**	Mumps hepatitis
Ø72.72	MUMPS POLYNEUROPATHY	➡	**B26.84**	Mumps polyneuropathy
Ø72.79	MUMPS WITH OTHER SPECIFIED COMPLICATIONS		**B26.82** **B26.83** **B26.85** **B26.89**	Mumps myocarditis Mumps nephritis Mumps arthritis Other mumps complications
Ø72.8	UNSPECIFIED MUMPS COMPLICATION		**B26.89**	Other mumps complications
Ø72.9	MUMPS WITHOUT MENTION OF COMPLICATION	➡	**B26.9**	Mumps without complication
Ø73.Ø	ORNITHOSIS WITH PNEUMONIA		**A7Ø** **J17**	Chlamydia psittaci infections *and* Pneumonia in diseases classified elsewhere
Ø73.7	ORNITHOSIS WITH OTHER SPECIFIED COMPLICATIONS		**A7Ø**	Chlamydia psittaci infections
Ø73.8	ORNITHOSIS WITH UNSPECIFIED COMPLICATION		**A7Ø**	Chlamydia psittaci infections
Ø73.9	UNSPECIFIED ORNITHOSIS		**A7Ø**	Chlamydia psittaci infections
Ø74.Ø	HERPANGINA	➡	**BØ8.5**	Enteroviral vesicular pharyngitis
Ø74.1	EPIDEMIC PLEURODYNIA	➡	**B33.Ø**	Epidemic myalgia
Ø74.2Ø	COXSACKIE CARDITIS, UNSPECIFIED		**B33.2Ø**	Viral carditis, unspecified
Ø74.21	COXSACKIE PERICARDITIS		**B33.23**	Viral pericarditis
Ø74.22	COXSACKIE ENDOCARDITIS		**B33.21**	Viral endocarditis
Ø74.23	COXSACKIE MYOCARDITIS		**B33.22**	Viral myocarditis
Ø74.3	HAND, FOOT, AND MOUTH DISEASE	➡	**BØ8.4**	Enteroviral vesicular stomatitis with exanthem
Ø74.8	OTHER SPECIFIED DISEASES DUE TO COXSACKIEVIRUS		**B34.1**	Enterovirus infection, unspecified
Ø75	INFECTIOUS MONONUCLEOSIS		**B27.ØØ** **B27.Ø1** **B27.Ø2** **B27.Ø9** **B27.1Ø** **B27.11** **B27.12** **B27.19** **B27.8Ø** **B27.81** **B27.82** **B27.89** **B27.9Ø** **B27.91** **B27.92** **B27.99**	Gammaherpesviral mononucleosis without complication Gammaherpesviral mononucleosis with polyneuropathy Gammaherpesviral mononucleosis with meningitis Gammaherpesviral mononucleosis with other complications Cytomegaloviral mononucleosis without complications Cytomegaloviral mononucleosis with polyneuropathy Cytomegaloviral mononucleosis with meningitis Cytomegaloviral mononucleosis with other complication Other infectious mononucleosis without complication Other infectious mononucleosis with polyneuropathy Other infectious mononucleosis with meningitis Other infectious mononucleosis with other complication Infectious mononucleosis, unspecified without complication Infectious mononucleosis, unspecified with polyneuropathy Infectious mononucleosis, unspecified with meningitis Infectious mononucleosis, unsp with other complication
Ø76.Ø	INITIAL STAGE TRACHOMA	➡	**A71.Ø**	Initial stage of trachoma
Ø76.1	ACTIVE STAGE TRACHOMA	➡	**A71.1**	Active stage of trachoma
Ø76.9	UNSPECIFIED TRACHOMA	➡	**A71.9**	Trachoma, unspecified
Ø77.Ø	INCLUSION CONJUNCTIVITIS		**A74.Ø**	Chlamydial conjunctivitis
Ø77.1	EPIDEMIC KERATOCONJUNCTIVITIS	➡	**B3Ø.Ø**	Keratoconjunctivitis due to adenovirus
Ø77.2	PHARYNGOCONJUNCTIVAL FEVER	➡	**B3Ø.2**	Viral pharyngoconjunctivitis
Ø77.3	OTHER ADENOVIRAL CONJUNCTIVITIS		**B3Ø.1**	Conjunctivitis due to adenovirus
Ø77.4	EPIDEMIC HEMORRHAGIC CONJUNCTIVITIS	➡	**B3Ø.3**	Acute epidemic hemorrhagic conjunctivitis (enteroviral)

ICD-9-CM			ICD-10-CM	
Ø77.8	OTHER VIRAL CONJUNCTIVITIS	➡	B3Ø.8	Other viral conjunctivitis
Ø77.98	UNSPECIFIED DISEASES CONJUNCTIVA DUE CHLAMYDIAE		A74.Ø A74.89	Chlamydial conjunctivitis Other chlamydial diseases
Ø77.99	UNSPECIFIED DISEASES CONJUNCTIVA DUE TO VIRUSES	➡	B3Ø.9	Viral conjunctivitis, unspecified
Ø78.Ø	MOLLUSCUM CONTAGIOSUM	➡	BØ8.1	Molluscum contagiosum
Ø78.1Ø	UNSPECIFIED VIRAL WARTS	➡	BØ7.9	Viral wart, unspecified
Ø78.11	CONDYLOMA ACUMINATUM	➡	A63.Ø	Anogenital (venereal) warts
Ø78.12	PLANTAR WART	➡	BØ7.Ø	Plantar wart
Ø78.19	OTHER SPECIFIED VIRAL WARTS	➡	BØ7.8	Other viral warts
Ø78.2	SWEATING FEVER		B33.8	Other specified viral diseases
Ø78.3	CAT-SCRATCH DISEASE	➡	A28.1	Cat-scratch disease
Ø78.4	FOOT AND MOUTH DISEASE		BØ8.8	Oth viral infections with skin and mucous membrane lesions
Ø78.5	CYTOMEGALOVIRAL DISEASE	◘ ◘ ◘	B25.Ø B25.1 B25.2 B25.8 B25.9	Cytomegaloviral pneumonitis Cytomegaloviral hepatitis Cytomegaloviral pancreatitis Other cytomegaloviral diseases Cytomegaloviral disease, unspecified
Ø78.6	HEMORRHAGIC NEPHROSONEPHRITIS	➡	A98.5	Hemorrhagic fever with renal syndrome
Ø78.7	ARENAVIRAL HEMORRHAGIC FEVER		A96.Ø A96.1 A96.8 A96.9	Junin hemorrhagic fever Machupo hemorrhagic fever Other arenaviral hemorrhagic fevers Arenaviral hemorrhagic fever, unspecified
Ø78.81	EPIDEMIC VERTIGO	➡	A88.1	Epidemic vertigo
Ø78.82	EPIDEMIC VOMITING SYNDROME		R11.11	Vomiting without nausea
Ø78.88	OTHER SPECIFIED DISEASES DUE TO CHLAMYDIAE		A74.89	Other chlamydial diseases
Ø78.89	OTHER SPECIFIED DISEASES DUE TO VIRUSES		A96.2 A98.3 A98.4 B33.24 B33.8	Lassa fever Marburg virus disease Ebola virus disease Viral cardiomyopathy Other specified viral diseases
Ø79.Ø	ADENOVIRUS INFECTION IN CCE & UNS SITE		B34.Ø B97.Ø	Adenovirus infection, unspecified Adenovirus as the cause of diseases classified elsewhere
Ø79.1	ECHO VIRUS INFECTION IN CCE & UNS SITE	 ◘	B97.12 J2Ø.7	Echovirus as the cause of diseases classified elsewhere Acute bronchitis due to echovirus
Ø79.2	COXSACKIEVIRUS INFECTION IN CCE & UNS SITE	 ◘	B97.11 J2Ø.3	Coxsackievirus as the cause of diseases classified elsewhere Acute bronchitis due to coxsackievirus
Ø79.3	RHINOVIRUS INFECTION IN CCE & UNS SITE	 ◘	B97.89 J2Ø.6	Oth viral agents as the cause of diseases classd elswhr Acute bronchitis due to rhinovirus
Ø79.4	HUMAN PAPILLOMA VIRUS IN CCE & UNS SITE	➡	B97.7	Papillomavirus as the cause of diseases classified elsewhere
Ø79.5Ø	UNSPECIFIED RETROVIRUS IN CCE & UNS SITE	➡	B97.3Ø	Unsp retrovirus as the cause of diseases classd elswhr
Ø79.51	HTLVTYPE I CCE & UNS SITE	➡	B97.33	HTLV-I as the cause of diseases classified elsewhere
Ø79.52	HTLV TYPE II CCE & UNS SITE	➡	B97.34	HTLV-II as the cause of diseases classified elsewhere
Ø79.53	HIV TYPE 2 IN CCE & UNS SITE	➡	B97.35	HIV 2 as the cause of diseases classified elsewhere
Ø79.59	OTHER SPECIFIED RETROVIRUS IN CCE & UNS SITE		B33.3 B97.31 B97.32 B97.39	Retrovirus infections, not elsewhere classified Lentivirus as the cause of diseases classified elsewhere Oncovirus as the cause of diseases classified elsewhere Oth retrovirus as the cause of diseases classified elsewhere
Ø79.6	RESPIRATORY SYNCYTIAL VIRUS	 ◘	B97.4 J2Ø.5	Respiratory syncytial virus causing diseases classd elswhr Acute bronchitis due to respiratory syncytial virus
Ø79.81	HANTAVIRUS INFECTION		B33.4	Hantavirus (cardio)-pulmonary syndrome [HPS] [HCPS]
Ø79.82	SARS-ASSOCIATED CORONAVIRUS	➡	B97.21	SARS-associated coronavirus causing diseases classd elswhr
Ø79.83	PARVOVIRUS B19		B34.3	Parvovirus infection, unspecified
Ø79.88	OTHER SPEC CHLAMYDIAL INFECTION CCE & UNS SITE		A74.81 A74.89	Chlamydial peritonitis Other chlamydial diseases
Ø79.89	OTHER SPECIFIED VIRAL INFECTION CCE & UNS SITE	 ◘	B33.8 B34.1 B34.2 B34.4 B34.8 B97.19 B97.29 B97.5 B97.6 B97.81 B97.89 J2Ø.4	Other specified viral diseases Enterovirus infection, unspecified Coronavirus infection, unspecified Papovavirus infection, unspecified Other viral infections of unspecified site Oth enterovirus as the cause of diseases classd elswhr Oth coronavirus as the cause of diseases classd elswhr Reovirus as the cause of diseases classified elsewhere Parvovirus as the cause of diseases classified elsewhere Human metapneumovirus as the cause of diseases classd elswhr Oth viral agents as the cause of diseases classd elswhr Acute bronchitis due to parainfluenza virus
Ø79.98	UNSPECIFIED CHLAMYDIAL INFECTION CCE & UNS SITE		A74.9	Chlamydial infection, unspecified
Ø79.99	UNSPECIFIED VIRAL INFECTION IN CCE & UNS SITE		B97.1Ø B97.89	Unsp enterovirus as the cause of diseases classd elswhr Oth viral agents as the cause of diseases classd elswhr
Ø8Ø	LOUSE-BORNE TYPHUS	➡	A75.Ø	Epidemic louse-borne typhus fever d/t Rickettsia prowazekii
Ø81.Ø	MURINE TYPHUS	➡	A75.2	Typhus fever due to Rickettsia typhi
Ø81.1	BRILLS DISEASE	➡	A75.1	Recrudescent typhus [Brill's disease]
Ø81.2	SCRUB TYPHUS	➡	A75.3	Typhus fever due to Rickettsia tsutsugamushi

[Brackets] indicate valid character values for each code. Character value meanings provided for each code grouping.

ICD-9-CM			ICD-10-CM	
Ø81.9	UNSPECIFIED TYPHUS	➡	**A75.9**	Typhus fever, unspecified
Ø82.Ø	SPOTTED FEVERS		**A77.Ø** **A77.9**	Spotted fever due to Rickettsia rickettsii Spotted fever, unspecified
Ø82.1	BOUTONNEUSE FEVER	➡	**A77.1**	Spotted fever due to Rickettsia conorii
Ø82.2	NORTH ASIAN TICK FEVER	➡	**A77.2**	Spotted fever due to Rickettsia siberica
Ø82.3	QUEENSLAND TICK TYPHUS	➡	**A77.3**	Spotted fever due to Rickettsia australis
Ø82.4Ø	EHRLICHIOSIS, UNSPECIFIED	➡	**A77.4Ø**	Ehrlichiosis, unspecified
Ø82.41	EHRLICHIOSIS CHAFEENSIS [E CHAFEENSIS]	➡	**A77.41**	Ehrlichiosis chafeensis [E. chafeensis]
Ø82.49	OTHER EHRLICHIOSIS	➡	**A77.49**	Other ehrlichiosis
Ø82.8	OTHER SPECIFIED TICK-BORNE RICKETTSIOSES		**A77.8**	Other spotted fevers
Ø82.9	UNSPECIFIED TICK-BORNE RICKETTSIOSIS		**A79.9**	Rickettsiosis, unspecified
Ø83.Ø	Q FEVER	➡	**A78**	Q fever
Ø83.1	TRENCH FEVER	➡	**A79.Ø**	Trench fever
Ø83.2	RICKETTSIALPOX		**A79.1**	Rickettsialpox due to Rickettsia akari
Ø83.8	OTHER SPECIFIED RICKETTSIOSES		**A79.81** **A79.89**	Rickettsiosis due to Ehrlichia sennetsu Other specified rickettsioses
Ø83.9	UNSPECIFIED RICKETTSIOSIS		**A79.9**	Rickettsiosis, unspecified
Ø84.Ø	FALCIPARUM MALARIA		**B5Ø.8** **B5Ø.9**	Other severe and complicated Plasmodium falciparum malaria Plasmodium falciparum malaria, unspecified
Ø84.1	VIVAX MALARIA		**B51.9**	Plasmodium vivax malaria without complication
Ø84.2	QUARTAN MALARIA		**B52.9**	Plasmodium malariae malaria without complication
Ø84.3	OVALE MALARIA	➡	**B53.Ø**	Plasmodium ovale malaria
Ø84.4	OTHER MALARIA		**B53.1** **B53.8**	Malaria due to simian plasmodia Other malaria, not elsewhere classified
Ø84.5	MIXED MALARIA		**B5Ø.9** **B51.9** **B52.9**	Plasmodium falciparum malaria, unspecified Plasmodium vivax malaria without complication Plasmodium malariae malaria without complication
Ø84.6	UNSPECIFIED MALARIA	➡	**B54**	Unspecified malaria
Ø84.7	INDUCED MALARIA		**B53.8**	Other malaria, not elsewhere classified
Ø84.8	BLACKWATER FEVER		**B5Ø.8**	Other severe and complicated Plasmodium falciparum malaria
Ø84.9	OTHER PERNICIOUS COMPLICATIONS OF MALARIA	 ■	**B5Ø.Ø** **B5Ø.8** **B51.Ø** **B51.8** **B52.Ø** **B52.8**	Plasmodium falciparum malaria with cerebral complications Other severe and complicated Plasmodium falciparum malaria Plasmodium vivax malaria with rupture of spleen Plasmodium vivax malaria with other complications Plasmodium malariae malaria with nephropathy Plasmodium malariae malaria with other complications
Ø85.Ø	VISCERAL LEISHMANIASIS	➡	**B55.Ø**	Visceral leishmaniasis
Ø85.1	CUTANEOUS LEISHMANIASIS, URBAN		**B55.1**	Cutaneous leishmaniasis
Ø85.2	CUTANEOUS LEISHMANIASIS ASIAN DESERT		**B55.1**	Cutaneous leishmaniasis
Ø85.3	CUTANEOUS LEISHMANIASIS, ETHIOPIAN		**B55.1**	Cutaneous leishmaniasis
Ø85.4	CUTANEOUS LEISHMANIASIS, AMERICAN		**B55.1**	Cutaneous leishmaniasis
Ø85.5	MUCOCUTANEOUS LEISHMANIASIS,	➡	**B55.2**	Mucocutaneous leishmaniasis
Ø85.9	UNSPECIFIED LEISHMANIASIS	➡	**B55.9**	Leishmaniasis, unspecified
Ø86.Ø	CHAGAS DISEASE WITH HEART INVOLVEMENT		**B57.Ø** **B57.2**	Acute Chagas' disease with heart involvement Chagas' disease (chronic) with heart involvement
Ø86.1	CHAGAS DISEASE WITH OTHER ORGAN INVOLVEMENT		**B57.3Ø** **B57.31** **B57.32** **B57.39** **B57.4Ø** **B57.41** **B57.42** **B57.49** **B57.5**	Chagas' disease with digestive system involvement, unsp Megaesophagus in Chagas' disease Megacolon in Chagas' disease Other digestive system involvement in Chagas' disease Chagas' disease with nervous system involvement, unspecified Meningitis in Chagas' disease Meningoencephalitis in Chagas' disease Other nervous system involvement in Chagas' disease Chagas' disease (chronic) with other organ involvement
Ø86.2	CHAGAS DISEASE WITHOUT MENTION ORGAN INVOLVEMENT		**B57.1**	Acute Chagas' disease without heart involvement
Ø86.3	GAMBIAN TRYPANOSOMIASIS	➡	**B56.Ø**	Gambiense trypanosomiasis
Ø86.4	RHODESIAN TRYPANOSOMIASIS	➡	**B56.1**	Rhodesiense trypanosomiasis
Ø86.5	AFRICAN TRYPANOSOMIASIS UNSPECIFIED		**B56.9**	African trypanosomiasis, unspecified
Ø86.9	UNSPECIFIED TRYPANOSOMIASIS		**B56.9**	African trypanosomiasis, unspecified
Ø87.Ø	LOUSE-BORNE RELAPSING FEVER	➡	**A68.Ø**	Louse-borne relapsing fever
Ø87.1	TICK-BORNE RELAPSING FEVER	➡	**A68.1**	Tick-borne relapsing fever
Ø87.9	UNSPECIFIED RELAPSING FEVER	➡	**A68.9**	Relapsing fever, unspecified
Ø88.Ø	BARTONELLOSIS		**A44.Ø** **A44.1** **A44.8** **A44.9**	Systemic bartonellosis Cutaneous and mucocutaneous bartonellosis Other forms of bartonellosis Bartonellosis, unspecified
Ø88.81	LYME DISEASE		**A69.2Ø** **A69.21** **A69.22** **A69.23** **A69.29**	Lyme disease, unspecified Meningitis due to Lyme disease Other neurologic disorders in Lyme disease Arthritis due to Lyme disease Other conditions associated with Lyme disease
Ø88.82	BABESIOSIS	➡	**B6Ø.Ø**	Babesiosis

ICD-9-CM			ICD-10-CM	
Ø88.89	OTHER SPECIFIED ARTHROPOD-BORNE DISEASES		**B6Ø.8**	Other specified protozoal diseases
Ø88.9	UNSPECIFIED ARTHROPOD-BORNE DISEASE		**B64**	Unspecified protozoal disease
Ø9Ø.Ø	EARLY CONGENITAL SYPHILIS SYMPTOMATIC		**A5Ø.Ø1**	Early congenital syphilitic oculopathy
			A5Ø.Ø2	Early congenital syphilitic osteochondropathy
			A5Ø.Ø3	Early congenital syphilitic pharyngitis
			A5Ø.Ø4	Early congenital syphilitic pneumonia
			A5Ø.Ø5	Early congenital syphilitic rhinitis
			A5Ø.Ø6	Early cutaneous congenital syphilis
			A5Ø.Ø7	Early mucocutaneous congenital syphilis
			A5Ø.Ø8	Early visceral congenital syphilis
			A5Ø.Ø9	Other early congenital syphilis, symptomatic
Ø9Ø.1	EARLY CONGENITAL SYPHILIS, LATENT	➡	**A5Ø.1**	Early congenital syphilis, latent
Ø9Ø.2	UNSPECIFIED EARLY CONGENITAL SYPHILIS	➡	**A5Ø.2**	Early congenital syphilis, unspecified
Ø9Ø.3	SYPHILITIC INTERSTITIAL KERATITIS		**A5Ø.31**	Late congenital syphilitic interstitial keratitis
Ø9Ø.4Ø	UNSPECIFIED JUVENILE NEUROSYPHILIS		**A5Ø.4Ø**	Late congenital neurosyphilis, unspecified
			A5Ø.43	Late congenital syphilitic polyneuropathy
			A5Ø.45	Juvenile general paresis
Ø9Ø.41	CONGENITAL SYPHILITIC ENCEPHALITIS		**A5Ø.42**	Late congenital syphilitic encephalitis
Ø9Ø.42	CONGENITAL SYPHILITIC MENINGITIS		**A5Ø.41**	Late congenital syphilitic meningitis
Ø9Ø.49	OTHER JUVENILE NEUROSYPHILIS		**A5Ø.49**	Other late congenital neurosyphilis
Ø9Ø.5	OTHER LATE CONGENITAL SYPHILIS SYMPTOMATIC		**A5Ø.3Ø**	Late congenital syphilitic oculopathy, unspecified
			A5Ø.32	Late congenital syphilitic chorioretinitis
			A5Ø.39	Other late congenital syphilitic oculopathy
			A5Ø.44	Late congenital syphilitic optic nerve atrophy
			A5Ø.51	Clutton's joints
			A5Ø.52	Hutchinson's teeth
			A5Ø.53	Hutchinson's triad
			A5Ø.54	Late congenital cardiovascular syphilis
			A5Ø.55	Late congenital syphilitic arthropathy
			A5Ø.56	Late congenital syphilitic osteochondropathy
			A5Ø.57	Syphilitic saddle nose
			A5Ø.59	Other late congenital syphilis, symptomatic
Ø9Ø.6	LATE CONGENITAL SYPHILIS, LATENT	➡	**A5Ø.6**	Late congenital syphilis, latent
Ø9Ø.7	LATE CONGENITAL SYPHILIS UNSPECIFIED	➡	**A5Ø.7**	Late congenital syphilis, unspecified
Ø9Ø.9	CONGENITAL SYPHILIS, UNSPECIFIED	➡	**A5Ø.9**	Congenital syphilis, unspecified
Ø91.Ø	GENITAL SYPHILIS	➡	**A51.Ø**	Primary genital syphilis
Ø91.1	PRIMARY ANAL SYPHILIS	➡	**A51.1**	Primary anal syphilis
Ø91.2	OTHER PRIMARY SYPHILIS	➡	**A51.2**	Primary syphilis of other sites
Ø91.3	SECONDARY SYPHILIS OF SKIN OR MUCOUS MEMBRANES		**A51.31**	Condyloma latum
			A51.39	Other secondary syphilis of skin
Ø91.4	ADENOPATHY DUE TO SECONDARY SYPHILIS		**A51.49**	Other secondary syphilitic conditions
Ø91.5Ø	EARLY SYPHILIS SYPHILITIC UVEITIS UNSPECIFIED		**A51.43**	Secondary syphilitic oculopathy
Ø91.51	EARLY SYPHILIS SYPHILITIC CHORIORETINITIS		**A51.43**	Secondary syphilitic oculopathy
Ø91.52	EARLY SYPHILIS SYPHILITIC IRIDOCYCLITIS		**A51.43**	Secondary syphilitic oculopathy
Ø91.61	EARLY SYPHILIS SECONDARY SYPHILITIC PERIOSTITIS		**A51.46**	Secondary syphilitic osteopathy
Ø91.62	EARLY SYPHILIS SECONDARY SYPHILITIC HEPATITIS	➡	**A51.45**	Secondary syphilitic hepatitis
Ø91.69	EARLY SYPHILIS SEC SYPHILIS OF OTHER VISCERA		**A51.49**	Other secondary syphilitic conditions
Ø91.7	EARLY SYPHILIS SECONDARY SYPHILIS RELAPSE		**A51.49**	Other secondary syphilitic conditions
Ø91.81	EARLY SYPHILIS ACUTE SYPHILITIC MENINGITIS		**A51.41**	Secondary syphilitic meningitis
Ø91.82	EARLY SYPHILIS, SYPHILITIC ALOPECIA	➡	**A51.32**	Syphilitic alopecia
Ø91.89	EARLY SYPHILIS OTHER FORMS OF SECONDARY SYPHILIS		**A51.42**	Secondary syphilitic female pelvic disease
			A51.44	Secondary syphilitic nephritis
			A51.49	Other secondary syphilitic conditions
Ø91.9	EARLY SYPHILIS UNSPECIFIED SECONDARY SYPHILIS		**A51.49**	Other secondary syphilitic conditions
Ø92.Ø	EARLY SYPH LATENT SEROLOGICAL RELAPSE AFTER TX		**A51.5**	Early syphilis, latent
Ø92.9	EARLY SYPHILIS, LATENT, UNSPECIFIED		**A51.5**	Early syphilis, latent
			A51.9	Early syphilis, unspecified
Ø93.Ø	ANEURYSM OF AORTA SPECIFIED AS SYPHILITIC	➡	**A52.Ø1**	Syphilitic aneurysm of aorta
Ø93.1	SYPHILITIC AORTITIS	➡	**A52.Ø2**	Syphilitic aortitis
Ø93.2Ø	UNSPECIFIED SYPHILITIC ENDOCARDITIS OF VALVE		**A52.Ø3**	Syphilitic endocarditis
Ø93.21	SYPHILITIC ENDOCARDITIS MITRAL VALVE		**A52.Ø3**	Syphilitic endocarditis
Ø93.22	SYPHILITIC ENDOCARDITIS AORTIC VALVE		**A52.Ø3**	Syphilitic endocarditis
Ø93.23	SYPHILITIC ENDOCARDITIS TRICUSPID VALVE		**A52.Ø3**	Syphilitic endocarditis
Ø93.24	SYPHILITIC ENDOCARDITIS PULMONARY VALVE		**A52.Ø3**	Syphilitic endocarditis
Ø93.81	SYPHILITIC PERICARDITIS		**A52.Ø6**	Other syphilitic heart involvement
Ø93.82	SYPHILITIC MYOCARDITIS		**A52.Ø6**	Other syphilitic heart involvement
Ø93.89	OTHER SPECIFIED CARDIOVASCULAR SYPHILIS		**A52.Ø4**	Syphilitic cerebral arteritis
			A52.Ø5	Other cerebrovascular syphilis
			A52.Ø9	Other cardiovascular syphilis
Ø93.9	UNSPECIFIED CARDIOVASCULAR SYPHILIS	➡	**A52.ØØ**	Cardiovascular syphilis, unspecified
Ø94.Ø	TABES DORSALIS		**A52.11**	Tabes dorsalis
			A52.16	Charcot's arthropathy (tabetic)

[Brackets] indicate valid character values for each code. Character value meanings provided for each code grouping.

ICD-9-CM		ICD-10-CM	
Ø94.1	GENERAL PARESIS	➡ A52.17	General paresis
Ø94.2	SYPHILITIC MENINGITIS	A52.13	Late syphilitic meningitis
Ø94.3	ASYMPTOMATIC NEUROSYPHILIS	➡ A52.2	Asymptomatic neurosyphilis
Ø94.81	SYPHILITIC ENCEPHALITIS	A52.14	Late syphilitic encephalitis
Ø94.82	SYPHILITIC PARKINSONISM	A52.19	Other symptomatic neurosyphilis
Ø94.83	SYPHILITIC DISSEMINATED RETINOCHOROIDITIS	A52.19	Other symptomatic neurosyphilis
Ø94.84	SYPHILITIC OPTIC ATROPHY	A52.15	Late syphilitic neuropathy
Ø94.85	SYPHILITIC RETROBULBAR NEURITIS	A52.15	Late syphilitic neuropathy
Ø94.86	SYPHILITIC ACOUSTIC NEURITIS	A52.15	Late syphilitic neuropathy
Ø94.87	SYPHILITIC RUPTURED CEREBRAL ANEURYSM	A52.19	Other symptomatic neurosyphilis
Ø94.89	OTHER SPECIFIED NEUROSYPHILIS	A52.12 ◘ A52.15 A52.19	Other cerebrospinal syphilis Late syphilitic neuropathy Other symptomatic neurosyphilis
Ø94.9	UNSPECIFIED NEUROSYPHILIS	A52.1Ø A52.3	Symptomatic neurosyphilis, unspecified Neurosyphilis, unspecified
Ø95.Ø	SYPHILITIC EPISCLERITIS	A52.71	Late syphilitic oculopathy
Ø95.1	SYPHILIS OF LUNG	A52.72	Syphilis of lung and bronchus
Ø95.2	SYPHILITIC PERITONITIS	A52.74	Syphilis of liver and other viscera
Ø95.3	SYPHILIS OF LIVER	A52.74	Syphilis of liver and other viscera
Ø95.4	SYPHILIS OF KIDNEY	A52.75	Syphilis of kidney and ureter
Ø95.5	SYPHILIS OF BONE	A52.77	Syphilis of bone and joint
Ø95.6	SYPHILIS OF MUSCLE	A52.78	Syphilis of other musculoskeletal tissue
Ø95.7	SYPHILIS OF SYNOVIUM TENDON AND BURSA	A52.78	Syphilis of other musculoskeletal tissue
Ø95.8	OTHER SPECIFIED FORMS LATE SYMPTOMATIC SYPHILIS	A52.73 A52.76 A52.79	Symptomatic late syphilis of other respiratory organs Other genitourinary symptomatic late syphilis Other symptomatic late syphilis
Ø95.9	UNSPECIFIED LATE SYMPTOMATIC SYPHILIS	A52.79	Other symptomatic late syphilis
Ø96	LATE SYPHILIS, LATENT	➡ A52.8	Late syphilis, latent
Ø97.Ø	UNSPECIFIED LATE SYPHILIS	➡ A52.9	Late syphilis, unspecified
Ø97.1	UNSPECIFIED LATENT SYPHILIS	➡ A53.Ø	Latent syphilis, unspecified as early or late
Ø97.9	UNSPECIFIED SYPHILIS	➡ A53.9	Syphilis, unspecified
Ø98.Ø	GONOCOCCAL INFECTION LOWER GENITOURINARY TRACT	A54.ØØ A54.Ø2 A54.Ø9 A54.1	Gonococcal infection of lower genitourinary tract, unsp Gonococcal vulvovaginitis, unspecified Other gonococcal infection of lower genitourinary tract Gonocl infct of lower GU tract w periureth and acc glnd abcs
Ø98.1Ø	GONOCOCCAL INFECTION UPPER GU TRACT SITE UNSPEC	A54.29	Other gonococcal genitourinary infections
Ø98.11	GONOCOCCAL CYSTITIS	A54.Ø1	Gonococcal cystitis and urethritis, unspecified
Ø98.12	GONOCOCCAL PROSTATITIS	A54.22	Gonococcal prostatitis
Ø98.13	GONOCOCCAL EPIDIDYMO-ORCHITIS	A54.23	Gonococcal infection of other male genital organs
Ø98.14	GONOCOCCAL SEMINAL VESICULITIS	A54.23	Gonococcal infection of other male genital organs
Ø98.15	GONOCOCCAL CERVICITIS	A54.Ø3	Gonococcal cervicitis, unspecified
Ø98.16	GONOCOCCAL ENDOMETRITIS	A54.24	Gonococcal female pelvic inflammatory disease
Ø98.17	GONOCOCCAL SALPINGITIS SPECIFIED AS ACUTE	A54.29	Other gonococcal genitourinary infections
Ø98.19	OTH GONOCOCCAL INFECTIONS UPPER GU TRACT	A54.21 A54.29	Gonococcal infection of kidney and ureter Other gonococcal genitourinary infections
Ø98.2	GONOCOCCAL INFECTIONS CHRONIC LOWER GU TRACT	A54.ØØ	Gonococcal infection of lower genitourinary tract, unsp
Ø98.3Ø	CHRONIC GONOCCL INF UPPER GU TRACT SITE UNSPEC	A54.29	Other gonococcal genitourinary infections
Ø98.31	GONOCOCCAL CYSTITIS, CHRONIC	A54.Ø1	Gonococcal cystitis and urethritis, unspecified
Ø98.32	GONOCOCCAL PROSTATITIS, CHRONIC	A54.22	Gonococcal prostatitis
Ø98.33	GONOCOCCAL EPIDIDYMO-ORCHITIS CHRONIC	A54.23	Gonococcal infection of other male genital organs
Ø98.34	GONOCOCCAL SEMINAL VESICULITIS CHRONIC	A54.23	Gonococcal infection of other male genital organs
Ø98.35	GONOCOCCAL CERVICITIS, CHRONIC	A54.Ø3	Gonococcal cervicitis, unspecified
Ø98.36	GONOCOCCAL ENDOMETRITIS, CHRONIC	A54.24	Gonococcal female pelvic inflammatory disease
Ø98.37	GONOCOCCAL SALPINGITIS	A54.29	Other gonococcal genitourinary infections
Ø98.39	OTH CHRONIC GONOCOCCAL INFECTIONS UPPER GU TRACT	A54.29	Other gonococcal genitourinary infections
Ø98.4Ø	GONOCOCCAL CONJUNCTIVITIS	➡ A54.31	Gonococcal conjunctivitis
Ø98.41	GONOCOCCAL IRIDOCYCLITIS	➡ A54.32	Gonococcal iridocyclitis
Ø98.42	GONOCOCCAL ENDOPHTHALMIA	A54.39	Other gonococcal eye infection
Ø98.43	GONOCOCCAL KERATITIS	➡ A54.33	Gonococcal keratitis
Ø98.49	OTHER GONOCOCCAL INFECTION OF EYE	A54.3Ø A54.39	Gonococcal infection of eye, unspecified Other gonococcal eye infection
Ø98.5Ø	GONOCOCCAL ARTHRITIS	➡ A54.42	Gonococcal arthritis
Ø98.51	GONOCOCCAL SYNOVITIS AND TENOSYNOVITIS	A54.49	Gonococcal infection of other musculoskeletal tissue
Ø98.52	GONOCOCCAL BURSITIS	A54.49	Gonococcal infection of other musculoskeletal tissue
Ø98.53	GONOCOCCAL SPONDYLITIS	➡ A54.41	Gonococcal spondylopathy
Ø98.59	OTHER GONOCOCCAL INFECTION OF JOINT	A54.4Ø A54.43	Gonococcal infection of musculoskeletal system, unspecified Gonococcal osteomyelitis
Ø98.6	GONOCOCCAL INFECTION OF PHARYNX	➡ A54.5	Gonococcal pharyngitis
Ø98.7	GONOCOCCAL INFECTION OF ANUS AND RECTUM	➡ A54.6	Gonococcal infection of anus and rectum

ICD-9-CM		ICD-10-CM		
Ø98.81	GONOCOCCAL KERATOSIS		**A54.89**	Other gonococcal infections
Ø98.82	GONOCOCCAL MENINGITIS	➡	**A54.81**	Gonococcal meningitis
Ø98.83	GONOCOCCAL PERICARDITIS		**A54.83**	Gonococcal heart infection
Ø98.84	GONOCOCCAL ENDOCARDITIS		**A54.83**	Gonococcal heart infection
Ø98.85	OTHER GONOCOCCAL HEART DISEASE		**A54.83**	Gonococcal heart infection
Ø98.86	GONOCOCCAL PERITONITIS	➡	**A54.85**	Gonococcal peritonitis
Ø98.89	GONOCOCCAL INFECTION OF OTHER SPECIFIED SITES	 ▣ 	**A54.82** **A54.84** **A54.86** **A54.89** **A54.9**	Gonococcal brain abscess Gonococcal pneumonia Gonococcal sepsis Other gonococcal infections Gonococcal infection, unspecified
Ø99.Ø	CHANCROID	➡	**A57**	Chancroid
Ø99.1	LYMPHOGRANULOMA VENEREUM	➡	**A55**	Chlamydial lymphogranuloma (venereum)
Ø99.2	GRANULOMA INGUINALE	➡	**A58**	Granuloma inguinale
Ø99.3	REITERS DISEASE	▣ ▣	**MØ2.3Ø** **MØ2.311** **MØ2.312** **MØ2.319** **MØ2.321** **MØ2.322** **MØ2.329** **MØ2.331** **MØ2.332** **MØ2.339** **MØ2.341** **MØ2.342** **MØ2.349** **MØ2.351** **MØ2.352** **MØ2.359** **MØ2.361** **MØ2.362** **MØ2.369** **MØ2.371** **MØ2.372** **MØ2.379** **MØ2.38** **MØ2.39**	Reiter's disease, unspecified site Reiter's disease, right shoulder Reiter's disease, left shoulder Reiter's disease, unspecified shoulder Reiter's disease, right elbow Reiter's disease, left elbow Reiter's disease, unspecified elbow Reiter's disease, right wrist Reiter's disease, left wrist Reiter's disease, unspecified wrist Reiter's disease, right hand Reiter's disease, left hand Reiter's disease, unspecified hand Reiter's disease, right hip Reiter's disease, left hip Reiter's disease, unspecified hip Reiter's disease, right knee Reiter's disease, left knee Reiter's disease, unspecified knee Reiter's disease, right ankle and foot Reiter's disease, left ankle and foot Reiter's disease, unspecified ankle and foot Reiter's disease, vertebrae Reiter's disease, multiple sites
Ø99.4Ø	UNSPECIFIED NONGONOCOCCAL URETHRITIS		**N34.1**	Nonspecific urethritis
Ø99.41	NONGONOCOCCAL URETHRITIS DUE CHLAMYDTRACHOMATIS		**N34.1**	Nonspecific urethritis
Ø99.49	NONGONOCOCCAL URETHRITIS DUE OTHER SPEC ORGANISM		**N34.1**	Nonspecific urethritis
Ø99.5Ø	CHLAMYDIA TRACHOMATIS INFECTION UNSPECIFIED SITE		**A56.19**	Other chlamydial genitourinary infection
Ø99.51	CHLAMYDIA TRACHOMATIS INFECTION OF PHARYNX	➡	**A56.4**	Chlamydial infection of pharynx
Ø99.52	CHLAMYDIA TRACHOMATIS INFECTION OF ANUS&RECTUM	➡	**A56.3**	Chlamydial infection of anus and rectum
Ø99.53	CHLAMYDTRACHOMATIS INFECTION LOWER GU SITES	 ▣ ▣ 	**A56.ØØ** **A56.Ø1** **A56.Ø2** **A56.Ø9**	Chlamydial infection of lower genitourinary tract, unsp Chlamydial cystitis and urethritis Chlamydial vulvovaginitis Other chlamydial infection of lower genitourinary tract
Ø99.54	CHLAMYDTRACHOMATIS INFECTION OTH GU SITES	▣ 	**A56.11** **A56.19**	Chlamydial female pelvic inflammatory disease Other chlamydial genitourinary infection
Ø99.55	CHLAMYDTRACHOMATIS INFECTION UNSPEC GU SITE	➡	**A56.2**	Chlamydial infection of genitourinary tract, unspecified
Ø99.56	CHLAMYDIA TRACHOMATIS INFECTION OF PERITONEUM		**A56.8**	Sexually transmitted chlamydial infection of other sites
Ø99.59	CHLAMYDIA TRACHOMATIS INFECTION OTHER SPEC SITE		**A56.8**	Sexually transmitted chlamydial infection of other sites
Ø99.8	OTHER SPECIFIED VENEREAL DISEASES		**A63.8**	Other specified predominantly sexually transmitted diseases
Ø99.9	UNSPECIFIED VENEREAL DISEASE	➡	**A64**	Unspecified sexually transmitted disease
1ØØ.Ø	LEPTOSPIROSIS ICTEROHEMORRHAGICA	➡	**A27.Ø**	Leptospirosis icterohemorrhagica
1ØØ.81	LEPTOSPIRAL MENINGITIS	➡	**A27.81**	Aseptic meningitis in leptospirosis
1ØØ.89	OTHER SPECIFIED LEPTOSPIRAL INFECTIONS		**A27.89**	Other forms of leptospirosis
1ØØ.9	UNSPECIFIED LEPTOSPIROSIS	➡	**A27.9**	Leptospirosis, unspecified
1Ø1	VINCENTS ANGINA		**A69.Ø** **A69.1**	Necrotizing ulcerative stomatitis Other Vincent's infections
1Ø2.Ø	INITIAL LESIONS OF YAWS	➡	**A66.Ø**	Initial lesions of yaws
1Ø2.1	MULTIPLE PAPILLOMATA&WET CRAB YAWS DUE TO YAWS	➡	**A66.1**	Multiple papillomata and wet crab yaws
1Ø2.2	OTHER EARLY SKIN LESIONS DUE TO YAWS	➡	**A66.2**	Other early skin lesions of yaws
1Ø2.3	HYPERKERATOSIS DUE TO YAWS	➡	**A66.3**	Hyperkeratosis of yaws
1Ø2.4	GUMMATA AND ULCERS DUE TO YAWS	➡	**A66.4**	Gummata and ulcers of yaws
1Ø2.5	GANGOSA DUE TO YAWS	➡	**A66.5**	Gangosa
1Ø2.6	BONE AND JOINT LESIONS DUE TO YAWS	➡	**A66.6**	Bone and joint lesions of yaws
1Ø2.7	OTHER MANIFESTATIONS DUE TO YAWS	➡	**A66.7**	Other manifestations of yaws
1Ø2.8	LATENT YAWS	➡	**A66.8**	Latent yaws
1Ø2.9	UNSPECIFIED YAWS	➡	**A66.9**	Yaws, unspecified
1Ø3.Ø	PRIMARY LESIONS OF PINTA	➡	**A67.Ø**	Primary lesions of pinta

ICD-9-CM			ICD-10-CM	
1Ø3.1	INTERMEDIATE LESIONS OF PINTA	➡	**A67.1**	Intermediate lesions of pinta
1Ø3.2	LATE LESIONS OF PINTA	➡	**A67.2**	Late lesions of pinta
1Ø3.3	MIXED LESIONS OF PINTA	➡	**A67.3**	Mixed lesions of pinta
1Ø3.9	UNSPECIFIED PINTA	➡	**A67.9**	Pinta, unspecified
1Ø4.Ø	NONVENEREAL ENDEMIC SYPHILIS	➡	**A65**	Nonvenereal syphilis
1Ø4.8	OTHER SPECIFIED SPIROCHETAL INFECTIONS	➡	**A69.8**	Other specified spirochetal infections
1Ø4.9	UNSPECIFIED SPIROCHETAL INFECTION	➡	**A69.9**	Spirochetal infection, unspecified
11Ø.Ø	DERMATOPHYTOSIS OF SCALP AND BEARD	➡	**B35.Ø**	Tinea barbae and tinea capitis
11Ø.1	DERMATOPHYTOSIS OF NAIL	➡	**B35.1**	Tinea unguium
11Ø.2	DERMATOPHYTOSIS OF HAND	➡	**B35.2**	Tinea manuum
11Ø.3	DERMATOPHYTOSIS OF GROIN AND PERIANAL AREA	➡	**B35.6**	Tinea cruris
11Ø.4	DERMATOPHYTOSIS OF FOOT	➡	**B35.3**	Tinea pedis
11Ø.5	DERMATOPHYTOSIS OF THE BODY		**B35.4** **B35.5**	Tinea corporis Tinea imbricata
11Ø.6	DEEP SEATED DERMATOPHYTOSIS		**B35.8**	Other dermatophytoses
11Ø.8	DERMATOPHYTOSIS OF OTHER SPECIFIED SITES		**B35.8**	Other dermatophytoses
11Ø.9	DERMATOPHYTOSIS OF UNSPECIFIED SITE	➡	**B35.9**	Dermatophytosis, unspecified
111.Ø	PITYRIASIS VERSICOLOR	➡	**B36.Ø**	Pityriasis versicolor
111.1	TINEA NIGRA	➡	**B36.1**	Tinea nigra
111.2	TINEA BLANCA	➡	**B36.2**	White piedra
111.3	BLACK PIEDRA	➡	**B36.3**	Black piedra
111.8	OTHER SPECIFIED DERMATOMYCOSES		**B36.8**	Other specified superficial mycoses
111.9	UNSPECIFIED DERMATOMYCOSIS		**B36.9**	Superficial mycosis, unspecified
112.Ø	CANDIDIASIS OF MOUTH		**B37.Ø** **B37.83**	Candidal stomatitis Candidal cheilitis
112.1	CANDIDIASIS OF VULVA AND VAGINA	➡	**B37.3**	Candidiasis of vulva and vagina
112.2	CANDIDIASIS OF OTHER UROGENITAL SITES		**B37.41** **B37.42** **B37.49**	Candidal cystitis and urethritis Candidal balanitis Other urogenital candidiasis
112.3	CANDIDIASIS OF SKIN AND NAILS	➡	**B37.2**	Candidiasis of skin and nail
112.4	CANDIDIASIS OF LUNG		**B37.1**	Pulmonary candidiasis
112.5	DISSEMINATED CANDIDIASIS	◘	**B37.7**	Candidal sepsis
112.81	CANDIDAL ENDOCARDITIS	➡	**B37.6**	Candidal endocarditis
112.82	CANDIDAL OTITIS EXTERNA	➡	**B37.84**	Candidal otitis externa
112.83	CANDIDAL MENINGITIS	➡	**B37.5**	Candidal meningitis
112.84	CANDIDIASIS OF THE ESOPHAGUS	➡	**B37.81**	Candidal esophagitis
112.85	CANDIDIASIS OF THE INTESTINE	➡	**B37.82**	Candidal enteritis
112.89	OTHER CANDIDIASIS OF OTHER SPECIFIED SITES		**B37.89**	Other sites of candidiasis
112.9	CANDIDIASIS OF UNSPECIFIED SITE	➡	**B37.9**	Candidiasis, unspecified
114.Ø	PRIMARY COCCIDIOIDOMYCOSIS		**B38.Ø**	Acute pulmonary coccidioidomycosis
114.1	PRIMARY EXTRAPULMONARY COCCIDIOIDOMYCOSIS		**B38.3** **B38.81**	Cutaneous coccidioidomycosis Prostatic coccidioidomycosis
114.2	COCCIDIOIDAL MENINGITIS	➡	**B38.4**	Coccidioidomycosis meningitis
114.3	OTHER FORMS OF PROGRESSIVE COCCIDIOIDOMYCOSIS		**B38.7** **B38.89**	Disseminated coccidioidomycosis Other forms of coccidioidomycosis
114.4	CHRONIC PULMONARY COCCIDIOIDOMYCOSIS	➡	**B38.1**	Chronic pulmonary coccidioidomycosis
114.5	UNSPECIFIED PULMONARY COCCIDIOIDOMYCOSIS	➡	**B38.2**	Pulmonary coccidioidomycosis, unspecified
114.9	UNSPECIFIED COCCIDIOIDOMYCOSIS	➡	**B38.9**	Coccidioidomycosis, unspecified
115.ØØ	HISTOPLASMA CAPSULATUM WITHOUT MENTION MANIFEST		**B39.4**	Histoplasmosis capsulati, unspecified
115.Ø1	HISTOPLASMA CAPSULATUM MENINGITIS		**B39.4** **GØ2**	Histoplasmosis capsulati, unspecified *and* Meningitis in oth infec/parastc diseases classd elswhr
115.Ø2	HISTOPLASMA CAPSULATUM RETINITIS		**B39.4** **H32**	Histoplasmosis capsulati, unspecified *and* Chorioretinal disorders in diseases classified elsewhere
115.Ø3	HISTOPLASMA CAPSULATUM PERICARDITIS		**B39.4** **I32**	Histoplasmosis capsulati, unspecified *and* Pericarditis in diseases classified elsewhere
115.Ø4	HISTOPLASMA CAPSULATUM ENDOCARDITIS		**B39.4** **I39**	Histoplasmosis capsulati, unspecified *and* Endocarditis and heart valve disord in dis classd elswhr
115.Ø5	HISTOPLASMA CAPSULATUM PNEUMONIA		**B39.Ø** **B39.1** **B39.2**	Acute pulmonary histoplasmosis capsulati Chronic pulmonary histoplasmosis capsulati Pulmonary histoplasmosis capsulati, unspecified
115.Ø9	HISTOPLASMA CAPSULATUM W/MENTION OTH MANIFEST		**B39.3**	Disseminated histoplasmosis capsulati
115.1Ø	HISTOPLASMA DUBOISII WITHOUT MENTION MANIFEST		**B39.5**	Histoplasmosis duboisii
115.11	HISTOPLASMA DUBOISII MENINGITIS		**B39.5** **GØ2**	Histoplasmosis duboisii *and* Meningitis in oth infec/parastc diseases classd elswhr
115.12	HISTOPLASMA DUBOISII RETINITIS		**B39.5** **H32**	Histoplasmosis duboisii *and* Chorioretinal disorders in diseases classified elsewhere

◘ See Appendix A ➡ Equivalent Mapping Scenario Scenario

ICD-9-CM		ICD-10-CM		
115.13	HISTOPLASMA DUBOISII PERICARDITIS	B39.5	Histoplasmosis duboisii	*and*
		I32	Pericarditis in diseases classified elsewhere	
115.14	HISTOPLASMA DUBOISII ENDOCARDITIS	B39.5	Histoplasmosis duboisii	*and*
		I39	Endocarditis and heart valve disord in dis classd elswhr	
115.15	HISTOPLASMA DUBOISII PNEUMONIA	B39.5	Histoplasmosis duboisii	*and*
		J17	Pneumonia in diseases classified elsewhere	
115.19	HISTOPLASMA DUBOISII W/MENTION OTH MANIFESTATION	B39.5	Histoplasmosis duboisii	
115.90	UNSPEC HISTOPLASMOSIS WITHOUT MENTION MANIFEST	B39.9	Histoplasmosis, unspecified	
115.91	UNSPECIFIED HISTOPLASMOSIS MENINGITIS	B39.9	Histoplasmosis, unspecified	*and*
		G02	Meningitis in oth infec/parastc diseases classd elswhr	
115.92	UNSPECIFIED HISTOPLASMOSIS RETINITIS	B39.9	Histoplasmosis, unspecified	*and*
		H32	Chorioretinal disorders in diseases classified elsewhere	
115.93	UNSPECIFIED HISTOPLASMOSIS PERICARDITIS	B39.9	Histoplasmosis, unspecified	*and*
		I32	Pericarditis in diseases classified elsewhere	
115.94	UNSPECIFIED HISTOPLASMOSIS ENDOCARDITIS	B39.9	Histoplasmosis, unspecified	*and*
		I39	Endocarditis and heart valve disord in dis classd elswhr	
115.95	UNSPECIFIED HISTOPLASMOSIS PNEUMONIA	B39.9	Histoplasmosis, unspecified	*and*
		J17	Pneumonia in diseases classified elsewhere	
115.99	UNSPEC HISTOPLASMOSIS W/MENTION OTH MANIFEST	B39.9	Histoplasmosis, unspecified	
116.0	BLASTOMYCOSIS	B40.0	Acute pulmonary blastomycosis	
		B40.1	Chronic pulmonary blastomycosis	
		B40.2	Pulmonary blastomycosis, unspecified	
		B40.3	Cutaneous blastomycosis	
		B40.7	Disseminated blastomycosis	
		B40.81	Blastomycotic meningoencephalitis	
		B40.89	Other forms of blastomycosis	
		B40.9	Blastomycosis, unspecified	
116.1	PARACOCCIDIOIDOMYCOSIS	B41.0	Pulmonary paracoccidioidomycosis	
		B41.7	Disseminated paracoccidioidomycosis	
		B41.8	Other forms of paracoccidioidomycosis	
		B41.9	Paracoccidioidomycosis, unspecified	
116.2	LOBOMYCOSIS	➡ B48.0	Lobomycosis	
117.0	RHINOSPORIDIOSIS	➡ B48.1	Rhinosporidiosis	
117.1	SPOROTRICHOSIS	B42.0	Pulmonary sporotrichosis	
		B42.1	Lymphocutaneous sporotrichosis	
		B42.7	Disseminated sporotrichosis	
		B42.81	Cerebral sporotrichosis	
		B42.82	Sporotrichosis arthritis	
		B42.89	Other forms of sporotrichosis	
		B42.9	Sporotrichosis, unspecified	
117.2	CHROMOBLASTOMYCOSIS	B43.0	Cutaneous chromomycosis	
		B43.1	Pheomycotic brain abscess	
		B43.2	Subcutaneous pheomycotic abscess and cyst	
		B43.8	Other forms of chromomycosis	
		B43.9	Chromomycosis, unspecified	
117.3	ASPERGILLOSIS	B44.0	Invasive pulmonary aspergillosis	
		B44.1	Other pulmonary aspergillosis	
		B44.2	Tonsillar aspergillosis	
		B44.7	Disseminated aspergillosis	
		B44.89	Other forms of aspergillosis	
		B44.9	Aspergillosis, unspecified	
		B48.4	Penicillosis	
117.4	MYCOTIC MYCETOMAS	B47.0	Eumycetoma	
117.5	CRYPTOCOCCOSIS	B45.0	Pulmonary cryptococcosis	
		B45.1	Cerebral cryptococcosis	
		B45.2	Cutaneous cryptococcosis	
		B45.3	Osseous cryptococcosis	
		B45.7	Disseminated cryptococcosis	
		B45.8	Other forms of cryptococcosis	
		B45.9	Cryptococcosis, unspecified	
117.6	ALLESCHERIOSIS	➡ B48.2	Allescheriasis	
117.7	ZYGOMYCOSIS	B46.0	Pulmonary mucormycosis	
		B46.1	Rhinocerebral mucormycosis	
		B46.2	Gastrointestinal mucormycosis	
		B46.3	Cutaneous mucormycosis	
		B46.4	Disseminated mucormycosis	
		B46.5	Mucormycosis, unspecified	
		B46.8	Other zygomycoses	
		B46.9	Zygomycosis, unspecified	
117.8	INFECTION BY DEMATIACIOUS FUNGI	B48.8	Other specified mycoses	
117.9	OTHER AND UNSPECIFIED MYCOSES	B48.3	Geotrichosis	
		B48.8	Other specified mycoses	
		B49	Unspecified mycosis	

[Brackets] indicate valid character values for each code. Character value meanings provided for each code grouping.

ICD-9-CM			ICD-10-CM	
118	OPPORTUNISTIC MYCOSES		B48.8	Other specified mycoses
12Ø.Ø	SCHISTOSOMIASIS DUE TO SCHISTOSOMA HAEMATOBIUM	➡	B65.Ø	Schistosomiasis due to Schistosoma haematobium
12Ø.1	SCHISTOSOMIASIS DUE TO SCHISTOSOMA MANSONI	➡	B65.1	Schistosomiasis due to Schistosoma mansoni
12Ø.2	SCHISTOSOMIASIS DUE TO SCHISTOSOMA JAPONICUM	➡	B65.2	Schistosomiasis due to Schistosoma japonicum
12Ø.3	CUTANEOUS SCHISTOSOMIASIS	➡	B65.3	Cercarial dermatitis
12Ø.8	OTHER SPECIFIED SCHISTOSOMIASIS	➡	B65.8	Other schistosomiasis
12Ø.9	UNSPECIFIED SCHISTOSOMIASIS	➡	B65.9	Schistosomiasis, unspecified
121.Ø	OPISTHORCHIASIS	➡	B66.Ø	Opisthorchiasis
121.1	CLONORCHIASIS	➡	B66.1	Clonorchiasis
121.2	PARAGONIMIASIS	➡	B66.4	Paragonimiasis
121.3	FASCIOLIASIS	➡	B66.3	Fascioliasis
121.4	FASCIOLOPSIASIS	➡	B66.5	Fasciolopsiasis
121.5	METAGONIMIASIS		B66.8	Other specified fluke infections
121.6	HETEROPHYIASIS		B66.8	Other specified fluke infections
121.8	OTHER SPECIFIED TREMATODE INFECTIONS		B66.2 B66.8	Dicroceliasis Other specified fluke infections
121.9	UNSPECIFIED TREMATODE INFECTION	➡	B66.9	Fluke infection, unspecified
122.Ø	ECHINOCOCCUS GRANULOSUS INFECTION OF LIVER	➡	B67.Ø	Echinococcus granulosus infection of liver
122.1	ECHINOCOCCUS GRANULOSUS INFECTION OF LUNG	➡	B67.1	Echinococcus granulosus infection of lung
122.2	ECHINOCOCCUS GRANULOSUS INFECTION OF THYROID	➡	B67.31	Echinococcus granulosus infection, thyroid gland
122.3	OTHER ECHINOCOCCUS GRANULOSUS INFECTION		B67.2 B67.32 B67.39	Echinococcus granulosus infection of bone Echinococcus granulosus infection, multiple sites Echinococcus granulosus infection, other sites
122.4	UNSPECIFIED ECHINOCOCCUS GRANULOSUS INFECTION	➡	B67.4	Echinococcus granulosus infection, unspecified
122.5	ECHINOCOCCUS MULTILOCULARIS INFECTION OF LIVER	➡	B67.5	Echinococcus multilocularis infection of liver
122.6	OTHER ECHINOCOCCUS MULTILOCULARIS INFECTION		B67.61 B67.69	Echinococcus multilocularis infection, multiple sites Echinococcus multilocularis infection, other sites
122.7	UNSPEC ECHINOCOCCUS MULTILOCULARIS INFECTION	➡	B67.7	Echinococcus multilocularis infection, unspecified
122.8	UNSPECIFIED ECHINOCOCCUS OF LIVER	➡	B67.8	Echinococcosis, unspecified, of liver
122.9	OTHER AND UNSPECIFIED ECHINOCOCCOSIS		B67.9Ø B67.99	Echinococcosis, unspecified Other echinococcosis
123.Ø	TAENIA SOLIUM INFECTION INTESTINAL FORM	➡	B68.Ø	Taenia solium taeniasis
123.1	CYSTICERCOSIS		B69.Ø B69.1 B69.81 B69.89 B69.9	Cysticercosis of central nervous system Cysticercosis of eye Myositis in cysticercosis Cysticercosis of other sites Cysticercosis, unspecified
123.2	TAENIA SAGINATA INFECTION	➡	B68.1	Taenia saginata taeniasis
123.3	TAENIASIS, UNSPECIFIED	➡	B68.9	Taeniasis, unspecified
123.4	DIPHYLLOBOTHRIASIS, INTESTINAL	➡	B7Ø.Ø	Diphyllobothriasis
123.5	SPARGANOSIS	➡	B7Ø.1	Sparganosis
123.6	HYMENOLEPIASIS	➡	B71.Ø	Hymenolepiasis
123.8	OTHER SPECIFIED CESTODE INFECTION		B71.1 B71.8	Dipylidiasis Other specified cestode infections
123.9	UNSPECIFIED CESTODE INFECTION	➡	B71.9	Cestode infection, unspecified
124	TRICHINOSIS	➡	B75	Trichinellosis
125.Ø	BANCROFTIAN FILARIASIS	➡	B74.Ø	Filariasis due to Wuchereria bancrofti
125.1	MALAYAN FILARIASIS	➡	B74.1	Filariasis due to Brugia malayi
125.2	LOIASIS	➡	B74.3	Loiasis
125.3	ONCHOCERCIASIS		B73.ØØ B73.Ø1 B73.Ø2 B73.Ø9 B73.1	Onchocerciasis with eye involvement, unspecified Onchocerciasis with endophthalmitis Onchocerciasis with glaucoma Onchocerciasis with other eye involvement Onchocerciasis without eye disease
125.4	DIPETALONEMIASIS		B74.8	Other filariases
125.5	MANSONELLA OZZARDI INFECTION	➡	B74.4	Mansonelliasis
125.6	OTHER SPECIFIED FILARIASIS		B74.2 B74.8	Filariasis due to Brugia timori Other filariases
125.7	DRACONTIASIS	➡	B72	Dracunculiasis
125.9	UNSPECIFIED FILARIASIS	➡	B74.9	Filariasis, unspecified
126.Ø	ANCYLOSTOMIASIS&NECATORIASIS-ANCYLOSTOMA DUODE		B76.Ø	Ancylostomiasis
126.1	ANCYLOSTOMIASIS&NECATORIASIS-NECATOR AMERICANUS	➡	B76.1	Necatoriasis
126.2	ANCYLOSTOMIASIS D/T ANCYLOSTOMA BRAZILIENSE		B76.Ø	Ancylostomiasis
126.3	ANCYLOSTOMIASIS D/T ANCYLOSTOMA CEYLANICUM		B76.Ø	Ancylostomiasis
126.8	ANCYLOSTOMIASIS&NECATORIASIS-OTH&UNS ANCYLOSTOMA		B76.Ø	Ancylostomiasis
126.9	UNSPECIFIED ANCYLOSTOMIASIS AND NECATORIASIS		B76.8 B76.9	Other hookworm diseases Hookworm disease, unspecified

ICD-9-CM		ICD-10-CM	
127.Ø	ASCARIASIS	**B77.Ø**	Ascariasis with intestinal complications
		B77.81	Ascariasis pneumonia
		B77.89	Ascariasis with other complications
		B77.9	Ascariasis, unspecified
127.1	ANISAKIASIS	➡ **B81.Ø**	Anisakiasis
127.2	STRONGYLOIDIASIS	**B78.Ø**	Intestinal strongyloidiasis
		B78.7	Disseminated strongyloidiasis
		B78.9	Strongyloidiasis, unspecified
127.3	TRICHURIASIS	➡ **B79**	Trichuriasis
127.4	ENTEROBIASIS	➡ **B8Ø**	Enterobiasis
127.5	CAPILLARIASIS	➡ **B81.1**	Intestinal capillariasis
127.6	TRICHOSTRONGYLIASIS	➡ **B81.2**	Trichostrongyliasis
127.7	OTHER SPECIFIED INTESTINAL HELMINTHIASIS	**B81.3**	Intestinal angiostrongyliasis
		B81.8	Other specified intestinal helminthiases
127.8	MIXED INTESTINAL HELMINTHIASIS	➡ **B81.4**	Mixed intestinal helminthiases
127.9	UNSPECIFIED INTESTINAL HELMINTHIASIS	➡ **B82.Ø**	Intestinal helminthiasis, unspecified
128.Ø	TOXOCARIASIS	➡ **B83.Ø**	Visceral larva migrans
128.1	GNATHOSTOMIASIS	➡ **B83.1**	Gnathostomiasis
128.8	OTHER SPECIFIED HELMINTHIASIS	**B83.2**	Angiostrongyliasis due to Parastrongylus cantonensis
		B83.3	Syngamiasis
		B83.8	Other specified helminthiases
128.9	UNSPECIFIED HELMINTH INFECTION	➡ **B83.9**	Helminthiasis, unspecified
129	UNSPECIFIED INTESTINAL PARASITISM	➡ **B82.9**	Intestinal parasitism, unspecified
13Ø.Ø	MENINGOENCEPHALITIS DUE TO TOXOPLASMOSIS	➡ **B58.2**	Toxoplasma meningoencephalitis
13Ø.1	CONJUNCTIVITIS DUE TO TOXOPLASMOSIS	**B58.Ø9**	Other toxoplasma oculopathy
13Ø.2	CHORIORETINITIS DUE TO TOXOPLASMOSIS	➡ **B58.Ø1**	Toxoplasma chorioretinitis
13Ø.3	MYOCARDITIS DUE TO TOXOPLASMOSIS	➡ **B58.81**	Toxoplasma myocarditis
13Ø.4	PNEUMONITIS DUE TO TOXOPLASMOSIS	**B58.3**	Pulmonary toxoplasmosis
13Ø.5	HEPATITIS DUE TO TOXOPLASMOSIS	➡ **B58.1**	Toxoplasma hepatitis
13Ø.7	TOXOPLASMOSIS OF OTHER SPECIFIED SITES	**B58.ØØ**	Toxoplasma oculopathy, unspecified
		B58.82	Toxoplasma myositis
		B58.83	Toxoplasma tubulo-interstitial nephropathy
		B58.89	Toxoplasmosis with other organ involvement
13Ø.8	MULTISYSTEMIC DISSEMINATED TOXOPLASMOSIS	**B58.89**	Toxoplasmosis with other organ involvement
13Ø.9	UNSPECIFIED TOXOPLASMOSIS	➡ **B58.9**	Toxoplasmosis, unspecified
131.ØØ	UNSPECIFIED UROGENITAL TRICHOMONIASIS	➡ **A59.ØØ**	Urogenital trichomoniasis, unspecified
131.Ø1	TRICHOMONAL VULVOVAGINITIS	➡ **A59.Ø1**	Trichomonal vulvovaginitis
131.Ø2	TRICHOMONAL URETHRITIS	**A59.Ø3**	Trichomonal cystitis and urethritis
131.Ø3	TRICHOMONAL PROSTATITIS	➡ **A59.Ø2**	Trichomonal prostatitis
131.Ø9	OTHER UROGENITAL TRICHOMONIASIS	➡ **A59.Ø9**	Other urogenital trichomoniasis
131.8	TRICHOMONIASIS OF OTHER SPECIFIED SITES	➡ **A59.8**	Trichomoniasis of other sites
131.9	UNSPECIFIED TRICHOMONIASIS	➡ **A59.9**	Trichomoniasis, unspecified
132.Ø	PEDICULUS CAPITIS	➡ **B85.Ø**	Pediculosis due to Pediculus humanus capitis
132.1	PEDICULUS CORPORIS	➡ **B85.1**	Pediculosis due to Pediculus humanus corporis
132.2	PHTHIRUS PUBIS	➡ **B85.3**	Phthiriasis
132.3	MIXED PEDICULOSIS AND PHTHIRUS INFESTATION	➡ **B85.4**	Mixed pediculosis and phthiriasis
132.9	UNSPECIFIED PEDICULOSIS	➡ **B85.2**	Pediculosis, unspecified
133.Ø	SCABIES	➡ **B86**	Scabies
133.8	OTHER ACARIASIS	**B88.Ø**	Other acariasis
133.9	UNSPECIFIED ACARIASIS	**B88.9**	Infestation, unspecified
134.Ø	MYIASIS	**B87.Ø**	Cutaneous myiasis
		B87.1	Wound myiasis
		B87.2	Ocular myiasis
		B87.3	Nasopharyngeal myiasis
		B87.4	Aural myiasis
		B87.81	Genitourinary myiasis
		B87.82	Intestinal myiasis
		B87.89	Myiasis of other sites
		B87.9	Myiasis, unspecified
134.1	OTHER ARTHROPOD INFESTATION	**B88.1**	Tungiasis [sandflea infestation]
		B88.2	Other arthropod infestations
134.2	HIRUDINIASIS	**B83.4**	Internal hirudiniasis
		B88.3	External hirudiniasis
134.8	OTHER SPECIFIED INFESTATIONS	**B88.8**	Other specified infestations
134.9	UNSPECIFIED INFESTATION	**B88.9**	Infestation, unspecified

ICD-9-CM			ICD-10-CM	
135	SARCOIDOSIS		**D86.Ø**	Sarcoidosis of lung
			D86.1	Sarcoidosis of lymph nodes
			D86.2	Sarcoidosis of lung with sarcoidosis of lymph nodes
			D86.3	Sarcoidosis of skin
			D86.81	Sarcoid meningitis
			D86.82	Multiple cranial nerve palsies in sarcoidosis
			D86.83	Sarcoid iridocyclitis
			D86.84	Sarcoid pyelonephritis
			D86.85	Sarcoid myocarditis
			D86.86	Sarcoid arthropathy
			D86.87	Sarcoid myositis
			D86.89	Sarcoidosis of other sites
			D86.9	Sarcoidosis, unspecified
136.Ø	AINHUM	➡	**L94.6**	Ainhum
136.1	BEHCETS SYNDROME	◘	**M35.2**	Behcet's disease
136.21	SPECIFIC INFECTION DUE TO ACANTHAMOEBA		**B6Ø.11**	Meningoencephalitis due to Acanthamoeba (culbertsoni)
		◘	**B6Ø.12**	Conjunctivitis due to Acanthamoeba
		◘	**B6Ø.13**	Keratoconjunctivitis due to Acanthamoeba
136.29	OTHER SPECIFIC INFECTIONS FREE-LIVING AMEBAE		**B6Ø.1Ø**	Acanthamebiasis, unspecified
			B6Ø.19	Other acanthamebic disease
			B6Ø.2	Naegleriasis
136.3	PNEUMOCYSTOSIS	➡	**B59**	Pneumocystosis
136.4	PSOROSPERMIASIS		**B6Ø.8**	Other specified protozoal diseases
136.5	SARCOSPORIDIOSIS		**AØ7.8**	Other specified protozoal intestinal diseases
136.8	OTHER SPECIFIED INFECTIOUS&PARASITIC DISEASES		**B6Ø.8**	Other specified protozoal diseases
			B99.8	Other infectious disease
136.9	UNSPECIFIED INFECTIOUS AND PARASITIC DISEASES		**B64**	Unspecified protozoal disease
			B89	Unspecified parasitic disease
			B99.9	Unspecified infectious disease
137.Ø	LATE EFFECTS RESPIRATORY/UNSPEC TUBERCULOSIS	➡	**B9Ø.9**	Sequelae of respiratory and unspecified tuberculosis
137.1	LATE EFFECTS OF CNTRL NERV SYS TUBERCULOSIS	➡	**B9Ø.Ø**	Sequelae of central nervous system tuberculosis
137.2	LATE EFFECTS OF GENITOURINARY TUBERCULOSIS	➡	**B9Ø.1**	Sequelae of genitourinary tuberculosis
137.3	LATE EFFECTS OF TUBERCULOSIS OF BONES AND JOINTS	➡	**B9Ø.2**	Sequelae of tuberculosis of bones and joints
137.4	LATE EFFECTS TUBERCULOSIS OTHER SPECIFIED ORGANS	➡	**B9Ø.8**	Sequelae of tuberculosis of other organs
138	LATE EFFECTS OF ACUTE POLIOMYELITIS		**B91**	Sequelae of poliomyelitis
			G14	Postpolio syndrome
139.Ø	LATE EFFECTS OF VIRAL ENCEPHALITIS	➡	**B94.1**	Sequelae of viral encephalitis
139.1	LATE EFFECTS OF TRACHOMA	➡	**B94.Ø**	Sequelae of trachoma
139.8	LATE EFFECTS OTH&UNSPEC INFECTIOUS&PARASITIC DZ		**B92**	Sequelae of leprosy
			B94.2	Sequelae of viral hepatitis
			B94.8	Sequelae of oth infectious and parasitic diseases
			B94.9	Sequelae of unspecified infectious and parasitic disease

Neoplasms

ICD-9-CM			ICD-10-CM	
140.0	MALIGNANT NEOPLASM OF UPPER LIP VERMILION BORDER	➡	C00.0	Malignant neoplasm of external upper lip
140.1	MALIGNANT NEOPLASM OF LOWER LIP VERMILION BORDER	➡	C00.1	Malignant neoplasm of external lower lip
140.3	MALIGNANT NEOPLASM OF UPPER LIP INNER ASPECT	➡	C00.3	Malignant neoplasm of upper lip, inner aspect
140.4	MALIGNANT NEOPLASM OF LOWER LIP INNER ASPECT	➡	C00.4	Malignant neoplasm of lower lip, inner aspect
140.5	MALIG NEOPLSM LIP INNR ASPECT UNS AS UPPER/LOW	➡	C00.5	Malignant neoplasm of lip, unspecified, inner aspect
140.6	MALIGNANT NEOPLASM OF COMMISSURE OF LIP	➡	C00.6	Malignant neoplasm of commissure of lip, unspecified
140.8	MALIGNANT NEOPLASM OF OTHER SITES OF LIP	➡	C00.8	Malignant neoplasm of overlapping sites of lip
140.9	MALIG NEOPLSM LIP VERMILION BORDR UNS AS UP/LOW		C00.2 C00.9	Malignant neoplasm of external lip, unspecified Malignant neoplasm of lip, unspecified
141.0	MALIGNANT NEOPLASM OF BASE OF TONGUE	➡	C01	Malignant neoplasm of base of tongue
141.1	MALIGNANT NEOPLASM OF DORSAL SURFACE OF TONGUE	➡	C02.0	Malignant neoplasm of dorsal surface of tongue
141.2	MALIGNANT NEOPLASM TIP&LATERAL BORDER TONGUE	➡	C02.1	Malignant neoplasm of border of tongue
141.3	MALIGNANT NEOPLASM OF VENTRAL SURFACE OF TONGUE	➡	C02.2	Malignant neoplasm of ventral surface of tongue
141.4	MALIG NEOPLASM ANTERIOR 2/3 TONGUE PART UNSPEC	➡	C02.3	Malig neoplasm of anterior two-thirds of tongue, part unsp
141.5	MALIGNANT NEOPLASM OF JUNCTIONAL ZONE OF TONGUE		C02.8	Malignant neoplasm of overlapping sites of tongue
141.6	MALIGNANT NEOPLASM OF LINGUAL TONSIL	➡	C02.4	Malignant neoplasm of lingual tonsil
141.8	MALIGNANT NEOPLASM OF OTHER SITES OF TONGUE		C02.8	Malignant neoplasm of overlapping sites of tongue
141.9	MALIGNANT NEOPLASM OF TONGUE UNSPECIFIED SITE	➡	C02.9	Malignant neoplasm of tongue, unspecified
142.0	MALIGNANT NEOPLASM OF PAROTID GLAND	➡	C07	Malignant neoplasm of parotid gland
142.1	MALIGNANT NEOPLASM OF SUBMANDIBULAR GLAND	➡	C08.0	Malignant neoplasm of submandibular gland
142.2	MALIGNANT NEOPLASM OF SUBLINGUAL GLAND	➡	C08.1	Malignant neoplasm of sublingual gland
142.8	MALIGNANT NEOPLASM OTHER MAJOR SALIVARY GLANDS		C08.9	Malignant neoplasm of major salivary gland, unspecified
142.9	MALIGNANT NEOPLASM OF SALIVARY GLAND UNSPECIFIED		C08.9	Malignant neoplasm of major salivary gland, unspecified
143.0	MALIGNANT NEOPLASM OF UPPER GUM	➡	C03.0	Malignant neoplasm of upper gum
143.1	MALIGNANT NEOPLASM OF LOWER GUM	➡	C03.1	Malignant neoplasm of lower gum
143.8	MALIGNANT NEOPLASM OF OTHER SITES OF GUM		C03.9	Malignant neoplasm of gum, unspecified
143.9	MALIGNANT NEOPLASM OF GUM UNSPECIFIED SITE		C03.9	Malignant neoplasm of gum, unspecified
144.0	MALIGNANT NEOPLASM ANTERIOR PORTION FLOOR MOUTH	➡	C04.0	Malignant neoplasm of anterior floor of mouth
144.1	MALIGNANT NEOPLASM LATERAL PORTION FLOOR MOUTH	➡	C04.1	Malignant neoplasm of lateral floor of mouth
144.8	MALIGNANT NEOPLASM OTHER SITES FLOOR MOUTH	➡	C04.8	Malignant neoplasm of overlapping sites of floor of mouth
144.9	MALIGNANT NEOPLASM FLOOR MOUTH PART UNSPECIFIED	➡	C04.9	Malignant neoplasm of floor of mouth, unspecified
145.0	MALIGNANT NEOPLASM OF CHEEK MUCOSA	➡	C06.0	Malignant neoplasm of cheek mucosa
145.1	MALIGNANT NEOPLASM OF VESTIBULE OF MOUTH	➡	C06.1	Malignant neoplasm of vestibule of mouth
145.2	MALIGNANT NEOPLASM OF HARD PALATE	➡	C05.0	Malignant neoplasm of hard palate
145.3	MALIGNANT NEOPLASM OF SOFT PALATE	➡	C05.1	Malignant neoplasm of soft palate
145.4	MALIGNANT NEOPLASM OF UVULA	➡	C05.2	Malignant neoplasm of uvula
145.5	MALIGNANT NEOPLASM OF PALATE UNSPECIFIED		C05.8 C05.9	Malignant neoplasm of overlapping sites of palate Malignant neoplasm of palate, unspecified
145.6	MALIGNANT NEOPLASM OF RETROMOLAR AREA	➡	C06.2	Malignant neoplasm of retromolar area
145.8	MALIGNANT NEOPLASM OTHER SPECIFIED PARTS MOUTH		C06.80 C06.89	Malignant neoplasm of ovrlp sites of unsp parts of mouth Malignant neoplasm of overlapping sites of oth prt mouth
145.9	MALIGNANT NEOPLASM OF MOUTH UNSPECIFIED SITE	➡	C06.9	Malignant neoplasm of mouth, unspecified
146.0	MALIGNANT NEOPLASM OF TONSIL		C09.8 C09.9	Malignant neoplasm of overlapping sites of tonsil Malignant neoplasm of tonsil, unspecified
146.1	MALIGNANT NEOPLASM OF TONSILLAR FOSSA	➡	C09.0	Malignant neoplasm of tonsillar fossa
146.2	MALIGNANT NEOPLASM OF TONSILLAR PILLARS	➡	C09.1	Malig neoplasm of tonsillar pillar (anterior) (posterior)
146.3	MALIGNANT NEOPLASM OF VALLECULA	➡	C10.0	Malignant neoplasm of vallecula
146.4	MALIGNANT NEOPLASM ANTERIOR ASPECT EPIGLOTTIS	➡	C10.1	Malignant neoplasm of anterior surface of epiglottis
146.5	MALIGNANT NEOPLASM JUNCTIONAL REGION OROPHARYNX		C10.8	Malignant neoplasm of overlapping sites of oropharynx
146.6	MALIGNANT NEOPLASM OF LATERAL WALL OF OROPHARYNX	➡	C10.2	Malignant neoplasm of lateral wall of oropharynx
146.7	MALIGNANT NEOPLASM POSTERIOR WALL OROPHARYNX	➡	C10.3	Malignant neoplasm of posterior wall of oropharynx
146.8	MALIGNANT NEOPLASM OTHER SPEC SITES OROPHARYNX		C10.4 C10.8	Malignant neoplasm of branchial cleft Malignant neoplasm of overlapping sites of oropharynx
146.9	MALIGNANT NEOPLASM OROPHARYNX UNSPECIFIED SITE	➡	C10.9	Malignant neoplasm of oropharynx, unspecified
147.0	MALIGNANT NEOPLASM SUPERIOR WALL NASOPHARYNX	➡	C11.0	Malignant neoplasm of superior wall of nasopharynx
147.1	MALIGNANT NEOPLASM POSTERIOR WALL NASOPHARYNX	➡	C11.1	Malignant neoplasm of posterior wall of nasopharynx
147.2	MALIGNANT NEOPLASM LATERAL WALL NASOPHARYNX	➡	C11.2	Malignant neoplasm of lateral wall of nasopharynx
147.3	MALIGNANT NEOPLASM ANTERIOR WALL NASOPHARYNX	➡	C11.3	Malignant neoplasm of anterior wall of nasopharynx
147.8	MALIGNANT NEOPLASM OTHER SPEC SITES NASOPHARYNX		C11.8	Malignant neoplasm of overlapping sites of nasopharynx
147.9	MALIGNANT NEOPLASM NASOPHARYNX UNSPECIFIED SITE	➡	C11.9	Malignant neoplasm of nasopharynx, unspecified
148.0	MALIG NEOPLASM POSTCRICOID REGION HYPOPHARYNX	➡	C13.0	Malignant neoplasm of postcricoid region
148.1	MALIGNANT NEOPLASM OF PYRIFORM SINUS	➡	C12	Malignant neoplasm of pyriform sinus
148.2	MAL NEO ARYEPIGLOTTIC FOLD HYPOPHARYNGEAL ASPECT	➡	C13.1	Malig neoplasm of aryepiglottic fold, hypopharyngeal aspect
148.3	MALIGNANT NEOPLASM POSTERIOR HYPOPHARYNGEAL WALL	➡	C13.2	Malignant neoplasm of posterior wall of hypopharynx
148.8	MALIGNANT NEOPLASM OTHER SPEC SITES HYPOPHARYNX		C13.8	Malignant neoplasm of overlapping sites of hypopharynx
148.9	MALIGNANT NEOPLASM HYPOPHARYNX UNSPECIFIED SITE	➡	C13.9	Malignant neoplasm of hypopharynx, unspecified
149.0	MALIGNANT NEOPLASM OF PHARYNX UNSPECIFIED	➡	C14.0	Malignant neoplasm of pharynx, unspecified
149.1	MALIGNANT NEOPLASM OF WALDEYERS RING	➡	C14.2	Malignant neoplasm of Waldeyer's ring

ICD-9-CM			ICD-10-CM	
149.8	MALIG NEOPLASM OTH SITES WITHIN LIP&ORAL CAVITY		C14.8	Malig neoplm of ovrlp sites of lip, oral cavity and pharynx
149.9	MALIG NEOPLASM ILL-DEFINED SITES LIP&ORAL CAVITY		C14.8	Malig neoplm of ovrlp sites of lip, oral cavity and pharynx
15Ø.Ø	MALIGNANT NEOPLASM OF CERVICAL ESOPHAGUS		C15.3	Malignant neoplasm of upper third of esophagus
15Ø.1	MALIGNANT NEOPLASM OF THORACIC ESOPHAGUS		C15.4	Malignant neoplasm of middle third of esophagus
15Ø.2	MALIGNANT NEOPLASM OF ABDOMINAL ESOPHAGUS		C15.5	Malignant neoplasm of lower third of esophagus
15Ø.3	MALIGNANT NEOPLASM OF UPPER THIRD OF ESOPHAGUS		C15.3	Malignant neoplasm of upper third of esophagus
15Ø.4	MALIGNANT NEOPLASM OF MIDDLE THIRD OF ESOPHAGUS		C15.4	Malignant neoplasm of middle third of esophagus
15Ø.5	MALIGNANT NEOPLASM OF LOWER THIRD OF ESOPHAGUS		C15.5	Malignant neoplasm of lower third of esophagus
15Ø.8	MALIGNANT NEOPLASM OTHER SPEC PART ESOPHAGUS		C15.8	Malignant neoplasm of overlapping sites of esophagus
15Ø.9	MALIGNANT NEOPLASM OF ESOPHAGUS UNSPECIFIED SITE	➡	C15.9	Malignant neoplasm of esophagus, unspecified
151.Ø	MALIGNANT NEOPLASM OF CARDIA	➡	C16.Ø	Malignant neoplasm of cardia
151.1	MALIGNANT NEOPLASM OF PYLORUS	➡	C16.4	Malignant neoplasm of pylorus
151.2	MALIGNANT NEOPLASM OF PYLORIC ANTRUM	➡	C16.3	Malignant neoplasm of pyloric antrum
151.3	MALIGNANT NEOPLASM OF FUNDUS OF STOMACH	➡	C16.1	Malignant neoplasm of fundus of stomach
151.4	MALIGNANT NEOPLASM OF BODY OF STOMACH	➡	C16.2	Malignant neoplasm of body of stomach
151.5	MALIGNANT NEOPLASM LESSER CURV STOMACH UNSPEC	➡	C16.5	Malignant neoplasm of lesser curvature of stomach, unsp
151.6	MALIGNANT NEOPLASM GREATER CURV STOMACH UNSPEC	➡	C16.6	Malignant neoplasm of greater curvature of stomach, unsp
151.8	MALIGNANT NEOPLASM OTHER SPECIFIED SITES STOMACH		C16.8	Malignant neoplasm of overlapping sites of stomach
151.9	MALIGNANT NEOPLASM OF STOMACH UNSPECIFIED SITE	➡	C16.9	Malignant neoplasm of stomach, unspecified
152.Ø	MALIGNANT NEOPLASM OF DUODENUM	➡	C17.Ø	Malignant neoplasm of duodenum
152.1	MALIGNANT NEOPLASM OF JEJUNUM	➡	C17.1	Malignant neoplasm of jejunum
152.2	MALIGNANT NEOPLASM OF ILEUM	➡	C17.2	Malignant neoplasm of ileum
152.3	MALIGNANT NEOPLASM OF MECKELS DIVERTICULUM	➡	C17.3	Meckel's diverticulum, malignant
152.8	MALIG NEOPLASM OTHER SPEC SITES SMALL INTESTINE		C17.8	Malignant neoplasm of overlapping sites of small intestine
152.9	MALIGNANT NEOPLASM SMALL INTESTINE UNSPEC SITE	➡	C17.9	Malignant neoplasm of small intestine, unspecified
153.Ø	MALIGNANT NEOPLASM OF HEPATIC FLEXURE	➡	C18.3	Malignant neoplasm of hepatic flexure
153.1	MALIGNANT NEOPLASM OF TRANSVERSE COLON	➡	C18.4	Malignant neoplasm of transverse colon
153.2	MALIGNANT NEOPLASM OF DESCENDING COLON	➡	C18.6	Malignant neoplasm of descending colon
153.3	MALIGNANT NEOPLASM OF SIGMOID COLON	➡	C18.7	Malignant neoplasm of sigmoid colon
153.4	MALIGNANT NEOPLASM OF CECUM	➡	C18.Ø	Malignant neoplasm of cecum
153.5	MALIGNANT NEOPLASM OF APPENDIX	➡	C18.1	Malignant neoplasm of appendix
153.6	MALIGNANT NEOPLASM OF ASCENDING COLON	➡	C18.2	Malignant neoplasm of ascending colon
153.7	MALIGNANT NEOPLASM OF SPLENIC FLEXURE	➡	C18.5	Malignant neoplasm of splenic flexure
153.8	MALIG NEOPLASM OTHER SPEC SITES LARGE INTESTINE		C18.8	Malignant neoplasm of overlapping sites of colon
153.9	MALIGNANT NEOPLASM OF COLON UNSPECIFIED SITE	➡	C18.9	Malignant neoplasm of colon, unspecified
154.Ø	MALIGNANT NEOPLASM OF RECTOSIGMOID JUNCTION	➡	C19	Malignant neoplasm of rectosigmoid junction
154.1	MALIGNANT NEOPLASM OF RECTUM	➡	C2Ø	Malignant neoplasm of rectum
154.2	MALIGNANT NEOPLASM OF ANAL CANAL	➡	C21.1	Malignant neoplasm of anal canal
154.3	MALIGNANT NEOPLASM OF ANUS UNSPECIFIED SITE	➡	C21.Ø	Malignant neoplasm of anus, unspecified
154.8	MAL NEOPLSM OTH SITE RECT RECTOSIGMOID JUNC&ANUS		C21.2 C21.8	Malignant neoplasm of cloacogenic zone Malig neoplasm of ovrlp sites of rectum, anus and anal canal
155.Ø	MALIGNANT NEOPLASM OF LIVER PRIMARY		C22.Ø C22.2 C22.3 C22.4 C22.7 C22.8	Liver cell carcinoma Hepatoblastoma Angiosarcoma of liver Other sarcomas of liver Other specified carcinomas of liver Malignant neoplasm of liver, primary, unspecified as to type
155.1	MALIGNANT NEOPLASM OF INTRAHEPATIC BILE DUCTS	➡	C22.1	Intrahepatic bile duct carcinoma
155.2	MALIGNANT NEOPLASM LIVER NOT SPEC AS PRIMARY/SEC	➡	C22.9	Malig neoplasm of liver, not specified as primary or sec
156.Ø	MALIGNANT NEOPLASM OF GALLBLADDER	➡	C23	Malignant neoplasm of gallbladder
156.1	MALIGNANT NEOPLASM OF EXTRAHEPATIC BILE DUCTS	➡	C24.Ø	Malignant neoplasm of extrahepatic bile duct
156.2	MALIGNANT NEOPLASM OF AMPULLA OF VATER	➡	C24.1	Malignant neoplasm of ampulla of Vater
156.8	MALIG NEOPLSM OTH SPEC SITE GB&XTRAHEP BDS	➡	C24.8	Malignant neoplasm of overlapping sites of biliary tract
156.9	MALIG NEOPLASM BILIARY TRACT PART UNSPEC SITE	➡	C24.9	Malignant neoplasm of biliary tract, unspecified
157.Ø	MALIGNANT NEOPLASM OF HEAD OF PANCREAS	➡	C25.Ø	Malignant neoplasm of head of pancreas
157.1	MALIGNANT NEOPLASM OF BODY OF PANCREAS	➡	C25.1	Malignant neoplasm of body of pancreas
157.2	MALIGNANT NEOPLASM OF TAIL OF PANCREAS	➡	C25.2	Malignant neoplasm of tail of pancreas
157.3	MALIGNANT NEOPLASM OF PANCREATIC DUCT	➡	C25.3	Malignant neoplasm of pancreatic duct
157.4	MALIGNANT NEOPLASM OF ISLETS OF LANGERHANS	➡	C25.4	Malignant neoplasm of endocrine pancreas
157.8	MALIGNANT NEOPLASM OTHER SPEC SITES PANCREAS		C25.7 C25.8	Malignant neoplasm of other parts of pancreas Malignant neoplasm of overlapping sites of pancreas
157.9	MALIGNANT NEOPLASM OF PANCREAS PART UNSPECIFIED	➡	C25.9	Malignant neoplasm of pancreas, unspecified
158.Ø	MALIGNANT NEOPLASM OF RETROPERITONEUM	➡	C48.Ø	Malignant neoplasm of retroperitoneum
158.8	MALIGNANT NEOPLASM SPECIFIED PARTS PERITONEUM		C45.1 C48.1 C48.8	Mesothelioma of peritoneum Malignant neoplasm of specified parts of peritoneum Malig neoplasm of ovrlp sites of retroperiton and peritoneum
158.9	MALIGNANT NEOPLASM OF PERITONEUM UNSPECIFIED	➡	C48.2	Malignant neoplasm of peritoneum, unspecified
159.Ø	MALIGNANT NEOPLASM INTESTINAL TRACT PART UNSPEC	➡	C26.Ø	Malignant neoplasm of intestinal tract, part unspecified

[Brackets] indicate valid character values for each code. Character value meanings provided for each code grouping.

ICD-9-CM			ICD-10-CM	
159.1	MALIGNANT NEOPLASM OF SPLEEN NEC	➡	**C26.1**	Malignant neoplasm of spleen
159.8	MAL NEOPLSM OTH SITE DIGESTV SYS&INTRA-ABD ORGN		**C26.9**	Malignant neoplasm of ill-defined sites within the dgstv sys
159.9	MAL NEOPLSM ILL-DEFIND SITE DIGESTV ORGN&PERITON		**C26.9**	Malignant neoplasm of ill-defined sites within the dgstv sys
160.0	MALIGNANT NEOPLASM OF NASAL CAVITIES	➡	**C30.0**	Malignant neoplasm of nasal cavity
160.1	MAL NEO AUDITRY TUBE MID EAR&MASTOID AIR CELLS	➡	**C30.1**	Malignant neoplasm of middle ear
160.2	MALIGNANT NEOPLASM OF MAXILLARY SINUS	➡	**C31.0**	Malignant neoplasm of maxillary sinus
160.3	MALIGNANT NEOPLASM OF ETHMOIDAL SINUS	➡	**C31.1**	Malignant neoplasm of ethmoidal sinus
160.4	MALIGNANT NEOPLASM OF FRONTAL SINUS	➡	**C31.2**	Malignant neoplasm of frontal sinus
160.5	MALIGNANT NEOPLASM OF SPHENOIDAL SINUS	➡	**C31.3**	Malignant neoplasm of sphenoid sinus
160.8	MAL NEO-OTH SITES-NASAL CAVITY-MIDDLE EAR-SINUS	➡	**C31.8**	Malignant neoplasm of overlapping sites of accessory sinuses
160.9	MAL NEO NASL CAV MID EAR&ACSS SINUS UNS SITE	➡	**C31.9**	Malignant neoplasm of accessory sinus, unspecified
161.0	MALIGNANT NEOPLASM OF GLOTTIS	➡	**C32.0**	Malignant neoplasm of glottis
161.1	MALIGNANT NEOPLASM OF SUPRAGLOTTIS	➡	**C32.1**	Malignant neoplasm of supraglottis
161.2	MALIGNANT NEOPLASM OF SUBGLOTTIS	➡	**C32.2**	Malignant neoplasm of subglottis
161.3	MALIGNANT NEOPLASM OF LARYNGEAL CARTILAGES	➡	**C32.3**	Malignant neoplasm of laryngeal cartilage
161.8	MALIGNANT NEOPLASM OTHER SPECIFIED SITES LARYNX	➡	**C32.8**	Malignant neoplasm of overlapping sites of larynx
161.9	MALIGNANT NEOPLASM OF LARYNX UNSPECIFIED SITE	➡	**C32.9**	Malignant neoplasm of larynx, unspecified
162.0	MALIGNANT NEOPLASM OF TRACHEA	➡	**C33**	Malignant neoplasm of trachea
162.2	MALIGNANT NEOPLASM OF MAIN BRONCHUS		**C34.00** **C34.01** **C34.02**	Malignant neoplasm of unspecified main bronchus Malignant neoplasm of right main bronchus Malignant neoplasm of left main bronchus
162.3	MALIGNANT NEOPLASM UPPER LOBE BRONCHUS OR LUNG		**C34.10** **C34.11** **C34.12**	Malignant neoplasm of upper lobe, unsp bronchus or lung Malignant neoplasm of upper lobe, right bronchus or lung Malignant neoplasm of upper lobe, left bronchus or lung
162.4	MALIGNANT NEOPLASM MIDDLE LOBE BRONCHUS OR LUNG	➡	**C34.2**	Malignant neoplasm of middle lobe, bronchus or lung
162.5	MALIGNANT NEOPLASM LOWER LOBE BRONCHUS OR LUNG		**C34.30** **C34.31** **C34.32**	Malignant neoplasm of lower lobe, unsp bronchus or lung Malignant neoplasm of lower lobe, right bronchus or lung Malignant neoplasm of lower lobe, left bronchus or lung
162.8	MALIGNANT NEOPLASM OTHER PARTS BRONCHUS OR LUNG		**C34.80** **C34.81** **C34.82**	Malignant neoplasm of ovrlp sites of unsp bronchus and lung Malignant neoplasm of ovrlp sites of right bronchus and lung Malignant neoplasm of ovrlp sites of left bronchus and lung
162.9	MALIGNANT NEOPLASM BRONCHUS&LUNG UNSPEC SITE		**C34.90** **C34.91** **C34.92**	Malignant neoplasm of unsp part of unsp bronchus or lung Malignant neoplasm of unsp part of right bronchus or lung Malignant neoplasm of unsp part of left bronchus or lung
163.0	MALIGNANT NEOPLASM OF PARIETAL PLEURA		**C38.4**	Malignant neoplasm of pleura
163.1	MALIGNANT NEOPLASM OF VISCERAL PLEURA		**C38.4**	Malignant neoplasm of pleura
163.8	MALIGNANT NEOPLASM OTHER SPECIFIED SITES PLEURA		**C38.4**	Malignant neoplasm of pleura
163.9	MALIGNANT NEOPLASM OF PLEURA UNSPECIFIED SITE		**C38.4** **C45.0**	Malignant neoplasm of pleura Mesothelioma of pleura
164.0	MALIGNANT NEOPLASM OF THYMUS	➡	**C37**	Malignant neoplasm of thymus
164.1	MALIGNANT NEOPLASM OF HEART		**C38.0** **C45.2**	Malignant neoplasm of heart Mesothelioma of pericardium
164.2	MALIGNANT NEOPLASM OF ANTERIOR MEDIASTINUM	➡	**C38.1**	Malignant neoplasm of anterior mediastinum
164.3	MALIGNANT NEOPLASM OF POSTERIOR MEDIASTINUM	➡	**C38.2**	Malignant neoplasm of posterior mediastinum
164.8	MALIGNANT NEOPLASM OF OTHER PARTS OF MEDIASTINUM	➡	**C38.8**	Malig neoplm of ovrlp sites of heart, mediastinum and pleura
164.9	MALIGNANT NEOPLASM MEDIASTINUM PART UNSPECIFIED	➡	**C38.3**	Malignant neoplasm of mediastinum, part unspecified
165.0	MALIG NEOPLASM UPPER RESP TRACT PART UNSPEC	➡	**C39.0**	Malignant neoplasm of upper respiratory tract, part unsp
165.8	MAL NEO OTH SITE WITHIN RESP SYS&INTRATHR ORGN		**C39.9**	Malignant neoplasm of lower respiratory tract, part unsp
165.9	MALIG NEOPLSM ILL-DEFIND SITE WITHIN RESP SYSTEM		**C39.9**	Malignant neoplasm of lower respiratory tract, part unsp
170.0	MALIG NEOPLASM BONES SKULL&FACE EXCEPT MANDIBLE	➡	**C41.0**	Malignant neoplasm of bones of skull and face
170.1	MALIGNANT NEOPLASM OF MANDIBLE	➡	**C41.1**	Malignant neoplasm of mandible
170.2	MALIG NEOPLASM VERT COLUMN EXCLD SACRUM&COCCYX	➡	**C41.2**	Malignant neoplasm of vertebral column
170.3	MALIGNANT NEOPLASM OF RIBS STERNUM AND CLAVICLE	➡	**C41.3**	Malignant neoplasm of ribs, sternum and clavicle
170.4	MALIGNANT NEOPLASM SCAPULA&LONG BONES UPPER LIMB		**C40.00** **C40.01** **C40.02**	Malig neoplasm of scapula and long bones of unsp upper limb Malig neoplasm of scapula and long bones of right upper limb Malig neoplasm of scapula and long bones of left upper limb
170.5	MALIGNANT NEOPLASM OF SHORT BONES OF UPPER LIMB		**C40.10** **C40.11** **C40.12**	Malignant neoplasm of short bones of unspecified upper limb Malignant neoplasm of short bones of right upper limb Malignant neoplasm of short bones of left upper limb
170.6	MALIGNANT NEOPLASM OF PELVIC BONES SACRUM&COCCYX	➡	**C41.4**	Malignant neoplasm of pelvic bones, sacrum and coccyx
170.7	MALIGNANT NEOPLASM OF LONG BONES OF LOWER LIMB		**C40.20** **C40.21** **C40.22**	Malignant neoplasm of long bones of unspecified lower limb Malignant neoplasm of long bones of right lower limb Malignant neoplasm of long bones of left lower limb
170.8	MALIGNANT NEOPLASM OF SHORT BONES OF LOWER LIMB		**C40.30** **C40.31** **C40.32**	Malignant neoplasm of short bones of unspecified lower limb Malignant neoplasm of short bones of right lower limb Malignant neoplasm of short bones of left lower limb

ICD-9-CM		ICD-10-CM	
170.9	MALIG NEOPLASM BONE&ARTICLR CART SITE UNSPEC	**C40.80**	Malig neoplm of ovrlp sites of bone/artic cartl of unsp limb
		C40.81	Malig neoplm of ovrlp sites of bone/artic cartl of r limb
		C40.82	Malig neoplm of ovrlp sites of bone/artic cartl of left limb
		C40.90	Malig neoplasm of unsp bones and artic cartlg of unsp limb
		C40.91	Malig neoplasm of unsp bones and artic cartlg of right limb
		C40.92	Malig neoplasm of unsp bones and artic cartlg of left limb
		C41.9	Malignant neoplasm of bone and articular cartilage, unsp
171.0	MALIG NEOPLSM CNCTV&OTH SOFT TISSUE HEAD FCE&NCK	**C47.0**	Malignant neoplasm of prph nerves of head, face and neck
		C49.0	Malig neoplm of conn and soft tissue of head, face and neck
171.2	MALIG NEOPLSM CNCTV&OTH SFT TISS UP LIMB W/SHLDR	**C47.10**	Malig neoplm of prph nerves of unsp upper limb, inc shoulder
		C47.11	Malig neoplm of prph nerves of right upper limb, inc shldr
		C47.12	Malig neoplm of prph nerves of left upper limb, inc shoulder
		C49.10	Malig neoplm of conn & soft tiss of unsp upr lmb, inc shldr
		C49.11	Malig neoplm of conn and soft tiss of r upr limb, inc shldr
		C49.12	Malig neoplm of conn and soft tiss of l upr limb, inc shldr
171.3	MALIG NEOPLSM CNCTV&OTH SFT TISS LOW LIMB W/HIP	**C47.20**	Malig neoplasm of prph nerves of unsp lower limb, inc hip
		C47.21	Malig neoplasm of prph nerves of right lower limb, inc hip
		C47.22	Malig neoplasm of prph nerves of left lower limb, inc hip
		C49.20	Malig neoplm of conn and soft tiss of unsp low limb, inc hip
		C49.21	Malig neoplm of conn and soft tiss of r low limb, inc hip
		C49.22	Malig neoplm of conn and soft tiss of left low limb, inc hip
171.4	MALIG NEOPLASM CONNECTIVE&OTH SOFT TISSUE THORAX	**C47.3**	Malignant neoplasm of peripheral nerves of thorax
		C49.3	Malignant neoplasm of connective and soft tissue of thorax
171.5	MALIG NEOPLASM CONNECTIVE&OTH SOFT TISSUE ABD	**C47.4**	Malignant neoplasm of peripheral nerves of abdomen
		C49.4	Malignant neoplasm of connective and soft tissue of abdomen
171.6	MALIG NEOPLASM CONNECTIVE&OTH SOFT TISSUE PELVIS	**C47.5**	Malignant neoplasm of peripheral nerves of pelvis
		C49.5	Malignant neoplasm of connective and soft tissue of pelvis
171.7	MALIG NEOPLSM CNCTV&OTH SFT TISS TRNK UNS SITE	**C47.6**	Malignant neoplasm of peripheral nerves of trunk, unsp
		C49.6	Malignant neoplasm of conn and soft tissue of trunk, unsp
171.8	MALIG NEOPLSM OTH SPEC SITE CNCTV&OTH SFT TISSUE	**C47.8**	Malig neoplm of ovrlp sites of prph nrv and autonm nrv sys
		C49.8	Malignant neoplasm of ovrlp sites of conn and soft tissue
171.9	MALIG NEOPLASM CNCTV&OTH SOFT TISSUE SITE UNSPEC	**C47.9**	Malig neoplasm of prph nerves and autonm nervous sys, unsp
		C49.9	Malignant neoplasm of connective and soft tissue, unsp
172.0	MALIGNANT MELANOMA OF SKIN OF LIP	**C43.0**	Malignant melanoma of lip
		D03.0	Melanoma in situ of lip
172.1	MALIGNANT MELANOMA SKIN EYELID INCLUDING CANTHUS	**C43.10**	Malignant melanoma of unspecified eyelid, including canthus
		C43.11	Malignant melanoma of right eyelid, including canthus
		C43.12	Malignant melanoma of left eyelid, including canthus
		D03.10	Melanoma in situ of unspecified eyelid, including canthus
		D03.11	Melanoma in situ of right eyelid, including canthus
		D03.12	Melanoma in situ of left eyelid, including canthus
172.2	MALIG MELANOMA SKIN EAR&EXTERNAL AUDITORY CANAL	**C43.20**	Malignant melanoma of unsp ear and external auricular canal
		C43.21	Malignant melanoma of right ear and external auricular canal
		C43.22	Malignant melanoma of left ear and external auricular canal
		D03.20	Melanoma in situ of unsp ear and external auricular canal
		D03.21	Melanoma in situ of right ear and external auricular canal
		D03.22	Melanoma in situ of left ear and external auricular canal
172.3	MALIGNANT MELANOMA SKIN OTHER&UNSPEC PARTS FACE	**C43.30**	Malignant melanoma of unspecified part of face
		C43.31	Malignant melanoma of nose
		C43.39	Malignant melanoma of other parts of face
		D03.30	Melanoma in situ of unspecified part of face
		D03.39	Melanoma in situ of other parts of face
172.4	MALIGNANT MELANOMA OF SKIN OF SCALP AND NECK	**C43.4**	Malignant melanoma of scalp and neck
		D03.4	Melanoma in situ of scalp and neck
172.5	MALIGNANT MELANOMA SKIN TRUNK EXCEPT SCROTUM	**C43.51**	Malignant melanoma of anal skin
		C43.52	Malignant melanoma of skin of breast
		C43.59	Malignant melanoma of other part of trunk
		D03.51	Melanoma in situ of anal skin
		D03.52	Melanoma in situ of breast (skin) (soft tissue)
		D03.59	Melanoma in situ of other part of trunk
172.6	MALIG MELANOMA SKIN UPPER LIMB INCL SHOULDER	**C43.60**	Malignant melanoma of unsp upper limb, including shoulder
		C43.61	Malignant melanoma of right upper limb, including shoulder
		C43.62	Malignant melanoma of left upper limb, including shoulder
		D03.60	Melanoma in situ of unsp upper limb, including shoulder
		D03.61	Melanoma in situ of right upper limb, including shoulder
		D03.62	Melanoma in situ of left upper limb, including shoulder
172.7	MALIGNANT MELANOMA SKIN LOWER LIMB INCLUDING HIP	**C43.70**	Malignant melanoma of unspecified lower limb, including hip
		C43.71	Malignant melanoma of right lower limb, including hip
		C43.72	Malignant melanoma of left lower limb, including hip
		D03.70	Melanoma in situ of unspecified lower limb, including hip
		D03.71	Melanoma in situ of right lower limb, including hip
		D03.72	Melanoma in situ of left lower limb, including hip
172.8	MALIGNANT MELANOMA OTHER SPECIFIED SITES SKIN	**C43.8**	Malignant melanoma of overlapping sites of skin
		D03.8	Melanoma in situ of other sites
172.9	MELANOMA OF SKIN, SITE UNSPECIFIED	**C43.9**	Malignant melanoma of skin, unspecified
		D03.9	Melanoma in situ, unspecified
173.00	UNSPECIFIED MALIGNANT NEOPLASM OF SKIN OF LIP	**C44.00**	Unspecified malignant neoplasm of skin of lip
173.01	BASAL CELL CARCINOMA OF SKIN OF LIP	**C44.01**	Basal cell carcinoma of skin of lip

[Brackets] indicate valid character values for each code. Character value meanings provided for each code grouping.

ICD-9-CM		ICD-10-CM	
173.02	SQUAMOUS CELL CARCINOMA OF SKIN OF LIP	C44.02	Squamous cell carcinoma of skin of lip
173.09	OTHER SPECIFIED MALIGNANT NEOPLASM SKIN OF LIP	C44.09	Other specified malignant neoplasm of skin of lip
173.10	UNS MALIGNANT NEOPLASM EYELID INCLUDING CANTHUS	C44.101	Unsp malignant neoplasm skin/ unsp eyelid, including canthus
		C44.102	Unsp malignant neoplasm skin/ right eyelid, inc canthus
		C44.109	Unsp malignant neoplasm skin/ left eyelid, including canthus
173.11	BASAL CELL CARCINOMA OF EYELID INCLUDING CANTHUS	C44.111	Basal cell carcinoma skin/ unsp eyelid, including canthus
		C44.112	Basal cell carcinoma skin/ right eyelid, including canthus
		C44.119	Basal cell carcinoma skin/ left eyelid, including canthus
173.12	SQUAMOUS CELL CARCINOMA EYELID INCLUDING CANTHUS	C44.121	Squamous cell carcinoma skin/ unsp eyelid, including canthus
		C44.122	Squamous cell carcinoma skin/ right eyelid, inc canthus
		C44.129	Squamous cell carcinoma skin/ left eyelid, including canthus
173.19	OTH SPEC MALIG NEOPLASM EYELID INCLUDING CANTHUS	C44.191	Oth malignant neoplasm skin/ unsp eyelid, including canthus
		C44.192	Oth malignant neoplasm skin/ right eyelid, including canthus
		C44.199	Oth malignant neoplasm skin/ left eyelid, including canthus
173.20	UNS MALIG NEOPLASM SKIN EAR EXT AUDITORY CANAL	C44.201	Unsp malig neoplasm skin/ unsp ear and external auric canal
		C44.202	Unsp malig neoplasm skin/ right ear and external auric canal
		C44.209	Unsp malig neoplasm skin/ left ear and external auric canal
173.21	BASAL CELL CARCINOMA SKIN EAR EXT AUDITORY CANAL	C44.211	Basal cell carcinoma skin/ unsp ear and external auric canal
		C44.212	Basal cell carcinoma skin/ r ear and external auric canal
		C44.219	Basal cell carcinoma skin/ left ear and external auric canal
173.22	SQUAMOUS CELL CARCINOMA SKIN EAR EXT AUD CANAL	C44.221	Squamous cell carcinoma skin/ unsp ear and extrn auric canal
		C44.222	Squamous cell carcinoma skin/ r ear and external auric canal
		C44.229	Squamous cell carcinoma skin/ left ear and extrn auric canal
173.29	OTH SPEC MALIG NEOPLASM SKIN EAR EXT AUD CANAL	C44.291	Oth malig neoplasm skin/ unsp ear and external auric canal
		C44.292	Oth malig neoplasm skin/ right ear and external auric canal
		C44.299	Oth malig neoplasm skin/ left ear and external auric canal
173.30	UNS MALIGNANT NEOPLASM SKIN OTHER UNS PARTS FACE	C44.300	Unsp malignant neoplasm of skin of unspecified part of face
		C44.301	Unspecified malignant neoplasm of skin of nose
		C44.309	Unsp malignant neoplasm of skin of other parts of face
173.31	BASAL CELL CARCINOMA SKIN OTHER & UNS PARTS FACE	C44.310	Basal cell carcinoma of skin of unspecified parts of face
		C44.311	Basal cell carcinoma of skin of nose
		C44.319	Basal cell carcinoma of skin of other parts of face
173.32	SQUAMOUS CELL CARCINOMA SKIN OTH UNS PARTS FACE	C44.320	Squamous cell carcinoma of skin of unspecified parts of face
		C44.321	Squamous cell carcinoma of skin of nose
		C44.329	Squamous cell carcinoma of skin of other parts of face
173.39	OTH SPEC MALIG NEOPLASM SKIN OTH UNS PARTS FACE	C44.390	Oth malignant neoplasm of skin of unspecified parts of face
		C44.391	Other specified malignant neoplasm of skin of nose
		C44.399	Oth malignant neoplasm of skin of other parts of face
173.40	UNSPECIFIED MALIGNANT NEOPLASM SCALP & SKIN NECK	C44.40	Unspecified malignant neoplasm of skin of scalp and neck
173.41	BASAL CELL CARCINOMA OF SCALP AND SKIN OF NECK	C44.41	Basal cell carcinoma of skin of scalp and neck
173.42	SQUAMOUS CELL CARCINOMA OF SCALP & SKIN OF NECK	C44.42	Squamous cell carcinoma of skin of scalp and neck
173.49	OTHER SPEC MALIGNANT NEOPLASM SCALP & SKIN NECK	C44.49	Other specified malignant neoplasm of skin of scalp and neck
173.50	UNS MALIGNANT NEOPLASM SKIN TRUNK EXCEPT SCROTUM	C44.500	Unspecified malignant neoplasm of anal skin
		C44.501	Unspecified malignant neoplasm of skin of breast
		C44.509	Unsp malignant neoplasm of skin of other part of trunk
173.51	BASAL CELL CARCINOMA SKIN TRUNK EXCEPT SCROTUM	C44.510	Basal cell carcinoma of anal skin
		C44.511	Basal cell carcinoma of skin of breast
		C44.519	Basal cell carcinoma of skin of other part of trunk
173.52	SQUAMOUS CELL CARCINOMA SKIN TRUNK EXCPT SCROTUM	C44.520	Squamous cell carcinoma of anal skin
		C44.521	Squamous cell carcinoma of skin of breast
		C44.529	Squamous cell carcinoma of skin of other part of trunk
173.59	OTH SPEC MALIG NEOPLASM SKIN TRUNK NO SCROTUM	C44.590	Other specified malignant neoplasm of anal skin
		C44.591	Other specified malignant neoplasm of skin of breast
		C44.599	Oth malignant neoplasm of skin of other part of trunk
173.60	UNS MALIG NEOPLASM SKIN UPPER LIMB INCL SHOULDER	C44.601	Unsp malignant neoplasm skin/ unsp upper limb, inc shoulder
		C44.602	Unsp malignant neoplasm skin/ right upper limb, inc shoulder
		C44.609	Unsp malignant neoplasm skin/ left upper limb, inc shoulder
173.61	BASAL CELL CARCINOMA SKIN UPPER LIMB INCL SHOULD	C44.611	Basal cell carcinoma skin/ unsp upper limb, inc shoulder
		C44.612	Basal cell carcinoma skin/ right upper limb, inc shoulder
		C44.619	Basal cell carcinoma skin/ left upper limb, inc shoulder
173.62	SQUAMOUS CELL CA SKIN UPPER LIMB INCL SHOULDER	C44.621	Squamous cell carcinoma skin/ unsp upper limb, inc shoulder
		C44.622	Squamous cell carcinoma skin/ right upper limb, inc shoulder
		C44.629	Squamous cell carcinoma skin/ left upper limb, inc shoulder
173.69	OTH SPEC MALIG NEOPLASM SKIN UP LIMB INCL SHLDR	C44.691	Oth malignant neoplasm skin/ unsp upper limb, inc shoulder
		C44.692	Oth malignant neoplasm skin/ right upper limb, inc shoulder
		C44.699	Oth malignant neoplasm skin/ left upper limb, inc shoulder
173.70	UNS MALIG NEOPLASM SKIN LOWER LIMB INCLUDING HIP	C44.701	Unsp malignant neoplasm skin/ unsp lower limb, including hip
		C44.702	Unsp malignant neoplasm skin/ right lower limb, inc hip
		C44.709	Unsp malignant neoplasm skin/ left lower limb, including hip
173.71	BASAL CELL CARCINOMA SKIN LOWER LIMB INCL HIP	C44.711	Basal cell carcinoma skin/ unsp lower limb, including hip
		C44.712	Basal cell carcinoma skin/ right lower limb, including hip
		C44.719	Basal cell carcinoma skin/ left lower limb, including hip
173.72	SQUAMOUS CELL CA SKIN LOWER LIMB INCLUDING HIP	C44.721	Squamous cell carcinoma skin/ unsp lower limb, including hip
		C44.722	Squamous cell carcinoma skin/ right lower limb, inc hip
		C44.729	Squamous cell carcinoma skin/ left lower limb, including hip

ICD-9-CM		ICD-10-CM	
173.79	OTH SPEC MALIG NEOPLASM SKIN LOWER LIMB INCL HIP	**C44.791**	Oth malignant neoplasm skin/ unsp lower limb, including hip
		C44.792	Oth malignant neoplasm skin/ right lower limb, including hip
		C44.799	Oth malignant neoplasm skin/ left lower limb, including hip
173.8Ø	UNS MALIGNANT NEOPLASM OTHER SPEC SITES SKIN	**C44.8Ø**	Unspecified malignant neoplasm of overlapping sites of skin
173.81	BASAL CELL CARCINOMA OTHER SPECIFIED SITES SKIN	**C44.81**	Basal cell carcinoma of overlapping sites of skin
173.82	SQUAMOUS CELL CARCINOMA OTHER SPEC SITES SKIN	**C44.82**	Squamous cell carcinoma of overlapping sites of skin
173.89	OTHER SPEC MALIG NEOPLASM OTHER SPEC SITES SKIN	**C44.89**	Oth malignant neoplasm of overlapping sites of skin
173.9Ø	UNS MALIGNANT NEOPLASM SKIN SITE UNSPECIFIED	**C44.9Ø**	Unspecified malignant neoplasm of skin, unspecified
173.91	BASAL CELL CARCINOMA OF SKIN SITE UNSPECIFIED	**C44.91**	Basal cell carcinoma of skin, unspecified
173.92	SQUAMOUS CELL CARCINOMA OF SKIN SITE UNSPECIFIED	**C44.92**	Squamous cell carcinoma of skin, unspecified
173.99	OTHER SPEC MALIGNANT NEOPLASM SKIN SITE UNS	**C44.99**	Other specified malignant neoplasm of skin, unspecified
174.Ø	MALIGNANT NEOPLASM NIPPLE&AREOLA FEMALE BREAST	**C5Ø.Ø11**	Malignant neoplasm of nipple and areola, right female breast
		C5Ø.Ø12	Malignant neoplasm of nipple and areola, left female breast
		C5Ø.Ø19	Malignant neoplasm of nipple and areola, unsp female breast
174.1	MALIGNANT NEOPLASM CENTRAL PORTION FEMALE BREAST	**C5Ø.111**	Malignant neoplasm of central portion of right female breast
		C5Ø.112	Malignant neoplasm of central portion of left female breast
		C5Ø.119	Malignant neoplasm of central portion of unsp female breast
174.2	MALIG NEOPLASM UPPER-INNER QUADRANT FE BREAST	**C5Ø.211**	Malig neoplm of upper-inner quadrant of right female breast
		C5Ø.212	Malig neoplasm of upper-inner quadrant of left female breast
		C5Ø.219	Malig neoplasm of upper-inner quadrant of unsp female breast
174.3	MALIG NEOPLASM LOWER-INNER QUADRANT FE BREAST	**C5Ø.311**	Malig neoplm of lower-inner quadrant of right female breast
		C5Ø.312	Malig neoplasm of lower-inner quadrant of left female breast
		C5Ø.319	Malig neoplasm of lower-inner quadrant of unsp female breast
174.4	MALIG NEOPLASM UPPER-OUTER QUADRANT FE BREAST	**C5Ø.411**	Malig neoplm of upper-outer quadrant of right female breast
		C5Ø.412	Malig neoplasm of upper-outer quadrant of left female breast
		C5Ø.419	Malig neoplasm of upper-outer quadrant of unsp female breast
174.5	MALIG NEOPLASM LOWER-OUTER QUADRANT FE BREAST	**C5Ø.511**	Malig neoplm of lower-outer quadrant of right female breast
		C5Ø.512	Malig neoplasm of lower-outer quadrant of left female breast
		C5Ø.519	Malig neoplasm of lower-outer quadrant of unsp female breast
174.6	MALIGNANT NEOPLASM AXILLARY TAIL FEMALE BREAST	**C5Ø.611**	Malignant neoplasm of axillary tail of right female breast
		C5Ø.612	Malignant neoplasm of axillary tail of left female breast
		C5Ø.619	Malignant neoplasm of axillary tail of unsp female breast
174.8	MALIG NEOPLASM OTHER SPEC SITES FEMALE BREAST	**C5Ø.811**	Malignant neoplasm of ovrlp sites of right female breast
		C5Ø.812	Malignant neoplasm of ovrlp sites of left female breast
		C5Ø.819	Malignant neoplasm of ovrlp sites of unsp female breast
174.9	MALIGNANT NEOPLASM OF BREAST UNSPECIFIED SITE	**C5Ø.911**	Malignant neoplasm of unsp site of right female breast
		C5Ø.912	Malignant neoplasm of unspecified site of left female breast
		C5Ø.919	Malignant neoplasm of unsp site of unspecified female breast
175.Ø	MALIGNANT NEOPLASM NIPPLE&AREOLA MALE BREAST	**C5Ø.Ø21**	Malignant neoplasm of nipple and areola, right male breast
		C5Ø.Ø22	Malignant neoplasm of nipple and areola, left male breast
		C5Ø.Ø29	Malignant neoplasm of nipple and areola, unsp male breast
175.9	MALIG NEOPLASM OTHER&UNSPEC SITES MALE BREAST	**C5Ø.121**	Malignant neoplasm of central portion of right male breast
		C5Ø.122	Malignant neoplasm of central portion of left male breast
		C5Ø.129	Malignant neoplasm of central portion of unsp male breast
		C5Ø.221	Malig neoplasm of upper-inner quadrant of right male breast
		C5Ø.222	Malig neoplasm of upper-inner quadrant of left male breast
		C5Ø.229	Malig neoplasm of upper-inner quadrant of unsp male breast
		C5Ø.321	Malig neoplasm of lower-inner quadrant of right male breast
		C5Ø.322	Malig neoplasm of lower-inner quadrant of left male breast
		C5Ø.329	Malig neoplasm of lower-inner quadrant of unsp male breast
		C5Ø.421	Malig neoplasm of upper-outer quadrant of right male breast
		C5Ø.422	Malig neoplasm of upper-outer quadrant of left male breast
		C5Ø.429	Malig neoplasm of upper-outer quadrant of unsp male breast
		C5Ø.521	Malig neoplasm of lower-outer quadrant of right male breast
		C5Ø.522	Malig neoplasm of lower-outer quadrant of left male breast
		C5Ø.529	Malig neoplasm of lower-outer quadrant of unsp male breast
		C5Ø.621	Malignant neoplasm of axillary tail of right male breast
		C5Ø.622	Malignant neoplasm of axillary tail of left male breast
		C5Ø.629	Malignant neoplasm of axillary tail of unsp male breast
		C5Ø.821	Malignant neoplasm of overlapping sites of right male breast
		C5Ø.822	Malignant neoplasm of overlapping sites of left male breast
		C5Ø.829	Malignant neoplasm of overlapping sites of unsp male breast
		C5Ø.921	Malignant neoplasm of unspecified site of right male breast
		C5Ø.922	Malignant neoplasm of unspecified site of left male breast
		C5Ø.929	Malignant neoplasm of unsp site of unspecified male breast
176.Ø	KAPOSIS SARCOMA OF SKIN	➡ **C46.Ø**	Kaposi's sarcoma of skin
176.1	KAPOSIS SARCOMA OF SOFT TISSUE	➡ **C46.1**	Kaposi's sarcoma of soft tissue
176.2	KAPOSIS SARCOMA OF PALATE	➡ **C46.2**	Kaposi's sarcoma of palate
176.3	KAPOSIS SARCOMA OF GASTROINTESTINAL SITES	➡ **C46.4**	Kaposi's sarcoma of gastrointestinal sites
176.4	KAPOSIS SARCOMA OF LUNG	**C46.5Ø**	Kaposi's sarcoma of unspecified lung
		C46.51	Kaposi's sarcoma of right lung
		C46.52	Kaposi's sarcoma of left lung
176.5	KAPOSIS SARCOMA OF LYMPH NODES	➡ **C46.3**	Kaposi's sarcoma of lymph nodes
176.8	KAPOSIS SARCOMA OF OTHER SPECIFIED SITES	➡ **C46.7**	Kaposi's sarcoma of other sites
176.9	KAPOSIS SARCOMA OF UNSPECIFIED SITE	➡ **C46.9**	Kaposi's sarcoma, unspecified
179	MALIGNANT NEOPLASM OF UTERUS PART UNSPECIFIED	➡ **C55**	Malignant neoplasm of uterus, part unspecified

ICD-9-CM			ICD-10-CM	
180.0	MALIGNANT NEOPLASM OF ENDOCERVIX	➡	C53.0	Malignant neoplasm of endocervix
180.1	MALIGNANT NEOPLASM OF EXOCERVIX	➡	C53.1	Malignant neoplasm of exocervix
180.8	MALIGNANT NEOPLASM OTHER SPECIFIED SITES CERVIX	➡	C53.8	Malignant neoplasm of overlapping sites of cervix uteri
180.9	MALIGNANT NEOPLASM CERVIX UTERI UNSPECIFIED SITE	➡	C53.9	Malignant neoplasm of cervix uteri, unspecified
181	MALIGNANT NEOPLASM OF PLACENTA	➡	C58	Malignant neoplasm of placenta
182.0	MALIGNANT NEOPLASM CORPUS UTERI EXCEPT ISTHMUS		C54.1	Malignant neoplasm of endometrium
			C54.2	Malignant neoplasm of myometrium
			C54.3	Malignant neoplasm of fundus uteri
			C54.9	Malignant neoplasm of corpus uteri, unspecified
182.1	MALIGNANT NEOPLASM OF ISTHMUS	➡	C54.0	Malignant neoplasm of isthmus uteri
182.8	MALIGNANT NEOPLASM OTHER SPEC SITES BODY UTERUS	➡	C54.8	Malignant neoplasm of overlapping sites of corpus uteri
183.0	MALIGNANT NEOPLASM OF OVARY		C56.1	Malignant neoplasm of right ovary
			C56.2	Malignant neoplasm of left ovary
			C56.9	Malignant neoplasm of unspecified ovary
183.2	MALIGNANT NEOPLASM OF FALLOPIAN TUBE		C57.00	Malignant neoplasm of unspecified fallopian tube
			C57.01	Malignant neoplasm of right fallopian tube
			C57.02	Malignant neoplasm of left fallopian tube
183.3	MALIGNANT NEOPLASM OF BROAD LIGAMENT OF UTERUS		C57.10	Malignant neoplasm of unspecified broad ligament
			C57.11	Malignant neoplasm of right broad ligament
			C57.12	Malignant neoplasm of left broad ligament
183.4	MALIGNANT NEOPLASM OF PARAMETRIUM OF UTERUS	➡	C57.3	Malignant neoplasm of parametrium
183.5	MALIGNANT NEOPLASM OF ROUND LIGAMENT OF UTERUS		C57.20	Malignant neoplasm of unspecified round ligament
			C57.21	Malignant neoplasm of right round ligament
			C57.22	Malignant neoplasm of left round ligament
183.8	MALIG NEOPLASM OTHER SPEC SITES UTERINE ADNEXA		C57.4	Malignant neoplasm of uterine adnexa, unspecified
183.9	MALIGNANT NEOPLASM UTERINE ADNEXA UNSPEC SITE		C57.4	Malignant neoplasm of uterine adnexa, unspecified
184.0	MALIGNANT NEOPLASM OF VAGINA	➡	C52	Malignant neoplasm of vagina
184.1	MALIGNANT NEOPLASM OF LABIA MAJORA	➡	C51.0	Malignant neoplasm of labium majus
184.2	MALIGNANT NEOPLASM OF LABIA MINORA	➡	C51.1	Malignant neoplasm of labium minus
184.3	MALIGNANT NEOPLASM OF CLITORIS	➡	C51.2	Malignant neoplasm of clitoris
184.4	MALIGNANT NEOPLASM OF VULVA UNSPECIFIED SITE	➡	C51.9	Malignant neoplasm of vulva, unspecified
184.8	MALIG NEOPLASM OTH SPEC SITES FE GENITAL ORGANS		C51.8	Malignant neoplasm of overlapping sites of vulva
			C57.7	Malignant neoplasm of other specified female genital organs
			C57.8	Malignant neoplasm of ovrlp sites of female genital organs
184.9	MALIG NEOPLASM FEMALE GENITAL ORGAN SITE UNSPEC	➡	C57.9	Malignant neoplasm of female genital organ, unspecified
185	MALIGNANT NEOPLASM OF PROSTATE	➡	C61	Malignant neoplasm of prostate
186.0	MALIGNANT NEOPLASM OF UNDESCENDED TESTIS		C62.00	Malignant neoplasm of unspecified undescended testis
			C62.01	Malignant neoplasm of undescended right testis
			C62.02	Malignant neoplasm of undescended left testis
186.9	MALIGNANT NEOPLASM OF OTHER&UNSPECIFIED TESTIS		C62.10	Malignant neoplasm of unspecified descended testis
			C62.11	Malignant neoplasm of descended right testis
			C62.12	Malignant neoplasm of descended left testis
			C62.90	Malig neoplasm of unsp testis, unsp descended or undescended
			C62.91	Malig neoplm of right testis, unsp descended or undescended
			C62.92	Malig neoplasm of left testis, unsp descended or undescended
187.1	MALIGNANT NEOPLASM OF PREPUCE	➡	C60.0	Malignant neoplasm of prepuce
187.2	MALIGNANT NEOPLASM OF GLANS PENIS	➡	C60.1	Malignant neoplasm of glans penis
187.3	MALIGNANT NEOPLASM OF BODY OF PENIS	➡	C60.2	Malignant neoplasm of body of penis
187.4	MALIGNANT NEOPLASM OF PENIS PART UNSPECIFIED	➡	C60.9	Malignant neoplasm of penis, unspecified
187.5	MALIGNANT NEOPLASM OF EPIDIDYMIS		C63.00	Malignant neoplasm of unspecified epididymis
			C63.01	Malignant neoplasm of right epididymis
			C63.02	Malignant neoplasm of left epididymis
187.6	MALIGNANT NEOPLASM OF SPERMATIC CORD		C63.10	Malignant neoplasm of unspecified spermatic cord
			C63.11	Malignant neoplasm of right spermatic cord
			C63.12	Malignant neoplasm of left spermatic cord
187.7	MALIGNANT NEOPLASM OF SCROTUM	➡	C63.2	Malignant neoplasm of scrotum
187.8	MALIG NEOPLASM OTH SPEC SITES MALE GENITAL ORGN		C60.8	Malignant neoplasm of overlapping sites of penis
			C63.7	Malignant neoplasm of other specified male genital organs
			C63.8	Malignant neoplasm of ovrlp sites of male genital organs
187.9	MALIG NEOPLASM MALE GENITAL ORGAN SITE UNSPEC	➡	C63.9	Malignant neoplasm of male genital organ, unspecified
188.0	MALIGNANT NEOPLASM OF TRIGONE OF URINARY BLADDER	➡	C67.0	Malignant neoplasm of trigone of bladder
188.1	MALIGNANT NEOPLASM OF DOME OF URINARY BLADDER	➡	C67.1	Malignant neoplasm of dome of bladder
188.2	MALIGNANT NEOPLASM LATERAL WALL URINARY BLADDER	➡	C67.2	Malignant neoplasm of lateral wall of bladder
188.3	MALIGNANT NEOPLASM ANTERIOR WALL URINARY BLADDER	➡	C67.3	Malignant neoplasm of anterior wall of bladder
188.4	MALIG NEOPLASM POSTERIOR WALL URINARY BLADDER	➡	C67.4	Malignant neoplasm of posterior wall of bladder
188.5	MALIGNANT NEOPLASM OF BLADDER NECK	➡	C67.5	Malignant neoplasm of bladder neck
188.6	MALIGNANT NEOPLASM OF URETERIC ORIFICE	➡	C67.6	Malignant neoplasm of ureteric orifice
188.7	MALIGNANT NEOPLASM OF URACHUS	➡	C67.7	Malignant neoplasm of urachus
188.8	MALIGNANT NEOPLASM OTHER SPECIFIED SITES BLADDER	➡	C67.8	Malignant neoplasm of overlapping sites of bladder
188.9	MALIGNANT NEOPLASM OF BLADDER PART UNSPECIFIED	➡	C67.9	Malignant neoplasm of bladder, unspecified

ICD-9-CM			ICD-10-CM	
189.Ø	MALIGNANT NEOPLASM OF KIDNEY EXCEPT PELVIS		**C64.1**	Malignant neoplasm of right kidney, except renal pelvis
			C64.2	Malignant neoplasm of left kidney, except renal pelvis
			C64.9	Malignant neoplasm of unsp kidney, except renal pelvis
189.1	MALIGNANT NEOPLASM OF RENAL PELVIS		**C65.1**	Malignant neoplasm of right renal pelvis
			C65.2	Malignant neoplasm of left renal pelvis
			C65.9	Malignant neoplasm of unspecified renal pelvis
189.2	MALIGNANT NEOPLASM OF URETER		**C66.1**	Malignant neoplasm of right ureter
			C66.2	Malignant neoplasm of left ureter
			C66.9	Malignant neoplasm of unspecified ureter
189.3	MALIGNANT NEOPLASM OF URETHRA	➡	**C68.Ø**	Malignant neoplasm of urethra
189.4	MALIGNANT NEOPLASM OF PARAURETHRAL GLANDS	➡	**C68.1**	Malignant neoplasm of paraurethral glands
189.8	MALIG NEOPLASM OTHER SPEC SITES URINARY ORGANS	➡	**C68.8**	Malignant neoplasm of overlapping sites of urinary organs
189.9	MALIGNANT NEOPLASM URINARY ORGAN SITE UNSPEC	➡	**C68.9**	Malignant neoplasm of urinary organ, unspecified
19Ø.Ø	MAL NEO EYEBALL NO CONJUNCT CORN RETINA&CHOROID		**C69.4Ø**	Malignant neoplasm of unspecified ciliary body
			C69.41	Malignant neoplasm of right ciliary body
			C69.42	Malignant neoplasm of left ciliary body
19Ø.1	MALIGNANT NEOPLASM OF ORBIT		**C69.6Ø**	Malignant neoplasm of unspecified orbit
			C69.61	Malignant neoplasm of right orbit
			C69.62	Malignant neoplasm of left orbit
19Ø.2	MALIGNANT NEOPLASM OF LACRIMAL GLAND		**C69.5Ø**	Malignant neoplasm of unspecified lacrimal gland and duct
			C69.51	Malignant neoplasm of right lacrimal gland and duct
			C69.52	Malignant neoplasm of left lacrimal gland and duct
19Ø.3	MALIGNANT NEOPLASM OF CONJUNCTIVA		**C69.ØØ**	Malignant neoplasm of unspecified conjunctiva
			C69.Ø1	Malignant neoplasm of right conjunctiva
			C69.Ø2	Malignant neoplasm of left conjunctiva
19Ø.4	MALIGNANT NEOPLASM OF CORNEA		**C69.1Ø**	Malignant neoplasm of unspecified cornea
			C69.11	Malignant neoplasm of right cornea
			C69.12	Malignant neoplasm of left cornea
19Ø.5	MALIGNANT NEOPLASM OF RETINA		**C69.2Ø**	Malignant neoplasm of unspecified retina
			C69.21	Malignant neoplasm of right retina
			C69.22	Malignant neoplasm of left retina
19Ø.6	MALIGNANT NEOPLASM OF CHOROID		**C69.3Ø**	Malignant neoplasm of unspecified choroid
			C69.31	Malignant neoplasm of right choroid
			C69.32	Malignant neoplasm of left choroid
19Ø.7	MALIGNANT NEOPLASM OF LACRIMAL DUCT		**C69.5Ø**	Malignant neoplasm of unspecified lacrimal gland and duct
			C69.51	Malignant neoplasm of right lacrimal gland and duct
			C69.52	Malignant neoplasm of left lacrimal gland and duct
19Ø.8	MALIGNANT NEOPLASM OTHER SPECIFIED SITES EYE		**C69.8Ø**	Malignant neoplasm of ovrlp sites of unsp eye and adnexa
			C69.81	Malignant neoplasm of ovrlp sites of right eye and adnexa
			C69.82	Malignant neoplasm of ovrlp sites of left eye and adnexa
19Ø.9	MALIGNANT NEOPLASM OF EYE PART UNSPECIFIED		**C69.9Ø**	Malignant neoplasm of unspecified site of unspecified eye
			C69.91	Malignant neoplasm of unspecified site of right eye
			C69.92	Malignant neoplasm of unspecified site of left eye
191.Ø	MALIG NEOPLASM CEREBRUM EXCEPT LOBES&VENTRICLES	➡	**C71.Ø**	Malignant neoplasm of cerebrum, except lobes and ventricles
191.1	MALIGNANT NEOPLASM OF FRONTAL LOBE OF BRAIN	➡	**C71.1**	Malignant neoplasm of frontal lobe
191.2	MALIGNANT NEOPLASM OF TEMPORAL LOBE OF BRAIN	➡	**C71.2**	Malignant neoplasm of temporal lobe
191.3	MALIGNANT NEOPLASM OF PARIETAL LOBE OF BRAIN	➡	**C71.3**	Malignant neoplasm of parietal lobe
191.4	MALIGNANT NEOPLASM OF OCCIPITAL LOBE OF BRAIN	➡	**C71.4**	Malignant neoplasm of occipital lobe
191.5	MALIGNANT NEOPLASM OF VENTRICLES OF BRAIN	➡	**C71.5**	Malignant neoplasm of cerebral ventricle
191.6	MALIGNANT NEOPLASM OF CEREBELLUM NOS	➡	**C71.6**	Malignant neoplasm of cerebellum
191.7	MALIGNANT NEOPLASM OF BRAIN STEM	➡	**C71.7**	Malignant neoplasm of brain stem
191.8	MALIGNANT NEOPLASM OF OTHER PARTS OF BRAIN	➡	**C71.8**	Malignant neoplasm of overlapping sites of brain
191.9	MALIGNANT NEOPLASM OF BRAIN UNSPECIFIED SITE	➡	**C71.9**	Malignant neoplasm of brain, unspecified
192.Ø	MALIGNANT NEOPLASM OF CRANIAL NERVES		**C72.2Ø**	Malignant neoplasm of unspecified olfactory nerve
			C72.21	Malignant neoplasm of right olfactory nerve
			C72.22	Malignant neoplasm of left olfactory nerve
			C72.3Ø	Malignant neoplasm of unspecified optic nerve
			C72.31	Malignant neoplasm of right optic nerve
			C72.32	Malignant neoplasm of left optic nerve
			C72.4Ø	Malignant neoplasm of unspecified acoustic nerve
			C72.41	Malignant neoplasm of right acoustic nerve
			C72.42	Malignant neoplasm of left acoustic nerve
			C72.5Ø	Malignant neoplasm of unspecified cranial nerve
			C72.59	Malignant neoplasm of other cranial nerves
192.1	MALIGNANT NEOPLASM OF CEREBRAL MENINGES		**C7Ø.Ø**	Malignant neoplasm of cerebral meninges
			C7Ø.9	Malignant neoplasm of meninges, unspecified
192.2	MALIGNANT NEOPLASM OF SPINAL CORD		**C72.Ø**	Malignant neoplasm of spinal cord
			C72.1	Malignant neoplasm of cauda equina
192.3	MALIGNANT NEOPLASM OF SPINAL MENINGES	➡	**C7Ø.1**	Malignant neoplasm of spinal meninges
192.8	MALIG NEOPLASM OTHER SPEC SITES NERVOUS SYSTEM		**C72.9**	Malignant neoplasm of central nervous system, unspecified
192.9	MALIGNANT NEOPLASM NERVOUS SYSTEM PART UNSPEC		**C72.9**	Malignant neoplasm of central nervous system, unspecified
193	MALIGNANT NEOPLASM OF THYROID GLAND	➡	**C73**	Malignant neoplasm of thyroid gland

ICD-9-CM			ICD-10-CM	
194.Ø	MALIGNANT NEOPLASM OF ADRENAL GLAND		**C74.ØØ** **C74.Ø1** **C74.Ø2** **C74.1Ø** **C74.11** **C74.12** **C74.9Ø** **C74.91** **C74.92**	Malignant neoplasm of cortex of unspecified adrenal gland Malignant neoplasm of cortex of right adrenal gland Malignant neoplasm of cortex of left adrenal gland Malignant neoplasm of medulla of unspecified adrenal gland Malignant neoplasm of medulla of right adrenal gland Malignant neoplasm of medulla of left adrenal gland Malignant neoplasm of unsp part of unspecified adrenal gland Malignant neoplasm of unsp part of right adrenal gland Malignant neoplasm of unspecified part of left adrenal gland
194.1	MALIGNANT NEOPLASM OF PARATHYROID GLAND	➡	**C75.Ø**	Malignant neoplasm of parathyroid gland
194.3	MAL NEO PITUITARY GLAND&CRANIOPHARYNGEAL DUCT		**C75.1** **C75.2**	Malignant neoplasm of pituitary gland Malignant neoplasm of craniopharyngeal duct
194.4	MALIGNANT NEOPLASM OF PINEAL GLAND	➡	**C75.3**	Malignant neoplasm of pineal gland
194.5	MALIGNANT NEOPLASM OF CAROTID BODY	➡	**C75.4**	Malignant neoplasm of carotid body
194.6	MALIGNANT NEOPLASM AORTIC BODY&OTHER PARAGANGLIA	➡	**C75.5**	Malignant neoplasm of aortic body and other paraganglia
194.8	MALIG NEOPLASM OTH ENDOCRN GLANDS&RELATED STRCT	➡	**C75.8**	Malignant neoplasm with pluriglandular involvement, unsp
194.9	MALIGNANT NEOPLASM ENDOCRINE GLAND SITE UNSPEC	➡	**C75.9**	Malignant neoplasm of endocrine gland, unspecified
195.Ø	MALIGNANT NEOPLASM OF HEAD FACE AND NECK	➡	**C76.Ø**	Malignant neoplasm of head, face and neck
195.1	MALIGNANT NEOPLASM OF THORAX	➡	**C76.1**	Malignant neoplasm of thorax
195.2	MALIGNANT NEOPLASM OF ABDOMEN	➡	**C76.2**	Malignant neoplasm of abdomen
195.3	MALIGNANT NEOPLASM OF PELVIS	➡	**C76.3**	Malignant neoplasm of pelvis
195.4	MALIGNANT NEOPLASM OF UPPER LIMB		**C76.4Ø** **C76.41** **C76.42**	Malignant neoplasm of unspecified upper limb Malignant neoplasm of right upper limb Malignant neoplasm of left upper limb
195.5	MALIGNANT NEOPLASM OF LOWER LIMB		**C76.5Ø** **C76.51** **C76.52**	Malignant neoplasm of unspecified lower limb Malignant neoplasm of right lower limb Malignant neoplasm of left lower limb
195.8	MALIGNANT NEOPLASM OF OTHER SPECIFIED SITES		**C45.7** **C76.8**	Mesothelioma of other sites Malignant neoplasm of other specified ill-defined sites
196.Ø	SEC&UNSPEC MALIG NEOPLASM NODES HEAD FACE&NECK	➡	**C77.Ø**	Sec and unsp malig neoplasm of nodes of head, face and neck
196.1	SEC&UNSPEC MALIG NEOPLASM INTRATHORACIC NODES	➡	**C77.1**	Secondary and unsp malignant neoplasm of intrathorac nodes
196.2	SEC&UNSPEC MALIG NEOPLASM INTRA-ABD LYMPH NODES	➡	**C77.2**	Secondary and unsp malignant neoplasm of intra-abd nodes
196.3	SEC&UNSPEC MALIG NEOPLASM NODES AX&UPPER LIMB	➡	**C77.3**	Sec and unsp malig neoplasm of axilla and upper limb nodes
196.5	SEC&UNSPEC MALIG NEOPLSM NODES ING RGN&LOW LIMB	➡	**C77.4**	Sec and unsp malig neoplasm of inguinal and lower limb nodes
196.6	SEC&UNSPEC MALIG NEOPLASM INTRAPELVIC NODES	➡	**C77.5**	Secondary and unsp malignant neoplasm of intrapelv nodes
196.8	SEC&UNSPEC MALIG NEOPLASM NODES MULTIPLE SITES	➡	**C77.8**	Sec and unsp malig neoplasm of nodes of multiple regions
196.9	SEC&UNSPEC MALIG NEOPLASM NODES SITE UNSPEC	➡	**C77.9**	Secondary and unsp malignant neoplasm of lymph node, unsp
197.Ø	SECONDARY MALIGNANT NEOPLASM OF LUNG		**C78.ØØ** **C78.Ø1** **C78.Ø2**	Secondary malignant neoplasm of unspecified lung Secondary malignant neoplasm of right lung Secondary malignant neoplasm of left lung
197.1	SECONDARY MALIGNANT NEOPLASM OF MEDIASTINUM	➡	**C78.1**	Secondary malignant neoplasm of mediastinum
197.2	SECONDARY MALIGNANT NEOPLASM OF PLEURA	➡	**C78.2**	Secondary malignant neoplasm of pleura
197.3	SEC MALIGNANT NEOPLASM OTHER RESPIRATORY ORGANS		**C78.3Ø** **C78.39**	Secondary malignant neoplasm of unsp respiratory organ Secondary malignant neoplasm of other respiratory organs
197.4	SEC MALIG NEOPLASM SMALL INTESTINE INCL DUODENUM	➡	**C78.4**	Secondary malignant neoplasm of small intestine
197.5	SEC MALIGNANT NEOPLASM OF LARGE INTESTINE&RECTUM	➡	**C78.5**	Secondary malignant neoplasm of large intestine and rectum
197.6	SEC MALIG NEOPLASM RETROPERITONEUM&PERITONEUM	➡	**C78.6**	Secondary malignant neoplasm of retroperiton and peritoneum
197.7	SECONDARY MALIGNANT NEOPLASM OF LIVER		**C78.7**	Secondary malig neoplasm of liver and intrahepatic bile duct
197.8	SEC MALIG NEOPLASM OTHER DIGESTIVE ORGANS&SPLEEN		**C78.7** **C78.8Ø** **C78.89**	Secondary malig neoplasm of liver and intrahepatic bile duct Secondary malignant neoplasm of unspecified digestive organ Secondary malignant neoplasm of other digestive organs
198.Ø	SECONDARY MALIGNANT NEOPLASM OF KIDNEY		**C79.ØØ** **C79.Ø1** **C79.Ø2**	Secondary malignant neoplasm of unsp kidney and renal pelvis Secondary malignant neoplasm of r kidney and renal pelvis Secondary malignant neoplasm of left kidney and renal pelvis
198.1	SEC MALIGNANT NEOPLASM OF OTHER URINARY ORGANS		**C79.1Ø** **C79.11** **C79.19**	Secondary malignant neoplasm of unspecified urinary organs Secondary malignant neoplasm of bladder Secondary malignant neoplasm of other urinary organs
198.2	SECONDARY MALIGNANT NEOPLASM OF SKIN	➡	**C79.2**	Secondary malignant neoplasm of skin
198.3	SEC MALIGNANT NEOPLASM OF BRAIN AND SPINAL CORD		**C79.31**	Secondary malignant neoplasm of brain
198.4	SEC MALIG NEOPLASM OTHER PARTS NERVOUS SYSTEM		**C79.32** **C79.4Ø** **C79.49**	Secondary malignant neoplasm of cerebral meninges Secondary malignant neoplasm of unsp part of nervous system Secondary malignant neoplasm of oth parts of nervous system
198.5	SEC MALIGNANT NEOPLASM OF BONE AND BONE MARROW		**C79.51** **C79.52**	Secondary malignant neoplasm of bone Secondary malignant neoplasm of bone marrow
198.6	SECONDARY MALIGNANT NEOPLASM OF OVARY		**C79.6Ø** **C79.61** **C79.62**	Secondary malignant neoplasm of unspecified ovary Secondary malignant neoplasm of right ovary Secondary malignant neoplasm of left ovary
198.7	SECONDARY MALIGNANT NEOPLASM OF ADRENAL GLAND		**C79.7Ø** **C79.71** **C79.72**	Secondary malignant neoplasm of unspecified adrenal gland Secondary malignant neoplasm of right adrenal gland Secondary malignant neoplasm of left adrenal gland
198.81	SECONDARY MALIGNANT NEOPLASM OF BREAST	➡	**C79.81**	Secondary malignant neoplasm of breast
198.82	SECONDARY MALIGNANT NEOPLASM OF GENITAL ORGANS	➡	**C79.82**	Secondary malignant neoplasm of genital organs

ICD-9-CM			ICD-10-CM	
198.89	SEC MALIGNANT NEOPLASM OF OTHER SPECIFIED SITES		**C79.89**	Secondary malignant neoplasm of other specified sites
			C79.9	Secondary malignant neoplasm of unspecified site
199.Ø	DISSEMINATED MALIGNANT NEOPLASM	➡	**C8Ø.Ø**	Disseminated malignant neoplasm, unspecified
199.1	OTHER MALIGNANT NEOPLASM OF UNSPECIFIED SITE		**C45.9**	Mesothelioma, unspecified
			C8Ø.1	Malignant (primary) neoplasm, unspecified
199.2	MALIGNANT NEOPLASM ASSOC W/TRANSPLANTED ORGAN	➡	**C8Ø.2**	Malignant neoplasm associated with transplanted organ
2ØØ.ØØ	RETICULOSARCOMA UNSPEC SITE XTRANOD&SOLID ORGN		**C83.3Ø**	Diffuse large B-cell lymphoma, unspecified site
			C83.39	Diffuse large B-cell lymphoma, extrnod and solid organ sites
2ØØ.Ø1	RETICULOSARCOMA OF LYMPH NODES OF HEAD FACE&NECK		**C83.31**	Diffuse large B-cell lymphoma, nodes of head, face, and neck
2ØØ.Ø2	RETICULOSARCOMA OF INTRATHORACIC LYMPH NODES		**C83.32**	Diffuse large B-cell lymphoma, intrathoracic lymph nodes
2ØØ.Ø3	RETICULOSARCOMA OF INTRA-ABDOMINAL LYMPH NODES		**C83.33**	Diffuse large B-cell lymphoma, intra-abdominal lymph nodes
2ØØ.Ø4	RETICULOSARCOMA LYMPH NODES AXILLA&UPPER LIMB		**C83.34**	Diffuse large B-cell lymph, nodes of axilla and upper limb
2ØØ.Ø5	RETICULOSARCOMA NODES ING REGION&LOWER LIMB		**C83.35**	Diffus large B-cell lymph, nodes of ing rgn and lower limb
2ØØ.Ø6	RETICULOSARCOMA OF INTRAPELVIC LYMPH NODES		**C83.36**	Diffuse large B-cell lymphoma, intrapelvic lymph nodes
2ØØ.Ø7	RETICULOSARCOMA OF SPLEEN		**C83.37**	Diffuse large B-cell lymphoma, spleen
2ØØ.Ø8	RETICULOSARCOMA OF LYMPH NODES OF MULTIPLE SITES		**C83.38**	Diffuse large B-cell lymphoma, lymph nodes of multiple sites
2ØØ.1Ø	LYMPHOSARCOMA UNSPEC SITE EXTRANODAL&SOLID ORGN		**C83.5Ø**	Lymphoblastic (diffuse) lymphoma, unspecified site
			C83.59	Lymphoblastic lymphoma, extrnod and solid organ sites
2ØØ.11	LYMPHOSARCOMA OF LYMPH NODES OF HEAD FACE&NECK		**C83.51**	Lymphoblastic lymphoma, nodes of head, face, and neck
2ØØ.12	LYMPHOSARCOMA OF INTRATHORACIC LYMPH NODES		**C83.52**	Lymphoblastic (diffuse) lymphoma, intrathoracic lymph nodes
2ØØ.13	LYMPHOSARCOMA OF INTRA-ABDOMINAL LYMPH NODES		**C83.53**	Lymphoblastic (diffuse) lymphoma, intra-abd lymph nodes
2ØØ.14	LYMPHOSARCOMA LYMPH NODES AXILLA&UPPER LIMB		**C83.54**	Lymphoblastic lymphoma, nodes of axilla and upper limb
2ØØ.15	LYMPHOSARCOMA LYMPH NODES ING REGION&LOWER LIMB		**C83.55**	Lymphoblastic lymphoma, nodes of ing region and lower limb
2ØØ.16	LYMPHOSARCOMA OF INTRAPELVIC LYMPH NODES		**C83.56**	Lymphoblastic (diffuse) lymphoma, intrapelvic lymph nodes
2ØØ.17	LYMPHOSARCOMA OF SPLEEN		**C83.57**	Lymphoblastic (diffuse) lymphoma, spleen
2ØØ.18	LYMPHOSARCOMA OF LYMPH NODES OF MULTIPLE SITES		**C83.58**	Lymphoblastic (diffuse) lymphoma, lymph nodes mult site
2ØØ.2Ø	BURKITTS TUMR/LYMPHOM UNS SITE XTRANOD&SOLID ORG		**C83.7Ø**	Burkitt lymphoma, unspecified site
			C83.79	Burkitt lymphoma, extranodal and solid organ sites
2ØØ.21	BURKITTS TUMOR/LYMPHOMA NODES HEAD FACE&NECK	➡	**C83.71**	Burkitt lymphoma, lymph nodes of head, face, and neck
2ØØ.22	BURKITTS TUMOR/LYMPHOMA INTRATHORACIC NODES	➡	**C83.72**	Burkitt lymphoma, intrathoracic lymph nodes
2ØØ.23	BURKITTS TUMOR/LYMPHOMA INTRA-ABD LYMPH NODES	➡	**C83.73**	Burkitt lymphoma, intra-abdominal lymph nodes
2ØØ.24	BURKITTS TUMOR/LYMPHOMA NODES AXILLA&UPPER LIMB	➡	**C83.74**	Burkitt lymphoma, lymph nodes of axilla and upper limb
2ØØ.25	BURKITTS TUMR/LYMPHOMA NODES ING REGION&LOW LIMB	➡	**C83.75**	Burkitt lymphoma, nodes of inguinal region and lower limb
2ØØ.26	BURKITTS TUMOR/LYMPHOMA INTRAPELVIC LYMPH NODES	➡	**C83.76**	Burkitt lymphoma, intrapelvic lymph nodes
2ØØ.27	BURKITTS TUMOR OR LYMPHOMA OF SPLEEN	➡	**C83.77**	Burkitt lymphoma, spleen
2ØØ.28	BURKITTS TUMOR/LYMPHOMA NODES MULTIPLE SITES	➡	**C83.78**	Burkitt lymphoma, lymph nodes of multiple sites
2ØØ.3Ø	MZ LYMPHOMA UNS SITE EXTRANODAL&SOLID ORGAN SITE		**C83.8Ø**	Other non-follicular lymphoma, unspecified site
			C83.89	Oth non-follic lymphoma, extranodal and solid organ sites
			C88.4	Extrnod mrgnl zn B-cell lymph of mucosa-assoc lymphoid tiss
2ØØ.31	MARGINAL ZONE LYMPHOMA LYMPH NODES HEAD FACE&NCK		**C83.81**	Oth non-follic lymphoma, lymph nodes of head, face, and neck
2ØØ.32	MARGINAL ZONE LYMPHOMA INTRATHORACIC LYMPH NODES		**C83.82**	Other non-follicular lymphoma, intrathoracic lymph nodes
2ØØ.33	MARGINAL ZONE LYMPHOMA INTRA-ABDOMINAL NODES		**C83.83**	Other non-follicular lymphoma, intra-abdominal lymph nodes
2ØØ.34	MARGINAL ZONE LYMPHOMA NODES AXILLA&UPPER LIMB		**C83.84**	Oth non-follic lymphoma, nodes of axilla and upper limb
2ØØ.35	MARGINAL ZONE LYMPHOMA NODES ING REGION&LOW LIMB		**C83.85**	Oth non-follic lymphoma, nodes of ing region and lower limb
2ØØ.36	MARGINAL ZONE LYMPHOMA INTRAPELVIC LYMPH NODES		**C83.86**	Other non-follicular lymphoma, intrapelvic lymph nodes
2ØØ.37	MARGINAL ZONE LYMPHOMA SPLEEN		**C83.87**	Other non-follicular lymphoma, spleen
2ØØ.38	MARGINAL ZONE LYMPHOMA LYMPH NODES MULTI SITES		**C83.88**	Other non-follicular lymphoma, lymph nodes of multiple sites
2ØØ.4Ø	MCL UNS SITE EXTRANODAL&SOLID ORGAN SITE		**C83.1Ø**	Mantle cell lymphoma, unspecified site
			C83.19	Mantle cell lymphoma, extranodal and solid organ sites
2ØØ.41	MANTLE CELL LYMPHOMA LYMPH NODES HEAD FACE&NECK	➡	**C83.11**	Mantle cell lymphoma, lymph nodes of head, face, and neck
2ØØ.42	MANTLE CELL LYMPHOMA INTRATHORACIC LYMPH NODES	➡	**C83.12**	Mantle cell lymphoma, intrathoracic lymph nodes
2ØØ.43	MANTLE CELL LYMPHOMA INTRA-ABDOMINAL LYMPH NODES	➡	**C83.13**	Mantle cell lymphoma, intra-abdominal lymph nodes
2ØØ.44	MANTLE CELL LYMPHOMA NODES AXILLA&UPPER LIMB	➡	**C83.14**	Mantle cell lymphoma, lymph nodes of axilla and upper limb
2ØØ.45	MANTLE CELL LYMPHOMA NODES ING REGION&LOWER LIMB	➡	**C83.15**	Mantle cell lymphoma, nodes of ing region and lower limb
2ØØ.46	MANTLE CELL LYMPHOMA INTRAPELVIC LYMPH NODES	➡	**C83.16**	Mantle cell lymphoma, intrapelvic lymph nodes
2ØØ.47	MANTLE CELL LYMPHOMA SPLEEN	➡	**C83.17**	Mantle cell lymphoma, spleen
2ØØ.48	MANTLE CELL LYMPHOMA LYMPH NODES MULTIPLE SITES	➡	**C83.18**	Mantle cell lymphoma, lymph nodes of multiple sites
2ØØ.5Ø	PRIM CNS LYMPHOMA UNS SITE EXTRANODL&SOLID ORGAN		**C83.39**	Diffuse large B-cell lymphoma, extrnod and solid organ sites
			C83.8Ø	Other non-follicular lymphoma, unspecified site
			C83.89	Oth non-follic lymphoma, extranodal and solid organ sites
2ØØ.51	PRIMARY CNS LYMPHOMA LYMPH NODES HEAD FACE&NECK		**C83.31**	Diffuse large B-cell lymphoma, nodes of head, face, and neck
			C83.81	Oth non-follic lymphoma, lymph nodes of head, face, and neck
2ØØ.52	PRIMARY CNS LYMPHOMA INTRATHORACIC LYMPH NODES		**C83.32**	Diffuse large B-cell lymphoma, intrathoracic lymph nodes
			C83.82	Other non-follicular lymphoma, intrathoracic lymph nodes
2ØØ.53	PRIMARY CNS LYMPHOMA INTRA-ABDOMINAL LYMPH NODES		**C83.33**	Diffuse large B-cell lymphoma, intra-abdominal lymph nodes
			C83.83	Other non-follicular lymphoma, intra-abdominal lymph nodes
2ØØ.54	PRIMARY CNS LYMPHOMA NODES AXILLA&UPPER LIMB		**C83.34**	Diffuse large B-cell lymph, nodes of axilla and upper limb
			C83.84	Oth non-follic lymphoma, nodes of axilla and upper limb

ICD-9-CM		ICD-10-CM	
200.55	PRIMARY CNS LYMPHOMA NODES INGUINAL&LOWER LIMB	**C83.35** **C83.85**	Diffus large B-cell lymph, nodes of ing rgn and lower limb Oth non-follic lymphoma, nodes of ing region and lower limb
200.56	PRIMARY CNS LYMPHOMA INTRAPELVIC LYMPH NODES	**C83.36** **C83.86**	Diffuse large B-cell lymphoma, intrapelvic lymph nodes Other non-follicular lymphoma, intrapelvic lymph nodes
200.57	PRIMARY CENTRAL NERVOUS SYSTEM LYMPHOMA SPLEEN	**C83.37** **C83.87**	Diffuse large B-cell lymphoma, spleen Other non-follicular lymphoma, spleen
200.58	PRIMARY CNS LYMPHOMA LYMPH NODES MULTIPLE SITES	**C83.38** **C83.88**	Diffuse large B-cell lymphoma, lymph nodes of multiple sites Other non-follicular lymphoma, lymph nodes of multiple sites
200.60	ALC LYMPHOMA UNS SITE EXTRANODAL&SOLID ORGAN	**C84.60** **C84.69** **C84.70** **C84.79**	Anaplastic large cell lymphoma, ALK-positive, unsp site Anaplstc lg cell lymph, ALK-pos, extrnod and solid org sites Anaplastic large cell lymphoma, ALK-negative, unsp site Anaplstc lg cell lymph, ALK-neg, extrnod and solid org sites
200.61	ANAPLASTIC LRG CELL LYMPHOMA NODES HEAD FACE&NCK	**C84.61** **C84.71**	Anaplstc lg cell lymph, ALK-pos, nodes of head, face, and nk Anaplstc lg cell lymph, ALK-neg, nodes of head, face, and nk
200.62	ANAPLASTIC LRG CELL LYMPHOMA INTRATHORACIC NODES	**C84.62** **C84.72**	Anaplastic large cell lymphoma, ALK-pos, intrathorac nodes Anaplastic large cell lymphoma, ALK-neg, intrathorac nodes
200.63	ANAPLASTIC LRG CELL LYMPHOMA INTRA-ABD NODES	**C84.63** **C84.73**	Anaplastic large cell lymphoma, ALK-pos, intra-abd nodes Anaplastic large cell lymphoma, ALK-neg, intra-abd nodes
200.64	ANAPLASTIC LRG CELL LYMPHOMA AXILLA&UPPER LIMB	**C84.64** **C84.74**	Anaplstc lg cell lymph, ALK-pos, nodes of axla and upr limb Anaplstc lg cell lymph, ALK-neg, nodes of axla and upr limb
200.65	ANAPLASTIC LRG CELL LYMPHOMA NODES ING&LOW LIMB	**C84.65** **C84.75**	Anaplstc lg cell lymph, ALK-pos, nodes of ing rgn & low lmb Anaplstc lg cell lymph, ALK-neg, nodes of ing rgn & low lmb
200.66	ANAPLASTIC LARGE CELL LYMPHOMA INTRAPELVIC NODES	**C84.66** **C84.76**	Anaplastic large cell lymphoma, ALK-pos, intrapelv nodes Anaplastic large cell lymphoma, ALK-neg, intrapelv nodes
200.67	ANAPLASTIC LARGE CELL LYMPHOMA SPLEEN	**C84.67** **C84.77**	Anaplastic large cell lymphoma, ALK-positive, spleen Anaplastic large cell lymphoma, ALK-negative, spleen
200.68	ANAPLASTIC LRG CELL LYMPHOMA NODES MULTIPLE SITE	**C84.68** **C84.78**	Anaplastic large cell lymphoma, ALK-pos, nodes mult site Anaplastic large cell lymphoma, ALK-neg, nodes mult site
200.70	LARGE CELL LYMPHOMA UNS SITE EXTRANODL&SOLID ORG	**C83.39** **C85.20** **C85.29**	Diffuse large B-cell lymphoma, extrnod and solid organ sites Mediastinal (thymic) large B-cell lymphoma, unspecified site Mediastnl large B-cell lymph, extrnod and solid organ sites
200.71	LARGE CELL LYMPHOMA LYMPH NODES HEAD FACE&NECK	**C83.31** **C85.21**	Diffuse large B-cell lymphoma, nodes of head, face, and neck Mediastnl large B-cell lymph, nodes of head, face, and neck
200.72	LARGE CELL LYMPHOMA INTRATHORACIC LYMPH NODES	**C83.32** **C85.22**	Diffuse large B-cell lymphoma, intrathoracic lymph nodes Mediastnl (thymic) large B-cell lymphoma, intrathorac nodes
200.73	LARGE CELL LYMPHOMA INTRA-ABDOMINAL LYMPH NODES	**C83.33** **C85.23**	Diffuse large B-cell lymphoma, intra-abdominal lymph nodes Mediastinal (thymic) large B-cell lymphoma, intra-abd nodes
200.74	LARGE CELL LYMPHOMA NODES AXILLA&UPPER LIMB	**C83.34** **C85.24**	Diffuse large B-cell lymph, nodes of axilla and upper limb Mediastnl large B-cell lymph, nodes of axilla and upper limb
200.75	LARGE CELL LYMPHOMA NODES INGUINAL&LOWER LIMB	**C83.35** **C85.25**	Diffus large B-cell lymph, nodes of ing rgn and lower limb Mediastnl lg B-cell lymph, nodes of ing rgn and lower limb
200.76	LARGE CELL LYMPHOMA INTRAPELVIC LYMPH NODES	**C83.36** **C85.26**	Diffuse large B-cell lymphoma, intrapelvic lymph nodes Mediastinal (thymic) large B-cell lymphoma, intrapelv nodes
200.77	LARGE CELL LYMPHOMA SPLEEN	**C83.37** **C85.27**	Diffuse large B-cell lymphoma, spleen Mediastinal (thymic) large B-cell lymphoma, spleen
200.78	LARGE CELL LYMPHOMA LYMPH NODES MULTIPLE SITES	**C83.38** **C85.28**	Diffuse large B-cell lymphoma, lymph nodes of multiple sites Mediastinal (thymic) large B-cell lymphoma, nodes mult site
200.80	VARIANTS UNSPECIFIED SITE EXTRANODAL&SOLID ORGN	**C83.00** **C83.09** **C83.80** **C83.89** **C83.90** **C83.99** **C86.5** **C86.6**	Small cell B-cell lymphoma, unspecified site Small cell B-cell lymphoma, extranodal and solid organ sites Other non-follicular lymphoma, unspecified site Oth non-follic lymphoma, extranodal and solid organ sites Non-follicular (diffuse) lymphoma, unsp, unspecified site Non-follic lymphoma, unsp, extrnod and solid organ sites Angioimmunoblastic T-cell lymphoma Primary cutaneous CD30-positive T-cell proliferations
200.81	OTH VARNTS LYMPHO&RETICULOSRCOM NODES HEAD&NCK	**C83.01** **C83.81** **C83.91**	Small cell B-cell lymphoma, nodes of head, face, and neck Oth non-follic lymphoma, lymph nodes of head, face, and neck Non-follic lymphoma, unsp, nodes of head, face, and neck
200.82	OTH VARNTS LYMPHO&RETICULOSRCOM INTRATHR NODES	**C83.02** **C83.82** **C83.92**	Small cell B-cell lymphoma, intrathoracic lymph nodes Other non-follicular lymphoma, intrathoracic lymph nodes Non-follic (diffuse) lymphoma, unsp, intrathorac lymph nodes
200.83	OTH VARNTS LYMPHO&RETICULOSRCOM INTRA-ABD NODES	**C83.03** **C83.83** **C83.93**	Small cell B-cell lymphoma, intra-abdominal lymph nodes Other non-follicular lymphoma, intra-abdominal lymph nodes Non-follic (diffuse) lymphoma, unsp, intra-abd lymph nodes
200.84	OTH VARNTS LYMPHO&RETICULOSRCOM NODES AX&UP LIMB	**C83.04** **C83.84** **C83.94**	Small cell B-cell lymphoma, nodes of axilla and upper limb Oth non-follic lymphoma, nodes of axilla and upper limb Non-follic lymphoma, unsp, nodes of axilla and upper limb
200.85	OTH VARNTS LYMPHO&RETICULOSRCOM ING REG&LW LIM	**C83.05** **C83.85** **C83.95**	Small cell B-cell lymph, nodes of ing region and lower limb Oth non-follic lymphoma, nodes of ing region and lower limb Non-follic lymph, unsp, nodes of ing region and lower limb
200.86	OTH VARNTS LYMPHO&RETICULOSRCOM INTRAPELV NODES	**C83.06** **C83.86** **C83.96**	Small cell B-cell lymphoma, intrapelvic lymph nodes Other non-follicular lymphoma, intrapelvic lymph nodes Non-follic (diffuse) lymphoma, unsp, intrapelvic lymph nodes
200.87	OTH VARIANT LYMPHOSARCOMA&RETICULOSARCOMA SPLEEN	**C83.07** **C83.87** **C83.97**	Small cell B-cell lymphoma, spleen Other non-follicular lymphoma, spleen Non-follicular (diffuse) lymphoma, unspecified, spleen

ICD-9-CM			ICD-10-CM	
2ØØ.88	OTH VARIANTS LYMPHOSRCOM&RETICULOSRCOM NODES MX		**C83.Ø8** **C83.88** **C83.98**	Small cell B-cell lymphoma, lymph nodes of multiple sites Other non-follicular lymphoma, lymph nodes of multiple sites Non-follic (diffuse) lymphoma, unsp, lymph nodes mult site
2Ø1.ØØ	HODGKINS PARAGRNULOM UNS SITE XTRANOD&SOLID ORGN		**C81.7Ø** **C81.79**	Other classical Hodgkin lymphoma, unspecified site Oth class Hodgkin lymphoma, extrnod and solid organ sites
2Ø1.Ø1	HODGKINS PARAGRANULOMA NODES HEAD FACE&NECK		**C81.71**	Oth class Hodgkin lymphoma, nodes of head, face, and neck
2Ø1.Ø2	HODGKINS PARAGRANULOMA INTRATHORACIC LYMPH NODES		**C81.72**	Other classical Hodgkin lymphoma, intrathoracic lymph nodes
2Ø1.Ø3	HODGKINS PARAGRANULOMA INTRA-ABD LYMPH NODES		**C81.73**	Oth classical Hodgkin lymphoma, intra-abdominal lymph nodes
2Ø1.Ø4	HODGKINS PARAGRANULOMA NODES AXILLA&UPPER LIMB		**C81.74**	Oth class Hodgkin lymphoma, nodes of axilla and upper limb
2Ø1.Ø5	HODGKINS PARAGRNULOM NODES ING REGION&LOWER LIMB		**C81.75**	Oth class Hodgkin lymph, nodes of ing region and lower limb
2Ø1.Ø6	HODGKINS PARAGRANULOMA INTRAPELVIC LYMPH NODES		**C81.76**	Other classical Hodgkin lymphoma, intrapelvic lymph nodes
2Ø1.Ø7	HODGKINS PARAGRANULOMA OF SPLEEN		**C81.77**	Other classical Hodgkin lymphoma, spleen
2Ø1.Ø8	HODGKINS PARAGRANULOMA NODES MULTIPLE SITES		**C81.78**	Oth classical Hodgkin lymphoma, lymph nodes mult site
2Ø1.1Ø	HODGKINS GRANULOMA UNS SITE XTRANOD&SOLID ORGN		**C81.7Ø** **C81.79**	Other classical Hodgkin lymphoma, unspecified site Oth class Hodgkin lymphoma, extrnod and solid organ sites
2Ø1.11	HODGKINS GRANULOMA LYMPH NODES HEAD FACE&NECK		**C81.71**	Oth class Hodgkin lymphoma, nodes of head, face, and neck
2Ø1.12	HODGKINS GRANULOMA OF INTRATHORACIC LYMPH NODES		**C81.72**	Other classical Hodgkin lymphoma, intrathoracic lymph nodes
2Ø1.13	HODGKINS GRANULOMA INTRA-ABDOMINAL LYMPH NODES		**C81.73**	Oth classical Hodgkin lymphoma, intra-abdominal lymph nodes
2Ø1.14	HODGKINS GRANULOMA LYMPH NODES AXILLA&UPPER LIMB		**C81.74**	Oth class Hodgkin lymphoma, nodes of axilla and upper limb
2Ø1.15	HODGKINS GRANULOMA NODES ING REGION&LOWER LIMB		**C81.75**	Oth class Hodgkin lymph, nodes of ing region and lower limb
2Ø1.16	HODGKINS GRANULOMA OF INTRAPELVIC LYMPH NODES		**C81.76**	Other classical Hodgkin lymphoma, intrapelvic lymph nodes
2Ø1.17	HODGKINS GRANULOMA OF SPLEEN		**C81.77**	Other classical Hodgkin lymphoma, spleen
2Ø1.18	HODGKINS GRANULOMA LYMPH NODES MULTIPLE SITES		**C81.78**	Oth classical Hodgkin lymphoma, lymph nodes mult site
2Ø1.2Ø	HODGKINS SARCOMA UNSPEC SITE XTRANOD&SOLID ORGN		**C81.7Ø** **C81.79**	Other classical Hodgkin lymphoma, unspecified site Oth class Hodgkin lymphoma, extrnod and solid organ sites
2Ø1.21	HODGKINS SARCOMA LYMPH NODES HEAD FACE&NECK		**C81.71**	Oth class Hodgkin lymphoma, nodes of head, face, and neck
2Ø1.22	HODGKINS SARCOMA OF INTRATHORACIC LYMPH NODES		**C81.72**	Other classical Hodgkin lymphoma, intrathoracic lymph nodes
2Ø1.23	HODGKINS SARCOMA OF INTRA-ABDOMINAL LYMPH NODES		**C81.73**	Oth classical Hodgkin lymphoma, intra-abdominal lymph nodes
2Ø1.24	HODGKINS SARCOMA LYMPH NODES AXILLA&UPPER LIMB		**C81.74**	Oth class Hodgkin lymphoma, nodes of axilla and upper limb
2Ø1.25	HODGKINS SARCOMA NODES ING REGION&LOWER LIMB		**C81.75**	Oth class Hodgkin lymph, nodes of ing region and lower limb
2Ø1.26	HODGKINS SARCOMA OF INTRAPELVIC LYMPH NODES		**C81.76**	Other classical Hodgkin lymphoma, intrapelvic lymph nodes
2Ø1.27	HODGKINS SARCOMA OF SPLEEN		**C81.77**	Other classical Hodgkin lymphoma, spleen
2Ø1.28	HODGKINS SARCOMA LYMPH NODES MULTIPLE SITES		**C81.78**	Oth classical Hodgkin lymphoma, lymph nodes mult site
2Ø1.4Ø	HODG LYMPHCYT-HISTCYT UNS SITE XTRANOD&SOLID ORG		**C81.ØØ** **C81.Ø9** **C81.4Ø** **C81.49**	Nodular lymphocyte predominant Hodgkin lymphoma, unsp site Nodlr lymphocy predom Hdgkn lymph, extrnod & solid org site Lymphocyte-rich classical Hodgkin lymphoma, unspecified site Lymp-rich class Hodgkin lymph, extrnod and solid organ sites
2Ø1.41	HODGKIN LYMPHCYT-HISTCYT NODES HEAD FCE&NCK		**C81.Ø1** **C81.41**	Nodlr lymphocy predom Hdgkn lymph, nodes of head, face, & nk Lymp-rich class Hodgkin lymph, nodes of head, face, and neck
2Ø1.42	HODGKIN LYMPHCYT-HISTCYT INTRATHR NODES		**C81.Ø2** **C81.42**	Nodular lymphocy predom Hodgkin lymphoma, intrathorac nodes Lymp-rich classical Hodgkin lymphoma, intrathorac nodes
2Ø1.43	HODGKIN LYMPHCYT-HISTCYT INTRA-ABD NODES		**C81.Ø3** **C81.43**	Nodular lymphocyte predom Hodgkin lymphoma, intra-abd nodes Lymp-rich classical Hodgkin lymphoma, intra-abd lymph nodes
2Ø1.44	HODGKIN LYMPHCYT-HISTCYT NODES AX&UP LIMB		**C81.Ø4** **C81.44**	Nodlr lymphocy predom Hdgkn lymph, nodes of axla and upr lmb Lymp-rich class Hdgkn lymph, nodes of axilla and upper limb
2Ø1.45	HODGKIN LYMPHCYT-HISTCYT NODES ING RGN&LW LIMB		**C81.Ø5** **C81.45**	Nodlr lymphocy predom Hdgkn lymph,nodes of ing rgn & low lmb Lymp-rich class Hdgkn lymph, nodes of ing rgn and lower limb
2Ø1.46	HODGKIN LYMPHCYT-HISTCYT INTRAPELV NODES		**C81.Ø6** **C81.46**	Nodular lymphocyte predom Hodgkin lymphoma, intrapelv nodes Lymp-rich classical Hodgkin lymphoma, intrapelv lymph nodes
2Ø1.47	HODGKINS LYMPHCYT-HISTCYT PREDOMINANCE SPLEEN		**C81.Ø7** **C81.47**	Nodular lymphocyte predominant Hodgkin lymphoma, spleen Lymphocyte-rich classical Hodgkin lymphoma, spleen
2Ø1.48	HODGKIN LYMPHCYT-HISTCYT NODES MX SITE		**C81.Ø8** **C81.48**	Nodular lymphocyte predom Hodgkin lymphoma, nodes mult site Lymp-rich classical Hodgkin lymphoma, lymph nodes mult site
2Ø1.5Ø	HODGKIN NODULR SCLER UNS SITE XTRANOD&SOLID ORGN		**C81.1Ø** **C81.19**	Nodular sclerosis classical Hodgkin lymphoma, unsp site Nodlr scler class Hdgkn lymph, extrnod and solid organ sites
2Ø1.51	HODGKINS NODULAR SCLEROSIS NODES HEAD FACE&NECK	➡	**C81.11**	Nodlr scler class Hdgkn lymph, nodes of head, face, and neck
2Ø1.52	HODGKINS NODULAR SCLEROSIS INTRATHORACIC NODES	➡	**C81.12**	Nodular sclerosis class Hodgkin lymphoma, intrathorac nodes
2Ø1.53	HODGKINS NODULAR SCLEROSIS INTRA-ABD LYMPH NODES	➡	**C81.13**	Nodular sclerosis class Hodgkin lymphoma, intra-abd nodes
2Ø1.54	HODGKINS NODULAR SCLEROSIS NODES AX&UPPER LIMB	➡	**C81.14**	Nodlr scler class Hdgkn lymph, nodes of axla and upper limb
2Ø1.55	HODGKINS NODULR SCLEROSIS NODES ING RGN&LOW LIMB	➡	**C81.15**	Nodlr scler class Hdgkn lymph, nodes of ing rgn and low limb
2Ø1.56	HODGKINS NODULAR SCLEROSIS INTRAPELVIC NODES	➡	**C81.16**	Nodular sclerosis class Hodgkin lymphoma, intrapelv nodes
2Ø1.57	HODGKINS DISEASE NODULAR SCLEROSIS OF SPLEEN	➡	**C81.17**	Nodular sclerosis classical Hodgkin lymphoma, spleen
2Ø1.58	HODGKINS NODULAR SCLEROSIS NODES MULTIPLE SITES	➡	**C81.18**	Nodular sclerosis class Hodgkin lymphoma, nodes mult site
2Ø1.6Ø	HODGKINS MIX CELLR UNS SITE XTRANOD&SOLID ORGN		**C81.2Ø** **C81.29**	Mixed cellularity classical Hodgkin lymphoma, unsp site Mix cellular class Hdgkn lymph, extrnod and solid org sites
2Ø1.61	HODGKINS MIXED CELLR INVLV NODES HEAD FACE&NECK	➡	**C81.21**	Mix cellular class Hdgkn lymph, nodes of head, face, and nk
2Ø1.62	HODGKINS MIXED CELLR INTRATHORACIC LYMPH NODES	➡	**C81.22**	Mixed cellular classical Hodgkin lymphoma, intrathorac nodes
2Ø1.63	HODGKINS MIXED CELLULARITY INTRA-ABD LYMPH NODES	➡	**C81.23**	Mixed cellular classical Hodgkin lymphoma, intra-abd nodes
2Ø1.64	HODGKINS MIXED CELLR NODES AXILLA&UPPER LIMB	➡	**C81.24**	Mix cellular class Hdgkn lymph, nodes of axla and upper limb
2Ø1.65	HODGKINS MIXED CELLR NODES ING REGION&LOWER LIMB	➡	**C81.25**	Mix cellular class Hdgkn lymph, nodes of ing rgn and low lmb

ICD-9-CM			ICD-10-CM	
201.66	HODGKINS MIXED CELLR INTRAPELVIC LYMPH NODES	➡	C81.26	Mixed cellular classical Hodgkin lymphoma, intrapelv nodes
201.67	HODGKINS DISEASE MIXED CELLULARITY OF SPLEEN	➡	C81.27	Mixed cellularity classical Hodgkin lymphoma, spleen
201.68	HODGKINS MIXED CELLR LYMPH NODES MULTIPLE SITES	➡	C81.28	Mixed cellular classical Hodgkin lymphoma, nodes mult site
201.70	HODGKIN LYMPHCYT DEPLET XTRANOD&SOLID ORGN		C81.30 C81.39	Lymphocyte depleted classical Hodgkin lymphoma, unsp site Lymphocy deplet class Hdgkn lymph, extrnod & solid org site
201.71	HODGKINS LYMPHOCYTIC DEPLET NODES HEAD FACE&NECK	➡	C81.31	Lymphocy deplet class Hdgkn lymph, nodes of head, face, & nk
201.72	HODGKINS LYMPHOCYTIC DEPLET INTRATHORACIC NODES	➡	C81.32	Lymphocy depleted class Hodgkin lymphoma, intrathorac nodes
201.73	HODGKINS LYMPHOCYTIC DEPLET INTRA-ABD NODES	➡	C81.33	Lymphocy depleted class Hodgkin lymphoma, intra-abd nodes
201.74	HODGKINS LYMPHCYT DEPLET NODES AXILLA&UPPER LIMB	➡	C81.34	Lymphocy deplet class Hdgkn lymph, nodes of axla and upr lmb
201.75	HODGKINS LYMPHCYT DEPLET NODES ING RGN&LOW LIMB	➡	C81.35	Lymphocy deplet class Hdgkn lymph,nodes of ing rgn & low lmb
201.76	HODGKINS LYMPHOCYTIC DEPLET INTRAPELVIC NODES	➡	C81.36	Lymphocy depleted class Hodgkin lymphoma, intrapelv nodes
201.77	HODGKINS DISEASE LYMPHOCYTIC DEPLETION OF SPLEEN	➡	C81.37	Lymphocyte depleted classical Hodgkin lymphoma, spleen
201.78	HODGKINS LYMPHOCYTIC DEPLET NODES MULTIPLE SITES	➡	C81.38	Lymphocy depleted class Hodgkin lymphoma, nodes mult site
201.90	HODGKINS UNS TYPE/SITE EXTRANODAL&SOLID ORGN		C81.90 C81.99	Hodgkin lymphoma, unspecified, unspecified site Hodgkin lymphoma, unsp, extranodal and solid organ sites
201.91	HODGKINS UNSPEC TYPE LYMPH NODES HEAD FACE&NECK	➡	C81.91	Hodgkin lymphoma, unsp, lymph nodes of head, face, and neck
201.92	HODGKINS UNSPEC TYPE INTRATHORACIC LYMPH NODES	➡	C81.92	Hodgkin lymphoma, unspecified, intrathoracic lymph nodes
201.93	HODGKINS UNSPEC TYPE INTRA-ABDOMINAL LYMPH NODES	➡	C81.93	Hodgkin lymphoma, unspecified, intra-abdominal lymph nodes
201.94	HODGKINS UNSPEC TYPE NODES AXILLA&UPPER LIMB	➡	C81.94	Hodgkin lymphoma, unsp, lymph nodes of axilla and upper limb
201.95	HODGKINS UNSPEC TYPE NODES ING REGION&LOWER LIMB	➡	C81.95	Hodgkin lymphoma, unsp, nodes of ing region and lower limb
201.96	HODGKINS UNSPEC TYPE INTRAPELVIC LYMPH NODES	➡	C81.96	Hodgkin lymphoma, unspecified, intrapelvic lymph nodes
201.97	HODGKINS DISEASE UNSPECIFIED TYPE OF SPLEEN	➡	C81.97	Hodgkin lymphoma, unspecified, spleen
201.98	HODGKINS UNSPEC TYPE LYMPH NODES MULTIPLE SITES	➡	C81.98	Hodgkin lymphoma, unspecified, lymph nodes of multiple sites
202.00	NODULAR LYMPHOMA UNSPEC SITE XTRANOD&SOLID ORGN		C82.00 C82.09 C82.10 C82.19 C82.20 C82.29 C82.30 C82.39 C82.40 C82.49 C82.60 C82.69 C82.80 C82.89 C82.90 C82.99	Follicular lymphoma grade I, unspecified site Follicular lymphoma grade I, extrnod and solid organ sites Follicular lymphoma grade II, unspecified site Follicular lymphoma grade II, extrnod and solid organ sites Follicular lymphoma grade III, unspecified, unspecified site Foliclar lymph grade III, unsp, extrnod and solid org sites Follicular lymphoma grade IIIa, unspecified site Foliclar lymphoma grade IIIa, extrnod and solid organ sites Follicular lymphoma grade IIIb, unspecified site Foliclar lymphoma grade IIIb, extrnod and solid organ sites Cutaneous follicle center lymphoma, unspecified site Cutan folicl center lymphoma, extrnod and solid organ sites Other types of follicular lymphoma, unspecified site Oth types of foliclar lymph, extrnod and solid organ sites Follicular lymphoma, unspecified, unspecified site Follicular lymphoma, unsp, extranodal and solid organ sites
202.01	NODULAR LYMPHOMA LYMPH NODES HEAD FACE&NECK		C82.01 C82.11 C82.21 C82.31 C82.41 C82.61 C82.81 C82.91	Follicular lymphoma grade I, nodes of head, face, and neck Follicular lymphoma grade II, nodes of head, face, and neck Foliclar lymph grade III, unsp, nodes of head, face, and nk Foliclar lymphoma grade IIIa, nodes of head, face, and neck Foliclar lymphoma grade IIIb, nodes of head, face, and neck Cutan folicl center lymphoma, nodes of head, face, and neck Oth types of foliclar lymph, nodes of head, face, and neck Follicular lymphoma, unsp, nodes of head, face, and neck
202.02	NODULAR LYMPHOMA OF INTRATHORACIC LYMPH NODES		C82.02 C82.12 C82.22 C82.32 C82.42 C82.62 C82.82 C82.92	Follicular lymphoma grade I, intrathoracic lymph nodes Follicular lymphoma grade II, intrathoracic lymph nodes Follicular lymphoma grade III, unsp, intrathorac lymph nodes Follicular lymphoma grade IIIa, intrathoracic lymph nodes Follicular lymphoma grade IIIb, intrathoracic lymph nodes Cutaneous follicle center lymphoma, intrathorac lymph nodes Oth types of follicular lymphoma, intrathoracic lymph nodes Follicular lymphoma, unspecified, intrathoracic lymph nodes
202.03	NODULAR LYMPHOMA OF INTRA-ABDOMINAL LYMPH NODES		C82.03 C82.13 C82.23 C82.33 C82.43 C82.63 C82.83 C82.93	Follicular lymphoma grade I, intra-abdominal lymph nodes Follicular lymphoma grade II, intra-abdominal lymph nodes Follicular lymphoma grade III, unsp, intra-abd lymph nodes Follicular lymphoma grade IIIa, intra-abdominal lymph nodes Follicular lymphoma grade IIIb, intra-abdominal lymph nodes Cutaneous follicle center lymphoma, intra-abd lymph nodes Oth types of follicular lymphoma, intra-abd lymph nodes Follicular lymphoma, unsp, intra-abdominal lymph nodes
202.04	NODULAR LYMPHOMA LYMPH NODES AXILLA&UPPER LIMB		C82.04 C82.14 C82.24 C82.34 C82.44 C82.64 C82.84 C82.94	Follicular lymphoma grade I, nodes of axilla and upper limb Follicular lymphoma grade II, nodes of axilla and upper limb Foliclar lymph grade III, unsp, nodes of axla and upper limb Foliclar lymphoma grade IIIa, nodes of axilla and upper limb Foliclar lymphoma grade IIIb, nodes of axilla and upper limb Cutan folicl center lymphoma, nodes of axilla and upper limb Oth types of foliclar lymph, nodes of axilla and upper limb Follicular lymphoma, unsp, nodes of axilla and upper limb

ICD-9-CM		ICD-10-CM	
202.05	NODULAR LYMPHOMA NODES ING REGION&LOWER LIMB	**C82.05**	Foliclar lymph grade I, nodes of ing region and lower limb
		C82.15	Foliclar lymph grade II, nodes of ing region and lower limb
		C82.25	Foliclar lymph grade III, unsp, nodes of ing rgn and low lmb
		C82.35	Foliclar lymph grade IIIa, nodes of ing rgn and lower limb
		C82.45	Foliclar lymph grade IIIb, nodes of ing rgn and lower limb
		C82.65	Cutan folicl cntr lymph, nodes of ing region and lower limb
		C82.85	Oth types of foliclar lymph, nodes of ing rgn and lower limb
		C82.95	Foliclar lymphoma, unsp, nodes of ing region and lower limb
202.06	NODULAR LYMPHOMA OF INTRAPELVIC LYMPH NODES	**C82.06**	Follicular lymphoma grade I, intrapelvic lymph nodes
		C82.16	Follicular lymphoma grade II, intrapelvic lymph nodes
		C82.26	Follicular lymphoma grade III, unsp, intrapelvic lymph nodes
		C82.36	Follicular lymphoma grade IIIa, intrapelvic lymph nodes
		C82.46	Follicular lymphoma grade IIIb, intrapelvic lymph nodes
		C82.66	Cutaneous follicle center lymphoma, intrapelvic lymph nodes
		C82.86	Other types of follicular lymphoma, intrapelvic lymph nodes
		C82.96	Follicular lymphoma, unspecified, intrapelvic lymph nodes
202.07	NODULAR LYMPHOMA OF SPLEEN	**C82.07**	Follicular lymphoma grade I, spleen
		C82.17	Follicular lymphoma grade II, spleen
		C82.27	Follicular lymphoma grade III, unspecified, spleen
		C82.37	Follicular lymphoma grade IIIa, spleen
		C82.47	Follicular lymphoma grade IIIb, spleen
		C82.67	Cutaneous follicle center lymphoma, spleen
		C82.87	Other types of follicular lymphoma, spleen
		C82.97	Follicular lymphoma, unspecified, spleen
202.08	NODULAR LYMPHOMA LYMPH NODES MULTIPLE SITES	**C82.08**	Follicular lymphoma grade I, lymph nodes of multiple sites
		C82.18	Follicular lymphoma grade II, lymph nodes of multiple sites
		C82.28	Follicular lymphoma grade III, unsp, lymph nodes mult site
		C82.38	Follicular lymphoma grade IIIa, lymph nodes mult site
		C82.48	Follicular lymphoma grade IIIb, lymph nodes mult site
		C82.68	Cutaneous follicle center lymphoma, lymph nodes mult site
		C82.88	Oth types of follicular lymphoma, lymph nodes mult site
		C82.98	Follicular lymphoma, unsp, lymph nodes of multiple sites
202.10	MYCOSIS FUNGOIDES UNSPEC SITE XTRANOD&SOLID ORGN	**C84.00**	Mycosis fungoides, unspecified site
		C84.09	Mycosis fungoides, extranodal and solid organ sites
202.11	MYCOSIS FUNGOIDES LYMPH NODES HEAD FACE&NECK	**C84.01**	Mycosis fungoides, lymph nodes of head, face, and neck
202.12	MYCOSIS FUNGOIDES OF INTRATHORACIC LYMPH NODES	**C84.02**	Mycosis fungoides, intrathoracic lymph nodes
202.13	MYCOSIS FUNGOIDES OF INTRA-ABDOMINAL LYMPH NODES	**C84.03**	Mycosis fungoides, intra-abdominal lymph nodes
202.14	MYCOSIS FUNGOIDES LYMPH NODES AXILLA&UPPER LIMB	**C84.04**	Mycosis fungoides, lymph nodes of axilla and upper limb
202.15	MYCOSIS FUNGOIDES NODES ING REGION&LOWER LIMB	**C84.05**	Mycosis fungoides, nodes of inguinal region and lower limb
202.16	MYCOSIS FUNGOIDES OF INTRAPELVIC LYMPH NODES	**C84.06**	Mycosis fungoides, intrapelvic lymph nodes
202.17	MYCOSIS FUNGOIDES OF SPLEEN	**C84.07**	Mycosis fungoides, spleen
202.18	MYCOSIS FUNGOIDES LYMPH NODES MULTIPLE SITES	**C84.08**	Mycosis fungoides, lymph nodes of multiple sites
202.20	SEZARYS DISEASE UNSPEC SITE XTRANOD&SOLID ORGN	**C84.10**	Sezary disease, unspecified site
		C84.19	Sezary disease, extranodal and solid organ sites
202.21	SEZARYS DISEASE OF LYMPH NODES OF HEAD FACE&NECK	➡ **C84.11**	Sezary disease, lymph nodes of head, face, and neck
202.22	SEZARYS DISEASE OF INTRATHORACIC LYMPH NODES	➡ **C84.12**	Sezary disease, intrathoracic lymph nodes
202.23	SEZARYS DISEASE OF INTRA-ABDOMINAL LYMPH NODES	➡ **C84.13**	Sezary disease, intra-abdominal lymph nodes
202.24	SEZARYS DISEASE LYMPH NODES AXILLA&UPPER LIMB	➡ **C84.14**	Sezary disease, lymph nodes of axilla and upper limb
202.25	SEZARYS DISEASE NODES ING REGION&LOWER LIMB	➡ **C84.15**	Sezary disease, nodes of inguinal region and lower limb
202.26	SEZARYS DISEASE OF INTRAPELVIC LYMPH NODES	➡ **C84.16**	Sezary disease, intrapelvic lymph nodes
202.27	SEZARYS DISEASE OF SPLEEN	➡ **C84.17**	Sezary disease, spleen
202.28	SEZARYS DISEASE OF LYMPH NODES OF MULTIPLE SITES	➡ **C84.18**	Sezary disease, lymph nodes of multiple sites
202.30	MALIG HISTIOCYTOSIS UNS SITE XTRANOD&SOLID ORGN	**C96.A**	Histiocytic sarcoma
202.31	MALIG HISTIOCYTOSIS LYMPH NODES HEAD FACE&NECK	**C96.A**	Histiocytic sarcoma
202.32	MALIG HISTIOCYTOSIS INTRATHORACIC LYMPH NODES	**C96.A**	Histiocytic sarcoma
202.33	MALIG HISTIOCYTOSIS INTRA-ABDOMINAL LYMPH NODES	**C96.A**	Histiocytic sarcoma
202.34	MALIG HISTIOCYTOSIS NODES AXILLA&UPPER LIMB	**C96.A**	Histiocytic sarcoma
202.35	MALIG HISTIOCYTOSIS NODES ING REGION&LOWER LIMB	**C96.A**	Histiocytic sarcoma
202.36	MALIGNANT HISTIOCYTOSIS INTRAPELVIC LYMPH NODES	**C96.A**	Histiocytic sarcoma
202.37	MALIGNANT HISTIOCYTOSIS OF SPLEEN	**C96.A**	Histiocytic sarcoma
202.38	MALIG HISTIOCYTOSIS LYMPH NODES MULTIPLE SITES	**C96.A**	Histiocytic sarcoma
202.40	LEUKEM RETICULOENDOTHELIOS XTRANOD&SOLID ORGN	**C91.40**	Hairy cell leukemia not having achieved remission
		C91.41	Hairy cell leukemia, in remission
		C91.42	Hairy cell leukemia, in relapse
202.41	LEUKEMIC RETICULOENDOTHELIOS NODES HEAD FCE&NECK	**C91.40**	Hairy cell leukemia not having achieved remission
202.42	LEUKEMIC RETICULOENDOTHELIOS INTRATHORACIC NODES	**C91.40**	Hairy cell leukemia not having achieved remission
202.43	LEUKEMIC RETICULOENDOTHELIOSIS INTRA-ABD NODES	**C91.40**	Hairy cell leukemia not having achieved remission
202.44	LEUKEMIC RETICULOENDOTHELIOS NODES AX&UPPER LIMB	**C91.40**	Hairy cell leukemia not having achieved remission
202.45	LEUKEM RETICULOENDOTHELIOS NODES ING RGN&LW LIMB	**C91.40**	Hairy cell leukemia not having achieved remission
202.46	LEUKEMIC RETICULOENDOTHELIOSIS INTRAPELVIC NODES	**C91.40**	Hairy cell leukemia not having achieved remission
202.47	LEUKEMIC RETICULOENDOTHELIOSIS OF SPLEEN	**C91.40**	Hairy cell leukemia not having achieved remission
202.48	LEUKEM RETICULOENDOTHELIOS NODES MULTIPES SITES	**C91.40**	Hairy cell leukemia not having achieved remission
202.50	LETTERER-SIWE DZ UNSPEC SITE XTRANOD&SOLID ORGN	**C96.0**	Multifocal and multisystemic Langerhans-cell histiocytosis

ICD-9-CM		ICD-10-CM	
2Ø2.51	LETTERER-SIWE DISEASE LYMPH NODES HEAD FACE&NECK	**C96.Ø**	Multifocal and multisystemic Langerhans-cell histiocytosis
2Ø2.52	LETTERER-SIWE DISEASE INTRATHORACIC LYMPH NODES	**C96.Ø**	Multifocal and multisystemic Langerhans-cell histiocytosis
2Ø2.53	LETTERER-SIWE DISEASE INTRA-ABD LYMPH NODES	**C96.Ø**	Multifocal and multisystemic Langerhans-cell histiocytosis
2Ø2.54	LETTERER-SIWE DISEASE NODES AXILLA&UPPER LIMB	**C96.Ø**	Multifocal and multisystemic Langerhans-cell histiocytosis
2Ø2.55	LETTERER-SIWE DISEASE NODES ING REGION&LOW LIMB	**C96.Ø**	Multifocal and multisystemic Langerhans-cell histiocytosis
2Ø2.56	LETTERER-SIWE DISEASE OF INTRAPELVIC LYMPH NODES	**C96.Ø**	Multifocal and multisystemic Langerhans-cell histiocytosis
2Ø2.57	LETTERER-SIWE DISEASE OF SPLEEN	**C96.Ø**	Multifocal and multisystemic Langerhans-cell histiocytosis
2Ø2.58	LETTERER-SIWE DISEASE LYMPH NODES MULTIPLE SITES	**C96.Ø**	Multifocal and multisystemic Langerhans-cell histiocytosis
2Ø2.6Ø	MAL MAST CELL TUMRS UNS SITE XTRANOD&SOLID ORGN	**C96.2**	Malignant mast cell tumor
2Ø2.61	MALIG MAST CELL TUMORS NODES HEAD FACE&NECK	**C96.2**	Malignant mast cell tumor
2Ø2.62	MALIG MAST CELL TUMORS INTRATHORACIC LYMPH NODES	**C96.2**	Malignant mast cell tumor
2Ø2.63	MALIG MAST CELL TUMORS INTRA-ABD LYMPH NODES	**C96.2**	Malignant mast cell tumor
2Ø2.64	MALIG MAST CELL TUMORS NODES AXILLA&UPPER LIMB	**C96.2**	Malignant mast cell tumor
2Ø2.65	MALIG MAST CELL TUMRS NODES ING REGION&LOW LIMB	**C96.2**	Malignant mast cell tumor
2Ø2.66	MALIG MAST CELL TUMORS INTRAPELVIC LYMPH NODES	**C96.2**	Malignant mast cell tumor
2Ø2.67	MALIGNANT MAST CELL TUMORS OF SPLEEN	**C96.2**	Malignant mast cell tumor
2Ø2.68	MALIG MAST CELL TUMORS NODES MULTIPLE SITES	**C96.2**	Malignant mast cell tumor
2Ø2.7Ø	PTL UNS SITE EXTRANODAL&SOLID ORGAN SITES	**C84.4Ø** **C84.49**	Peripheral T-cell lymphoma, not classified, unspecified site Prph T-cell lymph, not class, extrnod and solid organ sites
2Ø2.71	PERIPHERAL T-CELL LYMPHOMA NODES HEAD FACE&NECK	**C84.41**	Prph T-cell lymph, not class, nodes of head, face, and neck
2Ø2.72	PERIPHERAL T-CELL LYMPHOMA INTRATHORACIC NODES	**C84.42**	Peripheral T-cell lymphoma, not class, intrathorac nodes
2Ø2.73	PERIPHERAL T-CELL LYMPHOMA INTRA-ABDOMINAL NODES	**C84.43**	Peripheral T-cell lymphoma, not classified, intra-abd nodes
2Ø2.74	PERIPH T-CELL LYMPHOMA NODES AXILLA&UPPER LIMB	**C84.44**	Prph T-cell lymph, not class, nodes of axilla and upper limb
2Ø2.75	PERIPH T-CELL LYMPHOMA NODES INGUINAL&LOWER LIMB	**C84.45**	Prph T-cell lymph, not class, nodes of ing rgn and low limb
2Ø2.76	PERIPHERAL T-CELL LYMPHOMA INTRAPELVIC NODES	**C84.46**	Peripheral T-cell lymphoma, not classified, intrapelv nodes
2Ø2.77	PERIPHERAL T-CELL LYMPHOMA SPLEEN	**C84.47**	Peripheral T-cell lymphoma, not classified, spleen
2Ø2.78	PERIPHERAL T-CELL LYMPHOMA LYMPH NODES MX SITES	**C84.48**	Peripheral T-cell lymphoma, not classified, nodes mult site
2Ø2.8Ø	OTH MALIG LYMPHOMAS UNS SITE XTRANOD&SOLID ORGN	**C82.5Ø** **C82.59** **C84.9Ø** **C84.99** **C84.AØ** **C84.A9** **C84.ZØ** **C84.Z9** **C85.1Ø** **C85.19** **C85.2Ø** **C85.29** **C85.8Ø** **C85.89** **C85.9Ø** **C85.99** **C86.4**	Diffuse follicle center lymphoma, unspecified site Diffuse folicl center lymph, extrnod and solid organ sites Mature T/NK-cell lymphomas, unspecified, unspecified site Mature T/NK-cell lymph, unsp, extrnod and solid organ sites Cutaneous T-cell lymphoma, unspecified, unspecified site Cutan T-cell lymphoma, unsp, extrnod and solid organ sites Other mature T/NK-cell lymphomas, unspecified site Oth mature T/NK-cell lymph, extrnod and solid organ sites Unspecified B-cell lymphoma, unspecified site Unsp B-cell lymphoma, extranodal and solid organ sites Mediastinal (thymic) large B-cell lymphoma, unspecified site Mediastnl large B-cell lymph, extrnod and solid organ sites Oth types of non-Hodgkin lymphoma, unspecified site Oth types of non-hodg lymph, extrnod and solid organ sites Non-Hodgkin lymphoma, unspecified, unspecified site Non-Hodgkin lymphoma, unsp, extranodal and solid organ sites Blastic NK-cell lymphoma
2Ø2.81	OTHER MALIG LYMPHOMAS LYMPH NODES HEAD FACE&NECK	**C82.51** **C84.91** **C84.A1** **C84.Z1** **C85.11** **C85.21** **C85.81** **C85.91** **C86.Ø**	Diffuse folicl center lymph, nodes of head, face, and neck Mature T/NK-cell lymph, unsp, nodes of head, face, and neck Cutan T-cell lymphoma, unsp nodes of head, face, and neck Oth mature T/NK-cell lymph, nodes of head, face, and neck Unsp B-cell lymphoma, lymph nodes of head, face, and neck Mediastnl large B-cell lymph, nodes of head, face, and neck Oth types of non-hodg lymph, nodes of head, face, and neck Non-Hodgkin lymphoma, unsp, nodes of head, face, and neck Extranodal NK/T-cell lymphoma, nasal type
2Ø2.82	OTHER MALIG LYMPHOMAS INTRATHORACIC LYMPH NODES	**C82.52** **C84.92** **C84.A2** **C84.Z2** **C85.12** **C85.22** **C85.82** **C85.92**	Diffuse follicle center lymphoma, intrathoracic lymph nodes Mature T/NK-cell lymphomas, unsp, intrathoracic lymph nodes Cutaneous T-cell lymphoma, unsp, intrathoracic lymph nodes Other mature T/NK-cell lymphomas, intrathoracic lymph nodes Unspecified B-cell lymphoma, intrathoracic lymph nodes Mediastnl (thymic) large B-cell lymphoma, intrathorac nodes Oth types of non-Hodgkin lymphoma, intrathoracic lymph nodes Non-Hodgkin lymphoma, unspecified, intrathoracic lymph nodes
2Ø2.83	OTH MALIG LYMPHOMAS INTRA-ABDOMINAL LYMPH NODES	**C82.53** **C84.93** **C84.A3** **C84.Z3** **C85.13** **C85.23** **C85.83** **C85.93** **C86.2** **C86.3**	Diffuse follicle center lymphoma, intra-abd lymph nodes Mature T/NK-cell lymphomas, unsp, intra-abd lymph nodes Cutaneous T-cell lymphoma, unsp, intra-abdominal lymph nodes Oth mature T/NK-cell lymphomas, intra-abdominal lymph nodes Unspecified B-cell lymphoma, intra-abdominal lymph nodes Mediastinal (thymic) large B-cell lymphoma, intra-abd nodes Oth types of non-Hodgkin lymphoma, intra-abd lymph nodes Non-Hodgkin lymphoma, unsp, intra-abdominal lymph nodes Enteropathy-type (intestinal) T-cell lymphoma Subcutaneous panniculitis-like T-cell lymphoma

ICD-9-CM			ICD-10-CM	
202.84	OTH MALIG LYMPHOMAS NODES AXILLA&UPPER LIMB		**C82.54**	Diffuse folicl center lymph, nodes of axilla and upper limb
			C84.94	Mature T/NK-cell lymph, unsp, nodes of axilla and upper limb
			C84.A4	Cutan T-cell lymphoma, unsp, nodes of axilla and upper limb
			C84.Z4	Oth mature T/NK-cell lymph, nodes of axilla and upper limb
			C85.14	Unsp B-cell lymphoma, lymph nodes of axilla and upper limb
			C85.24	Mediastnl large B-cell lymph, nodes of axilla and upper limb
			C85.84	Oth types of non-hodg lymph, nodes of axilla and upper limb
			C85.94	Non-Hodgkin lymphoma, unsp, nodes of axilla and upper limb
202.85	OTH MALIG LYMPHOMAS NODES ING REGION&LOWER LIMB		**C82.55**	Diffus folicl cntr lymph, nodes of ing region and lower limb
			C84.95	Mature T/NK-cell lymph, unsp, nodes of ing rgn and low limb
			C84.A5	Cutan T-cell lymph, unsp, nodes of ing region and lower limb
			C84.Z5	Oth mature T/NK-cell lymph, nodes of ing rgn and lower limb
			C85.15	Unsp B-cell lymphoma, nodes of ing region and lower limb
			C85.25	Mediastnl lg B-cell lymph, nodes of ing rgn and lower limb
			C85.85	Oth types of non-hodg lymph, nodes of ing rgn and lower limb
			C85.95	Non-hodg lymphoma, unsp, nodes of ing region and lower limb
202.86	OTHER MALIG LYMPHOMAS INTRAPELVIC LYMPH NODES		**C82.56**	Diffuse follicle center lymphoma, intrapelvic lymph nodes
			C84.96	Mature T/NK-cell lymphomas, unsp, intrapelvic lymph nodes
			C84.A6	Cutaneous T-cell lymphoma, unsp, intrapelvic lymph nodes
			C84.Z6	Other mature T/NK-cell lymphomas, intrapelvic lymph nodes
			C85.16	Unspecified B-cell lymphoma, intrapelvic lymph nodes
			C85.26	Mediastinal (thymic) large B-cell lymphoma, intrapelv nodes
			C85.86	Oth types of non-Hodgkin lymphoma, intrapelvic lymph nodes
			C85.96	Non-Hodgkin lymphoma, unspecified, intrapelvic lymph nodes
202.87	OTHER MALIGNANT LYMPHOMAS OF SPLEEN		**C82.57**	Diffuse follicle center lymphoma, spleen
			C84.97	Mature T/NK-cell lymphomas, unspecified, spleen
			C84.A7	Cutaneous T-cell lymphoma, unspecified, spleen
			C84.Z7	Other mature T/NK-cell lymphomas, spleen
			C85.17	Unspecified B-cell lymphoma, spleen
			C85.27	Mediastinal (thymic) large B-cell lymphoma, spleen
			C85.87	Other specified types of non-Hodgkin lymphoma, spleen
			C85.97	Non-Hodgkin lymphoma, unspecified, spleen
			C86.1	Hepatosplenic T-cell lymphoma
202.88	OTHER MALIG LYMPHOMAS LYMPH NODES MULTIPLE SITES		**C82.58**	Diffuse follicle center lymphoma, lymph nodes mult site
			C84.98	Mature T/NK-cell lymphomas, unsp, lymph nodes mult site
			C84.A8	Cutaneous T-cell lymphoma, unsp, lymph nodes mult site
			C84.Z8	Oth mature T/NK-cell lymphomas, lymph nodes mult site
			C85.18	Unspecified B-cell lymphoma, lymph nodes of multiple sites
			C85.28	Mediastinal (thymic) large B-cell lymphoma, nodes mult site
			C85.88	Oth types of non-Hodgkin lymphoma, lymph nodes mult site
			C85.98	Non-Hodgkin lymphoma, unsp, lymph nodes of multiple sites
202.90	OTH-UNS MAL LYMPHOID-HISTIO TISS-UNS-EXTRANODAL		**C96.4**	Sarcoma of dendritic cells (accessory cells)
			C96.9	Malig neoplm of lymphoid, hematpoetc and rel tissue, unsp
			C96.Z	Oth malig neoplm of lymphoid, hematpoetc and related tissue
202.91	OTH&UNS MAL NEO LYMPHOID&HISTCYT TISS HEAD&NCK		**C96.9**	Malig neoplm of lymphoid, hematpoetc and rel tissue, unsp
			C96.Z	Oth malig neoplm of lymphoid, hematpoetc and related tissue
202.92	OTH&UNS MAL NEO LYMPHOID&HISTCYT TISS INTRATHR		**C96.9**	Malig neoplm of lymphoid, hematpoetc and rel tissue, unsp
			C96.Z	Oth malig neoplm of lymphoid, hematpoetc and related tissue
202.93	OTH-UNS MAL LYMPHOID-HISTIO TISS-INTRA-ABD NODES		**C96.9**	Malig neoplm of lymphoid, hematpoetc and rel tissue, unsp
			C96.Z	Oth malig neoplm of lymphoid, hematpoetc and related tissue
202.94	OTH-UNS MAL LYMPHOID-HISTIO TISS-AXILLARY NODES		**C96.9**	Malig neoplm of lymphoid, hematpoetc and rel tissue, unsp
			C96.Z	Oth malig neoplm of lymphoid, hematpoetc and related tissue
202.95	OTH-UNS MAL LYMPHOID-HISTIO TISS-INGUINAL NODES		**C96.9**	Malig neoplm of lymphoid, hematpoetc and rel tissue, unsp
			C96.Z	Oth malig neoplm of lymphoid, hematpoetc and related tissue
202.96	OTH-UNS MAL LYMPHOID-HISTIO TISSUE-PELVIC NODES		**C96.9**	Malig neoplm of lymphoid, hematpoetc and rel tissue, unsp
			C96.Z	Oth malig neoplm of lymphoid, hematpoetc and related tissue
202.97	OTH&UNS MAL NEOPLSM LYMPHOID&HISTCYT TISS SPLEEN		**C96.9**	Malig neoplm of lymphoid, hematpoetc and rel tissue, unsp
			C96.Z	Oth malig neoplm of lymphoid, hematpoetc and related tissue
202.98	UNS MAL NEO LYMPHOID&HISTCYT TISS NODES MX SITE		**C96.9**	Malig neoplm of lymphoid, hematpoetc and rel tissue, unsp
			C96.Z	Oth malig neoplm of lymphoid, hematpoetc and related tissue
203.00	MULTIPLE MYELOMA W/O MENTION ACHIEVED REMISSION	➡	**C90.00**	Multiple myeloma not having achieved remission
203.01	MULTIPLE MYELOMA IN REMISSION	➡	**C90.01**	Multiple myeloma in remission
203.02	MULTIPLE MYELOMA IN RELAPSE	➡	**C90.02**	Multiple myeloma in relapse
203.10	PLASMA CELL LEUKEMIA W/O ACHIEVED REMISSION	➡	**C90.10**	Plasma cell leukemia not having achieved remission
203.11	PLASMA CELL LEUKEMIA IN REMISSION	➡	**C90.11**	Plasma cell leukemia in remission
203.12	PLASMA CELL LEUKEMIA IN RELAPSE	➡	**C90.12**	Plasma cell leukemia in relapse
203.80	OTH IMMUNOPROLIF NEOPLASM W/O ACHIEVED REMISSION		**C88.2**	Heavy chain disease
			C88.3	Immunoproliferative small intestinal disease
			C88.8	Other malignant immunoproliferative diseases
			C88.9	Malignant immunoproliferative disease, unspecified
			C90.20	Extramedullary plasmacytoma not having achieved remission
			C90.30	Solitary plasmacytoma not having achieved remission
203.81	OTHER IMMUNOPROLIFERATIVE NEOPLASMS IN REMISSION		**C88.2**	Heavy chain disease
			C90.21	Extramedullary plasmacytoma in remission
			C90.31	Solitary plasmacytoma in remission
203.82	OTHER IMMUNOPROLIFERATIVE NEOPLASMS IN RELAPSE		**C88.8**	Other malignant immunoproliferative diseases
			C90.22	Extramedullary plasmacytoma in relapse
			C90.32	Solitary plasmacytoma in relapse

ICD-9-CM			ICD-10-CM	
204.00	ACUTE LYMPHOID LEUKEMIA W/O ACHIEVED REMISSION	➡	C91.00	Acute lymphoblastic leukemia not having achieved remission
204.01	ACUTE LYMPHOID LEUKEMIA IN REMISSION	➡	C91.01	Acute lymphoblastic leukemia, in remission
204.02	ACUTE LYMPHOID LEUKEMIA IN RELAPSE	➡	C91.02	Acute lymphoblastic leukemia, in relapse
204.10	CHRONIC LYMPHOID LEUKEMIA W/O ACHIEVED REMISSION	➡	C91.10	Chronic lymphocytic leuk of B-cell type not achieve remis
204.11	CHRONIC LYMPHOID LEUKEMIA IN REMISSION	➡	C91.11	Chronic lymphocytic leukemia of B-cell type in remission
204.12	CHRONIC LYMPHOID LEUKEMIA IN RELAPSE	➡	C91.12	Chronic lymphocytic leukemia of B-cell type in relapse
204.20	SUBACUTE LYMPHOID LEUKEMIA W/O ACHIEVD REMISSION		C91.Z0	Other lymphoid leukemia not having achieved remission
204.21	SUBACUTE LYMPHOID LEUKEMIA IN REMISSION		C91.Z1	Other lymphoid leukemia, in remission
204.22	SUBACUTE LYMPHOID LEUKEMIA IN RELAPSE		C91.Z2	Other lymphoid leukemia, in relapse
204.80	OTH LYMPHOID LEUKEMIA W/O ACHIEVED REMISSION		C91.30	Prolymphocytic leukemia of B-cell type not achieve remission
			C91.50	Adult T-cell lymph/leuk (HTLV-1-assoc) not achieve remission
			C91.60	Prolymphocytic leukemia of T-cell type not achieve remission
			C91.A0	Mature B-cell leukemia Burkitt-type not achieve remission
			C91.Z0	Other lymphoid leukemia not having achieved remission
204.81	OTHER LYMPHOID LEUKEMIA IN REMISSION		C91.31	Prolymphocytic leukemia of B-cell type, in remission
			C91.51	Adult T-cell lymphoma/leukemia (HTLV-1-assoc), in remission
			C91.61	Prolymphocytic leukemia of T-cell type, in remission
			C91.A1	Mature B-cell leukemia Burkitt-type, in remission
			C91.Z1	Other lymphoid leukemia, in remission
204.82	OTHER LYMPHOID LEUKEMIA IN RELAPSE		C91.32	Prolymphocytic leukemia of B-cell type, in relapse
			C91.52	Adult T-cell lymphoma/leukemia (HTLV-1-assoc), in relapse
			C91.62	Prolymphocytic leukemia of T-cell type, in relapse
			C91.A2	Mature B-cell leukemia Burkitt-type, in relapse
			C91.Z2	Other lymphoid leukemia, in relapse
204.90	UNS LYMPHOID LEUKEMIA W/O ACHIEVED REMISSION	➡	C91.90	Lymphoid leukemia, unspecified not having achieved remission
204.91	UNSPECIFIED LYMPHOID LEUKEMIA IN REMISSION	➡	C91.91	Lymphoid leukemia, unspecified, in remission
204.92	UNSPECIFIED LYMPHOID LEUKEMIA IN RELAPSE	➡	C91.92	Lymphoid leukemia, unspecified, in relapse
205.00	ACUTE MYELOID LEUKEMIA W/O ACHIEVED REMISSION		C92.00	Acute myeloblastic leukemia, not having achieved remission
			C92.40	Acute promyelocytic leukemia, not having achieved remission
			C92.50	Acute myelomonocytic leukemia, not having achieved remission
			C92.60	Acute myeloid leukemia w 11q23-abnormality not achieve remis
			C92.A0	Acute myeloid leuk w multilin dysplasia, not achieve remis
205.01	ACUTE MYELOID LEUKEMIA IN REMISSION		C92.01	Acute myeloblastic leukemia, in remission
			C92.41	Acute promyelocytic leukemia, in remission
			C92.51	Acute myelomonocytic leukemia, in remission
			C92.61	Acute myeloid leukemia with 11q23-abnormality in remission
			C92.A1	Acute myeloid leukemia w multilin dysplasia, in remission
205.02	ACUTE MYELOID LEUKEMIA IN RELAPSE		C92.02	Acute myeloblastic leukemia, in relapse
			C92.42	Acute promyelocytic leukemia, in relapse
			C92.52	Acute myelomonocytic leukemia, in relapse
			C92.62	Acute myeloid leukemia with 11q23-abnormality in relapse
			C92.A2	Acute myeloid leukemia w multilineage dysplasia, in relapse
205.10	CHRON MYELOID LEUKEMIA W/O ACHIEVED REMISSION		C92.10	Chronic myeloid leuk, BCR/ABL-positive, not achieve remis
205.11	CHRONIC MYELOID LEUKEMIA IN REMISSION		C92.11	Chronic myeloid leukemia, BCR/ABL-positive, in remission
205.12	CHRONIC MYELOID LEUKEMIA IN RELAPSE		C92.12	Chronic myeloid leukemia, BCR/ABL-positive, in relapse
205.20	SUBACUTE MYELOID LEUKEMIA W/O ACHIEVED REMISSION		C92.20	Atyp chronic myeloid leuk, BCR/ABL-neg, not achieve remis
205.21	SUBACUTE MYELOID LEUKEMIA IN REMISSION		C92.21	Atypical chronic myeloid leukemia, BCR/ABL-neg, in remission
205.22	SUBACUTE MYELOID LEUKEMIA IN RELAPSE		C92.22	Atypical chronic myeloid leukemia, BCR/ABL-neg, in relapse
205.30	MYELOID SARCOMA W/O MENTION ACHIEVED REMISSION	➡	C92.30	Myeloid sarcoma, not having achieved remission
205.31	MYELOID SARCOMA IN REMISSION	➡	C92.31	Myeloid sarcoma, in remission
205.32	MYELOID SARCOMA IN RELAPSE	➡	C92.32	Myeloid sarcoma, in relapse
205.80	OTHER MYELOID LEUKEMIA W/O ACHIEVED REMISSION		C92.Z0	Other myeloid leukemia not having achieved remission
205.81	OTHER MYELOID LEUKEMIA IN REMISSION		C92.Z1	Other myeloid leukemia, in remission
205.82	OTHER MYELOID LEUKEMIA IN RELAPSE		C92.Z2	Other myeloid leukemia, in relapse
205.90	UNS MYELOID LEUKEMIA W/O ACHIEVED REMISSION	➡	C92.90	Myeloid leukemia, unspecified, not having achieved remission
205.91	UNSPECIFIED MYELOID LEUKEMIA IN REMISSION	➡	C92.91	Myeloid leukemia, unspecified in remission
205.92	UNSPECIFIED MYELOID LEUKEMIA IN RELAPSE	➡	C92.92	Myeloid leukemia, unspecified in relapse
206.00	ACUTE MONOCYTIC LEUKEMIA W/O ACHIEVED REMISSION	➡	C93.00	Acute monoblastic/monocytic leukemia, not achieve remission
206.01	ACUTE MONOCYTIC LEUKEMIA IN REMISSION	➡	C93.01	Acute monoblastic/monocytic leukemia, in remission
206.02	ACUTE MONOCYTIC LEUKEMIA IN RELAPSE	➡	C93.02	Acute monoblastic/monocytic leukemia, in relapse
206.10	CHRON MONOCYTIC LEUKEMIA W/O ACHIEVED REMISSION	➡	C93.10	Chronic myelomonocytic leukemia not achieve remission
206.11	CHRONIC MONOCYTIC LEUKEMIA IN REMISSION	➡	C93.11	Chronic myelomonocytic leukemia, in remission
206.12	CHRONIC MONOCYTIC LEUKEMIA IN RELAPSE	➡	C93.12	Chronic myelomonocytic leukemia, in relapse
206.20	SUBACUT MONOCYTC LEUKEMIA W/O ACHIEVED REMISSION		C93.90	Monocytic leukemia, unsp, not having achieved remission
206.21	SUBACUTE MONOCYTIC LEUKEMIA IN REMISSION		C93.91	Monocytic leukemia, unspecified in remission
206.22	SUBACUTE MONOCYTIC LEUKEMIA IN RELAPSE		C93.92	Monocytic leukemia, unspecified in relapse
206.80	OTH MONOCYTIC LEUKEMIA W/O ACHIEVED REMISSION		C93.30	Juvenile myelomonocytic leukemia, not achieve remission
			C93.Z0	Other monocytic leukemia, not having achieved remission
206.81	OTHER MONOCYTIC LEUKEMIA IN REMISSION		C93.31	Juvenile myelomonocytic leukemia, in remission
			C93.Z1	Other monocytic leukemia, in remission
206.82	OTHER MONOCYTIC LEUKEMIA IN RELAPSE		C93.32	Juvenile myelomonocytic leukemia, in relapse
			C93.Z2	Other monocytic leukemia, in relapse

ICD-9-CM			ICD-10-CM	
206.90	UNS MONOCYTIC LEUKEMIA W/O ACHIEVED REMISSION		**C93.90**	Monocytic leukemia, unsp, not having achieved remission
206.91	UNSPECIFIED MONOCYTIC LEUKEMIA IN REMISSION		**C93.91**	Monocytic leukemia, unspecified in remission
206.92	UNSPECIFIED MONOCYTIC LEUKEMIA IN RELAPSE		**C93.92**	Monocytic leukemia, unspecified in relapse
207.00	ACUTE ERYTHREMIA & EL W/O ACHIEVED REMISSION	➡	**C94.00**	Acute erythroid leukemia, not having achieved remission
207.01	ACUTE ERYTHREMIA&ERYTHROLEUKEMIA IN REMISSION	➡	**C94.01**	Acute erythroid leukemia, in remission
207.02	ACUTE ERYTHREMIA AND ERYTHROLEUKEMIA IN RELAPSE	➡	**C94.02**	Acute erythroid leukemia, in relapse
207.10	CHRON ERYTHREMIA W/O MENTION ACHIEVED REMISSION		**D45**	Polycythemia vera
207.11	CHRONIC ERYTHREMIA IN REMISSION		**D45**	Polycythemia vera
207.12	CHRONIC ERYTHREMIA IN RELAPSE		**D45**	Polycythemia vera
207.20	MEGAKARYOCTIC LEUKEMIA W/O ACHIEVED REMISSION		**C94.20**	Acute megakaryoblastic leukemia not achieve remission
207.21	MEGAKARYOCYTIC LEUKEMIA IN REMISSION		**C94.21**	Acute megakaryoblastic leukemia, in remission
207.22	MEGAKARYOCYTIC LEUKEMIA IN RELAPSE		**C94.22**	Acute megakaryoblastic leukemia, in relapse
207.80	OTHER SPEC LEUKEMIA W/O ACHIEVED REMISSION		**C94.30** **C94.80**	Mast cell leukemia not having achieved remission Other specified leukemias not having achieved remission
207.81	OTHER SPECIFIED LEUKEMIA IN REMISSION		**C94.31** **C94.81**	Mast cell leukemia, in remission Other specified leukemias, in remission
207.82	OTHER SPECIFIED LEUKEMIA IN RELAPSE		**C94.32** **C94.82**	Mast cell leukemia, in relapse Other specified leukemias, in relapse
208.00	ACUTE LEUKEMIA UNS CELL W/O ACHIEVED REMISSION	➡	**C95.00**	Acute leukemia of unsp cell type not achieve remission
208.01	ACUTE LEUKEMIA UNSPECIFIED CELL TYPE REMISSION	➡	**C95.01**	Acute leukemia of unspecified cell type, in remission
208.02	ACUTE LEUKEMIA UNSPECIFIED CELL TYPE IN RELAPSE	➡	**C95.02**	Acute leukemia of unspecified cell type, in relapse
208.10	CHRON LEUKEMIA UNS CELL W/O ACHIEVED REMISSION	➡	**C95.10**	Chronic leukemia of unsp cell type not achieve remission
208.11	CHRONIC LEUKEMIA UNSPECIFIED CELL TYPE REMISSION	➡	**C95.11**	Chronic leukemia of unspecified cell type, in remission
208.12	CHRONIC LEUKEMIA UNS CELL TYPE IN RELAPSE	➡	**C95.12**	Chronic leukemia of unspecified cell type, in relapse
208.20	SUBACUTE LEUKEMIA UNS CELL W/O ACHIEVD REMISSION		**C95.90**	Leukemia, unspecified not having achieved remission
208.21	SUBACTUE LEUKEMIA UNSPEC CELL TYPE REMISSION		**C95.91**	Leukemia, unspecified, in remission
208.22	SUBACUTE LEUKEMIA UNS CELL TYPE IN RELAPSE		**C95.92**	Leukemia, unspecified, in relapse
208.80	OTH LEUKEMIA UNS CELL W/O ACHIEVED REMISSION		**C95.90**	Leukemia, unspecified not having achieved remission
208.81	OTHER LEUKEMIA UNSPECIFIED CELL TYPE REMISSION		**C95.91**	Leukemia, unspecified, in remission
208.82	OTHER LEUKEMIA UNSPECIFIED CELL TYPE IN RELAPSE		**C95.92**	Leukemia, unspecified, in relapse
208.90	UNS LEUKEMIA W/O MENTION ACHIEVED REMISSION		**C95.90**	Leukemia, unspecified not having achieved remission
208.91	UNSPECIFIED LEUKEMIA IN REMISSION		**C95.91**	Leukemia, unspecified, in remission
208.92	UNSPECIFIED LEUKEMIA IN RELAPSE		**C95.92**	Leukemia, unspecified, in relapse
209.00	MALIG CARCINOID TUMOR SMALL INTEST UNS PORTION	➡	**C7A.019**	Malignant carcinoid tumor of the sm int, unsp portion
209.01	MALIGNANT CARCINOID TUMOR OF THE DUODENUM	➡	**C7A.010**	Malignant carcinoid tumor of the duodenum
209.02	MALIGNANT CARCINOID TUMOR OF THE JEJUNUM	➡	**C7A.011**	Malignant carcinoid tumor of the jejunum
209.03	MALIGNANT CARCINOID TUMOR OF THE ILEUM	➡	**C7A.012**	Malignant carcinoid tumor of the ileum
209.10	MALIG CARCINOID TUMOR LARGE INTEST UNS PORTION	➡	**C7A.029**	Malignant carcinoid tumor of the lg int, unsp portion
209.11	MALIGNANT CARCINOID TUMOR OF THE APPENDIX	➡	**C7A.020**	Malignant carcinoid tumor of the appendix
209.12	MALIGNANT CARCINOID TUMOR OF THE CECUM	➡	**C7A.021**	Malignant carcinoid tumor of the cecum
209.13	MALIGNANT CARCINOID TUMOR OF THE ASCENDING COLON	➡	**C7A.022**	Malignant carcinoid tumor of the ascending colon
209.14	MALIGNANT CARCINOID TUMOR OF TRANSVERSE COLON	➡	**C7A.023**	Malignant carcinoid tumor of the transverse colon
209.15	MALIGNANT CARCINOID TUMOR OF DESCENDING COLON	➡	**C7A.024**	Malignant carcinoid tumor of the descending colon
209.16	MALIGNANT CARCINOID TUMOR OF THE SIGMOID COLON	➡	**C7A.025**	Malignant carcinoid tumor of the sigmoid colon
209.17	MALIGNANT CARCINOID TUMOR OF THE RECTUM	➡	**C7A.026**	Malignant carcinoid tumor of the rectum
209.20	MALIGNANT CARCINOID TUMOR UNKNOWN PRIMARY SITE	➡	**C7A.00**	Malignant carcinoid tumor of unspecified site
209.21	MALIGNANT CARCINOID TUMOR OF BRONCHUS AND LUNG	➡	**C7A.090**	Malignant carcinoid tumor of the bronchus and lung
209.22	MALIGNANT CARCINOID TUMOR OF THE THYMUS	➡	**C7A.091**	Malignant carcinoid tumor of the thymus
209.23	MALIGNANT CARCINOID TUMOR OF THE STOMACH	➡	**C7A.092**	Malignant carcinoid tumor of the stomach
209.24	MALIGNANT CARCINOID TUMOR OF THE KIDNEY	➡	**C7A.093**	Malignant carcinoid tumor of the kidney
209.25	MALIGNANT CARCINOID TUMOR OF FOREGUT NOS	➡	**C7A.094**	Malignant carcinoid tumor of the foregut NOS
209.26	MALIGNANT CARCINOID TUMOR OF MIDGUT NOS	➡	**C7A.095**	Malignant carcinoid tumor of the midgut NOS
209.27	MALIGNANT CARCINOID TUMOR OF HINDGUT NOS	➡	**C7A.096**	Malignant carcinoid tumor of the hindgut NOS
209.29	MALIGNANT CARCINOID TUMOR OF OTHER SITES	➡	**C7A.098**	Malignant carcinoid tumors of other sites
209.30	MALIG POORLY DIFF NEUROENDOCRINE CA ANY SITE		**C7A.1** **C7A.8**	Malignant poorly differentiated neuroendocrine tumors Other malignant neuroendocrine tumors
209.31	MERKEL CELL CARCINOMA OF THE FACE		**C4A.0** **C4A.10** **C4A.11** **C4A.12** **C4A.20** **C4A.21** **C4A.22** **C4A.30** **C4A.31** **C4A.39**	Merkel cell carcinoma of lip Merkel cell carcinoma of unsp eyelid, including canthus Merkel cell carcinoma of right eyelid, including canthus Merkel cell carcinoma of left eyelid, including canthus Merkel cell carcinoma of unsp ear and external auric canal Merkel cell carcinoma of right ear and external auric canal Merkel cell carcinoma of left ear and external auric canal Merkel cell carcinoma of unspecified part of face Merkel cell carcinoma of nose Merkel cell carcinoma of other parts of face
209.32	MERKEL CELL CARCINOMA OF THE SCALP AND NECK	➡	**C4A.4**	Merkel cell carcinoma of scalp and neck

[Brackets] indicate valid character values for each code. Character value meanings provided for each code grouping.

ICD-9-CM			ICD-10-CM	
2Ø9.33	MERKEL CELL CARCINOMA OF THE UPPER LIMB		**C4A.6Ø** **C4A.61** **C4A.62**	Merkel cell carcinoma of unsp upper limb, including shoulder Merkel cell carcinoma of right upper limb, inc shoulder Merkel cell carcinoma of left upper limb, including shoulder
2Ø9.34	MERKEL CELL CARCINOMA OF THE LOWER LIMB		**C4A.7Ø** **C4A.71** **C4A.72**	Merkel cell carcinoma of unsp lower limb, including hip Merkel cell carcinoma of right lower limb, including hip Merkel cell carcinoma of left lower limb, including hip
2Ø9.35	MERKEL CELL CARCINOMA OF THE TRUNK		**C4A.51** **C4A.52** **C4A.59**	Merkel cell carcinoma of anal skin Merkel cell carcinoma of skin of breast Merkel cell carcinoma of other part of trunk
2Ø9.36	MERKEL CELL CARCINOMA OF OTHER SITES		**C4A.8** **C4A.9**	Merkel cell carcinoma of overlapping sites Merkel cell carcinoma, unspecified
2Ø9.4Ø	BENIGN CARCINOID TUMOR SMALL INTEST UNS PORTION	➡	**D3A.Ø19**	Benign carcinoid tumor of the small intestine, unsp portion
2Ø9.41	BENIGN CARCINOID TUMOR OF THE DUODENUM	➡	**D3A.Ø1Ø**	Benign carcinoid tumor of the duodenum
2Ø9.42	BENIGN CARCINOID TUMOR OF THE JEJUNUM	➡	**D3A.Ø11**	Benign carcinoid tumor of the jejunum
2Ø9.43	BENIGN CARCINOID TUMOR OF THE ILEUM	➡	**D3A.Ø12**	Benign carcinoid tumor of the ileum
2Ø9.5Ø	BENIGN CARCINOID TUMOR LARGE INTEST UNS PORTION	➡	**D3A.Ø29**	Benign carcinoid tumor of the large intestine, unsp portion
2Ø9.51	BENIGN CARCINOID TUMOR OF THE APPENDIX	➡	**D3A.Ø2Ø**	Benign carcinoid tumor of the appendix
2Ø9.52	BENIGN CARCINOID TUMOR OF THE CECUM	➡	**D3A.Ø21**	Benign carcinoid tumor of the cecum
2Ø9.53	BENIGN CARCINOID TUMOR OF THE ASCENDING COLON	➡	**D3A.Ø22**	Benign carcinoid tumor of the ascending colon
2Ø9.54	BENIGN CARCINOID TUMOR OF THE TRANSVERSE COLON	➡	**D3A.Ø23**	Benign carcinoid tumor of the transverse colon
2Ø9.55	BENIGN CARCINOID TUMOR OF THE DESCENDING COLON	➡	**D3A.Ø24**	Benign carcinoid tumor of the descending colon
2Ø9.56	BENIGN CARCINOID TUMOR OF THE SIGMOID COLON	➡	**D3A.Ø25**	Benign carcinoid tumor of the sigmoid colon
2Ø9.57	BENIGN CARCINOID TUMOR OF THE RECTUM	➡	**D3A.Ø26**	Benign carcinoid tumor of the rectum
2Ø9.6Ø	BENIGN CARCINOID TUMOR UNKNOWN PRIMARY SITE		**D3A.ØØ** **D3A.8**	Benign carcinoid tumor of unspecified site Other benign neuroendocrine tumors
2Ø9.61	BENIGN CARCINOID TUMOR OF THE BRONCHUS AND LUNG	➡	**D3A.Ø9Ø**	Benign carcinoid tumor of the bronchus and lung
2Ø9.62	BENIGN CARCINOID TUMOR OF THE THYMUS	➡	**D3A.Ø91**	Benign carcinoid tumor of the thymus
2Ø9.63	BENIGN CARCINOID TUMOR OF THE STOMACH	➡	**D3A.Ø92**	Benign carcinoid tumor of the stomach
2Ø9.64	BENIGN CARCINOID TUMOR OF THE KIDNEY	➡	**D3A.Ø93**	Benign carcinoid tumor of the kidney
2Ø9.65	BENIGN CARCINOID TUMOR OF FOREGUT NOS	➡	**D3A.Ø94**	Benign carcinoid tumor of the foregut NOS
2Ø9.66	BENIGN CARCINOID TUMOR OF MIDGUT NOS	➡	**D3A.Ø95**	Benign carcinoid tumor of the midgut NOS
2Ø9.67	BENIGN CARCINOID TUMOR OF HINDGUT NOS	➡	**D3A.Ø96**	Benign carcinoid tumor of the hindgut NOS
2Ø9.69	BENIGN CARCINOID TUMOR OF OTHER SITES	➡	**D3A.Ø98**	Benign carcinoid tumors of other sites
2Ø9.7Ø	SECONDARY NEUROENDOCRINE TUMOR UNSPECIFIED SITE		**C7B.ØØ**	Secondary carcinoid tumors, unspecified site
2Ø9.71	SEC NEUROENDOCRINE TUMOR OF DISTANT LYMPH NODES		**C7B.Ø1**	Secondary carcinoid tumors of distant lymph nodes
2Ø9.72	SECONDARY NEUROENDOCRINE TUMOR OF LIVER		**C7B.Ø2**	Secondary carcinoid tumors of liver
2Ø9.73	SECONDARY NEUROENDOCRINE TUMOR OF BONE		**C7B.Ø3**	Secondary carcinoid tumors of bone
2Ø9.74	SECONDARY NEUROENDOCRINE TUMOR OF PERITONEUM		**C7B.Ø4**	Secondary carcinoid tumors of peritoneum
2Ø9.75	SECONDARY MERKEL CELL CARCINOMA		**C7B.1**	Secondary Merkel cell carcinoma
2Ø9.79	SECONDARY NEUROENDOCRINE TUMOR OF OTHER SITES		**C7B.Ø9** **C7B.8**	Secondary carcinoid tumors of other sites Other secondary neuroendocrine tumors
21Ø.Ø	BENIGN NEOPLASM OF LIP	➡	**D1Ø.Ø**	Benign neoplasm of lip
21Ø.1	BENIGN NEOPLASM OF TONGUE	➡	**D1Ø.1**	Benign neoplasm of tongue
21Ø.2	BENIGN NEOPLASM OF MAJOR SALIVARY GLANDS		**D11.Ø** **D11.7** **D11.9**	Benign neoplasm of parotid gland Benign neoplasm of other major salivary glands Benign neoplasm of major salivary gland, unspecified
21Ø.3	BENIGN NEOPLASM OF FLOOR OF MOUTH	➡	**D1Ø.2**	Benign neoplasm of floor of mouth
21Ø.4	BENIGN NEOPLASM OTHER&UNSPECIFIED PARTS MOUTH		**D1Ø.3Ø** **D1Ø.39**	Benign neoplasm of unspecified part of mouth Benign neoplasm of other parts of mouth
21Ø.5	BENIGN NEOPLASM OF TONSIL	➡	**D1Ø.4**	Benign neoplasm of tonsil
21Ø.6	BENIGN NEOPLASM OF OTHER PARTS OF OROPHARYNX	➡	**D1Ø.5**	Benign neoplasm of other parts of oropharynx
21Ø.7	BENIGN NEOPLASM OF NASOPHARYNX	➡	**D1Ø.6**	Benign neoplasm of nasopharynx
21Ø.8	BENIGN NEOPLASM OF HYPOPHARYNX	➡	**D1Ø.7**	Benign neoplasm of hypopharynx
21Ø.9	BENIGN NEOPLASM OF PHARYNX UNSPECIFIED	➡	**D1Ø.9**	Benign neoplasm of pharynx, unspecified
211.Ø	BENIGN NEOPLASM OF ESOPHAGUS	➡	**D13.Ø**	Benign neoplasm of esophagus
211.1	BENIGN NEOPLASM OF STOMACH		**D13.1** **K31.7**	Benign neoplasm of stomach Polyp of stomach and duodenum
211.2	BENIGN NEOPLASM OF DUODENUM JEJUNUM AND ILEUM		**D13.2** **D13.3Ø** **D13.39**	Benign neoplasm of duodenum Benign neoplasm of unspecified part of small intestine Benign neoplasm of other parts of small intestine
211.3	BENIGN NEOPLASM OF COLON		**D12.Ø** **D12.1** **D12.2** **D12.3** **D12.4** **D12.5** **D12.6** **K63.5**	Benign neoplasm of cecum Benign neoplasm of appendix Benign neoplasm of ascending colon Benign neoplasm of transverse colon Benign neoplasm of descending colon Benign neoplasm of sigmoid colon Benign neoplasm of colon, unspecified Polyp of colon
211.4	BENIGN NEOPLASM OF RECTUM AND ANAL CANAL		**D12.7** **D12.8** **D12.9**	Benign neoplasm of rectosigmoid junction Benign neoplasm of rectum Benign neoplasm of anus and anal canal

ICD-9-CM			ICD-10-CM	
211.5	BENIGN NEOPLASM OF LIVER AND BILIARY PASSAGES		D13.4	Benign neoplasm of liver
			D13.5	Benign neoplasm of extrahepatic bile ducts
211.6	BEN NEOPLASM PANCREAS EXCEPT ISLETS LANGERHANS	➡	D13.6	Benign neoplasm of pancreas
211.7	BENIGN NEOPLASM OF ISLETS OF LANGERHANS	➡	D13.7	Benign neoplasm of endocrine pancreas
211.8	BENIGN NEOPLASM OF RETROPERITONEUM&PERITONEUM		D19.1	Benign neoplasm of mesothelial tissue of peritoneum
			D20.0	Benign neoplasm of soft tissue of retroperitoneum
			D20.1	Benign neoplasm of soft tissue of peritoneum
211.9	BENIGN NEOPLASM OTH&UNSPEC SITE DIGESTIVE SYSTEM		D13.9	Benign neoplasm of ill-defined sites within the dgstv sys
212.0	BEN NEOPLASM NASL CAVITIES MID EAR&ACSS SINUSES	➡	D14.0	Benign neoplasm of mid ear, nasl cav and accessory sinuses
212.1	BENIGN NEOPLASM OF LARYNX	➡	D14.1	Benign neoplasm of larynx
212.2	BENIGN NEOPLASM OF TRACHEA	➡	D14.2	Benign neoplasm of trachea
212.3	BENIGN NEOPLASM OF BRONCHUS AND LUNG		D14.30	Benign neoplasm of unspecified bronchus and lung
			D14.31	Benign neoplasm of right bronchus and lung
			D14.32	Benign neoplasm of left bronchus and lung
212.4	BENIGN NEOPLASM OF PLEURA		D19.0	Benign neoplasm of mesothelial tissue of pleura
212.5	BENIGN NEOPLASM OF MEDIASTINUM	➡	D15.2	Benign neoplasm of mediastinum
212.6	BENIGN NEOPLASM OF THYMUS	➡	D15.0	Benign neoplasm of thymus
212.7	BENIGN NEOPLASM OF HEART	➡	D15.1	Benign neoplasm of heart
212.8	BEN NEOPLASM OTH SPEC SITES RESP&INTRATHOR ORGN		D15.7	Benign neoplasm of other specified intrathoracic organs
212.9	BEN NEOPLASM RESP&INTRATHORACIC ORGN SITE UNSPEC		D14.4	Benign neoplasm of respiratory system, unspecified
			D15.9	Benign neoplasm of intrathoracic organ, unspecified
213.0	BENIGN NEOPLASM OF BONES OF SKULL AND FACE	➡	D16.4	Benign neoplasm of bones of skull and face
213.1	BENIGN NEOPLASM OF LOWER JAW BONE	➡	D16.5	Benign neoplasm of lower jaw bone
213.2	BEN NEOPLASM VERT COLUMN EXCLD SACRUM&COCCYX	➡	D16.6	Benign neoplasm of vertebral column
213.3	BENIGN NEOPLASM OF RIBS STERNUM AND CLAVICLE	➡	D16.7	Benign neoplasm of ribs, sternum and clavicle
213.4	BENIGN NEOPLASM SCAPULA&LONG BONES UPPER LIMB		D16.00	Benign neoplasm of scapula and long bones of unsp upper limb
			D16.01	Benign neoplm of scapula and long bones of right upper limb
			D16.02	Benign neoplasm of scapula and long bones of left upper limb
213.5	BENIGN NEOPLASM OF SHORT BONES OF UPPER LIMB		D16.10	Benign neoplasm of short bones of unspecified upper limb
			D16.11	Benign neoplasm of short bones of right upper limb
			D16.12	Benign neoplasm of short bones of left upper limb
213.6	BENIGN NEOPLASM OF PELVIC BONES SACRUM&COCCYX	➡	D16.8	Benign neoplasm of pelvic bones, sacrum and coccyx
213.7	BENIGN NEOPLASM OF LONG BONES OF LOWER LIMB		D16.20	Benign neoplasm of long bones of unspecified lower limb
			D16.21	Benign neoplasm of long bones of right lower limb
			D16.22	Benign neoplasm of long bones of left lower limb
213.8	BENIGN NEOPLASM OF SHORT BONES OF LOWER LIMB		D16.30	Benign neoplasm of short bones of unspecified lower limb
			D16.31	Benign neoplasm of short bones of right lower limb
			D16.32	Benign neoplasm of short bones of left lower limb
213.9	BEN NEOPLASM BONE&ARTICLR CARTILAGE SITE UNSPEC	➡	D16.9	Benign neoplasm of bone and articular cartilage, unspecified
214.0	LIPOMA OF SKIN AND SUBCUTANEOUS TISSUE OF FACE		D17.0	Ben lipomatous neoplm of skin, subcu of head, face and neck
214.1	LIPOMA OF OTHER SKIN AND SUBCUTANEOUS TISSUE		D17.1	Benign lipomatous neoplasm of skin, subcu of trunk
			D17.20	Benign lipomatous neoplasm of skin, subcu of unsp limb
			D17.21	Benign lipomatous neoplasm of skin, subcu of right arm
			D17.22	Benign lipomatous neoplasm of skin, subcu of left arm
			D17.23	Benign lipomatous neoplasm of skin, subcu of right leg
			D17.24	Benign lipomatous neoplasm of skin, subcu of left leg
			D17.30	Benign lipomatous neoplasm of skin, subcu of unsp sites
			D17.39	Benign lipomatous neoplasm of skin, subcu of sites
214.2	LIPOMA OF INTRATHORACIC ORGANS	➡	D17.4	Benign lipomatous neoplasm of intrathoracic organs
214.3	LIPOMA OF INTRA-ABDOMINAL ORGANS		D17.5	Benign lipomatous neoplasm of intra-abdominal organs
			D17.71	Benign lipomatous neoplasm of kidney
214.4	LIPOMA OF SPERMATIC CORD	➡	D17.6	Benign lipomatous neoplasm of spermatic cord
214.8	LIPOMA OF OTHER SPECIFIED SITES		D17.72	Benign lipomatous neoplasm of other genitourinary organ
			D17.79	Benign lipomatous neoplasm of other sites
214.9	LIPOMA OF UNSPECIFIED SITE	➡	D17.9	Benign lipomatous neoplasm, unspecified
215.0	OTH BEN NEOPLSM CNCTV&OTH SFT TISS HEAD FCE&NCK	➡	D21.0	Benign neoplasm of connctv/soft tiss of head, face and neck
215.2	OTH BEN NEO CNCTV&OTH SFT TISS UP LIMB W/SHLDR		D21.10	Ben neoplm of connctv/soft tiss of unsp upr limb, inc shldr
			D21.11	Ben neoplm of connctv/soft tiss of r upper limb, inc shldr
			D21.12	Ben neoplm of connctv/soft tiss of left upr limb, inc shldr
215.3	OTH BEN NEOPLSM CNCTV&OTH SFT TISS LW LIMB W/HIP		D21.20	Ben neoplm of connctv/soft tiss of unsp lower limb, inc hip
			D21.21	Ben neoplm of connctv/soft tiss of right lower limb, inc hip
			D21.22	Ben neoplm of connctv/soft tiss of left lower limb, inc hip
215.4	OTH BEN NEOPLASM CONNECTIVE&OTH SOFT TISSUE THOR	➡	D21.3	Benign neoplasm of connective and oth soft tissue of thorax
215.5	OTH BEN NEOPLASM CONNECTIVE&OTH SOFT TISSUE ABD	➡	D21.4	Benign neoplasm of connective and oth soft tissue of abdomen
215.6	OTH BEN NEOPLASM CONNECTIVE&OTH SOFT TISSUE PELV	➡	D21.5	Benign neoplasm of connective and oth soft tissue of pelvis
215.7	OTH BEN NEOPLSM CNCTV&OTH SFT TISSUE TRNK UNSPEC	➡	D21.6	Benign neoplasm of connctv/soft tiss of trunk, unsp
215.8	OTH BEN NEOPLSM CNCTV&OTH SFT TISS OTH SPEC SITE		D21.9	Benign neoplasm of connective and other soft tissue, unsp

ICD-9-CM			ICD-10-CM	
215.9	OTH BEN NEOPLSM CNCTV&OTH SFT TISSUE UNSPEC SITE		**D21.9**	Benign neoplasm of connective and other soft tissue, unsp
			D36.1Ø	Benign neoplasm of prph nerves and autonm nervous sys, unsp
			D36.11	Ben neoplm of prph nerves and autonm nrv sys of face/hed/nk
			D36.12	Ben neoplm of prph nrv & autonm nrv sys, upr lmb, inc shldr
			D36.13	Ben neoplm of prph nrv & autonm nrv sys of low lmb, inc hip
			D36.14	Benign neoplm of prph nerves and autonm nrv sys of thorax
			D36.15	Benign neoplm of prph nerves and autonm nervous sys of abd
			D36.16	Benign neoplm of prph nerves and autonm nrv sys of pelvis
			D36.17	Ben neoplm of prph nerves and autonm nrv sys of trunk, unsp
216.Ø	BENIGN NEOPLASM OF SKIN OF LIP		**D22.Ø**	Melanocytic nevi of lip
			D23.Ø	Other benign neoplasm of skin of lip
216.1	BENIGN NEOPLASM OF EYELID INCLUDING CANTHUS		**D22.1Ø**	Melanocytic nevi of unspecified eyelid, including canthus
			D22.11	Melanocytic nevi of right eyelid, including canthus
			D22.12	Melanocytic nevi of left eyelid, including canthus
			D23.1Ø	Oth benign neoplasm skin/ unsp eyelid, including canthus
			D23.11	Oth benign neoplasm skin/ right eyelid, including canthus
			D23.12	Oth benign neoplasm skin/ left eyelid, including canthus
216.2	BENIGN NEOPLASM OF EAR&EXTERNAL AUDITORY CANAL		**D22.2Ø**	Melanocytic nevi of unsp ear and external auricular canal
			D22.21	Melanocytic nevi of right ear and external auricular canal
			D22.22	Melanocytic nevi of left ear and external auricular canal
			D23.2Ø	Oth benign neoplasm skin/ unsp ear and external auric canal
			D23.21	Oth benign neoplasm skin/ right ear and external auric canal
			D23.22	Oth benign neoplasm skin/ left ear and external auric canal
216.3	BENIGN NEOPLASM SKIN OTHER&UNSPEC PARTS FACE		**D22.3Ø**	Melanocytic nevi of unspecified part of face
			D22.39	Melanocytic nevi of other parts of face
			D23.3Ø	Other benign neoplasm of skin of unspecified part of face
			D23.39	Other benign neoplasm of skin of other parts of face
216.4	BENIGN NEOPLASM OF SCALP AND SKIN OF NECK		**D22.4**	Melanocytic nevi of scalp and neck
			D23.4	Other benign neoplasm of skin of scalp and neck
216.5	BENIGN NEOPLASM OF SKIN OF TRUNK EXCEPT SCROTUM		**D22.5**	Melanocytic nevi of trunk
			D23.5	Other benign neoplasm of skin of trunk
216.6	BEN NEOPLASM SKIN UPPER LIMB INCLUDING SHOULDER		**D22.6Ø**	Melanocytic nevi of unsp upper limb, including shoulder
			D22.61	Melanocytic nevi of right upper limb, including shoulder
			D22.62	Melanocytic nevi of left upper limb, including shoulder
			D23.6Ø	Oth benign neoplasm skin/ unsp upper limb, inc shoulder
			D23.61	Oth benign neoplasm skin/ right upper limb, inc shoulder
			D23.62	Oth benign neoplasm skin/ left upper limb, inc shoulder
216.7	BENIGN NEOPLASM SKIN LOWER LIMB INCLUDING HIP		**D22.7Ø**	Melanocytic nevi of unspecified lower limb, including hip
			D22.71	Melanocytic nevi of right lower limb, including hip
			D22.72	Melanocytic nevi of left lower limb, including hip
			D23.7Ø	Oth benign neoplasm skin/ unsp lower limb, including hip
			D23.71	Oth benign neoplasm skin/ right lower limb, including hip
			D23.72	Oth benign neoplasm skin/ left lower limb, including hip
216.8	BENIGN NEOPLASM OF OTHER SPECIFIED SITES OF SKIN		**D22.9**	Melanocytic nevi, unspecified
			D23.9	Other benign neoplasm of skin, unspecified
216.9	BENIGN NEOPLASM OF SKIN SITE UNSPECIFIED		**D22.9**	Melanocytic nevi, unspecified
			D23.9	Other benign neoplasm of skin, unspecified
217	BENIGN NEOPLASM OF BREAST		**D24.1**	Benign neoplasm of right breast
			D24.2	Benign neoplasm of left breast
			D24.9	Benign neoplasm of unspecified breast
218.Ø	SUBMUCOUS LEIOMYOMA OF UTERUS	➡	**D25.Ø**	Submucous leiomyoma of uterus
218.1	INTRAMURAL LEIOMYOMA OF UTERUS	➡	**D25.1**	Intramural leiomyoma of uterus
218.2	SUBSEROUS LEIOMYOMA OF UTERUS	➡	**D25.2**	Subserosal leiomyoma of uterus
218.9	LEIOMYOMA OF UTERUS, UNSPECIFIED	➡	**D25.9**	Leiomyoma of uterus, unspecified
219.Ø	BENIGN NEOPLASM OF CERVIX UTERI	➡	**D26.Ø**	Other benign neoplasm of cervix uteri
219.1	BENIGN NEOPLASM OF CORPUS UTERI	➡	**D26.1**	Other benign neoplasm of corpus uteri
219.8	BENIGN NEOPLASM OTHER SPECIFIED PARTS UTERUS	➡	**D26.7**	Other benign neoplasm of other parts of uterus
219.9	BENIGN NEOPLASM OF UTERUS PART UNSPECIFIED	➡	**D26.9**	Other benign neoplasm of uterus, unspecified
22Ø	BENIGN NEOPLASM OF OVARY		**D27.Ø**	Benign neoplasm of right ovary
			D27.1	Benign neoplasm of left ovary
			D27.9	Benign neoplasm of unspecified ovary
221.Ø	BENIGN NEOPLASM FALLOPIAN TUBE&UTERINE LIGAMENTS	➡	**D28.2**	Benign neoplasm of uterine tubes and ligaments
221.1	BENIGN NEOPLASM OF VAGINA	➡	**D28.1**	Benign neoplasm of vagina
221.2	BENIGN NEOPLASM OF VULVA	➡	**D28.Ø**	Benign neoplasm of vulva
221.8	BEN NEOPLASM OTH SPEC SITES FE GENITAL ORGANS	➡	**D28.7**	Benign neoplasm of other specified female genital organs
221.9	BENIGN NEOPLASM FEMALE GENITAL ORGAN SITE UNSPEC	➡	**D28.9**	Benign neoplasm of female genital organ, unspecified
222.Ø	BENIGN NEOPLASM OF TESTIS		**D29.2Ø**	Benign neoplasm of unspecified testis
			D29.21	Benign neoplasm of right testis
			D29.22	Benign neoplasm of left testis
222.1	BENIGN NEOPLASM OF PENIS	➡	**D29.Ø**	Benign neoplasm of penis
222.2	BENIGN NEOPLASM OF PROSTATE	➡	**D29.1**	Benign neoplasm of prostate
222.3	BENIGN NEOPLASM OF EPIDIDYMIS		**D29.3Ø**	Benign neoplasm of unspecified epididymis
			D29.31	Benign neoplasm of right epididymis
			D29.32	Benign neoplasm of left epididymis
222.4	BENIGN NEOPLASM OF SCROTUM	➡	**D29.4**	Benign neoplasm of scrotum

ICD-9-CM			ICD-10-CM	
222.8	BEN NEOPLASM OTH SPEC SITES MALE GENITAL ORGANS	➡	D29.8	Benign neoplasm of other specified male genital organs
222.9	BENIGN NEOPLASM MALE GENITAL ORGAN SITE UNSPEC	➡	D29.9	Benign neoplasm of male genital organ, unspecified
223.Ø	BENIGN NEOPLASM OF KIDNEY EXCEPT PELVIS		D3Ø.ØØ D3Ø.Ø1 D3Ø.Ø2	Benign neoplasm of unspecified kidney Benign neoplasm of right kidney Benign neoplasm of left kidney
223.1	BENIGN NEOPLASM OF RENAL PELVIS		D3Ø.1Ø D3Ø.11 D3Ø.12	Benign neoplasm of unspecified renal pelvis Benign neoplasm of right renal pelvis Benign neoplasm of left renal pelvis
223.2	BENIGN NEOPLASM OF URETER		D3Ø.2Ø D3Ø.21 D3Ø.22	Benign neoplasm of unspecified ureter Benign neoplasm of right ureter Benign neoplasm of left ureter
223.3	BENIGN NEOPLASM OF BLADDER	➡	D3Ø.3	Benign neoplasm of bladder
223.81	BENIGN NEOPLASM OF URETHRA	➡	D3Ø.4	Benign neoplasm of urethra
223.89	BENIGN NEOPLASM OTHER SPEC SITES URINARY ORGANS	➡	D3Ø.8	Benign neoplasm of other specified urinary organs
223.9	BENIGN NEOPLASM URINARY ORGAN SITE UNSPECIFIED	➡	D3Ø.9	Benign neoplasm of urinary organ, unspecified
224.Ø	BEN NEO EYEBALL NO CONJUNCT CORN RETINA&CHOROID		D31.4Ø D31.41 D31.42	Benign neoplasm of unspecified ciliary body Benign neoplasm of right ciliary body Benign neoplasm of left ciliary body
224.1	BENIGN NEOPLASM OF ORBIT		D31.6Ø D31.61 D31.62	Benign neoplasm of unspecified site of unspecified orbit Benign neoplasm of unspecified site of right orbit Benign neoplasm of unspecified site of left orbit
224.2	BENIGN NEOPLASM OF LACRIMAL GLAND		D31.5Ø D31.51 D31.52	Benign neoplasm of unspecified lacrimal gland and duct Benign neoplasm of right lacrimal gland and duct Benign neoplasm of left lacrimal gland and duct
224.3	BENIGN NEOPLASM OF CONJUNCTIVA		D31.ØØ D31.Ø1 D31.Ø2	Benign neoplasm of unspecified conjunctiva Benign neoplasm of right conjunctiva Benign neoplasm of left conjunctiva
224.4	BENIGN NEOPLASM OF CORNEA		D31.1Ø D31.11 D31.12	Benign neoplasm of unspecified cornea Benign neoplasm of right cornea Benign neoplasm of left cornea
224.5	BENIGN NEOPLASM OF RETINA		D31.2Ø D31.21 D31.22	Benign neoplasm of unspecified retina Benign neoplasm of right retina Benign neoplasm of left retina
224.6	BENIGN NEOPLASM OF CHOROID		D31.3Ø D31.31 D31.32	Benign neoplasm of unspecified choroid Benign neoplasm of right choroid Benign neoplasm of left choroid
224.7	BENIGN NEOPLASM OF LACRIMAL DUCT		D31.5Ø D31.51 D31.52	Benign neoplasm of unspecified lacrimal gland and duct Benign neoplasm of right lacrimal gland and duct Benign neoplasm of left lacrimal gland and duct
224.8	BENIGN NEOPLASM OF OTHER SPECIFIED PARTS OF EYE		D31.9Ø D31.91 D31.92	Benign neoplasm of unspecified part of unspecified eye Benign neoplasm of unspecified part of right eye Benign neoplasm of unspecified part of left eye
224.9	BENIGN NEOPLASM OF EYE PART UNSPECIFIED		D31.9Ø D31.91 D31.92	Benign neoplasm of unspecified part of unspecified eye Benign neoplasm of unspecified part of right eye Benign neoplasm of unspecified part of left eye
225.Ø	BENIGN NEOPLASM OF BRAIN		D33.Ø D33.1 D33.2	Benign neoplasm of brain, supratentorial Benign neoplasm of brain, infratentorial Benign neoplasm of brain, unspecified
225.1	BENIGN NEOPLASM OF CRANIAL NERVES	➡	D33.3	Benign neoplasm of cranial nerves
225.2	BENIGN NEOPLASM OF CEREBRAL MENINGES		D32.Ø D32.9	Benign neoplasm of cerebral meninges Benign neoplasm of meninges, unspecified
225.3	BENIGN NEOPLASM OF SPINAL CORD	➡	D33.4	Benign neoplasm of spinal cord
225.4	BENIGN NEOPLASM OF SPINAL MENINGES	➡	D32.1	Benign neoplasm of spinal meninges
225.8	BENIGN NEOPLASM OTHER SPEC SITES NERVOUS SYSTEM	➡	D33.7	Benign neoplasm of oth parts of central nervous system
225.9	BENIGN NEOPLASM NERVOUS SYSTEM PART UNSPECIFIED		D33.9	Benign neoplasm of central nervous system, unspecified
226	BENIGN NEOPLASM OF THYROID GLANDS	➡	D34	Benign neoplasm of thyroid gland
227.Ø	BENIGN NEOPLASM OF ADRENAL GLAND		D35.ØØ D35.Ø1 D35.Ø2	Benign neoplasm of unspecified adrenal gland Benign neoplasm of right adrenal gland Benign neoplasm of left adrenal gland
227.1	BENIGN NEOPLASM OF PARATHYROID GLAND	➡	D35.1	Benign neoplasm of parathyroid gland
227.3	BEN NEO PITUITARY GLAND&CRANIOPHARYNGEAL DUCT		D35.2 D35.3	Benign neoplasm of pituitary gland Benign neoplasm of craniopharyngeal duct
227.4	BENIGN NEOPLASM OF PINEAL GLAND	➡	D35.4	Benign neoplasm of pineal gland
227.5	BENIGN NEOPLASM OF CAROTID BODY	➡	D35.5	Benign neoplasm of carotid body
227.6	BENIGN NEOPLASM OF AORTIC BODY&OTHER PARAGANGLIA	➡	D35.6	Benign neoplasm of aortic body and other paraganglia
227.8	BEN NEOPLASM OTH ENDOCRN GLANDS&RELATED STRCT		D35.7	Benign neoplasm of other specified endocrine glands
227.9	BENIGN NEOPLASM ENDOCRINE GLAND SITE UNSPECIFIED	➡	D35.9	Benign neoplasm of endocrine gland, unspecified
228.ØØ	HEMANGIOMA OF UNSPECIFIED SITE	➡	D18.ØØ	Hemangioma unspecified site
228.Ø1	HEMANGIOMA OF SKIN AND SUBCUTANEOUS TISSUE	➡	D18.Ø1	Hemangioma of skin and subcutaneous tissue
228.Ø2	HEMANGIOMA OF INTRACRANIAL STRUCTURES	➡	D18.Ø2	Hemangioma of intracranial structures
228.Ø3	HEMANGIOMA OF RETINA		D18.Ø9	Hemangioma of other sites
228.Ø4	HEMANGIOMA OF INTRA-ABDOMINAL STRUCTURES	➡	D18.Ø3	Hemangioma of intra-abdominal structures
228.Ø9	HEMANGIOMA OF OTHER SITES		D18.Ø9	Hemangioma of other sites

ICD-9-CM		ICD-10-CM	
228.1	LYMPHANGIOMA, ANY SITE	➡ **D18.1**	Lymphangioma, any site
229.0	BENIGN NEOPLASM OF LYMPH NODES	➡ **D36.0**	Benign neoplasm of lymph nodes
229.8	BENIGN NEOPLASM OF OTHER SPECIFIED SITES	**D19.7** **D36.7**	Benign neoplasm of mesothelial tissue of other sites Benign neoplasm of other specified sites
229.9	BENIGN NEOPLASM OF UNSPECIFIED SITE	**D19.9** **D36.9**	Benign neoplasm of mesothelial tissue, unspecified Benign neoplasm, unspecified site
230.0	CARCINOMA IN SITU OF LIP ORAL CAVITY AND PHARYNX	**D00.00** **D00.01** **D00.02** **D00.03** **D00.04** **D00.05** **D00.06** **D00.07** **D00.08**	Carcinoma in situ of oral cavity, unspecified site Carcinoma in situ of labial mucosa and vermilion border Carcinoma in situ of buccal mucosa Carcinoma in situ of gingiva and edentulous alveolar ridge Carcinoma in situ of soft palate Carcinoma in situ of hard palate Carcinoma in situ of floor of mouth Carcinoma in situ of tongue Carcinoma in situ of pharynx
230.1	CARCINOMA IN SITU OF ESOPHAGUS	➡ **D00.1**	Carcinoma in situ of esophagus
230.2	CARCINOMA IN SITU OF STOMACH	➡ **D00.2**	Carcinoma in situ of stomach
230.3	CARCINOMA IN SITU OF COLON	➡ **D01.0**	Carcinoma in situ of colon
230.4	CARCINOMA IN SITU OF RECTUM	**D01.1** **D01.2**	Carcinoma in situ of rectosigmoid junction Carcinoma in situ of rectum
230.5	CARCINOMA IN SITU OF ANAL CANAL	**D01.3**	Carcinoma in situ of anus and anal canal
230.6	CARCINOMA IN SITU OF ANUS UNSPECIFIED	**D01.3**	Carcinoma in situ of anus and anal canal
230.7	CARCINOMA SITU OTHER&UNSPECIFIED PARTS INTESTINE	**D01.40** **D01.49**	Carcinoma in situ of unspecified part of intestine Carcinoma in situ of other parts of intestine
230.8	CARCINOMA IN SITU OF LIVER AND BILIARY SYSTEM	➡ **D01.5**	Carcinoma in situ of liver, gallbladder and bile ducts
230.9	CARCINOMA SITU OTHER&UNSPEC DIGESTIVE ORGANS	**D01.7** **D01.9**	Carcinoma in situ of other specified digestive organs Carcinoma in situ of digestive organ, unspecified
231.0	CARCINOMA IN SITU OF LARYNX	➡ **D02.0**	Carcinoma in situ of larynx
231.1	CARCINOMA IN SITU OF TRACHEA	➡ **D02.1**	Carcinoma in situ of trachea
231.2	CARCINOMA IN SITU OF BRONCHUS AND LUNG	**D02.20** **D02.21** **D02.22**	Carcinoma in situ of unspecified bronchus and lung Carcinoma in situ of right bronchus and lung Carcinoma in situ of left bronchus and lung
231.8	CARCINOMA SITU OTH SPEC PARTS RESPIRATORY SYSTEM	**D02.3**	Carcinoma in situ of other parts of respiratory system
231.9	CARCINOMA SITU RESPIRATORY SYSTEM PART UNSPEC	➡ **D02.4**	Carcinoma in situ of respiratory system, unspecified
232.0	CARCINOMA IN SITU OF SKIN OF LIP	**D04.0**	Carcinoma in situ of skin of lip
232.1	CARCINOMA IN SITU OF EYELID INCLUDING CANTHUS	**D04.10** **D04.11** **D04.12**	Carcinoma in situ of skin of unsp eyelid, including canthus Carcinoma in situ of skin of right eyelid, including canthus Carcinoma in situ of skin of left eyelid, including canthus
232.2	CARCINOMA SITU SKIN EAR&EXTERNAL AUDITORY CANAL	**D04.20** **D04.21** **D04.22**	Ca in situ skin of unsp ear and external auricular canal Ca in situ skin of right ear and external auricular canal Ca in situ skin of left ear and external auricular canal
232.3	CARCINOMA SITU SKIN OTHER&UNSPECIFIED PARTS FACE	**D04.30** **D04.39**	Carcinoma in situ of skin of unspecified part of face Carcinoma in situ of skin of other parts of face
232.4	CARCINOMA IN SITU OF SCALP AND SKIN OF NECK	**D04.4**	Carcinoma in situ of skin of scalp and neck
232.5	CARCINOMA SITU OF SKIN OF TRUNK EXCEPT SCROTUM	**D04.5**	Carcinoma in situ of skin of trunk
232.6	CA SITU SKIN UPPER LIMB INCLUDING SHOULDER	**D04.60** **D04.61** **D04.62**	Ca in situ skin of unsp upper limb, including shoulder Ca in situ skin of right upper limb, including shoulder Ca in situ skin of left upper limb, including shoulder
232.7	CARCINOMA SITU SKIN LOWER LIMB INCLUDING HIP	**D04.70** **D04.71** **D04.72**	Carcinoma in situ of skin of unsp lower limb, including hip Carcinoma in situ of skin of right lower limb, including hip Carcinoma in situ of skin of left lower limb, including hip
232.8	CARCINOMA SITU OF OTHER SPECIFIED SITES OF SKIN	**D04.8**	Carcinoma in situ of skin of other sites
232.9	CARCINOMA IN SITU OF SKIN SITE UNSPECIFIED	**D04.9**	Carcinoma in situ of skin, unspecified
233.0	CARCINOMA IN SITU OF BREAST	**D05.00** **D05.01** **D05.02** **D05.10** **D05.11** **D05.12** **D05.80** **D05.81** **D05.82** **D05.90** **D05.91** **D05.92**	Lobular carcinoma in situ of unspecified breast Lobular carcinoma in situ of right breast Lobular carcinoma in situ of left breast Intraductal carcinoma in situ of unspecified breast Intraductal carcinoma in situ of right breast Intraductal carcinoma in situ of left breast Oth type of carcinoma in situ of unspecified breast Other specified type of carcinoma in situ of right breast Other specified type of carcinoma in situ of left breast Unspecified type of carcinoma in situ of unspecified breast Unspecified type of carcinoma in situ of right breast Unspecified type of carcinoma in situ of left breast
233.1	CARCINOMA IN SITU OF CERVIX UTERI	**D06.0** **D06.1** **D06.7** **D06.9**	Carcinoma in situ of endocervix Carcinoma in situ of exocervix Carcinoma in situ of other parts of cervix Carcinoma in situ of cervix, unspecified
233.2	CARCINOMA SITU OTHER&UNSPECIFIED PARTS UTERUS	**D07.0**	Carcinoma in situ of endometrium
233.30	CARCINOMA IN SITU UNS FEMALE GENITAL ORGAN	➡ **D07.30**	Carcinoma in situ of unspecified female genital organs
233.31	CARCINOMA IN SITU VAGINA	➡ **D07.2**	Carcinoma in situ of vagina
233.32	CARCINOMA IN SITU VULVA	➡ **D07.1**	Carcinoma in situ of vulva
233.39	CARCINOMA IN SITU OTHER FEMALE GENITAL ORGAN	**D07.39**	Carcinoma in situ of other female genital organs

ICD-9-CM		ICD-10-CM		
233.4	CARCINOMA IN SITU OF PROSTATE	➡	**DØ7.5**	Carcinoma in situ of prostate
233.5	CARCINOMA IN SITU OF PENIS	➡	**DØ7.4**	Carcinoma in situ of penis
233.6	CARCINOMA SITU OTHER&UNSPEC MALE GENITAL ORGANS		**DØ7.6Ø**	Carcinoma in situ of unspecified male genital organs
			DØ7.61	Carcinoma in situ of scrotum
			DØ7.69	Carcinoma in situ of other male genital organs
233.7	CARCINOMA IN SITU OF BLADDER	➡	**DØ9.Ø**	Carcinoma in situ of bladder
233.9	CARCINOMA SITU OTHER&UNSPECIFIED URINARY ORGANS		**DØ9.1Ø**	Carcinoma in situ of unspecified urinary organ
			DØ9.19	Carcinoma in situ of other urinary organs
234.Ø	CARCINOMA IN SITU OF EYE		**DØ9.2Ø**	Carcinoma in situ of unspecified eye
			DØ9.21	Carcinoma in situ of right eye
			DØ9.22	Carcinoma in situ of left eye
234.8	CARCINOMA IN SITU OF OTHER SPECIFIED SITES		**DØ9.3**	Carcinoma in situ of thyroid and other endocrine glands
			DØ9.8	Carcinoma in situ of other specified sites
234.9	CARCINOMA IN SITU, SITE UNSPECIFIED	➡	**DØ9.9**	Carcinoma in situ, unspecified
235.Ø	NEOPLASM UNCERTAIN BEHAVIOR MAJOR SALIV GLANDS		**D37.Ø3Ø**	Neoplasm of uncertain behavior of the parotid salivary gland
			D37.Ø31	Neoplasm of uncrt behavior of the sublingual salivary gland
			D37.Ø32	Neoplasm of uncrt behav of the submandibular salivary gland
			D37.Ø39	Neoplasm of uncrt behavior of the major salivary gland, unsp
235.1	NEOPLASM UNCERTAIN BHV LIP ORAL CAVITY&PHARYNX		**D37.Ø1**	Neoplasm of uncertain behavior of lip
			D37.Ø2	Neoplasm of uncertain behavior of tongue
			D37.Ø4	Neoplasm of uncertain behavior of the minor salivary glands
			D37.Ø5	Neoplasm of uncertain behavior of pharynx
			D37.Ø9	Neoplasm of uncertain behavior of sites of the oral cavity
235.2	NEOPLASM UNCERTAIN BEHAVIOR STOMACH INTEST&RECT		**D37.1**	Neoplasm of uncertain behavior of stomach
			D37.2	Neoplasm of uncertain behavior of small intestine
			D37.3	Neoplasm of uncertain behavior of appendix
			D37.4	Neoplasm of uncertain behavior of colon
			D37.5	Neoplasm of uncertain behavior of rectum
235.3	NEOPLASM UNCERTAIN BEHAVIOR LIVER&BILI PASSAGES	➡	**D37.6**	Neoplasm of uncertain behavior of liver, GB & bile duct
235.4	NEOPLASM UNCERTAIN BEHAVIOR RETROPERITON&PERITON		**D48.3**	Neoplasm of uncertain behavior of retroperitoneum
			D48.4	Neoplasm of uncertain behavior of peritoneum
235.5	NEOPLASM UNCERTAIN BHV OTH&UNSPEC DIGESTIVE ORGN		**D37.8**	Neoplasm of uncertain behavior of oth digestive organs
			D37.9	Neoplasm of uncertain behavior of digestive organ, unsp
235.6	NEOPLASM OF UNCERTAIN BEHAVIOR OF LARYNX	➡	**D38.Ø**	Neoplasm of uncertain behavior of larynx
235.7	NEOPLASM UNCERTAIN BEHAVIOR TRACH BRONCHUS&LUNG	➡	**D38.1**	Neoplasm of uncertain behavior of trachea, bronchus and lung
235.8	NEOPLASM UNCERTAIN BEHAVIOR PLEU THYMUS&MEDIAST		**D38.2**	Neoplasm of uncertain behavior of pleura
			D38.3	Neoplasm of uncertain behavior of mediastinum
			D38.4	Neoplasm of uncertain behavior of thymus
235.9	NEOPLASM UNCERTAIN BEHAVIOR OTH&UNSPEC RESP ORGN		**D38.5**	Neoplasm of uncertain behavior of other respiratory organs
			D38.6	Neoplasm of uncertain behavior of respiratory organ, unsp
236.Ø	NEOPLASM OF UNCERTAIN BEHAVIOR OF UTERUS	➡	**D39.Ø**	Neoplasm of uncertain behavior of uterus
236.1	NEOPLASM OF UNCERTAIN BEHAVIOR OF PLACENTA	➡	**D39.2**	Neoplasm of uncertain behavior of placenta
236.2	NEOPLASM OF UNCERTAIN BEHAVIOR OF OVARY		**D39.1Ø**	Neoplasm of uncertain behavior of unspecified ovary
			D39.11	Neoplasm of uncertain behavior of right ovary
			D39.12	Neoplasm of uncertain behavior of left ovary
236.3	NEOPLASM UNCERTAIN BHV OTH&UNSPEC FE GENIT ORGN		**D39.8**	Neoplasm of uncertain behavior of oth female genital organs
			D39.9	Neoplasm of uncertain behavior of female genital organ, unsp
236.4	NEOPLASM OF UNCERTAIN BEHAVIOR OF TESTIS		**D4Ø.1Ø**	Neoplasm of uncertain behavior of unspecified testis
			D4Ø.11	Neoplasm of uncertain behavior of right testis
			D4Ø.12	Neoplasm of uncertain behavior of left testis
236.5	NEOPLASM OF UNCERTAIN BEHAVIOR OF PROSTATE	➡	**D4Ø.Ø**	Neoplasm of uncertain behavior of prostate
236.6	NEOPLSM UNCERTAIN BHV OTH&UNSPEC MALE GENIT ORGN		**D4Ø.8**	Neoplasm of uncertain behavior of oth male genital organs
			D4Ø.9	Neoplasm of uncertain behavior of male genital organ, unsp
236.7	NEOPLASM OF UNCERTAIN BEHAVIOR OF BLADDER	➡	**D41.4**	Neoplasm of uncertain behavior of bladder
236.9Ø	NEOPLASM UNCERTAIN BEHAVIOR URINARY ORGAN UNSPEC	➡	**D41.9**	Neoplasm of uncertain behavior of unspecified urinary organ
236.91	NEOPLASM OF UNCERTAIN BEHAVIOR OF KIDNEY&URETER		**D41.ØØ**	Neoplasm of uncertain behavior of unspecified kidney
			D41.Ø1	Neoplasm of uncertain behavior of right kidney
			D41.Ø2	Neoplasm of uncertain behavior of left kidney
			D41.1Ø	Neoplasm of uncertain behavior of unspecified renal pelvis
			D41.11	Neoplasm of uncertain behavior of right renal pelvis
			D41.12	Neoplasm of uncertain behavior of left renal pelvis
			D41.2Ø	Neoplasm of uncertain behavior of unspecified ureter
			D41.21	Neoplasm of uncertain behavior of right ureter
			D41.22	Neoplasm of uncertain behavior of left ureter
236.99	NEOPLASM UNCERTAIN BEHAVIOR OTH&UNSPEC URIN ORGN		**D41.3**	Neoplasm of uncertain behavior of urethra
			D41.8	Neoplasm of uncertain behavior of oth urinary organs
237.Ø	NEO UNCRT BHV PITUIT GLAND&CRANIOPHARYNGEAL DUCT		**D44.3**	Neoplasm of uncertain behavior of pituitary gland
			D44.4	Neoplasm of uncertain behavior of craniopharyngeal duct
237.1	NEOPLASM OF UNCERTAIN BEHAVIOR OF PINEAL GLAND	➡	**D44.5**	Neoplasm of uncertain behavior of pineal gland
237.2	NEOPLASM OF UNCERTAIN BEHAVIOR OF ADRENAL GLAND		**D44.1Ø**	Neoplasm of uncertain behavior of unspecified adrenal gland
			D44.11	Neoplasm of uncertain behavior of right adrenal gland
			D44.12	Neoplasm of uncertain behavior of left adrenal gland
237.3	NEOPLASM OF UNCERTAIN BEHAVIOR OF PARAGANGLIA		**D44.6**	Neoplasm of uncertain behavior of carotid body
			D44.7	Neoplasm of uncrt behav of aortic body and oth paraganglia

ICD-9-CM			ICD-10-CM	
237.4	NEOPLASM UNCERTAIN BHV OTH&UNSPEC ENDOCRN GLANDS		D44.Ø	Neoplasm of uncertain behavior of thyroid gland
			D44.2	Neoplasm of uncertain behavior of parathyroid gland
			D44.9	Neoplasm of uncertain behavior of unsp endocrine gland
237.5	NEOPLASM UNCERTAIN BEHAVIOR BRAIN&SPINAL CORD		D43.Ø	Neoplasm of uncertain behavior of brain, supratentorial
			D43.1	Neoplasm of uncertain behavior of brain, infratentorial
			D43.2	Neoplasm of uncertain behavior of brain, unspecified
			D43.4	Neoplasm of uncertain behavior of spinal cord
237.6	NEOPLASM OF UNCERTAIN BEHAVIOR OF MENINGES		D42.Ø	Neoplasm of uncertain behavior of cerebral meninges
			D42.1	Neoplasm of uncertain behavior of spinal meninges
			D42.9	Neoplasm of uncertain behavior of meninges, unspecified
237.7Ø	NEUROFIBROMATOSIS, UNSPECIFIED	➡	Q85.ØØ	Neurofibromatosis, unspecified
237.71	NEUROFIBROMATOSIS, TYPE 1	➡	Q85.Ø1	Neurofibromatosis, type 1
237.72	NEUROFIBROMATOSIS, TYPE 2	➡	Q85.Ø2	Neurofibromatosis, type 2
237.73	SCHWANNOMATOSIS	➡	Q85.Ø3	Schwannomatosis
237.79	OTHER NEUROFIBROMATOSIS	➡	Q85.Ø9	Other neurofibromatosis
237.9	NEOPLSM UNCERTAIN BHV OTH&UNSPEC PART NERV SYS		D43.3	Neoplasm of uncertain behavior of cranial nerves
			D43.8	Neoplasm of uncertain behavior of prt central nervous system
			D43.9	Neoplasm of uncertain behavior of cnsl, unsp
238.Ø	NEOPLASM UNCERTAIN BEHAVIOR BONE&ARTICLR CART	➡	D48.Ø	Neoplasm of uncertain behavior of bone/artic cartl
238.1	NEOPLASM UNCERTAIN BHV CNCTV&OTH SOFT TISSUE		D48.1	Neoplasm of uncertain behavior of connctv/soft tiss
			D48.2	Neoplm of uncrt behav of prph nerves and autonm nervous sys
238.2	NEOPLASM OF UNCERTAIN BEHAVIOR OF SKIN	➡	D48.5	Neoplasm of uncertain behavior of skin
238.3	NEOPLASM OF UNCERTAIN BEHAVIOR OF BREAST		D48.6Ø	Neoplasm of uncertain behavior of unspecified breast
			D48.61	Neoplasm of uncertain behavior of right breast
			D48.62	Neoplasm of uncertain behavior of left breast
238.4	NEOPLASM UNCERTAIN BEHAVIOR POLYCYTHEMIA VERA		D45	Polycythemia vera
238.5	NEOPLASM UNCERTAIN BHV HISTIOCYTIC&MAST CELLS	➡	D47.Ø	Histiocytic and mast cell tumors of uncertain behavior
238.6	NEOPLASM OF UNCERTAIN BEHAVIOR OF PLASMA CELLS		D47.Z9	Oth neoplm of uncrt behav of lymphoid, hematpoetc & rel tiss
238.71	ESSENTIAL THROMBOCYTHEMIA		D47.3	Essential (hemorrhagic) thrombocythemia
238.72	LOW GRADE MYELODYSPLASTIC SYNDROME LESIONS		D46.Ø	Refractory anemia without ring sideroblasts, so stated
			D46.1	Refractory anemia with ring sideroblasts
			D46.2Ø	Refractory anemia with excess of blasts, unspecified
			D46.21	Refractory anemia with excess of blasts 1
			D46.4	Refractory anemia, unspecified
			D46.A	Refractory cytopenia with multilineage dysplasia
			D46.B	Refract cytopenia w multilin dysplasia and ring sideroblasts
238.73	HIGH GRADE MYELODYSPLASTIC SYNDROME LESIONS		D46.22	Refractory anemia with excess of blasts 2
238.74	MYELODYSPLASTIC SYNDROME WITH 5Q DELETION	➡	D46.C	Myelodysplastic syndrome w isolated del(5q) chromsoml abnlt
238.75	MYELODYSPLASTIC SYNDROME UNSPECIFIED		D46.9	Myelodysplastic syndrome, unspecified
			D46.Z	Other myelodysplastic syndromes
238.76	MYELOFIBROSIS WITH MYELOID METAPLASIA		D47.1	Chronic myeloproliferative disease
238.77	POST-TRANSPLANT LYMPHOPROLIFERATE DISORDER	➡	D47.Z1	Post-transplant lymphoproliferative disorder (PTLD)
238.79	OTHER LYMPHATIC AND HEMATOPOIETIC TISSUES		C88.8	Other malignant immunoproliferative diseases
			C94.4Ø	Acute panmyelosis w myelofibrosis not achieve remission
			C94.41	Acute panmyelosis with myelofibrosis, in remission
			C94.42	Acute panmyelosis with myelofibrosis, in relapse
			C94.6	Myelodysplastic disease, not classified
			D47.1	Chronic myeloproliferative disease
			D47.9	Neoplm of uncrt behav of lymphoid,hematpoetc & rel tiss,unsp
			D47.Z9	Oth neoplm of uncrt behav of lymphoid, hematpoetc & rel tiss
238.8	NEOPLASM UNCERTAIN BEHAVIOR OTHER SPEC SITES	➡	D48.7	Neoplasm of uncertain behavior of other specified sites
238.9	NEOPLASM OF UNCERTAIN BEHAVIOR SITE UNSPECIFIED	➡	D48.9	Neoplasm of uncertain behavior, unspecified
239.Ø	NEOPLASM UNSPECIFIED NATURE DIGESTIVE SYSTEM	➡	D49.Ø	Neoplasm of unspecified behavior of digestive system
239.1	NEOPLASM UNSPECIFIED NATURE RESPIRATORY SYSTEM	➡	D49.1	Neoplasm of unspecified behavior of respiratory system
239.2	NEOPLASMS UNSPEC NATURE BONE SOFT TISSUE&SKIN	➡	D49.2	Neoplasm of unsp behavior of bone, soft tissue, and skin
239.3	NEOPLASM OF UNSPECIFIED NATURE OF BREAST	➡	D49.3	Neoplasm of unspecified behavior of breast
239.4	NEOPLASM OF UNSPECIFIED NATURE OF BLADDER	➡	D49.4	Neoplasm of unspecified behavior of bladder
239.5	NEOPLASM UNSPEC NATURE OTH GENITOURINARY ORGANS	➡	D49.5	Neoplasm of unsp behavior of other genitourinary organs
239.6	NEOPLASM OF UNSPECIFIED NATURE OF BRAIN	➡	D49.6	Neoplasm of unspecified behavior of brain
239.7	NEOPLSM UNS NATR ENDOCRN GLND&OTH PART NERV SYS	➡	D49.7	Neoplm of unsp behav of endo glands and oth prt nervous sys
239.81	NEOPLASMS UNSPECIFIED NATURE RETINA AND CHOROID	➡	D49.81	Neoplasm of unspecified behavior of retina and choroid
239.89	NEOPLASMS UNSPECIFIED NATURE OTH SPECIFIED SITES	➡	D49.89	Neoplasm of unspecified behavior of other specified sites
239.9	NEOPLASM OF UNSPECIFIED NATURE SITE UNSPECIFIED	➡	D49.9	Neoplasm of unspecified behavior of unspecified site

Endocrine, Nutritional and Metabolic, and Immunity

ICD-9-CM		ICD-10-CM	
240.0	GOITER, SPECIFIED AS SIMPLE	E04.0	Nontoxic diffuse goiter
240.9	GOITER, UNSPECIFIED	E01.0 E01.2 E04.9	Iodine-deficiency related diffuse (endemic) goiter Iodine-deficiency related (endemic) goiter, unspecified Nontoxic goiter, unspecified
241.0	NONTOXIC UNINODULAR GOITER	E04.1	Nontoxic single thyroid nodule
241.1	NONTOXIC MULTINODULAR GOITER	E01.1 E04.2	Iodine-deficiency related multinodular (endemic) goiter Nontoxic multinodular goiter
241.9	UNSPECIFIED NONTOXIC NODULAR GOITER	E04.8 E04.9	Other specified nontoxic goiter Nontoxic goiter, unspecified
242.00	TOX DIFFUSE GOITER W/O THYROTOX CRISIS/STORM	➡ E05.00	Thyrotoxicosis w diffuse goiter w/o thyrotoxic crisis
242.01	TOX DIFFUSE GOITER W/ THYROTOX CRISIS/STORM	➡ E05.01	Thyrotoxicosis w diffuse goiter w thyrotoxic crisis or storm
242.10	TOX UNINODULR GOITER W/O THYROTOX CRISIS/STORM	➡ E05.10	Thyrotxcosis w toxic sing thyroid nodule w/o thyrotxc crisis
242.11	TOX UNINODULR GOITER W/ THYROTOX CRISIS/STORM	➡ E05.11	Thyrotxcosis w toxic single thyroid nodule w thyrotxc crisis
242.20	TOX MULTINODULR GOITER W/O THYROTOX CRISIS/STORM	E05.20	Thyrotxcosis w toxic multinod goiter w/o thyrotoxic crisis
242.21	TOX MULTINODULR GOITER W/ THYROTOX CRISIS/STORM	E05.21	Thyrotxcosis w toxic multinodular goiter w thyrotoxic crisis
242.30	TOXIC NODULAR GOITER UNS TYPE W/O CRISIS/STORM	E05.20	Thyrotxcosis w toxic multinod goiter w/o thyrotoxic crisis
242.31	TOXIC NODULAR GOITER UNS TYPE W/CRISIS/STORM	E05.21	Thyrotxcosis w toxic multinodular goiter w thyrotoxic crisis
242.40	THYROTOX-ECTOPIC THYROID NODULE W/O CRISIS	➡ E05.30	Thyrotxcosis from ectopic thyroid tissue w/o thyrotxc crisis
242.41	THYROTOX-ECTOPIC THYROID NODULE W/CRISIS	➡ E05.31	Thyrotxcosis from ectopic thyroid tissue w thyrotoxic crisis
242.80	THYROTOXICOS-OTH SPEC ORIGIN WO CRISIS/STORM	E05.40 E05.80	Thyrotoxicosis factitia without thyrotoxic crisis or storm Other thyrotoxicosis without thyrotoxic crisis or storm
242.81	THYROTOXICOS OTH ORIGIN W/ THYROTOX CRISIS/STORM	E05.41 E05.81	Thyrotoxicosis factitia with thyrotoxic crisis or storm Other thyrotoxicosis with thyrotoxic crisis or storm
242.90	THYROTOX W/O GOITER/OTH CAUSE W/O CRISIS	➡ E05.90	Thyrotoxicosis, unsp without thyrotoxic crisis or storm
242.91	THYROTOX W/O GOITER/OTH CAUSE W/CRISIS	➡ E05.91	Thyrotoxicosis, unspecified with thyrotoxic crisis or storm
243	CONGENITAL HYPOTHYROIDISM	E00.0 E00.1 E00.2 E00.9 E03.0 E03.1	Congenital iodine-deficiency syndrome, neurological type Congenital iodine-deficiency syndrome, myxedematous type Congenital iodine-deficiency syndrome, mixed type Congenital iodine-deficiency syndrome, unspecified Congenital hypothyroidism with diffuse goiter Congenital hypothyroidism without goiter
244.0	POSTSURGICAL HYPOTHYROIDISM	E89.0	Postprocedural hypothyroidism
244.1	OTHER POSTABLATIVE HYPOTHYROIDISM	E89.0	Postprocedural hypothyroidism
244.2	IODINE HYPOTHYROIDISM	E03.2	Hypothyroidism due to meds and oth exogenous substances
244.3	OTHER IATROGENIC HYPOTHYROIDISM	E03.2	Hypothyroidism due to meds and oth exogenous substances
244.8	OTHER SPECIFIED ACQUIRED HYPOTHYROIDISM	E01.8 E02 E03.3 E03.8	Oth iodine-deficiency related thyroid disord and allied cond Subclinical iodine-deficiency hypothyroidism Postinfectious hypothyroidism Other specified hypothyroidism
244.9	UNSPECIFIED HYPOTHYROIDISM	➡ E03.9	Hypothyroidism, unspecified
245.0	ACUTE THYROIDITIS	➡ E06.0	Acute thyroiditis
245.1	SUBACUTE THYROIDITIS	➡ E06.1	Subacute thyroiditis
245.2	CHRONIC LYMPHOCYTIC THYROIDITIS	➡ E06.3	Autoimmune thyroiditis
245.3	CHRONIC FIBROUS THYROIDITIS	E06.5	Other chronic thyroiditis
245.4	IATROGENIC THYROIDITIS	E06.4	Drug-induced thyroiditis
245.8	OTHER AND UNSPECIFIED CHRONIC THYROIDITIS	E06.2 E06.5	Chronic thyroiditis with transient thyrotoxicosis Other chronic thyroiditis
245.9	UNSPECIFIED THYROIDITIS	➡ E06.9	Thyroiditis, unspecified
246.0	DISORDERS OF THYROCALCITONIN SECRETION	➡ E07.0	Hypersecretion of calcitonin
246.1	DYSHORMONOGENIC GOITER	➡ E07.1	Dyshormogenetic goiter
246.2	CYST OF THYROID	E04.1	Nontoxic single thyroid nodule
246.3	HEMORRHAGE AND INFARCTION OF THYROID	E07.89	Other specified disorders of thyroid
246.8	OTHER SPECIFIED DISORDERS OF THYROID	E03.4 E07.89 E35	Atrophy of thyroid (acquired) Other specified disorders of thyroid Disorders of endocrine glands in diseases classd elswhr
246.9	UNSPECIFIED DISORDER OF THYROID	➡ E07.9	Disorder of thyroid, unspecified
249.00	SECONDARY DM W/O COMPL NOT UNCONTROLLED OR UNS	E08.9 E09.9 E13.9	Diabetes due to underlying condition w/o complications Drug or chemical induced diabetes mellitus w/o complications Other specified diabetes mellitus without complications
249.01	SECONDARY DM W/O COMPLICATION UNCONTROLLED	E08.65 E09.65	Diabetes due to underlying condition w hyperglycemia Drug or chemical induced diabetes mellitus w hyperglycemia
249.10	SECONDARY DM W/KETOACIDOSIS NOT UNCONTROLLED/UNS	E08.10 E09.10 E13.10	Diabetes due to underlying condition w ketoacidosis w/o coma Drug/chem diabetes mellitus w ketoacidosis w/o coma Oth diabetes mellitus with ketoacidosis without coma
249.11	SECONDARY DM WITH KETOACIDOSIS UNCONTROLLED	E08.10 E09.10 E08.65	Diabetes due to underlying condition w ketoacidosis w/o coma *or* Drug/chem diabetes mellitus w ketoacidosis w/o coma *and* Diabetes due to underlying condition w hyperglycemia

ICD-9-CM		ICD-10-CM		
249.20	SECONDARY DM W/HYPEROSMOLARITY NOT UNCONTROL/UNS	E08.00	Diab d/t undrl cond w hyprosm w/o nonket hyprgly-hypros coma	
		E08.01	Diabetes due to underlying condition w hyprosm w coma	
		E09.00	Drug/chem diab w hyprosm w/o nonket hyprgly-hypros coma	
		E09.01	Drug/chem diabetes mellitus w hyperosmolarity w coma	
		E13.00	Oth diab w hyprosm w/o nonket hyprgly-hypros coma (NKHHC)	
		E13.01	Oth diabetes mellitus with hyperosmolarity with coma	
249.21	SECONDARY DM WITH HYPEROSMOLARITY UNCONTROLLED	E08.01	Diabetes due to underlying condition w hyprosm w coma	*or*
		E09.01	Drug/chem diabetes mellitus w hyperosmolarity w coma	*and*
		E08.65	Diabetes due to underlying condition w hyperglycemia	
249.30	SECONDARY DM W/OTHER COMA NOT UNCONTROLLED/UNS	E08.11	Diabetes due to underlying condition w ketoacidosis w coma	
		E08.641	Diabetes due to underlying condition w hypoglycemia w coma	
		E09.11	Drug/chem diabetes mellitus w ketoacidosis w coma	
		E09.641	Drug/chem diabetes mellitus w hypoglycemia w coma	
		E13.11	Oth diabetes mellitus with ketoacidosis with coma	
		E13.641	Oth diabetes mellitus with hypoglycemia with coma	
249.31	SECONDARY DM WITH OTHER COMA UNCONTROLLED	E08.11	Diabetes due to underlying condition w ketoacidosis w coma	*or*
		E09.11	Drug/chem diabetes mellitus w ketoacidosis w coma	*and*
		E08.65	Diabetes due to underlying condition w hyperglycemia	
249.40	SECONDARY DM W/RENAL MANIFEST NOT UNCONTROL/UNS	E08.21	Diabetes due to underlying condition w diabetic nephropathy	
		E08.22	Diabetes due to undrl cond w diabetic chronic kidney disease	
		E08.29	Diabetes due to undrl condition w oth diabetic kidney comp	
		E09.21	Drug/chem diabetes mellitus w diabetic nephropathy	
		E09.22	Drug/chem diabetes w diabetic chronic kidney disease	
		E09.29	Drug/chem diabetes w oth diabetic kidney complication	
		E13.21	Other specified diabetes mellitus with diabetic nephropathy	
		E13.22	Oth diabetes mellitus with diabetic chronic kidney disease	
		E13.29	Oth diabetes mellitus with oth diabetic kidney complication	
249.41	SECONDARY DM W/RENAL MANIFESTATIONS UNCONTROLLED	E08.21	Diabetes due to underlying condition w diabetic nephropathy	*or*
		E09.21	Drug/chem diabetes mellitus w diabetic nephropathy	*and*
		E08.65	Diabetes due to underlying condition w hyperglycemia	
249.50	SECONDARY DM OPHTHALMIC MANIFEST NOT UNCNTRL/UNS	E08.311	Diab due to undrl cond w unsp diabetic rtnop w macular edema	
		E08.319	Diab due to undrl cond w unsp diab rtnop w/o macular edema	
		E08.321	Diab d/t undrl cond w mild nonprlf diab rtnop w mclr edema	
		E08.329	Diab d/t undrl cond w mild nonprlf diab rtnop w/o mclr edema	
		E08.331	Diab due to undrl cond w mod nonprlf diab rtnop w mclr edema	
		E08.339	Diab d/t undrl cond w mod nonprlf diab rtnop w/o mclr edema	
		E08.341	Diab d/t undrl cond w severe nonprlf diab rtnop w mclr edema	
		E08.349	Diab d/t undrl cond w sev nonprlf diab rtnop w/o mclr edema	
		E08.351	Diab due to undrl cond w prolif diab rtnop w macular edema	
		E08.359	Diab due to undrl cond w prolif diab rtnop w/o macular edema	
		E08.36	Diabetes due to underlying condition w diabetic cataract	
		E08.39	Diabetes due to undrl condition w oth diabetic opth comp	
		E09.311	Drug/chem diabetes w unsp diabetic rtnop w macular edema	
		E09.319	Drug/chem diabetes w unsp diabetic rtnop w/o macular edema	
		E09.321	Drug/chem diab w mild nonprlf diabetic rtnop w macular edema	
		E09.329	Drug/chem diab w mild nonprlf diab rtnop w/o macular edema	
		E09.331	Drug/chem diab w moderate nonprlf diab rtnop w macular edema	
		E09.339	Drug/chem diab w mod nonprlf diab rtnop w/o macular edema	
		E09.341	Drug/chem diab w severe nonprlf diab rtnop w macular edema	
		E09.349	Drug/chem diab w severe nonprlf diab rtnop w/o macular edema	
		E09.351	Drug/chem diabetes w prolif diabetic rtnop w macular edema	
		E09.359	Drug/chem diabetes w prolif diabetic rtnop w/o macular edema	
		E09.36	Drug/chem diabetes mellitus w diabetic cataract	
		E09.39	Drug/chem diabetes w oth diabetic ophthalmic complication	
		E13.311	Oth diabetes w unsp diabetic retinopathy w macular edema	
		E13.319	Oth diabetes w unsp diabetic retinopathy w/o macular edema	
		E13.321	Oth diabetes w mild nonprlf diabetic rtnop w macular edema	
		E13.329	Oth diabetes w mild nonprlf diabetic rtnop w/o macular edema	
		E13.331	Oth diab w moderate nonprlf diabetic rtnop w macular edema	
		E13.339	Oth diab w moderate nonprlf diabetic rtnop w/o macular edema	
		E13.341	Oth diabetes w severe nonprlf diabetic rtnop w macular edema	
		E13.349	Oth diab w severe nonprlf diabetic rtnop w/o macular edema	
		E13.351	Oth diabetes w prolif diabetic retinopathy w macular edema	
		E13.359	Oth diabetes w prolif diabetic retinopathy w/o macular edema	
		E13.36	Other specified diabetes mellitus with diabetic cataract	
		E13.39	Oth diabetes mellitus w oth diabetic ophthalmic complication	
249.51	SECONDARY DM W/OPHTHALMIC MANIFEST UNCONTROLLED	E08.39	Diabetes due to undrl condition w oth diabetic opth comp	
		E09.39	Drug/chem diabetes w oth diabetic ophthalmic complication	
		E08.311	Diab due to undrl cond w unsp diabetic rtnop w macular edema	*or*
		E08.319	Diab due to undrl cond w unsp diab rtnop w/o macular edema	*or*
		E08.36	Diabetes due to underlying condition w diabetic cataract	*or*
		E09.311	Drug/chem diabetes w unsp diabetic rtnop w macular edema	*or*
		E09.319	Drug/chem diabetes w unsp diabetic rtnop w/o macular edema	*or*
		E09.36	Drug/chem diabetes mellitus w diabetic cataract	*and*
		E08.65	Diabetes due to underlying condition w hyperglycemia	

ICD-9-CM		ICD-10-CM		
249.60	SECONDARY DM NEUROLOGICAL MANIFEST NOT UNCONTROL	**E08.40**	Diabetes due to underlying condition w diabetic neurop, unsp	
		E08.41	Diabetes due to undrl condition w diabetic mononeuropathy	
		E08.42	Diabetes due to underlying condition w diabetic polyneurop	
		E08.43	Diab due to undrl cond w diabetic autonm (poly)neuropathy	
		E08.44	Diabetes due to underlying condition w diabetic amyotrophy	
		E08.49	Diabetes due to undrl condition w oth diabetic neuro comp	
		E08.610	Diabetes due to undrl cond w diabetic neuropathic arthrop	
		E09.40	Drug/chem diabetes w neuro comp w diabetic neuropathy, unsp	
		E09.41	Drug/chem diabetes w neuro comp w diabetic mononeuropathy	
		E09.42	Drug/chem diabetes w neurological comp w diabetic polyneurop	
		E09.43	Drug/chem diab w neuro comp w diab autonm (poly)neuropathy	
		E09.44	Drug/chem diabetes w neurological comp w diabetic amyotrophy	
		E09.49	Drug/chem diabetes w neuro comp w oth diabetic neuro comp	
		E09.610	Drug/chem diabetes w diabetic neuropathic arthropathy	
		E13.40	Oth diabetes mellitus with diabetic neuropathy, unspecified	
		E13.41	Oth diabetes mellitus with diabetic mononeuropathy	
		E13.42	Oth diabetes mellitus with diabetic polyneuropathy	
		E13.43	Oth diabetes mellitus w diabetic autonomic (poly)neuropathy	
		E13.44	Other specified diabetes mellitus with diabetic amyotrophy	
		E13.49	Oth diabetes w oth diabetic neurological complication	
		E13.610	Oth diabetes mellitus with diabetic neuropathic arthropathy	
249.61	SECONDARY DM W/NEUROLOGICAL MANIFEST UNCONTROL	**E08.40**	Diabetes due to underlying condition w diabetic neurop, unsp	*or*
		E09.40	Drug/chem diabetes w neuro comp w diabetic neuropathy, unsp	*and*
		E08.65	Diabetes due to underlying condition w hyperglycemia	
249.70	SECONDARY DM W/PERIPHERAL CIRC D/O NOT UNCONTROL	**E08.51**	Diab due to undrl cond w diab prph angiopath w/o gangrene	
		E08.52	Diab due to undrl cond w diabetic prph angiopath w gangrene	
		E08.59	Diabetes due to underlying condition w oth circulatory comp	
		E09.51	Drug/chem diabetes w diabetic prph angiopath w/o gangrene	
		E09.52	Drug/chem diabetes w diabetic prph angiopath w gangrene	
		E09.59	Drug/chem diabetes mellitus w oth circulatory complications	
		E13.51	Oth diabetes w diabetic peripheral angiopathy w/o gangrene	
		E13.52	Oth diabetes w diabetic peripheral angiopathy w gangrene	
		E13.59	Oth diabetes mellitus with other circulatory complications	
249.71	SECONDARY DM W/PERIPHERAL CIRC D/O UNCONTROLLED	**E08.51**	Diab due to undrl cond w diab prph angiopath w/o gangrene	*or*
		E09.51	Drug/chem diabetes w diabetic prph angiopath w/o gangrene	*and*
		E08.65	Diabetes due to underlying condition w hyperglycemia	
249.80	SECONDARY DM W/OTH SPEC MANIFEST NOT UNCONTROL	**E08.618**	Diabetes due to underlying condition w oth diabetic arthrop	
		E08.620	Diabetes due to underlying condition w diabetic dermatitis	
		E08.621	Diabetes mellitus due to underlying condition w foot ulcer	
		E08.622	Diabetes due to underlying condition w oth skin ulcer	
		E08.628	Diabetes due to underlying condition w oth skin comp	
		E08.630	Diabetes due to underlying condition w periodontal disease	
		E08.638	Diabetes due to underlying condition w oth oral comp	
		E08.649	Diabetes due to underlying condition w hypoglycemia w/o coma	
		E08.65	Diabetes due to underlying condition w hyperglycemia	
		E08.69	Diabetes due to underlying condition w oth complication	
		E09.618	Drug/chem diabetes mellitus w oth diabetic arthropathy	
		E09.620	Drug/chem diabetes mellitus w diabetic dermatitis	
		E09.621	Drug or chemical induced diabetes mellitus with foot ulcer	
		E09.622	Drug or chemical induced diabetes mellitus w oth skin ulcer	
		E09.628	Drug/chem diabetes mellitus w oth skin complications	
		E09.630	Drug/chem diabetes mellitus w periodontal disease	
		E09.638	Drug/chem diabetes mellitus w oth oral complications	
		E09.649	Drug/chem diabetes mellitus w hypoglycemia w/o coma	
		E09.65	Drug or chemical induced diabetes mellitus w hyperglycemia	
		E09.69	Drug/chem diabetes mellitus w oth complication	
		E13.618	Oth diabetes mellitus with other diabetic arthropathy	
		E13.620	Other specified diabetes mellitus with diabetic dermatitis	
		E13.621	Other specified diabetes mellitus with foot ulcer	
		E13.622	Other specified diabetes mellitus with other skin ulcer	
		E13.628	Oth diabetes mellitus with other skin complications	
		E13.630	Other specified diabetes mellitus with periodontal disease	
		E13.638	Oth diabetes mellitus with other oral complications	
		E13.649	Oth diabetes mellitus with hypoglycemia without coma	
		E13.65	Other specified diabetes mellitus with hyperglycemia	
		E13.69	Oth diabetes mellitus with other specified complication	
249.81	SECONDARY DM W/OTH SPECIFIED MANIFEST UNCONTROL	**E08.69**	Diabetes due to underlying condition w oth complication	*or*
		E09.69	Drug/chem diabetes mellitus w oth complication	*and*
		E08.65	Diabetes due to underlying condition w hyperglycemia	
249.90	SECONDARY DM W/UNS COMPL NOT UNCONTROLLED/UNS	**E08.8**	Diabetes due to underlying condition w unsp complications	
		E09.8	Drug/chem diabetes mellitus w unsp complications	
		E13.8	Oth diabetes mellitus with unspecified complications	
249.91	SECONDARY DM W/UNS COMPLICATION UNCONTROLLED	**E08.8**	Diabetes due to underlying condition w unsp complications	*or*
		E09.8	Drug/chem diabetes mellitus w unsp complications	*and*
		E08.65	Diabetes due to underlying condition w hyperglycemia	
250.00	DIAB W/O COMP TYPE II/UNS NOT STATED UNCNTRL	**E11.9**	Type 2 diabetes mellitus without complications	
		E13.9	Other specified diabetes mellitus without complications	

ICD-9-CM		ICD-10-CM		
250.01	DIAB W/O COMP TYPE I [JUV] NOT STATED UNCNTRL	E10.9	Type 1 diabetes mellitus without complications	
250.02	DIAB W/O MENTION COMP TYPE II/UNS TYPE UNCNTRL	E11.65	Type 2 diabetes mellitus with hyperglycemia	
250.03	DIAB W/O MENTION COMP TYPE I [JUV TYPE] UNCNTRL	E10.65	Type 1 diabetes mellitus with hyperglycemia	
250.10	DIAB W/KETOACIDOS TYPE II/UNS NOT STATED UNCNTRL	E11.69	Type 2 diabetes mellitus with other specified complication	
		E13.10	Oth diabetes mellitus with ketoacidosis without coma	
250.11	DIAB W/KETOACIDOS TYPE I [JUV] NOT STATE UNCNTRL	E10.10	Type 1 diabetes mellitus with ketoacidosis without coma	
250.12	DIABETES W/KETOACIDOSIS TYPE II/UNS TYPE UNCNTRL	E11.69	Type 2 diabetes mellitus with other specified complication	or
		E13.10	Oth diabetes mellitus with ketoacidosis without coma	and
		E11.65	Type 2 diabetes mellitus with hyperglycemia	
250.13	DIABETES W/KETOACIDOSIS TYPE I [JUV] UNCNTRL	E10.10	Type 1 diabetes mellitus with ketoacidosis without coma	and
		E10.65	Type 1 diabetes mellitus with hyperglycemia	
250.20	DIAB W/HYPEROSMOLARITY TYPE II/UNS NOT UNCNTRL	E11.00	Type 2 diab w hyprosm w/o nonket hyprgly-hypros coma (NKHHC)	
		E11.01	Type 2 diabetes mellitus with hyperosmolarity with coma	
		E13.00	Oth diab w hyprosm w/o nonket hyprgly-hypros coma (NKHHC)	
		E13.01	Oth diabetes mellitus with hyperosmolarity with coma	
250.21	DIAB W/HYPEROSMOLARITY TYPE I [JUV] NOT UNCNTRL	E10.69	Type 1 diabetes mellitus with other specified complication	
250.22	DIAB W/HYPEROSMOLARITY TYPE II/UNS TYPE UNCNTRL	E11.00	Type 2 diab w hyprosm w/o nonket hyprgly-hypros coma (NKHHC)	and
		E11.65	Type 2 diabetes mellitus with hyperglycemia	
250.23	DIAB W/HYPEROSMOLARITY TYPE I [JUV TYPE] UNCNTRL	E10.69	Type 1 diabetes mellitus with other specified complication	and
		E10.65	Type 1 diabetes mellitus with hyperglycemia	
250.30	DIAB W/OTH COMA TYPE II/UNS NOT STATED UNCNTRL	E11.641	Type 2 diabetes mellitus with hypoglycemia with coma	
		E13.11	Oth diabetes mellitus with ketoacidosis with coma	
		E13.641	Oth diabetes mellitus with hypoglycemia with coma	
250.31	DIAB W/OTH COMA TYPE I [JUV] NOT STATED UNCNTRL	E10.11	Type 1 diabetes mellitus with ketoacidosis with coma	
		E10.641	Type 1 diabetes mellitus with hypoglycemia with coma	
250.32	DIABETES W/OTH COMA TYPE II/UNS UNCONTROLLED	E11.01	Type 2 diabetes mellitus with hyperosmolarity with coma	and
		E11.65	Type 2 diabetes mellitus with hyperglycemia	
250.33	DIABETES W/OTH COMA TYPE I [JUV] UNCONTROLLED	E10.11	Type 1 diabetes mellitus with ketoacidosis with coma	and
		E10.65	Type 1 diabetes mellitus with hyperglycemia	
250.40	DIAB W/RENAL MANIFESTS TYPE II/UNS NOT UNCNTRL	E11.21	Type 2 diabetes mellitus with diabetic nephropathy	
		E11.22	Type 2 diabetes mellitus w diabetic chronic kidney disease	
		E11.29	Type 2 diabetes mellitus w oth diabetic kidney complication	
		E13.21	Other specified diabetes mellitus with diabetic nephropathy	
		E13.22	Oth diabetes mellitus with diabetic chronic kidney disease	
		E13.29	Oth diabetes mellitus with oth diabetic kidney complication	
250.41	DIAB W/RENAL MANIFESTS TYPE I [JUV] NOT UNCNTRL	E10.21	Type 1 diabetes mellitus with diabetic nephropathy	
		E10.22	Type 1 diabetes mellitus w diabetic chronic kidney disease	
		E10.29	Type 1 diabetes mellitus w oth diabetic kidney complication	
250.42	DIAB W/RENAL MANIFESTS TYPE II/UNS TYPE UNCNTRL	E11.21	Type 2 diabetes mellitus with diabetic nephropathy	and
		E11.65	Type 2 diabetes mellitus with hyperglycemia	
250.43	DIAB W/RENAL MANIFESTS TYPE I [JUV TYPE] UNCNTRL	E10.21	Type 1 diabetes mellitus with diabetic nephropathy	and
		E10.65	Type 1 diabetes mellitus with hyperglycemia	
250.50	DIAB W/OPHTH MANIFESTS TYPE II/UNS NOT UNCNTRL	E11.311	Type 2 diabetes w unsp diabetic retinopathy w macular edema	
		E11.319	Type 2 diabetes w unsp diabetic rtnop w/o macular edema	
		E11.321	Type 2 diab w mild nonprlf diabetic rtnop w macular edema	
		E11.329	Type 2 diab w mild nonprlf diabetic rtnop w/o macular edema	
		E11.331	Type 2 diab w moderate nonprlf diab rtnop w macular edema	
		E11.339	Type 2 diab w moderate nonprlf diab rtnop w/o macular edema	
		E11.341	Type 2 diab w severe nonprlf diabetic rtnop w macular edema	
		E11.349	Type 2 diab w severe nonprlf diab rtnop w/o macular edema	
		E11.351	Type 2 diabetes w prolif diabetic rtnop w macular edema	
		E11.359	Type 2 diabetes w prolif diabetic rtnop w/o macular edema	
		E11.36	Type 2 diabetes mellitus with diabetic cataract	
		E11.39	Type 2 diabetes w oth diabetic ophthalmic complication	
		E13.311	Oth diabetes w unsp diabetic retinopathy w macular edema	
		E13.319	Oth diabetes w unsp diabetic retinopathy w/o macular edema	
		E13.321	Oth diabetes w mild nonprlf diabetic rtnop w macular edema	
		E13.329	Oth diabetes w mild nonprlf diabetic rtnop w/o macular edema	
		E13.331	Oth diab w moderate nonprlf diabetic rtnop w macular edema	
		E13.339	Oth diab w moderate nonprlf diabetic rtnop w/o macular edema	
		E13.341	Oth diabetes w severe nonprlf diabetic rtnop w macular edema	
		E13.349	Oth diab w severe nonprlf diabetic rtnop w/o macular edema	
		E13.351	Oth diabetes w prolif diabetic retinopathy w macular edema	
		E13.359	Oth diabetes w prolif diabetic retinopathy w/o macular edema	
		E13.36	Other specified diabetes mellitus with diabetic cataract	
		E13.39	Oth diabetes mellitus w oth diabetic ophthalmic complication	

ICD-9-CM		ICD-10-CM		
250.51	DIAB W/OPHTH MANIFESTS TYPE I [JUV] NOT UNCNTRL	**E10.311**	Type 1 diabetes w unsp diabetic retinopathy w macular edema	
		E10.319	Type 1 diabetes w unsp diabetic rtnop w/o macular edema	
		E10.321	Type 1 diab w mild nonprlf diabetic rtnop w macular edema	
		E10.329	Type 1 diab w mild nonprlf diabetic rtnop w/o macular edema	
		E10.331	Type 1 diab w moderate nonprlf diab rtnop w macular edema	
		E10.339	Type 1 diab w moderate nonprlf diab rtnop w/o macular edema	
		E10.341	Type 1 diab w severe nonprlf diabetic rtnop w macular edema	
		E10.349	Type 1 diab w severe nonprlf diab rtnop w/o macular edema	
		E10.351	Type 1 diabetes w prolif diabetic rtnop w macular edema	
		E10.359	Type 1 diabetes w prolif diabetic rtnop w/o macular edema	
		E10.36	Type 1 diabetes mellitus with diabetic cataract	
		E10.39	Type 1 diabetes w oth diabetic ophthalmic complication	
250.52	DIAB W/OPHTH MANIFESTS TYPE II/UNS TYPE UNCNTRL	**E11.311**	Type 2 diabetes w unsp diabetic retinopathy w macular edema	*or*
		E11.319	Type 2 diabetes w unsp diabetic rtnop w/o macular edema	*or*
		E11.36	Type 2 diabetes mellitus with diabetic cataract	*or*
		E11.39	Type 2 diabetes w oth diabetic ophthalmic complication	*and*
		E11.65	Type 2 diabetes mellitus with hyperglycemia	
250.53	DIAB W/OPHTH MANIFESTS TYPE I [JUV TYPE] UNCNTRL	**E10.311**	Type 1 diabetes w unsp diabetic retinopathy w macular edema	*or*
		E10.319	Type 1 diabetes w unsp diabetic rtnop w/o macular edema	*or*
		E10.36	Type 1 diabetes mellitus with diabetic cataract	*or*
		E10.39	Type 1 diabetes w oth diabetic ophthalmic complication	*and*
		E10.65	Type 1 diabetes mellitus with hyperglycemia	
250.60	DIAB W/NEURO MANIFESTS TYPE II/UNS NOT UNCNTRL	**E11.40**	Type 2 diabetes mellitus with diabetic neuropathy, unsp	
		E11.41	Type 2 diabetes mellitus with diabetic mononeuropathy	
		E11.42	Type 2 diabetes mellitus with diabetic polyneuropathy	
		E11.43	Type 2 diabetes w diabetic autonomic (poly)neuropathy	
		E11.44	Type 2 diabetes mellitus with diabetic amyotrophy	
		E11.49	Type 2 diabetes w oth diabetic neurological complication	
		E11.610	Type 2 diabetes mellitus w diabetic neuropathic arthropathy	
		E13.40	Oth diabetes mellitus with diabetic neuropathy, unspecified	
		E13.41	Oth diabetes mellitus with diabetic mononeuropathy	
		E13.42	Oth diabetes mellitus with diabetic polyneuropathy	
		E13.43	Oth diabetes mellitus w diabetic autonomic (poly)neuropathy	
		E13.44	Other specified diabetes mellitus with diabetic amyotrophy	
		E13.49	Oth diabetes w oth diabetic neurological complication	
		E13.610	Oth diabetes mellitus with diabetic neuropathic arthropathy	
250.61	DIAB W/NEURO MANIFESTS TYPE I [JUV] NOT UNCNTRL	**E10.40**	Type 1 diabetes mellitus with diabetic neuropathy, unsp	
		E10.41	Type 1 diabetes mellitus with diabetic mononeuropathy	
		E10.42	Type 1 diabetes mellitus with diabetic polyneuropathy	
		E10.43	Type 1 diabetes w diabetic autonomic (poly)neuropathy	
		E10.44	Type 1 diabetes mellitus with diabetic amyotrophy	
		E10.49	Type 1 diabetes w oth diabetic neurological complication	
		E10.610	Type 1 diabetes mellitus w diabetic neuropathic arthropathy	
250.62	DIAB W/NEURO MANIFESTS TYPE II/UNS TYPE UNCNTRL	**E11.40**	Type 2 diabetes mellitus with diabetic neuropathy, unsp	*and*
		E11.65	Type 2 diabetes mellitus with hyperglycemia	
250.63	DIAB W/NEURO MANIFESTS TYPE I [JUV TYPE] UNCNTRL	**E10.40**	Type 1 diabetes mellitus with diabetic neuropathy, unsp	*and*
		E10.65	Type 1 diabetes mellitus with hyperglycemia	
250.70	DIAB W/PERIPH CIRC D/O TYPE II/UNS NOT UNCNTRL	**E11.51**	Type 2 diabetes w diabetic peripheral angiopath w/o gangrene	
		E11.52	Type 2 diabetes w diabetic peripheral angiopathy w gangrene	
		E11.59	Type 2 diabetes mellitus with oth circulatory complications	
		E13.51	Oth diabetes w diabetic peripheral angiopathy w/o gangrene	
		E13.52	Oth diabetes w diabetic peripheral angiopathy w gangrene	
		E13.59	Oth diabetes mellitus with other circulatory complications	
250.71	DIAB W/PERIPH CIRC D/O TYPE I [JUV] NOT UNCNTRL	**E10.51**	Type 1 diabetes w diabetic peripheral angiopath w/o gangrene	
		E10.52	Type 1 diabetes w diabetic peripheral angiopathy w gangrene	
		E10.59	Type 1 diabetes mellitus with oth circulatory complications	
250.72	DIAB W/PERIPH CIRC D/O TYPE II/UNS TYPE UNCNTRL	**E11.51**	Type 2 diabetes w diabetic peripheral angiopath w/o gangrene	*and*
		E11.65	Type 2 diabetes mellitus with hyperglycemia	
250.73	DIAB W/PERIPH CIRC D/O TYPE I [JUV TYPE] UNCNTRL	**E10.51**	Type 1 diabetes w diabetic peripheral angiopath w/o gangrene	*and*
		E10.65	Type 1 diabetes mellitus with hyperglycemia	

ICD-9-CM		ICD-10-CM		
25Ø.8Ø	DIAB W/OTH MANIFESTS TYPE II/UNS NOT UNCNTRL	E11.618 E11.62Ø E11.621 E11.622 E11.628 E11.63Ø E11.638 E11.649 E11.65 E11.69 E13.618 E13.62Ø E13.621 E13.622 E13.628 E13.63Ø E13.638 E13.649 E13.65 E13.69	Type 2 diabetes mellitus with other diabetic arthropathy Type 2 diabetes mellitus with diabetic dermatitis Type 2 diabetes mellitus with foot ulcer Type 2 diabetes mellitus with other skin ulcer Type 2 diabetes mellitus with other skin complications Type 2 diabetes mellitus with periodontal disease Type 2 diabetes mellitus with other oral complications Type 2 diabetes mellitus with hypoglycemia without coma Type 2 diabetes mellitus with hyperglycemia Type 2 diabetes mellitus with other specified complication Oth diabetes mellitus with other diabetic arthropathy Other specified diabetes mellitus with diabetic dermatitis Other specified diabetes mellitus with foot ulcer Other specified diabetes mellitus with other skin ulcer Oth diabetes mellitus with other skin complications Other specified diabetes mellitus with periodontal disease Oth diabetes mellitus with other oral complications Oth diabetes mellitus with hypoglycemia without coma Other specified diabetes mellitus with hyperglycemia Oth diabetes mellitus with other specified complication	
25Ø.81	DIAB W/OTH MANIFESTS TYPE I [JUV] NOT UNCNTRL	E1Ø.618 E1Ø.62Ø E1Ø.621 E1Ø.622 E1Ø.628 E1Ø.63Ø E1Ø.638 E1Ø.649 E1Ø.65 E1Ø.69	Type 1 diabetes mellitus with other diabetic arthropathy Type 1 diabetes mellitus with diabetic dermatitis Type 1 diabetes mellitus with foot ulcer Type 1 diabetes mellitus with other skin ulcer Type 1 diabetes mellitus with other skin complications Type 1 diabetes mellitus with periodontal disease Type 1 diabetes mellitus with other oral complications Type 1 diabetes mellitus with hypoglycemia without coma Type 1 diabetes mellitus with hyperglycemia Type 1 diabetes mellitus with other specified complication	
25Ø.82	DIAB W/OTH MANIFESTS TYPE II/UNS TYPE UNCNTRL	E11.69	Type 2 diabetes mellitus with other specified complication	*and*
		E11.65	Type 2 diabetes mellitus with hyperglycemia	
25Ø.83	DIAB W/OTH MANIFESTS TYPE I [JUV TYPE] UNCNTRL	E1Ø.69	Type 1 diabetes mellitus with other specified complication	*and*
		E1Ø.65	Type 1 diabetes mellitus with hyperglycemia	
25Ø.9Ø	DIAB W/UNS COMP TYPE II/UNS NOT STATED UNCNTRL	E11.8 E13.8	Type 2 diabetes mellitus with unspecified complications Oth diabetes mellitus with unspecified complications	
25Ø.91	DIAB W/UNS COMP TYPE I [JUV] NOT STATED UNCNTRL	E1Ø.8	Type 1 diabetes mellitus with unspecified complications	
25Ø.92	DIAB W/UNSPEC COMP TYPE II/UNSPEC TYPE UNCNTRL	E11.8	Type 2 diabetes mellitus with unspecified complications	*and*
		E11.65	Type 2 diabetes mellitus with hyperglycemia	
25Ø.93	DIAB W/UNSPEC COMP TYPE I [JUV TYPE] UNCNTRL	E1Ø.8	Type 1 diabetes mellitus with unspecified complications	*and*
		E1Ø.65	Type 1 diabetes mellitus with hyperglycemia	
251.Ø	HYPOGLYCEMIC COMA	E15	Nondiabetic hypoglycemic coma	
251.1	OTHER SPECIFIED HYPOGLYCEMIA	EØ8.649 E16.Ø E16.1	Diabetes due to underlying condition w hypoglycemia w/o coma Drug-induced hypoglycemia without coma Other hypoglycemia	
251.2	HYPOGLYCEMIA, UNSPECIFIED	E16.2	Hypoglycemia, unspecified	
251.3	POSTSURGICAL HYPOINSULINEMIA	E89.1	Postprocedural hypoinsulinemia	
251.4	ABNORMALITY OF SECRETION OF GLUCAGON	E16.3	Increased secretion of glucagon	
251.5	ABNORMALITY OF SECRETION OF GASTRIN	E16.4	Increased secretion of gastrin	
251.8	OTH SPEC DISORDERS PANCREATIC INTERNAL SECRETION	E16.8	Other specified disorders of pancreatic internal secretion	
251.9	UNSPEC DISORDER PANCREATIC INTERNAL SECRETION	E16.9	Disorder of pancreatic internal secretion, unspecified	
252.ØØ	HYPERPARATHYROIDISM UNSPECIFIED	E21.3	Hyperparathyroidism, unspecified	
252.Ø1	PRIMARY HYPERPARATHYROIDISM	E21.Ø	Primary hyperparathyroidism	
252.Ø2	SECONDARY HYPERPARATHYROIDISM NON-RENAL	E21.1	Secondary hyperparathyroidism, not elsewhere classified	
252.Ø8	OTHER HYPERPARATHYROIDISM	E21.2	Other hyperparathyroidism	
252.1	HYPOPARATHYROIDISM	E2Ø.Ø E2Ø.8 E2Ø.9 E89.2	Idiopathic hypoparathyroidism Other hypoparathyroidism Hypoparathyroidism, unspecified Postprocedural hypoparathyroidism	
252.8	OTHER SPECIFIED DISORDERS OF PARATHYROID GLAND	E21.4	Other specified disorders of parathyroid gland	
252.9	UNSPECIFIED DISORDER OF PARATHYROID GLAND	E21.5	Disorder of parathyroid gland, unspecified	
253.Ø	ACROMEGALY AND GIGANTISM	E22.Ø E34.4	Acromegaly and pituitary gigantism Constitutional tall stature	
253.1	OTHER&UNSPEC ANTERIOR PITUITARY HYPERFUNCTION	E22.1 E22.8 E22.9	Hyperprolactinemia Other hyperfunction of pituitary gland Hyperfunction of pituitary gland, unspecified	
253.2	PANHYPOPITUITARISM	E23.Ø	Hypopituitarism	
253.3	PITUITARY DWARFISM	E23.Ø	Hypopituitarism	
253.4	OTHER ANTERIOR PITUITARY DISORDERS	E23.6	Other disorders of pituitary gland	
253.5	DIABETES INSIPIDUS	E23.2	Diabetes insipidus	
253.6	OTHER DISORDERS OF NEUROHYPOPHYSIS	E22.2	Syndrome of inappropriate secretion of antidiuretic hormone	
253.7	IATROGENIC PITUITARY DISORDERS	E23.1 E89.3	Drug-induced hypopituitarism Postprocedural hypopituitarism	

 [Brackets] indicate valid character values for each code. Character value meanings provided for each code grouping.

ICD-9-CM		ICD-10-CM	
253.8	OTH PITUITARY DISORDERS & SYNDROMES	E23.6 E24.1	Other disorders of pituitary gland Nelson's syndrome
253.9	UNS D/O PITUITARY GLAND&ITS HYPOTHALAMIC CNTRL	E23.3 E23.7	Hypothalamic dysfunction, not elsewhere classified Disorder of pituitary gland, unspecified
254.0	PERSISTENT HYPERPLASIA OF THYMUS	➡ E32.0	Persistent hyperplasia of thymus
254.1	ABSCESS OF THYMUS	➡ E32.1	Abscess of thymus
254.8	OTHER SPECIFIED DISEASES OF THYMUS GLAND	➡ E32.8	Other diseases of thymus
254.9	UNSPECIFIED DISEASE OF THYMUS GLAND	➡ E32.9	Disease of thymus, unspecified
255.0	CUSHINGS SYNDROME	E24.0 E24.2 E24.3 E24.4 E24.8 E24.9	Pituitary-dependent Cushing's disease Drug-induced Cushing's syndrome Ectopic ACTH syndrome Alcohol-induced pseudo-Cushing's syndrome Other Cushing's syndrome Cushing's syndrome, unspecified
255.10	HYPERALDOSTERONISM UNSPECIFIED	E26.09 E26.9	Other primary hyperaldosteronism Hyperaldosteronism, unspecified
255.11	GLUCOCORTICOID-REMEDIABLE ALDOSTERONISM	➡ E26.02	Glucocorticoid-remediable aldosteronism
255.12	CONNS SYNDROME	➡ E26.01	Conn's syndrome
255.13	BARTTERS SYNDROME	➡ E26.81	Bartter's syndrome
255.14	OTHER SECONDARY ALDOSTERONISM	E26.1 E26.89	Secondary hyperaldosteronism Other hyperaldosteronism
255.2	ADRENOGENITAL DISORDERS	E25.0 E25.8 E25.9	Congenital adrenogenital disorders assoc w enzyme deficiency Other adrenogenital disorders Adrenogenital disorder, unspecified
255.3	OTHER CORTICOADRENAL OVERACTIVITY	E27.0	Other adrenocortical overactivity
255.41	GLUCOCORTICOID DEFICIENCY	E27.1 E27.2 E27.3 E27.40 E27.49 E89.6	Primary adrenocortical insufficiency Addisonian crisis Drug-induced adrenocortical insufficiency Unspecified adrenocortical insufficiency Other adrenocortical insufficiency Postprocedural adrenocortical (-medullary) hypofunction
255.42	MINERALOCORTICOID DEFICIENCY	E27.49	Other adrenocortical insufficiency
255.5	OTHER ADRENAL HYPOFUNCTION	E27.49	Other adrenocortical insufficiency
255.6	MEDULLOADRENAL HYPERFUNCTION	➡ E27.5	Adrenomedullary hyperfunction
255.8	OTHER SPECIFIED DISORDERS OF ADRENAL GLANDS	E27.8 E35	Other specified disorders of adrenal gland Disorders of endocrine glands in diseases classd elswhr
255.9	UNSPECIFIED DISORDER OF ADRENAL GLANDS	➡ E27.9	Disorder of adrenal gland, unspecified
256.0	HYPERESTROGENISM	➡ E28.0	Estrogen excess
256.1	OTHER OVARIAN HYPERFUNCTION	E28.1 N98.1	Androgen excess Hyperstimulation of ovaries
256.2	POSTABLATIVE OVARIAN FAILURE	E89.40 E89.41	Asymptomatic postprocedural ovarian failure Symptomatic postprocedural ovarian failure
256.31	PREMATURE MENOPAUSE	E28.310 E28.319	Symptomatic premature menopause Asymptomatic premature menopause
256.39	OTHER OVARIAN FAILURE	➡ E28.39	Other primary ovarian failure
256.4	POLYCYSTIC OVARIES	➡ E28.2	Polycystic ovarian syndrome
256.8	OTHER OVARIAN DYSFUNCTION	➡ E28.8	Other ovarian dysfunction
256.9	UNSPECIFIED OVARIAN DYSFUNCTION	➡ E28.9	Ovarian dysfunction, unspecified
257.0	TESTICULAR HYPERFUNCTION	➡ E29.0	Testicular hyperfunction
257.1	POSTABLATIVE TESTICULAR HYPOFUNCTION	➡ E89.5	Postprocedural testicular hypofunction
257.2	OTHER TESTICULAR HYPOFUNCTION	➡ E29.1	Testicular hypofunction
257.8	OTHER TESTICULAR DYSFUNCTION	➡ E29.8	Other testicular dysfunction
257.9	UNSPECIFIED TESTICULAR DYSFUNCTION	➡ E29.9	Testicular dysfunction, unspecified
258.01	MULTIPLE ENDOCRINE NEOPLASIA MEN TYPE I	➡ E31.21	Multiple endocrine neoplasia [MEN] type I
258.02	MULTIPLE ENDOCRINE NEOPLASIA MEN TYPE IIA	➡ E31.22	Multiple endocrine neoplasia [MEN] type IIA
258.03	MULTIPLE ENDOCRINE NEOPLASIA MEN TYPE IIB	➡ E31.23	Multiple endocrine neoplasia [MEN] type IIB
258.1	OTHER COMBINATIONS OF ENDOCRINE DYSFUNCTION	E31.0	Autoimmune polyglandular failure
258.8	OTHER SPECIFIED POLYGLANDULAR DYSFUNCTION	E31.1 E31.20 E31.8	Polyglandular hyperfunction Multiple endocrine neoplasia [MEN] syndrome, unspecified Other polyglandular dysfunction
258.9	UNSPECIFIED POLYGLANDULAR DYSFUNCTION	➡ E31.9	Polyglandular dysfunction, unspecified
259.0	DELAY IN SEXUAL DEVELOPMENT AND PUBERTY NEC	➡ E30.0	Delayed puberty
259.1	PRECOCIOUS SEXUAL DEVELOPMENT AND PUBERTY NEC	E30.1 E30.8	Precocious puberty Other disorders of puberty
259.2	CARCINOID SYNDROME	➡ E34.0	Carcinoid syndrome
259.3	ECTOPIC HORMONE SECRETION NEC	➡ E34.2	Ectopic hormone secretion, not elsewhere classified
259.4	DWARFISM, NOT ELSEWHERE CLASSIFIED	➡ E34.3	Short stature due to endocrine disorder
259.50	ANDROGEN INSENSITIVITY UNSPECIFIED	➡ E34.50	Androgen insensitivity syndrome, unspecified
259.51	ANDROGEN INSENSITIVITY SYNDROME	➡ E34.51	Complete androgen insensitivity syndrome
259.52	PARTIAL ANDROGEN INSENSITIVITY	➡ E34.52	Partial androgen insensitivity syndrome

ICD-9-CM		ICD-10-CM	
259.8	OTHER SPECIFIED ENDOCRINE DISORDERS	E34.1	Other hypersecretion of intestinal hormones
		E34.8	Other specified endocrine disorders
		E35	Disorders of endocrine glands in diseases classd elswhr
259.9	UNSPECIFIED ENDOCRINE DISORDER	E30.9	Disorder of puberty, unspecified
		E34.9	Endocrine disorder, unspecified
260	KWASHIORKOR	E40	Kwashiorkor
		E42	Marasmic kwashiorkor
261	NUTRITIONAL MARASMUS	E41	Nutritional marasmus
		E43	Unspecified severe protein-calorie malnutrition
262	OTHER SEVERE PROTEIN-CALORIE MALNUTRITION	E43	Unspecified severe protein-calorie malnutrition
263.0	MALNUTRITION OF MODERATE DEGREE	➡ E44.0	Moderate protein-calorie malnutrition
263.1	MALNUTRITION OF MILD DEGREE	➡ E44.1	Mild protein-calorie malnutrition
263.2	ARRESTED DVLP FOLLOW PROTEIN-CALORIE MLNUTRIT	E45	Retarded development following protein-calorie malnutrition
263.8	OTHER PROTEIN-CALORIE MALNUTRITION	E46	Unspecified protein-calorie malnutrition
263.9	UNSPECIFIED PROTEIN-CALORIE MALNUTRITION	E46	Unspecified protein-calorie malnutrition
		E64.0	Sequelae of protein-calorie malnutrition
264.0	VITAMIN A DEFICIENCY WITH CONJUNCTIVAL XEROSIS	➡ E50.0	Vitamin A deficiency with conjunctival xerosis
264.1	VITAMIN DEFIC W/CONJUNCTIVAL XEROSIS&BITOTS SPOT	➡ E50.1	Vitamin A deficiency w Bitot's spot and conjunctival xerosis
264.2	VITAMIN A DEFICIENCY WITH CORNEAL XEROSIS	➡ E50.2	Vitamin A deficiency with corneal xerosis
264.3	VITAMIN DEFICIENCY W/CORNEAL ULCERATION&XEROSIS	➡ E50.3	Vitamin A deficiency with corneal ulceration and xerosis
264.4	VITAMIN A DEFICIENCY WITH KERATOMALACIA	➡ E50.4	Vitamin A deficiency with keratomalacia
264.5	VITAMIN A DEFICIENCY WITH NIGHT BLINDNESS	➡ E50.5	Vitamin A deficiency with night blindness
264.6	VITAMIN DEFICIENCY W/XEROPHTHALMIC SCARS CORNEA	➡ E50.6	Vitamin A deficiency with xerophthalmic scars of cornea
264.7	OTHER OCULAR MANIFESTATIONS VITAMIN DEFICIENCY	➡ E50.7	Other ocular manifestations of vitamin A deficiency
264.8	OTHER MANIFESTATIONS OF VITAMIN A DEFICIENCY	➡ E50.8	Other manifestations of vitamin A deficiency
264.9	UNSPECIFIED VITAMIN A DEFICIENCY	E50.9	Vitamin A deficiency, unspecified
		E64.1	Sequelae of vitamin A deficiency
265.0	BERIBERI	E51.11	Dry beriberi
		E51.12	Wet beriberi
265.1	OTHER&UNSPEC MANIFESTATIONS THIAMINE DEFICIENCY	E51.2	Wernicke's encephalopathy
		E51.8	Other manifestations of thiamine deficiency
		E51.9	Thiamine deficiency, unspecified
265.2	PELLAGRA	➡ E52	Niacin deficiency [pellagra]
266.0	ARIBOFLAVINOSIS	➡ E53.0	Riboflavin deficiency
266.1	VITAMIN B6 DEFICIENCY	➡ E53.1	Pyridoxine deficiency
266.2	OTHER B-COMPLEX DEFICIENCIES	D81.818	Other biotin-dependent carboxylase deficiency
		D81.819	Biotin-dependent carboxylase deficiency, unspecified
		E53.8	Deficiency of other specified B group vitamins
266.9	UNSPECIFIED VITAMIN B DEFICIENCY	E53.9	Vitamin B deficiency, unspecified
267	ASCORBIC ACID DEFICIENCY	E54	Ascorbic acid deficiency
		E64.2	Sequelae of vitamin C deficiency
268.0	RICKETS, ACTIVE	➡ E55.0	Rickets, active
268.1	RICKETS, LATE EFFECT	E64.3	Sequelae of rickets
268.2	OSTEOMALACIA, UNSPECIFIED	M83.0	Puerperal osteomalacia
		M83.1	Senile osteomalacia
		M83.2	Adult osteomalacia due to malabsorption
		M83.3	Adult osteomalacia due to malnutrition
		M83.4	Aluminum bone disease
		M83.5	Other drug-induced osteomalacia in adults
		M83.8	Other adult osteomalacia
		M83.9	Adult osteomalacia, unspecified
268.9	UNSPECIFIED VITAMIN D DEFICIENCY	➡ E55.9	Vitamin D deficiency, unspecified
269.0	DEFICIENCY OF VITAMIN K	➡ E56.1	Deficiency of vitamin K
269.1	DEFICIENCY OF OTHER VITAMINS	E56.0	Deficiency of vitamin E
		E56.8	Deficiency of other vitamins
269.2	UNSPECIFIED VITAMIN DEFICIENCY	E56.9	Vitamin deficiency, unspecified
269.3	MINERAL DEFICIENCY NOT ELSEWHERE CLASSIFIED	E58	Dietary calcium deficiency
		E59	Dietary selenium deficiency
		E60	Dietary zinc deficiency
		E61.0	Copper deficiency
		E61.1	Iron deficiency
		E61.2	Magnesium deficiency
		E61.3	Manganese deficiency
		E61.4	Chromium deficiency
		E61.5	Molybdenum deficiency
		E61.6	Vanadium deficiency
269.8	OTHER NUTRITIONAL DEFICIENCY	E61.7	Deficiency of multiple nutrient elements
		E61.8	Deficiency of other specified nutrient elements
		E63.0	Essential fatty acid [EFA] deficiency
		E63.1	Imbalance of constituents of food intake
		E63.8	Other specified nutritional deficiencies
		E64.8	Sequelae of other nutritional deficiencies

ICD-9-CM		ICD-10-CM	
269.9	UNSPECIFIED NUTRITIONAL DEFICIENCY	**E61.9**	Deficiency of nutrient element, unspecified
		E63.9	Nutritional deficiency, unspecified
		E64.9	Sequelae of unspecified nutritional deficiency
270.0	DISTURBANCES OF AMINO-ACID TRANSPORT	**E72.00**	Disorders of amino-acid transport, unspecified
		E72.01	Cystinuria
		E72.02	Hartnup's disease
		E72.04	Cystinosis
		E72.09	Other disorders of amino-acid transport
270.1	PHENYLKETONURIA	**E70.0**	Classical phenylketonuria
		E70.1	Other hyperphenylalaninemias
270.2	OTH DISTURBANCES AROMATIC AMINO-ACID METABOLISM	**E70.20**	Disorder of tyrosine metabolism, unspecified
		E70.21	Tyrosinemia
		E70.29	Other disorders of tyrosine metabolism
		E70.30	Albinism, unspecified
		E70.310	X-linked ocular albinism
		E70.311	Autosomal recessive ocular albinism
		E70.318	Other ocular albinism
		E70.319	Ocular albinism, unspecified
		E70.320	Tyrosinase negative oculocutaneous albinism
		E70.321	Tyrosinase positive oculocutaneous albinism
		E70.328	Other oculocutaneous albinism
		E70.329	Oculocutaneous albinism, unspecified
		E70.330	Chediak-Higashi syndrome
		E70.331	Hermansky-Pudlak syndrome
		E70.338	Other albinism with hematologic abnormality
		E70.339	Albinism with hematologic abnormality, unspecified
		E70.39	Other specified albinism
		E70.5	Disorders of tryptophan metabolism
		E70.8	Other disorders of aromatic amino-acid metabolism
		E70.9	Disorder of aromatic amino-acid metabolism, unspecified
270.3	DISTURB BRANCHED-CHAIN AMINO-ACID METABOLISM	**E71.0**	Maple-syrup-urine disease
		E71.110	Isovaleric acidemia
		E71.111	3-methylglutaconic aciduria
		E71.118	Other branched-chain organic acidurias
		E71.120	Methylmalonic acidemia
		E71.121	Propionic acidemia
		E71.128	Other disorders of propionate metabolism
		E71.19	Other disorders of branched-chain amino-acid metabolism
		E71.2	Disorder of branched-chain amino-acid metabolism, unsp
270.4	DISTURBANCES SULPHUR-BEAR AMINO-ACID METABOLISM	**E72.10**	Disorders of sulfur-bearing amino-acid metabolism, unsp
		E72.11	Homocystinuria
		E72.12	Methylenetetrahydrofolate reductase deficiency
		E72.19	Other disorders of sulfur-bearing amino-acid metabolism
270.5	DISTURBANCES OF HISTIDINE METABOLISM	**E70.40**	Disorders of histidine metabolism, unspecified
		E70.41	Histidinemia
		E70.49	Other disorders of histidine metabolism
270.6	DISORDERS OF UREA CYCLE METABOLISM	**E72.20**	Disorder of urea cycle metabolism, unspecified
		E72.21	Argininemia
		E72.22	Arginosuccinic aciduria
		E72.23	Citrullinemia
		E72.29	Other disorders of urea cycle metabolism
		E72.4	Disorders of ornithine metabolism
270.7	OTH DISTURB STRAIGHT-CHAIN AMINO-ACID METABOLISM	**E71.120**	Methylmalonic acidemia
		E72.3	Disorders of lysine and hydroxylysine metabolism
		E72.50	Disorder of glycine metabolism, unspecified
		E72.51	Non-ketotic hyperglycinemia
		E72.59	Other disorders of glycine metabolism
		E72.8	Other specified disorders of amino-acid metabolism
270.8	OTHER SPECIFIED DISORDERS AMINO-ACID METABOLISM	**E72.03**	Lowe's syndrome
		E72.8	Other specified disorders of amino-acid metabolism
270.9	UNSPECIFIED DISORDER OF AMINO-ACID METABOLISM	➡ **E72.9**	Disorder of amino-acid metabolism, unspecified
271.0	GLYCOGENOSIS	**E74.00**	Glycogen storage disease, unspecified
		E74.01	von Gierke disease
		E74.02	Pompe disease
		E74.03	Cori disease
		E74.04	McArdle disease
		E74.09	Other glycogen storage disease
		E74.4	Disorders of pyruvate metabolism and gluconeogenesis
271.1	GALACTOSEMIA	**E74.20**	Disorders of galactose metabolism, unspecified
		E74.21	Galactosemia
		E74.29	Other disorders of galactose metabolism
271.2	HEREDITARY FRUCTOSE INTOLERANCE	**E74.10**	Disorder of fructose metabolism, unspecified
		E74.11	Essential fructosuria
		E74.12	Hereditary fructose intolerance
		E74.19	Other disorders of fructose metabolism

ICD-9-CM		ICD-10-CM	
271.3	INTEST DISACCHARIDASE DEFIC&DISACCHARIDE MALAB	**E73.0**	Congenital lactase deficiency
		E73.1	Secondary lactase deficiency
		E73.8	Other lactose intolerance
		E73.9	Lactose intolerance, unspecified
		E74.31	Sucrase-isomaltase deficiency
		E74.39	Other disorders of intestinal carbohydrate absorption
271.4	RENAL GLYCOSURIA	**E74.8**	Other specified disorders of carbohydrate metabolism
271.8	OTH SPEC D/O CARBOHYDRATE TRANSPORT&METABOLISM	**E72.52**	Trimethylaminuria
		E72.53	Hyperoxaluria
		E74.4	Disorders of pyruvate metabolism and gluconeogenesis
		E74.8	Other specified disorders of carbohydrate metabolism
		E77.1	Defects in glycoprotein degradation
271.9	UNSPEC DISORDER CARBOHYDRATE TRANSPORT&METAB	➡ **E74.9**	Disorder of carbohydrate metabolism, unspecified
272.0	PURE HYPERCHOLESTEROLEMIA	➡ **E78.0**	Pure hypercholesterolemia
272.1	PURE HYPERGLYCERIDEMIA	➡ **E78.1**	Pure hyperglyceridemia
272.2	MIXED HYPERLIPIDEMIA	➡ **E78.2**	Mixed hyperlipidemia
272.3	HYPERCHYLOMICRONEMIA	➡ **E78.3**	Hyperchylomicronemia
272.4	OTHER AND UNSPECIFIED HYPERLIPIDEMIA	**E78.4**	Other hyperlipidemia
		E78.5	Hyperlipidemia, unspecified
272.5	LIPOPROTEIN DEFICIENCIES	➡ **E78.6**	Lipoprotein deficiency
272.6	LIPODYSTROPHY	➡ **E88.1**	Lipodystrophy, not elsewhere classified
272.7	LIPIDOSES	**E75.21**	Fabry (-Anderson) disease
		E75.22	Gaucher disease
		E75.240	Niemann-Pick disease type A
		E75.241	Niemann-Pick disease type B
		E75.242	Niemann-Pick disease type C
		E75.243	Niemann-Pick disease type D
		E75.248	Other Niemann-Pick disease
		E75.249	Niemann-Pick disease, unspecified
		E75.3	Sphingolipidosis, unspecified
		E77.0	Defects in post-translational mod of lysosomal enzymes
		E77.1	Defects in glycoprotein degradation
		E77.8	Other disorders of glycoprotein metabolism
		E77.9	Disorder of glycoprotein metabolism, unspecified
272.8	OTHER DISORDERS OF LIPOID METABOLISM	**E71.30**	Disorder of fatty-acid metabolism, unspecified
		E75.5	Other lipid storage disorders
		E78.79	Other disorders of bile acid and cholesterol metabolism
		E78.81	Lipoid dermatoarthritis
		E78.89	Other lipoprotein metabolism disorders
		E88.2	Lipomatosis, not elsewhere classified
		E88.89	Other specified metabolic disorders
272.9	UNSPECIFIED DISORDER OF LIPOID METABOLISM	**E75.6**	Lipid storage disorder, unspecified
		E78.70	Disorder of bile acid and cholesterol metabolism, unsp
		E78.9	Disorder of lipoprotein metabolism, unspecified
273.0	POLYCLONAL HYPERGAMMAGLOBULINEMIA	➡ **D89.0**	Polyclonal hypergammaglobulinemia
273.1	MONOCLONAL PARAPROTEINEMIA	**D47.2**	Monoclonal gammopathy
		D89.2	Hypergammaglobulinemia, unspecified
273.2	OTHER PARAPROTEINEMIAS	➡ **D89.1**	Cryoglobulinemia
273.3	MACROGLOBULINEMIA	**C88.0**	Waldenstrom macroglobulinemia
273.4	ALPHA-1-ANTITRYPSIN DEFICIENCY	➡ **E88.01**	Alpha-1-antitrypsin deficiency
273.8	OTHER DISORDERS OF PLASMA PROTEIN METABOLISM	**E88.09**	Oth disorders of plasma-protein metabolism, NEC
273.9	UNSPECIFIED DISORDER PLASMA PROTEIN METABOLISM	**E88.09**	Oth disorders of plasma-protein metabolism, NEC
274.00	GOUTY ARTHROPATHY UNSPECIFIED	**M10.00**	Idiopathic gout, unspecified site
		M10.01[1,2,9]	Idiopathic gout, shoulder
		M10.02[1,2,9]	Idiopathic gout, elbow
		M10.03[1,2,9]	Idiopathic gout, wrist
		M10.04[1,2,9]	Idiopathic gout, hand
		M10.05[1,2,9]	Idiopathic gout, hip
		M10.06[1,2,9]	Idiopathic gout, knee
		M10.07[1,2,9]	Idiopathic gout, ankle and foot
		M10.08	Idiopathic gout, vertebrae
		M10.09	Idiopathic gout, multiple sites
		M10.10	Lead-induced gout, unspecified site
		M10.11[1,2,9]	Lead-induced gout, shoulder
		M10.12[1,2,9]	Lead-induced gout, elbow
		M10.13[1,2,9]	Lead-induced gout, wrist
		M10.14[1,2,9]	Lead-induced gout, hand
		M10.15[1,2,9]	Lead-induced gout, hip
		M10.16[1,2,9]	Lead-induced gout, knee
		M10.17[1,2,9]	Lead-induced gout, ankle and foot
		M10.18	Lead-induced gout, vertebrae
		M10.19	Lead-induced gout, multiple sites
		M10.20	Drug-induced gout, unspecified site
		M10.21[1,2,9]	Drug-induced gout, shoulder
		M10.22[1,2,9]	Drug-induced gout, elbow

(Continued on next page)

6th Character meanings for codes as indicated
1 Right ***2 Left*** ***9 Unspecified***

[Brackets] indicate valid character values for each code. Character value meanings provided for each code grouping.

ICD-9-CM		ICD-10-CM	
274.00	GOUTY ARTHROPATHY UNSPECIFIED **(Continued)**	**M10.23**[1,2,9]	Drug-induced gout, wrist
		M10.24[1,2,9]	Drug-induced gout, hand
		M10.25[1,2,9]	Drug-induced gout, hip
		M10.26[1,2,9]	Drug-induced gout, knee
		M10.27[1,2,9]	Drug-induced gout, ankle and foot
		M10.28	Drug-induced gout, vertebrae
		M10.29	Drug-induced gout, multiple sites
			6th Character meanings for codes as indicated *1 Right 2 Left 9 Unspecified*
274.01	ACUTE GOUTY ARTHROPATHY	**M10.00**	Idiopathic gout, unspecified site
		M10.01[1,2,9]	Idiopathic gout, shoulder
		M10.02[1,2,9]	Idiopathic gout, elbow
		M10.03[1,2,9]	Idiopathic gout, wrist
		M10.04[1,2,9]	Idiopathic gout, hand
		M10.05[1,2,9]	Idiopathic gout, hip
		M10.06[1,2,9]	Idiopathic gout, knee
		M10.07[1,2,9]	Idiopathic gout, ankle and foot
		M10.08	Idiopathic gout, vertebrae
		M10.09	Idiopathic gout, multiple sites
		M10.20	Drug-induced gout, unspecified site
		M10.21[1,2,9]	Drug-induced gout, shoulder
		M10.22[1,2,9]	Drug-induced gout, elbow
		M10.23[1,2,9]	Drug-induced gout, wrist
		M10.24[1,2,9]	Drug-induced gout, hand
		M10.25[1,2,9]	Drug-induced gout, hip
		M10.26[1,2,9]	Drug-induced gout, knee
		M10.27[1,2,9]	Drug-induced gout, ankle and foot
		M10.28	Drug-induced gout, vertebrae
		M10.29	Drug-induced gout, multiple sites
			6th Character meanings for codes as indicated *1 Right 2 Left 9 Unspecified*
274.02	CHRONIC GOUTY ARTHROPATHY W/O MENTION TOPHUS	**M1A.00X0**	Idiopathic chronic gout, unspecified site, without tophus
		M1A.01[1,2,9]	Idiopathic chronic gout, shoulder, without tophus
		M1A.02[1,2,9]	Idiopathic chronic gout, elbow, without tophus (tophi)
		M1A.03[1,2,9]	Idiopathic chronic gout, wrist, without tophus (tophi)
		M1A.04[1,2,9]	Idiopathic chronic gout, hand, without tophus (tophi)
		M1A.05[1,2,9]	Idiopathic chronic gout, hip, without tophus (tophi)
		M1A.06[1,2,9]	Idiopathic chronic gout, knee, without tophus (tophi)
		M1A.07[1,2,9]	Idiopathic chronic gout, ankle and foot, w/o tophus
		M1A.08X0	Idiopathic chronic gout, vertebrae, without tophus (tophi)
		M1A.09X0	Idiopathic chronic gout, multiple sites, without tophus
		M1A.20X0	Drug-induced chronic gout, unspecified site, without tophus
		M1A.21[1,2,9]	Drug-induced chronic gout, shoulder, without tophus
		M1A.22[1,2,9]	Drug-induced chronic gout, elbow, without tophus
		M1A.23[1,2,9]	Drug-induced chronic gout, wrist, without tophus
		M1A.24[1,2,9]	Drug-induced chronic gout, hand, without tophus
		M1A.25[1,2,9]	Drug-induced chronic gout, hip, without tophus (tophi)
		M1A.26[1,2,9]	Drug-induced chronic gout, knee, without tophus
		M1A.27[1,2,9]	Drug-induced chronic gout, ankle and foot, w/o tophus
		M1A.28X0	Drug-induced chronic gout, vertebrae, without tophus (tophi)
		M1A.29X0	Drug-induced chronic gout, multiple sites, without tophus
		M1A.30X0	Chronic gout due to renal impairment, unsp site, w/o tophus
		M1A.31[1,2,9]	Chronic gout due to renal impairment, r shoulder, w/o toph
		M1A.32[1,2,9]	Chronic gout due to renal impairment, elbow, w/o toph
		M1A.33[1,2,9]	Chronic gout due to renal impairment, wrist, w/o toph
		M1A.34[1,2,9]	Chronic gout due to renal impairment, hand, w/o tophus
		M1A.35[1,2,9]	Chronic gout due to renal impairment, hip, w/o tophus
		M1A.36[1,2,9]	Chronic gout due to renal impairment, knee, w/o tophus
		M1A.37[1,2,9]	Chronic gout due to renal impairment, ank/ft, w/o toph
		M1A.38X0	Chronic gout due to renal impairment, vertebrae, w/o tophus
		M1A.39X0	Chronic gout due to renal impairment, mult sites, w/o toph
		M1A.40X0	Other secondary chronic gout, unsp site, without tophus
		M1A.41[1,2,9]	Other secondary chronic gout, shoulder, without tophus
		M1A.42[1,2,9]	Other secondary chronic gout, elbow, without tophus
		M1A.43[1,2,9]	Other secondary chronic gout, wrist, without tophus
		M1A.44[1,2,9]	Other secondary chronic gout, hand, without tophus
		M1A.45[1,2,9]	Other secondary chronic gout, hip, without tophus
		M1A.46[1,2,9]	Other secondary chronic gout, knee, without tophus
		M1A.47[1,2,9]	Oth secondary chronic gout, ankle and foot, w/o tophus
		M1A.48X0	Other secondary chronic gout, vertebrae, without tophus
		M1A.49X0	Other secondary chronic gout, multiple sites, without tophus
		M1A.9XX0	Chronic gout, unspecified, without tophus (tophi)
			6th Character meanings for codes as indicated *1 Right 2 Left 9 Unspecified*

ICD-9-CM		ICD-10-CM	
274.Ø3	CHRONIC GOUTY ARTHROPATHY WITH TOPHUS	M1A.ØØX1	Idiopathic chronic gout, unspecified site, with tophus
		M1A.Ø1[1,2,9]	Idiopathic chronic gout, shoulder, with tophus (tophi)
		M1A.Ø2[1,2,9]	Idiopathic chronic gout, elbow, with tophus (tophi)
		M1A.Ø3[1,2,9]	Idiopathic chronic gout, wrist, with tophus (tophi)
		M1A.Ø4[1,2,9]	Idiopathic chronic gout, hand, with tophus (tophi)
		M1A.Ø5[1,2,9]	Idiopathic chronic gout, hip, with tophus (tophi)
		M1A.Ø6[1,2,9]	Idiopathic chronic gout, knee, with tophus (tophi)
		M1A.Ø7[1,2,9]	Idiopathic chronic gout, ankle and foot, with tophus
		M1A.Ø8X1	Idiopathic chronic gout, vertebrae, with tophus (tophi)
		M1A.Ø9X1	Idiopathic chronic gout, multiple sites, with tophus (tophi)
		M1A.2ØX1	Drug-induced chronic gout, unspecified site, with tophus
		M1A.21[1,2,9]	Drug-induced chronic gout, shoulder, with tophus
		M1A.22[1,2,9]	Drug-induced chronic gout, elbow, with tophus (tophi)
		M1A.23[1,2,9]	Drug-induced chronic gout, wrist, with tophus (tophi)
		M1A.24[1,2,9]	Drug-induced chronic gout, hand, with tophus (tophi)
		M1A.25[1,2,9]	Drug-induced chronic gout, hip, with tophus (tophi)
		M1A.26[1,2,9]	Drug-induced chronic gout, knee, with tophus (tophi)
		M1A.27[1,2,9]	Drug-induced chronic gout, ankle and foot, with tophus
		M1A.28X1	Drug-induced chronic gout, vertebrae, with tophus (tophi)
		M1A.29X1	Drug-induced chronic gout, multiple sites, with tophus
		M1A.3ØX1	Chronic gout due to renal impairment, unsp site, with tophus
		M1A.31[1,2,9]	Chronic gout due to renal impairment, shoulder, w toph
		M1A.32[1,2,9]	Chronic gout due to renal impairment, elbow, w tophus
		M1A.33[1,2,9]	Chronic gout due to renal impairment, wrist, w tophus
		M1A.34[1,2,9]	Chronic gout due to renal impairment, hand, w tophus
		M1A.35[1,2,9]	Chronic gout due to renal impairment, hip, with tophus
		M1A.36[1,2,9]	Chronic gout due to renal impairment, knee, w tophus
		M1A.37[1,2,9]	Chronic gout due to renal impairment, ank/ft, w toph
		M1A.38X1	Chronic gout due to renal impairment, vertebrae, with tophus
		M1A.39X1	Chronic gout due to renal impairment, multiple sites, w toph
		M1A.4ØX1	Other secondary chronic gout, unspecified site, with tophus
		M1A.41[1,2,9]	Other secondary chronic gout, shoulder, with tophus
		M1A.42[1,2,9]	Other secondary chronic gout, elbow, with tophus
		M1A.43[1,2,9]	Other secondary chronic gout, wrist, with tophus
		M1A.44[1,2,9]	Other secondary chronic gout, hand, with tophus
		M1A.45[1,2,9]	Other secondary chronic gout, hip, with tophus (tophi)
		M1A.46[1,2,9]	Other secondary chronic gout, knee, with tophus
		M1A.47[1,2,9]	Oth secondary chronic gout, ankle and foot, w tophus
		M1A.48X1	Other secondary chronic gout, vertebrae, with tophus (tophi)
		M1A.49X1	Other secondary chronic gout, multiple sites, with tophus
		M1A.9XX1	Chronic gout, unspecified, with tophus (tophi)
			6th Character meanings for codes as indicated ***1 Right*** ***2 Left*** ***9 Unspecified***
274.1Ø	GOUTY NEPHROPATHY, UNSPECIFIED	M1Ø.3Ø	Gout due to renal impairment, unspecified site
		M1Ø.31[1,2,9]	Gout due to renal impairment, shoulder
		M1Ø.32[1,2,9]	Gout due to renal impairment, elbow
		M1Ø.33[1,2,9]	Gout due to renal impairment, wrist
		M1Ø.34[1,2,9]	Gout due to renal impairment, hand
		M1Ø.35[1,2,9]	Gout due to renal impairment, hip
		M1Ø.36[1,2,9]	Gout due to renal impairment, knee
		M1Ø.37[1,2,9]	Gout due to renal impairment, ankle and foot
		M1Ø.38	Gout due to renal impairment, vertebrae
		M1Ø.39	Gout due to renal impairment, multiple sites
			6th Character meanings for codes as indicated ***1 Right*** ***2 Left*** ***9 Unspecified***
274.11	URIC ACID NEPHROLITHIASIS	N2Ø.Ø	Calculus of kidney
274.19	OTHER GOUTY NEPHROPATHY	M1Ø.3Ø	Gout due to renal impairment, unspecified site
274.81	GOUTY TOPHI OF EAR	M1Ø.9	Gout, unspecified
274.82	GOUTY TOPHI OF OTHER SITES	M1Ø.9	Gout, unspecified
274.89	GOUT WITH OTHER SPECIFIED MANIFESTATIONS	M1Ø.4Ø	Other secondary gout, unspecified site
		M1Ø.41[1,2,9]	Other secondary gout, shoulder
		M1Ø.42[1,2,9]	Other secondary gout, elbow
		M1Ø.43[1,2,9]	Other secondary gout, wrist
		M1Ø.44[1,2,9]	Other secondary gout, hand
		M1Ø.45[1,2,9]	Other secondary gout, hip
		M1Ø.46[1,2,9]	Other secondary gout, knee
		M1Ø.47[1,2,9]	Other secondary gout, ankle and foot
		M1Ø.48	Other secondary gout, vertebrae
		M1Ø.49	Other secondary gout, multiple sites
			6th Character meanings for codes as indicated ***1 Right*** ***2 Left*** ***9 Unspecified***
274.9	GOUT, UNSPECIFIED	M1Ø.9	Gout, unspecified
275.Ø1	HEREDITARY HEMOCHROMATOSIS	➡ E83.11Ø	Hereditary hemochromatosis
275.Ø2	HEMOCHROMATOSIS D/T REPEATED RBC TRANSFUSIONS	➡ E83.111	Hemochromatosis due to repeated red blood cell transfusions
275.Ø3	OTHER HEMOCHROMATOSIS	E83.118	Other hemochromatosis
		E83.119	Hemochromatosis, unspecified

[Brackets] indicate valid character values for each code. Character value meanings provided for each code grouping.

ICD-9-CM		ICD-10-CM	
275.09	OTHER DISORDERS OF IRON METABOLISM	E83.10	Disorder of iron metabolism, unspecified
		E83.19	Other disorders of iron metabolism
275.1	DISORDERS OF COPPER METABOLISM	E83.00	Disorder of copper metabolism, unspecified
		E83.01	Wilson's disease
		E83.09	Other disorders of copper metabolism
275.2	DISORDERS OF MAGNESIUM METABOLISM	E83.40	Disorders of magnesium metabolism, unspecified
		E83.41	Hypermagnesemia
		E83.42	Hypomagnesemia
		E83.49	Other disorders of magnesium metabolism
275.3	DISORDERS OF PHOSPHORUS METABOLISM	E83.30	Disorder of phosphorus metabolism, unspecified
		E83.31	Familial hypophosphatemia
		E83.32	Hereditary vitamin D-dependent rickets (type 1) (type 2)
		E83.39	Other disorders of phosphorus metabolism
275.40	UNSPECIFIED DISORDER OF CALCIUM METABOLISM	➡ E83.50	Unspecified disorder of calcium metabolism
275.41	HYPOCALCEMIA	➡ E83.51	Hypocalcemia
275.42	HYPERCALCEMIA	➡ E83.52	Hypercalcemia
275.49	OTHER DISORDERS OF CALCIUM METABOLISM	E20.1	Pseudohypoparathyroidism
		E83.59	Other disorders of calcium metabolism
275.5	HUNGRY BONE SYNDROME	➡ E83.81	Hungry bone syndrome
275.8	OTHER SPECIFIED DISORDERS OF MINERAL METABOLISM	➡ E83.89	Other disorders of mineral metabolism
275.9	UNSPECIFIED DISORDER OF MINERAL METABOLISM	➡ E83.9	Disorder of mineral metabolism, unspecified
276.0	HYPEROSMOLALITY AND/OR HYPERNATREMIA	➡ E87.0	Hyperosmolality and hypernatremia
276.1	HYPOSMOLALITY AND/OR HYPONATREMIA	➡ E87.1	Hypo-osmolality and hyponatremia
276.2	ACIDOSIS	➡ E87.2	Acidosis
276.3	ALKALOSIS	➡ E87.3	Alkalosis
276.4	MIXED ACID-BASE BALANCE DISORDER	➡ E87.4	Mixed disorder of acid-base balance
276.50	VOLUME DEPLETION UNSPECIFIED	➡ E86.9	Volume depletion, unspecified
276.51	DEHYDRATION	➡ E86.0	Dehydration
276.52	HYPOVOLEMIA	➡ E86.1	Hypovolemia
276.61	TRANSFUSION ASSOCIATED CIRCULATORY OVERLOAD	➡ E87.71	Transfusion associated circulatory overload
276.69	OTHER FLUID OVERLOAD	E87.70	Fluid overload, unspecified
		E87.79	Other fluid overload
276.7	HYPERPOTASSEMIA	➡ E87.5	Hyperkalemia
276.8	HYPOPOTASSEMIA	➡ E87.6	Hypokalemia
276.9	ELECTROLYTE AND FLUID DISORDERS NEC	➡ E87.8	Oth disorders of electrolyte and fluid balance, NEC
277.00	CYSTIC FIBROSIS WITHOUT MENTION MECONIUM ILEUS	➡ E84.9	Cystic fibrosis, unspecified
277.01	CYSTIC FIBROSIS WITH MECONIUM ILEUS	➡ E84.11	Meconium ileus in cystic fibrosis
277.02	CYSTIC FIBROSIS WITH PULMONARY MANIFESTATIONS	➡ E84.0	Cystic fibrosis with pulmonary manifestations
277.03	CF WITH GASTROINTESTINAL MANIFESTATIONS	E84.19	Cystic fibrosis with other intestinal manifestations
277.09	CYSTIC FIBROSIS WITH OTHER MANIFESTATIONS	➡ E84.8	Cystic fibrosis with other manifestations
277.1	DISORDERS OF PORPHYRIN METABOLISM	E80.0	Hereditary erythropoietic porphyria
		E80.1	Porphyria cutanea tarda
		E80.20	Unspecified porphyria
		E80.21	Acute intermittent (hepatic) porphyria
		E80.29	Other porphyria
277.2	OTHER DISORDERS OF PURINE&PYRIMIDINE METABOLISM	D81.3	Adenosine deaminase [ADA] deficiency
		D81.5	Purine nucleoside phosphorylase [PNP] deficiency
		E79.1	Lesch-Nyhan syndrome
		E79.2	Myoadenylate deaminase deficiency
		E79.8	Other disorders of purine and pyrimidine metabolism
		E79.9	Disorder of purine and pyrimidine metabolism, unspecified
277.30	AMYLOIDOSIS UNSPECIFIED	E85.9	Amyloidosis, unspecified
277.31	FAMILIAL MEDITERRANEAN FEVER	E85.0	Non-neuropathic heredofamilial amyloidosis
277.39	OTHER AMYLOIDOSIS	E85.1	Neuropathic heredofamilial amyloidosis
		E85.2	Heredofamilial amyloidosis, unspecified
		E85.3	Secondary systemic amyloidosis
		E85.4	Organ-limited amyloidosis
		E85.8	Other amyloidosis
277.4	DISORDERS OF BILIRUBIN EXCRETION	E80.4	Gilbert syndrome
		E80.5	Crigler-Najjar syndrome
		E80.6	Other disorders of bilirubin metabolism
		E80.7	Disorder of bilirubin metabolism, unspecified
277.5	MUCOPOLYSACCHARIDOSIS	E76.01	Hurler's syndrome
		E76.02	Hurler-Scheie syndrome
		E76.03	Scheie's syndrome
		E76.1	Mucopolysaccharidosis, type II
		E76.210	Morquio A mucopolysaccharidoses
		E76.211	Morquio B mucopolysaccharidoses
		E76.219	Morquio mucopolysaccharidoses, unspecified
		E76.22	Sanfilippo mucopolysaccharidoses
		E76.29	Other mucopolysaccharidoses
		E76.3	Mucopolysaccharidosis, unspecified
		E76.8	Other disorders of glucosaminoglycan metabolism
		E76.9	Glucosaminoglycan metabolism disorder, unspecified

ICD-9-CM		ICD-10-CM	
277.6	OTHER DEFICIENCIES OF CIRCULATING ENZYMES	D81.810	Biotinidase deficiency
		D84.1	Defects in the complement system
277.7	DYSMETABOLIC SYNDROME X	➡ E88.81	Metabolic syndrome
277.81	PRIMARY CARNITINE DEFICIENCY	➡ E71.41	Primary carnitine deficiency
277.82	CARNITINE DEFIC DUE INBORN ERRORS METABOLISM	➡ E71.42	Carnitine deficiency due to inborn errors of metabolism
277.83	IATROGENIC CARNITINE DEFICIENCY	➡ E71.43	Iatrogenic carnitine deficiency
277.84	OTHER SECONDARY CARNITINE DEFICIENCY	E71.40	Disorder of carnitine metabolism, unspecified
		E71.440	Ruvalcaba-Myhre-Smith syndrome
		E71.448	Other secondary carnitine deficiency
277.85	DISORDERS OF FATTY ACID OXIDATION	E71.310	Long chain/very long chain acyl CoA dehydrogenase deficiency
		E71.311	Medium chain acyl CoA dehydrogenase deficiency
		E71.312	Short chain acyl CoA dehydrogenase deficiency
		E71.313	Glutaric aciduria type II
		E71.314	Muscle carnitine palmitoyltransferase deficiency
		E71.318	Other disorders of fatty-acid oxidation
		E71.32	Disorders of ketone metabolism
277.86	PEROXISOMAL DISORDERS	E71.50	Peroxisomal disorder, unspecified
		E71.510	Zellweger syndrome
		E71.511	Neonatal adrenoleukodystrophy
		E71.518	Other disorders of peroxisome biogenesis
		E71.520	Childhood cerebral X-linked adrenoleukodystrophy
		E71.521	Adolescent X-linked adrenoleukodystrophy
		E71.522	Adrenomyeloneuropathy
		E71.528	Other X-linked adrenoleukodystrophy
		E71.529	X-linked adrenoleukodystrophy, unspecified type
		E71.53	Other group 2 peroxisomal disorders
		E71.540	Rhizomelic chondrodysplasia punctata
		E71.541	Zellweger-like syndrome
		E71.542	Other group 3 peroxisomal disorders
		E71.548	Other peroxisomal disorders
277.87	DISORDERS OF MITOCHONDRIAL METABOLISM	E88.40	Mitochondrial metabolism disorder, unspecified
		E88.41	MELAS syndrome
		E88.42	MERRF syndrome
		E88.49	Other mitochondrial metabolism disorders
		H49.811	Kearns-Sayre syndrome, right eye
		H49.812	Kearns-Sayre syndrome, left eye
		H49.813	Kearns-Sayre syndrome, bilateral
		H49.819	Kearns-Sayre syndrome, unspecified eye
277.88	TUMOR LYSIS SYNDROME	➡ E88.3	Tumor lysis syndrome
277.89	OTHER SPECIFIED DISORDERS OF METABOLISM	C96.5	Multifocal and unisystemic Langerhans-cell histiocytosis
		C96.6	Unifocal Langerhans-cell histiocytosis
		E71.39	Other disorders of fatty-acid metabolism
		E80.3	Defects of catalase and peroxidase
		E88.89	Other specified metabolic disorders
		E88.9	Metabolic disorder, unspecified
277.9	UNSPECIFIED DISORDER OF METABOLISM	E88.9	Metabolic disorder, unspecified
278.00	OBESITY, UNSPECIFIED	E66.09	Other obesity due to excess calories
		E66.1	Drug-induced obesity
		E66.8	Other obesity
		E66.9	Obesity, unspecified
278.01	MORBID OBESITY	E66.01	Morbid (severe) obesity due to excess calories
278.02	OVERWEIGHT	➡ E66.3	Overweight
278.03	OBESITY HYPOVENTILATION SYNDROME	➡ E66.2	Morbid (severe) obesity with alveolar hypoventilation
278.1	LOCALIZED ADIPOSITY	➡ E65	Localized adiposity
278.2	HYPERVITAMINOSIS A	➡ E67.0	Hypervitaminosis A
278.3	HYPERCAROTINEMIA	➡ E67.1	Hypercarotinemia
278.4	HYPERVITAMINOSIS D	➡ E67.3	Hypervitaminosis D
278.8	OTHER HYPERALIMENTATION	E67.2	Megavitamin-B6 syndrome
		E67.8	Other specified hyperalimentation
		E68	Sequelae of hyperalimentation
279.00	UNSPECIFIED HYPOGAMMAGLOBULINEMIA	➡ D80.1	Nonfamilial hypogammaglobulinemia
279.01	SELECTIVE IGA IMMUNODEFICIENCY	➡ D80.2	Selective deficiency of immunoglobulin A [IgA]
279.02	SELECTIVE IGM IMMUNODEFICIENCY	➡ D80.4	Selective deficiency of immunoglobulin M [IgM]
279.03	OTHER SELECTIVE IMMUNOGLOBULIN DEFICIENCIES	D80.3	Selective deficiency of immunoglobulin G [IgG] subclasses
279.04	CONGENITAL HYPOGAMMAGLOBULINEMIA	➡ D80.0	Hereditary hypogammaglobulinemia
279.05	IMMUNODEFICIENCY WITH INCREASED IGM	➡ D80.5	Immunodeficiency with increased immunoglobulin M [IgM]
279.06	COMMON VARIABLE IMMUNODEFICIENCY	D83.0	Com variab immunodef w predom abnlt of B-cell nums & functn
		D83.2	Common variable immunodef w autoantibodies to B- or T-cells
		D83.8	Other common variable immunodeficiencies
		D83.9	Common variable immunodeficiency, unspecified
279.09	OTHER DEFICIENCY OF HUMORAL IMMUNITY	D80.7	Transient hypogammaglobulinemia of infancy
279.10	UNSPEC IMMUNODEFIC W/PREDOMINANT T-CELL DEFECT	D83.1	Com variab immunodef w predom immunoreg T-cell disorders
279.11	DIGEORGES SYNDROME	➡ D82.1	Di George's syndrome
279.12	WISKOTT-ALDRICH SYNDROME	➡ D82.0	Wiskott-Aldrich syndrome
279.13	NEZELOFS SYNDROME	➡ D81.4	Nezelof's syndrome

ICD-9-CM			ICD-10-CM	
279.19	OTHER DEFICIENCY OF CELL-MEDIATED IMMUNITY		**D8Ø.6**	Antibody defic w near-norm immunoglob or w hyperimmunoglob
			D8Ø.8	Other immunodeficiencies with predominantly antibody defects
			D8Ø.9	Immunodeficiency with predominantly antibody defects, unsp
279.2	COMBINED IMMUNITY DEFICIENCY		**D81.Ø**	Severe combined immunodeficiency with reticular dysgenesis
			D81.1	Severe combined immunodeficiency w low T- and B-cell numbers
			D81.2	Severe combined immunodef w low or normal B-cell numbers
			D81.6	Major histocompatibility complex class I deficiency
			D81.7	Major histocompatibility complex class II deficiency
			D81.89	Other combined immunodeficiencies
			D81.9	Combined immunodeficiency, unspecified
279.3	UNSPECIFIED IMMUNITY DEFICIENCY		**D84.8**	Other specified immunodeficiencies
			D84.9	Immunodeficiency, unspecified
279.41	AUTOIMMUNE LYMPHOPROLIFERATIVE SYNDROME	➡	**D89.82**	Autoimmune lymphoproliferative syndrome [ALPS]
279.49	AUTOIMMUNE DISEASE NOT ELSEWHERE CLASSIFIED		**D89.89**	Oth disrd involving the immune mechanism, NEC
279.5Ø	GRAFT-VERSUS-HOST DISEASE UNSPECIFIED	➡	**D89.813**	Graft-versus-host disease, unspecified
279.51	ACUTE GRAFT-VERSUS-HOST DISEASE	➡	**D89.81Ø**	Acute graft-versus-host disease
279.52	CHRONIC GRAFT-VERSUS-HOST DISEASE	➡	**D89.811**	Chronic graft-versus-host disease
279.53	ACUTE ON CHRONIC GRAFT-VERSUS-HOST DISEASE	➡	**D89.812**	Acute on chronic graft-versus-host disease
279.8	OTHER SPEC DISORDERS INVOLVING IMMUNE MECHANISM		**D82.2**	Immunodeficiency with short-limbed stature
			D82.3	Immunodef fol heredit defctv response to Epstein-Barr virus
			D82.4	Hyperimmunoglobulin E [IgE] syndrome
			D82.8	Immunodeficiency associated with oth major defects
			D82.9	Immunodeficiency associated with major defect, unspecified
			D84.Ø	Lymphocyte function antigen-1 [LFA-1] defect
			D84.1	Defects in the complement system
			D89.3	Immune reconstitution syndrome
			D89.89	Oth disrd involving the immune mechanism, NEC
			M35.9	Systemic involvement of connective tissue, unspecified
279.9	UNSPECIFIED DISORDER OF IMMUNE MECHANISM	➡	**D89.9**	Disorder involving the immune mechanism, unspecified

279.19–279.9

Blood and Blood-Forming Organs

ICD-9-CM			ICD-10-CM	
280.0	IRON DEFICIENCY ANEMIA SECONDARY TO BLOOD LOSS	➡	D50.0	Iron deficiency anemia secondary to blood loss (chronic)
280.1	IRON DEFIC ANEMIA SEC DIET IRON INTAKE		D50.8	Other iron deficiency anemias
280.8	OTHER SPECIFIED IRON DEFICIENCY ANEMIAS		D50.1 D50.8	Sideropenic dysphagia Other iron deficiency anemias
280.9	UNSPECIFIED IRON DEFICIENCY ANEMIA	➡	D50.9	Iron deficiency anemia, unspecified
281.0	PERNICIOUS ANEMIA		D51.0	Vitamin B12 defic anemia due to intrinsic factor deficiency
281.1	OTHER VITAMIN B12 DEFICIENCY ANEMIA		D51.1 D51.2 D51.3 D51.8 D51.9	Vit B12 defic anemia d/t slctv vit B12 malabsorp w protein Transcobalamin II deficiency Other dietary vitamin B12 deficiency anemia Other vitamin B12 deficiency anemias Vitamin B12 deficiency anemia, unspecified
281.2	FOLATE-DEFICIENCY ANEMIA		D52.0 D52.1 D52.8 D52.9	Dietary folate deficiency anemia Drug-induced folate deficiency anemia Other folate deficiency anemias Folate deficiency anemia, unspecified
281.3	OTHER SPECIFIED MEGALOBLASTIC ANEMIAS NEC	➡	D53.1	Other megaloblastic anemias, not elsewhere classified
281.4	PROTEIN-DEFICIENCY ANEMIA	➡	D53.0	Protein deficiency anemia
281.8	ANEMIA ASSOCIATED W/OTHER SPEC NUTRITIONAL DEFIC		D53.2 D53.8	Scorbutic anemia Other specified nutritional anemias
281.9	UNSPECIFIED DEFICIENCY ANEMIA		D53.9	Nutritional anemia, unspecified
282.0	HEREDITARY SPHEROCYTOSIS	➡	D58.0	Hereditary spherocytosis
282.1	HEREDITARY ELLIPTOCYTOSIS	➡	D58.1	Hereditary elliptocytosis
282.2	ANEMIAS DUE TO DISORDERS GLUTATHIONE METABOLISM		D55.0 D55.1	Anemia due to glucose-6-phosphate dehydrogenase deficiency Anemia due to other disorders of glutathione metabolism
282.3	OTHER HEMOLYTIC ANEMIAS DUE TO ENZYME DEFICIENCY		D55.2 D55.3 D55.8 D55.9	Anemia due to disorders of glycolytic enzymes Anemia due to disorders of nucleotide metabolism Other anemias due to enzyme disorders Anemia due to enzyme disorder, unspecified
282.40	THALASSEMIA UNSPECIFIED		D56.9	Thalassemia, unspecified
282.41	SICKLE-CELL THALASSEMIA WITHOUT CRISIS	➡	D57.40	Sickle-cell thalassemia without crisis
282.42	SICKLE-CELL THALASSEMIA WITH CRISIS	▣ ▣	D57.411 D57.412 D57.419	Sickle-cell thalassemia with acute chest syndrome Sickle-cell thalassemia with splenic sequestration Sickle-cell thalassemia with crisis, unspecified
282.43	ALPHA THALASSEMIA		D56.0	Alpha thalassemia
282.44	BETA THALASSEMIA		D56.1	Beta thalassemia
282.45	DELTA-BETA THALASSEMIA		D56.2	Delta-beta thalassemia
282.46	THALASSEMIA MINOR		D56.3	Thalassemia minor
282.47	HEMOGLOBIN E-BETA THALASSEMIA		D56.5	Hemoglobin E-beta thalassemia
282.49	OTHER THALASSEMIA		D56.8	Other thalassemias
282.5	SICKLE-CELL TRAIT	➡	D57.3	Sickle-cell trait
282.60	SICKLE-CELL DISEASE UNSPECIFIED		D57.1	Sickle-cell disease without crisis
282.61	HB-SS DISEASE WITHOUT CRISIS		D57.1	Sickle-cell disease without crisis
282.62	HB-SS DISEASE WITH CRISIS	 ▣ ▣	D57.00 D57.01 D57.02	Hb-SS disease with crisis, unspecified Hb-SS disease with acute chest syndrome Hb-SS disease with splenic sequestration
282.63	SICKLE-CELL/HB-C DISEASE WITHOUT CRISIS	➡	D57.20	Sickle-cell/Hb-C disease without crisis
282.64	SICKLE-CELL/HB-C DISEASE WITH CRISIS	▣ ▣	D57.211 D57.212 D57.219	Sickle-cell/Hb-C disease with acute chest syndrome Sickle-cell/Hb-C disease with splenic sequestration Sickle-cell/Hb-C disease with crisis, unspecified
282.68	OTHER SICKLE-CELL DISEASE WITHOUT CRISIS	➡	D57.80	Other sickle-cell disorders without crisis
282.69	OTHER SICKLE-CELL DISEASE WITH CRISIS	▣ ▣	D57.811 D57.812 D57.819	Other sickle-cell disorders with acute chest syndrome Other sickle-cell disorders with splenic sequestration Other sickle-cell disorders with crisis, unspecified
282.7	OTHER HEMOGLOBINOPATHIES		D56.4 D58.2	Hereditary persistence of fetal hemoglobin [HPFH] Other hemoglobinopathies
282.8	OTHER SPECIFIED HEREDITARY HEMOLYTIC ANEMIAS	➡	D58.8	Other specified hereditary hemolytic anemias
282.9	UNSPECIFIED HEREDITARY HEMOLYTIC ANEMIA	➡	D58.9	Hereditary hemolytic anemia, unspecified
283.0	AUTOIMMUNE HEMOLYTIC ANEMIAS		D59.0 D59.1	Drug-induced autoimmune hemolytic anemia Other autoimmune hemolytic anemias
283.10	UNSPECIFIED NON-AUTOIMMUNE HEMOLYTIC ANEMIA		D59.4	Other nonautoimmune hemolytic anemias
283.11	HEMOLYTIC-UREMIC SYNDROME	➡	D59.3	Hemolytic-uremic syndrome
283.19	OTHER NON-AUTOIMMUNE HEMOLYTIC ANEMIAS		D59.2 D59.4	Drug-induced nonautoimmune hemolytic anemia Other nonautoimmune hemolytic anemias
283.2	HGBURIA DUE HEMOLYSIS FROM EXTERNAL CAUSES		D59.5 D59.6 D59.8	Paroxysmal nocturnal hemoglobinuria [Marchiafava-Micheli] Hemoglobinuria due to hemolysis from other external causes Other acquired hemolytic anemias
283.9	ACQUIRED HEMOLYTIC ANEMIA UNSPECIFIED	➡	D59.9	Acquired hemolytic anemia, unspecified
284.01	CONSTITUTIONAL RED BLOOD CELL APLASIA	➡	D61.01	Constitutional (pure) red blood cell aplasia
284.09	OTHER CONSTITUTIONAL APLASTIC ANEMIA	➡	D61.09	Other constitutional aplastic anemia
284.11	ANTINEOPLASTIC CHEMOTHERAPY INDUCED PANCYTOPENIA		D61.810	Antineoplastic chemotherapy induced pancytopenia
284.12	OTHER DRUG INDUCED PANCYTOPENIA		D61.811	Other drug-induced pancytopenia
284.19	OTHER PANCYTOPENIA		D61.818	Other pancytopenia

ICD-9-CM			ICD-10-CM	
284.2	MYELOPHTHISIS	➡	D61.82	Myelophthisis
284.81	RED CELL APLASIA ACQUIRED ADULT WITH THYMOMA		D60.0 D60.1 D60.8 D60.9	Chronic acquired pure red cell aplasia Transient acquired pure red cell aplasia Other acquired pure red cell aplasias Acquired pure red cell aplasia, unspecified
284.89	OTHER SPECIFIED APLASTIC ANEMIAS		D61.1 D61.2 D61.3 D61.89	Drug-induced aplastic anemia Aplastic anemia due to other external agents Idiopathic aplastic anemia Oth aplastic anemias and other bone marrow failure syndromes
284.9	UNSPECIFIED APLASTIC ANEMIA		D61.9	Aplastic anemia, unspecified
285.0	SIDEROBLASTIC ANEMIA		D64.0 D64.1 D64.2 D64.3	Hereditary sideroblastic anemia Secondary sideroblastic anemia due to disease Secondary sideroblastic anemia due to drugs and toxins Other sideroblastic anemias
285.1	ACUTE POSTHEMORRHAGIC ANEMIA	➡	D62	Acute posthemorrhagic anemia
285.21	ANEMIA IN CHRONIC KIDNEY DISEASE		D63.1	Anemia in chronic kidney disease
285.22	ANEMIA IN NEOPLASTIC DISEASE	➡	D63.0	Anemia in neoplastic disease
285.29	ANEMIA OF OTHER CHRONIC DISEASE		D63.8	Anemia in other chronic diseases classified elsewhere
285.3	ANTINEOPLASTIC CHEMOTHERAPY INDUCED ANEMIA	➡	D64.81	Anemia due to antineoplastic chemotherapy
285.8	OTHER SPECIFIED ANEMIAS		D64.4 D64.89	Congenital dyserythropoietic anemia Other specified anemias
285.9	UNSPECIFIED ANEMIA	➡	D64.9	Anemia, unspecified
286.0	CONGENITAL FACTOR VIII DISORDER	➡	D66	Hereditary factor VIII deficiency
286.1	CONGENITAL FACTOR IX DISORDER	➡	D67	Hereditary factor IX deficiency
286.2	CONGENITAL FACTOR XI DEFICIENCY	➡	D68.1	Hereditary factor XI deficiency
286.3	CONGENITAL DEFICIENCY OF OTHER CLOTTING FACTORS	➡	D68.2	Hereditary deficiency of other clotting factors
286.4	VON WILLEBRANDS DISEASE	➡	D68.0	Von Willebrand's disease
286.52	ACQUIRED HEMOPHILIA		D68.311	Acquired hemophilia
286.53	ANTIPHOSPHOLIPID ANTIBODY W/HEMORRHAGIC D/O		D68.312	Antiphospholipid antibody with hemorrhagic disorder
286.59	OTH HEMMORRHAGIC D/O INTRINSIC CIRC AC AB/INHIB		D68.318	Oth hemorrhagic disord d/t intrns circ anticoag,antib,inhib
286.6	DEFIBRINATION SYNDROME	➡	D65	Disseminated intravascular coagulation
286.7	ACQUIRED COAGULATION FACTOR DEFICIENCY		D68.32 D68.4	Hemorrhagic disord d/t extrinsic circulating anticoagulants Acquired coagulation factor deficiency
286.9	OTHER AND UNSPECIFIED COAGULATION DEFECTS		D68.8 D68.9	Other specified coagulation defects Coagulation defect, unspecified
287.0	ALLERGIC PURPURA	➡	D69.0	Allergic purpura
287.1	QUALITATIVE PLATELET DEFECTS	➡	D69.1	Qualitative platelet defects
287.2	OTHER NONTHROMBOCYTOPENIC PURPURAS	➡	D69.2	Other nonthrombocytopenic purpura
287.30	PRIMARY THROMBOCYTOPENIA UNSPECIFIED		D69.49	Other primary thrombocytopenia
287.31	IMMUNE THROMBOCYTOPENIC PURPURA	➡	D69.3	Immune thrombocytopenic purpura
287.32	EVANS SYNDROME	➡	D69.41	Evans syndrome
287.33	CONGENITAL & HEREDITARY THROMBOCYTOPENIC PURPURA	➡	D69.42	Congenital and hereditary thrombocytopenia purpura
287.39	OTHER PRIMARY THROMBOCYTOPENIA		D69.3 D69.49	Immune thrombocytopenic purpura Other primary thrombocytopenia
287.41	POSTTRANSFUSION PURPURA	➡	D69.51	Posttransfusion purpura
287.49	OTHER SECONDARY THROMBOCYTOPENIA	➡	D69.59	Other secondary thrombocytopenia
287.5	UNSPECIFIED THROMBOCYTOPENIA	➡	D69.6	Thrombocytopenia, unspecified
287.8	OTHER SPECIFIED HEMORRHAGIC CONDITIONS	➡	D69.8	Other specified hemorrhagic conditions
287.9	UNSPECIFIED HEMORRHAGIC CONDITIONS	➡	D69.9	Hemorrhagic condition, unspecified
288.00	NEUTROPENIA UNSPECIFIED	➡	D70.9	Neutropenia, unspecified
288.01	CONGENITAL NEUTROPENIA	➡	D70.0	Congenital agranulocytosis
288.02	CYCLIC NEUTROPENIA	➡	D70.4	Cyclic neutropenia
288.03	DRUG INDUCED NEUTROPENIA		D70.1 D70.2	Agranulocytosis secondary to cancer chemotherapy Other drug-induced agranulocytosis
288.04	NEUTROPENIA DUE TO INFECTION	➡	D70.3	Neutropenia due to infection
288.09	OTHER NEUTROPENIA	➡	D70.8	Other neutropenia
288.1	FUNCTIONAL D/O POLYMORPHONUCLEAR NEUTROPHILS	➡	D71	Functional disorders of polymorphonuclear neutrophils
288.2	GENETIC ANOMALIES OF LEUKOCYTES	➡	D72.0	Genetic anomalies of leukocytes
288.3	EOSINOPHILIA	➡	D72.1	Eosinophilia
288.4	HEMOPHAGOCYTIC SYNDROMES		D76.1 D76.2 D76.3	Hemophagocytic lymphohistiocytosis Hemophagocytic syndrome, infection-associated Other histiocytosis syndromes
288.50	LEUKOCYTOPENIA UNSPECIFIED		D72.819	Decreased white blood cell count, unspecified
288.51	LYMPHOCYTOPENIA	➡	D72.810	Lymphocytopenia
288.59	OTHER DECREASED WHITE BLOOD CELL COUNT	➡	D72.818	Other decreased white blood cell count
288.60	LEUKOCYTOSIS UNSPECIFIED	➡	D72.829	Elevated white blood cell count, unspecified
288.61	LYMPHOCYTOSIS SYMPTOMATIC	➡	D72.820	Lymphocytosis (symptomatic)
288.62	LEUKEMOID REACTION	➡	D72.823	Leukemoid reaction
288.63	MONOCYTOSIS SYMPTOMATIC	➡	D72.821	Monocytosis (symptomatic)
288.64	PLASMACYTOSIS	➡	D72.822	Plasmacytosis

[Brackets] indicate valid character values for each code. Character value meanings provided for each code grouping.

ICD-9-CM		ICD-10-CM		
288.65	BASOPHILIA	➡	**D72.824**	Basophilia
288.66	BANDEMIA	➡	**D72.825**	Bandemia
288.69	OTHER ELEVATED WHITE BLOOD CELL COUNT	➡	**D72.828**	Other elevated white blood cell count
288.8	OTHER SPECIFIED DISEASE OF WHITE BLOOD CELLS	➡	**D72.89**	Other specified disorders of white blood cells
288.9	UNSPECIFIED DISEASE OF WHITE BLOOD CELLS	➡	**D72.9**	Disorder of white blood cells, unspecified
289.0	POLYCYTHEMIA, SECONDARY	➡	**D75.1**	Secondary polycythemia
289.1	CHRONIC LYMPHADENITIS	➡	**I88.1**	Chronic lymphadenitis, except mesenteric
289.2	NONSPECIFIC MESENTERIC LYMPHADENITIS	➡	**I88.0**	Nonspecific mesenteric lymphadenitis
289.3	LYMPHADENITIS UNSPECIFIED EXCEPT MESENTERIC		**I88.8** **I88.9**	Other nonspecific lymphadenitis Nonspecific lymphadenitis, unspecified
289.4	HYPERSPLENISM	➡	**D73.1**	Hypersplenism
289.50	UNSPECIFIED DISEASE OF SPLEEN	➡	**D73.9**	Disease of spleen, unspecified
289.51	CHRONIC CONGESTIVE SPLENOMEGALY	➡	**D73.2**	Chronic congestive splenomegaly
289.52	SPLENIC SEQUESTRATION	◘ ◘ ◘ ◘	**D57.02** **D57.212** **D57.412** **D57.812**	Hb-SS disease with splenic sequestration Sickle-cell/Hb-C disease with splenic sequestration Sickle-cell thalassemia with splenic sequestration Other sickle-cell disorders with splenic sequestration
289.53	NEUTROPENIC SPLENOMEGALY	➡	**D73.81**	Neutropenic splenomegaly
289.59	OTHER DISEASES OF SPLEEN		**D73.0** **D73.3** **D73.4** **D73.5** **D73.89**	Hyposplenism Abscess of spleen Cyst of spleen Infarction of spleen Other diseases of spleen
289.6	FAMILIAL POLYCYTHEMIA	➡	**D75.0**	Familial erythrocytosis
289.7	METHEMOGLOBINEMIA		**D74.0** **D74.8** **D74.9**	Congenital methemoglobinemia Other methemoglobinemias Methemoglobinemia, unspecified
289.81	PRIMARY HYPERCOAGULABLE STATE		**D68.51** **D68.52** **D68.59** **D68.61** **D68.62**	Activated protein C resistance Prothrombin gene mutation Other primary thrombophilia Antiphospholipid syndrome Lupus anticoagulant syndrome
289.82	SECONDARY HYPERCOAGULABLE STATE		**D68.69**	Other thrombophilia
289.83	MYELOFIBROSIS	➡	**D75.81**	Myelofibrosis
289.84	HEPARIN-INDUCED THROMBOCYTOPENIA	➡	**D75.82**	Heparin induced thrombocytopenia (HIT)
289.89	OTHER SPEC DISEASES BLOOD&BLOOD-FORMING ORGANS		**D47.4** **D75.89** **D77** **D89.2**	Osteomyelofibrosis Other specified diseases of blood and blood-forming organs Oth disord of bld/bld-frm organs in diseases classd elswhr Hypergammaglobulinemia, unspecified
289.9	UNSPECIFIED DISEASES BLOOD&BLOOD-FORMING ORGANS		**D75.9**	Disease of blood and blood-forming organs, unspecified

Mental, Behavioral, and Neurodevelopmental Disorders

ICD-9-CM		ICD-10-CM			
290.Ø	SENILE DEMENTIA, UNCOMPLICATED		F03.90	Unspecified dementia without behavioral disturbance	
290.10	PRESENILE DEMENTIA, UNCOMPLICATED		F03.90	Unspecified dementia without behavioral disturbance	
290.11	PRESENILE DEMENTIA WITH DELIRIUM		F03.90	Unspecified dementia without behavioral disturbance	
290.12	PRESENILE DEMENTIA WITH DELUSIONAL FEATURES		F03.90	Unspecified dementia without behavioral disturbance	*and*
			F05	Delirium due to known physiological condition	
290.13	PRESENILE DEMENTIA WITH DEPRESSIVE FEATURES		F03.90	Unspecified dementia without behavioral disturbance	
290.20	SENILE DEMENTIA WITH DELUSIONAL FEATURES		F03.90	Unspecified dementia without behavioral disturbance	*and*
			F05	Delirium due to known physiological condition	
290.21	SENILE DEMENTIA WITH DEPRESSIVE FEATURES		F03.90	Unspecified dementia without behavioral disturbance	
290.3	SENILE DEMENTIA WITH DELIRIUM		F03.90	Unspecified dementia without behavioral disturbance	*and*
			F05	Delirium due to known physiological condition	
290.40	VASCULAR DEMENTIA UNCOMPLICATED		F01.50	Vascular dementia without behavioral disturbance	
290.41	VASCULAR DEMENTIA WITH DELIRIUM		F01.51	Vascular dementia with behavioral disturbance	
290.42	VASCULAR DEMENTIA WITH DELUSIONS		F01.51	Vascular dementia with behavioral disturbance	
290.43	VASCULAR DEMENTIA WITH DEPRESSED MOOD		F01.51	Vascular dementia with behavioral disturbance	
290.8	OTHER SPECIFIED SENILE PSYCHOTIC CONDITIONS		F03.90	Unspecified dementia without behavioral disturbance	
290.9	UNSPECIFIED SENILE PSYCHOTIC CONDITION		F03.90	Unspecified dementia without behavioral disturbance	
291.0	ALCOHOL WITHDRAWAL DELIRIUM		F10.121	Alcohol abuse with intoxication delirium	
			F10.221	Alcohol dependence with intoxication delirium	
			F10.231	Alcohol dependence with withdrawal delirium	
			F10.921	Alcohol use, unspecified with intoxication delirium	
291.1	ALCOHOL-INDUCED PERSISTING AMNESTIC DISORDER		F10.26	Alcohol depend w alcoh-induce persisting amnestic disorder	
			F10.96	Alcohol use, unsp w alcoh-induce persist amnestic disorder	
			F10.97	Alcohol use, unsp with alcohol-induced persisting dementia	
291.2	ALCOHOL-INDUCED PERSISTING DEMENTIA		F10.27	Alcohol dependence with alcohol-induced persisting dementia	
291.3	ALCOHOL-INDUCED PSYCHOT DISORDER W/HALLUCINATION		F10.151	Alcohol abuse w alcoh-induce psychotic disorder w hallucin	
			F10.251	Alcohol depend w alcoh-induce psychotic disorder w hallucin	
			F10.951	Alcohol use, unsp w alcoh-induce psych disorder w hallucin	
291.4	IDIOSYNCRATIC ALCOHOL INTOXICATION		F10.920	Alcohol use, unspecified with intoxication, uncomplicated	
			F10.929	Alcohol use, unspecified with intoxication, unspecified	
291.5	ALCOHOL-INDUCED PSYCHOTIC DISORDER W/DELUSIONS		F10.150	Alcohol abuse w alcoh-induce psychotic disorder w delusions	
			F10.250	Alcohol depend w alcoh-induce psychotic disorder w delusions	
			F10.950	Alcohol use, unsp w alcoh-induce psych disorder w delusions	
291.81	ALCOHOL WITHDRAWAL		F10.230	Alcohol dependence with withdrawal, uncomplicated	
			F10.232	Alcohol dependence w withdrawal with perceptual disturbance	
			F10.239	Alcohol dependence with withdrawal, unspecified	
291.82	ALCOHOL INDUCED SLEEP DISORDERS		F10.182	Alcohol abuse with alcohol-induced sleep disorder	
			F10.282	Alcohol dependence with alcohol-induced sleep disorder	
			F10.982	Alcohol use, unspecified with alcohol-induced sleep disorder	
291.89	OTHER SPECIFIED ALCOHOL-INDUCED MENTAL DISORDERS		F10.14	Alcohol abuse with alcohol-induced mood disorder	
			F10.159	Alcohol abuse with alcohol-induced psychotic disorder, unsp	
			F10.180	Alcohol abuse with alcohol-induced anxiety disorder	
			F10.181	Alcohol abuse with alcohol-induced sexual dysfunction	
			F10.188	Alcohol abuse with other alcohol-induced disorder	
			F10.24	Alcohol dependence with alcohol-induced mood disorder	
			F10.259	Alcohol dependence w alcoh-induce psychotic disorder, unsp	
			F10.280	Alcohol dependence with alcohol-induced anxiety disorder	
			F10.281	Alcohol dependence with alcohol-induced sexual dysfunction	
			F10.288	Alcohol dependence with other alcohol-induced disorder	
			F10.959	Alcohol use, unsp w alcohol-induced psychotic disorder, unsp	
			F10.980	Alcohol use, unsp with alcohol-induced anxiety disorder	
			F10.981	Alcohol use, unsp with alcohol-induced sexual dysfunction	
			F10.988	Alcohol use, unspecified with other alcohol-induced disorder	
291.9	UNSPECIFIED ALCOHOL-INDUCED MENTAL DISORDERS		F10.19	Alcohol abuse with unspecified alcohol-induced disorder	
			F10.29	Alcohol dependence with unspecified alcohol-induced disorder	
			F10.94	Alcohol use, unspecified with alcohol-induced mood disorder	
			F10.99	Alcohol use, unsp with unspecified alcohol-induced disorder	
292.0	DRUG WITHDRAWAL	▣	F11.23	Opioid dependence with withdrawal	
			F11.93	Opioid use, unspecified with withdrawal	
		▣	F13.230	Sedatv/hyp/anxiolytc dependence w withdrawal, uncomplicated	
		▣	F13.231	Sedatv/hyp/anxiolytc dependence w withdrawal delirium	
		▣	F13.232	Sedatv/hyp/anxiolytc depend w w/drawal w perceptual disturb	
		▣	F13.239	Sedatv/hyp/anxiolytc dependence w withdrawal, unsp	
			F13.930	Sedatv/hyp/anxiolytc use, unsp w withdrawal, uncomplicated	
			F13.931	Sedatv/hyp/anxiolytc use, unsp w withdrawal delirium	
			F13.932	Sedatv/hyp/anxiolytc use, unsp w w/drawal w perceptl disturb	
			F13.939	Sedatv/hyp/anxiolytc use, unsp w withdrawal, unsp	
		▣	F14.23	Cocaine dependence with withdrawal	
		▣	F15.23	Other stimulant dependence with withdrawal	
			F15.93	Other stimulant use, unspecified with withdrawal	
			F17.203	Nicotine dependence unspecified, with withdrawal	
			F17.213	Nicotine dependence, cigarettes, with withdrawal	
			F17.223	Nicotine dependence, chewing tobacco, with withdrawal	
			F17.293	Nicotine dependence, other tobacco product, with withdrawal	
		▣	F19.230	Oth psychoactive substance dependence w withdrawal, uncomp	
		▣	F19.231	Oth psychoactive substance dependence w withdrawal delirium	

(Continued on next page)

ICD-9-CM		ICD-10-CM	
292.Ø	DRUG WITHDRAWAL (Continued)	F19.232	Oth psychoactv sub depend w w/drawal w perceptl disturb
		F19.239	Oth psychoactive substance dependence with withdrawal, unsp
		F19.93Ø	Oth psychoactive substance use, unsp w withdrawal, uncomp
		F19.931	Oth psychoactive substance use, unsp w withdrawal delirium
		F19.932	Oth psychoactv sub use, unsp w w/drawal w perceptl disturb
		F19.939	Other psychoactive substance use, unsp with withdrawal, unsp
292.11	DRUG-INDUCED PSYCHOTIC DISORDER WITH DELUSIONS	F11.15Ø	Opioid abuse w opioid-induced psychotic disorder w delusions
		F11.25Ø	Opioid depend w opioid-induc psychotic disorder w delusions
		F11.95Ø	Opioid use, unsp w opioid-induc psych disorder w delusions
		F12.15Ø	Cannabis abuse with psychotic disorder with delusions
		F12.25Ø	Cannabis dependence with psychotic disorder with delusions
		F12.95Ø	Cannabis use, unsp with psychotic disorder with delusions
		F13.15Ø	Sedatv/hyp/anxiolytc abuse w psychotic disorder w delusions
		F13.25Ø	Sedatv/hyp/anxiolytc depend w psychotic disorder w delusions
		F13.95Ø	Sedatv/hyp/anxiolytc use, unsp w psych disorder w delusions
		F14.15Ø	Cocaine abuse w cocaine-induc psychotic disorder w delusions
		F14.25Ø	Cocaine depend w cocaine-induc psych disorder w delusions
		F14.95Ø	Cocaine use, unsp w cocaine-induc psych disorder w delusions
		F15.15Ø	Oth stimulant abuse w stim-induce psych disorder w delusions
		F15.25Ø	Oth stim depend w stim-induce psych disorder w delusions
		F15.95Ø	Oth stim use, unsp w stim-induce psych disorder w delusions
		F16.15Ø	Hallucinogen abuse w psychotic disorder w delusions
		F16.25Ø	Hallucinogen dependence w psychotic disorder w delusions
		F16.95Ø	Hallucinogen use, unsp w psychotic disorder w delusions
		F18.15Ø	Inhalant abuse w inhalnt-induce psych disorder w delusions
		F18.25Ø	Inhalant depend w inhalnt-induce psych disorder w delusions
		F18.95Ø	Inhalant use, unsp w inhalnt-induce psych disord w delusions
		F19.15Ø	Oth psychoactv substance abuse w psych disorder w delusions
		F19.25Ø	Oth psychoactv substance depend w psych disorder w delusions
		F19.95Ø	Oth psychoactv sub use, unsp w psych disorder w delusions
292.12	DRUG-INDUCED PSYCHOTIC DISORDER W/HALLUCINATIONS	F11.151	Opioid abuse w opioid-induced psychotic disorder w hallucin
		F11.251	Opioid depend w opioid-induc psychotic disorder w hallucin
		F11.951	Opioid use, unsp w opioid-induc psych disorder w hallucin
		F12.151	Cannabis abuse with psychotic disorder with hallucinations
		F12.251	Cannabis dependence w psychotic disorder with hallucinations
		F12.951	Cannabis use, unsp w psychotic disorder with hallucinations
		F13.151	Sedatv/hyp/anxiolytc abuse w psychotic disorder w hallucin
		F13.251	Sedatv/hyp/anxiolytc depend w psychotic disorder w hallucin
		F13.951	Sedatv/hyp/anxiolytc use, unsp w psych disorder w hallucin
		F14.151	Cocaine abuse w cocaine-induc psychotic disorder w hallucin
		F14.251	Cocaine depend w cocaine-induc psychotic disorder w hallucin
		F14.951	Cocaine use, unsp w cocaine-induc psych disorder w hallucin
		F15.151	Oth stimulant abuse w stim-induce psych disorder w hallucin
		F15.251	Oth stimulant depend w stim-induce psych disorder w hallucin
		F15.951	Oth stim use, unsp w stim-induce psych disorder w hallucin
		F16.151	Hallucinogen abuse w psychotic disorder w hallucinations
		F16.251	Hallucinogen dependence w psychotic disorder w hallucin
		F16.951	Hallucinogen use, unsp w psychotic disorder w hallucinations
		F18.151	Inhalant abuse w inhalnt-induce psych disorder w hallucin
		F18.251	Inhalant depend w inhalnt-induce psych disorder w hallucin
		F18.951	Inhalant use, unsp w inhalnt-induce psych disord w hallucin
		F19.151	Oth psychoactv substance abuse w psych disorder w hallucin
		F19.251	Oth psychoactv substance depend w psych disorder w hallucin
		F19.951	Oth psychoactv sub use, unsp w psych disorder w hallucin
292.2	PATHOLOGICAL DRUG INTOXICATION	F11.22Ø	Opioid dependence with intoxication, uncomplicated
		F11.229	Opioid dependence with intoxication, unspecified
		F11.92Ø	Opioid use, unspecified with intoxication, uncomplicated
		F11.929	Opioid use, unspecified with intoxication, unspecified
		F12.12Ø	Cannabis abuse with intoxication, uncomplicated
		F12.129	Cannabis abuse with intoxication, unspecified
		F12.22Ø	Cannabis dependence with intoxication, uncomplicated
		F12.229	Cannabis dependence with intoxication, unspecified
		F12.92Ø	Cannabis use, unspecified with intoxication, uncomplicated
		F12.929	Cannabis use, unspecified with intoxication, unspecified
		F13.129	Sedative, hypnotic or anxiolytic abuse w intoxication, unsp
		F13.22Ø	Sedatv/hyp/anxiolytc dependence w intoxication, uncomp
		F13.229	Sedatv/hyp/anxiolytc dependence w intoxication, unsp
		F13.92Ø	Sedatv/hyp/anxiolytc use, unsp w intoxication, uncomplicated
		F13.929	Sedatv/hyp/anxiolytc use, unsp w intoxication, unsp
		F14.129	Cocaine abuse with intoxication, unspecified
		F14.22Ø	Cocaine dependence with intoxication, uncomplicated
		F14.229	Cocaine dependence with intoxication, unspecified
		F14.92Ø	Cocaine use, unspecified with intoxication, uncomplicated
		F14.929	Cocaine use, unspecified with intoxication, unspecified
		F15.129	Other stimulant abuse with intoxication, unspecified
		F15.22Ø	Other stimulant dependence with intoxication, uncomplicated
		F15.229	Other stimulant dependence with intoxication, unspecified
		F15.92Ø	Other stimulant use, unsp with intoxication, uncomplicated
		F15.929	Other stimulant use, unsp with intoxication, unspecified
	(Continued on next page)	F16.129	Hallucinogen abuse with intoxication, unspecified

ICD-9-CM		ICD-10-CM	
292.2	PATHOLOGICAL DRUG INTOXICATION **(Continued)**	**F16.220**	Hallucinogen dependence with intoxication, uncomplicated
		F16.229	Hallucinogen dependence with intoxication, unspecified
		F16.920	Hallucinogen use, unsp with intoxication, uncomplicated
		F16.929	Hallucinogen use, unspecified with intoxication, unspecified
		F18.120	Inhalant abuse with intoxication, uncomplicated
		F18.129	Inhalant abuse with intoxication, unspecified
		F18.220	Inhalant dependence with intoxication, uncomplicated
		F18.229	Inhalant dependence with intoxication, unspecified
		F18.920	Inhalant use, unspecified with intoxication, uncomplicated
		F18.929	Inhalant use, unspecified with intoxication, unspecified
		F19.129	Other psychoactive substance abuse with intoxication, unsp
		F19.220	Oth psychoactive substance dependence w intoxication, uncomp
		F19.229	Oth psychoactive substance dependence w intoxication, unsp
		F19.920	Oth psychoactive substance use, unsp w intoxication, uncomp
		F19.929	Oth psychoactive substance use, unsp with intoxication, unsp
292.81	DRUG-INDUCED DELIRIUM	**F11.121**	Opioid abuse with intoxication delirium
		F11.221	Opioid dependence with intoxication delirium
		F11.921	Opioid use, unspecified with intoxication delirium
		F12.121	Cannabis abuse with intoxication delirium
		F12.221	Cannabis dependence with intoxication delirium
		F12.921	Cannabis use, unspecified with intoxication delirium
		F13.121	Sedatv/hyp/anxiolytc abuse w intoxication delirium
		F13.221	Sedatv/hyp/anxiolytc dependence w intoxication delirium
		F13.921	Sedatv/hyp/anxiolytc use, unsp w intoxication delirium
		F14.121	Cocaine abuse with intoxication with delirium
		F14.221	Cocaine dependence with intoxication delirium
		F14.921	Cocaine use, unspecified with intoxication delirium
		F15.121	Other stimulant abuse with intoxication delirium
		F15.221	Other stimulant dependence with intoxication delirium
		F15.921	Other stimulant use, unspecified with intoxication delirium
		F16.121	Hallucinogen abuse with intoxication with delirium
		F16.221	Hallucinogen dependence with intoxication with delirium
		F16.921	Hallucinogen use, unsp with intoxication with delirium
		F18.121	Inhalant abuse with intoxication delirium
		F18.221	Inhalant dependence with intoxication delirium
		F18.921	Inhalant use, unspecified with intoxication with delirium
		F19.121	Oth psychoactive substance abuse with intoxication delirium
		F19.221	Oth psychoactive substance dependence w intox delirium
		F19.921	Oth psychoactive substance use, unsp w intox w delirium
292.82	DRUG-INDUCED PERSISTING DEMENTIA	**F13.27**	Sedatv/hyp/anxiolytc dependence w persisting dementia
		F13.97	Sedatv/hyp/anxiolytc use, unsp w persisting dementia
		F18.17	Inhalant abuse with inhalant-induced dementia
		F18.27	Inhalant dependence with inhalant-induced dementia
		F18.97	Inhalant use, unsp with inhalant-induced persisting dementia
		F19.17	Oth psychoactive substance abuse w persisting dementia
		F19.27	Oth psychoactive substance dependence w persisting dementia
		F19.97	Oth psychoactive substance use, unsp w persisting dementia
292.83	DRUG-INDUCED PERSISTING AMNESTIC DISORDER	**F13.26**	Sedatv/hyp/anxiolytc depend w persisting amnestic disorder
		F13.96	Sedatv/hyp/anxiolytc use, unsp w persist amnestic disorder
		F19.16	Oth psychoactv substance abuse w persist amnestic disorder
		F19.26	Oth psychoactv substance depend w persist amnestic disorder
		F19.96	Oth psychoactv sub use, unsp w persist amnestic disorder
292.84	DRUG-INDUCED MOOD DISORDER	**F11.14**	Opioid abuse with opioid-induced mood disorder
		F11.24	Opioid dependence with opioid-induced mood disorder
		F11.94	Opioid use, unspecified with opioid-induced mood disorder
		F13.14	Sedative, hypnotic or anxiolytic abuse w mood disorder
		F13.24	Sedative, hypnotic or anxiolytic dependence w mood disorder
		F13.94	Sedative, hypnotic or anxiolytic use, unsp w mood disorder
		F14.14	Cocaine abuse with cocaine-induced mood disorder
		F14.24	Cocaine dependence with cocaine-induced mood disorder
		F14.94	Cocaine use, unspecified with cocaine-induced mood disorder
		F15.14	Other stimulant abuse with stimulant-induced mood disorder
		F15.24	Oth stimulant dependence w stimulant-induced mood disorder
		F15.94	Oth stimulant use, unsp with stimulant-induced mood disorder
		F16.14	Hallucinogen abuse with hallucinogen-induced mood disorder
		F16.24	Hallucinogen dependence w hallucinogen-induced mood disorder
		F16.94	Hallucinogen use, unsp w hallucinogen-induced mood disorder
		F18.14	Inhalant abuse with inhalant-induced mood disorder
		F18.24	Inhalant dependence with inhalant-induced mood disorder
		F18.94	Inhalant use, unsp with inhalant-induced mood disorder
		F19.14	Oth psychoactive substance abuse w mood disorder
		F19.24	Oth psychoactive substance dependence w mood disorder
		F19.94	Oth psychoactive substance use, unsp w mood disorder

ICD-9-CM		ICD-10-CM	
292.85	DRUG INDUCED SLEEP DISORDERS	**F11.182**	Opioid abuse with opioid-induced sleep disorder
		F11.282	Opioid dependence with opioid-induced sleep disorder
		F11.982	Opioid use, unspecified with opioid-induced sleep disorder
		F13.182	Sedative, hypnotic or anxiolytic abuse w sleep disorder
		F13.282	Sedative, hypnotic or anxiolytic dependence w sleep disorder
		F13.982	Sedative, hypnotic or anxiolytic use, unsp w sleep disorder
		F14.182	Cocaine abuse with cocaine-induced sleep disorder
		F14.282	Cocaine dependence with cocaine-induced sleep disorder
		F14.982	Cocaine use, unspecified with cocaine-induced sleep disorder
		F15.182	Other stimulant abuse with stimulant-induced sleep disorder
		F15.282	Oth stimulant dependence w stimulant-induced sleep disorder
		F15.982	Oth stimulant use, unsp w stimulant-induced sleep disorder
		F19.182	Oth psychoactive substance abuse w sleep disorder
		F19.21	Other psychoactive substance dependence, in remission
		F19.282	Oth psychoactive substance dependence w sleep disorder
		F19.982	Oth psychoactive substance use, unsp w sleep disorder
292.89	OTHER SPECIFIED DRUG-INDUCED MENTAL DISORDER	**F11.122**	Opioid abuse with intoxication with perceptual disturbance
		F11.159	Opioid abuse with opioid-induced psychotic disorder, unsp
		F11.18[1,8]	Opioid abuse with opioid-induced disorder
		F11.222	Opioid dependence w intoxication with perceptual disturbance
		F11.259	Opioid dependence w opioid-induced psychotic disorder, unsp
		F11.28[1,8]	Opioid dependence with opioid-induced disorder
		F11.922	Opioid use, unsp w intoxication with perceptual disturbance
		F11.959	Opioid use, unsp w opioid-induced psychotic disorder, unsp
		F11.98[1,8]	Opioid use, unsp with opioid-induced disorder
		F12.122	Cannabis abuse with intoxication with perceptual disturbance
		F12.159	Cannabis abuse with psychotic disorder, unspecified
		F12.180	Cannabis abuse with cannabis-induced anxiety disorder
		F12.188	Cannabis abuse with other cannabis-induced disorder
		F12.222	Cannabis dependence w intoxication w perceptual disturbance
		F12.259	Cannabis dependence with psychotic disorder, unspecified
		F12.280	Cannabis dependence with cannabis-induced anxiety disorder
		F12.288	Cannabis dependence with other cannabis-induced disorder
		F12.922	Cannabis use, unsp w intoxication w perceptual disturbance
		F12.959	Cannabis use, unsp with psychotic disorder, unspecified
		F12.980	Cannabis use, unspecified with anxiety disorder
		F12.988	Cannabis use, unsp with other cannabis-induced disorder
		F13.159	Sedatv/hyp/anxiolytc abuse w psychotic disorder, unsp
		F13.18[0,1,8]	Sedative, hypnotic or anxiolytic abuse w induced disorder
		F13.259	Sedative/hyp/anxiolytc dependence w psychotic disorder, unsp
		F13.28[0,1,8]	Sedative/hyp/anxiolytc dependence disorder
		F13.959	Sedative/hyp/anxiolytc use, unsp w psychotic disorder, unsp
		F13.98[0,1,8]	Sedative/hyp/anxiolytc use, unsp w induced disorder
		F14.122	Cocaine abuse with intoxication with perceptual disturbance
		F14.159	Cocaine abuse with cocaine-induced psychotic disorder, unsp
		F14.18[0,1,8]	Cocaine abuse with cocaine-induced disorder
		F14.222	Cocaine dependence w intoxication w perceptual disturbance
		F14.259	Cocaine dependence w cocaine-induc psychotic disorder, unsp
		F14.28[0,1,8]	Cocaine dependence with cocaine-induced disorder
		F14.922	Cocaine use, unsp w intoxication with perceptual disturbance
		F14.959	Cocaine use, unsp w cocaine-induced psychotic disorder, unsp
		F14.98[0,1,8]	Cocaine use, unsp with cocaine-induced disorder
		F15.122	Oth stimulant abuse w intoxication w perceptual disturbance
		F15.159	Oth stimulant abuse w stim-induce psychotic disorder, unsp
		F15.18[0,1,8]	Oth stimulant abuse with stimulant-induced disorder
		F15.222	Oth stimulant dependence w intox w perceptual disturbance
		F15.259	Oth stimulant depend w stim-induce psychotic disorder, unsp
		F15.28[0,1,8]	Oth stimulant dependence w stim-induce disorder
		F15.922	Oth stimulant use, unsp w intox w perceptual disturbance
		F15.959	Oth stimulant use, unsp w stim-induce psych disorder, unsp
		F15.98[0,1,8]	Oth stimulant use, unsp w stimulant-induced disorder
		F16.122	Hallucinogen abuse w intoxication w perceptual disturbance
		F16.159	Hallucinogen abuse w psychotic disorder, unsp
		F16.180	Hallucinogen abuse w hallucinogen-induced anxiety disorder
		F16.183	Hallucign abuse w hallucign persisting perception disorder
		F16.188	Hallucinogen abuse with other hallucinogen-induced disorder
		F16.259	Hallucinogen dependence w psychotic disorder, unsp
		F16.280	Hallucinogen dependence w anxiety disorder
		F16.283	Hallucign depend w hallucign persisting perception disorder
		F16.288	Hallucinogen dependence w oth hallucinogen-induced disorder
		F16.959	Hallucinogen use, unsp w psychotic disorder, unsp
		F16.980	Hallucinogen use, unsp w anxiety disorder
		F16.983	Hallucign use, unsp w hallucign persist perception disorder
		F16.988	Hallucinogen use, unsp w oth hallucinogen-induced disorder

6th Character meanings for codes as indicated

- ***0*** ***Anxiety Disorder***
- ***1*** ***Sexual Dysfunction***
- ***2*** ***Sleep Disorder***
- ***8*** ***Other Psychoactive Subs-induced Disorder***

Note: For 6th character 8, refer to subcategory for specific psychoactive substance

(Continued on next page)

[Brackets] indicate valid character values for each code. Character value meanings provided for each code grouping.

ICD-9-CM			ICD-10-CM	
292.89	OTHER SPECIFIED DRUG-INDUCED MENTAL DISORDER **(Continued)**		**F17.208**	Nicotine dependence, unsp, w oth nicotine-induced disorders
			F17.218	Nicotine dependence, cigarettes, w oth disorders
			F17.228	Nicotine dependence, chewing tobacco, w oth disorders
			F17.298	Nicotine dependence, oth tobacco product, w oth disorders
			F18.159	Inhalant abuse w inhalant-induced psychotic disorder, unsp
			F18.180	Inhalant abuse with inhalant-induced anxiety disorder
			F18.188	Inhalant abuse with other inhalant-induced disorder
		◙	**F18.259**	Inhalant depend w inhalnt-induce psychotic disorder, unsp
		◙	**F18.280**	Inhalant dependence with inhalant-induced anxiety disorder
		◙	**F18.288**	Inhalant dependence with other inhalant-induced disorder
			F18.959	Inhalant use, unsp w inhalnt-induce psychotic disorder, unsp
			F18.980	Inhalant use, unsp with inhalant-induced anxiety disorder
			F18.988	Inhalant use, unsp with other inhalant-induced disorder
			F19.122	Oth psychoactv substance abuse w intox w perceptual disturb
			F19.159	Oth psychoactive substance abuse w psychotic disorder, unsp
			F19.18[0,1,8]	Oth psychoactive substance abuse w disorder
		◙	**F19.222**	Oth psychoactv substance depend w intox w perceptual disturb
		◙	**F19.259**	Oth psychoactv substance depend w psychotic disorder, unsp
		◙	**F19.28[0,1,8]**	Oth psychoactive substance dependence w disorder
			F19.922	Oth psychoactv sub use, unsp w intox w perceptl disturb
			F19.959	Oth psychoactv substance use, unsp w psych disorder, unsp
			F19.980	Oth psychoactive substance use, unsp w anxiety disorder
			F19.981	Oth psychoactive substance use, unsp w sexual dysfunction
			F19.988	Oth psychoactive substance use, unsp w oth disorder
				6th Character meanings for codes as indicated ***0 Anxiety Disorder*** ***1 Sexual Dysfunction*** ***2 Sleep Disorder*** ***8 Other Psychoactive Subs-induced Disorder*** ***Note: For 6th character 8, refer to subcategory for specific psychoactive substance***
292.9	UNSPECIFIED DRUG-INDUCED MENTAL DISORDER		**F11.19**	Opioid abuse with unspecified opioid-induced disorder
		◙	**F11.29**	Opioid dependence with unspecified opioid-induced disorder
			F11.99	Opioid use, unsp with unspecified opioid-induced disorder
			F12.19	Cannabis abuse with unspecified cannabis-induced disorder
		◙	**F12.29**	Cannabis dependence with unsp cannabis-induced disorder
			F12.99	Cannabis use, unsp with unsp cannabis-induced disorder
			F13.19	Sedative, hypnotic or anxiolytic abuse w unsp disorder
		◙	**F13.29**	Sedative, hypnotic or anxiolytic dependence w unsp disorder
			F13.99	Sedative, hypnotic or anxiolytic use, unsp w unsp disorder
			F14.19	Cocaine abuse with unspecified cocaine-induced disorder
		◙	**F14.29**	Cocaine dependence with unspecified cocaine-induced disorder
			F14.99	Cocaine use, unsp with unspecified cocaine-induced disorder
			F15.19	Other stimulant abuse with unsp stimulant-induced disorder
		◙	**F15.29**	Oth stimulant dependence w unsp stimulant-induced disorder
			F15.99	Oth stimulant use, unsp with unsp stimulant-induced disorder
			F16.19	Hallucinogen abuse with unsp hallucinogen-induced disorder
		◙	**F16.29**	Hallucinogen dependence w unsp hallucinogen-induced disorder
			F16.99	Hallucinogen use, unsp w unsp hallucinogen-induced disorder
			F17.209	Nicotine dependence, unsp, w unsp nicotine-induced disorders
			F17.219	Nicotine dependence, cigarettes, w unsp disorders
			F17.229	Nicotine dependence, chewing tobacco, w unsp disorders
			F17.299	Nicotine dependence, oth tobacco product, w unsp disorders
			F18.19	Inhalant abuse with unspecified inhalant-induced disorder
		◙	**F18.29**	Inhalant dependence with unsp inhalant-induced disorder
			F18.99	Inhalant use, unsp with unsp inhalant-induced disorder
			F19.19	Oth psychoactive substance abuse w unsp disorder
		◙	**F19.29**	Oth psychoactive substance dependence w unsp disorder
			F19.99	Oth psychoactive substance use, unsp w unsp disorder
293.0	DELIRIUM DUE TO CONDITIONS CLASSIFIED ELSEWHERE		**F05**	Delirium due to known physiological condition
293.1	SUBACUTE DELIRIUM		**F05**	Delirium due to known physiological condition
293.81	PSYCHOTIC DISORDER W/DELUSIONS CONDS CLASS ELSW	➡	**F06.2**	Psychotic disorder w delusions due to known physiol cond
293.82	PSYCHOTIC D/O W/HALLUCINATIONS CONDS CLASS ELSW		**F06.0**	Psychotic disorder w hallucin due to known physiol condition
293.83	MOOD DISORDER IN CONDITIONS CLASSIFIED ELSEWHERE		**F06.30**	Mood disorder due to known physiological condition, unsp
			F06.31	Mood disorder due to known physiol cond w depressv features
			F06.32	Mood disord d/t physiol cond w major depressive-like epsd
			F06.33	Mood disorder due to known physiol cond w manic features
			F06.34	Mood disorder due to known physiol cond w mixed features
293.84	ANXIETY DISORDER CONDITIONS CLASSIFIED ELSEWHERE	➡	**F06.4**	Anxiety disorder due to known physiological condition
293.89	OTH TRANSIENT MENTAL D/O DUE CONDS CLASS ELSW		**F06.1**	Catatonic disorder due to known physiological condition
			F53	Puerperal psychosis
293.9	UNSPEC TRANSIENT MENTL DISORDER CONDS CLASS ELSW		**F06.8**	Oth mental disorders due to known physiological condition
294.0	AMNESTIC DISORDER CONDS CLASSIFIED ELSEWHERE		**F04**	Amnestic disorder due to known physiological condition
294.10	DEMENTIA CONDS CLASS ELSW W/O BHVAL DISTURBANCE	➡	**F02.80**	Dementia in oth diseases classd elswhr w/o behavrl disturb
294.11	DEMENTIA CCE W/BEHAVIORAL DISTURBANCES	➡	**F02.81**	Dementia in oth diseases classd elswhr w behavioral disturb
294.20	DEMENTIA UNSPECIFIED W/O BEHAVIORAL DISTURBANCE		**F03.90**	Unspecified dementia without behavioral disturbance
294.21	DEMENTIA UNSPECIFIED WITH BEHAVIORAL DISTURBANCE		**F03.91**	Unspecified dementia with behavioral disturbance

ICD-9-CM		ICD-10-CM	
294.8	OTH PERSISTENT MENTAL D/O DUE CONDS CLASS ELSW	**F06.0** **F06.1** **F06.8**	Psychotic disorder w hallucin due to known physiol condition Catatonic disorder due to known physiological condition Oth mental disorders due to known physiological condition
294.9	UNSPEC PERSISTENT MENTL D/O DUE CONDS CLASS ELSW	**F06.8**	Oth mental disorders due to known physiological condition
295.00	SIMPLE SCHIZOPHRENIA UNSPECIFIED CONDITION	**F20.89**	Other schizophrenia
295.01	SIMPLE SCHIZOPHRENIA SUBCHRONIC CONDITION	**F20.89**	Other schizophrenia
295.02	SIMPLE SCHIZOPHRENIA CHRONIC CONDITION	**F20.89**	Other schizophrenia
295.03	SIMPLE SCHIZO SUBCHRONIC COND W/ACUTE EXACERBAT	**F20.89**	Other schizophrenia
295.04	SIMPLE SCHIZO CHRONIC COND W/ACUTE EXACERBAT	**F20.89**	Other schizophrenia
295.05	SIMPLE SCHIZOPHRENIA, IN REMISSION	**F20.89**	Other schizophrenia
295.10	DISORGANIZED SCHIZOPHRENIA UNSPECIFIED CONDITION	**F20.1**	Disorganized schizophrenia
295.11	DISORGANIZED SCHIZOPHRENIA SUBCHRONIC CONDITION	**F20.1**	Disorganized schizophrenia
295.12	DISORGANIZED SCHIZOPHRENIA CHRONIC CONDITION	**F20.1**	Disorganized schizophrenia
295.13	DISORG SCHIZO SUBCHRONIC COND W/ACUTE EXACERBAT	**F20.1**	Disorganized schizophrenia
295.14	DISORG SCHIZO CHRONIC COND W/ACUTE EXACERBAT	**F20.1**	Disorganized schizophrenia
295.15	DISORGANIZED SCHIZOPHRENIA IN REMISSION	**F20.1**	Disorganized schizophrenia
295.20	CATATONIC SCHIZOPHRENIA UNSPECIFIED CONDITION	**F20.2**	Catatonic schizophrenia
295.21	CATATONIC SCHIZOPHRENIA SUBCHRONIC CONDITION	**F20.2**	Catatonic schizophrenia
295.22	CATATONIC SCHIZOPHRENIA CHRONIC CONDITION	**F20.2**	Catatonic schizophrenia
295.23	CATATONIC SCHIZO SUBCHRON COND W/ACUT EXACERBAT	**F20.2**	Catatonic schizophrenia
295.24	CATATONIC SCHIZO CHRONIC COND W/ACUTE EXACERBAT	**F20.2**	Catatonic schizophrenia
295.25	CATATONIC SCHIZOPHRENIA IN REMISSION	**F20.2**	Catatonic schizophrenia
295.30	PARANOID SCHIZOPHRENIA UNSPECIFIED CONDITION	**F20.0**	Paranoid schizophrenia
295.31	PARANOID SCHIZOPHRENIA SUBCHRONIC CONDITION	**F20.0**	Paranoid schizophrenia
295.32	PARANOID SCHIZOPHRENIA CHRONIC CONDITION	**F20.0**	Paranoid schizophrenia
295.33	PARANOID SCHIZO SUBCHRONIC COND W/ACUT EXACERBAT	**F20.0**	Paranoid schizophrenia
295.34	PARANOID SCHIZO CHRONIC COND W/ACUTE EXACERBAT	**F20.0**	Paranoid schizophrenia
295.35	PARANOID SCHIZOPHRENIA IN REMISSION	**F20.0**	Paranoid schizophrenia
295.40	SCHIZOPHRENIFORM DISORDER UNSPECIFIED	**F20.81**	Schizophreniform disorder
295.41	SCHIZOPHRENIFORM DISORDER SUBCHRONIC	**F20.81**	Schizophreniform disorder
295.42	SCHIZOPHRENIFORM DISORDER CHRONIC	**F20.81**	Schizophreniform disorder
295.43	SCHIZOPHRENIFORM D/O SUBCHRON W/ACUT EXACERBAT	**F20.81**	Schizophreniform disorder
295.44	SCHIZOPHRENIFORM DISORDER CHRON W/ACUT EXACERBAT	**F20.81**	Schizophreniform disorder
295.45	SCHIZOPHRENIFORM DISORDER IN REMISSION	**F20.81**	Schizophreniform disorder
295.50	LATENT SCHIZOPHRENIA UNSPECIFIED CONDITION	**F20.89**	Other schizophrenia
295.51	LATENT SCHIZOPHRENIA SUBCHRONIC CONDITION	**F20.89**	Other schizophrenia
295.52	LATENT SCHIZOPHRENIA CHRONIC CONDITION	**F20.89**	Other schizophrenia
295.53	LATENT SCHIZO SUBCHRONIC COND W/ACUTE EXACERBAT	**F20.89**	Other schizophrenia
295.54	LATENT SCHIZO CHRONIC COND W/ACUTE EXACERBAT	**F20.89**	Other schizophrenia
295.55	LATENT SCHIZOPHRENIA, IN REMISSION	**F20.89**	Other schizophrenia
295.60	SCHIZOPHRENIC DISORDERS RESIDUAL TYPE UNSPEC	**F20.5**	Residual schizophrenia
295.61	SCHIZOPHRENIC DISORDERS RESIDUAL TYPE SUBCHRONIC	**F20.5**	Residual schizophrenia
295.62	SCHIZOPHRENIC DISORDERS RESIDUAL TYPE CHRONIC	**F20.5**	Residual schizophrenia
295.63	SCHIZO D/O RESIDUL TYPE SUBCHRN W/ACUT XACRBAT	**F20.5**	Residual schizophrenia
295.64	SCHIZO D/O RESIDUL TYPE CHRN W/ACUT XACRBAT	**F20.5**	Residual schizophrenia
295.65	SCHIZOPHRENIC DISORDERS RESIDUAL TYPE REMISSION	**F20.5**	Residual schizophrenia
295.70	SCHIZOAFFECTIVE DISORDER UNSPECIFIED	**F25.0** **F25.1** **F25.8** **F25.9**	Schizoaffective disorder, bipolar type Schizoaffective disorder, depressive type Other schizoaffective disorders Schizoaffective disorder, unspecified
295.71	SCHIZOAFFECTIVE DISORDER SUBCHRONIC	**F25.9**	Schizoaffective disorder, unspecified
295.72	SCHIZOAFFECTIVE DISORDER CHRONIC	**F25.9**	Schizoaffective disorder, unspecified
295.73	SCHIZOAFFCT DISORDER SUBCHRONIC W/ACUT EXACERBAT	**F25.9**	Schizoaffective disorder, unspecified
295.74	SCHIZOAFFECT DISORDER CHRONIC W/ACUTE EXACERBAT	**F25.9**	Schizoaffective disorder, unspecified
295.75	SCHIZOAFFECTIVE DISORDER IN REMISSION	**F25.9**	Schizoaffective disorder, unspecified
295.80	OTHER SPEC TYPES SCHIZOPHRENIA UNSPEC CONDITION	**F20.89**	Other schizophrenia
295.81	OTHER SPEC TYPES SCHIZOPHRENIA SUBCHRONIC COND	**F20.89**	Other schizophrenia
295.82	OTHER SPEC TYPES SCHIZOPHRENIA CHRONIC CONDITION	**F20.89**	Other schizophrenia
295.83	OTH SPEC TYPES SCHIZO SUBCHRONW/ACUT EXACERBAT	**F20.89**	Other schizophrenia
295.84	OTH SPEC TYPES SCHIZO CHRONW/ACUT EXACERBAT	**F20.89**	Other schizophrenia
295.85	OTHER SPECIFIED TYPES OF SCHIZOPHRENIA REMISSION	**F20.89**	Other schizophrenia
295.90	UNSPECIFIED SCHIZOPHRENIA UNSPECIFIED CONDITION	**F20.3** **F20.9**	Undifferentiated schizophrenia Schizophrenia, unspecified
295.91	UNSPECIFIED SCHIZOPHRENIA SUBCHRONIC CONDITION	**F20.9**	Schizophrenia, unspecified
295.92	UNSPECIFIED SCHIZOPHRENIA CHRONIC CONDITION	**F20.9**	Schizophrenia, unspecified
295.93	UNSPEC SCHIZO SUBCHRONIC COND W/ACUTE EXACERBAT	**F20.9**	Schizophrenia, unspecified
295.94	UNSPEC SCHIZO CHRONIC COND W/ACUTE EXACERBAT	**F20.9**	Schizophrenia, unspecified
295.95	UNSPECIFIED SCHIZOPHRENIA IN REMISSION	**F20.9**	Schizophrenia, unspecified

[Brackets] indicate valid character values for each code. Character value meanings provided for each code grouping.

ICD-9-CM			ICD-10-CM	
296.00	BIPOLAR I DISORDER SINGLE MANIC EPISODE UNSPEC		**F30.10** **F30.9**	Manic episode without psychotic symptoms, unspecified Manic episode, unspecified
296.01	BIPOLAR I DISORDER SINGLE MANIC EPISODE MILD		**F30.11**	Manic episode without psychotic symptoms, mild
296.02	BIPOLAR I DISORDER SINGLE MANIC EPISODE MODERATE		**F30.12**	Manic episode without psychotic symptoms, moderate
296.03	BIPOLAR I D/O 1 MANIC EPIS SEV W/O PSYCHOT BHV		**F30.13**	Manic episode, severe, without psychotic symptoms
296.04	BIPOLAR I D/O 1 MANIC EPIS SEV W/PSYCHOT BHV		**F30.2**	Manic episode, severe with psychotic symptoms
296.05	BIPOLAR I D/O 1 MANIC EPIS PART/UNS REMISSION		**F30.3**	Manic episode in partial remission
296.06	BIPOLAR I D/O SINGLE MANIC EPIS FULL REMISSION		**F30.4**	Manic episode in full remission
296.10	MANIC DISORDER RECURRENT EPISODE UNSPECIFIED		**F30.10**	Manic episode without psychotic symptoms, unspecified
296.11	MANIC DISORDER RECURRENT EPISODE MILD		**F30.11**	Manic episode without psychotic symptoms, mild
296.12	MANIC DISORDER RECURRENT EPISODE MODERATE		**F30.12**	Manic episode without psychotic symptoms, moderate
296.13	MANIC D/O RECUR EPIS SEV W/O MENTION PSYCHOT BHV		**F30.13**	Manic episode, severe, without psychotic symptoms
296.14	MANIC D/O RECUR EPIS SEV SPEC AS W/PSYCHOT BHV		**F30.2**	Manic episode, severe with psychotic symptoms
296.15	MANIC DISORDER RECUR EPIS PART/UNSPEC REMISSION		**F30.3**	Manic episode in partial remission
296.16	MANIC DISORDER RECURRENT EPISODE FULL REMISSION		**F30.4**	Manic episode in full remission
296.20	MAJOR DEPRESSIVE DISORDER SINGLE EPISODE UNSPEC		**F32.9**	Major depressive disorder, single episode, unspecified
296.21	MAJOR DEPRESSIVE DISORDER SINGLE EPISODE MILD	➡	**F32.0**	Major depressive disorder, single episode, mild
296.22	MAJOR DPRSV DISORDER SINGLE EPISODE MODERATE	➡	**F32.1**	Major depressive disorder, single episode, moderate
296.23	MAJ DPRSV D/O 1 EPIS SEV W/O MENTION PSYCHOT BHV	➡	**F32.2**	Major depressv disord, single epsd, sev w/o psych features
296.24	MAJ DPRSV D/O 1 EPIS SEV SPEC AS W/PSYCHOT BHV		**F32.3**	Major depressv disord, single epsd, severe w psych features
296.25	MAJ DPRSV D/O SINGLE EPIS PART/UNSPEC REMISSION	➡	**F32.4**	Major depressv disorder, single episode, in partial remis
296.26	MAJOR DPRSV DISORDER SINGLE EPIS FULL REMISSION	➡	**F32.5**	Major depressive disorder, single episode, in full remission
296.30	MAJOR DPRSV DISORDER RECURRENT EPISODE UNSPEC		**F33.40** **F33.9**	Major depressive disorder, recurrent, in remission, unsp Major depressive disorder, recurrent, unspecified
296.31	MAJOR DEPRESSIVE DISORDER RECURRENT EPISODE MILD	➡	**F33.0**	Major depressive disorder, recurrent, mild
296.32	MAJOR DPRSV DISORDER RECURRENT EPISODE MODERATE	➡	**F33.1**	Major depressive disorder, recurrent, moderate
296.33	MAJ DPRSV D/O RECUR EPIS SEV W/O PSYCHOT BHV	➡	**F33.2**	Major depressv disorder, recurrent severe w/o psych features
296.34	MAJ DPRSV D/O RECUR EPIS SEV SPEC W/PSYCHOT BHV		**F33.3**	Major depressv disorder, recurrent, severe w psych symptoms
296.35	MAJ DPRSV D/O RECUR EPIS PART/UNSPEC REMISSION	➡	**F33.41**	Major depressive disorder, recurrent, in partial remission
296.36	MAJOR DPRSV DISORDER RECUR EPIS FULL REMISSION	➡	**F33.42**	Major depressive disorder, recurrent, in full remission
296.40	BIPOLAR I DISORDER MOST RECENT EPIS MANIC UNSPEC		**F31.0** **F31.10** **F31.89**	Bipolar disorder, current episode hypomanic Bipolar disord, crnt episode manic w/o psych features, unsp Other bipolar disorder
296.41	BIPOLAR I DISORDER MOST RECENT EPIS MANIC MILD	➡	**F31.11**	Bipolar disord, crnt episode manic w/o psych features, mild
296.42	BIPOLAR I DISORDER MOST RECENT EPIS MANIC MOD	➡	**F31.12**	Bipolar disord, crnt episode manic w/o psych features, mod
296.43	BIPLR I MOST RECENT EPIS MNIC SEV NO PSYCHOT BHV	➡	**F31.13**	Bipolar disord, crnt epsd manic w/o psych features, severe
296.44	BIPLR I MOST RECENT EPIS MNIC SEV W/PSYCHOT BHV	➡	**F31.2**	Bipolar disord, crnt episode manic severe w psych features
296.45	BIPLR I D/O MOST RECENT EPIS MNIC PART/UNS REMIS		**F31.73**	Bipolar disord, in partial remis, most recent episode manic
296.46	BIPLR I D/O MOST RECENT EPIS MNIC FULL REMISSION		**F31.74**	Bipolar disorder, in full remis, most recent episode manic
296.50	BIPOLAR I D/O MOST RECENT EPIS DEPRESSED UNS		**F31.30**	Bipolar disord, crnt epsd depress, mild or mod severt, unsp
296.51	BIPOLAR I D/O MOST RECENT EPIS DEPRESSED MILD	➡	**F31.31**	Bipolar disorder, current episode depressed, mild
296.52	BIPOLAR I D/O MOST RECENT EPIS DEPRESSED MOD	➡	**F31.32**	Bipolar disorder, current episode depressed, moderate
296.53	BIPLR I MOST RECENT EPIS DPRS SEV NO PSYCHOT BHV	➡	**F31.4**	Bipolar disord, crnt epsd depress, sev, w/o psych features
296.54	BIPLR I MOST RECENT EPIS DPRSD SEV W/PSYCHOT BHV	➡	**F31.5**	Bipolar disord, crnt epsd depress, severe, w psych features
296.55	BIPLR I MOST RECENT EPIS DPRSD PART/UNS REMISS	➡	**F31.75**	Bipolar disord, in partial remis, most recent epsd depress
296.56	BIPLR I D/O MOST RECENT EPIS DPRSD FULL REMISS	➡	**F31.76**	Bipolar disorder, in full remis, most recent episode depress
296.60	BIPOLAR I DISORDER MOST RECENT EPIS MIXED UNSPEC	➡	**F31.60**	Bipolar disorder, current episode mixed, unspecified
296.61	BIPOLAR I DISORDER MOST RECENT EPIS MIXED MILD	➡	**F31.61**	Bipolar disorder, current episode mixed, mild
296.62	BIPOLAR I DISORDER MOST RECENT EPIS MIX MODERATE	➡	**F31.62**	Bipolar disorder, current episode mixed, moderate
296.63	BIPLR I MOST RECENT EPIS MIX SEV W/O PSYCHOT BHV	➡	**F31.63**	Bipolar disord, crnt epsd mixed, severe, w/o psych features
296.64	BIPLR I MOST RECENT EPIS MIX SEV W/PSYCHOT BHV	➡	**F31.64**	Bipolar disord, crnt episode mixed, severe, w psych features
296.65	BIPLR I D/O MOST RECENT EPIS MIX PART/UNS REMISS	➡	**F31.77**	Bipolar disord, in partial remis, most recent episode mixed
296.66	BIPLR I D/O MOST RECENT EPIS MIX FULL REMISSION	➡	**F31.78**	Bipolar disorder, in full remis, most recent episode mixed
296.7	BIPOLAR I DISORDER MOST RECENT EPISODE UNSPEC		**F31.70** **F31.71** **F31.72** **F31.9**	Bipolar disord, currently in remis, most recent episode unsp Bipolar disord, in partial remis, most recent epsd hypomanic Bipolar disord, in full remis, most recent episode hypomanic Bipolar disorder, unspecified
296.80	BIPOLAR DISORDER UNSPECIFIED		**F31.9**	Bipolar disorder, unspecified
296.81	ATYPICAL MANIC DISORDER		**F30.8**	Other manic episodes
296.82	ATYPICAL DEPRESSIVE DISORDER		**F32.8**	Other depressive episodes
296.89	OTHER AND UNSPECIFIED BIPOLAR DISORDERS		**F31.81**	Bipolar II disorder
296.90	UNSPECIFIED EPISODIC MOOD DISORDER		**F39**	Unspecified mood [affective] disorder
296.99	OTHER SPECIFIED EPISODIC MOOD DISORDER		**F33.8** **F34.8** **F34.9**	Other recurrent depressive disorders Other persistent mood [affective] disorders Persistent mood [affective] disorder, unspecified
297.0	PARANOID STATE, SIMPLE		**F22**	Delusional disorders
297.1	DELUSIONAL DISORDER		**F22**	Delusional disorders
297.2	PARAPHRENIA		**F22**	Delusional disorders

ICD-9-CM		ICD-10-CM	
297.3	SHARED PSYCHOTIC DISORDER	➡ F24	Shared psychotic disorder
297.8	OTHER SPECIFIED PARANOID STATES	F22	Delusional disorders
297.9	UNSPECIFIED PARANOID STATE	F23	Brief psychotic disorder
298.0	DEPRESSIVE TYPE PSYCHOSIS	F32.3 F33.3	Major depressv disord, single epsd, severe w psych features Major depressv disorder, recurrent, severe w psych symptoms
298.1	EXCITATIVE TYPE PSYCHOSIS	F28	Oth psych disorder not due to a sub or known physiol cond
298.2	REACTIVE CONFUSION	F44.89	Other dissociative and conversion disorders
298.3	ACUTE PARANOID REACTION	F23	Brief psychotic disorder
298.4	PSYCHOGENIC PARANOID PSYCHOSIS	F23	Brief psychotic disorder
298.8	OTHER AND UNSPECIFIED REACTIVE PSYCHOSIS	F23	Brief psychotic disorder
298.9	UNSPECIFIED PSYCHOSIS	F28 F29	Oth psych disorder not due to a sub or known physiol cond Unsp psychosis not due to a substance or known physiol cond
299.00	AUTISTIC DISORDER CURRENT OR ACTIVE STATE	F84.0	Autistic disorder
299.01	AUTISTIC DISORDER RESIDUAL STATE	F84.0	Autistic disorder
299.10	CHLD DISINTEGRATIVE DISORDER CURRENT/ACTV STATE	F84.3	Other childhood disintegrative disorder
299.11	CHILDHOOD DISINTEGRATIVE DISORDER RESIDUAL STATE	F84.3	Other childhood disintegrative disorder
299.80	OTH SPEC PERVASIVE DVLPMENTL D/O CURR/ACTV STATE	F84.5 F84.8	Asperger's syndrome Other pervasive developmental disorders
299.81	OTH SPEC PERVASIVE DVLPMENTL D/O RESIDUAL STATE	F84.5 F84.8	Asperger's syndrome Other pervasive developmental disorders
299.90	UNSPEC PERVASIVE DVLPMENTL D/O CURRNT/ACTV STATE	F84.9	Pervasive developmental disorder, unspecified
299.91	UNSPEC PERVASIVE DVLPMENTL D/O RESIDUAL STATE	F84.9	Pervasive developmental disorder, unspecified
300.00	ANXIETY STATE, UNSPECIFIED	➡ F41.9	Anxiety disorder, unspecified
300.01	PANIC DISORDER WITHOUT AGORAPHOBIA	➡ F41.0	Panic disorder without agoraphobia
300.02	GENERALIZED ANXIETY DISORDER	➡ F41.1	Generalized anxiety disorder
300.09	OTHER ANXIETY STATES	F41.3 F41.8	Other mixed anxiety disorders Other specified anxiety disorders
300.10	HYSTERIA, UNSPECIFIED	F44.9	Dissociative and conversion disorder, unspecified
300.11	CONVERSION DISORDER	F44.4 F44.5 F44.6 F44.7	Conversion disorder with motor symptom or deficit Conversion disorder with seizures or convulsions Conversion disorder with sensory symptom or deficit Conversion disorder with mixed symptom presentation
300.12	DISSOCIATIVE AMNESIA	➡ F44.0	Dissociative amnesia
300.13	DISSOCIATIVE FUGUE	➡ F44.1	Dissociative fugue
300.14	DISSOCIATIVE IDENTITY DISORDER	➡ F44.81	Dissociative identity disorder
300.15	DISSOCIATIVE DISORDER OR REACTION UNSPECIFIED	F44.9	Dissociative and conversion disorder, unspecified
300.16	FACTITIOUS D/O W/PREDOM PSYCHOLOGICAL SIGNS&SX	F44.89 F68.11 F68.13	Other dissociative and conversion disorders Factitious disorder w predom psych signs and symptoms Factitious disord w comb psych and physcl signs and symptoms
300.19	OTHER AND UNSPECIFIED FACTITIOUS ILLNESS	F44.2 F68.8	Dissociative stupor Other specified disorders of adult personality and behavior
300.20	PHOBIA, UNSPECIFIED	F40.9	Phobic anxiety disorder, unspecified
300.21	AGORAPHOBIA WITH PANIC DISORDER	➡ F40.01	Agoraphobia with panic disorder
300.22	AGORAPHOBIA WITHOUT MENTION OF PANIC ATTACKS	F40.00 F40.02	Agoraphobia, unspecified Agoraphobia without panic disorder
300.23	SOCIAL PHOBIA	F40.10 F40.11	Social phobia, unspecified Social phobia, generalized
300.29	OTHER ISOLATED OR SPECIFIC PHOBIAS	F40.210 F40.218 F40.220 F40.228 F40.230 F40.231 F40.232 F40.233 F40.240 F40.241 F40.242 F40.243 F40.248 F40.290 F40.291 F40.298 F40.8	Arachnophobia Other animal type phobia Fear of thunderstorms Other natural environment type phobia Fear of blood Fear of injections and transfusions Fear of other medical care Fear of injury Claustrophobia Acrophobia Fear of bridges Fear of flying Other situational type phobia Androphobia Gynephobia Other specified phobia Other phobic anxiety disorders
300.3	OBSESSIVE-COMPULSIVE DISORDERS	➡ F42	Obsessive-compulsive disorder
300.4	DYSTHYMIC DISORDER	F34.1	Dysthymic disorder
300.5	NEURASTHENIA	F48.8	Other specified nonpsychotic mental disorders
300.6	DEPERSONALIZATION DISORDER	➡ F48.1	Depersonalization-derealization syndrome
300.7	HYPOCHONDRIASIS	F45.20 F45.21 F45.22 F45.29	Hypochondriacal disorder, unspecified Hypochondriasis Body dysmorphic disorder Other hypochondriacal disorders
300.81	SOMATIZATION DISORDER	➡ F45.0	Somatization disorder

[Brackets] indicate valid character values for each code. Character value meanings provided for each code grouping.

ICD-9-CM			ICD-10-CM	
300.82	UNDIFFERENTIATED SOMATOFORM DISORDER		**F45.1**	Undifferentiated somatoform disorder
			F45.9	Somatoform disorder, unspecified
300.89	OTHER SOMATOFORM DISORDERS		**F45.8**	Other somatoform disorders
			F48.8	Other specified nonpsychotic mental disorders
300.9	UNSPECIFIED NONPSYCHOTIC MENTAL DISORDER		**F48.9**	Nonpsychotic mental disorder, unspecified
			F99	Mental disorder, not otherwise specified
			R45.2	Unhappiness
			R45.5	Hostility
			R45.6	Violent behavior
301.0	PARANOID PERSONALITY DISORDER	➡	**F60.0**	Paranoid personality disorder
301.10	AFFECTIVE PERSONALITY DISORDER UNSPECIFIED		**F34.0**	Cyclothymic disorder
301.11	CHRONIC HYPOMANIC PERSONALITY DISORDER		**F60.89**	Other specific personality disorders
301.12	CHRONIC DEPRESSIVE PERSONALITY DISORDER		**F34.1**	Dysthymic disorder
301.13	CYCLOTHYMIC DISORDER		**F34.0**	Cyclothymic disorder
301.20	SCHIZOID PERSONALITY DISORDER UNSPECIFIED		**F60.1**	Schizoid personality disorder
301.21	INTROVERTED PERSONALITY		**F60.1**	Schizoid personality disorder
301.22	SCHIZOTYPAL PERSONALITY DISORDER	➡	**F21**	Schizotypal disorder
301.3	EXPLOSIVE PERSONALITY DISORDER		**F60.3**	Borderline personality disorder
301.4	OBSESSIVE-COMPULSIVE PERSONALITY DISORDER	➡	**F60.5**	Obsessive-compulsive personality disorder
301.50	HISTRIONIC PERSONALITY DISORDER UNSPECIFIED		**F60.4**	Histrionic personality disorder
301.51	CHRONIC FACTITIOUS ILLNESS W/PHYSICAL SYMPTOMS		**F68.10**	Factitious disorder, unspecified
			F68.12	Factitious disorder w predom physical signs and symptoms
		▣	**F68.13**	Factitious disord w comb psych and physcl signs and symptoms
301.59	OTHER HISTRIONIC PERSONALITY DISORDER		**F60.4**	Histrionic personality disorder
301.6	DEPENDENT PERSONALITY DISORDER	➡	**F60.7**	Dependent personality disorder
301.7	ANTISOCIAL PERSONALITY DISORDER	➡	**F60.2**	Antisocial personality disorder
301.81	NARCISSISTIC PERSONALITY DISORDER	➡	**F60.81**	Narcissistic personality disorder
301.82	AVOIDANT PERSONALITY DISORDER	➡	**F60.6**	Avoidant personality disorder
301.83	BORDERLINE PERSONALITY DISORDER		**F60.3**	Borderline personality disorder
301.84	PASSIVE-AGGRESSIVE PERSONALITY		**F60.89**	Other specific personality disorders
301.89	OTHER PERSONALITY DISORDER		**F60.89**	Other specific personality disorders
301.9	UNSPECIFIED PERSONALITY DISORDER		**F60.9**	Personality disorder, unspecified
			F69	Unspecified disorder of adult personality and behavior
302.0	EGO-DYSTONIC SEXUAL ORIENTATION		**F66**	Other sexual disorders
302.1	ZOOPHILIA		**F65.89**	Other paraphilias
302.2	PEDOPHILIA	➡	**F65.4**	Pedophilia
302.3	TRANSVESTIC FETISHISM	➡	**F65.1**	Transvestic fetishism
302.4	EXHIBITIONISM	➡	**F65.2**	Exhibitionism
302.50	TRANS-SEXUALISM WITH UNSPECIFIED SEXUAL HISTORY		**F64.1**	Gender identity disorder in adolescence and adulthood
			Z87.890	Personal history of sex reassignment
302.51	TRANS-SEXUALISM WITH ASEXUAL HISTORY		**F64.1**	Gender identity disorder in adolescence and adulthood
302.52	TRANS-SEXUALISM WITH HOMOSEXUAL HISTORY		**F64.1**	Gender identity disorder in adolescence and adulthood
302.53	TRANS-SEXUALISM WITH HETEROSEXUAL HISTORY		**F64.1**	Gender identity disorder in adolescence and adulthood
302.6	GENDER IDENTITY DISORDER IN CHILDREN		**F64.2**	Gender identity disorder of childhood
			F64.8	Other gender identity disorders
			F64.9	Gender identity disorder, unspecified
302.70	PSYCHOSEXUAL DYSFUNCTION UNSPECIFIED		**F52.9**	Unsp sexual dysfnct not due to a sub or known physiol cond
			R37	Sexual dysfunction, unspecified
302.71	HYPOACTIVE SEXUAL DESIRE DISORDER	➡	**F52.0**	Hypoactive sexual desire disorder
302.72	PSYCHOSEXUAL DYSF W/INHIBITED SEXUAL EXCITEMENT		**F52.21**	Male erectile disorder
			F52.22	Female sexual arousal disorder
			F52.8	Oth sexual dysfnct not due to a sub or known physiol cond
302.73	FEMALE ORGASMIC DISORDER	➡	**F52.31**	Female orgasmic disorder
302.74	MALE ORGASMIC DISORDER	➡	**F52.32**	Male orgasmic disorder
302.75	PREMATURE EJACULATION	➡	**F52.4**	Premature ejaculation
302.76	DYSPAREUNIA PSYCHOGENIC	➡	**F52.6**	Dyspareunia not due to a substance or known physiol cond
302.79	PSYCHOSEXUAL DYSF W/OTH SPEC PSYCHOSEXUAL DYSFS		**F52.1**	Sexual aversion disorder
			F52.8	Oth sexual dysfnct not due to a sub or known physiol cond
302.81	FETISHISM	➡	**F65.0**	Fetishism
302.82	VOYEURISM	➡	**F65.3**	Voyeurism
302.83	SEXUAL MASOCHISM	➡	**F65.51**	Sexual masochism
302.84	SEXUAL SADISM		**F65.50**	Sadomasochism, unspecified
			F65.52	Sexual sadism
302.85	GENDER IDENTITY DISORDER ADOLESCENTS OR ADULTS		**F64.1**	Gender identity disorder in adolescence and adulthood
302.89	OTHER SPECIFIED PSYCHOSEXUAL DISORDER		**F65.81**	Frotteurism
			F65.89	Other paraphilias
			F66	Other sexual disorders
302.9	UNSPECIFIED PSYCHOSEXUAL DISORDER		**F65.9**	Paraphilia, unspecified
303.00	ACUTE ALCOHOLIC INTOXICATION UNSPEC DRUNKENNESS		**F10.220**	Alcohol dependence with intoxication, uncomplicated
			F10.229	Alcohol dependence with intoxication, unspecified

ICD-9-CM			ICD-10-CM	
303.01	ACUTE ALCOHOLIC INTOXICATION CONT DRUNKENNESS		**F10.220**	Alcohol dependence with intoxication, uncomplicated
			F10.229	Alcohol dependence with intoxication, unspecified
303.02	ACUT ALCOHOLIC INTOXICATION EPISODIC DRUNKENNESS		**F10.220**	Alcohol dependence with intoxication, uncomplicated
			F10.229	Alcohol dependence with intoxication, unspecified
303.03	ACUTE ALCOHOLIC INTOXICATION IN REMISSION		**F10.220**	Alcohol dependence with intoxication, uncomplicated
			F10.229	Alcohol dependence with intoxication, unspecified
303.90	OTH&UNSPEC ALCOHOL DEPENDENCE UNSPEC DRUNKENNESS		**F10.20**	Alcohol dependence, uncomplicated
303.91	OTHER&UNSPEC ALCOHOL DEPENDENCE CONT DRUNKENNESS		**F10.20**	Alcohol dependence, uncomplicated
303.92	OTH&UNSPEC ALCOHOL DEPEND EPISODIC DRUNKENNESS		**F10.20**	Alcohol dependence, uncomplicated
303.93	OTHER&UNSPECIFIED ALCOHOL DEPENDENCE REMISSION	➡	**F10.21**	Alcohol dependence, in remission
304.00	OPIOID TYPE DEPENDENCE UNSPECIFIED ABUSE		**F11.20**	Opioid dependence, uncomplicated
		▣	**F11.220**	Opioid dependence with intoxication, uncomplicated
		▣	**F11.221**	Opioid dependence with intoxication delirium
		▣	**F11.222**	Opioid dependence w intoxication with perceptual disturbance
		▣	**F11.229**	Opioid dependence with intoxication, unspecified
		▣	**F11.23**	Opioid dependence with withdrawal
		▣	**F11.24**	Opioid dependence with opioid-induced mood disorder
		▣	**F11.250**	Opioid depend w opioid-induc psychotic disorder w delusions
		▣	**F11.251**	Opioid depend w opioid-induc psychotic disorder w hallucin
		▣	**F11.259**	Opioid dependence w opioid-induced psychotic disorder, unsp
		▣	**F11.281**	Opioid dependence with opioid-induced sexual dysfunction
		▣	**F11.282**	Opioid dependence with opioid-induced sleep disorder
		▣	**F11.288**	Opioid dependence with other opioid-induced disorder
		▣	**F11.29**	Opioid dependence with unspecified opioid-induced disorder
304.01	OPIOID TYPE DEPENDENCE CONTINUOUS ABUSE		**F11.20**	Opioid dependence, uncomplicated
304.02	OPIOID TYPE DEPENDENCE EPISODIC ABUSE		**F11.20**	Opioid dependence, uncomplicated
304.03	OPIOID TYPE DEPENDENCE IN REMISSION	➡	**F11.21**	Opioid dependence, in remission
304.10	SEDATIVE HYPNOTIC/ANXIOLYTIC DEPENDENCE UNSPEC		**F13.20**	Sedative, hypnotic or anxiolytic dependence, uncomplicated
		▣	**F13.220**	Sedatv/hyp/anxiolytc dependence w intoxication, uncomp
		▣	**F13.221**	Sedatv/hyp/anxiolytc dependence w intoxication delirium
		▣	**F13.229**	Sedatv/hyp/anxiolytc dependence w intoxication, unsp
		▣	**F13.230**	Sedatv/hyp/anxiolytc dependence w withdrawal, uncomplicated
		▣	**F13.231**	Sedatv/hyp/anxiolytc dependence w withdrawal delirium
		▣	**F13.232**	Sedatv/hyp/anxiolytc depend w w/drawal w perceptual disturb
		▣	**F13.239**	Sedatv/hyp/anxiolytc dependence w withdrawal, unsp
		▣	**F13.24**	Sedative, hypnotic or anxiolytic dependence w mood disorder
		▣	**F13.250**	Sedatv/hyp/anxiolytc depend w psychotic disorder w delusions
		▣	**F13.251**	Sedatv/hyp/anxiolytc depend w psychotic disorder w hallucin
		▣	**F13.259**	Sedatv/hyp/anxiolytc dependence w psychotic disorder, unsp
		▣	**F13.26**	Sedatv/hyp/anxiolytc depend w persisting amnestic disorder
		▣	**F13.27**	Sedatv/hyp/anxiolytc dependence w persisting dementia
		▣	**F13.280**	Sedatv/hyp/anxiolytc dependence w anxiety disorder
		▣	**F13.281**	Sedatv/hyp/anxiolytc dependence w sexual dysfunction
		▣	**F13.282**	Sedative, hypnotic or anxiolytic dependence w sleep disorder
		▣	**F13.288**	Sedative, hypnotic or anxiolytic dependence w oth disorder
		▣	**F13.29**	Sedative, hypnotic or anxiolytic dependence w unsp disorder
304.11	SEDATIVE HYPNOTIC/ANXIOLYTIC DEPENDENCE CONT		**F13.20**	Sedative, hypnotic or anxiolytic dependence, uncomplicated
304.12	SEDATIVE HYPNOTIC/ANXIOLYTIC DEPENDENCE EPISODIC		**F13.20**	Sedative, hypnotic or anxiolytic dependence, uncomplicated
304.13	SEDATIVE HYPNOTIC/ANXIOLYTIC DEPEND REMISSION	➡	**F13.21**	Sedative, hypnotic or anxiolytic dependence, in remission
304.20	COCAINE DEPENDENCE UNSPECIFIED ABUSE		**F14.20**	Cocaine dependence, uncomplicated
		▣	**F14.220**	Cocaine dependence with intoxication, uncomplicated
		▣	**F14.221**	Cocaine dependence with intoxication delirium
		▣	**F14.222**	Cocaine dependence w intoxication w perceptual disturbance
		▣	**F14.229**	Cocaine dependence with intoxication, unspecified
		▣	**F14.23**	Cocaine dependence with withdrawal
		▣	**F14.24**	Cocaine dependence with cocaine-induced mood disorder
		▣	**F14.250**	Cocaine depend w cocaine-induc psych disorder w delusions
		▣	**F14.251**	Cocaine depend w cocaine-induc psychotic disorder w hallucin
		▣	**F14.259**	Cocaine dependence w cocaine-induc psychotic disorder, unsp
		▣	**F14.280**	Cocaine dependence with cocaine-induced anxiety disorder
		▣	**F14.281**	Cocaine dependence with cocaine-induced sexual dysfunction
		▣	**F14.282**	Cocaine dependence with cocaine-induced sleep disorder
		▣	**F14.288**	Cocaine dependence with other cocaine-induced disorder
		▣	**F14.29**	Cocaine dependence with unspecified cocaine-induced disorder
304.21	COCAINE DEPENDENCE CONTINUOUS ABUSE		**F14.20**	Cocaine dependence, uncomplicated
304.22	COCAINE DEPENDENCE, EPISODIC ABUSE		**F14.20**	Cocaine dependence, uncomplicated
304.23	COCAINE DEPENDENCE, IN REMISSION	➡	**F14.21**	Cocaine dependence, in remission

[Brackets] indicate valid character values for each code. Character value meanings provided for each code grouping.

ICD-9-CM		ICD-10-CM		
304.30	CANNABIS DEPENDENCE UNSPECIFIED ABUSE		**F12.20**	Cannabis dependence, uncomplicated
		▣	**F12.220**	Cannabis dependence with intoxication, uncomplicated
		▣	**F12.221**	Cannabis dependence with intoxication delirium
		▣	**F12.222**	Cannabis dependence w intoxication w perceptual disturbance
		▣	**F12.229**	Cannabis dependence with intoxication, unspecified
		▣	**F12.250**	Cannabis dependence with psychotic disorder with delusions
		▣	**F12.251**	Cannabis dependence w psychotic disorder with hallucinations
		▣	**F12.259**	Cannabis dependence with psychotic disorder, unspecified
		▣	**F12.280**	Cannabis dependence with cannabis-induced anxiety disorder
		▣	**F12.288**	Cannabis dependence with other cannabis-induced disorder
		▣	**F12.29**	Cannabis dependence with unsp cannabis-induced disorder
304.31	CANNABIS DEPENDENCE CONTINUOUS ABUSE		**F12.20**	Cannabis dependence, uncomplicated
304.32	CANNABIS DEPENDENCE, EPISODIC ABUSE		**F12.20**	Cannabis dependence, uncomplicated
304.33	CANNABIS DEPENDENCE, IN REMISSION	➡	**F12.21**	Cannabis dependence, in remission
304.40	AMPHET&OTH PSYCHOSTIMULANT DEPENDENCE UNSPEC ABS		**F15.20**	Other stimulant dependence, uncomplicated
		▣	**F15.220**	Other stimulant dependence with intoxication, uncomplicated
		▣	**F15.221**	Other stimulant dependence with intoxication delirium
		▣	**F15.222**	Oth stimulant dependence w intox w perceptual disturbance
		▣	**F15.229**	Other stimulant dependence with intoxication, unspecified
		▣	**F15.23**	Other stimulant dependence with withdrawal
		▣	**F15.24**	Oth stimulant dependence w stimulant-induced mood disorder
		▣	**F15.250**	Oth stim depend w stim-induce psych disorder w delusions
		▣	**F15.251**	Oth stimulant depend w stim-induce psych disorder w hallucin
		▣	**F15.259**	Oth stimulant depend w stim-induce psychotic disorder, unsp
		▣	**F15.280**	Oth stimulant dependence w stim-induce anxiety disorder
		▣	**F15.281**	Oth stimulant dependence w stim-induce sexual dysfunction
		▣	**F15.282**	Oth stimulant dependence w stimulant-induced sleep disorder
		▣	**F15.288**	Oth stimulant dependence with oth stimulant-induced disorder
		▣	**F15.29**	Oth stimulant dependence w unsp stimulant-induced disorder
304.41	AMPHET&OTH PSYCHOSTIMULANT DEPENDENCE CONT ABS		**F15.20**	Other stimulant dependence, uncomplicated
304.42	AMPHET&OTH PSYCHOSTIMULANT DEPEND EPISODIC ABS		**F15.20**	Other stimulant dependence, uncomplicated
304.43	AMPHET&OTH PSYCHOSTIMULANT DEPENDENCE REMISSION		**F15.21**	Other stimulant dependence, in remission
304.50	HALLUCINOGEN DEPENDENCE UNSPECIFIED ABUSE		**F16.20**	Hallucinogen dependence, uncomplicated
		▣	**F16.220**	Hallucinogen dependence with intoxication, uncomplicated
		▣	**F16.221**	Hallucinogen dependence with intoxication with delirium
		▣	**F16.229**	Hallucinogen dependence with intoxication, unspecified
		▣	**F16.24**	Hallucinogen dependence w hallucinogen-induced mood disorder
		▣	**F16.250**	Hallucinogen dependence w psychotic disorder w delusions
		▣	**F16.251**	Hallucinogen dependence w psychotic disorder w hallucin
		▣	**F16.259**	Hallucinogen dependence w psychotic disorder, unsp
		▣	**F16.280**	Hallucinogen dependence w anxiety disorder
		▣	**F16.283**	Hallucign depend w hallucign persisting perception disorder
		▣	**F16.288**	Hallucinogen dependence w oth hallucinogen-induced disorder
		▣	**F16.29**	Hallucinogen dependence w unsp hallucinogen-induced disorder
304.51	HALLUCINOGEN DEPENDENCE CONTINUOUS ABUSE		**F16.20**	Hallucinogen dependence, uncomplicated
304.52	HALLUCINOGEN DEPENDENCE EPISODIC ABUSE		**F16.20**	Hallucinogen dependence, uncomplicated
304.53	HALLUCINOGEN DEPENDENCE IN REMISSION	➡	**F16.21**	Hallucinogen dependence, in remission
304.60	OTHER SPEC DRUG DEPENDENCE UNSPEC ABUSE		**F18.20**	Inhalant dependence, uncomplicated
		▣	**F18.220**	Inhalant dependence with intoxication, uncomplicated
		▣	**F18.221**	Inhalant dependence with intoxication delirium
		▣	**F18.229**	Inhalant dependence with intoxication, unspecified
		▣	**F18.24**	Inhalant dependence with inhalant-induced mood disorder
		▣	**F18.250**	Inhalant depend w inhalnt-induce psych disorder w delusions
		▣	**F18.251**	Inhalant depend w inhalnt-induce psych disorder w hallucin
		▣	**F18.259**	Inhalant depend w inhalnt-induce psychotic disorder, unsp
		▣	**F18.27**	Inhalant dependence with inhalant-induced dementia
		▣	**F18.280**	Inhalant dependence with inhalant-induced anxiety disorder
		▣	**F18.288**	Inhalant dependence with other inhalant-induced disorder
		▣	**F18.29**	Inhalant dependence with unsp inhalant-induced disorder
			F19.20	Other psychoactive substance dependence, uncomplicated
		▣	**F19.220**	Oth psychoactive substance dependence w intoxication, uncomp
		▣	**F19.221**	Oth psychoactive substance dependence w intox delirium
		▣	**F19.222**	Oth psychoactv substance depend w intox w perceptual disturb
		▣	**F19.229**	Oth psychoactive substance dependence w intoxication, unsp
		▣	**F19.230**	Oth psychoactive substance dependence w withdrawal, uncomp
		▣	**F19.231**	Oth psychoactive substance dependence w withdrawal delirium
		▣	**F19.232**	Oth psychoactv sub depend w w/drawal w perceptl disturb
		▣	**F19.239**	Oth psychoactive substance dependence with withdrawal, unsp
		▣	**F19.24**	Oth psychoactive substance dependence w mood disorder
		▣	**F19.250**	Oth psychoactv substance depend w psych disorder w delusions
		▣	**F19.251**	Oth psychoactv substance depend w psych disorder w hallucin
		▣	**F19.259**	Oth psychoactv substance depend w psychotic disorder, unsp
		▣	**F19.26**	Oth psychoactv substance depend w persist amnestic disorder
		▣	**F19.27**	Oth psychoactive substance dependence w persisting dementia
		▣	**F19.280**	Oth psychoactive substance dependence w anxiety disorder
		▣	**F19.281**	Oth psychoactive substance dependence w sexual dysfunction

(Continued on next page)

ICD-9-CM		ICD-10-CM	
304.60	OTHER SPEC DRUG DEPENDENCE UNSPEC ABUSE **(Continued)**	**F19.282**	Oth psychoactive substance dependence w sleep disorder
		F19.288	Oth psychoactive substance dependence w oth disorder
		F19.29	Oth psychoactive substance dependence w unsp disorder
304.61	OTHER SPECIFIED DRUG DEPENDENCE CONTINUOUS ABUSE	**F19.20**	Other psychoactive substance dependence, uncomplicated
304.62	OTHER SPECIFIED DRUG DEPENDENCE EPISODIC ABUSE	**F19.20**	Other psychoactive substance dependence, uncomplicated
304.63	OTHER SPECIFIED DRUG DEPENDENCE IN REMISSION	**F18.21**	Inhalant dependence, in remission
		F19.21	Other psychoactive substance dependence, in remission
304.70	COMB OPIOID RX W/ANY OTH RX DEPEND UNSPEC ABS	**F19.20**	Other psychoactive substance dependence, uncomplicated
304.71	COMB OPIOID DRUG W/ANY OTH DRUG DEPEND CONT ABS	**F19.20**	Other psychoactive substance dependence, uncomplicated
304.72	COMB OPIOID RX W/ANY OTH RX DEPEND EPISODIC ABS	**F19.20**	Other psychoactive substance dependence, uncomplicated
304.73	COMB OPIOID DRUG W/ANY OTH DRUG DEPEND REMISSION	**F19.21**	Other psychoactive substance dependence, in remission
304.80	COMB DRUG DEPEND EXCLD OPIOID DRUG UNSPEC ABS	**F19.20**	Other psychoactive substance dependence, uncomplicated
304.81	COMB DRUG DEPEND EXCLUDING OPIOID DRUG CONT ABS	**F19.20**	Other psychoactive substance dependence, uncomplicated
304.82	COMB DRUG DEPEND EXCLD OPIOID DRUG EPISODIC ABS	**F19.20**	Other psychoactive substance dependence, uncomplicated
304.83	COMB DRUG DEPEND EXCLUDING OPIOID DRUG REMISSION	**F19.21**	Other psychoactive substance dependence, in remission
304.90	UNSPECIFIED DRUG DEPENDENCE UNSPECIFIED ABUSE	**F19.20**	Other psychoactive substance dependence, uncomplicated
304.91	UNSPECIFIED DRUG DEPENDENCE CONTINUOUS ABUSE	**F19.20**	Other psychoactive substance dependence, uncomplicated
304.92	UNSPECIFIED DRUG DEPENDENCE EPISODIC ABUSE	**F19.20**	Other psychoactive substance dependence, uncomplicated
304.93	UNSPECIFIED DRUG DEPENDENCE IN REMISSION	**F19.21**	Other psychoactive substance dependence, in remission
305.00	NONDEPENDENT ALCOHOL ABUSE UNSPEC PATTERN OF USE	**F10.10**	Alcohol abuse, uncomplicated
		F10.120	Alcohol abuse with intoxication, uncomplicated
		F10.129	Alcohol abuse with intoxication, unspecified
305.01	NONDEPENDENT ALCOHOL ABUSE CONT PATTERN OF USE	**F10.10**	Alcohol abuse, uncomplicated
		F10.120	Alcohol abuse with intoxication, uncomplicated
		F10.129	Alcohol abuse with intoxication, unspecified
305.02	NONDEPEND ALCOHOL ABUSE EPISODIC PATTERN OF USE	**F10.10**	Alcohol abuse, uncomplicated
		F10.120	Alcohol abuse with intoxication, uncomplicated
		F10.129	Alcohol abuse with intoxication, unspecified
305.03	NONDEPENDENT ALCOHOL ABUSE IN REMISSION	**F10.10**	Alcohol abuse, uncomplicated
		F10.120	Alcohol abuse with intoxication, uncomplicated
		F10.129	Alcohol abuse with intoxication, unspecified
305.1	NONDEPENDENT TOBACCO USE DISORDER	**F17.200**	Nicotine dependence, unspecified, uncomplicated
		F17.201	Nicotine dependence, unspecified, in remission
		F17.210	Nicotine dependence, cigarettes, uncomplicated
		F17.211	Nicotine dependence, cigarettes, in remission
		F17.220	Nicotine dependence, chewing tobacco, uncomplicated
		F17.221	Nicotine dependence, chewing tobacco, in remission
		F17.290	Nicotine dependence, other tobacco product, uncomplicated
		F17.291	Nicotine dependence, other tobacco product, in remission
305.20	NONDEPEND CANNABIS ABUSE UNSPEC PATTERN OF USE	**F12.10**	Cannabis abuse, uncomplicated
		F12.90	Cannabis use, unspecified, uncomplicated
305.21	NONDEP CANNABIS ABUSE CONTINUOUS PATTERN OF USE	**F12.10**	Cannabis abuse, uncomplicated
		F12.90	Cannabis use, unspecified, uncomplicated
305.22	NONDEP CANNABIS ABUSE EPISODIC PATTERN OF USE	**F12.10**	Cannabis abuse, uncomplicated
		F12.90	Cannabis use, unspecified, uncomplicated
305.23	NONDEPENDENT CANNABIS ABUSE IN REMISSION	**F12.10**	Cannabis abuse, uncomplicated
		F12.90	Cannabis use, unspecified, uncomplicated
305.30	NONDEP HALLUCINOGEN ABUSE UNSPEC PATTERN OF USE	**F16.10**	Hallucinogen abuse, uncomplicated
		F16.120	Hallucinogen abuse with intoxication, uncomplicated
		F16.90	Hallucinogen use, unspecified, uncomplicated
305.31	NONDEP HALLUCINOGEN ABUSE CONTIN PATTERN OF USE	**F16.10**	Hallucinogen abuse, uncomplicated
		F16.120	Hallucinogen abuse with intoxication, uncomplicated
305.32	NONDEP HALLUCINOGEN ABUSE EPSODIC PATTERN OF USE	**F16.10**	Hallucinogen abuse, uncomplicated
		F16.120	Hallucinogen abuse with intoxication, uncomplicated
305.33	NONDEPENDENT HALLUCINOGEN ABUSE IN REMISSION	**F16.10**	Hallucinogen abuse, uncomplicated
		F16.120	Hallucinogen abuse with intoxication, uncomplicated
305.40	NONDEP SEDATIVE HYPNOT/ANXLYTIC ABS UNSP PAT USE	**F13.10**	Sedative, hypnotic or anxiolytic abuse, uncomplicated
		F13.120	Sedatv/hyp/anxiolytc abuse w intoxication, uncomplicated
		F13.90	Sedative, hypnotic, or anxiolytic use, unsp, uncomplicated
305.41	NONDEP SEDATVE HYPNOTC/ANXLYTIC ABS CONT PAT USE	**F13.10**	Sedative, hypnotic or anxiolytic abuse, uncomplicated
		F13.120	Sedatv/hyp/anxiolytc abuse w intoxication, uncomplicated
305.42	NONDEP SEDAT HYPNOT/ANXLYTIC ABS EPISOD PAT USE	**F13.10**	Sedative, hypnotic or anxiolytic abuse, uncomplicated
		F13.120	Sedatv/hyp/anxiolytc abuse w intoxication, uncomplicated
305.43	NONDEPEND SEDAT HYPNOT/ANXIOLYTIC ABS REMISSION	**F13.10**	Sedative, hypnotic or anxiolytic abuse, uncomplicated
		F13.120	Sedatv/hyp/anxiolytc abuse w intoxication, uncomplicated
305.50	NONDEP OPIOID ABUSE UNSPEC PATTERN OF USE	**F11.10**	Opioid abuse, uncomplicated
		F11.120	Opioid abuse with intoxication, uncomplicated
		F11.129	Opioid abuse with intoxication, unspecified
		F11.90	Opioid use, unspecified, uncomplicated
305.51	NONDEP OPIOID ABUSE CONTIN PATTERN OF USE	**F11.10**	Opioid abuse, uncomplicated
		F11.120	Opioid abuse with intoxication, uncomplicated
		F11.129	Opioid abuse with intoxication, unspecified

[Brackets] indicate valid character values for each code. Character value meanings provided for each code grouping.

ICD-9-CM		ICD-10-CM	
305.52	NONDEP OPIOID ABUSE EPISODIC PATTERN OF USE	**F11.10** **F11.120** **F11.129**	Opioid abuse, uncomplicated Opioid abuse with intoxication, uncomplicated Opioid abuse with intoxication, unspecified
305.53	NONDEPENDENT OPIOID ABUSE IN REMISSION	**F11.10** **F11.120** **F11.129**	Opioid abuse, uncomplicated Opioid abuse with intoxication, uncomplicated Opioid abuse with intoxication, unspecified
305.60	NONDEP COCAINE ABUSE UNSPEC PATTERN OF USE	**F14.10** **F14.120** **F14.90**	Cocaine abuse, uncomplicated Cocaine abuse with intoxication, uncomplicated Cocaine use, unspecified, uncomplicated
305.61	NONDEP COCAINE ABUSE CONTIN PATTERN OF USE	**F14.10** **F14.120**	Cocaine abuse, uncomplicated Cocaine abuse with intoxication, uncomplicated
305.62	NONDEP COCAINE ABUSE EPISOD PATTERN OF USE	**F14.10** **F14.120**	Cocaine abuse, uncomplicated Cocaine abuse with intoxication, uncomplicated
305.63	NONDEPENDENT COCAINE ABUSE IN REMISSION	**F14.10** **F14.120**	Cocaine abuse, uncomplicated Cocaine abuse with intoxication, uncomplicated
305.70	NONDEPEND AMPHET/REL ACT SYMPATH ABS UNS PAT USE	**F15.10** **F15.120** **F15.90**	Other stimulant abuse, uncomplicated Other stimulant abuse with intoxication, uncomplicated Other stimulant use, unspecified, uncomplicated
305.71	NONDEP AMPHET/REL ACT SYMPTH ABS CONT PAT OF USE	**F15.10** **F15.120**	Other stimulant abuse, uncomplicated Other stimulant abuse with intoxication, uncomplicated
305.72	AMPHET/RELATED DRUG ABUSE-EPISOD PATTERN OF USE	**F15.10** **F15.120**	Other stimulant abuse, uncomplicated Other stimulant abuse with intoxication, uncomplicated
305.73	NONDPND AMPHET/REL ACT SYMPATHOMIMET ABS REMISS	**F15.10** **F15.120**	Other stimulant abuse, uncomplicated Other stimulant abuse with intoxication, uncomplicated
305.80	NONDEP ANTIDEPRES TYPE ABUSE UNSPEC PAT OF USE	**F19.10** **F19.120** **F19.90**	Other psychoactive substance abuse, uncomplicated Oth psychoactive substance abuse w intoxication, uncomp Other psychoactive substance use, unspecified, uncomplicated
305.81	NONDEP ANTIDEPRESS TYPE ABUSE CONT PATTRN OF USE	**F19.10** **F19.120**	Other psychoactive substance abuse, uncomplicated Oth psychoactive substance abuse w intoxication, uncomp
305.82	NONDEP ANTIDEPRSSNT TYPE ABUS EPISOD PATTRN USE	**F19.10** **F19.120**	Other psychoactive substance abuse, uncomplicated Oth psychoactive substance abuse w intoxication, uncomp
305.83	NONDEPENDENT ANTIDEPRESSANT TYPE ABUSE REMISSION	**F19.10** **F19.120**	Other psychoactive substance abuse, uncomplicated Oth psychoactive substance abuse w intoxication, uncomp
305.90	OTH MIXED/UNSP NONDEP DRUG ABUSE UNSPEC PAT USE	**F18.10** **F18.120** **F18.90** **F55.0** **F55.1** **F55.2** **F55.3** **F55.4** **F55.8**	Inhalant abuse, uncomplicated Inhalant abuse with intoxication, uncomplicated Inhalant use, unspecified, uncomplicated Abuse of antacids Abuse of herbal or folk remedies Abuse of laxatives Abuse of steroids or hormones Abuse of vitamins Abuse of other non-psychoactive substances
305.91	OTH MIXED/UNSP NONDEP DRUG ABUSE CONT PAT OF USE	**F18.10** **F18.120** **F55.0** **F55.1** **F55.2** **F55.3** **F55.4** **F55.8**	Inhalant abuse, uncomplicated Inhalant abuse with intoxication, uncomplicated Abuse of antacids Abuse of herbal or folk remedies Abuse of laxatives Abuse of steroids or hormones Abuse of vitamins Abuse of other non-psychoactive substances
305.92	OTH MIXED/UNSP NONDEP DRUG ABS EPISODIC PAT USE	**F18.10** **F18.120** **F55.0** **F55.1** **F55.2** **F55.3** **F55.4** **F55.8**	Inhalant abuse, uncomplicated Inhalant abuse with intoxication, uncomplicated Abuse of antacids Abuse of herbal or folk remedies Abuse of laxatives Abuse of steroids or hormones Abuse of vitamins Abuse of other non-psychoactive substances
305.93	OTH MIXED/UNSPEC NONDEPENDENT DRUG ABS REMISSION	**F18.10** **F18.120** **F55.0** **F55.1** **F55.2** **F55.3** **F55.4** **F55.8**	Inhalant abuse, uncomplicated Inhalant abuse with intoxication, uncomplicated Abuse of antacids Abuse of herbal or folk remedies Abuse of laxatives Abuse of steroids or hormones Abuse of vitamins Abuse of other non-psychoactive substances
306.0	MUSCULOSKEL MALFUNCTION ARISE FROM MENTAL FCT	**F45.8**	Other somatoform disorders
306.1	RESPIRATORY MALFUNCTION ARISE FROM MENTAL FCT	**F45.8**	Other somatoform disorders
306.2	CV MALFUNCTION ARISE FROM MENTAL FACTORS	**F45.8**	Other somatoform disorders
306.3	SKIN MALFUNCTION ARISING FROM MENTAL FACTORS	**F45.8**	Other somatoform disorders
306.4	GI MALFUNCTION ARISE FROM MENTAL FCT	**F45.8**	Other somatoform disorders
306.50	PSYCHOGENIC GENITOURINARY MALFUNCTION UNSPEC	**F45.8**	Other somatoform disorders
306.51	PSYCHOGENIC VAGINISMUS	➡ **F52.5**	Vaginismus not due to a substance or known physiol condition
306.52	PSYCHOGENIC DYSMENORRHEA	**F45.8**	Other somatoform disorders
306.53	PSYCHOGENIC DYSURIA	**F45.8**	Other somatoform disorders
306.59	OTH GU MALFUNCTION ARISE FROM MENTAL FCT	**F45.8**	Other somatoform disorders

ICD-9-CM			ICD-10-CM	
306.6	ENDOCRINE MALFUNCTION ARISE FROM MENTAL FACTORS		F45.8	Other somatoform disorders
306.7	MALFUNCTION ORGN SPCL SENSE ARISE FROM MENTL FCT		F45.8	Other somatoform disorders
306.8	OTHER SPECIFIED PSYCHOPHYSIOLOGICAL MALFUNCTION		F45.8 F59	Other somatoform disorders Unsp behavrl synd assoc w physiol disturb and physcl factors
306.9	UNSPECIFIED PSYCHOPHYSIOLOGICAL MALFUNCTION		F45.9	Somatoform disorder, unspecified
307.0	ADULT ONSET FLUENCY DISORDER	➡	F98.5	Adult onset fluency disorder
307.1	ANOREXIA NERVOSA		F50.00 F50.01 F50.02	Anorexia nervosa, unspecified Anorexia nervosa, restricting type Anorexia nervosa, binge eating/purging type
307.20	TIC DISORDER, UNSPECIFIED		F95.8 F95.9	Other tic disorders Tic disorder, unspecified
307.21	TRANSIENT TIC DISORDER	➡	F95.0	Transient tic disorder
307.22	CHRONIC MOTOR OR VOCAL TIC DISORDER	➡	F95.1	Chronic motor or vocal tic disorder
307.23	TOURETTE'S DISORDER	➡	F95.2	Tourette's disorder
307.3	STEREOTYPIC MOVEMENT DISORDER	➡	F98.4	Stereotyped movement disorders
307.40	NONORGANIC SLEEP DISORDER UNSPECIFIED	➡	F51.9	Sleep disorder not due to a sub or known physiol cond, unsp
307.41	TRANSIENT DISORDER INITIATING/MAINTAINING SLEEP		F51.02 F51.09	Adjustment insomnia Oth insomnia not due to a substance or known physiol cond
307.42	PERSISTENT DISORDER INITIATING/MAINTAINING SLEEP		F51.01 F51.03 F51.09	Primary insomnia Paradoxical insomnia Oth insomnia not due to a substance or known physiol cond
307.43	TRANSIENT DISORDER INIT/MAINTAINING WAKEFULNESS		F51.19	Oth hypersomnia not due to a substance or known physiol cond
307.44	PERSISTENT DISORDER INIT/MAINTAINING WAKEFULNESS		F51.11 F51.12 F51.19	Primary hypersomnia Insufficient sleep syndrome Oth hypersomnia not due to a substance or known physiol cond
307.45	CIRCADIAN RHYTHM SLEEP D/O NONORGANIC ORIGIN		F51.8	Oth sleep disord not due to a sub or known physiol cond
307.46	SLEEP AROUSAL DISORDER		F51.3 F51.4	Sleepwalking [somnambulism] Sleep terrors [night terrors]
307.47	OTH DYSFUNCTIONS SLEEP STAGES/AROUSAL FROM SLEEP		F51.5 F51.8	Nightmare disorder Oth sleep disord not due to a sub or known physiol cond
307.48	REPETITIVE INTRUSIONS OF SLEEP		F51.8	Oth sleep disord not due to a sub or known physiol cond
307.49	OTHER SPECIFIC DISORDER SLEEP NONORGANIC ORIGIN		F51.8	Oth sleep disord not due to a sub or known physiol cond
307.50	EATING DISORDER, UNSPECIFIED	➡	F50.9	Eating disorder, unspecified
307.51	BULIMIA NERVOSA	➡	F50.2	Bulimia nervosa
307.52	PICA		F98.3	Pica of infancy and childhood
307.53	RUMINATION DISORDER		F98.21	Rumination disorder of infancy
307.54	PSYCHOGENIC VOMITING		F50.8	Other eating disorders
307.59	OTHER DISORDER OF EATING		F50.8 F98.29	Other eating disorders Other feeding disorders of infancy and early childhood
307.6	ENURESIS	➡	F98.0	Enuresis not due to a substance or known physiol condition
307.7	ENCOPRESIS	➡	F98.1	Encopresis not due to a substance or known physiol condition
307.80	PSYCHOGENIC PAIN, SITE UNSPECIFIED		F45.41	Pain disorder exclusively related to psychological factors
307.81	TENSION HEADACHE		G44.209	Tension-type headache, unspecified, not intractable
307.89	OTH PAIN DISORDER RELATED PSYCHOLOGICAL FACTORS		F45.42	Pain disorder with related psychological factors
307.9	OTHER&UNSPECIFIED SPECIAL SYMPTOM/SYNDROME NEC		F63.3 R45.1 R45.81 R45.82	Trichotillomania Restlessness and agitation Low self-esteem Worries
308.0	PREDOMINANT DISTURBANCE OF EMOTIONS		F43.0	Acute stress reaction
308.1	PREDOM DISTURBANCE CONSCIOUSNESS AS REACT STRESS		F43.0	Acute stress reaction
308.2	PREDOM PSYCHOMOTOR DISTURBANCE AS REACT STRESS		F43.0	Acute stress reaction
308.3	OTHER ACUTE REACTIONS TO STRESS		F43.0	Acute stress reaction
308.4	MIXED DISORDERS AS REACTION TO STRESS		F43.0	Acute stress reaction
308.9	UNSPECIFIED ACUTE REACTION TO STRESS		F43.0 R45.7	Acute stress reaction State of emotional shock and stress, unspecified
309.0	ADJUSTMENT DISORDER WITH DEPRESSED MOOD		F43.21	Adjustment disorder with depressed mood
309.1	PROLONGED DEPRESSIVE REACTION AS ADJ REACTION		F43.21	Adjustment disorder with depressed mood
309.21	SEPARATION ANXIETY DISORDER	➡	F93.0	Separation anxiety disorder of childhood
309.22	EMANCIPATION D/O ADOLESCENCE&EARLY ADLT LIFE		F94.8	Other childhood disorders of social functioning
309.23	SPECIFIC ACADEMIC/WORK INHIBITION AS ADJ REACT		F94.8	Other childhood disorders of social functioning
309.24	ADJUSTMENT DISORDER WITH ANXIETY	➡	F43.22	Adjustment disorder with anxiety
309.28	ADJ DISORDER WITH MIXED ANXIETY & DEPRESSED MOOD	➡	F43.23	Adjustment disorder with mixed anxiety and depressed mood
309.29	OTH ADJ REACT W/PREDOM DISTURBANCE OTH EMOTIONS		F43.29 F94.8	Adjustment disorder with other symptoms Other childhood disorders of social functioning
309.3	ADJUSTMENT DISORDER WITH DISTURBANCE OF CONDUCT	➡	F43.24	Adjustment disorder with disturbance of conduct
309.4	ADJ DISORDER W/MIXED DISTURBANCE EMOTION&CONDUCT	➡	F43.25	Adjustment disorder w mixed disturb of emotions and conduct
309.81	POSTTRAUMATIC STRESS DISORDER		F43.10 F43.11 F43.12	Post-traumatic stress disorder, unspecified Post-traumatic stress disorder, acute Post-traumatic stress disorder, chronic
309.82	ADJUSTMENT REACTION WITH PHYSICAL SYMPTOMS		F43.8	Other reactions to severe stress

 [Brackets] indicate valid character values for each code. Character value meanings provided for each code grouping.

ICD-9-CM			ICD-10-CM	
3Ø9.83	ADJUSTMENT REACTION WITH WITHDRAWAL		**F43.8**	Other reactions to severe stress
3Ø9.89	OTHER SPECIFIED ADJUSTMENT REACTION		**F43.8**	Other reactions to severe stress
3Ø9.9	UNSPECIFIED ADJUSTMENT REACTION		**F43.2Ø** **F43.9**	Adjustment disorder, unspecified Reaction to severe stress, unspecified
31Ø.Ø	FRONTAL LOBE SYNDROME		**FØ7.Ø**	Personality change due to known physiological condition
31Ø.1	PERSONALITY CHG DUE CONDS CLASSIFIED ELSEWHERE		**FØ7.Ø**	Personality change due to known physiological condition
31Ø.2	POSTCONCUSSION SYNDROME	➡	**FØ7.81**	Postconcussional syndrome
31Ø.81	PSEUDOBULBAR AFFECT		**F48.2**	Pseudobulbar affect
31Ø.89	OTH NONPSYCHOT MENTL D/O FLW ORGANIC BRAIN DAMGE		**FØ7.89**	Oth personality & behavrl disord due to known physiol cond
31Ø.9	UNS NONPSYCHOT MENTL D/O FLW ORGNIC BRAIN DAMGE		**FØ7.9** **FØ9**	Unsp personality & behavrl disord due to known physiol cond Unsp mental disorder due to known physiological condition
311	DEPRESSIVE DISORDER NOT ELSEWHERE CLASSIFIED		**F32.9**	Major depressive disorder, single episode, unspecified
312.ØØ	UNDERSOCIALIZED CONDUCT D/O AGRESSIVE UNSPEC		**F91.1**	Conduct disorder, childhood-onset type
312.Ø1	UNDERSOCIALIZED CONDUCT DISORDER AGRESSIVE MILD		**F91.1**	Conduct disorder, childhood-onset type
312.Ø2	UNDERSOCIALIZED CONDUCT DISORDER AGRESSIVE MOD		**F91.1**	Conduct disorder, childhood-onset type
312.Ø3	UNDERSOCIALIZED CONDUCT D/O AGRESSIVE SEVERE		**F91.1**	Conduct disorder, childhood-onset type
312.1Ø	UNDERSOCIALIZED CONDUCT D/O UNAGRESSIVE UNSPEC		**F91.8**	Other conduct disorders
312.11	UNDERSOCIALIZED CONDUCT D/O UNAGRESSIVE MILD		**F91.8**	Other conduct disorders
312.12	UNDERSOCIALIZED CONDUCT DISORDER UNAGRESSIVE MOD		**F91.8**	Other conduct disorders
312.13	UNDERSOCIALIZED CONDUCT D/O UNAGRESSIVE SEVERE		**F91.8**	Other conduct disorders
312.2Ø	SOCIALIZED CONDUCT DISORDER UNSPECIFIED		**F91.2**	Conduct disorder, adolescent-onset type
312.21	SOCIALIZED CONDUCT DISORDER, MILD		**F91.2**	Conduct disorder, adolescent-onset type
312.22	SOCIALIZED CONDUCT DISORDER MODERATE		**F91.2**	Conduct disorder, adolescent-onset type
312.23	SOCIALIZED CONDUCT DISORDER, SEVERE		**F91.2**	Conduct disorder, adolescent-onset type
312.3Ø	IMPULSE CONTROL DISORDER UNSPECIFIED	➡	**F63.9**	Impulse disorder, unspecified
312.31	PATHOLOGICAL GAMBLING	➡	**F63.Ø**	Pathological gambling
312.32	KLEPTOMANIA	➡	**F63.2**	Kleptomania
312.33	PYROMANIA	➡	**F63.1**	Pyromania
312.34	INTERMITTENT EXPLOSIVE DISORDER		**F63.81**	Intermittent explosive disorder
312.35	ISOLATED EXPLOSIVE DISORDER		**F63.81**	Intermittent explosive disorder
312.39	OTHER DISORDER OF IMPULSE CONTROL		**F63.3** **F63.89**	Trichotillomania Other impulse disorders
312.4	MIXED DISTURBANCE OF CONDUCT AND EMOTIONS		**F91.8**	Other conduct disorders
312.81	CONDUCT DISORDER CHILDHOOD ONSET TYPE		**F91.1**	Conduct disorder, childhood-onset type
312.82	CONDUCT DISORDER ADOLESCENT ONSET TYPE		**F91.2**	Conduct disorder, adolescent-onset type
312.89	OTHER SPECIFIED DISTURBANCE OF CONDUCT NEC		**F91.Ø** **F91.8**	Conduct disorder confined to family context Other conduct disorders
312.9	UNSPECIFIED DISTURBANCE OF CONDUCT	➡	**F91.9**	Conduct disorder, unspecified
313.Ø	OVERANXIOUS DISORDER SPECIFIC CHLD&ADOLESCENCE		**F93.8**	Other childhood emotional disorders
313.1	MISERY&UNHAPPINESS D/O SPECIFIC CHLD&ADOLESCENCE		**F93.8**	Other childhood emotional disorders
313.21	SHYNESS DISORDER OF CHILDHOOD		**F93.8**	Other childhood emotional disorders
313.22	INTROVERTED DISORDER OF CHILDHOOD		**F93.8**	Other childhood emotional disorders
313.23	SELECTIVE MUTISM	➡	**F94.Ø**	Selective mutism
313.3	RELATIONSHIP PROBLEMS SPECIFIC CHLD&ADOLESCENCE		**F93.8**	Other childhood emotional disorders
313.81	OPPOSITIONAL DEFIANT DISORDER	➡	**F91.3**	Oppositional defiant disorder
313.82	IDENTITY DISORDER OF CHILDHOOD OR ADOLESCENCE		**F93.8**	Other childhood emotional disorders
313.83	ACADEMIC UNDERACHIEVEMENT D/O CHLD/ADOLESCENCE		**F93.8**	Other childhood emotional disorders
313.89	OTH EMOTIONAL DISTURBANCE CHILDHOOD/ADOLESCENCE		**F93.8** **F94.1** **F94.2** **F94.9** **F98.8**	Other childhood emotional disorders Reactive attachment disorder of childhood Disinhibited attachment disorder of childhood Childhood disorder of social functioning, unspecified Oth behav/emotn disord w onset usly occur in chldhd and adol
313.9	UNSPEC EMOTIONAL DISTURBANCE CHLD/ADOLESCENCE		**F93.9** **F94.8** **F98.9**	Childhood emotional disorder, unspecified Other childhood disorders of social functioning Unsp behav/emotn disord w onst usly occur in chldhd and adol
314.ØØ	ADD CHILDHOOD WITHOUT MENTION HYPERACTIVITY		**F9Ø.Ø** **F9Ø.9**	Attn-defct hyperactivity disorder, predom inattentive type Attention-deficit hyperactivity disorder, unspecified type
314.Ø1	ADD OF CHILDHOOD WITH HYPERACTIVITY		**F9Ø.Ø** **F9Ø.1** **F9Ø.2** **F9Ø.8**	Attn-defct hyperactivity disorder, predom inattentive type Attn-defct hyperactivity disorder, predom hyperactive type Attention-deficit hyperactivity disorder, combined type Attention-deficit hyperactivity disorder, other type
314.1	HYPERKINESIS OF CHILDHOOD W/DEVELOPMENTAL DELAY		**F9Ø.8**	Attention-deficit hyperactivity disorder, other type
314.2	HYPERKINETIC CONDUCT DISORDER OF CHILDHOOD		**F9Ø.8**	Attention-deficit hyperactivity disorder, other type
314.8	OTH SPEC MANIFESTS HYPERKINETIC SYNDROME CHLD		**F9Ø.8**	Attention-deficit hyperactivity disorder, other type
314.9	UNSPECIFIED HYPERKINETIC SYNDROME OF CHILDHOOD		**F9Ø.9**	Attention-deficit hyperactivity disorder, unspecified type
315.ØØ	DEVELOPMENTAL READING DISORDER UNSPECIFIED		**F81.Ø**	Specific reading disorder
315.Ø1	ALEXIA		**R48.Ø**	Dyslexia and alexia
315.Ø2	DEVELOPMENTAL DYSLEXIA		**F81.Ø**	Specific reading disorder
315.Ø9	OTHER SPECIFIC DEVELOPMENTAL READING DISORDER		**F81.81**	Disorder of written expression

ICD-9-CM			ICD-10-CM	
315.1	MATHEMATICS DISORDER	➡	F81.2	Mathematics disorder
315.2	OTHER SPECIFIC DVLPMENTL LEARNING DIFFICULTIES		F81.81 F81.89	Disorder of written expression Other developmental disorders of scholastic skills
315.31	EXPRESSIVE LANGUAGE DISORDER	➡	F80.1	Expressive language disorder
315.32	MIXED RECEPTIVE-EXPRESSIVE LANGUAGE DISORDER		F80.2 H93.25	Mixed receptive-expressive language disorder Central auditory processing disorder
315.34	SPEECH&LANGUAGE DVLPMENTL DELAY D/T HEARING LOSS	➡	F80.4	Speech and language development delay due to hearing loss
315.35	CHILDHOOD ONSET FLUENCY DISORDER	➡	F80.81	Childhood onset fluency disorder
315.39	OTHER DEVELOPMENTAL SPEECH OR LANGUAGE DISORDER		F80.0 F80.89 F80.9	Phonological disorder Other developmental disorders of speech and language Developmental disorder of speech and language, unspecified
315.4	DEVELOPMENTAL COORDINATION DISORDER		F82	Specific developmental disorder of motor function
315.5	MIXED DEVELOPMENT DISORDER		F82	Specific developmental disorder of motor function
315.8	OTHER SPECIFIED DELAY IN DEVELOPMENT		F88	Other disorders of psychological development
315.9	UNSPECIFIED DELAY IN DEVELOPMENT		F81.9 F89	Developmental disorder of scholastic skills, unspecified Unspecified disorder of psychological development
316	PSYCHIC FACTORS ASSOC W/DISEASES CLASSIFIED ELSW	➡	F54	Psych & behavrl factors assoc w disord or dis classd elswhr
317	MILD INTELLECTUAL DISABILITIES	➡	F70	Mild intellectual disabilities
318.0	MODERATE INTELLECTUAL DISABILITIES	➡	F71	Moderate intellectual disabilities
318.1	SEVERE INTELLECTUAL DISABILITIES	➡	F72	Severe intellectual disabilities
318.2	PROFOUND INTELLECTUAL DISABILITIES	➡	F73	Profound intellectual disabilities
319	UNSPECIFIED INTELLECTUAL DISABILITIES		F78 F79	Other intellectual disabilities Unspecified intellectual disabilities

Nervous System and Sense Organs

ICD-9-CM			ICD-10-CM	
320.0	HEMOPHILUS MENINGITIS	➡	G00.0	Hemophilus meningitis
320.1	PNEUMOCOCCAL MENINGITIS	➡	G00.1	Pneumococcal meningitis
320.2	STREPTOCOCCAL MENINGITIS	➡	G00.2	Streptococcal meningitis
320.3	STAPHYLOCOCCAL MENINGITIS	➡	G00.3	Staphylococcal meningitis
320.7	MENINGITIS OTH BACTERL DISEASES CLASSIFIED ELSW	➡	G01	Meningitis in bacterial diseases classified elsewhere
320.81	ANAEROBIC MENINGITIS		G00.8	Other bacterial meningitis
320.82	MENINGITIS DUE TO GRAM-NEGATIVE BACTERIA NEC		G00.9	Bacterial meningitis, unspecified
320.89	MENINGITIS DUE TO OTHER SPECIFIED BACTERIA		G00.8	Other bacterial meningitis
320.9	MENINGITIS DUE TO UNSPECIFIED BACTERIUM		G00.9 G04.2	Bacterial meningitis, unspecified Bacterial meningoencephalitis and meningomyelitis, NEC
321.0	CRYPTOCOCCAL MENINGITIS	▣	B45.1	Cerebral cryptococcosis
321.1	MENINGITIS IN OTHER FUNGAL DISEASES		G02	Meningitis in oth infec/parastc diseases classd elswhr
321.2	MENINGITIS DUE TO VIRUSES NEC		G02	Meningitis in oth infec/parastc diseases classd elswhr
321.3	MENINGITIS DUE TO TRYPANOSOMIASIS		G02	Meningitis in oth infec/parastc diseases classd elswhr
321.4	MENINGITIS IN SARCOIDOSIS		G02	Meningitis in oth infec/parastc diseases classd elswhr
321.8	MENINGITIS DUE OTH NONBACTERL ORGNSMS CLASS ELSW		G02	Meningitis in oth infec/parastc diseases classd elswhr
322.0	NONPYOGENIC MENINGITIS	➡	G03.0	Nonpyogenic meningitis
322.1	EOSINOPHILIC MENINGITIS		G03.8	Meningitis due to other specified causes
322.2	CHRONIC MENINGITIS	➡	G03.1	Chronic meningitis
322.9	UNSPECIFIED MENINGITIS	➡	G03.9	Meningitis, unspecified
323.01	ENCEPHALITIS & ENCEPHALOMYELIT VIR DZ CLSS ELSW		G05.3	Encephalitis and encephalomyelitis in diseases classd elswhr
323.02	MYELITIS IN VIRAL DISEASES CLASSIFIED ELSEWHERE		G05.4	Myelitis in diseases classified elsewhere
323.1	ENCEPHALITIS MYELITIS & EM RICKETTS DZ CLSS ELSW		G05.3	Encephalitis and encephalomyelitis in diseases classd elswhr
323.2	ENCEPHALITIS MYELITIS & EM PROTOZOL DZ CLSS ELSW		G05.3	Encephalitis and encephalomyelitis in diseases classd elswhr
323.41	OTH ENCEPHALIT ENCEPHALOMYELIT OTH INF CLSS ELSW		G05.3	Encephalitis and encephalomyelitis in diseases classd elswhr
323.42	OTH MYELITIS D/T OTH INFECTION CLASS ELSEWHERE		G05.4	Myelitis in diseases classified elsewhere
323.51	ENCEPHALITIS & ENCEPHALOMYELITIS FLW IMMUN PROC		G04.02 G04.32	Postimmun ac dissem encphlts, myelitis and encephalomyelitis Postimmun acute necrotizing hemorrhagic encephalopathy
323.52	MYELITIS FOLLOWING IMMUNIZATION PROCEDURES		G04.02	Postimmun ac dissem encphlts, myelitis and encephalomyelitis
323.61	INFECTIOUS ACUTE DISSEMINATED ENCEPHALOMYELITIS		G04.00 G04.01 G04.39	Acute disseminated encephalitis and encephalomyelitis, unsp Postinfect acute dissem encephalitis and encephalomyelitis Other acute necrotizing hemorrhagic encephalopathy
323.62	OTH POSTINFECT ENCEPHALITIS & ENCEPHALOMYELITIS		G04.30 G04.31	Acute necrotizing hemorrhagic encephalopathy, unspecified Postinfectious acute necrotizing hemorrhagic encephalopathy
323.63	POSTINFECTIOUS MYELITIS		G05.4	Myelitis in diseases classified elsewhere
323.71	TOXIC ENCEPHALITIS AND ENCEPHALOMYELITIS		G92	Toxic encephalopathy
323.72	TOXIC MYELITIS		G92	Toxic encephalopathy
323.81	OTHER CAUSES OF ENCEPHALITIS & ENCEPHALOMYELITIS		G04.81	Other encephalitis and encephalomyelitis
323.82	OTHER CAUSES OF MYELITIS		G04.89	Other myelitis
323.9	UNS CAUS ENCEPHALITIS MYELITIS & ENCEPHALOMYELIT		G04.90 G04.91 G37.4	Encephalitis and encephalomyelitis, unspecified Myelitis, unspecified Subacute necrotizing myelitis of central nervous system
324.0	INTRACRANIAL ABSCESS		G06.0	Intracranial abscess and granuloma
324.1	INTRASPINAL ABSCESS		G06.1	Intraspinal abscess and granuloma
324.9	INTRACRANIAL&INTRASPINAL ABSCESS UNSPEC SITE		G06.2 G07	Extradural and subdural abscess, unspecified Intcrn & intraspinal abscs & granuloma in dis classd elswhr
325	PHLEBITIS&THROMBOPHLEB INTRACRAN VENOUS SINUSES	➡	G08	Intracranial and intraspinal phlebitis and thrombophlebitis
326	LATE EFF INTRACRANIAL ABSC/PYOGENIC INFECTION		G09	Sequelae of inflammatory diseases of central nervous system
327.00	ORGANIC INSOMNIA UNSPECIFIED		G47.01	Insomnia due to medical condition
327.01	INSOMNIA D/T MEDICAL COND CLASSIFIED ELSEWHERE		G47.01	Insomnia due to medical condition
327.02	INSOMNIA DUE TO MENTAL DISORDER		F51.04 F51.05	Psychophysiologic insomnia Insomnia due to other mental disorder
327.09	OTHER ORGANIC INSOMNIA		G47.09	Other insomnia
327.10	ORGANIC HYPERSOMNIA UNSPECIFIED		G47.10	Hypersomnia, unspecified
327.11	IDIOPATHIC HYPERSOMNIA WITH LONG SLEEP TIME	➡	G47.11	Idiopathic hypersomnia with long sleep time
327.12	IDIOPATHIC HYPERSOMNIA WITHOUT LONG SLEEP TIME	➡	G47.12	Idiopathic hypersomnia without long sleep time
327.13	RECURRENT HYPERSOMNIA	➡	G47.13	Recurrent hypersomnia
327.14	HYPERSOMNIA D/T MEDICAL COND CLASS ELSEWHERE	➡	G47.14	Hypersomnia due to medical condition
327.15	HYPERSOMNIA DUE TO MENTAL DISORDER		F51.13	Hypersomnia due to other mental disorder
327.19	OTHER ORGANIC HYPERSOMNIA		G47.19	Other hypersomnia
327.20	ORGANIC SLEEP APNEA UNSPECIFIED		G47.30	Sleep apnea, unspecified
327.21	PRIMARY CENTRAL SLEEP APNEA	➡	G47.31	Primary central sleep apnea
327.22	HIGH ALTITUDE PERIODIC BREATHING	➡	G47.32	High altitude periodic breathing
327.23	OBSTRUCTIVE SLEEP APNEA	➡	G47.33	Obstructive sleep apnea (adult) (pediatric)
327.24	IDIOPATH SLEEP REL NONOBST ALVEOLAR HYPOVENT	➡	G47.34	Idio sleep related nonobstructive alveolar hypoventilation
327.25	CONGNTAL CENTRAL ALVEOL HYPOVENTILATION SYNDROME	➡	G47.35	Congenital central alveolar hypoventilation syndrome
327.26	SLEEP RELATED HYPOVENTILATION/HYPOXEMIA CCE	➡	G47.36	Sleep related hypoventilation in conditions classd elswhr
327.27	CENTRAL SLEEP APNEA CONDS CLASSIFIED ELSEWHERE	➡	G47.37	Central sleep apnea in conditions classified elsewhere
327.29	OTHER ORGANIC SLEEP APNEA		G47.39	Other sleep apnea

▣ See Appendix A ➡ Equivalent Mapping Scenario Scenario

ICD-9-CM			ICD-10-CM	
327.30	CIRCADIAN RHYTHM SLEEP DISORDER UNSPECIFIED		G47.20	Circadian rhythm sleep disorder, unspecified type
327.31	CIRCADIAN RHYTHM SLEEP D/O DELAY SLEEP PHSE TYPE	➡	G47.21	Circadian rhythm sleep disorder, delayed sleep phase type
327.32	CIRCADIAN RHYTHM SLEEP D/O ADVD SLEEP PHASE TYPE	➡	G47.22	Circadian rhythm sleep disorder, advanced sleep phase type
327.33	CIRCADIAN RHYTHM SLEEP D/O IRREG SLEEPWAKE TYPE	➡	G47.23	Circadian rhythm sleep disorder, irregular sleep wake type
327.34	CIRCADIAN RHYTHM SLEEP DISORDER FREERUNNING TYPE	➡	G47.24	Circadian rhythm sleep disorder, free running type
327.35	CIRCADIAN RHYTHM SLEEP DISORDER JET LAG TYPE	➡	G47.25	Circadian rhythm sleep disorder, jet lag type
327.36	CIRCADIAN RHYTHM SLEEP DISORDER SHIFT WORK TYPE	➡	G47.26	Circadian rhythm sleep disorder, shift work type
327.37	CIRCADIAN RHYTHM SLEEP DISORDER CONDS CLASS ELSW	➡	G47.27	Circadian rhythm sleep disorder in conditions classd elswhr
327.39	OTHER CIRCADIAN RHYTHM SLEEP DISORDER	➡	G47.29	Other circadian rhythm sleep disorder
327.40	ORGANIC PARASOMNIA UNSPECIFIED	➡	G47.50	Parasomnia, unspecified
327.41	CONFUSIONAL AROUSALS		G47.51	Confusional arousals
327.42	REM SLEEP BEHAVIOR DISORDER		G47.52	REM sleep behavior disorder
327.43	RECURRENT ISOLATED SLEEP PARALYSIS	➡	G47.53	Recurrent isolated sleep paralysis
327.44	PARASOMNIA IN CONDITIONS CLASSIFIED ELSEWHERE	➡	G47.54	Parasomnia in conditions classified elsewhere
327.49	OTHER ORGANIC PARASOMNIA	➡	G47.59	Other parasomnia
327.51	PERIODIC LIMB MOVEMENT DISORDER	➡	G47.61	Periodic limb movement disorder
327.52	SLEEP RELATED LEG CRAMPS	➡	G47.62	Sleep related leg cramps
327.53	SLEEP RELATED BRUXISM	➡	G47.63	Sleep related bruxism
327.59	OTHER ORGANIC SLEEP RELATED MOVEMENT DISORDERS		G47.69	Other sleep related movement disorders
327.8	OTHER ORGANIC SLEEP DISORDERS		G47.8	Other sleep disorders
330.0	LEUKODYSTROPHY		E75.23 E75.25 E75.29	Krabbe disease Metachromatic leukodystrophy Other sphingolipidosis
330.1	CEREBRAL LIPIDOSES		E75.00 E75.01 E75.02 E75.09 E75.10 E75.11 E75.19 E75.4	GM2 gangliosidosis, unspecified Sandhoff disease Tay-Sachs disease Other GM2 gangliosidosis Unspecified gangliosidosis Mucolipidosis IV Other gangliosidosis Neuronal ceroid lipofuscinosis
330.2	CEREBRAL DEGENERATION IN GENERALIZED LIPIDOSES		G93.89	Other specified disorders of brain
330.3	CERBRL DEGENERATION CHLD OTH DISEASES CLASS ELSW		G93.9	Disorder of brain, unspecified
330.8	OTHER SPECIFIED CEREBRAL DEGENERATIONS CHILDHOOD		F84.2 G31.81 G31.82	Rett's syndrome Alpers disease Leigh's disease
330.9	UNSPECIFIED CEREBRAL DEGENERATION IN CHILDHOOD		G31.9	Degenerative disease of nervous system, unspecified
331.0	ALZHEIMERS DISEASE		G30.0 G30.1 G30.8 G30.9	Alzheimer's disease with early onset Alzheimer's disease with late onset Other Alzheimer's disease Alzheimer's disease, unspecified
331.11	PICKS DISEASE	➡	G31.01	Pick's disease
331.19	OTHER FRONTOTEMPORAL DEMENTIA	➡	G31.09	Other frontotemporal dementia
331.2	SENILE DEGENERATION OF BRAIN	➡	G31.1	Senile degeneration of brain, not elsewhere classified
331.3	COMMUNICATING HYDROCEPHALUS	➡	G91.0	Communicating hydrocephalus
331.4	OBSTRUCTIVE HYDROCEPHALUS		G91.1 G91.3 G91.8 G91.9	Obstructive hydrocephalus Post-traumatic hydrocephalus, unspecified Other hydrocephalus Hydrocephalus, unspecified
331.5	IDIOPATHIC NORMAL PRESSURE HYDROCEPHALUS	➡	G91.2	(Idiopathic) normal pressure hydrocephalus
331.6	CORTICOBASAL DEGENERATION		G31.85	Corticobasal degeneration
331.7	CEREBRAL DEGENERATION DISEASES CLASSIFIED ELSW		G13.2 G13.8 G31.2 G91.4 G94	Systemic atrophy primarily affecting the cnsl in myxedema Systemic atrophy aff cnsl in oth diseases classd elswhr Degeneration of nervous system due to alcohol Hydrocephalus in diseases classified elsewhere Other disorders of brain in diseases classified elsewhere
331.81	REYES SYNDROME	➡	G93.7	Reye's syndrome
331.82	DEMENTIA WITH LEWY BODIES	➡	G31.83	Dementia with Lewy bodies
331.83	MILD COGNITIVE IMPAIRMENT SO STATED	➡	G31.84	Mild cognitive impairment, so stated
331.89	OTHER CEREBRAL DEGENERATION		G31.89	Other specified degenerative diseases of nervous system
331.9	UNSPECIFIED CEREBRAL DEGENERATION		G31.9	Degenerative disease of nervous system, unspecified
332.0	PARALYSIS AGITANS		G20 G21.4	Parkinson's disease Vascular parkinsonism
332.1	SECONDARY PARKINSONISM		G21.11 G21.19 G21.2 G21.3 G21.8 G21.9	Neuroleptic induced parkinsonism Other drug induced secondary parkinsonism Secondary parkinsonism due to other external agents Postencephalitic parkinsonism Other secondary parkinsonism Secondary parkinsonism, unspecified

ICD-9-CM			ICD-10-CM	
333.Ø	OTHER DEGENERATIVE DISEASES OF THE BASAL GANGLIA		G23.Ø G23.1 G23.2 G23.8 G23.9 G9Ø.3	Hallervorden-Spatz disease Progressive supranuclear ophthalmoplegia Striatonigral degeneration Other specified degenerative diseases of basal ganglia Degenerative disease of basal ganglia, unspecified Multi-system degeneration of the autonomic nervous system
333.1	ESSENTIAL AND OTHER SPECIFIED FORMS OF TREMOR		G25.Ø G25.1 G25.2	Essential tremor Drug-induced tremor Other specified forms of tremor
333.2	MYOCLONUS	➡	G25.3	Myoclonus
333.3	TICS OF ORGANIC ORIGIN		G25.61 G25.69	Drug induced tics Other tics of organic origin
333.4	HUNTINGTONS CHOREA	➡	G1Ø	Huntington's disease
333.5	OTHER CHOREAS		G25.4 G25.5	Drug-induced chorea Other chorea
333.6	GENETIC TORSION DYSTONIA	➡	G24.1	Genetic torsion dystonia
333.71	ATHETOID CEREBRAL PALSY	➡	G8Ø.3	Athetoid cerebral palsy
333.72	ACUTE DYSTONIA DUE TO DRUGS	➡	G24.Ø2	Drug induced acute dystonia
333.79	OTHER ACQUIRED TORSION DYSTONIA		G24.Ø9 G24.2 G24.8	Other drug induced dystonia Idiopathic nonfamilial dystonia Other dystonia
333.81	BLEPHAROSPASM	➡	G24.5	Blepharospasm
333.82	OROFACIAL DYSKINESIA	➡	G24.4	Idiopathic orofacial dystonia
333.83	SPASMODIC TORTICOLLIS	➡	G24.3	Spasmodic torticollis
333.84	ORGANIC WRITERS CRAMP		G25.89	Other specified extrapyramidal and movement disorders
333.85	SUBACUTE DYSKINESIA DUE TO DRUGS	➡	G24.Ø1	Drug induced subacute dyskinesia
333.89	OTHER FRAGMENTS OF TORSION DYSTONIA		G24.9	Dystonia, unspecified
333.9Ø	UNSPEC EXTRAPYRAMIDAL DZ&ABNORM MOVMNT DISORDER		G25.9	Extrapyramidal and movement disorder, unspecified
333.91	STIFF-MAN SYNDROME	➡	G25.82	Stiff-man syndrome
333.92	NEUROLEPTIC MALIGNANT SYNDROME	➡	G21.Ø	Malignant neuroleptic syndrome
333.93	BENIGN SHUDDERING ATTACKS		G25.83	Benign shuddering attacks
333.94	RESTLESS LEGS SYNDROME	➡	G25.81	Restless legs syndrome
333.99	OTH EXTRAPYRAMIDAL DZ&ABNORM MOVMNT DISORDER		G25.7Ø G25.71 G25.79 G25.89 G25.9 G26	Drug induced movement disorder, unspecified Drug induced akathisia Other drug induced movement disorders Other specified extrapyramidal and movement disorders Extrapyramidal and movement disorder, unspecified Extrapyramidal and movement disord in diseases classd elswhr
334.Ø	FRIEDREICHS ATAXIA		G11.1	Early-onset cerebellar ataxia
334.1	HEREDITARY SPASTIC PARAPLEGIA		G11.4	Hereditary spastic paraplegia
334.2	PRIMARY CEREBELLAR DEGENERATION		G11.Ø G11.2	Congenital nonprogressive ataxia Late-onset cerebellar ataxia
334.3	OTHER CEREBELLAR ATAXIA		G11.1	Early-onset cerebellar ataxia
334.4	CEREBELLAR ATAXIA DISEASES CLASSIFIED ELSEWHERE		G32.81	Cerebellar ataxia in diseases classified elsewhere
334.8	OTHER SPINOCEREBELLAR DISEASES		G11.3 G11.8	Cerebellar ataxia with defective DNA repair Other hereditary ataxias
334.9	UNSPECIFIED SPINOCEREBELLAR DISEASE		G11.9	Hereditary ataxia, unspecified
335.Ø	WERDNIG-HOFFMANN DISEASE	➡	G12.Ø	Infantile spinal muscular atrophy, type I [Werdnig-Hoffman]
335.1Ø	UNSPECIFIED SPINAL MUSCULAR ATROPHY		G12.9	Spinal muscular atrophy, unspecified
335.11	KUGELBERG-WELANDER DISEASE		G12.1	Other inherited spinal muscular atrophy
335.19	OTHER SPINAL MUSCULAR ATROPHY		G12.8	Other spinal muscular atrophies and related syndromes
335.2Ø	AMYOTROPHIC LATERAL SCLEROSIS		G12.21	Amyotrophic lateral sclerosis
335.21	PROGRESSIVE MUSCULAR ATROPHY		G12.21	Amyotrophic lateral sclerosis
335.22	PROGRESSIVE BULBAR PALSY	➡	G12.22	Progressive bulbar palsy
335.23	PSEUDOBULBAR PALSY		G12.8	Other spinal muscular atrophies and related syndromes
335.24	PRIMARY LATERAL SCLEROSIS		G12.29	Other motor neuron disease
335.29	OTHER MOTOR NEURON DISEASES		G12.2Ø G12.29	Motor neuron disease, unspecified Other motor neuron disease
335.8	OTHER ANTERIOR HORN CELL DISEASES		G12.8	Other spinal muscular atrophies and related syndromes
335.9	UNSPECIFIED ANTERIOR HORN CELL DISEASE		G12.9	Spinal muscular atrophy, unspecified
336.Ø	SYRINGOMYELIA AND SYRINGOBULBIA	➡	G95.Ø	Syringomyelia and syringobulbia
336.1	VASCULAR MYELOPATHIES		G95.11 G95.19	Acute infarction of spinal cord (embolic) (nonembolic) Other vascular myelopathies
336.2	SUBACUTE COMB DEGEN SPINAL CORD DZ CLASS ELSW	➡	G32.Ø	Subac comb degeneration of spinal cord in dis classd elswhr
336.3	MYELOPATHY OTHER DISEASES CLASSIFIED ELSEWHERE		G99.2	Myelopathy in diseases classified elsewhere
336.8	OTHER MYELOPATHY		G95.81 G95.89	Conus medullaris syndrome Other specified diseases of spinal cord
336.9	UNSPECIFIED DISEASE OF SPINAL CORD		G95.2Ø G95.29 G95.9	Unspecified cord compression Other cord compression Disease of spinal cord, unspecified
337.ØØ	IDIOPATHIC PERIPHERAL AUTONOMIC NEUROPATHY UNSP		G9Ø.Ø9	Other idiopathic peripheral autonomic neuropathy

ICD-9-CM		ICD-10-CM	
337.Ø1	CAROTID SINUS SYNDROME	**G9Ø.Ø1**	Carotid sinus syncope
337.Ø9	OTHER IDIOPATHIC PERIPHERAL AUTONOMIC NEUROPATHY	**G9Ø.Ø9**	Other idiopathic peripheral autonomic neuropathy
337.1	PERIPHERAL AUTONOMIC NEUROPATHY D/O CLASS ELSW	➡ **G99.Ø**	Autonomic neuropathy in diseases classified elsewhere
337.2Ø	UNSPECIFIED REFLEX SYMPATHETIC DYSTROPHY	**G9Ø.5Ø** **G9Ø.59**	Complex regional pain syndrome I, unspecified Complex regional pain syndrome I of other specified site
337.21	REFLEX SYMPATHETIC DYSTROPHY OF THE UPPER LIMB	**G9Ø.511** **G9Ø.512** **G9Ø.513** **G9Ø.519**	Complex regional pain syndrome I of right upper limb Complex regional pain syndrome I of left upper limb Complex regional pain syndrome I of upper limb, bilateral Complex regional pain syndrome I of unspecified upper limb
337.22	REFLEX SYMPATHETIC DYSTROPHY OF THE LOWER LIMB	**G9Ø.521** **G9Ø.522** **G9Ø.523** **G9Ø.529**	Complex regional pain syndrome I of right lower limb Complex regional pain syndrome I of left lower limb Complex regional pain syndrome I of lower limb, bilateral Complex regional pain syndrome I of unspecified lower limb
337.29	REFLEX SYMPATHETIC DYSTROPHY OTHER SPEC SITE	**G9Ø.59**	Complex regional pain syndrome I of other specified site
337.3	AUTONOMIC DYSREFLEXIA	➡ **G9Ø.4**	Autonomic dysreflexia
337.9	UNSPECIFIED DISORDER OF AUTONOMIC NERVOUS SYSTEM	**G9Ø.2** **G9Ø.8** **G9Ø.9**	Horner's syndrome Other disorders of autonomic nervous system Disorder of the autonomic nervous system, unspecified
338.Ø	CENTRAL PAIN SYNDROME	➡ **G89.Ø**	Central pain syndrome
338.11	ACUTE PAIN DUE TO TRAUMA	➡ **G89.11**	Acute pain due to trauma
338.12	ACUTE POSTTHORACOTOMY PAIN	➡ **G89.12**	Acute post-thoracotomy pain
338.18	OTHER ACUTE POSTOPERATIVE PAIN	➡ **G89.18**	Other acute postprocedural pain
338.19	OTHER ACUTE PAIN	**R52**	Pain, unspecified
338.21	CHRONIC PAIN DUE TO TRAUMA	➡ **G89.21**	Chronic pain due to trauma
338.22	CHRONIC POSTTHORACOTOMY PAIN	➡ **G89.22**	Chronic post-thoracotomy pain
338.28	OTHER CHRONIC POSTOPERATIVE PAIN	➡ **G89.28**	Other chronic postprocedural pain
338.29	OTHER CHRONIC PAIN	**G89.29**	Other chronic pain
338.3	NEOPLASM RELATED PAIN ACUTE CHRONIC	➡ **G89.3**	Neoplasm related pain (acute) (chronic)
338.4	CHRONIC PAIN SYNDROME	➡ **G89.4**	Chronic pain syndrome
339.ØØ	CLUSTER HEADACHE SYNDROME UNSPECIFIED	**G44.ØØ1** **G44.ØØ9**	Cluster headache syndrome, unspecified, intractable Cluster headache syndrome, unspecified, not intractable
339.Ø1	EPISODIC CLUSTER HEADACHE	**G44.Ø11** **G44.Ø19**	Episodic cluster headache, intractable Episodic cluster headache, not intractable
339.Ø2	CHRONIC CLUSTER HEADACHE	**G44.Ø21** **G44.Ø29**	Chronic cluster headache, intractable Chronic cluster headache, not intractable
339.Ø3	EPISODIC PAROXYSMAL HEMICRANIA	**G44.Ø31** **G44.Ø39**	Episodic paroxysmal hemicrania, intractable Episodic paroxysmal hemicrania, not intractable
339.Ø4	CHRONIC PAROXYSMAL HEMICRANIA	**G44.Ø41** **G44.Ø49**	Chronic paroxysmal hemicrania, intractable Chronic paroxysmal hemicrania, not intractable
339.Ø5	SHORT LASTING UNI NEURALGIFORM HEADACHE CONJ INJ	**G44.Ø51** **G44.Ø59**	Shrt lst unil nerlgif hdache w cnjnct inject/tear, ntrct Shrt lst unil nerlgif hdache w cnjnct inject/tear, not ntrct
339.Ø9	OTHER TRIGEMINAL AUTONOMIC CEPHALGIAS	**G44.Ø91** **G44.Ø99**	Other trigeminal autonomic cephalgias (TAC), intractable Other trigeminal autonomic cephalgias (TAC), not intractable
339.1Ø	TENSION TYPE HEADACHE UNSPECIFIED	**G44.2Ø1** **G44.2Ø9**	Tension-type headache, unspecified, intractable Tension-type headache, unspecified, not intractable
339.11	EPISODIC TENSION TYPE HEADACHE	**G44.211** **G44.219**	Episodic tension-type headache, intractable Episodic tension-type headache, not intractable
339.12	CHRONIC TENSION TYPE HEADACHE	**G44.221** **G44.229**	Chronic tension-type headache, intractable Chronic tension-type headache, not intractable
339.2Ø	POST-TRAUMATIC HEADACHE UNSPECIFIED	**G44.3Ø1** **G44.3Ø9**	Post-traumatic headache, unspecified, intractable Post-traumatic headache, unspecified, not intractable
339.21	ACUTE POST-TRAUMATIC HEADACHE	**G44.311** **G44.319**	Acute post-traumatic headache, intractable Acute post-traumatic headache, not intractable
339.22	CHRONIC POST-TRAUMATIC HEADACHE	**G44.321** **G44.329**	Chronic post-traumatic headache, intractable Chronic post-traumatic headache, not intractable
339.3	DRUG INDUCED HEADACHE NOT ELSEWHERE CLASSIFIED	**G44.4Ø** **G44.41**	Drug-induced headache, NEC, not intractable Drug-induced headache, not elsewhere classified, intractable
339.41	HEMICRANIA CONTINUA	➡ **G44.51**	Hemicrania continua
339.42	NEW DAILY PERSISTENT HEADACHE	➡ **G44.52**	New daily persistent headache (NDPH)
339.43	PRIMARY THUNDERCLAP HEADACHE	➡ **G44.53**	Primary thunderclap headache
339.44	OTHER COMPLICATED HEADACHE SYNDROME	➡ **G44.59**	Other complicated headache syndrome
339.81	HYPNIC HEADACHE	➡ **G44.81**	Hypnic headache
339.82	HEADACHE ASSOCIATED WITH SEXUAL ACTIVITY	➡ **G44.82**	Headache associated with sexual activity
339.83	PRIMARY COUGH HEADACHE	➡ **G44.83**	Primary cough headache
339.84	PRIMARY EXERTIONAL HEADACHE	➡ **G44.84**	Primary exertional headache
339.85	PRIMARY STABBING HEADACHE	➡ **G44.85**	Primary stabbing headache
339.89	OTHER SPECIFIED HEADACHE SYNDROMES	➡ **G44.89**	Other headache syndrome
34Ø	MULTIPLE SCLEROSIS	➡ **G35**	Multiple sclerosis
341.Ø	NEUROMYELITIS OPTICA	➡ **G36.Ø**	Neuromyelitis optica [Devic]
341.1	SCHILDERS DISEASE	**G37.Ø** **G37.5**	Diffuse sclerosis of central nervous system Concentric sclerosis [Balo] of central nervous system

 [Brackets] indicate valid character values for each code. Character value meanings provided for each code grouping.

ICD-9-CM			ICD-10-CM	
341.20	ACUTE TRANSVERSE MYELITIS NOS		**G37.3**	Acute transverse myelitis in demyelinating disease of cnsl
341.21	ACUTE TRANSVERSE MYELITIS CONDS CLASSIFIED ELSW		**G37.3**	Acute transverse myelitis in demyelinating disease of cnsl
341.22	IDIOPATHIC TRANSVERSE MYELITIS		**G37.3**	Acute transverse myelitis in demyelinating disease of cnsl
341.8	OTHER DEMYELINATING DISEASES OF CNTRL NERV SYS		**G36.1** **G36.8** **G37.1** **G37.2** **G37.4** **G37.8**	Acute and subacute hemorrhagic leukoencephalitis [Hurst] Other specified acute disseminated demyelination Central demyelination of corpus callosum Central pontine myelinolysis Subacute necrotizing myelitis of central nervous system Oth demyelinating diseases of central nervous system
341.9	UNSPECIFIED DEMYELINATING DISEASE CNTRL NERV SYS		**G36.9** **G37.9**	Acute disseminated demyelination, unspecified Demyelinating disease of central nervous system, unspecified
342.00	FLACID HEMIPLEGIA AFFECTING UNSPECIFIED SIDE		**G81.00**	Flaccid hemiplegia affecting unspecified side
342.01	FLACID HEMIPLEGIA AFFECTING DOMINANT SIDE		**G81.01** **G81.02**	Flaccid hemiplegia affecting right dominant side Flaccid hemiplegia affecting left dominant side
342.02	FLACID HEMIPLEGIA AFFECTING NONDOMINANT SIDE		**G81.03** **G81.04**	Flaccid hemiplegia affecting right nondominant side Flaccid hemiplegia affecting left nondominant side
342.10	SPASTIC HEMIPLEGIA AFFECTING UNSPECIFIED SIDE		**G81.10**	Spastic hemiplegia affecting unspecified side
342.11	SPASTIC HEMIPLEGIA AFFECTING DOMINANT SIDE		**G81.11** **G81.12**	Spastic hemiplegia affecting right dominant side Spastic hemiplegia affecting left dominant side
342.12	SPASTIC HEMIPLEGIA AFFECTING NONDOMINANT SIDE		**G81.13** **G81.14**	Spastic hemiplegia affecting right nondominant side Spastic hemiplegia affecting left nondominant side
342.80	OTHER SPEC HEMIPLEGIA AFFECTING UNSPEC SIDE		**G81.90**	Hemiplegia, unspecified affecting unspecified side
342.81	OTHER SPEC HEMIPLEGIA AFFECTING DOMINANT SIDE		**G81.91** **G81.92**	Hemiplegia, unspecified affecting right dominant side Hemiplegia, unspecified affecting left dominant side
342.82	OTHER SPEC HEMIPLEGIA AFFECTING NONDOMINANT SIDE		**G81.93** **G81.94**	Hemiplegia, unspecified affecting right nondominant side Hemiplegia, unspecified affecting left nondominant side
342.90	UNSPEC HEMIPLEGIA AFFECTING UNSPEC SIDE		**G81.90**	Hemiplegia, unspecified affecting unspecified side
342.91	UNSPECIFIED HEMIPLEGIA AFFECTING DOMINANT SIDE		**G81.91** **G81.92**	Hemiplegia, unspecified affecting right dominant side Hemiplegia, unspecified affecting left dominant side
342.92	UNSPEC HEMIPLEGIA AFFECTING NONDOMINANT SIDE		**G81.93** **G81.94**	Hemiplegia, unspecified affecting right nondominant side Hemiplegia, unspecified affecting left nondominant side
343.0	DIPLEGIC INFANTILE CEREBRAL PALSY	➡	**G80.1**	Spastic diplegic cerebral palsy
343.1	HEMIPLEGIC INFANTILE CEREBRAL PALSY		**G80.2**	Spastic hemiplegic cerebral palsy
343.2	QUADRIPLEGIC INFANTILE CEREBRAL PALSY	➡	**G80.0**	Spastic quadriplegic cerebral palsy
343.3	MONOPLEGIC INFANTILE CEREBRAL PALSY		**G80.8**	Other cerebral palsy
343.4	INFANTILE HEMIPLEGIA		**G80.2**	Spastic hemiplegic cerebral palsy
343.8	OTHER SPECIFIED INFANTILE CEREBRAL PALSY		**G80.4** **G80.8**	Ataxic cerebral palsy Other cerebral palsy
343.9	UNSPECIFIED INFANTILE CEREBRAL PALSY	➡	**G80.9**	Cerebral palsy, unspecified
344.00	UNSPECIFIED QUADRIPLEGIA		**G82.50**	Quadriplegia, unspecified
344.01	QUADRIPLEGIA AND QUADRIPARESIS C1-C4 COMPLETE	➡	**G82.51**	Quadriplegia, C1-C4 complete
344.02	QUADRIPLEGIA AND QUADRIPARESIS C1-C4 INCOMPLETE	➡	**G82.52**	Quadriplegia, C1-C4 incomplete
344.03	QUADRIPLEGIA AND QUADRIPARESIS C5-C7 COMPLETE	➡	**G82.53**	Quadriplegia, C5-C7 complete
344.04	C5-C7, INCOMPLETE	➡	**G82.54**	Quadriplegia, C5-C7 incomplete
344.09	OTHER QUADRIPLEGIA AND QUADRIPARESIS		**G82.50**	Quadriplegia, unspecified
344.1	PARAPLEGIA		**G04.1** **G82.20** **G82.21** **G82.22**	Tropical spastic paraplegia Paraplegia, unspecified Paraplegia, complete Paraplegia, incomplete
344.2	DIPLEGIA OF UPPER LIMBS	➡	**G83.0**	Diplegia of upper limbs
344.30	MONOPLEGIA LOWER LIMB AFFECTING UNSPECIFIED SIDE		**G83.10**	Monoplegia of lower limb affecting unspecified side
344.31	MONOPLEGIA OF LOWER LIMB AFFECTING DOMINANT SIDE		**G83.11** **G83.12**	Monoplegia of lower limb affecting right dominant side Monoplegia of lower limb affecting left dominant side
344.32	MONOPLEGIA LOWER LIMB AFFECTING NONDOMINANT SIDE		**G83.13** **G83.14**	Monoplegia of lower limb affecting right nondominant side Monoplegia of lower limb affecting left nondominant side
344.40	MONOPLEGIA UPPER LIMB AFFECTING UNSPECIFIED SIDE		**G83.20**	Monoplegia of upper limb affecting unspecified side
344.41	MONOPLEGIA OF UPPER LIMB AFFECTING DOMINANT SIDE		**G83.21** **G83.22**	Monoplegia of upper limb affecting right dominant side Monoplegia of upper limb affecting left dominant side
344.42	MONOPLEGIA UPPER LIMB AFFECTING NONDOMINANT SIDE		**G83.23** **G83.24**	Monoplegia of upper limb affecting right nondominant side Monoplegia of upper limb affecting left nondominant side
344.5	UNSPECIFIED MONOPLEGIA		**G83.30** **G83.31** **G83.32** **G83.33** **G83.34**	Monoplegia, unspecified affecting unspecified side Monoplegia, unspecified affecting right dominant side Monoplegia, unspecified affecting left dominant side Monoplegia, unspecified affecting right nondominant side Monoplegia, unspecified affecting left nondominant side
344.60	CAUDA EQUINA SYND WITHOUT MENTION NEUROGEN BLADD		**G83.4**	Cauda equina syndrome
344.61	CAUDA EQUINA SYNDROME WITH NEUROGENIC BLADDER		**G83.4**	Cauda equina syndrome
344.81	LOCKED-IN STATE	➡	**G83.5**	Locked-in state

ICD-9-CM		ICD-10-CM	
344.89	OTHER SPECIFIED PARALYTIC SYNDROME	**G83.81**	Brown-Sequard syndrome
		G83.82	Anterior cord syndrome
		G83.83	Posterior cord syndrome
		G83.84	Todd's paralysis (postepileptic)
		G83.89	Other specified paralytic syndromes
344.9	UNSPECIFIED PARALYSIS	**G83.9**	Paralytic syndrome, unspecified
345.00	GEN NONCONVUL EPILEPSY W/O INTRACT EPILEPSY	**G40.A01**	Absence epileptic syndrome, not intractable, w stat epi
		G40.A09	Absence epileptic syndrome, not intractable, w/o stat epi
345.01	GEN NONCONVUL EPILEPSY W/INTRACTABLE EPILEPSY	**G40.A11**	Absence epileptic syndrome, intractable, w stat epi
		G40.A19	Absence epileptic syndrome, intractable, w/o stat epi
345.10	GEN CONVUL EPILEPSY W/O MENTION INTRACT EPILEPSY	**G40.309**	Gen idiopathic epilepsy, not intractable, w/o stat epi
		G40.401	Oth generalized epilepsy, not intractable, w stat epi
		G40.409	Oth generalized epilepsy, not intractable, w/o stat epi
345.11	GEN CONVUL EPILEPSY W/INTRACTABLE EPILEPSY	**G40.311**	Generalized idiopathic epilepsy, intractable, w stat epi
		G40.319	Generalized idiopathic epilepsy, intractable, w/o stat epi
		G40.411	Oth generalized epilepsy, intractable, w status epilepticus
		G40.419	Oth generalized epilepsy, intractable, w/o stat epi
345.2	EPILEPTIC PETIT MAL STATUS	**G40.A01**	Absence epileptic syndrome, not intractable, w stat epi
		G40.A09	Absence epileptic syndrome, not intractable, w/o stat epi
		G40.A11	Absence epileptic syndrome, intractable, w stat epi
		G40.A19	Absence epileptic syndrome, intractable, w/o stat epi
345.3	EPILEPTIC GRAND MAL STATUS	**G40.301**	Gen idiopathic epilepsy, not intractable, w stat epi
		G40.311	Generalized idiopathic epilepsy, intractable, w stat epi
		G40.319	Generalized idiopathic epilepsy, intractable, w/o stat epi
345.40	LOC-REL EPILEPSY & ES W/CPS W/O INTRACTABLE EPIL	**G40.201**	Local-rel sympte epi w cmplx prt seiz, not ntrct, w stat epi
		G40.209	Local-rel symptc epi w cmplx prt seiz,not ntrct,w/o stat epi
345.41	LOC-REL EPILEPSY & ES W/CPS W/INTRACTABLE EPIL	**G40.211**	Local-rel symptc epi w cmplx partial seiz, ntrct, w stat epi
		G40.219	Local-rel symptc epi w cmplx part seiz, ntrct, w/o stat epi
345.50	LOC-REL EPILEPSY & ES W/SPS W/O INTRACTABL EPIL	**G40.001**	Local-rel idio epi w seiz of loc onst, not ntrct, w stat epi
		G40.009	Local-rel idio epi w seiz of loc onst,not ntrct,w/o stat epi
		G40.101	Local-rel symptc epi w simp part seiz, not ntrct, w stat epi
		G40.109	Local-rel symptc epi w simp prt seiz,not ntrct, w/o stat epi
345.51	LOC-REL EPILEPSY & ES W/SPS W/INTRACTABLE EPIL	**G40.011**	Local-rel idio epi w seiz of loc onset, ntrct, w stat epi
		G40.019	Local-rel idio epi w seiz of loc onset, ntrct, w/o stat epi
		G40.111	Local-rel symptc epi w simple part seiz, ntrct, w stat epi
		G40.119	Local-rel symptc epi w simple part seiz, ntrct, w/o stat epi
345.60	INFNTILE SPASMS WITHOUT MENTION INTRACT EPILEPSY	**G40.821**	Epileptic spasms, not intractable, with status epilepticus
		G40.822	Epileptic spasms, not intractable, w/o status epilepticus
345.61	INFANTILE SPASMS WITH INTRACTABLE EPILEPSY	**G40.823**	Epileptic spasms, intractable, with status epilepticus
		G40.824	Epileptic spasms, intractable, without status epilepticus
345.70	EPILEPSIA PARTIS CONTINUA W/O INTRACT EPILEPSY	**G40.101**	Local-rel symptc epi w simp part seiz, not ntrct, w stat epi
		G40.109	Local-rel symptc epi w simp prt seiz,not ntrct, w/o stat epi
345.71	EPILEPSIA PARTIALIS CONTINUA W/INTRACT EPILEPSY	**G40.111**	Local-rel symptc epi w simple part seiz, ntrct, w stat epi
		G40.119	Local-rel symptc epi w simple part seiz, ntrct, w/o stat epi
345.80	OTH FORM EPILEPSY & RECUR SEIZUR NO INTRACT EPIL	**G40.101**	Local-rel symptc epi w simp part seiz, not ntrct, w stat epi
		G40.109	Local-rel symptc epi w simp prt seiz,not ntrct, w/o stat epi
		G40.501	Epileptic seiz rel to extrn causes, not ntrct, w stat epi
		G40.509	Epileptic seiz rel to extrn causes, not ntrct, w/o stat epi
		G40.801	Other epilepsy, not intractable, with status epilepticus
		G40.802	Other epilepsy, not intractable, without status epilepticus
		G40.811	Lennox-Gastaut syndrome, not intractable, w stat epi
		G40.812	Lennox-Gastaut syndrome, not intractable, w/o stat epi
		G40.89	Other seizures
		G40.B01	Juvenile myoclonic epilepsy, not intractable, w stat epi
		G40.B09	Juvenile myoclonic epilepsy, not intractable, w/o stat epi
345.81	OTH FORM EPILEPSY & RECUR SEIZUR W/INTRACT EPIL	**G40.111**	Local-rel symptc epi w simple part seiz, ntrct, w stat epi
		G40.119	Local-rel symptc epi w simple part seiz, ntrct, w/o stat epi
		G40.803	Other epilepsy, intractable, with status epilepticus
		G40.804	Other epilepsy, intractable, without status epilepticus
		G40.813	Lennox-Gastaut syndrome, intractable, w status epilepticus
		G40.814	Lennox-Gastaut syndrome, intractable, w/o status epilepticus
		G40.89	Other seizures
		G40.B11	Juvenile myoclonic epilepsy, intractable, w stat epi
		G40.B19	Juvenile myoclonic epilepsy, intractable, w/o stat epi
345.90	UNSPEC EPILEPSY WITHOUT MENTION INTRACT EPILEPSY	**G40.901**	Epilepsy, unsp, not intractable, with status epilepticus
		G40.909	Epilepsy, unsp, not intractable, without status epilepticus
345.91	UNSPECIFIED EPILEPSY WITH INTRACTABLE EPILEPSY	**G40.911**	Epilepsy, unspecified, intractable, with status epilepticus
		G40.919	Epilepsy, unsp, intractable, without status epilepticus
346.00	MIGRAINE W/AURA W/O INTRACT W/O STATUS MIGRNOSUS	➡ **G43.109**	Migraine with aura, not intractable, w/o status migrainosus
346.01	MIGRAINE W/AURA W/INTRACTABLE MIGRAINE W/O SM	➡ **G43.119**	Migraine with aura, intractable, without status migrainosus
346.02	MIGRAINE W/AURA W/O INTRACT W/STATUS MIGRAINOSUS	➡ **G43.101**	Migraine with aura, not intractable, with status migrainosus
346.03	MIGRAINE W/AURA W/INTRACTBL W/STATUS MIGRAINOSUS	➡ **G43.111**	Migraine with aura, intractable, with status migrainosus
346.10	MIGRAINE W/O AURA W/O INTRACT W/O STAT MIGRNOSUS	➡ **G43.009**	Migraine w/o aura, not intractable, w/o status migrainosus
346.11	MIGRAINE W/O AURA INTRACT W/O STATUS MIGRAINOSUS	➡ **G43.019**	Migraine w/o aura, intractable, without status migrainosus
346.12	MIGRAINE W/O AURA W/O INTRACT W/STATUS MIGRNOSUS	➡ **G43.001**	Migraine w/o aura, not intractable, with status migrainosus
346.13	MIGRAINE W/O AURA W/INTRACT W/STATUS MIGRAINOSUS	➡ **G43.011**	Migraine without aura, intractable, with status migrainosus

[Brackets] indicate valid character values for each code. Character value meanings provided for each code grouping.

ICD-9-CM			ICD-10-CM	
346.20	VAR MIGRAINE NEC W/O INTRACT W/O STAT MIGRNOSUS		**G43.809**	Other migraine, not intractable, without status migrainosus
			G43.A0	Cyclical vomiting, not intractable
			G43.B0	Ophthalmoplegic migraine, not intractable
			G43.C0	Periodic headache syndromes in chld/adlt, not intractable
			G43.D0	Abdominal migraine, not intractable
346.21	VARIANTS MIGRAINE NEC INTRACT MIGRAINE W/O SM		**G43.819**	Other migraine, intractable, without status migrainosus
			G43.A1	Cyclical vomiting, intractable
			G43.B1	Ophthalmoplegic migraine, intractable
			G43.C1	Periodic headache syndromes in child or adult, intractable
			G43.D1	Abdominal migraine, intractable
346.22	VAR MIGRAINE NEC W/O INTRACT W/STATUS MIGRNOSUS		**G43.801**	Other migraine, not intractable, with status migrainosus
346.23	VAR MIGRAINE NEC W/INTRACT W/STATUS MIGRAINOSUS		**G43.811**	Other migraine, intractable, with status migrainosus
346.30	HEMI MIGRAINE W/O INTRACT W/O STATUS MIGRAINOSUS	➡	**G43.409**	Hemiplegic migraine, not intractable, w/o status migrainosus
346.31	HEMIPLEGIC MIGRAINE W/INTRACTABLE W/O SM	➡	**G43.419**	Hemiplegic migraine, intractable, without status migrainosus
346.32	HEMI MIGRAINE W/O INTRACTBL W/STATUS MIGRAINOSUS	➡	**G43.401**	Hemiplegic migraine, not intractable, w status migrainosus
346.33	HEMI MIGRAINE W/INTRACTABLE W/STATUS MIGRAINOSUS	➡	**G43.411**	Hemiplegic migraine, intractable, with status migrainosus
346.40	MENST MIGRAINE W/O INTRACT W/O STATUS MIGRNOSUS		**G43.829**	Menstrual migraine, not intractable, w/o status migrainosus
346.41	MENSTRUAL MIGRAINE W/INTRACTABLE W/O SM		**G43.839**	Menstrual migraine, intractable, without status migrainosus
346.42	MENST MIGRAINE W/O INTRACT W/STATUS MIGRAINOSUS		**G43.821**	Menstrual migraine, not intractable, with status migrainosus
346.43	MENST MIGRAINE W/INTRACTBL W/STATUS MIGRAINOSUS		**G43.831**	Menstrual migraine, intractable, with status migrainosus
346.50	PERSIST MIGRAINE AURA W/O CI W/O INTRACT W/O SM	➡	**G43.509**	Perst migrn aura w/o cereb infrc, not ntrct, w/o stat migr
346.51	PMA W/O CI W/INTRACTABLE W/O SM	➡	**G43.519**	Perst migraine aura w/o cerebral infrc, ntrct, w/o stat migr
346.52	PERSISTENT MIGRAINE AURA W/O CI W/O INTRACT W/SM	➡	**G43.501**	Perst migraine aura w/o cereb infrc, not ntrct, w stat migr
346.53	PERSISTENT MIGRAINE AURA W/O CI W/INTRACTBL W/SM	➡	**G43.511**	Perst migraine aura w/o cerebral infrc, ntrct, w stat migr
346.60	PERSISTENT MIGRAINE AURA W/CI W/O INTRACT W/O SM	➡	**G43.609**	Perst migraine aura w cereb infrc, not ntrct, w/o stat migr
346.61	PERSISTENT MIGRAINE AURA W/CI W/INTRACT W/O SM	➡	**G43.619**	Perst migraine aura w cerebral infrc, ntrct, w/o stat migr
346.62	PERSISTENT MIGRAINE AURA W/CI W/O INTRACTBL W/SM	➡	**G43.601**	Perst migraine aura w cerebral infrc, not ntrct, w stat migr
346.63	PERSISTENT MIGRAINE AURA W/CI W/INTRACTABLE W/SM	➡	**G43.611**	Perst migraine aura w cerebral infrc, ntrct, w stat migr
346.70	CHRONIC MIGRAINE W/O AURA W/O INTRACTABLE W/O SM	➡	**G43.709**	Chronic migraine w/o aura, not intractable, w/o stat migr
346.71	CHRONIC MIGRAINE W/O W/INTRACTABLE W/O SM	➡	**G43.719**	Chronic migraine w/o aura, intractable, w/o stat migr
346.72	CHRONIC MIGRAINE W/O AURA W/O INTRACTABLE W/SM	➡	**G43.701**	Chronic migraine w/o aura, not intractable, w stat migr
346.73	CHRONIC MIGRAINE W/O AURA W/INTRACTABLE W/SM	➡	**G43.711**	Chronic migraine w/o aura, intractable, w status migrainosus
346.80	OTH MIGRAINE W/O INTRACT W/O STATUS MIGRAINOSUS		**G43.809**	Other migraine, not intractable, without status migrainosus
346.81	OTH FORMS MIGRAINE INTRACT NO STATUS MIGRAINOSUS		**G43.819**	Other migraine, intractable, without status migrainosus
346.82	OTH MIGRAINE W/O INTRACTABL W/STATUS MIGRAINOSUS		**G43.801**	Other migraine, not intractable, with status migrainosus
346.83	OTH MIGRAINE W/INTRACTABLE W/STATUS MIGRAINOSUS		**G43.811**	Other migraine, intractable, with status migrainosus
346.90	MIGRAINE UNSP W/O INTRACT W/O STATUS MIGRAINOSUS	➡	**G43.909**	Migraine, unsp, not intractable, without status migrainosus
346.91	MIGRAINE UNS W/INTRACTABL W/O STATUS MIGRAINOSUS	➡	**G43.919**	Migraine, unsp, intractable, without status migrainosus
346.92	MIGRAINE UNSP W/O INTRACTBL W/STATUS MIGRAINOSUS	➡	**G43.901**	Migraine, unsp, not intractable, with status migrainosus
346.93	MIGRAINE UNSP W/INTRACTABLE W/STATUS MIGRAINOSUS	➡	**G43.911**	Migraine, unspecified, intractable, with status migrainosus
347.00	NARCOLEPSY WITHOUT CATAPLEXY	➡	**G47.419**	Narcolepsy without cataplexy
347.01	NARCOLEPSY WITH CATAPLEXY	➡	**G47.411**	Narcolepsy with cataplexy
347.10	NARCOLEPSY CONDS CLASS ELSW WITHOUT CATAPLEXY	➡	**G47.429**	Narcolepsy in conditions classified elsewhere w/o cataplexy
347.11	NARCOLEPSY CONDS CLASSIFIED ELSW W/CATAPLEXY	➡	**G47.421**	Narcolepsy in conditions classified elsewhere with cataplexy
348.0	CEREBRAL CYSTS	➡	**G93.0**	Cerebral cysts
348.1	ANOXIC BRAIN DAMAGE	➡	**G93.1**	Anoxic brain damage, not elsewhere classified
348.2	BENIGN INTRACRANIAL HYPERTENSION	➡	**G93.2**	Benign intracranial hypertension
348.30	ENCEPHALOPATHY, UNSPECIFIED	➡	**G93.40**	Encephalopathy, unspecified
348.31	METABOLIC ENCEPHALOPATHY	➡	**G93.41**	Metabolic encephalopathy
348.39	OTHER ENCEPHALOPATHY		**G93.49**	Other encephalopathy
			I67.83	Posterior reversible encephalopathy syndrome
348.4	COMPRESSION OF BRAIN	➡	**G93.5**	Compression of brain
348.5	CEREBRAL EDEMA		**G93.6**	Cerebral edema
		🕮	**S06.1X0A**	Traumatic cerebral edema w/o loss of consciousness, init
		🕮	**S06.1X1A**	Traumatic cerebral edema w LOC of 30 minutes or less, init
		🕮	**S06.1X2A**	Traumatic cerebral edema w LOC of 31-59 min, init
		🕮	**S06.1X3A**	Traumatic cerebral edema w LOC of 1-5 hrs 59 min, init
		🕮	**S06.1X4A**	Traumatic cerebral edema w LOC of 6 hours to 24 hours, init
		🕮	**S06.1X5A**	Traumatic cerebral edema w LOC >24 hr w ret consc lev, init
		🕮	**S06.1X6A**	Traum cerebral edema w LOC >24 hr w/o ret consc w surv, init
		🕮	**S06.1X7A**	Traum cereb edema w LOC w death d/t brain inj bf consc, init
		🕮	**S06.1X8A**	Traum cereb edema w LOC w death d/t oth cause bf consc, init
		🕮	**S06.1X9A**	Traumatic cerebral edema w LOC of unsp duration, init
348.81	TEMPORAL SCLEROSIS	➡	**G93.81**	Temporal sclerosis
348.82	BRAIN DEATH		**G93.82**	Brain death
348.89	OTHER CONDITIONS OF BRAIN		**G93.89**	Other specified disorders of brain
348.9	UNSPECIFIED CONDITION OF BRAIN		**G93.9**	Disorder of brain, unspecified
349.0	REACTION TO SPINAL OR LUMBAR PUNCTURE		**G97.1**	Other reaction to spinal and lumbar puncture
349.1	NERVOUS SYSTEM COMPS FROM SURGICALLY IMPL DEVICE		**G97.82**	Oth postproc complications and disorders of nervous sys

 🕮 See Appendix A ➡ Equivalent Mapping Scenario Scenario

ICD-9-CM		ICD-10-CM	
349.2	DISORDERS OF MENINGES NOT ELSEWHERE CLASSIFIED	**G96.12**	Meningeal adhesions (cerebral) (spinal)
		G96.19	Other disorders of meninges, not elsewhere classified
349.31	ACCIDENTAL PUNCTURE/LACERATION DURA DURING PROC	**G97.41**	Accidental puncture or laceration of dura during a procedure
349.39	OTHER DURAL TEAR	**G96.11**	Dural tear
349.81	CEREBROSPINAL FLUID RHINORRHEA	**G96.0**	Cerebrospinal fluid leak
349.82	TOXIC ENCEPHALOPATHY	**G92**	Toxic encephalopathy
349.89	OTHER SPECIFIED DISORDER OF NERVOUS SYSTEM	**E08.49**	Diabetes due to undrl condition w oth diabetic neuro comp
		E09.49	Drug/chem diabetes w neuro comp w oth diabetic neuro comp
		E10.49	Type 1 diabetes w oth diabetic neurological complication
		E11.49	Type 2 diabetes w oth diabetic neurological complication
		E13.49	Oth diabetes w oth diabetic neurological complication
		G32.89	Oth degeneratv disord of nervous sys in dis classd elswhr
		G96.8	Other specified disorders of central nervous system
		G98.0	Neurogenic arthritis, not elsewhere classified
		G98.8	Other disorders of nervous system
		G99.8	Oth disrd of nervous system in diseases classified elsewhere
349.9	UNSPECIFIED DISORDERS OF NERVOUS SYSTEM	**G96.9**	Disorder of central nervous system, unspecified
		G98.8	Other disorders of nervous system
350.1	TRIGEMINAL NEURALGIA	**G50.0**	Trigeminal neuralgia
350.2	ATYPICAL FACE PAIN	**G50.1**	Atypical facial pain
350.8	OTHER SPECIFIED TRIGEMINAL NERVE DISORDERS	**G50.8**	Other disorders of trigeminal nerve
350.9	UNSPECIFIED TRIGEMINAL NERVE DISORDER	**G50.9**	Disorder of trigeminal nerve, unspecified
351.0	BELLS PALSY	**G51.0**	Bell's palsy
351.1	GENICULATE GANGLIONITIS	**G51.1**	Geniculate ganglionitis
351.8	OTHER FACIAL NERVE DISORDERS	**G51.2**	Melkersson's syndrome
		G51.3	Clonic hemifacial spasm
		G51.4	Facial myokymia
		G51.8	Other disorders of facial nerve
351.9	UNSPECIFIED FACIAL NERVE DISORDER	**G51.9**	Disorder of facial nerve, unspecified
352.0	DISORDERS OF OLFACTORY NERVE	**G52.0**	Disorders of olfactory nerve
352.1	GLOSSOPHARYNGEAL NEURALGIA	**G52.1**	Disorders of glossopharyngeal nerve
352.2	OTHER DISORDERS OF GLOSSOPHARYNGEAL NERVE	**G52.1**	Disorders of glossopharyngeal nerve
352.3	DISORDERS OF PNEUMOGASTRIC NERVE	**G52.2**	Disorders of vagus nerve
352.4	DISORDERS OF ACCESSORY NERVE	**G52.8**	Disorders of other specified cranial nerves
352.5	DISORDERS OF HYPOGLOSSAL NERVE	**G52.3**	Disorders of hypoglossal nerve
352.6	MULTIPLE CRANIAL NERVE PALSIES	**G52.7**	Disorders of multiple cranial nerves
352.9	UNSPECIFIED DISORDER OF CRANIAL NERVES	**G52.9**	Cranial nerve disorder, unspecified
		G53	Cranial nerve disorders in diseases classified elsewhere
353.0	BRACHIAL PLEXUS LESIONS	**G54.0**	Brachial plexus disorders
353.1	LUMBOSACRAL PLEXUS LESIONS	**G54.1**	Lumbosacral plexus disorders
353.2	CERVICAL ROOT LESIONS NOT ELSEWHERE CLASSIFIED	**G54.2**	Cervical root disorders, not elsewhere classified
353.3	THORACIC ROOT LESIONS NOT ELSEWHERE CLASSIFIED	**G54.3**	Thoracic root disorders, not elsewhere classified
353.4	LUMBOSACRAL ROOT LESIONS NEC	**G54.4**	Lumbosacral root disorders, not elsewhere classified
353.5	NEURALGIC AMYOTROPHY	**E08.44**	Diabetes due to underlying condition w diabetic amyotrophy
		E09.44	Drug/chem diabetes w neurological comp w diabetic amyotrophy
		E10.44	Type 1 diabetes mellitus with diabetic amyotrophy
		E11.44	Type 2 diabetes mellitus with diabetic amyotrophy
		E13.44	Other specified diabetes mellitus with diabetic amyotrophy
		G54.5	Neuralgic amyotrophy
353.6	PHANTOM LIMB	**G54.6**	Phantom limb syndrome with pain
		G54.7	Phantom limb syndrome without pain
353.8	OTHER NERVE ROOT AND PLEXUS DISORDERS	**G54.8**	Other nerve root and plexus disorders
		G55	Nerve root and plexus compressions in diseases classd elswhr
353.9	UNSPECIFIED NERVE ROOT AND PLEXUS DISORDER	**G54.9**	Nerve root and plexus disorder, unspecified
354.0	CARPAL TUNNEL SYNDROME	**G56.00**	Carpal tunnel syndrome, unspecified upper limb
		G56.01	Carpal tunnel syndrome, right upper limb
		G56.02	Carpal tunnel syndrome, left upper limb
354.1	OTHER LESION OF MEDIAN NERVE	**G56.10**	Other lesions of median nerve, unspecified upper limb
		G56.11	Other lesions of median nerve, right upper limb
		G56.12	Other lesions of median nerve, left upper limb
354.2	LESION OF ULNAR NERVE	**G56.20**	Lesion of ulnar nerve, unspecified upper limb
		G56.21	Lesion of ulnar nerve, right upper limb
		G56.22	Lesion of ulnar nerve, left upper limb
354.3	LESION OF RADIAL NERVE	**G56.30**	Lesion of radial nerve, unspecified upper limb
		G56.31	Lesion of radial nerve, right upper limb
		G56.32	Lesion of radial nerve, left upper limb
354.4	CAUSALGIA OF UPPER LIMB	**G56.40**	Causalgia of unspecified upper limb
		G56.41	Causalgia of right upper limb
		G56.42	Causalgia of left upper limb
354.5	MONONEURITIS MULTIPLEX	**G58.7**	Mononeuritis multiplex

ICD-9-CM		ICD-10-CM	
354.8	OTHER MONONEURITIS OF UPPER LIMB	**G56.8Ø**	Other specified mononeuropathies of unspecified upper limb
		G56.81	Other specified mononeuropathies of right upper limb
		G56.82	Other specified mononeuropathies of left upper limb
		G58.Ø	Intercostal neuropathy
354.9	UNSPECIFIED MONONEURITIS OF UPPER LIMB	**G56.9Ø**	Unspecified mononeuropathy of unspecified upper limb
		G56.91	Unspecified mononeuropathy of right upper limb
		G56.92	Unspecified mononeuropathy of left upper limb
355.Ø	LESION OF SCIATIC NERVE	**G57.ØØ**	Lesion of sciatic nerve, unspecified lower limb
		G57.Ø1	Lesion of sciatic nerve, right lower limb
		G57.Ø2	Lesion of sciatic nerve, left lower limb
355.1	MERALGIA PARESTHETICA	**G57.1Ø**	Meralgia paresthetica, unspecified lower limb
		G57.11	Meralgia paresthetica, right lower limb
		G57.12	Meralgia paresthetica, left lower limb
355.2	OTHER LESION OF FEMORAL NERVE	**G57.2Ø**	Lesion of femoral nerve, unspecified lower limb
		G57.21	Lesion of femoral nerve, right lower limb
		G57.22	Lesion of femoral nerve, left lower limb
355.3	LESION OF LATERAL POPLITEAL NERVE	**G57.3Ø**	Lesion of lateral popliteal nerve, unspecified lower limb
		G57.31	Lesion of lateral popliteal nerve, right lower limb
		G57.32	Lesion of lateral popliteal nerve, left lower limb
355.4	LESION OF MEDIAL POPLITEAL NERVE	**G57.4Ø**	Lesion of medial popliteal nerve, unspecified lower limb
		G57.41	Lesion of medial popliteal nerve, right lower limb
		G57.42	Lesion of medial popliteal nerve, left lower limb
355.5	TARSAL TUNNEL SYNDROME	**G57.5Ø**	Tarsal tunnel syndrome, unspecified lower limb
		G57.51	Tarsal tunnel syndrome, right lower limb
		G57.52	Tarsal tunnel syndrome, left lower limb
355.6	LESION OF PLANTAR NERVE	**G57.6Ø**	Lesion of plantar nerve, unspecified lower limb
		G57.61	Lesion of plantar nerve, right lower limb
		G57.62	Lesion of plantar nerve, left lower limb
355.71	CAUSALGIA OF LOWER LIMB	**G57.7Ø**	Causalgia of unspecified lower limb
		G57.71	Causalgia of right lower limb
		G57.72	Causalgia of left lower limb
355.79	OTHER MONONEURITIS OF LOWER LIMB	**G57.8Ø**	Other specified mononeuropathies of unspecified lower limb
		G57.81	Other specified mononeuropathies of right lower limb
		G57.82	Other specified mononeuropathies of left lower limb
355.8	UNSPECIFIED MONONEURITIS OF LOWER LIMB	**G57.9Ø**	Unspecified mononeuropathy of unspecified lower limb
		G57.91	Unspecified mononeuropathy of right lower limb
		G57.92	Unspecified mononeuropathy of left lower limb
355.9	MONONEURITIS OF UNSPECIFIED SITE	◘ **EØ8.41**	Diabetes due to undrl condition w diabetic mononeuropathy
		◘ **EØ9.41**	Drug/chem diabetes w neuro comp w diabetic mononeuropathy
		◘ **E1Ø.41**	Type 1 diabetes mellitus with diabetic mononeuropathy
		◘ **E11.41**	Type 2 diabetes mellitus with diabetic mononeuropathy
		◘ **E13.41**	Oth diabetes mellitus with diabetic mononeuropathy
		G58.8	Other specified mononeuropathies
		G58.9	Mononeuropathy, unspecified
		G59	Mononeuropathy in diseases classified elsewhere
356.Ø	HEREDITARY PERIPHERAL NEUROPATHY	**G6Ø.Ø**	Hereditary motor and sensory neuropathy
		G6Ø.2	Neuropathy in association with hereditary ataxia
356.1	PERONEAL MUSCULAR ATROPHY	**G6Ø.Ø**	Hereditary motor and sensory neuropathy
356.2	HEREDITARY SENSORY NEUROPATHY	**G6Ø.Ø**	Hereditary motor and sensory neuropathy
356.3	REFSUMS DISEASE	➡ **G6Ø.1**	Refsum's disease
356.4	IDIOPATHIC PROGRESSIVE POLYNEUROPATHY	➡ **G6Ø.3**	Idiopathic progressive neuropathy
356.8	OTHER SPECIFIED IDIOPATHIC PERIPHERAL NEUROPATHY	**G6Ø.8**	Other hereditary and idiopathic neuropathies
356.9	UNSPEC HEREDIT&IDIOPATHIC PERIPHERAL NEUROPATHY	**G6Ø.9**	Hereditary and idiopathic neuropathy, unspecified
357.Ø	ACUTE INFECTIVE POLYNEURITIS	➡ **G61.Ø**	Guillain-Barre syndrome
357.1	POLYNEUROPATHY IN COLLAGEN VASCULAR DISEASE	**G63**	Polyneuropathy in diseases classified elsewhere
		◘ **MØ5.5Ø**	Rheumatoid polyneurop w rheumatoid arthritis of unsp site
		◘ **MØ5.511**	Rheumatoid polyneurop w rheumatoid arthritis of r shoulder
		◘ **MØ5.512**	Rheumatoid polyneurop w rheumatoid arthritis of l shoulder
		◘ **MØ5.519**	Rheu polyneurop w rheumatoid arthritis of unsp shoulder
		◘ **MØ5.521**	Rheumatoid polyneurop w rheumatoid arthritis of right elbow
		◘ **MØ5.522**	Rheumatoid polyneurop w rheumatoid arthritis of left elbow
		◘ **MØ5.529**	Rheumatoid polyneurop w rheumatoid arthritis of unsp elbow
		◘ **MØ5.531**	Rheumatoid polyneurop w rheumatoid arthritis of right wrist
		◘ **MØ5.532**	Rheumatoid polyneurop w rheumatoid arthritis of left wrist
		◘ **MØ5.539**	Rheumatoid polyneurop w rheumatoid arthritis of unsp wrist
		◘ **MØ5.541**	Rheumatoid polyneurop w rheumatoid arthritis of right hand
		◘ **MØ5.542**	Rheumatoid polyneurop w rheumatoid arthritis of left hand
		◘ **MØ5.549**	Rheumatoid polyneurop w rheumatoid arthritis of unsp hand
		◘ **MØ5.551**	Rheumatoid polyneurop w rheumatoid arthritis of right hip
		◘ **MØ5.552**	Rheumatoid polyneuropathy w rheumatoid arthritis of left hip
		◘ **MØ5.559**	Rheumatoid polyneuropathy w rheumatoid arthritis of unsp hip
		◘ **MØ5.561**	Rheumatoid polyneurop w rheumatoid arthritis of right knee
		◘ **MØ5.562**	Rheumatoid polyneurop w rheumatoid arthritis of left knee
		◘ **MØ5.569**	Rheumatoid polyneurop w rheumatoid arthritis of unsp knee
		◘ **MØ5.571**	Rheumatoid polyneurop w rheumatoid arthritis of right ank/ft
		◘ **MØ5.572**	Rheumatoid polyneurop w rheumatoid arthritis of left ank/ft

(Continued on next page)

ICD-9-CM		ICD-10-CM	
357.1	POLYNEUROPATHY IN COLLAGEN VASCULAR DISEASE (Continued)	M05.579	Rheumatoid polyneurop w rheumatoid arthritis of unsp ank/ft
		M05.59	Rheumatoid polyneuropathy w rheumatoid arthritis mult site
357.2	POLYNEUROPATHY IN DIABETES	E08.40	Diabetes due to underlying condition w diabetic neurop, unsp
		E08.42	Diabetes due to underlying condition w diabetic polyneurop
		E09.40	Drug/chem diabetes w neuro comp w diabetic neuropathy, unsp
		E09.42	Drug/chem diabetes w neurological comp w diabetic polyneurop
		E10.40	Type 1 diabetes mellitus with diabetic neuropathy, unsp
		E10.42	Type 1 diabetes mellitus with diabetic polyneuropathy
		E11.40	Type 2 diabetes mellitus with diabetic neuropathy, unsp
		E11.42	Type 2 diabetes mellitus with diabetic polyneuropathy
		E13.40	Oth diabetes mellitus with diabetic neuropathy, unspecified
		E13.42	Oth diabetes mellitus with diabetic polyneuropathy
357.3	POLYNEUROPATHY IN MALIGNANT DISEASE	G13.0	Paraneoplastic neuromyopathy and neuropathy
		G13.1	Oth systemic atrophy aff cnsl in neoplastic disease
		G63	Polyneuropathy in diseases classified elsewhere
357.4	POLYNEUROPATHY OTHER DISEASES CLASSIFIED ELSW	A52.15	Late syphilitic neuropathy
		G63	Polyneuropathy in diseases classified elsewhere
		G65.0	Sequelae of Guillain-Barre syndrome
		G65.1	Sequelae of other inflammatory polyneuropathy
		G65.2	Sequelae of toxic polyneuropathy
		M34.83	Systemic sclerosis with polyneuropathy
357.5	ALCOHOLIC POLYNEUROPATHY	G62.1	Alcoholic polyneuropathy
357.6	POLYNEUROPATHY DUE TO DRUGS	G62.0	Drug-induced polyneuropathy
357.7	POLYNEUROPATHY DUE TO OTHER TOXIC AGENTS	G61.1	Serum neuropathy
		G62.2	Polyneuropathy due to other toxic agents
		G62.82	Radiation-induced polyneuropathy
357.81	CHRONIC INFLAMMATORY DEMYELINATING POLYNEURITIS	G61.81	Chronic inflammatory demyelinating polyneuritis
357.82	CRITICAL ILLNESS POLYNEUROPATHY	G62.81	Critical illness polyneuropathy
357.89	OTHER INFLAMMATORY AND TOXIC NEUROPATHY	G61.89	Other inflammatory polyneuropathies
		G62.89	Other specified polyneuropathies
		G64	Other disorders of peripheral nervous system
357.9	UNSPECIFIED INFLAMMATORY AND TOXIC NEUROPATHY	G61.9	Inflammatory polyneuropathy, unspecified
		G62.9	Polyneuropathy, unspecified
358.00	MYASTHENIA GRAVIS WITHOUT EXACERBATION	G70.00	Myasthenia gravis without (acute) exacerbation
358.01	MYASTHENIA GRAVIS WITH EXACERBATION	G70.01	Myasthenia gravis with (acute) exacerbation
358.1	MYASTHENIC SYNDROMES DISEASES CLASSIFIED ELSW	G73.3	Myasthenic syndromes in other diseases classified elsewhere
358.2	TOXIC MYONEURAL DISORDERS	G70.1	Toxic myoneural disorders
358.30	LAMBERT-EATON SYNDROME UNSPECIFIED	G70.80	Lambert-Eaton syndrome, unspecified
358.31	LAMBERT-EATON SYNDROME IN NEOPLASTIC DISEASE	G73.1	Lambert-Eaton syndrome in neoplastic disease
358.39	LAMBERT-EATON SYNDROME OTH DISEASES CLASS ELSW	G70.81	Lambert-Eaton syndrome in disease classified elsewhere
358.8	OTHER SPECIFIED MYONEURAL DISORDERS	G70.2	Congenital and developmental myasthenia
		G70.89	Other specified myoneural disorders
358.9	UNSPECIFIED MYONEURAL DISORDERS	G70.9	Myoneural disorder, unspecified
359.0	CONGENITAL HEREDITARY MUSCULAR DYSTROPHY	G71.2	Congenital myopathies
359.1	HEREDITARY PROGRESSIVE MUSCULAR DYSTROPHY	G71.0	Muscular dystrophy
359.21	MYOTONIC MUSCULAR DYSTROPHY	G71.11	Myotonic muscular dystrophy
359.22	MYOTONIA CONGENITA	G71.12	Myotonia congenita
359.23	MYOTONIC CHONDRODYSTROPHY	G71.13	Myotonic chondrodystrophy
359.24	DRUG-INDUCED MYOTONIA	G71.14	Drug induced myotonia
359.29	OTHER SPECIFIED MYOTONIC DISORDER	G71.19	Other specified myotonic disorders
359.3	PERIODIC PARALYSIS	G72.3	Periodic paralysis
359.4	TOXIC MYOPATHY	G72.0	Drug-induced myopathy
		G72.1	Alcoholic myopathy
		G72.2	Myopathy due to other toxic agents
359.5	MYOPATHY ENDOCRINE DISEASES CLASSIFIED ELSEWHERE	G73.7	Myopathy in diseases classified elsewhere
359.6	SYMPTOMATIC INFLAMMATORY MYOPATHY DZ CLASS ELSW	G73.7	Myopathy in diseases classified elsewhere
		M05.40	Rheumatoid myopathy with rheumatoid arthritis of unsp site
		M05.411	Rheumatoid myopathy w rheumatoid arthritis of right shoulder
		M05.412	Rheumatoid myopathy w rheumatoid arthritis of left shoulder
		M05.419	Rheumatoid myopathy w rheumatoid arthritis of unsp shoulder
		M05.421	Rheumatoid myopathy with rheumatoid arthritis of right elbow
		M05.422	Rheumatoid myopathy with rheumatoid arthritis of left elbow
		M05.429	Rheumatoid myopathy with rheumatoid arthritis of unsp elbow
		M05.431	Rheumatoid myopathy with rheumatoid arthritis of right wrist
		M05.432	Rheumatoid myopathy with rheumatoid arthritis of left wrist
		M05.439	Rheumatoid myopathy with rheumatoid arthritis of unsp wrist
		M05.441	Rheumatoid myopathy with rheumatoid arthritis of right hand
		M05.442	Rheumatoid myopathy with rheumatoid arthritis of left hand
		M05.449	Rheumatoid myopathy with rheumatoid arthritis of unsp hand
		M05.451	Rheumatoid myopathy with rheumatoid arthritis of right hip
		M05.452	Rheumatoid myopathy with rheumatoid arthritis of left hip
		M05.459	Rheumatoid myopathy with rheumatoid arthritis of unsp hip
	(Continued on next page)	M05.461	Rheumatoid myopathy with rheumatoid arthritis of right knee

ICD-9-CM		ICD-10-CM		
359.6	SYMPTOMATIC INFLAMMATORY MYOPATHY DZ CLASS ELSW (Continued)	◻	M05.462	Rheumatoid myopathy with rheumatoid arthritis of left knee
		◻	M05.469	Rheumatoid myopathy with rheumatoid arthritis of unsp knee
		◻	M05.471	Rheumatoid myopathy w rheumatoid arthritis of right ank/ft
		◻	M05.472	Rheumatoid myopathy w rheumatoid arthritis of left ank/ft
		◻	M05.479	Rheumatoid myopathy w rheumatoid arthritis of unsp ank/ft
		◻	M05.49	Rheumatoid myopathy w rheumatoid arthritis of multiple sites
		◻	M33.02	Juvenile dermatopolymyositis with myopathy
		◻	M33.12	Other dermatopolymyositis with myopathy
		◻	M33.22	Polymyositis with myopathy
		◻	M33.92	Dermatopolymyositis, unspecified with myopathy
		◻	M34.82	Systemic sclerosis with myopathy
		◻	M35.03	Sicca syndrome with myopathy
359.71	INCLUSION BODY MYOSITIS	➡	G72.41	Inclusion body myositis [IBM]
359.79	OTHER INFLAMMATORY AND IMMUNE MYOPATHIES NEC		G72.49	Oth inflammatory and immune myopathies, NEC
359.81	CRITICAL ILLNESS MYOPATHY	➡	G72.81	Critical illness myopathy
359.89	OTHER MYOPATHIES		G71.3	Mitochondrial myopathy, not elsewhere classified
			G71.8	Other primary disorders of muscles
			G72.89	Other specified myopathies
359.9	UNSPECIFIED MYOPATHY		G71.9	Primary disorder of muscle, unspecified
			G72.9	Myopathy, unspecified
360.00	UNSPECIFIED PURULENT ENDOPHTHALMITIS		H44.001	Unspecified purulent endophthalmitis, right eye
			H44.002	Unspecified purulent endophthalmitis, left eye
			H44.003	Unspecified purulent endophthalmitis, bilateral
			H44.009	Unspecified purulent endophthalmitis, unspecified eye
360.01	ACUTE ENDOPHTHALMITIS		H44.001	Unspecified purulent endophthalmitis, right eye
			H44.002	Unspecified purulent endophthalmitis, left eye
			H44.003	Unspecified purulent endophthalmitis, bilateral
			H44.009	Unspecified purulent endophthalmitis, unspecified eye
360.02	PANOPHTHALMITIS		H44.011	Panophthalmitis (acute), right eye
			H44.012	Panophthalmitis (acute), left eye
			H44.013	Panophthalmitis (acute), bilateral
			H44.019	Panophthalmitis (acute), unspecified eye
360.03	CHRONIC ENDOPHTHALMITIS		H44.001	Unspecified purulent endophthalmitis, right eye
			H44.002	Unspecified purulent endophthalmitis, left eye
			H44.003	Unspecified purulent endophthalmitis, bilateral
			H44.009	Unspecified purulent endophthalmitis, unspecified eye
360.04	VITREOUS ABSCESS		H44.021	Vitreous abscess (chronic), right eye
			H44.022	Vitreous abscess (chronic), left eye
			H44.023	Vitreous abscess (chronic), bilateral
			H44.029	Vitreous abscess (chronic), unspecified eye
360.11	SYMPATHETIC UVEITIS		H44.131	Sympathetic uveitis, right eye
			H44.132	Sympathetic uveitis, left eye
			H44.133	Sympathetic uveitis, bilateral
			H44.139	Sympathetic uveitis, unspecified eye
360.12	PANUVEITIS		H44.111	Panuveitis, right eye
			H44.112	Panuveitis, left eye
			H44.113	Panuveitis, bilateral
			H44.119	Panuveitis, unspecified eye
360.13	PARASITIC ENDOPHTHALMITIS NOS		H21.331	Parastc cyst of iris, ciliary body or ant chamber, right eye
			H21.332	Parastc cyst of iris, ciliary body or ant chamber, left eye
			H21.333	Parasitic cyst of iris, ciliary body or ant chamber, bi
			H21.339	Parastc cyst of iris, ciliary body or ant chamber, unsp eye
			H33.121	Parasitic cyst of retina, right eye
			H33.122	Parasitic cyst of retina, left eye
			H33.123	Parasitic cyst of retina, bilateral
			H33.129	Parasitic cyst of retina, unspecified eye
			H44.121	Parasitic endophthalmitis, unspecified, right eye
			H44.122	Parasitic endophthalmitis, unspecified, left eye
			H44.123	Parasitic endophthalmitis, unspecified, bilateral
			H44.129	Parasitic endophthalmitis, unspecified, unspecified eye
360.14	OPHTHALMIA NODOSA		H16.241	Ophthalmia nodosa, right eye
			H16.242	Ophthalmia nodosa, left eye
			H16.243	Ophthalmia nodosa, bilateral
			H16.249	Ophthalmia nodosa, unspecified eye
360.19	OTHER ENDOPHTHALMITIS	➡	H44.19	Other endophthalmitis
360.20	UNSPECIFIED DEGENERATIVE DISORDER OF GLOBE	➡	H44.30	Unspecified degenerative disorder of globe
360.21	PROGRESSIVE HIGH MYOPIA		H44.20	Degenerative myopia, unspecified eye
			H44.21	Degenerative myopia, right eye
			H44.22	Degenerative myopia, left eye
			H44.23	Degenerative myopia, bilateral
360.23	SIDEROSIS OF GLOBE		H44.321	Siderosis of eye, right eye
			H44.322	Siderosis of eye, left eye
			H44.323	Siderosis of eye, bilateral
			H44.329	Siderosis of eye, unspecified eye
360.24	OTHER METALLOSIS OF GLOBE		H44.311	Chalcosis, right eye
			H44.312	Chalcosis, left eye
			H44.313	Chalcosis, bilateral
			H44.319	Chalcosis, unspecified eye

ICD-9-CM		ICD-10-CM	
360.29	OTHER DEGENERATIVE DISORDERS OF GLOBE	**H44.391**	Other degenerative disorders of globe, right eye
		H44.392	Other degenerative disorders of globe, left eye
		H44.393	Other degenerative disorders of globe, bilateral
		H44.399	Other degenerative disorders of globe, unspecified eye
360.30	UNSPECIFIED HYPOTONY OF EYE	➡ **H44.40**	Unspecified hypotony of eye
360.31	PRIMARY HYPOTONY OF EYE	**H44.441**	Primary hypotony of right eye
		H44.442	Primary hypotony of left eye
		H44.443	Primary hypotony of eye, bilateral
		H44.449	Primary hypotony of unspecified eye
360.32	OCULAR FISTULA CAUSING HYPOTONY	**H44.421**	Hypotony of right eye due to ocular fistula
		H44.422	Hypotony of left eye due to ocular fistula
		H44.423	Hypotony of eye due to ocular fistula, bilateral
		H44.429	Hypotony of unspecified eye due to ocular fistula
360.33	HYPOTONY ASSOCIATED WITH OTHER OCULAR DISORDERS	**H44.431**	Hypotony of eye due to other ocular disorders, right eye
		H44.432	Hypotony of eye due to other ocular disorders, left eye
		H44.433	Hypotony of eye due to other ocular disorders, bilateral
		H44.439	Hypotony of eye due to other ocular disorders, unsp eye
360.34	FLAT ANTERIOR CHAMBER OF EYE	**H44.411**	Flat anterior chamber hypotony of right eye
		H44.412	Flat anterior chamber hypotony of left eye
		H44.413	Flat anterior chamber hypotony of eye, bilateral
		H44.419	Flat anterior chamber hypotony of unspecified eye
360.40	UNSPECIFIED DEGENERATED GLOBE OR EYE	➡ **H44.50**	Unspecified degenerated conditions of globe
360.41	BLIND HYPOTENSIVE EYE	**H44.521**	Atrophy of globe, right eye
		H44.522	Atrophy of globe, left eye
		H44.523	Atrophy of globe, bilateral
		H44.529	Atrophy of globe, unspecified eye
360.42	BLIND HYPERTENSIVE EYE	**H44.511**	Absolute glaucoma, right eye
		H44.512	Absolute glaucoma, left eye
		H44.513	Absolute glaucoma, bilateral
		H44.519	Absolute glaucoma, unspecified eye
360.43	HEMOPHTHALMOS EXCEPT CURRENT INJURY	**H44.811**	Hemophthalmos, right eye
		H44.812	Hemophthalmos, left eye
		H44.813	Hemophthalmos, bilateral
		H44.819	Hemophthalmos, unspecified eye
360.44	LEUCOCORIA	**H44.531**	Leucocoria, right eye
		H44.532	Leucocoria, left eye
		H44.533	Leucocoria, bilateral
		H44.539	Leucocoria, unspecified eye
360.50	RETAINED (OLD) FB MAGNET INTRAOCULR UNSPEC	**H44.601**	Unsp retained (old) intraocular fb, magnetic, right eye
		H44.602	Unsp retained (old) intraocular fb, magnetic, left eye
		H44.603	Unsp retained (old) intraocular fb, magnetic, bilateral
		H44.609	Unsp retained (old) intraocular fb, magnetic, unsp eye
360.51	RETAINED (OLD) FB MAGNETIC, ANT CHAMBER OF EYE	**H44.611**	Retained (old) magnetic fb in ant chamber, right eye
		H44.612	Retained (old) magnetic fb in ant chamber, left eye
		H44.613	Retained (old) magnetic fb in ant chamber, bilateral
		H44.619	Retained (old) magnetic fb in ant chamber, unsp eye
360.52	RETAINED (OLD) FB MAG IN IRIS OR CILIARY BODY	**H44.621**	Retained (old) magnetic fb in iris or ciliary body, r eye
		H44.622	Retained (old) magnetic fb in iris or ciliary body, left eye
		H44.623	Retained (old) magnetic fb in iris or ciliary body, bi
		H44.629	Retained (old) magnetic fb in iris or ciliary body, unsp eye
360.53	RETAINED (OLD) FOREIGN BODY, MAGNETIC, IN LENS	**H44.631**	Retained (old) magnetic foreign body in lens, right eye
		H44.632	Retained (old) magnetic foreign body in lens, left eye
		H44.633	Retained (old) magnetic foreign body in lens, bilateral
		H44.639	Retained (old) magnetic foreign body in lens, unsp eye
360.54	RETAINED (OLD) FB, MAGNETIC, IN VITREOUS	**H44.651**	Retained (old) magnetic fb in vitreous body, right eye
		H44.652	Retained (old) magnetic fb in vitreous body, left eye
		H44.653	Retained (old) magnetic fb in vitreous body, bilateral
		H44.659	Retained (old) magnetic fb in vitreous body, unsp eye
360.55	RETAINED (OLD) FB MAGNETIC IN POSTERIOR WALL	**H44.641**	Retained (old) magnetic fb in post wall of globe, right eye
		H44.642	Retained (old) magnetic fb in post wall of globe, left eye
		H44.643	Retained (old) magnetic fb in posterior wall of globe, bi
		H44.649	Retained (old) magnetic fb in post wall of globe, unsp eye
360.59	RET (OLD) INTRAOC FB MAGNETIC OTH/MULTIPLE SITES	**H44.691**	Retain (old) intraoc fb, magnet, in oth or mult sites, r eye
		H44.692	Retain (old) intraoc fb, magnet, in oth or mult sites, l eye
		H44.693	Retained (old) intraoc fb, magnet, in oth or mult sites, bi
		H44.699	Retain intraoc fb, magnet, in oth or mult sites, unsp eye
360.60	RETAINED (OLD) FB INTRAOCULAR UNSPECIFIED	**H44.701**	Unsp retained (old) intraocular fb, nonmagnetic, right eye
		H44.702	Unsp retained (old) intraocular fb, nonmagnetic, left eye
		H44.703	Unsp retained (old) intraocular fb, nonmagnetic, bilateral
		H44.709	Unsp retained (old) intraocular fb, nonmagnetic, unsp eye
360.61	RETAINED (OLD) FOREIGN BODY IN ANTERIOR CHAMBER	**H44.711**	Retained (old) foreign body in ant chamber, right eye
		H44.712	Retained (old) foreign body in ant chamber, left eye
		H44.713	Retained (old) foreign body in ant chamber, bilateral
		H44.719	Retained (old) foreign body in ant chamber, unsp eye
360.62	RETAINED (OLD) FB IN IRIS OR CILIARY BODY	**H44.721**	Retained (old) fb in iris or ciliary body, right eye
		H44.722	Retained (old) fb in iris or ciliary body, left eye
		H44.723	Retained (old) fb in iris or ciliary body, bilateral
		H44.729	Retained (old) fb in iris or ciliary body, unsp eye

ICD-9-CM		ICD-10-CM		
360.63	RETAINED (OLD) FOREIGN BODY IN LENS		H44.731	Retained (nonmagnetic) (old) foreign body in lens, right eye
			H44.732	Retained (nonmagnetic) (old) foreign body in lens, left eye
			H44.733	Retained (nonmagnetic) (old) foreign body in lens, bilateral
			H44.739	Retained (nonmagnetic) (old) foreign body in lens, unsp eye
360.64	RETAINED (OLD) FOREIGN BODY IN VITREOUS		H44.751	Retained (old) foreign body in vitreous body, right eye
			H44.752	Retained (old) foreign body in vitreous body, left eye
			H44.753	Retained (old) foreign body in vitreous body, bilateral
			H44.759	Retained (old) foreign body in vitreous body, unsp eye
360.65	RETAINED (OLD) FB IN POSTERIOR WALL OF EYE		H44.741	Retained (old) fb in posterior wall of globe, right eye
			H44.742	Retained (old) fb in posterior wall of globe, left eye
			H44.743	Retained (old) fb in posterior wall of globe, bilateral
			H44.749	Retained (old) fb in posterior wall of globe, unsp eye
360.69	RETAINED (OLD) FB IN OTHER OR MULT SITES OF EYE		H44.791	Retain (old) intraoc fb, nonmag, in oth or mult sites, r eye
			H44.792	Retain (old) intraoc fb, nonmag, in oth or mult sites, l eye
			H44.793	Retained (old) intraoc fb, nonmag, in oth or mult sites, bi
			H44.799	Retain intraoc fb, nonmag, in oth or mult sites, unsp eye
360.81	LUXATION OF GLOBE		H44.821	Luxation of globe, right eye
			H44.822	Luxation of globe, left eye
			H44.823	Luxation of globe, bilateral
			H44.829	Luxation of globe, unspecified eye
360.89	OTHER DISORDERS OF GLOBE	➡	H44.89	Other disorders of globe
360.9	UNSPECIFIED DISORDER OF GLOBE	➡	H44.9	Unspecified disorder of globe
361.00	RETINAL DETACHMENT W/RETINAL DEFECT UNSPECIFIED		H33.001	Unspecified retinal detachment with retinal break, right eye
			H33.002	Unspecified retinal detachment with retinal break, left eye
			H33.003	Unspecified retinal detachment with retinal break, bilateral
			H33.009	Unsp retinal detachment with retinal break, unspecified eye
361.01	RECENT RET DETACH PARTIAL W/SINGLE DEFECT		H33.011	Retinal detachment with single break, right eye
			H33.012	Retinal detachment with single break, left eye
			H33.013	Retinal detachment with single break, bilateral
			H33.019	Retinal detachment with single break, unspecified eye
361.02	RECENT RET DETACH PARTIAL W/MULTIPLE DEFECTS		H33.021	Retinal detachment with multiple breaks, right eye
			H33.022	Retinal detachment with multiple breaks, left eye
			H33.023	Retinal detachment with multiple breaks, bilateral
			H33.029	Retinal detachment with multiple breaks, unspecified eye
361.03	RECENT RETINAL DETACHMENT PARTIAL W/GIANT TEAR		H33.031	Retinal detachment with giant retinal tear, right eye
			H33.032	Retinal detachment with giant retinal tear, left eye
			H33.033	Retinal detachment with giant retinal tear, bilateral
			H33.039	Retinal detachment with giant retinal tear, unspecified eye
361.04	RECENT RET DETACH PARTIAL W/RETINAL DIALYSIS		H33.041	Retinal detachment with retinal dialysis, right eye
			H33.042	Retinal detachment with retinal dialysis, left eye
			H33.043	Retinal detachment with retinal dialysis, bilateral
			H33.049	Retinal detachment with retinal dialysis, unspecified eye
361.05	RECENT RETINAL DETACHMENT TOTAL OR SUBTOTAL		H33.051	Total retinal detachment, right eye
			H33.052	Total retinal detachment, left eye
			H33.053	Total retinal detachment, bilateral
			H33.059	Total retinal detachment, unspecified eye
361.06	OLD RETINAL DETACHMENT, PARTIAL		H33.8	Other retinal detachments
361.07	OLD RETINAL DETACHMENT TOTAL OR SUBTOTAL		H33.051	Total retinal detachment, right eye
			H33.052	Total retinal detachment, left eye
			H33.053	Total retinal detachment, bilateral
			H33.059	Total retinal detachment, unspecified eye
361.10	UNSPECIFIED RETINOSCHISIS		H33.101	Unspecified retinoschisis, right eye
			H33.102	Unspecified retinoschisis, left eye
			H33.103	Unspecified retinoschisis, bilateral
			H33.109	Unspecified retinoschisis, unspecified eye
361.11	FLAT RETINOSCHISIS		H33.199	Other retinoschisis and retinal cysts, unspecified eye
361.12	BULLOUS RETINOSCHISIS		H33.199	Other retinoschisis and retinal cysts, unspecified eye
361.13	PRIMARY RETINAL CYSTS		H33.199	Other retinoschisis and retinal cysts, unspecified eye
361.14	SECONDARY RETINAL CYSTS		H33.199	Other retinoschisis and retinal cysts, unspecified eye
361.19	OTHER RETINOSCHISIS AND RETINAL CYSTS		H33.111	Cyst of ora serrata, right eye
			H33.112	Cyst of ora serrata, left eye
			H33.113	Cyst of ora serrata, bilateral
			H33.119	Cyst of ora serrata, unspecified eye
			H33.191	Other retinoschisis and retinal cysts, right eye
			H33.192	Other retinoschisis and retinal cysts, left eye
			H33.193	Other retinoschisis and retinal cysts, bilateral
			H33.199	Other retinoschisis and retinal cysts, unspecified eye
361.2	SEROUS RETINAL DETACHMENT		H33.20	Serous retinal detachment, unspecified eye
			H33.21	Serous retinal detachment, right eye
			H33.22	Serous retinal detachment, left eye
			H33.23	Serous retinal detachment, bilateral
361.30	UNSPECIFIED RETINAL DEFECT		H33.301	Unspecified retinal break, right eye
			H33.302	Unspecified retinal break, left eye
			H33.303	Unspecified retinal break, bilateral
			H33.309	Unspecified retinal break, unspecified eye

ICD-9-CM		ICD-10-CM	
361.31	ROUND HOLE OF RETINA WITHOUT DETACHMENT	**H33.321**	Round hole, right eye
		H33.322	Round hole, left eye
		H33.323	Round hole, bilateral
		H33.329	Round hole, unspecified eye
361.32	HORSESHOE TEAR OF RETINA WITHOUT DETACHMENT	**H33.311**	Horseshoe tear of retina without detachment, right eye
		H33.312	Horseshoe tear of retina without detachment, left eye
		H33.313	Horseshoe tear of retina without detachment, bilateral
		H33.319	Horseshoe tear of retina without detachment, unspecified eye
361.33	MULTIPLE DEFECTS OF RETINA WITHOUT DETACHMENT	**H33.331**	Multiple defects of retina without detachment, right eye
		H33.332	Multiple defects of retina without detachment, left eye
		H33.333	Multiple defects of retina without detachment, bilateral
		H33.339	Multiple defects of retina without detachment, unsp eye
361.81	TRACTION DETACHMENT OF RETINA	**H33.4Ø**	Traction detachment of retina, unspecified eye
		H33.41	Traction detachment of retina, right eye
		H33.42	Traction detachment of retina, left eye
		H33.43	Traction detachment of retina, bilateral
361.89	OTHER FORMS OF RETINAL DETACHMENT	**H33.8**	Other retinal detachments
361.9	UNSPECIFIED RETINAL DETACHMENT	**H33.2Ø**	Serous retinal detachment, unspecified eye
362.Ø1	BACKGROUND DIABETIC RETINOPATHY	**EØ8.311**	Diab due to undrl cond w unsp diabetic rtnop w macular edema
		EØ8.319	Diab due to undrl cond w unsp diab rtnop w/o macular edema
		EØ8.321	Diab d/t undrl cond w mild nonprlf diab rtnop w mclr edema
		EØ8.329	Diab d/t undrl cond w mild nonprlf diab rtnop w/o mclr edema
		EØ8.331	Diab due to undrl cond w mod nonprlf diab rtnop w mclr edema
		EØ8.339	Diab d/t undrl cond w mod nonprlf diab rtnop w/o mclr edema
		EØ8.341	Diab d/t undrl cond w severe nonprlf diab rtnop w mclr edema
		EØ8.349	Diab d/t undrl cond w sev nonprlf diab rtnop w/o mclr edema
		EØ9.311	Drug/chem diabetes w unsp diabetic rtnop w macular edema
		EØ9.319	Drug/chem diabetes w unsp diabetic rtnop w/o macular edema
		EØ9.321	Drug/chem diab w mild nonprlf diabetic rtnop w macular edema
		EØ9.329	Drug/chem diab w mild nonprlf diab rtnop w/o macular edema
		EØ9.331	Drug/chem diab w moderate nonprlf diab rtnop w macular edema
		EØ9.339	Drug/chem diab w mod nonprlf diab rtnop w/o macular edema
		EØ9.341	Drug/chem diab w severe nonprlf diab rtnop w macular edema
		EØ9.349	Drug/chem diab w severe nonprlf diab rtnop w/o macular edema
		E1Ø.311	Type 1 diabetes w unsp diabetic retinopathy w macular edema
		E1Ø.319	Type 1 diabetes w unsp diabetic rtnop w/o macular edema
		E11.311	Type 2 diabetes w unsp diabetic retinopathy w macular edema
		E11.319	Type 2 diabetes w unsp diabetic rtnop w/o macular edema
		E13.311	Oth diabetes w unsp diabetic retinopathy w macular edema
		E13.319	Oth diabetes w unsp diabetic retinopathy w/o macular edema
362.Ø2	PROLIFERATIVE DIABETIC RETINOPATHY	**EØ8.351**	Diab due to undrl cond w prolif diab rtnop w macular edema
		EØ8.359	Diab due to undrl cond w prolif diab rtnop w/o macular edema
		EØ9.351	Drug/chem diabetes w prolif diabetic rtnop w macular edema
		EØ9.359	Drug/chem diabetes w prolif diabetic rtnop w/o macular edema
		E1Ø.351	Type 1 diabetes w prolif diabetic rtnop w macular edema
		E1Ø.359	Type 1 diabetes w prolif diabetic rtnop w/o macular edema
		E11.351	Type 2 diabetes w prolif diabetic rtnop w macular edema
		E11.359	Type 2 diabetes w prolif diabetic rtnop w/o macular edema
		E13.351	Oth diabetes w prolif diabetic retinopathy w macular edema
		E13.359	Oth diabetes w prolif diabetic retinopathy w/o macular edema
362.Ø3	NONPROLIFERATIVE DIABETIC RETINOPATHY NOS	**E11.329**	Type 2 diab w mild nonprlf diabetic rtnop w/o macular edema
362.Ø4	MILD NONPROLIFERATIVE DIABETIC RETINOPATHY	**EØ8.321**	Diab d/t undrl cond w mild nonprlf diab rtnop w mclr edema
		EØ8.329	Diab d/t undrl cond w mild nonprlf diab rtnop w/o mclr edema
		EØ9.321	Drug/chem diab w mild nonprlf diabetic rtnop w macular edema
		EØ9.329	Drug/chem diab w mild nonprlf diab rtnop w/o macular edema
		E1Ø.321	Type 1 diab w mild nonprlf diabetic rtnop w macular edema
		E1Ø.329	Type 1 diab w mild nonprlf diabetic rtnop w/o macular edema
		E11.321	Type 2 diab w mild nonprlf diabetic rtnop w macular edema
		E11.329	Type 2 diab w mild nonprlf diabetic rtnop w/o macular edema
		E13.321	Oth diabetes w mild nonprlf diabetic rtnop w macular edema
		E13.329	Oth diabetes w mild nonprlf diabetic rtnop w/o macular edema
362.Ø5	MODERATE NONPROLIFERATIVE DIABETIC RETINOPATHY	**E1Ø.331**	Type 1 diab w moderate nonprlf diab rtnop w macular edema
		E1Ø.339	Type 1 diab w moderate nonprlf diab rtnop w/o macular edema
		E11.331	Type 2 diab w moderate nonprlf diab rtnop w macular edema
		E11.339	Type 2 diab w moderate nonprlf diab rtnop w/o macular edema
		E13.331	Oth diab w moderate nonprlf diabetic rtnop w macular edema
		E13.339	Oth diab w moderate nonprlf diabetic rtnop w/o macular edema
362.Ø6	SEVERE NONPROLIFERATIVE DIABETIC RETINOPATHY	**E1Ø.341**	Type 1 diab w severe nonprlf diabetic rtnop w macular edema
		E1Ø.349	Type 1 diab w severe nonprlf diab rtnop w/o macular edema
		E11.341	Type 2 diab w severe nonprlf diabetic rtnop w macular edema
		E11.349	Type 2 diab w severe nonprlf diab rtnop w/o macular edema
		E13.341	Oth diabetes w severe nonprlf diabetic rtnop w macular edema
		E13.349	Oth diab w severe nonprlf diabetic rtnop w/o macular edema

ICD-9-CM			ICD-10-CM	
362.07	DIABETIC MACULAR EDEMA	▣	E08.311	Diab due to undrl cond w unsp diabetic rtnop w macular edema
		▣	E08.321	Diab d/t undrl cond w mild nonprlf diab rtnop w mclr edema
		▣	E08.331	Diab due to undrl cond w mod nonprlf diab rtnop w mclr edema
		▣	E08.341	Diab d/t undrl cond w severe nonprlf diab rtnop w mclr edema
		▣	E08.351	Diab due to undrl cond w prolif diab rtnop w macular edema
		▣	E09.311	Drug/chem diabetes w unsp diabetic rtnop w macular edema
		▣	E09.321	Drug/chem diab w mild nonprlf diabetic rtnop w macular edema
		▣	E09.331	Drug/chem diab w moderate nonprlf diab rtnop w macular edema
		▣	E09.341	Drug/chem diab w severe nonprlf diab rtnop w macular edema
		▣	E09.351	Drug/chem diabetes w prolif diabetic rtnop w macular edema
		▣	E10.311	Type 1 diabetes w unsp diabetic retinopathy w macular edema
		▣	E10.321	Type 1 diab w mild nonprlf diabetic rtnop w macular edema
		▣	E10.331	Type 1 diab w moderate nonprlf diab rtnop w macular edema
		▣	E10.341	Type 1 diab w severe nonprlf diabetic rtnop w macular edema
		▣	E10.351	Type 1 diabetes w prolif diabetic rtnop w macular edema
		▣	E11.311	Type 2 diabetes w unsp diabetic retinopathy w macular edema
		▣	E11.321	Type 2 diab w mild nonprlf diabetic rtnop w macular edema
		▣	E11.331	Type 2 diab w moderate nonprlf diab rtnop w macular edema
		▣	E11.341	Type 2 diab w severe nonprlf diabetic rtnop w macular edema
		▣	E11.351	Type 2 diabetes w prolif diabetic rtnop w macular edema
		▣	E13.311	Oth diabetes w unsp diabetic retinopathy w macular edema
		▣	E13.321	Oth diabetes w mild nonprlf diabetic rtnop w macular edema
		▣	E13.331	Oth diab w moderate nonprlf diabetic rtnop w macular edema
		▣	E13.341	Oth diabetes w severe nonprlf diabetic rtnop w macular edema
		▣	E13.351	Oth diabetes w prolif diabetic retinopathy w macular edema
362.10	UNSPECIFIED BACKGROUND RETINOPATHY	➡	H35.00	Unspecified background retinopathy
362.11	HYPERTENSIVE RETINOPATHY		H35.031	Hypertensive retinopathy, right eye
			H35.032	Hypertensive retinopathy, left eye
			H35.033	Hypertensive retinopathy, bilateral
			H35.039	Hypertensive retinopathy, unspecified eye
362.12	EXUDATIVE RETINOPATHY		H35.021	Exudative retinopathy, right eye
			H35.022	Exudative retinopathy, left eye
			H35.023	Exudative retinopathy, bilateral
			H35.029	Exudative retinopathy, unspecified eye
362.13	CHANGES IN VASCULAR APPEARANCE OF RETINA		H35.011	Changes in retinal vascular appearance, right eye
			H35.012	Changes in retinal vascular appearance, left eye
			H35.013	Changes in retinal vascular appearance, bilateral
			H35.019	Changes in retinal vascular appearance, unspecified eye
362.14	RETINAL MICROANEURYSMS NOS		H35.041	Retinal micro-aneurysms, unspecified, right eye
			H35.042	Retinal micro-aneurysms, unspecified, left eye
			H35.043	Retinal micro-aneurysms, unspecified, bilateral
			H35.049	Retinal micro-aneurysms, unspecified, unspecified eye
362.15	RETINAL TELANGIECTASIA		H35.071	Retinal telangiectasis, right eye
			H35.072	Retinal telangiectasis, left eye
			H35.073	Retinal telangiectasis, bilateral
			H35.079	Retinal telangiectasis, unspecified eye
362.16	RETINAL NEOVASCULARIZATION NOS		H35.051	Retinal neovascularization, unspecified, right eye
			H35.052	Retinal neovascularization, unspecified, left eye
			H35.053	Retinal neovascularization, unspecified, bilateral
			H35.059	Retinal neovascularization, unspecified, unspecified eye
362.17	OTHER INTRARETINAL MICROVASCULAR ABNORMALITIES	➡	H35.09	Other intraretinal microvascular abnormalities
362.18	RETINAL VASCULITIS		H35.061	Retinal vasculitis, right eye
			H35.062	Retinal vasculitis, left eye
			H35.063	Retinal vasculitis, bilateral
			H35.069	Retinal vasculitis, unspecified eye
362.20	RETINOPATHY OF PREMATURITY UNSPECIFIED		H35.101	Retinopathy of prematurity, unspecified, right eye
			H35.102	Retinopathy of prematurity, unspecified, left eye
			H35.103	Retinopathy of prematurity, unspecified, bilateral
			H35.109	Retinopathy of prematurity, unspecified, unspecified eye
362.21	RETROLENTAL FIBROPLASIA		H35.171	Retrolental fibroplasia, right eye
			H35.172	Retrolental fibroplasia, left eye
			H35.173	Retrolental fibroplasia, bilateral
			H35.179	Retrolental fibroplasia, unspecified eye
362.22	RETINOPATHY OF PREMATURITY STAGE 0		H35.111	Retinopathy of prematurity, stage 0, right eye
			H35.112	Retinopathy of prematurity, stage 0, left eye
			H35.113	Retinopathy of prematurity, stage 0, bilateral
			H35.119	Retinopathy of prematurity, stage 0, unspecified eye
362.23	RETINOPATHY OF PREMATURITY STAGE 1		H35.121	Retinopathy of prematurity, stage 1, right eye
			H35.122	Retinopathy of prematurity, stage 1, left eye
			H35.123	Retinopathy of prematurity, stage 1, bilateral
			H35.129	Retinopathy of prematurity, stage 1, unspecified eye
362.24	RETINOPATHY OF PREMATURITY STAGE 2		H35.131	Retinopathy of prematurity, stage 2, right eye
			H35.132	Retinopathy of prematurity, stage 2, left eye
			H35.133	Retinopathy of prematurity, stage 2, bilateral
			H35.139	Retinopathy of prematurity, stage 2, unspecified eye

ICD-9-CM		ICD-10-CM	
362.25	RETINOPATHY OF PREMATURITY STAGE 3	**H35.141**	Retinopathy of prematurity, stage 3, right eye
		H35.142	Retinopathy of prematurity, stage 3, left eye
		H35.143	Retinopathy of prematurity, stage 3, bilateral
		H35.149	Retinopathy of prematurity, stage 3, unspecified eye
362.26	RETINOPATHY OF PREMATURITY STAGE 4	**H35.151**	Retinopathy of prematurity, stage 4, right eye
		H35.152	Retinopathy of prematurity, stage 4, left eye
		H35.153	Retinopathy of prematurity, stage 4, bilateral
		H35.159	Retinopathy of prematurity, stage 4, unspecified eye
362.27	RETINOPATHY OF PREMATURITY STAGE 5	**H35.161**	Retinopathy of prematurity, stage 5, right eye
		H35.162	Retinopathy of prematurity, stage 5, left eye
		H35.163	Retinopathy of prematurity, stage 5, bilateral
		H35.169	Retinopathy of prematurity, stage 5, unspecified eye
362.29	OTHER NONDIABETIC PROLIFERATIVE RETINOPATHY	**H35.20**	Other non-diabetic proliferative retinopathy, unsp eye
		H35.21	Other non-diabetic proliferative retinopathy, right eye
		H35.22	Other non-diabetic proliferative retinopathy, left eye
		H35.23	Other non-diabetic proliferative retinopathy, bilateral
362.30	UNSPECIFIED RETINAL VASCULAR OCCLUSION	➡ **H34.9**	Unspecified retinal vascular occlusion
362.31	CENTRAL ARTERY OCCLUSION OF RETINA	**H34.10**	Central retinal artery occlusion, unspecified eye
		H34.11	Central retinal artery occlusion, right eye
		H34.12	Central retinal artery occlusion, left eye
		H34.13	Central retinal artery occlusion, bilateral
362.32	ARTERIAL BRANCH OCCLUSION OF RETINA	**H34.231**	Retinal artery branch occlusion, right eye
		H34.232	Retinal artery branch occlusion, left eye
		H34.233	Retinal artery branch occlusion, bilateral
		H34.239	Retinal artery branch occlusion, unspecified eye
362.33	PARTIAL ARTERIAL OCCLUSION OF RETINA	**H34.211**	Partial retinal artery occlusion, right eye
		H34.212	Partial retinal artery occlusion, left eye
		H34.213	Partial retinal artery occlusion, bilateral
		H34.219	Partial retinal artery occlusion, unspecified eye
362.34	TRANSIENT ARTERIAL OCCLUSION OF RETINA	**G45.3**	Amaurosis fugax
		H34.00	Transient retinal artery occlusion, unspecified eye
		H34.01	Transient retinal artery occlusion, right eye
		H34.02	Transient retinal artery occlusion, left eye
		H34.03	Transient retinal artery occlusion, bilateral
362.35	CENTRAL VEIN OCCLUSION OF RETINA	**H34.811**	Central retinal vein occlusion, right eye
		H34.812	Central retinal vein occlusion, left eye
		H34.813	Central retinal vein occlusion, bilateral
		H34.819	Central retinal vein occlusion, unspecified eye
362.36	VENOUS TRIBUTARY OCCLUSION OF RETINA	**H34.831**	Tributary (branch) retinal vein occlusion, right eye
		H34.832	Tributary (branch) retinal vein occlusion, left eye
		H34.833	Tributary (branch) retinal vein occlusion, bilateral
		H34.839	Tributary (branch) retinal vein occlusion, unspecified eye
362.37	VENOUS ENGORGEMENT OF RETINA	**H34.821**	Venous engorgement, right eye
		H34.822	Venous engorgement, left eye
		H34.823	Venous engorgement, bilateral
		H34.829	Venous engorgement, unspecified eye
362.40	UNSPECIFIED RETINAL LAYER SEPARATION	➡ **H35.70**	Unspecified separation of retinal layers
362.41	CENTRAL SEROUS RETINOPATHY	**H35.711**	Central serous chorioretinopathy, right eye
		H35.712	Central serous chorioretinopathy, left eye
		H35.713	Central serous chorioretinopathy, bilateral
		H35.719	Central serous chorioretinopathy, unspecified eye
362.42	SEROUS DETACHMENT OF RETINAL PIGMENT EPITHELIUM	**H35.721**	Serous detachment of retinal pigment epithelium, right eye
		H35.722	Serous detachment of retinal pigment epithelium, left eye
		H35.723	Serous detachment of retinal pigment epithelium, bilateral
		H35.729	Serous detachment of retinal pigment epithelium, unsp eye
362.43	HEMORRHAGIC DETACHMENT RETINAL PIGMENT EPITHEL	**H35.731**	Hemorrhagic detach of retinal pigment epithelium, right eye
		H35.732	Hemorrhagic detach of retinal pigment epithelium, left eye
		H35.733	Hemorrhagic detach of retinal pigment epithelium, bilateral
		H35.739	Hemorrhagic detach of retinal pigment epithelium, unsp eye
362.50	MACULAR DEGENERATION OF RETINA UNSPECIFIED	➡ **H35.30**	Unspecified macular degeneration
362.51	NONEXUDATIVE SENILE MACULAR DEGENERATION RETINA	➡ **H35.31**	Nonexudative age-related macular degeneration
362.52	EXUDATIVE SENILE MACULAR DEGENERATION OF RETINA	➡ **H35.32**	Exudative age-related macular degeneration
362.53	CYSTOID MACULAR DEGENERATION OF RETINA	**H35.351**	Cystoid macular degeneration, right eye
		H35.352	Cystoid macular degeneration, left eye
		H35.353	Cystoid macular degeneration, bilateral
		H35.359	Cystoid macular degeneration, unspecified eye
362.54	MACULAR CYST HOLE OR PSEUDOHOLE OF RETINA	**H35.341**	Macular cyst, hole, or pseudohole, right eye
		H35.342	Macular cyst, hole, or pseudohole, left eye
		H35.343	Macular cyst, hole, or pseudohole, bilateral
		H35.349	Macular cyst, hole, or pseudohole, unspecified eye
362.55	TOXIC MACULOPATHY OF RETINA	**H35.381**	Toxic maculopathy, right eye
		H35.382	Toxic maculopathy, left eye
		H35.383	Toxic maculopathy, bilateral
		H35.389	Toxic maculopathy, unspecified eye
362.56	MACULAR PUCKERING OF RETINA	**H35.371**	Puckering of macula, right eye
		H35.372	Puckering of macula, left eye
		H35.373	Puckering of macula, bilateral
		H35.379	Puckering of macula, unspecified eye

ICD-9-CM			ICD-10-CM	
362.57	DRUSEN OF RETINA		**H35.361**	Drusen (degenerative) of macula, right eye
			H35.362	Drusen (degenerative) of macula, left eye
			H35.363	Drusen (degenerative) of macula, bilateral
			H35.369	Drusen (degenerative) of macula, unspecified eye
362.6Ø	UNSPECIFIED PERIPHERAL RETINAL DEGENERATION	➡	**H35.4Ø**	Unspecified peripheral retinal degeneration
362.61	PAVING STONE DEGENERATION OF PERIPHERAL RETINA		**H35.431**	Paving stone degeneration of retina, right eye
			H35.432	Paving stone degeneration of retina, left eye
			H35.433	Paving stone degeneration of retina, bilateral
			H35.439	Paving stone degeneration of retina, unspecified eye
362.62	MICROCYSTOID DEGENERATION OF PERIPHERAL RETINA		**H35.421**	Microcystoid degeneration of retina, right eye
			H35.422	Microcystoid degeneration of retina, left eye
			H35.423	Microcystoid degeneration of retina, bilateral
			H35.429	Microcystoid degeneration of retina, unspecified eye
362.63	LATTICE DEGENERATION OF PERIPHERAL RETINA		**H35.411**	Lattice degeneration of retina, right eye
			H35.412	Lattice degeneration of retina, left eye
			H35.413	Lattice degeneration of retina, bilateral
			H35.419	Lattice degeneration of retina, unspecified eye
362.64	SENILE RETICULAR DEGENERATION PERIPHERAL RETINA		**H35.441**	Age-related reticular degeneration of retina, right eye
			H35.442	Age-related reticular degeneration of retina, left eye
			H35.443	Age-related reticular degeneration of retina, bilateral
			H35.449	Age-related reticular degeneration of retina, unsp eye
362.65	SEC PIGMENTARY DEGENERATION OF PERIPHERAL RETINA		**H35.451**	Secondary pigmentary degeneration, right eye
			H35.452	Secondary pigmentary degeneration, left eye
			H35.453	Secondary pigmentary degeneration, bilateral
			H35.459	Secondary pigmentary degeneration, unspecified eye
362.66	SEC VITREORETINAL DEGENS PERIPHERAL RETINA		**H35.461**	Secondary vitreoretinal degeneration, right eye
			H35.462	Secondary vitreoretinal degeneration, left eye
			H35.463	Secondary vitreoretinal degeneration, bilateral
			H35.469	Secondary vitreoretinal degeneration, unspecified eye
362.7Ø	UNSPECIFIED HEREDITARY RETINAL DYSTROPHY	➡	**H35.5Ø**	Unspecified hereditary retinal dystrophy
362.71	RETINAL DYSTROPHY SYS/CEREBRORETINAL LIPIDOSES		**H36**	Retinal disorders in diseases classified elsewhere
362.72	RETINAL DYSTROPHY OTH SYSTEMIC D/O&SYNDROMES		**H36**	Retinal disorders in diseases classified elsewhere
362.73	VITREORETINAL DYSTROPHIES	➡	**H35.51**	Vitreoretinal dystrophy
362.74	PIGMENTARY RETINAL DYSTROPHY	➡	**H35.52**	Pigmentary retinal dystrophy
362.75	OTH DYSTROPHIES PRIMARILY INVLV SENSORY RETINA	➡	**H35.53**	Other dystrophies primarily involving the sensory retina
362.76	DYSTROPHIES PRIM INVLV RETINAL PIGMENT EPITHEL	➡	**H35.54**	Dystrophies primarily w the retinal pigment epithelium
362.77	RETINAL DYSTROPHIES PRIM INVLV BRUCHS MEMBRANE		**H31.1Ø1**	Choroidal degeneration, unspecified, right eye
			H31.1Ø2	Choroidal degeneration, unspecified, left eye
			H31.1Ø3	Choroidal degeneration, unspecified, bilateral
			H31.1Ø9	Choroidal degeneration, unspecified, unspecified eye
			H31.111	Age-related choroidal atrophy, right eye
			H31.112	Age-related choroidal atrophy, left eye
			H31.113	Age-related choroidal atrophy, bilateral
			H31.119	Age-related choroidal atrophy, unspecified eye
			H31.121	Diffuse secondary atrophy of choroid, right eye
			H31.122	Diffuse secondary atrophy of choroid, left eye
			H31.123	Diffuse secondary atrophy of choroid, bilateral
			H31.129	Diffuse secondary atrophy of choroid, unspecified eye
362.81	RETINAL HEMORRHAGE		**H35.6Ø**	Retinal hemorrhage, unspecified eye
			H35.61	Retinal hemorrhage, right eye
			H35.62	Retinal hemorrhage, left eye
			H35.63	Retinal hemorrhage, bilateral
362.82	RETINAL EXUDATES AND DEPOSITS		**H35.89**	Other specified retinal disorders
362.83	RETINAL EDEMA	➡	**H35.81**	Retinal edema
362.84	RETINAL ISCHEMIA	➡	**H35.82**	Retinal ischemia
362.85	RETINAL NERVE FIBER BUNDLE DEFECTS		**H35.89**	Other specified retinal disorders
362.89	OTHER RETINAL DISORDERS		**H35.89**	Other specified retinal disorders
362.9	UNSPECIFIED RETINAL DISORDER	➡	**H35.9**	Unspecified retinal disorder
363.ØØ	UNSPECIFIED FOCAL CHORIORETINITIS		**H3Ø.ØØ1**	Unspecified focal chorioretinal inflammation, right eye
			H3Ø.ØØ2	Unspecified focal chorioretinal inflammation, left eye
			H3Ø.ØØ3	Unspecified focal chorioretinal inflammation, bilateral
			H3Ø.ØØ9	Unsp focal chorioretinal inflammation, unspecified eye
363.Ø1	FOCAL CHOROIDITIS&CHORIORETINITIS JUXTAPAPILLARY		**H3Ø.Ø11**	Focal chorioretinal inflammation, juxtapapillary, right eye
			H3Ø.Ø12	Focal chorioretinal inflammation, juxtapapillary, left eye
			H3Ø.Ø13	Focal chorioretinal inflammation, juxtapapillary, bilateral
			H3Ø.Ø19	Focal chorioretinal inflammation, juxtapapillary, unsp eye
363.Ø3	FOCAL CHOROIDITIS&CHORIORETINITIS OTH POST POLE		**H3Ø.Ø21**	Focal chorioretin inflammation of posterior pole, right eye
			H3Ø.Ø22	Focal chorioretinal inflammation of posterior pole, left eye
			H3Ø.Ø23	Focal chorioretin inflammation of posterior pole, bilateral
			H3Ø.Ø29	Focal chorioretinal inflammation of posterior pole, unsp eye
363.Ø4	FOCAL CHOROIDITIS AND CHORIORETINITIS PERIPHERAL		**H3Ø.Ø31**	Focal chorioretinal inflammation, peripheral, right eye
			H3Ø.Ø32	Focal chorioretinal inflammation, peripheral, left eye
			H3Ø.Ø33	Focal chorioretinal inflammation, peripheral, bilateral
			H3Ø.Ø39	Focal chorioretinal inflammation, peripheral, unsp eye

ICD-9-CM		ICD-10-CM	
363.Ø5	FOCAL RETINITIS&RETINOCHOROIDITIS JUXTAPAPILLARY	**H3Ø.Ø11**	Focal chorioretinal inflammation, juxtapapillary, right eye
		H3Ø.Ø12	Focal chorioretinal inflammation, juxtapapillary, left eye
		H3Ø.Ø13	Focal chorioretinal inflammation, juxtapapillary, bilateral
		H3Ø.Ø19	Focal chorioretinal inflammation, juxtapapillary, unsp eye
363.Ø6	FOCAL RETINIT&RETINOCHOROID MACULAR/PARAMACULAR	**H3Ø.Ø41**	Focal chorioretin inflam, macular or paramacular, right eye
		H3Ø.Ø42	Focal chorioretin inflam, macular or paramacular, left eye
		H3Ø.Ø43	Focal chorioretin inflam, macular or paramacular, bilateral
		H3Ø.Ø49	Focal chorioretin inflam, macular or paramacular, unsp eye
363.Ø7	FOCAL RETINITIS&RETINOCHOROIDITIS OTH POST POLE	**H3Ø.Ø21**	Focal chorioretin inflammation of posterior pole, right eye
		H3Ø.Ø22	Focal chorioretinal inflammation of posterior pole, left eye
		H3Ø.Ø23	Focal chorioretin inflammation of posterior pole, bilateral
		H3Ø.Ø29	Focal chorioretinal inflammation of posterior pole, unsp eye
363.Ø8	FOCAL RETINITIS AND RETINOCHOROIDITIS PERIPHERAL	**H3Ø.Ø31**	Focal chorioretinal inflammation, peripheral, right eye
		H3Ø.Ø32	Focal chorioretinal inflammation, peripheral, left eye
		H3Ø.Ø33	Focal chorioretinal inflammation, peripheral, bilateral
		H3Ø.Ø39	Focal chorioretinal inflammation, peripheral, unsp eye
363.1Ø	UNSPECIFIED DISSEMINATED CHORIORETINITIS	**H3Ø.1Ø1**	Unsp disseminated chorioretinal inflammation, right eye
		H3Ø.1Ø2	Unsp disseminated chorioretinal inflammation, left eye
		H3Ø.1Ø3	Unsp disseminated chorioretinal inflammation, bilateral
		H3Ø.1Ø9	Unsp disseminated chorioretinal inflammation, unsp eye
363.11	DISSEMIN CHOROIDITIS&CHORIORETINITIS POST POLE	**H3Ø.111**	Dissem chorioretin inflammation of posterior pole, right eye
		H3Ø.112	Dissem chorioretin inflammation of posterior pole, left eye
		H3Ø.113	Dissem chorioretin inflammation of posterior pole, bilateral
		H3Ø.119	Dissem chorioretin inflammation of posterior pole, unsp eye
363.12	DISSEMIN CHOROIDITIS&CHORIORETINITIS PERIPHERAL	**H3Ø.121**	Disseminated chorioretin inflammation, peripheral right eye
		H3Ø.122	Disseminated chorioretin inflammation, peripheral, left eye
		H3Ø.123	Disseminated chorioretin inflammation, peripheral, bilateral
		H3Ø.129	Disseminated chorioretin inflammation, peripheral, unsp eye
363.13	DISSEMIN CHOROIDITIS&CHORIORETINITIS GENERALIZED	**A18.53**	Tuberculous chorioretinitis
		H3Ø.131	Dissem chorioretin inflammation, generalized, right eye
		H3Ø.132	Disseminated chorioretin inflammation, generalized, left eye
		H3Ø.133	Dissem chorioretin inflammation, generalized, bilateral
		H3Ø.139	Disseminated chorioretin inflammation, generalized, unsp eye
363.14	DISSEMIN RETINITIS&RETINOCHOROIDITIS METASTATIC	**H3Ø.1Ø1**	Unsp disseminated chorioretinal inflammation, right eye
		H3Ø.1Ø2	Unsp disseminated chorioretinal inflammation, left eye
		H3Ø.1Ø3	Unsp disseminated chorioretinal inflammation, bilateral
		H3Ø.1Ø9	Unsp disseminated chorioretinal inflammation, unsp eye
363.15	DISSEMIN RETINIT&RETINOCHOROID PIG EPITHLIPATH	**H3Ø.141**	Acute post multifoc placoid pigment epitheliopathy, r eye
		H3Ø.142	Acute post multifoc placoid pigment epitheliopathy, left eye
		H3Ø.143	Acute posterior multifoc placoid pigment epitheliopathy, bi
		H3Ø.149	Acute post multifoc placoid pigment epitheliopathy, unsp eye
363.2Ø	UNSPECIFIED CHORIORETINITIS	**H3Ø.891**	Other chorioretinal inflammations, right eye
		H3Ø.892	Other chorioretinal inflammations, left eye
		H3Ø.893	Other chorioretinal inflammations, bilateral
		H3Ø.899	Other chorioretinal inflammations, unspecified eye
		H3Ø.9Ø	Unspecified chorioretinal inflammation, unspecified eye
		H3Ø.91	Unspecified chorioretinal inflammation, right eye
		H3Ø.92	Unspecified chorioretinal inflammation, left eye
		H3Ø.93	Unspecified chorioretinal inflammation, bilateral
363.21	PARS PLANITIS	**H3Ø.2Ø**	Posterior cyclitis, unspecified eye
		H3Ø.21	Posterior cyclitis, right eye
		H3Ø.22	Posterior cyclitis, left eye
		H3Ø.23	Posterior cyclitis, bilateral
363.22	HARADAS DISEASE	**H3Ø.811**	Harada's disease, right eye
		H3Ø.812	Harada's disease, left eye
		H3Ø.813	Harada's disease, bilateral
		H3Ø.819	Harada's disease, unspecified eye
363.3Ø	UNSPECIFIED CHORIORETINAL SCAR	**H31.ØØ1**	Unspecified chorioretinal scars, right eye
		H31.ØØ2	Unspecified chorioretinal scars, left eye
		H31.ØØ3	Unspecified chorioretinal scars, bilateral
		H31.ØØ9	Unspecified chorioretinal scars, unspecified eye
363.31	SOLAR RETINOPATHY	**H31.Ø21**	Solar retinopathy, right eye
		H31.Ø22	Solar retinopathy, left eye
		H31.Ø23	Solar retinopathy, bilateral
		H31.Ø29	Solar retinopathy, unspecified eye
363.32	OTH MACULAR CHORIORETINAL SCARS	**H31.Ø11**	Macula scars of posterior pole (post-traumatic), right eye
		H31.Ø12	Macula scars of posterior pole (post-traumatic), left eye
		H31.Ø13	Macula scars of posterior pole (post-traumatic), bilateral
		H31.Ø19	Macula scars of posterior pole (post-traumatic), unsp eye
363.33	OTHER CHORIORETINAL SCARS POSTERIOR POLE	**H31.Ø11**	Macula scars of posterior pole (post-traumatic), right eye
		H31.Ø12	Macula scars of posterior pole (post-traumatic), left eye
		H31.Ø13	Macula scars of posterior pole (post-traumatic), bilateral
		H31.Ø19	Macula scars of posterior pole (post-traumatic), unsp eye
363.34	PERIPH CHORIORETINAL SCARS	**H31.Ø91**	Other chorioretinal scars, right eye
		H31.Ø92	Other chorioretinal scars, left eye
		H31.Ø93	Other chorioretinal scars, bilateral
		H31.Ø99	Other chorioretinal scars, unspecified eye

[Brackets] indicate valid character values for each code. Character value meanings provided for each code grouping.

ICD-9-CM			ICD-10-CM	
363.35	DISSEMIN CHORIORETINAL SCARS		H31.091	Other chorioretinal scars, right eye
			H31.092	Other chorioretinal scars, left eye
			H31.093	Other chorioretinal scars, bilateral
			H31.099	Other chorioretinal scars, unspecified eye
363.40	UNSPECIFIED CHOROIDAL DEGENERATION		H31.101	Choroidal degeneration, unspecified, right eye
			H31.102	Choroidal degeneration, unspecified, left eye
			H31.103	Choroidal degeneration, unspecified, bilateral
			H31.109	Choroidal degeneration, unspecified, unspecified eye
363.41	SENILE ATROPHY OF CHOROID		H31.111	Age-related choroidal atrophy, right eye
			H31.112	Age-related choroidal atrophy, left eye
			H31.113	Age-related choroidal atrophy, bilateral
			H31.119	Age-related choroidal atrophy, unspecified eye
363.42	DIFFUSE SECONDARY ATROPHY OF CHOROID		H31.121	Diffuse secondary atrophy of choroid, right eye
			H31.122	Diffuse secondary atrophy of choroid, left eye
			H31.123	Diffuse secondary atrophy of choroid, bilateral
			H31.129	Diffuse secondary atrophy of choroid, unspecified eye
363.43	ANGIOID STREAKS OF CHOROID	➡	H35.33	Angioid streaks of macula
363.50	UNSPEC HEREDITARY CHOROIDAL DYSTROPHY/ATROPHY	➡	H31.20	Hereditary choroidal dystrophy, unspecified
363.51	CIRCUMPAPILLARY DYSTROPHY OF CHOROID PARTIAL		H31.29	Other hereditary choroidal dystrophy
363.52	CIRCUMPAPILLARY DYSTROPHY OF CHOROID TOTAL		H31.29	Other hereditary choroidal dystrophy
363.53	CENTRAL DYSTROPHY OF CHOROID PARTIAL		H31.22	Choroidal dystrophy (central areolar) (peripapillary)
363.54	CENTRAL CHOROIDAL ATROPHY, TOTAL		H31.22	Choroidal dystrophy (central areolar) (peripapillary)
363.55	CHOROIDEREMIA	➡	H31.21	Choroideremia
363.56	OTH DIFFUSE/GEN DYSTROPHY CHOROID PARTIAL		H31.29	Other hereditary choroidal dystrophy
363.57	OTH DIFFUSE/GENERALIZED DYSTROPHY CHOROID TOTAL	➡	H31.23	Gyrate atrophy, choroid
363.61	UNSPECIFIED CHOROIDAL HEMORRHAGE		H31.301	Unspecified choroidal hemorrhage, right eye
			H31.302	Unspecified choroidal hemorrhage, left eye
			H31.303	Unspecified choroidal hemorrhage, bilateral
			H31.309	Unspecified choroidal hemorrhage, unspecified eye
363.62	EXPULSIVE CHOROIDAL HEMORRHAGE		H31.311	Expulsive choroidal hemorrhage, right eye
			H31.312	Expulsive choroidal hemorrhage, left eye
			H31.313	Expulsive choroidal hemorrhage, bilateral
			H31.319	Expulsive choroidal hemorrhage, unspecified eye
363.63	CHOROIDAL RUPTURE		H31.321	Choroidal rupture, right eye
			H31.322	Choroidal rupture, left eye
			H31.323	Choroidal rupture, bilateral
			H31.329	Choroidal rupture, unspecified eye
363.70	UNSPECIFIED CHOROIDAL DETACHMENT		H31.401	Unspecified choroidal detachment, right eye
			H31.402	Unspecified choroidal detachment, left eye
			H31.403	Unspecified choroidal detachment, bilateral
			H31.409	Unspecified choroidal detachment, unspecified eye
363.71	SEROUS CHOROIDAL DETACHMENT		H31.421	Serous choroidal detachment, right eye
			H31.422	Serous choroidal detachment, left eye
			H31.423	Serous choroidal detachment, bilateral
			H31.429	Serous choroidal detachment, unspecified eye
363.72	HEMORRHAGIC CHOROIDAL DETACHMENT		H31.411	Hemorrhagic choroidal detachment, right eye
			H31.412	Hemorrhagic choroidal detachment, left eye
			H31.413	Hemorrhagic choroidal detachment, bilateral
			H31.419	Hemorrhagic choroidal detachment, unspecified eye
363.8	OTHER DISORDERS OF CHOROID		H31.8	Other specified disorders of choroid
			H32	Chorioretinal disorders in diseases classified elsewhere
363.9	UNSPECIFIED DISORDER OF CHOROID	➡	H31.9	Unspecified disorder of choroid
364.00	UNSPECIFIED ACUTE AND SUBACUTE IRIDOCYCLITIS	➡	H20.00	Unspecified acute and subacute iridocyclitis
364.01	PRIMARY IRIDOCYCLITIS		H20.011	Primary iridocyclitis, right eye
			H20.012	Primary iridocyclitis, left eye
			H20.013	Primary iridocyclitis, bilateral
			H20.019	Primary iridocyclitis, unspecified eye
364.02	RECURRENT IRIDOCYCLITIS		H20.021	Recurrent acute iridocyclitis, right eye
			H20.022	Recurrent acute iridocyclitis, left eye
			H20.023	Recurrent acute iridocyclitis, bilateral
			H20.029	Recurrent acute iridocyclitis, unspecified eye
364.03	SECONDARY IRIDOCYCLITIS, INFECTIOUS		H20.031	Secondary infectious iridocyclitis, right eye
			H20.032	Secondary infectious iridocyclitis, left eye
			H20.033	Secondary infectious iridocyclitis, bilateral
			H20.039	Secondary infectious iridocyclitis, unspecified eye
364.04	SECONDARY IRIDOCYCLITIS NONINFECTIOUS		H20.041	Secondary noninfectious iridocyclitis, right eye
			H20.042	Secondary noninfectious iridocyclitis, left eye
			H20.043	Secondary noninfectious iridocyclitis, bilateral
			H20.049	Secondary noninfectious iridocyclitis, unspecified eye
364.05	HYPOPYON		H20.051	Hypopyon, right eye
			H20.052	Hypopyon, left eye
			H20.053	Hypopyon, bilateral
			H20.059	Hypopyon, unspecified eye

ICD-9-CM		ICD-10-CM	
364.10	UNSPECIFIED CHRONIC IRIDOCYCLITIS	H20.10	Chronic iridocyclitis, unspecified eye
		H20.11	Chronic iridocyclitis, right eye
		H20.12	Chronic iridocyclitis, left eye
		H20.13	Chronic iridocyclitis, bilateral
364.11	CHRONIC IRIDOCYCLITIS DISEASES CLASSIFIED ELSW	A18.54	Tuberculous iridocyclitis
		H20.9	Unspecified iridocyclitis
364.21	FUCHS HETEROCHROMIC CYCLITIS	H20.811	Fuchs' heterochromic cyclitis, right eye
		H20.812	Fuchs' heterochromic cyclitis, left eye
		H20.813	Fuchs' heterochromic cyclitis, bilateral
		H20.819	Fuchs' heterochromic cyclitis, unspecified eye
364.22	GLAUCOMATOCYCLITIC CRISES	H40.40X0	Glaucoma secondary to eye inflammation, unsp eye, stage unsp
364.23	LENS-INDUCED IRIDOCYCLITIS	H20.20	Lens-induced iridocyclitis, unspecified eye
		H20.21	Lens-induced iridocyclitis, right eye
		H20.22	Lens-induced iridocyclitis, left eye
		H20.23	Lens-induced iridocyclitis, bilateral
364.24	VOGT-KOYANAGI SYNDROME	H20.821	Vogt-Koyanagi syndrome, right eye
		H20.822	Vogt-Koyanagi syndrome, left eye
		H20.823	Vogt-Koyanagi syndrome, bilateral
		H20.829	Vogt-Koyanagi syndrome, unspecified eye
364.3	UNSPECIFIED IRIDOCYCLITIS	H20.9	Unspecified iridocyclitis
364.41	HYPHEMA	H21.00	Hyphema, unspecified eye
		H21.01	Hyphema, right eye
		H21.02	Hyphema, left eye
		H21.03	Hyphema, bilateral
364.42	RUBEOSIS IRIDIS	H21.1X1	Other vascular disorders of iris and ciliary body, right eye
		H21.1X2	Other vascular disorders of iris and ciliary body, left eye
		H21.1X3	Other vascular disorders of iris and ciliary body, bilateral
		H21.1X9	Other vascular disorders of iris and ciliary body, unsp eye
364.51	ESSENTIAL OR PROGRESSIVE IRIS ATROPHY	H21.261	Iris atrophy (essential) (progressive), right eye
		H21.262	Iris atrophy (essential) (progressive), left eye
		H21.263	Iris atrophy (essential) (progressive), bilateral
		H21.269	Iris atrophy (essential) (progressive), unspecified eye
364.52	IRIDOSCHISIS	H21.251	Iridoschisis, right eye
		H21.252	Iridoschisis, left eye
		H21.253	Iridoschisis, bilateral
		H21.259	Iridoschisis, unspecified eye
364.53	PIGMENTARY IRIS DEGENERATION	H21.231	Degeneration of iris (pigmentary), right eye
		H21.232	Degeneration of iris (pigmentary), left eye
		H21.233	Degeneration of iris (pigmentary), bilateral
		H21.239	Degeneration of iris (pigmentary), unspecified eye
364.54	DEGENERATION OF PUPILLARY MARGIN	H21.241	Degeneration of pupillary margin, right eye
		H21.242	Degeneration of pupillary margin, left eye
		H21.243	Degeneration of pupillary margin, bilateral
		H21.249	Degeneration of pupillary margin, unspecified eye
364.55	MIOTIC CYSTS OF PUPILLARY MARGIN	H21.271	Miotic pupillary cyst, right eye
		H21.272	Miotic pupillary cyst, left eye
		H21.273	Miotic pupillary cyst, bilateral
		H21.279	Miotic pupillary cyst, unspecified eye
364.56	DEGENERATIVE CHANGES OF CHAMBER ANGLE	H21.211	Degeneration of chamber angle, right eye
		H21.212	Degeneration of chamber angle, left eye
		H21.213	Degeneration of chamber angle, bilateral
		H21.219	Degeneration of chamber angle, unspecified eye
364.57	DEGENERATIVE CHANGES OF CILIARY BODY	H21.221	Degeneration of ciliary body, right eye
		H21.222	Degeneration of ciliary body, left eye
		H21.223	Degeneration of ciliary body, bilateral
		H21.229	Degeneration of ciliary body, unspecified eye
364.59	OTHER IRIS ATROPHY	H21.29	Other iris atrophy
364.60	IDIOPATHIC CYSTS IRIS CILIARY BODY&ANT CHAMBER	H21.301	Idio cysts of iris, ciliary body or ant chamber, right eye
		H21.302	Idio cysts of iris, ciliary body or ant chamber, left eye
		H21.303	Idio cysts of iris, ciliary body or ant chamber, bilateral
		H21.309	Idio cysts of iris, ciliary body or ant chamber, unsp eye
364.61	IMPLANTATION CYSTS IRIS CILIARY BODY&ANT CHAMBER	H21.321	Implant cysts of iris, ciliary body or ant chamber, r eye
		H21.322	Implant cysts of iris, ciliary body or ant chamber, left eye
		H21.323	Implant cysts of iris, ciliary body or ant chamber, bi
		H21.329	Implant cysts of iris, ciliary body or ant chamber, unsp eye
364.62	EXUDATIVE CYSTS OF IRIS OR ANTERIOR CHAMBER	H21.311	Exudative cysts of iris or anterior chamber, right eye
		H21.312	Exudative cysts of iris or anterior chamber, left eye
		H21.313	Exudative cysts of iris or anterior chamber, bilateral
		H21.319	Exudative cysts of iris or anterior chamber, unspecified eye
364.63	PRIMARY CYST OF PARS PLANA	H21.341	Primary cyst of pars plana, right eye
		H21.342	Primary cyst of pars plana, left eye
		H21.343	Primary cyst of pars plana, bilateral
		H21.349	Primary cyst of pars plana, unspecified eye
364.64	EXUDATIVE CYST OF PARS PLANA	H21.351	Exudative cyst of pars plana, right eye
		H21.352	Exudative cyst of pars plana, left eye
		H21.353	Exudative cyst of pars plana, bilateral
		H21.359	Exudative cyst of pars plana, unspecified eye

ICD-9-CM		ICD-10-CM	
364.70	UNSPECIFIED ADHESIONS OF IRIS	**H21.501**	Unspecified adhesions of iris, right eye
		H21.502	Unspecified adhesions of iris, left eye
		H21.503	Unspecified adhesions of iris, bilateral
		H21.509	Unsp adhesions of iris and ciliary body, unspecified eye
364.71	POSTERIOR SYNECHIAE	**H21.541**	Posterior synechiae (iris), right eye
		H21.542	Posterior synechiae (iris), left eye
		H21.543	Posterior synechiae (iris), bilateral
		H21.549	Posterior synechiae (iris), unspecified eye
364.72	ANTERIOR SYNECHIAE	**H21.511**	Anterior synechiae (iris), right eye
		H21.512	Anterior synechiae (iris), left eye
		H21.513	Anterior synechiae (iris), bilateral
		H21.519	Anterior synechiae (iris), unspecified eye
364.73	GONIOSYNECHIAE	**H21.521**	Goniosynechiae, right eye
		H21.522	Goniosynechiae, left eye
		H21.523	Goniosynechiae, bilateral
		H21.529	Goniosynechiae, unspecified eye
364.74	ADHESIONS AND DISRUPTIONS OF PUPILLARY MEMBRANES	**H21.40**	Pupillary membranes, unspecified eye
		H21.41	Pupillary membranes, right eye
		H21.42	Pupillary membranes, left eye
		H21.43	Pupillary membranes, bilateral
364.75	PUPILLARY ABNORMALITIES	**H21.561**	Pupillary abnormality, right eye
		H21.562	Pupillary abnormality, left eye
		H21.563	Pupillary abnormality, bilateral
		H21.569	Pupillary abnormality, unspecified eye
364.76	IRIDODIALYSIS	**H21.531**	Iridodialysis, right eye
		H21.532	Iridodialysis, left eye
		H21.533	Iridodialysis, bilateral
		H21.539	Iridodialysis, unspecified eye
364.77	RECESSION OF CHAMBER ANGLE OF EYE	**H21.551**	Recession of chamber angle, right eye
		H21.552	Recession of chamber angle, left eye
		H21.553	Recession of chamber angle, bilateral
		H21.559	Recession of chamber angle, unspecified eye
364.81	FLOPPY IRIS SYNDROME	➡ **H21.81**	Floppy iris syndrome
364.82	PLATEAU IRIS SYNDROME	➡ **H21.82**	Plateau iris syndrome (post-iridectomy) (postprocedural)
364.89	OTHER DISORDERS OF IRIS AND CILIARY BODY	**H21.89**	Other specified disorders of iris and ciliary body
		H22	Disorders of iris and ciliary body in diseases classd elswhr
364.9	UNSPECIFIED DISORDER OF IRIS AND CILIARY BODY	➡ **H21.9**	Unspecified disorder of iris and ciliary body
365.00	UNSPECIFIED PREGLAUCOMA	**H40.001**	Preglaucoma, unspecified, right eye
		H40.002	Preglaucoma, unspecified, left eye
		H40.003	Preglaucoma, unspecified, bilateral
		H40.009	Preglaucoma, unspecified, unspecified eye
365.01	BORDERLINE GLAUC OPEN ANGLE BL FINDINGS LOW RSK	**H40.011**	Open angle with borderline findings, low risk, right eye
		H40.012	Open angle with borderline findings, low risk, left eye
		H40.013	Open angle with borderline findings, low risk, bilateral
		H40.019	Open angle with borderline findings, low risk, unsp eye
365.02	BORDERLINE GLAUCOMA WITH ANATOMICAL NARROW ANGLE	**H40.031**	Anatomical narrow angle, right eye
		H40.032	Anatomical narrow angle, left eye
		H40.033	Anatomical narrow angle, bilateral
		H40.039	Anatomical narrow angle, unspecified eye
365.03	BORDERLINE GLAUCOMA WITH STEROID RESPONDERS	**H40.041**	Steroid responder, right eye
		H40.042	Steroid responder, left eye
		H40.043	Steroid responder, bilateral
		H40.049	Steroid responder, unspecified eye
365.04	BORDERLINE GLAUCOMA WITH OCULAR HYPERTENSION	**H40.051**	Ocular hypertension, right eye
		H40.052	Ocular hypertension, left eye
		H40.053	Ocular hypertension, bilateral
		H40.059	Ocular hypertension, unspecified eye
365.05	OPEN ANGLE WITH BORDERLINE FINDINGS HIGH RISK	**H40.021**	Open angle with borderline findings, high risk, right eye
		H40.022	Open angle with borderline findings, high risk, left eye
		H40.023	Open angle with borderline findings, high risk, bilateral
		H40.029	Open angle with borderline findings, high risk, unsp eye
365.06	PRIMARY ANGLE CLOSURE WITHOUT GLAUCOMA DAMAGE	**H40.061**	Primary angle closure without glaucoma damage, right eye
		H40.062	Primary angle closure without glaucoma damage, left eye
		H40.063	Primary angle closure without glaucoma damage, bilateral
		H40.069	Primary angle closure without glaucoma damage, unsp eye
365.10	UNSPECIFIED OPEN-ANGLE GLAUCOMA	⊡ **H40.10X0**	Unspecified open-angle glaucoma, stage unspecified
		⊡ **H40.10X1**	Unspecified open-angle glaucoma, mild stage
		⊡ **H40.10X2**	Unspecified open-angle glaucoma, moderate stage
		⊡ **H40.10X3**	Unspecified open-angle glaucoma, severe stage
		⊡ **H40.10X4**	Unspecified open-angle glaucoma, indeterminate stage
365.11	PRIMARY OPEN-ANGLE GLAUCOMA	⊡ **H40.11X0**	Primary open-angle glaucoma, stage unspecified
		⊡ **H40.11X1**	Primary open-angle glaucoma, mild stage
		⊡ **H40.11X2**	Primary open-angle glaucoma, moderate stage
		⊡ **H40.11X3**	Primary open-angle glaucoma, severe stage
		⊡ **H40.11X4**	Primary open-angle glaucoma, indeterminate stage

ICD-9-CM		ICD-10-CM	
365.12	LOW TENSION OPEN-ANGLE GLAUCOMA	H40.1210	Low-tension glaucoma, right eye, stage unspecified
		H40.1211	Low-tension glaucoma, right eye, mild stage
		H40.1212	Low-tension glaucoma, right eye, moderate stage
		H40.1213	Low-tension glaucoma, right eye, severe stage
		H40.1214	Low-tension glaucoma, right eye, indeterminate stage
		H40.1220	Low-tension glaucoma, left eye, stage unspecified
		H40.1221	Low-tension glaucoma, left eye, mild stage
		H40.1222	Low-tension glaucoma, left eye, moderate stage
		H40.1223	Low-tension glaucoma, left eye, severe stage
		H40.1224	Low-tension glaucoma, left eye, indeterminate stage
		H40.1230	Low-tension glaucoma, bilateral, stage unspecified
		H40.1231	Low-tension glaucoma, bilateral, mild stage
		H40.1232	Low-tension glaucoma, bilateral, moderate stage
		H40.1233	Low-tension glaucoma, bilateral, severe stage
		H40.1234	Low-tension glaucoma, bilateral, indeterminate stage
		H40.1290	Low-tension glaucoma, unspecified eye, stage unspecified
		H40.1291	Low-tension glaucoma, unspecified eye, mild stage
		H40.1292	Low-tension glaucoma, unspecified eye, moderate stage
		H40.1293	Low-tension glaucoma, unspecified eye, severe stage
		H40.1294	Low-tension glaucoma, unspecified eye, indeterminate stage
365.13	PIGMENTARY OPEN-ANGLE GLAUCOMA	H40.1310	Pigmentary glaucoma, right eye, stage unspecified
		H40.1311	Pigmentary glaucoma, right eye, mild stage
		H40.1312	Pigmentary glaucoma, right eye, moderate stage
		H40.1313	Pigmentary glaucoma, right eye, severe stage
		H40.1314	Pigmentary glaucoma, right eye, indeterminate stage
		H40.1320	Pigmentary glaucoma, left eye, stage unspecified
		H40.1321	Pigmentary glaucoma, left eye, mild stage
		H40.1322	Pigmentary glaucoma, left eye, moderate stage
		H40.1323	Pigmentary glaucoma, left eye, severe stage
		H40.1324	Pigmentary glaucoma, left eye, indeterminate stage
		H40.1330	Pigmentary glaucoma, bilateral, stage unspecified
		H40.1331	Pigmentary glaucoma, bilateral, mild stage
		H40.1332	Pigmentary glaucoma, bilateral, moderate stage
		H40.1333	Pigmentary glaucoma, bilateral, severe stage
		H40.1334	Pigmentary glaucoma, bilateral, indeterminate stage
		H40.1390	Pigmentary glaucoma, unspecified eye, stage unspecified
		H40.1391	Pigmentary glaucoma, unspecified eye, mild stage
		H40.1392	Pigmentary glaucoma, unspecified eye, moderate stage
		H40.1393	Pigmentary glaucoma, unspecified eye, severe stage
		H40.1394	Pigmentary glaucoma, unspecified eye, indeterminate stage
365.14	OPEN-ANGLE GLAUCOMA OF CHILDHOOD	Q15.0	Congenital glaucoma
365.15	RESIDUAL STAGE OF OPEN ANGLE GLAUCOMA	H40.151	Residual stage of open-angle glaucoma, right eye
		H40.152	Residual stage of open-angle glaucoma, left eye
		H40.153	Residual stage of open-angle glaucoma, bilateral
		H40.159	Residual stage of open-angle glaucoma, unspecified eye
365.20	UNSPECIFIED PRIMARY ANGLE-CLOSURE GLAUCOMA	H40.20X0	Unsp primary angle-closure glaucoma, stage unspecified
		H40.20X1	Unspecified primary angle-closure glaucoma, mild stage
		H40.20X2	Unspecified primary angle-closure glaucoma, moderate stage
		H40.20X3	Unspecified primary angle-closure glaucoma, severe stage
		H40.20X4	Unsp primary angle-closure glaucoma, indeterminate stage
365.21	INTERMITTENT ANGLE-CLOSURE GLAUCOMA	H40.231	Intermittent angle-closure glaucoma, right eye
		H40.232	Intermittent angle-closure glaucoma, left eye
		H40.233	Intermittent angle-closure glaucoma, bilateral
		H40.239	Intermittent angle-closure glaucoma, unspecified eye
365.22	ACUTE ANGLE-CLOSURE GLAUCOMA	H40.211	Acute angle-closure glaucoma, right eye
		H40.212	Acute angle-closure glaucoma, left eye
		H40.213	Acute angle-closure glaucoma, bilateral
		H40.219	Acute angle-closure glaucoma, unspecified eye
365.23	CHRONIC ANGLE-CLOSURE GLAUCOMA	H40.2210	Chronic angle-closure glaucoma, right eye, stage unspecified
		H40.2211	Chronic angle-closure glaucoma, right eye, mild stage
		H40.2212	Chronic angle-closure glaucoma, right eye, moderate stage
		H40.2213	Chronic angle-closure glaucoma, right eye, severe stage
		H40.2214	Chronic angle-closure glaucoma, r eye, indeterminate stage
		H40.2220	Chronic angle-closure glaucoma, left eye, stage unspecified
		H40.2221	Chronic angle-closure glaucoma, left eye, mild stage
		H40.2222	Chronic angle-closure glaucoma, left eye, moderate stage
		H40.2223	Chronic angle-closure glaucoma, left eye, severe stage
		H40.2224	Chronic angle-closure glaucoma, l eye, indeterminate stage
		H40.2230	Chronic angle-closure glaucoma, bilateral, stage unspecified
		H40.2231	Chronic angle-closure glaucoma, bilateral, mild stage
		H40.2232	Chronic angle-closure glaucoma, bilateral, moderate stage
		H40.2233	Chronic angle-closure glaucoma, bilateral, severe stage
		H40.2234	Chronic angle-closure glaucoma, bi, indeterminate stage
		H40.2290	Chronic angle-closure glaucoma, unsp eye, stage unspecified
		H40.2291	Chronic angle-closure glaucoma, unspecified eye, mild stage
		H40.2292	Chronic angle-closure glaucoma, unsp eye, moderate stage
		H40.2293	Chronic angle-closure glaucoma, unsp eye, severe stage
		H40.2294	Chr angle-closure glaucoma, unsp eye, indeterminate stage

ICD-9-CM		ICD-10-CM		
365.24	RESIDUAL STAGE OF ANGLE-CLOSURE GLAUCOMA		**H40.241**	Residual stage of angle-closure glaucoma, right eye
			H40.242	Residual stage of angle-closure glaucoma, left eye
			H40.243	Residual stage of angle-closure glaucoma, bilateral
			H40.249	Residual stage of angle-closure glaucoma, unspecified eye
365.31	CORTICOSTEROID-INDUCED GLAUC GLAUCTOUS STAGE	☐	**H40.60X0**	Glaucoma secondary to drugs, unsp eye, stage unspecified
		☐	**H40.60X1**	Glaucoma secondary to drugs, unspecified eye, mild stage
		☐	**H40.60X2**	Glaucoma secondary to drugs, unspecified eye, moderate stage
		☐	**H40.60X3**	Glaucoma secondary to drugs, unspecified eye, severe stage
		☐	**H40.60X4**	Glaucoma secondary to drugs, unsp eye, indeterminate stage
		☐	**H40.61X0**	Glaucoma secondary to drugs, right eye, stage unspecified
		☐	**H40.61X1**	Glaucoma secondary to drugs, right eye, mild stage
		☐	**H40.61X2**	Glaucoma secondary to drugs, right eye, moderate stage
		☐	**H40.61X3**	Glaucoma secondary to drugs, right eye, severe stage
		☐	**H40.61X4**	Glaucoma secondary to drugs, right eye, indeterminate stage
		☐	**H40.62X0**	Glaucoma secondary to drugs, left eye, stage unspecified
		☐	**H40.62X1**	Glaucoma secondary to drugs, left eye, mild stage
		☐	**H40.62X2**	Glaucoma secondary to drugs, left eye, moderate stage
		☐	**H40.62X3**	Glaucoma secondary to drugs, left eye, severe stage
		☐	**H40.62X4**	Glaucoma secondary to drugs, left eye, indeterminate stage
		☐	**H40.63X0**	Glaucoma secondary to drugs, bilateral, stage unspecified
		☐	**H40.63X1**	Glaucoma secondary to drugs, bilateral, mild stage
		☐	**H40.63X2**	Glaucoma secondary to drugs, bilateral, moderate stage
		☐	**H40.63X3**	Glaucoma secondary to drugs, bilateral, severe stage
		☐	**H40.63X4**	Glaucoma secondary to drugs, bilateral, indeterminate stage
365.32	CORTICOSTEROID-INDUCED GLAUCOMA RESIDUAL STAGE	☐	**H40.60X0**	Glaucoma secondary to drugs, unsp eye, stage unspecified
		☐	**H40.60X1**	Glaucoma secondary to drugs, unspecified eye, mild stage
		☐	**H40.60X2**	Glaucoma secondary to drugs, unspecified eye, moderate stage
		☐	**H40.60X3**	Glaucoma secondary to drugs, unspecified eye, severe stage
		☐	**H40.60X4**	Glaucoma secondary to drugs, unsp eye, indeterminate stage
		☐	**H40.61X0**	Glaucoma secondary to drugs, right eye, stage unspecified
		☐	**H40.61X1**	Glaucoma secondary to drugs, right eye, mild stage
		☐	**H40.61X2**	Glaucoma secondary to drugs, right eye, moderate stage
		☐	**H40.61X3**	Glaucoma secondary to drugs, right eye, severe stage
		☐	**H40.61X4**	Glaucoma secondary to drugs, right eye, indeterminate stage
		☐	**H40.62X0**	Glaucoma secondary to drugs, left eye, stage unspecified
		☐	**H40.62X1**	Glaucoma secondary to drugs, left eye, mild stage
		☐	**H40.62X2**	Glaucoma secondary to drugs, left eye, moderate stage
		☐	**H40.62X3**	Glaucoma secondary to drugs, left eye, severe stage
		☐	**H40.62X4**	Glaucoma secondary to drugs, left eye, indeterminate stage
		☐	**H40.63X0**	Glaucoma secondary to drugs, bilateral, stage unspecified
		☐	**H40.63X1**	Glaucoma secondary to drugs, bilateral, mild stage
		☐	**H40.63X2**	Glaucoma secondary to drugs, bilateral, moderate stage
		☐	**H40.63X3**	Glaucoma secondary to drugs, bilateral, severe stage
		☐	**H40.63X4**	Glaucoma secondary to drugs, bilateral, indeterminate stage
365.41	GLAUCOMA ASSOCIATED WITH CHAMBER ANGLE ANOMALIES		**H40.89**	Other specified glaucoma
365.42	GLAUCOMA ASSOCIATED WITH ANOMALIES OF IRIS		**H40.89**	Other specified glaucoma
365.43	GLAUCOMA ASSOCIATED W/OTH ANT SEGMENT ANOMALIES		**H40.89**	Other specified glaucoma
365.44	GLAUCOMA ASSOCIATED WITH SYSTEMIC SYNDROMES		**H42**	Glaucoma in diseases classified elsewhere
365.51	PHACOLYTIC GLAUCOMA		**H40.89**	Other specified glaucoma
365.52	PSEUDOEXFOLIATION GLAUCOMA	☐	**H40.1410**	Capslr glaucoma w/pseudxf lens, right eye, stage unsp
		☐	**H40.1411**	Capslr glaucoma w/pseudxf lens, right eye, mild stage
		☐	**H40.1412**	Capslr glaucoma w/pseudxf lens, right eye, moderate stage
		☐	**H40.1413**	Capslr glaucoma w/pseudxf lens, right eye, severe stage
		☐	**H40.1414**	Capslr glaucoma w/pseudxf lens, r eye, indeterminate stage
		☐	**H40.1420**	Capslr glaucoma w/pseudxf lens, left eye, stage unsp
		☐	**H40.1421**	Capslr glaucoma w/pseudxf lens, left eye, mild stage
		☐	**H40.1422**	Capslr glaucoma w/pseudxf lens, left eye, moderate stage
		☐	**H40.1423**	Capslr glaucoma w/pseudxf lens, left eye, severe stage
		☐	**H40.1424**	Capslr glaucoma w/pseudxf lens, l eye, indeterminate stage
		☐	**H40.1430**	Capslr glaucoma w/pseudxf lens, bilateral, stage unsp
		☐	**H40.1431**	Capslr glaucoma w/pseudxf lens, bilateral, mild stage
		☐	**H40.1432**	Capslr glaucoma w/pseudxf lens, bilateral, moderate stage
		☐	**H40.1433**	Capslr glaucoma w/pseudxf lens, bilateral, severe stage
		☐	**H40.1434**	Capslr glaucoma w/pseudxf lens, bi, indeterminate stage
		☐	**H40.1490**	Capslr glaucoma w/pseudxf lens, unsp eye, stage unsp
		☐	**H40.1491**	Capslr glaucoma w/pseudxf lens, unsp eye, mild stage
		☐	**H40.1492**	Capslr glaucoma w/pseudxf lens, unsp eye, moderate stage
		☐	**H40.1493**	Capslr glaucoma w/pseudxf lens, unsp eye, severe stage
		☐	**H40.1494**	Capslr glaucoma w/pseudxf lens, unsp eye, indeterminate stg

ICD-9-CM	ICD-10-CM	
365.59 GLAUCOMA ASSOCIATED WITH OTHER LENS DISORDERS	**H4Ø.5ØXØ**	Glaucoma secondary to oth eye disord, unsp eye, stage unsp
	H4Ø.5ØX1	Glaucoma secondary to oth eye disord, unsp eye, mild stage
	H4Ø.5ØX2	Glaucoma sec to oth eye disord, unsp eye, moderate stage
	H4Ø.5ØX3	Glaucoma secondary to oth eye disord, unsp eye, severe stage
	H4Ø.5ØX4	Glaucoma sec to oth eye disord, unsp eye, indeterminate stg
	H4Ø.51XØ	Glaucoma secondary to oth eye disord, right eye, stage unsp
	H4Ø.51X1	Glaucoma secondary to oth eye disord, right eye, mild stage
	H4Ø.51X2	Glaucoma secondary to oth eye disord, r eye, moderate stage
	H4Ø.51X3	Glaucoma secondary to oth eye disord, r eye, severe stage
	H4Ø.51X4	Glaucoma sec to oth eye disord, r eye, indeterminate stage
	H4Ø.52XØ	Glaucoma secondary to oth eye disord, left eye, stage unsp
	H4Ø.52X1	Glaucoma secondary to oth eye disord, left eye, mild stage
	H4Ø.52X2	Glaucoma sec to oth eye disord, left eye, moderate stage
	H4Ø.52X3	Glaucoma secondary to oth eye disord, left eye, severe stage
	H4Ø.52X4	Glaucoma sec to oth eye disord, l eye, indeterminate stage
	H4Ø.53XØ	Glaucoma secondary to oth eye disorders, bi, stage unsp
	H4Ø.53X1	Glaucoma secondary to oth eye disorders, bi, mild stage
	H4Ø.53X2	Glaucoma secondary to oth eye disorders, bi, moderate stage
	H4Ø.53X3	Glaucoma secondary to oth eye disorders, bi, severe stage
	H4Ø.53X4	Glaucoma sec to oth eye disord, bi, indeterminate stage
365.6Ø GLAUCOMA ASSOCIATED W/UNSPEC OCULAR DISORDER	**H4Ø.5ØXØ**	Glaucoma secondary to oth eye disord, unsp eye, stage unsp
	H4Ø.5ØX1	Glaucoma secondary to oth eye disord, unsp eye, mild stage
	H4Ø.5ØX2	Glaucoma sec to oth eye disord, unsp eye, moderate stage
	H4Ø.5ØX3	Glaucoma secondary to oth eye disord, unsp eye, severe stage
	H4Ø.5ØX4	Glaucoma sec to oth eye disord, unsp eye, indeterminate stg
	H4Ø.51XØ	Glaucoma secondary to oth eye disord, right eye, stage unsp
	H4Ø.51X1	Glaucoma secondary to oth eye disord, right eye, mild stage
	H4Ø.51X2	Glaucoma secondary to oth eye disord, r eye, moderate stage
	H4Ø.51X3	Glaucoma secondary to oth eye disord, r eye, severe stage
	H4Ø.51X4	Glaucoma sec to oth eye disord, r eye, indeterminate stage
	H4Ø.52XØ	Glaucoma secondary to oth eye disord, left eye, stage unsp
	H4Ø.52X1	Glaucoma secondary to oth eye disord, left eye, mild stage
	H4Ø.52X2	Glaucoma sec to oth eye disord, left eye, moderate stage
	H4Ø.52X3	Glaucoma secondary to oth eye disord, left eye, severe stage
	H4Ø.52X4	Glaucoma sec to oth eye disord, l eye, indeterminate stage
	H4Ø.53XØ	Glaucoma secondary to oth eye disorders, bi, stage unsp
	H4Ø.53X1	Glaucoma secondary to oth eye disorders, bi, mild stage
	H4Ø.53X2	Glaucoma secondary to oth eye disorders, bi, moderate stage
	H4Ø.53X3	Glaucoma secondary to oth eye disorders, bi, severe stage
	H4Ø.53X4	Glaucoma sec to oth eye disord, bi, indeterminate stage
365.61 GLAUCOMA ASSOCIATED WITH PUPILLARY BLOCK	**H4Ø.5ØXØ**	Glaucoma secondary to oth eye disord, unsp eye, stage unsp
	H4Ø.5ØX1	Glaucoma secondary to oth eye disord, unsp eye, mild stage
	H4Ø.5ØX2	Glaucoma sec to oth eye disord, unsp eye, moderate stage
	H4Ø.5ØX3	Glaucoma secondary to oth eye disord, unsp eye, severe stage
	H4Ø.5ØX4	Glaucoma sec to oth eye disord, unsp eye, indeterminate stg
	H4Ø.51XØ	Glaucoma secondary to oth eye disord, right eye, stage unsp
	H4Ø.51X1	Glaucoma secondary to oth eye disord, right eye, mild stage
	H4Ø.51X2	Glaucoma secondary to oth eye disord, r eye, moderate stage
	H4Ø.51X3	Glaucoma secondary to oth eye disord, r eye, severe stage
	H4Ø.51X4	Glaucoma sec to oth eye disord, r eye, indeterminate stage
	H4Ø.52XØ	Glaucoma secondary to oth eye disord, left eye, stage unsp
	H4Ø.52X1	Glaucoma secondary to oth eye disord, left eye, mild stage
	H4Ø.52X2	Glaucoma sec to oth eye disord, left eye, moderate stage
	H4Ø.52X3	Glaucoma secondary to oth eye disord, left eye, severe stage
	H4Ø.52X4	Glaucoma sec to oth eye disord, l eye, indeterminate stage
	H4Ø.53XØ	Glaucoma secondary to oth eye disorders, bi, stage unsp
	H4Ø.53X1	Glaucoma secondary to oth eye disorders, bi, mild stage
	H4Ø.53X2	Glaucoma secondary to oth eye disorders, bi, moderate stage
	H4Ø.53X3	Glaucoma secondary to oth eye disorders, bi, severe stage
	H4Ø.53X4	Glaucoma sec to oth eye disord, bi, indeterminate stage
365.62 GLAUCOMA ASSOCIATED WITH OCULAR INFLAMMATIONS	**H4Ø.4ØXØ**	Glaucoma secondary to eye inflammation, unsp eye, stage unsp
	H4Ø.4ØX1	Glaucoma secondary to eye inflammation, unsp eye, mild stage
	H4Ø.4ØX2	Glaucoma secondary to eye inflam, unsp eye, moderate stage
	H4Ø.4ØX3	Glaucoma secondary to eye inflam, unsp eye, severe stage
	H4Ø.4ØX4	Glaucoma sec to eye inflam, unsp eye, indeterminate stage
	H4Ø.41XØ	Glaucoma secondary to eye inflam, right eye, stage unsp
	H4Ø.41X1	Glaucoma secondary to eye inflam, right eye, mild stage
	H4Ø.41X2	Glaucoma secondary to eye inflam, right eye, moderate stage
	H4Ø.41X3	Glaucoma secondary to eye inflam, right eye, severe stage
	H4Ø.41X4	Glaucoma secondary to eye inflam, r eye, indeterminate stage
	H4Ø.42XØ	Glaucoma secondary to eye inflammation, left eye, stage unsp
	H4Ø.42X1	Glaucoma secondary to eye inflammation, left eye, mild stage
	H4Ø.42X2	Glaucoma secondary to eye inflam, left eye, moderate stage
	H4Ø.42X3	Glaucoma secondary to eye inflam, left eye, severe stage
	H4Ø.42X4	Glaucoma sec to eye inflam, left eye, indeterminate stage
	H4Ø.43XØ	Glaucoma secondary to eye inflam, bilateral, stage unsp
	H4Ø.43X1	Glaucoma secondary to eye inflam, bilateral, mild stage
	H4Ø.43X2	Glaucoma secondary to eye inflam, bilateral, moderate stage
	H4Ø.43X3	Glaucoma secondary to eye inflam, bilateral, severe stage
	H4Ø.43X4	Glaucoma secondary to eye inflam, bi, indeterminate stage

ICD-9-CM		ICD-10-CM	
365.63	GLAUCOMA ASSOCIATED W/VASCULAR DISORDERS OF EYE	**H4Ø.89**	Other specified glaucoma
365.64	GLAUCOMA ASSOCIATED WITH TUMORS OR CYSTS	**H4Ø.5ØXØ**	Glaucoma secondary to oth eye disord, unsp eye, stage unsp
		H4Ø.5ØX1	Glaucoma secondary to oth eye disord, unsp eye, mild stage
		H4Ø.5ØX2	Glaucoma sec to oth eye disord, unsp eye, moderate stage
		H4Ø.5ØX3	Glaucoma secondary to oth eye disord, unsp eye, severe stage
		H4Ø.5ØX4	Glaucoma sec to oth eye disord, unsp eye, indeterminate stg
		H4Ø.51XØ	Glaucoma secondary to oth eye disord, right eye, stage unsp
		H4Ø.51X1	Glaucoma secondary to oth eye disord, right eye, mild stage
		H4Ø.51X2	Glaucoma secondary to oth eye disord, r eye, moderate stage
		H4Ø.51X3	Glaucoma secondary to oth eye disord, r eye, severe stage
		H4Ø.51X4	Glaucoma sec to oth eye disord, r eye, indeterminate stage
		H4Ø.52XØ	Glaucoma secondary to oth eye disord, left eye, stage unsp
		H4Ø.52X1	Glaucoma secondary to oth eye disord, left eye, mild stage
		H4Ø.52X2	Glaucoma sec to oth eye disord, left eye, moderate stage
		H4Ø.52X3	Glaucoma secondary to oth eye disord, left eye, severe stage
		H4Ø.52X4	Glaucoma sec to oth eye disord, l eye, indeterminate stage
		H4Ø.53XØ	Glaucoma secondary to oth eye disorders, bi, stage unsp
		H4Ø.53X1	Glaucoma secondary to oth eye disorders, bi, mild stage
		H4Ø.53X2	Glaucoma secondary to oth eye disorders, bi, moderate stage
		H4Ø.53X3	Glaucoma secondary to oth eye disorders, bi, severe stage
		H4Ø.53X4	Glaucoma sec to oth eye disord, bi, indeterminate stage
365.65	GLAUCOMA ASSOCIATED WITH OCULAR TRAUMA	**H4Ø.3ØXØ**	Glaucoma secondary to eye trauma, unsp eye, stage unsp
		H4Ø.3ØX1	Glaucoma secondary to eye trauma, unsp eye, mild stage
		H4Ø.3ØX2	Glaucoma secondary to eye trauma, unsp eye, moderate stage
		H4Ø.3ØX3	Glaucoma secondary to eye trauma, unsp eye, severe stage
		H4Ø.3ØX4	Glaucoma sec to eye trauma, unsp eye, indeterminate stage
		H4Ø.31XØ	Glaucoma secondary to eye trauma, right eye, stage unsp
		H4Ø.31X1	Glaucoma secondary to eye trauma, right eye, mild stage
		H4Ø.31X2	Glaucoma secondary to eye trauma, right eye, moderate stage
		H4Ø.31X3	Glaucoma secondary to eye trauma, right eye, severe stage
		H4Ø.31X4	Glaucoma secondary to eye trauma, r eye, indeterminate stage
		H4Ø.32XØ	Glaucoma secondary to eye trauma, left eye, stage unsp
		H4Ø.32X1	Glaucoma secondary to eye trauma, left eye, mild stage
		H4Ø.32X2	Glaucoma secondary to eye trauma, left eye, moderate stage
		H4Ø.32X3	Glaucoma secondary to eye trauma, left eye, severe stage
		H4Ø.32X4	Glaucoma sec to eye trauma, left eye, indeterminate stage
		H4Ø.33XØ	Glaucoma secondary to eye trauma, bilateral, stage unsp
		H4Ø.33X1	Glaucoma secondary to eye trauma, bilateral, mild stage
		H4Ø.33X2	Glaucoma secondary to eye trauma, bilateral, moderate stage
		H4Ø.33X3	Glaucoma secondary to eye trauma, bilateral, severe stage
		H4Ø.33X4	Glaucoma secondary to eye trauma, bi, indeterminate stage
365.7Ø	GLAUCOMA STAGE UNSPECIFIED	**H4Ø.1ØXØ**	Unspecified open-angle glaucoma, stage unspecified
		H4Ø.11XØ	Primary open-angle glaucoma, stage unspecified
		H4Ø.121Ø	Low-tension glaucoma, right eye, stage unspecified
		H4Ø.122Ø	Low-tension glaucoma, left eye, stage unspecified
		H4Ø.123Ø	Low-tension glaucoma, bilateral, stage unspecified
		H4Ø.129Ø	Low-tension glaucoma, unspecified eye, stage unspecified
		H4Ø.131Ø	Pigmentary glaucoma, right eye, stage unspecified
		H4Ø.132Ø	Pigmentary glaucoma, left eye, stage unspecified
		H4Ø.133Ø	Pigmentary glaucoma, bilateral, stage unspecified
		H4Ø.139Ø	Pigmentary glaucoma, unspecified eye, stage unspecified
		H4Ø.141Ø	Capslr glaucoma w/pseudxf lens, right eye, stage unsp
		H4Ø.142Ø	Capslr glaucoma w/pseudxf lens, left eye, stage unsp
		H4Ø.143Ø	Capslr glaucoma w/pseudxf lens, bilateral, stage unsp
		H4Ø.149Ø	Capslr glaucoma w/pseudxf lens, unsp eye, stage unsp
		H4Ø.2ØXØ	Unsp primary angle-closure glaucoma, stage unspecified
		H4Ø.221Ø	Chronic angle-closure glaucoma, right eye, stage unspecified
		H4Ø.222Ø	Chronic angle-closure glaucoma, left eye, stage unspecified
		H4Ø.223Ø	Chronic angle-closure glaucoma, bilateral, stage unspecified
		H4Ø.229Ø	Chronic angle-closure glaucoma, unsp eye, stage unspecified
		H4Ø.3ØXØ	Glaucoma secondary to eye trauma, unsp eye, stage unsp
		H4Ø.31XØ	Glaucoma secondary to eye trauma, right eye, stage unsp
		H4Ø.32XØ	Glaucoma secondary to eye trauma, left eye, stage unsp
		H4Ø.33XØ	Glaucoma secondary to eye trauma, bilateral, stage unsp
		H4Ø.4ØXØ	Glaucoma secondary to eye inflammation, unsp eye, stage unsp
		H4Ø.41XØ	Glaucoma secondary to eye inflam, right eye, stage unsp
		H4Ø.42XØ	Glaucoma secondary to eye inflammation, left eye, stage unsp
		H4Ø.43XØ	Glaucoma secondary to eye inflam, bilateral, stage unsp
		H4Ø.5ØXØ	Glaucoma secondary to oth eye disord, unsp eye, stage unsp
		H4Ø.51XØ	Glaucoma secondary to oth eye disord, right eye, stage unsp
		H4Ø.52XØ	Glaucoma secondary to oth eye disord, left eye, stage unsp
		H4Ø.53XØ	Glaucoma secondary to oth eye disorders, bi, stage unsp
		H4Ø.6ØXØ	Glaucoma secondary to drugs, unsp eye, stage unspecified
		H4Ø.61XØ	Glaucoma secondary to drugs, right eye, stage unspecified
		H4Ø.62XØ	Glaucoma secondary to drugs, left eye, stage unspecified
		H4Ø.63XØ	Glaucoma secondary to drugs, bilateral, stage unspecified

ICD-9-CM	ICD-10-CM	
365.71 MILD STAGE GLAUCOMA	**H40.10X1**	Unspecified open-angle glaucoma, mild stage
	H40.11X1	Primary open-angle glaucoma, mild stage
	H40.1211	Low-tension glaucoma, right eye, mild stage
	H40.1221	Low-tension glaucoma, left eye, mild stage
	H40.1231	Low-tension glaucoma, bilateral, mild stage
	H40.1291	Low-tension glaucoma, unspecified eye, mild stage
	H40.1311	Pigmentary glaucoma, right eye, mild stage
	H40.1321	Pigmentary glaucoma, left eye, mild stage
	H40.1331	Pigmentary glaucoma, bilateral, mild stage
	H40.1391	Pigmentary glaucoma, unspecified eye, mild stage
	H40.1411	Capslr glaucoma w/pseudxf lens, right eye, mild stage
	H40.1421	Capslr glaucoma w/pseudxf lens, left eye, mild stage
	H40.1431	Capslr glaucoma w/pseudxf lens, bilateral, mild stage
	H40.1491	Capslr glaucoma w/pseudxf lens, unsp eye, mild stage
	H40.20X1	Unspecified primary angle-closure glaucoma, mild stage
	H40.2211	Chronic angle-closure glaucoma, right eye, mild stage
	H40.2221	Chronic angle-closure glaucoma, left eye, mild stage
	H40.2231	Chronic angle-closure glaucoma, bilateral, mild stage
	H40.2291	Chronic angle-closure glaucoma, unspecified eye, mild stage
	H40.30X1	Glaucoma secondary to eye trauma, unsp eye, mild stage
	H40.31X1	Glaucoma secondary to eye trauma, right eye, mild stage
	H40.32X1	Glaucoma secondary to eye trauma, left eye, mild stage
	H40.33X1	Glaucoma secondary to eye trauma, bilateral, mild stage
	H40.40X1	Glaucoma secondary to eye inflammation, unsp eye, mild stage
	H40.41X1	Glaucoma secondary to eye inflam, right eye, mild stage
	H40.42X1	Glaucoma secondary to eye inflammation, left eye, mild stage
	H40.43X1	Glaucoma secondary to eye inflam, bilateral, mild stage
	H40.50X1	Glaucoma secondary to oth eye disord, unsp eye, mild stage
	H40.51X1	Glaucoma secondary to oth eye disord, right eye, mild stage
	H40.52X1	Glaucoma secondary to oth eye disord, left eye, mild stage
	H40.53X1	Glaucoma secondary to oth eye disorders, bi, mild stage
	H40.60X1	Glaucoma secondary to drugs, unspecified eye, mild stage
	H40.61X1	Glaucoma secondary to drugs, right eye, mild stage
	H40.62X1	Glaucoma secondary to drugs, left eye, mild stage
	H40.63X1	Glaucoma secondary to drugs, bilateral, mild stage
365.72 MODERATE STAGE GLAUCOMA	**H40.10X2**	Unspecified open-angle glaucoma, moderate stage
	H40.11X2	Primary open-angle glaucoma, moderate stage
	H40.1212	Low-tension glaucoma, right eye, moderate stage
	H40.1222	Low-tension glaucoma, left eye, moderate stage
	H40.1232	Low-tension glaucoma, bilateral, moderate stage
	H40.1292	Low-tension glaucoma, unspecified eye, moderate stage
	H40.1312	Pigmentary glaucoma, right eye, moderate stage
	H40.1322	Pigmentary glaucoma, left eye, moderate stage
	H40.1332	Pigmentary glaucoma, bilateral, moderate stage
	H40.1392	Pigmentary glaucoma, unspecified eye, moderate stage
	H40.1412	Capslr glaucoma w/pseudxf lens, right eye, moderate stage
	H40.1422	Capslr glaucoma w/pseudxf lens, left eye, moderate stage
	H40.1432	Capslr glaucoma w/pseudxf lens, bilateral, moderate stage
	H40.1492	Capslr glaucoma w/pseudxf lens, unsp eye, moderate stage
	H40.20X2	Unspecified primary angle-closure glaucoma, moderate stage
	H40.2212	Chronic angle-closure glaucoma, right eye, moderate stage
	H40.2222	Chronic angle-closure glaucoma, left eye, moderate stage
	H40.2232	Chronic angle-closure glaucoma, bilateral, moderate stage
	H40.2292	Chronic angle-closure glaucoma, unsp eye, moderate stage
	H40.30X2	Glaucoma secondary to eye trauma, unsp eye, moderate stage
	H40.31X2	Glaucoma secondary to eye trauma, right eye, moderate stage
	H40.32X2	Glaucoma secondary to eye trauma, left eye, moderate stage
	H40.33X2	Glaucoma secondary to eye trauma, bilateral, moderate stage
	H40.40X2	Glaucoma secondary to eye inflam, unsp eye, moderate stage
	H40.41X2	Glaucoma secondary to eye inflam, right eye, moderate stage
	H40.42X2	Glaucoma secondary to eye inflam, left eye, moderate stage
	H40.43X2	Glaucoma secondary to eye inflam, bilateral, moderate stage
	H40.50X2	Glaucoma sec to oth eye disord, unsp eye, moderate stage
	H40.51X2	Glaucoma secondary to oth eye disord, r eye, moderate stage
	H40.52X2	Glaucoma sec to oth eye disord, left eye, moderate stage
	H40.53X2	Glaucoma secondary to oth eye disorders, bi, moderate stage
	H40.60X2	Glaucoma secondary to drugs, unspecified eye, moderate stage
	H40.61X2	Glaucoma secondary to drugs, right eye, moderate stage
	H40.62X2	Glaucoma secondary to drugs, left eye, moderate stage
	H40.63X2	Glaucoma secondary to drugs, bilateral, moderate stage

ICD-9-CM		ICD-10-CM	
365.73	SEVERE STAGE GLAUCOMA	H40.10X3	Unspecified open-angle glaucoma, severe stage
		H40.11X3	Primary open-angle glaucoma, severe stage
		H40.1213	Low-tension glaucoma, right eye, severe stage
		H40.1223	Low-tension glaucoma, left eye, severe stage
		H40.1233	Low-tension glaucoma, bilateral, severe stage
		H40.1293	Low-tension glaucoma, unspecified eye, severe stage
		H40.1313	Pigmentary glaucoma, right eye, severe stage
		H40.1323	Pigmentary glaucoma, left eye, severe stage
		H40.1333	Pigmentary glaucoma, bilateral, severe stage
		H40.1393	Pigmentary glaucoma, unspecified eye, severe stage
		H40.1413	Capslr glaucoma w/pseudxf lens, right eye, severe stage
		H40.1423	Capslr glaucoma w/pseudxf lens, left eye, severe stage
		H40.1433	Capslr glaucoma w/pseudxf lens, bilateral, severe stage
		H40.1493	Capslr glaucoma w/pseudxf lens, unsp eye, severe stage
		H40.20X3	Unspecified primary angle-closure glaucoma, severe stage
		H40.2213	Chronic angle-closure glaucoma, right eye, severe stage
		H40.2223	Chronic angle-closure glaucoma, left eye, severe stage
		H40.2233	Chronic angle-closure glaucoma, bilateral, severe stage
		H40.2293	Chronic angle-closure glaucoma, unsp eye, severe stage
		H40.30X3	Glaucoma secondary to eye trauma, unsp eye, severe stage
		H40.31X3	Glaucoma secondary to eye trauma, right eye, severe stage
		H40.32X3	Glaucoma secondary to eye trauma, left eye, severe stage
		H40.33X3	Glaucoma secondary to eye trauma, bilateral, severe stage
		H40.40X3	Glaucoma secondary to eye inflam, unsp eye, severe stage
		H40.41X3	Glaucoma secondary to eye inflam, right eye, severe stage
		H40.42X3	Glaucoma secondary to eye inflam, left eye, severe stage
		H40.43X3	Glaucoma secondary to eye inflam, bilateral, severe stage
		H40.50X3	Glaucoma secondary to oth eye disord, unsp eye, severe stage
		H40.51X3	Glaucoma secondary to oth eye disord, r eye, severe stage
		H40.52X3	Glaucoma secondary to oth eye disord, left eye, severe stage
		H40.53X3	Glaucoma secondary to oth eye disorders, bi, severe stage
		H40.60X3	Glaucoma secondary to drugs, unspecified eye, severe stage
		H40.61X3	Glaucoma secondary to drugs, right eye, severe stage
		H40.62X3	Glaucoma secondary to drugs, left eye, severe stage
		H40.63X3	Glaucoma secondary to drugs, bilateral, severe stage
365.74	INDETERMINATE STAGE GLAUCOMA	H40.10X4	Unspecified open-angle glaucoma, indeterminate stage
		H40.11X4	Primary open-angle glaucoma, indeterminate stage
		H40.1214	Low-tension glaucoma, right eye, indeterminate stage
		H40.1224	Low-tension glaucoma, left eye, indeterminate stage
		H40.1234	Low-tension glaucoma, bilateral, indeterminate stage
		H40.1294	Low-tension glaucoma, unspecified eye, indeterminate stage
		H40.1314	Pigmentary glaucoma, right eye, indeterminate stage
		H40.1324	Pigmentary glaucoma, left eye, indeterminate stage
		H40.1334	Pigmentary glaucoma, bilateral, indeterminate stage
		H40.1394	Pigmentary glaucoma, unspecified eye, indeterminate stage
		H40.1414	Capslr glaucoma w/pseudxf lens, r eye, indeterminate stage
		H40.1424	Capslr glaucoma w/pseudxf lens, l eye, indeterminate stage
		H40.1434	Capslr glaucoma w/pseudxf lens, bi, indeterminate stage
		H40.1494	Capslr glaucoma w/pseudxf lens, unsp eye, indeterminate stg
		H40.20X4	Unsp primary angle-closure glaucoma, indeterminate stage
		H40.2214	Chronic angle-closure glaucoma, r eye, indeterminate stage
		H40.2224	Chronic angle-closure glaucoma, l eye, indeterminate stage
		H40.2234	Chronic angle-closure glaucoma, bi, indeterminate stage
		H40.2294	Chr angle-closure glaucoma, unsp eye, indeterminate stage
		H40.30X4	Glaucoma sec to eye trauma, unsp eye, indeterminate stage
		H40.31X4	Glaucoma secondary to eye trauma, r eye, indeterminate stage
		H40.32X4	Glaucoma sec to eye trauma, left eye, indeterminate stage
		H40.33X4	Glaucoma secondary to eye trauma, bi, indeterminate stage
		H40.40X4	Glaucoma sec to eye inflam, unsp eye, indeterminate stage
		H40.41X4	Glaucoma secondary to eye inflam, r eye, indeterminate stage
		H40.42X4	Glaucoma sec to eye inflam, left eye, indeterminate stage
		H40.43X4	Glaucoma secondary to eye inflam, bi, indeterminate stage
		H40.50X4	Glaucoma sec to oth eye disord, unsp eye, indeterminate stg
		H40.51X4	Glaucoma sec to oth eye disord, r eye, indeterminate stage
		H40.52X4	Glaucoma sec to oth eye disord, l eye, indeterminate stage
		H40.53X4	Glaucoma sec to oth eye disord, bi, indeterminate stage
		H40.60X4	Glaucoma secondary to drugs, unsp eye, indeterminate stage
		H40.61X4	Glaucoma secondary to drugs, right eye, indeterminate stage
		H40.62X4	Glaucoma secondary to drugs, left eye, indeterminate stage
		H40.63X4	Glaucoma secondary to drugs, bilateral, indeterminate stage
365.81	HYPERSECRETION GLAUCOMA	H40.821	Hypersecretion glaucoma, right eye
		H40.822	Hypersecretion glaucoma, left eye
		H40.823	Hypersecretion glaucoma, bilateral
		H40.829	Hypersecretion glaucoma, unspecified eye
365.82	GLAUCOMA W/INCREASED EPISCLERAL VENOUS PRESSURE	H40.811	Glaucoma w increased episcleral venous pressure, right eye
		H40.812	Glaucoma with increased episcleral venous pressure, left eye
		H40.813	Glaucoma w increased episcleral venous pressure, bilateral
		H40.819	Glaucoma with increased episcleral venous pressure, unsp eye

ICD-9-CM		ICD-10-CM	
365.83	AQUEOUS MISDIRECTION	**H40.831**	Aqueous misdirection, right eye
		H40.832	Aqueous misdirection, left eye
		H40.833	Aqueous misdirection, bilateral
		H40.839	Aqueous misdirection, unspecified eye
365.89	OTHER SPECIFIED GLAUCOMA	**H40.89**	Other specified glaucoma
365.9	UNSPECIFIED GLAUCOMA	➡ **H40.9**	Unspecified glaucoma
366.00	UNSPECIFIED NONSENILE CATARACT	**H26.001**	Unspecified infantile and juvenile cataract, right eye
		H26.002	Unspecified infantile and juvenile cataract, left eye
		H26.003	Unspecified infantile and juvenile cataract, bilateral
		H26.009	Unspecified infantile and juvenile cataract, unspecified eye
366.01	ANTERIOR SUBCAPSULAR POLAR CATARACT NONSENILE	**H26.041**	Ant subcapsular polar infantile and juvenile cataract, r eye
		H26.042	Ant subcapsular polar infantile and juv cataract, left eye
		H26.043	Ant subcapsular polar infantile and juvenile cataract, bi
		H26.049	Ant subcapsular polar infantile and juv cataract, unsp eye
366.02	POSTERIOR SUBCAPSULAR POLAR CATARACT NONSENILE	**H26.051**	Post subcapsular polar infantile and juv cataract, r eye
		H26.052	Post subcapsular polar infantile and juv cataract, left eye
		H26.053	Post subcapsular polar infantile and juvenile cataract, bi
		H26.059	Post subcapsular polar infantile and juv cataract, unsp eye
366.03	CORTICAL LAMELLAR OR ZONULAR CATARACT NONSENILE	**H26.011**	Infantile and juv cortical/lamellar/zonular cataract, r eye
		H26.012	Infantile and juv cortical/lamellar/zonular cataract, l eye
		H26.013	Infantile and juv cortical/lamellar/zonular cataract, bi
		H26.019	Infantile & juv cortical/lamellar/zonular cataract, unsp eye
366.04	NUCLEAR CATARACT, NONSENILE	**H26.031**	Infantile and juvenile nuclear cataract, right eye
		H26.032	Infantile and juvenile nuclear cataract, left eye
		H26.033	Infantile and juvenile nuclear cataract, bilateral
		H26.039	Infantile and juvenile nuclear cataract, unspecified eye
366.09	OTHER AND COMBINED FORMS OF NONSENILE CATARACT	**H26.061**	Combined forms of infantile and juvenile cataract, right eye
		H26.062	Combined forms of infantile and juvenile cataract, left eye
		H26.063	Combined forms of infantile and juvenile cataract, bilateral
		H26.069	Combined forms of infantile and juvenile cataract, unsp eye
		H26.09	Other infantile and juvenile cataract
366.10	UNSPECIFIED SENILE CATARACT	➡ **H25.9**	Unspecified age-related cataract
366.11	PSEUDOEXFOLIATION OF LENS CAPSULE	**H25.89**	Other age-related cataract
366.12	INCIPIENT CATARACT	**H25.091**	Other age-related incipient cataract, right eye
		H25.092	Other age-related incipient cataract, left eye
		H25.093	Other age-related incipient cataract, bilateral
		H25.099	Other age-related incipient cataract, unspecified eye
366.13	ANTERIOR SUBCAPSULAR POLAR SENILE CATARACT	**H25.031**	Anterior subcapsular polar age-related cataract, right eye
		H25.032	Anterior subcapsular polar age-related cataract, left eye
		H25.033	Anterior subcapsular polar age-related cataract, bilateral
		H25.039	Anterior subcapsular polar age-related cataract, unsp eye
366.14	POSTERIOR SUBCAPSULAR POLAR SENILE CATARACT	**H25.041**	Posterior subcapsular polar age-related cataract, right eye
		H25.042	Posterior subcapsular polar age-related cataract, left eye
		H25.043	Posterior subcapsular polar age-related cataract, bilateral
		H25.049	Posterior subcapsular polar age-related cataract, unsp eye
366.15	CORTICAL SENILE CATARACT	**H25.011**	Cortical age-related cataract, right eye
		H25.012	Cortical age-related cataract, left eye
		H25.013	Cortical age-related cataract, bilateral
		H25.019	Cortical age-related cataract, unspecified eye
366.16	NUCLEAR SCLEROSIS	**H25.10**	Age-related nuclear cataract, unspecified eye
		H25.11	Age-related nuclear cataract, right eye
		H25.12	Age-related nuclear cataract, left eye
		H25.13	Age-related nuclear cataract, bilateral
366.17	TOTAL OR MATURE SENILE CATARACT	**H25.89**	Other age-related cataract
366.18	HYPERMATURE SENILE CATARACT	**H25.20**	Age-related cataract, morgagnian type, unspecified eye
		H25.21	Age-related cataract, morgagnian type, right eye
		H25.22	Age-related cataract, morgagnian type, left eye
		H25.23	Age-related cataract, morgagnian type, bilateral
366.19	OTHER AND COMBINED FORMS OF SENILE CATARACT	**H25.811**	Combined forms of age-related cataract, right eye
		H25.812	Combined forms of age-related cataract, left eye
		H25.813	Combined forms of age-related cataract, bilateral
		H25.819	Combined forms of age-related cataract, unspecified eye
		H25.89	Other age-related cataract
366.20	UNSPECIFIED TRAUMATIC CATARACT	**H26.101**	Unspecified traumatic cataract, right eye
		H26.102	Unspecified traumatic cataract, left eye
		H26.103	Unspecified traumatic cataract, bilateral
		H26.109	Unspecified traumatic cataract, unspecified eye
366.21	LOCALIZED TRAUMATIC OPACITIES OF CATARACT	**H26.111**	Localized traumatic opacities, right eye
		H26.112	Localized traumatic opacities, left eye
		H26.113	Localized traumatic opacities, bilateral
		H26.119	Localized traumatic opacities, unspecified eye
366.22	TOTAL TRAUMATIC CATARACT	**H26.131**	Total traumatic cataract, right eye
		H26.132	Total traumatic cataract, left eye
		H26.133	Total traumatic cataract, bilateral
		H26.139	Total traumatic cataract, unspecified eye

ICD-9-CM			ICD-10-CM	
366.23	PARTIALLY RESOLVED TRAUMATIC CATARACT		**H26.121**	Partially resolved traumatic cataract, right eye
			H26.122	Partially resolved traumatic cataract, left eye
			H26.123	Partially resolved traumatic cataract, bilateral
			H26.129	Partially resolved traumatic cataract, unspecified eye
366.30	UNSPECIFIED CATARACTA COMPLICATA	➡	**H26.20**	Unspecified complicated cataract
366.31	CATARACT SECONDARY TO GLAUCOMATOUS FLECKS		**H26.231**	Glaucomatous flecks (subcapsular), right eye
			H26.232	Glaucomatous flecks (subcapsular), left eye
			H26.233	Glaucomatous flecks (subcapsular), bilateral
			H26.239	Glaucomatous flecks (subcapsular), unspecified eye
366.32	CATARACT IN INFLAMMATORY OCULAR DISORDERS		**H26.221**	Cataract secondary to ocular disorders, right eye
			H26.222	Cataract secondary to ocular disorders, left eye
			H26.223	Cataract secondary to ocular disorders, bilateral
			H26.229	Cataract secondary to ocular disorders, unsp eye
366.33	CATARACT WITH OCULAR NEOVASCULARIZATION		**H26.211**	Cataract with neovascularization, right eye
			H26.212	Cataract with neovascularization, left eye
			H26.213	Cataract with neovascularization, bilateral
			H26.219	Cataract with neovascularization, unspecified eye
366.34	CATARACT IN DEGENERATIVE OCULAR DISORDERS		**H26.221**	Cataract secondary to ocular disorders, right eye
			H26.222	Cataract secondary to ocular disorders, left eye
			H26.223	Cataract secondary to ocular disorders, bilateral
			H26.229	Cataract secondary to ocular disorders, unsp eye
366.41	DIABETIC CATARACT	▣	**E08.36**	Diabetes due to underlying condition w diabetic cataract
		▣	**E09.36**	Drug/chem diabetes mellitus w diabetic cataract
		▣	**E10.36**	Type 1 diabetes mellitus with diabetic cataract
		▣	**E11.36**	Type 2 diabetes mellitus with diabetic cataract
		▣	**E13.36**	Other specified diabetes mellitus with diabetic cataract
366.42	TETANIC CATARACT		**H28**	Cataract in diseases classified elsewhere
366.43	MYOTONIC CATARACT		**H28**	Cataract in diseases classified elsewhere
366.44	CATARACT ASSOCIATED WITH OTHER SYNDROMES		**H28**	Cataract in diseases classified elsewhere
366.45	TOXIC CATARACT		**H26.30**	Drug-induced cataract, unspecified eye
			H26.31	Drug-induced cataract, right eye
			H26.32	Drug-induced cataract, left eye
			H26.33	Drug-induced cataract, bilateral
366.46	CATARACT ASSOC W/RAD&OTH PHYSICAL INFLUENCES		**H26.8**	Other specified cataract
366.50	UNSPECIFIED AFTER-CATARACT	➡	**H26.40**	Unspecified secondary cataract
366.51	SOEMMERINGS RING		**H26.411**	Soemmering's ring, right eye
			H26.412	Soemmering's ring, left eye
			H26.413	Soemmering's ring, bilateral
			H26.419	Soemmering's ring, unspecified eye
366.52	OTHER AFTER-CATARACT NOT OBSCURING VISION		**H26.491**	Other secondary cataract, right eye
			H26.492	Other secondary cataract, left eye
			H26.493	Other secondary cataract, bilateral
			H26.499	Other secondary cataract, unspecified eye
366.53	AFTER-CATARACT, OBSCURING VISION		**H26.491**	Other secondary cataract, right eye
			H26.492	Other secondary cataract, left eye
			H26.493	Other secondary cataract, bilateral
			H26.499	Other secondary cataract, unspecified eye
366.8	OTHER CATARACT		**H26.8**	Other specified cataract
366.9	UNSPECIFIED CATARACT	➡	**H26.9**	Unspecified cataract
367.0	HYPERMETROPIA		**H52.00**	Hypermetropia, unspecified eye
			H52.01	Hypermetropia, right eye
			H52.02	Hypermetropia, left eye
			H52.03	Hypermetropia, bilateral
367.1	MYOPIA		**H52.10**	Myopia, unspecified eye
			H52.11	Myopia, right eye
			H52.12	Myopia, left eye
			H52.13	Myopia, bilateral
367.20	UNSPECIFIED ASTIGMATISM		**H52.201**	Unspecified astigmatism, right eye
			H52.202	Unspecified astigmatism, left eye
			H52.203	Unspecified astigmatism, bilateral
			H52.209	Unspecified astigmatism, unspecified eye
367.21	REGULAR ASTIGMATISM		**H52.221**	Regular astigmatism, right eye
			H52.222	Regular astigmatism, left eye
			H52.223	Regular astigmatism, bilateral
			H52.229	Regular astigmatism, unspecified eye
367.22	IRREGULAR ASTIGMATISM		**H52.211**	Irregular astigmatism, right eye
			H52.212	Irregular astigmatism, left eye
			H52.213	Irregular astigmatism, bilateral
			H52.219	Irregular astigmatism, unspecified eye
367.31	ANISOMETROPIA	➡	**H52.31**	Anisometropia
367.32	ANISEIKONIA	➡	**H52.32**	Aniseikonia
367.4	PRESBYOPIA	➡	**H52.4**	Presbyopia
367.51	PARESIS OF ACCOMMODATION		**H52.521**	Paresis of accommodation, right eye
			H52.522	Paresis of accommodation, left eye
			H52.523	Paresis of accommodation, bilateral
			H52.529	Paresis of accommodation, unspecified eye

ICD-9-CM		ICD-10-CM	
367.52	TOTAL OR COMPLETE INTERNAL OPHTHALMOPLEGIA	**H52.511**	Internal ophthalmoplegia (complete) (total), right eye
		H52.512	Internal ophthalmoplegia (complete) (total), left eye
		H52.513	Internal ophthalmoplegia (complete) (total), bilateral
		H52.519	Internal ophthalmoplegia (complete) (total), unspecified eye
367.53	SPASM OF ACCOMMODATION	**H52.531**	Spasm of accommodation, right eye
		H52.532	Spasm of accommodation, left eye
		H52.533	Spasm of accommodation, bilateral
		H52.539	Spasm of accommodation, unspecified eye
367.81	TRANSIENT REFRACTIVE CHANGE	**H52.6**	Other disorders of refraction
367.89	OTHER DISORDERS OF REFRACTION AND ACCOMMODATION	**H52.6**	Other disorders of refraction
367.9	UNSPECIFIED DISORDER OF REFRACTION&ACCOMMODATION	➡ **H52.7**	Unspecified disorder of refraction
368.00	UNSPECIFIED AMBLYOPIA	**H53.001**	Unspecified amblyopia, right eye
		H53.002	Unspecified amblyopia, left eye
		H53.003	Unspecified amblyopia, bilateral
		H53.009	Unspecified amblyopia, unspecified eye
368.01	STRABISMIC AMBLYOPIA	**H53.031**	Strabismic amblyopia, right eye
		H53.032	Strabismic amblyopia, left eye
		H53.033	Strabismic amblyopia, bilateral
		H53.039	Strabismic amblyopia, unspecified eye
368.02	DEPRIVATION AMBLYOPIA	**H53.011**	Deprivation amblyopia, right eye
		H53.012	Deprivation amblyopia, left eye
		H53.013	Deprivation amblyopia, bilateral
		H53.019	Deprivation amblyopia, unspecified eye
368.03	REFRACTIVE AMBLYOPIA	**H53.021**	Refractive amblyopia, right eye
		H53.022	Refractive amblyopia, left eye
		H53.023	Refractive amblyopia, bilateral
		H53.029	Refractive amblyopia, unspecified eye
368.10	UNSPECIFIED SUBJECTIVE VISUAL DISTURBANCE	**H53.10**	Unspecified subjective visual disturbances
		H53.11	Day blindness
368.11	SUDDEN VISUAL LOSS	**H53.131**	Sudden visual loss, right eye
		H53.132	Sudden visual loss, left eye
		H53.133	Sudden visual loss, bilateral
		H53.139	Sudden visual loss, unspecified eye
368.12	TRANSIENT VISUAL LOSS	**H53.121**	Transient visual loss, right eye
		H53.122	Transient visual loss, left eye
		H53.123	Transient visual loss, bilateral
		H53.129	Transient visual loss, unspecified eye
368.13	VISUAL DISCOMFORT	**H53.141**	Visual discomfort, right eye
		H53.142	Visual discomfort, left eye
		H53.143	Visual discomfort, bilateral
		H53.149	Visual discomfort, unspecified
368.14	VISUAL DISTORTIONS OF SHAPE AND SIZE	➡ **H53.15**	Visual distortions of shape and size
368.15	OTHER VISUAL DISTORTIONS AND ENTOPTIC PHENOMENA	**H53.19**	Other subjective visual disturbances
368.16	PSYCHOPHYSICAL VISUAL DISTURBANCES	**H53.16**	Psychophysical visual disturbances
		R44.1	Visual hallucinations
		R48.3	Visual agnosia
368.2	DIPLOPIA	➡ **H53.2**	Diplopia
368.30	UNSPECIFIED BINOCULAR VISION DISORDER	➡ **H53.30**	Unspecified disorder of binocular vision
368.31	SUPPRESSION OF BINOCULAR VISION	➡ **H53.34**	Suppression of binocular vision
368.32	SIMULTANEOUS VISUAL PERCEPTION WITHOUT FUSION	➡ **H53.33**	Simultaneous visual perception without fusion
368.33	FUSION WITH DEFECTIVE STEREOPSIS	➡ **H53.32**	Fusion with defective stereopsis
368.34	ABNORMAL RETINAL CORRESPONDENCE	➡ **H53.31**	Abnormal retinal correspondence
368.40	UNSPECIFIED VISUAL FIELD DEFECT	➡ **H53.40**	Unspecified visual field defects
368.41	SCOTOMA INVOLVING CENTRAL AREA IN VISUAL FIELD	**H53.411**	Scotoma involving central area, right eye
		H53.412	Scotoma involving central area, left eye
		H53.413	Scotoma involving central area, bilateral
		H53.419	Scotoma involving central area, unspecified eye
368.42	SCOTOMA OF BLIND SPOT AREA IN VISUAL FIELD	**H53.421**	Scotoma of blind spot area, right eye
		H53.422	Scotoma of blind spot area, left eye
		H53.423	Scotoma of blind spot area, bilateral
		H53.429	Scotoma of blind spot area, unspecified eye
368.43	SECTOR OR ARCUATE DEFECTS IN VISUAL FIELD	**H53.431**	Sector or arcuate defects, right eye
		H53.432	Sector or arcuate defects, left eye
		H53.433	Sector or arcuate defects, bilateral
		H53.439	Sector or arcuate defects, unspecified eye
368.44	OTHER LOCALIZED VISUAL FIELD DEFECT	**H53.451**	Other localized visual field defect, right eye
		H53.452	Other localized visual field defect, left eye
		H53.453	Other localized visual field defect, bilateral
		H53.459	Other localized visual field defect, unspecified eye
368.45	GEN CONTRACTION/CONSTRICTION VISUAL FIELD	**H53.481**	Generalized contraction of visual field, right eye
		H53.482	Generalized contraction of visual field, left eye
		H53.483	Generalized contraction of visual field, bilateral
		H53.489	Generalized contraction of visual field, unspecified eye
368.46	HOMONYMOUS BILATERAL FIELD DEFECTS VISUAL FIELD	**H53.461**	Homonymous bilateral field defects, right side
		H53.462	Homonymous bilateral field defects, left side
		H53.469	Homonymous bilateral field defects, unspecified side

[Brackets] indicate valid character values for each code. Character value meanings provided for each code grouping.

ICD-9-CM			ICD-10-CM	
368.47	HETERONYMOUS BILATERAL FIELD DEFEC VISUAL FIELD	➡	H53.47	Heteronymous bilateral field defects
368.51	PROTAN DEFECT IN COLOR VISION	➡	H53.54	Protanomaly
368.52	DEUTAN DEFECT IN COLOR VISION	➡	H53.53	Deuteranomaly
368.53	TRITAN DEFECT IN COLOR VISION	➡	H53.55	Tritanomaly
368.54	ACHROMATOPSIA	➡	H53.51	Achromatopsia
368.55	ACQUIRED COLOR VISION DEFICIENCIES	➡	H53.52	Acquired color vision deficiency
368.59	OTHER COLOR VISION DEFICIENCIES		H53.50 H53.59	Unspecified color vision deficiencies Other color vision deficiencies
368.60	UNSPECIFIED NIGHT BLINDNESS	➡	H53.60	Unspecified night blindness
368.61	CONGENITAL NIGHT BLINDNESS	➡	H53.63	Congenital night blindness
368.62	ACQUIRED NIGHT BLINDNESS	➡	H53.62	Acquired night blindness
368.63	ABNORMAL DARK ADAPTATION CURVE	➡	H53.61	Abnormal dark adaptation curve
368.69	OTHER NIGHT BLINDNESS	➡	H53.69	Other night blindness
368.8	OTHER SPECIFIED VISUAL DISTURBANCES		H53.71 H53.72 H53.8	Glare sensitivity Impaired contrast sensitivity Other visual disturbances
368.9	UNSPECIFIED VISUAL DISTURBANCE	➡	H53.9	Unspecified visual disturbance
369.00	BLINDNESS BOTH EYES IMPAIR LEVL NOT FURTHER SPEC		H54.0	Blindness, both eyes
369.01	BETR EYE: TOTIMPAIR; LESR EYE: TOT IMPAIR		H54.0	Blindness, both eyes
369.02	BETR EYE: NEAR-TOT IMPAIR; LESR EYE: NFS		H54.10	Blindness, one eye, low vision other eye, unspecified eyes
369.03	BETR EYE: NEAR-TOT IMPAIR; LESR EYE: TOT IMPAIR		H54.10	Blindness, one eye, low vision other eye, unspecified eyes
369.04	BETR EYE: NR-TOTIMPAIR; LESR EYE: NR-TOTIMPAIR		H54.10	Blindness, one eye, low vision other eye, unspecified eyes
369.05	BETR EYE: PROFND IMPAIR; LESR EYE: NFS		H54.10	Blindness, one eye, low vision other eye, unspecified eyes
369.06	BETR EYE: PROFND IMPAIR; LESR EYE: TOT IMPAIR		H54.10	Blindness, one eye, low vision other eye, unspecified eyes
369.07	BETR EYE: PROFND IMPAIR; LESR EYE: NR-TOT IMPAIR		H54.10	Blindness, one eye, low vision other eye, unspecified eyes
369.08	BETR EYE: PROFND IMPAIR; LESR EYE: PROFND IMPAIR		H54.10	Blindness, one eye, low vision other eye, unspecified eyes
369.10	PROFND MOD/SEVERE VISION IMPAIR NOT FURTHER SPEC		H54.10 H54.11 H54.12	Blindness, one eye, low vision other eye, unspecified eyes Blindness, right eye, low vision left eye Blindness, left eye, low vision right eye
369.11	BETR EYE: SEV IMPAIR; LESR EYE: BLIND NFS		H54.10	Blindness, one eye, low vision other eye, unspecified eyes
369.12	BETR EYE: SEV IMPAIR; LESR EYE: TOT IMPAIR		H54.10	Blindness, one eye, low vision other eye, unspecified eyes
369.13	BETR EYE: SEV IMPAIR; LESR EYE: NEAR-TOT IMPAIR		H54.10	Blindness, one eye, low vision other eye, unspecified eyes
369.14	BETR EYE: SEV IMPAIR; LESR EYE: PROFND IMPAIR		H54.10	Blindness, one eye, low vision other eye, unspecified eyes
369.15	BETR EYE: MOD IMPAIR; LESR EYE: BLIND NFS		H54.10	Blindness, one eye, low vision other eye, unspecified eyes
369.16	BETR EYE: MOD IMPAIR; LESR EYE: TOT IMPAIR		H54.10	Blindness, one eye, low vision other eye, unspecified eyes
369.17	BETR EYE: MOD IMPAIR; LESR EYE: NEAR-TOT IMPAIR		H54.10	Blindness, one eye, low vision other eye, unspecified eyes
369.18	BETR EYE: MOD IMPAIR; LESR EYE: PROFND IMPAIR		H54.10	Blindness, one eye, low vision other eye, unspecified eyes
369.20	VISION IMPAIR BOTH EYES IMPAIR LEVEL NFS		H54.2	Low vision, both eyes
369.21	BETR EYE: SEV IMPAIR; LESR EYE; IMPAIR NFS		H54.10	Blindness, one eye, low vision other eye, unspecified eyes
369.22	BETR EYE: SEV IMPAIR; LESR EYE: SEV IMPAIR		H54.10	Blindness, one eye, low vision other eye, unspecified eyes
369.23	BETR EYE: MOD IMPAIR; LESR EYE: IMPAIR NFS		H54.10	Blindness, one eye, low vision other eye, unspecified eyes
369.24	BETR EYE: MOD IMPAIR; LESR EYE: SEV IMPAIR		H54.10	Blindness, one eye, low vision other eye, unspecified eyes
369.25	BETR EYE: MOD IMPAIR; LESR EYE: MOD IMPAIR		H54.2	Low vision, both eyes
369.3	UNQUALIFIED VISUAL LOSS, BOTH EYES	➡	H54.3	Unqualified visual loss, both eyes
369.4	LEGAL BLINDNESS, AS DEFINED IN USA		H54.8	Legal blindness, as defined in USA
369.60	IMPAIRMENT LEVEL NOT FURTHER SPECIFIED		H54.40	Blindness, one eye, unspecified eye
369.61	ONE EYE: TOTAL VISION IMPAIR; OTH EYE: NOT SPEC		H54.41 H54.42	Blindness, right eye, normal vision left eye Blindness, left eye, normal vision right eye
369.62	ONE EYE: TOT VISN IMPAIR; OTH EYE: NR-NL VISN		H54.41 H54.42	Blindness, right eye, normal vision left eye Blindness, left eye, normal vision right eye
369.63	ONE EYE: TOTAL VISION IMPAIR; OTH EYE: NL VISION		H54.41 H54.42	Blindness, right eye, normal vision left eye Blindness, left eye, normal vision right eye
369.64	ONE EYE: NEAR-TOT IMPAIR; OTH EYE: NOT SPEC		H54.41 H54.42	Blindness, right eye, normal vision left eye Blindness, left eye, normal vision right eye
369.65	ONE EYE: NR-TOT VISN IMPAIR; OTH EYE: NR-NL VISN		H54.41 H54.42	Blindness, right eye, normal vision left eye Blindness, left eye, normal vision right eye
369.66	ONE EYE: NR-TOT VISN IMPAIR; OTH EYE: NL VISN		H54.41 H54.42	Blindness, right eye, normal vision left eye Blindness, left eye, normal vision right eye
369.67	ONE EYE: PROFND IMPAIR; OTH EYE:NOT SPEC		H54.41 H54.42	Blindness, right eye, normal vision left eye Blindness, left eye, normal vision right eye
369.68	ONE EYE: PROFND VISN IMPAIR; OTH EYE: NR-NL VISN		H54.41 H54.42	Blindness, right eye, normal vision left eye Blindness, left eye, normal vision right eye
369.69	ONE EYE: PROFND VISN IMPAIR; OTH EYE: NL VISN		H54.41 H54.42	Blindness, right eye, normal vision left eye Blindness, left eye, normal vision right eye
369.70	LOW VISION ONE EYE NOT OTHERWISE SPECIFIED		H54.50 H54.51 H54.52	Low vision, one eye, unspecified eye Low vision, right eye, normal vision left eye Low vision, left eye, normal vision right eye
369.71	ONE EYE: SEV VISN IMPAIR; OTH EYE: VISN NOT SPEC		H54.40	Blindness, one eye, unspecified eye
369.72	ONE EYE: SEV VISN IMPAIR; OTH EYE: NR-NL VISN		H54.40	Blindness, one eye, unspecified eye
369.73	ONE EYE: SEV VISION IMPAIR; OTH EYE: NL VISION		H54.40	Blindness, one eye, unspecified eye

ICD-9-CM		ICD-10-CM	
369.74	ONE EYE: MOD VISN IMPAIR; OTH EYE: VISN NOT SPEC	**H54.50**	Low vision, one eye, unspecified eye
369.75	ONE EYE: MOD VISN IMPAIR; OTH EYE: NR-NL VISN	**H54.50**	Low vision, one eye, unspecified eye
369.76	ONE EYE: MOD VISION IMPAIR; OTH EYE: NL VISION	**H54.50**	Low vision, one eye, unspecified eye
369.8	UNQUALIFIED VISUAL LOSS, ONE EYE	**H54.60**	Unqualified visual loss, one eye, unspecified
		H54.61	Unqualified visual loss, right eye, normal vision left eye
		H54.62	Unqualified visual loss, left eye, normal vision right eye
369.9	UNSPECIFIED VISUAL LOSS	**H54.7**	Unspecified visual loss
370.00	UNSPECIFIED CORNEAL ULCER	**H16.001**	Unspecified corneal ulcer, right eye
		H16.002	Unspecified corneal ulcer, left eye
		H16.003	Unspecified corneal ulcer, bilateral
		H16.009	Unspecified corneal ulcer, unspecified eye
370.01	MARGINAL CORNEAL ULCER	**H16.041**	Marginal corneal ulcer, right eye
		H16.042	Marginal corneal ulcer, left eye
		H16.043	Marginal corneal ulcer, bilateral
		H16.049	Marginal corneal ulcer, unspecified eye
370.02	RING CORNEAL ULCER	**H16.021**	Ring corneal ulcer, right eye
		H16.022	Ring corneal ulcer, left eye
		H16.023	Ring corneal ulcer, bilateral
		H16.029	Ring corneal ulcer, unspecified eye
370.03	CENTRAL CORNEAL ULCER	**H16.011**	Central corneal ulcer, right eye
		H16.012	Central corneal ulcer, left eye
		H16.013	Central corneal ulcer, bilateral
		H16.019	Central corneal ulcer, unspecified eye
370.04	HYPOPYON ULCER	**H16.031**	Corneal ulcer with hypopyon, right eye
		H16.032	Corneal ulcer with hypopyon, left eye
		H16.033	Corneal ulcer with hypopyon, bilateral
		H16.039	Corneal ulcer with hypopyon, unspecified eye
370.05	MYCOTIC CORNEAL ULCER	**H16.061**	Mycotic corneal ulcer, right eye
		H16.062	Mycotic corneal ulcer, left eye
		H16.063	Mycotic corneal ulcer, bilateral
		H16.069	Mycotic corneal ulcer, unspecified eye
370.06	PERFORATED CORNEAL ULCER	**H16.071**	Perforated corneal ulcer, right eye
		H16.072	Perforated corneal ulcer, left eye
		H16.073	Perforated corneal ulcer, bilateral
		H16.079	Perforated corneal ulcer, unspecified eye
370.07	MOORENS ULCER	**H16.051**	Mooren's corneal ulcer, right eye
		H16.052	Mooren's corneal ulcer, left eye
		H16.053	Mooren's corneal ulcer, bilateral
		H16.059	Mooren's corneal ulcer, unspecified eye
370.20	UNSPECIFIED SUPERFICIAL KERATITIS	**H16.101**	Unspecified superficial keratitis, right eye
		H16.102	Unspecified superficial keratitis, left eye
		H16.103	Unspecified superficial keratitis, bilateral
		H16.109	Unspecified superficial keratitis, unspecified eye
370.21	PUNCTATE KERATITIS	**H16.141**	Punctate keratitis, right eye
		H16.142	Punctate keratitis, left eye
		H16.143	Punctate keratitis, bilateral
		H16.149	Punctate keratitis, unspecified eye
370.22	MACULAR KERATITIS	**H16.111**	Macular keratitis, right eye
		H16.112	Macular keratitis, left eye
		H16.113	Macular keratitis, bilateral
		H16.119	Macular keratitis, unspecified eye
370.23	FILAMENTARY KERATITIS	**H16.121**	Filamentary keratitis, right eye
		H16.122	Filamentary keratitis, left eye
		H16.123	Filamentary keratitis, bilateral
		H16.129	Filamentary keratitis, unspecified eye
370.24	PHOTOKERATITIS	**H16.131**	Photokeratitis, right eye
		H16.132	Photokeratitis, left eye
		H16.133	Photokeratitis, bilateral
		H16.139	Photokeratitis, unspecified eye
370.31	PHLYCTENULAR KERATOCONJUNCTIVITIS	**A18.52**	Tuberculous keratitis
		H16.251	Phlyctenular keratoconjunctivitis, right eye
		H16.252	Phlyctenular keratoconjunctivitis, left eye
		H16.253	Phlyctenular keratoconjunctivitis, bilateral
		H16.259	Phlyctenular keratoconjunctivitis, unspecified eye
370.32	LIMBAR&CORNEAL INVOLVEMENT VERNAL CONJUNCTIVITIS	**H16.261**	Vernal keratoconjunct, w limbar and corneal involv, r eye
		H16.262	Vernal keratoconjunct, w limbar and corneal involv, left eye
		H16.263	Vernal keratoconjunct, w limbar and corneal involv, bi
		H16.269	Vernal keratoconjunct, w limbar and corneal involv, unsp eye
370.33	KERATOCONJUNCTIVITIS SICCA NOT SPEC AS SJOGRENS	**H16.221**	Keratoconjunct sicca, not specified as Sjogren's, right eye
		H16.222	Keratoconjunct sicca, not specified as Sjogren's, left eye
		H16.223	Keratoconjunct sicca, not specified as Sjogren's, bilateral
		H16.229	Keratoconjunct sicca, not specified as Sjogren's, unsp eye
370.34	EXPOSURE KERATOCONJUNCTIVITIS	**H16.211**	Exposure keratoconjunctivitis, right eye
		H16.212	Exposure keratoconjunctivitis, left eye
		H16.213	Exposure keratoconjunctivitis, bilateral
		H16.219	Exposure keratoconjunctivitis, unspecified eye

[Brackets] indicate valid character values for each code. Character value meanings provided for each code grouping.

ICD-9-CM			ICD-10-CM	
370.35	NEUROTROPHIC KERATOCONJUNCTIVITIS		**H16.231**	Neurotrophic keratoconjunctivitis, right eye
			H16.232	Neurotrophic keratoconjunctivitis, left eye
			H16.233	Neurotrophic keratoconjunctivitis, bilateral
			H16.239	Neurotrophic keratoconjunctivitis, unspecified eye
370.40	UNSPECIFIED KERATOCONJUNCTIVITIS		**H16.201**	Unspecified keratoconjunctivitis, right eye
			H16.202	Unspecified keratoconjunctivitis, left eye
			H16.203	Unspecified keratoconjunctivitis, bilateral
			H16.209	Unspecified keratoconjunctivitis, unspecified eye
370.44	KERATITIS OR KERATOCONJUNCTIVITIS IN EXANTHEMA		**H16.291**	Other keratoconjunctivitis, right eye
			H16.292	Other keratoconjunctivitis, left eye
			H16.293	Other keratoconjunctivitis, bilateral
			H16.299	Other keratoconjunctivitis, unspecified eye
370.49	OTHER UNSPECIFIED KERATOCONJUNCTIVITIS		**H16.291**	Other keratoconjunctivitis, right eye
			H16.292	Other keratoconjunctivitis, left eye
			H16.293	Other keratoconjunctivitis, bilateral
			H16.299	Other keratoconjunctivitis, unspecified eye
370.50	UNSPECIFIED INTERSTITIAL KERATITIS		**H16.301**	Unspecified interstitial keratitis, right eye
			H16.302	Unspecified interstitial keratitis, left eye
			H16.303	Unspecified interstitial keratitis, bilateral
			H16.309	Unspecified interstitial keratitis, unspecified eye
370.52	DIFFUSE INTERSTITIAL KERATITIS		**H16.321**	Diffuse interstitial keratitis, right eye
			H16.322	Diffuse interstitial keratitis, left eye
			H16.323	Diffuse interstitial keratitis, bilateral
			H16.329	Diffuse interstitial keratitis, unspecified eye
370.54	SCLEROSING KERATITIS		**H16.331**	Sclerosing keratitis, right eye
			H16.332	Sclerosing keratitis, left eye
			H16.333	Sclerosing keratitis, bilateral
			H16.339	Sclerosing keratitis, unspecified eye
370.55	CORNEAL ABSCESS		**H16.311**	Corneal abscess, right eye
			H16.312	Corneal abscess, left eye
			H16.313	Corneal abscess, bilateral
			H16.319	Corneal abscess, unspecified eye
370.59	OTHER INTERSTITIAL AND DEEP KERATITIS	◻	**A18.52**	Tuberculous keratitis
			H16.391	Other interstitial and deep keratitis, right eye
			H16.392	Other interstitial and deep keratitis, left eye
			H16.393	Other interstitial and deep keratitis, bilateral
			H16.399	Other interstitial and deep keratitis, unspecified eye
370.60	UNSPECIFIED CORNEAL NEOVASCULARIZATION		**H16.401**	Unspecified corneal neovascularization, right eye
			H16.402	Unspecified corneal neovascularization, left eye
			H16.403	Unspecified corneal neovascularization, bilateral
			H16.409	Unspecified corneal neovascularization, unspecified eye
370.61	LOCALIZED VASCULARIZATION OF CORNEA		**H16.431**	Localized vascularization of cornea, right eye
			H16.432	Localized vascularization of cornea, left eye
			H16.433	Localized vascularization of cornea, bilateral
			H16.439	Localized vascularization of cornea, unspecified eye
370.62	PANNUS		**H16.421**	Pannus (corneal), right eye
			H16.422	Pannus (corneal), left eye
			H16.423	Pannus (corneal), bilateral
			H16.429	Pannus (corneal), unspecified eye
370.63	DEEP VASCULARIZATION OF CORNEA		**H16.441**	Deep vascularization of cornea, right eye
			H16.442	Deep vascularization of cornea, left eye
			H16.443	Deep vascularization of cornea, bilateral
			H16.449	Deep vascularization of cornea, unspecified eye
370.64	GHOST VESSELS IN CORNEAL NEOVASCULARIZATION		**H16.411**	Ghost vessels (corneal), right eye
			H16.412	Ghost vessels (corneal), left eye
			H16.413	Ghost vessels (corneal), bilateral
			H16.419	Ghost vessels (corneal), unspecified eye
370.8	OTHER FORMS OF KERATITIS	◻	**B60.13**	Keratoconjunctivitis due to Acanthamoeba
			H16.8	Other keratitis
370.9	UNSPECIFIED KERATITIS	➡	**H16.9**	Unspecified keratitis
371.00	UNSPECIFIED CORNEAL OPACITY		**H17.89**	Other corneal scars and opacities
			H17.9	Unspecified corneal scar and opacity
371.01	MINOR OPACITY OF CORNEA		**H17.811**	Minor opacity of cornea, right eye
			H17.812	Minor opacity of cornea, left eye
			H17.813	Minor opacity of cornea, bilateral
			H17.819	Minor opacity of cornea, unspecified eye
371.02	PERIPHERAL OPACITY OF CORNEA		**H17.821**	Peripheral opacity of cornea, right eye
			H17.822	Peripheral opacity of cornea, left eye
			H17.823	Peripheral opacity of cornea, bilateral
			H17.829	Peripheral opacity of cornea, unspecified eye
371.03	CENTRAL OPACITY OF CORNEA		**H17.10**	Central corneal opacity, unspecified eye
			H17.11	Central corneal opacity, right eye
			H17.12	Central corneal opacity, left eye
			H17.13	Central corneal opacity, bilateral
371.04	ADHERENT LEUCOMA		**H17.00**	Adherent leukoma, unspecified eye
			H17.01	Adherent leukoma, right eye
			H17.02	Adherent leukoma, left eye
			H17.03	Adherent leukoma, bilateral

ICD-9-CM		ICD-10-CM	
371.05	PHTHISICAL CORNEA	A18.59	Other tuberculosis of eye
371.10	UNSPECIFIED CORNEAL DEPOSIT	H18.001	Unspecified corneal deposit, right eye
		H18.002	Unspecified corneal deposit, left eye
		H18.003	Unspecified corneal deposit, bilateral
		H18.009	Unspecified corneal deposit, unspecified eye
371.11	ANTERIOR PIGMENTATIONS OF CORNEA	H18.011	Anterior corneal pigmentations, right eye
		H18.012	Anterior corneal pigmentations, left eye
		H18.013	Anterior corneal pigmentations, bilateral
		H18.019	Anterior corneal pigmentations, unspecified eye
371.12	STROMAL PIGMENTATIONS OF CORNEA	H18.061	Stromal corneal pigmentations, right eye
		H18.062	Stromal corneal pigmentations, left eye
		H18.063	Stromal corneal pigmentations, bilateral
		H18.069	Stromal corneal pigmentations, unspecified eye
371.13	POSTERIOR PIGMENTATIONS OF CORNEA	H18.051	Posterior corneal pigmentations, right eye
		H18.052	Posterior corneal pigmentations, left eye
		H18.053	Posterior corneal pigmentations, bilateral
		H18.059	Posterior corneal pigmentations, unspecified eye
371.14	KAYSER-FLEISCHER RING	H18.041	Kayser-Fleischer ring, right eye
		H18.042	Kayser-Fleischer ring, left eye
		H18.043	Kayser-Fleischer ring, bilateral
		H18.049	Kayser-Fleischer ring, unspecified eye
371.15	OTH DEPOSITS CORNEA ASSOC W/METABOLIC DISORDERS	H18.031	Corneal deposits in metabolic disorders, right eye
		H18.032	Corneal deposits in metabolic disorders, left eye
		H18.033	Corneal deposits in metabolic disorders, bilateral
		H18.039	Corneal deposits in metabolic disorders, unspecified eye
371.16	ARGENTOUS DEPOSITS OF CORNEA	H18.021	Argentous corneal deposits, right eye
		H18.022	Argentous corneal deposits, left eye
		H18.023	Argentous corneal deposits, bilateral
		H18.029	Argentous corneal deposits, unspecified eye
371.20	UNSPECIFIED CORNEAL EDEMA	➡ H18.20	Unspecified corneal edema
371.21	IDIOPATHIC CORNEAL EDEMA	H18.221	Idiopathic corneal edema, right eye
		H18.222	Idiopathic corneal edema, left eye
		H18.223	Idiopathic corneal edema, bilateral
		H18.229	Idiopathic corneal edema, unspecified eye
371.22	SECONDARY CORNEAL EDEMA	H18.231	Secondary corneal edema, right eye
		H18.232	Secondary corneal edema, left eye
		H18.233	Secondary corneal edema, bilateral
		H18.239	Secondary corneal edema, unspecified eye
371.23	BULLOUS KERATOPATHY	H18.10	Bullous keratopathy, unspecified eye
		H18.11	Bullous keratopathy, right eye
		H18.12	Bullous keratopathy, left eye
		H18.13	Bullous keratopathy, bilateral
371.24	CORNEAL EDEMA DUE TO WEARING OF CONTACT LENSES	H18.211	Corneal edema secondary to contact lens, right eye
		H18.212	Corneal edema secondary to contact lens, left eye
		H18.213	Corneal edema secondary to contact lens, bilateral
		H18.219	Corneal edema secondary to contact lens, unspecified eye
371.30	UNSPECIFIED CORNEAL MEMBRANE CHANGE	➡ H18.30	Unspecified corneal membrane change
371.31	FOLDS AND RUPTURE OF BOWMANS MEMBRANE	H18.311	Folds and rupture in Bowman's membrane, right eye
		H18.312	Folds and rupture in Bowman's membrane, left eye
		H18.313	Folds and rupture in Bowman's membrane, bilateral
		H18.319	Folds and rupture in Bowman's membrane, unspecified eye
371.32	FOLDS IN DESCEMETS MEMBRANE	H18.321	Folds in Descemet's membrane, right eye
		H18.322	Folds in Descemet's membrane, left eye
		H18.323	Folds in Descemet's membrane, bilateral
		H18.329	Folds in Descemet's membrane, unspecified eye
371.33	RUPTURE IN DESCEMETS MEMBRANE	H18.331	Rupture in Descemet's membrane, right eye
		H18.332	Rupture in Descemet's membrane, left eye
		H18.333	Rupture in Descemet's membrane, bilateral
		H18.339	Rupture in Descemet's membrane, unspecified eye
371.40	UNSPECIFIED CORNEAL DEGENERATION	➡ H18.40	Unspecified corneal degeneration
371.41	SENILE CORNEAL CHANGES	H18.411	Arcus senilis, right eye
		H18.412	Arcus senilis, left eye
		H18.413	Arcus senilis, bilateral
		H18.419	Arcus senilis, unspecified eye
371.42	RECURRENT EROSION OF CORNEA	H18.831	Recurrent erosion of cornea, right eye
		H18.832	Recurrent erosion of cornea, left eye
		H18.833	Recurrent erosion of cornea, bilateral
		H18.839	Recurrent erosion of cornea, unspecified eye
371.43	BAND-SHAPED KERATOPATHY	H18.421	Band keratopathy, right eye
		H18.422	Band keratopathy, left eye
		H18.423	Band keratopathy, bilateral
		H18.429	Band keratopathy, unspecified eye
371.44	OTHER CALCEROUS DEGENERATIONS OF CORNEA	➡ H18.43	Other calcerous corneal degeneration
371.45	KERATOMALACIA NOS	H18.441	Keratomalacia, right eye
		H18.442	Keratomalacia, left eye
		H18.443	Keratomalacia, bilateral
		H18.449	Keratomalacia, unspecified eye

ICD-9-CM			ICD-10-CM	
371.46	NODULAR DEGENERATION OF CORNEA		**H18.451**	Nodular corneal degeneration, right eye
			H18.452	Nodular corneal degeneration, left eye
			H18.453	Nodular corneal degeneration, bilateral
			H18.459	Nodular corneal degeneration, unspecified eye
371.48	PERIPHERAL DEGENERATIONS OF CORNEA		**H18.461**	Peripheral corneal degeneration, right eye
			H18.462	Peripheral corneal degeneration, left eye
			H18.463	Peripheral corneal degeneration, bilateral
			H18.469	Peripheral corneal degeneration, unspecified eye
371.49	OTHER CORNEAL DEGENERATIONS		**H18.49**	Other corneal degeneration
371.50	UNSPECIFIED HEREDITARY CORNEAL DYSTROPHY	➡	**H18.50**	Unspecified hereditary corneal dystrophies
371.51	JUVENILE EPITHELIAL CORNEAL DYSTROPHY	➡	**H18.52**	Epithelial (juvenile) corneal dystrophy
371.52	OTHER ANTERIOR CORNEAL DYSTROPHIES		**H18.59**	Other hereditary corneal dystrophies
371.53	GRANULAR CORNEAL DYSTROPHY	➡	**H18.53**	Granular corneal dystrophy
371.54	LATTICE CORNEAL DYSTROPHY	➡	**H18.54**	Lattice corneal dystrophy
371.55	MACULAR CORNEAL DYSTROPHY	➡	**H18.55**	Macular corneal dystrophy
371.56	OTHER STROMAL CORNEAL DYSTROPHIES		**H18.59**	Other hereditary corneal dystrophies
371.57	ENDOTHELIAL CORNEAL DYSTROPHY	➡	**H18.51**	Endothelial corneal dystrophy
371.58	OTHER POSTERIOR CORNEAL DYSTROPHIES		**H18.59**	Other hereditary corneal dystrophies
371.60	UNSPECIFIED KERATOCONUS		**H18.601**	Keratoconus, unspecified, right eye
			H18.602	Keratoconus, unspecified, left eye
			H18.603	Keratoconus, unspecified, bilateral
			H18.609	Keratoconus, unspecified, unspecified eye
371.61	KERATOCONUS, STABLE CONDITION		**H18.611**	Keratoconus, stable, right eye
			H18.612	Keratoconus, stable, left eye
			H18.613	Keratoconus, stable, bilateral
			H18.619	Keratoconus, stable, unspecified eye
371.62	KERATOCONUS, ACUTE HYDROPS		**H18.621**	Keratoconus, unstable, right eye
			H18.622	Keratoconus, unstable, left eye
			H18.623	Keratoconus, unstable, bilateral
			H18.629	Keratoconus, unstable, unspecified eye
371.70	UNSPECIFIED CORNEAL DEFORMITY		**H18.70**	Unspecified corneal deformity
			H18.791	Other corneal deformities, right eye
			H18.792	Other corneal deformities, left eye
			H18.793	Other corneal deformities, bilateral
			H18.799	Other corneal deformities, unspecified eye
371.71	CORNEAL ECTASIA		**H18.711**	Corneal ectasia, right eye
			H18.712	Corneal ectasia, left eye
			H18.713	Corneal ectasia, bilateral
			H18.719	Corneal ectasia, unspecified eye
371.72	DESCEMETOCELE		**H18.731**	Descemetocele, right eye
			H18.732	Descemetocele, left eye
			H18.733	Descemetocele, bilateral
			H18.739	Descemetocele, unspecified eye
371.73	CORNEAL STAPHYLOMA		**H18.721**	Corneal staphyloma, right eye
			H18.722	Corneal staphyloma, left eye
			H18.723	Corneal staphyloma, bilateral
			H18.729	Corneal staphyloma, unspecified eye
371.81	CORNEAL ANESTHESIA AND HYPOESTHESIA		**H18.811**	Anesthesia and hypoesthesia of cornea, right eye
			H18.812	Anesthesia and hypoesthesia of cornea, left eye
			H18.813	Anesthesia and hypoesthesia of cornea, bilateral
			H18.819	Anesthesia and hypoesthesia of cornea, unspecified eye
371.82	CORNEAL DISORDER DUE TO CONTACT LENS		**H18.821**	Corneal disorder due to contact lens, right eye
			H18.822	Corneal disorder due to contact lens, left eye
			H18.823	Corneal disorder due to contact lens, bilateral
			H18.829	Corneal disorder due to contact lens, unspecified eye
371.89	OTHER CORNEAL DISORDER		**H18.891**	Other specified disorders of cornea, right eye
			H18.892	Other specified disorders of cornea, left eye
			H18.893	Other specified disorders of cornea, bilateral
			H18.899	Other specified disorders of cornea, unspecified eye
371.9	UNSPECIFIED CORNEAL DISORDER	➡	**H18.9**	Unspecified disorder of cornea
372.00	UNSPECIFIED ACUTE CONJUNCTIVITIS		**H10.30**	Unspecified acute conjunctivitis, unspecified eye
			H10.31	Unspecified acute conjunctivitis, right eye
			H10.32	Unspecified acute conjunctivitis, left eye
			H10.33	Unspecified acute conjunctivitis, bilateral
372.01	SEROUS CONJUNCTIVITIS, EXCEPT VIRAL		**H10.231**	Serous conjunctivitis, except viral, right eye
			H10.232	Serous conjunctivitis, except viral, left eye
			H10.233	Serous conjunctivitis, except viral, bilateral
			H10.239	Serous conjunctivitis, except viral, unspecified eye
372.02	ACUTE FOLLICULAR CONJUNCTIVITIS		**H10.011**	Acute follicular conjunctivitis, right eye
			H10.012	Acute follicular conjunctivitis, left eye
			H10.013	Acute follicular conjunctivitis, bilateral
			H10.019	Acute follicular conjunctivitis, unspecified eye
372.03	OTHER MUCOPURULENT CONJUNCTIVITIS		**H10.021**	Other mucopurulent conjunctivitis, right eye
			H10.022	Other mucopurulent conjunctivitis, left eye
			H10.023	Other mucopurulent conjunctivitis, bilateral
			H10.029	Other mucopurulent conjunctivitis, unspecified eye

ICD-9-CM		ICD-10-CM	
372.04	PSEUDOMEMBRANOUS CONJUNCTIVITIS	**H10.221**	Pseudomembranous conjunctivitis, right eye
		H10.222	Pseudomembranous conjunctivitis, left eye
		H10.223	Pseudomembranous conjunctivitis, bilateral
		H10.229	Pseudomembranous conjunctivitis, unspecified eye
372.05	ACUTE ATOPIC CONJUNCTIVITIS	**H10.10**	Acute atopic conjunctivitis, unspecified eye
		H10.11	Acute atopic conjunctivitis, right eye
		H10.12	Acute atopic conjunctivitis, left eye
		H10.13	Acute atopic conjunctivitis, bilateral
372.06	ACUTE CHEMICAL CONJUNCTIVITIS	**H10.211**	Acute toxic conjunctivitis, right eye
		H10.212	Acute toxic conjunctivitis, left eye
		H10.213	Acute toxic conjunctivitis, bilateral
		H10.219	Acute toxic conjunctivitis, unspecified eye
372.10	UNSPECIFIED CHRONIC CONJUNCTIVITIS	**H10.401**	Unspecified chronic conjunctivitis, right eye
		H10.402	Unspecified chronic conjunctivitis, left eye
		H10.403	Unspecified chronic conjunctivitis, bilateral
		H10.409	Unspecified chronic conjunctivitis, unspecified eye
372.11	SIMPLE CHRONIC CONJUNCTIVITIS	**H10.421**	Simple chronic conjunctivitis, right eye
		H10.422	Simple chronic conjunctivitis, left eye
		H10.423	Simple chronic conjunctivitis, bilateral
		H10.429	Simple chronic conjunctivitis, unspecified eye
372.12	CHRONIC FOLLICULAR CONJUNCTIVITIS	**H10.431**	Chronic follicular conjunctivitis, right eye
		H10.432	Chronic follicular conjunctivitis, left eye
		H10.433	Chronic follicular conjunctivitis, bilateral
		H10.439	Chronic follicular conjunctivitis, unspecified eye
372.13	VERNAL CONJUNCTIVITIS	**H10.44**	Vernal conjunctivitis
		H16.261	Vernal keratoconjunct, w limbar and corneal involv, r eye
		H16.262	Vernal keratoconjunct, w limbar and corneal involv, left eye
		H16.263	Vernal keratoconjunct, w limbar and corneal involv, bi
		H16.269	Vernal keratoconjunct, w limbar and corneal involv, unsp eye
372.14	OTHER CHRONIC ALLERGIC CONJUNCTIVITIS	**H10.411**	Chronic giant papillary conjunctivitis, right eye
		H10.412	Chronic giant papillary conjunctivitis, left eye
		H10.413	Chronic giant papillary conjunctivitis, bilateral
		H10.419	Chronic giant papillary conjunctivitis, unspecified eye
		H10.45	Other chronic allergic conjunctivitis
372.15	PARASITIC CONJUNCTIVITIS	**B60.12**	Conjunctivitis due to Acanthamoeba
		H10.89	Other conjunctivitis
372.20	UNSPECIFIED BLEPHAROCONJUNCTIVITIS	**H10.501**	Unspecified blepharoconjunctivitis, right eye
		H10.502	Unspecified blepharoconjunctivitis, left eye
		H10.503	Unspecified blepharoconjunctivitis, bilateral
		H10.509	Unspecified blepharoconjunctivitis, unspecified eye
372.21	ANGULAR BLEPHAROCONJUNCTIVITIS	**H10.521**	Angular blepharoconjunctivitis, right eye
		H10.522	Angular blepharoconjunctivitis, left eye
		H10.523	Angular blepharoconjunctivitis, bilateral
		H10.529	Angular blepharoconjunctivitis, unspecified eye
372.22	CONTACT BLEPHAROCONJUNCTIVITIS	**H10.531**	Contact blepharoconjunctivitis, right eye
		H10.532	Contact blepharoconjunctivitis, left eye
		H10.533	Contact blepharoconjunctivitis, bilateral
		H10.539	Contact blepharoconjunctivitis, unspecified eye
372.30	UNSPECIFIED CONJUNCTIVITIS	**H10.9**	Unspecified conjunctivitis
372.31	ROSACEA CONJUNCTIVITIS	**H10.89**	Other conjunctivitis
372.33	CONJUNCTIVITIS IN MUCOCUTANEOUS DISEASE	**H10.89**	Other conjunctivitis
372.34	PINGUECULITIS	**H10.811**	Pingueculitis, right eye
		H10.812	Pingueculitis, left eye
		H10.813	Pingueculitis, bilateral
		H10.819	Pingueculitis, unspecified eye
372.39	OTHER AND UNSPECIFIED CONJUNCTIVITIS	**H10.511**	Ligneous conjunctivitis, right eye
		H10.512	Ligneous conjunctivitis, left eye
		H10.513	Ligneous conjunctivitis, bilateral
		H10.519	Ligneous conjunctivitis, unspecified eye
		H10.89	Other conjunctivitis
372.40	UNSPECIFIED PTERYGIUM	**H11.001**	Unspecified pterygium of right eye
		H11.002	Unspecified pterygium of left eye
		H11.003	Unspecified pterygium of eye, bilateral
		H11.009	Unspecified pterygium of unspecified eye
		H11.011	Amyloid pterygium of right eye
		H11.012	Amyloid pterygium of left eye
		H11.013	Amyloid pterygium of eye, bilateral
		H11.019	Amyloid pterygium of unspecified eye
372.41	PERIPHERAL PTERGIUM, STATIONARY	**H11.041**	Peripheral pterygium, stationary, right eye
		H11.042	Peripheral pterygium, stationary, left eye
		H11.043	Peripheral pterygium, stationary, bilateral
		H11.049	Peripheral pterygium, stationary, unspecified eye
372.42	PERIPHERAL PTERYGIUM, PROGRESSIVE	**H11.051**	Peripheral pterygium, progressive, right eye
		H11.052	Peripheral pterygium, progressive, left eye
		H11.053	Peripheral pterygium, progressive, bilateral
		H11.059	Peripheral pterygium, progressive, unspecified eye

ICD-9-CM		ICD-10-CM	
372.43	CENTRAL PTERYGIUM	**H11.021**	Central pterygium of right eye
		H11.022	Central pterygium of left eye
		H11.023	Central pterygium of eye, bilateral
		H11.029	Central pterygium of unspecified eye
372.44	DOUBLE PTERYGIUM	**H11.031**	Double pterygium of right eye
		H11.032	Double pterygium of left eye
		H11.033	Double pterygium of eye, bilateral
		H11.039	Double pterygium of unspecified eye
372.45	RECURRENT PTERYGIUM	**H11.061**	Recurrent pterygium of right eye
		H11.062	Recurrent pterygium of left eye
		H11.063	Recurrent pterygium of eye, bilateral
		H11.069	Recurrent pterygium of unspecified eye
372.50	UNSPECIFIED CONJUNCTIVAL DEGENERATION	➡ **H11.10**	Unspecified conjunctival degenerations
372.51	PINGUECULA	**H11.151**	Pinguecula, right eye
		H11.152	Pinguecula, left eye
		H11.153	Pinguecula, bilateral
		H11.159	Pinguecula, unspecified eye
372.52	PSEUDOPTERYGIUM	**H11.811**	Pseudopterygium of conjunctiva, right eye
		H11.812	Pseudopterygium of conjunctiva, left eye
		H11.813	Pseudopterygium of conjunctiva, bilateral
		H11.819	Pseudopterygium of conjunctiva, unspecified eye
372.53	CONJUNCTIVAL XEROSIS	**H11.141**	Conjunctival xerosis, unspecified, right eye
		H11.142	Conjunctival xerosis, unspecified, left eye
		H11.143	Conjunctival xerosis, unspecified, bilateral
		H11.149	Conjunctival xerosis, unspecified, unspecified eye
372.54	CONJUNCTIVAL CONCRETIONS	**H11.121**	Conjunctival concretions, right eye
		H11.122	Conjunctival concretions, left eye
		H11.123	Conjunctival concretions, bilateral
		H11.129	Conjunctival concretions, unspecified eye
372.55	CONJUNCTIVAL PIGMENTATIONS	**H11.131**	Conjunctival pigmentations, right eye
		H11.132	Conjunctival pigmentations, left eye
		H11.133	Conjunctival pigmentations, bilateral
		H11.139	Conjunctival pigmentations, unspecified eye
372.56	CONJUNCTIVAL DEPOSITS	**H11.111**	Conjunctival deposits, right eye
		H11.112	Conjunctival deposits, left eye
		H11.113	Conjunctival deposits, bilateral
		H11.119	Conjunctival deposits, unspecified eye
372.61	GRANULOMA OF CONJUNCTIVA	**H11.221**	Conjunctival granuloma, right eye
		H11.222	Conjunctival granuloma, left eye
		H11.223	Conjunctival granuloma, bilateral
		H11.229	Conjunctival granuloma, unspecified
372.62	LOCALIZED ADHESIONS AND STRANDS OF CONJUNCTIVA	**H11.211**	Conjunctival adhesions and strands (localized), right eye
		H11.212	Conjunctival adhesions and strands (localized), left eye
		H11.213	Conjunctival adhesions and strands (localized), bilateral
		H11.219	Conjunctival adhesions and strands (localized), unsp eye
372.63	SYMBLEPHARON	**H11.231**	Symblepharon, right eye
		H11.232	Symblepharon, left eye
		H11.233	Symblepharon, bilateral
		H11.239	Symblepharon, unspecified eye
372.64	SCARRING OF CONJUNCTIVA	**H11.241**	Scarring of conjunctiva, right eye
		H11.242	Scarring of conjunctiva, left eye
		H11.243	Scarring of conjunctiva, bilateral
		H11.249	Scarring of conjunctiva, unspecified eye
372.71	HYPEREMIA OF CONJUNCTIVA	**H11.431**	Conjunctival hyperemia, right eye
		H11.432	Conjunctival hyperemia, left eye
		H11.433	Conjunctival hyperemia, bilateral
		H11.439	Conjunctival hyperemia, unspecified eye
372.72	CONJUNCTIVAL HEMORRHAGE	**H11.30**	Conjunctival hemorrhage, unspecified eye
		H11.31	Conjunctival hemorrhage, right eye
		H11.32	Conjunctival hemorrhage, left eye
		H11.33	Conjunctival hemorrhage, bilateral
372.73	CONJUNCTIVAL EDEMA	**H11.421**	Conjunctival edema, right eye
		H11.422	Conjunctival edema, left eye
		H11.423	Conjunctival edema, bilateral
		H11.429	Conjunctival edema, unspecified eye
372.74	VASCULAR ABNORMALITIES OF CONJUNCTIVA	**H11.411**	Vascular abnormalities of conjunctiva, right eye
		H11.412	Vascular abnormalities of conjunctiva, left eye
		H11.413	Vascular abnormalities of conjunctiva, bilateral
		H11.419	Vascular abnormalities of conjunctiva, unspecified eye
372.75	CONJUNCTIVAL CYSTS	**H11.441**	Conjunctival cysts, right eye
		H11.442	Conjunctival cysts, left eye
		H11.443	Conjunctival cysts, bilateral
		H11.449	Conjunctival cysts, unspecified eye
372.81	CONJUNCTIVOCHALASIS	**H11.821**	Conjunctivochalasis, right eye
		H11.822	Conjunctivochalasis, left eye
		H11.823	Conjunctivochalasis, bilateral
		H11.829	Conjunctivochalasis, unspecified eye
372.89	OTHER DISORDERS OF CONJUNCTIVA	**H11.89**	Other specified disorders of conjunctiva

ICD-9-CM		ICD-10-CM	
372.9	UNSPECIFIED DISORDER OF CONJUNCTIVA	➡ H11.9	Unspecified disorder of conjunctiva
373.00	BLEPHARITIS, UNSPECIFIED	H01.001	Unspecified blepharitis right upper eyelid
		H01.002	Unspecified blepharitis right lower eyelid
		H01.003	Unspecified blepharitis right eye, unspecified eyelid
		H01.004	Unspecified blepharitis left upper eyelid
		H01.005	Unspecified blepharitis left lower eyelid
		H01.006	Unspecified blepharitis left eye, unspecified eyelid
		H01.009	Unspecified blepharitis unspecified eye, unspecified eyelid
373.01	ULCERATIVE BLEPHARITIS	H01.011	Ulcerative blepharitis right upper eyelid
		H01.012	Ulcerative blepharitis right lower eyelid
		H01.013	Ulcerative blepharitis right eye, unspecified eyelid
		H01.014	Ulcerative blepharitis left upper eyelid
		H01.015	Ulcerative blepharitis left lower eyelid
		H01.016	Ulcerative blepharitis left eye, unspecified eyelid
		H01.019	Ulcerative blepharitis unspecified eye, unspecified eyelid
373.02	SQUAMOUS BLEPHARITIS	H01.021	Squamous blepharitis right upper eyelid
		H01.022	Squamous blepharitis right lower eyelid
		H01.023	Squamous blepharitis right eye, unspecified eyelid
		H01.024	Squamous blepharitis left upper eyelid
		H01.025	Squamous blepharitis left lower eyelid
		H01.026	Squamous blepharitis left eye, unspecified eyelid
		H01.029	Squamous blepharitis unspecified eye, unspecified eyelid
373.11	HORDEOLUM EXTERNUM	H00.011	Hordeolum externum right upper eyelid
		H00.012	Hordeolum externum right lower eyelid
		H00.013	Hordeolum externum right eye, unspecified eyelid
		H00.014	Hordeolum externum left upper eyelid
		H00.015	Hordeolum externum left lower eyelid
		H00.016	Hordeolum externum left eye, unspecified eyelid
		H00.019	Hordeolum externum unspecified eye, unspecified eyelid
373.12	HORDEOLUM INTERNUM	H00.021	Hordeolum internum right upper eyelid
		H00.022	Hordeolum internum right lower eyelid
		H00.023	Hordeolum internum right eye, unspecified eyelid
		H00.024	Hordeolum internum left upper eyelid
		H00.025	Hordeolum internum left lower eyelid
		H00.026	Hordeolum internum left eye, unspecified eyelid
		H00.029	Hordeolum internum unspecified eye, unspecified eyelid
373.13	ABSCESS OF EYELID	H00.031	Abscess of right upper eyelid
		H00.032	Abscess of right lower eyelid
		H00.033	Abscess of eyelid right eye, unspecified eyelid
		H00.034	Abscess of left upper eyelid
		H00.035	Abscess of left lower eyelid
		H00.036	Abscess of eyelid left eye, unspecified eyelid
		H00.039	Abscess of eyelid unspecified eye, unspecified eyelid
373.2	CHALAZION	H00.11	Chalazion right upper eyelid
		H00.12	Chalazion right lower eyelid
		H00.13	Chalazion right eye, unspecified eyelid
		H00.14	Chalazion left upper eyelid
		H00.15	Chalazion left lower eyelid
		H00.16	Chalazion left eye, unspecified eyelid
		H00.19	Chalazion unspecified eye, unspecified eyelid
373.31	ECZEMATOUS DERMATITIS OF EYELID	H01.131	Eczematous dermatitis of right upper eyelid
		H01.132	Eczematous dermatitis of right lower eyelid
		H01.133	Eczematous dermatitis of right eye, unspecified eyelid
		H01.134	Eczematous dermatitis of left upper eyelid
		H01.135	Eczematous dermatitis of left lower eyelid
		H01.136	Eczematous dermatitis of left eye, unspecified eyelid
		H01.139	Eczematous dermatitis of unspecified eye, unspecified eyelid
373.32	CONTACT AND ALLERGIC DERMATITIS OF EYELID	H01.111	Allergic dermatitis of right upper eyelid
		H01.112	Allergic dermatitis of right lower eyelid
		H01.113	Allergic dermatitis of right eye, unspecified eyelid
		H01.114	Allergic dermatitis of left upper eyelid
		H01.115	Allergic dermatitis of left lower eyelid
		H01.116	Allergic dermatitis of left eye, unspecified eyelid
		H01.119	Allergic dermatitis of unspecified eye, unspecified eyelid
373.33	XERODERMA OF EYELID	H01.141	Xeroderma of right upper eyelid
		H01.142	Xeroderma of right lower eyelid
		H01.143	Xeroderma of right eye, unspecified eyelid
		H01.144	Xeroderma of left upper eyelid
		H01.145	Xeroderma of left lower eyelid
		H01.146	Xeroderma of left eye, unspecified eyelid
		H01.149	Xeroderma of unspecified eye, unspecified eyelid
373.34	DISCOID LUPUS ERYTHEMATOSUS OF EYELID	H01.121	Discoid lupus erythematosus of right upper eyelid
		H01.122	Discoid lupus erythematosus of right lower eyelid
		H01.123	Discoid lupus erythematosus of right eye, unspecified eyelid
		H01.124	Discoid lupus erythematosus of left upper eyelid
		H01.125	Discoid lupus erythematosus of left lower eyelid
		H01.126	Discoid lupus erythematosus of left eye, unspecified eyelid
		H01.129	Discoid lupus erythematosus of unsp eye, unspecified eyelid
373.4	INFECTIVE DERMATITIS EYELID TYPES RESULT DEFORM	H01.8	Other specified inflammations of eyelid
373.5	OTHER INFECTIVE DERMATITIS OF EYELID	H01.8	Other specified inflammations of eyelid

[Brackets] indicate valid character values for each code. Character value meanings provided for each code grouping.

ICD-9-CM		ICD-10-CM	
373.6	PARASITIC INFESTATION OF EYELID	HØ1.8	Other specified inflammations of eyelid
373.8	OTHER INFLAMMATIONS OF EYELIDS	HØ1.8	Other specified inflammations of eyelid
373.9	UNSPECIFIED INFLAMMATION OF EYELID	➡ HØ1.9	Unspecified inflammation of eyelid
374.ØØ	UNSPECIFIED ENTROPION	HØ2.ØØ1	Unspecified entropion of right upper eyelid
		HØ2.ØØ2	Unspecified entropion of right lower eyelid
		HØ2.ØØ3	Unspecified entropion of right eye, unspecified eyelid
		HØ2.ØØ4	Unspecified entropion of left upper eyelid
		HØ2.ØØ5	Unspecified entropion of left lower eyelid
		HØ2.ØØ6	Unspecified entropion of left eye, unspecified eyelid
		HØ2.ØØ9	Unspecified entropion of unspecified eye, unspecified eyelid
374.Ø1	SENILE ENTROPION	HØ2.Ø31	Senile entropion of right upper eyelid
		HØ2.Ø32	Senile entropion of right lower eyelid
		HØ2.Ø33	Senile entropion of right eye, unspecified eyelid
		HØ2.Ø34	Senile entropion of left upper eyelid
		HØ2.Ø35	Senile entropion of left lower eyelid
		HØ2.Ø36	Senile entropion of left eye, unspecified eyelid
		HØ2.Ø39	Senile entropion of unspecified eye, unspecified eyelid
374.Ø2	MECHANICAL ENTROPION	HØ2.Ø21	Mechanical entropion of right upper eyelid
		HØ2.Ø22	Mechanical entropion of right lower eyelid
		HØ2.Ø23	Mechanical entropion of right eye, unspecified eyelid
		HØ2.Ø24	Mechanical entropion of left upper eyelid
		HØ2.Ø25	Mechanical entropion of left lower eyelid
		HØ2.Ø26	Mechanical entropion of left eye, unspecified eyelid
		HØ2.Ø29	Mechanical entropion of unspecified eye, unspecified eyelid
374.Ø3	SPASTIC ENTROPION	HØ2.Ø41	Spastic entropion of right upper eyelid
		HØ2.Ø42	Spastic entropion of right lower eyelid
		HØ2.Ø43	Spastic entropion of right eye, unspecified eyelid
		HØ2.Ø44	Spastic entropion of left upper eyelid
		HØ2.Ø45	Spastic entropion of left lower eyelid
		HØ2.Ø46	Spastic entropion of left eye, unspecified eyelid
		HØ2.Ø49	Spastic entropion of unspecified eye, unspecified eyelid
374.Ø4	CICATRICIAL ENTROPION	HØ2.Ø11	Cicatricial entropion of right upper eyelid
		HØ2.Ø12	Cicatricial entropion of right lower eyelid
		HØ2.Ø13	Cicatricial entropion of right eye, unspecified eyelid
		HØ2.Ø14	Cicatricial entropion of left upper eyelid
		HØ2.Ø15	Cicatricial entropion of left lower eyelid
		HØ2.Ø16	Cicatricial entropion of left eye, unspecified eyelid
		HØ2.Ø19	Cicatricial entropion of unspecified eye, unspecified eyelid
374.Ø5	TRICHIASIS OF EYELID WITHOUT ENTROPION	HØ2.Ø51	Trichiasis without entropian right upper eyelid
		HØ2.Ø52	Trichiasis without entropian right lower eyelid
		HØ2.Ø53	Trichiasis without entropian right eye, unspecified eyelid
		HØ2.Ø54	Trichiasis without entropian left upper eyelid
		HØ2.Ø55	Trichiasis without entropian left lower eyelid
		HØ2.Ø56	Trichiasis without entropian left eye, unspecified eyelid
		HØ2.Ø59	Trichiasis without entropian unsp eye, unspecified eyelid
374.1Ø	UNSPECIFIED ECTROPION	HØ2.1Ø1	Unspecified ectropion of right upper eyelid
		HØ2.1Ø2	Unspecified ectropion of right lower eyelid
		HØ2.1Ø3	Unspecified ectropion of right eye, unspecified eyelid
		HØ2.1Ø4	Unspecified ectropion of left upper eyelid
		HØ2.1Ø5	Unspecified ectropion of left lower eyelid
		HØ2.1Ø6	Unspecified ectropion of left eye, unspecified eyelid
		HØ2.1Ø9	Unspecified ectropion of unspecified eye, unspecified eyelid
374.11	SENILE ECTROPION	HØ2.131	Senile ectropion of right upper eyelid
		HØ2.132	Senile ectropion of right lower eyelid
		HØ2.133	Senile ectropion of right eye, unspecified eyelid
		HØ2.134	Senile ectropion of left upper eyelid
		HØ2.135	Senile ectropion of left lower eyelid
		HØ2.136	Senile ectropion of left eye, unspecified eyelid
		HØ2.139	Senile ectropion of unspecified eye, unspecified eyelid
374.12	MECHANICAL ECTROPION	HØ2.121	Mechanical ectropion of right upper eyelid
		HØ2.122	Mechanical ectropion of right lower eyelid
		HØ2.123	Mechanical ectropion of right eye, unspecified eyelid
		HØ2.124	Mechanical ectropion of left upper eyelid
		HØ2.125	Mechanical ectropion of left lower eyelid
		HØ2.126	Mechanical ectropion of left eye, unspecified eyelid
		HØ2.129	Mechanical ectropion of unspecified eye, unspecified eyelid
374.13	SPASTIC ECTROPION	HØ2.141	Spastic ectropion of right upper eyelid
		HØ2.142	Spastic ectropion of right lower eyelid
		HØ2.143	Spastic ectropion of right eye, unspecified eyelid
		HØ2.144	Spastic ectropion of left upper eyelid
		HØ2.145	Spastic ectropion of left lower eyelid
		HØ2.146	Spastic ectropion of left eye, unspecified eyelid
		HØ2.149	Spastic ectropion of unspecified eye, unspecified eyelid
374.14	CICATRICIAL ECTROPION	HØ2.111	Cicatricial ectropion of right upper eyelid
		HØ2.112	Cicatricial ectropion of right lower eyelid
		HØ2.113	Cicatricial ectropion of right eye, unspecified eyelid
		HØ2.114	Cicatricial ectropion of left upper eyelid
		HØ2.115	Cicatricial ectropion of left lower eyelid
		HØ2.116	Cicatricial ectropion of left eye, unspecified eyelid
		HØ2.119	Cicatricial ectropion of unspecified eye, unspecified eyelid

ICD-9-CM		ICD-10-CM	
374.20	UNSPECIFIED LAGOPHTHALMOS	**H02.201**	Unspecified lagophthalmos right upper eyelid
		H02.202	Unspecified lagophthalmos right lower eyelid
		H02.203	Unspecified lagophthalmos right eye, unspecified eyelid
		H02.204	Unspecified lagophthalmos left upper eyelid
		H02.205	Unspecified lagophthalmos left lower eyelid
		H02.206	Unspecified lagophthalmos left eye, unspecified eyelid
		H02.209	Unsp lagophthalmos unspecified eye, unspecified eyelid
374.21	PARALYTIC LAGOPHTHALMOS	**H02.231**	Paralytic lagophthalmos right upper eyelid
		H02.232	Paralytic lagophthalmos right lower eyelid
		H02.233	Paralytic lagophthalmos right eye, unspecified eyelid
		H02.234	Paralytic lagophthalmos left upper eyelid
		H02.235	Paralytic lagophthalmos left lower eyelid
		H02.236	Paralytic lagophthalmos left eye, unspecified eyelid
		H02.239	Paralytic lagophthalmos unspecified eye, unspecified eyelid
374.22	MECHANICAL LAGOPHTHALMOS	**H02.221**	Mechanical lagophthalmos right upper eyelid
		H02.222	Mechanical lagophthalmos right lower eyelid
		H02.223	Mechanical lagophthalmos right eye, unspecified eyelid
		H02.224	Mechanical lagophthalmos left upper eyelid
		H02.225	Mechanical lagophthalmos left lower eyelid
		H02.226	Mechanical lagophthalmos left eye, unspecified eyelid
		H02.229	Mechanical lagophthalmos unspecified eye, unspecified eyelid
374.23	CICATRICIAL LAGOPHTHALMOS	**H02.211**	Cicatricial lagophthalmos right upper eyelid
		H02.212	Cicatricial lagophthalmos right lower eyelid
		H02.213	Cicatricial lagophthalmos right eye, unspecified eyelid
		H02.214	Cicatricial lagophthalmos left upper eyelid
		H02.215	Cicatricial lagophthalmos left lower eyelid
		H02.216	Cicatricial lagophthalmos left eye, unspecified eyelid
		H02.219	Cicatricial lagophthalmos unsp eye, unspecified eyelid
374.30	UNSPECIFIED PTOSIS OF EYELID	**H02.401**	Unspecified ptosis of right eyelid
		H02.402	Unspecified ptosis of left eyelid
		H02.403	Unspecified ptosis of bilateral eyelids
		H02.409	Unspecified ptosis of unspecified eyelid
374.31	PARALYTIC PTOSIS	**H02.431**	Paralytic ptosis of right eyelid
		H02.432	Paralytic ptosis of left eyelid
		H02.433	Paralytic ptosis of bilateral eyelids
		H02.439	Paralytic ptosis unspecified eyelid
374.32	MYOGENIC PTOSIS	**H02.421**	Myogenic ptosis of right eyelid
		H02.422	Myogenic ptosis of left eyelid
		H02.423	Myogenic ptosis of bilateral eyelids
		H02.429	Myogenic ptosis of unspecified eyelid
374.33	MECHANICAL PTOSIS	**H02.411**	Mechanical ptosis of right eyelid
		H02.412	Mechanical ptosis of left eyelid
		H02.413	Mechanical ptosis of bilateral eyelids
		H02.419	Mechanical ptosis of unspecified eyelid
374.34	BLEPHAROCHALASIS	**H02.30**	Blepharochalasis unspecified eye, unspecified eyelid
		H02.31	Blepharochalasis right upper eyelid
		H02.32	Blepharochalasis right lower eyelid
		H02.33	Blepharochalasis right eye, unspecified eyelid
		H02.34	Blepharochalasis left upper eyelid
		H02.35	Blepharochalasis left lower eyelid
		H02.36	Blepharochalasis left eye, unspecified eyelid
374.41	EYELID RETRACTION OR LAG	**H02.531**	Eyelid retraction right upper eyelid
		H02.532	Eyelid retraction right lower eyelid
		H02.533	Eyelid retraction right eye, unspecified eyelid
		H02.534	Eyelid retraction left upper eyelid
		H02.535	Eyelid retraction left lower eyelid
		H02.536	Eyelid retraction left eye, unspecified eyelid
		H02.539	Eyelid retraction unspecified eye, unspecified lid
374.43	ABNORMAL INNERVATION SYNDROME OF EYELID	**H02.511**	Abnormal innervation syndrome right upper eyelid
		H02.512	Abnormal innervation syndrome right lower eyelid
		H02.513	Abnormal innervation syndrome right eye, unspecified eyelid
		H02.514	Abnormal innervation syndrome left upper eyelid
		H02.515	Abnormal innervation syndrome left lower eyelid
		H02.516	Abnormal innervation syndrome left eye, unspecified eyelid
		H02.519	Abnormal innervation syndrome unsp eye, unspecified eyelid
374.44	SENSORY DISORDERS OF EYELID	**H02.59**	Other disorders affecting eyelid function
374.45	OTHER SENSORIMOTOR DISORDERS OF EYELID	**H02.59**	Other disorders affecting eyelid function
374.46	BLEPHAROPHIMOSIS	**H02.521**	Blepharophimosis right upper eyelid
		H02.522	Blepharophimosis right lower eyelid
		H02.523	Blepharophimosis right eye, unspecified eyelid
		H02.524	Blepharophimosis left upper eyelid
		H02.525	Blepharophimosis left lower eyelid
		H02.526	Blepharophimosis left eye, unspecified eyelid
		H02.529	Blepharophimosis unspecified eye, unspecified lid
374.50	UNSPECIFIED DEGENERATIVE DISORDER OF EYELID	➡ **H02.70**	Unsp degenerative disorders of eyelid and periocular area

ICD-9-CM		ICD-10-CM	
374.51	XANTHELASMA OF EYELID	**HØ2.6Ø**	Xanthelasma of unspecified eye, unspecified eyelid
		HØ2.61	Xanthelasma of right upper eyelid
		HØ2.62	Xanthelasma of right lower eyelid
		HØ2.63	Xanthelasma of right eye, unspecified eyelid
		HØ2.64	Xanthelasma of left upper eyelid
		HØ2.65	Xanthelasma of left lower eyelid
		HØ2.66	Xanthelasma of left eye, unspecified eyelid
374.52	HYPERPIGMENTATION OF EYELID	**HØ2.711**	Chloasma of right upper eyelid and periocular area
		HØ2.712	Chloasma of right lower eyelid and periocular area
		HØ2.713	Chloasma of right eye, unsp eyelid and periocular area
		HØ2.714	Chloasma of left upper eyelid and periocular area
		HØ2.715	Chloasma of left lower eyelid and periocular area
		HØ2.716	Chloasma of left eye, unspecified eyelid and periocular area
		HØ2.719	Chloasma of unsp eye, unspecified eyelid and periocular area
374.53	HYPOPIGMENTATION OF EYELID	**HØ2.731**	Vitiligo of right upper eyelid and periocular area
		HØ2.732	Vitiligo of right lower eyelid and periocular area
		HØ2.733	Vitiligo of right eye, unsp eyelid and periocular area
		HØ2.734	Vitiligo of left upper eyelid and periocular area
		HØ2.735	Vitiligo of left lower eyelid and periocular area
		HØ2.736	Vitiligo of left eye, unspecified eyelid and periocular area
		HØ2.739	Vitiligo of unsp eye, unspecified eyelid and periocular area
374.54	HYPERTRICHOSIS OF EYELID	**HØ2.861**	Hypertrichosis of right upper eyelid
		HØ2.862	Hypertrichosis of right lower eyelid
		HØ2.863	Hypertrichosis of right eye, unspecified eyelid
		HØ2.864	Hypertrichosis of left upper eyelid
		HØ2.865	Hypertrichosis of left lower eyelid
		HØ2.866	Hypertrichosis of left eye, unspecified eyelid
		HØ2.869	Hypertrichosis of unspecified eye, unspecified eyelid
374.55	HYPOTRICHOSIS OF EYELID	**HØ2.721**	Madarosis of right upper eyelid and periocular area
		HØ2.722	Madarosis of right lower eyelid and periocular area
		HØ2.723	Madarosis of right eye, unsp eyelid and periocular area
		HØ2.724	Madarosis of left upper eyelid and periocular area
		HØ2.725	Madarosis of left lower eyelid and periocular area
		HØ2.726	Madarosis of left eye, unsp eyelid and periocular area
		HØ2.729	Madarosis of unsp eye, unsp eyelid and periocular area
374.56	OTH DEGENERATIVE DISORDERS SKIN AFFECTING EYELID	**HØ2.79**	Other degenerative disorders of eyelid and periocular area
374.81	HEMORRHAGE OF EYELID	**HØ2.89**	Other specified disorders of eyelid
374.82	EDEMA OF EYELID	**HØ2.841**	Edema of right upper eyelid
		HØ2.842	Edema of right lower eyelid
		HØ2.843	Edema of right eye, unspecified eyelid
		HØ2.844	Edema of left upper eyelid
		HØ2.845	Edema of left lower eyelid
		HØ2.846	Edema of left eye, unspecified eyelid
		HØ2.849	Edema of unspecified eye, unspecified eyelid
374.83	ELEPHANTIASIS OF EYELID	**HØ2.851**	Elephantiasis of right upper eyelid
		HØ2.852	Elephantiasis of right lower eyelid
		HØ2.853	Elephantiasis of right eye, unspecified eyelid
		HØ2.854	Elephantiasis of left upper eyelid
		HØ2.855	Elephantiasis of left lower eyelid
		HØ2.856	Elephantiasis of left eye, unspecified eyelid
		HØ2.859	Elephantiasis of unspecified eye, unspecified eyelid
374.84	CYSTS OF EYELIDS	**HØ2.821**	Cysts of right upper eyelid
		HØ2.822	Cysts of right lower eyelid
		HØ2.823	Cysts of right eye, unspecified eyelid
		HØ2.824	Cysts of left upper eyelid
		HØ2.825	Cysts of left lower eyelid
		HØ2.826	Cysts of left eye, unspecified eyelid
		HØ2.829	Cysts of unspecified eye, unspecified eyelid
374.85	VASCULAR ANOMALIES OF EYELID	**HØ2.871**	Vascular anomalies of right upper eyelid
		HØ2.872	Vascular anomalies of right lower eyelid
		HØ2.873	Vascular anomalies of right eye, unspecified eyelid
		HØ2.874	Vascular anomalies of left upper eyelid
		HØ2.875	Vascular anomalies of left lower eyelid
		HØ2.876	Vascular anomalies of left eye, unspecified eyelid
		HØ2.879	Vascular anomalies of unspecified eye, unspecified eyelid
374.86	RETAINED FOREIGN BODY OF EYELID	**HØ2.811**	Retained foreign body in right upper eyelid
		HØ2.812	Retained foreign body in right lower eyelid
		HØ2.813	Retained foreign body in right eye, unspecified eyelid
		HØ2.814	Retained foreign body in left upper eyelid
		HØ2.815	Retained foreign body in left lower eyelid
		HØ2.816	Retained foreign body in left eye, unspecified eyelid
		HØ2.819	Retained foreign body in unspecified eye, unspecified eyelid
374.87	DERMATOCHALASIS	**HØ2.831**	Dermatochalasis of right upper eyelid
		HØ2.832	Dermatochalasis of right lower eyelid
		HØ2.833	Dermatochalasis of right eye, unspecified eyelid
		HØ2.834	Dermatochalasis of left upper eyelid
		HØ2.835	Dermatochalasis of left lower eyelid
		HØ2.836	Dermatochalasis of left eye, unspecified eyelid
		HØ2.839	Dermatochalasis of unspecified eye, unspecified eyelid
374.89	OTHER DISORDERS OF EYELID	**HØ2.89**	Other specified disorders of eyelid

ICD-9-CM		ICD-10-CM	
374.9	UNSPECIFIED DISORDER OF EYELID	➡ H02.9	Unspecified disorder of eyelid
375.00	UNSPECIFIED DACRYOADENITIS	H04.001	Unspecified dacryoadenitis, right lacrimal gland
		H04.002	Unspecified dacryoadenitis, left lacrimal gland
		H04.003	Unspecified dacryoadenitis, bilateral lacrimal glands
		H04.009	Unspecified dacryoadenitis, unspecified lacrimal gland
375.01	ACUTE DACRYOADENITIS	H04.011	Acute dacryoadenitis, right lacrimal gland
		H04.012	Acute dacryoadenitis, left lacrimal gland
		H04.013	Acute dacryoadenitis, bilateral lacrimal glands
		H04.019	Acute dacryoadenitis, unspecified lacrimal gland
375.02	CHRONIC DACRYOADENITIS	H04.021	Chronic dacryoadenitis, right lacrimal gland
		H04.022	Chronic dacryoadenitis, left lacrimal gland
		H04.023	Chronic dacryoadenitis, bilateral lacrimal gland
		H04.029	Chronic dacryoadenitis, unspecified lacrimal gland
375.03	CHRONIC ENLARGEMENT OF LACRIMAL GLAND	H04.031	Chronic enlargement of right lacrimal gland
		H04.032	Chronic enlargement of left lacrimal gland
		H04.033	Chronic enlargement of bilateral lacrimal glands
		H04.039	Chronic enlargement of unspecified lacrimal gland
375.11	DACRYOPS	H04.111	Dacryops of right lacrimal gland
		H04.112	Dacryops of left lacrimal gland
		H04.113	Dacryops of bilateral lacrimal glands
		H04.119	Dacryops of unspecified lacrimal gland
375.12	OTHER LACRIMAL CYSTS AND CYSTIC DEGENERATION	H04.131	Lacrimal cyst, right lacrimal gland
		H04.132	Lacrimal cyst, left lacrimal gland
		H04.133	Lacrimal cyst, bilateral lacrimal glands
		H04.139	Lacrimal cyst, unspecified lacrimal gland
375.13	PRIMARY LACRIMAL ATROPHY	H04.141	Primary lacrimal gland atrophy, right lacrimal gland
		H04.142	Primary lacrimal gland atrophy, left lacrimal gland
		H04.143	Primary lacrimal gland atrophy, bilateral lacrimal glands
		H04.149	Primary lacrimal gland atrophy, unspecified lacrimal gland
375.14	SECONDARY LACRIMAL ATROPHY	H04.151	Secondary lacrimal gland atrophy, right lacrimal gland
		H04.152	Secondary lacrimal gland atrophy, left lacrimal gland
		H04.153	Secondary lacrimal gland atrophy, bilateral lacrimal glands
		H04.159	Secondary lacrimal gland atrophy, unspecified lacrimal gland
375.15	UNSPECIFIED TEAR FILM INSUFFICIENCY	H04.121	Dry eye syndrome of right lacrimal gland
		H04.122	Dry eye syndrome of left lacrimal gland
		H04.123	Dry eye syndrome of bilateral lacrimal glands
		H04.129	Dry eye syndrome of unspecified lacrimal gland
375.16	DISLOCATION OF LACRIMAL GLAND	H04.161	Lacrimal gland dislocation, right lacrimal gland
		H04.162	Lacrimal gland dislocation, left lacrimal gland
		H04.163	Lacrimal gland dislocation, bilateral lacrimal glands
		H04.169	Lacrimal gland dislocation, unspecified lacrimal gland
375.20	EPIPHORA, UNSPECIFIED AS TO CAUSE	H04.201	Unspecified epiphora, right lacrimal gland
		H04.202	Unspecified epiphora, left lacrimal gland
		H04.203	Unspecified epiphora, bilateral lacrimal glands
		H04.209	Unspecified epiphora, unspecified lacrimal gland
375.21	EPIPHORA DUE TO EXCESS LACRIMATION	H04.211	Epiphora due to excess lacrimation, right lacrimal gland
		H04.212	Epiphora due to excess lacrimation, left lacrimal gland
		H04.213	Epiphora due to excess lacrimation, bi lacrimal glands
		H04.219	Epiphora due to excess lacrimation, unsp lacrimal gland
375.22	EPIPHORA DUE TO INSUFFICIENT DRAINAGE	H04.221	Epiphora due to insufficient drainage, right lacrimal gland
		H04.222	Epiphora due to insufficient drainage, left lacrimal gland
		H04.223	Epiphora due to insufficient drainage, bi lacrimal glands
		H04.229	Epiphora due to insufficient drainage, unsp lacrimal gland
375.30	UNSPECIFIED DACRYOCYSTITIS	H04.301	Unspecified dacryocystitis of right lacrimal passage
		H04.302	Unspecified dacryocystitis of left lacrimal passage
		H04.303	Unspecified dacryocystitis of bilateral lacrimal passages
		H04.309	Unspecified dacryocystitis of unspecified lacrimal passage
375.31	ACUTE CANALICULITIS, LACRIMAL	H04.331	Acute lacrimal canaliculitis of right lacrimal passage
		H04.332	Acute lacrimal canaliculitis of left lacrimal passage
		H04.333	Acute lacrimal canaliculitis of bilateral lacrimal passages
		H04.339	Acute lacrimal canaliculitis of unspecified lacrimal passage
375.32	ACUTE DACRYOCYSTITIS	H04.321	Acute dacryocystitis of right lacrimal passage
		H04.322	Acute dacryocystitis of left lacrimal passage
		H04.323	Acute dacryocystitis of bilateral lacrimal passages
		H04.329	Acute dacryocystitis of unspecified lacrimal passage
375.33	PHLEGMONOUS DACRYOCYSTITIS	H04.311	Phlegmonous dacryocystitis of right lacrimal passage
		H04.312	Phlegmonous dacryocystitis of left lacrimal passage
		H04.313	Phlegmonous dacryocystitis of bilateral lacrimal passages
		H04.319	Phlegmonous dacryocystitis of unspecified lacrimal passage
375.41	CHRONIC CANALICULITIS	H04.421	Chronic lacrimal canaliculitis of right lacrimal passage
		H04.422	Chronic lacrimal canaliculitis of left lacrimal passage
		H04.423	Chronic lacrimal canaliculitis of bi lacrimal passages
		H04.429	Chronic lacrimal canaliculitis of unsp lacrimal passage
375.42	CHRONIC DACRYOCYSTITIS	H04.411	Chronic dacryocystitis of right lacrimal passage
		H04.412	Chronic dacryocystitis of left lacrimal passage
		H04.413	Chronic dacryocystitis of bilateral lacrimal passages
		H04.419	Chronic dacryocystitis of unspecified lacrimal passage

ICD-9-CM			ICD-10-CM	
375.43	LACRIMAL MUCOCELE		**HØ4.431**	Chronic lacrimal mucocele of right lacrimal passage
			HØ4.432	Chronic lacrimal mucocele of left lacrimal passage
			HØ4.433	Chronic lacrimal mucocele of bilateral lacrimal passages
			HØ4.439	Chronic lacrimal mucocele of unspecified lacrimal passage
375.51	EVERSION OF LACRIMAL PUNCTUM		**HØ4.521**	Eversion of right lacrimal punctum
			HØ4.522	Eversion of left lacrimal punctum
			HØ4.523	Eversion of bilateral lacrimal punctum
			HØ4.529	Eversion of unspecified lacrimal punctum
375.52	STENOSIS OF LACRIMAL PUNCTUM		**HØ4.561**	Stenosis of right lacrimal punctum
			HØ4.562	Stenosis of left lacrimal punctum
			HØ4.563	Stenosis of bilateral lacrimal punctum
			HØ4.569	Stenosis of unspecified lacrimal punctum
375.53	STENOSIS OF LACRIMAL CANALICULI		**HØ4.541**	Stenosis of right lacrimal canaliculi
			HØ4.542	Stenosis of left lacrimal canaliculi
			HØ4.543	Stenosis of bilateral lacrimal canaliculi
			HØ4.549	Stenosis of unspecified lacrimal canaliculi
375.54	STENOSIS OF LACRIMAL SAC		**HØ4.571**	Stenosis of right lacrimal sac
			HØ4.572	Stenosis of left lacrimal sac
			HØ4.573	Stenosis of bilateral lacrimal sac
			HØ4.579	Stenosis of unspecified lacrimal sac
375.55	OBSTRUCTION OF NASOLACRIMAL DUCT NEONATAL		**HØ4.531**	Neonatal obstruction of right nasolacrimal duct
			HØ4.532	Neonatal obstruction of left nasolacrimal duct
			HØ4.533	Neonatal obstruction of bilateral nasolacrimal duct
			HØ4.539	Neonatal obstruction of unspecified nasolacrimal duct
375.56	STENOSIS OF NASOLACRIMAL DUCT ACQUIRED		**HØ4.551**	Acquired stenosis of right nasolacrimal duct
			HØ4.552	Acquired stenosis of left nasolacrimal duct
			HØ4.553	Acquired stenosis of bilateral nasolacrimal duct
			HØ4.559	Acquired stenosis of unspecified nasolacrimal duct
375.57	DACRYOLITH		**HØ4.511**	Dacryolith of right lacrimal passage
			HØ4.512	Dacryolith of left lacrimal passage
			HØ4.513	Dacryolith of bilateral lacrimal passages
			HØ4.519	Dacryolith of unspecified lacrimal passage
375.61	LACRIMAL FISTULA		**HØ4.611**	Lacrimal fistula right lacrimal passage
			HØ4.612	Lacrimal fistula left lacrimal passage
			HØ4.613	Lacrimal fistula bilateral lacrimal passages
			HØ4.619	Lacrimal fistula unspecified lacrimal passage
375.69	OTHER CHANGE OF LACRIMAL PASSAGES	➡	**HØ4.69**	Other changes of lacrimal passages
375.81	GRANULOMA OF LACRIMAL PASSAGES		**HØ4.811**	Granuloma of right lacrimal passage
			HØ4.812	Granuloma of left lacrimal passage
			HØ4.813	Granuloma of bilateral lacrimal passages
			HØ4.819	Granuloma of unspecified lacrimal passage
375.89	OTHER DISORDER OF LACRIMAL SYSTEM		**HØ4.19**	Other specified disorders of lacrimal gland
			HØ4.89	Other disorders of lacrimal system
375.9	UNSPECIFIED DISORDER OF LACRIMAL SYSTEM	➡	**HØ4.9**	Disorder of lacrimal system, unspecified
376.ØØ	UNSPECIFIED ACUTE INFLAMMATION OF ORBIT	➡	**HØ5.ØØ**	Unspecified acute inflammation of orbit
376.Ø1	ORBITAL CELLULITIS		**HØ5.Ø11**	Cellulitis of right orbit
			HØ5.Ø12	Cellulitis of left orbit
			HØ5.Ø13	Cellulitis of bilateral orbits
			HØ5.Ø19	Cellulitis of unspecified orbit
376.Ø2	ORBITAL PERIOSTITIS		**HØ5.Ø31**	Periostitis of right orbit
			HØ5.Ø32	Periostitis of left orbit
			HØ5.Ø33	Periostitis of bilateral orbits
			HØ5.Ø39	Periostitis of unspecified orbit
376.Ø3	ORBITAL OSTEOMYELITIS		**HØ5.Ø21**	Osteomyelitis of right orbit
			HØ5.Ø22	Osteomyelitis of left orbit
			HØ5.Ø23	Osteomyelitis of bilateral orbits
			HØ5.Ø29	Osteomyelitis of unspecified orbit
376.Ø4	ORBITAL TENONITIS		**HØ5.Ø41**	Tenonitis of right orbit
			HØ5.Ø42	Tenonitis of left orbit
			HØ5.Ø43	Tenonitis of bilateral orbits
			HØ5.Ø49	Tenonitis of unspecified orbit
376.1Ø	UNSPECIFIED CHRONIC INFLAMMATION OF ORBIT	➡	**HØ5.1Ø**	Unspecified chronic inflammatory disorders of orbit
376.11	ORBITAL GRANULOMA		**HØ5.111**	Granuloma of right orbit
			HØ5.112	Granuloma of left orbit
			HØ5.113	Granuloma of bilateral orbits
			HØ5.119	Granuloma of unspecified orbit
376.12	ORBITAL MYOSITIS		**HØ5.121**	Orbital myositis, right orbit
			HØ5.122	Orbital myositis, left orbit
			HØ5.123	Orbital myositis, bilateral
			HØ5.129	Orbital myositis, unspecified orbit
376.13	PARASITIC INFESTATION OF ORBIT		**HØ5.89**	Other disorders of orbit
376.21	THYROTOXIC EXOPHTHALMOS		**HØ5.89**	Other disorders of orbit
376.22	EXOPHTHALMIC OPHTHALMOPLEGIA		**HØ5.89**	Other disorders of orbit
376.3Ø	UNSPECIFIED EXOPHTHALMOS	➡	**HØ5.2Ø**	Unspecified exophthalmos

ICD-9-CM			ICD-10-CM	
376.31	CONSTANT EXOPHTHALMOS		HØ5.241	Constant exophthalmos, right eye
			HØ5.242	Constant exophthalmos, left eye
			HØ5.243	Constant exophthalmos, bilateral
			HØ5.249	Constant exophthalmos, unspecified eye
376.32	ORBITAL HEMORRHAGE		HØ5.231	Hemorrhage of right orbit
			HØ5.232	Hemorrhage of left orbit
			HØ5.233	Hemorrhage of bilateral orbit
			HØ5.239	Hemorrhage of unspecified orbit
376.33	ORBITAL EDEMA OR CONGESTION		HØ5.221	Edema of right orbit
			HØ5.222	Edema of left orbit
			HØ5.223	Edema of bilateral orbit
			HØ5.229	Edema of unspecified orbit
376.34	INTERMITTENT EXOPHTHALMOS		HØ5.251	Intermittent exophthalmos, right eye
			HØ5.252	Intermittent exophthalmos, left eye
			HØ5.253	Intermittent exophthalmos, bilateral
			HØ5.259	Intermittent exophthalmos, unspecified eye
376.35	PULSATING EXOPHTHALMOS		HØ5.261	Pulsating exophthalmos, right eye
			HØ5.262	Pulsating exophthalmos, left eye
			HØ5.263	Pulsating exophthalmos, bilateral
			HØ5.269	Pulsating exophthalmos, unspecified eye
376.36	LATERAL DISPLACEMENT OF GLOBE OF EYE		HØ5.211	Displacement (lateral) of globe, right eye
			HØ5.212	Displacement (lateral) of globe, left eye
			HØ5.213	Displacement (lateral) of globe, bilateral
			HØ5.219	Displacement (lateral) of globe, unspecified eye
376.4Ø	UNSPECIFIED DEFORMITY OF ORBIT	➡	HØ5.3Ø	Unspecified deformity of orbit
376.41	HYPERTELORISM OF ORBIT		HØ5.89	Other disorders of orbit
376.42	EXOSTOSIS OF ORBIT		HØ5.351	Exostosis of right orbit
			HØ5.352	Exostosis of left orbit
			HØ5.353	Exostosis of bilateral orbits
			HØ5.359	Exostosis of unspecified orbit
376.43	LOCAL DEFORMITIES OF ORBIT DUE TO BONE DISEASE		HØ5.321	Deformity of right orbit due to bone disease
			HØ5.322	Deformity of left orbit due to bone disease
			HØ5.323	Deformity of bilateral orbits due to bone disease
			HØ5.329	Deformity of unspecified orbit due to bone disease
376.44	ORBITAL DEFORM ASSOC W/CRANIOFACIAL DEFORM		HØ5.89	Other disorders of orbit
376.45	ATROPHY OF ORBIT		HØ5.311	Atrophy of right orbit
			HØ5.312	Atrophy of left orbit
			HØ5.313	Atrophy of bilateral orbit
			HØ5.319	Atrophy of unspecified orbit
376.46	ENLARGEMENT OF ORBIT		HØ5.341	Enlargement of right orbit
			HØ5.342	Enlargement of left orbit
			HØ5.343	Enlargement of bilateral orbits
			HØ5.349	Enlargement of unspecified orbit
376.47	DEFORMITY OF ORBIT DUE TO TRAUMA OR SURGERY		HØ5.331	Deformity of right orbit due to trauma or surgery
			HØ5.332	Deformity of left orbit due to trauma or surgery
			HØ5.333	Deformity of bilateral orbits due to trauma or surgery
			HØ5.339	Deformity of unspecified orbit due to trauma or surgery
376.5Ø	ENOPHTHALMOS UNSPECIFIED AS TO CAUSE		HØ5.4Ø1	Unspecified enophthalmos, right eye
			HØ5.4Ø2	Unspecified enophthalmos, left eye
			HØ5.4Ø3	Unspecified enophthalmos, bilateral
			HØ5.4Ø9	Unspecified enophthalmos, unspecified eye
376.51	ENOPHTHALMOS DUE TO ATROPHY OF ORBITAL TISSUE		HØ5.411	Enophthalmos due to atrophy of orbital tissue, right eye
			HØ5.412	Enophthalmos due to atrophy of orbital tissue, left eye
			HØ5.413	Enophthalmos due to atrophy of orbital tissue, bilateral
			HØ5.419	Enophthalmos due to atrophy of orbital tissue, unsp eye
376.52	ENOPHTHALMOS DUE TO TRAUMA OR SURGERY		HØ5.421	Enophthalmos due to trauma or surgery, right eye
			HØ5.422	Enophthalmos due to trauma or surgery, left eye
			HØ5.423	Enophthalmos due to trauma or surgery, bilateral
			HØ5.429	Enophthalmos due to trauma or surgery, unspecified eye
376.6	RETAINED FB FOLLOW PENETRATING WOUND ORBIT		HØ5.5Ø	Retained (old) fb following penetrating wound of unsp orbit
			HØ5.51	Retained (old) fb following penetrating wound of right orbit
			HØ5.52	Retained (old) fb following penetrating wound of left orbit
			HØ5.53	Retained (old) fb following penetrating wound of bi orbit
376.81	ORBITAL CYSTS		HØ5.811	Cyst of right orbit
			HØ5.812	Cyst of left orbit
			HØ5.813	Cyst of bilateral orbits
			HØ5.819	Cyst of unspecified orbit
376.82	MYOPATHY OF EXTRAOCULAR MUSCLES		HØ5.821	Myopathy of extraocular muscles, right orbit
			HØ5.822	Myopathy of extraocular muscles, left orbit
			HØ5.823	Myopathy of extraocular muscles, bilateral
			HØ5.829	Myopathy of extraocular muscles, unspecified orbit
376.89	OTHER ORBITAL DISORDER		HØ5.89	Other disorders of orbit
376.9	UNSPECIFIED DISORDER OF ORBIT	➡	HØ5.9	Unspecified disorder of orbit
377.ØØ	UNSPECIFIED PAPILLEDEMA	➡	H47.1Ø	Unspecified papilledema
377.Ø1	PAPILLEDEMA ASSOC W/INCR INTRACRANIAL PRESSURE	➡	H47.11	Papilledema associated with increased intracranial pressure
377.Ø2	PAPILLEDEMA ASSOC W/DECREASED OCULAR PRESSURE	➡	H47.12	Papilledema associated with decreased ocular pressure
377.Ø3	PAPILLEDEMA ASSOCIATED WITH RETINAL DISORDER	➡	H47.13	Papilledema associated with retinal disorder

[Brackets] indicate valid character values for each code. Character value meanings provided for each code grouping.

ICD-9-CM			ICD-10-CM	
377.04	FOSTER-KENNEDY SYNDROME		**H47.141**	Foster-Kennedy syndrome, right eye
			H47.142	Foster-Kennedy syndrome, left eye
			H47.143	Foster-Kennedy syndrome, bilateral
			H47.149	Foster-Kennedy syndrome, unspecified eye
377.10	UNSPECIFIED OPTIC ATROPHY	➡	**H47.20**	Unspecified optic atrophy
377.11	PRIMARY OPTIC ATROPHY		**H47.211**	Primary optic atrophy, right eye
			H47.212	Primary optic atrophy, left eye
			H47.213	Primary optic atrophy, bilateral
			H47.219	Primary optic atrophy, unspecified eye
377.12	POSTINFLAMMATORY OPTIC ATROPHY		**H47.291**	Other optic atrophy, right eye
			H47.292	Other optic atrophy, left eye
			H47.293	Other optic atrophy, bilateral
			H47.299	Other optic atrophy, unspecified eye
377.13	OPTIC ATROPHY ASSOCIATED W/RETINAL DYSTROPHIES		**H47.291**	Other optic atrophy, right eye
			H47.292	Other optic atrophy, left eye
			H47.293	Other optic atrophy, bilateral
			H47.299	Other optic atrophy, unspecified eye
377.14	GLAUCOMATOUS ATROPHY OF OPTIC DISC		**H47.231**	Glaucomatous optic atrophy, right eye
			H47.232	Glaucomatous optic atrophy, left eye
			H47.233	Glaucomatous optic atrophy, bilateral
			H47.239	Glaucomatous optic atrophy, unspecified eye
377.15	PARTIAL OPTIC ATROPHY		**H47.291**	Other optic atrophy, right eye
			H47.292	Other optic atrophy, left eye
			H47.293	Other optic atrophy, bilateral
			H47.299	Other optic atrophy, unspecified eye
377.16	HEREDITARY OPTIC ATROPHY	➡	**H47.22**	Hereditary optic atrophy
377.21	DRUSEN OF OPTIC DISC		**H47.321**	Drusen of optic disc, right eye
			H47.322	Drusen of optic disc, left eye
			H47.323	Drusen of optic disc, bilateral
			H47.329	Drusen of optic disc, unspecified eye
377.22	CRATER-LIKE HOLES OF OPTIC DISC		**H47.391**	Other disorders of optic disc, right eye
			H47.392	Other disorders of optic disc, left eye
			H47.393	Other disorders of optic disc, bilateral
			H47.399	Other disorders of optic disc, unspecified eye
377.23	COLOBOMA OF OPTIC DISC		**H47.311**	Coloboma of optic disc, right eye
			H47.312	Coloboma of optic disc, left eye
			H47.313	Coloboma of optic disc, bilateral
			H47.319	Coloboma of optic disc, unspecified eye
377.24	PSEUDOPAPILLEDEMA		**H47.331**	Pseudopapilledema of optic disc, right eye
			H47.332	Pseudopapilledema of optic disc, left eye
			H47.333	Pseudopapilledema of optic disc, bilateral
			H47.339	Pseudopapilledema of optic disc, unspecified eye
377.30	UNSPECIFIED OPTIC NEURITIS	➡	**H46.9**	Unspecified optic neuritis
377.31	OPTIC PAPILLITIS		**H46.00**	Optic papillitis, unspecified eye
			H46.01	Optic papillitis, right eye
			H46.02	Optic papillitis, left eye
			H46.03	Optic papillitis, bilateral
377.32	RETROBULBAR NEURITIS		**H46.10**	Retrobulbar neuritis, unspecified eye
			H46.11	Retrobulbar neuritis, right eye
			H46.12	Retrobulbar neuritis, left eye
			H46.13	Retrobulbar neuritis, bilateral
377.33	NUTRITIONAL OPTIC NEUROPATHY	➡	**H46.2**	Nutritional optic neuropathy
377.34	TOXIC OPTIC NEUROPATHY	➡	**H46.3**	Toxic optic neuropathy
377.39	OTHER OPTIC NEURITIS	➡	**H46.8**	Other optic neuritis
377.41	ISCHEMIC OPTIC NEUROPATHY		**H47.011**	Ischemic optic neuropathy, right eye
			H47.012	Ischemic optic neuropathy, left eye
			H47.013	Ischemic optic neuropathy, bilateral
			H47.019	Ischemic optic neuropathy, unspecified eye
377.42	HEMORRHAGE IN OPTIC NERVE SHEATHS		**H47.021**	Hemorrhage in optic nerve sheath, right eye
			H47.022	Hemorrhage in optic nerve sheath, left eye
			H47.023	Hemorrhage in optic nerve sheath, bilateral
			H47.029	Hemorrhage in optic nerve sheath, unspecified eye
377.43	OPTIC NERVE HYPOPLASIA		**H47.031**	Optic nerve hypoplasia, right eye
			H47.032	Optic nerve hypoplasia, left eye
			H47.033	Optic nerve hypoplasia, bilateral
			H47.039	Optic nerve hypoplasia, unspecified eye
377.49	OTHER DISORDER OF OPTIC NERVE		**H47.091**	Oth disorders of optic nerve, NEC, right eye
			H47.092	Oth disorders of optic nerve, NEC, left eye
			H47.093	Oth disorders of optic nerve, NEC, bilateral
			H47.099	Oth disorders of optic nerve, NEC, unsp eye
377.51	D/O OPTIC CHIASM ASSOC W/PITUITARY NEOPLASMS&D/O		**H47.49**	Disorders of optic chiasm in (due to) other disorders
377.52	DISORDERS OPTIC CHIASM ASSOC W/OTH NEOPLASMS		**H47.42**	Disorders of optic chiasm in (due to) neoplasm
377.53	D/O OPTIC CHIASM ASSOC W/VASCULAR D/O	➡	**H47.43**	Disorders of optic chiasm in (due to) vascular disorders
377.54	D/O OPTIC CHIASM ASSOC W/INFLAMMATORY D/O	➡	**H47.41**	Disorders of optic chiasm in (due to) inflammatory disorders
377.61	DISORDERS OTH VISUAL PATHWAYS ASSOC W/NEOPLASMS		**H47.521**	Disord of visual pathways in (due to) neoplasm, right side
			H47.522	Disorders of visual pathways in (due to) neoplasm, left side
			H47.529	Disorders of visual pathways in (due to) neoplasm, unsp side

ICD-9-CM		ICD-10-CM	
377.62	D/O OTH VISUAL PATHWAYS ASSOC W/VASCULAR D/O	**H47.531**	Disord of visual pathways in vascular disord, right side
		H47.532	Disord of visual pathways in vascular disord, left side
		H47.539	Disord of visual pathways in vascular disord, unsp side
377.63	D/O OTH VISUAL PATHWAYS ASSOC W/INFLAMMATORY D/O	**H47.511**	Disord of visual pathways in inflam disord, right side
		H47.512	Disord of visual pathways in inflam disord, left side
		H47.519	Disord of visual pathways in inflam disord, unsp side
377.71	DISORDERS VISUAL CORTEX ASSOCIATED W/NEOPLASMS	**H47.631**	Disord of visual cortex in neoplasm, right side of brain
		H47.632	Disord of visual cortex in neoplasm, left side of brain
		H47.639	Disord of visual cortex in neoplasm, unsp side of brain
377.72	D/O VISUAL CORTEX ASSOC W/VASCULAR D/O	**H47.641**	Disord of visual cortex in vasc disord, right side of brain
		H47.642	Disord of visual cortex in vasc disord, left side of brain
		H47.649	Disord of visual cortex in vasc disord, unsp side of brain
377.73	D/O VISUAL CORTEX ASSOC W/INFLAMMATORY D/O	**H47.621**	Disord of visual cortex in inflam disord, r side of brain
		H47.622	Disord of visual cortex in inflam disord, left side of brain
		H47.629	Disord of visual cortex in inflam disord, unsp side of brain
377.75	D/O VISUAL CORTEX ASSOC W/CORTICAL BLINDNESS	**H47.611**	Cortical blindness, right side of brain
		H47.612	Cortical blindness, left side of brain
		H47.619	Cortical blindness, unspecified side of brain
377.9	UNSPECIFIED DISORDER OPTIC NERVE&VISUAL PATHWAYS	**H47.9**	Unspecified disorder of visual pathways
378.ØØ	UNSPECIFIED ESOTROPIA	➡ **H5Ø.ØØ**	Unspecified esotropia
378.Ø1	MONOCULAR ESOTROPIA	**H5Ø.Ø11**	Monocular esotropia, right eye
		H5Ø.Ø12	Monocular esotropia, left eye
378.Ø2	MONOCULAR ESOTROPIA WITH A PATTERN	**H5Ø.Ø21**	Monocular esotropia with A pattern, right eye
		H5Ø.Ø22	Monocular esotropia with A pattern, left eye
378.Ø3	MONOCULAR ESOTROPIA WITH V PATTERN	**H5Ø.Ø31**	Monocular esotropia with V pattern, right eye
		H5Ø.Ø32	Monocular esotropia with V pattern, left eye
378.Ø4	MONOCULAR ESOTROPIA WITH OTHER NONCOMITANCIES	**H5Ø.Ø41**	Monocular esotropia with other noncomitancies, right eye
		H5Ø.Ø42	Monocular esotropia with other noncomitancies, left eye
378.Ø5	ALTERNATING ESOTROPIA	➡ **H5Ø.Ø5**	Alternating esotropia
378.Ø6	ALTERNATING ESOTROPIA WITH A PATTERN	➡ **H5Ø.Ø6**	Alternating esotropia with A pattern
378.Ø7	ALTERNATING ESOTROPIA WITH V PATTERN	➡ **H5Ø.Ø7**	Alternating esotropia with V pattern
378.Ø8	ALTERNATING ESOTROPIA WITH OTHER NONCOMITANCIES	➡ **H5Ø.Ø8**	Alternating esotropia with other noncomitancies
378.1Ø	UNSPECIFIED EXOTROPIA	➡ **H5Ø.1Ø**	Unspecified exotropia
378.11	MONOCULAR EXOTROPIA	**H5Ø.111**	Monocular exotropia, right eye
		H5Ø.112	Monocular exotropia, left eye
378.12	MONOCULAR EXOTROPIA WITH A PATTERN	**H5Ø.121**	Monocular exotropia with A pattern, right eye
		H5Ø.122	Monocular exotropia with A pattern, left eye
378.13	MONOCULAR EXOTROPIA WITH V PATTERN	**H5Ø.131**	Monocular exotropia with V pattern, right eye
		H5Ø.132	Monocular exotropia with V pattern, left eye
378.14	MONOCULAR EXOTROPIA WITH OTHER NONCOMITANCIES	**H5Ø.141**	Monocular exotropia with other noncomitancies, right eye
		H5Ø.142	Monocular exotropia with other noncomitancies, left eye
378.15	ALTERNATING EXOTROPIA	➡ **H5Ø.15**	Alternating exotropia
378.16	ALTERNATING EXOTROPIA WITH A PATTERN	➡ **H5Ø.16**	Alternating exotropia with A pattern
378.17	ALTERNATING EXOTROPIA WITH V PATTERN	➡ **H5Ø.17**	Alternating exotropia with V pattern
378.18	ALTERNATING EXOTROPIA WITH OTHER NONCOMITANCIES	➡ **H5Ø.18**	Alternating exotropia with other noncomitancies
378.2Ø	UNSPECIFIED INTERMITTENT HETEROTROPIA	➡ **H5Ø.3Ø**	Unspecified intermittent heterotropia
378.21	INTERMITTENT ESOTROPIA, MONOCULAR	**H5Ø.311**	Intermittent monocular esotropia, right eye
		H5Ø.312	Intermittent monocular esotropia, left eye
378.22	INTERMITTENT ESOTROPIA, ALTERNATING	➡ **H5Ø.32**	Intermittent alternating esotropia
378.23	INTERMITTENT EXOTROPIA, MONOCULAR	**H5Ø.331**	Intermittent monocular exotropia, right eye
		H5Ø.332	Intermittent monocular exotropia, left eye
378.24	INTERMITTENT EXOTROPIA, ALTERNATING	➡ **H5Ø.34**	Intermittent alternating exotropia
378.3Ø	UNSPECIFIED HETEROTROPIA	➡ **H5Ø.4Ø**	Unspecified heterotropia
378.31	HYPERTROPIA	**H5Ø.21**	Vertical strabismus, right eye
		H5Ø.22	Vertical strabismus, left eye
378.32	HYPOTROPIA	**H5Ø.21**	Vertical strabismus, right eye
		H5Ø.22	Vertical strabismus, left eye
378.33	CYCLOTROPIA	**H5Ø.411**	Cyclotropia, right eye
		H5Ø.412	Cyclotropia, left eye
378.34	MONOFIXATION SYNDROME	➡ **H5Ø.42**	Monofixation syndrome
378.35	ACCOMMODATIVE COMPONENT IN ESOTROPIA	➡ **H5Ø.43**	Accommodative component in esotropia
378.4Ø	UNSPECIFIED HETEROPHORIA	➡ **H5Ø.5Ø**	Unspecified heterophoria
378.41	ESOPHORIA	➡ **H5Ø.51**	Esophoria
378.42	EXOPHORIA	➡ **H5Ø.52**	Exophoria
378.43	VERTICAL HETEROPHORIA	➡ **H5Ø.53**	Vertical heterophoria
378.44	CYCLOPHORIA	➡ **H5Ø.54**	Cyclophoria
378.45	ALTERNATING HYPERPHORIA	➡ **H5Ø.55**	Alternating heterophoria
378.5Ø	UNSPECIFIED PARALYTIC STRABISMUS	**H49.881**	Other paralytic strabismus, right eye
		H49.882	Other paralytic strabismus, left eye
		H49.883	Other paralytic strabismus, bilateral
		H49.889	Other paralytic strabismus, unspecified eye
		H49.9	Unspecified paralytic strabismus

ICD-9-CM		ICD-10-CM	
378.51	PARALYTIC STRAB THIRD/OCULOMOTR NERVE PALSY PART	**H49.00**	Third [oculomotor] nerve palsy, unspecified eye
		H49.01	Third [oculomotor] nerve palsy, right eye
		H49.02	Third [oculomotor] nerve palsy, left eye
		H49.03	Third [oculomotor] nerve palsy, bilateral
378.52	PARALYTIC STRAB THIRD/OCULOMOTR NERV PALSY TOTAL	**H49.00**	Third [oculomotor] nerve palsy, unspecified eye
		H49.01	Third [oculomotor] nerve palsy, right eye
		H49.02	Third [oculomotor] nerve palsy, left eye
		H49.03	Third [oculomotor] nerve palsy, bilateral
378.53	PARALYTIC STRABISMUS 1/4/TROCHLEAR NERVE PALSY	**H49.10**	Fourth [trochlear] nerve palsy, unspecified eye
		H49.11	Fourth [trochlear] nerve palsy, right eye
		H49.12	Fourth [trochlear] nerve palsy, left eye
		H49.13	Fourth [trochlear] nerve palsy, bilateral
378.54	PARALYTIC STRABISMUS SIXTH/ABDUCENS NERVE PALSY	**H49.20**	Sixth [abducent] nerve palsy, unspecified eye
		H49.21	Sixth [abducent] nerve palsy, right eye
		H49.22	Sixth [abducent] nerve palsy, left eye
		H49.23	Sixth [abducent] nerve palsy, bilateral
378.55	PARALYTIC STRABISMUS EXTERNAL OPHTHALMOPLEGIA	**H49.40**	Progressive external ophthalmoplegia, unspecified eye
		H49.41	Progressive external ophthalmoplegia, right eye
		H49.42	Progressive external ophthalmoplegia, left eye
		H49.43	Progressive external ophthalmoplegia, bilateral
378.56	PARALYTIC STRABISMUS TOTAL OPHTHALMOPLEGIA	**H49.30**	Total (external) ophthalmoplegia, unspecified eye
		H49.31	Total (external) ophthalmoplegia, right eye
		H49.32	Total (external) ophthalmoplegia, left eye
		H49.33	Total (external) ophthalmoplegia, bilateral
378.60	UNSPECIFIED MECHANICAL STRABISMUS	➡ **H50.60**	Mechanical strabismus, unspecified
378.61	MECH STRABISMUS FROM BROWNS SHEATH SYNDROME	**H50.611**	Brown's sheath syndrome, right eye
		H50.612	Brown's sheath syndrome, left eye
378.62	MECH STRABISMUS FROM OTH MUSCULOFASCIAL D/O	**H50.69**	Other mechanical strabismus
378.63	MECH STRAB FROM LTD DUCTION ASSOC W/OTH CONDS	**H50.69**	Other mechanical strabismus
378.71	DUANES SYNDROME	**H50.811**	Duane's syndrome, right eye
		H50.812	Duane's syndrome, left eye
378.72	PROGRESSIVE EXTERNAL OPHTHALMOPLEGIA	**H50.89**	Other specified strabismus
378.73	STRABISMUS IN OTHER NEUROMUSCULAR DISORDERS	**H50.89**	Other specified strabismus
378.81	PALSY OF CONJUGATE GAZE	**H51.0**	Palsy (spasm) of conjugate gaze
378.82	SPASM OF CONJUGATE GAZE	**H51.0**	Palsy (spasm) of conjugate gaze
378.83	CONVERGENCE INSUFF/PALSY BINOCULAR EYE MOVEMENT	➡ **H51.11**	Convergence insufficiency
378.84	CONVERGENCE EXCESS/SPASM BINOCULAR EYE MOVEMENT	➡ **H51.12**	Convergence excess
378.85	ANOMALIES OF DIVERGENCE BINOCULAR EYE MOVEMENT	**H51.8**	Other specified disorders of binocular movement
378.86	INTERNUCLEAR OPHTHALMOPLEGIA	**H51.20**	Internuclear ophthalmoplegia, unspecified eye
		H51.21	Internuclear ophthalmoplegia, right eye
		H51.22	Internuclear ophthalmoplegia, left eye
		H51.23	Internuclear ophthalmoplegia, bilateral
378.87	OTHER DISSOCIATED DEVIATION OF EYE MOVEMENTS	**H51.8**	Other specified disorders of binocular movement
378.9	UNSPECIFIED DISORDER OF EYE MOVEMENTS	**H50.9**	Unspecified strabismus
		H51.9	Unspecified disorder of binocular movement
379.00	UNSPECIFIED SCLERITIS	**H15.001**	Unspecified scleritis, right eye
		H15.002	Unspecified scleritis, left eye
		H15.003	Unspecified scleritis, bilateral
		H15.009	Unspecified scleritis, unspecified eye
		H15.101	Unspecified episcleritis, right eye
		H15.102	Unspecified episcleritis, left eye
		H15.103	Unspecified episcleritis, bilateral
		H15.109	Unspecified episcleritis, unspecified eye
379.01	EPISCLERITIS PERIODICA FUGAX	**H15.111**	Episcleritis periodica fugax, right eye
		H15.112	Episcleritis periodica fugax, left eye
		H15.113	Episcleritis periodica fugax, bilateral
		H15.119	Episcleritis periodica fugax, unspecified eye
379.02	NODULAR EPISCLERITIS	**H15.121**	Nodular episcleritis, right eye
		H15.122	Nodular episcleritis, left eye
		H15.123	Nodular episcleritis, bilateral
		H15.129	Nodular episcleritis, unspecified eye
379.03	ANTERIOR SCLERITIS	**H15.011**	Anterior scleritis, right eye
		H15.012	Anterior scleritis, left eye
		H15.013	Anterior scleritis, bilateral
		H15.019	Anterior scleritis, unspecified eye
379.04	SCLEROMALACIA PERFORANS	**H15.051**	Scleromalacia perforans, right eye
		H15.052	Scleromalacia perforans, left eye
		H15.053	Scleromalacia perforans, bilateral
		H15.059	Scleromalacia perforans, unspecified eye
379.05	SCLERITIS WITH CORNEAL INVOLVEMENT	**H15.041**	Scleritis with corneal involvement, right eye
		H15.042	Scleritis with corneal involvement, left eye
		H15.043	Scleritis with corneal involvement, bilateral
		H15.049	Scleritis with corneal involvement, unspecified eye

ICD-9-CM		ICD-10-CM	
379.Ø6	BRAWNY SCLERITIS	**H15.Ø21**	Brawny scleritis, right eye
		H15.Ø22	Brawny scleritis, left eye
		H15.Ø23	Brawny scleritis, bilateral
		H15.Ø29	Brawny scleritis, unspecified eye
379.Ø7	POSTERIOR SCLERITIS	**H15.Ø31**	Posterior scleritis, right eye
		H15.Ø32	Posterior scleritis, left eye
		H15.Ø33	Posterior scleritis, bilateral
		H15.Ø39	Posterior scleritis, unspecified eye
379.Ø9	OTHER SCLERITIS AND EPISCLERITIS	**A18.51**	Tuberculous episcleritis
		H15.Ø91	Other scleritis, right eye
		H15.Ø92	Other scleritis, left eye
		H15.Ø93	Other scleritis, bilateral
		H15.Ø99	Other scleritis, unspecified eye
379.11	SCLERAL ECTASIA	**H15.841**	Scleral ectasia, right eye
		H15.842	Scleral ectasia, left eye
		H15.843	Scleral ectasia, bilateral
		H15.849	Scleral ectasia, unspecified eye
379.12	STAPHYLOMA POSTICUM	**H15.831**	Staphyloma posticum, right eye
		H15.832	Staphyloma posticum, left eye
		H15.833	Staphyloma posticum, bilateral
		H15.839	Staphyloma posticum, unspecified eye
379.13	EQUATORIAL STAPHYLOMA	**H15.811**	Equatorial staphyloma, right eye
		H15.812	Equatorial staphyloma, left eye
		H15.813	Equatorial staphyloma, bilateral
		H15.819	Equatorial staphyloma, unspecified eye
379.14	ANTERIOR STAPHYLOMA, LOCALIZED	**H15.821**	Localized anterior staphyloma, right eye
		H15.822	Localized anterior staphyloma, left eye
		H15.823	Localized anterior staphyloma, bilateral
		H15.829	Localized anterior staphyloma, unspecified eye
379.15	RING STAPHYLOMA	**H15.851**	Ring staphyloma, right eye
		H15.852	Ring staphyloma, left eye
		H15.853	Ring staphyloma, bilateral
		H15.859	Ring staphyloma, unspecified eye
379.16	OTHER DEGENERATIVE DISORDERS OF SCLERA	**H15.89**	Other disorders of sclera
379.19	OTHER SCLERAL DISORDER	**H15.89**	Other disorders of sclera
		H15.9	Unspecified disorder of sclera
379.21	VITREOUS DEGENERATION	**H43.811**	Vitreous degeneration, right eye
		H43.812	Vitreous degeneration, left eye
		H43.813	Vitreous degeneration, bilateral
		H43.819	Vitreous degeneration, unspecified eye
379.22	CRYSTALLINE DEPOSITS IN VITREOUS	**H43.2Ø**	Crystalline deposits in vitreous body, unspecified eye
		H43.21	Crystalline deposits in vitreous body, right eye
		H43.22	Crystalline deposits in vitreous body, left eye
		H43.23	Crystalline deposits in vitreous body, bilateral
379.23	VITREOUS HEMORRHAGE	**H43.1Ø**	Vitreous hemorrhage, unspecified eye
		H43.11	Vitreous hemorrhage, right eye
		H43.12	Vitreous hemorrhage, left eye
		H43.13	Vitreous hemorrhage, bilateral
379.24	OTHER VITREOUS OPACITIES	**H43.391**	Other vitreous opacities, right eye
		H43.392	Other vitreous opacities, left eye
		H43.393	Other vitreous opacities, bilateral
		H43.399	Other vitreous opacities, unspecified eye
379.25	VITREOUS MEMBRANES AND STRANDS	**H43.311**	Vitreous membranes and strands, right eye
		H43.312	Vitreous membranes and strands, left eye
		H43.313	Vitreous membranes and strands, bilateral
		H43.319	Vitreous membranes and strands, unspecified eye
379.26	VITREOUS PROLAPSE	**H43.ØØ**	Vitreous prolapse, unspecified eye
		H43.Ø1	Vitreous prolapse, right eye
		H43.Ø2	Vitreous prolapse, left eye
		H43.Ø3	Vitreous prolapse, bilateral
379.27	VITREOMACULAR ADHESION	**H43.821**	Vitreomacular adhesion, right eye
		H43.822	Vitreomacular adhesion, left eye
		H43.823	Vitreomacular adhesion, bilateral
		H43.829	Vitreomacular adhesion, unspecified eye
379.29	OTHER DISORDERS OF VITREOUS	**H43.89**	Other disorders of vitreous body
		H43.9	Unspecified disorder of vitreous body
379.31	APHAKIA	**H27.ØØ**	Aphakia, unspecified eye
		H27.Ø1	Aphakia, right eye
		H27.Ø2	Aphakia, left eye
		H27.Ø3	Aphakia, bilateral
379.32	SUBLUXATION OF LENS	**H27.1Ø**	Unspecified dislocation of lens
		H27.111	Subluxation of lens, right eye
		H27.112	Subluxation of lens, left eye
		H27.113	Subluxation of lens, bilateral
		H27.119	Subluxation of lens, unspecified eye

ICD-9-CM			ICD-10-CM	
379.33	ANTERIOR DISLOCATION OF LENS		**H27.121** **H27.122** **H27.123** **H27.129**	Anterior dislocation of lens, right eye Anterior dislocation of lens, left eye Anterior dislocation of lens, bilateral Anterior dislocation of lens, unspecified eye
379.34	POSTERIOR DISLOCATION OF LENS		**H27.131** **H27.132** **H27.133** **H27.139**	Posterior dislocation of lens, right eye Posterior dislocation of lens, left eye Posterior dislocation of lens, bilateral Posterior dislocation of lens, unspecified eye
379.39	OTHER DISORDERS OF LENS		**H27.8** **H27.9**	Other specified disorders of lens Unspecified disorder of lens
379.4Ø	UNSPECIFIED ABNORMAL PUPILLARY FUNCTION		**H57.ØØ** **H57.9**	Unspecified anomaly of pupillary function Unspecified disorder of eye and adnexa
379.41	ANISOCORIA	➡	**H57.Ø2**	Anisocoria
379.42	MIOSIS , NOT DUE TO MIOTICS	➡	**H57.Ø3**	Miosis
379.43	MYDRIASIS , NOT DUE TO MYDRIATICS	➡	**H57.Ø4**	Mydriasis
379.45	ARGYLL ROBERTSON PUPIL, ATYPICAL	➡	**H57.Ø1**	Argyll Robertson pupil, atypical
379.46	TONIC PUPILLARY REACTION		**H57.Ø51** **H57.Ø52** **H57.Ø53** **H57.Ø59**	Tonic pupil, right eye Tonic pupil, left eye Tonic pupil, bilateral Tonic pupil, unspecified eye
379.49	OTHER ANOMALY OF PUPILLARY FUNCTION	➡	**H57.Ø9**	Other anomalies of pupillary function
379.5Ø	UNSPECIFIED NYSTAGMUS	➡	**H55.ØØ**	Unspecified nystagmus
379.51	CONGENITAL NYSTAGMUS	➡	**H55.Ø1**	Congenital nystagmus
379.52	LATENT NYSTAGMUS	➡	**H55.Ø2**	Latent nystagmus
379.53	VISUAL DEPRIVATION NYSTAGMUS	➡	**H55.Ø3**	Visual deprivation nystagmus
379.54	NYSTAGMUS ASSOC W/DISORDERS VESTIBULAR SYSTEM		**H55.Ø9**	Other forms of nystagmus
379.55	DISSOCIATED NYSTAGMUS	➡	**H55.Ø4**	Dissociated nystagmus
379.56	OTHER FORMS OF NYSTAGMUS		**H55.Ø9**	Other forms of nystagmus
379.57	NYSTAGMUS W/DEFICIENCIES SACCADIC EYE MOVEMENTS	➡	**H55.81**	Saccadic eye movements
379.58	NYSTAGMUS W/DEFIC SMOOTH PURSUIT MOVEMENTS		**H55.89**	Other irregular eye movements
379.59	OTHER IRREGULARITIES OF EYE MOVEMENTS		**H55.89**	Other irregular eye movements
379.6Ø	INFLAMMATION INFECTION POSTPROCEDURAL BLEB UNS	➡	**H59.4Ø**	Inflammation (infection) of postprocedural bleb, unspecified
379.61	INFLAMMATION INF POSTPROCEDURAL BLEB STAGE 1	➡	**H59.41**	Inflammation (infection) of postprocedural bleb, stage 1
379.62	INFLAMMATION INF POSTPROCEDURAL BLEB STAGE 2	➡	**H59.42**	Inflammation (infection) of postprocedural bleb, stage 2
379.63	INFLAMMATION INF POSTPROCEDURAL BLEB STAGE 3	➡	**H59.43**	Inflammation (infection) of postprocedural bleb, stage 3
379.8	OTHER SPECIFIED DISORDERS OF EYE AND ADNEXA		**H57.8**	Other specified disorders of eye and adnexa
379.9Ø	UNSPECIFIED DISORDER OF EYE		**H57.9**	Unspecified disorder of eye and adnexa
379.91	PAIN IN OR AROUND EYE		**H57.1Ø** **H57.11** **H57.12** **H57.13**	Ocular pain, unspecified eye Ocular pain, right eye Ocular pain, left eye Ocular pain, bilateral
379.92	SWELLING OR MASS OF EYE		**H57.8**	Other specified disorders of eye and adnexa
379.93	REDNESS OR DISCHARGE OF EYE		**H57.8**	Other specified disorders of eye and adnexa
379.99	OTHER ILL-DEFINED DISORDER OF EYE		**H57.8**	Other specified disorders of eye and adnexa
38Ø.ØØ	UNSPECIFIED PERICHONDRITIS OF PINNA		**H61.ØØ1** **H61.ØØ2** **H61.ØØ3** **H61.ØØ9**	Unspecified perichondritis of right external ear Unspecified perichondritis of left external ear Unspecified perichondritis of external ear, bilateral Unspecified perichondritis of external ear, unspecified ear
38Ø.Ø1	ACUTE PERICHONDRITIS OF PINNA		**H61.Ø11** **H61.Ø12** **H61.Ø13** **H61.Ø19**	Acute perichondritis of right external ear Acute perichondritis of left external ear Acute perichondritis of external ear, bilateral Acute perichondritis of external ear, unspecified ear
38Ø.Ø2	CHRONIC PERICHONDRITIS OF PINNA		**H61.Ø21** **H61.Ø22** **H61.Ø23** **H61.Ø29**	Chronic perichondritis of right external ear Chronic perichondritis of left external ear Chronic perichondritis of external ear, bilateral Chronic perichondritis of external ear, unspecified ear
38Ø.Ø3	CHONDRITIS OF PINNA		**H61.Ø31** **H61.Ø32** **H61.Ø33** **H61.Ø39**	Chondritis of right external ear Chondritis of left external ear Chondritis of external ear, bilateral Chondritis of external ear, unspecified ear

ICD-9-CM		ICD-10-CM	
380.10	UNSPECIFIED INFECTIVE OTITIS EXTERNA	**H60.00**	Abscess of external ear, unspecified ear
		H60.01	Abscess of right external ear
		H60.02	Abscess of left external ear
		H60.03	Abscess of external ear, bilateral
		H60.10	Cellulitis of external ear, unspecified ear
		H60.11	Cellulitis of right external ear
		H60.12	Cellulitis of left external ear
		H60.13	Cellulitis of external ear, bilateral
		H60.311	Diffuse otitis externa, right ear
		H60.312	Diffuse otitis externa, left ear
		H60.313	Diffuse otitis externa, bilateral
		H60.319	Diffuse otitis externa, unspecified ear
		H60.321	Hemorrhagic otitis externa, right ear
		H60.322	Hemorrhagic otitis externa, left ear
		H60.323	Hemorrhagic otitis externa, bilateral
		H60.329	Hemorrhagic otitis externa, unspecified ear
		H60.391	Other infective otitis externa, right ear
		H60.392	Other infective otitis externa, left ear
		H60.393	Other infective otitis externa, bilateral
		H60.399	Other infective otitis externa, unspecified ear
380.11	ACUTE INFECTION OF PINNA	**H61.90**	Disorder of external ear, unspecified, unspecified ear
		H61.91	Disorder of right external ear, unspecified
		H61.92	Disorder of left external ear, unspecified
		H61.93	Disorder of external ear, unspecified, bilateral
380.12	ACUTE SWIMMERS EAR	**H60.331**	Swimmer's ear, right ear
		H60.332	Swimmer's ear, left ear
		H60.333	Swimmer's ear, bilateral
		H60.339	Swimmer's ear, unspecified ear
380.13	OTHER ACUTE INFECTIONS OF EXTERNAL EAR	**H62.40**	Otitis externa in oth diseases classd elswhr, unsp ear
		H62.41	Otitis externa in oth diseases classd elswhr, right ear
		H62.42	Otitis externa in oth diseases classd elswhr, left ear
		H62.43	Otitis externa in oth diseases classd elswhr, bilateral
		H62.8X1	Oth disorders of r ext ear in diseases classd elswhr
		H62.8X2	Oth disorders of left external ear in diseases classd elswhr
		H62.8X3	Oth disorders of ext ear in diseases classd elswhr, bi
		H62.8X9	Oth disorders of ext ear in diseases classd elswhr, unsp ear
380.14	MALIGNANT OTITIS EXTERNA	**H60.20**	Malignant otitis externa, unspecified ear
		H60.21	Malignant otitis externa, right ear
		H60.22	Malignant otitis externa, left ear
		H60.23	Malignant otitis externa, bilateral
380.15	CHRONIC MYCOTIC OTITIS EXTERNA	**H62.8X1**	Oth disorders of r ext ear in diseases classd elswhr
		H62.8X2	Oth disorders of left external ear in diseases classd elswhr
		H62.8X3	Oth disorders of ext ear in diseases classd elswhr, bi
		H62.8X9	Oth disorders of ext ear in diseases classd elswhr, unsp ear
380.16	OTHER CHRONIC INFECTIVE OTITIS EXTERNA	**H60.399**	Other infective otitis externa, unspecified ear
380.21	CHOLESTEATOMA OF EXTERNAL EAR	**H60.40**	Cholesteatoma of external ear, unspecified ear
		H60.41	Cholesteatoma of right external ear
		H60.42	Cholesteatoma of left external ear
		H60.43	Cholesteatoma of external ear, bilateral
380.22	OTHER ACUTE OTITIS EXTERNA	**H60.501**	Unspecified acute noninfective otitis externa, right ear
		H60.502	Unspecified acute noninfective otitis externa, left ear
		H60.503	Unspecified acute noninfective otitis externa, bilateral
		H60.509	Unsp acute noninfective otitis externa, unspecified ear
		H60.511	Acute actinic otitis externa, right ear
		H60.512	Acute actinic otitis externa, left ear
		H60.513	Acute actinic otitis externa, bilateral
		H60.519	Acute actinic otitis externa, unspecified ear
		H60.521	Acute chemical otitis externa, right ear
		H60.522	Acute chemical otitis externa, left ear
		H60.523	Acute chemical otitis externa, bilateral
		H60.529	Acute chemical otitis externa, unspecified ear
		H60.531	Acute contact otitis externa, right ear
		H60.532	Acute contact otitis externa, left ear
		H60.533	Acute contact otitis externa, bilateral
		H60.539	Acute contact otitis externa, unspecified ear
		H60.541	Acute eczematoid otitis externa, right ear
		H60.542	Acute eczematoid otitis externa, left ear
		H60.543	Acute eczematoid otitis externa, bilateral
		H60.549	Acute eczematoid otitis externa, unspecified ear
		H60.551	Acute reactive otitis externa, right ear
		H60.552	Acute reactive otitis externa, left ear
		H60.553	Acute reactive otitis externa, bilateral
		H60.559	Acute reactive otitis externa, unspecified ear
		H60.591	Other noninfective acute otitis externa, right ear
		H60.592	Other noninfective acute otitis externa, left ear
		H60.593	Other noninfective acute otitis externa, bilateral
		H60.599	Other noninfective acute otitis externa, unspecified ear

ICD-9-CM		ICD-10-CM	
380.23	OTHER CHRONIC OTITIS EXTERNA	**H60.60**	Unspecified chronic otitis externa, unspecified ear
		H60.61	Unspecified chronic otitis externa, right ear
		H60.62	Unspecified chronic otitis externa, left ear
		H60.63	Unspecified chronic otitis externa, bilateral
		H60.8X1	Other otitis externa, right ear
		H60.8X2	Other otitis externa, left ear
		H60.8X3	Other otitis externa, bilateral
		H60.8X9	Other otitis externa, unspecified ear
		H60.90	Unspecified otitis externa, unspecified ear
		H60.91	Unspecified otitis externa, right ear
		H60.92	Unspecified otitis externa, left ear
		H60.93	Unspecified otitis externa, bilateral
380.30	UNSPECIFIED DISORDER OF PINNA	**H61.101**	Unspecified noninfective disorders of pinna, right ear
		H61.102	Unspecified noninfective disorders of pinna, left ear
		H61.103	Unspecified noninfective disorders of pinna, bilateral
		H61.109	Unspecified noninfective disorders of pinna, unspecified ear
380.31	HEMATOMA OF AURICLE OR PINNA	**H61.121**	Hematoma of pinna, right ear
		H61.122	Hematoma of pinna, left ear
		H61.123	Hematoma of pinna, bilateral
		H61.129	Hematoma of pinna, unspecified ear
380.32	ACQUIRED DEFORMITIES OF AURICLE OR PINNA	**H61.111**	Acquired deformity of pinna, right ear
		H61.112	Acquired deformity of pinna, left ear
		H61.113	Acquired deformity of pinna, bilateral
		H61.119	Acquired deformity of pinna, unspecified ear
380.39	OTHER NONINFECTIOUS DISORDER OF PINNA	**H61.191**	Noninfective disorders of pinna, right ear
		H61.192	Noninfective disorders of pinna, left ear
		H61.193	Noninfective disorders of pinna, bilateral
		H61.199	Noninfective disorders of pinna, unspecified ear
380.4	IMPACTED CERUMEN	**H61.20**	Impacted cerumen, unspecified ear
		H61.21	Impacted cerumen, right ear
		H61.22	Impacted cerumen, left ear
		H61.23	Impacted cerumen, bilateral
380.50	ACQ STENOSIS EXTERNAL EAR CANAL UNSPEC AS CAUSE	**H61.301**	Acquired stenosis of right external ear canal, unspecified
		H61.302	Acquired stenosis of left external ear canal, unspecified
		H61.303	Acquired stenosis of external ear canal, unsp, bilateral
		H61.309	Acquired stenosis of external ear canal, unsp, unsp ear
		H61.391	Other acquired stenosis of right external ear canal
		H61.392	Other acquired stenosis of left external ear canal
		H61.393	Other acquired stenosis of external ear canal, bilateral
		H61.399	Other acquired stenosis of external ear canal, unsp ear
380.51	ACQUIRED STENOSIS EXTERNAL EAR CANAL SEC TRAUMA	**H61.311**	Acquired stenosis of r ext ear canal secondary to trauma
		H61.312	Acquired stenosis of l ext ear canal secondary to trauma
		H61.313	Acquired stenosis of ext ear canal secondary to trauma, bi
		H61.319	Acquired stenosis of ext ear canal sec to trauma, unsp ear
380.52	ACQUIRED STENOSIS EXTERNAL EAR CANAL SEC SURGERY	**H61.391**	Other acquired stenosis of right external ear canal
		H61.392	Other acquired stenosis of left external ear canal
		H61.393	Other acquired stenosis of external ear canal, bilateral
		H61.399	Other acquired stenosis of external ear canal, unsp ear
380.53	ACQ STENOSIS EXTERNAL EAR CANAL SEC INFLAMMATION	**H61.321**	Acquired stenosis of r ext ear canal sec to inflam and infct
		H61.322	Acquired stenosis of l ext ear canal sec to inflam and infct
		H61.323	Acq stenosis of ext ear canal sec to inflam and infct, bi
		H61.329	Acq stenos of ext ear canal sec to inflam & infct, unsp ear
380.81	EXOSTOSIS OF EXTERNAL EAR CANAL	**H61.811**	Exostosis of right external canal
		H61.812	Exostosis of left external canal
		H61.813	Exostosis of external canal, bilateral
		H61.819	Exostosis of external canal, unspecified ear
380.89	OTHER DISORDER OF EXTERNAL EAR	**H61.891**	Other specified disorders of right external ear
		H61.892	Other specified disorders of left external ear
		H61.893	Other specified disorders of external ear, bilateral
		H61.899	Other specified disorders of external ear, unspecified ear
380.9	UNSPECIFIED DISORDER OF EXTERNAL EAR	**H61.90**	Disorder of external ear, unspecified, unspecified ear
		H61.91	Disorder of right external ear, unspecified
		H61.92	Disorder of left external ear, unspecified
		H61.93	Disorder of external ear, unspecified, bilateral
381.00	UNSPECIFIED ACUTE NONSUPPURATIVE OTITIS MEDIA	**H65.191**	Other acute nonsuppurative otitis media, right ear
		H65.192	Other acute nonsuppurative otitis media, left ear
		H65.193	Other acute nonsuppurative otitis media, bilateral
		H65.194	Oth acute nonsuppurative otitis media, recurrent, right ear
		H65.195	Other acute nonsuppurative otitis media, recurrent, left ear
		H65.196	Oth acute nonsuppurative otitis media, recurrent, bilateral
		H65.197	Other acute nonsuppurative otitis media recurrent, unsp ear
		H65.199	Other acute nonsuppurative otitis media, unspecified ear

ICD-9-CM		ICD-10-CM	
381.Ø1	ACUTE SEROUS OTITIS MEDIA	**H65.ØØ**	Acute serous otitis media, unspecified ear
		H65.Ø1	Acute serous otitis media, right ear
		H65.Ø2	Acute serous otitis media, left ear
		H65.Ø3	Acute serous otitis media, bilateral
		H65.Ø4	Acute serous otitis media, recurrent, right ear
		H65.Ø5	Acute serous otitis media, recurrent, left ear
		H65.Ø6	Acute serous otitis media, recurrent, bilateral
		H65.Ø7	Acute serous otitis media, recurrent, unspecified ear
381.Ø2	ACUTE MUCOID OTITIS MEDIA	**H65.111**	Acute and subacute allergic otitis media (serous), r ear
		H65.112	Acute and subacute allergic otitis media (serous), left ear
		H65.113	Acute and subacute allergic otitis media (serous), bi
		H65.114	Acute and subacute allergic otitis media, recur, r ear
		H65.115	Acute and subacute allergic otitis media, recur, left ear
		H65.116	Acute and subacute allergic otitis media (serous), recur, bi
		H65.117	Acute and subacute allergic otitis media, recur, unsp ear
		H65.119	Acute and subacute allergic otitis media (serous), unsp ear
381.Ø3	ACUTE SANGUINOUS OTITIS MEDIA	**H65.111**	Acute and subacute allergic otitis media (serous), r ear
		H65.112	Acute and subacute allergic otitis media (serous), left ear
		H65.113	Acute and subacute allergic otitis media (serous), bi
		H65.114	Acute and subacute allergic otitis media, recur, r ear
		H65.115	Acute and subacute allergic otitis media, recur, left ear
		H65.116	Acute and subacute allergic otitis media (serous), recur, bi
		H65.117	Acute and subacute allergic otitis media, recur, unsp ear
		H65.119	Acute and subacute allergic otitis media (serous), unsp ear
381.Ø4	ACUTE ALLERGIC SEROUS OTITIS MEDIA	**H65.111**	Acute and subacute allergic otitis media (serous), r ear
		H65.112	Acute and subacute allergic otitis media (serous), left ear
		H65.113	Acute and subacute allergic otitis media (serous), bi
		H65.114	Acute and subacute allergic otitis media, recur, r ear
		H65.115	Acute and subacute allergic otitis media, recur, left ear
		H65.116	Acute and subacute allergic otitis media (serous), recur, bi
		H65.117	Acute and subacute allergic otitis media, recur, unsp ear
		H65.119	Acute and subacute allergic otitis media (serous), unsp ear
381.Ø5	ACUTE ALLERGIC MUCOID OTITIS MEDIA	**H65.111**	Acute and subacute allergic otitis media (serous), r ear
		H65.112	Acute and subacute allergic otitis media (serous), left ear
		H65.113	Acute and subacute allergic otitis media (serous), bi
		H65.114	Acute and subacute allergic otitis media, recur, r ear
		H65.115	Acute and subacute allergic otitis media, recur, left ear
		H65.116	Acute and subacute allergic otitis media (serous), recur, bi
		H65.117	Acute and subacute allergic otitis media, recur, unsp ear
		H65.119	Acute and subacute allergic otitis media (serous), unsp ear
381.Ø6	ACUTE ALLERGIC SANGUINOUS OTITIS MEDIA	**H65.111**	Acute and subacute allergic otitis media (serous), r ear
		H65.112	Acute and subacute allergic otitis media (serous), left ear
		H65.113	Acute and subacute allergic otitis media (serous), bi
		H65.114	Acute and subacute allergic otitis media, recur, r ear
		H65.115	Acute and subacute allergic otitis media, recur, left ear
		H65.116	Acute and subacute allergic otitis media (serous), recur, bi
		H65.117	Acute and subacute allergic otitis media, recur, unsp ear
		H65.119	Acute and subacute allergic otitis media (serous), unsp ear
381.1Ø	SIMPLE/UNSPECIFIED CHRONIC SEROUS OTITIS MEDIA	**H65.2Ø**	Chronic serous otitis media, unspecified ear
		H65.21	Chronic serous otitis media, right ear
		H65.22	Chronic serous otitis media, left ear
		H65.23	Chronic serous otitis media, bilateral
381.19	OTHER CHRONIC SEROUS OTITIS MEDIA	**H65.2Ø**	Chronic serous otitis media, unspecified ear
		H65.21	Chronic serous otitis media, right ear
		H65.22	Chronic serous otitis media, left ear
		H65.23	Chronic serous otitis media, bilateral
381.2Ø	SIMPLE/UNSPECIFIED CHRONIC MUCOID OTITIS MEDIA	**H65.3Ø**	Chronic mucoid otitis media, unspecified ear
		H65.31	Chronic mucoid otitis media, right ear
		H65.32	Chronic mucoid otitis media, left ear
		H65.33	Chronic mucoid otitis media, bilateral
381.29	OTHER CHRONIC MUCOID OTITIS MEDIA	**H65.3Ø**	Chronic mucoid otitis media, unspecified ear
		H65.31	Chronic mucoid otitis media, right ear
		H65.32	Chronic mucoid otitis media, left ear
		H65.33	Chronic mucoid otitis media, bilateral
381.3	OTHER&UNSPEC CHRONIC NONSUPPURATIVE OTITIS MEDIA	**H65.411**	Chronic allergic otitis media, right ear
		H65.412	Chronic allergic otitis media, left ear
		H65.413	Chronic allergic otitis media, bilateral
		H65.419	Chronic allergic otitis media, unspecified ear
		H65.491	Other chronic nonsuppurative otitis media, right ear
		H65.492	Other chronic nonsuppurative otitis media, left ear
		H65.493	Other chronic nonsuppurative otitis media, bilateral
		H65.499	Other chronic nonsuppurative otitis media, unspecified ear
381.4	NONSUPPRATV OTITIS MEDIA NOT SPEC AS ACUT/CHRON	**H65.9Ø**	Unspecified nonsuppurative otitis media, unspecified ear
		H65.91	Unspecified nonsuppurative otitis media, right ear
		H65.92	Unspecified nonsuppurative otitis media, left ear
		H65.93	Unspecified nonsuppurative otitis media, bilateral
381.5Ø	UNSPECIFIED EUSTACHIAN SALPINGITIS	**H68.ØØ1**	Unspecified Eustachian salpingitis, right ear
		H68.ØØ2	Unspecified Eustachian salpingitis, left ear
		H68.ØØ3	Unspecified Eustachian salpingitis, bilateral
		H68.ØØ9	Unspecified Eustachian salpingitis, unspecified ear

ICD-9-CM		ICD-10-CM	
381.51	ACUTE EUSTACHIAN SALPINGITIS	**H68.Ø11**	Acute Eustachian salpingitis, right ear
		H68.Ø12	Acute Eustachian salpingitis, left ear
		H68.Ø13	Acute Eustachian salpingitis, bilateral
		H68.Ø19	Acute Eustachian salpingitis, unspecified ear
381.52	CHRONIC EUSTACHIAN SALPINGITIS	**H68.Ø21**	Chronic Eustachian salpingitis, right ear
		H68.Ø22	Chronic Eustachian salpingitis, left ear
		H68.Ø23	Chronic Eustachian salpingitis, bilateral
		H68.Ø29	Chronic Eustachian salpingitis, unspecified ear
381.6Ø	UNSPECIFIED OBSTRUCTION OF EUSTACHIAN TUBE	**H68.1Ø1**	Unspecified obstruction of Eustachian tube, right ear
		H68.1Ø2	Unspecified obstruction of Eustachian tube, left ear
		H68.1Ø3	Unspecified obstruction of Eustachian tube, bilateral
		H68.1Ø9	Unspecified obstruction of Eustachian tube, unspecified ear
381.61	OSSEOUS OBSTRUCTION OF EUSTACHIAN TUBE	**H68.111**	Osseous obstruction of Eustachian tube, right ear
		H68.112	Osseous obstruction of Eustachian tube, left ear
		H68.113	Osseous obstruction of Eustachian tube, bilateral
		H68.119	Osseous obstruction of Eustachian tube, unspecified ear
381.62	INTRINSIC CARTNOUS OBSTRUCTION EUSTACHIAN TUBE	**H68.121**	Intrinsic cartilagenous obst of eustach tube, right ear
		H68.122	Intrinsic cartilagenous obst of eustach tube, left ear
		H68.123	Intrinsic cartilagenous obst of eustach tube, bilateral
		H68.129	Intrinsic cartilagenous obst of eustach tube, unsp ear
381.63	EXTRINSIC CARTNOUS OBSTRUCTION EUSTACHIAN TUBE	**H68.131**	Extrinsic cartilagenous obst of eustach tube, right ear
		H68.132	Extrinsic cartilagenous obst of eustach tube, left ear
		H68.133	Extrinsic cartilagenous obst of eustach tube, bilateral
		H68.139	Extrinsic cartilagenous obst of eustach tube, unsp ear
381.7	PATULOUS EUSTACHIAN TUBE	**H69.ØØ**	Patulous Eustachian tube, unspecified ear
		H69.Ø1	Patulous Eustachian tube, right ear
		H69.Ø2	Patulous Eustachian tube, left ear
		H69.Ø3	Patulous Eustachian tube, bilateral
381.81	DYSFUNCTION OF EUSTACHIAN TUBE	**H69.8Ø**	Oth disrd of Eustachian tube, unspecified ear
		H69.81	Other specified disorders of Eustachian tube, right ear
		H69.82	Other specified disorders of Eustachian tube, left ear
		H69.83	Other specified disorders of Eustachian tube, bilateral
381.89	OTHER DISORDERS OF EUSTACHIAN TUBE	**H69.8Ø**	Oth disrd of Eustachian tube, unspecified ear
		H69.81	Other specified disorders of Eustachian tube, right ear
		H69.82	Other specified disorders of Eustachian tube, left ear
		H69.83	Other specified disorders of Eustachian tube, bilateral
381.9	UNSPECIFIED EUSTACHIAN TUBE DISORDER	**H69.9Ø**	Unspecified Eustachian tube disorder, unspecified ear
		H69.91	Unspecified Eustachian tube disorder, right ear
		H69.92	Unspecified Eustachian tube disorder, left ear
		H69.93	Unspecified Eustachian tube disorder, bilateral
382.ØØ	ACUT SUPPRATV OTITIS MEDIA W/O SPONT RUP EARDRUM	**H66.ØØ1**	Acute suppr otitis media w/o spon rupt ear drum, right ear
		H66.ØØ2	Acute suppr otitis media w/o spon rupt ear drum, left ear
		H66.ØØ3	Acute suppr otitis media w/o spon rupt ear drum, bilateral
		H66.ØØ4	Ac suppr otitis media w/o spon rupt ear drum, recur, r ear
		H66.ØØ5	Ac suppr otitis media w/o spon rupt ear drum, recur, l ear
		H66.ØØ6	Acute suppr otitis media w/o spon rupt ear drum, recur, bi
		H66.ØØ7	Ac suppr otitis media w/o spon rupt ear drum,recur, unsp ear
		H66.ØØ9	Acute suppr otitis media w/o spon rupt ear drum, unsp ear
382.Ø1	ACUT SUPPRATV OTITIS MEDIA W/SPONT RUP EARDRUM	**H66.Ø11**	Acute suppr otitis media w spon rupt ear drum, right ear
		H66.Ø12	Acute suppr otitis media w spon rupt ear drum, left ear
		H66.Ø13	Acute suppr otitis media w spon rupt ear drum, bilateral
		H66.Ø14	Acute suppr otitis media w spon rupt ear drum, recur, r ear
		H66.Ø15	Acute suppr otitis media w spon rupt ear drum, recur, l ear
		H66.Ø16	Acute suppr otitis media w spon rupt ear drum, recurrent, bi
		H66.Ø17	Ac suppr otitis media w spon rupt ear drum, recur, unsp ear
		H66.Ø19	Acute suppr otitis media w spon rupt ear drum, unsp ear
382.Ø2	ACUTE SUPPURATIVE OTITIS MEDIA DZ CLASS ELSW	**H67.1**	Otitis media in diseases classified elsewhere, right ear
		H67.2	Otitis media in diseases classified elsewhere, left ear
		H67.3	Otitis media in diseases classified elsewhere, bilateral
		H67.9	Otitis media in diseases classified elsewhere, unsp ear
382.1	CHRONIC TUBOTYMPANIC SUPPURATIVE OTITIS MEDIA	**H66.1Ø**	Chronic tubotympanic suppurative otitis media, unspecified
		H66.11	Chronic tubotympanic suppurative otitis media, right ear
		H66.12	Chronic tubotympanic suppurative otitis media, left ear
		H66.13	Chronic tubotympanic suppurative otitis media, bilateral
382.2	CHRONIC ATTICOANTRAL SUPPURATIVE OTITIS MEDIA	**H66.2Ø**	Chronic atticoantral suppurative otitis media, unsp ear
		H66.21	Chronic atticoantral suppurative otitis media, right ear
		H66.22	Chronic atticoantral suppurative otitis media, left ear
		H66.23	Chronic atticoantral suppurative otitis media, bilateral
382.3	UNSPECIFIED CHRONIC SUPPURATIVE OTITIS MEDIA	**H66.3X1**	Other chronic suppurative otitis media, right ear
		H66.3X2	Other chronic suppurative otitis media, left ear
		H66.3X3	Other chronic suppurative otitis media, bilateral
		H66.3X9	Other chronic suppurative otitis media, unspecified ear
382.4	UNSPECIFIED SUPPURATIVE OTITIS MEDIA	**H66.4Ø**	Suppurative otitis media, unspecified, unspecified ear
		H66.41	Suppurative otitis media, unspecified, right ear
		H66.42	Suppurative otitis media, unspecified, left ear
		H66.43	Suppurative otitis media, unspecified, bilateral

ICD-9-CM		ICD-10-CM	
382.9	UNSPECIFIED OTITIS MEDIA	**H66.90**	Otitis media, unspecified, unspecified ear
		H66.91	Otitis media, unspecified. right ear
		H66.92	Otitis media, unspecified, left ear
		H66.93	Otitis media, unspecified, bilateral
383.00	ACUTE MASTOIDITIS WITHOUT COMPLICATIONS	**H70.001**	Acute mastoiditis without complications, right ear
		H70.002	Acute mastoiditis without complications, left ear
		H70.003	Acute mastoiditis without complications, bilateral
		H70.009	Acute mastoiditis without complications, unspecified ear
383.01	SUBPERIOSTEAL ABSCESS OF MASTOID	**H70.011**	Subperiosteal abscess of mastoid, right ear
		H70.012	Subperiosteal abscess of mastoid, left ear
		H70.013	Subperiosteal abscess of mastoid, bilateral
		H70.019	Subperiosteal abscess of mastoid, unspecified ear
383.02	ACUTE MASTOIDITIS WITH OTHER COMPLICATIONS	**H70.091**	Acute mastoiditis with other complications, right ear
		H70.092	Acute mastoiditis with other complications, left ear
		H70.093	Acute mastoiditis with other complications, bilateral
		H70.099	Acute mastoiditis with other complications, unspecified ear
383.1	CHRONIC MASTOIDITIS	**H70.10**	Chronic mastoiditis, unspecified ear
		H70.11	Chronic mastoiditis, right ear
		H70.12	Chronic mastoiditis, left ear
		H70.13	Chronic mastoiditis, bilateral
383.20	UNSPECIFIED PETROSITIS	**H70.201**	Unspecified petrositis, right ear
		H70.202	Unspecified petrositis, left ear
		H70.203	Unspecified petrositis, bilateral
		H70.209	Unspecified petrositis, unspecified ear
383.21	ACUTE PETROSITIS	**H70.211**	Acute petrositis, right ear
		H70.212	Acute petrositis, left ear
		H70.213	Acute petrositis, bilateral
		H70.219	Acute petrositis, unspecified ear
383.22	CHRONIC PETROSITIS	**H70.221**	Chronic petrositis, right ear
		H70.222	Chronic petrositis, left ear
		H70.223	Chronic petrositis, bilateral
		H70.229	Chronic petrositis, unspecified ear
383.30	UNSPECIFIED POSTMASTOIDECTOMY COMPLICATION	**H95.111**	Chronic inflammation of postmastoidectomy cavity, right ear
		H95.112	Chronic inflammation of postmastoidectomy cavity, left ear
		H95.113	Chronic inflam of postmastoidectomy cavity, bilateral ears
		H95.119	Chronic inflammation of postmastoidectomy cavity, unsp ear
		H95.191	Other disorders following mastoidectomy, right ear
		H95.192	Other disorders following mastoidectomy, left ear
		H95.193	Other disorders following mastoidectomy, bilateral ears
		H95.199	Other disorders following mastoidectomy, unspecified ear
383.31	MUCOSAL CYST OF POSTMASTOIDECTOMY CAVITY	**H95.131**	Mucosal cyst of postmastoidectomy cavity, right ear
		H95.132	Mucosal cyst of postmastoidectomy cavity, left ear
		H95.133	Mucosal cyst of postmastoidectomy cavity, bilateral ears
		H95.139	Mucosal cyst of postmastoidectomy cavity, unspecified ear
383.32	RECURRENT CHOLESTEATOMA POSTMASTOIDECTOMY CAVITY	**H95.00**	Recur cholesteatoma of postmastoidectomy cavity, unsp ear
		H95.01	Recur cholesteatoma of postmastoidectomy cavity, right ear
		H95.02	Recur cholesteatoma of postmastoidectomy cavity, left ear
		H95.03	Recurrent cholesteatoma of postmastoidectomy cavity, bi ears
383.33	GRANULATIONS OF POSTMASTOIDECTOMY CAVITY	**H95.121**	Granulation of postmastoidectomy cavity, right ear
		H95.122	Granulation of postmastoidectomy cavity, left ear
		H95.123	Granulation of postmastoidectomy cavity, bilateral ears
		H95.129	Granulation of postmastoidectomy cavity, unspecified ear
383.81	POSTAURICULAR FISTULA	**H70.811**	Postauricular fistula, right ear
		H70.812	Postauricular fistula, left ear
		H70.813	Postauricular fistula, bilateral
		H70.819	Postauricular fistula, unspecified ear
383.89	OTHER DISORDER OF MASTOID	**H70.891**	Other mastoiditis and related conditions, right ear
		H70.892	Other mastoiditis and related conditions, left ear
		H70.893	Other mastoiditis and related conditions, bilateral
		H70.899	Other mastoiditis and related conditions, unspecified ear
		H75.00	Mastoiditis in infec/parastc dis classd elswhr, unsp ear
		H75.01	Mastoiditis in infec/parastc diseases classd elswhr, r ear
		H75.02	Mastoiditis in infec/parastc dis classd elswhr, left ear
		H75.03	Mastoiditis in infec/parastc diseases classd elswhr, bi
		H75.80	Oth disrd of mid ear and mast in dis classd elswhr, unsp ear
		H75.81	Oth disrd of r mid ear and mastoid in diseases classd elswhr
		H75.82	Oth disrd of l mid ear and mastoid in diseases classd elswhr
		H75.83	Oth disrd of mid ear and mastoid in dis classd elswhr, bi
383.9	UNSPECIFIED MASTOIDITIS	**H70.90**	Unspecified mastoiditis, unspecified ear
		H70.91	Unspecified mastoiditis, right ear
		H70.92	Unspecified mastoiditis, left ear
		H70.93	Unspecified mastoiditis, bilateral

ICD-9-CM		ICD-10-CM	
384.00	UNSPECIFIED ACUTE MYRINGITIS	**H73.001**	Acute myringitis, right ear
		H73.002	Acute myringitis, left ear
		H73.003	Acute myringitis, bilateral
		H73.009	Acute myringitis, unspecified ear
		H73.20	Unspecified myringitis, unspecified ear
		H73.21	Unspecified myringitis, right ear
		H73.22	Unspecified myringitis, left ear
		H73.23	Unspecified myringitis, bilateral
384.01	BULLOUS MYRINGITIS	**H73.011**	Bullous myringitis, right ear
		H73.012	Bullous myringitis, left ear
		H73.013	Bullous myringitis, bilateral
		H73.019	Bullous myringitis, unspecified ear
384.09	OTH ACUTE MYRINGITIS W/O MENTION OTITIS MEDIA	**H73.091**	Other acute myringitis, right ear
		H73.092	Other acute myringitis, left ear
		H73.093	Other acute myringitis, bilateral
		H73.099	Other acute myringitis, unspecified ear
384.1	CHRONIC MYRINGITIS WITHOUT MENTION OTITIS MEDIA	**H73.10**	Chronic myringitis, unspecified ear
		H73.11	Chronic myringitis, right ear
		H73.12	Chronic myringitis, left ear
		H73.13	Chronic myringitis, bilateral
384.20	UNSPECIFIED PERFORATION OF TYMPANIC MEMBRANE	**H72.90**	Unsp perforation of tympanic membrane, unspecified ear
		H72.91	Unspecified perforation of tympanic membrane, right ear
		H72.92	Unspecified perforation of tympanic membrane, left ear
		H72.93	Unspecified perforation of tympanic membrane, bilateral
384.21	CENTRAL PERFORATION OF TYMPANIC MEMBRANE	**H72.00**	Central perforation of tympanic membrane, unspecified ear
		H72.01	Central perforation of tympanic membrane, right ear
		H72.02	Central perforation of tympanic membrane, left ear
		H72.03	Central perforation of tympanic membrane, bilateral
384.22	ATTIC PERFORATION OF TYMPANIC MEMBRANE	**H72.10**	Attic perforation of tympanic membrane, unspecified ear
		H72.11	Attic perforation of tympanic membrane, right ear
		H72.12	Attic perforation of tympanic membrane, left ear
		H72.13	Attic perforation of tympanic membrane, bilateral
384.23	OTHER MARGINAL PERFORATION OF TYMPANIC MEMBRANE	**H72.2X1**	Other marginal perforations of tympanic membrane, right ear
		H72.2X2	Other marginal perforations of tympanic membrane, left ear
		H72.2X3	Other marginal perforations of tympanic membrane, bilateral
		H72.2X9	Other marginal perforations of tympanic membrane, unsp ear
384.24	MULTIPLE PERFORATIONS OF TYMPANIC MEMBRANE	**H72.811**	Multiple perforations of tympanic membrane, right ear
		H72.812	Multiple perforations of tympanic membrane, left ear
		H72.813	Multiple perforations of tympanic membrane, bilateral
		H72.819	Multiple perforations of tympanic membrane, unspecified ear
384.25	TOTAL PERFORATION OF TYMPANIC MEMBRANE	**H72.821**	Total perforations of tympanic membrane, right ear
		H72.822	Total perforations of tympanic membrane, left ear
		H72.823	Total perforations of tympanic membrane, bilateral
		H72.829	Total perforations of tympanic membrane, unspecified ear
384.81	ATROPHIC FLACCID TYMPANIC MEMBRANE	**H73.811**	Atrophic flaccid tympanic membrane, right ear
		H73.812	Atrophic flaccid tympanic membrane, left ear
		H73.813	Atrophic flaccid tympanic membrane, bilateral
		H73.819	Atrophic flaccid tympanic membrane, unspecified ear
384.82	ATROPHIC NONFLACCID TYMPANIC MEMBRANE	**H73.821**	Atrophic nonflaccid tympanic membrane, right ear
		H73.822	Atrophic nonflaccid tympanic membrane, left ear
		H73.823	Atrophic nonflaccid tympanic membrane, bilateral
		H73.829	Atrophic nonflaccid tympanic membrane, unspecified ear
384.9	UNSPECIFIED DISORDER OF TYMPANIC MEMBRANE	**H73.891**	Other specified disorders of tympanic membrane, right ear
		H73.892	Other specified disorders of tympanic membrane, left ear
		H73.893	Other specified disorders of tympanic membrane, bilateral
		H73.899	Oth disrd of tympanic membrane, unspecified ear
		H73.90	Unspecified disorder of tympanic membrane, unspecified ear
		H73.91	Unspecified disorder of tympanic membrane, right ear
		H73.92	Unspecified disorder of tympanic membrane, left ear
		H73.93	Unspecified disorder of tympanic membrane, bilateral
385.00	TYMPANOSCLEROSIS UNSPECIFIED AS TO INVOLVEMENT	**H74.01**	Tympanosclerosis, right ear
		H74.02	Tympanosclerosis, left ear
		H74.03	Tympanosclerosis, bilateral
		H74.09	Tympanosclerosis, unspecified ear
385.01	TYMPANOSCLEROSIS INVLV TYMPANIC MEMBRANE ONLY	**H74.01**	Tympanosclerosis, right ear
		H74.02	Tympanosclerosis, left ear
		H74.03	Tympanosclerosis, bilateral
		H74.09	Tympanosclerosis, unspecified ear
385.02	TYMPANOSCLEROS INVLV TYMPANIC MEMB&EAR OSSICLES	**H74.01**	Tympanosclerosis, right ear
		H74.02	Tympanosclerosis, left ear
		H74.03	Tympanosclerosis, bilateral
		H74.09	Tympanosclerosis, unspecified ear
385.03	TYMPANOSCLEROSIS OF TM-EAR OSSICLES & MIDDLE EAR	**H74.01**	Tympanosclerosis, right ear
		H74.02	Tympanosclerosis, left ear
		H74.03	Tympanosclerosis, bilateral
		H74.09	Tympanosclerosis, unspecified ear

ICD-9-CM		ICD-10-CM	
385.Ø9	TYMPANOSCLEROSIS INVLV OTH COMBINATION STRCT	**H74.Ø1**	Tympanosclerosis, right ear
		H74.Ø2	Tympanosclerosis, left ear
		H74.Ø3	Tympanosclerosis, bilateral
		H74.Ø9	Tympanosclerosis, unspecified ear
385.1Ø	ADHES MIDDLE EAR DISEASE UNSPEC AS INVOLVEMENT	**H74.11**	Adhesive right middle ear disease
		H74.12	Adhesive left middle ear disease
		H74.13	Adhesive middle ear disease, bilateral
		H74.19	Adhesive middle ear disease, unspecified ear
385.11	ADHESIONS OF DRUM HEAD TO INCUS	**H74.11**	Adhesive right middle ear disease
		H74.12	Adhesive left middle ear disease
		H74.13	Adhesive middle ear disease, bilateral
		H74.19	Adhesive middle ear disease, unspecified ear
385.12	ADHESIONS OF DRUM HEAD TO STAPES	**H74.11**	Adhesive right middle ear disease
		H74.12	Adhesive left middle ear disease
		H74.13	Adhesive middle ear disease, bilateral
		H74.19	Adhesive middle ear disease, unspecified ear
385.13	ADHESIONS OF DRUM HEAD TO PROMONTORIUM	**H74.11**	Adhesive right middle ear disease
		H74.12	Adhesive left middle ear disease
		H74.13	Adhesive middle ear disease, bilateral
		H74.19	Adhesive middle ear disease, unspecified ear
385.19	OTHER MIDDLE EAR ADHESIONS AND COMBINATIONS	**H74.11**	Adhesive right middle ear disease
		H74.12	Adhesive left middle ear disease
		H74.13	Adhesive middle ear disease, bilateral
		H74.19	Adhesive middle ear disease, unspecified ear
385.21	IMPAIRED MOBILITY OF MALLEUS	**H74.311**	Ankylosis of ear ossicles, right ear
		H74.312	Ankylosis of ear ossicles, left ear
		H74.313	Ankylosis of ear ossicles, bilateral
		H74.319	Ankylosis of ear ossicles, unspecified ear
385.22	IMPAIRED MOBILITY OF OTHER EAR OSSICLES	**H74.311**	Ankylosis of ear ossicles, right ear
		H74.312	Ankylosis of ear ossicles, left ear
		H74.313	Ankylosis of ear ossicles, bilateral
		H74.319	Ankylosis of ear ossicles, unspecified ear
385.23	DISCONTINUITY OR DISLOCATION OF EAR OSSICLES	**H74.2Ø**	Discontinuity and dislocation of ear ossicles, unsp ear
		H74.21	Discontinuity and dislocation of right ear ossicles
		H74.22	Discontinuity and dislocation of left ear ossicles
		H74.23	Discontinuity and dislocation of ear ossicles, bilateral
		H74.391	Other acquired abnormalities of right ear ossicles
		H74.392	Other acquired abnormalities of left ear ossicles
		H74.393	Other acquired abnormalities of ear ossicles, bilateral
		H74.399	Other acquired abnormalities of ear ossicles, unsp ear
385.24	PARTIAL LOSS OR NECROSIS OF EAR OSSICLES	**H74.321**	Partial loss of ear ossicles, right ear
		H74.322	Partial loss of ear ossicles, left ear
		H74.323	Partial loss of ear ossicles, bilateral
		H74.329	Partial loss of ear ossicles, unspecified ear
385.3Ø	UNSPECIFIED CHOLESTEATOMA	**H71.9Ø**	Unspecified cholesteatoma, unspecified ear
		H71.91	Unspecified cholesteatoma, right ear
		H71.92	Unspecified cholesteatoma, left ear
		H71.93	Unspecified cholesteatoma, bilateral
385.31	CHOLESTEATOMA OF ATTIC	**H71.ØØ**	Cholesteatoma of attic, unspecified ear
		H71.Ø1	Cholesteatoma of attic, right ear
		H71.Ø2	Cholesteatoma of attic, left ear
		H71.Ø3	Cholesteatoma of attic, bilateral
385.32	CHOLESTEATOMA OF MIDDLE EAR	**H71.1Ø**	Cholesteatoma of tympanum, unspecified ear
		H71.11	Cholesteatoma of tympanum, right ear
		H71.12	Cholesteatoma of tympanum, left ear
		H71.13	Cholesteatoma of tympanum, bilateral
		H74.4Ø	Polyp of middle ear, unspecified ear
		H74.41	Polyp of right middle ear
		H74.42	Polyp of left middle ear
		H74.43	Polyp of middle ear, bilateral
385.33	CHOLESTEATOMA OF MIDDLE EAR AND MASTOID	**H71.2Ø**	Cholesteatoma of mastoid, unspecified ear
		H71.21	Cholesteatoma of mastoid, right ear
		H71.22	Cholesteatoma of mastoid, left ear
		H71.23	Cholesteatoma of mastoid, bilateral
385.35	DIFFUSE CHOLESTEATOSIS OF MIDDLE EAR AND MASTOID	**H71.3Ø**	Diffuse cholesteatosis, unspecified ear
		H71.31	Diffuse cholesteatosis, right ear
		H71.32	Diffuse cholesteatosis, left ear
		H71.33	Diffuse cholesteatosis, bilateral
385.82	CHOLESTERIN GRANULOMA OF MIDDLE EAR	**H74.8X9**	Oth disrd of middle ear and mastoid, unspecified ear
385.83	RETAINED FOREIGN BODY OF MIDDLE EAR	**H74.8X9**	Oth disrd of middle ear and mastoid, unspecified ear
385.89	OTHER DISORDERS OF MIDDLE EAR AND MASTOID	**H74.8X1**	Other specified disorders of right middle ear and mastoid
		H74.8X2	Other specified disorders of left middle ear and mastoid
		H74.8X3	Oth disrd of middle ear and mastoid, bilateral
		H74.8X9	Oth disrd of middle ear and mastoid, unspecified ear
385.9	UNSPECIFIED DISORDER OF MIDDLE EAR AND MASTOID	**H74.9Ø**	Unsp disorder of middle ear and mastoid, unspecified ear
		H74.91	Unspecified disorder of right middle ear and mastoid
		H74.92	Unspecified disorder of left middle ear and mastoid
		H74.93	Unspecified disorder of middle ear and mastoid, bilateral

ICD-9-CM		ICD-10-CM	
386.00	UNSPECIFIED MENIERES DISEASE	**H81.01**	Meniere's disease, right ear
		H81.02	Meniere's disease, left ear
		H81.03	Meniere's disease, bilateral
		H81.09	Meniere's disease, unspecified ear
386.01	ACTIVE MENIERES DISEASE COCHLEOVESTIBULAR	**H81.01**	Meniere's disease, right ear
		H81.02	Meniere's disease, left ear
		H81.03	Meniere's disease, bilateral
		H81.09	Meniere's disease, unspecified ear
386.02	ACTIVE MENIERES DISEASE, COCHLEAR	**H81.01**	Meniere's disease, right ear
		H81.02	Meniere's disease, left ear
		H81.03	Meniere's disease, bilateral
		H81.09	Meniere's disease, unspecified ear
386.03	ACTIVE MENIERES DISEASE VESTIBULAR	**H81.01**	Meniere's disease, right ear
		H81.02	Meniere's disease, left ear
		H81.03	Meniere's disease, bilateral
		H81.09	Meniere's disease, unspecified ear
386.04	INACTIVE MENIERES DISEASE	**H81.01**	Meniere's disease, right ear
		H81.02	Meniere's disease, left ear
		H81.03	Meniere's disease, bilateral
		H81.09	Meniere's disease, unspecified ear
386.10	UNSPECIFIED PERIPHERAL VERTIGO	**H81.391**	Other peripheral vertigo, right ear
		H81.392	Other peripheral vertigo, left ear
		H81.393	Other peripheral vertigo, bilateral
		H81.399	Other peripheral vertigo, unspecified ear
386.11	BENIGN PAROXYSMAL POSITIONAL VERTIGO	**H81.10**	Benign paroxysmal vertigo, unspecified ear
		H81.11	Benign paroxysmal vertigo, right ear
		H81.12	Benign paroxysmal vertigo, left ear
		H81.13	Benign paroxysmal vertigo, bilateral
386.12	VESTIBULAR NEURONITIS	**H81.20**	Vestibular neuronitis, unspecified ear
		H81.21	Vestibular neuronitis, right ear
		H81.22	Vestibular neuronitis, left ear
		H81.23	Vestibular neuronitis, bilateral
386.19	OTHER AND UNSPECIFIED PERIPHERAL VERTIGO	**H81.311**	Aural vertigo, right ear
		H81.312	Aural vertigo, left ear
		H81.313	Aural vertigo, bilateral
		H81.319	Aural vertigo, unspecified ear
386.2	VERTIGO OF CENTRAL ORIGIN	**H81.41**	Vertigo of central origin, right ear
		H81.42	Vertigo of central origin, left ear
		H81.43	Vertigo of central origin, bilateral
		H81.49	Vertigo of central origin, unspecified ear
386.30	UNSPECIFIED LABYRINTHITIS	**H83.01**	Labyrinthitis, right ear
		H83.02	Labyrinthitis, left ear
		H83.03	Labyrinthitis, bilateral
		H83.09	Labyrinthitis, unspecified ear
386.31	SEROUS LABYRINTHITIS	**H83.01**	Labyrinthitis, right ear
		H83.02	Labyrinthitis, left ear
		H83.03	Labyrinthitis, bilateral
		H83.09	Labyrinthitis, unspecified ear
386.32	CIRCUMSCRIBED LABYRINTHITIS	**H83.01**	Labyrinthitis, right ear
		H83.02	Labyrinthitis, left ear
		H83.03	Labyrinthitis, bilateral
		H83.09	Labyrinthitis, unspecified ear
386.33	SUPPURATIVE LABYRINTHITIS	**H83.01**	Labyrinthitis, right ear
		H83.02	Labyrinthitis, left ear
		H83.03	Labyrinthitis, bilateral
		H83.09	Labyrinthitis, unspecified ear
386.34	TOXIC LABYRINTHITIS	**H83.01**	Labyrinthitis, right ear
		H83.02	Labyrinthitis, left ear
		H83.03	Labyrinthitis, bilateral
		H83.09	Labyrinthitis, unspecified ear
386.35	VIRAL LABYRINTHITIS	**H83.01**	Labyrinthitis, right ear
		H83.02	Labyrinthitis, left ear
		H83.03	Labyrinthitis, bilateral
		H83.09	Labyrinthitis, unspecified ear
386.40	UNSPECIFIED LABYRINTHINE FISTULA	**H83.11**	Labyrinthine fistula, right ear
		H83.12	Labyrinthine fistula, left ear
		H83.13	Labyrinthine fistula, bilateral
		H83.19	Labyrinthine fistula, unspecified ear
386.41	ROUND WINDOW FISTULA	**H83.11**	Labyrinthine fistula, right ear
		H83.12	Labyrinthine fistula, left ear
		H83.13	Labyrinthine fistula, bilateral
		H83.19	Labyrinthine fistula, unspecified ear
386.42	OVAL WINDOW FISTULA	**H83.11**	Labyrinthine fistula, right ear
		H83.12	Labyrinthine fistula, left ear
		H83.13	Labyrinthine fistula, bilateral
		H83.19	Labyrinthine fistula, unspecified ear

ICD-9-CM		ICD-10-CM	
386.43	SEMICIRCULAR CANAL FISTULA	**H83.11**	Labyrinthine fistula, right ear
		H83.12	Labyrinthine fistula, left ear
		H83.13	Labyrinthine fistula, bilateral
		H83.19	Labyrinthine fistula, unspecified ear
386.48	LABYRINTHINE FISTULA OF COMBINED SITES	**H83.11**	Labyrinthine fistula, right ear
		H83.12	Labyrinthine fistula, left ear
		H83.13	Labyrinthine fistula, bilateral
		H83.19	Labyrinthine fistula, unspecified ear
386.50	UNSPECIFIED LABYRINTHINE DYSFUNCTION	**H83.2X1**	Labyrinthine dysfunction, right ear
		H83.2X2	Labyrinthine dysfunction, left ear
		H83.2X3	Labyrinthine dysfunction, bilateral
		H83.2X9	Labyrinthine dysfunction, unspecified ear
386.51	HYPERACTIVE LABYRINTH, UNILATERAL	**H83.2X1**	Labyrinthine dysfunction, right ear
		H83.2X2	Labyrinthine dysfunction, left ear
		H83.2X9	Labyrinthine dysfunction, unspecified ear
386.52	HYPERACTIVE LABYRINTH, BILATERAL	**H83.2X3**	Labyrinthine dysfunction, bilateral
		H83.2X9	Labyrinthine dysfunction, unspecified ear
386.53	HYPOACTIVE LABYRINTH, UNILATERAL	**H83.2X1**	Labyrinthine dysfunction, right ear
		H83.2X2	Labyrinthine dysfunction, left ear
		H83.2X9	Labyrinthine dysfunction, unspecified ear
386.54	HYPOACTIVE LABYRINTH, BILATERAL	**H83.2X3**	Labyrinthine dysfunction, bilateral
		H83.2X9	Labyrinthine dysfunction, unspecified ear
386.55	LOSS OF LABYRINTHINE REACTIVITY UNILATERAL	**H83.2X1**	Labyrinthine dysfunction, right ear
		H83.2X2	Labyrinthine dysfunction, left ear
		H83.2X9	Labyrinthine dysfunction, unspecified ear
386.56	LOSS OF LABYRINTHINE REACTIVITY BILATERAL	**H83.2X3**	Labyrinthine dysfunction, bilateral
		H83.2X9	Labyrinthine dysfunction, unspecified ear
386.58	OTH FORMS&COMBINATIONS LABYRINTHINE DYSFUNCTION	**H83.2X1**	Labyrinthine dysfunction, right ear
		H83.2X2	Labyrinthine dysfunction, left ear
		H83.2X3	Labyrinthine dysfunction, bilateral
		H83.2X9	Labyrinthine dysfunction, unspecified ear
386.8	OTHER DISORDERS OF LABYRINTH	**H81.8X1**	Other disorders of vestibular function, right ear
		H81.8X2	Other disorders of vestibular function, left ear
		H81.8X3	Other disorders of vestibular function, bilateral
		H81.8X9	Other disorders of vestibular function, unspecified ear
		H82.1	Vertiginous syndromes in diseases classd elswhr, right ear
		H82.2	Vertiginous syndromes in diseases classd elswhr, left ear
		H82.3	Vertiginous syndromes in diseases classd elswhr, bilateral
		H82.9	Vertiginous syndromes in diseases classd elswhr, unsp ear
		H83.8X1	Other specified diseases of right inner ear
		H83.8X2	Other specified diseases of left inner ear
		H83.8X3	Other specified diseases of inner ear, bilateral
		H83.8X9	Other specified diseases of inner ear, unspecified ear
386.9	UNSPEC VERTIGINOUS SYNDROMES&LABYRINTHINE D/O	**H81.90**	Unspecified disorder of vestibular function, unspecified ear
		H81.91	Unspecified disorder of vestibular function, right ear
		H81.92	Unspecified disorder of vestibular function, left ear
		H81.93	Unspecified disorder of vestibular function, bilateral
		H83.90	Unspecified disease of inner ear, unspecified ear
		H83.91	Unspecified disease of right inner ear
		H83.92	Unspecified disease of left inner ear
		H83.93	Unspecified disease of inner ear, bilateral
387.0	OTOSCLEROSIS INVLV OVAL WINDOW NONOBLITERATIVE	**H80.00**	Otosclerosis w oval window, nonobliterative, unsp ear
		H80.01	Otosclerosis w oval window, nonobliterative, right ear
		H80.02	Otosclerosis w oval window, nonobliterative, left ear
		H80.03	Otosclerosis involving oval window, nonobliterative, bi
387.1	OTOSCLEROSIS INVOLVING OVAL WINDOW OBLITERATIVE	**H80.10**	Otosclerosis involving oval window, obliterative, unsp ear
		H80.11	Otosclerosis involving oval window, obliterative, right ear
		H80.12	Otosclerosis involving oval window, obliterative, left ear
		H80.13	Otosclerosis involving oval window, obliterative, bilateral
387.2	COCHLEAR OTOSCLEROSIS	**H80.20**	Cochlear otosclerosis, unspecified ear
		H80.21	Cochlear otosclerosis, right ear
		H80.22	Cochlear otosclerosis, left ear
		H80.23	Cochlear otosclerosis, bilateral
387.8	OTHER OTOSCLEROSIS	**H80.80**	Other otosclerosis, unspecified ear
		H80.81	Other otosclerosis, right ear
		H80.82	Other otosclerosis, left ear
		H80.83	Other otosclerosis, bilateral
387.9	UNSPECIFIED OTOSCLEROSIS	**H80.90**	Unspecified otosclerosis, unspecified ear
		H80.91	Unspecified otosclerosis, right ear
		H80.92	Unspecified otosclerosis, left ear
		H80.93	Unspecified otosclerosis, bilateral
388.00	UNSPECIFIED DEGENERATIVE AND VASCULAR DISORDERS	**H93.091**	Unspecified degenerative and vascular disorders of right ear
		H93.092	Unspecified degenerative and vascular disorders of left ear
		H93.093	Unsp degenerative and vascular disorders of ear, bilateral
		H93.099	Unsp degenerative and vascular disorders of unspecified ear
388.01	PRESBYACUSIS	**H91.10**	Presbycusis, unspecified ear
		H91.11	Presbycusis, right ear
		H91.12	Presbycusis, left ear
		H91.13	Presbycusis, bilateral

ICD-9-CM		ICD-10-CM	
388.02	TRANSIENT ISCHEMIC DEAFNESS	**H93.011**	Transient ischemic deafness, right ear
		H93.012	Transient ischemic deafness, left ear
		H93.013	Transient ischemic deafness, bilateral
		H93.019	Transient ischemic deafness, unspecified ear
388.10	UNSPECIFIED NOISE EFFECTS ON INNER EAR	**H83.3X1**	Noise effects on right inner ear
		H83.3X2	Noise effects on left inner ear
		H83.3X3	Noise effects on inner ear, bilateral
		H83.3X9	Noise effects on inner ear, unspecified ear
388.11	ACOUSTIC TRAUMA TO EAR	**H91.8X1**	Other specified hearing loss, right ear
		H91.8X2	Other specified hearing loss, left ear
		H91.8X3	Other specified hearing loss, bilateral
		H91.8X9	Other specified hearing loss, unspecified ear
388.12	NOISE-INDUCED HEARING LOSS	**H83.3X1**	Noise effects on right inner ear
		H83.3X2	Noise effects on left inner ear
		H83.3X3	Noise effects on inner ear, bilateral
		H83.3X9	Noise effects on inner ear, unspecified ear
388.2	UNSPECIFIED SUDDEN HEARING LOSS	**H91.20**	Sudden idiopathic hearing loss, unspecified ear
		H91.21	Sudden idiopathic hearing loss, right ear
		H91.22	Sudden idiopathic hearing loss, left ear
		H91.23	Sudden idiopathic hearing loss, bilateral
388.30	UNSPECIFIED TINNITUS	**H93.11**	Tinnitus, right ear
		H93.12	Tinnitus, left ear
		H93.13	Tinnitus, bilateral
		H93.19	Tinnitus, unspecified ear
388.31	SUBJECTIVE TINNITUS	**H93.11**	Tinnitus, right ear
		H93.12	Tinnitus, left ear
		H93.13	Tinnitus, bilateral
		H93.19	Tinnitus, unspecified ear
388.32	OBJECTIVE TINNITUS	**H93.11**	Tinnitus, right ear
		H93.12	Tinnitus, left ear
		H93.13	Tinnitus, bilateral
		H93.19	Tinnitus, unspecified ear
388.40	UNSPECIFIED ABNORMAL AUDITORY PERCEPTION	**H93.241**	Temporary auditory threshold shift, right ear
		H93.242	Temporary auditory threshold shift, left ear
		H93.243	Temporary auditory threshold shift, bilateral
		H93.249	Temporary auditory threshold shift, unspecified ear
		H93.291	Other abnormal auditory perceptions, right ear
		H93.292	Other abnormal auditory perceptions, left ear
		H93.293	Other abnormal auditory perceptions, bilateral
		H93.299	Other abnormal auditory perceptions, unspecified ear
388.41	DIPLACUSIS	**H93.221**	Diplacusis, right ear
		H93.222	Diplacusis, left ear
		H93.223	Diplacusis, bilateral
		H93.229	Diplacusis, unspecified ear
388.42	HYPERACUSIS	**H93.231**	Hyperacusis, right ear
		H93.232	Hyperacusis, left ear
		H93.233	Hyperacusis, bilateral
		H93.239	Hyperacusis, unspecified ear
388.43	IMPAIRMENT OF AUDITORY DISCRIMINATION	**H93.299**	Other abnormal auditory perceptions, unspecified ear
388.44	OTHER ABNORMAL AUDITORY PERCEPTION RECRUITMENT	**H93.211**	Auditory recruitment, right ear
		H93.212	Auditory recruitment, left ear
		H93.213	Auditory recruitment, bilateral
		H93.219	Auditory recruitment, unspecified ear
388.45	ACQUIRED AUDITORY PROCESSING DISORDER	**H93.299**	Other abnormal auditory perceptions, unspecified ear
388.5	DISORDERS OF ACOUSTIC NERVE	**H93.3X1**	Disorders of right acoustic nerve
		H93.3X2	Disorders of left acoustic nerve
		H93.3X3	Disorders of bilateral acoustic nerves
		H93.3X9	Disorders of unspecified acoustic nerve
		H94.00	Acustc neuritis in infec/parastc dis classd elswhr, unsp ear
		H94.01	Acustc neuritis in infec/parastc dis classd elswhr, r ear
		H94.02	Acustc neuritis in infec/parastc dis classd elswhr, left ear
		H94.03	Acustc neuritis in infec/parastc diseases classd elswhr, bi
388.60	UNSPECIFIED OTORRHEA	**H92.10**	Otorrhea, unspecified ear
		H92.11	Otorrhea, right ear
		H92.12	Otorrhea, left ear
		H92.13	Otorrhea, bilateral
388.61	CEREBROSPINAL FLUID OTORRHEA	**G96.0**	Cerebrospinal fluid leak
388.69	OTHER OTORRHEA	**H92.20**	Otorrhagia, unspecified ear
		H92.21	Otorrhagia, right ear
		H92.22	Otorrhagia, left ear
		H92.23	Otorrhagia, bilateral
388.70	UNSPECIFIED OTALGIA	**H92.01**	Otalgia, right ear
		H92.02	Otalgia, left ear
		H92.03	Otalgia, bilateral
		H92.09	Otalgia, unspecified ear
388.71	OTOGENIC PAIN	**H92.09**	Otalgia, unspecified ear
388.72	REFERRED OTOGENIC PAIN	**H92.09**	Otalgia, unspecified ear

ICD-9-CM		ICD-10-CM	
388.8	OTHER DISORDERS OF EAR	**H93.8X1**	Other specified disorders of right ear
		H93.8X2	Other specified disorders of left ear
		H93.8X3	Other specified disorders of ear, bilateral
		H93.8X9	Other specified disorders of ear, unspecified ear
		H94.80	Oth disrd of ear in diseases classified elsewhere, unsp ear
		H94.81	Oth disrd of right ear in diseases classified elsewhere
		H94.82	Oth disrd of left ear in diseases classified elsewhere
		H94.83	Oth disrd of ear in diseases classified elsewhere, bilateral
388.9	UNSPECIFIED DISORDER OF EAR	**H93.90**	Unspecified disorder of ear, unspecified ear
		H93.91	Unspecified disorder of right ear
		H93.92	Unspecified disorder of left ear
		H93.93	Unspecified disorder of ear, bilateral
389.00	UNSPECIFIED CONDUCTIVE HEARING LOSS	**H90.2**	Conductive hearing loss, unspecified
389.01	CONDUCTIVE HEARING LOSS EXTERNAL EAR	**H90.0**	Conductive hearing loss, bilateral
		H90.11	Condctv hear loss, uni, right ear, w unrestr hear cntra side
		H90.12	Condctv hear loss, uni, left ear, w unrestr hear cntra side
		H90.2	Conductive hearing loss, unspecified
389.02	CONDUCTIVE HEARING LOSS TYMPANIC MEMBRANE	**H90.0**	Conductive hearing loss, bilateral
		H90.11	Condctv hear loss, uni, right ear, w unrestr hear cntra side
		H90.12	Condctv hear loss, uni, left ear, w unrestr hear cntra side
		H90.2	Conductive hearing loss, unspecified
389.03	CONDUCTIVE HEARING LOSS, MIDDLE EAR	**H90.0**	Conductive hearing loss, bilateral
		H90.11	Condctv hear loss, uni, right ear, w unrestr hear cntra side
		H90.12	Condctv hear loss, uni, left ear, w unrestr hear cntra side
		H90.2	Conductive hearing loss, unspecified
389.04	CONDUCTIVE HEARING LOSS, INNER EAR	**H90.0**	Conductive hearing loss, bilateral
		H90.11	Condctv hear loss, uni, right ear, w unrestr hear cntra side
		H90.12	Condctv hear loss, uni, left ear, w unrestr hear cntra side
		H90.2	Conductive hearing loss, unspecified
389.05	CONDUCTIVE HEARING LOSS UNILATERAL	**H90.11**	Condctv hear loss, uni, right ear, w unrestr hear cntra side
		H90.12	Condctv hear loss, uni, left ear, w unrestr hear cntra side
389.06	CONDUCTIVE HEARING LOSS BILATERAL	**H90.0**	Conductive hearing loss, bilateral
389.08	CONDUCTIVE HEARING LOSS OF COMBINED TYPES	**H90.0**	Conductive hearing loss, bilateral
		H90.11	Condctv hear loss, uni, right ear, w unrestr hear cntra side
		H90.12	Condctv hear loss, uni, left ear, w unrestr hear cntra side
		H90.2	Conductive hearing loss, unspecified
389.10	UNSPECIFIED SENSORINEURAL HEARING LOSS	**H90.5**	Unspecified sensorineural hearing loss
389.11	SENSORY HEARING LOSS BILATERAL	**H90.3**	Sensorineural hearing loss, bilateral
389.12	NEURAL HEARING LOSS BILATERAL	**H90.3**	Sensorineural hearing loss, bilateral
389.13	NEURAL HEARING LOSS UNILATERAL	**H90.41**	Snsrnrl hear loss, uni, right ear, w unrestr hear cntra side
		H90.42	Snsrnrl hear loss, uni, left ear, w unrestr hear cntra side
389.14	CENTRAL HEARING LOSS	**H90.3**	Sensorineural hearing loss, bilateral
		H90.41	Snsrnrl hear loss, uni, right ear, w unrestr hear cntra side
		H90.42	Snsrnrl hear loss, uni, left ear, w unrestr hear cntra side
		H90.5	Unspecified sensorineural hearing loss
389.15	SENSORINEURAL HEARING LOSS UNILATERAL	**H90.41**	Snsrnrl hear loss, uni, right ear, w unrestr hear cntra side
		H90.42	Snsrnrl hear loss, uni, left ear, w unrestr hear cntra side
389.16	SENSORINEURAL HEARING LOSS ASYMMETRICAL	**H90.5**	Unspecified sensorineural hearing loss
389.17	SENSORY HEARING LOSS UNILATERAL	**H90.41**	Snsrnrl hear loss, uni, right ear, w unrestr hear cntra side
		H90.42	Snsrnrl hear loss, uni, left ear, w unrestr hear cntra side
389.18	SENSORINEURAL HEARING LOSS BILATERAL	**H90.3**	Sensorineural hearing loss, bilateral
389.20	MIXED HEARING LOSS UNSPECIFIED	➡ **H90.8**	Mixed conductive and sensorineural hearing loss, unspecified
389.21	MIXED HEARING LOSS UNILATERAL	**H90.71**	Mix cndct/snrl hear loss,uni,r ear,w unrestr hear cntra side
		H90.72	Mix cndct/snrl hear loss,uni,l ear,w unrestr hear cntra side
389.22	MIXED HEARING LOSS BILATERAL	➡ **H90.6**	Mixed conductive and sensorineural hearing loss, bilateral
389.7	DEAF NONSPEAKING NOT ELSEWHERE CLASSIFIABLE	➡ **H91.3**	Deaf nonspeaking, not elsewhere classified
389.8	OTHER SPECIFIED FORMS OF HEARING LOSS	**H91.01**	Ototoxic hearing loss, right ear
		H91.02	Ototoxic hearing loss, left ear
		H91.03	Ototoxic hearing loss, bilateral
		H91.09	Ototoxic hearing loss, unspecified ear
		H91.8X1	Other specified hearing loss, right ear
		H91.8X2	Other specified hearing loss, left ear
		H91.8X3	Other specified hearing loss, bilateral
		H91.8X9	Other specified hearing loss, unspecified ear
389.9	UNSPECIFIED HEARING LOSS	**H91.90**	Unspecified hearing loss, unspecified ear
		H91.91	Unspecified hearing loss, right ear
		H91.92	Unspecified hearing loss, left ear
		H91.93	Unspecified hearing loss, bilateral

Diseases of the Circulatory System

ICD-9-CM			ICD-10-CM	
390	RHEUMATIC FEVER WITHOUT MENTION HEART INVLV	➡	I00	Rheumatic fever without heart involvement
391.0	ACUTE RHEUMATIC PERICARDITIS	➡	I01.0	Acute rheumatic pericarditis
391.1	ACUTE RHEUMATIC ENDOCARDITIS	➡	I01.1	Acute rheumatic endocarditis
391.2	ACUTE RHEUMATIC MYOCARDITIS	➡	I01.2	Acute rheumatic myocarditis
391.8	OTHER ACUTE RHEUMATIC HEART DISEASE	➡	I01.8	Other acute rheumatic heart disease
391.9	UNSPECIFIED ACUTE RHEUMATIC HEART DISEASE	➡	I01.9	Acute rheumatic heart disease, unspecified
392.0	RHEUMATIC CHOREA WITH HEART INVOLVEMENT	➡	I02.0	Rheumatic chorea with heart involvement
392.9	RHEUMATIC CHOREA WITHOUT MENTION HEART INVLV	➡	I02.9	Rheumatic chorea without heart involvement
393	CHRONIC RHEUMATIC PERICARDITIS	➡	I09.2	Chronic rheumatic pericarditis
394.0	MITRAL STENOSIS	➡	I05.0	Rheumatic mitral stenosis
394.1	RHEUMATIC MITRAL INSUFFICIENCY	➡	I05.1	Rheumatic mitral insufficiency
394.2	MITRAL STENOSIS WITH INSUFFICIENCY	➡	I05.2	Rheumatic mitral stenosis with insufficiency
394.9	OTHER AND UNSPECIFIED MITRAL VALVE DISEASES		I05.8 I05.9	Other rheumatic mitral valve diseases Rheumatic mitral valve disease, unspecified
395.0	RHEUMATIC AORTIC STENOSIS	➡	I06.0	Rheumatic aortic stenosis
395.1	RHEUMATIC AORTIC INSUFFICIENCY	➡	I06.1	Rheumatic aortic insufficiency
395.2	RHEUMATIC AORTIC STENOSIS WITH INSUFFICIENCY	➡	I06.2	Rheumatic aortic stenosis with insufficiency
395.9	OTHER AND UNSPECIFIED RHEUMATIC AORTIC DISEASES		I06.8 I06.9	Other rheumatic aortic valve diseases Rheumatic aortic valve disease, unspecified
396.0	MITRAL VALVE STENOSIS AND AORTIC VALVE STENOSIS		I08.0	Rheumatic disorders of both mitral and aortic valves
396.1	MITRAL VALVE STENOSIS&AORTIC VALVE INSUFFICIENCY		I08.0	Rheumatic disorders of both mitral and aortic valves
396.2	MITRAL VALVE INSUFFICIENCY&AORTIC VALVE STENOSIS		I08.0	Rheumatic disorders of both mitral and aortic valves
396.3	MITRAL VALVE INSUFF&AORTIC VALVE INSUFF		I08.0	Rheumatic disorders of both mitral and aortic valves
396.8	MULTIPLE INVOLVEMENT OF MITRAL AND AORTIC VALVES		I08.8	Other rheumatic multiple valve diseases
396.9	UNSPECIFIED MITRAL AND AORTIC VALVE DISEASES		I08.9	Rheumatic multiple valve disease, unspecified
397.0	DISEASES OF TRICUSPID VALVE		I07.0 I07.1 I07.2 I07.8 I07.9	Rheumatic tricuspid stenosis Rheumatic tricuspid insufficiency Rheumatic tricuspid stenosis and insufficiency Other rheumatic tricuspid valve diseases Rheumatic tricuspid valve disease, unspecified
397.1	RHEUMATIC DISEASES OF PULMONARY VALVE		I09.89	Other specified rheumatic heart diseases
397.9	RHEUMATIC DISEASES ENDOCARDIUM VALVE UNSPECIFIED		I08.1 I08.2 I08.3 I08.8 I08.9 I09.1	Rheumatic disorders of both mitral and tricuspid valves Rheumatic disorders of both aortic and tricuspid valves Comb rheumatic disord of mitral, aortic and tricuspid valves Other rheumatic multiple valve diseases Rheumatic multiple valve disease, unspecified Rheumatic diseases of endocardium, valve unspecified
398.0	RHEUMATIC MYOCARDITIS	➡	I09.0	Rheumatic myocarditis
398.90	UNSPECIFIED RHEUMATIC HEART DISEASE	➡	I09.9	Rheumatic heart disease, unspecified
398.91	RHEUMATIC HEART FAILURE	➡	I09.81	Rheumatic heart failure
398.99	OTHER AND UNSPECIFIED RHEUMATIC HEART DISEASES		I09.89	Other specified rheumatic heart diseases
401.0	ESSENTIAL HYPERTENSION, MALIGNANT		I10	Essential (primary) hypertension
401.1	ESSENTIAL HYPERTENSION, BENIGN		I10	Essential (primary) hypertension
401.9	UNSPECIFIED ESSENTIAL HYPERTENSION		I10	Essential (primary) hypertension
402.00	MALIG HTN HEART DISEASE WITHOUT HEART FAIL		I11.9	Hypertensive heart disease without heart failure
402.01	MALIG HYPERTENSIVE HEART DISEASE W/HEART FAILURE		I11.0	Hypertensive heart disease with heart failure
402.10	BEN HTN HEART DISEASE WITHOUT HEART FAIL		I11.9	Hypertensive heart disease without heart failure
402.11	BEN HYPERTENSIVE HEART DISEASE W/HEART FAILURE		I11.0	Hypertensive heart disease with heart failure
402.90	UNSPEC HTN HEART DISEASE WITHOUT HEART FAIL		I11.9	Hypertensive heart disease without heart failure
402.91	HYPERTENSIVE HEART DISEASE UNSPEC W/HEART FAIL		I11.0	Hypertensive heart disease with heart failure
403.00	HTN CHRN KID DZ MALIG CHRN KID DZ STAGE I-IV/UNS		I12.9	Hypertensive chronic kidney disease w stg 1-4/unsp chr kdny
403.01	HTN CHRN KID DZ MALIG W/CHRN KID DZ STAGE V/ESRD		I12.0	Hyp chr kidney disease w stage 5 chr kidney disease or ESRD
403.10	HTN CKD BEN W/CKD STAGE I THRU STAGE IV/UNSPEC		I12.9	Hypertensive chronic kidney disease w stg 1-4/unsp chr kdny
403.11	HTN CKD BEN W/CKD STAGE V/ESRD		I12.0	Hyp chr kidney disease w stage 5 chr kidney disease or ESRD
403.90	HTN CKD UNS W/CKD STAGE I THRU STAGE IV/UNS		I12.9	Hypertensive chronic kidney disease w stg 1-4/unsp chr kdny
403.91	HTN CKD UNSPEC W/CKD STAGE V/ESRD		I12.0	Hyp chr kidney disease w stage 5 chr kidney disease or ESRD
404.00	HTN HRT & CKD MAL W/O HF & W/CKD STAGE I-IV/UNS		I13.10	Hyp hrt & chr kdny dis w/o hrt fail, w stg 1-4/unsp chr kdny
404.01	HTN HRT & CKD MAL W/HF & W/CKD STAGE 1-IV/UNS		I13.0	Hyp hrt & chr kdny dis w hrt fail and stg 1-4/unsp chr kdny
404.02	HTN HEART & CKD MAL W/O HF & CKD STAGE V/ESRD		I13.11	Hyp hrt and chr kdny dis w/o hrt fail, w stg 5 chr kdny/ESRD
404.03	HTN HRT & CKD MALIG W/HF & W/CKD STAGE V/ESRD		I13.2	Hyp hrt & chr kdny dis w hrt fail and w stg 5 chr kdny/ESRD
404.10	HTN HRT & CKD BEN W/O HF & W/CKD STAGE I-IV/UNS		I13.10	Hyp hrt & chr kdny dis w/o hrt fail, w stg 1-4/unsp chr kdny
404.11	HTN HRT & CKD BEN W/HF & W/CKD STAGE I-IV/UNS		I13.0	Hyp hrt & chr kdny dis w hrt fail and stg 1-4/unsp chr kdny
404.12	HTN HRT & CKD BEN W/O HF & W/CKD STAGE V/ESRD		I13.11	Hyp hrt and chr kdny dis w/o hrt fail, w stg 5 chr kdny/ESRD
404.13	HTN HEART & CKD BEN W/HF & CKD STAGE V/ESRD		I13.2	Hyp hrt & chr kdny dis w hrt fail and w stg 5 chr kdny/ESRD
404.90	HTN HRT & CKD UNS W/O HF & W/CDK STAGE I-IV/UNS		I13.10	Hyp hrt & chr kdny dis w/o hrt fail, w stg 1-4/unsp chr kdny
404.91	HTN HRT & CKD UNS W/HF & W/CKD STAGE I - IV/UNS		I13.0	Hyp hrt & chr kdny dis w hrt fail and stg 1-4/unsp chr kdny
404.92	HTN HRT & CKD UNS W/O HF & W/CKD STAGE V/ESRD		I13.11	Hyp hrt and chr kdny dis w/o hrt fail, w stg 5 chr kdny/ESRD
404.93	HTN HEART & CKD UNSPEC W/HF & CKD STAGE V/ESRD		I13.2	Hyp hrt & chr kdny dis w hrt fail and w stg 5 chr kdny/ESRD
405.01	SECONDARY RENOVASCULAR HYPERTENSION MALIGNANT		I15.0	Renovascular hypertension

ICD-9-CM		ICD-10-CM	
405.09	OTHER SECONDARY HYPERTENSION MALIGNANT	I15.8	Other secondary hypertension
405.11	SECONDARY RENOVASCULAR HYPERTENSION BENIGN	I15.0	Renovascular hypertension
405.19	OTHER SECONDARY HYPERTENSION BENIGN	I15.8	Other secondary hypertension
405.91	SECONDARY RENOVASCULAR HYPERTENSION UNSPECIFIED	I15.0	Renovascular hypertension
		I15.1	Hypertension secondary to other renal disorders
		N26.2	Page kidney
405.99	OTHER SECONDARY HYPERTENSION UNSPECIFIED	I15.2	Hypertension secondary to endocrine disorders
		I15.8	Other secondary hypertension
		I15.9	Secondary hypertension, unspecified
410.00	ACUT MI ANTEROLAT WALL EPIS CARE UNS	I21.09	STEMI involving oth coronary artery of anterior wall
410.01	ACUT MI ANTEROLAT WALL INIT EPIS CARE	I21.09	STEMI involving oth coronary artery of anterior wall
		I22.0	Subsequent STEMI of anterior wall
410.02	ACUT MI ANTEROLAT WALL SUBSQT EPIS CARE	I21.09	STEMI involving oth coronary artery of anterior wall
410.10	ACUT MYOCARD INFARCT OTH ANT WALL EPIS CARE UNS	I21.09	STEMI involving oth coronary artery of anterior wall
410.11	ACUT MYOCARD INFARCT OTH ANT WALL INIT EPIS CARE	I21.01	STEMI involving left main coronary artery
		I21.02	STEMI involving left anterior descending coronary artery
		I21.09	STEMI involving oth coronary artery of anterior wall
		I22.0	Subsequent STEMI of anterior wall
410.12	ACUT MI OTH ANT WALL SUBSQT EPIS CARE	I21.09	STEMI involving oth coronary artery of anterior wall
410.20	ACUT MI INFEROLAT WALL EPIS CARE UNS	I21.19	STEMI involving oth coronary artery of inferior wall
410.21	ACUT MI INFEROLAT WALL INIT EPIS CARE	I21.19	STEMI involving oth coronary artery of inferior wall
		I22.1	Subsequent STEMI of inferior wall
410.22	ACUT MI INFEROLAT WALL SUBSQT EPIS CARE	I21.19	STEMI involving oth coronary artery of inferior wall
410.30	ACUT MI INFEROPOST WALL EPIS CARE UNS	I21.11	STEMI involving right coronary artery
410.31	ACUT MI INFEROPOST WALL INIT EPIS CARE	I21.11	STEMI involving right coronary artery
		I22.1	Subsequent STEMI of inferior wall
410.32	ACUT MI INFEROPOST WALL SUBSQT EPIS CARE	I21.11	STEMI involving right coronary artery
410.40	ACUT MYOCARD INFARCT OTH INF WALL EPIS CARE UNS	I21.19	STEMI involving oth coronary artery of inferior wall
410.41	ACUT MYOCARD INFARCT OTH INF WALL INIT EPIS CARE	I21.19	STEMI involving oth coronary artery of inferior wall
		I22.1	Subsequent STEMI of inferior wall
410.42	ACUT MI OTH INF WALL SUBSQT EPIS CARE	I21.19	STEMI involving oth coronary artery of inferior wall
410.50	ACUT MYOCARD INFARCT OTH LAT WALL EPIS CARE UNS	I21.29	STEMI involving oth sites
410.51	ACUT MYOCARD INFARCT OTH LAT WALL INIT EPIS CARE	I21.29	STEMI involving oth sites
		I22.8	Subsequent STEMI of sites
410.52	ACUT MI OTH LAT WALL SUBSQT EPIS CARE	I21.29	STEMI involving oth sites
410.60	ACUT MI TRUE POST WALL INFARCT EPIS CARE UNS	I21.29	STEMI involving oth sites
410.61	ACUT MI TRUE POST WALL INFARCT INIT EPIS CARE	I21.29	STEMI involving oth sites
		I22.8	Subsequent STEMI of sites
410.62	ACUT MI TRUE POST WALL INFARCT SUBSQT EPIS CARE	I21.29	STEMI involving oth sites
410.70	ACUT MI SUBENDOCARDIAL INFARCT EPIS CARE UNS	I21.4	Non-ST elevation (NSTEMI) myocardial infarction
410.71	ACUT MI SUBENDOCARDIAL INFARCT INIT EPIS CARE	I21.4	Non-ST elevation (NSTEMI) myocardial infarction
		I22.2	Subsequent non-ST elevation (NSTEMI) myocardial infarction
410.72	ACUT MI SUBENDOCARDIAL INFARCT SUBSQT EPIS CARE	I21.4	Non-ST elevation (NSTEMI) myocardial infarction
410.80	ACUT MYOCARD INFARCT OTH SPEC SITE EPIS CARE UNS	I21.29	STEMI involving oth sites
410.81	ACUT MYOCARD INFARCT OTH SITE INIT EPIS CARE	I21.21	STEMI involving left circumflex coronary artery
		I21.29	STEMI involving oth sites
		I22.8	Subsequent STEMI of sites
410.82	ACUT MYOCARD INFARCT OTH SITE SUBSQT EPIS CARE	I21.29	STEMI involving oth sites
410.90	ACUT MYOCARD INFARCT UNS SITE EPIS CARE UNS	I21.3	ST elevation (STEMI) myocardial infarction of unsp site
410.91	ACUTE MYOCARD INFARCT UNSPEC SITE INIT EPIS CARE	I21.3	ST elevation (STEMI) myocardial infarction of unsp site
		I22.9	Subsequent STEMI of unsp site
410.92	ACUT MYOCARD INFARCT UNS SITE SUBSQT EPIS CARE	I21.3	ST elevation (STEMI) myocardial infarction of unsp site
411.0	POSTMYOCARDIAL INFARCTION SYNDROME	➡ I24.1	Dressler's syndrome
411.1	INTERMEDIATE CORONARY SYNDROME	I20.0	Unstable angina
		◘ I25.110	Athscl heart disease of native cor art w unstable ang pctrs
		◘ I25.700	Atherosclerosis of CABG, unsp, w unstable angina pectoris
		◘ I25.710	Athscl autologous vein CABG w unstable angina pectoris
		◘ I25.720	Athscl autologous artery CABG w unstable angina pectoris
		◘ I25.730	Athscl nonautologous biological CABG w unstable ang pctrs
		◘ I25.750	Athscl native cor art of txplt heart w unstable angina
		◘ I25.760	Athscl bypass of cor art of txplt heart w unstable angina
		◘ I25.790	Atherosclerosis of CABG w unstable angina pectoris
411.81	ACUTE COR OCCLUSION WITHOUT MYOCARDIAL INFARCT	➡ I24.0	Acute coronary thrombosis not resulting in myocardial infrc
411.89	OTHER ACUTE&SUBACUTE FORM ISCHEMIC HEART DISEASE	I24.8	Other forms of acute ischemic heart disease
		I24.9	Acute ischemic heart disease, unspecified
412	OLD MYOCARDIAL INFARCTION	➡ I25.2	Old myocardial infarction
413.0	ANGINA DECUBITUS	I20.8	Other forms of angina pectoris
413.1	PRINZMETAL ANGINA	➡ I20.1	Angina pectoris with documented spasm

ICD-9-CM			ICD-10-CM	
413.9	OTHER AND UNSPECIFIED ANGINA PECTORIS		**I20.8**	Other forms of angina pectoris
			I20.9	Angina pectoris, unspecified
		☐	**I25.111**	Athscl heart disease of native cor art w ang pctrs w spasm
		☐	**I25.118**	Athscl heart disease of native cor art w oth ang pctrs
		☐	**I25.119**	Athscl heart disease of native cor art w unsp ang pctrs
		☐	**I25.701**	Athscl CABG, unsp, w angina pectoris w documented spasm
		☐	**I25.708**	Atherosclerosis of CABG, unsp, w oth angina pectoris
		☐	**I25.709**	Atherosclerosis of CABG, unsp, w unsp angina pectoris
		☐	**I25.711**	Athscl autologous vein CABG w ang pctrs w documented spasm
		☐	**I25.718**	Athscl autologous vein CABG w oth angina pectoris
		☐	**I25.719**	Athscl autologous vein CABG w unsp angina pectoris
		☐	**I25.721**	Athscl autologous artery CABG w ang pctrs w documented spasm
		☐	**I25.728**	Athscl autologous artery CABG w oth angina pectoris
		☐	**I25.729**	Athscl autologous artery CABG w unsp angina pectoris
		☐	**I25.731**	Athscl nonaut biological CABG w ang pctrs w documented spasm
		☐	**I25.738**	Athscl nonautologous biological CABG w oth angina pectoris
		☐	**I25.739**	Athscl nonautologous biological CABG w unsp angina pectoris
		☐	**I25.751**	Athscl native cor art of txplt heart w ang pctrs w spasm
		☐	**I25.758**	Athscl native cor art of transplanted heart w oth ang pctrs
		☐	**I25.759**	Athscl native cor art of transplanted heart w unsp ang pctrs
		☐	**I25.761**	Athscl bypass of cor art of txplt heart w ang pctrs w spasm
		☐	**I25.768**	Athscl bypass of cor art of txplt heart w oth ang pctrs
		☐	**I25.769**	Athscl bypass of cor art of txplt heart w unsp ang pctrs
		☐	**I25.791**	Atherosclerosis of CABG w angina pectoris w documented spasm
		☐	**I25.798**	Atherosclerosis of CABG w oth angina pectoris
		☐	**I25.799**	Atherosclerosis of CABG w unsp angina pectoris
414.00	COR ATHEROSLERO UNSPEC TYPE VESSEL NATIVE/GRAFT		**I25.10**	Athscl heart disease of native coronary artery w/o ang pctrs
414.01	CORONARY ATHEROSCLEROSIS NATIVE CORONARY ARTERY		**I25.10**	Athscl heart disease of native coronary artery w/o ang pctrs
		☐	**I25.110**	Athscl heart disease of native cor art w unstable ang pctrs
		☐	**I25.111**	Athscl heart disease of native cor art w ang pctrs w spasm
		☐	**I25.118**	Athscl heart disease of native cor art w oth ang pctrs
		☐	**I25.119**	Athscl heart disease of native cor art w unsp ang pctrs
414.02	CORONARY ATHEROSLERO AUTOL VEIN BYPASS GRAFT	☐	**I25.710**	Athscl autologous vein CABG w unstable angina pectoris
		☐	**I25.711**	Athscl autologous vein CABG w ang pctrs w documented spasm
		☐	**I25.718**	Athscl autologous vein CABG w oth angina pectoris
		☐	**I25.719**	Athscl autologous vein CABG w unsp angina pectoris
			I25.810	Atherosclerosis of CABG w/o angina pectoris
414.03	COR ATHEROSLERO NONAUTOL BIOLOGICAL BYPS GRAFT	☐	**I25.730**	Athscl nonautologous biological CABG w unstable ang pctrs
		☐	**I25.731**	Athscl nonaut biological CABG w ang pctrs w documented spasm
		☐	**I25.738**	Athscl nonautologous biological CABG w oth angina pectoris
		☐	**I25.739**	Athscl nonautologous biological CABG w unsp angina pectoris
			I25.810	Atherosclerosis of CABG w/o angina pectoris
414.04	CORONARY ATHEROSCLEROSIS OF ARTERY BYPASS GRAFT	☐	**I25.720**	Athscl autologous artery CABG w unstable angina pectoris
		☐	**I25.721**	Athscl autologous artery CABG w ang pctrs w documented spasm
		☐	**I25.728**	Athscl autologous artery CABG w oth angina pectoris
		☐	**I25.729**	Athscl autologous artery CABG w unsp angina pectoris
		☐	**I25.790**	Atherosclerosis of CABG w unstable angina pectoris
		☐	**I25.791**	Atherosclerosis of CABG w angina pectoris w documented spasm
		☐	**I25.798**	Atherosclerosis of CABG w oth angina pectoris
		☐	**I25.799**	Atherosclerosis of CABG w unsp angina pectoris
			I25.810	Atherosclerosis of CABG w/o angina pectoris
414.05	CORONARY ATHEROSLERO UNSPEC TYPE BYPASS GRAFT	☐	**I25.700**	Atherosclerosis of CABG, unsp, w unstable angina pectoris
		☐	**I25.701**	Athscl CABG, unsp, w angina pectoris w documented spasm
		☐	**I25.708**	Atherosclerosis of CABG, unsp, w oth angina pectoris
		☐	**I25.709**	Atherosclerosis of CABG, unsp, w unsp angina pectoris
		☐	**I25.790**	Atherosclerosis of CABG w unstable angina pectoris
		☐	**I25.791**	Atherosclerosis of CABG w angina pectoris w documented spasm
		☐	**I25.798**	Atherosclerosis of CABG w oth angina pectoris
		☐	**I25.799**	Atherosclerosis of CABG w unsp angina pectoris
			I25.810	Atherosclerosis of CABG w/o angina pectoris
414.06	COR ATHEROSLERO COR ART TRANSPLANTED HEART	☐	**I25.750**	Athscl native cor art of txplt heart w unstable angina
		☐	**I25.751**	Athscl native cor art of txplt heart w ang pctrs w spasm
		☐	**I25.758**	Athscl native cor art of transplanted heart w oth ang pctrs
		☐	**I25.759**	Athscl native cor art of transplanted heart w unsp ang pctrs
			I25.811	Athscl native cor art of transplanted heart w/o ang pctrs
414.07	COR ATHEROSLERO BYPS GRAFT TRANSPLANTED HEART	☐	**I25.760**	Athscl bypass of cor art of txplt heart w unstable angina
		☐	**I25.761**	Athscl bypass of cor art of txplt heart w ang pctrs w spasm
		☐	**I25.768**	Athscl bypass of cor art of txplt heart w oth ang pctrs
		☐	**I25.769**	Athscl bypass of cor art of txplt heart w unsp ang pctrs
			I25.812	Athscl bypass of cor art of transplanted heart w/o ang pctrs
414.10	ANEURYSM OF HEART		**I25.3**	Aneurysm of heart
414.11	ANEURYSM OF CORONARY VESSELS	➡	**I25.41**	Coronary artery aneurysm
414.12	DISSECTION OF CORONARY ARTERY	➡	**I25.42**	Coronary artery dissection
414.19	OTHER ANEURYSM OF HEART		**I25.3**	Aneurysm of heart
414.2	CHRONIC TOTAL OCCLUSION OF CORONARY ARTERY	➡	**I25.82**	Chronic total occlusion of coronary artery
414.3	CORONARY ATHEROSCLEROSIS D/T LIPID RICH PLAQUE	➡	**I25.83**	Coronary atherosclerosis due to lipid rich plaque
414.4	CORONARY ATHEROSCL DUE TO CALCIFIED CORON LESION		**I25.84**	Coronary atherosclerosis due to calcified coronary lesion

ICD-9-CM		ICD-10-CM		
414.8	OTHER SPEC FORMS CHRONIC ISCHEMIC HEART DISEASE	**I25.5**	Ischemic cardiomyopathy	
		I25.6	Silent myocardial ischemia	
		I25.89	Other forms of chronic ischemic heart disease	
		I25.9	Chronic ischemic heart disease, unspecified	
414.9	UNSPECIFIED CHRONIC ISCHEMIC HEART DISEASE	**I25.9**	Chronic ischemic heart disease, unspecified	
415.Ø	ACUTE COR PULMONALE	**I26.Ø1**	Septic pulmonary embolism with acute cor pulmonale	
		I26.Ø2	Saddle embolus of pulmonary artery with acute cor pulmonale	
		I26.Ø9	Other pulmonary embolism with acute cor pulmonale	
415.11	IATROGENIC PULMONARY EMBOLISM AND INFARCTION	**T8Ø.ØXXA**	Air embolism fol infusion, tranfs and theraputc inject, init	*or*
		T81.718A	Complication of artery following a procedure, NEC, init	*or*
		T81.72XA	Complication of vein following a procedure, NEC, init	*or*
		T82.817A	Embolism of cardiac prosth dev/grft, init	*or*
		T82.818A	Embolism of vascular prosth dev/grft, init	*and*
		I26.9Ø	Septic pulmonary embolism without acute cor pulmonale	*or*
		I26.99	Other pulmonary embolism without acute cor pulmonale	
415.12	SEPTIC PULMONARY EMBOLISM	**I26.Ø1**	Septic pulmonary embolism with acute cor pulmonale	
		I26.9Ø	Septic pulmonary embolism without acute cor pulmonale	
415.13	SADDLE EMBOLUS OF PULMONARY ARTERY	**I26.Ø2**	Saddle embolus of pulmonary artery with acute cor pulmonale	
		I26.92	Saddle embolus of pulmonary artery w/o acute cor pulmonale	
415.19	OTHER PULMONARY EMBOLISM AND INFARCTION	**I26.Ø9**	Other pulmonary embolism with acute cor pulmonale	
		I26.99	Other pulmonary embolism without acute cor pulmonale	
416.Ø	PRIMARY PULMONARY HYPERTENSION	**I27.Ø**	Primary pulmonary hypertension	
416.1	KYPHOSCOLIOTIC HEART DISEASE	**I27.1**	Kyphoscoliotic heart disease	
416.2	CHRONIC PULMONARY EMBOLISM	**I27.82**	Chronic pulmonary embolism	
416.8	OTHER CHRONIC PULMONARY HEART DISEASES	**I27.2**	Other secondary pulmonary hypertension	
		I27.89	Other specified pulmonary heart diseases	
416.9	UNSPECIFIED CHRONIC PULMONARY HEART DISEASE	**I27.81**	Cor pulmonale (chronic)	
		I27.9	Pulmonary heart disease, unspecified	
417.Ø	ARTERIOVENOUS FISTULA OF PULMONARY VESSELS	**I28.Ø**	Arteriovenous fistula of pulmonary vessels	
417.1	ANEURYSM OF PULMONARY ARTERY	**I28.1**	Aneurysm of pulmonary artery	
417.8	OTHER SPECIFIED DISEASE OF PULMONARY CIRCULATION	**I28.8**	Other diseases of pulmonary vessels	
417.9	UNSPECIFIED DISEASE OF PULMONARY CIRCULATION	**I28.9**	Disease of pulmonary vessels, unspecified	
42Ø.Ø	ACUTE PERICARDITIS DISEASES CLASSIFIED ELSEWHERE	**A18.84**	Tuberculosis of heart	
		I32	Pericarditis in diseases classified elsewhere	
		M32.12	Pericarditis in systemic lupus erythematosus	
42Ø.9Ø	UNSPECIFIED ACUTE PERICARDITIS	**I3Ø.1**	Infective pericarditis	
		I3Ø.9	Acute pericarditis, unspecified	
42Ø.91	ACUTE IDIOPATHIC PERICARDITIS	**I3Ø.Ø**	Acute nonspecific idiopathic pericarditis	
42Ø.99	OTHER ACUTE PERICARDITIS	**I3Ø.8**	Other forms of acute pericarditis	
		I3Ø.9	Acute pericarditis, unspecified	
421.Ø	ACUTE AND SUBACUTE BACTERIAL ENDOCARDITIS	**I33.Ø**	Acute and subacute infective endocarditis	
421.1	ACUT&SUBACUT INFECTV ENDOCARDITIS DZ CLASS ELSW	**I39**	Endocarditis and heart valve disord in dis classd elswhr	
421.9	UNSPECIFIED ACUTE ENDOCARDITIS	**I33.9**	Acute and subacute endocarditis, unspecified	
422.Ø	ACUTE MYOCARDITIS DISEASES CLASSIFIED ELSEWHERE	**A18.84**	Tuberculosis of heart	
		I41	Myocarditis in diseases classified elsewhere	
422.9Ø	UNSPECIFIED ACUTE MYOCARDITIS	**I4Ø.9**	Acute myocarditis, unspecified	
422.91	IDIOPATHIC MYOCARDITIS	**I4Ø.Ø**	Infective myocarditis	
		I4Ø.1	Isolated myocarditis	
422.92	SEPTIC MYOCARDITIS	**I4Ø.Ø**	Infective myocarditis	
422.93	TOXIC MYOCARDITIS	**I4Ø.8**	Other acute myocarditis	
422.99	OTHER ACUTE MYOCARDITIS	**I4Ø.8**	Other acute myocarditis	
423.Ø	HEMOPERICARDIUM	**I31.2**	Hemopericardium, not elsewhere classified	
423.1	ADHESIVE PERICARDITIS	**I31.Ø**	Chronic adhesive pericarditis	
423.2	CONSTRICTIVE PERICARDITIS	**I31.1**	Chronic constrictive pericarditis	
423.3	CARDIAC TAMPONADE	**I31.4**	Cardiac tamponade	
423.8	OTHER SPECIFIED DISEASES OF PERICARDIUM	**I31.8**	Other specified diseases of pericardium	
423.9	UNSPECIFIED DISEASE OF PERICARDIUM	**I31.3**	Pericardial effusion (noninflammatory)	
		I31.9	Disease of pericardium, unspecified	
424.Ø	MITRAL VALVE DISORDERS	**I34.Ø**	Nonrheumatic mitral (valve) insufficiency	
		I34.1	Nonrheumatic mitral (valve) prolapse	
		I34.2	Nonrheumatic mitral (valve) stenosis	
		I34.8	Other nonrheumatic mitral valve disorders	
		I34.9	Nonrheumatic mitral valve disorder, unspecified	
424.1	AORTIC VALVE DISORDERS	**I35.Ø**	Nonrheumatic aortic (valve) stenosis	
		I35.1	Nonrheumatic aortic (valve) insufficiency	
		I35.2	Nonrheumatic aortic (valve) stenosis with insufficiency	
		I35.8	Other nonrheumatic aortic valve disorders	
		I35.9	Nonrheumatic aortic valve disorder, unspecified	

ICD-9-CM			ICD-10-CM	
424.2	TRICUSPID VALVE DISORDERS SPEC AS NONRHEUMATIC		I36.Ø	Nonrheumatic tricuspid (valve) stenosis
			I36.1	Nonrheumatic tricuspid (valve) insufficiency
			I36.2	Nonrheumatic tricuspid (valve) stenosis with insufficiency
			I36.8	Other nonrheumatic tricuspid valve disorders
			I36.9	Nonrheumatic tricuspid valve disorder, unspecified
424.3	PULMONARY VALVE DISORDERS		I37.Ø	Nonrheumatic pulmonary valve stenosis
			I37.1	Nonrheumatic pulmonary valve insufficiency
			I37.2	Nonrheumatic pulmonary valve stenosis with insufficiency
			I37.8	Other nonrheumatic pulmonary valve disorders
			I37.9	Nonrheumatic pulmonary valve disorder, unspecified
424.9Ø	ENDOCARDITIS VALVE UNSPECIFIED UNSPECIFIED CAUSE		I38	Endocarditis, valve unspecified
424.91	ENDOCARDITIS IN DISEASES CLASSIFIED ELSEWHERE	◘	A18.84	Tuberculosis of heart
			I39	Endocarditis and heart valve disord in dis classd elswhr
		◘	M32.11	Endocarditis in systemic lupus erythematosus
424.99	OTHER ENDOCARDITIS VALVE UNSPECIFIED		I38	Endocarditis, valve unspecified
425.Ø	ENDOMYOCARDIAL FIBROSIS		I42.3	Endomyocardial (eosinophilic) disease
425.11	HYPERTROPHIC OBSTRUCTIVE CARDIOMYOPATHY		I42.1	Obstructive hypertrophic cardiomyopathy
425.18	OTHER HYPERTROPHIC CARDIOMYOPATHY		I42.2	Other hypertrophic cardiomyopathy
425.2	OBSCURE CARDIOMYOPATHY OF AFRICA		I42.8	Other cardiomyopathies
425.3	ENDOCARDIAL FIBROELASTOSIS	➡	I42.4	Endocardial fibroelastosis
425.4	OTHER PRIMARY CARDIOMYOPATHIES		I42.Ø	Dilated cardiomyopathy
			I42.5	Other restrictive cardiomyopathy
			I42.8	Other cardiomyopathies
			I42.9	Cardiomyopathy, unspecified
425.5	ALCOHOLIC CARDIOMYOPATHY	➡	I42.6	Alcoholic cardiomyopathy
425.7	NUTRITIONAL AND METABOLIC CARDIOMYOPATHY		I43	Cardiomyopathy in diseases classified elsewhere
425.8	CARDIOMYOPATHY OTHER DISEASES CLASSIFIED ELSW	◘	A18.84	Tuberculosis of heart
			I43	Cardiomyopathy in diseases classified elsewhere
425.9	UNSPECIFIED SECONDARY CARDIOMYOPATHY		I42.7	Cardiomyopathy due to drug and external agent
			I42.9	Cardiomyopathy, unspecified
426.Ø	ATRIOVENTRICULAR BLOCK, COMPLETE	➡	I44.2	Atrioventricular block, complete
426.1Ø	UNSPECIFIED ATRIOVENTRICULAR BLOCK		I44.3Ø	Unspecified atrioventricular block
426.11	FIRST DEGREE ATRIOVENTRICULAR BLOCK	➡	I44.Ø	Atrioventricular block, first degree
426.12	MOBITZ II ATRIOVENTRICULAR BLOCK		I44.1	Atrioventricular block, second degree
426.13	OTHER SECOND DEGREE ATRIOVENTRICULAR BLOCK		I44.1	Atrioventricular block, second degree
426.2	LEFT BUNDLE BRANCH HEMIBLOCK		I44.4	Left anterior fascicular block
			I44.5	Left posterior fascicular block
			I44.6Ø	Unspecified fascicular block
			I44.69	Other fascicular block
426.3	OTHER LEFT BUNDLE BRANCH BLOCK		I44.7	Left bundle-branch block, unspecified
426.4	RIGHT BUNDLE BRANCH BLOCK		I45.Ø	Right fascicular block
			I45.1Ø	Unspecified right bundle-branch block
			I45.19	Other right bundle-branch block
426.5Ø	UNSPECIFIED BUNDLE BRANCH BLOCK		I44.3Ø	Unspecified atrioventricular block
			I44.39	Other atrioventricular block
			I45.4	Nonspecific intraventricular block
426.51	RT BUNDLE BRANCH BLOCK< POST FASCICULAR BLOCK		I45.2	Bifascicular block
426.52	RT BUNDLE BRANCH BLOCK< ANT FASCICULAR BLOCK		I45.2	Bifascicular block
426.53	OTHER BILATERAL BUNDLE BRANCH BLOCK		I45.2	Bifascicular block
426.54	TRIFASCICULAR BLOCK	➡	I45.3	Trifascicular block
426.6	OTHER HEART BLOCK	➡	I45.5	Other specified heart block
426.7	ANOMALOUS ATRIOVENTRICULAR EXCITATION		I45.6	Pre-excitation syndrome
426.81	LOWN-GANONG-LEVINE SYNDROME		I45.6	Pre-excitation syndrome
426.82	LONG QT SYNDROME	➡	I45.81	Long QT syndrome
426.89	OTHER SPECIFIED CONDUCTION DISORDER	➡	I45.89	Other specified conduction disorders
426.9	UNSPECIFIED CONDUCTION DISORDER	➡	I45.9	Conduction disorder, unspecified
427.Ø	PAROXYSMAL SUPRAVENTRICULAR TACHYCARDIA		I47.1	Supraventricular tachycardia
			I49.2	Junctional premature depolarization
427.1	PAROXYSMAL VENTRICULAR TACHYCARDIA		I47.Ø	Re-entry ventricular arrhythmia
			I47.2	Ventricular tachycardia
427.2	UNSPECIFIED PAROXYSMAL TACHYCARDIA	➡	I47.9	Paroxysmal tachycardia, unspecified
427.31	ATRIAL FIBRILLATION		I48.Ø	Paroxysmal arterial fibrillation
			I48.1	Persistent atrial fibrillation
			I48.2	Chronic atrial fibrillation
			I48.91	Unspecified atrial fibrillation
427.32	ATRIAL FLUTTER		I48.3	Typical atrial flutter
			I48.4	Atypical atrial flutter
			I48.92	Unspecified atrial flutter
427.41	VENTRICULAR FIBRILLATION	➡	I49.Ø1	Ventricular fibrillation
427.42	VENTRICULAR FLUTTER	➡	I49.Ø2	Ventricular flutter
427.5	CARDIAC ARREST		I46.2	Cardiac arrest due to underlying cardiac condition
			I46.8	Cardiac arrest due to other underlying condition
			I46.9	Cardiac arrest, cause unspecified

ICD-9-CM		ICD-10-CM	
427.60	UNSPECIFIED PREMATURE BEATS	I49.40	Unspecified premature depolarization
427.61	SUPRAVENTRICULAR PREMATURE BEATS	I49.1	Atrial premature depolarization
427.69	OTHER PREMATURE BEATS	I49.3	Ventricular premature depolarization
		I49.49	Other premature depolarization
427.81	SINOATRIAL NODE DYSFUNCTION	I49.5	Sick sinus syndrome
		R00.1	Bradycardia, unspecified
427.89	OTHER SPECIFIED CARDIAC DYSRHYTHMIAS	I49.8	Other specified cardiac arrhythmias
		R00.1	Bradycardia, unspecified
427.9	UNSPECIFIED CARDIAC DYSRHYTHMIA	I49.9	Cardiac arrhythmia, unspecified
428.0	CONGESTIVE HEART FAILURE UNSPECIFIED	I50.20	Unspecified systolic (congestive) heart failure
		I50.21	Acute systolic (congestive) heart failure
		I50.22	Chronic systolic (congestive) heart failure
		I50.23	Acute on chronic systolic (congestive) heart failure
		I50.30	Unspecified diastolic (congestive) heart failure
		I50.31	Acute diastolic (congestive) heart failure
		I50.32	Chronic diastolic (congestive) heart failure
		I50.33	Acute on chronic diastolic (congestive) heart failure
		I50.40	Unsp combined systolic and diastolic (congestive) hrt fail
		I50.41	Acute combined systolic and diastolic (congestive) hrt fail
		I50.42	Chronic combined systolic and diastolic hrt fail
		I50.43	Acute on chronic combined systolic and diastolic hrt fail
		I50.9	Heart failure, unspecified
428.1	LEFT HEART FAILURE	I50.1	Left ventricular failure
428.20	UNSPECIFIED SYSTOLIC HEART FAILURE	I50.20	Unspecified systolic (congestive) heart failure
428.21	ACUTE SYSTOLIC HEART FAILURE	I50.21	Acute systolic (congestive) heart failure
428.22	CHRONIC SYSTOLIC HEART FAILURE	I50.22	Chronic systolic (congestive) heart failure
428.23	ACUTE ON CHRONIC SYSTOLIC HEART FAILURE	I50.23	Acute on chronic systolic (congestive) heart failure
428.30	UNSPECIFIED DIASTOLIC HEART FAILURE	I50.30	Unspecified diastolic (congestive) heart failure
428.31	ACUTE DIASTOLIC HEART FAILURE	I50.31	Acute diastolic (congestive) heart failure
428.32	CHRONIC DIASTOLIC HEART FAILURE	I50.32	Chronic diastolic (congestive) heart failure
428.33	ACUTE ON CHRONIC DIASTOLIC HEART FAILURE	I50.33	Acute on chronic diastolic (congestive) heart failure
428.40	UNSPEC COMBINED SYSTOLIC&DIASTOLIC HEART FAILURE	I50.40	Unsp combined systolic and diastolic (congestive) hrt fail
428.41	ACUTE COMBINED SYSTOLIC&DIASTOLIC HEART FAILURE	I50.41	Acute combined systolic and diastolic (congestive) hrt fail
428.42	CHRONIC COMB SYSTOLIC&DIASTOLIC HEART FAILURE	I50.42	Chronic combined systolic and diastolic hrt fail
428.43	ACUTE CHRONIC COMB SYSTOLIC&DIASTOLIC HEART FAIL	I50.43	Acute on chronic combined systolic and diastolic hrt fail
428.9	UNSPECIFIED HEART FAILURE	I50.9	Heart failure, unspecified
429.0	UNSPECIFIED MYOCARDITIS	I51.4	Myocarditis, unspecified
429.1	MYOCARDIAL DEGENERATION	I51.5	Myocardial degeneration
429.2	UNSPECIFIED CARDIOVASCULAR DISEASE	I25.10	Athscl heart disease of native coronary artery w/o ang pctrs
429.3	CARDIOMEGALY	I51.7	Cardiomegaly
429.4	FUNCTIONAL DISTURBANCES FOLLOWING CARD SURGERY	I97.0	Postcardiotomy syndrome
		I97.110	Postproc cardiac insufficiency following cardiac surgery
		I97.111	Postprocedural cardiac insufficiency following other surgery
		I97.120	Postprocedural cardiac arrest following cardiac surgery
		I97.121	Postprocedural cardiac arrest following other surgery
		I97.130	Postprocedural heart failure following cardiac surgery
		I97.131	Postprocedural heart failure following other surgery
		I97.190	Oth postproc cardiac functn disturb fol cardiac surgery
		I97.191	Oth postproc cardiac functn disturb following oth surgery
429.5	RUPTURE OF CHORDAE TENDINEAE	I23.4	Rupture of chord tendne as current comp following AMI
		I51.1	Rupture of chordae tendineae, not elsewhere classified
429.6	RUPTURE OF PAPILLARY MUSCLE	I23.5	Rupture of papillary muscle as current comp following AMI
		I51.2	Rupture of papillary muscle, not elsewhere classified
429.71	ACQUIRED CARDIAC SEPTAL DEFECT	I23.1	Atrial septal defect as current complication following AMI
		I23.2	Ventricular septal defect as current comp following AMI
		I51.0	Cardiac septal defect, acquired
429.79	OTHER CERTAIN SEQUELAE MYOCARDIAL INFARCTION NEC	I23.0	Hemopericardium as current complication following AMI
		I23.3	Rupture of card wall w/o hemoperic as current comp fol AMI
		I23.6	Thombos of atrium/auric append/ventr as current comp fol AMI
		I23.7	Postinfarction angina
		I23.8	Oth current complications following AMI
429.81	OTHER DISORDERS PAPILLARY MUSCLE	I51.89	Other ill-defined heart diseases
429.82	HYPERKINETIC HEART DISEASE	I51.89	Other ill-defined heart diseases
429.83	TAKOTSUBO SYNDROME	I51.81	Takotsubo syndrome
429.89	OTHER ILL-DEFINED HEART DISEASE	I51.3	Intracardiac thrombosis, not elsewhere classified
		I51.89	Other ill-defined heart diseases
429.9	UNSPECIFIED HEART DISEASE	I51.9	Heart disease, unspecified
		I52	Other heart disorders in diseases classified elsewhere

ICD-9-CM		ICD-10-CM	
430	SUBARACHNOID HEMORRHAGE	I60.00	Ntrm subarach hemorrhage from unsp carotid siphon and bifurc
		I60.01	Ntrm subarach hemor from right carotid siphon and bifurc
		I60.02	Ntrm subarach hemorrhage from left carotid siphon and bifurc
		I60.10	Ntrm subarach hemorrhage from unsp middle cerebral artery
		I60.11	Ntrm subarach hemorrhage from right middle cerebral artery
		I60.12	Ntrm subarach hemorrhage from left middle cerebral artery
		I60.20	Ntrm subarach hemor from unsp anterior communicating artery
		I60.21	Ntrm subarach hemor from right anterior communicating artery
		I60.22	Ntrm subarach hemor from left anterior communicating artery
		I60.30	Ntrm subarach hemor from unsp posterior communicating artery
		I60.31	Ntrm subarach hemor from right post communicating artery
		I60.32	Ntrm subarach hemor from left posterior communicating artery
		I60.4	Nontraumatic subarachnoid hemorrhage from basilar artery
		I60.50	Nontraumatic subarachnoid hemorrhage from unsp verteb art
		I60.51	Nontraumatic subarachnoid hemorrhage from r verteb art
		I60.52	Nontraumatic subarachnoid hemorrhage from l verteb art
		I60.6	Nontraumatic subarachnoid hemorrhage from oth intracran art
		I60.7	Nontraumatic subarachnoid hemorrhage from unsp intracran art
		I60.8	Other nontraumatic subarachnoid hemorrhage
		I60.9	Nontraumatic subarachnoid hemorrhage, unspecified
431	INTRACEREBRAL HEMORRHAGE	I61.0	Nontraumatic intcrbl hemorrhage in hemisphere, subcortical
		I61.1	Nontraumatic intcrbl hemorrhage in hemisphere, cortical
		I61.2	Nontraumatic intracerebral hemorrhage in hemisphere, unsp
		I61.3	Nontraumatic intracerebral hemorrhage in brain stem
		I61.4	Nontraumatic intracerebral hemorrhage in cerebellum
		I61.5	Nontraumatic intracerebral hemorrhage, intraventricular
		I61.6	Nontraumatic intracerebral hemorrhage, multiple localized
		I61.8	Other nontraumatic intracerebral hemorrhage
		I61.9	Nontraumatic intracerebral hemorrhage, unspecified
432.0	NONTRAUMATIC EXTRADURAL HEMORRHAGE	➡ I62.1	Nontraumatic extradural hemorrhage
432.1	SUBDURAL HEMORRHAGE	I62.00	Nontraumatic subdural hemorrhage, unspecified
		I62.01	Nontraumatic acute subdural hemorrhage
		I62.02	Nontraumatic subacute subdural hemorrhage
		I62.03	Nontraumatic chronic subdural hemorrhage
432.9	UNSPECIFIED INTRACRANIAL HEMORRHAGE	➡ I62.9	Nontraumatic intracranial hemorrhage, unspecified
433.00	OCCLUSION&STENOS BASILAR ART W/O MENTION INFARCT	➡ I65.1	Occlusion and stenosis of basilar artery
433.01	OCCLUSION&STENOSIS BASILAR ARTERY W/INFARCT	I63.02	Cerebral infarction due to thrombosis of basilar artery
		I63.12	Cerebral infarction due to embolism of basilar artery
		I63.22	Cerebral infrc due to unsp occls or stenosis of basilar art
433.10	OCCLUSION&STENOS CAROTID ART W/O MENTION INFARCT	I65.21	Occlusion and stenosis of right carotid artery
		I65.22	Occlusion and stenosis of left carotid artery
		I65.23	Occlusion and stenosis of bilateral carotid arteries
		I65.29	Occlusion and stenosis of unspecified carotid artery
433.11	OCCLUSION&STENOSIS CAROTID ARTERY W/INFARCT	I63.031	Cerebral infrc due to thrombosis of right carotid artery
		I63.032	Cerebral infarction due to thrombosis of left carotid artery
		I63.039	Cerebral infarction due to thrombosis of unsp carotid artery
		I63.131	Cerebral infarction due to embolism of right carotid artery
		I63.132	Cerebral infarction due to embolism of left carotid artery
		I63.139	Cerebral infarction due to embolism of unsp carotid artery
		I63.231	Cereb infrc due to unsp occls or stenos of right carotid art
		I63.232	Cereb infrc due to unsp occls or stenos of left carotid art
		I63.239	Cereb infrc due to unsp occls or stenos of unsp carotid art
433.20	OCCLUSION&STENOS VERT ART W/O MENTION INFARCT	I65.01	Occlusion and stenosis of right vertebral artery
		I65.02	Occlusion and stenosis of left vertebral artery
		I65.03	Occlusion and stenosis of bilateral vertebral arteries
		I65.09	Occlusion and stenosis of unspecified vertebral artery
433.21	OCCLUSION&STENOSIS VERTEBRAL ARTERY W/INFARCT	I63.011	Cerebral infarction due to thrombosis of r verteb art
		I63.012	Cerebral infarction due to thrombosis of l verteb art
		I63.019	Cerebral infarction due to thombos unsp vertebral artery
		I63.111	Cerebral infarction due to embolism of r verteb art
		I63.112	Cerebral infarction due to embolism of left vertebral artery
		I63.119	Cerebral infarction due to embolism of unsp vertebral artery
		I63.211	Cereb infrc due to unsp occls or stenos of right verteb art
		I63.212	Cereb infrc due to unsp occls or stenosis of left verteb art
		I63.219	Cereb infrc due to unsp occls or stenosis of unsp verteb art
433.30	OCCL&STENOS MX&BILAT PRECERBRL ART W/O INFARCT	I65.8	Occlusion and stenosis of other precerebral arteries
433.31	OCCL&STENOS MX&BILAT PRECERBRL ART W/INFARCT	I63.59	Cereb infrc due to unsp occls or stenosis of cerebral artery
433.80	OCCL&STENOS OTH SPEC PRECERBRL ART W/O INFARCT	I65.8	Occlusion and stenosis of other precerebral arteries
433.81	OCCL&STENOS OTH SPEC PRECERBRL ART W/INFARCT	I63.09	Cerebral infarction due to thrombosis of precerebral artery
		I63.19	Cerebral infarction due to embolism of precerebral artery
		I63.59	Cereb infrc due to unsp occls or stenosis of cerebral artery
433.90	OCCL&STENOS UNS PRECERBRL ART W/O INFARCT	I65.9	Occlusion and stenosis of unspecified precerebral artery
433.91	OCCLUSION&STENOS UNSPEC PRECERBRL ART W/INFARCT	I63.00	Cerebral infarction due to thombos unsp precerebral artery
		I63.10	Cerebral infarction due to embolism of unsp precerb artery
		I63.20	Cereb infrc due to unsp occls or stenos of unsp precerb art
		I63.29	Cerebral infrc due to unsp occls or stenosis of precerb art

ICD-9-CM		ICD-10-CM	
434.00	CEREBRAL THROMBOSIS WITHOUT MENTION INFARCT	**I66.01**	Occlusion and stenosis of right middle cerebral artery
		I66.02	Occlusion and stenosis of left middle cerebral artery
		I66.03	Occlusion and stenosis of bilateral middle cerebral arteries
		I66.09	Occlusion and stenosis of unspecified middle cerebral artery
		I66.11	Occlusion and stenosis of right anterior cerebral artery
		I66.12	Occlusion and stenosis of left anterior cerebral artery
		I66.13	Occlusion and stenosis of bi anterior cerebral arteries
		I66.19	Occlusion and stenosis of unsp anterior cerebral artery
		I66.21	Occlusion and stenosis of right posterior cerebral artery
		I66.22	Occlusion and stenosis of left posterior cerebral artery
		I66.23	Occlusion and stenosis of bi posterior cerebral arteries
		I66.29	Occlusion and stenosis of unsp posterior cerebral artery
		I66.3	Occlusion and stenosis of cerebellar arteries
434.01	CEREBRAL THROMBOSIS WITH CEREBRAL INFARCTION	**I63.30**	Cerebral infarction due to thombos unsp cerebral artery
		I63.311	Cereb infrc due to thombos of right middle cerebral artery
		I63.312	Cerebral infrc due to thombos of left middle cerebral artery
		I63.319	Cerebral infrc due to thombos unsp middle cerebral artery
		I63.321	Cerebral infrc due to thombos of right ant cerebral artery
		I63.322	Cerebral infrc due to thombos of left ant cerebral artery
		I63.329	Cerebral infrc due to thombos unsp anterior cerebral artery
		I63.331	Cerebral infrc due to thombos of right post cerebral artery
		I63.332	Cerebral infrc due to thombos of left post cerebral artery
		I63.339	Cerebral infrc due to thombos unsp posterior cerebral artery
		I63.341	Cerebral infrc due to thrombosis of right cereblr artery
		I63.342	Cerebral infarction due to thrombosis of left cereblr artery
		I63.349	Cerebral infarction due to thombos unsp cerebellar artery
		I63.39	Cerebral infarction due to thrombosis of oth cerebral artery
		I63.6	Cerebral infrc due to cerebral venous thombos, nonpyogenic
434.10	CEREBRAL EMBOLISM WITHOUT MENTION INFARCT	**I66.01**	Occlusion and stenosis of right middle cerebral artery
		I66.02	Occlusion and stenosis of left middle cerebral artery
		I66.03	Occlusion and stenosis of bilateral middle cerebral arteries
		I66.09	Occlusion and stenosis of unspecified middle cerebral artery
		I66.11	Occlusion and stenosis of right anterior cerebral artery
		I66.12	Occlusion and stenosis of left anterior cerebral artery
		I66.13	Occlusion and stenosis of bi anterior cerebral arteries
		I66.19	Occlusion and stenosis of unsp anterior cerebral artery
		I66.21	Occlusion and stenosis of right posterior cerebral artery
		I66.22	Occlusion and stenosis of left posterior cerebral artery
		I66.23	Occlusion and stenosis of bi posterior cerebral arteries
		I66.29	Occlusion and stenosis of unsp posterior cerebral artery
		I66.3	Occlusion and stenosis of cerebellar arteries
		I66.9	Occlusion and stenosis of unspecified cerebral artery
434.11	CEREBRAL EMBOLISM WITH CEREBRAL INFARCTION	**I63.40**	Cerebral infarction due to embolism of unsp cerebral artery
		I63.411	Cereb infrc due to embolism of right middle cerebral artery
		I63.412	Cereb infrc due to embolism of left middle cerebral artery
		I63.419	Cereb infrc due to embolism of unsp middle cerebral artery
		I63.421	Cerebral infrc due to embolism of right ant cerebral artery
		I63.422	Cerebral infrc due to embolism of left ant cerebral artery
		I63.429	Cerebral infrc due to embolism of unsp ant cerebral artery
		I63.431	Cerebral infrc due to embolism of right post cerebral artery
		I63.432	Cerebral infrc due to embolism of left post cerebral artery
		I63.439	Cerebral infrc due to embolism of unsp post cerebral artery
		I63.441	Cerebral infarction due to embolism of right cereblr artery
		I63.442	Cerebral infarction due to embolism of left cereblr artery
		I63.449	Cerebral infarction due to embolism of unsp cereblr artery
		I63.49	Cerebral infarction due to embolism of other cerebral artery
434.90	UNSPEC CERBRL ART OCCLUSION W/O MENTION INFARCT	**I66.01**	Occlusion and stenosis of right middle cerebral artery
		I66.02	Occlusion and stenosis of left middle cerebral artery
		I66.03	Occlusion and stenosis of bilateral middle cerebral arteries
		I66.09	Occlusion and stenosis of unspecified middle cerebral artery
		I66.11	Occlusion and stenosis of right anterior cerebral artery
		I66.12	Occlusion and stenosis of left anterior cerebral artery
		I66.13	Occlusion and stenosis of bi anterior cerebral arteries
		I66.19	Occlusion and stenosis of unsp anterior cerebral artery
		I66.21	Occlusion and stenosis of right posterior cerebral artery
		I66.22	Occlusion and stenosis of left posterior cerebral artery
		I66.23	Occlusion and stenosis of bi posterior cerebral arteries
		I66.29	Occlusion and stenosis of unsp posterior cerebral artery
		I66.3	Occlusion and stenosis of cerebellar arteries
		I66.8	Occlusion and stenosis of other cerebral arteries
		I66.9	Occlusion and stenosis of unspecified cerebral artery

ICD-9-CM			ICD-10-CM	
434.91	UNSPECIFIED CEREBRAL ARTERY OCCLUSION W/INFARCT		I63.50	Cereb infrc due to unsp occls or stenos of unsp cereb artery
			I63.511	Cereb infrc d/t unsp occls or stenos of right mid cereb art
			I63.512	Cereb infrc d/t unsp occls or stenos of left mid cereb art
			I63.519	Cereb infrc d/t unsp occls or stenos of unsp mid cereb art
			I63.521	Cereb infrc d/t unsp occls or stenos of right ant cereb art
			I63.522	Cereb infrc d/t unsp occls or stenos of left ant cereb art
			I63.529	Cereb infrc d/t unsp occls or stenos of unsp ant cereb art
			I63.531	Cereb infrc d/t unsp occls or stenos of right post cereb art
			I63.532	Cereb infrc d/t unsp occls or stenos of left post cereb art
			I63.539	Cereb infrc d/t unsp occls or stenos of unsp post cereb art
			I63.541	Cereb infrc due to unsp occls or stenos of right cereblr art
			I63.542	Cereb infrc due to unsp occls or stenos of left cereblr art
			I63.549	Cereb infrc due to unsp occls or stenos of unsp cereblr art
			I63.59	Cereb infrc due to unsp occls or stenosis of cerebral artery
			I63.8	Other cerebral infarction
			I63.9	Cerebral infarction, unspecified
435.0	BASILAR ARTERY SYNDROME		G45.0	Vertebro-basilar artery syndrome
435.1	VERTEBRAL ARTERY SYNDROME		G45.0	Vertebro-basilar artery syndrome
435.2	SUBCLAVIAN STEAL SYNDROME		G45.8	Oth transient cerebral ischemic attacks and related synd
435.3	VERTEBROBASILAR ARTERY SYNDROME		G45.0	Vertebro-basilar artery syndrome
435.8	OTHER SPECIFIED TRANSIENT CEREBRAL ISCHEMIAS		G45.1	Carotid artery syndrome (hemispheric)
			G45.2	Multiple and bilateral precerebral artery syndromes
			G45.8	Oth transient cerebral ischemic attacks and related synd
			G46.0	Middle cerebral artery syndrome
			G46.1	Anterior cerebral artery syndrome
			G46.2	Posterior cerebral artery syndrome
435.9	UNSPECIFIED TRANSIENT CEREBRAL ISCHEMIA		G45.9	Transient cerebral ischemic attack, unspecified
			I67.841	Reversible cerebrovascular vasoconstriction syndrome
			I67.848	Other cerebrovascular vasospasm and vasoconstriction
436	ACUTE BUT ILL-DEFINED CEREBROVASCULAR DISEASE		I67.89	Other cerebrovascular disease
437.0	CEREBRAL ATHEROSCLEROSIS	➡	I67.2	Cerebral atherosclerosis
437.1	OTH GENERALIZED ISCHEMIC CEREBROVASCULAR DISEASE		I67.81	Acute cerebrovascular insufficiency
			I67.82	Cerebral ischemia
			I67.89	Other cerebrovascular disease
437.2	HYPERTENSIVE ENCEPHALOPATHY	➡	I67.4	Hypertensive encephalopathy
437.3	CEREBRAL ANEURYSM, NONRUPTURED		I67.1	Cerebral aneurysm, nonruptured
437.4	CEREBRAL ARTERITIS		I67.7	Cerebral arteritis, not elsewhere classified
			I68.2	Cerebral arteritis in other diseases classified elsewhere
437.5	MOYAMOYA DISEASE	➡	I67.5	Moyamoya disease
437.6	NONPYOGENIC THROMBOSIS INTRACRANIAL VENOUS SINUS	➡	I67.6	Nonpyogenic thrombosis of intracranial venous system
437.7	TRANSIENT GLOBAL AMNESIA	➡	G45.4	Transient global amnesia
437.8	OTHER ILL-DEFINED CEREBROVASCULAR DISEASE		G46.3	Brain stem stroke syndrome
			G46.4	Cerebellar stroke syndrome
			G46.5	Pure motor lacunar syndrome
			G46.6	Pure sensory lacunar syndrome
			G46.7	Other lacunar syndromes
			G46.8	Oth vascular syndromes of brain in cerebrovascular diseases
			I67.89	Other cerebrovascular disease
			I68.0	Cerebral amyloid angiopathy
			I68.8	Oth cerebrovascular disorders in diseases classd elswhr
437.9	UNSPECIFIED CEREBROVASCULAR DISEASE	➡	I67.9	Cerebrovascular disease, unspecified
438.0	COGNITIVE DEFICITS DUE CEREBROVASCULAR DISEASE		I69.01	Cognitive deficits following ntrm subarachnoid hemorrhage
			I69.11	Cognitive deficits following nontraumatic intcrbl hemorrhage
			I69.21	Cognitive deficits following oth ntrm intcrn hemorrhage
			I69.31	Cognitive deficits following cerebral infarction
			I69.81	Cognitive deficits following other cerebrovascular disease
			I69.91	Cognitive deficits following unsp cerebrovascular disease
438.10	UNSPEC SPCH&LANGE DEFICIT DUE CEREBRVASC DISEASE		I69.928	Oth speech/lang deficits following unsp cerebvasc disease
438.11	APHASIA DUE TO CEREBROVASCULAR DISEASE		I69.020	Aphasia following nontraumatic subarachnoid hemorrhage
			I69.120	Aphasia following nontraumatic intracerebral hemorrhage
			I69.220	Aphasia following other nontraumatic intracranial hemorrhage
			I69.320	Aphasia following cerebral infarction
			I69.820	Aphasia following other cerebrovascular disease
			I69.920	Aphasia following unspecified cerebrovascular disease
438.12	DYSPHASIA DUE TO CEREBROVASCULAR DISEASE		I69.021	Dysphasia following nontraumatic subarachnoid hemorrhage
			I69.121	Dysphasia following nontraumatic intracerebral hemorrhage
			I69.221	Dysphasia following oth nontraumatic intracranial hemorrhage
			I69.321	Dysphasia following cerebral infarction
			I69.821	Dysphasia following other cerebrovascular disease
			I69.921	Dysphasia following unspecified cerebrovascular disease
438.13	LATE EFF CVD SPEECH & LANG DEFICITS DYSARTHRIA		I69.022	Dysarthria following nontraumatic subarachnoid hemorrhage
			I69.122	Dysarthria following nontraumatic intracerebral hemorrhage
			I69.222	Dysarthria following oth nontraumatic intcrn hemorrhage
			I69.322	Dysarthria following cerebral infarction
			I69.822	Dysarthria following other cerebrovascular disease
			I69.922	Dysarthria following unspecified cerebrovascular disease

ICD-9-CM		ICD-10-CM	
438.14	LATE EFF CVD SPCH AND LANGE DEFICITS FLUENCY D/O	**I69.Ø23**	Fluency disorder following ntrm subarachnoid hemorrhage
		I69.123	Fluency disorder following nontraumatic intcrbl hemorrhage
		I69.223	Fluency disorder following oth ntrm intcrn hemorrhage
		I69.323	Fluency disorder following cerebral infarction
		I69.823	Fluency disorder following other cerebrovascular disease
		I69.923	Fluency disorder following unsp cerebrovascular disease
438.19	OTH SPCH&LANGE DEFICITS DUE CEREBRVASC DISEASE	**I69.Ø28**	Oth speech/lang deficits following ntrm subarach hemorrhage
		I69.128	Oth speech/lang deficits following ntrm intcrbl hemorrhage
		I69.228	Oth speech/lang deficits following oth ntrm intcrn hemor
		I69.328	Oth speech/lang deficits following cerebral infarction
		I69.828	Oth speech/lang deficits following oth cerebvasc disease
		I69.928	Oth speech/lang deficits following unsp cerebvasc disease
438.2Ø	HEMIPL AFFECT UNSPEC SIDE DUE CEREBRVASC DISEASE	**I69.Ø59**	Hemiplga following ntrm subarach hemor affecting unsp side
		I69.159	Hemiplga following ntrm intcrbl hemor affecting unsp side
		I69.259	Hemiplga following oth ntrm intcrn hemor affecting unsp side
		I69.359	Hemiplga following cerebral infarction affecting unsp side
		I69.859	Hemiplga following oth cerebvasc disease affecting unsp side
		I69.959	Hemiplga following unsp cerebvasc disease aff unsp side
438.21	HEMIPL AFFCT DOMINANT SIDE DUE CEREBRVASC DZ	**I69.Ø51**	Hemiplga fol ntrm subarach hemor aff right dominant side
		I69.Ø52	Hemiplga fol ntrm subarach hemor aff left dominant side
		I69.151	Hemiplga fol ntrm intcrbl hemor aff right dominant side
		I69.152	Hemiplga following ntrm intcrbl hemor aff left dominant side
		I69.251	Hemiplga fol oth ntrm intcrn hemor aff right dominant side
		I69.252	Hemiplga fol oth ntrm intcrn hemor aff left dominant side
		I69.351	Hemiplga following cerebral infrc aff right dominant side
		I69.352	Hemiplga following cerebral infrc aff left dominant side
		I69.851	Hemiplga fol oth cerebvasc disease aff right dominant side
		I69.852	Hemiplga fol oth cerebvasc disease aff left dominant side
		I69.951	Hemiplga fol unsp cerebvasc disease aff right dominant side
		I69.952	Hemiplga fol unsp cerebvasc disease aff left dominant side
438.22	HEMIPL AFFCT NONDOMINANT SIDE DUE CEREBRVASC DZ	**I69.Ø53**	Hemiplga following ntrm subarach hemor aff right nondom side
		I69.Ø54	Hemiplga following ntrm subarach hemor aff left nondom side
		I69.153	Hemiplga following ntrm intcrbl hemor aff right nondom side
		I69.154	Hemiplga following ntrm intcrbl hemor aff left nondom side
		I69.253	Hemiplga fol oth ntrm intcrn hemor aff right nondom side
		I69.254	Hemiplga fol oth ntrm intcrn hemor aff left nondom side
		I69.353	Hemiplga following cerebral infrc aff right nondom side
		I69.354	Hemiplga following cerebral infrc affecting left nondom side
		I69.853	Hemiplga fol oth cerebvasc disease aff right nondom side
		I69.854	Hemiplga fol oth cerebvasc disease aff left nondom side
		I69.953	Hemiplga fol unsp cerebvasc disease aff right nondom side
		I69.954	Hemiplga fol unsp cerebvasc disease aff left nondom side
438.3Ø	MONOPLEG UPPER LIMB UNS SIDE DUE CEREBRVASC DZ	**I69.Ø39**	Monoplg upr lmb following ntrm subarach hemor aff unsp side
		I69.139	Monoplg upr lmb following ntrm intcrbl hemor aff unsp side
		I69.239	Monoplg upr lmb fol oth ntrm intcrn hemor aff unsp side
		I69.339	Monoplg upr lmb following cerebral infrc affecting unsp side
		I69.839	Monoplg upr lmb fol oth cerebvasc disease aff unsp side
		I69.939	Monoplg upr lmb fol unsp cerebvasc disease aff unsp side
438.31	MONOPLEG UPPER LIMB DOM SIDE DUE CEREBRVASC DZ	**I69.Ø31**	Monoplg upr lmb fol ntrm subarach hemor aff right dom side
		I69.Ø32	Monoplg upr lmb fol ntrm subarach hemor aff left dom side
		I69.131	Monoplg upr lmb fol ntrm intcrbl hemor aff right dom side
		I69.132	Monoplg upr lmb fol ntrm intcrbl hemor aff left dom side
		I69.231	Monoplg upr lmb fol oth ntrm intcrn hemor aff right dom side
		I69.232	Monoplg upr lmb fol oth ntrm intcrn hemor aff left dom side
		I69.331	Monoplg upr lmb fol cerebral infrc aff right dominant side
		I69.332	Monoplg upr lmb fol cerebral infrc aff left dominant side
		I69.831	Monoplg upr lmb fol oth cerebvasc disease aff right dom side
		I69.832	Monoplg upr lmb fol oth cerebvasc disease aff left dom side
		I69.931	Monoplg upr lmb fol unsp cerebvasc dis aff right dom side
		I69.932	Monoplg upr lmb fol unsp cerebvasc disease aff left dom side
438.32	MONOPLEG UP LIMB NONDOM SIDE DUE CEREBRVASC DZ	**I69.Ø33**	Monoplg upr lmb fol ntrm subarach hemor aff r nondom side
		I69.Ø34	Monoplg upr lmb fol ntrm subarach hemor aff left nondom side
		I69.133	Monoplg upr lmb fol ntrm intcrbl hemor aff right nondom side
		I69.134	Monoplg upr lmb fol ntrm intcrbl hemor aff left nondom side
		I69.233	Monoplg upr lmb fol oth ntrm intcrn hemor aff r nondom side
		I69.234	Monoplg upr lmb fol oth ntrm intcrn hemor aff l nondom side
		I69.333	Monoplg upr lmb fol cerebral infrc aff right nondom side
		I69.334	Monoplg upr lmb fol cerebral infrc aff left nondom side
		I69.833	Monoplg upr lmb fol oth cerebvasc dis aff right nondom side
		I69.834	Monoplg upr lmb fol oth cerebvasc dis aff left nondom side
		I69.933	Monoplg upr lmb fol unsp cerebvasc dis aff right nondom side
		I69.934	Monoplg upr lmb fol unsp cerebvasc dis aff left nondom side
438.4Ø	MONOPLEG LOW LIMB UNSPEC SIDE DUE CEREBRVASC DZ	**I69.Ø49**	Monoplg low lmb following ntrm subarach hemor aff unsp side
		I69.149	Monoplg low lmb following ntrm intcrbl hemor aff unsp side
		I69.249	Monoplg low lmb fol oth ntrm intcrn hemor aff unsp side
		I69.349	Monoplg low lmb following cerebral infrc affecting unsp side
		I69.849	Monoplg low lmb fol oth cerebvasc disease aff unsp side
		I69.949	Monoplg low lmb fol unsp cerebvasc disease aff unsp side

ICD-9-CM		ICD-10-CM	
438.41	MONOPLEG LOW LIMB DOM SIDE DUE CEREBRVASC DZ	**I69.041**	Monoplg low lmb fol ntrm subarach hemor aff right dom side
		I69.042	Monoplg low lmb fol ntrm subarach hemor aff left dom side
		I69.141	Monoplg low lmb fol ntrm intcrbl hemor aff right dom side
		I69.142	Monoplg low lmb fol ntrm intcrbl hemor aff left dom side
		I69.241	Monoplg low lmb fol oth ntrm intcrn hemor aff right dom side
		I69.242	Monoplg low lmb fol oth ntrm intcrn hemor aff left dom side
		I69.341	Monoplg low lmb fol cerebral infrc aff right dominant side
		I69.342	Monoplg low lmb fol cerebral infrc aff left dominant side
		I69.841	Monoplg low lmb fol oth cerebvasc disease aff right dom side
		I69.842	Monoplg low lmb fol oth cerebvasc disease aff left dom side
		I69.941	Monoplg low lmb fol unsp cerebvasc dis aff right dom side
		I69.942	Monoplg low lmb fol unsp cerebvasc disease aff left dom side
438.42	MONOPLEG LOW LIMB NONDOM SIDE DUE CEREBRVASC DZ	**I69.043**	Monoplg low lmb fol ntrm subarach hemor aff r nondom side
		I69.044	Monoplg low lmb fol ntrm subarach hemor aff left nondom side
		I69.143	Monoplg low lmb fol ntrm intcrbl hemor aff right nondom side
		I69.144	Monoplg low lmb fol ntrm intcrbl hemor aff left nondom side
		I69.243	Monoplg low lmb fol oth ntrm intcrn hemor aff r nondom side
		I69.244	Monoplg low lmb fol oth ntrm intcrn hemor aff l nondom side
		I69.343	Monoplg low lmb fol cerebral infrc aff right nondom side
		I69.344	Monoplg low lmb fol cerebral infrc aff left nondom side
		I69.843	Monoplg low lmb fol oth cerebvasc dis aff right nondom side
		I69.844	Monoplg low lmb fol oth cerebvasc dis aff left nondom side
		I69.943	Monoplg low lmb fol unsp cerebvasc dis aff right nondom side
		I69.944	Monoplg low lmb fol unsp cerebvasc dis aff left nondom side
438.50	OTH PARALYT SYND AFFCT UNS SIDE-CEREBRVASC DZ	**I69.069**	Oth paralytic syndrome fol ntrm subarach hemor aff unsp side
		I69.169	Oth paralytic syndrome fol ntrm intcrbl hemor aff unsp side
		I69.269	Oth parlyt syndrome fol oth ntrm intcrn hemor aff unsp side
		I69.369	Oth paralytic syndrome fol cerebral infrc aff unsp side
		I69.869	Oth parlyt syndrome fol oth cerebvasc disease aff unsp side
		I69.969	Oth parlyt syndrome fol unsp cerebvasc disease aff unsp side
438.51	OTH PARALYT SYND AFFCT DOM SIDE-CEREBRVASC DZ	**I69.061**	Oth parlyt synd fol ntrm subarach hemor aff right dom side
		I69.062	Oth parlyt synd fol ntrm subarach hemor aff left dom side
		I69.161	Oth parlyt synd fol ntrm intcrbl hemor aff right dom side
		I69.162	Oth parlyt syndrome fol ntrm intcrbl hemor aff left dom side
		I69.261	Oth parlyt synd fol oth ntrm intcrn hemor aff right dom side
		I69.262	Oth parlyt synd fol oth ntrm intcrn hemor aff left dom side
		I69.361	Oth parlyt syndrome fol cereb infrc aff right dominant side
		I69.362	Oth parlyt syndrome fol cereb infrc aff left dominant side
		I69.861	Oth parlyt synd fol oth cerebvasc disease aff right dom side
		I69.862	Oth parlyt synd fol oth cerebvasc disease aff left dom side
		I69.961	Oth parlyt synd fol unsp cerebvasc dis aff right dom side
		I69.962	Oth parlyt synd fol unsp cerebvasc disease aff left dom side
438.52	OTH PARALYT SYND AFFCT NONDOM SIDE-CEREBRVASC DZ	**I69.063**	Oth parlyt synd fol ntrm subarach hemor aff r nondom side
		I69.064	Oth parlyt synd fol ntrm subarach hemor aff left nondom side
		I69.163	Oth parlyt synd fol ntrm intcrbl hemor aff right nondom side
		I69.164	Oth parlyt synd fol ntrm intcrbl hemor aff left nondom side
		I69.263	Oth parlyt synd fol oth ntrm intcrn hemor aff r nondom side
		I69.264	Oth parlyt synd fol oth ntrm intcrn hemor aff l nondom side
		I69.363	Oth parlyt syndrome fol cerebral infrc aff right nondom side
		I69.364	Oth parlyt syndrome fol cerebral infrc aff left nondom side
		I69.863	Oth parlyt synd fol oth cerebvasc dis aff right nondom side
		I69.864	Oth parlyt synd fol oth cerebvasc dis aff left nondom side
		I69.963	Oth parlyt synd fol unsp cerebvasc dis aff right nondom side
		I69.964	Oth parlyt synd fol unsp cerebvasc dis aff left nondom side
438.53	OTHER PARALYTIC SYNDROME, BILATERAL	**I69.065**	Oth paralytic syndrome following ntrm subarach hemor, bi
		I69.165	Oth paralytic syndrome following ntrm intcrbl hemor, bi
		I69.265	Oth paralytic syndrome following oth ntrm intcrn hemor, bi
		I69.365	Oth paralytic syndrome following cerebral infrc, bilateral
		I69.865	Oth paralytic syndrome following oth cerebvasc disease, bi
		I69.965	Oth paralytic syndrome following unsp cerebvasc disease, bi
438.6	ALTERATION SENSATIONS AS LATE EFF CEREBRVASC DZ	**I69.998**	Other sequelae following unspecified cerebrovascular disease
438.7	DISTURBANCE VISION AS LATE EFFECT CEREBRVASC DZ	**I69.998**	Other sequelae following unspecified cerebrovascular disease
438.81	APRAXIA DUE TO CEREBROVASCULAR DISEASE	**I69.090**	Apraxia following nontraumatic subarachnoid hemorrhage
		I69.190	Apraxia following nontraumatic intracerebral hemorrhage
		I69.290	Apraxia following other nontraumatic intracranial hemorrhage
		I69.390	Apraxia following cerebral infarction
		I69.890	Apraxia following other cerebrovascular disease
		I69.990	Apraxia following unspecified cerebrovascular disease
438.82	DYSPHAGIA DUE TO CEREBROVASCULAR DISEASE	**I69.091**	Dysphagia following nontraumatic subarachnoid hemorrhage
		I69.191	Dysphagia following nontraumatic intracerebral hemorrhage
		I69.291	Dysphagia following oth nontraumatic intracranial hemorrhage
		I69.391	Dysphagia following cerebral infarction
		I69.891	Dysphagia following other cerebrovascular disease
		I69.991	Dysphagia following unspecified cerebrovascular disease
438.83	FACIAL WEAKNESS LATE EFFECT CEREBROVASCULAR DZ	**I69.092**	Facial weakness following ntrm subarachnoid hemorrhage
		I69.192	Facial weakness following nontraumatic intcrbl hemorrhage
		I69.292	Facial weakness following oth nontraumatic intcrn hemorrhage
		I69.392	Facial weakness following cerebral infarction
		I69.892	Facial weakness following other cerebrovascular disease
		I69.992	Facial weakness following unsp cerebrovascular disease

ICD-9-CM		ICD-10-CM	
438.84	ATAXIA AS LATE EFFECT OF CEREBROVASCULAR DISEASE	I69.093	Ataxia following nontraumatic subarachnoid hemorrhage
		I69.193	Ataxia following nontraumatic intracerebral hemorrhage
		I69.293	Ataxia following other nontraumatic intracranial hemorrhage
		I69.393	Ataxia following cerebral infarction
		I69.893	Ataxia following other cerebrovascular disease
		I69.993	Ataxia following unspecified cerebrovascular disease
438.85	VERTIGO AS LATE EFFECT CEREBROVASCULAR DISEASE	I69.998	Other sequelae following unspecified cerebrovascular disease
438.89	OTHER LATE EFFECTS OF CEREBROVASCULAR DISEASE	I69.098	Oth sequelae following nontraumatic subarachnoid hemorrhage
		I69.198	Other sequelae of nontraumatic intracerebral hemorrhage
		I69.298	Other sequelae of other nontraumatic intracranial hemorrhage
		I69.398	Other sequelae of cerebral infarction
		I69.898	Other sequelae of other cerebrovascular disease
		I69.998	Other sequelae following unspecified cerebrovascular disease
438.9	UNSPEC LATE EFF CEREBRVASC DZ DUE CEREBRVASC DZ	I69.00	Unspecified sequelae of nontraumatic subarachnoid hemorrhage
		I69.10	Unsp sequelae of nontraumatic intracerebral hemorrhage
		I69.20	Unsp sequelae of other nontraumatic intracranial hemorrhage
		I69.30	Unspecified sequelae of cerebral infarction
		I69.80	Unspecified sequelae of other cerebrovascular disease
		I69.90	Unspecified sequelae of unspecified cerebrovascular disease
440.0	ATHEROSCLEROSIS OF AORTA	➡ I70.0	Atherosclerosis of aorta
440.1	ATHEROSCLEROSIS OF RENAL ARTERY	➡ I70.1	Atherosclerosis of renal artery
440.20	ATHEROSCLEROSIS NATIVE ART EXTREMITIES UNSPEC	I70.201	Unsp athscl native arteries of extremities, right leg
		I70.202	Unsp athscl native arteries of extremities, left leg
		I70.203	Unsp athscl native arteries of extremities, bilateral legs
		I70.208	Unsp athscl native arteries of extremities, oth extremity
		I70.209	Unsp athscl native arteries of extremities, unsp extremity
440.21	ATHEROSLERO NATV ART EXTREM W/INTERMIT CLAUDICAT	I70.211	Athscl native arteries of extrm w intrmt claud, right leg
		I70.212	Athscl native arteries of extrm w intrmt claud, left leg
		I70.213	Athscl native arteries of extrm w intrmt claud, bi legs
		I70.218	Athscl native arteries of extrm w intrmt claud, oth extrm
		I70.219	Athscl native arteries of extrm w intrmt claud, unsp extrm
440.22	ATHEROSLERO NATIVE ART EXTREMITIES W/REST PAIN	I70.221	Athscl native arteries of extremities w rest pain, right leg
		I70.222	Athscl native arteries of extremities w rest pain, left leg
		I70.223	Athscl native arteries of extrm w rest pain, bilateral legs
		I70.228	Athscl native arteries of extrm w rest pain, oth extremity
		I70.229	Athscl native arteries of extrm w rest pain, unsp extremity
440.23	ATHEROSLERO NATIVE ART EXTREMITIES W/ULCERATION	I70.231	Athscl native arteries of right leg w ulceration of thigh
		I70.232	Athscl native arteries of right leg w ulceration of calf
		I70.233	Athscl native arteries of right leg w ulceration of ankle
		I70.234	Athscl native art of right leg w ulcer of heel and midfoot
		I70.235	Athscl native arteries of right leg w ulcer oth prt foot
		I70.238	Athscl natv art of right leg w ulcer oth prt lower right leg
		I70.239	Athscl native arteries of right leg w ulcer of unsp site
		I70.241	Athscl native arteries of left leg w ulceration of thigh
		I70.242	Athscl native arteries of left leg w ulceration of calf
		I70.243	Athscl native arteries of left leg w ulceration of ankle
		I70.244	Athscl native art of left leg w ulcer of heel and midfoot
		I70.245	Athscl native arteries of left leg w ulceration oth prt foot
		I70.248	Athscl native art of left leg w ulcer oth prt lower left leg
		I70.249	Athscl native arteries of left leg w ulceration of unsp site
		I70.25	Athscl native arteries of extremities w ulceration
440.24	ATHEROSLERO NATIVE ART EXTREMITIES W/GANGRENE	I70.261	Athscl native arteries of extremities w gangrene, right leg
		I70.262	Athscl native arteries of extremities w gangrene, left leg
		I70.263	Athscl native arteries of extrm w gangrene, bilateral legs
		I70.268	Athscl native arteries of extrm w gangrene, oth extremity
		I70.269	Athscl native arteries of extrm w gangrene, unsp extremity
440.29	OTH ATHEROSCLEROSIS NATIVE ARTERIES EXTREMITIES	I70.291	Oth athscl native arteries of extremities, right leg
		I70.292	Oth athscl native arteries of extremities, left leg
		I70.293	Oth athscl native arteries of extremities, bilateral legs
		I70.298	Oth athscl native arteries of extremities, oth extremity
		I70.299	Oth athscl native arteries of extremities, unsp extremity

[Brackets] indicate valid character values for each code. Character value meanings provided for each code grouping.

ICD-9-CM		ICD-10-CM	
44Ø.3Ø	ATHEROSCLEROSIS UNSPEC BYPASS GRAFT EXTREMITIES	**I7Ø.3Ø1**	Unsp athscl unsp type bypass of the extremities, right leg
		I7Ø.3Ø2	Unsp athscl unsp type bypass of the extremities, left leg
		I7Ø.3Ø3	Unsp athscl unsp type bypass of the extrm, bilateral legs
		I7Ø.3Ø8	Unsp athscl unsp type bypass of the extrm, oth extremity
		I7Ø.3Ø9	Unsp athscl unsp type bypass of the extrm, unsp extremity
		I7Ø.311	Athscl unsp type bypass of extrm w intrmt claud, right leg
		I7Ø.312	Athscl unsp type bypass of extrm w intrmt claud, left leg
		I7Ø.313	Athscl unsp type bypass of the extrm w intrmt claud, bi legs
		I7Ø.318	Athscl unsp type bypass of extrm w intrmt claud, oth extrm
		I7Ø.319	Athscl unsp type bypass of extrm w intrmt claud, unsp extrm
		I7Ø.321	Athscl unsp type bypass of the extrm w rest pain, right leg
		I7Ø.322	Athscl unsp type bypass of the extrm w rest pain, left leg
		I7Ø.323	Athscl unsp type bypass of the extrm w rest pain, bi legs
		I7Ø.328	Athscl unsp type bypass of the extrm w rest pain, oth extrm
		I7Ø.329	Athscl unsp type bypass of the extrm w rest pain, unsp extrm
		I7Ø.331	Athscl unsp type bypass of the right leg w ulcer of thigh
		I7Ø.332	Athscl unsp type bypass of the right leg w ulcer of calf
		I7Ø.333	Athscl unsp type bypass of the right leg w ulcer of ankle
		I7Ø.334	Athscl unsp type bypass of r leg w ulcer of heel and midft
		I7Ø.335	Athscl unsp type bypass of right leg w ulcer oth prt foot
		I7Ø.338	Athscl unsp type bypass of right leg w ulcer oth prt low leg
		I7Ø.339	Athscl unsp type bypass of right leg w ulcer of unsp site
		I7Ø.341	Athscl unsp type bypass of the left leg w ulcer of thigh
		I7Ø.342	Athscl unsp type bypass of the left leg w ulceration of calf
		I7Ø.343	Athscl unsp type bypass of the left leg w ulcer of ankle
		I7Ø.344	Athscl unsp type bypass of left leg w ulc of heel and midft
		I7Ø.345	Athscl unsp type bypass of the left leg w ulcer oth prt foot
		I7Ø.348	Athscl unsp type bypass of left leg w ulcer oth prt low leg
		I7Ø.349	Athscl unsp type bypass of the left leg w ulcer of unsp site
		I7Ø.35	Athscl unsp type bypass graft(s) of extremity w ulceration
		I7Ø.361	Athscl unsp type bypass of the extrm w gangrene, right leg
		I7Ø.362	Athscl unsp type bypass of the extrm w gangrene, left leg
		I7Ø.363	Athscl unsp type bypass of the extrm w gangrene, bi legs
		I7Ø.368	Athscl unsp type bypass of the extrm w gangrene, oth extrm
		I7Ø.369	Athscl unsp type bypass of the extrm w gangrene, unsp extrm
		I7Ø.391	Oth athscl unsp type bypass of the extremities, right leg
		I7Ø.392	Oth athscl unsp type bypass of the extremities, left leg
		I7Ø.393	Oth athscl unsp type bypass of the extrm, bilateral legs
		I7Ø.398	Oth athscl unsp type bypass of the extrm, oth extremity
		I7Ø.399	Oth athscl unsp type bypass of the extrm, unsp extremity
		I7Ø.6Ø1	Unsp athscl nonbiol bypass of the extremities, right leg
		I7Ø.6Ø2	Unsp athscl nonbiol bypass of the extremities, left leg
		I7Ø.6Ø3	Unsp athscl nonbiol bypass of the extrm, bilateral legs
		I7Ø.6Ø8	Unsp athscl nonbiol bypass of the extremities, oth extremity
		I7Ø.6Ø9	Unsp athscl nonbiol bypass of the extrm, unsp extremity
		I7Ø.611	Athscl nonbiol bypass of the extrm w intrmt claud, right leg
		I7Ø.612	Athscl nonbiol bypass of the extrm w intrmt claud, left leg
		I7Ø.613	Athscl nonbiol bypass of the extrm w intrmt claud, bi legs
		I7Ø.618	Athscl nonbiol bypass of the extrm w intrmt claud, oth extrm
		I7Ø.619	Athscl nonbiol bypass of extrm w intrmt claud, unsp extrm
		I7Ø.621	Athscl nonbiol bypass of the extrm w rest pain, right leg
		I7Ø.622	Athscl nonbiol bypass of the extrm w rest pain, left leg
		I7Ø.623	Athscl nonbiol bypass of the extrm w rest pain, bi legs
		I7Ø.628	Athscl nonbiol bypass of the extrm w rest pain, oth extrm
		I7Ø.629	Athscl nonbiol bypass of the extrm w rest pain, unsp extrm
		I7Ø.631	Athscl nonbiol bypass of the right leg w ulceration of thigh
		I7Ø.632	Athscl nonbiol bypass of the right leg w ulceration of calf
		I7Ø.633	Athscl nonbiol bypass of the right leg w ulceration of ankle
		I7Ø.634	Athscl nonbiol bypass of right leg w ulcer of heel and midft
		I7Ø.635	Athscl nonbiol bypass of the right leg w ulcer oth prt foot
		I7Ø.638	Athscl nonbiol bypass of right leg w ulcer oth prt low leg
		I7Ø.639	Athscl nonbiol bypass of the right leg w ulcer of unsp site
		I7Ø.641	Athscl nonbiol bypass of the left leg w ulceration of thigh
		I7Ø.642	Athscl nonbiol bypass of the left leg w ulceration of calf
		I7Ø.643	Athscl nonbiol bypass of the left leg w ulceration of ankle
		I7Ø.644	Athscl nonbiol bypass of left leg w ulcer of heel and midft
		I7Ø.645	Athscl nonbiol bypass of the left leg w ulcer oth prt foot
		I7Ø.648	Athscl nonbiol bypass of left leg w ulcer oth prt low leg
		I7Ø.649	Athscl nonbiol bypass of the left leg w ulcer of unsp site
		I7Ø.65	Athscl nonbiological bypass of extremity w ulceration
		I7Ø.661	Athscl nonbiol bypass of the extrm w gangrene, right leg
		I7Ø.662	Athscl nonbiol bypass of the extrm w gangrene, left leg
		I7Ø.663	Athscl nonbiol bypass of the extrm w gangrene, bi legs
		I7Ø.668	Athscl nonbiol bypass of the extrm w gangrene, oth extremity
		I7Ø.669	Athscl nonbiol bypass of the extrm w gangrene, unsp extrm
		I7Ø.691	Oth athscl nonbiol bypass of the extremities, right leg
		I7Ø.692	Oth athscl nonbiological bypass of the extremities, left leg
		I7Ø.693	Oth athscl nonbiol bypass of the extremities, bilateral legs
		I7Ø.698	Oth athscl nonbiol bypass of the extremities, oth extremity
		I7Ø.699	Oth athscl nonbiol bypass of the extremities, unsp extremity
		I7Ø.7Ø1	Unsp athscl type of bypass of the extremities, right leg

(Continued on next page)

ICD-9-CM		ICD-10-CM	
440.30	ATHEROSCLEROSIS UNSPEC BYPASS GRAFT EXTREMITIES **(Continued)**	**I70.702**	Unsp athscl type of bypass of the extremities, left leg
		I70.703	Unsp athscl type of bypass of the extrm, bilateral legs
		I70.708	Unsp athscl type of bypass of the extremities, oth extremity
		I70.709	Unsp athscl type of bypass of the extrm, unsp extremity
		I70.711	Athscl type of bypass of the extrm w intrmt claud, right leg
		I70.712	Athscl type of bypass of the extrm w intrmt claud, left leg
		I70.713	Athscl type of bypass of the extrm w intrmt claud, bi legs
		I70.718	Athscl type of bypass of the extrm w intrmt claud, oth extrm
		I70.719	Athscl type of bypass of extrm w intrmt claud, unsp extrm
		I70.721	Athscl type of bypass of the extrm w rest pain, right leg
		I70.722	Athscl type of bypass of the extrm w rest pain, left leg
		I70.723	Athscl type of bypass of the extrm w rest pain, bi legs
		I70.728	Athscl type of bypass of the extrm w rest pain, oth extrm
		I70.729	Athscl type of bypass of the extrm w rest pain, unsp extrm
		I70.731	Athscl type of bypass of the right leg w ulceration of thigh
		I70.732	Athscl type of bypass of the right leg w ulceration of calf
		I70.733	Athscl type of bypass of the right leg w ulceration of ankle
		I70.734	Athscl type of bypass of right leg w ulcer of heel and midft
		I70.735	Athscl type of bypass of the right leg w ulcer oth prt foot
		I70.738	Athscl type of bypass of right leg w ulcer oth prt low leg
		I70.739	Athscl type of bypass of the right leg w ulcer of unsp site
		I70.741	Athscl type of bypass of the left leg w ulceration of thigh
		I70.742	Athscl type of bypass of the left leg w ulceration of calf
		I70.743	Athscl type of bypass of the left leg w ulceration of ankle
		I70.744	Athscl type of bypass of left leg w ulcer of heel and midft
		I70.745	Athscl type of bypass of the left leg w ulcer oth prt foot
		I70.748	Athscl type of bypass of left leg w ulcer oth prt low leg
		I70.749	Athscl type of bypass of the left leg w ulcer of unsp site
		I70.75	Athscl type of bypass graft(s) of extremity w ulceration
		I70.761	Athscl type of bypass of the extrm w gangrene, right leg
		I70.762	Athscl type of bypass of the extrm w gangrene, left leg
		I70.763	Athscl type of bypass of the extrm w gangrene, bi legs
		I70.768	Athscl type of bypass of the extrm w gangrene, oth extremity
		I70.769	Athscl type of bypass of the extrm w gangrene, unsp extrm
		I70.791	Oth athscl type of bypass of the extremities, right leg
		I70.792	Oth athscl type of bypass of the extremities, left leg
		I70.793	Oth athscl type of bypass of the extremities, bilateral legs
		I70.798	Oth athscl type of bypass of the extremities, oth extremity
		I70.799	Oth athscl type of bypass of the extremities, unsp extremity
440.31	ATHEROSLEROSIS AUTOL VEIN BYPS GRAFT EXTREMITIES	**I70.401**	Unsp athscl autologous vein bypass of the extrm, right leg
		I70.402	Unsp athscl autologous vein bypass of the extrm, left leg
		I70.403	Unsp athscl autol vein bypass of the extrm, bilateral legs
		I70.408	Unsp athscl autol vein bypass of the extrm, oth extremity
		I70.409	Unsp athscl autol vein bypass of the extrm, unsp extremity
		I70.411	Athscl autol vein bypass of extrm w intrmt claud, right leg
		I70.412	Athscl autol vein bypass of extrm w intrmt claud, left leg
		I70.413	Athscl autol vein bypass of extrm w intrmt claud, bi legs
		I70.418	Athscl autol vein bypass of extrm w intrmt claud, oth extrm
		I70.419	Athscl autol vein bypass of extrm w intrmt claud, unsp extrm
		I70.421	Athscl autol vein bypass of the extrm w rest pain, right leg
		I70.422	Athscl autol vein bypass of the extrm w rest pain, left leg
		I70.423	Athscl autol vein bypass of the extrm w rest pain, bi legs
		I70.428	Athscl autol vein bypass of the extrm w rest pain, oth extrm
		I70.429	Athscl autol vein bypass of extrm w rest pain, unsp extrm
		I70.431	Athscl autol vein bypass of the right leg w ulcer of thigh
		I70.432	Athscl autol vein bypass of the right leg w ulcer of calf
		I70.433	Athscl autol vein bypass of the right leg w ulcer of ankle
		I70.434	Athscl autol vein bypass of r leg w ulcer of heel and midft
		I70.435	Athscl autol vein bypass of right leg w ulcer oth prt foot
		I70.438	Athscl autol vein bypass of r leg w ulcer oth prt low leg
		I70.439	Athscl autol vein bypass of right leg w ulcer of unsp site
		I70.441	Athscl autol vein bypass of the left leg w ulcer of thigh
		I70.442	Athscl autol vein bypass of the left leg w ulcer of calf
		I70.443	Athscl autol vein bypass of the left leg w ulcer of ankle
		I70.444	Athscl autol vein bypass of left leg w ulc of heel and midft
		I70.445	Athscl autol vein bypass of left leg w ulcer oth prt foot
		I70.448	Athscl autol vein bypass of left leg w ulcer oth prt low leg
		I70.449	Athscl autol vein bypass of left leg w ulcer of unsp site
		I70.45	Athscl autologous vein bypass of extremity w ulceration
		I70.461	Athscl autol vein bypass of the extrm w gangrene, right leg
		I70.462	Athscl autol vein bypass of the extrm w gangrene, left leg
		I70.463	Athscl autol vein bypass of the extrm w gangrene, bi legs
		I70.468	Athscl autol vein bypass of the extrm w gangrene, oth extrm
		I70.469	Athscl autol vein bypass of the extrm w gangrene, unsp extrm
		I70.491	Oth athscl autologous vein bypass of the extrm, right leg
		I70.492	Oth athscl autologous vein bypass of the extrm, left leg
		I70.493	Oth athscl autol vein bypass of the extrm, bilateral legs
		I70.498	Oth athscl autol vein bypass of the extrm, oth extremity
		I70.499	Oth athscl autol vein bypass of the extrm, unsp extremity

[Brackets] indicate valid character values for each code. Character value meanings provided for each code grouping.

ICD-9-CM			ICD-10-CM	
44Ø.32	ATHEROSLEROSIS NONAUTOL BIOLOGIC BYPS GFT EXTREM		**I7Ø.5Ø1**	Unsp athscl nonaut bio bypass of the extremities, right leg
			I7Ø.5Ø2	Unsp athscl nonaut bio bypass of the extremities, left leg
			I7Ø.5Ø3	Unsp athscl nonaut bio bypass of the extrm, bilateral legs
			I7Ø.5Ø8	Unsp athscl nonaut bio bypass of the extrm, oth extremity
			I7Ø.5Ø9	Unsp athscl nonaut bio bypass of the extrm, unsp extremity
			I7Ø.511	Athscl nonaut bio bypass of extrm w intrmt claud, right leg
			I7Ø.512	Athscl nonaut bio bypass of extrm w intrmt claud, left leg
			I7Ø.513	Athscl nonaut bio bypass of extrm w intrmt claud, bi legs
			I7Ø.518	Athscl nonaut bio bypass of extrm w intrmt claud, oth extrm
			I7Ø.519	Athscl nonaut bio bypass of extrm w intrmt claud, unsp extrm
			I7Ø.521	Athscl nonaut bio bypass of the extrm w rest pain, right leg
			I7Ø.522	Athscl nonaut bio bypass of the extrm w rest pain, left leg
			I7Ø.523	Athscl nonaut bio bypass of the extrm w rest pain, bi legs
			I7Ø.528	Athscl nonaut bio bypass of the extrm w rest pain, oth extrm
			I7Ø.529	Athscl nonaut bio bypass of extrm w rest pain, unsp extrm
		🔖	**I7Ø.531**	Athscl nonaut bio bypass of the right leg w ulcer of thigh
		🔖	**I7Ø.532**	Athscl nonaut bio bypass of the right leg w ulcer of calf
		🔖	**I7Ø.533**	Athscl nonaut bio bypass of the right leg w ulcer of ankle
		🔖	**I7Ø.534**	Athscl nonaut bio bypass of r leg w ulcer of heel and midft
		🔖	**I7Ø.535**	Athscl nonaut bio bypass of right leg w ulcer oth prt foot
		🔖	**I7Ø.538**	Athscl nonaut bio bypass of r leg w ulcer oth prt low leg
		🔖	**I7Ø.539**	Athscl nonaut bio bypass of right leg w ulcer of unsp site
		🔖	**I7Ø.541**	Athscl nonaut bio bypass of the left leg w ulcer of thigh
		🔖	**I7Ø.542**	Athscl nonaut bio bypass of the left leg w ulcer of calf
		🔖	**I7Ø.543**	Athscl nonaut bio bypass of the left leg w ulcer of ankle
		🔖	**I7Ø.544**	Athscl nonaut bio bypass of left leg w ulc of heel and midft
		🔖	**I7Ø.545**	Athscl nonaut bio bypass of left leg w ulcer oth prt foot
		🔖	**I7Ø.548**	Athscl nonaut bio bypass of left leg w ulcer oth prt low leg
		🔖	**I7Ø.549**	Athscl nonaut bio bypass of left leg w ulcer of unsp site
		🔖	**I7Ø.55**	Athscl nonautologous bio bypass of extremity w ulceration
		🔖	**I7Ø.561**	Athscl nonaut bio bypass of the extrm w gangrene, right leg
		🔖	**I7Ø.562**	Athscl nonaut bio bypass of the extrm w gangrene, left leg
		🔖	**I7Ø.563**	Athscl nonaut bio bypass of the extrm w gangrene, bi legs
		🔖	**I7Ø.568**	Athscl nonaut bio bypass of the extrm w gangrene, oth extrm
		🔖	**I7Ø.569**	Athscl nonaut bio bypass of the extrm w gangrene, unsp extrm
			I7Ø.591	Oth athscl nonaut bio bypass of the extremities, right leg
			I7Ø.592	Oth athscl nonaut bio bypass of the extremities, left leg
			I7Ø.593	Oth athscl nonaut bio bypass of the extrm, bilateral legs
			I7Ø.598	Oth athscl nonaut bio bypass of the extrm, oth extremity
			I7Ø.599	Oth athscl nonaut bio bypass of the extrm, unsp extremity
44Ø.4	CHRONIC TOTAL OCCLUSION ARTERY EXTREMITIES	➡	**I7Ø.92**	Chronic total occlusion of artery of the extremities
44Ø.8	ATHEROSCLEROSIS OF OTHER SPECIFIED ARTERIES		**I7Ø.8**	Atherosclerosis of other arteries
44Ø.9	GENERALIZED AND UNSPECIFIED ATHEROSCLEROSIS		**I7Ø.9Ø**	Unspecified atherosclerosis
			I7Ø.91	Generalized atherosclerosis
441.ØØ	DISSECTING AORTIC ANEURYSM UNSPECIFIED SITE	➡	**I71.ØØ**	Dissection of unspecified site of aorta
441.Ø1	DISSECTING AORTIC ANEURYSM THORACIC	➡	**I71.Ø1**	Dissection of thoracic aorta
441.Ø2	DISSECTING AORTIC ANEURYSM ABDOMINAL	➡	**I71.Ø2**	Dissection of abdominal aorta
441.Ø3	DISSECTING AORTIC ANEURYSM THORACOABDOMINAL	➡	**I71.Ø3**	Dissection of thoracoabdominal aorta
441.1	THORACIC ANEURYSM, RUPTURED	➡	**I71.1**	Thoracic aortic aneurysm, ruptured
441.2	THORACIC ANEURYSM WITHOUT MENTION OF RUPTURE	➡	**I71.2**	Thoracic aortic aneurysm, without rupture
441.3	ABDOMINAL ANEURYSM, RUPTURED	➡	**I71.3**	Abdominal aortic aneurysm, ruptured
441.4	ABDOMINAL ANEURYSM WITHOUT MENTION OF RUPTURE	➡	**I71.4**	Abdominal aortic aneurysm, without rupture
441.5	AORTIC ANEURYSM OF UNSPECIFIED SITE RUPTURED	➡	**I71.8**	Aortic aneurysm of unspecified site, ruptured
441.6	THORACOABDOMINAL ANEURYSM, RUPTURED	➡	**I71.5**	Thoracoabdominal aortic aneurysm, ruptured
441.7	THORACOABD ANEURYSM WITHOUT MENTION RUPTURE	➡	**I71.6**	Thoracoabdominal aortic aneurysm, without rupture
441.9	AORTIC ANEUR UNSPEC SITE WITHOUT MENTION RUPTURE		**I71.9**	Aortic aneurysm of unspecified site, without rupture
			I79.Ø	Aneurysm of aorta in diseases classified elsewhere
442.Ø	ANEURYSM OF ARTERY OF UPPER EXTREMITY	➡	**I72.1**	Aneurysm of artery of upper extremity
442.1	ANEURYSM OF RENAL ARTERY	➡	**I72.2**	Aneurysm of renal artery
442.2	ANEURYSM OF ILIAC ARTERY	➡	**I72.3**	Aneurysm of iliac artery
442.3	ANEURYSM OF ARTERY OF LOWER EXTREMITY	➡	**I72.4**	Aneurysm of artery of lower extremity
442.81	ANEURYSM OF ARTERY OF NECK	➡	**I72.Ø**	Aneurysm of carotid artery
442.82	ANEURYSM OF SUBCLAVIAN ARTERY		**I72.8**	Aneurysm of other specified arteries
442.83	ANEURYSM OF SPLENIC ARTERY		**I72.8**	Aneurysm of other specified arteries
442.84	ANEURYSM OF OTHER VISCERAL ARTERY		**I72.8**	Aneurysm of other specified arteries
442.89	ANEURYSM OF OTHER SPECIFIED ARTERY		**I72.8**	Aneurysm of other specified arteries
442.9	OTHER ANEURYSM OF UNSPECIFIED SITE	➡	**I72.9**	Aneurysm of unspecified site
443.Ø	RAYNAUDS SYNDROME		**I73.ØØ**	Raynaud's syndrome without gangrene
		🔖	**I73.Ø1**	Raynaud's syndrome with gangrene
443.1	THROMBOANGIITIS OBLITERANS	➡	**I73.1**	Thromboangiitis obliterans [Buerger's disease]
443.21	DISSECTION OF CAROTID ARTERY	➡	**I77.71**	Dissection of carotid artery
443.22	DISSECTION OF ILIAC ARTERY	➡	**I77.72**	Dissection of iliac artery
443.23	DISSECTION OF RENAL ARTERY	➡	**I77.73**	Dissection of renal artery
443.24	DISSECTION OF VERTEBRAL ARTERY	➡	**I77.74**	Dissection of vertebral artery

ICD-9-CM			ICD-10-CM	
443.29	DISSECTION OF OTHER ARTERY		**I67.Ø**	Dissection of cerebral arteries, nonruptured
			I77.79	Dissection of other artery
443.81	PERIPHERAL ANGIOPATHY DISEASES CLASSIFIED ELSW		**EØ8.51**	Diab due to undrl cond w diab prph angiopath w/o gangrene
			EØ8.52	Diab due to undrl cond w diabetic prph angiopath w gangrene
			EØ9.51	Drug/chem diabetes w diabetic prph angiopath w/o gangrene
			EØ9.52	Drug/chem diabetes w diabetic prph angiopath w gangrene
			E1Ø.51	Type 1 diabetes w diabetic peripheral angiopath w/o gangrene
			E1Ø.52	Type 1 diabetes w diabetic peripheral angiopathy w gangrene
			E11.51	Type 2 diabetes w diabetic peripheral angiopath w/o gangrene
			E11.52	Type 2 diabetes w diabetic peripheral angiopathy w gangrene
			E13.51	Oth diabetes w diabetic peripheral angiopathy w/o gangrene
			E13.52	Oth diabetes w diabetic peripheral angiopathy w gangrene
			I79.1	Aortitis in diseases classified elsewhere
			I79.8	Oth disord of art,arterioles & capilare in dis classd elswhr
443.82	ERYTHROMELALGIA	➡	**I73.81**	Erythromelalgia
443.89	OTHER PERIPHERAL VASCULAR DISEASE		**I73.89**	Other specified peripheral vascular diseases
443.9	UNSPECIFIED PERIPHERAL VASCULAR DISEASE	➡	**I73.9**	Peripheral vascular disease, unspecified
444.Ø1	SADDLE EMBOLUS OF ABDOMINAL AORTA		**I74.Ø1**	Saddle embolus of abdominal aorta
444.Ø9	OTH ARTERIAL EMBOLISM THROMBOSIS ABDOMINAL AORTA		**I74.Ø9**	Other arterial embolism and thrombosis of abdominal aorta
			I74.1Ø	Embolism and thrombosis of unspecified parts of aorta
			I74.19	Embolism and thrombosis of other parts of aorta
444.1	EMBOLISM AND THROMBOSIS OF THORACIC AORTA	➡	**I74.11**	Embolism and thrombosis of thoracic aorta
444.21	EMBOLISM&THROMBOSIS ARTERIES UPPER EXTREMITY	➡	**I74.2**	Embolism and thrombosis of arteries of the upper extremities
444.22	EMBOLISM&THROMBOSIS ARTERIES LOWER EXTREMITY		**I74.3**	Embolism and thrombosis of arteries of the lower extremities
			I74.4	Embolism and thrombosis of arteries of extremities, unsp
444.81	EMBOLISM AND THROMBOSIS OF ILIAC ARTERY	➡	**I74.5**	Embolism and thrombosis of iliac artery
444.89	EMBOLISM&THROMBOSIS OF OTHER SPECIFIED ARTERY	➡	**I74.8**	Embolism and thrombosis of other arteries
444.9	EMBOLISM AND THROMBOSIS OF UNSPECIFIED ARTERY	➡	**I74.9**	Embolism and thrombosis of unspecified artery
445.Ø1	ATHEROEMBOLISM OF UPPER EXTREMITY		**I75.Ø11**	Atheroembolism of right upper extremity
			I75.Ø12	Atheroembolism of left upper extremity
			I75.Ø13	Atheroembolism of bilateral upper extremities
			I75.Ø19	Atheroembolism of unspecified upper extremity
445.Ø2	ATHEROEMBOLISM OF LOWER EXTREMITY		**I75.Ø21**	Atheroembolism of right lower extremity
			I75.Ø22	Atheroembolism of left lower extremity
			I75.Ø23	Atheroembolism of bilateral lower extremities
			I75.Ø29	Atheroembolism of unspecified lower extremity
445.81	ATHEROEMBOLISM OF KIDNEY	➡	**I75.81**	Atheroembolism of kidney
445.89	ATHEROEMBOLISM OF OTHER SITE	➡	**I75.89**	Atheroembolism of other site
446.Ø	POLYARTERITIS NODOSA		**M3Ø.Ø**	Polyarteritis nodosa
			M3Ø.2	Juvenile polyarteritis
			M3Ø.8	Other conditions related to polyarteritis nodosa
			M31.7	Microscopic polyangiitis
446.1	ACUTE FEBRILE MUCOCUTANEOUS LYMPH NODE SYNDROME	➡	**M3Ø.3**	Mucocutaneous lymph node syndrome [Kawasaki]
446.2Ø	UNSPECIFIED HYPERSENSITIVITY ANGIITIS		**M31.Ø**	Hypersensitivity angiitis
446.21	GOODPASTURES SYNDROME		**M31.Ø**	Hypersensitivity angiitis
446.29	OTHER SPECIFIED HYPERSENSITIVITY ANGIITIS		**M31.Ø**	Hypersensitivity angiitis
446.3	LETHAL MIDLINE GRANULOMA	➡	**M31.2**	Lethal midline granuloma
446.4	WEGENERS GRANULOMATOSIS		**M3Ø.1**	Polyarteritis with lung involvement [Churg-Strauss]
			M31.3Ø	Wegener's granulomatosis without renal involvement
			M31.31	Wegener's granulomatosis with renal involvement
446.5	GIANT CELL ARTERITIS		**M31.5**	Giant cell arteritis with polymyalgia rheumatica
			M31.6	Other giant cell arteritis
446.6	THROMBOTIC MICROANGIOPATHY	➡	**M31.1**	Thrombotic microangiopathy
446.7	TAKAYASUS DISEASE	➡	**M31.4**	Aortic arch syndrome [Takayasu]
447.Ø	ARTERIOVENOUS FISTULA, ACQUIRED	➡	**I77.Ø**	Arteriovenous fistula, acquired
447.1	STRICTURE OF ARTERY	➡	**I77.1**	Stricture of artery
447.2	RUPTURE OF ARTERY	➡	**I77.2**	Rupture of artery
447.3	HYPERPLASIA OF RENAL ARTERY		**I77.3**	Arterial fibromuscular dysplasia
447.4	CELIAC ARTERY COMPRESSION SYNDROME	➡	**I77.4**	Celiac artery compression syndrome
447.5	NECROSIS OF ARTERY		**I77.5**	Necrosis of artery
			M31.8	Other specified necrotizing vasculopathies
			M31.9	Necrotizing vasculopathy, unspecified
447.6	UNSPECIFIED ARTERITIS	➡	**I77.6**	Arteritis, unspecified
447.7Ø	AORTIC ECTASIA UNSPECIFIED SITE	➡	**I77.819**	Aortic ectasia, unspecified site
447.71	THORACIC AORTIC ECTASIA	➡	**I77.81Ø**	Thoracic aortic ectasia
447.72	ABDOMINAL AORTIC ECTASIA	➡	**I77.811**	Abdominal aortic ectasia
447.73	THORACOABDOMINAL AORTIC ECTASIA	➡	**I77.812**	Thoracoabdominal aortic ectasia
447.8	OTHER SPECIFIED DISORDERS OF ARTERIES&ARTERIOLES		**I77.3**	Arterial fibromuscular dysplasia
			I77.89	Other specified disorders of arteries and arterioles
447.9	UNSPECIFIED DISORDERS OF ARTERIES AND ARTERIOLES	➡	**I77.9**	Disorder of arteries and arterioles, unspecified
448.Ø	HEREDITARY HEMORRHAGIC TELANGIECTASIA	➡	**I78.Ø**	Hereditary hemorrhagic telangiectasia
448.1	NEVUS, NON-NEOPLASTIC	➡	**I78.1**	Nevus, non-neoplastic

[Brackets] indicate valid character values for each code. Character value meanings provided for each code grouping.

ICD-9-CM		ICD-10-CM	
448.9	OTHER AND UNSPECIFIED CAPILLARY DISEASES	I78.8	Other diseases of capillaries
		I78.9	Disease of capillaries, unspecified
449	SEPTIC ARTERIAL EMBOLISM	➡ I76	Septic arterial embolism
451.Ø	PHLEBITIS&THROMBOPHLEB SUP VESSELS LOWER EXTREM	I8Ø.ØØ	Phlbts and thombophlb of superfic vessels of unsp low extrm
		I8Ø.Ø1	Phlebitis and thombophlb of superfic vessels of r low extrem
		I8Ø.Ø2	Phlebitis and thombophlb of superfic vessels of l low extrem
		I8Ø.Ø3	Phlbts and thombophlb of superfic vessels of low extrm, bi
451.11	PHLEBITIS AND THROMBOPHLEBITIS OF FEMORAL VEIN	I8Ø.1Ø	Phlebitis and thrombophlebitis of unspecified femoral vein
		I8Ø.11	Phlebitis and thrombophlebitis of right femoral vein
		I8Ø.12	Phlebitis and thrombophlebitis of left femoral vein
		I8Ø.13	Phlebitis and thrombophlebitis of femoral vein, bilateral
451.19	PHLEBITIS&THROMBOPHLEB OTH DEEP VES LOWER EXTREM	I8Ø.2Ø1	Phlbts and thombophlb of unsp deep vessels of r low extrem
		I8Ø.2Ø2	Phlbts and thombophlb of unsp deep vessels of l low extrem
		I8Ø.2Ø3	Phlbts and thombophlb of unsp deep vessels of low extrm, bi
		I8Ø.2Ø9	Phlbts and thombophlb of unsp deep vessels of unsp low extrm
		I8Ø.221	Phlebitis and thrombophlebitis of right popliteal vein
		I8Ø.222	Phlebitis and thrombophlebitis of left popliteal vein
		I8Ø.223	Phlebitis and thrombophlebitis of popliteal vein, bilateral
		I8Ø.229	Phlebitis and thrombophlebitis of unspecified popliteal vein
		I8Ø.231	Phlebitis and thrombophlebitis of right tibial vein
		I8Ø.232	Phlebitis and thrombophlebitis of left tibial vein
		I8Ø.233	Phlebitis and thrombophlebitis of tibial vein, bilateral
		I8Ø.239	Phlebitis and thrombophlebitis of unspecified tibial vein
		I8Ø.291	Phlebitis and thombophlb of deep vessels of r low extrem
		I8Ø.292	Phlebitis and thombophlb of deep vessels of l low extrem
		I8Ø.293	Phlebitis and thombophlb of deep vessels of low extrm, bi
		I8Ø.299	Phlebitis and thombophlb of deep vessels of unsp low extrm
451.2	PHLEBITIS&THROMBOPHLEBITIS LOWER EXTREM UNSPEC	➡ I8Ø.3	Phlebitis and thrombophlebitis of lower extremities, unsp
451.81	PHLEBITIS AND THROMBOPHLEBITIS OF ILIAC VEIN	I8Ø.211	Phlebitis and thrombophlebitis of right iliac vein
		I8Ø.212	Phlebitis and thrombophlebitis of left iliac vein
		I8Ø.213	Phlebitis and thrombophlebitis of iliac vein, bilateral
		I8Ø.219	Phlebitis and thrombophlebitis of unspecified iliac vein
451.82	PHLEBITIS&THROMBOPHLEB SUP VEINS UPPER EXTREM	I8Ø.8	Phlebitis and thrombophlebitis of other sites
451.83	PHLEBITIS&THROMBOPHLEB DEEP VEINS UPPER EXTREM	I8Ø.8	Phlebitis and thrombophlebitis of other sites
451.84	PHLEBITIS&THROMBOPHLEBITIS UPPER EXTREM UNSPEC	I8Ø.8	Phlebitis and thrombophlebitis of other sites
451.89	PHLEBITIS AND THROMBOPHLEBITIS OF OTHER SITE	I8Ø.8	Phlebitis and thrombophlebitis of other sites
451.9	PHLEBITIS&THROMBOPHLEBITIS OF UNSPECIFIED SITE	➡ I8Ø.9	Phlebitis and thrombophlebitis of unspecified site
452	PORTAL VEIN THROMBOSIS	➡ I81	Portal vein thrombosis
453.Ø	BUDD-CHIARI SYNDROME	➡ I82.Ø	Budd-Chiari syndrome
453.1	THROMBOPHLEBITIS MIGRANS	➡ I82.1	Thrombophlebitis migrans
453.2	OTH VENOUS EMBO & THROMBOSIS INFERIOR VENA CAVA	I82.22Ø	Acute embolism and thrombosis of inferior vena cava
		I82.221	Chronic embolism and thrombosis of inferior vena cava
453.3	EMBOLISM AND THROMBOSIS OF RENAL VEIN	➡ I82.3	Embolism and thrombosis of renal vein
453.4Ø	AC VENUS EMBO & THROMB UNSPEC DEEP VES LOWER EXT	I82.4Ø1	Acute embolism and thombos unsp deep veins of r low extrem
		I82.4Ø2	Acute embolism and thombos unsp deep veins of l low extrem
		I82.4Ø3	Acute embolism and thombos unsp deep veins of low extrm, bi
		I82.4Ø9	Acute embolism and thombos unsp deep vn unsp lower extremity
453.41	ACUT VENUS EMBO&THROMB DEEP VES PROX LOWR EXTREM	I82.411	Acute embolism and thrombosis of right femoral vein
		I82.412	Acute embolism and thrombosis of left femoral vein
		I82.413	Acute embolism and thrombosis of femoral vein, bilateral
		I82.419	Acute embolism and thrombosis of unspecified femoral vein
		I82.421	Acute embolism and thrombosis of right iliac vein
		I82.422	Acute embolism and thrombosis of left iliac vein
		I82.423	Acute embolism and thrombosis of iliac vein, bilateral
		I82.429	Acute embolism and thrombosis of unspecified iliac vein
		I82.431	Acute embolism and thrombosis of right popliteal vein
		I82.432	Acute embolism and thrombosis of left popliteal vein
		I82.433	Acute embolism and thrombosis of popliteal vein, bilateral
		I82.439	Acute embolism and thrombosis of unspecified popliteal vein
		I82.4Y1	Ac emblsm and thombos unsp deep veins of r prox low extrm
		I82.4Y2	Ac emblsm and thombos unsp deep veins of left prox low extrm
		I82.4Y3	Ac emblsm and thombos unsp deep veins of prox low extrm, bi
		I82.4Y9	Acute emblsm and thombos unsp deep vn unsp prox low extrm
453.42	ACUT VENUS EMBO&THROMB DEEP VES DIST LOWR EXTREM	I82.441	Acute embolism and thrombosis of right tibial vein
		I82.442	Acute embolism and thrombosis of left tibial vein
		I82.443	Acute embolism and thrombosis of tibial vein, bilateral
		I82.449	Acute embolism and thrombosis of unspecified tibial vein
		I82.491	Acute embolism and thrombosis of deep vein of r low extrem
		I82.492	Acute embolism and thrombosis of deep vein of l low extrem
		I82.493	Acute embolism and thombos of deep vein of low extrm, bi
		I82.499	Acute embolism and thrombosis of deep vein of unsp low extrm
		I82.4Z1	Ac emblsm and thombos unsp deep veins of r dist low extrm
		I82.4Z2	Ac emblsm and thombos unsp deep veins of left dist low extrm
		I82.4Z3	Ac emblsm and thombos unsp deep veins of dist low extrm, bi
		I82.4Z9	Acute emblsm and thombos unsp deep vn unsp distal low extrm

ICD-9-CM		ICD-10-CM	
453.5Ø	CHRON VNUS EMB & THROMB UNSPEC DEEP VES LOWR EXT	**I82.5Ø1**	Chronic embolism and thombos unsp deep veins of r low extrem
		I82.5Ø2	Chronic embolism and thombos unsp deep veins of l low extrem
		I82.5Ø3	Chronic emblsm and thombos unsp deep veins of low extrm, bi
		I82.5Ø9	Chronic embolism and thombos unsp deep vn unsp low extrm
		I82.591	Chronic embolism and thrombosis of deep vein of r low extrem
		I82.592	Chronic embolism and thrombosis of deep vein of l low extrem
		I82.593	Chronic embolism and thombos of deep vein of low extrm, bi
		I82.599	Chronic embolism and thombos of deep vein of unsp low extrm
453.51	CHRN VNUS EMB & THROMB DEEP VES PROX LOWR EXTREM	**I82.511**	Chronic embolism and thrombosis of right femoral vein
		I82.512	Chronic embolism and thrombosis of left femoral vein
		I82.513	Chronic embolism and thrombosis of femoral vein, bilateral
		I82.519	Chronic embolism and thrombosis of unspecified femoral vein
		I82.521	Chronic embolism and thrombosis of right iliac vein
		I82.522	Chronic embolism and thrombosis of left iliac vein
		I82.523	Chronic embolism and thrombosis of iliac vein, bilateral
		I82.529	Chronic embolism and thrombosis of unspecified iliac vein
		I82.531	Chronic embolism and thrombosis of right popliteal vein
		I82.532	Chronic embolism and thrombosis of left popliteal vein
		I82.533	Chronic embolism and thrombosis of popliteal vein, bilateral
		I82.539	Chronic embolism and thrombosis of unsp popliteal vein
		I82.5Y1	Chr emblsm and thombos unsp deep veins of r prox low extrm
		I82.5Y2	Chr emblsm and thombos unsp deep vn of left prox low extrm
		I82.5Y3	Chr emblsm and thombos unsp deep veins of prox low extrm, bi
		I82.5Y9	Chronic emblsm and thombos unsp deep vn unsp prox low extrm
453.52	CHRN VNUS EMBO & THROMB DP VES DISTL LOWR EXTREM	**I82.541**	Chronic embolism and thrombosis of right tibial vein
		I82.542	Chronic embolism and thrombosis of left tibial vein
		I82.543	Chronic embolism and thrombosis of tibial vein, bilateral
		I82.549	Chronic embolism and thrombosis of unspecified tibial vein
		I82.5Z1	Chr emblsm and thombos unsp deep veins of r dist low extrm
		I82.5Z2	Chr emblsm and thombos unsp deep vn of left dist low extrm
		I82.5Z3	Chr emblsm and thombos unsp deep veins of dist low extrm, bi
		I82.5Z9	Chr emblsm and thombos unsp deep vn unsp distal low extrm
453.6	VENOUS EMBO & THROMB SUPERFICIAL VES LOWR EXTREM	**I82.811**	Embolism and thrombosis of superfic veins of right low extrm
		I82.812	Embolism and thrombosis of superfic veins of left low extrm
		I82.813	Embolism and thombos of superfic veins of low extrm, bi
		I82.819	Embolism and thrombosis of superficial vn unsp low extrm
453.71	CHRON VENOUS EMBO & THROMB SUP VEINS UPPER EXT	**I82.711**	Chronic emblsm and thombos of superfic veins of r up extrem
		I82.712	Chronic emblsm and thombos of superfic veins of l up extrem
		I82.713	Chr emblsm and thombos of superfic veins of up extrem, bi
		I82.719	Chronic embolism and thombos of superfic vn unsp up extrem
453.72	CHRONIC VENOUS EMBO & THROMB DP VEINS UPPER EXT	**I82.721**	Chronic embolism and thrombosis of deep veins of r up extrem
		I82.722	Chronic embolism and thrombosis of deep veins of l up extrem
		I82.723	Chronic embolism and thombos of deep veins of up extrem, bi
		I82.729	Chronic embolism and thrombosis of deep vn unsp up extrem
453.73	CHRONIC VENOUS EMBO & THROMB UPPER EXTREMITY UNS	**I82.7Ø1**	Chronic embolism and thombos unsp veins of r up extrem
		I82.7Ø2	Chronic embolism and thombos unsp veins of l up extrem
		I82.7Ø3	Chronic embolism and thombos unsp veins of up extrem, bi
		I82.7Ø9	Chronic embolism and thombos unsp vn unsp upper extremity
453.74	CHRON VENUS EMBOLISM & THROMBOSIS AXILLARY VEINS	**I82.A21**	Chronic embolism and thrombosis of right axillary vein
		I82.A22	Chronic embolism and thrombosis of left axillary vein
		I82.A23	Chronic embolism and thrombosis of axillary vein, bilateral
		I82.A29	Chronic embolism and thrombosis of unspecified axillary vein
453.75	CHRONIC VENOUS EMBO & THROMB SUBCLAVIAN VEINS	**I82.B21**	Chronic embolism and thrombosis of right subclavian vein
		I82.B22	Chronic embolism and thrombosis of left subclavian vein
		I82.B23	Chronic embolism and thrombosis of subclav vein, bilateral
		I82.B29	Chronic embolism and thrombosis of unsp subclavian vein
453.76	CHRON VENUS EMBO & THROMB INTERNAL JUGULAR VEINS	**I82.C21**	Chronic embolism and thrombosis of r int jugular vein
		I82.C22	Chronic embolism and thrombosis of l int jugular vein
		I82.C23	Chronic embolism and thombos of int jugular vein, bilateral
		I82.C29	Chronic embolism and thombos unsp internal jugular vein
453.77	CHRON VENOUS EMBO AND THROMB OTH THORACIC VEINS	**I82.211**	Chronic embolism and thrombosis of superior vena cava
		I82.291	Chronic embolism and thrombosis of other thoracic veins
453.79	CHRN VENOUS EMBOLISM & THROMBOSIS OTH SPEC VEINS	**I82.891**	Chronic embolism and thrombosis of other specified veins
		I82.91	Chronic embolism and thrombosis of unspecified vein
453.81	ACUTE VENOUS EMBO & THROMB SUP VEINS UPPER EXT	**I82.611**	Acute embolism and thombos of superfic veins of r up extrem
		I82.612	Acute embolism and thombos of superfic veins of l up extrem
		I82.613	Acute emblsm and thombos of superfic veins of up extrem, bi
		I82.619	Acute embolism and thrombosis of superfic vn unsp up extrem
453.82	ACUTE VENOUS EMBO & THROMB DEEP VEINS UPPER EXT	**I82.621**	Acute embolism and thrombosis of deep veins of r up extrem
		I82.622	Acute embolism and thrombosis of deep veins of l up extrem
		I82.623	Acute embolism and thombos of deep veins of up extrem, bi
		I82.629	Acute embolism and thrombosis of deep vn unsp up extrem
453.83	ACUTE VENOUS EMBO AND THROMB UPPER EXTREM UNS	**I82.6Ø1**	Acute embolism and thombos unsp veins of r up extrem
		I82.6Ø2	Acute embolism and thombos unsp veins of l up extrem
		I82.6Ø3	Acute embolism and thombos unsp veins of up extrem, bi
		I82.6Ø9	Acute embolism and thombos unsp vn unsp upper extremity

ICD-9-CM		ICD-10-CM	
453.84	ACUT VENOUS EMBOLISM & THROMBOSIS AXILLARY VEINS	**I82.A11**	Acute embolism and thrombosis of right axillary vein
		I82.A12	Acute embolism and thrombosis of left axillary vein
		I82.A13	Acute embolism and thrombosis of axillary vein, bilateral
		I82.A19	Acute embolism and thrombosis of unspecified axillary vein
453.85	ACUTE VENOUS EMBO & THROMBOSIS SUBCLAVIAN VEINS	**I82.B11**	Acute embolism and thrombosis of right subclavian vein
		I82.B12	Acute embolism and thrombosis of left subclavian vein
		I82.B13	Acute embolism and thrombosis of subclavian vein, bilateral
		I82.B19	Acute embolism and thrombosis of unspecified subclavian vein
453.86	ACUTE VENOUS EMBO & THROMB INTRL JUGULAR VEINS	**I82.C11**	Acute embolism and thrombosis of right internal jugular vein
		I82.C12	Acute embolism and thrombosis of left internal jugular vein
		I82.C13	Acute embolism and thrombosis of int jugular vein, bilateral
		I82.C19	Acute embolism and thrombosis of unsp internal jugular vein
453.87	ACUT VENOUS EMBO & THROMBOSIS OTH THORACIC VEINS	**I82.21Ø**	Acute embolism and thrombosis of superior vena cava
		I82.29Ø	Acute embolism and thrombosis of other thoracic veins
453.89	ACUT VENOUS EMBOLISM & THROMBOSIS OTH SPEC VEINS	**I82.89Ø**	Acute embolism and thrombosis of other specified veins
		I82.9Ø	Acute embolism and thrombosis of unspecified vein
453.9	EMBOLISM AND THROMBOSIS OF UNSPECIFIED SITE	**I82.91**	Chronic embolism and thrombosis of unspecified vein
454.Ø	VARICOSE VEINS OF LOWER EXTREMITIES WITH ULCER	**I83.ØØ1**	Varicose veins of unsp lower extremity with ulcer of thigh
		I83.ØØ2	Varicose veins of unsp lower extremity with ulcer of calf
		I83.ØØ3	Varicose veins of unsp lower extremity with ulcer of ankle
		I83.ØØ4	Varicos vn unsp lower extremity w ulcer of heel and midfoot
		I83.ØØ5	Varicos vn unsp lower extremity w ulcer oth part of foot
		I83.ØØ8	Varicos vn unsp low extrm w ulcer oth part of lower leg
		I83.ØØ9	Varicose veins of unsp lower extremity w ulcer of unsp site
		I83.Ø11	Varicose veins of right lower extremity with ulcer of thigh
		I83.Ø12	Varicose veins of right lower extremity with ulcer of calf
		I83.Ø13	Varicose veins of right lower extremity with ulcer of ankle
		I83.Ø14	Varicose veins of r low extrem w ulcer of heel and midfoot
		I83.Ø15	Varicose veins of r low extrem w ulcer oth part of foot
		I83.Ø18	Varicose veins of r low extrem w ulcer oth part of lower leg
		I83.Ø19	Varicose veins of right lower extremity w ulcer of unsp site
		I83.Ø21	Varicose veins of left lower extremity with ulcer of thigh
		I83.Ø22	Varicose veins of left lower extremity with ulcer of calf
		I83.Ø23	Varicose veins of left lower extremity with ulcer of ankle
		I83.Ø24	Varicose veins of l low extrem w ulcer of heel and midfoot
		I83.Ø25	Varicose veins of l low extrem w ulcer oth part of foot
		I83.Ø28	Varicose veins of l low extrem w ulcer oth part of lower leg
		I83.Ø29	Varicose veins of left lower extremity w ulcer of unsp site
454.1	VARICOSE VEINS LOWER EXTREMITIES W/INFLAMMATION	**I83.1Ø**	Varicose veins of unsp lower extremity with inflammation
		I83.11	Varicose veins of right lower extremity with inflammation
		I83.12	Varicose veins of left lower extremity with inflammation
454.2	VARICOSE VEINS LOWER EXTREM W/ULCER&INFLAMMATION	**I83.2Ø1**	Varicos vn unsp low extrm w ulc of thigh and inflammation
		I83.2Ø2	Varicos vn unsp low extrm w ulc of calf and inflammation
		I83.2Ø3	Varicos vn unsp low extrm w ulc of ankle and inflammation
		I83.2Ø4	Varicos vn unsp low extrm w ulc of heel and midft and inflam
		I83.2Ø5	Varicos vn unsp low extrm w ulc oth part of foot and inflam
		I83.2Ø8	Varicos vn unsp low extrm w ulc oth prt low extrm and inflam
		I83.2Ø9	Varicos vn unsp low extrm w ulc of unsp site and inflam
		I83.211	Varicos vn of r low extrem w ulc of thigh and inflammation
		I83.212	Varicos vn of r low extrem w ulc of calf and inflammation
		I83.213	Varicos vn of r low extrem w ulc of ankle and inflammation
		I83.214	Varicos vn of r low extrem w ulc of heel & midft and inflam
		I83.215	Varicos vn of r low extrem w ulc oth part of foot and inflam
		I83.218	Varicos vn of r low extrem w ulc oth prt low extrm & inflam
		I83.219	Varicos vn of r low extrem w ulc of unsp site and inflam
		I83.221	Varicos vn of l low extrem w ulc of thigh and inflammation
		I83.222	Varicos vn of l low extrem w ulc of calf and inflammation
		I83.223	Varicos vn of l low extrem w ulc of ankle and inflammation
		I83.224	Varicos vn of l low extrem w ulc of heel & midft and inflam
		I83.225	Varicos vn of l low extrem w ulc oth part of foot and inflam
		I83.228	Varicos vn of l low extrem w ulc oth prt low extrm & inflam
		I83.229	Varicos vn of l low extrem w ulc of unsp site and inflam
454.8	VARICOSE VEINS LOWER EXTREMITIES W/OTH COMPS	**I83.811**	Varicose veins of right lower extremities with pain
		I83.812	Varicose veins of left lower extremities with pain
		I83.813	Varicose veins of bilateral lower extremities with pain
		I83.819	Varicose veins of unspecified lower extremities with pain
		I83.891	Varicose veins of right low extrm w oth complications
		I83.892	Varicose veins of left lower extremities w oth complications
		I83.893	Varicose veins of bi low extrem w oth complications
		I83.899	Varicose veins of unsp lower extremities w oth complications
454.9	ASYMPTOMATIC VARICOSE VEINS	**I83.9Ø**	Asymptomatic varicose veins of unspecified lower extremity
		I83.91	Asymptomatic varicose veins of right lower extremity
		I83.92	Asymptomatic varicose veins of left lower extremity
		I83.93	Asymptomatic varicose veins of bilateral lower extremities
455.Ø	INTERNAL HEMORRHOIDS WITHOUT MENTION COMP	**K64.Ø**	First degree hemorrhoids
		K64.1	Second degree hemorrhoids
		K64.2	Third degree hemorrhoids
		K64.3	Fourth degree hemorrhoids
		K64.8	Other hemorrhoids

ICD-9-CM		ICD-10-CM		
455.1	INTERNAL THROMBOSED HEMORRHOIDS		K64.Ø	First degree hemorrhoids
			K64.1	Second degree hemorrhoids
			K64.2	Third degree hemorrhoids
			K64.3	Fourth degree hemorrhoids
			K64.8	Other hemorrhoids
455.2	INTERNAL HEMORRHOIDS WITH OTHER COMPLICATION		K64.Ø	First degree hemorrhoids
			K64.1	Second degree hemorrhoids
			K64.2	Third degree hemorrhoids
			K64.3	Fourth degree hemorrhoids
			K64.8	Other hemorrhoids
455.3	EXTERNAL HEMORRHOIDS WITHOUT MENTION COMP		K64.4	Residual hemorrhoidal skin tags
455.4	EXTERNAL THROMBOSED HEMORRHOIDS		K64.5	Perianal venous thrombosis
455.5	EXTERNAL HEMORRHOIDS WITH OTHER COMPLICATION		K64.Ø	First degree hemorrhoids
			K64.1	Second degree hemorrhoids
			K64.2	Third degree hemorrhoids
			K64.3	Fourth degree hemorrhoids
			K64.4	Residual hemorrhoidal skin tags
455.6	UNSPEC HEMORRHOIDS WITHOUT MENTION COMPLICATION		K64.Ø	First degree hemorrhoids
			K64.1	Second degree hemorrhoids
			K64.2	Third degree hemorrhoids
			K64.3	Fourth degree hemorrhoids
			K64.9	Unspecified hemorrhoids
455.7	UNSPECIFIED THROMBOSED HEMORRHOIDS		K64.Ø	First degree hemorrhoids
			K64.1	Second degree hemorrhoids
			K64.2	Third degree hemorrhoids
			K64.3	Fourth degree hemorrhoids
			K64.5	Perianal venous thrombosis
455.8	UNSPECIFIED HEMORRHOIDS WITH OTHER COMPLICATION		K64.Ø	First degree hemorrhoids
			K64.1	Second degree hemorrhoids
			K64.2	Third degree hemorrhoids
			K64.3	Fourth degree hemorrhoids
			K64.8	Other hemorrhoids
455.9	RESIDUAL HEMORRHOIDAL SKIN TAGS		K64.4	Residual hemorrhoidal skin tags
456.Ø	ESOPHAGEAL VARICES WITH BLEEDING	➡	I85.Ø1	Esophageal varices with bleeding
456.1	ESOPHAGEAL VARICES WITHOUT MENTION OF BLEEDING	➡	I85.ØØ	Esophageal varices without bleeding
456.2Ø	ESOPHAGEAL VARICES W/BLEED DISEASES CLASS ELSW	➡	I85.11	Secondary esophageal varices with bleeding
456.21	ESOPH VARICES W/O MENTION BLEED DZ CLASS ELSW	➡	I85.1Ø	Secondary esophageal varices without bleeding
456.3	SUBLINGUAL VARICES	➡	I86.Ø	Sublingual varices
456.4	SCROTAL VARICES	➡	I86.1	Scrotal varices
456.5	PELVIC VARICES	➡	I86.2	Pelvic varices
456.6	VULVAL VARICES	➡	I86.3	Vulval varices
456.8	VARICES OF OTHER SITES		I86.4	Gastric varices
			I86.8	Varicose veins of other specified sites
457.Ø	POSTMASTECTOMY LYMPHEDEMA SYNDROME	➡	I97.2	Postmastectomy lymphedema syndrome
457.1	OTHER NONINFECTIOUS LYMPHEDEMA	➡	I89.Ø	Lymphedema, not elsewhere classified
457.2	LYMPHANGITIS	➡	I89.1	Lymphangitis
457.8	OTHER NONINFECTIOUS DISORDERS LYMPHATIC CHANNELS	➡	I89.8	Oth noninfective disorders of lymphatic vessels and nodes
457.9	UNSPEC NONINFECTIOUS DISORDER LYMPHATIC CHANNELS	➡	I89.9	Noninfective disorder of lymphatic vessels and nodes, unsp
458.Ø	ORTHOSTATIC HYPOTENSION	➡	I95.1	Orthostatic hypotension
458.1	CHRONIC HYPOTENSION		I95.Ø	Idiopathic hypotension
			I95.89	Other hypotension
458.21	HYPOTENSION OF HEMODIALYSIS	➡	I95.3	Hypotension of hemodialysis
458.29	OTHER IATROGENIC HYPOTENSION		I95.2	Hypotension due to drugs
			I95.81	Postprocedural hypotension
458.8	OTHER SPECIFIED HYPOTENSION		I95.89	Other hypotension
458.9	UNSPECIFIED HYPOTENSION	➡	I95.9	Hypotension, unspecified
459.Ø	UNSPECIFIED HEMORRHAGE	➡	R58	Hemorrhage, not elsewhere classified
459.1Ø	POSTPHLEBITIC SYNDROME WITHOUT COMPLICATIONS		I87.ØØ1	Postthrombotic syndrome w/o complications of r low extrem
			I87.ØØ2	Postthrombotic syndrome w/o complications of l low extrem
			I87.ØØ3	Postthrom syndrome w/o complications of bilateral low extrm
			I87.ØØ9	Postthrombotic syndrome w/o complications of unsp extremity
459.11	POSTPHLEBITIC SYNDROME WITH ULCER		I87.Ø11	Postthrombotic syndrome with ulcer of right lower extremity
			I87.Ø12	Postthrombotic syndrome with ulcer of left lower extremity
			I87.Ø13	Postthrombotic syndrome w ulcer of bilateral lower extremity
			I87.Ø19	Postthrombotic syndrome with ulcer of unsp lower extremity
459.12	POSTPHLEBITIC SYNDROME WITH INFLAMMATION		I87.Ø21	Postthrombotic syndrome w inflammation of r low extrem
			I87.Ø22	Postthrombotic syndrome w inflammation of l low extrem
			I87.Ø23	Postthrom syndrome w inflammation of bilateral low extrm
			I87.Ø29	Postthrombotic syndrome w inflammation of unsp low extrm
459.13	POSTPHLEBITIC SYNDROME W/ULCER AND INFLAMMATION		I87.Ø31	Postthrom syndrome w ulcer and inflammation of r low extrem
			I87.Ø32	Postthrom syndrome w ulcer and inflammation of l low extrem
			I87.Ø33	Postthrom syndrome w ulcer and inflam of bilateral low extrm
			I87.Ø39	Postthrom syndrome w ulcer and inflam of unsp low extrm

[Brackets] indicate valid character values for each code. Character value meanings provided for each code grouping.

ICD-9-CM		ICD-10-CM	
459.19	POSTPHLEBITIC SYNDROME WITH OTHER COMPLICATION	**I87.Ø91**	Postthrombotic syndrome w oth complications of r low extrem
		I87.Ø92	Postthrombotic syndrome w oth complications of l low extrem
		I87.Ø93	Postthrom syndrome w oth comp of bilateral low extrm
		I87.Ø99	Postthrom syndrome w oth complications of unsp low extrm
459.2	COMPRESSION OF VEIN	➡ **I87.1**	Compression of vein
459.3Ø	CHRONIC VENOUS HYPERTENSION WITHOUT COMPS	**I87.3Ø1**	Chronic venous hypertension w/o comp of r low extrem
		I87.3Ø2	Chronic venous hypertension w/o comp of l low extrem
		I87.3Ø3	Chronic venous hypertension w/o comp of bilateral low extrm
		I87.3Ø9	Chronic venous hypertension w/o comp of unsp low extrm
459.31	CHRONIC VENOUS HYPERTENSION WITH ULCER	**I87.311**	Chronic venous hypertension w ulcer of r low extrem
		I87.312	Chronic venous hypertension w ulcer of l low extrem
		I87.313	Chronic venous hypertension w ulcer of bilateral low extrm
		I87.319	Chronic venous hypertension w ulcer of unsp low extrm
459.32	CHRONIC VENOUS HYPERTENSION WITH INFLAMMATION	**I87.321**	Chronic venous hypertension w inflammation of r low extrem
		I87.322	Chronic venous hypertension w inflammation of l low extrem
		I87.323	Chronic venous htn w inflammation of bilateral low extrm
		I87.329	Chronic venous hypertension w inflammation of unsp low extrm
459.33	CHRONIC VENOUS HYPERTENSION W/ULCER&INFLAMMATION	**I87.331**	Chronic venous htn w ulcer and inflammation of r low extrem
		I87.332	Chronic venous htn w ulcer and inflammation of l low extrem
		I87.333	Chronic venous htn w ulcer and inflam of bilateral low extrm
		I87.339	Chronic venous htn w ulcer and inflam of unsp low extrm
459.39	CHRONIC VENOUS HYPERTENSION W/OTHER COMPLICATION	**I87.391**	Chronic venous hypertension w oth comp of r low extrem
		I87.392	Chronic venous hypertension w oth comp of l low extrem
		I87.393	Chronic venous htn w oth comp of bilateral low extrm
		I87.399	Chronic venous hypertension w oth comp of unsp low extrm
459.81	UNSPECIFIED VENOUS INSUFFICIENCY	**I87.2**	Venous insufficiency (chronic) (peripheral)
459.89	OTHER SPECIFIED CIRCULATORY SYSTEM DISORDERS	**I87.8**	Other specified disorders of veins
		I99.8	Other disorder of circulatory system
459.9	UNSPECIFIED CIRCULATORY SYSTEM DISORDER	**I87.9**	Disorder of vein, unspecified
		I99.9	Unspecified disorder of circulatory system

Diseases of the Respiratory System

ICD-9-CM			ICD-10-CM	
460	ACUTE NASOPHARYNGITIS	➡	J00	Acute nasopharyngitis [common cold]
461.0	ACUTE MAXILLARY SINUSITIS		J01.00 J01.01	Acute maxillary sinusitis, unspecified Acute recurrent maxillary sinusitis
461.1	ACUTE FRONTAL SINUSITIS		J01.10 J01.11	Acute frontal sinusitis, unspecified Acute recurrent frontal sinusitis
461.2	ACUTE ETHMOIDAL SINUSITIS		J01.20 J01.21	Acute ethmoidal sinusitis, unspecified Acute recurrent ethmoidal sinusitis
461.3	ACUTE SPHENOIDAL SINUSITIS		J01.30 J01.31	Acute sphenoidal sinusitis, unspecified Acute recurrent sphenoidal sinusitis
461.8	OTHER ACUTE SINUSITIS		J01.40 J01.41 J01.80 J01.81	Acute pansinusitis, unspecified Acute recurrent pansinusitis Other acute sinusitis Other acute recurrent sinusitis
461.9	ACUTE SINUSITIS, UNSPECIFIED		J01.90 J01.91	Acute sinusitis, unspecified Acute recurrent sinusitis, unspecified
462	ACUTE PHARYNGITIS		J02.8 J02.9	Acute pharyngitis due to other specified organisms Acute pharyngitis, unspecified
463	ACUTE TONSILLITIS		J03.80 J03.81 J03.90 J03.91	Acute tonsillitis due to other specified organisms Acute recurrent tonsillitis due to other specified organisms Acute tonsillitis, unspecified Acute recurrent tonsillitis, unspecified
464.00	ACUTE LARYNGITIS, WITHOUT MENTION OF OBSTRUCTIO	➡	J04.0	Acute laryngitis
464.01	ACUTE LARYNGITIS, WITH OBSTRUCTION		J05.0	Acute obstructive laryngitis [croup]
464.10	ACUTE TRACHEITIS WITHOUT MENTION OF OBSTRUCTION	➡	J04.10	Acute tracheitis without obstruction
464.11	ACUTE TRACHEITIS WITH OBSTRUCTION	➡	J04.11	Acute tracheitis with obstruction
464.20	ACUTE LARYNGOTRACHEITIS W/O MENTION OBSTRUCTION	➡	J04.2	Acute laryngotracheitis
464.21	ACUTE LARYNGOTRACHEITIS WITH OBSTRUCTION		J05.0	Acute obstructive laryngitis [croup]
464.30	ACUTE EPIGLOTTITIS WITHOUT MENTION OBSTRUCTION	➡	J05.10	Acute epiglottitis without obstruction
464.31	ACUTE EPIGLOTTITIS WITH OBSTRUCTION	➡	J05.11	Acute epiglottitis with obstruction
464.4	CROUP		J05.0	Acute obstructive laryngitis [croup]
464.50	UNSPEC SUPRAGLOTTIS WITHOUT MENTION OBSTRUCTION	➡	J04.30	Supraglottitis, unspecified, without obstruction
464.51	UNSPECIFIED SUPRAGLOTTIS, WITH OBSTRUCTION	➡	J04.31	Supraglottitis, unspecified, with obstruction
465.0	ACUTE LARYNGOPHARYNGITIS	➡	J06.0	Acute laryngopharyngitis
465.8	ACUTE URIS OF OTHER MULTIPLE SITES		J06.9	Acute upper respiratory infection, unspecified
465.9	ACUTE URIS OF UNSPECIFIED SITE		J06.9	Acute upper respiratory infection, unspecified
466.0	ACUTE BRONCHITIS	◘ ◘ ◘ ◘ ◘ ◘ ◘ ◘	J20.0 J20.1 J20.2 J20.3 J20.4 J20.5 J20.6 J20.7 J20.8 J20.9	Acute bronchitis due to Mycoplasma pneumoniae Acute bronchitis due to Hemophilus influenzae Acute bronchitis due to streptococcus Acute bronchitis due to coxsackievirus Acute bronchitis due to parainfluenza virus Acute bronchitis due to respiratory syncytial virus Acute bronchitis due to rhinovirus Acute bronchitis due to echovirus Acute bronchitis due to other specified organisms Acute bronchitis, unspecified
466.11	ACUTE BRONCHIOLITIS DUE TO RSV	➡	J21.0	Acute bronchiolitis due to respiratory syncytial virus
466.19	ACUTE BRONCHIOLITIS DUE OTH INFECTIOUS ORGANISMS		J21.1 J21.8 J21.9	Acute bronchiolitis due to human metapneumovirus Acute bronchiolitis due to other specified organisms Acute bronchiolitis, unspecified
470	DEVIATED NASAL SEPTUM	➡	J34.2	Deviated nasal septum
471.0	POLYP OF NASAL CAVITY	➡	J33.0	Polyp of nasal cavity
471.1	POLYPOID SINUS DEGENERATION	➡	J33.1	Polypoid sinus degeneration
471.8	OTHER POLYP OF SINUS	➡	J33.8	Other polyp of sinus
471.9	UNSPECIFIED NASAL POLYP	➡	J33.9	Nasal polyp, unspecified
472.0	CHRONIC RHINITIS	➡	J31.0	Chronic rhinitis
472.1	CHRONIC PHARYNGITIS	➡	J31.2	Chronic pharyngitis
472.2	CHRONIC NASOPHARYNGITIS	➡	J31.1	Chronic nasopharyngitis
473.0	CHRONIC MAXILLARY SINUSITIS	➡	J32.0	Chronic maxillary sinusitis
473.1	CHRONIC FRONTAL SINUSITIS	➡	J32.1	Chronic frontal sinusitis
473.2	CHRONIC ETHMOIDAL SINUSITIS	➡	J32.2	Chronic ethmoidal sinusitis
473.3	CHRONIC SPHENOIDAL SINUSITIS	➡	J32.3	Chronic sphenoidal sinusitis
473.8	OTHER CHRONIC SINUSITIS		J32.4 J32.8	Chronic pansinusitis Other chronic sinusitis
473.9	UNSPECIFIED SINUSITIS	➡	J32.9	Chronic sinusitis, unspecified
474.00	CHRONIC TONSILLITIS	➡	J35.01	Chronic tonsillitis
474.01	CHRONIC ADENOIDITIS	➡	J35.02	Chronic adenoiditis
474.02	CHRONIC TONSILLITIS AND ADENOIDITIS	➡	J35.03	Chronic tonsillitis and adenoiditis
474.10	HYPERTROPHY OF TONSIL WITH ADENOIDS	➡	J35.3	Hypertrophy of tonsils with hypertrophy of adenoids
474.11	HYPERTROPHY OF TONSILS ALONE	➡	J35.1	Hypertrophy of tonsils
474.12	HYPERTROPHY OF ADENOIDS ALONE	➡	J35.2	Hypertrophy of adenoids
474.2	ADENOID VEGETATIONS		J35.8	Other chronic diseases of tonsils and adenoids
474.8	OTHER CHRONIC DISEASE OF TONSILS AND ADENOIDS		J35.8	Other chronic diseases of tonsils and adenoids

ICD-9-CM		ICD-10-CM	
474.9	UNSPECIFIED CHRONIC DISEASE OF T&A	➡ J35.9	Chronic disease of tonsils and adenoids, unspecified
475	PERITONSILLAR ABSCESS	➡ J36	Peritonsillar abscess
476.0	CHRONIC LARYNGITIS	➡ J37.0	Chronic laryngitis
476.1	CHRONIC LARYNGOTRACHEITIS	➡ J37.1	Chronic laryngotracheitis
477.0	ALLERGIC RHINITIS DUE TO POLLEN	➡ J30.1	Allergic rhinitis due to pollen
477.1	ALLERGIC RHINITIS, DUE TO FOOD	➡ J30.5	Allergic rhinitis due to food
477.2	ALLERGIC RHINITIS DUE TO ANIMAL HAIR AND DANDER	➡ J30.81	Allergic rhinitis due to animal (cat) (dog) hair and dander
477.8	ALLERGIC RHINITIS DUE TO OTHER ALLERGEN	J30.2 J30.89	Other seasonal allergic rhinitis Other allergic rhinitis
477.9	ALLERGIC RHINITIS CAUSE UNSPECIFIED	J30.0 J30.9	Vasomotor rhinitis Allergic rhinitis, unspecified
478.0	HYPERTROPHY OF NASAL TURBINATES	➡ J34.3	Hypertrophy of nasal turbinates
478.11	NASAL MUCOSITIS ULCERATIVE	➡ J34.81	Nasal mucositis (ulcerative)
478.19	OTHER DISEASES OF NASAL CAVITY AND SINUSES	J34.0 J34.1 J34.89 J34.9 R09.81	Abscess, furuncle and carbuncle of nose Cyst and mucocele of nose and nasal sinus Other specified disorders of nose and nasal sinuses Unspecified disorder of nose and nasal sinuses Nasal congestion
478.20	UNSPECIFIED DISEASE OF PHARYNX	J39.2	Other diseases of pharynx
478.21	CELLULITIS OF PHARYNX OR NASOPHARYNX	J39.1	Other abscess of pharynx
478.22	PARAPHARYNGEAL ABSCESS	J39.0	Retropharyngeal and parapharyngeal abscess
478.24	RETROPHARYNGEAL ABSCESS	J39.0	Retropharyngeal and parapharyngeal abscess
478.25	EDEMA OF PHARYNX OR NASOPHARYNX	J39.2	Other diseases of pharynx
478.26	CYST OF PHARYNX OR NASOPHARYNX	J39.2	Other diseases of pharynx
478.29	OTHER DISEASE OF PHARYNX OR NASOPHARYNX	J39.2	Other diseases of pharynx
478.30	UNSPECIFIED PARALYSIS OF VOCAL CORDS OR LARYNX	➡ J38.00	Paralysis of vocal cords and larynx, unspecified
478.31	UNILATERAL PARTIAL PARALYSIS VOCAL CORDS/LARYNX	J38.01	Paralysis of vocal cords and larynx, unilateral
478.32	UNILATERAL COMPLETE PARALYSIS VOCAL CORDS/LARYNX	J38.01	Paralysis of vocal cords and larynx, unilateral
478.33	BILATERAL PARTIAL PARALYSIS VOCAL CORDS/LARYNX	J38.02	Paralysis of vocal cords and larynx, bilateral
478.34	BILATERAL COMPLETE PARALYSIS VOCAL CORDS/LARYNX	J38.02	Paralysis of vocal cords and larynx, bilateral
478.4	POLYP OF VOCAL CORD OR LARYNX	➡ J38.1	Polyp of vocal cord and larynx
478.5	OTHER DISEASES OF VOCAL CORDS	J38.2 J38.3	Nodules of vocal cords Other diseases of vocal cords
478.6	EDEMA OF LARYNX	➡ J38.4	Edema of larynx
478.70	UNSPECIFIED DISEASE OF LARYNX	J38.7	Other diseases of larynx
478.71	CELLULITIS AND PERICHONDRITIS OF LARYNX	J38.7	Other diseases of larynx
478.74	STENOSIS OF LARYNX	➡ J38.6	Stenosis of larynx
478.75	LARYNGEAL SPASM	➡ J38.5	Laryngeal spasm
478.79	OTHER DISEASES OF LARYNX	J38.7	Other diseases of larynx
478.8	UPPER RESP TRACT HYPERSENS REACT SITE UNSPEC	➡ J39.3	Upper respiratory tract hypersensitivity reaction, site unsp
478.9	OTHER&UNSPEC DISEASES UPPER RESPIRATORY TRACT	J39.8 J39.9	Other specified diseases of upper respiratory tract Disease of upper respiratory tract, unspecified
480.0	PNEUMONIA DUE TO ADENOVIRUS	➡ J12.0	Adenoviral pneumonia
480.1	PNEUMONIA DUE TO RESPIRATORY SYNCYTIAL VIRUS	➡ J12.1	Respiratory syncytial virus pneumonia
480.2	PNEUMONIA DUE TO PARAINFLUENZA VIRUS	➡ J12.2	Parainfluenza virus pneumonia
480.3	PNEUMONIA DUE TO SARS-ASSOCIATED CORONAVIRUS	➡ J12.81	Pneumonia due to SARS-associated coronavirus
480.8	PNEUMONIA DUE TO OTHER VIRUS NEC	J12.3 J12.89	Human metapneumovirus pneumonia Other viral pneumonia
480.9	UNSPECIFIED VIRAL PNEUMONIA	J12.9	Viral pneumonia, unspecified
481	PNEUMOCOCCAL PNEUMONIA	J13 J18.1	Pneumonia due to Streptococcus pneumoniae Lobar pneumonia, unspecified organism
482.0	PNEUMONIA DUE TO KLEBSIELLA PNEUMONIAE	➡ J15.0	Pneumonia due to Klebsiella pneumoniae
482.1	PNEUMONIA DUE TO PSEUDOMONAS	➡ J15.1	Pneumonia due to Pseudomonas
482.2	PNEUMONIA DUE TO HEMOPHILUS INFLUENZAE	➡ J14	Pneumonia due to Hemophilus influenzae
482.30	PNEUMONIA DUE TO UNSPECIFIED STREPTOCOCCUS	J15.4	Pneumonia due to other streptococci
482.31	PNEUMONIA DUE TO STREPTOCOCCUS GROUP A	J15.4	Pneumonia due to other streptococci
482.32	PNEUMONIA DUE TO STREPTOCOCCUS GROUP B	➡ J15.3	Pneumonia due to streptococcus, group B
482.39	PNEUMONIA DUE TO OTHER STREPTOCOCCUS	J15.4	Pneumonia due to other streptococci
482.40	PNEUMONIA DUE TO STAPHYLOCOCCUS UNSPECIFIED	➡ J15.20	Pneumonia due to staphylococcus, unspecified
482.41	METHICILLIN SUSECPTIBLE PNEUMONIA STAPH AUREUS	J15.211	Pneumonia due to methicillin suscep staph
482.42	METHICILLIN RESISTANT PNEUMONIA D/T STAPH AUREUS	J15.212	Pneumonia due to Methicillin resistant Staphylococcus aureus
482.49	OTHER STAPHYLOCOCCUS PNEUMONIA	➡ J15.29	Pneumonia due to other staphylococcus
482.81	PNEUMONIA DUE TO ANAEROBES	J15.8	Pneumonia due to other specified bacteria
482.82	PNEUMONIA DUE TO ESCHERICHIA COLI	➡ J15.5	Pneumonia due to Escherichia coli
482.83	PNEUMONIA DUE TO OTHER GRAM-NEGATIVE BACTERIA	➡ J15.6	Pneumonia due to other aerobic Gram-negative bacteria
482.84	LEGIONNAIRES+ DISEASE	➡ A48.1	Legionnaires' disease
482.89	PNEUMONIA DUE TO OTHER SPECIFIED BACTERIA	J15.8	Pneumonia due to other specified bacteria
482.9	UNSPECIFIED BACTERIAL PNEUMONIA	➡ J15.9	Unspecified bacterial pneumonia

ICD-9-CM			ICD-10-CM	
483.0	PNEUMONIA DUE TO MYCOPLASMA PNEUMONIAE	➡	**J15.7**	Pneumonia due to Mycoplasma pneumoniae
483.1	PNEUMONIA DUE TO CHLAMYDIA	➡	**J16.0**	Chlamydial pneumonia
483.8	PNEUMONIA DUE TO OTHER SPECIFIED ORGANISM	➡	**J16.8**	Pneumonia due to other specified infectious organisms
484.1	PNEUMONIA IN CYTOMEGALIC INCLUSION DISEASE	▣	**B25.0**	Cytomegaloviral pneumonitis
484.3	PNEUMONIA IN WHOOPING COUGH	▣ ▣ ▣ ▣	**A37.01** **A37.11** **A37.81** **A37.91**	Whooping cough due to Bordetella pertussis with pneumonia Whooping cough due to Bordetella parapertussis w pneumonia Whooping cough due to oth Bordetella species with pneumonia Whooping cough, unspecified species with pneumonia
484.5	PNEUMONIA IN ANTHRAX	▣	**A22.1**	Pulmonary anthrax
484.6	PNEUMONIA IN ASPERGILLOSIS	▣	**B44.0**	Invasive pulmonary aspergillosis
484.7	PNEUMONIA IN OTHER SYSTEMIC MYCOSES		**J17**	Pneumonia in diseases classified elsewhere
484.8	PNEUMONIA OTH INFECTIOUS DISEASES CLASS ELSW	▣	**B77.81** **J17**	Ascariasis pneumonia Pneumonia in diseases classified elsewhere
485	BRONCHOPNEUMONIA ORGANISM UNSPECIFIED	➡	**J18.0**	Bronchopneumonia, unspecified organism
486	PNEUMONIA, ORGANISM UNSPECIFIED		**J18.8** **J18.9**	Other pneumonia, unspecified organism Pneumonia, unspecified organism
487.0	INFLUENZA WITH PNEUMONIA		**J10.00** **J10.01** **J10.08** **J11.00** **J11.08** **J12.9**	Flu due to oth ident flu virus w unsp type of pneumonia Flu due to oth ident flu virus w same oth ident flu virus pn Influenza due to oth ident influenza virus w oth pneumonia Flu due to unidentified flu virus w unsp type of pneumonia Flu due to unidentified flu virus w specified pneumonia Viral pneumonia, unspecified
487.1	INFLUENZA WITH OTHER RESPIRATORY MANIFESTATIONS		**J10.1** **J11.1**	Flu due to oth ident influenza virus w oth resp manifest Flu due to unidentified influenza virus w oth resp manifest
487.8	INFLUENZA WITH OTHER MANIFESTATIONS		**J10.2** **J10.81** **J10.82** **J10.83** **J10.89** **J11.2** **J11.81** **J11.82** **J11.83** **J11.89**	Influenza due to oth ident influenza virus w GI manifest Influenza due to oth ident influenza virus w encephalopathy Influenza due to oth ident influenza virus w myocarditis Influenza due to oth ident influenza virus w otitis media Influenza due to oth ident influenza virus w oth manifest Influenza due to unidentified influenza virus w GI manifest Flu due to unidentified influenza virus w encephalopathy Influenza due to unidentified influenza virus w myocarditis Influenza due to unidentified influenza virus w otitis media Influenza due to unidentified influenza virus w oth manifest
488.01	INFLUENZA D/T ID AVIAN INFLUENZA VIRUS PNEUMONIA		**J09.X1**	Influenza due to ident novel influenza A virus w pneumonia
488.02	INFLUENZA D/T ID AVIAN FLU VIRUS OTH RESP MANIF		**J09.X2**	Flu due to ident novel influenza A virus w oth resp manifest
488.09	INFLUENZA D/T ID AVIAN FLU VIRUS W/OTH MANIF		**J09.X3** **J09.X9**	Influenza due to ident novel influenza A virus w GI manifest Flu due to ident novel influenza A virus w oth manifest
488.11	FLU D/T ID 2009 NOVEL H1N1 VIRUS W/PNEUMONIA		**J10.08**	Influenza due to oth ident influenza virus w oth pneumonia
488.12	FLU D/T ID 2009 H1N1 VIRUS OTH RESP MANIF		**J10.1**	Flu due to oth ident influenza virus w oth resp manifest
488.19	FLU D/T ID 2009 H1N1 VIRUS W/OTH MANIF		**J09.X9**	Flu due to ident novel influenza A virus w oth manifest
488.81	INFLUENZA IDENT NOVEL INFLUENZA A W/PNEUMONIA		**J09.X1**	Influenza due to ident novel influenza A virus w pneumonia
488.82	INFLUENZA IDENT NOVEL INFLUENZA A RESP MANIFEST		**J09.X2**	Flu due to ident novel influenza A virus w oth resp manifest
488.89	INFLUENZA IDENT NOVEL INFLUENZA A OTH MANIFEST		**J09.X3** **J09.X9**	Influenza due to ident novel influenza A virus w GI manifest Flu due to ident novel influenza A virus w oth manifest
490	BRONCHITIS NOT SPECIFIED AS ACUTE OR CHRONIC	➡	**J40**	Bronchitis, not specified as acute or chronic
491.0	SIMPLE CHRONIC BRONCHITIS	➡	**J41.0**	Simple chronic bronchitis
491.1	MUCOPURULENT CHRONIC BRONCHITIS	➡	**J41.1**	Mucopurulent chronic bronchitis
491.20	OBSTRUCTIVE CHRONIC BRONCHITIS WITHOUT EXACERBAT		**J44.9**	Chronic obstructive pulmonary disease, unspecified
491.21	OBSTRUCTIVE CHRONIC BRONCHITIS WITH EXACERBATION		**J44.1**	Chronic obstructive pulmonary disease w (acute) exacerbation
491.22	OBST CHRONIC BRONCHITIS W/ACUTE BRONCHITIS		**J44.0**	Chronic obstructive pulmon disease w acute lower resp infct
491.8	OTHER CHRONIC BRONCHITIS		**J41.8**	Mixed simple and mucopurulent chronic bronchitis
491.9	UNSPECIFIED CHRONIC BRONCHITIS	➡	**J42**	Unspecified chronic bronchitis
492.0	EMPHYSEMATOUS BLEB		**J43.9**	Emphysema, unspecified
492.8	OTHER EMPHYSEMA		**J43.0** **J43.1** **J43.2** **J43.8** **J43.9**	Unilateral pulmonary emphysema [MacLeod's syndrome] Panlobular emphysema Centrilobular emphysema Other emphysema Emphysema, unspecified
493.00	EXTRINSIC ASTHMA, UNSPECIFIED		**J45.20** **J45.30** **J45.40** **J45.50**	Mild intermittent asthma, uncomplicated Mild persistent asthma, uncomplicated Moderate persistent asthma, uncomplicated Severe persistent asthma, uncomplicated
493.01	EXTRINSIC ASTHMA WITH STATUS ASTHMATICUS		**J45.22** **J45.32** **J45.42** **J45.52**	Mild intermittent asthma with status asthmaticus Mild persistent asthma with status asthmaticus Moderate persistent asthma with status asthmaticus Severe persistent asthma with status asthmaticus
493.02	EXTRINSIC ASTHMA, WITH EXACERBATION		**J45.21** **J45.31** **J45.41** **J45.51**	Mild intermittent asthma with (acute) exacerbation Mild persistent asthma with (acute) exacerbation Moderate persistent asthma with (acute) exacerbation Severe persistent asthma with (acute) exacerbation

ICD-9-CM		ICD-10-CM	
493.10	INTRINSIC ASTHMA, UNSPECIFIED	**J45.20** **J45.30** **J45.40** **J45.50**	Mild intermittent asthma, uncomplicated Mild persistent asthma, uncomplicated Moderate persistent asthma, uncomplicated Severe persistent asthma, uncomplicated
493.11	INTRINSIC ASTHMA WITH STATUS ASTHMATICUS	**J45.22** **J45.32** **J45.42** **J45.52**	Mild intermittent asthma with status asthmaticus Mild persistent asthma with status asthmaticus Moderate persistent asthma with status asthmaticus Severe persistent asthma with status asthmaticus
493.12	INTRINSIC ASTHMA, WITH EXACERBATION	**J45.21** **J45.31** **J45.41** **J45.51**	Mild intermittent asthma with (acute) exacerbation Mild persistent asthma with (acute) exacerbation Moderate persistent asthma with (acute) exacerbation Severe persistent asthma with (acute) exacerbation
493.20	CHRONIC OBSTRUCTIVE ASTHMA UNSPECIFIED	**J44.9**	Chronic obstructive pulmonary disease, unspecified
493.21	CHRONIC OBSTRUCTIVE ASTHMA W/STATUS ASTHMATICUS	**J44.0**	Chronic obstructive pulmon disease w acute lower resp infct
493.22	CHRONIC OBSTRUCTIVE ASTHMA WITH EXACERBATION	**J44.1**	Chronic obstructive pulmonary disease w (acute) exacerbation
493.81	EXERCISE INDUCED BRONCHOSPASM	➡ **J45.990**	Exercise induced bronchospasm
493.82	COUGH VARIANT ASTHMA	➡ **J45.991**	Cough variant asthma
493.90	ASTHMA, UNSPECIFIED, UNSPECIFIED STATUS	**J45.909** **J45.998**	Unspecified asthma, uncomplicated Other asthma
493.91	ASTHMA UNSPECIFIED WITH STATUS ASTHMATICUS	➡ **J45.902**	Unspecified asthma with status asthmaticus
493.92	ASTHMA UNSPECIFIED WITH EXACERBATION	➡ **J45.901**	Unspecified asthma with (acute) exacerbation
494.0	BRONCHIECTASIS WITHOUT ACUTE EXACERBATION	➡ **J47.9**	Bronchiectasis, uncomplicated
494.1	BRONCHIECTASIS WITH ACUTE EXACERBATION	**J47.0** **J47.1**	Bronchiectasis with acute lower respiratory infection Bronchiectasis with (acute) exacerbation
495.0	FARMERS LUNG	➡ **J67.0**	Farmer's lung
495.1	BAGASSOSIS	➡ **J67.1**	Bagassosis
495.2	BIRD-FANCIERS LUNG	➡ **J67.2**	Bird fancier's lung
495.3	SUBEROSIS	➡ **J67.3**	Suberosis
495.4	MALT WORKERS LUNG	➡ **J67.4**	Maltworker's lung
495.5	MUSHROOM WORKERS LUNG	➡ **J67.5**	Mushroom-worker's lung
495.6	MAPLE BARK-STRIPPERS LUNG	➡ **J67.6**	Maple-bark-stripper's lung
495.7	VENTILATION PNEUMONITIS	➡ **J67.7**	Air conditioner and humidifier lung
495.8	OTHER SPECIFIED ALLERGIC ALVEOLITIS&PNEUMONITIS	➡ **J67.8**	Hypersensitivity pneumonitis due to other organic dusts
495.9	UNSPECIFIED ALLERGIC ALVEOLITIS AND PNEUMONITIS	➡ **J67.9**	Hypersensitivity pneumonitis due to unspecified organic dust
496	CHRONIC AIRWAY OBSTRUCTION NEC	**J44.9**	Chronic obstructive pulmonary disease, unspecified
500	COAL WORKERS PNEUMOCONIOSIS	➡ **J60**	Coalworker's pneumoconiosis
501	ASBESTOSIS	**J61**	Pneumoconiosis due to asbestos and other mineral fibers
502	PNEUMOCONIOSIS DUE TO OTHER SILICA OR SILICATES	**J62.0** **J62.8**	Pneumoconiosis due to talc dust Pneumoconiosis due to other dust containing silica
503	PNEUMOCONIOSIS DUE TO OTHER INORGANIC DUST	**J63.0** **J63.1** **J63.2** **J63.3** **J63.4** **J63.5** **J63.6**	Aluminosis (of lung) Bauxite fibrosis (of lung) Berylliosis Graphite fibrosis (of lung) Siderosis Stannosis Pneumoconiosis due to other specified inorganic dusts
504	PNEUMONOPATHY DUE TO INHALATION OF OTHER DUST	**J66.0** **J66.1** **J66.2** **J66.8**	Byssinosis Flax-dressers' disease Cannabinosis Airway disease due to other specific organic dusts
505	UNSPECIFIED PNEUMOCONIOSIS	**J64** **J65**	Unspecified pneumoconiosis Pneumoconiosis associated with tuberculosis
506.0	BRONCHITIS&PNEUMONITIS DUE TO FUMES&VAPORS	➡ **J68.0**	Bronchitis & pneumonitis d/t chemicals, gas, fumes & vapors
506.1	ACUTE PULMONARY EDEMA DUE TO FUMES AND VAPORS	➡ **J68.1**	Pulmonary edema due to chemicals, gases, fumes and vapors
506.2	UPPER RESPIRATORY INFLAMMATION DUE FUMES&VAPORS	➡ **J68.2**	Upper resp inflam d/t chemicals, gas, fumes and vapors, NEC
506.3	OTH ACUTE&SUBACUTE RESP CONDS DUE FUMES&VAPORS	➡ **J68.3**	Oth ac & subac resp cond d/t chemicals, gas, fumes & vapors
506.4	CHRONIC RESPIRATORY CONDITIONS DUE FUMES&VAPORS	**J68.4**	Chronic resp cond due to chemicals, gases, fumes and vapors
506.9	UNSPEC RESPIRATORY CONDITIONS DUE FUMES&VAPORS	**J68.8** **J68.9**	Oth resp cond due to chemicals, gases, fumes and vapors Unsp resp cond due to chemicals, gases, fumes and vapors
507.0	PNEUMONITIS DUE TO INHALATION OF FOOD OR VOMITUS	➡ **J69.0**	Pneumonitis due to inhalation of food and vomit
507.1	PNEUMONITIS DUE TO INHALATION OF OILS&ESSENCES	➡ **J69.1**	Pneumonitis due to inhalation of oils and essences
507.8	PNEUMONITIS DUE TO OTHER SOLIDS AND LIQUIDS	➡ **J69.8**	Pneumonitis due to inhalation of other solids and liquids
508.0	ACUTE PULMONARY MANIFESTATIONS DUE TO RADIATION	➡ **J70.0**	Acute pulmonary manifestations due to radiation
508.1	CHRONIC&OTH PULMONARY MANIFESTS DUE RADIATION	➡ **J70.1**	Chronic and other pulmonary manifestations due to radiation
508.2	RESPIRATORY CONDITIONS DUE TO SMOKE INHALATION	**J70.5**	Respiratory conditions due to smoke inhalation
508.8	RESPIRATORY CONDS DUE OTHER SPEC EXTERNAL AGENTS	**J70.2** **J70.3** **J70.4** **J70.8**	Acute drug-induced interstitial lung disorders Chronic drug-induced interstitial lung disorders Drug-induced interstitial lung disorders, unspecified Respiratory conditions due to oth external agents
508.9	RESPIRATORY CONDITIONS DUE UNSPEC EXTERNAL AGENT	➡ **J70.9**	Respiratory conditions due to unspecified external agent
510.0	EMPYEMA WITH FISTULA	**J86.0**	Pyothorax with fistula
510.9	EMPYEMA WITHOUT MENTION OF FISTULA	**J86.9**	Pyothorax without fistula

ICD-9-CM		ICD-10-CM	
511.Ø	PLEURISY WITHOUT MENTION EFFUS/CURRENT TB	J86.9	Pyothorax without fistula
		J92.Ø	Pleural plaque with presence of asbestos
		J92.9	Pleural plaque without asbestos
		J94.1	Fibrothorax
		J94.8	Other specified pleural conditions
		J94.9	Pleural condition, unspecified
		RØ9.1	Pleurisy
511.1	PLEURISY W/EFFUS W/BACTERL CAUSE OTH THAN TB	J9Ø	Pleural effusion, not elsewhere classified
		J94.2	Hemothorax
511.81	MALIGNANT PLEURAL EFFUSION	➡ J91.Ø	Malignant pleural effusion
511.89	OTHER SPEC FORMS OF EFFUSION EXCEPT TUBERCULOUS	J9Ø	Pleural effusion, not elsewhere classified
		J94.Ø	Chylous effusion
		J94.2	Hemothorax
		J94.8	Other specified pleural conditions
511.9	UNSPECIFIED PLEURAL EFFUSION	J91.8	Pleural effusion in other conditions classified elsewhere
512.Ø	SPONTANEOUS TENSION PNEUMOTHORAX	➡ J93.Ø	Spontaneous tension pneumothorax
512.1	IATROGENIC PNEUMOTHROAX	J95.811	Postprocedural pneumothorax
512.2	POSTOPERATIVE AIR LEAK	J95.812	Postprocedural air leak
512.81	PRIMARY SPONTANEOUS PNEUMOTHORAX	J93.11	Primary spontaneous pneumothorax
512.82	SECONDARY SPONTANEOUS PNEUMOTHORAX	J93.12	Secondary spontaneous pneumothorax
512.83	CHRONIC PNEUMOTHORAX	J93.81	Chronic pneumothorax
512.84	OTHER AIR LEAK	J93.82	Other air leak
512.89	OTHER PNEUMOTHORAX	J93.83	Other pneumothorax
		J93.9	Pneumothorax, unspecified
513.Ø	ABSCESS OF LUNG	J85.Ø	Gangrene and necrosis of lung
		J85.1	Abscess of lung with pneumonia
		J85.2	Abscess of lung without pneumonia
513.1	ABSCESS OF MEDIASTINUM	➡ J85.3	Abscess of mediastinum
514	PULMONARY CONGESTION AND HYPOSTASIS	J18.2	Hypostatic pneumonia, unspecified organism
		J81.1	Chronic pulmonary edema
515	POSTINFLAMMATORY PULMONARY FIBROSIS	J84.1Ø	Pulmonary fibrosis, unspecified
		J84.17	Oth interstit pulmon dis w fibrosis in dis classd elswhr
		J84.89	Other specified interstitial pulmonary diseases
516.Ø	PULMONARY ALVEOLAR PROTEINOSIS	J84.Ø1	Alveolar proteinosis
516.1	IDIOPATHIC PULMONARY HEMOSIDEROSIS	J84.Ø3	Idiopathic pulmonary hemosiderosis
516.2	PULMONARY ALVEOLAR MICROLITHIASIS	J84.Ø2	Pulmonary alveolar microlithiasis
516.3Ø	IDIOPATHIC INTERSTITIAL PNEUMONIA NOS	J84.111	Idiopathic interstitial pneumonia, not otherwise specified
516.31	IDIOPATHIC PULMONARY FIBROSIS	J84.112	Idiopathic pulmonary fibrosis
516.32	IDIOPATHIC NON-SPECIFIC INTERSTITIAL PNEUMONITIS	J84.113	Idiopathic non-specific interstitial pneumonitis
516.33	ACUTE INTERSTITIAL PNEUMONITIS	J84.114	Acute interstitial pneumonitis
516.34	RESPIRATORY BRONCHIOLITIS INTERST LUNG DISEASE	J84.115	Respiratory bronchiolitis interstitial lung disease
516.35	IDIOPATHIC LYMPHOID INTERSTITIAL PNEUMONIA	J84.2	Lymphoid interstitial pneumonia
516.36	CRYPTOGENIC ORGANIZING PNEUMONIA	J84.116	Cryptogenic organizing pneumonia
516.37	DESQUAMATIVE INTERSTITIAL PNEUMONIA	J84.117	Desquamative interstitial pneumonia
516.4	LYMPHANGIOLEIOMYOMATOSIS	J84.81	Lymphangioleiomyomatosis
516.5	ADULT PULMONARY LANGERHANS CELL HISTIOCYTOSIS	J84.82	Adult pulmonary Langerhans cell histiocytosis
516.61	NEUROENDOCRINE CELL HYPERPLASIA OF INFANCY	J84.841	Neuroendocrine cell hyperplasia of infancy
516.62	PULMONARY INTERSTITIAL GLYCOGENOSIS	J84.842	Pulmonary interstitial glycogenosis
516.63	SURFACTANT MUTATIONS OF THE LUNG	J84.83	Surfactant mutations of the lung
516.64	ALVEOL CAPILLARY DYSPLASIA W/VEIN MISALIGNMENT	J84.843	Alveolar capillary dysplasia with vein misalignment
516.69	OTHER INTERSTITIAL LUNG DISEASES OF CHILDHOOD	J84.848	Other interstitial lung diseases of childhood
516.8	OTH SPEC ALVEOL&PARIETOALVEOL PNEUMONOPATHIES	J84.Ø9	Other alveolar and parieto-alveolar conditions
516.9	UNSPEC ALVEOLAR&PARIETOALVEOLAR PNEUMONOPATHY	J84.9	Interstitial pulmonary disease, unspecified
517.1	RHEUMATIC PNEUMONIA	J17	Pneumonia in diseases classified elsewhere
517.2	LUNG INVOLVEMENT IN SYSTEMIC SCLEROSIS	◘ M34.81	Systemic sclerosis with lung involvement
517.3	ACUTE CHEST SYNDROME	◘ D57.Ø1	Hb-SS disease with acute chest syndrome
		◘ D57.211	Sickle-cell/Hb-C disease with acute chest syndrome
		◘ D57.411	Sickle-cell thalassemia with acute chest syndrome
		◘ D57.811	Other sickle-cell disorders with acute chest syndrome
		J99	Respiratory disorders in diseases classified elsewhere
517.8	LUNG INVOLVEMENT OTHER DISEASES CLASSIFIED ELSW	J99	Respiratory disorders in diseases classified elsewhere
		◘ M32.13	Lung involvement in systemic lupus erythematosus
		◘ M33.Ø1	Juvenile dermatopolymyositis with respiratory involvement
		◘ M33.11	Other dermatopolymyositis with respiratory involvement
		◘ M33.21	Polymyositis with respiratory involvement
		◘ M33.91	Dermatopolymyositis, unsp with respiratory involvement
		◘ M35.Ø2	Sicca syndrome with lung involvement
518.Ø	PULMONARY COLLAPSE	J98.11	Atelectasis
		J98.19	Other pulmonary collapse
518.1	INTERSTITIAL EMPHYSEMA	➡ J98.2	Interstitial emphysema
518.2	COMPENSATORY EMPHYSEMA	➡ J98.3	Compensatory emphysema

ICD-9-CM			ICD-10-CM	
518.3	PULMONARY EOSINOPHILIA	➡	J82	Pulmonary eosinophilia, not elsewhere classified
518.4	UNSPECIFIED ACUTE EDEMA OF LUNG	➡	J81.Ø	Acute pulmonary edema
518.51	ACUTE RESPIRATORY FAILURE FLW TRAUMA & SURGERY		J95.821 J96.ØØ J96.Ø1 J96.Ø2	Acute postprocedural respiratory failure Acute respiratory failure, unsp w hypoxia or hypercapnia Acute respiratory failure with hypoxia Acute respiratory failure with hypercapnia
518.52	OTH PULM INSUFF NOT ELSW CLASS FLW TRAUMA & SURG		J95.1 J95.2 J95.3	Acute pulmonary insufficiency following thoracic surgery Acute pulmonary insufficiency following nonthoracic surgery Chronic pulmonary insufficiency following surgery
518.53	ACUTE & CHRONIC RESP FAILURE FOLW TRAUMA & SURG		J95.822 J96.2Ø J96.21 J96.22	Acute and chronic postprocedural respiratory failure Acute and chr resp failure, unsp w hypoxia or hypercapnia Acute and chronic respiratory failure with hypoxia Acute and chronic respiratory failure with hypercapnia
518.6	ALLERGIC BRONCHOPULMONARY ASPERGILLOSIS	➡	B44.81	Allergic bronchopulmonary aspergillosis
518.7	TRANSFUSION RELATED ACUTE LUNG INJURY	➡	J95.84	Transfusion-related acute lung injury (TRALI)
518.81	ACUTE RESPIRATORY FAILURE		J96.ØØ J96.Ø1 J96.Ø2 J96.9Ø J96.91 J96.92	Acute respiratory failure, unsp w hypoxia or hypercapnia Acute respiratory failure with hypoxia Acute respiratory failure with hypercapnia Respiratory failure, unsp, unsp w hypoxia or hypercapnia Respiratory failure, unspecified with hypoxia Respiratory failure, unspecified with hypercapnia
518.82	OTHER PULMONARY INSUFFICIENCY NEC		J8Ø	Acute respiratory distress syndrome
518.83	CHRONIC RESPIRATORY FAILURE		J96.1Ø J96.11 J96.12	Chronic respiratory failure, unsp w hypoxia or hypercapnia Chronic respiratory failure with hypoxia Chronic respiratory failure with hypercapnia
518.84	ACUTE AND CHRONIC RESPIRATORY FAILURE		J96.2Ø J96.21 J96.22	Acute and chr resp failure, unsp w hypoxia or hypercapnia Acute and chronic respiratory failure with hypoxia Acute and chronic respiratory failure with hypercapnia
518.89	OTHER DISEASES OF LUNG NOT ELSEWHERE CLASSIFIED	➡	J98.4	Other disorders of lung
519.ØØ	UNSPECIFIED TRACHEOSTOMY COMPLICATION	➡	J95.ØØ	Unspecified tracheostomy complication
519.Ø1	INFECTION OF TRACHEOSTOMY	➡	J95.Ø2	Infection of tracheostomy stoma
519.Ø2	MECHANICAL COMPLICATION OF TRACHEOSTOMY		J95.Ø3	Malfunction of tracheostomy stoma
519.Ø9	OTHER TRACHEOSTOMY COMPLICATIONS		J95.Ø1 J95.Ø3 J95.Ø4 J95.Ø9	Hemorrhage from tracheostomy stoma Malfunction of tracheostomy stoma Tracheo-esophageal fistula following tracheostomy Other tracheostomy complication
519.11	ACUTE BRONCHOSPASM	➡	J98.Ø1	Acute bronchospasm
519.19	OTHER DISEASES OF TRACHEA AND BRONCHUS		J39.8 J98.Ø9	Other specified diseases of upper respiratory tract Other diseases of bronchus, not elsewhere classified
519.2	MEDIASTINITIS		J98.5	Diseases of mediastinum, not elsewhere classified
519.3	OTHER DISEASES OF MEDIASTINUM NEC		J98.5	Diseases of mediastinum, not elsewhere classified
519.4	DISORDERS OF DIAPHRAGM	➡	J98.6	Disorders of diaphragm
519.8	OTHER DISEASES OF RESPIRATORY SYSTEM NEC		J22 J98.8	Unspecified acute lower respiratory infection Other specified respiratory disorders
519.9	UNSPECIFIED DISEASE OF RESPIRATORY SYSTEM	➡	J98.9	Respiratory disorder, unspecified

[Brackets] indicate valid character values for each code. Character value meanings provided for each code grouping.

Diseases of the Digestive System

ICD-9-CM			ICD-10-CM	
520.0	ANODONTIA	➡	**K00.0**	Anodontia
520.1	SUPERNUMERARY TEETH	➡	**K00.1**	Supernumerary teeth
520.2	ABNORMALITIES OF SIZE AND FORM OF TEETH	➡	**K00.2**	Abnormalities of size and form of teeth
520.3	MOTTLED TEETH	➡	**K00.3**	Mottled teeth
520.4	DISTURBANCES OF TOOTH FORMATION	➡	**K00.4**	Disturbances in tooth formation
520.5	HEREDITARY DISTURBANCES IN TOOTH STRUCTURE NEC	➡	**K00.5**	Hereditary disturbances in tooth structure, NEC
520.6	DISTURBANCES IN TOOTH ERUPTION		**K00.6**	Disturbances in tooth eruption
			K01.0	Embedded teeth
			K01.1	Impacted teeth
520.7	TEETHING SYNDROME	➡	**K00.7**	Teething syndrome
520.8	OTHER SPEC DISORDERS TOOTH DEVELOPMENT&ERUPTION		**K00.8**	Other disorders of tooth development
520.9	UNSPECIFIED DISORDER TOOTH DEVELOPMENT&ERUPTION	➡	**K00.9**	Disorder of tooth development, unspecified
521.00	UNSPECIFIED DENTAL CARIES		**K02.9**	Dental caries, unspecified
521.01	DENTAL CARIES LIMITED TO ENAMEL	▣	**K02.51**	Dental caries on pit and fissure surface limited to enamel
		▣	**K02.61**	Dental caries on smooth surface limited to enamel
521.02	DENTAL CARIES EXTENDING INTO DENTINE	▣	**K02.52**	Dental caries on pit and fissure surfc penetrat into dentin
		▣	**K02.62**	Dental caries on smooth surface penetrating into dentin
521.03	DENTAL CARIES EXTENDING INTO PULP	▣	**K02.53**	Dental caries on pit and fissure surface penetrat into pulp
		▣	**K02.63**	Dental caries on smooth surface penetrating into pulp
521.04	ARRESTED DENTAL CARIES	➡	**K02.3**	Arrested dental caries
521.05	ODONTOCLASIA		**K03.89**	Other specified diseases of hard tissues of teeth
521.06	DENTAL CARIES PIT AND FISSURE	▣	**K02.51**	Dental caries on pit and fissure surface limited to enamel
		▣	**K02.52**	Dental caries on pit and fissure surfc penetrat into dentin
		▣	**K02.53**	Dental caries on pit and fissure surface penetrat into pulp
521.07	DENTAL CARIES OF SMOOTH SURFACE	▣	**K02.61**	Dental caries on smooth surface limited to enamel
		▣	**K02.62**	Dental caries on smooth surface penetrating into dentin
		▣	**K02.63**	Dental caries on smooth surface penetrating into pulp
521.08	DENTAL CARIES OF ROOT SURFACE	➡	**K02.7**	Dental root caries
521.09	OTHER DENTAL CARIES		**K02.9**	Dental caries, unspecified
521.10	DZ HARD TISSUES TEETH EXCESSIVE ATTRITION UNSPEC		**K03.0**	Excessive attrition of teeth
521.11	DZ HARD TISS TEETH EXCESS ATTRITION LTD ENAMEL		**K03.0**	Excessive attrition of teeth
521.12	DZ HARD TISS TEETH EXCESS ATTRITN EXT IN DENTINE		**K03.0**	Excessive attrition of teeth
521.13	DZ HARD TISS TEETH EXCESS ATTRITION EXT IN PULP		**K03.0**	Excessive attrition of teeth
521.14	DZ HARD TISSUES TEETH EXCESS ATTRITION LOCALIZED		**K03.0**	Excessive attrition of teeth
521.15	DZ HARD TISSUES TEETH EXCESS ATTRITION GEN		**K03.0**	Excessive attrition of teeth
521.20	DISEASES HARD TISSUES TEETH ABRASION UNSPECIFIED		**K03.1**	Abrasion of teeth
521.21	DISEASES HARD TISSUES TEETH ABRASION LTD ENAMEL		**K03.1**	Abrasion of teeth
521.22	DZ HARD TISSUES TEETH ABRASION EXT INTO DENTINE		**K03.1**	Abrasion of teeth
521.23	DZ HARD TISSUES TEETH ABRASION EXT INTO PULP		**K03.1**	Abrasion of teeth
521.24	DISEASES HARD TISSUES TEETH ABRASION LOCALIZED		**K03.1**	Abrasion of teeth
521.25	DISEASES HARD TISSUES TEETH ABRASION GENERALIZED		**K03.1**	Abrasion of teeth
521.30	DISEASES HARD TISSUES TEETH EROSION UNSPECIFIED		**K03.2**	Erosion of teeth
521.31	DISEASES HARD TISSUES TEETH EROSION LTD ENAMEL		**K03.2**	Erosion of teeth
521.32	DZ HARD TISSUES TEETH EROSION EXT INTO DENTINE		**K03.2**	Erosion of teeth
521.33	DZ HARD TISSUES TEETH EROSION EXT INTO PULP		**K03.2**	Erosion of teeth
521.34	DISEASES HARD TISSUES TEETH EROSION LOCALIZED		**K03.2**	Erosion of teeth
521.35	DISEASES HARD TISSUES TEETH EROSION GENERALIZED		**K03.2**	Erosion of teeth
521.40	DISEASES HARD TISSUES TEETH PATH RESORPTION UNS		**K03.3**	Pathological resorption of teeth
521.41	DZ HARD TISSUES TEETH PATH RESORPTION INTERNAL		**K03.3**	Pathological resorption of teeth
521.42	DZ HARD TISSUES TEETH PATH RESORPTION EXTERNAL		**K03.3**	Pathological resorption of teeth
521.49	DISEASES HARD TISSUES TEETH OTH PATH RESORPTION		**K03.3**	Pathological resorption of teeth
521.5	HYPERCEMENTOSIS	➡	**K03.4**	Hypercementosis
521.6	ANKYLOSIS OF TEETH	➡	**K03.5**	Ankylosis of teeth
521.7	INTRINSIC POSTERUPTIVE COLOR CHANGES		**K03.7**	Posteruptive color changes of dental hard tissues
521.81	CRACKED TOOTH	➡	**K03.81**	Cracked tooth
521.89	OTHER SPECIFIC DISEASES OF HARD TISSUES OF TEETH		**K03.89**	Other specified diseases of hard tissues of teeth
521.9	UNSPECIFIED DISEASE OF HARD TISSUES OF TEETH	➡	**K03.9**	Disease of hard tissues of teeth, unspecified
522.0	PULPITIS	➡	**K04.0**	Pulpitis
522.1	NECROSIS OF DENTAL PULP	➡	**K04.1**	Necrosis of pulp
522.2	DENTAL PULP DEGENERATION	➡	**K04.2**	Pulp degeneration
522.3	ABNORMAL HARD TISSUE FORMATION IN DENTAL PULP	➡	**K04.3**	Abnormal hard tissue formation in pulp
522.4	ACUTE APICAL PERIODONTITIS OF PULPAL ORIGIN	➡	**K04.4**	Acute apical periodontitis of pulpal origin
522.5	PERIAPICAL ABSCESS WITHOUT SINUS	➡	**K04.7**	Periapical abscess without sinus
522.6	CHRONIC APICAL PERIODONTITIS	➡	**K04.5**	Chronic apical periodontitis
522.7	PERIAPICAL ABSCESS WITH SINUS	➡	**K04.6**	Periapical abscess with sinus
522.8	RADICULAR CYST OF DENTAL PULP	➡	**K04.8**	Radicular cyst
522.9	OTHER&UNSPEC DISEASES PULP&PERIAPICAL TISSUES		**K04.90**	Unspecified diseases of pulp and periapical tissues
			K04.99	Other diseases of pulp and periapical tissues

ICD-9-CM			ICD-10-CM	
523.00	ACUTE GINGIVITIS PLAQUE INDUCED	➡	**K05.00**	Acute gingivitis, plaque induced
523.01	ACUTE GINGIVITIS NONPLAQUE INDUCED	➡	**K05.01**	Acute gingivitis, non-plaque induced
523.10	CHRONIC GINGIVITIS PLAQUE INDUCED	➡	**K05.10**	Chronic gingivitis, plaque induced
523.11	CHRONIC GINGIVITIS NONPLAQUE INDUCED	➡	**K05.11**	Chronic gingivitis, non-plaque induced
523.20	GINGIVAL RECESSION UNSPECIFIED		**K06.0**	Gingival recession
523.21	GINGIVAL RECESSION MINIMAL		**K06.0**	Gingival recession
523.22	GINGIVAL RECESSION MODERATE		**K06.0**	Gingival recession
523.23	GINGIVAL RECESSION SEVERE		**K06.0**	Gingival recession
523.24	GINGIVAL RECESSION LOCALIZED		**K06.0**	Gingival recession
523.25	GINGIVAL RECESSION GENERALIZED		**K06.0**	Gingival recession
523.30	AGGRESSIVE PERIODONTITIS UNSPECIFIED		**K05.20**	Aggressive periodontitis, unspecified
523.31	AGGRESSIVE PERIODONTITIS LOCALIZED	➡	**K05.21**	Aggressive periodontitis, localized
523.32	AGGRESSIVE PERIODONTITIS GENERALIZED	➡	**K05.22**	Aggressive periodontitis, generalized
523.33	ACUTE PERIODONTITIS		**K05.20**	Aggressive periodontitis, unspecified
523.40	CHRONIC PERIODONTITIS UNSPECIFIED	➡	**K05.30**	Chronic periodontitis, unspecified
523.41	CHRONIC PERIODONTITIS LOCALIZED	➡	**K05.31**	Chronic periodontitis, localized
523.42	CHRONIC PERIODONTITIS GENERALIZED	➡	**K05.32**	Chronic periodontitis, generalized
523.5	PERIODONTOSIS	➡	**K05.4**	Periodontosis
523.6	ACCRETIONS ON TEETH	➡	**K03.6**	Deposits [accretions] on teeth
523.8	OTHER SPECIFIED PERIODONTAL DISEASES		**E08.630** **E09.630** **E10.630** **E11.630** **E13.630** **K05.5** **K06.1** **K06.2** **K06.8**	Diabetes due to underlying condition w periodontal disease Drug/chem diabetes mellitus w periodontal disease Type 1 diabetes mellitus with periodontal disease Type 2 diabetes mellitus with periodontal disease Other specified diabetes mellitus with periodontal disease Other periodontal diseases Gingival enlargement Gingival & edentulous alveolar ridge lesions assoc w trauma Oth disrd of gingiva and edentulous alveolar ridge
523.9	UNSPECIFIED GINGIVAL AND PERIODONTAL DISEASE		**K05.6** **K06.9**	Periodontal disease, unspecified Disorder of gingiva and edentulous alveolar ridge, unsp
524.00	UNSPECIFIED MAJOR ANOMALY OF JAW SIZE	➡	**M26.00**	Unspecified anomaly of jaw size
524.01	MAXILLARY HYPERPLASIA	➡	**M26.01**	Maxillary hyperplasia
524.02	MANDIBULAR HYPERPLASIA	➡	**M26.03**	Mandibular hyperplasia
524.03	MAXILLARY HYPOPLASIA	➡	**M26.02**	Maxillary hypoplasia
524.04	MANDIBULAR HYPOPLASIA	➡	**M26.04**	Mandibular hypoplasia
524.05	MACROGENIA	➡	**M26.05**	Macrogenia
524.06	MICROGENIA	➡	**M26.06**	Microgenia
524.07	EXCESSIVE TUBEROSITY OF JAW	➡	**M26.07**	Excessive tuberosity of jaw
524.09	OTHER SPECIFIED MAJOR ANOMALY OF JAW SIZE		**M26.09**	Other specified anomalies of jaw size
524.10	UNSPEC ANOMALY RELATIONSHIP JAW CRANIAL BASE	➡	**M26.10**	Unspecified anomaly of jaw-cranial base relationship
524.11	MAXILLARY ASYMMETRY	➡	**M26.11**	Maxillary asymmetry
524.12	OTHER JAW ASYMMETRY	➡	**M26.12**	Other jaw asymmetry
524.19	OTHER SPEC ANOMALY RELATIONSHIP JAW CRANIAL BASE	➡	**M26.19**	Other specified anomalies of jaw-cranial base relationship
524.20	UNSPECIFIED ANOMALY OF DENTAL ARCH RELATIONSHIP	➡	**M26.20**	Unspecified anomaly of dental arch relationship
524.21	MALOCCLUSION ANGLES CLASS I	➡	**M26.211**	Malocclusion, Angle's class I
524.22	MALOCCLUSION ANGLES CLASS II	➡	**M26.212**	Malocclusion, Angle's class II
524.23	MALOCCLUSION ANGLES CLASS III	➡	**M26.213**	Malocclusion, Angle's class III
524.24	ANOMALY DENTAL ARCH REL OPEN ANT OCCLUSAL REL	➡	**M26.220**	Open anterior occlusal relationship
524.25	ANOMALY DENTAL ARCH REL OPEN POST OCCLUSAL REL	➡	**M26.221**	Open posterior occlusal relationship
524.26	ANOMALY DENTAL ARCH REL EXCESS HORIZONTAL OVRLAP	➡	**M26.23**	Excessive horizontal overlap
524.27	ANOMALY DENTAL ARCH RELATIONSHIP REVERSE ARTIC	➡	**M26.24**	Reverse articulation
524.28	ANOMALY DENTAL ARCH REL ANOM INTERARCH DISTANCE	➡	**M26.25**	Anomalies of interarch distance
524.29	OTHER ANOMALIES OF DENTAL ARCH RELATIONSHIP	➡	**M26.29**	Other anomalies of dental arch relationship
524.30	ANOMALY OF TOOTH POSITION UNSPECIFIED	➡	**M26.30**	Unsp anomaly of tooth position of fully erupted tooth/teeth
524.31	CROWDING OF TEETH	➡	**M26.31**	Crowding of fully erupted teeth
524.32	EXCESSIVE SPACING OF TEETH	➡	**M26.32**	Excessive spacing of fully erupted teeth
524.33	HORIZONTAL DISPLACEMENT OF TEETH	➡	**M26.33**	Horizontal displacement of fully erupted tooth or teeth
524.34	VERTICAL DISPLACEMENT OF TEETH	➡	**M26.34**	Vertical displacement of fully erupted tooth or teeth
524.35	ROTATION OF TOOTH/TEETH	➡	**M26.35**	Rotation of fully erupted tooth or teeth
524.36	INSUFFICIENT INTEROCCLUSAL DISTANCE OF TEETH	➡	**M26.36**	Insufficient interocclusal distance of fully erupted teeth
524.37	EXCESSIVE INTEROCCLUSAL DISTANCE OF TEETH	➡	**M26.37**	Excessive interocclusal distance of fully erupted teeth
524.39	OTHER ANOMALIES OF TOOTH POSITION	➡	**M26.39**	Oth anomalies of tooth position of fully erupted tooth/teeth
524.4	UNSPECIFIED MALOCCLUSION		**M26.219** **M26.4**	Malocclusion, Angle's class, unspecified Malocclusion, unspecified
524.50	DENTOFACIAL FUNCTIONAL ABNORMALITY UNSPECIFIED	➡	**M26.50**	Dentofacial functional abnormalities, unspecified
524.51	ABNORMAL JAW CLOSURE	➡	**M26.51**	Abnormal jaw closure
524.52	LIMITED MANDIBULAR RANGE OF MOTION	➡	**M26.52**	Limited mandibular range of motion
524.53	DEVIATION IN OPENING AND CLOSING OF THE MANDIBLE	➡	**M26.53**	Deviation in opening and closing of the mandible

ICD-9-CM			ICD-10-CM	
524.54	INSUFFICIENT ANTERIOR GUIDANCE	➡	M26.54	Insufficient anterior guidance
524.55	CENTRIC OCCL MAXIMUM INTERCUSPATION DISCREPANCY	➡	M26.55	Centric occlusion maximum intercuspation discrepancy
524.56	NON-WORKING SIDE INTERFERENCE	➡	M26.56	Non-working side interference
524.57	LACK OF POSTERIOR OCCLUSAL SUPPORT	➡	M26.57	Lack of posterior occlusal support
524.59	OTHER DENTOFACIAL FUNCTIONAL ABNORMALITIES	➡	M26.59	Other dentofacial functional abnormalities
524.60	UNSPECIFIED TEMPOROMANDIBULAR JOINT DISORDERS		M26.60 M26.69	Temporomandibular joint disorder, unspecified Other specified disorders of temporomandibular joint
524.61	ADHESIONS AND ANKYLOSIS OF TMJ	➡	M26.61	Adhesions and ankylosis of temporomandibular joint
524.62	ARTHRALGIA OF TEMPOROMANDIBULAR JOINT	➡	M26.62	Arthralgia of temporomandibular joint
524.63	ARTICULAR DISC DISORDER OF TMJ	➡	M26.63	Articular disc disorder of temporomandibular joint
524.64	TMJ SOUNDS ON OPENING AND/OR CLOSING THE JAW		M26.69	Other specified disorders of temporomandibular joint
524.69	OTHER SPECIFIED TMJ DISORDERS		M26.69	Other specified disorders of temporomandibular joint
524.70	UNSPECIFIED ALVEOLAR ANOMALY	➡	M26.70	Unspecified alveolar anomaly
524.71	ALVEOLAR MAXILLARY HYPERPLASIA	➡	M26.71	Alveolar maxillary hyperplasia
524.72	ALVEOLAR MANDIBULAR HYPERPLASIA	➡	M26.72	Alveolar mandibular hyperplasia
524.73	ALVEOLAR MAXILLARY HYPOPLASIA	➡	M26.73	Alveolar maxillary hypoplasia
524.74	ALVEOLAR MANDIBULAR HYPOPLASIA	➡	M26.74	Alveolar mandibular hypoplasia
524.75	VERTICAL DISPLACEMENT OF ALVEOLUS AND TEETH		M26.79	Other specified alveolar anomalies
524.76	OCCLUSAL PLANE DEVIATION		M26.79	Other specified alveolar anomalies
524.79	OTHER SPECIFIED ALVEOLAR ANOMALY		M26.79	Other specified alveolar anomalies
524.81	ANTERIOR SOFT TISSUE IMPINGEMENT	➡	M26.81	Anterior soft tissue impingement
524.82	POSTERIOR SOFT TISSUE IMPINGEMENT	➡	M26.82	Posterior soft tissue impingement
524.89	OTHER SPECIFIED DENTOFACIAL ANOMALIES		M26.4 M26.89	Malocclusion, unspecified Other dentofacial anomalies
524.9	UNSPECIFIED DENTOFACIAL ANOMALIES	➡	M26.9	Dentofacial anomaly, unspecified
525.0	EXFOLIATION OF TEETH DUE TO SYSTEMIC CAUSES	➡	K08.0	Exfoliation of teeth due to systemic causes
525.10	UNSPECIFIED ACQUIRED ABSENCE OF TEETH	◘ ◘ ◘ ◘ ◘ ◘ ◘ ◘ ◘ ◘	K08.101 K08.102 K08.103 K08.104 K08.109 K08.401 K08.402 K08.403 K08.404 K08.409	Complete loss of teeth, unspecified cause, class I Complete loss of teeth, unspecified cause, class II Complete loss of teeth, unspecified cause, class III Complete loss of teeth, unspecified cause, class IV Complete loss of teeth, unspecified cause, unspecified class Partial loss of teeth, unspecified cause, class I Partial loss of teeth, unspecified cause, class II Partial loss of teeth, unspecified cause, class III Partial loss of teeth, unspecified cause, class IV Partial loss of teeth, unspecified cause, unspecified class
525.11	LOSS OF TEETH DUE TO TRAUMA	◘ ◘ ◘ ◘ ◘ ◘ ◘ ◘ ◘ ◘	K08.111 K08.112 K08.113 K08.114 K08.119 K08.411 K08.412 K08.413 K08.414 K08.419	Complete loss of teeth due to trauma, class I Complete loss of teeth due to trauma, class II Complete loss of teeth due to trauma, class III Complete loss of teeth due to trauma, class IV Complete loss of teeth due to trauma, unspecified class Partial loss of teeth due to trauma, class I Partial loss of teeth due to trauma, class II Partial loss of teeth due to trauma, class III Partial loss of teeth due to trauma, class IV Partial loss of teeth due to trauma, unspecified class
525.12	LOSS OF TEETH DUE TO PERIODONTAL DISEASE	◘ ◘ ◘ ◘ ◘ ◘ ◘ ◘ ◘ ◘	K08.121 K08.122 K08.123 K08.124 K08.129 K08.421 K08.422 K08.423 K08.424 K08.429	Complete loss of teeth due to periodontal diseases, class I Complete loss of teeth due to periodontal diseases, class II Complete loss of teeth due to periodontal dis, class III Complete loss of teeth due to periodontal diseases, class IV Complete loss of teeth due to periodontal dis, unsp class Partial loss of teeth due to periodontal diseases, class I Partial loss of teeth due to periodontal diseases, class II Partial loss of teeth due to periodontal diseases, class III Partial loss of teeth due to periodontal diseases, class IV Partial loss of teeth due to periodontal dis, unsp class
525.13	LOSS OF TEETH DUE TO CARIES	◘ ◘ ◘ ◘ ◘ ◘ ◘ ◘ ◘ ◘	K08.131 K08.132 K08.133 K08.134 K08.139 K08.431 K08.432 K08.433 K08.434 K08.439	Complete loss of teeth due to caries, class I Complete loss of teeth due to caries, class II Complete loss of teeth due to caries, class III Complete loss of teeth due to caries, class IV Complete loss of teeth due to caries, unspecified class Partial loss of teeth due to caries, class I Partial loss of teeth due to caries, class II Partial loss of teeth due to caries, class III Partial loss of teeth due to caries, class IV Partial loss of teeth due to caries, unspecified class

ICD-9-CM		ICD-10-CM	
525.19	OTHER LOSS OF TEETH	K08.191	Complete loss of teeth due to other specified cause, class I
		K08.192	Complete loss of teeth due to oth cause, class II
		K08.193	Complete loss of teeth due to oth cause, class III
		K08.194	Complete loss of teeth due to oth cause, class IV
		K08.199	Complete loss of teeth due to oth cause, unspecified class
		K08.491	Partial loss of teeth due to other specified cause, class I
		K08.492	Partial loss of teeth due to other specified cause, class II
		K08.493	Partial loss of teeth due to oth cause, class III
		K08.494	Partial loss of teeth due to other specified cause, class IV
		K08.499	Partial loss of teeth due to oth cause, unspecified class
525.20	UNSPECIFIED ATROPHY OF EDENTULOUS ALVEOLAR RIDGE	K08.20	Unspecified atrophy of edentulous alveolar ridge
525.21	MINIMAL ATROPHY OF THE MANDIBLE	K08.21	Minimal atrophy of the mandible
525.22	MODERATE ATROPHY OF THE MANDIBLE	K08.22	Moderate atrophy of the mandible
525.23	SEVERE ATROPHY OF THE MANDIBLE	K08.23	Severe atrophy of the mandible
525.24	MINIMAL ATROPHY OF THE MAXILLA	K08.24	Minimal atrophy of maxilla
525.25	MODERATE ATROPHY OF THE MAXILLA	K08.25	Moderate atrophy of the maxilla
525.26	SEVERE ATROPHY OF THE MAXILLA	K08.26	Severe atrophy of the maxilla
525.3	RETAINED DENTAL ROOT	K08.3	Retained dental root
525.40	COMPLETE EDENTULISM UNSPECIFIED	K08.109	Complete loss of teeth, unspecified cause, unspecified class
		K08.119	Complete loss of teeth due to trauma, unspecified class
		K08.129	Complete loss of teeth due to periodontal dis, unsp class
		K08.139	Complete loss of teeth due to caries, unspecified class
		K08.199	Complete loss of teeth due to oth cause, unspecified class
525.41	COMPLETE EDENTULISM CLASS I	K08.101	Complete loss of teeth, unspecified cause, class I
		K08.111	Complete loss of teeth due to trauma, class I
		K08.121	Complete loss of teeth due to periodontal diseases, class I
		K08.131	Complete loss of teeth due to caries, class I
		K08.191	Complete loss of teeth due to other specified cause, class I
525.42	COMPLETE EDENTULISM CLASS II	K08.102	Complete loss of teeth, unspecified cause, class II
		K08.112	Complete loss of teeth due to trauma, class II
		K08.122	Complete loss of teeth due to periodontal diseases, class II
		K08.132	Complete loss of teeth due to caries, class II
		K08.192	Complete loss of teeth due to oth cause, class II
525.43	COMPLETE EDENTULISM CLASS III	K08.103	Complete loss of teeth, unspecified cause, class III
		K08.113	Complete loss of teeth due to trauma, class III
		K08.123	Complete loss of teeth due to periodontal dis, class III
		K08.133	Complete loss of teeth due to caries, class III
		K08.193	Complete loss of teeth due to oth cause, class III
525.44	COMPLETE EDENTULISM CLASS IV	K08.104	Complete loss of teeth, unspecified cause, class IV
		K08.114	Complete loss of teeth due to trauma, class IV
		K08.124	Complete loss of teeth due to periodontal diseases, class IV
		K08.134	Complete loss of teeth due to caries, class IV
		K08.194	Complete loss of teeth due to oth cause, class IV
525.50	PARTIAL EDENTULISM UNSPECIFIED	K08.409	Partial loss of teeth, unspecified cause, unspecified class
		K08.419	Partial loss of teeth due to trauma, unspecified class
		K08.429	Partial loss of teeth due to periodontal dis, unsp class
		K08.439	Partial loss of teeth due to caries, unspecified class
		K08.499	Partial loss of teeth due to oth cause, unspecified class
525.51	PARTIAL EDENTULISM CLASS I	K08.401	Partial loss of teeth, unspecified cause, class I
		K08.411	Partial loss of teeth due to trauma, class I
		K08.421	Partial loss of teeth due to periodontal diseases, class I
		K08.431	Partial loss of teeth due to caries, class I
		K08.491	Partial loss of teeth due to other specified cause, class I
525.52	PARTIAL EDENTULISM CLASS II	K08.402	Partial loss of teeth, unspecified cause, class II
		K08.412	Partial loss of teeth due to trauma, class II
		K08.422	Partial loss of teeth due to periodontal diseases, class II
		K08.432	Partial loss of teeth due to caries, class II
		K08.492	Partial loss of teeth due to other specified cause, class II
525.53	PARTIAL EDENTULISM CLASS III	K08.403	Partial loss of teeth, unspecified cause, class III
		K08.413	Partial loss of teeth due to trauma, class III
		K08.423	Partial loss of teeth due to periodontal diseases, class III
		K08.433	Partial loss of teeth due to caries, class III
		K08.493	Partial loss of teeth due to oth cause, class III
525.54	PARTIAL EDENTULISM CLASS IV	K08.404	Partial loss of teeth, unspecified cause, class IV
		K08.414	Partial loss of teeth due to trauma, class IV
		K08.424	Partial loss of teeth due to periodontal diseases, class IV
		K08.434	Partial loss of teeth due to caries, class IV
		K08.494	Partial loss of teeth due to other specified cause, class IV
525.60	UNSPECIFIED UNSATISFACTORY RESTORATION OF TOOTH	K08.50	Unsatisfactory restoration of tooth, unspecified
525.61	OPEN RESTORATION MARGINS	K08.51	Open restoration margins of tooth
525.62	UNREPAIRABLE OVERHANGING DENTAL RESTORATIVE MATL	K08.52	Unrepairable overhanging of dental restorative materials
525.63	FX DENTAL RESTORATIVE MATERIAL W/O LOSS MATERIAL	K08.530	Fractured dental restorative material w/o loss of material
525.64	FX DENTAL RESTORATIVE MATERIAL W/LOSS MATERIAL	K08.531	Fractured dental restorative material with loss of material
525.65	CONTOUR EXIST REST TOOTH BIOL INCOMPAT ORAL HEA	K08.54	Contour of exist restor of tooth biolog incompat w oral hlth

[Brackets] indicate valid character values for each code. Character value meanings provided for each code grouping.

ICD-9-CM			ICD-10-CM	
525.66	ALLERGY TO EXISTING DENTAL RESTORATIVE MATERIAL	➡	**K08.55**	Allergy to existing dental restorative material
525.67	POOR AESTHETICS OF EXISTING RESTORATION	➡	**K08.56**	Poor aesthetic of existing restoration of tooth
525.69	OTHER UNSATISFACTORY RESTORATION OF EXIST TOOTH		**K08.539** **K08.59**	Fractured dental restorative material, unspecified Other unsatisfactory restoration of tooth
525.71	OSSEOINTEGRATION FAILURE OF DENTAL IMPLANT	➡	**M27.61**	Osseointegration failure of dental implant
525.72	POST-OSSEOINTGR BIOLOGICAL FAIL DENTAL IMPLANT	➡	**M27.62**	Post-osseointegration biological failure of dental implant
525.73	POST-OSSEOINTGR MECH FAIL DENTAL IMPLANT	➡	**M27.63**	Post-osseointegration mechanical failure of dental implant
525.79	OTHER ENDOSSEOUS DENTAL IMPLANT FAILURE	➡	**M27.69**	Other endosseous dental implant failure
525.8	OTHER SPEC DISORDERS TEETH&SUPPORTING STRUCTURES		**K08.8** **M26.79**	Other specified disorders of teeth and supporting structures Other specified alveolar anomalies
525.9	UNSPECIFIED DISORDER TEETH&SUPPORTING STRUCTURES	➡	**K08.9**	Disorder of teeth and supporting structures, unspecified
526.0	DEVELOPMENTAL ODONTOGENIC CYSTS	➡	**K09.0**	Developmental odontogenic cysts
526.1	FISSURAL CYSTS OF JAW		**K09.1**	Developmental (nonodontogenic) cysts of oral region
526.2	OTHER CYSTS OF JAWS		**M27.40** **M27.49**	Unspecified cyst of jaw Other cysts of jaw
526.3	CENTRAL GIANT CELL GRANULOMA	➡	**M27.1**	Giant cell granuloma, central
526.4	INFLAMMATORY CONDITIONS OF JAW	➡	**M27.2**	Inflammatory conditions of jaws
526.5	ALVEOLITIS OF JAW	➡	**M27.3**	Alveolitis of jaws
526.61	PERFORATION OF ROOT CANAL SPACE	➡	**M27.51**	Perforation of root canal space due to endodontic treatment
526.62	ENDODONTIC OVERFILL	➡	**M27.52**	Endodontic overfill
526.63	ENDODONTIC UNDERFILL	➡	**M27.53**	Endodontic underfill
526.69	OTH PERIRADICULAR PATH ASSOC W/PREVIOUS ENDO TX	➡	**M27.59**	Oth periradicular pathology assoc w prev endodontic trtmt
526.81	EXOSTOSIS OF JAW		**M27.8**	Other specified diseases of jaws
526.89	OTHER SPECIFIED DISEASE OF THE JAWS		**M27.8**	Other specified diseases of jaws
526.9	UNSPECIFIED DISEASE OF THE JAWS		**M27.0** **M27.9**	Developmental disorders of jaws Disease of jaws, unspecified
527.0	ATROPHY OF SALIVARY GLAND	➡	**K11.0**	Atrophy of salivary gland
527.1	HYPERTROPHY OF SALIVARY GLAND	➡	**K11.1**	Hypertrophy of salivary gland
527.2	SIALOADENITIS		**K11.20** **K11.21** **K11.22** **K11.23**	Sialoadenitis, unspecified Acute sialoadenitis Acute recurrent sialoadenitis Chronic sialoadenitis
527.3	ABSCESS OF SALIVARY GLAND	➡	**K11.3**	Abscess of salivary gland
527.4	FISTULA OF SALIVARY GLAND	➡	**K11.4**	Fistula of salivary gland
527.5	SIALOLITHIASIS	➡	**K11.5**	Sialolithiasis
527.6	MUCOCELE OF SALIVARY GLAND	➡	**K11.6**	Mucocele of salivary gland
527.7	DISTURBANCE OF SALIVARY SECRETION		**K11.7** **R68.2**	Disturbances of salivary secretion Dry mouth, unspecified
527.8	OTHER SPECIFIED DISEASES OF THE SALIVARY GLANDS		**K11.8**	Other diseases of salivary glands
527.9	UNSPECIFIED DISEASE OF THE SALIVARY GLANDS	➡	**K11.9**	Disease of salivary gland, unspecified
528.00	STOMATITIS AND MUCOSITIS UNSPECIFIED		**K12.2** **K12.30**	Cellulitis and abscess of mouth Oral mucositis (ulcerative), unspecified
528.01	MUCOSITIS DUE TO ANTINEOPLASTIC THERAPY		**K12.31** **K12.33**	Oral mucositis (ulcerative) due to antineoplastic therapy Oral mucositis (ulcerative) due to radiation
528.02	MUCOSITIS ULCERATIVE DUE TO OTHER DRUGS	➡	**K12.32**	Oral mucositis (ulcerative) due to other drugs
528.09	OTHER STOMATITIS AND MUCOSITIS ULCERATIVE		**K12.1** **K12.39**	Other forms of stomatitis Other oral mucositis (ulcerative)
528.1	CANCRUM ORIS		**A69.0**	Necrotizing ulcerative stomatitis
528.2	ORAL APHTHAE	➡	**K12.0**	Recurrent oral aphthae
528.3	CELLULITIS AND ABSCESS OF ORAL SOFT TISSUES		**K12.2**	Cellulitis and abscess of mouth
528.4	CYSTS OF ORAL SOFT TISSUES		**K09.8** **K09.9**	Other cysts of oral region, not elsewhere classified Cyst of oral region, unspecified
528.5	DISEASES OF LIPS	➡	**K13.0**	Diseases of lips
528.6	LEUKOPLAKIA OF ORAL MUCOSA INCLUDING TONGUE		**K13.21** **K13.3**	Leukoplakia of oral mucosa, including tongue Hairy leukoplakia
528.71	MINIMAL KERATINIZED RESIDUAL RIDGE MUCOSA	➡	**K13.22**	Minimal keratinized residual ridge mucosa
528.72	EXCESSIVE KERATINIZED RESIDUAL RIDGE MUCOSA	➡	**K13.23**	Excessive keratinized residual ridge mucosa
528.79	OTH DISTURB ORAL EPITHELIUM INCLUDING TONGUE		**K13.24** **K13.29**	Leukokeratosis nicotina palati Other disturbances of oral epithelium, including tongue
528.8	ORAL SUBMUCOSAL FIBROSIS INCLUDING OF TONGUE	➡	**K13.5**	Oral submucous fibrosis
528.9	OTHER&UNSPECIFIED DISEASES THE ORAL SOFT TISSUES	▣ ▣	**E08.638** **E09.638** **K13.1** **K13.4** **K13.6** **K13.70** **K13.79**	Diabetes due to underlying condition w oth oral comp Drug/chem diabetes mellitus w oth oral complications Cheek and lip biting Granuloma and granuloma-like lesions of oral mucosa Irritative hyperplasia of oral mucosa Unspecified lesions of oral mucosa Other lesions of oral mucosa
529.0	GLOSSITIS	➡	**K14.0**	Glossitis
529.1	GEOGRAPHIC TONGUE	➡	**K14.1**	Geographic tongue
529.2	MEDIAN RHOMBOID GLOSSITIS	➡	**K14.2**	Median rhomboid glossitis

ICD-9-CM			ICD-10-CM		
529.3	HYPERTROPHY OF TONGUE PAPILLAE	➡	**K14.3**	Hypertrophy of tongue papillae	
529.4	ATROPHY OF TONGUE PAPILLAE	➡	**K14.4**	Atrophy of tongue papillae	
529.5	PLICATED TONGUE	➡	**K14.5**	Plicated tongue	
529.6	GLOSSODYNIA	➡	**K14.6**	Glossodynia	
529.8	OTHER SPECIFIED CONDITIONS OF THE TONGUE	➡	**K14.8**	Other diseases of tongue	
529.9	UNSPECIFIED CONDITION OF THE TONGUE	➡	**K14.9**	Disease of tongue, unspecified	
530.0	ACHALASIA AND CARDIOSPASM		**K22.0**	Achalasia of cardia	
530.10	UNSPECIFIED ESOPHAGITIS		**K20.9**	Esophagitis, unspecified	
530.11	REFLUX ESOPHAGITIS	➡	**K21.0**	Gastro-esophageal reflux disease with esophagitis	
530.12	ACUTE ESOPHAGITIS		**K20.9**	Esophagitis, unspecified	
530.13	EOSINOPHILIC ESOPHAGITIS	➡	**K20.0**	Eosinophilic esophagitis	
530.19	OTHER ESOPHAGITIS	➡	**K20.8**	Other esophagitis	
530.20	ULCER OF ESOPHAGUS WITHOUT BLEEDING	➡	**K22.10**	Ulcer of esophagus without bleeding	
530.21	ULCER OF ESOPHAGUS WITH BLEEDING	➡	**K22.11**	Ulcer of esophagus with bleeding	
530.3	STRICTURE AND STENOSIS OF ESOPHAGUS	➡	**K22.2**	Esophageal obstruction	
530.4	PERFORATION OF ESOPHAGUS	➡	**K22.3**	Perforation of esophagus	
530.5	DYSKINESIA OF ESOPHAGUS	➡	**K22.4**	Dyskinesia of esophagus	
530.6	DIVERTICULUM OF ESOPHAGUS, ACQUIRED	➡	**K22.5**	Diverticulum of esophagus, acquired	
530.7	GASTROESOPHAGEAL LACERATION-HEMORRHAGE SYNDROME	➡	**K22.6**	Gastro-esophageal laceration-hemorrhage syndrome	
530.81	ESOPHAGEAL REFLUX	➡	**K21.9**	Gastro-esophageal reflux disease without esophagitis	
530.82	ESOPHAGEAL HEMORRHAGE		**K22.8**	Other specified diseases of esophagus	
530.83	ESOPHAGEAL LEUKOPLAKIA		**K22.8**	Other specified diseases of esophagus	
530.84	TRACHEOESOPHAGEAL FISTULA		**J86.0**	Pyothorax with fistula	
530.85	BARRETTS ESOPHAGUS		**K22.70** **K22.710** **K22.711** **K22.719**	Barrett's esophagus without dysplasia Barrett's esophagus with low grade dysplasia Barrett's esophagus with high grade dysplasia Barrett's esophagus with dysplasia, unspecified	
530.86	INFECTION OF ESOPHAGOSTOMY	➡	**K94.32**	Esophagostomy infection	
530.87	MECHANICAL COMPLICATION OF ESOPHAGOSTOMY		**K94.30** **K94.31** **K94.33** **K94.39**	Esophagostomy complications, unspecified Esophagostomy hemorrhage Esophagostomy malfunction Other complications of esophagostomy	
530.89	OTHER SPECIFIED DISORDER OF THE ESOPHAGUS		**K22.8** **K23**	Other specified diseases of esophagus Disorders of esophagus in diseases classified elsewhere	
530.9	UNSPECIFIED DISORDER OF ESOPHAGUS	➡	**K22.9**	Disease of esophagus, unspecified	
531.00	ACUT GASTR ULCER W/HEMORR W/O MENTION OBST		**K25.0**	Acute gastric ulcer with hemorrhage	
531.01	ACUTE GASTRIC ULCER W/HEMORRHAGE AND OBSTRUCTION		**K25.0** **K56.60**	Acute gastric ulcer with hemorrhage Unspecified intestinal obstruction	*and*
531.10	ACUT GASTR ULCER W/PERF W/O MENTION OBSTRUCTION		**K25.1**	Acute gastric ulcer with perforation	
531.11	ACUTE GASTRIC ULCER W/PERFORATION&OBSTRUCTION		**K25.1** **K56.60**	Acute gastric ulcer with perforation Unspecified intestinal obstruction	*and*
531.20	ACUT GASTR ULCER W/HEMORR&PERF W/O MENTION OBST		**K25.2**	Acute gastric ulcer with both hemorrhage and perforation	
531.21	ACUTE GASTRIC ULCER W/HEMORR PERF&OBSTRUCTION		**K25.2** **K56.60**	Acute gastric ulcer with both hemorrhage and perforation Unspecified intestinal obstruction	*and*
531.30	ACUT GASTR ULCER W/O MENTION HEMORR PERF/OBST		**K25.3**	Acute gastric ulcer without hemorrhage or perforation	
531.31	ACUT GASTR ULCER W/O MENTION HEMORR/PERF W/OBST		**K25.3** **K56.60**	Acute gastric ulcer without hemorrhage or perforation Unspecified intestinal obstruction	*and*
531.40	CHRON/UNS GASTR ULCR W/HEMORR W/O MENTION OBST		**K25.4**	Chronic or unspecified gastric ulcer with hemorrhage	
531.41	CHRON/UNSPEC GASTRIC ULCER W/HEMORR&OBSTRUCTION		**K25.4** **K56.60**	Chronic or unspecified gastric ulcer with hemorrhage Unspecified intestinal obstruction	*and*
531.50	CHRON/UNSPEC GASTR ULCER W/PERF W/O MENTION OBST		**K25.5**	Chronic or unspecified gastric ulcer with perforation	
531.51	CHRONIC/UNSPEC GASTRIC ULCER W/PERF&OBSTRUCTION		**K25.5** **K56.60**	Chronic or unspecified gastric ulcer with perforation Unspecified intestinal obstruction	*and*
531.60	CHRN/UNS GASTR ULCR W/HEMORR&PERF W/O OBST		**K25.6**	Chronic or unsp gastric ulcer w both hemorrhage and perf	
531.61	CHRON/UNSPEC GASTR ULCER W/HEMORR PERF&OBST		**K25.6** **K56.60**	Chronic or unsp gastric ulcer w both hemorrhage and perf Unspecified intestinal obstruction	*and*
531.70	CHRN GASTR ULCR W/O HEMOR PERF W/O OBST		**K25.7**	Chronic gastric ulcer without hemorrhage or perforation	
531.71	CHRON GASTR ULCER W/O MENTION HEMORR/PERF W/OBST		**K25.7** **K56.60**	Chronic gastric ulcer without hemorrhage or perforation Unspecified intestinal obstruction	*and*
531.90	GASTR ULCR UNS ACUT/CHRN W/O HEMOR PERF/OBST		**K25.9**	Gastric ulcer, unsp as acute or chronic, w/o hemor or perf	
531.91	GASTR ULCR UNS ACUT/CHRN W/O HEMOR/PERF W/OBST		**K25.9** **K56.60**	Gastric ulcer, unsp as acute or chronic, w/o hemor or perf Unspecified intestinal obstruction	*and*
532.00	ACUT DUOD ULCER W/HEMORR W/O MENTION OBSTRUCTION		**K26.0**	Acute duodenal ulcer with hemorrhage	
532.01	ACUTE DUODENAL ULCER W/HEMORRHAGE&OBSTRUCTION		**K26.0** **K56.60**	Acute duodenal ulcer with hemorrhage Unspecified intestinal obstruction	*and*
532.10	ACUT DUODEN ULCER W/PERF W/O MENTION OBSTRUCTION		**K26.1**	Acute duodenal ulcer with perforation	

[Brackets] indicate valid character values for each code. Character value meanings provided for each code grouping.

ICD-9-CM		ICD-10-CM		
532.11	ACUTE DUODENAL ULCER W/PERFORATION&OBSTRUCTION	**K26.1**	Acute duodenal ulcer with perforation	*and*
		K56.6Ø	Unspecified intestinal obstruction	
532.2Ø	ACUT DUOD ULCER W/HEMORR&PERF W/O MENTION OBST	**K26.2**	Acute duodenal ulcer with both hemorrhage and perforation	
532.21	ACUTE DUODEN ULCER W/HEMORR PERF&OBSTRUCTION	**K26.2**	Acute duodenal ulcer with both hemorrhage and perforation	*and*
		K56.6Ø	Unspecified intestinal obstruction	
532.3Ø	ACUT DUOD ULCER W/O MENTION HEMORR PERF/OBST	**K26.3**	Acute duodenal ulcer without hemorrhage or perforation	
532.31	ACUT DUOD ULCER W/O MENTION HEMORR/PERF W/OBST	**K26.3**	Acute duodenal ulcer without hemorrhage or perforation	*and*
		K56.6Ø	Unspecified intestinal obstruction	
532.4Ø	CHRON/UNSPEC DUOD ULCR W/HEMORR W/O MENTION OBST	**K26.4**	Chronic or unspecified duodenal ulcer with hemorrhage	
532.41	CHRONIC/UNSPEC DUODEN ULCER W/HEMORR&OBSTRUCTION	**K26.4**	Chronic or unspecified duodenal ulcer with hemorrhage	*and*
		K56.6Ø	Unspecified intestinal obstruction	
532.5Ø	CHRON/UNSPEC DUOD ULCER W/PERF W/O MENTION OBST	**K26.5**	Chronic or unspecified duodenal ulcer with perforation	
532.51	CHRONIC/UNSPEC DUODEN ULCER W/PERF&OBSTRUCTION	**K26.5**	Chronic or unspecified duodenal ulcer with perforation	*and*
		K56.6Ø	Unspecified intestinal obstruction	
532.6Ø	CHRN/UNS DUOD ULCR W/HEMORR&PERF W/O OBST	**K26.6**	Chronic or unsp duodenal ulcer w both hemorrhage and perf	
532.61	CHRON/UNSPEC DUOD ULCER W/HEMORR PERF&OBST	**K26.6**	Chronic or unsp duodenal ulcer w both hemorrhage and perf	*and*
		K56.6Ø	Unspecified intestinal obstruction	
532.7Ø	CHRON DUOD ULCER W/O MENTION HEMORR PERF/OBST	**K26.7**	Chronic duodenal ulcer without hemorrhage or perforation	
532.71	CHRON DUOD ULCER W/O MENTION HEMORR/PERF W/OBST	**K26.7**	Chronic duodenal ulcer without hemorrhage or perforation	*and*
		K56.6Ø	Unspecified intestinal obstruction	
532.9Ø	DUOD ULCR UNS AS ACUT/CHRON W/O HEMORR PERF/OBST	**K26.9**	Duodenal ulcer, unsp as acute or chronic, w/o hemor or perf	
532.91	DUOD ULCR UNS ACUT/CHRN W/O HEMOR/PERF W/OBST	**K26.9**	Duodenal ulcer, unsp as acute or chronic, w/o hemor or perf	*and*
		K56.6Ø	Unspecified intestinal obstruction	
533.ØØ	ACUT PEPTC ULCR UNS SITE W/HEM W/O MENTION OBST	**K27.Ø**	Acute peptic ulcer, site unspecified, with hemorrhage	
533.Ø1	ACUT PEPTIC ULCER UNSPEC SITE W/HEMORR&OBST	**K27.Ø**	Acute peptic ulcer, site unspecified, with hemorrhage	
533.1Ø	ACUT PEPTC ULCR UNS SITE W/PERF W/O MENTION OBST	**K27.1**	Acute peptic ulcer, site unspecified, with perforation	
533.11	ACUT PEPTIC ULCER UNSPEC SITE W/PERF&OBSTRUCTION	**K27.1**	Acute peptic ulcer, site unspecified, with perforation	
533.2Ø	ACUT PEPTC ULCR UNS SITE W/HEMORR&PERF W/O OBST	**K27.2**	Acute peptic ulcer, site unsp, w both hemorrhage and perf	
533.21	ACUT PEPTIC ULCER UNSPEC SITE W/HEMORR PERF&OBST	**K27.2**	Acute peptic ulcer, site unsp, w both hemorrhage and perf	
533.3Ø	ACUT PEPTC ULCR UNS SITE W/O HEMOR PERF/OBST	**K27.3**	Acute peptic ulcer, site unsp, w/o hemorrhage or perforation	
533.31	ACUT PEPTC ULCR UNS SITE W/O HEMOR&PERF W/OBST	**K27.3**	Acute peptic ulcer, site unsp, w/o hemorrhage or perforation	
533.4Ø	CHRN/UNS PEPTC ULCR UNS SITE W/HEM W/O OBST	**K27.4**	Chronic or unsp peptic ulcer, site unsp, with hemorrhage	
533.41	CHRON/UNS PEPTC ULCR UNS SITE W/HEMORR&OBST	**K27.4**	Chronic or unsp peptic ulcer, site unsp, with hemorrhage	
533.5Ø	CHRN/UNS PEPTC ULCR UNS SITE W/PERF W/O OBST	**K27.5**	Chronic or unsp peptic ulcer, site unsp, with perforation	
533.51	CHRON/UNSPEC PEPTC ULCER UNSPEC SITE W/PERF&OBST	**K27.5**	Chronic or unsp peptic ulcer, site unsp, with perforation	
533.6Ø	CHRN/UNS PEPTC ULCR W/HEMORR&PERF W/O OBST	**K27.6**	Chr or unsp peptic ulcer, site unsp, w both hemor and perf	
533.61	CHRON/UNS PEPTC ULCR UNS SITE W/HEMORR PERF&OBST	**K27.6**	Chr or unsp peptic ulcer, site unsp, w both hemor and perf	
533.7Ø	CHRN PEPTC ULCR UNS SITE W/O HEMOR PERF/OBST	**K27.7**	Chronic peptic ulcer, site unsp, w/o hemorrhage or perf	
533.71	CHRN PEPTC ULCR UNS SITE W/O HEMOR/PERF W/OBST	**K27.7**	Chronic peptic ulcer, site unsp, w/o hemorrhage or perf	
533.9Ø	PEPTC ULCR UNS ACUT/CHRN W/O HEMOR PERF/OBST	**K27.9**	Peptic ulc, site unsp, unsp as ac or chr, w/o hemor or perf	
533.91	PEPTC ULCR UNS ACUT/CHRN W/O HEMOR/PERF W/OBST	**K27.9**	Peptic ulc, site unsp, unsp as ac or chr, w/o hemor or perf	
534.ØØ	ACUT GASTROJEJUN ULCER W/HEMORR W/O MENTION OBST	**K28.Ø**	Acute gastrojejunal ulcer with hemorrhage	
534.Ø1	ACUTE GASTROJEJUN ULCER W/HEMORRHAGE&OBSTRUCTION	**K28.Ø**	Acute gastrojejunal ulcer with hemorrhage	
534.1Ø	ACUT GASTROJEJUN ULCER W/PERF W/O MENTION OBST	**K28.1**	Acute gastrojejunal ulcer with perforation	
534.11	ACUTE GASTROJEJUN ULCER W/PERF&OBSTRUCTION	**K28.1**	Acute gastrojejunal ulcer with perforation	
534.2Ø	ACUT GASTROJEJ ULCR W/HEMORR&PERF W/O OBST	**K28.2**	Acute gastrojejunal ulcer w both hemorrhage and perforation	
534.21	ACUT GASTROJEJUN ULCER W/HEMORR PERF&OBSTRUCTION	**K28.2**	Acute gastrojejunal ulcer w both hemorrhage and perforation	
534.3Ø	ACUT GASTROJEJ ULCR W/O MENTION HEMOR PERF/OBST	**K28.3**	Acute gastrojejunal ulcer without hemorrhage or perforation	
534.31	ACUT GASTROJEJ ULCR W/O HEMOR/PERF W/OBST	**K28.3**	Acute gastrojejunal ulcer without hemorrhage or perforation	
534.4Ø	CHRN/UNS GASTROJEJ ULCR W/HEM W/O MENTION OBST	**K28.4**	Chronic or unspecified gastrojejunal ulcer with hemorrhage	
534.41	CHRON/UNSPEC GASTROJEJUN ULCER W/HEMORR&OBST	**K28.4**	Chronic or unspecified gastrojejunal ulcer with hemorrhage	
534.5Ø	CHRN/UNS GASTROJEJ ULCR W/PERF W/O MENTION OBST	**K28.5**	Chronic or unspecified gastrojejunal ulcer with perforation	
534.51	CHRON/UNSPEC GASTROJEJUN ULCER W/PERF&OBST	**K28.5**	Chronic or unspecified gastrojejunal ulcer with perforation	
534.6Ø	CHRN/UNS GASTROJEJ ULCR W/HEMORR&PERF W/O OBST	**K28.6**	Chronic or unsp gastrojejunal ulcer w both hemor and perf	
534.61	CHRON/UNSPEC GASTROJEJUN ULCR W/HEMORR PERF&OBST	**K28.6**	Chronic or unsp gastrojejunal ulcer w both hemor and perf	
534.7Ø	CHRN GASTROJEJ ULCR W/O MENTION HEMOR PERF/OBST	**K28.7**	Chronic gastrojejunal ulcer w/o hemorrhage or perforation	
534.71	CHRN GASTROJEJ ULCR W/O HEMOR/PERF W/OBST	**K28.7**	Chronic gastrojejunal ulcer w/o hemorrhage or perforation	
534.9Ø	GASTROJEJ ULCR UNS ACUT/CHRN W/O HEMOR PERF/OBST	**K28.9**	Gastrojejunal ulcer, unsp as acute or chr, w/o hemor or perf	
534.91	GASTROJEJ ULCR UNS AC/CHRN W/O HEMOR/PERF W/OBST	**K28.9**	Gastrojejunal ulcer, unsp as acute or chr, w/o hemor or perf	
535.ØØ	ACUTE GASTRITIS WITHOUT MENTION OF HEMORRHAGE	➡ **K29.ØØ**	Acute gastritis without bleeding	
535.Ø1	ACUTE GASTRITIS WITH HEMORRHAGE	➡ **K29.Ø1**	Acute gastritis with bleeding	
535.1Ø	ATROPHIC GASTRITIS WITHOUT MENTION OF HEMORRHAGE	**K29.3Ø**	Chronic superficial gastritis without bleeding	
		K29.4Ø	Chronic atrophic gastritis without bleeding	
		K29.5Ø	Unspecified chronic gastritis without bleeding	

ICD-9-CM			ICD-10-CM	
535.11	ATROPHIC GASTRITIS WITH HEMORRHAGE		K29.31 K29.41 K29.51	Chronic superficial gastritis with bleeding Chronic atrophic gastritis with bleeding Unspecified chronic gastritis with bleeding
535.20	GASTRIC MUCOS HYPERTROPHY WITHOUT MENTION HEMORR		K29.60	Other gastritis without bleeding
535.21	GASTRIC MUCOSAL HYPERTROPHY WITH HEMORRHAGE		K29.61	Other gastritis with bleeding
535.30	ALCOHOLIC GASTRITIS WITHOUT MENTION HEMORRHAGE	➡	K29.20	Alcoholic gastritis without bleeding
535.31	ALCOHOLIC GASTRITIS WITH HEMORRHAGE	➡	K29.21	Alcoholic gastritis with bleeding
535.40	OTHER SPEC GASTRITIS WITHOUT MENTION HEMORRHAGE		K29.30 K29.60	Chronic superficial gastritis without bleeding Other gastritis without bleeding
535.41	OTHER SPECIFIED GASTRITIS WITH HEMORRHAGE		K29.31 K29.61	Chronic superficial gastritis with bleeding Other gastritis with bleeding
535.50	UNS GASTRITIS&GASTRODUODITIS W/O MENTION HEMORR		K29.70 K29.90	Gastritis, unspecified, without bleeding Gastroduodenitis, unspecified, without bleeding
535.51	UNSPEC GASTRITIS&GASTRODUODENITIS W/HEMORRHAGE		K29.71 K29.91	Gastritis, unspecified, with bleeding Gastroduodenitis, unspecified, with bleeding
535.60	DUODENITIS WITHOUT MENTION OF HEMORRHAGE	➡	K29.80	Duodenitis without bleeding
535.61	DUODENITIS WITH HEMORRHAGE	➡	K29.81	Duodenitis with bleeding
535.70	EOSINOPHILIC GASTRITIS W/O MENTION OF HEMORRHAGE		K52.81	Eosinophilic gastritis or gastroenteritis
535.71	EOSINOPHILIC GASTRITIS WITH HEMORRHAGE		K52.81	Eosinophilic gastritis or gastroenteritis
536.0	ACHLORHYDRIA	➡	K31.83	Achlorhydria
536.1	ACUTE DILATATION OF STOMACH	➡	K31.0	Acute dilatation of stomach
536.2	PERSISTENT VOMITING		R11.10	Vomiting, unspecified
536.3	GASTROPARESIS	⚑ ⚑ ⚑ ⚑ ⚑	E08.43 E09.43 E10.43 E11.43 E13.43 K31.84	Diab due to undrl cond w diabetic autonm (poly)neuropathy Drug/chem diab w neuro comp w diab autonm (poly)neuropathy Type 1 diabetes w diabetic autonomic (poly)neuropathy Type 2 diabetes w diabetic autonomic (poly)neuropathy Oth diabetes mellitus w diabetic autonomic (poly)neuropathy Gastroparesis
536.40	UNSPECIFIED GASTROSTOMY COMPLICATION	➡	K94.20	Gastrostomy complication, unspecified
536.41	INFECTION OF GASTROSTOMY	➡	K94.22	Gastrostomy infection
536.42	MECHANICAL COMPLICATION OF GASTROSTOMY	➡	K94.23	Gastrostomy malfunction
536.49	OTHER GASTROSTOMY COMPLICATIONS		K94.21 K94.29	Gastrostomy hemorrhage Other complications of gastrostomy
536.8	DYSPEPSIA&OTHER SPEC DISORDERS FUNCTION STOMACH	➡	K30	Functional dyspepsia
536.9	UNSPECIFIED FUNCTIONAL DISORDER OF STOMACH		K31.89 K31.9	Other diseases of stomach and duodenum Disease of stomach and duodenum, unspecified
537.0	ACQUIRED HYPERTROPHIC PYLORIC STENOSIS	➡	K31.1	Adult hypertrophic pyloric stenosis
537.1	GASTRIC DIVERTICULUM	➡	K31.4	Gastric diverticulum
537.2	CHRONIC DUODENAL ILEUS		K31.5	Obstruction of duodenum
537.3	OTHER OBSTRUCTION OF DUODENUM		K31.5	Obstruction of duodenum
537.4	FISTULA OF STOMACH OR DUODENUM	➡	K31.6	Fistula of stomach and duodenum
537.5	GASTROPTOSIS		K31.89	Other diseases of stomach and duodenum
537.6	HOURGLASS STRICTURE OR STENOSIS OF STOMACH	➡	K31.2	Hourglass stricture and stenosis of stomach
537.81	PYLOROSPASM	➡	K31.3	Pylorospasm, not elsewhere classified
537.82	ANGIODYSPLASIA OF STOMACH AND DUODENUM	➡	K31.819	Angiodysplasia of stomach and duodenum without bleeding
537.83	ANGIODYSPLASIA OF STOMACH&DUODENUM W/HEMORRHAGE	➡	K31.811	Angiodysplasia of stomach and duodenum with bleeding
537.84	DIEULAFOY LESION OF STOMACH AND DUODENUM	➡	K31.82	Dieulafoy lesion (hemorrhagic) of stomach and duodenum
537.89	OTHER SPECIFIED DISORDER OF STOMACH AND DUODENUM		K31.89	Other diseases of stomach and duodenum
537.9	UNSPECIFIED DISORDER OF STOMACH AND DUODENUM		K31.9	Disease of stomach and duodenum, unspecified
538	GASTROINTESTINAL MUCOSITIS ULCERATIVE	➡	K92.81	Gastrointestinal mucositis (ulcerative)
539.01	INFECTION DUE TO GASTRIC BAND PROCEDURE		K95.01	Infection due to gastric band procedure
539.09	OTHER COMPLICATIONS OF GASTRIC BAND PROCEDURE		K95.09	Other complications of gastric band procedure
539.81	INFECTION DUE TO OTHER BARIATRIC PROCEDURE		K95.81	Infection due to other bariatric procedure
539.89	OTHER COMPLICATIONS OF OTHER BARIATRIC PROCEDURE		K95.89	Other complications of other bariatric procedure
540.0	ACUTE APPENDICITIS WITH GENERALIZED PERITONITIS	➡	K35.2	Acute appendicitis with generalized peritonitis
540.1	ACUTE APPENDICITIS WITH PERITONEAL ABSCESS		K35.3	Acute appendicitis with localized peritonitis
540.9	ACUTE APPENDICITIS WITHOUT MENTION PERITONITIS		K35.80 K35.89	Unspecified acute appendicitis Other acute appendicitis
541	APPENDICITIS, UNQUALIFIED	➡	K37	Unspecified appendicitis
542	OTHER APPENDICITIS	➡	K36	Other appendicitis
543.0	HYPERPLASIA OF APPENDIX	➡	K38.0	Hyperplasia of appendix
543.9	OTHER AND UNSPECIFIED DISEASES OF APPENDIX		K38.1 K38.2 K38.3 K38.8 K38.9	Appendicular concretions Diverticulum of appendix Fistula of appendix Other specified diseases of appendix Disease of appendix, unspecified
550.00	INGUINAL HERNIA W/GANGRENE UNILATERAL/UNSPEC	➡	K40.40	Unil inguinal hernia, w gangrene, not specified as recurrent
550.01	ING HERN W/GANGREN RECUR UNILAT/UNSPEC ING HERN	➡	K40.41	Unilateral inguinal hernia, with gangrene, recurrent
550.02	INGUINAL HERNIA WITH GANGRENE BILATERAL	➡	K40.10	Bi inguinal hernia, w gangrene, not specified as recurrent
550.03	INGUINAL HERNIA W/GANGRENE RECURRENT BILATERAL	➡	K40.11	Bilateral inguinal hernia, with gangrene, recurrent

[Brackets] indicate valid character values for each code. Character value meanings provided for each code grouping.

ICD-9-CM			ICD-10-CM	
550.10	ING HERN W/OBST W/O MENTION GANGREN UNILAT/UNS	➡	**K40.30**	Unil inguinal hernia, w obst, w/o gangr, not spcf as recur
550.11	ING HERN W/OBST W/O GANGREN RECUR UNILAT/UNS	➡	**K40.31**	Unilateral inguinal hernia, w obst, w/o gangrene, recurrent
550.12	ING HERN W/OBSTRUCTION W/O MENTION GANGREN BILAT	➡	**K40.00**	Bi inguinal hernia, w obst, w/o gangrene, not spcf as recur
550.13	ING HERN W/OBST W/O MENTION GANGREN RECUR BILAT	➡	**K40.01**	Bilateral inguinal hernia, w obst, w/o gangrene, recurrent
550.90	ING HERN W/O MENTION OBST/GANGREN UNILAT/UNSPEC	➡	**K40.90**	Unil inguinal hernia, w/o obst or gangr, not spcf as recur
550.91	ING HERN W/O OBST/GANGREN RECUR UNILAT/UNS	➡	**K40.91**	Unilateral inguinal hernia, w/o obst or gangrene, recurrent
550.92	ING HERNIA W/O MENTION OBSTRUCTION/GANGREN BILAT	➡	**K40.20**	Bi inguinal hernia, w/o obst or gangrene, not spcf as recur
550.93	ING HERN W/O MENTION OBST/GANGREN RECUR BILAT	➡	**K40.21**	Bilateral inguinal hernia, w/o obst or gangrene, recurrent
551.00	FEMORAL HERNIA W/GANGRENE UNILATERAL/UNSPECIFIED	➡	**K41.40**	Unil femoral hernia, w gangrene, not specified as recurrent
551.01	FEMORAL HERNIA W/GANGRENE RECUR UNILAT/UNSPEC	➡	**K41.41**	Unilateral femoral hernia, with gangrene, recurrent
551.02	FEMORAL HERNIA WITH GANGRENE BILATERAL	➡	**K41.10**	Bi femoral hernia, w gangrene, not specified as recurrent
551.03	FEMORAL HERNIA WITH GANGRENE RECURRENT BILATERAL	➡	**K41.11**	Bilateral femoral hernia, with gangrene, recurrent
551.1	UMBILICAL HERNIA WITH GANGRENE	➡	**K42.1**	Umbilical hernia with gangrene
551.20	UNSPECIFIED VENTRAL HERNIA WITH GANGRENE		**K43.7**	Other and unspecified ventral hernia with gangrene
551.21	INCISIONAL VENTRAL HERNIA WITH GANGRENE		**K43.1**	Incisional hernia with gangrene
551.29	OTHER VENTRAL HERNIA WITH GANGRENE		**K43.4**	Parastomal hernia with gangrene
			K43.7	Other and unspecified ventral hernia with gangrene
551.3	DIAPHRAGMATIC HERNIA WITH GANGRENE	➡	**K44.1**	Diaphragmatic hernia with gangrene
551.8	HERNIA OF OTHER SPECIFIED SITES WITH GANGRENE	➡	**K45.1**	Other specified abdominal hernia with gangrene
551.9	HERNIA OF UNSPECIFIED SITE WITH GANGRENE	➡	**K46.1**	Unspecified abdominal hernia with gangrene
552.00	UNILATERAL/UNSPEC FEMORAL HERNIA W/OBSTRUCTION	➡	**K41.30**	Unil femoral hernia, w obst, w/o gangrene, not spcf as recur
552.01	RECUR UNILAT/UNSPEC FEMORAL HERNIA W/OBSTRUCTION	➡	**K41.31**	Unilateral femoral hernia, w obst, w/o gangrene, recurrent
552.02	BILATERAL FEMORAL HERNIA WITH OBSTRUCTION	➡	**K41.00**	Bi femoral hernia, w obst, w/o gangrene, not spcf as recur
552.03	RECURRENT BILATERAL FEMORAL HERNIA W/OBSTRUCTION	➡	**K41.01**	Bilateral femoral hernia, w obst, w/o gangrene, recurrent
552.1	UMBILICAL HERNIA WITH OBSTRUCTION	➡	**K42.0**	Umbilical hernia with obstruction, without gangrene
552.20	UNSPECIFIED VENTRAL HERNIA WITH OBSTRUCTION		**K43.6**	Other and unsp ventral hernia with obstruction, w/o gangrene
552.21	INCISIONAL HERNIA WITH OBSTRUCTION		**K43.0**	Incisional hernia with obstruction, without gangrene
552.29	OTHER VENTRAL HERNIA WITH OBSTRUCTION		**K43.3**	Parastomal hernia with obstruction, without gangrene
			K43.6	Other and unsp ventral hernia with obstruction, w/o gangrene
552.3	DIAPHRAGMATIC HERNIA WITH OBSTRUCTION	➡	**K44.0**	Diaphragmatic hernia with obstruction, without gangrene
552.8	HERNIA OF OTHER SPECIFIED SITE WITH OBSTRUCTION	➡	**K45.0**	Oth abdominal hernia with obstruction, without gangrene
552.9	HERNIA OF UNSPECIFIED SITE WITH OBSTRUCTION	➡	**K46.0**	Unsp abdominal hernia with obstruction, without gangrene
553.00	UNILAT/UNS FEM HERN W/O OBST/GANGREN UNILAT/UNS	➡	**K41.90**	Unil femoral hernia, w/o obst or gangrene, not spcf as recur
553.01	FEM HERN W/O OBST/GANGREN RECUR UNILAT/UNS	➡	**K41.91**	Unilateral femoral hernia, w/o obst or gangrene, recurrent
553.02	FEM HERNIA W/O MENTION OBSTRUCTION/GANGREN BILAT	➡	**K41.20**	Bi femoral hernia, w/o obst or gangrene, not spcf as recur
553.03	FEM HERN W/O MENTION OBST/GANGREN RECUR BILAT	➡	**K41.21**	Bilateral femoral hernia, w/o obst or gangrene, recurrent
553.1	UMB HERNIA WITHOUT MENTION OBSTRUCTION/GANGRENE	➡	**K42.9**	Umbilical hernia without obstruction or gangrene
553.20	UNSPEC VENTRAL HERN W/O MENTION OBST/GANGREN		**K43.9**	Ventral hernia without obstruction or gangrene
553.21	INCI HERNIA WITHOUT MENTION OBSTRUCTION/GANGRENE		**K43.2**	Incisional hernia without obstruction or gangrene
553.29	OTH VENTRAL HERN W/O MENTION OBSTRUCTION/GANGREN		**K43.5**	Parastomal hernia without obstruction or gangrene
			K43.9	Ventral hernia without obstruction or gangrene
			K46.9	Unspecified abdominal hernia without obstruction or gangrene
553.3	DIAPHRAGMAT HERN W/O MENTION OBSTRUCTION/GANGREN	➡	**K44.9**	Diaphragmatic hernia without obstruction or gangrene
553.8	HERN OTH SPEC SITE ABD CAV W/O OBST/GANGREN	➡	**K45.8**	Oth abdominal hernia without obstruction or gangrene
553.9	HERN UNS SITE ABD CAV W/O MENTION OBST/GANGREN		**K46.9**	Unspecified abdominal hernia without obstruction or gangrene
555.0	REGIONAL ENTERITIS OF SMALL INTESTINE		**K50.00**	Crohn's disease of small intestine without complications
			K50.011	Crohn's disease of small intestine with rectal bleeding
		⊡	**K50.012**	Crohn's disease of small intestine w intestinal obstruction
		⊡	**K50.013**	Crohn's disease of small intestine with fistula
		⊡	**K50.014**	Crohn's disease of small intestine with abscess
			K50.018	Crohn's disease of small intestine with other complication
			K50.019	Crohn's disease of small intestine with unsp complications
555.1	REGIONAL ENTERITIS OF LARGE INTESTINE		**K50.10**	Crohn's disease of large intestine without complications
			K50.111	Crohn's disease of large intestine with rectal bleeding
		⊡	**K50.112**	Crohn's disease of large intestine w intestinal obstruction
		⊡	**K50.113**	Crohn's disease of large intestine with fistula
		⊡	**K50.114**	Crohn's disease of large intestine with abscess
			K50.118	Crohn's disease of large intestine with other complication
			K50.119	Crohn's disease of large intestine with unsp complications
555.2	RGN ENTERITIS SMALL INTESTINE W/LG INTESTINE		**K50.80**	Crohn's disease of both small and lg int w/o complications
			K50.811	Crohn's disease of both small and lg int w rectal bleeding
		⊡	**K50.812**	Crohn's disease of both small and lg int w intestinal obst
		⊡	**K50.813**	Crohn's disease of both small and large intestine w fistula
		⊡	**K50.814**	Crohn's disease of both small and large intestine w abscess
			K50.818	Crohn's disease of both small and lg int w oth complication
			K50.819	Crohn's disease of both small and lg int w unsp comp

ICD-9-CM		ICD-10-CM	
555.9	REGIONAL ENTERITIS OF UNSPECIFIED SITE	K50.90	Crohn's disease, unspecified, without complications
		K50.911	Crohn's disease, unspecified, with rectal bleeding
		K50.912	Crohn's disease, unspecified, with intestinal obstruction
		K50.913	Crohn's disease, unspecified, with fistula
		K50.914	Crohn's disease, unspecified, with abscess
		K50.918	Crohn's disease, unspecified, with other complication
		K50.919	Crohn's disease, unspecified, with unspecified complications
556.0	ULCERATIVE ENTEROCOLITIS	K51.80	Other ulcerative colitis without complications
556.1	ULCERATIVE ILEOCOLITIS	K51.80	Other ulcerative colitis without complications
556.2	ULCERATIVE PROCTITIS	K51.20	Ulcerative (chronic) proctitis without complications
		K51.211	Ulcerative (chronic) proctitis with rectal bleeding
		K51.212	Ulcerative (chronic) proctitis with intestinal obstruction
		K51.213	Ulcerative (chronic) proctitis with fistula
		K51.214	Ulcerative (chronic) proctitis with abscess
		K51.218	Ulcerative (chronic) proctitis with other complication
		K51.219	Ulcerative (chronic) proctitis with unsp complications
556.3	ULCERATIVE PROCTOSIGMOIDITIS	K51.30	Ulcerative (chronic) rectosigmoiditis without complications
		K51.311	Ulcerative (chronic) rectosigmoiditis with rectal bleeding
		K51.312	Ulcerative (chronic) rectosigmoiditis w intestinal obst
		K51.313	Ulcerative (chronic) rectosigmoiditis with fistula
		K51.314	Ulcerative (chronic) rectosigmoiditis with abscess
		K51.318	Ulcerative (chronic) rectosigmoiditis with oth complication
		K51.319	Ulcerative (chronic) rectosigmoiditis w unsp complications
556.4	PSEUDOPOLYPOSIS OF COLON	K51.40	Inflammatory polyps of colon without complications
		K51.411	Inflammatory polyps of colon with rectal bleeding
		K51.412	Inflammatory polyps of colon with intestinal obstruction
		K51.413	Inflammatory polyps of colon with fistula
		K51.414	Inflammatory polyps of colon with abscess
		K51.418	Inflammatory polyps of colon with other complication
		K51.419	Inflammatory polyps of colon with unspecified complications
556.5	LEFT SIDED ULCERATIVE COLITIS	K51.50	Left sided colitis without complications
		K51.511	Left sided colitis with rectal bleeding
		K51.512	Left sided colitis with intestinal obstruction
		K51.513	Left sided colitis with fistula
		K51.514	Left sided colitis with abscess
		K51.518	Left sided colitis with other complication
		K51.519	Left sided colitis with unspecified complications
556.6	UNIVERSAL ULCERATIVE COLITIS	K51.00	Ulcerative (chronic) pancolitis without complications
		K51.011	Ulcerative (chronic) pancolitis with rectal bleeding
		K51.012	Ulcerative (chronic) pancolitis with intestinal obstruction
		K51.013	Ulcerative (chronic) pancolitis with fistula
		K51.014	Ulcerative (chronic) pancolitis with abscess
		K51.018	Ulcerative (chronic) pancolitis with other complication
		K51.019	Ulcerative (chronic) pancolitis with unsp complications
556.8	OTHER ULCERATIVE COLITIS	K51.80	Other ulcerative colitis without complications
		K51.811	Other ulcerative colitis with rectal bleeding
		K51.812	Other ulcerative colitis with intestinal obstruction
		K51.813	Other ulcerative colitis with fistula
		K51.814	Other ulcerative colitis with abscess
		K51.818	Other ulcerative colitis with other complication
		K51.819	Other ulcerative colitis with unspecified complications
556.9	UNSPECIFIED ULCERATIVE COLITIS	K51.90	Ulcerative colitis, unspecified, without complications
		K51.911	Ulcerative colitis, unspecified with rectal bleeding
		K51.912	Ulcerative colitis, unspecified with intestinal obstruction
		K51.913	Ulcerative colitis, unspecified with fistula
		K51.914	Ulcerative colitis, unspecified with abscess
		K51.918	Ulcerative colitis, unspecified with other complication
		K51.919	Ulcerative colitis, unsp with unspecified complications
557.0	ACUTE VASCULAR INSUFFICIENCY OF INTESTINE	K55.0	Acute vascular disorders of intestine
557.1	CHRONIC VASCULAR INSUFFICIENCY OF INTESTINE	K55.1	Chronic vascular disorders of intestine
557.9	UNSPECIFIED VASCULAR INSUFFICIENCY OF INTESTINE	K55.8	Other vascular disorders of intestine
		K55.9	Vascular disorder of intestine, unspecified
558.1	GASTROENTERITIS AND COLITIS DUE TO RADIATION	K52.0	Gastroenteritis and colitis due to radiation
558.2	TOXIC GASTROENTERITIS AND COLITIS	K52.1	Toxic gastroenteritis and colitis
558.3	GASTROENTERITIS AND COLITIS ALLERGIC	K52.2	Allergic and dietetic gastroenteritis and colitis
558.41	EOSINOPHILIC GASTROENTERITIS	K52.81	Eosinophilic gastritis or gastroenteritis
558.42	EOSINOPHILIC COLITIS	K52.82	Eosinophilic colitis
558.9	OTH&UNSPEC NONINFECTIOUS GASTROENTERITIS&COLITIS	K52.89	Other specified noninfective gastroenteritis and colitis
		K52.9	Noninfective gastroenteritis and colitis, unspecified
560.0	INTUSSUSCEPTION	K56.1	Intussusception
560.1	PARALYTIC ILEUS	K56.0	Paralytic ileus
		K56.7	Ileus, unspecified
560.2	VOLVULUS	K56.2	Volvulus
560.30	UNSPECIFIED IMPACTION OF INTESTINE	K56.49	Other impaction of intestine
560.31	GALLSTONE ILEUS	K56.3	Gallstone ileus
560.32	FECAL IMPACTION	K56.41	Fecal impaction

ICD-9-CM			ICD-10-CM	
56Ø.39	OTHER IMPACTION OF INTESTINE	➡	K56.49	Other impaction of intestine
56Ø.81	INTESTINAL OR PERITONEAL ADHESIONS W/OBSTRUCTION	➡	K56.5	Intestinal adhesions w obst (postprocedural) (postinfection)
56Ø.89	OTHER SPECIFIED INTESTINAL OBSTRUCTION	◙	K51.Ø12	Ulcerative (chronic) pancolitis with intestinal obstruction
		◙	K51.212	Ulcerative (chronic) proctitis with intestinal obstruction
		◙	K51.312	Ulcerative (chronic) rectosigmoiditis w intestinal obst
		◙	K51.412	Inflammatory polyps of colon with intestinal obstruction
		◙	K51.512	Left sided colitis with intestinal obstruction
		◙	K51.812	Other ulcerative colitis with intestinal obstruction
		◙	K51.912	Ulcerative colitis, unspecified with intestinal obstruction
			K56.69	Other intestinal obstruction
56Ø.9	UNSPECIFIED INTESTINAL OBSTRUCTION	◙	K5Ø.Ø12	Crohn's disease of small intestine w intestinal obstruction
		◙	K5Ø.112	Crohn's disease of large intestine w intestinal obstruction
		◙	K5Ø.812	Crohn's disease of both small and lg int w intestinal obst
		◙	K5Ø.912	Crohn's disease, unspecified, with intestinal obstruction
			K56.6Ø	Unspecified intestinal obstruction
562.ØØ	DIVERTICULOSIS OF SMALL INTESTINE		K57.1Ø	Dvrtclos of sm int w/o perforation or abscess w/o bleeding
		◙	K57.5Ø	Dvrtclos of both sm and lg int w/o perf or abscs w/o bleed
562.Ø1	DIVERTICULITIS OF SMALL INTESTINE	◙	K57.ØØ	Dvtrcli of sm int w perforation and abscess w/o bleeding
			K57.12	Dvtrcli of sm int w/o perforation or abscess w/o bleeding
		◙	K57.4Ø	Dvtrcli of both small and lg int w perf and abscs w/o bleed
		◙	K57.52	Dvtrcli of both small and lg int w/o perf or abscs w/o bleed
562.Ø2	DIVERTICULOSIS OF SMALL INTESTINE W/HEMORRHAGE		K57.11	Dvrtclos of sm int w/o perforation or abscess w bleeding
		◙	K57.51	Dvrtclos of both small and lg int w/o perf or abscs w bleed
562.Ø3	DIVERTULITIS OF SMALL INTESTINE WITH HEMORRHAGE	◙	K57.Ø1	Dvtrcli of sm int w perforation and abscess w bleeding
			K57.13	Dvtrcli of sm int w/o perforation or abscess w bleeding
		◙	K57.41	Dvtrcli of both small and lg int w perf and abscess w bleed
		◙	K57.53	Dvtrcli of both small and lg int w/o perf or abscess w bleed
562.1Ø	DIVERTICULOSIS OF COLON		K57.3Ø	Dvrtclos of lg int w/o perforation or abscess w/o bleeding
		◙	K57.5Ø	Dvrtclos of both sm and lg int w/o perf or abscs w/o bleed
			K57.9Ø	Dvrtclos of intest, part unsp, w/o perf or abscess w/o bleed
562.11	DIVERTICULITIS OF COLON	◙	K57.2Ø	Dvtrcli of lg int w perforation and abscess w/o bleeding
			K57.32	Dvtrcli of lg int w/o perforation or abscess w/o bleeding
		◙	K57.4Ø	Dvtrcli of both small and lg int w perf and abscs w/o bleed
		◙	K57.52	Dvtrcli of both small and lg int w/o perf or abscs w/o bleed
		◙	K57.8Ø	Dvtrcli of intest, part unsp, w perf and abscess w/o bleed
			K57.92	Dvtrcli of intest, part unsp, w/o perf or abscess w/o bleed
562.12	DIVERTICULOSIS OF COLON WITH HEMORRHAGE		K57.31	Dvrtclos of lg int w/o perforation or abscess w bleeding
		◙	K57.51	Dvrtclos of both small and lg int w/o perf or abscs w bleed
			K57.91	Dvrtclos of intest, part unsp, w/o perf or abscess w bleed
562.13	DIVERTICULITIS OF COLON WITH HEMORRHAGE	◙	K57.21	Dvtrcli of lg int w perforation and abscess w bleeding
			K57.33	Dvtrcli of lg int w/o perforation or abscess w bleeding
		◙	K57.41	Dvtrcli of both small and lg int w perf and abscess w bleed
		◙	K57.53	Dvtrcli of both small and lg int w/o perf or abscess w bleed
		◙	K57.81	Dvtrcli of intest, part unsp, w perf and abscess w bleeding
			K57.93	Dvtrcli of intest, part unsp, w/o perf or abscess w bleeding
564.ØØ	UNSPECIFIED CONSTIPATION	➡	K59.ØØ	Constipation, unspecified
564.Ø1	SLOW TRANSIT CONSTIPATION	➡	K59.Ø1	Slow transit constipation
564.Ø2	OUTLET DYSFUNCTION CONSTIPATION	➡	K59.Ø2	Outlet dysfunction constipation
564.Ø9	OTHER CONSTIPATION	➡	K59.Ø9	Other constipation
564.1	IRRITABLE BOWEL SYNDROME		K58.Ø	Irritable bowel syndrome with diarrhea
			K58.9	Irritable bowel syndrome without diarrhea
564.2	POSTGASTRIC SURGERY SYNDROMES	➡	K91.1	Postgastric surgery syndromes
564.3	VOMITING FOLLOWING GASTROINTESTINAL SURGERY	➡	K91.Ø	Vomiting following gastrointestinal surgery
564.4	OTHER POSTOPERATIVE FUNCTIONAL DISORDERS		K91.89	Oth postprocedural complications and disorders of dgstv sys
564.5	FUNCTIONAL DIARRHEA	➡	K59.1	Functional diarrhea
564.6	ANAL SPASM	➡	K59.4	Anal spasm
564.7	MEGACOLON OTHER THAN HIRSCHSPRUNGS	➡	K59.3	Megacolon, not elsewhere classified
564.81	NEUROGENIC BOWEL	➡	K59.2	Neurogenic bowel, not elsewhere classified
564.89	OTHER FUNCTIONAL DISORDERS OF INTESTINE	➡	K59.8	Other specified functional intestinal disorders
564.9	UNSPECIFIED FUNCTIONAL DISORDER OF INTESTINE	➡	K59.9	Functional intestinal disorder, unspecified
565.Ø	ANAL FISSURE		K6Ø.Ø	Acute anal fissure
			K6Ø.1	Chronic anal fissure
			K6Ø.2	Anal fissure, unspecified
565.1	ANAL FISTULA		K6Ø.3	Anal fistula
			K6Ø.4	Rectal fistula
			K6Ø.5	Anorectal fistula
566	ABSCESS OF ANAL AND RECTAL REGIONS		K61.Ø	Anal abscess
			K61.1	Rectal abscess
			K61.2	Anorectal abscess
			K61.3	Ischiorectal abscess
			K61.4	Intrasphincteric abscess
567.Ø	PERITONITIS INFECTIOUS DISEASES CLASSIFIED ELSW	➡	K67	Disorders of peritoneum in infectious diseases classd elswhr
567.1	PNEUMOCOCCAL PERITONITIS		K65.8	Other peritonitis
567.21	PERITONITIS (ACUTE) GENERALIZED		K65.Ø	Generalized (acute) peritonitis

56Ø.39–567.21

ICD-9-CM		ICD-10-CM	
567.22	PERITONEAL ABSCESS	➡ K65.1	Peritoneal abscess
567.23	SPONTANEOUS BACTERIAL PERITONITIS	➡ K65.2	Spontaneous bacterial peritonitis
567.29	OTHER SUPPURATIVE PERITONITIS	K65.Ø	Generalized (acute) peritonitis
567.31	PSOAS MUSCLE ABSCESS	➡ K68.12	Psoas muscle abscess
567.38	OTHER RETROPERITONEAL ABSCESS	➡ K68.19	Other retroperitoneal abscess
567.39	OTHER RETROPERITONEAL INFECTIONS	K68.9	Other disorders of retroperitoneum
567.81	CHOLEPERITONITIS	➡ K65.3	Choleperitonitis
567.82	SCLEROSING MESENTERITIS	➡ K65.4	Sclerosing mesenteritis
567.89	OTHER SPECIFIED PERITONITIS	K65.8	Other peritonitis
567.9	UNSPECIFIED PERITONITIS	➡ K65.9	Peritonitis, unspecified
568.Ø	PERITONEAL ADHESIONS	K66.Ø N99.4	Peritoneal adhesions (postprocedural) (postinfection) Postprocedural pelvic peritoneal adhesions
568.81	HEMOPERITONEUM	➡ K66.1	Hemoperitoneum
568.82	PERITONEAL EFFUSION	R18.8	Other ascites
568.89	OTHER SPECIFIED DISORDER OF PERITONEUM	K66.8 K68.9	Other specified disorders of peritoneum Other disorders of retroperitoneum
568.9	UNSPECIFIED DISORDER OF PERITONEUM	➡ K66.9	Disorder of peritoneum, unspecified
569.Ø	ANAL AND RECTAL POLYP	K62.Ø K62.1	Anal polyp Rectal polyp
569.1	RECTAL PROLAPSE	K62.2 K62.3	Anal prolapse Rectal prolapse
569.2	STENOSIS OF RECTUM AND ANUS	➡ K62.4	Stenosis of anus and rectum
569.3	HEMORRHAGE OF RECTUM AND ANUS	➡ K62.5	Hemorrhage of anus and rectum
569.41	ULCER OF ANUS AND RECTUM	➡ K62.6	Ulcer of anus and rectum
569.42	ANAL OR RECTAL PAIN	K62.89	Other specified diseases of anus and rectum
569.43	ANAL SPHINCTER TEAR HEALED OLD	➡ K62.81	Anal sphincter tear (healed) (nontraumatic) (old)
569.44	DYSPLASIA OF ANUS	➡ K62.82	Dysplasia of anus
569.49	OTHER SPECIFIED DISORDER OF RECTUM AND ANUS	K62.7 K62.89 K62.9	Radiation proctitis Other specified diseases of anus and rectum Disease of anus and rectum, unspecified
569.5	ABSCESS OF INTESTINE	K5Ø.Ø14 K5Ø.114 K5Ø.814 K5Ø.914 K51.Ø14 K51.214 K51.314 K51.414 K51.514 K51.814 K51.914 K57.ØØ K57.Ø1 K57.2Ø K57.21 K57.4Ø K57.41 K57.8Ø K57.81 K63.Ø	Crohn's disease of small intestine with abscess Crohn's disease of large intestine with abscess Crohn's disease of both small and large intestine w abscess Crohn's disease, unspecified, with abscess Ulcerative (chronic) pancolitis with abscess Ulcerative (chronic) proctitis with abscess Ulcerative (chronic) rectosigmoiditis with abscess Inflammatory polyps of colon with abscess Left sided colitis with abscess Other ulcerative colitis with abscess Ulcerative colitis, unspecified with abscess Dvtrcli of sm int w perforation and abscess w/o bleeding Dvtrcli of sm int w perforation and abscess w bleeding Dvtrcli of lg int w perforation and abscess w/o bleeding Dvtrcli of lg int w perforation and abscess w bleeding Dvtrcli of both small and lg int w perf and abscs w/o bleed Dvtrcli of both small and lg int w perf and abscess w bleed Dvtrcli of intest, part unsp, w perf and abscess w/o bleed Dvtrcli of intest, part unsp, w perf and abscess w bleeding Abscess of intestine
569.6Ø	UNSPECIFIED COMPLICATION COLOSTOMY/ENTEROSTOMY	K94.ØØ K94.1Ø	Colostomy complication, unspecified Enterostomy complication, unspecified
569.61	INFECTION OF COLOSTOMY OR ENTEROSTOMY	K94.Ø2 K94.12	Colostomy infection Enterostomy infection
569.62	MECHANICAL COMPLICATION OF COLOSTOMY&ENTEROSTOMY	K94.Ø3 K94.13	Colostomy malfunction Enterostomy malfunction
569.69	OTHER COMPLICATION OF COLOSTOMY OR ENTEROSTOMY	K94.Ø1 K94.Ø9 K94.11 K94.19	Colostomy hemorrhage Other complications of colostomy Enterostomy hemorrhage Other complications of enterostomy
569.71	POUCHITIS	➡ K91.85Ø	Pouchitis
569.79	OTHER COMPLICATIONS OF INTESTINAL POUCH	➡ K91.858	Other complications of intestinal pouch
569.81	FISTULA OF INTESTINE EXCLUDING RECTUM AND ANUS	K5Ø.Ø13 K5Ø.113 K5Ø.813 K5Ø.913 K51.Ø13 K51.213 K51.313 K51.413 K51.513 K51.813 K51.913 K63.2	Crohn's disease of small intestine with fistula Crohn's disease of large intestine with fistula Crohn's disease of both small and large intestine w fistula Crohn's disease, unspecified, with fistula Ulcerative (chronic) pancolitis with fistula Ulcerative (chronic) proctitis with fistula Ulcerative (chronic) rectosigmoiditis with fistula Inflammatory polyps of colon with fistula Left sided colitis with fistula Other ulcerative colitis with fistula Ulcerative colitis, unspecified with fistula Fistula of intestine

 [Brackets] indicate valid character values for each code. Character value meanings provided for each code grouping.

ICD-9-CM			ICD-10-CM	
569.82	ULCERATION OF INTESTINE	➡	K63.3	Ulcer of intestine
569.83	PERFORATION OF INTESTINE	➡	K63.1	Perforation of intestine (nontraumatic)
569.84	ANGIODYSPLASIA OF INTESTINE	➡	K55.20	Angiodysplasia of colon without hemorrhage
569.85	ANGIODYSPLASIA OF INTESTINE WITH HEMORRHAGE	➡	K55.21	Angiodysplasia of colon with hemorrhage
569.86	DIEULAFOY LESION OF INTESTINE	➡	K63.81	Dieulafoy lesion of intestine
569.87	VOMITING OF FECAL MATTER	➡	R11.13	Vomiting of fecal matter
569.89	OTHER SPECIFIED DISORDER OF INTESTINES		K63.4	Enteroptosis
			K63.89	Other specified diseases of intestine
			K92.89	Other specified diseases of the digestive system
569.9	UNSPECIFIED DISORDER OF INTESTINE		K63.9	Disease of intestine, unspecified
			K92.9	Disease of digestive system, unspecified
570	ACUTE AND SUBACUTE NECROSIS OF LIVER		K72.00	Acute and subacute hepatic failure without coma
		◘	K72.01	Acute and subacute hepatic failure with coma
			K76.2	Central hemorrhagic necrosis of liver
571.0	ALCOHOLIC FATTY LIVER	➡	K70.0	Alcoholic fatty liver
571.1	ACUTE ALCOHOLIC HEPATITIS		K70.10	Alcoholic hepatitis without ascites
			K70.11	Alcoholic hepatitis with ascites
571.2	ALCOHOLIC CIRRHOSIS OF LIVER		K70.2	Alcoholic fibrosis and sclerosis of liver
			K70.30	Alcoholic cirrhosis of liver without ascites
			K70.31	Alcoholic cirrhosis of liver with ascites
571.3	UNSPECIFIED ALCOHOLIC LIVER DAMAGE		K70.40	Alcoholic hepatic failure without coma
		◘	K70.41	Alcoholic hepatic failure with coma
			K70.9	Alcoholic liver disease, unspecified
571.40	UNSPECIFIED CHRONIC HEPATITIS	➡	K73.9	Chronic hepatitis, unspecified
571.41	CHRONIC PERSISTENT HEPATITIS	➡	K73.0	Chronic persistent hepatitis, not elsewhere classified
571.42	AUTOIMMUNE HEPATITIS	➡	K75.4	Autoimmune hepatitis
571.49	OTHER CHRONIC HEPATITIS		K73.1	Chronic lobular hepatitis, not elsewhere classified
			K73.2	Chronic active hepatitis, not elsewhere classified
			K73.8	Other chronic hepatitis, not elsewhere classified
571.5	CIRRHOSIS OF LIVER WITHOUT MENTION OF ALCOHOL		K74.0	Hepatic fibrosis
			K74.60	Unspecified cirrhosis of liver
			K74.69	Other cirrhosis of liver
571.6	BILIARY CIRRHOSIS		K74.3	Primary biliary cirrhosis
			K74.4	Secondary biliary cirrhosis
			K74.5	Biliary cirrhosis, unspecified
571.8	OTHER CHRONIC NONALCOHOLIC LIVER DISEASE		K75.81	Nonalcoholic steatohepatitis (NASH)
			K76.0	Fatty (change of) liver, not elsewhere classified
			K76.89	Other specified diseases of liver
571.9	UNSPEC CHRONIC LIVER DISEASE W/O MENTION ALCOHOL		K74.1	Hepatic sclerosis
			K74.2	Hepatic fibrosis with hepatic sclerosis
			K76.9	Liver disease, unspecified
572.0	ABSCESS OF LIVER	➡	K75.0	Abscess of liver
572.1	PORTAL PYEMIA		K75.1	Phlebitis of portal vein
572.2	HEPATIC ENCEPHALOPATHY	◘	K70.41	Alcoholic hepatic failure with coma
		◘	K71.11	Toxic liver disease with hepatic necrosis, with coma
		◘	K72.01	Acute and subacute hepatic failure with coma
		◘	K72.11	Chronic hepatic failure with coma
			K72.90	Hepatic failure, unspecified without coma
		◘	K72.91	Hepatic failure, unspecified with coma
572.3	PORTAL HYPERTENSION	➡	K76.6	Portal hypertension
572.4	HEPATORENAL SYNDROME	➡	K76.7	Hepatorenal syndrome
572.8	OTHER SEQUELAE OF CHRONIC LIVER DISEASE		K72.10	Chronic hepatic failure without coma
		◘	K72.11	Chronic hepatic failure with coma
			K72.90	Hepatic failure, unspecified without coma
		◘	K72.91	Hepatic failure, unspecified with coma
573.0	CHRONIC PASSIVE CONGESTION OF LIVER	➡	K76.1	Chronic passive congestion of liver
573.1	HEPATITIS IN VIRAL DISEASES CLASSIFIED ELSEWHERE	◘	B25.1	Cytomegaloviral hepatitis
			K77	Liver disorders in diseases classified elsewhere
573.2	HEPATITIS OTH INFECTIOUS DISEASES CLASS ELSW		K77	Liver disorders in diseases classified elsewhere

ICD-9-CM			ICD-10-CM	
573.3	UNSPECIFIED HEPATITIS		**K71.Ø**	Toxic liver disease with cholestasis
			K71.1Ø	Toxic liver disease with hepatic necrosis, without coma
		⚑	**K71.11**	Toxic liver disease with hepatic necrosis, with coma
			K71.2	Toxic liver disease with acute hepatitis
			K71.3	Toxic liver disease with chronic persistent hepatitis
			K71.4	Toxic liver disease with chronic lobular hepatitis
			K71.5Ø	Toxic liver disease w chronic active hepatitis w/o ascites
			K71.51	Toxic liver disease w chronic active hepatitis with ascites
			K71.6	Toxic liver disease with hepatitis, not elsewhere classified
			K71.7	Toxic liver disease with fibrosis and cirrhosis of liver
			K71.8	Toxic liver disease with other disorders of liver
			K71.9	Toxic liver disease, unspecified
			K75.2	Nonspecific reactive hepatitis
			K75.3	Granulomatous hepatitis, not elsewhere classified
			K75.81	Nonalcoholic steatohepatitis (NASH)
			K75.89	Other specified inflammatory liver diseases
			K75.9	Inflammatory liver disease, unspecified
			K76.4	Peliosis hepatis
573.4	HEPATIC INFARCTION	➡	**K76.3**	Infarction of liver
573.5	HEPATOPULMONARY SYNDROME		**K76.81**	Hepatopulmonary syndrome
573.8	OTHER SPECIFIED DISORDERS OF LIVER		**K76.1**	Chronic passive congestion of liver
			K76.5	Hepatic veno-occlusive disease
			K76.89	Other specified diseases of liver
			K77	Liver disorders in diseases classified elsewhere
573.9	UNSPECIFIED DISORDER OF LIVER		**K76.9**	Liver disease, unspecified
574.ØØ	CALCU GALLBLADD W/ACUT CHOLCYST W/O MENTION OBST		**K8Ø.ØØ**	Calculus of gallbladder w acute cholecyst w/o obstruction
		⚑	**K8Ø.12**	Calculus of GB w acute and chronic cholecyst w/o obstruction
574.Ø1	CALCU GALLBLADD W/ACUTE CHOLECYST&OBSTRUCTION		**K8Ø.Ø1**	Calculus of gallbladder w acute cholecystitis w obstruction
		⚑	**K8Ø.13**	Calculus of GB w acute and chronic cholecyst w obstruction
574.1Ø	CALCU GALLBLADD W/OTH CHOLECYST W/O MENTION OBST		**K8Ø.1Ø**	Calculus of gallbladder w chronic cholecyst w/o obstruction
		⚑	**K8Ø.12**	Calculus of GB w acute and chronic cholecyst w/o obstruction
			K8Ø.18	Calculus of gallbladder w oth cholecystitis w/o obstruction
574.11	CALCU GALLBLADD W/OTH CHOLECYSTITIS&OBSTRUCTION		**K8Ø.11**	Calculus of gallbladder w chronic cholecyst w obstruction
		⚑	**K8Ø.13**	Calculus of GB w acute and chronic cholecyst w obstruction
			K8Ø.19	Calculus of gallbladder w oth cholecystitis with obstruction
574.2Ø	CALCU GALLBLADD W/O MENTION CHOLECYST/OBST		**K8Ø.2Ø**	Calculus of gallbladder w/o cholecystitis w/o obstruction
			K8Ø.8Ø	Other cholelithiasis without obstruction
574.21	CALCU GALLBLADD W/O MENTION CHOLECYST W/OBST	➡	**K8Ø.21**	Calculus of gallbladder w/o cholecystitis with obstruction
574.3Ø	CALCU BD W/ACUT CHOLECYST W/O MENTION OBST		**K8Ø.42**	Calculus of bile duct w acute cholecystitis w/o obstruction
		⚑	**K8Ø.46**	Calculus of bile duct w acute and chronic cholecyst w/o obst
574.31	CALCULUS OF BD W/ACUTE CHOLECYSTITIS&OBSTRUCTION		**K8Ø.43**	Calculus of bile duct w acute cholecystitis with obstruction
		⚑	**K8Ø.47**	Calculus of bile duct w acute and chronic cholecyst w obst
574.4Ø	CALCU BD W/OTH CHOLECYST W/O MENTION OBSTRUCTION		**K8Ø.4Ø**	Calculus of bile duct w cholecystitis, unsp, w/o obstruction
			K8Ø.44	Calculus of bile duct w chronic cholecyst w/o obstruction
		⚑	**K8Ø.46**	Calculus of bile duct w acute and chronic cholecyst w/o obst
574.41	CALCULUS OF BD W/OTHER CHOLECYSTITIS&OBSTRUCTION		**K8Ø.41**	Calculus of bile duct w cholecystitis, unsp, w obstruction
			K8Ø.45	Calculus of bile duct w chronic cholecystitis w obstruction
		⚑	**K8Ø.47**	Calculus of bile duct w acute and chronic cholecyst w obst
			K8Ø.81	Other cholelithiasis with obstruction
574.5Ø	CALCU BD WITHOUT MENTION CHOLECYST/OBSTRUCTION	⚑	**K8Ø.3Ø**	Calculus of bile duct w cholangitis, unsp, w/o obstruction
		⚑	**K8Ø.32**	Calculus of bile duct with acute cholangitis w/o obstruction
		⚑	**K8Ø.34**	Calculus of bile duct w chronic cholangitis w/o obstruction
		⚑	**K8Ø.36**	Calculus of bile duct w acute and chr cholangitis w/o obst
			K8Ø.5Ø	Calculus of bile duct w/o cholangitis or cholecyst w/o obst
574.51	CALCU BD WITHOUT MENTION CHOLECYST W/OBSTRUCTION	⚑	**K8Ø.31**	Calculus of bile duct w cholangitis, unsp, with obstruction
		⚑	**K8Ø.33**	Calculus of bile duct w acute cholangitis with obstruction
		⚑	**K8Ø.35**	Calculus of bile duct w chronic cholangitis with obstruction
		⚑	**K8Ø.37**	Calculus of bile duct w acute and chronic cholangitis w obst
			K8Ø.51	Calculus of bile duct w/o cholangitis or cholecyst w obst
574.6Ø	CALCU GB&BD W/ACUT CHOLCYST W/O MENTION OBST	➡	**K8Ø.62**	Calculus of GB and bile duct w acute cholecyst w/o obst
574.61	CALCU GALLBLADD&BD W/ACUT CHOLECYST W/OBST	➡	**K8Ø.63**	Calculus of GB and bile duct w acute cholecyst w obstruction
574.7Ø	CALCU GB&BD W/OTH CHOLCYST W/O MENTION OBST		**K8Ø.6Ø**	Calculus of GB and bile duct w cholecyst, unsp, w/o obst
			K8Ø.64	Calculus of GB and bile duct w chronic cholecyst w/o obst
574.71	CALCU GALLBLADD&BD W/OTH CHOLECYST W/OBSTRUCTION		**K8Ø.61**	Calculus of GB and bile duct w cholecyst, unsp, w obst
			K8Ø.65	Calculus of GB and bile duct w chronic cholecyst w obst
574.8Ø	CALCU GB&BD W/ACUT&CHRN CHOLCYST W/O OBST	➡	**K8Ø.66**	Calculus of GB and bile duct w ac and chr cholecyst w/o obst
574.81	CALCU GALLBLADD&BD W/ACUT&CHRON CHOLECYST W/OBST	➡	**K8Ø.67**	Calculus of GB and bile duct w ac and chr cholecyst w obst
574.9Ø	CALCU GALLBLADD&BD W/O CHOLCYST W/O MENTION OBST	➡	**K8Ø.7Ø**	Calculus of GB and bile duct w/o cholecyst w/o obstruction
574.91	CALCU GALLBLADD&BD W/O CHOLECYST W/OBSTRUCTION	➡	**K8Ø.71**	Calculus of GB and bile duct w/o cholecyst w obstruction
575.Ø	ACUTE CHOLECYSTITIS	➡	**K81.Ø**	Acute cholecystitis
575.1Ø	CHOLECYSTITIS, UNSPECIFIED	➡	**K81.9**	Cholecystitis, unspecified
575.11	CHRONIC CHOLECYSTITIS	➡	**K81.1**	Chronic cholecystitis
575.12	ACUTE AND CHRONIC CHOLECYSTITIS	➡	**K81.2**	Acute cholecystitis with chronic cholecystitis
575.2	OBSTRUCTION OF GALLBLADDER	➡	**K82.Ø**	Obstruction of gallbladder
575.3	HYDROPS OF GALLBLADDER	➡	**K82.1**	Hydrops of gallbladder

 [Brackets] indicate valid character values for each code. Character value meanings provided for each code grouping.

ICD-9-CM			ICD-10-CM	
575.4	PERFORATION OF GALLBLADDER	➡	K82.2	Perforation of gallbladder
575.5	FISTULA OF GALLBLADDER	➡	K82.3	Fistula of gallbladder
575.6	CHOLESTEROLOSIS OF GALLBLADDER	➡	K82.4	Cholesterolosis of gallbladder
575.8	OTHER SPECIFIED DISORDER OF GALLBLADDER	➡	K82.8	Other specified diseases of gallbladder
575.9	UNSPECIFIED DISORDER OF GALLBLADDER	➡	K82.9	Disease of gallbladder, unspecified
576.0	POSTCHOLECYSTECTOMY SYNDROME	➡	K91.5	Postcholecystectomy syndrome
576.1	CHOLANGITIS	▣	K80.30	Calculus of bile duct w cholangitis, unsp, w/o obstruction
		▣	K80.31	Calculus of bile duct w cholangitis, unsp, with obstruction
		▣	K80.32	Calculus of bile duct with acute cholangitis w/o obstruction
		▣	K80.33	Calculus of bile duct w acute cholangitis with obstruction
		▣	K80.34	Calculus of bile duct w chronic cholangitis w/o obstruction
		▣	K80.35	Calculus of bile duct w chronic cholangitis with obstruction
		▣	K80.36	Calculus of bile duct w acute and chr cholangitis w/o obst
		▣	K80.37	Calculus of bile duct w acute and chronic cholangitis w obst
			K83.0	Cholangitis
576.2	OBSTRUCTION OF BILE DUCT	➡	K83.1	Obstruction of bile duct
576.3	PERFORATION OF BILE DUCT	➡	K83.2	Perforation of bile duct
576.4	FISTULA OF BILE DUCT	➡	K83.3	Fistula of bile duct
576.5	SPASM OF SPHINCTER OF ODDI	➡	K83.4	Spasm of sphincter of Oddi
576.8	OTHER SPECIFIED DISORDERS OF BILIARY TRACT		K83.5	Biliary cyst
			K83.8	Other specified diseases of biliary tract
			K87	Disord of GB, biliary trac and pancreas in dis classd elswhr
576.9	UNSPECIFIED DISORDER OF BILIARY TRACT	➡	K83.9	Disease of biliary tract, unspecified
577.0	ACUTE PANCREATITIS	▣	B25.2	Cytomegaloviral pancreatitis
			K85.0	Idiopathic acute pancreatitis
			K85.1	Biliary acute pancreatitis
			K85.2	Alcohol induced acute pancreatitis
			K85.3	Drug induced acute pancreatitis
			K85.8	Other acute pancreatitis
			K85.9	Acute pancreatitis, unspecified
577.1	CHRONIC PANCREATITIS		K86.0	Alcohol-induced chronic pancreatitis
			K86.1	Other chronic pancreatitis
577.2	CYST AND PSEUDOCYST OF PANCREAS		K86.2	Cyst of pancreas
			K86.3	Pseudocyst of pancreas
577.8	OTHER SPECIFIED DISEASE OF PANCREAS		K86.1	Other chronic pancreatitis
			K86.8	Other specified diseases of pancreas
			K87	Disord of GB, biliary trac and pancreas in dis classd elswhr
577.9	UNSPECIFIED DISEASE OF PANCREAS	➡	K86.9	Disease of pancreas, unspecified
578.0	HEMATEMESIS	➡	K92.0	Hematemesis
578.1	BLOOD IN STOOL	➡	K92.1	Melena
578.9	UNSPECIFIED HEMORRHAGE OF GASTROINTESTINAL TRACT	➡	K92.2	Gastrointestinal hemorrhage, unspecified
579.0	CELIAC DISEASE	➡	K90.0	Celiac disease
579.1	TROPICAL SPRUE	➡	K90.1	Tropical sprue
579.2	BLIND LOOP SYNDROME	➡	K90.2	Blind loop syndrome, not elsewhere classified
579.3	OTHER AND UNSPECIFIED POSTSURGICAL NONABSORPTION	➡	K91.2	Postsurgical malabsorption, not elsewhere classified
579.4	PANCREATIC STEATORRHEA	➡	K90.3	Pancreatic steatorrhea
579.8	OTHER SPECIFIED INTESTINAL MALABSORPTION		K90.4	Malabsorption due to intolerance, not elsewhere classified
			K90.89	Other intestinal malabsorption
579.9	UNSPECIFIED INTESTINAL MALABSORPTION	➡	K90.9	Intestinal malabsorption, unspecified

Diseases of the Genitourinary System

ICD-9-CM			ICD-10-CM	
580.Ø	ACUTE GLN W/LESION PROLIFERATIVE GLN		NØØ.Ø	Acute nephritic syndrome with minor glomerular abnormality
			NØØ.1	Acute neph syndrome w focal and segmental glomerular lesions
			NØØ.2	Acute nephritic syndrome w diffuse membranous glomrlneph
			NØØ.3	Acute neph syndrome w diffuse mesangial prolif glomrlneph
			NØØ.4	Acute neph syndrome w diffuse endocaplry prolif glomrlneph
			NØØ.5	Acute nephritic syndrome w diffuse mesangiocap glomrlneph
			NØØ.6	Acute nephritic syndrome with dense deposit disease
			NØØ.7	Acute nephritic syndrome w diffuse crescentic glomrlneph
580.4	ACUTE GLN W/LESION RAPIDLY PROGRESSIVE GLN		NØ1.Ø	Rapidly progr nephritic syndrome w minor glomerular abnlt
			NØ1.1	Rapidly progr neph synd w focal and seg glomerular lesions
			NØ1.2	Rapidly progr neph syndrome w diffuse membranous glomrlneph
			NØ1.3	Rapidly progr neph synd w diffus mesangial prolif glomrlneph
			NØ1.4	Rapid progr neph synd w diffus endocaplry prolif glomrlneph
			NØ1.5	Rapidly progr neph syndrome w diffuse mesangiocap glomrlneph
			NØ1.6	Rapidly progr nephritic syndrome w dense deposit disease
			NØ1.7	Rapidly progr neph syndrome w diffuse crescentic glomrlneph
			NØ1.8	Rapidly progr nephritic syndrome w oth morphologic changes
			NØ1.9	Rapidly progr nephritic syndrome w unsp morphologic changes
580.81	ACUT GLN W/OTH PATHAL LES KIDNEY DZ CLASS ELSW		NØ8	Glomerular disorders in diseases classified elsewhere
580.89	OTH ACUT GLOMERULONEPHRIT W/OTH PATH LES KIDNEY		NØØ.8	Acute nephritic syndrome with other morphologic changes
580.9	ACUT GLOMERULONEPHRITIS W/UNSPEC PATH LES KIDNEY		NØØ.9	Acute nephritic syndrome with unsp morphologic changes
581.Ø	NEPHROTIC SYNDROME W/LESION PROLIFERATIVE GLN		NØ4.4	Nephrotic syndrome w diffuse endocaplry prolif glomrlneph
581.1	NEPHROTIC SYNDROME W/LESION MEMBRANOUS GLN		NØ2.1	Recur and perst hematur w focal and seg glomerular lesions
			NØ2.2	Recurrent and perst hematur w diffuse membranous glomrlneph
			NØ2.3	Recur and perst hematur w diffus mesangial prolif glomrlneph
			NØ4.1	Nephrotic syndrome w focal and segmental glomerular lesions
			NØ4.2	Nephrotic syndrome w diffuse membranous glomerulonephritis
581.2	NEPHROTIC SYND W/LESION MEMBRANOPROLIFERAT GLN		NØ2.4	Recur & perst hematur w diffus endocaplry prolif glomrlneph
			NØ2.5	Recurrent and perst hematur w diffuse mesangiocap glomrlneph
			NØ2.6	Recurrent and persistent hematuria w dense deposit disease
			NØ2.7	Recurrent and perst hematur w diffuse crescentic glomrlneph
			NØ4.3	Nephrotic syndrome w diffuse mesangial prolif glomrlneph
			NØ4.4	Nephrotic syndrome w diffuse endocaplry prolif glomrlneph
			NØ4.5	Nephrotic syndrome w diffuse mesangiocapillary glomrlneph
			NØ4.6	Nephrotic syndrome with dense deposit disease
581.3	NEPHROTIC SYND W/LES MIN CHG GLOMERULONEPHRIT		NØ2.Ø	Recurrent and persistent hematuria w minor glomerular abnlt
			NØ4.Ø	Nephrotic syndrome with minor glomerular abnormality
581.81	NEPHROTIC SYND W/OTH PATHAL LES DZ CLASS ELSW	◘	B52.Ø	Plasmodium malariae malaria with nephropathy
		◘	EØ8.21	Diabetes due to underlying condition w diabetic nephropathy
		◘	EØ8.22	Diabetes due to undrl cond w diabetic chronic kidney disease
		◘	EØ8.29	Diabetes due to undrl condition w oth diabetic kidney comp
		◘	EØ9.21	Drug/chem diabetes mellitus w diabetic nephropathy
		◘	EØ9.22	Drug/chem diabetes w diabetic chronic kidney disease
		◘	EØ9.29	Drug/chem diabetes w oth diabetic kidney complication
			NØ8	Glomerular disorders in diseases classified elsewhere
581.89	OTH NEPHROTIC SYND W/SPEC PATHAL LESION KIDNEY		NØ2.8	Recurrent and persistent hematuria w oth morphologic changes
			NØ4.7	Nephrotic syndrome w diffuse crescentic glomerulonephritis
			NØ4.8	Nephrotic syndrome with other morphologic changes
581.9	NEPHROTIC SYNDROME W/UNSPEC PATHAL LESION KIDNEY		NØ2.9	Recurrent and perst hematuria w unsp morphologic changes
			NØ4.9	Nephrotic syndrome with unspecified morphologic changes
582.Ø	CHRONIC GLN W/LESION PROLIFERATIVE GLN		NØ3.2	Chronic nephritic syndrome w diffuse membranous glomrlneph
582.1	CHRON GLOMERULONEPHRIT W/LES MEMBRANOUS GLN		NØ3.1	Chronic neph syndrome w focal and seg glomerular lesions
			NØ3.3	Chronic neph syndrome w diffuse mesangial prolif glomrlneph
582.2	CHRONIC GLN W/LESION MEMBRANOPROLIFERATIVE GLN		NØ3.4	Chronic neph syndrome w diffuse endocaplry prolif glomrlneph
			NØ3.5	Chronic nephritic syndrome w diffuse mesangiocap glomrlneph
			NØ3.6	Chronic nephritic syndrome with dense deposit disease
			NØ3.7	Chronic nephritic syndrome w diffuse crescentic glomrlneph
582.4	CHRONIC GLN W/LESION RAPIDLY PROGRESSIVE GLN		NØ3.8	Chronic nephritic syndrome with other morphologic changes
582.81	CHRN GLN W/OTH PATHAL LES KIDNEY DZ CLASS ELSW		NØ8	Glomerular disorders in diseases classified elsewhere
582.89	CHR GLOMERULONEPHRITIS W/PATH KIDNEY LES DZ CE		NØ3.Ø	Chronic nephritic syndrome with minor glomerular abnormality
			NØ3.8	Chronic nephritic syndrome with other morphologic changes
582.9	CHRONIC GLN W/UNSPEC PATHOLOGICAL LESION KIDNEY		NØ3.9	Chronic nephritic syndrome with unsp morphologic changes
583.Ø	NEPHRITIS&NEPHRPATH NOT AC/CHRN W/LES PROLIF GLN		NØ5.9	Unsp nephritic syndrome with unspecified morphologic changes
583.1	NEPHRITIS&NEPHRPATH NOT ACUT/CHRN W/LES MEMB GLN		NØ5.2	Unsp nephritic syndrome w diffuse membranous glomrlneph
			NØ6.2	Isolated proteinuria w diffuse membranous glomerulonephritis
			NØ7.2	Hereditary nephropathy, NEC w diffuse membranous glomrlneph
583.2	NEPHRITIS&NEPHROPATHY W/LES MEMBRANOPROLIFER GLN		NØ5.3	Unsp neph syndrome w diffuse mesangial prolif glomrlneph
			NØ5.4	Unsp neph syndrome w diffuse endocaplry prolif glomrlneph
			NØ5.5	Unsp nephritic syndrome w diffuse mesangiocap glomrlneph
			NØ6.3	Isolated proteinuria w diffuse mesangial prolif glomrlneph
			NØ6.4	Isolated proteinuria w diffuse endocaplry prolif glomrlneph
			NØ6.5	Isolated proteinuria w diffuse mesangiocapillary glomrlneph
			NØ7.3	Heredit neuropath, NEC w diffuse mesangial prolif glomrlneph
			NØ7.4	Heredit neuropath, NEC w diffus endocaplry prolif glomrlneph
			NØ7.5	Hereditary nephropathy, NEC w diffuse mesangiocap glomrlneph
583.4	NEPHRITIS&NEPHROPATHY W/LES RAPIDLY PROGRESS GLN		NØ5.9	Unsp nephritic syndrome with unspecified morphologic changes
583.6	NEPHRITIS&NEPHROPATH W/LES RENL CORTICL NECROSIS		N17.1	Acute kidney failure with acute cortical necrosis

ICD-9-CM		ICD-10-CM		
583.7	NEPHRITIS&NEPHROPATHY W/LES MEDULLARY NECROSIS		**N17.2**	Acute kidney failure with medullary necrosis
583.81	NEPHRITIS&NEPHROPATHY-OTH SPEC PATH LES DZ CE	■	**EØ9.21**	Drug/chem diabetes mellitus w diabetic nephropathy
		■	**EØ9.22**	Drug/chem diabetes w diabetic chronic kidney disease
		■	**EØ9.29**	Drug/chem diabetes w oth diabetic kidney complication
		■	**M32.14**	Glomerular disease in systemic lupus erythematosus
		■	**M32.15**	Tubulo-interstitial neuropath in sys lupus erythematosus
		■	**M35.Ø4**	Sicca syndrome with tubulo-interstitial nephropathy
			NØ8	Glomerular disorders in diseases classified elsewhere
			N16	Renal tubulo-interstitial disord in diseases classd elswhr
583.89	NEPHRITIS&NEPHROPATHY W/OTH PATHOLOG KIDNEY LES		**NØ5.Ø**	Unsp nephritic syndrome with minor glomerular abnormality
			NØ5.1	Unsp neph syndrome w focal and segmental glomerular lesions
			NØ5.6	Unspecified nephritic syndrome with dense deposit disease
			NØ5.7	Unsp nephritic syndrome w diffuse crescentic glomrlneph
			NØ5.8	Unsp nephritic syndrome with other morphologic changes
			NØ6.Ø	Isolated proteinuria with minor glomerular abnormality
			NØ6.1	Isolated protein w focal and segmental glomerular lesions
			NØ6.6	Isolated proteinuria with dense deposit disease
			NØ6.7	Isolated proteinuria w diffuse crescentic glomerulonephritis
			NØ6.8	Isolated proteinuria with other morphologic lesion
			NØ7.Ø	Hereditary nephropathy, NEC w minor glomerular abnormality
			NØ7.1	Heredit neuropath, NEC w focal and seg glomerular lesions
			NØ7.6	Hereditary nephropathy, NEC w dense deposit disease
			NØ7.7	Hereditary nephropathy, NEC w diffuse crescentic glomrlneph
			NØ7.8	Hereditary nephropathy, NEC w oth morphologic lesions
			N14.Ø	Analgesic nephropathy
			N14.1	Nephropathy induced by oth drug/meds/biol subst
			N14.2	Neuropath induced by unsp drug, medicament or biolg sub
			N14.3	Nephropathy induced by heavy metals
			N14.4	Toxic nephropathy, not elsewhere classified
			N15.Ø	Balkan nephropathy
			N15.8	Other specified renal tubulo-interstitial diseases
583.9	NEPHRITIS&NEPHRPATH NOT AC/CHRN W/UNS PATHAL LES		**NØ5.9**	Unsp nephritic syndrome with unspecified morphologic changes
			NØ6.9	Isolated proteinuria with unspecified morphologic lesion
			NØ7.9	Hereditary nephropathy, NEC w unsp morphologic lesions
			N15.9	Renal tubulo-interstitial disease, unspecified
584.5	ACUTE KIDNEY FAILURE W/LESION TUBULAR NECROSIS	➡	**N17.Ø**	Acute kidney failure with tubular necrosis
584.6	ACUTE KIDNEY FAILURE W/LES RENAL CORTICAL NECRO		**N17.1**	Acute kidney failure with acute cortical necrosis
584.7	ACUTE KIDNEY FAILURE W/LESION MEDULLARY NECROSIS		**N17.2**	Acute kidney failure with medullary necrosis
584.8	AC KIDNEY FAIL OTH SPEC PATHOLOGICAL LES KIDNEY	➡	**N17.8**	Other acute kidney failure
584.9	ACUTE KIDNEY FAILURE UNSPECIFIED	➡	**N17.9**	Acute kidney failure, unspecified
585.1	CHRONIC KIDNEY DISEASE STAGE I	➡	**N18.1**	Chronic kidney disease, stage 1
585.2	CHRONIC KIDNEY DISEASE STAGE II (MILD)	➡	**N18.2**	Chronic kidney disease, stage 2 (mild)
585.3	CHRONIC KIDNEY DISEASE STAGE III (MODERATE)	➡	**N18.3**	Chronic kidney disease, stage 3 (moderate)
585.4	CHRONIC KIDNEY DISEASE STAGE IV (SEVERE)	➡	**N18.4**	Chronic kidney disease, stage 4 (severe)
585.5	CHRONIC KIDNEY DISEASE STAGE V	➡	**N18.5**	Chronic kidney disease, stage 5
585.6	END STAGE RENAL DISEASE	➡	**N18.6**	End stage renal disease
585.9	CHRONIC KIDNEY DISEASE UNSPECIFIED	➡	**N18.9**	Chronic kidney disease, unspecified
586	UNSPECIFIED RENAL FAILURE	➡	**N19**	Unspecified kidney failure
587	UNSPECIFIED RENAL SCLEROSIS		**N26.1**	Atrophy of kidney (terminal)
			N26.9	Renal sclerosis, unspecified
588.Ø	RENAL OSTEODYSTROPHY	➡	**N25.Ø**	Renal osteodystrophy
588.1	NEPHROGENIC DIABETES INSIPIDUS	➡	**N25.1**	Nephrogenic diabetes insipidus
588.81	SECONDARY HYPERPARATHYROIDISM	➡	**N25.81**	Secondary hyperparathyroidism of renal origin
588.89	OTH SPEC D/O RESULT FROM IMPAIRED RENAL FUNCTION	➡	**N25.89**	Oth disorders resulting from impaired renal tubular function
588.9	UNSPEC D/O RESULT FROM IMPAIRED RENAL FUNCTION	➡	**N25.9**	Disorder rslt from impaired renal tubular function, unsp
589.Ø	UNILATERAL SMALL KIDNEY	➡	**N27.Ø**	Small kidney, unilateral
589.1	BILATERAL SMALL KIDNEYS	➡	**N27.1**	Small kidney, bilateral
589.9	UNSPECIFIED SMALL KIDNEY	➡	**N27.9**	Small kidney, unspecified
59Ø.ØØ	CHRON PYELONEPHRITIS W/O LES RENL MEDULRY NECROS		**N11.Ø**	Nonobstructive reflux-associated chronic pyelonephritis
59Ø.Ø1	CHRON PYELONEPHRITIS W/LES RENAL MEDULRY NECROS		**N11.Ø**	Nonobstructive reflux-associated chronic pyelonephritis
		■	**N11.1**	Chronic obstructive pyelonephritis
			N11.8	Other chronic tubulo-interstitial nephritis
59Ø.1Ø	ACUT PYELONEPHRITIS W/O LES RENAL MEDULRY NECROS		**N1Ø**	Acute tubulo-interstitial nephritis
59Ø.11	ACUT PYELONEPHRITIS W/LES RENAL MEDULRY NECROS		**N1Ø**	Acute tubulo-interstitial nephritis
59Ø.2	RENAL AND PERINEPHRIC ABSCESS	➡	**N15.1**	Renal and perinephric abscess
59Ø.3	PYELOURETERITIS CYSTICA		**N28.84**	Pyelitis cystica
			N28.85	Pyeloureteritis cystica
			N28.86	Ureteritis cystica
59Ø.8Ø	UNSPECIFIED PYELONEPHRITIS		**N11.9**	Chronic tubulo-interstitial nephritis, unspecified
			N12	Tubulo-interstitial nephritis, not spcf as acute or chronic
			N13.6	Pyonephrosis
59Ø.81	PYELITIS/PYELONEPHRITIS DISEASES CLASSIFIED ELSW		**N16**	Renal tubulo-interstitial disord in diseases classd elswhr
59Ø.9	UNSPECIFIED INFECTION OF KIDNEY		**N15.9**	Renal tubulo-interstitial disease, unspecified

[Brackets] indicate valid character values for each code. Character value meanings provided for each code grouping.

ICD-9-CM			ICD-10-CM	
591	HYDRONEPHROSIS	☐[1]	N13.1	Hydronephrosis w ureteral stricture, NEC
		☐[1]	N13.2	Hydronephrosis with renal and ureteral calculous obstruction
			N13.30	Unspecified hydronephrosis
			N13.39	Other hydronephrosis
592.0	CALCULUS OF KIDNEY	☐[1]	N13.2	Hydronephrosis with renal and ureteral calculous obstruction
			N20.0	Calculus of kidney
			N20.2	Calculus of kidney with calculus of ureter
592.1	CALCULUS OF URETER	☐[1]	N13.2	Hydronephrosis with renal and ureteral calculous obstruction
		➡	N20.1	Calculus of ureter
		☐	N20.2	Calculus of kidney with calculus of ureter
592.9	UNSPECIFIED URINARY CALCULUS	☐[2]	N13.9	Obstructive and reflux uropathy, unspecified
			N20.9	Urinary calculus, unspecified
			N22	Calculus of urinary tract in diseases classified elsewhere
593.0	NEPHROPTOSIS		N28.83	Nephroptosis
593.1	HYPERTROPHY OF KIDNEY	➡	N28.81	Hypertrophy of kidney
593.2	ACQUIRED CYST OF KIDNEY	➡	N28.1	Cyst of kidney, acquired
593.3	STRICTURE OR KINKING OF URETER	☐	N11.1	Chronic obstructive pyelonephritis
		☐[1]	N13.1	Hydronephrosis w ureteral stricture, NEC
			N13.5	Crossing vessel and stricture of ureter w/o hydronephrosis
593.4	OTHER URETERIC OBSTRUCTION	☐	N11.1	Chronic obstructive pyelonephritis
			N13.8	Other obstructive and reflux uropathy
593.5	HYDROURETER	➡	N13.4	Hydroureter
593.6	POSTURAL PROTEINURIA		R80.2	Orthostatic proteinuria, unspecified
593.70	VESICOURETRL REFLUX UNS/NO REFLUX NEPHROPATHY		N13.70	Vesicoureteral-reflux, unspecified
			N13.71	Vesicoureteral-reflux without reflux nephropathy
593.71	VESICOURETRL REFLUX W/REFLUX NEPHROPATHY UNILAT		N13.721	Vesicoureter-reflux w reflux neuropath w/o hydrourt, unil
			N13.731	Vesicoureter-reflux w reflux neuropath w hydrourt, unil
593.72	VESICOURETERAL REFLUX W/REFLUX NEPHROPATHY BILAT		N13.722	Vesicoureter-reflux w reflux neuropath w/o hydrourt, bi
			N13.732	Vesicoureter-reflux w reflux neuropath w hydrourt, bilateral
593.73	VESICOURETERAL REFLUX W/REFLUX NEPHROPATHY NOS		N13.729	Vesicoureter-reflux w reflux nephropathy w/o hydrourt, unsp
			N13.739	Vesicoureter-reflux w reflux nephropathy w hydroureter, unsp
			N13.9	Obstructive and reflux uropathy, unspecified
593.81	VASCULAR DISORDERS OF KIDNEY		N28.0	Ischemia and infarction of kidney
593.82	URETERAL FISTULA		N28.89	Other specified disorders of kidney and ureter
593.89	OTHER SPECIFIED DISORDER OF KIDNEY AND URETER		N28.82	Megaloureter
			N28.89	Other specified disorders of kidney and ureter
593.9	UNSPECIFIED DISORDER OF KIDNEY AND URETER		N28.9	Disorder of kidney and ureter, unspecified
			N29	Oth disorders of kidney and ureter in diseases classd elswhr
594.0	CALCULUS IN DIVERTICULUM OF BLADDER		N21.0	Calculus in bladder
594.1	OTHER CALCULUS IN BLADDER		N21.0	Calculus in bladder
594.2	CALCULUS IN URETHRA	➡	N21.1	Calculus in urethra
594.8	OTHER LOWER URINARY TRACT CALCULUS	➡	N21.8	Other lower urinary tract calculus
594.9	UNSPECIFIED CALCULUS OF LOWER URINARY TRACT	➡	N21.9	Calculus of lower urinary tract, unspecified
595.0	ACUTE CYSTITIS		N30.00	Acute cystitis without hematuria
			N30.01	Acute cystitis with hematuria
595.1	CHRONIC INTERSTITIAL CYSTITIS		N30.10	Interstitial cystitis (chronic) without hematuria
			N30.11	Interstitial cystitis (chronic) with hematuria
595.2	OTHER CHRONIC CYSTITIS		N30.20	Other chronic cystitis without hematuria
			N30.21	Other chronic cystitis with hematuria
595.3	TRIGONITIS		N30.30	Trigonitis without hematuria
			N30.31	Trigonitis with hematuria
595.4	CYSTITIS IN DISEASES CLASSIFIED ELSEWHERE	☐	A56.01	Chlamydial cystitis and urethritis
			N30.80	Other cystitis without hematuria
			N30.81	Other cystitis with hematuria
595.81	CYSTITIS CYSTICA		N30.80	Other cystitis without hematuria
			N30.81	Other cystitis with hematuria
595.82	IRRADIATION CYSTITIS		N30.40	Irradiation cystitis without hematuria
			N30.41	Irradiation cystitis with hematuria
595.89	OTHER SPECIFIED TYPES OF CYSTITIS		N30.80	Other cystitis without hematuria
			N30.81	Other cystitis with hematuria
595.9	UNSPECIFIED CYSTITIS		N30.90	Cystitis, unspecified without hematuria
			N30.91	Cystitis, unspecified with hematuria
596.0	BLADDER NECK OBSTRUCTION	➡	N32.0	Bladder-neck obstruction
596.1	INTESTINOVESICAL FISTULA	➡	N32.1	Vesicointestinal fistula
596.2	VESICAL FISTULA NOT ELSEWHERE CLASSIFIED	➡	N32.2	Vesical fistula, not elsewhere classified
596.3	DIVERTICULUM OF BLADDER	➡	N32.3	Diverticulum of bladder
596.4	ATONY OF BLADDER		N31.2	Flaccid neuropathic bladder, not elsewhere classified
596.51	HYPERTONICITY OF BLADDER	➡	N32.81	Overactive bladder

1. Official ICD-10-CM GEM update summary indicates ICD-9-CM code 592.9 should be included in Choice List 2 with GEM flag 10112 for the cluster/combination map for ICD-10-CM code N13.2, but this is not included in the Official ICD-10-CM GEM file as of date of publication.
2. Official ICD-10-CM GEM files show ICD-10-CM code N13.9 mapped to ICD-9-CM code 592.9 as a cluster/combination Choice List 2 GEM flag 10112 without an option for a Choice List 1 GEM flag 10111 as of date of publication.

ICD-9-CM			ICD-10-CM	
596.52	LOW BLADDER COMPLIANCE		**N31.8**	Other neuromuscular dysfunction of bladder
596.53	PARALYSIS OF BLADDER		**N31.2**	Flaccid neuropathic bladder, not elsewhere classified
596.54	NEUROGENIC BLADDER, NOS		**N31.Ø**	Uninhibited neuropathic bladder, not elsewhere classified
			N31.1	Reflex neuropathic bladder, not elsewhere classified
			N31.9	Neuromuscular dysfunction of bladder, unspecified
596.55	DETRUSOR SPHINCTER DYSSYNERGIA	➡	**N36.44**	Muscular disorders of urethra
596.59	OTHER FUNCTIONAL DISORDER OF BLADDER		**N31.9**	Neuromuscular dysfunction of bladder, unspecified
596.6	NONTRAUMATIC RUPTURE OF BLADDER		**N32.89**	Other specified disorders of bladder
596.7	HEMORRHAGE INTO BLADDER WALL		**N32.89**	Other specified disorders of bladder
596.81	INFECTION OF CYSTOSTOMY		**N99.511**	Cystostomy infection
596.82	MECHANICAL COMPLICATION OF CYSTOSTOMY		**N99.512**	Cystostomy malfunction
596.83	OTHER COMPLICATION OF CYSTOSTOMY		**N99.51Ø**	Cystostomy hemorrhage
			N99.518	Other cystostomy complication
596.89	OTHER SPECIFIED DISORDERS OF BLADDER		**N32.89**	Other specified disorders of bladder
			N33	Bladder disorders in diseases classified elsewhere
596.9	UNSPECIFIED DISORDER OF BLADDER	➡	**N32.9**	Bladder disorder, unspecified
597.Ø	URETHRAL ABSCESS	➡	**N34.Ø**	Urethral abscess
597.8Ø	UNSPECIFIED URETHRITIS		**N34.1**	Nonspecific urethritis
			N34.2	Other urethritis
597.81	URETHRAL SYNDROME NOS	➡	**N34.3**	Urethral syndrome, unspecified
597.89	OTHER URETHRITIS		**N34.2**	Other urethritis
598.ØØ	URETHRAL STRICTURE DUE TO UNSPECIFIED INFECTION		**N35.111**	Postinfective urethral stricture, NEC, male, meatal
			N35.112	Postinfective bulbous urethral stricture, NEC
			N35.113	Postinfective membranous urethral stricture, NEC
			N35.114	Postinfective anterior urethral stricture, NEC
			N35.119	Postinfective urethral stricture, NEC, male, unsp
			N35.12	Postinfective urethral stricture, NEC, female
598.Ø1	URETHRAL STRICTURE DUE INFECTIVE DZ CLASS ELSW		**N37**	Urethral disorders in diseases classified elsewhere
598.1	TRAUMATIC URETHRAL STRICTURE		**N35.Ø1Ø**	Post-traumatic urethral stricture, male, meatal
			N35.Ø11	Post-traumatic bulbous urethral stricture
			N35.Ø12	Post-traumatic membranous urethral stricture
			N35.Ø13	Post-traumatic anterior urethral stricture
			N35.Ø14	Post-traumatic urethral stricture, male, unspecified
			N35.Ø21	Urethral stricture due to childbirth
			N35.Ø28	Other post-traumatic urethral stricture, female
598.2	POSTOPERATIVE URETHRAL STRICTURE		**N99.11Ø**	Postprocedural urethral stricture, male, meatal
			N99.111	Postprocedural bulbous urethral stricture
			N99.112	Postprocedural membranous urethral stricture
			N99.113	Postprocedural anterior urethral stricture
			N99.114	Postprocedural urethral stricture, male, unspecified
			N99.12	Postprocedural urethral stricture, female
598.8	OTHER SPECIFIED CAUSES OF URETHRAL STRICTURE	➡	**N35.8**	Other urethral stricture
598.9	UNSPECIFIED URETHRAL STRICTURE	➡	**N35.9**	Urethral stricture, unspecified
599.Ø	URINARY TRACT INFECTION SITE NOT SPECIFIED	➡	**N39.Ø**	Urinary tract infection, site not specified
599.1	URETHRAL FISTULA		**N36.Ø**	Urethral fistula
599.2	URETHRAL DIVERTICULUM	➡	**N36.1**	Urethral diverticulum
599.3	URETHRAL CARUNCLE	➡	**N36.2**	Urethral caruncle
599.4	URETHRAL FALSE PASSAGE		**N36.5**	Urethral false passage
599.5	PROLAPSED URETHRAL MUCOSA		**N36.8**	Other specified disorders of urethra
599.6Ø	URINARY OBSTRUCTION UNSPECIFIED		**N13.9**	Obstructive and reflux uropathy, unspecified
599.69	URINARY OBSTRUCTION NOT ELSEWHERE CLASSIFIED		**N13.9**	Obstructive and reflux uropathy, unspecified
599.7Ø	HEMATURIA UNSPECIFIED	➡	**R31.9**	Hematuria, unspecified
599.71	GROSS HEMATURIA	➡	**R31.Ø**	Gross hematuria
599.72	MICROSCOPIC HEMATURIA		**R31.1**	Benign essential microscopic hematuria
			R31.2	Other microscopic hematuria
599.81	URETHRAL HYPERMOBILITY		**N36.41**	Hypermobility of urethra
		▣	**N36.43**	Combined hypermobility of urethra and intrns sphincter defic
599.82	INTRINSIC SPHINCTER DEFICIENCY		**N36.42**	Intrinsic sphincter deficiency (ISD)
		▣	**N36.43**	Combined hypermobility of urethra and intrns sphincter defic
599.83	URETHRAL INSTABILITY		**N36.8**	Other specified disorders of urethra
599.84	OTHER SPECIFIED DISORDERS OF URETHRA		**N36.8**	Other specified disorders of urethra
599.89	OTHER SPECIFIED DISORDERS OF URINARY TRACT	➡	**N39.8**	Other specified disorders of urinary system
599.9	UNSPECIFIED DISORDER OF URETHRA&URINARY TRACT		**N36.9**	Urethral disorder, unspecified
			N39.9	Disorder of urinary system, unspecified
6ØØ.ØØ	HYPERTROPHY PROSTATE W/O UR OBST & OTH LUTS		**N4Ø.Ø**	Enlarged prostate without lower urinary tract symptoms
6ØØ.Ø1	HYPERTROPHY PROSTATE W/UR OBST & OTH LUTS		**N4Ø.1**	Enlarged prostate with lower urinary tract symptoms
6ØØ.1Ø	NODULAR PROSTATE WITHOUT URINARY OBSTRUCTION		**N4Ø.2**	Nodular prostate without lower urinary tract symptoms
6ØØ.11	NODULAR PROSTATE WITH URINARY OBSTRUCTION		**N4Ø.3**	Nodular prostate with lower urinary tract symptoms
6ØØ.2Ø	BEN LOC HYPERPLASIA PROS W/O UR OBST & OTH LUTS		**N4Ø.Ø**	Enlarged prostate without lower urinary tract symptoms
6ØØ.21	BEN LOC HYPERPLASIA PROS W/UR OBST & OTH LUTS		**N4Ø.1**	Enlarged prostate with lower urinary tract symptoms
6ØØ.3	CYST OF PROSTATE		**N42.83**	Cyst of prostate

 [Brackets] indicate valid character values for each code. Character value meanings provided for each code grouping.

ICD-9-CM			ICD-10-CM	
600.90	HYPERPLASIA PROSTATE UNS W/O UR OBST & OTH LUTS		N40.0	Enlarged prostate without lower urinary tract symptoms
600.91	HYPERPLASIA PROSTATE UNS W/UR OBST & OTH LUTS		N40.1	Enlarged prostate with lower urinary tract symptoms
601.0	ACUTE PROSTATITIS		N41.0	Acute prostatitis
601.1	CHRONIC PROSTATITIS		N41.1	Chronic prostatitis
601.2	ABSCESS OF PROSTATE	➡	N41.2	Abscess of prostate
601.3	PROSTATOCYSTITIS	➡	N41.3	Prostatocystitis
601.4	PROSTATITIS IN DISEASES CLASSIFIED ELSEWHERE	◘	A18.14 N51	Tuberculosis of prostate Disorders of male genital organs in diseases classd elswhr
601.8	OTHER SPECIFIED INFLAMMATORY DISEASE OF PROSTATE		N41.4 N41.8	Granulomatous prostatitis Other inflammatory diseases of prostate
601.9	UNSPECIFIED PROSTATITIS	➡	N41.9	Inflammatory disease of prostate, unspecified
602.0	CALCULUS OF PROSTATE	➡	N42.0	Calculus of prostate
602.1	CONGESTION OR HEMORRHAGE OF PROSTATE	➡	N42.1	Congestion and hemorrhage of prostate
602.2	ATROPHY OF PROSTATE		N42.89	Other specified disorders of prostate
602.3	DYSPLASIA OF PROSTATE	➡	N42.3	Dysplasia of prostate
602.8	OTHER SPECIFIED DISORDER OF PROSTATE		N42.81 N42.82 N42.89	Prostatodynia syndrome Prostatosis syndrome Other specified disorders of prostate
602.9	UNSPECIFIED DISORDER OF PROSTATE	➡	N42.9	Disorder of prostate, unspecified
603.0	ENCYSTED HYDROCELE	➡	N43.0	Encysted hydrocele
603.1	INFECTED HYDROCELE	➡	N43.1	Infected hydrocele
603.8	OTHER SPECIFIED TYPE OF HYDROCELE	➡	N43.2	Other hydrocele
603.9	UNSPECIFIED HYDROCELE	➡	N43.3	Hydrocele, unspecified
604.0	ORCHITIS EPIDIDYMITIS&EPIDIDYMO-ORCHITIS W/ABSC		N45.4	Abscess of epididymis or testis
604.90	UNSPECIFIED ORCHITIS AND EPIDIDYMITIS		N45.1 N45.2 N45.3	Epididymitis Orchitis Epididymo-orchitis
604.91	ORCHITIS&EPIDIDYMITIS DISEASE CLASSIFIED ELSW		N51	Disorders of male genital organs in diseases classd elswhr
604.99	OTH ORCHIT EPIDIDYMIT&EPIDIDYMO-ORCHIT W/O ABSC		N45.1 N45.2 N45.3	Epididymitis Orchitis Epididymo-orchitis
605	REDUNDANT PREPUCE AND PHIMOSIS		N47.0 N47.1 N47.2 N47.3 N47.4 N47.5 N47.7 N47.8	Adherent prepuce, newborn Phimosis Paraphimosis Deficient foreskin Benign cyst of prepuce Adhesions of prepuce and glans penis Other inflammatory diseases of prepuce Other disorders of prepuce
606.0	AZOOSPERMIA		N46.01 N46.021 N46.022 N46.023 N46.024 N46.025	Organic azoospermia Azoospermia due to drug therapy Azoospermia due to infection Azoospermia due to obstruction of efferent ducts Azoospermia due to radiation Azoospermia due to systemic disease
606.1	OLIGOSPERMIA		N46.11 N46.121 N46.122 N46.123 N46.124 N46.125 N46.129	Organic oligospermia Oligospermia due to drug therapy Oligospermia due to infection Oligospermia due to obstruction of efferent ducts Oligospermia due to radiation Oligospermia due to systemic disease Oligospermia due to other extratesticular causes
606.8	INFERTILITY DUE TO EXTRATESTICULAR CAUSES		N46.029 N46.8	Azoospermia due to other extratesticular causes Other male infertility
606.9	UNSPECIFIED MALE INFERTILITY	➡	N46.9	Male infertility, unspecified
607.0	LEUKOPLAKIA OF PENIS		N48.0	Leukoplakia of penis
607.1	BALANOPOSTHITIS		N47.6 N48.1	Balanoposthitis Balanitis
607.2	OTHER INFLAMMATORY DISORDERS OF PENIS		N48.21 N48.22 N48.29	Abscess of corpus cavernosum and penis Cellulitis of corpus cavernosum and penis Other inflammatory disorders of penis
607.3	PRIAPISM		N48.30 N48.31 N48.32 N48.33 N48.39	Priapism, unspecified Priapism due to trauma Priapism due to disease classified elsewhere Priapism, drug-induced Other priapism
607.81	BALANITIS XEROTICA OBLITERANS		N48.0	Leukoplakia of penis
607.82	VASCULAR DISORDERS OF PENIS		N50.1	Vascular disorders of male genital organs
607.83	EDEMA OF PENIS		N48.89	Other specified disorders of penis

ICD-9-CM			ICD-10-CM	
607.84	IMPOTENCE OF ORGANIC ORIGIN		N52.01	Erectile dysfunction due to arterial insufficiency
			N52.02	Corporo-venous occlusive erectile dysfunction
			N52.03	Comb artrl insuff & corporo-venous occlusv erectile dysfnct
			N52.1	Erectile dysfunction due to diseases classified elsewhere
			N52.2	Drug-induced erectile dysfunction
			N52.31	Erectile dysfunction following radical prostatectomy
			N52.32	Erectile dysfunction following radical cystectomy
			N52.33	Erectile dysfunction following urethral surgery
			N52.34	Erectile dysfunction following simple prostatectomy
			N52.39	Other post-surgical erectile dysfunction
			N52.8	Other male erectile dysfunction
			N52.9	Male erectile dysfunction, unspecified
607.85	PEYRONIES DISEASE		N48.6	Induration penis plastica
607.89	OTHER SPECIFIED DISORDER OF PENIS		N48.5	Ulcer of penis
			N48.81	Thrombosis of superficial vein of penis
			N48.82	Acquired torsion of penis
			N48.83	Acquired buried penis
			N48.89	Other specified disorders of penis
607.9	UNSPECIFIED DISORDER OF PENIS	➡	N48.9	Disorder of penis, unspecified
608.0	SEMINAL VESICULITIS	➡	N49.0	Inflammatory disorders of seminal vesicle
608.1	SPERMATOCELE		N43.40	Spermatocele of epididymis, unspecified
			N43.41	Spermatocele of epididymis, single
			N43.42	Spermatocele of epididymis, multiple
608.20	TORSION OF TESTIS UNSPECIFIED	➡	N44.00	Torsion of testis, unspecified
608.21	EXTRAVAGINAL TORSION OF SPERMATIC CORD	➡	N44.01	Extravaginal torsion of spermatic cord
608.22	INTRAVAGINAL TORSION OF SPERMATIC CORD	➡	N44.02	Intravaginal torsion of spermatic cord
608.23	TORSION OF APPENDIX TESTIS	➡	N44.03	Torsion of appendix testis
608.24	TORSION OF APPENDIX EPIDIDYMIS	➡	N44.04	Torsion of appendix epididymis
608.3	ATROPHY OF TESTIS	➡	N50.0	Atrophy of testis
608.4	OTHER INFLAMMATORY DISORDER MALE GENITAL ORGANS		N49.1	Inflam disorders of sperm cord, tunica vaginalis and vas def
			N49.2	Inflammatory disorders of scrotum
			N49.3	Fournier gangrene
			N49.8	Inflammatory disorders of oth male genital organs
			N49.9	Inflammatory disorder of unspecified male genital organ
608.81	SPEC DISORDER MALE GENITAL ORGANS DZ CLASS ELSW		N51	Disorders of male genital organs in diseases classd elswhr
608.82	HEMATOSPERMIA	➡	R36.1	Hematospermia
608.83	SPECIFIED VASCULAR DISORDER MALE GENITAL ORGANS		N50.1	Vascular disorders of male genital organs
608.84	CHYLOCELE OF TUNICA VAGINALIS		N50.8	Other specified disorders of male genital organs
608.85	STRICTURE OF MALE GENITAL ORGANS		N50.8	Other specified disorders of male genital organs
608.86	EDEMA OF MALE GENITAL ORGANS		N50.8	Other specified disorders of male genital organs
608.87	RETROGRADE EJACULATION		N53.11	Retarded ejaculation
			N53.13	Anejaculatory orgasm
			N53.14	Retrograde ejaculation
			N53.19	Other ejaculatory dysfunction
608.89	OTHER SPECIFIED DISORDER OF MALE GENITAL ORGANS		N44.1	Cyst of tunica albuginea testis
			N44.2	Benign cyst of testis
			N44.8	Other noninflammatory disorders of the testis
			N50.3	Cyst of epididymis
			N50.8	Other specified disorders of male genital organs
			N53.12	Painful ejaculation
			N53.8	Other male sexual dysfunction
			N53.9	Unspecified male sexual dysfunction
608.9	UNSPECIFIED DISORDER OF MALE GENITAL ORGANS		N50.9	Disorder of male genital organs, unspecified
			R10.2	Pelvic and perineal pain
610.0	SOLITARY CYST OF BREAST		N60.01	Solitary cyst of right breast
			N60.02	Solitary cyst of left breast
			N60.09	Solitary cyst of unspecified breast
610.1	DIFFUSE CYSTIC MASTOPATHY		N60.11	Diffuse cystic mastopathy of right breast
			N60.12	Diffuse cystic mastopathy of left breast
			N60.19	Diffuse cystic mastopathy of unspecified breast
610.2	FIBROADENOSIS OF BREAST		N60.21	Fibroadenosis of right breast
			N60.22	Fibroadenosis of left breast
			N60.29	Fibroadenosis of unspecified breast
610.3	FIBROSCLEROSIS OF BREAST		N60.31	Fibrosclerosis of right breast
			N60.32	Fibrosclerosis of left breast
			N60.39	Fibrosclerosis of unspecified breast
610.4	MAMMARY DUCT ECTASIA		N60.41	Mammary duct ectasia of right breast
			N60.42	Mammary duct ectasia of left breast
			N60.49	Mammary duct ectasia of unspecified breast
610.8	OTHER SPECIFIED BENIGN MAMMARY DYSPLASIAS		N60.81	Other benign mammary dysplasias of right breast
			N60.82	Other benign mammary dysplasias of left breast
			N60.89	Other benign mammary dysplasias of unspecified breast
610.9	UNSPECIFIED BENIGN MAMMARY DYSPLASIA		N60.91	Unspecified benign mammary dysplasia of right breast
			N60.92	Unspecified benign mammary dysplasia of left breast
			N60.99	Unspecified benign mammary dysplasia of unspecified breast
611.0	INFLAMMATORY DISEASE OF BREAST	➡	N61	Inflammatory disorders of breast

ICD-9-CM			ICD-10-CM	
611.1	HYPERTROPHY OF BREAST	➡	**N62**	Hypertrophy of breast
611.2	FISSURE OF NIPPLE		**N64.Ø**	Fissure and fistula of nipple
611.3	FAT NECROSIS OF BREAST	➡	**N64.1**	Fat necrosis of breast
611.4	ATROPHY OF BREAST	➡	**N64.2**	Atrophy of breast
611.5	GALACTOCELE		**N64.89**	Other specified disorders of breast
611.6	GALACTORRHEA NOT ASSOCIATED WITH CHILDBIRTH	➡	**N64.3**	Galactorrhea not associated with childbirth
611.71	MASTODYNIA	➡	**N64.4**	Mastodynia
611.72	LUMP OR MASS IN BREAST	➡	**N63**	Unspecified lump in breast
611.79	OTHER SIGN AND SYMPTOM IN BREAST		**N64.51** **N64.52** **N64.53** **N64.59**	Induration of breast Nipple discharge Retraction of nipple Other signs and symptoms in breast
611.81	PTOSIS OF BREAST	➡	**N64.81**	Ptosis of breast
611.82	HYPOPLASIA OF BREAST	➡	**N64.82**	Hypoplasia of breast
611.83	CAPSULAR CONTRACTURE OF BREAST IMPLANT		**N64.89**	Other specified disorders of breast
611.89	OTHER SPECIFIED DISORDERS OF BREAST		**N64.89**	Other specified disorders of breast
611.9	UNSPECIFIED BREAST DISORDER	➡	**N64.9**	Disorder of breast, unspecified
612.Ø	DEFORMITY OF RECONSTRUCTED BREAST	➡	**N65.Ø**	Deformity of reconstructed breast
612.1	DISPROPORTION OF RECONSTRUCTED BREAST	➡	**N65.1**	Disproportion of reconstructed breast
614.Ø	ACUTE SALPINGITIS AND OOPHORITIS		**N7Ø.Ø1** **N7Ø.Ø2** **N7Ø.Ø3**	Acute salpingitis Acute oophoritis Acute salpingitis and oophoritis
614.1	CHRONIC SALPINGITIS AND OOPHORITIS		**N7Ø.11** **N7Ø.12** **N7Ø.13**	Chronic salpingitis Chronic oophoritis Chronic salpingitis and oophoritis
614.2	SALPINGITIS&OOPHORITIS NOT ACUT SUBACUT/CHRN		**N7Ø.91** **N7Ø.92** **N7Ø.93**	Salpingitis, unspecified Oophoritis, unspecified Salpingitis and oophoritis, unspecified
614.3	ACUTE PARAMETRITIS AND PELVIC CELLULITIS	➡	**N73.Ø**	Acute parametritis and pelvic cellulitis
614.4	CHRONIC/UNSPEC PARAMETRITIS&PELVIC CELLULITIS		**N73.1** **N73.2**	Chronic parametritis and pelvic cellulitis Unspecified parametritis and pelvic cellulitis
614.5	ACUTE OR UNSPECIFIED PELVIC PERITONITIS FEMALE	➡	**N73.3**	Female acute pelvic peritonitis
614.6	PELVIC PERITONEAL ADHESIONS, FEMALE	➡	**N73.6**	Female pelvic peritoneal adhesions (postinfective)
614.7	OTHER CHRONIC PELVIC PERITONITIS FEMALE	➡	**N73.4**	Female chronic pelvic peritonitis
614.8	OTH SPEC INFLAM DISEASE FE PELVIC ORGANS&TISSUES		**N73.8** **N74**	Other specified female pelvic inflammatory diseases Female pelvic inflam disorders in diseases classd elswhr
614.9	UNSPEC INFLAM DISEASE FE PELVIC ORGANS&TISSUES	📖	**A56.11** **N73.5** **N73.9**	Chlamydial female pelvic inflammatory disease Female pelvic peritonitis, unspecified Female pelvic inflammatory disease, unspecified
615.Ø	ACUTE INFLAMMATORY DISEASE UTERUS EXCEPT CERVIX	➡	**N71.Ø**	Acute inflammatory disease of uterus
615.1	CHRONIC INFLAMMATORY DISEASE UTERUS EXCEPT CERV	➡	**N71.1**	Chronic inflammatory disease of uterus
615.9	UNSPECIFIED INFLAMMATORY DISEASE OF UTERUS	➡	**N71.9**	Inflammatory disease of uterus, unspecified
616.Ø	CERVICITIS AND ENDOCERVICITIS	➡	**N72**	Inflammatory disease of cervix uteri
616.1Ø	UNSPECIFIED VAGINITIS AND VULVOVAGINITIS		**N76.Ø** **N76.1** **N76.2** **N76.3**	Acute vaginitis Subacute and chronic vaginitis Acute vulvitis Subacute and chronic vulvitis
616.11	VAGINITIS&VULVOVAGINITIS DISEASES CLASS ELSW	📖	**A56.Ø2** **N77.1**	Chlamydial vulvovaginitis Vaginitis, vulvitis and vulvovaginitis in dis classd elswhr
616.2	CYST OF BARTHOLINS GLAND		**N75.Ø** **N75.8**	Cyst of Bartholin's gland Other diseases of Bartholin's gland
616.3	ABSCESS OF BARTHOLINS GLAND	➡	**N75.1**	Abscess of Bartholin's gland
616.4	OTHER ABSCESS OF VULVA	➡	**N76.4**	Abscess of vulva
616.5Ø	UNSPECIFIED ULCERATION OF VULVA	➡	**N76.6**	Ulceration of vulva
616.51	ULCERATION OF VULVA DISEASE CLASSIFIED ELSEWHERE	➡	**N77.Ø**	Ulceration of vulva in diseases classified elsewhere
616.81	MUCOSITIS ULCERATIVE OF CERVIX VAGINA AND VULVA	➡	**N76.81**	Mucositis (ulcerative) of vagina and vulva
616.89	OTHER INFLAMMATORY DISEASE CERVIX VAGINA&VULVA		**N75.9** **N76.5** **N76.89**	Disease of Bartholin's gland, unspecified Ulceration of vagina Other specified inflammation of vagina and vulva
616.9	UNSPEC INFLAMMATORY DISEASE CERVIX VAGINA&VULVA		**N73.9**	Female pelvic inflammatory disease, unspecified
617.Ø	ENDOMETRIOSIS OF UTERUS	➡	**N8Ø.Ø**	Endometriosis of uterus
617.1	ENDOMETRIOSIS OF OVARY	➡	**N8Ø.1**	Endometriosis of ovary
617.2	ENDOMETRIOSIS OF FALLOPIAN TUBE	➡	**N8Ø.2**	Endometriosis of fallopian tube
617.3	ENDOMETRIOSIS OF PELVIC PERITONEUM	➡	**N8Ø.3**	Endometriosis of pelvic peritoneum
617.4	ENDOMETRIOSIS OF RECTOVAGINAL SEPTUM AND VAGINA	➡	**N8Ø.4**	Endometriosis of rectovaginal septum and vagina
617.5	ENDOMETRIOSIS OF INTESTINE	➡	**N8Ø.5**	Endometriosis of intestine
617.6	ENDOMETRIOSIS IN SCAR OF SKIN	➡	**N8Ø.6**	Endometriosis in cutaneous scar
617.8	ENDOMETRIOSIS OF OTHER SPECIFIED SITES	➡	**N8Ø.8**	Other endometriosis
617.9	ENDOMETRIOSIS, SITE UNSPECIFIED	➡	**N8Ø.9**	Endometriosis, unspecified
618.ØØ	UNS PROLAPS VAG WALLS W/O MENTION UTERN PROLAPS		**N81.9**	Female genital prolapse, unspecified

ICD-9-CM			ICD-10-CM	
618.01	CYSTOCELE WITHOUT MENTION UTERINE PROLAPSE MIDLN		**N81.10** **N81.11**	Cystocele, unspecified Cystocele, midline
618.02	CYSTOCELE WITHOUT MENTION UTERINE PROLAPSE LAT	➡	**N81.12**	Cystocele, lateral
618.03	URETHROCELE WITHOUT MENTION OF UTERINE PROLAPSE	➡	**N81.0**	Urethrocele
618.04	RECTOCELE WITHOUT MENTION OF UTERINE PROLAPSE	➡	**N81.6**	Rectocele
618.05	PERINEOCELE WITHOUT MENTION OF UTERINE PROLAPSE	➡	**N81.81**	Perineocele
618.09	OTH PROLAPS VAG WALLS W/O MENTION UTERN PROLAPS		**N81.89**	Other female genital prolapse
618.1	UTERINE PROLAPSE W/O MENTION VAG WALL PROLAPSE		**N81.2**	Incomplete uterovaginal prolapse
618.2	UTEROVAGINAL PROLAPSE, INCOMPLETE		**N81.2**	Incomplete uterovaginal prolapse
618.3	UTEROVAGINAL PROLAPSE, COMPLETE	➡	**N81.3**	Complete uterovaginal prolapse
618.4	UTEROVAGINAL PROLAPSE, UNSPECIFIED	➡	**N81.4**	Uterovaginal prolapse, unspecified
618.5	PROLAPSE OF VAGINAL VAULT AFTER HYSTERECTOMY	➡	**N99.3**	Prolapse of vaginal vault after hysterectomy
618.6	VAGINAL ENTEROCELE CONGENITAL OR ACQUIRED	➡	**N81.5**	Vaginal enterocele
618.7	GENITAL PROLAPSE OLD LACERATION MUSC PELVIC FLR		**N81.89**	Other female genital prolapse
618.81	INCOMPETENCE OR WEAKENING OF PUBOCERVICAL TISSUE	➡	**N81.82**	Incompetence or weakening of pubocervical tissue
618.82	INCOMPETENCE OR WEAKENING OF RECTOVAGINAL TISSUE	➡	**N81.83**	Incompetence or weakening of rectovaginal tissue
618.83	PELVIC MUSCLE WASTING	➡	**N81.84**	Pelvic muscle wasting
618.84	CERVICAL STUMP PROLAPSE		**N81.2** **N81.85**	Incomplete uterovaginal prolapse Cervical stump prolapse
618.89	OTHER SPECIFIED GENITAL PROLAPSE		**N81.89**	Other female genital prolapse
618.9	UNSPECIFIED GENITAL PROLAPSE		**N81.9**	Female genital prolapse, unspecified
619.0	URINARY-GENITAL TRACT FISTULA FEMALE		**N82.0** **N82.1**	Vesicovaginal fistula Other female urinary-genital tract fistulae
619.1	DIGESTIVE-GENITAL TRACT FISTULA FEMALE		**N82.2** **N82.3** **N82.4**	Fistula of vagina to small intestine Fistula of vagina to large intestine Other female intestinal-genital tract fistulae
619.2	GENITAL TRACT-SKIN FISTULA, FEMALE	➡	**N82.5**	Female genital tract-skin fistulae
619.8	OTH SPEC FISTULA INVOLVING FEMALE GENITAL TRACT		**N82.8**	Other female genital tract fistulae
619.9	UNSPEC FISTULA INVOLVING FEMALE GENITAL TRACT	➡	**N82.9**	Female genital tract fistula, unspecified
620.0	FOLLICULAR CYST OF OVARY	➡	**N83.0**	Follicular cyst of ovary
620.1	CORPUS LUTEUM CYST OR HEMATOMA	➡	**N83.1**	Corpus luteum cyst
620.2	OTHER AND UNSPECIFIED OVARIAN CYST		**N83.20** **N83.29**	Unspecified ovarian cysts Other ovarian cysts
620.3	ACQUIRED ATROPHY OF OVARY AND FALLOPIAN TUBE		**N83.31** **N83.32** **N83.33**	Acquired atrophy of ovary Acquired atrophy of fallopian tube Acquired atrophy of ovary and fallopian tube
620.4	PROLAPSE OR HERNIA OF OVARY AND FALLOPIAN TUBE	➡	**N83.4**	Prolapse and hernia of ovary and fallopian tube
620.5	TORSION OVARY OVARIAN PEDICLE OR FALLOPIAN TUBE		**N83.51** **N83.52** **N83.53**	Torsion of ovary and ovarian pedicle Torsion of fallopian tube Torsion of ovary, ovarian pedicle and fallopian tube
620.6	BROAD LIGAMENT LACERATION SYNDROME		**N83.8**	Oth noninflammatory disord of ovary, fallop and broad ligmt
620.7	HEMATOMA OF BROAD LIGAMENT	➡	**N83.7**	Hematoma of broad ligament
620.8	OTH NONINFLAM D/O OVRY FALLOP TUBE&BROAD LIG		**N83.6** **N83.8** **N99.83**	Hematosalpinx Oth noninflammatory disord of ovary, fallop and broad ligmt Residual ovary syndrome
620.9	UNSPEC NONINFLAM D/O OVRY FALLOP TUBE&BROAD LIG	➡	**N83.9**	Noninflammatory disord of ovary, fallop & broad ligmt, unsp
621.0	POLYP OF CORPUS UTERI		**N84.0** **N84.8** **N84.9**	Polyp of corpus uteri Polyp of other parts of female genital tract Polyp of female genital tract, unspecified
621.1	CHRONIC SUBINVOLUTION OF UTERUS		**N85.3**	Subinvolution of uterus
621.2	HYPERTROPHY OF UTERUS	➡	**N85.2**	Hypertrophy of uterus
621.30	ENDOMETRIAL HYPERPLASIA UNSPECIFIED	➡	**N85.00**	Endometrial hyperplasia, unspecified
621.31	SIMPLE ENDOMETRIAL HYPERPLASIA WITHOUT ATYPIA		**N85.01**	Benign endometrial hyperplasia
621.32	COMPLEX ENDOMETRIAL HYPERPLASIA WITHOUT ATYPIA		**N85.01**	Benign endometrial hyperplasia
621.33	ENDOMETRIAL HYPERPLASIA WITH ATYPIA		**N85.02**	Endometrial intraepithelial neoplasia [EIN]
621.34	BENIGN ENDOMETRIAL HYPERPLASIA		**N85.01**	Benign endometrial hyperplasia
621.35	ENDOMETRIAL INTRAEPITHELIAL NEOPLASIA		**N85.02**	Endometrial intraepithelial neoplasia [EIN]
621.4	HEMATOMETRA	➡	**N85.7**	Hematometra
621.5	INTRAUTERINE SYNECHIAE	➡	**N85.6**	Intrauterine synechiae
621.6	MALPOSITION OF UTERUS	➡	**N85.4**	Malposition of uterus
621.7	CHRONIC INVERSION OF UTERUS		**N85.5**	Inversion of uterus
621.8	OTHER SPECIFIED DISORDERS OF UTERUS NEC		**N85.8**	Other specified noninflammatory disorders of uterus
621.9	UNSPECIFIED DISORDER OF UTERUS	➡	**N85.9**	Noninflammatory disorder of uterus, unspecified
622.0	EROSION AND ECTROPION OF CERVIX	➡	**N86**	Erosion and ectropion of cervix uteri
622.10	DYSPLASIA OF CERVIX UNSPECIFIED	➡	**N87.9**	Dysplasia of cervix uteri, unspecified
622.11	MILD DYSPLASIA OF CERVIX	➡	**N87.0**	Mild cervical dysplasia
622.12	MODERATE DYSPLASIA OF CERVIX	➡	**N87.1**	Moderate cervical dysplasia
622.2	LEUKOPLAKIA OF CERVIX	➡	**N88.0**	Leukoplakia of cervix uteri
622.3	OLD LACERATION OF CERVIX	➡	**N88.1**	Old laceration of cervix uteri

[Brackets] indicate valid character values for each code. Character value meanings provided for each code grouping.

ICD-9-CM			ICD-10-CM	
622.4	STRICTURE AND STENOSIS OF CERVIX	➡	N88.2	Stricture and stenosis of cervix uteri
622.5	INCOMPETENCE OF CERVIX	➡	N88.3	Incompetence of cervix uteri
622.6	HYPERTROPHIC ELONGATION OF CERVIX	➡	N88.4	Hypertrophic elongation of cervix uteri
622.7	MUCOUS POLYP OF CERVIX	➡	N84.1	Polyp of cervix uteri
622.8	OTHER SPECIFIED NONINFLAMMATORY DISORDER CERVIX	➡	N88.8	Other specified noninflammatory disorders of cervix uteri
622.9	UNSPECIFIED NONINFLAMMATORY DISORDER OF CERVIX	➡	N88.9	Noninflammatory disorder of cervix uteri, unspecified
623.Ø	DYSPLASIA OF VAGINA		N89.Ø N89.1 N89.3	Mild vaginal dysplasia Moderate vaginal dysplasia Dysplasia of vagina, unspecified
623.1	LEUKOPLAKIA OF VAGINA	➡	N89.4	Leukoplakia of vagina
623.2	STRICTURE OR ATRESIA OF VAGINA		N89.5 N99.2	Stricture and atresia of vagina Postprocedural adhesions of vagina
623.3	TIGHT HYMENAL RING	➡	N89.6	Tight hymenal ring
623.4	OLD VAGINAL LACERATION		N89.8	Other specified noninflammatory disorders of vagina
623.5	LEUKORRHEA NOT SPECIFIED AS INFECTIVE		N89.8	Other specified noninflammatory disorders of vagina
623.6	VAGINAL HEMATOMA		N89.8	Other specified noninflammatory disorders of vagina
623.7	POLYP OF VAGINA	➡	N84.2	Polyp of vagina
623.8	OTHER SPECIFIED NONINFLAMMATORY DISORDER VAGINA		N89.8	Other specified noninflammatory disorders of vagina
623.9	UNSPECIFIED NONINFLAMMATORY DISORDER OF VAGINA	➡	N89.9	Noninflammatory disorder of vagina, unspecified
624.Ø1	VULVAR INTRAEPITHELIAL NEOPLASIA I [VIN I]	➡	N9Ø.Ø	Mild vulvar dysplasia
624.Ø2	VULVAR INTRAEPITHELIAL NEOPLASIA II [VIN II]	➡	N9Ø.1	Moderate vulvar dysplasia
624.Ø9	OTHER DYSTROPHY OF VULVA		N9Ø.4	Leukoplakia of vulva
624.1	ATROPHY OF VULVA	➡	N9Ø.5	Atrophy of vulva
624.2	HYPERTROPHY OF CLITORIS		N9Ø.89	Oth noninflammatory disorders of vulva and perineum
624.3	HYPERTROPHY OF LABIA		N9Ø.6	Hypertrophy of vulva
624.4	OLD LACERATION OR SCARRING OF VULVA		N9Ø.89	Oth noninflammatory disorders of vulva and perineum
624.5	HEMATOMA OF VULVA		N9Ø.89	Oth noninflammatory disorders of vulva and perineum
624.6	POLYP OF LABIA AND VULVA	➡	N84.3	Polyp of vulva
624.8	OTH SPEC NONINFLAMMATORY DISORDER VULVA&PERINEUM		N9Ø.3 N9Ø.7 N9Ø.89	Dysplasia of vulva, unspecified Vulvar cyst Oth noninflammatory disorders of vulva and perineum
624.9	UNSPEC NONINFLAMMATORY DISORDER VULVA&PERINEUM	➡	N9Ø.9	Noninflammatory disorder of vulva and perineum, unspecified
625.Ø	DYSPAREUNIA	➡	N94.1	Dyspareunia
625.1	VAGINISMUS	➡	N94.2	Vaginismus
625.2	MITTELSCHMERZ	➡	N94.Ø	Mittelschmerz
625.3	DYSMENORRHEA		N94.4 N94.5 N94.6	Primary dysmenorrhea Secondary dysmenorrhea Dysmenorrhea, unspecified
625.4	PREMENSTRUAL TENSION SYNDROMES	➡	N94.3	Premenstrual tension syndrome
625.5	PELVIC CONGESTION SYNDROME		N94.89	Oth cond assoc w female genital organs and menstrual cycle
625.6	FEMALE STRESS INCONTINENCE		N39.3	Stress incontinence (female) (male)
625.7Ø	VULVODYNIA UNSPECIFIED	➡	N94.819	Vulvodynia, unspecified
625.71	VULVAR VESTIBULITIS	➡	N94.81Ø	Vulvar vestibulitis
625.79	OTHER VULVODYNIA	➡	N94.818	Other vulvodynia
625.8	OTH SPEC SYMPTOM ASSOC W/FEMALE GENITAL ORGANS		N94.89	Oth cond assoc w female genital organs and menstrual cycle
625.9	UNSPEC SYMPTOM ASSOC W/FEMALE GENITAL ORGANS		N94.89 R1Ø.2	Oth cond assoc w female genital organs and menstrual cycle Pelvic and perineal pain
626.Ø	ABSENCE OF MENSTRUATION		N91.Ø N91.1 N91.2	Primary amenorrhea Secondary amenorrhea Amenorrhea, unspecified
626.1	SCANTY OR INFREQUENT MENSTRUATION		N91.3 N91.4 N91.5	Primary oligomenorrhea Secondary oligomenorrhea Oligomenorrhea, unspecified
626.2	EXCESSIVE OR FREQUENT MENSTRUATION	➡	N92.Ø	Excessive and frequent menstruation with regular cycle
626.3	PUBERTY BLEEDING	➡	N92.2	Excessive menstruation at puberty
626.4	IRREGULAR MENSTRUAL CYCLE		N92.5 N92.6	Other specified irregular menstruation Irregular menstruation, unspecified
626.5	OVULATION BLEEDING	➡	N92.3	Ovulation bleeding
626.6	METRORRHAGIA	➡	N92.1	Excessive and frequent menstruation with irregular cycle
626.7	POSTCOITAL BLEEDING	➡	N93.Ø	Postcoital and contact bleeding
626.8	OTH D/O MENSTRUATION&OTH ABN BLEED FE GNT TRACT		N89.7 N92.5 N93.8	Hematocolpos Other specified irregular menstruation Other specified abnormal uterine and vaginal bleeding
626.9	UNS D/O MENSTRUATION&OTH ABN BLEED FE GNT TRACT		N92.6 N93.9	Irregular menstruation, unspecified Abnormal uterine and vaginal bleeding, unspecified
627.Ø	PREMENOPAUSAL MENORRHAGIA	➡	N92.4	Excessive bleeding in the premenopausal period
627.1	POSTMENOPAUSAL BLEEDING	➡	N95.Ø	Postmenopausal bleeding
627.2	SYMPTOMATIC MENOPAUSAL/FEMALE CLIMACTERIC STATES	➡	N95.1	Menopausal and female climacteric states
627.3	POSTMENOPAUSAL ATROPHIC VAGINITIS	➡	N95.2	Postmenopausal atrophic vaginitis
627.4	SYMPTOMATIC STATES ASSOC W/ARTFICL MENOPAUSE		N95.8	Other specified menopausal and perimenopausal disorders

ICD-9-CM		ICD-10-CM		
627.8	OTHER SPEC MENOPAUSAL&POSTMENOPAUSAL DISORDER		**N95.8**	Other specified menopausal and perimenopausal disorders
627.9	UNSPECIFIED MENOPAUSAL&POSTMENOPAUSAL DISORDER		**N95.9**	Unspecified menopausal and perimenopausal disorder
628.Ø	FEMALE INFERTILITY ASSOCIATED WITH ANOVULATION	➡	**N97.Ø**	Female infertility associated with anovulation
628.1	FEMALE INFERTILITY PITUITARY-HYPOTHALAMIC ORIGIN		**E23.Ø**	Hypopituitarism
628.2	FEMALE INFERTILITY OF TUBAL ORIGIN	➡	**N97.1**	Female infertility of tubal origin
628.3	FEMALE INFERTILITY OF UTERINE ORIGIN	➡	**N97.2**	Female infertility of uterine origin
628.4	FEMALE INFERTILITY OF CERVICAL OR VAGINAL ORIGIN		**N97.8**	Female infertility of other origin
628.8	FEMALE INFERTILITY OF OTHER SPECIFIED ORIGIN		**N97.8**	Female infertility of other origin
628.9	FEMALE INFERTILITY OF UNSPECIFIED ORIGIN	➡	**N97.9**	Female infertility, unspecified
629.Ø	HEMATOCELE FEMALE NOT ELSEWHERE CLASSIFIED		**N94.89**	Oth cond assoc w female genital organs and menstrual cycle
629.1	HYDROCELE, CANAL OF NUCK		**N94.89**	Oth cond assoc w female genital organs and menstrual cycle
629.2Ø	FEMALE GENITAL MUTILATION STATUS UNSPECIFIED	➡	**N9Ø.81Ø**	Female genital mutilation status, unspecified
629.21	FEMALE GENITAL MUTILATION TYPE I STATUS	➡	**N9Ø.811**	Female genital mutilation Type I status
629.22	FEMALE GENITAL MUTILATION TYPE II STATUS	➡	**N9Ø.812**	Female genital mutilation Type II status
629.23	FEMALE GENITAL MUTILATION TYPE III STATUS	➡	**N9Ø.813**	Female genital mutilation Type III status
629.29	OTHER FEMALE GENITAL MUTILATION STATUS	➡	**N9Ø.818**	Other female genital mutilation status
629.31	EROSION IMPL VAG MESH OTH MATL SURROUND ORG/TISS		**T83.711A**	Erosion of implnt vag prstht mtrl to surrnd org/tiss, init
629.32	EXPOSURE IMPL VAG MESH OTH PROSTH MATL VAGINA		**T83.721A**	Exposure of implnt vag prstht mtrl into vagina, init encntr
629.81	RECURRENT PREGNANCY LOSS W/O CURRENT PREGNANCY	➡	**N96**	Recurrent pregnancy loss
629.89	OTH SPECIFIED DISORDERS OF FEMALE GENITAL ORGANS		**N94.89**	Oth cond assoc w female genital organs and menstrual cycle
629.9	UNSPECIFIED DISORDER OF FEMALE GENITAL ORGANS		**N94.9**	Unsp cond assoc w female genital organs and menstrual cycle

[Brackets] indicate valid character values for each code. Character value meanings provided for each code grouping.

Complications of Pregnancy, Childbirth, and the Puerperium

ICD-9-CM			ICD-10-CM	
630	HYDATIDIFORM MOLE		**O01.0** **O01.1** **O01.9**	Classical hydatidiform mole Incomplete and partial hydatidiform mole Hydatidiform mole, unspecified
631.0	INAPPROPRIATE CHANGE QUAN HCG EARLY PREGNANCY		**O02.81**	Inapprop chg quantitav hCG in early pregnancy
631.8	OTHER ABNORMAL PRODUCTS OF CONCEPTION		**O02.0** **O02.89** **O02.9**	Blighted ovum and nonhydatidiform mole Other abnormal products of conception Abnormal product of conception, unspecified
632	MISSED ABORTION	➡	**O02.1**	Missed abortion
633.00	ABD PREGNANCY WITHOUT INTRAUTERINE PREGNANCY		**O00.0**	Abdominal pregnancy
633.01	ABDOMINAL PREGNANCY WITH INTRAUTERINE PREGNANCY		**O00.0**	Abdominal pregnancy
633.10	TUBAL PREGNANCY WITHOUT INTRAUTERINE PREGNANCY		**O00.1**	Tubal pregnancy
633.11	TUBAL PREGNANCY WITH INTRAUTERINE PREGNANCY		**O00.1**	Tubal pregnancy
633.20	OVARIAN PREGNANCY WITHOUT INTRAUTERINE PREGNANCY		**O00.2**	Ovarian pregnancy
633.21	OVARIAN PREGNANCY WITH INTRAUTERINE PREGNANCY		**O00.2**	Ovarian pregnancy
633.80	OTH ECTOPIC PG WITHOUT INTRAUTERINE PG		**O00.8**	Other ectopic pregnancy
633.81	OTHER ECTOPIC PREGNANCY W/INTRAUTERINE PREGNANCY		**O00.8**	Other ectopic pregnancy
633.90	UNSPEC ECTOPIC PG WITHOUT INTRAUTERINE PG		**O00.9**	Ectopic pregnancy, unspecified
633.91	UNSPEC ECTOPIC PG W/INTRAUTERINE PG		**O00.9**	Ectopic pregnancy, unspecified
634.00	UNSPEC SPONT AB COMP GENITAL TRACT&PELV INF		**O03.5** **O03.87**	Genitl trct and pelvic infct fol complete or unsp spon abort Sepsis following complete or unsp spontaneous abortion
634.01	INCPL SPONTANEOUS AB COMP GENITAL TRACT&PELV INF		**O03.0** **O03.37**	Genitl trct and pelvic infection fol incmpl spon abortion Sepsis following incomplete spontaneous abortion
634.02	COMPLETE SPONT AB COMP GENITAL TRACT&PELV INF		**O03.5** **O03.87**	Genitl trct and pelvic infct fol complete or unsp spon abort Sepsis following complete or unsp spontaneous abortion
634.10	UNSPEC SPONTANEOUS AB COMP DELAY/EXCESS HEMORR		**O03.6**	Delayed or excess hemor fol complete or unsp spon abortion
634.11	INCPL SPONTANEOUS AB COMP DELAY/EXCESS HEMORR	➡	**O03.1**	Delayed or excessive hemor following incmpl spon abortion
634.12	COMPLETE SPONTANEOUS AB COMP DELAY/EXCESS HEMORR		**O03.6**	Delayed or excess hemor fol complete or unsp spon abortion
634.20	UNSPEC SPONT AB COMP DAMGE PELV ORGN/TISSUES		**O03.84**	Damage to pelvic organs fol complete or unsp spon abortion
634.21	INCPL SPONT AB COMP DAMGE PELV ORGN/TISSUES	➡	**O03.34**	Damage to pelvic organs following incomplete spon abortion
634.22	COMPLETE SPONT AB COMP DAMGE PELV ORGN/TISSUES		**O03.84**	Damage to pelvic organs fol complete or unsp spon abortion
634.30	UNSPEC SPONTANEOUS AB COMPLICATED RENAL FAILURE		**O03.82**	Renal failure following complete or unsp spon abortion
634.31	INCOMPLETE SPONTANEOUS AB COMP RENAL FAILURE	➡	**O03.32**	Renal failure following incomplete spontaneous abortion
634.32	COMPLETE SPONTANEOUS AB COMP RENAL FAILURE		**O03.82**	Renal failure following complete or unsp spon abortion
634.40	UNSPEC SPONTANEOUS AB COMP METABOLIC DISORDER		**O03.83**	Metabolic disorder following complete or unsp spon abortion
634.41	INCPL SPONTANEOUS AB COMP METABOLIC DISORDER	➡	**O03.33**	Metabolic disorder following incomplete spontaneous abortion
634.42	COMPLETE SPONTANEOUS AB COMP METABOLIC DISORDER		**O03.83**	Metabolic disorder following complete or unsp spon abortion
634.50	UNSPEC SPONTANEOUS ABORTION COMPLICATED SHOCK		**O03.81**	Shock following complete or unspecified spontaneous abortion
634.51	INCOMPLETE SPONTANEOUS AB COMPLICATED SHOCK	➡	**O03.31**	Shock following incomplete spontaneous abortion
634.52	COMPLETE SPONTANEOUS ABORTION COMPLICATED SHOCK		**O03.81**	Shock following complete or unspecified spontaneous abortion
634.60	UNSPEC SPONTANEOUS ABORTION COMPLICATED EMBOLISM		**O03.7**	Embolism following complete or unsp spontaneous abortion
634.61	INCOMPLETE SPONTANEOUS AB COMPLICATED EMBOLISM	➡	**O03.2**	Embolism following incomplete spontaneous abortion
634.62	COMPLETE SPONTANEOUS AB COMPLICATED EMBOLISM		**O03.7**	Embolism following complete or unsp spontaneous abortion
634.70	UNSPEC SPONTANEOUS AB W/OTH SPEC COMPLICATIONS		**O03.85** **O03.86** **O03.88** **O03.89**	Oth venous comp following complete or unsp spon abortion Cardiac arrest following complete or unsp spon abortion Urinary tract infection fol complete or unsp spon abortion Complete or unsp spontaneous abortion with oth complicat
634.71	INCOMPLETE SPONTANEOUS AB W/OTH SPEC COMPS		**O03.35** **O03.36** **O03.38** **O03.39**	Oth venous comp following incomplete spontaneous abortion Cardiac arrest following incomplete spontaneous abortion Urinary tract infection following incomplete spon abortion Incomplete spontaneous abortion with other complications
634.72	COMPLETE SPONTANEOUS AB W/OTH SPEC COMPLICATIONS		**O03.85** **O03.86** **O03.88** **O03.89**	Oth venous comp following complete or unsp spon abortion Cardiac arrest following complete or unsp spon abortion Urinary tract infection fol complete or unsp spon abortion Complete or unsp spontaneous abortion with oth complicat
634.80	UNSPEC SPONTANEOUS AB W/UNSPEC COMPLICATION		**O03.80**	Unsp comp following complete or unsp spontaneous abortion
634.81	INCOMPLETE SPONTANEOUS AB W/UNSPEC COMPLICATION		**O03.30**	Unsp complication following incomplete spontaneous abortion
634.82	COMPLETE SPONTANEOUS AB W/UNSPEC COMPLICATION		**O03.80**	Unsp comp following complete or unsp spontaneous abortion
634.90	UNSPEC SPONTANEOUS AB WITHOUT MENTION COMP		**O03.9**	Complete or unsp spontaneous abortion without complication
634.91	INCOMPLETE SPONTANEOUS AB WITHOUT MENTION COMP		**O03.4**	Incomplete spontaneous abortion without complication
634.92	COMPLETE SPONTANEOUS AB WITHOUT MENTION COMP		**O03.9**	Complete or unsp spontaneous abortion without complication
635.00	UNSPEC LEGL INDUCD AB COMPL GENIT TRACT&PELV INF		**O04.5** **O04.87**	Genitl trct and pelvic infct fol (induced) term of pregnancy Sepsis following (induced) termination of pregnancy
635.01	INCOMPL LEGL INDUCD AB COMPL GENIT TRCT&PELV INF		**O04.5** **O04.87**	Genitl trct and pelvic infct fol (induced) term of pregnancy Sepsis following (induced) termination of pregnancy
635.02	CMPL LEGL INDUCD AB COMPL GENITAL TRACT&PELV INF		**O04.5** **O04.87**	Genitl trct and pelvic infct fol (induced) term of pregnancy Sepsis following (induced) termination of pregnancy
635.10	UNSPEC LEGL INDUCD AB COMPL DELAY/EXCESS HEMORR		**O04.6**	Delayed or excess hemor fol (induced) term of pregnancy
635.11	INCOMPL LEGL INDUCD AB COMPL DELAY/EXCESS HEMORR		**O04.6**	Delayed or excess hemor fol (induced) term of pregnancy
635.12	CMPL LEGL INDUCD AB COMPL DELAY/EXCESS HEMORR		**O04.6**	Delayed or excess hemor fol (induced) term of pregnancy
635.20	UNSPEC LEGL INDUCD AB COMPL DAMGE PELV ORGN/TISS		**O04.84**	Damage to pelvic organs fol (induced) term of pregnancy
635.21	LEGL INDUCD AB COMPL DAMGE PELV ORGN/TISS INCMPL		**O04.84**	Damage to pelvic organs fol (induced) term of pregnancy

ICD-9-CM		ICD-10-CM	
635.22	CMPL LEGL INDUCD AB COMPL DAMGE PELV ORGN/TISS	O04.84	Damage to pelvic organs fol (induced) term of pregnancy
635.30	UNSPEC LEGALLY INDUCED AB COMP RENAL FAILURE	O04.82	Renal failure following (induced) termination of pregnancy
635.31	INCOMPLETE LEGALLY INDUCED AB COMP RENAL FAILURE	O04.82	Renal failure following (induced) termination of pregnancy
635.32	COMPLETE LEGALLY INDUCED AB COMP RENAL FAILURE	O04.82	Renal failure following (induced) termination of pregnancy
635.40	UNSPEC LEGALLY INDUCD AB COMP METABOLIC DISORDER	O04.83	Metabolic disorder following (induced) term of pregnancy
635.41	INCPL LEGALLY INDUCED AB COMP METABOLIC DISORDER	O04.83	Metabolic disorder following (induced) term of pregnancy
635.42	COMPLETE LEGL INDUCD AB COMP METABOLIC DISORDER	O04.83	Metabolic disorder following (induced) term of pregnancy
635.50	UNSPEC LEGALLY INDUCED AB COMPLICATED SHOCK	O04.81	Shock following (induced) termination of pregnancy
635.51	LEGALLY INDUCED AB COMPLICATED SHOCK INCOMPLETE	O04.81	Shock following (induced) termination of pregnancy
635.52	COMPLETE LEGALLY INDUCED AB COMPLICATED SHOCK	O04.81	Shock following (induced) termination of pregnancy
635.60	UNSPEC LEGALLY INDUCED AB COMPLICATED EMBOLISM	O04.7	Embolism following (induced) termination of pregnancy
635.61	INCOMPLETE LEGALLY INDUCED AB COMP EMBOLISM	O04.7	Embolism following (induced) termination of pregnancy
635.62	COMPLETE LEGALLY INDUCED AB COMPLICATED EMBOLISM	O04.7	Embolism following (induced) termination of pregnancy
635.70	UNSPEC LEGALLY INDUCED AB W/OTH SPEC COMPS	O04.85 O04.86 O04.88 O04.89	Oth venous comp following (induced) termination of preg Cardiac arrest following (induced) termination of pregnancy Urinary tract infection fol (induced) term of pregnancy (Induced) termination of pregnancy with other complications
635.71	INCOMPLETE LEGALLY INDUCED AB W/OTH SPEC COMPS	O04.85 O04.86 O04.88 O04.89	Oth venous comp following (induced) termination of preg Cardiac arrest following (induced) termination of pregnancy Urinary tract infection fol (induced) term of pregnancy (Induced) termination of pregnancy with other complications
635.72	COMPLETE LEGALLY INDUCED AB W/OTH SPEC COMPS	O04.85 O04.86 O04.88 O04.89	Oth venous comp following (induced) termination of preg Cardiac arrest following (induced) termination of pregnancy Urinary tract infection fol (induced) term of pregnancy (Induced) termination of pregnancy with other complications
635.80	UNSPEC LEGALLY INDUCED AB W/UNSPEC COMPLICATION	O04.80	(Induced) termination of pregnancy with unsp complications
635.81	INCOMPLETE LEGALLY INDUCED AB W/UNSPEC COMP	O04.80	(Induced) termination of pregnancy with unsp complications
635.82	COMPLETE LEGALLY INDUCED AB W/UNSPEC COMP	O04.80	(Induced) termination of pregnancy with unsp complications
635.90	UNSPEC LEGALLY INDUCED AB WITHOUT MENTION COMP	Z33.2	Encounter for elective termination of pregnancy
635.91	INCPL LEGALLY INDUCED AB WITHOUT MENTION COMP	Z33.2	Encounter for elective termination of pregnancy
635.92	COMPLETE LEGALLY INDUCED AB WITHOUT MENTION COMP	Z33.2	Encounter for elective termination of pregnancy
636.00	UNS ILEG AB COMPL GENIT TRACT&PELV INF	O04.5	Genitl trct and pelvic infct fol (induced) term of pregnancy
636.01	INCOMPL ILEG AB COMPL GEN TRACT&PELV INF	O04.5	Genitl trct and pelvic infct fol (induced) term of pregnancy
636.02	CMPL ILEG INDUCD AB COMPL GENITAL TRACT&PELV INF	O04.5	Genitl trct and pelvic infct fol (induced) term of pregnancy
636.10	UNSPEC ILEG INDUCED AB COMPL DELAY/EXCESS HEMORR	O04.6	Delayed or excess hemor fol (induced) term of pregnancy
636.11	INCOMPL ILEG INDUCD AB COMPL DELAY/EXCESS HEMORR	O04.6	Delayed or excess hemor fol (induced) term of pregnancy
636.12	CMPL ILEG INDUCD AB COMPL DELAY/EXCESS HEMORR	O04.6	Delayed or excess hemor fol (induced) term of pregnancy
636.20	UNSPEC ILEG INDUCD AB COMPL DAMGE PELV ORGN/TISS	O04.84	Damage to pelvic organs fol (induced) term of pregnancy
636.21	INCMPL ILEG INDUCD AB COMPL DAMGE PELV ORGN/TISS	O04.84	Damage to pelvic organs fol (induced) term of pregnancy
636.22	CMPL ILEG INDUCD AB COMPL DAMGE PELV ORGN/TISS	O04.84	Damage to pelvic organs fol (induced) term of pregnancy
636.30	UNSPEC ILLEGALLY INDUCED AB COMP RENAL FAILURE	O04.82	Renal failure following (induced) termination of pregnancy
636.31	INCOMPLETE ILLEGALLY INDUCED AB COMP RENAL FAIL	O04.82	Renal failure following (induced) termination of pregnancy
636.32	COMPLETE ILLEGALLY INDUCED AB COMP RENAL FAILURE	O04.82	Renal failure following (induced) termination of pregnancy
636.40	UNSPEC ILEG INDUCED AB COMPL METABOLIC D/O	O04.83	Metabolic disorder following (induced) term of pregnancy
636.41	INCOMPL ILEG INDUCED AB COMPL METABOLIC DISORDER	O04.83	Metabolic disorder following (induced) term of pregnancy
636.42	COMPLETE ILEG INDUCED AB COMP METABOLIC DISORDER	O04.83	Metabolic disorder following (induced) term of pregnancy
636.50	UNSPEC ILLEGALLY INDUCED AB COMPLICATED SHOCK	O04.81	Shock following (induced) termination of pregnancy
636.51	INCOMPLETE ILLEGALLY INDUCED AB COMP SHOCK	O04.81	Shock following (induced) termination of pregnancy
636.52	COMPLETE ILLEGALLY INDUCED AB COMPLICATED SHOCK	O04.81	Shock following (induced) termination of pregnancy
636.60	UNSPEC ILLEGALLY INDUCED AB COMPLICATED EMBOLISM	O04.7	Embolism following (induced) termination of pregnancy
636.61	INCOMPLETE ILLEGALLY INDUCED AB COMP EMBOLISM	O04.7	Embolism following (induced) termination of pregnancy
636.62	COMPLETE ILLEGALLY INDUCED AB COMP EMBOLISM	O04.7	Embolism following (induced) termination of pregnancy
636.70	UNSPEC ILLEGALLY INDUCED AB W/OTH SPEC COMPS	O04.89	(Induced) termination of pregnancy with other complications
636.71	INCOMPLETE ILLEGALLY INDUCED AB W/OTH SPEC COMPS	O04.89	(Induced) termination of pregnancy with other complications
636.72	COMPLETE ILLEGALLY INDUCED AB W/OTH SPEC COMPS	O04.89	(Induced) termination of pregnancy with other complications
636.80	UNSPEC ILLEGALLY INDUCED AB W/UNSPEC COMP	O04.80	(Induced) termination of pregnancy with unsp complications
636.81	INCOMPLETE ILLEGALLY INDUCED AB W/UNSPEC COMP	O04.80	(Induced) termination of pregnancy with unsp complications
636.82	COMPLETE ILLEGALLY INDUCED AB W/UNSPEC COMP	O04.80	(Induced) termination of pregnancy with unsp complications
636.90	UNSPEC ILLEGALLY INDUCED AB WITHOUT MENTION COMP	Z33.2	Encounter for elective termination of pregnancy
636.91	INCOMPLETE ILEG INDUCED AB WITHOUT MENTION COMP	Z33.2	Encounter for elective termination of pregnancy
636.92	COMPLETE ILEG INDUCED AB WITHOUT MENTION COMP	Z33.2	Encounter for elective termination of pregnancy
637.00	ABORTION UNS AS CMPL/LEGL COMPL GT & PELV INF	O04.5	Genitl trct and pelvic infct fol (induced) term of pregnancy
637.01	ABORTION UNS LEGL INCOMPL COMPL GT & PELV INF	O04.5	Genitl trct and pelvic infct fol (induced) term of pregnancy
637.02	ABORTION UNS LEGL CMPL COMP GT & PELV INF	O04.5	Genitl trct and pelvic infct fol (induced) term of pregnancy
637.10	ABORTION UNS CMPL/LEGL COMPL DLAY/EXCESS HEMORR	O04.6	Delayed or excess hemor fol (induced) term of pregnancy
637.11	ABORTION UNS LEGL INCMPL COMP DLAY/EXCESS HEMORR	O04.6	Delayed or excess hemor fol (induced) term of pregnancy
637.12	ABORTION UNS LEGL CMPL COMP DLAY/EXCESS HEMORR	O04.6	Delayed or excess hemor fol (induced) term of pregnancy
637.20	ABORTION UNS CMPL/LEGL COMPL DMG PELV ORG/TISS	O04.84	Damage to pelvic organs fol (induced) term of pregnancy

[Brackets] indicate valid character values for each code. Character value meanings provided for each code grouping.

ICD-9-CM		ICD-10-CM	
637.21	ABORTIION UNS LEGL INCMPL COMP DMG PELV ORG/TISS	**OØ4.84**	Damage to pelvic organs fol (induced) term of pregnancy
637.22	ABORTION UNS LEGL CMPL COMP DAMAGE PELV ORG/TISS	**OØ4.84**	Damage to pelvic organs fol (induced) term of pregnancy
637.3Ø	ABORTION UNS CMPL/LEGALITY COMP RENAL FAILURE	**OØ4.82**	Renal failure following (induced) termination of pregnancy
637.31	ABORTION UNS LEGL INCMPL COMP BY RENAL FAILURE	**OØ4.82**	Renal failure following (induced) termination of pregnancy
637.32	ABORTION UNS LEGL CMPL COMP BY RENAL FAILURE	**OØ4.82**	Renal failure following (induced) termination of pregnancy
637.4Ø	ABORTION UNS CMPL/LEGL COMP METABOLIC DISORDER	**OØ4.83**	Metabolic disorder following (induced) term of pregnancy
637.41	ABORTION UNS LEGL INCMPL COMP METABOLIC DISORDER	**OØ4.83**	Metabolic disorder following (induced) term of pregnancy
637.42	ABORTION UNS LEGL CMPL COMP METABOLIC DISORDER	**OØ4.83**	Metabolic disorder following (induced) term of pregnancy
637.5Ø	ABORTION UNS AS CMPL/LEGALITY COMPLICATED SHOCK	**OØ4.81**	Shock following (induced) termination of pregnancy
637.51	ABORTION UNS LEGL INCMPL COMPLICATED BY SHOCK	**OØ4.81**	Shock following (induced) termination of pregnancy
637.52	ABORTION UNS LEGALITY CMPL COMPLICATED BY SHOCK	**OØ4.81**	Shock following (induced) termination of pregnancy
637.6Ø	ABORTION UNS CMPL/LEGALITY COMPLICATED EMBOLISM	**OØ4.7**	Embolism following (induced) termination of pregnancy
637.61	ABORTION UNS LEGALITY INCMPL COMP EMBOLISM	**OØ4.7**	Embolism following (induced) termination of pregnancy
637.62	ABORTION UNS LEGALITY CMPL COMP BY EMBOLISM	**OØ4.7**	Embolism following (induced) termination of pregnancy
637.7Ø	ABORTION UNS CMPL/LEGL W/OTH SPEC COMPLICATIONS	**OØ4.89**	(Induced) termination of pregnancy with other complications
637.71	ABORTION UNS LEGALITY INCMPL W/OTH SPEC COMPS	**OØ4.89**	(Induced) termination of pregnancy with other complications
637.72	ABORTION UNS LEGALITY CMPL W/OTH SPEC COMPS	**OØ4.89**	(Induced) termination of pregnancy with other complications
637.8Ø	ABORTION UNS CMPL/LEGALITY W/UNSP COMPLICATION	**OØ4.8Ø**	(Induced) termination of pregnancy with unsp complications
637.81	ABORTION UNS LEGALITY INCMPL W/UNS COMPLICATION	**OØ4.8Ø**	(Induced) termination of pregnancy with unsp complications
637.82	ABORTION UNS LEGALITY CMPL W/UNS COMPLICATION	**OØ4.8Ø**	(Induced) termination of pregnancy with unsp complications
637.9Ø	UNS TYPE AB UNS AS CMPL/LEGL W/O MENTION COMP	**Z33.2**	Encounter for elective termination of pregnancy
637.91	ABORTION UNS LEGL INCMPL NO MENTION COMPLICATION	**Z33.2**	Encounter for elective termination of pregnancy
637.92	ABORTION UNS LEGL CMPL NO MENTION COMPLICATION	**Z33.2**	Encounter for elective termination of pregnancy
638.Ø	FAILD ATTEMP AB COMP GENITAL TRACT&PELVIC INF	**OØ7.Ø** **OØ7.37**	Genitl trct and pelvic infct fol failed attempt term of preg Sepsis following failed attempted termination of pregnancy
638.1	FAILED ATTEMP AB COMP DELAY/EXCESSIVE HEMORRHAGE	➡ **OØ7.1**	Delayed or excess hemor fol failed attempt term of pregnancy
638.2	FAILD ATTEMP AB COMP DAMGE PELVIC ORGANS/TISSUES	➡ **OØ7.34**	Damage to pelvic organs fol failed attempt term of pregnancy
638.3	FAILED ATTEMPTED AB COMPLICATED RENAL FAILURE	➡ **OØ7.32**	Renal failure following failed attempted term of pregnancy
638.4	FAILED ATTEMP AB COMPLICATED METABOLIC DISORDER	➡ **OØ7.33**	Metabolic disorder fol failed attempt term of pregnancy
638.5	FAILED ATTEMPTED ABORTION COMPLICATED BY SHOCK	➡ **OØ7.31**	Shock following failed attempted termination of pregnancy
638.6	FAILED ATTEMPTED ABORTION COMPLICATED EMBOLISM	➡ **OØ7.2**	Embolism following failed attempted termination of pregnancy
638.7	FAILED ATTEMPTED AB W/OTH SPEC COMPLICATION	**OØ7.35** **OØ7.36** **OØ7.38** **OØ7.39**	Oth venous comp following failed attempted term of preg Cardiac arrest following failed attempted term of pregnancy Urinary tract infection fol failed attempt term of pregnancy Failed attempted termination of pregnancy w oth comp
638.8	FAILED ATTEMPTED ABORTION W/UNSPEC COMPLICATION	➡ **OØ7.3Ø**	Failed attempted termination of pregnancy w unsp comp
638.9	FAILED ATTEMPTED AB WITHOUT MENTION COMPLICATION	➡ **OØ7.4**	Failed attempted termination of pregnancy w/o complication
639.Ø	GENIT TRACT&PELV INF FOLLOW AB/ECTOPIC&MOLAR PG	**A34** **OØ8.Ø** **OØ8.82**	Obstetrical tetanus Genitl trct and pelvic infct fol ectopic and molar pregnancy Sepsis following ectopic and molar pregnancy
639.1	DELAY/EXCESS HEMORR FOLLOW AB/ECTOPIC&MOLAR PG	➡ **OØ8.1**	Delayed or excess hemor fol ectopic and molar pregnancy
639.2	DAMGE PELV ORGN&TISS FOLLOW AB/ECTOPIC&MOLAR PG	➡ **OØ8.6**	Damage to pelvic organs and tiss fol an ect and molar preg
639.3	COMP FLW AB & ECTOPIC & MOLAR PG KIDNEY FAILURE	➡ **OØ8.4**	Renal failure following ectopic and molar pregnancy
639.4	METAB D/O FOLLOW AB/ECTOPIC&MOLAR PREGNANCIES	➡ **OØ8.5**	Metabolic disorders following an ectopic and molar pregnancy
639.5	SHOCK FOLLOWING AB/ECTOPIC&MOLAR PREGNANCIES	➡ **OØ8.3**	Shock following ectopic and molar pregnancy
639.6	EMBOLISM FOLLOWING AB/ECTOPIC&MOLAR PREGNANCIES	➡ **OØ8.2**	Embolism following ectopic and molar pregnancy
639.8	OTH SPEC COMP FOLLOW AB/ECTOPIC&MOLAR PG	**OØ8.7** **OØ8.81** **OØ8.83** **OØ8.89**	Oth venous comp following an ectopic and molar pregnancy Cardiac arrest following an ectopic and molar pregnancy Urinary tract infection fol an ectopic and molar pregnancy Other complications following an ectopic and molar pregnancy
639.9	UNSPEC COMP FOLLOW AB/ECTOPIC&MOLAR PREGNANCIES	**OØ8.9**	Unsp complication following an ectopic and molar pregnancy
64Ø.ØØ	THREATENED ABORTION UNSPECIFIED AS EPISODE CARE	**O2Ø.Ø**	Threatened abortion
64Ø.Ø1	THREATENED ABORTION, DELIVERED	**O2Ø.Ø**	Threatened abortion
64Ø.Ø3	THREATENED ABORTION, ANTEPARTUM	**O2Ø.Ø**	Threatened abortion
64Ø.8Ø	OTH SPEC HEMORR EARLY PG UNSPEC AS EPIS CARE	**O2Ø.8**	Other hemorrhage in early pregnancy
64Ø.81	OTHER SPEC HEMORRHAGE EARLY PREGNANCY DELIVERED	**O2Ø.8**	Other hemorrhage in early pregnancy
64Ø.83	OTHER SPEC HEMORRHAGE EARLY PREGNANCY ANTEPARTUM	**O2Ø.8**	Other hemorrhage in early pregnancy
64Ø.9Ø	UNSPEC HEMORR EARLY PG UNSPEC AS EPIS CARE	**O2Ø.9**	Hemorrhage in early pregnancy, unspecified
64Ø.91	UNSPECIFIED HEMORRHAGE EARLY PREGNANCY DELIVERED	**O2Ø.9**	Hemorrhage in early pregnancy, unspecified
64Ø.93	UNSPEC HEMORRHAGE EARLY PREGNANCY ANTEPARTUM	**O2Ø.9**	Hemorrhage in early pregnancy, unspecified
641.ØØ	PLACENTA PREVIA W/O HEMORR UNSPEC AS EPIS CARE	**O44.ØØ**	Placenta previa specified as w/o hemorrhage, unsp trimester
641.Ø1	PLACENTA PREVIA WITHOUT HEMORRHAGE WITH DELIVERY	**O44.Ø1** **O44.Ø2** **O44.Ø3**	Placenta previa specified as w/o hemorrhage, first trimester Placenta previa specified as w/o hemor, second trimester Placenta previa specified as w/o hemorrhage, third trimester
641.Ø3	PLACENTA PREVIA WITHOUT HEMORRHAGE ANTEPARTUM	**O44.Ø1** **O44.Ø2** **O44.Ø3**	Placenta previa specified as w/o hemorrhage, first trimester Placenta previa specified as w/o hemor, second trimester Placenta previa specified as w/o hemorrhage, third trimester
641.1Ø	HEMORR FROM PLACENTA PREVIA UNSPEC AS EPIS CARE	**O44.1Ø**	Placenta previa with hemorrhage, unspecified trimester

ICD-9-CM		ICD-10-CM	
641.11	HEMORRHAGE FROM PLACENTA PREVIA WITH DELIVERY	**O44.11**	Placenta previa with hemorrhage, first trimester
		O44.12	Placenta previa with hemorrhage, second trimester
		O44.13	Placenta previa with hemorrhage, third trimester
641.13	HEMORRHAGE FROM PLACENTA PREVIA ANTEPARTUM	**O44.11**	Placenta previa with hemorrhage, first trimester
		O44.12	Placenta previa with hemorrhage, second trimester
		O44.13	Placenta previa with hemorrhage, third trimester
641.2Ø	PRMAT SEPARATION PLACENTA UNSPEC AS EPIS CARE	**O45.8X9**	Other premature separation of placenta, unsp trimester
		O45.9Ø	Premature separation of placenta, unsp, unsp trimester
641.21	PREMATURE SEPARATION OF PLACENTA WITH DELIVERY	**O45.8X1**	Other premature separation of placenta, first trimester
		O45.8X2	Other premature separation of placenta, second trimester
		O45.8X3	Other premature separation of placenta, third trimester
		O45.91	Premature separation of placenta, unsp, first trimester
		O45.92	Premature separation of placenta, unsp, second trimester
		O45.93	Premature separation of placenta, unsp, third trimester
641.23	PREMATURE SEPARATION OF PLACENTA ANTEPARTUM	**O45.8X1**	Other premature separation of placenta, first trimester
		O45.8X2	Other premature separation of placenta, second trimester
		O45.8X3	Other premature separation of placenta, third trimester
		O45.91	Premature separation of placenta, unsp, first trimester
		O45.92	Premature separation of placenta, unsp, second trimester
		O45.93	Premature separation of placenta, unsp, third trimester
641.3Ø	ANTPRTM HEMORR W/COAGULAT DEFEC UNS EPIS CARE	**O45.ØØ9**	Prem separtn of placenta w coag defect, unsp, unsp trimester
		O45.Ø19	Prem separtn of placenta w afibrinogenemia, unsp trimester
		O45.Ø29	Prem separtn of placenta w dissem intravasc coag, unsp tri
		O45.Ø99	Prem separtn of placenta w oth coag defect, unsp trimester
		O46.ØØ9	Antepartum hemorrhage w coag defect, unsp, unsp trimester
		O46.Ø19	Antepartum hemorrhage with afibrinogenemia, unsp trimester
		O46.Ø29	Antepart hemorrhage w dissem intravasc coag, unsp trimester
		O46.Ø99	Antepartum hemorrhage w oth coag defect, unsp trimester
641.31	ANTPRTM HEMORR ASSOC W/COAGULAT DEFEC W/DELIV	**O45.ØØ1**	Prem separtn of placenta w coag defect, unsp, first tri
		O45.ØØ2	Prem separtn of placenta w coag defect, unsp, second tri
		O45.ØØ3	Prem separtn of placenta w coag defect, unsp, third tri
		O45.Ø11	Prem separtn of placenta w afibrinogenemia, first trimester
		O45.Ø12	Prem separtn of placenta w afibrinogenemia, second trimester
		O45.Ø13	Prem separtn of placenta w afibrinogenemia, third trimester
		O45.Ø21	Prem separtn of placenta w dissem intravasc coag, first tri
		O45.Ø22	Prem separtn of placenta w dissem intravasc coag, second tri
		O45.Ø23	Prem separtn of placenta w dissem intravasc coag, third tri
		O45.Ø91	Prem separtn of placenta w oth coag defect, first trimester
		O45.Ø92	Prem separtn of placenta w oth coag defect, second trimester
		O45.Ø93	Prem separtn of placenta w oth coag defect, third trimester
		O46.ØØ1	Antepartum hemorrhage w coag defect, unsp, first trimester
		O46.ØØ2	Antepartum hemorrhage w coag defect, unsp, second trimester
		O46.ØØ3	Antepartum hemorrhage w coag defect, unsp, third trimester
		O46.Ø11	Antepartum hemorrhage with afibrinogenemia, first trimester
		O46.Ø12	Antepartum hemorrhage with afibrinogenemia, second tri
		O46.Ø13	Antepartum hemorrhage with afibrinogenemia, third trimester
		O46.Ø21	Antepart hemorrhage w dissem intravasc coag, first trimester
		O46.Ø22	Antepart hemor w dissem intravasc coag, second trimester
		O46.Ø23	Antepart hemorrhage w dissem intravasc coag, third trimester
		O46.Ø91	Antepartum hemorrhage w oth coag defect, first trimester
		O46.Ø92	Antepartum hemorrhage w oth coag defect, second trimester
		O46.Ø93	Antepartum hemorrhage w oth coag defect, third trimester
		O67.Ø	Intrapartum hemorrhage with coagulation defect
641.33	ANTPRTM HEMORR ASSOC W/COAGULAT DEFECT ANTPRTM	**O45.ØØ1**	Prem separtn of placenta w coag defect, unsp, first tri
		O45.ØØ2	Prem separtn of placenta w coag defect, unsp, second tri
		O45.ØØ3	Prem separtn of placenta w coag defect, unsp, third tri
		O45.Ø11	Prem separtn of placenta w afibrinogenemia, first trimester
		O45.Ø12	Prem separtn of placenta w afibrinogenemia, second trimester
		O45.Ø13	Prem separtn of placenta w afibrinogenemia, third trimester
		O45.Ø21	Prem separtn of placenta w dissem intravasc coag, first tri
		O45.Ø22	Prem separtn of placenta w dissem intravasc coag, second tri
		O45.Ø23	Prem separtn of placenta w dissem intravasc coag, third tri
		O45.Ø91	Prem separtn of placenta w oth coag defect, first trimester
		O45.Ø92	Prem separtn of placenta w oth coag defect, second trimester
		O45.Ø93	Prem separtn of placenta w oth coag defect, third trimester
		O46.ØØ1	Antepartum hemorrhage w coag defect, unsp, first trimester
		O46.ØØ2	Antepartum hemorrhage w coag defect, unsp, second trimester
		O46.ØØ3	Antepartum hemorrhage w coag defect, unsp, third trimester
		O46.Ø11	Antepartum hemorrhage with afibrinogenemia, first trimester
		O46.Ø12	Antepartum hemorrhage with afibrinogenemia, second tri
		O46.Ø13	Antepartum hemorrhage with afibrinogenemia, third trimester
		O46.Ø21	Antepart hemorrhage w dissem intravasc coag, first trimester
		O46.Ø22	Antepart hemor w dissem intravasc coag, second trimester
		O46.Ø23	Antepart hemorrhage w dissem intravasc coag, third trimester
		O46.Ø91	Antepartum hemorrhage w oth coag defect, first trimester
		O46.Ø92	Antepartum hemorrhage w oth coag defect, second trimester
		O46.Ø93	Antepartum hemorrhage w oth coag defect, third trimester
641.8Ø	OTH ANTEPARTUM HEMORRHAGE UNSPEC AS EPISODE CARE	**O46.8X9**	Other antepartum hemorrhage, unspecified trimester

[Brackets] indicate valid character values for each code. Character value meanings provided for each code grouping.

ICD-9-CM		ICD-10-CM	
641.81	OTHER ANTEPARTUM HEMORRHAGE WITH DELIVERY	**O46.8X1**	Other antepartum hemorrhage, first trimester
		O46.8X2	Other antepartum hemorrhage, second trimester
		O46.8X3	Other antepartum hemorrhage, third trimester
		O67.8	Other intrapartum hemorrhage
641.83	OTHER ANTEPARTUM HEMORRHAGE ANTEPARTUM	**O46.8X1**	Other antepartum hemorrhage, first trimester
		O46.8X2	Other antepartum hemorrhage, second trimester
		O46.8X3	Other antepartum hemorrhage, third trimester
641.90	UNSPEC ANTPRTM HEMORRHAGE UNSPEC AS EPISODE CARE	**O46.90**	Antepartum hemorrhage, unspecified, unspecified trimester
641.91	UNSPECIFIED ANTEPARTUM HEMORRHAGE WITH DELIVERY	**O46.91**	Antepartum hemorrhage, unspecified, first trimester
		O46.92	Antepartum hemorrhage, unspecified, second trimester
		O46.93	Antepartum hemorrhage, unspecified, third trimester
		O67.9	Intrapartum hemorrhage, unspecified
641.93	UNSPECIFIED ANTEPARTUM HEMORRHAGE ANTEPARTUM	**O46.91**	Antepartum hemorrhage, unspecified, first trimester
		O46.92	Antepartum hemorrhage, unspecified, second trimester
		O46.93	Antepartum hemorrhage, unspecified, third trimester
642.00	BEN HTN COMP PG CHLDBRTH&THE PUERPERIUM UNS EOC	**O10.019**	Pre-existing essential htn comp pregnancy, unsp trimester
		O10.919	Unsp pre-existing htn comp pregnancy, unsp trimester
642.01	BENIGN ESSENTIAL HYPERTENSION WITH DELIVERY	**O10.011**	Pre-existing essential htn comp pregnancy, first trimester
		O10.012	Pre-existing essential htn comp pregnancy, second trimester
		O10.013	Pre-existing essential htn comp pregnancy, third trimester
		O10.02	Pre-existing essential hypertension complicating childbirth
		O10.911	Unsp pre-existing htn comp pregnancy, first trimester
		O10.912	Unsp pre-existing htn comp pregnancy, second trimester
		O10.913	Unsp pre-existing htn comp pregnancy, third trimester
		O10.92	Unsp pre-existing hypertension complicating childbirth
642.02	BEN ESSENTIAL HYPERTENSION W/DELIV W/CURRENT PPC	**O10.03**	Pre-existing essential hypertension comp the puerperium
642.03	BENIGN ESSENTIAL HYPERTENSION ANTEPARTUM	**O10.011**	Pre-existing essential htn comp pregnancy, first trimester
		O10.012	Pre-existing essential htn comp pregnancy, second trimester
		O10.013	Pre-existing essential htn comp pregnancy, third trimester
		O10.911	Unsp pre-existing htn comp pregnancy, first trimester
		O10.912	Unsp pre-existing htn comp pregnancy, second trimester
		O10.913	Unsp pre-existing htn comp pregnancy, third trimester
642.04	BENIGN ESSENTIAL HYPERTENSION PP COND/COMPL	**O10.03**	Pre-existing essential hypertension comp the puerperium
		O10.93	Unsp pre-existing hypertension complicating the puerperium
642.10	HTN SEC RENL DZ COMPL PG BRTH&PP UNS EOC	**O10.419**	Pre-existing secondary htn comp pregnancy, unsp trimester
642.11	HYPERTENSION SEC TO RENAL DISEASE WITH DELIVERY	**O10.411**	Pre-existing secondary htn comp pregnancy, first trimester
		O10.412	Pre-existing secondary htn comp pregnancy, second trimester
		O10.413	Pre-existing secondary htn comp pregnancy, third trimester
		O10.42	Pre-existing secondary hypertension complicating childbirth
642.12	HTN SEC RENAL DISEASE W/DELIV W/CURRENT PP COMPL	**O10.43**	Pre-existing secondary hypertension comp the puerperium
642.13	HYPERTENSION SEC TO RENAL DISEASE ANTEPARTUM	**O10.411**	Pre-existing secondary htn comp pregnancy, first trimester
		O10.412	Pre-existing secondary htn comp pregnancy, second trimester
		O10.413	Pre-existing secondary htn comp pregnancy, third trimester
642.14	HTN SEC RENAL DISEASE POSTPARTUM COND/COMPL	**O10.43**	Pre-existing secondary hypertension comp the puerperium
642.20	OTH PRE-XST HTN COMPL PG BRTH&PP UNS EOC	**O10.119**	Pre-exist hyp heart disease comp pregnancy, unsp trimester
		O10.219	Pre-exist hyp chronic kidney disease comp preg, unsp tri
		O10.319	Pre-exist hyp heart and chr kidney dis comp preg, unsp tri
		O11.9	Pre-existing hypertension with pre-eclampsia, unsp trimester
642.21	OTHER PRE-EXISTING HYPERTENSION WITH DELIVERY	**O10.111**	Pre-exist hyp heart disease comp pregnancy, first trimester
		O10.112	Pre-exist hyp heart disease comp pregnancy, second trimester
		O10.113	Pre-exist hyp heart disease comp pregnancy, third trimester
		O10.12	Pre-existing hypertensive heart disease comp childbirth
		O10.211	Pre-exist hyp chronic kidney disease comp preg, first tri
		O10.212	Pre-exist hyp chronic kidney disease comp preg, second tri
		O10.213	Pre-exist hyp chronic kidney disease comp preg, third tri
		O10.22	Pre-existing hyp chronic kidney disease comp childbirth
		O10.311	Pre-exist hyp heart and chr kidney dis comp preg, first tri
		O10.312	Pre-exist hyp heart and chr kidney dis comp preg, second tri
		O10.313	Pre-exist hyp heart and chr kidney dis comp preg, third tri
		O10.32	Pre-exist hyp heart and chronic kidney disease comp chldbrth
		O11.1	Pre-existing hypertension w pre-eclampsia, first trimester
		O11.2	Pre-existing hypertension w pre-eclampsia, second trimester
		O11.3	Pre-existing hypertension w pre-eclampsia, third trimester
642.22	OTH PRE-EXISTING HTN W/DELIV W/CURRENT PP COMPL	**O10.13**	Pre-existing hypertensive heart disease comp the puerperium
642.23	OTHER PRE-EXISTING HYPERTENSION ANTEPARTUM	**O10.111**	Pre-exist hyp heart disease comp pregnancy, first trimester
		O10.112	Pre-exist hyp heart disease comp pregnancy, second trimester
		O10.113	Pre-exist hyp heart disease comp pregnancy, third trimester
		O10.211	Pre-exist hyp chronic kidney disease comp preg, first tri
		O10.212	Pre-exist hyp chronic kidney disease comp preg, second tri
		O10.213	Pre-exist hyp chronic kidney disease comp preg, third tri
		O10.311	Pre-exist hyp heart and chr kidney dis comp preg, first tri
		O10.312	Pre-exist hyp heart and chr kidney dis comp preg, second tri
		O10.313	Pre-exist hyp heart and chr kidney dis comp preg, third tri
		O11.1	Pre-existing hypertension w pre-eclampsia, first trimester
		O11.2	Pre-existing hypertension w pre-eclampsia, second trimester
		O11.3	Pre-existing hypertension w pre-eclampsia, third trimester

ICD-9-CM		ICD-10-CM	
642.24	OTH PRE-EXISTING HTN POSTPARTUM COND/COMPL	O10.13	Pre-existing hypertensive heart disease comp the puerperium
		O10.23	Pre-existing hyp chronic kidney disease comp the puerperium
		O10.33	Pre-exist hyp heart and chr kidney disease comp the puerp
642.30	TRANSIENT HTN PREGNANCY UNSPEC AS EPIS CARE	O13.9	Gestational htn w/o significant proteinuria, unsp trimester
642.31	TRANSIENT HYPERTENSION OF PREGNANCY W/DELIVERY	O13.1	Gestational htn w/o significant proteinuria, first trimester
		O13.2	Gestatnl htn w/o significant proteinuria, second trimester
		O13.3	Gestational htn w/o significant proteinuria, third trimester
		O16.1	Unspecified maternal hypertension, first trimester
		O16.2	Unspecified maternal hypertension, second trimester
		O16.3	Unspecified maternal hypertension, third trimester
642.32	TRANSIENT HTN PG W/DELIV W/CURRENT PP COMPL	O13.1	Gestational htn w/o significant proteinuria, first trimester
		O13.2	Gestatnl htn w/o significant proteinuria, second trimester
		O13.3	Gestational htn w/o significant proteinuria, third trimester
642.33	TRANSIENT HYPERTENSION OF PREGNANCY ANTEPARTUM	O13.1	Gestational htn w/o significant proteinuria, first trimester
		O13.2	Gestatnl htn w/o significant proteinuria, second trimester
		O13.3	Gestational htn w/o significant proteinuria, third trimester
		O16.1	Unspecified maternal hypertension, first trimester
		O16.2	Unspecified maternal hypertension, second trimester
		O16.3	Unspecified maternal hypertension, third trimester
642.34	TRANSIENT HTN PREGNANCY POSTPARTUM COND/COMPL	O13.1	Gestational htn w/o significant proteinuria, first trimester
		O13.2	Gestatnl htn w/o significant proteinuria, second trimester
		O13.3	Gestational htn w/o significant proteinuria, third trimester
642.40	MILD/UNSPEC PRE-ECLAMPSIA UNSPEC AS EPISODE CARE	O14.00	Mild to moderate pre-eclampsia, unspecified trimester
		O14.90	Unspecified pre-eclampsia, unspecified trimester
642.41	MILD OR UNSPECIFIED PRE-ECLAMPSIA WITH DELIVERY	O14.02	Mild to moderate pre-eclampsia, second trimester
		O14.03	Mild to moderate pre-eclampsia, third trimester
		O14.92	Unspecified pre-eclampsia, second trimester
		O14.93	Unspecified pre-eclampsia, third trimester
642.42	MILD/UNSPEC PRE-ECLAMPSIA W/DELIV W/CURRENT PPC	O14.02	Mild to moderate pre-eclampsia, second trimester
		O14.03	Mild to moderate pre-eclampsia, third trimester
642.43	MILD OR UNSPECIFIED PRE-ECLAMPSIA ANTEPARTUM	O14.02	Mild to moderate pre-eclampsia, second trimester
		O14.03	Mild to moderate pre-eclampsia, third trimester
		O14.92	Unspecified pre-eclampsia, second trimester
		O14.93	Unspecified pre-eclampsia, third trimester
642.44	MILD/UNSPEC PRE-ECLAMPSIA PP COND/COMPL	O15.2	Eclampsia in the puerperium
642.50	SEVERE PRE-ECLAMPSIA UNSPECIFIED AS EPISODE CARE	O14.10	Severe pre-eclampsia, unspecified trimester
		O14.20	HELLP syndrome (HELLP), unspecified trimester
642.51	SEVERE PRE-ECLAMPSIA, WITH DELIVERY	O14.12	Severe pre-eclampsia, second trimester
		O14.13	Severe pre-eclampsia, third trimester
		O14.22	HELLP syndrome (HELLP), second trimester
		O14.23	HELLP syndrome (HELLP), third trimester
642.52	SEVERE PRE-ECLAMPSIA W/DELIVERY W/CURRENT PPC	O14.12	Severe pre-eclampsia, second trimester
		O14.13	Severe pre-eclampsia, third trimester
		O14.22	HELLP syndrome (HELLP), second trimester
		O14.23	HELLP syndrome (HELLP), third trimester
642.53	SEVERE PRE-ECLAMPSIA, ANTEPARTUM	O14.12	Severe pre-eclampsia, second trimester
		O14.13	Severe pre-eclampsia, third trimester
		O14.22	HELLP syndrome (HELLP), second trimester
		O14.23	HELLP syndrome (HELLP), third trimester
642.54	SEVERE PRE-ECLAMPSIA POSTPARTUM COND/COMPL	O14.12	Severe pre-eclampsia, second trimester
		O14.13	Severe pre-eclampsia, third trimester
		O14.22	HELLP syndrome (HELLP), second trimester
		O14.23	HELLP syndrome (HELLP), third trimester
642.60	ECLAMPSIA-UNS EOC	O15.00	Eclampsia in pregnancy, unspecified trimester
		O15.9	Eclampsia, unspecified as to time period
642.61	ECLAMPSIA, WITH DELIVERY	O15.02	Eclampsia in pregnancy, second trimester
		O15.03	Eclampsia in pregnancy, third trimester
		O15.1	Eclampsia in labor
642.62	ECLAMPSIA W/DELIVERY W/CURRENT PPC	O15.2	Eclampsia in the puerperium
642.63	ECLAMPSIA, ANTEPARTUM	O15.02	Eclampsia in pregnancy, second trimester
		O15.03	Eclampsia in pregnancy, third trimester
642.64	ECLAMPSIA POSTPARTUM CONDITION/COMPLICATION	O15.2	Eclampsia in the puerperium
642.70	PRE-ECLAMPSIA/ECLAMPSIA W/PRE-EXIST HTN-UNS EOC	O11.9	Pre-existing hypertension with pre-eclampsia, unsp trimester
642.71	PRE-ECLAMP/ECLAMPSIA SUPERIMPS PRE-XST HTN DELIV	O11.1	Pre-existing hypertension w pre-eclampsia, first trimester
		O11.2	Pre-existing hypertension w pre-eclampsia, second trimester
		O11.3	Pre-existing hypertension w pre-eclampsia, third trimester
642.72	PRE-ECLAMPSIA/ECLMPSIA W/PRE-EXIST HTN-DEL W/PPC	O15.2	Eclampsia in the puerperium
642.73	PRE-ECLAMPSIA/ECLAMPSIA PRE-EXIST HTN ANTEPARTUM	O11.1	Pre-existing hypertension w pre-eclampsia, first trimester
		O11.2	Pre-existing hypertension w pre-eclampsia, second trimester
		O11.3	Pre-existing hypertension w pre-eclampsia, third trimester
642.74	PRE-ECLAMP/ECLAMPSIA SUPRMPSD PRE-XST HTN PP CON	O15.2	Eclampsia in the puerperium
642.90	UNS HTN COMP PG CHLDBRTH/THE PUERPERIUM UNS EOC	O16.9	Unspecified maternal hypertension, unspecified trimester
642.91	UNSPECIFIED HYPERTENSION WITH DELIVERY	O16.1	Unspecified maternal hypertension, first trimester
		O16.2	Unspecified maternal hypertension, second trimester
		O16.3	Unspecified maternal hypertension, third trimester
642.92	UNSPEC HYPERTENSION W/DELIVERY W/CURRENT PPC	O16.9	Unspecified maternal hypertension, unspecified trimester

ICD-9-CM		ICD-10-CM	
642.93	UNSPECIFIED HYPERTENSION ANTEPARTUM	O16.1 O16.2 O16.3	Unspecified maternal hypertension, first trimester Unspecified maternal hypertension, second trimester Unspecified maternal hypertension, third trimester
642.94	UNSPEC HYPERTENSION POSTPARTUM COND/COMPL	O16.1 O16.2 O16.3	Unspecified maternal hypertension, first trimester Unspecified maternal hypertension, second trimester Unspecified maternal hypertension, third trimester
643.00	MILD HYPEREMESIS GRAVIDARUM UNSPEC AS EPIS CARE	O21.0	Mild hyperemesis gravidarum
643.01	MILD HYPEREMESIS GRAVIDARUM DELIVERED	O21.0	Mild hyperemesis gravidarum
643.03	MILD HYPEREMESIS GRAVIDARUM ANTEPARTUM	O21.0	Mild hyperemesis gravidarum
643.10	HYPEREMESIS GRAVIDA W/METAB DSTUR UNS EPIS CARE	O21.1	Hyperemesis gravidarum with metabolic disturbance
643.11	HYPEREMESIS GRAVIDA W/METAB DISTURBANCE DELIV	O21.1	Hyperemesis gravidarum with metabolic disturbance
643.13	HYPEREMESIS GRAVIDA W/METAB DISTURBANCE ANTPRTM	O21.1	Hyperemesis gravidarum with metabolic disturbance
643.20	LATE VOMITING PREGNANCY UNSPEC AS EPISODE CARE	O21.2	Late vomiting of pregnancy
643.21	LATE VOMITING OF PREGNANCY DELIVERED	O21.2	Late vomiting of pregnancy
643.23	LATE VOMITING OF PREGNANCY ANTEPARTUM	O21.2	Late vomiting of pregnancy
643.80	OTH VOMITING COMP PREGNANCY UNSPEC AS EPIS CARE	O21.8	Other vomiting complicating pregnancy
643.81	OTHER VOMITING COMPLICATING PREGNANCY DELIVERED	O21.8	Other vomiting complicating pregnancy
643.83	OTHER VOMITING COMPLICATING PREGNANCY ANTEPARTUM	O21.8	Other vomiting complicating pregnancy
643.90	UNSPEC VOMITING PREGNANCY UNSPEC AS EPISODE CARE	O21.9	Vomiting of pregnancy, unspecified
643.91	UNSPECIFIED VOMITING OF PREGNANCY DELIVERED	O21.9	Vomiting of pregnancy, unspecified
643.93	UNSPECIFIED VOMITING OF PREGNANCY ANTEPARTUM	O21.9	Vomiting of pregnancy, unspecified
644.00	THREATENED PREMATURE LABOR UNSPEC AS EPIS CARE	O60.00	Preterm labor without delivery, unspecified trimester
644.03	THREATENED PREMATURE LABOR ANTEPARTUM	O60.02 O60.03	Preterm labor without delivery, second trimester Preterm labor without delivery, third trimester
644.10	OTHER THREATENED LABOR UNSPEC AS EPISODE CARE	O47.00 O47.9	False labor before 37 completed weeks of gest, unsp tri False labor, unspecified
644.13	OTHER THREATENED LABOR, ANTEPARTUM	O47.02 O47.03 O47.1	False labor before 37 completed weeks of gest, second tri False labor before 37 completed weeks of gest, third tri False labor at or after 37 completed weeks of gestation
644.20	EARLY ONSET DELIVERY UNSPECIFIED AS EPISODE CARE	O60.10X0 O60.10X[1,2,3,4,5] O60.10X9 O60.20X0 O60.20X[1,2,3,4,5] O60.20X9	Preterm labor w preterm delivery, unsp trimester, unsp Preterm labor with preterm delivery, unsp trimester Preterm labor w preterm delivery, unsp trimester, oth fetus Term delivery w preterm labor, unsp trimester, unsp Term delivery with preterm labor, unsp trimester Term delivery with preterm labor, unsp trimester, oth fetus ***7th Character meanings for codes as indicated*** ***1 Fetus 1 2 Fetus 2 3 Fetus 3 4 Fetus 4 5 Fetus 5***
644.21	ERLY ONSET DELIV DELIV W/WO MENTION ANTPRTM COND	O60.12X0 O60.12X[1,2,3,4,5] O60.12X9 O60.13X0 O60.13X[1,2,3,4,5] O60.13X9 O60.14X0 O60.14X[1,2,3,4,5] O60.14X9 O60.22X0 O60.22X[1,2,3,4,5] O60.22X9 O60.23X0 O60.23X[1,2,3,4,5] O60.23X9	Preterm labor second tri w preterm delivery second tri, unsp Preterm labor second tri w preterm del second tri Preterm labor second tri w preterm delivery second tri, oth Preterm labor second tri w preterm delivery third tri, unsp Preterm labor second tri w preterm del third tri Preterm labor second tri w preterm delivery third tri, oth Preterm labor third tri w preterm delivery third tri, unsp Preterm labor third tri w preterm del third tri Preterm labor third tri w preterm delivery third tri, oth Term delivery w preterm labor, second trimester, unsp Term delivery with preterm labor, second trimester Term delivery w preterm labor, second trimester, oth fetus Term delivery w preterm labor, third trimester, unsp Term delivery with preterm labor, third trimester Term delivery with preterm labor, third trimester, oth fetus ***7th Character meanings for codes as indicated*** ***1 Fetus 1 2 Fetus 2 3 Fetus 3 4 Fetus 4 5 Fetus 5***
645.10	POST TERM PG UNSPEC AS EPIS CARE/NOT APPLIC	O48.0	Post-term pregnancy
645.11	POST TERM PG DELIV W/WO MENTION ANTPRTM COND	O48.0	Post-term pregnancy
645.13	POST TERM PREGNANCY ANTEPARTUM COND/COMPLICATION	O48.0	Post-term pregnancy
645.20	PROLONGED PG UNSPEC AS EPIS CARE/NOT APPLIC	O48.1	Prolonged pregnancy
645.21	PROLONGED PG DELIV W/WO MENTION ANTPRTM COND	O48.1	Prolonged pregnancy
645.23	PROLONGED PREGNANCY ANTPRTM COND/COMP	O48.1	Prolonged pregnancy
646.00	PAPYRACEOUS FETUS UNSPECIFIED AS TO EPISODE CARE	O31.00X0 O31.00X1 O31.00X2 O31.00X3 O31.00X4 O31.00X5 O31.00X9	Papyraceous fetus, unsp trimester, not applicable or unsp Papyraceous fetus, unspecified trimester, fetus 1 Papyraceous fetus, unspecified trimester, fetus 2 Papyraceous fetus, unspecified trimester, fetus 3 Papyraceous fetus, unspecified trimester, fetus 4 Papyraceous fetus, unspecified trimester, fetus 5 Papyraceous fetus, unspecified trimester, other fetus

ICD-9-CM		ICD-10-CM	
646.01	PAPYRACEOUS FETUS DELIV W/WO ANTPRTM COND	**O31.01X0**	Papyraceous fetus, first trimester, not applicable or unsp
		O31.01X[1,2,3,4,5]	Papyraceous fetus, first trimester
		O31.01X9	Papyraceous fetus, first trimester, other fetus
		O31.02X0	Papyraceous fetus, second trimester, not applicable or unsp
		O31.02X[1,2,3,4,5]	Papyraceous fetus, second trimester
		O31.02X9	Papyraceous fetus, second trimester, other fetus
		O31.03X0	Papyraceous fetus, third trimester, not applicable or unsp
		O31.03X[1,2,3,4,5]	Papyraceous fetus, third trimester, fetus 1
		O31.03X9	Papyraceous fetus, third trimester, other fetus
			7th Character meanings for codes as indicated ***1 Fetus 1 2 Fetus 2 3 Fetus 3 4 Fetus 4 5 Fetus 5***
646.03	PAPYRACEOUS FETUS, ANTEPARTUM	**O31.01X0**	Papyraceous fetus, first trimester, not applicable or unsp
		O31.01X[1,2,3,4,5]	Papyraceous fetus, first trimester
		O31.01X9	Papyraceous fetus, first trimester, other fetus
		O31.02X0	Papyraceous fetus, second trimester, not applicable or unsp
		O31.02X[1,2,3,4,5]	Papyraceous fetus, second trimester
		O31.02X9	Papyraceous fetus, second trimester, other fetus
		O31.03X0	Papyraceous fetus, third trimester, not applicable or unsp
		O31.03X[1,2,3,4,5]	Papyraceous fetus, third trimester
		O31.03X9	Papyraceous fetus, third trimester, other fetus
			7th Character meanings for codes as indicated ***1 Fetus 1 2 Fetus 2 3 Fetus 3 4 Fetus 4 5 Fetus 5***
646.10	EDEMA/EXCESS WEIGHT GAIN PG UNSPEC AS EPIS CARE	**O12.00**	Gestational edema, unspecified trimester
		O12.20	Gestational edema with proteinuria, unspecified trimester
		O26.00	Excessive weight gain in pregnancy, unspecified trimester
646.11	EDEMA/XCESS WT GAIN PG DELIV W/WO ANTPRTM COMP	**O12.01**	Gestational edema, first trimester
		O12.02	Gestational edema, second trimester
		O12.03	Gestational edema, third trimester
		O12.21	Gestational edema with proteinuria, first trimester
		O12.22	Gestational edema with proteinuria, second trimester
		O12.23	Gestational edema with proteinuria, third trimester
		O26.01	Excessive weight gain in pregnancy, first trimester
		O26.02	Excessive weight gain in pregnancy, second trimester
		O26.03	Excessive weight gain in pregnancy, third trimester
646.12	EDEMA/EXCESS WEIGHT GAIN PG DELIV W/CURRENT PPC	**O12.01**	Gestational edema, first trimester
		O12.02	Gestational edema, second trimester
		O12.03	Gestational edema, third trimester
646.13	EDEMA OR EXCESSIVE WEIGHT GAIN ANTEPARTUM	**O12.01**	Gestational edema, first trimester
		O12.02	Gestational edema, second trimester
		O12.03	Gestational edema, third trimester
		O12.21	Gestational edema with proteinuria, first trimester
		O12.22	Gestational edema with proteinuria, second trimester
		O12.23	Gestational edema with proteinuria, third trimester
		O26.01	Excessive weight gain in pregnancy, first trimester
		O26.02	Excessive weight gain in pregnancy, second trimester
		O26.03	Excessive weight gain in pregnancy, third trimester
646.14	EDEMA/EXCESS WEIGHT GAIN NO HTN PP COND/COMPL	**O12.01**	Gestational edema, first trimester
		O12.02	Gestational edema, second trimester
		O12.03	Gestational edema, third trimester
646.20	UNSPEC RENAL DISEASE PG UNSPEC AS EPIS CARE	**O12.10**	Gestational proteinuria, unspecified trimester
		O12.20	Gestational edema with proteinuria, unspecified trimester
		O26.839	Pregnancy related renal disease, unspecified trimester
646.21	UNSPECIFIED RENAL DISEASE PREGNANCY W/DELIVERY	**O12.11**	Gestational proteinuria, first trimester
		O12.12	Gestational proteinuria, second trimester
		O12.13	Gestational proteinuria, third trimester
		O12.21	Gestational edema with proteinuria, first trimester
		O12.22	Gestational edema with proteinuria, second trimester
		O12.23	Gestational edema with proteinuria, third trimester
		O26.831	Pregnancy related renal disease, first trimester
		O26.832	Pregnancy related renal disease, second trimester
		O26.833	Pregnancy related renal disease, third trimester
646.22	UNSPEC RENAL DISEASE PG W/DELIV W/CURRENT PPC	**O26.831**	Pregnancy related renal disease, first trimester
		O26.832	Pregnancy related renal disease, second trimester
		O26.833	Pregnancy related renal disease, third trimester
646.23	UNSPECIFIED ANTEPARTUM RENAL DISEASE	**O12.11**	Gestational proteinuria, first trimester
		O12.12	Gestational proteinuria, second trimester
		O12.13	Gestational proteinuria, third trimester
		O12.21	Gestational edema with proteinuria, first trimester
		O12.22	Gestational edema with proteinuria, second trimester
		O12.23	Gestational edema with proteinuria, third trimester
		O26.831	Pregnancy related renal disease, first trimester
		O26.832	Pregnancy related renal disease, second trimester
		O26.833	Pregnancy related renal disease, third trimester
646.24	UNSPEC RENAL DZ NO HTN POSTPARTUM COND/COMPL	**O90.89**	Oth complications of the puerperium, NEC
646.30	PREGNANCY COMP RECURRENT PREG LOSS UNS EPIS CARE	**O26.20**	Preg care for patient w recurrent preg loss, unsp trimester

[Brackets] indicate valid character values for each code. Character value meanings provided for each code grouping.

ICD-9-CM		ICD-10-CM	
646.31	PREGNANCY COMP RECUR PREG LOSS W/WO ANTPRTM COND	**O26.21**	Preg care for patient w recurrent preg loss, first trimester
		O26.22	Preg care for patient w recur preg loss, second trimester
		O26.23	Preg care for patient w recurrent preg loss, third trimester
646.33	PREGNANCY COMP RECUR PREG LOSS ANTPRTM COND/COMP	**O26.21**	Preg care for patient w recurrent preg loss, first trimester
		O26.22	Preg care for patient w recurrent preg loss, second trimester
		O26.23	Preg care for patient w recurrent preg loss, third trimester
646.40	PERIPH NEURITIS PREGNANCY UNSPEC AS EPIS CARE	**O26.829**	Pregnancy related peripheral neuritis, unspecified trimester
646.41	PERIPHERAL NEURITIS IN PREGNANCY WITH DELIVERY	**O26.821**	Pregnancy related peripheral neuritis, first trimester
		O26.822	Pregnancy related peripheral neuritis, second trimester
		O26.823	Pregnancy related peripheral neuritis, third trimester
646.42	PERIPH NEURITIS PREGNANCY W/DELIV W/CURRENT PPC	**O26.821**	Pregnancy related peripheral neuritis, first trimester
		O26.822	Pregnancy related peripheral neuritis, second trimester
		O26.823	Pregnancy related peripheral neuritis, third trimester
646.43	PERIPHERAL NEURITIS ANTEPARTUM	**O26.821**	Pregnancy related peripheral neuritis, first trimester
		O26.822	Pregnancy related peripheral neuritis, second trimester
		O26.823	Pregnancy related peripheral neuritis, third trimester
646.44	PERIPHERAL NEURITIS POSTPARTUM COND/COMPL	**O90.89**	Oth complications of the puerperium, NEC
646.50	ASYMPTOMATIC BACTERIURIA PG UNSPEC AS EPIS CARE	**O23.40**	Unsp infection of urinary tract in pregnancy, unsp trimester
646.51	ASYMPTOMATIC BACTERIURIA IN PREGNANCY W/DELIVERY	**O23.41**	Unsp infct of urinary tract in pregnancy, first trimester
		O23.42	Unsp infct of urinary tract in pregnancy, second trimester
		O23.43	Unsp infct of urinary tract in pregnancy, third trimester
646.52	ASX BACTERIURIA PG W/DELIV W/CURRENT PPC	**O23.91**	Unsp GU tract infection in pregnancy, first trimester
		O23.92	Unsp GU tract infection in pregnancy, second trimester
		O23.93	Unsp GU tract infection in pregnancy, third trimester
646.53	ASYMPTOMATIC BACTERIURIA ANTEPARTUM	**O23.41**	Unsp infct of urinary tract in pregnancy, first trimester
		O23.42	Unsp infct of urinary tract in pregnancy, second trimester
		O23.43	Unsp infct of urinary tract in pregnancy, third trimester
646.54	ASYMPTOMATIC BACTERIURIA PP COND/COMPL	**O90.89**	Oth complications of the puerperium, NEC
646.60	INFS GU TRACT PREGNANCY UNSPEC AS EPIS CARE	**O23.00**	Infections of kidney in pregnancy, unspecified trimester
		O23.10	Infections of bladder in pregnancy, unspecified trimester
		O23.20	Infections of urethra in pregnancy, unspecified trimester
		O23.30	Infections of prt urinary tract in pregnancy, unsp trimester
		O23.40	Unsp infection of urinary tract in pregnancy, unsp trimester
		O23.519	Infections of cervix in pregnancy, unspecified trimester
		O23.529	Salpingo-oophoritis in pregnancy, unspecified trimester
		O23.599	Infection oth prt genital tract in pregnancy, unsp trimester
		O23.90	Unsp GU tract infection in pregnancy, unsp trimester
646.61	INFECTIONS GENITOURINARY TRACT PREGNANCY W/DELIV	**O23.01**	Infections of kidney in pregnancy, first trimester
		O23.02	Infections of kidney in pregnancy, second trimester
		O23.03	Infections of kidney in pregnancy, third trimester
		O23.11	Infections of bladder in pregnancy, first trimester
		O23.12	Infections of bladder in pregnancy, second trimester
		O23.13	Infections of bladder in pregnancy, third trimester
		O23.21	Infections of urethra in pregnancy, first trimester
		O23.22	Infections of urethra in pregnancy, second trimester
		O23.23	Infections of urethra in pregnancy, third trimester
		O23.31	Infect of prt urinary tract in pregnancy, first trimester
		O23.32	Infect of prt urinary tract in pregnancy, second trimester
		O23.33	Infect of prt urinary tract in pregnancy, third trimester
		O23.41	Unsp infct of urinary tract in pregnancy, first trimester
		O23.42	Unsp infct of urinary tract in pregnancy, second trimester
		O23.43	Unsp infct of urinary tract in pregnancy, third trimester
		O23.511	Infections of cervix in pregnancy, first trimester
		O23.512	Infections of cervix in pregnancy, second trimester
		O23.513	Infections of cervix in pregnancy, third trimester
		O23.521	Salpingo-oophoritis in pregnancy, first trimester
		O23.522	Salpingo-oophoritis in pregnancy, second trimester
		O23.523	Salpingo-oophoritis in pregnancy, third trimester
		O23.591	Infection oth prt genitl trct in pregnancy, first trimester
		O23.592	Infection oth prt genitl trct in pregnancy, second trimester
		O23.593	Infection oth prt genitl trct in pregnancy, third trimester
		O23.91	Unsp GU tract infection in pregnancy, first trimester
		O23.92	Unsp GU tract infection in pregnancy, second trimester
		O23.93	Unsp GU tract infection in pregnancy, third trimester
646.62	INFS GU TRACT PREGNANCY W/DELIV W/CURRENT PPC	**O23.91**	Unsp GU tract infection in pregnancy, first trimester
		O23.92	Unsp GU tract infection in pregnancy, second trimester
		O23.93	Unsp GU tract infection in pregnancy, third trimester

ICD-9-CM		ICD-10-CM	
646.63	INFECTIONS OF GENITOURINARY TRACT ANTEPARTUM	**O23.Ø1**	Infections of kidney in pregnancy, first trimester
		O23.Ø2	Infections of kidney in pregnancy, second trimester
		O23.Ø3	Infections of kidney in pregnancy, third trimester
		O23.11	Infections of bladder in pregnancy, first trimester
		O23.12	Infections of bladder in pregnancy, second trimester
		O23.13	Infections of bladder in pregnancy, third trimester
		O23.21	Infections of urethra in pregnancy, first trimester
		O23.22	Infections of urethra in pregnancy, second trimester
		O23.23	Infections of urethra in pregnancy, third trimester
		O23.31	Infect of prt urinary tract in pregnancy, first trimester
		O23.32	Infect of prt urinary tract in pregnancy, second trimester
		O23.33	Infect of prt urinary tract in pregnancy, third trimester
		O23.41	Unsp infct of urinary tract in pregnancy, first trimester
		O23.42	Unsp infct of urinary tract in pregnancy, second trimester
		O23.43	Unsp infct of urinary tract in pregnancy, third trimester
		O23.511	Infections of cervix in pregnancy, first trimester
		O23.512	Infections of cervix in pregnancy, second trimester
		O23.513	Infections of cervix in pregnancy, third trimester
		O23.521	Salpingo-oophoritis in pregnancy, first trimester
		O23.522	Salpingo-oophoritis in pregnancy, second trimester
		O23.523	Salpingo-oophoritis in pregnancy, third trimester
		O23.591	Infection oth prt genitl trct in pregnancy, first trimester
		O23.592	Infection oth prt genitl trct in pregnancy, second trimester
		O23.593	Infection oth prt genitl trct in pregnancy, third trimester
		O23.91	Unsp GU tract infection in pregnancy, first trimester
		O23.92	Unsp GU tract infection in pregnancy, second trimester
		O23.93	Unsp GU tract infection in pregnancy, third trimester
646.64	INFECTIONS GU TRACT POSTPARTUM COND/COMPL	**O86.11**	Cervicitis following delivery
		O86.13	Vaginitis following delivery
		O86.19	Other infection of genital tract following delivery
		O86.2Ø	Urinary tract infection following delivery, unspecified
		O86.21	Infection of kidney following delivery
		O86.22	Infection of bladder following delivery
		O86.29	Other urinary tract infection following delivery
646.7Ø	LIVER BILIARY TRACT D/O PREG UNS AS EPIS CARE/NA	**O26.619**	Liver and biliary tract disord in pregnancy, unsp trimester
646.71	LIVER BILIARY TRACT D/O PREG DEL W/WO ANTPRTM	**O26.611**	Liver and biliary tract disord in pregnancy, first trimester
		O26.612	Liver and biliary tract disord in preg, second trimester
		O26.613	Liver and biliary tract disord in pregnancy, third trimester
		O26.62	Liver and biliary tract disorders in childbirth
646.73	LIVER BILIARY TRACT D/O PREG ANTEPARTM COND/COMP	**O26.611**	Liver and biliary tract disord in pregnancy, first trimester
		O26.612	Liver and biliary tract disord in preg, second trimester
		O26.613	Liver and biliary tract disord in pregnancy, third trimester
646.8Ø	OTH SPEC COMP PREGNANCY UNSPEC AS EPISODE CARE	**O26.1Ø**	Low weight gain in pregnancy, unspecified trimester
		O26.3Ø	Retained uterin contracep dev in pregnancy, unsp trimester
		O26.4Ø	Herpes gestationis, unspecified trimester
		O26.719	Sublux of symphysis (pubis) in pregnancy, unsp trimester
		O26.819	Pregnancy related exhaustion and fatigue, unsp trimester
		O26.899	Oth pregnancy related conditions, unspecified trimester
		O29.Ø19	Aspirat pneumonitis due to anesth during preg, unsp tri
		O29.Ø29	Pressr collapse of lung due to anesth during preg, unsp tri
		O29.Ø99	Oth pulmonary comp of anesth during preg, unsp trimester
		O29.119	Cardiac arrest due to anesth during preg, unsp trimester
		O29.129	Cardiac failure due to anesth during preg, unsp trimester
		O29.199	Oth cardiac comp of anesth during pregnancy, unsp trimester
		O29.219	Cerebral anoxia due to anesth during preg, unsp trimester
		O29.299	Oth cnsl comp of anesthesia during pregnancy, unsp trimester
		O29.3X9	Toxic reaction to local anesth during preg, unsp trimester
		O29.4Ø	Spinal and epidur anesth induce hdache during preg, unsp tri
		O29.5X9	Oth comp of spinal and epidural anesth during preg, unsp tri
		O29.6Ø	Failed or difficult intubation for anesth dur preg, unsp tri
		O29.8X9	Oth comp of anesthesia during pregnancy, unsp trimester
		O29.9Ø	Unsp comp of anesthesia during pregnancy, unsp trimester
		O99.35Ø	Diseases of the nervous sys comp pregnancy, unsp trimester
		O99.89	Oth diseases and conditions compl preg/chldbrth

ICD-9-CM		ICD-10-CM	
646.81	OTHER SPEC COMPLICATION PREGNANCY W/DELIVERY	**O26.11**	Low weight gain in pregnancy, first trimester
		O26.12	Low weight gain in pregnancy, second trimester
		O26.13	Low weight gain in pregnancy, third trimester
		O26.31	Retained uterin contracep dev in pregnancy, first trimester
		O26.32	Retained uterin contracep dev in pregnancy, second trimester
		O26.33	Retained uterin contracep dev in pregnancy, third trimester
		O26.41	Herpes gestationis, first trimester
		O26.42	Herpes gestationis, second trimester
		O26.43	Herpes gestationis, third trimester
		O26.711	Sublux of symphysis (pubis) in pregnancy, first trimester
		O26.712	Sublux of symphysis (pubis) in pregnancy, second trimester
		O26.713	Sublux of symphysis (pubis) in pregnancy, third trimester
		O26.72	Subluxation of symphysis (pubis) in childbirth
		O26.811	Pregnancy related exhaustion and fatigue, first trimester
		O26.812	Pregnancy related exhaustion and fatigue, second trimester
		O26.813	Pregnancy related exhaustion and fatigue, third trimester
		O26.86	Pruritic urticarial papules and plaques of pregnancy (PUPPP)
		O26.891	Oth pregnancy related conditions, first trimester
		O26.892	Oth pregnancy related conditions, second trimester
		O26.893	Oth pregnancy related conditions, third trimester
		O26.91	Pregnancy related conditions, unspecified, first trimester
		O26.92	Pregnancy related conditions, unspecified, second trimester
		O26.93	Pregnancy related conditions, unspecified, third trimester
		O29.Ø11	Aspirat pneumonitis due to anesth during preg, first tri
		O29.Ø12	Aspirat pneumonitis due to anesth during preg, second tri
		O29.Ø13	Aspirat pneumonitis due to anesth during preg, third tri
		O29.Ø21	Pressr collapse of lung due to anesth during preg, first tri
		O29.Ø22	Pressr collapse of lung d/t anesth during preg, second tri
		O29.Ø23	Pressr collapse of lung due to anesth during preg, third tri
		O29.Ø91	Oth pulmonary comp of anesth during preg, first trimester
		O29.Ø92	Oth pulmonary comp of anesth during preg, second trimester
		O29.Ø93	Oth pulmonary comp of anesth during preg, third trimester
		O29.111	Cardiac arrest due to anesth during preg, first trimester
		O29.112	Cardiac arrest due to anesth during preg, second trimester
		O29.113	Cardiac arrest due to anesth during preg, third trimester
		O29.121	Cardiac failure due to anesth during preg, first trimester
		O29.122	Cardiac failure due to anesth during preg, second trimester
		O29.123	Cardiac failure due to anesth during preg, third trimester
		O29.191	Oth cardiac comp of anesth during pregnancy, first trimester
		O29.192	Oth cardiac comp of anesth during preg, second trimester
		O29.193	Oth cardiac comp of anesth during pregnancy, third trimester
		O29.211	Cerebral anoxia due to anesth during preg, first trimester
		O29.212	Cerebral anoxia due to anesth during preg, second trimester
		O29.213	Cerebral anoxia due to anesth during preg, third trimester
		O29.291	Oth cnsl comp of anesth during pregnancy, first trimester
		O29.292	Oth cnsl comp of anesth during pregnancy, second trimester
		O29.293	Oth cnsl comp of anesth during pregnancy, third trimester
		O29.3X1	Toxic reaction to local anesth during preg, first trimester
		O29.3X2	Toxic reaction to local anesth during preg, second trimester
		O29.3X3	Toxic reaction to local anesth during preg, third trimester
		O29.41	Spinal and epidur anesth induce hdache dur preg, first tri
		O29.42	Spinal and epidur anesth induce hdache dur preg, second tri
		O29.43	Spinal and epidur anesth induce hdache dur preg, third tri
		O29.5X1	Oth comp of spinal and epidur anesth during preg, first tri
		O29.5X2	Oth comp of spinal and epidur anesth during preg, second tri
		O29.5X3	Oth comp of spinal and epidur anesth during preg, third tri
		O29.61	Fail or difficult intubation for anesth dur preg, first tri
		O29.62	Fail or difficult intubation for anesth dur preg, second tri
		O29.63	Fail or difficult intubation for anesth dur preg, third tri
		O29.8X1	Oth comp of anesthesia during pregnancy, first trimester
		O29.8X2	Oth comp of anesthesia during pregnancy, second trimester
		O29.8X3	Oth comp of anesthesia during pregnancy, third trimester
		O29.91	Unsp comp of anesthesia during pregnancy, first trimester
		O29.92	Unsp comp of anesthesia during pregnancy, second trimester
		O29.93	Unsp comp of anesthesia during pregnancy, third trimester
		O99.351	Diseases of the nervous sys comp pregnancy, first trimester
		O99.352	Diseases of the nervous sys comp pregnancy, second trimester
		O99.353	Diseases of the nervous sys comp pregnancy, third trimester
		O99.354	Diseases of the nervous system complicating childbirth
		O99.89	Oth diseases and conditions compl preg/chldbrth
646.82	OTH SPEC COMPS PREGNANCY W/DELIV W/CURRENT PPC	**O26.891**	Oth pregnancy related conditions, first trimester
		O26.892	Oth pregnancy related conditions, second trimester
		O26.893	Oth pregnancy related conditions, third trimester
		O99.355	Diseases of the nervous system complicating the puerperium

ICD-9-CM		ICD-10-CM	
646.83	OTHER SPECIFED COMPLICATION ANTEPARTUM	**O26.1**[1,2,3]	Low weight gain in pregnancy
		O26.3[1,2,3]	Retained uterin contracep dev in pregnancy
		O26.4[1,2,3]	Herpes gestationis
		O26.71[1,2,3]	Sublux of symphysis (pubis) in pregnancy
		O26.81[1,2,3]	Pregnancy related exhaustion and fatigue
		O26.86	Pruritic urticarial papules and plaques of pregnancy (PUPPP)
		O26.89[1,2,3]	Oth pregnancy related conditions
		O26.9[1,2,3]	Pregnancy related conditions, unspecified
		O29.Ø1[1,2,3]	Aspirat pneumonitis due to anesth during preg
		O29.Ø2[1,2,3]	Pressr collapse of lung due to anesth during preg
		O29.Ø9[1,2,3]	Oth pulmonary comp of anesth during preg
		O29.11[1,2,3]	Cardiac arrest due to anesth during preg
		O29.12[1,2,3]	Cardiac failure due to anesth during preg
		O29.19[1,2,3]	Oth cardiac comp of anesth during pregnancy
		O29.21[1,2,3]	Cerebral anoxia due to anesth during preg
		O29.29[1,2,3]	Oth cnsl comp of anesth during pregnancy
		O29.3X[1,2,3]	Toxic reaction to local anesth during preg
		O29.4[1,2,3]	Spinal and epidur anesth induce hdache dur preg
		O29.5X[1,2,3]	Oth comp of spinal and epidur anesth during preg
		O29.6[1,2,3]	Fail or difficult intubation for anesth dur preg
		O29.8X[1,2,3]	Oth comp of anesthesia during pregnancy
		O29.91	Unsp comp of anesthesia during pregnancy, first trimester
		O29.92	Unsp comp of anesthesia during pregnancy, second trimester
		O29.93	Unsp comp of anesthesia during pregnancy, third trimester
		O99.351	Diseases of the nervous sys comp pregnancy, first trimester
		O99.352	Diseases of the nervous sys comp pregnancy, second trimester
		O99.353	Diseases of the nervous sys comp pregnancy, third trimester
		O99.89	Oth diseases and conditions compl preg/chldbrth
			5th and 6th Character meanings for codes as indicated ***1 1st Trimester*** ***2 2nd Trimester*** ***3 3rd Trimester***
646.84	OTH SPEC COMPLICATIONS POSTPARTUM COND/COMPL	**O26.63**	Liver and biliary tract disorders in the puerperium
		O26.73	Subluxation of symphysis (pubis) in the puerperium
		O9Ø.89	Oth complications of the puerperium, NEC
		O99.355	Diseases of the nervous system complicating the puerperium
646.9Ø	UNSPEC COMP PREGNANCY UNSPEC AS EPISODE CARE	**O26.9Ø**	Pregnancy related conditions, unsp, unspecified trimester
646.91	UNSPECIFIED COMPLICATION OF PREGNANCY W/DELIVERY	**O99.89**	Oth diseases and conditions compl preg/chldbrth
646.93	UNSPECIFIED COMPLICATION OF PREGNANCY ANTEPARTUM	**O99.89**	Oth diseases and conditions compl preg/chldbrth
647.ØØ	MATERNAL SYPHILIS-COMPLICATING PC/P-UNS EOC	**O98.119**	Syphilis complicating pregnancy, unspecified trimester
647.Ø1	MATERNAL SYPHILIS COMP PREGNANCY W/DELIVERY	**O98.111**	Syphilis complicating pregnancy, first trimester
		O98.112	Syphilis complicating pregnancy, second trimester
		O98.113	Syphilis complicating pregnancy, third trimester
		O98.12	Syphilis complicating childbirth
647.Ø2	MTRN SYPHILIS COMP PG W/DELIV W/CURRENT PPC	**O98.13**	Syphilis complicating the puerperium
647.Ø3	MATERNAL SYPHILIS, ANTEPARTUM	**O98.111**	Syphilis complicating pregnancy, first trimester
		O98.112	Syphilis complicating pregnancy, second trimester
		O98.113	Syphilis complicating pregnancy, third trimester
647.Ø4	MATERNAL SYPHILIS POSTPARTUM CONDITION/COMPLICAT	**O98.13**	Syphilis complicating the puerperium
647.1Ø	MATERNAL GONORRHEA-COMPLICATING PC/P-UNS EOC	**O98.219**	Gonorrhea complicating pregnancy, unspecified trimester
647.11	MATERNAL GONORRHEA WITH DELIVERY	**O98.211**	Gonorrhea complicating pregnancy, first trimester
		O98.212	Gonorrhea complicating pregnancy, second trimester
		O98.213	Gonorrhea complicating pregnancy, third trimester
		O98.22	Gonorrhea complicating childbirth
647.12	MATERNAL GONORRHEA W/DELIVERY W/CURRENT PPC	**O98.23**	Gonorrhea complicating the puerperium
647.13	MATERNAL GONORRHEA, ANTEPARTUM	**O98.211**	Gonorrhea complicating pregnancy, first trimester
		O98.212	Gonorrhea complicating pregnancy, second trimester
		O98.213	Gonorrhea complicating pregnancy, third trimester
647.14	MATERNAL GONORRHEA POSTPART CONDITION/COMPLICAT	**O98.23**	Gonorrhea complicating the puerperium
647.2Ø	OTH MATERNAL VENEREAL DZ-COMPLICAT PC/P-UNS EOC	**O98.319**	Oth infect w sexl mode of transmiss comp preg, unsp tri
647.21	OTHER MATERNAL VENEREAL DISEASES WITH DELIVERY	**O98.311**	Oth infect w sexl mode of transmiss comp preg, first tri
		O98.312	Oth infect w sexl mode of transmiss comp preg, second tri
		O98.313	Oth infect w sexl mode of transmiss comp preg, third tri
		O98.32	Oth infections w sexl mode of transmiss comp childbirth
647.22	OTH MATERNAL VENEREAL DZ W/DELIV W/CURRENT PPC	**O98.33**	Oth infections w sexl mode of transmiss comp the puerperium
647.23	OTH MATERNAL VENEREAL DISEASE ANTPRTM COND/COMPL	**O98.311**	Oth infect w sexl mode of transmiss comp preg, first tri
		O98.312	Oth infect w sexl mode of transmiss comp preg, second tri
		O98.313	Oth infect w sexl mode of transmiss comp preg, third tri
647.24	OTHER VENEREAL DISEASES POSTPARTUM COND/COMPL	**O98.33**	Oth infections w sexl mode of transmiss comp the puerperium
647.3Ø	MTRN TB COMP PG CHLDBRTH/THE PUERPERIUM UNS EOC	**O98.Ø19**	Tuberculosis complicating pregnancy, unspecified trimester
647.31	MATERNAL TUBERCULOSIS WITH DELIVERY	**O98.Ø11**	Tuberculosis complicating pregnancy, first trimester
		O98.Ø12	Tuberculosis complicating pregnancy, second trimester
		O98.Ø13	Tuberculosis complicating pregnancy, third trimester
		O98.Ø2	Tuberculosis complicating childbirth
647.32	MATERNAL TUBERCULOSIS W/DELIVERY W/CURRENT PPC	**O98.Ø3**	Tuberculosis complicating the puerperium

[Brackets] indicate valid character values for each code. Character value meanings provided for each code grouping.

ICD-9-CM		ICD-10-CM	
647.33	MATERNAL TUBERCULOSIS, ANTEPARTUM	**O98.Ø11**	Tuberculosis complicating pregnancy, first trimester
		O98.Ø12	Tuberculosis complicating pregnancy, second trimester
		O98.Ø13	Tuberculosis complicating pregnancy, third trimester
647.34	MATERNAL TUBERCULOSIS POSTPARTUM COND/COMPL	**O98.Ø3**	Tuberculosis complicating the puerperium
647.4Ø	MATERNAL MALARIA-COMPLICATING PC/P-UNS EOC	**O98.619**	Protozoal diseases complicating pregnancy, unsp trimester
647.41	MATERNAL MALARIA WITH DELIVERY	**O98.611**	Protozoal diseases complicating pregnancy, first trimester
		O98.612	Protozoal diseases complicating pregnancy, second trimester
		O98.613	Protozoal diseases complicating pregnancy, third trimester
		O98.62	Protozoal diseases complicating childbirth
647.42	MATERNAL MALARIA W/DELIVERY W/CURRENT PPC	**O98.63**	Protozoal diseases complicating the puerperium
647.43	MATERNAL MALARIA, ANTEPARTUM	**O98.611**	Protozoal diseases complicating pregnancy, first trimester
		O98.612	Protozoal diseases complicating pregnancy, second trimester
		O98.613	Protozoal diseases complicating pregnancy, third trimester
647.44	MATERNAL MALARIA POSTPARTUM CONDITION/COMPLICAT	**O98.63**	Protozoal diseases complicating the puerperium
647.5Ø	MAT RUBELLA COMPL PG BRTH/PP UNS EOC	**O98.519**	Other viral diseases complicating pregnancy, unsp trimester
647.51	MATERNAL RUBELLA WITH DELIVERY	**O98.511**	Other viral diseases complicating pregnancy, first trimester
		O98.512	Oth viral diseases complicating pregnancy, second trimester
		O98.513	Other viral diseases complicating pregnancy, third trimester
		O98.52	Other viral diseases complicating childbirth
647.52	MATERNAL RUBELLA W/DELIVERY W/CURRENT PPC	**O98.53**	Other viral diseases complicating the puerperium
647.53	MATERNAL RUBELLA, ANTEPARTUM	**O98.511**	Other viral diseases complicating pregnancy, first trimester
		O98.512	Oth viral diseases complicating pregnancy, second trimester
		O98.513	Other viral diseases complicating pregnancy, third trimester
647.54	MATERNAL RUBELLA POSTPARTUM CONDITION/COMPLICAT	**O98.53**	Other viral diseases complicating the puerperium
647.6Ø	OTH MATERNAL VIRAL DZ-COMPLICATING PC/P-UNS EOC	**O98.419**	Viral hepatitis complicating pregnancy, unsp trimester
		O98.519	Other viral diseases complicating pregnancy, unsp trimester
		O98.719	Human immunodef virus disease comp pregnancy, unsp tri
647.61	OTHER MATERNAL VIRAL DISEASE WITH DELIVERY	**O98.411**	Viral hepatitis complicating pregnancy, first trimester
		O98.412	Viral hepatitis complicating pregnancy, second trimester
		O98.413	Viral hepatitis complicating pregnancy, third trimester
		O98.42	Viral hepatitis complicating childbirth
		O98.511	Other viral diseases complicating pregnancy, first trimester
		O98.512	Oth viral diseases complicating pregnancy, second trimester
		O98.513	Other viral diseases complicating pregnancy, third trimester
		O98.52	Other viral diseases complicating childbirth
		O98.711	Human immunodef virus disease comp preg, first trimester
		O98.712	Human immunodef virus disease comp preg, second trimester
		O98.713	Human immunodef virus disease comp preg, third trimester
		O98.72	Human immunodeficiency virus disease complicating childbirth
647.62	OTH MATERNAL VIRAL DISEASE W/DELIV W/CURRENT PPC	**O98.43**	Viral hepatitis complicating the puerperium
		O98.53	Other viral diseases complicating the puerperium
647.63	OTHER MATERNAL VIRAL DISEASE ANTEPARTUM	**O98.411**	Viral hepatitis complicating pregnancy, first trimester
		O98.412	Viral hepatitis complicating pregnancy, second trimester
		O98.413	Viral hepatitis complicating pregnancy, third trimester
		O98.511	Other viral diseases complicating pregnancy, first trimester
		O98.512	Oth viral diseases complicating pregnancy, second trimester
		O98.513	Other viral diseases complicating pregnancy, third trimester
		O98.711	Human immunodef virus disease comp preg, first trimester
		O98.712	Human immunodef virus disease comp preg, second trimester
		O98.713	Human immunodef virus disease comp preg, third trimester
647.64	OTH MTRN VIRAL DISEASE POSTPARTUM COND/COMPLICAT	**O98.43**	Viral hepatitis complicating the puerperium
		O98.53	Other viral diseases complicating the puerperium
		O98.73	Human immunodef virus disease complicating the puerperium
647.8Ø	OTH MATERN INFECT-PARASIT DZ-COMPLI PC/P-UNS EOC	**O98.819**	Oth maternal infec/parastc diseases comp preg, unsp tri
647.81	OTH SPEC MATERNAL INF&PARASITIC DISEASE W/DELIV	**O98.611**	Protozoal diseases complicating pregnancy, first trimester
		O98.612	Protozoal diseases complicating pregnancy, second trimester
		O98.613	Protozoal diseases complicating pregnancy, third trimester
		O98.811	Oth maternal infec/parastc diseases comp preg, first tri
		O98.812	Oth maternal infec/parastc diseases comp preg, second tri
		O98.813	Oth maternal infec/parastc diseases comp preg, third tri
		O98.82	Oth maternal infec/parastc diseases complicating childbirth
		O99.83Ø	Other infection carrier state complicating pregnancy
		O99.834	Other infection carrier state complicating childbirth
647.82	OTH SPEC MTRN INF&PARASITIC DZ DELIV W/CURR PPC	**O98.83**	Oth maternal infec/parastc diseases comp the puerperium
		O99.835	Other infection carrier state complicating the puerperium
647.83	OTH SPEC MATERNAL INF&PARASITIC DISEASE ANTPRTM	**O98.611**	Protozoal diseases complicating pregnancy, first trimester
		O98.612	Protozoal diseases complicating pregnancy, second trimester
		O98.613	Protozoal diseases complicating pregnancy, third trimester
		O98.811	Oth maternal infec/parastc diseases comp preg, first tri
		O98.812	Oth maternal infec/parastc diseases comp preg, second tri
		O98.813	Oth maternal infec/parastc diseases comp preg, third tri
		O99.83Ø	Other infection carrier state complicating pregnancy
647.84	OTH SPEC MTRN INF&PARASITIC DZ PP COND/COMPL	**O98.83**	Oth maternal infec/parastc diseases comp the puerperium
		O99.835	Other infection carrier state complicating the puerperium
647.9Ø	UNS MATERN INFECT/INFESTAT-COMPLI PC/P-UNS EOC	**O98.919**	Unsp maternal infec/parastc disease comp preg, unsp tri

ICD-9-CM		ICD-10-CM	
647.91	UNSPEC MATERNAL INFECTION/INFESTATION W/DELIVERY	**O98.911**	Unsp maternal infec/parastc disease comp preg, first tri
		O98.912	Unsp maternal infec/parastc disease comp preg, second tri
		O98.913	Unsp maternal infec/parastc disease comp preg, third tri
		O98.92	Unsp maternal infec/parastc disease complicating childbirth
647.92	UNSPEC MATERNAL INF/INFEST W/DELIV W/CURRENT PPC	**O98.93**	Unsp maternal infec/parastc disease comp the puerperium
647.93	UNSPEC MATERNAL INFECTION/INFESTATION ANTEPARTUM	**O98.911**	Unsp maternal infec/parastc disease comp preg, first tri
		O98.912	Unsp maternal infec/parastc disease comp preg, second tri
		O98.913	Unsp maternal infec/parastc disease comp preg, third tri
647.94	UNSPEC MTRN INF/INFEST POSTPARTUM COND/COMPLICAT	**O98.93**	Unsp maternal infec/parastc disease comp the puerperium
648.ØØ	MTRN DM COMP PG CHLDBRTH/THE PUERPERIUM UNS EOC	**O24.Ø19**	Pre-existing diabetes, type 1, in pregnancy, unsp trimester
		O24.119	Pre-existing diabetes, type 2, in pregnancy, unsp trimester
		O24.319	Unsp pre-existing diabetes in pregnancy, unsp trimester
		O24.819	Oth pre-existing diabetes in pregnancy, unsp trimester
		O24.919	Unsp diabetes mellitus in pregnancy, unspecified trimester
648.Ø1	MATERNAL DIABETES MELLITUS WITH DELIVERY	**O24.Ø11**	Pre-existing diabetes, type 1, in pregnancy, first trimester
		O24.Ø12	Pre-exist diabetes, type 1, in pregnancy, second trimester
		O24.Ø13	Pre-existing diabetes, type 1, in pregnancy, third trimester
		O24.Ø2	Pre-existing diabetes mellitus, type 1, in childbirth
		O24.111	Pre-existing diabetes, type 2, in pregnancy, first trimester
		O24.112	Pre-exist diabetes, type 2, in pregnancy, second trimester
		O24.113	Pre-existing diabetes, type 2, in pregnancy, third trimester
		O24.12	Pre-existing diabetes mellitus, type 2, in childbirth
		O24.311	Unsp pre-existing diabetes in pregnancy, first trimester
		O24.312	Unsp pre-existing diabetes in pregnancy, second trimester
		O24.313	Unsp pre-existing diabetes in pregnancy, third trimester
		O24.32	Unspecified pre-existing diabetes mellitus in childbirth
		O24.811	Oth pre-existing diabetes in pregnancy, first trimester
		O24.812	Oth pre-existing diabetes in pregnancy, second trimester
		O24.813	Oth pre-existing diabetes in pregnancy, third trimester
		O24.82	Other pre-existing diabetes mellitus in childbirth
		O24.911	Unspecified diabetes mellitus in pregnancy, first trimester
		O24.912	Unspecified diabetes mellitus in pregnancy, second trimester
		O24.913	Unspecified diabetes mellitus in pregnancy, third trimester
		O24.92	Unspecified diabetes mellitus in childbirth
648.Ø2	MATERNAL DM W/DELIVERY W/CURRENT PPC	**O24.93**	Unspecified diabetes mellitus in the puerperium
648.Ø3	MATERNAL DIABETES MELLITUS ANTEPARTUM	**O24.Ø11**	Pre-existing diabetes, type 1, in pregnancy, first trimester
		O24.Ø12	Pre-exist diabetes, type 1, in pregnancy, second trimester
		O24.Ø13	Pre-existing diabetes, type 1, in pregnancy, third trimester
		O24.111	Pre-existing diabetes, type 2, in pregnancy, first trimester
		O24.112	Pre-exist diabetes, type 2, in pregnancy, second trimester
		O24.113	Pre-existing diabetes, type 2, in pregnancy, third trimester
		O24.311	Unsp pre-existing diabetes in pregnancy, first trimester
		O24.312	Unsp pre-existing diabetes in pregnancy, second trimester
		O24.313	Unsp pre-existing diabetes in pregnancy, third trimester
		O24.811	Oth pre-existing diabetes in pregnancy, first trimester
		O24.812	Oth pre-existing diabetes in pregnancy, second trimester
		O24.813	Oth pre-existing diabetes in pregnancy, third trimester
		O24.911	Unspecified diabetes mellitus in pregnancy, first trimester
		O24.912	Unspecified diabetes mellitus in pregnancy, second trimester
		O24.913	Unspecified diabetes mellitus in pregnancy, third trimester
648.Ø4	MATERNAL DM POSTPARTUM COND/COMPLICATION	**O24.Ø3**	Pre-existing diabetes mellitus, type 1, in the puerperium
		O24.13	Pre-existing diabetes mellitus, type 2, in the puerperium
		O24.33	Unspecified pre-existing diabetes mellitus in the puerperium
		O24.83	Other pre-existing diabetes mellitus in the puerperium
		O24.93	Unspecified diabetes mellitus in the puerperium
648.1Ø	MATERNAL THYROID DYSFUNCTION-COMPLI PC/P-UNS EOC	**O99.28Ø**	Endo, nutritional and metab diseases comp preg, unsp tri
648.11	MTRN THYROID DYSF DELIV W/WO ANTPRTM COND	**O99.281**	Endo, nutritional and metab diseases comp preg, first tri
		O99.282	Endo, nutritional and metab diseases comp preg, second tri
		O99.283	Endo, nutritional and metab diseases comp preg, third tri
		O99.284	Endocrine, nutritional and metabolic diseases comp chldbrth
648.12	MATERNAL THYROID DYSF W/DELIV W/CURRENT PPC	**O9Ø.5**	Postpartum thyroiditis
		O99.285	Endocrine, nutritional and metabolic diseases comp the puerp
648.13	MATERNAL THYROID DYSFUNCTION ANTPRTM COND/COMP	**O99.281**	Endo, nutritional and metab diseases comp preg, first tri
		O99.282	Endo, nutritional and metab diseases comp preg, second tri
		O99.283	Endo, nutritional and metab diseases comp preg, third tri
648.14	MTRN THYROID DYSF POSTPARTUM COND/COMPL	**O9Ø.5**	Postpartum thyroiditis
		O99.285	Endocrine, nutritional and metabolic diseases comp the puerp
648.2Ø	MATERNAL ANEMIA MOM COMPL PG CB/PP UNS EOC	**O99.Ø19**	Anemia complicating pregnancy, unspecified trimester
648.21	MATERNAL ANEMIA, WITH DELIVERY	**O99.Ø11**	Anemia complicating pregnancy, first trimester
		O99.Ø12	Anemia complicating pregnancy, second trimester
		O99.Ø13	Anemia complicating pregnancy, third trimester
		O99.Ø2	Anemia complicating childbirth
648.22	MATERNAL ANEMIA W/DELIVERY W/CURRENT PPC	**O99.Ø3**	Anemia complicating the puerperium
648.23	MATERNAL ANEMIA, ANTEPARTUM	**O99.Ø11**	Anemia complicating pregnancy, first trimester
		O99.Ø12	Anemia complicating pregnancy, second trimester
		O99.Ø13	Anemia complicating pregnancy, third trimester
648.24	MATERNAL ANEMIA POSTPARTUM CONDITION/COMPLICAT	**O9Ø.81**	Anemia of the puerperium
		O99.Ø3	Anemia complicating the puerperium

ICD-9-CM		ICD-10-CM	
648.30	MATERNAL RX DEPEND COMPL PG CB/PP UNS EOC	O99.320	Drug use complicating pregnancy, unspecified trimester
648.31	MATERNAL DRUG DEPENDENCE WITH DELIVERY	O99.321	Drug use complicating pregnancy, first trimester
		O99.322	Drug use complicating pregnancy, second trimester
		O99.323	Drug use complicating pregnancy, third trimester
		O99.324	Drug use complicating childbirth
648.32	MATERNAL DRUG DEPENDENCE W/DELIV W/CURRENT PPC	O99.325	Drug use complicating the puerperium
648.33	MATERNAL DRUG DEPENDENCE ANTEPARTUM	O99.321	Drug use complicating pregnancy, first trimester
		O99.322	Drug use complicating pregnancy, second trimester
		O99.323	Drug use complicating pregnancy, third trimester
648.34	MATERNAL DRUG DEPEND POSTPARTUM COND/COMPL	O99.325	Drug use complicating the puerperium
648.40	MATERNAL MENTAL D/O COMPL PG CB/PP UNS EOC	O99.310	Alcohol use complicating pregnancy, unspecified trimester
		O99.340	Oth mental disorders complicating pregnancy, unsp trimester
648.41	MATERNAL MENTAL DISORDERS WITH DELIVERY	O99.311	Alcohol use complicating pregnancy, first trimester
		O99.312	Alcohol use complicating pregnancy, second trimester
		O99.313	Alcohol use complicating pregnancy, third trimester
		O99.314	Alcohol use complicating childbirth
		O99.341	Oth mental disorders complicating pregnancy, first trimester
		O99.342	Oth mental disorders comp pregnancy, second trimester
		O99.343	Oth mental disorders complicating pregnancy, third trimester
		O99.344	Other mental disorders complicating childbirth
648.42	MATERNAL MENTAL DISORDERS W/DELIV W/CURRENT PPC	O90.6	Postpartum mood disturbance
		O99.345	Other mental disorders complicating the puerperium
648.43	MATERNAL MENTAL DISORDERS ANTEPARTUM	O99.311	Alcohol use complicating pregnancy, first trimester
		O99.312	Alcohol use complicating pregnancy, second trimester
		O99.313	Alcohol use complicating pregnancy, third trimester
		O99.341	Oth mental disorders complicating pregnancy, first trimester
		O99.342	Oth mental disorders comp pregnancy, second trimester
		O99.343	Oth mental disorders complicating pregnancy, third trimester
648.44	MATERNAL MENTAL D/O POSTPARTUM COND/COMPLICATION	O90.6	Postpartum mood disturbance
		O99.315	Alcohol use complicating the puerperium
		O99.345	Other mental disorders complicating the puerperium
648.50	MATERNAL CONGENITAL CV DIS-COMPLI PC/P-UNS EOC	O99.419	Diseases of the circ sys comp pregnancy, unsp trimester
648.51	MATERNAL CONGENITAL CV DISORDERS W/DELIVERY	O99.411	Diseases of the circ sys comp pregnancy, first trimester
		O99.412	Diseases of the circ sys comp pregnancy, second trimester
		O99.413	Diseases of the circ sys comp pregnancy, third trimester
		O99.42	Diseases of the circulatory system complicating childbirth
648.52	MATERNAL CONGEN CV D/O W/DELIV W/CURRENT PPC	O99.43	Diseases of the circ sys complicating the puerperium
648.53	MATERNAL CONGENITAL CV DISORDERS ANTPRTM	O99.411	Diseases of the circ sys comp pregnancy, first trimester
		O99.412	Diseases of the circ sys comp pregnancy, second trimester
		O99.413	Diseases of the circ sys comp pregnancy, third trimester
648.54	MATERNAL CONGEN CV D/O POSTPARTUM COND/COMPL	O99.43	Diseases of the circ sys complicating the puerperium
648.60	OTH MATERNAL CV DZ-COMPLICATING PC/P-UNS EOC	O99.419	Diseases of the circ sys comp pregnancy, unsp trimester
648.61	OTH MATERNAL CARDIOVASCULAR DISEASES W/DELIVERY	O99.411	Diseases of the circ sys comp pregnancy, first trimester
		O99.412	Diseases of the circ sys comp pregnancy, second trimester
		O99.413	Diseases of the circ sys comp pregnancy, third trimester
		O99.42	Diseases of the circulatory system complicating childbirth
648.62	OTH MATERNAL CV DISEASES W/DELIV W/CURRENT PPC	O99.43	Diseases of the circ sys complicating the puerperium
648.63	OTH MATERNAL CARDIOVASCULAR DISEASES ANTEPARTUM	O99.411	Diseases of the circ sys comp pregnancy, first trimester
		O99.412	Diseases of the circ sys comp pregnancy, second trimester
		O99.413	Diseases of the circ sys comp pregnancy, third trimester
648.64	OTH MATERNAL CV DZ POSTPARTUM COND/COMPL	O99.43	Diseases of the circ sys complicating the puerperium
648.70	BN&JNT D/O MAT BACK & LW LMB-COMPL PG CB/PP UNS	O33.0	Matern care for disproprtn d/t deformity of matern pelv bone
648.71	BN&JNT D/O MAT BACK PELVIS&LW LMB W/DEL	O33.0	Matern care for disproprtn d/t deformity of matern pelv bone
648.72	BN&JNT D/O MAT BACK PELV&LW LMB W/DEL W/PP COMPL	O33.0	Matern care for disproprtn d/t deformity of matern pelv bone
648.73	BN&JNT D/O MAT BACK PELVIS&LW LIMBS ANTEPARTUM	O33.0	Matern care for disproprtn d/t deformity of matern pelv bone
648.74	BN&JNT D/O MAT BACK PELVIS&LW LIMBS PP COND/COMP	O33.0	Matern care for disproprtn d/t deformity of matern pelv bone
648.80	ABN MAT GLUCOSE TOLERANCE COMPL PG CB/PP UNS EOC	O99.810	Abnormal glucose complicating pregnancy
648.81	ABNORMAL MATERNAL GLUCOSE TOLERANCE W/DELIVERY	O24.410	Gestational diabetes mellitus in pregnancy, diet controlled
		O24.414	Gestational diabetes in pregnancy, insulin controlled
		O24.419	Gestational diabetes mellitus in pregnancy, unsp control
		O24.420	Gestational diabetes mellitus in childbirth, diet controlled
		O24.424	Gestational diabetes in childbirth, insulin controlled
		O24.429	Gestational diabetes mellitus in childbirth, unsp control
		O99.810	Abnormal glucose complicating pregnancy
		O99.814	Abnormal glucose complicating childbirth
648.82	ABNORMAL MTRN GLU TOLERNC W/DELIV W/CURRENT PPC	O99.815	Abnormal glucose complicating the puerperium
648.83	ABNORMAL MATERNAL GLUCOSE TOLERANCE ANTEPARTUM	O24.410	Gestational diabetes mellitus in pregnancy, diet controlled
		O24.414	Gestational diabetes in pregnancy, insulin controlled
		O24.419	Gestational diabetes mellitus in pregnancy, unsp control
		O99.810	Abnormal glucose complicating pregnancy
648.84	ABNORMAL MTRN GLU TOLERANCE PP COND/COMPL	O24.430	Gestational diabetes in the puerperium, diet controlled
		O24.434	Gestational diabetes in the puerperium, insulin controlled
		O24.439	Gestational diabetes in the puerperium, unsp control
		O99.815	Abnormal glucose complicating the puerperium

ICD-9-CM		ICD-10-CM	
648.9Ø	OTH CURRENT MATERNAL CCE-COMPL PG CB/PP-UNS EOC	O25.1Ø	Malnutrition in pregnancy, unspecified trimester
		O99.28Ø	Endo, nutritional and metab diseases comp preg, unsp tri
		O99.519	Diseases of the resp sys comp pregnancy, unsp trimester
		O99.619	Diseases of the dgstv sys comp pregnancy, unsp trimester
		O99.719	Diseases of the skin, subcu comp pregnancy, unsp trimester
		O9A.119	Malignant neoplasm complicating pregnancy, unsp trimester
		O9A.219	Inj/poisn/oth conseq of external causes comp preg, unsp tri
		O9A.319	Physical abuse complicating pregnancy, unspecified trimester
		O9A.419	Sexual abuse complicating pregnancy, unspecified trimester
		O9A.519	Psychological abuse complicating pregnancy, unsp trimester
648.91	OTH CURRENT MATERNAL CCE W/DELIVERY	O25.11	Malnutrition in pregnancy, first trimester
		O25.12	Malnutrition in pregnancy, second trimester
		O25.13	Malnutrition in pregnancy, third trimester
		O25.2	Malnutrition in childbirth
		O99.281	Endo, nutritional and metab diseases comp preg, first tri
		O99.282	Endo, nutritional and metab diseases comp preg, second tri
		O99.283	Endo, nutritional and metab diseases comp preg, third tri
		O99.284	Endocrine, nutritional and metabolic diseases comp chldbrth
		O99.511	Diseases of the resp sys comp pregnancy, first trimester
		O99.512	Diseases of the resp sys comp pregnancy, second trimester
		O99.513	Diseases of the resp sys comp pregnancy, third trimester
		O99.52	Diseases of the respiratory system complicating childbirth
		O99.611	Diseases of the dgstv sys comp pregnancy, first trimester
		O99.612	Diseases of the dgstv sys comp pregnancy, second trimester
		O99.613	Diseases of the dgstv sys comp pregnancy, third trimester
		O99.62	Diseases of the digestive system complicating childbirth
		O99.711	Diseases of the skin, subcu comp pregnancy, first trimester
		O99.712	Diseases of the skin, subcu comp pregnancy, second trimester
		O99.713	Diseases of the skin, subcu comp pregnancy, third trimester
		O99.72	Diseases of the skin, subcu complicating childbirth
		O99.824	Streptococcus B carrier state complicating childbirth
		O9A.111	Malignant neoplasm complicating pregnancy, first trimester
		O9A.112	Malignant neoplasm complicating pregnancy, second trimester
		O9A.113	Malignant neoplasm complicating pregnancy, third trimester
		O9A.12	Malignant neoplasm complicating childbirth
		O9A.211	Inj/poisn/oth conseq of external causes comp preg, first tri
		O9A.212	Inj/poisn/oth conseq of extrn causes comp preg, second tri
		O9A.213	Inj/poisn/oth conseq of external causes comp preg, third tri
		O9A.22	Inj/poisn/oth conseq of external causes comp childbirth
		O9A.311	Physical abuse complicating pregnancy, first trimester
		O9A.312	Physical abuse complicating pregnancy, second trimester
		O9A.313	Physical abuse complicating pregnancy, third trimester
		O9A.32	Physical abuse complicating childbirth
		O9A.411	Sexual abuse complicating pregnancy, first trimester
		O9A.412	Sexual abuse complicating pregnancy, second trimester
		O9A.413	Sexual abuse complicating pregnancy, third trimester
		O9A.42	Sexual abuse complicating childbirth
		O9A.511	Psychological abuse complicating pregnancy, first trimester
		O9A.512	Psychological abuse complicating pregnancy, second trimester
		O9A.513	Psychological abuse complicating pregnancy, third trimester
		O9A.52	Psychological abuse complicating childbirth
648.92	OTH CURRENT MATERNAL CCE W/DEL W/CURRNT PP COMPL	O99.285	Endocrine, nutritional and metabolic diseases comp the puerp
648.93	OTH CURRENT MAT CONDS CLASSIFIABLE ELSW ANTPRTM	O25.11	Malnutrition in pregnancy, first trimester
		O25.12	Malnutrition in pregnancy, second trimester
		O25.13	Malnutrition in pregnancy, third trimester
		O99.281	Endo, nutritional and metab diseases comp preg, first tri
		O99.282	Endo, nutritional and metab diseases comp preg, second tri
		O99.283	Endo, nutritional and metab diseases comp preg, third tri
		O99.511	Diseases of the resp sys comp pregnancy, first trimester
		O99.512	Diseases of the resp sys comp pregnancy, second trimester
		O99.513	Diseases of the resp sys comp pregnancy, third trimester
		O99.611	Diseases of the dgstv sys comp pregnancy, first trimester
		O99.612	Diseases of the dgstv sys comp pregnancy, second trimester
		O99.613	Diseases of the dgstv sys comp pregnancy, third trimester
		O99.711	Diseases of the skin, subcu comp pregnancy, first trimester
		O99.712	Diseases of the skin, subcu comp pregnancy, second trimester
		O99.713	Diseases of the skin, subcu comp pregnancy, third trimester
		O99.82Ø	Streptococcus B carrier state complicating pregnancy
		O9A.111	Malignant neoplasm complicating pregnancy, first trimester
		O9A.112	Malignant neoplasm complicating pregnancy, second trimester
		O9A.113	Malignant neoplasm complicating pregnancy, third trimester
		O9A.211	Inj/poisn/oth conseq of external causes comp preg, first tri
		O9A.212	Inj/poisn/oth conseq of extrn causes comp preg, second tri
		O9A.213	Inj/poisn/oth conseq of external causes comp preg, third tri
		O9A.311	Physical abuse complicating pregnancy, first trimester
		O9A.312	Physical abuse complicating pregnancy, second trimester
		O9A.313	Physical abuse complicating pregnancy, third trimester
		O9A.411	Sexual abuse complicating pregnancy, first trimester
		O9A.412	Sexual abuse complicating pregnancy, second trimester
		O9A.413	Sexual abuse complicating pregnancy, third trimester

(Continued on next page)

ICD-9-CM		ICD-10-CM	
648.93	OTH CURRENT MAT CONDS CLASSIFIABLE ELSW ANTPRTM **(Continued)**	**O9A.511** **O9A.512** **O9A.513**	Psychological abuse complicating pregnancy, first trimester Psychological abuse complicating pregnancy, second trimester Psychological abuse complicating pregnancy, third trimester
648.94	OTH CURRENT MATERNAL CCE PP CONDITION/COMPL	**O25.3** **O99.285** **O99.53** **O99.63** **O99.73** **O99.825** **O9A.13** **O9A.23** **O9A.33** **O9A.43** **O9A.53**	Malnutrition in the puerperium Endocrine, nutritional and metabolic diseases comp the puerp Diseases of the resp sys complicating the puerperium Diseases of the digestive system complicating the puerperium Diseases of the skin, subcu complicating the puerperium Streptococcus B carrier state complicating the puerperium Malignant neoplasm complicating the puerperium Inj/poisn/oth conseq of external causes comp the puerperium Physical abuse complicating the puerperium Sexual abuse complicating the puerperium Psychological abuse complicating the puerperium
649.00	TOB USE D/O COMP PG BIRTH/PP UNSPEC EPIS CARE/NA	**O99.330**	Smoking (tobacco) complicating pregnancy, unsp trimester
649.01	TOBACCO USE D/O COMP PG CHILDBIRTH/PP DELIVERED	**O99.331** **O99.332** **O99.333** **O99.334**	Smoking (tobacco) complicating pregnancy, first trimester Smoking (tobacco) complicating pregnancy, second trimester Smoking (tobacco) complicating pregnancy, third trimester Smoking (tobacco) complicating childbirth
649.02	TOB USE D/O COMP PG BIRTH/PP DEL W/MEN PP COMP	**O99.335**	Smoking (tobacco) complicating the puerperium
649.03	TOB USE D/O COMP PG BIRTH/PP ANTEPARTM COND/COMP	**O99.331** **O99.332** **O99.333**	Smoking (tobacco) complicating pregnancy, first trimester Smoking (tobacco) complicating pregnancy, second trimester Smoking (tobacco) complicating pregnancy, third trimester
649.04	TOB USE D/O COMP PG BIRTH/THE PP PP COND/COMP	**O99.335**	Smoking (tobacco) complicating the puerperium
649.10	OBES COMP PG BIRH/PP UNSPEC AS TO EPIS CARE/NA	**O99.210**	Obesity complicating pregnancy, unspecified trimester
649.11	OBESITY COMP PG CHILDBIRTH/THE PP DELIVERED	**O99.211** **O99.212** **O99.213** **O99.214**	Obesity complicating pregnancy, first trimester Obesity complicating pregnancy, second trimester Obesity complicating pregnancy, third trimester Obesity complicating childbirth
649.12	OBESITY COMP PG CHILDBIRTH/THE PP DEL W/PP COMP	**O99.215**	Obesity complicating the puerperium
649.13	OBES COMP PG BIRTH/THE PP ANTEPARTUM COND/COMP	**O99.211** **O99.212** **O99.213**	Obesity complicating pregnancy, first trimester Obesity complicating pregnancy, second trimester Obesity complicating pregnancy, third trimester
649.14	OBES COMP PG BIRTH/THE PP POSTPARTUM COND/COMP	**O99.215**	Obesity complicating the puerperium
649.20	BARIATRIC SURG COMP PG BIRTH/PP UNSPC EPIS CARE	**O99.840**	Bariatric surgery status comp pregnancy, unsp trimester
649.21	BARIATRIC SURG STS COMP PG BIRTH/PP DELIVERED	**O99.841** **O99.842** **O99.843** **O99.844**	Bariatric surgery status comp pregnancy, first trimester Bariatric surgery status comp pregnancy, second trimester Bariatric surgery status comp pregnancy, third trimester Bariatric surgery status complicating childbirth
649.22	BARIATRC SURG STS COMP PG BIRTH/PP DEL W/PP COMP	**O99.845**	Bariatric surgery status complicating the puerperium
649.23	BARIATRIC SURG STS COMP PG BIRTH/PP AP COND/COMP	**O99.841** **O99.842** **O99.843**	Bariatric surgery status comp pregnancy, first trimester Bariatric surgery status comp pregnancy, second trimester Bariatric surgery status comp pregnancy, third trimester
649.24	BARIATRIC SURG STS COMP PG BIRTH/PP PP COND/COMP	**O99.845**	Bariatric surgery status complicating the puerperium
649.30	COAG DEFEC COMP PG BIRTH/PP UNSPEC EPIS CARE/NA	**O99.119**	Oth dis of bld/bld-form org/immun mech comp preg,unsp tri
649.31	COAGULATION DEFECTS COMP PG BIRTH/THE PP DEL	**O99.111** **O99.112** **O99.113** **O99.12**	Oth dis of bld/bld-form org/immun mech comp preg, 1st tri Oth dis of bld/bld-form org/immun mech comp preg, 2nd tri Oth dis of bld/bld-form org/immun mech comp preg, 3rd tri Oth dis of the bld/bld-form org/immun mech comp chldbrth
649.32	COAGULATION DEFEC COMP PG BIRTH/PP DEL W/PP COMP	**O99.13**	Oth dis of the bld/bld-form org/immun mech comp the puerp
649.33	COAGULAT DEFEC COMP PG BIRTH/THE PP AP COND/COMP	**O99.111** **O99.112** **O99.113**	Oth dis of bld/bld-form org/immun mech comp preg, 1st tri Oth dis of bld/bld-form org/immun mech comp preg, 2nd tri Oth dis of bld/bld-form org/immun mech comp preg, 3rd tri
649.34	COAGULATION DEFEC COMP PG BIRTH/PP PP COND/COMP	**O99.13**	Oth dis of the bld/bld-form org/immun mech comp the puerp
649.40	EPILEPSY COMP PG BIRTH/PP UNSPEC EPIS CARE/NA	**O99.350**	Diseases of the nervous sys comp pregnancy, unsp trimester
649.41	EPILEPSY COMP PG CHILDBIRTH/THE PP DELIVERED	**O99.351** **O99.352** **O99.353** **O99.354**	Diseases of the nervous sys comp pregnancy, first trimester Diseases of the nervous sys comp pregnancy, second trimester Diseases of the nervous sys comp pregnancy, third trimester Diseases of the nervous system complicating childbirth
649.42	EPILEPSY COMP PG CHILDBIRTH/THE PP DEL W/PP COMP	**O99.355**	Diseases of the nervous system complicating the puerperium
649.43	EPILEPSY COMP PG BIRTH/PP ANTEPARTUM COND/COMP	**O99.351** **O99.352** **O99.353**	Diseases of the nervous sys comp pregnancy, first trimester Diseases of the nervous sys comp pregnancy, second trimester Diseases of the nervous sys comp pregnancy, third trimester
649.44	EPILEPSY COMP PG CHILDBIRTH/THE PP PP COND/COMP	**O99.355**	Diseases of the nervous system complicating the puerperium
649.50	SPOTTING COMP PREGNANCY UNS EPIS CARE/NOT APPLIC	**O26.859**	Spotting complicating pregnancy, unspecified trimester
649.51	SPOTTING COMPLICATING PREGNANCY DELIVERED	**O26.851** **O26.852** **O26.853**	Spotting complicating pregnancy, first trimester Spotting complicating pregnancy, second trimester Spotting complicating pregnancy, third trimester
649.53	SPOTTING COMP PREGNANCY ANTEPARTUM COND/COMP	**O26.851** **O26.852** **O26.853**	Spotting complicating pregnancy, first trimester Spotting complicating pregnancy, second trimester Spotting complicating pregnancy, third trimester
649.60	UTERN SIZE DATE DISCREPANCY UNSPEC EPIS CARE/NA	**O26.849**	Uterine size-date discrepancy, unspecified trimester
649.61	UTERINE SIZE DATE DISCREPANCY DELIVERED	**O26.841** **O26.842** **O26.843**	Uterine size-date discrepancy, first trimester Uterine size-date discrepancy, second trimester Uterine size-date discrepancy, third trimester

ICD-9-CM		ICD-10-CM	
649.62	UTERINE SZ DATE DISCREPANCY DEL W/MEN PP COMPL	O26.841	Uterine size-date discrepancy, first trimester
		O26.842	Uterine size-date discrepancy, second trimester
		O26.843	Uterine size-date discrepancy, third trimester
649.63	UTERINE SIZE DATE DISCREPANCY ANTPRTM COND/COMPL	O26.841	Uterine size-date discrepancy, first trimester
		O26.842	Uterine size-date discrepancy, second trimester
		O26.843	Uterine size-date discrepancy, third trimester
649.64	UTERINE SIZE DATE DISCREPANCY PP COND/COMPL	O26.841	Uterine size-date discrepancy, first trimester
		O26.842	Uterine size-date discrepancy, second trimester
		O26.843	Uterine size-date discrepancy, third trimester
649.70	CERVICAL SHORTENING UNSPECIFIED AS TO EOC/NA	O26.879	Cervical shortening, unspecified trimester
649.71	CERVICAL SHORTENING DELIVERED W/WO ANTPRTM COND	O26.872	Cervical shortening, second trimester
		O26.873	Cervical shortening, third trimester
649.73	CERVICAL SHORTENING ANTEPARTUM CONDITION OR COMP	O26.872	Cervical shortening, second trimester
		O26.873	Cervical shortening, third trimester
649.81	ONSET LABR AFTR 37 BEFOR 39 CMPL WK GEST C/S DEL	O75.82	Onset labor 37-39 weeks, w del by (planned) cesarean section
649.82	ONSET LABR AFTR 37 BFOR 39 WK GEST C/S DEL W/PPC	O75.82	Onset labor 37-39 weeks, w del by (planned) cesarean section
650	NORMAL DELIVERY	➡ O80	Encounter for full-term uncomplicated delivery
651.00	TWIN PREGNANCY UNSPECIFIED AS TO EPISODE OF CARE	O30.009	Twin pregnancy, unsp num plcnta & amnio sacs, unsp trimester
		O30.019	Twin pregnancy, monochorionic/monoamniotic, unsp trimester
		O30.039	Twin pregnancy, monochorionic/diamniotic, unsp trimester
		O30.049	Twin pregnancy, dichorionic/diamniotic, unsp trimester
		O30.099	Twin preg, unable to dtrm num plcnta & amnio sacs, unsp tri
651.01	TWIN PREGNANCY, DELIVERED	O30.001	Twin preg, unsp num plcnta & amnio sacs, first trimester
		O30.002	Twin preg, unsp num plcnta & amnio sacs, second trimester
		O30.003	Twin preg, unsp num plcnta & amnio sacs, third trimester
		O30.011	Twin pregnancy, monochorionic/monoamniotic, first trimester
		O30.012	Twin pregnancy, monochorionic/monoamniotic, second tri
		O30.013	Twin pregnancy, monochorionic/monoamniotic, third trimester
		O30.031	Twin pregnancy, monochorionic/diamniotic, first trimester
		O30.032	Twin pregnancy, monochorionic/diamniotic, second trimester
		O30.033	Twin pregnancy, monochorionic/diamniotic, third trimester
		O30.041	Twin pregnancy, dichorionic/diamniotic, first trimester
		O30.042	Twin pregnancy, dichorionic/diamniotic, second trimester
		O30.043	Twin pregnancy, dichorionic/diamniotic, third trimester
		O30.091	Twin preg, unable to dtrm num plcnta & amnio sacs, first tri
		O30.092	Twin preg, unable to dtrm num plcnta & amnio sacs, 2nd tri
		O30.093	Twin preg, unable to dtrm num plcnta & amnio sacs, third tri
651.03	TWIN PREGNANCY, ANTEPARTUM	O30.001	Twin preg, unsp num plcnta & amnio sacs, first trimester
		O30.002	Twin preg, unsp num plcnta & amnio sacs, second trimester
		O30.003	Twin preg, unsp num plcnta & amnio sacs, third trimester
		O30.011	Twin pregnancy, monochorionic/monoamniotic, first trimester
		O30.012	Twin pregnancy, monochorionic/monoamniotic, second tri
		O30.013	Twin pregnancy, monochorionic/monoamniotic, third trimester
		O30.031	Twin pregnancy, monochorionic/diamniotic, first trimester
		O30.032	Twin pregnancy, monochorionic/diamniotic, second trimester
		O30.033	Twin pregnancy, monochorionic/diamniotic, third trimester
		O30.041	Twin pregnancy, dichorionic/diamniotic, first trimester
		O30.042	Twin pregnancy, dichorionic/diamniotic, second trimester
		O30.043	Twin pregnancy, dichorionic/diamniotic, third trimester
		O30.091	Twin preg, unable to dtrm num plcnta & amnio sacs, first tri
		O30.092	Twin preg, unable to dtrm num plcnta & amnio sacs, 2nd tri
		O30.093	Twin preg, unable to dtrm num plcnta & amnio sacs, third tri
651.10	TRIPLET PREGNANCY UNSPECIFIED AS TO EPISODE CARE	O30.109	Triplet preg, unsp num plcnta & amnio sacs, unsp trimester
		O30.119	Triplet preg w two or more monochorionic fetuses, unsp tri
		O30.129	Triplet preg w two or more monoamnio fetuses, unsp trimester
		O30.199	Trp preg, unable to dtrm num plcnta & amnio sacs, unsp tri
651.11	TRIPLET PREGNANCY, DELIVERED	O30.101	Triplet preg, unsp num plcnta & amnio sacs, first trimester
		O30.102	Triplet preg, unsp num plcnta & amnio sacs, second trimester
		O30.103	Triplet preg, unsp num plcnta & amnio sacs, third trimester
		O30.111	Triplet preg w two or more monochorionic fetuses, first tri
		O30.112	Triplet preg w two or more monochorionic fetuses, second tri
		O30.113	Triplet preg w two or more monochorionic fetuses, third tri
		O30.121	Triplet preg w two or more monoamnio fetuses, first tri
		O30.122	Triplet preg w two or more monoamnio fetuses, second tri
		O30.123	Triplet preg w two or more monoamnio fetuses, third tri
		O30.191	Trp preg, unable to dtrm num plcnta & amnio sacs, first tri
		O30.192	Trp preg, unable to dtrm num plcnta & amnio sacs, second tri
		O30.193	Trp preg, unable to dtrm num plcnta & amnio sacs, third tri

ICD-9-CM		ICD-10-CM	
651.13	TRIPLET PREGNANCY, ANTEPARTUM	O3Ø.1Ø1	Triplet preg, unsp num plcnta & amnio sacs, first trimester
		O3Ø.1Ø2	Triplet preg, unsp num plcnta & amnio sacs, second trimester
		O3Ø.1Ø3	Triplet preg, unsp num plcnta & amnio sacs, third trimester
		O3Ø.111	Triplet preg w two or more monochorionic fetuses, first tri
		O3Ø.112	Triplet preg w two or more monochorionic fetuses, second tri
		O3Ø.113	Triplet preg w two or more monochorionic fetuses, third tri
		O3Ø.121	Triplet preg w two or more monoamnio fetuses, first tri
		O3Ø.122	Triplet preg w two or more monoamnio fetuses, second tri
		O3Ø.123	Triplet preg w two or more monoamnio fetuses, third tri
		O3Ø.191	Trp preg, unable to dtrm num plcnta & amnio sacs, first tri
		O3Ø.192	Trp preg, unable to dtrm num plcnta & amnio sacs, second tri
		O3Ø.193	Trp preg, unable to dtrm num plcnta & amnio sacs, third tri
651.2Ø	QUADRUPLET PREGNANCY UNSPECIFIED AS EPISODE CARE	O3Ø.2Ø9	Quad pregnancy, unsp num plcnta & amnio sacs, unsp trimester
		O3Ø.219	Quad preg w two or more monochorionic fetuses, unsp tri
		O3Ø.229	Quad preg w two or more monoamnio fetuses, unsp trimester
		O3Ø.299	Quad preg, unable to dtrm num plcnta & amnio sacs, unsp tri
651.21	QUADRUPLET PREGNANCY, DELIVERED	O3Ø.2Ø1	Quad preg, unsp num plcnta & amnio sacs, first trimester
		O3Ø.2Ø2	Quad preg, unsp num plcnta & amnio sacs, second trimester
		O3Ø.2Ø3	Quad preg, unsp num plcnta & amnio sacs, third trimester
		O3Ø.211	Quad preg w two or more monochorionic fetuses, first tri
		O3Ø.212	Quad preg w two or more monochorionic fetuses, second tri
		O3Ø.213	Quad preg w two or more monochorionic fetuses, third tri
		O3Ø.221	Quad preg w two or more monoamnio fetuses, first trimester
		O3Ø.222	Quad preg w two or more monoamnio fetuses, second trim
		O3Ø.223	Quad preg w two or more monoamnio fetuses, third trimester
		O3Ø.291	Quad preg, unable to dtrm num plcnta & amnio sacs, first tri
		O3Ø.292	Quad preg, unable to dtrm num plcnta & amnio sacs, 2nd tri
		O3Ø.293	Quad preg, unable to dtrm num plcnta & amnio sacs, third tri
651.23	QUADRUPLET PREGNANCY, ANTEPARTUM	O3Ø.2Ø1	Quad preg, unsp num plcnta & amnio sacs, first trimester
		O3Ø.2Ø2	Quad preg, unsp num plcnta & amnio sacs, second trimester
		O3Ø.2Ø3	Quad preg, unsp num plcnta & amnio sacs, third trimester
		O3Ø.211	Quad preg w two or more monochorionic fetuses, first tri
		O3Ø.212	Quad preg w two or more monochorionic fetuses, second tri
		O3Ø.213	Quad preg w two or more monochorionic fetuses, third tri
		O3Ø.221	Quad preg w two or more monoamnio fetuses, first trimester
		O3Ø.222	Quad preg w two or more monoamnio fetuses, second trim
		O3Ø.223	Quad preg w two or more monoamnio fetuses, third trimester
		O3Ø.291	Quad preg, unable to dtrm num plcnta & amnio sacs, first tri
		O3Ø.292	Quad preg, unable to dtrm num plcnta & amnio sacs, 2nd tri
		O3Ø.293	Quad preg, unable to dtrm num plcnta & amnio sacs, third tri
651.3Ø	TWIN PREG W/FETL LOSS&RETAIN 1 FETUS-UNS EOC	O31.1ØXØ	Cont preg aft spon abort of one fts or more, unsp tri, unsp
		O31.1ØX1	Cont preg aft spon abort of one fts or more, unsp tri, fts1
		O31.1ØX2	Cont preg aft spon abort of one fts or more, unsp tri, fts2
		O31.2ØXØ	Cont preg aft uterin dth of one fts or more, unsp tri, unsp
		O31.2ØX1	Cont preg aft uterin dth of one fts or more, unsp tri, fts1
		O31.2ØX2	Cont preg aft uterin dth of one fts or more, unsp tri, fts2
651.31	TWIN PG W/FETAL LOSS&RETENTION 1 FETUS DELIV	O31.11XØ	Cont preg aft spon abort of one fts or more, first tri, unsp
		O31.11X1	Cont preg aft spon abort of one fts or more, first tri, fts1
		O31.11X2	Cont preg aft spon abort of one fts or more, first tri, fts2
		O31.12XØ	Cont preg aft spon abort of one fetus or more, 2nd tri, unsp
		O31.12X1	Cont preg aft spon abort of one fetus or more, 2nd tri, fts1
		O31.12X2	Cont preg aft spon abort of one fetus or more, 2nd tri, fts2
		O31.13XØ	Cont preg aft spon abort of one fts or more, third tri, unsp
		O31.13X1	Cont preg aft spon abort of one fts or more, third tri, fts1
		O31.13X2	Cont preg aft spon abort of one fts or more, third tri, fts2
		O31.21XØ	Cont preg aft uterin dth of one fts or more, first tri, unsp
		O31.21X1	Cont preg aft uterin dth of one fts or more, first tri, fts1
		O31.21X2	Cont preg aft uterin dth of one fts or more, first tri, fts2
		O31.22XØ	Cont preg aft uterin dth of one fetus or more, 2nd tri, unsp
		O31.22X1	Cont preg aft uterin dth of one fetus or more, 2nd tri, fts1
		O31.22X2	Cont preg aft uterin dth of one fetus or more, 2nd tri, fts2
		O31.23XØ	Cont preg aft uterin dth of one fts or more, third tri, unsp
		O31.23X1	Cont preg aft uterin dth of one fts or more, third tri, fts1
		O31.23X2	Cont preg aft uterin dth of one fts or more, third tri, fts2

ICD-9-CM		ICD-10-CM	
651.33	TWIN PG W/FETAL LOSS&RETENTION 1 FETUS ANTPRTM	**O31.11XØ**	Cont preg aft spon abort of one fts or more, first tri, unsp
		O31.11X1	Cont preg aft spon abort of one fts or more, first tri, fts1
		O31.11X2	Cont preg aft spon abort of one fts or more, first tri, fts2
		O31.12XØ	Cont preg aft spon abort of one fetus or more, 2nd tri, unsp
		O31.12X1	Cont preg aft spon abort of one fetus or more, 2nd tri, fts1
		O31.12X2	Cont preg aft spon abort of one fetus or more, 2nd tri, fts2
		O31.13XØ	Cont preg aft spon abort of one fts or more, third tri, unsp
		O31.13X1	Cont preg aft spon abort of one fts or more, third tri, fts1
		O31.13X2	Cont preg aft spon abort of one fts or more, third tri, fts2
		O31.21XØ	Cont preg aft uterin dth of one fts or more, first tri, unsp
		O31.21X1	Cont preg aft uterin dth of one fts or more, first tri, fts1
		O31.21X2	Cont preg aft uterin dth of one fts or more, first tri, fts2
		O31.22XØ	Cont preg aft uterin dth of one fetus or more, 2nd tri, unsp
		O31.22X1	Cont preg aft uterin dth of one fetus or more, 2nd tri, fts1
		O31.22X2	Cont preg aft uterin dth of one fetus or more, 2nd tri, fts2
		O31.23XØ	Cont preg aft uterin dth of one fts or more, third tri, unsp
		O31.23X1	Cont preg aft uterin dth of one fts or more, third tri, fts1
		O31.23X2	Cont preg aft uterin dth of one fts or more, third tri, fts2
651.4Ø	TRIPLET PREG W/FETAL LOSS&RETN 1/> FETUS-UNS EOC	**O31.1ØXØ**	Cont preg aft spon abort of one fts or more, unsp tri, unsp
651.41	TRIPLET PG W/FETAL LOSS&RETENTION 1/MORE DELIV	**O31.11XØ**	Cont preg aft spon abort of one fts or more, first tri, unsp
651.43	TRIPLET PG W/FETAL LOSS&RETENTION 1/MORE ANTPRTM	**O31.11XØ**	Cont preg aft spon abort of one fts or more, first tri, unsp
651.5Ø	QUAD PREG W/FETAL LOSS&RETN 1/> FETUS-UNS EOC	**O31.1ØXØ**	Cont preg aft spon abort of one fts or more, unsp tri, unsp
651.51	QUADRUPLET PG W/FETAL LOSS&RETN 1/MORE DELIV	**O31.11XØ**	Cont preg aft spon abort of one fts or more, first tri, unsp
651.53	QUADRUPLET PG W/FETAL LOSS&RETN 1/MORE ANTPRTM	**O31.11XØ**	Cont preg aft spon abort of one fts or more, first tri, unsp
651.6Ø	OTH MULT PREG W/FETAL-RETAIN >= 1 FETUS-UNS EOC	**O31.1ØXØ**	Cont preg aft spon abort of one fts or more, unsp tri, unsp
		O31.1ØX[1,2,3,4,5]	Cont preg aft spon abort of one fts or more, unsp tri
		O31.1ØX9	Cont preg aft spon abort of one fetus or more, unsp tri, oth
		O31.2ØXØ	Cont preg aft uterin dth of one fts or more, unsp tri, unsp
		O31.2ØX[1,2,3,4,5]	Cont preg aft uterin dth of one fts or more, unsp tri
		O31.2ØX9	Cont preg aft uterin dth of one fetus or more, unsp tri, oth
			7th Character meanings for codes as indicated *1 Fetus 1; 2 Fetus 2; 3 Fetus 3; 4 Fetus 4; 5 Fetus 5*
651.61	OTH MX PG W/FETAL LOSS&RETN 1/MORE FETUS DELIV	**O31.11XØ**	Cont preg aft spon abort of one fts or more, first tri, unsp
		O31.11X[1,2,3,4,5]	Cont preg aft spon abort of one fts or more, first tri
		O31.11X9	Cont preg aft spon abort of one fts or more, first tri, oth
		O31.12XØ	Cont preg aft spon abort of one fetus or more, 2nd tri, unsp
		O31.12X[1,2,3,4,5]	Cont preg aft spon abort of one fetus or more, 2nd tri
		O31.12X9	Cont preg aft spon abort of one fetus or more, 2nd tri, oth
		O31.13XØ	Cont preg aft spon abort of one fts or more, third tri, unsp
		O31.13X[1,2,3,4,5]	Cont preg aft spon abort of one fts or more, third tri
		O31.13X9	Cont preg aft spon abort of one fts or more, third tri, oth
		O31.21XØ	Cont preg aft uterin dth of one fts or more, first tri, unsp
		O31.21X[1,2,3,4,5]	Cont preg aft uterin dth of one fts or more, first tri
		O31.21X9	Cont preg aft uterin dth of one fts or more, first tri, oth
		O31.22XØ	Cont preg aft uterin dth of one fetus or more, 2nd tri, unsp
		O31.22X[1,2,3,4,5]	Cont preg aft uterin dth of one fetus or more, 2nd tri
		O31.22X9	Cont preg aft uterin dth of one fetus or more, 2nd tri, oth
		O31.23XØ	Cont preg aft uterin dth of one fts or more, third tri, unsp
		O31.23X[1,2,3,4,5]	Cont preg aft uterin dth of one fts or more, third tri
		O31.23X9	Cont preg aft uterin dth of one fts or more, third tri, oth
			7th Character meanings for codes as indicated *1 Fetus 1; 2 Fetus 2; 3 Fetus 3; 4 Fetus 4; 5 Fetus 5*
651.63	OTH MX PG W/FETAL LOSS&RETN 1/MORE FETUS ANTPRTM	**O31.11XØ**	Cont preg aft spon abort of one fts or more, first tri, unsp
		O31.11X[1,2,3,4,5]	Cont preg aft spon abort of one fts or more, first tri
		O31.11X9	Cont preg aft spon abort of one fts or more, first tri, oth
		O31.12XØ	Cont preg aft spon abort of one fetus or more, 2nd tri, unsp
		O31.12X[1,2,3,4,5]	Cont preg aft spon abort of one fetus or more, 2nd tri
		O31.12X9	Cont preg aft spon abort of one fetus or more, 2nd tri, oth
		O31.13XØ	Cont preg aft spon abort of one fts or more, third tri, unsp
		O31.13X[1,2,3,4,5]	Cont preg aft spon abort of one fts or more, third tri
		O31.13X9	Cont preg aft spon abort of one fts or more, third tri, oth
		O31.21XØ	Cont preg aft uterin dth of one fts or more, first tri, unsp
		O31.21X[1,2,3,4,5]	Cont preg aft uterin dth of one fts or more, first tri
		O31.21X9	Cont preg aft uterin dth of one fts or more, first tri, oth
		O31.22XØ	Cont preg aft uterin dth of one fetus or more, 2nd tri, unsp
		O31.22X[1,2,3,4,5]	Cont preg aft uterin dth of one fetus or more, 2nd tri
		O31.22X9	Cont preg aft uterin dth of one fetus or more, 2nd tri, oth
		O31.23XØ	Cont preg aft uterin dth of one fts or more, third tri, unsp
		O31.23X[1,2,3,4,5]	Cont preg aft uterin dth of one fts or more, third tri
		O31.23X9	Cont preg aft uterin dth of one fts or more, third tri, oth
			7th Character meanings for codes as indicated *1 Fetus 1; 2 Fetus 2; 3 Fetus 3; 4 Fetus 4; 5 Fetus 5*

[Brackets] indicate valid character values for each code. Character value meanings provided for each code grouping.

ICD-9-CM		ICD-10-CM	
651.7Ø	MX GEST FLW ELCTV FETAL RDUC UNS EPIS CARE/NA	**O31.3ØXØ**	Cont preg aft elctv fetl rdct of 1 fts or more,unsp tri,unsp
		O31.3ØX1	Cont preg aft elctv fetl rdct of 1 fts or more,unsp tri,fts1
		O31.3ØX2	Cont preg aft elctv fetl rdct of 1 fts or more,unsp tri,fts2
		O31.3ØX3	Cont preg aft elctv fetl rdct of 1 fts or more,unsp tri,fts3
		O31.3ØX4	Cont preg aft elctv fetl rdct of 1 fts or more,unsp tri,fts4
		O31.3ØX5	Cont preg aft elctv fetl rdct of 1 fts or more,unsp tri,fts5
		O31.3ØX9	Cont preg aft elctv fetl rdct of 1 fts or more,unsp tri, oth
651.71	MX GEST FLW ELCTV FETAL RDUC DEL W/WO AP COND	**O31.31XØ**	Cont preg aft elctv fetl rdct of 1 fts or more,1st tri, unsp
		O31.31X[1,2,3,4,5]	Cont preg aft elctv fetl rdct of 1 fts or more,1st tri
		O31.31X9	Cont preg aft elctv fetl rdct of 1 fts or more, 1st tri, oth
		O31.32XØ	Cont preg aft elctv fetl rdct of 1 fts or more, 2nd tri, unsp
		O31.32X[1,2,3,4,5]	Cont preg aft elctv fetl rdct of 1 fts or more, 2nd tri
		O31.32X9	Cont preg aft elctv fetl rdct of 1 fts or more, 2nd tri, oth
		O31.33XØ	Cont preg aft elctv fetl rdct of 1 fts or more, 3rd tri, unsp
		O31.33X[1,2,3,4,5]	Cont preg aft elctv fetl rdct of 1 fts or more, 3rd tri
		O31.33X9	Cont preg aft elctv fetl rdct of 1 fts or more, 3rd tri, oth
			7th Character meanings for codes as indicated *1 Fetus 1; 2 Fetus 2; 3 Fetus 3; 4 Fetus 4; 5 Fetus 5*
651.73	MX GEST FLW ELCTV FETAL RDUC ANTPRTM COND/COMPL	**O31.31XØ**	Cont preg aft elctv fetl rdct of 1 fts or more,1st tri, unsp
		O31.31X[1,2,3,4,5]	Cont preg aft elctv fetl rdct of 1 fts or more,1st tr
		O31.31X9	Cont preg aft elctv fetl rdct of 1 fts or more, 1st tri, oth
		O31.32XØ	Cont preg aft elctv fetl rdct of 1 fts or more,2nd tri, unsp
		O31.32X[1,2,3,4,5]	Cont preg aft elctv fetl rdct of 1 fts or more,2nd tri
		O31.32X9	Cont preg aft elctv fetl rdct of 1 fts or more, 2nd tri, oth
		O31.33XØ	Cont preg aft elctv fetl rdct of 1 fts or more,3rd tri, unsp
		O31.33X[1,2,3,4,5]	Cont preg aft elctv fetl rdct of 1 fts or more,3rd tri
		O31.33X9	Cont preg aft elctv fetl rdct of 1 fts or more, 3rd tri, oth
			7th Character meanings for codes as indicated *1 Fetus 1; 2 Fetus 2; 3 Fetus 3; 4 Fetus 4; 5 Fetus 5*
651.8Ø	OTH SPEC MULTIPLE GESTATION UNSPEC AS EPIS CARE	**O3Ø.8Ø9**	Oth multiple gest, unsp num plcnta & amnio sacs, unsp tri
		O3Ø.819	Oth mult gest w two or more monochorionic fetuses, unsp tri
		O3Ø.829	Oth multiple gest w two or more monoamnio fetuses, unsp tri
		O3Ø.899	Oth mult gest,unab to dtrm num plcnta & amnio sacs, unsp tri
651.81	OTHER SPECIFIED MULTIPLE GESTATION DELIVERED	**O3Ø.8Ø1**	Oth multiple gest, unsp num plcnta & amnio sacs, first tri
		O3Ø.8Ø2	Oth multiple gest, unsp num plcnta & amnio sacs, second tri
		O3Ø.8Ø3	Oth multiple gest, unsp num plcnta & amnio sacs, third tri
		O3Ø.811	Oth mult gest w two or more monochorionic fetuses, first tri
		O3Ø.812	Oth mult gest w two or more monochorionic fetuses, 2nd tri
		O3Ø.813	Oth mult gest w two or more monochorionic fetuses, third tri
		O3Ø.821	Oth multiple gest w two or more monoamnio fetuses, first tri
		O3Ø.822	Oth mult gest w two or more monoamnio fetuses, second tri
		O3Ø.823	Oth multiple gest w two or more monoamnio fetuses, third tri
		O3Ø.891	Oth mult gest, unab to dtrm num plcnta & amnio sacs, 1st tri
		O3Ø.892	Oth mult gest, unab to dtrm num plcnta & amnio sacs, 2nd tri
		O3Ø.893	Oth mult gest, unab to dtrm num plcnta & amnio sacs, 3rd tri
		O31.8X1Ø	Oth comp specific to multiple gest, first trimester, unsp
		O31.8X1[1,2,3,4,5]	Oth comp specific to multiple gest, first trimester
		O31.8X19	Oth comp specific to multiple gest, first trimester, oth
		O31.8X2Ø	Oth comp specific to multiple gest, second trimester, unsp
		O31.8X2[1,2,3,4,5]	Oth comp specific to multiple gest, second tri
		O31.8X29	Oth comp specific to multiple gest, second trimester, oth
		O31.8X3Ø	Oth comp specific to multiple gest, third trimester, unsp
		O31.8X3[1,2,3,4,5]	Oth comp specific to multiple gest, third trimester
		O31.8X39	Oth comp specific to multiple gest, third trimester, oth
			7th Character meanings for codes as indicated *1 Fetus 1; 2 Fetus 2; 3 Fetus 3; 4 Fetus 4; 5 Fetus 5*

ICD-9-CM		ICD-10-CM	
651.83	OTHER SPECIFIED MULTIPLE GESTATION ANTEPARTUM	**O3Ø.8Ø1**	Oth multiple gest, unsp num plcnta & amnio sacs, first tri
		O3Ø.8Ø2	Oth multiple gest, unsp num plcnta & amnio sacs, second tri
		O3Ø.8Ø3	Oth multiple gest, unsp num plcnta & amnio sacs, third tri
		O3Ø.811	Oth mult gest w two or more monochorionic fetuses, first tri
		O3Ø.812	Oth mult gest w two or more monochorionic fetuses, 2nd tri
		O3Ø.813	Oth mult gest w two or more monochorionic fetuses, third tri
		O3Ø.821	Oth multiple gest w two or more monoamnio fetuses, first tri
		O3Ø.822	Oth mult gest w two or more monoamnio fetuses, second tri
		O3Ø.823	Oth multiple gest w two or more monoamnio fetuses, third tri
		O3Ø.891	Oth mult gest, unab to dtrm num plcnta & amnio sacs, 1st tri
		O3Ø.892	Oth mult gest, unab to dtrm num plcnta & amnio sacs, 2nd tri
		O3Ø.893	Oth mult gest, unab to dtrm num plcnta & amnio sacs, 3rd tri
		O31.8X1Ø	Oth comp specific to multiple gest, first trimester, unsp
		O31.8X1[1,2,3,4,5]	Oth comp specific to multiple gest, first trimester
		O31.8X19	Oth comp specific to multiple gest, first trimester, oth
		O31.8X2Ø	Oth comp specific to multiple gest, second trimester, unsp
		O31.8X2[1,2,3,4,5]	Oth comp specific to multiple gest, second tri
		O31.8X29	Oth comp specific to multiple gest, second trimester, oth
		O31.8X3Ø	Oth comp specific to multiple gest, third trimester, unsp
		O31.8X3[1,2,3,4,5]	Oth comp specific to multiple gest, third trimester
		O31.8X39	Oth comp specific to multiple gest, third trimester, oth
			7th Character meanings for codes as indicated *1 Fetus 1; 2 Fetus 2; 3 Fetus 3; 4 Fetus 4; 5 Fetus 5*
651.9Ø	UNSPEC MULTIPLE GESTATION UNSPEC AS EPISODE CARE	**O3Ø.9Ø**	Multiple gestation, unspecified, unspecified trimester
		O31.8X9Ø	Oth comp specific to multiple gest, unsp trimester, unsp
		O31.8X91	Oth comp specific to multiple gest, unsp trimester, fetus 1
		O31.8X92	Oth comp specific to multiple gest, unsp trimester, fetus 2
		O31.8X93	Oth comp specific to multiple gest, unsp trimester, fetus 3
		O31.8X94	Oth comp specific to multiple gest, unsp trimester, fetus 4
		O31.8X95	Oth comp specific to multiple gest, unsp trimester, fetus 5
		O31.8X99	Oth comp specific to multiple gestation, unsp trimester, oth
651.91	UNSPECIFIED MULTIPLE GESTATION DELIVERED	**O3Ø.91**	Multiple gestation, unspecified, first trimester
		O3Ø.92	Multiple gestation, unspecified, second trimester
		O3Ø.93	Multiple gestation, unspecified, third trimester
651.93	UNSPECIFIED MULTIPLE GESTATION ANTEPARTUM	**O3Ø.91**	Multiple gestation, unspecified, first trimester
		O3Ø.92	Multiple gestation, unspecified, second trimester
		O3Ø.93	Multiple gestation, unspecified, third trimester
652.ØØ	UNSTABLE LIE FETUS UNSPECIFIED AS EPISODE CARE	**O32.ØXXØ**	Maternal care for unstable lie, not applicable or unsp
652.Ø1	UNSTABLE LIE OF FETUS, DELIVERED	**O32.ØXXØ**	Maternal care for unstable lie, not applicable or unsp
		O32.ØXX1	Maternal care for unstable lie, fetus 1
		O32.ØXX2	Maternal care for unstable lie, fetus 2
		O32.ØXX3	Maternal care for unstable lie, fetus 3
		O32.ØXX4	Maternal care for unstable lie, fetus 4
		O32.ØXX5	Maternal care for unstable lie, fetus 5
		O32.ØXX9	Maternal care for unstable lie, other fetus
652.Ø3	UNSTABLE LIE OF FETUS, ANTEPARTUM	**O32.ØXXØ**	Maternal care for unstable lie, not applicable or unsp
		O32.ØXX1	Maternal care for unstable lie, fetus 1
		O32.ØXX2	Maternal care for unstable lie, fetus 2
		O32.ØXX3	Maternal care for unstable lie, fetus 3
		O32.ØXX4	Maternal care for unstable lie, fetus 4
		O32.ØXX5	Maternal care for unstable lie, fetus 5
		O32.ØXX9	Maternal care for unstable lie, other fetus
652.1Ø	BREECH/MALPRESENT CONVERTED TO CEPHALIC-UNS EOC	**O32.1XXØ**	Maternal care for breech presentation, unsp
652.11	BREECH/ MALPRSATION CONVRT CEPHALIC PRSATION DEL	**O32.1XXØ**	Maternal care for breech presentation, unsp
		O32.1XX1	Maternal care for breech presentation, fetus 1
		O32.1XX2	Maternal care for breech presentation, fetus 2
		O32.1XX3	Maternal care for breech presentation, fetus 3
		O32.1XX4	Maternal care for breech presentation, fetus 4
		O32.1XX5	Maternal care for breech presentation, fetus 5
		O32.1XX9	Maternal care for breech presentation, other fetus
652.13	BREECH/MALPRESENT CONVERTED TO CEPHALIC-APC/C	**O32.1XXØ**	Maternal care for breech presentation, unsp
652.2Ø	BREECH PRESENTATION W/O VERSION UNS EPIS CARE	**O32.1XXØ**	Maternal care for breech presentation, unsp
652.21	BREECH PRESENTATION W/O MENTION VERSION DELIV	**O32.1XXØ**	Maternal care for breech presentation, unsp
		O32.1XX[1,2,3,4,5]	Maternal care for breech presentation
		O32.1XX9	Maternal care for breech presentation, other fetus
		O64.1XXØ	Obstructed labor due to breech presentation, unsp
		O64.1XX[1,2,3,4,5]	Obstructed labor due to breech presentation
		O64.1XX9	Obstructed labor due to breech presentation, other fetus
			7th Character meanings for codes as indicated *1 Fetus 1; 2 Fetus 2; 3 Fetus 3; 4 Fetus 4; 5 Fetus 5*

[Brackets] indicate valid character values for each code. Character value meanings provided for each code grouping.

ICD-9-CM		ICD-10-CM	
652.23	BREECH PRESENTATION W/O MENTION VERSION ANTPRTM	**O32.1XXØ**	Maternal care for breech presentation, unsp
		O32.1XX1	Maternal care for breech presentation, fetus 1
		O32.1XX2	Maternal care for breech presentation, fetus 2
		O32.1XX3	Maternal care for breech presentation, fetus 3
		O32.1XX4	Maternal care for breech presentation, fetus 4
		O32.1XX5	Maternal care for breech presentation, fetus 5
		O32.1XX9	Maternal care for breech presentation, other fetus
652.3Ø	TRNS/OBL FETAL PRESENTATION UNSPEC AS EPIS CARE	**O32.2XXØ**	Maternal care for transverse and oblique lie, unsp
652.31	TRANSVERSE/OBLIQUE FETAL PRESENTATION DELIVERED	**O32.2XXØ**	Maternal care for transverse and oblique lie, unsp
		O32.2XX1	Maternal care for transverse and oblique lie, fetus 1
		O32.2XX2	Maternal care for transverse and oblique lie, fetus 2
		O32.2XX3	Maternal care for transverse and oblique lie, fetus 3
		O32.2XX4	Maternal care for transverse and oblique lie, fetus 4
		O32.2XX5	Maternal care for transverse and oblique lie, fetus 5
		O32.2XX9	Maternal care for transverse and oblique lie, other fetus
652.33	TRANSVERSE/OBLIQUE FETAL PRESENTATION ANTEPARTUM	**O32.2XXØ**	Maternal care for transverse and oblique lie, unsp
		O32.2XX1	Maternal care for transverse and oblique lie, fetus 1
		O32.2XX2	Maternal care for transverse and oblique lie, fetus 2
		O32.2XX3	Maternal care for transverse and oblique lie, fetus 3
		O32.2XX4	Maternal care for transverse and oblique lie, fetus 4
		O32.2XX5	Maternal care for transverse and oblique lie, fetus 5
		O32.2XX9	Maternal care for transverse and oblique lie, other fetus
652.4Ø	FETAL FACE/BROW PRESENTATION UNSPEC AS EPIS CARE	**O32.3XXØ**	Maternal care for face, brow and chin presentation, unsp
652.41	FETAL FACE OR BROW PRESENTATION DELIVERED	**O32.3XXØ**	Maternal care for face, brow and chin presentation, unsp
		O32.3XX[1,2,3,4,5]	Maternal care for face, brow and chin presentation
		O32.3XX9	Maternal care for face, brow and chin presentation, oth
		O64.2XXØ	Obstructed labor due to face presentation, unsp
		O64.2XX[1,2,3,4,5]	Obstructed labor due to face presentation
		O64.2XX9	Obstructed labor due to face presentation, other fetus
		O64.3XXØ	Obstructed labor due to brow presentation, unsp
		O64.3XX[1,2,3,4,5]	Obstructed labor due to brow presentation
		O64.3XX9	Obstructed labor due to brow presentation, other fetus
			7th Character meanings for codes as indicated *1 Fetus 1* *3 Fetus 3* *5 Fetus 5* *2 Fetus 2* *4 Fetus 4*
652.43	FETAL FACE OR BROW PRESENTATION ANTEPARTUM	**O32.3XXØ**	Maternal care for face, brow and chin presentation, unsp
		O32.3XX1	Maternal care for face, brow and chin presentation, fetus 1
		O32.3XX2	Maternal care for face, brow and chin presentation, fetus 2
		O32.3XX3	Maternal care for face, brow and chin presentation, fetus 3
		O32.3XX4	Maternal care for face, brow and chin presentation, fetus 4
		O32.3XX5	Maternal care for face, brow and chin presentation, fetus 5
		O32.3XX9	Maternal care for face, brow and chin presentation, oth
652.5Ø	HIGH FETAL HEAD@TERM UNSPECIFIED AS EPISODE CARE	**O32.4XXØ**	Maternal care for high head at term, not applicable or unsp
652.51	HIGH FETAL HEAD AT TERM, DELIVERED	**O32.4XXØ**	Maternal care for high head at term, not applicable or unsp
		O32.4XX1	Maternal care for high head at term, fetus 1
		O32.4XX2	Maternal care for high head at term, fetus 2
		O32.4XX3	Maternal care for high head at term, fetus 3
		O32.4XX4	Maternal care for high head at term, fetus 4
		O32.4XX5	Maternal care for high head at term, fetus 5
		O32.4XX9	Maternal care for high head at term, other fetus
652.53	HIGH FETAL HEAD AT TERM, ANTEPARTUM	**O32.4XXØ**	Maternal care for high head at term, not applicable or unsp
		O32.4XX1	Maternal care for high head at term, fetus 1
		O32.4XX2	Maternal care for high head at term, fetus 2
		O32.4XX3	Maternal care for high head at term, fetus 3
		O32.4XX4	Maternal care for high head at term, fetus 4
		O32.4XX5	Maternal care for high head at term, fetus 5
		O32.4XX9	Maternal care for high head at term, other fetus
652.6Ø	MX GEST W/MALPRSATION 1 FETUS/MORE UNS EPIS CARE	**O32.9XXØ**	Maternal care for malpresentation of fetus, unsp, unsp
652.61	MX GEST W/MALPRESENTATION 1 FETUS/MORE DELIV	**O32.9XXØ**	Maternal care for malpresentation of fetus, unsp, unsp
		O32.9XX1	Maternal care for malpresentation of fetus, unsp, fetus 1
		O32.9XX2	Maternal care for malpresentation of fetus, unsp, fetus 2
		O32.9XX3	Maternal care for malpresentation of fetus, unsp, fetus 3
		O32.9XX4	Maternal care for malpresentation of fetus, unsp, fetus 4
		O32.9XX5	Maternal care for malpresentation of fetus, unsp, fetus 5
		O32.9XX9	Maternal care for malpresentation of fetus, unsp, oth fetus
		O66.6	Obstructed labor due to other multiple fetuses
652.63	MX GEST W/MALPRESENTATION 1 FETUS/MORE ANTPRTM	**O32.9XXØ**	Maternal care for malpresentation of fetus, unsp, unsp
652.7Ø	PROLAPSED ARM FETUS UNSPECIFIED AS EPISODE CARE	**O32.8XXØ**	Maternal care for oth malpresentation of fetus, unsp
652.71	PROLAPSED ARM OF FETUS, DELIVERED	**O32.8XXØ**	Maternal care for oth malpresentation of fetus, unsp
652.73	PROLAPSED ARM FETUS ANTEPARTUM COND/COMPLICATION	**O32.8XXØ**	Maternal care for oth malpresentation of fetus, unsp
652.8Ø	OTH SPEC MALPSTN/MALPRSATION FETUS UNS EPIS CARE	**O32.8XXØ**	Maternal care for oth malpresentation of fetus, unsp

ICD-9-CM		ICD-10-CM	
652.81	OTH SPEC MALPOSITION/MALPRESENTATION FETUS DELIV	**O32.6XXØ**	Maternal care for compound presentation, unsp
		O32.6XX[1,2,3,4,5]	Maternal care for compound presentation
		O32.6XX9	Maternal care for compound presentation, other fetus
		O32.8XXØ	Maternal care for oth malpresentation of fetus, unsp
		O32.8XX[1,2,3,4,5]	Maternal care for other malpresentation of fetus
		O32.8XX9	Maternal care for oth malpresentation of fetus, other fetus
		O64.4XXØ	Obstructed labor due to shoulder presentation, unsp
		O64.4XX[1,2,3,4,5]	Obstructed labor due to shoulder presentation
		O64.4XX9	Obstructed labor due to shoulder presentation, other fetus
		O64.5XXØ	Obstructed labor due to compound presentation, unsp
		O64.5XX[1,2,3,4,5]	Obstructed labor due to compound presentation
		O64.5XX9	Obstructed labor due to compound presentation, other fetus
		O64.8XXØ	Obstructed labor due to oth malposition and malpresent, unsp
		O64.8XX[1,2,3,4,5]	Obstructed labor due to oth malpos and malpresent
		O64.8XX9	Obstructed labor due to oth malposition and malpresent, oth
			7th Character meanings for codes as indicated *1 Fetus 1; 2 Fetus 2; 3 Fetus 3; 4 Fetus 4; 5 Fetus 5*
652.83	OTH SPEC MALPSTN/MALPRESENTATION FETUS ANTPRTM	**O32.6XXØ**	Maternal care for compound presentation, unsp
		O32.6XX[1,2,3,4,5]	Maternal care for compound presentation
		O32.6XX9	Maternal care for compound presentation, other fetus
		O32.8XXØ	Maternal care for oth malpresentation of fetus, unsp
		O32.8XX[1,2,3,4,5]	Maternal care for other malpresentation of fetus
		O32.8XX9	Maternal care for oth malpresentation of fetus, other fetus
			7th Character meanings for codes as indicated *1 Fetus 1; 2 Fetus 2; 3 Fetus 3; 4 Fetus 4; 5 Fetus 5*
652.9Ø	UNS MALPSTN/MALPRESENTATION FETUS UNS EPIS CARE	**O32.9XXØ**	Maternal care for malpresentation of fetus, unsp, unsp
652.91	UNSPEC MALPOSITION/MALPRESENTATION FETUS DELIV	**O32.9XXØ**	Maternal care for malpresentation of fetus, unsp, unsp
		O32.9XX[1,2,3,4,5	Maternal care for malpresentation of fetus, unsp
		O32.9XX9	Maternal care for malpresentation of fetus, unsp, oth fetus
		O64.9XXØ	Obstructed labor due to malpos and malpresent, unsp, unsp
		O64.9XX[1,2,3,4,5	Obstructed labor due to malpos and malpresent, unsp
		O64.9XX9	Obstructed labor due to malpos and malpresent, unsp, oth
			7th Character meanings for codes as indicated *1 Fetus 1; 2 Fetus 2; 3 Fetus 3; 4 Fetus 4; 5 Fetus 5*
652.93	UNSPEC MALPOSITION/MALPRESENTATION FETUS ANTPRTM	**O32.9XXØ**	Maternal care for malpresentation of fetus, unsp, unsp
		O32.9XX1	Maternal care for malpresentation of fetus, unsp, fetus 1
		O32.9XX2	Maternal care for malpresentation of fetus, unsp, fetus 2
		O32.9XX3	Maternal care for malpresentation of fetus, unsp, fetus 3
		O32.9XX4	Maternal care for malpresentation of fetus, unsp, fetus 4
		O32.9XX5	Maternal care for malpresentation of fetus, unsp, fetus 5
		O32.9XX9	Maternal care for malpresentation of fetus, unsp, oth fetus
653.ØØ	MAJ ABN BONY PELV NOT FURTHER SPEC PG UNS EOC	**O33.Ø**	Matern care for disproprtn d/t deformity of matern pelv bone
653.Ø1	MAJOR ABNORM BONY PELVIS NOT FURTHER SPEC DELIV	**O33.Ø**	Matern care for disproprtn d/t deformity of matern pelv bone
		O65.Ø	Obstructed labor due to deformed pelvis
653.Ø3	MAJOR ABNORM BONY PELV NOT FURTHER SPEC ANTPRTM	**O33.Ø**	Matern care for disproprtn d/t deformity of matern pelv bone
653.1Ø	GENLY CONTRACTED PELV PG UNSPEC AS EPIS CARE PG	**O33.1**	Matern care for disproprtn d/t generally contracted pelvis
653.11	GENERALLY CONTRACTED PELVIS PREGNANCY DELIVERED	**O33.1**	Matern care for disproprtn d/t generally contracted pelvis
		O65.1	Obstructed labor due to generally contracted pelvis
653.13	GENERALLY CONTRACTED PELVIS PREGNANCY ANTEPARTUM	**O33.1**	Matern care for disproprtn d/t generally contracted pelvis
653.2Ø	INLET CONTRACTION PELV PG UNSPEC AS EPIS CARE PG	**O33.2**	Maternal care for disproprtn due to inlet contrctn of pelvis
653.21	INLET CONTRACTION OF PELVIS PREGNANCY DELIVERED	**O33.2**	Maternal care for disproprtn due to inlet contrctn of pelvis
		O65.2	Obstructed labor due to pelvic inlet contraction
653.23	INLET CONTRACTION OF PELVIS PREGNANCY ANTEPARTUM	**O33.2**	Maternal care for disproprtn due to inlet contrctn of pelvis
653.3Ø	OUTLET CONTRAC PELV PG UNSPEC AS EPIS CARE PG	**O33.3XXØ**	Matern care for disproprtn d/t outlet contrctn of pelv, unsp
653.31	OUTLET CONTRACTION OF PELVIS PREGNANCY DELIVERED	**O33.3XXØ**	Matern care for disproprtn d/t outlet contrctn of pelv, unsp
		O33.3XX1	Matern care for disproprtn d/t outlet contrctn of pelv, fts1
		O33.3XX2	Matern care for disproprtn d/t outlet contrctn of pelv, fts2
		O33.3XX3	Matern care for disproprtn d/t outlet contrctn of pelv, fts3
		O33.3XX4	Matern care for disproprtn d/t outlet contrctn of pelv, fts4
		O33.3XX5	Matern care for disproprtn d/t outlet contrctn of pelv, fts5
		O33.3XX9	Matern care for disproprtn d/t outlet contrctn of pelv, oth
		O65.3	Obst labor due to pelvic outlet and mid-cavity contrctn
653.33	OUTLET CONTRACTION PELVIS PREGNANCY ANTEPARTUM	**O33.3XXØ**	Matern care for disproprtn d/t outlet contrctn of pelv, unsp
		O33.3XX1	Matern care for disproprtn d/t outlet contrctn of pelv, fts1
		O33.3XX2	Matern care for disproprtn d/t outlet contrctn of pelv, fts2
		O33.3XX3	Matern care for disproprtn d/t outlet contrctn of pelv, fts3
		O33.3XX4	Matern care for disproprtn d/t outlet contrctn of pelv, fts4
		O33.3XX5	Matern care for disproprtn d/t outlet contrctn of pelv, fts5
		O33.3XX9	Matern care for disproprtn d/t outlet contrctn of pelv, oth
653.4Ø	FETOPELVIC DISPROPORTION UNSPEC AS EPISODE CARE	**O33.4XXØ**	Matern care for disproprtn of mix matern & fetl origin, unsp

[Brackets] indicate valid character values for each code. Character value meanings provided for each code grouping.

ICD-9-CM		ICD-10-CM	
653.41	FETOPELVIC DISPROPORTION, DELIVERED	**O33.4XX0**	Matern care for disproprtn of mix matern & fetl origin, unsp
		O33.4XX1	Matern care for disproprtn of mix matern & fetl origin, fts1
		O33.4XX2	Matern care for disproprtn of mix matern & fetl origin, fts2
		O33.4XX3	Matern care for disproprtn of mix matern & fetl origin, fts3
		O33.4XX4	Matern care for disproprtn of mix matern & fetl origin, fts4
		O33.4XX5	Matern care for disproprtn of mix matern & fetl origin, fts5
		O33.4XX9	Matern care for disproprtn of mix matern & fetl origin, oth
		O65.4	Obstructed labor due to fetopelvic disproportion, unsp
653.43	FETOPELVIC DISPROPORTION ANTEPARTUM	**O33.4XX0**	Matern care for disproprtn of mix matern & fetl origin, unsp
		O33.4XX1	Matern care for disproprtn of mix matern & fetl origin, fts1
		O33.4XX2	Matern care for disproprtn of mix matern & fetl origin, fts2
		O33.4XX3	Matern care for disproprtn of mix matern & fetl origin, fts3
		O33.4XX4	Matern care for disproprtn of mix matern & fetl origin, fts4
		O33.4XX5	Matern care for disproprtn of mix matern & fetl origin, fts5
		O33.4XX9	Matern care for disproprtn of mix matern & fetl origin, oth
653.50	UNUSULLY LG FETUS CAUS DISPROPRTN UNS EPIS CARE	**O33.5XX0**	Matern care for disproprtn d/t unusually large fetus, unsp
653.51	UNUSUALLY LARGE FETUS CAUS DISPROPRTN DELIVERED	**O33.5XX0**	Matern care for disproprtn d/t unusually large fetus, unsp
		O33.5XX1	Matern care for disproprtn d/t unusually large fetus, fts1
		O33.5XX2	Matern care for disproprtn d/t unusually large fetus, fts2
		O33.5XX3	Matern care for disproprtn d/t unusually large fetus, fts3
		O33.5XX4	Matern care for disproprtn d/t unusually large fetus, fts4
		O33.5XX5	Matern care for disproprtn d/t unusually large fetus, fts5
		O33.5XX9	Matern care for disproprtn due to unusually large fetus, oth
		O66.2	Obstructed labor due to unusually large fetus
653.53	UNUSUALLY LARGE FETUS CAUSING DISPROPRTN ANTPRTM	**O33.5XX0**	Matern care for disproprtn d/t unusually large fetus, unsp
		O33.5XX1	Matern care for disproprtn d/t unusually large fetus, fts1
		O33.5XX2	Matern care for disproprtn d/t unusually large fetus, fts2
		O33.5XX3	Matern care for disproprtn d/t unusually large fetus, fts3
		O33.5XX4	Matern care for disproprtn d/t unusually large fetus, fts4
		O33.5XX5	Matern care for disproprtn d/t unusually large fetus, fts5
		O33.5XX9	Matern care for disproprtn due to unusually large fetus, oth
653.60	HYDROCEPHALIC FETUS CAUS DISPROPRTN UNS EOC	**O33.6XX0**	Matern care for disproprtn due to hydrocephalic fetus, unsp
653.61	HYDROCEPHALIC FETUS CAUSING DISPROPRTN DELIVERED	**O33.6XX0**	Matern care for disproprtn due to hydrocephalic fetus, unsp
		O33.6XX1	Matern care for disproprtn due to hydrocephalic fetus, fts1
		O33.6XX2	Matern care for disproprtn due to hydrocephalic fetus, fts2
		O33.6XX3	Matern care for disproprtn due to hydrocephalic fetus, fts3
		O33.6XX4	Matern care for disproprtn due to hydrocephalic fetus, fts4
		O33.6XX5	Matern care for disproprtn due to hydrocephalic fetus, fts5
		O33.6XX9	Maternal care for disproprtn due to hydrocephalic fetus, oth
653.63	HYDROCEPHALIC FETUS CAUSING DISPROPRTN ANTPRTM	**O33.6XX0**	Matern care for disproprtn due to hydrocephalic fetus, unsp
		O33.6XX1	Matern care for disproprtn due to hydrocephalic fetus, fts1
		O33.6XX2	Matern care for disproprtn due to hydrocephalic fetus, fts2
		O33.6XX3	Matern care for disproprtn due to hydrocephalic fetus, fts3
		O33.6XX4	Matern care for disproprtn due to hydrocephalic fetus, fts4
		O33.6XX5	Matern care for disproprtn due to hydrocephalic fetus, fts5
		O33.6XX9	Maternal care for disproprtn due to hydrocephalic fetus, oth
653.70	OTH FETAL ABNORM CAUS DISPROPRTN UNS EPIS CARE	**O33.7**	Maternal care for disproportion due to oth fetal deformities
653.71	OTH FETAL ABNORM CAUSING DISPROPRTN DELIVERED	**O33.7**	Maternal care for disproportion due to oth fetal deformities
653.73	OTH FETAL ABNORM CAUSING DISPROPRTN ANTEPARTUM	**O33.7**	Maternal care for disproportion due to oth fetal deformities
653.80	FETAL DISPROPRTN OTH ORIGIN UNSPEC AS EPIS CARE	**O33.8**	Maternal care for disproportion of other origin
653.81	FETAL DISPROPORTION OF OTHER ORIGIN DELIVERED	**O33.8**	Maternal care for disproportion of other origin
653.83	FETAL DISPROPORTION OF OTHER ORIGIN ANTEPARTUM	**O33.8**	Maternal care for disproportion of other origin
653.90	UNSPEC FETAL DISPROPRTN UNSPEC AS EPISODE CARE	**O33.9**	Maternal care for disproportion, unspecified
653.91	UNSPECIFIED FETAL DISPROPORTION DELIVERED	**O33.9**	Maternal care for disproportion, unspecified
653.93	UNSPECIFIED FETAL DISPROPORTION ANTEPARTUM	**O33.9**	Maternal care for disproportion, unspecified
654.00	CONGEN ABNORM PG UTERUS UNSPEC AS EPIS CARE	**O34.00**	Maternal care for unsp congen malform of uterus, unsp tri
654.01	CONGENITAL ABNORM PREGNANT UTERUS DELIVERED	**O34.01**	Maternal care for unsp congen malform of uterus, first tri
		O34.02	Maternal care for unsp congen malform of uterus, second tri
		O34.03	Maternal care for unsp congen malform of uterus, third tri
654.02	CONGEN ABNORM PG UTERUS DELIV W/MENTION PPC	**O34.01**	Maternal care for unsp congen malform of uterus, first tri
		O34.02	Maternal care for unsp congen malform of uterus, second tri
		O34.03	Maternal care for unsp congen malform of uterus, third tri
654.03	CONGENITAL ABNORM PREGNANT UTERUS ANTEPARTUM	**O34.01**	Maternal care for unsp congen malform of uterus, first tri
		O34.02	Maternal care for unsp congen malform of uterus, second tri
		O34.03	Maternal care for unsp congen malform of uterus, third tri
654.04	CONGENITAL ABNORMALITIES OF UTERUS PP COND/COMP	**O34.01**	Maternal care for unsp congen malform of uterus, first tri
		O34.02	Maternal care for unsp congen malform of uterus, second tri
		O34.03	Maternal care for unsp congen malform of uterus, third tri
654.10	TUMORS BODY PG UTERUS UNSPEC AS EPIS CARE PG	**O34.10**	Maternal care for benign tumor of corpus uteri, unsp tri
654.11	TUMORS OF BODY OF UTERUS, DELIVERED	**O34.11**	Maternal care for benign tumor of corpus uteri, first tri
		O34.12	Maternal care for benign tumor of corpus uteri, second tri
		O34.13	Maternal care for benign tumor of corpus uteri, third tri
654.12	TUMORS BODY UTERUS DELIVERED W/MENTION PPC	**O34.11**	Maternal care for benign tumor of corpus uteri, first tri
		O34.12	Maternal care for benign tumor of corpus uteri, second tri
		O34.13	Maternal care for benign tumor of corpus uteri, third tri

ICD-9-CM		ICD-10-CM	
654.13	TUMORS BODY UTERUS ANTEPARTUM COND/COMPLICATION	**O34.11**	Maternal care for benign tumor of corpus uteri, first tri
		O34.12	Maternal care for benign tumor of corpus uteri, second tri
		O34.13	Maternal care for benign tumor of corpus uteri, third tri
654.14	TUMORS BODY UTERUS POSTPARTUM COND/COMPLICATION	**O34.11**	Maternal care for benign tumor of corpus uteri, first tri
		O34.12	Maternal care for benign tumor of corpus uteri, second tri
		O34.13	Maternal care for benign tumor of corpus uteri, third tri
654.2Ø	PREV C/S DELIV UNSPEC AS EPIS CARE/NOT APPLIC	**O34.21**	Maternal care for scar from previous cesarean delivery
654.21	PREV C/S DELIV DELIV W/WO MENTION ANTPRTM COND	**O34.21**	Maternal care for scar from previous cesarean delivery
654.23	PREVIOUS C-SECT DELIVERY ANTPRTM COND/COMP	**O34.21**	Maternal care for scar from previous cesarean delivery
654.3Ø	RETROVRT&INCARCERAT GRAVID UTRUS UNS EPIS CARE	**O34.519**	Maternal care for incarceration of gravid uterus, unsp tri
		O34.539	Maternal care for retroversion of gravid uterus, unsp tri
654.31	RETROVERTED&INCARCERATED GRAVID UTERUS DELIVERED	**O34.511**	Maternal care for incarceration of gravid uterus, first tri
		O34.512	Maternal care for incarceration of gravid uterus, second tri
		O34.513	Maternal care for incarceration of gravid uterus, third tri
		O34.531	Maternal care for retroversion of gravid uterus, first tri
		O34.532	Maternal care for retroversion of gravid uterus, second tri
		O34.533	Maternal care for retroversion of gravid uterus, third tri
654.32	RETROVRT&INCARCERAT GRAVD UTRUS DELIV W/ PPC	**O34.511**	Maternal care for incarceration of gravid uterus, first tri
		O34.512	Maternal care for incarceration of gravid uterus, second tri
		O34.513	Maternal care for incarceration of gravid uterus, third tri
		O34.531	Maternal care for retroversion of gravid uterus, first tri
		O34.532	Maternal care for retroversion of gravid uterus, second tri
		O34.533	Maternal care for retroversion of gravid uterus, third tri
654.33	RETROVERTED&INCARCERATED GRAVID UTERUS ANTPRTM	**O34.511**	Maternal care for incarceration of gravid uterus, first tri
		O34.512	Maternal care for incarceration of gravid uterus, second tri
		O34.513	Maternal care for incarceration of gravid uterus, third tri
		O34.531	Maternal care for retroversion of gravid uterus, first tri
		O34.532	Maternal care for retroversion of gravid uterus, second tri
		O34.533	Maternal care for retroversion of gravid uterus, third tri
654.34	RETROVRT & INCARCERAT GRAVID UTERUS PP COND/COMP	**O34.511**	Maternal care for incarceration of gravid uterus, first tri
		O34.512	Maternal care for incarceration of gravid uterus, second tri
		O34.513	Maternal care for incarceration of gravid uterus, third tri
		O34.531	Maternal care for retroversion of gravid uterus, first tri
		O34.532	Maternal care for retroversion of gravid uterus, second tri
		O34.533	Maternal care for retroversion of gravid uterus, third tri
654.4Ø	OTH ABNORMAL SHAPE/POSITON GRAVID UTERUS-UNS EOC	**O34.529**	Maternal care for prolapse of gravid uterus, unsp trimester
		O34.599	Maternal care for oth abnlt of gravid uterus, unsp trimester
654.41	OTH ABN SHAPE/PSTN GRAVD UTRUS&NGHBR STRCT DELIV	**O34.521**	Maternal care for prolapse of gravid uterus, first trimester
		O34.522	Maternal care for prolapse of gravid uterus, second tri
		O34.523	Maternal care for prolapse of gravid uterus, third trimester
		O34.591	Maternal care for oth abnlt of gravid uterus, first tri
		O34.592	Maternal care for oth abnlt of gravid uterus, second tri
		O34.593	Maternal care for oth abnlt of gravid uterus, third tri
654.42	OTH ABN SHAPE/POS GRAVID UTERUS DEL W/PP COMPL	**O34.591**	Maternal care for oth abnlt of gravid uterus, first tri
		O34.592	Maternal care for oth abnlt of gravid uterus, second tri
		O34.593	Maternal care for oth abnlt of gravid uterus, third tri
654.43	OTH ABN SHAPE/POSITION GRAVID UTERUS ANTEPARTUM	**O34.521**	Maternal care for prolapse of gravid uterus, first trimester
		O34.522	Maternal care for prolapse of gravid uterus, second tri
		O34.523	Maternal care for prolapse of gravid uterus, third trimester
		O34.591	Maternal care for oth abnlt of gravid uterus, first tri
		O34.592	Maternal care for oth abnlt of gravid uterus, second tri
		O34.593	Maternal care for oth abnlt of gravid uterus, third tri
654.44	OTH ABN SHAP/PSTN GRAV UT NB STRCT PP COND/COMPL	**O34.591**	Maternal care for oth abnlt of gravid uterus, first tri
		O34.592	Maternal care for oth abnlt of gravid uterus, second tri
		O34.593	Maternal care for oth abnlt of gravid uterus, third tri
654.5Ø	CERV INCOMPETENCE UNSPEC AS EPIS CARE PREGNANCY	**O34.3Ø**	Maternal care for cervical incompetence, unsp trimester
654.51	CERVICAL INCOMPETENCE, DELIVERED	**O34.31**	Maternal care for cervical incompetence, first trimester
		O34.32	Maternal care for cervical incompetence, second trimester
		O34.33	Maternal care for cervical incompetence, third trimester
654.52	CERVICAL INCOMPETENCE DELIVERED W/MENTION PPC	**O34.31**	Maternal care for cervical incompetence, first trimester
		O34.32	Maternal care for cervical incompetence, second trimester
		O34.33	Maternal care for cervical incompetence, third trimester
654.53	CERVICAL INCOMPETENCE ANTPRTM COND/COMPLICATION	**O34.31**	Maternal care for cervical incompetence, first trimester
		O34.32	Maternal care for cervical incompetence, second trimester
		O34.33	Maternal care for cervical incompetence, third trimester
654.54	CERV INCOMPETENCE POSTPARTUM COND/COMPLICATION	**O34.31**	Maternal care for cervical incompetence, first trimester
		O34.32	Maternal care for cervical incompetence, second trimester
		O34.33	Maternal care for cervical incompetence, third trimester
654.6Ø	OTH CONGN/ACQ ABNORM CERV UNSPEC AS EPIS CARE PG	**O34.4Ø**	Maternal care for oth abnlt of cervix, unsp trimester
654.61	OTH CONGENITAL/ACQUIRED ABNORM CERVIX W/DELIVERY	**O34.41**	Maternal care for oth abnlt of cervix, first trimester
		O34.42	Maternal care for oth abnlt of cervix, second trimester
		O34.43	Maternal care for oth abnlt of cervix, third trimester
654.62	OTH CONGEN/ACQ ABNORM CERV DELIV W/MENTION PPC	**O34.41**	Maternal care for oth abnlt of cervix, first trimester
		O34.42	Maternal care for oth abnlt of cervix, second trimester
		O34.43	Maternal care for oth abnlt of cervix, third trimester

[Brackets] indicate valid character values for each code. Character value meanings provided for each code grouping.

ICD-9-CM		ICD-10-CM	
654.63	OTH CONGENITAL/ACQ ABNORM CERV ANTPRTM COND/COMP	**O34.41**	Maternal care for oth abnlt of cervix, first trimester
		O34.42	Maternal care for oth abnlt of cervix, second trimester
		O34.43	Maternal care for oth abnlt of cervix, third trimester
654.64	OTH CONGEN/ACQ ABNORM CERV POSTPARTUM COND/COMP	**O34.41**	Maternal care for oth abnlt of cervix, first trimester
		O34.42	Maternal care for oth abnlt of cervix, second trimester
		O34.43	Maternal care for oth abnlt of cervix, third trimester
654.7Ø	CONGEN/ACQ ABNORM VAGINA UNSPEC AS EPIS CARE PG	**O34.6Ø**	Maternal care for abnormality of vagina, unsp trimester
654.71	CONGENITAL/ACQUIRED ABNORM VAGINA W/DELIVERY	**O34.61**	Maternal care for abnormality of vagina, first trimester
		O34.62	Maternal care for abnormality of vagina, second trimester
		O34.63	Maternal care for abnormality of vagina, third trimester
654.72	CONGEN/ACQ ABNORM VAGINA DELIVERED W/MENTION PPC	**O34.61**	Maternal care for abnormality of vagina, first trimester
		O34.62	Maternal care for abnormality of vagina, second trimester
		O34.63	Maternal care for abnormality of vagina, third trimester
654.73	CONGENITAL/ACQ ABNORM VAGINA ANTPRTM COND/COMP	**O34.61**	Maternal care for abnormality of vagina, first trimester
		O34.62	Maternal care for abnormality of vagina, second trimester
		O34.63	Maternal care for abnormality of vagina, third trimester
654.74	CONGEN/ACQ ABNORM VAGINA POSTPARTUM COND/COMP	**O34.61**	Maternal care for abnormality of vagina, first trimester
		O34.62	Maternal care for abnormality of vagina, second trimester
		O34.63	Maternal care for abnormality of vagina, third trimester
654.8Ø	CONGEN/ACQ ABNORM VULVA UNSPEC AS EPIS CARE PG	**O34.7Ø**	Maternal care for abnlt of vulva and perineum, unsp tri
654.81	CONGENITAL/ACQUIRED ABNORMALITY VULVA W/DELIVERY	**O34.71**	Maternal care for abnlt of vulva and perineum, first tri
		O34.72	Maternal care for abnlt of vulva and perineum, second tri
		O34.73	Maternal care for abnlt of vulva and perineum, third tri
654.82	CONGEN/ACQ ABNORM VULVA DELIVERED W/MENTION PPC	**O34.71**	Maternal care for abnlt of vulva and perineum, first tri
		O34.72	Maternal care for abnlt of vulva and perineum, second tri
		O34.73	Maternal care for abnlt of vulva and perineum, third tri
654.83	CONGENITAL/ACQ ABNORM VULVA ANTPRTM COND/COMP	**O34.71**	Maternal care for abnlt of vulva and perineum, first tri
		O34.72	Maternal care for abnlt of vulva and perineum, second tri
		O34.73	Maternal care for abnlt of vulva and perineum, third tri
654.84	CONGENITAL/ACQ ABNORM VULVA POSTPARTUM COND/COMP	**O34.71**	Maternal care for abnlt of vulva and perineum, first tri
		O34.72	Maternal care for abnlt of vulva and perineum, second tri
		O34.73	Maternal care for abnlt of vulva and perineum, third tri
654.9Ø	OTH&UNS ABN ORGANS&SOFT TISS PELVIS UNS EOC PG	**O34.8Ø**	Maternal care for oth abnlt of pelvic organs, unsp trimester
		O34.9Ø	Maternal care for abnlt of pelvic organ, unsp, unsp tri
654.91	OTH&UNSPEC ABNORM ORGN&SOFT TISSUES PELV W/DELIV	**O34.29**	Maternal care due to uterine scar from oth previous surgery
		O34.81	Maternal care for oth abnlt of pelvic organs, first tri
		O34.82	Maternal care for oth abnlt of pelvic organs, second tri
		O34.83	Maternal care for oth abnlt of pelvic organs, third tri
		O34.91	Maternal care for abnlt of pelvic organ, unsp, first tri
		O34.92	Maternal care for abnlt of pelvic organ, unsp, second tri
		O34.93	Maternal care for abnlt of pelvic organ, unsp, third tri
		O65.8	Obstructed labor due to other maternal pelvic abnormalities
		O65.9	Obstructed labor due to maternal pelvic abnormality, unsp
654.92	OTH&UNS ABN ORGN&SOFT TISS PELVIS DEL W/PP COMPL	**O34.81**	Maternal care for oth abnlt of pelvic organs, first tri
		O34.82	Maternal care for oth abnlt of pelvic organs, second tri
		O34.83	Maternal care for oth abnlt of pelvic organs, third tri
		O34.91	Maternal care for abnlt of pelvic organ, unsp, first tri
		O34.92	Maternal care for abnlt of pelvic organ, unsp, second tri
		O34.93	Maternal care for abnlt of pelvic organ, unsp, third tri
654.93	OTH&UNS ABN ORGN&PELVIS ANTPRTM COND/COMPL	**O34.29**	Maternal care due to uterine scar from oth previous surgery
		O34.81	Maternal care for oth abnlt of pelvic organs, first tri
		O34.82	Maternal care for oth abnlt of pelvic organs, second tri
		O34.83	Maternal care for oth abnlt of pelvic organs, third tri
		O34.91	Maternal care for abnlt of pelvic organ, unsp, first tri
		O34.92	Maternal care for abnlt of pelvic organ, unsp, second tri
		O34.93	Maternal care for abnlt of pelvic organ, unsp, third tri
654.94	OTH&UNS ABN ORGAN&SOFT TISS PELVIS PP COND/COMPL	**O34.81**	Maternal care for oth abnlt of pelvic organs, first tri
		O34.82	Maternal care for oth abnlt of pelvic organs, second tri
		O34.83	Maternal care for oth abnlt of pelvic organs, third tri
		O34.91	Maternal care for abnlt of pelvic organ, unsp, first tri
		O34.92	Maternal care for abnlt of pelvic organ, unsp, second tri
		O34.93	Maternal care for abnlt of pelvic organ, unsp, third tri
655.ØØ	CNTRL NERV SYS MALFORM FETUS UNS AS EPIS CARE PG	**O35.ØXXØ**	Maternal care for (suspected) cnsl malform in fetus, unsp
655.Ø1	CNTRL NERV SYS MALFORMATION IN FETUS W/DELIVERY	**O35.ØXXØ**	Maternal care for (suspected) cnsl malform in fetus, unsp
		O35.ØXX1	Maternal care for (suspected) cnsl malform in fetus, fetus 1
		O35.ØXX2	Maternal care for (suspected) cnsl malform in fetus, fetus 2
		O35.ØXX3	Maternal care for (suspected) cnsl malform in fetus, fetus 3
		O35.ØXX4	Maternal care for (suspected) cnsl malform in fetus, fetus 4
		O35.ØXX5	Maternal care for (suspected) cnsl malform in fetus, fetus 5
		O35.ØXX9	Maternal care for (suspected) cnsl malform in fetus, oth
655.Ø3	CNTRL NERV SYS MALFORMATION IN FETUS ANTEPARTUM	**O35.ØXXØ**	Maternal care for (suspected) cnsl malform in fetus, unsp
		O35.ØXX1	Maternal care for (suspected) cnsl malform in fetus, fetus 1
		O35.ØXX2	Maternal care for (suspected) cnsl malform in fetus, fetus 2
		O35.ØXX3	Maternal care for (suspected) cnsl malform in fetus, fetus 3
		O35.ØXX4	Maternal care for (suspected) cnsl malform in fetus, fetus 4
		O35.ØXX5	Maternal care for (suspected) cnsl malform in fetus, fetus 5
		O35.ØXX9	Maternal care for (suspected) cnsl malform in fetus, oth
655.1Ø	CHROMOSM ABNORM FETUS MGMT MOTH UNS EPIS CARE PG	**O35.1XXØ**	Maternal care for chromosomal abnormality in fetus, unsp

ICD-9-CM		ICD-10-CM	
655.11	CHROMOSM ABNORM FETUS AFFECT MGMT MOTH W/DELIV	O35.1XXØ	Maternal care for chromosomal abnormality in fetus, unsp
		O35.1XX1	Maternal care for chromosomal abnormality in fetus, fetus 1
		O35.1XX2	Maternal care for chromosomal abnormality in fetus, fetus 2
		O35.1XX3	Maternal care for chromosomal abnormality in fetus, fetus 3
		O35.1XX4	Maternal care for chromosomal abnormality in fetus, fetus 4
		O35.1XX5	Maternal care for chromosomal abnormality in fetus, fetus 5
		O35.1XX9	Maternal care for chromosomal abnormality in fetus, oth
655.13	CHROMOSOM ABNORM FETUS AFFECT MGMT MOM ANTPRTM	O35.1XXØ	Maternal care for chromosomal abnormality in fetus, unsp
		O35.1XX1	Maternal care for chromosomal abnormality in fetus, fetus 1
		O35.1XX2	Maternal care for chromosomal abnormality in fetus, fetus 2
		O35.1XX3	Maternal care for chromosomal abnormality in fetus, fetus 3
		O35.1XX4	Maternal care for chromosomal abnormality in fetus, fetus 4
		O35.1XX5	Maternal care for chromosomal abnormality in fetus, fetus 5
		O35.1XX9	Maternal care for chromosomal abnormality in fetus, oth
655.2Ø	HEREDITARY DZ POSS AFFECT FETUS UNS EOC PG	O35.2XXØ	Maternal care for hereditary disease in fetus, unsp
655.21	HEREDITARY DZ POSS AFFECT FETUS MGMT MOM W/DEL	O35.2XXØ	Maternal care for hereditary disease in fetus, unsp
		O35.2XX1	Maternal care for hereditary disease in fetus, fetus 1
		O35.2XX2	Maternal care for hereditary disease in fetus, fetus 2
		O35.2XX3	Maternal care for hereditary disease in fetus, fetus 3
		O35.2XX4	Maternal care for hereditary disease in fetus, fetus 4
		O35.2XX5	Maternal care for hereditary disease in fetus, fetus 5
		O35.2XX9	Maternal care for hereditary disease in fetus, oth
655.23	HEREDITRY DZ POSS AFFCT FETUS ANTPRTM COND/COMPL	O35.2XXØ	Maternal care for hereditary disease in fetus, unsp
		O35.2XX1	Maternal care for hereditary disease in fetus, fetus 1
		O35.2XX2	Maternal care for hereditary disease in fetus, fetus 2
		O35.2XX3	Maternal care for hereditary disease in fetus, fetus 3
		O35.2XX4	Maternal care for hereditary disease in fetus, fetus 4
		O35.2XX5	Maternal care for hereditary disease in fetus, fetus 5
		O35.2XX9	Maternal care for hereditary disease in fetus, oth
655.3Ø	SUSPECTED DAMAGE FETUS MATERNL VIRUS-UNS EOC	O35.3XXØ	Matern care for damag to fts from viral dis in mother, unsp
655.31	SPCT DAMGE FETUS VIRL DZ MOM AFFCT MGMT MOM DEL	O35.3XXØ	Matern care for damag to fts from viral dis in mother, unsp
		O35.3XX1	Matern care for damag to fts from viral dis in mother, fts1
		O35.3XX2	Matern care for damag to fts from viral dis in mother, fts2
		O35.3XX3	Matern care for damag to fts from viral dis in mother, fts3
		O35.3XX4	Matern care for damag to fts from viral dis in mother, fts4
		O35.3XX5	Matern care for damag to fts from viral dis in mother, fts5
		O35.3XX9	Matern care for damag to fetus from viral dis in mother, oth
655.33	SPCT DAMGE FETUS VIRAL DZ MOM ANTPRTM COMPL	O35.3XXØ	Matern care for damag to fts from viral dis in mother, unsp
		O35.3XX1	Matern care for damag to fts from viral dis in mother, fts1
		O35.3XX2	Matern care for damag to fts from viral dis in mother, fts2
		O35.3XX3	Matern care for damag to fts from viral dis in mother, fts3
		O35.3XX4	Matern care for damag to fts from viral dis in mother, fts4
		O35.3XX5	Matern care for damag to fts from viral dis in mother, fts5
		O35.3XX9	Matern care for damag to fetus from viral dis in mother, oth
655.4Ø	SPCT DAMGE FETUS OTH DZ MOM UNS EOC PG	O35.4XXØ	Maternal care for damage to fetus from alcohol, unsp
655.41	SPCT DAMGE FETUS OTH DZ MOM AFFCT MGMT MOM DEL	O35.4XXØ	Maternal care for damage to fetus from alcohol, unsp
		O35.4XX1	Maternal care for damage to fetus from alcohol, fetus 1
		O35.4XX2	Maternal care for damage to fetus from alcohol, fetus 2
		O35.4XX3	Maternal care for damage to fetus from alcohol, fetus 3
		O35.4XX4	Maternal care for damage to fetus from alcohol, fetus 4
		O35.4XX5	Maternal care for damage to fetus from alcohol, fetus 5
		O35.4XX9	Maternal care for damage to fetus from alcohol, oth
655.43	SPCT DAMGE FETUS OTH DZ MOM ANTPRTM COND/COMPL	O35.4XXØ	Maternal care for damage to fetus from alcohol, unsp
		O35.4XX1	Maternal care for damage to fetus from alcohol, fetus 1
		O35.4XX2	Maternal care for damage to fetus from alcohol, fetus 2
		O35.4XX3	Maternal care for damage to fetus from alcohol, fetus 3
		O35.4XX4	Maternal care for damage to fetus from alcohol, fetus 4
		O35.4XX5	Maternal care for damage to fetus from alcohol, fetus 5
		O35.4XX9	Maternal care for damage to fetus from alcohol, oth
655.5Ø	SPCT DAMGE FETUS FROM RX MGMT MOTH UNS EPIS CARE	O35.5XXØ	Maternal care for (suspected) damage to fetus by drugs, unsp
655.51	SPCT DAMGE FETUS FROM RX AFFECT MGMT MOTH DELIV	O35.5XXØ	Maternal care for (suspected) damage to fetus by drugs, unsp
		O35.5XX1	Maternal care for damage to fetus by drugs, fetus 1
		O35.5XX2	Maternal care for damage to fetus by drugs, fetus 2
		O35.5XX3	Maternal care for damage to fetus by drugs, fetus 3
		O35.5XX4	Maternal care for damage to fetus by drugs, fetus 4
		O35.5XX5	Maternal care for damage to fetus by drugs, fetus 5
		O35.5XX9	Maternal care for (suspected) damage to fetus by drugs, oth
655.53	SPCT DAMGE FETUS FROM RX AFFCT MGMT MOTH ANTPRTM	O35.5XXØ	Maternal care for (suspected) damage to fetus by drugs, unsp
		O35.5XX1	Maternal care for damage to fetus by drugs, fetus 1
		O35.5XX2	Maternal care for damage to fetus by drugs, fetus 2
		O35.5XX3	Maternal care for damage to fetus by drugs, fetus 3
		O35.5XX4	Maternal care for damage to fetus by drugs, fetus 4
		O35.5XX5	Maternal care for damage to fetus by drugs, fetus 5
		O35.5XX9	Maternal care for (suspected) damage to fetus by drugs, oth
655.6Ø	SPCT DAMGE FETUS RAD MGMT MOTH UNS EPIS CARE	O35.6XXØ	Maternal care for damage to fetus by radiation, unsp

[Brackets] indicate valid character values for each code. Character value meanings provided for each code grouping.

ICD-9-CM		ICD-10-CM	
655.61	SPCT DAMGE FETUS FROM RAD AFFECT MGMT MOTH DELIV	**O35.6XXØ**	Maternal care for damage to fetus by radiation, unsp
		O35.6XX1	Maternal care for damage to fetus by radiation, fetus 1
		O35.6XX2	Maternal care for damage to fetus by radiation, fetus 2
		O35.6XX3	Maternal care for damage to fetus by radiation, fetus 3
		O35.6XX4	Maternal care for damage to fetus by radiation, fetus 4
		O35.6XX5	Maternal care for damage to fetus by radiation, fetus 5
		O35.6XX9	Maternal care for damage to fetus by radiation, oth
655.63	SPCT DAMGE FETUS RAD MGMT MOTH ANTPRTM COND/COMP	**O35.6XXØ**	Maternal care for damage to fetus by radiation, unsp
		O35.6XX1	Maternal care for damage to fetus by radiation, fetus 1
		O35.6XX2	Maternal care for damage to fetus by radiation, fetus 2
		O35.6XX3	Maternal care for damage to fetus by radiation, fetus 3
		O35.6XX4	Maternal care for damage to fetus by radiation, fetus 4
		O35.6XX5	Maternal care for damage to fetus by radiation, fetus 5
		O35.6XX9	Maternal care for damage to fetus by radiation, oth
655.7Ø	DECREASED FETAL MOVEMENTS UNSPEC AS EPISODE CARE	**O36.819Ø**	Decreased fetal movements, unsp trimester, unsp
655.71	DECR FETAL MOVEMENTS AFFECT MGMT MOTH DELIV	**O36.812Ø**	Decreased fetal movements, second trimester, unsp
		O36.812[1,2,3,4,5]	Decreased fetal movements, second trimester
		O36.8129	Decreased fetal movements, second trimester, other fetus
		O36.813Ø	Decreased fetal movements, third trimester, unsp
		O36.813[1,2,3,4,5]	Decreased fetal movements, third trimester
		O36.8139	Decreased fetal movements, third trimester, other fetus
			7th Character meanings for codes as indicated *1 Fetus 1; 2 Fetus 2; 3 Fetus 3; 4 Fetus 4; 5 Fetus 5*
655.73	DECR FETAL MOVMNTS MGMT MOTH ANTPRTM COND/COMP	**O36.812Ø**	Decreased fetal movements, second trimester, unsp
		O36.812[1,2,3,4,5]	Decreased fetal movements, second trimester
		O36.8129	Decreased fetal movements, second trimester, other fetus
		O36.813Ø	Decreased fetal movements, third trimester, unsp
		O36.813[1,2,3,4,5]	Decreased fetal movements, third trimester
		O36.8139	Decreased fetal movements, third trimester, other fetus
		O36.819Ø	Decreased fetal movements, unsp trimester, unsp
		O36.819[1,2,3,4,5]	Decreased fetal movements, unspecified trimester
		O36.8199	Decreased fetal movements, unsp trimester, other fetus
			7th Character meanings for codes as indicated *1 Fetus 1; 2 Fetus 2; 3 Fetus 3; 4 Fetus 4; 5 Fetus 5*
655.8Ø	OTH KNOWN/SPCT FETL ABN NEC MGMT MOTH UNS EOC	**O35.8XXØ**	Maternal care for oth fetal abnormality and damage, unsp
655.81	OTH KNOWN/SPCT FETAL ABNORM NEC MGMT MOTH DELIV	**O35.8XXØ**	Maternal care for oth fetal abnormality and damage, unsp
		O35.8XX1	Maternal care for oth fetal abnormality and damage, fetus 1
		O35.8XX2	Maternal care for oth fetal abnormality and damage, fetus 2
		O35.8XX3	Maternal care for oth fetal abnormality and damage, fetus 3
		O35.8XX4	Maternal care for oth fetal abnormality and damage, fetus 4
		O35.8XX5	Maternal care for oth fetal abnormality and damage, fetus 5
		O35.8XX9	Maternal care for oth fetal abnormality and damage, oth
655.83	OTH KNOWN/SUSPECTED FETAL ABNORMALITY-NEC-APC/C	**O35.8XXØ**	Maternal care for oth fetal abnormality and damage, unsp
		O35.8XX1	Maternal care for oth fetal abnormality and damage, fetus 1
		O35.8XX2	Maternal care for oth fetal abnormality and damage, fetus 2
		O35.8XX3	Maternal care for oth fetal abnormality and damage, fetus 3
		O35.8XX4	Maternal care for oth fetal abnormality and damage, fetus 4
		O35.8XX5	Maternal care for oth fetal abnormality and damage, fetus 5
		O35.8XX9	Maternal care for oth fetal abnormality and damage, oth
655.9Ø	UNS FETAL ABNORM MGMT MOTH UNS AS EPIS CARE	**O35.9XXØ**	Maternal care for fetal abnormality and damage, unsp, unsp
655.91	UNSPEC FETAL ABNORM AFFECT MANAGEMENT MOTH DELIV	**O35.9XXØ**	Maternal care for fetal abnormality and damage, unsp, unsp
		O35.9XX1	Maternal care for fetal abnlt and damage, unsp, fetus 1
		O35.9XX2	Maternal care for fetal abnlt and damage, unsp, fetus 2
		O35.9XX3	Maternal care for fetal abnlt and damage, unsp, fetus 3
		O35.9XX4	Maternal care for fetal abnlt and damage, unsp, fetus 4
		O35.9XX5	Maternal care for fetal abnlt and damage, unsp, fetus 5
		O35.9XX9	Maternal care for fetal abnormality and damage, unsp, oth
655.93	UNS FETAL ABNORM MGMT MOTH ANTPRTM COND/COMP	**O35.9XXØ**	Maternal care for fetal abnormality and damage, unsp, unsp
		O35.9XX1	Maternal care for fetal abnlt and damage, unsp, fetus 1
		O35.9XX2	Maternal care for fetal abnlt and damage, unsp, fetus 2
		O35.9XX3	Maternal care for fetal abnlt and damage, unsp, fetus 3
		O35.9XX4	Maternal care for fetal abnlt and damage, unsp, fetus 4
		O35.9XX5	Maternal care for fetal abnlt and damage, unsp, fetus 5
		O35.9XX9	Maternal care for fetal abnormality and damage, unsp, oth
656.ØØ	FETAL-MTRN HEMORR UNSPEC AS EPIS CARE PREGNANCY	**O43.Ø19**	Fetomaternal placental transfusion syndrome, unsp trimester
656.Ø1	FETAL-MATERNAL HEMORRHAGE WITH DELIVERY	**O43.Ø11**	Fetomaternal placental transfusion syndrome, first trimester
		O43.Ø12	Fetomaternal placental transfuse syndrome, second trimester
		O43.Ø13	Fetomaternal placental transfusion syndrome, third trimester
656.Ø3	FETAL-MATERNAL HEMORRHAGE ANTPRTM COND/COMP	**O43.Ø11**	Fetomaternal placental transfusion syndrome, first trimester
		O43.Ø12	Fetomaternal placental transfuse syndrome, second trimester
		O43.Ø13	Fetomaternal placental transfusion syndrome, third trimester

ICD-9-CM		ICD-10-CM	
656.10	RHESUS ISOIMMUNIZATION UNSPEC AS EPIS CARE PG	**O36.0190**	Maternal care for anti-D antibodies, unsp trimester, unsp
		O36.019[1,2,3,4,5]	Maternal care for anti-D antibodies, unsp trimester
		O36.0199	Maternal care for anti-D antibodies, unsp trimester, oth
		O36.0990	Maternal care for oth rhesus isoimmun, unsp trimester, unsp
		O36.099[1,2,3,4,5]	Maternal care for oth rhesus isoimmun, unsp tri
		O36.0999	Maternal care for oth rhesus isoimmun, unsp trimester, oth
			7th Character meanings for codes as indicated *1 Fetus 1* *2 Fetus 2* *3 Fetus 3* *4 Fetus 4* *5 Fetus 5*
656.11	RHESUS ISOIMMUNIZATION AFFECT MGMT MOTH DELIV	**O36.0110**	Maternal care for anti-D antibodies, first trimester, unsp
		O36.011[1,2,3,4,5]	Maternal care for anti-D antibodies, first tri
		O36.0119	Maternal care for anti-D antibodies, first trimester, oth
		O36.0120	Maternal care for anti-D antibodies, second trimester, unsp
		O36.012[1,2,3,4,5]	Maternal care for anti-D antibodies, second tri
		O36.0129	Maternal care for anti-D antibodies, second trimester, oth
		O36.0130	Maternal care for anti-D antibodies, third trimester, unsp
		O36.013[1,2,3,4,5]	Maternal care for anti-D antibodies, third tri
		O36.0139	Maternal care for anti-D antibodies, third trimester, oth
		O36.0910	Maternal care for oth rhesus isoimmun, first trimester, unsp
		O36.091[1,2,3,4,5]	Maternal care for oth rhesus isoimmun, first tri
		O36.0919	Maternal care for oth rhesus isoimmun, first trimester, oth
		O36.0920	Maternal care for oth rhesus isoimmun, second tri, unsp
		O36.092[1,2,3,4,5]	Maternal care for oth rhesus isoimmun, second tri
		O36.0929	Maternal care for oth rhesus isoimmun, second trimester, oth
		O36.0930	Maternal care for oth rhesus isoimmun, third trimester, unsp
		O36.093[1,2,3,4,5]	Maternal care for oth rhesus isoimmun, third tri
		O36.0939	Maternal care for oth rhesus isoimmun, third trimester, oth
			7th Character meanings for codes as indicated *1 Fetus 1* *2 Fetus 2* *3 Fetus 3* *4 Fetus 4* *5 Fetus 5*
656.13	RHESUS ISOIMMUN AFFCT MGMT MOTH ANTPRTM COND	**O36.0110**	Maternal care for anti-D antibodies, first trimester, unsp
		O36.011[1,2,3,4,5]	Maternal care for anti-D antibodies, first tri
		O36.0119	Maternal care for anti-D antibodies, first trimester, oth
		O36.0120	Maternal care for anti-D antibodies, second trimester, unsp
		O36.012[1,2,3,4,5]	Maternal care for anti-D antibodies, second tri
		O36.0129	Maternal care for anti-D antibodies, second trimester, oth
		O36.0130	Maternal care for anti-D antibodies, third trimester, unsp
		O36.013[1,2,3,4,5]	Maternal care for anti-D antibodies, third tri
		O36.0139	Maternal care for anti-D antibodies, third trimester, oth
		O36.0910	Maternal care for oth rhesus isoimmun, first trimester, unsp
		O36.091[1,2,3,4,5]	Maternal care for oth rhesus isoimmun, first tri
		O36.0919	Maternal care for oth rhesus isoimmun, first trimester, oth
		O36.0920	Maternal care for oth rhesus isoimmun, second tri, unsp
		O36.092[1,2,3,4,5]	Maternal care for oth rhesus isoimmun, second tri
		O36.0929	Maternal care for oth rhesus isoimmun, second trimester, oth
		O36.0930	Maternal care for oth rhesus isoimmun, third trimester, unsp
		O36.093[1,2,3,4,5]	Maternal care for oth rhesus isoimmun, third tri
		O36.0939	Maternal care for oth rhesus isoimmun, third trimester, oth
			7th Character meanings for codes as indicated *1 Fetus 1* *2 Fetus 2* *3 Fetus 3* *4 Fetus 4* *5 Fetus 5*
656.20	ISOIMMU UNS BLD-GRP INCOMPAT UNS EPIS CARE PG	**O36.1190**	Maternal care for Anti-A sensitization, unsp trimester, unsp
		O36.119[1,2,3,4,5]	Maternal care for Anti-A sensitization, unsp tri
		O36.1199	Maternal care for Anti-A sensitization, unsp trimester, oth
		O36.1990	Maternal care for oth isoimmunization, unsp trimester, unsp
		O36.199[1,2,3,4,5]	Maternal care for oth isoimmun, unsp trimester
		O36.1999	Maternal care for oth isoimmunization, unsp trimester, oth
			7th Character meanings for codes as indicated *1 Fetus 1* *2 Fetus 2* *3 Fetus 3* *4 Fetus 4* *5 Fetus 5*

[Brackets] indicate valid character values for each code. Character value meanings provided for each code grouping.

ICD-9-CM		ICD-10-CM	
656.21	ISOIMMU OTH&UNS BLD-GRP INCOMPAT MGMT MOTH DELIV	**O36.111Ø**	Maternal care for Anti-A sensitization, first tri, unsp
		O36.111[1,2,3,4,5]	Maternal care for Anti-A sensitization, first tri
		O36.1119	Maternal care for Anti-A sensitization, first trimester, oth
		O36.112Ø	Maternal care for Anti-A sensitization, second tri, unsp
		O36.112[1,2,3,4,5]	Maternal care for Anti-A sensitization, second tri
		O36.1129	Maternal care for Anti-A sensitization, second tri, oth
		O36.113Ø	Maternal care for Anti-A sensitization, third tri, unsp
		O36.113[1,2,3,4,5]	Maternal care for Anti-A sensitization, third tri
		O36.1139	Maternal care for Anti-A sensitization, third trimester, oth
		O36.191Ø	Maternal care for oth isoimmunization, first trimester, unsp
		O36.191[1,2,3,4,5]	Maternal care for oth isoimmun, first trimester
		O36.1919	Maternal care for oth isoimmunization, first trimester, oth
		O36.192Ø	Maternal care for oth isoimmun, second trimester, unsp
		O36.192[1,2,3,4,5]	Maternal care for oth isoimmun, second trimester
		O36.1929	Maternal care for oth isoimmunization, second trimester, oth
		O36.193Ø	Maternal care for oth isoimmunization, third trimester, unsp
		O36.193[1,2,3,4,5]	Maternal care for oth isoimmun, third trimester
		O36.1939	Maternal care for oth isoimmunization, third trimester, oth
			7th Character meanings for codes as indicated *1 Fetus 1; 2 Fetus 2; 3 Fetus 3; 4 Fetus 4; 5 Fetus 5*
656.23	ISOIMMU UNS BLD-GRP INCOMPAT MGMT MOTH ANTPRTM	**O36.111Ø**	Maternal care for Anti-A sensitization, first tri, unsp
		O36.111[1,2,3,4,5]	Maternal care for Anti-A sensitization, first tri
		O36.1119	Maternal care for Anti-A sensitization, first trimester, oth
		O36.112Ø	Maternal care for Anti-A sensitization, second tri, unsp
		O36.112[1,2,3,4,5]	Maternal care for Anti-A sensitization, second tri
		O36.1129	Maternal care for Anti-A sensitization, second tri, oth
		O36.113Ø	Maternal care for Anti-A sensitization, third tri, unsp
		O36.113[1,2,3,4,5]	Maternal care for Anti-A sensitization, third tri
		O36.1139	Maternal care for Anti-A sensitization, third trimester, oth
		O36.191Ø	Maternal care for oth isoimmunization, first trimester, unsp
		O36.191[1,2,3,4,5]	Maternal care for oth isoimmun, first trimester
		O36.1919	Maternal care for oth isoimmunization, first trimester, oth
		O36.192Ø	Maternal care for oth isoimmun, second trimester, unsp
		O36.192[1,2,3,4,5]	Maternal care for oth isoimmun, second trimester
		O36.1929	Maternal care for oth isoimmunization, second trimester, oth
		O36.193Ø	Maternal care for oth isoimmunization, third trimester, unsp
		O36.193[1,2,3,4,5]	Maternal care for oth isoimmun, third trimester
		O36.1939	Maternal care for oth isoimmunization, third trimester, oth
			7th Character meanings for codes as indicated *1 Fetus 1; 2 Fetus 2; 3 Fetus 3; 4 Fetus 4; 5 Fetus 5*
656.3Ø	FETAL DISTRESS AFFCT MGMT MOTH UNS AS EPIS CARE	**O68**	Labor and delivery comp by abnlt of fetal acid-base balance
656.31	FETAL DISTRESS AFFECT MANAGEMENT MOTH DELIVERED	**O68**	Labor and delivery comp by abnlt of fetal acid-base balance
656.33	FETAL DISTRESS AFFECT MANAGEMENT MOTH ANTEPARTUM	**O68**	Labor and delivery comp by abnlt of fetal acid-base balance
656.4Ø	INTRAUTERN DEATH MGMT MOTH UNS AS EPIS CARE	**O36.4XXØ**	Maternal care for intrauterine death, not applicable or unsp
656.41	INTRAUTERINE DEATH AFFECT MANAGEMENT MOTH DELIV	**O36.4XXØ**	Maternal care for intrauterine death, not applicable or unsp
		O36.4XX1	Maternal care for intrauterine death, fetus 1
		O36.4XX2	Maternal care for intrauterine death, fetus 2
		O36.4XX3	Maternal care for intrauterine death, fetus 3
		O36.4XX4	Maternal care for intrauterine death, fetus 4
		O36.4XX5	Maternal care for intrauterine death, fetus 5
		O36.4XX9	Maternal care for intrauterine death, other fetus
656.43	INTRAUTERINE DEATH AFFECT MGMT MOTH ANTPRTM	**O36.4XXØ**	Maternal care for intrauterine death, not applicable or unsp
		O36.4XX1	Maternal care for intrauterine death, fetus 1
		O36.4XX2	Maternal care for intrauterine death, fetus 2
		O36.4XX3	Maternal care for intrauterine death, fetus 3
		O36.4XX4	Maternal care for intrauterine death, fetus 4
		O36.4XX5	Maternal care for intrauterine death, fetus 5
		O36.4XX9	Maternal care for intrauterine death, other fetus
656.5Ø	POOR FETAL GROWTH MGMT MOTH UNS AS EPIS CARE	**O36.519Ø**	Matern care for known or susp placntl insuff, unsp tri, unsp
		O36.519[1,2,3,4,5]	Matern care for known or susp placntl insuff, unsp tri
		O36.5199	Matern care for known or susp placntl insuff, unsp tri, oth
		O36.599Ø	Matern care for oth or susp poor fetl grth, unsp tri, unsp
		O36.599[1,2,3,4,5]	Matern care for oth or susp poor fetl grth, unsp tri
		O36.5999	Matern care for oth or susp poor fetl grth, unsp tri, oth
			7th Character meanings for codes as indicated *1 Fetus 1; 2 Fetus 2; 3 Fetus 3; 4 Fetus 4; 5 Fetus 5*

ICD-9-CM		ICD-10-CM	
656.51	POOR FETAL GROWTH AFFECT MANAGEMENT MOTH DELIV	**O36.5110**	Matern care for known or susp placntl insuff, 1st tri, unsp
		O36.511[1,2,3,4,5]	Matern care for known or susp placntl insuff, 1st tri
		O36.5119	Matern care for known or susp placntl insuff, first tri, oth
		O36.5120	Matern care for known or susp placntl insuff, 2nd tri, unsp
		O36.512[1,2,3,4,5]	Matern care for known or susp placntl insuff, 2nd tri
		O36.5129	Matern care for known or susp placntl insuff, 2nd tri, oth
		O36.5130	Matern care for or susp placntl insuff, third tri, unsp
		O36.513[1,2,3,4,5]	Matern care for or susp placntl insuff, third tri
		O36.5139	Matern care for known or susp placntl insuff, third tri, oth
		O36.5910	Matern care for oth or susp poor fetl grth, 1st tri, unsp
		O36.591[1,2,3,4,5]	Matern care for oth or susp poor fetl grth, 1st tri
		O36.5919	Matern care for oth or susp poor fetl grth, 1st tri, oth
		O36.5920	Matern care for oth or susp poor fetl grth, 2nd tri, unsp
		O36.592[1,2,3,4,5]	Matern care for oth or susp poor fetl grth, 2nd tri
		O36.5929	Matern care for oth or susp poor fetl grth, 2nd tri, oth
		O36.5930	Matern care for oth or susp poor fetl grth, third tri, unsp
		O36.593[1,2,3,4,5]	Matern care for oth or susp poor fetl grth, third tri
		O36.5939	Matern care for oth or susp poor fetl grth, third tri, oth
			7th Character meanings for codes as indicated ***1 Fetus 1*** ***2 Fetus 2*** ***3 Fetus 3*** ***4 Fetus 4*** ***5 Fetus 5***
656.53	POOR FETAL GROWTH MGMT MOTH ANTPRTM COND/COMP	**O36.5110**	Matern care for known or susp placntl insuff, 1st tri, unsp
		O36.511[1,2,3,4,5]	Matern care for known or susp placntl insuff, 1st tri
		O36.5119	Matern care for known or susp placntl insuff, first tri, oth
		O36.5120	Matern care for known or susp placntl insuff, 2nd tri, unsp
		O36.512[1,2,3,4,5]	Matern care for known or susp placntl insuff, 2nd tri
		O36.5129	Matern care for known or susp placntl insuff, 2nd tri, oth
		O36.5130	Matern care for or susp placntl insuff, third tri, unsp
		O36.513[1,2,3,4,5]	Matern care for or susp placntl insuff, third tri
		O36.5139	Matern care for known or susp placntl insuff, third tri, oth
		O36.5910	Matern care for oth or susp poor fetl grth, 1st tri, unsp
		O36.591[1,2,3,4,5]	Matern care for oth or susp poor fetl grth, 1st tri
		O36.5919	Matern care for oth or susp poor fetl grth, 1st tri, oth
		O36.5920	Matern care for oth or susp poor fetl grth, 2nd tri, unsp
		O36.592[1,2,3,4,5]	Matern care for oth or susp poor fetl grth, 2nd tri
		O36.5929	Matern care for oth or susp poor fetl grth, 2nd tri, oth
		O36.5930	Matern care for oth or susp poor fetl grth, third tri, unsp
		O36.593[1,2,3,4,5]	Matern care for oth or susp poor fetl grth, third tri
		O36.5939	Matern care for oth or susp poor fetl grth, third tri, oth
			7th Character meanings for codes as indicated ***1 Fetus 1*** ***2 Fetus 2*** ***3 Fetus 3*** ***4 Fetus 4*** ***5 Fetus 5***
656.60	XCESS FETAL GROWTH MGMT MOTH UNS AS EPIS CARE	**O36.60X0**	Maternal care for excess fetal growth, unsp trimester, unsp
		O36.60X1	Maternal care for excess fetal growth, unsp tri, fetus 1
		O36.60X2	Maternal care for excess fetal growth, unsp tri, fetus 2
		O36.60X3	Maternal care for excess fetal growth, unsp tri, fetus 3
		O36.60X4	Maternal care for excess fetal growth, unsp tri, fetus 4
		O36.60X5	Maternal care for excess fetal growth, unsp tri, fetus 5
		O36.60X9	Maternal care for excess fetal growth, unsp trimester, oth
656.61	EXCESS FETAL GROWTH AFFECT MANAGEMENT MOTH DELIV	**O36.61X0**	Maternal care for excess fetal growth, first trimester, unsp
		O36.61X[1,2,3,4,5]	Maternal care for excess fetal growth, first tri
		O36.61X9	Maternal care for excess fetal growth, first trimester, oth
		O36.62X0	Maternal care for excess fetal growth, second tri, unsp
		O36.62X[1,2,3,4,5]	Maternal care for excess fetal growth, second tri
		O36.62X9	Maternal care for excess fetal growth, second trimester, oth
		O36.63X0	Maternal care for excess fetal growth, third trimester, unsp
		O36.63X[1,2,3,4,5]	Maternal care for excess fetal growth, third tri
		O36.63X9	Maternal care for excess fetal growth, third trimester, oth
			7th Character meanings for codes as indicated ***1 Fetus 1*** ***2 Fetus 2*** ***3 Fetus 3*** ***4 Fetus 4*** ***5 Fetus 5***
656.63	EXCESS FETAL GROWTH AFFECT MGMT MOTH ANTPRTM	**O36.61X0**	Maternal care for excess fetal growth, first trimester, unsp
		O36.61X[1,2,3,4,5]	Maternal care for excess fetal growth, first tri
		O36.61X9	Maternal care for excess fetal growth, first trimester, oth
		O36.62X0	Maternal care for excess fetal growth, second tri, unsp
		O36.62X[1,2,3,4,5]	Maternal care for excess fetal growth, second tri
		O36.62X9	Maternal care for excess fetal growth, second trimester, oth
		O36.63X0	Maternal care for excess fetal growth, third trimester, unsp
		O36.63X[1,2,3,4,5]	Maternal care for excess fetal growth, third tri
		O36.63X9	Maternal care for excess fetal growth, third trimester, oth
			7th Character meanings for codes as indicated ***1 Fetus 1*** ***2 Fetus 2*** ***3 Fetus 3*** ***4 Fetus 4*** ***5 Fetus 5***

[Brackets] indicate valid character values for each code. Character value meanings provided for each code grouping.

ICD-9-CM		ICD-10-CM	
656.70	OTH PLACNTL CONDS MGMT MOTH UNS AS EPIS CARE	**O43.029**	Fetus-to-fetus placental transfuse syndrome, unsp trimester
		O43.109	Malformation of placenta, unspecified, unspecified trimester
		O43.119	Circumvallate placenta, unspecified trimester
		O43.199	Other malformation of placenta, unspecified trimester
		O43.819	Placental infarction, unspecified trimester
		O43.90	Unspecified placental disorder, unspecified trimester
656.71	OTH PLACENTAL CONDS AFFECT MANAGEMENT MOTH DELIV	**O43.021**	Fetus-to-fetus placental transfuse syndrome, first trimester
		O43.022	Fetus-to-fetus placntl transfuse syndrome, second trimester
		O43.023	Fetus-to-fetus placental transfuse syndrome, third trimester
		O43.101	Malformation of placenta, unspecified, first trimester
		O43.102	Malformation of placenta, unspecified, second trimester
		O43.103	Malformation of placenta, unspecified, third trimester
		O43.111	Circumvallate placenta, first trimester
		O43.112	Circumvallate placenta, second trimester
		O43.113	Circumvallate placenta, third trimester
		O43.191	Other malformation of placenta, first trimester
		O43.192	Other malformation of placenta, second trimester
		O43.193	Other malformation of placenta, third trimester
		O43.811	Placental infarction, first trimester
		O43.812	Placental infarction, second trimester
		O43.813	Placental infarction, third trimester
		O43.91	Unspecified placental disorder, first trimester
		O43.92	Unspecified placental disorder, second trimester
		O43.93	Unspecified placental disorder, third trimester
656.73	OTH PLACENTAL CONDS AFFECT MGMT MOTH ANTPRTM	**O43.021**	Fetus-to-fetus placental transfuse syndrome, first trimester
		O43.022	Fetus-to-fetus placntl transfuse syndrome, second trimester
		O43.023	Fetus-to-fetus placental transfuse syndrome, third trimester
		O43.101	Malformation of placenta, unspecified, first trimester
		O43.102	Malformation of placenta, unspecified, second trimester
		O43.103	Malformation of placenta, unspecified, third trimester
		O43.111	Circumvallate placenta, first trimester
		O43.112	Circumvallate placenta, second trimester
		O43.113	Circumvallate placenta, third trimester
		O43.191	Other malformation of placenta, first trimester
		O43.192	Other malformation of placenta, second trimester
		O43.193	Other malformation of placenta, third trimester
		O43.811	Placental infarction, first trimester
		O43.812	Placental infarction, second trimester
		O43.813	Placental infarction, third trimester
		O43.91	Unspecified placental disorder, first trimester
		O43.92	Unspecified placental disorder, second trimester
		O43.93	Unspecified placental disorder, third trimester
656.80	OTH SPEC FETL&PLACNTL PROBS MGMT MOTH UNS EOC	**O36.20X0**	Maternal care for hydrops fetalis, unsp trimester, unsp
		O36.20X[1,2,3,4,5]	Maternal care for hydrops fetalis, unsp trimester
		O36.20X9	Maternal care for hydrops fetalis, unsp trimester, oth fetus
		O36.70X0	Maternal care for viable fetus in abd preg, unsp tri, unsp
		O36.70X[1,2,3,4,5]	Matern care for viable fetus in abd preg, unsp tri
		O36.70X9	Maternal care for viable fetus in abd preg, unsp tri, oth
		O36.8990	Maternal care for oth fetal problems, unsp trimester, unsp
		O36.899[1,2,3,4,5]	Maternal care for oth fetal problems, unsp tri
		O36.8999	Maternal care for oth fetal problems, unsp trimester, oth
		O43.899	Other placental disorders, unspecified trimester
		O68	Labor and delivery comp by abnlt of fetal acid-base balance
		O77.0	Labor and delivery complicated by meconium in amniotic fluid

7th Character meanings for codes as indicated

1 Fetus 1 *2 Fetus 2* *3 Fetus 3* *4 Fetus 4* *5 Fetus 5*

ICD-9-CM		ICD-10-CM	
656.81	OTH SPEC FETAL&PLACNTL PROBS MGMT MOTH DELIV	**O36.21XØ**	Maternal care for hydrops fetalis, first trimester, unsp
		O36.21X[1,2,3,4,5]	Maternal care for hydrops fetalis, first trimester
		O36.21X9	Maternal care for hydrops fetalis, first trimester, oth
		O36.22XØ	Maternal care for hydrops fetalis, second trimester, unsp
		O36.22X[1,2,3,4,5]	Maternal care for hydrops fetalis, second trimester
		O36.22X9	Maternal care for hydrops fetalis, second trimester, oth
		O36.23XØ	Maternal care for hydrops fetalis, third trimester, unsp
		O36.23X[1,2,3,4,5]	Maternal care for hydrops fetalis, third trimester
		O36.23X9	Maternal care for hydrops fetalis, third trimester, oth
		O36.71XØ	Maternal care for viable fetus in abd preg, first tri, unsp
		O36.71X[1,2,3,4,5]	Matern care for viable fetus in abd preg, first tri
		O36.71X9	Maternal care for viable fetus in abd preg, first tri, oth
		O36.72XØ	Maternal care for viable fetus in abd preg, second tri, unsp
		O36.72X[1,2,3,4,5]	Matern care for viable fetus in abd preg, second tri, fts1
		O36.72X9	Maternal care for viable fetus in abd preg, second tri, oth
		O36.73XØ	Maternal care for viable fetus in abd preg, third tri, unsp
		O36.73X[1,2,3,4,5]	Matern care for viable fetus in abd preg, third tri
		O36.73X9	Maternal care for viable fetus in abd preg, third tri, oth
		O36.891Ø	Maternal care for oth fetal problems, first trimester, unsp
		O36.891[1,2,3,4,5]	Maternal care for oth fetal problems, first tri
		O36.8919	Maternal care for oth fetal problems, first trimester, oth
		O36.892Ø	Maternal care for oth fetal problems, second trimester, unsp
		O36.892[1,2,3,4,5]	Maternal care for oth fetal problems, second tri
		O36.8929	Maternal care for oth fetal problems, second trimester, oth
		O36.893Ø	Maternal care for oth fetal problems, third trimester, unsp
		O36.893[1,2,3,4,5]	Maternal care for oth fetal problems, third tri
		O36.8939	Maternal care for oth fetal problems, third trimester, oth
		O43.891	Other placental disorders, first trimester
		O43.892	Other placental disorders, second trimester
		O43.893	Other placental disorders, third trimester
		O68	Labor and delivery comp by abnlt of fetal acid-base balance
		O77.Ø	Labor and delivery complicated by meconium in amniotic fluid
		O77.1	Fetal stress in labor or delivery due to drug administration
		O77.8	Labor and delivery comp by oth evidence of fetal stress
		O77.9	Labor and delivery complicated by fetal stress, unspecified
			7th Character meanings for codes as indicated ***1 Fetus 1*** ***2 Fetus 2*** ***3 Fetus 3*** ***4 Fetus 4*** ***5 Fetus 5***
656.83	OTH SPEC FETAL&PLACNTL PROBS MGMT MOTH ANTPRTM	**O36.21XØ**	Maternal care for hydrops fetalis, first trimester, unsp
		O36.21X[1,2,3,4,5]	Maternal care for hydrops fetalis, first trimester
		O36.21X9	Maternal care for hydrops fetalis, first trimester, oth
		O36.22XØ	Maternal care for hydrops fetalis, second trimester, unsp
		O36.22X[1,2,3,4,5]	Maternal care for hydrops fetalis, second trimester
		O36.22X9	Maternal care for hydrops fetalis, second trimester, oth
		O36.23XØ	Maternal care for hydrops fetalis, third trimester, unsp
		O36.23X[1,2,3,4,5]	Maternal care for hydrops fetalis, third trimester
		O36.23X9	Maternal care for hydrops fetalis, third trimester, oth
		O36.71XØ	Maternal care for viable fetus in abd preg, first tri, unsp
		O36.71X[1,2,3,4,5]	Matern care for viable fetus in abd preg, first tri
		O36.71X9	Maternal care for viable fetus in abd preg, first tri, oth
		O36.72XØ	Maternal care for viable fetus in abd preg, second tri, unsp
		O36.72X[1,2,3,4,5]	Matern care for viable fetus in abd preg, second tri, fts1
		O36.72X9	Maternal care for viable fetus in abd preg, second tri, oth
		O36.73XØ	Maternal care for viable fetus in abd preg, third tri, unsp
		O36.73X[1,2,3,4,5]	Matern care for viable fetus in abd preg, third tri
		O36.73X9	Maternal care for viable fetus in abd preg, third tri, oth
		O36.891Ø	Maternal care for oth fetal problems, first trimester, unsp
		O36.891[1,2,3,4,5]	Maternal care for oth fetal problems, first tri
		O36.8919	Maternal care for oth fetal problems, first trimester, oth
		O36.892Ø	Maternal care for oth fetal problems, second trimester, unsp
		O36.892[1,2,3,4,5]	Maternal care for oth fetal problems, second tri
		O36.8929	Maternal care for oth fetal problems, second trimester, oth
		O36.893Ø	Maternal care for oth fetal problems, third trimester, unsp
		O36.893[1,2,3,4,5]	Maternal care for oth fetal problems, third tri
		O36.8939	Maternal care for oth fetal problems, third trimester, oth
		O43.891	Other placental disorders, first trimester
		O43.892	Other placental disorders, second trimester
		O43.893	Other placental disorders, third trimester
		O68	Labor and delivery comp by abnlt of fetal acid-base balance
			7th Character meanings for codes as indicated ***1 Fetus 1*** ***2 Fetus 2*** ***3 Fetus 3*** ***4 Fetus 4*** ***5 Fetus 5***
656.9Ø	UNS FETAL&PLACNTL PROB MGMT MOTH UNS EPIS CARE	**O36.9ØXØ**	Maternal care for fetal problem, unsp, unsp trimester, unsp
		O36.9ØX1	Maternal care for fetal problem, unsp, unsp tri, fetus 1
		O36.9ØX2	Maternal care for fetal problem, unsp, unsp tri, fetus 2
		O36.9ØX3	Maternal care for fetal problem, unsp, unsp tri, fetus 3
		O36.9ØX4	Maternal care for fetal problem, unsp, unsp tri, fetus 4
		O36.9ØX5	Maternal care for fetal problem, unsp, unsp tri, fetus 5
		O36.9ØX9	Maternal care for fetal problem, unsp, unsp trimester, oth

 [Brackets] indicate valid character values for each code. Character value meanings provided for each code grouping.

ICD-9-CM		ICD-10-CM	
656.91	UNSPEC FETAL&PLACNTL PROB AFFECT MGMT MOTH DELIV	**O36.91X0**	Maternal care for fetal problem, unsp, first trimester, unsp
		O36.91X[1,2,3,4,5]	Maternal care for fetal problem, unsp, first tri
		O36.91X9	Maternal care for fetal problem, unsp, first trimester, oth
		O36.92X0	Maternal care for fetal problem, unsp, second tri, unsp
		O36.92X[1,2,3,4,5]	Maternal care for fetal problem, unsp, second tri
		O36.92X9	Maternal care for fetal problem, unsp, second trimester, oth
		O36.93X0	Maternal care for fetal problem, unsp, third trimester, unsp
		O36.93X[1,2,3,4,5]	Maternal care for fetal problem, unsp, third tri
		O36.93X9	Maternal care for fetal problem, unsp, third trimester, oth
			7th Character meanings for codes as indicated 1 Fetus 1; 2 Fetus 2; 3 Fetus 3; 4 Fetus 4; 5 Fetus 5
656.93	UNS FETAL&PLACNTL PROB AFFCT MGMT MOTH ANTPRTM	**O36.91X0**	Maternal care for fetal problem, unsp, first trimester, unsp
		O36.91X[1,2,3,4,5]	Maternal care for fetal problem, unsp, first tri
		O36.91X9	Maternal care for fetal problem, unsp, first trimester, oth
		O36.92X0	Maternal care for fetal problem, unsp, second tri, unsp
		O36.92X[1,2,3,4,5]	Maternal care for fetal problem, unsp, second tri
		O36.92X9	Maternal care for fetal problem, unsp, second trimester, oth
		O36.93X0	Maternal care for fetal problem, unsp, third trimester, unsp
		O36.93X[1,2,3,4,5]	Maternal care for fetal problem, unsp, third tri
		O36.93X9	Maternal care for fetal problem, unsp, third trimester, oth
			7th Character meanings for codes as indicated 1 Fetus 1; 2 Fetus 2; 3 Fetus 3; 4 Fetus 4; 5 Fetus 5
657.00	POLYHYDRAMNIOS UNSPECIFIED AS TO EPISODE OF CARE	**O40.9XX0**	Polyhydramnios, unsp trimester, not applicable or unsp
		O40.9XX1	Polyhydramnios, unspecified trimester, fetus 1
		O40.9XX2	Polyhydramnios, unspecified trimester, fetus 2
		O40.9XX3	Polyhydramnios, unspecified trimester, fetus 3
		O40.9XX4	Polyhydramnios, unspecified trimester, fetus 4
		O40.9XX5	Polyhydramnios, unspecified trimester, fetus 5
		O40.9XX9	Polyhydramnios, unspecified trimester, other fetus
657.01	POLYHYDRAMNIOS, WITH DELIVERY	**O40.1XX0**	Polyhydramnios, first trimester, not applicable or unsp
		O40.1XX[1,2,3,4,5]	Polyhydramnios, first trimester
		O40.1XX9	Polyhydramnios, first trimester, other fetus
		O40.2XX0	Polyhydramnios, second trimester, not applicable or unsp
		O40.2XX[1,2,3,4,5]	Polyhydramnios, second trimester
		O40.2XX9	Polyhydramnios, second trimester, other fetus
		O40.3XX0	Polyhydramnios, third trimester, not applicable or unsp
		O40.3XX[1,2,3,4,5]	Polyhydramnios, third trimester
		O40.3XX9	Polyhydramnios, third trimester, other fetus
			7th Character meanings for codes as indicated 1 Fetus 1; 2 Fetus 2; 3 Fetus 3; 4 Fetus 4; 5 Fetus 5
657.03	POLYHYDRAMNIOS ANTEPARTUM COMPLICATION	**O40.1XX0**	Polyhydramnios, first trimester, not applicable or unsp
		O40.1XX[1,2,3,4,5]	Polyhydramnios, first trimester
		O40.1XX9	Polyhydramnios, first trimester, other fetus
		O40.2XX0	Polyhydramnios, second trimester, not applicable or unsp
		O40.2XX[1,2,3,4,5]	Polyhydramnios, second trimester
		O40.2XX9	Polyhydramnios, second trimester, other fetus
		O40.3XX0	Polyhydramnios, third trimester, not applicable or unsp
		O40.3XX[1,2,3,4,5]	Polyhydramnios, third trimester
		O40.3XX9	Polyhydramnios, third trimester, other fetus
			7th Character meanings for codes as indicated 1 Fetus 1; 2 Fetus 2; 3 Fetus 3; 4 Fetus 4; 5 Fetus 5
658.00	OLIGOHYDRAMNIOS UNSPECIFIED AS TO EPISODE CARE	**O41.00X0**	Oligohydramnios, unsp trimester, not applicable or unsp
		O41.00X1	Oligohydramnios, unspecified trimester, fetus 1
		O41.00X2	Oligohydramnios, unspecified trimester, fetus 2
		O41.00X3	Oligohydramnios, unspecified trimester, fetus 3
		O41.00X4	Oligohydramnios, unspecified trimester, fetus 4
		O41.00X5	Oligohydramnios, unspecified trimester, fetus 5
		O41.00X9	Oligohydramnios, unspecified trimester, other fetus
658.01	OLIGOHYDRAMNIOS, DELIVERED	**O41.01X0**	Oligohydramnios, first trimester, not applicable or unsp
		O41.01X[1,2,3,4,5]	Oligohydramnios, first trimester
		O41.01X9	Oligohydramnios, first trimester, other fetus
		O41.02X0	Oligohydramnios, second trimester, not applicable or unsp
		O41.02X[1,2,3,4,5]	Oligohydramnios, second trimester
		O41.02X9	Oligohydramnios, second trimester, other fetus
		O41.03X0	Oligohydramnios, third trimester, not applicable or unsp
		O41.03X[1,2,3,4,5]	Oligohydramnios, third trimester
		O41.03X9	Oligohydramnios, third trimester, other fetus
			7th Character meanings for codes as indicated 1 Fetus 1; 2 Fetus 2; 3 Fetus 3; 4 Fetus 4; 5 Fetus 5

ICD-9-CM		ICD-10-CM	
658.Ø3	OLIGOHYDRAMNIOS, ANTEPARTUM	**O41.Ø1XØ**	Oligohydramnios, first trimester, not applicable or unsp
		O41.Ø1X[1,2,3,4,5]	Oligohydramnios, first trimester
		O41.Ø1X9	Oligohydramnios, first trimester, other fetus
		O41.Ø2XØ	Oligohydramnios, second trimester, not applicable or unsp
		O41.Ø2X[1,2,3,4,5]	Oligohydramnios, second trimester
		O41.Ø2X9	Oligohydramnios, second trimester, other fetus
		O41.Ø3XØ	Oligohydramnios, third trimester, not applicable or unsp
		O41.Ø3X[1,2,3,4,5]	Oligohydramnios, third trimester
		O41.Ø3X9	Oligohydramnios, third trimester, other fetus
			7th Character meanings for codes as indicated ***1 Fetus 1 3 Fetus 3 5 Fetus 5*** ***2 Fetus 2 4 Fetus 4***
658.1Ø	PREMATURE RUPTURE MEMB PG UNSPEC AS EPIS CARE	**O42.ØØ**	Prem ROM, onset labor w/n 24 hr of rupt, unsp weeks of gest
		O42.Ø19	Pretrm prem ROM, onset labor w/n 24 hours of rupt, unsp tri
		O42.9Ø	Prem ROM, 7thØ betw rupt & onst labr, unsp weeks of gest
		O42.919	Pretrm prem ROM, unsp time betw rupt and onst labr, unsp tri
658.11	PREMATURE RUPTURE MEMBRANES PREGNANCY DELIVERED	**O42.ØØ**	Prem ROM, onset labor w/n 24 hr of rupt, unsp weeks of gest
		O42.Ø11	Pretrm prem ROM, onset labor w/n 24 hours of rupt, first tri
		O42.Ø12	Pretrm prem ROM, onset labor w/n 24 hours of rupt, 2nd tri
		O42.Ø13	Pretrm prem ROM, onset labor w/n 24 hours of rupt, third tri
		O42.Ø2	Full-term prem ROM, onset labor within 24 hours of rupture
		O42.911	Pretrm prem ROM, unsp time betw rupt and onset labr, 1st tri
		O42.912	Pretrm prem ROM, unsp time betw rupt and onset labr, 2nd tri
		O42.913	Pretrm prem ROM, unsp time betw rupt and onst labr, 3rd tri
		O42.92	Full-term prem ROM, unsp time betw rupture and onset labor
658.13	PREMATURE RUPTURE MEMBRANES PREGNANCY ANTEPARTUM	**O42.Ø11**	Pretrm prem ROM, onset labor w/n 24 hours of rupt, first tri
		O42.Ø12	Pretrm prem ROM, onset labor w/n 24 hours of rupt, 2nd tri
		O42.Ø13	Pretrm prem ROM, onset labor w/n 24 hours of rupt, third tri
		O42.911	Pretrm prem ROM, unsp time betw rupt and onset labr, 1st tri
		O42.912	Pretrm prem ROM, unsp time betw rupt and onset labr, 2nd tri
		O42.913	Pretrm prem ROM, unsp time betw rupt and onst labr, 3rd tri
658.2Ø	DELAY DELIV AFTER SPONT/UNS RUP MEMB UNS EOC	**O42.1Ø**	Prem ROM, onset labor > 24 hr fol rupt, unsp weeks of gest
		O42.119	Pretrm prem ROM, onset labor > 24 hours fol rupt, unsp tri
658.21	DELAY DELIV AFTER SPONT/UNSPEC RUP MEMB DELIV	**O42.1Ø**	Prem ROM, onset labor > 24 hr fol rupt, unsp weeks of gest
		O42.111	Pretrm prem ROM, onset labor > 24 hours fol rupt, first tri
		O42.112	Pretrm prem ROM, onset labor > 24 hours fol rupt, second tri
		O42.113	Pretrm prem ROM, onset labor > 24 hours fol rupt, third tri
		O42.12	Full-term premature ROM, onset labor > 24 hours fol rupture
658.23	DELAY DELIV AFTER SPONT/UNSPEC RUP MEMB ANTPRTM	**O42.111**	Pretrm prem ROM, onset labor > 24 hours fol rupt, first tri
		O42.112	Pretrm prem ROM, onset labor > 24 hours fol rupt, second tri
		O42.113	Pretrm prem ROM, onset labor > 24 hours fol rupt, third tri
658.3Ø	DELAY DELIV AFTER ARTFICL RUP MEMB UNS EPIS CARE	**O75.5**	Delayed delivery after artificial rupture of membranes
658.31	DELAY DELIV AFTER ARTFICL RUPTURE MEMB DELIV	**O75.5**	Delayed delivery after artificial rupture of membranes
658.33	DELAY DELIV AFTER ARTFICL RUPTURE MEMB ANTPRTM	**O75.5**	Delayed delivery after artificial rupture of membranes
658.4Ø	INFECTION AMNIOTIC CAVITY UNSPEC AS EPISODE CARE	**O41.1Ø9Ø**	Infct of amniotic sac and membrns, unsp, unsp tri, unsp
		O41.1Ø9[1,2,3,4,5]	Infct of amniotic sac and membrns, unsp, unsp tri
		O41.1Ø99	Infct of amniotic sac and membrns, unsp, unsp trimester, oth
		O41.129Ø	Chorioamnionitis, unsp trimester, not applicable or unsp
		O41.129[1,2,3,4,5]	Chorioamnionitis, unspecified trimester
		O41.1299	Chorioamnionitis, unspecified trimester, other fetus
		O41.149Ø	Placentitis, unsp trimester, not applicable or unspecified
		O41.149[1,2,3,4,5]	Placentitis, unspecified trimester
		O41.1499	Placentitis, unspecified trimester, other fetus
			7th Character meanings for codes as indicated ***1 Fetus 1 3 Fetus 3 5 Fetus 5*** ***2 Fetus 2 4 Fetus 4***
658.41	INFECTION OF AMNIOTIC CAVITY DELIVERED	**O41.1Ø1Ø**	Infct of amniotic sac and membrns, unsp, first tri, unsp
		O41.1Ø1[1,2,3,4,5]	Infct of amniotic sac and membrns, unsp, first tri
		O41.1Ø19	Infct of amniotic sac and membrns, unsp, first tri, oth
		O41.1Ø2Ø	Infct of amniotic sac and membrns, unsp, second tri, unsp
		O41.1Ø2[1,2,3,4,5]	Infct of amniotic sac and membrns, unsp, second tri
		O41.1Ø29	Infct of amniotic sac and membrns, unsp, second tri, oth
		O41.1Ø3Ø	Infct of amniotic sac and membrns, unsp, third tri, unsp
		O41.1Ø3[1,2,3,4,5]	Infct of amniotic sac and membrns, unsp, third tri
		O41.1Ø39	Infct of amniotic sac and membrns, unsp, third tri, oth
		O41.121Ø	Chorioamnionitis, first trimester, not applicable or unsp
		O41.121[1,2,3,4,5]	Chorioamnionitis, first trimester
		O41.1219	Chorioamnionitis, first trimester, other fetus
		O41.122Ø	Chorioamnionitis, second trimester, not applicable or unsp
		O41.122[1,2,3,4,5]	Chorioamnionitis, second trimester
		O41.1229	Chorioamnionitis, second trimester, other fetus
		O41.123Ø	Chorioamnionitis, third trimester, not applicable or unsp
		O41.123[1,2,3,4,5]	Chorioamnionitis, third trimester
			7th Character meanings for codes as indicated ***1 Fetus 1 3 Fetus 3 5 Fetus 5*** ***2 Fetus 2 4 Fetus 4***

(Continued on next page)

ICD-9-CM		ICD-10-CM	
658.41	INFECTION OF AMNIOTIC CAVITY DELIVERED **(Continued)**	**O41.1239**	Chorioamnionitis, third trimester, other fetus
		O41.1410	Placentitis, first trimester, not applicable or unspecified
		O41.141[1,2,3,4,5]	Placentitis, first trimester
		O41.1419	Placentitis, first trimester, other fetus
		O41.1420	Placentitis, second trimester, not applicable or unspecified
		O41.142[1,2,3,4,5]	Placentitis, second trimester
		O41.1429	Placentitis, second trimester, other fetus
		O41.1430	Placentitis, third trimester, not applicable or unspecified
		O41.143[1,2,3,4,5]	Placentitis, third trimester
		O41.1439	Placentitis, third trimester, other fetus
			7th Character meanings for codes as indicated 1 Fetus 1; 2 Fetus 2; 3 Fetus 3; 4 Fetus 4; 5 Fetus 5
658.43	INFECTION OF AMNIOTIC CAVITY ANTEPAR	**O41.1010**	Infct of amniotic sac and membrns, unsp, first tri, unsp
		O41.101[1,2,3,4,5]	Infct of amniotic sac and membrns, unsp, first tri
		O41.1019	Infct of amniotic sac and membrns, unsp, first tri, oth
		O41.1020	Infct of amniotic sac and membrns, unsp, second tri, unsp
		O41.102[1,2,3,4,5]	Infct of amniotic sac and membrns, unsp, second tri
		O41.1029	Infct of amniotic sac and membrns, unsp, second tri, oth
		O41.1030	Infct of amniotic sac and membrns, unsp, third tri, unsp
		O41.103[1,2,3,4,5]	Infct of amniotic sac and membrns, unsp, third tri
		O41.1039	Infct of amniotic sac and membrns, unsp, third tri, oth
		O41.1210	Chorioamnionitis, first trimester, not applicable or unsp
		O41.121[1,2,3,4,5]	Chorioamnionitis, first trimester
		O41.1219	Chorioamnionitis, first trimester, other fetus
		O41.1220	Chorioamnionitis, second trimester, not applicable or unsp
		O41.122[1,2,3,4,5]	Chorioamnionitis, second trimester
		O41.1229	Chorioamnionitis, second trimester, other fetus
		O41.1230	Chorioamnionitis, third trimester, not applicable or unsp
		O41.123[1,2,3,4,5]	Chorioamnionitis, third trimester
		O41.1239	Chorioamnionitis, third trimester, other fetus
		O41.1410	Placentitis, first trimester, not applicable or unspecified
		O41.141[1,2,3,4,5]	Placentitis, first trimester
		O41.1419	Placentitis, first trimester, other fetus
		O41.1420	Placentitis, second trimester, not applicable or unspecified
		O41.142[1,2,3,4,5]	Placentitis, second trimester
		O41.1429	Placentitis, second trimester, other fetus
		O41.1430	Placentitis, third trimester, not applicable or unspecified
		O41.143[1,2,3,4,5]	Placentitis, third trimester
		O41.1439	Placentitis, third trimester, other fetu
			7th Character meanings for codes as indicated 1 Fetus 1; 2 Fetus 2; 3 Fetus 3; 4 Fetus 4; 5 Fetus 5
658.80	OTH PROB ASSOC W/AMNIOTIC CAV&MEMB UNS EPIS CARE	**O41.8X90**	Oth disrd of amniotic fluid and membrns, unsp tri, unsp
		O41.8X91	Oth disrd of amniotic fluid and membrns, unsp tri, fetus 1
		O41.8X92	Oth disrd of amniotic fluid and membrns, unsp tri, fetus 2
		O41.8X93	Oth disrd of amniotic fluid and membrns, unsp tri, fetus 3
		O41.8X94	Oth disrd of amniotic fluid and membrns, unsp tri, fetus 4
		O41.8X95	Oth disrd of amniotic fluid and membrns, unsp tri, fetus 5
		O41.8X99	Oth disrd of amniotic fluid and membrns, unsp trimester, oth
658.81	OTH PROBLEM ASSOC W/AMNIOTIC CAVITY&MEMB DELIV	**O41.8X10**	Oth disrd of amniotic fluid and membrns, first tri, unsp
		O41.8X1[1,2,3,4,5]	Oth disrd of amniotic fluid and membrns, first tri
		O41.8X19	Oth disrd of amniotic fluid and membrns, first tri, oth
		O41.8X20	Oth disrd of amniotic fluid and membrns, second tri, unsp
		O41.8X2[1,2,3,4,5]	Oth disrd of amniotic fluid and membrns, second tri
		O41.8X29	Oth disrd of amniotic fluid and membrns, second tri, oth
		O41.8X30	Oth disrd of amniotic fluid and membrns, third tri, unsp
		O41.8X3[1,2,3,4,5]	Oth disrd of amniotic fluid and membrns, third tri
		O41.8X39	Oth disrd of amniotic fluid and membrns, third tri, oth
			7th Character meanings for codes as indicated 1 Fetus 1; 2 Fetus 2; 3 Fetus 3; 4 Fetus 4; 5 Fetus 5
658.83	OTH PROBLEM ASSOC W/AMNIOTIC CAVITY&MEMB ANTPRTM	**O41.8X10**	Oth disrd of amniotic fluid and membrns, first tri, unsp
		O41.8X1[1,2,3,4,5]	Oth disrd of amniotic fluid and membrns, first tri
		O41.8X19	Oth disrd of amniotic fluid and membrns, first tri, oth
		O41.8X20	Oth disrd of amniotic fluid and membrns, second tri, unsp
		O41.8X2[1,2,3,4,5]	Oth disrd of amniotic fluid and membrns, second tri
		O41.8X29	Oth disrd of amniotic fluid and membrns, second tri, oth
		O41.8X30	Oth disrd of amniotic fluid and membrns, third tri, unsp
		O41.8X3[1,2,3,4,5]	Oth disrd of amniotic fluid and membrns, third tri
		O41.8X39	Oth disrd of amniotic fluid and membrns, third tri, oth
			7th Character meanings for codes as indicated 1 Fetus 1; 2 Fetus 2; 3 Fetus 3; 4 Fetus 4; 5 Fetus 5

ICD-9-CM		ICD-10-CM	
658.9Ø	UNS PROB ASSOC W/AMNIOTIC CAV&MEMB UNS EPIS CARE	**O41.9ØXØ**	Disorder of amniotic fluid and membrns, unsp, unsp tri, unsp
		O41.9ØX1	Disorder of amnio fluid and membrns, unsp, unsp tri, fetus 1
		O41.9ØX2	Disorder of amnio fluid and membrns, unsp, unsp tri, fetus 2
		O41.9ØX3	Disorder of amnio fluid and membrns, unsp, unsp tri, fetus 3
		O41.9ØX4	Disorder of amnio fluid and membrns, unsp, unsp tri, fetus 4
		O41.9ØX5	Disorder of amnio fluid and membrns, unsp, unsp tri, fetus 5
		O41.9ØX9	Disorder of amniotic fluid and membrns, unsp, unsp tri, oth
658.91	UNSPEC PROB ASSOC W/AMNIOTIC CAVITY&MEMB DELIV	**O41.91XØ**	Disorder of amnio fluid and membrns, unsp, first tri, unsp
		O41.91X[1,2,3,4,5]	Disord of amnio fluid and membrns, unsp, first tri
		O41.91X9	Disorder of amniotic fluid and membrns, unsp, first tri, oth
		O41.92XØ	Disorder of amnio fluid and membrns, unsp, second tri, unsp
		O41.92X[1,2,3,4,5]	Disord of amnio fluid and membrns, unsp, second tri
		O41.92X9	Disorder of amnio fluid and membrns, unsp, second tri, oth
		O41.93XØ	Disorder of amnio fluid and membrns, unsp, third tri, unsp
		O41.93X[1,2,3,4,5]	Disord of amnio fluid and membrns, unsp, third tri
		O41.93X9	Disorder of amniotic fluid and membrns, unsp, third tri, oth
			7th Character meanings for codes as indicated ***1 Fetus 1*** ***3 Fetus 3*** ***5 Fetus 5*** ***2 Fetus 2*** ***4 Fetus 4***
658.93	UNSPEC PROB ASSOC W/AMNIOTIC CAVITY&MEMB ANTPRTM	**O41.91XØ**	Disorder of amnio fluid and membrns, unsp, first tri, unsp
		O41.91X[1,2,3,4,5]	Disord of amnio fluid and membrns, unsp, first tri
		O41.91X9	Disorder of amniotic fluid and membrns, unsp, first tri, oth
		O41.92XØ	Disorder of amnio fluid and membrns, unsp, second tri, unsp
		O41.92X[1,2,3,4,5]	Disord of amnio fluid and membrns, unsp, second tri
		O41.92X9	Disorder of amnio fluid and membrns, unsp, second tri, oth
		O41.93XØ	Disorder of amnio fluid and membrns, unsp, third tri, unsp
		O41.93X[1,2,3,4,5]	Disord of amnio fluid and membrns, unsp, third tri
		O41.93X9	Disorder of amniotic fluid and membrns, unsp, third tri, oth
			7th Character meanings for codes as indicated ***1 Fetus 1*** ***3 Fetus 3*** ***5 Fetus 5*** ***2 Fetus 2*** ***4 Fetus 4***
659.ØØ	FAILED MECH INDUCTION LABOR UNSPEC AS EPIS CARE	**O61.1**	Failed instrumental induction of labor
659.Ø1	FAILED MECHANICAL INDUCTION OF LABOR DELIVERED	**O61.1**	Failed instrumental induction of labor
659.Ø3	FAILED MECHANICAL INDUCTION OF LABOR ANTEPARTUM	**O61.1**	Failed instrumental induction of labor
659.1Ø	FAILMED/UNSPEC INDUCT LABR UNSPEC AS EPIS CARE	**O61.Ø**	Failed medical induction of labor
659.11	FAILED MEDICAL/UNSPEC INDUCTION LABOR DELIVERED	**O61.Ø**	Failed medical induction of labor
		O61.8	Other failed induction of labor
		O61.9	Failed induction of labor, unspecified
659.13	FAILED MEDICAL/UNSPEC INDUCTION LABOR ANTEPARTUM	**O61.Ø**	Failed medical induction of labor
659.2Ø	UNSPEC MTRN PYREXIA DUR LABR UNSPEC AS EPIS CARE	**O75.2**	Pyrexia during labor, not elsewhere classified
659.21	UNSPEC MATERNAL PYREXIA DURING LABOR DELIVERED	**O75.2**	Pyrexia during labor, not elsewhere classified
659.23	UNSPECIFIED MATERNAL PYREXIA ANTEPARTUM	**O75.2**	Pyrexia during labor, not elsewhere classified
659.3Ø	GEN INFECTION DURING LABOR UNSPEC AS EPIS CARE	**O75.3**	Other infection during labor
659.31	GENERALIZED INFECTION DURING LABOR DELIVERED	**O75.3**	Other infection during labor
659.33	GENERALIZED INFECTION DURING LABOR ANTEPARTUM	**O75.3**	Other infection during labor
659.4Ø	GRAND MULTIPARITY W/CURRNT PG UNS AS EPIS CARE	**OØ9.4Ø**	Supervision of pregnancy w grand multiparity, unsp trimester
659.41	GRAND MULTIPARITY DELIV W/WO ANTPRTM COND	**OØ9.41**	Suprvsn of pregnancy w grand multiparity, first trimester
		OØ9.42	Suprvsn of pregnancy w grand multiparity, second trimester
		OØ9.43	Suprvsn of pregnancy w grand multiparity, third trimester
659.43	GRAND MULTIPARITY W/CURRENT PREGNANCY ANTEPARTUM	**OØ9.41**	Suprvsn of pregnancy w grand multiparity, first trimester
		OØ9.42	Suprvsn of pregnancy w grand multiparity, second trimester
		OØ9.43	Suprvsn of pregnancy w grand multiparity, third trimester
659.5Ø	ELDERLY PRIMIGRAVIDA UNSPECIFIED AS EPISODE CARE	**OØ9.519**	Supervision of elderly primigravida, unspecified trimester
659.51	ELDERLY PRIMIGRAVIDA, DELIVERED	**OØ9.511**	Supervision of elderly primigravida, first trimester
		OØ9.512	Supervision of elderly primigravida, second trimester
		OØ9.513	Supervision of elderly primigravida, third trimester
659.53	ELDERLY PRIMIGRAVIDA, ANTEPARTUM	**OØ9.511**	Supervision of elderly primigravida, first trimester
		OØ9.512	Supervision of elderly primigravida, second trimester
		OØ9.513	Supervision of elderly primigravida, third trimester
659.6Ø	ELDER MULTIGRAVIDA UNS AS EPIS CARE/NOT APPLIC	**OØ9.529**	Supervision of elderly multigravida, unspecified trimester
659.61	ELDER MULTIGRAVIDA DELIV W/MENTION ANTPRTM COND	**OØ9.521**	Supervision of elderly multigravida, first trimester
		OØ9.522	Supervision of elderly multigravida, second trimester
		OØ9.523	Supervision of elderly multigravida, third trimester
659.63	ELDERLY MULTIGRAVIDA W/ANTPRTM COND/COMPLICATION	**OØ9.521**	Supervision of elderly multigravida, first trimester
		OØ9.522	Supervision of elderly multigravida, second trimester
		OØ9.523	Supervision of elderly multigravida, third trimester
659.7Ø	ABN FETL HRT RATE/RHYTHM UNS EOC/NOT APPLIC	**O76**	Abnlt in fetal heart rate and rhythm comp labor and delivery
659.71	ABN FETL HRT RATE/RHYTHM DELIV W/WO ANTPRTM COND	**O76**	Abnlt in fetal heart rate and rhythm comp labor and delivery
659.73	ABNORM FETAL HEART RATE/RHYTHM ANTPRTM COND/COMP	**O76**	Abnlt in fetal heart rate and rhythm comp labor and delivery
659.8Ø	OTH SPEC INDICAT CARE/INTRVN REL L&D UNS EOC	**O75.89**	Other specified complications of labor and delivery
659.81	OTH SPEC INDICAT CARE/INTERVEN RELATED L&D DELIV	**O75.89**	Other specified complications of labor and delivery
659.83	OTH SPEC INDICAT CARE/INTERVEN REL L&D ANTPRTM	**O75.89**	Other specified complications of labor and delivery
659.9Ø	UNS INDICAT CARE/INTERVEN REL L&D UNS EPIS CARE	**O75.9**	Complication of labor and delivery, unspecified

[Brackets] indicate valid character values for each code. Character value meanings provided for each code grouping.

ICD-9-CM		ICD-10-CM	
659.91	UNSPEC INDICAT CARE/INTERVEN RELATED L&D DELIV	**O75.9**	Complication of labor and delivery, unspecified
659.93	UNSPEC INDICAT CARE/INTERVEN RELATED L&D ANTPRTM	**O75.9**	Complication of labor and delivery, unspecified
660.00	OBST CAUS MALPSTN FETUS@ONSET LABR UNS EPIS CARE	**O64.9XX0**	Obstructed labor due to malpos and malpresent, unsp, unsp
660.01	OBST CAUS MALPOSITION FETUS@ONSET LABR DELIV	**O64.1XX0**	Obstructed labor due to breech presentation, unsp
		O64.1XX[1,2,3,4,5]	Obstructed labor due to breech presentation
		O64.1XX9	Obstructed labor due to breech presentation, other fetus
		O64.2XX0	Obstructed labor due to face presentation, unsp
		O64.2XX[1,2,3,4,5]	Obstructed labor due to face presentation
		O64.2XX9	Obstructed labor due to face presentation, other fetus
		O64.3XX0	Obstructed labor due to brow presentation, unsp
		O64.3XX[1,2,3,4,5]	Obstructed labor due to brow presentation
		O64.3XX9	Obstructed labor due to brow presentation, other fetus
		O64.4XX0	Obstructed labor due to shoulder presentation, unsp
		O64.4XX[1,2,3,4,5]	Obstructed labor due to shoulder presentation
		O64.4XX9	Obstructed labor due to shoulder presentation, other fetus
		O64.5XX0	Obstructed labor due to compound presentation, unsp
		O64.5XX[1,2,3,4,5]	Obstructed labor due to compound presentation
		O64.5XX9	Obstructed labor due to compound presentation, other fetus
		O64.8XX0	Obstructed labor due to oth malposition and malpresent, unsp
		O64.8XX[1,2,3,4,5]	Obstructed labor due to oth malpos and malpresent
		O64.8XX9	Obstructed labor due to oth malposition and malpresent, oth
		O64.9XX0	Obstructed labor due to malpos and malpresent, unsp, unsp
		O64.9XX[1,2,3,4,5]	Obstructed labor due to malpos and malpresent, unsp
		O64.9XX9	Obstructed labor due to malpos and malpresent, unsp, oth
			7th Character meanings for codes as indicated ***1 Fetus 1*** ***3 Fetus 3*** ***5 Fetus 5*** ***2 Fetus 2*** ***4 Fetus 4***
660.03	OBST CAUS MALPOSITION FETUS@ONSET LABR ANTPRTM	**O64.9XX0**	Obstructed labor due to malpos and malpresent, unsp, unsp
660.10	OBST BONY PELV DUR L&D UNSPEC AS EPIS CARE	**O65.4**	Obstructed labor due to fetopelvic disproportion, unsp
660.11	OBSTRUCTION BY BONY PELVIS DURING L&D DELIVERED	**O65.0**	Obstructed labor due to deformed pelvis
		O65.1	Obstructed labor due to generally contracted pelvis
		O65.2	Obstructed labor due to pelvic inlet contraction
		O65.3	Obst labor due to pelvic outlet and mid-cavity contrctn
		O65.4	Obstructed labor due to fetopelvic disproportion, unsp
660.13	OBSTRUCTION BY BONY PELVIS DURING L&D ANTEPARTUM	**O65.4**	Obstructed labor due to fetopelvic disproportion, unsp
660.20	OBST ABNORM PELV SFT TISS DUR L&D UNS EPIS CARE	**O65.9**	Obstructed labor due to maternal pelvic abnormality, unsp
660.21	OBST ABN PELV SFT TISS DUR LABRAND DELIV DELIV	**O65.5**	Obstructed labor due to abnlt of maternal pelvic organs
		O65.8	Obstructed labor due to other maternal pelvic abnormalities
		O65.9	Obstructed labor due to maternal pelvic abnormality, unsp
660.23	OBST ABNORM PELV SOFT TISS DUR L&D ANTPRTM	**O65.9**	Obstructed labor due to maternal pelvic abnormality, unsp
660.30	DEEP TRNSVRSE ARREST-OCCIPITOPOST POSIT-UNS EOC	**O64.0XX0**	Obstructed labor due to incmpl rotation of fetal head, unsp
660.31	DEEP TRNSVRSE ARREST-OCCIPITOPOSTER-DEL-UNS APC	**O64.0XX0**	Obstructed labor due to incmpl rotation of fetal head, unsp
		O64.0XX1	Obst labor due to incmpl rotation of fetal head, fetus 1
		O64.0XX2	Obst labor due to incmpl rotation of fetal head, fetus 2
		O64.0XX3	Obst labor due to incmpl rotation of fetal head, fetus 3
		O64.0XX4	Obst labor due to incmpl rotation of fetal head, fetus 4
		O64.0XX5	Obst labor due to incmpl rotation of fetal head, fetus 5
		O64.0XX9	Obstructed labor due to incmpl rotation of fetal head, oth
660.33	DEEP TRANSVERSE ARREST-OCCIPITOPOST POSIT-APC/C	**O64.0XX0**	Obstructed labor due to incmpl rotation of fetal head, unsp
660.40	SHOULDER DYSTOCIA DURING L&D UNSPEC AS EPIS CARE	**O66.0**	Obstructed labor due to shoulder dystocia
660.41	SHOULDER DYSTOCIA DURING LABOR&DELIVER DELIVERED	**O66.0**	Obstructed labor due to shoulder dystocia
660.43	SHOULDER DYSTOCIA DURING L&D ANTEPARTUM	**O66.0**	Obstructed labor due to shoulder dystocia
660.50	LOCKED TWINS DURING L&D UNSPEC AS EPIS CARE PG	**O66.1**	Obstructed labor due to locked twins
660.51	LOCKED TWINS, DELIVERED	**O66.1**	Obstructed labor due to locked twins
660.53	LOCKED TWINS, ANTEPARTUM	**O66.1**	Obstructed labor due to locked twins
660.60	UNSPEC FAILED TRIAL LABOR UNSPECIFED AS EPISODE	**O66.40**	Failed trial of labor, unspecified
660.61	UNSPECIFIED FAILED TRIAL OF LABOR DELIVERED	**O66.40**	Failed trial of labor, unspecified
		O66.41	Failed attempt vaginal birth after previous cesarean del
660.63	UNSPECIFIED FAILED TRIAL OF LABOR ANTEPARTUM	**O66.40**	Failed trial of labor, unspecified
660.70	UNS FAILD FORCEP/VAC EXTRACTOR UNS AS EPIS CARE	**O66.5**	Attempted application of vacuum extractor and forceps
660.71	UNSPEC FAILED FORCEPS/VACUUM EXTRACTOR DELIVERED	**O66.5**	Attempted application of vacuum extractor and forceps
660.73	FAILED FORCEPS/VAC EXT UNSPEC ANTEPARTUM	**O66.5**	Attempted application of vacuum extractor and forceps
660.80	OTH CAUSES OBSTRUCTED LABOR UNSPEC AS EPIS CARE	**O66.8**	Other specified obstructed labor
660.81	OTHER CAUSES OF OBSTRUCTED LABOR DELIVERED	**O66.2**	Obstructed labor due to unusually large fetus
		O66.3	Obstructed labor due to other abnormalities of fetus
		O66.6	Obstructed labor due to other multiple fetuses
		O66.8	Other specified obstructed labor
660.83	OTHER CAUSES OF OBSTRUCTED LABOR ANTEPARTUM	**O66.8**	Other specified obstructed labor
660.90	UNSPEC OBSTRUCTED LABOR UNSPEC AS EPISODE CARE	**O66.9**	Obstructed labor, unspecified
660.91	UNSPECIFIED OBSTRUCTED LABOR WITH DELIVERY	**O66.9**	Obstructed labor, unspecified
660.93	UNSPECIFIED OBSTRUCTED LABOR ANTEPARTUM	**O66.9**	Obstructed labor, unspecified
661.00	PRIMARY UTERINE INERTIA UNSPEC AS EPISODE CARE	**O62.0**	Primary inadequate contractions
661.01	PRIMARY UTERINE INERTIA WITH DELIVERY	**O62.0**	Primary inadequate contractions

ICD-9-CM		ICD-10-CM	
661.Ø3	PRIMARY UTERINE INERTIA, ANTEPARTUM	**O62.Ø**	Primary inadequate contractions
661.1Ø	SEC UTERINE INERTIA UNSPECIFIED AS EPISODE CARE	**O62.1**	Secondary uterine inertia
661.11	SECONDARY UTERINE INERTIA WITH DELIVERY	**O62.1**	Secondary uterine inertia
661.13	SECONDARY UTERINE INERTIA ANTEPARTUM	**O62.1**	Secondary uterine inertia
661.2Ø	OTH&UNSPEC UTERINE INERTIA UNSPEC AS EPIS CARE	**O62.2**	Other uterine inertia
661.21	OTHER AND UNSPECIFIED UTERINE INERTIA W/DELIVERY	**O62.2**	Other uterine inertia
661.23	OTHER AND UNSPECIFIED UTERINE INERTIA ANTEPARTUM	**O62.2**	Other uterine inertia
661.3Ø	PRECIPITATE LABOR UNSPECIFIED AS TO EPISODE CARE	**O62.3**	Precipitate labor
661.31	PRECIPITATE LABOR, WITH DELIVERY	**O62.3**	Precipitate labor
661.33	PRECIPITATE LABOR, ANTEPARTUM	**O62.3**	Precipitate labor
661.4Ø	HYPERTON INCOORD/PROLNG UTERN CONTRACS UNS EOC	**O62.4**	Hypertonic, incoordinate, and prolonged uterine contractions
661.41	HYPERTON INCOORD/PROLONG UTERINE CONTRACS DELIV	**O62.4**	Hypertonic, incoordinate, and prolonged uterine contractions
661.43	HYPERTON INCOORD/PROLNG UTERINE CONTRACS ANTPRTM	**O62.4**	Hypertonic, incoordinate, and prolonged uterine contractions
661.9Ø	UNSPEC ABNORMALITY LABOR UNSPEC AS EPISODE CARE	**O62.9**	Abnormality of forces of labor, unspecified
661.91	UNSPECIFIED ABNORMALITY OF LABOR WITH DELIVERY	**O62.8**	Other abnormalities of forces of labor
		O62.9	Abnormality of forces of labor, unspecified
661.93	UNSPECIFIED ABNORMALITY OF LABOR ANTEPARTUM	**O62.9**	Abnormality of forces of labor, unspecified
662.ØØ	PROLONGED 1 STAGE LABOR UNSPEC AS EPISODE CARE	**O63.Ø**	Prolonged first stage (of labor)
662.Ø1	PROLONGED FIRST STAGE OF LABOR DELIVERED	**O63.Ø**	Prolonged first stage (of labor)
662.Ø3	PROLONGED FIRST STAGE OF LABOR ANTEPARTUM	**O63.Ø**	Prolonged first stage (of labor)
662.1Ø	UNSPEC PROLONGED LABOR UNSPEC AS EPISODE CARE	**O63.9**	Long labor, unspecified
662.11	UNSPECIFIED PROLONGED LABOR DELIVERED	**O63.9**	Long labor, unspecified
662.13	UNSPECIFIED PROLONGED LABOR ANTEPARTUM	**O63.9**	Long labor, unspecified
662.2Ø	PROLONGED 2 STAGE LABOR UNSPEC AS EPISODE CARE	**O63.1**	Prolonged second stage (of labor)
662.21	PROLONGED SECOND STAGE OF LABOR DELIVERED	**O63.1**	Prolonged second stage (of labor)
662.23	PROLONGED SECOND STAGE OF LABOR ANTEPARTUM	**O63.1**	Prolonged second stage (of labor)
662.3Ø	DELAY DELIV 2 TWIN TRIPLT ETC UNS AS EPIS CARE	**O63.2**	Delayed delivery of second twin, triplet, etc.
662.31	DELAYED DELIVERY 2 TWIN TRIPLET ETC DELIVERED	**O63.2**	Delayed delivery of second twin, triplet, etc.
662.33	DELAYED DELIVERY 2 TWIN TRIPLET ETC ANTEPARTUM	**O63.2**	Delayed delivery of second twin, triplet, etc.
663.ØØ	PROLAPSE CORD COMP L&D UNSPEC AS EPISODE CARE	**O69.ØXXØ**	Labor and delivery complicated by prolapse of cord, unsp
663.Ø1	PROLAPSE OF CORD COMPLICATING L&D DELIVERED	**O69.ØXXØ**	Labor and delivery complicated by prolapse of cord, unsp
		O69.ØXX1	Labor and delivery complicated by prolapse of cord, fetus 1
		O69.ØXX2	Labor and delivery complicated by prolapse of cord, fetus 2
		O69.ØXX3	Labor and delivery complicated by prolapse of cord, fetus 3
		O69.ØXX4	Labor and delivery complicated by prolapse of cord, fetus 4
		O69.ØXX5	Labor and delivery complicated by prolapse of cord, fetus 5
		O69.ØXX9	Labor and delivery complicated by prolapse of cord, oth
663.Ø3	PROLAPSE OF CORD COMPLICATING L&D ANTEPARTUM	**O69.ØXXØ**	Labor and delivery complicated by prolapse of cord, unsp
663.1Ø	CORD AROUND NCK W/COMPRS COMP L&D UNS EPIS CARE	**O69.1XXØ**	Labor and del comp by cord around neck, w comprsn, unsp
663.11	CORD AROUND NECK W/COMPRS COMP L&D DELIVERED	**O69.1XXØ**	Labor and del comp by cord around neck, w comprsn, unsp
		O69.1XX1	Labor and del comp by cord around neck, w comprsn, fetus 1
		O69.1XX2	Labor and del comp by cord around neck, w comprsn, fetus 2
		O69.1XX3	Labor and del comp by cord around neck, w comprsn, fetus 3
		O69.1XX4	Labor and del comp by cord around neck, w comprsn, fetus 4
		O69.1XX5	Labor and del comp by cord around neck, w comprsn, fetus 5
		O69.1XX9	Labor and delivery comp by cord around neck, w comprsn, oth
663.13	CORD AROUND NECK W/COMPRESSION COMP L&D ANTPRTM	**O69.1XXØ**	Labor and del comp by cord aroundnd neck, w comprsn, unsp
663.2Ø	UNS CRD ENTANGL W/COMPRS COMP L&D UNS EPIS CARE	**O69.2XXØ**	Labor and del comp by oth cord entangle, w comprsn, unsp
663.21	OTH&UNSPEC CORD ENTANGL W/COMPRS COMP L&D DELIV	**O69.2XXØ**	Labor and del comp by oth cord entangle, w comprsn, unsp
		O69.2XX1	Labor and del comp by oth cord entangle, w comprsn, fetus 1
		O69.2XX2	Labor and del comp by oth cord entangle, w comprsn, fetus 2
		O69.2XX3	Labor and del comp by oth cord entangle, w comprsn, fetus 3
		O69.2XX4	Labor and del comp by oth cord entangle, w comprsn, fetus 4
		O69.2XX5	Labor and del comp by oth cord entangle, w comprsn, fetus 5
		O69.2XX9	Labor and delivery comp by oth cord entangle, w comprsn, oth
663.23	OTH&UNS CORD ENTANGL W/COMPRS COMP L&D ANTPRTM	**O69.2XXØ**	Labor and del comp by oth cord entangle, w comprsn, unsp
663.3Ø	UNS CRD ENTANGL W/O COMPRS COMP L&D UNS EOC	**O69.81XØ**	Labor and del comp by cord around neck, w/o comprsn, unsp
		O69.82XØ	Labor and del comp by oth cord entangle, w/o comprsn, unsp
		O69.89XØ	Labor and delivery complicated by oth cord comp, unsp
663.31	OTH&UNS CRD ENTANGL W/O COMPRS COMP L&D DELIV	**O69.81XØ**	Labor and del comp by cord around neck, w/o comprsn, unsp
		O69.81X[1,2,3,4,5]	Labor and del comp by cord around neck, w/o comprsn
		O69.81X9	Labor and del comp by cord around neck, w/o comprsn, oth
		O69.82XØ	Labor and del comp by oth cord entangle, w/o comprsn, unsp
		O69.82X[1,2,3,4,5]	Labor and del comp by oth cord entangle, w/o comprsn
		O69.82X9	Labor and del comp by oth cord entangle, w/o comprsn, oth
		O69.89XØ	Labor and delivery complicated by oth cord comp, unsp
		O69.89X[1,2,3,4,5]	Labor and delivery complicated by oth cord comp
		O69.89X9	Labor and delivery complicated by oth cord comp, oth

7th Character meanings for codes as indicated

1 Fetus 1	***3 Fetus 3***	***5 Fetus 5***
2 Fetus 2	***4 Fetus 4***	

[Brackets] indicate valid character values for each code. Character value meanings provided for each code grouping.

ICD-9-CM		ICD-10-CM	
663.33	OTH&UNS CRD ENTANGL W/O COMPRS COMP L&D ANTPRTM	**O69.81XØ**	Labor and del comp by cord around neck, w/o comprsn, unsp
		O69.82XØ	Labor and del comp by oth cord entangle, w/o comprsn, unsp
		O69.89XØ	Labor and delivery complicated by oth cord comp, unsp
663.4Ø	SHORT CORD COMP L&D UNSPEC AS EPISODE CARE	**O69.3XXØ**	Labor and delivery complicated by short cord, unsp
663.41	SHORT CORD COMPLICATING L&D DELIVERED	**O69.3XXØ**	Labor and delivery complicated by short cord, unsp
		O69.3XX1	Labor and delivery complicated by short cord, fetus 1
		O69.3XX2	Labor and delivery complicated by short cord, fetus 2
		O69.3XX3	Labor and delivery complicated by short cord, fetus 3
		O69.3XX4	Labor and delivery complicated by short cord, fetus 4
		O69.3XX5	Labor and delivery complicated by short cord, fetus 5
		O69.3XX9	Labor and delivery complicated by short cord, other fetus
663.43	SHORT CORD COMPLICATING L&D ANTEPARTUM	**O69.3XXØ**	Labor and delivery complicated by short cord, unsp
663.5Ø	VASA PREVIA COMP L&D UNSPEC AS EPISODE CARE	**O69.4XXØ**	Labor and delivery complicated by vasa previa, unsp
663.51	VASA PREVIA COMPLICATING L&D DELIVERED	**O69.4XXØ**	Labor and delivery complicated by vasa previa, unsp
		O69.4XX1	Labor and delivery complicated by vasa previa, fetus 1
		O69.4XX2	Labor and delivery complicated by vasa previa, fetus 2
		O69.4XX3	Labor and delivery complicated by vasa previa, fetus 3
		O69.4XX4	Labor and delivery complicated by vasa previa, fetus 4
		O69.4XX5	Labor and delivery complicated by vasa previa, fetus 5
		O69.4XX9	Labor and delivery complicated by vasa previa, other fetus
663.53	VASA PREVIA COMPLICATING L&D ANTEPARTUM	**O69.4XXØ**	Labor and delivery complicated by vasa previa, unsp
663.6Ø	VASCULAR LES CORD COMP L&D UNSPEC AS EPIS CARE	**O69.5XXØ**	Labor and delivery comp by vascular lesion of cord, unsp
663.61	VASCULAR LESIONS CORD COMPLICATING L&D DELIVERED	**O69.5XXØ**	Labor and delivery comp by vascular lesion of cord, unsp
		O69.5XX1	Labor and delivery comp by vascular lesion of cord, fetus 1
		O69.5XX2	Labor and delivery comp by vascular lesion of cord, fetus 2
		O69.5XX3	Labor and delivery comp by vascular lesion of cord, fetus 3
		O69.5XX4	Labor and delivery comp by vascular lesion of cord, fetus 4
		O69.5XX5	Labor and delivery comp by vascular lesion of cord, fetus 5
		O69.5XX9	Labor and delivery comp by vascular lesion of cord, oth
663.63	VASCULAR LESIONS CORD COMPLICATING L&D ANTPRTM	**O69.5XXØ**	Labor and delivery comp by vascular lesion of cord, unsp
663.8Ø	OTH UMB CORD COMPS DUR L&D UNSPEC AS EPIS CARE	**O43.129**	Velamentous insertion of umbilical cord, unsp trimester
		O69.89XØ	Labor and delivery complicated by oth cord comp, unsp
663.81	OTH UMBILICAL CORD COMPS DURING L&D DELIVERED	**O43.121**	Velamentous insertion of umbilical cord, first trimester
		O43.122	Velamentous insertion of umbilical cord, second trimester
		O43.123	Velamentous insertion of umbilical cord, third trimester
		O69.89XØ	Labor and delivery complicated by oth cord comp, unsp
		O69.89X1	Labor and delivery complicated by oth cord comp, fetus 1
		O69.89X2	Labor and delivery complicated by oth cord comp, fetus 2
		O69.89X3	Labor and delivery complicated by oth cord comp, fetus 3
		O69.89X4	Labor and delivery complicated by oth cord comp, fetus 4
		O69.89X5	Labor and delivery complicated by oth cord comp, fetus 5
		O69.89X9	Labor and delivery complicated by oth cord comp, oth
663.83	OTH UMBILICAL CORD COMPS DURING L&D ANTPRTM	**O69.89XØ**	Labor and delivery complicated by oth cord comp, unsp
663.9Ø	UNSPEC UMB CORD COMP DUR L&D UNSPEC AS EPIS CARE	**O69.9XXØ**	Labor and delivery complicated by cord comp, unsp, unsp
663.91	UNSPEC UMBILICAL CORD COMP DURING L&D DELIVERED	**O69.9XXØ**	Labor and delivery complicated by cord comp, unsp, unsp
		O69.9XX1	Labor and delivery complicated by cord comp, unsp, fetus 1
		O69.9XX2	Labor and delivery complicated by cord comp, unsp, fetus 2
		O69.9XX3	Labor and delivery complicated by cord comp, unsp, fetus 3
		O69.9XX4	Labor and delivery complicated by cord comp, unsp, fetus 4
		O69.9XX5	Labor and delivery complicated by cord comp, unsp, fetus 5
		O69.9XX9	Labor and delivery complicated by cord comp, unsp, oth
663.93	UNSPEC UMBILICAL CORD COMP DURING L&D ANTPRTM	**O69.9XXØ**	Labor and delivery complicated by cord comp, unsp, unsp
664.ØØ	1-DEG PERINL LACERATION UNSPEC AS EPIS CARE PG	**O7Ø.Ø**	First degree perineal laceration during delivery
664.Ø1	FIRST-DEGREE PERINEAL LACERATION WITH DELIVERY	**O7Ø.Ø**	First degree perineal laceration during delivery
664.Ø4	FIRST-DEGREE PERINEAL LAC POSTPARTUM COND/COMPL	**O7Ø.Ø**	First degree perineal laceration during delivery
664.1Ø	2-DEG PERINL LACERATION UNSPEC AS EPIS CARE PG	**O7Ø.1**	Second degree perineal laceration during delivery
664.11	SECOND-DEGREE PERINEAL LACERATION WITH DELIVERY	**O7Ø.1**	Second degree perineal laceration during delivery
664.14	SECOND-DEGREE PERINEAL LAC POSTPARTUM COND/COMPL	**O7Ø.1**	Second degree perineal laceration during delivery
664.2Ø	THIRD-DEG PERINL LAC UNSPEC AS EPIS CARE PG	**O7Ø.2**	Third degree perineal laceration during delivery
664.21	THIRD-DEGREE PERINEAL LACERATION WITH DELIVERY	**O7Ø.2**	Third degree perineal laceration during delivery
664.24	THIRD-DEGREE PERINEAL LAC POSTPARTUM COND/COMPL	**O7Ø.2**	Third degree perineal laceration during delivery
664.3Ø	FOURTH-DEG PERINL LAC UNSPEC AS EPIS CARE PG	**O7Ø.3**	Fourth degree perineal laceration during delivery
664.31	FOURTH-DEGREE PERINEAL LACERATION WITH DELIVERY	**O7Ø.3**	Fourth degree perineal laceration during delivery
664.34	FOURTH-DEGREE PERINEAL LAC POSTPARTUM COND/COMPL	**O7Ø.3**	Fourth degree perineal laceration during delivery
664.4Ø	UNSPEC PERINL LACERATION UNSPEC AS EPIS CARE PG	**O7Ø.9**	Perineal laceration during delivery, unspecified
664.41	UNSPECIFIED PERINEAL LACERATION WITH DELIVERY	**O7Ø.9**	Perineal laceration during delivery, unspecified
664.44	UNSPECIFIED PERINEAL LAC POSTPARTUM COND/COMPL	**O7Ø.9**	Perineal laceration during delivery, unspecified
664.5Ø	VULVAR&PERINL HEMAT UNSPEC AS EPIS CARE PG	**O71.7**	Obstetric hematoma of pelvis
664.51	VULVAR AND PERINEAL HEMATOMA WITH DELIVERY	**O71.7**	Obstetric hematoma of pelvis
664.54	VULVAR & PERINEAL HEMATOMA POSTPARTUM COND/COMPL	**O71.7**	Obstetric hematoma of pelvis
664.6Ø	ANAL SPHINCTER TEAR COMP DELIVERY UNS EOC/NA	**O7Ø.4**	Anal sphincter tear comp del, not assoc w third degree lac
664.61	ANAL SPHINCT TEAR COMP DELIVERY W OR W/O AP COND	**O7Ø.4**	Anal sphincter tear comp del, not assoc w third degree lac
664.64	ANAL SPHINCT TEAR COMP DELIVERY PP COND/COMP	**O7Ø.4**	Anal sphincter tear comp del, not assoc w third degree lac
664.8Ø	OTH SPEC TRAUMA PERIN&VULVA UNS AS EPIS CARE PG	**O71.82**	Other specified trauma to perineum and vulva

ICD-9-CM		ICD-10-CM		
664.81	OTHER SPECIFIED TRAUMA PERINEUM&VULVA W/DELIVERY	**O71.82**	Other specified trauma to perineum and vulva	
664.84	OTHER SPEC TRAUMA PERINEUM&VULVA PP COND/COMPL	**O71.82**	Other specified trauma to perineum and vulva	
664.90	UNSPEC TRAUMA PERIN&VULVA UNSPEC AS EPIS CARE PG	**O71.9**	Obstetric trauma, unspecified	
664.91	UNSPECIFIED TRAUMA TO PERINEUM&VULVA W/DELIVERY	**O71.9**	Obstetric trauma, unspecified	
664.94	UNSPEC TRAUMA TO PERINEUM & VULVA PP COND/COMPL	**O71.9**	Obstetric trauma, unspecified	
665.00	RUP UTERUS BEFORE ONSET LABR UNSPEC AS EPIS CARE	**O71.00**	Rupture of uterus before onset of labor, unsp trimester	
665.01	RUPTURE UTERUS BEFORE ONSET LABOR W/DELIVERY	**O71.02** **O71.03**	Rupture of uterus before onset of labor, second trimester Rupture of uterus before onset of labor, third trimester	
665.03	RUPTURE UTERUS BEFORE ONSET LABOR ANTEPARTUM	**O71.02** **O71.03**	Rupture of uterus before onset of labor, second trimester Rupture of uterus before onset of labor, third trimester	
665.10	RUPTURE UTERUS DURING LABOR UNSPEC AS EPISODE	**O71.1**	Rupture of uterus during labor	
665.11	RUPTURE OF UTERUS DURING LABOR WITH DELIVERY	**O71.1**	Rupture of uterus during labor	
665.20	INVERSION UTERUS UNSPEC AS EPIS CARE PREGNANCY	**O71.2**	Postpartum inversion of uterus	
665.22	INVERSION UTERUS DELIVERED W/PPC	**O71.2**	Postpartum inversion of uterus	
665.24	INVERSION OF UTERUS, POSTPARTUM COND/COMPL	**O71.2**	Postpartum inversion of uterus	
665.30	LACERATION CERV UNSPEC AS EPISODE CARE PREGNANCY	**O71.3**	Obstetric laceration of cervix	
665.31	LACERATION OF CERVIX, WITH DELIVERY	**O71.3**	Obstetric laceration of cervix	
665.34	LACERATION OF CERVIX, POSTPARTUM COND/COMPL	**O71.3**	Obstetric laceration of cervix	
665.40	HIGH VAGINAL LACERATION UNSPEC AS EPIS CARE PG	**O71.4**	Obstetric high vaginal laceration alone	
665.41	HIGH VAGINAL LACERATION WITH DELIVERY	**O71.4**	Obstetric high vaginal laceration alone	
665.44	HIGH VAGINAL LACERATION POSTPARTUM COND/COMPL	**O71.4**	Obstetric high vaginal laceration alone	
665.50	OTH INJURY PELV ORGN UNSPEC AS EPIS CARE PG	**O71.5**	Other obstetric injury to pelvic organs	
665.51	OTHER INJURY TO PELVIC ORGANS WITH DELIVERY	**O71.5**	Other obstetric injury to pelvic organs	
665.54	OTHER INJURY TO PELVIC ORG POSTPARTUM COND/COMP	**O71.5**	Other obstetric injury to pelvic organs	
665.60	DAMGE PELV JNT&LIG UNSPEC AS EPIS CARE PREGNANCY	**O71.6**	Obstetric damage to pelvic joints and ligaments	
665.61	DAMAGE TO PELVIC JOINTS AND LIGAMENTS W/DELIVERY	**O71.6**	Obstetric damage to pelvic joints and ligaments	
665.64	DAMAGE TO PELVIC JOINTS & LIGAMENTS PP COND/COMP	**O71.6**	Obstetric damage to pelvic joints and ligaments	
665.70	PELVIC HEMATOMA UNSPECIFIED AS TO EPISODE CARE	**O71.7**	Obstetric hematoma of pelvis	
665.71	PELVIC HEMATOMA, WITH DELIVERY	**O71.7**	Obstetric hematoma of pelvis	
665.72	PELVIC HEMATOMA DELIVERED W/PPC	**O71.7**	Obstetric hematoma of pelvis	
665.74	PELVIC HEMATOMA, POSTPARTUM COND/COMPL	**O71.7**	Obstetric hematoma of pelvis	
665.80	OTH SPEC OBSTETRICAL TRAUMA UNSPEC AS EPIS CARE	**O71.89**	Other specified obstetric trauma	
665.81	OTHER SPECIFIED OBSTETRICAL TRAUMA WITH DELIVERY	**O71.81** **O71.89**	Laceration of uterus, not elsewhere classified Other specified obstetric trauma	
665.82	OTH SPEC OBSTETRICAL TRAUMA DELIV W/POSTPARTUM	**O71.81** **O71.89**	Laceration of uterus, not elsewhere classified Other specified obstetric trauma	
665.83	OTHER SPECIFIED OBSTETRICAL TRAUMA ANTEPARTUM	**O71.89**	Other specified obstetric trauma	
665.84	OTHER SPECIFIED OB TRAUMA POSTPARTUM COND/COMPL	**O71.89**	Other specified obstetric trauma	
665.90	UNSPEC OBSTETRICAL TRAUMA UNSPEC AS EPISODE CARE	**O71.9**	Obstetric trauma, unspecified	
665.91	UNSPECIFIED OBSTETRICAL TRAUMA WITH DELIVERY	**O71.9**	Obstetric trauma, unspecified	
665.92	UNSPECIFIED OBSTETRICAL TRAUMA DELIVERED W/PPC	**O71.9**	Obstetric trauma, unspecified	
665.93	UNSPECIFIED OBSTETRICAL TRAUMA ANTEPARTUM	**O71.9**	Obstetric trauma, unspecified	
665.94	UNSPECIFIED OB TRAUMA POSTPARTUM COND/COMPL	**O71.9**	Obstetric trauma, unspecified	
666.00	THIRD-STAGE PP HEMORR UNSPEC AS EPIS CARE	**O72.0**	Third-stage hemorrhage	
666.02	THIRD-STAGE POSTPARTUM HEMORRHAGE WITH DELIVERY	**O72.0**	Third-stage hemorrhage	
		O72.0	Third-stage hemorrhage	*and*
		O43.211	Placenta accreta, first trimester	*or*
		O43.212	Placenta accreta, second trimester	*or*
		O43.213	Placenta accreta, third trimester	*or*
		O43.221	Placenta increta, first trimester	*or*
		O43.222	Placenta increta, second trimester	*or*
		O43.223	Placenta increta, third trimester	*or*
		O43.231	Placenta percreta, first trimester	*or*
		O43.232	Placenta percreta, second trimester	*or*
		O43.233	Placenta percreta, third trimester	
666.04	THIRD-STAGE POSTPARTUM HEM POSTPARTUM COND/COMPL	**O72.0**	Third-stage hemorrhage	
		O72.0	Third-stage hemorrhage	*and*
		O43.211	Placenta accreta, first trimester	*or*
		O43.212	Placenta accreta, second trimester	*or*
		O43.213	Placenta accreta, third trimester	*or*
		O43.221	Placenta increta, first trimester	*or*
		O43.222	Placenta increta, second trimester	*or*
		O43.223	Placenta increta, third trimester	*or*
		O43.231	Placenta percreta, first trimester	*or*
		O43.232	Placenta percreta, second trimester	*or*
		O43.233	Placenta percreta, third trimester	
666.10	OTH IMMEDIATE PP HEMORR UNSPEC AS EPIS CARE	**O72.1**	Other immediate postpartum hemorrhage	
666.12	OTHER IMMEDIATE POSTPARTUM HEMORRHAGE W/DELIVERY	**O72.1**	Other immediate postpartum hemorrhage	
666.14	OTHER IMMED PP HEMORRHAGE POSTPARTUM COND/COMPL	**O72.1**	Other immediate postpartum hemorrhage	
666.20	DELAY&SEC POSTPARTUM HEMORR UNSPEC AS EPIS CARE	**O72.2**	Delayed and secondary postpartum hemorrhage	

[Brackets] indicate valid character values for each code. Character value meanings provided for each code grouping.

ICD-9-CM		ICD-10-CM	
666.22	DELAYED AND SEC POSTPARTUM HEMORRHAGE W/DELIVERY	**O72.2**	Delayed and secondary postpartum hemorrhage
666.24	DELAYED & SEC PP HEMORRHAGE POSTPARTUM COND/COMP	**O72.2**	Delayed and secondary postpartum hemorrhage
666.30	POSTPARTUM COAGULAT DEFEC UNSPEC AS EPISODE CARE	**O72.3**	Postpartum coagulation defects
666.32	POSTPARTUM COAGULATION DEFECTS WITH DELIVERY	**O72.3**	Postpartum coagulation defects
666.34	POSTPARTUM COAG DEFECTS POSTPARTUM COND/COMPL	**O72.3**	Postpartum coagulation defects
667.00	RETAIN PLACENTA W/O HEMORR UNSPEC AS EPIS CARE	**O43.219** **O43.229** **O43.239** **O73.0**	Placenta accreta, unspecified trimester Placenta increta, unspecified trimester Placenta percreta, unspecified trimester Retained placenta without hemorrhage
667.02	RETN PLACNTA W/O HEMORR DEL W/MENTION PP COMPL	**O43.211** **O43.212** **O43.213** **O43.221** **O43.222** **O43.223** **O43.231** **O43.232** **O43.233** **O73.0**	Placenta accreta, first trimester Placenta accreta, second trimester Placenta accreta, third trimester Placenta increta, first trimester Placenta increta, second trimester Placenta increta, third trimester Placenta percreta, first trimester Placenta percreta, second trimester Placenta percreta, third trimester Retained placenta without hemorrhage
667.04	RETAINED PLACENTA WITHOUT HEMORR PP COND/COMP	**O43.211** **O43.212** **O43.213** **O43.221** **O43.222** **O43.223** **O43.231** **O43.232** **O43.233** **O73.0**	Placenta accreta, first trimester Placenta accreta, second trimester Placenta accreta, third trimester Placenta increta, first trimester Placenta increta, second trimester Placenta increta, third trimester Placenta percreta, first trimester Placenta percreta, second trimester Placenta percreta, third trimester Retained placenta without hemorrhage
667.10	RETN PORTIONS PLACNTA/MEMB W/O HEMORR UNS EOC	**O73.1**	Retained portions of placenta and membranes, w/o hemorr
667.12	RETN PORTIONS PLCNTA/MEMB W/O HEMORR DEL W/COMPL	**O73.1**	Retained portions of placenta and membranes, w/o hemorr
667.14	RETN PORTIONS PLACNTA/MEMB W/O HEMOR PP COMPL	**O73.1**	Retained portions of placenta and membranes, w/o hemorr
668.00	PULM COMPL ADMN ANES/OTH SEDATION L&D UNS EOC	**O74.1**	Oth pulmonary comp of anesthesia during labor and delivery
668.01	PULM COMPL ADMN ANES/OTH SEDATION L&D DEL	**O74.0** **O74.1**	Aspirat pneumonitis due to anesth during labor and delivery Oth pulmonary comp of anesthesia during labor and delivery
668.02	PULM COMPL ADMN ANES/OTH SEDAT DEL W/PP COMPL	**O74.0** **O74.1** **O89.09**	Aspirat pneumonitis due to anesth during labor and delivery Oth pulmonary comp of anesthesia during labor and delivery Oth pulmonary comp of anesthesia during the puerperium
668.03	PULM COMPL ADMN ANES/OTH SEDATION L&D ANTPRTM	**O74.1**	Oth pulmonary comp of anesthesia during labor and delivery
668.04	PULM COMPL ADMIN ANES/OTH SED L&D PP COND/COMPL	**O89.01** **O89.09**	Aspiration pneumonitis due to anesth during the puerperium Oth pulmonary comp of anesthesia during the puerperium
668.10	CARD COMPL ADMN ANES/OTH SEDAT L&D UNS EOC	**O74.2**	Cardiac comp of anesthesia during labor and delivery
668.11	CARD COMPL ADMIN ANES/OTH SEDATION L&D DEL	**O74.2**	Cardiac comp of anesthesia during labor and delivery
668.12	CARD COMPL ADMIN ANES/SEDAT L&D-DEL W/PP COMPL	**O74.2**	Cardiac comp of anesthesia during labor and delivery
668.13	CARD COMPL ADMN ANES/OTH SEDAT L&D ANTPARTUM	**O74.2**	Cardiac comp of anesthesia during labor and delivery
668.14	CARD COMPL ADMN ANES/OTH SEDAT L&D PP COND/COMP	**O89.1**	Cardiac complications of anesthesia during the puerperium
668.20	CNA COMPL ADMN ANES/OTH SEDAT L&D DEL UNS EOC	**O74.3**	Cnsl complications of anesthesia during labor and delivery
668.21	CNA COMPL ADMN ANES/OTH SEDATION L&D DEL	**O74.3**	Cnsl complications of anesthesia during labor and delivery
668.22	CNA COMPL ADMN ANES/SEDAT L&D DEL W/PP COMPL	**O74.3**	Cnsl complications of anesthesia during labor and delivery
668.23	CNA COMPL ADMN ANES/OTH SEDAT L&D ANTEPARTUM	**O74.3**	Cnsl complications of anesthesia during labor and delivery
668.24	CNS COMPL ADMIN ANES/OTH SEDAT L&D PP COND/COMPL	**O89.2**	Cnsl complications of anesthesia during the puerperium
668.80	OTH COMPL ADMN ANES/OTH SEDAT L&D UNS EOC	**O74.8**	Other complications of anesthesia during labor and delivery
668.81	OTH COMPL ADMN ANES/OTH SEDATION L&D DEL	**O74.4** **O74.5** **O74.6** **O74.7** **O74.8**	Toxic reaction to local anesthesia during labor and delivery Spinal and epidur anesthesia-induced hdache dur labr and del Oth comp of spinal and epidural anesth during labor and del Failed or difficult intubation for anesth dur labor and del Other complications of anesthesia during labor and delivery
668.82	OTH COMPL ADMN ANES/OTH SEDAT DEL W/PP COMPL	**O74.4** **O74.5** **O74.6** **O74.7** **O74.8** **O89.8**	Toxic reaction to local anesthesia during labor and delivery Spinal and epidur anesthesia-induced hdache dur labr and del Oth comp of spinal and epidural anesth during labor and del Failed or difficult intubation for anesth dur labor and del Other complications of anesthesia during labor and delivery Other complications of anesthesia during the puerperium
668.83	OTH COMPL ADMN ANES/OTH SEDAT L&D ANTEPARTUM	**O74.8**	Other complications of anesthesia during labor and delivery
668.84	OTH COMPL ADMN ANES/OTH SEDAT L&D PP COND/COMPL	**O89.3** **O89.4** **O89.5** **O89.6** **O89.8**	Toxic reaction to local anesthesia during the puerperium Spinal and epidur anesthesia-induced hdache during the puerp Oth comp of spinal and epidural anesth during the puerperium Failed or difficult intubation for anesth during the puerp Other complications of anesthesia during the puerperium
668.90	UNS COMPL ADMN ANES/OTH SEDATION L&D UNS EOC	**O74.9**	Complication of anesthesia during labor and delivery, unsp
668.91	UNS COMPL ADMN ANES/OTH SEDATION L&D DEL	**O74.9**	Complication of anesthesia during labor and delivery, unsp
668.92	UNS COMP ADMN ANESTHESIA/OTH SEDAT L&D DEL W/PPC	**O74.9** **O89.9**	Complication of anesthesia during labor and delivery, unsp Complication of anesthesia during the puerperium, unsp
668.93	UNS COMPL ADMN ANES/OTH SEDAT L&D ANTEPARTUM	**O74.9**	Complication of anesthesia during labor and delivery, unsp

ICD-9-CM		ICD-10-CM	
668.94	UNS COMPL ADMIN ANES/OTH SEDAT L&D PP COND/COMPL	**O89.9**	Complication of anesthesia during the puerperium, unsp
669.ØØ	MATERNAL DISTRESS COMP L&D UNSPEC AS EPIS CARE	**O75.Ø**	Maternal distress during labor and delivery
669.Ø1	MTRN DISTRESS W/DELIV W/WO MENTION ANTPRTM COND	**O75.Ø**	Maternal distress during labor and delivery
669.Ø2	MATERNAL DISTRESS W/DELIVERY W/MENTION PPC	**O75.Ø**	Maternal distress during labor and delivery
669.Ø3	MATERNAL DISTRESS COMP L&D ANTPRTM COND/COMP	**O75.Ø**	Maternal distress during labor and delivery
669.Ø4	MATERNAL DISTRESS COMP L&D POSTPARTUM COND/COMP	**O75.Ø**	Maternal distress during labor and delivery
669.1Ø	SHOCK DURING/FOLLOWING L&D UNSPEC AS EPIS CARE	**O75.1**	Shock during or following labor and delivery
669.11	SHOCK DURING/FOLLOW L&D W/DEL W/W/O ANTPRTM COND	**O75.1**	Shock during or following labor and delivery
669.12	SHOCK DURING/FOLLOWING L&D W/DELIV W/MENTION PPC	**O75.1**	Shock during or following labor and delivery
669.13	SHOCK DURING OR FOLLOWING L&D ANTEPARTUM SHOCK	**O75.1**	Shock during or following labor and delivery
669.14	SHOCK DURNG/ FOLLOWING L&D POSTPARTUM COND/COMPL	**O75.1**	Shock during or following labor and delivery
669.2Ø	MTRN HYPOTENS SYND COMP L&D UNSPEC AS EPIS CARE	**O26.5Ø**	Maternal hypotension syndrome, unspecified trimester
669.21	MAT HYPOTENSION SYND W/DEL W/W/O ANTPRTM COND	**O26.51** **O26.52** **O26.53**	Maternal hypotension syndrome, first trimester Maternal hypotension syndrome, second trimester Maternal hypotension syndrome, third trimester
669.22	MATERNAL HYPOTENS SYNDROME W/DELIV W/MENTION PPC	**O26.51** **O26.52** **O26.53**	Maternal hypotension syndrome, first trimester Maternal hypotension syndrome, second trimester Maternal hypotension syndrome, third trimester
669.23	MATERNAL HYPOTENSION SYNDROME ANTEPARTUM	**O26.51** **O26.52** **O26.53**	Maternal hypotension syndrome, first trimester Maternal hypotension syndrome, second trimester Maternal hypotension syndrome, third trimester
669.24	MATERNAL HYPOTENSION SYND POSTPARTUM COND/COMPL	**O26.51** **O26.52** **O26.53**	Maternal hypotension syndrome, first trimester Maternal hypotension syndrome, second trimester Maternal hypotension syndrome, third trimester
669.3Ø	ACUTE KIDNEY FAIL FOLLOW L&D UNSPEC AS EOC/N/A	**O9Ø.4**	Postpartum acute kidney failure
669.32	ACUTE KIDNEY FAILURE FOLLOW L&D DELIV W/MEN PPC	**O9Ø.4**	Postpartum acute kidney failure
669.34	ACUTE KIDNEY FAIL FOLLOWING L&D PP COND OR COMP	**O9Ø.4**	Postpartum acute kidney failure
669.4Ø	OTH COMPS OB SURGERY&PROC UNSPEC AS EPIS CARE	**O75.4**	Other complications of obstetric surgery and procedures
669.41	OTH COMPL OB SURG&PROC DELIV W/WO ANTPRTM COND	**O75.4**	Other complications of obstetric surgery and procedures
669.42	OTH COMPL OB SURG&PROC W/DEL W/MENTION PP COMPL	**O75.4**	Other complications of obstetric surgery and procedures
669.43	OTH COMPS OB SURGERY&PROC ANTPRTM COND/COMP	**O75.4**	Other complications of obstetric surgery and procedures
669.44	OTH COMPS OB SURGERY&PROC POSTPARTUM COND/COMP	**O75.4**	Other complications of obstetric surgery and procedures
669.5Ø	FORCEPS/VAC EXT DELIV W/O INDICAT UNS EPIS CARE	**O66.5**	Attempted application of vacuum extractor and forceps
669.51	FORCEPS/EXTRACTOR DEL W/O INDICATION-DELIVERED	**O66.5**	Attempted application of vacuum extractor and forceps
669.6Ø	BREECH XTRAC W/O MENTION INDICAT UNS EPIS CARE	**O64.1XXØ**	Obstructed labor due to breech presentation, unsp
669.61	BREECH XTRAC W/O INDICAT DELIV W/WO ANTPRTM COND	**O64.1XXØ**	Obstructed labor due to breech presentation, unsp
669.7Ø	C/S DELIV W/O MENTION INDICAT UNS AS EPIS CARE	**O82**	Encounter for cesarean delivery without indication
669.71	C/S DELIV W/O INDICAT DELIV W/WO ANTPRTM COND	**O82**	Encounter for cesarean delivery without indication
669.8Ø	OTHER COMPLICATION L&D UNSPEC AS EPISODE CARE	**O75.81** **O75.89**	Maternal exhaustion complicating labor and delivery Other specified complications of labor and delivery
669.81	OTH COMP L&D DELIVERED W/WO MENTION ANTPRTM COND	**O75.81** **O75.89**	Maternal exhaustion complicating labor and delivery Other specified complications of labor and delivery
669.82	OTHER COMPLICATION L&D DELIVERED W/MENTION PPC	**O75.81** **O75.89**	Maternal exhaustion complicating labor and delivery Other specified complications of labor and delivery
669.83	OTH COMPLICATION L&D ANTPRTM COND/COMPLICATION	**O75.81** **O75.89**	Maternal exhaustion complicating labor and delivery Other specified complications of labor and delivery
669.84	OTH COMP L&D POSTPARTUM COND/COMP	**O75.81** **O75.89**	Maternal exhaustion complicating labor and delivery Other specified complications of labor and delivery
669.9Ø	UNSPEC COMPLICATION L&D UNSPEC AS EPISODE CARE	**O75.9**	Complication of labor and delivery, unspecified
669.91	UNSPEC COMP L&D DELIV W/WO MENTION ANTPRTM COND	**O75.9**	Complication of labor and delivery, unspecified
669.92	UNSPEC COMPLICATION L&D W/DELIVERY W/MENTION PPC	**O75.9**	Complication of labor and delivery, unspecified
669.93	UNSPEC COMP L&D ANTPRTM COND/COMP	**O75.9**	Complication of labor and delivery, unspecified
669.94	UNSPEC COMP L&D POSTPARTUM COND/COMP	**O75.9**	Complication of labor and delivery, unspecified
67Ø.ØØ	MAJOR PUERPERAL INFECTION UNS UNS AS TO EOC/NA	**O86.89**	Other specified puerperal infections
67Ø.Ø2	MAJOR PUERPERAL INFECTION, UNSPECIFIED, DELIVERE	**O86.89**	Other specified puerperal infections
67Ø.Ø4	MAJOR PUERPERAL INFECTION UNSPEC PP COND/COMP	**O86.89**	Other specified puerperal infections
67Ø.1Ø	PUERPERAL ENDOMETRITIS UNSPECIFIED AS TO EOC/N/A	**O86.12**	Endometritis following delivery
67Ø.12	PUERPERAL ENDOMETRITIS DELIVERED W/MEN PP COMP	**O86.12**	Endometritis following delivery
67Ø.14	PUERPERAL ENDOMETRITIS PP CONDITION/COMPLICATION	**O86.12**	Endometritis following delivery
67Ø.2Ø	PUERPERAL SEPSIS UNSPEC AS TO EOC/NOT APPLICABLE	**O85**	Puerperal sepsis
67Ø.22	PUERPERAL SEPSIS DELIVERED W/MENTION OF PP COMP	**O85**	Puerperal sepsis
67Ø.24	PUERPERAL SEPSIS PP CONDITION OR COMPLICATION	**O85**	Puerperal sepsis
67Ø.3Ø	PUERPERAL SEPTIC THROMBOPHLEBITIS UNS AS EOC/N/A	**O86.81**	Puerperal septic thrombophlebitis
67Ø.32	PUERPERAL SEPTIC THROMBOPHLEBITS DEL MEN PP COMP	**O86.81**	Puerperal septic thrombophlebitis
67Ø.34	PUERPERAL SEPTIC THROMBOPHLEBITIS PP COND/COMP	**O86.81**	Puerperal septic thrombophlebitis
67Ø.8Ø	OTH MAJOR PUERPERAL INFECTION UNSPEC AS EOC/N/A	**O86.89**	Other specified puerperal infections
67Ø.82	OTHER MAJOR PUERPERAL INFECTION DEL MEN PP COMP	**O86.89**	Other specified puerperal infections
67Ø.84	OTHER MAJOR PUERPERAL INFECTION PP COND/COMP	**O86.89**	Other specified puerperal infections
671.ØØ	VARICOSE VNS LEGS COMP PG&THE PUERPERIUM UNS EOC	**O22.ØØ**	Varicose veins of low extrm in pregnancy, unsp trimester

[Brackets] indicate valid character values for each code. Character value meanings provided for each code grouping.

ICD-9-CM		ICD-10-CM	
671.01	VARICOSE VNS LEGS DELIV W/WO ANTPRTM COND	O22.01 O22.02 O22.03	Varicose veins of low extrm in pregnancy, first trimester Varicose veins of low extrm in pregnancy, second trimester Varicose veins of low extrm in pregnancy, third trimester
671.02	VARICOSE VEINS LEGS W/DELIVERY W/MENTION PPC	O87.4	Varicose veins of lower extremity in the puerperium
671.03	VARICOSE VEINS OF LEGS, ANTEPARTUM	O22.01 O22.02 O22.03	Varicose veins of low extrm in pregnancy, first trimester Varicose veins of low extrm in pregnancy, second trimester Varicose veins of low extrm in pregnancy, third trimester
671.04	VARICOSE VEINS OF LEGS, POSTPARTUM COND/COMPL	O87.4	Varicose veins of lower extremity in the puerperium
671.10	VARICOS VNS VULVA&PERIN COMP PG&PP UNS EOC	O22.10	Genital varices in pregnancy, unspecified trimester
671.11	VARICOSE VNS VULVA&PERIN DELIV W/WO ANTPRTM COND	O22.11 O22.12 O22.13	Genital varices in pregnancy, first trimester Genital varices in pregnancy, second trimester Genital varices in pregnancy, third trimester
671.12	VARICOSE VEINS VULVA&PERIN W/DELIV W/MENTION PPC	O22.11 O22.12 O22.13	Genital varices in pregnancy, first trimester Genital varices in pregnancy, second trimester Genital varices in pregnancy, third trimester
671.13	VARICOSE VEINS OF VULVA AND PERINEUM ANTEPARTUM	O22.11 O22.12 O22.13	Genital varices in pregnancy, first trimester Genital varices in pregnancy, second trimester Genital varices in pregnancy, third trimester
671.14	VARICSE VEINS VULVA & PERINEUM POSTPRT COND/COMP	O22.11 O22.12 O22.13	Genital varices in pregnancy, first trimester Genital varices in pregnancy, second trimester Genital varices in pregnancy, third trimester
671.20	SUP THROMBOPHLEB COMP PG&THE PUERPERIUM UNS EOC	O22.20	Superficial thrombophlebitis in pregnancy, unsp trimester
671.21	SUP THROMBOPHLEB DELIV W/WO MENTION ANTPRTM COND	O22.21 O22.22 O22.23	Superficial thrombophlebitis in pregnancy, first trimester Superficial thrombophlebitis in pregnancy, second trimester Superficial thrombophlebitis in pregnancy, third trimester
671.22	SUP THROMBOPHLEBITIS W/DELIV W/MENTION PPC	O87.0	Superficial thrombophlebitis in the puerperium
671.23	SUPERFICIAL THROMBOPHLEBITIS ANTEPARTUM	O22.21 O22.22 O22.23	Superficial thrombophlebitis in pregnancy, first trimester Superficial thrombophlebitis in pregnancy, second trimester Superficial thrombophlebitis in pregnancy, third trimester
671.24	SUPERFICIAL THROMBOPHLEBITIS PP COND/COMPL	O87.0	Superficial thrombophlebitis in the puerperium
671.30	DEEP PHLEBOTHROMB ANTPRTM UNSPEC AS EPIS CARE	O22.30	Deep phlebothrombosis in pregnancy, unspecified trimester
671.31	DEEP PHLEBOTHROMBOSIS ANTEPARTUM WITH DELIVERY	O22.31 O22.32 O22.33	Deep phlebothrombosis in pregnancy, first trimester Deep phlebothrombosis in pregnancy, second trimester Deep phlebothrombosis in pregnancy, third trimester
671.33	DEEP PHLEBOTHROMBOSIS ANTPRTM-ANTPRTM COND/COMP	O22.31 O22.32 O22.33	Deep phlebothrombosis in pregnancy, first trimester Deep phlebothrombosis in pregnancy, second trimester Deep phlebothrombosis in pregnancy, third trimester
671.40	DEEP PHLEBOTHROMBOSIS PP UNSPEC AS EPIS CARE	O87.1	Deep phlebothrombosis in the puerperium
671.42	DEEP PHLEBOTHROMBOSIS POSTPARTUM WITH DELIVERY	O87.1	Deep phlebothrombosis in the puerperium
671.44	DEEP PHLEBOTHROMBOSIS POSTPARTUM COND/COMPL	O87.1	Deep phlebothrombosis in the puerperium
671.50	OTH PHLEBITIS&THROMB COMP PG&PP UNS EOC	O22.50	Cerebral venous thrombosis in pregnancy, unsp trimester
671.51	OTH PHLEBITIS&THROMB DELIV W/WO ANTPRTM COND	O22.51 O22.52 O22.53 O22.91 O22.92 O22.93	Cerebral venous thrombosis in pregnancy, first trimester Cerebral venous thrombosis in pregnancy, second trimester Cerebral venous thrombosis in pregnancy, third trimester Venous complication in pregnancy, unsp, first trimester Venous complication in pregnancy, unsp, second trimester Venous complication in pregnancy, unsp, third trimester
671.52	OTH PHLEBITIS&THROMBOSIS W/DELIV W/MENTION PPC	O87.3	Cerebral venous thrombosis in the puerperium
671.53	OTHER ANTEPARTUM PHLEBITIS AND THROMBOSIS	O22.51 O22.52 O22.53 O22.91 O22.92 O22.93	Cerebral venous thrombosis in pregnancy, first trimester Cerebral venous thrombosis in pregnancy, second trimester Cerebral venous thrombosis in pregnancy, third trimester Venous complication in pregnancy, unsp, first trimester Venous complication in pregnancy, unsp, second trimester Venous complication in pregnancy, unsp, third trimester
671.54	OTHER PHLEBITIS AND THROMBOSIS PP COND/COMPL	O87.3	Cerebral venous thrombosis in the puerperium
671.80	OTH VENUS COMP PG&THE PUERPERIUM UNS EPIS CARE	O22.40 O22.8X9	Hemorrhoids in pregnancy, unspecified trimester Other venous complications in pregnancy, unsp trimester
671.81	OTH VENOUS COMP DELIV W/WO MENTION ANTPRTM COND	O22.41 O22.42 O22.43 O22.8X1 O22.8X2 O22.8X3	Hemorrhoids in pregnancy, first trimester Hemorrhoids in pregnancy, second trimester Hemorrhoids in pregnancy, third trimester Other venous complications in pregnancy, first trimester Other venous complications in pregnancy, second trimester Other venous complications in pregnancy, third trimester
671.82	OTH VENOUS COMPLICATION W/DELIVERY W/MENTION PPC	O87.2 O87.8	Hemorrhoids in the puerperium Other venous complications in the puerperium
671.83	OTHER VENOUS COMPLICATION ANTEPARTUM	O22.41 O22.42 O22.43 O22.8X1 O22.8X2 O22.8X3	Hemorrhoids in pregnancy, first trimester Hemorrhoids in pregnancy, second trimester Hemorrhoids in pregnancy, third trimester Other venous complications in pregnancy, first trimester Other venous complications in pregnancy, second trimester Other venous complications in pregnancy, third trimester
671.84	OTHER VENOUS COMPLICATION POSTPARTUM COND/COMPL	O87.2 O87.8	Hemorrhoids in the puerperium Other venous complications in the puerperium
671.90	UNS VENUS COMP PG&THE PUERPERIUM UNS EPIS CARE	O22.90	Venous complication in pregnancy, unsp, unsp trimester

ICD-9-CM		ICD-10-CM	
671.91	UNS VENOUS COMP DELIV W/WO MENTION ANTPRTM COND	**O22.91**	Venous complication in pregnancy, unsp, first trimester
		O22.92	Venous complication in pregnancy, unsp, second trimester
		O22.93	Venous complication in pregnancy, unsp, third trimester
671.92	UNSPEC VENOUS COMP W/DELIVERY W/MENTION PPC	**O87.9**	Venous complication in the puerperium, unspecified
671.93	UNSPECIFIED VENOUS COMPLICATION ANTEPARTUM	**O22.91**	Venous complication in pregnancy, unsp, first trimester
		O22.92	Venous complication in pregnancy, unsp, second trimester
		O22.93	Venous complication in pregnancy, unsp, third trimester
671.94	UNSPECIFIED VENOUS COMPLICATION PP COND/COMPL	**O87.9**	Venous complication in the puerperium, unspecified
672.00	PUERPERAL PYREXIA UNKN ORIGIN UNS AS EPIS CARE	**O86.4**	Pyrexia of unknown origin following delivery
672.02	PUERPERAL PYREXIA UNKN ORIGIN DELIV W/ PPC	**O86.4**	Pyrexia of unknown origin following delivery
672.04	PUERPERAL PYREXIA OF UNKN ORIGIN PP COND/COMPL	**O86.4**	Pyrexia of unknown origin following delivery
673.00	OBSTETRICAL AIR EMBOLISM UNSPEC AS EPISODE CARE	**O88.019**	Air embolism in pregnancy, unspecified trimester
673.01	OB AIR EMBO W/DELIV W/WO MENTION ANTPRTM COND	**O88.011**	Air embolism in pregnancy, first trimester
		O88.012	Air embolism in pregnancy, second trimester
		O88.013	Air embolism in pregnancy, third trimester
		O88.02	Air embolism in childbirth
673.02	OBSTETRICAL AIR EMBOLISM W/DELIV W/MENTION PPC	**O88.02**	Air embolism in childbirth
		O88.03	Air embolism in the puerperium
673.03	OBSTETRICAL AIR EMBOLISM ANTPRTM COND/COMP	**O88.011**	Air embolism in pregnancy, first trimester
		O88.012	Air embolism in pregnancy, second trimester
		O88.013	Air embolism in pregnancy, third trimester
673.04	OBSTETRICAL AIR EMBOLISM POSTPARTUM COND/COMP	**O88.03**	Air embolism in the puerperium
673.10	AMNIOTIC FLUID EMBOLISM UNSPEC AS EPISODE CARE	**O88.119**	Amniotic fluid embolism in pregnancy, unspecified trimester
673.11	AMNIOTIC FLUID EMBOLISM DEL W/WO ANTEPARTUM COND	**O88.111**	Amniotic fluid embolism in pregnancy, first trimester
		O88.112	Amniotic fluid embolism in pregnancy, second trimester
		O88.113	Amniotic fluid embolism in pregnancy, third trimester
		O88.12	Amniotic fluid embolism in childbirth
673.12	AMNIOTIC FLUID EMBOLISM W/DELIVERY W/MENTION PPC	**O88.12**	Amniotic fluid embolism in childbirth
		O88.13	Amniotic fluid embolism in the puerperium
673.13	AMNIOTIC FLUID EMBOLISM ANTPRTM COND/COMP	**O88.111**	Amniotic fluid embolism in pregnancy, first trimester
		O88.112	Amniotic fluid embolism in pregnancy, second trimester
		O88.113	Amniotic fluid embolism in pregnancy, third trimester
673.14	AMNIOTIC FLUID EMBOLISM POSTPARTUM COND/COMP	**O88.13**	Amniotic fluid embolism in the puerperium
673.20	OBSTETRICAL BLD-CLOT EMBO UNSPEC AS EPISODE CARE	**O88.219**	Thromboembolism in pregnancy, unspecified trimester
673.21	OB BLD-CLOT EMBOLISM DEL W/WO ANTEPARTUM COND	**O88.211**	Thromboembolism in pregnancy, first trimester
		O88.212	Thromboembolism in pregnancy, second trimester
		O88.213	Thromboembolism in pregnancy, third trimester
		O88.22	Thromboembolism in childbirth
673.22	OBSTETRICAL BLOOD-CLOT EMBOLISM W/MENTION PPC	**O88.22**	Thromboembolism in childbirth
		O88.23	Thromboembolism in the puerperium
673.23	OBSTETRICAL BLOOD-CLOT EMBOLISM ANTEPARTUM	**O88.211**	Thromboembolism in pregnancy, first trimester
		O88.212	Thromboembolism in pregnancy, second trimester
		O88.213	Thromboembolism in pregnancy, third trimester
673.24	OBSTETRICAL BLOOD-CLOT EMBOLISM PP COND/COMPL	**O88.23**	Thromboembolism in the puerperium
673.30	OB PYEMIC&SEPTIC EMBO UNSPEC AS EPIS CARE	**O88.319**	Pyemic and septic embolism in pregnancy, unsp trimester
673.31	OB PYEMIC&SEPTIC EMBOLISM DEL W/WO ANTPRTM COND	**O88.311**	Pyemic and septic embolism in pregnancy, first trimester
		O88.312	Pyemic and septic embolism in pregnancy, second trimester
		O88.313	Pyemic and septic embolism in pregnancy, third trimester
		O88.32	Pyemic and septic embolism in childbirth
673.32	OB PYEMIC&SEPTIC EMBOLISM DELIVERY W/PP COMPL	**O88.32**	Pyemic and septic embolism in childbirth
		O88.33	Pyemic and septic embolism in the puerperium
673.33	OBSTETRICAL PYEMIC&SEPTIC EMBOLISM ANTEPARTUM	**O88.311**	Pyemic and septic embolism in pregnancy, first trimester
		O88.312	Pyemic and septic embolism in pregnancy, second trimester
		O88.313	Pyemic and septic embolism in pregnancy, third trimester
673.34	OBSTETRICAL PYEMIC&SEPTIC EMBOLISM PP COND/COMPL	**O88.33**	Pyemic and septic embolism in the puerperium
673.80	OTH OB PULMONARY EMBO UNSPEC AS EPIS CARE	**O88.819**	Other embolism in pregnancy, unspecified trimester
673.81	OTH OB PULMARY EMBOLSIM DEL W/WO ANTEPARTUM COND	**O88.811**	Other embolism in pregnancy, first trimester
		O88.812	Other embolism in pregnancy, second trimester
		O88.813	Other embolism in pregnancy, third trimester
		O88.82	Other embolism in childbirth
673.82	OTH OB PULMONARY EMBO W/DELIV W/MENTION PPC	**O88.811**	Other embolism in pregnancy, first trimester
		O88.812	Other embolism in pregnancy, second trimester
		O88.813	Other embolism in pregnancy, third trimester
		O88.82	Other embolism in childbirth
		O88.83	Other embolism in the puerperium
673.83	OTHER OBSTETRICAL PULMONARY EMBOLISM ANTEPARTUM	**O88.811**	Other embolism in pregnancy, first trimester
		O88.812	Other embolism in pregnancy, second trimester
		O88.813	Other embolism in pregnancy, third trimester
673.84	OTHER OBSTET PULMONARY EMBOLISM PP COND/COMPL	**O88.83**	Other embolism in the puerperium
674.00	CERBROVASCULAR D/O OCCURRING PG CB/PP UNS EOC	**O99.419**	Diseases of the circ sys comp pregnancy, unsp trimester
674.01	CERBROVASC D/O DELIV W/WO MENTION ANTPRTM COND	**O99.411**	Diseases of the circ sys comp pregnancy, first trimester
		O99.412	Diseases of the circ sys comp pregnancy, second trimester
		O99.413	Diseases of the circ sys comp pregnancy, third trimester
		O99.42	Diseases of the circulatory system complicating childbirth

[Brackets] indicate valid character values for each code. Character value meanings provided for each code grouping.

ICD-9-CM		ICD-10-CM	
674.02	CEREBRVASC DISORDER W/DELIVERY W/MENTION PPC	O99.42 O99.43	Diseases of the circulatory system complicating childbirth Diseases of the circ sys complicating the puerperium
674.03	CEREBROVASCULAR DISORDER ANTEPARTUM	O99.411 O99.412 O99.413	Diseases of the circ sys comp pregnancy, first trimester Diseases of the circ sys comp pregnancy, second trimester Diseases of the circ sys comp pregnancy, third trimester
674.04	CEREBROVASCULAR DISRD PUERP PP COND/COMPL	O99.43	Diseases of the circ sys complicating the puerperium
674.10	DISRUPTION CESAREAN WOUND UNSPEC AS EPISODE CARE	O90.0	Disruption of cesarean delivery wound
674.12	DISRUPTION C-SECT WOUND W/DELIVERY W/MENTION PPC	O90.0	Disruption of cesarean delivery wound
674.14	DISRUPTION OF CESAREAN WOUND PP COND/COMPL	O90.0	Disruption of cesarean delivery wound
674.20	DISRUPT PERINL WOUND UNSPEC AS EPIS CARE PG	O90.1	Disruption of perineal obstetric wound
674.22	DISRUPTRUPT PERINL WOUND W/DEL W/PP COMPLICATON	O90.1	Disruption of perineal obstetric wound
674.24	DISRUPTION PERINEAL WOUND POSTPARTUM COND/COMPL	O90.1	Disruption of perineal obstetric wound
674.30	OTH COMP OB SURGICAL WOUNDS UNSPEC AS EPIS CARE	O86.0 O90.2	Infection of obstetric surgical wound Hematoma of obstetric wound
674.32	OTH COMP OB SURG WOUNDS W/DELIV W/MENTION PPC	O86.0 O90.2	Infection of obstetric surgical wound Hematoma of obstetric wound
674.34	OTH COMP OB SURGICAL WOUNDS POSTPARTUM COND/COMP	O86.0 O90.2	Infection of obstetric surgical wound Hematoma of obstetric wound
674.40	PLACENTAL POLYP UNSPECIFIED AS TO EPISODE CARE	O90.89	Oth complications of the puerperium, NEC
674.42	PLACENTAL POLYP W/DELIVERY W/MENTION PPC	O90.89	Oth complications of the puerperium, NEC
674.44	PLACENTAL POLYP, POSTPARTUM COND/COMPL	O90.89	Oth complications of the puerperium, NEC
674.50	PERIPARTUM CARDIOMYPATH UNS EPIS CARE/NOT APPLIC	O90.3	Peripartum cardiomyopathy
674.51	PERIPARTUM CARDIOMYPATH DELIV W/WO ANTPRTM COND	O90.3	Peripartum cardiomyopathy
674.52	PERIPARTUM CARDIOMYPATH DELIV W/MENTION PP COND	O90.3	Peripartum cardiomyopathy
674.53	PERIPARTUM CARDIOMYOPATHY ANTPRTM COND/COMP	O90.3	Peripartum cardiomyopathy
674.54	PERIPARTUM CARDIOMYOPATHY POSTPARTUM COND/COMP	O90.3	Peripartum cardiomyopathy
674.80	OTH COMP PUERPERIUM UNSPEC AS EPISODE CARE	O90.89	Oth complications of the puerperium, NEC
674.82	OTH COMP PUERPERIUM W/DELIVERY W/MENTION PPC	O90.89	Oth complications of the puerperium, NEC
674.84	OTHER COMPL OF PUERPERIUM PP COND/COMPL	O90.89	Oth complications of the puerperium, NEC
674.90	UNSPEC COMPS PUERPERIUM UNSPEC AS EPISODE CARE	O90.9	Complication of the puerperium, unspecified
674.92	UNSPEC COMPS PUERPERIUM W/DELIVERY W/MENTION PPC	O90.9	Complication of the puerperium, unspecified
674.94	UNSPECIFIED COMPL OF PUERPERIUM PP COND/COMPL	O90.9	Complication of the puerperium, unspecified
675.00	INF NIPPLE ASSOC W/CHILDBRTH UNSPEC AS EPIS CARE	O91.019	Infection of nipple associated w pregnancy, unsp trimester
675.01	INF NIPPLE W/CHLDBRTH DEL W/WO ANTEPARTUM COND	O91.011 O91.012 O91.013	Infection of nipple associated w pregnancy, first trimester Infection of nipple associated w pregnancy, second trimester Infection of nipple associated w pregnancy, third trimester
675.02	INF NIPPLE ASSOC W/CHILDBRTH DELIV W/MENTION PPC	O91.02	Infection of nipple associated with the puerperium
675.03	INFECTION OF NIPPLE, ANTEPARTUM	O91.011 O91.012 O91.013	Infection of nipple associated w pregnancy, first trimester Infection of nipple associated w pregnancy, second trimester Infection of nipple associated w pregnancy, third trimester
675.04	INFECTION OF NIPPLE POSTPARTUM COND/COMPL	O91.02 O91.03	Infection of nipple associated with the puerperium Infection of nipple associated with lactation
675.10	ABSC BRST ASSOC W/CHILDBIRTH UNSPEC AS EPIS CARE	O91.119	Abscess of breast associated with pregnancy, unsp trimester
675.11	ABSCESS BREAST W/CHLDBRTH DEL W/WO ANTPRTM COND	O91.111 O91.112 O91.113	Abscess of breast associated with pregnancy, first trimester Abscess of breast associated w pregnancy, second trimester Abscess of breast associated with pregnancy, third trimester
675.12	ABSC BRST ASSOC W/CHILDBIRTH DELIV W/MENTION PPC	O91.12	Abscess of breast associated with the puerperium
675.13	ABSCESS OF BREAST, ANTEPARTUM	O91.111 O91.112 O91.113	Abscess of breast associated with pregnancy, first trimester Abscess of breast associated w pregnancy, second trimester Abscess of breast associated with pregnancy, third trimester
675.14	ABSCESS OF BREAST POSTPARTUM COND/COMPL	O91.12 O91.13	Abscess of breast associated with the puerperium Abscess of breast associated with lactation
675.20	NONPURULENT MASTITIS-UNS EPIS PRE/POSTNATAL CARE	O91.219	Nonpurulent mastitis associated w pregnancy, unsp trimester
675.21	NONPURULENT MASTITIS DELIV W/WO ANTPRTM COND	O91.211 O91.212 O91.213	Nonpurulent mastitis associated w pregnancy, first trimester Nonpurulent mastitis assoc w pregnancy, second trimester Nonpurulent mastitis associated w pregnancy, third trimester
675.22	NONPURULENT MASTITIS DELIVERED W/MENTION PPC	O91.22	Nonpurulent mastitis associated with the puerperium
675.23	NONPURULENT MASTITIS, ANTEPARTUM	O91.211 O91.212 O91.213	Nonpurulent mastitis associated w pregnancy, first trimester Nonpurulent mastitis assoc w pregnancy, second trimester Nonpurulent mastitis associated w pregnancy, third trimester
675.24	NONPURULENT MASTITIS, POSTPARTUM COND/COMPL	O91.22	Nonpurulent mastitis associated with the puerperium
675.80	OTH SPEC INF BREAST&NIPPLE W/CHILDBIRTH UNS EOC	O91.23	Nonpurulent mastitis associated with lactation
675.81	OTH SPEC BREAST-NIPPLE INFECT ASSOC W/CB DELIVER	O91.23	Nonpurulent mastitis associated with lactation
675.82	OTH INF BRST&NIPPLE W/CHLDBRTH DEL W/PP COMPL	O91.23	Nonpurulent mastitis associated with lactation
675.83	OTHER SPEC INFECTION BREAST&NIPPLE ANTEPARTUM	O91.23	Nonpurulent mastitis associated with lactation
675.84	OTHER SPEC INFECTION BREAST&NIPPLE PP COND/COMPL	O91.23	Nonpurulent mastitis associated with lactation
675.90	UNS INF BRST&NIPPLE UNS PRENATAL/POSTNATAL EOC	O91.23	Nonpurulent mastitis associated with lactation
675.91	UNS INF BRST&NIPPLE DELIV W/WO ANTPRTM COND	O91.23	Nonpurulent mastitis associated with lactation
675.92	UNSPEC INF BREAST&NIPPLE DELIV W/MENTION PPC	O91.23	Nonpurulent mastitis associated with lactation
675.93	UNSPECIFIED INFECTION BREAST&NIPPLE ANTEPARTUM	O91.23	Nonpurulent mastitis associated with lactation

ICD-9-CM		ICD-10-CM	
675.94	UNS INFECT BREAST NIPPLE POSTPARTUM COND/COMPL	**O91.23**	Nonpurulent mastitis associated with lactation
676.ØØ	RETRACTED NIPPLE UNS PRENATAL/POSTNATAL EOC	**O92.Ø19**	Retracted nipple associated with pregnancy, unsp trimester
676.Ø1	RETRACTED NIPPLE DELIV W/WO MENTION ANTPRTM COND	**O92.Ø11** **O92.Ø12** **O92.Ø13**	Retracted nipple associated with pregnancy, first trimester Retracted nipple associated with pregnancy, second trimester Retracted nipple associated with pregnancy, third trimester
676.Ø2	RETRACTED NIPPLE DELIVERED W/MENTION PPC	**O92.Ø3**	Retracted nipple associated with lactation
676.Ø3	RETRACTED NIPPLE ANTEPARTUM COND/COMPLICATION	**O92.Ø11** **O92.Ø12** **O92.Ø13**	Retracted nipple associated with pregnancy, first trimester Retracted nipple associated with pregnancy, second trimester Retracted nipple associated with pregnancy, third trimester
676.Ø4	RETRACTED NIPPLE POSTPARTUM COND/COMPLICATION	**O92.Ø2** **O92.Ø3**	Retracted nipple associated with the puerperium Retracted nipple associated with lactation
676.1Ø	CRACKED NIPPLE UNS PRENATAL/POSTNATAL EPIS CARE	**O92.119**	Cracked nipple associated with pregnancy, unsp trimester
676.11	CRACKED NIPPLE DELIV W/WO MENTION ANTPRTM COND	**O92.111** **O92.112** **O92.113**	Cracked nipple associated with pregnancy, first trimester Cracked nipple associated with pregnancy, second trimester Cracked nipple associated with pregnancy, third trimester
676.12	CRACKED NIPPLE DELIVERED W/MENTION PPC	**O92.13**	Cracked nipple associated with lactation
676.13	CRACKED NIPPLE ANTEPARTUM CONDITION/COMPLICATION	**O92.111** **O92.112** **O92.113**	Cracked nipple associated with pregnancy, first trimester Cracked nipple associated with pregnancy, second trimester Cracked nipple associated with pregnancy, third trimester
676.14	CRACKED NIPPLE POSTPARTUM CONDITION/COMPLICATION	**O92.12** **O92.13**	Cracked nipple associated with the puerperium Cracked nipple associated with lactation
676.2Ø	ENGORGEMENT BRSTS UNS PRENATAL/POSTNATAL EOC	**O92.29**	Oth disorders of breast assoc w pregnancy and the puerperium
676.21	ENGORGEMENT BREASTS DEL W/WO ANTEPARTUM COND	**O92.29**	Oth disorders of breast assoc w pregnancy and the puerperium
676.22	ENGORGEMENT BREASTS DELIVERED W/MENTION PPC	**O92.29**	Oth disorders of breast assoc w pregnancy and the puerperium
676.23	ENGORGEMENT OF BREAST, ANTEPARTUM	**O92.29**	Oth disorders of breast assoc w pregnancy and the puerperium
676.24	ENGORGEMENT OF BREASTS, POSTPARTUM COND/COMPL	**O92.29**	Oth disorders of breast assoc w pregnancy and the puerperium
676.3Ø	OTH&UNS D/O BRST ASSOC W/CHLDBRTH UNS EPIS CARE	**O92.2Ø** **O92.29**	Unsp disorder of breast assoc w pregnancy and the puerperium Oth disorders of breast assoc w pregnancy and the puerperium
676.31	UNS D/O BREAST W/CHLDBRTH DEL W/WO ANTPRTM COND	**O92.2Ø** **O92.29**	Unsp disorder of breast assoc w pregnancy and the puerperium Oth disorders of breast assoc w pregnancy and the puerperium
676.32	OTH&UNS D/O BREAST W/CHILDBIRTH DEL W/PP COMPL	**O92.2Ø** **O92.29**	Unsp disorder of breast assoc w pregnancy and the puerperium Oth disorders of breast assoc w pregnancy and the puerperium
676.33	OTH&UNS D/O BRSTW/CHLDBRTH ANTPRTM COND/COMP	**O92.2Ø**	Unsp disorder of breast assoc w pregnancy and the puerperium
676.34	OTH&UNS D/O BRST ASSOC W/CHLDBRTH PP COND/COMP	**O92.2Ø** **O92.29**	Unsp disorder of breast assoc w pregnancy and the puerperium Oth disorders of breast assoc w pregnancy and the puerperium
676.4Ø	FAILURE LACTATION UNSPECIFIED AS TO EPISODE CARE	**O92.3**	Agalactia
676.41	FAILED LACTATION W/DEL W/WO MENTION ANTPRTM COND	**O92.3**	Agalactia
676.42	FAILURE LACTATION W/DELIVERY W/MENTION PPC	**O92.3**	Agalactia
676.43	FAILURE LACTATION ANTEPARTUM COND/COMPLICATION	**O92.3**	Agalactia
676.44	FAILURE LACTATION POSTPARTUM COND/COMPLICATION	**O92.3**	Agalactia
676.5Ø	SUPPRESSED LACTATION UNSPECIFIED AS EPISODE CARE	**O92.5**	Suppressed lactation
676.51	SUPPRESSED LACTATION DELIV W/WO ANTPRTM COND	**O92.5**	Suppressed lactation
676.52	SUPPRESSED LACTATION W/DELIVERY W/MENTION PPC	**O92.5**	Suppressed lactation
676.53	SUPPRESSED LACTATION ANTPRTM COND/COMPLICATION	**O92.5**	Suppressed lactation
676.54	SUPPRESSED LACTATION POSTPARTUM COND/COMP	**O92.5**	Suppressed lactation
676.6Ø	GALACTORRHEA ASSOC W/CHLDBRTH UNS AS EPIS CARE	**O92.6**	Galactorrhea
676.61	GALACTORRHEA W/DELIV W/WO MENTION ANTPRTM COND	**O92.6**	Galactorrhea
676.62	GALACTORRHEA W/DELIVERY W/MENTION PPC	**O92.6**	Galactorrhea
676.63	GALACTORRHEA ANTEPARTUM CONDITION/COMPLICATION	**O92.6**	Galactorrhea
676.64	GALACTORRHEA POSTPARTUM CONDITION/COMPLICATION	**O92.6**	Galactorrhea
676.8Ø	OTHER DISORDER LACTATION UNSPEC AS EPISODE CARE	**O92.79**	Other disorders of lactation
676.81	OTH D/O LACTATION DELIV W/WO ANTPRTM COND	**O92.79**	Other disorders of lactation
676.82	OTH DISORDER LACTATION W/DELIVERY W/MENTION PPC	**O92.79**	Other disorders of lactation
676.83	OTH DISORDER LACTATION ANTPRTM COND/COMPLICATION	**O92.79**	Other disorders of lactation
676.84	OTH DISORDERS LACTATION POSTPARTUM COND/COMP	**O92.4** **O92.79**	Hypogalactia Other disorders of lactation
676.9Ø	UNSPEC DISORDER LACTATION UNSPEC AS EPISODE CARE	**O92.7Ø**	Unspecified disorders of lactation
676.91	UNS D/O LACTATION DELIV W/WO ANTPRTM COND	**O92.7Ø**	Unspecified disorders of lactation
676.92	UNSPEC DISORDER LACTATION W/DELIV W/MENTION PPC	**O92.7Ø**	Unspecified disorders of lactation
676.93	UNSPEC DISORDER LACTATION ANTPRTM COND/COMP	**O92.7Ø**	Unspecified disorders of lactation
676.94	UNSPEC DISORDER LACTATION POSTPARTUM COND/COMP	**O92.7Ø**	Unspecified disorders of lactation
677	LATE EFFECT COMP PG CHILDBIRTH&THE PUERPERIUM	➡ **O94**	Sequelae of comp of pregnancy, chldbrth, and the puerperium
678.ØØ	FETAL HEMATOLOGIC CONDITIONS UNSPEC AS TO EOC/NA	**O35.8XXØ** **O36.829Ø** **O36.8291** **O36.8292** **O36.8293** **O36.8294** **O36.8295** **O36.8299**	Maternal care for oth fetal abnormality and damage, unsp Fetal anemia and thrombocytopenia, unsp trimester, unsp Fetal anemia and thrombocytopenia, unsp trimester, fetus 1 Fetal anemia and thrombocytopenia, unsp trimester, fetus 2 Fetal anemia and thrombocytopenia, unsp trimester, fetus 3 Fetal anemia and thrombocytopenia, unsp trimester, fetus 4 Fetal anemia and thrombocytopenia, unsp trimester, fetus 5 Fetal anemia and thrombocytopenia, unsp trimester, oth fetus

ICD-9-CM		ICD-10-CM	
678.01	FETAL HEMATOLOGIC COND DELIV W/WO ANTPRTM COND	**O35.8XX0**	Maternal care for oth fetal abnormality and damage, unsp
		O35.8XX[1,2,3,4,5]	Maternal care for oth fetal abnormality and damage
		O35.8XX9	Maternal care for oth fetal abnormality and damage, oth
		O36.8210	Fetal anemia and thrombocytopenia, first trimester, unsp
		O36.821[1,2,3,4,5]	Fetal anemia and thrombocytopenia, first trimester
		O36.8219	Fetal anemia and thrombocytopenia, first trimester, oth
		O36.8220	Fetal anemia and thrombocytopenia, second trimester, unsp
		O36.822[1,2,3,4,5]	Fetal anemia and thrombocytopenia, second trimester
		O36.8229	Fetal anemia and thrombocytopenia, second trimester, oth
		O36.8230	Fetal anemia and thrombocytopenia, third trimester, unsp
		O36.823[1,2,3,4,5]	Fetal anemia and thrombocytopenia, third trimester
		O36.8239	Fetal anemia and thrombocytopenia, third trimester, oth
			7th Character meanings for codes as indicated *1 Fetus 1; 2 Fetus 2; 3 Fetus 3; 4 Fetus 4; 5 Fetus 5*
678.03	FETAL HEMATOLOGIC CONDITIONS ANTEPARTM COND/COMP	**O35.8XX0**	Maternal care for oth fetal abnormality and damage, unsp
		O36.8210	Fetal anemia and thrombocytopenia, first trimester, unsp
		O36.8211	Fetal anemia and thrombocytopenia, first trimester, fetus 1
		O36.8212	Fetal anemia and thrombocytopenia, first trimester, fetus 2
		O36.8213	Fetal anemia and thrombocytopenia, first trimester, fetus 3
		O36.8214	Fetal anemia and thrombocytopenia, first trimester, fetus 4
		O36.8215	Fetal anemia and thrombocytopenia, first trimester, fetus 5
		O36.8219	Fetal anemia and thrombocytopenia, first trimester, oth
		O36.8220	Fetal anemia and thrombocytopenia, second trimester, unsp
		O36.8221	Fetal anemia and thrombocytopenia, second trimester, fetus 1
		O36.8222	Fetal anemia and thrombocytopenia, second trimester, fetus 2
		O36.8223	Fetal anemia and thrombocytopenia, second trimester, fetus 3
		O36.8224	Fetal anemia and thrombocytopenia, second trimester, fetus 4
		O36.8225	Fetal anemia and thrombocytopenia, second trimester, fetus 5
		O36.8229	Fetal anemia and thrombocytopenia, second trimester, oth
		O36.8230	Fetal anemia and thrombocytopenia, third trimester, unsp
		O36.8231	Fetal anemia and thrombocytopenia, third trimester, fetus 1
		O36.8232	Fetal anemia and thrombocytopenia, third trimester, fetus 2
		O36.8233	Fetal anemia and thrombocytopenia, third trimester, fetus 3
		O36.8234	Fetal anemia and thrombocytopenia, third trimester, fetus 4
		O36.8235	Fetal anemia and thrombocytopenia, third trimester, fetus 5
		O36.8239	Fetal anemia and thrombocytopenia, third trimester, oth
678.10	FETAL CONJOINED TWINS UNSPECIFIED AS TO EOC/NA	**O30.029**	Conjoined twin pregnancy, unspecified trimester
678.11	FETAL CONJOINED TWINS DELIV W/WO ANTPRTM COND	**O30.021**	Conjoined twin pregnancy, first trimester
		O30.022	Conjoined twin pregnancy, second trimester
		O30.023	Conjoined twin pregnancy, third trimester
678.13	FETAL CONJOINED TWINS ANTEPARTUM COND OR COMP	**O30.021**	Conjoined twin pregnancy, first trimester
		O30.022	Conjoined twin pregnancy, second trimester
		O30.023	Conjoined twin pregnancy, third trimester
679.00	MATERNAL COMP FROM IN UTERO PROC UNSPEC EOC/NA	**O26.899**	Oth pregnancy related conditions, unspecified trimester
679.01	MATERNAL COMP FROM IU PROC DEL W/WO ANTPRTM COND	**O75.89**	Other specified complications of labor and delivery
679.02	MATERNAL COMP FROM IN UTERO PROC DEL W/PP COMP	**O75.89**	Other specified complications of labor and delivery
679.03	MATERNAL COMP FROM IU PROC ANTPRTM COND/COMP	**O26.891**	Oth pregnancy related conditions, first trimester
		O26.892	Oth pregnancy related conditions, second trimester
		O26.893	Oth pregnancy related conditions, third trimester
679.04	MATERNAL COMP FROM IN UTERO PROC PP COND/COMP	**O90.89**	Oth complications of the puerperium, NEC
679.10	FETAL COMP FROM IN UTERO PROCEDURE UNS EOC/NA	**O35.7XX0**	Maternal care for damage to fetus by oth medical proc, unsp
		O35.7XX1	Matern care for damage to fetus by oth medical proc, fetus 1
		O35.7XX2	Matern care for damage to fetus by oth medical proc, fetus 2
		O35.7XX3	Matern care for damage to fetus by oth medical proc, fetus 3
		O35.7XX4	Matern care for damage to fetus by oth medical proc, fetus 4
		O35.7XX5	Matern care for damage to fetus by oth medical proc, fetus 5
		O35.7XX9	Maternal care for damage to fetus by oth medical proc, oth
679.11	FETAL COMP FROM IN UTERO PROCEDURE DELIVERED	**O35.7XX0**	Maternal care for damage to fetus by oth medical proc, unsp
		O35.7XX1	Matern care for damage to fetus by oth medical proc, fetus 1
		O35.7XX2	Matern care for damage to fetus by oth medical proc, fetus 2
		O35.7XX3	Matern care for damage to fetus by oth medical proc, fetus 3
		O35.7XX4	Matern care for damage to fetus by oth medical proc, fetus 4
		O35.7XX5	Matern care for damage to fetus by oth medical proc, fetus 5
		O35.7XX9	Maternal care for damage to fetus by oth medical proc, oth
679.12	FETAL COMP FROM IN UTERO PROC DELIVERY W/PP COMP	**O35.7XX0**	Maternal care for damage to fetus by oth medical proc, unsp
		O35.7XX1	Matern care for damage to fetus by oth medical proc, fetus 1
		O35.7XX2	Matern care for damage to fetus by oth medical proc, fetus 2
		O35.7XX3	Matern care for damage to fetus by oth medical proc, fetus 3
		O35.7XX4	Matern care for damage to fetus by oth medical proc, fetus 4
		O35.7XX5	Matern care for damage to fetus by oth medical proc, fetus 5
		O35.7XX9	Maternal care for damage to fetus by oth medical proc, oth

ICD-9-CM		ICD-10-CM	
679.13	FETAL COMP FROM IN UTERO PROC ANTPRTM COND/COMP	**O35.7XXØ**	Maternal care for damage to fetus by oth medical proc, unsp
		O35.7XX1	Matern care for damage to fetus by oth medical proc, fetus 1
		O35.7XX2	Matern care for damage to fetus by oth medical proc, fetus 2
		O35.7XX3	Matern care for damage to fetus by oth medical proc, fetus 3
		O35.7XX4	Matern care for damage to fetus by oth medical proc, fetus 4
		O35.7XX5	Matern care for damage to fetus by oth medical proc, fetus 5
		O35.7XX9	Maternal care for damage to fetus by oth medical proc, oth
679.14	FETAL COMP FROM IN UTERO PROC PP COND/COMP	**O35.7XXØ**	Maternal care for damage to fetus by oth medical proc, unsp
		O35.7XX1	Matern care for damage to fetus by oth medical proc, fetus 1
		O35.7XX2	Matern care for damage to fetus by oth medical proc, fetus 2
		O35.7XX3	Matern care for damage to fetus by oth medical proc, fetus 3
		O35.7XX4	Matern care for damage to fetus by oth medical proc, fetus 4
		O35.7XX5	Matern care for damage to fetus by oth medical proc, fetus 5
		O35.7XX9	Maternal care for damage to fetus by oth medical proc, oth

680.0	CARBUNCLE AND FURUNCLE OF FACE	L02.02	Furuncle of face
		L02.03	Carbuncle of face
680.1	CARBUNCLE AND FURUNCLE OF NECK	L02.12	Furuncle of neck
		L02.13	Carbuncle of neck
680.2	CARBUNCLE AND FURUNCLE OF TRUNK	L02.221	Furuncle of abdominal wall
		L02.222	Furuncle of back [any part, except buttock]
		L02.223	Furuncle of chest wall
		L02.224	Furuncle of groin
		L02.225	Furuncle of perineum
		L02.226	Furuncle of umbilicus
		L02.229	Furuncle of trunk, unspecified
		L02.231	Carbuncle of abdominal wall
		L02.232	Carbuncle of back [any part, except buttock]
		L02.233	Carbuncle of chest wall
		L02.234	Carbuncle of groin
		L02.235	Carbuncle of perineum
		L02.236	Carbuncle of umbilicus
		L02.239	Carbuncle of trunk, unspecified
680.3	CARBUNCLE AND FURUNCLE OF UPPER ARM AND FOREARM	L02.421	Furuncle of right axilla
		L02.422	Furuncle of left axilla
		L02.423	Furuncle of right upper limb
		L02.424	Furuncle of left upper limb
		L02.429	Furuncle of limb, unspecified
		L02.431	Carbuncle of right axilla
		L02.432	Carbuncle of left axilla
		L02.433	Carbuncle of right upper limb
		L02.434	Carbuncle of left upper limb
		L02.439	Carbuncle of limb, unspecified
680.4	CARBUNCLE AND FURUNCLE OF HAND	L02.521	Furuncle right hand
		L02.522	Furuncle left hand
		L02.529	Furuncle unspecified hand
		L02.531	Carbuncle of right hand
		L02.532	Carbuncle of left hand
		L02.539	Carbuncle of unspecified hand
680.5	CARBUNCLE AND FURUNCLE OF BUTTOCK	L02.32	Furuncle of buttock
		L02.33	Carbuncle of buttock
680.6	CARBUNCLE AND FURUNCLE OF LEG EXCEPT FOOT	L02.425	Furuncle of right lower limb
		L02.426	Furuncle of left lower limb
		L02.429	Furuncle of limb, unspecified
		L02.435	Carbuncle of right lower limb
		L02.436	Carbuncle of left lower limb
		L02.439	Carbuncle of limb, unspecified
680.7	CARBUNCLE AND FURUNCLE OF FOOT	L02.621	Furuncle of right foot
		L02.622	Furuncle of left foot
		L02.629	Furuncle of unspecified foot
		L02.631	Carbuncle of right foot
		L02.632	Carbuncle of left foot
		L02.639	Carbuncle of unspecified foot
680.8	CARBUNCLE AND FURUNCLE OF OTHER SPECIFIED SITES	L02.821	Furuncle of head [any part, except face]
		L02.828	Furuncle of other sites
		L02.831	Carbuncle of head [any part, except face]
		L02.838	Carbuncle of other sites
680.9	CARBUNCLE AND FURUNCLE OF UNSPECIFIED SITE	L02.92	Furuncle, unspecified
		L02.93	Carbuncle, unspecified
681.00	UNSPECIFIED CELLULITIS AND ABSCESS OF FINGER	L02.511	Cutaneous abscess of right hand
		L02.512	Cutaneous abscess of left hand
		L02.519	Cutaneous abscess of unspecified hand
		L03.011	Cellulitis of right finger
		L03.012	Cellulitis of left finger
		L03.019	Cellulitis of unspecified finger
		L03.021	Acute lymphangitis of right finger
		L03.022	Acute lymphangitis of left finger
		L03.029	Acute lymphangitis of unspecified finger
681.01	FELON	L03.011	Cellulitis of right finger
		L03.012	Cellulitis of left finger
		L03.019	Cellulitis of unspecified finger
681.02	ONYCHIA AND PARONYCHIA OF FINGER	L03.011	Cellulitis of right finger
		L03.012	Cellulitis of left finger
		L03.019	Cellulitis of unspecified finger
681.10	UNSPECIFIED CELLULITIS AND ABSCESS OF TOE	L02.611	Cutaneous abscess of right foot
		L02.612	Cutaneous abscess of left foot
		L02.619	Cutaneous abscess of unspecified foot
		L03.031	Cellulitis of right toe
		L03.032	Cellulitis of left toe
		L03.039	Cellulitis of unspecified toe
		L03.041	Acute lymphangitis of right toe
		L03.042	Acute lymphangitis of left toe
		L03.049	Acute lymphangitis of unspecified toe

ICD-9-CM		ICD-10-CM	
681.11	ONYCHIA AND PARONYCHIA OF TOE	L03.031	Cellulitis of right toe
		L03.032	Cellulitis of left toe
		L03.039	Cellulitis of unspecified toe
681.9	CELLULITIS AND ABSCESS OF UNSPECIFIED DIGIT	L03.019	Cellulitis of unspecified finger
		L03.029	Acute lymphangitis of unspecified finger
		L03.039	Cellulitis of unspecified toe
		L03.049	Acute lymphangitis of unspecified toe
682.0	CELLULITIS AND ABSCESS OF FACE	K12.2	Cellulitis and abscess of mouth
		L02.01	Cutaneous abscess of face
		L03.211	Cellulitis of face
		L03.212	Acute lymphangitis of face
682.1	CELLULITIS AND ABSCESS OF NECK	L02.11	Cutaneous abscess of neck
		L03.221	Cellulitis of neck
		L03.222	Acute lymphangitis of neck
682.2	CELLULITIS AND ABSCESS OF TRUNK	L02.211	Cutaneous abscess of abdominal wall
		L02.212	Cutaneous abscess of back [any part, except buttock]
		L02.213	Cutaneous abscess of chest wall
		L02.214	Cutaneous abscess of groin
		L02.215	Cutaneous abscess of perineum
		L02.216	Cutaneous abscess of umbilicus
		L02.219	Cutaneous abscess of trunk, unspecified
		L03.311	Cellulitis of abdominal wall
		L03.312	Cellulitis of back [any part except buttock]
		L03.313	Cellulitis of chest wall
		L03.314	Cellulitis of groin
		L03.315	Cellulitis of perineum
		L03.316	Cellulitis of umbilicus
		L03.319	Cellulitis of trunk, unspecified
		L03.321	Acute lymphangitis of abdominal wall
		L03.322	Acute lymphangitis of back [any part except buttock]
		L03.323	Acute lymphangitis of chest wall
		L03.324	Acute lymphangitis of groin
		L03.325	Acute lymphangitis of perineum
		L03.326	Acute lymphangitis of umbilicus
		L03.329	Acute lymphangitis of trunk, unspecified
682.3	CELLULITIS AND ABSCESS OF UPPER ARM AND FOREARM	L02.411	Cutaneous abscess of right axilla
		L02.412	Cutaneous abscess of left axilla
		L02.413	Cutaneous abscess of right upper limb
		L02.414	Cutaneous abscess of left upper limb
		L02.419	Cutaneous abscess of limb, unspecified
		L03.111	Cellulitis of right axilla
		L03.112	Cellulitis of left axilla
		L03.113	Cellulitis of right upper limb
		L03.114	Cellulitis of left upper limb
		L03.119	Cellulitis of unspecified part of limb
		L03.121	Acute lymphangitis of right axilla
		L03.122	Acute lymphangitis of left axilla
		L03.123	Acute lymphangitis of right upper limb
		L03.124	Acute lymphangitis of left upper limb
		L03.129	Acute lymphangitis of unspecified part of limb
682.4	CELLULITIS&ABSCESS OF HAND EXCEPT FINGERS&THUMB	L02.511	Cutaneous abscess of right hand
		L02.512	Cutaneous abscess of left hand
		L02.519	Cutaneous abscess of unspecified hand
		L03.113	Cellulitis of right upper limb
		L03.114	Cellulitis of left upper limb
		L03.119	Cellulitis of unspecified part of limb
		L03.123	Acute lymphangitis of right upper limb
		L03.124	Acute lymphangitis of left upper limb
		L03.129	Acute lymphangitis of unspecified part of limb
682.5	CELLULITIS AND ABSCESS OF BUTTOCK	L02.31	Cutaneous abscess of buttock
		L03.317	Cellulitis of buttock
		L03.327	Acute lymphangitis of buttock
682.6	CELLULITIS AND ABSCESS OF LEG EXCEPT FOOT	L02.415	Cutaneous abscess of right lower limb
		L02.416	Cutaneous abscess of left lower limb
		L02.419	Cutaneous abscess of limb, unspecified
		L03.115	Cellulitis of right lower limb
		L03.116	Cellulitis of left lower limb
		L03.119	Cellulitis of unspecified part of limb
		L03.125	Acute lymphangitis of right lower limb
		L03.126	Acute lymphangitis of left lower limb
		L03.129	Acute lymphangitis of unspecified part of limb
682.7	CELLULITIS AND ABSCESS OF FOOT EXCEPT TOES	L02.611	Cutaneous abscess of right foot
		L02.612	Cutaneous abscess of left foot
		L02.619	Cutaneous abscess of unspecified foot
		L03.115	Cellulitis of right lower limb
		L03.116	Cellulitis of left lower limb
		L03.119	Cellulitis of unspecified part of limb
		L03.125	Acute lymphangitis of right lower limb
		L03.126	Acute lymphangitis of left lower limb
		L03.129	Acute lymphangitis of unspecified part of limb

ICD-9-CM	Description		ICD-10-CM	Description
682.8	CELLULITIS AND ABSCESS OF OTHER SPECIFIED SITE		**LØ2.811**	Cutaneous abscess of head [any part, except face]
			LØ2.818	Cutaneous abscess of other sites
			LØ3.811	Cellulitis of head [any part, except face]
			LØ3.818	Cellulitis of other sites
			LØ3.891	Acute lymphangitis of head [any part, except face]
			LØ3.898	Acute lymphangitis of other sites
682.9	CELLULITIS AND ABSCESS OF UNSPECIFIED SITE		**LØ2.91**	Cutaneous abscess, unspecified
			LØ3.9Ø	Cellulitis, unspecified
			LØ3.91	Acute lymphangitis, unspecified
			L98.3	Eosinophilic cellulitis [Wells]
683	ACUTE LYMPHADENITIS		**LØ4.Ø**	Acute lymphadenitis of face, head and neck
			LØ4.1	Acute lymphadenitis of trunk
			LØ4.2	Acute lymphadenitis of upper limb
			LØ4.3	Acute lymphadenitis of lower limb
			LØ4.8	Acute lymphadenitis of other sites
			LØ4.9	Acute lymphadenitis, unspecified
684	IMPETIGO		**LØ1.ØØ**	Impetigo, unspecified
			LØ1.Ø1	Non-bullous impetigo
			LØ1.Ø2	Bockhart's impetigo
			LØ1.Ø3	Bullous impetigo
			LØ1.Ø9	Other impetigo
			LØ1.1	Impetiginization of other dermatoses
685.Ø	PILONIDAL CYST WITH ABSCESS		**LØ5.Ø1**	Pilonidal cyst with abscess
			LØ5.Ø2	Pilonidal sinus with abscess
685.1	PILONIDAL CYST WITHOUT MENTION OF ABSCESS		**LØ5.91**	Pilonidal cyst without abscess
			LØ5.92	Pilonidal sinus without abscess
686.ØØ	UNSPECIFIED PYODERMA		**LØ8.Ø**	Pyoderma
686.Ø1	PYODERMA GANGRENOSUM	➡	**L88**	Pyoderma gangrenosum
686.Ø9	OTHER PYODERMA		**LØ8.81**	Pyoderma vegetans
			LØ8.89	Oth local infections of the skin and subcutaneous tissue
686.1	PYOGENIC GRANULOMA OF SKIN&SUBCUTANEOUS TISSUE		**L92.8**	Oth granulomatous disorders of the skin, subcu
			L98.Ø	Pyogenic granuloma
686.8	OTH SPEC LOCAL INFECTIONS SKIN&SUBCUT TISSUE		**B78.1**	Cutaneous strongyloidiasis
			E83.2	Disorders of zinc metabolism
			LØ8.82	Omphalitis not of newborn
			LØ8.89	Oth local infections of the skin and subcutaneous tissue
686.9	UNSPEC LOCAL INFECTION SKIN&SUBCUTANEOUS TISSUE	➡	**LØ8.9**	Local infection of the skin and subcutaneous tissue, unsp
69Ø.1Ø	UNSPECIFIED SEBORRHEIC DERMATITIS		**L21.9**	Seborrheic dermatitis, unspecified
69Ø.11	SEBORRHEA CAPITIS	➡	**L21.Ø**	Seborrhea capitis
69Ø.12	SEBORRHEIC INFANTILE DERMATITIS		**L2Ø.83**	Infantile (acute) (chronic) eczema
			L21.1	Seborrheic infantile dermatitis
69Ø.18	OTHER SEBORRHEIC DERMATITIS	➡	**L21.8**	Other seborrheic dermatitis
69Ø.8	OTHER ERYTHEMATOSQUAMOUS DERMATOSIS		**L3Ø.3**	Infective dermatitis
691.Ø	DIAPER OR NAPKIN RASH	➡	**L22**	Diaper dermatitis
691.8	OTHER ATOPIC DERMATITIS AND RELATED CONDITIONS		**L2Ø.Ø**	Besnier's prurigo
			L2Ø.81	Atopic neurodermatitis
			L2Ø.82	Flexural eczema
			L2Ø.84	Intrinsic (allergic) eczema
			L2Ø.89	Other atopic dermatitis
			L2Ø.9	Atopic dermatitis, unspecified
692.Ø	CONTACT DERMATITIS&OTHER ECZEMA DUE DETERGENTS	➡	**L24.Ø**	Irritant contact dermatitis due to detergents
692.1	CONTACT DERMATITIS&OTHER ECZEMA DUE OILS&GREASES	➡	**L24.1**	Irritant contact dermatitis due to oils and greases
692.2	CONTACT DERMATITIS&OTHER ECZEMA DUE TO SOLVENTS	➡	**L24.2**	Irritant contact dermatitis due to solvents
692.3	CNTC DERMATITIS&OTH ECZEMA-RX&MEDS CNTC W/SKN		**L23.3**	Allergic contact dermatitis due to drugs in contact w skin
			L24.4	Irritant contact dermatitis due to drugs in contact w skin
			L25.1	Unsp contact dermatitis due to drugs in contact with skin
692.4	CNTC DERMATITIS&OTH ECZEMA DUE OTH CHEM PRODUCTS		**L23.1**	Allergic contact dermatitis due to adhesives
			L23.5	Allergic contact dermatitis due to other chemical products
			L24.5	Irritant contact dermatitis due to other chemical products
			L25.3	Unsp contact dermatitis due to other chemical products
692.5	CNTC DERMATITIS&OTH ECZEMA DUE FOOD CNTC W/SKIN		**L23.6**	Allergic contact dermatitis due to food in contact w skin
			L24.6	Irritant contact dermatitis due to food in contact with skin
			L25.4	Unsp contact dermatitis due to food in contact with skin
692.6	CONTACT DERMATITIS&OTHER ECZEMA DUE TO PLANTS		**L23.7**	Allergic contact dermatitis due to plants, except food
			L24.7	Irritant contact dermatitis due to plants, except food
			L25.5	Unspecified contact dermatitis due to plants, except food
692.7Ø	UNSPECIFIED DERMATITIS DUE TO SUN		**L57.8**	Oth skin changes due to chr expsr to nonionizing radiation
692.71	CONTACT DERMATITIS&OTHER ECZEMA DUE TO SUNBURN		**L55.Ø**	Sunburn of first degree
			L55.9	Sunburn, unspecified
692.72	ACUTE DERMATITIS DUE TO SOLAR RADIATION		**L56.Ø**	Drug phototoxic response
			L56.1	Drug photoallergic response
			L56.2	Photocontact dermatitis [berloque dermatitis]
			L56.3	Solar urticaria
692.73	ACTINIC RETICULOID AND ACTINIC GRANULOMA		**L57.1**	Actinic reticuloid
			L57.5	Actinic granuloma

ICD-9-CM	Description		ICD-10-CM	Description
692.74	OTHER CHRONIC DERMATITIS DUE TO SOLAR RADIATION		L57.8	Oth skin changes due to chr expsr to nonionizing radiation
			L57.9	Skin changes due to chr expsr to nonionizing radiation, unsp
692.75	DISSEMINATED SUPERFICIAL ACTINIC POROKERATOSIS	➡	L56.5	Disseminated superficial actinic porokeratosis (DSAP)
692.76	SUNBURN OF SECOND DEGREE	➡	L55.1	Sunburn of second degree
692.77	SUNBURN OF THIRD DEGREE	➡	L55.2	Sunburn of third degree
692.79	OTHER DERMATITIS DUE TO SOLAR RADIATION		L56.8	Oth acute skin changes due to ultraviolet radiation
			L56.9	Acute skin change due to ultraviolet radiation, unspecified
692.81	DERMATITIS DUE TO COSMETICS		L23.2	Allergic contact dermatitis due to cosmetics
			L24.3	Irritant contact dermatitis due to cosmetics
			L25.0	Unspecified contact dermatitis due to cosmetics
692.82	DERMATITIS DUE TO OTHER RADIATION		L56.4	Polymorphous light eruption
			L58.0	Acute radiodermatitis
			L58.1	Chronic radiodermatitis
			L58.9	Radiodermatitis, unspecified
			L59.0	Erythema ab igne [dermatitis ab igne]
			L59.8	Oth disrd of the skin, subcu related to radiation
			L59.9	Disorder of the skin, subcu related to radiation, unsp
692.83	DERMATITIS DUE TO METALS		L23.0	Allergic contact dermatitis due to metals
			L24.81	Irritant contact dermatitis due to metals
692.84	CONTACT DERMATITIS&OTH ECZEMA DUE ANIMAL DANDER		L23.81	Allergic contact dermatitis due to animal (cat) (dog) dander
692.89	CONTACT DERMATITIS&OTH ECZEMA DUE OTH SPEC AGENT		L23.4	Allergic contact dermatitis due to dyes
			L23.89	Allergic contact dermatitis due to other agents
			L24.89	Irritant contact dermatitis due to other agents
			L25.2	Unspecified contact dermatitis due to dyes
			L25.8	Unspecified contact dermatitis due to other agents
692.9	CONTACT DERMATITIS&OTHER ECZEMA DUE UNSPEC CAUSE		L23.9	Allergic contact dermatitis, unspecified cause
			L24.9	Irritant contact dermatitis, unspecified cause
			L25.9	Unspecified contact dermatitis, unspecified cause
			L30.0	Nummular dermatitis
			L30.2	Cutaneous autosensitization
			L30.8	Other specified dermatitis
			L30.9	Dermatitis, unspecified
693.0	DERMATITIS DUE DRUGS&MEDICINES TAKEN INTERNALLY		L27.0	Gen skin eruption due to drugs and meds taken internally
			L27.1	Loc skin eruption due to drugs and meds taken internally
693.1	DERMATITIS DUE TO FOOD TAKEN INTERNALLY	➡	L27.2	Dermatitis due to ingested food
693.8	DERMATITIS DUE OTH SPEC SUBSTANCES TAKEN INTRLLY	➡	L27.8	Dermatitis due to other substances taken internally
693.9	DERMATITIS DUE UNSPEC SUBSTANCE TAKEN INTERNALLY	➡	L27.9	Dermatitis due to unspecified substance taken internally
694.0	DERMATITIS HERPETIFORMIS	➡	L13.0	Dermatitis herpetiformis
694.1	SUBCORNEAL PUSTULAR DERMATOSIS	➡	L13.1	Subcorneal pustular dermatitis
694.2	JUVENILE DERMATITIS HERPETIFORMIS	➡	L12.2	Chronic bullous disease of childhood
694.3	IMPETIGO HERPETIFORMIS		L40.1	Generalized pustular psoriasis
694.4	PEMPHIGUS		L10.0	Pemphigus vulgaris
			L10.1	Pemphigus vegetans
			L10.2	Pemphigus foliaceous
			L10.3	Brazilian pemphigus [fogo selvagem]
			L10.4	Pemphigus erythematosus
			L10.5	Drug-induced pemphigus
			L10.81	Paraneoplastic pemphigus
			L10.89	Other pemphigus
			L10.9	Pemphigus, unspecified
694.5	PEMPHIGOID		L12.0	Bullous pemphigoid
			L12.8	Other pemphigoid
			L12.9	Pemphigoid, unspecified
694.60	BEN MUCOS MEMB PEMPHIGOID W/O OCULR INVLV		L12.1	Cicatricial pemphigoid
694.61	BEN MUCOUS MEMBRANE PEMPHIGOID W/OCULAR INVLV		L12.1	Cicatricial pemphigoid
694.8	OTHER SPECIFIED BULLOUS DERMATOSIS		L13.8	Other specified bullous disorders
			L14	Bullous disorders in diseases classified elsewhere
694.9	UNSPECIFIED BULLOUS DERMATOSIS	➡	L13.9	Bullous disorder, unspecified
695.0	TOXIC ERYTHEMA		L53.0	Toxic erythema
			L53.1	Erythema annulare centrifugum
			L53.2	Erythema marginatum
			L53.3	Other chronic figurate erythema
695.10	ERYTHEMA MULTIFORME UNSPECIFIED		L51.0	Nonbullous erythema multiforme
			L51.9	Erythema multiforme, unspecified
695.11	ERYTHEMA MULTIFORME MINOR		L51.8	Other erythema multiforme
695.12	ERYTHEMA MULTIFORME MAJOR		L51.8	Other erythema multiforme
695.13	STEVENS-JOHNSON SYNDROME	➡	L51.1	Stevens-Johnson syndrome
695.14	STEVENS-JOHNSON SYNDROME-TEN OVERLAP SYNDROME	➡	L51.3	Stevens-Johnson synd-tox epdrml necrolysis overlap syndrome
695.15	TOXIC EPIDERMAL NECROLYSIS		L12.30	Acquired epidermolysis bullosa, unspecified
			L12.31	Epidermolysis bullosa due to drug
			L12.35	Other acquired epidermolysis bullosa
			L51.2	Toxic epidermal necrolysis [Lyell]
695.19	OTHER ERYTHEMA MULTIFORME		L51.8	Other erythema multiforme
695.2	ERYTHEMA NODOSUM	➡	L52	Erythema nodosum

ICD-9	Description		ICD-10	Description
695.3	ROSACEA		L71.0	Perioral dermatitis
			L71.1	Rhinophyma
			L71.8	Other rosacea
			L71.9	Rosacea, unspecified
695.4	LUPUS ERYTHEMATOSUS		L93.0	Discoid lupus erythematosus
			L93.1	Subacute cutaneous lupus erythematosus
			L93.2	Other local lupus erythematosus
695.50	EXFOLIATION D/T ERYTHEMATOUS < 10% BODY SURFACE	➡	L49.0	Exfoliatn due to erythemat cond w < 10 pct of body surface
695.51	EXFOLIATION D/T ERYTHEMATOUS 10-19% BODY SURFACE	➡	L49.1	Exfoliatn due to erythemat cond w 10-19 pct of body surface
695.52	EXFOLIATION D/T ERYTHEMATOUS 20-29% BODY SURFACE	➡	L49.2	Exfoliatn due to erythemat cond w 20-29 pct of body surface
695.53	EXFOLIATION D/T ERYTHEMATOUS 30-39% BODY SURFACE	➡	L49.3	Exfoliatn due to erythemat cond w 30-39 pct of body surface
695.54	EXFOLIATION D/T ERYTHEMATOUS 40-49% BODY SURFACE	➡	L49.4	Exfoliatn due to erythemat cond w 40-49 pct of body surface
695.55	EXFOLIATION D/T ERYTHEMATOUS 50-59% BODY SURFACE	➡	L49.5	Exfoliatn due to erythemat cond w 50-59 pct of body surface
695.56	EXFOLIATION D/T ERYTHEMATOUS 60-69% BODY SURFACE	➡	L49.6	Exfoliatn due to erythemat cond w 60-69 pct of body surface
695.57	EXFOLIATION D/T ERYTHEMATOUS 70-79% BODY SURFACE	➡	L49.7	Exfoliatn due to erythemat cond w 70-79 pct of body surface
695.58	EXFOLIATION D/T ERYTHEMATOUS 80-89% BODY SURFACE	➡	L49.8	Exfoliatn due to erythemat cond w 80-89 pct of body surface
695.59	EXFOLIATION D/T ERYTHEMATOUS 90% > BODY SURFACE	➡	L49.9	Exfoliatn d/t erythemat cond w 90 or more pct of body surfc
695.81	RITTERS DISEASE		L00	Staphylococcal scalded skin syndrome
695.89	OTHER SPECIFIED ERYTHEMATOUS CONDITION OTHER		L26	Exfoliative dermatitis
			L30.4	Erythema intertrigo
			L53.8	Other specified erythematous conditions
			L54	Erythema in diseases classified elsewhere
			L92.0	Granuloma annulare
			L95.1	Erythema elevatum diutinum
			L98.2	Febrile neutrophilic dermatosis [Sweet]
695.9	UNSPECIFIED ERYTHEMATOUS CONDITION	➡	L53.9	Erythematous condition, unspecified
696.0	PSORIATIC ARTHROPATHY		L40.50	Arthropathic psoriasis, unspecified
			L40.51	Distal interphalangeal psoriatic arthropathy
			L40.52	Psoriatic arthritis mutilans
			L40.53	Psoriatic spondylitis
			L40.54	Psoriatic juvenile arthropathy
			L40.59	Other psoriatic arthropathy
696.1	OTHER PSORIASIS AND SIMILAR DISORDERS		L40.0	Psoriasis vulgaris
			L40.1	Generalized pustular psoriasis
			L40.2	Acrodermatitis continua
			L40.3	Pustulosis palmaris et plantaris
			L40.4	Guttate psoriasis
			L40.8	Other psoriasis
			L40.9	Psoriasis, unspecified
696.2	PARAPSORIASIS		L41.0	Pityriasis lichenoides et varioliformis acuta
			L41.1	Pityriasis lichenoides chronica
			L41.3	Small plaque parapsoriasis
			L41.4	Large plaque parapsoriasis
			L41.5	Retiform parapsoriasis
			L41.8	Other parapsoriasis
			L41.9	Parapsoriasis, unspecified
			L94.5	Poikiloderma vasculare atrophicans
696.3	PITYRIASIS ROSEA	➡	L42	Pityriasis rosea
696.4	PITYRIASIS RUBRA PILARIS		L44.0	Pityriasis rubra pilaris
696.5	OTHER AND UNSPECIFIED PITYRIASIS		L30.5	Pityriasis alba
696.8	OTH PSORIASIS & SIMILAR DISORDERS OTH		L44.0	Pityriasis rubra pilaris
			L44.8	Other specified papulosquamous disorders
			L45	Papulosquamous disorders in diseases classified elsewhere
697.0	LICHEN PLANUS		L43.0	Hypertrophic lichen planus
			L43.1	Bullous lichen planus
			L43.2	Lichenoid drug reaction
			L43.3	Subacute (active) lichen planus
			L43.8	Other lichen planus
			L43.9	Lichen planus, unspecified
			L66.1	Lichen planopilaris
697.1	LICHEN NITIDUS	➡	L44.1	Lichen nitidus
697.8	OTHER LICHEN NOT ELSEWHERE CLASSIFIED		L44.2	Lichen striatus
			L44.3	Lichen ruber moniliformis
697.9	UNSPECIFIED LICHEN		L44.9	Papulosquamous disorder, unspecified
698.0	PRURITUS ANI	➡	L29.0	Pruritus ani
698.1	PRURITUS OF GENITAL ORGANS		L29.1	Pruritus scroti
			L29.2	Pruritus vulvae
			L29.3	Anogenital pruritus, unspecified
698.2	PRURIGO	➡	L28.2	Other prurigo
698.3	LICHENIFICATION AND LICHEN SIMPLEX CHRONICUS		L28.0	Lichen simplex chronicus
			L28.1	Prurigo nodularis
698.4	DERMATITIS FACTITIA	➡	L98.1	Factitial dermatitis
698.8	OTHER SPECIFIED PRURITIC CONDITIONS		L29.8	Other pruritus
698.9	UNSPECIFIED PRURITIC DISORDER	➡	L29.9	Pruritus, unspecified
700	CORNS AND CALLOSITIES	➡	L84	Corns and callosities

ICD-9-CM	Description		ICD-10-CM	Description
701.0	CIRCUMSCRIBED SCLERODERMA		L90.0	Lichen sclerosus et atrophicus
			L94.0	Localized scleroderma [morphea]
			L94.1	Linear scleroderma
			L94.3	Sclerodactyly
701.1	ACQUIRED KERATODERMA		L11.0	Acquired keratosis follicularis
			L85.0	Acquired ichthyosis
			L85.1	Acquired keratosis [keratoderma] palmaris et plantaris
			L85.2	Keratosis punctata (palmaris et plantaris)
			L86	Keratoderma in diseases classified elsewhere
			L87.0	Keratos follicularis et parafollicularis in cutem penetrans
			L87.2	Elastosis perforans serpiginosa
701.2	ACQUIRED ACANTHOSIS NIGRICANS	➡	L83	Acanthosis nigricans
701.3	STRIAE ATROPHICAE		L90.1	Anetoderma of Schweninger-Buzzi
			L90.2	Anetoderma of Jadassohn-Pellizzari
			L90.6	Striae atrophicae
701.4	KELOID SCAR	➡	L91.0	Hypertrophic scar
701.5	OTHER ABNORMAL GRANULATION TISSUE		L92.9	Granulomatous disorder of the skin, subcu, unsp
701.8	OTHER SPEC HYPERTROPHIC&ATROPHIC CONDITION SKIN		L11.8	Other specified acantholytic disorders
			L11.9	Acantholytic disorder, unspecified
			L57.2	Cutis rhomboidalis nuchae
			L57.4	Cutis laxa senilis
			L66.4	Folliculitis ulerythematosa reticulata
			L85.8	Other specified epidermal thickening
			L87.1	Reactive perforating collagenosis
			L87.8	Other transepidermal elimination disorders
			L90.3	Atrophoderma of Pasini and Pierini
			L90.4	Acrodermatitis chronica atrophicans
			L90.8	Other atrophic disorders of skin
			L91.8	Other hypertrophic disorders of the skin
			L92.2	Granuloma faciale [eosinophilic granuloma of skin]
			L94.8	Other specified localized connective tissue disorders
			L98.5	Mucinosis of the skin
			L98.6	Oth infiltrative disorders of the skin, subcu
			L99	Oth disorders of skin, subcu in diseases classd elswhr
701.9	UNSPECIFIED HYPERTROPHIC&ATROPHIC CONDITION SKIN		L85.9	Epidermal thickening, unspecified
			L87.9	Transepidermal elimination disorder, unspecified
			L90.9	Atrophic disorder of skin, unspecified
			L91.9	Hypertrophic disorder of the skin, unspecified
			L94.9	Localized connective tissue disorder, unspecified
702.0	ACTINIC KERATOSIS	➡	L57.0	Actinic keratosis
702.11	INFLAMED SEBORRHEIC KERATOSIS	➡	L82.0	Inflamed seborrheic keratosis
702.19	OTHER SEBORRHEIC KERATOSIS	➡	L82.1	Other seborrheic keratosis
702.8	OTHER SPECIFIED DERMATOSES		L11.1	Transient acantholytic dermatosis [Grover]
			L98.8	Oth disrd of the skin and subcutaneous tissue
703.0	INGROWING NAIL	➡	L60.0	Ingrowing nail
703.8	OTHER SPECIFIED DISEASE OF NAIL		L60.1	Onycholysis
			L60.2	Onychogryphosis
			L60.3	Nail dystrophy
			L60.4	Beau's lines
			L60.5	Yellow nail syndrome
			L60.8	Other nail disorders
			L62	Nail disorders in diseases classified elsewhere
703.9	UNSPECIFIED DISEASE OF NAIL	➡	L60.9	Nail disorder, unspecified
704.00	UNSPECIFIED ALOPECIA		L64.9	Androgenic alopecia, unspecified
			L65.9	Nonscarring hair loss, unspecified
704.01	ALOPECIA AREATA		L63.2	Ophiasis
			L63.8	Other alopecia areata
			L63.9	Alopecia areata, unspecified
704.02	TELOGEN EFFLUVIUM	➡	L65.0	Telogen effluvium
704.09	OTHER ALOPECIA		L63.0	Alopecia (capitis) totalis
			L63.1	Alopecia universalis
			L64.0	Drug-induced androgenic alopecia
			L64.8	Other androgenic alopecia
			L65.1	Anagen effluvium
			L65.2	Alopecia mucinosa
			L65.8	Other specified nonscarring hair loss
			L66.0	Pseudopelade
			L66.2	Folliculitis decalvans
			L66.8	Other cicatricial alopecia
			L66.9	Cicatricial alopecia, unspecified
704.1	HIRSUTISM		L68.0	Hirsutism
			L68.1	Acquired hypertrichosis lanuginosa
			L68.2	Localized hypertrichosis
			L68.3	Polytrichia
			L68.8	Other hypertrichosis
			L68.9	Hypertrichosis, unspecified

ICD-9-CM	Description		ICD-10-CM	Description
704.2	ABNORMALITIES OF THE HAIR		**L67.0**	Trichorrhexis nodosa
			L67.8	Other hair color and hair shaft abnormalities
			L67.9	Hair color and hair shaft abnormality, unspecified
704.3	VARIATIONS IN HAIR COLOR	➡	**L67.1**	Variations in hair color
704.41	PILAR CYST		**L72.11**	Pilar cyst
704.42	TRICHILEMMAL CYST		**L72.12**	Trichodermal cyst
704.8	OTHER SPECIFIED DISEASE OF HAIR&HAIR FOLLICLES		**L66.3**	Perifolliculitis capitis abscedens
			L73.1	Pseudofolliculitis barbae
			L73.8	Other specified follicular disorders
704.9	UNSPECIFIED DISEASE OF HAIR AND HAIR FOLLICLES		**L73.9**	Follicular disorder, unspecified
705.0	ANHIDROSIS	➡	**L74.4**	Anhidrosis
705.1	PRICKLY HEAT		**L74.0**	Miliaria rubra
			L74.1	Miliaria crystallina
			L74.2	Miliaria profunda
			L74.3	Miliaria, unspecified
705.21	PRIMARY FOCAL HYPERHIDROSIS		**L74.510**	Primary focal hyperhidrosis, axilla
			L74.511	Primary focal hyperhidrosis, face
			L74.512	Primary focal hyperhidrosis, palms
			L74.513	Primary focal hyperhidrosis, soles
			L74.519	Primary focal hyperhidrosis, unspecified
705.22	SECONDARY FOCAL HYPERHIDROSIS	➡	**L74.52**	Secondary focal hyperhidrosis
705.81	DYSHIDROSIS	➡	**L30.1**	Dyshidrosis [pompholyx]
705.82	FOX-FORDYCE DISEASE	➡	**L75.2**	Apocrine miliaria
705.83	HIDRADENITIS	➡	**L73.2**	Hidradenitis suppurativa
705.89	OTHER SPECIFIED DISORDER OF SWEAT GLANDS		**L74.8**	Other eccrine sweat disorders
			L75.0	Bromhidrosis
			L75.1	Chromhidrosis
			L75.8	Other apocrine sweat disorders
705.9	UNSPECIFIED DISORDER OF SWEAT GLANDS		**L74.9**	Eccrine sweat disorder, unspecified
			L75.9	Apocrine sweat disorder, unspecified
706.0	ACNE VARIOLIFORMIS	➡	**L70.2**	Acne varioliformis
706.1	OTHER ACNE		**L70.0**	Acne vulgaris
			L70.1	Acne conglobata
			L70.3	Acne tropica
			L70.4	Infantile acne
			L70.5	Acne excoriee des jeunes filles
			L70.8	Other acne
			L70.9	Acne, unspecified
			L73.0	Acne keloid
706.2	SEBACEOUS CYST		**L72.0**	Epidermal cyst
			L72.2	Steatocystoma multiplex
			L72.3	Sebaceous cyst
			L72.8	Other follicular cysts of the skin and subcutaneous tissue
			L72.9	Follicular cyst of the skin and subcutaneous tissue, unsp
706.3	SEBORRHEA		**L21.9**	Seborrheic dermatitis, unspecified
706.8	OTHER SPECIFIED DISEASE OF SEBACEOUS GLANDS		**L85.3**	Xerosis cutis
706.9	UNSPECIFIED DISEASE OF SEBACEOUS GLANDS		**L73.9**	Follicular disorder, unspecified
707.00	PRESSURE ULCER UNSPECIFIED SITE	▣	**L89.90**	Pressure ulcer of unspecified site, unspecified stage
		▣	**L89.91**	Pressure ulcer of unspecified site, stage 1
		▣	**L89.92**	Pressure ulcer of unspecified site, stage 2
		▣	**L89.93**	Pressure ulcer of unspecified site, stage 3
		▣	**L89.94**	Pressure ulcer of unspecified site, stage 4
		▣	**L89.95**	Pressure ulcer of unspecified site, unstageable
707.01	PRESSURE ULCER ELBOW	▣	**L89.000**	Pressure ulcer of unspecified elbow, unstageable
		▣	**L89.001**	Pressure ulcer of unspecified elbow, stage 1
		▣	**L89.002**	Pressure ulcer of unspecified elbow, stage 2
		▣	**L89.003**	Pressure ulcer of unspecified elbow, stage 3
		▣	**L89.004**	Pressure ulcer of unspecified elbow, stage 4
		▣	**L89.009**	Pressure ulcer of unspecified elbow, unspecified stage
		▣	**L89.010**	Pressure ulcer of right elbow, unstageable
		▣	**L89.011**	Pressure ulcer of right elbow, stage 1
		▣	**L89.012**	Pressure ulcer of right elbow, stage 2
		▣	**L89.013**	Pressure ulcer of right elbow, stage 3
		▣	**L89.014**	Pressure ulcer of right elbow, stage 4
		▣	**L89.019**	Pressure ulcer of right elbow, unspecified stage
		▣	**L89.020**	Pressure ulcer of left elbow, unstageable
		▣	**L89.021**	Pressure ulcer of left elbow, stage 1
		▣	**L89.022**	Pressure ulcer of left elbow, stage 2
		▣	**L89.023**	Pressure ulcer of left elbow, stage 3
		▣	**L89.024**	Pressure ulcer of left elbow, stage 4
		▣	**L89.029**	Pressure ulcer of left elbow, unspecified stage

ICD-9-CM	ICD-10-CM	
707.02 PRESSURE ULCER UPPER BACK	**L89.100**	Pressure ulcer of unspecified part of back, unstageable
	L89.101	Pressure ulcer of unspecified part of back, stage 1
	L89.102	Pressure ulcer of unspecified part of back, stage 2
	L89.103	Pressure ulcer of unspecified part of back, stage 3
	L89.104	Pressure ulcer of unspecified part of back, stage 4
	L89.109	Pressure ulcer of unsp part of back, unspecified stage
	L89.110	Pressure ulcer of right upper back, unstageable
	L89.111	Pressure ulcer of right upper back, stage 1
	L89.112	Pressure ulcer of right upper back, stage 2
	L89.113	Pressure ulcer of right upper back, stage 3
	L89.114	Pressure ulcer of right upper back, stage 4
	L89.119	Pressure ulcer of right upper back, unspecified stage
	L89.120	Pressure ulcer of left upper back, unstageable
	L89.121	Pressure ulcer of left upper back, stage 1
	L89.122	Pressure ulcer of left upper back, stage 2
	L89.123	Pressure ulcer of left upper back, stage 3
	L89.124	Pressure ulcer of left upper back, stage 4
	L89.129	Pressure ulcer of left upper back, unspecified stage
707.03 PRESSURE ULCER LOWER BACK	**L89.130**	Pressure ulcer of right lower back, unstageable
	L89.131	Pressure ulcer of right lower back, stage 1
	L89.132	Pressure ulcer of right lower back, stage 2
	L89.133	Pressure ulcer of right lower back, stage 3
	L89.134	Pressure ulcer of right lower back, stage 4
	L89.139	Pressure ulcer of right lower back, unspecified stage
	L89.140	Pressure ulcer of left lower back, unstageable
	L89.141	Pressure ulcer of left lower back, stage 1
	L89.142	Pressure ulcer of left lower back, stage 2
	L89.143	Pressure ulcer of left lower back, stage 3
	L89.144	Pressure ulcer of left lower back, stage 4
	L89.149	Pressure ulcer of left lower back, unspecified stage
	L89.150	Pressure ulcer of sacral region, unstageable
	L89.151	Pressure ulcer of sacral region, stage 1
	L89.152	Pressure ulcer of sacral region, stage 2
	L89.153	Pressure ulcer of sacral region, stage 3
	L89.154	Pressure ulcer of sacral region, stage 4
	L89.159	Pressure ulcer of sacral region, unspecified stage
	L89.40	Pressr ulc of contig site of back, buttock and hip, unsp stg
	L89.41	Pressr ulcer of contig site of back, buttock and hip, stg 1
	L89.42	Pressr ulcer of contig site of back, buttock and hip, stg 2
	L89.43	Pressr ulcer of contig site of back, buttock and hip, stg 3
	L89.44	Pressr ulcer of contig site of back, buttock and hip, stg 4
	L89.45	Pressr ulc of contig site of back,buttock & hip, unstageable
707.04 PRESSURE ULCER HIP	**L89.200**	Pressure ulcer of unspecified hip, unstageable
	L89.201	Pressure ulcer of unspecified hip, stage 1
	L89.202	Pressure ulcer of unspecified hip, stage 2
	L89.203	Pressure ulcer of unspecified hip, stage 3
	L89.204	Pressure ulcer of unspecified hip, stage 4
	L89.209	Pressure ulcer of unspecified hip, unspecified stage
	L89.210	Pressure ulcer of right hip, unstageable
	L89.211	Pressure ulcer of right hip, stage 1
	L89.212	Pressure ulcer of right hip, stage 2
	L89.213	Pressure ulcer of right hip, stage 3
	L89.214	Pressure ulcer of right hip, stage 4
	L89.219	Pressure ulcer of right hip, unspecified stage
	L89.220	Pressure ulcer of left hip, unstageable
	L89.221	Pressure ulcer of left hip, stage 1
	L89.222	Pressure ulcer of left hip, stage 2
	L89.223	Pressure ulcer of left hip, stage 3
	L89.224	Pressure ulcer of left hip, stage 4
	L89.229	Pressure ulcer of left hip, unspecified stage
	L89.40	Pressr ulc of contig site of back, buttock and hip, unsp stg
	L89.41	Pressr ulcer of contig site of back, buttock and hip, stg 1
	L89.42	Pressr ulcer of contig site of back, buttock and hip, stg 2
	L89.43	Pressr ulcer of contig site of back, buttock and hip, stg 3
	L89.44	Pressr ulcer of contig site of back, buttock and hip, stg 4
	L89.45	Pressr ulc of contig site of back,buttock & hip, unstageable

ICD-9-CM	ICD-10-CM	Description
707.05 PRESSURE ULCER BUTTOCK	**L89.300**	Pressure ulcer of unspecified buttock, unstageable
	L89.301	Pressure ulcer of unspecified buttock, stage 1
	L89.302	Pressure ulcer of unspecified buttock, stage 2
	L89.303	Pressure ulcer of unspecified buttock, stage 3
	L89.304	Pressure ulcer of unspecified buttock, stage 4
	L89.309	Pressure ulcer of unspecified buttock, unspecified stage
	L89.310	Pressure ulcer of right buttock, unstageable
	L89.311	Pressure ulcer of right buttock, stage 1
	L89.312	Pressure ulcer of right buttock, stage 2
	L89.313	Pressure ulcer of right buttock, stage 3
	L89.314	Pressure ulcer of right buttock, stage 4
	L89.319	Pressure ulcer of right buttock, unspecified stage
	L89.320	Pressure ulcer of left buttock, unstageable
	L89.321	Pressure ulcer of left buttock, stage 1
	L89.322	Pressure ulcer of left buttock, stage 2
	L89.323	Pressure ulcer of left buttock, stage 3
	L89.324	Pressure ulcer of left buttock, stage 4
	L89.329	Pressure ulcer of left buttock, unspecified stage
	L89.40	Pressr ulc of contig site of back, buttock and hip, unsp stg
	L89.41	Pressr ulcer of contig site of back, buttock and hip, stg 1
	L89.42	Pressr ulcer of contig site of back, buttock and hip, stg 2
	L89.43	Pressr ulcer of contig site of back, buttock and hip, stg 3
	L89.44	Pressr ulcer of contig site of back, buttock and hip, stg 4
	L89.45	Pressr ulc of contig site of back,buttock & hip, unstageable
707.06 PRESSURE ULCER ANKLE	**L89.500**	Pressure ulcer of unspecified ankle, unstageable
	L89.501	Pressure ulcer of unspecified ankle, stage 1
	L89.502	Pressure ulcer of unspecified ankle, stage 2
	L89.503	Pressure ulcer of unspecified ankle, stage 3
	L89.504	Pressure ulcer of unspecified ankle, stage 4
	L89.509	Pressure ulcer of unspecified ankle, unspecified stage
	L89.510	Pressure ulcer of right ankle, unstageable
	L89.511	Pressure ulcer of right ankle, stage 1
	L89.512	Pressure ulcer of right ankle, stage 2
	L89.513	Pressure ulcer of right ankle, stage 3
	L89.514	Pressure ulcer of right ankle, stage 4
	L89.519	Pressure ulcer of right ankle, unspecified stage
	L89.520	Pressure ulcer of left ankle, unstageable
	L89.521	Pressure ulcer of left ankle, stage 1
	L89.522	Pressure ulcer of left ankle, stage 2
	L89.523	Pressure ulcer of left ankle, stage 3
	L89.524	Pressure ulcer of left ankle, stage 4
	L89.529	Pressure ulcer of left ankle, unspecified stage
707.07 PRESSURE ULCER HEEL	**L89.600**	Pressure ulcer of unspecified heel, unstageable
	L89.601	Pressure ulcer of unspecified heel, stage 1
	L89.602	Pressure ulcer of unspecified heel, stage 2
	L89.603	Pressure ulcer of unspecified heel, stage 3
	L89.604	Pressure ulcer of unspecified heel, stage 4
	L89.609	Pressure ulcer of unspecified heel, unspecified stage
	L89.610	Pressure ulcer of right heel, unstageable
	L89.611	Pressure ulcer of right heel, stage 1
	L89.612	Pressure ulcer of right heel, stage 2
	L89.613	Pressure ulcer of right heel, stage 3
	L89.614	Pressure ulcer of right heel, stage 4
	L89.619	Pressure ulcer of right heel, unspecified stage
	L89.620	Pressure ulcer of left heel, unstageable
	L89.621	Pressure ulcer of left heel, stage 1
	L89.622	Pressure ulcer of left heel, stage 2
	L89.623	Pressure ulcer of left heel, stage 3
	L89.624	Pressure ulcer of left heel, stage 4
	L89.629	Pressure ulcer of left heel, unspecified stage
707.09 PRESSURE ULCER OTHER SITE	**L89.810**	Pressure ulcer of head, unstageable
	L89.811	Pressure ulcer of head, stage 1
	L89.812	Pressure ulcer of head, stage 2
	L89.813	Pressure ulcer of head, stage 3
	L89.814	Pressure ulcer of head, stage 4
	L89.819	Pressure ulcer of head, unspecified stage
	L89.890	Pressure ulcer of other site, unstageable
	L89.891	Pressure ulcer of other site, stage 1
	L89.892	Pressure ulcer of other site, stage 2
	L89.893	Pressure ulcer of other site, stage 3
	L89.894	Pressure ulcer of other site, stage 4
	L89.899	Pressure ulcer of other site, unspecified stage

707.10 ULCER OF LOWER LIMB, UNSPECIFIED	**L97.901**	Non-prs chr ulc unsp prt of unsp low leg lmt to brkdwn skin
	L97.902	Non-prs chr ulc unsp prt of unsp low leg w fat layer exposed
	L97.903	Non-prs chronic ulc unsp prt of unsp low leg w necros muscle
	L97.904	Non-prs chronic ulc unsp prt of unsp lower leg w necros bone
	L97.909	Non-prs chronic ulc unsp prt of unsp low leg w unsp severity
	L97.911	Non-prs chr ulc unsp prt of r low leg limited to brkdwn skin
	L97.912	Non-prs chr ulc unsp prt of r low leg w fat layer exposed
	L97.913	Non-prs chronic ulc unsp prt of r low leg w necros muscle
	L97.914	Non-prs chronic ulc unsp prt of r low leg w necrosis of bone
	L97.919	Non-prs chronic ulc unsp prt of r low leg w unsp severity
	L97.921	Non-prs chr ulc unsp prt of l low leg limited to brkdwn skin
	L97.922	Non-prs chr ulc unsp prt of l low leg w fat layer exposed
	L97.923	Non-prs chronic ulc unsp prt of l low leg w necros muscle
	L97.924	Non-prs chronic ulc unsp prt of l low leg w necrosis of bone
	L97.929	Non-prs chronic ulc unsp prt of l low leg w unsp severity
707.11 ULCER OF THIGH	◘ **I70.231**	Athscl native arteries of right leg w ulceration of thigh
	◘ **I70.241**	Athscl native arteries of left leg w ulceration of thigh
	◘ **I70.331**	Athscl unsp type bypass of the right leg w ulcer of thigh
	◘ **I70.341**	Athscl unsp type bypass of the left leg w ulcer of thigh
	◘ **I70.431**	Athscl autol vein bypass of the right leg w ulcer of thigh
	◘ **I70.441**	Athscl autol vein bypass of the left leg w ulcer of thigh
	◘ **I70.531**	Athscl nonaut bio bypass of the right leg w ulcer of thigh
	◘ **I70.541**	Athscl nonaut bio bypass of the left leg w ulcer of thigh
	◘ **I70.631**	Athscl nonbiol bypass of the right leg w ulceration of thigh
	◘ **I70.641**	Athscl nonbiol bypass of the left leg w ulceration of thigh
	◘ **I70.731**	Athscl type of bypass of the right leg w ulceration of thigh
	◘ **I70.741**	Athscl type of bypass of the left leg w ulceration of thigh
	L97.101	Non-prs chronic ulcer of unsp thigh limited to brkdwn skin
	L97.102	Non-pressure chronic ulcer of unsp thigh w fat layer exposed
	L97.103	Non-prs chronic ulcer of unsp thigh w necrosis of muscle
	L97.104	Non-pressure chronic ulcer of unsp thigh w necrosis of bone
	L97.109	Non-pressure chronic ulcer of unsp thigh with unsp severity
	L97.111	Non-prs chronic ulcer of right thigh limited to brkdwn skin
	L97.112	Non-prs chronic ulcer of right thigh w fat layer exposed
	L97.113	Non-prs chronic ulcer of right thigh w necrosis of muscle
	L97.114	Non-pressure chronic ulcer of right thigh w necrosis of bone
	L97.119	Non-pressure chronic ulcer of right thigh with unsp severity
	L97.121	Non-prs chronic ulcer of left thigh limited to brkdwn skin
	L97.122	Non-pressure chronic ulcer of left thigh w fat layer exposed
	L97.123	Non-prs chronic ulcer of left thigh w necrosis of muscle
	L97.124	Non-pressure chronic ulcer of left thigh w necrosis of bone
	L97.129	Non-pressure chronic ulcer of left thigh with unsp severity
707.12 ULCER OF CALF	◘ **I70.232**	Athscl native arteries of right leg w ulceration of calf
	◘ **I70.242**	Athscl native arteries of left leg w ulceration of calf
	◘ **I70.332**	Athscl unsp type bypass of the right leg w ulcer of calf
	◘ **I70.342**	Athscl unsp type bypass of the left leg w ulceration of calf
	◘ **I70.432**	Athscl autol vein bypass of the right leg w ulcer of calf
	◘ **I70.442**	Athscl autol vein bypass of the left leg w ulcer of calf
	◘ **I70.532**	Athscl nonaut bio bypass of the right leg w ulcer of calf
	◘ **I70.542**	Athscl nonaut bio bypass of the left leg w ulcer of calf
	◘ **I70.632**	Athscl nonbiol bypass of the right leg w ulceration of calf
	◘ **I70.642**	Athscl nonbiol bypass of the left leg w ulceration of calf
	◘ **I70.732**	Athscl type of bypass of the right leg w ulceration of calf
	◘ **I70.742**	Athscl type of bypass of the left leg w ulceration of calf
	L97.201	Non-prs chronic ulcer of unsp calf limited to brkdwn skin
	L97.202	Non-pressure chronic ulcer of unsp calf w fat layer exposed
	L97.203	Non-pressure chronic ulcer of unsp calf w necrosis of muscle
	L97.204	Non-pressure chronic ulcer of unsp calf w necrosis of bone
	L97.209	Non-pressure chronic ulcer of unsp calf with unsp severity
	L97.211	Non-prs chronic ulcer of right calf limited to brkdwn skin
	L97.212	Non-pressure chronic ulcer of right calf w fat layer exposed
	L97.213	Non-prs chronic ulcer of right calf w necrosis of muscle
	L97.214	Non-pressure chronic ulcer of right calf w necrosis of bone
	L97.219	Non-pressure chronic ulcer of right calf with unsp severity
	L97.221	Non-prs chronic ulcer of left calf limited to brkdwn skin
	L97.222	Non-pressure chronic ulcer of left calf w fat layer exposed
	L97.223	Non-pressure chronic ulcer of left calf w necrosis of muscle
	L97.224	Non-pressure chronic ulcer of left calf w necrosis of bone
	L97.229	Non-pressure chronic ulcer of left calf with unsp severity

ICD-9-CM		ICD-10-CM	
707.13 ULCER OF ANKLE	◻	**I70.233**	Athscl native arteries of right leg w ulceration of ankle
	◻	**I70.243**	Athscl native arteries of left leg w ulceration of ankle
	◻	**I70.333**	Athscl unsp type bypass of the right leg w ulcer of ankle
	◻	**I70.343**	Athscl unsp type bypass of the left leg w ulcer of ankle
	◻	**I70.433**	Athscl autol vein bypass of the right leg w ulcer of ankle
	◻	**I70.443**	Athscl autol vein bypass of the left leg w ulcer of ankle
	◻	**I70.533**	Athscl nonaut bio bypass of the right leg w ulcer of ankle
	◻	**I70.543**	Athscl nonaut bio bypass of the left leg w ulcer of ankle
	◻	**I70.633**	Athscl nonbiol bypass of the right leg w ulceration of ankle
	◻	**I70.643**	Athscl nonbiol bypass of the left leg w ulceration of ankle
	◻	**I70.733**	Athscl type of bypass of the right leg w ulceration of ankle
	◻	**I70.743**	Athscl type of bypass of the left leg w ulceration of ankle
		L97.301	Non-prs chronic ulcer of unsp ankle limited to brkdwn skin
		L97.302	Non-pressure chronic ulcer of unsp ankle w fat layer exposed
		L97.303	Non-prs chronic ulcer of unsp ankle w necrosis of muscle
		L97.304	Non-pressure chronic ulcer of unsp ankle w necrosis of bone
		L97.309	Non-pressure chronic ulcer of unsp ankle with unsp severity
		L97.311	Non-prs chronic ulcer of right ankle limited to brkdwn skin
		L97.312	Non-prs chronic ulcer of right ankle w fat layer exposed
		L97.313	Non-prs chronic ulcer of right ankle w necrosis of muscle
		L97.314	Non-pressure chronic ulcer of right ankle w necrosis of bone
		L97.319	Non-pressure chronic ulcer of right ankle with unsp severity
		L97.321	Non-prs chronic ulcer of left ankle limited to brkdwn skin
		L97.322	Non-pressure chronic ulcer of left ankle w fat layer exposed
		L97.323	Non-prs chronic ulcer of left ankle w necrosis of muscle
		L97.324	Non-pressure chronic ulcer of left ankle w necrosis of bone
		L97.329	Non-pressure chronic ulcer of left ankle with unsp severity
707.14 ULCER OF HEEL AND MIDFOOT	◻	**I70.234**	Athscl native art of right leg w ulcer of heel and midfoot
	◻	**I70.244**	Athscl native art of left leg w ulcer of heel and midfoot
	◻	**I70.334**	Athscl unsp type bypass of r leg w ulcer of heel and midft
	◻	**I70.344**	Athscl unsp type bypass of left leg w ulc of heel and midft
	◻	**I70.434**	Athscl autol vein bypass of r leg w ulcer of heel and midft
	◻	**I70.444**	Athscl autol vein bypass of left leg w ulc of heel and midft
	◻	**I70.534**	Athscl nonaut bio bypass of r leg w ulcer of heel and midft
	◻	**I70.544**	Athscl nonaut bio bypass of left leg w ulc of heel and midft
	◻	**I70.634**	Athscl nonbiol bypass of right leg w ulcer of heel and midft
	◻	**I70.644**	Athscl nonbiol bypass of left leg w ulcer of heel and midft
	◻	**I70.734**	Athscl type of bypass of right leg w ulcer of heel and midft
	◻	**I70.744**	Athscl type of bypass of left leg w ulcer of heel and midft
		L97.401	Non-prs chr ulcer of unsp heel and midft lmt to brkdwn skin
		L97.402	Non-prs chr ulcer of unsp heel and midfoot w fat layer expos
		L97.403	Non-prs chr ulcer of unsp heel and midfoot w necros muscle
		L97.404	Non-prs chronic ulcer of unsp heel and midfoot w necros bone
		L97.409	Non-prs chronic ulcer of unsp heel and midfoot w unsp severt
		L97.411	Non-prs chr ulcer of right heel and midft lmt to brkdwn skin
		L97.412	Non-prs chr ulcer of right heel and midft w fat layer expos
		L97.413	Non-prs chr ulcer of right heel and midfoot w necros muscle
		L97.414	Non-prs chr ulcer of right heel and midfoot w necros bone
		L97.419	Non-prs chr ulcer of right heel and midfoot w unsp severt
		L97.421	Non-prs chr ulcer of left heel and midft lmt to brkdwn skin
		L97.422	Non-prs chr ulcer of left heel and midfoot w fat layer expos
		L97.423	Non-prs chr ulcer of left heel and midfoot w necros muscle
		L97.424	Non-prs chronic ulcer of left heel and midfoot w necros bone
		L97.429	Non-prs chronic ulcer of left heel and midfoot w unsp severt
707.15 ULCER OF OTHER PART OF FOOT	◻	**I70.235**	Athscl native arteries of right leg w ulcer oth prt foot
	◻	**I70.245**	Athscl native arteries of left leg w ulceration oth prt foot
	◻	**I70.335**	Athscl unsp type bypass of right leg w ulcer oth prt foot
	◻	**I70.345**	Athscl unsp type bypass of the left leg w ulcer oth prt foot
	◻	**I70.435**	Athscl autol vein bypass of right leg w ulcer oth prt foot
	◻	**I70.445**	Athscl autol vein bypass of left leg w ulcer oth prt foot
	◻	**I70.535**	Athscl nonaut bio bypass of right leg w ulcer oth prt foot
	◻	**I70.545**	Athscl nonaut bio bypass of left leg w ulcer oth prt foot
	◻	**I70.635**	Athscl nonbiol bypass of the right leg w ulcer oth prt foot
	◻	**I70.645**	Athscl nonbiol bypass of the left leg w ulcer oth prt foot
	◻	**I70.735**	Athscl type of bypass of the right leg w ulcer oth prt foot
	◻	**I70.745**	Athscl type of bypass of the left leg w ulcer oth prt foot
		L97.501	Non-prs chr ulcer oth prt unsp foot limited to brkdwn skin
		L97.502	Non-prs chronic ulcer oth prt unsp foot w fat layer exposed
		L97.503	Non-prs chronic ulcer oth prt unsp foot w necrosis of muscle
		L97.504	Non-prs chronic ulcer oth prt unsp foot w necrosis of bone
		L97.509	Non-pressure chronic ulcer oth prt unsp foot w unsp severity
		L97.511	Non-prs chronic ulcer oth prt r foot limited to brkdwn skin
		L97.512	Non-prs chronic ulcer oth prt right foot w fat layer exposed
		L97.513	Non-prs chronic ulcer oth prt right foot w necros muscle
		L97.514	Non-prs chronic ulcer oth prt right foot w necrosis of bone
		L97.519	Non-prs chronic ulcer oth prt right foot w unsp severity
		L97.521	Non-prs chronic ulcer oth prt l foot limited to brkdwn skin
		L97.522	Non-prs chronic ulcer oth prt left foot w fat layer exposed
		L97.523	Non-prs chronic ulcer oth prt left foot w necrosis of muscle
		L97.524	Non-prs chronic ulcer oth prt left foot w necrosis of bone
		L97.529	Non-pressure chronic ulcer oth prt left foot w unsp severity

ICD-9-CM		ICD-10-CM	
707.19	ULCER OF OTHER PART OF LOWER LIMB	**I70.238**	Athscl natv art of right leg w ulcer oth prt lower right leg
		I70.239	Athscl native arteries of right leg w ulcer of unsp site
		I70.248	Athscl native art of left leg w ulcer oth prt lower left leg
		I70.249	Athscl native arteries of left leg w ulceration of unsp site
		I70.338	Athscl unsp type bypass of right leg w ulcer oth prt low leg
		I70.339	Athscl unsp type bypass of right leg w ulcer of unsp site
		I70.348	Athscl unsp type bypass of left leg w ulcer oth prt low leg
		I70.349	Athscl unsp type bypass of the left leg w ulcer of unsp site
		I70.438	Athscl autol vein bypass of r leg w ulcer oth prt low leg
		I70.439	Athscl autol vein bypass of right leg w ulcer of unsp site
		I70.448	Athscl autol vein bypass of left leg w ulcer oth prt low leg
		I70.449	Athscl autol vein bypass of left leg w ulcer of unsp site
		I70.538	Athscl nonaut bio bypass of r leg w ulcer oth prt low leg
		I70.539	Athscl nonaut bio bypass of right leg w ulcer of unsp site
		I70.548	Athscl nonaut bio bypass of left leg w ulcer oth prt low leg
		I70.549	Athscl nonaut bio bypass of left leg w ulcer of unsp site
		I70.638	Athscl nonbiol bypass of right leg w ulcer oth prt low leg
		I70.639	Athscl nonbiol bypass of the right leg w ulcer of unsp site
		I70.648	Athscl nonbiol bypass of left leg w ulcer oth prt low leg
		I70.649	Athscl nonbiol bypass of the left leg w ulcer of unsp site
		I70.738	Athscl type of bypass of right leg w ulcer oth prt low leg
		I70.739	Athscl type of bypass of the right leg w ulcer of unsp site
		I70.748	Athscl type of bypass of left leg w ulcer oth prt low leg
		I70.749	Athscl type of bypass of the left leg w ulcer of unsp site
		L97.801	Non-prs chr ulcer oth prt unsp low leg lmt to brkdwn skin
		L97.802	Non-prs chr ulcer oth prt unsp low leg w fat layer exposed
		L97.803	Non-prs chronic ulcer oth prt unsp lower leg w necros muscle
		L97.804	Non-prs chronic ulcer oth prt unsp lower leg w necros bone
		L97.809	Non-prs chronic ulcer oth prt unsp lower leg w unsp severity
		L97.811	Non-prs chr ulcer oth prt r low leg limited to brkdwn skin
		L97.812	Non-prs chronic ulcer oth prt r low leg w fat layer exposed
		L97.813	Non-prs chronic ulcer oth prt r low leg w necrosis of muscle
		L97.814	Non-prs chronic ulcer oth prt r low leg w necrosis of bone
		L97.819	Non-pressure chronic ulcer oth prt r low leg w unsp severity
		L97.821	Non-prs chr ulcer oth prt l low leg limited to brkdwn skin
		L97.822	Non-prs chronic ulcer oth prt l low leg w fat layer exposed
		L97.823	Non-prs chronic ulcer oth prt l low leg w necrosis of muscle
		L97.824	Non-prs chronic ulcer oth prt l low leg w necrosis of bone
		L97.829	Non-pressure chronic ulcer oth prt l low leg w unsp severity
707.20	PRESSURE ULCER UNSPECIFIED STAGE	**L89.009**	Pressure ulcer of unspecified elbow, unspecified stage
		L89.019	Pressure ulcer of right elbow, unspecified stage
		L89.029	Pressure ulcer of left elbow, unspecified stage
		L89.109	Pressure ulcer of unsp part of back, unspecified stage
		L89.119	Pressure ulcer of right upper back, unspecified stage
		L89.129	Pressure ulcer of left upper back, unspecified stage
		L89.139	Pressure ulcer of right lower back, unspecified stage
		L89.149	Pressure ulcer of left lower back, unspecified stage
		L89.159	Pressure ulcer of sacral region, unspecified stage
		L89.209	Pressure ulcer of unspecified hip, unspecified stage
		L89.219	Pressure ulcer of right hip, unspecified stage
		L89.229	Pressure ulcer of left hip, unspecified stage
		L89.309	Pressure ulcer of unspecified buttock, unspecified stage
		L89.319	Pressure ulcer of right buttock, unspecified stage
		L89.329	Pressure ulcer of left buttock, unspecified stage
		L89.40	Pressr ulc of contig site of back, buttock and hip, unsp stg
		L89.509	Pressure ulcer of unspecified ankle, unspecified stage
		L89.519	Pressure ulcer of right ankle, unspecified stage
		L89.529	Pressure ulcer of left ankle, unspecified stage
		L89.609	Pressure ulcer of unspecified heel, unspecified stage
		L89.619	Pressure ulcer of right heel, unspecified stage
		L89.629	Pressure ulcer of left heel, unspecified stage
		L89.819	Pressure ulcer of head, unspecified stage
		L89.899	Pressure ulcer of other site, unspecified stage
		L89.90	Pressure ulcer of unspecified site, unspecified stage

ICD-9-CM	ICD-10-CM	Description
7Ø7.21 PRESSURE ULCER STAGE I	**L89.ØØ1**	Pressure ulcer of unspecified elbow, stage 1
	L89.Ø11	Pressure ulcer of right elbow, stage 1
	L89.Ø21	Pressure ulcer of left elbow, stage 1
	L89.1Ø1	Pressure ulcer of unspecified part of back, stage 1
	L89.111	Pressure ulcer of right upper back, stage 1
	L89.121	Pressure ulcer of left upper back, stage 1
	L89.131	Pressure ulcer of right lower back, stage 1
	L89.141	Pressure ulcer of left lower back, stage 1
	L89.151	Pressure ulcer of sacral region, stage 1
	L89.2Ø1	Pressure ulcer of unspecified hip, stage 1
	L89.211	Pressure ulcer of right hip, stage 1
	L89.221	Pressure ulcer of left hip, stage 1
	L89.3Ø1	Pressure ulcer of unspecified buttock, stage 1
	L89.311	Pressure ulcer of right buttock, stage 1
	L89.321	Pressure ulcer of left buttock, stage 1
	L89.41	Pressr ulcer of contig site of back, buttock and hip, stg 1
	L89.5Ø1	Pressure ulcer of unspecified ankle, stage 1
	L89.511	Pressure ulcer of right ankle, stage 1
	L89.521	Pressure ulcer of left ankle, stage 1
	L89.6Ø1	Pressure ulcer of unspecified heel, stage 1
	L89.611	Pressure ulcer of right heel, stage 1
	L89.621	Pressure ulcer of left heel, stage 1
	L89.811	Pressure ulcer of head, stage 1
	L89.891	Pressure ulcer of other site, stage 1
	L89.91	Pressure ulcer of unspecified site, stage 1
7Ø7.22 PRESSURE ULCER STAGE II	**L89.ØØ2**	Pressure ulcer of unspecified elbow, stage 2
	L89.Ø12	Pressure ulcer of right elbow, stage 2
	L89.Ø22	Pressure ulcer of left elbow, stage 2
	L89.1Ø2	Pressure ulcer of unspecified part of back, stage 2
	L89.112	Pressure ulcer of right upper back, stage 2
	L89.122	Pressure ulcer of left upper back, stage 2
	L89.132	Pressure ulcer of right lower back, stage 2
	L89.142	Pressure ulcer of left lower back, stage 2
	L89.152	Pressure ulcer of sacral region, stage 2
	L89.2Ø2	Pressure ulcer of unspecified hip, stage 2
	L89.212	Pressure ulcer of right hip, stage 2
	L89.222	Pressure ulcer of left hip, stage 2
	L89.3Ø2	Pressure ulcer of unspecified buttock, stage 2
	L89.312	Pressure ulcer of right buttock, stage 2
	L89.322	Pressure ulcer of left buttock, stage 2
	L89.42	Pressr ulcer of contig site of back, buttock and hip, stg 2
	L89.5Ø2	Pressure ulcer of unspecified ankle, stage 2
	L89.512	Pressure ulcer of right ankle, stage 2
	L89.522	Pressure ulcer of left ankle, stage 2
	L89.6Ø2	Pressure ulcer of unspecified heel, stage 2
	L89.612	Pressure ulcer of right heel, stage 2
	L89.622	Pressure ulcer of left heel, stage 2
	L89.812	Pressure ulcer of head, stage 2
	L89.892	Pressure ulcer of other site, stage 2
	L89.92	Pressure ulcer of unspecified site, stage 2
7Ø7.23 PRESSURE ULCER STAGE III	**L89.ØØ3**	Pressure ulcer of unspecified elbow, stage 3
	L89.Ø13	Pressure ulcer of right elbow, stage 3
	L89.Ø23	Pressure ulcer of left elbow, stage 3
	L89.1Ø3	Pressure ulcer of unspecified part of back, stage 3
	L89.113	Pressure ulcer of right upper back, stage 3
	L89.123	Pressure ulcer of left upper back, stage 3
	L89.133	Pressure ulcer of right lower back, stage 3
	L89.143	Pressure ulcer of left lower back, stage 3
	L89.153	Pressure ulcer of sacral region, stage 3
	L89.2Ø3	Pressure ulcer of unspecified hip, stage 3
	L89.213	Pressure ulcer of right hip, stage 3
	L89.223	Pressure ulcer of left hip, stage 3
	L89.3Ø3	Pressure ulcer of unspecified buttock, stage 3
	L89.313	Pressure ulcer of right buttock, stage 3
	L89.323	Pressure ulcer of left buttock, stage 3
	L89.43	Pressr ulcer of contig site of back, buttock and hip, stg 3
	L89.5Ø3	Pressure ulcer of unspecified ankle, stage 3
	L89.513	Pressure ulcer of right ankle, stage 3
	L89.523	Pressure ulcer of left ankle, stage 3
	L89.6Ø3	Pressure ulcer of unspecified heel, stage 3
	L89.613	Pressure ulcer of right heel, stage 3
	L89.623	Pressure ulcer of left heel, stage 3
	L89.813	Pressure ulcer of head, stage 3
	L89.893	Pressure ulcer of other site, stage 3
	L89.93	Pressure ulcer of unspecified site, stage 3

ICD-9-CM		ICD-10-CM		
7Ø7.24	PRESSURE ULCER STAGE IV	◻	L89.ØØ4	Pressure ulcer of unspecified elbow, stage 4
		◻	L89.Ø14	Pressure ulcer of right elbow, stage 4
		◻	L89.Ø24	Pressure ulcer of left elbow, stage 4
		◻	L89.1Ø4	Pressure ulcer of unspecified part of back, stage 4
		◻	L89.114	Pressure ulcer of right upper back, stage 4
		◻	L89.124	Pressure ulcer of left upper back, stage 4
		◻	L89.134	Pressure ulcer of right lower back, stage 4
		◻	L89.144	Pressure ulcer of left lower back, stage 4
		◻	L89.154	Pressure ulcer of sacral region, stage 4
		◻	L89.2Ø4	Pressure ulcer of unspecified hip, stage 4
		◻	L89.214	Pressure ulcer of right hip, stage 4
		◻	L89.224	Pressure ulcer of left hip, stage 4
		◻	L89.3Ø4	Pressure ulcer of unspecified buttock, stage 4
		◻	L89.314	Pressure ulcer of right buttock, stage 4
		◻	L89.324	Pressure ulcer of left buttock, stage 4
		◻	L89.44	Pressr ulcer of contig site of back, buttock and hip, stg 4
		◻	L89.5Ø4	Pressure ulcer of unspecified ankle, stage 4
		◻	L89.514	Pressure ulcer of right ankle, stage 4
		◻	L89.524	Pressure ulcer of left ankle, stage 4
		◻	L89.6Ø4	Pressure ulcer of unspecified heel, stage 4
		◻	L89.614	Pressure ulcer of right heel, stage 4
		◻	L89.624	Pressure ulcer of left heel, stage 4
		◻	L89.814	Pressure ulcer of head, stage 4
		◻	L89.894	Pressure ulcer of other site, stage 4
		◻	L89.94	Pressure ulcer of unspecified site, stage 4
7Ø7.25	PRESSURE ULCER UNSTAGEABLE	◻	L89.ØØØ	Pressure ulcer of unspecified elbow, unstageable
		◻	L89.Ø1Ø	Pressure ulcer of right elbow, unstageable
		◻	L89.Ø2Ø	Pressure ulcer of left elbow, unstageable
		◻	L89.1ØØ	Pressure ulcer of unspecified part of back, unstageable
		◻	L89.11Ø	Pressure ulcer of right upper back, unstageable
		◻	L89.12Ø	Pressure ulcer of left upper back, unstageable
		◻	L89.13Ø	Pressure ulcer of right lower back, unstageable
		◻	L89.14Ø	Pressure ulcer of left lower back, unstageable
		◻	L89.15Ø	Pressure ulcer of sacral region, unstageable
		◻	L89.2ØØ	Pressure ulcer of unspecified hip, unstageable
		◻	L89.21Ø	Pressure ulcer of right hip, unstageable
		◻	L89.22Ø	Pressure ulcer of left hip, unstageable
		◻	L89.3ØØ	Pressure ulcer of unspecified buttock, unstageable
		◻	L89.31Ø	Pressure ulcer of right buttock, unstageable
		◻	L89.32Ø	Pressure ulcer of left buttock, unstageable
		◻	L89.45	Pressr ulc of contig site of back,buttock & hip, unstageable
		◻	L89.5ØØ	Pressure ulcer of unspecified ankle, unstageable
		◻	L89.51Ø	Pressure ulcer of right ankle, unstageable
		◻	L89.52Ø	Pressure ulcer of left ankle, unstageable
		◻	L89.6ØØ	Pressure ulcer of unspecified heel, unstageable
		◻	L89.61Ø	Pressure ulcer of right heel, unstageable
		◻	L89.62Ø	Pressure ulcer of left heel, unstageable
		◻	L89.81Ø	Pressure ulcer of head, unstageable
		◻	L89.89Ø	Pressure ulcer of other site, unstageable
		◻	L89.95	Pressure ulcer of unspecified site, unstageable
7Ø7.8	CHRONIC ULCER OF OTHER SPECIFIED SITE		L98.411	Non-pressure chronic ulcer of buttock limited to brkdwn skin
			L98.412	Non-pressure chronic ulcer of buttock with fat layer exposed
			L98.413	Non-pressure chronic ulcer of buttock w necrosis of muscle
			L98.414	Non-pressure chronic ulcer of buttock with necrosis of bone
			L98.419	Non-pressure chronic ulcer of buttock with unsp severity
			L98.421	Non-pressure chronic ulcer of back limited to brkdwn skin
			L98.422	Non-pressure chronic ulcer of back with fat layer exposed
			L98.423	Non-pressure chronic ulcer of back with necrosis of muscle
			L98.424	Non-pressure chronic ulcer of back with necrosis of bone
			L98.429	Non-pressure chronic ulcer of back with unspecified severity
7Ø7.9	CHRONIC ULCER OF UNSPECIFIED SITE	◻	I7Ø.25	Athscl native arteries of extremities w ulceration
		◻	I7Ø.35	Athscl unsp type bypass graft(s) of extremity w ulceration
		◻	I7Ø.45	Athscl autologous vein bypass of extremity w ulceration
		◻	I7Ø.55	Athscl nonautologous bio bypass of extremity w ulceration
		◻	I7Ø.65	Athscl nonbiological bypass of extremity w ulceration
		◻	I7Ø.75	Athscl type of bypass graft(s) of extremity w ulceration
			L98.491	Non-prs chronic ulcer skin/ sites limited to brkdwn skin
			L98.492	Non-prs chronic ulcer of skin of sites w fat layer exposed
			L98.493	Non-prs chronic ulcer of skin of sites w necrosis of muscle
			L98.494	Non-prs chronic ulcer of skin of sites w necrosis of bone
			L98.499	Non-pressure chronic ulcer of skin of sites w unsp severity
7Ø8.Ø	ALLERGIC URTICARIA	➡	L5Ø.Ø	Allergic urticaria
7Ø8.1	IDIOPATHIC URTICARIA	➡	L5Ø.1	Idiopathic urticaria
7Ø8.2	URTICARIA DUE TO COLD AND HEAT	➡	L5Ø.2	Urticaria due to cold and heat
7Ø8.3	DERMATOGRAPHIC URTICARIA	➡	L5Ø.3	Dermatographic urticaria
7Ø8.4	VIBRATORY URTICARIA	➡	L5Ø.4	Vibratory urticaria
7Ø8.5	CHOLINERGIC URTICARIA	➡	L5Ø.5	Cholinergic urticaria

ICD-9-CM			ICD-10-CM	
708.8	OTHER SPECIFIED URTICARIA		L50.6	Contact urticaria
			L50.8	Other urticaria
708.9	UNSPECIFIED URTICARIA	➡	L50.9	Urticaria, unspecified
709.00	DYSCHROMIA, UNSPECIFIED	➡	L81.9	Disorder of pigmentation, unspecified
709.01	VITILIGO	➡	L80	Vitiligo
709.09	OTHER DYSCHROMIA		L57.3	Poikiloderma of Civatte
			L81.0	Postinflammatory hyperpigmentation
			L81.1	Chloasma
			L81.2	Freckles
			L81.3	Cafe au lait spots
			L81.4	Other melanin hyperpigmentation
			L81.5	Leukoderma, not elsewhere classified
			L81.6	Other disorders of diminished melanin formation
			L81.7	Pigmented purpuric dermatosis
			L81.8	Other specified disorders of pigmentation
709.1	VASCULAR DISORDER OF SKIN		L95.0	Livedoid vasculitis
			L95.8	Other vasculitis limited to the skin
			L95.9	Vasculitis limited to the skin, unspecified
709.2	SCAR CONDITION AND FIBROSIS OF SKIN	➡	L90.5	Scar conditions and fibrosis of skin
709.3	DEGENERATIVE SKIN DISORDER		L92.1	Necrobiosis lipoidica, not elsewhere classified
			L94.2	Calcinosis cutis
			L98.8	Oth disrd of the skin and subcutaneous tissue
709.4	FOREIGN BODY GRANULOMA SKIN&SUBCUTANEOUS TISSUE	➡	L92.3	Foreign body granuloma of the skin and subcutaneous tissue
709.8	OTHER SPECIFIED DISORDER OF SKIN	◘	E08.628	Diabetes due to underlying condition w oth skin comp
		◘	E09.628	Drug/chem diabetes mellitus w oth skin complications
			L44.8	Other specified papulosquamous disorders
			L44.9	Papulosquamous disorder, unspecified
			L45	Papulosquamous disorders in diseases classified elsewhere
			L94.2	Calcinosis cutis
			L94.4	Gottron's papules
			L98.8	Oth disrd of the skin and subcutaneous tissue
			L99	Oth disorders of skin, subcu in diseases classd elswhr
709.9	UNSPECIFIED DISORDER OF SKIN&SUBCUTANEOUS TISSUE		L98.9	Disorder of the skin and subcutaneous tissue, unspecified

Musculoskeletal System and Connective Tissue

ICD-9-CM			ICD-10-CM	
71Ø.Ø	SYSTEMIC LUPUS ERYTHEMATOSUS		**M32.Ø**	Drug-induced systemic lupus erythematosus
			M32.1Ø	Systemic lupus erythematosus, organ or system involv unsp
		◘	**M32.11**	Endocarditis in systemic lupus erythematosus
		◘	**M32.12**	Pericarditis in systemic lupus erythematosus
		◘	**M32.13**	Lung involvement in systemic lupus erythematosus
		◘	**M32.14**	Glomerular disease in systemic lupus erythematosus
		◘	**M32.15**	Tubulo-interstitial neuropath in sys lupus erythematosus
			M32.19	Oth organ or system involv in systemic lupus erythematosus
			M32.8	Other forms of systemic lupus erythematosus
			M32.9	Systemic lupus erythematosus, unspecified
71Ø.1	SYSTEMIC SCLEROSIS		**M34.Ø**	Progressive systemic sclerosis
			M34.1	CR(E)ST syndrome
			M34.2	Systemic sclerosis induced by drug and chemical
		◘	**M34.81**	Systemic sclerosis with lung involvement
		◘	**M34.82**	Systemic sclerosis with myopathy
		◘	**M34.83**	Systemic sclerosis with polyneuropathy
			M34.89	Other systemic sclerosis
			M34.9	Systemic sclerosis, unspecified
71Ø.2	SICCA SYNDROME		**M35.ØØ**	Sicca syndrome, unspecified
			M35.Ø1	Sicca syndrome with keratoconjunctivitis
		◘	**M35.Ø2**	Sicca syndrome with lung involvement
		◘	**M35.Ø3**	Sicca syndrome with myopathy
		◘	**M35.Ø4**	Sicca syndrome with tubulo-interstitial nephropathy
			M35.Ø9	Sicca syndrome with other organ involvement
71Ø.3	DERMATOMYOSITIS		**M33.ØØ**	Juvenile dermatopolymyositis, organ involvement unspecified
		◘	**M33.Ø1**	Juvenile dermatopolymyositis with respiratory involvement
		◘	**M33.Ø2**	Juvenile dermatopolymyositis with myopathy
			M33.Ø9	Juvenile dermatopolymyositis with other organ involvement
			M33.1Ø	Other dermatopolymyositis, organ involvement unspecified
		◘	**M33.11**	Other dermatopolymyositis with respiratory involvement
		◘	**M33.12**	Other dermatopolymyositis with myopathy
			M33.19	Other dermatopolymyositis with other organ involvement
			M33.9Ø	Dermatopolymyositis, unsp, organ involvement unspecified
		◘	**M33.91**	Dermatopolymyositis, unsp with respiratory involvement
		◘	**M33.92**	Dermatopolymyositis, unspecified with myopathy
			M33.99	Dermatopolymyositis, unsp with other organ involvement
			M36.Ø	Dermato(poly)myositis in neoplastic disease
71Ø.4	POLYMYOSITIS		**M33.2Ø**	Polymyositis, organ involvement unspecified
		◘	**M33.21**	Polymyositis with respiratory involvement
		◘	**M33.22**	Polymyositis with myopathy
			M33.29	Polymyositis with other organ involvement
71Ø.5	EOSINOPHILIA MYALGIA SYNDROME		**M35.8**	Other specified systemic involvement of connective tissue
71Ø.8	OTHER SPEC DIFFUSE DISEASE CONNECTIVE TISSUE		**M35.1**	Other overlap syndromes
			M35.5	Multifocal fibrosclerosis
			M35.8	Other specified systemic involvement of connective tissue
71Ø.9	UNSPECIFIED DIFFUSE CONNECTIVE TISSUE DISEASE		**M35.9**	Systemic involvement of connective tissue, unspecified
			M36.8	Systemic disord of conn tiss in oth diseases classd elswhr
711.ØØ	PYOGENIC ARTHRITIS SITE UNSPECIFIED	◘	**MØØ.ØØ**	Staphylococcal arthritis, unspecified joint
		◘	**MØØ.1Ø**	Pneumococcal arthritis, unspecified joint
		◘	**MØØ.2Ø**	Other streptococcal arthritis, unspecified joint
		◘	**MØØ.8Ø**	Arthritis due to other bacteria, unspecified joint
			MØØ.9	Pyogenic arthritis, unspecified
711.Ø1	PYOGENIC ARTHRITIS, SHOULDER REGION	◘	**MØØ.Ø11**	Staphylococcal arthritis, right shoulder
		◘	**MØØ.Ø12**	Staphylococcal arthritis, left shoulder
		◘	**MØØ.Ø19**	Staphylococcal arthritis, unspecified shoulder
		◘	**MØØ.111**	Pneumococcal arthritis, right shoulder
		◘	**MØØ.112**	Pneumococcal arthritis, left shoulder
		◘	**MØØ.119**	Pneumococcal arthritis, unspecified shoulder
		◘	**MØØ.211**	Other streptococcal arthritis, right shoulder
		◘	**MØØ.212**	Other streptococcal arthritis, left shoulder
		◘	**MØØ.219**	Other streptococcal arthritis, unspecified shoulder
		◘	**MØØ.811**	Arthritis due to other bacteria, right shoulder
		◘	**MØØ.812**	Arthritis due to other bacteria, left shoulder
		◘	**MØØ.819**	Arthritis due to other bacteria, unspecified shoulder
711.Ø2	PYOGENIC ARTHRITIS, UPPER ARM	◘	**MØØ.Ø21**	Staphylococcal arthritis, right elbow
		◘	**MØØ.Ø22**	Staphylococcal arthritis, left elbow
		◘	**MØØ.Ø29**	Staphylococcal arthritis, unspecified elbow
		◘	**MØØ.121**	Pneumococcal arthritis, right elbow
		◘	**MØØ.122**	Pneumococcal arthritis, left elbow
		◘	**MØØ.129**	Pneumococcal arthritis, unspecified elbow
		◘	**MØØ.221**	Other streptococcal arthritis, right elbow
		◘	**MØØ.222**	Other streptococcal arthritis, left elbow
		◘	**MØØ.229**	Other streptococcal arthritis, unspecified elbow
		◘	**MØØ.821**	Arthritis due to other bacteria, right elbow
		◘	**MØØ.822**	Arthritis due to other bacteria, left elbow
		◘	**MØØ.829**	Arthritis due to other bacteria, unspecified elbow

ICD-9-CM		ICD-10-CM	
711.Ø3	PYOGENIC ARTHRITIS, FOREARM	**MØØ.Ø31**	Staphylococcal arthritis, right wrist
		MØØ.Ø32	Staphylococcal arthritis, left wrist
		MØØ.Ø39	Staphylococcal arthritis, unspecified wrist
		MØØ.131	Pneumococcal arthritis, right wrist
		MØØ.132	Pneumococcal arthritis, left wrist
		MØØ.139	Pneumococcal arthritis, unspecified wrist
		MØØ.231	Other streptococcal arthritis, right wrist
		MØØ.232	Other streptococcal arthritis, left wrist
		MØØ.239	Other streptococcal arthritis, unspecified wrist
		MØØ.831	Arthritis due to other bacteria, right wrist
		MØØ.832	Arthritis due to other bacteria, left wrist
		MØØ.839	Arthritis due to other bacteria, unspecified wrist
711.Ø4	PYOGENIC ARTHRITIS, HAND	**MØØ.Ø41**	Staphylococcal arthritis, right hand
		MØØ.Ø42	Staphylococcal arthritis, left hand
		MØØ.Ø49	Staphylococcal arthritis, unspecified hand
		MØØ.141	Pneumococcal arthritis, right hand
		MØØ.142	Pneumococcal arthritis, left hand
		MØØ.149	Pneumococcal arthritis, unspecified hand
		MØØ.241	Other streptococcal arthritis, right hand
		MØØ.242	Other streptococcal arthritis, left hand
		MØØ.249	Other streptococcal arthritis, unspecified hand
		MØØ.841	Arthritis due to other bacteria, right hand
		MØØ.842	Arthritis due to other bacteria, left hand
		MØØ.849	Arthritis due to other bacteria, unspecified hand
711.Ø5	PYOGENIC ARTHRITIS PELVIC REGION AND THIGH	**MØØ.Ø51**	Staphylococcal arthritis, right hip
		MØØ.Ø52	Staphylococcal arthritis, left hip
		MØØ.Ø59	Staphylococcal arthritis, unspecified hip
		MØØ.151	Pneumococcal arthritis, right hip
		MØØ.152	Pneumococcal arthritis, left hip
		MØØ.159	Pneumococcal arthritis, unspecified hip
		MØØ.251	Other streptococcal arthritis, right hip
		MØØ.252	Other streptococcal arthritis, left hip
		MØØ.259	Other streptococcal arthritis, unspecified hip
		MØØ.851	Arthritis due to other bacteria, right hip
		MØØ.852	Arthritis due to other bacteria, left hip
		MØØ.859	Arthritis due to other bacteria, unspecified hip
711.Ø6	PYOGENIC ARTHRITIS, LOWER LEG	**MØØ.Ø61**	Staphylococcal arthritis, right knee
		MØØ.Ø62	Staphylococcal arthritis, left knee
		MØØ.Ø69	Staphylococcal arthritis, unspecified knee
		MØØ.161	Pneumococcal arthritis, right knee
		MØØ.162	Pneumococcal arthritis, left knee
		MØØ.169	Pneumococcal arthritis, unspecified knee
		MØØ.261	Other streptococcal arthritis, right knee
		MØØ.262	Other streptococcal arthritis, left knee
		MØØ.269	Other streptococcal arthritis, unspecified knee
		MØØ.861	Arthritis due to other bacteria, right knee
		MØØ.862	Arthritis due to other bacteria, left knee
		MØØ.869	Arthritis due to other bacteria, unspecified knee
711.Ø7	PYOGENIC ARTHRITIS, ANKLE AND FOOT	**MØØ.Ø71**	Staphylococcal arthritis, right ankle and foot
		MØØ.Ø72	Staphylococcal arthritis, left ankle and foot
		MØØ.Ø79	Staphylococcal arthritis, unspecified ankle and foot
		MØØ.171	Pneumococcal arthritis, right ankle and foot
		MØØ.172	Pneumococcal arthritis, left ankle and foot
		MØØ.179	Pneumococcal arthritis, unspecified ankle and foot
		MØØ.271	Other streptococcal arthritis, right ankle and foot
		MØØ.272	Other streptococcal arthritis, left ankle and foot
		MØØ.279	Other streptococcal arthritis, unspecified ankle and foot
		MØØ.871	Arthritis due to other bacteria, right ankle and foot
		MØØ.872	Arthritis due to other bacteria, left ankle and foot
		MØØ.879	Arthritis due to other bacteria, unspecified ankle and foot
711.Ø8	PYOGENIC ARTHRITIS OTHER SPECIFIED SITES	**MØØ.Ø8**	Staphylococcal arthritis, vertebrae
		MØØ.Ø9	Staphylococcal polyarthritis
		MØØ.18	Pneumococcal arthritis, vertebrae
		MØØ.28	Other streptococcal arthritis, vertebrae
		MØØ.88	Arthritis due to other bacteria, vertebrae
		MØØ.9	Pyogenic arthritis, unspecified
711.Ø9	PYOGENIC ARTHRITIS, MULTIPLE SITES	**MØØ.Ø9**	Staphylococcal polyarthritis
		MØØ.19	Pneumococcal polyarthritis
		MØØ.29	Other streptococcal polyarthritis
		MØØ.89	Polyarthritis due to other bacteria
711.1Ø	ARTHROPATHY W/REITERS DZ & URETHRITIS-SITE UNS	**MØ2.3Ø**	Reiter's disease, unspecified site
711.11	ARTHROPATHY W/REITERS DZ & URETHRITIS-SHOULDER	**MØ2.311**	Reiter's disease, right shoulder
		MØ2.312	Reiter's disease, left shoulder
		MØ2.319	Reiter's disease, unspecified shoulder
711.12	ARTHRPATHW/REITERS DZ&NONSPEC URETHRITIS UP ARM	**MØ2.321**	Reiter's disease, right elbow
		MØ2.322	Reiter's disease, left elbow
		MØ2.329	Reiter's disease, unspecified elbow

[Brackets] indicate valid character values for each code. Character value meanings provided for each code grouping.

ICD-9-CM		ICD-10-CM		
711.13	ARTHRPATHW/REITERS DZ&NONSPEC URETHRITIS FORARM	▣	MØ2.331	Reiter's disease, right wrist
		▣	MØ2.332	Reiter's disease, left wrist
		▣	MØ2.339	Reiter's disease, unspecified wrist
711.14	ARTHRPATHW/REITERS DZ&NONSPEC URETHRITIS HND	▣	MØ2.341	Reiter's disease, right hand
		▣	MØ2.342	Reiter's disease, left hand
		▣	MØ2.349	Reiter's disease, unspecified hand
711.15	ARTHROPATHY W/REITERS DZ & URETHRITIS-PELVIS	▣	MØ2.351	Reiter's disease, right hip
		▣	MØ2.352	Reiter's disease, left hip
		▣	MØ2.359	Reiter's disease, unspecified hip
711.16	ARTHRPATHW/REITERS DZ&NONSPEC URETHRITIS LOW LEG	▣	MØ2.361	Reiter's disease, right knee
		▣	MØ2.362	Reiter's disease, left knee
		▣	MØ2.369	Reiter's disease, unspecified knee
711.17	ARTHROPATHY W/REITERS DZ & URETHRITIS-ANKLE	▣	MØ2.371	Reiter's disease, right ankle and foot
		▣	MØ2.372	Reiter's disease, left ankle and foot
		▣	MØ2.379	Reiter's disease, unspecified ankle and foot
711.18	ARTHROPATHY W/REITERS DZ & URETHRITIS-OTH SITES	▣	MØ2.38	Reiter's disease, vertebrae
711.19	ARTHRPATHW/REITERS DZ&NONSPEC URETHRITIS MX SITE	▣	MØ2.39	Reiter's disease, multiple sites
711.2Ø	ARTHROPATHY IN BEHCETS SYNDROME SITE UNSPECIFIED	▣	M35.2	Behcet's disease
711.21	ARTHROPATHY IN BEHCETS SYNDROME SHOULDER REGION		M35.2	Behcet's disease
711.22	ARTHROPATHY IN BEHCETS SYNDROMEUPPER ARM		M35.2	Behcet's disease
711.23	ARTHROPATHY IN BEHCETS SYNDROME FOREARM		M35.2	Behcet's disease
711.24	ARTHROPATHY IN BEHCETS SYNDROME HAND		M35.2	Behcet's disease
711.25	ARTHROPATHY BEHCETS SYNDROME PELVIC REGION&THIGH		M35.2	Behcet's disease
711.26	ARTHROPATHY IN BEHCETS SYNDROME LOWER LEG		M35.2	Behcet's disease
711.27	ARTHROPATHY IN BEHCETS SYNDROME ANKLE AND FOOT		M35.2	Behcet's disease
711.28	ARTHROPATHY BEHCETS SYNDROME OTHER SPEC SITES		M35.2	Behcet's disease
711.29	ARTHROPATHY IN BEHCETS SYNDROME MULTIPLE SITES		M35.2	Behcet's disease
711.3Ø	POSTDYSENTERIC ARTHROPATHY SITE UNSPECIFIED	➡	MØ2.1Ø	Postdysenteric arthropathy, unspecified site
711.31	POSTDYSENTERIC ARTHROPATHY SHOULDER REGION		MØ2.111	Postdysenteric arthropathy, right shoulder
			MØ2.112	Postdysenteric arthropathy, left shoulder
			MØ2.119	Postdysenteric arthropathy, unspecified shoulder
711.32	POSTDYSENTERIC ARTHROPATHY UPPER ARM		MØ2.121	Postdysenteric arthropathy, right elbow
			MØ2.122	Postdysenteric arthropathy, left elbow
			MØ2.129	Postdysenteric arthropathy, unspecified elbow
711.33	POSTDYSENTERIC ARTHROPATHY, FOREARM		MØ2.131	Postdysenteric arthropathy, right wrist
			MØ2.132	Postdysenteric arthropathy, left wrist
			MØ2.139	Postdysenteric arthropathy, unspecified wrist
711.34	POSTDYSENTERIC ARTHROPATHY, HAND		MØ2.141	Postdysenteric arthropathy, right hand
			MØ2.142	Postdysenteric arthropathy, left hand
			MØ2.149	Postdysenteric arthropathy, unspecified hand
711.35	POSTDYSENTERIC ARTHROPATHY PELVIC REGION&THIGH		MØ2.151	Postdysenteric arthropathy, right hip
			MØ2.152	Postdysenteric arthropathy, left hip
			MØ2.159	Postdysenteric arthropathy, unspecified hip
711.36	POSTDYSENTERIC ARTHROPATHY LOWER LEG		MØ2.161	Postdysenteric arthropathy, right knee
			MØ2.162	Postdysenteric arthropathy, left knee
			MØ2.169	Postdysenteric arthropathy, unspecified knee
711.37	POSTDYSENTERIC ARTHROPATHY ANKLE AND FOOT		MØ2.171	Postdysenteric arthropathy, right ankle and foot
			MØ2.172	Postdysenteric arthropathy, left ankle and foot
			MØ2.179	Postdysenteric arthropathy, unspecified ankle and foot
711.38	POSTDYSENTERIC ARTHROPATHY OTHER SPECIFIED SITES		MØ2.18	Postdysenteric arthropathy, vertebrae
711.39	POSTDYSENTERIC ARTHROPATHY MULTIPLE SITES	➡	MØ2.19	Postdysenteric arthropathy, multiple sites
711.4Ø	ARTHRPATH W/OTH BACTERIAL DISEASES SITE UNSPEC		MØ1.XØ	Dir infct of unsp joint in infec/parastc dis classd elswhr
			MØ2.8Ø	Other reactive arthropathies, unspecified site
711.41	ARTHRPATH W/OTH BACTERL DISEASES SHOULDER REGION		MØ1.X11	Direct infct of r shldr in infec/parastc dis classd elswhr
			MØ1.X12	Direct infct of l shldr in infec/parastc dis classd elswhr
			MØ1.X19	Dir infct of unsp shldr in infec/parastc dis classd elswhr
			MØ2.811	Other reactive arthropathies, right shoulder
			MØ2.812	Other reactive arthropathies, left shoulder
			MØ2.819	Other reactive arthropathies, unspecified shoulder
711.42	ARTHRPATH W/OTH BACTERIAL DISEASES UPPER ARM		MØ1.X21	Direct infct of r elbow in infec/parastc dis classd elswhr
			MØ1.X22	Direct infct of l elbow in infec/parastc dis classd elswhr
			MØ1.X29	Dir infct of unsp elbow in infec/parastc dis classd elswhr
			MØ2.821	Other reactive arthropathies, right elbow
			MØ2.822	Other reactive arthropathies, left elbow
			MØ2.829	Other reactive arthropathies, unspecified elbow
711.43	ARTHRPATH W/OTH BACTERIAL DISEASES FOREARM		MØ1.X31	Direct infct of r wrist in infec/parastc dis classd elswhr
			MØ1.X32	Direct infct of l wrist in infec/parastc dis classd elswhr
			MØ1.X39	Dir infct of unsp wrist in infec/parastc dis classd elswhr
			MØ2.831	Other reactive arthropathies, right wrist
			MØ2.832	Other reactive arthropathies, left wrist
			MØ2.839	Other reactive arthropathies, unspecified wrist

ICD-9-CM		ICD-10-CM	
711.44	ARTHRPATH W/OTH BACTERIAL DISEASES HAND	MØ1.X41	Direct infct of r hand in infec/parastc dis classd elswhr
		MØ1.X42	Direct infct of l hand in infec/parastc dis classd elswhr
		MØ1.X49	Direct infct of unsp hand in infec/parastc dis classd elswhr
		MØ2.841	Other reactive arthropathies, right hand
		MØ2.842	Other reactive arthropathies, left hand
		MØ2.849	Other reactive arthropathies, unspecified hand
711.45	ARTHRPATH W/OTH BACTERL DZ PELVIC REGION&THIGH	A18.Ø2	Tuberculous arthritis of other joints
		MØ1.X51	Direct infct of r hip in infec/parastc dis classd elswhr
		MØ1.X52	Direct infct of left hip in infec/parastc dis classd elswhr
		MØ1.X59	Direct infct of unsp hip in infec/parastc dis classd elswhr
		MØ2.851	Other reactive arthropathies, right hip
		MØ2.852	Other reactive arthropathies, left hip
		MØ2.859	Other reactive arthropathies, unspecified hip
711.46	ARTHRPATH W/OTH BACTERIAL DISEASES LOWER LEG	A18.Ø2	Tuberculous arthritis of other joints
		MØ1.X61	Direct infct of r knee in infec/parastc dis classd elswhr
		MØ1.X62	Direct infct of l knee in infec/parastc dis classd elswhr
		MØ1.X69	Direct infct of unsp knee in infec/parastc dis classd elswhr
		MØ2.861	Other reactive arthropathies, right knee
		MØ2.862	Other reactive arthropathies, left knee
		MØ2.869	Other reactive arthropathies, unspecified knee
711.47	ARTHRPATH W/OTH BACTERIAL DISEASE ANKLE AND FOOT	MØ1.X71	Dir infct of right ank/ft in infec/parastc dis classd elswhr
		MØ1.X72	Dir infct of left ank/ft in infec/parastc dis classd elswhr
		MØ1.X79	Dir infct of unsp ank/ft in infec/parastc dis classd elswhr
		MØ2.871	Other reactive arthropathies, right ankle and foot
		MØ2.872	Other reactive arthropathies, left ankle and foot
		MØ2.879	Other reactive arthropathies, unspecified ankle and foot
711.48	ARTHRPATH W/OTH BACTERL DZ OTH SPECIFIC SITES	A18.Ø1	Tuberculosis of spine
		A18.Ø2	Tuberculous arthritis of other joints
		MØ1.X8	Direct infct of verteb in infec/parastc dis classd elswhr
		MØ2.88	Other reactive arthropathies, vertebrae
711.49	ARTHRPATH W/OTH BACTERL DISEASES MULTIPLE SITES	MØ1.X9	Dir infct of mult joints in infec/parastc dis classd elswhr
		MØ2.89	Other reactive arthropathies, multiple sites
711.5Ø	ARTHRPATH W/OTH VIRAL DISEASES SITE UNSPECIFIED	MØ1.XØ	Dir infct of unsp joint in infec/parastc dis classd elswhr
		MØ2.8Ø	Other reactive arthropathies, unspecified site
711.51	ARTHRPATH W/OTH VIRAL DISEASES SHOULDER REGION	MØ1.X11	Direct infct of r shldr in infec/parastc dis classd elswhr
		MØ1.X12	Direct infct of l shldr in infec/parastc dis classd elswhr
		MØ1.X19	Dir infct of unsp shldr in infec/parastc dis classd elswhr
		MØ2.811	Other reactive arthropathies, right shoulder
		MØ2.812	Other reactive arthropathies, left shoulder
		MØ2.819	Other reactive arthropathies, unspecified shoulder
711.52	ARTHRPATH W/OTH VIRAL DISEASES UPPER ARM	MØ1.X21	Direct infct of r elbow in infec/parastc dis classd elswhr
		MØ1.X22	Direct infct of l elbow in infec/parastc dis classd elswhr
		MØ1.X29	Dir infct of unsp elbow in infec/parastc dis classd elswhr
		MØ2.821	Other reactive arthropathies, right elbow
		MØ2.822	Other reactive arthropathies, left elbow
		MØ2.829	Other reactive arthropathies, unspecified elbow
711.53	ARTHRPATH W/OTH VIRAL DISEASES FOREARM	MØ1.X31	Direct infct of r wrist in infec/parastc dis classd elswhr
		MØ1.X32	Direct infct of l wrist in infec/parastc dis classd elswhr
		MØ1.X39	Dir infct of unsp wrist in infec/parastc dis classd elswhr
		MØ2.831	Other reactive arthropathies, right wrist
		MØ2.832	Other reactive arthropathies, left wrist
		MØ2.839	Other reactive arthropathies, unspecified wrist
711.54	ARTHRPATH W/OTH VIRAL DISEASES HAND	MØ1.X41	Direct infct of r hand in infec/parastc dis classd elswhr
		MØ1.X42	Direct infct of l hand in infec/parastc dis classd elswhr
		MØ1.X49	Direct infct of unsp hand in infec/parastc dis classd elswhr
		MØ2.841	Other reactive arthropathies, right hand
		MØ2.842	Other reactive arthropathies, left hand
		MØ2.849	Other reactive arthropathies, unspecified hand
711.55	ARTHRPATH W/OTH VIRAL DZ PELVIC REGION&THIGH	MØ1.X51	Direct infct of r hip in infec/parastc dis classd elswhr
		MØ1.X52	Direct infct of left hip in infec/parastc dis classd elswhr
		MØ1.X59	Direct infct of unsp hip in infec/parastc dis classd elswhr
		MØ2.851	Other reactive arthropathies, right hip
		MØ2.852	Other reactive arthropathies, left hip
		MØ2.859	Other reactive arthropathies, unspecified hip
711.56	ARTHRPATH W/OTH VIRAL DISEASES LOWER LEG	MØ1.X61	Direct infct of r knee in infec/parastc dis classd elswhr
		MØ1.X62	Direct infct of l knee in infec/parastc dis classd elswhr
		MØ1.X69	Direct infct of unsp knee in infec/parastc dis classd elswhr
		MØ2.861	Other reactive arthropathies, right knee
		MØ2.862	Other reactive arthropathies, left knee
		MØ2.869	Other reactive arthropathies, unspecified knee
711.57	ARTHRPATH W/OTH VIRAL DISEASES ANKLE AND FOOT	MØ1.X71	Dir infct of right ank/ft in infec/parastc dis classd elswhr
		MØ1.X72	Dir infct of left ank/ft in infec/parastc dis classd elswhr
		MØ1.X79	Dir infct of unsp ank/ft in infec/parastc dis classd elswhr
		MØ2.871	Other reactive arthropathies, right ankle and foot
		MØ2.872	Other reactive arthropathies, left ankle and foot
		MØ2.879	Other reactive arthropathies, unspecified ankle and foot
711.58	ARTHRPATH W/OTH VIRAL DISEASES OTHER SPEC SITES	MØ1.X8	Direct infct of verteb in infec/parastc dis classd elswhr
		MØ2.88	Other reactive arthropathies, vertebrae

[Brackets] indicate valid character values for each code. Character value meanings provided for each code grouping.

ICD-9-CM		ICD-10-CM	
711.59	ARTHRPATH W/OTH VIRAL DISEASES OF MULTIPLE SITES	**M01.X9**	Dir infct of mult joints in infec/parastc dis classd elswhr
		M02.89	Other reactive arthropathies, multiple sites
711.60	ARTHRPATH W/MYCOSES SITE UNSPECIFIED	**M01.X0**	Dir infct of unsp joint in infec/parastc dis classd elswhr
711.61	ARTHRPATH W/MYCOSES SHOULDER REGION	**M01.X11**	Direct infct of r shldr in infec/parastc dis classd elswhr
		M01.X12	Direct infct of l shldr in infec/parastc dis classd elswhr
		M01.X19	Dir infct of unsp shldr in infec/parastc dis classd elswhr
711.62	ARTHROPATHY ASSOCIATED WITH MYCOSES UPPER ARM	**M01.X21**	Direct infct of r elbow in infec/parastc dis classd elswhr
		M01.X22	Direct infct of l elbow in infec/parastc dis classd elswhr
		M01.X29	Dir infct of unsp elbow in infec/parastc dis classd elswhr
711.63	ARTHROPATHY ASSOCIATED WITH MYCOSES FOREARM	**M01.X31**	Direct infct of r wrist in infec/parastc dis classd elswhr
		M01.X32	Direct infct of l wrist in infec/parastc dis classd elswhr
		M01.X39	Dir infct of unsp wrist in infec/parastc dis classd elswhr
711.64	ARTHROPATHY ASSOCIATED WITH MYCOSES HAND	**M01.X41**	Direct infct of r hand in infec/parastc dis classd elswhr
		M01.X42	Direct infct of l hand in infec/parastc dis classd elswhr
		M01.X49	Direct infct of unsp hand in infec/parastc dis classd elswhr
711.65	ARTHRPATH W/MYCOSES PELVIC REGION AND THIGH	**M01.X51**	Direct infct of r hip in infec/parastc dis classd elswhr
		M01.X52	Direct infct of left hip in infec/parastc dis classd elswhr
		M01.X59	Direct infct of unsp hip in infec/parastc dis classd elswhr
711.66	ARTHROPATHY ASSOCIATED WITH MYCOSES LOWER LEG	**M01.X61**	Direct infct of r knee in infec/parastc dis classd elswhr
		M01.X62	Direct infct of l knee in infec/parastc dis classd elswhr
		M01.X69	Direct infct of unsp knee in infec/parastc dis classd elswhr
711.67	ARTHRPATH W/MYCOSES ANKLE AND FOOT	**M01.X71**	Dir infct of right ank/ft in infec/parastc dis classd elswhr
		M01.X72	Dir infct of left ank/ft in infec/parastc dis classd elswhr
		M01.X79	Dir infct of unsp ank/ft in infec/parastc dis classd elswhr
711.68	ARTHRPATH W/MYCOSES OTHER SPECIFIED SITE	**M01.X8**	Direct infct of verteb in infec/parastc dis classd elswhr
711.69	ARTHRPATH W/MYCOSES MULTIPLE SITES	**M01.X9**	Dir infct of mult joints in infec/parastc dis classd elswhr
711.70	ARTHRPATH W/HELMINTHIASIS SITE UNSPECIFIED	**M01.X0**	Dir infct of unsp joint in infec/parastc dis classd elswhr
711.71	ARTHRPATH W/HELMINTHIASIS SHOULDER REGION	**M01.X11**	Direct infct of r shldr in infec/parastc dis classd elswhr
		M01.X12	Direct infct of l shldr in infec/parastc dis classd elswhr
		M01.X19	Dir infct of unsp shldr in infec/parastc dis classd elswhr
711.72	ARTHRPATH W/HELMINTHIASIS UPPER ARM	**M01.X21**	Direct infct of r elbow in infec/parastc dis classd elswhr
		M01.X22	Direct infct of l elbow in infec/parastc dis classd elswhr
		M01.X29	Dir infct of unsp elbow in infec/parastc dis classd elswhr
711.73	ARTHRPATH W/HELMINTHIASIS FOREARM	**M01.X31**	Direct infct of r wrist in infec/parastc dis classd elswhr
		M01.X32	Direct infct of l wrist in infec/parastc dis classd elswhr
		M01.X39	Dir infct of unsp wrist in infec/parastc dis classd elswhr
711.74	ARTHROPATHY ASSOCIATED WITH HELMINTHIASIS HAND	**M01.X41**	Direct infct of r hand in infec/parastc dis classd elswhr
		M01.X42	Direct infct of l hand in infec/parastc dis classd elswhr
		M01.X49	Direct infct of unsp hand in infec/parastc dis classd elswhr
711.75	ARTHRPATH W/HELMINTHIASIS PELVIC REGION&THIGH	**M01.X51**	Direct infct of r hip in infec/parastc dis classd elswhr
		M01.X52	Direct infct of left hip in infec/parastc dis classd elswhr
		M01.X59	Direct infct of unsp hip in infec/parastc dis classd elswhr
711.76	ARTHRPATH W/HELMINTHIASIS LOWER LEG	**M01.X61**	Direct infct of r knee in infec/parastc dis classd elswhr
		M01.X62	Direct infct of l knee in infec/parastc dis classd elswhr
		M01.X69	Direct infct of unsp knee in infec/parastc dis classd elswhr
711.77	ARTHRPATH W/HELMINTHIASIS ANKLE AND FOOT	**M01.X71**	Dir infct of right ank/ft in infec/parastc dis classd elswhr
		M01.X72	Dir infct of left ank/ft in infec/parastc dis classd elswhr
		M01.X79	Dir infct of unsp ank/ft in infec/parastc dis classd elswhr
711.78	ARTHRPATH W/HELMINTHIASIS OTHER SPECIFIED SITE	**M01.X8**	Direct infct of verteb in infec/parastc dis classd elswhr
711.79	ARTHRPATH W/HELMINTHIASIS MULTIPLE SITES	**M01.X9**	Dir infct of mult joints in infec/parastc dis classd elswhr
711.80	ARTHRPATH W/OTH INF&PARASITIC DZ-SITE UNSPEC	**M01.X0**	Dir infct of unsp joint in infec/parastc dis classd elswhr
		M02.80	Other reactive arthropathies, unspecified site
711.81	ARTHRPATH W/OTH INF&PARASITIC DZ-SHOULDER REGION	**M01.X11**	Direct infct of r shldr in infec/parastc dis classd elswhr
		M01.X12	Direct infct of l shldr in infec/parastc dis classd elswhr
		M01.X19	Dir infct of unsp shldr in infec/parastc dis classd elswhr
		M02.811	Other reactive arthropathies, right shoulder
		M02.812	Other reactive arthropathies, left shoulder
		M02.819	Other reactive arthropathies, unspecified shoulder
711.82	ARTHRPATH W/OTH INF&PARASITIC DZ-UPPER ARM	**M01.X21**	Direct infct of r elbow in infec/parastc dis classd elswhr
		M01.X22	Direct infct of l elbow in infec/parastc dis classd elswhr
		M01.X29	Dir infct of unsp elbow in infec/parastc dis classd elswhr
		M02.821	Other reactive arthropathies, right elbow
		M02.822	Other reactive arthropathies, left elbow
		M02.829	Other reactive arthropathies, unspecified elbow
711.83	ARTHRPATH W/OTH INFECTIOUS&PARASITIC DZ-FOREARM	**M01.X31**	Direct infct of r wrist in infec/parastc dis classd elswhr
		M01.X32	Direct infct of l wrist in infec/parastc dis classd elswhr
		M01.X39	Dir infct of unsp wrist in infec/parastc dis classd elswhr
		M02.831	Other reactive arthropathies, right wrist
		M02.832	Other reactive arthropathies, left wrist
		M02.839	Other reactive arthropathies, unspecified wrist
711.84	ARTHRPATH W/OTH INFECTIOUS&PARASITIC DZ-HAND	**M01.X41**	Direct infct of r hand in infec/parastc dis classd elswhr
		M01.X42	Direct infct of l hand in infec/parastc dis classd elswhr
		M01.X49	Direct infct of unsp hand in infec/parastc dis classd elswhr
		M02.841	Other reactive arthropathies, right hand
		M02.842	Other reactive arthropathies, left hand
		M02.849	Other reactive arthropathies, unspecified hand

ICD-9-CM		ICD-10-CM	
711.85	ARTHRPATH W/OTH INF&PARASITIC DZ-PELV REGION&THI	M01.X51	Direct infct of r hip in infec/parastc dis classd elswhr
		M01.X52	Direct infct of left hip in infec/parastc dis classd elswhr
		M01.X59	Direct infct of unsp hip in infec/parastc dis classd elswhr
		M02.851	Other reactive arthropathies, right hip
		M02.852	Other reactive arthropathies, left hip
		M02.859	Other reactive arthropathies, unspecified hip
711.86	ARTHRPATH W/OTH INF&PARASITIC DZ-LOWER LEG	M01.X61	Direct infct of r knee in infec/parastc dis classd elswhr
		M01.X62	Direct infct of l knee in infec/parastc dis classd elswhr
		M01.X69	Direct infct of unsp knee in infec/parastc dis classd elswhr
		M02.861	Other reactive arthropathies, right knee
		M02.862	Other reactive arthropathies, left knee
		M02.869	Other reactive arthropathies, unspecified knee
711.87	ARTHRPATH W/OTH INFECTIOUS&PARASITIC DZ-ANK&FOOT	M01.X71	Dir infct of right ank/ft in infec/parastc dis classd elswhr
		M01.X72	Dir infct of left ank/ft in infec/parastc dis classd elswhr
		M01.X79	Dir infct of unsp ank/ft in infec/parastc dis classd elswhr
		M02.871	Other reactive arthropathies, right ankle and foot
		M02.872	Other reactive arthropathies, left ankle and foot
		M02.879	Other reactive arthropathies, unspecified ankle and foot
711.88	ARTHRPATH W/OTH INF&PARASITIC DZ-OTH SPEC SITE	M01.X8	Direct infct of verteb in infec/parastc dis classd elswhr
		M02.88	Other reactive arthropathies, vertebrae
711.89	ARTHRPATH W/OTH INF&PARASITIC DZ-MULTIPLE SITES	M01.X9	Dir infct of mult joints in infec/parastc dis classd elswhr
		M02.89	Other reactive arthropathies, multiple sites
711.90	UNSPECIFIED INFECTIVE ARTHRITIS SITE UNSPECIFIED	M01.X0	Dir infct of unsp joint in infec/parastc dis classd elswhr
711.91	UNSPECIFIED INFECTIVE ARTHRITIS SHOULDER REGION	M01.X19	Dir infct of unsp shldr in infec/parastc dis classd elswhr
711.92	UNSPECIFIED INFECTIVE ARTHRITIS UPPER ARM	M01.X29	Dir infct of unsp elbow in infec/parastc dis classd elswhr
711.93	UNSPECIFIED INFECTIVE ARTHRITIS FOREARM	M01.X39	Dir infct of unsp wrist in infec/parastc dis classd elswhr
711.94	UNSPECIFIED INFECTIVE ARTHRITIS HAND	M01.X49	Direct infct of unsp hand in infec/parastc dis classd elswhr
711.95	UNSPEC INFECTIVE ARTHRITIS PELVIC REGION&THIGH	M01.X59	Direct infct of unsp hip in infec/parastc dis classd elswhr
711.96	UNSPECIFIED INFECTIVE ARTHRITIS LOWER LEG	M01.X69	Direct infct of unsp knee in infec/parastc dis classd elswhr
711.97	UNSPECIFIED INFECTIVE ARTHRITIS ANKLE AND FOOT	M01.X79	Dir infct of unsp ank/ft in infec/parastc dis classd elswhr
711.98	UNSPEC INFECTIVE ARTHRITIS OTHER SPEC SITES	M01.X8	Direct infct of verteb in infec/parastc dis classd elswhr
711.99	UNSPECIFIED INFECTIVE ARTHRITIS MULTIPLE SITES	M01.X9	Dir infct of mult joints in infec/parastc dis classd elswhr
712.10	CHONDROCALCINOS DUE DICALCM PHOSHATE CRYSTLS	M11.80	Other specified crystal arthropathies, unspecified site
712.11	CHONDROCALCINOSIS-DICALCM PO4 CRYSTALS SHOULDER	M11.819	Other specified crystal arthropathies, unspecified shoulder
712.12	CHONDROCALCINOS-DICALCM PHOSHATE CRYSTLS UP ARM	M11.829	Other specified crystal arthropathies, unspecified elbow
712.13	CHONDROCALCINOS-DICALCM PHOSHATE CRYSTLS FORARM	M11.839	Other specified crystal arthropathies, unspecified wrist
712.14	CHONDROCALCINOS DUE DICALCM PHOSHATE CRYSTLS HND	M11.849	Other specified crystal arthropathies, unspecified hand
712.15	CHONDROCALCINOSIS-DICALCM PO4 CRYSTALS PELVC REG	M11.859	Other specified crystal arthropathies, unspecified hip
712.16	CHONDROCALCINOS-DICALCM PHOSHATE CRYSTLS LW LEG	M11.869	Other specified crystal arthropathies, unspecified knee
712.17	CHONDROCALCINOSIS-DICALCM PO4 CRYSTALS ANKLE	M11.879	Oth crystal arthropathies, unspecified ankle and foot
712.18	CHONDROCALCIN-DICALCM PO4 CRYSTALS OTH SITES	M11.88	Other specified crystal arthropathies, vertebrae
712.19	CHONDROCALCINOS-DICALCM PHOSHATE CRYSTLS MX SITE	M11.89	Other specified crystal arthropathies, multiple sites
712.20	CHONDROCALCINOS DUE PYROPHOSHATE CRYSTLS	M11.80	Other specified crystal arthropathies, unspecified site
712.21	CHONDROCALCINOS-PYROPHOSHATE CRYSTLS SHLDR RGN	M11.819	Other specified crystal arthropathies, unspecified shoulder
712.22	CHONDROCALCINOS DUE PYROPHOSPHATE CRYSTLS UP ARM	M11.829	Other specified crystal arthropathies, unspecified elbow
712.23	CHONDROCALCINOS DUE PYROPHOSPHATE CRYSTLS FORARM	M11.839	Other specified crystal arthropathies, unspecified wrist
712.24	CHONDROCALCINOS DUE PYROPHOSPHATE CRYSTALS HAND	M11.849	Other specified crystal arthropathies, unspecified hand
712.25	CHONDROCALCINOSIS-PYROPO4 CRYSTALS PELVIC REG	M11.859	Other specified crystal arthropathies, unspecified hip
712.26	CHONDROCALCINOS DUE PYROPHOSHATE CRYSTLS LOW LEG	M11.869	Other specified crystal arthropathies, unspecified knee
712.27	CHONDROCALCINOS-PYROPHOSHATE CRYSTLS ANK&FOOT	M11.879	Oth crystal arthropathies, unspecified ankle and foot
712.28	CHONDROCALCINOS-PYROPHOSHATE CRYSTLS OTH SITE	M11.88	Other specified crystal arthropathies, vertebrae
712.29	CHONDROCALCINOS DUE PYROPHOSHATE CRYSTLS MX SITE	M11.89	Other specified crystal arthropathies, multiple sites
712.30	CHONDROCALCINOS CAUSE UNSPEC INVLV UNSPEC SITE	M11.10	Familial chondrocalcinosis, unspecified site
		M11.20	Other chondrocalcinosis, unspecified site
712.31	CHONDROCALCINOS CAUSE UNSPEC INVLV SHLDR REGION	M11.111	Familial chondrocalcinosis, right shoulder
		M11.112	Familial chondrocalcinosis, left shoulder
		M11.119	Familial chondrocalcinosis, unspecified shoulder
		M11.211	Other chondrocalcinosis, right shoulder
		M11.212	Other chondrocalcinosis, left shoulder
		M11.219	Other chondrocalcinosis, unspecified shoulder
712.32	CHONDROCALCINOS CAUSE UNSPEC INVOLVING UPPER ARM	M11.121	Familial chondrocalcinosis, right elbow
		M11.122	Familial chondrocalcinosis, left elbow
		M11.129	Familial chondrocalcinosis, unspecified elbow
		M11.221	Other chondrocalcinosis, right elbow
		M11.222	Other chondrocalcinosis, left elbow
		M11.229	Other chondrocalcinosis, unspecified elbow
712.33	CHONDROCALCINOSIS CAUSE UNSPEC INVOLVING FOREARM	M11.131	Familial chondrocalcinosis, right wrist
		M11.132	Familial chondrocalcinosis, left wrist
		M11.139	Familial chondrocalcinosis, unspecified wrist
		M11.231	Other chondrocalcinosis, right wrist
		M11.232	Other chondrocalcinosis, left wrist
		M11.239	Other chondrocalcinosis, unspecified wrist

ICD-9-CM		ICD-10-CM	
712.34	CHONDROCALCINOSIS CAUSE UNSPEC INVOLVING HAND	**M11.141**	Familial chondrocalcinosis, right hand
		M11.142	Familial chondrocalcinosis, left hand
		M11.149	Familial chondrocalcinosis, unspecified hand
		M11.241	Other chondrocalcinosis, right hand
		M11.242	Other chondrocalcinosis, left hand
		M11.249	Other chondrocalcinosis, unspecified hand
712.35	CHONDROCALCINOS CAUSE UNSPEC INVLV PELV RGN&THI	**M11.151**	Familial chondrocalcinosis, right hip
		M11.152	Familial chondrocalcinosis, left hip
		M11.159	Familial chondrocalcinosis, unspecified hip
		M11.251	Other chondrocalcinosis, right hip
		M11.252	Other chondrocalcinosis, left hip
		M11.259	Other chondrocalcinosis, unspecified hip
712.36	CHONDROCALCINOS CAUSE UNSPEC INVOLVING LOWER LEG	**M11.161**	Familial chondrocalcinosis, right knee
		M11.162	Familial chondrocalcinosis, left knee
		M11.169	Familial chondrocalcinosis, unspecified knee
		M11.261	Other chondrocalcinosis, right knee
		M11.262	Other chondrocalcinosis, left knee
		M11.269	Other chondrocalcinosis, unspecified knee
712.37	CHONDROCALCINOS CAUSE UNSPEC INVOLVING ANK&FOOT	**M11.171**	Familial chondrocalcinosis, right ankle and foot
		M11.172	Familial chondrocalcinosis, left ankle and foot
		M11.179	Familial chondrocalcinosis, unspecified ankle and foot
		M11.271	Other chondrocalcinosis, right ankle and foot
		M11.272	Other chondrocalcinosis, left ankle and foot
		M11.279	Other chondrocalcinosis, unspecified ankle and foot
712.38	CHONDROCALCINOS CAUSE UNSPEC INVLV OTH SPEC SITE	**M11.18**	Familial chondrocalcinosis, vertebrae
		M11.28	Other chondrocalcinosis, vertebrae
712.39	CHONDROCALCINOS CAUSE UNSPEC INVLV MX SITES	**M11.19**	Familial chondrocalcinosis, multiple sites
		M11.29	Other chondrocalcinosis, multiple sites
712.80	OTHER SPEC CRYSTAL ARTHROPATHIES SITE UNSPEC	**M11.00**	Hydroxyapatite deposition disease, unspecified site
		M11.80	Other specified crystal arthropathies, unspecified site
712.81	OTHER SPEC CRYSTAL ARTHROPATHIES SHOULDER REGION	**M11.011**	Hydroxyapatite deposition disease, right shoulder
		M11.012	Hydroxyapatite deposition disease, left shoulder
		M11.019	Hydroxyapatite deposition disease, unspecified shoulder
		M11.811	Other specified crystal arthropathies, right shoulder
		M11.812	Other specified crystal arthropathies, left shoulder
		M11.819	Other specified crystal arthropathies, unspecified shoulder
712.82	OTHER SPECIFIED CRYSTAL ARTHROPATHIES UPPER ARM	**M11.021**	Hydroxyapatite deposition disease, right elbow
		M11.022	Hydroxyapatite deposition disease, left elbow
		M11.029	Hydroxyapatite deposition disease, unspecified elbow
		M11.821	Other specified crystal arthropathies, right elbow
		M11.822	Other specified crystal arthropathies, left elbow
		M11.829	Other specified crystal arthropathies, unspecified elbow
712.83	OTHER SPECIFIED CRYSTAL ARTHROPATHIES FOREARM	**M11.031**	Hydroxyapatite deposition disease, right wrist
		M11.032	Hydroxyapatite deposition disease, left wrist
		M11.039	Hydroxyapatite deposition disease, unspecified wrist
		M11.831	Other specified crystal arthropathies, right wrist
		M11.832	Other specified crystal arthropathies, left wrist
		M11.839	Other specified crystal arthropathies, unspecified wrist
712.84	OTHER SPECIFIED CRYSTAL ARTHROPATHIES HAND	**M11.041**	Hydroxyapatite deposition disease, right hand
		M11.042	Hydroxyapatite deposition disease, left hand
		M11.049	Hydroxyapatite deposition disease, unspecified hand
		M11.841	Other specified crystal arthropathies, right hand
		M11.842	Other specified crystal arthropathies, left hand
		M11.849	Other specified crystal arthropathies, unspecified hand
712.85	OTH SPEC CRYSTAL ARTHROPATHIES PELV REGION&THIGH	**M11.051**	Hydroxyapatite deposition disease, right hip
		M11.052	Hydroxyapatite deposition disease, left hip
		M11.059	Hydroxyapatite deposition disease, unspecified hip
		M11.851	Other specified crystal arthropathies, right hip
		M11.852	Other specified crystal arthropathies, left hip
		M11.859	Other specified crystal arthropathies, unspecified hip
712.86	OTHER SPECIFIED CRYSTAL ARTHROPATHIES LOWER LEG	**M11.061**	Hydroxyapatite deposition disease, right knee
		M11.062	Hydroxyapatite deposition disease, left knee
		M11.069	Hydroxyapatite deposition disease, unspecified knee
		M11.861	Other specified crystal arthropathies, right knee
		M11.862	Other specified crystal arthropathies, left knee
		M11.869	Other specified crystal arthropathies, unspecified knee
712.87	OTHER SPECIFIED CRYSTAL ARTHROPATHIES ANKLE&FOOT	**M11.071**	Hydroxyapatite deposition disease, right ankle and foot
		M11.072	Hydroxyapatite deposition disease, left ankle and foot
		M11.079	Hydroxyapatite deposition disease, unsp ankle and foot
		M11.871	Other specified crystal arthropathies, right ankle and foot
		M11.872	Other specified crystal arthropathies, left ankle and foot
		M11.879	Oth crystal arthropathies, unspecified ankle and foot
712.88	OTH SPEC CRYSTAL ARTHROPATHIES OTH SPEC SITES	**M11.08**	Hydroxyapatite deposition disease, vertebrae
		M11.88	Other specified crystal arthropathies, vertebrae
712.89	OTHER SPEC CRYSTAL ARTHROPATHIES MULTIPLE SITES	**M11.09**	Hydroxyapatite deposition disease, multiple sites
		M11.89	Other specified crystal arthropathies, multiple sites
712.90	UNSPECIFIED CRYSTAL ARTHROPATHY SITE UNSPECIFIED	**M11.80**	Other specified crystal arthropathies, unspecified site
		M11.9	Crystal arthropathy, unspecified
712.91	UNSPECIFIED CRYSTAL ARTHROPATHY SHOULDER REGION	**M11.819**	Other specified crystal arthropathies, unspecified shoulder

ICD-9-CM		ICD-10-CM	
712.92	UNSPECIFIED CRYSTAL ARTHROPATHY UPPER ARM	M11.829	Other specified crystal arthropathies, unspecified elbow
712.93	UNSPECIFIED CRYSTAL ARTHROPATHY FOREARM	M11.839	Other specified crystal arthropathies, unspecified wrist
712.94	UNSPECIFIED CRYSTAL ARTHROPATHY HAND	M11.849	Other specified crystal arthropathies, unspecified hand
712.95	UNSPEC CRYSTAL ARTHROPATHY PELVIC REGION&THIGH	M11.859	Other specified crystal arthropathies, unspecified hip
712.96	UNSPECIFIED CRYSTAL ARTHROPATHY LOWER LEG	M11.869	Other specified crystal arthropathies, unspecified knee
712.97	UNSPECIFIED CRYSTAL ARTHROPATHY ANKLE AND FOOT	M11.879	Oth crystal arthropathies, unspecified ankle and foot
712.98	UNSPEC CRYSTAL ARTHROPATHY OTHER SPEC SITES	M11.88	Other specified crystal arthropathies, vertebrae
712.99	UNSPECIFIED CRYSTAL ARTHROPATHY MULTIPLE SITES	M11.89	Other specified crystal arthropathies, multiple sites
713.Ø	ARTHRPATH W/OTH ENDOCRINE&METABOLIC DISORDERS	M14.8Ø	Arthropathies in oth diseases classd elswhr, unsp site
713.1	ARTHROPATHY ASSOC W/GI CONDS OTH THAN INFECTIONS	MØ2.ØØ	Arthropathy following intestinal bypass, unspecified site
		MØ2.Ø1[1,2,9]	Arthropathy following intestinal bypass, shoulder
		MØ2.Ø2[1,2,9]	Arthropathy following intestinal bypass, elbow
		MØ2.Ø3[1,2,9]	Arthropathy following intestinal bypass, wrist
		MØ2.Ø4[1,2,9]	Arthropathy following intestinal bypass, hand
		MØ2.Ø5[1,2,9]	Arthropathy following intestinal bypass, hip
		MØ2.Ø6[1,2,9]	Arthropathy following intestinal bypass, knee
		MØ2.Ø7[1,2,9]	Arthropathy following intestinal bypass, ank/ft
		MØ2.Ø8	Arthropathy following intestinal bypass, vertebrae
		MØ2.Ø9	Arthropathy following intestinal bypass, multiple sites
		MØ7.6Ø	Enteropathic arthropathies, unspecified site
		MØ7.61[1,2,9]	Enteropathic arthropathies, shoulder
		MØ7.62[1,2,9]	Enteropathic arthropathies, elbow
		MØ7.63[1,2,9]	Enteropathic arthropathies, wrist
		MØ7.64[1,2,9]	Enteropathic arthropathies, hand
		MØ7.65[1,2,9]	Enteropathic arthropathies, hip
		MØ7.66[1,2,9]	Enteropathic arthropathies, knee
		MØ7.67[1,2,9]	Enteropathic arthropathies, ankle and foot
		MØ7.68	Enteropathic arthropathies, vertebrae
		MØ7.69	Enteropathic arthropathies, multiple sites
			6th Character meanings for codes as indicated ***1 Right 2 Left 9 Unspecified***
713.2	ARTHROPATHY ASSOCIATED W/HEMATOLOGICAL DISORDERS	M36.2	Hemophilic arthropathy
		M36.3	Arthropathy in other blood disorders
713.3	ARTHROPATHY ASSOC W/DERMATOLOGICAL DISORDERS	M12.8Ø	Oth specific arthropathies, NEC, unsp site
713.4	ARTHROPATHY ASSOCIATED W/RESPIRATORY DISORDERS	M12.8Ø	Oth specific arthropathies, NEC, unsp site
713.5	ARTHROPATHY ASSOCIATED W/NEUROLOGICAL DISORDERS	A52.16	Charcot's arthropathy (tabetic)
		EØ8.61Ø	Diabetes due to undrl cond w diabetic neuropathic arthrop
		EØ9.61Ø	Drug/chem diabetes w diabetic neuropathic arthropathy
		E1Ø.61Ø	Type 1 diabetes mellitus w diabetic neuropathic arthropathy
		E11.61Ø	Type 2 diabetes mellitus w diabetic neuropathic arthropathy
		E13.61Ø	Oth diabetes mellitus with diabetic neuropathic arthropathy
		M14.6Ø	Charcot's joint, unspecified site
		M14.61[1,2,9]	Charcot's joint, shoulder
		M14.62[1,2,9]	Charcot's joint, elbow
		M14.63[1,2,9]	Charcot's joint, wrist
		M14.64[1,2,9]	Charcot's joint, hand
		M14.65[1,2,9]	Charcot's joint, hip
		M14.66[1,2,9]	Charcot's joint, knee
		M14.67[1,2,9]	Charcot's joint, ankle and foot
		M14.68	Charcot's joint, vertebrae
		M14.69	Charcot's joint, multiple sites
			6th Character meanings for codes as indicated ***1 Right 2 Left 9 Unspecified***
713.6	ARTHROPATHY ASSOC W/HYPERSENSITIVITY REACTION	MØ2.2Ø	Postimmunization arthropathy, unspecified site
		MØ2.21[1,2,9]	Postimmunization arthropathy, shoulder
		MØ2.22[1,2,9]	Postimmunization arthropathy, elbow
		MØ2.23[1,2,9]	Postimmunization arthropathy, wrist
		MØ2.24[1,2,9]	Postimmunization arthropathy, hand
		MØ2.25[1,2,9]	Postimmunization arthropathy, hip
		MØ2.26[1,2,9]	Postimmunization arthropathy, knee
		MØ2.27[1,2,9]	Postimmunization arthropathy, ankle and foot
		MØ2.28	Postimmunization arthropathy, vertebrae
		MØ2.29	Postimmunization arthropathy, multiple sites
		M36.4	Arthropathy in hypersensitivity reactions classd elswhr
			6th Character meanings for codes as indicated ***1 Right 2 Left 9 Unspecified***
713.7	OTHER GENERAL DISEASES W/ARTICULAR INVOLVEMENT	MØ2.9	Reactive arthropathy, unspecified

ICD-9-CM		ICD-10-CM	
713.8	ARTHRPATH W/OTH CONDS CLASSIFIABLE ELSEWHERE	**M14.8Ø**	Arthropathies in oth diseases classd elswhr, unsp site
		M14.81[1,2,9]	Arthropathies in oth diseases classd elswhr, shoulder
		M14.82[1,2,9]	Arthropathies in oth diseases classd elswhr, elbow
		M14.83[1,2,9]	Arthropathies in oth diseases classd elswhr, wrist
		M14.84[1,2,9]	Arthropathies in oth diseases classd elswhr, hand
		M14.85[1,2,9]	Arthropathies in oth diseases classd elswhr, hip
		M14.86[1,2,9]	Arthropathies in oth diseases classd elswhr, knee
		M14.87[1,2,9]	Arthropathies in oth diseases classd elswhr, ank/ft
		M14.88	Arthropathies in oth diseases classd elswhr, vertebrae
		M14.89	Arthropathies in oth diseases classd elswhr, multiple sites
		M36.1	Arthropathy in neoplastic disease
			6th Character meanings for codes as indicated ***1 Right*** ***2 Left*** ***9 Unspecified***
714.Ø	RHEUMATOID ARTHRITIS	**MØ5.4Ø**	Rheumatoid myopathy with rheumatoid arthritis of unsp site
		MØ5.41[1,2,9]	Rheumatoid myopathy w rheumatoid arthritis of shoulder
		MØ5.42[1,2,9]	Rheumatoid myopathy with rheumatoid arthritis of elbow
		MØ5.43[1,2,9]	Rheumatoid myopathy with rheumatoid arthritis of wrist
		MØ5.44[1,2,9]	Rheumatoid myopathy with rheumatoid arthritis of hand
		MØ5.45[1,2,9]	Rheumatoid myopathy with rheumatoid arthritis of hip
		MØ5.46[1,2,9]	Rheumatoid myopathy with rheumatoid arthritis of knee
		MØ5.47[1,2,9]	Rheumatoid myopathy w rheumatoid arthritis of ank/ft
		MØ5.49	Rheumatoid myopathy w rheumatoid arthritis of multiple sites
		MØ5.5Ø	Rheumatoid polyneurop w rheumatoid arthritis of unsp site
		MØ5.51[1,2,9]	Rheumatoid polyneurop w rheumatoid arthritis of shoulder
		MØ5.52[1,2,9]	Rheumatoid polyneurop w rheumatoid arthritis of elbow
		MØ5.53[1,2,9]	Rheumatoid polyneurop w rheumatoid arthritis of wrist
		MØ5.54[1,2,9]	Rheumatoid polyneurop w rheumatoid arthritis of hand
		MØ5.55[1,2,9]	Rheumatoid polyneurop w rheumatoid arthritis of hip
		MØ5.56[1,2,9]	Rheumatoid polyneurop w rheumatoid arthritis of knee
		MØ5.57[1,2,9]	Rheumatoid polyneurop w rheumatoid arthritis of ank/ft
		MØ5.59	Rheumatoid polyneuropathy w rheumatoid arthritis mult site
		MØ5.7Ø	Rheu arthritis w rheu factor of unsp site w/o org/sys involv
		MØ5.71[1,2,9]	Rheu arthrit w rheu factor of r shoulder w/o org/sys involv
		MØ5.72[1,2,9]	Rheu arthritis w rheu factor of elbow w/o org/sys involv
		MØ5.73[1,2,9]	Rheu arthritis w rheu factor of wrist w/o org/sys involv
		MØ5.74[1,2,9]	Rheu arthritis w rheu factor of hand w/o org/sys involv
		MØ5.75[1,2,9]	Rheu arthritis w rheu factor of hip w/o org/sys involv
		MØ5.76[1,2,9]	Rheu arthritis w rheu factor of knee w/o org/sys involv
		MØ5.77[1,2,9]	Rheu arthrit w rheu fctr of ank/ft w/o org/sys involv
		MØ5.79	Rheu arthritis w rheu factor mult site w/o org/sys involv
		MØ5.8Ø	Oth rheumatoid arthritis with rheumatoid factor of unsp site
		MØ5.81[1,2,9]	Oth rheumatoid arthritis w rheumatoid factor of shoulder
		MØ5.82[1,2,9]	Oth rheumatoid arthritis w rheumatoid factor of elbow
		MØ5.83[1,2,9]	Oth rheumatoid arthritis w rheumatoid factor of wrist
		MØ5.84[1,2,9]	Oth rheumatoid arthritis w rheumatoid factor of hand
		MØ5.85[1,2,9]	Oth rheumatoid arthritis with rheumatoid factor of hip
		MØ5.86[1,2,9]	Oth rheumatoid arthritis w rheumatoid factor of knee
		MØ5.87[1,2,9]	Oth rheumatoid arthritis w rheumatoid factor of ank/ft
		MØ5.89	Oth rheumatoid arthritis w rheumatoid factor mult site
		MØ5.9	Rheumatoid arthritis with rheumatoid factor, unspecified
		MØ6.ØØ	Rheumatoid arthritis without rheumatoid factor, unsp site
		MØ6.Ø1[1,2,9]	Rheumatoid arthritis w/o rheumatoid factor, shoulder
		MØ6.Ø2[1,2,9]	Rheumatoid arthritis without rheumatoid factor, elbow
		MØ6.Ø3[1,2,9]	Rheumatoid arthritis without rheumatoid factor, wrist
		MØ6.Ø4[1,2,9]	Rheumatoid arthritis without rheumatoid factor, hand
		MØ6.Ø5[1,2,9]	Rheumatoid arthritis without rheumatoid factor, hip
		MØ6.Ø6[1,2,9]	Rheumatoid arthritis without rheumatoid factor, knee
		MØ6.Ø7[1,2,9]	Rheumatoid arthritis w/o rheumatoid factor, ank/ft
		MØ6.Ø8	Rheumatoid arthritis without rheumatoid factor, vertebrae
		MØ6.Ø9	Rheumatoid arthritis w/o rheumatoid factor, multiple sites
		MØ6.2Ø	Rheumatoid bursitis, unspecified site
		MØ6.21[1,2,9]	Rheumatoid bursitis, shoulder
		MØ6.22[1,2,9]	Rheumatoid bursitis, elbow
		MØ6.23[1,2,9]	Rheumatoid bursitis, wrist
		MØ6.24[1,2,9]	Rheumatoid bursitis, hand
		MØ6.25[1,2,9]	Rheumatoid bursitis, hip
		MØ6.26[1,2,9]	Rheumatoid bursitis, knee
		MØ6.27[1,2,9]	Rheumatoid bursitis, ankle and foot
		MØ6.28	Rheumatoid bursitis, vertebrae
		MØ6.29	Rheumatoid bursitis, multiple sites
		MØ6.3Ø	Rheumatoid nodule, unspecified site
		MØ6.31[1,2,9]	Rheumatoid nodule, shoulder
		MØ6.32[1,2,9]	Rheumatoid nodule, elbow
		MØ6.33[1,2,9]	Rheumatoid nodule, wrist
		MØ6.34[1,2,9]	Rheumatoid nodule, hand
		MØ6.35[1,2,9]	Rheumatoid nodule, hip
		MØ6.36[1,2,9]	Rheumatoid nodule, knee
		MØ6.37[1,2,9]	Rheumatoid nodule, ankle and foot
			6th Character meanings for codes as indicated ***1 Right*** ***2 Left*** ***9 Unspecified***

(Continued on next page)

ICD-9-CM		ICD-10-CM	
714.Ø	RHEUMATOID ARTHRITIS **(Continued)**	**MØ6.38**	Rheumatoid nodule, vertebrae
		MØ6.39	Rheumatoid nodule, multiple sites
		MØ6.8Ø	Other specified rheumatoid arthritis, unspecified site
		MØ6.81[1,2,9]	Other specified rheumatoid arthritis, shoulder
		MØ6.82[1,2,9]	Other specified rheumatoid arthritis, elbow
		MØ6.83[1,2,9]	Other specified rheumatoid arthritis, wrist
		MØ6.84[1,2,9]	Other specified rheumatoid arthritis, hand
		MØ6.85[1,2,9]	Other specified rheumatoid arthritis, hip
		MØ6.86[1,2,9]	Other specified rheumatoid arthritis, knee
		MØ6.87[1,2,9]	Other specified rheumatoid arthritis, ankle and foot
		MØ6.88	Other specified rheumatoid arthritis, vertebrae
		MØ6.89	Other specified rheumatoid arthritis, multiple sites
		MØ6.9	Rheumatoid arthritis, unspecified
			6th Character meanings for codes as indicated *1 Right* *2 Left* *9 Unspecified*
714.1	FELTYS SYNDROME	**MØ5.ØØ**	Felty's syndrome, unspecified site
		MØ5.Ø1[1,2,9]	Felty's syndrome, shoulder
		MØ5.Ø2[1,2,9]	Felty's syndrome, elbow
		MØ5.Ø3[1,2,9]	Felty's syndrome, wrist
		MØ5.Ø4[1,2,9]	Felty's syndrome, hand
		MØ5.Ø5[1,2,9]	Felty's syndrome, hip
		MØ5.Ø6[1,2,9]	Felty's syndrome, knee
		MØ5.Ø7[1,2,9]	Felty's syndrome, ankle and foot
		MØ5.Ø9	Felty's syndrome, multiple sites
			6th Character meanings for codes as indicated *1 Right* *2 Left* *9 Unspecified*
714.2	OTHER RA WITH VISCERAL OR SYSTEMIC INVOLVEMENT	**MØ5.2Ø**	Rheumatoid vasculitis with rheumatoid arthritis of unsp site
		MØ5.21[1,2,9]	Rheumatoid vasculitis w rheumatoid arthritis of shoulder
		MØ5.22[1,2,9]	Rheumatoid vasculitis w rheumatoid arthritis of elbow
		MØ5.23[1,2,9]	Rheumatoid vasculitis w rheumatoid arthritis of wrist
		MØ5.24[1,2,9]	Rheumatoid vasculitis w rheumatoid arthritis of hand
		MØ5.25[1,2,9]	Rheumatoid vasculitis with rheumatoid arthritis of hip
		MØ5.26[1,2,9]	Rheumatoid vasculitis w rheumatoid arthritis of knee
		MØ5.27[1,2,9]	Rheumatoid vasculitis w rheumatoid arthritis of ank/ft
		MØ5.29	Rheumatoid vasculitis w rheumatoid arthritis mult site
		MØ5.3Ø	Rheumatoid heart disease w rheumatoid arthritis of unsp site
		MØ5.31[1,2,9]	Rheu heart disease w rheumatoid arthritis of shoulder
		MØ5.32[1,2,9]	Rheumatoid heart disease w rheumatoid arthritis of elbow
		MØ5.33[1,2,9]	Rheumatoid heart disease w rheumatoid arthritis of wrist
		MØ5.34[1,2,9]	Rheu heart disease w rheumatoid arthritis of hand
		MØ5.35[1,2,9]	Rheumatoid heart disease w rheumatoid arthritis of hip
		MØ5.36[1,2,9]	Rheu heart disease w rheumatoid arthritis of knee
		MØ5.37[1,2,9]	Rheu heart disease w rheumatoid arthritis of ank/ft
		MØ5.39	Rheumatoid heart disease w rheumatoid arthritis mult site
		MØ5.6Ø	Rheu arthritis of unsp site w involv of organs and systems
		MØ5.61[1,2,9]	Rheu arthritis of shoulder w involv of organs and systems
		MØ5.62[1,2,9]	Rheu arthritis of elbow w involv of organs and systems
		MØ5.63[1,2,9]	Rheu arthritis of wrist w involv of organs and systems
		MØ5.64[1,2,9]	Rheu arthritis of hand w involv of organs and systems
		MØ5.65[1,2,9]	Rheu arthritis of hip w involv of organs and systems
		MØ5.66[1,2,9]	Rheu arthritis of knee w involv of organs and systems
		MØ5.67[1,2,9]	Rheu arthrit of ank/ft w involv of organs and systems
		MØ5.69	Rheu arthritis mult site w involv of organs and systems
		MØ6.1	Adult-onset Still's disease
			6th Character meanings for codes as indicated *1 Right* *2 Left* *9 Unspecified*
714.3Ø	POLYARTICULAR JUVENILE RA CHRONIC OR UNSPECIFIED	**MØ8.ØØ**	Unsp juvenile rheumatoid arthritis of unspecified site
		MØ8.Ø1[1,2,9]	Unspecified juvenile rheumatoid arthritis, shoulder
		MØ8.Ø2[1,2,9]	Unspecified juvenile rheumatoid arthritis, elbow
		MØ8.Ø3[1,2,9]	Unspecified juvenile rheumatoid arthritis, wrist
		MØ8.Ø4[1,2,9]	Unspecified juvenile rheumatoid arthritis, hand
		MØ8.Ø5[1,2,9]	Unspecified juvenile rheumatoid arthritis, hip
		MØ8.Ø6[1,2,9]	Unspecified juvenile rheumatoid arthritis, knee
		MØ8.Ø7[1,2,9]	Unsp juvenile rheumatoid arthritis, ankle and foot
		MØ8.Ø8	Unspecified juvenile rheumatoid arthritis, vertebrae
		MØ8.Ø9	Unspecified juvenile rheumatoid arthritis, multiple sites
		MØ8.2Ø	Juvenile rheumatoid arthritis with systemic onset, unsp site
		MØ8.21[1,2,9]	Juvenile rheumatoid arthritis w systemic onset, shoulder
		MØ8.22[1,2,9]	Juvenile rheumatoid arthritis w systemic onset, elbow
		MØ8.23[1,2,9]	Juvenile rheumatoid arthritis w systemic onset, wrist
		MØ8.24[1,2,9]	Juvenile rheumatoid arthritis w systemic onset, hand
		MØ8.25[1,2,9]	Juvenile rheumatoid arthritis with systemic onset, hip
		MØ8.26[1,2,9]	Juvenile rheumatoid arthritis w systemic onset, knee
		MØ8.27[1,2,9]	Juvenile rheumatoid arthritis w systemic onset, ank/ft
		MØ8.28	Juvenile rheumatoid arthritis with systemic onset, vertebrae
		MØ8.29	Juvenile rheu arthritis w systemic onset, multiple sites
			6th Character meanings for codes as indicated *1 Right* *2 Left* *9 Unspecified*

(Continued on next page)

[Brackets] indicate valid character values for each code. Character value meanings provided for each code grouping.

ICD-9-CM		ICD-10-CM	
714.3Ø	POLYARTICULAR JUVENILE RA CHRONIC OR UNSPECIFIED (Continued)	MØ8.3	Juvenile rheumatoid polyarthritis (seronegative)
		MØ8.8Ø	Other juvenile arthritis, unspecified site
		MØ8.81[1,2,9]	Other juvenile arthritis, shoulder
		MØ8.82[1,2,9]	Other juvenile arthritis, elbow
		MØ8.83[1,2,9]	Other juvenile arthritis, wrist
		MØ8.84[1,2,9]	Other juvenile arthritis, hand
		MØ8.85[1,2,9]	Other juvenile arthritis, hip
		MØ8.86[1,2,9]	Other juvenile arthritis, knee
		MØ8.87[1,2,9]	Other juvenile arthritis, ankle and foot
		MØ8.88	Other juvenile arthritis, oth spec site
		MØ8.89	Other juvenile arthritis, multiple sites
		MØ8.9Ø	Juvenile arthritis, unspecified, unspecified site
		MØ8.91[1,2,9]	Juvenile arthritis, unspecified, shoulder
		MØ8.92[1,2,9]	Juvenile arthritis, unspecified, elbow
		MØ8.93[1,2,9]	Juvenile arthritis, unspecified, wrist
		MØ8.94[1,2,9]	Juvenile arthritis, unspecified, hand
		MØ8.95[1,2,9]	Juvenile arthritis, unspecified, hip
		MØ8.96[1,2,9]	Juvenile arthritis, unspecified, knee
		MØ8.97[1,2,9]	Juvenile arthritis, unspecified, ankle and foot
		MØ8.98	Juvenile arthritis, unspecified, vertebrae
		MØ8.99	Juvenile arthritis, unspecified, multiple sites
			6th Character meanings for codes as indicated 1 Right 2 Left 9 Unspecified
714.31	POLYARTICULAR JUVENILE RA ACUTE	MØ8.3	Juvenile rheumatoid polyarthritis (seronegative)
714.32	PAUCIARTICULAR JUVENILE RHEUMATOID ARTHRITIS	MØ8.4Ø	Pauciarticular juvenile rheumatoid arthritis, unsp site
		MØ8.41[1,2,9]	Pauciarticular juvenile rheumatoid arthritis, shoulder
		MØ8.42[1,2,9]	Pauciarticular juvenile rheumatoid arthritis, elbow
		MØ8.43[1,2,9]	Pauciarticular juvenile rheumatoid arthritis, wrist
		MØ8.44[1,2,9]	Pauciarticular juvenile rheumatoid arthritis, hand
		MØ8.45[1,2,9]	Pauciarticular juvenile rheumatoid arthritis, hip
		MØ8.46[1,2,9]	Pauciarticular juvenile rheumatoid arthritis, knee
		MØ8.47[1,2,9]	Pauciarticular juvenile rheumatoid arthritis, ank/ft
		MØ8.48	Pauciarticular juvenile rheumatoid arthritis, vertebrae
			6th Character meanings for codes as indicated 1 Right 2 Left 9 Unspecified
714.33	MONOARTICULAR JUVENILE RHEUMATOID ARTHRITIS	MØ8.4Ø	Pauciarticular juvenile rheumatoid arthritis, unsp site
714.4	CHRONIC POSTRHEUMATIC ARTHROPATHY	M12.ØØ	Chronic postrheumatic arthropathy, unspecified site
		M12.Ø1[1,2,9]	Chronic postrheumatic arthropathy [Jaccoud], shoulder
		M12.Ø2[1,2,9]	Chronic postrheumatic arthropathy [Jaccoud], elbow
		M12.Ø3[1,2,9]	Chronic postrheumatic arthropathy [Jaccoud], wrist
		M12.Ø4[1,2,9]	Chronic postrheumatic arthropathy [Jaccoud], hand
		M12.Ø5[1,2,9]	Chronic postrheumatic arthropathy [Jaccoud], hip
		M12.Ø6[1,2,9]	Chronic postrheumatic arthropathy [Jaccoud], knee
		M12.Ø7[1,2,9]	Chronic postrheumatic arthropathy, ankle and foot
		M12.Ø8	Chronic postrheumatic arthropathy [Jaccoud], oth spec site
		M12.Ø9	Chronic postrheumatic arthropathy [Jaccoud], multiple sites
			6th Character meanings for codes as indicated 1 Right 2 Left 9 Unspecified
714.81	RHEUMATOID LUNG	MØ5.1Ø	Rheumatoid lung disease w rheumatoid arthritis of unsp site
		MØ5.11[1,2,9]	Rheumatoid lung disease w rheumatoid arthritis of shoulder
		MØ5.12[1,2,9]	Rheumatoid lung disease w rheumatoid arthritis of elbow
		MØ5.13[1,2,9]	Rheumatoid lung disease w rheumatoid arthritis of wrist
		MØ5.14[1,2,9]	Rheumatoid lung disease w rheumatoid arthritis of hand
		MØ5.15[1,2,9]	Rheumatoid lung disease w rheumatoid arthritis of hip
		MØ5.16[1,2,9]	Rheumatoid lung disease w rheumatoid arthritis of knee
		MØ5.17[1,2,9]	Rheu lung disease w rheumatoid arthritis of ank/ft
		MØ5.19	Rheumatoid lung disease w rheumatoid arthritis mult site
			6th Character meanings for codes as indicated 1 Right 2 Left 9 Unspecified
714.89	OTH SPECIFIED INFLAMMATORY POLYARTHROPATHIES OTH	MØ6.4	Inflammatory polyarthropathy
714.9	UNSPECIFIED INFLAMMATORY POLYARTHROPATHY	MØ6.4	Inflammatory polyarthropathy
715.ØØ	GENERALIZED OSTEOARTHROSIS UNSPECIFIED SITE	M15.Ø	Primary generalized (osteo)arthritis
		M15.9	Polyosteoarthritis, unspecified
715.Ø4	GENERALIZED OSTEOARTHROSIS INVOLVING HAND	M15.1	Heberden's nodes (with arthropathy)
		M15.2	Bouchard's nodes (with arthropathy)
715.Ø9	GEN OSTEOARTHROSIS INVOLVING MULTIPLE SITES	M15.Ø	Primary generalized (osteo)arthritis
715.1Ø	PRIMARY LOCALIZED OSTEOARTHROSIS SPECIFIED SITE	M19.91	Primary osteoarthritis, unspecified site
715.11	PRIMARY LOCALIZED OSTEOARTHROSIS SHOULDER REGION	M19.Ø11	Primary osteoarthritis, right shoulder
		M19.Ø12	Primary osteoarthritis, left shoulder
		M19.Ø19	Primary osteoarthritis, unspecified shoulder
715.12	PRIMARY LOCALIZED OSTEOARTHROSIS UPPER ARM	M19.Ø21	Primary osteoarthritis, right elbow
		M19.Ø22	Primary osteoarthritis, left elbow
		M19.Ø29	Primary osteoarthritis, unspecified elbow

ICD-9-CM		ICD-10-CM	
715.13	PRIMARY LOCALIZED OSTEOARTHROSIS FOREARM	**M19.Ø31**	Primary osteoarthritis, right wrist
		M19.Ø32	Primary osteoarthritis, left wrist
		M19.Ø39	Primary osteoarthritis, unspecified wrist
715.14	PRIMARY LOCALIZED OSTEOARTHROSIS HAND	**M18.Ø**	Bilateral primary osteoarth of first carpometacarp joints
		M18.1Ø	Unil prim osteoarth of first carpometacarp joint, unsp hand
		M18.11	Unil primary osteoarth of first carpometacarp joint, r hand
		M18.12	Unil primary osteoarth of first carpometacarp joint, l hand
		M19.Ø41	Primary osteoarthritis, right hand
		M19.Ø42	Primary osteoarthritis, left hand
		M19.Ø49	Primary osteoarthritis, unspecified hand
715.15	PRIMARY LOC OSTEOARTHROSIS PELVIC REGION&THIGH	**M16.Ø**	Bilateral primary osteoarthritis of hip
		M16.1Ø	Unilateral primary osteoarthritis, unspecified hip
		M16.11	Unilateral primary osteoarthritis, right hip
		M16.12	Unilateral primary osteoarthritis, left hip
715.16	PRIMARY LOCALIZED OSTEOARTHROSIS LOWER LEG	**M17.Ø**	Bilateral primary osteoarthritis of knee
		M17.1Ø	Unilateral primary osteoarthritis, unspecified knee
		M17.11	Unilateral primary osteoarthritis, right knee
		M17.12	Unilateral primary osteoarthritis, left knee
715.17	PRIMARY LOCALIZED OSTEOARTHROSIS ANKLE AND FOOT	**M19.Ø71**	Primary osteoarthritis, right ankle and foot
		M19.Ø72	Primary osteoarthritis, left ankle and foot
		M19.Ø79	Primary osteoarthritis, unspecified ankle and foot
715.18	PRIMARY LOCALIZED OSTEOARTHROSIS OTH SPEC SITES	**M19.91**	Primary osteoarthritis, unspecified site
715.2Ø	SEC LOCALIZED OSTEOARTHROSIS UNSPECIFIED SITE	**M19.92**	Post-traumatic osteoarthritis, unspecified site
		M19.93	Secondary osteoarthritis, unspecified site
715.21	SEC LOCALIZED OSTEOARTHROSIS SHOULDER REGION	**M19.111**	Post-traumatic osteoarthritis, right shoulder
		M19.112	Post-traumatic osteoarthritis, left shoulder
		M19.119	Post-traumatic osteoarthritis, unspecified shoulder
		M19.211	Secondary osteoarthritis, right shoulder
		M19.212	Secondary osteoarthritis, left shoulder
		M19.219	Secondary osteoarthritis, unspecified shoulder
715.22	SECONDARY LOCALIZED OSTEOARTHROSIS UPPER ARM	**M19.121**	Post-traumatic osteoarthritis, right elbow
		M19.122	Post-traumatic osteoarthritis, left elbow
		M19.129	Post-traumatic osteoarthritis, unspecified elbow
		M19.221	Secondary osteoarthritis, right elbow
		M19.222	Secondary osteoarthritis, left elbow
		M19.229	Secondary osteoarthritis, unspecified elbow
715.23	SECONDARY LOCALIZED OSTEOARTHROSIS FOREARM	**M19.131**	Post-traumatic osteoarthritis, right wrist
		M19.132	Post-traumatic osteoarthritis, left wrist
		M19.139	Post-traumatic osteoarthritis, unspecified wrist
		M19.231	Secondary osteoarthritis, right wrist
		M19.232	Secondary osteoarthritis, left wrist
		M19.239	Secondary osteoarthritis, unspecified wrist
715.24	SEC LOCALIZED OSTEOARTHROSIS INVOLVING HAND	**M18.2**	Bi post-trauma osteoarth of first carpometacarp joints
		M18.3Ø	Unil post-trauma osteoarth of 1st carpometacarp jt, unsp hand
		M18.3[1,2]	Unil post-trauma osteoarth of 1st carpometacarp jt, hand
		M18.4	Oth bi secondary osteoarth of first carpometacarp joints
		M18.5Ø	Oth unil sec osteoarth of 1st carpometacarp joint, unsp hand
		M18.5[1,2]	Oth unil sec osteoarth of first carpometacarp joint, hand
		M19.14[1,2,9]	Post-traumatic osteoarthritis, hand
		M19.24[1,2,9]	Secondary osteoarthritis, hand
			6th Character meanings for codes as indicated ***1 Right 2 Left 9 Unspecified***
715.25	SEC LOCALIZED OSTEOARTHROSIS PELVIC REGION&THIGH	**M16.2**	Bilateral osteoarthritis resulting from hip dysplasia
		M16.3Ø	Unilateral osteoarth resulting from hip dysplasia, unsp hip
		M16.31	Unilateral osteoarth resulting from hip dysplasia, right hip
		M16.32	Unilateral osteoarth resulting from hip dysplasia, left hip
		M16.4	Bilateral post-traumatic osteoarthritis of hip
		M16.5Ø	Unilateral post-traumatic osteoarthritis, unspecified hip
		M16.51	Unilateral post-traumatic osteoarthritis, right hip
		M16.52	Unilateral post-traumatic osteoarthritis, left hip
		M16.6	Other bilateral secondary osteoarthritis of hip
		M16.7	Other unilateral secondary osteoarthritis of hip
715.26	SECONDARY LOCALIZED OSTEOARTHROSIS LOWER LEG	**M17.2**	Bilateral post-traumatic osteoarthritis of knee
		M17.3Ø	Unilateral post-traumatic osteoarthritis, unspecified knee
		M17.31	Unilateral post-traumatic osteoarthritis, right knee
		M17.32	Unilateral post-traumatic osteoarthritis, left knee
		M17.4	Other bilateral secondary osteoarthritis of knee
		M17.5	Other unilateral secondary osteoarthritis of knee
715.27	SEC LOCALIZED OSTEOARTHROSIS ANKLE AND FOOT	**M19.171**	Post-traumatic osteoarthritis, right ankle and foot
		M19.172	Post-traumatic osteoarthritis, left ankle and foot
		M19.179	Post-traumatic osteoarthritis, unspecified ankle and foot
		M19.271	Secondary osteoarthritis, right ankle and foot
		M19.272	Secondary osteoarthritis, left ankle and foot
		M19.279	Secondary osteoarthritis, unspecified ankle and foot
715.28	SEC LOCALIZED OSTEOARTHROSIS OTHER SPEC SITE	**M19.92**	Post-traumatic osteoarthritis, unspecified site
		M19.93	Secondary osteoarthritis, unspecified site
715.3Ø	LOC OSTEOARTHROS NOT SPEC PRIM/SEC UNSPEC SITE	**M19.9Ø**	Unspecified osteoarthritis, unspecified site
715.31	LOC OSTEOARTHROS NOT SPEC PRIM/SEC SHLDR REGION	**M19.9Ø**	Unspecified osteoarthritis, unspecified site

[Brackets] indicate valid character values for each code. Character value meanings provided for each code grouping.

ICD-9-CM		ICD-10-CM	
715.32	LOC OSTEOARTHROS NOT SPEC PRIM/SEC UPPER ARM	**M19.90**	Unspecified osteoarthritis, unspecified site
715.33	LOC OSTEOARTHROS NOT SPEC PRIM/SEC FOREARM	**M19.90**	Unspecified osteoarthritis, unspecified site
715.34	LOC OSTEOARTHROS NOT SPEC WHETHER PRIM/SEC HAND	**M18.9**	Osteoarthritis of first carpometacarpal joint, unspecified
715.35	LOC OSTEOARTHROS NOT SPEC PRIM/SEC PELV RGN&THI	**M16.9**	Osteoarthritis of hip, unspecified
715.36	LOC OSTEOARTHROS NOT SPEC PRIM/SEC LOWER LEG	**M17.9**	Osteoarthritis of knee, unspecified
715.37	LOC OSTEOARTHROS NOT SPEC PRIM/SEC ANK&FOOT	**M19.90**	Unspecified osteoarthritis, unspecified site
715.38	LOC OSTEOARTHROS NOT SPEC PRIM/SEC OTH SPEC SITE	**M19.90**	Unspecified osteoarthritis, unspecified site
715.80	OSTEOARTHROS INVLV > 1 SITE BUT NOT SPEC GEN	**M15.4** **M15.8**	Erosive (osteo)arthritis Other polyosteoarthritis
715.89	OSTEOARTHROS INVLV MX SITES BUT NOT SPEC AS GEN	**M15.3** **M15.8**	Secondary multiple arthritis Other polyosteoarthritis
715.90	OSTEOARTHROS UNSPEC WHETHER GEN/LOC UNSPEC SITE	**M15.9** **M19.90**	Polyosteoarthritis, unspecified Unspecified osteoarthritis, unspecified site
715.91	OSTEOARTHROS UNSPEC WHETHER GEN/LOC SHLDR REGION	**M19.90**	Unspecified osteoarthritis, unspecified site
715.92	OSTEOARTHROSIS UNSPEC WHETHER GEN/LOC UPPER ARM	**M19.90**	Unspecified osteoarthritis, unspecified site
715.93	OSTEOARTHROSIS UNSPEC WHETHER GEN/LOC FOREARM	**M19.90**	Unspecified osteoarthritis, unspecified site
715.94	OSTEOARTHROSIS UNSPEC WHETHER GEN/LOCALIZED HAND	**M18.9**	Osteoarthritis of first carpometacarpal joint, unspecified
715.95	OSTEOARTHROS UNSPEC GEN/LOC PELV REGION&THIGH	**M16.9**	Osteoarthritis of hip, unspecified
715.96	OSTEOARTHROSIS UNSPEC WHETHER GEN/LOC LOWER LEG	**M17.9**	Osteoarthritis of knee, unspecified
715.97	OSTEOARTHROSIS UNSPEC WHETHER GEN/LOC ANK&FOOT	**M19.90**	Unspecified osteoarthritis, unspecified site
715.98	OSTEOARTHROS UNSPEC GEN/LOC OTH SPEC SITES	**M19.90**	Unspecified osteoarthritis, unspecified site
716.00	KASCHIN-BECK DISEASE SITE UNSPECIFIED	➡ **M12.10**	Kaschin-Beck disease, unspecified site
716.01	KASCHIN-BECK DISEASE SHOULDER REGION	**M12.111** **M12.112** **M12.119**	Kaschin-Beck disease, right shoulder Kaschin-Beck disease, left shoulder Kaschin-Beck disease, unspecified shoulder
716.02	KASCHIN-BECK DISEASE, UPPER ARM	**M12.121** **M12.122** **M12.129**	Kaschin-Beck disease, right elbow Kaschin-Beck disease, left elbow Kaschin-Beck disease, unspecified elbow
716.03	KASCHIN-BECK DISEASE, FOREARM	**M12.131** **M12.132** **M12.139**	Kaschin-Beck disease, right wrist Kaschin-Beck disease, left wrist Kaschin-Beck disease, unspecified wrist
716.04	KASCHIN-BECK DISEASE, HAND	**M12.141** **M12.142** **M12.149**	Kaschin-Beck disease, right hand Kaschin-Beck disease, left hand Kaschin-Beck disease, unspecified hand
716.05	KASCHIN-BECK DISEASE PELVIC REGION AND THIGH	**M12.151** **M12.152** **M12.159**	Kaschin-Beck disease, right hip Kaschin-Beck disease, left hip Kaschin-Beck disease, unspecified hip
716.06	KASCHIN-BECK DISEASE, LOWER LEG	**M12.161** **M12.162** **M12.169**	Kaschin-Beck disease, right knee Kaschin-Beck disease, left knee Kaschin-Beck disease, unspecified knee
716.07	KASCHIN-BECK DISEASE ANKLE AND FOOT	**M12.171** **M12.172** **M12.179**	Kaschin-Beck disease, right ankle and foot Kaschin-Beck disease, left ankle and foot Kaschin-Beck disease, unspecified ankle and foot
716.08	KASCHIN-BECK DISEASE OTHER SPECIFIED SITES	**M12.18**	Kaschin-Beck disease, vertebrae
716.09	KASCHIN-BECK DISEASE MULTIPLE SITES	➡ **M12.19**	Kaschin-Beck disease, multiple sites
716.10	TRAUMATIC ARTHROPATHY SITE UNSPECIFIED	➡ **M12.50**	Traumatic arthropathy, unspecified site
716.11	TRAUMATIC ARTHROPATHY SHOULDER REGION	**M12.511** **M12.512** **M12.519**	Traumatic arthropathy, right shoulder Traumatic arthropathy, left shoulder Traumatic arthropathy, unspecified shoulder
716.12	TRAUMATIC ARTHROPATHY, UPPER ARM	**M12.521** **M12.522** **M12.529**	Traumatic arthropathy, right elbow Traumatic arthropathy, left elbow Traumatic arthropathy, unspecified elbow
716.13	TRAUMATIC ARTHROPATHY, FOREARM	**M12.531** **M12.532** **M12.539**	Traumatic arthropathy, right wrist Traumatic arthropathy, left wrist Traumatic arthropathy, unspecified wrist
716.14	TRAUMATIC ARTHROPATHY, HAND	**M12.541** **M12.542** **M12.549**	Traumatic arthropathy, right hand Traumatic arthropathy, left hand Traumatic arthropathy, unspecified hand
716.15	TRAUMATIC ARTHROPATHY PELVIC REGION AND THIGH	**M12.551** **M12.552** **M12.559**	Traumatic arthropathy, right hip Traumatic arthropathy, left hip Traumatic arthropathy, unspecified hip
716.16	TRAUMATIC ARTHROPATHY, LOWER LEG	**M12.561** **M12.562** **M12.569**	Traumatic arthropathy, right knee Traumatic arthropathy, left knee Traumatic arthropathy, unspecified knee
716.17	TRAUMATIC ARTHROPATHY ANKLE AND FOOT	**M12.571** **M12.572** **M12.579**	Traumatic arthropathy, right ankle and foot Traumatic arthropathy, left ankle and foot Traumatic arthropathy, unspecified ankle and foot
716.18	TRAUMATIC ARTHROPATHY OTHER SPECIFIED SITES	➡ **M12.58**	Traumatic arthropathy, oth spec site
716.19	TRAUMATIC ARTHROPATHY MULTIPLE SITES	➡ **M12.59**	Traumatic arthropathy, multiple sites
716.20	ALLERGIC ARTHRITIS SITE UNSPECIFIED	**M13.80**	Other specified arthritis, unspecified site
716.21	ALLERGIC ARTHRITIS, SHOULDER REGION	**M13.811** **M13.812** **M13.819**	Other specified arthritis, right shoulder Other specified arthritis, left shoulder Other specified arthritis, unspecified shoulder

ICD-9-CM		ICD-10-CM	
716.22	ALLERGIC ARTHRITIS, UPPER ARM	M13.821	Other specified arthritis, right elbow
		M13.822	Other specified arthritis, left elbow
		M13.829	Other specified arthritis, unspecified elbow
716.23	ALLERGIC ARTHRITIS, FOREARM	M13.831	Other specified arthritis, right wrist
		M13.832	Other specified arthritis, left wrist
		M13.839	Other specified arthritis, unspecified wrist
716.24	ALLERGIC ARTHRITIS, HAND	M13.841	Other specified arthritis, right hand
		M13.842	Other specified arthritis, left hand
		M13.849	Other specified arthritis, unspecified hand
716.25	ALLERGIC ARTHRITIS PELVIC REGION AND THIGH	M13.851	Other specified arthritis, right hip
		M13.852	Other specified arthritis, left hip
		M13.859	Other specified arthritis, unspecified hip
716.26	ALLERGIC ARTHRITIS, LOWER LEG	M13.861	Other specified arthritis, right knee
		M13.862	Other specified arthritis, left knee
		M13.869	Other specified arthritis, unspecified knee
716.27	ALLERGIC ARTHRITIS, ANKLE AND FOOT	M13.871	Other specified arthritis, right ankle and foot
		M13.872	Other specified arthritis, left ankle and foot
		M13.879	Other specified arthritis, unspecified ankle and foot
716.28	ALLERGIC ARTHRITIS OTHER SPECIFIED SITES	M13.88	Other specified arthritis, other site
716.29	ALLERGIC ARTHRITIS, MULTIPLE SITES	M13.89	Other specified arthritis, multiple sites
716.30	CLIMACTERIC ARTHRITIS SITE UNSPECIFIED	M13.80	Other specified arthritis, unspecified site
716.31	CLIMACTERIC ARTHRITIS SHOULDER REGION	M13.819	Other specified arthritis, unspecified shoulder
716.32	CLIMACTERIC ARTHRITIS, UPPER ARM	M13.829	Other specified arthritis, unspecified elbow
716.33	CLIMACTERIC ARTHRITIS, FOREARM	M13.839	Other specified arthritis, unspecified wrist
716.34	CLIMACTERIC ARTHRITIS, HAND	M13.849	Other specified arthritis, unspecified hand
716.35	CLIMACTERIC ARTHRITIS PELVIC REGION AND THIGH	M13.859	Other specified arthritis, unspecified hip
716.36	CLIMACTERIC ARTHRITIS, LOWER LEG	M13.869	Other specified arthritis, unspecified knee
716.37	CLIMACTERIC ARTHRITIS INVOLVING ANKLE AND FOOT	M13.879	Other specified arthritis, unspecified ankle and foot
716.38	CLIMACTERIC ARTHRITIS INVOLVING OTHER SPEC SITES	M13.88	Other specified arthritis, other site
716.39	CLIMACTERIC ARTHRITIS INVOLVING MULTIPLE SITES	M13.89	Other specified arthritis, multiple sites
716.40	TRANSIENT ARTHROPATHY SITE UNSPECIFIED	M12.80	Oth specific arthropathies, NEC, unsp site
716.41	TRANSIENT ARTHROPATHY SHOULDER REGION	M12.811	Oth specific arthropathies, NEC, right shoulder
		M12.812	Oth specific arthropathies, NEC, left shoulder
		M12.819	Oth specific arthropathies, NEC, unsp shoulder
716.42	TRANSIENT ARTHROPATHY, UPPER ARM	M12.821	Oth specific arthropathies, NEC, right elbow
		M12.822	Oth specific arthropathies, NEC, left elbow
		M12.829	Oth specific arthropathies, NEC, unsp elbow
716.43	TRANSIENT ARTHROPATHY, FOREARM	M12.831	Oth specific arthropathies, NEC, right wrist
		M12.832	Oth specific arthropathies, NEC, left wrist
		M12.839	Oth specific arthropathies, NEC, unsp wrist
716.44	TRANSIENT ARTHROPATHY, HAND	M12.841	Oth specific arthropathies, NEC, right hand
		M12.842	Oth specific arthropathies, NEC, left hand
		M12.849	Oth specific arthropathies, NEC, unsp hand
716.45	TRANSIENT ARTHROPATHY PELVIC REGION AND THIGH	M12.851	Oth specific arthropathies, NEC, right hip
		M12.852	Oth specific arthropathies, NEC, left hip
		M12.859	Oth specific arthropathies, NEC, unsp hip
716.46	TRANSIENT ARTHROPATHY, LOWER LEG	M12.861	Oth specific arthropathies, NEC, right knee
		M12.862	Oth specific arthropathies, NEC, left knee
		M12.869	Oth specific arthropathies, NEC, unsp knee
716.47	TRANSIENT ARTHROPATHY ANKLE AND FOOT	M12.871	Oth specific arthropathies, NEC, right ankle and foot
		M12.872	Oth specific arthropathies, NEC, left ankle and foot
		M12.879	Oth specific arthropathies, NEC, unsp ankle and foot
716.48	TRANSIENT ARTHROPATHY OTHER SPECIFIED SITE	M12.88	Oth specific arthropathies, NEC, oth spec site
716.49	TRANSIENT ARTHROPATHY MULTIPLE SITES	M12.89	Oth specific arthropathies, NEC, multiple sites
716.50	UNSPEC POLYARTHROPATHY/POLYARTHRITIS SITE UNSPEC	M13.0	Polyarthritis, unspecified
716.51	UNSPEC POLYARTHROPATHY/POLYARTHRIT SHLDR REGION	M13.0	Polyarthritis, unspecified
716.52	UNSPEC POLYARTHROPATHY/POLYARTHRITIS UPPER ARM	M13.0	Polyarthritis, unspecified
716.53	UNSPEC POLYARTHROPATHY/POLYARTHRITIS FOREARM	M13.0	Polyarthritis, unspecified
716.54	UNSPECIFIED POLYARTHROPATHY/POLYARTHRITIS HAND	M13.0	Polyarthritis, unspecified
716.55	UNSPEC POLYARTHROPATHY/POLYARTHRIT PELV RGN&THI	M13.0	Polyarthritis, unspecified
716.56	UNSPEC POLYARTHROPATHY/POLYARTHRITIS LOWER LEG	M13.0	Polyarthritis, unspecified
716.57	UNSPEC POLYARTHROPATHY/POLYARTHRITIS ANKLE&FOOT	M13.0	Polyarthritis, unspecified
716.58	UNSPEC POLYARTHROPATHY/POLYARTHRIT OTH SPEC SITE	M13.0	Polyarthritis, unspecified
716.59	UNSPEC POLYARTHROPATHY/POLYARTHRIT MX SITES	M13.0	Polyarthritis, unspecified
716.60	UNSPECIFIED MONOARTHRITIS SITE UNSPECIFIED	M13.10	Monoarthritis, not elsewhere classified, unspecified site
716.61	UNSPECIFIED MONOARTHRITIS SHOULDER REGION	M13.111	Monoarthritis, not elsewhere classified, right shoulder
		M13.112	Monoarthritis, not elsewhere classified, left shoulder
		M13.119	Monoarthritis, not elsewhere classified, unsp shoulder
716.62	UNSPECIFIED MONOARTHRITIS UPPER ARM	M13.121	Monoarthritis, not elsewhere classified, right elbow
		M13.122	Monoarthritis, not elsewhere classified, left elbow
		M13.129	Monoarthritis, not elsewhere classified, unspecified elbow

ICD-9-CM		ICD-10-CM	
716.63	UNSPECIFIED MONOARTHRITIS, FOREARM	**M13.131**	Monoarthritis, not elsewhere classified, right wrist
		M13.132	Monoarthritis, not elsewhere classified, left wrist
		M13.139	Monoarthritis, not elsewhere classified, unspecified wrist
716.64	UNSPECIFIED MONOARTHRITIS, HAND	**M13.141**	Monoarthritis, not elsewhere classified, right hand
		M13.142	Monoarthritis, not elsewhere classified, left hand
		M13.149	Monoarthritis, not elsewhere classified, unspecified hand
716.65	UNSPECIFIED MONOARTHRITIS PELVIC REGION&THIGH	**M13.151**	Monoarthritis, not elsewhere classified, right hip
		M13.152	Monoarthritis, not elsewhere classified, left hip
		M13.159	Monoarthritis, not elsewhere classified, unspecified hip
716.66	UNSPECIFIED MONOARTHRITIS LOWER LEG	**M13.161**	Monoarthritis, not elsewhere classified, right knee
		M13.162	Monoarthritis, not elsewhere classified, left knee
		M13.169	Monoarthritis, not elsewhere classified, unspecified knee
716.67	UNSPECIFIED MONOARTHRITIS ANKLE AND FOOT	**M13.171**	Monoarthritis, NEC, right ankle and foot
		M13.172	Monoarthritis, not elsewhere classified, left ankle and foot
		M13.179	Monoarthritis, not elsewhere classified, unsp ankle and foot
716.68	UNSPECIFIED MONOARTHRITIS OTHER SPECIFIED SITES	**M13.10**	Monoarthritis, not elsewhere classified, unspecified site
716.80	OTHER SPECIFIED ARTHROPATHY SITE UNSPECIFIED	**E08.618**	Diabetes due to underlying condition w oth diabetic arthrop
		E09.618	Drug/chem diabetes mellitus w oth diabetic arthropathy
		E10.618	Type 1 diabetes mellitus with other diabetic arthropathy
		E11.618	Type 2 diabetes mellitus with other diabetic arthropathy
		E13.618	Oth diabetes mellitus with other diabetic arthropathy
		M07.60	Enteropathic arthropathies, unspecified site
		M12.80	Oth specific arthropathies, NEC, unsp site
716.81	OTHER SPECIFIED ARTHROPATHY SHOULDER REGION	**M07.611**	Enteropathic arthropathies, right shoulder
		M07.612	Enteropathic arthropathies, left shoulder
		M07.619	Enteropathic arthropathies, unspecified shoulder
		M12.811	Oth specific arthropathies, NEC, right shoulder
		M12.812	Oth specific arthropathies, NEC, left shoulder
		M12.819	Oth specific arthropathies, NEC, unsp shoulder
716.82	OTHER SPECIFIED ARTHROPATHY UPPER ARM	**M07.621**	Enteropathic arthropathies, right elbow
		M07.622	Enteropathic arthropathies, left elbow
		M07.629	Enteropathic arthropathies, unspecified elbow
		M12.821	Oth specific arthropathies, NEC, right elbow
		M12.822	Oth specific arthropathies, NEC, left elbow
		M12.829	Oth specific arthropathies, NEC, unsp elbow
716.83	OTHER SPECIFIED ARTHROPATHY FOREARM	**M07.631**	Enteropathic arthropathies, right wrist
		M07.632	Enteropathic arthropathies, left wrist
		M07.639	Enteropathic arthropathies, unspecified wrist
		M12.831	Oth specific arthropathies, NEC, right wrist
		M12.832	Oth specific arthropathies, NEC, left wrist
		M12.839	Oth specific arthropathies, NEC, unsp wrist
716.84	OTHER SPECIFIED ARTHROPATHY, HAND	**M07.641**	Enteropathic arthropathies, right hand
		M07.642	Enteropathic arthropathies, left hand
		M07.649	Enteropathic arthropathies, unspecified hand
		M12.841	Oth specific arthropathies, NEC, right hand
		M12.842	Oth specific arthropathies, NEC, left hand
		M12.849	Oth specific arthropathies, NEC, unsp hand
716.85	OTHER SPECIFIED ARTHROPATHY PELVIC REGION&THIGH	**M07.651**	Enteropathic arthropathies, right hip
		M07.652	Enteropathic arthropathies, left hip
		M07.659	Enteropathic arthropathies, unspecified hip
		M12.851	Oth specific arthropathies, NEC, right hip
		M12.852	Oth specific arthropathies, NEC, left hip
		M12.859	Oth specific arthropathies, NEC, unsp hip
716.86	OTHER SPECIFIED ARTHROPATHY LOWER LEG	**M07.661**	Enteropathic arthropathies, right knee
		M07.662	Enteropathic arthropathies, left knee
		M07.669	Enteropathic arthropathies, unspecified knee
		M12.861	Oth specific arthropathies, NEC, right knee
		M12.862	Oth specific arthropathies, NEC, left knee
		M12.869	Oth specific arthropathies, NEC, unsp knee
716.87	OTHER SPECIFIED ARTHROPATHY ANKLE AND FOOT	**M07.671**	Enteropathic arthropathies, right ankle and foot
		M07.672	Enteropathic arthropathies, left ankle and foot
		M07.679	Enteropathic arthropathies, unspecified ankle and foot
		M12.871	Oth specific arthropathies, NEC, right ankle and foot
		M12.872	Oth specific arthropathies, NEC, left ankle and foot
		M12.879	Oth specific arthropathies, NEC, unsp ankle and foot
716.88	OTHER SPEC ARTHROPATHY OTHER SPEC SITES	**M07.68**	Enteropathic arthropathies, vertebrae
		M12.88	Oth specific arthropathies, NEC, vertebrae
716.89	OTHER SPECIFIED ARTHROPATHY MULTIPLE SITES	**M07.69**	Enteropathic arthropathies, multiple sites
		M12.89	Oth specific arthropathies, NEC, multiple sites
716.90	UNSPECIFIED ARTHROPATHY SITE UNSPECIFIED	**M12.9**	Arthropathy, unspecified
716.91	UNSPECIFIED ARTHROPATHY SHOULDER REGION	**M12.9**	Arthropathy, unspecified
716.92	UNSPECIFIED ARTHROPATHY, UPPER ARM	**M12.9**	Arthropathy, unspecified
716.93	UNSPECIFIED ARTHROPATHY, FOREARM	**M12.9**	Arthropathy, unspecified
716.94	UNSPECIFIED ARTHOPATHY, HAND	**M12.9**	Arthropathy, unspecified
716.95	UNSPECIFIED ARTHROPATHY PELVIC REGION AND THIGH	**M12.9**	Arthropathy, unspecified
716.96	UNSPECIFIED ARTHROPATHY, LOWER LEG	**M12.9**	Arthropathy, unspecified

ICD-9-CM		ICD-10-CM	
716.97	UNSPECIFIED ARTHROPATHY ANKLE AND FOOT	**M12.9**	Arthropathy, unspecified
716.98	UNSPECIFIED ARTHROPATHY OTHER SPECIFIED SITES	**M12.9**	Arthropathy, unspecified
716.99	UNSPECIFIED ARTHROPATHY MULTIPLE SITES	**M12.9**	Arthropathy, unspecified
717.Ø	OLD BUCKET HANDLE TEAR OF MEDIAL MENISCUS	**M23.2Ø5**	Derang of unsp medial mensc due to old tear/inj, unsp knee
717.1	DERANGEMENT OF ANTERIOR HORN OF MEDIAL MENISCUS	**M23.Ø11**	Cystic meniscus, anterior horn of medial meniscus, r knee
		M23.Ø12	Cystic meniscus, anterior horn of medial meniscus, left knee
		M23.Ø19	Cystic meniscus, anterior horn of medial meniscus, unsp knee
		M23.211	Derang of ant horn of medial mensc d/t old tear/inj, r knee
		M23.212	Derang of ant horn of medial mensc d/t old tear/inj, l knee
		M23.219	Derang of ant horn of med mensc d/t old tear/inj, unsp knee
		M23.311	Oth meniscus derang, ant horn of medial meniscus, r knee
		M23.312	Oth meniscus derang, ant horn of medial meniscus, l knee
		M23.319	Oth meniscus derang, ant horn of medial meniscus, unsp knee
717.2	DERANGEMENT OF POSTERIOR HORN OF MEDIAL MENISCUS	**M23.Ø21**	Cystic meniscus, posterior horn of medial meniscus, r knee
		M23.Ø22	Cystic meniscus, posterior horn of medial meniscus, l knee
		M23.Ø29	Cystic meniscus, post horn of medial meniscus, unsp knee
		M23.221	Derang of post horn of medial mensc d/t old tear/inj, r knee
		M23.222	Derang of post horn of medial mensc d/t old tear/inj, l knee
		M23.229	Derang of post horn of med mensc d/t old tear/inj, unsp knee
		M23.321	Oth meniscus derang, post horn of medial meniscus, r knee
		M23.322	Oth meniscus derang, post horn of medial meniscus, l knee
		M23.329	Oth meniscus derang, post horn of medial meniscus, unsp knee
717.3	OTHER&UNSPECIFIED DERANGEMENT OF MEDIAL MENISCUS	**M23.Ø3**[1,2,9]	Cystic meniscus, other medial meniscus, knee
		M23.2Ø3	Derang of unsp medial meniscus due to old tear/inj, r knee
		M23.2Ø4	Derang of unsp medial meniscus due to old tear/inj, l knee
		M23.2Ø5	Derang of unsp medial mensc due to old tear/inj, unsp knee
		M23.23[1,2,9]	Derang of medial meniscus due to old tear/inj, knee
		M23.3Ø3	Oth meniscus derangements, unsp medial meniscus, right knee
		M23.3Ø4	Other meniscus derangements, unsp medial meniscus, left knee
		M23.3Ø5	Other meniscus derangements, unsp medial meniscus, unsp knee
		M23.33[1,2,9]	Oth meniscus derangements, other medial meniscus, knee
			6th Character meanings for codes as indicated ***1 Right*** ***2 Left*** ***9 Unspecified***
717.4Ø	UNSPECIFIED DERANGEMENT OF LATERAL MENISCUS	**M23.2ØØ**	Derang of unsp lat mensc due to old tear/inj, right knee
		M23.2Ø1	Derangement of unsp lat mensc due to old tear/inj, left knee
		M23.2Ø2	Derangement of unsp lat mensc due to old tear/inj, unsp knee
		M23.261	Derangement of lat mensc due to old tear/inj, right knee
		M23.262	Derangement of lat mensc due to old tear/inj, left knee
		M23.269	Derangement of lat mensc due to old tear/inj, unsp knee
		M23.3ØØ	Oth meniscus derangements, unsp lateral meniscus, right knee
		M23.3Ø1	Oth meniscus derangements, unsp lateral meniscus, left knee
		M23.3Ø2	Oth meniscus derangements, unsp lateral meniscus, unsp knee
717.41	BUCKET HANDLE TEAR OF LATERAL MENISCUS	**M23.2Ø2**	Derangement of unsp lat mensc due to old tear/inj, unsp knee
717.42	DERANGEMENT OF ANTERIOR HORN OF LATERAL MENISCUS	**M23.Ø41**	Cystic meniscus, anterior horn of lat mensc, right knee
		M23.Ø42	Cystic meniscus, anterior horn of lat mensc, left knee
		M23.Ø49	Cystic meniscus, anterior horn of lat mensc, unsp knee
		M23.241	Derang of ant horn of lat mensc due to old tear/inj, r knee
		M23.242	Derang of ant horn of lat mensc due to old tear/inj, l knee
		M23.249	Derang of ant horn of lat mensc d/t old tear/inj, unsp knee
		M23.341	Oth meniscus derang, anterior horn of lat mensc, right knee
		M23.342	Oth meniscus derang, anterior horn of lat mensc, left knee
		M23.349	Oth meniscus derang, anterior horn of lat mensc, unsp knee
717.43	DERANGEMENT POSTERIOR HORN LATERAL MENISCUS	**M23.Ø51**	Cystic meniscus, posterior horn of lat mensc, right knee
		M23.Ø52	Cystic meniscus, posterior horn of lat mensc, left knee
		M23.Ø59	Cystic meniscus, posterior horn of lat mensc, unsp knee
		M23.251	Derang of post horn of lat mensc due to old tear/inj, r knee
		M23.252	Derang of post horn of lat mensc due to old tear/inj, l knee
		M23.259	Derang of post horn of lat mensc d/t old tear/inj, unsp knee
		M23.351	Oth meniscus derang, posterior horn of lat mensc, right knee
		M23.352	Oth meniscus derang, posterior horn of lat mensc, left knee
		M23.359	Oth meniscus derang, posterior horn of lat mensc, unsp knee
717.49	OTHER DERANGEMENT OF LATERAL MENISCUS	**M23.Ø61**	Cystic meniscus, other lateral meniscus, right knee
		M23.Ø62	Cystic meniscus, other lateral meniscus, left knee
		M23.Ø69	Cystic meniscus, other lateral meniscus, unspecified knee
		M23.3ØØ	Oth meniscus derangements, unsp lateral meniscus, right knee
		M23.3Ø1	Oth meniscus derangements, unsp lateral meniscus, left knee
		M23.3Ø2	Oth meniscus derangements, unsp lateral meniscus, unsp knee
		M23.361	Oth meniscus derangements, oth lateral meniscus, right knee
		M23.362	Oth meniscus derangements, other lateral meniscus, left knee
		M23.369	Oth meniscus derangements, other lateral meniscus, unsp knee

[Brackets] indicate valid character values for each code. Character value meanings provided for each code grouping.

ICD-9-CM		ICD-10-CM	
717.5	DERANGEMENT OF MENISCUS NOT ELSEWHERE CLASSIFIED	**M23.000**	Cystic meniscus, unspecified lateral meniscus, right knee
		M23.001	Cystic meniscus, unspecified lateral meniscus, left knee
		M23.002	Cystic meniscus, unsp lateral meniscus, unspecified knee
		M23.003	Cystic meniscus, unspecified medial meniscus, right knee
		M23.004	Cystic meniscus, unspecified medial meniscus, left knee
		M23.005	Cystic meniscus, unsp medial meniscus, unspecified knee
		M23.006	Cystic meniscus, unspecified meniscus, right knee
		M23.007	Cystic meniscus, unspecified meniscus, left knee
		M23.009	Cystic meniscus, unspecified meniscus, unspecified knee
		M23.206	Derangement of unsp meniscus due to old tear/inj, right knee
		M23.207	Derangement of unsp meniscus due to old tear/inj, left knee
		M23.209	Derangement of unsp meniscus due to old tear/inj, unsp knee
		M23.306	Other meniscus derangements, unsp meniscus, right knee
		M23.307	Other meniscus derangements, unspecified meniscus, left knee
		M23.309	Other meniscus derangements, unsp meniscus, unspecified knee
		Q68.6	Discoid meniscus
717.6	LOOSE BODY IN KNEE	**M23.40**	Loose body in knee, unspecified knee
		M23.41	Loose body in knee, right knee
		M23.42	Loose body in knee, left knee
717.7	CHONDROMALACIA OF PATELLA	**M22.40**	Chondromalacia patellae, unspecified knee
		M22.41	Chondromalacia patellae, right knee
		M22.42	Chondromalacia patellae, left knee
717.81	OLD DISRUPTION OF LATERAL COLLATERAL LIGAMENT	**M23.50**	Chronic instability of knee, unspecified knee
717.82	OLD DISRUPTION OF MEDIAL COLLATERAL LIGAMENT	**M23.50**	Chronic instability of knee, unspecified knee
717.83	OLD DISRUPTION OF ANTERIOR CRUCIATE LIGAMENT	**M23.50**	Chronic instability of knee, unspecified knee
717.84	OLD DISRUPTION OF POSTERIOR CRUCIATE LIGAMENT	**M23.50**	Chronic instability of knee, unspecified knee
717.85	OLD DISRUPTION OF OTHER LIGAMENT OF KNEE	**M23.50**	Chronic instability of knee, unspecified knee
		M23.51	Chronic instability of knee, right knee
		M23.52	Chronic instability of knee, left knee
717.89	OTHER INTERNAL DERANGEMENT OF KNEE OTHER	**M22.2X**[1,2,9]	Patellofemoral disorders, knee
		M22.3X[1,2,9]	Other derangements of patella, knee
		M22.8X[1,2,9]	Other disorders of patella, knee
		M23.60[1,2,9]	Other spontaneous disruption of unsp ligament, knee
		M23.61[1,2,9]	Oth spon disrupt of anterior cruciate ligament, knee
		M23.62[1,2,9]	Oth spon disrupt of posterior cruciate ligament, knee
		M23.63[1,2,9]	Oth spon disruption of medial collat ligament, knee
		M23.64[1,2,9]	Oth spon disruption of lateral collat ligament, knee
		M23.67[1,2,9]	Oth spon disruption of capsular ligament, knee
		M23.8X[1,2,9]	Other internal derangements, knee
			6th Character meanings for codes as indicated ***1 Right*** ***2 Left*** ***9 Unspecified***
717.9	UNSPECIFIED INTERNAL DERANGEMENT OF KNEE	**M22.90**	Unspecified disorder of patella, unspecified knee
		M22.91	Unspecified disorder of patella, right knee
		M22.92	Unspecified disorder of patella, left knee
		M23.90	Unspecified internal derangement of unspecified knee
		M23.91	Unspecified internal derangement of right knee
		M23.92	Unspecified internal derangement of left knee
718.00	ARTICULAR CARTILAGE DISORDER SITE UNSPECIFIED	**M24.10**	Other articular cartilage disorders, unspecified site
718.01	ARTICULAR CARTILAGE DISORDER SHOULDER REGION	**M24.111**	Other articular cartilage disorders, right shoulder
		M24.112	Other articular cartilage disorders, left shoulder
		M24.119	Other articular cartilage disorders, unspecified shoulder
718.02	ARTICULAR CARTILAGE DISORDER UPPER ARM	**M24.121**	Other articular cartilage disorders, right elbow
		M24.122	Other articular cartilage disorders, left elbow
		M24.129	Other articular cartilage disorders, unspecified elbow
718.03	ARTICULAR CARTILAGE DISORDER FOREARM	**M24.131**	Other articular cartilage disorders, right wrist
		M24.132	Other articular cartilage disorders, left wrist
		M24.139	Other articular cartilage disorders, unspecified wrist
718.04	ARTICULAR CARTILAGE DISORDER, HAND	**M24.141**	Other articular cartilage disorders, right hand
		M24.142	Other articular cartilage disorders, left hand
		M24.149	Other articular cartilage disorders, unspecified hand
718.05	ARTICULAR CARTILAGE DISORDER PELVIC REGION&THIGH	**M24.151**	Other articular cartilage disorders, right hip
		M24.152	Other articular cartilage disorders, left hip
		M24.159	Other articular cartilage disorders, unspecified hip
718.07	ARTICULAR CARTILAGE DISORDER ANKLE AND FOOT	**M24.171**	Other articular cartilage disorders, right ankle
		M24.172	Other articular cartilage disorders, left ankle
		M24.173	Other articular cartilage disorders, unspecified ankle
		M24.174	Other articular cartilage disorders, right foot
		M24.175	Other articular cartilage disorders, left foot
		M24.176	Other articular cartilage disorders, unspecified foot
718.08	ARTICULAR CARTILAGE DISORDER OTHER SPEC SITE	**M24.10**	Other articular cartilage disorders, unspecified site
718.09	ARTICULAR CARTILAGE DISORDER MULTIPLE SITES	**M24.10**	Other articular cartilage disorders, unspecified site
718.10	LOOSE BODY IN JOINT SITE UNSPECIFIED	**M24.00**	Loose body in unspecified joint
718.11	LOOSE BODY IN SHOULDER JOINT	**M24.011**	Loose body in right shoulder
		M24.012	Loose body in left shoulder
		M24.019	Loose body in unspecified shoulder

ICD-9-CM		ICD-10-CM	
718.12	LOOSE BODY IN UPPER ARM JOINT	**M24.021**	Loose body in right elbow
		M24.022	Loose body in left elbow
		M24.029	Loose body in unspecified elbow
718.13	LOOSE BODY IN FOREARM JOINT	**M24.031**	Loose body in right wrist
		M24.032	Loose body in left wrist
		M24.039	Loose body in unspecified wrist
718.14	LOOSE BODY IN HAND JOINT	**M24.041**	Loose body in right finger joint(s)
		M24.042	Loose body in left finger joint(s)
		M24.049	Loose body in unspecified finger joint(s)
718.15	LOOSE BODY IN PELVIC JOINT	**M24.051**	Loose body in right hip
		M24.052	Loose body in left hip
		M24.059	Loose body in unspecified hip
718.17	LOOSE BODY IN ANKLE AND FOOT JOINT	**M24.071**	Loose body in right ankle
		M24.072	Loose body in left ankle
		M24.073	Loose body in unspecified ankle
		M24.074	Loose body in right toe joint(s)
		M24.075	Loose body in left toe joint(s)
		M24.076	Loose body in unspecified toe joints
718.18	LOOSE BODY IN JOINT OF OTHER SPECIFIED SITE	➡ **M24.08**	Loose body, other site
718.19	LOOSE BODY IN JOINT OF MULTIPLE SITES	**M24.00**	Loose body in unspecified joint
718.20	PATHOLOGICAL DISLOCATION JOINT SITE UNSPECIFIED	**M24.30**	Pathological dislocation of unsp joint, NEC
718.21	PATHOLOGICAL DISLOCATION OF SHOULDER JOINT	**M24.311**	Pathological dislocation of right shoulder, NEC
		M24.312	Pathological dislocation of left shoulder, NEC
		M24.319	Pathological dislocation of unsp shoulder, NEC
718.22	PATHOLOGICAL DISLOCATION OF UPPER ARM JOINT	**M24.321**	Pathological dislocation of right elbow, NEC
		M24.322	Pathological dislocation of left elbow, NEC
		M24.329	Pathological dislocation of unsp elbow, NEC
718.23	PATHOLOGICAL DISLOCATION OF FOREARM JOINT	**M24.331**	Pathological dislocation of right wrist, NEC
		M24.332	Pathological dislocation of left wrist, NEC
		M24.339	Pathological dislocation of unsp wrist, NEC
718.24	PATHOLOGICAL DISLOCATION OF HAND JOINT	**M24.341**	Pathological dislocation of right hand, NEC
		M24.342	Pathological dislocation of left hand, NEC
		M24.349	Pathological dislocation of unsp hand, NEC
718.25	PATHOLOGICAL DISLOC PELVIC REGION&THIGH JOINT	**M24.351**	Pathological dislocation of right hip, NEC
		M24.352	Pathological dislocation of left hip, NEC
		M24.359	Pathological dislocation of unsp hip, NEC
718.26	PATHOLOGICAL DISLOCATION OF LOWER LEG JOINT	**M24.361**	Pathological dislocation of right knee, NEC
		M24.362	Pathological dislocation of left knee, NEC
		M24.369	Pathological dislocation of unsp knee, NEC
718.27	PATHOLOGICAL DISLOCATION OF ANKLE AND FOOT JOINT	**M24.371**	Pathological dislocation of right ankle, NEC
		M24.372	Pathological dislocation of left ankle, NEC
		M24.373	Pathological dislocation of unsp ankle, NEC
		M24.374	Pathological dislocation of right foot, NEC
		M24.375	Pathological dislocation of left foot, NEC
		M24.376	Pathological dislocation of unsp foot, NEC
718.28	PATHOLOGICAL DISLOCATION JOINT OTHER SPEC SITE	**M24.30**	Pathological dislocation of unsp joint, NEC
718.29	PATHOLOGICAL DISLOCATION JOINT MULTIPLE SITES	**M24.30**	Pathological dislocation of unsp joint, NEC
718.30	RECURRENT DISLOCATION OF JOINT SITE UNSPECIFIED	➡ **M24.40**	Recurrent dislocation, unspecified joint
718.31	RECURRENT DISLOCATION OF SHOULDER JOINT	**M24.411**	Recurrent dislocation, right shoulder
		M24.412	Recurrent dislocation, left shoulder
		M24.419	Recurrent dislocation, unspecified shoulder
718.32	RECURRENT DISLOCATION OF UPPER ARM JOINT	**M24.421**	Recurrent dislocation, right elbow
		M24.422	Recurrent dislocation, left elbow
		M24.429	Recurrent dislocation, unspecified elbow
718.33	RECURRENT DISLOCATION OF FOREARM JOINT	**M24.431**	Recurrent dislocation, right wrist
		M24.432	Recurrent dislocation, left wrist
		M24.439	Recurrent dislocation, unspecified wrist
718.34	RECURRENT DISLOCATION OF HAND JOINT	**M24.441**	Recurrent dislocation, right hand
		M24.442	Recurrent dislocation, left hand
		M24.443	Recurrent dislocation, unspecified hand
		M24.444	Recurrent dislocation, right finger
		M24.445	Recurrent dislocation, left finger
		M24.446	Recurrent dislocation, unspecified finger
718.35	RECURRENT DISLOCATION PELVIC REGION&THIGH JOINT	**M24.451**	Recurrent dislocation, right hip
		M24.452	Recurrent dislocation, left hip
		M24.459	Recurrent dislocation, unspecified hip
718.36	RECURRENT DISLOCATION OF LOWER LEG JOINT	**M22.00**	Recurrent dislocation of patella, unspecified knee
		M22.01	Recurrent dislocation of patella, right knee
		M22.02	Recurrent dislocation of patella, left knee
		M22.10	Recurrent subluxation of patella, unspecified knee
		M22.11	Recurrent subluxation of patella, right knee
		M22.12	Recurrent subluxation of patella, left knee
		M24.461	Recurrent dislocation, right knee
		M24.462	Recurrent dislocation, left knee
		M24.469	Recurrent dislocation, unspecified knee

ICD-9-CM		ICD-10-CM	
718.37	RECURRENT DISLOCATION OF ANKLE AND FOOT JOINT	**M24.471**	Recurrent dislocation, right ankle
		M24.472	Recurrent dislocation, left ankle
		M24.473	Recurrent dislocation, unspecified ankle
		M24.474	Recurrent dislocation, right foot
		M24.475	Recurrent dislocation, left foot
		M24.476	Recurrent dislocation, unspecified foot
		M24.477	Recurrent dislocation, right toe(s)
		M24.478	Recurrent dislocation, left toe(s)
		M24.479	Recurrent dislocation, unspecified toe(s)
718.38	RECURRENT DISLOCATION JOINT OTHER SPECIFIED SITE	**M43.3**	Recurrent atlantoaxial dislocation with myelopathy
		M43.4	Other recurrent atlantoaxial dislocation
		M43.5X2	Other recurrent vertebral dislocation, cervical region
		M43.5X3	Oth recurrent vertebral dislocation, cervicothoracic region
		M43.5X4	Other recurrent vertebral dislocation, thoracic region
		M43.5X5	Other recurrent vertebral dislocation, thoracolumbar region
		M43.5X6	Other recurrent vertebral dislocation, lumbar region
		M43.5X7	Other recurrent vertebral dislocation, lumbosacral region
		M43.5X8	Oth recurrent vertebral dislocation, sacr/sacrocygl region
		M43.5X9	Other recurrent vertebral dislocation, site unspecified
718.39	RECURRENT DISLOCATION OF JOINT OF MULTIPLE SITES	**M43.5X9**	Other recurrent vertebral dislocation, site unspecified
718.4Ø	CONTRACTURE OF JOINT SITE UNSPECIFIED	**M24.5Ø**	Contracture, unspecified joint
718.41	CONTRACTURE OF SHOULDER JOINT	**M24.511**	Contracture, right shoulder
		M24.512	Contracture, left shoulder
		M24.519	Contracture, unspecified shoulder
718.42	CONTRACTURE OF UPPER ARM JOINT	**M24.521**	Contracture, right elbow
		M24.522	Contracture, left elbow
		M24.529	Contracture, unspecified elbow
718.43	CONTRACTURE OF FOREARM JOINT	**M24.531**	Contracture, right wrist
		M24.532	Contracture, left wrist
		M24.539	Contracture, unspecified wrist
718.44	CONTRACTURE OF HAND JOINT	**M24.541**	Contracture, right hand
		M24.542	Contracture, left hand
		M24.549	Contracture, unspecified hand
718.45	CONTRACTURE OF PELVIC JOINT	**M24.551**	Contracture, right hip
		M24.552	Contracture, left hip
		M24.559	Contracture, unspecified hip
718.46	CONTRACTURE OF LOWER LEG JOINT	**M24.561**	Contracture, right knee
		M24.562	Contracture, left knee
		M24.569	Contracture, unspecified knee
718.47	CONTRACTURE OF ANKLE AND FOOT JOINT	**M24.571**	Contracture, right ankle
		M24.572	Contracture, left ankle
		M24.573	Contracture, unspecified ankle
		M24.574	Contracture, right foot
		M24.575	Contracture, left foot
		M24.576	Contracture, unspecified foot
718.48	CONTRACTURE OF JOINT OF OTHER SPECIFIED SITE	**M24.5Ø**	Contracture, unspecified joint
718.49	CONTRACTURE OF JOINT OF MULTIPLE SITES	**M24.5Ø**	Contracture, unspecified joint
718.5Ø	ANKYLOSIS OF JOINT SITE UNSPECIFIED	**M24.6Ø**	Ankylosis, unspecified joint
718.51	ANKYLOSIS OF JOINT OF SHOULDER REGION	**M24.611**	Ankylosis, right shoulder
		M24.612	Ankylosis, left shoulder
		M24.619	Ankylosis, unspecified shoulder
718.52	ANKYLOSIS OF UPPER ARM JOINT	**M24.621**	Ankylosis, right elbow
		M24.622	Ankylosis, left elbow
		M24.629	Ankylosis, unspecified elbow
718.53	ANKYLOSIS OF FOREARM JOINT	**M24.631**	Ankylosis, right wrist
		M24.632	Ankylosis, left wrist
		M24.639	Ankylosis, unspecified wrist
718.54	ANKYLOSIS OF HAND JOINT	**M24.641**	Ankylosis, right hand
		M24.642	Ankylosis, left hand
		M24.649	Ankylosis, unspecified hand
718.55	ANKYLOSIS OF PELVIC REGION AND THIGH JOINT	**M24.651**	Ankylosis, right hip
		M24.652	Ankylosis, left hip
		M24.659	Ankylosis, unspecified hip
718.56	ANKYLOSIS OF LOWER LEG JOINT	**M24.661**	Ankylosis, right knee
		M24.662	Ankylosis, left knee
		M24.669	Ankylosis, unspecified knee
718.57	ANKYLOSIS OF ANKLE AND FOOT JOINT	**M24.671**	Ankylosis, right ankle
		M24.672	Ankylosis, left ankle
		M24.673	Ankylosis, unspecified ankle
		M24.674	Ankylosis, right foot
		M24.675	Ankylosis, left foot
		M24.676	Ankylosis, unspecified foot
718.58	ANKYLOSIS OF JOINT OF OTHER SPECIFIED SITE	**M24.6Ø**	Ankylosis, unspecified joint
718.59	ANKYLOSIS OF JOINT OF MULTIPLE SITES	**M24.6Ø**	Ankylosis, unspecified joint
718.65	UNSPEC INTRAPELV PROTRUSION ACETAB PELV RGN&THI	**M24.7**	Protrusio acetabuli
718.7Ø	DEVELOPMENTAL DISLOCATION JOINT SITE UNSPECIFIED	**M24.8Ø**	Oth specific joint derangements of unsp joint, NEC

ICD-9-CM		ICD-10-CM	
718.71	DEVELOPMENTAL DISLOCATION JOINT SHOULDER REGION	**M24.811**	Oth specific joint derangements of right shoulder, NEC
		M24.812	Oth specific joint derangements of left shoulder, NEC
		M24.819	Oth specific joint derangements of unsp shoulder, NEC
718.72	DEVELOPMENTAL DISLOCATION OF JOINT, UPPER ARM	**M24.821**	Oth specific joint derangements of right elbow, NEC
		M24.822	Oth specific joint derangements of left elbow, NEC
		M24.829	Oth specific joint derangements of unsp elbow, NEC
718.73	DEVELOPMENTAL DISLOCATION OF JOINT, FOREARM	**M24.831**	Oth specific joint derangements of right wrist, NEC
		M24.832	Oth specific joint derangements of left wrist, NEC
		M24.839	Oth specific joint derangements of unsp wrist, NEC
718.74	DEVELOPMENTAL DISLOCATION OF JOINT, HAND	**M24.841**	Oth specific joint derangements of right hand, NEC
		M24.842	Oth specific joint derangements of left hand, NEC
		M24.849	Oth specific joint derangements of unsp hand, NEC
718.75	DVLPMNTL DISLOCATION JOINT PELV REGION&THIGH	**M24.851**	Oth specific joint derangements of right hip, NEC
		M24.852	Oth specific joint derangements of left hip, NEC
		M24.859	Oth specific joint derangements of unsp hip, NEC
718.76	DEVELOPMENTAL DISLOCATION OF JOINT, LOWER LEG	**M24.80**	Oth specific joint derangements of unsp joint, NEC
718.77	DEVELOPMENTAL DISLOCATION OF JOINT ANKLE&FOOT	**M24.871**	Oth specific joint derangements of right ankle, NEC
		M24.872	Oth specific joint derangements of left ankle, NEC
		M24.873	Oth specific joint derangements of unsp ankle, NEC
		M24.874	Oth specific joint derangements of right foot, NEC
		M24.875	Oth specific joint derangements left foot, NEC
		M24.876	Oth specific joint derangements of unsp foot, NEC
718.78	DEVELOPMENTAL DISLOCATION JOINT OTHER SPEC SITES	**M24.80**	Oth specific joint derangements of unsp joint, NEC
718.79	DEVELOPMENTAL DISLOCATION JOINT MULTIPLE SITES	**M24.80**	Oth specific joint derangements of unsp joint, NEC
718.80	OTHER JOINT DERANGEMENT NEC UNSPECIFIED SITE	**M24.80**	Oth specific joint derangements of unsp joint, NEC
		M25.20	Flail joint, unspecified joint
		M25.30	Other instability, unspecified joint
		M53.2X9	Spinal instabilities, site unspecified
718.81	OTHER JOINT DERANGEMENT NEC SHOULDER REGION	**M24.811**	Oth specific joint derangements of right shoulder, NEC
		M24.812	Oth specific joint derangements of left shoulder, NEC
		M24.819	Oth specific joint derangements of unsp shoulder, NEC
		M25.211	Flail joint, right shoulder
		M25.212	Flail joint, left shoulder
		M25.219	Flail joint, unspecified shoulder
		M25.311	Other instability, right shoulder
		M25.312	Other instability, left shoulder
		M25.319	Other instability, unspecified shoulder
718.82	OTHER JOINT DERANGEMENT NEC UPPER ARM	**M24.821**	Oth specific joint derangements of right elbow, NEC
		M24.822	Oth specific joint derangements of left elbow, NEC
		M24.829	Oth specific joint derangements of unsp elbow, NEC
		M25.221	Flail joint, right elbow
		M25.222	Flail joint, left elbow
		M25.229	Flail joint, unspecified elbow
		M25.321	Other instability, right elbow
		M25.322	Other instability, left elbow
		M25.329	Other instability, unspecified elbow
718.83	OTHER JOINT DERANGEMENT NEC FOREARM	**M24.831**	Oth specific joint derangements of right wrist, NEC
		M24.832	Oth specific joint derangements of left wrist, NEC
		M24.839	Oth specific joint derangements of unsp wrist, NEC
		M25.231	Flail joint, right wrist
		M25.232	Flail joint, left wrist
		M25.239	Flail joint, unspecified wrist
		M25.331	Other instability, right wrist
		M25.332	Other instability, left wrist
		M25.339	Other instability, unspecified wrist
718.84	OTHER JOINT DERANGEMENT NEC HAND	**M24.841**	Oth specific joint derangements of right hand, NEC
		M24.842	Oth specific joint derangements of left hand, NEC
		M24.849	Oth specific joint derangements of unsp hand, NEC
		M25.241	Flail joint, right hand
		M25.242	Flail joint, left hand
		M25.249	Flail joint, unspecified hand
		M25.341	Other instability, right hand
		M25.342	Other instability, left hand
		M25.349	Other instability, unspecified hand
718.85	OTHER JOINT DERANGEMENT NEC PELVIC REGION&THIGH	**M24.851**	Oth specific joint derangements of right hip, NEC
		M24.852	Oth specific joint derangements of left hip, NEC
		M24.859	Oth specific joint derangements of unsp hip, NEC
		M25.251	Flail joint, right hip
		M25.252	Flail joint, left hip
		M25.259	Flail joint, unspecified hip
		M25.351	Other instability, right hip
		M25.352	Other instability, left hip
		M25.359	Other instability, unspecified hip

ICD-9-CM		ICD-10-CM	
718.86	OTHER JOINT DERANGEMENT NEC LOWER LEG	M23.5Ø	Chronic instability of knee, unspecified knee
		M23.51	Chronic instability of knee, right knee
		M23.52	Chronic instability of knee, left knee
		M23.8X9	Other internal derangements of unspecified knee
		M25.261	Flail joint, right knee
		M25.262	Flail joint, left knee
		M25.269	Flail joint, unspecified knee
		M25.361	Other instability, right knee
		M25.362	Other instability, left knee
		M25.369	Other instability, unspecified knee
718.87	OTHER JOINT DERANGEMENT NEC ANKLE AND FOOT	M24.871	Oth specific joint derangements of right ankle, NEC
		M24.872	Oth specific joint derangements of left ankle, NEC
		M24.873	Oth specific joint derangements of unsp ankle, NEC
		M24.874	Oth specific joint derangements of right foot, NEC
		M24.875	Oth specific joint derangements left foot, NEC
		M24.876	Oth specific joint derangements of unsp foot, NEC
		M25.271	Flail joint, right ankle and foot
		M25.272	Flail joint, left ankle and foot
		M25.279	Flail joint, unspecified ankle and foot
		M25.371	Other instability, right ankle
		M25.372	Other instability, left ankle
		M25.373	Other instability, unspecified ankle
		M25.374	Other instability, right foot
		M25.375	Other instability, left foot
		M25.376	Other instability, unspecified foot
718.88	OTHER JOINT DERANGEMENT NEC OTHER SPECIFIED SITE	M24.8Ø	Oth specific joint derangements of unsp joint, NEC
		M25.28	Flail joint, other site
		M53.2X1	Spinal instabilities, occipito-atlanto-axial region
		M53.2X2	Spinal instabilities, cervical region
		M53.2X3	Spinal instabilities, cervicothoracic region
		M53.2X4	Spinal instabilities, thoracic region
		M53.2X5	Spinal instabilities, thoracolumbar region
		M53.2X6	Spinal instabilities, lumbar region
718.89	OTHER JOINT DERANGEMENT NEC MULTIPLE SITES	M24.8Ø	Oth specific joint derangements of unsp joint, NEC
718.9Ø	UNSPECIFIED DERANGEMENT JOINT SITE UNSPECIFIED	M24.9	Joint derangement, unspecified
718.91	UNSPECIFIED DERANGEMENT SHOULDER REGION	M24.9	Joint derangement, unspecified
718.92	UNSPECIFIED DERANGEMENT UPPER ARM JOINT	M24.9	Joint derangement, unspecified
718.93	UNSPECIFIED DERANGEMENT FOREARM JOINT	M24.9	Joint derangement, unspecified
718.94	UNSPECIFIED DERANGEMENT OF HAND JOINT	M24.9	Joint derangement, unspecified
718.95	UNSPECIFIED PELVIC JOINT DERANGEMENT	M24.9	Joint derangement, unspecified
718.97	UNSPECIFIED ANKLE AND FOOT JOINT DERANGEMENT	M24.9	Joint derangement, unspecified
718.98	UNSPEC DERANGEMENT JOINT OTHER SPEC SITES	M24.9	Joint derangement, unspecified
718.99	UNSPECIFIED DERANGEMENT OF JOINT MULTIPLE SITES	M24.9	Joint derangement, unspecified
719.ØØ	EFFUSION OF JOINT, SITE UNSPECIFIED	M25.4Ø	Effusion, unspecified joint
719.Ø1	EFFUSION OF SHOULDER JOINT	M25.411	Effusion, right shoulder
		M25.412	Effusion, left shoulder
		M25.419	Effusion, unspecified shoulder
719.Ø2	EFFUSION OF UPPER ARM JOINT	M25.421	Effusion, right elbow
		M25.422	Effusion, left elbow
		M25.429	Effusion, unspecified elbow
719.Ø3	EFFUSION OF FOREARM JOINT	M25.431	Effusion, right wrist
		M25.432	Effusion, left wrist
		M25.439	Effusion, unspecified wrist
719.Ø4	EFFUSION OF HAND JOINT	M25.441	Effusion, right hand
		M25.442	Effusion, left hand
		M25.449	Effusion, unspecified hand
719.Ø5	EFFUSION OF PELVIC JOINT	M25.451	Effusion, right hip
		M25.452	Effusion, left hip
		M25.459	Effusion, unspecified hip
719.Ø6	EFFUSION OF LOWER LEG JOINT	M25.461	Effusion, right knee
		M25.462	Effusion, left knee
		M25.469	Effusion, unspecified knee
719.Ø7	EFFUSION OF ANKLE AND FOOT JOINT	M25.471	Effusion, right ankle
		M25.472	Effusion, left ankle
		M25.473	Effusion, unspecified ankle
		M25.474	Effusion, right foot
		M25.475	Effusion, left foot
		M25.476	Effusion, unspecified foot
719.Ø8	EFFUSION OF JOINT OTHER SPECIFIED SITE	➡ M25.48	Effusion, other site
719.Ø9	EFFUSION OF JOINT, MULTIPLE SITES	M25.4Ø	Effusion, unspecified joint
719.1Ø	HEMARTHROSIS, SITE UNSPECIFIED	M25.ØØ	Hemarthrosis, unspecified joint
719.11	HERARTHROSIS, SHOULDER REGION	M25.Ø11	Hemarthrosis, right shoulder
		M25.Ø12	Hemarthrosis, left shoulder
		M25.Ø19	Hemarthrosis, unspecified shoulder
719.12	HEMARTHORSIS, UPPER ARM	M25.Ø21	Hemarthrosis, right elbow
		M25.Ø22	Hemarthrosis, left elbow
		M25.Ø29	Hemarthrosis, unspecified elbow

ICD-9-CM		ICD-10-CM	
719.13	HEMARTHROSIS, FOREARM	**M25.Ø31**	Hemarthrosis, right wrist
		M25.Ø32	Hemarthrosis, left wrist
		M25.Ø39	Hemarthrosis, unspecified wrist
719.14	HEMARTHROSIS, HAND	**M25.Ø41**	Hemarthrosis, right hand
		M25.Ø42	Hemarthrosis, left hand
		M25.Ø49	Hemarthrosis, unspecified hand
719.15	HEMARTHROSIS PELVIC REGION AND THIGH	**M25.Ø51**	Hemarthrosis, right hip
		M25.Ø52	Hemarthrosis, left hip
		M25.Ø59	Hemarthrosis, unspecified hip
719.16	HEMARTHROSIS, LOWER LEG	**M25.Ø61**	Hemarthrosis, right knee
		M25.Ø62	Hemarthrosis, left knee
		M25.Ø69	Hemarthrosis, unspecified knee
719.17	HEMARTHROSIS, ANKLE AND FOOT	**M25.Ø71**	Hemarthrosis, right ankle
		M25.Ø72	Hemarthrosis, left ankle
		M25.Ø73	Hemarthrosis, unspecified ankle
		M25.Ø74	Hemarthrosis, right foot
		M25.Ø75	Hemarthrosis, left foot
		M25.Ø76	Hemarthrosis, unspecified foot
719.18	HEMARTHROSIS, OTHER SPECIFIED SITE	➡ **M25.Ø8**	Hemarthrosis, oth spec site
719.19	HEMARTHROSIS, MULTIPLE SITES	**M25.ØØ**	Hemarthrosis, unspecified joint
719.2Ø	VILLONODULAR SYNOVITIS SITE UNSPECIFIED	➡ **M12.2Ø**	Villonodular synovitis (pigmented), unspecified site
719.21	VILLONODULAR SYNOVITIS SHOULDER REGION	**M12.211**	Villonodular synovitis (pigmented), right shoulder
		M12.212	Villonodular synovitis (pigmented), left shoulder
		M12.219	Villonodular synovitis (pigmented), unspecified shoulder
719.22	VILLONODULAR SYNOVITIS, UPPER ARM	**M12.221**	Villonodular synovitis (pigmented), right elbow
		M12.222	Villonodular synovitis (pigmented), left elbow
		M12.229	Villonodular synovitis (pigmented), unspecified elbow
719.23	VILLONODULAR SYNOVITIS, FOREARM	**M12.231**	Villonodular synovitis (pigmented), right wrist
		M12.232	Villonodular synovitis (pigmented), left wrist
		M12.239	Villonodular synovitis (pigmented), unspecified wrist
719.24	VILLONODULAR SYNOVITIS, HAND	**M12.241**	Villonodular synovitis (pigmented), right hand
		M12.242	Villonodular synovitis (pigmented), left hand
		M12.249	Villonodular synovitis (pigmented), unspecified hand
719.25	VILLONODULAR SYNOVITIS PELVIC REGION AND THIGH	**M12.251**	Villonodular synovitis (pigmented), right hip
		M12.252	Villonodular synovitis (pigmented), left hip
		M12.259	Villonodular synovitis (pigmented), unspecified hip
719.26	VILLONODULAR SYNOVITIS, LOWER LEG	**M12.261**	Villonodular synovitis (pigmented), right knee
		M12.262	Villonodular synovitis (pigmented), left knee
		M12.269	Villonodular synovitis (pigmented), unspecified knee
719.27	VILLONODULAR SYNOVITIS ANKLE AND FOOT	**M12.271**	Villonodular synovitis (pigmented), right ankle and foot
		M12.272	Villonodular synovitis (pigmented), left ankle and foot
		M12.279	Villonodular synovitis (pigmented), unsp ankle and foot
719.28	VILLONODULAR SYNOVITIS OTHER SPECIFIED SITES	➡ **M12.28**	Villonodular synovitis (pigmented), oth spec site
719.29	VILLONODULAR SYNOVITIS MULTIPLE SITES	➡ **M12.29**	Villonodular synovitis (pigmented), multiple sites
719.3Ø	PALINDROMIC RHEUMATISM SITE UNSPECIFIED	**M12.3Ø**	Palindromic rheumatism, unspecified site
		M12.4Ø	Intermittent hydrarthrosis, unspecified site
719.31	PALINDROMIC RHEUMATISM SHOULDER REGION	**M12.311**	Palindromic rheumatism, right shoulder
		M12.312	Palindromic rheumatism, left shoulder
		M12.319	Palindromic rheumatism, unspecified shoulder
		M12.411	Intermittent hydrarthrosis, right shoulder
		M12.412	Intermittent hydrarthrosis, left shoulder
		M12.419	Intermittent hydrarthrosis, unspecified shoulder
719.32	PALINDROMIC RHEUMATISM, UPPER ARM	**M12.321**	Palindromic rheumatism, right elbow
		M12.322	Palindromic rheumatism, left elbow
		M12.329	Palindromic rheumatism, unspecified elbow
		M12.421	Intermittent hydrarthrosis, right elbow
		M12.422	Intermittent hydrarthrosis, left elbow
		M12.429	Intermittent hydrarthrosis, unspecified elbow
719.33	PALINDROMIC RHEUMATISM, FOREARM	**M12.331**	Palindromic rheumatism, right wrist
		M12.332	Palindromic rheumatism, left wrist
		M12.339	Palindromic rheumatism, unspecified wrist
		M12.431	Intermittent hydrarthrosis, right wrist
		M12.432	Intermittent hydrarthrosis, left wrist
		M12.439	Intermittent hydrarthrosis, unspecified wrist
719.34	PALINDROMIC RHEUMATISM, HAND	**M12.341**	Palindromic rheumatism, right hand
		M12.342	Palindromic rheumatism, left hand
		M12.349	Palindromic rheumatism, unspecified hand
		M12.441	Intermittent hydrarthrosis, right hand
		M12.442	Intermittent hydrarthrosis, left hand
		M12.449	Intermittent hydrarthrosis, unspecified hand
719.35	PALINDROMIC RHEUMATISM PELVIC REGION AND THIGH	**M12.351**	Palindromic rheumatism, right hip
		M12.352	Palindromic rheumatism, left hip
		M12.359	Palindromic rheumatism, unspecified hip
		M12.451	Intermittent hydrarthrosis, right hip
		M12.452	Intermittent hydrarthrosis, left hip
		M12.459	Intermittent hydrarthrosis, unspecified hip

ICD-9-CM		ICD-10-CM	
719.36	PALINDROMIC RHEUMATISM, LOWER LEG	**M12.361**	Palindromic rheumatism, right knee
		M12.362	Palindromic rheumatism, left knee
		M12.369	Palindromic rheumatism, unspecified knee
		M12.461	Intermittent hydrarthrosis, right knee
		M12.462	Intermittent hydrarthrosis, left knee
		M12.469	Intermittent hydrarthrosis, unspecified knee
719.37	PALINDROMIC RHEUMATISM ANKLE AND FOOT	**M12.371**	Palindromic rheumatism, right ankle and foot
		M12.372	Palindromic rheumatism, left ankle and foot
		M12.379	Palindromic rheumatism, unspecified ankle and foot
		M12.471	Intermittent hydrarthrosis, right ankle and foot
		M12.472	Intermittent hydrarthrosis, left ankle and foot
		M12.479	Intermittent hydrarthrosis, unspecified ankle and foot
719.38	PALINDROMIC RHEUMATISM OTHER SPECIFIED SITES	**M12.38**	Palindromic rheumatism, oth spec site
		M12.48	Intermittent hydrarthrosis, other site
719.39	PALINDROMIC RHEUMATISM MULTIPLE SITES	**M12.39**	Palindromic rheumatism, multiple sites
		M12.49	Intermittent hydrarthrosis, multiple sites
719.4Ø	PAIN IN JOINT, SITE UNSPECIFIED	**M25.5Ø**	Pain in unspecified joint
719.41	PAIN IN JOINT, SHOULDER REGION	**M25.511**	Pain in right shoulder
		M25.512	Pain in left shoulder
		M25.519	Pain in unspecified shoulder
719.42	PAIN IN JOINT, UPPER ARM	**M25.521**	Pain in right elbow
		M25.522	Pain in left elbow
		M25.529	Pain in unspecified elbow
719.43	PAIN IN JOINT, FOREARM	**M25.531**	Pain in right wrist
		M25.532	Pain in left wrist
		M25.539	Pain in unspecified wrist
719.44	PAIN IN JOINT, HAND	**M79.643**	Pain in unspecified hand
		M79.646	Pain in unspecified finger(s)
719.45	PAIN IN JOINT PELVIC REGION AND THIGH	**M25.551**	Pain in right hip
		M25.552	Pain in left hip
		M25.559	Pain in unspecified hip
719.46	PAIN IN JOINT, LOWER LEG	**M25.561**	Pain in right knee
		M25.562	Pain in left knee
		M25.569	Pain in unspecified knee
719.47	PAIN IN JOINT, ANKLE AND FOOT	**M25.571**	Pain in right ankle
		M25.572	Pain in left ankle
		M25.579	Pain in unspecified ankle
719.48	PAIN IN JOINT OTHER SPECIFIED SITES	**M25.5Ø**	Pain in unspecified joint
719.49	PAIN IN JOINT, MULTIPLE SITES	**M25.5Ø**	Pain in unspecified joint
719.5Ø	STIFFNESS OF JOINT NEC UNSPECIFIED SITE	**M25.6Ø**	Stiffness of unspecified joint, not elsewhere classified
719.51	STIFFNESS OF JOINT NEC SHOULDER REGION	**M25.611**	Stiffness of right shoulder, not elsewhere classified
		M25.612	Stiffness of left shoulder, not elsewhere classified
		M25.619	Stiffness of unspecified shoulder, not elsewhere classified
719.52	STIFFNESS OF JOINT NEC UPPER ARM	**M25.621**	Stiffness of right elbow, not elsewhere classified
		M25.622	Stiffness of left elbow, not elsewhere classified
		M25.629	Stiffness of unspecified elbow, not elsewhere classified
719.53	STIFFNESS OF JOINT NEC FOREARM	**M25.631**	Stiffness of right wrist, not elsewhere classified
		M25.632	Stiffness of left wrist, not elsewhere classified
		M25.639	Stiffness of unspecified wrist, not elsewhere classified
719.54	STIFFNESS OF JOINT NOT ELSEWHERE CLASSIFIED HAND	**M25.641**	Stiffness of right hand, not elsewhere classified
		M25.642	Stiffness of left hand, not elsewhere classified
		M25.649	Stiffness of unspecified hand, not elsewhere classified
719.55	STIFFNESS OF JOINT NEC PELVIC REGION AND THIGH	**M25.651**	Stiffness of right hip, not elsewhere classified
		M25.652	Stiffness of left hip, not elsewhere classified
		M25.659	Stiffness of unspecified hip, not elsewhere classified
719.56	STIFFNESS OF JOINT NEC LOWER LEG	**M25.661**	Stiffness of right knee, not elsewhere classified
		M25.662	Stiffness of left knee, not elsewhere classified
		M25.669	Stiffness of unspecified knee, not elsewhere classified
719.57	STIFFNESS OF JOINT NEC ANKLE AND FOOT	**M25.671**	Stiffness of right ankle, not elsewhere classified
		M25.672	Stiffness of left ankle, not elsewhere classified
		M25.673	Stiffness of unspecified ankle, not elsewhere classified
		M25.674	Stiffness of right foot, not elsewhere classified
		M25.675	Stiffness of left foot, not elsewhere classified
		M25.676	Stiffness of unspecified foot, not elsewhere classified
719.58	STIFFNESS OF JOINT NEC OTHER SPECIFIED SITE	**M25.6Ø**	Stiffness of unspecified joint, not elsewhere classified
719.59	STIFFNESS OF JOINTS NEC MULTIPLE SITES	**M25.6Ø**	Stiffness of unspecified joint, not elsewhere classified
719.6Ø	OTHER SYMPTOMS REFERABLE JOINT SITE UNSPECIFIED	**R29.898**	Oth symptoms and signs involving the musculoskeletal system
719.61	OTHER SYMPTOMS REFERABLE TO SHOULDER JOINT	**R29.898**	Oth symptoms and signs involving the musculoskeletal system
719.62	OTHER SYMPTOMS REFERABLE TO UPPER ARM JOINT	**R29.898**	Oth symptoms and signs involving the musculoskeletal system
719.63	OTHER SYMPTOMS REFERABLE TO FOREARM JOINT	**R29.898**	Oth symptoms and signs involving the musculoskeletal system
719.64	OTHER SYMPTOMS REFERABLE TO HAND JOINT	**R29.898**	Oth symptoms and signs involving the musculoskeletal system
719.65	OTHER SYMPTOMS REFERABLE TO PELVIC JOINT	**R29.4**	Clicking hip
719.66	OTHER SYMPTOMS REFERABLE TO LOWER LEG JOINT	**R29.898**	Oth symptoms and signs involving the musculoskeletal system
719.67	OTHER SYMPTOMS REFERABLE TO ANKLE AND FOOT JOINT	**R29.898**	Oth symptoms and signs involving the musculoskeletal system
719.68	OTHER SYMPTOMS REFERABLE JOINT OTHER SPEC SITE	**R29.898**	Oth symptoms and signs involving the musculoskeletal system

ICD-9-CM		ICD-10-CM	
719.69	OTHER SYMPTOMS REFERABLE JOINTS MULTIPLE SITES	**R29.898**	Oth symptoms and signs involving the musculoskeletal system
719.7	DIFFICULTY IN WALKING	➡ **R26.2**	Difficulty in walking, not elsewhere classified
719.80	OTHER SPECIFIED DISORDERS JOINT SITE UNSPECIFIED	**M25.10**	Fistula, unspecified joint
		M25.80	Other specified joint disorders, unspecified joint
719.81	OTHER SPECIFIED DISORDERS OF SHOULDER JOINT	**M25.111**	Fistula, right shoulder
		M25.112	Fistula, left shoulder
		M25.119	Fistula, unspecified shoulder
		M25.811	Other specified joint disorders, right shoulder
		M25.812	Other specified joint disorders, left shoulder
		M25.819	Other specified joint disorders, unspecified shoulder
719.82	OTHER SPECIFIED DISORDERS OF UPPER ARM JOINT	**M25.121**	Fistula, right elbow
		M25.122	Fistula, left elbow
		M25.129	Fistula, unspecified elbow
		M25.821	Other specified joint disorders, right elbow
		M25.822	Other specified joint disorders, left elbow
		M25.829	Other specified joint disorders, unspecified elbow
719.83	OTHER SPECIFIED DISORDERS OF FOREARM JOINT	**M25.131**	Fistula, right wrist
		M25.132	Fistula, left wrist
		M25.139	Fistula, unspecified wrist
		M25.831	Other specified joint disorders, right wrist
		M25.832	Other specified joint disorders, left wrist
		M25.839	Other specified joint disorders, unspecified wrist
719.84	OTHER SPECIFIED DISORDERS OF HAND JOINT	**M25.141**	Fistula, right hand
		M25.142	Fistula, left hand
		M25.149	Fistula, unspecified hand
		M25.841	Other specified joint disorders, right hand
		M25.842	Other specified joint disorders, left hand
		M25.849	Other specified joint disorders, unspecified hand
719.85	OTHER SPECIFIED DISORDERS OF PELVIC JOINT	**M25.151**	Fistula, right hip
		M25.152	Fistula, left hip
		M25.159	Fistula, unspecified hip
		M25.851	Other specified joint disorders, right hip
		M25.852	Other specified joint disorders, left hip
		M25.859	Other specified joint disorders, unspecified hip
719.86	OTHER SPECIFIED DISORDERS OF LOWER LEG JOINT	**M25.161**	Fistula, right knee
		M25.162	Fistula, left knee
		M25.169	Fistula, unspecified knee
		M25.861	Other specified joint disorders, right knee
		M25.862	Other specified joint disorders, left knee
		M25.869	Other specified joint disorders, unspecified knee
719.87	OTHER SPECIFIED DISORDERS OF ANKLE&FOOT JOINT	**M25.171**	Fistula, right ankle
		M25.172	Fistula, left ankle
		M25.173	Fistula, unspecified ankle
		M25.174	Fistula, right foot
		M25.175	Fistula, left foot
		M25.176	Fistula, unspecified foot
		M25.871	Other specified joint disorders, right ankle and foot
		M25.872	Other specified joint disorders, left ankle and foot
		M25.879	Other specified joint disorders, unspecified ankle and foot
719.88	OTHER SPEC DISORDERS JOINT OTHER SPEC SITE	**M25.18**	Fistula, oth spec site
719.89	OTHER SPECIFIED DISORDERS JOINTS MULTIPLE SITES	**M25.10**	Fistula, unspecified joint
		M25.80	Other specified joint disorders, unspecified joint
719.90	UNSPECIFIED DISORDER OF JOINT SITE UNSPECIFIED	**M25.9**	Joint disorder, unspecified
719.91	UNSPECIFIED DISORDER OF SHOULDER JOINT	**M25.9**	Joint disorder, unspecified
719.92	UNSPECIFIED DISORDER OF UPPER ARM JOINT	**M25.9**	Joint disorder, unspecified
719.93	UNSPECIFIED DISORDER OF FOREARM JOINT	**M25.9**	Joint disorder, unspecified
719.94	UNSPECIFIED DISORDER OF HAND JOINT	**M25.9**	Joint disorder, unspecified
719.95	UNSPECIFIED DISORDER JOINT PELVIC REGION&THIGH	**M25.9**	Joint disorder, unspecified
719.96	UNSPECIFIED DISORDER OF LOWER LEG JOINT	**M25.9**	Joint disorder, unspecified
719.97	UNSPECIFIED DISORDER OF ANKLE AND FOOT JOINT	**M25.9**	Joint disorder, unspecified
719.98	UNSPECIFIED JOINT DISORDER OTHER SPECIFIED SITE	**M25.9**	Joint disorder, unspecified
719.99	UNSPECIFIED JOINT DISORDER OF MULTIPLE SITES	**M25.9**	Joint disorder, unspecified

ICD-9-CM		ICD-10-CM	
720.Ø	ANKYLOSING SPONDYLITIS	MØ8.1	Juvenile ankylosing spondylitis
		M45.Ø	Ankylosing spondylitis of multiple sites in spine
		M45.1	Ankylosing spondylitis of occipito-atlanto-axial region
		M45.2	Ankylosing spondylitis of cervical region
		M45.3	Ankylosing spondylitis of cervicothoracic region
		M45.4	Ankylosing spondylitis of thoracic region
		M45.5	Ankylosing spondylitis of thoracolumbar region
		M45.6	Ankylosing spondylitis lumbar region
		M45.7	Ankylosing spondylitis of lumbosacral region
		M45.8	Ankylosing spondylitis sacral and sacrococcygeal region
		M45.9	Ankylosing spondylitis of unspecified sites in spine
		M48.8X1	Oth spondylopathies, occipito-atlanto-axial region
		M48.8X2	Other specified spondylopathies, cervical region
		M48.8X3	Other specified spondylopathies, cervicothoracic region
		M48.8X4	Other specified spondylopathies, thoracic region
		M48.8X5	Other specified spondylopathies, thoracolumbar region
		M48.8X6	Other specified spondylopathies, lumbar region
		M48.8X7	Other specified spondylopathies, lumbosacral region
		M48.8X8	Oth spondylopathies, sacral and sacrococcygeal region
		M48.8X9	Other specified spondylopathies, site unspecified
720.1	SPINAL ENTHESOPATHY	M46.ØØ	Spinal enthesopathy, site unspecified
		M46.Ø1	Spinal enthesopathy, occipito-atlanto-axial region
		M46.Ø2	Spinal enthesopathy, cervical region
		M46.Ø3	Spinal enthesopathy, cervicothoracic region
		M46.Ø4	Spinal enthesopathy, thoracic region
		M46.Ø5	Spinal enthesopathy, thoracolumbar region
		M46.Ø6	Spinal enthesopathy, lumbar region
		M46.Ø7	Spinal enthesopathy, lumbosacral region
		M46.Ø8	Spinal enthesopathy, sacral and sacrococcygeal region
		M46.Ø9	Spinal enthesopathy, multiple sites in spine
720.2	SACROILIITIS NOT ELSEWHERE CLASSIFIED	➡ M46.1	Sacroiliitis, not elsewhere classified
720.81	INFLAMMATORY SPONDYLOPATHIES DISEASES CLASS ELSW	◘ A18.Ø1	Tuberculosis of spine
		M49.8Ø	Spondylopathy in diseases classified elsewhere, site unsp
		M49.81	Spond in diseases classd elswhr, occipt-atlan-ax region
		M49.82	Spondylopathy in diseases classd elswhr, cervical region
		M49.83	Spondylopathy in diseases classd elswhr, cervicothor region
		M49.84	Spondylopathy in diseases classd elswhr, thoracic region
		M49.85	Spond in diseases classd elswhr, thoracolumbar region
		M49.86	Spondylopathy in diseases classd elswhr, lumbar region
		M49.87	Spondylopathy in diseases classd elswhr, lumbosacral region
		M49.88	Spond in diseases classd elswhr, sacr/sacrocygl region
		M49.89	Spond in diseases classd elswhr, multiple sites in spine
720.89	OTHER INFLAMMATORY SPONDYLOPATHIES OTHER	M46.5Ø	Other infective spondylopathies, site unspecified
		M46.51	Oth infective spondylopathies, occipito-atlanto-axial region
		M46.52	Other infective spondylopathies, cervical region
		M46.53	Other infective spondylopathies, cervicothoracic region
		M46.54	Other infective spondylopathies, thoracic region
		M46.55	Other infective spondylopathies, thoracolumbar region
		M46.56	Other infective spondylopathies, lumbar region
		M46.57	Other infective spondylopathies, lumbosacral region
		M46.58	Oth infective spondylopathies, sacr/sacrocygl region
		M46.59	Other infective spondylopathies, multiple sites in spine
		M46.8Ø	Oth inflammatory spondylopathies, site unspecified
		M46.81	Oth inflammatory spondylopathies, occipt-atlan-ax region
		M46.82	Oth inflammatory spondylopathies, cervical region
		M46.83	Oth inflammatory spondylopathies, cervicothoracic region
		M46.84	Oth inflammatory spondylopathies, thoracic region
		M46.85	Oth inflammatory spondylopathies, thoracolumbar region
		M46.86	Other specified inflammatory spondylopathies, lumbar region
		M46.87	Oth inflammatory spondylopathies, lumbosacral region
		M46.88	Oth inflammatory spondylopathies, sacr/sacrocygl region
		M46.89	Oth inflammatory spondylopathies, multiple sites in spine
720.9	UNSPECIFIED INFLAMMATORY SPONDYLOPATHY	M46.9Ø	Unspecified inflammatory spondylopathy, site unspecified
		M46.91	Unsp inflammatory spondylopathy, occipt-atlan-ax region
		M46.92	Unspecified inflammatory spondylopathy, cervical region
		M46.93	Unsp inflammatory spondylopathy, cervicothoracic region
		M46.94	Unspecified inflammatory spondylopathy, thoracic region
		M46.95	Unspecified inflammatory spondylopathy, thoracolumbar region
		M46.96	Unspecified inflammatory spondylopathy, lumbar region
		M46.97	Unspecified inflammatory spondylopathy, lumbosacral region
		M46.98	Unsp inflammatory spondylopathy, sacr/sacrocygl region
		M46.99	Unsp inflammatory spondylopathy, multiple sites in spine
721.Ø	CERVICAL SPONDYLOSIS WITHOUT MYELOPATHY	M47.21	Oth spondylosis w radiculopathy, occipt-atlan-ax region
		M47.22	Other spondylosis with radiculopathy, cervical region
		M47.23	Other spondylosis with radiculopathy, cervicothoracic region
		M47.811	Spondyls w/o myelpath or radiculopathy, occipt-atlan-ax rgn
		M47.812	Spondylosis w/o myelopathy or radiculopathy, cervical region
		M47.813	Spondyls w/o myelopathy or radiculopathy, cervicothor region
		M47.891	Other spondylosis, occipito-atlanto-axial region
		M47.892	Other spondylosis, cervical region
		M47.893	Other spondylosis, cervicothoracic region

ICD-9-CM		ICD-10-CM	
721.1	CERVICAL SPONDYLOSIS WITH MYELOPATHY	**M47.011**	Anterior spinal artery comprsn synd, occipt-atlan-ax region
		M47.012	Anterior spinal artery comprsn syndromes, cervical region
		M47.013	Anterior spinal artery comprsn syndromes, cervicothor region
		M47.014	Anterior spinal artery comprsn syndromes, thoracic region
		M47.015	Anterior spinal artery comprsn syndromes, thoracolum region
		M47.016	Anterior spinal artery compression syndromes, lumbar region
		M47.019	Anterior spinal artery compression syndromes, site unsp
		M47.021	Verteb art compression syndromes, occipt-atlan-ax region
		M47.022	Vertebral artery compression syndromes, cervical region
		M47.029	Vertebral artery compression syndromes, site unspecified
		M47.11	Oth spondylosis w myelopathy, occipito-atlanto-axial region
		M47.12	Other spondylosis with myelopathy, cervical region
		M47.13	Other spondylosis with myelopathy, cervicothoracic region
721.2	THORACIC SPONDYLOSIS WITHOUT MYELOPATHY	**M47.24**	Other spondylosis with radiculopathy, thoracic region
		M47.25	Other spondylosis with radiculopathy, thoracolumbar region
		M47.814	Spondylosis w/o myelopathy or radiculopathy, thoracic region
		M47.815	Spondyls w/o myelopathy or radiculopathy, thoracolum region
		M47.894	Other spondylosis, thoracic region
		M47.895	Other spondylosis, thoracolumbar region
721.3	LUMBOSACRAL SPONDYLOSIS WITHOUT MYELOPATHY	**M47.26**	Other spondylosis with radiculopathy, lumbar region
		M47.27	Other spondylosis with radiculopathy, lumbosacral region
		M47.28	Oth spondylosis w radiculopathy, sacr/sacrocygl region
		M47.816	Spondylosis w/o myelopathy or radiculopathy, lumbar region
		M47.817	Spondyls w/o myelopathy or radiculopathy, lumbosacr region
		M47.818	Spondyls w/o myelpath or radiculopathy, sacr/sacrocygl rgn
		M47.896	Other spondylosis, lumbar region
		M47.897	Other spondylosis, lumbosacral region
		M47.898	Other spondylosis, sacral and sacrococcygeal region
721.41	SPONDYLOSIS WITH MYELOPATHY THORACIC REGION	**M47.14**	Other spondylosis with myelopathy, thoracic region
		M47.15	Other spondylosis with myelopathy, thoracolumbar region
721.42	SPONDYLOSIS WITH MYELOPATHY LUMBAR REGION	**M47.16**	Other spondylosis with myelopathy, lumbar region
721.5	KISSING SPINE	**M48.20**	Kissing spine, site unspecified
		M48.21	Kissing spine, occipito-atlanto-axial region
		M48.22	Kissing spine, cervical region
		M48.23	Kissing spine, cervicothoracic region
		M48.24	Kissing spine, thoracic region
		M48.25	Kissing spine, thoracolumbar region
		M48.26	Kissing spine, lumbar region
		M48.27	Kissing spine, lumbosacral region
721.6	ANKYLOSING VERTEBRAL HYPEROSTOSIS	**M48.10**	Ankylosing hyperostosis [Forestier], site unspecified
		M48.11	Ankylosing hyperostosis, occipito-atlanto-axial region
		M48.12	Ankylosing hyperostosis [Forestier], cervical region
		M48.13	Ankylosing hyperostosis [Forestier], cervicothoracic region
		M48.14	Ankylosing hyperostosis [Forestier], thoracic region
		M48.15	Ankylosing hyperostosis [Forestier], thoracolumbar region
		M48.16	Ankylosing hyperostosis [Forestier], lumbar region
		M48.17	Ankylosing hyperostosis [Forestier], lumbosacral region
		M48.18	Ankylosing hyperostosis, sacral and sacrococcygeal region
		M48.19	Ankylosing hyperostosis [Forestier], multiple sites in spine
721.7	TRAUMATIC SPONDYLOPATHY	**M48.30**	Traumatic spondylopathy, site unspecified
		M48.31	Traumatic spondylopathy, occipito-atlanto-axial region
		M48.32	Traumatic spondylopathy, cervical region
		M48.33	Traumatic spondylopathy, cervicothoracic region
		M48.34	Traumatic spondylopathy, thoracic region
		M48.35	Traumatic spondylopathy, thoracolumbar region
		M48.36	Traumatic spondylopathy, lumbar region
		M48.37	Traumatic spondylopathy, lumbosacral region
		M48.38	Traumatic spondylopathy, sacral and sacrococcygeal region
721.8	OTHER ALLIED DISORDERS OF SPINE	**M25.78**	Osteophyte, vertebrae
		M48.9	Spondylopathy, unspecified
721.90	SPONDYLOSIS UNSPEC SITE W/O MENTION MYELOPATHY	**M47.20**	Other spondylosis with radiculopathy, site unspecified
		M47.819	Spondylosis without myelopathy or radiculopathy, site unsp
		M47.899	Other spondylosis, site unspecified
		M47.9	Spondylosis, unspecified
721.91	SPONDYLOSIS OF UNSPECIFIED SITE WITH MYELOPATHY	**M47.10**	Other spondylosis with myelopathy, site unspecified
722.0	DISPLCMT CERV INTERVERT DISC WITHOUT MYELOPATHY	**M50.20**	Other cervical disc displacement, unsp cervical region
		M50.21	Oth cervical disc displacement, high cervical region
		M50.22	Other cervical disc displacement, mid-cervical region
		M50.23	Other cervical disc displacement, cervicothoracic region
722.10	DISPLCMT LUMBAR INTERVERT DISC W/O MYELOPATHY	**M51.26**	Other intervertebral disc displacement, lumbar region
		M51.27	Other intervertebral disc displacement, lumbosacral region
722.11	DISPLCMT THOR INTERVERT DISC WITHOUT MYELOPATHY	**M51.24**	Other intervertebral disc displacement, thoracic region
		M51.25	Other intervertebral disc displacement, thoracolumbar region
722.2	DISPLCMT INTERVERT DISC SITE UNS W/O MYELOPATHY	**M51.9**	Unsp thoracic, thoracolum and lumbosacr intvrt disc disorder
722.30	SCHMORLS NODES, UNSPECIFIED REGION	**M51.9**	Unsp thoracic, thoracolum and lumbosacr intvrt disc disorder
722.31	SCHMORLS NODES, THORACIC REGION	**M51.44**	Schmorl's nodes, thoracic region
		M51.45	Schmorl's nodes, thoracolumbar region
722.32	SCHMORLS NODES, LUMBAR REGION	**M51.46**	Schmorl's nodes, lumbar region
		M51.47	Schmorl's nodes, lumbosacral region

[Brackets] indicate valid character values for each code. Character value meanings provided for each code grouping.

ICD-9-CM		ICD-10-CM	
722.39	SCHMORLS NODES OTHER SPINAL REGION	**M51.9**	Unsp thoracic, thoracolum and lumbosacr intvrt disc disorder
722.4	DEGENERATION OF CERVICAL INTERVERTEBRAL DISC	**M5Ø.3Ø**	Other cervical disc degeneration, unsp cervical region
		M5Ø.31	Oth cervical disc degeneration, high cervical region
		M5Ø.32	Other cervical disc degeneration, mid-cervical region
		M5Ø.33	Other cervical disc degeneration, cervicothoracic region
722.51	DEGEN THORACIC/THORACOLUMBAR INTERVERTEBRAL DISC	**M51.34**	Other intervertebral disc degeneration, thoracic region
		M51.35	Other intervertebral disc degeneration, thoracolumbar region
722.52	DEGEN LUMBAR/LUMBOSACRAL INTERVERTEBRAL DISC	**M51.36**	Other intervertebral disc degeneration, lumbar region
		M51.37	Other intervertebral disc degeneration, lumbosacral region
722.6	DEGENERATION INTERVERTEBRAL DISC SITE UNSPEC	**M51.34**	Other intervertebral disc degeneration, thoracic region
		M51.35	Other intervertebral disc degeneration, thoracolumbar region
		M51.36	Other intervertebral disc degeneration, lumbar region
		M51.37	Other intervertebral disc degeneration, lumbosacral region
722.7Ø	INTERVERT DISC D/O W/MYELOPATHY UNSPEC REGION	**M51.9**	Unsp thoracic, thoracolum and lumbosacr intvrt disc disorder
722.71	INTERVERT CERV DISC D/O W/MYELOPATHY CERV REGION	**M5Ø.ØØ**	Cervical disc disorder with myelopathy, unsp cervical region
		M5Ø.Ø1	Cervical disc disorder w myelopathy, high cervical region
		M5Ø.Ø2	Cervical disc disorder with myelopathy, mid-cervical region
		M5Ø.Ø3	Cervical disc disorder w myelopathy, cervicothoracic region
722.72	INTERVERT THOR DISC D/O W/MYELOPATHY THOR REGION	**M51.Ø4**	Intervertebral disc disorders w myelopathy, thoracic region
		M51.Ø5	Intvrt disc disorders w myelopathy, thoracolumbar region
722.73	INTERVERT LUMB DISC D/O W/MYELOPATHY LUMB REGION	➡ **M51.Ø6**	Intervertebral disc disorders with myelopathy, lumbar region
722.8Ø	POSTLAMINECTOMY SYNDROME UNSPECIFIED REGION	**M96.1**	Postlaminectomy syndrome, not elsewhere classified
722.81	POSTLAMINECTOMY SYNDROME CERVICAL REGION	**M96.1**	Postlaminectomy syndrome, not elsewhere classified
722.82	POSTLAMINECTOMY SYNDROME THORACIC REGION	**M96.1**	Postlaminectomy syndrome, not elsewhere classified
722.83	POSTLAMINECTOMY SYNDROME LUMBAR REGION	**M96.1**	Postlaminectomy syndrome, not elsewhere classified
722.9Ø	OTHER&UNSPEC DISC DISORDER UNSPEC REGION	**M46.4Ø**	Discitis, unspecified, site unspecified
		M46.48	Discitis, unspecified, sacral and sacrococcygeal region
		M46.49	Discitis, unspecified, multiple sites in spine
		M51.9	Unsp thoracic, thoracolum and lumbosacr intvrt disc disorder
722.91	OTHER&UNSPECIFIED DISC DISORDER CERVICAL REGION	**M46.41**	Discitis, unspecified, occipito-atlanto-axial region
		M46.42	Discitis, unspecified, cervical region
		M46.43	Discitis, unspecified, cervicothoracic region
		M5Ø.1Ø	Cervical disc disorder w radiculopathy, unsp cervical region
		M5Ø.11	Cerv disc disorder w radiculopathy, high cervical region
		M5Ø.12	Cervical disc disorder w radiculopathy, mid-cervical region
		M5Ø.13	Cervical disc disorder w radiculopathy, cervicothor region
		M5Ø.8Ø	Other cervical disc disorders, unspecified cervical region
		M5Ø.81	Other cervical disc disorders, high cervical region
		M5Ø.82	Other cervical disc disorders, mid-cervical region
		M5Ø.83	Other cervical disc disorders, cervicothoracic region
		M5Ø.9Ø	Cervical disc disorder, unsp, unspecified cervical region
		M5Ø.91	Cervical disc disorder, unspecified, high cervical region
		M5Ø.92	Cervical disc disorder, unspecified, mid-cervical region
		M5Ø.93	Cervical disc disorder, unspecified, cervicothoracic region
722.92	OTHER&UNSPECIFIED DISC DISORDER THORACIC REGION	**M46.44**	Discitis, unspecified, thoracic region
		M46.45	Discitis, unspecified, thoracolumbar region
		M51.14	Intvrt disc disorders w radiculopathy, thoracic region
		M51.15	Intvrt disc disorders w radiculopathy, thoracolumbar region
		M51.84	Other intervertebral disc disorders, thoracic region
		M51.85	Other intervertebral disc disorders, thoracolumbar region
722.93	OTHER&UNSPECIFIED DISC DISORDER OF LUMBAR REGION	**M46.46**	Discitis, unspecified, lumbar region
		M46.47	Discitis, unspecified, lumbosacral region
		M51.16	Intervertebral disc disorders w radiculopathy, lumbar region
		M51.17	Intvrt disc disorders w radiculopathy, lumbosacral region
		M51.86	Other intervertebral disc disorders, lumbar region
		M51.87	Other intervertebral disc disorders, lumbosacral region
723.Ø	SPINAL STENOSIS IN CERVICAL REGION	**M48.Ø1**	Spinal stenosis, occipito-atlanto-axial region
		M48.Ø2	Spinal stenosis, cervical region
		M48.Ø3	Spinal stenosis, cervicothoracic region
		M99.2Ø	Subluxation stenosis of neural canal of head region
		M99.21	Subluxation stenosis of neural canal of cervical region
		M99.3Ø	Osseous stenosis of neural canal of head region
		M99.31	Osseous stenosis of neural canal of cervical region
		M99.4Ø	Connective tissue stenosis of neural canal of head region
		M99.41	Connective tiss stenosis of neural canal of cervical region
		M99.5Ø	Intervertebral disc stenosis of neural canal of head region
		M99.51	Intvrt disc stenosis of neural canal of cervical region
		M99.6Ø	Osseous and sublux stenosis of intvrt foramin of head region
		M99.61	Osseous and sublux stenosis of intvrt foramin of cerv region
		M99.7Ø	Conn tiss and disc stenosis of intvrt foramin of head region
		M99.71	Conn tiss and disc stenosis of intvrt foramin of cerv region
723.1	CERVICALGIA	➡ **M54.2**	Cervicalgia
723.2	CERVICOCRANIAL SYNDROME	➡ **M53.Ø**	Cervicocranial syndrome
723.3	CERVICOBRACHIAL SYNDROME	➡ **M53.1**	Cervicobrachial syndrome
723.4	BRACHIAL NEURITIS OR RADICULITIS NOS	**M54.11**	Radiculopathy, occipito-atlanto-axial region
		M54.12	Radiculopathy, cervical region
		M54.13	Radiculopathy, cervicothoracic region
723.5	TORTICOLLIS, UNSPECIFIED	➡ **M43.6**	Torticollis

ICD-9-CM		ICD-10-CM	
723.6	PANNICULITIS SPECIFIED AS AFFECTING NECK	**M54.ØØ**	Panniculitis affecting regions of neck and back, site unsp
		M54.Ø1	Panniculitis aff regions of neck/bk, occipt-atlan-ax region
		M54.Ø2	Panniculitis affecting regions of neck/bk, cervical region
723.7	OSSIFICATION POST LONGITUDINAL LIGAMENT CERV REG	**M67.88**	Other specified disorders of synovium and tendon, other site
723.8	OTHER SYNDROMES AFFECTING CERVICAL REGION	**M53.81**	Other specified dorsopathies, occipito-atlanto-axial region
		M53.82	Other specified dorsopathies, cervical region
		M53.83	Other specified dorsopathies, cervicothoracic region
		M54.81	Occipital neuralgia
723.9	UNSPEC MUSCULOSKEL D/O&SYMPTOMS REFERABLE NECK	**M53.82**	Other specified dorsopathies, cervical region
724.ØØ	SPINAL STENOSIS UNSPEC REGION OTH THAN CERVICAL	➡ **M48.ØØ**	Spinal stenosis, site unspecified
724.Ø1	SPINAL STENOSIS OF THORACIC REGION	**M48.Ø4**	Spinal stenosis, thoracic region
		M48.Ø5	Spinal stenosis, thoracolumbar region
		M99.22	Subluxation stenosis of neural canal of thoracic region
		M99.32	Osseous stenosis of neural canal of thoracic region
		M99.42	Connective tiss stenosis of neural canal of thoracic region
		M99.52	Intvrt disc stenosis of neural canal of thoracic region
		M99.62	Osseous and sublux stenos of intvrt foramin of thor region
		M99.72	Conn tiss and disc stenos of intvrt foramin of thor region
724.Ø2	SPINAL STEN LUMB REG W/O NEUROGENIC CLAUDICATION	**M48.Ø6**	Spinal stenosis, lumbar region
		M48.Ø7	Spinal stenosis, lumbosacral region
		M99.23	Subluxation stenosis of neural canal of lumbar region
		M99.33	Osseous stenosis of neural canal of lumbar region
		M99.43	Connective tissue stenosis of neural canal of lumbar region
		M99.53	Intvrt disc stenosis of neural canal of lumbar region
		M99.63	Osseous and sublux stenos of intvrt foramin of lumbar region
		M99.73	Conn tiss and disc stenos of intvrt foramin of lumbar region
724.Ø3	SPINAL STENOS LUMB REGION NEUROGEN CLAUDICATION	**M48.Ø6**	Spinal stenosis, lumbar region
724.Ø9	SPINAL STENOSIS OTHER REGION OTHER THAN CERVICAL	**M48.Ø8**	Spinal stenosis, sacral and sacrococcygeal region
		M99.24	Subluxation stenosis of neural canal of sacral region
		M99.25	Subluxation stenosis of neural canal of pelvic region
		M99.26	Subluxation stenosis of neural canal of lower extremity
		M99.27	Subluxation stenosis of neural canal of upper extremity
		M99.28	Subluxation stenosis of neural canal of rib cage
		M99.29	Sublux stenosis of neural canal of abdomen and oth regions
		M99.34	Osseous stenosis of neural canal of sacral region
		M99.35	Osseous stenosis of neural canal of pelvic region
		M99.36	Osseous stenosis of neural canal of lower extremity
		M99.37	Osseous stenosis of neural canal of upper extremity
		M99.38	Osseous stenosis of neural canal of rib cage
		M99.39	Osseous stenosis of neural canal of abdomen and oth regions
		M99.44	Connective tissue stenosis of neural canal of sacral region
		M99.45	Connective tissue stenosis of neural canal of pelvic region
		M99.46	Connective tiss stenosis of neural canal of lower extremity
		M99.47	Connective tiss stenosis of neural canal of upper extremity
		M99.48	Connective tissue stenosis of neural canal of rib cage
		M99.49	Conn tiss stenos of neural canal of abdomen and oth regions
		M99.54	Intvrt disc stenosis of neural canal of sacral region
		M99.55	Intvrt disc stenosis of neural canal of pelvic region
		M99.56	Intervertebral disc stenosis of neural canal of low extrm
		M99.57	Intervertebral disc stenosis of neural canal of up extrem
		M99.58	Intervertebral disc stenosis of neural canal of rib cage
		M99.59	Intvrt disc stenos of neural canal of abd and oth regions
		M99.64	Osseous and sublux stenos of intvrt foramin of sacral region
		M99.65	Osseous and sublux stenos of intvrt foramin of pelvic region
		M99.66	Osseous and sublux stenosis of intvrt foramina of low extrm
		M99.67	Osseous and sublux stenosis of intvrt foramina of up extrem
		M99.68	Osseous and sublux stenosis of intvrt foramina of rib cage
		M99.69	Osseous & sublux stenos of intvrt foramin of abd and oth rgn
		M99.74	Conn tiss and disc stenos of intvrt foramin of sacral region
		M99.75	Conn tiss and disc stenos of intvrt foramin of pelvic region
		M99.76	Conn tiss and disc stenosis of intvrt foramina of low extrm
		M99.77	Conn tiss and disc stenosis of intvrt foramina of up extrem
		M99.78	Conn tiss and disc stenosis of intvrt foramina of rib cage
		M99.79	Conn tiss & disc stenos of intvrt foramin of abd and oth rgn
724.1	PAIN IN THORACIC SPINE	➡ **M54.6**	Pain in thoracic spine
724.2	LUMBAGO	➡ **M54.5**	Low back pain
724.3	SCIATICA	**M54.3Ø**	Sciatica, unspecified side
		M54.31	Sciatica, right side
		M54.32	Sciatica, left side
		M54.4Ø	Lumbago with sciatica, unspecified side
		M54.41	Lumbago with sciatica, right side
		M54.42	Lumbago with sciatica, left side
724.4	THORACIC/LUMBOSACRAL NEURITIS/RADICULITIS UNSPEC	**M54.14**	Radiculopathy, thoracic region
		M54.15	Radiculopathy, thoracolumbar region
		M54.16	Radiculopathy, lumbar region
		M54.17	Radiculopathy, lumbosacral region
724.5	UNSPECIFIED BACKACHE	**M54.89**	Other dorsalgia
		M54.9	Dorsalgia, unspecified

ICD-9-CM		ICD-10-CM	
724.6	DISORDERS OF SACRUM	**M43.27**	Fusion of spine, lumbosacral region
		M43.28	Fusion of spine, sacral and sacrococcygeal region
		M53.2X7	Spinal instabilities, lumbosacral region
		M53.2X8	Spinal instabilities, sacral and sacrococcygeal region
		M53.3	Sacrococcygeal disorders, not elsewhere classified
		M53.86	Other specified dorsopathies, lumbar region
		M53.87	Other specified dorsopathies, lumbosacral region
		M53.88	Oth dorsopathies, sacral and sacrococcygeal region
724.70	UNSPECIFIED DISORDER OF COCCYX	**M53.3**	Sacrococcygeal disorders, not elsewhere classified
724.71	HYPERMOBILITY OF COCCYX	**M53.2X8**	Spinal instabilities, sacral and sacrococcygeal region
724.79	OTHER DISORDER OF COCCYX	**M53.3**	Sacrococcygeal disorders, not elsewhere classified
724.8	OTHER SYMPTOMS REFERABLE TO BACK	**M54.03**	Panniculitis aff regions of neck/bk, cervicothor region
		M54.04	Panniculitis affecting regions of neck/bk, thoracic region
		M54.05	Panniculitis affecting regions of neck/bk, thoracolum region
		M54.06	Panniculitis affecting regions of neck/bk, lumbar region
		M54.07	Panniculitis affecting regions of neck/bk, lumbosacr region
		M54.08	Panniculitis aff regions of neck/bk, sacr/sacrocygl region
		M54.09	Panniculitis aff regions, neck/bk, multiple sites in spine
		M62.830	Muscle spasm of back
724.9	OTHER UNSPECIFIED BACK DISORDER	**M43.20**	Fusion of spine, site unspecified
		M43.21	Fusion of spine, occipito-atlanto-axial region
		M43.22	Fusion of spine, cervical region
		M43.23	Fusion of spine, cervicothoracic region
		M43.24	Fusion of spine, thoracic region
		M43.25	Fusion of spine, thoracolumbar region
		M43.26	Fusion of spine, lumbar region
		M43.27	Fusion of spine, lumbosacral region
		M43.28	Fusion of spine, sacral and sacrococcygeal region
		M43.8X9	Other specified deforming dorsopathies, site unspecified
		M53.80	Other specified dorsopathies, site unspecified
		M53.84	Other specified dorsopathies, thoracic region
		M53.85	Other specified dorsopathies, thoracolumbar region
		M53.9	Dorsopathy, unspecified
725	POLYMYALGIA RHEUMATICA	➡ **M35.3**	Polymyalgia rheumatica
726.0	ADHESIVE CAPSULITIS OF SHOULDER	**M75.00**	Adhesive capsulitis of unspecified shoulder
		M75.01	Adhesive capsulitis of right shoulder
		M75.02	Adhesive capsulitis of left shoulder
726.10	UNSPEC DISORDERS BURSAE&TENDONS SHOULDER REGION	**M66.211**	Spontaneous rupture of extensor tendons, right shoulder
		M66.212	Spontaneous rupture of extensor tendons, left shoulder
		M66.219	Spontaneous rupture of extensor tendons, unsp shoulder
		M66.811	Spontaneous rupture of other tendons, right shoulder
		M66.812	Spontaneous rupture of other tendons, left shoulder
		M66.819	Spontaneous rupture of other tendons, unspecified shoulder
		M75.100	Unsp rotatr-cuff tear/ruptr of unsp shoulder, not trauma
		M75.101	Unsp rotatr-cuff tear/ruptr of right shoulder, not trauma
		M75.102	Unsp rotatr-cuff tear/ruptr of left shoulder, not trauma
		M75.50	Bursitis of unspecified shoulder
		M75.51	Bursitis of right shoulder
		M75.52	Bursitis of left shoulder
726.11	CALCIFYING TENDINITIS OF SHOULDER	**M75.30**	Calcific tendinitis of unspecified shoulder
		M75.31	Calcific tendinitis of right shoulder
		M75.32	Calcific tendinitis of left shoulder
726.12	BICIPITAL TENOSYNOVITIS	**M75.20**	Bicipital tendinitis, unspecified shoulder
		M75.21	Bicipital tendinitis, right shoulder
		M75.22	Bicipital tendinitis, left shoulder
726.13	PARTIAL TEAR OF ROTATOR CUFF	**M75.110**	Incmpl rotatr-cuff tear/ruptr of unsp shoulder, not trauma
		M75.111	Incomplete rotatr-cuff tear/ruptr of r shoulder, not trauma
		M75.112	Incomplete rotatr-cuff tear/ruptr of l shoulder, not trauma
726.19	OTH SPEC D/O ROTATOR CUFF SYND SHLDR&ALLIED D/O	**M75.80**	Other shoulder lesions, unspecified shoulder
		M75.81	Other shoulder lesions, right shoulder
		M75.82	Other shoulder lesions, left shoulder
726.2	OTHER AFFECTIONS OF SHOULDER REGION NEC	**M25.711**	Osteophyte, right shoulder
		M25.712	Osteophyte, left shoulder
		M25.719	Osteophyte, unspecified shoulder
		M75.30	Calcific tendinitis of unspecified shoulder
		M75.31	Calcific tendinitis of right shoulder
		M75.32	Calcific tendinitis of left shoulder
		M75.40	Impingement syndrome of unspecified shoulder
		M75.41	Impingement syndrome of right shoulder
		M75.42	Impingement syndrome of left shoulder
		M75.80	Other shoulder lesions, unspecified shoulder
		M75.81	Other shoulder lesions, right shoulder
		M75.82	Other shoulder lesions, left shoulder
		M75.90	Shoulder lesion, unspecified, unspecified shoulder
		M75.91	Shoulder lesion, unspecified, right shoulder
		M75.92	Shoulder lesion, unspecified, left shoulder
726.30	UNSPECIFIED ENTHESOPATHY OF ELBOW	**M25.721**	Osteophyte, right elbow
		M25.722	Osteophyte, left elbow
		M25.729	Osteophyte, unspecified elbow

ICD-9-CM		ICD-10-CM	
726.31	MEDIAL EPICONDYLITIS OF ELBOW	**M77.00**	Medial epicondylitis, unspecified elbow
		M77.01	Medial epicondylitis, right elbow
		M77.02	Medial epicondylitis, left elbow
726.32	LATERAL EPICONDYLITIS OF ELBOW	**M77.10**	Lateral epicondylitis, unspecified elbow
		M77.11	Lateral epicondylitis, right elbow
		M77.12	Lateral epicondylitis, left elbow
726.33	OLECRANON BURSITIS	**M70.20**	Olecranon bursitis, unspecified elbow
		M70.21	Olecranon bursitis, right elbow
		M70.22	Olecranon bursitis, left elbow
726.39	OTHER ENTHESOPATHY OF ELBOW REGION	**M70.30**	Other bursitis of elbow, unspecified elbow
		M70.31	Other bursitis of elbow, right elbow
		M70.32	Other bursitis of elbow, left elbow
726.4	ENTHESOPATHY OF WRIST AND CARPUS	**M25.731**	Osteophyte, right wrist
		M25.732	Osteophyte, left wrist
		M25.739	Osteophyte, unspecified wrist
		M25.741	Osteophyte, right hand
		M25.742	Osteophyte, left hand
		M25.749	Osteophyte, unspecified hand
		M70.10	Bursitis, unspecified hand
		M70.11	Bursitis, right hand
		M70.12	Bursitis, left hand
		M77.20	Periarthritis, unspecified wrist
		M77.21	Periarthritis, right wrist
		M77.22	Periarthritis, left wrist
726.5	ENTHESOPATHY OF HIP REGION	**M25.751**	Osteophyte, right hip
		M25.752	Osteophyte, left hip
		M25.759	Osteophyte, unspecified hip
		M70.60	Trochanteric bursitis, unspecified hip
		M70.61	Trochanteric bursitis, right hip
		M70.62	Trochanteric bursitis, left hip
		M70.70	Other bursitis of hip, unspecified hip
		M70.71	Other bursitis of hip, right hip
		M70.72	Other bursitis of hip, left hip
		M76.00	Gluteal tendinitis, unspecified hip
		M76.01	Gluteal tendinitis, right hip
		M76.02	Gluteal tendinitis, left hip
		M76.10	Psoas tendinitis, unspecified hip
		M76.11	Psoas tendinitis, right hip
		M76.12	Psoas tendinitis, left hip
		M76.20	Iliac crest spur, unspecified hip
		M76.21	Iliac crest spur, right hip
		M76.22	Iliac crest spur, left hip
		M76.30	Iliotibial band syndrome, unspecified leg
		M76.31	Iliotibial band syndrome, right leg
		M76.32	Iliotibial band syndrome, left leg
726.60	UNSPECIFIED ENTHESOPATHY OF KNEE	**M25.761**	Osteophyte, right knee
		M25.762	Osteophyte, left knee
		M25.769	Osteophyte, unspecified knee
		M70.50	Other bursitis of knee, unspecified knee
		M70.51	Other bursitis of knee, right knee
		M70.52	Other bursitis of knee, left knee
726.61	PES ANSERINUS TENDINITIS OR BURSITIS	**M76.899**	Oth enthesopathies of unspecified lower limb, excluding foot
726.62	TIBIAL COLLATERAL LIGAMENT BURSITIS	**M76.40**	Tibial collateral bursitis, unspecified leg
		M76.41	Tibial collateral bursitis [Pellegrini-Stieda], right leg
		M76.42	Tibial collateral bursitis [Pellegrini-Stieda], left leg
726.63	FIBULAR COLLATERAL LIGAMENT BURSITIS	**M76.899**	Oth enthesopathies of unspecified lower limb, excluding foot
726.64	PATELLAR TENDINITIS	**M76.50**	Patellar tendinitis, unspecified knee
		M76.51	Patellar tendinitis, right knee
		M76.52	Patellar tendinitis, left knee
726.65	PREPATELLAR BURSITIS	**M70.40**	Prepatellar bursitis, unspecified knee
		M70.41	Prepatellar bursitis, right knee
		M70.42	Prepatellar bursitis, left knee
726.69	OTHER ENTHESOPATHY OF KNEE	**M76.899**	Oth enthesopathies of unspecified lower limb, excluding foot
726.70	UNSPECIFIED ENTHESOPATHY OF ANKLE AND TARSUS	**M25.771**	Osteophyte, right ankle
		M25.772	Osteophyte, left ankle
		M25.773	Osteophyte, unspecified ankle
		M25.774	Osteophyte, right foot
		M25.775	Osteophyte, left foot
		M25.776	Osteophyte, unspecified foot
		M76.899	Oth enthesopathies of unspecified lower limb, excluding foot
		M77.40	Metatarsalgia, unspecified foot
		M77.41	Metatarsalgia, right foot
		M77.42	Metatarsalgia, left foot
726.71	ACHILLES BURSITIS OR TENDINITIS	**M76.60**	Achilles tendinitis, unspecified leg
		M76.61	Achilles tendinitis, right leg
		M76.62	Achilles tendinitis, left leg

ICD-9-CM		ICD-10-CM	
726.72	TIBIALIS TENDINITIS	**M76.811**	Anterior tibial syndrome, right leg
		M76.812	Anterior tibial syndrome, left leg
		M76.819	Anterior tibial syndrome, unspecified leg
		M76.821	Posterior tibial tendinitis, right leg
		M76.822	Posterior tibial tendinitis, left leg
		M76.829	Posterior tibial tendinitis, unspecified leg
726.73	CALCANEAL SPUR	**M77.3Ø**	Calcaneal spur, unspecified foot
		M77.31	Calcaneal spur, right foot
		M77.32	Calcaneal spur, left foot
726.79	OTHER ENTHESOPATHY OF ANKLE AND TARSUS	**M76.7Ø**	Peroneal tendinitis, unspecified leg
		M76.71	Peroneal tendinitis, right leg
		M76.72	Peroneal tendinitis, left leg
		M77.5Ø	Other enthesopathy of unspecified foot
		M77.51	Other enthesopathy of right foot
		M77.52	Other enthesopathy of left foot
726.8	OTHER PERIPHERAL ENTHESOPATHIES	**M76.891**	Oth enthesopathies of right lower limb, excluding foot
		M76.892	Oth enthesopathies of left lower limb, excluding foot
		M76.9	Unspecified enthesopathy, lower limb, excluding foot
		M77.8	Other enthesopathies, not elsewhere classified
726.9Ø	ENTHESOPATHY OF UNSPECIFIED SITE	➡ **M77.9**	Enthesopathy, unspecified
726.91	EXOSTOSIS OF UNSPECIFIED SITE	➡ **M25.7Ø**	Osteophyte, unspecified joint
727.ØØ	UNSPECIFIED SYNOVITIS AND TENOSYNOVITIS	➡ **M65.9**	Synovitis and tenosynovitis, unspecified
727.Ø1	SYNOVITIS&TENOSYNOVITIS DISEASES CLASSIFIED ELSW	**M65.8Ø**	Other synovitis and tenosynovitis, unspecified site
727.Ø2	GIANT CELL TUMOR OF TENDON SHEATH	**D48.1**	Neoplasm of uncertain behavior of connctv/soft tiss
727.Ø3	TRIGGER FINGER	**M65.3Ø**	Trigger finger, unspecified finger
		M65.311	Trigger thumb, right thumb
		M65.312	Trigger thumb, left thumb
		M65.319	Trigger thumb, unspecified thumb
		M65.321	Trigger finger, right index finger
		M65.322	Trigger finger, left index finger
		M65.329	Trigger finger, unspecified index finger
		M65.331	Trigger finger, right middle finger
		M65.332	Trigger finger, left middle finger
		M65.339	Trigger finger, unspecified middle finger
		M65.341	Trigger finger, right ring finger
		M65.342	Trigger finger, left ring finger
		M65.349	Trigger finger, unspecified ring finger
		M65.351	Trigger finger, right little finger
		M65.352	Trigger finger, left little finger
		M65.359	Trigger finger, unspecified little finger
727.Ø4	RADIAL STYLOID TENOSYNOVITIS	➡ **M65.4**	Radial styloid tenosynovitis [de Quervain]
727.Ø5	OTHER TENOSYNOVITIS OF HAND AND WRIST	**M65.831**	Other synovitis and tenosynovitis, right forearm
		M65.832	Other synovitis and tenosynovitis, left forearm
		M65.839	Other synovitis and tenosynovitis, unspecified forearm
		M65.841	Other synovitis and tenosynovitis, right hand
		M65.842	Other synovitis and tenosynovitis, left hand
		M65.849	Other synovitis and tenosynovitis, unspecified hand
727.Ø6	TENOSYNOVITIS OF FOOT AND ANKLE	**M65.871**	Other synovitis and tenosynovitis, right ankle and foot
		M65.872	Other synovitis and tenosynovitis, left ankle and foot
		M65.879	Other synovitis and tenosynovitis, unsp ankle and foot
727.Ø9	OTHER SYNOVITIS AND TENOSYNOVITIS	**M65.1Ø**	Other infective (teno)synovitis, unspecified site
		M65.11[1,2,9]	Other infective (teno)synovitis, shoulder
		M65.12[1,2,9]	Other infective (teno)synovitis, elbow
		M65.13[1,2,9]	Other infective (teno)synovitis, wrist
		M65.14[1,2,9]	Other infective (teno)synovitis, hand
		M65.15[1,2,9]	Other infective (teno)synovitis, hip
		M65.16[1,2,9]	Other infective (teno)synovitis, knee
		M65.17[1,2,9]	Other infective (teno)synovitis, ankle and foot
		M65.18	Other infective (teno)synovitis, other site
		M65.19	Other infective (teno)synovitis, multiple sites
		M65.8Ø	Other synovitis and tenosynovitis, unspecified site
		M65.81[1,2,9]	Other synovitis and tenosynovitis, shoulder
		M65.82[1,2,9]	Other synovitis and tenosynovitis, upper arm
		M65.85[1,2,9]	Other synovitis and tenosynovitis, thigh
		M65.86[1,2,9]	Other synovitis and tenosynovitis, lower leg
		M65.88	Other synovitis and tenosynovitis, other site
		M65.89	Other synovitis and tenosynovitis, multiple sites
		M67.3Ø	Transient synovitis, unspecified site
		M67.31[1,2,9]	Transient synovitis, shoulder
		M67.32[1,2,9]	Transient synovitis, elbow
		M67.33[1,2,9]	Transient synovitis, wrist
		M67.34[1,2,9]	Transient synovitis, hand
		M67.35[1,2,9]	Transient synovitis, hip
		M67.36[1,2,9]	Transient synovitis, knee
		M67.37[1,2,9]	Transient synovitis, ankle and foot
		M67.38	Transient synovitis, other site
		M67.39	Transient synovitis, multiple sites

6th Character meanings for codes as indicated
1 Right   2 Left   9 Unspecified

ICD-9-CM		ICD-10-CM	
727.1	BUNION	**M2Ø.1Ø**	Hallux valgus (acquired), unspecified foot
727.2	SPECIFIC BURSITIDES OFTEN OF OCCUPATIONAL ORIGIN	**M7Ø.Ø31**	Crepitant synovitis (acute) (chronic), right wrist
		M7Ø.Ø32	Crepitant synovitis (acute) (chronic), left wrist
		M7Ø.Ø39	Crepitant synovitis (acute) (chronic), unspecified wrist
		M7Ø.Ø41	Crepitant synovitis (acute) (chronic), right hand
		M7Ø.Ø42	Crepitant synovitis (acute) (chronic), left hand
		M7Ø.Ø49	Crepitant synovitis (acute) (chronic), unspecified hand
		M7Ø.1Ø	Bursitis, unspecified hand
		M7Ø.11	Bursitis, right hand
		M7Ø.12	Bursitis, left hand
		M7Ø.3Ø	Other bursitis of elbow, unspecified elbow
		M7Ø.31	Other bursitis of elbow, right elbow
		M7Ø.32	Other bursitis of elbow, left elbow
		M7Ø.4Ø	Prepatellar bursitis, unspecified knee
		M7Ø.41	Prepatellar bursitis, right knee
		M7Ø.42	Prepatellar bursitis, left knee
727.3	OTHER BURSITIS DISORDERS	**M71.1Ø**	Other infective bursitis, unspecified site
		M71.11[1,2,9]	Other infective bursitis, shoulder
		M71.12[1,2,9]	Other infective bursitis, elbow
		M71.13[1,2,9]	Other infective bursitis, wrist
		M71.14[1,2,9]	Other infective bursitis, hand
		M71.15[1,2,9]	Other infective bursitis, hip
		M71.16[1,2,9]	Other infective bursitis, knee
		M71.17[1,2,9]	Other infective bursitis, ankle and foot
		M71.18	Other infective bursitis, other site
		M71.19	Other infective bursitis, multiple sites
		M71.5Ø	Other bursitis, not elsewhere classified, unspecified site
		M71.52[1,2,9]	Other bursitis, not elsewhere classified, elbow
		M71.53[1,2,9]	Other bursitis, not elsewhere classified, wrist
		M71.54[1,2,9]	Other bursitis, not elsewhere classified, hand
		M71.55[1,2,9]	Other bursitis, not elsewhere classified, hip
		M71.56[1,2,9]	Other bursitis, not elsewhere classified, knee
		M71.57[1,2,9]	Oth bursitis, not elsewhere classified, ankle and foot
		M71.58	Other bursitis, not elsewhere classified, other site
			6th Character meanings for codes as indicated ***1 Right 2 Left 9 Unspecified***
727.4Ø	UNSPECIFIED SYNOVIAL CYST	**M71.3Ø**	Other bursal cyst, unspecified site
727.41	GANGLION OF JOINT	**M67.41**[1,2,9]	Ganglion, shoulder
		M67.42[1,2,9]	Ganglion, elbow
		M67.43[1,2,9]	Ganglion, wrist
		M67.44[1,2,9]	Ganglion, hand
		M67.45[1,2,9]	Ganglion, hip
		M67.46[1,2,9]	Ganglion, knee
		M67.47[1,2,9]	Ganglion, ankle and foot
		M67.48	Ganglion, other site
		M67.49	Ganglion, multiple sites
			6th Character meanings for codes as indicated ***1 Right 2 Left 9 Unspecified***
727.42	GANGLION OF TENDON SHEATH	**M67.41**[1,2,9]	Ganglion, shoulder
		M67.42[1,2,9]	Ganglion, elbow
		M67.43[1,2,9]	Ganglion, wrist
		M67.44[1,2,9]	Ganglion, hand
		M67.45[1,2,9]	Ganglion, hip
		M67.46[1,2,9]	Ganglion, knee
		M67.47[1,2,9]	Ganglion, ankle and foot
		M67.48	Ganglion, other site
		M67.49	Ganglion, multiple sites
			6th Character meanings for codes as indicated ***1 Right 2 Left 9 Unspecified***
727.43	UNSPECIFIED GANGLION	**M67.4Ø**	Ganglion, unspecified site
727.49	OTHER GANGLION&CYST OF SYNOVIUM TENDON&BURSA	**M71.3Ø**	Other bursal cyst, unspecified site
		M71.31[1,2,9]	Other bursal cyst, shoulder
		M71.32[1,2,9]	Other bursal cyst, elbow
		M71.33[1,2,9]	Other bursal cyst, wrist
		M71.34[1,2,9]	Other bursal cyst, hand
		M71.35[1,2,9]	Other bursal cyst, hip
		M71.37[1,2,9]	Other bursal cyst, ankle and foot
		M71.38	Other bursal cyst, other site
		M71.39	Other bursal cyst, multiple sites
			6th Character meanings for codes as indicated ***1 Right 2 Left 9 Unspecified***
727.5Ø	UNSPECIFIED RUPTURE OF SYNOVIUM	➡ **M66.1Ø**	Rupture of synovium, unspecified joint
727.51	SYNOVIAL CYST OF POPLITEAL SPACE	**M66.Ø**	Rupture of popliteal cyst
		M71.2Ø	Synovial cyst of popliteal space [Baker], unspecified knee
		M71.21	Synovial cyst of popliteal space [Baker], right knee
		M71.22	Synovial cyst of popliteal space [Baker], left knee

[Brackets] indicate valid character values for each code. Character value meanings provided for each code grouping.

ICD-9-CM		ICD-10-CM	
727.59	OTHER RUPTURE OF SYNOVIUM	**M66.Ø**	Rupture of popliteal cyst
		M66.11[1,2,9]	Rupture of synovium, shoulder
		M66.12[1,2,9]	Rupture of synovium, elbow
		M66.13[1,2,9]	Rupture of synovium, wrist
		M66.14[1,2]	Rupture of synovium, hand
		M66.143	Rupture of synovium, unspecified hand
		M66.144	Rupture of synovium, right finger(s)
		M66.145	Rupture of synovium, left finger(s)
		M66.146	Rupture of synovium, unspecified finger(s)
		M66.15[1,2,9]	Rupture of synovium, hip
		M66.171	Rupture of synovium, right ankle
		M66.172	Rupture of synovium, left ankle
		M66.173	Rupture of synovium, unspecified ankle
		M66.174	Rupture of synovium, right foot
		M66.175	Rupture of synovium, left foot
		M66.176	Rupture of synovium, unspecified foot
		M66.177	Rupture of synovium, right toe(s)
		M66.178	Rupture of synovium, left toe(s)
		M66.179	Rupture of synovium, unspecified toe(s)
		M66.18	Rupture of synovium, other site
			6th Character meanings for codes as indicated ***1 Right 2 Left 9 Unspecified***
727.6Ø	NONTRAUMATIC RUPTURE OF UNSPECIFIED TENDON	**M66.2Ø**	Spontaneous rupture of extensor tendons, unspecified site
		M66.9	Spontaneous rupture of unspecified tendon
727.61	COMPLETE RUPTURE OF ROTATOR CUFF	**M75.12Ø**	Complete rotatr-cuff tear/ruptr of unsp shoulder, not trauma
		M75.121	Complete rotatr-cuff tear/ruptr of r shoulder, not trauma
		M75.122	Complete rotatr-cuff tear/ruptr of left shoulder, not trauma
727.62	NONTRAUMATIC RUPTURE OF TENDONS OF BICEPS	**M66.22**[1,2,9]	Spontaneous rupture of extensor tendons, upper arm
		M66.3Ø	Spontaneous rupture of flexor tendons, unspecified site
		M66.31[1,2,9]	Spontaneous rupture of flexor tendons, shoulder
		M66.32[1,2,9]	Spontaneous rupture of flexor tendons, upper arm
		M66.82[1,2,9]	Spontaneous rupture of other tendons, upper arm
		M66.83[1,2,9]	Spontaneous rupture of other tendons, forearm
			6th Character meanings for codes as indicated ***1 Right 2 Left 9 Unspecified***
727.63	NONTRAUMATIC RUPTURE EXTENSOR TENDONS HAND&WRIST	**M66.23**[1,2,9]	Spontaneous rupture of extensor tendons, forearm
		M66.24[1,2,9]	Spontaneous rupture of extensor tendons, hand
			6th Character meanings for codes as indicated ***1 Right 2 Left 9 Unspecified***
727.64	NONTRAUMATIC RUPTURE FLEXOR TENDONS HAND&WRIST	**M66.33**[1,2,9]	Spontaneous rupture of flexor tendons, forearm
		M66.34[1,2,9]	Spontaneous rupture of flexor tendons, hand
		M66.84[1,2,9]	Spontaneous rupture of other tendons, hand
			6th Character meanings for codes as indicated ***1 Right 2 Left 9 Unspecified***
727.65	NONTRAUMATIC RUPTURE OF QUADRICEPS TENDON	**M66.251**	Spontaneous rupture of extensor tendons, right thigh
		M66.252	Spontaneous rupture of extensor tendons, left thigh
		M66.259	Spontaneous rupture of extensor tendons, unspecified thigh
727.66	NONTRAUMATIC RUPTURE OF PATELLAR TENDON	**M66.261**	Spontaneous rupture of extensor tendons, right lower leg
		M66.262	Spontaneous rupture of extensor tendons, left lower leg
		M66.269	Spontaneous rupture of extensor tendons, unsp lower leg
727.67	NONTRAUMATIC RUPTURE OF ACHILLES TENDON	**M66.36**[1,2,9]	Spontaneous rupture of flexor tendons, lower leg
		M66.86[1,2,9]	Spontaneous rupture of other tendons, lower leg
			6th Character meanings for codes as indicated ***1 Right 2 Left 9 Unspecified***
727.68	NONTRAUMATIC RUPTURE OTHER TENDONS FOOT&ANKLE	**M66.27**[1,2,9]	Spontaneous rupture of extensor tendons, ank/ft
		M66.37[1,2,9]	Spontaneous rupture of flexor tendons, ankle and foot
		M66.87[1,2,9]	Spontaneous rupture of other tendons, ankle and foot
			6th Character meanings for codes as indicated ***1 Right 2 Left 9 Unspecified***
727.69	NONTRAUMATIC RUPTURE OF OTHER TENDON	**M66.28**	Spontaneous rupture of extensor tendons, other site
		M66.29	Spontaneous rupture of extensor tendons, multiple sites
		M66.35[1,2,9]	Spontaneous rupture of flexor tendons, thigh
		M66.38	Spontaneous rupture of flexor tendons, other site
		M66.39	Spontaneous rupture of flexor tendons, multiple sites
		M66.8Ø	Spontaneous rupture of other tendons, unspecified site
		M66.85[1,2,9]	Spontaneous rupture of other tendons, thigh
		M66.88	Spontaneous rupture of other tendons, other
		M66.89	Spontaneous rupture of other tendons, multiple sites
			6th Character meanings for codes as indicated ***1 Right 2 Left 9 Unspecified***

ICD-9-CM		ICD-10-CM	
727.81	CONTRACTURE OF TENDON	**M67.00**	Short Achilles tendon (acquired), unspecified ankle
		M67.01	Short Achilles tendon (acquired), right ankle
		M67.02	Short Achilles tendon (acquired), left ankle
727.82	CALCIUM DEPOSITS IN TENDON AND BURSA	**M65.20**	Calcific tendinitis, unspecified site
		M65.22[1,2,9]	Calcific tendinitis, upper arm
		M65.23[1,2,9]	Calcific tendinitis, forearm
		M65.24[1,2,9]	Calcific tendinitis, hand
		M65.25[1,2,9]	Calcific tendinitis, thigh
		M65.26[1,2,9]	Calcific tendinitis, lower leg
		M65.27[1,2,9]	Calcific tendinitis, ankle and foot
		M65.28	Calcific tendinitis, other site
		M65.29	Calcific tendinitis, multiple sites
		M71.40	Calcium deposit in bursa, unspecified site
		M71.42[1,2,9]	Calcium deposit in bursa, elbow
		M71.43[1,2,9]	Calcium deposit in bursa, wrist
		M71.44[1,2,9]	Calcium deposit in bursa, hand
		M71.45[1,2,9]	Calcium deposit in bursa, hip
		M71.46[1,2,9]	Calcium deposit in bursa, knee
		M71.47[1,2,9]	Calcium deposit in bursa, ankle and foot
		M71.48	Calcium deposit in bursa, other site
		M71.49	Calcium deposit in bursa, multiple sites
			6th Character meanings for codes as indicated ***1 Right*** ***2 Left*** ***9 Unspecified***
727.83	PLICA SYNDROME	**M67.50**	Plica syndrome, unspecified knee
		M67.51	Plica syndrome, right knee
		M67.52	Plica syndrome, left knee
727.89	OTHER DISORDERS SYNOVIUM TENDON AND BURSA OTHER	**M65.00**	Abscess of tendon sheath, unspecified site
		M65.01[1,2,9]	Abscess of tendon sheath, shoulder
		M65.02[1,2,9]	Abscess of tendon sheath, upper arm
		M65.03[1,2,9]	Abscess of tendon sheath, forearm
		M65.04[1,2,9]	Abscess of tendon sheath, hand
		M65.05[1,2,9]	Abscess of tendon sheath, thigh
		M65.06[1,2,9]	Abscess of tendon sheath, lower leg
		M65.07[1,2,9]	Abscess of tendon sheath, ankle and foot
		M65.08	Abscess of tendon sheath, other site
		M67.20	Synovial hypertrophy, not elsewhere classified, unsp site
		M67.21[1,2,9]	Synovial hypertrophy, NEC, shoulder
		M67.22[1,2,9]	Synovial hypertrophy, NEC, upper arm
		M67.23[1,2,9]	Synovial hypertrophy, NEC, forearm
		M67.24[1,2,9]	Synovial hypertrophy, not elsewhere classified, hand
		M67.25[1,2,9]	Synovial hypertrophy, not elsewhere classified, thigh
		M67.26[1,2,9]	Synovial hypertrophy, NEC, lower leg
		M67.27[1,2,9]	Synovial hypertrophy, NEC, ankle and foot
		M67.28	Synovial hypertrophy, not elsewhere classified, other site
		M67.29	Synovial hypertrophy, NEC, multiple sites
		M67.80	Oth disrd of synovium and tendon, unspecified site
		M67.811	Other specified disorders of synovium, right shoulder
		M67.812	Other specified disorders of synovium, left shoulder
		M67.813	Other specified disorders of tendon, right shoulder
		M67.814	Other specified disorders of tendon, left shoulder
		M67.819	Oth disrd of synovium and tendon, unspecified shoulder
		M67.821	Other specified disorders of synovium, right elbow
		M67.822	Other specified disorders of synovium, left elbow
		M67.823	Other specified disorders of tendon, right elbow
		M67.824	Other specified disorders of tendon, left elbow
		M67.829	Oth disrd of synovium and tendon, unspecified elbow
		M67.831	Other specified disorders of synovium, right wrist
		M67.832	Other specified disorders of synovium, left wrist
		M67.833	Other specified disorders of tendon, right wrist
		M67.834	Other specified disorders of tendon, left wrist
		M67.839	Oth disrd of synovium and tendon, unspecified forearm
		M67.841	Other specified disorders of synovium, right hand
		M67.842	Other specified disorders of synovium, left hand
		M67.843	Other specified disorders of tendon, right hand
		M67.844	Other specified disorders of tendon, left hand
		M67.849	Oth disrd of synovium and tendon, unspecified hand
		M67.851	Other specified disorders of synovium, right hip
		M67.852	Other specified disorders of synovium, left hip
		M67.853	Other specified disorders of tendon, right hip
		M67.854	Other specified disorders of tendon, left hip
		M67.859	Oth disrd of synovium and tendon, unspecified hip
		M67.861	Other specified disorders of synovium, right knee
		M67.862	Other specified disorders of synovium, left knee
		M67.863	Other specified disorders of tendon, right knee
		M67.864	Other specified disorders of tendon, left knee
		M67.869	Oth disrd of synovium and tendon, unspecified knee
		M67.871	Other specified disorders of synovium, right ankle and foot
		M67.872	Other specified disorders of synovium, left ankle and foot
			6th Character meanings for codes as indicated ***1 Right*** ***2 Left*** ***9 Unspecified***

(Continued on next page)

ICD-9-CM		ICD-10-CM	
727.89	OTHER DISORDERS SYNOVIUM TENDON AND BURSA OTHER **(Continued)**	**M67.873**	Other specified disorders of tendon, right ankle and foot
		M67.874	Other specified disorders of tendon, left ankle and foot
		M67.879	Oth disrd of synovium and tendon, unspecified ankle and foot
		M67.88	Other specified disorders of synovium and tendon, other site
		M67.89	Oth disrd of synovium and tendon, multiple sites
		M71.ØØ	Abscess of bursa, unspecified site
		M71.Ø1[1,2,9]	Abscess of bursa, shoulder
		M71.Ø2[1,2,9]	Abscess of bursa, elbow
		M71.Ø3[1,2,9]	Abscess of bursa, wrist
		M71.Ø4[1,2,9]	Abscess of bursa, hand
		M71.Ø5[1,2,9]	Abscess of bursa, hip
		M71.Ø6[1,2,9]	Abscess of bursa, knee
		M71.Ø7[1,2,9]	Abscess of bursa, ankle and foot
		M71.Ø8	Abscess of bursa, other site
		M71.Ø9	Abscess of bursa, multiple sites
		M71.8Ø	Other specified bursopathies, unspecified site
		M71.81[1,2,9]	Other specified bursopathies, shoulder
		M71.82[1,2,9]	Other specified bursopathies, elbow
		M71.83[1,2,9]	Other specified bursopathies, wrist
		M71.84[1,2,9]	Other specified bursopathies, hand
		M71.85[1,2,9]	Other specified bursopathies, hip
		M71.86[1,2,9]	Other specified bursopathies, knee
		M71.87[1,2,9]	Other specified bursopathies, ankle and foot
		M71.88	Other specified bursopathies, other site
		M71.89	Other specified bursopathies, multiple sites
			6th Character meanings for codes as indicated ***1 Right 2 Left 9 Unspecified***
727.9	UNSPECIFIED DISORDER OF SYNOVIUM TENDON&BURSA	**M67.9Ø**	Unsp disorder of synovium and tendon, unspecified site
		M67.91[1,2,9]	Unspecified disorder of synovium and tendon, shoulder
		M67.92[1,2,9]	Unspecified disorder of synovium and tendon, upper arm
		M67.93[1,2,9]	Unspecified disorder of synovium and tendon, forearm
		M67.94[1,2,9]	Unspecified disorder of synovium and tendon, hand
		M67.95[1,2,9]	Unspecified disorder of synovium and tendon, thigh
		M67.96[1,2,9]	Unspecified disorder of synovium and tendon, lower leg
		M67.97[1,2,9]	Unsp disorder of synovium and tendon, ankle and foot
		M67.98	Unspecified disorder of synovium and tendon, other site
		M67.99	Unspecified disorder of synovium and tendon, multiple sites
		M71.9	Bursopathy, unspecified
			6th Character meanings for codes as indicated ***1 Right 2 Left 9 Unspecified***
728.Ø	INFECTIVE MYOSITIS	**M6Ø.ØØØ**	Infective myositis, unspecified right arm
		M6Ø.ØØ1	Infective myositis, unspecified left arm
		M6Ø.ØØ2	Infective myositis, unspecified arm
		M6Ø.ØØ3	Infective myositis, unspecified right leg
		M6Ø.ØØ4	Infective myositis, unspecified left leg
		M6Ø.ØØ5	Infective myositis, unspecified leg
		M6Ø.ØØ9	Infective myositis, unspecified site
		M6Ø.Ø1[1,2,9]	Infective myositis, shoulder
		M6Ø.Ø2[1,2,9]	Infective myositis, upper arm
		M6Ø.Ø3[1,2,9]	Infective myositis, forearm
		M6Ø.Ø41	Infective myositis, right hand
		M6Ø.Ø42	Infective myositis, left hand
		M6Ø.Ø43	Infective myositis, unspecified hand
		M6Ø.Ø44	Infective myositis, right finger(s)
		M6Ø.Ø45	Infective myositis, left finger(s)
		M6Ø.Ø46	Infective myositis, unspecified finger(s)
		M6Ø.Ø5[1,2,9]	Infective myositis, thigh
		M6Ø.Ø6[1,2,9]	Infective myositis, lower leg
		M6Ø.Ø7Ø	Infective myositis, right ankle
		M6Ø.Ø71	Infective myositis, left ankle
		M6Ø.Ø72	Infective myositis, unspecified ankle
		M6Ø.Ø73	Infective myositis, right foot
		M6Ø.Ø74	Infective myositis, left foot
		M6Ø.Ø75	Infective myositis, unspecified foot
		M6Ø.Ø76	Infective myositis, right toe(s)
		M6Ø.Ø77	Infective myositis, left toe(s)
		M6Ø.Ø78	Infective myositis, unspecified toe(s)
		M6Ø.Ø8	Infective myositis, other site
		M6Ø.Ø9	Infective myositis, multiple sites
			6th Character meanings for codes as indicated ***1 Right 2 Left 9 Unspecified***

ICD-9-CM		ICD-10-CM	
728.10	UNSPECIFIED CALCIFICATION AND OSSIFICATION	**M61.20**	Paralytic calcifcn and ossification of muscle, unsp site
		M61.21[1,2,9]	Paralytic calcifcn and ossification of muscle, shoulder
		M61.22[1,2,9]	Paralytic calcification and ossification of muscle, up arm
		M61.23[1,2,9]	Paralytic calcifcn and ossification of muscle, forearm
		M61.24[1,2,9]	Paralytic calcifcn and ossification of muscle, hand
		M61.25[1,2,9]	Paralytic calcifcn and ossification of muscle, thigh
		M61.26[1,2,9]	Paralytic calcifcn and ossification of muscle, low leg
		M61.27[1,2,9]	Paralytic calcifcn and ossification of muscle, ank/ft
		M61.28	Paralytic calcification and ossification of muscle, oth site
		M61.29	Paralytic calcifcn and ossifictn of muscle, multiple sites
		M61.9	Calcification and ossification of muscle, unspecified
			6th Character meanings for codes as indicated ***1 Right*** ***2 Left*** ***9 Unspecified***
728.11	PROGRESSIVE MYOSITIS OSSIFICANS	**M61.10**	Myositis ossificans progressiva, unspecified site
		M61.11[1,2,9]	Myositis ossificans progressiva, shoulder
		M61.12[1,2,9]	Myositis ossificans progressiva, upper arm
		M61.13[1,2,9]	Myositis ossificans progressiva, forearm
		M61.141	Myositis ossificans progressiva, right hand
		M61.142	Myositis ossificans progressiva, left hand
		M61.143	Myositis ossificans progressiva, unspecified hand
		M61.144	Myositis ossificans progressiva, right finger(s)
		M61.145	Myositis ossificans progressiva, left finger(s)
		M61.146	Myositis ossificans progressiva, unspecified finger(s)
		M61.15[1,2,9]	Myositis ossificans progressiva, thigh
		M61.16[1,2,9]	Myositis ossificans progressiva, lower leg
		M61.171	Myositis ossificans progressiva, right ankle
		M61.172	Myositis ossificans progressiva, left ankle
		M61.173	Myositis ossificans progressiva, unspecified ankle
		M61.174	Myositis ossificans progressiva, right foot
		M61.175	Myositis ossificans progressiva, left foot
		M61.176	Myositis ossificans progressiva, unspecified foot
		M61.177	Myositis ossificans progressiva, right toe(s)
		M61.178	Myositis ossificans progressiva, left toe(s)
		M61.179	Myositis ossificans progressiva, unspecified toe(s)
		M61.18	Myositis ossificans progressiva, other site
		M61.19	Myositis ossificans progressiva, multiple sites
			6th Character meanings for codes as indicated ***1 Right*** ***2 Left*** ***9 Unspecified***
728.12	TRAUMATIC MYOSITIS OSSIFICANS	**M61.00**	Myositis ossificans traumatica, unspecified site
		M61.01[1,2,9]	Myositis ossificans traumatica, shoulder
		M61.02[1,2,9]	Myositis ossificans traumatica, upper arm
		M61.03[1,2,9]	Myositis ossificans traumatica, forearm
		M61.04[1,2,9]	Myositis ossificans traumatica, hand
		M61.05[1,2,9]	Myositis ossificans traumatica, thigh
		M61.06[1,2,9]	Myositis ossificans traumatica, lower leg
		M61.07[1,2,9]	Myositis ossificans traumatica, ankle and foot
		M61.08	Myositis ossificans traumatica, other site
		M61.09	Myositis ossificans traumatica, multiple sites
			6th Character meanings for codes as indicated ***1 Right*** ***2 Left*** ***9 Unspecified***
728.13	POSTOPERATIVE HETEROTOPIC CALCIFICATION	**M61.40**	Other calcification of muscle, unspecified site
728.19	OTHER MUSCULAR CALCIFICATION AND OSSIFICATION	**M61.30**	Calcifcn and ossifictn of muscles assoc w burns, unsp site
		M61.31[1,2,9]	Calcifcn and ossifictn of muscles assoc w burns, shoulder
		M61.32[1,2,9]	Calcifcn and ossifictn of muscles assoc w burns, up arm
		M61.33[1,2,9]	Calcifcn and ossifictn of muscles assoc w burns, forearm
		M61.34[1,2,9]	Calcifcn and ossifictn of muscles assoc w burns, hand
		M61.35[1,2,9]	Calcifcn and ossifictn of muscles assoc w burns, thigh
		M61.36[1,2,9]	Calcifcn and ossifictn of muscles assoc w burns, low leg
		M61.37[1,2,9]	Calcifcn and ossifictn of musc assoc w burns, ank/ft
		M61.38	Calcifcn and ossifictn of muscles assoc w burns, oth site
		M61.39	Calcifcn and ossifictn of muscles assoc w burns, mult sites
		M61.40	Other calcification of muscle, unspecified site
		M61.41[1,2,9]	Other calcification of muscle, shoulder
		M61.42[1,2,9]	Other calcification of muscle, upper arm
		M61.43[1,2,9]	Other calcification of muscle, forearm
		M61.44[1,2,9]	Other calcification of muscle, hand
		M61.45[1,2,9]	Other calcification of muscle, thigh
		M61.46[1,2,9]	Other calcification of muscle, lower leg
		M61.47[1,2,9]	Other calcification of muscle, ankle and foot
		M61.48	Other calcification of muscle, other site
		M61.49	Other calcification of muscle, multiple sites
		M61.50	Other ossification of muscle, unspecified site
		M61.51[1,2,9]	Other ossification of muscle, shoulder
		M61.52[1,2,9]	Other ossification of muscle, upper arm
		M61.53[1,2,9]	Other ossification of muscle, forearm
			6th Character meanings for codes as indicated ***1 Right*** ***2 Left*** ***9 Unspecified***

(Continued on next page)

ICD-9-CM		ICD-10-CM	
728.19	OTHER MUSCULAR CALCIFICATION AND OSSIFICATION (Continued)	M61.54[1,2,9]	Other ossification of muscle, hand
		M61.55[1,2,9]	Other ossification of muscle, thigh
		M61.56[1,2,9]	Other ossification of muscle, lower leg
		M61.57[1,2,9]	Other ossification of muscle, ankle and foot
		M61.58	Other ossification of muscle, other site
		M61.59	Other ossification of muscle, multiple sites
			6th Character meanings for codes as indicated *1 Right 2 Left 9 Unspecified*
728.2	MUSCULAR WASTING AND DISUSE ATROPHY NEC	M62.50	Muscle wasting and atrophy, NEC, unsp site
		M62.51[1,2,9]	Muscle wasting and atrophy, NEC, shoulder
		M62.52[1,2,9]	Muscle wasting and atrophy, NEC, upper arm
		M62.53[1,2,9]	Muscle wasting and atrophy, NEC, forearm
		M62.54[1,2,9]	Muscle wasting and atrophy, NEC, hand
		M62.55[1,2,9]	Muscle wasting and atrophy, NEC, thigh
		M62.56[1,2,9]	Muscle wasting and atrophy, NEC, lower leg
		M62.57[1,2,9]	Muscle wasting and atrophy, NEC, ankle and foot
		M62.58	Muscle wasting and atrophy, NEC, oth site
		M62.59	Muscle wasting and atrophy, NEC, multiple sites
			6th Character meanings for codes as indicated *1 Right 2 Left 9 Unspecified*
728.3	OTHER SPECIFIC MUSCLE DISORDERS	M62.3	Immobility syndrome (paraplegic)
		M62.89	Other specified disorders of muscle
728.4	LAXITY OF LIGAMENT	M24.20	Disorder of ligament, unspecified site
		M24.21[1,2,9]	Disorder of ligament, shoulder
		M24.22[1,2,9]	Disorder of ligament, elbow
		M24.23[1,2,9]	Disorder of ligament, wrist
		M24.24[1,2,9]	Disorder of ligament, hand
		M24.25[1,2,9]	Disorder of ligament, hip
		M24.27[1,2,3]	Disorder of ligament, ankle
		M24.274	Disorder of ligament, right foot
		M24.275	Disorder of ligament, left foot
		M24.276	Disorder of ligament, unspecified foot
		M24.28	Disorder of ligament, vertebrae
			6th Character meanings for codes as indicated *1 Right 2 Left 3 or 9 Unspecified*
728.5	HYPERMOBILITY SYNDROME	➡ M35.7	Hypermobility syndrome
728.6	CONTRACTURE OF PALMAR FASCIA	➡ M72.0	Palmar fascial fibromatosis [Dupuytren]
728.71	PLANTAR FASCIAL FIBROMATOSIS	➡ M72.2	Plantar fascial fibromatosis
728.79	OTH FIBROMATOSES MUSCLE LIGAMENT AND FASCIA OTH	M72.1	Knuckle pads
		M72.4	Pseudosarcomatous fibromatosis
		M72.9	Fibroblastic disorder, unspecified
728.81	INTERSTITIAL MYOSITIS	M60.10	Interstitial myositis of unspecified site
		M60.11[1,2,9]	Interstitial myositis, shoulder
		M60.12[1,2,9]	Interstitial myositis, upper arm
		M60.13[1,2,9]	Interstitial myositis, forearm
		M60.14[1,2,9]	Interstitial myositis, hand
		M60.15[1,2,9]	Interstitial myositis, thigh
		M60.16[1,2,9]	Interstitial myositis, lower leg
		M60.17[1,2,9]	Interstitial myositis, ankle and foot
		M60.18	Interstitial myositis, other site
		M60.19	Interstitial myositis, multiple sites
			6th Character meanings for codes as indicated *1 Right 2 Left 9 Unspecified*
728.82	FOREIGN BODY GRANULOMA OF MUSCLE	M60.20	Foreign body granuloma of soft tissue, NEC, unsp site
		M60.21[1,2,9]	Foreign body granuloma of soft tissue, NEC, shoulder
		M60.22[1,2,9]	Foreign body granuloma of soft tissue, NEC, upper arm
		M60.23[1,2,9]	Foreign body granuloma of soft tissue, NEC, forearm
		M60.24[1,2,9]	Foreign body granuloma of soft tissue, NEC, hand
		M60.25[1,2,9]	Foreign body granuloma of soft tissue, NEC, thigh
		M60.26[1,2,9]	Foreign body granuloma of soft tissue, NEC, lower leg
		M60.27[1,2,9]	Foreign body granuloma of soft tissue, NEC, ank/ft
		M60.28	Foreign body granuloma of soft tissue, NEC, oth site
			6th Character meanings for codes as indicated *1 Right 2 Left 9 Unspecified*

ICD-9-CM		ICD-10-CM	
728.83	RUPTURE OF MUSCLE, NONTRAUMATIC	**M62.1Ø**	Other rupture of muscle (nontraumatic), unspecified site
		M62.11[1,2,9]	Other rupture of muscle (nontraumatic), shoulder
		M62.12[1,2,9]	Other rupture of muscle (nontraumatic), upper arm
		M62.13[1,2,9]	Other rupture of muscle (nontraumatic), forearm
		M62.14[1,2,9]	Other rupture of muscle (nontraumatic), hand
		M62.15[1,2,9]	Other rupture of muscle (nontraumatic), thigh
		M62.16[1,2,9]	Other rupture of muscle (nontraumatic), lower leg
		M62.17[1,2,9]	Other rupture of muscle (nontraumatic), ankle and foot
		M62.18	Other rupture of muscle (nontraumatic), other site
			6th Character meanings for codes as indicated ***1 Right*** ***2 Left*** ***9 Unspecified***
728.84	DIASTASIS OF MUSCLE	**M62.ØØ**	Separation of muscle (nontraumatic), unspecified site
		M62.Ø1[1,2,9]	Separation of muscle (nontraumatic), shoulder
		M62.Ø2[1,2,9]	Separation of muscle (nontraumatic), upper arm
		M62.Ø3[1,2,9]	Separation of muscle (nontraumatic), forearm
		M62.Ø4[1,2,9]	Separation of muscle (nontraumatic), hand
		M62.Ø5[1,2,9]	Separation of muscle (nontraumatic), thigh
		M62.Ø6[1,2,9]	Separation of muscle (nontraumatic), lower leg
		M62.Ø7[1,2,9]	Separation of muscle (nontraumatic), ankle and foot
		M62.Ø8	Separation of muscle (nontraumatic), other site
			6th Character meanings for codes as indicated ***1 Right*** ***2 Left*** ***9 Unspecified***
728.85	SPASM OF MUSCLE	**M62.4Ø**	Contracture of muscle, unspecified site
		M62.41[1,2,9]	Contracture of muscle, shoulder
		M62.42[1,2,9]	Contracture of muscle, upper arm
		M62.43[1,2,9]	Contracture of muscle, forearm
		M62.44[1,2,9]	Contracture of muscle, hand
		M62.45[1,2,9]	Contracture of muscle, thigh
		M62.46[1,2,9]	Contracture of muscle, lower leg
		M62.47[1,2,9]	Contracture of muscle, ankle and foot
		M62.48	Contracture of muscle, other site
		M62.49	Contracture of muscle, multiple sites
		M62.831	Muscle spasm of calf
		M62.838	Other muscle spasm
			6th Character meanings for codes as indicated ***1 Right*** ***2 Left*** ***9 Unspecified***
728.86	NECROTIZING FASCIITIS	➡ **M72.6**	Necrotizing fasciitis
728.87	MUSCLE WEAKNESS (GENERALIZED)	➡ **M62.81**	Muscle weakness (generalized)
728.88	RHABDOMYOLYSIS	➡ **M62.82**	Rhabdomyolysis
728.89	OTHER DISORDER OF MUSCLE LIGAMENT AND FASCIA	**M35.4**	Diffuse (eosinophilic) fasciitis
		M62.2Ø	Nontraumatic ischemic infarction of muscle, unspecified site
		M62.21[1,2,9]	Nontraumatic ischemic infarction of muscle, shoulder
		M62.22[1,2,9]	Nontraumatic ischemic infarction of muscle, upper arm
		M62.23[1,2,9]	Nontraumatic ischemic infarction of muscle, forearm
		M62.24[1,2,9]	Nontraumatic ischemic infarction of muscle, hand
		M62.25[1,2,9]	Nontraumatic ischemic infarction of muscle, thigh
		M62.26[1,2,9]	Nontraumatic ischemic infarction of muscle, lower leg
		M62.27[1,2,9]	Nontraumatic ischemic infarction of muscle, ank/ft
		M62.28	Nontraumatic ischemic infarction of muscle, other site
		M62.89	Other specified disorders of muscle
		M72.8	Other fibroblastic disorders
			6th Character meanings for codes as indicated ***1 Right*** ***2 Left*** ***9 Unspecified***
728.9	UNSPECIFIED DISORDER OF MUSCLE LIGAMENT&FASCIA	**M62.9**	Disorder of muscle, unspecified
		M63.8Ø	Disorders of muscle in diseases classd elswhr, unsp site
		M63.81[1,2,9]	Disorders of muscle in diseases classd elswhr, shoulder
		M63.82[1,2,9]	Disorders of muscle in diseases classd elswhr, up arm
		M63.83[1,2,9]	Disorders of muscle in diseases classd elswhr, forearm
		M63.84[1,2,9]	Disorders of muscle in diseases classd elswhr, hand
		M63.85[1,2,9]	Disorders of muscle in diseases classd elswhr, thigh
		M63.86[1,2,9]	Disorders of muscle in diseases classd elswhr, low leg
		M63.87[1,2,9]	Disorders of muscle in diseases classd elswhr, ank/ft
		M63.88	Disorders of muscle in diseases classd elswhr, oth site
		M63.89	Disord of muscle in diseases classd elswhr, multiple sites
			6th Character meanings for codes as indicated ***1 Right*** ***2 Left*** ***9 Unspecified***
729.Ø	RHEUMATISM UNSPECIFIED AND FIBROSITIS	➡ **M79.Ø**	Rheumatism, unspecified

ICD-9-CM		ICD-10-CM	
729.1	UNSPECIFIED MYALGIA AND MYOSITIS	M60.80	Other myositis, unspecified site
		M60.81[1,2,9]	Other myositis, shoulder
		M60.82[1,2,9]	Other myositis, upper arm
		M60.83[1,2,9]	Other myositis, forearm
		M60.84[1,2,9]	Other myositis, hand
		M60.85[1,2,9]	Other myositis, thigh
		M60.86[1,2,9]	Other myositis, lower leg
		M60.87[1,2,9]	Other myositis, ankle and foot
		M60.88	Other myositis, other site
		M60.89	Other myositis, multiple sites
		M60.9	Myositis, unspecified
		M79.1	Myalgia
		M79.7	Fibromyalgia
			6th Character meanings for codes as indicated *1 Right* *2 Left* *9 Unspecified*
729.2	UNSPECIFIED NEURALGIA NEURITIS AND RADICULITIS	M54.10	Radiculopathy, site unspecified
		M54.18	Radiculopathy, sacral and sacrococcygeal region
		M79.2	Neuralgia and neuritis, unspecified
729.30	PANNICULITIS, UNSPECIFIED SITE	M35.6	Relapsing panniculitis [Weber-Christian]
		M79.3	Panniculitis, unspecified
729.31	HYPERTROPHY OF FAT PAD, KNEE	➡ M79.4	Hypertrophy of (infrapatellar) fat pad
729.39	PANNICULITIS OF OTHER SITES	M79.3	Panniculitis, unspecified
729.4	UNSPECIFIED FASCIITIS	M72.9	Fibroblastic disorder, unspecified
729.5	PAIN IN SOFT TISSUES OF LIMB	M79.601	Pain in right arm
		M79.602	Pain in left arm
		M79.603	Pain in arm, unspecified
		M79.604	Pain in right leg
		M79.605	Pain in left leg
		M79.606	Pain in leg, unspecified
		M79.609	Pain in unspecified limb
		M79.62[1,2,9]	Pain in upper arm
		M79.63[1,2,9]	Pain in forearm
		M79.641	Pain in right hand
		M79.642	Pain in left hand
		M79.643	Pain in unspecified hand
		M79.644	Pain in right finger(s)
		M79.645	Pain in left finger(s)
		M79.646	Pain in unspecified finger(s)
		M79.65[1,2,9]	Pain in thigh
		M79.66[1,2,9]	Pain in lower leg
		M79.671	Pain in right foot
		M79.672	Pain in left foot
		M79.673	Pain in unspecified foot
		M79.674	Pain in right toe(s)
		M79.675	Pain in left toe(s)
		M79.676	Pain in unspecified toe(s)
			6th Character meanings for codes as indicated *1 Right* *2 Left* *9 Unspecified*
729.6	RESIDUAL FOREIGN BODY IN SOFT TISSUE	➡ M79.5	Residual foreign body in soft tissue
729.71	NONTRAUMATIC COMPARTMENT SYNDROME UPPER EXTREM	M79.A11	Nontraumatic compartment syndrome of right upper extremity
		M79.A12	Nontraumatic compartment syndrome of left upper extremity
		M79.A19	Nontraumatic compartment syndrome of unsp upper extremity
729.72	NONTRAUMATIC COMPARTMENT SYNDROME LOWER EXTREM	M79.A21	Nontraumatic compartment syndrome of right lower extremity
		M79.A22	Nontraumatic compartment syndrome of left lower extremity
		M79.A29	Nontraumatic compartment syndrome of unsp lower extremity
729.73	NONTRAUMATIC COMPARTMENT SYNDROME OF ABDOMEN	➡ M79.A3	Nontraumatic compartment syndrome of abdomen
729.79	NONTRAUMATIC COMPARTMENT SYNDROME OF OTHER SITES	➡ M79.A9	Nontraumatic compartment syndrome of other sites
729.81	SWELLING OF LIMB	M79.89	Other specified soft tissue disorders
729.82	CRAMP OF LIMB	R25.2	Cramp and spasm
729.89	OTH MUSCULOSKELETAL SX REFERABLE LIMBS OTH	R29.898	Oth symptoms and signs involving the musculoskeletal system
729.90	DISORDERS OF SOFT TISSUE UNSPECIFIED	M70.90	Unsp soft tissue disord related to use/pressure of unsp site
		M70.91[1,2,9]	Unsp soft tissue disord related to use/pressure, shoulder
		M70.92[1,2,9]	Unsp soft tissue disorder related to use/pressure, up arm
		M70.93[1,2,9]	Unsp soft tissue disorder related to use/pressure, forearm
		M70.94[1,2,9]	Unsp soft tissue disorder related to use/pressure, hand
		M70.95[1,2,9]	Unsp soft tissue disord related to use/pressure, thigh
		M70.96[1,2,9]	Unsp soft tissue disorder related to use/pressure, low leg
		M70.97[1,2,9]	Unsp soft tissue disord rel to use/pressure, ank/ft
		M70.98	Unsp soft tissue disorder related to use/pressure oth
		M70.99	Unsp soft tissue disord related to use/pressure mult sites
		M79.9	Soft tissue disorder, unspecified
			6th Character meanings for codes as indicated *1 Right* *2 Left* *9 Unspecified*
729.91	POST-TRAUMATIC SEROMA	M70.98	Unsp soft tissue disorder related to use/pressure oth
729.92	NONTRAUMATIC HEMATOMA OF SOFT TISSUE	➡ M79.81	Nontraumatic hematoma of soft tissue

ICD-9-CM		ICD-10-CM	
729.99	OTHER DISORDERS OF SOFT TISSUE	**M70.80**	Oth soft tissue disord related to use/pressure of unsp site
		M70.81[1,2,9]	Oth soft tissue disord related to use/pressure, shoulder
		M70.82[1,2,9]	Oth soft tissue disorders related to use/pressure, up arm
		M70.83[1,2,9]	Oth soft tissue disorders related to use/pressure, forearm
		M70.84[1,2,9]	Oth soft tissue disorders related to use/pressure, hand
		M70.85[1,2,9]	Oth soft tissue disord related to use/pressure, thigh
		M70.86[1,2,9]	Oth soft tissue disorders related to use/pressure, low leg
		M70.87[1,2,9]	Oth soft tissue disord related to use/pressure, ank/ft
		M70.88	Oth soft tissue disorders related to use/pressure oth site
		M70.89	Oth soft tissue disord related to use/pressure mult sites
		M79.89	Other specified soft tissue disorders
			6th Character meanings for codes as indicated ***1 Right 2 Left 9 Unspecified***
730.00	ACUTE OSTEOMYELITIS SITE UNSPECIFIED	**M86.00**	Acute hematogenous osteomyelitis, unspecified site
		M86.10	Other acute osteomyelitis, unspecified site
		M86.20	Subacute osteomyelitis, unspecified site
730.01	ACUTE OSTEOMYELITIS SHOULDER REGION	**M86.011**	Acute hematogenous osteomyelitis, right shoulder
		M86.012	Acute hematogenous osteomyelitis, left shoulder
		M86.019	Acute hematogenous osteomyelitis, unspecified shoulder
		M86.111	Other acute osteomyelitis, right shoulder
		M86.112	Other acute osteomyelitis, left shoulder
		M86.119	Other acute osteomyelitis, unspecified shoulder
		M86.211	Subacute osteomyelitis, right shoulder
		M86.212	Subacute osteomyelitis, left shoulder
		M86.219	Subacute osteomyelitis, unspecified shoulder
730.02	ACUTE OSTEOMYELITIS, UPPER ARM	**M86.021**	Acute hematogenous osteomyelitis, right humerus
		M86.022	Acute hematogenous osteomyelitis, left humerus
		M86.029	Acute hematogenous osteomyelitis, unspecified humerus
		M86.121	Other acute osteomyelitis, right humerus
		M86.122	Other acute osteomyelitis, left humerus
		M86.129	Other acute osteomyelitis, unspecified humerus
		M86.221	Subacute osteomyelitis, right humerus
		M86.222	Subacute osteomyelitis, left humerus
		M86.229	Subacute osteomyelitis, unspecified humerus
730.03	ACUTE OSTEOMYELITIS, FOREARM	**M86.031**	Acute hematogenous osteomyelitis, right radius and ulna
		M86.032	Acute hematogenous osteomyelitis, left radius and ulna
		M86.039	Acute hematogenous osteomyelitis, unsp radius and ulna
		M86.131	Other acute osteomyelitis, right radius and ulna
		M86.132	Other acute osteomyelitis, left radius and ulna
		M86.139	Other acute osteomyelitis, unspecified radius and ulna
		M86.231	Subacute osteomyelitis, right radius and ulna
		M86.232	Subacute osteomyelitis, left radius and ulna
		M86.239	Subacute osteomyelitis, unspecified radius and ulna
730.04	ACUTE OSTEOMYELITIS, HAND	**M86.041**	Acute hematogenous osteomyelitis, right hand
		M86.042	Acute hematogenous osteomyelitis, left hand
		M86.049	Acute hematogenous osteomyelitis, unspecified hand
		M86.141	Other acute osteomyelitis, right hand
		M86.142	Other acute osteomyelitis, left hand
		M86.149	Other acute osteomyelitis, unspecified hand
		M86.241	Subacute osteomyelitis, right hand
		M86.242	Subacute osteomyelitis, left hand
		M86.249	Subacute osteomyelitis, unspecified hand
730.05	ACUTE OSTEOMYELITIS PELVIC REGION AND THIGH	**M86.051**	Acute hematogenous osteomyelitis, right femur
		M86.052	Acute hematogenous osteomyelitis, left femur
		M86.059	Acute hematogenous osteomyelitis, unspecified femur
		M86.151	Other acute osteomyelitis, right femur
		M86.152	Other acute osteomyelitis, left femur
		M86.159	Other acute osteomyelitis, unspecified femur
		M86.251	Subacute osteomyelitis, right femur
		M86.252	Subacute osteomyelitis, left femur
		M86.259	Subacute osteomyelitis, unspecified femur
730.06	ACUTE OSTEOMYELITIS, LOWER LEG	**M86.061**	Acute hematogenous osteomyelitis, right tibia and fibula
		M86.062	Acute hematogenous osteomyelitis, left tibia and fibula
		M86.069	Acute hematogenous osteomyelitis, unsp tibia and fibula
		M86.161	Other acute osteomyelitis, right tibia and fibula
		M86.162	Other acute osteomyelitis, left tibia and fibula
		M86.169	Other acute osteomyelitis, unspecified tibia and fibula
		M86.261	Subacute osteomyelitis, right tibia and fibula
		M86.262	Subacute osteomyelitis, left tibia and fibula
		M86.269	Subacute osteomyelitis, unspecified tibia and fibula
730.07	ACUTE OSTEOMYELITIS, ANKLE AND FOOT	**M86.071**	Acute hematogenous osteomyelitis, right ankle and foot
		M86.072	Acute hematogenous osteomyelitis, left ankle and foot
		M86.079	Acute hematogenous osteomyelitis, unspecified ankle and foot
		M86.171	Other acute osteomyelitis, right ankle and foot
		M86.172	Other acute osteomyelitis, left ankle and foot
		M86.179	Other acute osteomyelitis, unspecified ankle and foot
		M86.271	Subacute osteomyelitis, right ankle and foot
		M86.272	Subacute osteomyelitis, left ankle and foot
		M86.279	Subacute osteomyelitis, unspecified ankle and foot

[Brackets] indicate valid character values for each code. Character value meanings provided for each code grouping.

ICD-9-CM		ICD-10-CM	
73Ø.Ø8	ACUTE OSTEOMYELITIS OTHER SPECIFIED SITE	**M86.Ø8**	Acute hematogenous osteomyelitis, other sites
		M86.18	Other acute osteomyelitis, other site
		M86.28	Subacute osteomyelitis, other site
73Ø.Ø9	ACUTE OSTEOMYELITIS, MULTIPLE SITES	**M86.Ø9**	Acute hematogenous osteomyelitis, multiple sites
		M86.19	Other acute osteomyelitis, multiple sites
		M86.29	Subacute osteomyelitis, multiple sites
73Ø.1Ø	CHRONIC OSTEOMYELITIS SITE UNSPECIFIED	**M86.3Ø**	Chronic multifocal osteomyelitis, unspecified site
		M86.4Ø	Chronic osteomyelitis with draining sinus, unspecified site
		M86.5Ø	Other chronic hematogenous osteomyelitis, unspecified site
		M86.6Ø	Other chronic osteomyelitis, unspecified site
		M86.8X9	Other osteomyelitis, unspecified sites
73Ø.11	CHRONIC OSTEOMYELITIS SHOULDER REGION	**M86.311**	Chronic multifocal osteomyelitis, right shoulder
		M86.312	Chronic multifocal osteomyelitis, left shoulder
		M86.319	Chronic multifocal osteomyelitis, unspecified shoulder
		M86.411	Chronic osteomyelitis with draining sinus, right shoulder
		M86.412	Chronic osteomyelitis with draining sinus, left shoulder
		M86.419	Chronic osteomyelitis with draining sinus, unsp shoulder
		M86.511	Other chronic hematogenous osteomyelitis, right shoulder
		M86.512	Other chronic hematogenous osteomyelitis, left shoulder
		M86.519	Other chronic hematogenous osteomyelitis, unsp shoulder
		M86.611	Other chronic osteomyelitis, right shoulder
		M86.612	Other chronic osteomyelitis, left shoulder
		M86.619	Other chronic osteomyelitis, unspecified shoulder
		M86.8X1	Other osteomyelitis, shoulder
73Ø.12	CHRONIC OSTEOMYELITIS, UPPER ARM	**M86.321**	Chronic multifocal osteomyelitis, right humerus
		M86.322	Chronic multifocal osteomyelitis, left humerus
		M86.329	Chronic multifocal osteomyelitis, unspecified humerus
		M86.421	Chronic osteomyelitis with draining sinus, right humerus
		M86.422	Chronic osteomyelitis with draining sinus, left humerus
		M86.429	Chronic osteomyelitis with draining sinus, unsp humerus
		M86.521	Other chronic hematogenous osteomyelitis, right humerus
		M86.522	Other chronic hematogenous osteomyelitis, left humerus
		M86.529	Other chronic hematogenous osteomyelitis, unsp humerus
		M86.621	Other chronic osteomyelitis, right humerus
		M86.622	Other chronic osteomyelitis, left humerus
		M86.629	Other chronic osteomyelitis, unspecified humerus
		M86.8X2	Other osteomyelitis, upper arm
73Ø.13	CHRONIC OSTEOMYELITIS, FOREARM	**M86.331**	Chronic multifocal osteomyelitis, right radius and ulna
		M86.332	Chronic multifocal osteomyelitis, left radius and ulna
		M86.339	Chronic multifocal osteomyelitis, unsp radius and ulna
		M86.431	Chronic osteomyelit w draining sinus, right radius and ulna
		M86.432	Chronic osteomyelitis w draining sinus, left radius and ulna
		M86.439	Chronic osteomyelitis w draining sinus, unsp radius and ulna
		M86.531	Oth chronic hematogenous osteomyelit, right radius and ulna
		M86.532	Oth chronic hematogenous osteomyelitis, left radius and ulna
		M86.539	Oth chronic hematogenous osteomyelitis, unsp radius and ulna
		M86.631	Other chronic osteomyelitis, right radius and ulna
		M86.632	Other chronic osteomyelitis, left radius and ulna
		M86.639	Other chronic osteomyelitis, unspecified radius and ulna
		M86.8X3	Other osteomyelitis, forearm
73Ø.14	CHRONIC OSTEOMYELITIS, HAND	**M86.341**	Chronic multifocal osteomyelitis, right hand
		M86.342	Chronic multifocal osteomyelitis, left hand
		M86.349	Chronic multifocal osteomyelitis, unspecified hand
		M86.441	Chronic osteomyelitis with draining sinus, right hand
		M86.442	Chronic osteomyelitis with draining sinus, left hand
		M86.449	Chronic osteomyelitis with draining sinus, unspecified hand
		M86.541	Other chronic hematogenous osteomyelitis, right hand
		M86.542	Other chronic hematogenous osteomyelitis, left hand
		M86.549	Other chronic hematogenous osteomyelitis, unspecified hand
		M86.641	Other chronic osteomyelitis, right hand
		M86.642	Other chronic osteomyelitis, left hand
		M86.649	Other chronic osteomyelitis, unspecified hand
		M86.8X4	Other osteomyelitis, hand
73Ø.15	CHRONIC OSTEOMYELITIS PELVIC REGION AND THIGH	**M86.351**	Chronic multifocal osteomyelitis, right femur
		M86.352	Chronic multifocal osteomyelitis, left femur
		M86.359	Chronic multifocal osteomyelitis, unspecified femur
		M86.451	Chronic osteomyelitis with draining sinus, right femur
		M86.452	Chronic osteomyelitis with draining sinus, left femur
		M86.459	Chronic osteomyelitis with draining sinus, unspecified femur
		M86.551	Other chronic hematogenous osteomyelitis, right femur
		M86.552	Other chronic hematogenous osteomyelitis, left femur
		M86.559	Other chronic hematogenous osteomyelitis, unspecified femur
		M86.651	Other chronic osteomyelitis, right thigh
		M86.652	Other chronic osteomyelitis, left thigh
		M86.659	Other chronic osteomyelitis, unspecified thigh
		M86.8X5	Other osteomyelitis, thigh

ICD-9-CM		ICD-10-CM	
730.16	CHRONIC OSTEOMYELITIS, LOWER LEG	**M86.361**	Chronic multifocal osteomyelitis, right tibia and fibula
		M86.362	Chronic multifocal osteomyelitis, left tibia and fibula
		M86.369	Chronic multifocal osteomyelitis, unsp tibia and fibula
		M86.461	Chronic osteomyelit w draining sinus, right tibia and fibula
		M86.462	Chronic osteomyelit w draining sinus, left tibia and fibula
		M86.469	Chronic osteomyelit w draining sinus, unsp tibia and fibula
		M86.561	Oth chronic hematogenous osteomyelit, right tibia and fibula
		M86.562	Oth chronic hematogenous osteomyelit, left tibia and fibula
		M86.569	Oth chronic hematogenous osteomyelit, unsp tibia and fibula
		M86.661	Other chronic osteomyelitis, right tibia and fibula
		M86.662	Other chronic osteomyelitis, left tibia and fibula
		M86.669	Other chronic osteomyelitis, unspecified tibia and fibula
		M86.8X6	Other osteomyelitis, lower leg
730.17	CHRONIC OSTEOMYELITIS ANKLE AND FOOT	**M86.371**	Chronic multifocal osteomyelitis, right ankle and foot
		M86.372	Chronic multifocal osteomyelitis, left ankle and foot
		M86.379	Chronic multifocal osteomyelitis, unspecified ankle and foot
		M86.471	Chronic osteomyelitis w draining sinus, right ankle and foot
		M86.472	Chronic osteomyelitis w draining sinus, left ankle and foot
		M86.479	Chronic osteomyelitis w draining sinus, unsp ankle and foot
		M86.571	Oth chronic hematogenous osteomyelitis, right ankle and foot
		M86.572	Oth chronic hematogenous osteomyelitis, left ankle and foot
		M86.579	Oth chronic hematogenous osteomyelitis, unsp ankle and foot
		M86.671	Other chronic osteomyelitis, right ankle and foot
		M86.672	Other chronic osteomyelitis, left ankle and foot
		M86.679	Other chronic osteomyelitis, unspecified ankle and foot
		M86.8X7	Other osteomyelitis, ankle and foot
730.18	CHRONIC OSTEOMYELITIS OTHER SPECIFIED SITES	**M86.38**	Chronic multifocal osteomyelitis, other site
		M86.48	Chronic osteomyelitis with draining sinus, other site
		M86.58	Other chronic hematogenous osteomyelitis, other site
		M86.68	Other chronic osteomyelitis, other site
		M86.8X8	Other osteomyelitis, other site
730.19	CHRONIC OSTEOMYELITIS MULTIPLE SITES	**M86.39**	Chronic multifocal osteomyelitis, multiple sites
		M86.49	Chronic osteomyelitis with draining sinus, multiple sites
		M86.59	Other chronic hematogenous osteomyelitis, multiple sites
		M86.69	Other chronic osteomyelitis, multiple sites
		M86.8X0	Other osteomyelitis, multiple sites
730.20	UNSPECIFIED OSTEOMYELITIS SITE UNSPECIFIED	**M86.9**	Osteomyelitis, unspecified
730.21	UNSPECIFIED OSTEOMYELITIS SHOULDER REGION	**M86.9**	Osteomyelitis, unspecified
730.22	UNSPECIFIED OSTEOMYELITIS UPPER ARM	**M86.9**	Osteomyelitis, unspecified
730.23	UNSPECIFIED OSTEOMYELITIS, FOREARM	**M86.9**	Osteomyelitis, unspecified
730.24	UNSPECIFIED OSTEOMYELITIS, HAND	**M86.9**	Osteomyelitis, unspecified
730.25	UNSPECIFIED OSTEOMYELITIS PELVIC REGION&THIGH	**M86.9**	Osteomyelitis, unspecified
730.26	UNSPECIFIED OSTEOMYELITIS LOWER LEG	**M86.9**	Osteomyelitis, unspecified
730.27	UNSPECIFIED OSTEOMYELITIS ANKLE AND FOOT	**M86.9**	Osteomyelitis, unspecified
730.28	UNSPECIFIED OSTEOMYELITIS OTHER SPECIFIED SITES	**M46.20**	Osteomyelitis of vertebra, site unspecified
		M46.21	Osteomyelitis of vertebra, occipito-atlanto-axial region
		M46.22	Osteomyelitis of vertebra, cervical region
		M46.23	Osteomyelitis of vertebra, cervicothoracic region
		M46.24	Osteomyelitis of vertebra, thoracic region
		M46.25	Osteomyelitis of vertebra, thoracolumbar region
		M46.26	Osteomyelitis of vertebra, lumbar region
		M46.27	Osteomyelitis of vertebra, lumbosacral region
		M46.28	Osteomyelitis of vertebra, sacral and sacrococcygeal region
730.29	UNSPECIFIED OSTEOMYELITIS MULTIPLE SITES	**M86.9**	Osteomyelitis, unspecified
730.30	PERIOSTITIS W/O MENTION OSTEOMYEL UNSPEC SITE	**M86.9**	Osteomyelitis, unspecified
730.31	PERIOSTITIS W/O MENTION OSTEOMYEL SHLDR REGION	**M86.9**	Osteomyelitis, unspecified
730.32	PERIOSTITIS WITHOUT MENTION OSTEOMYEL UPPER ARM	**M86.9**	Osteomyelitis, unspecified
730.33	PERIOSTITIS WITHOUT MENTION OSTEOMYEL FOREARM	**M86.9**	Osteomyelitis, unspecified
730.34	PERIOSTITIS WITHOUT MENTION OSTEOMYELITIS HAND	**M86.9**	Osteomyelitis, unspecified
730.35	PERIOSTITIS W/O MENTION OSTEOMYEL PELV RGN&THI	**M86.9**	Osteomyelitis, unspecified
730.36	PERIOSTITIS WITHOUT MENTION OSTEOMYEL LOWER LEG	**M86.9**	Osteomyelitis, unspecified
730.37	PERIOSTITIS WITHOUT MENTION OSTEOMYEL ANK&FOOT	**M86.9**	Osteomyelitis, unspecified
730.38	PERIOSTITIS W/O MENTION OSTEOMYEL OTH SPEC SITES	**M86.9**	Osteomyelitis, unspecified
730.39	PERIOSTITIS WITHOUT MENTION OSTEOMYEL MX SITES	**M86.9**	Osteomyelitis, unspecified
730.70	OSTEOPATHY RESULTING FROM POLIOMYEL UNSPEC SITE	➡ **M89.60**	Osteopathy after poliomyelitis, unspecified site
730.71	OSTEOPATHY RESULT FROM POLIOMYEL SHOULDER REGION	**M89.611**	Osteopathy after poliomyelitis, right shoulder
		M89.612	Osteopathy after poliomyelitis, left shoulder
		M89.619	Osteopathy after poliomyelitis, unspecified shoulder
730.72	OSTEOPATHY RESULTING FROM POLIOMYEL UPPER ARM	**M89.621**	Osteopathy after poliomyelitis, right upper arm
		M89.622	Osteopathy after poliomyelitis, left upper arm
		M89.629	Osteopathy after poliomyelitis, unspecified upper arm
730.73	OSTEOPATHY RESULTING FROM POLIOMYELITIS FOREARM	**M89.631**	Osteopathy after poliomyelitis, right forearm
		M89.632	Osteopathy after poliomyelitis, left forearm
		M89.639	Osteopathy after poliomyelitis, unspecified forearm

ICD-9-CM		ICD-10-CM		
730.74	OSTEOPATHY RESULTING FROM POLIOMYELITIS HAND		M89.641	Osteopathy after poliomyelitis, right hand
			M89.642	Osteopathy after poliomyelitis, left hand
			M89.649	Osteopathy after poliomyelitis, unspecified hand
730.75	OSTEOPATHY RESULT FROM POLIOMYEL PELV REGION&THI		M89.651	Osteopathy after poliomyelitis, right thigh
			M89.652	Osteopathy after poliomyelitis, left thigh
			M89.659	Osteopathy after poliomyelitis, unspecified thigh
730.76	OSTEOPATHY RESULTING FROM POLIOMYEL LOWER LEG		M89.661	Osteopathy after poliomyelitis, right lower leg
			M89.662	Osteopathy after poliomyelitis, left lower leg
			M89.669	Osteopathy after poliomyelitis, unspecified lower leg
730.77	OSTEOPATHY RESULTING FROM POLIOMYELITIS ANK&FOOT		M89.671	Osteopathy after poliomyelitis, right ankle and foot
			M89.672	Osteopathy after poliomyelitis, left ankle and foot
			M89.679	Osteopathy after poliomyelitis, unspecified ankle and foot
730.78	OSTEOPATHY RESULT FROM POLIOMYEL OTH SPEC SITES	➡	M89.68	Osteopathy after poliomyelitis, other site
730.79	OSTEOPATHY RESULTING FROM POLIOMYELITIS MX SITES	➡	M89.69	Osteopathy after poliomyelitis, multiple sites
730.80	OTH INFS INVLV BONE DZ CLASS ELSW SITE UNSPEC		M90.80	Osteopathy in diseases classified elsewhere, unsp site
730.81	OTH INFS INVLV BONE DZ CLASS ELSW SHLDR REGION		M90.811	Osteopathy in diseases classified elsewhere, right shoulder
			M90.812	Osteopathy in diseases classified elsewhere, left shoulder
			M90.819	Osteopathy in diseases classified elsewhere, unsp shoulder
730.82	OTH INFS INVOLVING BONE DZ CLASS ELSW UPPER ARM		M90.821	Osteopathy in diseases classified elsewhere, right upper arm
			M90.822	Osteopathy in diseases classified elsewhere, left upper arm
			M90.829	Osteopathy in diseases classified elsewhere, unsp upper arm
730.83	OTH INFS INVOLVING BONE DZ CLASS ELSW FOREARM		M90.831	Osteopathy in diseases classified elsewhere, right forearm
			M90.832	Osteopathy in diseases classified elsewhere, left forearm
			M90.839	Osteopathy in diseases classified elsewhere, unsp forearm
730.84	OTH INFECTIONS INVOLVING DZ CLASS ELSW HAND BONE		M90.841	Osteopathy in diseases classified elsewhere, right hand
			M90.842	Osteopathy in diseases classified elsewhere, left hand
			M90.849	Osteopathy in diseases classified elsewhere, unsp hand
730.85	OTH INFS INVLV BN DZ CLASS ELSW PELV REGION&THI		M90.851	Osteopathy in diseases classified elsewhere, right thigh
			M90.852	Osteopathy in diseases classified elsewhere, left thigh
			M90.859	Osteopathy in diseases classified elsewhere, unsp thigh
730.86	OTH INFS INVOLVING BONE DZ CLASS ELSW LOWER LEG		M90.861	Osteopathy in diseases classified elsewhere, right lower leg
			M90.862	Osteopathy in diseases classified elsewhere, left lower leg
			M90.869	Osteopathy in diseases classified elsewhere, unsp lower leg
730.87	OTH INFS INVOLVING BONE DZ CLASS ELSW ANK&FOOT		M90.871	Osteopathy in diseases classd elswhr, right ankle and foot
			M90.872	Osteopathy in diseases classd elswhr, left ankle and foot
			M90.879	Osteopathy in diseases classd elswhr, unsp ankle and foot
730.88	OTH INFS INVLV BONE DZ CLASS ELSW OTH SPEC SITES	▣	A18.01	Tuberculosis of spine
		▣	A18.03	Tuberculosis of other bones
			M90.88	Osteopathy in diseases classified elsewhere, other site
730.89	OTH INFS INVLV BONE DZ CLASS ELSW MULTIPLE SITES		M90.89	Osteopathy in diseases classified elsewhere, multiple sites
730.90	UNSPECIFIED INFECTION OF BONE SITE UNSPECIFIED		M86.9	Osteomyelitis, unspecified
730.91	UNSPECIFIED INFECTION OF BONE SHOULDER REGION		M86.9	Osteomyelitis, unspecified
730.92	UNSPECIFIED INFECTION OF BONE UPPER ARM		M86.9	Osteomyelitis, unspecified
730.93	UNSPECIFIED INFECTION OF BONE FOREARM		M86.9	Osteomyelitis, unspecified
730.94	UNSPECIFIED INFECTION OF BONE, HAND		M86.9	Osteomyelitis, unspecified
730.95	UNSPECIFIED INFECTION BONE PELVIC REGION&THIGH		M86.9	Osteomyelitis, unspecified
730.96	UNSPECIFIED INFECTION OF BONE LOWER LEG		M86.9	Osteomyelitis, unspecified
730.97	UNSPECIFIED INFECTION OF BONE ANKLE AND FOOT		M86.9	Osteomyelitis, unspecified
730.98	UNSPECIFIED INFECTION BONE OTHER SPECIFIED SITE		M46.30	Infection of intervertebral disc (pyogenic), site unsp
			M46.31	Infection of intvrt disc (pyogenic), occipt-atlan-ax region
			M46.32	Infection of intervertebral disc (pyogenic), cervical region
			M46.33	Infection of intvrt disc (pyogenic), cervicothor region
			M46.34	Infection of intervertebral disc (pyogenic), thoracic region
			M46.35	Infection of intvrt disc (pyogenic), thoracolumbar region
			M46.36	Infection of intervertebral disc (pyogenic), lumbar region
			M46.37	Infection of intvrt disc (pyogenic), lumbosacral region
			M46.38	Infection of intvrt disc (pyogenic), sacr/sacrocygl region
			M46.39	Infection of intvrt disc (pyogenic), multiple sites in spine
			M86.9	Osteomyelitis, unspecified
730.99	UNSPECIFIED INFECTION OF BONE IN MULTIPLE SITES		M86.9	Osteomyelitis, unspecified
731.0	OSTEITIS DEFORMANS WITHOUT MENTION OF BONE TUMOR		M88.0	Osteitis deformans of skull
			M88.1	Osteitis deformans of vertebrae
			M88.81[1,2,9]	Osteitis deformans of shoulder
			M88.82[1,2,9]	Osteitis deformans of upper arm
			M88.83[1,2,9]	Osteitis deformans of forearm
			M88.84[1,2,9]	Osteitis deformans of hand
			M88.85[1,2,9]	Osteitis deformans of thigh
			M88.86[1,2,9]	Osteitis deformans of lower leg
			M88.87[1,2,9]	Osteitis deformans of ankle and foot
			M88.88	Osteitis deformans of other bones
			M88.89	Osteitis deformans of multiple sites
			M88.9	Osteitis deformans of unspecified bone

6th Character meanings for codes as indicated
1 Right 2 Left 9 Unspecified

ICD-9-CM		ICD-10-CM	
731.1	OSTEITIS DEFORMANS DISEASES CLASSIFIED ELSEWHERE	**M9Ø.6Ø**	Osteitis deformans in neoplastic diseases, unspecified site
		M9Ø.61[1,2,9]	Osteitis deformans in neoplastic diseases, shoulder
		M9Ø.62[1,2,9]	Osteitis deformans in neoplastic diseases, upper arm
		M9Ø.63[1,2,9]	Osteitis deformans in neoplastic diseases, forearm
		M9Ø.64[1,2,9]	Osteitis deformans in neoplastic diseases, hand
		M9Ø.65[1,2,9]	Osteitis deformans in neoplastic diseases, thigh
		M9Ø.66[1,2,9]	Osteitis deformans in neoplastic diseases, lower leg
		M9Ø.67[1,2,9]	Osteitis deformans in neoplastic diseases, ank/ft
		M9Ø.68	Osteitis deformans in neoplastic diseases, other site
		M9Ø.69	Osteitis deformans in neoplastic diseases, multiple sites
			6th Character meanings for codes as indicated ***1 Right 2 Left 9 Unspecified***
731.2	HYPERTROPHIC PULMONARY OSTEOARTHROPATHY	**M89.4Ø**	Other hypertrophic osteoarthropathy, unspecified site
		M89.41[1,2,9]	Other hypertrophic osteoarthropathy, shoulder
		M89.42[1,2,9]	Other hypertrophic osteoarthropathy, upper arm
		M89.43[1,2,9]	Other hypertrophic osteoarthropathy, forearm
		M89.44[1,2,9]	Other hypertrophic osteoarthropathy, hand
		M89.45[1,2,9]	Other hypertrophic osteoarthropathy, thigh
		M89.46[1,2,9]	Other hypertrophic osteoarthropathy, lower leg
		M89.47[1,2,9]	Other hypertrophic osteoarthropathy, ankle and foot
		M89.48	Other hypertrophic osteoarthropathy, other site
		M89.49	Other hypertrophic osteoarthropathy, multiple sites
			6th Character meanings for codes as indicated ***1 Right 2 Left 9 Unspecified***
731.3	MAJOR OSSEOUS DEFECTS	**M89.7Ø**	Major osseous defect, unspecified site
		M89.71[1,2,9]	Major osseous defect, shoulder region
		M89.72[1,2,9]	Major osseous defect, humerus
		M89.73[1,2,9]	Major osseous defect, forearm
		M89.74[1,2,9]	Major osseous defect, hand
		M89.75[1,2,9]	Major osseous defect, pelvic region and thigh
		M89.76[1,2,9]	Major osseous defect, lower leg
		M89.77[1,2,9]	Major osseous defect, ankle and foot
		M89.78	Major osseous defect, other site
		M89.79	Major osseous defect, multiple sites
			6th Character meanings for codes as indicated ***1 Right 2 Left 9 Unspecified***
731.8	OTHER BONE INVOLVEMENT DISEASES CLASSIFIED ELSW	**M9Ø.5Ø**	Osteonecrosis in diseases classified elsewhere, unsp site
		M9Ø.51[1,2,9]	Osteonecrosis in diseases classd elswhr, shoulder
		M9Ø.52[1,2,9]	Osteonecrosis in diseases classd elswhr, upper arm
		M9Ø.53[1,2,9]	Osteonecrosis in diseases classd elswhr, forearm
		M9Ø.54[1,2,9]	Osteonecrosis in diseases classified elsewhere, hand
		M9Ø.55[1,2,9]	Osteonecrosis in diseases classified elsewhere, thigh
		M9Ø.56[1,2,9]	Osteonecrosis in diseases classd elswhr, lower leg
		M9Ø.57[1,2,9]	Osteonecrosis in diseases classd elswhr, ank/ft
		M9Ø.58	Osteonecrosis in diseases classified elsewhere, other site
		M9Ø.59	Osteonecrosis in diseases classd elswhr, multiple sites
		M9Ø.8Ø	Osteopathy in diseases classified elsewhere, unsp site
		M9Ø.81[1,2,9]	Osteopathy in diseases classified elsewhere, shoulder
		M9Ø.82[1,2,9]	Osteopathy in diseases classified elsewhere, upper arm
		M9Ø.83[1,2,9]	Osteopathy in diseases classified elsewhere, forearm
		M9Ø.84[1,2,9]	Osteopathy in diseases classified elsewhere, hand
		M9Ø.85[1,2,9]	Osteopathy in diseases classified elsewhere, thigh
		M9Ø.86[1,2,9]	Osteopathy in diseases classified elsewhere, lower leg
		M9Ø.87[1,2,9]	Osteopathy in diseases classd elswhr, right ankle and foot
		M9Ø.88	Osteopathy in diseases classified elsewhere, other site
		M9Ø.89	Osteopathy in diseases classified elsewhere, multiple sites
			6th Character meanings for codes as indicated ***1 Right 2 Left 9 Unspecified***
732.Ø	JUVENILE OSTEOCHONDROSIS OF SPINE	**M42.ØØ**	Juvenile osteochondrosis of spine, site unspecified
		M42.Ø1	Juvenile osteochondrosis of spine, occipt-atlan-ax region
		M42.Ø2	Juvenile osteochondrosis of spine, cervical region
		M42.Ø3	Juvenile osteochondrosis of spine, cervicothoracic region
		M42.Ø4	Juvenile osteochondrosis of spine, thoracic region
		M42.Ø5	Juvenile osteochondrosis of spine, thoracolumbar region
		M42.Ø6	Juvenile osteochondrosis of spine, lumbar region
		M42.Ø7	Juvenile osteochondrosis of spine, lumbosacral region
		M42.Ø8	Juvenile osteochondrosis of spine, sacr/sacrocygl region
		M42.Ø9	Juvenile osteochondrosis of spine, multiple sites in spine

[Brackets] indicate valid character values for each code. Character value meanings provided for each code grouping.

ICD-9-CM		ICD-10-CM	
732.1	JUVENILE OSTEOCHONDROSIS OF HIP AND PELVIS	M91.Ø	Juvenile osteochondrosis of pelvis
		M91.1Ø	Juvenile osteochondrosis of head of femur, unspecified leg
		M91.11	Juvenile osteochondrosis of head of femur, right leg
		M91.12	Juvenile osteochondrosis of head of femur, left leg
		M91.2Ø	Coxa plana, unspecified hip
		M91.21	Coxa plana, right hip
		M91.22	Coxa plana, left hip
		M91.3Ø	Pseudocoxalgia, unspecified hip
		M91.31	Pseudocoxalgia, right hip
		M91.32	Pseudocoxalgia, left hip
		M91.4Ø	Coxa magna, unspecified hip
		M91.41	Coxa magna, right hip
		M91.42	Coxa magna, left hip
		M91.8Ø	Other juvenile osteochondrosis of hip and pelvis, unsp leg
		M91.81	Other juvenile osteochondrosis of hip and pelvis, right leg
		M91.82	Other juvenile osteochondrosis of hip and pelvis, left leg
		M91.9Ø	Juvenile osteochondrosis of hip and pelvis, unsp, unsp leg
		M91.91	Juvenile osteochondrosis of hip and pelvis, unsp, right leg
		M91.92	Juvenile osteochondrosis of hip and pelvis, unsp, left leg
732.2	NONTRAUMATIC SLIPPED UPPER FEMORAL EPIPHYSIS	M93.ØØ1	Unsp slipped upper femoral epiphysis, right hip
		M93.ØØ2	Unsp slipped upper femoral epiphysis, left hip
		M93.ØØ3	Unsp slipped upper femoral epiphysis, unsp hip
		M93.Ø11	Acute slipped upper femoral epiphysis, right hip
		M93.Ø12	Acute slipped upper femoral epiphysis, left hip
		M93.Ø13	Acute slipped upper femoral epiphysis, unsp hip
		M93.Ø21	Chronic slipped upper femoral epiphysis, right hip
		M93.Ø22	Chronic slipped upper femoral epiphysis, left hip
		M93.Ø23	Chronic slipped upper femoral epiphysis, unsp hip
		M93.Ø31	Acute on chronic slipped upper femoral epiphysis, right hip
		M93.Ø32	Acute on chronic slipped upper femoral epiphysis, left hip
		M93.Ø33	Acute on chronic slipped upper femoral epiphysis, unsp hip
732.3	JUVENILE OSTEOCHONDROSIS OF UPPER EXTREMITY	M92.ØØ	Juvenile osteochondrosis of humerus, unspecified arm
		M92.Ø1	Juvenile osteochondrosis of humerus, right arm
		M92.Ø2	Juvenile osteochondrosis of humerus, left arm
		M92.1Ø	Juvenile osteochondrosis of radius and ulna, unspecified arm
		M92.11	Juvenile osteochondrosis of radius and ulna, right arm
		M92.12	Juvenile osteochondrosis of radius and ulna, left arm
		M92.2Ø[1,2,9]	Unspecified juvenile osteochondrosis, hand
		M92.21[1,2,9]	Osteochondrosis (juvenile) of carpal lunate, hand
		M92.22[1,2,9]	Osteochondrosis (juvenile) of metacarpal heads, hand
		M92.29[1,2,9]	Other juvenile osteochondrosis, hand
		M92.3Ø	Other juvenile osteochondrosis, unspecified upper limb
		M92.31	Other juvenile osteochondrosis, right upper limb
		M92.32	Other juvenile osteochondrosis, left upper limb
			6th Character meanings for codes as indicated ***1 Right 2 Left 9 Unspecified***
732.4	JUVENILE OSTEOCHONDROSIS LOWER EXTREM EXCLD FOOT	M92.4Ø	Juvenile osteochondrosis of patella, unspecified knee
		M92.41	Juvenile osteochondrosis of patella, right knee
		M92.42	Juvenile osteochondrosis of patella, left knee
		M92.5Ø	Juvenile osteochondrosis of tibia and fibula, unsp leg
		M92.51	Juvenile osteochondrosis of tibia and fibula, right leg
		M92.52	Juvenile osteochondrosis of tibia and fibula, left leg
732.5	JUVENILE OSTEOCHONDROSIS OF FOOT	M92.6Ø	Juvenile osteochondrosis of tarsus, unspecified ankle
		M92.61	Juvenile osteochondrosis of tarsus, right ankle
		M92.62	Juvenile osteochondrosis of tarsus, left ankle
		M92.7Ø	Juvenile osteochondrosis of metatarsus, unspecified foot
		M92.71	Juvenile osteochondrosis of metatarsus, right foot
		M92.72	Juvenile osteochondrosis of metatarsus, left foot
732.6	OTHER JUVENILE OSTEOCHONDROSIS	M92.8	Other specified juvenile osteochondrosis
		M92.9	Juvenile osteochondrosis, unspecified
732.7	OSTEOCHONDRITIS DISSECANS	M93.2Ø	Osteochondritis dissecans of unspecified site
		M93.21[1,2,9]	Osteochondritis dissecans, shoulder
		M93.22[1,2,9]	Osteochondritis dissecans, elbow
		M93.23[1,2,9]	Osteochondritis dissecans, wrist
		M93.24[1,2,9]	Osteochondritis dissecans, joints of hand
		M93.25[1,2,9]	Osteochondritis dissecans, hip
		M93.26[1,2,9]	Osteochondritis dissecans, knee
		M93.27[1,2,9]	Osteochondritis dissecans, ankle and joints of foot
		M93.28	Osteochondritis dissecans other site
		M93.29	Osteochondritis dissecans multiple sites
			6th Character meanings for codes as indicated ***1 Right 2 Left 9 Unspecified***

ICD-9-CM		ICD-10-CM	
732.8	OTHER SPECIFIED FORMS OF OSTEOCHONDROPATHY	**M42.1Ø**	Adult osteochondrosis of spine, site unspecified
		M42.11	Adult osteochondrosis of spine, occipt-atlan-ax region
		M42.12	Adult osteochondrosis of spine, cervical region
		M42.13	Adult osteochondrosis of spine, cervicothoracic region
		M42.14	Adult osteochondrosis of spine, thoracic region
		M42.15	Adult osteochondrosis of spine, thoracolumbar region
		M42.16	Adult osteochondrosis of spine, lumbar region
		M42.17	Adult osteochondrosis of spine, lumbosacral region
		M42.18	Adult osteochondrosis of spine, sacr/sacrocygl region
		M42.19	Adult osteochondrosis of spine, multiple sites in spine
		M93.1	Kienbock's disease of adults
		M93.8Ø	Other specified osteochondropathies of unspecified site
		M93.81[1,2,9]	Other specified osteochondropathies, shoulder
		M93.82[1,2,9]	Other specified osteochondropathies, upper arm
		M93.83[1,2,9]	Other specified osteochondropathies, forearm
		M93.84[1,2,9]	Other specified osteochondropathies, hand
		M93.85[1,2,9]	Other specified osteochondropathies, thigh
		M93.86[1,2,9]	Other specified osteochondropathies, lower leg
		M93.87[1,2,9]	Other specified osteochondropathies, ankle and foot
		M93.88	Other specified osteochondropathies other
		M93.89	Other specified osteochondropathies multiple sites
			6th Character meanings for codes as indicated ***1 Right*** ***2 Left*** ***9 Unspecified***
732.9	UNSPECIFIED OSTEOCHONDROPATHY	**M42.9**	Spinal osteochondrosis, unspecified
		M93.9Ø	Osteochondropathy, unspecified of unspecified site
		M93.91[1,2,9]	Osteochondropathy, unspecified, shoulder
		M93.92[1,2,9]	Osteochondropathy, unspecified, upper arm
		M93.93[1,2,9]	Osteochondropathy, unspecified, forearm
		M93.94[1,2,9]	Osteochondropathy, unspecified, hand
		M93.95[1,2,9]	Osteochondropathy, unspecified, thigh
		M93.96[1,2,9]	Osteochondropathy, unspecified, lower leg
		M93.97[1,2,9]	Osteochondropathy, unspecified, ankle and foot
		M93.98	Osteochondropathy, unspecified other
		M93.99	Osteochondropathy, unspecified multiple sites
			6th Character meanings for codes as indicated ***1 Right*** ***2 Left*** ***9 Unspecified***
733.ØØ	UNSPECIFIED OSTEOPOROSIS	**M81.Ø**	Age-related osteoporosis w/o current pathological fracture
733.Ø1	SENILE OSTEOPOROSIS	➡ **M81.Ø**	Age-related osteoporosis w/o current pathological fracture
733.Ø2	IDIOPATHIC OSTEOPOROSIS	**M81.8**	Other osteoporosis without current pathological fracture
733.Ø3	DISUSE OSTEOPOROSIS	**M81.8**	Other osteoporosis without current pathological fracture
733.Ø9	OTHER OSTEOPOROSIS	**M81.6**	Localized osteoporosis [Lequesne]
		M81.8	Other osteoporosis without current pathological fracture
733.1Ø	PATHOLOGIC FRACTURE UNSPECIFIED SITE	**M8Ø.ØØXA**	Age-rel osteopor w current path fracture, unsp site, init
		M8Ø.8ØXA	Oth osteopor w current path fracture, unsp site, init
		M84.4ØXA	Pathological fracture, unsp site, init encntr for fracture
		M84.5ØXA	Pathological fracture in neoplastic disease, unsp site, init
		M84.6ØXA	Pathological fracture in oth disease, unsp site, init for fx
733.11	PATHOLOGIC FRACTURE OF HUMERUS	**M8Ø.Ø2**[1,2,9]**A**	Age-rel osteopor w current path fracture, humerus, init
		M8Ø.82[1,2,9]**A**	Oth osteopor w current path fracture, humerus, init
		M84.42[1,2,9]**A**	Pathological fracture, humerus, init for fx
		M84.52[1,2,9]**A**	Pathological fracture in neoplastic disease, humerus, init
		M84.62[1,2,9]**A**	Pathological fracture in oth disease, humerus, init
			6th Character meanings for codes as indicated ***1 Right*** ***2 Left*** ***9 Unspecified***
733.12	PATHOLOGIC FRACTURE OF DISTAL RADIUS AND ULNA	**M8Ø.Ø3**[1,2,9]**A**	Age-rel osteopor w current path fracture, forearm, init
		M8Ø.83[1,2,9]**A**	Oth osteopor w current path fracture, forearm, init
		M84.431A	Pathological fracture, right ulna, init encntr for fracture
		M84.432A	Pathological fracture, left ulna, init encntr for fracture
		M84.433A	Pathological fracture, right radius, init for fx
		M84.434A	Pathological fracture, left radius, init encntr for fracture
		M84.439A	Pathological fracture, unsp ulna and radius, init for fx
		M84.531A	Path fracture in neoplastic disease, right ulna, init
		M84.532A	Pathological fracture in neoplastic disease, left ulna, init
		M84.533A	Path fracture in neoplastic disease, right radius, init
		M84.534A	Path fracture in neoplastic disease, left radius, init
		M84.539A	Path fracture in neopltc disease, unsp ulna and radius, init
		M84.631A	Pathological fracture in oth disease, right ulna, init
		M84.632A	Pathological fracture in oth disease, left ulna, init for fx
		M84.633A	Pathological fracture in oth disease, right radius, init
		M84.634A	Pathological fracture in oth disease, left radius, init
		M84.639A	Path fracture in oth disease, unsp ulna and radius, init
			6th Character meanings for codes as indicated ***1 Right*** ***2 Left*** ***9 Unspecified***

[Brackets] indicate valid character values for each code. Character value meanings provided for each code grouping.

ICD-9-CM	ICD-10-CM	
733.13 PATHOLOGIC FRACTURE OF VERTEBRAE	**M48.5ØXA**	Collapsed vertebra, NEC, site unsp, init
	M48.51XA	Collapsed vertebra, NEC, occipito-atlanto-axial region, init
	M48.52XA	Collapsed vertebra, NEC, cervical region, init
	M48.53XA	Collapsed vertebra, NEC, cervicothoracic region, init
	M48.54XA	Collapsed vertebra, NEC, thoracic region, init
	M48.55XA	Collapsed vertebra, NEC, thoracolumbar region, init
	M48.56XA	Collapsed vertebra, NEC, lumbar region, init
	M48.57XA	Collapsed vertebra, NEC, lumbosacral region, init
	M48.58XA	Collapsed vertebra, NEC, sacr/sacrocygl region, init
	M8Ø.Ø8XA	Age-rel osteopor w current path fracture, vertebra(e), init
	M8Ø.88XA	Oth osteopor w current path fracture, vertebra(e), init
	M84.48XA	Pathological fracture, other site, init encntr for fracture
	M84.58XA	Path fracture in neoplastic disease, oth spec site, init
	M84.68XA	Pathological fracture in oth disease, oth site, init for fx
733.14 PATHOLOGIC FRACTURE OF NECK OF FEMUR	**M8Ø.Ø51A**	Age-rel osteopor w current path fracture, right femur, init
	M8Ø.Ø52A	Age-rel osteopor w current path fracture, left femur, init
	M8Ø.Ø59A	Age-rel osteopor w current path fracture, unsp femur, init
	M8Ø.851A	Oth osteopor w current path fracture, right femur, init
	M8Ø.852A	Oth osteopor w current path fracture, left femur, init
	M8Ø.859A	Oth osteopor w current path fracture, unsp femur, init
	M84.451A	Pathological fracture, right femur, init encntr for fracture
	M84.452A	Pathological fracture, left femur, init encntr for fracture
	M84.459A	Pathological fracture, hip, unsp, init encntr for fracture
	M84.551A	Path fracture in neoplastic disease, right femur, init
	M84.552A	Path fracture in neoplastic disease, left femur, init
	M84.553A	Path fracture in neoplastic disease, unsp femur, init
	M84.559A	Pathological fracture in neoplastic disease, hip, unsp, init
	M84.651A	Pathological fracture in oth disease, right femur, init
	M84.652A	Pathological fracture in oth disease, left femur, init
	M84.653A	Pathological fracture in oth disease, unsp femur, init
	M84.659A	Pathological fracture in oth disease, hip, unsp, init for fx
733.15 PATHOLOGIC FRACTURE OTHER SPECIFIED PART FEMUR	**M8Ø.Ø51A**	Age-rel osteopor w current path fracture, right femur, init
	M8Ø.Ø52A	Age-rel osteopor w current path fracture, left femur, init
	M8Ø.Ø59A	Age-rel osteopor w current path fracture, unsp femur, init
	M8Ø.851A	Oth osteopor w current path fracture, right femur, init
	M8Ø.852A	Oth osteopor w current path fracture, left femur, init
	M8Ø.859A	Oth osteopor w current path fracture, unsp femur, init
	M84.451A	Pathological fracture, right femur, init encntr for fracture
	M84.452A	Pathological fracture, left femur, init encntr for fracture
	M84.453A	Pathological fracture, unsp femur, init encntr for fracture
	M84.551A	Path fracture in neoplastic disease, right femur, init
	M84.552A	Path fracture in neoplastic disease, left femur, init
	M84.553A	Path fracture in neoplastic disease, unsp femur, init
	M84.559A	Pathological fracture in neoplastic disease, hip, unsp, init
	M84.651A	Pathological fracture in oth disease, right femur, init
	M84.652A	Pathological fracture in oth disease, left femur, init
	M84.653A	Pathological fracture in oth disease, unsp femur, init
	M84.659A	Pathological fracture in oth disease, hip, unsp, init for fx
733.16 PATHOLOGIC FRACTURE OF TIBIA AND FIBULA	**M8Ø.Ø6**[1,2,9]**A**	Age-rel osteopor w current path fracture, low leg, init
	M8Ø.Ø7[1,2,9]**A**	Age-rel osteopor w current path fracture, ank/ft, init
	M8Ø.86[1,2,9]**A**	Oth osteopor w current path fracture, low leg, init
	M8Ø.87[1,2,9]**A**	Oth osteopor w current path fracture, ank/ft, init
	M84.461A	Pathological fracture, right tibia, init encntr for fracture
	M84.462A	Pathological fracture, left tibia, init encntr for fracture
	M84.463A	Pathological fracture, right fibula, init for fx
	M84.464A	Pathological fracture, left fibula, init encntr for fracture
	M84.469A	Pathological fracture, unsp tibia and fibula, init for fx
	M84.471A	Pathological fracture, right ankle, init encntr for fracture
	M84.472A	Pathological fracture, left ankle, init encntr for fracture
	M84.473A	Pathological fracture, unsp ankle, init encntr for fracture
	M84.561A	Path fracture in neoplastic disease, right tibia, init
	M84.562A	Path fracture in neoplastic disease, left tibia, init
	M84.563A	Path fracture in neoplastic disease, right fibula, init
	M84.564A	Path fracture in neoplastic disease, left fibula, init
	M84.569A	Path fx in neopltc disease, unsp tibia and fibula, init
	M84.571A	Path fracture in neoplastic disease, right ankle, init
	M84.572A	Path fracture in neoplastic disease, left ankle, init
	M84.573A	Path fracture in neoplastic disease, unsp ankle, init
	M84.661A	Pathological fracture in oth disease, right tibia, init
	M84.662A	Pathological fracture in oth disease, left tibia, init
	M84.663A	Pathological fracture in oth disease, right fibula, init
	M84.664A	Pathological fracture in oth disease, left fibula, init
	M84.669A	Path fracture in oth disease, unsp tibia and fibula, init
	M84.671A	Pathological fracture in oth disease, right ankle, init
	M84.672A	Pathological fracture in oth disease, left ankle, init
	M84.673A	Pathological fracture in oth disease, unsp ankle, init

6th Character meanings for codes as indicated
1 Right 2 Left 9 Unspecified

ICD-9-CM		ICD-10-CM	
733.19	PATHOLOGIC FRACTURE OF OTHER SPECIFIED SITE	**M8Ø.Ø1**[1,2,9]**A**	Age-rel osteopor w current path fracture, shoulder, init
		M8Ø.Ø4[1,2,9]**A**	Age-rel osteopor w current path fracture, hand, init
		M8Ø.81[1,2,9]**A**	Oth osteopor w current path fracture, shoulder, init
		M8Ø.84[1,2,9]**A**	Oth osteopor w current path fracture, hand, init
		M84.41[1,2,9]**A**	Pathological fracture, shoulder, init for fx
		M84.441A	Pathological fracture, right hand, init encntr for fracture
		M84.442A	Pathological fracture, left hand, init encntr for fracture
		M84.443A	Pathological fracture, unsp hand, init encntr for fracture
		M84.444A	Pathological fracture, right finger(s), init for fx
		M84.445A	Pathological fracture, left finger(s), init for fx
		M84.446A	Pathological fracture, unsp finger(s), init for fx
		M84.454A	Pathological fracture, pelvis, init encntr for fracture
		M84.474A	Pathological fracture, right foot, init encntr for fracture
		M84.475A	Pathological fracture, left foot, init encntr for fracture
		M84.476A	Pathological fracture, unsp foot, init encntr for fracture
		M84.477A	Pathological fracture, right toe(s), init for fx
		M84.478A	Pathological fracture, left toe(s), init encntr for fracture
		M84.479A	Pathological fracture, unsp toe(s), init encntr for fracture
		M84.48XA	Pathological fracture, other site, init encntr for fracture
		M84.51[1,2,9]**A**	Path fracture in neoplastic disease, shoulder, init
		M84.54[1,2,9]**A**	Path fracture in neoplastic disease, hand, init
		M84.55ØA	Pathological fracture in neoplastic disease, pelvis, init
		M84.574A	Path fracture in neoplastic disease, right foot, init
		M84.575A	Pathological fracture in neoplastic disease, left foot, init
		M84.576A	Pathological fracture in neoplastic disease, unsp foot, init
		M84.61[1,2,9]**A**	Pathological fracture in oth disease, shoulder, init
		M84.64[1,2,9]**A**	Pathological fracture in oth disease, hand, init
		M84.65ØA	Pathological fracture in oth disease, pelvis, init for fx
		M84.674A	Pathological fracture in oth disease, right foot, init
		M84.675A	Pathological fracture in oth disease, left foot, init for fx
		M84.676A	Pathological fracture in oth disease, unsp foot, init for fx
		M84.68XA	Pathological fracture in oth disease, oth site, init for fx
			6th Character meanings for codes as indicated ***1 Right*** ***2 Left*** ***9 Unspecified***
733.2Ø	UNSPECIFIED CYST OF BONE	**M85.6Ø**	Other cyst of bone, unspecified site
733.21	SOLITARY BONE CYST	**M85.4Ø**	Solitary bone cyst, unspecified site
		M85.41[1,2,9]	Solitary bone cyst, shoulder
		M85.42[1,2,9]	Solitary bone cyst, humerus
		M85.43[1,2,9]	Solitary bone cyst, ulna and radius
		M85.44[1,2,9]	Solitary bone cyst, hand
		M85.45[1,2,9]	Solitary bone cyst, pelvis
		M85.46[1,2,9]	Solitary bone cyst, tibia and fibula
		M85.47[1,2,9]	Solitary bone cyst, ankle and foot
		M85.48	Solitary bone cyst, other site
			6th Character meanings for codes as indicated ***1 Right*** ***2 Left*** ***9 Unspecified***
733.22	ANEURYSMAL BONE CYST	**M85.5Ø**	Aneurysmal bone cyst, unspecified site
		M85.51[1,2,9]	Aneurysmal bone cyst, shoulder
		M85.52[1,2,9]	Aneurysmal bone cyst, upper arm
		M85.53[1,2,9]	Aneurysmal bone cyst, forearm
		M85.54[1,2,9]	Aneurysmal bone cyst, hand
		M85.55[1,2,9]	Aneurysmal bone cyst, thigh
		M85.56[1,2,9]	Aneurysmal bone cyst, lower leg
		M85.57[1,2,9]	Aneurysmal bone cyst, ankle and foot
		M85.58	Aneurysmal bone cyst, other site
		M85.59	Aneurysmal bone cyst, multiple sites
			6th Character meanings for codes as indicated ***1 Right*** ***2 Left*** ***9 Unspecified***

ICD-9-CM		ICD-10-CM	
733.29	OTHER CYST OF BONE	**M85.ØØ**	Fibrous dysplasia (monostotic), unspecified site
		M85.Ø1[1,2,9]	Fibrous dysplasia (monostotic), shoulder
		M85.Ø2[1,2,9]	Fibrous dysplasia (monostotic), upper arm
		M85.Ø3[1,2,9]	Fibrous dysplasia (monostotic), forearm
		M85.Ø4[1,2,9]	Fibrous dysplasia (monostotic), hand
		M85.Ø5[1,2,9]	Fibrous dysplasia (monostotic), thigh
		M85.Ø6[1,2,9]	Fibrous dysplasia (monostotic), lower leg
		M85.Ø7[1,2,9]	Fibrous dysplasia (monostotic), ankle and foot
		M85.Ø8	Fibrous dysplasia (monostotic), other site
		M85.Ø9	Fibrous dysplasia (monostotic), multiple sites
		M85.6Ø	Other cyst of bone, unspecified site
		M85.61[1,2,9]	Other cyst of bone, shoulder
		M85.62[1,2,9]	Other cyst of bone, upper arm
		M85.63[1,2,9]	Other cyst of bone, forearm
		M85.64[1,2,9]	Other cyst of bone, hand
		M85.65[1,2,9]	Other cyst of bone, thigh
		M85.66[1,2,9]	Other cyst of bone, lower leg
		M85.67[1,2,9]	Other cyst of bone, ankle and foot
		M85.68	Other cyst of bone, other site
		M85.69	Other cyst of bone, multiple sites
			6th Character meanings for codes as indicated ***1 Right 2 Left 9 Unspecified***
733.3	HYPEROSTOSIS OF SKULL	➡ **M85.2**	Hyperostosis of skull
733.4Ø	ASEPTIC NECROSIS OF BONE SITE UNSPECIFIED	**M87.ØØ**	Idiopathic aseptic necrosis of unspecified bone
		M87.1Ø	Osteonecrosis due to drugs, unspecified bone
		M87.2Ø	Osteonecrosis due to previous trauma, unspecified bone
		M87.3Ø	Other secondary osteonecrosis, unspecified bone
		M87.8Ø	Other osteonecrosis, unspecified bone
		M87.9	Osteonecrosis, unspecified
		◘ **M9Ø.5Ø**	Osteonecrosis in diseases classified elsewhere, unsp site
733.41	ASEPTIC NECROSIS OF HEAD OF HUMERUS	**M87.Ø1**[1,2,9]	Idiopathic aseptic necrosis of shoulder
		M87.Ø2[1,2,9]	Idiopathic aseptic necrosis of humerus
		M87.12[1,2,9]	Osteonecrosis due to drugs, humerus
		M87.22[1,2,9]	Osteonecrosis due to previous trauma, humerus
		M87.32[1,2,9]	Other secondary osteonecrosis, humerus
		M87.82[1,2,9]	Other osteonecrosis, humerus
		◘ **M9Ø.51**[1,2,9]	Osteonecrosis in diseases classd elswhr, shoulder
			6th Character meanings for codes as indicated ***1 Right 2 Left 9 Unspecified***
733.42	ASEPTIC NECROSIS OF HEAD AND NECK OF FEMUR	**M87.Ø5**[1,2,9]	Idiopathic aseptic necrosis of femur
		M87.15Ø	Osteonecrosis due to drugs, pelvis
		M87.15[1,2,9]	Osteonecrosis due to drugs, femur
		M87.251	Osteonecrosis due to previous trauma, right femur
		M87.252	Osteonecrosis due to previous trauma, left femur
		M87.256	Osteonecrosis due to previous trauma, unspecified femur
		M87.35Ø	Other secondary osteonecrosis, pelvis
		M87.351	Other secondary osteonecrosis, right femur
		M87.352	Other secondary osteonecrosis, left femur
		M87.353	Other secondary osteonecrosis, unspecified femur
		M87.85Ø	Other osteonecrosis, pelvis
		M87.85[1,2,9]	Other osteonecrosis, femur
		◘ **M9Ø.55**[1,2,9]	Osteonecrosis in diseases classified elsewhere, thigh
			6th Character meanings for codes as indicated ***1 Right 2 Left 9 Unspecified***
733.43	ASEPTIC NECROSIS OF MEDIAL FEMORAL CONDYLE	**M87.Ø5**[1,2,9]	Idiopathic aseptic necrosis of femur
		M87.15Ø	Osteonecrosis due to drugs, pelvis
		M87.15[1,2,9]	Osteonecrosis due to drugs, femur
		M87.251	Osteonecrosis due to previous trauma, right femur
		M87.252	Osteonecrosis due to previous trauma, left femur
		M87.256	Osteonecrosis due to previous trauma, unspecified femur
		M87.35Ø	Other secondary osteonecrosis, pelvis
		M87.351	Other secondary osteonecrosis, right femur
		M87.352	Other secondary osteonecrosis, left femur
		M87.353	Other secondary osteonecrosis, unspecified femur
		M87.85[1,2,9]	Other osteonecrosis, femur
			6th Character meanings for codes as indicated ***1 Right 2 Left 9 Unspecified***

ICD-9-CM		ICD-10-CM	
733.44	ASEPTIC NECROSIS OF TALUS	**M87.Ø74**	Idiopathic aseptic necrosis of right foot
		M87.Ø75	Idiopathic aseptic necrosis of left foot
		M87.Ø76	Idiopathic aseptic necrosis of unspecified foot
		M87.174	Osteonecrosis due to drugs, right foot
		M87.175	Osteonecrosis due to drugs, left foot
		M87.176	Osteonecrosis due to drugs, unspecified foot
		M87.274	Osteonecrosis due to previous trauma, right foot
		M87.275	Osteonecrosis due to previous trauma, left foot
		M87.276	Osteonecrosis due to previous trauma, unspecified foot
		M87.374	Other secondary osteonecrosis, right foot
		M87.375	Other secondary osteonecrosis, left foot
		M87.376	Other secondary osteonecrosis, unspecified foot
		M87.874	Other osteonecrosis, right foot
		M87.875	Other osteonecrosis, left foot
		M87.876	Other osteonecrosis, unspecified foot
733.45	ASEPTIC NECROSIS OF BONE JAW	**M87.Ø8**	Idiopathic aseptic necrosis of bone, other site
		M87.18Ø	Osteonecrosis due to drugs, jaw
733.49	ASEPTIC NECROSIS OF OTHER BONE SITE	**M87.Ø3**[1,2,3]	Idiopathic aseptic necrosis of radius
		M87.Ø3[4,5,6]	Idiopathic aseptic necrosis of ulna
		M87.Ø3[7,8,9]	Idiopathic aseptic necrosis of carpus
		M87.Ø4[1,2,3]	Idiopathic aseptic necrosis of hand
		M87.Ø4[4,5,6]	Idiopathic aseptic necrosis of finger(s)
		M87.Ø5Ø	Idiopathic aseptic necrosis of pelvis
		M87.Ø6[1,2,3]	Idiopathic aseptic necrosis of tibia
		M87.Ø6[4,5,6]	Idiopathic aseptic necrosis of fibula
		M87.Ø7[1,2,3]	Idiopathic aseptic necrosis of ankle
		M87.Ø7[7,8,9]	Idiopathic aseptic necrosis of toe(s)
		M87.Ø8	Idiopathic aseptic necrosis of bone, other site
		M87.Ø9	Idiopathic aseptic necrosis of bone, multiple sites
		M87.11[1,2,9]	Osteonecrosis due to drugs, shoulder
		M87.13[1,2,3]	Osteonecrosis due to drugs of radius
		M87.13[4,5,6]	Osteonecrosis due to drugs of ulna
		M87.13[7,8,9]	Osteonecrosis due to drugs of carpus
		M87.14[1,2,3]	Osteonecrosis due to drugs, hand
		M87.14[4,5,6]	Osteonecrosis due to drugs, finger(s)
		M87.16[1,2,3]	Osteonecrosis due to drugs, tibia
		M87.16[4,5,6]	Osteonecrosis due to drugs, fibula
		M87.17[1,2,3]	Osteonecrosis due to drugs, ankle
		M87.17[7,8,9]	Osteonecrosis due to drugs, toe(s)
		M87.188	Osteonecrosis due to drugs, other site
		M87.19	Osteonecrosis due to drugs, multiple sites
		M87.21[1,2,9]	Osteonecrosis due to previous trauma, shoulder
		M87.23[1,2,3]	Osteonecrosis due to previous trauma of radius
		M87.23[4,5,6]	Osteonecrosis due to previous trauma of ulna
		M87.23[7,8,9]	Osteonecrosis due to previous trauma of carpus
		M87.24[1,2,3]	Osteonecrosis due to previous trauma, hand
		M87.24[4,5,6]	Osteonecrosis due to previous trauma, finger(s)
		M87.25Ø	Osteonecrosis due to previous trauma, pelvis
		M87.26[1,2,3]	Osteonecrosis due to previous trauma, tibia
		M87.26[4,5,6]	Osteonecrosis due to previous trauma, fibula
		M87.27[1,2,3]	Osteonecrosis due to previous trauma, ankle
		M87.27[7,8,9]	Osteonecrosis due to previous trauma, toe(s)
		M87.28	Osteonecrosis due to previous trauma, other site
		M87.29	Osteonecrosis due to previous trauma, multiple sites
		M87.31[1,2,9]	Other secondary osteonecrosis, shoulder
		M87.33[1,2,3]	Other secondary osteonecrosis of radius
		M87.33[4,5,6]	Other secondary osteonecrosis of ulna
		M87.33[7,8,9]	Other secondary osteonecrosis of carpus
		M87.34[1,2,3]	Other secondary osteonecrosis, hand
		M87.34[4,5,6]	Other secondary osteonecrosis, finger(s)
		M87.36[1,2,3]	Other secondary osteonecrosis, tibia
		M87.36[4,5,6]	Other secondary osteonecrosis, fibula
		M87.37[1,2,3]	Other secondary osteonecrosis, ankle
		M87.37[7,8,9]	Other secondary osteonecrosis, toe(s)
		M87.38	Other secondary osteonecrosis, other site
		M87.39	Other secondary osteonecrosis, multiple sites
		M87.81[1,2,9]	Other osteonecrosis, shoulder
		M87.83[1,2,3]	Other osteonecrosis of radius
		M87.83[4,5,6]	Other osteonecrosis of ulna
		M87.83[7,8,9]	Other osteonecrosis of carpus
		M87.84[1,2,3]	Other osteonecrosis, hand
		M87.84[4,5]	Other osteonecrosis, finger(s)
		M87.849	Other osteonecrosis, unspecified finger(s)
		M87.86[1,2,3]	Other osteonecrosis, tibia
		M87.86[4,5,6]	Other osteonecrosis, fibula
		M87.87[1,2,3]	Other osteonecrosis, right ankle
		M87.87[7,8,9]	Other osteonecrosis, right toe(s)

6th Character meanings for codes as indicated		
1 Right	***4 Right***	***7 Right***
2 Left	***5 Left***	***8 Left***
3 Unspecified	***6 Unspecified***	***9 Unspecified***

(Continued on next page)

[Brackets] indicate valid character values for each code. Character value meanings provided for each code grouping.

ICD-9-CM		ICD-10-CM		
733.49	ASEPTIC NECROSIS OF OTHER BONE SITE **(Continued)**		**M87.88**	Other osteonecrosis, other site
			M87.89	Other osteonecrosis, multiple sites
		◘	**M9Ø.521**	Osteonecrosis in diseases classd elswhr, right upper arm
		◘	**M9Ø.522**	Osteonecrosis in diseases classd elswhr, left upper arm
		◘	**M9Ø.529**	Osteonecrosis in diseases classd elswhr, unsp upper arm
		◘	**M9Ø.531**	Osteonecrosis in diseases classd elswhr, right forearm
		◘	**M9Ø.532**	Osteonecrosis in diseases classified elsewhere, left forearm
		◘	**M9Ø.539**	Osteonecrosis in diseases classified elsewhere, unsp forearm
		◘	**M9Ø.541**	Osteonecrosis in diseases classified elsewhere, right hand
		◘	**M9Ø.542**	Osteonecrosis in diseases classified elsewhere, left hand
		◘	**M9Ø.549**	Osteonecrosis in diseases classified elsewhere, unsp hand
		◘	**M9Ø.561**	Osteonecrosis in diseases classd elswhr, right lower leg
		◘	**M9Ø.562**	Osteonecrosis in diseases classd elswhr, left lower leg
		◘	**M9Ø.569**	Osteonecrosis in diseases classd elswhr, unsp lower leg
		◘	**M9Ø.571**	Osteonecrosis in diseases classd elswhr, right ank/ft
		◘	**M9Ø.572**	Osteonecrosis in diseases classd elswhr, left ankle and foot
		◘	**M9Ø.579**	Osteonecrosis in diseases classd elswhr, unsp ankle and foot
		◘	**M9Ø.58**	Osteonecrosis in diseases classified elsewhere, other site
		◘	**M9Ø.59**	Osteonecrosis in diseases classd elswhr, multiple sites
733.5	OSTEITIS CONDENSANS		**M85.3Ø**	Osteitis condensans, unspecified site
			M85.31[1,2,9]	Osteitis condensans, shoulder
			M85.32[1,2,9]	Osteitis condensans, upper arm
			M85.33[1,2,9]	Osteitis condensans, forearm
			M85.34[1,2,9]	Osteitis condensans, hand
			M85.35[1,2,9]	Osteitis condensans, thigh
			M85.36[1,2,9]	Osteitis condensans, lower leg
			M85.37[1,2,9]	Osteitis condensans, ankle and foot
			M85.38	Osteitis condensans, other site
			M85.39	Osteitis condensans, multiple sites
				6th Character meanings for codes as indicated ***1 Right 2 Left 9 Unspecified***
733.6	TIETZES DISEASE	➡	**M94.Ø**	Chondrocostal junction syndrome [Tietze]
733.7	ALGONEURODYSTROPHY		**M89.ØØ**	Algoneurodystrophy, unspecified site
			M89.Ø1[1,2,9]	Algoneurodystrophy, shoulder
			M89.Ø2[1,2,9]	Algoneurodystrophy, upper arm
			M89.Ø3[1,2,9]	Algoneurodystrophy, forearm
			M89.Ø4[1,2,9]	Algoneurodystrophy, hand
			M89.Ø5[1,2,9]	Algoneurodystrophy, thigh
			M89.Ø6[1,2,9]	Algoneurodystrophy, lower leg
			M89.Ø7[1,2,9]	Algoneurodystrophy, ankle and foot
			M89.Ø8	Algoneurodystrophy, other site
			M89.Ø9	Algoneurodystrophy, multiple sites
				6th Character meanings for codes as indicated ***1 Right 2 Left 9 Unspecified***
733.81	MALUNION OF FRACTURE		**M8Ø.ØØXP**	Age-rel osteopor w crnt path fx, unsp site, sub for fx w malun
			M8Ø.Ø1[1,2,9]**P**	Age-rel osteopor w crnt path fx, shldr, sub for fx w malun
			M8Ø.Ø2[1,2,9]**P**	Age-rel osteopor w crnt path fx, humer, sub for fx w malun
			M8Ø.Ø3[1,2,9]**P**	Age-rel osteopor w crnt path fx, forearm, sub for fx w malun
			M8Ø.Ø4[1,2,9]**P**	Age-rel osteopor w crnt path fx, hand, sub for fx w malun
			M8Ø.Ø5[1,2,9]**P**	Age-rel osteopor w crnt path fx, femr, sub for fx w malun
			M8Ø.Ø6[1,2,9]**P**	Age-rel osteopor w crnt path fx, low leg, sub for fx w malun
			M8Ø.Ø7[1,2,9]**P**	Age-rel osteopor w crnt path fx, ank/ft, sub for fx w malun
			M8Ø.Ø8XP	Age-rel osteopor w crnt path fx, verteb, sub for fx w malun
			M8Ø.8ØXP	Oth osteopor w crnt path fx, unsp site, sub for fx w malun
			M8Ø.81[1,2,9]**P**	Oth osteopor w crnt path fx, shldr, subs for fx w malunion
			M8Ø.82[1,2,9]**P**	Oth osteopor w crnt path fx, humer, subs for fx w malunion
			M8Ø.83[1,2,9]**P**	Oth osteopor w crnt path fx, forearm, sub for fx w malun
			M8Ø.84[1,2,9]**P**	Oth osteopor w crnt path fx, hand, subs for fx w malunion
			M8Ø.85[1,2,9]**P**	Oth osteopor w crnt path fx, femur, subs for fx w malunion
			M8Ø.86[1,2,9]**P**	Oth osteopor w crnt path fx, low leg, sub for fx w malun
			M8Ø.87[1,2,9]**P**	Oth osteopor w crnt path fx, ank/ft, sub for fx w malun
			M8Ø.88XP	Oth osteopor w crnt path fx, verteb, subs for fx w malunion
			M84.3ØXP	Stress fracture, unsp site, subs for fx w malunion
			M84.31[1,2,9]**P**	Stress fracture, shoulder, subs for fx w malunion
			M84.32[1,2,9]**P**	Stress fracture, humerus, subs for fx w malunion
			M84.331P	Stress fracture, right ulna, subs for fx w malunion
			M84.332P	Stress fracture, left ulna, subs for fx w malunion
			M84.333P	Stress fracture, right radius, subs for fx w malunion
			M84.334P	Stress fracture, left radius, subs for fx w malunion
			M84.339P	Stress fx, unsp ulna and radius, subs for fx w malunion
			M84.341P	Stress fracture, right hand, subs for fx w malunion
			M84.342P	Stress fracture, left hand, subs for fx w malunion
			M84.343P	Stress fracture, unsp hand, subs for fx w malunion
			M84.344P	Stress fracture, right finger(s), subs for fx w malunion
			M84.345P	Stress fracture, left finger(s), subs for fx w malunion
	(Continued on next page)			***6th Character meanings for codes as indicated*** ***1 Right 2 Left 9 Unspecified***

ICD-9-CM		ICD-10-CM	
733.81	MALUNION OF FRACTURE **(Continued)**	**M84.346P**	Stress fracture, unsp finger(s), subs for fx w malunion
		M84.35ØP	Stress fracture, pelvis, subs encntr for fracture w malunion
		M84.351P	Stress fracture, right femur, subs for fx w malunion
		M84.352P	Stress fracture, left femur, subs for fx w malunion
		M84.353P	Stress fracture, unsp femur, subs for fx w malunion
		M84.359P	Stress fracture, hip, unsp, subs for fx w malunion
		M84.361P	Stress fracture, right tibia, subs for fx w malunion
		M84.362P	Stress fracture, left tibia, subs for fx w malunion
		M84.363P	Stress fracture, right fibula, subs for fx w malunion
		M84.364P	Stress fracture, left fibula, subs for fx w malunion
		M84.369P	Stress fx, unsp tibia and fibula, subs for fx w malunion
		M84.371P	Stress fracture, right ankle, subs for fx w malunion
		M84.372P	Stress fracture, left ankle, subs for fx w malunion
		M84.373P	Stress fracture, unsp ankle, subs for fx w malunion
		M84.374P	Stress fracture, right foot, subs for fx w malunion
		M84.375P	Stress fracture, left foot, subs for fx w malunion
		M84.376P	Stress fracture, unsp foot, subs for fx w malunion
		M84.377P	Stress fracture, right toe(s), subs for fx w malunion
		M84.378P	Stress fracture, left toe(s), subs for fx w malunion
		M84.379P	Stress fracture, unsp toe(s), subs for fx w malunion
		M84.38XP	Stress fracture, oth site, subs for fx w malunion
		M84.4ØXP	Pathological fracture, unsp site, subs for fx w malunion
		M84.41[1,2,9]P	Pathological fracture, shoulder, subs for fx w malunion
		M84.42[1,2,9]P	Pathological fracture, humerus, subs for fx w malunion
		M84.431P	Pathological fracture, right ulna, subs for fx w malunion
		M84.432P	Pathological fracture, left ulna, subs for fx w malunion
		M84.433P	Pathological fracture, right radius, subs for fx w malunion
		M84.434P	Pathological fracture, left radius, subs for fx w malunion
		M84.439P	Path fracture, unsp ulna and radius, subs for fx w malunion
		M84.441P	Pathological fracture, right hand, subs for fx w malunion
		M84.442P	Pathological fracture, left hand, subs for fx w malunion
		M84.443P	Pathological fracture, unsp hand, subs for fx w malunion
		M84.444P	Path fracture, right finger(s), subs for fx w malunion
		M84.445P	Path fracture, left finger(s), subs for fx w malunion
		M84.446P	Path fracture, unsp finger(s), subs for fx w malunion
		M84.451P	Pathological fracture, right femur, subs for fx w malunion
		M84.452P	Pathological fracture, left femur, subs for fx w malunion
		M84.453P	Pathological fracture, unsp femur, subs for fx w malunion
		M84.454P	Pathological fracture, pelvis, subs for fx w malunion
		M84.459P	Pathological fracture, hip, unsp, subs for fx w malunion
		M84.461P	Pathological fracture, right tibia, subs for fx w malunion
		M84.462P	Pathological fracture, left tibia, subs for fx w malunion
		M84.463P	Pathological fracture, right fibula, subs for fx w malunion
		M84.464P	Pathological fracture, left fibula, subs for fx w malunion
		M84.469P	Path fracture, unsp tibia and fibula, subs for fx w malunion
		M84.471P	Pathological fracture, right ankle, subs for fx w malunion
		M84.472P	Pathological fracture, left ankle, subs for fx w malunion
		M84.473P	Pathological fracture, unsp ankle, subs for fx w malunion
		M84.474P	Pathological fracture, right foot, subs for fx w malunion
		M84.475P	Pathological fracture, left foot, subs for fx w malunion
		M84.476P	Pathological fracture, unsp foot, subs for fx w malunion
		M84.477P	Pathological fracture, right toe(s), subs for fx w malunion
		M84.478P	Pathological fracture, left toe(s), subs for fx w malunion
		M84.479P	Pathological fracture, unsp toe(s), subs for fx w malunion
		M84.48XP	Pathological fracture, oth site, subs for fx w malunion
		M84.5ØXP	Path fx in neopltc dis, unsp site, subs for fx w malunion
		M84.51[1,2,9]P	Path fx in neopltc disease, shldr, subs for fx w malunion
		M84.52[1,2,9]P	Path fx in neopltc dis, humerus, subs for fx w malunion
		M84.531P	Path fx in neopltc disease, r ulna, subs for fx w malunion
		M84.532P	Path fx in neopltc disease, l ulna, subs for fx w malunion
		M84.533P	Path fx in neopltc disease, r radius, subs for fx w malunion
		M84.534P	Path fx in neopltc dis, left radius, subs for fx w malunion
		M84.539P	Path fx in neopltc dis, unsp ulna & rad, sub for fx w malun
		M84.54[1,2,9]P	Path fx in neopltc disease, hand, subs for fx w malunion
		M84.55ØP	Path fx in neopltc disease, pelvis, subs for fx w malunion
		M84.551P	Path fx in neopltc disease, r femur, subs for fx w malunion
		M84.552P	Path fx in neopltc disease, l femur, subs for fx w malunion
		M84.553P	Path fx in neopltc dis, unsp femur, subs for fx w malunion
		M84.559P	Path fx in neopltc dis, hip, unsp, subs for fx w malunion
		M84.561P	Path fx in neopltc disease, r tibia, subs for fx w malunion
		M84.562P	Path fx in neopltc disease, l tibia, subs for fx w malunion
		M84.563P	Path fx in neopltc disease, r fibula, subs for fx w malunion
		M84.564P	Path fx in neopltc disease, l fibula, subs for fx w malunion
		M84.569P	Path fx in neopltc dis, unsp tibia & fibula, sub for fx w malun
		M84.571P	Path fx in neopltc disease, r ankle, subs for fx w malunion
		M84.572P	Path fx in neopltc disease, l ankle, subs for fx w malunion
		M84.573P	Path fx in neopltc dis, unsp ankle, subs for fx w malunion
		M84.574P	Path fx in neopltc disease, r foot, subs for fx w malunion
		M84.575P	Path fx in neopltc disease, l foot, subs for fx w malunion
		M84.576P	Path fx in neopltc dis, unsp foot, subs for fx w malunion

6th Character meanings for codes as indicated
1 Right ***2 Left*** ***9 Unspecified***

(Continued on next page)

ICD-9-CM		ICD-10-CM	
733.81	MALUNION OF FRACTURE **(Continued)**	**M84.58XP**	Path fx in neopltc disease, oth spec site
		M84.6ØXP	Path fx in oth disease, unsp site
		M84.61[1,2,9]**P**	Path fx in oth disease, shoulder, subs for fx w malunion
		M84.62[1,2,9]**P**	Path fx in oth disease, humerus, subs for fx w malunion
		M84.631P	Path fracture in oth disease, r ulna, subs for fx w malunion
		M84.632P	Path fracture in oth disease, l ulna, subs for fx w malunion
		M84.633P	Path fx in oth disease, r radius, subs for fx w malunion
		M84.634P	Path fx in oth disease, left radius, subs for fx w malunion
		M84.639P	Path fx in oth dis, unsp ulna & rad, subs for fx w malunion
		M84.64[1,2,9]**P**	Path fracture in oth disease, hand, subs for fx w malunion
		M84.65ØP	Path fracture in oth disease, pelvis, subs for fx w malunion
		M84.651P	Path fx in oth disease, r femur, subs for fx w malunion
		M84.652P	Path fx in oth disease, l femur, subs for fx w malunion
		M84.653P	Path fx in oth disease, unsp femur, subs for fx w malunion
		M84.659P	Path fx in oth disease, hip, unsp, subs for fx w malunion
		M84.661P	Path fx in oth disease, r tibia, subs for fx w malunion
		M84.662P	Path fx in oth disease, l tibia, subs for fx w malunion
		M84.663P	Path fx in oth disease, r fibula, subs for fx w malunion
		M84.664P	Path fx in oth disease, l fibula, subs for fx w malunion
		M84.669P	Path fx in oth dis, unsp tibia & fibula, sub for fx w malun
		M84.671P	Path fx in oth disease, r ankle, subs for fx w malunion
		M84.672P	Path fx in oth disease, l ankle, subs for fx w malunion
		M84.673P	Path fx in oth disease, unsp ankle, subs for fx w malunion
		M84.674P	Path fracture in oth disease, r foot, subs for fx w malunion
		M84.675P	Path fracture in oth disease, l foot, subs for fx w malunion
		M84.676P	Path fx in oth disease, unsp foot, subs for fx w malunion
		M84.68XP	Path fx in oth disease, oth site, subs for fx w malunion
		S42.ØØ[1,2,9]**P**	Fracture of unsp part of clavicle, subs for fx w malunion
		S42.Ø11P	Ant disp fx of sternal end r clavicle, sub for fx w malun
		S42.Ø12P	Ant disp fx of sternal end l clavicle, sub for fx w malun
		S42.Ø13P	Ant disp fx of sternal end unsp clavicle, sub for fx w malun
		S42.Ø14P	Post disp fx of sternal end r clavicle, sub for fx w malun
		S42.Ø15P	Post disp fx of sternal end l clavicle, sub for fx w malun
		S42.Ø16P	Post disp fx of sternal end unsp clavicle, sub for fx w malun
		S42.Ø17P	Nondisp fx of sternal end r clavicle, subs for fx w malunion
		S42.Ø18P	Nondisp fx of sternal end l clavicle, subs for fx w malunion
		S42.Ø19P	Nondisp fx of sternal end unsp clavicle, sub for fx w malun
		S42.Ø21P	Disp fx of shaft of right clavicle, subs for fx w malunion
		S42.Ø22P	Disp fx of shaft of left clavicle, subs for fx w malunion
		S42.Ø23P	Disp fx of shaft of unsp clavicle, subs for fx w malunion
		S42.Ø24P	Nondisp fx of shaft of r clavicle, subs for fx w malunion
		S42.Ø25P	Nondisp fx of shaft of left clavicle, subs for fx w malunion
		S42.Ø26P	Nondisp fx of shaft of unsp clavicle, subs for fx w malunion
		S42.Ø31P	Disp fx of lateral end of r clavicle, subs for fx w malunion
		S42.Ø32P	Disp fx of lateral end of l clavicle, subs for fx w malunion
		S42.Ø33P	Disp fx of lateral end unsp clavicle, subs for fx w malunion
		S42.Ø34P	Nondisp fx of lateral end r clavicle, subs for fx w malunion
		S42.Ø35P	Nondisp fx of lateral end l clavicle, subs for fx w malunion
		S42.Ø36P	Nondisp fx of lateral end unsp clavicle, sub for fx w malun
		S42.1Ø[1,2,9]**P**	Fx unsp part of scapula, shoulder, subs for fx w malunion
		S42.111P	Disp fx of body of scapula, r shldr, subs for fx w malunion
		S42.112P	Disp fx of body of scapula, l shldr, subs for fx w malunion
		S42.113P	Disp fx of body of scapula, unsp shldr, sub for fx w malun
		S42.114P	Nondisp fx of body of scapula, r shldr, sub for fx w malun
		S42.115P	Nondisp fx of body of scapula, l shldr, sub for fx w malun
		S42.116P	Nondisp fx of body of scapula, unsp shldr, sub for fx w malun
		S42.121P	Disp fx of acromial process, r shldr, subs for fx w malunion
		S42.122P	Disp fx of acromial process, l shldr, subs for fx w malunion
		S42.123P	Disp fx of acromial pro, unsp shldr, subs for fx w malunion
		S42.124P	Nondisp fx of acromial pro, r shldr, subs for fx w malunion
		S42.125P	Nondisp fx of acromial pro, l shldr, subs for fx w malunion
		S42.126P	Nondisp fx of acromial pro, unsp shldr, sub for fx w malun
		S42.131P	Disp fx of coracoid process, r shldr, subs for fx w malunion
		S42.132P	Disp fx of coracoid process, l shldr, subs for fx w malunion
		S42.133P	Disp fx of coracoid pro, unsp shldr, subs for fx w malunion
		S42.134P	Nondisp fx of coracoid pro, r shldr, subs for fx w malunion
		S42.135P	Nondisp fx of coracoid pro, l shldr, subs for fx w malunion
		S42.136P	Nondisp fx of coracoid pro, unsp shldr, subs for fx w malunion
		S42.141P	Disp fx of glenoid cav of scapula, r shldr, sub for fx w malun
		S42.142P	Disp fx of glenoid cav of scapula, l shldr, sub for fx w malun
		S42.143P	Disp fx of glenoid cav of scapula, unsp shldr, sub for fx w malun
		S42.144P	Nondisp fx of glenoid cav of scapula, r shldr,sub for fx w malun
		S42.145P	Nondisp fx of glenoid cav of scapula, l shldr, sub for fx w malun
		S42.146P	Nondisp fx of glenoid cav of scapula, unsp shldr, sub for fx w malun
		S42.151P	Disp fx of neck of scapula, r shldr, subs for fx w malunion
		S42.152P	Disp fx of neck of scapula, l shldr, subs for fx w malunion
		S42.153P	Disp fx of nk of scapula, unsp shldr, subs for fx w malunion
		S42.154P	Nondisp fx of nk of scapula, r shldr, subs for fx w malunion
		S42.155P	Nondisp fx of nk of scapula, l shldr, subs for fx w malunion

6th Character meanings for codes as indicated
1 Right ***2 Left*** ***9 Unspecified***

(Continued on next page)

ICD-9-CM		ICD-10-CM	
733.81	MALUNION OF FRACTURE **(Continued)**	**S42.156P**	Nondisp fx of nk of scapula, unsp shldr, sub for fx w malun
		S42.19[1,2,9]P	Fracture oth prt scapula, shoulder, subs for fx w malunion
		S42.2Ø[1,2,9]P	Unsp fx upper end of humerus, subs for fx w malunion
		S42.211P	Unsp disp fx of surg neck of r humer, subs for fx w malunion
		S42.212P	Unsp disp fx of surg neck of l humer, subs for fx w malunion
		S42.213P	Unsp disp fx of surg nk of unsp humer, sub for fx w malun
		S42.214P	Unsp nondisp fx of surg nk of r humer, sub for fx w malun
		S42.215P	Unsp nondisp fx of surg nk of l humer, sub for fx w malun
		S42.216P	Unsp nondisp fx of surg nk of unsp humer, sub for fx w malun
		S42.221P	2-part disp fx of surg nk of r humer, subs for fx w malunion
		S42.222P	2-part disp fx of surg nk of l humer, subs for fx w malunion
		S42.223P	2-part disp fx of surg nk of unsp humer, sub for fx w malun
		S42.224P	2-part nondisp fx of surg nk of r humer, sub for fx w malun
		S42.225P	2-part nondisp fx of surg nk of l humer, sub for fx w malun
		S42.226P	2-part nondisp fx of surg nk of unsp humer, sub for fx w malun
		S42.23[1,2,9]P	3-part fx surgical neck of humerus, subs for fx w malunion
		S42.24[1,2,9]P	4-part fx surgical neck of humerus, subs for fx w malunion
		S42.251P	Disp fx of greater tuberosity of r humer, sub for fx w malun
		S42.252P	Disp fx of greater tuberosity of l humer, sub for fx w malun
		S42.253P	Disp fx of greater tuberosity of unsp humer, sub for fx w malun
		S42.254P	Nondisp fx of greater tuberosity of r humer, sub for fx w malun
		S42.255P	Nondisp fx of greater tuberosity of l humer, sub for fx w malun
		S42.256P	Nondisp fx of greater tuberosity of unsp humer, sub for fx w malun
		S42.261P	Disp fx of less tuberosity of r humer, sub for fx w malun
		S42.262P	Disp fx of less tuberosity of l humer, sub for fx w malun
		S42.263P	Disp fx of less tuberosity of unsp humer, sub for fx w malun
		S42.264P	Nondisp fx of less tuberosity of r humer, sub for fx w malun
		S42.265P	Nondisp fx of less tuberosity of l humer, sub for fx w malun
		S42.266P	Nondisp fx of less tuberosity of unsp humer, sub for fx w malun
		S42.27[1,2,9]P	Torus fx upper end of humerus, subs for fx w malunion
		S42.291P	Oth disp fx of upper end of r humer, subs for fx w malunion
		S42.292P	Oth disp fx of upper end of l humer, subs for fx w malunion
		S42.293P	Oth disp fx of upper end unsp humer, subs for fx w malunion
		S42.294P	Oth nondisp fx of upper end r humer, subs for fx w malunion
		S42.295P	Oth nondisp fx of upper end l humer, subs for fx w malunion
		S42.296P	Oth nondisp fx of upr end unsp humer, subs for fx w malunion
		S42.3Ø[1,2,9]P	Unsp fx shaft of humerus, arm, subs for fx w malunion
		S42.31[1,2,9]P	Greenstick fx shaft of humer, arm, subs for fx w malunion
		S42.321P	Displ transverse fx shaft of humer, r arm, sub for fx w malun
		S42.322P	Displ transverse fx shaft of humer, l arm, sub for fx w malun
		S42.323P	Displ transverse fx shaft of humer, unsp arm, sub for fx w malun
		S42.324P	Nondisp transverse fx shaft of humer, r arm, sub for fx w malun
		S42.325P	Nondisp transverse fx shaft of humer, l arm, sub for fx w malun
		S42.326P	Nondisp transverse fx shaft of humer, unsp arm, sub for fx w malun
		S42.331P	Displ oblique fx shaft of humer, r arm, sub for fx w malun
		S42.332P	Displ oblique fx shaft of humer, l arm, sub for fx w malun
		S42.333P	Displ oblique fx shaft of humer, unsp arm, sub for fx w malun
		S42.334P	Nondisp oblique fx shaft of humer, r arm, sub for fx w malun
		S42.335P	Nondisp oblique fx shaft of humer, l arm, sub for fx w malun
		S42.336P	Nondisp oblique fx shaft of humer, unsp arm, sub for fx w malun
		S42.341P	Displ spiral fx shaft of humer, r arm, sub for fx w malun
		S42.342P	Displ spiral fx shaft of humer, l arm, sub for fx w malun
		S42.343P	Displ spiral fx shaft of humer, unsp arm, sub for fx w malun
		S42.344P	Nondisp spiral fx shaft of humer, r arm, sub for fx w malun
		S42.345P	Nondisp spiral fx shaft of humer, l arm, sub for fx w malun
		S42.346P	Nondisp spiral fx shaft of humer, unsp arm, sub for fx w malun
		S42.351P	Displ commnt fx shaft of humer, r arm, sub for fx w malun
		S42.352P	Displ commnt fx shaft of humer, l arm, sub for fx w malun
		S42.353P	Displ commnt fx shaft of humer, unsp arm, sub for fx w malun
		S42.354P	Nondisp commnt fx shaft of humer, r arm, sub for fx w malun
		S42.355P	Nondisp commnt fx shaft of humer, l arm, sub for fx w malun
		S42.356P	Nondisp commnt fx shaft of humer, unsp arm, sub for fx w malun
		S42.361P	Displ seg fx shaft of humer, r arm, subs for fx w malunion
		S42.362P	Displ seg fx shaft of humer, l arm, subs for fx w malunion
		S42.363P	Displ seg fx shaft of humer, unsp arm, sub for fx w malun
		S42.364P	Nondisp seg fx shaft of humer, r arm, subs for fx w malunion
		S42.365P	Nondisp seg fx shaft of humer, l arm, subs for fx w malunion
		S42.366P	Nondisp seg fx shaft of humer, unsp arm, sub for fx w malun
		S42.391P	Oth fracture of shaft of r humerus, subs for fx w malunion
		S42.392P	Oth fracture of shaft of l humerus, subs for fx w malunion
		S42.399P	Oth fx shaft of unsp humerus, subs for fx w malunion
		S42.4Ø[1,2,9]P	Unsp fx lower end of humerus, subs for fx w malunion
		S42.411P	Displ simp suprcndl fx w/o intrcndl fx humer, sub for fx w malun
		S42.412P	Displ simp suprcndl fx w/o intrcndl fx l humer, sub for fx w malun
		S42.413P	Displ simp suprcndl fx w/o intrcndl fx unsp humer, sub for fx w malun
		S42.414P	Nondisp simp suprcndl fx w/o intrcndl fx r humer, sub for fx w malun
		S42.415P	Nondisp simp suprcndl fx w/o intrcndl fx l humer, sub for fx w malun
		S42.416P	Nondisp simp suprcndl fx w/o intrcndl fx unsp humer, sub for fx w malun
		S42.421P	Displ commnt suprcndl fx w/o intrcndl fx r humer, sub for fx w malun
		S42.422P	Displ commnt suprcndl fx w/o intrcndl fx l humer, sub for fx w malun

6th Character meanings for codes as indicated
1 Right ***2 Left*** ***9 Unspecified***

(Continued on next page)

[Brackets] indicate valid character values for each code. Character value meanings provided for each code grouping.

ICD-9-CM		ICD-10-CM	
733.81	MALUNION OF FRACTURE (Continued)	S42.423P	Displ commnt suprcndl fx w/o intrcndl fx unsp humer, sub for fx w malun
		S42.424P	Nondisp commnt suprcndl fx w/o intrcndl fx r humer, sub for fx w malun
		S42.425P	Nondisp commnt suprcndl fx w/o intrcndl fx l humer, sub for fx w malun
		S42.426P	Nondisp commnt suprcndl fx w/o intrcndl fx unsp humer, sub for fx w malun
		S42.431P	Disp fx of lateral epicondyl of r humer, sub for fx w malun
		S42.432P	Disp fx of lateral epicondyl of l humer, sub for fx w malun
		S42.433P	Disp fx of lateral epicondyl of unsp humer, sub for fx w malun
		S42.434P	Nondisp fx of lateral epicondyl of r humer, sub for fx w malun
		S42.435P	Nondisp fx of lateral epicondyl of l humer, sub for fx w malun
		S42.436P	Nondisp fx of lateral epicondyl of unsp humer, sub for fx w malun
		S42.441P	Disp fx of med epicondyl of r humer, subs for fx w malunion
		S42.442P	Disp fx of med epicondyl of l humer, subs for fx w malunion
		S42.443P	Disp fx of med epicondyl of unsp humer, sub for fx w malun
		S42.444P	Nondisp fx of med epicondyl of r humer, sub for fx w malun
		S42.445P	Nondisp fx of med epicondyl of l humer, sub for fx w malun
		S42.446P	Nondisp fx of med epicondyl of unsp humer, sub for fx w malun
		S42.447P	Incarcerated fx of med epicondyl of r humer, sub for fx w malun
		S42.448P	Incarcerated fx of med epicondyl of l humer, sub for fx w malun
		S42.449P	Incarcerated fx of med epicondyl of unsp humer, sub for fx w malun
		S42.451P	Disp fx of lateral condyle of r humer, sub for fx w malun
		S42.452P	Disp fx of lateral condyle of l humer, sub for fx w malun
		S42.453P	Disp fx of lateral condyle of unsp humer, sub for fx w malun
		S42.454P	Nondisp fx of lateral condyle of r humer, sub for fx w malun
		S42.455P	Nondisp fx of lateral condyle of l humer, sub for fx w malun
		S42.456P	Nondisp fx of lateral condyle of unsp humer, sub for fx w malun
		S42.461P	Disp fx of medial condyle of r humer, subs for fx w malunion
		S42.462P	Disp fx of medial condyle of l humer, subs for fx w malunion
		S42.463P	Disp fx of med condyle of unsp humer, subs for fx w malunion
		S42.464P	Nondisp fx of med condyle of r humer, subs for fx w malunion
		S42.465P	Nondisp fx of med condyle of l humer, subs for fx w malunion
		S42.466P	Nondisp fx of med condyle of unsp humer, sub for fx w malun
		S42.471P	Displaced transcondy fx r humerus, subs for fx w malunion
		S42.472P	Displaced transcondy fx l humerus, subs for fx w malunion
		S42.473P	Displaced transcondy fx unsp humerus, subs for fx w malunion
		S42.474P	Nondisp transcondy fx r humerus, subs for fx w malunion
		S42.475P	Nondisp transcondy fx l humerus, subs for fx w malunion
		S42.476P	Nondisp transcondy fx unsp humerus, subs for fx w malunion
		S42.481P	Torus fx lower end of r humerus, subs for fx w malunion
		S42.482P	Torus fx lower end of l humerus, subs for fx w malunion
		S42.489P	Torus fx lower end of unsp humerus, subs for fx w malunion
		S42.491P	Oth disp fx of lower end of r humer, subs for fx w malunion
		S42.492P	Oth disp fx of lower end of l humer, subs for fx w malunion
		S42.493P	Oth disp fx of lower end unsp humer, subs for fx w malunion
		S42.494P	Oth nondisp fx of lower end r humer, subs for fx w malunion
		S42.495P	Oth nondisp fx of lower end l humer, subs for fx w malunion
		S42.496P	Oth nondisp fx of low end unsp humer, subs for fx w malunion
		S42.9ØXP	Fx unsp shoulder girdle, part unsp, subs for fx w malunion
		S42.91XP	Fx r shoulder girdle, part unsp, subs for fx w malunion
		S42.92XP	Fx l shoulder girdle, part unsp, subs for fx w malunion
		S49.ØØ[1,2,9]P	Unsp physl fx upper end humer, arm, subs for fx w malunion
		S49.Ø1[1,2,9]P	Sltr-haris Type I physl fx upr end humer, arm, sub for fx w malun
		S49.Ø2[1,2,9]P	Sltr-haris Type II physl fx upr end humer, arm, sub for fx w malun
		S49.Ø3[1,2,9]P	Sltr-haris Type III physl fx upr end humer, arm, sub for fx w malun
		S49.Ø4[1,2,9]P	Sltr-haris Type IV physl fx upr end humer, arm, sub for fx w malun
		S49.Ø9[1,2,9]P	Oth physl fx upper end humer, arm, subs for fx w malunion
		S49.1Ø[1,2,9]P	Unsp physl fx low end humer, arm, subs for fx w malunion
		S49.11[1,2,9]P	Sltr-haris Type I physl fx low end humer, arm, sub for fx w malun
		S49.12[1,2,9]P	Sltr-haris Type II physl fx low end humer, arm, sub for fx w malun
		S49.13[1,2,9]P	Sltr-haris Type III physl fx low end humer, arm, sub for fx w malun
		S49.14[1,2,9]P	Sltr-haris Type IV physl fx low end humer, arm, sub for fx w malun
		S49.19[1,2,9]P	Oth physl fx low end humer, arm, subs for fx w malunion
		S52.ØØ1[P,Q,R]	Unsp fx upper end of right ulna
		S52.ØØ2[P,Q,R]	Unsp fx upper end of left ulna
		S52.ØØ9[P,Q,R]	Unsp fx upper end of unsp ulna
		S52.Ø1[1,2,9]P	Torus fx upper end of ulna, subs for fx w malunion
		S52.Ø21[P,Q,R]	Disp fx of olecran pro w/o intartic extn r ulna
		S52.Ø22[P,Q,R]	Disp fx of olecran pro w/o intartic extn l ulna
		S52.Ø23[P,Q,R]	Disp fx of olecran pro w/o intartic extn unsp ulna
		S52.Ø24[P,Q,R]	Nondisp fx of olecran pro w/o intartic extn r ulna
		S52.Ø25[P,Q,R]	Nondisp fx of olecran pro w/o intartic extn l ulna
		S52.Ø26[P,Q,R]	Nondisp fx of olecran pro w/o intartic extn unsp ulna
		S52.Ø31[P,Q,R]	Disp fx of olecran pro w intartic extn r ulna
		S52.Ø32[P,Q,R]	Disp fx of olecran pro w intartic extn l ulna
		S52.Ø33[P,Q,R]	Disp fx of olecran pro w intartic extn unsp ulna

(Continued on next page)

6th Character meanings for codes as indicated
1 Right ***2 Left*** ***9 Unspecified***

7th Character meanins for codes S52.-
P Sub Enc Closed FX Malunion
Q Sub Enc Open FX Type I/II Malunion
R Sub Enc Open IIIA/B/C Malunion

ICD-9-CM	ICD-10-CM
733.81 MALUNION OF FRACTURE **(Continued)**	**S52.Ø34**[P,Q,R] Nondisp fx of olecran pro w intartic extn r ulna
	S52.Ø35[P,Q,R] Nondisp fx of olecran pro w intartic extn l ulna
	S52.Ø36[P,Q,R] Nondisp fx of olecran pro w intartic extn unsp ulna
	S52.Ø41[P,Q,R] Disp fx of coronoid pro of r ulna
	S52.Ø42[P,Q,R] Disp fx of coronoid pro of l ulna
	S52.Ø43[P,Q,R] Disp fx of coronoid pro of unsp ulna
	S52.Ø44[P,Q,R] Nondisp fx of coronoid pro of r ulna
	S52.Ø45[P,Q,R] Nondisp fx of coronoid pro of l ulna
	S52.Ø46[P,Q,R] Nondisp fx of coronoid pro of unsp ulna
	S52.Ø91[P,Q,R] Oth fx upper end of right ulna
	S52.Ø92[P,Q,R] Oth fx upper end of left ulna
	S52.Ø99[P,Q,R] Oth fx upper end of unsp ulna
	S52.1Ø1[P,Q,R] Unsp fx upper end of r radius
	S52.1Ø2[P,Q,R] Unsp fx upper end left radius
	S52.1Ø9[P,Q,R] Unsp fx upper end unsp radius
	S52.11[1,2,9]**P** Torus fx upper end of radius, subs for fx w malunion
	S52.121[P,Q,R] Disp fx of head of right radius
	S52.122[P,Q,R] Disp fx of head of left radius
	S52.123[P,Q,R] Disp fx of head of unsp radius
	S52.124[P,Q,R] Nondisp fx of head of r radius
	S52.125[P,Q,R] Nondisp fx of head of left rad
	S52.126[P,Q,R] Nondisp fx of head of unsp rad
	S52.131[P,Q,R] Disp fx of neck of right radius
	S52.132[P,Q,R] Disp fx of neck of left radius
	S52.133[P,Q,R] Disp fx of neck of unsp radius
	S52.134[P,Q,R] Nondisp fx of neck of r radius
	S52.135[P,Q,R] Nondisp fx of neck of left rad
	S52.136[P,Q,R] Nondisp fx of neck of unsp rad
	S52.181[P,Q,R] Oth fx upper end of r radius
	S52.182[P,Q,R] Oth fx upper end of left radius
	S52.189[P,Q,R] Oth fx upper end of unsp radius
	S52.2Ø1[P,Q,R] Unsp fx shaft of right ulna
	S52.2Ø2[P,Q,R] Unsp fx shaft of left ulna
	S52.2Ø9[P,Q,R] Unsp fx shaft of unsp ulna
	S52.21[1,2,9]**P** Greenstick fx shaft of ulna, subs for fx w malunion
	S52.221[P,Q,R] Displ transverse fx shaft of r ulna
	S52.222[P,Q,R] Displ transverse fx shaft of l ulna
	S52.223[P,Q,R] Displ transverse fx shaft of unsp ulna
	S52.224[P,Q,R] Nondisp transverse fx shaft of r ulna
	S52.225[P,Q,R] Nondisp transverse fx shaft of l ulna
	S52.226[P,Q,R] Nondisp transverse fx shaft of unsp ulna
	S52.231[P,Q,R] Displ oblique fx shaft of r ulna
	S52.232[P,Q,R] Displ oblique fx shaft of l ulna
	S52.233[P,Q,R] Displ oblique fx shaft of unsp ulna
	S52.234[P,Q,R] Nondisp oblique fx shaft of r ulna
	S52.235[P,Q,R] Nondisp oblique fx shaft of l ulna
	S52.236[P,Q,R] Nondisp oblique fx shaft of unsp ulna
	S52.241[P,Q,R] Displ spiral fx shaft of ulna, r arm
	S52.242[P,Q,R] Displ spiral fx shaft of ulna, l arm
	S52.243[P,Q,R] Displ spiral fx shaft of ulna, unsp arm
	S52.244[P,Q,R] Nondisp spiral fx shaft of ulna, r arm
	S52.245[P,Q,R] Nondisp spiral fx shaft of ulna, l arm
	S52.246[P,Q,R] Nondisp spiral fx shaft of ulna, unsp arm
	S52.251[P,Q,R] Displ commnt fx shaft of ulna, r arm
	S52.252[P,Q,R] Displ commnt fx shaft of ulna, l arm
	S52.253[P,Q,R] Displ commnt fx shaft of ulna, unsp arm
	S52.254[P,Q,R] Nondisp commnt fx shaft of ulna, r arm
	S52.255[P,Q,R] Nondisp commnt fx shaft of ulna, l arm
	S52.256[P,Q,R] Nondisp commnt fx shaft of ulna, unsp arm
	S52.261[P,Q,R] Displ seg fx shaft of ulna, r arm
	S52.262[P,Q,R] Displ seg fx shaft of ulna, l arm
	S52.263[P,Q,R] Displ seg fx shaft of ulna, unsp arm
	S52.264[P,Q,R] Nondisp seg fx shaft of ulna, r arm
	S52.265[P,Q,R] Nondisp seg fx shaft of ulna, l arm
	S52.266[P,Q,R] Nondisp seg fx shaft of ulna, unsp arm
	S52.271[P,Q,R] Monteggia's fx right ulna
	S52.272[P,Q,R] Monteggia's fx left ulna
	S52.279[P,Q,R] Monteggia's fx unsp ulna
	S52.281[P,Q,R] Bent bone of right ulna
	S52.282[P,Q,R] Bent bone of left ulna
	S52.283[P,Q,R] Bent bone of unsp ulna
	S52.291[P,Q,R] Oth fx shaft of right ulna
	S52.292[P,Q,R] Oth fx shaft of left ulna
	S52.299[P,Q,R] Oth fx shaft of unsp ulna

6th Character meanings for codes as indicated
1 Right ***2 Left*** ***9 Unspecified***

7th Character meanins for codes S52.-
P Sub Enc Closed FX Malunion
Q Sub Enc Open FX Type I/II Malunion
R Sub Enc Open IIIA/B/C Malunion

(Continued on next page)

[Brackets] indicate valid character values for each code. Character value meanings provided for each code grouping.

ICD-9-CM		ICD-10-CM	
733.81	MALUNION OF FRACTURE (Continued)	**S52.301[P,Q,R]**	Unsp fx shaft of r radius
		S52.302[P,Q,R]	Unsp fx shaft of left radius
		S52.309[P,Q,R]	Unsp fx shaft of unsp radius
		S52.31[1,2,9]P	Greenstick fx shaft of rad, arm, subs for fx w malunion
		S52.321[P,Q,R]	Displ transverse fx shaft of r rad
		S52.322[P,Q,R]	Displ transverse fx shaft of l rad
		S52.323[P,Q,R]	Displ transverse fx shaft of unsp rad
		S52.324[P,Q,R]	Nondisp transverse fx shaft of r rad
		S52.325[P,Q,R]	Nondisp transverse fx shaft of l rad
		S52.326[P,Q,R]	Nondisp transverse fx shaft of unsp rad
		S52.331[P,Q,R]	Displ oblique fx shaft of r rad
		S52.332[P,Q,R]	Displ oblique fx shaft of l rad
		S52.333[P,Q,R]	Displ oblique fx shaft of unsp rad
		S52.334[P,Q,R]	Nondisp oblique fx shaft of r rad
		S52.335[P,Q,R]	Nondisp oblique fx shaft of l rad
		S52.336[P,Q,R]	Nondisp oblique fx shaft of unsp rad
		S52.341[P,Q,R]	Displ spiral fx shaft of rad, r arm
		S52.342[P,Q,R]	Displ spiral fx shaft of rad, l arm
		S52.343[P,Q,R]	Displ spiral fx shaft of rad, unsp arm
		S52.344[P,Q,R]	Nondisp spiral fx shaft of rad, r arm
		S52.345[P,Q,R]	Nondisp spiral fx shaft of rad, l arm
		S52.346[P,Q,R]	Nondisp spiral fx shaft of rad, unsp arm
		S52.351[P,Q,R]	Displ commnt fx shaft of rad, r arm
		S52.352[P,Q,R]	Displ commnt fx shaft of rad, l arm
		S52.353[P,Q,R]	Displ commnt fx shaft of rad, unsp arm
		S52.354[P,Q,R]	Nondisp commnt fx shaft of rad, r arm
		S52.355[P,Q,R]	Nondisp commnt fx shaft of rad, l arm
		S52.356[P,Q,R]	Nondisp commnt fx shaft of rad, unsp arm
		S52.361[P,Q,R]	Displ seg fx shaft of rad, r arm
		S52.362[P,Q,R]	Displ seg fx shaft of rad, l arm
		S52.363[P,Q,R]	Displ seg fx shaft of rad, unsp arm
		S52.364[P,Q,R]	Nondisp seg fx shaft of rad, r arm
		S52.365[P,Q,R]	Nondisp seg fx shaft of rad, l arm
		S52.366[P,Q,R]	Nondisp seg fx shaft of rad, unsp arm
		S52.371[P,Q,R]	Galeazzi's fracture of r radius
		S52.372[P,Q,R]	Galeazzi's fx left radius
		S52.379[P,Q,R]	Galeazzi's fx unsp radius
		S52.381[P,Q,R]	Bent bone of right radius
		S52.382[P,Q,R]	Bent bone of left radius
		S52.389[P,Q,R]	Bent bone of unsp radius
		S52.391[P,Q,R]	Oth fx shaft of rad, right arm
		S52.392[P,Q,R]	Oth fx shaft of rad, left arm
		S52.399[P,Q,R]	Oth fx shaft of rad, unsp arm
		S52.501[P,Q,R]	Unsp fx the lower end r radius
		S52.502[P,Q,R]	Unsp fx the lower end left rad
		S52.509[P,Q,R]	Unsp fx the lower end unsp rad
		S52.511[P,Q,R]	Disp fx of r radial styloid pro
		S52.512[P,Q,R]	Disp fx of l radial styloid pro
		S52.513[P,Q,R]	Disp fx of unsp radial styloid pro
		S52.514[P,Q,R]	Nondisp fx of r radial styloid pro
		S52.515[P,Q,R]	Nondisp fx of l radial styloid pro
		S52.516[P,Q,R]	Nondisp fx of unsp radial styloid pro
		S52.521P	Torus fx lower end of radius
		S52.522P	Torus fx lower end of left radius, subs for fx w malunion
		S52.529P	Torus fx lower end of unsp radius, subs for fx w malunion
		S52.531[P,Q,R]	Colles' fracture of r radius
		S52.532[P,Q,R]	Colles' fracture of left radius
		S52.539[P,Q,R]	Colles' fracture of unsp radius
		S52.541[P,Q,R]	Smith's fracture of r radius
		S52.542[P,Q,R]	Smith's fracture of left radius
		S52.549[P,Q,R]	Smith's fracture of unsp radius
		S52.551[P,Q,R]	Oth extrartic fx low end r rad
		S52.552[P,Q,R]	Oth extrartic fx low end l rad
		S52.559[P,Q,R]	Oth extrartic fx low end unsp rad
		S52.561[P,Q,R]	Barton's fracture of r radius
		S52.562[P,Q,R]	Barton's fx left radius
		S52.569[P,Q,R]	Barton's fx unsp radius
		S52.571[P,Q,R]	Oth intartic fx lower end r rad
		S52.572[P,Q,R]	Oth intartic fx low end l rad
		S52.579[P,Q,R]	Oth intartic fx low end unsp rad
		S52.591[P,Q,R]	Oth fx of lower end of r radius
		S52.592[P,Q,R]	Oth fx of lower end left radius
		S52.599[P,Q,R]	Oth fx of lower end unsp radius
		S52.601[P,Q,R]	Unsp fx lower end of right ulna
		S52.602[P,Q,R]	Unsp fx lower end of left ulna
		S52.609[P,Q,R]	Unsp fx lower end of unsp ulna

6th Character meanings for codes as indicated
1 Right ***2 Left*** ***9 Unspecified***

7th Character meanins for codes S52.-
P Sub Enc Closed FX Malunion
Q Sub Enc Open FX Type I/II Malunion
R Sub Enc Open IIIA/B/C Malunion

(Continued on next page)

ICD-9-CM		ICD-10-CM	
733.81	MALUNION OF FRACTURE **(Continued)**	**S52.611**[P,Q,R]	Disp fx of r ulna styloid pro
		S52.612[P,Q,R]	Disp fx of l ulna styloid pro
		S52.613[P,Q,R]	Disp fx of unsp ulna styloid pro
		S52.614[P,Q,R]	Nondisp fx of r ulna styloid pro
		S52.615[P,Q,R]	Nondisp fx of l ulna styloid pro
		S52.616[P,Q,R]	Nondisp fx of unsp ulna styloid pro
		S52.62[1,2,9]**P**	Torus fx lower end of ulna, subs for fx w malunion
		S52.691[P,Q,R]	Oth fx lower end of right ulna
		S52.692[P,Q,R]	Oth fx lower end of left ulna
		S52.699[P,Q,R]	Oth fx lower end of unsp ulna
		S52.9ØX[P,Q,R]	Unsp fracture of unsp forearm
		S52.91X[P,Q,R]	Unsp fracture of right forearm
		S52.92X[P,Q,R]	Unsp fracture of left forearm
		S59.ØØ[1,2,9]**P**	Unsp physl fx low end ulna, arm, subs for fx w malunion
		S59.Ø1[1,2,9]**P**	Sltr-haris Type I physl fx low end ulna, arm, sub for fx w malun
		S59.Ø2[1,2,9]**P**	Sltr-haris Type II physl fx low end ulna, arm, sub for fx w malun
		S59.Ø3[1,2,9]**P**	Sltr-haris Type III physl fx low end ulna, arm, sub for fx w malun
		S59.Ø4[1,2,9]**P**	Sltr-haris Type IV physl fx low end ulna, arm, sub for fx w malun
		S59.Ø9[1,2,9]**P**	Oth physl fx low end ulna, arm, subs for fx w malunion
		S59.1Ø[1,2,9]**P**	Unsp physl fx upper end rad, arm, subs for fx w malunion
		S59.11[1,2,9]**P**	Sltr-haris Type I physl fx upr end rad, arm, sub for fx w malun
		S59.12[1,2,9]**P**	Sltr-haris Type II physl fx upr end rad, arm, sub for fx w malun
		S59.13[1,2,9]**P**	Sltr-haris Type III physl fx upr end rad, arm, sub for fx w malun
		S59.14[1,2,9]**P**	Sltr-haris Type IV physl fx upr end rad, arm, sub for fx w malun
		S59.19[1,2,9]**P**	Oth physl fx upper end rad, arm, subs for fx w malunion
		S59.2Ø[1,2,9]**P**	Unsp physl fx low end rad, right arm, subs for fx w malunion
		S59.21[1,2,9]**P**	Sltr-haris Type I physl fx low end rad, arm, sub for fx w malun
		S59.22[1,2,9]**P**	Sltr-haris Type II physl fx low end rad, arm, sub for fx w malun
		S59.23[1,2,9]**P**	Sltr-haris Type III physl fx low end rad, arm, sub for fx w malun
		S59.24[1,2,9]**P**	Sltr-haris Type IV physl fx low end rad, arm, sub for fx w malun
		S59.29[1,2,9]**P**	Oth physl fx low end rad, arm, subs for fx w malunion
		S62.ØØ[1,2,9]**P**	Unsp fx navicular bone of wrist, subs for fx w malunion
		S62.Ø11P	Disp fx of dist pole of navic bone of r wrs, sub for fx w malun
		S62.Ø12P	Disp fx of dist pole of navic bone of l wrs, sub for fx w malun
		S62.Ø13P	Disp fx of dist pole of navic bone of unsp wrs, sub for fx w malun
		S62.Ø14P	Nondisp fx of dist pole of navic bone of r wrs, sub for fx w malun
		S62.Ø15P	Nondisp fx of dist pole of navic bone of l wrs, sub for fx w malun
		S62.Ø16P	Nondisp fx of dist pole of navic bone of unsp wrs, sub for fx w malun
		S62.Ø21P	Disp fx of mid 3rd of navic bone of r wrs, sub for fx w malun
		S62.Ø22P	Disp fx of mid 3rd of navic bone of l wrs, sub for fx w malun
		S62.Ø23P	Disp fx of mid 3rd of navic bone of unsp wrs, sub for fx w malun
		S62.Ø24P	Nondisp fx of mid 3rd of navic bone of r wrs, sub for fx w malun
		S62.Ø25P	Nondisp fx of mid 3rd of navic bone of l wrs, sub for fx w malun
		S62.Ø26P	Nondisp fx of mid 3rd of navic bone of unsp wrs, sub for fx w malun
		S62.Ø31P	Disp fx of prox 3rd of navic bone of r wrs, sub for fx w malun
		S62.Ø32P	Disp fx of prox 3rd of navic bone of l wrs, sub for fx w malun
		S62.Ø33P	Disp fx of prox 3rd of navic bone of unsp wrs, sub for fx w malun
		S62.Ø34P	Nondisp fx of prox 3rd of navic bone of r wrs, sub for fx w malun
		S62.Ø35P	Nondisp fx of prox 3rd of navic bone of l wrs, sub for fx w malun
		S62.Ø36P	Nondisp fx of prox 3rd of navic bone of unsp wrs, sub for fx w malun
		S62.1Ø[1,2,9]**P**	Fx unsp carpal bone, wrist, subs for fx w malunion
		S62.111P	Disp fx of triquetrum bone, r wrist, subs for fx w malunion
		S62.112P	Disp fx of triquetrum bone, l wrist, subs for fx w malunion
		S62.113P	Disp fx of triquetrum bone, unsp wrs, subs for fx w malunion
		S62.114P	Nondisp fx of triquetrum bone, r wrs, subs for fx w malunion
		S62.115P	Nondisp fx of triquetrum bone, l wrs, subs for fx w malunion
		S62.116P	Nondisp fx of triquetrum bone, unsp wrs, sub for fx w malun
		S62.121P	Disp fx of lunate, right wrist, subs for fx w malunion
		S62.122P	Disp fx of lunate, left wrist, subs for fx w malunion
		S62.123P	Disp fx of lunate, unsp wrist, subs for fx w malunion
		S62.124P	Nondisp fx of lunate, right wrist, subs for fx w malunion
		S62.125P	Nondisp fx of lunate, left wrist, subs for fx w malunion
		S62.126P	Nondisp fx of lunate, unsp wrist, subs for fx w malunion
		S62.131P	Disp fx of capitate bone, r wrist, subs for fx w malunion
		S62.132P	Disp fx of capitate bone, left wrist, subs for fx w malunion
		S62.133P	Disp fx of capitate bone, unsp wrist, subs for fx w malunion
		S62.134P	Nondisp fx of capitate bone, r wrist, subs for fx w malunion
		S62.135P	Nondisp fx of capitate bone, l wrist, subs for fx w malunion
		S62.136P	Nondisp fx of capitate bone, unsp wrs, sub for fx w malun
		S62.141P	Disp fx of body of hamate bone, r wrs, sub for fx w malun
		S62.142P	Disp fx of body of hamate bone, l wrs, sub for fx w malun
		S62.143P	Disp fx of body of hamate bone, unsp wrs, sub for fx w malun
		S62.144P	Nondisp fx of body of hamate bone, r wrs, sub for fx w malun
		S62.145P	Nondisp fx of body of hamate bone, l wrs, sub for fx w malun
		S62.146P	Nondisp fx of body of hamate bone, unsp wrs, sub for fx w malun
		S62.151P	Disp fx of hook pro of hamate bone, r wrs, sub for fx w malun
		S62.152P	Disp fx of hook pro of hamate bone, l wrs, sub for fx w malun
		S62.153P	Disp fx of hook pro of hamate bone, unsp wrs, sub for fx w malun

6th Character meanings for codes as indicated
1 Right ***2 Left*** ***9 Unspecified***

7th Character meanins for codes S52.-
P Sub Enc Closed FX Malunion
Q Sub Enc Open FX Type I/II Malunion
R Sub Enc Open IIIA/B/C Malunion

(Continued on next page)

ICD-9-CM		ICD-10-CM	
733.81	MALUNION OF FRACTURE **(Continued)**	**S62.154P**	Nondisp fx of hook pro of hamate bone, r wrs, sub for fx w malun
		S62.155P	Nondisp fx of hook pro of hamate bone, l wrs, sub for fx w malun
		S62.156P	Nondisp fx of hook pro of hamate bone, unsp wrs, sub for fx w malun
		S62.161P	Disp fx of pisiform, right wrist, subs for fx w malunion
		S62.162P	Disp fx of pisiform, left wrist, subs for fx w malunion
		S62.163P	Disp fx of pisiform, unsp wrist, subs for fx w malunion
		S62.164P	Nondisp fx of pisiform, right wrist, subs for fx w malunion
		S62.165P	Nondisp fx of pisiform, left wrist, subs for fx w malunion
		S62.166P	Nondisp fx of pisiform, unsp wrist, subs for fx w malunion
		S62.171P	Disp fx of trapezium, right wrist, subs for fx w malunion
		S62.172P	Disp fx of trapezium, left wrist, subs for fx w malunion
		S62.173P	Disp fx of trapezium, unsp wrist, subs for fx w malunion
		S62.174P	Nondisp fx of trapezium, right wrist, subs for fx w malunion
		S62.175P	Nondisp fx of trapezium, left wrist, subs for fx w malunion
		S62.176P	Nondisp fx of trapezium, unsp wrist, subs for fx w malunion
		S62.181P	Disp fx of trapezoid, right wrist, subs for fx w malunion
		S62.182P	Disp fx of trapezoid, left wrist, subs for fx w malunion
		S62.183P	Disp fx of trapezoid, unsp wrist, subs for fx w malunion
		S62.184P	Nondisp fx of trapezoid, right wrist, subs for fx w malunion
		S62.185P	Nondisp fx of trapezoid, left wrist, subs for fx w malunion
		S62.186P	Nondisp fx of trapezoid, unsp wrist, subs for fx w malunion
		S62.2Ø[1,2,9]P	Unsp fx first MC bone, hand, subs for fx w malunion
		S62.211P	Bennett's fracture, right hand, subs for fx w malunion
		S62.212P	Bennett's fracture, left hand, subs for fx w malunion
		S62.213P	Bennett's fracture, unsp hand, subs for fx w malunion
		S62.221P	Displaced Rolando's fracture, r hand, subs for fx w malunion
		S62.222P	Displ Rolando's fracture, left hand, subs for fx w malunion
		S62.223P	Displ Rolando's fracture, unsp hand, subs for fx w malunion
		S62.224P	Nondisp Rolando's fracture, r hand, subs for fx w malunion
		S62.225P	Nondisp Rolando's fracture, l hand, subs for fx w malunion
		S62.226P	Nondisp Rolando's fx, unsp hand, subs for fx w malunion
		S62.231P	Oth disp fx of base of 1st MC bone, r hand, sub for fx w malun
		S62.232P	Oth disp fx of base of 1st MC bone, l hand, sub for fx w malun
		S62.233P	Oth disp fx of base of 1st MC bone, unsp hand, sub for fx w malun
		S62.234P	Oth nondisp fx of base of 1st MC bone, r hand, sub for fx w malun
		S62.235P	Oth nondisp fx of base of 1st MC bone, l hand, sub for fx w malun
		S62.236P	Oth nondisp fx of base of 1st MC bone, unsp hand, sub for fx w malun
		S62.241P	Disp fx of shaft of 1st MC bone, r hand, sub for fx w malun
		S62.242P	Disp fx of shaft of 1st MC bone, l hand, sub for fx w malun
		S62.243P	Disp fx of shaft of 1st MC bone, unsp hand, sub for fx w malun
		S62.244P	Nondisp fx of shaft of 1st MC bone, r hand, sub for fx w malun
		S62.245P	Nondisp fx of shaft of 1st MC bone, l hand, sub for fx w malun
		S62.246P	Nondisp fx of shaft of 1st MC bone, unsp hand, sub for fx w malun
		S62.251P	Disp fx of nk of 1st MC bone, r hand, subs for fx w malunion
		S62.252P	Disp fx of nk of 1st MC bone, l hand, subs for fx w malunion
		S62.253P	Disp fx of nk of 1st MC bone, unsp hand, subs for fx w malunion
		S62.254P	Nondisp fx of nk of 1st MC bone, r hand, sub for fx w malun
		S62.255P	Nondisp fx of nk of 1st MC bone, l hand, sub for fx w malun
		S62.256P	Nondisp fx of nk of 1st MC bone, unsp hand, sub for fx w malun
		S62.29[1,2,9]P	Oth fx first MC bone, right hand, subs for fx w malunion
		S62.3ØØP	Unsp fx second MC bone, right hand, subs for fx w malunion
		S62.3Ø1P	Unsp fx second MC bone, left hand, subs for fx w malunion
		S62.3Ø2P	Unsp fx third MC bone, right hand, subs for fx w malunion
		S62.3Ø3P	Unsp fx third MC bone, left hand, subs for fx w malunion
		S62.3Ø4P	Unsp fx fourth MC bone, right hand, subs for fx w malunion
		S62.3Ø5P	Unsp fx fourth MC bone, left hand, subs for fx w malunion
		S62.3Ø6P	Unsp fx fifth MC bone, right hand, subs for fx w malunion
		S62.3Ø7P	Unsp fx fifth MC bone, left hand, subs for fx w malunion
		S62.3Ø8P	Unsp fracture of oth metacarpal bone, subs for fx w malunion
		S62.3Ø9P	Unsp fx unsp metacarpal bone, subs for fx w malunion
		S62.31ØP	Disp fx of base of 2nd MC bone, r hand, sub for fx w malun
		S62.311P	Disp fx of base of 2nd MC bone. l hand, sub for fx w malun
		S62.312P	Disp fx of base of 3rd MC bone, r hand, sub for fx w malun
		S62.313P	Disp fx of base of 3rd MC bone, l hand, sub for fx w malun
		S62.314P	Disp fx of base of 4th MC bone, r hand, sub for fx w malun
		S62.315P	Disp fx of base of 4th MC bone, l hand, sub for fx w malun
		S62.316P	Disp fx of base of 5th MC bone, r hand, sub for fx w malun
		S62.317P	Disp fx of base of 5th MC bone. l hand, sub for fx w malun
		S62.318P	Disp fx of base of metacarpal bone, subs for fx w malunion
		S62.319P	Disp fx of base of unsp MC bone, subs for fx w malunion
		S62.32ØP	Disp fx of shaft of 2nd MC bone, r hand, sub for fx w malun
		S62.321P	Disp fx of shaft of 2nd MC bone, l hand, sub for fx w malun
		S62.322P	Disp fx of shaft of 3rd MC bone, r hand, sub for fx w malun
		S62.323P	Disp fx of shaft of 3rd MC bone, l hand, sub for fx w malun
		S62.324P	Disp fx of shaft of 4th MC bone, r hand, sub for fx w malun
		S62.325P	Disp fx of shaft of 4th MC bone, l hand, sub for fx w malun
		S62.326P	Disp fx of shaft of 5th MC bone, r hand, sub for fx w malun
		S62.327P	Disp fx of shaft of 5th MC bone, l hand, sub for fx w malun
		S62.328P	Disp fx of shaft of metacarpal bone, subs for fx w malunion

6th Character meanings for codes as indicated
1 Right ***2 Left*** ***9 Unspecified***

(Continued on next page)

ICD-9-CM		ICD-10-CM	
733.81	MALUNION OF FRACTURE **(Continued)**	**S62.329P**	Disp fx of shaft of unsp MC bone, subs for fx w malunion
		S62.330P	Disp fx of nk of 2nd MC bone, r hand, subs for fx w malunion
		S62.331P	Disp fx of nk of 2nd MC bone, l hand, subs for fx w malunion
		S62.332P	Disp fx of nk of 3rd MC bone, r hand, subs for fx w malunion
		S62.333P	Disp fx of nk of 3rd MC bone, l hand, subs for fx w malunion
		S62.334P	Disp fx of nk of 4th MC bone, r hand, subs for fx w malunion
		S62.335P	Disp fx of nk of 4th MC bone, l hand, subs for fx w malunion
		S62.336P	Disp fx of nk of 5th MC bone, r hand, subs for fx w malunion
		S62.337P	Disp fx of nk of 5th MC bone, l hand, subs for fx w malunion
		S62.338P	Disp fx of neck of metacarpal bone, subs for fx w malunion
		S62.339P	Disp fx of neck of unsp MC bone, subs for fx w malunion
		S62.340P	Nondisp fx of base of 2nd MC bone, r hand, sub for fx w malun
		S62.341P	Nondisp fx of base of 2nd MC bone. l hand, sub for fx w malun
		S62.342P	Nondisp fx of base of 3rd MC bone, r hand, sub for fx w malun
		S62.343P	Nondisp fx of base of 3rd MC bone, l hand, sub for fx w malun
		S62.344P	Nondisp fx of base of 4th MC bone, r hand, sub for fx w malun
		S62.345P	Nondisp fx of base of 4th MC bone, l hand, sub for fx w malun
		S62.346P	Nondisp fx of base of 5th MC bone, r hand, sub for fx w malun
		S62.347P	Nondisp fx of base of 5th MC bone. l hand, sub for fx w malun
		S62.348P	Nondisp fx of base of MC bone, subs for fx w malunion
		S62.349P	Nondisp fx of base of unsp MC bone, subs for fx w malunion
		S62.350P	Nondisp fx of shaft of 2nd MC bone, r hand, sub for fx w malun
		S62.351P	Nondisp fx of shaft of 2nd MC bone, l hand, sub for fx w malun
		S62.352P	Nondisp fx of shaft of 3rd MC bone, r hand, sub for fx w malun
		S62.353P	Nondisp fx of shaft of 3rd MC bone, l hand, sub for fx w malun
		S62.354P	Nondisp fx of shaft of 4th MC bone, r hand, sub for fx w malun
		S62.355P	Nondisp fx of shaft of 4th MC bone, l hand, sub for fx w malun
		S62.356P	Nondisp fx of shaft of 5th MC bone, r hand, sub for fx w malun
		S62.357P	Nondisp fx of shaft of 5th MC bone, l hand, sub for fx w malun
		S62.358P	Nondisp fx of shaft of MC bone, subs for fx w malunion
		S62.359P	Nondisp fx of shaft of unsp MC bone, subs for fx w malunion
		S62.360P	Nondisp fx of nk of 2nd MC bone, r hand, sub for fx w malun
		S62.361P	Nondisp fx of nk of 2nd MC bone, l hand, sub for fx w malun
		S62.362P	Nondisp fx of nk of 3rd MC bone, r hand, sub for fx w malun
		S62.363P	Nondisp fx of nk of 3rd MC bone, l hand, sub for fx w malun
		S62.364P	Nondisp fx of nk of 4th MC bone, r hand, sub for fx w malun
		S62.365P	Nondisp fx of nk of 4th MC bone, l hand, sub for fx w malun
		S62.366P	Nondisp fx of nk of 5th MC bone, r hand, sub for fx w malun
		S62.367P	Nondisp fx of nk of 5th MC bone, l hand, sub for fx w malun
		S62.368P	Nondisp fx of neck of MC bone, subs for fx w malunion
		S62.369P	Nondisp fx of neck of unsp MC bone, subs for fx w malunion
		S62.390P	Oth fx second MC bone, right hand, subs for fx w malunion
		S62.391P	Oth fx second MC bone, left hand, subs for fx w malunion
		S62.392P	Oth fx third MC bone, right hand, subs for fx w malunion
		S62.393P	Oth fx third MC bone, left hand, subs for fx w malunion
		S62.394P	Oth fx fourth MC bone, right hand, subs for fx w malunion
		S62.395P	Oth fx fourth MC bone, left hand, subs for fx w malunion
		S62.396P	Oth fx fifth MC bone, right hand, subs for fx w malunion
		S62.397P	Oth fx fifth MC bone, left hand, subs for fx w malunion
		S62.398P	Oth fracture of oth metacarpal bone, subs for fx w malunion
		S62.399P	Oth fracture of unsp metacarpal bone, subs for fx w malunion
		S62.50[1,2,9]P	Fx unsp phalanx of thumb, subs for fx w malunion
		S62.511P	Disp fx of proximal phalanx of r thm, subs for fx w malunion
		S62.512P	Disp fx of proximal phalanx of l thm, subs for fx w malunion
		S62.513P	Disp fx of proximal phalanx of thmb, subs for fx w malunion
		S62.514P	Nondisp fx of prox phalanx of r thm, subs for fx w malunion
		S62.515P	Nondisp fx of prox phalanx of l thm, subs for fx w malunion
		S62.516P	Nondisp fx of prox phalanx of thmb, subs for fx w malunion
		S62.521P	Disp fx of distal phalanx of r thm, subs for fx w malunion
		S62.522P	Disp fx of distal phalanx of l thm, subs for fx w malunion
		S62.523P	Disp fx of distal phalanx of thmb, subs for fx w malunion
		S62.524P	Nondisp fx of dist phalanx of r thm, subs for fx w malunion
		S62.525P	Nondisp fx of dist phalanx of l thm, subs for fx w malunion
		S62.526P	Nondisp fx of distal phalanx of thmb, subs for fx w malunion
		S62.600P	Fx unsp phalanx of r idx fngr, subs for fx w malunion
		S62.601P	Fx unsp phalanx of l idx fngr, subs for fx w malunion
		S62.602P	Fx unsp phalanx of r mid finger, subs for fx w malunion
		S62.603P	Fx unsp phalanx of l mid finger, subs for fx w malunion
		S62.604P	Fx unsp phalanx of r rng fngr, subs for fx w malunion
		S62.605P	Fx unsp phalanx of l rng fngr, subs for fx w malunion
		S62.606P	Fx unsp phalanx of r little finger, subs for fx w malunion
		S62.607P	Fx unsp phalanx of l little finger, subs for fx w malunion
		S62.608P	Fracture of unsp phalanx of finger, subs for fx w malunion
		S62.609P	Fx unsp phalanx of unsp finger, subs for fx w malunion
		S62.610P	Disp fx of prox phalanx of r idx fngr, sub for fx w malun
		S62.611P	Disp fx of prox phalanx of l idx fngr, sub for fx w malun
		S62.612P	Disp fx of prox phalanx of r mid fngr, sub for fx w malun
		S62.613P	Disp fx of prox phalanx of l mid fngr, sub for fx w malun
		S62.614P	Disp fx of prox phalanx of r rng fngr, sub for fx w malun

6th Character meanings for codes as indicated
1 Right *2 Left* *9 Unspecified*

(Continued on next page)

ICD-9-CM		ICD-10-CM	
733.81	MALUNION OF FRACTURE **(Continued)**	**S62.615P**	Disp fx of prox phalanx of l rng fngr, sub for fx w malun
		S62.616P	Disp fx of prox phalanx of r lit fngr, sub for fx w malun
		S62.617P	Disp fx of prox phalanx of l lit fngr, sub for fx w malun
		S62.618P	Disp fx of prox phalanx of finger, subs for fx w malunion
		S62.619P	Disp fx of prox phalanx of unsp fngr, subs for fx w malunion
		S62.62ØP	Disp fx of med phalanx of r idx fngr, subs for fx w malunion
		S62.621P	Disp fx of med phalanx of l idx fngr, subs for fx w malunion
		S62.622P	Disp fx of med phalanx of r mid fngr, subs for fx w malunion
		S62.623P	Disp fx of med phalanx of l mid fngr, subs for fx w malunion
		S62.624P	Disp fx of med phalanx of r rng fngr, subs for fx w malunion
		S62.625P	Disp fx of med phalanx of l rng fngr, subs for fx w malunion
		S62.626P	Disp fx of med phalanx of r lit fngr, subs for fx w malunion
		S62.627P	Disp fx of med phalanx of l lit fngr, subs for fx w malunion
		S62.628P	Disp fx of medial phalanx of finger, subs for fx w malunion
		S62.629P	Disp fx of med phalanx of unsp fngr, subs for fx w malunion
		S62.63ØP	Disp fx of dist phalanx of r idx fngr, sub for fx w malun
		S62.631P	Disp fx of dist phalanx of l idx fngr, sub for fx w malun
		S62.632P	Disp fx of dist phalanx of r mid fngr, sub for fx w malun
		S62.633P	Disp fx of dist phalanx of l mid fngr, sub for fx w malun
		S62.634P	Disp fx of dist phalanx of r rng fngr, sub for fx w malun
		S62.635P	Disp fx of dist phalanx of l rng fngr, sub for fx w malun
		S62.636P	Disp fx of dist phalanx of r lit fngr, sub for fx w malun
		S62.637P	Disp fx of dist phalanx of l lit fngr, sub for fx w malun
		S62.638P	Disp fx of distal phalanx of finger, subs for fx w malunion
		S62.639P	Disp fx of dist phalanx of unsp fngr, subs for fx w malunion
		S62.64ØP	Nondisp fx of prox phalanx of r idx fngr, sub for fx w malun
		S62.641P	Nondisp fx of prox phalanx of l idx fngr, sub for fx w malun
		S62.642P	Nondisp fx of prox phalanx of r mid fngr, sub for fx w malun
		S62.643P	Nondisp fx of prox phalanx of l mid fngr, sub for fx w malun
		S62.644P	Nondisp fx of prox phalanx of r rng fngr, sub for fx w malun
		S62.645P	Nondisp fx of prox phalanx of l rng fngr, sub for fx w malun
		S62.646P	Nondisp fx of prox phalanx of r lit fngr, sub for fx w malun
		S62.647P	Nondisp fx of prox phalanx of l lit fngr, sub for fx w malun
		S62.648P	Nondisp fx of prox phalanx of finger, subs for fx w malunion
		S62.649P	Nondisp fx of prox phalanx of unsp fngr, sub for fx w malun
		S62.65ØP	Nondisp fx of med phalanx of r idx fngr, sub for fx w malun
		S62.651P	Nondisp fx of med phalanx of l idx fngr, sub for fx w malun
		S62.652P	Nondisp fx of med phalanx of r mid fngr, sub for fx w malun
		S62.653P	Nondisp fx of med phalanx of l mid fngr, sub for fx w malun
		S62.654P	Nondisp fx of med phalanx of r rng fngr, sub for fx w malun
		S62.655P	Nondisp fx of med phalanx of l rng fngr, sub for fx w malun
		S62.656P	Nondisp fx of med phalanx of r lit fngr, sub for fx w malun
		S62.657P	Nondisp fx of med phalanx of l lit fngr, sub for fx w malun
		S62.658P	Nondisp fx of medial phalanx of fngr, subs for fx w malunion
		S62.659P	Nondisp fx of med phalanx of unsp fngr, sub for fx w malun
		S62.66ØP	Nondisp fx of dist phalanx of r idx fngr, sub for fx w malun
		S62.661P	Nondisp fx of dist phalanx of l idx fngr, sub for fx w malun
		S62.662P	Nondisp fx of dist phalanx of r mid fngr, sub for fx w malun
		S62.663P	Nondisp fx of dist phalanx of l mid fngr, sub for fx w malun
		S62.664P	Nondisp fx of dist phalanx of r rng fngr, sub for fx w malun
		S62.665P	Nondisp fx of dist phalanx of l rng fngr, sub for fx w malun
		S62.666P	Nondisp fx of dist phalanx of r lit fngr, sub for fx w malun
		S62.667P	Nondisp fx of dist phalanx of l lit fngr, sub for fx w malun
		S62.668P	Nondisp fx of dist phalanx of finger, subs for fx w malunion
		S62.669P	Nondisp fx of dist phalanx of unsp fngr, sub for fx w malun
		S62.9ØXP	Unsp fracture of unsp wrist and hand, subs for fx w malunion
		S62.91XP	Unsp fracture of right wrs/hnd, subs for fx w malunion
		S62.92XP	Unsp fracture of left wrist and hand, subs for fx w malunion
		S72.ØØ1[P,Q,R]	Fx unsp part of neck of r femur
		S72.ØØ2[P,Q,R]	Fx unsp part of neck of l femur
		S72.ØØ9[P,Q,R]	Fx unsp part of nk of unsp femr
		S72.Ø11[P,Q,R]	Unsp intracap fx right femur
		S72.Ø12[P,Q,R]	Unsp intracap fx left femur
		S72.Ø19[P,Q,R]	Unsp intracap fx unsp femur
		S72.Ø21[P,Q,R]	Disp fx of epiphy (separation) (upper) of r femr
		S72.Ø22[P,Q,R]	Disp fx of epiphy (separation) (upper) of l femr
		S72.Ø23[P,Q,R]	Disp fx of epiphy (separation) (upper) of unsp femr
		S72.Ø24[P,Q,R]	Nondisp fx of epiphy (separation) (upper) of r femr
		S72.Ø25[P,Q,R]	Nondisp fx of epiphy (separation) (upper) of l femr
		S72.Ø26[P,Q,R]	Nondisp fx of epiphy (separation) (upper) of unsp femr
		S72.Ø31[P,Q,R]	Displ midcervical fx r femur
		S72.Ø32[P,Q,R]	Displ midcervical fx l femur
		S72.Ø33[P,Q,R]	Displ midcervical fx unsp femur
		S72.Ø34[P,Q,R]	Nondisp midcervical fx r femur
		S72.Ø35[P,Q,R]	Nondisp midcervical fx l femur
		S72.Ø36[P,Q,R]	Nondisp midcervical fx unsp femr
		S72.Ø41[P,Q,R]	Disp fx of base of nk of r femr

7th Character meanins for codes S72.-
P Sub Enc Closed FX Malunion
Q Sub Enc Open FX Type I/II Malunion
R Sub Enc Open IIIA/B/C Malunion

(Continued on next page)

ICD-9-CM		ICD-10-CM
733.81	MALUNION OF FRACTURE **(Continued)**	**S72.Ø42**[P,Q,R] Disp fx of base of nk of l femr **S72.Ø43**[P,Q,R] Disp fx of base of nk of unsp femr **S72.Ø44**[P,Q,R] Nondisp fx of base of nk of r femr **S72.Ø45**[P,Q,R] Nondisp fx of base of nk of l femr **S72.Ø46**[P,Q,R] Nondisp fx of base of nk of unsp femr **S72.Ø51**[P,Q,R] Unsp fx head of right femur **S72.Ø52**[P,Q,R] Unsp fx head of left femur **S72.Ø59**[P,Q,R] Unsp fx head of unsp femur **S72.Ø61**[P,Q,R] Displ artic fx head of r femur **S72.Ø62**[P,Q,R] Displ artic fx head of l femur **S72.Ø63**[P,Q,R] Displ artic fx head of unsp femr **S72.Ø64**[P,Q,R] Nondisp artic fx head of r femr **S72.Ø65**[P,Q,R] Nondisp artic fx head of l femr **S72.Ø66**[P,Q,R] Nondisp artic fx head of unsp femr **S72.Ø91**[P,Q,R] Oth fx head/neck of right femur **S72.Ø92**[P,Q,R] Oth fx head/neck of left femur **S72.Ø99**[P,Q,R] Oth fx head/neck of unsp femur **S72.1Ø1**[P,Q,R] Unsp trochan fx right femur **S72.1Ø2**[P,Q,R] Unsp trochan fx left femur **S72.1Ø9**[P,Q,R] Unsp trochan fx unsp femur **S72.111**[P,Q,R] Disp fx of greater trochanter of r femr **S72.112**[P,Q,R] Disp fx of greater trochanter of l femr **S72.113**[P,Q,R] Disp fx of greater trochanter of unsp femr **S72.114**[P,Q,R] Nondisp fx of greater trochanter of r femr **S72.115**[P,Q,R] Nondisp fx of greater trochanter of l femr **S72.116**[P,Q,R] Nondisp fx of greater trochanter of unsp femr **S72.121**[P,Q,R] Disp fx of less trochanter of r femr **S72.122**[P,Q,R] Disp fx of less trochanter of l femr **S72.123**[P,Q,R] Disp fx of less trochanter of unsp femr **S72.124**[P,Q,R] Nondisp fx of less trochanter of r femr **S72.125**[P,Q,R] Nondisp fx of less trochanter of l femr **S72.126**[P,Q,R] Nondisp fx of less trochanter of unsp femr **S72.131**[P,Q,R] Displaced apophyseal fx r femur **S72.132**[P,Q,R] Displaced apophyseal fx l femur **S72.133**[P,Q,R] Displ apophyseal fx unsp femur **S72.134**[P,Q,R] Nondisp apophyseal fx r femur **S72.135**[P,Q,R] Nondisp apophyseal fx l femur **S72.136**[P,Q,R] Nondisp apophyseal fx unsp femr **S72.141**[P,Q,R] Displaced intertroch fx r femur **S72.142**[P,Q,R] Displaced intertroch fx l femur **S72.143**[P,Q,R] Displ intertroch fx unsp femur **S72.144**[P,Q,R] Nondisp intertroch fx r femur **S72.145**[P,Q,R] Nondisp intertroch fx l femur **S72.146**[P,Q,R] Nondisp intertroch fx unsp femr **S72.21X**[P,Q,R] Displaced subtrochnt fx r femur **S72.22X**[P,Q,R] Displaced subtrochnt fx l femur **S72.23X**[P,Q,R] Displ subtrochnt fx unsp femur **S72.24X**[P,Q,R] Nondisp subtrochnt fx r femur **S72.25X**[P,Q,R] Nondisp subtrochnt fx l femur **S72.26X**[P,Q,R] Nondisp subtrochnt fx unsp femr **S72.3Ø1**[P,Q,R] Unsp fx shaft of right femur **S72.3Ø2**[P,Q,R] Unsp fx shaft of left femur **S72.3Ø9**[P,Q,R] Unsp fx shaft of unsp femur **S72.321**[P,Q,R] Displ transverse fx shaft of r femr **S72.322**[P,Q,R] Displ transverse fx shaft of l femr **S72.323**[P,Q,R] Displ transverse fx shaft of unsp femr **S72.324**[P,Q,R] Nondisp transverse fx shaft of r femr **S72.325**[P,Q,R] Nondisp transverse fx shaft of l femr **S72.326**[P,Q,R] Nondisp transverse fx shaft of unsp femr **S72.331**[P,Q,R] Displ oblique fx shaft of r femr **S72.332**[P,Q,R] Displ oblique fx shaft of l femr **S72.333**[P,Q,R] Displ oblique fx shaft of unsp femr **S72.334**[P,Q,R] Nondisp oblique fx shaft of r femr **S72.335**[P,Q,R] Nondisp oblique fx shaft of l femr **S72.336**[P,Q,R] Nondisp oblique fx shaft of unsp femr **S72.341**[P,Q,R] Displ spiral fx shaft of r femr **S72.342**[P,Q,R] Displ spiral fx shaft of l femr **S72.343**[P,Q,R] Displ spiral fx shaft of unsp femr **S72.344**[P,Q,R] Nondisp spiral fx shaft of r femr **S72.345**[P,Q,R] Nondisp spiral fx shaft of l femr **S72.346**[P,Q,R] Nondisp spiral fx shaft of unsp femr **S72.351**[P,Q,R] Displ commnt fx shaft of r femr **S72.352**[P,Q,R] Displ commnt fx shaft of l femr **S72.353**[P,Q,R] Displ commnt fx shaft of unsp femr **S72.354**[P,Q,R] Nondisp commnt fx shaft of r femr **S72.355**[P,Q,R] Nondisp commnt fx shaft of l femr **S72.356**[P,Q,R] Nondisp commnt fx shaft of unsp femr

7th Character meanins for codes S72.-
P Sub Enc Closed FX Malunion
Q Sub Enc Open FX Type I/II Malunion
R Sub Enc Open IIIA/B/C Malunion

(Continued on next page)

 [Brackets] indicate valid character values for each code. Character value meanings provided for each code grouping.

ICD-9-CM		ICD-10-CM	
733.81	MALUNION OF FRACTURE (Continued)	S72.361[P,Q,R]	Displ seg fx shaft of r femur
		S72.362[P,Q,R]	Displ seg fx shaft of l femur
		S72.363[P,Q,R]	Displ seg fx shaft of unsp femr
		S72.364[P,Q,R]	Nondisp seg fx shaft of r femur
		S72.365[P,Q,R]	Nondisp seg fx shaft of l femur
		S72.366[P,Q,R]	Nondisp seg fx shaft of unsp femr
		S72.391[P,Q,R]	Oth fx shaft of right femur
		S72.392[P,Q,R]	Oth fx shaft of left femur
		S72.399[P,Q,R]	Oth fx shaft of unsp femur
		S72.4Ø1[P,Q,R]	Unsp fx lower end of r femur
		S72.4Ø2[P,Q,R]	Unsp fx lower end of left femur
		S72.4Ø9[P,Q,R]	Unsp fx lower end of unsp femur
		S72.411[P,Q,R]	Displ unsp condyle fx low end r femr
		S72.412[P,Q,R]	Displ unsp condyle fx low end l femr
		S72.413[P,Q,R]	Displ unsp condyle fx low end unsp femr
		S72.414[P,Q,R]	Nondisp unsp condyle fx low end r femr
		S72.415[P,Q,R]	Nondisp unsp condyle fx low end l femr
		S72.416[P,Q,R]	Nondisp unsp condyle fx low end unsp femr
		S72.421[P,Q,R]	Disp fx of lateral condyle of r femr
		S72.422[P,Q,R]	Disp fx of lateral condyle of l femr
		S72.423[P,Q,R]	Disp fx of lateral condyle of unsp femr
		S72.424[P,Q,R]	Nondisp fx of lateral condyle of r femr
		S72.425[P,Q,R]	Nondisp fx of lateral condyle of l femr
		S72.426[P,Q,R]	Nondisp fx of lateral condyle of unsp femr
		S72.431[P,Q,R]	Disp fx of med condyle of r femr
		S72.432[P,Q,R]	Disp fx of med condyle of l femr
		S72.433[P,Q,R]	Disp fx of med condyle of unsp femr
		S72.434[P,Q,R]	Nondisp fx of med condyle of r femr
		S72.435[P,Q,R]	Nondisp fx of med condyle of l femr
		S72.436[P,Q,R]	Nondisp fx of med condyle of unsp femr
		S72.441[P,Q,R]	Disp fx of low epiphy (separation) of r femr
		S72.442[P,Q,R]	Disp fx of low epiphy (separation) of l femr
		S72.443[P,Q,R]	Disp fx of low epiphy (separation) of unsp femr
		S72.444[P,Q,R]	Nondisp fx of low epiphy (separation) of r femr
		S72.445[P,Q,R]	Nondisp fx of low epiphy (separation) of l femr
		S72.446[P,Q,R]	Nondisp fx of low epiphy (separation) of unsp femr
		S72.451[P,Q,R]	Displ suprcndl fx w/o intrcndl extn low end r femr
		S72.452[P,Q,R]	Displ suprcndl fx w/o intrcndl extn low end l femr
		S72.453[P,Q,R]	Displ suprcndl fx w/o intrcndl extn low end unsp femr
		S72.454[P,Q,R]	Nondisp suprcndl fx w/o intrcndl extn low end r femr
		S72.455[P,Q,R]	Nondisp suprcndl fx w/o intrcndl extn low end l femr
		S72.456[P,Q,R]	Nondisp suprcndl fx w/o intrcndl extn low end unsp femr
		S72.461[P,Q,R]	Displ suprcndl fx w intrcndl extn low end r femr
		S72.462[P,Q,R]	Displ suprcndl fx w intrcndl extn low end l femr
		S72.463[P,Q,R]	Displ suprcndl fx w intrcndl extn low end unsp femr
		S72.464[P,Q,R]	Nondisp suprcndl fx w intrcndl extn low end r femr
		S72.465[P,Q,R]	Nondisp suprcndl fx w intrcndl extn low end l femr
		S72.466[P,Q,R]	Nondisp suprcndl fx w intrcndl extn low end unsp femr
		S72.47[1,2,9]P	Torus fx lower end of femur, subs for fx w malunion
		S72.491[P,Q,R]	Oth fx lower end of right femur
		S72.492[P,Q,R]	Oth fx lower end of left femur
		S72.499[P,Q,R]	Oth fx lower end of unsp femur
		S72.8X1[P,Q,R]	Oth fracture of right femur
		S72.8X2[P,Q,R]	Oth fracture of left femur
		S72.8X9[P,Q,R]	Oth fracture of unsp femur
		S72.9ØX[P,Q,R]	Unsp fracture of unsp femur
		S72.91X[P,Q,R]	Unsp fracture of right femur
		S72.92X[P,Q,R]	Unsp fracture of left femur
		S79.ØØ[1,2,9]P	Unsp physeal fx upper end of femur, subs for fx w malunion
		S79.Ø1[1,2,9]P	Sltr-haris Type I physl fx upr end femr, sub for fx w malun
		S79.Ø9[1,2,9]P	Oth physeal fx upper end of femur, subs for fx w malunion
		S79.1Ø[1,2,9]P	Unsp physeal fx lower end of femur, subs for fx w malunion
		S79.11[1,2,9]P	Sltr-haris Type I physl fx low end femr, sub for fx w malun
		S79.12[1,2,9]P	Sltr-haris Type II physl fx low end femr, sub for fx w malun
		S79.13[1,2,9]P	Sltr-haris Type III physl fx low end femr, sub for fx w malun
		S79.14[1,2,9]P	Sltr-haris Type IV physl fx low end femr, sub for fx w malun
		S79.19[1,2,9]P	Oth physeal fx lower end of femur, subs for fx w malunion
		S82.ØØ1[P,Q,R]	Unsp fracture of right patella
		S82.ØØ2[P,Q,R]	Unsp fracture of left patella
		S82.ØØ9[P,Q,R]	Unsp fracture of unsp patella
		S82.Ø11[P,Q,R]	Displ osteochon fx r patella
		S82.Ø12[P,Q,R]	Displ osteochon fx left patella
		S82.Ø13[P,Q,R]	Displ osteochon fx unsp patella
		S82.Ø14[P,Q,R]	Nondisp osteochon fx r patella
		S82.Ø15[P,Q,R]	Nondisp osteochon fx l patella

6th Character meanings for codes as indicated
1 Right ***2 Left*** ***9 Unspecified***

7th Character meanins for codes S72.-, S82.-
P Sub Enc Closed FX Malunion
Q Sub Enc Open FX Type I/II Malunion
R Sub Enc Open IIIA/B/C Malunion

(Continued on next page)

ICD-9-CM		ICD-10-CM
733.81	MALUNION OF FRACTURE **(Continued)**	**S82.016**[P,Q,R] Nondisp osteochon fx unsp patella, sub for fx w malun
		S82.021[P,Q,R] Displ longitud fx right patella
		S82.022[P,Q,R] Displ longitud fx left patella
		S82.023[P,Q,R] Displ longitud fx unsp patella
		S82.024[P,Q,R] Nondisp longitud fx r patella
		S82.025[P,Q,R] Nondisp longitud fx l patella
		S82.026[P,Q,R] Nondisp longitud fx unsp patella, sub for fx w malun
		S82.031[P,Q,R] Displ transverse fx r patella
		S82.032[P,Q,R] Displ transverse fx l patella
		S82.033[P,Q,R] Displ transverse fx unsp patella, sub for fx w malun
		S82.034[P,Q,R] Nondisp transverse fx r patella
		S82.035[P,Q,R] Nondisp transverse fx l patella
		S82.036[P,Q,R] Nondisp transverse fx unsp patella, sub for fx w malun
		S82.041[P,Q,R] Displ commnt fx right patella
		S82.042[P,Q,R] Displ commnt fx left patella
		S82.043[P,Q,R] Displ commnt fx unsp patella
		S82.044[P,Q,R] Nondisp commnt fx right patella
		S82.045[P,Q,R] Nondisp commnt fx left patella
		S82.046[P,Q,R] Nondisp commnt fx unsp patella
		S82.091[P,Q,R] Oth fracture of right patella
		S82.092[P,Q,R] Oth fracture of left patella
		S82.099[P,Q,R] Oth fracture of unsp patella
		S82.101[P,Q,R] Unsp fx upper end of r tibia
		S82.102[P,Q,R] Unsp fx upper end of left tibia
		S82.109[P,Q,R] Unsp fx upper end of unsp tibia
		S82.111[P,Q,R] Disp fx of right tibial spine
		S82.112[P,Q,R] Disp fx of left tibial spine
		S82.113[P,Q,R] Disp fx of unsp tibial spine
		S82.114[P,Q,R] Nondisp fx of r tibial spine
		S82.115[P,Q,R] Nondisp fx of left tibial spine
		S82.116[P,Q,R] Nondisp fx of unsp tibial spine
		S82.121[P,Q,R] Disp fx of lateral condyle of r tibia, sub for fx w malun
		S82.122[P,Q,R] Disp fx of lateral condyle of l tibia, sub for fx w malun
		S82.123[P,Q,R] Disp fx of lateral condyle of unsp tibia, sub for fx w malun
		S82.124[P,Q,R] Nondisp fx of lateral condyle of r tibia, sub for fx w malun
		S82.125[P,Q,R] Nondisp fx of lateral condyle of l tibia, sub for fx w malun
		S82.126[P,Q,R] Nondisp fx of lateral condyle of unsp tibia, sub for fx w malun
		S82.131[P,Q,R] Disp fx of med condyle of r tibia, sub for fx w malun
		S82.132[P,Q,R] Disp fx of med condyle of l tibia, sub for fx w malun
		S82.133[P,Q,R] Disp fx of med condyle of unsp tibia, sub for fx w malun
		S82.134[P,Q,R] Nondisp fx of med condyle of r tibia, sub for fx w malun
		S82.135[P,Q,R] Nondisp fx of med condyle of l tibia, sub for fx w malun
		S82.136[P,Q,R] Nondisp fx of med condyle of unsp tibia, sub for fx w malun
		S82.141[P,Q,R] Displaced bicondylar fx r tibia
		S82.142[P,Q,R] Displaced bicondylar fx l tibia
		S82.143[P,Q,R] Displ bicondylar fx unsp tibia
		S82.144[P,Q,R] Nondisp bicondylar fx r tibia
		S82.145[P,Q,R] Nondisp bicondylar fx l tibia
		S82.146[P,Q,R] Nondisp bicondylar fx unsp tibia, sub for fx w malun
		S82.151[P,Q,R] Disp fx of r tibial tuberosity
		S82.152[P,Q,R] Disp fx of l tibial tuberosity
		S82.153[P,Q,R] Disp fx of unsp tibial tuberosity, sub for fx w malun
		S82.154[P,Q,R] Nondisp fx of r tibial tuberosity, sub for fx w malun
		S82.155[P,Q,R] Nondisp fx of l tibial tuberosity, sub for fx w malun
		S82.156[P,Q,R] Nondisp fx of unsp tibial tuberosity, sub for fx w malun
		S82.16[1,2,9]**P** Torus fx upper end of tibia, subs for fx w malunion
		S82.191[P,Q,R] Oth fx upper end of right tibia
		S82.192[P,Q,R] Oth fx upper end of left tibia
		S82.199[P,Q,R] Oth fx upper end of unsp tibia
		S82.201[P,Q,R] Unsp fx shaft of right tibia
		S82.202[P,Q,R] Unsp fx shaft of left tibia
		S82.209[P,Q,R] Unsp fx shaft of unsp tibia
		S82.221[P,Q,R] Displ transverse fx shaft of r tibia, sub for fx w malun
		S82.222[P,Q,R] Displ transverse fx shaft of l tibia, sub for fx w malun
		S82.223[P,Q,R] Displ transverse fx shaft of unsp tibia, sub for fx w malun
		S82.224[P,Q,R] Nondisp transverse fx shaft of r tibia, sub for fx w malun
		S82.225[P,Q,R] Nondisp transverse fx shaft of l tibia, sub for fx w malun
		S82.226[P,Q,R] Nondisp transverse fx shaft of unsp tibia, sub for fx w malun
		S82.231[P,Q,R] Displ oblique fx shaft of r tibia, sub for fx w malun
		S82.232[P,Q,R] Displ oblique fx shaft of l tibia, sub for fx w malun
		S82.233[P,Q,R] Displ oblique fx shaft of unsp tibia, sub for fx w malun
		S82.234[P,Q,R] Nondisp oblique fx shaft of r tibia, sub for fx w malun
		S82.235[P,Q,R] Nondisp oblique fx shaft of l tibia, sub for fx w malun
		S82.236[P,Q,R] Nondisp oblique fx shaft of unsp tibia, sub for fx w malun
		S82.241[P,Q,R] Displ spiral fx shaft of r tibia, sub for fx w malun

6th Character meanings for codes as indicated
1 Right ***2 Left*** ***9 Unspecified***

7th Character meanins for codes S82.-
P Sub Enc Closed FX Malunion
Q Sub Enc Open FX Type I/II Malunion
R Sub Enc Open IIIA/B/C Malunion

(Continued on next page)

ICD-9-CM		ICD-10-CM	
733.81	MALUNION OF FRACTURE (Continued)	S82.242[P,Q,R]	Displ spiral fx shaft of l tibia
		S82.243[P,Q,R]	Displ spiral fx shaft of unsp tibia
		S82.244[P,Q,R]	Nondisp spiral fx shaft of r tibiaP
		S82.245[P,Q,R]	Nondisp spiral fx shaft of l tibia
		S82.246[P,Q,R]	Nondisp spiral fx shaft of unsp tibia
		S82.251[P,Q,R]	Displ commnt fx shaft of r tibia
		S82.252[P,Q,R]	Displ commnt fx shaft of l tibia
		S82.253[P,Q,R]	Displ commnt fx shaft of unsp tibia
		S82.254[P,Q,R]	Nondisp commnt fx shaft of r tibia
		S82.255[P,Q,R]	Nondisp commnt fx shaft of l tibia
		S82.256[P,Q,R]	Nondisp commnt fx shaft of unsp tibia
		S82.261[P,Q,R]	Displ seg fx shaft of r tibia
		S82.262[P,Q,R]	Displ seg fx shaft of l tibia
		S82.263[P,Q,R]	Displ seg fx shaft of unsp tibia
		S82.264[P,Q,R]	Nondisp seg fx shaft of r tibia
		S82.265[P,Q,R]	Nondisp seg fx shaft of l tibia
		S82.266[P,Q,R]	Nondisp seg fx shaft of unsp tibia
		S82.291[P,Q,R]	Oth fx shaft of right tibia
		S82.292[P,Q,R]	Oth fx shaft of left tibia
		S82.299[P,Q,R]	Oth fx shaft of unsp tibia
		S82.301[P,Q,R]	Unsp fx lower end of r tibia
		S82.302[P,Q,R]	Unsp fx lower end of left tibia
		S82.309[P,Q,R]	Unsp fx lower end of unsp tibia
		S82.31[1,2,9]P	Torus fx lower end of tibia, subs for fx w malunion
		S82.391[P,Q,R]	Oth fx lower end of right tibia
		S82.392[P,Q,R]	Oth fx lower end of left tibia
		S82.399[P,Q,R]	Oth fx lower end of unsp tibia
		S82.401[P,Q,R]	Unsp fx shaft of r fibula
		S82.402[P,Q,R]	Unsp fx shaft of left fibula
		S82.409[P,Q,R]	Unsp fx shaft of unsp fibula
		S82.421[P,Q,R]	Displ transverse fx shaft of r fibula
		S82.422[P,Q,R]	Displ transverse fx shaft of l fibula
		S82.423[P,Q,R]	Displ transverse fx shaft of unsp fibula
		S82.424[P,Q,R]	Nondisp transverse fx shaft of r fibula
		S82.425[P,Q,R]	Nondisp transverse fx shaft of l fibula
		S82.426[P,Q,R]	Nondisp transverse fx shaft of unsp fibula
		S82.431[P,Q,R]	Displ oblique fx shaft of r fibula
		S82.432[P,Q,R]	Displ oblique fx shaft of l fibula
		S82.433[P,Q,R]	Displ oblique fx shaft of unsp fibula
		S82.434[P,Q,R]	Nondisp oblique fx shaft of r fibula
		S82.435[P,Q,R]	Nondisp oblique fx shaft of l fibula
		S82.436[P,Q,R]	Nondisp oblique fx shaft of unsp fibula
		S82.441[P,Q,R]	Displ spiral fx shaft of r fibula
		S82.442[P,Q,R]	Displ spiral fx shaft of l fibula
		S82.443[P,Q,R]	Displ spiral fx shaft of unsp fibula
		S82.444[P,Q,R]	Nondisp spiral fx shaft of r fibula
		S82.445[P,Q,R]	Nondisp spiral fx shaft of l fibula
		S82.446[P,Q,R]	Nondisp spiral fx shaft of unsp fibula
		S82.451[P,Q,R]	Displ commnt fx shaft of r fibula
		S82.452[P,Q,R]	Displ commnt fx shaft of l fibula
		S82.453[P,Q,R]	Displ commnt fx shaft of unsp fibula
		S82.454[P,Q,R]	Nondisp commnt fx shaft of r fibula
		S82.455[P,Q,R]	Nondisp commnt fx shaft of l fibula
		S82.456[P,Q,R]	Nondisp commnt fx shaft of unsp fibula
		S82.461[P,Q,R]	Displ seg fx shaft of r fibula
		S82.462[P,Q,R]	Displ seg fx shaft of l fibula
		S82.463[P,Q,R]	Displ seg fx shaft of unsp fibula
		S82.464[P,Q,R]	Nondisp seg fx shaft of r fibula
		S82.465[P,Q,R]	Nondisp seg fx shaft of l fibula
		S82.466[P,Q,R]	Nondisp seg fx shaft of unsp fibula
		S82.491[P,Q,R]	Oth fx shaft of r fibula
		S82.492[P,Q,R]	Oth fx shaft of left fibula
		S82.499[P,Q,R]	Oth fx shaft of unsp fibula
		S82.51X[P,Q,R]	Disp fx of med malleolus of r tibia
		S82.52X[P,Q,R]	Disp fx of med malleolus of l tibia
		S82.53X[P,Q,R]	Disp fx of med malleolus of unsp tibia
		S82.54X[P,Q,R]	Nondisp fx of med malleolus of r tibia
		S82.55X[P,Q,R]	Nondisp fx of med malleolus of l tibia
		S82.56X[P,Q,R]	Nondisp fx of med malleolus of unsp tibia
		S82.61X[P,Q,R]	Disp fx of lateral malleolus of r fibula
		S82.62X[P,Q,R]	Disp fx of lateral malleolus of l fibula
		S82.63X[P,Q,R]	Disp fx of lateral malleolus of unsp fibula
		S82.64X[P,Q,R]	Nondisp fx of lateral malleolus of r fibula
		S82.65X[P,Q,R]	Nondisp fx of lateral malleolus of l fibula
		S82.66X[P,Q,R]	Nondisp fx of lateral malleolus of unsp fibula

6th Character meanings for codes as indicated
1 Right 2 Left 9 Unspecified

7th Character meanins for codes S82.-
P Sub Enc Closed FX Malunion
Q Sub Enc Open FX Type I/II Malunion
R Sub Enc Open IIIA/B/C Malunion

(Continued on next page)

ICD-9-CM		ICD-10-CM	
733.81	MALUNION OF FRACTURE **(Continued)**	**S82.81**[1,2,9]**P**	Torus fx upper end of r fibula, subs for fx w malunion
		S82.82[1,2,9]**P**	Torus fx lower end of r fibula, subs for fx w malunion
		S82.831[P,Q,R]	Oth fx upr and low end r fibula
		S82.832[P,Q,R]	Oth fx upr and low end l fibula
		S82.839[P,Q,R]	Oth fx upr & low end unsp fibula
		S82.841[P,Q,R]	Displ bimalleol fx r low leg
		S82.842[P,Q,R]	Displ bimalleol fx l low leg
		S82.843[P,Q,R]	Displ bimalleol fx unsp low leg
		S82.844[P,Q,R]	Nondisp bimalleol fx r low leg
		S82.845[P,Q,R]	Nondisp bimalleol fx l low leg
		S82.846[P,Q,R]	Nondisp bimalleol fx unsp low leg
		S82.851[P,Q,R]	Displ trimalleol fx r low leg
		S82.852[P,Q,R]	Displ trimalleol fx l low leg
		S82.853[P,Q,R]	Displ trimalleol fx unsp low leg
		S82.854[P,Q,R]	Nondisp trimalleol fx r low leg
		S82.855[P,Q,R]	Nondisp trimalleol fx l low leg
		S82.856[P,Q,R]	Nondisp trimalleol fx unsp low leg
		S82.861[P,Q,R]	Displ Maisonneuve's fx r leg
		S82.862[P,Q,R]	Displ Maisonneuve's fx left leg
		S82.863[P,Q,R]	Displ Maisonneuve's fx unsp leg
		S82.864[P,Q,R]	Nondisp Maisonneuve's fx r leg
		S82.865[P,Q,R]	Nondisp Maisonneuve's fx l leg
		S82.866[P,Q,R]	Nondisp Maisonneuve's fx unsp leg
		S82.871[P,Q,R]	Displaced pilon fx right tibia
		S82.872[P,Q,R]	Displaced pilon fx left tibia
		S82.873[P,Q,R]	Displaced pilon fx unsp tibia
		S82.874[P,Q,R]	Nondisp pilon fx right tibia
		S82.875[P,Q,R]	Nondisp pilon fx left tibia
		S82.876[P,Q,R]	Nondisp pilon fx unsp tibia
		S82.891[P,Q,R]	Oth fracture of right lower leg
		S82.892[P,Q,R]	Oth fracture of left lower leg
		S82.899[P,Q,R]	Oth fracture of unsp lower leg
		S82.90X[P,Q,R]	Unsp fracture of unsp lower leg
		S82.91X[P,Q,R]	Unsp fracture of r low leg
		S82.92X[P,Q,R]	Unsp fracture of left lower leg
		S89.00[1,2,9]**P**	Unsp physeal fx upper end of tibia, subs for fx w malunion
		S89.01[1,2,9]**P**	Sltr-haris Type I physl fx upr end tibia, sub for fx w malun
		S89.02[1,2,9]**P**	Sltr-haris Type II physl fx upr end tibia, sub for fx w malun
		S89.03[1,2,9]**P**	Sltr-haris Type III physl fx upr end tibia, sub for fx w malun
		S89.04[1,2,9]**P**	Sltr-haris Type IV physl fx upr end tibia, sub for fx w malun
		S89.09[1,2,9]**P**	Oth physeal fx upper end of tibia, subs for fx w malunion
		S89.10[1,2,9]**P**	Unsp physeal fx lower end of tibia, subs for fx w malunion
		S89.11[1,2,9]**P**	Sltr-haris Type I physl fx low end tibia, sub for fx w malun
		S89.12[1,2,9]**P**	Sltr-haris Type II physl fx low end tibia, sub for fx w malun
		S89.13[1,2,9]**P**	Sltr-haris Type III physl fx low end tibia, sub for fx w malun
		S89.14[1,2,9]**P**	Sltr-haris Type IV physl fx low end tibia, sub for fx w malun
		S89.19[1,2,9]**P**	Oth physeal fx lower end of tibia, subs for fx w malunion
		S89.20[1,2,9]**P**	Unsp physl fx upper end of fibula, subs for fx w malunion
		S89.21[1,2,9]**P**	Sltr-haris Type I physl fx upr end fibula, sub for fx w malun
		S89.22[1,2,9]**P**	Sltr-haris Type II physl fx upr end fibula, sub for fx w malun
		S89.29[1,2,9]**P**	Oth physeal fx upper end of fibula, subs for fx w malunion
		S89.30[1,2,9]**P**	Unsp physl fx lower end of fibula, subs for fx w malunion
		S89.31[1,2,9]**P**	Sltr-haris Type I physl fx low end fibula, sub for fx w malun
		S89.32[1,2,9]**P**	Sltr-haris Type II physl fx low end fibula, sub for fx w malun
		S89.39[1,2,9]**P**	Oth physeal fx lower end of fibula, subs for fx w malunion
		S92.00[1,2,9]**P**	Unsp fracture of right calcaneus, subs for fx w malunion
		S92.011P	Disp fx of body of right calcaneus, subs for fx w malunion
		S92.012P	Disp fx of body of left calcaneus, subs for fx w malunion
		S92.013P	Disp fx of body of unsp calcaneus, subs for fx w malunion
		S92.014P	Nondisp fx of body of r calcaneus, subs for fx w malunion
		S92.015P	Nondisp fx of body of left calcaneus, subs for fx w malunion
		S92.016P	Nondisp fx of body of unsp calcaneus, subs for fx w malunion
		S92.021P	Disp fx of ant pro of r calcaneus, subs for fx w malunion
		S92.022P	Disp fx of ant pro of l calcaneus, subs for fx w malunion
		S92.023P	Disp fx of ant pro of unsp calcaneus, subs for fx w malunion
		S92.024P	Nondisp fx of ant pro of r calcaneus, subs for fx w malunion
		S92.025P	Nondisp fx of ant pro of l calcaneus, subs for fx w malunion
		S92.026P	Nondisp fx of ant pro of unsp calcaneus, sub for fx w malun
		S92.031P	Displ avuls fx tuberosity of r calcaneus, sub for fx w malun
		S92.032P	Displ avuls fx tuberosity of l calcaneus, sub for fx w malun
		S92.033P	Displ avuls fx tuberosity of unsp calcaneus, sub for fx w malun
		S92.034P	Nondisp avuls fx tuberosity of r calcaneus, sub for fx w malun
		S92.035P	Nondisp avuls fx tuberosity of l calcaneus, sub for fx w malun
		S92.036P	Nondisp avuls fx tuberosity of unsp calcaneus, sub for fx w malun
		S92.041P	Displ oth fx tuberosity of r calcaneus, sub for fx w malun

6th Character meanings for codes as indicated
1 Right ***2 Left*** ***9 Unspecified***

7th Character meanins for codes S82.-
P Sub Enc Closed FX Malunion
Q Sub Enc Open FX Type I/II Malunion
R Sub Enc Open IIIA/B/C Malunion

(Continued on next page)

ICD-9-CM		ICD-10-CM	
733.81	MALUNION OF FRACTURE **(Continued)**	**S92.Ø42P**	Displ oth fx tuberosity of l calcaneus, sub for fx w malun
		S92.Ø43P	Displ oth fx tuberosity of unsp calcaneus, sub for fx w malun
		S92.Ø44P	Nondisp oth fx tuberosity of r calcaneus, sub for fx w malun
		S92.Ø45P	Nondisp oth fx tuberosity of l calcaneus, sub for fx w malun
		S92.Ø46P	Nondisp oth fx tuberosity of unsp calcaneus, sub for fx w malun
		S92.Ø51P	Displ oth extrartic fx r calcaneus, subs for fx w malunion
		S92.Ø52P	Displ oth extrartic fx l calcaneus, subs for fx w malunion
		S92.Ø53P	Displ oth extrartic fx unsp calcaneus, sub for fx w malun
		S92.Ø54P	Nondisp oth extrartic fx r calcaneus, subs for fx w malunion
		S92.Ø55P	Nondisp oth extrartic fx l calcaneus, subs for fx w malunion
		S92.Ø56P	Nondisp oth extrartic fx unsp calcaneus, sub for fx w malun
		S92.Ø61P	Displaced intartic fx r calcaneus, subs for fx w malunion
		S92.Ø62P	Displaced intartic fx l calcaneus, subs for fx w malunion
		S92.Ø63P	Displaced intartic fx unsp calcaneus, subs for fx w malunion
		S92.Ø64P	Nondisp intartic fx r calcaneus, subs for fx w malunion
		S92.Ø65P	Nondisp intartic fx l calcaneus, subs for fx w malunion
		S92.Ø66P	Nondisp intartic fx unsp calcaneus, subs for fx w malunion
		S92.1Ø[1,2,9]P	Unsp fracture of right talus, subs for fx w malunion
		S92.111P	Disp fx of neck of right talus, subs for fx w malunion
		S92.112P	Disp fx of neck of left talus, subs for fx w malunion
		S92.113P	Disp fx of neck of unsp talus, subs for fx w malunion
		S92.114P	Nondisp fx of neck of right talus, subs for fx w malunion
		S92.115P	Nondisp fx of neck of left talus, subs for fx w malunion
		S92.116P	Nondisp fx of neck of unsp talus, subs for fx w malunion
		S92.121P	Disp fx of body of right talus, subs for fx w malunion
		S92.122P	Disp fx of body of left talus, subs for fx w malunion
		S92.123P	Disp fx of body of unsp talus, subs for fx w malunion
		S92.124P	Nondisp fx of body of right talus, subs for fx w malunion
		S92.125P	Nondisp fx of body of left talus, subs for fx w malunion
		S92.126P	Nondisp fx of body of unsp talus, subs for fx w malunion
		S92.131P	Disp fx of post pro of right talus, subs for fx w malunion
		S92.132P	Disp fx of post pro of left talus, subs for fx w malunion
		S92.133P	Disp fx of post pro of unsp talus, subs for fx w malunion
		S92.134P	Nondisp fx of post pro of r talus, subs for fx w malunion
		S92.135P	Nondisp fx of post pro of left talus, subs for fx w malunion
		S92.136P	Nondisp fx of post pro of unsp talus, subs for fx w malunion
		S92.141P	Displaced dome fx right talus, subs for fx w malunion
		S92.142P	Displaced dome fx left talus, subs for fx w malunion
		S92.143P	Displaced dome fx unsp talus, subs for fx w malunion
		S92.144P	Nondisp dome fracture of right talus, subs for fx w malunion
		S92.145P	Nondisp dome fracture of left talus, subs for fx w malunion
		S92.146P	Nondisp dome fracture of unsp talus, subs for fx w malunion
		S92.151P	Displ avuls fx (chip fracture) of r talus, sub for fx w malun
		S92.152P	Displ avuls fx (chip fracture) of l talus, sub for fx w malun
		S92.153P	Displ avuls fx (chip fracture) of unsp talus, sub for fx w malun
		S92.154P	Nondisp avuls fx (chip fracture) of r talus, sub for fx w malun
		S92.155P	Nondisp avuls fx (chip fracture) of l talus, sub for fx w malun
		S92.156P	Nondisp avuls fx (chip fracture) of unsp talus, sub for fx w malun
		S92.19[1,2,9]P	Oth fracture of talus, subs for fx w malunion
		S92.2Ø[1,2,9]P	Fx unsp tarsal bone(s) of foot, subs for fx w malunion
		S92.211P	Disp fx of cuboid bone of right foot, subs for fx w malunion
		S92.212P	Disp fx of cuboid bone of left foot, subs for fx w malunion
		S92.213P	Disp fx of cuboid bone of unsp foot, subs for fx w malunion
		S92.214P	Nondisp fx of cuboid bone of r foot, subs for fx w malunion
		S92.215P	Nondisp fx of cuboid bone of l foot, subs for fx w malunion
		S92.216P	Nondisp fx of cuboid bone of unsp ft, subs for fx w malunion
		S92.221P	Disp fx of lateral cuneiform of r ft, subs for fx w malunion
		S92.222P	Disp fx of lateral cuneiform of l ft, subs for fx w malunion
		S92.223P	Disp fx of lateral cuneiform of unsp ft, sub for fx w malun
		S92.224P	Nondisp fx of lateral cuneiform of r ft, sub for fx w malun
		S92.225P	Nondisp fx of lateral cuneiform of l ft, sub for fx w malun
		S92.226P	Nondisp fx of lateral cuneiform of unsp ft, sub for fx w malun
		S92.231P	Disp fx of intermed cuneiform of r ft, sub for fx w malun
		S92.232P	Disp fx of intermed cuneiform of l ft, sub for fx w malun
		S92.233P	Disp fx of intermed cuneiform of unsp ft, sub for fx w malun
		S92.234P	Nondisp fx of intermed cuneiform of r ft, sub for fx w malun
		S92.235P	Nondisp fx of intermed cuneiform of l ft, sub for fx w malun
		S92.236P	Nondisp fx of intermed cuneiform of unsp ft, sub for fx w malun
		S92.241P	Disp fx of med cuneiform of r foot, subs for fx w malunion
		S92.242P	Disp fx of med cuneiform of l foot, subs for fx w malunion
		S92.243P	Disp fx of med cuneiform of unsp ft, subs for fx w malunion
		S92.244P	Nondisp fx of med cuneiform of r ft, subs for fx w malunion
		S92.245P	Nondisp fx of med cuneiform of l ft, subs for fx w malunion
		S92.246P	Nondisp fx of med cuneiform of unsp ft, sub for fx w malun
		S92.251P	Disp fx of navicular of right foot, subs for fx w malunion
		S92.252P	Disp fx of navicular of left foot, subs for fx w malunion
		S92.253P	Disp fx of navicular of unsp foot, subs for fx w malunion
		S92.254P	Nondisp fx of navicular of r foot, subs for fx w malunion
		S92.255P	Nondisp fx of navicular of left foot, subs for fx w malunion

6th Character meanings for codes as indicated
1 Right 2 Left 9 Unspecified

(Continued on next page)

ICD-9-CM		ICD-10-CM	
733.81	MALUNION OF FRACTURE **(Continued)**	**S92.256P**	Nondisp fx of navicular of unsp foot, subs for fx w malunion
		S92.3Ø[1,2,9]P	Fx unsp metatarsal bone(s), foot, subs for fx w malunion
		S92.311P	Disp fx of 1st metatarsal bone, r ft, subs for fx w malunion
		S92.312P	Disp fx of 1st metatarsal bone, l ft, subs for fx w malunion
		S92.313P	Disp fx of 1st metatarsal bone, unsp ft, sub for fx w malun
		S92.314P	Nondisp fx of 1st metatarsal bone, r ft, sub for fx w malun
		S92.315P	Nondisp fx of 1st metatarsal bone, l ft, sub for fx w malun
		S92.316P	Nondisp fx of 1st metatarsal bone, unsp ft, sub for fx w malun
		S92.321P	Disp fx of 2nd metatarsal bone, r ft, subs for fx w malunion
		S92.322P	Disp fx of 2nd metatarsal bone, l ft, subs for fx w malunion
		S92.323P	Disp fx of 2nd metatarsal bone, unsp ft, sub for fx w malun
		S92.324P	Nondisp fx of 2nd metatarsal bone, r ft, sub for fx w malun
		S92.325P	Nondisp fx of 2nd metatarsal bone, l ft, sub for fx w malun
		S92.326P	Nondisp fx of 2nd metatarsal bone, unsp ft, sub for fx w malun
		S92.331P	Disp fx of 3rd metatarsal bone, r ft, subs for fx w malunion
		S92.332P	Disp fx of 3rd metatarsal bone, l ft, subs for fx w malunion
		S92.333P	Disp fx of 3rd metatarsal bone, unsp ft, sub for fx w malun
		S92.334P	Nondisp fx of 3rd metatarsal bone, r ft, sub for fx w malun
		S92.335P	Nondisp fx of 3rd metatarsal bone, l ft, sub for fx w malun
		S92.336P	Nondisp fx of 3rd metatarsal bone, unsp ft, sub for fx w malun
		S92.341P	Disp fx of 4th metatarsal bone, r ft, subs for fx w malunion
		S92.342P	Disp fx of 4th metatarsal bone, l ft, subs for fx w malunion
		S92.343P	Disp fx of 4th metatarsal bone, unsp ft, sub for fx w malun
		S92.344P	Nondisp fx of 4th metatarsal bone, r ft, sub for fx w malun
		S92.345P	Nondisp fx of 4th metatarsal bone, l ft, sub for fx w malun
		S92.346P	Nondisp fx of 4th metatarsal bone, unsp ft, sub for fx w malun
		S92.351P	Disp fx of 5th metatarsal bone, r ft, subs for fx w malunion
		S92.352P	Disp fx of 5th metatarsal bone, l ft, subs for fx w malunion
		S92.353P	Disp fx of 5th metatarsal bone, unsp ft, sub for fx w malun
		S92.354P	Nondisp fx of 5th metatarsal bone, r ft, sub for fx w malun
		S92.355P	Nondisp fx of 5th metatarsal bone, l ft, sub for fx w malun
		S92.356P	Nondisp fx of 5th metatarsal bone, unsp ft, sub for fx w malun
		S92.4Ø1P	Displaced unsp fx right great toe, subs for fx w malunion
		S92.4Ø2P	Displaced unsp fx left great toe, subs for fx w malunion
		S92.4Ø3P	Displaced unsp fx unsp great toe, subs for fx w malunion
		S92.4Ø4P	Nondisp unsp fx right great toe, subs for fx w malunion
		S92.4Ø5P	Nondisp unsp fx left great toe, subs for fx w malunion
		S92.4Ø6P	Nondisp unsp fx unsp great toe, subs for fx w malunion
		S92.411P	Disp fx of prox phalanx of r great toe, sub for fx w malun
		S92.412P	Disp fx of prox phalanx of l great toe, sub for fx w malun
		S92.413P	Disp fx of prox phalanx of unsp great toe, sub for fx w malun
		S92.414P	Nondisp fx of prox phalanx of r great toe, sub for fx w malun
		S92.415P	Nondisp fx of prox phalanx of l great toe, sub for fx w malun
		S92.416P	Nondisp fx of prox phalanx of unsp great toe, sub for fx w malun
		S92.421P	Disp fx of dist phalanx of r great toe, sub for fx w malun
		S92.422P	Disp fx of dist phalanx of l great toe, sub for fx w malun
		S92.423P	Disp fx of dist phalanx of unsp great toe, sub for fx w malun
		S92.424P	Nondisp fx of dist phalanx of r great toe, sub for fx w malun
		S92.425P	Nondisp fx of dist phalanx of l great toe, sub for fx w malun
		S92.426P	Nondisp fx of dist phalanx of unsp great toe, sub for fx w malun
		S92.49[1,2,9]P	Oth fracture of great toe, subs for fx w malunion
		S92.5Ø1P	Displ unsp fx right lesser toe(s), subs for fx w malunion
		S92.5Ø2P	Displaced unsp fx left lesser toe(s), subs for fx w malunion
		S92.5Ø3P	Displaced unsp fx unsp lesser toe(s), subs for fx w malunion
		S92.5Ø4P	Nondisp unsp fx right lesser toe(s), subs for fx w malunion
		S92.5Ø5P	Nondisp unsp fx left lesser toe(s), subs for fx w malunion
		S92.5Ø6P	Nondisp unsp fx unsp lesser toe(s), subs for fx w malunion
		S92.511P	Disp fx of prox phalanx of r less toe(s), sub for fx w malun
		S92.512P	Disp fx of prox phalanx of l less toe(s), sub for fx w malun
		S92.513P	Disp fx of prox phalanx of unsp less toe(s), sub for fx w malun
		S92.514P	Nondisp fx of prox phalanx of r less toe(s), sub for fx w malun
		S92.515P	Nondisp fx of prox phalanx of l less toe(s), sub for fx w malun
		S92.516P	Nondisp fx of prox phalanx of unsp less toe(s), sub for fx w malun
		S92.521P	Disp fx of med phalanx of r less toe(s), sub for fx w malun
		S92.522P	Disp fx of med phalanx of l less toe(s), sub for fx w malun
		S92.523P	Disp fx of med phalanx of unsp less toe(s), sub for fx w malun
		S92.524P	Nondisp fx of med phalanx of r less toe(s), sub for fx w malun
		S92.525P	Nondisp fx of med phalanx of l less toe(s), sub for fx w malun
		S92.526P	Nondisp fx of med phalanx of unsp less toe(s), sub for fx w malun
		S92.531P	Disp fx of dist phalanx of r less toe(s), sub for fx w malun
		S92.532P	Disp fx of dist phalanx of l less toe(s), sub for fx w malun
		S92.533P	Disp fx of dist phalanx of unsp less toe(s), sub for fx w malun
		S92.534P	Nondisp fx of dist phalanx of r less toe(s), sub for fx w malun
		S92.535P	Nondisp fx of dist phalanx of l less toe(s), sub for fx w malun
		S92.536P	Nondisp fx of dist phalanx of unsp less toe(s), sub for fx w malun
		S92.59[1,2,9]P	Oth fracture of lesser toe(s), subs for fx w malunion
		S92.9Ø[1,2,9]P	Unsp fracture of foot, subs for fx w malunion
		S92.91[1,2,9]P	Unsp fracture of toe(s), subs for fx w malunion

6th Character meanings for codes as indicated
1 Right 2 Left 9 Unspecified

ICD-9-CM		ICD-10-CM	
733.82	NONUNION OF FRACTURE	M80.00XK	Age-rel osteopor w crnt path fx, unsp site, sub for fx w nonun
		M80.01[1,2,9]K	Age-rel osteopor w crnt path fx, shldr, sub for fx w nonun
		M80.02[1,2,9]K	Age-rel osteopor w crnt path fx, humer, sub for fx w nonun
		M80.03[1,2,9]K	Age-rel osteopor w crnt path fx, forearm, sub for fx w nonun
		M80.04[1,2,9]K	Age-rel osteopor w crnt path fx, hand, sub for fx w nonun
		M80.05[1,2,9]K	Age-rel osteopor w crnt path fx, femr, sub for fx w nonun
		M80.06[1,2,9]K	Age-rel osteopor w crnt path fx, low leg, sub for fx w nonun
		M80.07[1,2,9]K	Age-rel osteopor w crnt path fx, ank/ft, sub for fx w nonun
		M80.08XK	Age-rel osteopor w crnt path fx, verteb, sub for fx w nonun
		M80.80XK	Oth osteopor w crnt path fx, unsp site, sub for fx w nonun
		M80.81[1,2,9]K	Oth osteopor w crnt path fx, shldr, subs for fx w nonunion
		M80.82[1,2,9]K	Oth osteopor w crnt path fx, humer, subs for fx w nonunion
		M80.83[1,2,9]K	Oth osteopor w crnt path fx, forearm, sub for fx w nonun
		M80.84[1,2,9]K	Oth osteopor w crnt path fx, hand, subs for fx w nonunion
		M80.85[1,2,9]K	Oth osteopor w crnt path fx, femur, subs for fx w nonunion
		M80.86[1,2,9]K	Oth osteopor w crnt path fx, low leg, sub for fx w nonun
		M80.87[1,2,9]K	Oth osteopor w crnt path fx, ank/ft, sub for fx w nonun
		M80.88XK	Oth osteopor w crnt path fx, verteb, subs for fx w nonunion
		M84.30XK	Stress fracture, unsp site, subs for fx w nonunion
		M84.31[1,2,9]K	Stress fracture, shoulder, subs for fx w nonunion
		M84.32[1,2,9]K	Stress fracture, humerus, subs for fx w nonunion
		M84.331K	Stress fracture, right ulna, subs for fx w nonunion
		M84.332K	Stress fracture, left ulna, subs for fx w nonunion
		M84.333K	Stress fracture, right radius, subs for fx w nonunion
		M84.334K	Stress fracture, left radius, subs for fx w nonunion
		M84.339K	Stress fx, unsp ulna and radius, subs for fx w nonunion
		M84.341K	Stress fracture, right hand, subs for fx w nonunion
		M84.342K	Stress fracture, left hand, subs for fx w nonunion
		M84.343K	Stress fracture, unsp hand, subs for fx w nonunion
		M84.344K	Stress fracture, right finger(s), subs for fx w nonunion
		M84.345K	Stress fracture, left finger(s), subs for fx w nonunion
		M84.346K	Stress fracture, unsp finger(s), subs for fx w nonunion
		M84.350K	Stress fracture, pelvis, subs encntr for fracture w nonunion
		M84.351K	Stress fracture, right femur, subs for fx w nonunion
		M84.352K	Stress fracture, left femur, subs for fx w nonunion
		M84.353K	Stress fracture, unsp femur, subs for fx w nonunion
		M84.359K	Stress fracture, hip, unsp, subs for fx w nonunion
		M84.361K	Stress fracture, right tibia, subs for fx w nonunion
		M84.362K	Stress fracture, left tibia, subs for fx w nonunion
		M84.363K	Stress fracture, right fibula, subs for fx w nonunion
		M84.364K	Stress fracture, left fibula, subs for fx w nonunion
		M84.369K	Stress fx, unsp tibia and fibula, subs for fx w nonunion
		M84.371K	Stress fracture, right ankle, subs for fx w nonunion
		M84.372K	Stress fracture, left ankle, subs for fx w nonunion
		M84.373K	Stress fracture, unsp ankle, subs for fx w nonunion
		M84.374K	Stress fracture, right foot, subs for fx w nonunion
		M84.375K	Stress fracture, left foot, subs for fx w nonunion
		M84.376K	Stress fracture, unsp foot, subs for fx w nonunion
		M84.377K	Stress fracture, right toe(s), subs for fx w nonunion
		M84.378K	Stress fracture, left toe(s), subs for fx w nonunion
		M84.379K	Stress fracture, unsp toe(s), subs for fx w nonunion
		M84.38XK	Stress fracture, oth site, subs for fx w nonunion
		M84.40XK	Pathological fracture, unsp site, subs for fx w nonunion
		M84.41[1,2,9]K	Pathological fracture, shoulder, subs for fx w nonunion
		M84.42[1,2,9]K	Pathological fracture, humerus, subs for fx w nonunion
		M84.431K	Pathological fracture, right ulna, subs for fx w nonunion
		M84.432K	Pathological fracture, left ulna, subs for fx w nonunion
		M84.433K	Pathological fracture, right radius, subs for fx w nonunion
		M84.434K	Pathological fracture, left radius, subs for fx w nonunion
		M84.439K	Path fracture, unsp ulna and radius, subs for fx w nonunion
		M84.441K	Pathological fracture, right hand, subs for fx w nonunion
		M84.442K	Pathological fracture, left hand, subs for fx w nonunion
		M84.443K	Pathological fracture, unsp hand, subs for fx w nonunion
		M84.444K	Path fracture, right finger(s), subs for fx w nonunion
		M84.445K	Path fracture, left finger(s), subs for fx w nonunion
		M84.446K	Path fracture, unsp finger(s), subs for fx w nonunion
		M84.451K	Pathological fracture, right femur, subs for fx w nonunion
		M84.452K	Pathological fracture, left femur, subs for fx w nonunion
		M84.453K	Pathological fracture, unsp femur, subs for fx w nonunion
		M84.454K	Pathological fracture, pelvis, subs for fx w nonunion
		M84.459K	Pathological fracture, hip, unsp, subs for fx w nonunion
		M84.461K	Pathological fracture, right tibia, subs for fx w nonunion
		M84.462K	Pathological fracture, left tibia, subs for fx w nonunion
		M84.463K	Pathological fracture, right fibula, subs for fx w nonunion
		M84.464K	Pathological fracture, left fibula, subs for fx w nonunion
		M84.469K	Path fracture, unsp tibia and fibula, subs for fx w nonunion
		M84.471K	Pathological fracture, right ankle, subs for fx w nonunion
		M84.472K	Pathological fracture, left ankle, subs for fx w nonunion
		M84.473K	Pathological fracture, unsp ankle, subs for fx w nonunion

6th Character meanings for codes as indicated
1 Right 2 Left 9 Unspecified

(Continued on next page)

ICD-9-CM		ICD-10-CM	
733.82	NONUNION OF FRACTURE **(Continued)**	**M84.474K**	Pathological fracture, right foot, subs for fx w nonunion
		M84.475K	Pathological fracture, left foot, subs for fx w nonunion
		M84.476K	Pathological fracture, unsp foot, subs for fx w nonunion
		M84.477K	Pathological fracture, right toe(s), subs for fx w nonunion
		M84.478K	Pathological fracture, left toe(s), subs for fx w nonunion
		M84.479K	Pathological fracture, unsp toe(s), subs for fx w nonunion
		M84.48XK	Pathological fracture, oth site, subs for fx w nonunion
		M84.5ØXK	Path fx in neopltc dis, unsp site, subs for fx w nonunion
		M84.51[1,2,9]K	Path fx in neopltc disease, r shldr, subs for fx w nonunion
		M84.52[1,2,9]K	Path fx in neopltc dis, r humerus, subs for fx w nonunion
		M84.531K	Path fx in neopltc disease, r ulna, subs for fx w nonunion
		M84.532K	Path fx in neopltc disease, l ulna, subs for fx w nonunion
		M84.533K	Path fx in neopltc disease, r radius, subs for fx w nonunion
		M84.534K	Path fx in neopltc dis, left radius, subs for fx w nonunion
		M84.539K	Path fx in neopltc dis, unsp ulna & rad, sub for fx w nonun
		M84.54[1,2,9]K	Path fx in neopltc disease, r hand, subs for fx w nonunion
		M84.55ØK	Path fx in neopltc disease, pelvis, subs for fx w nonunion
		M84.551K	Path fx in neopltc disease, r femur, subs for fx w nonunion
		M84.552K	Path fx in neopltc disease, l femur, subs for fx w nonunion
		M84.553K	Path fx in neopltc dis, unsp femur, subs for fx w nonunion
		M84.559K	Path fx in neopltc dis, hip, unsp, subs for fx w nonunion
		M84.561K	Path fx in neopltc disease, r tibia, subs for fx w nonunion
		M84.562K	Path fx in neopltc disease, l tibia, subs for fx w nonunion
		M84.563K	Path fx in neopltc disease, r fibula, subs for fx w nonunion
		M84.564K	Path fx in neopltc disease, l fibula, subs for fx w nonunion
		M84.569K	Path fx in neopltc dis, unsp tibia & fibula, sub for fx w nonun
		M84.571K	Path fx in neopltc disease, r ankle, subs for fx w nonunion
		M84.572K	Path fx in neopltc disease, l ankle, subs for fx w nonunion
		M84.573K	Path fx in neopltc dis, unsp ankle, subs for fx w nonunion
		M84.574K	Path fx in neopltc disease, r foot, subs for fx w nonunion
		M84.575K	Path fx in neopltc disease, l foot, subs for fx w nonunion
		M84.576K	Path fx in neopltc dis, unsp foot, subs for fx w nonunion
		M84.58XK	Path fx in neopltc dis, oth spec site, subs for fx w nonun
		M84.6ØXK	Path fx in oth disease, unsp site, subs for fx w nonunion
		M84.61[1,2,9]K	Path fx in oth disease, r shoulder, subs for fx w nonunion
		M84.62[1,2,9]K	Path fx in oth disease, r humerus, subs for fx w nonunion
		M84.631K	Path fracture in oth disease, r ulna, subs for fx w nonunion
		M84.632K	Path fracture in oth disease, l ulna, subs for fx w nonunion
		M84.633K	Path fx in oth disease, r radius, subs for fx w nonunion
		M84.634K	Path fx in oth disease, left radius, subs for fx w nonunion
		M84.639K	Path fx in oth dis, unsp ulna & rad, subs for fx w nonunion
		M84.64[1,2,9]K	Path fracture in oth disease, r hand, subs for fx w nonunion
		M84.65ØK	Path fracture in oth disease, pelvis, subs for fx w nonunion
		M84.651K	Path fx in oth disease, r femur, subs for fx w nonunion
		M84.652K	Path fx in oth disease, l femur, subs for fx w nonunion
		M84.653K	Path fx in oth disease, unsp femur, subs for fx w nonunion
		M84.659K	Path fx in oth disease, hip, unsp, subs for fx w nonunion
		M84.661K	Path fx in oth disease, r tibia, subs for fx w nonunion
		M84.662K	Path fx in oth disease, l tibia, subs for fx w nonunion
		M84.663K	Path fx in oth disease, r fibula, subs for fx w nonunion
		M84.664K	Path fx in oth disease, l fibula, subs for fx w nonunion
		M84.669K	Path fx in oth dis, unsp tibia & fibula, sub for fx w nonun
		M84.671K	Path fx in oth disease, r ankle, subs for fx w nonunion
		M84.672K	Path fx in oth disease, l ankle, subs for fx w nonunion
		M84.673K	Path fx in oth disease, unsp ankle, subs for fx w nonunion
		M84.674K	Path fracture in oth disease, r foot, subs for fx w nonunion
		M84.675K	Path fracture in oth disease, l foot, subs for fx w nonunion
		M84.676K	Path fx in oth disease, unsp foot, subs for fx w nonunion
		M84.68XK	Path fx in oth disease, oth site, subs for fx w nonunion
		SØ2.ØXXK	Fracture of vault of skull, subs for fx w nonunion
		SØ2.1ØXK	Unsp fracture of base of skull, subs for fx w nonunion
		SØ2.11ØK	Type I occipital condyle fracture, subs for fx w nonunion
		SØ2.111K	Type II occipital condyle fracture, subs for fx w nonunion
		SØ2.112K	Type III occipital condyle fracture, subs for fx w nonunion
		SØ2.113K	Unsp occipital condyle fracture, subs for fx w nonunion
		SØ2.118K	Oth fracture of occiput, subs encntr for fracture w nonunion
		SØ2.119K	Unsp fracture of occiput, subs for fx w nonunion
		SØ2.19XK	Oth fracture of base of skull, subs for fx w nonunion
		SØ2.2XXK	Fracture of nasal bones, subs encntr for fracture w nonunion
		SØ2.3XXK	Fracture of orbital floor, subs for fx w nonunion
		SØ2.4ØØK	Malar fracture unsp, subs encntr for fracture with nonunion
		SØ2.4Ø1K	Maxillary fracture, unsp, subs for fx w nonunion
		SØ2.4Ø2K	Zygomatic fracture, unsp, subs for fx w nonunion
		SØ2.411K	LeFort I fracture, subs encntr for fracture with nonunion
		SØ2.412K	LeFort II fracture, subs encntr for fracture with nonunion
		SØ2.413K	LeFort III fracture, subs encntr for fracture with nonunion
		SØ2.42XK	Fracture of alveolus of maxilla, subs for fx w nonunion
		SØ2.5XXK	Fracture of tooth (traumatic), subs for fx w nonunion
		SØ2.6ØØK	Fx unsp part of body of mandible, subs for fx w nonunion

6th Character meanings for codes as indicated
1 Right 2 Left 9 Unspecified

(Continued on next page)

ICD-9-CM		ICD-10-CM	
733.82	NONUNION OF FRACTURE **(Continued)**	**S02.609K**	Fracture of mandible, unsp, subs for fx w nonunion
		S02.61XK	Fx condylar process of mandible, subs for fx w nonunion
		S02.62XK	Fx subcondylar process of mandible, subs for fx w nonunion
		S02.63XK	Fx coronoid process of mandible, subs for fx w nonunion
		S02.64XK	Fracture of ramus of mandible, subs for fx w nonunion
		S02.65XK	Fracture of angle of mandible, subs for fx w nonunion
		S02.66XK	Fracture of symphysis of mandible, subs for fx w nonunion
		S02.67XK	Fracture of alveolus of mandible, subs for fx w nonunion
		S02.69XK	Fracture of mandible of oth site, subs for fx w nonunion
		S02.8XXK	Fractures of skull and facial bones, subs for fx w nonunion
		S02.91XK	Unsp fracture of skull, subs encntr for fracture w nonunion
		S02.92XK	Unsp fracture of facial bones, subs for fx w nonunion
		S12.000K	Unsp disp fx of first cervcal vert, subs for fx w nonunion
		S12.001K	Unsp nondisp fx of 1st cervcal vert, subs for fx w nonunion
		S12.01XK	Stable burst fx first cervcal vert, subs for fx w nonunion
		S12.02XK	Unstbl burst fx first cervcal vert, subs for fx w nonunion
		S12.030K	Displ post arch fx 1st cervcal vert, subs for fx w nonunion
		S12.031K	Nondisp post arch fx 1st cervcal vert, sub for fx w nonun
		S12.040K	Displ lateral mass fx 1st cervcal vert, sub for fx w nonun
		S12.041K	Nondisp lateral mass fx 1st cervcal vert, sub for fx w nonun
		S12.090K	Oth disp fx of first cervcal vert, subs for fx w nonunion
		S12.091K	Oth nondisp fx of first cervcal vert, subs for fx w nonunion
		S12.100K	Unsp disp fx of second cervcal vert, subs for fx w nonunion
		S12.101K	Unsp nondisp fx of 2nd cervcal vert, subs for fx w nonunion
		S12.110K	Anterior displ Type II dens fracture, subs for fx w nonunion
		S12.111K	Post displ Type II dens fracture, subs for fx w nonunion
		S12.112K	Nondisplaced Type II dens fracture, subs for fx w nonunion
		S12.120K	Oth displaced dens fracture, subs for fx w nonunion
		S12.121K	Oth nondisplaced dens fracture, subs for fx w nonunion
		S12.130K	Unsp traum displ spondylolysis of 2nd cervcal vert, sub for fx w nonun
		S12.131K	Unsp traum nondisp spondylolysis of 2nd cervcal vert, sub for fx w nonun
		S12.14XK	Type III traum spondylolysis of 2nd cervcal vert, sub for fx w nonun
		S12.150K	Oth traum displ spondylolysis of 2nd cervcal vert, sub for fx w nonun
		S12.151K	Oth traum nondisp spondylolysis of 2nd cervcal vert, sub for fx w nonun
		S12.190K	Oth disp fx of second cervcal vert, subs for fx w nonunion
		S12.191K	Oth nondisp fx of 2nd cervcal vert, subs for fx w nonunion
		S12.200K	Unsp disp fx of third cervcal vert, subs for fx w nonunion
		S12.201K	Unsp nondisp fx of 3rd cervcal vert, subs for fx w nonunion
		S12.230K	Unsp traum displ spondylolysis of 3rd cervcal vert, sub for fx w nonun
		S12.231K	Unsp traum nondisp spondylolysis of 3rd cervcal vert, sub for fx w nonun
		S12.24XK	Type III traum spondylolysis of 3rd cervcal vert, sub for fx w nonun
		S12.250K	Oth traum displ spondylolysis of 3rd cervcal vert, sub for fx w nonun
		S12.251K	Oth traum nondisp spondylolysis of 3rd cervcal vert, sub for fx w nonun
		S12.290K	Oth disp fx of third cervcal vert, subs for fx w nonunion
		S12.291K	Oth nondisp fx of third cervcal vert, subs for fx w nonunion
		S12.300K	Unsp disp fx of fourth cervcal vert, subs for fx w nonunion
		S12.301K	Unsp nondisp fx of 4th cervcal vert, subs for fx w nonunion
		S12.330K	Unsp traum displ spondylolysis of 4th cervcal vert, sub for fx w nonun
		S12.331K	Unsp traum nondisp spondylolysis of 4th cervcal vert, sub for fx w nonun
		S12.34XK	Type III traum spondylolysis of 4th cervcal vert, sub for fx w nonun
		S12.350K	Oth traum displ spondylolysis of 4th cervcal vert, sub for fx w nonun
		S12.351K	Oth traum nondisp spondylolysis of 4th cervcal vert, sub for fx w nonun
		S12.390K	Oth disp fx of fourth cervcal vert, subs for fx w nonunion
		S12.391K	Oth nondisp fx of 4th cervcal vert, subs for fx w nonunion
		S12.400K	Unsp disp fx of fifth cervcal vert, subs for fx w nonunion
		S12.401K	Unsp nondisp fx of 5th cervcal vert, subs for fx w nonunion
		S12.430K	Unsp traum displ spondylolysis of 5th cervcal vert, sub for fx w nonun
		S12.431K	Unsp traum nondisp spondylolysis of 5th cervcal vert, sub for fx w nonun
		S12.44XK	Type III traum spondylolysis of 5th cervcal vert, sub for fx w nonun
		S12.450K	Oth traum displ spondylolysis of 5th cervcal vert, sub for fx w nonun
		S12.451K	Oth traum nondisp spondylolysis of 5th cervcal vert, sub for fx w nonun
		S12.490K	Oth disp fx of fifth cervcal vert, subs for fx w nonunion
		S12.491K	Oth nondisp fx of fifth cervcal vert, subs for fx w nonunion
		S12.500K	Unsp disp fx of sixth cervcal vert, subs for fx w nonunion
		S12.501K	Unsp nondisp fx of sixth cervcal vert, sub for fx w nonun
		S12.530K	Unsp traum displ spondylolysis of sixth cervcal vert, sub for fx w nonun
		S12.531K	Unsp traum nondisp spondylolysis of sixth cervcal vert, sub for fx w nonun
		S12.54XK	Type III traum spondylolysis of sixth cervcal vert, sub for fx w nonun
		S12.550K	Oth traum displ spondylolysis of sixth cervcal vert, sub for fx w nonun
		S12.551K	Oth traum nondisp spondylolysis of sixth cervcal vert, sub for fx w nonun
		S12.590K	Oth disp fx of sixth cervcal vert, subs for fx w nonunion
		S12.591K	Oth nondisp fx of sixth cervcal vert, subs for fx w nonunion
		S12.600K	Unsp disp fx of seventh cervcal vert, subs for fx w nonunion
		S12.601K	Unsp nondisp fx of 7th cervcal vert, subs for fx w nonunion
		S12.630K	Unsp traum displ spondylolysis of 7th cervcal vert, sub for fx w nonun
		S12.631K	Unsp traum nondisp spondylolysis of 7th cervcal vert, sub for fx w nonun
		S12.64XK	Type III traum spondylolysis of 7th cervcal vert, sub for fx w nonun
		S12.650K	Oth traum displ spondylolysis of 7th cervcal vert, sub for fx w nonun
		S12.651K	Oth traum nondisp spondylolysis of 7th cervcal vert, sub for fx w nonun
		S12.690K	Oth disp fx of seventh cervcal vert, subs for fx w nonunion
		S12.691K	Oth nondisp fx of 7th cervcal vert, subs for fx w nonunion
	(Continued on next page)	**S22.000K**	Wedge comprsn fx unsp thor vertebra, subs for fx w nonunion

ICD-9-CM		ICD-10-CM	
733.82	NONUNION OF FRACTURE **(Continued)**	**S22.001K**	Stable burst fx unsp thor vertebra, subs for fx w nonunion
		S22.002K	Unstable burst fx unsp thor vertebra, subs for fx w nonunion
		S22.008K	Oth fracture of unsp thor vertebra, subs for fx w nonunion
		S22.009K	Unsp fracture of unsp thor vertebra, subs for fx w nonunion
		S22.010K	Wedge comprsn fx first thor vertebra, subs for fx w nonunion
		S22.011K	Stable burst fx first thor vertebra, subs for fx w nonunion
		S22.012K	Unstbl burst fx first thor vertebra, subs for fx w nonunion
		S22.018K	Oth fracture of first thor vertebra, subs for fx w nonunion
		S22.019K	Unsp fracture of first thor vertebra, subs for fx w nonunion
		S22.020K	Wedge comprsn fx second thor vert, subs for fx w nonunion
		S22.021K	Stable burst fx second thor vertebra, subs for fx w nonunion
		S22.022K	Unstbl burst fx second thor vertebra, subs for fx w nonunion
		S22.028K	Oth fracture of second thor vertebra, subs for fx w nonunion
		S22.029K	Unsp fx second thor vertebra, subs for fx w nonunion
		S22.030K	Wedge comprsn fx third thor vertebra, subs for fx w nonunion
		S22.031K	Stable burst fx third thor vertebra, subs for fx w nonunion
		S22.032K	Unstbl burst fx third thor vertebra, subs for fx w nonunion
		S22.038K	Oth fracture of third thor vertebra, subs for fx w nonunion
		S22.039K	Unsp fracture of third thor vertebra, subs for fx w nonunion
		S22.040K	Wedge comprsn fx fourth thor vert, subs for fx w nonunion
		S22.041K	Stable burst fx fourth thor vertebra, subs for fx w nonunion
		S22.042K	Unstbl burst fx fourth thor vertebra, subs for fx w nonunion
		S22.048K	Oth fracture of fourth thor vertebra, subs for fx w nonunion
		S22.049K	Unsp fx fourth thor vertebra, subs for fx w nonunion
		S22.050K	Wedge comprsn fx T5-T6 vertebra, subs for fx w nonunion
		S22.051K	Stable burst fx T5-T6 vertebra, subs for fx w nonunion
		S22.052K	Unstable burst fx T5-T6 vertebra, subs for fx w nonunion
		S22.058K	Oth fracture of T5-T6 vertebra, subs for fx w nonunion
		S22.059K	Unsp fracture of T5-T6 vertebra, subs for fx w nonunion
		S22.060K	Wedge comprsn fx T7-T8 vertebra, subs for fx w nonunion
		S22.061K	Stable burst fx T7-T8 vertebra, subs for fx w nonunion
		S22.062K	Unstable burst fx T7-T8 vertebra, subs for fx w nonunion
		S22.068K	Oth fracture of T7-T8 thor vertebra, subs for fx w nonunion
		S22.069K	Unsp fracture of T7-T8 vertebra, subs for fx w nonunion
		S22.070K	Wedge comprsn fx T9-T10 vertebra, subs for fx w nonunion
		S22.071K	Stable burst fx T9-T10 vertebra, subs for fx w nonunion
		S22.072K	Unstable burst fx T9-T10 vertebra, subs for fx w nonunion
		S22.078K	Oth fracture of T9-T10 vertebra, subs for fx w nonunion
		S22.079K	Unsp fracture of T9-T10 vertebra, subs for fx w nonunion
		S22.080K	Wedge comprsn fx T11-T12 vertebra, subs for fx w nonunion
		S22.081K	Stable burst fx T11-T12 vertebra, subs for fx w nonunion
		S22.082K	Unstable burst fx T11-T12 vertebra, subs for fx w nonunion
		S22.088K	Oth fracture of T11-T12 vertebra, subs for fx w nonunion
		S22.089K	Unsp fracture of T11-T12 vertebra, subs for fx w nonunion
		S22.20XK	Unsp fracture of sternum, subs for fx w nonunion
		S22.21XK	Fracture of manubrium, subs encntr for fracture w nonunion
		S22.22XK	Fracture of body of sternum, subs for fx w nonunion
		S22.23XK	Sternal manubrial dissociation, subs for fx w nonunion
		S22.24XK	Fracture of xiphoid process, subs for fx w nonunion
		S22.31XK	Fracture of one rib, right side, subs for fx w nonunion
		S22.32XK	Fracture of one rib, left side, subs for fx w nonunion
		S22.39XK	Fracture of one rib, unsp side, subs for fx w nonunion
		S22.41XK	Multiple fx of ribs, right side, subs for fx w nonunion
		S22.42XK	Multiple fx of ribs, left side, subs for fx w nonunion
		S22.43XK	Multiple fractures of ribs, bi, subs for fx w nonunion
		S22.49XK	Multiple fx of ribs, unsp side, subs for fx w nonunion
		S22.5XXK	Flail chest, subsequent encounter for fracture with nonunion
		S22.9XXK	Fracture of bony thorax, part unsp, subs for fx w nonunion
		S32.000K	Wedge comprsn fx unsp lum vertebra, subs for fx w nonunion
		S32.001K	Stable burst fx unsp lum vertebra, subs for fx w nonunion
		S32.002K	Unstable burst fx unsp lum vertebra, subs for fx w nonunion
		S32.008K	Oth fracture of unsp lumbar vertebra, subs for fx w nonunion
		S32.009K	Unsp fracture of unsp lum vertebra, subs for fx w nonunion
		S32.010K	Wedge comprsn fx first lum vertebra, subs for fx w nonunion
		S32.011K	Stable burst fx first lum vertebra, subs for fx w nonunion
		S32.012K	Unstable burst fx first lum vertebra, subs for fx w nonunion
		S32.018K	Oth fracture of first lum vertebra, subs for fx w nonunion
		S32.019K	Unsp fracture of first lum vertebra, subs for fx w nonunion
		S32.020K	Wedge comprsn fx second lum vertebra, subs for fx w nonunion
		S32.021K	Stable burst fx second lum vertebra, subs for fx w nonunion
		S32.022K	Unstbl burst fx second lum vertebra, subs for fx w nonunion
		S32.028K	Oth fracture of second lum vertebra, subs for fx w nonunion
		S32.029K	Unsp fracture of second lum vertebra, subs for fx w nonunion
		S32.030K	Wedge comprsn fx third lum vertebra, subs for fx w nonunion
		S32.031K	Stable burst fx third lum vertebra, subs for fx w nonunion
		S32.032K	Unstable burst fx third lum vertebra, subs for fx w nonunion
		S32.038K	Oth fracture of third lum vertebra, subs for fx w nonunion
		S32.039K	Unsp fracture of third lum vertebra, subs for fx w nonunion
		S32.040K	Wedge comprsn fx fourth lum vertebra, subs for fx w nonunion
		S32.041K	Stable burst fx fourth lum vertebra, subs for fx w nonunion
		S32.042K	Unstbl burst fx fourth lum vertebra, subs for fx w nonunion
		S32.048K	Oth fracture of fourth lum vertebra, subs for fx w nonunion
	(Continued on next page)	**S32.049K**	Unsp fracture of fourth lum vertebra, subs for fx w nonunion

ICD-9-CM		ICD-10-CM	
733.82	NONUNION OF FRACTURE **(Continued)**	**S32.Ø5ØK**	Wedge comprsn fx fifth lum vertebra, subs for fx w nonunion
		S32.Ø51K	Stable burst fx fifth lum vertebra, subs for fx w nonunion
		S32.Ø52K	Unstable burst fx fifth lum vertebra, subs for fx w nonunion
		S32.Ø58K	Oth fracture of fifth lum vertebra, subs for fx w nonunion
		S32.Ø59K	Unsp fracture of fifth lum vertebra, subs for fx w nonunion
		S32.1ØXK	Unsp fracture of sacrum, subs encntr for fracture w nonunion
		S32.11ØK	Nondisp Zone I fracture of sacrum, subs for fx w nonunion
		S32.111K	Minimally displaced Zone I fx sacrum, subs for fx w nonunion
		S32.112K	Severely displaced Zone I fx sacrum, subs for fx w nonunion
		S32.119K	Unsp Zone I fracture of sacrum, subs for fx w nonunion
		S32.12ØK	Nondisp Zone II fracture of sacrum, subs for fx w nonunion
		S32.121K	Minimally displ Zone II fx sacrum, subs for fx w nonunion
		S32.122K	Severely displaced Zone II fx sacrum, subs for fx w nonunion
		S32.129K	Unsp Zone II fracture of sacrum, subs for fx w nonunion
		S32.13ØK	Nondisp Zone III fracture of sacrum, subs for fx w nonunion
		S32.131K	Minimally displ Zone III fx sacrum, subs for fx w nonunion
		S32.132K	Severely displ Zone III fx sacrum, subs for fx w nonunion
		S32.139K	Unsp Zone III fracture of sacrum, subs for fx w nonunion
		S32.14XK	Type 1 fracture of sacrum, subs for fx w nonunion
		S32.15XK	Type 2 fracture of sacrum, subs for fx w nonunion
		S32.16XK	Type 3 fracture of sacrum, subs for fx w nonunion
		S32.17XK	Type 4 fracture of sacrum, subs for fx w nonunion
		S32.19XK	Oth fracture of sacrum, subs encntr for fracture w nonunion
		S32.2XXK	Fracture of coccyx, subs encntr for fracture with nonunion
		S32.3Ø[1,2,9]K	Unsp fracture of ilium, subs for fx w nonunion
		S32.311K	Displaced avulsion fx right ilium, subs for fx w nonunion
		S32.312K	Displaced avulsion fx left ilium, subs for fx w nonunion
		S32.313K	Displaced avulsion fx unsp ilium, subs for fx w nonunion
		S32.314K	Nondisp avulsion fx right ilium, subs for fx w nonunion
		S32.315K	Nondisp avulsion fx left ilium, subs for fx w nonunion
		S32.316K	Nondisp avulsion fx unsp ilium, subs for fx w nonunion
		S32.39[1,2,9]K	Oth fracture of ilium, subs for fx w nonunion
		S32.4Ø[1,2,9]K	Unsp fracture of acetabulum, subs for fx w nonunion
		S32.411K	Disp fx of ant wall of right acetab, subs for fx w nonunion
		S32.412K	Disp fx of ant wall of left acetab, subs for fx w nonunion
		S32.413K	Disp fx of ant wall of unsp acetab, subs for fx w nonunion
		S32.414K	Nondisp fx of ant wall of r acetab, subs for fx w nonunion
		S32.415K	Nondisp fx of ant wall of l acetab, subs for fx w nonunion
		S32.416K	Nondisp fx of ant wl of unsp acetab, subs for fx w nonunion
		S32.421K	Disp fx of post wall of right acetab, subs for fx w nonunion
		S32.422K	Disp fx of post wall of left acetab, subs for fx w nonunion
		S32.423K	Disp fx of post wall of unsp acetab, subs for fx w nonunion
		S32.424K	Nondisp fx of post wall of r acetab, subs for fx w nonunion
		S32.425K	Nondisp fx of post wall of l acetab, subs for fx w nonunion
		S32.426K	Nondisp fx of post wl of unsp acetab, subs for fx w nonunion
		S32.431K	Disp fx of ant column of r acetab, subs for fx w nonunion
		S32.432K	Disp fx of ant column of left acetab, subs for fx w nonunion
		S32.433K	Disp fx of ant column of unsp acetab, subs for fx w nonunion
		S32.434K	Nondisp fx of ant column of r acetab, subs for fx w nonunion
		S32.435K	Nondisp fx of ant column of l acetab, subs for fx w nonunion
		S32.436K	Nondisp fx of ant column of unsp acetab, sub for fx w nonun
		S32.441K	Disp fx of post column of r acetab, subs for fx w nonunion
		S32.442K	Disp fx of post column of l acetab, subs for fx w nonunion
		S32.443K	Disp fx of post column of unsp acetab, sub for fx w nonun
		S32.444K	Nondisp fx of post column of r acetab, sub for fx w nonun
		S32.445K	Nondisp fx of post column of l acetab, sub for fx w nonun
		S32.446K	Nondisp fx of post column of unsp acetab, sub for fx w nonun
		S32.451K	Displaced transverse fx right acetab, subs for fx w nonunion
		S32.452K	Displaced transverse fx left acetab, subs for fx w nonunion
		S32.453K	Displaced transverse fx unsp acetab, subs for fx w nonunion
		S32.454K	Nondisp transverse fx right acetab, subs for fx w nonunion
		S32.455K	Nondisp transverse fx left acetab, subs for fx w nonunion
		S32.456K	Nondisp transverse fx unsp acetab, subs for fx w nonunion
		S32.461K	Displ assoc transv/post fx r acetab, subs for fx w nonunion
		S32.462K	Displ assoc transv/post fx l acetab, subs for fx w nonunion
		S32.463K	Displ assoc transv/post fx unsp acetab, sub for fx w nonun
		S32.464K	Nondisp assoc transv/post fx r acetab, sub for fx w nonun
		S32.465K	Nondisp assoc transv/post fx l acetab, sub for fx w nonun
		S32.466K	Nondisp assoc transv/post fx unsp acetab, sub for fx w nonun
		S32.471K	Disp fx of med wall of right acetab, subs for fx w nonunion
		S32.472K	Disp fx of med wall of left acetab, subs for fx w nonunion
		S32.473K	Disp fx of med wall of unsp acetab, subs for fx w nonunion
		S32.474K	Nondisp fx of med wall of r acetab, subs for fx w nonunion
		S32.475K	Nondisp fx of med wall of l acetab, subs for fx w nonunion
		S32.476K	Nondisp fx of med wl of unsp acetab, subs for fx w nonunion
		S32.481K	Displaced dome fx right acetabulum, subs for fx w nonunion
		S32.482K	Displaced dome fx left acetabulum, subs for fx w nonunion
		S32.483K	Displaced dome fx unsp acetabulum, subs for fx w nonunion
		S32.484K	Nondisp dome fx right acetabulum, subs for fx w nonunion
		S32.485K	Nondisp dome fx left acetabulum, subs for fx w nonunion

6th Character meanings for codes as indicated
1 Right ***2 Left*** ***9 Unspecified***

(Continued on next page)

ICD-9-CM		ICD-10-CM	
733.82	NONUNION OF FRACTURE **(Continued)**	**S32.486K**	Nondisp dome fx unsp acetabulum, subs for fx w nonunion
		S32.49[1,2,9]K	Oth fracture of acetabulum, subs for fx w nonunion
		S32.5Ø[1,2,9]K	Unsp fracture of pubis, subs for fx w nonunion
		S32.51[1,2,9]K	Fx superior rim of pubis, subs for fx w nonunion
		S32.59[1,2,9]K	Oth fracture of right pubis, subs for fx w nonunion
		S32.6Ø[1,2,9]K	Unsp fracture of ischium, subs for fx w nonunion
		S32.611K	Displaced avulsion fx right ischium, subs for fx w nonunion
		S32.612K	Displaced avulsion fx left ischium, subs for fx w nonunion
		S32.613K	Displaced avulsion fx unsp ischium, subs for fx w nonunion
		S32.614K	Nondisp avulsion fx right ischium, subs for fx w nonunion
		S32.615K	Nondisp avulsion fx left ischium, subs for fx w nonunion
		S32.616K	Nondisp avulsion fx unsp ischium, subs for fx w nonunion
		S32.69[1,2,9]K	Oth fracture of ischium, subs for fx w nonunion
		S32.81ØK	Mult fx of pelv w stable disrupt of pelv ring, sub for fx w nonun
		S32.811K	Mult fx of pelv w unstbl disrupt of pelv ring, sub for fx w nonun
		S32.82XK	Mult fx of pelv w/o disrupt of pelv ring, sub for fx w nonun
		S32.89XK	Fracture of oth parts of pelvis, subs for fx w nonunion
		S32.9XXK	Fx unsp parts of lumbosacr spin & pelv, sub for fx w nonun
		S42.ØØ[1,2,9]K	Fracture of unsp part of clavicle, subs for fx w nonunion
		S42.Ø11K	Ant disp fx of sternal end r clavicle, sub for fx w nonun
		S42.Ø12K	Ant disp fx of sternal end l clavicle, sub for fx w nonun
		S42.Ø13K	Ant disp fx of sternal end unsp clavicle, sub for fx w nonun
		S42.Ø14K	Post disp fx of sternal end r clavicle, sub for fx w nonun
		S42.Ø15K	Post disp fx of sternal end l clavicle, sub for fx w nonun
		S42.Ø16K	Post disp fx of sternal end unsp clavicle, sub for fx w nonun
		S42.Ø17K	Nondisp fx of sternal end r clavicle, subs for fx w nonunion
		S42.Ø18K	Nondisp fx of sternal end l clavicle, subs for fx w nonunion
		S42.Ø19K	Nondisp fx of sternal end unsp clavicle, sub for fx w nonun
		S42.Ø21K	Disp fx of shaft of right clavicle, subs for fx w nonunion
		S42.Ø22K	Disp fx of shaft of left clavicle, subs for fx w nonunion
		S42.Ø23K	Disp fx of shaft of unsp clavicle, subs for fx w nonunion
		S42.Ø24K	Nondisp fx of shaft of r clavicle, subs for fx w nonunion
		S42.Ø25K	Nondisp fx of shaft of left clavicle, subs for fx w nonunion
		S42.Ø26K	Nondisp fx of shaft of unsp clavicle, subs for fx w nonunion
		S42.Ø31K	Disp fx of lateral end of r clavicle, subs for fx w nonunion
		S42.Ø32K	Disp fx of lateral end of l clavicle, subs for fx w nonunion
		S42.Ø33K	Disp fx of lateral end unsp clavicle, subs for fx w nonunion
		S42.Ø34K	Nondisp fx of lateral end r clavicle, subs for fx w nonunion
		S42.Ø35K	Nondisp fx of lateral end l clavicle, subs for fx w nonunion
		S42.Ø36K	Nondisp fx of lateral end unsp clavicle, sub for fx w nonun
		S42.1Ø[1,2,9]K	Fx unsp part of scapula, shoulder, subs for fx w nonunion
		S42.111K	Disp fx of body of scapula, r shldr, subs for fx w nonunion
		S42.112K	Disp fx of body of scapula, l shldr, subs for fx w nonunion
		S42.113K	Disp fx of body of scapula, unsp shldr, sub for fx w nonun
		S42.114K	Nondisp fx of body of scapula, r shldr, sub for fx w nonun
		S42.115K	Nondisp fx of body of scapula, l shldr, sub for fx w nonun
		S42.116K	Nondisp fx of body of scapula, unsp shldr, 7thK
		S42.121K	Disp fx of acromial process, r shldr, subs for fx w nonunion
		S42.122K	Disp fx of acromial process, l shldr, subs for fx w nonunion
		S42.123K	Disp fx of acromial pro, unsp shldr, subs for fx w nonunion
		S42.124K	Nondisp fx of acromial pro, r shldr, subs for fx w nonunion
		S42.125K	Nondisp fx of acromial pro, l shldr, subs for fx w nonunion
		S42.126K	Nondisp fx of acromial pro, unsp shldr, 7thK
		S42.131K	Disp fx of coracoid process, r shldr, subs for fx w nonunion
		S42.132K	Disp fx of coracoid process, l shldr, subs for fx w nonunion
		S42.133K	Disp fx of coracoid pro, unsp shldr, subs for fx w nonunion
		S42.134K	Nondisp fx of coracoid pro, r shldr, subs for fx w nonunion
		S42.135K	Nondisp fx of coracoid pro, l shldr, subs for fx w nonunion
		S42.136K	Nondisp fx of coracoid pro, unsp shldr, sub for fx w nonun
		S42.141K	Disp fx of glenoid cav of scapula, r shldr, sub for fx w nonun
		S42.142K	Disp fx of glenoid cav of scapula, l shldr, sub for fx w nonun
		S42.143K	Disp fx of glenoid cav of scapula, unsp shldr, sub for fx w nonun
		S42.144K	Nondisp fx of glenoid cav of scapula, r shldr, sub for fx w nonun
		S42.145K	Nondisp fx of glenoid cav of scapula, l shldr, sub for fx w nonun
		S42.146K	Nondisp fx of glenoid cav of scapula, unsp shldr, sub for fx w nonun
		S42.151K	Disp fx of neck of scapula, r shldr, subs for fx w nonunion
		S42.152K	Disp fx of neck of scapula, l shldr, subs for fx w nonunion
		S42.153K	Disp fx of nk of scapula, unsp shldr, subs for fx w nonunion
		S42.154K	Nondisp fx of nk of scapula, r shldr, subs for fx w nonunion
		S42.155K	Nondisp fx of nk of scapula, l shldr, subs for fx w nonunion
		S42.156K	Nondisp fx of nk of scapula, unsp shldr, sub for fx w nonun
		S42.19[1,2,9]K	Fracture oth prt scapula, shoulder, subs for fx w nonunion
		S42.2Ø[1,2,9]K	Unsp fx upper end of humerus, subs for fx w nonunion
		S42.211K	Unsp disp fx of surg neck of r humer, subs for fx w nonunion
		S42.212K	Unsp disp fx of surg neck of l humer, subs for fx w nonunion
		S42.213K	Unsp disp fx of surg nk of unsp humer, sub for fx w nonun
		S42.214K	Unsp nondisp fx of surg nk of r humer, sub for fx w nonun
		S42.215K	Unsp nondisp fx of surg nk of l humer, sub for fx w nonun
		S42.216K	Unsp nondisp fx of surg nk of unsp humer, sub for fx w nonun

6th Character meanings for codes as indicated
1 Right *2 Left* *9 Unspecified*

(Continued on next page)

ICD-9-CM		ICD-10-CM	
733.82	NONUNION OF FRACTURE **(Continued)**	**S42.221K**	2-part disp fx of surg nk of r humer, subs for fx w nonunion
		S42.222K	2-part disp fx of surg nk of l humer, subs for fx w nonunion
		S42.223K	2-part disp fx of surg nk of unsp humer, sub for fx w nonun
		S42.224K	2-part nondisp fx of surg nk of r humer, sub for fx w nonun
		S42.225K	2-part nondisp fx of surg nk of l humer, sub for fx w nonun
		S42.226K	2-part nondisp fx of surg nk of unsp humer, sub for fx w nonun
		S42.23[1,2,9]K	3-part fx surgical neck of humerus, subs for fx w nonunion
		S42.24[1,2,9]K	4-part fx surgical neck of humerus, subs for fx w nonunion
		S42.251K	Disp fx of greater tuberosity of r humer, sub for fx w nonun
		S42.252K	Disp fx of greater tuberosity of l humer, sub for fx w nonun
		S42.253K	Disp fx of greater tuberosity of unsp humer, sub for fx w nonun
		S42.254K	Nondisp fx of greater tuberosity of r humer, sub for fx w nonun
		S42.255K	Nondisp fx of greater tuberosity of l humer, sub for fx w nonun
		S42.256K	Nondisp fx of greater tuberosity of unsp humer, sub for fx w nonun
		S42.261K	Disp fx of less tuberosity of r humer, sub for fx w nonun
		S42.262K	Disp fx of less tuberosity of l humer, sub for fx w nonun
		S42.263K	Disp fx of less tuberosity of unsp humer, sub for fx w nonun
		S42.264K	Nondisp fx of less tuberosity of r humer, sub for fx w nonun
		S42.265K	Nondisp fx of less tuberosity of l humer, sub for fx w nonun
		S42.266K	Nondisp fx of less tuberosity of unsp humer, sub for fx w nonun
		S42.27[1,2,9]K	Torus fx upper end of humerus, subs for fx w nonunion
		S42.291K	Oth disp fx of upper end of r humer, subs for fx w nonunion
		S42.292K	Oth disp fx of upper end of l humer, subs for fx w nonunion
		S42.293K	Oth disp fx of upper end unsp humer, subs for fx w nonunion
		S42.294K	Oth nondisp fx of upper end r humer, subs for fx w nonunion
		S42.295K	Oth nondisp fx of upper end l humer, subs for fx w nonunion
		S42.296K	Oth nondisp fx of upr end unsp humer, subs for fx w nonunion
		S42.3Ø1K	Unsp fx shaft of humerus, right arm, subs for fx w nonunion
		S42.3Ø2K	Unsp fx shaft of humerus, left arm, subs for fx w nonunion
		S42.3Ø9K	Unsp fx shaft of humerus, unsp arm, subs for fx w nonunion
		S42.31[1,2,9]K	Greenstick fx shaft of humer, r arm, subs for fx w nonunion
		S42.321K	Displ transverse fx shaft of humer, r arm, sub for fx w nonun
		S42.322K	Displ transverse fx shaft of humer, l arm, sub for fx w nonun
		S42.323K	Displ transverse fx shaft of humer, unsp arm, sub for fx w nonun
		S42.324K	Nondisp transverse fx shaft of humer, r arm, sub for fx w nonun
		S42.325K	Nondisp transverse fx shaft of humer, l arm, sub for fx w nonun
		S42.326K	Nondisp transverse fx shaft of humer, unsp arm, sub for fx w nonun
		S42.331K	Displ oblique fx shaft of humer, r arm, sub for fx w nonun
		S42.332K	Displ oblique fx shaft of humer, l arm, sub for fx w nonun
		S42.333K	Displ oblique fx shaft of humer, unsp arm, sub for fx w nonun
		S42.334K	Nondisp oblique fx shaft of humer, r arm, sub for fx w nonun
		S42.335K	Nondisp oblique fx shaft of humer, l arm, sub for fx w nonun
		S42.336K	Nondisp oblique fx shaft of humer, unsp arm, sub for fx w nonun
		S42.341K	Displ spiral fx shaft of humer, r arm, sub for fx w nonun
		S42.342K	Displ spiral fx shaft of humer, l arm, sub for fx w nonun
		S42.343K	Displ spiral fx shaft of humer, unsp arm, sub for fx w nonun
		S42.344K	Nondisp spiral fx shaft of humer, r arm, sub for fx w nonun
		S42.345K	Nondisp spiral fx shaft of humer, l arm, sub for fx w nonun
		S42.346K	Nondisp spiral fx shaft of humer, unsp arm, sub for fx w nonun
		S42.351K	Displ commnt fx shaft of humer, r arm, sub for fx w nonun
		S42.352K	Displ commnt fx shaft of humer, l arm, sub for fx w nonun
		S42.353K	Displ commnt fx shaft of humer, unsp arm, sub for fx w nonun
		S42.354K	Nondisp commnt fx shaft of humer, r arm, sub for fx w nonun
		S42.355K	Nondisp commnt fx shaft of humer, l arm, sub for fx w nonun
		S42.356K	Nondisp commnt fx shaft of humer, unsp arm, sub for fx w nonun
		S42.361K	Displ seg fx shaft of humer, r arm, subs for fx w nonunion
		S42.362K	Displ seg fx shaft of humer, l arm, subs for fx w nonunion
		S42.363K	Displ seg fx shaft of humer, unsp arm, sub for fx w nonun
		S42.364K	Nondisp seg fx shaft of humer, r arm, subs for fx w nonunion
		S42.365K	Nondisp seg fx shaft of humer, l arm, subs for fx w nonunion
		S42.366K	Nondisp seg fx shaft of humer, unsp arm, sub for fx w nonun
		S42.39[1,2,9]K	Oth fracture of shaft of humerus, subs for fx w nonunion
		S42.4Ø[1,2,9]K	Unsp fx lower end of humerus, subs for fx w nonunion
		S42.411K	Displ simp suprcndl fx w/o intrcndl fx r humer, sub for fx w nonun
		S42.412K	Displ simp suprcndl fx w/o intrcndl fx l humer, sub for fx w nonun
		S42.413K	Displ simp suprcndl fx w/o intrcndl fx unsp humer, sub for fx w nonun
		S42.414K	Nondisp simp suprcndl fx w/o intrcndl fx r humer, sub for fx w nonun
		S42.415K	Nondisp simp suprcndl fx w/o intrcndl fx l humer, sub for fx w nonun
		S42.416K	Nondisp simp suprcndl fx w/o intrcndl fx unsp humer, sub for fx w nonun
		S42.421K	Displ commnt suprcndl fx w/o intrcndl fx r humer, sub for fx w nonun
		S42.422K	Displ commnt suprcndl fx w/o intrcndl fx l humer, sub for fx w nonun
		S42.423K	Displ commnt suprcndl fx w/o intrcndl fx unsp humer, sub for fx w nonun
		S42.424K	Nondisp commnt suprcndl fx w/o intrcndl fx r humer, sub for fx w nonun
		S42.425K	Nondisp commnt suprcndl fx w/o intrcndl fx l humer, sub for fx w nonun
		S42.426K	Nondis commnt suprcndl fx w/o intrcndl fx unsp humer, sub for fx w nonu
		S42.431K	Disp fx of lateral epicondyl of r humer, sub for fx w nonun
		S42.432K	Disp fx of lateral epicondyl of l humer, sub for fx w nonun
		S42.433K	Disp fx of lateral epicondyl of unsp humer, sub for fx w nonun
		S42.434K	Nondisp fx of lateral epicondyl of r humer, sub for fx w nonun

6th Character meanings for codes as indicated
1 Right ***2 Left*** ***9 Unspecified***

(Continued on next page)

ICD-9-CM		ICD-10-CM	
733.82	NONUNION OF FRACTURE **(Continued)**	**S42.435K**	Nondisp fx of lateral epicondyl of l humer, sub for fx w nonun
		S42.436K	Nondisp fx of lateral epicondyl of unsp humer, sub for fx w nonun
		S42.441K	Disp fx of med epicondyl of r humer, subs for fx w nonunion
		S42.442K	Disp fx of med epicondyl of l humer, subs for fx w nonunion
		S42.443K	Disp fx of med epicondyl of unsp humer, sub for fx w nonun
		S42.444K	Nondisp fx of med epicondyl of r humer, sub for fx w nonun
		S42.445K	Nondisp fx of med epicondyl of l humer, sub for fx w nonun
		S42.446K	Nondisp fx of med epicondyl of unsp humer, sub for fx w nonun
		S42.447K	Incarcerated fx of med epicondyl of r humer, sub for fx w nonun
		S42.448K	Incarcerated fx of med epicondyl of l humer, sub for fx w nonun
		S42.449K	Incarcerated fx of med epicondyl of unsp humer, sub for fx w nonun
		S42.451K	Disp fx of lateral condyle of r humer, sub for fx w nonun
		S42.452K	Disp fx of lateral condyle of l humer, sub for fx w nonun
		S42.453K	Disp fx of lateral condyle of unsp humer, sub for fx w nonun
		S42.454K	Nondisp fx of lateral condyle of r humer, sub for fx w nonun
		S42.455K	Nondisp fx of lateral condyle of l humer, sub for fx w nonun
		S42.456K	Nondisp fx of lateral condyle of unsp humer, sub for fx w nonun
		S42.461K	Disp fx of medial condyle of r humer, subs for fx w nonunion
		S42.462K	Disp fx of medial condyle of l humer, subs for fx w nonunion
		S42.463K	Disp fx of med condyle of unsp humer, subs for fx w nonunion
		S42.464K	Nondisp fx of med condyle of r humer, subs for fx w nonunion
		S42.465K	Nondisp fx of med condyle of l humer, subs for fx w nonunion
		S42.466K	Nondisp fx of med condyle of unsp humer, sub for fx w nonun
		S42.471K	Displaced transcondy fx r humerus, subs for fx w nonunion
		S42.472K	Displaced transcondy fx l humerus, subs for fx w nonunion
		S42.473K	Displaced transcondy fx unsp humerus, subs for fx w nonunion
		S42.474K	Nondisp transcondy fx r humerus, subs for fx w nonunion
		S42.475K	Nondisp transcondy fx l humerus, subs for fx w nonunion
		S42.476K	Nondisp transcondy fx unsp humerus, subs for fx w nonunion
		S42.48[1,2,9]**K**	Torus fx lower end of humerus, subs for fx w nonunion
		S42.491K	Oth disp fx of lower end of r humer, subs for fx w nonunion
		S42.492K	Oth disp fx of lower end of l humer, subs for fx w nonunion
		S42.493K	Oth disp fx of lower end unsp humer, subs for fx w nonunion
		S42.494K	Oth nondisp fx of lower end r humer, subs for fx w nonunion
		S42.495K	Oth nondisp fx of lower end l humer, subs for fx w nonunion
		S42.496K	Oth nondisp fx of low end unsp humer, subs for fx w nonunion
		S42.9ØXK	Fx unsp shoulder girdle, part unsp, subs for fx w nonunion
		S42.91XK	Fx r shoulder girdle, part unsp, subs for fx w nonunion
		S42.92XK	Fx l shoulder girdle, part unsp, subs for fx w nonunion
		S49.ØØ[1,2,9]**K**	Unsp physl fx upper end humer, arm, subs for fx w nonunion
		S49.Ø1[1,2,9]**K**	Sltr-haris Type I physl fx upr end humer, arm, sub for fx w nonun
		S49.Ø2[1,2,9]**K**	Sltr-haris Type II physl fx upr end humer, arm, sub for fx w nonun
		S49.Ø3[1,2,9]**K**	Sltr-haris Type III physl fx upr end humer, arm, sub for fx w nonun
		S49.Ø4[1,2,9]**K**	Sltr-haris Type IV physl fx upr end humer, arm, sub for fx w nonun
		S49.Ø9[1,2,9]**K**	Oth physl fx upper end humer, arm, subs for fx w nonunion
		S49.1Ø[1,2,9]**K**	Unsp physl fx low end humer, arm, subs for fx w nonunion
		S49.11[1,2,9]**K**	Sltr-haris Type I physl fx low end humer, arm, sub for fx w nonun
		S49.12[1,2,9]**K**	Sltr-haris Type II physl fx low end humer, arm, sub for fx w nonun
		S49.13[1,2,9]**K**	Sltr-haris Type III physl fx low end humer, arm, sub for fx w nonun
		S49.14[1,2,9]**K**	Sltr-haris Type IV physl fx low end humer, arm, sub for fx w nonun
		S49.19[1,2,9]**K**	Oth physl fx low end humer, arm, subs for fx w nonunion
		S52.ØØ1[K,M,N]	Unsp fx upper end of right ulna
		S52.ØØ2[K,M,N]	Unsp fx upper end of left ulna
		S52.ØØ9[K,M,N]	Unsp fx upper end of unsp ulna
		S52.Ø1[1,2,9]**K**	Torus fx upper end of ulna, subs for fx w nonunion
		S52.Ø21[K,M,N]	Disp fx of olecran pro w/o intartic extn r ulna
		S52.Ø22[K,M,N]	Disp fx of olecran pro w/o intartic extn l ulna
		S52.Ø23[K,M,N]	Disp fx of olecran pro w/o intartic extn unsp ulna
		S52.Ø24[K,M,N]	Nondisp fx of olecran pro w/o intartic extn r ulna
		S52.Ø25[K,M,N]	Nondisp fx of olecran pro w/o intartic extn l ulna,
		S52.Ø26[K,M,N]	Nondisp fx of olecran pro w/o intartic extn unsp ulna,
		S52.Ø31[K,M,N]	Disp fx of olecran pro w intartic extn r ulna
		S52.Ø32[K,M,N]	Disp fx of olecran pro w intartic extn l ulna
		S52.Ø33[K,M,N]	Disp fx of olecran pro w intartic extn unsp ulna
		S52.Ø34[K,M,N]	Nondisp fx of olecran pro w intartic extn r ulna
		S52.Ø35[K,M,N]	Nondisp fx of olecran pro w intartic extn l ulna
		S52.Ø36[K,M,N]	Nondisp fx of olecran pro w intartic extn unsp ulna
		S52.Ø41[K,M,N]	Disp fx of coronoid pro of r ulna
		S52.Ø42[K,M,N]	Disp fx of coronoid pro of l ulna
		S52.Ø43[K,M,N]	Disp fx of coronoid pro of unsp ulna
		S52.Ø44[K,M,N]	Nondisp fx of coronoid pro of r ulna
		S52.Ø45[K,M,N]	Nondisp fx of coronoid pro of l ulna
		S52.Ø46[K,M,N]	Nondisp fx of coronoid pro of unsp ulna
		S52.Ø91[K,M,N]	Oth fx upper end of right ulna

6th Character meanings for codes as indicated
1 Right ***2 Left*** ***9 Unspecified***

7th Character meanins for codes S52.-
K Sub Enc Closed FX Nonunion
M Sub Enc Open FX Type I/II Nonunion
N Sub Enc Open IIIA/B/C Nonunion

(Continued on next page)

ICD-9-CM		ICD-10-CM
733.82	NONUNION OF FRACTURE **(Continued)**	**S52.092**[K,M,N] Oth fx upper end of left ulna **S52.099**[K,M,N] Oth fx upper end of unsp ulna **S52.101**[K,M,N] Unsp fx upper end of r radius **S52.102**[K,M,N] Unsp fx upper end left radius **S52.109**[K,M,N] Unsp fx upper end unsp radius **S52.11**[1,2,9]**K** Torus fx upper end of radius **S52.121**[K,M,N] Disp fx of head of right radius **S52.122**[K,M,N] Disp fx of head of left radius **S52.123**[K,M,N] Disp fx of head of unsp radius **S52.124**[K,M,N] Nondisp fx of head of r radius **S52.125**[K,M,N] Nondisp fx of head of left rad **S52.126**[K,M,N] Nondisp fx of head of unsp rad **S52.131**[K,M,N] Disp fx of neck of right radius **S52.132**[K,M,N] Disp fx of neck of left radius **S52.133**[K,M,N] Disp fx of neck of unsp radius **S52.134**[K,M,N] Nondisp fx of neck of r radius **S52.135**[K,M,N] Nondisp fx of neck of left rad **S52.136**[K,M,N] Nondisp fx of neck of unsp rad **S52.181**[K,M,N] Oth fx upper end of r radius **S52.182**[K,M,N] Oth fx upper end of left radius **S52.189**[K,M,N] Oth fx upper end of unsp radius **S52.201**[K,M,N] Unsp fx shaft of right ulna **S52.202**[K,M,N] Unsp fx shaft of left ulna **S52.209**[K,M,N] Unsp fx shaft of unsp ulna **S52.21**[1,2,9]**K** Greenstick fx shaft of ulna, subs for fx w nonunion **S52.221**[K,M,N] Displ transverse fx shaft of r ulna **S52.222**[K,M,N] Displ transverse fx shaft of l ulna **S52.223**[K,M,N] Displ transverse fx shaft of unsp ulna **S52.224**[K,M,N] Nondisp transverse fx shaft of r ulna **S52.225**[K,M,N] Nondisp transverse fx shaft of l ulna **S52.226**[K,M,N] Nondisp transverse fx shaft of unsp ulna **S52.231**[K,M,N] Displ oblique fx shaft of r ulna **S52.232**[K,M,N] Displ oblique fx shaft of l ulna **S52.233**[K,M,N] Displ oblique fx shaft of unsp ulna **S52.234**[K,M,N] Nondisp oblique fx shaft of r ulna **S52.235**[K,M,N] Nondisp oblique fx shaft of l ulna **S52.236**[K,M,N] Nondisp oblique fx shaft of unsp ulna **S52.241**[K,M,N] Displ spiral fx shaft of ulna, r arm **S52.242**[K,M,N] Displ spiral fx shaft of ulna, l arm **S52.243**[K,M,N] Displ spiral fx shaft of ulna, unsp arm **S52.244**[K,M,N] Nondisp spiral fx shaft of ulna, r arm **S52.245**[K,M,N] Nondisp spiral fx shaft of ulna, l arm **S52.246**[K,M,N] Nondisp spiral fx shaft of ulna, unsp arm **S52.251**[K,M,N] Displ commnt fx shaft of ulna, r arm **S52.252**[K,M,N] Displ commnt fx shaft of ulna, l arm **S52.253**[K,M,N] Displ commnt fx shaft of ulna, unsp arm **S52.254**[K,M,N] Nondisp commnt fx shaft of ulna, r arm **S52.255**[K,M,N] Nondisp commnt fx shaft of ulna, l arm **S52.256**[K,M,N] Nondisp commnt fx shaft of ulna, unsp arm **S52.261**[K,M,N] Displ seg fx shaft of ulna, r arm **S52.262**[K,M,N] Displ seg fx shaft of ulna, l arm **S52.263**[K,M,N] Displ seg fx shaft of ulna, unsp arm **S52.264**[K,M,N] Nondisp seg fx shaft of ulna, r arm **S52.265**[K,M,N] Nondisp seg fx shaft of ulna, l arm **S52.266**[K,M,N] Nondisp seg fx shaft of ulna, unsp arm **S52.271**[K,M,N] Monteggia's fx right ulna **S52.272**[K,M,N] Monteggia's fx left ulna **S52.279**[K,M,N] Monteggia's fx unsp ulna **S52.281**[K,M,N] Bent bone of right ulna **S52.282**[K,M,N] Bent bone of left ulna **S52.283**[K,M,N] Bent bone of unsp ulna **S52.291**[K,M,N] Oth fx shaft of right ulna **S52.292**[K,M,N] Oth fx shaft of left ulna **S52.299**[K,M,N] Oth fx shaft of unsp ulna **S52.301**[K,M,N] Unsp fx shaft of r radius **S52.302**[K,M,N] Unsp fx shaft of left radius **S52.309**[K,M,N] Unsp fx shaft of unsp radius **S52.31**[1,2,9]**K** Greenstick fx shaft of rad, arm, subs for fx w nonunion **S52.321**[K,M,N] Displ transverse fx shaft of r rad **S52.322**[K,M,N] Displ transverse fx shaft of l rad **S52.323**[K,M,N] Displ transverse fx shaft of unsp rad **S52.324**[K,M,N] Nondisp transverse fx shaft of r rad **S52.325**[K,M,N] Nondisp transverse fx shaft of l rad **S52.326**[K,M,N] Nondisp transverse fx shaft of unsp rad **S52.331**[K,M,N] Displ oblique fx shaft of r rad
	(Continued on next page)	***6th Character meanings for codes as indicated*** *1 Right* *2 Left* *9 Unspecified* ***7th Character meanins for codes S52.-*** *K Sub Enc Closed FX Nonunion* *M Sub Enc Open FX Type I/II Nonunion* *N Sub Enc Open IIIA/B/C Nonunion*

ICD-9-CM		ICD-10-CM
733.82	NONUNION OF FRACTURE **(Continued)**	**S52.332**[K,M,N] Displ oblique fx shaft of l rad
		S52.333[K,M,N] Displ oblique fx shaft of unsp rad
		S52.334[K,M,N] Nondisp oblique fx shaft of r rad
		S52.335[K,M,N] Nondisp oblique fx shaft of l rad
		S52.336[K,M,N] Nondisp oblique fx shaft of unsp rad
		S52.341[K,M,N] Displ spiral fx shaft of rad, r arm
		S52.342[K,M,N] Displ spiral fx shaft of rad, l arm
		S52.343[K,M,N] Displ spiral fx shaft of rad, unsp arm
		S52.344[K,M,N] Nondisp spiral fx shaft of rad, r arm
		S52.345[K,M,N] Nondisp spiral fx shaft of rad, l arm
		S52.346[K,M,N] Nondisp spiral fx shaft of rad, unsp arm
		S52.351[K,M,N] Displ commnt fx shaft of rad, r arm
		S52.352[K,M,N] Displ commnt fx shaft of rad, l arm
		S52.353[K,M,N] Displ commnt fx shaft of rad, unsp arm
		S52.354[K,M,N] Nondisp commnt fx shaft of rad, r arm
		S52.355[K,M,N] Nondisp commnt fx shaft of rad, l arm
		S52.356[K,M,N] Nondisp commnt fx shaft of rad, unsp arm
		S52.361[K,M,N] Displ seg fx shaft of rad, r arm
		S52.362[K,M,N] Displ seg fx shaft of rad, l arm
		S52.363[K,M,N] Displ seg fx shaft of rad, unsp arm
		S52.364[K,M,N] Nondisp seg fx shaft of rad, r arm
		S52.365[K,M,N] Nondisp seg fx shaft of rad, l arm
		S52.366[K,M,N] Nondisp seg fx shaft of rad, unsp arm
		S52.371[K,M,N] Galeazzi's fracture of r radius
		S52.372[K,M,N] Galeazzi's fx left radius
		S52.379[K,M,N] Galeazzi's fx unsp radius
		S52.381[K,M,N] Bent bone of right radius
		S52.382 [K,M,N] Bent bone of left radius
		S52.389[K,M,N] Bent bone of unsp radius
		S52.391[K,M,N] Oth fx shaft of rad, right arm
		S52.392[K,M,N] Oth fx shaft of rad, left arm
		S52.399[K,M,N] Oth fx shaft of rad, unsp arm
		S52.501[K,M,N] Unsp fx the lower end r radius
		S52.502[K,M,N] Unsp fx the lower end left rad
		S52.509[K,M,N] Unsp fx the lower end unsp rad
		S52.511[K,M,N] Disp fx of r radial styloid pro
		S52.512[K,M,N] Disp fx of l radial styloid pro
		S52.513[K,M,N] Disp fx of unsp radial styloid pro
		S52.514[K,M,N] Nondisp fx of r radial styloid pro
		S52.515[K,M,N] Nondisp fx of l radial styloid pro
		S52.516[K,M,N] Nondisp fx of unsp radial styloid pro
		S52.52[1,2,9]**K** Torus fx lower end of radius, subs for fx w nonunion
		S52.531[K,M,N] Colles' fracture of r radius
		S52.532[K,M,N] Colles' fracture of left radius
		S52.539[K,M,N] Colles' fracture of unsp radius
		S52.541[K,M,N] Smith's fracture of r radius
		S52.542[K,M,N] Smith's fracture of left radius
		S52.549[K,M,N] Smith's fracture of unsp radius
		S52.551[K,M,N] Oth extrartic fx low end r rad
		S52.552[K,M,N] Oth extrartic fx low end l rad
		S52.559[K,M,N] Oth extrartic fx low end unsp rad
		S52.561[K,M,N] Barton's fracture of r radius
		S52.562[K,M,N] Barton's fx left radius
		S52.569[K,M,N] Barton's fx unsp radius
		S52.571[K,M,N] Oth intartic fx lower end r rad
		S52.572[K,M,N] Oth intartic fx low end l rad
		S52.579[K,M,N] Oth intartic fx low end unsp rad
		S52.591[K,M,N] Oth fx of lower end of r radius
		S52.592[K,M,N] Oth fx of lower end left radius
		S52.599[K,M,N] Oth fx of lower end unsp radius
		S52.601[K,M,N] Unsp fx lower end of right ulna
		S52.602[K,M,N] Unsp fx lower end of left ulna
		S52.609[K,M,N] Unsp fx lower end of unsp ulna
		S52.611[K,M,N] Disp fx of r ulna styloid pro
		S52.612[K,M,N] Disp fx of l ulna styloid pro
		S52.613[K,M,N] Disp fx of unsp ulna styloid pro
		S52.614[K,M,N] Nondisp fx of r ulna styloid pro
		S52.615[K,M,N] Nondisp fx of l ulna styloid pro
		S52.616[K,M,N] Nondisp fx of unsp ulna styloid pro
		S52.62[1,2,9]**K** Torus fx lower end of ulna, subs for fx w nonunion
		S52.691[K,M,N] Oth fx lower end of right ulna
		S52.692[K,M,N] Oth fx lower end of left ulna
		S52.699[K,M,N] Oth fx lower end of unsp ulna
		S52.90X[K,M,N] Unsp fracture of unsp forearm
		S52.91X[K,M,N] Unsp fracture of right forearm
	(Continued on next page)	***6th Character meanings for codes as indicated*** *1 Right 2 Left 9 Unspecified* ***7th Character meanins for codes S52.-*** *K Sub Enc Closed FX Nonunion; M Sub Enc Open FX Type I/II Nonunion; N Sub Enc Open IIIA/B/C Nonunion*

ICD-9-CM		ICD-10-CM	
733.82	NONUNION OF FRACTURE **(Continued)**	**S52.92X**[K,M,N]	Unsp fracture of left forearm
		S59.ØØ[1,2,9]**K**	Unsp physl fx low end ulna, arm, subs for fx w nonunion
		S59.Ø1[1,2,9]**K**	Sltr-haris Type I physl fx low end ulna, arm, sub for fx w nonun
		S59.Ø2[1,2,9]**K**	Sltr-haris Type II physl fx low end ulna, arm, sub for fx w nonun
		S59.Ø3[1,2,9]**K**	Sltr-haris Type III physl fx low end ulna, arm, sub for fx w nonun
		S59.Ø4[1,2,9]**K**	Sltr-haris Type IV physl fx low end ulna, arm, sub for fx w nonun
		S59.Ø9[1,2,9]**K**	Oth physl fx low end ulna, arm, subs for fx w nonunion
		S59.1Ø[1,2,9]**K**	Unsp physl fx upper end rad, arm, subs for fx w nonunion
		S59.11[1,2,9]**K**	Sltr-haris Type I physl fx upr end rad, arm, sub for fx w nonun
		S59.12[1,2,9]**K**	Sltr-haris Type II physl fx upr end rad, arm, sub for fx w nonun
		S59.13[1,2,9]**K**	Sltr-haris Type III physl fx upr end rad, arm, sub for fx w nonun
		S59.14[1,2,9]**K**	Sltr-haris Type IV physl fx upr end rad, arm, sub for fx w nonun
		S59.19[1,2,9]**K**	Oth physl fx upper end rad, arm, subs for fx w nonunion
		S59.2Ø[1,2,9]**K**	Unsp physl fx low end rad, arm, subs for fx w nonunion
		S59.21[1,2,9]**K**	Sltr-haris Type I physl fx low end rad, arm, sub for fx w nonun
		S59.22[1,2,9]**K**	Sltr-haris Type II physl fx low end rad, arm, sub for fx w nonun
		S59.23[1,2,9]**K**	Sltr-haris Type III physl fx low end rad, arm, sub for fx w nonun
		S59.24[1,2,9]**K**	Sltr-haris Type IV physl fx low end rad, arm, sub for fx w nonun
		S59.29[1,2,9]**K**	Oth physl fx low end rad, right arm, subs for fx w nonunion
		S62.ØØ[1,2,9]**K**	Unsp fx navicular bone of r wrist, subs for fx w nonunion
		S62.Ø11K	Disp fx of dist pole of navic bone of r wrs, sub for fx w nonun
		S62.Ø12K	Disp fx of dist pole of navic bone of l wrs, sub for fx w nonun
		S62.Ø13K	Disp fx of dist pole of navic bone of unsp wrs, sub for fx w nonun
		S62.Ø14K	Nondisp fx of dist pole of navic bone of r wrs, sub for fx w nonun
		S62.Ø15K	Nondisp fx of dist pole of navic bone of l wrs, sub for fx w nonun
		S62.Ø16K	Nondisp fx of dist pole of navic bone of unsp wrs, sub for fx w nonun
		S62.Ø21K	Disp fx of mid 3rd of navic bone of r wrs, sub for fx w nonun
		S62.Ø22K	Disp fx of mid 3rd of navic bone of l wrs, sub for fx w nonun
		S62.Ø23K	Disp fx of mid 3rd of navic bone of unsp wrs, sub for fx w nonun
		S62.Ø24K	Nondisp fx of mid 3rd of navic bone of r wrs, sub for fx w nonun
		S62.Ø25K	Nondisp fx of mid 3rd of navic bone of l wrs, sub for fx w nonun
		S62.Ø26K	Nondisp fx of mid 3rd of navic bone of unsp wrs, sub for fx w nonun
		S62.Ø31K	Disp fx of prox 3rd of navic bone of r wrs, sub for fx w nonun
		S62.Ø32K	Disp fx of prox 3rd of navic bone of l wrs, sub for fx w nonun
		S62.Ø33K	Disp fx of prox 3rd of navic bone of unsp wrs, sub for fx w nonun
		S62.Ø34K	Nondisp fx of prox 3rd of navic bone of r wrs, sub for fx w nonun
		S62.Ø35K	Nondisp fx of prox 3rd of navic bone of l wrs, sub for fx w nonun
		S62.Ø36K	Nondisp fx of prox 3rd of navic bone of unsp wrs, sub for fx w nonun
		S62.1Ø[1,2,9]**K**	Fx unsp carpal bone, wrist, subs for fx w nonunion
		S62.111K	Disp fx of triquetrum bone, r wrist, subs for fx w nonunion
		S62.112K	Disp fx of triquetrum bone, l wrist, subs for fx w nonunion
		S62.113K	Disp fx of triquetrum bone, unsp wrs, subs for fx w nonunion
		S62.114K	Nondisp fx of triquetrum bone, r wrs, subs for fx w nonunion
		S62.115K	Nondisp fx of triquetrum bone, l wrs, subs for fx w nonunion
		S62.116K	Nondisp fx of triquetrum bone, unsp wrs, sub for fx w nonun
		S62.121K	Disp fx of lunate, right wrist, subs for fx w nonunion
		S62.122K	Disp fx of lunate, left wrist, subs for fx w nonunion
		S62.123K	Disp fx of lunate, unsp wrist, subs for fx w nonunion
		S62.124K	Nondisp fx of lunate, right wrist, subs for fx w nonunion
		S62.125K	Nondisp fx of lunate, left wrist, subs for fx w nonunion
		S62.126K	Nondisp fx of lunate, unsp wrist, subs for fx w nonunion
		S62.131K	Disp fx of capitate bone, r wrist, subs for fx w nonunion
		S62.132K	Disp fx of capitate bone, left wrist, subs for fx w nonunion
		S62.133K	Disp fx of capitate bone, unsp wrist, subs for fx w nonunion
		S62.134K	Nondisp fx of capitate bone, r wrist, subs for fx w nonunion
		S62.135K	Nondisp fx of capitate bone, l wrist, subs for fx w nonunion
		S62.136K	Nondisp fx of capitate bone, unsp wrs, sub for fx w nonun
		S62.141K	Disp fx of body of hamate bone, r wrs, sub for fx w nonun
		S62.142K	Disp fx of body of hamate bone, l wrs, sub for fx w nonun
		S62.143K	Disp fx of body of hamate bone, unsp wrs, sub for fx w nonun
		S62.144K	Nondisp fx of body of hamate bone, r wrs, sub for fx w nonun
		S62.145K	Nondisp fx of body of hamate bone, l wrs, sub for fx w nonun
		S62.146K	Nondisp fx of body of hamate bone, unsp wrs, sub for fx w nonun
		S62.151K	Disp fx of hook pro of hamate bone, r wrs, sub for fx w nonun
		S62.152K	Disp fx of hook pro of hamate bone, l wrs, sub for fx w nonun
		S62.153K	Disp fx of hook pro of hamate bone, unsp wrs, sub for fx w nonun
		S62.154K	Nondisp fx of hook pro of hamate bone, r wrs, sub for fx w nonun
		S62.155K	Nondisp fx of hook pro of hamate bone, l wrs, sub for fx w nonun
		S62.156K	Nondisp fx of hook pro of hamate bone, unsp wrs, sub for fx w nonun
		S62.161K	Disp fx of pisiform, right wrist, subs for fx w nonunion
		S62.162K	Disp fx of pisiform, left wrist, subs for fx w nonunion
		S62.163K	Disp fx of pisiform, unsp wrist, subs for fx w nonunion
		S62.164K	Nondisp fx of pisiform, right wrist, subs for fx w nonunion
		S62.165K	Nondisp fx of pisiform, left wrist, subs for fx w nonunion
		S62.166K	Nondisp fx of pisiform, unsp wrist, subs for fx w nonunion
		S62.171K	Disp fx of trapezium, right wrist, subs for fx w nonunion
		S62.172K	Disp fx of trapezium, left wrist, subs for fx w nonunion
		S62.173K	Disp fx of trapezium, unsp wrist, subs for fx w nonunion
		S62.174K	Nondisp fx of trapezium, right wrist, subs for fx w nonunion

6th Character meanings for codes as indicated
1 Right   2 Left   9 Unspecified

(Continued on next page)

ICD-9-CM		ICD-10-CM	
733.82	NONUNION OF FRACTURE **(Continued)**	**S62.175K**	Nondisp fx of trapezium, left wrist, subs for fx w nonunion
		S62.176K	Nondisp fx of trapezium, unsp wrist, subs for fx w nonunion
		S62.181K	Disp fx of trapezoid, right wrist, subs for fx w nonunion
		S62.182K	Disp fx of trapezoid, left wrist, subs for fx w nonunion
		S62.183K	Disp fx of trapezoid, unsp wrist, subs for fx w nonunion
		S62.184K	Nondisp fx of trapezoid, right wrist, subs for fx w nonunion
		S62.185K	Nondisp fx of trapezoid, left wrist, subs for fx w nonunion
		S62.186K	Nondisp fx of trapezoid, unsp wrist, subs for fx w nonunion
		S62.2Ø[1,2,9]K	Unsp fx first MC bone, hand, subs for fx w nonunion
		S62.211K	Bennett's fracture, right hand, subs for fx w nonunion
		S62.212K	Bennett's fracture, left hand, subs for fx w nonunion
		S62.213K	Bennett's fracture, unsp hand, subs for fx w nonunion
		S62.221K	Displaced Rolando's fracture, r hand, subs for fx w nonunion
		S62.222K	Displ Rolando's fracture, left hand, subs for fx w nonunion
		S62.223K	Displ Rolando's fracture, unsp hand, subs for fx w nonunion
		S62.224K	Nondisp Rolando's fracture, r hand, subs for fx w nonunion
		S62.225K	Nondisp Rolando's fracture, l hand, subs for fx w nonunion
		S62.226K	Nondisp Rolando's fx, unsp hand, subs for fx w nonunion
		S62.231K	Oth disp fx of base of 1st MC bone, r hand, sub for fx w nonun
		S62.232K	Oth disp fx of base of 1st MC bone, l hand, sub for fx w nonun
		S62.233K	Oth disp fx of base of 1st MC bone, unsp hand, sub for fx w nonun
		S62.234K	Oth nondisp fx of base of 1st MC bone, r hand, sub for fx w nonun
		S62.235K	Oth nondisp fx of base of 1st MC bone, l hand, sub for fx w nonun
		S62.236K	Oth nondisp fx of base of 1st MC bone, unsp hand, sub for fx w nonu
		S62.241K	Disp fx of shaft of 1st MC bone, r hand, sub for fx w nonun
		S62.242K	Disp fx of shaft of 1st MC bone, l hand, sub for fx w nonun
		S62.243K	Disp fx of shaft of 1st MC bone, unsp hand, sub for fx w nonun
		S62.244K	Nondisp fx of shaft of 1st MC bone, r hand, sub for fx w nonun
		S62.245K	Nondisp fx of shaft of 1st MC bone, l hand, sub for fx w nonun
		S62.246K	Nondisp fx of shaft of 1st MC bone, unsp hand, sub for fx w nonun
		S62.251K	Disp fx of nk of 1st MC bone, r hand, subs for fx w nonunion
		S62.252K	Disp fx of nk of 1st MC bone, l hand, subs for fx w nonunion
		S62.253K	Disp fx of nk of 1st MC bone, unsp hand, sub for fx w nonun
		S62.254K	Nondisp fx of nk of 1st MC bone, r hand, sub for fx w nonun
		S62.255K	Nondisp fx of nk of 1st MC bone, l hand, sub for fx w nonun
		S62.256K	Nondisp fx of nk of 1st MC bone, unsp hand, sub for fx w nonun
		S62.29[1,2,9]K	Oth fx first MC bone, hand, subs for fx w nonunion
		S62.3ØØK	Unsp fx second MC bone, right hand, subs for fx w nonunion
		S62.3Ø1K	Unsp fx second MC bone, left hand, subs for fx w nonunion
		S62.3Ø2K	Unsp fx third MC bone, right hand, subs for fx w nonunion
		S62.3Ø3K	Unsp fx third MC bone, left hand, subs for fx w nonunion
		S62.3Ø4K	Unsp fx fourth MC bone, right hand, subs for fx w nonunion
		S62.3Ø5K	Unsp fx fourth MC bone, left hand, subs for fx w nonunion
		S62.3Ø6K	Unsp fx fifth MC bone, right hand, subs for fx w nonunion
		S62.3Ø7K	Unsp fx fifth MC bone, left hand, subs for fx w nonunion
		S62.3Ø8K	Unsp fracture of oth metacarpal bone, subs for fx w nonunion
		S62.3Ø9K	Unsp fx unsp metacarpal bone, subs for fx w nonunion
		S62.31ØK	Disp fx of base of 2nd MC bone, r hand, sub for fx w nonun
		S62.311K	Disp fx of base of 2nd MC bone. l hand, sub for fx w nonun
		S62.312K	Disp fx of base of 3rd MC bone, r hand, sub for fx w nonun
		S62.313K	Disp fx of base of 3rd MC bone, l hand, sub for fx w nonun
		S62.314K	Disp fx of base of 4th MC bone, r hand, sub for fx w nonun
		S62.315K	Disp fx of base of 4th MC bone, l hand, sub for fx w nonun
		S62.316K	Disp fx of base of 5th MC bone, r hand, sub for fx w nonun
		S62.317K	Disp fx of base of 5th MC bone. l hand, sub for fx w nonun
		S62.318K	Disp fx of base of metacarpal bone, subs for fx w nonunion
		S62.319K	Disp fx of base of unsp MC bone, subs for fx w nonunion
		S62.32ØK	Disp fx of shaft of 2nd MC bone, r hand, sub for fx w nonun
		S62.321K	Disp fx of shaft of 2nd MC bone, l hand, sub for fx w nonun
		S62.322K	Disp fx of shaft of 3rd MC bone, r hand, sub for fx w nonun
		S62.323K	Disp fx of shaft of 3rd MC bone, l hand, sub for fx w nonun
		S62.324K	Disp fx of shaft of 4th MC bone, r hand, sub for fx w nonun
		S62.325K	Disp fx of shaft of 4th MC bone, l hand, sub for fx w nonun
		S62.326K	Disp fx of shaft of 5th MC bone, r hand, sub for fx w nonun
		S62.327K	Disp fx of shaft of 5th MC bone, l hand, sub for fx w nonun
		S62.328K	Disp fx of shaft of metacarpal bone, subs for fx w nonunion
		S62.329K	Disp fx of shaft of unsp MC bone, subs for fx w nonunion
		S62.33ØK	Disp fx of nk of 2nd MC bone, r hand, subs for fx w nonunion
		S62.331K	Disp fx of nk of 2nd MC bone, l hand, subs for fx w nonunion
		S62.332K	Disp fx of nk of 3rd MC bone, r hand, subs for fx w nonunion
		S62.333K	Disp fx of nk of 3rd MC bone, l hand, subs for fx w nonunion
		S62.334K	Disp fx of nk of 4th MC bone, r hand, subs for fx w nonunion
		S62.335K	Disp fx of nk of 4th MC bone, l hand, subs for fx w nonunion
		S62.336K	Disp fx of nk of 5th MC bone, r hand, subs for fx w nonunion
		S62.337K	Disp fx of nk of 5th MC bone, l hand, subs for fx w nonunion
		S62.338K	Disp fx of neck of metacarpal bone, subs for fx w nonunion
		S62.339K	Disp fx of neck of unsp MC bone, subs for fx w nonunion
		S62.34ØK	Nondisp fx of base of 2nd MC bone, r hand, sub for fx w nonun

6th Character meanings for codes as indicated
1 Right ***2 Left*** ***9 Unspecified***

(Continued on next page)

ICD-9-CM		ICD-10-CM	
733.82	NONUNION OF FRACTURE **(Continued)**	**S62.341K**	Nondisp fx of base of 2nd MC bone. l hand, sub for fx w nonun
		S62.342K	Nondisp fx of base of 3rd MC bone, r hand, sub for fx w nonun
		S62.343K	Nondisp fx of base of 3rd MC bone, l hand, sub for fx w nonun
		S62.344K	Nondisp fx of base of 4th MC bone, r hand, sub for fx w nonun
		S62.345K	Nondisp fx of base of 4th MC bone, l hand, sub for fx w nonun
		S62.346K	Nondisp fx of base of 5th MC bone, r hand, sub for fx w nonun
		S62.347K	Nondisp fx of base of 5th MC bone. l hand, sub for fx w nonun
		S62.348K	Nondisp fx of base of MC bone, subs for fx w nonunion
		S62.349K	Nondisp fx of base of unsp MC bone, subs for fx w nonunion
		S62.350K	Nondisp fx of shaft of 2nd MC bone, r hand, sub for fx w nonun
		S62.351K	Nondisp fx of shaft of 2nd MC bone, l hand, sub for fx w nonun
		S62.352K	Nondisp fx of shaft of 3rd MC bone, r hand, sub for fx w nonun
		S62.353K	Nondisp fx of shaft of 3rd MC bone, l hand, sub for fx w nonun
		S62.354K	Nondisp fx of shaft of 4th MC bone, r hand, sub for fx w nonun
		S62.355K	Nondisp fx of shaft of 4th MC bone, l hand, sub for fx w nonun
		S62.356K	Nondisp fx of shaft of 5th MC bone, r hand, sub for fx w nonun
		S62.357K	Nondisp fx of shaft of 5th MC bone, l hand, sub for fx w nonun
		S62.358K	Nondisp fx of shaft of MC bone, subs for fx w nonunion
		S62.359K	Nondisp fx of shaft of unsp MC bone, subs for fx w nonunion
		S62.360K	Nondisp fx of nk of 2nd MC bone, r hand, sub for fx w nonun
		S62.361K	Nondisp fx of nk of 2nd MC bone, l hand, sub for fx w nonun
		S62.362K	Nondisp fx of nk of 3rd MC bone, r hand, sub for fx w nonun
		S62.363K	Nondisp fx of nk of 3rd MC bone, l hand, sub for fx w nonun
		S62.364K	Nondisp fx of nk of 4th MC bone, r hand, sub for fx w nonun
		S62.365K	Nondisp fx of nk of 4th MC bone, l hand, sub for fx w nonun
		S62.366K	Nondisp fx of nk of 5th MC bone, r hand, sub for fx w nonun
		S62.367K	Nondisp fx of nk of 5th MC bone, l hand, sub for fx w nonun
		S62.368K	Nondisp fx of neck of MC bone, subs for fx w nonunion
		S62.369K	Nondisp fx of neck of unsp MC bone, subs for fx w nonunion
		S62.390K	Oth fx second MC bone, right hand, subs for fx w nonunion
		S62.391K	Oth fx second MC bone, left hand, subs for fx w nonunion
		S62.392K	Oth fx third MC bone, right hand, subs for fx w nonunion
		S62.393K	Oth fx third MC bone, left hand, subs for fx w nonunion
		S62.394K	Oth fx fourth MC bone, right hand, subs for fx w nonunion
		S62.395K	Oth fx fourth MC bone, left hand, subs for fx w nonunion
		S62.396K	Oth fx fifth MC bone, right hand, subs for fx w nonunion
		S62.397K	Oth fx fifth MC bone, left hand, subs for fx w nonunion
		S62.398K	Oth fracture of oth metacarpal bone, subs for fx w nonunion
		S62.399K	Oth fracture of unsp metacarpal bone, subs for fx w nonunion
		S62.501K	Fx unsp phalanx of right thumb, subs for fx w nonunion
		S62.502K	Fx unsp phalanx of left thumb, subs for fx w nonunion
		S62.509K	Fracture of unsp phalanx of thmb, subs for fx w nonunion
		S62.511K	Disp fx of proximal phalanx of r thm, subs for fx w nonunion
		S62.512K	Disp fx of proximal phalanx of l thm, subs for fx w nonunion
		S62.513K	Disp fx of proximal phalanx of thmb, subs for fx w nonunion
		S62.514K	Nondisp fx of prox phalanx of r thm, subs for fx w nonunion
		S62.515K	Nondisp fx of prox phalanx of l thm, subs for fx w nonunion
		S62.516K	Nondisp fx of prox phalanx of thmb, subs for fx w nonunion
		S62.521K	Disp fx of distal phalanx of r thm, subs for fx w nonunion
		S62.522K	Disp fx of distal phalanx of l thm, subs for fx w nonunion
		S62.523K	Disp fx of distal phalanx of thmb, subs for fx w nonunion
		S62.524K	Nondisp fx of dist phalanx of r thm, subs for fx w nonunion
		S62.525K	Nondisp fx of dist phalanx of l thm, subs for fx w nonunion
		S62.526K	Nondisp fx of distal phalanx of thmb, subs for fx w nonunion
		S62.600K	Fx unsp phalanx of r idx fngr, subs for fx w nonunion
		S62.601K	Fx unsp phalanx of l idx fngr, subs for fx w nonunion
		S62.602K	Fx unsp phalanx of r mid finger, subs for fx w nonunion
		S62.603K	Fx unsp phalanx of l mid finger, subs for fx w nonunion
		S62.604K	Fx unsp phalanx of r rng fngr, subs for fx w nonunion
		S62.605K	Fx unsp phalanx of l rng fngr, subs for fx w nonunion
		S62.606K	Fx unsp phalanx of r little finger, subs for fx w nonunion
		S62.607K	Fx unsp phalanx of l little finger, subs for fx w nonunion
		S62.608K	Fracture of unsp phalanx of finger, subs for fx w nonunion
		S62.609K	Fx unsp phalanx of unsp finger, subs for fx w nonunion
		S62.610K	Disp fx of prox phalanx of r idx fngr, sub for fx w nonun
		S62.611K	Disp fx of prox phalanx of l idx fngr, sub for fx w nonun
		S62.612K	Disp fx of prox phalanx of r mid fngr, sub for fx w nonun
		S62.613K	Disp fx of prox phalanx of l mid fngr, sub for fx w nonun
		S62.614K	Disp fx of prox phalanx of r rng fngr, sub for fx w nonun
		S62.615K	Disp fx of prox phalanx of l rng fngr, sub for fx w nonun
		S62.616K	Disp fx of prox phalanx of r lit fngr, sub for fx w nonun
		S62.617K	Disp fx of prox phalanx of l lit fngr, sub for fx w nonun
		S62.618K	Disp fx of prox phalanx of finger, subs for fx w nonunion
		S62.619K	Disp fx of prox phalanx of unsp fngr, subs for fx w nonunion
		S62.620K	Disp fx of med phalanx of r idx fngr, subs for fx w nonunion
		S62.621K	Disp fx of med phalanx of l idx fngr, subs for fx w nonunion
		S62.622K	Disp fx of med phalanx of r mid fngr, subs for fx w nonunion
		S62.623K	Disp fx of med phalanx of l mid fngr, subs for fx w nonunion
		S62.624K	Disp fx of med phalanx of r rng fngr, subs for fx w nonunion
		S62.625K	Disp fx of med phalanx of l rng fngr, subs for fx w nonunion
		S62.626K	Disp fx of med phalanx of r lit fngr, subs for fx w nonunion
		S62.627K	Disp fx of med phalanx of l lit fngr, subs for fx w nonunion
	(Continued on next page)	**S62.628K**	Disp fx of medial phalanx of finger, subs for fx w nonunion

ICD-9-CM		ICD-10-CM	
733.82	NONUNION OF FRACTURE **(Continued)**	**S62.629K**	Disp fx of med phalanx of unsp fngr, subs for fx w nonunion
		S62.63ØK	Disp fx of dist phalanx of r idx fngr, sub for fx w nonun
		S62.631K	Disp fx of dist phalanx of l idx fngr, sub for fx w nonun
		S62.632K	Disp fx of dist phalanx of r mid fngr, sub for fx w nonun
		S62.633K	Disp fx of dist phalanx of l mid fngr, sub for fx w nonun
		S62.634K	Disp fx of dist phalanx of r rng fngr, sub for fx w nonun
		S62.635K	Disp fx of dist phalanx of l rng fngr, sub for fx w nonun
		S62.636K	Disp fx of dist phalanx of r lit fngr, sub for fx w nonun
		S62.637K	Disp fx of dist phalanx of l lit fngr, sub for fx w nonun
		S62.638K	Disp fx of distal phalanx of finger, subs for fx w nonunion
		S62.639K	Disp fx of dist phalanx of unsp fngr, subs for fx w nonunion
		S62.64ØK	Nondisp fx of prox phalanx of r idx fngr, sub for fx w nonun
		S62.641K	Nondisp fx of prox phalanx of l idx fngr, sub for fx w nonun
		S62.642K	Nondisp fx of prox phalanx of r mid fngr, sub for fx w nonun
		S62.643K	Nondisp fx of prox phalanx of l mid fngr, sub for fx w nonun
		S62.644K	Nondisp fx of prox phalanx of r rng fngr, sub for fx w nonun
		S62.645K	Nondisp fx of prox phalanx of l rng fngr, sub for fx w nonun
		S62.646K	Nondisp fx of prox phalanx of r lit fngr, sub for fx w nonun
		S62.647K	Nondisp fx of prox phalanx of l lit fngr, sub for fx w nonun
		S62.648K	Nondisp fx of prox phalanx of finger, subs for fx w nonunion
		S62.649K	Nondisp fx of prox phalanx of unsp fngr, sub for fx w nonun
		S62.65ØK	Nondisp fx of med phalanx of r idx fngr, sub for fx w nonun
		S62.651K	Nondisp fx of med phalanx of l idx fngr, sub for fx w nonun
		S62.652K	Nondisp fx of med phalanx of r mid fngr, sub for fx w nonun
		S62.653K	Nondisp fx of med phalanx of l mid fngr, sub for fx w nonun
		S62.654K	Nondisp fx of med phalanx of r rng fngr, sub for fx w nonun
		S62.655K	Nondisp fx of med phalanx of l rng fngr, sub for fx w nonun
		S62.656K	Nondisp fx of med phalanx of r lit fngr, sub for fx w nonun
		S62.657K	Nondisp fx of med phalanx of l lit fngr, sub for fx w nonun
		S62.658K	Nondisp fx of medial phalanx of fngr, subs for fx w nonunion
		S62.659K	Nondisp fx of med phalanx of unsp fngr, sub for fx w nonun
		S62.66ØK	Nondisp fx of dist phalanx of r idx fngr, sub for fx w nonun
		S62.661K	Nondisp fx of dist phalanx of l idx fngr, sub for fx w nonun
		S62.662K	Nondisp fx of dist phalanx of r mid fngr, sub for fx w nonun
		S62.663K	Nondisp fx of dist phalanx of l mid fngr, sub for fx w nonun
		S62.664K	Nondisp fx of dist phalanx of r rng fngr, sub for fx w nonun
		S62.665K	Nondisp fx of dist phalanx of l rng fngr, sub for fx w nonun
		S62.666K	Nondisp fx of dist phalanx of r lit fngr, sub for fx w nonun
		S62.667K	Nondisp fx of dist phalanx of l lit fngr, sub for fx w nonun
		S62.668K	Nondisp fx of dist phalanx of finger, subs for fx w nonunion
		S62.669K	Nondisp fx of dist phalanx of unsp fngr, sub for fx w nonun
		S62.9ØXK	Unsp fracture of unsp wrist and hand, subs for fx w nonunion
		S62.91XK	Unsp fracture of right wrs/hnd, subs for fx w nonunion
		S62.92XK	Unsp fracture of left wrist and hand, subs for fx w nonunion
		S72.ØØ1[K,M,N]	Fx unsp part of neck of r femur
		S72.ØØ2[K,M,N]	Fx unsp part of neck of l femur
		S72.ØØ9[K,M,N]	Fx unsp part of nk of unsp femr
		S72.Ø11[K,M,N]	Unsp intracap fx right femur
		S72.Ø12[K,M,N]	Unsp intracap fx left femur
		S72.Ø19[K,M,N]	Unsp intracap fx unsp femur
		S72.Ø21[K,M,N]	Disp fx of epiphy (separation) (upper) of r femr
		S72.Ø22[K,M,N]	Disp fx of epiphy (separation) (upper) of l femr
		S72.Ø23[K,M,N]	Disp fx of epiphy (separation) (upper) of unsp femr
		S72.Ø24[K,M,N]	Nondisp fx of epiphy (separation) (upper) of r femr
		S72.Ø25[K,M,N]	Nondisp fx of epiphy (separation) (upper) of l femr
		S72.Ø26[K,M,N]	Nondisp fx of epiphy (separation) (upper) of unsp femr
		S72.Ø31[K,M,N]	Displ midcervical fx r femur
		S72.Ø32[K,M,N]	Displ midcervical fx l femur
		S72.Ø33[K,M,N]	Displ midcervical fx unsp femur
		S72.Ø34[K,M,N]	Nondisp midcervical fx r femur
		S72.Ø35[K,M,N]	Nondisp midcervical fx l femur
		S72.Ø36[K,M,N]	Nondisp midcervical fx unsp femr
		S72.Ø41[K,M,N]	Disp fx of base of nk of r femr
		S72.Ø42[K,M,N]	Disp fx of base of nk of l femr
		S72.Ø43[K,M,N]	Disp fx of base of nk of unsp femr
		S72.Ø44[K,M,N]	Nondisp fx of base of nk of r femr
		S72.Ø45[K,M,N]	Nondisp fx of base of nk of l femr
		S72.Ø46[K,M,N]	Nondisp fx of base of nk of unsp femr
		S72.Ø51[K,M,N]	Unsp fx head of right femur
		S72.Ø52[K,M,N]	Unsp fx head of left femur
		S72.Ø59[K,M,N]	Unsp fx head of unsp femur
		S72.Ø61[K,M,N]	Displ artic fx head of r femur
		S72.Ø62[K,M,N]	Displ artic fx head of l femur
		S72.Ø63[K,M,N]	Displ artic fx head of unsp femr
		S72.Ø64[K,M,N]	Nondisp artic fx head of r femr
		S72.Ø65[K,M,N]	Nondisp artic fx head of l femr
		S72.Ø66[K,M,N]	Nondisp artic fx head of unsp femr
		S72.Ø91[K,M,N]	Oth fx head/neck of right femur

7th Character meanins for codes S72.-
K Sub Enc Closed FX Nonunion
M Sub Enc Open FX Type I/II Nonunion
N Sub Enc Open IIIA/B/C Nonunion

(Continued on next page)

[Brackets] indicate valid character values for each code. Character value meanings provided for each code grouping.

ICD-9-CM		ICD-10-CM
733.82	NONUNION OF FRACTURE (Continued)	S72.092[K,M,N] Oth fx head/neck of left femur
		S72.099[K,M,N] Oth fx head/neck of unsp femur
		S72.101[K,M,N] Unsp trochan fx right femur
		S72.102[K,M,N] Unsp trochan fx left femur
		S72.109[K,M,N] Unsp trochan fx unsp femur
		S72.111[K,M,N] Disp fx of greater trochanter of r femr
		S72.112[K,M,N] Disp fx of greater trochanter of l femr
		S72.113[K,M,N] Disp fx of greater trochanter of unsp femr
		S72.114[K,M,N] Nondisp fx of greater trochanter of r femr
		S72.115[K,M,N] Nondisp fx of greater trochanter of l femr
		S72.116[K,M,N] Nondisp fx of greater trochanter of unsp femr
		S72.121[K,M,N] Disp fx of less trochanter of r femr
		S72.122[K,M,N] Disp fx of less trochanter of l femr
		S72.123[K,M,N] Disp fx of less trochanter of unsp femr
		S72.124[K,M,N] Nondisp fx of less trochanter of r femr
		S72.125[K,M,N] Nondisp fx of less trochanter of l femr
		S72.126[K,M,N] Nondisp fx of less trochanter of unsp femr
		S72.131[K,M,N] Displaced apophyseal fx r femur
		S72.132[K,M,N] Displaced apophyseal fx l femur
		S72.133[K,M,N] Displ apophyseal fx unsp femur
		S72.134[K,M,N] Nondisp apophyseal fx r femur
		S72.135[K,M,N] Nondisp apophyseal fx l femur
		S72.136[K,M,N] Nondisp apophyseal fx unsp femr
		S72.141[K,M,N] Displaced intertroch fx r femur
		S72.142[K,M,N] Displaced intertroch fx l femur
		S72.143[K,M,N] Displ intertroch fx unsp femur
		S72.144[K,M,N] Nondisp intertroch fx r femur
		S72.145[K,M,N] Nondisp intertroch fx l femur
		S72.146[K,M,N] Nondisp intertroch fx unsp femr
		S72.21X[K,M,N] Displaced subtrochnt fx r femur
		S72.22X[K,M,N] Displaced subtrochnt fx l femur
		S72.23X[K,M,N] Displ subtrochnt fx unsp femur
		S72.24X[K,M,N] Nondisp subtrochnt fx r femur
		S72.25X[K,M,N] Nondisp subtrochnt fx l femur
		S72.26X[K,M,N] Nondisp subtrochnt fx unsp femr
		S72.301[K,M,N] Unsp fx shaft of right femur
		S72.302[K,M,N] Unsp fx shaft of left femur
		S72.309[K,M,N] Unsp fx shaft of unsp femur
		S72.321[K,M,N] Displ transverse fx shaft of r femr
		S72.322[K,M,N] Displ transverse fx shaft of l femr
		S72.323[K,M,N] Displ transverse fx shaft of unsp femr
		S72.324[K,M,N] Nondisp transverse fx shaft of r femr
		S72.325[K,M,N] Nondisp transverse fx shaft of l femr
		S72.326[K,M,N] Nondisp transverse fx shaft of unsp femr
		S72.331[K,M,N] Displ oblique fx shaft of r femr
		S72.332[K,M,N] Displ oblique fx shaft of l femr
		S72.333[K,M,N] Displ oblique fx shaft of unsp femr
		S72.334[K,M,N] Nondisp oblique fx shaft of r femr
		S72.335[K,M,N] Nondisp oblique fx shaft of l femr
		S72.336[K,M,N] Nondisp oblique fx shaft of unsp femr
		S72.341[K,M,N] Displ spiral fx shaft of r femr
		S72.342[K,M,N] Displ spiral fx shaft of l femr
		S72.343[K,M,N] Displ spiral fx shaft of unsp femr
		S72.344[K,M,N] Nondisp spiral fx shaft of r femr
		S72.345[K,M,N] Nondisp spiral fx shaft of l femr
		S72.346[K,M,N] Nondisp spiral fx shaft of unsp femr
		S72.351[K,M,N] Displ commnt fx shaft of r femr
		S72.352[K,M,N] Displ commnt fx shaft of l femr
		S72.353[K,M,N] Displ commnt fx shaft of unsp femr
		S72.354[K,M,N] Nondisp commnt fx shaft of r femr
		S72.355[K,M,N] Nondisp commnt fx shaft of l femr
		S72.356[K,M,N] Nondisp commnt fx shaft of unsp femr
		S72.361[K,M,N] Displ seg fx shaft of r femur
		S72.362[K,M,N] Displ seg fx shaft of l femur
		S72.363[K,M,N] Displ seg fx shaft of unsp femr
		S72.364[K,M,N] Nondisp seg fx shaft of r femur
		S72.365[K,M,N] Nondisp seg fx shaft of l femur
		S72.366[K,M,N] Nondisp seg fx shaft of unsp femr
		S72.391[K,M,N] Oth fx shaft of right femur
		S72.392[K,M,N] Oth fx shaft of left femur
		S72.399[K,M,N] Oth fx shaft of unsp femur
		S72.401[K,M,N] Unsp fx lower end of r femur
		S72.402[K,M,N] Unsp fx lower end of left femur
		S72.409[K,M,N] Unsp fx lower end of unsp femur
		S72.411[K,M,N] Displ unsp condyle fx low end r femr
		S72.412[K,M,N] Displ unsp condyle fx low end l femr
		S72.413[K,M,N] Displ unsp condyle fx low end unsp femr

7th Character meanins for codes S72.-
K Sub Enc Closed FX Nonunion
M Sub Enc Open FX Type I/II Nonunion
N Sub Enc Open IIIA/B/C Nonunion

(Continued on next page)

ICD-9-CM		ICD-10-CM
733.82	NONUNION OF FRACTURE **(Continued)**	**S72.414**[K,M,N] Nondisp unsp condyle fx low end r femr
		S72.415[K,M,N] Nondisp unsp condyle fx low end l femr
		S72.416[K,M,N] Nondisp unsp condyle fx low end unsp femr
		S72.421[K,M,N] Disp fx of lateral condyle of r femr
		S72.422[K,M,N] Disp fx of lateral condyle of l femr
		S72.423[K,M,N] Disp fx of lateral condyle of unsp femr
		S72.424[K,M,N] Nondisp fx of lateral condyle of r femr
		S72.425[K,M,N] Nondisp fx of lateral condyle of l femr
		S72.426[K,M,N] Nondisp fx of lateral condyle of unsp femr
		S72.431[K,M,N] Disp fx of med condyle of r femr
		S72.432[K,M,N] Disp fx of med condyle of l femr
		S72.433[K,M,N] Disp fx of med condyle of unsp femr
		S72.434[K,M,N] Nondisp fx of med condyle of r femr
		S72.435[K,M,N] Nondisp fx of med condyle of l femr
		S72.436[K,M,N] Nondisp fx of med condyle of unsp femr
		S72.441[K,M,N] Disp fx of low epiphy (separation) of r femr
		S72.442[K,M,N] Disp fx of low epiphy (separation) of l femr
		S72.443[K,M,N] Disp fx of low epiphy (separation) of unsp femr
		S72.444[K,M,N] Nondisp fx of low epiphy (separation) of r femr
		S72.445[K,M,N] Nondisp fx of low epiphy (separation) of l femr
		S72.446[K,M,N] Nondisp fx of low epiphy (separation) of unsp femr
		S72.451[K,M,N] Displ suprcndl fx w/o intrcndl extn low end r femr
		S72.452[K,M,N] Displ suprcndl fx w/o intrcndl extn low end l femr
		S72.453[K,M,N] Displ suprcndl fx w/o intrcndl extn low end unsp femr
		S72.454[K,M,N] Nondisp suprcndl fx w/o intrcndl extn low end r femr
		S72.455[K,M,N] Nondisp suprcndl fx w/o intrcndl extn low end l femr
		S72.456[K,M,N] Nondisp suprcndl fx w/o intrcndl extn low end unsp femr
		S72.461[K,M,N] Displ suprcndl fx w intrcndl extn low end r femr
		S72.462[K,M,N] Displ suprcndl fx w intrcndl extn low end l femr
		S72.463[K,M,N] Displ suprcndl fx w intrcndl extn low end unsp femr
		S72.464[K,M,N] Nondisp suprcndl fx w intrcndl extn low end r femr
		S72.465[K,M,N] Nondisp suprcndl fx w intrcndl extn low end l femr
		S72.466[K,M,N] Nondisp suprcndl fx w intrcndl extn low end unsp femr
		S72.47[1,2,9]**K** Torus fx lower end of right femur, subs for fx w nonunion
		S72.491[K,M,N] Oth fx lower end of right femur
		S72.492[K,M,N] Oth fx lower end of left femur
		S72.499[K,M,N] Oth fx lower end of unsp femur
		S72.8X1[K,M,N] Oth fracture of right femur
		S72.8X2[K,M,N] Oth fracture of left femur
		S72.8X9[K,M,N] Oth fracture of unsp femur
		S72.90X[K,M,N] Unsp fracture of unsp femur
		S72.91X[K,M,N] Unsp fracture of right femur
		S72.92X[K,M,N] Unsp fracture of left femur
		S79.00[1,2,9]**K** Unsp physeal fx upper end of r femur, subs for fx w nonunion
		S79.01[1,2,9]**K** Sltr-haris Type I physl fx upr end r femr, sub for fx w nonun
		S79.09[1,2,9]**K** Oth physeal fx upper end of r femur, subs for fx w nonunion
		S79.10[1,2,9]**K** Unsp physeal fx lower end of r femur, subs for fx w nonunion
		S79.11[1,2,9]**K** Sltr-haris Type I physl fx low end r femr, sub for fx w nonun
		S79.12[1,2,9]**K** Sltr-haris Type II physl fx low end r femr, sub for fx w nonun
		S79.13[1,2,9]**K** Sltr-haris Type III physl fx low end r femr, sub for fx w nonun
		S79.14[1,2,9]**K** Sltr-haris Type IV physl fx low end r femr, sub for fx w nonun
		S79.19[1,2,9]**K** Oth physeal fx lower end of r femur, subs for fx w nonunion
		S82.001[K,M,N] Unsp fracture of right patella
		S82.002[K,M,N] Unsp fracture of left patella
		S82.009[K,M,N] Unsp fracture of unsp patella
		S82.011[K,M,N] Displ osteochon fx r patella
		S82.012[K,M,N] Displ osteochon fx left patella
		S82.013[K,M,N] Displ osteochon fx unsp patella
		S82.014[K,M,N] Nondisp osteochon fx r patella
		S82.015[K,M,N] Nondisp osteochon fx l patella
		S82.016[K,M,N] Nondisp osteochon fx unsp patella
		S82.021[K,M,N] Displ longitud fx right patella
		S82.022[K,M,N] Displ longitud fx left patella
		S82.023[K,M,N] Displ longitud fx unsp patella
		S82.024[K,M,N] Nondisp longitud fx r patella
		S82.025[K,M,N] Nondisp longitud fx l patella
		S82.026[K,M,N] Nondisp longitud fx unsp patella
		S82.031[K,M,N] Displ transverse fx r patella
		S82.032[K,M,N] Displ transverse fx l patella
		S82.033[K,M,N] Displ transverse fx unsp patella
		S82.034[K,M,N] Nondisp transverse fx r patella
		S82.035[K,M,N] Nondisp transverse fx l patella
		S82.036[K,M,N] Nondisp transverse fx unsp patella
		S82.041[K,M,N] Displ commnt fx right patella

6th Character meanings for codes as indicated
1 Right ***2 Left*** ***9 Unspecified***

7th Character meanins for codes S72.-, S82.-
K Sub Enc Closed FX Nonunion
M Sub Enc Open FX Type I/II Nonunion
N Sub Enc Open IIIA/B/C Nonunion

(Continued on next page)

ICD-9-CM		ICD-10-CM
733.82	NONUNION OF FRACTURE **(Continued)**	**S82.Ø42**[K,M,N] Displ commnt fx left patella **S82.Ø43**[K,M,N] Displ commnt fx unsp patella **S82.Ø44**[K,M,N] Nondisp commnt fx right patella **S82.Ø45**[K,M,N] Nondisp commnt fx left patella **S82.Ø46**[K,M,N] Nondisp commnt fx unsp patella **S82.Ø91**[K,M,N] Oth fracture of right patella **S82.Ø92**[K,M,N] Oth fracture of left patella **S82.Ø99**[K,M,N] Oth fracture of unsp patella **S82.1Ø1**[K,M,N] Unsp fx upper end of r tibia **S82.1Ø2**[K,M,N] Unsp fx upper end of left tibia **S82.1Ø9**[K,M,N] Unsp fx upper end of unsp tibia **S82.111**[K,M,N] Disp fx of right tibial spine **S82.112**[K,M,N] Disp fx of left tibial spine **S82.113**[K,M,N] Disp fx of unsp tibial spine **S82.114**[K,M,N] Nondisp fx of r tibial spine **S82.115**[K,M,N] Nondisp fx of left tibial spine **S82.116**[K,M,N] Nondisp fx of unsp tibial spine **S82.121**[K,M,N] Disp fx of lateral condyle of r tibia **S82.122**[K,M,N] Disp fx of lateral condyle of l tibia **S82.123**[K,M,N] Disp fx of lateral condyle of unsp tibia **S82.124**[K,M,N] Nondisp fx of lateral condyle of r tibia **S82.125**[K,M,N] Nondisp fx of lateral condyle of l tibia **S82.126**[K,M,N] Nondisp fx of lateral condyle of unsp tibia **S82.131**[K,M,N] Disp fx of med condyle of r tibia **S82.132**[K,M,N] Disp fx of med condyle of l tibia **S82.133**[K,M,N] Disp fx of med condyle of unsp tibia **S82.134**[K,M,N] Nondisp fx of med condyle of r tibia **S82.135**[K,M,N] Nondisp fx of med condyle of l tibia **S82.136**[K,M,N] Nondisp fx of med condyle of unsp tibia **S82.141**[K,M,N] Displaced bicondylar fx r tibia **S82.142**[K,M,N] Displaced bicondylar fx l tibia **S82.143**[K,M,N] Displ bicondylar fx unsp tibia **S82.144**[K,M,N] Nondisp bicondylar fx r tibia **S82.145**[K,M,N] Nondisp bicondylar fx l tibia **S82.146**[K,M,N] Nondisp bicondylar fx unsp tibia **S82.151**[K,M,N] Disp fx of r tibial tuberosity **S82.152**[K,M,N] Disp fx of l tibial tuberosity **S82.153**[K,M,N] Disp fx of unsp tibial tuberosity **S82.154**[K,M,N] Nondisp fx of r tibial tuberosity **S82.155**[K,M,N] Nondisp fx of l tibial tuberosity **S82.156**[K,M,N] Nondisp fx of unsp tibial tuberosity **S82.16**[1,2,9]**K** Torus fx upper end of right tibia, subs for fx w nonunion **S82.191**[K,M,N] Oth fx upper end of right tibia **S82.192**[K,M,N] Oth fx upper end of left tibia **S82.199**[K,M,N] Oth fx upper end of unsp tibia **S82.2Ø1**[K,M,N] Unsp fx shaft of right tibia **S82.2Ø2**[K,M,N] Unsp fx shaft of left tibia **S82.2Ø9**[K,M,N] Unsp fx shaft of unsp tibia **S82.221**[K,M,N] Displ transverse fx shaft of r tibia **S82.222**[K,M,N] Displ transverse fx shaft of l tibia **S82.223**[K,M,N] Displ transverse fx shaft of unsp tibia **S82.224**[K,M,N] Nondisp transverse fx shaft of r tibia **S82.225**[K,M,N] Nondisp transverse fx shaft of l tibia **S82.226**[K,M,N] Nondisp transverse fx shaft of unsp tibia **S82.231**[K,M,N] Displ oblique fx shaft of r tibia **S82.232**[K,M,N] Displ oblique fx shaft of l tibia **S82.233**[K,M,N] Displ oblique fx shaft of unsp tibia **S82.234**[K,M,N] Nondisp oblique fx shaft of r tibia **S82.235**[K,M,N] Nondisp oblique fx shaft of l tibia **S82.236**[K,M,N] Nondisp oblique fx shaft of unsp tibia **S82.241**[K,M,N] Displ spiral fx shaft of r tibia **S82.242**[K,M,N] Displ spiral fx shaft of l tibia **S82.243**[K,M,N] Displ spiral fx shaft of unsp tibia **S82.244**[K,M,N] Nondisp spiral fx shaft of r tibia **S82.245**[K,M,N] Nondisp spiral fx shaft of l tibia **S82.246**[K,M,N] Nondisp spiral fx shaft of unsp tibia **S82.251**[K,M,N] Displ commnt fx shaft of r tibia **S82.252**[K,M,N] Displ commnt fx shaft of l tibia **S82.253**[K,M,N] Displ commnt fx shaft of unsp tibia **S82.254**[K,M,N] Nondisp commnt fx shaft of r tibia **S82.255**[K,M,N] Nondisp commnt fx shaft of l tibia **S82.256**[K,M,N] Nondisp commnt fx shaft of unsp tibia **S82.261**[K,M,N] Displ seg fx shaft of r tibia **S82.262**[K,M,N] Displ seg fx shaft of l tibia **S82.263**[K,M,N] Displ seg fx shaft of unsp tibia

6th Character meanings for codes as indicated
1 Right ***2 Left*** ***9 Unspecified***

7th Character meanins for codes S82.-
K Sub Enc Closed FX Nonunion
M Sub Enc Open FX Type I/II Nonunion
N Sub Enc Open IIIA/B/C Nonunion

(Continued on next page)

ICD-9-CM	ICD-10-CM
733.82 NONUNION OF FRACTURE **(Continued)**	**S82.264**[K,M,N] Nondisp seg fx shaft of r tibia
	S82.265[K,M,N] Nondisp seg fx shaft of l tibia
	S82.266[K,M,N] Nondisp seg fx shaft of unsp tibia
	S82.291[K,M,N] Oth fx shaft of right tibia
	S82.292[K,M,N] Oth fx shaft of left tibia
	S82.299[K,M,N] Oth fx shaft of unsp tibia
	S82.301[K,M,N] Unsp fx lower end of r tibia
	S82.302[K,M,N] Unsp fx lower end of left tibia
	S82.309[K,M,N] Unsp fx lower end of unsp tibia
	S82.31[1,2,9]**K** Torus fx lower end of tibia, subs for fx w nonunion
	S82.391[K,M,N] Oth fx lower end of right tibia
	S82.392[K,M,N] Oth fx lower end of left tibia
	S82.399[K,M,N] Oth fx lower end of unsp tibia
	S82.401[K,M,N] Unsp fx shaft of r fibula
	S82.402[K,M,N] Unsp fx shaft of left fibula
	S82.409[K,M,N] Unsp fx shaft of unsp fibula
	S82.421[K,M,N] Displ transverse fx shaft of r fibula
	S82.422[K,M,N] Displ transverse fx shaft of l fibula
	S82.423[K,M,N] Displ transverse fx shaft of unsp fibula
	S82.424[K,M,N] Nondisp transverse fx shaft of r fibula
	S82.425[K,M,N] Nondisp transverse fx shaft of l fibula
	S82.426[K,M,N] Nondisp transverse fx shaft of unsp fibula
	S82.431[K,M,N] Displ oblique fx shaft of r fibula
	S82.432[K,M,N] Displ oblique fx shaft of l fibula
	S82.433[K,M,N] Displ oblique fx shaft of unsp fibula
	S82.434[K,M,N] Nondisp oblique fx shaft of r fibula
	S82.435[K,M,N] Nondisp oblique fx shaft of l fibula
	S82.436[K,M,N] Nondisp oblique fx shaft of unsp fibula
	S82.441[K,M,N] Displ spiral fx shaft of r fibula
	S82.442[K,M,N] Displ spiral fx shaft of l fibula
	S82.443[K,M,N] Displ spiral fx shaft of unsp fibula
	S82.444[K,M,N] Nondisp spiral fx shaft of r fibula
	S82.445[K,M,N] Nondisp spiral fx shaft of l fibula
	S82.446[K,M,N] Nondisp spiral fx shaft of unsp fibula
	S82.451[K,M,N] Displ commnt fx shaft of r fibula
	S82.452[K,M,N] Displ commnt fx shaft of l fibula
	S82.453[K,M,N] Displ commnt fx shaft of unsp fibula
	S82.454[K,M,N] Nondisp commnt fx shaft of r fibula
	S82.455[K,M,N] Nondisp commnt fx shaft of l fibula
	S82.456[K,M,N] Nondisp commnt fx shaft of unsp fibula
	S82.461[K,M,N] Displ seg fx shaft of r fibula
	S82.462[K,M,N] Displ seg fx shaft of l fibula
	S82.463[K,M,N] Displ seg fx shaft of unsp fibula
	S82.464[K,M,N] Nondisp seg fx shaft of r fibula
	S82.465[K,M,N] Nondisp seg fx shaft of l fibula
	S82.466[K,M,N] Nondisp seg fx shaft of unsp fibula
	S82.491[K,M,N] Oth fx shaft of r fibula
	S82.492[K,M,N] Oth fx shaft of left fibula
	S82.499[K,M,N] Oth fx shaft of unsp fibula
	S82.51X[K,M,N] Disp fx of med malleolus of r tibia
	S82.52X[K,M,N] Disp fx of med malleolus of l tibia
	S82.53X[K,M,N] Disp fx of med malleolus of unsp tibia
	S82.54X[K,M,N] Nondisp fx of med malleolus of r tibia
	S82.55X[K,M,N] Nondisp fx of med malleolus of l tibia
	S82.56X[K,M,N] Nondisp fx of med malleolus of unsp tibia
	S82.61X[K,M,N] Disp fx of lateral malleolus of r fibula
	S82.62X[K,M,N] Disp fx of lateral malleolus of l fibula
	S82.63X[K,M,N] Disp fx of lateral malleolus of unsp fibula
	S82.64X[K,M,N] Nondisp fx of lateral malleolus of r fibula
	S82.65X[K,M,N] Nondisp fx of lateral malleolus of l fibula
	S82.66X[K,M,N] Nondisp fx of lateral malleolus of unsp fibula
	S82.81[1,2,9]**K** Torus fx upper end of fibula, subs for fx w nonunion
	S82.82[1,2,9]**K** Torus fx lower end of fibula, subs for fx w nonunion
	S82.831[K,M,N] Oth fx upr and low end r fibula
	S82.832[K,M,N] Oth fx upr and low end l fibula
	S82.839[K,M,N] Oth fx upr & low end unsp fibula
	S82.841[K,M,N] Displ bimalleol fx r low leg
	S82.842[K,M,N] Displ bimalleol fx l low leg
	S82.843[K,M,N] Displ bimalleol fx unsp low leg
	S82.844[K,M,N] Nondisp bimalleol fx r low leg
	S82.845[K,M,N] Nondisp bimalleol fx l low leg
	S82.846[K,M,N] Nondisp bimalleol fx unsp low leg
	S82.851[K,M,N] Displ trimalleol fx r low leg
	S82.852[K,M,N] Displ trimalleol fx l low leg
	S82.853[K,M,N] Displ trimalleol fx unsp low leg

6th Character meanings for codes as indicated
1 Right 2 Left 9 Unspecified

7th Character meanins for codes S82.-
K Sub Enc Closed FX Nonunion
M Sub Enc Open FX Type I/II Nonunion
N Sub Enc Open IIIA/B/C Nonunion

(Continued on next page)

ICD-9-CM		ICD-10-CM	
733.82	NONUNION OF FRACTURE **(Continued)**	**S82.854**[K,M,N]	Nondisp trimalleol fx r low leg
		S82.855[K,M,N]	Nondisp trimalleol fx l low leg
		S82.856[K,M,N]	Nondisp trimalleol fx unsp low leg
		S82.861[K,M,N]	Displ Maisonneuve's fx r leg
		S82.862[K,M,N]	Displ Maisonneuve's fx left leg
		S82.863[K,M,N]	Displ Maisonneuve's fx unsp leg
		S82.864[K,M,N]	Nondisp Maisonneuve's fx r leg
		S82.865[K,M,N]	Nondisp Maisonneuve's fx l leg
		S82.866[K,M,N]	Nondisp Maisonneuve's fx unsp leg
		S82.871[K,M,N]	Displaced pilon fx right tibia
		S82.872[K,M,N]	Displaced pilon fx left tibia
		S82.873[K,M,N]	Displaced pilon fx unsp tibia
		S82.874[K,M,N]	Nondisp pilon fx right tibia
		S82.875[K,M,N]	Nondisp pilon fx left tibia
		S82.876[K,M,N]	Nondisp pilon fx unsp tibia
		S82.891[K,M,N]	Oth fracture of right lower leg
		S82.892[K,M,N]	Oth fracture of left lower leg
		S82.899[K,M,N]	Oth fracture of unsp lower leg
		S82.90X[K,M,N]	Unsp fracture of unsp lower leg
		S82.91X[K,M,N]	Unsp fracture of r low leg
		S82.92X[K,M,N]	Unsp fracture of left lower leg
		S89.00[1,2,9]**K**	Unsp physeal fx upper end of tibia, subs for fx w nonunion
		S89.01[1,2,9]**K**	Sltr-haris Type I physl fx upr end tibia, sub for fx w nonun
		S89.02[1,2,9]**K**	Sltr-haris Type II physl fx upr end tibia, sub for fx w nonun
		S89.03[1,2,9]**K**	Sltr-haris Type III physl fx upr end tibia, sub for fx w nonun
		S89.04[1,2,9]**K**	Sltr-haris Type IV physl fx upr end tibia, sub for fx w nonun
		S89.09[1,2,9]**K**	Oth physeal fx upper end of tibia, subs for fx w nonunion
		S89.10[1,2,9]**K**	Unsp physeal fx lower end of tibia, subs for fx w nonunion
		S89.11[1,2,9]**K**	Sltr-haris Type I physl fx low end tibia, sub for fx w nonun
		S89.12[1,2,9]**K**	Sltr-haris Type II physl fx low end tibia, sub for fx w nonun
		S89.13[1,2,9]**K**	Sltr-haris Type III physl fx low end tibia, sub for fx w nonun
		S89.14[1,2,9]**K**	Sltr-haris Type IV physl fx low end tibia, sub for fx w nonun
		S89.19[1,2,9]**K**	Oth physeal fx lower end of tibia, subs for fx w nonunion
		S89.20[1,2,9]**K**	Unsp physl fx upper end of fibula, subs for fx w nonunion
		S89.21[1,2,9]**K**	Sltr-haris Type I physl fx upr end fibula, sub for fx w nonun
		S89.22[1,2,9]**K**	Sltr-haris Type II physl fx upr end fibula, sub for fx w nonun
		S89.29[1,2,9]**K**	Oth physeal fx upper end of fibula, subs for fx w nonunion
		S89.30[1,2,9]**K**	Unsp physl fx lower end of fibula, subs for fx w nonunion
		S89.31[1,2,9]**K**	Sltr-haris Type I physl fx low end fibula, sub for fx w nonun
		S89.32[1,2,9]**K**	Sltr-haris Type II physl fx low end fibula, sub for fx w nonun
		S89.39[1,2,9]**K**	Oth physeal fx lower end of fibula, subs for fx w nonunion
		S92.00[1,2,9]**K**	Unsp fracture of calcaneus, subs for fx w nonunion
		S92.011K	Disp fx of body of right calcaneus, subs for fx w nonunion
		S92.012K	Disp fx of body of left calcaneus, subs for fx w nonunion
		S92.013K	Disp fx of body of unsp calcaneus, subs for fx w nonunion
		S92.014K	Nondisp fx of body of r calcaneus, subs for fx w nonunion
		S92.015K	Nondisp fx of body of left calcaneus, subs for fx w nonunion
		S92.016K	Nondisp fx of body of unsp calcaneus, subs for fx w nonunion
		S92.021K	Disp fx of ant pro of r calcaneus, subs for fx w nonunion
		S92.022K	Disp fx of ant pro of l calcaneus, subs for fx w nonunion
		S92.023K	Disp fx of ant pro of unsp calcaneus, subs for fx w nonunion
		S92.024K	Nondisp fx of ant pro of r calcaneus, subs for fx w nonunion
		S92.025K	Nondisp fx of ant pro of l calcaneus, subs for fx w nonunion
		S92.026K	Nondisp fx of ant pro of unsp calcaneus, sub for fx w nonun
		S92.031K	Displ avuls fx tuberosity of r calcaneus, sub for fx w nonun
		S92.032K	Displ avuls fx tuberosity of l calcaneus, sub for fx w nonun
		S92.033K	Displ avuls fx tuberosity of unsp calcaneus, sub for fx w nonun
		S92.034K	Nondisp avuls fx tuberosity of r calcaneus, sub for fx w nonun
		S92.035K	Nondisp avuls fx tuberosity of l calcaneus, sub for fx w nonun
		S92.036K	Nondisp avuls fx tuberosity of unsp calcaneus, sub for fx w nonun
		S92.041K	Displ oth fx tuberosity of r calcaneus, sub for fx w nonun
		S92.042K	Displ oth fx tuberosity of l calcaneus, sub for fx w nonun
		S92.043K	Displ oth fx tuberosity of unsp calcaneus, sub for fx w nonun
		S92.044K	Nondisp oth fx tuberosity of r calcaneus, sub for fx w nonun
		S92.045K	Nondisp oth fx tuberosity of l calcaneus, sub for fx w nonun
		S92.046K	Nondisp oth fx tuberosity of unsp calcaneus, sub for rx w nonun
		S92.051K	Displ oth extrartic fx r calcaneus, subs for fx w nonunion
		S92.052K	Displ oth extrartic fx l calcaneus, subs for fx w nonunion
		S92.053K	Displ oth extrartic fx unsp calcaneus, sub for fx w nonun
		S92.054K	Nondisp oth extrartic fx r calcaneus, subs for fx w nonunion
		S92.055K	Nondisp oth extrartic fx l calcaneus, subs for fx w nonunion
		S92.056K	Nondisp oth extrartic fx unsp calcaneus, sub for fx w nonun
		S92.061K	Displaced intartic fx r calcaneus, subs for fx w nonunion
		S92.062K	Displaced intartic fx l calcaneus, subs for fx w nonunion

6th Character meanings for codes as indicated
1 Right ***2 Left*** ***9 Unspecified***

7th Character meanins for codes S82.-
K Sub Enc Closed FX Nonunion
M Sub Enc Open FX Type I/II Nonunion
N Sub Enc Open IIIA/B/C Nonunion

(Continued on next page)

ICD-9-CM		ICD-10-CM	
733.82	NONUNION OF FRACTURE **(Continued)**	**S92.Ø63K**	Displaced intartic fx unsp calcaneus, subs for fx w nonunion
		S92.Ø64K	Nondisp intartic fx r calcaneus, subs for fx w nonunion
		S92.Ø65K	Nondisp intartic fx l calcaneus, subs for fx w nonunion
		S92.Ø66K	Nondisp intartic fx unsp calcaneus, subs for fx w nonunion
		S92.1Ø[1,2,9]K	Unsp fracture of talus, subs for fx w nonunion
		S92.111K	Disp fx of neck of right talus, subs for fx w nonunion
		S92.112K	Disp fx of neck of left talus, subs for fx w nonunion
		S92.113K	Disp fx of neck of unsp talus, subs for fx w nonunion
		S92.114K	Nondisp fx of neck of right talus, subs for fx w nonunion
		S92.115K	Nondisp fx of neck of left talus, subs for fx w nonunion
		S92.116K	Nondisp fx of neck of unsp talus, subs for fx w nonunion
		S92.121K	Disp fx of body of right talus, subs for fx w nonunion
		S92.122K	Disp fx of body of left talus, subs for fx w nonunion
		S92.123K	Disp fx of body of unsp talus, subs for fx w nonunion
		S92.124K	Nondisp fx of body of right talus, subs for fx w nonunion
		S92.125K	Nondisp fx of body of left talus, subs for fx w nonunion
		S92.126K	Nondisp fx of body of unsp talus, subs for fx w nonunion
		S92.131K	Disp fx of post pro of right talus, subs for fx w nonunion
		S92.132K	Disp fx of post pro of left talus, subs for fx w nonunion
		S92.133K	Disp fx of post pro of unsp talus, subs for fx w nonunion
		S92.134K	Nondisp fx of post pro of r talus, subs for fx w nonunion
		S92.135K	Nondisp fx of post pro of left talus, subs for fx w nonunion
		S92.136K	Nondisp fx of post pro of unsp talus, subs for fx w nonunion
		S92.141K	Displaced dome fx right talus, subs for fx w nonunion
		S92.142K	Displaced dome fx left talus, subs for fx w nonunion
		S92.143K	Displaced dome fx unsp talus, subs for fx w nonunion
		S92.144K	Nondisp dome fracture of right talus, subs for fx w nonunion
		S92.145K	Nondisp dome fracture of left talus, subs for fx w nonunion
		S92.146K	Nondisp dome fracture of unsp talus, subs for fx w nonunion
		S92.151K	Displ avuls fx (chip fracture) of r talus, sub for fx w nonun
		S92.152K	Displ avuls fx (chip fracture) of l talus, sub for fx w nonun
		S92.153K	Displ avuls fx (chip fracture) of unsp talus, sub for fx w nonun
		S92.154K	Nondisp avuls fx (chip fracture) of r talus, sub for fx w nonun
		S92.155K	Nondisp avuls fx (chip fracture) of l talus, sub for fx w nonun
		S92.156K	Nondisp avuls fx (chip fracture) of unsp talus, sub for fx w nonun
		S92.19[1,2,9]K	Oth fracture of talus, subs for fx w nonunion
		S92.2Ø[1,2,9]K	Fx unsp tarsal bone(s) of foot, subs for fx w nonunion
		S92.211K	Disp fx of cuboid bone of right foot, subs for fx w nonunion
		S92.212K	Disp fx of cuboid bone of left foot, subs for fx w nonunion
		S92.213K	Disp fx of cuboid bone of unsp foot, subs for fx w nonunion
		S92.214K	Nondisp fx of cuboid bone of r foot, subs for fx w nonunion
		S92.215K	Nondisp fx of cuboid bone of l foot, subs for fx w nonunion
		S92.216K	Nondisp fx of cuboid bone of unsp ft, subs for fx w nonunion
		S92.221K	Disp fx of lateral cuneiform of r ft, subs for fx w nonunion
		S92.222K	Disp fx of lateral cuneiform of l ft, subs for fx w nonunion
		S92.223K	Disp fx of lateral cuneiform of unsp ft, sub for fx w nonun
		S92.224K	Nondisp fx of lateral cuneiform of r ft, sub for fx w nonun
		S92.225K	Nondisp fx of lateral cuneiform of l ft, sub for fx w nonun
		S92.226K	Nondisp fx of lateral cuneiform of unsp ft, sub for fx w nonun
		S92.231K	Disp fx of intermed cuneiform of r ft, sub for fx w nonun
		S92.232K	Disp fx of intermed cuneiform of l ft, sub for fx w nonun
		S92.233K	Disp fx of intermed cuneiform of unsp ft, sub for fx w nonun
		S92.234K	Nondisp fx of intermed cuneiform of r ft, sub for fx w nonun
		S92.235K	Nondisp fx of intermed cuneiform of l ft, sub for fx w nonun
		S92.236K	Nondisp fx of intermed cuneiform of unsp ft, sub for fx w nonun
		S92.241K	Disp fx of med cuneiform of r foot, subs for fx w nonunion
		S92.242K	Disp fx of med cuneiform of l foot, subs for fx w nonunion
		S92.243K	Disp fx of med cuneiform of unsp ft, subs for fx w nonunion
		S92.244K	Nondisp fx of med cuneiform of r ft, subs for fx w nonunion
		S92.245K	Nondisp fx of med cuneiform of l ft, subs for fx w nonunion
		S92.246K	Nondisp fx of med cuneiform of unsp ft, sub for fx w nonun
		S92.251K	Disp fx of navicular of right foot, subs for fx w nonunion
		S92.252K	Disp fx of navicular of left foot, subs for fx w nonunion
		S92.253K	Disp fx of navicular of unsp foot, subs for fx w nonunion
		S92.254K	Nondisp fx of navicular of r foot, subs for fx w nonunion
		S92.255K	Nondisp fx of navicular of left foot, subs for fx w nonunion
		S92.256K	Nondisp fx of navicular of unsp foot, subs for fx w nonunion
		S92.3Ø[1,2,9]K	Fx unsp metatarsal bone(s), foot, subs for fx w nonunion
		S92.311K	Disp fx of 1st metatarsal bone, r ft, subs for fx w nonunion
		S92.312K	Disp fx of 1st metatarsal bone, l ft, subs for fx w nonunion
		S92.313K	Disp fx of 1st metatarsal bone, unsp ft, sub for fx w nonun
		S92.314K	Nondisp fx of 1st metatarsal bone, r ft, sub for fx w nonun
		S92.315K	Nondisp fx of 1st metatarsal bone, l ft, sub for fx w nonun
		S92.316K	Nondisp fx of 1st metatarsal bone, unsp ft, sub for fx w nonun
		S92.321K	Disp fx of 2nd metatarsal bone, r ft, subs for fx w nonunion
		S92.322K	Disp fx of 2nd metatarsal bone, l ft, subs for fx w nonunion
		S92.323K	Disp fx of 2nd metatarsal bone, unsp ft, sub for fx w nonun
		S92.324K	Nondisp fx of 2nd metatarsal bone, r ft, sub for fx w nonun

6th Character meanings for codes as indicated
1 Right ***2 Left*** ***9 Unspecified***

(Continued on next page)

 [Brackets] indicate valid character values for each code. Character value meanings provided for each code grouping.

ICD-9-CM		ICD-10-CM	
733.82	NONUNION OF FRACTURE (Continued)	**S92.325K**	Nondisp fx of 2nd metatarsal bone, l ft, sub for fx w nonun
		S92.326K	Nondisp fx of 2nd metatarsal bone, unsp ft, sub for fx w nonun
		S92.331K	Disp fx of 3rd metatarsal bone, r ft, subs for fx w nonunion
		S92.332K	Disp fx of 3rd metatarsal bone, l ft, subs for fx w nonunion
		S92.333K	Disp fx of 3rd metatarsal bone, unsp ft, sub for fx w nonun
		S92.334K	Nondisp fx of 3rd metatarsal bone, r ft, sub for fx w nonun
		S92.335K	Nondisp fx of 3rd metatarsal bone, l ft, sub for fx w nonun
		S92.336K	Nondisp fx of 3rd metatarsal bone, unsp ft, sub for fx w nonun
		S92.341K	Disp fx of 4th metatarsal bone, r ft, subs for fx w nonunion
		S92.342K	Disp fx of 4th metatarsal bone, l ft, subs for fx w nonunion
		S92.343K	Disp fx of 4th metatarsal bone, unsp ft, sub for fx w nonun
		S92.344K	Nondisp fx of 4th metatarsal bone, r ft, sub for fx w nonun
		S92.345K	Nondisp fx of 4th metatarsal bone, l ft, sub for fx w nonun
		S92.346K	Nondisp fx of 4th metatarsal bone, unsp ft, sub for fx w nonun
		S92.351K	Disp fx of 5th metatarsal bone, r ft, subs for fx w nonunion
		S92.352K	Disp fx of 5th metatarsal bone, l ft, subs for fx w nonunion
		S92.353K	Disp fx of 5th metatarsal bone, unsp ft, sub for fx w nonun
		S92.354K	Nondisp fx of 5th metatarsal bone, r ft, sub for fx w nonun
		S92.355K	Nondisp fx of 5th metatarsal bone, l ft, sub for fx w nonun
		S92.356K	Nondisp fx of 5th metatarsal bone, unsp ft, sub for fx w nonun
		S92.4Ø1K	Displaced unsp fx right great toe, subs for fx w nonunion
		S92.4Ø2K	Displaced unsp fx left great toe, subs for fx w nonunion
		S92.4Ø3K	Displaced unsp fx unsp great toe, subs for fx w nonunion
		S92.4Ø4K	Nondisp unsp fx right great toe, subs for fx w nonunion
		S92.4Ø5K	Nondisp unsp fx left great toe, subs for fx w nonunion
		S92.4Ø6K	Nondisp unsp fx unsp great toe, subs for fx w nonunion
		S92.411K	Disp fx of prox phalanx of r great toe, sub for fx w nonun
		S92.412K	Disp fx of prox phalanx of l great toe, sub for fx w nonun
		S92.413K	Disp fx of prox phalanx of unsp great toe, sub for fx w nonun
		S92.414K	Nondisp fx of prox phalanx of r great toe, sub for fx w nonun
		S92.415K	Nondisp fx of prox phalanx of l great toe, sub for fx w nonun
		S92.416K	Nondisp fx of prox phalanx of unsp great toe, sub for fx w nonun
		S92.421K	Disp fx of dist phalanx of r great toe, sub for fx w nonun
		S92.422K	Disp fx of dist phalanx of l great toe, sub for fx w nonun
		S92.423K	Disp fx of dist phalanx of unsp great toe, sub for fx w nonun
		S92.424K	Nondisp fx of dist phalanx of r great toe, sub for fx w nonun
		S92.425K	Nondisp fx of dist phalanx of l great toe, sub for fx w nonun
		S92.426K	Nondisp fx of dist phalanx of unsp great toe, sub for fx w nonun
		S92.49[1,2,9]**K**	Oth fracture of great toe, subs for fx w nonunion
		S92.5Ø1K	Displ unsp fx right lesser toe(s), subs for fx w nonunion
		S92.5Ø2K	Displaced unsp fx left lesser toe(s), subs for fx w nonunion
		S92.5Ø3K	Displaced unsp fx unsp lesser toe(s), subs for fx w nonunion
		S92.5Ø4K	Nondisp unsp fx right lesser toe(s), subs for fx w nonunion
		S92.5Ø5K	Nondisp unsp fx left lesser toe(s), subs for fx w nonunion
		S92.5Ø6K	Nondisp unsp fx unsp lesser toe(s), subs for fx w nonunion
		S92.511K	Disp fx of prox phalanx of r less toe(s), sub for fx w nonun
		S92.512K	Disp fx of prox phalanx of l less toe(s), sub for fx w nonun
		S92.513K	Disp fx of prox phalanx of unsp less toe(s), sub for fx w nonun
		S92.514K	Nondisp fx of prox phalanx of r less toe(s), sub for fx w nonun
		S92.515K	Nondisp fx of prox phalanx of l less toe(s), sub for fx w nonun
		S92.516K	Nondisp fx of prox phalanx of unsp less toe(s), sub for fx w nonun
		S92.521K	Disp fx of med phalanx of r less toe(s), sub for fx w nonun
		S92.522K	Disp fx of med phalanx of l less toe(s), sub for fx w nonun
		S92.523K	Disp fx of med phalanx of unsp less toe(s), sub for fx w nonun
		S92.524K	Nondisp fx of med phalanx of r less toe(s), sub for fx w nonun
		S92.525K	Nondisp fx of med phalanx of l less toe(s), sub for fx w nonun
		S92.526K	Nondisp fx of med phalanx of unsp less toe(s), sub for fx w nonun
		S92.531K	Disp fx of dist phalanx of r less toe(s), sub for fx w nonun
		S92.532K	Disp fx of dist phalanx of l less toe(s), sub for fx w nonun
		S92.533K	Disp fx of dist phalanx of unsp less toe(s), sub for fx w nonun
		S92.534K	Nondisp fx of dist phalanx of r less toe(s), sub for fx w nonun
		S92.535K	Nondisp fx of dist phalanx of l less toe(s), sub for fx w nonun
		S92.536K	Nondisp fx of dist phalanx of unsp less toe(s), sub for fx w nonun
		S92.59[1,2,9]**K**	Oth fracture of lesser toe(s), subs for fx w nonunion
		S92.9Ø[1,2,9]**K**	Unsp fracture of foot, subs for fx w nonunion
		S92.91[1,2,9]**K**	Unsp fracture of toe(s), subs for fx w nonunion
			6th Character meanings for codes as indicated ***1 Right*** ***2 Left*** ***9 Unspecified***
733.9Ø	DISORDER OF BONE AND CARTILAGE UNSPECIFIED	**M85.9**	Disorder of bone density and structure, unspecified
		M89.9	Disorder of bone, unspecified
		M94.9	Disorder of cartilage, unspecified

ICD-9-CM		ICD-10-CM	
733.91	ARREST OF BONE DEVELOPMENT OR GROWTH	**M89.121**	Complete physeal arrest, right proximal humerus
		M89.122	Complete physeal arrest, left proximal humerus
		M89.123	Partial physeal arrest, right proximal humerus
		M89.124	Partial physeal arrest, left proximal humerus
		M89.125	Complete physeal arrest, right distal humerus
		M89.126	Complete physeal arrest, left distal humerus
		M89.127	Partial physeal arrest, right distal humerus
		M89.128	Partial physeal arrest, left distal humerus
		M89.129	Physeal arrest, humerus, unspecified
		M89.131	Complete physeal arrest, right distal radius
		M89.132	Complete physeal arrest, left distal radius
		M89.133	Partial physeal arrest, right distal radius
		M89.134	Partial physeal arrest, left distal radius
		M89.138	Other physeal arrest of forearm
		M89.139	Physeal arrest, forearm, unspecified
		M89.151	Complete physeal arrest, right proximal femur
		M89.152	Complete physeal arrest, left proximal femur
		M89.153	Partial physeal arrest, right proximal femur
		M89.154	Partial physeal arrest, left proximal femur
		M89.155	Complete physeal arrest, right distal femur
		M89.156	Complete physeal arrest, left distal femur
		M89.157	Partial physeal arrest, right distal femur
		M89.158	Partial physeal arrest, left distal femur
		M89.159	Physeal arrest, femur, unspecified
		M89.16Ø	Complete physeal arrest, right proximal tibia
		M89.161	Complete physeal arrest, left proximal tibia
		M89.162	Partial physeal arrest, right proximal tibia
		M89.163	Partial physeal arrest, left proximal tibia
		M89.164	Complete physeal arrest, right distal tibia
		M89.165	Complete physeal arrest, left distal tibia
		M89.166	Partial physeal arrest, right distal tibia
		M89.167	Partial physeal arrest, left distal tibia
		M89.168	Other physeal arrest of lower leg
		M89.169	Physeal arrest, lower leg, unspecified
		M89.18	Physeal arrest, other site
733.92	CHONDROMALACIA	**M94.2Ø**	Chondromalacia, unspecified site
		M94.211	Chondromalacia, right shoulder
		M94.212	Chondromalacia, left shoulder
		M94.219	Chondromalacia, unspecified shoulder
		M94.221	Chondromalacia, right elbow
		M94.222	Chondromalacia, left elbow
		M94.229	Chondromalacia, unspecified elbow
		M94.231	Chondromalacia, right wrist
		M94.232	Chondromalacia, left wrist
		M94.239	Chondromalacia, unspecified wrist
		M94.241	Chondromalacia, joints of right hand
		M94.242	Chondromalacia, joints of left hand
		M94.249	Chondromalacia, joints of unspecified hand
		M94.251	Chondromalacia, right hip
		M94.252	Chondromalacia, left hip
		M94.259	Chondromalacia, unspecified hip
		M94.261	Chondromalacia, right knee
		M94.262	Chondromalacia, left knee
		M94.269	Chondromalacia, unspecified knee
		M94.271	Chondromalacia, right ankle and joints of right foot
		M94.272	Chondromalacia, left ankle and joints of left foot
		M94.279	Chondromalacia, unspecified ankle and joints of foot
		M94.28	Chondromalacia, other site
		M94.29	Chondromalacia, multiple sites
733.93	STRESS FRACTURE OF TIBIA OR FIBULA	**M84.361A**	Stress fracture, right tibia, initial encounter for fracture
		M84.362A	Stress fracture, left tibia, initial encounter for fracture
		M84.363A	Stress fracture, right fibula, init encntr for fracture
		M84.364A	Stress fracture, left fibula, initial encounter for fracture
		M84.369A	Stress fracture, unsp tibia and fibula, init for fx
733.94	STRESS FRACTURE OF THE METATARSALS	**M84.374A**	Stress fracture, right foot, initial encounter for fracture
		M84.375A	Stress fracture, left foot, initial encounter for fracture
		M84.376A	Stress fracture, unspecified foot, init encntr for fracture
		M84.377A	Stress fracture, right toe(s), init encntr for fracture
		M84.378A	Stress fracture, left toe(s), initial encounter for fracture
		M84.379A	Stress fracture, unsp toe(s), init encntr for fracture
733.95	STRESS FRACTURE OF OTHER BONE	**M48.4ØXA**	Fatigue fracture of vertebra, site unsp, init for fx
		M48.41XA	Fatigue fracture of vertebra, occipt-atlan-ax region, init
		M48.42XA	Fatigue fracture of vertebra, cervical region, init for fx
		M48.43XA	Fatigue fracture of vertebra, cervicothoracic region, init
		M48.44XA	Fatigue fracture of vertebra, thoracic region, init for fx
		M48.45XA	Fatigue fracture of vertebra, thoracolumbar region, init
		M48.46XA	Fatigue fracture of vertebra, lumbar region, init for fx
		M48.47XA	Fatigue fracture of vertebra, lumbosacral region, init
		M48.48XA	Fatigue fracture of vertebra, sacr/sacrocygl region, init
		M84.3ØXA	Stress fracture, unspecified site, init encntr for fracture
	(Continued on next page)	**M84.311A**	Stress fracture, right shoulder, init encntr for fracture

ICD-9-CM		ICD-10-CM	
733.95	STRESS FRACTURE OF OTHER BONE **(Continued)**	**M84.312A**	Stress fracture, left shoulder, init encntr for fracture
		M84.319A	Stress fracture, unsp shoulder, init encntr for fracture
		M84.321A	Stress fracture, right humerus, init encntr for fracture
		M84.322A	Stress fracture, left humerus, init encntr for fracture
		M84.329A	Stress fracture, unsp humerus, init encntr for fracture
		M84.331A	Stress fracture, right ulna, initial encounter for fracture
		M84.332A	Stress fracture, left ulna, initial encounter for fracture
		M84.333A	Stress fracture, right radius, init encntr for fracture
		M84.334A	Stress fracture, left radius, initial encounter for fracture
		M84.339A	Stress fracture, unsp ulna and radius, init for fx
		M84.341A	Stress fracture, right hand, initial encounter for fracture
		M84.342A	Stress fracture, left hand, initial encounter for fracture
		M84.343A	Stress fracture, unspecified hand, init encntr for fracture
		M84.344A	Stress fracture, right finger(s), init encntr for fracture
		M84.345A	Stress fracture, left finger(s), init encntr for fracture
		M84.346A	Stress fracture, unsp finger(s), init encntr for fracture
		M84.371A	Stress fracture, right ankle, initial encounter for fracture
		M84.372A	Stress fracture, left ankle, initial encounter for fracture
		M84.373A	Stress fracture, unspecified ankle, init encntr for fracture
		M84.38XA	Stress fracture, other site, initial encounter for fracture
733.96	STRESS FRACTURE OF FEMORAL NECK	**M84.359A**	Stress fracture, hip, unspecified, init encntr for fracture
733.97	STRESS FRACTURE OF SHAFT OF FEMUR	**M84.351A**	Stress fracture, right femur, initial encounter for fracture
		M84.352A	Stress fracture, left femur, initial encounter for fracture
		M84.353A	Stress fracture, unspecified femur, init encntr for fracture
733.98	STRESS FRACTURE OF PELVIS	**M84.35ØA**	Stress fracture, pelvis, initial encounter for fracture
733.99	OTHER DISORDERS OF BONE AND CARTILAGE OTHER	**M84.8Ø**	Other disorders of continuity of bone, unspecified site
		M84.81[1,2,9]	Other disorders of continuity of bone, shoulder
		M84.82[1,2,9]	Other disorders of continuity of bone, humerus
		M84.831	Other disorders of continuity of bone, right ulna
		M84.832	Other disorders of continuity of bone, left ulna
		M84.833	Other disorders of continuity of bone, right radius
		M84.834	Other disorders of continuity of bone, left radius
		M84.839	Other disorders of continuity of bone, unsp ulna and radius
		M84.84[1,2,9]	Other disorders of continuity of bone, hand
		M84.85[1,2,9]	Oth disord of continuity of bone, pelv rgn and thigh
		M84.861	Other disorders of continuity of bone, right tibia
		M84.862	Other disorders of continuity of bone, left tibia
		M84.863	Other disorders of continuity of bone, right fibula
		M84.864	Other disorders of continuity of bone, left fibula
		M84.869	Other disorders of continuity of bone, unsp tibia and fibula
		M84.87[1,2,9]	Other disorders of continuity of bone, ankle and foot
		M84.88	Other disorders of continuity of bone, other site
		M84.9	Disorder of continuity of bone, unspecified
		M85.1Ø	Skeletal fluorosis, unspecified site
		M85.11[1,2,9]	Skeletal fluorosis, shoulder
		M85.12[1,2,9]	Skeletal fluorosis, upper arm
		M85.13[1,2,9]	Skeletal fluorosis, forearm
		M85.14[1,2,9]	Skeletal fluorosis, hand
		M85.15[1,2,9]	Skeletal fluorosis, thigh
		M85.16[1,2,9]	Skeletal fluorosis, lower leg
		M85.17[1,2,9]	Skeletal fluorosis, ankle and foot
		M85.18	Skeletal fluorosis, other site
		M85.19	Skeletal fluorosis, multiple sites
		M85.8Ø	Oth disrd of bone density and structure, unspecified site
		M85.81[1,2,9]	Oth disrd of bone density and structure, shoulder
		M85.82[1,2,9]	Oth disrd of bone density and structure, upper arm
		M85.83[1,2,9]	Oth disrd of bone density and structure, forearm
		M85.84[1,2,9]	Oth disrd of bone density and structure, hand
		M85.85[1,2,9]	Oth disrd of bone density and structure, thigh
		M85.86[1,2,9]	Oth disrd of bone density and structure, lower leg
		M85.87[1,2,9]	Oth disrd of bone density and structure, ank/ft
		M85.88	Oth disrd of bone density and structure, other site
		M85.89	Oth disrd of bone density and structure, multiple sites
		M89.2Ø	Other disorders of bone development and growth, unsp site
		M89.21[1,2,9]	Oth disorders of bone development and growth, shoulder
		M89.22[1,2,9]	Oth disorders of bone development and growth, humerus
		M89.231	Other disorders of bone development and growth, right ulna
		M89.232	Other disorders of bone development and growth, left ulna
		M89.233	Other disorders of bone development and growth, right radius
		M89.234	Other disorders of bone development and growth, left radius
		M89.239	Oth disorders of bone dev and growth, unsp ulna and radius
		M89.24[1,2,9]	Other disorders of bone development and growth, hand
		M89.25[1,2,9]	Other disorders of bone development and growth, femur
		M89.261	Other disorders of bone development and growth, right tibia
		M89.262	Other disorders of bone development and growth, left tibia
		M89.263	Other disorders of bone development and growth, right fibula
		M89.264	Other disorders of bone development and growth, left fibula
		M89.269	Oth disorders of bone development and growth, unsp lower leg

6th Character meanings for codes as indicated
1 Right 2 Left 9 Unspecified

(Continued on next page)

ICD-9-CM		ICD-10-CM	
733.99	OTHER DISORDERS OF BONE AND CARTILAGE OTHER **(Continued)**	**M89.27**[1,2,9]	Oth disorders of bone development and growth ank/ft
		M89.28	Other disorders of bone development and growth, other site
		M89.29	Oth disorders of bone development and growth, multiple sites
		M89.3Ø	Hypertrophy of bone, unspecified site
		M89.31[1,2,9]	Hypertrophy of bone, shoulder
		M89.32[1,2,9]	Hypertrophy of bone, humerus
		M89.331	Hypertrophy of bone, right ulna
		M89.332	Hypertrophy of bone, left ulna
		M89.333	Hypertrophy of bone, right radius
		M89.334	Hypertrophy of bone, left radius
		M89.339	Hypertrophy of bone, unspecified ulna and radius
		M89.34[1,2,9]	Hypertrophy of bone, hand
		M89.35[1,2,9]	Hypertrophy of bone, femur
		M89.361	Hypertrophy of bone, right tibia
		M89.362	Hypertrophy of bone, left tibia
		M89.363	Hypertrophy of bone, right fibula
		M89.364	Hypertrophy of bone, left fibula
		M89.369	Hypertrophy of bone, unspecified tibia and fibula
		M89.37[1,2,9]	Hypertrophy of bone, ankle and foot
		M89.38	Hypertrophy of bone, other site
		M89.39	Hypertrophy of bone, multiple sites
		M89.5Ø	Osteolysis, unspecified site
		M89.51[1,2,9]	Osteolysis, shoulder
		M89.52[1,2,9]	Osteolysis, upper arm
		M89.53[1,2,9]	Osteolysis, forearm
		M89.54[1,2,9]	Osteolysis, hand
		M89.55[1,2,9]	Osteolysis, thigh
		M89.56[1,2,9]	Osteolysis, lower leg
		M89.57[1,2,9]	Osteolysis, ankle and foot
		M89.58	Osteolysis, other site
		M89.59	Osteolysis, multiple sites
		M89.8XØ	Other specified disorders of bone, multiple sites
		M89.8X1	Other specified disorders of bone, shoulder
		M89.8X2	Other specified disorders of bone, upper arm
		M89.8X3	Other specified disorders of bone, forearm
		M89.8X4	Other specified disorders of bone, hand
		M89.8X5	Other specified disorders of bone, thigh
		M89.8X6	Other specified disorders of bone, lower leg
		M89.8X7	Other specified disorders of bone, ankle and foot
		M89.8X8	Other specified disorders of bone, other site
		M89.8X9	Other specified disorders of bone, unspecified site
		M94.1	Relapsing polychondritis
		M94.35[1,2,9]	Chondrolysis, hip
		M94.8XØ	Other specified disorders of cartilage, multiple sites
		M94.8X1	Other specified disorders of cartilage, shoulder
		M94.8X2	Other specified disorders of cartilage, upper arm
		M94.8X3	Other specified disorders of cartilage, forearm
		M94.8X4	Other specified disorders of cartilage, hand
		M94.8X5	Other specified disorders of cartilage, thigh
		M94.8X6	Other specified disorders of cartilage, lower leg
		M94.8X7	Other specified disorders of cartilage, ankle and foot
		M94.8X8	Other specified disorders of cartilage, other site
		M94.8X9	Other specified disorders of cartilage, unspecified sites
			6th Character meanings for codes as indicated ***1 Right 2 Left 9 Unspecified***
734	FLAT FOOT	**M21.4Ø**	Flat foot [pes planus] (acquired), unspecified foot
		M21.41	Flat foot [pes planus] (acquired), right foot
		M21.42	Flat foot [pes planus] (acquired), left foot
735.Ø	HALLUX VALGUS	**M2Ø.1Ø**	Hallux valgus (acquired), unspecified foot
		M2Ø.11	Hallux valgus (acquired), right foot
		M2Ø.12	Hallux valgus (acquired), left foot
735.1	HALLUX VARUS	**M2Ø.3Ø**	Hallux varus (acquired), unspecified foot
		M2Ø.31	Hallux varus (acquired), right foot
		M2Ø.32	Hallux varus (acquired), left foot
735.2	HALLUX RIGIDUS	**M2Ø.2Ø**	Hallux rigidus, unspecified foot
		M2Ø.21	Hallux rigidus, right foot
		M2Ø.22	Hallux rigidus, left foot
735.3	HALLUX MALLEUS	**M2Ø.4Ø**	Other hammer toe(s) (acquired), unspecified foot
735.4	OTHER HAMMER TOE	**M2Ø.4Ø**	Other hammer toe(s) (acquired), unspecified foot
		M2Ø.41	Other hammer toe(s) (acquired), right foot
		M2Ø.42	Other hammer toe(s) (acquired), left foot
735.5	CLAW TOE	**M2Ø.5X9**	Other deformities of toe(s) (acquired), unspecified foot
735.8	OTHER ACQUIRED DEFORMITY OF TOE	**M2Ø.5X1**	Other deformities of toe(s) (acquired), right foot
		M2Ø.5X2	Other deformities of toe(s) (acquired), left foot
		M2Ø.5X9	Other deformities of toe(s) (acquired), unspecified foot
735.9	UNSPECIFIED ACQUIRED DEFORMITY OF TOE	**M2Ø.6Ø**	Acquired deformities of toe(s), unsp, unspecified foot
		M2Ø.61	Acquired deformities of toe(s), unspecified, right foot
		M2Ø.62	Acquired deformities of toe(s), unspecified, left foot

[Brackets] indicate valid character values for each code. Character value meanings provided for each code grouping.

ICD-9-CM		ICD-10-CM	
736.ØØ	UNSPECIFIED DEFORMITY FOREARM EXCLUDING FINGERS	**M21.931**	Unspecified acquired deformity of right forearm
		M21.932	Unspecified acquired deformity of left forearm
		M21.939	Unspecified acquired deformity of unspecified forearm
		M21.941	Unspecified acquired deformity of hand, right hand
		M21.942	Unspecified acquired deformity of hand, left hand
		M21.949	Unspecified acquired deformity of hand, unspecified hand
736.Ø1	CUBITUS VALGUS	**M21.Ø21**	Valgus deformity, not elsewhere classified, right elbow
		M21.Ø22	Valgus deformity, not elsewhere classified, left elbow
		M21.Ø29	Valgus deformity, not elsewhere classified, unsp elbow
736.Ø2	CUBITUS VARUS	**M21.121**	Varus deformity, not elsewhere classified, right elbow
		M21.122	Varus deformity, not elsewhere classified, left elbow
		M21.129	Varus deformity, not elsewhere classified, unspecified elbow
736.Ø3	VALGUS DEFORMITY OF WRIST	**M21.839**	Other specified acquired deformities of unspecified forearm
736.Ø4	VARUS DEFORMITY OF WRIST	**M21.839**	Other specified acquired deformities of unspecified forearm
736.Ø5	WRIST DROP	**M21.331**	Wrist drop, right wrist
		M21.332	Wrist drop, left wrist
		M21.339	Wrist drop, unspecified wrist
736.Ø6	CLAW HAND	**M21.511**	Acquired clawhand, right hand
		M21.512	Acquired clawhand, left hand
		M21.519	Acquired clawhand, unspecified hand
736.Ø7	CLUB HAND, ACQUIRED	**M21.521**	Acquired clubhand, right hand
		M21.522	Acquired clubhand, left hand
		M21.529	Acquired clubhand, unspecified hand
736.Ø9	OTH ACQ DEFORMITIES FOREARM EXCLUDING FINGERS	**M21.831**	Other specified acquired deformities of right forearm
		M21.832	Other specified acquired deformities of left forearm
		M21.839	Other specified acquired deformities of unspecified forearm
736.1	MALLET FINGER	**M2Ø.Ø11**	Mallet finger of right finger(s)
		M2Ø.Ø12	Mallet finger of left finger(s)
		M2Ø.Ø19	Mallet finger of unspecified finger(s)
736.2Ø	UNSPECIFIED DEFORMITY OF FINGER	**M2Ø.ØØ1**	Unspecified deformity of right finger(s)
		M2Ø.ØØ2	Unspecified deformity of left finger(s)
		M2Ø.ØØ9	Unspecified deformity of unspecified finger(s)
736.21	BOUTONNIERE DEFORMITY	**M2Ø.Ø21**	Boutonniere deformity of right finger(s)
		M2Ø.Ø22	Boutonniere deformity of left finger(s)
		M2Ø.Ø29	Boutonniere deformity of unspecified finger(s)
736.22	SWAN-NECK DEFORMITY	**M2Ø.Ø31**	Swan-neck deformity of right finger(s)
		M2Ø.Ø32	Swan-neck deformity of left finger(s)
		M2Ø.Ø39	Swan-neck deformity of unspecified finger(s)
736.29	OTHER ACQUIRED DEFORMITY OF FINGER	**M2Ø.Ø91**	Other deformity of right finger(s)
		M2Ø.Ø92	Other deformity of left finger(s)
		M2Ø.Ø99	Other deformity of finger(s), unspecified finger(s)
736.3Ø	UNSPECIFIED ACQUIRED DEFORMITY OF HIP	**M21.951**	Unspecified acquired deformity of right thigh
		M21.952	Unspecified acquired deformity of left thigh
		M21.959	Unspecified acquired deformity of unspecified thigh
736.31	COXA VALGA	**M21.Ø51**	Valgus deformity, not elsewhere classified, right hip
		M21.Ø52	Valgus deformity, not elsewhere classified, left hip
		M21.Ø59	Valgus deformity, not elsewhere classified, unspecified hip
736.32	COXA VARA	**M21.151**	Varus deformity, not elsewhere classified, right hip
		M21.152	Varus deformity, not elsewhere classified, left hip
		M21.159	Varus deformity, not elsewhere classified, unspecified
736.39	OTHER ACQUIRED DEFORMITIES OF HIP	**M21.851**	Other specified acquired deformities of right thigh
		M21.852	Other specified acquired deformities of left thigh
		M21.859	Other specified acquired deformities of unspecified thigh
736.41	GENU VALGUM	**M21.Ø61**	Valgus deformity, not elsewhere classified, right knee
		M21.Ø62	Valgus deformity, not elsewhere classified, left knee
		M21.Ø69	Valgus deformity, not elsewhere classified, unspecified knee
736.42	GENU VARUM	**M21.161**	Varus deformity, not elsewhere classified, right knee
		M21.162	Varus deformity, not elsewhere classified, left knee
		M21.169	Varus deformity, not elsewhere classified, unspecified knee
736.5	GENU RECURVATUM	**M21.869**	Oth acquired deformities of unspecified lower leg
736.6	OTHER ACQUIRED DEFORMITIES OF KNEE	**M21.861**	Other specified acquired deformities of right lower leg
		M21.862	Other specified acquired deformities of left lower leg
		M21.869	Oth acquired deformities of unspecified lower leg
736.7Ø	UNSPECIFIED DEFORMITY OF ANKLE AND FOOT ACQUIRED	**M21.961**	Unspecified acquired deformity of right lower leg
		M21.962	Unspecified acquired deformity of left lower leg
		M21.969	Unspecified acquired deformity of unspecified lower leg
736.71	ACQUIRED EQUINOVARUS DEFORMITY	**M21.17**[1,2,9]	Varus deformity, not elsewhere classified, ankle
		M21.54[1,2,9]	Acquired clubfoot, foot
			6th Character meanings for codes as indicated ***1 Right*** ***2 Left*** ***9 Unspecified***
736.72	EQUINUS DEFORMITY OF FOOT, ACQUIRED	**M21.6X9**	Other acquired deformities of unspecified foot
736.73	CAVUS DEFORMITY OF FOOT, ACQUIRED	**M21.6X9**	Other acquired deformities of unspecified foot
736.74	CLAW FOOT, ACQUIRED	**M21.531**	Acquired clawfoot, right foot
		M21.532	Acquired clawfoot, left foot
		M21.539	Acquired clawfoot, unspecified foot

ICD-9-CM		ICD-10-CM	
736.75	CAVOVARUS DEFORMITY OF FOOT ACQUIRED	**M21.6X9**	Other acquired deformities of unspecified foot
736.76	OTHER ACQUIRED CALCANEUS DEFORMITY	**M21.6X9**	Other acquired deformities of unspecified foot
736.79	OTHER ACQUIRED DEFORMITY OF ANKLE AND FOOT OTHER	**M21.Ø7**[1,2,9]	Valgus deformity, not elsewhere classified, ankle
		M21.37[1,2,9]	Foot drop, foot
		M21.6X[1,2,9]	Other acquired deformities of foot
			6th Character meanings for codes as indicated ***1 Right*** ***2 Left*** ***9 Unspecified***
736.81	UNEQUAL LEG LENGTH	**M21.751**	Unequal limb length (acquired), right femur
		M21.752	Unequal limb length (acquired), left femur
		M21.759	Unequal limb length (acquired), unspecified femur
		M21.761	Unequal limb length (acquired), right tibia
		M21.762	Unequal limb length (acquired), left tibia
		M21.763	Unequal limb length (acquired), right fibula
		M21.764	Unequal limb length (acquired), left fibula
		M21.769	Unequal limb length (acquired), unspecified tibia and fibula
736.89	OTHER ACQUIRED DEFORMITY OF OTHER PARTS OF LIMB	**M21.2Ø**	Flexion deformity, unspecified site
		M21.21[1,2,9]	Flexion deformity, shoulder
		M21.22[1,2,9]	Flexion deformity, elbow
		M21.23[1,2,9]	Flexion deformity, wrist
		M21.24[1,2,9]	Flexion deformity, finger joints
		M21.25[1,2,9]	Flexion deformity, hip
		M21.26[1,2,9]	Flexion deformity, knee
		M21.27[1,2,9]	Flexion deformity, ankle and toes
		M21.7Ø	Unequal limb length (acquired), unspecified site
		M21.72[1,2,9]	Unequal limb length (acquired), humerus
		M21.731	Unequal limb length (acquired), right ulna
		M21.732	Unequal limb length (acquired), left ulna
		M21.733	Unequal limb length (acquired), right radius
		M21.734	Unequal limb length (acquired), left radius
		M21.739	Unequal limb length (acquired), unspecified ulna and radius
		M21.8Ø	Other specified acquired deformities of unspecified limb
		M21.82[1,2,9]	Other specified acquired deformities of upper arm
		M21.92[1,2,9]	Unspecified acquired deformity of upper arm
		M21.95[1,2,9]	Unspecified acquired deformity of thigh
		M21.96[1,2,9]	Unspecified acquired deformity of lower leg
			6th Character meanings for codes as indicated ***1 Right*** ***2 Left*** ***9 Unspecified***
736.9	ACQUIRED DEFORMITY OF LIMB SITE UNSPECIFIED	**M21.ØØ**	Valgus deformity, not elsewhere classified, unspecified site
		M21.1Ø	Varus deformity, not elsewhere classified, unspecified site
		M21.9Ø	Unspecified acquired deformity of unspecified limb
737.Ø	ADOLESCENT POSTURAL KYPHOSIS	**M4Ø.ØØ**	Postural kyphosis, site unspecified
737.1Ø	KYPHOSIS ACQUIRED POSTURAL	**M4Ø.ØØ**	Postural kyphosis, site unspecified
		M4Ø.Ø3	Postural kyphosis, cervicothoracic region
		M4Ø.Ø4	Postural kyphosis, thoracic region
		M4Ø.Ø5	Postural kyphosis, thoracolumbar region
		M4Ø.2Ø2	Unspecified kyphosis, cervical region
		M4Ø.2Ø3	Unspecified kyphosis, cervicothoracic region
		M4Ø.2Ø4	Unspecified kyphosis, thoracic region
		M4Ø.2Ø5	Unspecified kyphosis, thoracolumbar region
		M4Ø.2Ø9	Unspecified kyphosis, site unspecified
737.11	KYPHOSIS DUE TO RADIATION	➡ **M96.2**	Postradiation kyphosis
737.12	KYPHOSIS, POSTLAMINECTOMY	➡ **M96.3**	Postlaminectomy kyphosis
737.19	OTHER KYPHOSIS	**M4Ø.292**	Other kyphosis, cervical region
		M4Ø.293	Other kyphosis, cervicothoracic region
		M4Ø.294	Other kyphosis, thoracic region
		M4Ø.295	Other kyphosis, thoracolumbar region
		M4Ø.299	Other kyphosis, site unspecified
		M4Ø.3Ø	Flatback syndrome, site unspecified
		M4Ø.35	Flatback syndrome, thoracolumbar region
		M4Ø.36	Flatback syndrome, lumbar region
		M4Ø.37	Flatback syndrome, lumbosacral region
737.2Ø	LORDOSIS ACQUIRED POSTURAL	**M4Ø.4Ø**	Postural lordosis, site unspecified
		M4Ø.45	Postural lordosis, thoracolumbar region
		M4Ø.46	Postural lordosis, lumbar region
		M4Ø.47	Postural lordosis, lumbosacral region
737.21	LORDOSIS, POSTLAMINECTOMY	**M96.4**	Postsurgical lordosis
737.22	OTHER POSTSURGICAL LORDOSIS	**M96.4**	Postsurgical lordosis
737.29	OTHER LORDOSIS	**M4Ø.5Ø**	Lordosis, unspecified, site unspecified
		M4Ø.55	Lordosis, unspecified, thoracolumbar region
		M4Ø.56	Lordosis, unspecified, lumbar region
		M4Ø.57	Lordosis, unspecified, lumbosacral region

[Brackets] indicate valid character values for each code. Character value meanings provided for each code grouping.

ICD-9-CM		ICD-10-CM	
737.30	SCOLIOSIS , IDIOPATHIC	M41.112	Juvenile idiopathic scoliosis, cervical region
		M41.113	Juvenile idiopathic scoliosis, cervicothoracic region
		M41.114	Juvenile idiopathic scoliosis, thoracic region
		M41.115	Juvenile idiopathic scoliosis, thoracolumbar region
		M41.116	Juvenile idiopathic scoliosis, lumbar region
		M41.117	Juvenile idiopathic scoliosis, lumbosacral region
		M41.119	Juvenile idiopathic scoliosis, site unspecified
		M41.122	Adolescent idiopathic scoliosis, cervical region
		M41.123	Adolescent idiopathic scoliosis, cervicothoracic region
		M41.124	Adolescent idiopathic scoliosis, thoracic region
		M41.125	Adolescent idiopathic scoliosis, thoracolumbar region
		M41.126	Adolescent idiopathic scoliosis, lumbar region
		M41.127	Adolescent idiopathic scoliosis, lumbosacral region
		M41.129	Adolescent idiopathic scoliosis, site unspecified
		M41.20	Other idiopathic scoliosis, site unspecified
		M41.22	Other idiopathic scoliosis, cervical region
		M41.23	Other idiopathic scoliosis, cervicothoracic region
		M41.24	Other idiopathic scoliosis, thoracic region
		M41.25	Other idiopathic scoliosis, thoracolumbar region
		M41.26	Other idiopathic scoliosis, lumbar region
		M41.27	Other idiopathic scoliosis, lumbosacral region
737.31	RESOLVING INFANTILE IDIOPATHIC SCOLIOSIS	M41.00	Infantile idiopathic scoliosis, site unspecified
		M41.02	Infantile idiopathic scoliosis, cervical region
		M41.03	Infantile idiopathic scoliosis, cervicothoracic region
		M41.04	Infantile idiopathic scoliosis, thoracic region
		M41.05	Infantile idiopathic scoliosis, thoracolumbar region
		M41.06	Infantile idiopathic scoliosis, lumbar region
		M41.07	Infantile idiopathic scoliosis, lumbosacral region
		M41.08	Infantile idiopathic scoliosis, sacr/sacrocygl region
737.32	PROGRESSIVE INFANTILE IDIOPATHIC SCOLIOSIS	M41.00	Infantile idiopathic scoliosis, site unspecified
		M41.02	Infantile idiopathic scoliosis, cervical region
		M41.03	Infantile idiopathic scoliosis, cervicothoracic region
		M41.04	Infantile idiopathic scoliosis, thoracic region
		M41.05	Infantile idiopathic scoliosis, thoracolumbar region
		M41.06	Infantile idiopathic scoliosis, lumbar region
		M41.07	Infantile idiopathic scoliosis, lumbosacral region
		M41.08	Infantile idiopathic scoliosis, sacr/sacrocygl region
737.33	SCOLIOSIS DUE TO RADIATION	➡ M96.5	Postradiation scoliosis
737.34	THORACOGENIC SCOLIOSIS	M41.30	Thoracogenic scoliosis, site unspecified
		M41.34	Thoracogenic scoliosis, thoracic region
		M41.35	Thoracogenic scoliosis, thoracolumbar region
737.39	OTHER KYPHOSCOLIOSIS AND SCOLIOSIS	M41.80	Other forms of scoliosis, site unspecified
		M41.82	Other forms of scoliosis, cervical region
		M41.83	Other forms of scoliosis, cervicothoracic region
		M41.84	Other forms of scoliosis, thoracic region
		M41.85	Other forms of scoliosis, thoracolumbar region
		M41.86	Other forms of scoliosis, lumbar region
		M41.87	Other forms of scoliosis, lumbosacral region
		M41.9	Scoliosis, unspecified
737.40	UNSPEC CURVATURE SPINE ASSOCIATED W/OTHER COND	◘ A18.01	Tuberculosis of spine
		M43.8X9	Other specified deforming dorsopathies, site unspecified
737.41	KYPHOSIS ASSOCIATED WITH OTHER CONDITION	M40.10	Other secondary kyphosis, site unspecified
		M40.12	Other secondary kyphosis, cervical region
		M40.13	Other secondary kyphosis, cervicothoracic region
		M40.14	Other secondary kyphosis, thoracic region
		M40.15	Other secondary kyphosis, thoracolumbar region
737.42	LORDOSIS ASSOCIATED WITH OTHER CONDITION	M40.50	Lordosis, unspecified, site unspecified
		M40.55	Lordosis, unspecified, thoracolumbar region
		M40.56	Lordosis, unspecified, lumbar region
		M40.57	Lordosis, unspecified, lumbosacral region
737.43	SCOLIOSIS ASSOCIATED WITH OTHER CONDITION	M41.40	Neuromuscular scoliosis, site unspecified
		M41.41	Neuromuscular scoliosis, occipito-atlanto-axial region
		M41.42	Neuromuscular scoliosis, cervical region
		M41.43	Neuromuscular scoliosis, cervicothoracic region
		M41.44	Neuromuscular scoliosis, thoracic region
		M41.45	Neuromuscular scoliosis, thoracolumbar region
		M41.46	Neuromuscular scoliosis, lumbar region
		M41.47	Neuromuscular scoliosis, lumbosacral region
		M41.50	Other secondary scoliosis, site unspecified
		M41.52	Other secondary scoliosis, cervical region
		M41.53	Other secondary scoliosis, cervicothoracic region
		M41.54	Other secondary scoliosis, thoracic region
		M41.55	Other secondary scoliosis, thoracolumbar region
		M41.56	Other secondary scoliosis, lumbar region
		M41.57	Other secondary scoliosis, lumbosacral region

ICD-9-CM		ICD-10-CM	
737.8	OTHER CURVATURES SPINE ASSOCIATED W/OTHER CONDS	**M43.8X1**	Oth deforming dorsopathies, occipito-atlanto-axial region
		M43.8X2	Other specified deforming dorsopathies, cervical region
		M43.8X3	Oth deforming dorsopathies, cervicothoracic region
		M43.8X4	Other specified deforming dorsopathies, thoracic region
		M43.8X5	Other specified deforming dorsopathies, thoracolumbar region
		M43.8X6	Other specified deforming dorsopathies, lumbar region
		M43.8X7	Other specified deforming dorsopathies, lumbosacral region
		M43.8X8	Oth deforming dorsopathies, sacral and sacrococcygeal region
		M43.8X9	Other specified deforming dorsopathies, site unspecified
		M43.9	Deforming dorsopathy, unspecified
737.9	UNSPECIFIED CURVATURE OF SPINE	**M43.8X1**	Oth deforming dorsopathies, occipito-atlanto-axial region
		M43.8X2	Other specified deforming dorsopathies, cervical region
		M43.8X3	Oth deforming dorsopathies, cervicothoracic region
		M43.8X4	Other specified deforming dorsopathies, thoracic region
		M43.8X5	Other specified deforming dorsopathies, thoracolumbar region
		M43.8X6	Other specified deforming dorsopathies, lumbar region
		M43.8X7	Other specified deforming dorsopathies, lumbosacral region
		M43.8X8	Oth deforming dorsopathies, sacral and sacrococcygeal region
		M43.8X9	Other specified deforming dorsopathies, site unspecified
738.Ø	ACQUIRED DEFORMITY OF NOSE	➡ **M95.Ø**	Acquired deformity of nose
738.1Ø	UNSPECIFIED ACQUIRED DEFORMITY OF HEAD	**M95.2**	Other acquired deformity of head
738.11	ZYGOMATIC HYPERPLASIA	**M89.38**	Hypertrophy of bone, other site
738.12	ZYGOMATIC HYPOPLASIA	**M89.8X8**	Other specified disorders of bone, other site
738.19	OTHER SPECIFIED ACQUIRED DEFORMITY OF HEAD	**M95.2**	Other acquired deformity of head
		M99.8Ø	Other biomechanical lesions of head region
738.2	ACQUIRED DEFORMITY OF NECK	**M95.3**	Acquired deformity of neck
		M99.81	Other biomechanical lesions of cervical region
738.3	ACQUIRED DEFORMITY OF CHEST AND RIB	**M95.4**	Acquired deformity of chest and rib
		M99.82	Other biomechanical lesions of thoracic region
		M99.88	Other biomechanical lesions of rib cage
738.4	ACQUIRED SPONDYLOLISTHESIS	**M43.ØØ**	Spondylolysis, site unspecified
		M43.Ø1	Spondylolysis, occipito-atlanto-axial region
		M43.Ø2	Spondylolysis, cervical region
		M43.Ø3	Spondylolysis, cervicothoracic region
		M43.Ø4	Spondylolysis, thoracic region
		M43.Ø5	Spondylolysis, thoracolumbar region
		M43.Ø6	Spondylolysis, lumbar region
		M43.Ø7	Spondylolysis, lumbosacral region
		M43.Ø8	Spondylolysis, sacral and sacrococcygeal region
		M43.Ø9	Spondylolysis, multiple sites in spine
		M43.1Ø	Spondylolisthesis, site unspecified
		M43.11	Spondylolisthesis, occipito-atlanto-axial region
		M43.12	Spondylolisthesis, cervical region
		M43.13	Spondylolisthesis, cervicothoracic region
		M43.14	Spondylolisthesis, thoracic region
		M43.15	Spondylolisthesis, thoracolumbar region
		M43.16	Spondylolisthesis, lumbar region
		M43.17	Spondylolisthesis, lumbosacral region
		M43.18	Spondylolisthesis, sacral and sacrococcygeal region
		M43.19	Spondylolisthesis, multiple sites in spine
738.5	OTHER ACQUIRED DEFORMITY OF BACK OR SPINE	**M99.83**	Other biomechanical lesions of lumbar region
		M99.84	Other biomechanical lesions of sacral region
738.6	ACQUIRED DEFORMITY OF PELVIS	**M95.5**	Acquired deformity of pelvis
		M99.85	Other biomechanical lesions of pelvic region
		M99.89	Other biomechanical lesions of abdomen and other regions
738.7	CAULIFLOWER EAR	**M95.1Ø**	Cauliflower ear, unspecified ear
		M95.11	Cauliflower ear, right ear
		M95.12	Cauliflower ear, left ear
738.8	ACQUIRED MUSCULOSKELETAL DEFORMITY OTH SPEC SITE	**M95.8**	Oth acquired deformities of musculoskeletal system
		M99.86	Other biomechanical lesions of lower extremity
		M99.87	Other biomechanical lesions of upper extremity
		M99.89	Other biomechanical lesions of abdomen and other regions
738.9	ACQUIRED MUSCULOSKELETAL DEFORMITY UNSPEC SITE	**M95.9**	Acquired deformity of musculoskeletal system, unspecified
		M99.9	Biomechanical lesion, unspecified
739.Ø	NONALLOPATHIC LESION OF HEAD REGION NEC	**M99.ØØ**	Segmental and somatic dysfunction of head region
739.1	NONALLOPATHIC LESION OF CERVICAL REGION NEC	**M99.Ø1**	Segmental and somatic dysfunction of cervical region
739.2	NONALLOPATHIC LESION OF THORACIC REGION NEC	**M99.Ø2**	Segmental and somatic dysfunction of thoracic region
739.3	NONALLOPATHIC LESION OF LUMBAR REGION NEC	**M99.Ø3**	Segmental and somatic dysfunction of lumbar region
739.4	NONALLOPATHIC LESION OF SACRAL REGION NEC	**M99.Ø4**	Segmental and somatic dysfunction of sacral region
739.5	NONALLOPATHIC LESION OF PELVIC REGION NEC	**M99.Ø5**	Segmental and somatic dysfunction of pelvic region
739.6	NONALLOPATHIC LESION OF LOWER EXTREMITIES NEC	**M99.Ø6**	Segmental and somatic dysfunction of lower extremity
739.7	NONALLOPATHIC LESION OF UPPER EXTREMITIES NEC	**M99.Ø7**	Segmental and somatic dysfunction of upper extremity
739.8	NONALLOPATHIC LESION OF RIB CAGE NEC	**M99.Ø8**	Segmental and somatic dysfunction of rib cage
739.9	NONALLOPATHIC LESION OF ABDOMEN&OTHER SITES NEC	**M99.Ø9**	Segmental and somatic dysfunction of abdomen and oth regions

[Brackets] indicate valid character values for each code. Character value meanings provided for each code grouping.

Congenital Anomalies

ICD-9-CM			ICD-10-CM	
740.0	ANENCEPHALUS	➡	Q00.0	Anencephaly
740.1	CRANIORACHISCHISIS	➡	Q00.1	Craniorachischisis
740.2	INIENCEPHALY	➡	Q00.2	Iniencephaly
741.00	SPINA BIFIDA W/HYDROCEPHALUS UNSPECIFIED REGION		Q05.4 Q05.9 Q07.02 Q07.03	Unspecified spina bifida with hydrocephalus Spina bifida, unspecified Arnold-Chiari syndrome with hydrocephalus Arnold-Chiari syndrome with spina bifida and hydrocephalus
741.01	SPINA BIFIDA WITH HYDROCEPHALUS CERVICAL REGION	➡	Q05.0	Cervical spina bifida with hydrocephalus
741.02	SPINA BIFIDA WITH HYDROCEPHALUS DORSAL REGION	➡	Q05.1	Thoracic spina bifida with hydrocephalus
741.03	SPINA BIFIDA WITH HYDROCEPHALUS LUMBAR REGION		Q05.2 Q05.3	Lumbar spina bifida with hydrocephalus Sacral spina bifida with hydrocephalus
741.90	SPINA BIFIDA W/O MENTION HYDROCEPHALUS UNS RGN		Q05.8 Q05.9 Q07.00 Q07.01	Sacral spina bifida without hydrocephalus Spina bifida, unspecified Arnold-Chiari syndrome without spina bifida or hydrocephalus Arnold-Chiari syndrome with spina bifida
741.91	SPINA BIFIDA W/O MENTION HYDROCEPHALUS CERV RGN	➡	Q05.5	Cervical spina bifida without hydrocephalus
741.92	SPINA BIFIDA W/O MENTION HYDROCEPHALUS DORS RGN	➡	Q05.6	Thoracic spina bifida without hydrocephalus
741.93	SPINA BIFIDA W/O MENTION HYDROCEPHALUS LUMB RGN	➡	Q05.7	Lumbar spina bifida without hydrocephalus
742.0	ENCEPHALOCELE		Q01.0 Q01.1 Q01.2 Q01.8 Q01.9	Frontal encephalocele Nasofrontal encephalocele Occipital encephalocele Encephalocele of other sites Encephalocele, unspecified
742.1	MICROCEPHALUS	➡	Q02	Microcephaly
742.2	CONGENITAL REDUCTION DEFORMITIES OF BRAIN		Q04.0 Q04.1 Q04.2 Q04.3	Congenital malformations of corpus callosum Arhinencephaly Holoprosencephaly Other reduction deformities of brain
742.3	CONGENITAL HYDROCEPHALUS		Q03.0 Q03.1 Q03.8 Q03.9	Malformations of aqueduct of Sylvius Atresia of foramina of Magendie and Luschka Other congenital hydrocephalus Congenital hydrocephalus, unspecified
742.4	OTHER SPECIFIED CONGENITAL ANOMALIES OF BRAIN		Q04.4 Q04.5 Q04.6 Q04.8	Septo-optic dysplasia of brain Megalencephaly Congenital cerebral cysts Other specified congenital malformations of brain
742.51	DIASTEMATOMYELIA	➡	Q06.2	Diastematomyelia
742.53	HYDROMYELIA	➡	Q06.4	Hydromyelia
742.59	OTHER SPECIFIED CONGENITAL ANOMALY SPINAL CORD		Q06.0 Q06.1 Q06.3 Q06.8 Q06.9	Amyelia Hypoplasia and dysplasia of spinal cord Other congenital cauda equina malformations Other specified congenital malformations of spinal cord Congenital malformation of spinal cord, unspecified
742.8	OTHER SPEC CONGENITAL ANOMALIES NERVOUS SYSTEM		G90.1 Q07.8	Familial dysautonomia [Riley-Day] Other specified congenital malformations of nervous system
742.9	UNSPEC CONGN ANOMALY BRAIN SP CORD&NERV SYSTEM		Q04.9 Q06.9 Q07.9	Congenital malformation of brain, unspecified Congenital malformation of spinal cord, unspecified Congenital malformation of nervous system, unspecified
743.00	UNSPECIFIED CLINICAL ANOPHTHALMOS	➡	Q11.1	Other anophthalmos
743.03	CYSTIC EYEBALL, CONGENITAL	➡	Q11.0	Cystic eyeball
743.06	CRYPTOPHTHALMOS		Q11.2	Microphthalmos
743.10	UNSPECIFIED MICROPHTHALMOS		Q11.2	Microphthalmos
743.11	SIMPLE MICROPHTHALMOS		Q11.2	Microphthalmos
743.12	MICROPHTHALMOS ASSOC W/OTH ANOMALIES EYE&ADNEXA		Q11.2	Microphthalmos
743.20	UNSPECIFIED BUPHTHALMOS		Q15.0	Congenital glaucoma
743.21	SIMPLE BUPHTHALMOS		Q15.0	Congenital glaucoma
743.22	BUPHTHALMOS ASSOCIATED WITH OTHER OCULAR ANOMALY		Q15.0	Congenital glaucoma
743.30	UNSPECIFIED CONGENITAL CATARACT		Q12.0	Congenital cataract
743.31	CONGENITAL CAPSULAR AND SUBCAPSULAR CATARACT		Q12.0	Congenital cataract
743.32	CONGENITAL CORTICAL AND ZONULAR CATARACT		Q12.0	Congenital cataract
743.33	CONGENITAL NUCLEAR CATARACT		Q12.0	Congenital cataract
743.34	CONGENITAL TOTAL AND SUBTOTAL CATARACT		Q12.0	Congenital cataract
743.35	CONGENITAL APHAKIA	➡	Q12.3	Congenital aphakia
743.36	CONGENITAL ANOMALIES OF LENS SHAPE		Q12.2 Q12.4 Q12.8	Coloboma of lens Spherophakia Other congenital lens malformations
743.37	CONGENITAL ECTOPIC LENS	➡	Q12.1	Congenital displaced lens
743.39	OTHER CONGENITAL CATARACT AND LENS ANOMALIES		Q12.9	Congenital lens malformation, unspecified
743.41	CONGENITAL ANOMALY OF CORNEAL SIZE AND SHAPE		Q13.4	Other congenital corneal malformations
743.42	CONGENITAL CORNEAL OPACITY INTERFERING W/VISION		Q13.3	Congenital corneal opacity
743.43	OTHER CONGENITAL CORNEAL OPACITY		Q13.3	Congenital corneal opacity

ICD-9-CM		ICD-10-CM	
743.44	SPEC CONGN ANOMALY ANT CHAMB CHAMB ANG&REL STRCT	**Q13.4** **Q13.81** **Q13.9** **Q15.Ø**	Other congenital corneal malformations Rieger's anomaly Congenital malformation of anterior segment of eye, unsp Congenital glaucoma
743.45	ANIRIDIA	➡ **Q13.1**	Absence of iris
743.46	OTHER SPEC CONGENITAL ANOMALY IRIS&CILIARY BODY	**Q13.Ø** **Q13.2**	Coloboma of iris Other congenital malformations of iris
743.47	SPECIFIED CONGENITAL ANOMALY OF SCLERA	**Q13.5**	Blue sclera
743.48	MULTIPLE&COMB CONGEN ANOMALIES ANT SEGMENT EYE	**Q13.89**	Other congenital malformations of anterior segment of eye
743.49	OTHER CONGENITAL ANOMALY ANTERIOR SEGMENT EYE	**Q13.89** **Q13.9**	Other congenital malformations of anterior segment of eye Congenital malformation of anterior segment of eye, unsp
743.51	VITREOUS ANOMALY, CONGENITAL	➡ **Q14.Ø**	Congenital malformation of vitreous humor
743.52	FUNDUS COLOBOMA	**Q14.8**	Other congenital malformations of posterior segment of eye
743.53	CONGENITAL CHORIORETINAL DEGENERATION	**Q14.3**	Congenital malformation of choroid
743.54	CONGENITAL FOLDS&CYSTS POSTERIOR SEGMENT EYE	**Q14.8**	Other congenital malformations of posterior segment of eye
743.55	CONGENITAL MACULAR CHANGE	**Q14.8**	Other congenital malformations of posterior segment of eye
743.56	OTHER CONGENITAL RETINAL CHANGES	**Q14.1**	Congenital malformation of retina
743.57	SPECIFIED CONGENITAL ANOMALIES OF OPTIC DISC	**Q14.2**	Congenital malformation of optic disc
743.58	CONGEN VASCULAR ANOMALIES POSTERIOR SEGMENT EYE	**Q14.8**	Other congenital malformations of posterior segment of eye
743.59	OTHER CONGENITAL ANOMALIES POSTERIOR SEGMENT EYE	**Q14.8** **Q14.9**	Other congenital malformations of posterior segment of eye Congenital malformation of posterior segment of eye, unsp
743.61	CONGENITAL PTOSIS OF EYELID	➡ **Q1Ø.Ø**	Congenital ptosis
743.62	CONGENITAL DEFORMITY OF EYELID	**Q1Ø.1** **Q1Ø.2** **Q1Ø.3**	Congenital ectropion Congenital entropion Other congenital malformations of eyelid
743.63	OTHER SPECIFIED CONGENITAL ANOMALY OF EYELID	**Q1Ø.3**	Other congenital malformations of eyelid
743.64	SPECIFIED CONGENITAL ANOMALY OF LACRIMAL GLAND	**Q1Ø.6**	Other congenital malformations of lacrimal apparatus
743.65	SPECIFIED CONGENITAL ANOMALY LACRIMAL PASSAGES	**Q1Ø.4** **Q1Ø.5** **Q1Ø.6**	Absence and agenesis of lacrimal apparatus Congenital stenosis and stricture of lacrimal duct Other congenital malformations of lacrimal apparatus
743.66	SPECIFIED CONGENITAL ANOMALY OF ORBIT	**Q1Ø.7**	Congenital malformation of orbit
743.69	OTH CONGEN ANOMALIES EYELD LACRIMAL SYSTEM&ORBIT	**Q1Ø.3** **Q1Ø.6** **Q1Ø.7**	Other congenital malformations of eyelid Other congenital malformations of lacrimal apparatus Congenital malformation of orbit
743.8	OTHER SPECIFIED CONGENITAL ANOMALIES OF EYE	**Q11.3** **Q15.8**	Macrophthalmos Other specified congenital malformations of eye
743.9	UNSPECIFIED CONGENITAL ANOMALY OF EYE	➡ **Q15.9**	Congenital malformation of eye, unspecified
744.ØØ	UNSPEC CONGEN ANOMALY EAR CAUS IMPAIR HEARING	**Q16.9**	Congen malform of ear causing impairment of hearing, unsp
744.Ø1	CONGEN ABSENCE EXTERNAL EAR CAUS IMPAIR HEARING	➡ **Q16.Ø**	Congenital absence of (ear) auricle
744.Ø2	OTH CONGN ANOMALY EXT EAR CAUS IMPAIR HEARING	**Q16.1**	Congenital absence, atresia and stricture of auditory canal
744.Ø3	ANOMALY OF MIDDLE EAR-EXCEPT OSSICLES	➡ **Q16.4**	Other congenital malformations of middle ear
744.Ø4	CONGENITAL ANOMALIES OF EAR OSSICLES	➡ **Q16.3**	Congenital malformation of ear ossicles
744.Ø5	CONGENITAL ANOMALIES OF INNER EAR	➡ **Q16.5**	Congenital malformation of inner ear
744.Ø9	OTH CONGEN ANOMALIES EAR CAUS IMPAIRMENT HEARING	**Q16.9**	Congen malform of ear causing impairment of hearing, unsp
744.1	CONGENITAL ANOMALIES OF ACCESSORY AURICLE	➡ **Q17.Ø**	Accessory auricle
744.21	CONGENITAL ABSENCE OF EAR LOBE	**Q17.8**	Other specified congenital malformations of ear
744.22	MACROTIA	➡ **Q17.1**	Macrotia
744.23	MICROTIA	➡ **Q17.2**	Microtia
744.24	SPECIFIED CONGENITAL ANOMALY OF EUSTACHIAN TUBE	**Q16.2**	Absence of eustachian tube
744.29	OTHER CONGENITAL ANOMALY OF EAR	**Q17.3** **Q17.4** **Q17.5** **Q17.8**	Other misshapen ear Misplaced ear Prominent ear Other specified congenital malformations of ear
744.3	UNSPECIFIED CONGENITAL ANOMALY OF EAR	➡ **Q17.9**	Congenital malformation of ear, unspecified
744.41	CONGENITAL BRANCHIAL CLEFT SINUS OR FISTULA	**Q18.Ø**	Sinus, fistula and cyst of branchial cleft
744.42	CONGENITAL BRANCHIAL CLEFT CYST	**Q18.Ø**	Sinus, fistula and cyst of branchial cleft
744.43	CONGENITAL CERVICAL AURICLE	**Q18.2**	Other branchial cleft malformations
744.46	CONGENITAL PREAURICULAR SINUS OR FISTULA	**Q18.1**	Preauricular sinus and cyst
744.47	CONGENITAL PREAURICULAR CYST	**Q18.1**	Preauricular sinus and cyst
744.49	BRANCHIAL CLEFT CYST/FISTULA-PREAURICULAR SINUS	**Q18.2**	Other branchial cleft malformations
744.5	CONGENITAL WEBBING OF NECK	➡ **Q18.3**	Webbing of neck
744.81	MACROCHEILIA	➡ **Q18.6**	Macrocheilia
744.82	MICROCHEILIA	➡ **Q18.7**	Microcheilia
744.83	MACROSTOMIA	➡ **Q18.4**	Macrostomia
744.84	MICROSTOMIA	➡ **Q18.5**	Microstomia
744.89	OTHER SPECIFIED CONGENITAL ANOMALY OF FACE&NECK	➡ **Q18.8**	Other specified congenital malformations of face and neck
744.9	UNSPECIFIED CONGENITAL ANOMALY OF FACE AND NECK	➡ **Q18.9**	Congenital malformation of face and neck, unspecified
745.Ø	COMMON TRUNCUS	➡ **Q2Ø.Ø**	Common arterial trunk
745.1Ø	COMPLETE TRANSPOSITION OF GREAT VESSELS	**Q2Ø.3**	Discordant ventriculoarterial connection
745.11	TRANSPOSITION GREAT VES DBL OUTLET RIGHT VENT	➡ **Q2Ø.1**	Double outlet right ventricle

ICD-9-CM			ICD-10-CM	
745.12	CORRECTED TRANSPOSITION OF GREAT VESSELS		Q20.5	Discordant atrioventricular connection
745.19	OTHER TRANSPOSITION OF GREAT VESSELS		Q20.2	Double outlet left ventricle
			Q20.3	Discordant ventriculoarterial connection
			Q20.8	Oth congenital malform of cardiac chambers and connections
745.2	TETRALOGY OF FALLOT	➡	Q21.3	Tetralogy of Fallot
745.3	COMMON VENTRICLE ANOMALIES	➡	Q20.4	Double inlet ventricle
745.4	VENTRICULAR SEPTAL DEFECT	➡	Q21.0	Ventricular septal defect
745.5	OSTIUM SECUNDUM TYPE ATRIAL SEPTAL DEFECT	➡	Q21.1	Atrial septal defect
745.60	UNSPEC TYPE CONGENITAL ENDOCARDIAL CUSHN DEFECT		Q21.2	Atrioventricular septal defect
745.61	OSTIUM PRIMUM DEFECT		Q21.2	Atrioventricular septal defect
745.69	OTHER CONGENITAL ENDOCARDIAL CUSHION DEFECT		Q21.2	Atrioventricular septal defect
745.7	COR BILOCULARE		Q20.8	Oth congenital malform of cardiac chambers and connections
745.8	OTH DEFECTS OF SEPTAL CLOSURE		Q20.6	Isomerism of atrial appendages
			Q20.8	Oth congenital malform of cardiac chambers and connections
			Q21.4	Aortopulmonary septal defect
			Q21.8	Other congenital malformations of cardiac septa
745.9	UNSPECIFIED CONGENITAL DEFECT OF SEPTAL CLOSURE	➡	Q21.9	Congenital malformation of cardiac septum, unspecified
746.00	UNSPECIFIED CONGENITAL PULMONARY VALVE ANOMALY		Q22.3	Other congenital malformations of pulmonary valve
746.01	CONGENITAL ATRESIA OF PULMONARY VALVE	➡	Q22.0	Pulmonary valve atresia
746.02	CONGENITAL STENOSIS OF PULMONARY VALVE	➡	Q22.1	Congenital pulmonary valve stenosis
746.09	OTHER CONGENITAL ANOMALIES OF PULMONARY VALVE		Q22.2	Congenital pulmonary valve insufficiency
746.1	CONGENITAL TRICUSPID ATRESIA AND STENOSIS		Q22.4	Congenital tricuspid stenosis
			Q22.6	Hypoplastic right heart syndrome
			Q22.8	Other congenital malformations of tricuspid valve
			Q22.9	Congenital malformation of tricuspid valve, unspecified
746.2	EBSTEINS ANOMALY	➡	Q22.5	Ebstein's anomaly
746.3	CONGENITAL STENOSIS OF AORTIC VALVE	➡	Q23.0	Congenital stenosis of aortic valve
746.4	CONGENITAL INSUFFICIENCY OF AORTIC VALVE	➡	Q23.1	Congenital insufficiency of aortic valve
746.5	CONGENITAL MITRAL STENOSIS	➡	Q23.2	Congenital mitral stenosis
746.6	CONGENITAL MITRAL INSUFFICIENCY	➡	Q23.3	Congenital mitral insufficiency
746.7	HYPOPLASTIC LEFT HEART SYNDROME	➡	Q23.4	Hypoplastic left heart syndrome
746.81	CONGENITAL SUBAORTIC STENOSIS	➡	Q24.4	Congenital subaortic stenosis
746.82	COR TRIATRIATUM	➡	Q24.2	Cor triatriatum
746.83	CONGENITAL INFUNDIBULAR PULMONIC STENOSIS	➡	Q24.3	Pulmonary infundibular stenosis
746.84	CONGENITAL OBSTRUCTIVE ANOMALIES OF HEART NEC		Q24.8	Other specified congenital malformations of heart
746.85	CONGENITAL CORONARY ARTERY ANOMALY		Q24.5	Malformation of coronary vessels
746.86	CONGENITAL HEART BLOCK	➡	Q24.6	Congenital heart block
746.87	CONGENITAL MALPOSITION OF HEART AND CARDIAC APEX		Q24.0	Dextrocardia
			Q24.1	Levocardia
			Q24.8	Other specified congenital malformations of heart
746.89	OTHER SPECIFIED CONGENITAL ANOMALY HEART OTHER		Q23.8	Other congenital malformations of aortic and mitral valves
			Q23.9	Congenital malformation of aortic and mitral valves, unsp
			Q24.8	Other specified congenital malformations of heart
746.9	UNSPECIFIED CONGENITAL ANOMALY OF HEART		Q20.9	Congenital malform of cardiac chambers and connections, unsp
			Q24.9	Congenital malformation of heart, unspecified
747.0	PATENT DUCTUS ARTERIOSUS	➡	Q25.0	Patent ductus arteriosus
747.10	COARCTATION OF AORTA PREDUCTAL POSTDUCTAL	➡	Q25.1	Coarctation of aorta
747.11	CONGENITAL INTERRUPTION OF AORTIC ARCH		Q25.2	Atresia of aorta
747.20	UNSPECIFIED CONGENITAL ANOMALY OF AORTA		Q25.4	Other congenital malformations of aorta
747.21	CONGENITAL ANOMALY OF AORTIC ARCH		Q25.4	Other congenital malformations of aorta
747.22	CONGENITAL ATRESIA AND STENOSIS OF AORTA		Q25.2	Atresia of aorta
			Q25.3	Supravalvular aortic stenosis
747.29	OTHER CONGENITAL ANOMALY OF AORTA OTHER		Q25.4	Other congenital malformations of aorta
			Q25.8	Other congenital malformations of other great arteries
			Q25.9	Congenital malformation of great arteries, unspecified
747.31	PULMONARY ARTERY COARCTATION AND ATRESIA		Q25.5	Atresia of pulmonary artery
			Q25.71	Coarctation of pulmonary artery
747.32	PULMONARY ARTERIOVENOUS MALFORMATION		Q25.72	Congenital pulmonary arteriovenous malformation
747.39	OTH ANOMALIES PULMONARY ART PULMONARY CIRC		Q25.6	Stenosis of pulmonary artery
			Q25.79	Other congenital malformations of pulmonary artery
747.40	CONGENITAL ANOMALY OF GREAT VEINS UNSPECIFIED		Q26.9	Congenital malformation of great vein, unspecified
747.41	TOTAL CONGEN ANOMALOUS PULMONARY VENOUS CONNECT	➡	Q26.2	Total anomalous pulmonary venous connection
747.42	PART CONGEN ANOMALOUS PULMONARY VENOUS CONNECT		Q26.3	Partial anomalous pulmonary venous connection
			Q26.4	Anomalous pulmonary venous connection, unspecified
747.49	OTHER CONGENITAL ANOMALIES OF GREAT VEINS		Q26.0	Congenital stenosis of vena cava
			Q26.1	Persistent left superior vena cava
			Q26.8	Other congenital malformations of great veins
747.5	CONGENITAL ABSENCE/HYPOPLASIA UMBILICAL ARTERY	➡	Q27.0	Congenital absence and hypoplasia of umbilical artery
747.60	CONGEN ANOMALY PERIPH VASC SYSTEM UNSPEC SITE		Q27.9	Congenital malformation of peripheral vascular system, unsp

ICD-9-CM		ICD-10-CM	
747.61	CONGENITAL GASTROINTESTINAL VESSEL ANOMALY	Q26.5	Anomalous portal venous connection
		Q26.6	Portal vein-hepatic artery fistula
		Q27.33	Arteriovenous malformation of digestive system vessel
747.62	CONGENITAL RENAL VESSEL ANOMALY	Q27.1	Congenital renal artery stenosis
		Q27.2	Other congenital malformations of renal artery
		Q27.34	Arteriovenous malformation of renal vessel
747.63	CONGENITAL UPPER LIMB VESSEL ANOMALY	➡ Q27.31	Arteriovenous malformation of vessel of upper limb
747.64	CONGENITAL LOWER LIMB VESSEL ANOMALY	➡ Q27.32	Arteriovenous malformation of vessel of lower limb
747.69	CONGEN ANOMALY OTH SPEC SITE PERIPH VASC SYSTEM	Q27.39	Arteriovenous malformation, other site
		Q27.8	Oth congenital malformations of peripheral vascular system
747.81	CONGENITAL ANOMALY OF CEREBROVASCULAR SYSTEM	Q28.2	Arteriovenous malformation of cerebral vessels
		Q28.3	Other malformations of cerebral vessels
747.82	CONGENITAL SPINAL VESSEL ANOMALY	Q27.9	Congenital malformation of peripheral vascular system, unsp
747.83	PERSISTENT FETAL CIRCULATION	➡ P29.3	Persistent fetal circulation
747.89	OTHER SPEC CONGENITAL ANOMALY CIRCULATORY SYSTEM	Q27.3Ø	Arteriovenous malformation, site unspecified
		Q27.4	Congenital phlebectasia
		Q28.Ø	Arteriovenous malformation of precerebral vessels
		Q28.1	Other malformations of precerebral vessels
		Q28.8	Oth congenital malformations of circulatory system
747.9	UNSPEC CONGENITAL ANOMALY CIRCULATORY SYSTEM	➡ Q28.9	Congenital malformation of circulatory system, unspecified
748.Ø	CONGENITAL CHOANAL ATRESIA	➡ Q3Ø.Ø	Choanal atresia
748.1	OTHER CONGENITAL ANOMALY OF NOSE	Q3Ø.1	Agenesis and underdevelopment of nose
		Q3Ø.2	Fissured, notched and cleft nose
		Q3Ø.3	Congenital perforated nasal septum
		Q3Ø.8	Other congenital malformations of nose
		Q3Ø.9	Congenital malformation of nose, unspecified
748.2	CONGENITAL WEB OF LARYNX	➡ Q31.Ø	Web of larynx
748.3	OTHER CONGENITAL ANOMALY LARYNX TRACHEA&BRONCHUS	Q31.1	Congenital subglottic stenosis
		Q31.2	Laryngeal hypoplasia
		Q31.3	Laryngocele
		Q31.5	Congenital laryngomalacia
		Q31.8	Other congenital malformations of larynx
		Q31.9	Congenital malformation of larynx, unspecified
		Q32.Ø	Congenital tracheomalacia
		Q32.1	Other congenital malformations of trachea
		Q32.2	Congenital bronchomalacia
		Q32.3	Congenital stenosis of bronchus
		Q32.4	Other congenital malformations of bronchus
748.4	CONGENITAL CYSTIC LUNG	➡ Q33.Ø	Congenital cystic lung
748.5	CONGENITAL AGENESIS HYPOPLASIA&DYSPLASIA OF LUNG	Q33.2	Sequestration of lung
		Q33.3	Agenesis of lung
		Q33.6	Congenital hypoplasia and dysplasia of lung
748.6Ø	UNSPECIFIED CONGENITAL ANOMALY OF LUNG	➡ Q33.9	Congenital malformation of lung, unspecified
748.61	CONGENITAL BRONCHIECTASIS	➡ Q33.4	Congenital bronchiectasis
748.69	OTHER CONGENITAL ANOMALY OF LUNG	Q33.1	Accessory lobe of lung
		Q33.5	Ectopic tissue in lung
		Q33.8	Other congenital malformations of lung
748.8	OTHER SPEC CONGENITAL ANOMALY RESPIRATORY SYSTEM	Q34.Ø	Anomaly of pleura
		Q34.1	Congenital cyst of mediastinum
		Q34.8	Oth congenital malformations of respiratory system
748.9	UNSPEC CONGENITAL ANOMALY RESPIRATORY SYSTEM	➡ Q34.9	Congenital malformation of respiratory system, unspecified
749.ØØ	UNSPECIFIED CLEFT PALATE	Q35.1	Cleft hard palate
		Q35.3	Cleft soft palate
		Q35.5	Cleft hard palate with cleft soft palate
		Q35.9	Cleft palate, unspecified
749.Ø1	UNILATERAL CLEFT PALATE, COMPLETE	Q35.9	Cleft palate, unspecified
749.Ø2	UNILATERAL CLEFT PALATE, INCOMPLETE	Q35.7	Cleft uvula
		Q35.9	Cleft palate, unspecified
749.Ø3	BILATERAL CLEFT PALATE, COMPLETE	Q35.9	Cleft palate, unspecified
749.Ø4	BILATERAL CLEFT PALATE, INCOMPLETE	Q35.9	Cleft palate, unspecified
749.1Ø	UNSPECIFIED CLEFT LIP	Q36.9	Cleft lip, unilateral
749.11	UNILATERAL CLEFT LIP, COMPLETE	Q36.1	Cleft lip, median
		Q36.9	Cleft lip, unilateral
749.12	UNILATERAL CLEFT LIP, INCOMPLETE	Q36.9	Cleft lip, unilateral
749.13	BILATERAL CLEFT LIP, COMPLETE	Q36.Ø	Cleft lip, bilateral
749.14	BILATERAL CLEFT LIP, INCOMPLETE	Q36.Ø	Cleft lip, bilateral
749.2Ø	UNSPECIFIED CLEFT PALATE WITH CLEFT LIP	Q37.9	Unspecified cleft palate with unilateral cleft lip
749.21	UNILATERAL CLEFT PALATE WITH CLEFT LIP COMPLETE	Q37.1	Cleft hard palate with unilateral cleft lip
		Q37.3	Cleft soft palate with unilateral cleft lip
		Q37.5	Cleft hard and soft palate with unilateral cleft lip
		Q37.9	Unspecified cleft palate with unilateral cleft lip
749.22	UNILATERAL CLEFT PALATE W/CLEFT LIP INCOMPLETE	Q37.1	Cleft hard palate with unilateral cleft lip
		Q37.3	Cleft soft palate with unilateral cleft lip
		Q37.5	Cleft hard and soft palate with unilateral cleft lip
		Q37.9	Unspecified cleft palate with unilateral cleft lip

[Brackets] indicate valid character values for each code. Character value meanings provided for each code grouping.

ICD-9-CM		ICD-10-CM	
749.23	BILATERAL CLEFT PALATE WITH CLEFT LIP COMPLETE	Q37.Ø Q37.2 Q37.4 Q37.8	Cleft hard palate with bilateral cleft lip Cleft soft palate with bilateral cleft lip Cleft hard and soft palate with bilateral cleft lip Unspecified cleft palate with bilateral cleft lip
749.24	BILATERAL CLEFT PALATE WITH CLEFT LIP INCOMPLETE	Q37.Ø Q37.2 Q37.4 Q37.8	Cleft hard palate with bilateral cleft lip Cleft soft palate with bilateral cleft lip Cleft hard and soft palate with bilateral cleft lip Unspecified cleft palate with bilateral cleft lip
749.25	OTHER COMBINATIONS OF CLEFT PALATE W/CLEFT LIP	Q37.9	Unspecified cleft palate with unilateral cleft lip
75Ø.Ø	TONGUE TIE	➡ Q38.1	Ankyloglossia
75Ø.1Ø	CONGENITAL ANOMALY OF TONGUE UNSPECIFIED	Q38.3	Other congenital malformations of tongue
75Ø.11	AGLOSSIA	Q38.3	Other congenital malformations of tongue
75Ø.12	CONGENITAL ADHESIONS OF TONGUE	Q38.3	Other congenital malformations of tongue
75Ø.13	CONGENITAL FISSURE OF TONGUE	Q38.3	Other congenital malformations of tongue
75Ø.15	MACROGLOSSIA	➡ Q38.2	Macroglossia
75Ø.16	MICROGLOSSIA	Q38.3	Other congenital malformations of tongue
75Ø.19	OTHER CONGENITAL ANOMALY OF TONGUE	Q38.3	Other congenital malformations of tongue
75Ø.21	CONGENITAL ABSENCE OF SALIVARY GLAND	Q38.4	Congenital malformations of salivary glands and ducts
75Ø.22	CONGENITAL ACCESSORY SALIVARY GLAND	Q38.4	Congenital malformations of salivary glands and ducts
75Ø.23	CONGENITAL ATRESIA, SALIVARY DUCT	Q38.4	Congenital malformations of salivary glands and ducts
75Ø.24	CONGENITAL FISTULA OF SALIVARY GLAND	Q38.4	Congenital malformations of salivary glands and ducts
75Ø.25	CONGENITAL FISTULA OF LIP	Q38.Ø	Congenital malformations of lips, not elsewhere classified
75Ø.26	OTHER SPECIFIED CONGENITAL ANOMALIES OF MOUTH	Q38.6	Other congenital malformations of mouth
75Ø.27	CONGENITAL DIVERTICULUM OF PHARYNX	➡ Q38.7	Congenital pharyngeal pouch
75Ø.29	OTHER SPECIFIED CONGENITAL ANOMALY OF PHARYNX	➡ Q38.8	Other congenital malformations of pharynx
75Ø.3	CONGEN TRACHEOESOPH FIST ESOPH ATRESIA&STENOSIS	Q39.Ø Q39.1 Q39.2 Q39.3 Q39.4	Atresia of esophagus without fistula Atresia of esophagus with tracheo-esophageal fistula Congenital tracheo-esophageal fistula without atresia Congenital stenosis and stricture of esophagus Esophageal web
75Ø.4	OTHER SPECIFIED CONGENITAL ANOMALY OF ESOPHAGUS	Q39.5 Q39.6 Q39.8 Q39.9	Congenital dilatation of esophagus Congenital diverticulum of esophagus Other congenital malformations of esophagus Congenital malformation of esophagus, unspecified
75Ø.5	CONGENITAL HYPERTROPHIC PYLORIC STENOSIS	➡ Q4Ø.Ø	Congenital hypertrophic pyloric stenosis
75Ø.6	CONGENITAL HIATUS HERNIA	➡ Q4Ø.1	Congenital hiatus hernia
75Ø.7	OTHER SPECIFIED CONGENITAL ANOMALIES OF STOMACH	Q39.5 Q4Ø.2 Q4Ø.3	Congenital dilatation of esophagus Other specified congenital malformations of stomach Congenital malformation of stomach, unspecified
75Ø.8	OTH SPEC CONGEN ANOMALIES UPPER ALIMENTARY TRACT	➡ Q4Ø.8	Oth congenital malformations of upper alimentary tract
75Ø.9	UNSPEC CONGENITAL ANOMALY UPPER ALIMENTARY TRACT	Q38.5 Q4Ø.9	Congenital malformations of palate, not elsewhere classified Congenital malformation of upper alimentary tract, unsp
751.Ø	MECKELS DIVERTICULUM	➡ Q43.Ø	Meckel's diverticulum (displaced) (hypertrophic)
751.1	CONGENITAL ATRESIA&STENOSIS OF SMALL INTESTINE	Q41.Ø Q41.1 Q41.2 Q41.8 Q41.9	Congenital absence, atresia and stenosis of duodenum Congenital absence, atresia and stenosis of jejunum Congenital absence, atresia and stenosis of ileum Congenital absence, atresia and stenosis of prt sm int Congen absence, atresia and stenosis of sm int, part unsp
751.2	CONGN ATRESIA&STENOS LG INTEST RECT&ANAL CANAL	Q42.Ø Q42.1 Q42.2 Q42.3 Q42.8 Q42.9	Congenital absence, atresia and stenosis of rectum w fistula Congen absence, atresia and stenosis of rectum w/o fistula Congenital absence, atresia and stenosis of anus w fistula Congenital absence, atresia and stenosis of anus w/o fistula Congenital absence, atresia and stenosis of prt lg int Congen absence, atresia and stenosis of lg int, part unsp
751.3	HIRSCHSPRUNGS DISEASE&OTH CONGEN FUNC D/O COLON	Q43.1 Q43.2	Hirschsprung's disease Other congenital functional disorders of colon
751.4	CONGENITAL ANOMALIES OF INTESTINAL FIXATION	➡ Q43.3	Congenital malformations of intestinal fixation
751.5	OTHER CONGENITAL ANOMALIES OF INTESTINE	Q43.4 Q43.5 Q43.6 Q43.7 Q43.8 Q43.9	Duplication of intestine Ectopic anus Congenital fistula of rectum and anus Persistent cloaca Other specified congenital malformations of intestine Congenital malformation of intestine, unspecified
751.6Ø	UNSPEC CONGENITAL ANOMALY GALLBLADDER BDS&LIVER	Q44.1 Q44.5 Q44.7	Other congenital malformations of gallbladder Other congenital malformations of bile ducts Other congenital malformations of liver
751.61	CONGENITAL BILIARY ATRESIA	Q44.2 Q44.3	Atresia of bile ducts Congenital stenosis and stricture of bile ducts
751.62	CONGENITAL CYSTIC DISEASE OF LIVER	➡ Q44.6	Cystic disease of liver
751.69	OTHER CONGENITAL ANOMALY GALLBLADDER BDS&LIVER	Q44.Ø Q44.1 Q44.4 Q44.5 Q44.7	Agenesis, aplasia and hypoplasia of gallbladder Other congenital malformations of gallbladder Choledochal cyst Other congenital malformations of bile ducts Other congenital malformations of liver

ICD-9-CM		ICD-10-CM	
751.7	CONGENITAL ANOMALIES OF PANCREAS	**Q45.0** **Q45.1** **Q45.2** **Q45.3**	Agenesis, aplasia and hypoplasia of pancreas Annular pancreas Congenital pancreatic cyst Oth congenital malformations of pancreas and pancreatic duct
751.8	OTHER SPEC CONGENITAL ANOMALIES DIGESTIVE SYSTEM	➡ **Q45.8**	Other specified congenital malformations of digestive system
751.9	UNSPECIFIED CONGENITAL ANOMALY DIGESTIVE SYSTEM	➡ **Q45.9**	Congenital malformation of digestive system, unspecified
752.0	CONGENITAL ANOMALIES OF OVARIES	**Q50.01** **Q50.02** **Q50.1** **Q50.2** **Q50.31** **Q50.32** **Q50.39**	Congenital absence of ovary, unilateral Congenital absence of ovary, bilateral Developmental ovarian cyst Congenital torsion of ovary Accessory ovary Ovarian streak Other congenital malformation of ovary
752.10	UNSPEC CONGEN ANOMALY FALLOP TUBES&BROAD LIG	**Q50.6**	Oth congenital malformations of fallop and broad ligament
752.11	EMBRYONIC CYST FALLOPIAN TUBES&BROAD LIGAMENTS	**Q50.4** **Q50.5**	Embryonic cyst of fallopian tube Embryonic cyst of broad ligament
752.19	OTH CONGEN ANOMALY FALLOP TUBES&BROAD LIGAMENTS	**Q50.6**	Oth congenital malformations of fallop and broad ligament
752.2	CONGENITAL DOUBLING OF UTERUS	**Q51.10** **Q51.11** **Q51.2**	Doubling of uterus w doubling of cervix and vagina w/o obst Doubling of uterus w doubling of cervix and vagina w obst Other doubling of uterus
752.31	AGENESIS OF UTERUS	**Q51.0**	Agenesis and aplasia of uterus
752.32	HYPOPLASIA OF UTERUS	➡ **Q51.811**	Hypoplasia of uterus
752.33	UNICORNUATE UTERUS	➡ **Q51.4**	Unicornate uterus
752.34	BICORNUATE UTERUS	➡ **Q51.3**	Bicornate uterus
752.35	SEPTATE UTERUS	**Q51.2**	Other doubling of uterus
752.36	ARCUATE UTERUS	➡ **Q51.810**	Arcuate uterus
752.39	OTHER ANOMALIES OF UTERUS	**Q51.818** **Q51.9**	Other congenital malformations of uterus Congenital malformation of uterus and cervix, unspecified
752.40	UNSPEC CONGN ANOMALY CERV VAGINA&EXT FE GENIT	**Q52.9**	Congenital malformation of female genitalia, unspecified
752.41	EMBRYONIC CYST CERV VAGINA&EXTERNAL FE GENITALIA	**Q51.6** **Q52.4**	Embryonic cyst of cervix Other congenital malformations of vagina
752.42	IMPERFORATE HYMEN	➡ **Q52.3**	Imperforate hymen
752.43	CERVICAL AGENESIS	**Q51.5**	Agenesis and aplasia of cervix
752.44	CERVICAL DUPLICATION	➡ **Q51.820**	Cervical duplication
752.45	VAGINAL AGENESIS	➡ **Q52.0**	Congenital absence of vagina
752.46	TRANSVERSE VAGINAL SEPTUM	➡ **Q52.11**	Transverse vaginal septum
752.47	LONGITUDINAL VAGINAL SEPTUM	➡ **Q52.12**	Longitudinal vaginal septum
752.49	OTH CONGEN ANOMALY CERV VAGINA&EXTERNAL FE GENIT	**Q51.0** **Q51.5** **Q51.7** **Q51.821** **Q51.828** **Q51.9** **Q52.10** **Q52.2** **Q52.4** **Q52.5** **Q52.6** **Q52.70** **Q52.71** **Q52.79** **Q52.8**	Agenesis and aplasia of uterus Agenesis and aplasia of cervix Congen fistulae betw uterus and digestive and urinary tracts Hypoplasia of cervix Other congenital malformations of cervix Congenital malformation of uterus and cervix, unspecified Doubling of vagina, unspecified Congenital rectovaginal fistula Other congenital malformations of vagina Fusion of labia Congenital malformation of clitoris Unspecified congenital malformations of vulva Congenital absence of vulva Other congenital malformations of vulva Other specified congenital malformations of female genitalia
752.51	UNDESCENDED TESTIS	**Q53.00** **Q53.01** **Q53.02** **Q53.10** **Q53.11** **Q53.12** **Q53.20** **Q53.21** **Q53.22** **Q53.9**	Ectopic testis, unspecified Ectopic testis, unilateral Ectopic testes, bilateral Unspecified undescended testicle, unilateral Abdominal testis, unilateral Ectopic perineal testis, unilateral Undescended testicle, unspecified, bilateral Abdominal testis, bilateral Ectopic perineal testis, bilateral Undescended testicle, unspecified
752.52	RETRACTILE TESTIS	➡ **Q55.22**	Retractile testis
752.61	HYPOSPADIAS	**Q54.0** **Q54.1** **Q54.2** **Q54.3** **Q54.8** **Q54.9**	Hypospadias, balanic Hypospadias, penile Hypospadias, penoscrotal Hypospadias, perineal Other hypospadias Hypospadias, unspecified
752.62	EPISPADIAS	➡ **Q64.0**	Epispadias
752.63	CONGENITAL CHORDEE	➡ **Q54.4**	Congenital chordee
752.64	MICROPENIS	➡ **Q55.62**	Hypoplasia of penis
752.65	HIDDEN PENIS	**Q55.64**	Hidden penis

ICD-9-CM		ICD-10-CM	
752.69	OTHER PENILE ANOMALIES	**Q55.5**	Congenital absence and aplasia of penis
		Q55.61	Curvature of penis (lateral)
		Q55.63	Congenital torsion of penis
		Q55.69	Other congenital malformation of penis
752.7	INDETERMINATE SEX AND PSEUDOHERMAPHRODITISM	**Q56.Ø**	Hermaphroditism, not elsewhere classified
		Q56.1	Male pseudohermaphroditism, not elsewhere classified
		Q56.2	Female pseudohermaphroditism, not elsewhere classified
		Q56.3	Pseudohermaphroditism, unspecified
		Q56.4	Indeterminate sex, unspecified
752.81	SCROTAL TRANSPOSITION	➡ **Q55.23**	Scrotal transposition
752.89	OTHER SPECIFIED ANOMALIES OF GENITAL ORGANS	**Q52.8**	Other specified congenital malformations of female genitalia
		Q55.Ø	Absence and aplasia of testis
		Q55.1	Hypoplasia of testis and scrotum
		Q55.2Ø	Unspecified congenital malformations of testis and scrotum
		Q55.21	Polyorchism
		Q55.29	Other congenital malformations of testis and scrotum
		Q55.3	Atresia of vas deferens
		Q55.4	Oth congen malform of vas def,epidid, semnl vescl & prostate
		Q55.7	Congenital vasocutaneous fistula
		Q55.8	Oth congenital malformations of male genital organs
752.9	UNSPECIFIED CONGENITAL ANOMALY OF GENITAL ORGANS	**Q52.9**	Congenital malformation of female genitalia, unspecified
		Q55.9	Congenital malformation of male genital organ, unspecified
753.Ø	CONGENITAL RENAL AGENESIS AND DYSGENESIS	**Q6Ø.Ø**	Renal agenesis, unilateral
		Q6Ø.1	Renal agenesis, bilateral
		Q6Ø.2	Renal agenesis, unspecified
		Q6Ø.3	Renal hypoplasia, unilateral
		Q6Ø.4	Renal hypoplasia, bilateral
		Q6Ø.5	Renal hypoplasia, unspecified
		Q6Ø.6	Potter's syndrome
753.1Ø	UNSPECIFIED CONGENITAL CYSTIC KIDNEY DISEASE	**Q61.ØØ**	Congenital renal cyst, unspecified
		Q61.9	Cystic kidney disease, unspecified
753.11	CONGENITAL SINGLE RENAL CYST	➡ **Q61.Ø1**	Congenital single renal cyst
753.12	CONGENITAL POLYCYSTIC KIDNEY UNSPECIFIED TYPE	➡ **Q61.3**	Polycystic kidney, unspecified
753.13	CONGENITAL POLYCYSTIC KIDNEY AUTOSOMAL DOMINANT	➡ **Q61.2**	Polycystic kidney, adult type
753.14	CONGENITAL POLYCYSTIC KIDNEY AUTOSOMAL RECESSIVE	**Q61.11**	Cystic dilatation of collecting ducts
		Q61.19	Other polycystic kidney, infantile type
753.15	CONGENITAL RENAL DYSPLASIA	➡ **Q61.4**	Renal dysplasia
753.16	CONGENITAL MEDULLARY CYSTIC KIDNEY	**Q61.5**	Medullary cystic kidney
753.17	CONGENITAL MEDULLARY SPONGE KIDNEY	**Q61.5**	Medullary cystic kidney
753.19	OTHER SPECIFIED CONGENITAL CYSTIC KIDNEY DISEASE	**Q61.Ø2**	Congenital multiple renal cysts
		Q61.8	Other cystic kidney diseases
753.2Ø	UNSPEC OBSTRUCTIVE DEFECT RENAL PELVIS&URETER	**Q62.39**	Other obstructive defects of renal pelvis and ureter
753.21	CONGENITAL OBSTRUCTION OF URETEROPELVIC JUNCTION	**Q62.11**	Congenital occlusion of ureteropelvic junction
753.22	CONGENITAL OBSTRUCTION URETEROVESICAL JUNCTION	**Q62.12**	Congenital occlusion of ureterovesical orifice
		Q62.2	Congenital megaureter
753.23	CONGENITAL URETEROCELE	**Q62.31**	Congenital ureterocele, orthotopic
		Q62.32	Cecoureterocele
753.29	OTHER OBSTRUCTIVE DEFECT OF RENAL PELVIS&URETER	**Q62.Ø**	Congenital hydronephrosis
		Q62.1Ø	Congenital occlusion of ureter, unspecified
		Q62.11	Congenital occlusion of ureteropelvic junction
753.3	OTHER SPECIFIED CONGENITAL ANOMALIES OF KIDNEY	**Q63.Ø**	Accessory kidney
		Q63.1	Lobulated, fused and horseshoe kidney
		Q63.2	Ectopic kidney
		Q63.3	Hyperplastic and giant kidney
		Q63.8	Other specified congenital malformations of kidney
		Q63.9	Congenital malformation of kidney, unspecified
753.4	OTHER SPECIFIED CONGENITAL ANOMALIES OF URETER	**Q62.4**	Agenesis of ureter
		Q62.5	Duplication of ureter
		Q62.6Ø	Malposition of ureter, unspecified
		Q62.61	Deviation of ureter
		Q62.62	Displacement of ureter
		Q62.63	Anomalous implantation of ureter
		Q62.69	Other malposition of ureter
		Q62.7	Congenital vesico-uretero-renal reflux
		Q62.8	Other congenital malformations of ureter
753.5	EXSTROPHY OF URINARY BLADDER	**Q64.1Ø**	Exstrophy of urinary bladder, unspecified
		Q64.11	Supravesical fissure of urinary bladder
		Q64.12	Cloacal extrophy of urinary bladder
		Q64.19	Other exstrophy of urinary bladder
753.6	CONGENITAL ATRESIA&STENOSIS URETHRA&BLADDER NECK	**Q64.2**	Congenital posterior urethral valves
		Q64.31	Congenital bladder neck obstruction
		Q64.32	Congenital stricture of urethra
		Q64.33	Congenital stricture of urinary meatus
		Q64.39	Other atresia and stenosis of urethra and bladder neck
753.7	CONGENITAL ANOMALIES OF URACHUS	➡ **Q64.4**	Malformation of urachus

ICD-9-CM			ICD-10-CM	
753.8	OTHER SPEC CONGENITAL ANOMALY BLADDER&URETHRA		Q64.11	Supravesical fissure of urinary bladder
			Q64.5	Congenital absence of bladder and urethra
			Q64.6	Congenital diverticulum of bladder
			Q64.7Ø	Unspecified congenital malformation of bladder and urethra
			Q64.71	Congenital prolapse of urethra
			Q64.72	Congenital prolapse of urinary meatus
			Q64.73	Congenital urethrorectal fistula
			Q64.74	Double urethra
			Q64.75	Double urinary meatus
			Q64.79	Other congenital malformations of bladder and urethra
753.9	UNSPECIFIED CONGENITAL ANOMALY OF URINARY SYSTEM		Q64.8	Other specified congenital malformations of urinary system
			Q64.9	Congenital malformation of urinary system, unspecified
754.Ø	CONGEN MUSCULOSKELETAL DEFORM SKULL FACE&JAW		Q67.Ø	Congenital facial asymmetry
			Q67.1	Congenital compression facies
			Q67.2	Dolichocephaly
			Q67.3	Plagiocephaly
			Q67.4	Other congenital deformities of skull, face and jaw
754.1	CONGN MUSCULOSKEL DEFORM STRNOCLEIDOMSTOID MUSC	➡	Q68.Ø	Congenital deformity of sternocleidomastoid muscle
754.2	CONGENITAL MUSCULOSKELETAL DEFORMITY OF SPINE		Q67.5	Congenital deformity of spine
			Q76.3	Congenital scoliosis due to congenital bony malformation
			Q76.425	Congenital lordosis, thoracolumbar region
			Q76.426	Congenital lordosis, lumbar region
			Q76.427	Congenital lordosis, lumbosacral region
			Q76.428	Congenital lordosis, sacral and sacrococcygeal region
			Q76.429	Congenital lordosis, unspecified region
754.3Ø	CONGENITAL DISLOCATION OF HIP UNILATERAL		Q65.ØØ	Congenital dislocation of unspecified hip, unilateral
			Q65.Ø1	Congenital dislocation of right hip, unilateral
			Q65.Ø2	Congenital dislocation of left hip, unilateral
			Q65.2	Congenital dislocation of hip, unspecified
754.31	CONGENITAL DISLOCATION OF HIP BILATERAL	➡	Q65.1	Congenital dislocation of hip, bilateral
754.32	CONGENITAL SUBLUXATION OF HIP UNILATERAL		Q65.3Ø	Congenital partial dislocation of unsp hip, unilateral
			Q65.31	Congenital partial dislocation of right hip, unilateral
			Q65.32	Congenital partial dislocation of left hip, unilateral
			Q65.5	Congenital partial dislocation of hip, unspecified
			Q65.6	Congenital unstable hip
754.33	CONGENITAL SUBLUXATION OF HIP BILATERAL	➡	Q65.4	Congenital partial dislocation of hip, bilateral
754.35	CONGEN DISLOCATION 1 HIP W/SUBLUXATION OTH HIP		Q65.Ø1	Congenital dislocation of right hip, unilateral *and*
			Q65.32	Congenital partial dislocation of left hip, unilateral
			Q65.Ø2	Congenital dislocation of left hip, unilateral *and*
			Q65.31	Congenital partial dislocation of right hip, unilateral
754.4Ø	CONGENITAL GENU RECURVATUM		Q68.2	Congenital deformity of knee
754.41	CONGENITAL DISLOCATION OF KNEE		Q68.2	Congenital deformity of knee
754.42	CONGENITAL BOWING OF FEMUR	➡	Q68.3	Congenital bowing of femur
754.43	CONGENITAL BOWING OF TIBIA AND FIBULA	➡	Q68.4	Congenital bowing of tibia and fibula
754.44	CONGENITAL BOWING UNSPECIFIED LONG BONES LEG	➡	Q68.5	Congenital bowing of long bones of leg, unspecified
754.5Ø	CONGENITAL TALIPES VARUS		Q66.Ø	Congenital talipes equinovarus
754.51	CONGENITAL TALIPES EQUINOVARUS		Q66.Ø	Congenital talipes equinovarus
754.52	CONGENITAL METATARSUS PRIMUS VARUS		Q66.2	Congenital metatarsus (primus) varus
754.53	CONGENITAL METATARSUS VARUS		Q66.2	Congenital metatarsus (primus) varus
754.59	OTHER CONGENITAL VARUS DEFORMITY OF FEET		Q66.1	Congenital talipes calcaneovarus
			Q66.3	Other congenital varus deformities of feet
754.6Ø	CONGENITAL TALIPES VALGUS		Q66.4	Congenital talipes calcaneovalgus
754.61	CONGENITAL PES PLANUS		Q66.5Ø	Congenital pes planus, unspecified foot
			Q66.51	Congenital pes planus, right foot
			Q66.52	Congenital pes planus, left foot
			Q66.8Ø	Congenital vertical talus deformity, unspecified foot
			Q66.81	Congenital vertical talus deformity, right foot
			Q66.82	Congenital vertical talus deformity, left foot
754.62	TALIPES CALCANEOVALGUS		Q66.4	Congenital talipes calcaneovalgus
754.69	OTHER CONGENITAL VALGUS DEFORMITY OF FEET	➡	Q66.6	Other congenital valgus deformities of feet
754.7Ø	UNSPECIFIED TALIPES		Q66.89	Other specified congenital deformities of feet
754.71	TALIPES CAVUS	➡	Q66.7	Congenital pes cavus
754.79	OTHER CONGENITAL DEFORMITY OF FEET OTHER		Q66.89	Other specified congenital deformities of feet
			Q66.9	Congenital deformity of feet, unspecified
754.81	PECTUS EXCAVATUM	➡	Q67.6	Pectus excavatum
754.82	PECTUS CARINATUM	➡	Q67.7	Pectus carinatum
754.89	OTHER SPECIFIED NONTERATOGENIC ANOMALIES OTHER		Q67.8	Other congenital deformities of chest
			Q68.1	Congenital deformity of finger(s) and hand
			Q74.3	Arthrogryposis multiplex congenita
755.ØØ	POLYDACTYLY, UNSPECIFIED DIGITS		Q69.9	Polydactyly, unspecified
			Q7Ø.4	Polysyndactyly, unspecified
755.Ø1	POLYDACTYLY OF FINGERS		Q69.Ø	Accessory finger(s)
			Q69.1	Accessory thumb(s)
755.Ø2	POLYDACTYLY OF TOES	➡	Q69.2	Accessory toe(s)

ICD-9-CM		ICD-10-CM	
755.10	SYNDACTYLY OF MULTIPLE AND UNSPECIFIED SITES	**Q70.4**	Polysyndactyly, unspecified
		Q70.9	Syndactyly, unspecified
755.11	SYNDACTYLY OF FINGERS WITHOUT FUSION OF BONE	**Q70.10**	Webbed fingers, unspecified hand
		Q70.11	Webbed fingers, right hand
		Q70.12	Webbed fingers, left hand
		Q70.13	Webbed fingers, bilateral
755.12	SYNDACTYLY OF FINGERS WITH FUSION OF BONE	**Q70.00**	Fused fingers, unspecified hand
		Q70.01	Fused fingers, right hand
		Q70.02	Fused fingers, left hand
		Q70.03	Fused fingers, bilateral
755.13	SYNDACTYLY OF TOES WITHOUT FUSION OF BONE	**Q70.30**	Webbed toes, unspecified foot
		Q70.31	Webbed toes, right foot
		Q70.32	Webbed toes, left foot
		Q70.33	Webbed toes, bilateral
755.14	SYNDACTYLY OF TOES WITH FUSION OF BONE	**Q70.20**	Fused toes, unspecified foot
		Q70.21	Fused toes, right foot
		Q70.22	Fused toes, left foot
		Q70.23	Fused toes, bilateral
755.20	CONGENITAL UNSPEC REDUCTION DEFORMITY UPPER LIMB	**Q71.811**	Congenital shortening of right upper limb
		Q71.812	Congenital shortening of left upper limb
		Q71.813	Congenital shortening of upper limb, bilateral
		Q71.819	Congenital shortening of unspecified upper limb
		Q71.891	Other reduction defects of right upper limb
		Q71.892	Other reduction defects of left upper limb
		Q71.893	Other reduction defects of upper limb, bilateral
		Q71.899	Other reduction defects of unspecified upper limb
		Q71.90	Unspecified reduction defect of unspecified upper limb
		Q71.91	Unspecified reduction defect of right upper limb
		Q71.92	Unspecified reduction defect of left upper limb
		Q71.93	Unspecified reduction defect of upper limb, bilateral
755.21	CONGENITAL TRANSVERSE DEFICIENCY OF UPPER LIMB	**Q71.00**	Congenital complete absence of unspecified upper limb
		Q71.01	Congenital complete absence of right upper limb
		Q71.02	Congenital complete absence of left upper limb
		Q71.03	Congenital complete absence of upper limb, bilateral
755.22	CONGENITAL LONGITUDINAL DEFIC UPPER LIMB NEC	**Q71.00**	Congenital complete absence of unspecified upper limb
755.23	CONGN LONGTUDNL DEFIC COMB INVLV HUM RADIUS&ULNA	**Q71.10**	Congen absence of unsp upper arm and forearm w hand present
		Q71.11	Congenital absence of r up arm and forearm w hand present
		Q71.12	Congenital absence of l up arm and forearm w hand present
		Q71.13	Congen absence of upper arm and forearm w hand present, bi
755.24	CONGEN LONGITUDINAL DEFIC HUM COMPLETE/PARTIAL	**Q71.10**	Congen absence of unsp upper arm and forearm w hand present
755.25	CONGEN LONGTUDNL DEFIC RADIOULNAR COMPLETE/PART	**Q71.20**	Congenital absence of both forearm and hand, unsp upper limb
		Q71.21	Congen absence of both forearm and hand, right upper limb
		Q71.22	Congenital absence of both forearm and hand, left upper limb
		Q71.23	Congenital absence of both forearm and hand, bilateral
755.26	CONGEN LONGTUDNL DEFIC RADIAL COMPLETE/PARTIAL	**Q71.40**	Longitudinal reduction defect of unspecified radius
		Q71.41	Longitudinal reduction defect of right radius
		Q71.42	Longitudinal reduction defect of left radius
		Q71.43	Longitudinal reduction defect of radius, bilateral
755.27	CONGEN LONGITUDINAL DEFIC ULNAR COMPLETE/PARTIAL	**Q71.50**	Longitudinal reduction defect of unspecified ulna
		Q71.51	Longitudinal reduction defect of right ulna
		Q71.52	Longitudinal reduction defect of left ulna
		Q71.53	Longitudinal reduction defect of ulna, bilateral
755.28	CONGEN LONGTUDNL DEFIC CARPALS/MCS COMPLETE/PART	**Q71.30**	Congenital absence of unspecified hand and finger
		Q71.31	Congenital absence of right hand and finger
		Q71.32	Congenital absence of left hand and finger
		Q71.33	Congenital absence of hand and finger, bilateral
755.29	CONGEN LONGTUDNL DEFIC PHALANGES COMPLETE/PART	**Q71.30**	Congenital absence of unspecified hand and finger
		Q71.31	Congenital absence of right hand and finger
		Q71.32	Congenital absence of left hand and finger
		Q71.33	Congenital absence of hand and finger, bilateral
755.30	CONGENITAL UNSPEC REDUCTION DEFORMITY LOWER LIMB	**Q72.811**	Congenital shortening of right lower limb
		Q72.812	Congenital shortening of left lower limb
		Q72.813	Congenital shortening of lower limb, bilateral
		Q72.819	Congenital shortening of unspecified lower limb
		Q72.891	Other reduction defects of right lower limb
		Q72.892	Other reduction defects of left lower limb
		Q72.893	Other reduction defects of lower limb, bilateral
		Q72.899	Other reduction defects of unspecified lower limb
755.31	CONGENITAL TRANSVERSE DEFICIENCY OF LOWER LIMB	**Q72.00**	Congenital complete absence of unspecified lower limb
		Q72.01	Congenital complete absence of right lower limb
		Q72.02	Congenital complete absence of left lower limb
		Q72.03	Congenital complete absence of lower limb, bilateral
755.32	CONGENITAL LONGITUDINAL DEFIC LOWER LIMB NEC	**Q72.899**	Other reduction defects of unspecified lower limb
		Q72.90	Unspecified reduction defect of unspecified lower limb
		Q72.91	Unspecified reduction defect of right lower limb
		Q72.92	Unspecified reduction defect of left lower limb
		Q72.93	Unspecified reduction defect of lower limb, bilateral

ICD-9-CM		ICD-10-CM	
755.33	CONGEN LONGTUDNL DEFIC COMB INVLV FEM TIBIA&FIB	**Q72.1Ø**	Congen absence of unsp thigh and lower leg w foot present
		Q72.11	Congen absence of right thigh and lower leg w foot present
		Q72.12	Congen absence of left thigh and lower leg w foot present
		Q72.13	Congen absence of thigh and lower leg w foot present, bi
755.34	CONGEN LONGTUDNL DEFIC FEMORAL COMPLETE/PARTIAL	**Q72.4Ø**	Longitudinal reduction defect of unspecified femur
		Q72.41	Longitudinal reduction defect of right femur
		Q72.42	Longitudinal reduction defect of left femur
		Q72.43	Longitudinal reduction defect of femur, bilateral
755.35	CONGEN LONGTUDNL DEFIC TIBIOFIBR COMPLETE/PART	**Q72.2Ø**	Congen absence of both lower leg and foot, unsp lower limb
		Q72.21	Congen absence of both lower leg and foot, right lower limb
		Q72.22	Congen absence of both lower leg and foot, left lower limb
		Q72.23	Congenital absence of both lower leg and foot, bilateral
755.36	CONGEN LONGITUDINAL DEFIC TIBIA COMPLETE/PARTIAL	**Q72.5Ø**	Longitudinal reduction defect of unspecified tibia
		Q72.51	Longitudinal reduction defect of right tibia
		Q72.52	Longitudinal reduction defect of left tibia
		Q72.53	Longitudinal reduction defect of tibia, bilateral
755.37	CONGEN LONGITUDINAL DEFIC FIBR COMPLETE/PARTIAL	**Q72.6Ø**	Longitudinal reduction defect of unspecified fibula
		Q72.61	Longitudinal reduction defect of right fibula
		Q72.62	Longitudinal reduction defect of left fibula
		Q72.63	Longitudinal reduction defect of fibula, bilateral
755.38	CONGEN LONGTUDNL DEFIC TARSALS/MTS COMPLETE/PART	**Q72.3Ø**	Congenital absence of unspecified foot and toe(s)
		Q72.31	Congenital absence of right foot and toe(s)
		Q72.32	Congenital absence of left foot and toe(s)
		Q72.33	Congenital absence of foot and toe(s), bilateral
		Q72.7Ø	Split foot, unspecified lower limb
		Q72.71	Split foot, right lower limb
		Q72.72	Split foot, left lower limb
		Q72.73	Split foot, bilateral
755.39	CONGEN LONGTUDNL DEFIC PHALANGES COMPLETE/PART	**Q72.3Ø**	Congenital absence of unspecified foot and toe(s)
		Q72.31	Congenital absence of right foot and toe(s)
		Q72.32	Congenital absence of left foot and toe(s)
		Q72.33	Congenital absence of foot and toe(s), bilateral
		Q72.7Ø	Split foot, unspecified lower limb
		Q72.71	Split foot, right lower limb
		Q72.72	Split foot, left lower limb
		Q72.73	Split foot, bilateral
755.4	CONGENITAL REDUCTION DEFORMITIES UNSPEC LIMB	**Q73.Ø**	Congenital absence of unspecified limb(s)
		Q73.1	Phocomelia, unspecified limb(s)
		Q73.8	Other reduction defects of unspecified limb(s)
755.5Ø	UNSPECIFIED CONGENITAL ANOMALY OF UPPER LIMB	**Q74.9**	Unspecified congenital malformation of limb(s)
755.51	CONGENITAL DEFORMITY OF CLAVICLE	**Q68.8**	Other specified congenital musculoskeletal deformities
755.52	CONGENITAL ELEVATION OF SCAPULA	**Q68.8**	Other specified congenital musculoskeletal deformities
755.53	RADIOULNAR SYNOSTOSIS	**Q74.Ø**	Oth congen malform of upper limb(s), inc shoulder girdle
755.54	MADELUNGS DEFORMITY	**Q74.Ø**	Oth congen malform of upper limb(s), inc shoulder girdle
755.55	ACROCEPHALOSYNDACTYLY	**Q87.Ø**	Congen malform syndromes predom affecting facial appearance
755.56	ACCESSORY CARPAL BONES	**Q74.Ø**	Oth congen malform of upper limb(s), inc shoulder girdle
755.57	MACRODACTYLIA	**Q74.Ø**	Oth congen malform of upper limb(s), inc shoulder girdle
755.58	CONGENITAL CLEFT HAND	**Q71.6Ø**	Lobster-claw hand, unspecified hand
		Q71.61	Lobster-claw right hand
		Q71.62	Lobster-claw left hand
		Q71.63	Lobster-claw hand, bilateral
755.59	OTH CONGEN ANOMALY UPPER LIMB INCL SHLDR GIRDL	**Q74.Ø**	Oth congen malform of upper limb(s), inc shoulder girdle
755.6Ø	UNSPECIFIED CONGENITAL ANOMALY OF LOWER LIMB	**Q74.2**	Oth congen malform of lower limb(s), including pelvic girdle
755.61	CONGENITAL COXA VALGA	**Q65.81**	Congenital coxa valga
755.62	CONGENITAL COXA VARA	**Q65.82**	Congenital coxa vara
755.63	OTHER CONGENITAL DEFORMITY OF HIP	**Q65.89**	Other specified congenital deformities of hip
		Q65.9	Congenital deformity of hip, unspecified
755.64	CONGENITAL DEFORMITY OF KNEE	**Q68.2**	Congenital deformity of knee
		Q74.1	Congenital malformation of knee
755.65	MACRODACTYLIA OF TOES	**Q74.2**	Oth congen malform of lower limb(s), including pelvic girdle
755.66	OTHER CONGENITAL ANOMALY OF TOES	**Q66.89**	Other specified congenital deformities of feet
755.67	CONGENITAL ANOMALIES OF FOOT NEC	**Q66.89**	Other specified congenital deformities of feet
		Q72.7Ø	Split foot, unspecified lower limb
755.69	OTH CONGEN ANOMALY LOW LIMB INCL PELV GIRDL OTH	**Q72.7Ø**	Split foot, unspecified lower limb
		Q74.2	Oth congen malform of lower limb(s), including pelvic girdle
755.8	OTHER SPEC CONGENITAL ANOMALIES UNSPEC LIMB	➡ **Q74.8**	Other specified congenital malformations of limb(s)
755.9	UNSPECIFIED CONGENITAL ANOMALY UNSPECIFIED LIMB	**Q74.9**	Unspecified congenital malformation of limb(s)
756.Ø	CONGENITAL ANOMALIES OF SKULL AND FACE BONES	**Q75.Ø**	Craniosynostosis
		Q75.1	Craniofacial dysostosis
		Q75.2	Hypertelorism
		Q75.3	Macrocephaly
		Q75.4	Mandibulofacial dysostosis
		Q75.5	Oculomandibular dysostosis
		Q75.8	Oth congenital malformations of skull and face bones
		Q75.9	Congenital malformation of skull and face bones, unspecified
		Q87.Ø	Congen malform syndromes predom affecting facial appearance

ICD-9-CM		ICD-10-CM	
756.10	CONGENITAL ANOMALY OF SPINE UNSPECIFIED	Q76.49	Oth congenital malform of spine, not associated w scoliosis
756.11	CONGENITAL SPONDYLOLYSIS LUMBOSACRAL REGION	Q76.2	Congenital spondylolisthesis
756.12	CONGENITAL SPONDYLOLISTHESIS	Q76.2	Congenital spondylolisthesis
756.13	CONGENITAL ABSENCE OF VERTEBRA	Q76.49	Oth congenital malform of spine, not associated w scoliosis
756.14	HEMIVERTEBRA	Q76.49	Oth congenital malform of spine, not associated w scoliosis
756.15	CONGENITAL FUSION OF SPINE	Q76.49	Oth congenital malform of spine, not associated w scoliosis
756.16	KLIPPEL-FEIL SYNDROME	➡ Q76.1	Klippel-Feil syndrome
756.17	SPINA BIFIDA OCCULTA	➡ Q76.0	Spina bifida occulta
756.19	OTHER CONGENITAL ANOMALY OF SPINE	Q76.411	Congenital kyphosis, occipito-atlanto-axial region
		Q76.412	Congenital kyphosis, cervical region
		Q76.413	Congenital kyphosis, cervicothoracic region
		Q76.414	Congenital kyphosis, thoracic region
		Q76.415	Congenital kyphosis, thoracolumbar region
		Q76.419	Congenital kyphosis, unspecified region
		Q76.49	Oth congenital malform of spine, not associated w scoliosis
756.2	CERVICAL RIB	➡ Q76.5	Cervical rib
756.3	OTHER CONGENITAL ANOMALY OF RIBS AND STERNUM	Q76.6	Other congenital malformations of ribs
		Q76.7	Congenital malformation of sternum
		Q76.8	Other congenital malformations of bony thorax
		Q76.9	Congenital malformation of bony thorax, unspecified
		Q77.2	Short rib syndrome
756.4	CHONDRODYSTROPHY	Q77.0	Achondrogenesis
		Q77.1	Thanatophoric short stature
		Q77.4	Achondroplasia
		Q77.5	Diastrophic dysplasia
		Q77.7	Spondyloepiphyseal dysplasia
		Q77.8	Oth osteochndrdys w defct of growth of tublr bones and spine
		Q77.9	Osteochndrdys w defct of grth of tublr bones and spine, unsp
		Q78.4	Enchondromatosis
756.50	UNSPECIFIED CONGENITAL OSTEODYSTROPHY	Q78.9	Osteochondrodysplasia, unspecified
756.51	OSTEOGENESIS IMPERFECTA	➡ Q78.0	Osteogenesis imperfecta
756.52	OSTEOPETROSIS	➡ Q78.2	Osteopetrosis
756.53	OSTEOPOIKILOSIS	Q78.8	Other specified osteochondrodysplasias
756.54	POLYOSTOTIC FIBROUS DYSPLASIA OF BONE	➡ Q78.1	Polyostotic fibrous dysplasia
756.55	CHONDROECTODERMAL DYSPLASIA	➡ Q77.6	Chondroectodermal dysplasia
756.56	MULTIPLE EPIPHYSEAL DYSPLASIA	Q78.3	Progressive diaphyseal dysplasia
756.59	OTHER CONGENITAL OSTEODYSTROPHY	Q77.3	Chondrodysplasia punctata
		Q78.5	Metaphyseal dysplasia
		Q78.6	Multiple congenital exostoses
		Q78.8	Other specified osteochondrodysplasias
756.6	CONGENITAL ANOMALY OF DIAPHRAGM	Q79.0	Congenital diaphragmatic hernia
		Q79.1	Other congenital malformations of diaphragm
756.70	UNSPECIFIED CONGENITAL ANOMALY OF ABDOMINAL WALL	Q79.59	Other congenital malformations of abdominal wall
756.71	PRUNE BELLY SYNDROME	Q79.4	Prune belly syndrome
		Q79.51	Congenital hernia of bladder
756.72	OMPHALOCELE	➡ Q79.2	Exomphalos
756.73	GASTROSCHISIS	➡ Q79.3	Gastroschisis
756.79	OTHER CONGENITAL ANOMALIES OF ABDOMINAL WALL	Q79.59	Other congenital malformations of abdominal wall
756.81	CONGENITAL ABSENCE OF MUSCLE AND TENDON	Q79.8	Other congenital malformations of musculoskeletal system
756.82	ACCESSORY MUSCLE	Q79.8	Other congenital malformations of musculoskeletal system
756.83	EHLERS-DANLOS SYNDROME	➡ Q79.6	Ehlers-Danlos syndrome
756.89	OTH SPEC CONGN ANOMALY MUSC TEND FASC&CNCTV TISS	Q79.8	Other congenital malformations of musculoskeletal system
756.9	OTH&UNSPEC CONGEN ANOMALY MUSCULOSKELETAL SYSTEM	Q68.8	Other specified congenital musculoskeletal deformities
		Q79.8	Other congenital malformations of musculoskeletal system
		Q79.9	Congenital malformation of musculoskeletal system, unsp
757.0	HEREDITARY EDEMA OF LEGS	➡ Q82.0	Hereditary lymphedema
757.1	ICHTHYOSIS CONGENITA	Q80.0	Ichthyosis vulgaris
		Q80.1	X-linked ichthyosis
		Q80.2	Lamellar ichthyosis
		Q80.3	Congenital bullous ichthyosiform erythroderma
		Q80.4	Harlequin fetus
		Q80.8	Other congenital ichthyosis
		Q80.9	Congenital ichthyosis, unspecified
757.2	DERMATOGLYPHIC ANOMALIES	Q82.8	Other specified congenital malformations of skin
757.31	CONGENITAL ECTODERMAL DYSPLASIA	➡ Q82.4	Ectodermal dysplasia (anhidrotic)
757.32	CONGENITAL VASCULAR HAMARTOMAS	Q82.5	Congenital non-neoplastic nevus
757.33	CONGENITAL PIGMENTARY ANOMALY OF SKIN	Q82.1	Xeroderma pigmentosum
		Q82.2	Mastocytosis
		Q82.3	Incontinentia pigmenti

ICD-9-CM		ICD-10-CM	
757.39	OTHER SPECIFIED CONGENITAL ANOMALY OF SKIN	**Q81.Ø**	Epidermolysis bullosa simplex
		Q81.1	Epidermolysis bullosa letalis
		Q81.2	Epidermolysis bullosa dystrophica
		Q81.8	Other epidermolysis bullosa
		Q81.9	Epidermolysis bullosa, unspecified
		Q82.8	Other specified congenital malformations of skin
		Q82.9	Congenital malformation of skin, unspecified
757.4	SPECIFIED CONGENITAL ANOMALIES OF HAIR	**Q84.Ø**	Congenital alopecia
		Q84.1	Congenital morphological disturbances of hair, NEC
		Q84.2	Other congenital malformations of hair
757.5	SPECIFIED CONGENITAL ANOMALIES OF NAILS	**Q84.3**	Anonychia
		Q84.4	Congenital leukonychia
		Q84.5	Enlarged and hypertrophic nails
		Q84.6	Other congenital malformations of nails
757.6	SPECIFIED CONGENITAL ANOMALIES OF BREAST	**Q83.Ø**	Congenital absence of breast with absent nipple
		Q83.1	Accessory breast
		Q83.2	Absent nipple
		Q83.3	Accessory nipple
		Q83.8	Other congenital malformations of breast
		Q83.9	Congenital malformation of breast, unspecified
757.8	OTHER SPECIFIED CONGENITAL ANOMALIES INTEGUMENT	➡ **Q84.8**	Other specified congenital malformations of integument
757.9	UNSPECIFIED CONGENITAL ANOMALY OF THE INTEGUMENT	➡ **Q84.9**	Congenital malformation of integument, unspecified
758.Ø	DOWNS SYNDROME	**Q9Ø.Ø**	Trisomy 21, nonmosaicism (meiotic nondisjunction)
		Q9Ø.1	Trisomy 21, mosaicism (mitotic nondisjunction)
		Q9Ø.2	Trisomy 21, translocation
		Q9Ø.9	Down syndrome, unspecified
758.1	PATAUS SYNDROME	**Q91.4**	Trisomy 13, nonmosaicism (meiotic nondisjunction)
		Q91.5	Trisomy 13, mosaicism (mitotic nondisjunction)
		Q91.6	Trisomy 13, translocation
		Q91.7	Trisomy 13, unspecified
758.2	EDWARDS SYNDROME	**Q91.Ø**	Trisomy 18, nonmosaicism (meiotic nondisjunction)
		Q91.1	Trisomy 18, mosaicism (mitotic nondisjunction)
		Q91.2	Trisomy 18, translocation
		Q91.3	Trisomy 18, unspecified
758.31	CRI-DU-CHAT SYNDROME	➡ **Q93.4**	Deletion of short arm of chromosome 5
758.32	VELO-CARDIO-FACIAL SYNDROME	➡ **Q93.81**	Velo-cardio-facial syndrome
758.33	AUTOSOMAL DELETION SYNDROMES OTH MICRODELETIONS	➡ **Q93.88**	Other microdeletions
758.39	AUTOSOMAL DELETION SYNDROMES OTH AUTOSOMAL DELS	**Q93.3**	Deletion of short arm of chromosome 4
		Q93.5	Other deletions of part of a chromosome
		Q93.7	Deletions with other complex rearrangements
		Q93.89	Other deletions from the autosomes
		Q93.9	Deletion from autosomes, unspecified
758.4	BALANCED AUTOSOMAL TRNSLOCAT NORMAL INDIVIDUAL	**Q95.Ø**	Balanced translocation and insertion in normal individual
		Q95.1	Chromosome inversion in normal individual
		Q95.5	Individual with autosomal fragile site
		Q95.8	Other balanced rearrangements and structural markers
		Q95.9	Balanced rearrangement and structural marker, unspecified
758.5	OTHER CONDITIONS DUE TO AUTOSOMAL ANOMALIES	**Q92.Ø**	Whole chromosome trisomy, nonmosaic (meiotic nondisjunction)
		Q92.1	Whole chromosome trisomy, mosaicism (mitotic nondisjunction)
		Q92.2	Partial trisomy
		Q92.5	Duplications with other complex rearrangements
		Q92.61	Marker chromosomes in normal individual
		Q92.62	Marker chromosomes in abnormal individual
		Q92.7	Triploidy and polyploidy
		Q92.8	Other specified trisomies and partial trisomies of autosomes
		Q92.9	Trisomy and partial trisomy of autosomes, unspecified
		Q93.Ø	Whole chromosome monosomy,nonmosaic (meiotic nondisjunction)
		Q93.1	Whole chromosome monosomy, mosaic (mitotic nondisjunction)
		Q93.2	Chromosome replaced with ring, dicentric or isochromosome
		Q95.2	Balanced autosomal rearrangement in abnormal individual
		Q95.3	Balanced sex/autosomal rearrangement in abnormal individual
758.6	GONADAL DYSGENESIS	**Q96.Ø**	Karyotype 45, X
		Q96.1	Karyotype 46, X iso (Xq)
		Q96.2	Karyotype 46, X w abnormal sex chromosome, except iso (Xq)
		Q96.3	Mosaicism, 45, X/46, XX or XY
		Q96.4	Mosaic, 45, X/other cell line(s) w abnormal sex chromosome
		Q96.8	Other variants of Turner's syndrome
		Q96.9	Turner's syndrome, unspecified
758.7	KLINEFELTERS SYNDROME	**Q98.Ø**	Klinefelter syndrome karyotype 47, XXY
		Q98.1	Klinefelter syndrome, male with more than two X chromosomes
		Q98.3	Other male with 46, XX karyotype
		Q98.4	Klinefelter syndrome, unspecified

[Brackets] indicate valid character values for each code. Character value meanings provided for each code grouping.

ICD-9-CM			ICD-10-CM	
758.81	OTHER CONDITIONS DUE TO SEX CHROMOSOME ANOMALIES		**Q97.Ø**	Karyotype 47, XXX
			Q97.1	Female with more than three X chromosomes
			Q97.2	Mosaicism, lines with various numbers of X chromosomes
			Q97.3	Female with 46, XY karyotype
			Q97.8	Oth sex chromosome abnormalities, female phenotype
			Q97.9	Sex chromosome abnormality, female phenotype, unspecified
			Q98.5	Karyotype 47, XYY
			Q98.6	Male with structurally abnormal sex chromosome
			Q98.7	Male with sex chromosome mosaicism
			Q98.8	Other specified sex chromosome abnormalities, male phenotype
			Q98.9	Sex chromosome abnormality, male phenotype, unspecified
			Q99.Ø	Chimera 46, XX/46, XY
			Q99.1	46, XX true hermaphrodite
			Q99.8	Other specified chromosome abnormalities
758.89	OTHER CONDITIONS DUE TO CHROMOSOME ANOMALIES OTH		**Q99.8**	Other specified chromosome abnormalities
758.9	CONDITIONS DUE TO ANOMALY UNSPECIFIED CHROMOSOME	➡	**Q99.9**	Chromosomal abnormality, unspecified
759.Ø	CONGENITAL ANOMALIES OF SPLEEN		**Q89.Ø1**	Asplenia (congenital)
			Q89.Ø9	Congenital malformations of spleen
759.1	CONGENITAL ANOMALIES OF ADRENAL GLAND	➡	**Q89.1**	Congenital malformations of adrenal gland
759.2	CONGENITAL ANOMALIES OF OTHER ENDOCRINE GLANDS	➡	**Q89.2**	Congenital malformations of other endocrine glands
759.3	SITUS INVERSUS	➡	**Q89.3**	Situs inversus
759.4	CONJOINED TWINS	➡	**Q89.4**	Conjoined twins
759.5	TUBEROUS SCLEROSIS	➡	**Q85.1**	Tuberous sclerosis
759.6	OTHER CONGENITAL HAMARTOSES NEC		**Q85.8**	Other phakomatoses, not elsewhere classified
			Q85.9	Phakomatosis, unspecified
759.7	MULTIPLE CONGENITAL ANOMALIES SO DESCRIBED	➡	**Q89.7**	Multiple congenital malformations, not elsewhere classified
759.81	PRADER-WILLI SYNDROME		**Q87.1**	Congenital malform syndromes predom assoc w short stature
759.82	MARFANS SYNDROME		**Q87.4Ø**	Marfan's syndrome, unspecified
			Q87.41Ø	Marfan's syndrome with aortic dilation
			Q87.418	Marfan's syndrome with other cardiovascular manifestations
			Q87.42	Marfan's syndrome with ocular manifestations
			Q87.43	Marfan's syndrome with skeletal manifestation
759.83	FRAGILE X SYNDROME	➡	**Q99.2**	Fragile X chromosome
759.89	OTHER SPEC MULTIPLE CONGENITAL ANOMALIES SO DESC		**E78.71**	Barth syndrome
			E78.72	Smith-Lemli-Opitz syndrome
			Q87.2	Congenital malformation syndromes predom involving limbs
			Q87.3	Congenital malformation syndromes involving early overgrowth
			Q87.5	Oth congenital malformation syndromes w oth skeletal changes
			Q87.81	Alport syndrome
			Q87.89	Oth congenital malformation syndromes, NEC
			Q89.8	Other specified congenital malformations
759.9	UNSPECIFIED CONGENITAL ANOMALY	➡	**Q89.9**	Congenital malformation, unspecified

Conditions in the Perinatal Period

ICD-9-CM			ICD-10-CM	
760.Ø	FETUS/NEWBORN AFFECTED MATERNAL HYPERTENSIVE D/O	➡	**PØØ.Ø**	Newborn affected by maternal hypertensive disorders
760.1	FETUS/NB AFFECTED MTRN RENAL&URINARY TRACT DZ	➡	**PØØ.1**	Newborn aff by maternal renal and urinary tract diseases
760.2	FETUS OR NEWBORN AFFECTED BY MATERNAL INFECTIONS		**PØØ.2**	Newborn affected by maternal infec/parastc diseases
760.3	FETUS/NB AFFECTED OTH CHRONIC MTRN CIRC&RESP DZ		**PØØ.3**	Newborn affected by oth maternal circ and resp diseases
760.4	FETUS/NEWBORN AFFECTED MATERNAL NUTRITIONAL D/O	➡	**PØØ.4**	Newborn affected by maternal nutritional disorders
760.5	FETUS OR NEWBORN AFFECTED BY MATERNAL INJURY	➡	**PØØ.5**	Newborn (suspected to be) affected by maternal injury
760.61	NEWBORN AFFECTED BY AMNIOCENTESIS		**PØØ.7**	Newborn affected by oth medical procedures on mother, NEC
760.62	NEWBORN AFFECTED BY OTHER IN UTERO PROCEDURE		**PØØ.7**	Newborn affected by oth medical procedures on mother, NEC
760.63	NEWBORN AFFECTED BY OTHER OP ON MOTHER DUR PG		**PØØ.6**	Newborn affected by surgical procedure on mother
760.64	NB AFFECTED PREV SURG PROC ON MOM NOT ASSOC W/PG		**PØØ.6**	Newborn affected by surgical procedure on mother
760.7Ø	NOX INFLUENCE FETUS/NB VIA PLACNTA/BRST MILK UNS		**PØ4.9**	Newborn affected by maternal noxious substance, unsp
760.71	NOX INFLUENCE FETUS/NB VIA PLACNTA/BRST MILK ALC		**PØ4.3** **Q86.Ø**	Newborn affected by maternal use of alcohol Fetal alcohol syndrome (dysmorphic)
760.72	NOX INFLUNCE FETUS/NB VIA PLACNTA/BRST MILK NARC		**PØ4.49**	Newborn affected by maternal use of drugs of addiction
760.73	NOX INFLUENCE FETUS/NB PLACNTA/BRST MILK HALLUCN		**PØ4.49**	Newborn affected by maternal use of drugs of addiction
760.74	NOX INFLU FETUS/NB PLACNTA/BRST MILK ANTI-INFCTV		**PØ4.1**	Newborn affected by oth maternal medication
760.75	NOX INFLUENCE FETUS/NB PLACNTA/BRST MILK COCAINE	➡	**PØ4.41**	Newborn affected by maternal use of cocaine
760.76	NOX INFLUENCE FETUS/NB VIA PLACNTA/BRST MILK DES		**PØ4.8**	Newborn affected by oth maternal noxious substances
760.77	NOX INFLU FETUS/NB PLACNTA/BRST MILK ANTICONVUL		**PØ4.1** **Q86.1**	Newborn affected by oth maternal medication Fetal hydantoin syndrome
760.78	NOX INFLU FETUS/NB PLACNTA/BRST MILK ANTMETABOLC		**PØ4.1**	Newborn affected by oth maternal medication
760.79	NOX INFLUENCE FETUS/NB VIA PLACNTA/BRST MILK OTH		**PØ4.2** **PØ4.5** **PØ4.6** **PØ4.8** **PØ4.9** **Q86.2** **Q86.8**	Newborn affected by maternal use of tobacco Newborn aff by maternal use of nutritional chemical substnc Newborn aff by maternal exposure to environ chemical substnc Newborn affected by oth maternal noxious substances Newborn affected by maternal noxious substance, unsp Dysmorphism due to warfarin Oth congen malform syndromes due to known exogenous causes
760.8	OTH SPEC MATERNAL CONDS AFFECTING FETUS/NEWBORN		**PØØ.81** **PØØ.89** **P96.81**	Newborn affected by periodontal disease in mother Newborn affected by oth maternal conditions Expsr to (environmental) tobacco smoke in the perinat period
760.9	UNSPEC MATERNAL COND AFFECTING FETUS/NEWBORN		**PØØ.9**	Newborn affected by unsp maternal condition
761.Ø	FETUS/NEWBORN AFFECTED INCOMPETENT CERVIX MOTHER	➡	**PØ1.Ø**	Newborn (suspected to be) affected by incompetent cervix
761.1	FETUS/NB AFFECTED PREMATURE RUPTURE MEMB MOTH	➡	**PØ1.1**	Newborn (suspected to be) affected by premature ROM
761.2	FETUS OR NEWBORN AFFECTED BY OLIGOHYDRAMNIOS	➡	**PØ1.2**	Newborn (suspected to be) affected by oligohydramnios
761.3	FETUS OR NEWBORN AFFECTED BY POLYHYDRAMNIOS	➡	**PØ1.3**	Newborn (suspected to be) affected by polyhydramnios
761.4	FETUS/NEWBORN AFFECTED ECTOPIC PREGNANCY MOTHER	➡	**PØ1.4**	Newborn (suspected to be) affected by ectopic pregnancy
761.5	FETUS/NEWBORN AFFECTED MULTIPLE PREGNANCY MOTHER	➡	**PØ1.5**	Newborn (suspected to be) affected by multiple pregnancy
761.6	FETUS OR NEWBORN AFFECTED BY MATERNAL DEATH	➡	**PØ1.6**	Newborn (suspected to be) affected by maternal death
761.7	FETUS/NB AFFECTED MALPRESENTATION BEFORE LABOR	➡	**PØ1.7**	Newborn affected by malpresentation before labor
761.8	FETUS/NB AFFECTED OTH SPEC MTRN COMPS PREGNANCY	➡	**PØ1.8**	Newborn affected by oth maternal complications of pregnancy
761.9	FETUS/NB AFFECTED UNSPEC MTRN COMP PREGNANCY	➡	**PØ1.9**	Newborn affected by maternal complication of pregnancy, unsp
762.Ø	FETUS OR NEWBORN AFFECTED BY PLACENTA PREVIA	➡	**PØ2.Ø**	Newborn (suspected to be) affected by placenta previa
762.1	FETUS/NB AFFECTED OTH FORMS PLACNTL SEP&HEMORR	➡	**PØ2.1**	Newborn affected by oth placental separation and hemorrhage
762.2	F/NB AFFECT BY MORPHOLOG-FUNCT PLACENTA ABNORMAL		**PØ2.2Ø** **PØ2.29**	Newborn aff by unsp morpholog and functn abnlt of placenta Newborn aff by oth morpholog and functn abnlt of placenta
762.3	FETUS/NB AFFECTED PLACENTAL TRANSFUS SYNDROMES	➡	**PØ2.3**	Newborn affected by placental transfusion syndromes
762.4	FETUS OR NEWBORN AFFECTED BY PROLAPSED CORD	➡	**PØ2.4**	Newborn (suspected to be) affected by prolapsed cord
762.5	FETUS/NEWBORN AFFECTED OTH COMPRS UMBILICAL CORD	➡	**PØ2.5**	Newborn affected by oth compression of umbilical cord
762.6	FETUS/NB AFFECTED OTH&UNSPEC CONDS UMB CORD		**PØ2.6Ø** **PØ2.69**	Newborn affected by unsp conditions of umbilical cord Newborn affected by oth conditions of umbilical cord
762.7	FETUS OR NEWBORN AFFECTED BY CHORIOAMNIONITIS	➡	**PØ2.7**	Newborn (suspected to be) affected by chorioamnionitis
762.8	FETUS/NB AFFECTED OTH SPEC ABNORM CHORION&AMNION	➡	**PØ2.8**	Newborn affected by oth abnormalities of membranes
762.9	FETUS/NB AFFECTED UNSPEC ABNORM CHORION&AMNION	➡	**PØ2.9**	Newborn affected by abnormality of membranes, unsp
763.Ø	FETUS/NEWBORN AFFECTED BREECH DELIV&EXTRACTION	➡	**PØ3.Ø**	Newborn affected by breech delivery and extraction
763.1	FETUS/NB AFFECT BY OTH MALPRESENT&DISPROPOR-L&D	➡	**PØ3.1**	NB aff by oth malpresent, malpos & disproprtn dur labr & del
763.2	FETUS OR NEWBORN AFFECTED BY FORCEPS DELIVERY	➡	**PØ3.2**	Newborn (suspected to be) affected by forceps delivery
763.3	FETUS/NEWBORN AFFECTED DELIVERY VACUUM EXTRACTOR	➡	**PØ3.3**	Newborn affected by delivery by vacuum extractor
763.4	FETUS OR NEWBORN AFFECTED BY CESAREAN DELIVERY	➡	**PØ3.4**	Newborn (suspected to be) affected by Cesarean delivery
763.5	FETUS/NEWBORN AFFECTED MATERNAL ANESTHESIA&ANALG	➡	**PØ4.Ø**	NB aff by matern anesth and analgesia in preg, labor and del
763.6	FETUS OR NEWBORN AFFECTED PRECIPITATE DELIVERY	➡	**PØ3.5**	Newborn (suspected to be) affected by precipitate delivery
763.7	FETUS/NB AFFECTED ABNORMAL UTERINE CONTRACTIONS	➡	**PØ3.6**	Newborn affected by abnormal uterine contractions
763.81	ABNORM FETAL HRT RATE/RHYTHM BEFORE ONSET LABOR	➡	**PØ3.81Ø**	NB aff by abnlt in fetl heart rate or rhythm bef onset labor
763.82	ABNORMALITY FETAL HEART RATE/RHYTHM DURING LABOR	➡	**PØ3.811**	NB aff by abnlt in fetal heart rate or rhythm during labor
763.83	ABNORM FETAL HRT RATE/RHYTHM UNS AS TIME ONSET	➡	**PØ3.819**	NB aff by abnlt in fetl hrt rate or rhythm, unsp time onset
763.84	COMPL L&D AFFCT FETUS/NB MECON PASSAGE DUR DEL	➡	**PØ3.82**	Meconium passage during delivery
763.89	OTH SPEC COMPLICATIONS L&D AFFECT FETUS/NEWBORN	➡	**PØ3.89**	Newborn affected by oth complications of labor and delivery
763.9	UNSPEC COMPLICATION L&D AFFECTING FETUS/NEWBORN	➡	**PØ3.9**	Newborn affected by complication of labor and delivery, unsp
764.ØØ	LGHT-FOR-DATES W/O MENTION FETAL MLNUTRIT UNSPEC		**PØ5.ØØ** **PØ5.1Ø**	Newborn light for gestational age, unspecified weight Newborn small for gestational age, unspecified weight

ICD-9-CM		ICD-10-CM	
764.01	LGHT-FOR-DATES W/O FETL MLNUTRIT < 500 GMS	P05.01	Newborn light for gestational age, less than 500 grams
		P05.11	Newborn small for gestational age, less than 500 grams
764.02	LGHT-FOR-DATES W/O FETL MLNUTRIT 500-749 GMS	P05.02	Newborn light for gestational age, 500-749 grams
		P05.12	Newborn small for gestational age, 500-749 grams
764.03	LGHT-FOR-DATES W/O FETL MLNUTRIT 750-999 GMS	P05.03	Newborn light for gestational age, 750-999 grams
		P05.13	Newborn small for gestational age, 750-999 grams
764.04	LGHT-FOR-DATES W/O FETL MLNUTRIT 1000-1249 GMS	P05.04	Newborn light for gestational age, 1000-1249 grams
		P05.14	Newborn small for gestational age, 1000-1249 grams
764.05	LGHT-FOR-DATES W/O FETL MLNUTRIT 1250-1499 GMS	P05.05	Newborn light for gestational age, 1250-1499 grams
		P05.15	Newborn small for gestational age, 1250-1499 grams
764.06	LGHT-FOR-DATES W/O FETL MLNUTRIT 1500-1749 GMS	P05.06	Newborn light for gestational age, 1500-1749 grams
		P05.16	Newborn small for gestational age, 1500-1749 grams
764.07	LGHT-FOR-DATES W/O FETL MLNUTRIT 1750-1999 GMS	P05.07	Newborn light for gestational age, 1750-1999 grams
		P05.17	Newborn small for gestational age, 1750-1999 grams
764.08	LGHT-FOR-DATES W/O FETL MLNUTRIT 2000-2499 GMS	P05.08	Newborn light for gestational age, 2000-2499 grams
		P05.18	Newborn small for gestational age, 2000-2499 grams
764.09	LGHT-FOR-DATES W/O FETL MLNUTRIT 2500/MORE GMS	NO DIAGNOSIS	
764.10	LIGHT-FOR-DATES W/SIGNS FETAL MLNUTRIT UNSPEC	P05.00	Newborn light for gestational age, unspecified weight
		P05.10	Newborn small for gestational age, unspecified weight
764.11	LIGHT-FOR-DATES W/SIGNS FETAL MLNUTRIT < 500 GMS	P05.01	Newborn light for gestational age, less than 500 grams
		P05.11	Newborn small for gestational age, less than 500 grams
764.12	LT-F-D W/SIGNS FETL MLNUTRIT 500-749 GMS	P05.02	Newborn light for gestational age, 500-749 grams
		P05.12	Newborn small for gestational age, 500-749 grams
764.13	LT-F-D W/SIGNS FETL MLNUTRIT 750-999 GMS	P05.03	Newborn light for gestational age, 750-999 grams
		P05.13	Newborn small for gestational age, 750-999 grams
764.14	LGHT-FOR-DATES W/SIGNS FETL MLNUT 1000-1249 GMS	P05.04	Newborn light for gestational age, 1000-1249 grams
		P05.14	Newborn small for gestational age, 1000-1249 grams
764.15	LGHT-FOR-DATES W/SIGNS FETL MLNUT 1250-1499 GMS	P05.05	Newborn light for gestational age, 1250-1499 grams
		P05.15	Newborn small for gestational age, 1250-1499 grams
764.16	LGHT-FOR-DATES W/SIGNS FETL MLNUT 1500-1749 GMS	P05.06	Newborn light for gestational age, 1500-1749 grams
		P05.16	Newborn small for gestational age, 1500-1749 grams
764.17	LGHT-FOR-DATES W/SIGNS FETL MLNUT 1750-1999 GMS	P05.07	Newborn light for gestational age, 1750-1999 grams
		P05.17	Newborn small for gestational age, 1750-1999 grams
764.18	LGHT-FOR-DATES W/SIGNS FETL MLNUT 2000-2499 GMS	P05.08	Newborn light for gestational age, 2000-2499 grams
		P05.18	Newborn small for gestational age, 2000-2499 grams
764.19	LGHT-FOR-DATES W/SIGNS FETL MLNUT 2500/MORE GMS	NO DIAGNOSIS	
764.20	FETAL MLNUTRIT W/O MENTION LGHT-FOR-DATES+ UNS	P05.2	NB aff by fetal malnut not light or small for gestatnl age
764.21	FETL MLNUTRIT W/O LGHT-FOR-DATES+ < 500 GMS	P05.2	NB aff by fetal malnut not light or small for gestatnl age
764.22	FETL MLNUTRIT W/O LGHT-FOR-DATES+ 500-749 GMS	P05.2	NB aff by fetal malnut not light or small for gestatnl age
764.23	FETL MLNUTRIT W/O LGHT-FOR-DATES+ 750-999 GMS	P05.2	NB aff by fetal malnut not light or small for gestatnl age
764.24	FETL MLNUTRIT W/O LGHT-FOR-DATES 1000-1249 GMS	P05.2	NB aff by fetal malnut not light or small for gestatnl age
764.25	FETL MLNUTRIT W/O LGHT-FOR-DATES+ 1250-1499 GMS	P05.2	NB aff by fetal malnut not light or small for gestatnl age
764.26	FETL MLNUTRIT W/O LGHT-FOR-DATES+ 1500-1749 GMS	P05.2	NB aff by fetal malnut not light or small for gestatnl age
764.27	FETL MLNUTRIT W/O LGHT-FOR-DATES 1750-1999 GMS	P05.2	NB aff by fetal malnut not light or small for gestatnl age
764.28	FETL MLNUTRIT W/O LGHT-FOR-DATES 2000-2499 GMS	P05.2	NB aff by fetal malnut not light or small for gestatnl age
764.29	FETL MLNUTRIT W/O LGHT-FOR-DATES 2500/MORE GMS	P05.2	NB aff by fetal malnut not light or small for gestatnl age
764.90	UNSPECIFIED FETAL GROWTH RETARDATION UNSPECIFIED	P05.9	Newborn affected by slow intrauterine growth, unspecified
764.91	UNSPECIFIED FETAL GROWTH RETARDATION < 500 GRAMS	P05.9	Newborn affected by slow intrauterine growth, unspecified
764.92	UNSPEC FETAL GROWTH RETARDATION 500-749 GRAMS	P05.9	Newborn affected by slow intrauterine growth, unspecified
764.93	UNSPEC FETAL GROWTH RETARDATION 750-999 GRAMS	P05.9	Newborn affected by slow intrauterine growth, unspecified
764.94	UNSPEC FETAL GROWTH RETARDATION 1000-1249 GRAMS	P05.9	Newborn affected by slow intrauterine growth, unspecified
764.95	UNSPEC FETAL GROWTH RETARDATION 1250-1499 GRAMS	P05.9	Newborn affected by slow intrauterine growth, unspecified
764.96	UNSPEC FETAL GROWTH RETARDATION 1500-1749 GRAMS	P05.9	Newborn affected by slow intrauterine growth, unspecified
764.97	UNSPEC FETAL GROWTH RETARDATION 1750-1999 GRAMS	P05.9	Newborn affected by slow intrauterine growth, unspecified
764.98	UNSPEC FETAL GROWTH RETARDATION 2000-2499 GRAMS	P05.9	Newborn affected by slow intrauterine growth, unspecified
764.99	UNSPEC FETAL GROWTH RETARDATION 2500/MORE GRAMS	P05.9	Newborn affected by slow intrauterine growth, unspecified
765.00	EXTREME FETAL IMMATURITY UNSPECIFIED	P07.00	Extremely low birth weight newborn, unspecified weight
		P07.10	Other low birth weight newborn, unspecified weight
765.01	EXTREME FETAL IMMATURITY LESS THAN 500 GRAMS	P07.01	Extremely low birth weight newborn, less than 500 grams
765.02	EXTREME FETAL IMMATURITY 500-749 GRAMS	P07.02	Extremely low birth weight newborn, 500-749 grams
765.03	EXTREME FETAL IMMATURITY 750-999 GRAMS	P07.03	Extremely low birth weight newborn, 750-999 grams
765.04	EXTREME FETAL IMMATURITY 1000-1249 GRAMS	P07.14	Other low birth weight newborn, 1000-1249 grams
765.05	EXTREME FETAL IMMATURITY 1250-1499 GRAMS	P07.15	Other low birth weight newborn, 1250-1499 grams
765.06	EXTREME FETAL IMMATURITY 1500-1749 GRAMS	P07.16	Other low birth weight newborn, 1500-1749 grams
765.07	EXTREME FETAL IMMATURITY 1750-1999 GRAMS	P07.17	Other low birth weight newborn, 1750-1999 grams
765.08	EXTREME FETAL IMMATURITY 2000-2499 GRAMS	P07.18	Other low birth weight newborn, 2000-2499 grams
765.09	EXTREME FETAL IMMATURITY 2500 OR MORE GRAMS	P07.30	Preterm newborn, unspecified weeks of gestation
765.10	OTHER PRETERM INFANTS, UNSPECIFIED	P07.00	Extremely low birth weight newborn, unspecified weight
		P07.10	Other low birth weight newborn, unspecified weight
765.11	OTHER PRETERM INFANTS LESS THAN 500 GRAMS	P07.01	Extremely low birth weight newborn, less than 500 grams

 [Brackets] indicate valid character values for each code. Character value meanings provided for each code grouping.

ICD-9-CM		ICD-10-CM	
765.12	OTHER PRETERM INFANTS 500-749 GRAMS	**P07.Ø2**	Extremely low birth weight newborn, 500-749 grams
765.13	OTHER PRETERM INFANTS 750-999 GRAMS	**P07.Ø3**	Extremely low birth weight newborn, 750-999 grams
765.14	OTHER PRETERM INFANTS 1000-1249 GRAMS	**PØ7.14**	Other low birth weight newborn, 1000-1249 grams
765.15	OTHER PRETERM INFANTS 1250-1499 GRAMS	**PØ7.15**	Other low birth weight newborn, 1250-1499 grams
765.16	OTHER PRETERM INFANTS 1500-1749 GRAMS	**PØ7.16**	Other low birth weight newborn, 1500-1749 grams
765.17	OTHER PRETERM INFANTS 1750-1999 GRAMS	**PØ7.17**	Other low birth weight newborn, 1750-1999 grams
765.18	OTHER PRETERM INFANTS 2000-2499 GRAMS	**PØ7.18**	Other low birth weight newborn, 2000-2499 grams
765.19	OTHER PRETERM INFANTS 2500 OR MORE GRAMS	**PØ7.3Ø**	Preterm newborn, unspecified weeks of gestation
765.2Ø	UNSPECIFIED WEEKS OF GESTATION	**PØ7.2Ø** **PØ7.3Ø**	Extreme immaturity of newborn, unsp weeks of gestation Preterm newborn, unspecified weeks of gestation
765.21	LESS THAN 24 COMPLETED WEEKS OF GESTATION	**PØ7.21** **PØ7.22**	Extreme immaturity of NB, gestatnl age < 23 completed weeks Extreme immaturity of NB, gestatnl age 23 completed weeks
765.22	24 COMPLETED WEEKS OF GESTATION	**PØ7.23**	Extreme immaturity of NB, gestatnl age 24 completed weeks
765.23	25-26 COMPLETED WEEKS OF GESTATION	**PØ7.24** **PØ7.25**	Extreme immaturity of NB, gestatnl age 25 completed weeks Extreme immaturity of NB, gestatnl age 26 completed weeks
765.24	27-28 COMPLETED WEEKS OF GESTATION	**PØ7.26** **PØ7.31**	Extreme immaturity of NB, gestatnl age 27 completed weeks Preterm newborn, gestational age 28 completed weeks
765.25	29-30 COMPLETED WEEKS OF GESTATION	**PØ7.32** **PØ7.33**	Preterm newborn, gestational age 29 completed weeks Preterm newborn, gestational age 30 completed weeks
765.26	31-32 COMPLETED WEEKS OF GESTATION	**PØ7.34** **PØ7.35**	Preterm newborn, gestational age 31 completed weeks Preterm newborn, gestational age 32 completed weeks
765.27	33-34 COMPLETED WEEKS OF GESTATION	**PØ7.36** **PØ7.37**	Preterm newborn, gestational age 33 completed weeks Preterm newborn, gestational age 34 completed weeks
765.28	35-36 COMPLETED WEEKS OF GESTATION	**PØ7.38** **PØ7.39**	Preterm newborn, gestational age 35 completed weeks Preterm newborn, gestational age 36 completed weeks
765.29	37 OR MORE COMPLETED WEEKS OF GESTATION	NO DIAGNOSIS	
766.Ø	EXCEPTIONALLY LARGE BABY RELATING LONG GESTATION	➡ **PØ8.Ø**	Exceptionally large newborn baby
766.1	OTH HEVY-FOR-DATES INFNTS NOT RELATED GEST PRD	➡ **PØ8.1**	Other heavy for gestational age newborn
766.21	POST-TERM INFANT	➡ **PØ8.21**	Post-term newborn
766.22	PROLONGED GESTATION OF INFANT	➡ **PØ8.22**	Prolonged gestation of newborn
767.Ø	SUBDURAL AND CEREBRAL HEMORRHAGE BIRTH TRAUMA	**P1Ø.Ø** **P1Ø.1** **P1Ø.4** **P1Ø.8** **P1Ø.9** **P11.Ø** **P11.2** **P11.9** **P52.4** **P52.6** **P52.8** **P52.9**	Subdural hemorrhage due to birth injury Cerebral hemorrhage due to birth injury Tentorial tear due to birth injury Oth intcrn lacerations and hemorrhages due to birth injury Unsp intcrn laceration and hemorrhage due to birth injury Cerebral edema due to birth injury Unspecified brain damage due to birth injury Birth injury to central nervous system, unspecified Intracerebral (nontraumatic) hemorrhage of newborn Cerebellar and posterior fossa hemorrhage of newborn Other intracranial (nontraumatic) hemorrhages of newborn Intracranial (nontraumatic) hemorrhage of newborn, unsp
767.11	BIRTH TRAUMA, EPICRANIAL SUBAPONEURO HEMORRHAGE	➡ **P12.2**	Epicranial subaponeurotic hemorrhage due to birth injury
767.19	BIRTH TRAUMA, OTHER INJURIES TO SCALP	**P12.Ø** **P12.1** **P12.3** **P12.4** **P12.81** **P12.89** **P12.9**	Cephalhematoma due to birth injury Chignon (from vacuum extraction) due to birth injury Bruising of scalp due to birth injury Injury of scalp of newborn due to monitoring equipment Caput succedaneum Other birth injuries to scalp Birth injury to scalp, unspecified
767.2	FRACTURE OF CLAVICLE, BIRTH TRAUMA	➡ **P13.4**	Fracture of clavicle due to birth injury
767.3	OTHER INJURIES TO SKELETON BIRTH TRAUMA	**P13.Ø** **P13.1** **P13.2** **P13.3** **P13.8** **P13.9**	Fracture of skull due to birth injury Other birth injuries to skull Birth injury to femur Birth injury to other long bones Birth injuries to other parts of skeleton Birth injury to skeleton, unspecified
767.4	INJURY TO SPINE AND SPINAL CORD BIRTH TRAUMA	➡ **P11.5**	Birth injury to spine and spinal cord
767.5	FACIAL NERVE INJURY, BIRTH TRAUMA	➡ **P11.3**	Birth injury to facial nerve
767.6	INJURY TO BRACHIAL PLEXUS BIRTH TRAUMA	**P14.Ø** **P14.1** **P14.3**	Erb's paralysis due to birth injury Klumpke's paralysis due to birth injury Other brachial plexus birth injuries
767.7	OTH CRANIAL&PERIPH NERVE INJURIES BIRTH TRAUMA	**P11.4** **P14.2** **P14.8** **P14.9**	Birth injury to other cranial nerves Phrenic nerve paralysis due to birth injury Birth injuries to other parts of peripheral nervous system Birth injury to peripheral nervous system, unspecified
767.8	OTHER SPECIFIED BIRTH TRAUMA	**P11.1** **P15.Ø** **P15.1** **P15.2** **P15.3** **P15.4** **P15.5** **P15.6** **P15.8**	Other specified brain damage due to birth injury Birth injury to liver Birth injury to spleen Sternomastoid injury due to birth injury Birth injury to eye Birth injury to face Birth injury to external genitalia Subcutaneous fat necrosis due to birth injury Other specified birth injuries

ICD-9-CM			ICD-10-CM	
767.9	UNSPECIFIED BIRTH TRAUMA	➡	P15.9	Birth injury, unspecified
768.Ø	FETAL DEATH D/T ASPHYX/ANOXIA BFOR LABR/UNS TIME		P84	Other problems with newborn
768.1	FETAL DEATH FROM ASPHYXIA OR ANOXIA DURING LABOR		P84	Other problems with newborn
768.2	FETAL DISTRESS BEFORE ONSET LABOR LIVEBORN INFNT		P19.Ø	Metabolic acidemia in newborn first noted before onset labor
768.3	FETL DISTRSS FIRST NOTED DURING L&D LIVE NEWBORN		P19.1	Metabolic acidemia in newborn first noted during labor
768.4	FETAL DISTRESS UNSPEC AS TIME ONSET LIVEB INFNT		P19.2 P19.9	Metabolic acidemia noted at birth Metabolic acidemia, unspecified
768.5	SEVERE BIRTH ASPHYXIA		P84	Other problems with newborn
768.6	MILD OR MODERATE BIRTH ASPHYXIA		P84	Other problems with newborn
768.7Ø	HYPOXIC-ISCHEMIC ENCEPHALOPATHY UNSPECIFIED	➡	P91.6Ø	Hypoxic ischemic encephalopathy [HIE], unspecified
768.71	MILD HYPOXIC-ISCHEMIC ENCEPHALOPATHY	➡	P91.61	Mild hypoxic ischemic encephalopathy [HIE]
768.72	MODERATE HYPOXIC-ISCHEMIC ENCEPHALOPATHY	➡	P91.62	Moderate hypoxic ischemic encephalopathy [HIE]
768.73	SEVERE HYPOXIC-ISCHEMIC ENCEPHALOPATHY	➡	P91.63	Severe hypoxic ischemic encephalopathy [HIE]
768.9	UNSPECIFIED BIRTH ASPHYXIA IN LIVEBORN INFANT		P84	Other problems with newborn
769	RESPIRATORY DISTRESS SYNDROME IN NEWBORN	➡	P22.Ø	Respiratory distress syndrome of newborn
77Ø.Ø	CONGENITAL PNEUMONIA		P23.Ø P23.1 P23.2 P23.3 P23.4 P23.5 P23.6 P23.8 P23.9	Congenital pneumonia due to viral agent Congenital pneumonia due to Chlamydia Congenital pneumonia due to staphylococcus Congenital pneumonia due to streptococcus, group B Congenital pneumonia due to Escherichia coli Congenital pneumonia due to Pseudomonas Congenital pneumonia due to other bacterial agents Congenital pneumonia due to other organisms Congenital pneumonia, unspecified
77Ø.1Ø	FETAL AND NEWBORN ASPIRATION UNSPECIFIED		P24.9	Neonatal aspiration, unspecified
77Ø.11	MECONIUM ASPIRATION W/O RESPIRATORY SYMPTOMS	➡	P24.ØØ	Meconium aspiration without respiratory symptoms
77Ø.12	NB MECONIUM ASPIRATION WITH RESPIRATORY SYMPTOMS	➡	P24.Ø1	Meconium aspiration with respiratory symptoms
77Ø.13	ASPIRATION CLEAR AMNIO FLUID W/O RESP SYMPTOM	➡	P24.1Ø	Neonatal aspirat of amnio fluid and mucus w/o resp symp
77Ø.14	ASPIRATION CLEAR AMNIO FLUID W/RESP SYMPTOMS	➡	P24.11	Neonatal aspirat of amnio fluid and mucus w resp symp
77Ø.15	ASPIRATION OF BLOOD W/O RESPIRATORY SYMPTOMS	➡	P24.2Ø	Neonatal aspiration of blood without respiratory symptoms
77Ø.16	NB ASPIRATION OF BLOOD WITH RESPIRATORY SYMPTOMS	➡	P24.21	Neonatal aspiration of blood with respiratory symptoms
77Ø.17	OTH FETAL&NB ASPIRATION W/O RESPIRATORY SYMPTOMS	➡	P24.8Ø	Other neonatal aspiration without respiratory symptoms
77Ø.18	OTH FETAL&NB ASPIRATION W/RESPIRATORY SYMPTOMS	➡	P24.81	Other neonatal aspiration with respiratory symptoms
77Ø.2	INTERSTITIAL EMPHYSEMA&RELATED CONDS NEWBORN		P25.Ø P25.1 P25.2 P25.3 P25.8	Interstitial emphysema originating in the perinatal period Pneumothorax originating in the perinatal period Pneumomediastinum originating in the perinatal period Pneumopericardium originating in the perinatal period Oth cond rel to interstit emphysema origin in perinat period
77Ø.3	PULMONARY HEMORRHAGE OF FETUS OR NEWBORN		P26.Ø P26.1 P26.8 P26.9	Tracheobronchial hemorrhage origin in the perinatal period Massive pulmonary hemorrhage origin in the perinatal period Oth pulmonary hemorrhages origin in the perinatal period Unsp pulmonary hemorrhage origin in the perinatal period
77Ø.4	PRIMARY ATELECTASIS OF NEWBORN	➡	P28.Ø	Primary atelectasis of newborn
77Ø.5	OTHER AND UNSPECIFIED ATELECTASIS OF NEWBORN		P28.1Ø P28.11 P28.19	Unspecified atelectasis of newborn Resorption atelectasis without respiratory distress syndrome Other atelectasis of newborn
77Ø.6	TRANSITORY TACHYPNEA OF NEWBORN	➡	P22.1	Transient tachypnea of newborn
77Ø.7	CHRONIC RESPIRATORY DISEASE ARISE PERINTL PERIOD		P27.Ø P27.1 P27.8 P27.9	Wilson-Mikity syndrome Bronchopulmonary dysplasia origin in the perinatal period Oth chronic resp diseases origin in the perinatal period Unsp chronic resp disease origin in the perinatal period
77Ø.81	PRIMARY APNEA OF NEWBORN		P28.3	Primary sleep apnea of newborn
77Ø.82	OTHER APNEA OF NEWBORN	➡	P28.4	Other apnea of newborn
77Ø.83	CYANOTIC ATTACKS OF NEWBORN	➡	P28.2	Cyanotic attacks of newborn
77Ø.84	RESPIRATORY FAILURE OF NEWBORN	➡	P28.5	Respiratory failure of newborn
77Ø.85	ASPIRATION POSTNATAL STOMACH CONTENT W/O RESP SX	➡	P24.3Ø	Neonatal aspirat of milk and regurgitated food w/o resp symp
77Ø.86	ASPIRATION POSTNATAL STOMACH CONTENT W/RESP SX	➡	P24.31	Neonatal aspirat of milk and regurgitated food w resp symp
77Ø.87	RESPIRATORY ARREST OF NEWBORN	➡	P28.81	Respiratory arrest of newborn
77Ø.88	HYPOXEMIA OF NEWBORN		P84	Other problems with newborn
77Ø.89	OTHER RESPIRATORY PROBLEMS NEWBORN AFTER BIRTH		P22.8 P22.9 P28.89	Other respiratory distress of newborn Respiratory distress of newborn, unspecified Other specified respiratory conditions of newborn
77Ø.9	UNSPECIFIED RESPIRATORY CONDITION FETUS&NEWBORN		P28.9	Respiratory condition of newborn, unspecified
771.Ø	CONGENITAL RUBELLA	➡	P35.Ø	Congenital rubella syndrome
771.1	CONGENITAL CYTOMEGALOVIRUS INFECTION	➡	P35.1	Congenital cytomegalovirus infection

 [Brackets] indicate valid character values for each code. Character value meanings provided for each code grouping.

ICD-9-CM		ICD-10-CM	
771.2	OTH CONGEN INFECTION SPECIFIC PERINATAL PERIOD	**P35.2**	Congenital herpesviral [herpes simplex] infection
		P35.3	Congenital viral hepatitis
		P35.8	Other congenital viral diseases
		P35.9	Congenital viral disease, unspecified
		P37.Ø	Congenital tuberculosis
		P37.1	Congenital toxoplasmosis
		P37.2	Neonatal (disseminated) listeriosis
		P37.3	Congenital falciparum malaria
		P37.4	Other congenital malaria
		P37.8	Other specified congenital infectious and parasitic diseases
		P37.9	Congenital infectious or parasitic disease, unspecified
771.3	TETANUS NEONATORUM	➡ **A33**	Tetanus neonatorum
771.4	OMPHALITIS OF THE NEWBORN	**P38.1**	Omphalitis with mild hemorrhage
		P38.9	Omphalitis without hemorrhage
771.5	NEONATAL INFECTIVE MASTITIS	➡ **P39.Ø**	Neonatal infective mastitis
771.6	NEONATAL CONJUNCTIVITIS AND DACRYOCYSTITIS	➡ **P39.1**	Neonatal conjunctivitis and dacryocystitis
771.7	NEONATAL CANDIDA INFECTION	➡ **P37.5**	Neonatal candidiasis
771.81	SEPTICEMIA OF NEWBORN	**P36.Ø**	Sepsis of newborn due to streptococcus, group B
		P36.1Ø	Sepsis of newborn due to unspecified streptococci
		P36.19	Sepsis of newborn due to other streptococci
		P36.2	Sepsis of newborn due to Staphylococcus aureus
		P36.3Ø	Sepsis of newborn due to unspecified staphylococci
		P36.39	Sepsis of newborn due to other staphylococci
		P36.4	Sepsis of newborn due to Escherichia coli
		P36.5	Sepsis of newborn due to anaerobes
		P36.8	Other bacterial sepsis of newborn
		P36.9	Bacterial sepsis of newborn, unspecified
771.82	URINARY TRACT INFECTION OF NEWBORN	➡ **P39.3**	Neonatal urinary tract infection
771.83	BACTEREMIA OF NEWBORN	**R78.81**	Bacteremia
771.89	OTHER INFECTIONS SPECIFIC TO PERINATAL PERIOD	**P39.2**	Intra-amniotic infection affecting newborn, NEC
		P39.4	Neonatal skin infection
		P39.8	Other specified infections specific to the perinatal period
		P39.9	Infection specific to the perinatal period, unspecified
772.Ø	FETAL BLOOD LOSS AFFECTING NEWBORN	**P5Ø.Ø**	Newborn aff by uterin (fetal) blood loss from vasa previa
		P5Ø.1	Newborn aff by uterin (fetal) blood loss from ruptured cord
		P5Ø.2	Newborn affected by uterin (fetal) blood loss from placenta
		P5Ø.3	Newborn affected by hemorrhage into co-twin
		P5Ø.4	Newborn affected by hemorrhage into maternal circulation
		P5Ø.5	NB aff by uterin blood loss from cut end of co-twin's cord
		P5Ø.8	Newborn affected by other intrauterine (fetal) blood loss
		P5Ø.9	Newborn affected by intrauterine (fetal) blood loss, unsp
772.1Ø	INTRAVENTRICULAR HEMORRHAGE, UNSPECIFIED GRADE	**P1Ø.2**	Intraventricular hemorrhage due to birth injury
		P52.3	Unsp intraventricular (nontraumatic) hemorrhage of newborn
772.11	INTRAVENTRICULAR HEMORRHAGE, GRADE I	➡ **P52.Ø**	Intraventricular hemorrhage, grade 1, of newborn
772.12	INTRAVENTRICULAR HEMORRHAGE, GRADE II	➡ **P52.1**	Intraventricular hemorrhage, grade 2, of newborn
772.13	INTRAVENTRICULAR HEMORRHAGE, GRADE III	➡ **P52.21**	Intraventricular hemorrhage, grade 3, of newborn
772.14	INTRAVENTRICULAR HEMORRHAGE, GRADE IV	➡ **P52.22**	Intraventricular hemorrhage, grade 4, of newborn
772.2	FETAL&NEONATAL SUBARACHNOID HEMORRHAGE NEWBORN	**P1Ø.3**	Subarachnoid hemorrhage due to birth injury
		P52.5	Subarachnoid (nontraumatic) hemorrhage of newborn
772.3	UMBILICAL HEMORRHAGE AFTER BIRTH	**P51.Ø**	Massive umbilical hemorrhage of newborn
		P51.8	Other umbilical hemorrhages of newborn
		P51.9	Umbilical hemorrhage of newborn, unspecified
772.4	FETAL AND NEONATAL GASTROINTESTINAL HEMORRHAGE	**P54.1**	Neonatal melena
		P54.2	Neonatal rectal hemorrhage
		P54.3	Other neonatal gastrointestinal hemorrhage
772.5	FETAL AND NEONATAL ADRENAL HEMORRHAGE	➡ **P54.4**	Neonatal adrenal hemorrhage
772.6	FETAL AND NEONATAL CUTANEOUS HEMORRHAGE	➡ **P54.5**	Neonatal cutaneous hemorrhage
772.8	OTHER SPECIFIED HEMORRHAGE OF FETUS OR NEWBORN	**P54.Ø**	Neonatal hematemesis
		P54.6	Neonatal vaginal hemorrhage
		P54.8	Other specified neonatal hemorrhages
772.9	UNSPECIFIED HEMORRHAGE OF NEWBORN	➡ **P54.9**	Neonatal hemorrhage, unspecified
773.Ø	HEMOLYTIC DZ DUE RH ISOIMMUNIZATION FETUS/NB	➡ **P55.Ø**	Rh isoimmunization of newborn
773.1	HEMOLYTIC DZ DUE ABO ISOIMMUNIZATION FETUS/NB	**P55.1**	ABO isoimmunization of newborn
773.2	HEMOLYT DZ DUE OTH&UNSPEC ISOIMMUN FETUS/NB	**P55.8**	Other hemolytic diseases of newborn
		P55.9	Hemolytic disease of newborn, unspecified
773.3	HYDROPS FETALIS DUE TO ISOIMMUNIZATION	**P56.Ø**	Hydrops fetalis due to isoimmunization
		P56.9Ø	Hydrops fetalis due to unspecified hemolytic disease
		P56.99	Hydrops fetalis due to other hemolytic disease
773.4	KERNICTERUS DUE TO ISOIMMUNIZATION FETUS/NEWBORN	➡ **P57.Ø**	Kernicterus due to isoimmunization
773.5	LATE ANEMIA DUE TO ISOIMMUNIZATION FETUS/NEWBORN	**P55.1**	ABO isoimmunization of newborn
774.Ø	PERINTL JAUNDICE FROM HEREDIT HEMOLYTIC ANEMIAS	**P58.8**	Neonatal jaundice due to other specified excessive hemolysis

ICD-9-CM			ICD-10-CM	
774.1	PERINATAL JAUNDICE FROM OTH EXCESSIVE HEMOLYSIS		**P58.0** **P58.1** **P58.2** **P58.3** **P58.41** **P58.42** **P58.5** **P58.8** **P58.9**	Neonatal jaundice due to bruising Neonatal jaundice due to bleeding Neonatal jaundice due to infection Neonatal jaundice due to polycythemia NB jaund due to drugs or toxins transmitted from mother Neonatal jaundice due to drugs or toxins given to newborn Neonatal jaundice due to swallowed maternal blood Neonatal jaundice due to other specified excessive hemolysis Neonatal jaundice due to excessive hemolysis, unspecified
774.2	NEONATAL JAUNDICE ASSOCIATED W/PRETERM DELIVERY	➡	**P59.0**	Neonatal jaundice associated with preterm delivery
774.30	NEONAT JAUNDICE DUE DELAY CONJUGAT CAUSE UNSPEC		**P59.8**	Neonatal jaundice from other specified causes
774.31	NEONAT JAUNDICE DUE DELAY CONJUGAT DZ CLASS ELSW		**P59.8**	Neonatal jaundice from other specified causes
774.39	OTH NEONAT JAUNDCE DUE DELAY CONJUGAT OTH CAUS		**P59.3**	Neonatal jaundice from breast milk inhibitor
774.4	PERINATAL JAUNDICE DUE TO HEPATOCELLULAR DAMAGE		**P59.1** **P59.20** **P59.29**	Inspissated bile syndrome Neonatal jaundice from unspecified hepatocellular damage Neonatal jaundice from other hepatocellular damage
774.5	PERINATAL JAUNDICE FROM OTHER CAUSES		**P59.8**	Neonatal jaundice from other specified causes
774.6	UNSPECIFIED FETAL AND NEONATAL JAUNDICE		**P59.9**	Neonatal jaundice, unspecified
774.7	KERNICTERUS FETUS/NB NOT DUE ISOIMMUNIZATION		**P57.8** **P57.9**	Other specified kernicterus Kernicterus, unspecified
775.0	SYNDROME OF INFANT OF DIABETIC MOTHER		**P70.0** **P70.1**	Syndrome of infant of mother with gestational diabetes Syndrome of infant of a diabetic mother
775.1	NEONATAL DIABETES MELLITUS	➡	**P70.2**	Neonatal diabetes mellitus
775.2	NEONATAL MYASTHENIA GRAVIS		**P94.0**	Transient neonatal myasthenia gravis
775.3	NEONATAL THYROTOXICOSIS	➡	**P72.1**	Transitory neonatal hyperthyroidism
775.4	HYPOCALCEMIA AND HYPOMAGNESEMIA OF NEWBORN		**P71.0** **P71.1** **P71.2** **P71.3** **P71.4** **P71.8** **P71.9**	Cow's milk hypocalcemia in newborn Other neonatal hypocalcemia Neonatal hypomagnesemia Neonatal tetany without calcium or magnesium deficiency Transitory neonatal hypoparathyroidism Oth transitory neonatal disord of calcium & magnesium metab Transitory neonatal disord of calcium & magnesium metab,unsp
775.5	OTH TRANSITORY NEONATAL ELECTROLYTE DISTURBANCES		**P74.1** **P74.2** **P74.3** **P74.4**	Dehydration of newborn Disturbances of sodium balance of newborn Disturbances of potassium balance of newborn Other transitory electrolyte disturbances of newborn
775.6	NEONATAL HYPOGLYCEMIA		**P70.3** **P70.4**	Iatrogenic neonatal hypoglycemia Other neonatal hypoglycemia
775.7	LATE METABOLIC ACIDOSIS OF NEWBORN	➡	**P74.0**	Late metabolic acidosis of newborn
775.81	OTHER ACIDOSIS OF NEWBORN		**P84**	Other problems with newborn
775.89	OTH NEONATAL ENDOCRINE & METABOLIC DISTURBANCES		**P70.8** **P72.0** **P72.2** **P72.8** **P74.5** **P74.6** **P74.8**	Oth transitory disorders of carbohydrate metab of newborn Neonatal goiter, not elsewhere classified Oth transitory neonatal disorders of thyroid function, NEC Other specified transitory neonatal endocrine disorders Transitory tyrosinemia of newborn Transitory hyperammonemia of newborn Other transitory metabolic disturbances of newborn
775.9	UNSPEC ENDOCRN&METAB DISTURB SPECIFIC FETUS&NB		**P70.9** **P72.9** **P74.9**	Transitory disorder of carbohydrate metab of newborn, unsp Transitory neonatal endocrine disorder, unspecified Transitory metabolic disturbance of newborn, unspecified
776.0	HEMORRHAGIC DISEASE OF NEWBORN	➡	**P53**	Hemorrhagic disease of newborn
776.1	TRANSIENT NEONATAL THROMBOCYTOPENIA	➡	**P61.0**	Transient neonatal thrombocytopenia
776.2	DISSEMINATED INTRAVASCULAR COAGULATION NEWBORN	➡	**P60**	Disseminated intravascular coagulation of newborn
776.3	OTHER TRANSIENT NEONATAL DISORDERS COAGULATION	➡	**P61.6**	Other transient neonatal disorders of coagulation
776.4	POLYCYTHEMIA NEONATORUM	➡	**P61.1**	Polycythemia neonatorum
776.5	CONGENITAL ANEMIA		**P61.3** **P61.4**	Congenital anemia from fetal blood loss Other congenital anemias, not elsewhere classified
776.6	ANEMIA OF NEONATAL PREMATURITY	➡	**P61.2**	Anemia of prematurity
776.7	TRANSIENT NEONATAL NEUTROPENIA	➡	**P61.5**	Transient neonatal neutropenia
776.8	OTH SPEC TRANSIENT HEMATOLOGICAL D/O FETUS/NB	➡	**P61.8**	Other specified perinatal hematological disorders
776.9	UNS HEMATOLOGICAL DISORDER SPECIFIC TO NEWBORN	➡	**P61.9**	Perinatal hematological disorder, unspecified
777.1	FETAL AND NEWBORN MECONIUM OBSTRUCTION		**P76.0**	Meconium plug syndrome
777.2	NEONATAL INTEST OBSTRUCTION DUE INSPISSATED MILK	➡	**P76.2**	Intestinal obstruction due to inspissated milk
777.3	NEONAT HEMATEMESIS&MELENA DUE SWALLOWED MTRN BLD	➡	**P78.2**	Neonatal hematemesis and melena d/t swallowed matern blood
777.4	TRANSITORY ILEUS OF NEWBORN	➡	**P76.1**	Transitory ileus of newborn
777.50	NECROTIZING ENTEROCOLITIS IN NEWBORN UNSPECIFIED	➡	**P77.9**	Necrotizing enterocolitis in newborn, unspecified
777.51	STAGE I NECROTIZING ENTEROCOLITIS IN NEWBORN	➡	**P77.1**	Stage 1 necrotizing enterocolitis in newborn
777.52	STAGE II NECROTIZING ENTEROCOLITIS IN NEWBORN	➡	**P77.2**	Stage 2 necrotizing enterocolitis in newborn
777.53	STAGE III NECROTIZING ENTEROCOLITIES IN NEWBORN	➡	**P77.3**	Stage 3 necrotizing enterocolitis in newborn
777.6	PERINATAL INTESTINAL PERFORATION	➡	**P78.0**	Perinatal intestinal perforation

[Brackets] indicate valid character values for each code. Character value meanings provided for each code grouping.

ICD-9-CM		ICD-10-CM	
777.8	OTHER SPEC PERINATAL DISORDER DIGESTIVE SYSTEM	P76.8 P76.9 P78.1 P78.3 P78.81 P78.82 P78.83 P78.89	Other specified intestinal obstruction of newborn Intestinal obstruction of newborn, unspecified Other neonatal peritonitis Noninfective neonatal diarrhea Congenital cirrhosis (of liver) Peptic ulcer of newborn Newborn esophageal reflux Other specified perinatal digestive system disorders
777.9	UNSPECIFIED PERINATAL DISORDER DIGESTIVE SYSTEM	➡ P78.9	Perinatal digestive system disorder, unspecified
778.Ø	HYDROPS FETALIS NOT DUE TO ISOIMMUNIZATION	➡ P83.2	Hydrops fetalis not due to hemolytic disease
778.1	SCLEREMA NEONATORUM	➡ P83.Ø	Sclerema neonatorum
778.2	COLD INJURY SYNDROME OF NEWBORN	➡ P8Ø.Ø	Cold injury syndrome
778.3	OTHER HYPOTHERMIA OF NEWBORN	P8Ø.8 P8Ø.9	Other hypothermia of newborn Hypothermia of newborn, unspecified
778.4	OTHER DISTURBANCE TEMPERATURE REGULATION NEWBORN	P81.Ø P81.8 P81.9	Environmental hyperthermia of newborn Oth disturbances of temperature regulation of newborn Disturbance of temperature regulation of newborn, unsp
778.5	OTHER AND UNSPECIFIED EDEMA OF NEWBORN	P83.3Ø P83.39	Unspecified edema specific to newborn Other edema specific to newborn
778.6	CONGENITAL HYDROCELE	➡ P83.5	Congenital hydrocele
778.7	BREAST ENGORGEMENT IN NEWBORN	➡ P83.4	Breast engorgement of newborn
778.8	OTH SPEC COND INVOLVING INTEGUMENT FETUS&NEWBORN	P83.1 P83.6 P83.8	Neonatal erythema toxicum Umbilical polyp of newborn Other specified conditions of integument specific to newborn
778.9	UNSPEC COND INVLV INTEGUMENT&TEMP REG FETUS&NB	P83.9	Condition of the integument specific to newborn, unspecified
779.Ø	CONVULSIONS IN NEWBORN	➡ P9Ø	Convulsions of newborn
779.1	OTHER&UNSPECIFIED CEREBRAL IRRITABILITY NEWBORN	P91.8 P91.9	Other specified disturbances of cerebral status of newborn Disturbance of cerebral status of newborn, unspecified
779.2	CEREBRAL DEPRESS COMA&OTH CEREBRAL SIGN-FETUS/NB	P91.Ø P91.1 P91.3 P91.4 P91.5	Neonatal cerebral ischemia Acquired periventricular cysts of newborn Neonatal cerebral irritability Neonatal cerebral depression Neonatal coma
779.31	FEEDING PROBLEMS IN NEWBORN	P92.1 P92.2 P92.3 P92.4 P92.5 P92.8 P92.9	Regurgitation and rumination of newborn Slow feeding of newborn Underfeeding of newborn Overfeeding of newborn Neonatal difficulty in feeding at breast Other feeding problems of newborn Feeding problem of newborn, unspecified
779.32	BILIOUS VOMITING IN NEWBORN	➡ P92.Ø1	Bilious vomiting of newborn
779.33	OTHER VOMITING IN NEWBORN	P92.Ø9	Other vomiting of newborn
779.34	FAILURE TO THRIVE IN NEWBORN	➡ P92.6	Failure to thrive in newborn
779.4	DRUG REACTIONS&INTOXICATIONS SPECIFIC TO NEWBORN	P93.Ø P93.8	Grey baby syndrome Oth reactions and intoxications d/t drugs administered to NB
779.5	DRUG WITHDRAWAL SYNDROME IN NEWBORN	P96.1 P96.2	Neonatal w/drawal symp from matern use of drugs of addiction Withdrawal symptoms from therapeutic use of drugs in newborn
779.6	TERMINATION OF PREGNANCY	NO DIAGNOSIS	
779.7	PERIVENTRICULAR LEUKOMALACIA	P91.2	Neonatal cerebral leukomalacia
779.81	NEONATAL BRADYCARDIA	➡ P29.12	Neonatal bradycardia
779.82	NEONATAL TACHYCARDIA	➡ P29.11	Neonatal tachycardia
779.83	DELAYED SEPARATION OF UMBILICAL CORD	➡ P96.82	Delayed separation of umbilical cord
779.84	OTH SPEC CONDS ORIG PERINTAL PERIOD MEC STAINING	➡ P96.83	Meconium staining
779.85	CARDIAC ARREST OF NEWBORN	➡ P29.81	Cardiac arrest of newborn
779.89	OTHER SPEC CONDS ORIGINATING PERINATAL PERIOD	P29.Ø P29.2 P29.4 P29.89 P29.9 P94.1 P94.2 P94.8 P94.9 P96.Ø P96.3 P96.5 P96.89	Neonatal cardiac failure Neonatal hypertension Transient myocardial ischemia in newborn Oth cardiovasc disorders originating in the perinatal period Cardiovasc disorder origin in the perinatal period, unsp Congenital hypertonia Congenital hypotonia Other disorders of muscle tone of newborn Disorder of muscle tone of newborn, unspecified Congenital renal failure Wide cranial sutures of newborn Comp to newborn due to (fetal) intrauterine procedure Oth conditions originating in the perinatal period
779.9	UNSPEC CONDITION ORIGINATING PERINATAL PERIOD	P95 P96.9	Stillbirth Condition originating in the perinatal period, unspecified

Symptoms, Signs, and Ill-Defined Conditions

ICD-9-CM			ICD-10-CM	
780.01	COMA		**E03.5**	Myxedema coma
			R40.20	Unspecified coma
			R40.2110	Coma scale, eyes open, never, unspecified time
			R40.2111	Coma scale, eyes open, never, in the field
			R40.2112	Coma scale, eyes open, never, EMR
			R40.2113	Coma scale, eyes open, never, at hospital admission
			R40.2114	Coma scale, eyes open, never, 24+hrs
			R40.2120	Coma scale, eyes open, to pain, unspecified time
			R40.2121	Coma scale, eyes open, to pain, in the field
			R40.2122	Coma scale, eyes open, to pain, EMR
			R40.2123	Coma scale, eyes open, to pain, at hospital admission
			R40.2124	Coma scale, eyes open, to pain, 24+hrs
			R40.2210	Coma scale, best verbal response, none, unspecified time
			R40.2211	Coma scale, best verbal response, none, in the field
			R40.2212	Coma scale, best verbal response, none, EMR
			R40.2213	Coma scale, best verbal response, none, admit
			R40.2214	Coma scale, best verbal response, none, 24+hrs
			R40.2220	Coma scale, best verb, incomprehensible words, unsp time
			R40.2221	Coma scale, best verb, incomprehensible words, in the field
			R40.2222	Coma scale, best verb, incomprehensible words, EMR
			R40.2223	Coma scale, best verb, incomprehensible words, admit
			R40.2224	Coma scale, best verb, incomprehensible words, 24+hrs
			R40.2310	Coma scale, best motor response, none, unspecified time
			R40.2311	Coma scale, best motor response, none, in the field
			R40.2312	Coma scale, best motor response, none, EMR
			R40.2313	Coma scale, best motor response, none, at hospital admission
			R40.2314	Coma scale, best motor response, none, 24+hrs
			R40.2320	Coma scale, best motor response, extension, unspecified time
			R40.2321	Coma scale, best motor response, extension, in the field
			R40.2322	Coma scale, best motor response, extension, EMR
			R40.2323	Coma scale, best motor response, extension, admit
			R40.2324	Coma scale, best motor response, extension, 24+hrs
			R40.2340	Coma scale, best motor, flexion withdrawal, unsp time
			R40.2341	Coma scale, best motor, flexion withdrawal, in the field
			R40.2342	Coma scale, best motor response, flexion withdrawal, EMR
			R40.2343	Coma scale, best motor response, flexion withdrawal, admit
			R40.2344	Coma scale, best motor response, flexion withdrawal, 24+hrs
780.02	TRANSIENT ALTERATION OF AWARENESS	➡	**R40.4**	Transient alteration of awareness
780.03	PERSISTENT VEGETATIVE STATE	➡	**R40.3**	Persistent vegetative state
780.09	OTHER ALTERATION OF CONSCIOUSNESS		**R40.0**	Somnolence
			R40.1	Stupor
780.1	HALLUCINATIONS		**R44.0**	Auditory hallucinations
			R44.2	Other hallucinations
			R44.3	Hallucinations, unspecified
780.2	SYNCOPE AND COLLAPSE	➡	**R55**	Syncope and collapse
780.31	FEBRILE CONVULSIONS SIMPLE UNSPECIFIED	➡	**R56.00**	Simple febrile convulsions
780.32	COMPLEX FEBRILE CONVULSIONS	➡	**R56.01**	Complex febrile convulsions
780.33	POST TRAUMATIC SEIZURES	➡	**R56.1**	Post traumatic seizures
780.39	OTHER CONVULSIONS		**R56.9**	Unspecified convulsions
780.4	DIZZINESS AND GIDDINESS	➡	**R42**	Dizziness and giddiness
780.50	UNSPECIFIED SLEEP DISTURBANCE		**G47.9**	Sleep disorder, unspecified
780.51	INSOMNIA WITH SLEEP APNEA UNSPECIFIED		**G47.30**	Sleep apnea, unspecified
780.52	INSOMNIA UNSPECIFIED	➡	**G47.00**	Insomnia, unspecified
780.53	HYPERSOMNIA WITH SLEEP APNEA UNSPECIFIED		**G47.30**	Sleep apnea, unspecified
780.54	HYPERSOMNIA UNSPECIFIED		**G47.10**	Hypersomnia, unspecified
780.55	DISRUPTION 24 HOUR SLEEP WAKE CYCLE UNSPECIFIED		**G47.20**	Circadian rhythm sleep disorder, unspecified type
780.56	DYSFNCT ASSO W/SLEEP STGES/AROUSAL FRM SLEEP		**G47.8**	Other sleep disorders
780.57	UNSPECIFIED SLEEP APNEA		**G47.30**	Sleep apnea, unspecified
780.58	SLEEP RELATED MOVEMENT DISORDER UNSPECIFIED		**F51.8**	Oth sleep disord not due to a sub or known physiol cond
780.59	OTHER SLEEP DISTURBANCES		**G47.8**	Other sleep disorders
780.60	FEVER UNSPECIFIED	◘	**R50.2**	Drug induced fever
			R50.9	Fever, unspecified
780.61	FEVER PRESENTING CONDITIONS CLASSIFIED ELSEWHERE	➡	**R50.81**	Fever presenting with conditions classified elsewhere
780.62	POSTPROCEDURAL FEVER	➡	**R50.82**	Postprocedural fever
780.63	POSTVACCINATION FEVER	➡	**R50.83**	Postvaccination fever
780.64	CHILLS WITHOUT FEVER	➡	**R68.83**	Chills (without fever)
780.65	HYPOTHERMIA NOT ASSOC W/LOW ENVIRONMENTAL TEMP	➡	**R68.0**	Hypothermia, not associated w low environmental temperature
780.66	FEBRILE NONHEMOLYTIC TRANSFUSION REACTION	➡	**R50.84**	Febrile nonhemolytic transfusion reaction
780.71	CHRONIC FATIGUE SYNDROME	➡	**R53.82**	Chronic fatigue, unspecified
780.72	FUNCTIONAL QUADRIPLEGIA	➡	**R53.2**	Functional quadriplegia
780.79	OTHER MALAISE AND FATIGUE		**G93.3**	Postviral fatigue syndrome
			R53.0	Neoplastic (malignant) related fatigue
			R53.1	Weakness
			R53.81	Other malaise
			R53.83	Other fatigue
780.8	GENERALIZED HYPERHIDROSIS	➡	**R61**	Generalized hyperhidrosis

ICD-9-CM			ICD-10-CM	
780.91	FUSSY INFANT	➡	R68.12	Fussy infant (baby)
780.92	EXCESSIVE CRYING OF INFANT	➡	R68.11	Excessive crying of infant (baby)
780.93	MEMORY LOSS		R41.1 R41.2 R41.3	Anterograde amnesia Retrograde amnesia Other amnesia
780.94	EARLY SATIETY	➡	R68.81	Early satiety
780.95	EXCESSIVE CRYING OF CHILD ADOLESCENT OR ADULT	➡	R45.83	Excessive crying of child, adolescent or adult
780.96	GENERALIZED PAIN		R52	Pain, unspecified
780.97	ALTERED MENTAL STATUS		R41.0 R41.82	Disorientation, unspecified Altered mental status, unspecified
780.99	OTHER GENERAL SYMPTOMS		R41.9 R45.84 R68.89	Unsp symptoms and signs w cognitive functions and awareness Anhedonia Other general symptoms and signs
781.0	ABNORMAL INVOLUNTARY MOVEMENTS		R25.0 R25.1 R25.2 R25.3 R25.8 R25.9	Abnormal head movements Tremor, unspecified Cramp and spasm Fasciculation Other abnormal involuntary movements Unspecified abnormal involuntary movements
781.1	DISTURBANCES OF SENSATION OF SMELL AND TASTE		R43.0 R43.1 R43.2 R43.8 R43.9	Anosmia Parosmia Parageusia Other disturbances of smell and taste Unspecified disturbances of smell and taste
781.2	ABNORMALITY OF GAIT		R26.0 R26.1 R26.81 R26.89 R26.9	Ataxic gait Paralytic gait Unsteadiness on feet Other abnormalities of gait and mobility Unspecified abnormalities of gait and mobility
781.3	LACK OF COORDINATION		R27.0 R27.8 R27.9	Ataxia, unspecified Other lack of coordination Unspecified lack of coordination
781.4	TRANSIENT PARALYSIS OF LIMB		R29.5	Transient paralysis
781.5	CLUBBING OF FINGERS	➡	R68.3	Clubbing of fingers
781.6	MENINGISMUS	➡	R29.1	Meningismus
781.7	TETANY	➡	R29.0	Tetany
781.8	NEUROLOGICAL NEGLECT SYNDROME	➡	R41.4	Neurologic neglect syndrome
781.91	LOSS OF HEIGHT	➡	R29.890	Loss of height
781.92	ABNORMAL POSTURE	➡	R29.3	Abnormal posture
781.93	OCULAR TORTICOLLIS	➡	R29.891	Ocular torticollis
781.94	FACIAL WEAKNESS	➡	R29.810	Facial weakness
781.99	OTH SYMPTOMS INVLV NERV&MUSCULOSKELETAL SYSTEMS		R29.6 R29.818 R29.898 R29.90 R29.91	Repeated falls Other symptoms and signs involving the nervous system Oth symptoms and signs involving the musculoskeletal system Unspecified symptoms and signs involving the nervous system Unsp symptoms and signs involving the musculoskeletal system
782.0	DISTURBANCE OF SKIN SENSATION		R20.0 R20.1 R20.2 R20.3 R20.8 R20.9	Anesthesia of skin Hypoesthesia of skin Paresthesia of skin Hyperesthesia Other disturbances of skin sensation Unspecified disturbances of skin sensation
782.1	RASH AND OTHER NONSPECIFIC SKIN ERUPTION	➡	R21	Rash and other nonspecific skin eruption
782.2	LOCALIZED SUPERFICIAL SWELLING MASS OR LUMP		R22.0 R22.1 R22.2 R22.30 R22.31 R22.32 R22.33 R22.40 R22.41 R22.42 R22.43 R22.9	Localized swelling, mass and lump, head Localized swelling, mass and lump, neck Localized swelling, mass and lump, trunk Localized swelling, mass and lump, unspecified upper limb Localized swelling, mass and lump, right upper limb Localized swelling, mass and lump, left upper limb Localized swelling, mass and lump, upper limb, bilateral Localized swelling, mass and lump, unspecified lower limb Localized swelling, mass and lump, right lower limb Localized swelling, mass and lump, left lower limb Localized swelling, mass and lump, lower limb, bilateral Localized swelling, mass and lump, unspecified
782.3	EDEMA		R60.0 R60.1 R60.9	Localized edema Generalized edema Edema, unspecified
782.4	JAUNDICE UNSPECIFIED NOT OF NEWBORN	➡	R17	Unspecified jaundice
782.5	CYANOSIS	➡	R23.0	Cyanosis
782.61	PALLOR	➡	R23.1	Pallor
782.62	FLUSHING	➡	R23.2	Flushing
782.7	SPONTANEOUS ECCHYMOSES	➡	R23.3	Spontaneous ecchymoses
782.8	CHANGES IN SKIN TEXTURE	➡	R23.4	Changes in skin texture

ICD-9-CM			ICD-10-CM	
782.9	OTH SYMPTOMS INVOLVING SKIN&INTEG TISSUES		**R23.8**	Other skin changes
			R23.9	Unspecified skin changes
783.Ø	ANOREXIA	➡	**R63.Ø**	Anorexia
783.1	ABNORMAL WEIGHT GAIN	➡	**R63.5**	Abnormal weight gain
783.21	LOSS OF WEIGHT	➡	**R63.4**	Abnormal weight loss
783.22	UNDERWEIGHT	➡	**R63.6**	Underweight
783.3	FEEDING DIFFICULTIES AND MISMANAGEMENT	➡	**R63.3**	Feeding difficulties
783.4Ø	LACK NORMAL PHYSIOLOGICAL DEVELOPMENT UNSPEC		**R62.5Ø**	Unsp lack of expected normal physiol dev in childhood
			R62.59	Oth lack of expected normal physiol development in childhood
783.41	FAILURE TO THRIVE	➡	**R62.51**	Failure to thrive (child)
783.42	DELAYED MILESTONES	➡	**R62.Ø**	Delayed milestone in childhood
783.43	SHORT STATURE	➡	**R62.52**	Short stature (child)
783.5	POLYDIPSIA	➡	**R63.1**	Polydipsia
783.6	POLYPHAGIA	➡	**R63.2**	Polyphagia
783.7	ADULT FAILURE TO THRIVE	➡	**R62.7**	Adult failure to thrive
783.9	OTH SYMPTOMS CONCERNING NUTRITION METAB&DVLP		**R63.8**	Other symptoms and signs concerning food and fluid intake
784.Ø	HEADACHE		**G44.1**	Vascular headache, not elsewhere classified
			R51	Headache
784.1	THROAT PAIN	➡	**RØ7.Ø**	Pain in throat
784.2	SWELLING MASS OR LUMP IN HEAD AND NECK		**R22.Ø**	Localized swelling, mass and lump, head
			R22.1	Localized swelling, mass and lump, neck
			R9Ø.Ø	Intcrn space-occupying lesion found on dx imaging of cnsl
784.3	APHASIA	➡	**R47.Ø1**	Aphasia
784.4Ø	VOICE AND RESONANCE DISORDER UNSPECIFIED		**R49.9**	Unspecified voice and resonance disorder
784.41	APHONIA	➡	**R49.1**	Aphonia
784.42	DYSPHONIA	➡	**R49.Ø**	Dysphonia
784.43	HYPERNASALITY	➡	**R49.21**	Hypernasality
784.44	HYPONASALITY	➡	**R49.22**	Hyponasality
784.49	OTHER VOICE AND RESONANCE DISORDERS		**R49.8**	Other voice and resonance disorders
784.51	DYSARTHRIA	➡	**R47.1**	Dysarthria and anarthria
784.52	FLUENCY DISORDER CONDITIONS CLASSIFIED ELSEWHERE	➡	**R47.82**	Fluency disorder in conditions classified elsewhere
784.59	OTHER SPEECH DISTURBANCE		**R47.Ø2**	Dysphasia
			R47.81	Slurred speech
			R47.89	Other speech disturbances
			R47.9	Unspecified speech disturbances
784.6Ø	SYMBOLIC DYSFUNCTION, UNSPECIFIED	➡	**R48.9**	Unspecified symbolic dysfunctions
784.61	ALEXIA AND DYSLEXIA		**R48.Ø**	Dyslexia and alexia
784.69	OTHER SYMBOLIC DYSFUNCTION		**R48.1**	Agnosia
			R48.2	Apraxia
			R48.8	Other symbolic dysfunctions
784.7	EPISTAXIS	➡	**RØ4.Ø**	Epistaxis
784.8	HEMORRHAGE FROM THROAT	➡	**RØ4.1**	Hemorrhage from throat
784.91	POSTNASAL DRIP	➡	**RØ9.82**	Postnasal drip
784.92	JAW PAIN	➡	**R68.84**	Jaw pain
784.99	OTHER SYMPTOMS INVOLVING HEAD AND NECK		**RØ6.5**	Mouth breathing
			RØ6.7	Sneezing
			RØ6.89	Other abnormalities of breathing
			R19.6	Halitosis
785.Ø	UNSPECIFIED TACHYCARDIA	➡	**RØØ.Ø**	Tachycardia, unspecified
785.1	PALPITATIONS	➡	**RØØ.2**	Palpitations
785.2	UNDIAGNOSED CARDIAC MURMURS		**RØ1.Ø**	Benign and innocent cardiac murmurs
			RØ1.1	Cardiac murmur, unspecified
785.3	OTHER ABNORMAL HEART SOUNDS		**RØØ.8**	Other abnormalities of heart beat
			RØØ.9	Unspecified abnormalities of heart beat
			RØ1.2	Other cardiac sounds
785.4	GANGRENE	◘	**EØ8.52**	Diab due to undrl cond w diabetic prph angiopath w gangrene
		◘	**EØ9.52**	Drug/chem diabetes w diabetic prph angiopath w gangrene
		◘	**E1Ø.52**	Type 1 diabetes w diabetic peripheral angiopathy w gangrene
		◘	**E11.52**	Type 2 diabetes w diabetic peripheral angiopathy w gangrene
		◘	**E13.52**	Oth diabetes w diabetic peripheral angiopathy w gangrene
		◘	**I7Ø.361**	Athscl unsp type bypass of the extrm w gangrene, right leg
		◘	**I7Ø.362**	Athscl unsp type bypass of the extrm w gangrene, left leg
		◘	**I7Ø.363**	Athscl unsp type bypass of the extrm w gangrene, bi legs
		◘	**I7Ø.368**	Athscl unsp type bypass of the extrm w gangrene, oth extrm
		◘	**I7Ø.369**	Athscl unsp type bypass of the extrm w gangrene, unsp extrm
		◘	**I7Ø.461**	Athscl autol vein bypass of the extrm w gangrene, right leg
		◘	**I7Ø.462**	Athscl autol vein bypass of the extrm w gangrene, left leg
		◘	**I7Ø.463**	Athscl autol vein bypass of the extrm w gangrene, bi legs
		◘	**I7Ø.468**	Athscl autol vein bypass of the extrm w gangrene, oth extrm
		◘	**I7Ø.469**	Athscl autol vein bypass of the extrm w gangrene, unsp extrm
	(Continued on next page)	◘	**I7Ø.561**	Athscl nonaut bio bypass of the extrm w gangrene, right leg
		◘	**I7Ø.562**	Athscl nonaut bio bypass of the extrm w gangrene, left leg

ICD-9-CM			ICD-10-CM	
785.4	GANGRENE (Continued)		I70.563	Athscl nonaut bio bypass of the extrm w gangrene, bi legs
			I70.568	Athscl nonaut bio bypass of the extrm w gangrene, oth extrm
			I70.569	Athscl nonaut bio bypass of the extrm w gangrene, unsp extrm
			I70.661	Athscl nonbiol bypass of the extrm w gangrene, right leg
			I70.662	Athscl nonbiol bypass of the extrm w gangrene, left leg
			I70.663	Athscl nonbiol bypass of the extrm w gangrene, bi legs
			I70.668	Athscl nonbiol bypass of the extrm w gangrene, oth extremity
			I70.669	Athscl nonbiol bypass of the extrm w gangrene, unsp extrm
			I70.761	Athscl type of bypass of the extrm w gangrene, right leg
			I70.762	Athscl type of bypass of the extrm w gangrene, left leg
			I70.763	Athscl type of bypass of the extrm w gangrene, bi legs
			I70.768	Athscl type of bypass of the extrm w gangrene, oth extremity
			I70.769	Athscl type of bypass of the extrm w gangrene, unsp extrm
			I73.01	Raynaud's syndrome with gangrene
			I96	Gangrene, not elsewhere classified
785.50	UNSPECIFIED SHOCK	➡	R57.9	Shock, unspecified
785.51	CARDIOGENIC SHOCK	➡	R57.0	Cardiogenic shock
785.52	SEPTIC SHOCK		R65.21	Severe sepsis with septic shock
785.59	OTHER SHOCK WITHOUT MENTION OF TRAUMA		R57.1	Hypovolemic shock
			R57.8	Other shock
785.6	ENLARGEMENT OF LYMPH NODES		R59.0	Localized enlarged lymph nodes
			R59.1	Generalized enlarged lymph nodes
			R59.9	Enlarged lymph nodes, unspecified
785.9	OTHER SYMPTOMS INVOLVING CARDIOVASCULAR SYSTEM		R09.89	Oth symptoms and signs involving the circ and resp systems
786.00	UNSPECIFIED RESPIRATORY ABNORMALITY		R06.9	Unspecified abnormalities of breathing
786.01	HYPERVENTILATION	➡	R06.4	Hyperventilation
786.02	ORTHOPNEA	➡	R06.01	Orthopnea
786.03	APNEA	➡	R06.81	Apnea, not elsewhere classified
786.04	CHEYNE-STOKES RESPIRATION	➡	R06.3	Periodic breathing
786.05	SHORTNESS OF BREATH	➡	R06.02	Shortness of breath
786.06	TACHYPNEA	➡	R06.82	Tachypnea, not elsewhere classified
786.07	WHEEZING	➡	R06.2	Wheezing
786.09	OTHER DYSPNEA AND RESPIRATORY ABNORMALITIES		R06.00	Dyspnea, unspecified
			R06.09	Other forms of dyspnea
			R06.3	Periodic breathing
			R06.83	Snoring
			R06.89	Other abnormalities of breathing
786.1	STRIDOR	➡	R06.1	Stridor
786.2	COUGH	➡	R05	Cough
786.30	HEMOPTYSIS UNSPECIFIED		R04.2	Hemoptysis
			R04.9	Hemorrhage from respiratory passages, unspecified
786.31	ACUTE IDIOPATHIC PULMONARY HEMORR INFANTS AIPHI	➡	R04.81	Acute idiopathic pulmonary hemorrhage in infants
786.39	OTHER HEMOPTYSIS		R04.89	Hemorrhage from other sites in respiratory passages
786.4	ABNORMAL SPUTUM	➡	R09.3	Abnormal sputum
786.50	CHEST PAIN UNSPECIFIED	➡	R07.9	Chest pain, unspecified
786.51	PRECORDIAL PAIN	➡	R07.2	Precordial pain
786.52	PAINFUL RESPIRATION		R07.1	Chest pain on breathing
			R07.81	Pleurodynia
786.59	OTHER CHEST PAIN		R07.82	Intercostal pain
			R07.89	Other chest pain
786.6	SWELLING, MASS, OR LUMP IN CHEST		R22.2	Localized swelling, mass and lump, trunk
786.7	ABNORMAL CHEST SOUNDS		R09.89	Oth symptoms and signs involving the circ and resp systems
786.8	HICCOUGH	➡	R06.6	Hiccough
786.9	OTH SYMPTOMS INVOLVING RESPIRATORY SYSTEM&CHEST		R06.89	Other abnormalities of breathing
787.01	NAUSEA WITH VOMITING		R11.2	Nausea with vomiting, unspecified
787.02	NAUSEA ALONE	➡	R11.0	Nausea
787.03	VOMITING ALONE		R11.10	Vomiting, unspecified
			R11.11	Vomiting without nausea
			R11.12	Projectile vomiting
787.04	BILIOUS EMESIS	➡	R11.14	Bilious vomiting
787.1	HEARTBURN	➡	R12	Heartburn
787.20	DYSPHAGIA UNSPECIFIED		R13.0	Aphagia
			R13.10	Dysphagia, unspecified
787.21	DYSPHAGIA ORAL PHASE	➡	R13.11	Dysphagia, oral phase
787.22	DYSPHAGIA OROPHARYNGEAL PHASE	➡	R13.12	Dysphagia, oropharyngeal phase
787.23	DYSPHAGIA PHARYNGEAL PHASE	➡	R13.13	Dysphagia, pharyngeal phase
787.24	DYSPHAGIA PHARYNGOESOPHAGEAL PHASE	➡	R13.14	Dysphagia, pharyngoesophageal phase
787.29	OTHER DYSPHAGIA		R13.19	Other dysphagia
787.3	FLATULENCE ERUCTATION AND GAS PAIN		R14.0	Abdominal distension (gaseous)
			R14.1	Gas pain
			R14.2	Eructation
			R14.3	Flatulence

ICD-9-CM			ICD-10-CM	
787.4	VISIBLE PERISTALSIS	→	R19.2	Visible peristalsis
787.5	ABNORMAL BOWEL SOUNDS		R19.11 R19.12 R19.15	Absent bowel sounds Hyperactive bowel sounds Other abnormal bowel sounds
787.60	FULL INCONTINENCE OF FECES	→	R15.9	Full incontinence of feces
787.61	INCOMPLETE DEFECATION	→	R15.0	Incomplete defecation
787.62	FECAL SMEARING	→	R15.1	Fecal smearing
787.63	FECAL URGENCY	→	R15.2	Fecal urgency
787.7	ABNORMAL FECES		R19.5	Other fecal abnormalities
787.91	DIARRHEA		K52.2 K52.89 R19.7	Allergic and dietetic gastroenteritis and colitis Other specified noninfective gastroenteritis and colitis Diarrhea, unspecified
787.99	OTHER SYMPTOMS INVOLVING DIGESTIVE SYSTEM OTHER		R19.4 R19.8	Change in bowel habit Oth symptoms and signs involving the dgstv sys and abdomen
788.0	RENAL COLIC	→	N23	Unspecified renal colic
788.1	DYSURIA		R30.0 R30.9	Dysuria Painful micturition, unspecified
788.20	UNSPECIFIED RETENTION OF URINE	→	R33.9	Retention of urine, unspecified
788.21	INCOMPLETE BLADDER EMPTYING		R39.14	Feeling of incomplete bladder emptying
788.29	OTHER SPECIFIED RETENTION OF URINE		R33.0 R33.8	Drug induced retention of urine Other retention of urine
788.30	UNSPECIFIED URINARY INCONTINENCE	→	R32	Unspecified urinary incontinence
788.31	URGE INCONTINENCE	→	N39.41	Urge incontinence
788.32	STRESS INCONTINENCE, MALE		N39.3	Stress incontinence (female) (male)
788.33	MIXED INCONTINENCE URGE AND STRESS	→	N39.46	Mixed incontinence
788.34	INCONTINENCE WITHOUT SENSORY AWARENESS	→	N39.42	Incontinence without sensory awareness
788.35	POST-VOID DRIBBLING	→	N39.43	Post-void dribbling
788.36	NOCTURNAL ENURESIS	→	N39.44	Nocturnal enuresis
788.37	CONTINUOUS LEAKAGE	→	N39.45	Continuous leakage
788.38	OVERFLOW INCONTINENCE	→	N39.490	Overflow incontinence
788.39	OTHER URINARY INCONTINENCE	→	N39.498	Other specified urinary incontinence
788.41	URINARY FREQUENCY	→	R35.0	Frequency of micturition
788.42	POLYURIA	→	R35.8	Other polyuria
788.43	NOCTURIA	→	R35.1	Nocturia
788.5	OLIGURIA AND ANURIA	→	R34	Anuria and oliguria
788.61	SPLITTING OF URINARY STREAM	→	R39.13	Splitting of urinary stream
788.62	SLOWING OF URINARY STREAM		R39.12	Poor urinary stream
788.63	URGENCY OF URINATION	→	R39.15	Urgency of urination
788.64	URINARY HESITANCY	→	R39.11	Hesitancy of micturition
788.65	STRAINING ON URINATION	→	R39.16	Straining to void
788.69	OTHER ABNORMALITY OF URINATION	→	R39.19	Other difficulties with micturition
788.7	URETHRAL DISCHARGE		R36.0 R36.9	Urethral discharge without blood Urethral discharge, unspecified
788.8	EXTRAVASATION OF URINE	→	R39.0	Extravasation of urine
788.91	FUNCTIONAL URINARY INCONTINENCE	→	R39.81	Functional urinary incontinence
788.99	OTHER SYMPTOMS INVOLVING URINARY SYSTEM		R30.1 R39.2 R39.89 R39.9	Vesical tenesmus Extrarenal uremia Other symptoms and signs involving the genitourinary system Unsp symptoms and signs involving the genitourinary system
789.00	ABDOMINAL PAIN, UNSPECIFIED SITE		R10.0 R10.9	Acute abdomen Unspecified abdominal pain
789.01	ABDOMINAL PAIN RIGHT UPPER QUADRANT	→	R10.11	Right upper quadrant pain
789.02	ABDOMINAL PAIN, LEFT UPPER QUADRANT	→	R10.12	Left upper quadrant pain
789.03	ABDOMINAL PAIN RIGHT LOWER QUADRANT	→	R10.31	Right lower quadrant pain
789.04	ABDOMINAL PAIN, LEFT LOWER QUADRANT	→	R10.32	Left lower quadrant pain
789.05	ABDOMINAL PAIN, PERIUMBILIC	→	R10.33	Periumbilical pain
789.06	ABDOMINAL PAIN, EPIGASTRIC	→	R10.13	Epigastric pain
789.07	ABDOMINAL PAIN, GENERALIZED	→	R10.84	Generalized abdominal pain
789.09	ABDOMINAL PAIN OTHER SPECIFIED SITE		R10.10 R10.2 R10.30	Upper abdominal pain, unspecified Pelvic and perineal pain Lower abdominal pain, unspecified
789.1	HEPATOMEGALY	 ▣	R16.0 R16.2	Hepatomegaly, not elsewhere classified Hepatomegaly with splenomegaly, not elsewhere classified
789.2	SPLENOMEGALY	 ▣	R16.1 R16.2	Splenomegaly, not elsewhere classified Hepatomegaly with splenomegaly, not elsewhere classified
789.30	ABDOMINAL/PELVIC SWELLING MASS/LUMP UNSPEC SITE	→	R19.00	Intra-abd and pelvic swelling, mass and lump, unsp site
789.31	ABDOMINAL OR PELVIC SWELLING MASS OR LUMP RUQ	→	R19.01	Right upper quadrant abdominal swelling, mass and lump
789.32	ABDOMINAL OR PELVIC SWELLING MASS OR LUMP LUQ	→	R19.02	Left upper quadrant abdominal swelling, mass and lump
789.33	ABD/PELV SWELLING MASS/LUMP RIGHT LOWER QUADRANT	→	R19.03	Right lower quadrant abdominal swelling, mass and lump
789.34	ABDOMINAL OR PELVIC SWELLING MASS OR LUMP LLQ	→	R19.04	Left lower quadrant abdominal swelling, mass and lump

ICD-9-CM			ICD-10-CM	
789.35	ABDOMINAL/PELVIC SWELLING MASS/LUMP PERIUMBILIC	➡	**R19.Ø5**	Periumbilic swelling, mass or lump
789.36	ABDOMINAL/PELVIC SWELLING MASS/LUMP EPIGASTRIC	➡	**R19.Ø6**	Epigastric swelling, mass or lump
789.37	ABD/PELVIC SWELLING MASS/LUMP GEN	➡	**R19.Ø7**	Generalized intra-abd and pelvic swelling, mass and lump
789.39	ABD/PELVIC SWELLING MASS/LUMP OTH SPEC SITE		**R19.Ø9**	Other intra-abdominal and pelvic swelling, mass and lump
789.4Ø	ABDOMINAL RIGIDITY UNSPECIFIED SITE		**R19.3Ø**	Abdominal rigidity, unspecified site
789.41	ABDOMINAL RIGIDITY RIGHT UPPER QUADRANT	➡	**R19.31**	Right upper quadrant abdominal rigidity
789.42	ABDOMINAL RIGIDITY LEFT UPPER QUADRANT	➡	**R19.32**	Left upper quadrant abdominal rigidity
789.43	ABDOMINAL RIGIDITY RIGHT LOWER QUADRANT	➡	**R19.33**	Right lower quadrant abdominal rigidity
789.44	ABDOMINAL RIGIDITY LEFT LOWER QUADRANT	➡	**R19.34**	Left lower quadrant abdominal rigidity
789.45	ABDOMINAL RIGIDITY, PERIUMBILIC	➡	**R19.35**	Periumbilic abdominal rigidity
789.46	ABDOMINAL RIGIDITY, EPIGASTRIC	➡	**R19.36**	Epigastric abdominal rigidity
789.47	ABDOMINAL RIGIDITY, GENERALIZED	➡	**R19.37**	Generalized abdominal rigidity
789.49	ABDOMINAL RIGIDITY OTHER SPECIFIED SITE		**R19.3Ø**	Abdominal rigidity, unspecified site
789.51	MALIGNANT ASCITES	➡	**R18.Ø**	Malignant ascites
789.59	OTHER ASCITES	➡	**R18.8**	Other ascites
789.6Ø	ABDOMINAL TENDERNESS UNSPECIFIED SITE		**R1Ø.819** **R1Ø.829**	Abdominal tenderness, unspecified site Rebound abdominal tenderness, unspecified site
789.61	ABDOMINAL TENDERNESS RIGHT UPPER QUADRANT		**R1Ø.811** **R1Ø.821**	Right upper quadrant abdominal tenderness Right upper quadrant rebound abdominal tenderness
789.62	ABDOMINAL TENDERNESS LEFT UPPER QUADRANT		**R1Ø.812** **R1Ø.822**	Left upper quadrant abdominal tenderness Left upper quadrant rebound abdominal tenderness
789.63	ABDOMINAL TENDERNESS RIGHT LOWER QUADRANT		**R1Ø.813** **R1Ø.823**	Right lower quadrant abdominal tenderness Right lower quadrant rebound abdominal tenderness
789.64	ABDOMINAL TENDERNESS LEFT LOWER QUADRANT		**R1Ø.814** **R1Ø.824**	Left lower quadrant abdominal tenderness Left lower quadrant rebound abdominal tenderness
789.65	ABDOMINAL TENDERNESS, PERIUMBILIC		**R1Ø.815** **R1Ø.825**	Periumbilic abdominal tenderness Periumbilic rebound abdominal tenderness
789.66	ABDOMINAL TENDERNESS, EPIGASTRIC		**R1Ø.816** **R1Ø.826**	Epigastric abdominal tenderness Epigastric rebound abdominal tenderness
789.67	ABDOMINAL TENDERNESS, GENERALIZED		**R1Ø.817** **R1Ø.827**	Generalized abdominal tenderness Generalized rebound abdominal tenderness
789.69	ABDOMINAL TENDERNESS OTHER SPECIFIED SITE		**R1Ø.819** **R1Ø.829**	Abdominal tenderness, unspecified site Rebound abdominal tenderness, unspecified site
789.7	COLIC	➡	**R1Ø.83**	Colic
789.9	OTHER SYMPTOMS INVOLVING ABDOMEN AND PELVIS		**R19.8**	Oth symptoms and signs involving the dgstv sys and abdomen
79Ø.Ø1	PRECIPITOUS DROP IN HEMATOCRIT	➡	**R71.Ø**	Precipitous drop in hematocrit
79Ø.Ø9	OTHER ABNORMALITY OF RED BLOOD CELLS	➡	**R71.8**	Other abnormality of red blood cells
79Ø.1	ELEVATED SEDIMENTATION RATE	➡	**R7Ø.Ø**	Elevated erythrocyte sedimentation rate
79Ø.21	IMPAIRED FASTING GLUCOSE	➡	**R73.Ø1**	Impaired fasting glucose
79Ø.22	IMPAIRED GLUCOSE TOLERANCE TEST	➡	**R73.Ø2**	Impaired glucose tolerance (oral)
79Ø.29	OTHER ABNORMAL GLUCOSE		**R73.Ø9** **R73.9**	Other abnormal glucose Hyperglycemia, unspecified
79Ø.3	EXCESSIVE BLOOD LEVEL OF ALCOHOL		**R78.Ø**	Finding of alcohol in blood
79Ø.4	NONSPEC ELEVATION OF LEVELS OF TRANSAMINASE/LDH	➡	**R74.Ø**	Nonspec elev of levels of transamns & lactic acid dehydrgnse
79Ø.5	OTHER NONSPECIFIC ABNORMAL SERUM ENZYME LEVELS		**R74.8** **R74.9**	Abnormal levels of other serum enzymes Abnormal serum enzyme level, unspecified
79Ø.6	OTHER ABNORMAL BLOOD CHEMISTRY		**E79.Ø** **R78.71** **R78.79** **R78.89** **R79.Ø** **R79.89** **R79.9**	Hyperuricemia w/o signs of inflam arthrit and tophaceous dis Abnormal lead level in blood Finding of abnormal level of heavy metals in blood Finding of oth substances, not normally found in blood Abnormal level of blood mineral Other specified abnormal findings of blood chemistry Abnormal finding of blood chemistry, unspecified
79Ø.7	BACTEREMIA		**R78.81**	Bacteremia
79Ø.8	UNSPECIFIED VIREMIA		**B34.9**	Viral infection, unspecified
79Ø.91	ABNORMAL ARTERIAL BLOOD GASES		**R79.81**	Abnormal blood-gas level
79Ø.92	ABNORMAL COAGULATION PROFILE	➡	**R79.1**	Abnormal coagulation profile
79Ø.93	ELEVATED PROSTATE SPECIFIC ANTIGEN	➡	**R97.2**	Elevated prostate specific antigen [PSA]
79Ø.94	EUTHYROID SICK SYNDROME	➡	**EØ7.81**	Sick-euthyroid syndrome
79Ø.95	OTH NONSPECIFIC FIND EX BLD ELEVD C-REACTV PROT	➡	**R79.82**	Elevated C-reactive protein (CRP)

ICD-9-CM			ICD-10-CM	
79Ø.99	OTHER NONSPECIFIC FINDINGS EXAMINATION OF BLOOD		**R7Ø.1**	Abnormal plasma viscosity
			R77.Ø	Abnormality of albumin
			R77.1	Abnormality of globulin
			R77.2	Abnormality of alphafetoprotein
			R77.8	Other specified abnormalities of plasma proteins
			R77.9	Abnormality of plasma protein, unspecified
			R78.1	Finding of opiate drug in blood
			R78.2	Finding of cocaine in blood
			R78.3	Finding of hallucinogen in blood
			R78.4	Finding of other drugs of addictive potential in blood
			R78.5	Finding of other psychotropic drug in blood
			R78.6	Finding of steroid agent in blood
			R78.89	Finding of oth substances, not normally found in blood
			R78.9	Finding of unsp substance, not normally found in blood
			R79.89	Other specified abnormal findings of blood chemistry
791.Ø	PROTEINURIA		**R8Ø.Ø**	Isolated proteinuria
			R8Ø.1	Persistent proteinuria, unspecified
			R8Ø.3	Bence Jones proteinuria
			R8Ø.8	Other proteinuria
			R8Ø.9	Proteinuria, unspecified
791.1	CHYLURIA	➡	**R82.Ø**	Chyluria
791.2	HEMOGLOBINURIA	➡	**R82.3**	Hemoglobinuria
791.3	MYOGLOBINURIA	➡	**R82.1**	Myoglobinuria
791.4	BILIURIA	➡	**R82.2**	Biliuria
791.5	GLYCOSURIA	➡	**R81**	Glycosuria
791.6	ACETONURIA	➡	**R82.4**	Acetonuria
791.7	OTHER CELLS AND CASTS IN URINE		**R82.99**	Other abnormal findings in urine
791.9	OTHER NONSPECIFIC FINDING EXAMINATION OF URINE		**R82.5**	Elevated urine levels of drug/meds/biol subst
			R82.6	Abnormal urine levels of substances chiefly nonmed source
			R82.7	Abnormal findings on microbiological examination of urine
			R82.8	Abnormal findings on cytolog and histolog exam of urine
			R82.9Ø	Unspecified abnormal findings in urine
			R82.91	Other chromoabnormalities of urine
			R82.99	Other abnormal findings in urine
792.Ø	NONSPECIFIC ABNORMAL FINDING IN CEREBROSP FL		**R83.Ø**	Abnormal level of enzymes in cerebrospinal fluid
			R83.1	Abnormal level of hormones in cerebrospinal fluid
			R83.2	Abn lev drug/meds/biol subst in cerebrospinal fluid
			R83.3	Abn lev substances chiefly nonmedicinal as to source in CSF
			R83.4	Abnormal immunological findings in cerebrospinal fluid
			R83.5	Abnormal microbiological findings in cerebrospinal fluid
			R83.6	Abnormal cytological findings in cerebrospinal fluid
			R83.8	Other abnormal findings in cerebrospinal fluid
			R83.9	Unspecified abnormal finding in cerebrospinal fluid
792.1	NONSPECIFIC ABNORMAL FINDING IN STOOL CONTENTS		**R19.5**	Other fecal abnormalities
792.2	NONSPECIFIC ABNORMAL FINDING IN SEMEN		**R86.Ø**	Abn lev enzymes in specimens from male genital organs
			R86.1	Abn lev hormones in specimens from male genital organs
			R86.2	Abn lev drug/meds/biol subst in specmn from male gntl organs
			R86.3	Abn lev substnc nonmed source in specmn from male gntl org
			R86.4	Abn immunolog findings in specmn from male genital organs
			R86.5	Abn microbiolog findings in specmn from male genital organs
			R86.6	Abnormal cytolog findings in specmn from male genital organs
			R86.7	Abn histolog findings in specmn from male genital organs
			R86.8	Oth abnormal findings in specimens from male genital organs
			R86.9	Unsp abnormal finding in specimens from male genital organs
792.3	NONSPECIFIC ABNORMAL FINDING IN AMNIOTIC FLUID		**O28.9**	Unsp abnormal findings on antenatal screening of mother
792.4	NONSPECIFIC ABNORMAL FINDING IN SALIVA		**R85.Ø**	Abn lev enzymes in specimens from dgstv org/abd cav
			R85.1	Abn lev hormones in specimens from dgstv org/abd cav
			R85.2	Abn lev drug/meds/biol subst in specmn fr dgstv org/abd cav
			R85.3	Abn lev substnc nonmed source in specmn fr dgstv org/abd cav
			R85.4	Abnormal immunolog findings in specmn from dgstv org/abd cav
			R85.5	Abn microbiolog findings in specmn from dgstv org/abd cav
			R85.69	Abn cytolog findings in specmn from oth dgstv org/abd cav
			R85.7	Abnormal histolog findings in specmn from dgstv org/abd cav
			R85.89	Oth abnormal findings in specimens from dgstv org/abd cav
			R85.9	Unsp abnormal finding in specimens from dgstv org/abd cav
792.5	CLOUDY DIALYSIS AFFLUENT	➡	**R88.Ø**	Cloudy (hemodialysis) (peritoneal) dialysis effluent

ICD-9-CM			ICD-10-CM	
792.9	OTH NONSPECIFIC ABNORMAL FINDING BODY SUBSTANCES		**R84.Ø**	Abnormal level of enzymes in specimens from resp org/thrx
			R84.1	Abnormal level of hormones in specimens from resp org/thrx
			R84.2	Abn lev drug/meds/biol subst in specimens from resp org/thrx
			R84.3	Abn lev substnc nonmed source in specmn from resp org/thrx
			R84.4	Abnormal immunolog findings in specimens from resp org/thrx
			R84.5	Abnormal microbiolog findings in specmn from resp org/thrx
			R84.6	Abnormal cytolog findings in specimens from resp org/thrx
			R84.7	Abnormal histolog findings in specimens from resp org/thrx
			R84.8	Oth abnormal findings in specimens from resp org/thrx
			R84.9	Unsp abnormal finding in specimens from resp org/thrx
			R85.Ø	Abn lev enzymes in specimens from dgstv org/abd cav
			R85.1	Abn lev hormones in specimens from dgstv org/abd cav
			R85.2	Abn lev drug/meds/biol subst in specmn fr dgstv org/abd cav
			R85.3	Abn lev substnc nonmed source in specmn fr dgstv org/abd cav
			R85.4	Abnormal immunolog findings in specmn from dgstv org/abd cav
			R85.5	Abn microbiolog findings in specmn from dgstv org/abd cav
			R85.69	Abn cytolog findings in specmn from oth dgstv org/abd cav
			R85.7	Abnormal histolog findings in specmn from dgstv org/abd cav
			R85.89	Oth abnormal findings in specimens from dgstv org/abd cav
			R85.9	Unsp abnormal finding in specimens from dgstv org/abd cav
			R87.Ø	Abn lev enzymes in specimens from female genital organs
			R87.1	Abn lev hormones in specimens from female genital organs
			R87.2	Abn lev drug/meds/biol subst in specmn from fem gntl organs
			R87.3	Abn lev substnc nonmed source in specmn from fem gntl organs
			R87.4	Abn immunolog findings in specmn from female genital organs
			R87.5	Abn microbiolog find in specmn from female genital organs
			R87.69	Abn cytolog find in specmn from oth female genital organs
			R87.7	Abn histolog findings in specmn from female genital organs
			R87.89	Oth abnormal findings in specmn from female genital organs
			R87.9	Unsp abnormal finding in specmn from female genital organs
			R88.8	Abnormal findings in other body fluids and substances
			R89.Ø	Abnormal level of enzymes in specimens from oth org/tiss
			R89.1	Abnormal level of hormones in specimens from oth org/tiss
			R89.2	Abn lev drug/meds/biol subst in specimens from oth org/tiss
			R89.3	Abn lev substnc nonmed source in specmn from oth org/tiss
			R89.4	Abnormal immunolog findings in specimens from oth org/tiss
			R89.5	Abnormal microbiolog findings in specimens from oth org/tiss
			R89.6	Abnormal cytological findings in specimens from oth org/tiss
			R89.7	Abnormal histolog findings in specimens from oth org/tiss
			R89.8	Oth abnormal findings in specimens from oth org/tiss
			R89.9	Unsp abnormal finding in specimens from oth org/tiss
793.Ø	NONSPECIFIC ABN FNDNG RAD & OTH EXM SKULL & HEAD		**R9Ø.82**	White matter disease, unspecified
			R93.Ø	Abnormal findings on dx imaging of skull and head, NEC
793.11	SOLITARY PULMONARY NODULE	➡	**R91.1**	Solitary pulmonary nodule
793.19	OTHER NONSPECIFIC ABNORMAL FINDING OF LUNG FIELD	➡	**R91.8**	Other nonspecific abnormal finding of lung field
793.2	NONSPC ABN FINDNG RAD&OTH EXAM OTH INTRTHOR ORGN		**R93.1**	Abnormal findings on dx imaging of heart and cor circ
			R93.8	Abnormal findings on diagnostic imaging of body structures
793.3	NONSPECIFIC ABN FINDNG RAD&OTH EXAM BILARY TRCT		**R93.2**	Abnormal findings on dx imaging of liver and biliary tract
793.4	NONSPECIFIC ABN FINDING RAD & OTH EXAM GI TRACT		**R93.3**	Abnormal findings on dx imaging of prt digestive tract
793.5	NONSPECIFIC ABN FINDING RAD & OTH EXAM GU ORGAN		**R93.4**	Abnormal findings on diagnostic imaging of urinary organs
793.6	NONSPEC ABN FINDNG RAD & OTH EXAM ABDOMINAL AREA		**R93.5**	Abn findings on dx imaging of abd regions, inc retroperiton
793.7	NONSPC ABN FINDNG RAD & OTH EXM MUSCULSKELTL SYS		**R93.6**	Abnormal findings on diagnostic imaging of limbs
			R93.7	Abnormal findings on diagnostic imaging of prt ms sys
793.8Ø	UNSPECIFIED ABNORMAL MAMMOGRAM		**R92.8**	Oth abn and inconclusive findings on dx imaging of breast
793.81	MAMMOGRAPHIC MICROCALCIFICATION	➡	**R92.Ø**	Mammographic microcalcification found on dx imaging of brst
793.82	INCONCLUSIVE MAMMOGRAM	➡	**R92.2**	Inconclusive mammogram
793.89	OTHER ABNORMAL FINDING RADIOLOGICAL EXAM BREAST		**R92.1**	Mammographic calcifcn found on diagnostic imaging of breast
			R92.8	Oth abn and inconclusive findings on dx imaging of breast
793.91	IMAGE TEST INCONCLUSIVE DUE TO EXCESS BODY FAT	➡	**R93.9**	Dx imaging inconclusive due to excess body fat of patient
793.99	OTH NONSPC ABN FINDNG RAD&OTH EXM BODY STRUCTURE		**R9Ø.89**	Oth abnormal findings on diagnostic imaging of cnsl
			R93.8	Abnormal findings on diagnostic imaging of body structures
794.ØØ	UNSPEC ABNORM FUNCT STUDY BRAIN&CNTRL NERV SYS		**R94.Ø9**	Abnormal results of function studies of cnsl
794.Ø1	NONSPECIFIC ABNORMAL ECHOENCEPHALOGRAM	➡	**R9Ø.81**	Abnormal echoencephalogram
794.Ø2	NONSPECIFIC ABNORMAL ELECTROENCEPHALOGRAM	➡	**R94.Ø1**	Abnormal electroencephalogram [EEG]
794.Ø9	OTH ABNORMAL BRAIN & CNS FUNCTION STUDY		**R94.Ø2**	Abnormal brain scan
			R94.Ø9	Abnormal results of function studies of cnsl
794.1Ø	NONSPECIFIC ABNORMAL RESPONSE UNSPEC NERVE STIM	➡	**R94.13Ø**	Abnormal response to nerve stimulation, unspecified
794.11	NONSPECIFIC ABNORMAL RETINAL FUNCTION STUDIES	➡	**R94.111**	Abnormal electroretinogram [ERG]
794.12	NONSPECIFIC ABNORMAL ELECTRO-OCULOGRAM	➡	**R94.11Ø**	Abnormal electro-oculogram [EOG]
794.13	NONSPECIFIC ABNORMAL VISUALLY EVOKED POTENTIAL	➡	**R94.112**	Abnormal visually evoked potential [VEP]
794.14	NONSPECIFIC ABNORMAL OCULOMOTOR STUDIES	➡	**R94.113**	Abnormal oculomotor study
794.15	NONSPECIFIC ABNORMAL AUDITORY FUNCTION STUDIES	➡	**R94.12Ø**	Abnormal auditory function study
794.16	NONSPECIFIC ABNORMAL VESTIBULAR FUNCTION STUDIES	➡	**R94.121**	Abnormal vestibular function study
794.17	NONSPECIFIC ABNORMAL ELECTROMYOGRAM	➡	**R94.131**	Abnormal electromyogram [EMG]

ICD-9-CM			ICD-10-CM	
794.19	OTH ABNORMAL PERIPH NERVE-SPECIAL SENSES STUDIES		**R94.118** **R94.128** **R94.138**	Abnormal results of other function studies of eye Abn results of function studies of ear and oth sp senses Abnormal results of function studies of prph nervous sys
794.2	NONSPECIFIC ABNORM RSLTS PULM SYSTEM FUNCT STUDY	➡	**R94.2**	Abnormal results of pulmonary function studies
794.30	NONSPECIFIC ABNORMAL UNSPEC CV FUNCTION STUDY	➡	**R94.30**	Abnormal result of cardiovascular function study, unsp
794.31	NONSPECIFIC ABNORMAL ELECTROCARDIOGRAM	➡	**R94.31**	Abnormal electrocardiogram [ECG] [EKG]
794.39	OTH NONSPECIFIC ABNORM CV SYSTEM FUNCTION STUDY	➡	**R94.39**	Abnormal result of other cardiovascular function study
794.4	NONSPECIFIC ABNORM RESULTS KIDNEY FUNCTION STUDY	➡	**R94.4**	Abnormal results of kidney function studies
794.5	NONSPECIFIC ABNORM RESULTS THYROID FUNCT STUDY	➡	**R94.6**	Abnormal results of thyroid function studies
794.6	NONSPECIFIC ABNORM RSLTS OTH ENDOCRN FUNCT STUDY	➡	**R94.7**	Abnormal results of other endocrine function studies
794.7	NONSPECIFIC ABNORM RSLTS BASAL METAB FUNCT STUDY		**R94.8**	Abnormal results of function studies of organs and systems
794.8	NONSPECIFIC ABNORMAL RESULTS LIVR FUNCTION STUDY	➡	**R94.5**	Abnormal results of liver function studies
794.9	NONSPECIFIC ABNORM RESULTS OTH SPEC FUNCT STUDY		**R94.8**	Abnormal results of function studies of organs and systems
795.00	ABNORMAL GLANDULAR PAPANICOLAOU SMEAR OF CERVIX		**R87.619**	Unsp abnormal cytolog findings in specmn from cervix uteri
795.01	PAP SMER CERV W/ATYPICAL SQUAMOUS CELLS UNDET	➡	**R87.610**	Atyp squam cell of undet signfc cyto smr crvx (ASC-US)
795.02	PAP SMER W/ATYPCL SQAUMOUS CELL NOT EXCLD HI GRD	➡	**R87.611**	Atyp squam cell not excl hi grd intrepith lesn cyto smr crvx
795.03	PAP SMER CERV W/LW GRADE SQUAMOUS INTRAEPITH LES	➡	**R87.612**	Low grade intrepith lesion cyto smr crvx (LGSIL)
795.04	PAP SMER CERV W/HI GRADE SQUAMOUS INTRAEPITH LES	➡	**R87.613**	High grade intrepith lesion cyto smr crvx (HGSIL)
795.05	CERV HIGH RISK HUMAN PAPILLOMAVIRUS DNA TEST POS	➡	**R87.810**	Cervical high risk HPV DNA test positive
795.06	PAP SMEAR CERV W/CYTOL EVIDENCE MALIGNANCY	➡	**R87.614**	Cytologic evidence of malignancy on smear of cervix
795.07	SATISFACTORY CERVICAL SMEAR BUT LACKING T ZONE	➡	**R87.616**	Satisfactory cervical smear but lacking transformation zone
795.08	NONSPEC ABNORM PAP CERV UNSATISFACTORY CYTOLOGY	➡	**R87.615**	Unsatisfactory cytologic smear of cervix
795.09	OTH ABNORMAL PAPANICOLAOU SMEAR CERVIX&CERV HPV		**R87.820**	Cervical low risk HPV DNA test positive
795.10	ABNORMAL GLANDULAR PAPANICOLAOU SMEAR OF VAGINA		**R87.628**	Other abnormal cytological findings on specimens from vagina
795.11	PAPANICOLAOU SMEAR OF VAGINA WITH ASC-US	➡	**R87.620**	Atyp squam cell of undet signfc cyto smr vagn (ASC-US)
795.12	PAPANICOLAOU SMEAR OF VAGINA WITH ASH-H	➡	**R87.621**	Atyp squam cell not excl hi grd intrepith lesn cyto smr vagn
795.13	PAPANICOLAOU SMEAR OF VAGINA WITH LGSIL	➡	**R87.622**	Low grade intrepith lesion cyto smr vagn (LGSIL)
795.14	PAPANICOLAOU SMEAR OF VAGINA WITH HGSIL	➡	**R87.623**	High grade intrepith lesion cyto smr vagn (HGSIL)
795.15	VAG HIGH RISK HUMAN PAPILLOMAVIRUS DNA TEST POS		**R87.811**	Vaginal high risk HPV DNA test positive
795.16	PAP SMEAR VAG W/CYTOLOGIC EVIDENCE OF MALIGNANCY	➡	**R87.624**	Cytologic evidence of malignancy on smear of vagina
795.18	UNSATISFACTORY VAGINAL CYTOLOGY SMEAR	➡	**R87.625**	Unsatisfactory cytologic smear of vagina
795.19	OTH ABNORMAL PAP SMEAR OF VAGINA AND VAGINAL HPV		**R87.628** **R87.821**	Other abnormal cytological findings on specimens from vagina Vaginal low risk HPV DNA test positive
795.2	NONSPECIFIC ABNORMAL FINDINGS CHROMOSOMAL ANALY		**R89.8**	Oth abnormal findings in specimens from oth org/tiss
795.31	NONSPECIFIC POSITIVE FINDINGS FOR ANTHRAX		**R89.5**	Abnormal microbiolog findings in specimens from oth org/tiss
795.39	OTHER NONSPECIFIC POSITIVE CULTURE FINDINGS		**R89.9**	Unsp abnormal finding in specimens from oth org/tiss
795.4	OTHER NONSPECIFIC ABNORMAL HISTOLOGICAL FINDINGS		**R87.618** **R87.619** **R87.629** **R89.7**	Oth abnormal cytolog findings on specimens from cervix uteri Unsp abnormal cytolog findings in specmn from cervix uteri Unsp abnormal cytological findings in specimens from vagina Abnormal histolog findings in specimens from oth org/tiss
795.51	NONSPEC REACT TUBERCULIN SKIN TEST W/O ACTIVE TB	➡	**R76.11**	Nonspecific reaction to skin test w/o active tuberculosis
795.52	NONSPEC RXN CMI MSR G-IFN ANTIG RSPN NO ACT TB	➡	**R76.12**	Nonspec reaction to gamma intrfrn respns w/o actv tubrclosis
795.6	FALSE POSITIVE SEROLOGICAL TEST FOR SYPHILIS		**R76.8**	Other specified abnormal immunological findings in serum
795.71	NONSPECIFIC SEROLOGIC EVIDENCE OF HIV		**R75**	Inconclusive laboratory evidence of human immunodef virus
795.79	OTHER&UNSPEC NONSPECIFIC IMMUNOLOGICAL FINDINGS		**R76.0** **R76.8** **R76.9**	Raised antibody titer Other specified abnormal immunological findings in serum Abnormal immunological finding in serum, unspecified
795.81	ELEVATED CARCINOEMBRYONIC ANTIGEN	➡	**R97.0**	Elevated carcinoembryonic antigen [CEA]
795.82	ELEVATED CANCER ANTIGEN 125	➡	**R97.1**	Elevated cancer antigen 125 [CA 125]
795.89	OTHER ABNORMAL TUMOR MARKERS	➡	**R97.8**	Other abnormal tumor markers
796.0	NONSPECIFIC ABNORMAL TOXICOLOGICAL FINDINGS		**R82.5** **R82.6** **R89.2** **R89.3**	Elevated urine levels of drug/meds/biol subst Abnormal urine levels of substances chiefly nonmed source Abn lev drug/meds/biol subst in specimens from oth org/tiss Abn lev substnc nonmed source in specmn from oth org/tiss
796.1	ABNORMAL REFLEX	➡	**R29.2**	Abnormal reflex
796.2	ELEVATED BP READING WITHOUT DX HYPERTENSION	➡	**R03.0**	Elevated blood-pressure reading, w/o diagnosis of htn
796.3	NONSPECIFIC LOW BLOOD PRESSURE READING	➡	**R03.1**	Nonspecific low blood-pressure reading
796.4	OTHER ABNORMAL CLINICAL FINDING		**R68.89**	Other general symptoms and signs
796.5	ABNORMAL FINDING ON ANTENATAL SCREENING		**O28.0** **O28.1** **O28.2** **O28.3** **O28.4** **O28.5** **O28.8** **O28.9**	Abnormal hematolog finding on antenatal screening of mother Abnormal biochemical finding on antenat screening of mother Abnormal cytolog finding on antenatal screening of mother Abnormal ultrasonic finding on antenatal screening of mother Abnormal radiolog finding on antenatal screening of mother Abn chromsoml and genetic find on antenat screen of mother Other abnormal findings on antenatal screening of mother Unsp abnormal findings on antenatal screening of mother
796.6	NONSPECIFIC ABNORMAL FINDINGS NEONATAL SCREENING	➡	**P09**	Abnormal findings on neonatal screening
796.70	ABNORMAL GLANDULAR PAPANICOLAOU SMEAR OF ANUS	➡	**R85.619**	Unsp abnormal cytological findings in specimens from anus
796.71	PAPANICOLAOU SMEAR OF ANUS WITH ASC-US	➡	**R85.610**	Atyp squam cell of undet signfc cyto smr anus (ASC-US)
796.72	PAPANICOLAOU SMEAR OF ANUS WITH ASC-H	➡	**R85.611**	Atyp squam cell not excl hi grd intrepith lesn cyto smr anus

ICD-9-CM		ICD-10-CM		
796.73	PAPANICOLAOU SMEAR OF ANUS WITH LGSIL	➡	**R85.612**	Low grade intrepith lesion cyto smr anus (LGSIL)
796.74	PAPANICOLAOU SMEAR OF ANUS WITH HGSIL	➡	**R85.613**	High grade intrepith lesion cyto smr anus (HGSIL)
796.75	ANAL HIGH RISK HUMAN PAPILLOMAVIRUS DNA TEST POS	➡	**R85.81**	Anal high risk human papillomavirus (HPV) DNA test positive
796.76	PAP SMEAR ANUS W/CYTOLOGIC EVIDENCE OF MALIG	➡	**R85.614**	Cytologic evidence of malignancy on smear of anus
796.77	SAT ANAL SMEAR BUT LACKING TRANSFORMATION ZONE	➡	**R85.616**	Satisfactory anal smear but lacking transformation zone
796.78	UNSATISFACTORY ANAL CYTOLOGY SMEAR	➡	**R85.615**	Unsatisfactory cytologic smear of anus
796.79	OTHER ABNORMAL PAP SMEAR OF ANUS AND ANAL HPV		**R85.618** **R85.82**	Other abnormal cytological findings on specimens from anus Anal low risk human papillomavirus (HPV) DNA test positive
796.9	OTHER NONSPECIFIC ABNORMAL FINDING		**R68.89**	Other general symptoms and signs
797	SENILITY WITHOUT MENTION OF PSYCHOSIS		**R41.81** **R54**	Age-related cognitive decline Age-related physical debility
798.0	SUDDEN INFANT DEATH SYNDROME		**R99**	Ill-defined and unknown cause of mortality
798.1	INSTANTANEOUS DEATH		**R99**	Ill-defined and unknown cause of mortality
798.2	DEATH < 24 HRS AFTER SYMPTOMS ONSET-UNEXPLAINED		**R99**	Ill-defined and unknown cause of mortality
798.9	UNATTENDED DEATH		**R99**	Ill-defined and unknown cause of mortality
799.01	ASPHYXIA	➡	**R09.01**	Asphyxia
799.02	HYPOXEMIA	➡	**R09.02**	Hypoxemia
799.1	RESPIRATORY ARREST	➡	**R09.2**	Respiratory arrest
799.21	NERVOUSNESS	➡	**R45.0**	Nervousness
799.22	IRRITABILITY		**R45.4**	Irritability and anger
799.23	IMPULSIVENESS	➡	**R45.87**	Impulsiveness
799.24	EMOTIONAL LABILITY	➡	**R45.86**	Emotional lability
799.25	DEMORALIZATION AND APATHY	➡	**R45.3**	Demoralization and apathy
799.29	OTHER SIGNS AND SYMPTOMS INVOLV EMOTIONAL STATE		**R45.89**	Other symptoms and signs involving emotional state
799.3	UNSPECIFIED DEBILITY		**R53.81**	Other malaise
799.4	CACHEXIA	➡	**R64**	Cachexia
799.51	ATTENTION OR CONCENTRATION DEFICIT	➡	**R41.840**	Attention and concentration deficit
799.52	COGNITIVE COMMUNICATION DEFICIT	➡	**R41.841**	Cognitive communication deficit
799.53	VISUOSPATIAL DEFICIT	➡	**R41.842**	Visuospatial deficit
799.54	PSYCHOMOTOR DEFICIT	➡	**R41.843**	Psychomotor deficit
799.55	FRONTAL LOBE AND EXECUTIVE FUNCTION DEFICIT	➡	**R41.844**	Frontal lobe and executive function deficit
799.59	OTHER SIGNS AND SYMPTOMS INVOLVING COGNITION	➡	**R41.89**	Oth symptoms and signs w cognitive functions and awareness
799.81	DECREASED LIBIDO	➡	**R68.82**	Decreased libido
799.82	APPARENT LIFE THREATENING EVENT INFANT	➡	**R68.13**	Apparent life threatening event in infant (ALTE)
799.89	OTHER ILL-DEFINED CONDITIONS		**R44.8** **R44.9** **R46.0** **R46.1** **R46.2** **R46.3** **R46.4** **R46.5** **R46.6** **R46.7** **R46.81** **R46.89** **R68.19** **R69**	Oth symptoms and signs w general sensations and perceptions Unsp symptoms and signs w general sensations and perceptions Very low level of personal hygiene Bizarre personal appearance Strange and inexplicable behavior Overactivity Slowness and poor responsiveness Suspiciousness and marked evasiveness Undue concern and preoccupation with stressful events Verbosity and circumstantial detail obscuring rsn for cntct Obsessive-compulsive behavior Other symptoms and signs involving appearance and behavior Other nonspecific symptoms peculiar to infancy Illness, unspecified
799.9	OTHER UNKNOWN&UNSPEC CAUSE MORBIDITY/MORTALITY		**R69** **R99**	Illness, unspecified Ill-defined and unknown cause of mortality

Injury and Poisoning

ICD-9-CM		ICD-10-CM		
800.00	CLOS FX VALT SKUL W/O ICIR UNS STATE CONSCIOUS	**S02.0XXA**	Fracture of vault of skull, init encntr for closed fracture	
800.01	CLOS FX VALT SKUL W/O INTRACRAN INJR NO LOC	**S02.0XXA**	Fracture of vault of skull, init encntr for closed fracture	
800.02	CLOS FX VALT SKUL W/O INTRACRAN INJR BRF LOC	**S02.0XXA**	Fracture of vault of skull, init encntr for closed fracture	
800.03	CLOS FX VALT SKUL W/O INTRACRAN INJR MOD LOC	**S02.0XXA**	Fracture of vault of skull, init encntr for closed fracture	
800.04	CLOS FX VLT SKULL W/O ICI LOC>24 HR&RETURN	**S02.0XXA**	Fracture of vault of skull, init encntr for closed fracture	
800.05	CLOS FX VAULT SKULL W/O ICI-LOC>24 NO RETURN	**S02.0XXA**	Fracture of vault of skull, init encntr for closed fracture	
800.06	CLOS FX VLT SKUL NO ICI-LOSS CONSCOUSNSS UNS DUR	**S02.0XXA**	Fracture of vault of skull, init encntr for closed fracture	
800.09	CLOS FX VALT SKUL W/O INTRACRAN INJR UNS CONCUS	**S02.0XXA**	Fracture of vault of skull, init encntr for closed fracture	
800.10	CLOS FX VAULT SKULL W/CERBRL LAC&CONTUS UNS SOC	**S02.0XXA**	Fracture of vault of skull, init encntr for closed fracture	*and*
		S06.330A	Contus/lac cereb, w/o loss of consciousness, init	
800.11	CLOS FX VAULT SKULL W/CERBRL LAC&CONTUS NO LOC	**S02.0XXA**	Fracture of vault of skull, init encntr for closed fracture	*and*
		S06.330A	Contus/lac cereb, w/o loss of consciousness, init	
800.12	CLOS FX VALT SKUL W/CERBRL LAC&CONTUS BRIEF LOC	**S02.0XXA**	Fracture of vault of skull, init encntr for closed fracture	*and*
		S06.331A	Contus/lac cereb, w LOC of 30 minutes or less, init	*or*
		S06.332A	Contus/lac cereb, w loss of consciousness of 31-59 min, init	
800.13	CLOS FX VAULT SKUL W/CERBRL LAC&CONTUS MOD LOC	**S02.0XXA**	Fracture of vault of skull, init encntr for closed fracture	*and*
		S06.333A	Contus/lac cereb, w LOC of 1-5 hrs 59 min, init	*or*
		S06.334A	Contus/lac cereb, w LOC of 6 hours to 24 hours, init	
800.14	CLOS FX VAULT SKULL CEREB LAC LOC >24 HR &RETURN	**S02.0XXA**	Fracture of vault of skull, init encntr for closed fracture	*and*
		S06.335A	Contus/lac cereb, w LOC >24 hr w ret consc lev, init	
800.15	CLOSFX VAULT SKULL CEREB LAC LOS >24 W/O RETURN	**S02.0XXA**	Fracture of vault of skull, init encntr for closed fracture	*and*
		S06.336A	Contus/lac cereb, w LOC >24 hr w/o ret consc w surv, init	*or*
		S06.337A	Contus/lac cereb, w LOC w death d/t brain inj bf consc, init	*or*
		S06.338A	Contus/lac cereb, w LOC w death d/t oth cause bf consc, init	
800.16	CLOS FX VLT SKUL W/CERBRL LAC&CONTUS LOC UNS DUR	**S02.0XXA**	Fracture of vault of skull, init encntr for closed fracture	*and*
		S06.339A	Contus/lac cereb, w LOC of unsp duration, init	
800.19	CLOS FX VALT SKUL W/CERBRL LAC&CONTUS UNS CONCUS	**S02.0XXA**	Fracture of vault of skull, init encntr for closed fracture	*and*
		S06.330A	Contus/lac cereb, w/o loss of consciousness, init	
800.20	CLOSED SKULL VAULT FX-SUBARACH-DURAL HEM-UNS SOC	**S02.0XXA**	Fracture of vault of skull, init encntr for closed fracture	*and*
		S06.4X0A	Epidural hemorrhage w/o loss of consciousness, init encntr	*or*
		S06.5X0A	Traum subdr hem w/o loss of consciousness, init	*or*
		S06.6X0A	Traum subrac hem w/o loss of consciousness, init	
800.21	CLOS FX VAULT SKULL-SUBARACH-DURAL HEMORR-NO LOC	**S02.0XXA**	Fracture of vault of skull, init encntr for closed fracture	*and*
		S06.4X0A	Epidural hemorrhage w/o loss of consciousness, init encntr	*or*
		S06.5X0A	Traum subdr hem w/o loss of consciousness, init	*or*
		S06.6X0A	Traum subrac hem w/o loss of consciousness, init	
800.22	CLOS FX VALT SKUL-SUBARACH-DURAL HEM-BRF LOC	**S02.0XXA**	Fracture of vault of skull, init encntr for closed fracture	*and*
		S06.4X1A	Epidural hemorrhage w LOC of 30 minutes or less, init	*or*
		S06.4X2A	Epidural hemorrhage w LOC of 31-59 min, init	*or*
		S06.5X1A	Traum subdr hem w LOC of 30 minutes or less, init	*or*
		S06.5X2A	Traum subdr hem w loss of consciousness of 31-59 min, init	*or*
		S06.6X1A	Traum subrac hem w LOC of 30 minutes or less, init	*or*
		S06.6X2A	Traum subrac hem w loss of consciousness of 31-59 min, init	
800.23	CLOS FX VAULT SKULL W/SUBARACH-DURA HEM-MOD LOC	**S02.0XXA**	Fracture of vault of skull, init encntr for closed fracture	*and*
		S06.4X3A	Epidural hemorrhage w LOC of 1-5 hrs 59 min, init	*or*
		S06.4X4A	Epidural hemorrhage w LOC of 6 hours to 24 hours, init	*or*
		S06.5X3A	Traum subdr hem w LOC of 1-5 hrs 59 min, init	*or*
		S06.5X4A	Traum subdr hem w LOC of 6 hours to 24 hours, init	*or*
		S06.6X3A	Traum subrac hem w LOC of 1-5 hrs 59 min, init	*or*
		S06.6X4A	Traum subrac hem w LOC of 6 hours to 24 hours, init	
800.24	CLOS FX VAULT SKULL-DURAL HEM-LOC >24 HR & RETRN	**S02.0XXA**	Fracture of vault of skull, init encntr for closed fracture	*and*
		S06.4X5A	Epidural hemorrhage w LOC >24 hr w ret consc lev, init	*or*
		S06.5X5A	Traum subdr hem w LOC >24 hr w ret consc lev, init	*or*
		S06.6X5A	Traum subrac hem w LOC >24 hr w ret consc lev, init	
800.25	CLOS FX VAULT SKULL-DURAL HEM-LOC>24 & NO RETURN	**S02.0XXA**	Fracture of vault of skull, init encntr for closed fracture	*and*
		S06.4X6A	Epidural hemorrhage w LOC >24 hr w/o ret consc w surv, init	*or*
		S06.4X7A	Epidur hemor w LOC w death d/t brain injury bf consc, init	*or*
		S06.4X8A	Epidur hemor w LOC w death due to oth causes bf consc, init	*or*
		S06.5X6A	Traum subdr hem w LOC >24 hr w/o ret consc w surv, init	*or*
		S06.5X7A	Traum subdr hem w LOC w dth d/t brain inj bef reg consc,init	*or*
		S06.5X8A	Traum subdr hem w LOC w dth d/t oth cause bef reg consc,init	*or*
		S06.6X6A	Traum subrac hem w LOC >24 hr w/o ret consc w surv, init	*or*
		S06.6X7A	Traum subrac hem w LOC w death d/t brain inj bf consc, init	*or*
		S06.6X8A	Traum subrac hem w LOC w death d/t oth cause bf consc, init	
800.26	CLOS FX VAULT SKULL W/SUBARACH-DURAL HEM-LOC UNS	**S02.0XXA**	Fracture of vault of skull, init encntr for closed fracture	*and*
		S06.4X9A	Epidural hemorrhage w LOC of unsp duration, init	*or*
		S06.5X9A	Traum subdr hem w LOC of unsp duration, init	*or*
		S06.6X9A	Traum subrac hem w LOC of unsp duration, init	

ICD-9-CM		ICD-10-CM		
800.29	CLOS SKULL VAULT FX-SUBARACH-DUR HEM-UNS CONCUSS	**S02.0XXA**	Fracture of vault of skull, init encntr for closed fracture	*and*
		S06.4X0A	Epidural hemorrhage w/o loss of consciousness, init encntr	*or*
		S06.5X0A	Traum subdr hem w/o loss of consciousness, init	*or*
		S06.6X0A	Traum subrac hem w/o loss of consciousness, init	
800.30	CLOS FX VALT SKUL W/UNS INTRACRAN HEMOR UNS SOC	**S02.0XXA**	Fracture of vault of skull, init encntr for closed fracture	*and*
		S06.360A	Traum hemor cereb, w/o loss of consciousness, init	
800.31	CLOS FX VALT SKUL W/UNS INTRACRAN HEMOR NO LOC	**S02.0XXA**	Fracture of vault of skull, init encntr for closed fracture	*and*
		S06.360A	Traum hemor cereb, w/o loss of consciousness, init	
800.32	CLOS FX VAULT SKULL W/UNS ICH BRIEF LOC	**S02.0XXA**	Fracture of vault of skull, init encntr for closed fracture	*and*
		S06.361A	Traum hemor cereb, w LOC of 30 minutes or less, init	*or*
		S06.362A	Traum hemor cereb, w LOC of 31-59 min, init	
800.33	CLOS FX VALT SKUL W/UNS INTRACRAN HEMOR MOD LOC	**S02.0XXA**	Fracture of vault of skull, init encntr for closed fracture	*and*
		S06.363A	Traum hemor cereb, w LOC of 1-5 hrs 59 minutes, init	*or*
		S06.364A	Traum hemor cereb, w LOC of 6 hours to 24 hours, init	
800.34	CLOSED FX VAULT SKULL W/OTH ICH-LOC>24-RETURN	**S02.0XXA**	Fracture of vault of skull, init encntr for closed fracture	*and*
		S06.365A	Traum hemor cereb, w LOC >24 hr w ret consc lev, init	
800.35	CLOS FX VAULT SKULL W/OTH ICH-LOC>24 NO RETURN	**S02.0XXA**	Fracture of vault of skull, init encntr for closed fracture	*and*
		S06.366A	Traum hemor cereb, w LOC >24 hr w/o ret consc w surv, init	*or*
		S06.367A	Traum hemor cereb, w LOC w dth d/t brain inj bf consc, init	*or*
		S06.368A	Traum hemor cereb, w LOC w dth d/t oth cause bf consc, init	
800.36	CLOS FX VAULT SKULL W/UNS ICH LOC UNS DUR	**S02.0XXA**	Fracture of vault of skull, init encntr for closed fracture	*and*
		S06.369A	Traum hemor cereb, w LOC of unsp duration, init	
800.39	CLOS FX VAULT SKULL W/UNS ICH UNS CONCUSSION	**S02.0XXA**	Fracture of vault of skull, init encntr for closed fracture	*and*
		S06.360A	Traum hemor cereb, w/o loss of consciousness, init	
800.40	CLOS FX VAULT SKULLW/ICI UNS NATUR UNS SOC	**S02.0XXA**	Fracture of vault of skull, init encntr for closed fracture	*and*
		S06.890A	Intcran inj w/o loss of consciousness, init encntr	*or*
		S06.9X0A	Unsp intracranial injury w/o loss of consciousness, init	
800.41	CLOS FX VAULT SKULL W/ICI UNS NATUR NO LOC	**S02.0XXA**	Fracture of vault of skull, init encntr for closed fracture	*and*
		S06.890A	Intcran inj w/o loss of consciousness, init encntr	*or*
		S06.9X0A	Unsp intracranial injury w/o loss of consciousness, init	
800.42	CLOS FX VAULT SKULL W/ICI UNS NATUR BRIEF LOC	**S02.0XXA**	Fracture of vault of skull, init encntr for closed fracture	*and*
		S06.891A	Intcran inj w LOC of 30 minutes or less, init	*or*
		S06.892A	Intcran inj w loss of consciousness of 31-59 min, init	*or*
		S06.9X1A	Unsp intracranial injury w LOC of 30 minutes or less, init	*or*
		S06.9X2A	Unsp intracranial injury w LOC of 31-59 min, init	
800.43	CLOS FX VAULT SKULL W/ICI UNS NATUR MOD LOC	**S02.0XXA**	Fracture of vault of skull, init encntr for closed fracture	*and*
		S06.893A	Intcran inj w loss of consciousness of 1-5 hrs 59 min, init	*or*
		S06.894A	Intcran inj w LOC of 6 hours to 24 hours, init	*or*
		S06.9X3A	Unsp intracranial injury w LOC of 1-5 hrs 59 min, init	*or*
		S06.9X4A	Unsp intracranial injury w LOC of 6 hours to 24 hours, init	
800.44	CLOS FX VAULT SKULL W/OTH ICI-LOC >24 HR-RETURN	**S02.0XXA**	Fracture of vault of skull, init encntr for closed fracture	*and*
		S06.895A	Intcran inj w LOC >24 hr w ret consc lev, init	*or*
		S06.9X5A	Unsp intracranial injury w LOC >24 hr w ret consc lev, init	
800.45	CLOSED FX VAULT SKULL-OTH ICI-LOC >24 NO RETURN	**S02.0XXA**	Fracture of vault of skull, init encntr for closed fracture	*and*
		S06.896A	Intcran inj w LOC >24 hr w/o ret consc w surv, init	*or*
		S06.897A	Intcran inj w LOC w death due to brain injury bf consc, init	*or*
		S06.898A	Intcran inj w LOC w death due to oth cause bf consc, init	*or*
		S06.9X6A	Unsp intcrn injury w LOC >24 hr w/o ret consc w surv, init	*or*
		S06.9X7A	Unsp intcrn inj w LOC w death d/t brain inj bf consc, init	*or*
		S06.9X8A	Unsp intcrn inj w LOC w death d/t oth cause bf consc, init	
800.46	CLOS FX VAULT SKULL W ICI UNS NATUR LOC UNS DUR	**S02.0XXA**	Fracture of vault of skull, init encntr for closed fracture	*and*
		S06.899A	Intcran inj w loss of consciousness of unsp duration, init	*or*
		S06.9X9A	Unsp intracranial injury w LOC of unsp duration, init	
800.49	CLOS FX VAULT SKULL W/ICI UNS NATURE UNS CONCUS	**S02.0XXA**	Fracture of vault of skull, init encntr for closed fracture	*and*
		S06.890A	Intcran inj w/o loss of consciousness, init encntr	*or*
		S06.9X0A	Unsp intracranial injury w/o loss of consciousness, init	
800.50	OPEN FX VALT SKUL W/O ICI UNS STATE CONSCIOUS	**S02.0XXB**	Fracture of vault of skull, init encntr for open fracture	
800.51	OPEN FX VALT SKUL W/O INTRACRAN INJR NO LOC	**S02.0XXB**	Fracture of vault of skull, init encntr for open fracture	
800.52	OPEN FX VALT SKUL W/O INTRACRAN INJR BRF LOC	**S02.0XXB**	Fracture of vault of skull, init encntr for open fracture	
800.53	OPEN FX VALT SKUL W/O INTRACRAN INJR MOD LOC	**S02.0XXB**	Fracture of vault of skull, init encntr for open fracture	
800.54	OPEN SKULL VAULT FX W/O ICI-LOC>24 HR-RETURN	**S02.0XXB**	Fracture of vault of skull, init encntr for open fracture	
800.55	OPEN SKULL VAULT FX W/O ICI-LOC>24 HR NO RETURN	**S02.0XXB**	Fracture of vault of skull, init encntr for open fracture	
800.56	OPEN FX VALT SKUL W/O INTRACRAN INJR LOC UNS DUR	**S02.0XXB**	Fracture of vault of skull, init encntr for open fracture	
800.59	OPEN FX VALT SKUL W/O INTRACRAN INJR UNS CONCUS	**S02.0XXB**	Fracture of vault of skull, init encntr for open fracture	

ICD-9-CM		ICD-10-CM		
800.60	OPN FX VALT SKUL W/CERBRL LAC&CONTUS UNS SOC	S02.0XXB	Fracture of vault of skull, init encntr for open fracture	and
		S06.330A	Contus/lac cereb, w/o loss of consciousness, init	
800.61	OPN FX VAULT SKULL WITH CERBRL LAC&CONTUS NO LOC	S02.0XXB	Fracture of vault of skull, init encntr for open fracture	and
		S06.330A	Contus/lac cereb, w/o loss of consciousness, init	
800.62	OPN FX VAULT SKULL W/CERBRL LAC&CONTUS BRIEF LOC	S02.0XXB	Fracture of vault of skull, init encntr for open fracture	and
		S06.331A	Contus/lac cereb, w LOC of 30 minutes or less, init	or
		S06.332A	Contus/lac cereb, w loss of consciousness of 31-59 min, init	
800.63	OPN FX VAULT SKULL W/CEREBRAL LAC&CONTUS MOD LOC	S02.0XXB	Fracture of vault of skull, init encntr for open fracture	and
		S06.333A	Contus/lac cereb, w LOC of 1-5 hrs 59 min, init	or
		S06.334A	Contus/lac cereb, w LOC of 6 hours to 24 hours, init	
800.64	OPN FX VAULT SKUL-CEREB LAC&CONTUS LOC>24&RETURN	S02.0XXB	Fracture of vault of skull, init encntr for open fracture	and
		S06.335A	Contus/lac cereb, w LOC >24 hr w ret consc lev, init	
800.65	OPN FX VLT SKULL-CEREB LAC&CONTUS LOC>24 NO RTRN	S02.0XXB	Fracture of vault of skull, init encntr for open fracture	and
		S06.336A	Contus/lac cereb, w LOC >24 hr w/o ret consc w surv, init	or
		S06.337A	Contus/lac cereb, w LOC w death d/t brain inj bf consc, init	or
		S06.338A	Contus/lac cereb, w LOC w death d/t oth cause bf consc, init	
800.66	OPN FX VALT SKUL W/CERBRL LAC&CONTUS LOC UNS DUR	S02.0XXB	Fracture of vault of skull, init encntr for open fracture	and
		S06.339A	Contus/lac cereb, w LOC of unsp duration, init	
800.69	OPN FX VALT SKUL W/CERBRL LAC&CONTUS UNS CONCUSS	S02.0XXB	Fracture of vault of skull, init encntr for open fracture	and
		S06.330A	Contus/lac cereb, w/o loss of consciousness, init	
800.70	OPN FX VAULT SKULL-SUBARACH-DURAL HEMOR UNS SOC	S02.0XXB	Fracture of vault of skull, init encntr for open fracture	and
		S06.4X0A	Epidural hemorrhage w/o loss of consciousness, init encntr	or
		S06.5X0A	Traum subdr hem w/o loss of consciousness, init	or
		S06.6X0A	Traum subrac hem w/o loss of consciousness, init	
800.71	OPN FX VAULT SKUL-SUBARACH-DURAL HEMORR NO LOC	S02.0XXB	Fracture of vault of skull, init encntr for open fracture	and
		S06.4X0A	Epidural hemorrhage w/o loss of consciousness, init encntr	or
		S06.5X0A	Traum subdr hem w/o loss of consciousness, init	or
		S06.6X0A	Traum subrac hem w/o loss of consciousness, init	
800.72	OPN FX VAULT SKUL-SUBARACH DURAL HEM BRIEF LOC	S02.0XXB	Fracture of vault of skull, init encntr for open fracture	and
		S06.4X1A	Epidural hemorrhage w LOC of 30 minutes or less, init	or
		S06.4X2A	Epidural hemorrhage w LOC of 31-59 min, init	or
		S06.5X1A	Traum subdr hem w LOC of 30 minutes or less, init	or
		S06.5X2A	Traum subdr hem w loss of consciousness of 31-59 min, init	or
		S06.6X1A	Traum subrac hem w LOC of 30 minutes or less, init	or
		S06.6X2A	Traum subrac hem w loss of consciousness of 31-59 min, init	
800.73	OPN FX VAULT SKUL-SUBARACH DURAL HEM MOD LOC	S02.0XXB	Fracture of vault of skull, init encntr for open fracture	and
		S06.4X3A	Epidural hemorrhage w LOC of 1-5 hrs 59 min, init	or
		S06.4X4A	Epidural hemorrhage w LOC of 6 hours to 24 hours, init	or
		S06.5X3A	Traum subdr hem w LOC of 1-5 hrs 59 min, init	or
		S06.5X4A	Traum subdr hem w LOC of 6 hours to 24 hours, init	or
		S06.6X3A	Traum subrac hem w LOC of 1-5 hrs 59 min, init	or
		S06.6X4A	Traum subrac hem w LOC of 6 hours to 24 hours, init	
800.74	OPN FX VAULT SKUL-SUBARACH DURL HEM LOC>24&RETRN	S02.0XXB	Fracture of vault of skull, init encntr for open fracture	and
		S06.4X5A	Epidural hemorrhage w LOC >24 hr w ret consc lev, init	or
		S06.5X5A	Traum subdr hem w LOC >24 hr w ret consc lev, init	or
		S06.6X5A	Traum subrac hem w LOC >24 hr w ret consc lev, init	
800.75	OPN FX VAULT SKULL-SUBARACH DURL HEM LOC NO RTRN	S02.0XXB	Fracture of vault of skull, init encntr for open fracture	and
		S06.4X6A	Epidural hemorrhage w LOC >24 hr w/o ret consc w surv, init	or
		S06.4X7A	Epidur hemor w LOC w death d/t brain injury bf consc, init	or
		S06.4X8A	Epidur hemor w LOC w death due to oth causes bf consc, init	or
		S06.5X6A	Traum subdr hem w LOC >24 hr w/o ret consc w surv, init	or
		S06.5X7A	Traum subdr hem w LOC w dth d/t brain inj bef reg consc,init	or
		S06.5X8A	Traum subdr hem w LOC w dth d/t oth cause bef reg consc,init	or
		S06.6X6A	Traum subrac hem w LOC >24 hr w/o ret consc w surv, init	or
		S06.6X7A	Traum subrac hem w LOC w death d/t brain inj bf consc, init	or
		S06.6X8A	Traum subrac hem w LOC w death d/t oth cause bf consc, init	
800.76	OPN FX VAULT SKULL-SUBARACH DURL HEM LOC UNS DUR	S02.0XXB	Fracture of vault of skull, init encntr for open fracture	and
		S06.4X9A	Epidural hemorrhage w LOC of unsp duration, init	or
		S06.5X9A	Traum subdr hem w LOC of unsp duration, init	or
		S06.6X9A	Traum subrac hem w LOC of unsp duration, init	
800.79	OPN FX VAULT SKULL-SUBARACH DURL HEM UNS CONCUSS	S02.0XXB	Fracture of vault of skull, init encntr for open fracture	and
		S06.4X0A	Epidural hemorrhage w/o loss of consciousness, init encntr	or
		S06.5X0A	Traum subdr hem w/o loss of consciousness, init	or
		S06.6X0A	Traum subrac hem w/o loss of consciousness, init	
800.80	OPEN FX VAULT SKULL OTH&UNS ICH UNS SOC	S02.0XXB	Fracture of vault of skull, init encntr for open fracture	and
		S06.360A	Traum hemor cereb, w/o loss of consciousness, init	
800.81	OPEN FX VAULT SKULL OTH&UNS ICH NO LOC	S02.0XXB	Fracture of vault of skull, init encntr for open fracture	and
		S06.360A	Traum hemor cereb, w/o loss of consciousness, init	

ICD-9-CM		ICD-10-CM		
800.82	OPEN FX VALT SKUL W/UNS INTRACRAN HEMOR BRF LOC	**S02.0XXB**	Fracture of vault of skull, init encntr for open fracture	*and*
		S06.361A	Traum hemor cereb, w LOC of 30 minutes or less, init	*or*
		S06.362A	Traum hemor cereb, w LOC of 31-59 min, init	
800.83	OPEN FX VAULT SKULL OTH&UNS ICH MOD LOC	**S02.0XXB**	Fracture of vault of skull, init encntr for open fracture	*and*
		S06.363A	Traum hemor cereb, w LOC of 1-5 hrs 59 minutes, init	*or*
		S06.364A	Traum hemor cereb, w LOC of 6 hours to 24 hours, init	
800.84	OPEN FX VAULT SKULL W/OTH ICH-LOC >24 HR&RETURN	**S02.0XXB**	Fracture of vault of skull, init encntr for open fracture	*and*
		S06.365A	Traum hemor cereb, w LOC >24 hr w ret consc lev, init	
800.85	OPEN FX VAULT SKULL W/OTH ICH-LOC >24 NO RETURN	**S02.0XXB**	Fracture of vault of skull, init encntr for open fracture	*and*
		S06.366A	Traum hemor cereb, w LOC >24 hr w/o ret consc w surv, init	*or*
		S06.367A	Traum hemor cereb, w LOC w dth d/t brain inj bf consc, init	*or*
		S06.368A	Traum hemor cereb, w LOC w dth d/t oth cause bf consc, init	
800.86	OPEN FX VAULT SKULL OTH&UNS ICH LOC UNS DUR	**S02.0XXB**	Fracture of vault of skull, init encntr for open fracture	*and*
		S06.369A	Traum hemor cereb, w LOC of unsp duration, init	
800.89	OPN FX VAULT SKULL OTH&UNS ICH UNS CONCUSS	**S02.0XXB**	Fracture of vault of skull, init encntr for open fracture	*and*
		S06.360A	Traum hemor cereb, w/o loss of consciousness, init	
800.90	OPN FX VAULT SKULL W/ICI UNS NATURE UNS SOC	**S02.0XXB**	Fracture of vault of skull, init encntr for open fracture	*and*
		S06.890A	Intcran inj w/o loss of consciousness, init encntr	*or*
		S06.9X0A	Unsp intracranial injury w/o loss of consciousness, init	
800.91	OPN FX VAULT SKULL W/ICI UNS NATURE NO LOC	**S02.0XXB**	Fracture of vault of skull, init encntr for open fracture	*and*
		S06.890A	Intcran inj w/o loss of consciousness, init encntr	*or*
		S06.9X0A	Unsp intracranial injury w/o loss of consciousness, init	
800.92	OPN FX VAULT SKULL W/ICI UNS NATURE BRIEF LOC	**S02.0XXB**	Fracture of vault of skull, init encntr for open fracture	*and*
		S06.891A	Intcran inj w LOC of 30 minutes or less, init	*or*
		S06.892A	Intcran inj w loss of consciousness of 31-59 min, init	*or*
		S06.9X1A	Unsp intracranial injury w LOC of 30 minutes or less, init	*or*
		S06.9X2A	Unsp intracranial injury w LOC of 31-59 min, init	
800.93	OPN FX VAULT SKULL W/ICI UNS NATURE MOD LOC	**S02.0XXB**	Fracture of vault of skull, init encntr for open fracture	*and*
		S06.893A	Intcran inj w loss of consciousness of 1-5 hrs 59 min, init	*or*
		S06.894A	Intcran inj w LOC of 6 hours to 24 hours, init	*or*
		S06.9X3A	Unsp intracranial injury w LOC of 1-5 hrs 59 min, init	*or*
		S06.9X4A	Unsp intracranial injury w LOC of 6 hours to 24 hours, init	
800.94	OPEN FX VAULT SKULL W/OTH ICI LOC >24 HR&RETURN	**S02.0XXB**	Fracture of vault of skull, init encntr for open fracture	*and*
		S06.895A	Intcran inj w LOC >24 hr w ret consc lev, init	*or*
		S06.9X5A	Unsp intracranial injury w LOC >24 hr w ret consc lev, init	
800.95	OPEN FX VAULT SKULL W/OTH ICI LOC >24 NO RETURN	**S02.0XXB**	Fracture of vault of skull, init encntr for open fracture	*and*
		S06.896A	Intcran inj w LOC >24 hr w/o ret consc w surv, init	*or*
		S06.897A	Intcran inj w LOC w death due to brain injury bf consc, init	*or*
		S06.898A	Intcran inj w LOC w death due to oth cause bf consc, init	*or*
		S06.9X6A	Unsp intcrn injury w LOC >24 hr w/o ret consc w surv, init	*or*
		S06.9X7A	Unsp intcrn inj w LOC w death d/t brain inj bf consc, init	*or*
		S06.9X8A	Unsp intcrn inj w LOC w death d/t oth cause bf consc, init	
800.96	OPN FX VAULT SKULL W/ICI UNS NATURE LOC UNS DUR	**S02.0XXB**	Fracture of vault of skull, init encntr for open fracture	*and*
		S06.899A	Intcran inj w loss of consciousness of unsp duration, init	*or*
		S06.9X9A	Unsp intracranial injury w LOC of unsp duration, init	
800.99	OPN FX VAULT SKULL W/ICI UNS NATURE UNS CONCUS	**S02.0XXB**	Fracture of vault of skull, init encntr for open fracture	*and*
		S06.890A	Intcran inj w/o loss of consciousness, init encntr	*or*
		S06.9X0A	Unsp intracranial injury w/o loss of consciousness, init	
801.00	CLOS FX BASE SKUL W/O ICI UNS STATE CONSCIOUS	**S02.10XA**	Unsp fracture of base of skull, init for clos fx	
		S02.110A	Type I occipital condyle fracture, init for clos fx	
		S02.111A	Type II occipital condyle fracture, init for clos fx	
		S02.112A	Type III occipital condyle fracture, init for clos fx	
		S02.113A	Unsp occipital condyle fracture, init for clos fx	
		S02.118A	Other fracture of occiput, init encntr for closed fracture	
		S02.119A	Unsp fracture of occiput, init encntr for closed fracture	
		S02.19XA	Oth fracture of base of skull, init for clos fx	
801.01	CLOS FX BASE SKUL W/O INTRACRAN INJR NO LOC	**S02.10XA**	Unsp fracture of base of skull, init for clos fx	
801.02	CLOS FX BASE SKUL W/O INTRACRAN INJR BRF LOC	**S02.10XA**	Unsp fracture of base of skull, init for clos fx	
801.03	CLOS FX BASE SKUL W/O INTRACRAN INJR MOD LOC	**S02.10XA**	Unsp fracture of base of skull, init for clos fx	
801.04	CLOSED FX BASE SKULL W/O ICI-LOC >24 HR&RETURN	**S02.10XA**	Unsp fracture of base of skull, init for clos fx	
801.05	CLOSED FX BASE SKULL W/O ICI-LOC >24 NO RETURN	**S02.10XA**	Unsp fracture of base of skull, init for clos fx	
801.06	CLOS FX BASE SKULL W/O INTRACRAN INJ LOC UNS DUR	**S02.10XA**	Unsp fracture of base of skull, init for clos fx	
801.09	CLOS FX BASE SKUL W/O INTRACRAN INJR UNS CONCUS	**S02.10XA**	Unsp fracture of base of skull, init for clos fx	
801.10	CLOS FX BASE SKUL W/CERBRL LAC&CONTUS UNS SOC	**S02.10XA**	Unsp fracture of base of skull, init for clos fx	*and*
		S06.330A	Contus/lac cereb, w/o loss of consciousness, init	
801.11	CLOS FX BASE SKULL WITH CERBRL LAC&CONTUS NO LOC	**S02.10XA**	Unsp fracture of base of skull, init for clos fx	*and*
		S06.330A	Contus/lac cereb, w/o loss of consciousness, init	

ICD-9-CM		ICD-10-CM		
801.12	CLOS FX BASE SKUL W/CERBRL LAC&CONTUS BRIEF LOC	**S02.10XA**	Unsp fracture of base of skull, init for clos fx	*and*
		S06.331A	Contus/lac cereb, w LOC of 30 minutes or less, init	*or*
		S06.332A	Contus/lac cereb, w loss of consciousness of 31-59 min, init	
801.13	CLOS FX BASE SKULL W/CERBRL LAC&CONTUS MOD LOC	**S02.10XA**	Unsp fracture of base of skull, init for clos fx	*and*
		S06.333A	Contus/lac cereb, w LOC of 1-5 hrs 59 min, init	*or*
		S06.334A	Contus/lac cereb, w LOC of 6 hours to 24 hours, init	
801.14	CLOS FX BASE SKULL-CEREB LAC LOC >24 HR&RETURN	**S02.10XA**	Unsp fracture of base of skull, init for clos fx	*and*
		S06.335A	Contus/lac cereb, w LOC >24 hr w ret consc lev, init	
801.15	CLOS FX BASE SKULL-CEREB LAC LOC >24-NO RETURN	**S02.10XA**	Unsp fracture of base of skull, init for clos fx	*and*
		S06.336A	Contus/lac cereb, w LOC >24 hr w/o ret consc w surv, init	*or*
		S06.337A	Contus/lac cereb, w LOC w death d/t brain inj bf consc, init	*or*
		S06.338A	Contus/lac cereb, w LOC w death d/t oth cause bf consc, init	
801.16	CLOS FX BASE SKL W/CERBRL LAC&CONTUS LOC UNS DUR	**S02.10XA**	Unsp fracture of base of skull, init for clos fx	*and*
		S06.339A	Contus/lac cereb, w LOC of unsp duration, init	
801.19	CLOS FX BASE SKUL W/CERBRL LAC&CONTUS UNS CONCUS	**S02.10XA**	Unsp fracture of base of skull, init for clos fx	*and*
		S06.330A	Contus/lac cereb, w/o loss of consciousness, init	
801.20	CLOS FX BASE SKULL-SUBARACH DURAL HEMORR UNS SOC	**S02.10XA**	Unsp fracture of base of skull, init for clos fx	*and*
		S06.4X0A	Epidural hemorrhage w/o loss of consciousness, init encntr	*or*
		S06.5X0A	Traum subdr hem w/o loss of consciousness, init	*or*
		S06.6X0A	Traum subrac hem w/o loss of consciousness, init	
801.21	CLOS FX BASE SKULL W/SUBARACH DURAL HEM NO LOS	**S02.10XA**	Unsp fracture of base of skull, init for clos fx	*and*
		S06.4X0A	Epidural hemorrhage w/o loss of consciousness, init encntr	*or*
		S06.5X0A	Traum subdr hem w/o loss of consciousness, init	*or*
		S06.6X0A	Traum subrac hem w/o loss of consciousness, init	
801.22	CLOS FX BASE SKULL-SUBARACH DURL HEM BRIEF LOC	**S02.10XA**	Unsp fracture of base of skull, init for clos fx	*and*
		S06.4X1A	Epidural hemorrhage w LOC of 30 minutes or less, init	*or*
		S06.4X2A	Epidural hemorrhage w LOC of 31-59 min, init	*or*
		S06.5X1A	Traum subdr hem w LOC of 30 minutes or less, init	*or*
		S06.5X2A	Traum subdr hem w loss of consciousness of 31-59 min, init	*or*
		S06.6X1A	Traum subrac hem w LOC of 30 minutes or less, init	*or*
		S06.6X2A	Traum subrac hem w loss of consciousness of 31-59 min, init	
801.23	CLOS FX BASE SKULL-SUBARACH DURAL HEM MOD LOC	**S02.10XA**	Unsp fracture of base of skull, init for clos fx	*and*
		S06.4X3A	Epidural hemorrhage w LOC of 1-5 hrs 59 min, init	*or*
		S06.4X4A	Epidural hemorrhage w LOC of 6 hours to 24 hours, init	*or*
		S06.5X3A	Traum subdr hem w LOC of 1-5 hrs 59 min, init	*or*
		S06.5X4A	Traum subdr hem w LOC of 6 hours to 24 hours, init	*or*
		S06.6X3A	Traum subrac hem w LOC of 1-5 hrs 59 min, init	*or*
		S06.6X4A	Traum subrac hem w LOC of 6 hours to 24 hours, init	
801.24	CLOS FX BASE SKULL-DURAL HEMORR LOC >24&RETURN	**S02.10XA**	Unsp fracture of base of skull, init for clos fx	*and*
		S06.4X5A	Epidural hemorrhage w LOC >24 hr w ret consc lev, init	*or*
		S06.5X5A	Traum subdr hem w LOC >24 hr w ret consc lev, init	*or*
		S06.6X5A	Traum subrac hem w LOC >24 hr w ret consc lev, init	
801.25	CLOS FX BASE SKULL-DURAL HEMORR LOC>24-NO RETURN	**S02.10XA**	Unsp fracture of base of skull, init for clos fx	*and*
		S06.4X6A	Epidural hemorrhage w LOC >24 hr w/o ret consc w surv, init	*or*
		S06.4X7A	Epidur hemor w LOC w death d/t brain injury bf consc, init	*or*
		S06.4X8A	Epidur hemor w LOC w death due to oth causes bf consc, init	*or*
		S06.5X6A	Traum subdr hem w LOC >24 hr w/o ret consc w surv, init	*or*
		S06.5X7A	Traum subdr hem w LOC w dth d/t brain inj bef reg consc,init	*or*
		S06.5X8A	Traum subdr hem w LOC w dth d/t oth cause bef reg consc,init	*or*
		S06.6X6A	Traum subrac hem w LOC >24 hr w/o ret consc w surv, init	*or*
		S06.6X7A	Traum subrac hem w LOC w death d/t brain inj bf consc, init	*or*
		S06.6X8A	Traum subrac hem w LOC w death d/t oth cause bf consc, init	
801.26	CLOS FX BASE SKULL-SUBARACH DURAL HEMORR LOC UNS	**S02.10XA**	Unsp fracture of base of skull, init for clos fx	*and*
		S06.4X9A	Epidural hemorrhage w LOC of unsp duration, init	*or*
		S06.5X9A	Traum subdr hem w LOC of unsp duration, init	*or*
		S06.6X9A	Traum subrac hem w LOC of unsp duration, init	
801.29	CLOS FX BASE SKULL-SUBARACH DURA HEM UNS CONCUSS	**S02.10XA**	Unsp fracture of base of skull, init for clos fx	*and*
		S06.4X0A	Epidural hemorrhage w/o loss of consciousness, init encntr	*or*
		S06.5X0A	Traum subdr hem w/o loss of consciousness, init	*or*
		S06.6X0A	Traum subrac hem w/o loss of consciousness, init	
801.30	CLOS FX BASE SKULL OTH&UNS ICH UNS SOC	**S02.10XA**	Unsp fracture of base of skull, init for clos fx	*and*
		S06.360A	Traum hemor cereb, w/o loss of consciousness, init	
801.31	CLOS FX BASE SKULL OTH&UNS ICH NO LOC	**S02.10XA**	Unsp fracture of base of skull, init for clos fx	*and*
		S06.360A	Traum hemor cereb, w/o loss of consciousness, init	
801.32	CLOS FX BASE SKULL OTH&UNS ICH BRIEF LOC	**S02.10XA**	Unsp fracture of base of skull, init for clos fx	*and*
		S06.361A	Traum hemor cereb, w LOC of 30 minutes or less, init	*or*
		S06.362A	Traum hemor cereb, w LOC of 31-59 min, init	
801.33	CLOS FX BASE SKULL OTH&UNS ICH MOD LOC	**S02.10XA**	Unsp fracture of base of skull, init for clos fx	*and*
		S06.363A	Traum hemor cereb, w LOC of 1-5 hrs 59 minutes, init	*or*
		S06.364A	Traum hemor cereb, w LOC of 6 hours to 24 hours, init	

ICD-9-CM		ICD-10-CM		
801.34	CLOS FX BASE SKULL-OTH&UNS ICH LOC>24 HR&RETURN	**S02.10XA**	Unsp fracture of base of skull, init for clos fx	*and*
		S06.365A	Traum hemor cereb, w LOC >24 hr w ret consc lev, init	
801.35	CLOS FX BASE SKULL-OTH&UNS ICH LOC >24 NO RETURN	**S02.10XA**	Unsp fracture of base of skull, init for clos fx	*and*
		S06.366A	Traum hemor cereb, w LOC >24 hr w/o ret consc w surv, init	*or*
		S06.367A	Traum hemor cereb, w LOC w dth d/t brain inj bf consc, init	*or*
		S06.368A	Traum hemor cereb, w LOC w dth d/t oth cause bf consc, init	
801.36	CLOS FX BASE SKULL OTH&UNS ICH LOC UNS DUR	**S02.10XA**	Unsp fracture of base of skull, init for clos fx	*and*
		S06.369A	Traum hemor cereb, w LOC of unsp duration, init	
801.39	CLOS FX BASE SKULL OTH&UNS ICH UNS CONCUS	**S02.10XA**	Unsp fracture of base of skull, init for clos fx	*and*
		S06.360A	Traum hemor cereb, w/o loss of consciousness, init	
801.40	CLOS FX BASE SKULL W/ICI UNS NATURE UNS SOC	**S02.10XA**	Unsp fracture of base of skull, init for clos fx	*and*
		S06.890A	Intcran inj w/o loss of consciousness, init encntr	*or*
		S06.9X0A	Unsp intracranial injury w/o loss of consciousness, init	
801.41	CLOS FX BASE SKULL W/ICI UNS NATURE NO LOC	**S02.10XA**	Unsp fracture of base of skull, init for clos fx	*and*
		S06.890A	Intcran inj w/o loss of consciousness, init encntr	*or*
		S06.9X0A	Unsp intracranial injury w/o loss of consciousness, init	
801.42	CLOS FX BASE SKULL W/ICI UNS NATURE BRIEF LOC	**S02.10XA**	Unsp fracture of base of skull, init for clos fx	*and*
		S06.891A	Intcran inj w LOC of 30 minutes or less, init	*or*
		S06.892A	Intcran inj w loss of consciousness of 31-59 min, init	*or*
		S06.9X1A	Unsp intracranial injury w LOC of 30 minutes or less, init	*or*
		S06.9X2A	Unsp intracranial injury w LOC of 31-59 min, init	
801.43	CLOS FX BASE SKULL W/ICI UNS NATURE MOD LOC	**S02.10XA**	Unsp fracture of base of skull, init for clos fX	*and*
		S06.893A	Intcran inj w loss of consciousness of 1-5 hrs 59 min, init	*or*
		S06.894A	Intcran inj w LOC of 6 hours to 24 hours, init	*or*
		S06.9X3A	Unsp intracranial injury w LOC of 1-5 hrs 59 min, init	*or*
		S06.9X4A	Unsp intracranial injury w LOC of 6 hours t	
801.44	CLOS FX BASE SKULL-OTH&UNS ICI LOC >24 HR&RETURN	**S02.10XA**	Unsp fracture of base of skull, init for clos fx	*and*
		S06.895A	Intcran inj w LOC >24 hr w ret consc lev, init	*or*
		S06.9X5A	Unsp intracranial injury w LOC >24 hr w ret consc lev, init	
801.45	CLOS FX BASE SKULL-OTH&UNS ICI LOC >24-NO RETURN	**S02.10XA**	Unsp fracture of base of skull, init for clos fx	*and*
		S06.896A	Intcran inj w LOC >24 hr w/o ret consc w surv, init	*or*
		S06.897A	Intcran inj w LOC w death due to brain injury bf consc, init	*or*
		S06.898A	Intcran inj w LOC w death due to oth cause bf consc, init	*or*
		S06.9X6A	Unsp intcrn injury w LOC >24 hr w/o ret consc w surv, init	*or*
		S06.9X7A	Unsp intcrn inj w LOC w death d/t brain inj bf consc, init	*or*
		S06.9X8A	Unsp intcrn inj w LOC w death d/t oth cause bf consc, init	
801.46	CLOS FX BASE SKULL W/ICI UNS NATURE LOC UNS DUR	**S02.10XA**	Unsp fracture of base of skull, init for clos fx	*and*
		S06.899A	Intcran inj w loss of consciousness of unsp duration, init	*or*
		S06.9X9A	Unsp intracranial injury w LOC of unsp duration, init	
801.49	CLOS FX BASE SKULL W/ICI UNS NATURE UNS CONCUS	**S02.10XA**	Unsp fracture of base of skull, init for clos fX	*and*
		S06.890A	Intcran inj w/o loss of consciousness, init encntr	*or*
		S06.9X0A	Unsp intracranial injury w/o loss of consciousness, init	
801.50	OPEN FX BASE SKUL W/O ICIR UNS STATE CONSCIOUS	**S02.10XB**	Unsp fracture of base of skull, init for opn fx	
		S02.110B	Type I occipital condyle fracture, init for opn fx	
		S02.111B	Type II occipital condyle fracture, init for opn fx	
		S02.112B	Type III occipital condyle fracture, init for opn fx	
		S02.113B	Unsp occipital condyle fracture, init for opn fx	
		S02.118B	Other fracture of occiput, init encntr for open fracture	
		S02.119B	Unsp fracture of occiput, init encntr for open fracture	
		S02.19XB	Oth fracture of base of skull, init encntr for open fracture	
801.51	OPEN FX BASE SKUL W/O INTRACRAN INJR NO LOC	**S02.10XB**	Unsp fracture of base of skull, init for opn fx	
801.52	OPEN FX BASE SKUL W/O INTRACRAN INJR BRF LOC	**S02.10XB**	Unsp fracture of base of skull, init for opn fx	
801.53	OPEN FX BASE SKUL W/O INTRACRAN INJR MOD LOC	**S02.10XB**	Unsp fracture of base of skull, init for opn fx	
801.54	OPEN FX BASE SKULL W/O ICI-LOC >24 HR&RETURN	**S02.10XB**	Unsp fracture of base of skull, init for opn fx	
801.55	OPEN FX BASE SKULL W/O ICI-LOC >24 HR NO RETURN	**S02.10XB**	Unsp fracture of base of skull, init for opn fx	
801.56	OPEN FX BASE SKUL W/O INTRACRAN INJR LOC UNS DUR	**S02.10XB**	Unsp fracture of base of skull, init for opn fx	
801.59	OPEN FX BASE SKUL W/O INTRACRAN INJR UNS CONCUS	**S02.10XB**	Unsp fracture of base of skull, init for opn fx	
801.60	OPN FX BASE SKUL W/CERBRL LAC&CONTUS UNS SOC	**S02.10XB**	Unsp fracture of base of skull, init for opn fx	*and*
		S06.330A	Contus/lac cereb, w/o loss of consciousness, init	
801.61	OPN FX BASE SKULL WITH CERBRL LAC&CONTUS NO LOC	**S02.10XB**	Unsp fracture of base of skull, init for opn fx	*and*
		S06.330A	Contus/lac cereb, w/o loss of consciousness, init	
801.62	OPN FX BASE SKUL W/CERBRL LAC&CONTUS BRIEF LOC	**S02.10XB**	Unsp fracture of base of skull, init for opn fx	*and*
		S06.331A	Contus/lac cereb, w LOC of 30 minutes or less, init	*or*
		S06.332A	Contus/lac cereb, w loss of consciousness of 31-59 min, init	
801.63	OPN FX BASE SKULL WITH CERBRL LAC&CONTUS MOD LOC	**S02.10XB**	Unsp fracture of base of skull, init for opn fx	*and*
		S06.333A	Contus/lac cereb, w LOC of 1-5 hrs 59 min, init	*or*
		S06.334A	Contus/lac cereb, w LOC of 6 hours to 24 hours, init	

[Brackets] indicate valid character values for each code. Character value meanings provided for each code grouping.

ICD-9-CM		ICD-10-CM		
8Ø1.64	OPEN FX BASE SKULL-CEREB LAC-LOC >24 HR&RETURN	**SØ2.1ØXB**	Unsp fracture of base of skull, init for opn fx	*and*
		SØ6.335A	Contus/lac cereb, w LOC >24 hr w ret consc lev, init	
8Ø1.65	OPEN FX BASE SKULL-CEREB LAC-LOC>24 HR-NO RETURN	**SØ2.1ØXB**	Unsp fracture of base of skull, init for opn fx	*and*
		SØ6.336A	Contus/lac cereb, w LOC >24 hr w/o ret consc w surv, init	*or*
		SØ6.337A	Contus/lac cereb, w LOC w death d/t brain inj bf consc, init	*or*
		SØ6.338A	Contus/lac cereb, w LOC w death d/t oth cause bf consc, init	
8Ø1.66	OPN FX BASE SKUL W/CERBRL LAC&CONTUS LOC UNS DUR	**SØ2.1ØXB**	Unsp fracture of base of skull, init for opn fx	*and*
		SØ6.339A	Contus/lac cereb, w LOC of unsp duration, init	
8Ø1.69	OPN FX BASE SKUL W/CERBRL LAC&CONTUS UNS CONCUSS	**SØ2.1ØXB**	Unsp fracture of base of skull, init for opn fx	*and*
		SØ6.33ØA	Contus/lac cereb, w/o loss of consciousness, init	
8Ø1.7Ø	OPEN FX BASE SKULL-SUBARACH-DURAL HEMORR-UNS SOC	**SØ2.1ØXB**	Unsp fracture of base of skull, init for opn fx	*and*
		SØ6.4XØA	Epidural hemorrhage w/o loss of consciousness, init encntr	*or*
		SØ6.5XØA	Traum subdr hem w/o loss of consciousness, init	*or*
		SØ6.6XØA	Traum subrac hem w/o loss of consciousness, init	
8Ø1.71	OPEN FX BASE SKULL-SUBARACH-DURAL HEMORR-NO LOC	**SØ2.1ØXB**	Unsp fracture of base of skull, init for opn fx	*and*
		SØ6.4XØA	Epidural hemorrhage w/o loss of consciousness, init encntr	*or*
		SØ6.5XØA	Traum subdr hem w/o loss of consciousness, init	*or*
		SØ6.6XØA	Traum subrac hem w/o loss of consciousness, init	
8Ø1.72	OPN FX BASE SKUL-SUBARACH-DURAL HEMORR-BRIEF LOC	**SØ2.1ØXB**	Unsp fracture of base of skull, init for opn fx	*and*
		SØ6.4X1A	Epidural hemorrhage w LOC of 30 minutes or less, init	*or*
		SØ6.4X2A	Epidural hemorrhage w LOC of 31-59 min, init	*or*
		SØ6.5X1A	Traum subdr hem w LOC of 30 minutes or less, init	*or*
		SØ6.5X2A	Traum subdr hem w loss of consciousness of 31-59 min, init	*or*
		SØ6.6X1A	Traum subrac hem w LOC of 30 minutes or less, init	*or*
		SØ6.6X2A	Traum subrac hem w loss of consciousness of 31-59 min, init	
8Ø1.73	OPN FX BASE SKULL-SUBARACH-DURAL HEMORR-MOD LOC	**SØ2.1ØXB**	Unsp fracture of base of skull, init for opn fx	*and*
		SØ6.4X3A	Epidural hemorrhage w LOC of 1-5 hrs 59 min, init	*or*
		SØ6.4X4A	Epidural hemorrhage w LOC of 6 hours to 24 hours, init	*or*
		SØ6.5X3A	Traum subdr hem w LOC of 1-5 hrs 59 min, init	*or*
		SØ6.5X4A	Traum subdr hem w LOC of 6 hours to 24 hours, init	*or*
		SØ6.6X3A	Traum subrac hem w LOC of 1-5 hrs 59 min, init	*or*
		SØ6.6X4A	Traum subrac hem w LOC of 6 hours to 24 hours, init	
8Ø1.74	OPEN FX BASE SKULL-DURAL HEMORR-LOC >24&RETURN	**SØ2.1ØXB**	Unsp fracture of base of skull, init for opn fx	*and*
		SØ6.4X5A	Epidural hemorrhage w LOC >24 hr w ret consc lev, init	*or*
		SØ6.5X5A	Traum subdr hem w LOC >24 hr w ret consc lev, init	*or*
		SØ6.6X5A	Traum subrac hem w LOC >24 hr w ret consc lev, init	
8Ø1.75	OPEN FX BASE SKULL-DURAL HEMORR-LOC>24-NO RETURN	**SØ2.1ØXB**	Unsp fracture of base of skull, init for opn fx	*and*
		SØ6.4X6A	Epidural hemorrhage w LOC >24 hr w/o ret consc w surv, init	*or*
		SØ6.4X7A	Epidur hemor w LOC w death d/t brain injury bf consc, init	*or*
		SØ6.4X8A	Epidur hemor w LOC w death due to oth causes bf consc, init	*or*
		SØ6.5X6A	Traum subdr hem w LOC >24 hr w/o ret consc w surv, init	*or*
		SØ6.5X7A	Traum subdr hem w LOC w dth d/t brain inj bef reg consc,init	*or*
		SØ6.5X8A	Traum subdr hem w LOC w dth d/t oth cause bef reg consc,init	*or*
		SØ6.6X6A	Traum subrac hem w LOC >24 hr w/o ret consc w surv, init	*or*
		SØ6.6X7A	Traum subrac hem w LOC w death d/t brain inj bf consc, init	*or*
		SØ6.6X8A	Traum subrac hem w LOC w death d/t oth cause bf consc, init	
8Ø1.76	OPEN FX BASE SKULL-SUBARACH-DURAL HEMORR-LOC UNS	**SØ2.1ØXB**	Unsp fracture of base of skull, init for opn fx	*and*
		SØ6.4X9A	Epidural hemorrhage w LOC of unsp duration, init	*or*
		SØ6.5X9A	Traum subdr hem w LOC of unsp duration, init	*or*
		SØ6.6X9A	Traum subrac hem w LOC of unsp duration, init	
8Ø1.79	OPN FX BASE SKULL-SUBARACH-DURAL HEM-UNS CONCUSS	**SØ2.1ØXB**	Unsp fracture of base of skull, init for opn fx	*and*
		SØ6.4XØA	Epidural hemorrhage w/o loss of consciousness, init encntr	*or*
		SØ6.5XØA	Traum subdr hem w/o loss of consciousness, init	*or*
		SØ6.6XØA	Traum subrac hem w/o loss of consciousness, init	
8Ø1.8Ø	OPEN FX BASE SKULL- OTH&UNS ICH UNS SOC	**SØ2.1ØXB**	Unsp fracture of base of skull, init for opn fx	*and*
		SØ6.36ØA	Traum hemor cereb, w/o loss of consciousness, init	
8Ø1.81	OPEN FX BASE SKULL- OTH&UNS ICH NO LOC	**SØ2.1ØXB**	Unsp fracture of base of skull, init for opn fx	*and*
		SØ6.36ØA	Traum hemor cereb, w/o loss of consciousness, init	
8Ø1.82	OPEN FX BASE SKUL W/UNS INTRACRAN HEMOR BRF LOC	**SØ2.1ØXB**	Unsp fracture of base of skull, init for opn fx	*and*
		SØ6.361A	Traum hemor cereb, w LOC of 30 minutes or less, init	*or*
		SØ6.362A	Traum hemor cereb, w LOC of 31-59 min, init	
8Ø1.83	OPEN FX BASE SKUL W/UNS INTRACRAN HEMOR MOD LOC	**SØ2.1ØXB**	Unsp fracture of base of skull, init for opn fx	*and*
		SØ6.363A	Traum hemor cereb, w LOC of 1-5 hrs 59 minutes, init	*or*
		SØ6.364A	Traum hemor cereb, w LOC of 6 hours to 24 hours, init	
8Ø1.84	OPN FX BASE SKULL-OTH& UNS ICH LOC >24 HR&RETURN	**SØ2.1ØXB**	Unsp fracture of base of skull, init for opn fx	*and*
		SØ6.365A	Traum hemor cereb, w LOC >24 hr w ret consc lev, init	
8Ø1.85	OPEN FX BASE SKULL-OTH&UNS ICH-LOC >24 NO RETURN	**SØ2.1ØXB**	Unsp fracture of base of skull, init for opn fx	*and*
		SØ6.366A	Traum hemor cereb, w LOC >24 hr w/o ret consc w surv, init	*or*
		SØ6.367A	Traum hemor cereb, w LOC w dth d/t brain inj bf consc, init	*or*
		SØ6.368A	Traum hemor cereb, w LOC w dth d/t oth cause bf consc, init	

See Appendix A ➡ Equivalent Mapping Scenario Scenario

ICD-9-CM		ICD-10-CM		
801.86	OPN FX BASE SKULL-OTH&UNS ICH LOC UNS DUR	**S02.10XB**	Unsp fracture of base of skull, init for opn fx	*and*
		S06.369A	Traum hemor cereb, w LOC of unsp duration, init	
801.89	OPN FX BASE SKUL-OTH&UNS ICH UNS CONCUS	**S02.10XB**	Unsp fracture of base of skull, init for opn fx	*and*
		S06.360A	Traum hemor cereb, w/o loss of consciousness, init	
801.90	OPN FX BASE SKUL-ICI OTH&UNS NATURE UNS SOC	**S02.10XB**	Unsp fracture of base of skull, init for opn fx	*and*
		S06.890A	Intcran inj w/o loss of consciousness, init encntr	*or*
		S06.9X0A	Unsp intracranial injury w/o loss of consciousness, init	
801.91	OPN FX BASE SKUL-ICI OTH&UNS NATURE NO LOC	**S02.10XB**	Unsp fracture of base of skull, init for opn fx	*and*
		S06.890A	Intcran inj w/o loss of consciousness, init encntr	*or*
		S06.9X0A	Unsp intracranial injury w/o loss of consciousness, init	
801.92	OPN FX BASE SKULL-ICI OTH&UNS NATURE BRIEF LOC	**S02.10XB**	Unsp fracture of base of skull, init for opn fx	*and*
		S06.891A	Intcran inj w LOC of 30 minutes or less, init	*or*
		S06.892A	Intcran inj w loss of consciousness of 31-59 min, init	*or*
		S06.9X1A	Unsp intracranial injury w LOC of 30 minutes or less, init	*or*
		S06.9X2A	Unsp intracranial injury w LOC of 31-59 min, init	
801.93	OPN FX BASE SKULL-ICI OTH&UNS NATURE MOD LOC	**S02.10XB**	Unsp fracture of base of skull, init for opn fX	*and*
		S06.893A	Intcran inj w loss of consciousness of 1-5 hrs 59 min, init	*or*
		S06.894A	Intcran inj w LOC of 6 hours to 24 hours, init	*or*
		S06.9X3A	Unsp intracranial injury w LOC of 1-5 hrs 59 min, init	*or*
		S06.9X4A	Unsp intracranial injury w LOC of 6 hours to 24 hours, init	
801.94	OPN FX BASE SKULL-ICI OTH&UNS LOC >24 HR&RETURN	**S02.10XB**	Unsp fracture of base of skull, init for opn fx	*and*
		S06.895A	Intcran inj w LOC >24 hr w ret consc lev, init	*or*
		S06.9X5A	Unsp intracranial injury w LOC >24 hr w ret consc lev, init	
801.95	OPN FX BASE SKULL-ICI OTH&UNS LOC >24 NO RETURN	**S02.10XB**	Unsp fracture of base of skull, init for opn fx	*and*
		S06.896A	Intcran inj w LOC >24 hr w/o ret consc w surv, init	*or*
		S06.897A	Intcran inj w LOC w death due to brain injury bf consc, init	*or*
		S06.898A	Intcran inj w LOC w death due to oth cause bf consc, init	*or*
		S06.9X6A	Unsp intcrn injury w LOC >24 hr w/o ret consc w surv, init	*or*
		S06.9X7A	Unsp intcrn inj w LOC w death d/t brain inj bf consc, init	*or*
		S06.9X8A	Unsp intcrn inj w LOC w death d/t oth cause bf consc, init	
801.96	OPN FX BASE SKUL-ICI UNS NATURE LOC UNS DUR	**S02.10XB**	Unsp fracture of base of skull, init for opn fx	*and*
		S06.899A	Intcran inj w loss of consciousness of unsp duration, init	*or*
		S06.9X9A	Unsp intracranial injury w LOC of unsp duration, init	
801.99	OPN FX BASE SKUL-ICI UNS NATURE UNS CONCUS	**S02.10XB**	Unsp fracture of base of skull, init for opn fX	*and*
		S06.890A	Intcran inj w/o loss of consciousness, init encntr	*or*
		S06.9X0A	Unsp intracranial injury w/o loss of consciousness, init	
802.0	NASAL BONES, CLOSED FRACTURE	**S02.2XXA**	Fracture of nasal bones, init encntr for closed fracture	
802.1	NASAL BONES, OPEN FRACTURE	**S02.2XXB**	Fracture of nasal bones, initial encounter for open fracture	
802.20	CLOSED FRACTURE OF UNSPECIFIED SITE OF MANDIBLE	**S02.609A**	Fracture of mandible, unsp, init encntr for closed fracture	
		S02.69XA	Fracture of mandible of oth site, init for clos fx	
802.21	CLOSED FRACTURE OF CONDYLAR PROCESS OF MANDIBLE	**S02.61XA**	Fracture of condylar process of mandible, init for clos fx	
802.22	CLOSED FRACTURE SUBCONDYLAR PROCESS MANDIBLE	**S02.62XA**	Fracture of subcondylar process of mandible, init	
802.23	CLOSED FRACTURE OF CORONOID PROCESS OF MANDIBLE	**S02.63XA**	Fracture of coronoid process of mandible, init for clos fx	
802.24	CLOSED FRACTURE UNSPECIFIED PART RAMUS MANDIBLE	**S02.64XA**	Fracture of ramus of mandible, init for clos fx	
802.25	CLOSED FRACTURE OF ANGLE OF JAW	**S02.65XA**	Fracture of angle of mandible, init for clos fx	
802.26	CLOSED FRACTURE OF SYMPHYSIS OF BODY OF MANDIBLE	**S02.66XA**	Fracture of symphysis of mandible, init for clos fx	
802.27	CLOSED FRACTURE ALVEOLAR BORDER BODY MANDIBLE	**S02.67XA**	Fracture of alveolus of mandible, init for clos fx	
802.28	CLOSED FRACTURE OTHER&UNSPEC PART BODY MANDIBLE	**S02.600A**	Fracture of unsp part of body of mandible, init for clos fx	
802.29	CLOSED FRACTURE OF MULTIPLE SITES OF MANDIBLE	**S02.609A**	Fracture of mandible, unsp, init encntr for closed fracture	
		S02.69XA	Fracture of mandible of oth site, init for clos fx	
802.30	OPEN FRACTURE OF UNSPECIFIED SITE OF MANDIBLE	**S02.609B**	Fracture of mandible, unsp, init encntr for open fracture	
		S02.69XB	Fracture of mandible of oth site, init for opn fx	
802.31	OPEN FRACTURE OF CONDYLAR PROCESS OF MANDIBLE	**S02.61XB**	Fracture of condylar process of mandible, init for opn fx	
802.32	OPEN FRACTURE OF SUBCONDYLAR PROCESS OF MANDIBLE	**S02.62XB**	Fracture of subcondylar process of mandible, init for opn fx	
802.33	OPEN FRACTURE OF CORONOID PROCESS OF MANDIBLE	**S02.63XB**	Fracture of coronoid process of mandible, init for opn fx	
802.34	OPEN FRACTURE UNSPECIFIED PART RAMUS MANDIBLE	**S02.64XB**	Fracture of ramus of mandible, init encntr for open fracture	
802.35	OPEN FRACTURE OF ANGLE OF JAW	**S02.65XB**	Fracture of angle of mandible, init encntr for open fracture	
802.36	OPEN FRACTURE OF SYMPHYSIS OF BODY OF MANDIBLE	**S02.66XB**	Fracture of symphysis of mandible, init for opn fx	
802.37	OPEN FRACTURE ALVEOLAR BORDER BODY MANDIBLE	**S02.67XB**	Fracture of alveolus of mandible, init for opn fx	
802.38	OPEN FRACTURE OTHER&UNSPEC PART BODY MANDIBLE	**S02.600B**	Fracture of unsp part of body of mandible, init for opn fx	
802.39	OPEN FRACTURE OF MULTIPLE SITES OF MANDIBLE	**S02.609B**	Fracture of mandible, unsp, init encntr for open fracture	
		S02.69XB	Fracture of mandible of oth site, init for opn fx	
802.4	MALAR AND MAXILLARY BONES CLOSED FRACTURE	**S02.400A**	Malar fracture unspecified, init encntr for closed fracture	
		S02.401A	Maxillary fracture, unsp, init encntr for closed fracture	
		S02.402A	Zygomatic fracture, unsp, init encntr for closed fracture	
		S02.411A	LeFort I fracture, initial encounter for closed fracture	
		S02.412A	LeFort II fracture, initial encounter for closed fracture	
		S02.413A	LeFort III fracture, initial encounter for closed fracture	

[Brackets] indicate valid character values for each code. Character value meanings provided for each code grouping.

ICD-9-CM		ICD-10-CM		
802.5	MALAR AND MAXILLARY BONES OPEN FRACTURE	S02.400B	Malar fracture unspecified, init encntr for open fracture	
		S02.401B	Maxillary fracture, unsp, init encntr for open fracture	
		S02.402B	Zygomatic fracture, unsp, init encntr for open fracture	
		S02.411B	LeFort I fracture, initial encounter for open fracture	
		S02.412B	LeFort II fracture, initial encounter for open fracture	
		S02.413B	LeFort III fracture, initial encounter for open fracture	
802.6	ORBITAL FLOOR , CLOSED FRACTURE	S02.3XXA	Fracture of orbital floor, init encntr for closed fracture	
802.7	ORBITAL FLOOR , OPEN FRACTURE	S02.3XXB	Fracture of orbital floor, init encntr for open fracture	
802.8	OTHER FACIAL BONES CLOSED FRACTURE	S02.42XA	Fracture of alveolus of maxilla, init for clos fx	
		S02.8XXA	Fractures of oth skull and facial bones, init for clos fx	
		S02.92XA	Unsp fracture of facial bones, init for clos fx	
802.9	OTHER FACIAL BONES, OPEN FRACTURE	S02.42XB	Fracture of alveolus of maxilla, init for opn fx	
		S02.8XXB	Fractures of oth skull and facial bones, init for opn fx	
		S02.92XB	Unsp fracture of facial bones, init encntr for open fracture	
803.00	OTH CLO SKUL FX W/O ICIR UNS STATE CONSCIOUS	S02.91XA	Unsp fracture of skull, init encntr for closed fracture	
803.01	OTH CLO SKUL FX W/O INTRACRAN INJR NO LOC	S02.91XA	Unsp fracture of skull, init encntr for closed fracture	
803.02	OTH CLO SKUL FX W/O INTRACRAN INJR BRF LOC	S02.91XA	Unsp fracture of skull, init encntr for closed fracture	
803.03	OTH CLO SKUL FX W/O INTRACRAN INJR MOD LOC	S02.91XA	Unsp fracture of skull, init encntr for closed fracture	
803.04	OTH CLOSED SKULL FX W/O ICI-LOC >24 HR&RETURN	S02.91XA	Unsp fracture of skull, init encntr for closed fracture	
803.05	OTH CLOSED SKULL FX W/O ICI-LOC >24 NO RETURN	S02.91XA	Unsp fracture of skull, init encntr for closed fracture	
803.06	OTH CLO SKUL FX W/O INTRACRAN INJR LOC UNS DUR	S02.91XA	Unsp fracture of skull, init encntr for closed fracture	
803.09	OTH CLO SKUL FX W/O INTRACRAN INJR UNS CONCUS	S02.91XA	Unsp fracture of skull, init encntr for closed fracture	
803.10	OTH CLO SKUL FX W/CERBRL LAC&CONTUS UNS SOC	S02.91XA	Unsp fracture of skull, init encntr for closed fracture	*and*
		S06.330A	Contus/lac cereb, w/o loss of consciousness, init	
803.11	OTH CLOS SKULL FX W/CERBRL LAC&CONTUS NO LOC	S02.91XA	Unsp fracture of skull, init encntr for closed fracture	*and*
		S06.330A	Contus/lac cereb, w/o loss of consciousness, init	
803.12	OTH CLOS SKULL FX W/CERBRL LAC&CONTUS BRF LOC	S02.91XA	Unsp fracture of skull, init encntr for closed fracture	*and*
		S06.331A	Contus/lac cereb, w LOC of 30 minutes or less, init	*or*
		S06.332A	Contus/lac cereb, w loss of consciousness of 31-59 min, init	
803.13	OTH CLOS SKULL FX W/CERBRL LAC&CONTUS MOD LOC	S02.91XA	Unsp fracture of skull, init encntr for closed fracture	*and*
		S06.333A	Contus/lac cereb, w LOC of 1-5 hrs 59 min, init	*or*
		S06.334A	Contus/lac cereb, w LOC of 6 hours to 24 hours, init	
803.14	OTH CLOS SKULL FX-CERBRL LAC LOC >24 HR&RETURN	S02.91XA	Unsp fracture of skull, init encntr for closed fracture	*and*
		S06.335A	Contus/lac cereb, w LOC >24 hr w ret consc lev, init	
803.15	OTH CLOS SKULL FX-CERBRL LAC LOC >24 NO RETURN	S02.91XA	Unsp fracture of skull, init encntr for closed fracture	*and*
		S06.336A	Contus/lac cereb, w LOC >24 hr w/o ret consc w surv, init	*or*
		S06.337A	Contus/lac cereb, w LOC w death d/t brain inj bf consc, init	*or*
		S06.338A	Contus/lac cereb, w LOC w death d/t oth cause bf consc, init	
803.16	OTH CLOS SKUL FX W/CERBRL LAC&CONTUS LOC UNS DUR	S02.91XA	Unsp fracture of skull, init encntr for closed fracture	*and*
		S06.339A	Contus/lac cereb, w LOC of unsp duration, init	
803.19	OTH CLOS SKUL FX W/CERBRL LAC&CONTUS UNS CONCUSS	S02.91XA	Unsp fracture of skull, init encntr for closed fracture	*and*
		S06.330A	Contus/lac cereb, w/o loss of consciousness, init	
803.20	OTH CLOSED SKULL FX-SUBARACH-DURAL HEM-UNS SOC	S02.91XA	Unsp fracture of skull, init encntr for closed fracture	*and*
		S06.4X0A	Epidural hemorrhage w/o loss of consciousness, init encntr	*or*
		S06.5X0A	Traum subdr hem w/o loss of consciousness, init	*or*
		S06.6X0A	Traum subrac hem w/o loss of consciousness, init	
803.21	OTH CLOSED SKULL FX W/SUBARACH-DURAL HEM-NO LOC	S02.91XA	Unsp fracture of skull, init encntr for closed fracture	*and*
		S06.4X0A	Epidural hemorrhage w/o loss of consciousness, init encntr	*or*
		S06.5X0A	Traum subdr hem w/o loss of consciousness, init	*or*
		S06.6X0A	Traum subrac hem w/o loss of consciousness, init	
803.22	OTH CLOS SKULL FX SUBARACH-DURAL HEM-BRIEF LOC	S02.91XA	Unsp fracture of skull, init encntr for closed fracture	*and*
		S06.4X1A	Epidural hemorrhage w LOC of 30 minutes or less, init	*or*
		S06.4X2A	Epidural hemorrhage w LOC of 31-59 min, init	*or*
		S06.5X1A	Traum subdr hem w LOC of 30 minutes or less, init	*or*
		S06.5X2A	Traum subdr hem w loss of consciousness of 31-59 min, init	*or*
		S06.6X1A	Traum subrac hem w LOC of 30 minutes or less, init	*or*
		S06.6X2A	Traum subrac hem w loss of consciousness of 31-59 min, init	
803.23	OTH CLOS SKULL FX-SUBARACH-DURAL HEM-MOD LOC	S02.91XA	Unsp fracture of skull, init encntr for closed fracture	*and*
		S06.4X3A	Epidural hemorrhage w LOC of 1-5 hrs 59 min, init	*or*
		S06.4X4A	Epidural hemorrhage w LOC of 6 hours to 24 hours, init	*or*
		S06.5X3A	Traum subdr hem w LOC of 1-5 hrs 59 min, init	*or*
		S06.5X4A	Traum subdr hem w LOC of 6 hours to 24 hours, init	*or*
		S06.6X3A	Traum subrac hem w LOC of 1-5 hrs 59 min, init	*or*
		S06.6X4A	Traum subrac hem w LOC of 6 hours to 24 hours, init	
803.24	OTH CLOS SKULL FX-DURAL HEMORR-LOC >24 HR&RETURN	S02.91XA	Unsp fracture of skull, init encntr for closed fracture	*and*
		S06.4X5A	Epidural hemorrhage w LOC >24 hr w ret consc lev, init	*or*
		S06.5X5A	Traum subdr hem w LOC >24 hr w ret consc lev, init	*or*
		S06.6X5A	Traum subrac hem w LOC >24 hr w ret consc lev, init	

ICD-9-CM		ICD-10-CM		
803.25	OTH CLOS SKULL FX-DURAL HEMORR-LOC >24-NO RETURN	**S02.91XA**	Unsp fracture of skull, init encntr for closed fracture	*and*
		S06.4X6A	Epidural hemorrhage w LOC >24 hr w/o ret consc w surv, init	*or*
		S06.4X7A	Epidur hemor w LOC w death d/t brain injury bf consc, init	*or*
		S06.4X8A	Epidur hemor w LOC w death due to oth causes bf consc, init	*or*
		S06.5X6A	Traum subdr hem w LOC >24 hr w/o ret consc w surv, init	*or*
		S06.5X7A	Traum subdr hem w LOC w dth d/t brain inj bef reg consc,init	*or*
		S06.5X8A	Traum subdr hem w LOC w dth d/t oth cause bef reg consc,init	*or*
		S06.6X6A	Traum subrac hem w LOC >24 hr w/o ret consc w surv, init	*or*
		S06.6X7A	Traum subrac hem w LOC w death d/t brain inj bf consc, init	*or*
		S06.6X8A	Traum subrac hem w LOC w death d/t oth cause bf consc, init	
803.26	OTH CLOSED SKULL FX-SUBARACH-DURAL HEM-LOC UNS	**S02.91XA**	Unsp fracture of skull, init encntr for closed fracture	*and*
		S06.4X9A	Epidural hemorrhage w LOC of unsp duration, init	*or*
		S06.5X9A	Traum subdr hem w LOC of unsp duration, init	*or*
		S06.6X9A	Traum subrac hem w LOC of unsp duration, init	
803.29	OTH CLOS SKULL FX-SUBARACH-DURA HEM-UNS CONCUSS	**S02.91XA**	Unsp fracture of skull, init encntr for closed fracture	*and*
		S06.4X0A	Epidural hemorrhage w/o loss of consciousness, init encntr	*or*
		S06.5X0A	Traum subdr hem w/o loss of consciousness, init	*or*
		S06.6X0A	Traum subrac hem w/o loss of consciousness, init	
803.30	OTH CLOS SKUL FX W/OTH&UNS ICH UNS UNCONSCIOUS	**S02.91XA**	Unsp fracture of skull, init encntr for closed fracture	*and*
		S06.369A	Traum hemor cereb, w LOC of unsp duration, init	
803.31	OTH CLOS SKULL FX OTH&UNS ICH NO LOC	**S02.91XA**	Unsp fracture of skull, init encntr for closed fracture	*and*
		S06.360A	Traum hemor cereb, w/o loss of consciousness, init	
803.32	OTH CLOS SKULL FX OTH&UNS ICH BRIEF LOC	**S02.91XA**	Unsp fracture of skull, init encntr for closed fracture	*and*
		S06.361A	Traum hemor cereb, w LOC of 30 minutes or less, init	*or*
		S06.362A	Traum hemor cereb, w LOC of 31-59 min, init	
803.33	OTH CLOS SKULL FX OTH&UNS ICH MOD LOC	**S02.91XA**	Unsp fracture of skull, init encntr for closed fracture	*and*
		S06.363A	Traum hemor cereb, w LOC of 1-5 hrs 59 minutes, init	
		S06.364A	Traum hemor cereb, w LOC of 6 hours to 24 hours, init	
803.34	OTH CLOS SKULL FX-OTH&UNS ICH-LOC >24 HR&RETURN	**S02.91XA**	Unsp fracture of skull, init encntr for closed fracture	*and*
		S06.365A	Traum hemor cereb, w LOC >24 hr w ret consc lev, init	
803.35	OTH CLOS SKULL FX-OTH&UNS ICH LOC >24-NO RETURN	**S02.91XA**	Unsp fracture of skull, init encntr for closed fracture	*and*
		S06.366A	Traum hemor cereb, w LOC >24 hr w/o ret consc w surv, init	*or*
		S06.367A	Traum hemor cereb, w LOC w dth d/t brain inj bf consc, init	*or*
		S06.368A	Traum hemor cereb, w LOC w dth d/t oth cause bf consc, init	
803.36	OTH CLOS SKUL FX W/OTH&UNS ICH LOC UNS DUR	**S02.91XA**	Unsp fracture of skull, init encntr for closed fracture	*and*
		S06.369A	Traum hemor cereb, w LOC of unsp duration, init	
803.39	OTH CLOS SKUL FX W/OTH&UNS ICH UNS CONCUS	**S02.91XA**	Unsp fracture of skull, init encntr for closed fracture	*and*
		S06.360A	Traum hemor cereb, w/o loss of consciousness, init	
803.40	OTH CLOS SKUL FX W/ICI OTH&UNS NATURE UNS SOC	**S02.91XA**	Unsp fracture of skull, init encntr for closed fracture	*and*
		S06.890A	Intcran inj w/o loss of consciousness, init encntr	*or*
		S06.9X0A	Unsp intracranial injury w/o loss of consciousness, init	
803.41	OTH CLOS SKUL FX W/ICI OTH&UNS NATURE NO LOC	**S02.91XA**	Unsp fracture of skull, init encntr for closed fracture	*and*
		S06.890A	Intcran inj w/o loss of consciousness, init encntr	*or*
		S06.9X0A	Unsp intracranial injury w/o loss of consciousness, init	
803.42	OTH CLOS SKUL FX W/ICI OTH&UNS NATURE BRIEF LOC	**S02.91XA**	Unsp fracture of skull, init encntr for closed fracture	*and*
		S06.891A	Intcran inj w LOC of 30 minutes or less, init	*or*
		S06.892A	Intcran inj w loss of consciousness of 31-59 min, init	*or*
		S06.9X1A	Unsp intracranial injury w LOC of 30 minutes or less, init	*or*
		S06.9X2A	Unsp intracranial injury w LOC of 31-59 min, init	
803.43	OTH CLOS SKUL FX W/ICI OTH&UNS NATURE MOD LOC	**S02.91XA**	Unsp fracture of skull, init encntr for closed fracture	*and*
		S06.893A	Intcran inj w loss of consciousness of 1-5 hrs 59 min, init	*or*
		S06.894A	Intcran inj w LOC of 6 hours to 24 hours, init	*or*
		S06.9X3A	Unsp intracranial injury w LOC of 1-5 hrs 59 min, init	*or*
		S06.9X4A	Unsp intracranial injury w LOC of 6 hours to 24 hours, init	
803.44	OTH CLOS SKUL FX W/ICI OTH&UNS LOC>24 HR&RTRN	**S02.91XA**	Unsp fracture of skull, init encntr for closed fracture	*and*
		S06.895A	Intcran inj w LOC >24 hr w ret consc lev, init	*or*
		S06.9X5A	Unsp intracranial injury w LOC >24 hr w ret consc lev, init	
803.45	OTH CLOS SKUL FX W/ICI OTH&UNS LOC>24 NO RTRN	**S02.91XA**	Unsp fracture of skull, init encntr for closed fracture	*and*
		S06.896A	Intcran inj w LOC >24 hr w/o ret consc w surv, init	*or*
		S06.897A	Intcran inj w LOC w death due to brain injury bf consc, init	*or*
		S06.898A	Intcran inj w LOC w death due to oth cause bf consc, init	*or*
		S06.9X6A	Unsp intcrn injury w LOC >24 hr w/o ret consc w surv, init	*or*
		S06.9X7A	Unsp intcrn inj w LOC w death d/t brain inj bf consc, init	*or*
		S06.9X8A	Unsp intcrn inj w LOC w death d/t oth cause bf consc, init	

[Brackets] indicate valid character values for each code. Character value meanings provided for each code grouping.

ICD-9-CM		ICD-10-CM		
803.46	OTH CLO SKUL FX W/ICI UNS NATURE LOC UNS DUR	**S02.91XA**	Unsp fracture of skull, init encntr for closed fracture	*and*
		S06.899A	Intcran inj w loss of consciousness of unsp duration, init	*or*
		S06.9X9A	Unsp intracranial injury w LOC of unsp duration, init	
803.49	OTH CLO SKUL FX W/ICI UNS NATURE UNS CONCUS	**S02.91XA**	Unsp fracture of skull, init encntr for closed fracture	*and*
		S06.890A	Intcran inj w/o loss of consciousness, init encntr	*or*
		S06.9X0A	Unsp intracranial injury w/o loss of consciousness, init	
803.50	OTH OPEN SKULL FX W/O ICI STATE CONSCIOUS UNS	**S02.91XB**	Unspecified fracture of skull, init encntr for open fracture	
803.51	OTH OPEN SKULL FX W/O INTRACRAN INJR NO LOC	**S02.91XB**	Unspecified fracture of skull, init encntr for open fracture	
803.52	OTH OPEN SKULL FX W/O INTRACRAN INJR BRIEF LOC	**S02.91XB**	Unspecified fracture of skull, init encntr for open fracture	
803.53	OTH OPEN SKULL FX W/O INTRACRAN INJR MOD LOC	**S02.91XB**	Unspecified fracture of skull, init encntr for open fracture	
803.54	OTH OPEN SKULL FRACTURE W/O ICI LOC>24 HR-RETURN	**S02.91XB**	Unspecified fracture of skull, init encntr for open fracture	
803.55	OTH OPEN SKULL FRACTURE W/O ICI LOC>24 NO RETURN	**S02.91XB**	Unspecified fracture of skull, init encntr for open fracture	
803.56	OTH OPEN SKULL FX W/O INTRACRAN INJR LOC UNS DUR	**S02.91XB**	Unspecified fracture of skull, init encntr for open fracture	
803.59	OTH OPEN SKULL FX W/O INTRACRAN INJR UNS CONCUS	**S02.91XB**	Unspecified fracture of skull, init encntr for open fracture	
803.60	OTH OPN SKUL FX W/CERBRL LAC&CONTUS UNS SOC	**S02.91XB**	Unspecified fracture of skull, init encntr for open fracture	*and*
		S06.330A	Contus/lac cereb, w/o loss of consciousness, init	
803.61	OTH OPN SKULL FX WITH CERBRL LAC&CONTUS NO LOC	**S02.91XB**	Unspecified fracture of skull, init encntr for open fracture	*and*
		S06.330A	Contus/lac cereb, w/o loss of consciousness, init	
803.62	OTH OPN SKULL FX W/CERBRL LAC&CONTUS BRIEF LOC	**S02.91XB**	Unspecified fracture of skull, init encntr for open fracture	*and*
		S06.331A	Contus/lac cereb, w LOC of 30 minutes or less, init	*or*
		S06.332A	Contus/lac cereb, w loss of consciousness of 31-59 min, init	
803.63	OTH OPN SKULL FX WITH CERBRL LAC&CONTUS MOD LOC	**S02.91XB**	Unspecified fracture of skull, init encntr for open fracture	*and*
		S06.333A	Contus/lac cereb, w LOC of 1-5 hrs 59 min, init	*or*
		S06.334A	Contus/lac cereb, w LOC of 6 hours to 24 hours, init	
803.64	OTH OPEN SKULL FX-CEREB LAC LOC >24 HR&RETURN	**S02.91XB**	Unspecified fracture of skull, init encntr for open fracture	*and*
		S06.335A	Contus/lac cereb, w LOC >24 hr w ret consc lev, init	
803.65	OTH OPEN SKULL FX-CEREB LAC LOC >24 NO RETURN	**S02.91XB**	Unspecified fracture of skull, init encntr for open fracture	*and*
		S06.336A	Contus/lac cereb, w LOC >24 hr w/o ret consc w surv, init	*or*
		S06.337A	Contus/lac cereb, w LOC w death d/t brain inj bf consc, init	*or*
		S06.338A	Contus/lac cereb, w LOC w death d/t oth cause bf consc, init	
803.66	OTH OPN SKUL FX W/CERBRL LAC&CONTUS LOC UNS DUR	**S02.91XB**	Unspecified fracture of skull, init encntr for open fracture	*and*
		S06.339A	Contus/lac cereb, w LOC of unsp duration, init	
803.69	OTH OPN SKUL FX W/CERBRL LAC&CONTUS UNS CONCUSS	**S02.91XB**	Unspecified fracture of skull, init encntr for open fracture	*and*
		S06.330A	Contus/lac cereb, w/o loss of consciousness, init	
803.70	OTH OPEN SKULL FX-SUBARACH DURAL HEMORR UNS SOC	**S02.91XB**	Unspecified fracture of skull, init encntr for open fracture	*and*
		S06.4X0A	Epidural hemorrhage w/o loss of consciousness, init encntr	*or*
		S06.5X0A	Traum subdr hem w/o loss of consciousness, init	*or*
		S06.6X0A	Traum subrac hem w/o loss of consciousness, init	
803.71	OTH OPEN SKULL FX-SUBARACH DURAL HEMORR NO LOC	**S02.91XB**	Unspecified fracture of skull, init encntr for open fracture	*and*
		S06.4X0A	Epidural hemorrhage w/o loss of consciousness, init encntr	*or*
		S06.5X0A	Traum subdr hem w/o loss of consciousness, init	*or*
		S06.6X0A	Traum subrac hem w/o loss of consciousness, init	
803.72	OTH OPEN SKULL FX-SUBARACH DURAL HEM BRF LOC	**S02.91XB**	Unspecified fracture of skull, init encntr for open fracture	*and*
		S06.4X1A	Epidural hemorrhage w LOC of 30 minutes or less, init	*or*
		S06.4X2A	Epidural hemorrhage w LOC of 31-59 min, init	*or*
		S06.5X1A	Traum subdr hem w LOC of 30 minutes or less, init	*or*
		S06.5X2A	Traum subdr hem w loss of consciousness of 31-59 min, init	*or*
		S06.6X1A	Traum subrac hem w LOC of 30 minutes or less, init	*or*
		S06.6X2A	Traum subrac hem w loss of consciousness of 31-59 min, init	
803.73	OTH OPEN SKULL FX-SUBARCH DURAL HEM MOD LOC	**S02.91XB**	Unspecified fracture of skull, init encntr for open fracture	*and*
		S06.4X3A	Epidural hemorrhage w LOC of 1-5 hrs 59 min, init	*or*
		S06.4X4A	Epidural hemorrhage w LOC of 6 hours to 24 hours, init	*or*
		S06.5X3A	Traum subdr hem w LOC of 1-5 hrs 59 min, init	*or*
		S06.5X4A	Traum subdr hem w LOC of 6 hours to 24 hours, init	*or*
		S06.6X3A	Traum subrac hem w LOC of 1-5 hrs 59 min, init	*or*
		S06.6X4A	Traum subrac hem w LOC of 6 hours to 24 hours, init	
803.74	OTH OPN SKULL FX-SUBARACH DURA HEM LOC>24-RETURN	**S02.91XB**	Unspecified fracture of skull, init encntr for open fracture	*and*
		S06.4X5A	Epidural hemorrhage w LOC >24 hr w ret consc lev, init	*or*
		S06.5X5A	Traum subdr hem w LOC >24 hr w ret consc lev, init	*or*
		S06.6X5A	Traum subrac hem w LOC >24 hr w ret consc lev, init	

ICD-9-CM		ICD-10-CM		
8Ø3.75	OTH OPN SKUL FX-SUBARACH DURA HEMORR LOC NO RTRN	**SØ2.91XB**	Unspecified fracture of skull, init encntr for open fracture	*and*
		SØ6.4X6A	Epidural hemorrhage w LOC >24 hr w/o ret consc w surv, init	*or*
		SØ6.4X7A	Epidur hemor w LOC w death d/t brain injury bf consc, init	*or*
		SØ6.4X8A	Epidur hemor w LOC w death due to oth causes bf consc, init	*or*
		SØ6.5X6A	Traum subdr hem w LOC >24 hr w/o ret consc w surv, init	*or*
		SØ6.5X7A	Traum subdr hem w LOC w dth d/t brain inj bef reg consc,init	*or*
		SØ6.5X8A	Traum subdr hem w LOC w dth d/t oth cause bef reg consc,init	*or*
		SØ6.6X6A	Traum subrac hem w LOC >24 hr w/o ret consc w surv, init	*or*
		SØ6.6X7A	Traum subrac hem w LOC w death d/t brain inj bf consc, init	*or*
		SØ6.6X8A	Traum subrac hem w LOC w death d/t oth cause bf consc, init	
8Ø3.76	OTH OPEN SKULL FX-SUBARACH DURAL HEMORR LOC UNS	**SØ2.91XB**	Unspecified fracture of skull, init encntr for open fracture	*and*
		SØ6.4X9A	Epidural hemorrhage w LOC of unsp duration, init	*or*
		SØ6.5X9A	Traum subdr hem w LOC of unsp duration, init	*or*
		SØ6.6X9A	Traum subrac hem w LOC of unsp duration, init	
8Ø3.79	OTH OPEN SKULL FX-SUBARACH DURA HEM UNS CONCUSS	**SØ2.91XB**	Unspecified fracture of skull, init encntr for open fracture	*and*
		SØ6.4XØA	Epidural hemorrhage w/o loss of consciousness, init encntr	*or*
		SØ6.5XØA	Traum subdr hem w/o loss of consciousness, init	*or*
		SØ6.6XØA	Traum subrac hem w/o loss of consciousness, init	
8Ø3.8Ø	OTH OPN SKUL FX OTH&UNS INTRACRAN HEMORR UNS SOC	**SØ2.91XB**	Unspecified fracture of skull, init encntr for open fracture	*and*
		SØ6.36ØA	Traum hemor cereb, w/o loss of consciousness, init	
8Ø3.81	OTH OPN SKUL FX W/OTH&UNS INTRACRAN HEMOR NO LOC	**SØ2.91XB**	Unspecified fracture of skull, init encntr for open fracture	*and*
		SØ6.36ØA	Traum hemor cereb, w/o loss of consciousness, init	
8Ø3.82	OTH OPN SKUL FX OTH&UNS INTRACRAN HEMORR BRF LOC	**SØ2.91XB**	Unspecified fracture of skull, init encntr for open fracture	*and*
		SØ6.361A	Traum hemor cereb, w LOC of 30 minutes or less, init	*or*
		SØ6.362A	Traum hemor cereb, w LOC of 31-59 min, init	
8Ø3.83	OTH OPN SKUL FX OTH&UNS INTRACRAN HEMORR MOD LOC	**SØ2.91XB**	Unspecified fracture of skull, init encntr for open fracture	*and*
		SØ6.363A	Traum hemor cereb, w LOC of 1-5 hrs 59 minutes, init	*or*
		SØ6.364A	Traum hemor cereb, w LOC of 6 hours to 24 hours, init	
8Ø3.84	OTH OPEN SKULL FX-OTH UNS ICH LOC >24 HR&RETURN	**SØ2.91XB**	Unspecified fracture of skull, init encntr for open fracture	*and*
		SØ6.365A	Traum hemor cereb, w LOC >24 hr w ret consc lev, init	
8Ø3.85	OTH OPEN SKULL FX-OTH&UNS ICH LOC >24-NO RETURN	**SØ2.91XB**	Unspecified fracture of skull, init encntr for open fracture	*and*
		SØ6.366A	Traum hemor cereb, w LOC >24 hr w/o ret consc w surv, init	*or*
		SØ6.367A	Traum hemor cereb, w LOC w dth d/t brain inj bf consc, init	*or*
		SØ6.368A	Traum hemor cereb, w LOC w dth d/t oth cause bf consc, init	
8Ø3.86	OTH OPN SKUL FX W/OTH&UNS ICH LOC UNS DUR	**SØ2.91XB**	Unspecified fracture of skull, init encntr for open fracture	*and*
		SØ6.369A	Traum hemor cereb, w LOC of unsp duration, init	
8Ø3.89	OTH OPN SKUL FX W/UNS INTRACRAN HEMOR UNS CONCUS	**SØ2.91XB**	Unspecified fracture of skull, init encntr for open fracture	*and*
		SØ6.36ØA	Traum hemor cereb, w/o loss of consciousness, init	
8Ø3.9Ø	OTH OPN SKULL FX W/ICI UNS NATUR UNS SOC	**SØ2.91XB**	Unspecified fracture of skull, init encntr for open fracture	*and*
		SØ6.89ØA	Intcran inj w/o loss of consciousness, init encntr	*or*
		SØ6.9XØA	Unsp intracranial injury w/o loss of consciousness, init	
8Ø3.91	OTH OPN SKULL FX W/INTRACRAN INJ UNS NATR NO LOC	**SØ2.91XB**	Unspecified fracture of skull, init encntr for open fracture	*and*
		SØ6.89ØA	Intcran inj w/o loss of consciousness, init encntr	*or*
		SØ6.9XØA	Unsp intracranial injury w/o loss of consciousness, init	
8Ø3.92	OTH OPN SKULL FX W/ICI UNS NATURE BRIEF LOC	**SØ2.91XB**	Unspecified fracture of skull, init encntr for open fracture	*and*
		SØ6.891A	Intcran inj w LOC of 30 minutes or less, init	*or*
		SØ6.892A	Intcran inj w loss of consciousness of 31-59 min, init	*or*
		SØ6.9X1A	Unsp intracranial injury w LOC of 30 minutes or less, init	*or*
		SØ6.9X2A	Unsp intracranial injury w LOC of 31-59 min, init	
8Ø3.93	OTH OPN SKULL FX W/ICI UNS NATURE MODERATE LOC	**SØ2.91XB**	Unspecified fracture of skull, init encntr for open fracture	*and*
		SØ6.893A	Intcran inj w loss of consciousness of 1-5 hrs 59 min, init	*or*
		SØ6.894A	Intcran inj w LOC of 6 hours to 24 hours, init	*or*
		SØ6.9X3A	Unsp intracranial injury w LOC of 1-5 hrs 59 min, init	*or*
		SØ6.9X4A	Unsp intracranial injury w LOC of 6 hours to 24 hours, init	
8Ø3.94	OTH OPEN SKULL FX-OTH&UNS ICI LOC>24 HR&RETURN	**SØ2.91XB**	Unspecified fracture of skull, init encntr for open fracture	*and*
		SØ6.895A	Intcran inj w LOC >24 hr w ret consc lev, init	*or*
		SØ6.9X5A	Unsp intracranial injury w LOC >24 hr w ret consc lev, init	
8Ø3.95	OTH OPEN SKULL FX-OTH&UNS ICI LOC>24 NO RETURN	**SØ2.91XB**	Unspecified fracture of skull, init encntr for open fracture	*and*
		SØ6.896A	Intcran inj w LOC >24 hr w/o ret consc w surv, init	*or*
		SØ6.897A	Intcran inj w LOC w death due to brain injury bf consc, init	*or*
		SØ6.898A	Intcran inj w LOC w death due to oth cause bf consc, init	*or*
		SØ6.9X6A	Unsp intcrn injury w LOC >24 hr w/o ret consc w surv, init	*or*
		SØ6.9X7A	Unsp intcrn inj w LOC w death d/t brain inj bf consc, init	*or*
		SØ6.9X8A	Unsp intcrn inj w LOC w death d/t oth cause bf consc, init	
8Ø3.96	OTH OPN SKULL FX W/ICI UNS NATUR LOC UNS DUR	**SØ2.91XB**	Unspecified fracture of skull, init encntr for open fracture	*and*
		SØ6.899A	Intcran inj w loss of consciousness of unsp duration, init	*or*
		SØ6.9X9A	Unsp intracranial injury w LOC of unsp duration, init	

[Brackets] indicate valid character values for each code. Character value meanings provided for each code grouping.

ICD-9-CM		ICD-10-CM		
803.99	OTH OPN SKULL FX W/ICI UNS NATUR UNS CONCUS	**S02.91XB**	Unspecified fracture of skull, init encntr for open fracture	*and*
		S06.890A	Intcran inj w/o loss of consciousness, init encntr	*or*
		S06.9X0A	Unsp intracranial injury w/o loss of consciousness, init	
804.00	CLOS FXS INVOLV SKL/FCE W/OTH BNS NO ICI UNS SOC	**S02.91XA**	Unsp fracture of skull, init encntr for closed fracture	
804.01	CLOS FXS INVOLV SKUL/FCE W/OTH BNS NO ICI NO LOC	**S02.91XA**	Unsp fracture of skull, init encntr for closed fracture	
804.02	CLOS FXS SKULL/FACE-OTH BNS W/O ICI LOC<1 HR	**S02.91XA**	Unsp fracture of skull, init encntr for closed fracture	
804.03	CLOS FXS INVOLV SKL/FCE W/OTH BNS NO ICI MOD LOC	**S02.91XA**	Unsp fracture of skull, init encntr for closed fracture	
804.04	CLOS FXS SKULL/FACE-OTH BNS NO ICI LOC>24-RETURN	**S02.91XA**	Unsp fracture of skull, init encntr for closed fracture	
804.05	CLOS FXS SKULL/FACE-OTH BNS NO ICI LOC NO RTRN	**S02.91XA**	Unsp fracture of skull, init encntr for closed fracture	
804.06	CLOS FXS SKULL/FACE & OTH BNS NO ICI LOC UNS	**S02.91XA**	Unsp fracture of skull, init encntr for closed fracture	
804.09	CLOS FXS SKULL/FACE-OTH BNS NO ICI UNS CONCUSS	**S02.91XA**	Unsp fracture of skull, init encntr for closed fracture	
804.10	CLOS FXS SKULL/FACE-OTH BNS CEREB LAC UNS SOC	**S02.91XA**	Unsp fracture of skull, init encntr for closed fracture	*and*
		S06.330A	Contus/lac cereb, w/o loss of consciousness, init	
804.11	CLOS FXS SKULL/FACE-OTH BNS CERBRL LAC NO LOC	**S02.91XA**	Unsp fracture of skull, init encntr for closed fracture	*and*
		S06.330A	Contus/lac cereb, w/o loss of consciousness, init	
804.12	CLOS FXS SKULL/FACE-OTH BNS CERBR LAC BRIEF LOC	**S02.91XA**	Unsp fracture of skull, init encntr for closed fracture	*and*
		S06.331A	Contus/lac cereb, w LOC of 30 minutes or less, init	*or*
		S06.332A	Contus/lac cereb, w loss of consciousness of 31-59 min, init	
804.13	CLOS FXS SKULL/FACE-OTH BNS CERBRL LAC MOD LOC	**S02.91XA**	Unsp fracture of skull, init encntr for closed fracture	*and*
		S06.333A	Contus/lac cereb, w LOC of 1-5 hrs 59 min, init	*or*
		S06.334A	Contus/lac cereb, w LOC of 6 hours to 24 hours, init	
804.14	CLOS FXS SKULL/FACE-OTH BNS CERBRL LAC>24&RTRN	**S02.91XA**	Unsp fracture of skull, init encntr for closed fracture	*and*
		S06.335A	Contus/lac cereb, w LOC >24 hr w ret consc lev, init	
804.15	CLOS FXS SKULL/FACE-OTH BNS CERBRL LAC NO RTRN	**S02.91XA**	Unsp fracture of skull, init encntr for closed fracture	*and*
		S06.336A	Contus/lac cereb, w LOC >24 hr w/o ret consc w surv, init	*or*
		S06.337A	Contus/lac cereb, w LOC w death d/t brain inj bf consc, init	*or*
		S06.338A	Contus/lac cereb, w LOC w death d/t oth cause bf consc, init	
804.16	CLOS FXS SKULL/FACE-OTH BNS CERBRL LAC LOC UNS	**S02.91XA**	Unsp fracture of skull, init encntr for closed fracture	*and*
		S06.339A	Contus/lac cereb, w LOC of unsp duration, init	
804.19	CLOS FXS SKULL/FACE-OTH BNS CERBRL LAC UNS CNCUS	**S02.91XA**	Unsp fracture of skull, init encntr for closed fracture	*and*
		S06.330A	Contus/lac cereb, w/o loss of consciousness, init	
804.20	CLOS FXS SKULL/FACE-OTH BNS DURL HEM UNS SOC	**S02.91XA**	Unsp fracture of skull, init encntr for closed fracture	*and*
		S06.4X0A	Epidural hemorrhage w/o loss of consciousness, init encntr	*or*
		S06.5X0A	Traum subdr hem w/o loss of consciousness, init	*or*
		S06.6X0A	Traum subrac hem w/o loss of consciousness, init	
804.21	CLOS FXS SKULL/FACE-OTH BNS DURL HEM NO LOC	**S02.91XA**	Unsp fracture of skull, init encntr for closed fracture	*and*
		S06.4X0A	Epidural hemorrhage w/o loss of consciousness, init encntr	*or*
		S06.5X0A	Traum subdr hem w/o loss of consciousness, init	*or*
		S06.6X0A	Traum subrac hem w/o loss of consciousness, init	
804.22	CLOS FXS SKULL/FACE-OTH BNS DURL HEM BRF LOC	**S02.91XA**	Unsp fracture of skull, init encntr for closed fracture	*and*
		S06.4X1A	Epidural hemorrhage w LOC of 30 minutes or less, init	*or*
		S06.4X2A	Epidural hemorrhage w LOC of 31-59 min, init	*or*
		S06.5X1A	Traum subdr hem w LOC of 30 minutes or less, init	*or*
		S06.5X2A	Traum subdr hem w loss of consciousness of 31-59 min, init	*or*
		S06.6X1A	Traum subrac hem w LOC of 30 minutes or less, init	*or*
		S06.6X2A	Traum subrac hem w loss of consciousness of 31-59 min, init	
804.23	CLOS FXS SKULL/FACE-OTH BNS DURL HEM MOD LOC	**S02.91XA**	Unsp fracture of skull, init encntr for closed fracture	*and*
		S06.4X3A	Epidural hemorrhage w LOC of 1-5 hrs 59 min, init	*or*
		S06.4X4A	Epidural hemorrhage w LOC of 6 hours to 24 hours, init	*or*
		S06.5X3A	Traum subdr hem w LOC of 1-5 hrs 59 min, init	*or*
		S06.5X4A	Traum subdr hem w LOC of 6 hours to 24 hours, init	*or*
		S06.6X3A	Traum subrac hem w LOC of 1-5 hrs 59 min, init	*or*
		S06.6X4A	Traum subrac hem w LOC of 6 hours to 24 hours, init	
804.24	CLOS FXS SKULL/FACE-OTH BNS DURL HEM>24&RTRN	**S02.91XA**	Unsp fracture of skull, init encntr for closed fracture	*and*
		S06.4X5A	Epidural hemorrhage w LOC >24 hr w ret consc lev, init	*or*
		S06.5X5A	Traum subdr hem w LOC >24 hr w ret consc lev, init	*or*
		S06.6X5A	Traum subrac hem w LOC >24 hr w ret consc lev, init	
804.25	CLOS FXS SKULL/FACE-OTH BNS DURL HEM NO RTRN	**S02.91XA**	Unsp fracture of skull, init encntr for closed fracture	*and*
		S06.4X6A	Epidural hemorrhage w LOC >24 hr w/o ret consc w surv, init	*or*
		S06.4X7A	Epidur hemor w LOC w death d/t brain injury bf consc, init	*or*
		S06.4X8A	Epidur hemor w LOC w death due to oth causes bf consc, init	*or*
		S06.5X6A	Traum subdr hem w LOC >24 hr w/o ret consc w surv, init	*or*
		S06.5X7A	Traum subdr hem w LOC w dth d/t brain inj bef reg consc,init	*or*
		S06.5X8A	Traum subdr hem w LOC w dth d/t oth cause bef reg consc,init	*or*
		S06.6X6A	Traum subrac hem w LOC >24 hr w/o ret consc w surv, init	*or*
		S06.6X7A	Traum subrac hem w LOC w death d/t brain inj bf consc, init	*or*
		S06.6X8A	Traum subrac hem w LOC w death d/t oth cause bf consc, init	

ICD-9-CM		ICD-10-CM		
804.26	CLOS FXS SKULL/FACE-OTH BNS DURL HEM LOC UNS	**S02.91XA**	Unsp fracture of skull, init encntr for closed fracture	*and*
		S06.4X9A	Epidural hemorrhage w LOC of unsp duration, init	*or*
		S06.5X9A	Traum subdr hem w LOC of unsp duration, init	*or*
		S06.6X9A	Traum subrac hem w LOC of unsp duration, init	
804.29	CLOS FXS SKULL/FACE-OTH BNS DURL HEM UNS CONCUS	**S02.91XA**	Unsp fracture of skull, init encntr for closed fracture	*and*
		S06.4X0A	Epidural hemorrhage w/o loss of consciousness, init encntr	*or*
		S06.5X0A	Traum subdr hem w/o loss of consciousness, init	*or*
		S06.6X0A	Traum subrac hem w/o loss of consciousness, init	
804.30	CLOS FXS SKULL/FACE-OTH BNS-OTH&UNS ICH UNS SOC	**S02.91XA**	Unsp fracture of skull, init encntr for closed fracture	*and*
		S06.360A	Traum hemor cereb, w/o loss of consciousness, init	
804.31	CLOS FXS SKULL/FACE-OTH BNS-OTH&UNS ICH NO LOC	**S02.91XA**	Unsp fracture of skull, init encntr for closed fracture	*and*
		S06.360A	Traum hemor cereb, w/o loss of consciousness, init	
804.32	CLOS FXS SKULL/FACE-OTH BNS-OTH ICH BRIEF LOC	**S02.91XA**	Unsp fracture of skull, init encntr for closed fracture	*and*
		S06.361A	Traum hemor cereb, w LOC of 30 minutes or less, init	*or*
		S06.362A	Traum hemor cereb, w LOC of 31-59 min, init	
804.33	CLOS FXS SKULL/FACE-OTH BNS-OTH ICH MODERATE LOC	**S02.91XA**	Unsp fracture of skull, init encntr for closed fracture	*and*
		S06.363A	Traum hemor cereb, w LOC of 1-5 hrs 59 minutes, init	*or*
		S06.364A	Traum hemor cereb, w LOC of 6 hours to 24 hours, init	
804.34	CLOS FXS SKULL/FACE-OTH BNS-OTH ICH LOC&RTRN	**S02.91XA**	Unsp fracture of skull, init encntr for closed fracture	*and*
		S06.365A	Traum hemor cereb, w LOC >24 hr w ret consc lev, init	
804.35	CLOS FXS SKULL/FACE-OTH BNS-OTH ICH-LOC NO RTRN	**S02.91XA**	Unsp fracture of skull, init encntr for closed fracture	*and*
		S06.366A	Traum hemor cereb, w LOC >24 hr w/o ret consc w surv, init	*or*
		S06.367A	Traum hemor cereb, w LOC w dth d/t brain inj bf consc, init	*or*
		S06.368A	Traum hemor cereb, w LOC w dth d/t oth cause bf consc, init	
804.36	CLOS FXS SKULL/FACE-OTH BNS-OTH&UNS ICH LOC UNS	**S02.91XA**	Unsp fracture of skull, init encntr for closed fracture	*and*
		S06.369A	Traum hemor cereb, w LOC of unsp duration, init	
804.39	CLOS FXS SKULL/FACE-OTH BNS-OTH ICH UNS CONCUSS	**S02.91XA**	Unsp fracture of skull, init encntr for closed fracture	*and*
		S06.360A	Traum hemor cereb, w/o loss of consciousness, init	
804.40	CLOS FXS SKULL/FACE-OTH BNS-OTH ICI-UNS SOC	**S02.91XA**	Unsp fracture of skull, init encntr for closed fracture	*and*
		S06.890A	Intcran inj w/o loss of consciousness, init encntr	*or*
		S06.9X0A	Unsp intracranial injury w/o loss of consciousness, init	
804.41	CLOS FXS SKULL/FACE-OTH BNS-OTH&UNS ICI-NO LOC	**S02.91XA**	Unsp fracture of skull, init encntr for closed fracture	*and*
		S06.890A	Intcran inj w/o loss of consciousness, init encntr	*or*
		S06.9X0A	Unsp intracranial injury w/o loss of consciousness, init	
804.42	CLOS FXS SKULL/FACE-OTH BNS-OTH&UNS ICI-BRF LOC	**S02.91XA**	Unsp fracture of skull, init encntr for closed fracture	*and*
		S06.891A	Intcran inj w LOC of 30 minutes or less, init	*or*
		S06.892A	Intcran inj w loss of consciousness of 31-59 min, init	*or*
		S06.9X1A	Unsp intracranial injury w LOC of 30 minutes or less, init	*or*
		S06.9X2A	Unsp intracranial injury w LOC of 31-59 min, init	
804.43	CLOS FXS SKULL/FACE-OTH BNS-OTH&UNS ICI-MOD LOC	**S02.91XA**	Unsp fracture of skull, init encntr for closed fracture	*and*
		S06.893A	Intcran inj w loss of consciousness of 1-5 hrs 59 min, init	*or*
		S06.894A	Intcran inj w LOC of 6 hours to 24 hours, init	*or*
		S06.9X4A	Unsp intracranial injury w LOC of 6 hours to 24 hours, init	
804.44	CLOS FXS SKULL/FACE-OTH BNS-OTH ICI LOC&RETURN	**S02.91XA**	Unsp fracture of skull, init encntr for closed fracture	*and*
		S06.895A	Intcran inj w LOC >24 hr w ret consc lev, init	*or*
		S06.9X5A	Unsp intracranial injury w LOC >24 hr w ret consc lev, init	
804.45	CLOS FXS SKULL/FACE-OTH BNS-OTH ICI-LOC NO RETRN	**S02.91XA**	Unsp fracture of skull, init encntr for closed fracture	*and*
		S06.896A	Intcran inj w LOC >24 hr w/o ret consc w surv, init	*or*
		S06.897A	Intcran inj w LOC w death due to brain injury bf consc, init	*or*
		S06.898A	Intcran inj w LOC w death due to oth cause bf consc, init	*or*
		S06.9X6A	Unsp intcrn injury w LOC >24 hr w/o ret consc w surv, init	*or*
		S06.9X7A	Unsp intcrn inj w LOC w death d/t brain inj bf consc, init	*or*
		S06.9X8A	Unsp intcrn inj w LOC w death d/t oth cause bf consc, init	
804.46	CLOS FXS SKULL/FACE-OTH BNS-OTH&UNS ICI-LOC UNS	**S02.91XA**	Unsp fracture of skull, init encntr for closed fracture	*and*
		S06.899A	Intcran inj w loss of consciousness of unsp duration, init	*or*
		S06.9X9A	Unsp intracranial injury w LOC of unsp duration, init	
804.49	CLOS FXS SKULL/FACE-OTH BNS-OTH ICI UNS CONCUSS	**S02.91XA**	Unsp fracture of skull, init encntr for closed fracture	*and*
		S06.890A	Intcran inj w/o loss of consciousness, init encntr	*or*
		S06.9X9A	Unsp intracranial injury w LOC of unsp duration, init	
804.50	OPN FXS INVOLV SKUL/FCE W/OTH BNS NO ICI UNS SOC	**S02.91XB**	Unspecified fracture of skull, init encntr for open fracture	
804.51	OPN FXS INVOLV SKUL/FCE W/OTH BNS W/O ICI NO LOC	**S02.91XB**	Unspecified fracture of skull, init encntr for open fracture	
804.52	OPEN FXS SKULL/FACE-OTH BNS W/O ICI BRIEF LOC	**S02.91XB**	Unspecified fracture of skull, init encntr for open fracture	
804.53	OPN FXS INVOLV SKUL/FCE W/OTH BNS NO ICI MOD LOC	**S02.91XB**	Unspecified fracture of skull, init encntr for open fracture	
804.54	OPN FXS SKULL/FACE-OTH BNS W/O ICI LOC>24&RETURN	**S02.91XB**	Unspecified fracture of skull, init encntr for open fracture	
804.55	OPEN FXS SKULL/FACE-OTH BNS NO ICI LOC NO RTRN	**S02.91XB**	Unspecified fracture of skull, init encntr for open fracture	
804.56	OPEN FXS SKULL/FACE-OTH BNS NO ICI LOC UNS	**S02.91XB**	Unspecified fracture of skull, init encntr for open fracture	
804.59	OPEN FXS SKULL/FACE-OTH BNS NO ICI UNS CONCUSS	**S02.91XB**	Unspecified fracture of skull, init encntr for open fracture	

[Brackets] indicate valid character values for each code. Character value meanings provided for each code grouping.

ICD-9-CM		ICD-10-CM		
804.60	OPN SKULL/FACE-OTH BNS-CERBRL LAC UNS SOC	**S02.91XB**	Unspecified fracture of skull, init encntr for open fracture	*and*
		S06.330A	Contus/lac cereb, w/o loss of consciousness, init	
804.61	OPEN FXS SKULL/FACE-OTH BNS-CERBRL LAC NO LOC	**S02.91XB**	Unspecified fracture of skull, init encntr for open fracture	*and*
		S06.330A	Contus/lac cereb, w/o loss of consciousness, init	
804.62	OPN FXS SKULL/FACE-OTH BNS-CERBRL LAC BRF LOC	**S02.91XB**	Unspecified fracture of skull, init encntr for open fracture	*and*
		S06.331A	Contus/lac cereb, w LOC of 30 minutes or less, init	*or*
		S06.332A	Contus/lac cereb, w loss of consciousness of 31-59 min, init	
804.63	OPN FXS SKULL/FACE-OTH BNS-CERBRL LAC MOD LOC	**S02.91XB**	Unspecified fracture of skull, init encntr for open fracture	*and*
		S06.333A	Contus/lac cereb, w LOC of 1-5 hrs 59 min, init	*or*
		S06.334A	Contus/lac cereb, w LOC of 6 hours to 24 hours, init	
804.64	OPEN FXS SKULL/FACE-OTH BNS-CERBRL LAC LOC&RTRN	**S02.91XB**	Unspecified fracture of skull, init encntr for open fracture	*and*
		S06.335A	Contus/lac cereb, w LOC >24 hr w ret consc lev, init	
804.65	OPN FXS SKUL/FACE-OTH BNS-CERBRL LAC LOC NO RTRN	**S02.91XB**	Unspecified fracture of skull, init encntr for open fracture	*and*
		S06.336A	Contus/lac cereb, w LOC >24 hr w/o ret consc w surv, init	*or*
		S06.337A	Contus/lac cereb, w LOC w death d/t brain inj bf consc, init	*or*
		S06.338A	Contus/lac cereb, w LOC w death d/t oth cause bf consc, init	
804.66	OPN FXS SKULL/FACE-OTH BNS-CERBRL LAC LOC UNS	**S02.91XB**	Unspecified fracture of skull, init encntr for open fracture	*and*
		S06.339A	Contus/lac cereb, w LOC of unsp duration, init	
804.69	OPN SKULL/FACE-OTH BNS-CERBRL LAC UNS CONCUSS	**S02.91XB**	Unspecified fracture of skull, init encntr for open fracture	*and*
		S06.330A	Contus/lac cereb, w/o loss of consciousness, init	
804.70	OPN FXS SKULL/FACE-OTH BNS-DURAL HEMORR-UNS SOC	**S02.91XB**	Unspecified fracture of skull, init encntr for open fracture	*and*
		S06.4X0A	Epidural hemorrhage w/o loss of consciousness, init encntr	*or*
		S06.5X0A	Traum subdr hem w/o loss of consciousness, init	*or*
		S06.6X0A	Traum subrac hem w/o loss of consciousness, init	
804.71	OPN FXS SKULL/FACE-OTH BNS-DURAL HEMORR NO LOC	**S02.91XB**	Unspecified fracture of skull, init encntr for open fracture	*and*
		S06.4X0A	Epidural hemorrhage w/o loss of consciousness, init encntr	*or*
		S06.5X0A	Traum subdr hem w/o loss of consciousness, init	*or*
		S06.6X0A	Traum subrac hem w/o loss of consciousness, init	
804.72	OPN FXS SKULL/FACE-OTH BNS-DURAL HEMORR BRF LOC	**S02.91XB**	Unspecified fracture of skull, init encntr for open fracture	*and*
		S06.4X1A	Epidural hemorrhage w LOC of 30 minutes or less, init	*or*
		S06.4X2A	Epidural hemorrhage w LOC of 31-59 min, init	*or*
		S06.5X1A	Traum subdr hem w LOC of 30 minutes or less, init	*or*
		S06.5X2A	Traum subdr hem w loss of consciousness of 31-59 min, init	*or*
		S06.6X1A	Traum subrac hem w LOC of 30 minutes or less, init	*or*
		S06.6X2A	Traum subrac hem w loss of consciousness of 31-59 min, init	
804.73	OPN FXS SKULL/FACE-OTH BNS-DURAL HEM-MOD LOC	**S02.91XB**	Unspecified fracture of skull, init encntr for open fracture	*and*
		S06.4X3A	Epidural hemorrhage w LOC of 1-5 hrs 59 min, init	*or*
		S06.4X4A	Epidural hemorrhage w LOC of 6 hours to 24 hours, init	*or*
		S06.5X3A	Traum subdr hem w LOC of 1-5 hrs 59 min, init	*or*
		S06.5X4A	Traum subdr hem w LOC of 6 hours to 24 hours, init	*or*
		S06.6X3A	Traum subrac hem w LOC of 1-5 hrs 59 min, init	*or*
		S06.6X4A	Traum subrac hem w LOC of 6 hours to 24 hours, init	
804.74	OPN FXS SKULL/FACE-OTH BNS-DURAL HEM LOC&RTRN	**S02.91XB**	Unspecified fracture of skull, init encntr for open fracture	*and*
		S06.4X5A	Epidural hemorrhage w LOC >24 hr w ret consc lev, init	*or*
		S06.5X5A	Traum subdr hem w LOC >24 hr w ret consc lev, init	*or*
		S06.6X5A	Traum subrac hem w LOC >24 hr w ret consc lev, init	
804.75	OPN FXS SKULL/FACE-OTH BNS-DURAL HEM LOC NO RTRN	**S02.91XB**	Unspecified fracture of skull, init encntr for open fracture	*and*
		S06.4X6A	Epidural hemorrhage w LOC >24 hr w/o ret consc w surv, init	*or*
		S06.4X7A	Epidur hemor w LOC w death d/t brain injury bf consc, init	*or*
		S06.4X8A	Epidur hemor w LOC w death due to oth causes bf consc, init	*or*
		S06.5X6A	Traum subdr hem w LOC >24 hr w/o ret consc w surv, init	*or*
		S06.5X7A	Traum subdr hem w LOC w dth d/t brain inj bef reg consc,init	*or*
		S06.5X8A	Traum subdr hem w LOC w dth d/t oth cause bef reg consc,init	*or*
		S06.6X6A	Traum subrac hem w LOC >24 hr w/o ret consc w surv, init	*or*
		S06.6X7A	Traum subrac hem w LOC w death d/t brain inj bf consc, init	*or*
		S06.6X8A	Traum subrac hem w LOC w death d/t oth cause bf consc, init	
804.76	OPN FXS SKULL/FACE-OTH BNS-DURAL HEMORR LOC UNS	**S02.91XB**	Unspecified fracture of skull, init encntr for open fracture	*and*
		S06.4X9A	Epidural hemorrhage w LOC of unsp duration, init	*or*
		S06.5X9A	Traum subdr hem w LOC of unsp duration, init	*or*
		S06.6X9A	Traum subrac hem w LOC of unsp duration, init	
804.79	OPN FXS SKULL/FACE-OTH BNS-DURAL HEM UNS CONCUSS	**S02.91XB**	Unspecified fracture of skull, init encntr for open fracture	*and*
		S06.4X0A	Epidural hemorrhage w/o loss of consciousness, init encntr	*or*
		S06.5X0A	Traum subdr hem w/o loss of consciousness, init	*or*
		S06.6X0A	Traum subrac hem w/o loss of consciousness, init	
804.80	OPN FXS SKULL/FACE-OTH BNS-OTH&UNS ICH UNS SOC	**S02.91XB**	Unspecified fracture of skull, init encntr for open fracture	*and*
		S06.360A	Traum hemor cereb, w/o loss of consciousness, init	
804.81	OPN FXS SKULL/FACE-OTH BNS-OTH&UNS ICH NO LOC	**S02.91XB**	Unspecified fracture of skull, init encntr for open fracture	*and*
		S06.360A	Traum hemor cereb, w/o loss of consciousness, init	

ICD-9-CM		ICD-10-CM		
8Ø4.82	OPN FXS SKULL/FACE-OTH BNS-OTH&UNS ICH BRF LOC	**SØ2.91XB**	Unspecified fracture of skull, init encntr for open fracture	*and*
		SØ6.361A	Traum hemor cereb, w LOC of 30 minutes or less, init	*or*
		SØ6.362A	Traum hemor cereb, w LOC of 31-59 min, init	
8Ø4.83	OPN FXS SKULL/FACE-OTH BNS-OTH&UNS ICH MOD LOC	**SØ2.91XB**	Unspecified fracture of skull, init encntr for open fracture	*and*
		SØ6.363A	Traum hemor cereb, w LOC of 1-5 hrs 59 minutes, init	*or*
		SØ6.364A	Traum hemor cereb, w LOC of 6 hours to 24 hours, init	
8Ø4.84	OPN FXS SKULL/FACE-OTH BNS-OTH ICH LOC>24&RETURN	**SØ2.91XB**	Unspecified fracture of skull, init encntr for open fracture	*and*
		SØ6.365A	Traum hemor cereb, w LOC >24 hr w ret consc lev, init	
8Ø4.85	OPN FXS SKULL/FACE-OTH BNS-OTH&ICH LOC NO RTRN	**SØ2.91XB**	Unspecified fracture of skull, init encntr for open fracture	*and*
		SØ6.366A	Traum hemor cereb, w LOC >24 hr w/o ret consc w surv, init	*or*
		SØ6.367A	Traum hemor cereb, w LOC w dth d/t brain inj bf consc, init	*or*
		SØ6.368A	Traum hemor cereb, w LOC w dth d/t oth cause bf consc, init	
8Ø4.86	OPN FXS SKULL/FACE-OTH BNS-OTH&UNS ICH LOC UNS	**SØ2.91XB**	Unspecified fracture of skull, init encntr for open fracture	*and*
		SØ6.369A	Traum hemor cereb, w LOC of unsp duration, init	
8Ø4.89	OPN FXS SKULL/FACE-OTH BNS-OTH ICH UNS CONCUSS	**SØ2.91XB**	Unspecified fracture of skull, init encntr for open fracture	*and*
		SØ6.36ØA	Traum hemor cereb, w/o loss of consciousness, init	
8Ø4.9Ø	OPN FXS SKULL/FACE-OTH BNS-OTH&UNS ICI UNS SOC	**SØ2.91XB**	Unspecified fracture of skull, init encntr for open fracture	*and*
		SØ6.89ØA	Intcran inj w/o loss of consciousness, init encntr	*or*
		SØ6.9XØA	Unsp intracranial injury w/o loss of consciousness, init	
8Ø4.91	OPN FXS SKULL/FACE-OTH BNS-OTH&UNS ICI NO LOC	**SØ2.91XB**	Unspecified fracture of skull, init encntr for open fracture	*and*
		SØ6.89ØA	Intcran inj w/o loss of consciousness, init encntr	*or*
		SØ6.9XØA	Unsp intracranial injury w/o loss of consciousness, init	
8Ø4.92	OPN FXS SKULL/FACE-OTH BNS-OTH&UNS ICI BRIEF LOC	**SØ2.91XB**	Unspecified fracture of skull, init encntr for open fracture	*and*
		SØ6.891A	Intcran inj w LOC of 30 minutes or less, init	*or*
		SØ6.892A	Intcran inj w loss of consciousness of 31-59 min, init	*or*
		SØ6.9X1A	Unsp intracranial injury w LOC of 30 minutes or less, init	*or*
		SØ6.9X2A	Unsp intracranial injury w LOC of 31-59 min, init	
8Ø4.93	OPN FXS SKULL/FACE-OTH BNS-OTH&UNS ICI MOD LOC	**SØ2.91XB**	Unspecified fracture of skull, init encntr for open fracture	*and*
		SØ6.893A	Intcran inj w loss of consciousness of 1-5 hrs 59 min, init	*or*
		SØ6.894A	Intcran inj w LOC of 6 hours to 24 hours, init	*or*
		SØ6.9X4A	Unsp intracranial injury w LOC of 6 hours to 24 hours, init	
8Ø4.94	OPN FXS SKULL/FACE-OTH BNS-OTH ICI LOC&RTRN	**SØ2.91XB**	Unspecified fracture of skull, init encntr for open fracture	*and*
		SØ6.895A	Intcran inj w LOC >24 hr w ret consc lev, init	*or*
		SØ6.9X5A	Unsp intracranial injury w LOC >24 hr w ret consc lev, init	
8Ø4.95	OPN FXS SKULL/FACE-OTH BNS-OTH ICI LOC NO RTRN	**SØ2.91XB**	Unspecified fracture of skull, init encntr for open fracture	*and*
		SØ6.896A	Intcran inj w LOC >24 hr w/o ret consc w surv, init	*or*
		SØ6.897A	Intcran inj w LOC w death due to brain injury bf consc, init	*or*
		SØ6.898A	Intcran inj w LOC w death due to oth cause bf consc, init	*or*
		SØ6.9X6A	Unsp intcrn injury w LOC >24 hr w/o ret consc w surv, init	*or*
		SØ6.9X7A	Unsp intcrn inj w LOC w death d/t brain inj bf consc, init	*or*
		SØ6.9X8A	Unsp intcrn inj w LOC w death d/t oth cause bf consc, init	
8Ø4.96	OPN FXS SKULL/FACE-OTH BNS-OTH&UNS ICI LOC UNS	**SØ2.91XB**	Unspecified fracture of skull, init encntr for open fracture	*and*
		SØ6.899A	Intcran inj w loss of consciousness of unsp duration, init	*or*
		SØ6.9X9A	Unsp intracranial injury w LOC of unsp duration, init	
8Ø4.99	OPN FXS SKULL/FACE-OTH BNS-OTH ICI UNS CONCUSS	**SØ2.91XB**	Unspecified fracture of skull, init encntr for open fracture	*and*
		SØ6.89ØA	Intcran inj w/o loss of consciousness, init encntr	*or*
		SØ6.9XØA	Unsp intracranial injury w/o loss of consciousness, init	
8Ø5.ØØ	CLOS FX CERV VERTEBRA UNS LEVL W/O SP CRD INJURY	**S12.9XXA**	Fracture of neck, unspecified, initial encounter	
8Ø5.Ø1	CLOS FX C1 VERTEBRA W/O MENTION SP CRD INJURY	**S12.ØØØA**	Unsp disp fx of first cervical vertebra, init for clos fx	
		S12.ØØ1A	Unsp nondisp fx of first cervical vertebra, init for clos fx	
		S12.Ø1XA	Stable burst fracture of first cervical vertebra, init	
		S12.Ø2XA	Unstable burst fracture of first cervical vertebra, init	
		S12.Ø3ØA	Displaced posterior arch fx first cervcal vertebra, init	
		S12.Ø31A	Nondisp posterior arch fx first cervcal vertebra, init	
		S12.Ø4ØA	Displaced lateral mass fx first cervcal vertebra, init	
		S12.Ø41A	Nondisp lateral mass fx first cervcal vertebra, init	
		S12.Ø9ØA	Oth disp fx of first cervical vertebra, init for clos fx	
		S12.Ø91A	Oth nondisp fx of first cervical vertebra, init for clos fx	
8Ø5.Ø2	CLOS FX C2 VERTEBRA W/O MENTION SP CRD INJURY	**S12.1ØØA**	Unsp disp fx of second cervical vertebra, init for clos fx	
		S12.1Ø1A	Unsp nondisp fx of second cervical vertebra, init	
		S12.11ØA	Anterior displaced Type II dens fracture, init for clos fx	
		S12.111A	Posterior displaced Type II dens fracture, init for clos fx	
		S12.112A	Nondisplaced Type II dens fracture, init for clos fx	
		S12.12ØA	Oth displaced dens fracture, init encntr for closed fracture	
		S12.121A	Oth nondisplaced dens fracture, init for clos fx	
		S12.13ØA	Unsp traum displ spondylolysis of second cervcal vert, init	
		S12.131A	Unsp traum nondisp spondylolysis of 2nd cervcal vert, init	
		S12.14XA	Type III traum spondylolysis of second cervcal vert, init	
		S12.15ØA	Oth traum displ spondylolysis of second cervcal vert, init	
		S12.151A	Oth traum nondisp spondylolysis of second cervcal vert, init	
		S12.19ØA	Oth disp fx of second cervical vertebra, init for clos fx	
		S12.191A	Oth nondisp fx of second cervical vertebra, init for clos fx	

ICD-9-CM		ICD-10-CM	
805.03	CLOS FX C3 VERTEBRA W/O MENTION SP CRD INJURY	**S12.200A**	Unsp disp fx of third cervical vertebra, init for clos fx
		S12.201A	Unsp nondisp fx of third cervical vertebra, init for clos fx
		S12.230A	Unsp traum displ spondylolysis of third cervcal vert, init
		S12.231A	Unsp traum nondisp spondylolysis of third cervcal vert, init
		S12.24XA	Type III traum spondylolysis of third cervcal vertebra, init
		S12.250A	Oth traum displ spondylolysis of third cervcal vert, init
		S12.251A	Oth traum nondisp spondylolysis of third cervcal vert, init
		S12.290A	Oth disp fx of third cervical vertebra, init for clos fx
		S12.291A	Oth nondisp fx of third cervical vertebra, init for clos fx
805.04	CLOS FX C4 VERTEBRA W/O MENTION SP CRD INJURY	**S12.300A**	Unsp disp fx of fourth cervical vertebra, init for clos fx
		S12.301A	Unsp nondisp fx of fourth cervical vertebra, init
		S12.330A	Unsp traum displ spondylolysis of fourth cervcal vert, init
		S12.331A	Unsp traum nondisp spondylolysis of 4th cervcal vert, init
		S12.34XA	Type III traum spondylolysis of fourth cervcal vert, init
		S12.350A	Oth traum displ spondylolysis of fourth cervcal vert, init
		S12.351A	Oth traum nondisp spondylolysis of fourth cervcal vert, init
		S12.390A	Oth disp fx of fourth cervical vertebra, init for clos fx
		S12.391A	Oth nondisp fx of fourth cervical vertebra, init for clos fx
805.05	CLOS FX C5 VERTEBRA W/O MENTION SP CRD INJURY	**S12.400A**	Unsp disp fx of fifth cervical vertebra, init for clos fx
		S12.401A	Unsp nondisp fx of fifth cervical vertebra, init for clos fx
		S12.430A	Unsp traum displ spondylolysis of fifth cervcal vert, init
		S12.431A	Unsp traum nondisp spondylolysis of fifth cervcal vert, init
		S12.44XA	Type III traum spondylolysis of fifth cervcal vertebra, init
		S12.450A	Oth traum displ spondylolysis of fifth cervcal vert, init
		S12.451A	Oth traum nondisp spondylolysis of fifth cervcal vert, init
		S12.490A	Oth disp fx of fifth cervical vertebra, init for clos fx
		S12.491A	Oth nondisp fx of fifth cervical vertebra, init for clos fx
805.06	CLOS FX C6 VERTEBRA W/O MENTION SP CRD INJURY	**S12.500A**	Unsp disp fx of sixth cervical vertebra, init for clos fx
		S12.501A	Unsp nondisp fx of sixth cervical vertebra, init for clos fx
		S12.530A	Unsp traum displ spondylolysis of sixth cervcal vert, init
		S12.531A	Unsp traum nondisp spondylolysis of sixth cervcal vert, init
		S12.54XA	Type III traum spondylolysis of sixth cervcal vertebra, init
		S12.550A	Oth traum displ spondylolysis of sixth cervcal vert, init
		S12.551A	Oth traum nondisp spondylolysis of sixth cervcal vert, init
		S12.590A	Oth disp fx of sixth cervical vertebra, init for clos fx
		S12.591A	Oth nondisp fx of sixth cervical vertebra, init for clos fx
805.07	CLOS FX C7 VERTEBRA W/O MENTION SP CRD INJURY	**S12.600A**	Unsp disp fx of seventh cervical vertebra, init for clos fx
		S12.601A	Unsp nondisp fx of seventh cervical vertebra, init
		S12.630A	Unsp traum displ spondylolysis of seventh cervcal vert, init
		S12.631A	Unsp traum nondisp spondylolysis of 7th cervcal vert, init
		S12.64XA	Type III traum spondylolysis of seventh cervcal vert, init
		S12.650A	Oth traum displ spondylolysis of seventh cervcal vert, init
		S12.651A	Oth traum nondisp spondylolysis of 7th cervcal vert, init
		S12.690A	Oth disp fx of seventh cervical vertebra, init for clos fx
		S12.691A	Oth nondisp fx of seventh cervical vertebra, init
805.08	CLOS FX MULT CERV VERTEBRAE W/O SP CRD INJURY	**S12.9XXA**	Fracture of neck, unspecified, initial encounter
805.10	OPN FX CERV VERTEBRA UNS LEVL W/O SP CRD INJURY	**S12.9XXA**	Fracture of neck, unspecified, initial encounter
805.11	OPN FX C1 VERTEBRA W/O MENTION SP CORD INJURY	**S12.000B**	Unsp disp fx of first cervical vertebra, init for opn fx
		S12.001B	Unsp nondisp fx of first cervical vertebra, init for opn fx
		S12.01XB	Stable burst fx first cervcal vertebra, init for opn fx
		S12.02XB	Unstable burst fx first cervcal vertebra, init for opn fx
		S12.030B	Displ post arch fx first cervcal vertebra, init for opn fx
		S12.031B	Nondisp post arch fx first cervcal vertebra, init for opn fx
		S12.040B	Displ lateral mass fx first cervcal vert, init for opn fx
		S12.041B	Nondisp lateral mass fx first cervcal vert, init for opn fx
		S12.090B	Oth disp fx of first cervical vertebra, init for opn fx
		S12.091B	Oth nondisp fx of first cervical vertebra, init for opn fx
805.12	OPN FX C2 VERTEBRA W/O MENTION SP CORD INJURY	**S12.100B**	Unsp disp fx of second cervical vertebra, init for opn fx
		S12.101B	Unsp nondisp fx of second cervical vertebra, init for opn fx
		S12.110B	Anterior displaced Type II dens fracture, init for opn fx
		S12.111B	Posterior displaced Type II dens fracture, init for opn fx
		S12.112B	Nondisplaced Type II dens fracture, init for opn fx
		S12.120B	Other displaced dens fracture, init encntr for open fracture
		S12.121B	Oth nondisplaced dens fracture, init for opn fx
		S12.130B	Unsp traum displ spondylolysis of 2nd cervcal vert, init op fx
		S12.131B	Unsp traum nondisp spondylolysis of 2nd cervcal vert, init op fx
		S12.14XB	Type III traum spondylolysis of 2nd cervcal vert, init op fx
		S12.150B	Oth traum displ spondylolysis of 2nd cervcal vert, init op fx
		S12.151B	Oth traum nondisp spondylolysis of 2nd cervcal vert, init op fx
		S12.190B	Oth disp fx of second cervical vertebra, init for opn fx
		S12.191B	Oth nondisp fx of second cervical vertebra, init for opn fx
805.13	OPN FX C3 VERTEBRA W/O MENTION SP CORD INJURY	**S12.200B**	Unsp disp fx of third cervical vertebra, init for opn fx
		S12.201B	Unsp nondisp fx of third cervical vertebra, init for opn fx
		S12.230B	Unsp traum displ spondylolysis of 3rd cervcal vert, init op fx
		S12.231B	Unsp traum nondisp spondylolysis of 3rd cervcal vert, init op fx
		S12.24XB	Type III traum spondylolysis of 3rd cervcal vert, init op fx
		S12.250B	Oth traum displ spondylolysis of 3rd cervcal vert, init op fx
		S12.251B	Oth traum nondisp spondylolysis of 3rd cervcal vert, init op fx
		S12.290B	Oth disp fx of third cervical vertebra, init for opn fx
		S12.291B	Oth nondisp fx of third cervical vertebra, init for opn fx

ICD-9-CM		ICD-10-CM	
805.14	OPN FX C4 VERTEBRA W/O MENTION SP CORD INJURY	**S12.300B**	Unsp disp fx of fourth cervical vertebra, init for opn fx
		S12.301B	Unsp nondisp fx of fourth cervical vertebra, init for opn fx
		S12.330B	Unsp traum displ spondylolysis of 4th cervcal vert, init op fx
		S12.331B	Unsp traum nondisp spondylolysis of 4th cervcal vert, init op fx
		S12.34XB	Type III traum spondylolysis of 4th cervcal vert, init op fx
		S12.350B	Oth traum displ spondylolysis of 4th cervcal vert, init op fx
		S12.351B	Oth traum nondisp spondylolysis of 4th cervcal vert, init op fx
		S12.390B	Oth disp fx of fourth cervical vertebra, init for opn fx
		S12.391B	Oth nondisp fx of fourth cervical vertebra, init for opn fx
805.15	OPN FX C5 VERTEBRA W/O MENTION SP CORD INJURY	**S12.400B**	Unsp disp fx of fifth cervical vertebra, init for opn fx
		S12.401B	Unsp nondisp fx of fifth cervical vertebra, init for opn fx
		S12.430B	Unsp traum displ spondylolysis of 5th cervcal vert, init op fx
		S12.431B	Unsp traum nondisp spondylolysis of 5th cervcal vert, init op fx
		S12.44XB	Type III traum spondylolysis of 5th cervcal vert, init op fx
		S12.450B	Oth traum displ spondylolysis of 5th cervcal vert, init op fx
		S12.451B	Oth traum nondisp spondylolysis of 5th cervcal vert, init op fx
		S12.490B	Oth disp fx of fifth cervical vertebra, init for opn fx
		S12.491B	Oth nondisp fx of fifth cervical vertebra, init for opn fx
805.16	OPN FX C6 VERTEBRA W/O MENTION SP CORD INJURY	**S12.500B**	Unsp disp fx of sixth cervical vertebra, init for opn fx
		S12.501B	Unsp nondisp fx of sixth cervical vertebra, init for opn fx
		S12.530B	Unsp traum displ spondylolysis of sixth cervcal vert, init op fx
		S12.531B	Unsp traum nondisp spondylolysis of sixth cervcal vert, init op fx
		S12.54XB	Type III traum spondylolysis of sixth cervcal vert, init op fx
		S12.550B	Oth traum displ spondylolysis of sixth cervcal vert, init op fx
		S12.551B	Oth traum nondisp spondylolysis of sixth cervcal vert, init op fx
		S12.590B	Oth disp fx of sixth cervical vertebra, init for opn fx
		S12.591B	Oth nondisp fx of sixth cervical vertebra, init for opn fx
805.17	OPN FX C7 VERTEBRA W/O MENTION SP CORD INJURY	**S12.600B**	Unsp disp fx of seventh cervical vertebra, init for opn fx
		S12.601B	Unsp nondisp fx of seventh cervcal vertebra, init for opn fx
		S12.630B	Unsp traum displ spondylolysis of 7th cervcal vert, init op fx
		S12.631B	Unsp traum nondisp spondylolysis of 7th cervcal vert, init op fx
		S12.64XB	Type III traum spondylolysis of 7th cervcal vert, init op fx
		S12.650B	Oth traum displ spondylolysis of 7th cervcal vert, init op fx
		S12.651B	Oth traum nondisp spondylolysis of 7th cervcal vert, init op fx
		S12.690B	Oth disp fx of seventh cervical vertebra, init for opn fx
		S12.691B	Oth nondisp fx of seventh cervical vertebra, init for opn fx
805.18	OP FX MULT CERV VERTEBRAE W/O SP CRD INJURY	**S12.9XXA**	Fracture of neck, unspecified, initial encounter
805.2	CLOS FX DORS VERTEBRA W/O MENTION SP CORD INJURY	**S22.000A**	Wedge compression fracture of unsp thoracic vertebra, init
		S22.001A	Stable burst fracture of unsp thoracic vertebra, init
		S22.002A	Unstable burst fracture of unsp thoracic vertebra, init
		S22.008A	Oth fracture of unsp thoracic vertebra, init for clos fx
		S22.009A	Unsp fracture of unsp thoracic vertebra, init for clos fx
		S22.010A	Wedge compression fracture of first thoracic vertebra, init
		S22.011A	Stable burst fracture of first thoracic vertebra, init
		S22.012A	Unstable burst fracture of first thoracic vertebra, init
		S22.018A	Oth fracture of first thoracic vertebra, init for clos fx
		S22.019A	Unsp fracture of first thoracic vertebra, init for clos fx
		S22.020A	Wedge compression fracture of second thoracic vertebra, init
		S22.021A	Stable burst fracture of second thoracic vertebra, init
		S22.022A	Unstable burst fracture of second thoracic vertebra, init
		S22.028A	Oth fracture of second thoracic vertebra, init for clos fx
		S22.029A	Unsp fracture of second thoracic vertebra, init for clos fx
		S22.030A	Wedge compression fracture of third thoracic vertebra, init
		S22.031A	Stable burst fracture of third thoracic vertebra, init
		S22.032A	Unstable burst fracture of third thoracic vertebra, init
		S22.038A	Oth fracture of third thoracic vertebra, init for clos fx
		S22.039A	Unsp fracture of third thoracic vertebra, init for clos fx
		S22.040A	Wedge compression fracture of fourth thoracic vertebra, init
		S22.041A	Stable burst fracture of fourth thoracic vertebra, init
		S22.042A	Unstable burst fracture of fourth thoracic vertebra, init
		S22.048A	Oth fracture of fourth thoracic vertebra, init for clos fx
		S22.049A	Unsp fracture of fourth thoracic vertebra, init for clos fx
		S22.050A	Wedge compression fracture of T5-T6 vertebra, init
		S22.051A	Stable burst fracture of T5-T6 vertebra, init for clos fx
		S22.052A	Unstable burst fracture of T5-T6 vertebra, init for clos fx
		S22.058A	Oth fracture of T5-T6 vertebra, init for clos fx
		S22.059A	Unsp fracture of T5-T6 vertebra, init for clos fx
		S22.060A	Wedge compression fracture of T7-T8 vertebra, init
		S22.061A	Stable burst fracture of T7-T8 vertebra, init for clos fx
		S22.062A	Unstable burst fracture of T7-T8 vertebra, init for clos fx
		S22.068A	Oth fracture of T7-T8 thoracic vertebra, init for clos fx
		S22.069A	Unsp fracture of T7-T8 vertebra, init for clos fx
		S22.070A	Wedge compression fracture of T9-T10 vertebra, init
		S22.071A	Stable burst fracture of T9-T10 vertebra, init for clos fx
		S22.072A	Unstable burst fracture of T9-T10 vertebra, init for clos fx
		S22.078A	Oth fracture of T9-T10 vertebra, init for clos fx
		S22.079A	Unsp fracture of T9-T10 vertebra, init for clos fx
		S22.080A	Wedge compression fracture of T11-T12 vertebra, init
		S22.081A	Stable burst fracture of T11-T12 vertebra, init for clos fx
		S22.082A	Unstable burst fracture of T11-T12 vertebra, init
		S22.088A	Oth fracture of T11-T12 vertebra, init for clos fx
		S22.089A	Unsp fracture of T11-T12 vertebra, init for clos fx

[Brackets] indicate valid character values for each code. Character value meanings provided for each code grouping.

ICD-9-CM		ICD-10-CM	
8Ø5.3	OPEN FX DORS VERTEBRA W/O MENTION SP CORD INJURY	**S22.ØØØB**	Wedge comprsn fx unsp thor vertebra, init for opn fx
		S22.ØØ1B	Stable burst fracture of unsp thor vertebra, init for opn fx
		S22.ØØ2B	Unstable burst fx unsp thor vertebra, init for opn fx
		S22.ØØ8B	Oth fracture of unsp thoracic vertebra, init for opn fx
		S22.ØØ9B	Unsp fracture of unsp thoracic vertebra, init for opn fx
		S22.Ø1ØB	Wedge comprsn fx first thor vertebra, init for opn fx
		S22.Ø11B	Stable burst fx first thor vertebra, init for opn fx
		S22.Ø12B	Unstable burst fx first thor vertebra, init for opn fx
		S22.Ø18B	Oth fracture of first thoracic vertebra, init for opn fx
		S22.Ø19B	Unsp fracture of first thoracic vertebra, init for opn fx
		S22.Ø2ØB	Wedge comprsn fx second thor vertebra, init for opn fx
		S22.Ø21B	Stable burst fx second thor vertebra, init for opn fx
		S22.Ø22B	Unstable burst fx second thor vertebra, init for opn fx
		S22.Ø28B	Oth fracture of second thoracic vertebra, init for opn fx
		S22.Ø29B	Unsp fracture of second thoracic vertebra, init for opn fx
		S22.Ø3ØB	Wedge comprsn fx third thor vertebra, init for opn fx
		S22.Ø31B	Stable burst fx third thor vertebra, init for opn fx
		S22.Ø32B	Unstable burst fx third thor vertebra, init for opn fx
		S22.Ø38B	Oth fracture of third thoracic vertebra, init for opn fx
		S22.Ø39B	Unsp fracture of third thoracic vertebra, init for opn fx
		S22.Ø4ØB	Wedge comprsn fx fourth thor vertebra, init for opn fx
		S22.Ø41B	Stable burst fx fourth thor vertebra, init for opn fx
		S22.Ø42B	Unstable burst fx fourth thor vertebra, init for opn fx
		S22.Ø48B	Oth fracture of fourth thoracic vertebra, init for opn fx
		S22.Ø49B	Unsp fracture of fourth thoracic vertebra, init for opn fx
		S22.Ø5ØB	Wedge comprsn fracture of T5-T6 vertebra, init for opn fx
		S22.Ø51B	Stable burst fracture of T5-T6 vertebra, init for opn fx
		S22.Ø52B	Unstable burst fracture of T5-T6 vertebra, init for opn fx
		S22.Ø58B	Oth fracture of T5-T6 vertebra, init for opn fx
		S22.Ø59B	Unsp fracture of T5-T6 vertebra, init for opn fx
		S22.Ø6ØB	Wedge comprsn fracture of T7-T8 vertebra, init for opn fx
		S22.Ø61B	Stable burst fracture of T7-T8 vertebra, init for opn fx
		S22.Ø62B	Unstable burst fracture of T7-T8 vertebra, init for opn fx
		S22.Ø68B	Oth fracture of T7-T8 thoracic vertebra, init for opn fx
		S22.Ø69B	Unsp fracture of T7-T8 vertebra, init for opn fx
		S22.Ø7ØB	Wedge comprsn fracture of T9-T10 vertebra, init for opn fx
		S22.Ø71B	Stable burst fracture of T9-T10 vertebra, init for opn fx
		S22.Ø72B	Unstable burst fracture of T9-T10 vertebra, init for opn fx
		S22.Ø78B	Oth fracture of T9-T10 vertebra, init for opn fx
		S22.Ø79B	Unsp fracture of T9-T10 vertebra, init for opn fx
		S22.Ø8ØB	Wedge comprsn fracture of T11-T12 vertebra, init for opn fx
		S22.Ø81B	Stable burst fracture of T11-T12 vertebra, init for opn fx
		S22.Ø82B	Unstable burst fracture of T11-T12 vertebra, init for opn fx
		S22.Ø88B	Oth fracture of T11-T12 vertebra, init for opn fx
		S22.Ø89B	Unsp fracture of T11-T12 vertebra, init for opn fx
8Ø5.4	CLOS FX LUMB VERTEBRA W/O MENTION SP CORD INJURY	**S32.ØØØA**	Wedge compression fracture of unsp lumbar vertebra, init
		S32.ØØ1A	Stable burst fracture of unsp lumbar vertebra, init
		S32.ØØ2A	Unstable burst fracture of unsp lumbar vertebra, init
		S32.ØØ8A	Oth fracture of unsp lumbar vertebra, init for clos fx
		S32.ØØ9A	Unsp fracture of unsp lumbar vertebra, init for clos fx
		S32.Ø1ØA	Wedge compression fracture of first lumbar vertebra, init
		S32.Ø11A	Stable burst fracture of first lumbar vertebra, init
		S32.Ø12A	Unstable burst fracture of first lumbar vertebra, init
		S32.Ø18A	Oth fracture of first lumbar vertebra, init for clos fx
		S32.Ø19A	Unsp fracture of first lumbar vertebra, init for clos fx
		S32.Ø2ØA	Wedge compression fracture of second lumbar vertebra, init
		S32.Ø21A	Stable burst fracture of second lumbar vertebra, init
		S32.Ø22A	Unstable burst fracture of second lumbar vertebra, init
		S32.Ø28A	Oth fracture of second lumbar vertebra, init for clos fx
		S32.Ø29A	Unsp fracture of second lumbar vertebra, init for clos fx
		S32.Ø3ØA	Wedge compression fracture of third lumbar vertebra, init
		S32.Ø31A	Stable burst fracture of third lumbar vertebra, init
		S32.Ø32A	Unstable burst fracture of third lumbar vertebra, init
		S32.Ø38A	Oth fracture of third lumbar vertebra, init for clos fx
		S32.Ø39A	Unsp fracture of third lumbar vertebra, init for clos fx
		S32.Ø4ØA	Wedge compression fracture of fourth lumbar vertebra, init
		S32.Ø41A	Stable burst fracture of fourth lumbar vertebra, init
		S32.Ø42A	Unstable burst fracture of fourth lumbar vertebra, init
		S32.Ø48A	Oth fracture of fourth lumbar vertebra, init for clos fx
		S32.Ø49A	Unsp fracture of fourth lumbar vertebra, init for clos fx
		S32.Ø5ØA	Wedge compression fracture of fifth lumbar vertebra, init
		S32.Ø51A	Stable burst fracture of fifth lumbar vertebra, init
		S32.Ø52A	Unstable burst fracture of fifth lumbar vertebra, init
		S32.Ø58A	Oth fracture of fifth lumbar vertebra, init for clos fx
		S32.Ø59A	Unsp fracture of fifth lumbar vertebra, init for clos fx

ICD-9-CM		ICD-10-CM	
805.5	OPEN FX LUMB VERTEBRA W/O MENTION SP CORD INJURY	**S32.000B**	Wedge comprsn fracture of unsp lum vertebra, init for opn fx
		S32.001B	Stable burst fracture of unsp lum vertebra, init for opn fx
		S32.002B	Unstable burst fx unsp lum vertebra, init for opn fx
		S32.008B	Oth fracture of unsp lumbar vertebra, init for opn fx
		S32.009B	Unsp fracture of unsp lumbar vertebra, init for opn fx
		S32.010B	Wedge comprsn fx first lum vertebra, init for opn fx
		S32.011B	Stable burst fracture of first lum vertebra, init for opn fx
		S32.012B	Unstable burst fx first lum vertebra, init for opn fx
		S32.018B	Oth fracture of first lumbar vertebra, init for opn fx
		S32.019B	Unsp fracture of first lumbar vertebra, init for opn fx
		S32.020B	Wedge comprsn fx second lum vertebra, init for opn fx
		S32.021B	Stable burst fx second lum vertebra, init for opn fx
		S32.022B	Unstable burst fx second lum vertebra, init for opn fx
		S32.028B	Oth fracture of second lumbar vertebra, init for opn fx
		S32.029B	Unsp fracture of second lumbar vertebra, init for opn fx
		S32.030B	Wedge comprsn fx third lum vertebra, init for opn fx
		S32.031B	Stable burst fracture of third lum vertebra, init for opn fx
		S32.032B	Unstable burst fx third lum vertebra, init for opn fx
		S32.038B	Oth fracture of third lumbar vertebra, init for opn fx
		S32.039B	Unsp fracture of third lumbar vertebra, init for opn fx
		S32.040B	Wedge comprsn fx fourth lum vertebra, init for opn fx
		S32.041B	Stable burst fx fourth lum vertebra, init for opn fx
		S32.042B	Unstable burst fx fourth lum vertebra, init for opn fx
		S32.048B	Oth fracture of fourth lumbar vertebra, init for opn fx
		S32.049B	Unsp fracture of fourth lumbar vertebra, init for opn fx
		S32.050B	Wedge comprsn fx fifth lum vertebra, init for opn fx
		S32.051B	Stable burst fracture of fifth lum vertebra, init for opn fx
		S32.052B	Unstable burst fx fifth lum vertebra, init for opn fx
		S32.058B	Oth fracture of fifth lumbar vertebra, init for opn fx
		S32.059B	Unsp fracture of fifth lumbar vertebra, init for opn fx
805.6	CLOS FX SACRUM&COCCYX W/O MENTION SP CORD INJURY	**S32.10XA**	Unsp fracture of sacrum, init encntr for closed fracture
		S32.110A	Nondisplaced Zone I fracture of sacrum, init for clos fx
		S32.111A	Minimally displaced Zone I fracture of sacrum, init
		S32.112A	Severely displaced Zone I fracture of sacrum, init
		S32.119A	Unsp Zone I fracture of sacrum, init for clos fx
		S32.120A	Nondisplaced Zone II fracture of sacrum, init for clos fx
		S32.121A	Minimally displaced Zone II fracture of sacrum, init
		S32.122A	Severely displaced Zone II fracture of sacrum, init
		S32.129A	Unsp Zone II fracture of sacrum, init for clos fx
		S32.130A	Nondisplaced Zone III fracture of sacrum, init for clos fx
		S32.131A	Minimally displaced Zone III fracture of sacrum, init
		S32.132A	Severely displaced Zone III fracture of sacrum, init
		S32.139A	Unsp Zone III fracture of sacrum, init for clos fx
		S32.14XA	Type 1 fracture of sacrum, init encntr for closed fracture
		S32.15XA	Type 2 fracture of sacrum, init encntr for closed fracture
		S32.16XA	Type 3 fracture of sacrum, init encntr for closed fracture
		S32.17XA	Type 4 fracture of sacrum, init encntr for closed fracture
		S32.19XA	Other fracture of sacrum, init encntr for closed fracture
		S32.2XXA	Fracture of coccyx, initial encounter for closed fracture
805.7	OPEN FX SACRUM&COCCYX W/O MENTION SP CORD INJURY	**S32.10XB**	Unsp fracture of sacrum, init encntr for open fracture
		S32.110B	Nondisplaced Zone I fracture of sacrum, init for opn fx
		S32.111B	Minimally displaced Zone I fx sacrum, init for opn fx
		S32.112B	Severely displaced Zone I fx sacrum, init for opn fx
		S32.119B	Unsp Zone I fracture of sacrum, init for opn fx
		S32.120B	Nondisplaced Zone II fracture of sacrum, init for opn fx
		S32.121B	Minimally displaced Zone II fx sacrum, init for opn fx
		S32.122B	Severely displaced Zone II fx sacrum, init for opn fx
		S32.129B	Unsp Zone II fracture of sacrum, init for opn fx
		S32.130B	Nondisplaced Zone III fracture of sacrum, init for opn fx
		S32.131B	Minimally displaced Zone III fx sacrum, init for opn fx
		S32.132B	Severely displaced Zone III fx sacrum, init for opn fx
		S32.139B	Unsp Zone III fracture of sacrum, init for opn fx
		S32.14XB	Type 1 fracture of sacrum, init encntr for open fracture
		S32.15XB	Type 2 fracture of sacrum, init encntr for open fracture
		S32.16XB	Type 3 fracture of sacrum, init encntr for open fracture
		S32.17XB	Type 4 fracture of sacrum, init encntr for open fracture
		S32.19XB	Other fracture of sacrum, init encntr for open fracture
		S32.2XXB	Fracture of coccyx, initial encounter for open fracture
805.8	CLOS FX UNS PART VERT COLUMN W/O SP CRD INJURY	**S12.9XXA**	Fracture of neck, unspecified, initial encounter
		S22.009A	Unsp fracture of unsp thoracic vertebra, init for clos fx
		S32.009A	Unsp fracture of unsp lumbar vertebra, init for clos fx
		S32.10XA	Unsp fracture of sacrum, init encntr for closed fracture
		S32.2XXA	Fracture of coccyx, initial encounter for closed fracture
805.9	OPN FX UNS PART VERT COLUMN W/O SP CRD INJURY	**S12.9XXA**	Fracture of neck, unspecified, initial encounter
		S22.009B	Unsp fracture of unsp thoracic vertebra, init for opn fx
		S32.009B	Unsp fracture of unsp lumbar vertebra, init for opn fx
		S32.10XB	Unsp fracture of sacrum, init encntr for open fracture
		S32.2XXB	Fracture of coccyx, initial encounter for open fracture

ICD-9-CM		ICD-10-CM		
806.00	CLOS FX C1-C4 LEVEL W/UNSPEC SPINAL CORD INJURY	**S14.101A**	Unsp injury at C1 level of cervical spinal cord, init encntr	*and*
		S12.000A	Unsp disp fx of first cervical vertebra, init for clos fx	*or*
		S12.001A	Unsp nondisp fx of first cervical vertebra, init for clos fx	
		S14.102A	Unsp injury at C2 level of cervical spinal cord, init encntr	*and*
		S12.100A	Unsp disp fx of second cervical vertebra, init for clos fx	*or*
		S12.101A	Unsp nondisp fx of second cervical vertebra, init	
		S14.103A	Unsp injury at C3 level of cervical spinal cord, init encntr	*and*
		S12.200A	Unsp disp fx of third cervical vertebra, init for clos fx	*or*
		S12.201A	Unsp nondisp fx of third cervical vertebra, init for clos fx	
		S14.104A	Unsp injury at C4 level of cervical spinal cord, init encntr	*and*
		S12.300A	Unsp disp fx of fourth cervical vertebra, init for clos fx	*or*
		S12.301A	Unsp nondisp fx of fourth cervical vertebra, init	
806.01	CLOS FRACTURE C1-C4 LEVEL W/COMPLETE LESION CORD	**S14.111A**	Complete lesion at C1 level of cervical spinal cord, init	*and*
		S12.000A	Unsp disp fx of first cervical vertebra, init for clos fx	*or*
		S12.001A	Unsp nondisp fx of first cervical vertebra, init for clos fx	
		S14.112A	Complete lesion at C2 level of cervical spinal cord, init	*and*
		S12.100A	Unsp disp fx of second cervical vertebra, init for clos fx	*or*
		S12.101A	Unsp nondisp fx of second cervical vertebra, init	
		S14.113A	Complete lesion at C3 level of cervical spinal cord, init	*and*
		S12.200A	Unsp disp fx of third cervical vertebra, init for clos fx	*or*
		S12.201A	Unsp nondisp fx of third cervical vertebra, init for clos fx	
		S14.114A	Complete lesion at C4 level of cervical spinal cord, init	*and*
		S12.300A	Unsp disp fx of fourth cervical vertebra, init for clos fx	*or*
		S12.301A	Unsp nondisp fx of fourth cervical vertebra, init	
806.02	CLOSED FRACTURE C1-C4 LEVEL W/ANT CORD SYNDROME	**S14.131A**	Anterior cord syndrome at C1, init	*and*
		S12.000A	Unsp disp fx of first cervical vertebra, init for clos fx	*or*
		S12.001A	Unsp nondisp fx of first cervical vertebra, init for clos fx	
		S14.132A	Anterior cord syndrome at C2, init	*and*
		S12.100A	Unsp disp fx of second cervical vertebra, init for clos fx	*or*
		S12.101A	Unsp nondisp fx of second cervical vertebra, init	
		S14.133A	Anterior cord syndrome at C3, init	*and*
		S12.200A	Unsp disp fx of third cervical vertebra, init for clos fx	*or*
		S12.201A	Unsp nondisp fx of third cervical vertebra, init for clos fx	
		S14.134A	Anterior cord syndrome at C4, init	*and*
		S12.300A	Unsp disp fx of fourth cervical vertebra, init for clos fx	*or*
		S12.301A	Unsp nondisp fx of fourth cervical vertebra, init	
806.03	CLOS FRACTURE C1-C4 LEVEL W/CNTRL CORD SYNDROME	**S14.121A**	Central cord syndrome at C1, init	*and*
		S12.000A	Unsp disp fx of first cervical vertebra, init for clos fx	*or*
		S12.001A	Unsp nondisp fx of first cervical vertebra, init for clos fx	
		S14.122A	Central cord syndrome at C2, init	*and*
		S12.100A	Unsp disp fx of second cervical vertebra, init for clos fx	*or*
		S12.101A	Unsp nondisp fx of second cervical vertebra, init	
		S14.123A	Central cord syndrome at C3, init	*and*
		S12.200A	Unsp disp fx of third cervical vertebra, init for clos fx	*or*
		S12.201A	Unsp nondisp fx of third cervical vertebra, init for clos fx	
		S14.124A	Central cord syndrome at C4, init	*and*
		S12.300A	Unsp disp fx of fourth cervical vertebra, init for clos fx	*or*
		S12.301A	Unsp nondisp fx of fourth cervical vertebra, init	
806.04	CLOS FX C1-C4 LEVL W/OTH SPEC SPINAL CORD INJURY	**S14.151A**	Oth incomplete lesion at C1, init	*and*
		S12.000A	Unsp disp fx of first cervical vertebra, init for clos fx	*or*
		S12.001A	Unsp nondisp fx of first cervical vertebra, init for clos fx	
		S14.152A	Oth incomplete lesion at C2, init	*and*
		S12.100A	Unsp disp fx of second cervical vertebra, init for clos fx	*or*
		S12.101A	Unsp nondisp fx of second cervical vertebra, init	
		S14.153A	Oth incomplete lesion at C3, init	*and*
		S12.200A	Unsp disp fx of third cervical vertebra, init for clos fx	*or*
		S12.201A	Unsp nondisp fx of third cervical vertebra, init for clos fx	
		S14.154A	Oth incomplete lesion at C4, init	*and*
		S12.300A	Unsp disp fx of fourth cervical vertebra, init for clos fx	*or*
		S12.301A	Unsp nondisp fx of fourth cervical vertebra, init	

ICD-9-CM		ICD-10-CM		
806.05	CLOS FX C5-C7 LEVEL W/UNSPEC SPINAL CORD INJURY	**S14.105A**	Unsp injury at C5 level of cervical spinal cord, init encntr	*and*
		S12.400A **S12.401A**	Unsp disp fx of fifth cervical vertebra, init for clos fx Unsp nondisp fx of fifth cervical vertebra, init for clos fx	*or*
		S14.106A	Unsp injury at C6 level of cervical spinal cord, init encntr	*and*
		S12.500A **S12.501A**	Unsp disp fx of sixth cervical vertebra, init for clos fx Unsp nondisp fx of sixth cervical vertebra, init for clos fx	*or*
		S14.107A	Unsp injury at C7 level of cervical spinal cord, init encntr	*and*
		S12.600A **S12.601A**	Unsp disp fx of seventh cervical vertebra, init for clos fx Unsp nondisp fx of seventh cervical vertebra, init	*or*
806.06	CLOS FRACTURE C5-C7 LEVEL W/COMPLETE LESION CORD	**S14.115A**	Complete lesion at C5 level of cervical spinal cord, init	*and*
		S12.400A **S12.401A**	Unsp disp fx of fifth cervical vertebra, init for clos fx Unsp nondisp fx of fifth cervical vertebra, init for clos fx	*or*
		S14.116A	Complete lesion at C6 level of cervical spinal cord, init	*and*
		S12.500A **S12.501A**	Unsp disp fx of sixth cervical vertebra, init for clos fx Unsp nondisp fx of sixth cervical vertebra, init for clos fx	*or*
		S14.117A	Complete lesion at C7 level of cervical spinal cord, init	*and*
		S12.600A **S12.601A**	Unsp disp fx of seventh cervical vertebra, init for clos fx Unsp nondisp fx of seventh cervical vertebra, init	*or*
806.07	CLOSED FRACTURE C5-C7 LEVEL W/ANT CORD SYNDROME	**S14.135A**	Anterior cord syndrome at C5, init	*and*
		S12.400A **S12.401A**	Unsp disp fx of fifth cervical vertebra, init for clos fx Unsp nondisp fx of fifth cervical vertebra, init for clos fx	*or*
		S14.136A	Anterior cord syndrome at C6, init	*and*
		S12.500A **S12.501A**	Unsp disp fx of sixth cervical vertebra, init for clos fx Unsp nondisp fx of sixth cervical vertebra, init for clos fx	*or*
		S14.137A	Anterior cord syndrome at C7, init	*and*
		S12.600A **S12.601A**	Unsp disp fx of seventh cervical vertebra, init for clos fx Unsp nondisp fx of seventh cervical vertebra, init	*or*
806.08	CLOS FRACTURE C5-C7 LEVEL W/CNTRL CORD SYNDROME	**S14.125A**	Central cord syndrome at C5, init	*and*
		S12.400A **S12.401A**	Unsp disp fx of fifth cervical vertebra, init for clos fx Unsp nondisp fx of fifth cervical vertebra, init for clos fx	*or*
		S14.126A	Central cord syndrome at C6, init	*and*
		S12.500A **S12.501A**	Unsp disp fx of sixth cervical vertebra, init for clos fx Unsp nondisp fx of sixth cervical vertebra, init for clos fx	*or*
		S14.127A	Central cord syndrome at C7, init	*and*
		S12.600A **S12.601A**	Unsp disp fx of seventh cervical vertebra, init for clos fx Unsp nondisp fx of seventh cervical vertebra, init	*or*
806.09	CLOS FX C5-C7 LEVL W/OTH SPEC SPINAL CORD INJURY	**S14.155A**	Oth incomplete lesion at C5, init	*and*
		S12.400A **S12.401A**	Unsp disp fx of fifth cervical vertebra, init for clos fx Unsp nondisp fx of fifth cervical vertebra, init for clos fx	*or*
		S14.156A	Oth incomplete lesion at C6, init	*and*
		S12.500A **S12.501A**	Unsp disp fx of sixth cervical vertebra, init for clos fx Unsp nondisp fx of sixth cervical vertebra, init for clos fx	*or*
		S14.157A	Oth incomplete lesion at C7, init	*and*
		S12.600A **S12.601A**	Unsp disp fx of seventh cervical vertebra, init for clos fx Unsp nondisp fx of seventh cervical vertebra, init	*or*
806.10	OPEN FX C1-C4 LEVEL W/UNSPEC SPINAL CORD INJURY	**S14.101A**	Unsp injury at C1 level of cervical spinal cord, init encntr	*and*
		S12.000B **S12.001B**	Unsp disp fx of first cervical vertebra, init for opn fx Unsp nondisp fx of first cervical vertebra, init for opn fx	*or*
		S14.102A	Unsp injury at C2 level of cervical spinal cord, init encntr	*and*
		S12.100B **S12.101B**	Unsp disp fx of second cervical vertebra, init for opn fx Unsp nondisp fx of second cervical vertebra, init for opn fx	*or*
		S14.103A	Unsp injury at C3 level of cervical spinal cord, init encntr	*and*
		S12.200B **S12.201B**	Unsp disp fx of third cervical vertebra, init for opn fx Unsp nondisp fx of third cervical vertebra, init for opn fx	*or*
		S14.104A	Unsp injury at C4 level of cervical spinal cord, init encntr	*and*
		S12.300B **S12.301B**	Unsp disp fx of fourth cervical vertebra, init for opn fx Unsp nondisp fx of fourth cervical vertebra, init for opn fx	*or*

ICD-9-CM		ICD-10-CM		
806.11	OPEN FRACTURE C1-C4 LEVEL W/COMPLETE LESION CORD	**S14.111A**	Complete lesion at C1 level of cervical spinal cord, init	*and*
		S12.000B	Unsp disp fx of first cervical vertebra, init for opn fx	*or*
		S12.001B	Unsp nondisp fx of first cervical vertebra, init for opn fx	
		S14.112A	Complete lesion at C2 level of cervical spinal cord, init	*and*
		S12.100B	Unsp disp fx of second cervical vertebra, init for opn fx	*or*
		S12.101B	Unsp nondisp fx of second cervical vertebra, init for opn fx	
		S14.113A	Complete lesion at C3 level of cervical spinal cord, init	*and*
		S12.200B	Unsp disp fx of third cervical vertebra, init for opn fx	*or*
		S12.201B	Unsp nondisp fx of third cervical vertebra, init for opn fx	
		S14.114A	Complete lesion at C4 level of cervical spinal cord, init	*and*
		S12.300B	Unsp disp fx of fourth cervical vertebra, init for opn fx	*or*
		S12.301B	Unsp nondisp fx of fourth cervical vertebra, init for opn fx	
806.12	OPEN FRACTURE C1-C4 LEVEL W/ANT CORD SYNDROME	**S14.131A**	Anterior cord syndrome at C1, init	*and*
		S12.000B	Unsp disp fx of first cervical vertebra, init for opn fx	*or*
		S12.001B	Unsp nondisp fx of first cervical vertebra, init for opn fx	
		S14.132A	Anterior cord syndrome at C2, init	*and*
		S12.100B	Unsp disp fx of second cervical vertebra, init for opn fx	*or*
		S12.101B	Unsp nondisp fx of second cervical vertebra, init for opn fx	
		S14.133A	Anterior cord syndrome at C3, init	*and*
		S12.200B	Unsp disp fx of third cervical vertebra, init for opn fx	*or*
		S12.201B	Unsp nondisp fx of third cervical vertebra, init for opn fx	
		S14.134A	Anterior cord syndrome at C4, init	*and*
		S12.300B	Unsp disp fx of fourth cervical vertebra, init for opn fx	*or*
		S12.301B	Unsp nondisp fx of fourth cervical vertebra, init for opn fx	
806.13	OPEN FRACTURE C1-C4 LEVEL W/CNTRL CORD SYNDROME	**S14.121A**	Central cord syndrome at C1, init	*and*
		S12.000B	Unsp disp fx of first cervical vertebra, init for opn fx	*or*
		S12.001B	Unsp nondisp fx of first cervical vertebra, init for opn fx	
		S14.122A	Central cord syndrome at C2, init	*and*
		S12.100B	Unsp disp fx of second cervical vertebra, init for opn fx	*or*
		S12.101B	Unsp nondisp fx of second cervical vertebra, init for opn fx	
		S14.123A	Central cord syndrome at C3, init	*and*
		S12.200B	Unsp disp fx of third cervical vertebra, init for opn fx	*or*
		S12.201B	Unsp nondisp fx of third cervical vertebra, init for opn fx	
		S14.124A	Central cord syndrome at C4, init	*and*
		S12.300B	Unsp disp fx of fourth cervical vertebra, init for opn fx	*or*
		S12.301B	Unsp nondisp fx of fourth cervical vertebra, init for opn fx	
806.14	OPEN FX C1-C4 LEVL W/OTH SPEC SPINAL CORD INJURY	**S14.151A**	Oth incomplete lesion at C1, init	*and*
		S12.000B	Unsp disp fx of first cervical vertebra, init for opn fx	*or*
		S12.001B	Unsp nondisp fx of first cervical vertebra, init for opn fx	
		S14.152A	Oth incomplete lesion at C2, init	*and*
		S12.100B	Unsp disp fx of second cervical vertebra, init for opn fx	*or*
		S12.101B	Unsp nondisp fx of second cervical vertebra, init for opn fx	
		S14.153A	Oth incomplete lesion at C3, init	*and*
		S12.200B	Unsp disp fx of third cervical vertebra, init for opn fx	*or*
		S12.201B	Unsp nondisp fx of third cervical vertebra, init for opn fx	
		S14.154A	Oth incomplete lesion at C4, init	*and*
		S12.300B	Unsp disp fx of fourth cervical vertebra, init for opn fx	*or*
		S12.301B	Unsp nondisp fx of fourth cervical vertebra, init for opn fx	
806.15	OPEN FX C5-C7 LEVEL W/UNSPEC SPINAL CORD INJURY	**S14.105A**	Unsp injury at C5 level of cervical spinal cord, init encntr	*and*
		S12.400B	Unsp disp fx of fifth cervical vertebra, init for opn fx	*or*
		S12.401B	Unsp nondisp fx of fifth cervical vertebra, init for opn fx	
		S14.106A	Unsp injury at C6 level of cervical spinal cord, init encntr	*and*
		S12.500B	Unsp disp fx of sixth cervical vertebra, init for opn fx	*or*
		S12.501B	Unsp nondisp fx of sixth cervical vertebra, init for opn fx	
		S14.107A	Unsp injury at C7 level of cervical spinal cord, init encntr	*and*
		S12.600B	Unsp disp fx of seventh cervical vertebra, init for opn fx	*or*
		S12.601B	Unsp nondisp fx of seventh cervcal vertebra, init for opn fx	
806.16	OPEN FRACTURE C5-C7 LEVEL W/COMPLETE LESION CORD	**S14.115A**	Complete lesion at C5 level of cervical spinal cord, init	*and*
		S12.400B	Unsp disp fx of fifth cervical vertebra, init for opn fx	*or*
		S12.401B	Unsp nondisp fx of fifth cervical vertebra, init for opn fx	
		S14.116A	Complete lesion at C6 level of cervical spinal cord, init	*and*
		S12.500B	Unsp disp fx of sixth cervical vertebra, init for opn fx	*or*
		S12.501B	Unsp nondisp fx of sixth cervical vertebra, init for opn fx	
		S14.117A	Complete lesion at C7 level of cervical spinal cord, init	*and*
		S12.600B	Unsp disp fx of seventh cervical vertebra, init for opn fx	*or*
		S12.601B	Unsp nondisp fx of seventh cervcal vertebra, init for opn fx	

ICD-9-CM		ICD-10-CM		
8Ø6.17	OPEN FRACTURE C5-C7 LEVEL W/ANT CORD SYNDROME	**S14.135A**	Anterior cord syndrome at C5, init	*and*
		S12.4ØØB	Unsp disp fx of fifth cervical vertebra, init for opn fx	*or*
		S12.4Ø1B	Unsp nondisp fx of fifth cervical vertebra, init for opn fx	
		S14.136A	Anterior cord syndrome at C6, init	*and*
		S12.5ØØB	Unsp disp fx of sixth cervical vertebra, init for opn fx	*or*
		S12.5Ø1B	Unsp nondisp fx of sixth cervical vertebra, init for opn fx	
		S14.137A	Anterior cord syndrome at C7, init	*and*
		S12.6ØØB	Unsp disp fx of seventh cervical vertebra, init for opn fx	*or*
		S12.6Ø1B	Unsp nondisp fx of seventh cervcal vertebra, init for opn fx	
8Ø6.18	OPEN FRACTURE C5-C7 LEVEL W/CNTRL CORD SYNDROME	**S14.125A**	Central cord syndrome at C5, init	*and*
		S12.4ØØB	Unsp disp fx of fifth cervical vertebra, init for opn fx	*or*
		S12.4Ø1B	Unsp nondisp fx of fifth cervical vertebra, init for opn fx	
		S14.126A	Central cord syndrome at C6, init	*and*
		S12.5ØØB	Unsp disp fx of sixth cervical vertebra, init for opn fx	*or*
		S12.5Ø1B	Unsp nondisp fx of sixth cervical vertebra, init for opn fx	
		S14.127A	Central cord syndrome at C7, init	*and*
		S12.6ØØB	Unsp disp fx of seventh cervical vertebra, init for opn fx	*or*
		S12.6Ø1B	Unsp nondisp fx of seventh cervcal vertebra, init for opn fx	
8Ø6.19	OPEN FX C5-C7 LEVL W/OTH SPEC SPINAL CORD INJURY	**S14.155A**	Oth incomplete lesion at C5, init	*and*
		S12.4ØØB	Unsp disp fx of fifth cervical vertebra, init for opn fx	*or*
		S12.4Ø1B	Unsp nondisp fx of fifth cervical vertebra, init for opn fx	
		S14.156A	Oth incomplete lesion at C6, init	*and*
		S12.5ØØB	Unsp disp fx of sixth cervical vertebra, init for opn fx	*or*
		S12.5Ø1B	Unsp nondisp fx of sixth cervical vertebra, init for opn fx	
		S14.157A	Oth incomplete lesion at C7, init	*and*
		S12.6ØØB	Unsp disp fx of seventh cervical vertebra, init for opn fx	*or*
		S12.6Ø1B	Unsp nondisp fx of seventh cervcal vertebra, init for opn fx	
8Ø6.2Ø	CLOS FX T1-T6 LEVEL W/UNSPEC SPINAL CORD INJURY	**S24.1Ø1A**	Unsp injury at T1 level of thoracic spinal cord, init encntr	*and*
		S22.Ø19A	Unsp fracture of first thoracic vertebra, init for clos fx	
		S24.1Ø2A	Unsp injury at T2-T6 level of thoracic spinal cord, init	*and*
		S22.Ø29A	Unsp fracture of second thoracic vertebra, init for clos fx	*or*
		S22.Ø39A	Unsp fracture of third thoracic vertebra, init for clos fx	*or*
		S22.Ø49A	Unsp fracture of fourth thoracic vertebra, init for clos fx	*or*
		S22.Ø59A	Unsp fracture of T5-T6 vertebra, init for clos fx	
8Ø6.21	CLOS FRACTURE T1-T6 LEVEL W/COMPLETE LESION CORD	**S24.111A**	Complete lesion at T1 level of thoracic spinal cord, init	*and*
		S22.Ø19A	Unsp fracture of first thoracic vertebra, init for clos fx	
		S24.112A	Complete lesion at T2-T6 level of thoracic spinal cord, init	*and*
		S22.Ø29A	Unsp fracture of second thoracic vertebra, init for clos fx	*or*
		S22.Ø39A	Unsp fracture of third thoracic vertebra, init for clos fx	*or*
		S22.Ø49A	Unsp fracture of fourth thoracic vertebra, init for clos fx	*or*
		S22.Ø59A	Unsp fracture of T5-T6 vertebra, init for clos fx	
8Ø6.22	CLOSED FRACTURE T1-T6 LEVEL W/ANT CORD SYNDROME	**S24.131A**	Anterior cord syndrome at T1, init	*and*
		S22.Ø19A	Unsp fracture of first thoracic vertebra, init for clos fx	
		S24.132A	Anterior cord syndrome at T2-T6, init	*and*
		S22.Ø29A	Unsp fracture of second thoracic vertebra, init for clos fx	*or*
		S22.Ø39A	Unsp fracture of third thoracic vertebra, init for clos fx	*or*
		S22.Ø49A	Unsp fracture of fourth thoracic vertebra, init for clos fx	*or*
		S22.Ø59A	Unsp fracture of T5-T6 vertebra, init for clos fx	
8Ø6.23	CLOS FRACTURE T1-T6 LEVEL W/CNTRL CORD SYNDROME	**S24.151A**	Oth incomplete lesion at T1, init	*and*
		S22.Ø19A	Unsp fracture of first thoracic vertebra, init for clos fx	
		S24.152A	Oth incomplete lesion at T2-T6, init	*and*
		S22.Ø29A	Unsp fracture of second thoracic vertebra, init for clos fx	*or*
		S22.Ø39A	Unsp fracture of third thoracic vertebra, init for clos fx	*or*
		S22.Ø49A	Unsp fracture of fourth thoracic vertebra, init for clos fx	*or*
		S22.Ø59A	Unsp fracture of T5-T6 vertebra, init for clos fx	
8Ø6.24	CLOS FX T1-T6 LEVL W/OTH SPEC SPINAL CORD INJURY	**S24.151A**	Oth incomplete lesion at T1, init	*and*
		S22.Ø19A	Unsp fracture of first thoracic vertebra, init for clos fx	
		S24.152A	Oth incomplete lesion at T2-T6, init	*and*
		S22.Ø29A	Unsp fracture of second thoracic vertebra, init for clos fx	*or*
		S22.Ø39A	Unsp fracture of third thoracic vertebra, init for clos fx	*or*
		S22.Ø49A	Unsp fracture of fourth thoracic vertebra, init for clos fx	*or*
		S22.Ø59A	Unsp fracture of T5-T6 vertebra, init for clos fx	
8Ø6.25	CLOS FX T7-T12 LEVEL W/UNSPEC SPINAL CORD INJURY	**S24.1Ø3A**	Unsp injury at T7-T10 level of thoracic spinal cord, init	*and*
		S22.Ø69A	Unsp fracture of T7-T8 vertebra, init for clos fx	*or*
		S22.Ø79A	Unsp fracture of T9-T10 vertebra, init for clos fx	
		S24.1Ø4A	Unsp injury at T11-T12 level of thoracic spinal cord, init	*and*
		S22.Ø89A	Unsp fracture of T11-T12 vertebra, init for clos fx	

ICD-9-CM		ICD-10-CM		
806.26	CLOS FRACTURE T7-T12 LEVEL W/CMPL LESION CORD	**S24.113A**	Complete lesion at T7-T10, init	*and*
		S22.069A	Unsp fracture of T7-T8 vertebra, init for clos fx	*or*
		S22.079A	Unsp fracture of T9-T10 vertebra, init for clos fx	
		S24.114A	Complete lesion at T11-T12, init	*and*
		S22.089A	Unsp fracture of T11-T12 vertebra, init for clos fx	
806.27	CLOSED FRACTURE T7-T12 LEVEL W/ANT CORD SYNDROME	**S24.133A**	Anterior cord syndrome at T7-T10, init	*and*
		S22.069A	Unsp fracture of T7-T8 vertebra, init for clos fx	*or*
		S22.079A	Unsp fracture of T9-T10 vertebra, init for clos fx	
		S24.134A	Anterior cord syndrome at T11-T12, init	*and*
		S22.089A	Unsp fracture of T11-T12 vertebra, init for clos fx	
806.28	CLOS FRACTURE T7-T12 LEVEL W/CNTRL CORD SYNDROME	**S24.153A**	Oth incomplete lesion at T7-T10, init	*and*
		S22.069A	Unsp fracture of T7-T8 vertebra, init for clos fx	*or*
		S22.079A	Unsp fracture of T9-T10 vertebra, init for clos fx	
		S24.154A	Oth incomplete lesion at T11-T12, init	*and*
		S22.089A	Unsp fracture of T11-T12 vertebra, init for clos fx	
806.29	CLOS FX T7-T12 LEVL W/OTH SPEC SP CORD INJURY	**S24.153A**	Oth incomplete lesion at T7-T10, init	*and*
		S22.069A	Unsp fracture of T7-T8 vertebra, init for clos fx	*or*
		S22.079A	Unsp fracture of T9-T10 vertebra, init for clos fx	
		S24.154A	Oth incomplete lesion at T11-T12, init	*and*
		S22.089A	Unsp fracture of T11-T12 vertebra, init for clos fx	
806.30	OPEN FX T1-T6 LEVEL W/UNSPEC SPINAL CORD INJURY	**S24.101A**	Unsp injury at T1 level of thoracic spinal cord, init encntr	*and*
		S22.019B	Unsp fracture of first thoracic vertebra, init for opn fx	
		S24.102A	Unsp injury at T2-T6 level of thoracic spinal cord, init	*and*
		S22.029B	Unsp fracture of second thoracic vertebra, init for opn fx	*or*
		S22.039B	Unsp fracture of third thoracic vertebra, init for opn fx	*or*
		S22.049B	Unsp fracture of fourth thoracic vertebra, init for opn fx	*or*
		S22.059B	Unsp fracture of T5-T6 vertebra, init for opn fx	
806.31	OPEN FRACTURE T1-T6 LEVEL W/COMPLETE LESION CORD	**S24.111A**	Complete lesion at T1 level of thoracic spinal cord, init	*and*
		S22.019B	Unsp fracture of first thoracic vertebra, init for opn fx	
		S24.112A	Complete lesion at T2-T6 level of thoracic spinal cord, init	*and*
		S22.029B	Unsp fracture of second thoracic vertebra, init for opn fx	*or*
		S22.039B	Unsp fracture of third thoracic vertebra, init for opn fx	*or*
		S22.049B	Unsp fracture of fourth thoracic vertebra, init for opn fx	*or*
		S22.059B	Unsp fracture of T5-T6 vertebra, init for opn fx	
806.32	OPEN FRACTURE T1-T6 LEVEL W/ANT CORD SYNDROME	**S24.131A**	Anterior cord syndrome at T1, init	*and*
		S22.019B	Unsp fracture of first thoracic vertebra, init for opn fx	
		S24.132A	Anterior cord syndrome at T2-T6, init	*and*
		S22.029B	Unsp fracture of second thoracic vertebra, init for opn fx	*or*
		S22.039B	Unsp fracture of third thoracic vertebra, init for opn fx	*or*
		S22.049B	Unsp fracture of fourth thoracic vertebra, init for opn fx	*or*
		S22.059B	Unsp fracture of T5-T6 vertebra, init for opn fx	
806.33	OPEN FRACTURE T1-T6 LEVEL W/CNTRL CORD SYNDROME	**S24.151A**	Oth incomplete lesion at T1, init	*and*
		S22.019B	Unsp fracture of first thoracic vertebra, init for opn fx	
		S24.152A	Oth incomplete lesion at T2-T6, init	*and*
		S22.029B	Unsp fracture of second thoracic vertebra, init for opn fx	*or*
		S22.039B	Unsp fracture of third thoracic vertebra, init for opn fx	*or*
		S22.049B	Unsp fracture of fourth thoracic vertebra, init for opn fx	*or*
		S22.059B	Unsp fracture of T5-T6 vertebra, init for opn fx	
806.34	OPEN FX T1-T6 LEVL W/OTH SPEC SPINAL CORD INJURY	**S24.151A**	Oth incomplete lesion at T1, init	*and*
		S22.019B	Unsp fracture of first thoracic vertebra, init for opn fx	
		S24.152A	Oth incomplete lesion at T2-T6, init	*and*
		S22.029B	Unsp fracture of second thoracic vertebra, init for opn fx	*or*
		S22.039B	Unsp fracture of third thoracic vertebra, init for opn fx	*or*
		S22.049B	Unsp fracture of fourth thoracic vertebra, init for opn fx	*or*
		S22.059B	Unsp fracture of T5-T6 vertebra, init for opn fx	
806.35	OPEN FX T7-T12 LEVEL W/UNSPEC SPINAL CORD INJURY	**S24.103A**	Unsp injury at T7-T10 level of thoracic spinal cord, init	*and*
		S22.069B	Unsp fracture of T7-T8 vertebra, init for opn fx	*or*
		S22.079B	Unsp fracture of T9-T10 vertebra, init for opn fx	
		S24.104A	Unsp injury at T11-T12 level of thoracic spinal cord, init	*and*
		S22.089B	Unsp fracture of T11-T12 vertebra, init for opn fx	
806.36	OPEN FRACTURE T7-T12 LEVEL W/CMPL LESION CORD	**S24.113A**	Complete lesion at T7-T10, init	*and*
		S22.069B	Unsp fracture of T7-T8 vertebra, init for opn fx	*or*
		S22.079B	Unsp fracture of T9-T10 vertebra, init for opn fx	
		S24.114A	Complete lesion at T11-T12, init	*and*
		S22.089B	Unsp fracture of T11-T12 vertebra, init for opn fx	

Injury and Poisoning

806.26–806.36

ICD-9-CM		ICD-10-CM		
8Ø6.37	OPEN FRACTURE T7-T12 LEVEL W/ANT CORD SYNDROME	**S24.133A**	Anterior cord syndrome at T7-T10, init	*and*
		S22.Ø69B	Unsp fracture of T7-T8 vertebra, init for opn fx	*or*
		S22.Ø79B	Unsp fracture of T9-T10 vertebra, init for opn fx	
		S24.134A	Anterior cord syndrome at T11-T12, init	*and*
		S22.Ø89B	Unsp fracture of T11-T12 vertebra, init for opn fx	
8Ø6.38	OPEN FRACTURE T7-T12 LEVEL W/CNTRL CORD SYNDROME	**S24.153A**	Oth incomplete lesion at T7-T10, init	*and*
		S22.Ø69B	Unsp fracture of T7-T8 vertebra, init for opn fx	*or*
		S22.Ø79B	Unsp fracture of T9-T10 vertebra, init for opn fx	
		S24.154A	Oth incomplete lesion at T11-T12, init	*and*
		S22.Ø89B	Unsp fracture of T11-T12 vertebra, init for opn fx	
8Ø6.39	OPEN FX T7-T12 LEVL W/OTH SPEC SP CORD INJURY	**S24.153A**	Oth incomplete lesion at T7-T10, init	*and*
		S22.Ø69B	Unsp fracture of T7-T8 vertebra, init for opn fx	*or*
		S22.Ø79B	Unsp fracture of T9-T10 vertebra, init for opn fx	
		S24.154A	Oth incomplete lesion at T11-T12, init	*and*
		S22.Ø89B	Unsp fracture of T11-T12 vertebra, init for opn fx	
8Ø6.4	CLOS FRACTURE LUMBAR SPINE W/SPINAL CORD INJURY	**S32.ØØ9A**	Unsp fracture of unsp lumbar vertebra, init for clos fx	*and*
		S34.1Ø9A	Unsp injury to unsp level of lumbar spinal cord, init encntr	*or*
		S34.119A	Complete lesion of unsp level of lumbar spinal cord, init	*or*
		S34.129A	Incomplete lesion of unsp level of lumbar spinal cord, init	
		S32.Ø19A	Unsp fracture of first lumbar vertebra, init for clos fx	*and*
		S34.1Ø1A	Unsp injury to L1 level of lumbar spinal cord, init encntr	*or*
		S34.111A	Complete lesion of L1 level of lumbar spinal cord, init	*or*
		S34.121A	Incomplete lesion of L1 level of lumbar spinal cord, init	
		S32.Ø29A	Unsp fracture of second lumbar vertebra, init for clos fx	*and*
		S34.1Ø2A	Unsp injury to L2 level of lumbar spinal cord, init encntr	*or*
		S34.112A	Complete lesion of L2 level of lumbar spinal cord, init	*or*
		S34.122A	Incomplete lesion of L2 level of lumbar spinal cord, init	
		S32.Ø39A	Unsp fracture of third lumbar vertebra, init for clos fx	*and*
		S34.1Ø3A	Unsp injury to L3 level of lumbar spinal cord, init encntr	*or*
		S34.113A	Complete lesion of L3 level of lumbar spinal cord, init	*or*
		S34.123A	Incomplete lesion of L3 level of lumbar spinal cord, init	
		S32.Ø49A	Unsp fracture of fourth lumbar vertebra, init for clos fx	*and*
		S34.1Ø4A	Unsp injury to L4 level of lumbar spinal cord, init encntr	*or*
		S34.114A	Complete lesion of L4 level of lumbar spinal cord, init	*or*
		S34.124A	Incomplete lesion of L4 level of lumbar spinal cord, init	
		S32.Ø59A	Unsp fracture of fifth lumbar vertebra, init for clos fx	*and*
		S34.1Ø5A	Unsp injury to L5 level of lumbar spinal cord, init encntr	*or*
		S34.115A	Complete lesion of L5 level of lumbar spinal cord, init	*or*
		S34.125A	Incomplete lesion of L5 level of lumbar spinal cord, init	
8Ø6.5	OPEN FRACTURE LUMBAR SPINE W/SPINAL CORD INJURY	**S32.ØØ9B**	Unsp fracture of unsp lumbar vertebra, init for opn fx	*and*
		S34.1Ø9A	Unsp injury to unsp level of lumbar spinal cord, init encntr	*or*
		S34.119A	Complete lesion of unsp level of lumbar spinal cord, init	*or*
		S34.129A	Incomplete lesion of unsp level of lumbar spinal cord, init	
		S32.Ø19B	Unsp fracture of first lumbar vertebra, init for opn fx	*and*
		S34.1Ø1A	Unsp injury to L1 level of lumbar spinal cord, init encntr	*or*
		S34.111A	Complete lesion of L1 level of lumbar spinal cord, init	*or*
		S34.121A	Incomplete lesion of L1 level of lumbar spinal cord, init	
		S32.Ø29B	Unsp fracture of second lumbar vertebra, init for opn fx	*and*
		S34.1Ø2A	Unsp injury to L2 level of lumbar spinal cord, init encntr	*or*
		S34.112A	Complete lesion of L2 level of lumbar spinal cord, init	*or*
		S34.122A	Incomplete lesion of L2 level of lumbar spinal cord, init	
		S32.Ø39B	Unsp fracture of third lumbar vertebra, init for opn fx	*and*
		S34.1Ø3A	Unsp injury to L3 level of lumbar spinal cord, init encntr	*or*
		S34.113A	Complete lesion of L3 level of lumbar spinal cord, init	*or*
		S34.123A	Incomplete lesion of L3 level of lumbar spinal cord, init	
		S32.Ø49B	Unsp fracture of fourth lumbar vertebra, init for opn fx	*and*
		S34.1Ø4A	Unsp injury to L4 level of lumbar spinal cord, init encntr	*or*
		S34.114A	Complete lesion of L4 level of lumbar spinal cord, init	*or*
		S34.124A	Incomplete lesion of L4 level of lumbar spinal cord, init	
		S32.Ø59B	Unsp fracture of fifth lumbar vertebra, init for opn fx	*and*
		S34.1Ø5A	Unsp injury to L5 level of lumbar spinal cord, init encntr	*or*
		S34.115A	Complete lesion of L5 level of lumbar spinal cord, init	*or*
		S34.125A	Incomplete lesion of L5 level of lumbar spinal cord, init	
8Ø6.6Ø	CLOS FX SACRUM&COCCYX WITH UNSPEC SP CORD INJURY	**S34.139A**	Unspecified injury to sacral spinal cord, initial encounter	*and*
		S32.1ØXA	Unsp fracture of sacrum, init encntr for closed fracture	*or*
		S32.2XXA	Fracture of coccyx, initial encounter for closed fracture	

ICD-9-CM		ICD-10-CM		
806.61	CLOS FX SACRUM&COCCYX W/COMPLT CAUDA EQUINA LES	**S34.3XXA**	Injury of cauda equina, initial encounter	*and*
		S32.10XA	Unsp fracture of sacrum, init encntr for closed fracture	*or*
		S32.2XXA	Fracture of coccyx, initial encounter for closed fracture	
806.62	CLOS FX SACRUM&COCCYX W/OTH CAUDA EQUINA INJURY	**S34.3XXA**	Injury of cauda equina, initial encounter	*and*
		S32.10XA	Unsp fracture of sacrum, init encntr for closed fracture	*or*
		S32.2XXA	Fracture of coccyx, initial encounter for closed fracture	
806.69	CLOS FX SACRUM&COCCYX WITH OTH SPINAL CORD INJUR	**S34.131A**	Complete lesion of sacral spinal cord, initial encounter	*or*
		S34.132A	Incomplete lesion of sacral spinal cord, initial encounter	*and*
		S32.10XA	Unsp fracture of sacrum, init encntr for closed fracture	*or*
		S32.2XXA	Fracture of coccyx, initial encounter for closed fracture	
806.70	OPN FX SACRUM&COCCYX WITH UNSPEC SP CORD INJURY	**S34.139A**	Unspecified injury to sacral spinal cord, initial encounter	*and*
		S32.10XB	Unsp fracture of sacrum, init encntr for open fracture	*or*
		S32.2XXB	Fracture of coccyx, initial encounter for open fracture	
806.71	OPN FX SACRUM&COCCYX W/COMPLT CAUDA EQUINA LES	**S34.3XXA**	Injury of cauda equina, initial encounter	*and*
		S32.10XB	Unsp fracture of sacrum, init encntr for open fracture	*or*
		S32.2XXB	Fracture of coccyx, initial encounter for open fracture	
806.72	OPN FX SACRUM&COCCYX WITH OTH CAUDA EQUINA INJUR	**S34.3XXA**	Injury of cauda equina, initial encounter	*and*
		S32.10XB	Unsp fracture of sacrum, init encntr for open fracture	*or*
		S32.2XXB	Fracture of coccyx, initial encounter for open fracture	
806.79	OPN FX SACRUM&COCCYX WITH OTH SPINAL CORD INJURY	**S34.131A**	Complete lesion of sacral spinal cord, initial encounter	*or*
		S34.132A	Incomplete lesion of sacral spinal cord, initial encounter	*and*
		S32.10XB	Unsp fracture of sacrum, init encntr for open fracture	*or*
		S32.2XXB	Fracture of coccyx, initial encounter for open fracture	
806.8	CLOS FX UNSPEC VERTEBRA W/SPINAL CORD INJURY	**S14.109A**	Unsp injury at unsp level of cervical spinal cord, init	*and*
		S12.9XXA	Fracture of neck, unspecified, initial encounter	
		S24.109A	Unsp injury at unsp level of thoracic spinal cord, init	*and*
		S22.009A	Unsp fracture of unsp thoracic vertebra, init for clos fx	
		S34.109A	Unsp injury to unsp level of lumbar spinal cord, init encntr	*and*
		S32.009A	Unsp fracture of unsp lumbar vertebra, init for clos fx	
		S34.139A	Unspecified injury to sacral spinal cord, initial encounter	*and*
		S32.10XA	Unsp fracture of sacrum, init encntr for closed fracture	
806.9	OPEN FX UNSPEC VERTEBRA W/SPINAL CORD INJURY	**S14.109A**	Unsp injury at unsp level of cervical spinal cord, init	*and*
		S12.9XXA	Fracture of neck, unspecified, initial encounter	
		S24.109A	Unsp injury at unsp level of thoracic spinal cord, init	*and*
		S22.009B	Unsp fracture of unsp thoracic vertebra, init for opn fx	
		S34.109A	Unsp injury to unsp level of lumbar spinal cord, init encntr	*and*
		S32.009B	Unsp fracture of unsp lumbar vertebra, init for opn fx	
		S34.139A	Unspecified injury to sacral spinal cord, initial encounter	*and*
		S32.10XB	Unsp fracture of sacrum, init encntr for open fracture	
807.00	CLOSED FRACTURE OF RIB, UNSPECIFIED	**S22.39XA**	Fracture of one rib, unsp side, init for clos fx	
807.01	CLOSED FRACTURE OF ONE RIB	**S22.31XA**	Fracture of one rib, right side, init for clos fx	
		S22.32XA	Fracture of one rib, left side, init for clos fx	
		S22.39XA	Fracture of one rib, unsp side, init for clos fx	
807.02	CLOSED FRACTURE OF TWO RIBS	**S22.41XA**	Multiple fractures of ribs, right side, init for clos fx	
		S22.42XA	Multiple fractures of ribs, left side, init for clos fx	
		S22.43XA	Multiple fractures of ribs, bilateral, init for clos fx	
		S22.49XA	Multiple fractures of ribs, unsp side, init for clos fx	
807.03	CLOSED FRACTURE OF THREE RIBS	**S22.41XA**	Multiple fractures of ribs, right side, init for clos fx	
		S22.42XA	Multiple fractures of ribs, left side, init for clos fx	
		S22.43XA	Multiple fractures of ribs, bilateral, init for clos fx	
		S22.49XA	Multiple fractures of ribs, unsp side, init for clos fx	
807.04	CLOSED FRACTURE OF FOUR RIBS	**S22.41XA**	Multiple fractures of ribs, right side, init for clos fx	
		S22.42XA	Multiple fractures of ribs, left side, init for clos fx	
		S22.43XA	Multiple fractures of ribs, bilateral, init for clos fx	
		S22.49XA	Multiple fractures of ribs, unsp side, init for clos fx	
807.05	CLOSED FRACTURE OF FIVE RIBS	**S22.41XA**	Multiple fractures of ribs, right side, init for clos fx	
		S22.42XA	Multiple fractures of ribs, left side, init for clos fx	
		S22.43XA	Multiple fractures of ribs, bilateral, init for clos fx	
		S22.49XA	Multiple fractures of ribs, unsp side, init for clos fx	
807.06	CLOSED FRACTURE OF SIX RIBS	**S22.41XA**	Multiple fractures of ribs, right side, init for clos fx	
		S22.42XA	Multiple fractures of ribs, left side, init for clos fx	
		S22.43XA	Multiple fractures of ribs, bilateral, init for clos fx	
		S22.49XA	Multiple fractures of ribs, unsp side, init for clos fx	
807.07	CLOSED FRACTURE OF SEVEN RIBS	**S22.41XA**	Multiple fractures of ribs, right side, init for clos fx	
		S22.42XA	Multiple fractures of ribs, left side, init for clos fx	
		S22.43XA	Multiple fractures of ribs, bilateral, init for clos fx	
		S22.49XA	Multiple fractures of ribs, unsp side, init for clos fx	

ICD-9-CM		ICD-10-CM	
807.08	CLOSED FRACTURE OF EIGHT OR MORE RIBS	**S22.41XA**	Multiple fractures of ribs, right side, init for clos fx
		S22.42XA	Multiple fractures of ribs, left side, init for clos fx
		S22.43XA	Multiple fractures of ribs, bilateral, init for clos fx
		S22.49XA	Multiple fractures of ribs, unsp side, init for clos fx
807.09	CLOSED FRACTURE OF MULTIPLE RIBS UNSPECIFIED	**S22.41XA**	Multiple fractures of ribs, right side, init for clos fx
		S22.42XA	Multiple fractures of ribs, left side, init for clos fx
		S22.43XA	Multiple fractures of ribs, bilateral, init for clos fx
		S22.49XA	Multiple fractures of ribs, unsp side, init for clos fx
807.10	OPEN FRACTURE OF RIB, UNSPECIFIED	**S22.39XB**	Fracture of one rib, unsp side, init for opn fx
807.11	OPEN FRACTURE OF ONE RIB	**S22.31XB**	Fracture of one rib, right side, init for opn fx
		S22.32XB	Fracture of one rib, left side, init for opn fx
		S22.39XB	Fracture of one rib, unsp side, init for opn fx
807.12	OPEN FRACTURE OF TWO RIBS	**S22.41XB**	Multiple fractures of ribs, right side, init for opn fx
		S22.42XB	Multiple fractures of ribs, left side, init for opn fx
		S22.43XB	Multiple fractures of ribs, bilateral, init for opn fx
		S22.49XB	Multiple fractures of ribs, unsp side, init for opn fx
807.13	OPEN FRACTURE OF THREE RIBS	**S22.41XB**	Multiple fractures of ribs, right side, init for opn fx
		S22.42XB	Multiple fractures of ribs, left side, init for opn fx
		S22.43XB	Multiple fractures of ribs, bilateral, init for opn fx
		S22.49XB	Multiple fractures of ribs, unsp side, init for opn fx
807.14	OPEN FRACTURE OF FOUR RIBS	**S22.41XB**	Multiple fractures of ribs, right side, init for opn fx
		S22.42XB	Multiple fractures of ribs, left side, init for opn fx
		S22.43XB	Multiple fractures of ribs, bilateral, init for opn fx
		S22.49XB	Multiple fractures of ribs, unsp side, init for opn fx
807.15	OPEN FRACTURE OF FIVE RIBS	**S22.41XB**	Multiple fractures of ribs, right side, init for opn fx
		S22.42XB	Multiple fractures of ribs, left side, init for opn fx
		S22.43XB	Multiple fractures of ribs, bilateral, init for opn fx
		S22.49XB	Multiple fractures of ribs, unsp side, init for opn fx
807.16	OPEN FRACTURE OF SIX RIBS	**S22.41XB**	Multiple fractures of ribs, right side, init for opn fx
		S22.42XB	Multiple fractures of ribs, left side, init for opn fx
		S22.43XB	Multiple fractures of ribs, bilateral, init for opn fx
		S22.49XB	Multiple fractures of ribs, unsp side, init for opn fx
807.17	OPEN FRACTURE OF SEVEN RIBS	**S22.41XB**	Multiple fractures of ribs, right side, init for opn fx
		S22.42XB	Multiple fractures of ribs, left side, init for opn fx
		S22.43XB	Multiple fractures of ribs, bilateral, init for opn fx
		S22.49XB	Multiple fractures of ribs, unsp side, init for opn fx
807.18	OPEN FRACTURE OF EIGHT OR MORE RIBS	**S22.41XB**	Multiple fractures of ribs, right side, init for opn fx
		S22.42XB	Multiple fractures of ribs, left side, init for opn fx
		S22.43XB	Multiple fractures of ribs, bilateral, init for opn fx
		S22.49XB	Multiple fractures of ribs, unsp side, init for opn fx
807.19	OPEN FRACTURE OF MULTIPLE RIBS UNSPECIFIED	**S22.41XB**	Multiple fractures of ribs, right side, init for opn fx
		S22.42XB	Multiple fractures of ribs, left side, init for opn fx
		S22.43XB	Multiple fractures of ribs, bilateral, init for opn fx
		S22.49XB	Multiple fractures of ribs, unsp side, init for opn fx
807.2	CLOSED FRACTURE OF STERNUM	**S22.20XA**	Unsp fracture of sternum, init encntr for closed fracture
		S22.21XA	Fracture of manubrium, initial encounter for closed fracture
		S22.22XA	Fracture of body of sternum, init encntr for closed fracture
		S22.23XA	Sternal manubrial dissociation, init for clos fx
		S22.24XA	Fracture of xiphoid process, init encntr for closed fracture
807.3	OPEN FRACTURE OF STERNUM	**S22.20XB**	Unsp fracture of sternum, init encntr for open fracture
		S22.21XB	Fracture of manubrium, initial encounter for open fracture
		S22.22XB	Fracture of body of sternum, init encntr for open fracture
		S22.23XB	Sternal manubrial dissociation, init for opn fx
		S22.24XB	Fracture of xiphoid process, init encntr for open fracture
807.4	FLAIL CHEST	**S22.5XXA**	Flail chest, initial encounter for closed fracture
		S22.5XXB	Flail chest, initial encounter for open fracture
807.5	CLOSED FRACTURE OF LARYNX AND TRACHEA	**S12.8XXA**	Fracture of other parts of neck, initial encounter
807.6	OPEN FRACTURE OF LARYNX AND TRACHEA	**S12.8XXA**	Fracture of other parts of neck, initial encounter
808.0	CLOSED FRACTURE OF ACETABULUM	**S32.401A**	Unsp fracture of right acetabulum, init for clos fx
		S32.402A	Unsp fracture of left acetabulum, init for clos fx
		S32.409A	Unsp fracture of unsp acetabulum, init for clos fx
		S32.411A	Disp fx of anterior wall of right acetabulum, init
		S32.412A	Disp fx of anterior wall of left acetabulum, init
		S32.413A	Disp fx of anterior wall of unsp acetabulum, init
		S32.414A	Nondisp fx of anterior wall of right acetabulum, init
		S32.415A	Nondisp fx of anterior wall of left acetabulum, init
		S32.416A	Nondisp fx of anterior wall of unsp acetabulum, init
		S32.421A	Disp fx of posterior wall of right acetabulum, init
		S32.422A	Disp fx of posterior wall of left acetabulum, init
		S32.423A	Disp fx of posterior wall of unsp acetabulum, init
		S32.424A	Nondisp fx of posterior wall of right acetabulum, init
		S32.425A	Nondisp fx of posterior wall of left acetabulum, init
		S32.426A	Nondisp fx of posterior wall of unsp acetabulum, init
		S32.431A	Disp fx of anterior column of right acetabulum, init
		S32.432A	Disp fx of anterior column of left acetabulum, init
		S32.433A	Disp fx of anterior column of unsp acetabulum, init
		S32.434A	Nondisp fx of anterior column of right acetabulum, init
	(Continued on next page)	**S32.435A**	Nondisp fx of anterior column of left acetabulum, init

ICD-9-CM		ICD-10-CM	
808.Ø	CLOSED FRACTURE OF ACETABULUM **(Continued)**	**S32.436A**	Nondisp fx of anterior column of unsp acetabulum, init
		S32.441A	Disp fx of posterior column of right acetabulum, init
		S32.442A	Disp fx of posterior column of left acetabulum, init
		S32.443A	Disp fx of posterior column of unsp acetabulum, init
		S32.444A	Nondisp fx of posterior column of right acetabulum, init
		S32.445A	Nondisp fx of posterior column of left acetabulum, init
		S32.446A	Nondisp fx of posterior column of unsp acetabulum, init
		S32.451A	Displaced transverse fracture of right acetabulum, init
		S32.452A	Displaced transverse fracture of left acetabulum, init
		S32.453A	Displaced transverse fracture of unsp acetabulum, init
		S32.454A	Nondisplaced transverse fracture of right acetabulum, init
		S32.455A	Nondisplaced transverse fracture of left acetabulum, init
		S32.456A	Nondisplaced transverse fracture of unsp acetabulum, init
		S32.461A	Displaced associated transv/post fx right acetabulum, init
		S32.462A	Displaced associated transv/post fx left acetabulum, init
		S32.463A	Displaced associated transv/post fx unsp acetabulum, init
		S32.464A	Nondisp associated transv/post fx right acetabulum, init
		S32.465A	Nondisp associated transv/post fx left acetabulum, init
		S32.466A	Nondisp associated transv/post fx unsp acetabulum, init
		S32.471A	Disp fx of medial wall of right acetabulum, init for clos fx
		S32.472A	Disp fx of medial wall of left acetabulum, init for clos fx
		S32.473A	Disp fx of medial wall of unsp acetabulum, init for clos fx
		S32.474A	Nondisp fx of medial wall of right acetabulum, init
		S32.475A	Nondisp fx of medial wall of left acetabulum, init
		S32.476A	Nondisp fx of medial wall of unsp acetabulum, init
		S32.481A	Displaced dome fracture of right acetabulum, init
		S32.482A	Displaced dome fracture of left acetabulum, init for clos fx
		S32.483A	Displaced dome fracture of unsp acetabulum, init for clos fx
		S32.484A	Nondisplaced dome fracture of right acetabulum, init
		S32.485A	Nondisplaced dome fracture of left acetabulum, init
		S32.486A	Nondisplaced dome fracture of unsp acetabulum, init
		S32.491A	Oth fracture of right acetabulum, init for clos fx
		S32.492A	Oth fracture of left acetabulum, init for clos fx
		S32.499A	Oth fracture of unsp acetabulum, init for clos fx
808.1	OPEN FRACTURE OF ACETABULUM	**S32.4Ø1B**	Unsp fracture of right acetabulum, init for opn fx
		S32.4Ø2B	Unsp fracture of left acetabulum, init for opn fx
		S32.4Ø9B	Unsp fracture of unsp acetabulum, init for opn fx
		S32.411B	Disp fx of anterior wall of right acetab, init for opn fx
		S32.412B	Disp fx of anterior wall of left acetabulum, init for opn fx
		S32.413B	Disp fx of anterior wall of unsp acetabulum, init for opn fx
		S32.414B	Nondisp fx of anterior wall of right acetab, init for opn fx
		S32.415B	Nondisp fx of anterior wall of left acetab, init for opn fx
		S32.416B	Nondisp fx of anterior wall of unsp acetab, init for opn fx
		S32.421B	Disp fx of posterior wall of right acetab, init for opn fx
		S32.422B	Disp fx of posterior wall of left acetab, init for opn fx
		S32.423B	Disp fx of posterior wall of unsp acetab, init for opn fx
		S32.424B	Nondisp fx of post wall of right acetab, init for opn fx
		S32.425B	Nondisp fx of posterior wall of left acetab, init for opn fx
		S32.426B	Nondisp fx of posterior wall of unsp acetab, init for opn fx
		S32.431B	Disp fx of anterior column of right acetab, init for opn fx
		S32.432B	Disp fx of anterior column of left acetab, init for opn fx
		S32.433B	Disp fx of anterior column of unsp acetab, init for opn fx
		S32.434B	Nondisp fx of ant column of right acetab, init for opn fx
		S32.435B	Nondisp fx of ant column of left acetab, init for opn fx
		S32.436B	Nondisp fx of ant column of unsp acetab, init for opn fx
		S32.441B	Disp fx of posterior column of right acetab, init for opn fx
		S32.442B	Disp fx of posterior column of left acetab, init for opn fx
		S32.443B	Disp fx of posterior column of unsp acetab, init for opn fx
		S32.444B	Nondisp fx of post column of right acetab, init for opn fx
		S32.445B	Nondisp fx of post column of left acetab, init for opn fx
		S32.446B	Nondisp fx of post column of unsp acetab, init for opn fx
		S32.451B	Displaced transverse fx right acetabulum, init for opn fx
		S32.452B	Displaced transverse fx left acetabulum, init for opn fx
		S32.453B	Displaced transverse fx unsp acetabulum, init for opn fx
		S32.454B	Nondisp transverse fx right acetabulum, init for opn fx
		S32.455B	Nondisp transverse fx left acetabulum, init for opn fx
		S32.456B	Nondisp transverse fx unsp acetabulum, init for opn fx
		S32.461B	Displaced assoc transv/post fx right acetab, init for opn fx
		S32.462B	Displaced assoc transv/post fx left acetab, init for opn fx
		S32.463B	Displaced assoc transv/post fx unsp acetab, init for opn fx
		S32.464B	Nondisp assoc transv/post fx right acetab, init for opn fx
		S32.465B	Nondisp assoc transv/post fx left acetab, init for opn fx
		S32.466B	Nondisp assoc transv/post fx unsp acetab, init for opn fx
		S32.471B	Disp fx of medial wall of right acetabulum, init for opn fx
		S32.472B	Disp fx of medial wall of left acetabulum, init for opn fx
		S32.473B	Disp fx of medial wall of unsp acetabulum, init for opn fx
		S32.474B	Nondisp fx of medial wall of right acetab, init for opn fx
		S32.475B	Nondisp fx of medial wall of left acetab, init for opn fx
		S32.476B	Nondisp fx of medial wall of unsp acetab, init for opn fx
		S32.481B	Displaced dome fracture of right acetabulum, init for opn fx
		S32.482B	Displaced dome fracture of left acetabulum, init for opn fx
	(Continued on next page)	**S32.483B**	Displaced dome fracture of unsp acetabulum, init for opn fx

ICD-9-CM		ICD-10-CM	
808.1	OPEN FRACTURE OF ACETABULUM **(Continued)**	**S32.484B**	Nondisp dome fracture of right acetabulum, init for opn fx
		S32.485B	Nondisp dome fracture of left acetabulum, init for opn fx
		S32.486B	Nondisp dome fracture of unsp acetabulum, init for opn fx
		S32.491B	Oth fracture of right acetabulum, init for opn fx
		S32.492B	Oth fracture of left acetabulum, init for opn fx
		S32.499B	Oth fracture of unsp acetabulum, init for opn fx
808.2	CLOSED FRACTURE OF PUBIS	**S32.501A**	Unsp fracture of right pubis, init for clos fx
		S32.502A	Unsp fracture of left pubis, init encntr for closed fracture
		S32.509A	Unsp fracture of unsp pubis, init encntr for closed fracture
		S32.511A	Fracture of superior rim of right pubis, init for clos fx
		S32.512A	Fracture of superior rim of left pubis, init for clos fx
		S32.519A	Fracture of superior rim of unsp pubis, init for clos fx
		S32.591A	Oth fracture of right pubis, init encntr for closed fracture
		S32.592A	Oth fracture of left pubis, init encntr for closed fracture
		S32.599A	Oth fracture of unsp pubis, init encntr for closed fracture
808.3	OPEN FRACTURE OF PUBIS	**S32.501B**	Unsp fracture of right pubis, init encntr for open fracture
		S32.502B	Unsp fracture of left pubis, init encntr for open fracture
		S32.509B	Unsp fracture of unsp pubis, init encntr for open fracture
		S32.511B	Fracture of superior rim of right pubis, init for opn fx
		S32.512B	Fracture of superior rim of left pubis, init for opn fx
		S32.519B	Fracture of superior rim of unsp pubis, init for opn fx
		S32.591B	Oth fracture of right pubis, init encntr for open fracture
		S32.592B	Oth fracture of left pubis, init encntr for open fracture
		S32.599B	Oth fracture of unsp pubis, init encntr for open fracture
808.41	CLOSED FRACTURE OF ILIUM	**S32.301A**	Unsp fracture of right ilium, init for clos fx
		S32.302A	Unsp fracture of left ilium, init encntr for closed fracture
		S32.309A	Unsp fracture of unsp ilium, init encntr for closed fracture
		S32.311A	Displaced avulsion fracture of right ilium, init for clos fx
		S32.312A	Displaced avulsion fracture of left ilium, init for clos fx
		S32.313A	Displaced avulsion fracture of unsp ilium, init for clos fx
		S32.314A	Nondisplaced avulsion fracture of right ilium, init
		S32.315A	Nondisplaced avulsion fracture of left ilium, init
		S32.316A	Nondisplaced avulsion fracture of unsp ilium, init
		S32.391A	Oth fracture of right ilium, init encntr for closed fracture
		S32.392A	Oth fracture of left ilium, init encntr for closed fracture
		S32.399A	Oth fracture of unsp ilium, init encntr for closed fracture
808.42	CLOSED FRACTURE OF ISCHIUM	**S32.601A**	Unsp fracture of right ischium, init for clos fx
		S32.602A	Unsp fracture of left ischium, init for clos fx
		S32.609A	Unsp fracture of unsp ischium, init for clos fx
		S32.611A	Displaced avulsion fracture of right ischium, init
		S32.612A	Displaced avulsion fracture of left ischium, init
		S32.613A	Displaced avulsion fracture of unsp ischium, init
		S32.614A	Nondisplaced avulsion fracture of right ischium, init
		S32.615A	Nondisplaced avulsion fracture of left ischium, init
		S32.616A	Nondisplaced avulsion fracture of unsp ischium, init
		S32.691A	Oth fracture of right ischium, init for clos fx
		S32.692A	Oth fracture of left ischium, init for clos fx
		S32.699A	Oth fracture of unsp ischium, init for clos fx
808.43	MULTIPLE CLOSED PELVIC FX DISRUPT PELVIC CIRCLE	**S32.810A**	Multiple fx of pelvis w stable disrupt of pelvic ring, init
		S32.811A	Mult fx of pelvis w unstable disrupt of pelvic ring, init
808.44	MX CLOS PELVIC FX W/O DISRUPT PELVIC CIRCLE	**S32.82XA**	Multiple fx of pelvis w/o disrupt of pelvic ring, init
808.49	CLOSED FRACTURE OTH SPECIFIED PART PELVIS OTH	**S32.89XA**	Fracture of oth parts of pelvis, init for clos fx
		S32.9XXA	Fracture of unsp parts of lumbosacral spine and pelvis, init
808.51	OPEN FRACTURE OF ILIUM	**S32.301B**	Unsp fracture of right ilium, init encntr for open fracture
		S32.302B	Unsp fracture of left ilium, init encntr for open fracture
		S32.309B	Unsp fracture of unsp ilium, init encntr for open fracture
		S32.311B	Displaced avulsion fracture of right ilium, init for opn fx
		S32.312B	Displaced avulsion fracture of left ilium, init for opn fx
		S32.313B	Displaced avulsion fracture of unsp ilium, init for opn fx
		S32.314B	Nondisp avulsion fracture of right ilium, init for opn fx
		S32.315B	Nondisp avulsion fracture of left ilium, init for opn fx
		S32.316B	Nondisp avulsion fracture of unsp ilium, init for opn fx
		S32.391B	Other fracture of right ilium, init encntr for open fracture
		S32.392B	Other fracture of left ilium, init encntr for open fracture
		S32.399B	Other fracture of unsp ilium, init encntr for open fracture
808.52	OPEN FRACTURE OF ISCHIUM	**S32.601B**	Unsp fracture of right ischium, init for opn fx
		S32.602B	Unsp fracture of left ischium, init encntr for open fracture
		S32.609B	Unsp fracture of unsp ischium, init encntr for open fracture
		S32.611B	Displaced avulsion fx right ischium, init for opn fx
		S32.612B	Displaced avulsion fracture of left ischium, init for opn fx
		S32.613B	Displaced avulsion fracture of unsp ischium, init for opn fx
		S32.614B	Nondisp avulsion fracture of right ischium, init for opn fx
		S32.615B	Nondisp avulsion fracture of left ischium, init for opn fx
		S32.616B	Nondisp avulsion fracture of unsp ischium, init for opn fx
		S32.691B	Oth fracture of right ischium, init encntr for open fracture
		S32.692B	Oth fracture of left ischium, init encntr for open fracture
		S32.699B	Oth fracture of unsp ischium, init encntr for open fracture
808.53	MULTIPLE OPEN PELVIC FX W/DISRUPT PELVIC CIRCLE	**S32.810B**	Mult fx of pelv w stable disrupt of pelv ring, int for opn fx
		S32.811B	Mult fx of pelv w unstbl disrupt of pelv ring, int for opn fx
808.54	MX OPEN PELVIC FX W/O DISRUPT PELVIC CIRCLE	**S32.82XB**	Mult fx of pelvis w/o disrupt of pelv ring, init for opn fx

 [Brackets] indicate valid character values for each code. Character value meanings provided for each code grouping.

ICD-9-CM		ICD-10-CM	
8Ø8.59	OPEN FRACTURE OTHER SPECIFIED PART PELVIS OTHER	**S32.89XB**	Fracture of oth parts of pelvis, init for opn fx
		S32.9XXB	Fx unsp parts of lumbosacral spine & pelvis, init for opn fx
8Ø8.8	UNSPECIFIED CLOSED FRACTURE OF PELVIS	**S32.9XXA**	Fracture of unsp parts of lumbosacral spine and pelvis, init
8Ø8.9	UNSPECIFIED OPEN FRACTURE OF PELVIS	**S32.9XXB**	Fx unsp parts of lumbosacral spine & pelvis, init for opn fx
8Ø9.Ø	FRACTURE OF BONES OF TRUNK, CLOSED	**S22.9XXA**	Fracture of bony thorax, part unsp, init for clos fx
8Ø9.1	FRACTURE OF BONES OF TRUNK, OPEN	**S22.9XXB**	Fracture of bony thorax, part unsp, init for opn fx
81Ø.ØØ	UNSPECIFIED PART OF CLOSED FRACTURE OF CLAVICLE	**S42.ØØ1A**	Fracture of unsp part of right clavicle, init for clos fx
		S42.ØØ2A	Fracture of unsp part of left clavicle, init for clos fx
		S42.ØØ9A	Fracture of unsp part of unsp clavicle, init for clos fx
81Ø.Ø1	CLOSED FRACTURE OF STERNAL END OF CLAVICLE	**S42.Ø11A**	Anterior disp fx of sternal end of right clavicle, init
		S42.Ø12A	Anterior disp fx of sternal end of left clavicle, init
		S42.Ø13A	Anterior disp fx of sternal end of unsp clavicle, init
		S42.Ø14A	Posterior disp fx of sternal end of right clavicle, init
		S42.Ø15A	Posterior disp fx of sternal end of left clavicle, init
		S42.Ø16A	Posterior disp fx of sternal end of unsp clavicle, init
		S42.Ø17A	Nondisp fx of sternal end of right clavicle, init
		S42.Ø18A	Nondisp fx of sternal end of left clavicle, init for clos fx
		S42.Ø19A	Nondisp fx of sternal end of unsp clavicle, init for clos fx
81Ø.Ø2	CLOSED FRACTURE OF SHAFT OF CLAVICLE	**S42.Ø21A**	Disp fx of shaft of right clavicle, init for clos fx
		S42.Ø22A	Disp fx of shaft of left clavicle, init for clos fx
		S42.Ø23A	Disp fx of shaft of unsp clavicle, init for clos fx
		S42.Ø24A	Nondisp fx of shaft of right clavicle, init for clos fx
		S42.Ø25A	Nondisp fx of shaft of left clavicle, init for clos fx
		S42.Ø26A	Nondisp fx of shaft of unsp clavicle, init for clos fx
81Ø.Ø3	CLOSED FRACTURE OF ACROMIAL END OF CLAVICLE	**S42.Ø31A**	Disp fx of lateral end of right clavicle, init for clos fx
		S42.Ø32A	Disp fx of lateral end of left clavicle, init for clos fx
		S42.Ø33A	Disp fx of lateral end of unsp clavicle, init for clos fx
		S42.Ø34A	Nondisp fx of lateral end of right clavicle, init
		S42.Ø35A	Nondisp fx of lateral end of left clavicle, init for clos fx
		S42.Ø36A	Nondisp fx of lateral end of unsp clavicle, init for clos fx
81Ø.1Ø	UNSPECIFIED PART OF OPEN FRACTURE OF CLAVICLE	**S42.ØØ1B**	Fracture of unsp part of right clavicle, init for opn fx
		S42.ØØ2B	Fracture of unsp part of left clavicle, init for opn fx
		S42.ØØ9B	Fracture of unsp part of unsp clavicle, init for opn fx
81Ø.11	OPEN FRACTURE OF STERNAL END OF CLAVICLE	**S42.Ø11B**	Ant disp fx of sternal end of r clavicle, init for opn fx
		S42.Ø12B	Ant disp fx of sternal end of l clavicle, init for opn fx
		S42.Ø13B	Ant disp fx of sternal end of unsp clavicle, init for opn fx
		S42.Ø14B	Post disp fx of sternal end of r clavicle, init for opn fx
		S42.Ø15B	Post disp fx of sternal end of l clavicle, init for opn fx
		S42.Ø16B	Post disp fx of sternal end unsp clavicle, init for opn fx
		S42.Ø17B	Nondisp fx of sternal end of right clavicle, init for opn fx
		S42.Ø18B	Nondisp fx of sternal end of left clavicle, init for opn fx
		S42.Ø19B	Nondisp fx of sternal end of unsp clavicle, init for opn fx
81Ø.12	OPEN FRACTURE OF SHAFT OF CLAVICLE	**S42.Ø21B**	Disp fx of shaft of right clavicle, init for opn fx
		S42.Ø22B	Disp fx of shaft of left clavicle, init for opn fx
		S42.Ø23B	Disp fx of shaft of unsp clavicle, init for opn fx
		S42.Ø24B	Nondisp fx of shaft of right clavicle, init for opn fx
		S42.Ø25B	Nondisp fx of shaft of left clavicle, init for opn fx
		S42.Ø26B	Nondisp fx of shaft of unsp clavicle, init for opn fx
81Ø.13	OPEN FRACTURE OF ACROMIAL END OF CLAVICLE	**S42.Ø31B**	Disp fx of lateral end of right clavicle, init for opn fx
		S42.Ø32B	Disp fx of lateral end of left clavicle, init for opn fx
		S42.Ø33B	Disp fx of lateral end of unsp clavicle, init for opn fx
		S42.Ø34B	Nondisp fx of lateral end of right clavicle, init for opn fx
		S42.Ø35B	Nondisp fx of lateral end of left clavicle, init for opn fx
		S42.Ø36B	Nondisp fx of lateral end of unsp clavicle, init for opn fx
811.ØØ	CLOSED FRACTURE OF UNSPECIFIED PART OF SCAPULA	**S42.1Ø1A**	Fracture of unsp part of scapula, right shoulder, init
		S42.1Ø2A	Fracture of unsp part of scapula, left shoulder, init
		S42.1Ø9A	Fracture of unsp part of scapula, unsp shoulder, init
811.Ø1	CLOSED FRACTURE OF ACROMIAL PROCESS OF SCAPULA	**S42.121A**	Disp fx of acromial process, right shoulder, init
		S42.122A	Disp fx of acromial process, left shoulder, init for clos fx
		S42.123A	Disp fx of acromial process, unsp shoulder, init for clos fx
		S42.124A	Nondisp fx of acromial process, right shoulder, init
		S42.125A	Nondisp fx of acromial process, left shoulder, init
		S42.126A	Nondisp fx of acromial process, unsp shoulder, init
811.Ø2	CLOSED FRACTURE OF CORACOID PROCESS OF SCAPULA	**S42.131A**	Disp fx of coracoid process, right shoulder, init
		S42.132A	Disp fx of coracoid process, left shoulder, init for clos fx
		S42.133A	Disp fx of coracoid process, unsp shoulder, init for clos fx
		S42.134A	Nondisp fx of coracoid process, right shoulder, init
		S42.135A	Nondisp fx of coracoid process, left shoulder, init
		S42.136A	Nondisp fx of coracoid process, unsp shoulder, init
811.Ø3	CLOSED FRACTURE GLENOID CAVITY&NECK SCAPULA	**S42.141A**	Disp fx of glenoid cavity of scapula, right shoulder, init
		S42.142A	Disp fx of glenoid cavity of scapula, left shoulder, init
		S42.143A	Disp fx of glenoid cavity of scapula, unsp shoulder, init
		S42.144A	Nondisp fx of glenoid cav of scapula, right shoulder, init
		S42.145A	Nondisp fx of glenoid cavity of scapula, left shoulder, init
		S42.146A	Nondisp fx of glenoid cavity of scapula, unsp shoulder, init
		S42.151A	Disp fx of neck of scapula, right shoulder, init for clos fx
		S42.152A	Disp fx of neck of scapula, left shoulder, init for clos fx
	(Continued on next page)	**S42.153A**	Disp fx of neck of scapula, unsp shoulder, init for clos fx

ICD-9-CM		ICD-10-CM	
811.Ø3	CLOSED FRACTURE GLENOID CAVITY&NECK SCAPULA **(Continued)**	**S42.154A**	Nondisp fx of neck of scapula, right shoulder, init
		S42.155A	Nondisp fx of neck of scapula, left shoulder, init
		S42.156A	Nondisp fx of neck of scapula, unsp shoulder, init
811.Ø9	CLOSED FRACTURE OF OTHER PART OF SCAPULA	**S42.111A**	Disp fx of body of scapula, right shoulder, init for clos fx
		S42.112A	Disp fx of body of scapula, left shoulder, init for clos fx
		S42.113A	Disp fx of body of scapula, unsp shoulder, init for clos fx
		S42.114A	Nondisp fx of body of scapula, right shoulder, init
		S42.115A	Nondisp fx of body of scapula, left shoulder, init
		S42.116A	Nondisp fx of body of scapula, unsp shoulder, init
		S42.191A	Fracture of oth part of scapula, right shoulder, init
		S42.192A	Fracture of oth part of scapula, left shoulder, init
		S42.199A	Fracture of oth part of scapula, unsp shoulder, init
811.1Ø	OPEN FRACTURE OF UNSPECIFIED PART OF SCAPULA	**S42.1Ø1B**	Fx unsp part of scapula, r shoulder, init for opn fx
		S42.1Ø2B	Fx unsp part of scapula, l shoulder, init for opn fx
		S42.1Ø9B	Fx unsp part of scapula, unsp shoulder, init for opn fx
811.11	OPEN FRACTURE OF ACROMIAL PROCESS OF SCAPULA	**S42.121B**	Disp fx of acromial process, right shoulder, init for opn fx
		S42.122B	Disp fx of acromial process, left shoulder, init for opn fx
		S42.123B	Disp fx of acromial process, unsp shoulder, init for opn fx
		S42.124B	Nondisp fx of acromial process, r shoulder, init for opn fx
		S42.125B	Nondisp fx of acromial process, l shoulder, init for opn fx
		S42.126B	Nondisp fx of acromial process, unsp shldr, init for opn fx
811.12	OPEN FRACTURE OF CORACOID PROCESS	**S42.131B**	Disp fx of coracoid process, right shoulder, init for opn fx
		S42.132B	Disp fx of coracoid process, left shoulder, init for opn fx
		S42.133B	Disp fx of coracoid process, unsp shoulder, init for opn fx
		S42.134B	Nondisp fx of coracoid process, r shoulder, init for opn fx
		S42.135B	Nondisp fx of coracoid process, l shoulder, init for opn fx
		S42.136B	Nondisp fx of coracoid process, unsp shldr, init for opn fx
811.13	OPEN FRACTURE OF GLENOID CAVITY&NECK OF SCAPULA	**S42.141B**	Disp fx of glenoid cav of scapula, r shldr, init for opn fx
		S42.142B	Disp fx of glenoid cav of scapula, l shldr, init for opn fx
		S42.143B	Disp fx of glenoid cav of scapula, unsp shldr, init opn fx
		S42.144B	Nondisp fx of glenoid cav of scapula, r shldr, init opn fx
		S42.145B	Nondisp fx of glenoid cav of scapula, l shldr, init opn fx
		S42.146B	Nondisp fx of glenoid cav of scapula, unsp shldr, init opn fx
		S42.151B	Disp fx of neck of scapula, right shoulder, init for opn fx
		S42.152B	Disp fx of neck of scapula, left shoulder, init for opn fx
		S42.153B	Disp fx of neck of scapula, unsp shoulder, init for opn fx
		S42.154B	Nondisp fx of neck of scapula, r shoulder, init for opn fx
		S42.155B	Nondisp fx of neck of scapula, l shoulder, init for opn fx
		S42.156B	Nondisp fx of neck of scapula, unsp shldr, init for opn fx
811.19	OPEN FRACTURE OF OTHER PART OF SCAPULA	**S42.111B**	Disp fx of body of scapula, right shoulder, init for opn fx
		S42.112B	Disp fx of body of scapula, left shoulder, init for opn fx
		S42.113B	Disp fx of body of scapula, unsp shoulder, init for opn fx
		S42.114B	Nondisp fx of body of scapula, r shoulder, init for opn fx
		S42.115B	Nondisp fx of body of scapula, l shoulder, init for opn fx
		S42.116B	Nondisp fx of body of scapula, unsp shldr, init for opn fx
		S42.191B	Fracture oth prt scapula, right shoulder, init for opn fx
		S42.192B	Fracture oth prt scapula, left shoulder, init for opn fx
		S42.199B	Fracture oth prt scapula, unsp shoulder, init for opn fx
812.ØØ	CLOSED FRACTURE UNSPEC PART UPPER END HUMERUS	**S42.2Ø1A**	Unsp fracture of upper end of right humerus, init
		S42.2Ø2A	Unsp fracture of upper end of left humerus, init for clos fx
		S42.2Ø9A	Unsp fracture of upper end of unsp humerus, init for clos fx
812.Ø1	CLOSED FRACTURE OF SURGICAL NECK OF HUMERUS	**S42.211A**	Unsp disp fx of surgical neck of right humerus, init
		S42.212A	Unsp disp fx of surgical neck of left humerus, init
		S42.213A	Unsp disp fx of surgical neck of unsp humerus, init
		S42.214A	Unsp nondisp fx of surgical neck of right humerus, init
		S42.215A	Unsp nondisp fx of surgical neck of left humerus, init
		S42.216A	Unsp nondisp fx of surgical neck of unsp humerus, init
		S42.221A	2-part disp fx of surgical neck of right humerus, init
		S42.222A	2-part disp fx of surgical neck of left humerus, init
		S42.223A	2-part disp fx of surgical neck of unsp humerus, init
		S42.224A	2-part nondisp fx of surgical neck of right humerus, init
		S42.225A	2-part nondisp fx of surgical neck of left humerus, init
		S42.226A	2-part nondisp fx of surgical neck of unsp humerus, init
		S42.231A	3-part fracture of surgical neck of right humerus, init
		S42.232A	3-part fracture of surgical neck of left humerus, init
		S42.239A	3-part fracture of surgical neck of unsp humerus, init
		S42.241A	4-part fracture of surgical neck of right humerus, init
		S42.242A	4-part fracture of surgical neck of left humerus, init
		S42.249A	4-part fracture of surgical neck of unsp humerus, init
812.Ø2	CLOSED FRACTURE OF ANATOMICAL NECK OF HUMERUS	**S42.291A**	Oth disp fx of upper end of right humerus, init for clos fx
		S42.292A	Oth disp fx of upper end of left humerus, init for clos fx
		S42.293A	Oth disp fx of upper end of unsp humerus, init for clos fx
		S42.294A	Oth nondisp fx of upper end of right humerus, init
		S42.295A	Oth nondisp fx of upper end of left humerus, init
		S42.296A	Oth nondisp fx of upper end of unsp humerus, init
812.Ø3	CLOSED FRACTURE OF GREATER TUBEROSITY OF HUMERUS	**S42.251A**	Disp fx of greater tuberosity of right humerus, init
		S42.252A	Disp fx of greater tuberosity of left humerus, init
		S42.253A	Disp fx of greater tuberosity of unsp humerus, init
		S42.254A	Nondisp fx of greater tuberosity of right humerus, init
		S42.255A	Nondisp fx of greater tuberosity of left humerus, init
		S42.256A	Nondisp fx of greater tuberosity of unsp humerus, init

ICD-9-CM		ICD-10-CM	
812.09	OTHER CLOSED FRACTURES OF UPPER END OF HUMERUS	**S42.261A**	Disp fx of lesser tuberosity of right humerus, init
		S42.262A	Disp fx of lesser tuberosity of left humerus, init
		S42.263A	Disp fx of lesser tuberosity of unsp humerus, init
		S42.264A	Nondisp fx of lesser tuberosity of right humerus, init
		S42.265A	Nondisp fx of lesser tuberosity of left humerus, init
		S42.266A	Nondisp fx of lesser tuberosity of unsp humerus, init
		S42.271A	Torus fracture of upper end of right humerus, init
		S42.272A	Torus fracture of upper end of left humerus, init
		S42.279A	Torus fracture of upper end of unsp humerus, init
		S42.291A	Oth disp fx of upper end of right humerus, init for clos fx
		S42.292A	Oth disp fx of upper end of left humerus, init for clos fx
		S42.293A	Oth disp fx of upper end of unsp humerus, init for clos fx
		S42.294A	Oth nondisp fx of upper end of right humerus, init
		S42.295A	Oth nondisp fx of upper end of left humerus, init
		S42.296A	Oth nondisp fx of upper end of unsp humerus, init
		S49.001A	Unsp physeal fx upper end of humerus, right arm, init
		S49.002A	Unsp physeal fx upper end of humerus, left arm, init
		S49.009A	Unsp physeal fx upper end of humerus, unsp arm, init
		S49.011A	Sltr-haris Type I physl fx upper end humer, right arm, init
		S49.012A	Sltr-haris Type I physl fx upper end humer, left arm, init
		S49.019A	Sltr-haris Type I physl fx upper end humer, unsp arm, init
		S49.021A	Sltr-haris Type II physl fx upper end humer, right arm, init
		S49.022A	Sltr-haris Type II physl fx upper end humer, left arm, init
		S49.029A	Sltr-haris Type II physl fx upper end humer, unsp arm, init
		S49.031A	Sltr-haris Type III physl fx upper end humer, r arm, init
		S49.032A	Sltr-haris Type III physl fx upper end humer, left arm, init
		S49.039A	Sltr-haris Type III physl fx upper end humer, unsp arm, init
		S49.041A	Sltr-haris Type IV physl fx upper end humer, right arm, init
		S49.042A	Sltr-haris Type IV physl fx upper end humer, left arm, init
		S49.049A	Sltr-haris Type IV physl fx upper end humer, unsp arm, init
		S49.091A	Oth physeal fx upper end of humerus, right arm, init
		S49.092A	Oth physeal fracture of upper end of humerus, left arm, init
		S49.099A	Oth physeal fracture of upper end of humerus, unsp arm, init
812.10	OPEN FRACTURE UNSPECIFIED PART UPPER END HUMERUS	**S42.201B**	Unsp fracture of upper end of right humerus, init for opn fx
		S42.202B	Unsp fracture of upper end of left humerus, init for opn fx
		S42.209B	Unsp fracture of upper end of unsp humerus, init for opn fx
812.11	OPEN FRACTURE OF SURGICAL NECK OF HUMERUS	**S42.211B**	Unsp disp fx of surgical neck of r humerus, init for opn fx
		S42.212B	Unsp disp fx of surgical neck of l humerus, init for opn fx
		S42.213B	Unsp disp fx of surg neck of unsp humerus, init for opn fx
		S42.214B	Unsp nondisp fx of surg neck of r humerus, init for opn fx
		S42.215B	Unsp nondisp fx of surg neck of l humerus, init for opn fx
		S42.216B	Unsp nondisp fx of surg neck of unsp humer, init for opn fx
		S42.221B	2-part disp fx of surg neck of r humerus, init for opn fx
		S42.222B	2-part disp fx of surg neck of l humerus, init for opn fx
		S42.223B	2-part disp fx of surg neck of unsp humerus, init for opn fx
		S42.224B	2-part nondisp fx of surg neck of r humerus, init for opn fx
		S42.225B	2-part nondisp fx of surg neck of l humerus, init for opn fx
		S42.226B	2-part nondisp fx of surg nk of unsp humer, init for opn fx
		S42.231B	3-part fx surgical neck of r humerus, init for opn fx
		S42.232B	3-part fx surgical neck of l humerus, init for opn fx
		S42.239B	3-part fx surgical neck of unsp humerus, init for opn fx
		S42.241B	4-part fx surgical neck of r humerus, init for opn fx
		S42.242B	4-part fx surgical neck of l humerus, init for opn fx
		S42.249B	4-part fx surgical neck of unsp humerus, init for opn fx
812.12	OPEN FRACTURE OF ANATOMICAL NECK OF HUMERUS	**S42.291B**	Oth disp fx of upper end of right humerus, init for opn fx
		S42.292B	Oth disp fx of upper end of left humerus, init for opn fx
		S42.293B	Oth disp fx of upper end of unsp humerus, init for opn fx
		S42.294B	Oth nondisp fx of upper end of r humerus, init for opn fx
		S42.295B	Oth nondisp fx of upper end of left humerus, init for opn fx
		S42.296B	Oth nondisp fx of upper end of unsp humerus, init for opn fx
812.13	OPEN FRACTURE OF GREATER TUBEROSITY OF HUMERUS	**S42.251B**	Disp fx of greater tuberosity of r humerus, init for opn fx
		S42.252B	Disp fx of greater tuberosity of l humerus, init for opn fx
		S42.253B	Disp fx of greater tuberosity of unsp humer, init for opn fx
		S42.254B	Nondisp fx of greater tuberosity of r humer, init for opn fx
		S42.255B	Nondisp fx of greater tuberosity of l humer, init for opn fx
		S42.256B	Nondisp fx of greater tuberosity of unsp humer, init op fx
812.19	OTHER OPEN FRACTURE OF UPPER END OF HUMERUS	**S42.261B**	Disp fx of lesser tuberosity of r humerus, init for opn fx
		S42.262B	Disp fx of lesser tuberosity of l humerus, init for opn fx
		S42.263B	Disp fx of lesser tuberosity of unsp humer, init for opn fx
		S42.264B	Nondisp fx of lesser tuberosity of r humer, init for opn fx
		S42.265B	Nondisp fx of lesser tuberosity of l humer, init for opn fx
		S42.266B	Nondisp fx of less tuberosity of unsp humer, init for opn fx
		S42.291B	Oth disp fx of upper end of right humerus, init for opn fx
		S42.292B	Oth disp fx of upper end of left humerus, init for opn fx
		S42.293B	Oth disp fx of upper end of unsp humerus, init for opn fx
		S42.294B	Oth nondisp fx of upper end of r humerus, init for opn fx
		S42.295B	Oth nondisp fx of upper end of left humerus, init for opn fx
		S42.296B	Oth nondisp fx of upper end of unsp humerus, init for opn fx

ICD-9-CM		ICD-10-CM	
812.2Ø	CLOSED FRACTURE OF UNSPECIFIED PART OF HUMERUS	**S42.3Ø1A**	Unsp fracture of shaft of humerus, right arm, init
		S42.3Ø2A	Unsp fracture of shaft of humerus, left arm, init
		S42.3Ø9A	Unsp fracture of shaft of humerus, unsp arm, init
		S42.9ØXA	Fracture of unsp shoulder girdle, part unsp, init
		S42.91XA	Fracture of right shoulder girdle, part unsp, init
		S42.92XA	Fracture of left shoulder girdle, part unsp, init
812.21	CLOSED FRACTURE OF SHAFT OF HUMERUS	**S42.311A**	Greenstick fracture of shaft of humerus, right arm, init
		S42.312A	Greenstick fracture of shaft of humerus, left arm, init
		S42.319A	Greenstick fracture of shaft of humerus, unsp arm, init
		S42.321A	Displaced transverse fx shaft of humerus, right arm, init
		S42.322A	Displaced transverse fx shaft of humerus, left arm, init
		S42.323A	Displaced transverse fx shaft of humerus, unsp arm, init
		S42.324A	Nondisp transverse fx shaft of humerus, right arm, init
		S42.325A	Nondisp transverse fx shaft of humerus, left arm, init
		S42.326A	Nondisp transverse fx shaft of humerus, unsp arm, init
		S42.331A	Displaced oblique fx shaft of humerus, right arm, init
		S42.332A	Displaced oblique fx shaft of humerus, left arm, init
		S42.333A	Displaced oblique fx shaft of humerus, unsp arm, init
		S42.334A	Nondisp oblique fx shaft of humerus, right arm, init
		S42.335A	Nondisp oblique fracture of shaft of humerus, left arm, init
		S42.336A	Nondisp oblique fracture of shaft of humerus, unsp arm, init
		S42.341A	Displaced spiral fx shaft of humerus, right arm, init
		S42.342A	Displaced spiral fx shaft of humerus, left arm, init
		S42.343A	Displaced spiral fx shaft of humerus, unsp arm, init
		S42.344A	Nondisp spiral fracture of shaft of humerus, right arm, init
		S42.345A	Nondisp spiral fracture of shaft of humerus, left arm, init
		S42.346A	Nondisp spiral fracture of shaft of humerus, unsp arm, init
		S42.351A	Displaced comminuted fx shaft of humerus, right arm, init
		S42.352A	Displaced comminuted fx shaft of humerus, left arm, init
		S42.353A	Displaced comminuted fx shaft of humerus, unsp arm, init
		S42.354A	Nondisp comminuted fx shaft of humerus, right arm, init
		S42.355A	Nondisp comminuted fx shaft of humerus, left arm, init
		S42.356A	Nondisp comminuted fx shaft of humerus, unsp arm, init
		S42.361A	Displaced segmental fx shaft of humerus, right arm, init
		S42.362A	Displaced segmental fx shaft of humerus, left arm, init
		S42.363A	Displaced segmental fx shaft of humerus, unsp arm, init
		S42.364A	Nondisp segmental fx shaft of humerus, right arm, init
		S42.365A	Nondisp segmental fx shaft of humerus, left arm, init
		S42.366A	Nondisp segmental fx shaft of humerus, unsp arm, init
		S42.391A	Oth fracture of shaft of right humerus, init for clos fx
		S42.392A	Oth fracture of shaft of left humerus, init for clos fx
		S42.399A	Oth fracture of shaft of unsp humerus, init for clos fx
812.3Ø	OPEN FRACTURE OF UNSPECIFIED PART OF HUMERUS	**S42.3Ø1B**	Unsp fx shaft of humerus, right arm, init for opn fx
		S42.3Ø2B	Unsp fracture of shaft of humerus, left arm, init for opn fx
		S42.3Ø9B	Unsp fracture of shaft of humerus, unsp arm, init for opn fx
		S42.9ØXB	Fracture of unsp shoulder girdle, part unsp, init for opn fx
		S42.91XB	Fracture of r shoulder girdle, part unsp, init for opn fx
		S42.92XB	Fracture of left shoulder girdle, part unsp, init for opn fx
812.31	OPEN FRACTURE OF SHAFT OF HUMERUS	**S42.321B**	Displ transverse fx shaft of humer, r arm, init for opn fx
		S42.322B	Displ transverse fx shaft of humer, l arm, init for opn fx
		S42.323B	Displ transverse fx shaft of humer, unsp arm, init op fx
		S42.324B	Nondisp transverse fx shaft of humer, r arm, init for opn fx
		S42.325B	Nondisp transverse fx shaft of humer, l arm, init for opn fx
		S42.326B	Nondisp transverse fx shaft of humer, unsp arm, init op fx
		S42.331B	Displ oblique fx shaft of humer, right arm, init for opn fx
		S42.332B	Displ oblique fx shaft of humerus, left arm, init for opn fx
		S42.333B	Displ oblique fx shaft of humerus, unsp arm, init for opn fx
		S42.334B	Nondisp oblique fx shaft of humer, r arm, init for opn fx
		S42.335B	Nondisp oblique fx shaft of humer, left arm, init for opn fx
		S42.336B	Nondisp oblique fx shaft of humer, unsp arm, init for opn fx
		S42.341B	Displ spiral fx shaft of humerus, right arm, init for opn fx
		S42.342B	Displ spiral fx shaft of humerus, left arm, init for opn fx
		S42.343B	Displ spiral fx shaft of humerus, unsp arm, init for opn fx
		S42.344B	Nondisp spiral fx shaft of humer, right arm, init for opn fx
		S42.345B	Nondisp spiral fx shaft of humer, left arm, init for opn fx
		S42.346B	Nondisp spiral fx shaft of humer, unsp arm, init for opn fx
		S42.351B	Displ commnt fx shaft of humerus, right arm, init for opn fx
		S42.352B	Displ commnt fx shaft of humerus, left arm, init for opn fx
		S42.353B	Displ commnt fx shaft of humerus, unsp arm, init for opn fx
		S42.354B	Nondisp commnt fx shaft of humer, right arm, init for opn fx
		S42.355B	Nondisp commnt fx shaft of humer, left arm, init for opn fx
		S42.356B	Nondisp commnt fx shaft of humer, unsp arm, init for opn fx
		S42.361B	Displ seg fx shaft of humerus, right arm, init for opn fx
		S42.362B	Displ seg fx shaft of humerus, left arm, init for opn fx
		S42.363B	Displ seg fx shaft of humerus, unsp arm, init for opn fx
		S42.364B	Nondisp seg fx shaft of humerus, right arm, init for opn fx
		S42.365B	Nondisp seg fx shaft of humerus, left arm, init for opn fx
		S42.366B	Nondisp seg fx shaft of humerus, unsp arm, init for opn fx
		S42.391B	Oth fracture of shaft of right humerus, init for opn fx
		S42.392B	Oth fracture of shaft of left humerus, init for opn fx
		S42.399B	Oth fracture of shaft of unsp humerus, init for opn fx

ICD-9-CM		ICD-10-CM	
812.4Ø	CLOSED FRACTURE UNSPEC PART LOWER END HUMERUS	**S42.4Ø1A**	Unsp fracture of lower end of right humerus, init
		S42.4Ø2A	Unsp fracture of lower end of left humerus, init for clos fx
		S42.4Ø9A	Unsp fracture of lower end of unsp humerus, init for clos fx
812.41	CLOSED FRACTURE OF SUPRACONDYLAR HUMERUS	**S42.411A**	Displ simple suprcndl fx w/o intrcndl fx r humerus, init
		S42.412A	Displ simple suprcndl fx w/o intrcndl fx l humerus, init
		S42.413A	Displ simple suprcndl fx w/o intrcndl fx unsp humerus, init
		S42.414A	Nondisp simple suprcndl fx w/o intrcndl fx r humerus, init
		S42.415A	Nondisp simple suprcndl fx w/o intrcndl fx l humerus, init
		S42.416A	Nondisp simple suprcndl fx w/o intrcndl fx unsp humer, init
		S42.421A	Displ commnt suprcndl fx w/o intrcndl fx r humerus, init
		S42.422A	Displ commnt suprcndl fx w/o intrcndl fx l humerus, init
		S42.423A	Displ commnt suprcndl fx w/o intrcndl fx unsp humerus, init
		S42.424A	Nondisp commnt suprcndl fx w/o intrcndl fx r humerus, init
		S42.425A	Nondisp commnt suprcndl fx w/o intrcndl fx l humerus, init
		S42.426A	Nondisp commnt suprcndl fx w/o intrcndl fx unsp humer, init
812.42	CLOSED FRACTURE OF LATERAL CONDYLE OF HUMERUS	**S42.431A**	Disp fx (avulsion) of lateral epicondyle of r humerus, init
		S42.432A	Disp fx (avulsion) of lateral epicondyle of l humerus, init
		S42.433A	Disp fx of lateral epicondyle of unsp humerus, init
		S42.434A	Nondisp fx of lateral epicondyle of r humerus, init
		S42.435A	Nondisp fx of lateral epicondyle of l humerus, init
		S42.436A	Nondisp fx of lateral epicondyle of unsp humerus, init
		S42.451A	Disp fx of lateral condyle of right humerus, init
		S42.452A	Disp fx of lateral condyle of left humerus, init for clos fx
		S42.453A	Disp fx of lateral condyle of unsp humerus, init for clos fx
		S42.454A	Nondisp fx of lateral condyle of right humerus, init
		S42.455A	Nondisp fx of lateral condyle of left humerus, init
		S42.456A	Nondisp fx of lateral condyle of unsp humerus, init
812.43	CLOSED FRACTURE OF MEDIAL CONDYLE OF HUMERUS	**S42.441A**	Disp fx (avulsion) of medial epicondyle of r humerus, init
		S42.442A	Disp fx (avulsion) of medial epicondyle of l humerus, init
		S42.443A	Disp fx of medial epicondyle of unsp humerus, init
		S42.444A	Nondisp fx of medial epicondyle of r humerus, init
		S42.445A	Nondisp fx of medial epicondyle of l humerus, init
		S42.446A	Nondisp fx of medial epicondyle of unsp humerus, init
		S42.447A	Incarcerated fracture of medial epicondyl of r humerus, init
		S42.448A	Incarcerated fracture of medial epicondyl of l humerus, init
		S42.449A	Incarcerated fx of medial epicondyl of unsp humerus, init
		S42.461A	Disp fx of medial condyle of right humerus, init for clos fx
		S42.462A	Disp fx of medial condyle of left humerus, init for clos fx
		S42.463A	Disp fx of medial condyle of unsp humerus, init for clos fx
		S42.464A	Nondisp fx of medial condyle of right humerus, init
		S42.465A	Nondisp fx of medial condyle of left humerus, init
		S42.466A	Nondisp fx of medial condyle of unsp humerus, init
812.44	CLOSED FRACTURE UNSPECIFIED CONDYLE HUMERUS	**S42.471A**	Displaced transcondylar fracture of right humerus, init
		S42.472A	Displaced transcondylar fracture of left humerus, init
		S42.473A	Displaced transcondylar fracture of unsp humerus, init
		S42.474A	Nondisplaced transcondylar fracture of right humerus, init
		S42.475A	Nondisplaced transcondylar fracture of left humerus, init
		S42.476A	Nondisplaced transcondylar fracture of unsp humerus, init
		S49.1Ø1A	Unsp physeal fx lower end of humerus, right arm, init
		S49.1Ø2A	Unsp physeal fx lower end of humerus, left arm, init
		S49.1Ø9A	Unsp physeal fx lower end of humerus, unsp arm, init
		S49.111A	Sltr-haris Type I physl fx lower end humer, right arm, init
		S49.112A	Sltr-haris Type I physl fx lower end humer, left arm, init
		S49.119A	Sltr-haris Type I physl fx lower end humer, unsp arm, init
		S49.121A	Sltr-haris Type II physl fx lower end humer, right arm, init
		S49.122A	Sltr-haris Type II physl fx lower end humer, left arm, init
		S49.129A	Sltr-haris Type II physl fx lower end humer, unsp arm, init
		S49.131A	Sltr-haris Type III physl fx low end humer, right arm, init
		S49.132A	Sltr-haris Type III physl fx lower end humer, left arm, init
		S49.139A	Sltr-haris Type III physl fx lower end humer, unsp arm, init
		S49.141A	Sltr-haris Type IV physl fx lower end humer, right arm, init
		S49.142A	Sltr-haris Type IV physl fx lower end humer, left arm, init
		S49.149A	Sltr-haris Type IV physl fx lower end humer, unsp arm, init
		S49.191A	Oth physeal fx lower end of humerus, right arm, init
		S49.192A	Oth physeal fracture of lower end of humerus, left arm, init
		S49.199A	Oth physeal fracture of lower end of humerus, unsp arm, init
812.49	OTHER CLOSED FRACTURE OF LOWER END OF HUMERUS	**S42.481A**	Torus fracture of lower end of right humerus, init
		S42.482A	Torus fracture of lower end of left humerus, init
		S42.489A	Torus fracture of lower end of unsp humerus, init
		S42.491A	Oth disp fx of lower end of right humerus, init for clos fx
		S42.492A	Oth disp fx of lower end of left humerus, init for clos fx
		S42.493A	Oth disp fx of lower end of unsp humerus, init for clos fx
		S42.494A	Oth nondisp fx of lower end of right humerus, init
		S42.495A	Oth nondisp fx of lower end of left humerus, init
		S42.496A	Oth nondisp fx of lower end of unsp humerus, init
812.5Ø	OPEN FRACTURE UNSPECIFIED PART LOWER END HUMERUS	**S42.4Ø1B**	Unsp fracture of lower end of right humerus, init for opn fx
		S42.4Ø2B	Unsp fracture of lower end of left humerus, init for opn fx
		S42.4Ø9B	Unsp fracture of lower end of unsp humerus, init for opn fx

ICD-9-CM		ICD-10-CM	
812.51	OPEN FRACTURE OF SUPRACONDYLAR HUMERUS	S42.411B	Displ simp suprcndl fx w/o intrcndl fx r humer, init opn fx
		S42.412B	Displ simp suprcndl fx w/o intrcndl fx l humer, init opn fx
		S42.413B	Displ simp suprcndl fx w/o intrcndl fx unsp humer, init opn fx
		S42.414B	Nondisp simp suprcndl fx w/o intrcndl fx r humer, init opn fx
		S42.415B	Nondisp simp suprcndl fx w/o intrcndl fx l humer, init opn fx
		S42.416B	Nondisp simp suprcndl fx w/o intrcndl fx unsp humer, init opn fx
		S42.421B	Displ commnt suprcndl fx w/o intrcndl fx r humer, init opn fx
		S42.422B	Displ commnt suprcndl fx w/o intrcndl fx l humer, init opn fx
		S42.423B	Displ commnt suprcndl fx w/o intrcndl fx unsp humer, init opn fx
		S42.424B	Nondisp commnt suprcndl fx w/o intrcndl fx r humer, init opn fx
		S42.425B	Nondisp commnt suprcndl fx w/o intrcndl fx l humer, init opn fx
		S42.426B	Nondisp commnt suprcndl fx w/o intrcndl fx unsp humer, init opn fx
812.52	OPEN FRACTURE OF LATERAL CONDYLE OF HUMERUS	S42.431B	Disp fx of lateral epicondyle of r humerus, init for opn fx
		S42.432B	Disp fx of lateral epicondyle of l humerus, init for opn fx
		S42.433B	Disp fx of lateral epicondyl of unsp humer, init for opn fx
		S42.434B	Nondisp fx of lateral epicondyl of r humer, init for opn fx
		S42.435B	Nondisp fx of lateral epicondyl of l humer, init for opn fx
		S42.436B	Nondisp fx of lateral epicondyl of unsp humer, init opn fx
		S42.451B	Disp fx of lateral condyle of right humerus, init for opn fx
		S42.452B	Disp fx of lateral condyle of left humerus, init for opn fx
		S42.453B	Disp fx of lateral condyle of unsp humerus, init for opn fx
		S42.454B	Nondisp fx of lateral condyle of r humerus, init for opn fx
		S42.455B	Nondisp fx of lateral condyle of l humerus, init for opn fx
		S42.456B	Nondisp fx of lateral condyle of unsp humer, init for opn fx
812.53	OPEN FRACTURE OF MEDIAL CONDYLE OF HUMERUS	S42.441B	Disp fx of medial epicondyle of r humerus, init for opn fx
		S42.442B	Disp fx of medial epicondyle of l humerus, init for opn fx
		S42.443B	Disp fx of medial epicondyl of unsp humerus, init for opn fx
		S42.444B	Nondisp fx of medial epicondyl of r humerus, init for opn fx
		S42.445B	Nondisp fx of medial epicondyl of l humerus, init for opn fx
		S42.446B	Nondisp fx of med epicondyl of unsp humer, init for opn fx
		S42.447B	Incarcerated fx of med epicondyl of r humer, init for opn fx
		S42.448B	Incarcerated fx of med epicondyl of l humer, init for opn fx
		S42.449B	Incarcerated fx of med epicondyl of unsp humer, init opn fx
		S42.461B	Disp fx of medial condyle of right humerus, init for opn fx
		S42.462B	Disp fx of medial condyle of left humerus, init for opn fx
		S42.463B	Disp fx of medial condyle of unsp humerus, init for opn fx
		S42.464B	Nondisp fx of medial condyle of r humerus, init for opn fx
		S42.465B	Nondisp fx of medial condyle of l humerus, init for opn fx
		S42.466B	Nondisp fx of medial condyle of unsp humer, init for opn fx
812.54	OPEN FRACTURE OF UNSPECIFIED CONDYLE OF HUMERUS	S42.471B	Displaced transcondy fracture of r humerus, init for opn fx
		S42.472B	Displaced transcondy fracture of l humerus, init for opn fx
		S42.473B	Displaced transcondy fx unsp humerus, init for opn fx
		S42.474B	Nondisp transcondy fracture of r humerus, init for opn fx
		S42.475B	Nondisp transcondy fracture of l humerus, init for opn fx
		S42.476B	Nondisp transcondy fracture of unsp humerus, init for opn fx
812.59	OTHER OPEN FRACTURE OF LOWER END OF HUMERUS	S42.491B	Oth disp fx of lower end of right humerus, init for opn fx
		S42.492B	Oth disp fx of lower end of left humerus, init for opn fx
		S42.493B	Oth disp fx of lower end of unsp humerus, init for opn fx
		S42.494B	Oth nondisp fx of lower end of r humerus, init for opn fx
		S42.495B	Oth nondisp fx of lower end of left humerus, init for opn fx
		S42.496B	Oth nondisp fx of lower end of unsp humerus, init for opn fx
813.00	UNSPEC FX RADIUS&ULNA UPPER END FORARM CLOS	S52.90XA	Unsp fracture of unsp forearm, init for clos fx
813.01	CLOSED FRACTURE OF OLECRANON PROCESS OF ULNA	S52.021A	Disp fx of olecran pro w/o intartic extn right ulna, init
		S52.022A	Disp fx of olecran pro w/o intartic extn left ulna, init
		S52.023A	Disp fx of olecran pro w/o intartic extn unsp ulna, init
		S52.024A	Nondisp fx of olecran pro w/o intartic extn right ulna, init
		S52.025A	Nondisp fx of olecran pro w/o intartic extn left ulna, init
		S52.026A	Nondisp fx of olecran pro w/o intartic extn unsp ulna, init
		S52.031A	Disp fx of olecran pro w intartic extn right ulna, init
		S52.032A	Disp fx of olecran pro w intartic extn left ulna, init
		S52.033A	Disp fx of olecran pro w intartic extn unsp ulna, init
		S52.034A	Nondisp fx of olecran pro w intartic extn right ulna, init
		S52.035A	Nondisp fx of olecran pro w intartic extn left ulna, init
		S52.036A	Nondisp fx of olecran pro w intartic extn unsp ulna, init
813.02	CLOSED FRACTURE OF CORONOID PROCESS OF ULNA	S52.041A	Disp fx of coronoid process of right ulna, init for clos fx
		S52.042A	Disp fx of coronoid process of left ulna, init for clos fx
		S52.043A	Disp fx of coronoid process of unsp ulna, init for clos fx
		S52.044A	Nondisp fx of coronoid process of right ulna, init
		S52.045A	Nondisp fx of coronoid process of left ulna, init
		S52.046A	Nondisp fx of coronoid process of unsp ulna, init
813.03	CLOSED MONTEGGIAS FRACTURE	S52.271A	Monteggia's fracture of right ulna, init for clos fx
		S52.272A	Monteggia's fracture of left ulna, init for clos fx
		S52.279A	Monteggia's fracture of unsp ulna, init for clos fx
813.04	OTHER&UNSPEC CLOSED FRACTURES PROXIMAL END ULNA	S52.001A	Unsp fracture of upper end of right ulna, init for clos fx
		S52.002A	Unsp fracture of upper end of left ulna, init for clos fx
		S52.009A	Unsp fracture of upper end of unsp ulna, init for clos fx
		S52.091A	Oth fracture of upper end of right ulna, init for clos fx
		S52.092A	Oth fracture of upper end of left ulna, init for clos fx
		S52.099A	Oth fracture of upper end of unsp ulna, init for clos fx

[Brackets] indicate valid character values for each code. Character value meanings provided for each code grouping.

ICD-9-CM		ICD-10-CM		
813.05	CLOSED FRACTURE OF HEAD OF RADIUS	**S52.121A**	Disp fx of head of right radius, init for clos fx	
		S52.122A	Disp fx of head of left radius, init for clos fx	
		S52.123A	Disp fx of head of unsp radius, init for clos fx	
		S52.124A	Nondisp fx of head of right radius, init for clos fx	
		S52.125A	Nondisp fx of head of left radius, init for clos fx	
		S52.126A	Nondisp fx of head of unsp radius, init for clos fx	
813.06	CLOSED FRACTURE OF NECK OF RADIUS	**S52.131A**	Disp fx of neck of right radius, init for clos fx	
		S52.132A	Disp fx of neck of left radius, init for clos fx	
		S52.133A	Disp fx of neck of unsp radius, init for clos fx	
		S52.134A	Nondisp fx of neck of right radius, init for clos fx	
		S52.135A	Nondisp fx of neck of left radius, init for clos fx	
		S52.136A	Nondisp fx of neck of unsp radius, init for clos fx	
813.07	OTH&UNSPEC CLOSED FRACTURES PROXIMAL END RADIUS	**S52.101A**	Unsp fracture of upper end of right radius, init for clos fx	
		S52.102A	Unsp fracture of upper end of left radius, init for clos fx	
		S52.109A	Unsp fracture of upper end of unsp radius, init for clos fx	
		S52.181A	Oth fracture of upper end of right radius, init for clos fx	
		S52.182A	Oth fracture of upper end of left radius, init for clos fx	
		S52.189A	Oth fracture of upper end of unsp radius, init for clos fx	
		S59.101A	Unsp physeal fracture of upper end radius, right arm, init	
		S59.102A	Unsp physeal fracture of upper end of radius, left arm, init	
		S59.109A	Unsp physeal fracture of upper end of radius, unsp arm, init	
		S59.111A	Sltr-haris Type I physl fx upper end radius, right arm, init	
		S59.112A	Sltr-haris Type I physl fx upper end radius, left arm, init	
		S59.119A	Sltr-haris Type I physl fx upper end radius, unsp arm, init	
		S59.121A	Sltr-haris Type II physl fx upper end rad, right arm, init	
		S59.122A	Sltr-haris Type II physl fx upper end radius, left arm, init	
		S59.129A	Sltr-haris Type II physl fx upper end radius, unsp arm, init	
		S59.131A	Sltr-haris Type III physl fx upper end rad, right arm, init	
		S59.132A	Sltr-haris Type III physl fx upper end rad, left arm, init	
		S59.139A	Sltr-haris Type III physl fx upper end rad, unsp arm, init	
		S59.141A	Sltr-haris Type IV physl fx upper end rad, right arm, init	
		S59.142A	Sltr-haris Type IV physl fx upper end radius, left arm, init	
		S59.149A	Sltr-haris Type IV physl fx upper end radius, unsp arm, init	
		S59.191A	Oth physeal fracture of upper end of radius, right arm, init	
		S59.192A	Oth physeal fracture of upper end of radius, left arm, init	
		S59.199A	Oth physeal fracture of upper end of radius, unsp arm, init	
813.08	CLOSED FRACTURE OF RADIUS WITH ULNA UPPER END	**S52.109A**	Unsp fracture of upper end of unsp radius, init for clos fx	*and*
		S52.009A	Unsp fracture of upper end of unsp ulna, init for clos fx	
813.10	UNSPECIFIED OPEN FRACTURE UPPER END FOREARM	**S52.90XB**	Unsp fracture of unsp forearm, init for opn fx type I/2	
		S52.90XC	Unsp fracture of unsp forearm, init for opn fx type 3A/B/C	
813.11	OPEN FRACTURE OF OLECRANON PROCESS OF ULNA	**S52.021B**	Disp fx of olecran pro w/o intartic extn r ulna, init opn fx 1/2	
		S52.021C	Disp fx of olecran pro w/o intartic extn r ulna, init opn fx 3 A/B/C	
		S52.022B	Disp fx of olecran pro w/o intartic extn l ulna, init opn fx 1/2	
		S52.022C	Disp fx of olecran pro w/o intartic extn l ulna, init opn fx 3 A/B/C	
		S52.023B	Disp fx of olecran pro w/o intartic extn unsp ulna, init opn fx 1/2	
		S52.023C	Disp fx of olecran pro w/o intartic extn unsp ulna, init opn fx 3 A/B/C	
		S52.024B	Nondisp fx of olecran pro w/o intartic extn r ulna, init opn fx 1/2	
		S52.024C	Nondisp fx of olecran pro w/o intartic extn r ulna, init opn fx 3 A/B/C	
		S52.025B	Nondisp fx of olecran pro w/o intartic extn l ulna, init opn fx 1/2	
		S52.025C	Nondisp fx of olecran pro w/o intartic extn l ulna, init opn fx 3 A/B/C	
		S52.026B	Nondisp fx of olecran pro w/o intartic extn unsp ulna, init opn fx 1/2	
		S52.026C	Nondisp fx of olecran pro w/o intartic extn unsp ulna, init opn fx 3 A/B/C	
		S52.031B	Disp fx of olecran pro w intartic extn r ulna, init opn fx 1/2	
		S52.031C	Disp fx of olecran pro w intartic extn r ulna, init opn fx 3 A/B/C	
		S52.032B	Disp fx of olecran pro w Intartic extn l ulna, init opn fx 1/2	
		S52.032C	Disp fx of olecran pro w intartic extn l ulna, init opn fx 3 A/B/C	
		S52.033B	Disp fx of olecran pro w intartic extn unsp ulna, init opn fx 1/2	
		S52.033C	Disp fx of olecran pro w intartic extn unsp ulna, init opn fx 3 A/B/C	
		S52.034B	Nondisp fx of olecran pro w intartic extn r ulna, init opn fx 1/2	
		S52.034C	Nondisp fx of olecran pro w intartic extn r ulna, init opn fx 3 A/B/C	
		S52.035B	Nondisp fx of olecran pro w intartic extn l ulna, init opn fx 1/2	
		S52.035C	Nondisp fx of olecran pro w intartic extn l ulna, init opn fx 3 A/B/C	
		S52.036B	Nondisp fx of olecran pro w intartic extn unsp ulna, init opn fx 1/2	
		S52.036C	Nondisp fx of olecran pro w intartic extn unsp ulna, init opn fx 3 A/B/C	
813.12	OPEN FRACTURE OF CORONOID PROCESS OF ULNA	**S52.041B**	Disp fx of coronoid pro of r ulna, init for opn fx type I/2	
		S52.041C	Disp fx of coronoid pro of r ulna,init opn fx 3 A/B/C	
		S52.042B	Disp fx of coronoid pro of l ulna, init for opn fx type I/2	
		S52.042C	Disp fx of coronoid pro of l ulna, init opn fx 3 A/B/C	
		S52.043B	Disp fx of coronoid pro of unsp ulna, init opn fx 1/2	
		S52.043C	Disp fx of coronoid pro of unsp ulna, init opn fx 3 A/B/C	
		S52.044B	Nondisp fx of coronoid pro of r ulna, init opn fx 1/2	
		S52.044C	Nondisp fx of coronoid pro of r ulna, init opn fx 3 A/B/C	
		S52.045B	Nondisp fx of coronoid pro of l ulna, init opn fx 1/2	
		S52.045C	Nondisp fx of coronoid pro of l ulna, init opn fx 3 A/B/C	
		S52.046B	Nondisp fx of coronoid pro of unsp ulna, init opn fx 1/2	
		S52.046C	Nondisp fx of coronoid pro of unsp ulna, init opn fx 3 A/B/C	

ICD-9-CM		ICD-10-CM		
813.13	OPEN MONTEGGIAS FRACTURE	**S52.271B**	Monteggia's fracture of right ulna, init for opn fx type I/2	
		S52.271C	Monteggia's fx right ulna, init for opn fx type 3A/B/C	
		S52.272B	Monteggia's fracture of left ulna, init for opn fx type I/2	
		S52.272C	Monteggia's fx left ulna, init for opn fx type 3A/B/C	
		S52.279B	Monteggia's fracture of unsp ulna, init for opn fx type I/2	
		S52.279C	Monteggia's fx unsp ulna, init for opn fx type 3A/B/C	
813.14	OTHER&UNSPEC OPEN FRACTURES PROXIMAL END ULNA	**S52.001B**	Unsp fx upper end of right ulna, init for opn fx type I/2	
		S52.001C	Unsp fx upper end of right ulna, init for opn fx type 3A/B/C	
		S52.002B	Unsp fx upper end of left ulna, init for opn fx type I/2	
		S52.002C	Unsp fx upper end of left ulna, init for opn fx type 3A/B/C	
		S52.009B	Unsp fx upper end of unsp ulna, init for opn fx type I/2	
		S52.009C	Unsp fx upper end of unsp ulna, init for opn fx type 3A/B/C	
		S52.091B	Oth fx upper end of right ulna, init for opn fx type I/2	
		S52.091C	Oth fx upper end of right ulna, init for opn fx type 3A/B/C	
		S52.092B	Oth fx upper end of left ulna, init for opn fx type I/2	
		S52.092C	Oth fx upper end of left ulna, init for opn fx type 3A/B/C	
		S52.099B	Oth fx upper end of unsp ulna, init for opn fx type I/2	
		S52.099C	Oth fx upper end of unsp ulna, init for opn fx type 3A/B/C	
813.15	OPEN FRACTURE OF HEAD OF RADIUS	**S52.121B**	Disp fx of head of right radius, init for opn fx type I/2	
		S52.121C	Disp fx of head of right radius, init for opn fx type 3A/B/C	
		S52.122B	Disp fx of head of left radius, init for opn fx type I/2	
		S52.122C	Disp fx of head of left radius, init for opn fx type 3A/B/C	
		S52.123B	Disp fx of head of unsp radius, init for opn fx type I/2	
		S52.123C	Disp fx of head of unsp radius, init for opn fx type 3A/B/C	
		S52.124B	Nondisp fx of head of right radius, init for opn fx type I/2	
		S52.124C	Nondisp fx of head of r radius, init for opn fx type 3A/B/C	
		S52.125B	Nondisp fx of head of left radius, init for opn fx type I/2	
		S52.125C	Nondisp fx of head of left rad, init for opn fx type 3A/B/C	
		S52.126B	Nondisp fx of head of unsp radius, init for opn fx type I/2	
		S52.126C	Nondisp fx of head of unsp rad, init for opn fx type 3A/B/C	
813.16	OPEN FRACTURE OF NECK OF RADIUS	**S52.131B**	Disp fx of neck of right radius, init for opn fx type I/2	
		S52.131C	Disp fx of neck of right radius, init for opn fx type 3A/B/C	
		S52.132B	Disp fx of neck of left radius, init for opn fx type I/2	
		S52.132C	Disp fx of neck of left radius, init for opn fx type 3A/B/C	
		S52.133B	Disp fx of neck of unsp radius, init for opn fx type I/2	
		S52.133C	Disp fx of neck of unsp radius, init for opn fx type 3A/B/C	
		S52.134B	Nondisp fx of neck of right radius, init for opn fx type I/2	
		S52.134C	Nondisp fx of neck of r radius, init for opn fx type 3A/B/C	
		S52.135B	Nondisp fx of neck of left radius, init for opn fx type I/2	
		S52.135C	Nondisp fx of neck of left rad, init for opn fx type 3A/B/C	
		S52.136B	Nondisp fx of neck of unsp radius, init for opn fx type I/2	
		S52.136C	Nondisp fx of neck of unsp rad, init for opn fx type 3A/B/C	
813.17	OTHER&UNSPEC OPEN FRACTURES PROXIMAL END RADIUS	**S52.101B**	Unsp fx upper end of r radius, init for opn fx type I/2	
		S52.101C	Unsp fx upper end of r radius, init for opn fx type 3A/B/C	
		S52.102B	Unsp fx upper end of left radius, init for opn fx type I/2	
		S52.102C	Unsp fx upper end left radius, init for opn fx type 3A/B/C	
		S52.109B	Unsp fx upper end of unsp radius, init for opn fx type I/2	
		S52.109C	Unsp fx upper end unsp radius, init for opn fx type 3A/B/C	
		S52.181B	Oth fx upper end of r radius, init for opn fx type I/2	
		S52.181C	Oth fx upper end of r radius, init for opn fx type 3A/B/C	
		S52.182B	Oth fx upper end of left radius, init for opn fx type I/2	
		S52.182C	Oth fx upper end of left radius, init for opn fx type 3A/B/C	
		S52.189B	Oth fx upper end of unsp radius, init for opn fx type I/2	
		S52.189C	Oth fx upper end of unsp radius, init for opn fx type 3A/B/C	
813.18	OPEN FRACTURE OF RADIUS WITH ULNA UPPER END	**S52.109B**	Unsp fx upper end of unsp radius, init for opn fx type I/2	*and*
		S52.009B	Unsp fx upper end of unsp ulna, init for opn fx type I/2	*or*
		S52.009C	Unsp fx upper end of unsp ulna, init for opn fx type 3A/B/C	
		S52.109C	Unsp fx upper end unsp radius, init for opn fx type 3A/B/C	*and*
		S52.009B	Unsp fx upper end of unsp ulna, init for opn fx type I/2	*or*
		S52.009C	Unsp fx upper end of unsp ulna, init for opn fx type 3A/B/C	
813.20	UNSPECIFIED CLOSED FRACTURE SHAFT RADIUS OR ULNA	**S52.90XA**	Unsp fracture of unsp forearm, init for clos fx	
813.21	CLOSED FRACTURE OF SHAFT OF RADIUS	**S52.301A**	Unsp fracture of shaft of right radius, init for clos fx	
		S52.302A	Unsp fracture of shaft of left radius, init for clos fx	
		S52.309A	Unsp fracture of shaft of unsp radius, init for clos fx	
		S52.311A	Greenstick fracture of shaft of radius, right arm, init	
		S52.312A	Greenstick fracture of shaft of radius, left arm, init	
		S52.319A	Greenstick fracture of shaft of radius, unsp arm, init	
		S52.321A	Displaced transverse fracture of shaft of right radius, init	
		S52.322A	Displaced transverse fracture of shaft of left radius, init	
		S52.323A	Displaced transverse fracture of shaft of unsp radius, init	
		S52.324A	Nondisp transverse fracture of shaft of right radius, init	
		S52.325A	Nondisp transverse fracture of shaft of left radius, init	
		S52.326A	Nondisp transverse fracture of shaft of unsp radius, init	
		S52.331A	Displaced oblique fracture of shaft of right radius, init	
		S52.332A	Displaced oblique fracture of shaft of left radius, init	
		S52.333A	Displaced oblique fracture of shaft of unsp radius, init	
		S52.334A	Nondisplaced oblique fracture of shaft of right radius, init	
		S52.335A	Nondisplaced oblique fracture of shaft of left radius, init	
		S52.336A	Nondisplaced oblique fracture of shaft of unsp radius, init	
	(Continued on next page)	**S52.341A**	Displaced spiral fx shaft of radius, right arm, init	

ICD-9-CM		ICD-10-CM	
813.21	CLOSED FRACTURE OF SHAFT OF RADIUS **(Continued)**	**S52.342A**	Displaced spiral fracture of shaft of radius, left arm, init
		S52.343A	Displaced spiral fracture of shaft of radius, unsp arm, init
		S52.344A	Nondisp spiral fracture of shaft of radius, right arm, init
		S52.345A	Nondisp spiral fracture of shaft of radius, left arm, init
		S52.346A	Nondisp spiral fracture of shaft of radius, unsp arm, init
		S52.351A	Displaced comminuted fx shaft of radius, right arm, init
		S52.352A	Displaced comminuted fx shaft of radius, left arm, init
		S52.353A	Displaced comminuted fx shaft of radius, unsp arm, init
		S52.354A	Nondisp comminuted fx shaft of radius, right arm, init
		S52.355A	Nondisp comminuted fx shaft of radius, left arm, init
		S52.356A	Nondisp comminuted fx shaft of radius, unsp arm, init
		S52.361A	Displaced segmental fx shaft of radius, right arm, init
		S52.362A	Displaced segmental fx shaft of radius, left arm, init
		S52.363A	Displaced segmental fx shaft of radius, unsp arm, init
		S52.364A	Nondisp segmental fx shaft of radius, right arm, init
		S52.365A	Nondisp segmental fx shaft of radius, left arm, init
		S52.366A	Nondisp segmental fx shaft of radius, unsp arm, init
		S52.371A	Galeazzi's fracture of right radius, init for clos fx
		S52.372A	Galeazzi's fracture of left radius, init for clos fx
		S52.379A	Galeazzi's fracture of unsp radius, init for clos fx
		S52.381A	Bent bone of right radius, init encntr for closed fracture
		S52.382A	Bent bone of left radius, init encntr for closed fracture
		S52.389A	Bent bone of unsp radius, init encntr for closed fracture
		S52.391A	Oth fracture of shaft of radius, right arm, init for clos fx
		S52.392A	Oth fracture of shaft of radius, left arm, init for clos fx
		S52.399A	Oth fracture of shaft of radius, unsp arm, init for clos fx
813.22	CLOSED FRACTURE OF SHAFT OF ULNA	**S52.201A**	Unsp fracture of shaft of right ulna, init for clos fx
		S52.202A	Unsp fracture of shaft of left ulna, init for clos fx
		S52.209A	Unsp fracture of shaft of unsp ulna, init for clos fx
		S52.211A	Greenstick fracture of shaft of right ulna, init for clos fx
		S52.212A	Greenstick fracture of shaft of left ulna, init for clos fx
		S52.219A	Greenstick fracture of shaft of unsp ulna, init for clos fx
		S52.221A	Displaced transverse fracture of shaft of right ulna, init
		S52.222A	Displaced transverse fracture of shaft of left ulna, init
		S52.223A	Displaced transverse fracture of shaft of unsp ulna, init
		S52.224A	Nondisp transverse fracture of shaft of right ulna, init
		S52.225A	Nondisplaced transverse fracture of shaft of left ulna, init
		S52.226A	Nondisplaced transverse fracture of shaft of unsp ulna, init
		S52.231A	Displaced oblique fracture of shaft of right ulna, init
		S52.232A	Displaced oblique fracture of shaft of left ulna, init
		S52.233A	Displaced oblique fracture of shaft of unsp ulna, init
		S52.234A	Nondisplaced oblique fracture of shaft of right ulna, init
		S52.235A	Nondisplaced oblique fracture of shaft of left ulna, init
		S52.236A	Nondisplaced oblique fracture of shaft of unsp ulna, init
		S52.241A	Displaced spiral fracture of shaft of ulna, right arm, init
		S52.242A	Displaced spiral fracture of shaft of ulna, left arm, init
		S52.243A	Displaced spiral fracture of shaft of ulna, unsp arm, init
		S52.244A	Nondisp spiral fracture of shaft of ulna, right arm, init
		S52.245A	Nondisp spiral fracture of shaft of ulna, left arm, init
		S52.246A	Nondisp spiral fracture of shaft of ulna, unsp arm, init
		S52.251A	Displaced comminuted fx shaft of ulna, right arm, init
		S52.252A	Displaced comminuted fx shaft of ulna, left arm, init
		S52.253A	Displaced comminuted fx shaft of ulna, unsp arm, init
		S52.254A	Nondisp comminuted fx shaft of ulna, right arm, init
		S52.255A	Nondisp comminuted fracture of shaft of ulna, left arm, init
		S52.256A	Nondisp comminuted fracture of shaft of ulna, unsp arm, init
		S52.261A	Displaced segmental fx shaft of ulna, right arm, init
		S52.262A	Displaced segmental fx shaft of ulna, left arm, init
		S52.263A	Displaced segmental fx shaft of ulna, unsp arm, init
		S52.264A	Nondisp segmental fracture of shaft of ulna, right arm, init
		S52.265A	Nondisp segmental fracture of shaft of ulna, left arm, init
		S52.266A	Nondisp segmental fracture of shaft of ulna, unsp arm, init
		S52.281A	Bent bone of right ulna, init encntr for closed fracture
		S52.282A	Bent bone of left ulna, init encntr for closed fracture
		S52.283A	Bent bone of unsp ulna, init encntr for closed fracture
		S52.291A	Oth fracture of shaft of right ulna, init for clos fx
		S52.292A	Oth fracture of shaft of left ulna, init for clos fx
		S52.299A	Oth fracture of shaft of unsp ulna, init for clos fx
813.23	CLOSED FRACTURE OF SHAFT OF RADIUS WITH ULNA	**S52.209A**	Unsp fracture of shaft of unsp ulna, init for clos fx ***and***
		S52.309A	Unsp fracture of shaft of unsp radius, init for clos fx
813.30	UNSPECIFIED OPEN FRACTURE SHAFT RADIUS OR ULNA	**S52.90XB**	Unsp fracture of unsp forearm, init for opn fx type I/2
		S52.90XC	Unsp fracture of unsp forearm, init for opn fx type 3A/B/C
813.31	OPEN FRACTURE OF SHAFT OF RADIUS	**S52.301B**	Unsp fracture of shaft of r radius, init for opn fx type I/2
		S52.301C	Unsp fx shaft of r radius, init for opn fx type 3A/B/C
		S52.302B	Unsp fx shaft of left radius, init for opn fx type I/2
		S52.302C	Unsp fx shaft of left radius, init for opn fx type 3A/B/C
		S52.309B	Unsp fx shaft of unsp radius, init for opn fx type I/2
		S52.309C	Unsp fx shaft of unsp radius, init for opn fx type 3A/B/C
		S52.321B	Displ transverse fx shaft of r rad, init for opn fx type I/2
	(Continued on next page)	**S52.321C**	Displ transverse fx shaft of r rad, init op fx 3A/B/C

ICD-9-CM		ICD-10-CM	
813.31	OPEN FRACTURE OF SHAFT OF RADIUS **(Continued)**	**S52.322B**	Displ transverse fx shaft of l rad, init for opn fx type I/2
		S52.322C	Displ transverse fx shaft of l rad, init op fx 3A/B/C
		S52.323B	Displ transverse fx shaft of unsp rad, init op fx 1/2
		S52.323C	Displ transverse fx shaft of unsp rad, init op fx 3A/B/C
		S52.324B	Nondisp transverse fx shaft of r rad, init op fx 1/2
		S52.324C	Nondisp transverse fx shaft of r rad, init op fx 3A/B/C
		S52.325B	Nondisp transverse fx shaft of l rad, init op fx 1/2
		S52.325C	Nondisp transverse fx shaft of l rad, init op fx 3A/B/C
		S52.326B	Nondisp transverse fx shaft of unsp rad, init op fx 1/2
		S52.326C	Nondisp transverse fx shaft of unsp rad, init op fx 3A/B/C
		S52.331B	Displ oblique fx shaft of r radius, init for opn fx type I/2
		S52.331C	Displ oblique fx shaft of r rad, init for opn fx type 3A/B/C
		S52.332B	Displ oblique fx shaft of left rad, init for opn fx type I/2
		S52.332C	Displ oblique fx shaft of l rad, init for opn fx type 3A/B/C
		S52.333B	Displ oblique fx shaft of unsp rad, init for opn fx type I/2
		S52.333C	Displ oblique fx shaft of unsp rad, init op fx 3A/B/C
		S52.334B	Nondisp oblique fx shaft of r rad, init for opn fx type I/2
		S52.334C	Nondisp oblique fx shaft of r rad, init op fx 3A/B/C
		S52.335B	Nondisp oblique fx shaft of l rad, init for opn fx type I/2
		S52.335C	Nondisp oblique fx shaft of l rad, init op fx 3A/B/C
		S52.336B	Nondisp oblique fx shaft of unsp rad, init op fx 1/2
		S52.336C	Nondisp oblique fx shaft of unsp rad, init op fx 3A/B/C
		S52.341B	Displ spiral fx shaft of rad, r arm, init op fx 1/2
		S52.341C	Displ spiral fx shaft of rad, r arm, init op fx 3A/B/C
		S52.342B	Displ spiral fx shaft of rad, l arm, init op fx 1/2
		S52.342C	Displ spiral fx shaft of rad, l arm, init op fx 3A/B/C
		S52.343B	Displ spiral fx shaft of rad, unsp arm, init op fx 1/2
		S52.343C	Displ spiral fx shaft of rad, unsp arm, init op fx 3A/B/C
		S52.344B	Nondisp spiral fx shaft of rad, r arm, init op fx 1/2
		S52.344C	Nondisp spiral fx shaft of rad, r arm, init op fx 3A/B/C
		S52.345B	Nondisp spiral fx shaft of rad, l arm, init op fx 1/2
		S52.345C	Nondisp spiral fx shaft of rad, l arm, init op fx 3A/B/C
		S52.346B	Nondisp spiral fx shaft of rad, unsp arm, init op fx 1/2
		S52.346C	Nondisp spiral fx shaft of rad, unsp arm, init op fx 3A/B/C
		S52.351B	Displ commnt fx shaft of rad, r arm, init op fx 1/2
		S52.351C	Displ commnt fx shaft of rad, r arm, init op fx 3A/B/C
		S52.352B	Displ commnt fx shaft of rad, l arm, init op fx 1/2
		S52.352C	Displ commnt fx shaft of rad, l arm, init op fx 3A/B/C
		S52.353B	Displ commnt fx shaft of rad, unsp arm, init op fx 1/2
		S52.353C	Displ commnt fx shaft of rad, unsp arm, init op fx 3A/B/C
		S52.354B	Nondisp commnt fx shaft of rad, r arm, init op fx 1/2
		S52.354C	Nondisp commnt fx shaft of rad, r arm, init op fx 3A/B/C
		S52.355B	Nondisp commnt fx shaft of rad, l arm, init op fx 1/2
		S52.355C	Nondisp commnt fx shaft of rad, l arm, init op fx 3A/B/C
		S52.356B	Nondisp commnt fx shaft of rad, unsp arm, init op fx 1/2
		S52.356C	Nondisp commnt fx shaft of rad, unsp arm, init op fx 3A/B/C
		S52.361B	Displ seg fx shaft of rad, r arm, init for opn fx type I/2
		S52.361C	Displ seg fx shaft of rad, r arm, init op fx 3A/B/C
		S52.362B	Displ seg fx shaft of rad, l arm, init for opn fx type I/2
		S52.362C	Displ seg fx shaft of rad, l arm, init op fx 3A/B/C
		S52.363B	Displ seg fx shaft of rad, unsp arm, init op fx 1/2
		S52.363C	Displ seg fx shaft of rad, unsp arm, init op fx 3A/B/C
		S52.364B	Nondisp seg fx shaft of rad, r arm, init for opn fx type I/2
		S52.364C	Nondisp seg fx shaft of rad, r arm, init op fx 3A/B/C
		S52.365B	Nondisp seg fx shaft of rad, l arm, init for opn fx type I/2
		S52.365C	Nondisp seg fx shaft of rad, l arm, init op fx 3A/B/C
		S52.366B	Nondisp seg fx shaft of rad, unsp arm, init op fx 1/2
		S52.366C	Nondisp seg fx shaft of rad, unsp arm, init op fx 3A/B/C
		S52.371B	Galeazzi's fracture of r radius, init for opn fx type I/2
		S52.371C	Galeazzi's fracture of r radius, init for opn fx type 3A/B/C
		S52.372B	Galeazzi's fracture of left radius, init for opn fx type I/2
		S52.372C	Galeazzi's fx left radius, init for opn fx type 3A/B/C
		S52.379B	Galeazzi's fracture of unsp radius, init for opn fx type I/2
		S52.379C	Galeazzi's fx unsp radius, init for opn fx type 3A/B/C
		S52.381B	Bent bone of right radius, init for opn fx type I/2
		S52.381C	Bent bone of right radius, init for opn fx type 3A/B/C
		S52.382B	Bent bone of left radius, init for opn fx type I/2
		S52.382C	Bent bone of left radius, init for opn fx type 3A/B/C
		S52.389B	Bent bone of unsp radius, init for opn fx type I/2
		S52.389C	Bent bone of unsp radius, init for opn fx type 3A/B/C
		S52.391B	Oth fx shaft of radius, right arm, init for opn fx type I/2
		S52.391C	Oth fx shaft of rad, right arm, init for opn fx type 3A/B/C
		S52.392B	Oth fx shaft of radius, left arm, init for opn fx type I/2
		S52.392C	Oth fx shaft of rad, left arm, init for opn fx type 3A/B/C
		S52.399B	Oth fx shaft of radius, unsp arm, init for opn fx type I/2
		S52.399C	Oth fx shaft of rad, unsp arm, init for opn fx type 3A/B/C

ICD-9-CM	ICD-10-CM	
813.32 OPEN FRACTURE OF SHAFT OF ULNA	**S52.201B**	Unsp fx shaft of right ulna, init for opn fx type I/2
	S52.201C	Unsp fx shaft of right ulna, init for opn fx type 3A/B/C
	S52.202B	Unsp fx shaft of left ulna, init for opn fx type I/2
	S52.202C	Unsp fx shaft of left ulna, init for opn fx type 3A/B/C
	S52.209B	Unsp fx shaft of unsp ulna, init for opn fx type I/2
	S52.209C	Unsp fx shaft of unsp ulna, init for opn fx type 3A/B/C
	S52.221B	Displ transverse fx shaft of r ulna, init op fx 1/2
	S52.221C	Displ transverse fx shaft of r ulna, init op fx 3A/B/C
	S52.222B	Displ transverse fx shaft of l ulna, init op fx 1/2
	S52.222C	Displ transverse fx shaft of l ulna, init op fx 3A/B/C
	S52.223B	Displ transverse fx shaft of unsp ulna, init op fx 1/2
	S52.223C	Displ transverse fx shaft of unsp ulna, init op fx 3A/B/C
	S52.224B	Nondisp transverse fx shaft of r ulna, init op fx 1/2
	S52.224C	Nondisp transverse fx shaft of r ulna, init op fx 3A/B/C
	S52.225B	Nondisp transverse fx shaft of l ulna, init op fx 1/2
	S52.225C	Nondisp transverse fx shaft of l ulna, init op fx 3A/B/C
	S52.226B	Nondisp transverse fx shaft of unsp ulna, init op fx 1/2
	S52.226C	Nondisp transverse fx shaft of unsp ulna, init op fx 3A/B/C
	S52.231B	Displ oblique fx shaft of r ulna, init for opn fx type I/2
	S52.231C	Displ oblique fx shaft of r ulna, init op fx 3A/B/C
	S52.232B	Displ oblique fx shaft of l ulna, init for opn fx type I/2
	S52.232C	Displ oblique fx shaft of l ulna, init op fx 3A/B/C
	S52.233B	Displ oblique fx shaft of unsp ulna, init op fx 1/2
	S52.233C	Displ oblique fx shaft of unsp ulna, init op fx 3A/B/C
	S52.234B	Nondisp oblique fx shaft of r ulna, init for opn fx type I/2
	S52.234C	Nondisp oblique fx shaft of r ulna, init op fx 3A/B/C
	S52.235B	Nondisp oblique fx shaft of l ulna, init for opn fx type I/2
	S52.235C	Nondisp oblique fx shaft of l ulna, init op fx 3A/B/C
	S52.236B	Nondisp oblique fx shaft of unsp ulna, init op fx 1/2
	S52.236C	Nondisp oblique fx shaft of unsp ulna, init op fx 3A/B/C
	S52.241B	Displ spiral fx shaft of ulna, r arm, init op fx 1/2
	S52.241C	Displ spiral fx shaft of ulna, r arm, init op fx 3A/B/C
	S52.242B	Displ spiral fx shaft of ulna, l arm, init op fx 1/2
	S52.242C	Displ spiral fx shaft of ulna, l arm, init op fx 3A/B/C
	S52.243B	Displ spiral fx shaft of ulna, unsp arm,init op fx 1/2
	S52.243C	Displ spiral fx shaft of ulna, unsp arm, init op fx 3A/B/C
	S52.244B	Nondisp spiral fx shaft of ulna, r arm, init op fx 1/2
	S52.244C	Nondisp spiral fx shaft of ulna, r arm, init op fx 3A/B/C
	S52.245B	Nondisp spiral fx shaft of ulna, l arm, init op fx 1/2
	S52.245C	Nondisp spiral fx shaft of ulna, l arm, init op fx 3A/B/C
	S52.246B	Nondisp spiral fx shaft of ulna, unsp arm, init op fx 1/2
	S52.246C	Nondisp spiral fx shaft of ulna, unsp arm, init op fx 3A/B/C
	S52.251B	Displ commnt fx shaft of ulna, r arm, init op fx 1/2
	S52.251C	Displ commnt fx shaft of ulna, r arm, init op fx 3A/B/C
	S52.252B	Displ commnt fx shaft of ulna, l arm, init op fx 1/2
	S52.252C	Displ commnt fx shaft of ulna, l arm, init op fx 3A/B/C
	S52.253B	Displ commnt fx shaft of ulna, unsp arm, init op fx 1/2
	S52.253C	Displ commnt fx shaft of ulna, unsp arm, init op fx 3A/B/C
	S52.254B	Nondisp commnt fx shaft of ulna, r arm, init op fx 1/2
	S52.254C	Nondisp commnt fx shaft of ulna, r arm, init op fx 3A/B/C
	S52.255B	Nondisp commnt fx shaft of ulna, l arm, init op fx 1/2
	S52.255C	Nondisp commnt fx shaft of ulna, l arm, init op fx 3A/B/C
	S52.256B	Nondisp commnt fx shaft of ulna, unsp arm, init op fx 1/2
	S52.256C	Nondisp commnt fx shaft of ulna, unsp arm, init op fx 3A/B/C
	S52.261B	Displ seg fx shaft of ulna, r arm, init for opn fx type I/2
	S52.261C	Displ seg fx shaft of ulna, r arm, init op fx 3A/B/C
	S52.262B	Displ seg fx shaft of ulna, l arm, init for opn fx type I/2
	S52.262C	Displ seg fx shaft of ulna, l arm, init op fx 3A/B/C
	S52.263B	Displ seg fx shaft of ulna, unsp arm,init op fx 1/2
	S52.263C	Displ seg fx shaft of ulna, unsp arm, init op fx 3A/B/C
	S52.264B	Nondisp seg fx shaft of ulna, r arm, init op fx 1/2
	S52.264C	Nondisp seg fx shaft of ulna, r arm, init op fx 3A/B/C
	S52.265B	Nondisp seg fx shaft of ulna, l arm, init op fx 1/2
	S52.265C	Nondisp seg fx shaft of ulna, l arm, init op fx 3A/B/C
	S52.266B	Nondisp seg fx shaft of ulna, unsp arm, init op fx 1/2
	S52.266C	Nondisp seg fx shaft of ulna, unsp arm, init op fx 3A/B/C
	S52.281B	Bent bone of right ulna, init for opn fx type I/2
	S52.281C	Bent bone of right ulna, init for opn fx type 3A/B/C
	S52.282B	Bent bone of left ulna, init for opn fx type I/2
	S52.282C	Bent bone of left ulna, init for opn fx type 3A/B/C
	S52.283B	Bent bone of unsp ulna, init for opn fx type I/2
	S52.283C	Bent bone of unsp ulna, init for opn fx type 3A/B/C
	S52.291B	Oth fx shaft of right ulna, init for opn fx type I/2
	S52.291C	Oth fx shaft of right ulna, init for opn fx type 3A/B/C
	S52.292B	Oth fracture of shaft of left ulna, init for opn fx type I/2
	S52.292C	Oth fx shaft of left ulna, init for opn fx type 3A/B/C
	S52.299B	Oth fracture of shaft of unsp ulna, init for opn fx type I/2
	S52.299C	Oth fx shaft of unsp ulna, init for opn fx type 3A/B/C

ICD-9-CM		ICD-10-CM		
813.33	OPEN FRACTURE OF SHAFT OF RADIUS WITH ULNA	**S52.209B**	Unsp fx shaft of unsp ulna, init for opn fx type I/2	*and*
		S52.309B	Unsp fx shaft of unsp radius, init for opn fx type I/2	*or*
		S52.309C	Unsp fx shaft of unsp radius, init for opn fx type 3A/B/C	
		S52.209C	Unsp fx shaft of unsp ulna, init for opn fx type 3A/B/C	*and*
		S52.309B	Unsp fx shaft of unsp radius, init for opn fx type I/2	*or*
		S52.309C	Unsp fx shaft of unsp radius, init for opn fx type 3A/B/C	
813.40	UNSPECIFIED CLOSED FRACTURE LOWER END FOREARM	**S52.90XA**	Unsp fracture of unsp forearm, init for clos fx	
813.41	CLOSED COLLES FRACTURE	**S52.531A**	Colles' fracture of right radius, init for clos fx	
		S52.532A	Colles' fracture of left radius, init for clos fx	
		S52.539A	Colles' fracture of unsp radius, init for clos fx	
		S52.541A	Smith's fracture of right radius, init for clos fx	
		S52.542A	Smith's fracture of left radius, init for clos fx	
		S52.549A	Smith's fracture of unsp radius, init for clos fx	
813.42	OTHER CLOSED FRACTURES OF DISTAL END OF RADIUS	**S52.501A**	Unsp fracture of the lower end of right radius, init	
		S52.502A	Unsp fracture of the lower end of left radius, init	
		S52.509A	Unsp fracture of the lower end of unsp radius, init	
		S52.511A	Disp fx of right radial styloid process, init for clos fx	
		S52.512A	Disp fx of left radial styloid process, init for clos fx	
		S52.513A	Disp fx of unsp radial styloid process, init for clos fx	
		S52.514A	Nondisp fx of right radial styloid process, init for clos fx	
		S52.515A	Nondisp fx of left radial styloid process, init for clos fx	
		S52.516A	Nondisp fx of unsp radial styloid process, init for clos fx	
		S52.551A	Oth extrartic fracture of lower end of right radius, init	
		S52.552A	Oth extrartic fracture of lower end of left radius, init	
		S52.559A	Oth extrartic fracture of lower end of unsp radius, init	
		S52.561A	Barton's fracture of right radius, init for clos fx	
		S52.562A	Barton's fracture of left radius, init for clos fx	
		S52.569A	Barton's fracture of unsp radius, init for clos fx	
		S52.571A	Oth intartic fracture of lower end of right radius, init	
		S52.572A	Oth intartic fracture of lower end of left radius, init	
		S52.579A	Oth intartic fracture of lower end of unsp radius, init	
		S52.591A	Oth fractures of lower end of right radius, init for clos fx	
		S52.592A	Oth fractures of lower end of left radius, init for clos fx	
		S52.599A	Oth fractures of lower end of unsp radius, init for clos fx	
		S59.201A	Unsp physeal fracture of lower end radius, right arm, init	
		S59.202A	Unsp physeal fracture of lower end of radius, left arm, init	
		S59.209A	Unsp physeal fracture of lower end of radius, unsp arm, init	
		S59.211A	Sltr-haris Type I physl fx lower end radius, right arm, init	
		S59.212A	Sltr-haris Type I physl fx lower end radius, left arm, init	
		S59.219A	Sltr-haris Type I physl fx lower end radius, unsp arm, init	
		S59.221A	Sltr-haris Type II physl fx lower end rad, right arm, init	
		S59.222A	Sltr-haris Type II physl fx lower end radius, left arm, init	
		S59.229A	Sltr-haris Type II physl fx lower end radius, unsp arm, init	
		S59.231A	Sltr-haris Type III physl fx lower end rad, right arm, init	
		S59.232A	Sltr-haris Type III physl fx lower end rad, left arm, init	
		S59.239A	Sltr-haris Type III physl fx lower end rad, unsp arm, init	
		S59.241A	Sltr-haris Type IV physl fx lower end rad, right arm, init	
		S59.242A	Sltr-haris Type IV physl fx lower end radius, left arm, init	
		S59.249A	Sltr-haris Type IV physl fx lower end radius, unsp arm, init	
		S59.291A	Oth physeal fracture of lower end of radius, right arm, init	
		S59.292A	Oth physeal fracture of lower end of radius, left arm, init	
		S59.299A	Oth physeal fracture of lower end of radius, unsp arm, init	
813.43	CLOSED FRACTURE OF DISTAL END OF ULNA	**S52.601A**	Unsp fracture of lower end of right ulna, init for clos fx	
		S52.602A	Unsp fracture of lower end of left ulna, init for clos fx	
		S52.609A	Unsp fracture of lower end of unsp ulna, init for clos fx	
		S52.611A	Disp fx of right ulna styloid process, init for clos fx	
		S52.612A	Disp fx of left ulna styloid process, init for clos fx	
		S52.613A	Disp fx of unsp ulna styloid process, init for clos fx	
		S52.614A	Nondisp fx of right ulna styloid process, init for clos fx	
		S52.615A	Nondisp fx of left ulna styloid process, init for clos fx	
		S52.616A	Nondisp fx of unsp ulna styloid process, init for clos fx	
		S52.691A	Oth fracture of lower end of right ulna, init for clos fx	
		S52.692A	Oth fracture of lower end of left ulna, init for clos fx	
		S52.699A	Oth fracture of lower end of unsp ulna, init for clos fx	
		S59.001A	Unsp physeal fracture of lower end of ulna, right arm, init	
		S59.002A	Unsp physeal fracture of lower end of ulna, left arm, init	
		S59.009A	Unsp physeal fracture of lower end of ulna, unsp arm, init	
		S59.011A	Sltr-haris Type I physl fx lower end ulna, right arm, init	
		S59.012A	Sltr-haris Type I physl fx lower end of ulna, left arm, init	
		S59.019A	Sltr-haris Type I physl fx lower end of ulna, unsp arm, init	
		S59.021A	Sltr-haris Type II physl fx lower end ulna, right arm, init	
		S59.022A	Sltr-haris Type II physl fx lower end ulna, left arm, init	
		S59.029A	Sltr-haris Type II physl fx lower end ulna, unsp arm, init	
		S59.031A	Sltr-haris Type III physl fx lower end ulna, right arm, init	
		S59.032A	Sltr-haris Type III physl fx lower end ulna, left arm, init	
		S59.039A	Sltr-haris Type III physl fx lower end ulna, unsp arm, init	
		S59.041A	Sltr-haris Type IV physl fx lower end ulna, right arm, init	
		S59.042A	Sltr-haris Type IV physl fx lower end ulna, left arm, init	
		S59.049A	Sltr-haris Type IV physl fx lower end ulna, unsp arm, init	
	(Continued on next page)	**S59.091A**	Oth physeal fracture of lower end of ulna, right arm, init	

ICD-9-CM		ICD-10-CM		
813.43	CLOSED FRACTURE OF DISTAL END OF ULNA **(Continued)**	**S59.Ø92A**	Oth physeal fracture of lower end of ulna, left arm, init	
		S59.Ø99A	Oth physeal fracture of lower end of ulna, unsp arm, init	
813.44	CLOSED FRACTURE OF LOWER END OF RADIUS WITH ULNA	**S52.6Ø9A**	Unsp fracture of lower end of unsp ulna, init for clos fx	*and*
		S52.5Ø9A	Unsp fracture of the lower end of unsp radius, init	
813.45	TORUS FRACTURE RADIUS ALONE	**S52.111A**	Torus fracture of upper end of right radius, init	
		S52.112A	Torus fracture of upper end of left radius, init for clos fx	
		S52.119A	Torus fracture of upper end of unsp radius, init for clos fx	
		S52.521A	Torus fracture of lower end of right radius, init	
		S52.522A	Torus fracture of lower end of left radius, init for clos fx	
		S52.529A	Torus fracture of lower end of unsp radius, init for clos fx	
813.46	TORUS FRACTURE ULNA ALONE	**S52.Ø11A**	Torus fracture of upper end of right ulna, init for clos fx	
		S52.Ø12A	Torus fracture of upper end of left ulna, init for clos fx	
		S52.Ø19A	Torus fracture of upper end of unsp ulna, init for clos fx	
		S52.621A	Torus fracture of lower end of right ulna, init for clos fx	
		S52.622A	Torus fracture of lower end of left ulna, init for clos fx	
		S52.629A	Torus fracture of lower end of unsp ulna, init for clos fx	
813.47	TORUS FRACTURE OF RADIUS AND ULNA	**S52.621A**	Torus fracture of lower end of right ulna, init for clos fx	*and*
		S52.521A	Torus fracture of lower end of right radius, init	
		S52.Ø11A	Torus fracture of upper end of right ulna, init for clos fx	*and*
		S52.111A	Torus fracture of upper end of right radius, init	
		S52.622A	Torus fracture of lower end of left ulna, init for clos fx	*and*
		S52.522A	Torus fracture of lower end of left radius, init for clos fx	
		S52.Ø12A	Torus fracture of upper end of left ulna, init for clos fx	*and*
		S52.112A	Torus fracture of upper end of left radius, init for clos fx	
813.5Ø	UNSPECIFIED OPEN FRACTURE LOWER END FOREARM	**S52.9ØXB**	Unsp fracture of unsp forearm, init for opn fx type I/2	
		S52.9ØXC	Unsp fracture of unsp forearm, init for opn fx type 3A/B/C	
813.51	OPEN COLLES FRACTURE	**S52.531B**	Colles' fracture of right radius, init for opn fx type I/2	
		S52.531C	Colles' fracture of r radius, init for opn fx type 3A/B/C	
		S52.532B	Colles' fracture of left radius, init for opn fx type I/2	
		S52.532C	Colles' fracture of left radius, init for opn fx type 3A/B/C	
		S52.539B	Colles' fracture of unsp radius, init for opn fx type I/2	
		S52.539C	Colles' fracture of unsp radius, init for opn fx type 3A/B/C	
813.52	OTHER OPEN FRACTURES OF DISTAL END OF RADIUS	**S52.5Ø1B**	Unsp fx the lower end of r radius, init for opn fx type I/2	
		S52.5Ø1C	Unsp fx the lower end r radius, init for opn fx type 3A/B/C	
		S52.5Ø2B	Unsp fx the lower end left radius, init for opn fx type I/2	
		S52.5Ø2C	Unsp fx the lower end left rad, init for opn fx type 3A/B/C	
		S52.5Ø9B	Unsp fx the lower end unsp radius, init for opn fx type I/2	
		S52.5Ø9C	Unsp fx the lower end unsp rad, init for opn fx type 3A/B/C	
		S52.511B	Disp fx of r radial styloid pro, init for opn fx type I/2	
		S52.511C	Disp fx of r radial styloid pro, init for opn fx type 3A/B/C	
		S52.512B	Disp fx of left radial styloid pro, init for opn fx type I/2	
		S52.512C	Disp fx of l radial styloid pro, init for opn fx type 3A/B/C	
		S52.513B	Disp fx of unsp radial styloid pro, init for opn fx type I/2	
		S52.513C	Disp fx of unsp radial styloid pro, init op fx 3A/B/C	
		S52.514B	Nondisp fx of r radial styloid pro, init for opn fx type I/2	
		S52.514C	Nondisp fx of r radial styloid pro, init op fx 3A/B/C	
		S52.515B	Nondisp fx of l radial styloid pro, init for opn fx type I/2	
		S52.515C	Nondisp fx of l radial styloid pro, init op fx 3A/B/C	
		S52.516B	Nondisp fx of unsp radial styloid pro, init op fx 1/2	
		S52.516C	Nondisp fx of unsp radial styloid pro, init op fx 3A/B/C	
		S52.541B	Smith's fracture of right radius, init for opn fx type I/2	
		S52.541C	Smith's fracture of r radius, init for opn fx type 3A/B/C	
		S52.542B	Smith's fracture of left radius, init for opn fx type I/2	
		S52.542C	Smith's fracture of left radius, init for opn fx type 3A/B/C	
		S52.549B	Smith's fracture of unsp radius, init for opn fx type I/2	
		S52.549C	Smith's fracture of unsp radius, init for opn fx type 3A/B/C	
		S52.551B	Oth extrartic fx lower end r rad, init for opn fx type I/2	
		S52.551C	Oth extrartic fx low end r rad, init for opn fx type 3A/B/C	
		S52.552B	Oth extrartic fx low end left rad, init for opn fx type I/2	
		S52.552C	Oth extrartic fx low end l rad, init for opn fx type 3A/B/C	
		S52.559B	Oth extrartic fx low end unsp rad, init for opn fx type I/2	
		S52.559C	Oth extrartic fx low end unsp rad, init op fx 3A/B/C	
		S52.561B	Barton's fracture of right radius, init for opn fx type I/2	
		S52.561C	Barton's fracture of r radius, init for opn fx type 3A/B/C	
		S52.562B	Barton's fracture of left radius, init for opn fx type I/2	
		S52.562C	Barton's fx left radius, init for opn fx type 3A/B/C	
		S52.569B	Barton's fracture of unsp radius, init for opn fx type I/2	
		S52.569C	Barton's fx unsp radius, init for opn fx type 3A/B/C	
		S52.571B	Oth intartic fx lower end r radius, init for opn fx type I/2	
		S52.571C	Oth intartic fx lower end r rad, init for opn fx type 3A/B/C	
		S52.572B	Oth intartic fx lower end left rad, init for opn fx type I/2	
		S52.572C	Oth intartic fx low end l rad, init for opn fx type 3A/B/C	
		S52.579B	Oth intartic fx lower end unsp rad, init for opn fx type I/2	
		S52.579C	Oth intartic fx low end unsp rad, init op fx 3A/B/C	
		S52.591B	Oth fx of lower end of r radius, init for opn fx type I/2	
		S52.591C	Oth fx of lower end of r radius, init for opn fx type 3A/B/C	
	(Continued on next page)	**S52.592B**	Oth fx of lower end of left radius, init for opn fx type I/2	

ICD-9-CM		ICD-10-CM		
813.52	OTHER OPEN FRACTURES OF DISTAL END OF RADIUS **(Continued)**	**S52.592C**	Oth fx of lower end left radius, init for opn fx type 3A/B/C	
		S52.599B	Oth fx of lower end of unsp radius, init for opn fx type I/2	
		S52.599C	Oth fx of lower end unsp radius, init for opn fx type 3A/B/C	
813.53	OPEN FRACTURE OF DISTAL END OF ULNA	**S52.601B**	Unsp fx lower end of right ulna, init for opn fx type I/2	
		S52.601C	Unsp fx lower end of right ulna, init for opn fx type 3A/B/C	
		S52.602B	Unsp fx lower end of left ulna, init for opn fx type I/2	
		S52.602C	Unsp fx lower end of left ulna, init for opn fx type 3A/B/C	
		S52.609B	Unsp fx lower end of unsp ulna, init for opn fx type I/2	
		S52.609C	Unsp fx lower end of unsp ulna, init for opn fx type 3A/B/C	
		S52.611B	Disp fx of r ulna styloid process, init for opn fx type I/2	
		S52.611C	Disp fx of r ulna styloid pro, init for opn fx type 3A/B/C	
		S52.612B	Disp fx of l ulna styloid process, init for opn fx type I/2	
		S52.612C	Disp fx of l ulna styloid pro, init for opn fx type 3A/B/C	
		S52.613B	Disp fx of unsp ulna styloid pro, init for opn fx type I/2	
		S52.613C	Disp fx of unsp ulna styloid pro, init op fx 3A/B/C	
		S52.614B	Nondisp fx of r ulna styloid pro, init for opn fx type I/2	
		S52.614C	Nondisp fx of r ulna styloid pro, init op fx 3A/B/C	
		S52.615B	Nondisp fx of l ulna styloid pro, init for opn fx type I/2	
		S52.615C	Nondisp fx of l ulna styloid pro, init op fx 3A/B/C	
		S52.616B	Nondisp fx of unsp ulna styloid pro, init op fx 1/2	
		S52.616C	Nondisp fx of unsp ulna styloid pro, init op fx 3A/B/C	
		S52.691B	Oth fx lower end of right ulna, init for opn fx type I/2	
		S52.691C	Oth fx lower end of right ulna, init for opn fx type 3A/B/C	
		S52.692B	Oth fx lower end of left ulna, init for opn fx type I/2	
		S52.692C	Oth fx lower end of left ulna, init for opn fx type 3A/B/C	
		S52.699B	Oth fx lower end of unsp ulna, init for opn fx type I/2	
		S52.699C	Oth fx lower end of unsp ulna, init for opn fx type 3A/B/C	
813.54	OPEN FRACTURE OF LOWER END OF RADIUS WITH ULNA	**S52.609B**	Unsp fx lower end of unsp ulna, init for opn fx type I/2	***and***
		S52.509B	Unsp fx the lower end unsp radius, init for opn fx type I/2	***or***
		S52.509C	Unsp fx the lower end unsp rad, init for opn fx type 3A/B/C	
		S52.609C	Unsp fx lower end of unsp ulna, init for opn fx type 3A/B/C	***and***
		S52.509B	Unsp fx the lower end unsp radius, init for opn fx type I/2	***or***
		S52.509C	Unsp fx the lower end unsp rad, init for opn fx type 3A/B/C	
813.80	CLOSED FRACTURE OF UNSPECIFIED PART OF FOREARM	**S52.90XA**	Unsp fracture of unsp forearm, init for clos fx	
		S52.91XA	Unsp fracture of right forearm, init for clos fx	
		S52.92XA	Unsp fracture of left forearm, init for clos fx	
813.81	CLOSED FRACTURE OF UNSPECIFIED PART OF RADIUS	**S52.90XA**	Unsp fracture of unsp forearm, init for clos fx	
813.82	CLOSED FRACTURE OF UNSPECIFIED PART OF ULNA	**S52.90XA**	Unsp fracture of unsp forearm, init for clos fx	
813.83	CLOSED FRACTURE UNSPECIFIED PART RADIUS W/ULNA	**S52.90XA**	Unsp fracture of unsp forearm, init for clos fx	
813.90	OPEN FRACTURE OF UNSPECIFIED PART OF FOREARM	**S52.90XB**	Unsp fracture of unsp forearm, init for opn fx type I/2	
		S52.90XC	Unsp fracture of unsp forearm, init for opn fx type 3A/B/C	
		S52.91XB	Unsp fracture of right forearm, init for opn fx type I/2	
		S52.91XC	Unsp fracture of right forearm, init for opn fx type 3A/B/C	
		S52.92XB	Unsp fracture of left forearm, init for opn fx type I/2	
		S52.92XC	Unsp fracture of left forearm, init for opn fx type 3A/B/C	
813.91	OPEN FRACTURE OF UNSPECIFIED PART OF RADIUS	**S52.90XB**	Unsp fracture of unsp forearm, init for opn fx type I/2	
		S52.90XC	Unsp fracture of unsp forearm, init for opn fx type 3A/B/C	
813.92	OPEN FRACTURE OF UNSPECIFIED PART OF ULNA	**S52.90XB**	Unsp fracture of unsp forearm, init for opn fx type I/2	
		S52.90XC	Unsp fracture of unsp forearm, init for opn fx type 3A/B/C	
813.93	OPEN FRACTURE UNSPECIFIED PART RADIUS W/ULNA	**S52.90XB**	Unsp fracture of unsp forearm, init for opn fx type I/2	
		S52.90XC	Unsp fracture of unsp forearm, init for opn fx type 3A/B/C	
814.00	UNSPECIFIED CLOSED FRACTURE OF CARPAL BONE	**S62.101A**	Fracture of unsp carpal bone, right wrist, init for clos fx	
		S62.102A	Fracture of unsp carpal bone, left wrist, init for clos fx	
		S62.109A	Fracture of unsp carpal bone, unsp wrist, init for clos fx	
814.01	CLOSED FRACTURE OF NAVICULAR BONE OF WRIST	**S62.001A**	Unsp fracture of navicular bone of right wrist, init	
		S62.002A	Unsp fracture of navicular bone of left wrist, init	
		S62.009A	Unsp fracture of navicular bone of unsp wrist, init	
		S62.011A	Disp fx of distal pole of navicular bone of r wrist, init	
		S62.012A	Disp fx of distal pole of navicular bone of left wrist, init	
		S62.013A	Disp fx of distal pole of navicular bone of unsp wrist, init	
		S62.014A	Nondisp fx of distal pole of navicular bone of r wrist, init	
		S62.015A	Nondisp fx of distal pole of navicular bone of l wrist, init	
		S62.016A	Nondisp fx of distal pole of navic bone of unsp wrist, init	
		S62.021A	Disp fx of middle third of navicular bone of r wrist, init	
		S62.022A	Disp fx of middle third of navicular bone of l wrist, init	
		S62.023A	Disp fx of middle third of navic bone of unsp wrist, init	
		S62.024A	Nondisp fx of middle third of navic bone of r wrist, init	
		S62.025A	Nondisp fx of middle third of navic bone of l wrist, init	
		S62.026A	Nondisp fx of middle third of navic bone of unsp wrist, init	
		S62.031A	Disp fx of proximal third of navicular bone of r wrist, init	
		S62.032A	Disp fx of proximal third of navicular bone of l wrist, init	
		S62.033A	Disp fx of proximal third of navic bone of unsp wrist, init	
		S62.034A	Nondisp fx of proximal third of navic bone of r wrist, init	
		S62.035A	Nondisp fx of proximal third of navic bone of l wrist, init	
		S62.036A	Nondisp fx of prox third of navic bone of unsp wrist, init	

ICD-9-CM		ICD-10-CM	
814.Ø2	CLOSED FRACTURE OF LUNATE BONE OF WRIST	**S62.121A**	Disp fx of lunate, right wrist, init for clos fx
		S62.122A	Disp fx of lunate, left wrist, init for clos fx
		S62.123A	Disp fx of lunate, unsp wrist, init for clos fx
		S62.124A	Nondisp fx of lunate, right wrist, init for clos fx
		S62.125A	Nondisp fx of lunate, left wrist, init for clos fx
		S62.126A	Nondisp fx of lunate, unsp wrist, init for clos fx
814.Ø3	CLOSED FRACTURE OF TRIQUETRAL BONE OF WRIST	**S62.111A**	Disp fx of triquetrum bone, right wrist, init for clos fx
		S62.112A	Disp fx of triquetrum bone, left wrist, init for clos fx
		S62.113A	Disp fx of triquetrum bone, unsp wrist, init for clos fx
		S62.114A	Nondisp fx of triquetrum bone, right wrist, init for clos fx
		S62.115A	Nondisp fx of triquetrum bone, left wrist, init for clos fx
		S62.116A	Nondisp fx of triquetrum bone, unsp wrist, init for clos fx
814.Ø4	CLOSED FRACTURE OF PISIFORM BONE OF WRIST	**S62.161A**	Disp fx of pisiform, right wrist, init for clos fx
		S62.162A	Disp fx of pisiform, left wrist, init for clos fx
		S62.163A	Disp fx of pisiform, unsp wrist, init for clos fx
		S62.164A	Nondisp fx of pisiform, right wrist, init for clos fx
		S62.165A	Nondisp fx of pisiform, left wrist, init for clos fx
		S62.166A	Nondisp fx of pisiform, unsp wrist, init for clos fx
814.Ø5	CLOSED FRACTURE OF TRAPEZIUM BONE OF WRIST	**S62.171A**	Disp fx of trapezium, right wrist, init for clos fx
		S62.172A	Disp fx of trapezium, left wrist, init for clos fx
		S62.173A	Disp fx of trapezium, unsp wrist, init for clos fx
		S62.174A	Nondisp fx of trapezium, right wrist, init for clos fx
		S62.175A	Nondisp fx of trapezium, left wrist, init for clos fx
		S62.176A	Nondisp fx of trapezium, unsp wrist, init for clos fx
814.Ø6	CLOSED FRACTURE OF TRAPEZOID BONE OF WRIST	**S62.181A**	Disp fx of trapezoid, right wrist, init for clos fx
		S62.182A	Disp fx of trapezoid, left wrist, init for clos fx
		S62.183A	Disp fx of trapezoid, unsp wrist, init for clos fx
		S62.184A	Nondisp fx of trapezoid, right wrist, init for clos fx
		S62.185A	Nondisp fx of trapezoid, left wrist, init for clos fx
		S62.186A	Nondisp fx of trapezoid, unsp wrist, init for clos fx
814.Ø7	CLOSED FRACTURE OF CAPITATE BONE OF WRIST	**S62.131A**	Disp fx of capitate bone, right wrist, init for clos fx
		S62.132A	Disp fx of capitate bone, left wrist, init for clos fx
		S62.133A	Disp fx of capitate bone, unsp wrist, init for clos fx
		S62.134A	Nondisp fx of capitate bone, right wrist, init for clos fx
		S62.135A	Nondisp fx of capitate bone, left wrist, init for clos fx
		S62.136A	Nondisp fx of capitate bone, unsp wrist, init for clos fx
814.Ø8	CLOSED FRACTURE OF HAMATE BONE OF WRIST	**S62.141A**	Disp fx of body of hamate bone, right wrist, init
		S62.142A	Disp fx of body of hamate bone, left wrist, init for clos fx
		S62.143A	Disp fx of body of hamate bone, unsp wrist, init for clos fx
		S62.144A	Nondisp fx of body of hamate bone, right wrist, init
		S62.145A	Nondisp fx of body of hamate bone, left wrist, init
		S62.146A	Nondisp fx of body of hamate bone, unsp wrist, init
814.Ø9	CLOSED FRACTURE OF OTHER BONE OF WRIST	**S62.151A**	Disp fx of hook process of hamate bone, right wrist, init
		S62.152A	Disp fx of hook process of hamate bone, left wrist, init
		S62.153A	Disp fx of hook process of hamate bone, unsp wrist, init
		S62.154A	Nondisp fx of hook process of hamate bone, right wrist, init
		S62.155A	Nondisp fx of hook process of hamate bone, left wrist, init
		S62.156A	Nondisp fx of hook process of hamate bone, unsp wrist, init
814.1Ø	UNSPECIFIED OPEN FRACTURE OF CARPAL BONE	**S62.1Ø1B**	Fracture of unsp carpal bone, right wrist, init for opn fx
		S62.1Ø2B	Fracture of unsp carpal bone, left wrist, init for opn fx
		S62.1Ø9B	Fracture of unsp carpal bone, unsp wrist, init for opn fx
814.11	OPEN FRACTURE OF NAVICULAR BONE OF WRIST	**S62.ØØ1B**	Unsp fx navicular bone of right wrist, init for opn fx
		S62.ØØ2B	Unsp fx navicular bone of left wrist, init for opn fx
		S62.ØØ9B	Unsp fx navicular bone of unsp wrist, init for opn fx
		S62.Ø11B	Disp fx of dist pole of navic bone of r wrs, init for opn fx
		S62.Ø12B	Disp fx of dist pole of navic bone of l wrs, init for opn fx
		S62.Ø13B	Disp fx of dist pole of navic bone of unsp wrs, init op fx
		S62.Ø14B	Nondisp fx of dist pole of navic bone of r wrs, init op fx
		S62.Ø15B	Nondisp fx of dist pole of navic bone of l wrs, init op fx
		S62.Ø16B	Nondisp fx of dist pole of navic bone of unsp wrs, init op fx
		S62.Ø21B	Disp fx of mid 3rd of navic bone of r wrist, init for opn fx
		S62.Ø22B	Disp fx of mid 3rd of navic bone of l wrist, init for opn fx
		S62.Ø23B	Disp fx of mid 3rd of navic bone of unsp wrs, init op fx
		S62.Ø24B	Nondisp fx of mid 3rd of navic bone of r wrs, init op fx
		S62.Ø25B	Nondisp fx of mid 3rd of navic bone of l wrs, init op fx
		S62.Ø26B	Nondisp fx of mid 3rd of navic bone of unsp wrs, init op fx
		S62.Ø31B	Disp fx of prox 3rd of navic bone of r wrs, init for opn fx
		S62.Ø32B	Disp fx of prox 3rd of navic bone of l wrs, init for opn fx
		S62.Ø33B	Disp fx of prox 3rd of navic bone of unsp wrs, init op fx
		S62.Ø34B	Nondisp fx of prox 3rd of navic bone of r wrs, init op fx
		S62.Ø35B	Nondisp fx of prox 3rd of navic bone of l wrs, init op fx
		S62.Ø36B	Nondisp fx of prox 3rd of navic bone of unsp wrs, init op fx
814.12	OPEN FRACTURE OF LUNATE BONE OF WRIST	**S62.121B**	Disp fx of lunate, right wrist, init for opn fx
		S62.122B	Disp fx of lunate, left wrist, init encntr for open fracture
		S62.123B	Disp fx of lunate, unsp wrist, init encntr for open fracture
		S62.124B	Nondisp fx of lunate, right wrist, init for opn fx
		S62.125B	Nondisp fx of lunate, left wrist, init for opn fx
		S62.126B	Nondisp fx of lunate, unsp wrist, init for opn fx

ICD-9-CM		ICD-10-CM	
814.13	OPEN FRACTURE OF TRIQUETRAL BONE OF WRIST	**S62.111B**	Disp fx of triquetrum bone, right wrist, init for opn fx
		S62.112B	Disp fx of triquetrum bone, left wrist, init for opn fx
		S62.113B	Disp fx of triquetrum bone, unsp wrist, init for opn fx
		S62.114B	Nondisp fx of triquetrum bone, right wrist, init for opn fx
		S62.115B	Nondisp fx of triquetrum bone, left wrist, init for opn fx
		S62.116B	Nondisp fx of triquetrum bone, unsp wrist, init for opn fx
814.14	OPEN FRACTURE OF PISIFORM BONE OF WRIST	**S62.161B**	Disp fx of pisiform, right wrist, init for opn fx
		S62.162B	Disp fx of pisiform, left wrist, init for opn fx
		S62.163B	Disp fx of pisiform, unsp wrist, init for opn fx
		S62.164B	Nondisp fx of pisiform, right wrist, init for opn fx
		S62.165B	Nondisp fx of pisiform, left wrist, init for opn fx
		S62.166B	Nondisp fx of pisiform, unsp wrist, init for opn fx
814.15	OPEN FRACTURE OF TRAPEZIUM BONE OF WRIST	**S62.171B**	Disp fx of trapezium, right wrist, init for opn fx
		S62.172B	Disp fx of trapezium, left wrist, init for opn fx
		S62.173B	Disp fx of trapezium, unsp wrist, init for opn fx
		S62.174B	Nondisp fx of trapezium, right wrist, init for opn fx
		S62.175B	Nondisp fx of trapezium, left wrist, init for opn fx
		S62.176B	Nondisp fx of trapezium, unsp wrist, init for opn fx
814.16	OPEN FRACTURE OF TRAPEZOID BONE OF WRIST	**S62.181B**	Disp fx of trapezoid, right wrist, init for opn fx
		S62.182B	Disp fx of trapezoid, left wrist, init for opn fx
		S62.183B	Disp fx of trapezoid, unsp wrist, init for opn fx
		S62.184B	Nondisp fx of trapezoid, right wrist, init for opn fx
		S62.185B	Nondisp fx of trapezoid, left wrist, init for opn fx
		S62.186B	Nondisp fx of trapezoid, unsp wrist, init for opn fx
814.17	OPEN FRACTURE OF CAPITATE BONE OF WRIST	**S62.131B**	Disp fx of capitate bone, right wrist, init for opn fx
		S62.132B	Disp fx of capitate bone, left wrist, init for opn fx
		S62.133B	Disp fx of capitate bone, unsp wrist, init for opn fx
		S62.134B	Nondisp fx of capitate bone, right wrist, init for opn fx
		S62.135B	Nondisp fx of capitate bone, left wrist, init for opn fx
		S62.136B	Nondisp fx of capitate bone, unsp wrist, init for opn fx
814.18	OPEN FRACTURE OF HAMATE BONE OF WRIST	**S62.141B**	Disp fx of body of hamate bone, right wrist, init for opn fx
		S62.142B	Disp fx of body of hamate bone, left wrist, init for opn fx
		S62.143B	Disp fx of body of hamate bone, unsp wrist, init for opn fx
		S62.144B	Nondisp fx of body of hamate bone, r wrist, init for opn fx
		S62.145B	Nondisp fx of body of hamate bone, l wrist, init for opn fx
		S62.146B	Nondisp fx of body of hamate bone, unsp wrs, init for opn fx
814.19	OPEN FRACTURE OF OTHER BONE OF WRIST	**S62.151B**	Disp fx of hook pro of hamate bone, r wrist, init for opn fx
		S62.152B	Disp fx of hook pro of hamate bone, l wrist, init for opn fx
		S62.153B	Disp fx of hook pro of hamate bone, unsp wrs, init opn fx
		S62.154B	Nondisp fx of hook pro of hamate bone, r wrs, init opn fx
		S62.155B	Nondisp fx of hook pro of hamate bone, l wrs, init opn fx
		S62.156B	Nondisp fx of hook pro of hamate bone, unsp wrs, init opn fx
815.00	CLOSED FRACTURE METACARPAL BONE SITE UNSPECIFIED	**S62.309A**	Unsp fracture of unsp metacarpal bone, init for clos fx
		S62.319A	Disp fx of base of unsp metacarpal bone, init for clos fx
		S62.329A	Disp fx of shaft of unsp metacarpal bone, init for clos fx
		S62.339A	Disp fx of neck of unsp metacarpal bone, init for clos fx
		S62.349A	Nondisp fx of base of unsp metacarpal bone, init for clos fx
		S62.359A	Nondisp fx of shaft of unsp metacarpal bone, init
		S62.369A	Nondisp fx of neck of unsp metacarpal bone, init for clos fx
		S62.399A	Oth fracture of unsp metacarpal bone, init for clos fx
815.01	CLOSED FRACTURE OF BASE OF THUMB METACARPAL BONE	**S62.201A**	Unsp fracture of first metacarpal bone, right hand, init
		S62.202A	Unsp fracture of first metacarpal bone, left hand, init
		S62.209A	Unsp fracture of first metacarpal bone, unsp hand, init
		S62.211A	Bennett's fracture, right hand, init for clos fx
		S62.212A	Bennett's fracture, left hand, init for clos fx
		S62.213A	Bennett's fracture, unsp hand, init for clos fx
		S62.221A	Displaced Rolando's fracture, right hand, init for clos fx
		S62.222A	Displaced Rolando's fracture, left hand, init for clos fx
		S62.223A	Displaced Rolando's fracture, unsp hand, init for clos fx
		S62.224A	Nondisplaced Rolando's fracture, right hand, init
		S62.225A	Nondisplaced Rolando's fracture, left hand, init for clos fx
		S62.226A	Nondisplaced Rolando's fracture, unsp hand, init for clos fx
		S62.231A	Oth disp fx of base of first MC bone, right hand, init
		S62.232A	Oth disp fx of base of first MC bone, left hand, init
		S62.233A	Oth disp fx of base of first MC bone, unsp hand, init
		S62.234A	Oth nondisp fx of base of first MC bone, right hand, init
		S62.235A	Oth nondisp fx of base of first MC bone, left hand, init
		S62.236A	Oth nondisp fx of base of first MC bone, unsp hand, init
815.02	CLOSED FRACTURE OF BASE OF OTHER METACARPAL BONE	**S62.310A**	Disp fx of base of second metacarpal bone, right hand, init
		S62.311A	Disp fx of base of second metacarpal bone. left hand, init
		S62.312A	Disp fx of base of third metacarpal bone, right hand, init
		S62.313A	Disp fx of base of third metacarpal bone, left hand, init
		S62.314A	Disp fx of base of fourth metacarpal bone, right hand, init
		S62.315A	Disp fx of base of fourth metacarpal bone, left hand, init
		S62.316A	Disp fx of base of fifth metacarpal bone, right hand, init
		S62.317A	Disp fx of base of fifth metacarpal bone. left hand, init
		S62.318A	Disp fx of base of oth metacarpal bone, init for clos fx
		S62.319A	Disp fx of base of unsp metacarpal bone, init for clos fx
		S62.340A	Nondisp fx of base of second MC bone, right hand, init
		S62.341A	Nondisp fx of base of second MC bone. left hand, init
	(Continued on next page)	**S62.342A**	Nondisp fx of base of third MC bone, right hand, init

[Brackets] indicate valid character values for each code. Character value meanings provided for each code grouping.

ICD-9-CM		ICD-10-CM	
815.Ø2	CLOSED FRACTURE OF BASE OF OTHER METACARPAL BONE **(Continued)**	**S62.343A**	Nondisp fx of base of third metacarpal bone, left hand, init
		S62.344A	Nondisp fx of base of fourth MC bone, right hand, init
		S62.345A	Nondisp fx of base of fourth MC bone, left hand, init
		S62.346A	Nondisp fx of base of fifth MC bone, right hand, init
		S62.347A	Nondisp fx of base of fifth metacarpal bone. left hand, init
		S62.348A	Nondisp fx of base of oth metacarpal bone, init for clos fx
		S62.349A	Nondisp fx of base of unsp metacarpal bone, init for clos fx
815.Ø3	CLOSED FRACTURE OF SHAFT OF METACARPAL BONE	**S62.241A**	Disp fx of shaft of first metacarpal bone, right hand, init
		S62.242A	Disp fx of shaft of first metacarpal bone, left hand, init
		S62.243A	Disp fx of shaft of first metacarpal bone, unsp hand, init
		S62.244A	Nondisp fx of shaft of first MC bone, right hand, init
		S62.245A	Nondisp fx of shaft of first MC bone, left hand, init
		S62.246A	Nondisp fx of shaft of first MC bone, unsp hand, init
		S62.32ØA	Disp fx of shaft of second metacarpal bone, right hand, init
		S62.321A	Disp fx of shaft of second metacarpal bone, left hand, init
		S62.322A	Disp fx of shaft of third metacarpal bone, right hand, init
		S62.323A	Disp fx of shaft of third metacarpal bone, left hand, init
		S62.324A	Disp fx of shaft of fourth metacarpal bone, right hand, init
		S62.325A	Disp fx of shaft of fourth metacarpal bone, left hand, init
		S62.326A	Disp fx of shaft of fifth metacarpal bone, right hand, init
		S62.327A	Disp fx of shaft of fifth metacarpal bone, left hand, init
		S62.328A	Disp fx of shaft of oth metacarpal bone, init for clos fx
		S62.329A	Disp fx of shaft of unsp metacarpal bone, init for clos fx
		S62.35ØA	Nondisp fx of shaft of second MC bone, right hand, init
		S62.351A	Nondisp fx of shaft of second MC bone, left hand, init
		S62.352A	Nondisp fx of shaft of third MC bone, right hand, init
		S62.353A	Nondisp fx of shaft of third MC bone, left hand, init
		S62.354A	Nondisp fx of shaft of fourth MC bone, right hand, init
		S62.355A	Nondisp fx of shaft of fourth MC bone, left hand, init
		S62.356A	Nondisp fx of shaft of fifth MC bone, right hand, init
		S62.357A	Nondisp fx of shaft of fifth MC bone, left hand, init
		S62.358A	Nondisp fx of shaft of oth metacarpal bone, init for clos fx
		S62.359A	Nondisp fx of shaft of unsp metacarpal bone, init
815.Ø4	CLOSED FRACTURE OF NECK OF METACARPAL BONE	**S62.251A**	Disp fx of neck of first metacarpal bone, right hand, init
		S62.252A	Disp fx of neck of first metacarpal bone, left hand, init
		S62.253A	Disp fx of neck of first metacarpal bone, unsp hand, init
		S62.254A	Nondisp fx of neck of first MC bone, right hand, init
		S62.255A	Nondisp fx of neck of first metacarpal bone, left hand, init
		S62.256A	Nondisp fx of neck of first metacarpal bone, unsp hand, init
		S62.33ØA	Disp fx of neck of second metacarpal bone, right hand, init
		S62.331A	Disp fx of neck of second metacarpal bone, left hand, init
		S62.332A	Disp fx of neck of third metacarpal bone, right hand, init
		S62.333A	Disp fx of neck of third metacarpal bone, left hand, init
		S62.334A	Disp fx of neck of fourth metacarpal bone, right hand, init
		S62.335A	Disp fx of neck of fourth metacarpal bone, left hand, init
		S62.336A	Disp fx of neck of fifth metacarpal bone, right hand, init
		S62.337A	Disp fx of neck of fifth metacarpal bone, left hand, init
		S62.338A	Disp fx of neck of oth metacarpal bone, init for clos fx
		S62.339A	Disp fx of neck of unsp metacarpal bone, init for clos fx
		S62.36ØA	Nondisp fx of neck of second MC bone, right hand, init
		S62.361A	Nondisp fx of neck of second MC bone, left hand, init
		S62.362A	Nondisp fx of neck of third MC bone, right hand, init
		S62.363A	Nondisp fx of neck of third metacarpal bone, left hand, init
		S62.364A	Nondisp fx of neck of fourth MC bone, right hand, init
		S62.365A	Nondisp fx of neck of fourth MC bone, left hand, init
		S62.366A	Nondisp fx of neck of fifth MC bone, right hand, init
		S62.367A	Nondisp fx of neck of fifth metacarpal bone, left hand, init
		S62.368A	Nondisp fx of neck of oth metacarpal bone, init for clos fx
		S62.369A	Nondisp fx of neck of unsp metacarpal bone, init for clos fx
815.Ø9	CLOSED FRACTURE OF MULTIPLE SITES OF METACARPUS	**S62.291A**	Oth fracture of first metacarpal bone, right hand, init
		S62.292A	Oth fracture of first metacarpal bone, left hand, init
		S62.299A	Oth fracture of first metacarpal bone, unsp hand, init
		S62.3ØØA	Unsp fracture of second metacarpal bone, right hand, init
		S62.3Ø1A	Unsp fracture of second metacarpal bone, left hand, init
		S62.3Ø2A	Unsp fracture of third metacarpal bone, right hand, init
		S62.3Ø3A	Unsp fracture of third metacarpal bone, left hand, init
		S62.3Ø4A	Unsp fracture of fourth metacarpal bone, right hand, init
		S62.3Ø5A	Unsp fracture of fourth metacarpal bone, left hand, init
		S62.3Ø6A	Unsp fracture of fifth metacarpal bone, right hand, init
		S62.3Ø7A	Unsp fracture of fifth metacarpal bone, left hand, init
		S62.3Ø8A	Unsp fracture of oth metacarpal bone, init for clos fx
		S62.3Ø9A	Unsp fracture of unsp metacarpal bone, init for clos fx
		S62.39ØA	Oth fracture of second metacarpal bone, right hand, init
		S62.391A	Oth fracture of second metacarpal bone, left hand, init
		S62.392A	Oth fracture of third metacarpal bone, right hand, init
		S62.393A	Oth fracture of third metacarpal bone, left hand, init
		S62.394A	Oth fracture of fourth metacarpal bone, right hand, init
		S62.395A	Oth fracture of fourth metacarpal bone, left hand, init
		S62.396A	Oth fracture of fifth metacarpal bone, right hand, init
		S62.397A	Oth fracture of fifth metacarpal bone, left hand, init
		S62.398A	Oth fracture of oth metacarpal bone, init for clos fx
		S62.399A	Oth fracture of unsp metacarpal bone, init for clos fx

ICD-9-CM		ICD-10-CM	
815.10	OPEN FRACTURE METACARPAL BONE SITE UNSPECIFIED	**S62.309B**	Unsp fracture of unsp metacarpal bone, init for opn fx
815.11	OPEN FRACTURE OF BASE OF THUMB METACARPAL BONE	**S62.201B**	Unsp fx first metacarpal bone, right hand, init for opn fx
		S62.202B	Unsp fx first metacarpal bone, left hand, init for opn fx
		S62.209B	Unsp fx first metacarpal bone, unsp hand, init for opn fx
		S62.211B	Bennett's fracture, right hand, init for opn fx
		S62.212B	Bennett's fracture, left hand, init encntr for open fracture
		S62.213B	Bennett's fracture, unsp hand, init encntr for open fracture
		S62.221B	Displaced Rolando's fracture, right hand, init for opn fx
		S62.222B	Displaced Rolando's fracture, left hand, init for opn fx
		S62.223B	Displaced Rolando's fracture, unsp hand, init for opn fx
		S62.224B	Nondisplaced Rolando's fracture, right hand, init for opn fx
		S62.225B	Nondisplaced Rolando's fracture, left hand, init for opn fx
		S62.226B	Nondisplaced Rolando's fracture, unsp hand, init for opn fx
		S62.231B	Oth disp fx of base of 1st MC bone, r hand, init for opn fx
		S62.232B	Oth disp fx of base of 1st MC bone, l hand, init for opn fx
		S62.233B	Oth disp fx of base of 1st MC bone, unsp hand, init for op fx
		S62.234B	Oth nondisp fx of base of 1st MC bone, r hand, init for op fx
		S62.235B	Oth nondisp fx of base of 1st MC bone, l hand, init for op fx
		S62.236B	Oth nondisp fx of base of 1st MC bone, unsp hand, init for op fx
815.12	OPEN FRACTURE OF BASE OF OTHER METACARPAL BONE	**S62.310B**	Disp fx of base of second MC bone, r hand, init for opn fx
		S62.311B	Disp fx of base of second MC bone. l hand, init for opn fx
		S62.312B	Disp fx of base of third MC bone, r hand, init for opn fx
		S62.313B	Disp fx of base of third MC bone, left hand, init for opn fx
		S62.314B	Disp fx of base of fourth MC bone, r hand, init for opn fx
		S62.315B	Disp fx of base of fourth MC bone, l hand, init for opn fx
		S62.316B	Disp fx of base of fifth MC bone, r hand, init for opn fx
		S62.317B	Disp fx of base of fifth MC bone. left hand, init for opn fx
		S62.318B	Disp fx of base of oth metacarpal bone, init for opn fx
		S62.319B	Disp fx of base of unsp metacarpal bone, init for opn fx
		S62.340B	Nondisp fx of base of 2nd MC bone, r hand, init for opn fx
		S62.341B	Nondisp fx of base of 2nd MC bone. l hand, init for opn fx
		S62.342B	Nondisp fx of base of third MC bone, r hand, init for opn fx
		S62.343B	Nondisp fx of base of third MC bone, l hand, init for opn fx
		S62.344B	Nondisp fx of base of 4th MC bone, r hand, init for opn fx
		S62.345B	Nondisp fx of base of 4th MC bone, l hand, init for opn fx
		S62.346B	Nondisp fx of base of fifth MC bone, r hand, init for opn fx
		S62.347B	Nondisp fx of base of fifth MC bone. l hand, init for opn fx
		S62.348B	Nondisp fx of base of oth metacarpal bone, init for opn fx
		S62.349B	Nondisp fx of base of unsp metacarpal bone, init for opn fx
815.13	OPEN FRACTURE OF SHAFT OF METACARPAL BONE	**S62.241B**	Disp fx of shaft of first MC bone, r hand, init for opn fx
		S62.242B	Disp fx of shaft of first MC bone, l hand, init for opn fx
		S62.243B	Disp fx of shaft of 1st MC bone, unsp hand, init for opn fx
		S62.244B	Nondisp fx of shaft of 1st MC bone, r hand, init for opn fx
		S62.245B	Nondisp fx of shaft of 1st MC bone, l hand, init for opn fx
		S62.246B	Nondisp fx of shaft of 1st MC bone, unsp hand, init for op fx
		S62.320B	Disp fx of shaft of second MC bone, r hand, init for opn fx
		S62.321B	Disp fx of shaft of second MC bone, l hand, init for opn fx
		S62.322B	Disp fx of shaft of third MC bone, r hand, init for opn fx
		S62.323B	Disp fx of shaft of third MC bone, l hand, init for opn fx
		S62.324B	Disp fx of shaft of fourth MC bone, r hand, init for opn fx
		S62.325B	Disp fx of shaft of fourth MC bone, l hand, init for opn fx
		S62.326B	Disp fx of shaft of fifth MC bone, r hand, init for opn fx
		S62.327B	Disp fx of shaft of fifth MC bone, l hand, init for opn fx
		S62.328B	Disp fx of shaft of oth metacarpal bone, init for opn fx
		S62.329B	Disp fx of shaft of unsp metacarpal bone, init for opn fx
		S62.350B	Nondisp fx of shaft of 2nd MC bone, r hand, init for opn fx
		S62.351B	Nondisp fx of shaft of 2nd MC bone, l hand, init for opn fx
		S62.352B	Nondisp fx of shaft of 3rd MC bone, r hand, init for opn fx
		S62.353B	Nondisp fx of shaft of 3rd MC bone, l hand, init for opn fx
		S62.354B	Nondisp fx of shaft of 4th MC bone, r hand, init for opn fx
		S62.355B	Nondisp fx of shaft of 4th MC bone, l hand, init for opn fx
		S62.356B	Nondisp fx of shaft of 5th MC bone, r hand, init for opn fx
		S62.357B	Nondisp fx of shaft of 5th MC bone, l hand, init for opn fx
		S62.358B	Nondisp fx of shaft of oth metacarpal bone, init for opn fx
		S62.359B	Nondisp fx of shaft of unsp metacarpal bone, init for opn fx
815.14	OPEN FRACTURE OF NECK OF METACARPAL BONE	**S62.251B**	Disp fx of neck of first MC bone, r hand, init for opn fx
		S62.252B	Disp fx of neck of first MC bone, left hand, init for opn fx
		S62.253B	Disp fx of neck of first MC bone, unsp hand, init for opn fx
		S62.254B	Nondisp fx of neck of first MC bone, r hand, init for opn fx
		S62.255B	Nondisp fx of neck of first MC bone, l hand, init for opn fx
		S62.256B	Nondisp fx of nk of 1st MC bone, unsp hand, init for opn fx
		S62.330B	Disp fx of neck of second MC bone, r hand, init for opn fx
		S62.331B	Disp fx of neck of second MC bone, l hand, init for opn fx
		S62.332B	Disp fx of neck of third MC bone, r hand, init for opn fx
		S62.333B	Disp fx of neck of third MC bone, left hand, init for opn fx
		S62.334B	Disp fx of neck of fourth MC bone, r hand, init for opn fx
		S62.335B	Disp fx of neck of fourth MC bone, l hand, init for opn fx
		S62.336B	Disp fx of neck of fifth MC bone, r hand, init for opn fx
		S62.337B	Disp fx of neck of fifth MC bone, left hand, init for opn fx
		S62.338B	Disp fx of neck of oth metacarpal bone, init for opn fx
		S62.339B	Disp fx of neck of unsp metacarpal bone, init for opn fx
		S62.360B	Nondisp fx of neck of 2nd MC bone, r hand, init for opn fx

(Continued on next page)

[Brackets] indicate valid character values for each code. Character value meanings provided for each code grouping.

ICD-9-CM		ICD-10-CM	
815.14	OPEN FRACTURE OF NECK OF METACARPAL BONE **(Continued)**	**S62.361B**	Nondisp fx of neck of 2nd MC bone, l hand, init for opn fx
		S62.362B	Nondisp fx of neck of third MC bone, r hand, init for opn fx
		S62.363B	Nondisp fx of neck of third MC bone, l hand, init for opn fx
		S62.364B	Nondisp fx of neck of 4th MC bone, r hand, init for opn fx
		S62.365B	Nondisp fx of neck of 4th MC bone, l hand, init for opn fx
		S62.366B	Nondisp fx of neck of fifth MC bone, r hand, init for opn fx
		S62.367B	Nondisp fx of neck of fifth MC bone, l hand, init for opn fx
		S62.368B	Nondisp fx of neck of oth metacarpal bone, init for opn fx
		S62.369B	Nondisp fx of neck of unsp metacarpal bone, init for opn fx
815.19	OPEN FRACTURE OF MULTIPLE SITES OF METACARPUS	**S62.291B**	Oth fx first metacarpal bone, right hand, init for opn fx
		S62.292B	Oth fx first metacarpal bone, left hand, init for opn fx
		S62.299B	Oth fx first metacarpal bone, unsp hand, init for opn fx
		S62.300B	Unsp fx second metacarpal bone, right hand, init for opn fx
		S62.301B	Unsp fx second metacarpal bone, left hand, init for opn fx
		S62.302B	Unsp fx third metacarpal bone, right hand, init for opn fx
		S62.303B	Unsp fx third metacarpal bone, left hand, init for opn fx
		S62.304B	Unsp fx fourth metacarpal bone, right hand, init for opn fx
		S62.305B	Unsp fx fourth metacarpal bone, left hand, init for opn fx
		S62.306B	Unsp fx fifth metacarpal bone, right hand, init for opn fx
		S62.307B	Unsp fx fifth metacarpal bone, left hand, init for opn fx
		S62.308B	Unsp fracture of oth metacarpal bone, init for opn fx
		S62.309B	Unsp fracture of unsp metacarpal bone, init for opn fx
		S62.390B	Oth fx second metacarpal bone, right hand, init for opn fx
		S62.391B	Oth fx second metacarpal bone, left hand, init for opn fx
		S62.392B	Oth fx third metacarpal bone, right hand, init for opn fx
		S62.393B	Oth fx third metacarpal bone, left hand, init for opn fx
		S62.394B	Oth fx fourth metacarpal bone, right hand, init for opn fx
		S62.395B	Oth fx fourth metacarpal bone, left hand, init for opn fx
		S62.396B	Oth fx fifth metacarpal bone, right hand, init for opn fx
		S62.397B	Oth fx fifth metacarpal bone, left hand, init for opn fx
		S62.398B	Oth fracture of oth metacarpal bone, init for opn fx
		S62.399B	Oth fracture of unsp metacarpal bone, init for opn fx
816.00	CLOSED FRACTURE UNSPEC PHALANX/PHALANGES HAND	**S62.501A**	Fracture of unsp phalanx of right thumb, init for clos fx
		S62.502A	Fracture of unsp phalanx of left thumb, init for clos fx
		S62.509A	Fracture of unsp phalanx of unsp thumb, init for clos fx
		S62.600A	Fracture of unsp phalanx of right index finger, init
		S62.601A	Fracture of unsp phalanx of left index finger, init
		S62.602A	Fracture of unsp phalanx of right middle finger, init
		S62.603A	Fracture of unsp phalanx of left middle finger, init
		S62.604A	Fracture of unsp phalanx of right ring finger, init
		S62.605A	Fracture of unsp phalanx of left ring finger, init
		S62.606A	Fracture of unsp phalanx of right little finger, init
		S62.607A	Fracture of unsp phalanx of left little finger, init
		S62.608A	Fracture of unsp phalanx of oth finger, init for clos fx
		S62.609A	Fracture of unsp phalanx of unsp finger, init for clos fx
816.01	CLOS FRACTURE MID/PROXIMAL PHALANX/PHALANG HAND	**S62.511A**	Disp fx of proximal phalanx of right thumb, init for clos fx
		S62.512A	Disp fx of proximal phalanx of left thumb, init for clos fx
		S62.513A	Disp fx of proximal phalanx of unsp thumb, init for clos fx
		S62.514A	Nondisp fx of proximal phalanx of right thumb, init
		S62.515A	Nondisp fx of proximal phalanx of left thumb, init
		S62.516A	Nondisp fx of proximal phalanx of unsp thumb, init
		S62.610A	Disp fx of proximal phalanx of right index finger, init
		S62.611A	Disp fx of proximal phalanx of left index finger, init
		S62.612A	Disp fx of proximal phalanx of right middle finger, init
		S62.613A	Disp fx of proximal phalanx of left middle finger, init
		S62.614A	Disp fx of proximal phalanx of right ring finger, init
		S62.615A	Disp fx of proximal phalanx of left ring finger, init
		S62.616A	Disp fx of proximal phalanx of right little finger, init
		S62.617A	Disp fx of proximal phalanx of left little finger, init
		S62.618A	Disp fx of proximal phalanx of oth finger, init for clos fx
		S62.619A	Disp fx of proximal phalanx of unsp finger, init for clos fx
		S62.620A	Disp fx of medial phalanx of right index finger, init
		S62.621A	Disp fx of medial phalanx of left index finger, init
		S62.622A	Disp fx of medial phalanx of right middle finger, init
		S62.623A	Disp fx of medial phalanx of left middle finger, init
		S62.624A	Disp fx of medial phalanx of right ring finger, init
		S62.625A	Disp fx of medial phalanx of left ring finger, init
		S62.626A	Disp fx of medial phalanx of right little finger, init
		S62.627A	Disp fx of medial phalanx of left little finger, init
		S62.628A	Disp fx of medial phalanx of oth finger, init for clos fx
		S62.629A	Disp fx of medial phalanx of unsp finger, init for clos fx
		S62.640A	Nondisp fx of proximal phalanx of right index finger, init
		S62.641A	Nondisp fx of proximal phalanx of left index finger, init
		S62.642A	Nondisp fx of proximal phalanx of right middle finger, init
		S62.643A	Nondisp fx of proximal phalanx of left middle finger, init
		S62.644A	Nondisp fx of proximal phalanx of right ring finger, init
		S62.645A	Nondisp fx of proximal phalanx of left ring finger, init
		S62.646A	Nondisp fx of proximal phalanx of right little finger, init
		S62.647A	Nondisp fx of proximal phalanx of left little finger, init
		S62.648A	Nondisp fx of proximal phalanx of oth finger, init
		S62.649A	Nondisp fx of proximal phalanx of unsp finger, init

(Continued on next page)

ICD-9-CM		ICD-10-CM	
816.01	CLOS FRACTURE MID/PROXIMAL PHALANX/PHALANG HAND **(Continued)**	**S62.650A**	Nondisp fx of medial phalanx of right index finger, init
		S62.651A	Nondisp fx of medial phalanx of left index finger, init
		S62.652A	Nondisp fx of medial phalanx of right middle finger, init
		S62.653A	Nondisp fx of medial phalanx of left middle finger, init
		S62.654A	Nondisp fx of medial phalanx of right ring finger, init
		S62.655A	Nondisp fx of medial phalanx of left ring finger, init
		S62.656A	Nondisp fx of medial phalanx of right little finger, init
		S62.657A	Nondisp fx of medial phalanx of left little finger, init
		S62.658A	Nondisp fx of medial phalanx of oth finger, init for clos fx
		S62.659A	Nondisp fx of medial phalanx of unsp finger, init
816.02	CLOSED FRACTURE DISTAL PHALANX OR PHALANGES HAND	**S62.521A**	Disp fx of distal phalanx of right thumb, init for clos fx
		S62.522A	Disp fx of distal phalanx of left thumb, init for clos fx
		S62.523A	Disp fx of distal phalanx of unsp thumb, init for clos fx
		S62.524A	Nondisp fx of distal phalanx of right thumb, init
		S62.525A	Nondisp fx of distal phalanx of left thumb, init for clos fx
		S62.526A	Nondisp fx of distal phalanx of unsp thumb, init for clos fx
		S62.630A	Disp fx of distal phalanx of right index finger, init
		S62.631A	Disp fx of distal phalanx of left index finger, init
		S62.632A	Disp fx of distal phalanx of right middle finger, init
		S62.633A	Disp fx of distal phalanx of left middle finger, init
		S62.634A	Disp fx of distal phalanx of right ring finger, init
		S62.635A	Disp fx of distal phalanx of left ring finger, init
		S62.636A	Disp fx of distal phalanx of right little finger, init
		S62.637A	Disp fx of distal phalanx of left little finger, init
		S62.638A	Disp fx of distal phalanx of oth finger, init for clos fx
		S62.639A	Disp fx of distal phalanx of unsp finger, init for clos fx
		S62.660A	Nondisp fx of distal phalanx of right index finger, init
		S62.661A	Nondisp fx of distal phalanx of left index finger, init
		S62.662A	Nondisp fx of distal phalanx of right middle finger, init
		S62.663A	Nondisp fx of distal phalanx of left middle finger, init
		S62.664A	Nondisp fx of distal phalanx of right ring finger, init
		S62.665A	Nondisp fx of distal phalanx of left ring finger, init
		S62.666A	Nondisp fx of distal phalanx of right little finger, init
		S62.667A	Nondisp fx of distal phalanx of left little finger, init
		S62.668A	Nondisp fx of distal phalanx of oth finger, init for clos fx
		S62.669A	Nondisp fx of distal phalanx of unsp finger, init
816.03	CLOS FRACTURE MX SITES PHALANX/PHALANGES HAND	**S62.90XA**	Unsp fracture of unsp wrist and hand, init for clos fx
		S62.91XA	Unsp fracture of right wrist and hand, init for clos fx
		S62.92XA	Unsp fracture of left wrist and hand, init for clos fx
816.10	OPEN FRACTURE PHALANX/PHALANGES HAND UNSPECIFIED	**S62.501B**	Fracture of unsp phalanx of right thumb, init for opn fx
		S62.502B	Fracture of unsp phalanx of left thumb, init for opn fx
		S62.509B	Fracture of unsp phalanx of unsp thumb, init for opn fx
		S62.600B	Fracture of unsp phalanx of r idx fngr, init for opn fx
		S62.601B	Fracture of unsp phalanx of l idx fngr, init for opn fx
		S62.602B	Fracture of unsp phalanx of r mid finger, init for opn fx
		S62.603B	Fracture of unsp phalanx of l mid finger, init for opn fx
		S62.604B	Fracture of unsp phalanx of r rng fngr, init for opn fx
		S62.605B	Fracture of unsp phalanx of l rng fngr, init for opn fx
		S62.606B	Fracture of unsp phalanx of r little finger, init for opn fx
		S62.607B	Fracture of unsp phalanx of l little finger, init for opn fx
		S62.608B	Fracture of unsp phalanx of oth finger, init for opn fx
		S62.609B	Fracture of unsp phalanx of unsp finger, init for opn fx
816.11	OPEN FRACTURE MID/PROXIMAL PHALANX/PHALANG HAND	**S62.511B**	Disp fx of proximal phalanx of right thumb, init for opn fx
		S62.512B	Disp fx of proximal phalanx of left thumb, init for opn fx
		S62.513B	Disp fx of proximal phalanx of unsp thumb, init for opn fx
		S62.514B	Nondisp fx of proximal phalanx of r thm, init for opn fx
		S62.515B	Nondisp fx of proximal phalanx of l thm, init for opn fx
		S62.516B	Nondisp fx of proximal phalanx of thmb, init for opn fx
		S62.610B	Disp fx of proximal phalanx of r idx fngr, init for opn fx
		S62.611B	Disp fx of proximal phalanx of l idx fngr, init for opn fx
		S62.612B	Disp fx of proximal phalanx of r mid finger, init for opn fx
		S62.613B	Disp fx of proximal phalanx of l mid finger, init for opn fx
		S62.614B	Disp fx of proximal phalanx of r rng fngr, init for opn fx
		S62.615B	Disp fx of proximal phalanx of l rng fngr, init for opn fx
		S62.616B	Disp fx of prox phalanx of r little finger, init for opn fx
		S62.617B	Disp fx of prox phalanx of l little finger, init for opn fx
		S62.618B	Disp fx of proximal phalanx of oth finger, init for opn fx
		S62.619B	Disp fx of proximal phalanx of unsp finger, init for opn fx
		S62.620B	Disp fx of medial phalanx of r idx fngr, init for opn fx
		S62.621B	Disp fx of medial phalanx of l idx fngr, init for opn fx
		S62.622B	Disp fx of medial phalanx of r mid finger, init for opn fx
		S62.623B	Disp fx of medial phalanx of l mid finger, init for opn fx
		S62.624B	Disp fx of medial phalanx of r rng fngr, init for opn fx
		S62.625B	Disp fx of medial phalanx of l rng fngr, init for opn fx
		S62.626B	Disp fx of medial phalanx of r little fngr, init for opn fx
		S62.627B	Disp fx of medial phalanx of l little fngr, init for opn fx
		S62.628B	Disp fx of medial phalanx of oth finger, init for opn fx
		S62.629B	Disp fx of medial phalanx of unsp finger, init for opn fx
		S62.640B	Nondisp fx of prox phalanx of r idx fngr, init for opn fx
		S62.641B	Nondisp fx of prox phalanx of l idx fngr, init for opn fx
		S62.642B	Nondisp fx of prox phalanx of r mid finger, init for opn fx
	(Continued on next page)	**S62.643B**	Nondisp fx of prox phalanx of l mid finger, init for opn fx

ICD-9-CM		ICD-10-CM		
816.11	OPEN FRACTURE MID/PROXIMAL PHALANX/PHALANG HAND (Continued)	**S62.644B**	Nondisp fx of prox phalanx of r rng fngr, init for opn fx	
		S62.645B	Nondisp fx of prox phalanx of l rng fngr, init for opn fx	
		S62.646B	Nondisp fx of prox phalanx of r little fngr, init for opn fx	
		S62.647B	Nondisp fx of prox phalanx of l little fngr, init for opn fx	
		S62.648B	Nondisp fx of proximal phalanx of finger, init for opn fx	
		S62.649B	Nondisp fx of prox phalanx of unsp finger, init for opn fx	
		S62.650B	Nondisp fx of medial phalanx of r idx fngr, init for opn fx	
		S62.651B	Nondisp fx of medial phalanx of l idx fngr, init for opn fx	
		S62.652B	Nondisp fx of medial phalanx of r mid fngr, init for opn fx	
		S62.653B	Nondisp fx of medial phalanx of l mid fngr, init for opn fx	
		S62.654B	Nondisp fx of medial phalanx of r rng fngr, init for opn fx	
		S62.655B	Nondisp fx of medial phalanx of l rng fngr, init for opn fx	
		S62.656B	Nondisp fx of medial phalanx of r lit fngr, init for opn fx	
		S62.657B	Nondisp fx of medial phalanx of l lit fngr, init for opn fx	
		S62.658B	Nondisp fx of medial phalanx of oth finger, init for opn fx	
		S62.659B	Nondisp fx of medial phalanx of unsp finger, init for opn fx	
816.12	OPEN FRACTURE DISTAL PHALANX OR PHALANGES HAND	**S62.521B**	Disp fx of distal phalanx of right thumb, init for opn fx	
		S62.522B	Disp fx of distal phalanx of left thumb, init for opn fx	
		S62.523B	Disp fx of distal phalanx of unsp thumb, init for opn fx	
		S62.524B	Nondisp fx of distal phalanx of right thumb, init for opn fx	
		S62.525B	Nondisp fx of distal phalanx of left thumb, init for opn fx	
		S62.526B	Nondisp fx of distal phalanx of unsp thumb, init for opn fx	
		S62.630B	Disp fx of distal phalanx of r idx fngr, init for opn fx	
		S62.631B	Disp fx of distal phalanx of l idx fngr, init for opn fx	
		S62.632B	Disp fx of distal phalanx of r mid finger, init for opn fx	
		S62.633B	Disp fx of distal phalanx of l mid finger, init for opn fx	
		S62.634B	Disp fx of distal phalanx of r rng fngr, init for opn fx	
		S62.635B	Disp fx of distal phalanx of l rng fngr, init for opn fx	
		S62.636B	Disp fx of dist phalanx of r little finger, init for opn fx	
		S62.637B	Disp fx of dist phalanx of l little finger, init for opn fx	
		S62.638B	Disp fx of distal phalanx of oth finger, init for opn fx	
		S62.639B	Disp fx of distal phalanx of unsp finger, init for opn fx	
		S62.660B	Nondisp fx of distal phalanx of r idx fngr, init for opn fx	
		S62.661B	Nondisp fx of distal phalanx of l idx fngr, init for opn fx	
		S62.662B	Nondisp fx of dist phalanx of r mid finger, init for opn fx	
		S62.663B	Nondisp fx of dist phalanx of l mid finger, init for opn fx	
		S62.664B	Nondisp fx of distal phalanx of r rng fngr, init for opn fx	
		S62.665B	Nondisp fx of distal phalanx of l rng fngr, init for opn fx	
		S62.666B	Nondisp fx of dist phalanx of r little fngr, init for opn fx	
		S62.667B	Nondisp fx of dist phalanx of l little fngr, init for opn fx	
		S62.668B	Nondisp fx of distal phalanx of oth finger, init for opn fx	
		S62.669B	Nondisp fx of distal phalanx of unsp finger, init for opn fx	
816.13	OPEN FX MULTIPLE SITES PHALANX/PHALANGES HAND	**S62.90XB**	Unsp fracture of unsp wrist and hand, init for opn fx	
		S62.91XB	Unsp fracture of right wrist and hand, init for opn fx	
		S62.92XB	Unsp fracture of left wrist and hand, init for opn fx	
817.0	MULTIPLE CLOSED FRACTURES OF HAND BONES	**S62.90XA**	Unsp fracture of unsp wrist and hand, init for clos fx	
817.1	MULTIPLE OPEN FRACTURES OF HAND BONES	**S62.90XB**	Unsp fracture of unsp wrist and hand, init for opn fx	
818.0	ILL-DEFINED CLOSED FRACTURES OF UPPER LIMB	**S62.90XA**	Unsp fracture of unsp wrist and hand, init for clos fx	
818.1	ILL-DEFINED OPEN FRACTURES OF UPPER LIMB	**S62.90XB**	Unsp fracture of unsp wrist and hand, init for opn fx	
819.0	MULT CLOS FX BOTH UP LIMBS&UP LIMB W/RIB&STERNUM	**S42.91XA**	Fracture of right shoulder girdle, part unsp, init	*or*
		S52.91XA	Unsp fracture of right forearm, init for clos fx	*and*
		S42.92XA	Fracture of left shoulder girdle, part unsp, init	*or*
		S52.92XA	Unsp fracture of left forearm, init for clos fx	
		S42.90XA	Fracture of unsp shoulder girdle, part unsp, init	*or*
		S52.90XA	Unsp fracture of unsp forearm, init for clos fx	*and*
		S22.20XA	Unsp fracture of sternum, init encntr for closed fracture	*and*
		S22.49XA	Multiple fractures of ribs, unsp side, init for clos fx	
819.1	MULT OPEN FX BOTH UP LIMBS&UP LIMB W/RIB&STERNUM	**S22.9XXB**	Fracture of bony thorax, part unsp, init for opn fx	
820.00	CLOS FRACTURE UNSPEC INTRACAPSLR SECTION NCK FEM	**S72.011A**	Unsp intracapsular fracture of right femur, init for clos fx	
		S72.012A	Unsp intracapsular fracture of left femur, init for clos fx	
		S72.019A	Unsp intracapsular fracture of unsp femur, init for clos fx	
820.01	CLOSED FRACTURE OF EPIPHYSIS OF NECK OF FEMUR	**S72.021A**	Disp fx of epiphysis (separation) (upper) of r femur, init	
		S72.022A	Disp fx of epiphysis (separation) (upper) of l femur, init	
		S72.023A	Disp fx of epiphy (separation) (upper) of unsp femur, init	
		S72.024A	Nondisp fx of epiphy (separation) (upper) of r femur, init	
		S72.025A	Nondisp fx of epiphy (separation) (upper) of l femur, init	
		S72.026A	Nondisp fx of epiphy (separation) (upper) of unsp femr, init	
		S79.001A	Unsp physeal fracture of upper end of right femur, init	
		S79.002A	Unsp physeal fracture of upper end of left femur, init	
		S79.009A	Unsp physeal fracture of upper end of unsp femur, init	
		S79.011A	Sltr-haris Type I physeal fx upper end of right femur, init	
		S79.012A	Sltr-haris Type I physeal fx upper end of left femur, init	
		S79.019A	Sltr-haris Type I physeal fx upper end of unsp femur, init	
		S79.091A	Oth physeal fracture of upper end of right femur, init	
		S79.092A	Oth physeal fracture of upper end of left femur, init	
		S79.099A	Oth physeal fracture of upper end of unsp femur, init	

ICD-9-CM		ICD-10-CM	
82Ø.Ø2	CLOSED FRACTURE OF MIDCERVICAL SECTION OF FEMUR	**S72.Ø31A**	Displaced midcervical fracture of right femur, init
		S72.Ø32A	Displaced midcervical fracture of left femur, init
		S72.Ø33A	Displaced midcervical fracture of unsp femur, init
		S72.Ø34A	Nondisplaced midcervical fracture of right femur, init
		S72.Ø35A	Nondisplaced midcervical fracture of left femur, init
		S72.Ø36A	Nondisplaced midcervical fracture of unsp femur, init
82Ø.Ø3	CLOSED FRACTURE OF BASE OF NECK OF FEMUR	**S72.Ø41A**	Disp fx of base of neck of right femur, init for clos fx
		S72.Ø42A	Disp fx of base of neck of left femur, init for clos fx
		S72.Ø43A	Disp fx of base of neck of unsp femur, init for clos fx
		S72.Ø44A	Nondisp fx of base of neck of right femur, init for clos fx
		S72.Ø45A	Nondisp fx of base of neck of left femur, init for clos fx
		S72.Ø46A	Nondisp fx of base of neck of unsp femur, init for clos fx
82Ø.Ø9	OTHER CLOSED TRANSCERVICAL FRACTURE OF FEMUR	**S72.Ø51A**	Unsp fracture of head of right femur, init for clos fx
		S72.Ø52A	Unsp fracture of head of left femur, init for clos fx
		S72.Ø59A	Unsp fracture of head of unsp femur, init for clos fx
		S72.Ø61A	Displaced articular fracture of head of right femur, init
		S72.Ø62A	Displaced articular fracture of head of left femur, init
		S72.Ø63A	Displaced articular fracture of head of unsp femur, init
		S72.Ø64A	Nondisplaced articular fracture of head of right femur, init
		S72.Ø65A	Nondisplaced articular fracture of head of left femur, init
		S72.Ø66A	Nondisplaced articular fracture of head of unsp femur, init
		S72.Ø91A	Oth fracture of head and neck of right femur, init
		S72.Ø92A	Oth fracture of head and neck of left femur, init
		S72.Ø99A	Oth fracture of head and neck of unsp femur, init
82Ø.1Ø	OPEN FRACTURE UNSPEC INTRACAPSLR SECTION NCK FEM	**S72.Ø11B**	Unsp intracap fx right femur, init for opn fx type I/2
		S72.Ø11C	Unsp intracap fx right femur, init for opn fx type 3A/B/C
		S72.Ø12B	Unsp intracap fx left femur, init for opn fx type I/2
		S72.Ø12C	Unsp intracap fx left femur, init for opn fx type 3A/B/C
		S72.Ø19B	Unsp intracap fx unsp femur, init for opn fx type I/2
		S72.Ø19C	Unsp intracap fx unsp femur, init for opn fx type 3A/B/C
82Ø.11	OPEN FRACTURE OF EPIPHYSIS OF NECK OF FEMUR	**S72.Ø21B**	Disp fx of epiphy (separation) (upper) of r femr, init op fx 1/2
		S72.Ø21C	Disp fx of epiphy (separation) (upper) of r femr, init op fx 3A/B/C
		S72.Ø22B	Disp fx of epiphy (separation) (upper) of l femr, init op fx 1/2
		S72.Ø22C	Disp fx of epiphy (separation) (upper) of l femr, init op fx 3A/B/C
		S72.Ø23B	Disp fx of epiphy (separation) (upper) of unsp femr, init op fx 1/2
		S72.Ø23C	Disp fx of epiphy (separation) (upper) of unsp femr, init op fx 3A/B/C
		S72.Ø24B	Nondisp fx of epiphy (separation) (upper) of r femr, init op fx 1/2
		S72.Ø24C	Nondisp fx of epiphy (separation) (upper) of r femr, init op fx 3A/B/C
		S72.Ø25B	Nondisp fx of epiphy (separation) (upper) of l femr, init op fx 1/2
		S72.Ø25C	Nondisp fx of epiphy (separation) (upper) of l femr, init op fx 3A/B/C
		S72.Ø26B	Nondisp fx of epiphy (separation) (upper) of unsp femr, init op fx 1/2
		S72.Ø26C	Nondisp fx of epiphy (separation) (upper) of unsp femr, init op fx 3A/B/C
82Ø.12	OPEN FRACTURE OF MIDCERVICAL SECTION OF FEMUR	**S72.Ø31B**	Displaced midcervical fx r femur, init for opn fx type I/2
		S72.Ø31C	Displ midcervical fx r femur, init for opn fx type 3A/B/C
		S72.Ø32B	Displaced midcervical fx l femur, init for opn fx type I/2
		S72.Ø32C	Displ midcervical fx l femur, init for opn fx type 3A/B/C
		S72.Ø33B	Displ midcervical fx unsp femur, init for opn fx type I/2
		S72.Ø33C	Displ midcervical fx unsp femur, init for opn fx type 3A/B/C
		S72.Ø34B	Nondisp midcervical fx right femur, init for opn fx type I/2
		S72.Ø34C	Nondisp midcervical fx r femur, init for opn fx type 3A/B/C
		S72.Ø35B	Nondisp midcervical fx left femur, init for opn fx type I/2
		S72.Ø35C	Nondisp midcervical fx l femur, init for opn fx type 3A/B/C
		S72.Ø36B	Nondisp midcervical fx unsp femur, init for opn fx type I/2
		S72.Ø36C	Nondisp midcervical fx unsp femr, init op fx 3A/B/C
82Ø.13	OPEN FRACTURE OF BASE OF NECK OF FEMUR	**S72.Ø41B**	Disp fx of base of neck of r femur, init for opn fx type I/2
		S72.Ø41C	Disp fx of base of nk of r femr, init for opn fx type 3A/B/C
		S72.Ø42B	Disp fx of base of neck of l femur, init for opn fx type I/2
		S72.Ø42C	Disp fx of base of nk of l femr, init for opn fx type 3A/B/C
		S72.Ø43B	Disp fx of base of nk of unsp femr, init for opn fx type I/2
		S72.Ø43C	Disp fx of base of nk of unsp femr, init op fx 3A/B/C
		S72.Ø44B	Nondisp fx of base of nk of r femr, init for opn fx type I/2
		S72.Ø44C	Nondisp fx of base of nk of r femr, init op fx 3A/B/C
		S72.Ø45B	Nondisp fx of base of nk of l femr, init for opn fx type I/2
		S72.Ø45C	Nondisp fx of base of nk of l femr, init op fx 3A/B/C
		S72.Ø46B	Nondisp fx of base of nk of unsp femr, init op fx 1/2
		S72.Ø46C	Nondisp fx of base of nk of unsp femr, init op fx 3A/B/C
82Ø.19	OTHER OPEN TRANSCERVICAL FRACTURE OF FEMUR	**S72.Ø51B**	Unsp fx head of right femur, init for opn fx type I/2
		S72.Ø51C	Unsp fx head of right femur, init for opn fx type 3A/B/C
		S72.Ø52B	Unsp fx head of left femur, init for opn fx type I/2
		S72.Ø52C	Unsp fx head of left femur, init for opn fx type 3A/B/C
		S72.Ø59B	Unsp fx head of unsp femur, init for opn fx type I/2
		S72.Ø59C	Unsp fx head of unsp femur, init for opn fx type 3A/B/C
		S72.Ø61B	Displaced artic fx head of r femur, init for opn fx type I/2
		S72.Ø61C	Displ artic fx head of r femur, init for opn fx type 3A/B/C
		S72.Ø62B	Displaced artic fx head of l femur, init for opn fx type I/2
		S72.Ø62C	Displ artic fx head of l femur, init for opn fx type 3A/B/C
		S72.Ø63B	Displ artic fx head of unsp femur, init for opn fx type I/2
		S72.Ø63C	Displ artic fx head of unsp femr, init op fx 3A/B/C
		S72.Ø64B	Nondisp artic fx head of r femur, init for opn fx type I/2
		S72.Ø64C	Nondisp artic fx head of r femr, init for opn fx type 3A/B/C
		S72.Ø65B	Nondisp artic fx head of l femur, init for opn fx type I/2

(Continued on next page)

[Brackets] indicate valid character values for each code. Character value meanings provided for each code grouping.

ICD-9-CM		ICD-10-CM	
820.19	OTHER OPEN TRANSCERVICAL FRACTURE OF FEMUR (Continued)	S72.065C	Nondisp artic fx head of l femr, init for opn fx type 3A/B/C
		S72.066B	Nondisp artic fx head of unsp femr, init for opn fx type I/2
		S72.066C	Nondisp artic fx head of unsp femr, init op fx 3A/B/C
		S72.091B	Oth fx head/neck of right femur, init for opn fx type I/2
		S72.091C	Oth fx head/neck of right femur, init for opn fx type 3A/B/C
		S72.092B	Oth fx head/neck of left femur, init for opn fx type I/2
		S72.092C	Oth fx head/neck of left femur, init for opn fx type 3A/B/C
		S72.099B	Oth fx head/neck of unsp femur, init for opn fx type I/2
		S72.099C	Oth fx head/neck of unsp femur, init for opn fx type 3A/B/C
820.20	CLOS FRACTURE UNSPEC TROCHANTERIC SECTION FEMUR	S72.101A	Unsp trochanteric fracture of right femur, init for clos fx
		S72.102A	Unsp trochanteric fracture of left femur, init for clos fx
		S72.109A	Unsp trochanteric fracture of unsp femur, init for clos fx
		S72.111A	Disp fx of greater trochanter of right femur, init
		S72.112A	Disp fx of greater trochanter of left femur, init
		S72.113A	Disp fx of greater trochanter of unsp femur, init
		S72.114A	Nondisp fx of greater trochanter of right femur, init
		S72.115A	Nondisp fx of greater trochanter of left femur, init
		S72.116A	Nondisp fx of greater trochanter of unsp femur, init
		S72.121A	Disp fx of lesser trochanter of right femur, init
		S72.122A	Disp fx of lesser trochanter of left femur, init for clos fx
		S72.123A	Disp fx of lesser trochanter of unsp femur, init for clos fx
		S72.124A	Nondisp fx of lesser trochanter of right femur, init
		S72.125A	Nondisp fx of lesser trochanter of left femur, init
		S72.126A	Nondisp fx of lesser trochanter of unsp femur, init
		S72.131A	Displaced apophyseal fracture of right femur, init
		S72.132A	Displaced apophyseal fracture of left femur, init
		S72.133A	Displaced apophyseal fracture of unsp femur, init
		S72.134A	Nondisplaced apophyseal fracture of right femur, init
		S72.135A	Nondisplaced apophyseal fracture of left femur, init
		S72.136A	Nondisplaced apophyseal fracture of unsp femur, init
820.21	CLOSED FRACTURE INTERTROCHANTERIC SECTION FEMUR	S72.141A	Displaced intertrochanteric fracture of right femur, init
		S72.142A	Displaced intertrochanteric fracture of left femur, init
		S72.143A	Displaced intertrochanteric fracture of unsp femur, init
		S72.144A	Nondisplaced intertrochanteric fracture of right femur, init
		S72.145A	Nondisplaced intertrochanteric fracture of left femur, init
		S72.146A	Nondisplaced intertrochanteric fracture of unsp femur, init
820.22	CLOSED FRACTURE SUBTROCHANTERIC SECTION FEMUR	S72.21XA	Displaced subtrochanteric fracture of right femur, init
		S72.22XA	Displaced subtrochanteric fracture of left femur, init
		S72.23XA	Displaced subtrochanteric fracture of unsp femur, init
		S72.24XA	Nondisplaced subtrochanteric fracture of right femur, init
		S72.25XA	Nondisplaced subtrochanteric fracture of left femur, init
		S72.26XA	Nondisplaced subtrochanteric fracture of unsp femur, init
820.30	OPEN FRACTURE UNSPEC TROCHANTERIC SECTION FEMUR	S72.101B	Unsp trochan fx right femur, init for opn fx type I/2
		S72.101C	Unsp trochan fx right femur, init for opn fx type 3A/B/C
		S72.102B	Unsp trochan fx left femur, init for opn fx type I/2
		S72.102C	Unsp trochan fx left femur, init for opn fx type 3A/B/C
		S72.109B	Unsp trochan fx unsp femur, init for opn fx type I/2
		S72.109C	Unsp trochan fx unsp femur, init for opn fx type 3A/B/C
		S72.111B	Disp fx of greater trochanter of r femr, init op fx 1/2
		S72.111C	Disp fx of greater trochanter of r femr, init op fx 3A/B/C
		S72.112B	Disp fx of greater trochanter of l femr, init op fx 1/2
		S72.112C	Disp fx of greater trochanter of l femr, init op fx 3A/B/C
		S72.113B	Disp fx of greater trochanter of unsp femr, init op fx 1/2
		S72.113C	Disp fx of greater trochanter of unsp femr, init op fx 3A/B/C
		S72.114B	Nondisp fx of greater trochanter of r femr, init op fx 1/2
		S72.114C	Nondisp fx of greater trochanter of r femr, init op fx 3A/B/C
		S72.115B	Nondisp fx of greater trochanter of l femr, init op fx 1/2
		S72.115C	Nondisp fx of greater trochanter of l femr, init op fx 3A/B/C
		S72.116B	Nondisp fx of greater trochanter of unsp femr, init op fx 1/2
		S72.116C	Nondisp fx of greater trochanter of unsp femr, init op fx 3A/B/C
		S72.121B	Disp fx of less trochanter of r femr, init op fx 1/2
		S72.121C	Disp fx of less trochanter of r femr, init op fx 3A/B/C
		S72.122B	Disp fx of less trochanter of l femr, init op fx 1/2
		S72.122C	Disp fx of less trochanter of l femr, init op fx 3A/B/C
		S72.123B	Disp fx of less trochanter of unsp femr, init op fx 1/2
		S72.123C	Disp fx of less trochanter of unsp femr, init op fx 3A/B/C
		S72.124B	Nondisp fx of less trochanter of r femr, init op fx 1/2
		S72.124C	Nondisp fx of less trochanter of r femr, init op fx 3A/B/C
		S72.125B	Nondisp fx of less trochanter of l femr, init op fx 1/2
		S72.125C	Nondisp fx of less trochanter of l femr, init op fx 3A/B/C
		S72.126B	Nondisp fx of less trochanter of unsp femr, init op fx 1/2
		S72.126C	Nondisp fx of less trochanter of unsp femr, init op fx 3A/B/C
		S72.131B	Displaced apophyseal fx r femur, init for opn fx type I/2
		S72.131C	Displaced apophyseal fx r femur, init for opn fx type 3A/B/C
		S72.132B	Displaced apophyseal fx left femur, init for opn fx type I/2
		S72.132C	Displaced apophyseal fx l femur, init for opn fx type 3A/B/C
		S72.133B	Displaced apophyseal fx unsp femur, init for opn fx type I/2
		S72.133C	Displ apophyseal fx unsp femur, init for opn fx type 3A/B/C
		S72.134B	Nondisp apophyseal fx right femur, init for opn fx type I/2
		S72.134C	Nondisp apophyseal fx r femur, init for opn fx type 3A/B/C
		S72.135B	Nondisp apophyseal fx left femur, init for opn fx type I/2

(Continued on next page)

ICD-9-CM		ICD-10-CM	
82Ø.3Ø	OPEN FRACTURE UNSPEC TROCHANTERIC SECTION FEMUR **(Continued)**	**S72.135C**	Nondisp apophyseal fx l femur, init for opn fx type 3A/B/C
		S72.136B	Nondisp apophyseal fx unsp femur, init for opn fx type I/2
		S72.136C	Nondisp apophyseal fx unsp femr, init for opn fx type 3A/B/C
82Ø.31	OPEN FRACTURE INTERTROCHANTERIC SECTION FEMUR	**S72.141B**	Displaced intertroch fx r femur, init for opn fx type I/2
		S72.141C	Displaced intertroch fx r femur, init for opn fx type 3A/B/C
		S72.142B	Displaced intertroch fx left femur, init for opn fx type I/2
		S72.142C	Displaced intertroch fx l femur, init for opn fx type 3A/B/C
		S72.143B	Displaced intertroch fx unsp femur, init for opn fx type I/2
		S72.143C	Displ intertroch fx unsp femur, init for opn fx type 3A/B/C
		S72.144B	Nondisp intertroch fx right femur, init for opn fx type I/2
		S72.144C	Nondisp intertroch fx r femur, init for opn fx type 3A/B/C
		S72.145B	Nondisp intertroch fx left femur, init for opn fx type I/2
		S72.145C	Nondisp intertroch fx l femur, init for opn fx type 3A/B/C
		S72.146B	Nondisp intertroch fx unsp femur, init for opn fx type I/2
		S72.146C	Nondisp intertroch fx unsp femr, init for opn fx type 3A/B/C
82Ø.32	OPEN FRACTURE SUBTROCHANTERIC SECTION FEMUR	**S72.21XB**	Displaced subtrochnt fx r femur, init for opn fx type I/2
		S72.21XC	Displaced subtrochnt fx r femur, init for opn fx type 3A/B/C
		S72.22XB	Displaced subtrochnt fx left femur, init for opn fx type I/2
		S72.22XC	Displaced subtrochnt fx l femur, init for opn fx type 3A/B/C
		S72.23XB	Displaced subtrochnt fx unsp femur, init for opn fx type I/2
		S72.23XC	Displ subtrochnt fx unsp femur, init for opn fx type 3A/B/C
		S72.24XB	Nondisp subtrochnt fx right femur, init for opn fx type I/2
		S72.24XC	Nondisp subtrochnt fx r femur, init for opn fx type 3A/B/C
		S72.25XB	Nondisp subtrochnt fx left femur, init for opn fx type I/2
		S72.25XC	Nondisp subtrochnt fx l femur, init for opn fx type 3A/B/C
		S72.26XB	Nondisp subtrochnt fx unsp femur, init for opn fx type I/2
		S72.26XC	Nondisp subtrochnt fx unsp femr, init for opn fx type 3A/B/C
82Ø.8	CLOSED FRACTURE UNSPECIFIED PART NECK FEMUR	**S72.ØØ1A**	Fracture of unsp part of neck of right femur, init
		S72.ØØ2A	Fracture of unsp part of neck of left femur, init
		S72.ØØ9A	Fracture of unsp part of neck of unsp femur, init
82Ø.9	OPEN FRACTURE UNSPECIFIED PART NECK FEMUR	**S72.ØØ1B**	Fx unsp part of neck of r femur, init for opn fx type I/2
		S72.ØØ1C	Fx unsp part of neck of r femur, init for opn fx type 3A/B/C
		S72.ØØ2B	Fx unsp part of neck of left femur, init for opn fx type I/2
		S72.ØØ2C	Fx unsp part of neck of l femur, init for opn fx type 3A/B/C
		S72.ØØ9B	Fx unsp part of neck of unsp femur, init for opn fx type I/2
		S72.ØØ9C	Fx unsp part of nk of unsp femr, init for opn fx type 3A/B/C
821.ØØ	CLOSED FRACTURE OF UNSPECIFIED PART OF FEMUR	**S72.8X1A**	Oth fracture of right femur, init encntr for closed fracture
		S72.8X2A	Oth fracture of left femur, init encntr for closed fracture
		S72.8X9A	Oth fracture of unsp femur, init encntr for closed fracture
		S72.9ØXA	Unsp fracture of unsp femur, init encntr for closed fracture
		S72.91XA	Unsp fracture of right femur, init for clos fx
		S72.92XA	Unsp fracture of left femur, init encntr for closed fracture
821.Ø1	CLOSED FRACTURE OF SHAFT OF FEMUR	**S72.3Ø1A**	Unsp fracture of shaft of right femur, init for clos fx
		S72.3Ø2A	Unsp fracture of shaft of left femur, init for clos fx
		S72.3Ø9A	Unsp fracture of shaft of unsp femur, init for clos fx
		S72.321A	Displaced transverse fracture of shaft of right femur, init
		S72.322A	Displaced transverse fracture of shaft of left femur, init
		S72.323A	Displaced transverse fracture of shaft of unsp femur, init
		S72.324A	Nondisp transverse fracture of shaft of right femur, init
		S72.325A	Nondisp transverse fracture of shaft of left femur, init
		S72.326A	Nondisp transverse fracture of shaft of unsp femur, init
		S72.331A	Displaced oblique fracture of shaft of right femur, init
		S72.332A	Displaced oblique fracture of shaft of left femur, init
		S72.333A	Displaced oblique fracture of shaft of unsp femur, init
		S72.334A	Nondisplaced oblique fracture of shaft of right femur, init
		S72.335A	Nondisplaced oblique fracture of shaft of left femur, init
		S72.336A	Nondisplaced oblique fracture of shaft of unsp femur, init
		S72.341A	Displaced spiral fracture of shaft of right femur, init
		S72.342A	Displaced spiral fracture of shaft of left femur, init
		S72.343A	Displaced spiral fracture of shaft of unsp femur, init
		S72.344A	Nondisplaced spiral fracture of shaft of right femur, init
		S72.345A	Nondisplaced spiral fracture of shaft of left femur, init
		S72.346A	Nondisplaced spiral fracture of shaft of unsp femur, init
		S72.351A	Displaced comminuted fracture of shaft of right femur, init
		S72.352A	Displaced comminuted fracture of shaft of left femur, init
		S72.353A	Displaced comminuted fracture of shaft of unsp femur, init
		S72.354A	Nondisp comminuted fracture of shaft of right femur, init
		S72.355A	Nondisp comminuted fracture of shaft of left femur, init
		S72.356A	Nondisp comminuted fracture of shaft of unsp femur, init
		S72.361A	Displaced segmental fracture of shaft of right femur, init
		S72.362A	Displaced segmental fracture of shaft of left femur, init
		S72.363A	Displaced segmental fracture of shaft of unsp femur, init
		S72.364A	Nondisp segmental fracture of shaft of right femur, init
		S72.365A	Nondisplaced segmental fracture of shaft of left femur, init
		S72.366A	Nondisplaced segmental fracture of shaft of unsp femur, init
		S72.391A	Oth fracture of shaft of right femur, init for clos fx
		S72.392A	Oth fracture of shaft of left femur, init for clos fx
		S72.399A	Oth fracture of shaft of unsp femur, init for clos fx

[Brackets] indicate valid character values for each code. Character value meanings provided for each code grouping.

ICD-9-CM		ICD-10-CM	
821.1Ø	OPEN FRACTURE OF UNSPECIFIED PART OF FEMUR	**S72.8X1B**	Oth fracture of right femur, init for opn fx type I/2
		S72.8X1C	Oth fracture of right femur, init for opn fx type 3A/B/C
		S72.8X2B	Oth fracture of left femur, init for opn fx type I/2
		S72.8X2C	Oth fracture of left femur, init for opn fx type 3A/B/C
		S72.8X9B	Oth fracture of unsp femur, init for opn fx type I/2
		S72.8X9C	Oth fracture of unsp femur, init for opn fx type 3A/B/C
		S72.9ØXB	Unsp fracture of unsp femur, init for opn fx type I/2
		S72.9ØXC	Unsp fracture of unsp femur, init for opn fx type 3A/B/C
		S72.91XB	Unsp fracture of right femur, init for opn fx type I/2
		S72.91XC	Unsp fracture of right femur, init for opn fx type 3A/B/C
		S72.92XB	Unsp fracture of left femur, init for opn fx type I/2
		S72.92XC	Unsp fracture of left femur, init for opn fx type 3A/B/C
821.11	OPEN FRACTURE OF SHAFT OF FEMUR	**S72.3Ø1B**	Unsp fx shaft of right femur, init for opn fx type I/2
		S72.3Ø1C	Unsp fx shaft of right femur, init for opn fx type 3A/B/C
		S72.3Ø2B	Unsp fx shaft of left femur, init for opn fx type I/2
		S72.3Ø2C	Unsp fx shaft of left femur, init for opn fx type 3A/B/C
		S72.3Ø9B	Unsp fx shaft of unsp femur, init for opn fx type I/2
		S72.3Ø9C	Unsp fx shaft of unsp femur, init for opn fx type 3A/B/C
		S72.321B	Displ transverse fx shaft of r femr, init op fx 1/2
		S72.321C	Displ transverse fx shaft of r femr, init op fx 3A/B/C
		S72.322B	Displ transverse fx shaft of l femr, init op fx 1/2
		S72.322C	Displ transverse fx shaft of l femr, init op fx 3A/B/C
		S72.323B	Displ transverse fx shaft of unsp femr, init op fx 1/2
		S72.323C	Displ transverse fx shaft of unsp femr, init op fx 3A/B/C
		S72.324B	Nondisp transverse fx shaft of r femr, init op fx 1/2
		S72.324C	Nondisp transverse fx shaft of r femr, init op fx 3A/B/C
		S72.325B	Nondisp transverse fx shaft of l femr, init op fx 1/2
		S72.325C	Nondisp transverse fx shaft of l femr, init op fx 3A/B/C
		S72.326B	Nondisp transverse fx shaft of unsp femr, init op fx 1/2
		S72.326C	Nondisp transverse fx shaft of unsp femr, init op fx 3A/B/C
		S72.331B	Displ oblique fx shaft of r femur, init for opn fx type I/2
		S72.331C	Displ oblique fx shaft of r femr, init op fx 3A/B/C
		S72.332B	Displ oblique fx shaft of l femur, init for opn fx type I/2
		S72.332C	Displ oblique fx shaft of l femr, init op fx 3A/B/C
		S72.333B	Displ oblique fx shaft of unsp femr, init op fx 1/2
		S72.333C	Displ oblique fx shaft of unsp femr, init op fx 3A/B/C
		S72.334B	Nondisp oblique fx shaft of r femr, init for opn fx type I/2
		S72.334C	Nondisp oblique fx shaft of r femr, init op fx 3A/B/C
		S72.335B	Nondisp oblique fx shaft of l femr, init for opn fx type I/2
		S72.335C	Nondisp oblique fx shaft of l femr, init op fx 3A/B/C
		S72.336B	Nondisp oblique fx shaft of unsp femr, init op fx 1/2
		S72.336C	Nondisp oblique fx shaft of unsp femr, init op fx 3A/B/C
		S72.341B	Displ spiral fx shaft of r femur, init for opn fx type I/2
		S72.341C	Displ spiral fx shaft of r femr, init for opn fx type 3A/B/C
		S72.342B	Displ spiral fx shaft of l femur, init for opn fx type I/2
		S72.342C	Displ spiral fx shaft of l femr, init for opn fx type 3A/B/C
		S72.343B	Displ spiral fx shaft of unsp femr, init for opn fx type I/2
		S72.343C	Displ spiral fx shaft of unsp femr, init op fx 3A/B/C
		S72.344B	Nondisp spiral fx shaft of r femur, init for opn fx type I/2
		S72.344C	Nondisp spiral fx shaft of r femr, init op fx 3A/B/C
		S72.345B	Nondisp spiral fx shaft of l femur, init for opn fx type I/2
		S72.345C	Nondisp spiral fx shaft of l femr, init op fx 3A/B/C
		S72.346B	Nondisp spiral fx shaft of unsp femr, init op fx 1/2
		S72.346C	Nondisp spiral fx shaft of unsp femr, init op fx 3A/B/C
		S72.351B	Displ commnt fx shaft of r femur, init for opn fx type I/2
		S72.351C	Displ commnt fx shaft of r femr, init for opn fx type 3A/B/C
		S72.352B	Displ commnt fx shaft of l femur, init for opn fx type I/2
		S72.352C	Displ commnt fx shaft of l femr, init for opn fx type 3A/B/C
		S72.353B	Displ commnt fx shaft of unsp femr, init for opn fx type I/2
		S72.353C	Displ commnt fx shaft of unsp femr, init op fx 3A/B/C
		S72.354B	Nondisp commnt fx shaft of r femur, init for opn fx type I/2
		S72.354C	Nondisp commnt fx shaft of r femr, init op fx 3A/B/C
		S72.355B	Nondisp commnt fx shaft of l femur, init for opn fx type I/2
		S72.355C	Nondisp commnt fx shaft of l femr, init op fx 3A/B/C
		S72.356B	Nondisp commnt fx shaft of unsp femr, init op fx 1/2
		S72.356C	Nondisp commnt fx shaft of unsp femr, init op fx 3A/B/C
		S72.361B	Displ seg fx shaft of r femur, init for opn fx type I/2
		S72.361C	Displ seg fx shaft of r femur, init for opn fx type 3A/B/C
		S72.362B	Displ seg fx shaft of l femur, init for opn fx type I/2
		S72.362C	Displ seg fx shaft of l femur, init for opn fx type 3A/B/C
		S72.363B	Displ seg fx shaft of unsp femur, init for opn fx type I/2
		S72.363C	Displ seg fx shaft of unsp femr, init for opn fx type 3A/B/C
		S72.364B	Nondisp seg fx shaft of r femur, init for opn fx type I/2
		S72.364C	Nondisp seg fx shaft of r femur, init for opn fx type 3A/B/C
		S72.365B	Nondisp seg fx shaft of l femur, init for opn fx type I/2
		S72.365C	Nondisp seg fx shaft of l femur, init for opn fx type 3A/B/C
		S72.366B	Nondisp seg fx shaft of unsp femur, init for opn fx type I/2
		S72.366C	Nondisp seg fx shaft of unsp femr, init op fx 3A/B/C
		S72.391B	Oth fx shaft of right femur, init for opn fx type I/2
		S72.391C	Oth fx shaft of right femur, init for opn fx type 3A/B/C
		S72.392B	Oth fx shaft of left femur, init for opn fx type I/2

(Continued on next page)

ICD-9-CM		ICD-10-CM	
821.11	OPEN FRACTURE OF SHAFT OF FEMUR **(Continued)**	**S72.392C**	Oth fx shaft of left femur, init for opn fx type 3A/B/C
		S72.399B	Oth fx shaft of unsp femur, init for opn fx type I/2
		S72.399C	Oth fx shaft of unsp femur, init for opn fx type 3A/B/C
821.2Ø	CLOSED FRACTURE UNSPECIFIED PART LOWER END FEMUR	**S72.4Ø1A**	Unsp fracture of lower end of right femur, init for clos fx
		S72.4Ø2A	Unsp fracture of lower end of left femur, init for clos fx
		S72.4Ø9A	Unsp fracture of lower end of unsp femur, init for clos fx
821.21	CLOSED FRACTURE OF FEMORAL CONDYLE	**S72.411A**	Displaced unsp condyle fx lower end of right femur, init
		S72.412A	Displaced unsp condyle fx lower end of left femur, init
		S72.413A	Displaced unsp condyle fx lower end of unsp femur, init
		S72.414A	Nondisp unsp condyle fx lower end of right femur, init
		S72.415A	Nondisp unsp condyle fx lower end of left femur, init
		S72.416A	Nondisp unsp condyle fx lower end of unsp femur, init
		S72.421A	Disp fx of lateral condyle of right femur, init for clos fx
		S72.422A	Disp fx of lateral condyle of left femur, init for clos fx
		S72.423A	Disp fx of lateral condyle of unsp femur, init for clos fx
		S72.424A	Nondisp fx of lateral condyle of right femur, init
		S72.425A	Nondisp fx of lateral condyle of left femur, init
		S72.426A	Nondisp fx of lateral condyle of unsp femur, init
		S72.431A	Disp fx of medial condyle of right femur, init for clos fx
		S72.432A	Disp fx of medial condyle of left femur, init for clos fx
		S72.433A	Disp fx of medial condyle of unsp femur, init for clos fx
		S72.434A	Nondisp fx of medial condyle of right femur, init
		S72.435A	Nondisp fx of medial condyle of left femur, init for clos fx
		S72.436A	Nondisp fx of medial condyle of unsp femur, init for clos fx
821.22	CLOSED FRACTURE OF LOWER EPIPHYSIS OF FEMUR	**S72.441A**	Disp fx of lower epiphysis (separation) of right femur, init
		S72.442A	Disp fx of lower epiphysis (separation) of left femur, init
		S72.443A	Disp fx of lower epiphysis (separation) of unsp femur, init
		S72.444A	Nondisp fx of lower epiphysis (separation) of r femur, init
		S72.445A	Nondisp fx of lower epiphysis (separation) of l femur, init
		S72.446A	Nondisp fx of lower epiphy (separation) of unsp femur, init
		S79.1Ø1A	Unsp physeal fracture of lower end of right femur, init
		S79.1Ø2A	Unsp physeal fracture of lower end of left femur, init
		S79.1Ø9A	Unsp physeal fracture of lower end of unsp femur, init
		S79.111A	Sltr-haris Type I physeal fx lower end of right femur, init
		S79.112A	Sltr-haris Type I physeal fx lower end of left femur, init
		S79.119A	Sltr-haris Type I physeal fx lower end of unsp femur, init
		S79.121A	Sltr-haris Type II physeal fx lower end of right femur, init
		S79.122A	Sltr-haris Type II physeal fx lower end of left femur, init
		S79.129A	Sltr-haris Type II physeal fx lower end of unsp femur, init
		S79.131A	Sltr-haris Type III physeal fx lower end of r femur, init
		S79.132A	Sltr-haris Type III physeal fx lower end of left femur, init
		S79.139A	Sltr-haris Type III physeal fx lower end of unsp femur, init
		S79.141A	Sltr-haris Type IV physeal fx lower end of right femur, init
		S79.142A	Sltr-haris Type IV physeal fx lower end of left femur, init
		S79.149A	Sltr-haris Type IV physeal fx lower end of unsp femur, init
		S79.191A	Oth physeal fracture of lower end of right femur, init
		S79.192A	Oth physeal fracture of lower end of left femur, init
		S79.199A	Oth physeal fracture of lower end of unsp femur, init
821.23	CLOSED SUPRACONDYLAR FRACTURE OF FEMUR	**S72.451A**	Displ suprcndl fx w/o intrcndl extn lower end r femur, init
		S72.452A	Displ suprcndl fx w/o intrcndl extn lower end l femur, init
		S72.453A	Displ suprcndl fx w/o intrcndl extn low end unsp femr, init
		S72.454A	Nondisp suprcndl fx w/o intrcndl extn lower end r femr, init
		S72.455A	Nondisp suprcndl fx w/o intrcndl extn lower end l femr, init
		S72.456A	Nondisp suprcndl fx w/o intrcndl extn low end unsp femr,init
		S72.461A	Displ suprcndl fx w intrcndl extn lower end of r femur, init
		S72.462A	Displ suprcndl fx w intrcndl extn lower end of l femur, init
		S72.463A	Displ suprcndl fx w intrcndl extn lower end unsp femur, init
		S72.464A	Nondisp suprcndl fx w intrcndl extn lower end r femur, init
		S72.465A	Nondisp suprcndl fx w intrcndl extn lower end l femur, init
		S72.466A	Nondisp suprcndl fx w intrcndl extn low end unsp femr, init
821.29	OTHER CLOSED FRACTURE OF LOWER END OF FEMUR	**S72.471A**	Torus fracture of lower end of right femur, init for clos fx
		S72.472A	Torus fracture of lower end of left femur, init for clos fx
		S72.479A	Torus fracture of lower end of unsp femur, init for clos fx
		S72.491A	Oth fracture of lower end of right femur, init for clos fx
		S72.492A	Oth fracture of lower end of left femur, init for clos fx
		S72.499A	Oth fracture of lower end of unsp femur, init for clos fx
821.3Ø	OPEN FRACTURE UNSPECIFIED PART LOWER END FEMUR	**S72.4Ø1B**	Unsp fx lower end of right femur, init for opn fx type I/2
		S72.4Ø1C	Unsp fx lower end of r femur, init for opn fx type 3A/B/C
		S72.4Ø2B	Unsp fx lower end of left femur, init for opn fx type I/2
		S72.4Ø2C	Unsp fx lower end of left femur, init for opn fx type 3A/B/C
		S72.4Ø9B	Unsp fx lower end of unsp femur, init for opn fx type I/2
		S72.4Ø9C	Unsp fx lower end of unsp femur, init for opn fx type 3A/B/C

[Brackets] indicate valid character values for each code. Character value meanings provided for each code grouping.

ICD-9-CM		ICD-10-CM	
821.31	OPEN FRACTURE OF FEMORAL CONDYLE	**S72.411B**	Displ unsp condyle fx low end r femr, init op fx 1/2
		S72.411C	Displ unsp condyle fx low end r femr, init op fx 3A/B/C
		S72.412B	Displ unsp condyle fx low end l femr, init op fx 1/2
		S72.412C	Displ unsp condyle fx low end l femr, init op fx 3A/B/C
		S72.413B	Displ unsp condyle fx low end unsp femr, init op fx 1/2
		S72.413C	Displ unsp condyle fx low end unsp femr, init op fx 3A/B/C
		S72.414B	Nondisp unsp condyle fx low end r femr, init op fx 1/2
		S72.414C	Nondisp unsp condyle fx low end r femr, init op fx 3A/B/C
		S72.415B	Nondisp unsp condyle fx low end l femr, init op fx 1/2
		S72.415C	Nondisp unsp condyle fx low end l femr, init op fx 3A/B/C
		S72.416B	Nondisp unsp condyle fx low end unsp femr, init op fx 1/2
		S72.416C	Nondisp unsp condyle fx low end unsp femr, init op fx 3A/B/C
		S72.421B	Disp fx of lateral condyle of r femr, init op fx 1/2
		S72.421C	Disp fx of lateral condyle of r femr, init op fx 3A/B/C
		S72.422B	Disp fx of lateral condyle of l femr, init op fx 1/2
		S72.422C	Disp fx of lateral condyle of l femr, init op fx 3A/B/C
		S72.423B	Disp fx of lateral condyle of unsp femr, init op fx 1/2
		S72.423C	Disp fx of lateral condyle of unsp femr, init op fx 3A/B/C
		S72.424B	Nondisp fx of lateral condyle of r femr, init op fx 1/2
		S72.424C	Nondisp fx of lateral condyle of r femr, init op fx 3A/B/C
		S72.425B	Nondisp fx of lateral condyle of l femr, init op fx 1/2
		S72.425C	Nondisp fx of lateral condyle of l femr, init op fx 3A/B/C
		S72.426B	Nondisp fx of lateral condyle of unsp femr, init op fx 1/2
		S72.426C	Nondisp fx of lateral condyle of unsp femr, init op fx 3A/B/C
		S72.431B	Disp fx of med condyle of r femur, init for opn fx type I/2
		S72.431C	Disp fx of med condyle of r femr, init op fx 3A/B/C
		S72.432B	Disp fx of med condyle of l femur, init for opn fx type I/2
		S72.432C	Disp fx of med condyle of l femr, init op fx 3A/B/C
		S72.433B	Disp fx of med condyle of unsp femr, init op fx 1/2
		S72.433C	Disp fx of med condyle of unsp femr, init op fx 3A/B/C
		S72.434B	Nondisp fx of med condyle of r femr, init op fx 1/2
		S72.434C	Nondisp fx of med condyle of r femr, init op fx 3A/B/C
		S72.435B	Nondisp fx of med condyle of l femr, init op fx 1/2
		S72.435C	Nondisp fx of med condyle of l femr, init op fx 3A/B/C
		S72.436B	Nondisp fx of med condyle of unsp femr, init op fx 1/2
		S72.436C	Nondisp fx of med condyle of unsp femr, init op fx 3A/B/C
821.32	OPEN FRACTURE OF LOWER EPIPHYSIS OF FEMUR	**S72.441B**	Disp fx of low epiphy (separation) of r femr, init op fx 1/2
		S72.441C	Disp fx of low epiphy (separation) of r femr, init op fx 3A/B/C
		S72.442B	Disp fx of low epiphy (separation) of l femr, init op fx 1/2
		S72.442C	Disp fx of low epiphy (separation) of l femr, init op fx 3A/B/C
		S72.443B	Disp fx of low epiphy (separation) of unsp femr, init op fx 1/2
		S72.443C	Disp fx of low epiphy (separation) of unsp femr, init op fx 3A/B/C
		S72.444B	Nondisp fx of low epiphy (separation) of r femr, init op fx 1/2
		S72.444C	Nondisp fx of low epiphy (separation) of r femr, init op fx 3A/B/C
		S72.445B	Nondisp fx of low epiphy (separation) of l femr, init op fx 1/2
		S72.445C	Nondisp fx of low epiphy (separation) of l femr, init op fx 3A/B/C
		S72.446B	Nondisp fx of low epiphy (separation) of unsp femr, init op fx 1/2
		S72.446C	Nondisp fx of low epiphy (separation) of unsp femr, init op fx 3A/B/C
821.33	OPEN SUPRACONDYLAR FRACTURE OF FEMUR	**S72.451B**	Displ suprcndl fx w/o intrcndl extn low end r femr, init op fx 1/2
		S72.451C	Displ suprcndl fx w/o intrcndl extn low end r femr, init op fx 3A/B/C
		S72.452B	Displ suprcndl fx w/o intrcndl extn low end l femr, init op fx 1/2
		S72.452C	Displ suprcndl fx w/o intrcndl extn low end l femr, init op fx 3A/B/C
		S72.453B	Displ suprcndl fx w/o intrcndl extn low end unsp femr, init op fx 1/2
		S72.453C	Displ suprcndl fx w/o intrcndl extn low end unsp femr, init op fx 3A/B/C
		S72.454B	Nondisp suprcndl fx w/o intrcndl extn low end r femr, init op fx 1/2
		S72.454C	Nondisp suprcndl fx w/o intrcndl extn low end r femr, init op fx 3A/B/C
		S72.455B	Nondisp suprcndl fx w/o intrcndl extn low end l femr, init op fx 1/2
		S72.455C	Nondisp suprcndl fx w/o intrcndl extn low end l femr, init op fx 3A/B/C
		S72.456B	Nondisp suprcndl fx w/o intrcndl extn low end unsp femr,init op fx 1/2
		S72.456C	Nondisp suprcndl fx w/o intrcndl extn low end unsp femr, init op fx 3A/B/C
		S72.461B	Displ suprcndl fx w intrcndl extn low end r femr, init op fx 1/2
		S72.461C	Displ suprcndl fx w intrcndl extn low end r femr, init op fx 3A/B/C
		S72.462B	Displ suprcndl fx w intrcndl extn low end l femr, init op fx 1/2
		S72.462C	Displ suprcndl fx w intrcndl extn low end l femr, init op fx 3A/B/C
		S72.463B	Displ suprcndl fx w intrcndl extn low end unsp femr, init op fx 1/2
		S72.463C	Displ suprcndl fx w intrcndl extn low end unsp femr, init op fx 3A/B/C
		S72.464B	Nondisp suprcndl fx w intrcndl extn low end r femr, init op fx 1/2
		S72.464C	Nondisp suprcndl fx w intrcndl extn low end r femr, init op fx 3A/B/C
		S72.465B	Nondisp suprcndl fx w intrcndl extn low end l femr, init op fx 1/2
		S72.465C	Nondisp suprcndl fx w intrcndl extn low end l femr, init op fx 3A/B/C
		S72.466B	Nondisp suprcndl fx w intrcndl extn low end unsp femr, init op fx 1/2
		S72.466C	Nondisp suprcndl fx w intrcndl extn low end unsp femr, init op fx 3A/B/C
821.39	OTHER OPEN FRACTURE OF LOWER END OF FEMUR	**S72.491B**	Oth fx lower end of right femur, init for opn fx type I/2
		S72.491C	Oth fx lower end of right femur, init for opn fx type 3A/B/C
		S72.492B	Oth fx lower end of left femur, init for opn fx type I/2
		S72.492C	Oth fx lower end of left femur, init for opn fx type 3A/B/C
		S72.499B	Oth fx lower end of unsp femur, init for opn fx type I/2
		S72.499C	Oth fx lower end of unsp femur, init for opn fx type 3A/B/C

ICD-9-CM		ICD-10-CM	
822.Ø	CLOSED FRACTURE OF PATELLA	**S82.ØØ1A**	Unsp fracture of right patella, init for clos fx
		S82.ØØ2A	Unsp fracture of left patella, init for clos fx
		S82.ØØ9A	Unsp fracture of unsp patella, init for clos fx
		S82.Ø11A	Displaced osteochondral fracture of right patella, init
		S82.Ø12A	Displaced osteochondral fracture of left patella, init
		S82.Ø13A	Displaced osteochondral fracture of unsp patella, init
		S82.Ø14A	Nondisplaced osteochondral fracture of right patella, init
		S82.Ø15A	Nondisplaced osteochondral fracture of left patella, init
		S82.Ø16A	Nondisplaced osteochondral fracture of unsp patella, init
		S82.Ø21A	Displaced longitudinal fracture of right patella, init
		S82.Ø22A	Displaced longitudinal fracture of left patella, init
		S82.Ø23A	Displaced longitudinal fracture of unsp patella, init
		S82.Ø24A	Nondisplaced longitudinal fracture of right patella, init
		S82.Ø25A	Nondisplaced longitudinal fracture of left patella, init
		S82.Ø26A	Nondisplaced longitudinal fracture of unsp patella, init
		S82.Ø31A	Displaced transverse fracture of right patella, init
		S82.Ø32A	Displaced transverse fracture of left patella, init
		S82.Ø33A	Displaced transverse fracture of unsp patella, init
		S82.Ø34A	Nondisplaced transverse fracture of right patella, init
		S82.Ø35A	Nondisplaced transverse fracture of left patella, init
		S82.Ø36A	Nondisplaced transverse fracture of unsp patella, init
		S82.Ø41A	Displaced comminuted fracture of right patella, init
		S82.Ø42A	Displaced comminuted fracture of left patella, init
		S82.Ø43A	Displaced comminuted fracture of unsp patella, init
		S82.Ø44A	Nondisplaced comminuted fracture of right patella, init
		S82.Ø45A	Nondisplaced comminuted fracture of left patella, init
		S82.Ø46A	Nondisplaced comminuted fracture of unsp patella, init
		S82.Ø91A	Oth fracture of right patella, init for clos fx
		S82.Ø92A	Oth fracture of left patella, init for clos fx
		S82.Ø99A	Oth fracture of unsp patella, init for clos fx
822.1	OPEN FRACTURE OF PATELLA	**S82.ØØ1B**	Unsp fracture of right patella, init for opn fx type I/2
		S82.ØØ1C	Unsp fracture of right patella, init for opn fx type 3A/B/C
		S82.ØØ2B	Unsp fracture of left patella, init for opn fx type I/2
		S82.ØØ2C	Unsp fracture of left patella, init for opn fx type 3A/B/C
		S82.ØØ9B	Unsp fracture of unsp patella, init for opn fx type I/2
		S82.ØØ9C	Unsp fracture of unsp patella, init for opn fx type 3A/B/C
		S82.Ø11B	Displ osteochon fx right patella, init for opn fx type I/2
		S82.Ø11C	Displ osteochon fx r patella, init for opn fx type 3A/B/C
		S82.Ø12B	Displ osteochon fx left patella, init for opn fx type I/2
		S82.Ø12C	Displ osteochon fx left patella, init for opn fx type 3A/B/C
		S82.Ø13B	Displ osteochon fx unsp patella, init for opn fx type I/2
		S82.Ø13C	Displ osteochon fx unsp patella, init for opn fx type 3A/B/C
		S82.Ø14B	Nondisp osteochon fx right patella, init for opn fx type I/2
		S82.Ø14C	Nondisp osteochon fx r patella, init for opn fx type 3A/B/C
		S82.Ø15B	Nondisp osteochon fx left patella, init for opn fx type I/2
		S82.Ø15C	Nondisp osteochon fx l patella, init for opn fx type 3A/B/C
		S82.Ø16B	Nondisp osteochon fx unsp patella, init for opn fx type I/2
		S82.Ø16C	Nondisp osteochon fx unsp patella, init op fx 3A/B/C
		S82.Ø21B	Displ longitud fx right patella, init for opn fx type I/2
		S82.Ø21C	Displ longitud fx right patella, init for opn fx type 3A/B/C
		S82.Ø22B	Displaced longitud fx left patella, init for opn fx type I/2
		S82.Ø22C	Displ longitud fx left patella, init for opn fx type 3A/B/C
		S82.Ø23B	Displaced longitud fx unsp patella, init for opn fx type I/2
		S82.Ø23C	Displ longitud fx unsp patella, init for opn fx type 3A/B/C
		S82.Ø24B	Nondisp longitud fx right patella, init for opn fx type I/2
		S82.Ø24C	Nondisp longitud fx r patella, init for opn fx type 3A/B/C
		S82.Ø25B	Nondisp longitud fx left patella, init for opn fx type I/2
		S82.Ø25C	Nondisp longitud fx l patella, init for opn fx type 3A/B/C
		S82.Ø26B	Nondisp longitud fx unsp patella, init for opn fx type I/2
		S82.Ø26C	Nondisp longitud fx unsp patella, init op fx 3A/B/C
		S82.Ø31B	Displ transverse fx right patella, init for opn fx type I/2
		S82.Ø31C	Displ transverse fx r patella, init for opn fx type 3A/B/C
		S82.Ø32B	Displ transverse fx left patella, init for opn fx type I/2
		S82.Ø32C	Displ transverse fx l patella, init for opn fx type 3A/B/C
		S82.Ø33B	Displ transverse fx unsp patella, init for opn fx type I/2
		S82.Ø33C	Displ transverse fx unsp patella, init op fx 3A/B/C
		S82.Ø34B	Nondisp transverse fx r patella, init for opn fx type I/2
		S82.Ø34C	Nondisp transverse fx r patella, init for opn fx type 3A/B/C
		S82.Ø35B	Nondisp transverse fx left patella, init for opn fx type I/2
		S82.Ø35C	Nondisp transverse fx l patella, init for opn fx type 3A/B/C
		S82.Ø36B	Nondisp transverse fx unsp patella, init for opn fx type I/2
		S82.Ø36C	Nondisp transverse fx unsp patella, init op fx 3A/B/C
		S82.Ø41B	Displaced commnt fx right patella, init for opn fx type I/2
		S82.Ø41C	Displ commnt fx right patella, init for opn fx type 3A/B/C
		S82.Ø42B	Displaced commnt fx left patella, init for opn fx type I/2
		S82.Ø42C	Displ commnt fx left patella, init for opn fx type 3A/B/C
		S82.Ø43B	Displaced commnt fx unsp patella, init for opn fx type I/2
		S82.Ø43C	Displ commnt fx unsp patella, init for opn fx type 3A/B/C
		S82.Ø44B	Nondisp commnt fx right patella, init for opn fx type I/2
		S82.Ø44C	Nondisp commnt fx right patella, init for opn fx type 3A/B/C
		S82.Ø45B	Nondisp comminuted fx left patella, init for opn fx type I/2
	(Continued on next page)	**S82.Ø45C**	Nondisp commnt fx left patella, init for opn fx type 3A/B/C

[Brackets] indicate valid character values for each code. Character value meanings provided for each code grouping.

ICD-9-CM		ICD-10-CM		
822.1	OPEN FRACTURE OF PATELLA (Continued)	**S82.046B**	Nondisp comminuted fx unsp patella, init for opn fx type I/2	
		S82.046C	Nondisp commnt fx unsp patella, init for opn fx type 3A/B/C	
		S82.091B	Oth fracture of right patella, init for opn fx type I/2	
		S82.091C	Oth fracture of right patella, init for opn fx type 3A/B/C	
		S82.092B	Oth fracture of left patella, init for opn fx type I/2	
		S82.092C	Oth fracture of left patella, init for opn fx type 3A/B/C	
		S82.099B	Oth fracture of unsp patella, init for opn fx type I/2	
		S82.099C	Oth fracture of unsp patella, init for opn fx type 3A/B/C	
823.00	CLOSED FRACTURE OF UPPER END OF TIBIA	**S82.101A**	Unsp fracture of upper end of right tibia, init for clos fx	
		S82.102A	Unsp fracture of upper end of left tibia, init for clos fx	
		S82.109A	Unsp fracture of upper end of unsp tibia, init for clos fx	
		S82.111A	Disp fx of right tibial spine, init for clos fx	
		S82.112A	Disp fx of left tibial spine, init for clos fx	
		S82.113A	Disp fx of unsp tibial spine, init for clos fx	
		S82.114A	Nondisp fx of right tibial spine, init for clos fx	
		S82.115A	Nondisp fx of left tibial spine, init for clos fx	
		S82.116A	Nondisp fx of unsp tibial spine, init for clos fx	
		S82.121A	Disp fx of lateral condyle of right tibia, init for clos fx	
		S82.122A	Disp fx of lateral condyle of left tibia, init for clos fx	
		S82.123A	Disp fx of lateral condyle of unsp tibia, init for clos fx	
		S82.124A	Nondisp fx of lateral condyle of right tibia, init	
		S82.125A	Nondisp fx of lateral condyle of left tibia, init	
		S82.126A	Nondisp fx of lateral condyle of unsp tibia, init	
		S82.131A	Disp fx of medial condyle of right tibia, init for clos fx	
		S82.132A	Disp fx of medial condyle of left tibia, init for clos fx	
		S82.133A	Disp fx of medial condyle of unsp tibia, init for clos fx	
		S82.134A	Nondisp fx of medial condyle of right tibia, init	
		S82.135A	Nondisp fx of medial condyle of left tibia, init for clos fx	
		S82.136A	Nondisp fx of medial condyle of unsp tibia, init for clos fx	
		S82.141A	Displaced bicondylar fracture of right tibia, init	
		S82.142A	Displaced bicondylar fracture of left tibia, init	
		S82.143A	Displaced bicondylar fracture of unsp tibia, init	
		S82.144A	Nondisplaced bicondylar fracture of right tibia, init	
		S82.145A	Nondisplaced bicondylar fracture of left tibia, init	
		S82.146A	Nondisplaced bicondylar fracture of unsp tibia, init	
		S82.151A	Disp fx of right tibial tuberosity, init for clos fx	
		S82.152A	Disp fx of left tibial tuberosity, init for clos fx	
		S82.153A	Disp fx of unsp tibial tuberosity, init for clos fx	
		S82.154A	Nondisp fx of right tibial tuberosity, init for clos fx	
		S82.155A	Nondisp fx of left tibial tuberosity, init for clos fx	
		S82.156A	Nondisp fx of unsp tibial tuberosity, init for clos fx	
		S82.191A	Oth fracture of upper end of right tibia, init for clos fx	
		S82.192A	Oth fracture of upper end of left tibia, init for clos fx	
		S82.199A	Oth fracture of upper end of unsp tibia, init for clos fx	
		S89.001A	Unsp physeal fracture of upper end of right tibia, init	
		S89.002A	Unsp physeal fracture of upper end of left tibia, init	
		S89.009A	Unsp physeal fracture of upper end of unsp tibia, init	
		S89.011A	Sltr-haris Type I physeal fx upper end of right tibia, init	
		S89.012A	Sltr-haris Type I physeal fx upper end of left tibia, init	
		S89.019A	Sltr-haris Type I physeal fx upper end of unsp tibia, init	
		S89.021A	Sltr-haris Type II physeal fx upper end of right tibia, init	
		S89.022A	Sltr-haris Type II physeal fx upper end of left tibia, init	
		S89.029A	Sltr-haris Type II physeal fx upper end of unsp tibia, init	
		S89.031A	Sltr-haris Type III physeal fx upper end of r tibia, init	
		S89.032A	Sltr-haris Type III physeal fx upper end of left tibia, init	
		S89.039A	Sltr-haris Type III physeal fx upper end of unsp tibia, init	
		S89.041A	Sltr-haris Type IV physeal fx upper end of right tibia, init	
		S89.042A	Sltr-haris Type IV physeal fx upper end of left tibia, init	
		S89.049A	Sltr-haris Type IV physeal fx upper end of unsp tibia, init	
		S89.091A	Oth physeal fracture of upper end of right tibia, init	
		S89.092A	Oth physeal fracture of upper end of left tibia, init	
		S89.099A	Oth physeal fracture of upper end of unsp tibia, init	
823.01	CLOSED FRACTURE OF UPPER END OF FIBULA	**S82.831A**	Oth fracture of upper and lower end of right fibula, init	
		S82.832A	Oth fracture of upper and lower end of left fibula, init	
		S82.839A	Oth fracture of upper and lower end of unsp fibula, init	
		S89.201A	Unsp physeal fracture of upper end of right fibula, init	
		S89.202A	Unsp physeal fracture of upper end of left fibula, init	
		S89.209A	Unsp physeal fracture of upper end of unsp fibula, init	
		S89.211A	Sltr-haris Type I physeal fx upper end of r fibula, init	
		S89.212A	Sltr-haris Type I physeal fx upper end of left fibula, init	
		S89.219A	Sltr-haris Type I physeal fx upper end of unsp fibula, init	
		S89.221A	Sltr-haris Type II physeal fx upper end of r fibula, init	
		S89.222A	Sltr-haris Type II physeal fx upper end of left fibula, init	
		S89.229A	Sltr-haris Type II physeal fx upper end of unsp fibula, init	
		S89.291A	Oth physeal fracture of upper end of right fibula, init	
		S89.292A	Oth physeal fracture of upper end of left fibula, init	
		S89.299A	Oth physeal fracture of upper end of unsp fibula, init	
823.02	CLOSED FRACTURE OF UPPER END OF FIBULA W/TIBIA	**S82.101A**	Unsp fracture of upper end of right tibia, init for clos fx	*and*
		S82.831A	Oth fracture of upper and lower end of right fibula, init	
		S82.102A	Unsp fracture of upper end of left tibia, init for clos fx	*and*
		S82.832A	Oth fracture of upper and lower end of left fibula, init	

ICD-9-CM	ICD-10-CM	
823.10 OPEN FRACTURE OF UPPER END OF TIBIA	**S82.101B**	Unsp fx upper end of right tibia, init for opn fx type I/2
	S82.101C	Unsp fx upper end of r tibia, init for opn fx type 3A/B/C
	S82.102B	Unsp fx upper end of left tibia, init for opn fx type I/2
	S82.102C	Unsp fx upper end of left tibia, init for opn fx type 3A/B/C
	S82.109B	Unsp fx upper end of unsp tibia, init for opn fx type I/2
	S82.109C	Unsp fx upper end of unsp tibia, init for opn fx type 3A/B/C
	S82.111B	Disp fx of right tibial spine, init for opn fx type I/2
	S82.111C	Disp fx of right tibial spine, init for opn fx type 3A/B/C
	S82.112B	Disp fx of left tibial spine, init for opn fx type I/2
	S82.112C	Disp fx of left tibial spine, init for opn fx type 3A/B/C
	S82.113B	Disp fx of unsp tibial spine, init for opn fx type I/2
	S82.113C	Disp fx of unsp tibial spine, init for opn fx type 3A/B/C
	S82.114B	Nondisp fx of right tibial spine, init for opn fx type I/2
	S82.114C	Nondisp fx of r tibial spine, init for opn fx type 3A/B/C
	S82.115B	Nondisp fx of left tibial spine, init for opn fx type I/2
	S82.115C	Nondisp fx of left tibial spine, init for opn fx type 3A/B/C
	S82.116B	Nondisp fx of unsp tibial spine, init for opn fx type I/2
	S82.116C	Nondisp fx of unsp tibial spine, init for opn fx type 3A/B/C
	S82.121B	Disp fx of lateral condyle of r tibia, init op fx 1/2
	S82.121C	Disp fx of lateral condyle of r tibia, init op fx 3A/B/C
	S82.122B	Disp fx of lateral condyle of l tibia, init op fx 1/2
	S82.122C	Disp fx of lateral condyle of l tibia, init op fx 3A/B/C
	S82.123B	Disp fx of lateral condyle of unsp tibia, init op fx 1/2
	S82.123C	Disp fx of lateral condyle of unsp tibia, init op fx 3A/B/C
	S82.124B	Nondisp fx of lateral condyle of r tibia, init op fx 1/2
	S82.124C	Nondisp fx of lateral condyle of r tibia, init op fx 3A/B/C
	S82.125B	Nondisp fx of lateral condyle of l tibia, init op fx 1/2
	S82.125C	Nondisp fx of lateral condyle of l tibia, init op fx 3A/B/C
	S82.126B	Nondisp fx of lateral condyle of unsp tibia, init op fx 1/2
	S82.126C	Nondisp fx of lateral condyle of unsp tibia, init op fx 3A/B/C
	S82.131B	Disp fx of med condyle of r tibia, init for opn fx type I/2
	S82.131C	Disp fx of med condyle of r tibia, init op fx 3A/B/C
	S82.132B	Disp fx of med condyle of l tibia, init for opn fx type I/2
	S82.132C	Disp fx of med condyle of l tibia, init op fx 3A/B/C
	S82.133B	Disp fx of med condyle of unsp tibia, init op fx 1/2
	S82.133C	Disp fx of med condyle of unsp tibia, init op fx 3A/B/C
	S82.134B	Nondisp fx of med condyle of r tibia, init op fx 1/2
	S82.134C	Nondisp fx of med condyle of r tibia, init op fx 3A/B/C
	S82.135B	Nondisp fx of med condyle of l tibia, init op fx 1/2
	S82.135C	Nondisp fx of med condyle of l tibia, init op fx 3A/B/C
	S82.136B	Nondisp fx of med condyle of unsp tibia, init op fx 1/2
	S82.136C	Nondisp fx of med condyle of unsp tibia, init op fx 3A/B/C
	S82.141B	Displaced bicondylar fx r tibia, init for opn fx type I/2
	S82.141C	Displaced bicondylar fx r tibia, init for opn fx type 3A/B/C
	S82.142B	Displaced bicondylar fx left tibia, init for opn fx type I/2
	S82.142C	Displaced bicondylar fx l tibia, init for opn fx type 3A/B/C
	S82.143B	Displaced bicondylar fx unsp tibia, init for opn fx type I/2
	S82.143C	Displ bicondylar fx unsp tibia, init for opn fx type 3A/B/C
	S82.144B	Nondisp bicondylar fx right tibia, init for opn fx type I/2
	S82.144C	Nondisp bicondylar fx r tibia, init for opn fx type 3A/B/C
	S82.145B	Nondisp bicondylar fx left tibia, init for opn fx type I/2
	S82.145C	Nondisp bicondylar fx l tibia, init for opn fx type 3A/B/C
	S82.146B	Nondisp bicondylar fx unsp tibia, init for opn fx type I/2
	S82.146C	Nondisp bicondylar fx unsp tibia, init op fx 3A/B/C
	S82.151B	Disp fx of right tibial tuberosity, init for opn fx type I/2
	S82.151C	Disp fx of r tibial tuberosity, init for opn fx type 3A/B/C
	S82.152B	Disp fx of left tibial tuberosity, init for opn fx type I/2
	S82.152C	Disp fx of l tibial tuberosity, init for opn fx type 3A/B/C
	S82.153B	Disp fx of unsp tibial tuberosity, init for opn fx type I/2
	S82.153C	Disp fx of unsp tibial tuberosity, init op fx 3A/B/C
	S82.154B	Nondisp fx of r tibial tuberosity, init for opn fx type I/2
	S82.154C	Nondisp fx of r tibial tuberosity, init op fx 3A/B/C
	S82.155B	Nondisp fx of l tibial tuberosity, init for opn fx type I/2
	S82.155C	Nondisp fx of l tibial tuberosity, init op fx 3A/B/C
	S82.156B	Nondisp fx of unsp tibial tuberosity, init op fx 1/2
	S82.156C	Nondisp fx of unsp tibial tuberosity, init op fx 3A/B/C
	S82.191B	Oth fx upper end of right tibia, init for opn fx type I/2
	S82.191C	Oth fx upper end of right tibia, init for opn fx type 3A/B/C
	S82.192B	Oth fx upper end of left tibia, init for opn fx type I/2
	S82.192C	Oth fx upper end of left tibia, init for opn fx type 3A/B/C
	S82.199B	Oth fx upper end of unsp tibia, init for opn fx type I/2
	S82.199C	Oth fx upper end of unsp tibia, init for opn fx type 3A/B/C
823.11 OPEN FRACTURE OF UPPER END OF FIBULA	**S82.831B**	Oth fx upper and low end r fibula, init for opn fx type I/2
	S82.831C	Oth fx upr and low end r fibula, init for opn fx type 3A/B/C
	S82.832B	Oth fx upper and low end l fibula, init for opn fx type I/2
	S82.832C	Oth fx upr and low end l fibula, init for opn fx type 3A/B/C
	S82.839B	Oth fx upr and low end unsp fibula, init for opn fx type I/2
	S82.839C	Oth fx upr & low end unsp fibula, init op fx 3A/B/C

ICD-9-CM		ICD-10-CM		
823.12	OPEN FRACTURE OF UPPER END OF FIBULA WITH TIBIA	**S82.1Ø1B**	Unsp fx upper end of right tibia, init for opn fx type I/2	*and*
		S82.831B	Oth fx upper and low end r fibula, init for opn fx type I/2	
		S82.1Ø2B	Unsp fx upper end of left tibia, init for opn fx type I/2	*and*
		S82.832B	Oth fx upper and low end l fibula, init for opn fx type I/2	
823.2Ø	CLOSED FRACTURE OF SHAFT OF TIBIA	**S82.2Ø1A**	Unsp fracture of shaft of right tibia, init for clos fx	
		S82.2Ø2A	Unsp fracture of shaft of left tibia, init for clos fx	
		S82.2Ø9A	Unsp fracture of shaft of unsp tibia, init for clos fx	
		S82.221A	Displaced transverse fracture of shaft of right tibia, init	
		S82.222A	Displaced transverse fracture of shaft of left tibia, init	
		S82.223A	Displaced transverse fracture of shaft of unsp tibia, init	
		S82.224A	Nondisp transverse fracture of shaft of right tibia, init	
		S82.225A	Nondisp transverse fracture of shaft of left tibia, init	
		S82.226A	Nondisp transverse fracture of shaft of unsp tibia, init	
		S82.231A	Displaced oblique fracture of shaft of right tibia, init	
		S82.232A	Displaced oblique fracture of shaft of left tibia, init	
		S82.233A	Displaced oblique fracture of shaft of unsp tibia, init	
		S82.234A	Nondisplaced oblique fracture of shaft of right tibia, init	
		S82.235A	Nondisplaced oblique fracture of shaft of left tibia, init	
		S82.236A	Nondisplaced oblique fracture of shaft of unsp tibia, init	
		S82.241A	Displaced spiral fracture of shaft of right tibia, init	
		S82.242A	Displaced spiral fracture of shaft of left tibia, init	
		S82.243A	Displaced spiral fracture of shaft of unsp tibia, init	
		S82.244A	Nondisplaced spiral fracture of shaft of right tibia, init	
		S82.245A	Nondisplaced spiral fracture of shaft of left tibia, init	
		S82.246A	Nondisplaced spiral fracture of shaft of unsp tibia, init	
		S82.251A	Displaced comminuted fracture of shaft of right tibia, init	
		S82.252A	Displaced comminuted fracture of shaft of left tibia, init	
		S82.253A	Displaced comminuted fracture of shaft of unsp tibia, init	
		S82.254A	Nondisp comminuted fracture of shaft of right tibia, init	
		S82.255A	Nondisp comminuted fracture of shaft of left tibia, init	
		S82.256A	Nondisp comminuted fracture of shaft of unsp tibia, init	
		S82.261A	Displaced segmental fracture of shaft of right tibia, init	
		S82.262A	Displaced segmental fracture of shaft of left tibia, init	
		S82.263A	Displaced segmental fracture of shaft of unsp tibia, init	
		S82.264A	Nondisp segmental fracture of shaft of right tibia, init	
		S82.265A	Nondisplaced segmental fracture of shaft of left tibia, init	
		S82.266A	Nondisplaced segmental fracture of shaft of unsp tibia, init	
		S82.291A	Oth fracture of shaft of right tibia, init for clos fx	
		S82.292A	Oth fracture of shaft of left tibia, init for clos fx	
		S82.299A	Oth fracture of shaft of unsp tibia, init for clos fx	
823.21	CLOSED FRACTURE OF SHAFT OF FIBULA	**S82.4Ø1A**	Unsp fracture of shaft of right fibula, init for clos fx	
		S82.4Ø2A	Unsp fracture of shaft of left fibula, init for clos fx	
		S82.4Ø9A	Unsp fracture of shaft of unsp fibula, init for clos fx	
		S82.421A	Displaced transverse fracture of shaft of right fibula, init	
		S82.422A	Displaced transverse fracture of shaft of left fibula, init	
		S82.423A	Displaced transverse fracture of shaft of unsp fibula, init	
		S82.424A	Nondisp transverse fracture of shaft of right fibula, init	
		S82.425A	Nondisp transverse fracture of shaft of left fibula, init	
		S82.426A	Nondisp transverse fracture of shaft of unsp fibula, init	
		S82.431A	Displaced oblique fracture of shaft of right fibula, init	
		S82.432A	Displaced oblique fracture of shaft of left fibula, init	
		S82.433A	Displaced oblique fracture of shaft of unsp fibula, init	
		S82.434A	Nondisplaced oblique fracture of shaft of right fibula, init	
		S82.435A	Nondisplaced oblique fracture of shaft of left fibula, init	
		S82.436A	Nondisplaced oblique fracture of shaft of unsp fibula, init	
		S82.441A	Displaced spiral fracture of shaft of right fibula, init	
		S82.442A	Displaced spiral fracture of shaft of left fibula, init	
		S82.443A	Displaced spiral fracture of shaft of unsp fibula, init	
		S82.444A	Nondisplaced spiral fracture of shaft of right fibula, init	
		S82.445A	Nondisplaced spiral fracture of shaft of left fibula, init	
		S82.446A	Nondisplaced spiral fracture of shaft of unsp fibula, init	
		S82.451A	Displaced comminuted fracture of shaft of right fibula, init	
		S82.452A	Displaced comminuted fracture of shaft of left fibula, init	
		S82.453A	Displaced comminuted fracture of shaft of unsp fibula, init	
		S82.454A	Nondisp comminuted fracture of shaft of right fibula, init	
		S82.455A	Nondisp comminuted fracture of shaft of left fibula, init	
		S82.456A	Nondisp comminuted fracture of shaft of unsp fibula, init	
		S82.461A	Displaced segmental fracture of shaft of right fibula, init	
		S82.462A	Displaced segmental fracture of shaft of left fibula, init	
		S82.463A	Displaced segmental fracture of shaft of unsp fibula, init	
		S82.464A	Nondisp segmental fracture of shaft of right fibula, init	
		S82.465A	Nondisp segmental fracture of shaft of left fibula, init	
		S82.466A	Nondisp segmental fracture of shaft of unsp fibula, init	
		S82.491A	Oth fracture of shaft of right fibula, init for clos fx	
		S82.492A	Oth fracture of shaft of left fibula, init for clos fx	
		S82.499A	Oth fracture of shaft of unsp fibula, init for clos fx	
		S82.861A	Displaced Maisonneuve's fracture of right leg, init	
		S82.862A	Displaced Maisonneuve's fracture of left leg, init	

(Continued on next page)

ICD-9-CM		ICD-10-CM		
823.21	CLOSED FRACTURE OF SHAFT OF FIBULA (Continued)	S82.863A	Displaced Maisonneuve's fracture of unsp leg, init	
		S82.864A	Nondisplaced Maisonneuve's fracture of right leg, init	
		S82.865A	Nondisplaced Maisonneuve's fracture of left leg, init	
		S82.866A	Nondisplaced Maisonneuve's fracture of unsp leg, init	
823.22	CLOSED FRACTURE OF SHAFT OF FIBULA WITH TIBIA	S82.2Ø1A	Unsp fracture of shaft of right tibia, init for clos fx	and
		S82.4Ø1A	Unsp fracture of shaft of right fibula, init for clos fx	
		S82.2Ø2A	Unsp fracture of shaft of left tibia, init for clos fx	and
		S82.4Ø2A	Unsp fracture of shaft of left fibula, init for clos fx	
823.3Ø	OPEN FRACTURE OF SHAFT OF TIBIA	S82.2Ø1B	Unsp fx shaft of right tibia, init for opn fx type I/2	
		S82.2Ø1C	Unsp fx shaft of right tibia, init for opn fx type 3A/B/C	
		S82.2Ø2B	Unsp fx shaft of left tibia, init for opn fx type I/2	
		S82.2Ø2C	Unsp fx shaft of left tibia, init for opn fx type 3A/B/C	
		S82.2Ø9B	Unsp fx shaft of unsp tibia, init for opn fx type I/2	
		S82.2Ø9C	Unsp fx shaft of unsp tibia, init for opn fx type 3A/B/C	
		S82.221B	Displ transverse fx shaft of r tibia, init op fx 1/2	
		S82.221C	Displ transverse fx shaft of r tibia, init op fx 3A/B/C	
		S82.222B	Displ transverse fx shaft of l tibia, init op fx 1/2	
		S82.222C	Displ transverse fx shaft of l tibia, init op fx 3A/B/C	
		S82.223B	Displ transverse fx shaft of unsp tibia, init op fx 1/2	
		S82.223C	Displ transverse fx shaft of unsp tibia, init op fx 3A/B/C	
		S82.224B	Nondisp transverse fx shaft of r tibia, init op fx 1/2	
		S82.224C	Nondisp transverse fx shaft of r tibia, init op fx 3A/B/C	
		S82.225B	Nondisp transverse fx shaft of l tibia, init op fx 1/2	
		S82.225C	Nondisp transverse fx shaft of l tibia, init op fx 3A/B/C	
		S82.226B	Nondisp transverse fx shaft of unsp tibia, init op fx 1/2	
		S82.226C	Nondisp transverse fx shaft of unsp tibia, init op fx 3A/B/C	
		S82.231B	Displ oblique fx shaft of r tibia, init for opn fx type I/2	
		S82.231C	Displ oblique fx shaft of r tibia, init op fx 3A/B/C	
		S82.232B	Displ oblique fx shaft of l tibia, init for opn fx type I/2	
		S82.232C	Displ oblique fx shaft of l tibia, init op fx 3A/B/C	
		S82.233B	Displ oblique fx shaft of unsp tibia, init op fx 1/2	
		S82.233C	Displ oblique fx shaft of unsp tibia, init op fx 3A/B/C	
		S82.234B	Nondisp oblique fx shaft of r tibia, init op fx 1/2	
		S82.234C	Nondisp oblique fx shaft of r tibia, init op fx 3A/B/C	
		S82.235B	Nondisp oblique fx shaft of l tibia, init op fx 1/2	
		S82.235C	Nondisp oblique fx shaft of l tibia, init op fx 3A/B/C	
		S82.236B	Nondisp oblique fx shaft of unsp tibia, init op fx 1/2	
		S82.236C	Nondisp oblique fx shaft of unsp tibia, init op fx 3A/B/C	
		S82.241B	Displ spiral fx shaft of r tibia, init for opn fx type I/2	
		S82.241C	Displ spiral fx shaft of r tibia, init op fx 3A/B/C	
		S82.242B	Displ spiral fx shaft of l tibia, init for opn fx type I/2	
		S82.242C	Displ spiral fx shaft of l tibia, init op fx 3A/B/C	
		S82.243B	Displ spiral fx shaft of unsp tibia, init op fx 1/2	
		S82.243C	Displ spiral fx shaft of unsp tibia, init op fx 3A/B/C	
		S82.244B	Nondisp spiral fx shaft of r tibia, init for opn fx type I/2	
		S82.244C	Nondisp spiral fx shaft of r tibia, init op fx 3A/B/C	
		S82.245B	Nondisp spiral fx shaft of l tibia, init for opn fx type I/2	
		S82.245C	Nondisp spiral fx shaft of l tibia, init op fx 3A/B/C	
		S82.246B	Nondisp spiral fx shaft of unsp tibia, init op fx 1/2	
		S82.246C	Nondisp spiral fx shaft of unsp tibia, init op fx 3A/B/C	
		S82.251B	Displ commnt fx shaft of r tibia, init for opn fx type I/2	
		S82.251C	Displ commnt fx shaft of r tibia, init op fx 3A/B/C	
		S82.252B	Displ commnt fx shaft of l tibia, init for opn fx type I/2	
		S82.252C	Displ commnt fx shaft of l tibia, init op fx 3A/B/C	
		S82.253B	Displ commnt fx shaft of unsp tibia, init op fx 1/2	
		S82.253C	Displ commnt fx shaft of unsp tibia, init op fx 3A/B/C	
		S82.254B	Nondisp commnt fx shaft of r tibia, init for opn fx type I/2	
		S82.254C	Nondisp commnt fx shaft of r tibia, init op fx 3A/B/C	
		S82.255B	Nondisp commnt fx shaft of l tibia, init for opn fx type I/2	
		S82.255C	Nondisp commnt fx shaft of l tibia, init op fx 3A/B/C	
		S82.256B	Nondisp commnt fx shaft of unsp tibia, init op fx 1/2	
		S82.256C	Nondisp commnt fx shaft of unsp tibia, init op fx 3A/B/C	
		S82.261B	Displ seg fx shaft of r tibia, init for opn fx type I/2	
		S82.261C	Displ seg fx shaft of r tibia, init for opn fx type 3A/B/C	
		S82.262B	Displ seg fx shaft of l tibia, init for opn fx type I/2	
		S82.262C	Displ seg fx shaft of l tibia, init for opn fx type 3A/B/C	
		S82.263B	Displ seg fx shaft of unsp tibia, init for opn fx type I/2	
		S82.263C	Displ seg fx shaft of unsp tibia, init op fx 3A/B/C	
		S82.264B	Nondisp seg fx shaft of r tibia, init for opn fx type I/2	
		S82.264C	Nondisp seg fx shaft of r tibia, init for opn fx type 3A/B/C	
		S82.265B	Nondisp seg fx shaft of l tibia, init for opn fx type I/2	
		S82.265C	Nondisp seg fx shaft of l tibia, init for opn fx type 3A/B/C	
		S82.266B	Nondisp seg fx shaft of unsp tibia, init for opn fx type I/2	
		S82.266C	Nondisp seg fx shaft of unsp tibia, init op fx 3A/B/C	
		S82.291B	Oth fx shaft of right tibia, init for opn fx type I/2	
		S82.291C	Oth fx shaft of right tibia, init for opn fx type 3A/B/C	
		S82.292B	Oth fx shaft of left tibia, init for opn fx type I/2	
		S82.292C	Oth fx shaft of left tibia, init for opn fx type 3A/B/C	
		S82.299B	Oth fx shaft of unsp tibia, init for opn fx type I/2	
		S82.299C	Oth fx shaft of unsp tibia, init for opn fx type 3A/B/C	

ICD-9-CM		ICD-10-CM	
823.31	OPEN FRACTURE OF SHAFT OF FIBULA	**S82.401B**	Unsp fracture of shaft of r fibula, init for opn fx type I/2
		S82.401C	Unsp fx shaft of r fibula, init for opn fx type 3A/B/C
		S82.402B	Unsp fx shaft of left fibula, init for opn fx type I/2
		S82.402C	Unsp fx shaft of left fibula, init for opn fx type 3A/B/C
		S82.409B	Unsp fx shaft of unsp fibula, init for opn fx type I/2
		S82.409C	Unsp fx shaft of unsp fibula, init for opn fx type 3A/B/C
		S82.421B	Displ transverse fx shaft of r fibula, init op fx 1/2
		S82.421C	Displ transverse fx shaft of r fibula, init op fx 3A/B/C
		S82.422B	Displ transverse fx shaft of l fibula, init op fx 1/2
		S82.422C	Displ transverse fx shaft of l fibula, init op fx 3A/B/C
		S82.423B	Displ transverse fx shaft of unsp fibula, init op fx 1/2
		S82.423C	Displ transverse fx shaft of unsp fibula, init op fx 3A/B/C
		S82.424B	Nondisp transverse fx shaft of r fibula, init op fx 1/2
		S82.424C	Nondisp transverse fx shaft of r fibula, init op fx 3A/B/C
		S82.425B	Nondisp transverse fx shaft of l fibula, init op fx 1/2
		S82.425C	Nondisp transverse fx shaft of l fibula, init op fx 3A/B/C
		S82.426B	Nondisp transverse fx shaft of unsp fibula, init op fx 1/2
		S82.426C	Nondisp transverse fx shaft of unsp fibula, init op fx 3A/B/C
		S82.431B	Displ oblique fx shaft of r fibula, init for opn fx type I/2
		S82.431C	Displ oblique fx shaft of r fibula, init op fx 3A/B/C
		S82.432B	Displ oblique fx shaft of l fibula, init for opn fx type I/2
		S82.432C	Displ oblique fx shaft of l fibula, init op fx 3A/B/C
		S82.433B	Displ oblique fx shaft of unsp fibula, init op fx 1/2
		S82.433C	Displ oblique fx shaft of unsp fibula, init op fx 3A/B/C
		S82.434B	Nondisp oblique fx shaft of r fibula, init op fx 1/2
		S82.434C	Nondisp oblique fx shaft of r fibula, init op fx 3A/B/C
		S82.435B	Nondisp oblique fx shaft of l fibula, init op fx 1/2
		S82.435C	Nondisp oblique fx shaft of l fibula, init op fx 3A/B/C
		S82.436B	Nondisp oblique fx shaft of unsp fibula, init op fx 1/2
		S82.436C	Nondisp oblique fx shaft of unsp fibula, init op fx 3A/B/C
		S82.441B	Displ spiral fx shaft of r fibula, init for opn fx type I/2
		S82.441C	Displ spiral fx shaft of r fibula, init op fx 3A/B/C
		S82.442B	Displ spiral fx shaft of l fibula, init for opn fx type I/2
		S82.442C	Displ spiral fx shaft of l fibula, init op fx 3A/B/C
		S82.443B	Displ spiral fx shaft of unsp fibula, init op fx 1/2
		S82.443C	Displ spiral fx shaft of unsp fibula, init op fx 3A/B/C
		S82.444B	Nondisp spiral fx shaft of r fibula, init op fx 1/2
		S82.444C	Nondisp spiral fx shaft of r fibula, init op fx 3A/B/C
		S82.445B	Nondisp spiral fx shaft of l fibula, init op fx 1/2
		S82.445C	Nondisp spiral fx shaft of l fibula, init op fx 3A/B/C
		S82.446B	Nondisp spiral fx shaft of unsp fibula, init op fx 1/2
		S82.446C	Nondisp spiral fx shaft of unsp fibula, init op fx 3A/B/C
		S82.451B	Displ commnt fx shaft of r fibula, init for opn fx type I/2
		S82.451C	Displ commnt fx shaft of r fibula, init op fx 3A/B/C
		S82.452B	Displ commnt fx shaft of l fibula, init for opn fx type I/2
		S82.452C	Displ commnt fx shaft of l fibula, init op fx 3A/B/C
		S82.453B	Displ commnt fx shaft of unsp fibula, init op fx 1/2
		S82.453C	Displ commnt fx shaft of unsp fibula, init op fx 3A/B/C
		S82.454B	Nondisp commnt fx shaft of r fibula, init op fx 1/2
		S82.454C	Nondisp commnt fx shaft of r fibula, init op fx 3A/B/C
		S82.455B	Nondisp commnt fx shaft of l fibula, init op fx 1/2
		S82.455C	Nondisp commnt fx shaft of l fibula, init op fx 3A/B/C
		S82.456B	Nondisp commnt fx shaft of unsp fibula, init op fx 1/2
		S82.456C	Nondisp commnt fx shaft of unsp fibula, init op fx 3A/B/C
		S82.461B	Displ seg fx shaft of r fibula, init for opn fx type I/2
		S82.461C	Displ seg fx shaft of r fibula, init for opn fx type 3A/B/C
		S82.462B	Displ seg fx shaft of l fibula, init for opn fx type I/2
		S82.462C	Displ seg fx shaft of l fibula, init for opn fx type 3A/B/C
		S82.463B	Displ seg fx shaft of unsp fibula, init for opn fx type I/2
		S82.463C	Displ seg fx shaft of unsp fibula, init op fx 3A/B/C
		S82.464B	Nondisp seg fx shaft of r fibula, init for opn fx type I/2
		S82.464C	Nondisp seg fx shaft of r fibula, init op fx 3A/B/C
		S82.465B	Nondisp seg fx shaft of l fibula, init for opn fx type I/2
		S82.465C	Nondisp seg fx shaft of l fibula, init op fx 3A/B/C
		S82.466B	Nondisp seg fx shaft of unsp fibula, init op fx 1/2
		S82.466C	Nondisp seg fx shaft of unsp fibula, init op fx 3A/B/C
		S82.491B	Oth fracture of shaft of r fibula, init for opn fx type I/2
		S82.491C	Oth fx shaft of r fibula, init for opn fx type 3A/B/C
		S82.492B	Oth fx shaft of left fibula, init for opn fx type I/2
		S82.492C	Oth fx shaft of left fibula, init for opn fx type 3A/B/C
		S82.499B	Oth fx shaft of unsp fibula, init for opn fx type I/2
		S82.499C	Oth fx shaft of unsp fibula, init for opn fx type 3A/B/C
		S82.861B	Displ Maisonneuve's fx right leg, init for opn fx type I/2
		S82.861C	Displ Maisonneuve's fx r leg, init for opn fx type 3A/B/C
		S82.862B	Displ Maisonneuve's fx left leg, init for opn fx type I/2
		S82.862C	Displ Maisonneuve's fx left leg, init for opn fx type 3A/B/C
		S82.863B	Displ Maisonneuve's fx unsp leg, init for opn fx type I/2
		S82.863C	Displ Maisonneuve's fx unsp leg, init for opn fx type 3A/B/C
		S82.864B	Nondisp Maisonneuve's fx right leg, init for opn fx type I/2
		S82.864C	Nondisp Maisonneuve's fx r leg, init for opn fx type 3A/B/C
		S82.865B	Nondisp Maisonneuve's fx left leg, init for opn fx type I/2
		S82.865C	Nondisp Maisonneuve's fx l leg, init for opn fx type 3A/B/C
		S82.866B	Nondisp Maisonneuve's fx unsp leg, init for opn fx type I/2
		S82.866C	Nondisp Maisonneuve's fx unsp leg, init op fx 3A/B/C

ICD-9-CM		ICD-10-CM		
823.32	OPEN FRACTURE OF SHAFT OF FIBULA WITH TIBIA	**S82.201B**	Unsp fx shaft of right tibia, init for opn fx type I/2	*or*
		S82.401B	Unsp fracture of shaft of r fibula, init for opn fx type I/2	*and*
		S82.202B	Unsp fx shaft of left tibia, init for opn fx type I/2	*or*
		S82.402B	Unsp fx shaft of left fibula, init for opn fx type I/2	
823.40	TORUS FRACTURE OF TIBIA ALONE	**S82.161A**	Torus fracture of upper end of right tibia, init for clos fx	
		S82.162A	Torus fracture of upper end of left tibia, init for clos fx	
		S82.169A	Torus fracture of upper end of unsp tibia, init for clos fx	
		S82.311A	Torus fracture of lower end of right tibia, init for clos fx	
		S82.312A	Torus fracture of lower end of left tibia, init for clos fx	
		S82.319A	Torus fracture of lower end of unsp tibia, init for clos fx	
823.41	TORUS FRACTURE OF FIBULA ALONE	**S82.811A**	Torus fracture of upper end of right fibula, init	
		S82.812A	Torus fracture of upper end of left fibula, init for clos fx	
		S82.819A	Torus fracture of upper end of unsp fibula, init for clos fx	
		S82.821A	Torus fracture of lower end of right fibula, init	
		S82.822A	Torus fracture of lower end of left fibula, init for clos fx	
		S82.829A	Torus fracture of lower end of unsp fibula, init for clos fx	
823.42	TORUS FRACTURE OF FIBULA WITH TIBIA	**S82.161A**	Torus fracture of upper end of right tibia, init for clos fx	*and*
		S82.811A	Torus fracture of upper end of right fibula, init	
		S82.311A	Torus fracture of lower end of right tibia, init for clos fx	*and*
		S82.821A	Torus fracture of lower end of right fibula, init	
		S82.162A	Torus fracture of upper end of left tibia, init for clos fx	*and*
		S82.812A	Torus fracture of upper end of left fibula, init for clos fx	
		S82.312A	Torus fracture of lower end of left tibia, init for clos fx	*and*
		S82.822A	Torus fracture of lower end of left fibula, init for clos fx	
823.80	CLOSED FRACTURE OF UNSPECIFIED PART OF TIBIA	**S82.201A**	Unsp fracture of shaft of right tibia, init for clos fx	
		S82.202A	Unsp fracture of shaft of left tibia, init for clos fx	
		S82.209A	Unsp fracture of shaft of unsp tibia, init for clos fx	
823.81	CLOSED FRACTURE OF UNSPECIFIED PART OF FIBULA	**S82.401A**	Unsp fracture of shaft of right fibula, init for clos fx	
		S82.402A	Unsp fracture of shaft of left fibula, init for clos fx	
		S82.409A	Unsp fracture of shaft of unsp fibula, init for clos fx	
823.82	CLOSED FRACTURE UNSPECIFIED PART FIBULA W/TIBIA	**S82.201A**	Unsp fracture of shaft of right tibia, init for clos fx	*and*
		S82.401A	Unsp fracture of shaft of right fibula, init for clos fx	
		S82.202A	Unsp fracture of shaft of left tibia, init for clos fx	*and*
		S82.402A	Unsp fracture of shaft of left fibula, init for clos fx	
823.90	OPEN FRACTURE OF UNSPECIFIED PART OF TIBIA	**S82.201B**	Unsp fx shaft of right tibia, init for opn fx type I/2	
		S82.201C	Unsp fx shaft of right tibia, init for opn fx type 3A/B/C	
		S82.202B	Unsp fx shaft of left tibia, init for opn fx type I/2	
		S82.202C	Unsp fx shaft of left tibia, init for opn fx type 3A/B/C	
		S82.209B	Unsp fx shaft of unsp tibia, init for opn fx type I/2	
		S82.209C	Unsp fx shaft of unsp tibia, init for opn fx type 3A/B/C	
823.91	OPEN FRACTURE OF UNSPECIFIED PART OF FIBULA	**S82.401B**	Unsp fracture of shaft of r fibula, init for opn fx type I/2	
		S82.401C	Unsp fx shaft of r fibula, init for opn fx type 3A/B/C	
		S82.402B	Unsp fx shaft of left fibula, init for opn fx type I/2	
		S82.402C	Unsp fx shaft of left fibula, init for opn fx type 3A/B/C	
		S82.409B	Unsp fx shaft of unsp fibula, init for opn fx type I/2	
		S82.409C	Unsp fx shaft of unsp fibula, init for opn fx type 3A/B/C	
823.92	OPEN FRACTURE UNSPECIFIED PART FIBULA W/TIBIA	**S82.201B**	Unsp fx shaft of right tibia, init for opn fx type I/2	*and*
		S82.401B	Unsp fracture of shaft of r fibula, init for opn fx type I/2	
		S82.202B	Unsp fx shaft of left tibia, init for opn fx type I/2	*and*
		S82.402B	Unsp fx shaft of left fibula, init for opn fx type I/2	
824.0	CLOSED FRACTURE OF MEDIAL MALLEOLUS	**S82.51XA**	Disp fx of medial malleolus of right tibia, init for clos fx	
		S82.52XA	Disp fx of medial malleolus of left tibia, init for clos fx	
		S82.53XA	Disp fx of medial malleolus of unsp tibia, init for clos fx	
		S82.54XA	Nondisp fx of medial malleolus of right tibia, init	
		S82.55XA	Nondisp fx of medial malleolus of left tibia, init	
		S82.56XA	Nondisp fx of medial malleolus of unsp tibia, init	
		S82.871A	Displaced pilon fracture of right tibia, init for clos fx	
		S82.872A	Displaced pilon fracture of left tibia, init for clos fx	
		S82.873A	Displaced pilon fracture of unsp tibia, init for clos fx	
		S82.874A	Nondisplaced pilon fracture of right tibia, init for clos fx	
		S82.875A	Nondisplaced pilon fracture of left tibia, init for clos fx	
		S82.876A	Nondisplaced pilon fracture of unsp tibia, init for clos fx	
824.1	OPEN FRACTURE OF MEDIAL MALLEOLUS	**S82.51XB**	Disp fx of med malleolus of r tibia, init op fx 1/2	
		S82.51XC	Disp fx of med malleolus of r tibia, init op fx 3A/B/C	
		S82.52XB	Disp fx of med malleolus of l tibia, init op fx 1/2	
		S82.52XC	Disp fx of med malleolus of l tibia, init op fx 3A/B/C	
		S82.53XB	Disp fx of med malleolus of unsp tibia, init op fx 1/2	
		S82.53XC	Disp fx of med malleolus of unsp tibia, init op fx 3A/B/C	
		S82.54XB	Nondisp fx of med malleolus of r tibia, init op fx 1/2	
		S82.54XC	Nondisp fx of med malleolus of r tibia, init op fx 3A/B/C	
		S82.55XB	Nondisp fx of med malleolus of l tibia, init op fx 1/2	
	(Continued on next page)	**S82.55XC**	Nondisp fx of med malleolus of l tibia, init op fx 3A/B/C	

ICD-9-CM		ICD-10-CM	
824.1	OPEN FRACTURE OF MEDIAL MALLEOLUS **(Continued)**	**S82.56XB**	Nondisp fx of med malleolus of unsp tibia, init op fx 1/2
		S82.56XC	Nondisp fx of med malleolus of unsp tibia, init op fx 3A/B/C
		S82.871B	Displaced pilon fx right tibia, init for opn fx type I/2
		S82.871C	Displaced pilon fx right tibia, init for opn fx type 3A/B/C
		S82.872B	Displaced pilon fx left tibia, init for opn fx type I/2
		S82.872C	Displaced pilon fx left tibia, init for opn fx type 3A/B/C
		S82.873B	Displaced pilon fx unsp tibia, init for opn fx type I/2
		S82.873C	Displaced pilon fx unsp tibia, init for opn fx type 3A/B/C
		S82.874B	Nondisp pilon fx right tibia, init for opn fx type I/2
		S82.874C	Nondisp pilon fx right tibia, init for opn fx type 3A/B/C
		S82.875B	Nondisp pilon fx left tibia, init for opn fx type I/2
		S82.875C	Nondisp pilon fx left tibia, init for opn fx type 3A/B/C
		S82.876B	Nondisp pilon fx unsp tibia, init for opn fx type I/2
		S82.876C	Nondisp pilon fx unsp tibia, init for opn fx type 3A/B/C
824.2	CLOSED FRACTURE OF LATERAL MALLEOLUS	**S82.61XA**	Disp fx of lateral malleolus of right fibula, init
		S82.62XA	Disp fx of lateral malleolus of left fibula, init
		S82.63XA	Disp fx of lateral malleolus of unsp fibula, init
		S82.64XA	Nondisp fx of lateral malleolus of right fibula, init
		S82.65XA	Nondisp fx of lateral malleolus of left fibula, init
		S82.66XA	Nondisp fx of lateral malleolus of unsp fibula, init
824.3	OPEN FRACTURE OF LATERAL MALLEOLUS	**S82.61XB**	Disp fx of lateral malleolus of r fibula, init op fx 1/2
		S82.61XC	Disp fx of lateral malleolus of r fibula, init op fx 3A/B/C
		S82.62XB	Disp fx of lateral malleolus of l fibula, init op fx 1/2
		S82.62XC	Disp fx of lateral malleolus of l fibula, init op fx 3A/B/C
		S82.63XB	Disp fx of lateral malleolus of unsp fibula, init op fx 1/2
		S82.63XC	Disp fx of lateral malleolus of unsp fibula,init op fx 3A/B/C
		S82.64XB	Nondisp fx of lateral malleolus of r fibula, init op fx 1/2
		S82.64XC	Nondisp fx of lateral malleolus of r fibula, init op fx 3A/B/C
		S82.65XB	Nondisp fx of lateral malleolus of l fibula, init op fx 1/2
		S82.65XC	Nondisp fx of lateral malleolus of l fibula, init op fx 3A/B/C
		S82.66XB	Nondisp fx of lateral malleolus of unsp fibula, init op fx 1/2
		S82.66XC	Nondisp fx of lateral malleolus of unsp fibula, init op fx 3A/B/C
824.4	CLOSED BIMALLEOLAR FRACTURE	**S82.841A**	Displaced bimalleolar fracture of right lower leg, init
		S82.842A	Displaced bimalleolar fracture of left lower leg, init
		S82.843A	Displaced bimalleolar fracture of unsp lower leg, init
		S82.844A	Nondisplaced bimalleolar fracture of right lower leg, init
		S82.845A	Nondisplaced bimalleolar fracture of left lower leg, init
		S82.846A	Nondisplaced bimalleolar fracture of unsp lower leg, init
824.5	OPEN BIMALLEOLAR FRACTURE	**S82.841B**	Displaced bimalleol fx r low leg, init for opn fx type I/2
		S82.841C	Displ bimalleol fx r low leg, init for opn fx type 3A/B/C
		S82.842B	Displaced bimalleol fx l low leg, init for opn fx type I/2
		S82.842C	Displ bimalleol fx l low leg, init for opn fx type 3A/B/C
		S82.843B	Displ bimalleol fx unsp lower leg, init for opn fx type I/2
		S82.843C	Displ bimalleol fx unsp low leg, init for opn fx type 3A/B/C
		S82.844B	Nondisp bimalleol fx r low leg, init for opn fx type I/2
		S82.844C	Nondisp bimalleol fx r low leg, init for opn fx type 3A/B/C
		S82.845B	Nondisp bimalleol fx l low leg, init for opn fx type I/2
		S82.845C	Nondisp bimalleol fx l low leg, init for opn fx type 3A/B/C
		S82.846B	Nondisp bimalleol fx unsp low leg, init for opn fx type I/2
		S82.846C	Nondisp bimalleol fx unsp low leg, init op fx 3A/B/C
824.6	CLOSED TRIMALLEOLAR FRACTURE	**S82.851A**	Displaced trimalleolar fracture of right lower leg, init
		S82.852A	Displaced trimalleolar fracture of left lower leg, init
		S82.853A	Displaced trimalleolar fracture of unsp lower leg, init
		S82.854A	Nondisplaced trimalleolar fracture of right lower leg, init
		S82.855A	Nondisplaced trimalleolar fracture of left lower leg, init
		S82.856A	Nondisplaced trimalleolar fracture of unsp lower leg, init
824.7	OPEN TRIMALLEOLAR FRACTURE	**S82.851B**	Displaced trimalleol fx r low leg, init for opn fx type I/2
		S82.851C	Displ trimalleol fx r low leg, init for opn fx type 3A/B/C
		S82.852B	Displaced trimalleol fx l low leg, init for opn fx type I/2
		S82.852C	Displ trimalleol fx l low leg, init for opn fx type 3A/B/C
		S82.853B	Displ trimalleol fx unsp lower leg, init for opn fx type I/2
		S82.853C	Displ trimalleol fx unsp low leg, init op fx 3A/B/C
		S82.854B	Nondisp trimalleol fx r low leg, init for opn fx type I/2
		S82.854C	Nondisp trimalleol fx r low leg, init for opn fx type 3A/B/C
		S82.855B	Nondisp trimalleol fx l low leg, init for opn fx type I/2
		S82.855C	Nondisp trimalleol fx l low leg, init for opn fx type 3A/B/C
		S82.856B	Nondisp trimalleol fx unsp low leg, init for opn fx type I/2
		S82.856C	Nondisp trimalleol fx unsp low leg, init op fx 3A/B/C
824.8	UNSPECIFIED CLOSED FRACTURE OF ANKLE	**S82.301A**	Unsp fracture of lower end of right tibia, init for clos fx
		S82.302A	Unsp fracture of lower end of left tibia, init for clos fx
		S82.309A	Unsp fracture of lower end of unsp tibia, init for clos fx
		S82.391A	Oth fracture of lower end of right tibia, init for clos fx
		S82.392A	Oth fracture of lower end of left tibia, init for clos fx
		S82.399A	Oth fracture of lower end of unsp tibia, init for clos fx
		S82.891A	Oth fracture of right lower leg, init for clos fx
		S82.892A	Oth fracture of left lower leg, init for clos fx
		S82.899A	Oth fracture of unsp lower leg, init for clos fx
		S89.101A	Unsp physeal fracture of lower end of right tibia, init
		S89.102A	Unsp physeal fracture of lower end of left tibia, init
		S89.109A	Unsp physeal fracture of lower end of unsp tibia, init
	(Continued on next page)	**S89.111A**	Sltr-haris Type I physeal fx lower end of right tibia, init

ICD-9-CM		ICD-10-CM	
824.8	UNSPECIFIED CLOSED FRACTURE OF ANKLE **(Continued)**	**S89.112A**	Sltr-haris Type I physeal fx lower end of left tibia, init
		S89.119A	Sltr-haris Type I physeal fx lower end of unsp tibia, init
		S89.121A	Sltr-haris Type II physeal fx lower end of right tibia, init
		S89.122A	Sltr-haris Type II physeal fx lower end of left tibia, init
		S89.129A	Sltr-haris Type II physeal fx lower end of unsp tibia, init
		S89.131A	Sltr-haris Type III physeal fx lower end of r tibia, init
		S89.132A	Sltr-haris Type III physeal fx lower end of left tibia, init
		S89.139A	Sltr-haris Type III physeal fx lower end of unsp tibia, init
		S89.141A	Sltr-haris Type IV physeal fx lower end of right tibia, init
		S89.142A	Sltr-haris Type IV physeal fx lower end of left tibia, init
		S89.149A	Sltr-haris Type IV physeal fx lower end of unsp tibia, init
		S89.191A	Oth physeal fracture of lower end of right tibia, init
		S89.192A	Oth physeal fracture of lower end of left tibia, init
		S89.199A	Oth physeal fracture of lower end of unsp tibia, init
		S89.3Ø1A	Unsp physeal fracture of lower end of right fibula, init
		S89.3Ø2A	Unsp physeal fracture of lower end of left fibula, init
		S89.3Ø9A	Unsp physeal fracture of lower end of unsp fibula, init
		S89.311A	Sltr-haris Type I physeal fx lower end of r fibula, init
		S89.312A	Sltr-haris Type I physeal fx lower end of left fibula, init
		S89.319A	Sltr-haris Type I physeal fx lower end of unsp fibula, init
		S89.321A	Sltr-haris Type II physeal fx lower end of r fibula, init
		S89.322A	Sltr-haris Type II physeal fx lower end of left fibula, init
		S89.329A	Sltr-haris Type II physeal fx lower end of unsp fibula, init
		S89.391A	Oth physeal fracture of lower end of right fibula, init
		S89.392A	Oth physeal fracture of lower end of left fibula, init
		S89.399A	Oth physeal fracture of lower end of unsp fibula, init
824.9	UNSPECIFIED OPEN FRACTURE OF ANKLE	**S82.3Ø1B**	Unsp fx lower end of right tibia, init for opn fx type I/2
		S82.3Ø1C	Unsp fx lower end of r tibia, init for opn fx type 3A/B/C
		S82.3Ø2B	Unsp fx lower end of left tibia, init for opn fx type I/2
		S82.3Ø2C	Unsp fx lower end of left tibia, init for opn fx type 3A/B/C
		S82.3Ø9B	Unsp fx lower end of unsp tibia, init for opn fx type I/2
		S82.3Ø9C	Unsp fx lower end of unsp tibia, init for opn fx type 3A/B/C
		S82.391B	Oth fx lower end of right tibia, init for opn fx type I/2
		S82.391C	Oth fx lower end of right tibia, init for opn fx type 3A/B/C
		S82.392B	Oth fx lower end of left tibia, init for opn fx type I/2
		S82.392C	Oth fx lower end of left tibia, init for opn fx type 3A/B/C
		S82.399B	Oth fx lower end of unsp tibia, init for opn fx type I/2
		S82.399C	Oth fx lower end of unsp tibia, init for opn fx type 3A/B/C
		S82.891B	Oth fracture of right lower leg, init for opn fx type I/2
		S82.891C	Oth fracture of right lower leg, init for opn fx type 3A/B/C
		S82.892B	Oth fracture of left lower leg, init for opn fx type I/2
		S82.892C	Oth fracture of left lower leg, init for opn fx type 3A/B/C
		S82.899B	Oth fracture of unsp lower leg, init for opn fx type I/2
		S82.899C	Oth fracture of unsp lower leg, init for opn fx type 3A/B/C
825.Ø	CLOSED FRACTURE OF CALCANEUS	**S92.ØØ1A**	Unsp fracture of right calcaneus, init for clos fx
		S92.ØØ2A	Unsp fracture of left calcaneus, init for clos fx
		S92.ØØ9A	Unsp fracture of unsp calcaneus, init for clos fx
		S92.Ø11A	Disp fx of body of right calcaneus, init for clos fx
		S92.Ø12A	Disp fx of body of left calcaneus, init for clos fx
		S92.Ø13A	Disp fx of body of unsp calcaneus, init for clos fx
		S92.Ø14A	Nondisp fx of body of right calcaneus, init for clos fx
		S92.Ø15A	Nondisp fx of body of left calcaneus, init for clos fx
		S92.Ø16A	Nondisp fx of body of unsp calcaneus, init for clos fx
		S92.Ø21A	Disp fx of anterior process of right calcaneus, init
		S92.Ø22A	Disp fx of anterior process of left calcaneus, init
		S92.Ø23A	Disp fx of anterior process of unsp calcaneus, init
		S92.Ø24A	Nondisp fx of anterior process of right calcaneus, init
		S92.Ø25A	Nondisp fx of anterior process of left calcaneus, init
		S92.Ø26A	Nondisp fx of anterior process of unsp calcaneus, init
		S92.Ø31A	Displaced avulsion fx tuberosity of r calcaneus, init
		S92.Ø32A	Displaced avulsion fx tuberosity of l calcaneus, init
		S92.Ø33A	Displaced avulsion fx tuberosity of unsp calcaneus, init
		S92.Ø34A	Nondisp avulsion fracture of tuberosity of r calcaneus, init
		S92.Ø35A	Nondisp avulsion fracture of tuberosity of l calcaneus, init
		S92.Ø36A	Nondisp avulsion fx tuberosity of unsp calcaneus, init
		S92.Ø41A	Displaced oth fracture of tuberosity of r calcaneus, init
		S92.Ø42A	Displaced oth fracture of tuberosity of left calcaneus, init
		S92.Ø43A	Displaced oth fracture of tuberosity of unsp calcaneus, init
		S92.Ø44A	Nondisplaced oth fracture of tuberosity of r calcaneus, init
		S92.Ø45A	Nondisplaced oth fracture of tuberosity of l calcaneus, init
		S92.Ø46A	Nondisp oth fracture of tuberosity of unsp calcaneus, init
		S92.Ø51A	Displaced oth extraarticular fracture of r calcaneus, init
		S92.Ø52A	Displaced oth extrartic fracture of left calcaneus, init
		S92.Ø53A	Displaced oth extrartic fracture of unsp calcaneus, init
		S92.Ø54A	Nondisplaced oth extrartic fracture of r calcaneus, init
		S92.Ø55A	Nondisplaced oth extrartic fracture of left calcaneus, init
		S92.Ø56A	Nondisplaced oth extrartic fracture of unsp calcaneus, init
		S92.Ø61A	Displaced intraarticular fracture of right calcaneus, init
		S92.Ø62A	Displaced intraarticular fracture of left calcaneus, init
		S92.Ø63A	Displaced intraarticular fracture of unsp calcaneus, init
		S92.Ø64A	Nondisplaced intraarticular fracture of r calcaneus, init
		S92.Ø65A	Nondisplaced intraarticular fracture of left calcaneus, init
		S92.Ø66A	Nondisplaced intraarticular fracture of unsp calcaneus, init

ICD-9-CM		ICD-10-CM	
825.1	OPEN FRACTURE OF CALCANEUS	**S92.ØØ1B**	Unsp fracture of right calcaneus, init for opn fx
		S92.ØØ2B	Unsp fracture of left calcaneus, init for opn fx
		S92.ØØ9B	Unsp fracture of unsp calcaneus, init for opn fx
		S92.Ø11B	Disp fx of body of right calcaneus, init for opn fx
		S92.Ø12B	Disp fx of body of left calcaneus, init for opn fx
		S92.Ø13B	Disp fx of body of unsp calcaneus, init for opn fx
		S92.Ø14B	Nondisp fx of body of right calcaneus, init for opn fx
		S92.Ø15B	Nondisp fx of body of left calcaneus, init for opn fx
		S92.Ø16B	Nondisp fx of body of unsp calcaneus, init for opn fx
		S92.Ø21B	Disp fx of anterior process of r calcaneus, init for opn fx
		S92.Ø22B	Disp fx of anterior process of l calcaneus, init for opn fx
		S92.Ø23B	Disp fx of ant process of unsp calcaneus, init for opn fx
		S92.Ø24B	Nondisp fx of ant process of r calcaneus, init for opn fx
		S92.Ø25B	Nondisp fx of ant process of l calcaneus, init for opn fx
		S92.Ø26B	Nondisp fx of ant process of unsp calcaneus, init for opn fx
		S92.Ø31B	Displ avulsion fx tuberosity of r calcaneus, init for opn fx
		S92.Ø32B	Displ avulsion fx tuberosity of l calcaneus, init for opn fx
		S92.Ø33B	Displ avuls fx tuberosity of unsp calcaneus, init for opn fx
		S92.Ø34B	Nondisp avuls fx tuberosity of r calcaneus, init for opn fx
		S92.Ø35B	Nondisp avuls fx tuberosity of l calcaneus, init for opn fx
		S92.Ø36B	Nondisp avuls fx tuberosity of unsp calcaneus, init op fx
		S92.Ø41B	Displaced oth fx tuberosity of r calcaneus, init for opn fx
		S92.Ø42B	Displaced oth fx tuberosity of l calcaneus, init for opn fx
		S92.Ø43B	Displ oth fx tuberosity of unsp calcaneus, init for opn fx
		S92.Ø44B	Nondisp oth fx tuberosity of r calcaneus, init for opn fx
		S92.Ø45B	Nondisp oth fx tuberosity of l calcaneus, init for opn fx
		S92.Ø46B	Nondisp oth fx tuberosity of unsp calcaneus, init for opn fx
		S92.Ø51B	Displaced oth extrartic fx r calcaneus, init for opn fx
		S92.Ø52B	Displaced oth extrartic fx l calcaneus, init for opn fx
		S92.Ø53B	Displaced oth extrartic fx unsp calcaneus, init for opn fx
		S92.Ø54B	Nondisp oth extrartic fx r calcaneus, init for opn fx
		S92.Ø55B	Nondisp oth extrartic fx l calcaneus, init for opn fx
		S92.Ø56B	Nondisp oth extrartic fx unsp calcaneus, init for opn fx
		S92.Ø61B	Displaced intartic fracture of r calcaneus, init for opn fx
		S92.Ø62B	Displaced intartic fracture of l calcaneus, init for opn fx
		S92.Ø63B	Displaced intartic fx unsp calcaneus, init for opn fx
		S92.Ø64B	Nondisp intartic fracture of r calcaneus, init for opn fx
		S92.Ø65B	Nondisp intartic fracture of l calcaneus, init for opn fx
		S92.Ø66B	Nondisp intartic fracture of unsp calcaneus, init for opn fx
825.2Ø	CLOSED FRACTURE OF UNSPECIFIED BONE OF FOOT	**S92.9Ø1A**	Unsp fracture of right foot, init encntr for closed fracture
		S92.9Ø2A	Unsp fracture of left foot, init encntr for closed fracture
		S92.9Ø9A	Unsp fracture of unsp foot, init encntr for closed fracture
825.21	CLOSED FRACTURE OF ASTRAGALUS	**S92.1Ø1A**	Unsp fracture of right talus, init for clos fx
		S92.1Ø2A	Unsp fracture of left talus, init encntr for closed fracture
		S92.1Ø9A	Unsp fracture of unsp talus, init encntr for closed fracture
		S92.111A	Disp fx of neck of right talus, init for clos fx
		S92.112A	Disp fx of neck of left talus, init for clos fx
		S92.113A	Disp fx of neck of unsp talus, init for clos fx
		S92.114A	Nondisp fx of neck of right talus, init for clos fx
		S92.115A	Nondisp fx of neck of left talus, init for clos fx
		S92.116A	Nondisp fx of neck of unsp talus, init for clos fx
		S92.121A	Disp fx of body of right talus, init for clos fx
		S92.122A	Disp fx of body of left talus, init for clos fx
		S92.123A	Disp fx of body of unsp talus, init for clos fx
		S92.124A	Nondisp fx of body of right talus, init for clos fx
		S92.125A	Nondisp fx of body of left talus, init for clos fx
		S92.126A	Nondisp fx of body of unsp talus, init for clos fx
		S92.131A	Disp fx of posterior process of right talus, init
		S92.132A	Disp fx of posterior process of left talus, init for clos fx
		S92.133A	Disp fx of posterior process of unsp talus, init for clos fx
		S92.134A	Nondisp fx of posterior process of right talus, init
		S92.135A	Nondisp fx of posterior process of left talus, init
		S92.136A	Nondisp fx of posterior process of unsp talus, init
		S92.141A	Displaced dome fracture of right talus, init for clos fx
		S92.142A	Displaced dome fracture of left talus, init for clos fx
		S92.143A	Displaced dome fracture of unsp talus, init for clos fx
		S92.144A	Nondisplaced dome fracture of right talus, init for clos fx
		S92.145A	Nondisplaced dome fracture of left talus, init for clos fx
		S92.146A	Nondisplaced dome fracture of unsp talus, init for clos fx
		S92.151A	Displ avulsion fracture (chip fracture) of right talus, init
		S92.152A	Displ avulsion fracture (chip fracture) of left talus, init
		S92.153A	Displ avulsion fracture (chip fracture) of unsp talus, init
		S92.154A	Nondisp avuls fracture (chip fracture) of right talus, init
		S92.155A	Nondisp avuls fracture (chip fracture) of left talus, init
		S92.156A	Nondisp avuls fracture (chip fracture) of unsp talus, init
		S92.191A	Oth fracture of right talus, init encntr for closed fracture
		S92.192A	Oth fracture of left talus, init encntr for closed fracture
		S92.199A	Oth fracture of unsp talus, init encntr for closed fracture

ICD-9-CM		ICD-10-CM	
825.22	CLOSED FRACTURE OF NAVICULAR BONE OF FOOT	**S92.251A**	Disp fx of navicular of right foot, init for clos fx
		S92.252A	Disp fx of navicular of left foot, init for clos fx
		S92.253A	Disp fx of navicular of unsp foot, init for clos fx
		S92.254A	Nondisp fx of navicular of right foot, init for clos fx
		S92.255A	Nondisp fx of navicular of left foot, init for clos fx
		S92.256A	Nondisp fx of navicular of unsp foot, init for clos fx
825.23	CLOSED FRACTURE OF CUBOID BONE	**S92.211A**	Disp fx of cuboid bone of right foot, init for clos fx
		S92.212A	Disp fx of cuboid bone of left foot, init for clos fx
		S92.213A	Disp fx of cuboid bone of unsp foot, init for clos fx
		S92.214A	Nondisp fx of cuboid bone of right foot, init for clos fx
		S92.215A	Nondisp fx of cuboid bone of left foot, init for clos fx
		S92.216A	Nondisp fx of cuboid bone of unsp foot, init for clos fx
825.24	CLOSED FRACTURE OF CUNEIFORM BONE OF FOOT	**S92.221A**	Disp fx of lateral cuneiform of right foot, init for clos fx
		S92.222A	Disp fx of lateral cuneiform of left foot, init for clos fx
		S92.223A	Disp fx of lateral cuneiform of unsp foot, init for clos fx
		S92.224A	Nondisp fx of lateral cuneiform of right foot, init
		S92.225A	Nondisp fx of lateral cuneiform of left foot, init
		S92.226A	Nondisp fx of lateral cuneiform of unsp foot, init
		S92.231A	Disp fx of intermediate cuneiform of right foot, init
		S92.232A	Disp fx of intermediate cuneiform of left foot, init
		S92.233A	Disp fx of intermediate cuneiform of unsp foot, init
		S92.234A	Nondisp fx of intermediate cuneiform of right foot, init
		S92.235A	Nondisp fx of intermediate cuneiform of left foot, init
		S92.236A	Nondisp fx of intermediate cuneiform of unsp foot, init
		S92.241A	Disp fx of medial cuneiform of right foot, init for clos fx
		S92.242A	Disp fx of medial cuneiform of left foot, init for clos fx
		S92.243A	Disp fx of medial cuneiform of unsp foot, init for clos fx
		S92.244A	Nondisp fx of medial cuneiform of right foot, init
		S92.245A	Nondisp fx of medial cuneiform of left foot, init
		S92.246A	Nondisp fx of medial cuneiform of unsp foot, init
825.25	CLOSED FRACTURE OF METATARSAL BONE	**S92.301A**	Fracture of unsp metatarsal bone(s), right foot, init
		S92.302A	Fracture of unsp metatarsal bone(s), left foot, init
		S92.309A	Fracture of unsp metatarsal bone(s), unsp foot, init
		S92.311A	Disp fx of first metatarsal bone, right foot, init
		S92.312A	Disp fx of first metatarsal bone, left foot, init
		S92.313A	Disp fx of first metatarsal bone, unsp foot, init
		S92.314A	Nondisp fx of first metatarsal bone, right foot, init
		S92.315A	Nondisp fx of first metatarsal bone, left foot, init
		S92.316A	Nondisp fx of first metatarsal bone, unsp foot, init
		S92.321A	Disp fx of second metatarsal bone, right foot, init
		S92.322A	Disp fx of second metatarsal bone, left foot, init
		S92.323A	Disp fx of second metatarsal bone, unsp foot, init
		S92.324A	Nondisp fx of second metatarsal bone, right foot, init
		S92.325A	Nondisp fx of second metatarsal bone, left foot, init
		S92.326A	Nondisp fx of second metatarsal bone, unsp foot, init
		S92.331A	Disp fx of third metatarsal bone, right foot, init
		S92.332A	Disp fx of third metatarsal bone, left foot, init
		S92.333A	Disp fx of third metatarsal bone, unsp foot, init
		S92.334A	Nondisp fx of third metatarsal bone, right foot, init
		S92.335A	Nondisp fx of third metatarsal bone, left foot, init
		S92.336A	Nondisp fx of third metatarsal bone, unsp foot, init
		S92.341A	Disp fx of fourth metatarsal bone, right foot, init
		S92.342A	Disp fx of fourth metatarsal bone, left foot, init
		S92.343A	Disp fx of fourth metatarsal bone, unsp foot, init
		S92.344A	Nondisp fx of fourth metatarsal bone, right foot, init
		S92.345A	Nondisp fx of fourth metatarsal bone, left foot, init
		S92.346A	Nondisp fx of fourth metatarsal bone, unsp foot, init
		S92.351A	Disp fx of fifth metatarsal bone, right foot, init
		S92.352A	Disp fx of fifth metatarsal bone, left foot, init
		S92.353A	Disp fx of fifth metatarsal bone, unsp foot, init
		S92.354A	Nondisp fx of fifth metatarsal bone, right foot, init
		S92.355A	Nondisp fx of fifth metatarsal bone, left foot, init
		S92.356A	Nondisp fx of fifth metatarsal bone, unsp foot, init
825.29	OTHER CLOSED FRACTURE OF TARSAL&METATARSAL BONES	**S92.201A**	Fracture of unsp tarsal bone(s) of right foot, init
		S92.202A	Fracture of unsp tarsal bone(s) of left foot, init
		S92.209A	Fracture of unsp tarsal bone(s) of unsp foot, init
		S92.301A	Fracture of unsp metatarsal bone(s), right foot, init
		S92.302A	Fracture of unsp metatarsal bone(s), left foot, init
		S92.309A	Fracture of unsp metatarsal bone(s), unsp foot, init
825.30	OPEN FRACTURE OF UNSPECIFIED BONE OF FOOT	**S92.901B**	Unsp fracture of right foot, init encntr for open fracture
		S92.902B	Unsp fracture of left foot, init encntr for open fracture
		S92.909B	Unsp fracture of unsp foot, init encntr for open fracture

ICD-9-CM		ICD-10-CM	
825.31	OPEN FRACTURE OF ASTRAGALUS	**S92.101B**	Unsp fracture of right talus, init encntr for open fracture
		S92.102B	Unsp fracture of left talus, init encntr for open fracture
		S92.109B	Unsp fracture of unsp talus, init encntr for open fracture
		S92.111B	Disp fx of neck of right talus, init for opn fx
		S92.112B	Disp fx of neck of left talus, init encntr for open fracture
		S92.113B	Disp fx of neck of unsp talus, init encntr for open fracture
		S92.114B	Nondisp fx of neck of right talus, init for opn fx
		S92.115B	Nondisp fx of neck of left talus, init for opn fx
		S92.116B	Nondisp fx of neck of unsp talus, init for opn fx
		S92.121B	Disp fx of body of right talus, init for opn fx
		S92.122B	Disp fx of body of left talus, init encntr for open fracture
		S92.123B	Disp fx of body of unsp talus, init encntr for open fracture
		S92.124B	Nondisp fx of body of right talus, init for opn fx
		S92.125B	Nondisp fx of body of left talus, init for opn fx
		S92.126B	Nondisp fx of body of unsp talus, init for opn fx
		S92.131B	Disp fx of posterior process of right talus, init for opn fx
		S92.132B	Disp fx of posterior process of left talus, init for opn fx
		S92.133B	Disp fx of posterior process of unsp talus, init for opn fx
		S92.134B	Nondisp fx of post process of right talus, init for opn fx
		S92.135B	Nondisp fx of post process of left talus, init for opn fx
		S92.136B	Nondisp fx of post process of unsp talus, init for opn fx
		S92.141B	Displaced dome fracture of right talus, init for opn fx
		S92.142B	Displaced dome fracture of left talus, init for opn fx
		S92.143B	Displaced dome fracture of unsp talus, init for opn fx
		S92.144B	Nondisplaced dome fracture of right talus, init for opn fx
		S92.145B	Nondisplaced dome fracture of left talus, init for opn fx
		S92.146B	Nondisplaced dome fracture of unsp talus, init for opn fx
		S92.151B	Displ avuls fx (chip fracture) of r talus, init for opn fx
		S92.152B	Displ avuls fx (chip fracture) of l talus, init for opn fx
		S92.153B	Displ avuls fx (chip fracture) of unsp talus, init op fx
		S92.154B	Nondisp avuls fx (chip fracture) of r talus, init for opn fx
		S92.155B	Nondisp avuls fx (chip fracture) of l talus, init for opn fx
		S92.156B	Nondisp avuls fx (chip fracture) of unsp talus, init op fx
		S92.191B	Other fracture of right talus, init encntr for open fracture
		S92.192B	Other fracture of left talus, init encntr for open fracture
		S92.199B	Other fracture of unsp talus, init encntr for open fracture
825.32	OPEN FRACTURE OF NAVICULAR BONE OF FOOT	**S92.251B**	Disp fx of navicular of right foot, init for opn fx
		S92.252B	Disp fx of navicular of left foot, init for opn fx
		S92.253B	Disp fx of navicular of unsp foot, init for opn fx
		S92.254B	Nondisp fx of navicular of right foot, init for opn fx
		S92.255B	Nondisp fx of navicular of left foot, init for opn fx
		S92.256B	Nondisp fx of navicular of unsp foot, init for opn fx
825.33	OPEN FRACTURE OF CUBOID BONE	**S92.211B**	Disp fx of cuboid bone of right foot, init for opn fx
		S92.212B	Disp fx of cuboid bone of left foot, init for opn fx
		S92.213B	Disp fx of cuboid bone of unsp foot, init for opn fx
		S92.214B	Nondisp fx of cuboid bone of right foot, init for opn fx
		S92.215B	Nondisp fx of cuboid bone of left foot, init for opn fx
		S92.216B	Nondisp fx of cuboid bone of unsp foot, init for opn fx
825.34	OPEN FRACTURE OF CUNEIFORM BONE OF FOOT	**S92.221B**	Disp fx of lateral cuneiform of right foot, init for opn fx
		S92.222B	Disp fx of lateral cuneiform of left foot, init for opn fx
		S92.223B	Disp fx of lateral cuneiform of unsp foot, init for opn fx
		S92.224B	Nondisp fx of lateral cuneiform of r foot, init for opn fx
		S92.225B	Nondisp fx of lateral cuneiform of l foot, init for opn fx
		S92.226B	Nondisp fx of lateral cuneiform of unsp ft, init for opn fx
		S92.231B	Disp fx of intermed cuneiform of right foot, init for opn fx
		S92.232B	Disp fx of intermed cuneiform of left foot, init for opn fx
		S92.233B	Disp fx of intermed cuneiform of unsp foot, init for opn fx
		S92.234B	Nondisp fx of intermed cuneiform of r foot, init for opn fx
		S92.235B	Nondisp fx of intermed cuneiform of l foot, init for opn fx
		S92.236B	Nondisp fx of intermed cuneiform of unsp ft, init for opn fx
		S92.241B	Disp fx of medial cuneiform of right foot, init for opn fx
		S92.242B	Disp fx of medial cuneiform of left foot, init for opn fx
		S92.243B	Disp fx of medial cuneiform of unsp foot, init for opn fx
		S92.244B	Nondisp fx of medial cuneiform of r foot, init for opn fx
		S92.245B	Nondisp fx of medial cuneiform of left foot, init for opn fx
		S92.246B	Nondisp fx of medial cuneiform of unsp foot, init for opn fx
825.35	OPEN FRACTURE OF METATARSAL BONE	**S92.301B**	Fx unsp metatarsal bone(s), right foot, init for opn fx
		S92.302B	Fx unsp metatarsal bone(s), left foot, init for opn fx
		S92.309B	Fx unsp metatarsal bone(s), unsp foot, init for opn fx
		S92.311B	Disp fx of first metatarsal bone, r foot, init for opn fx
		S92.312B	Disp fx of first metatarsal bone, left foot, init for opn fx
		S92.313B	Disp fx of first metatarsal bone, unsp foot, init for opn fx
		S92.314B	Nondisp fx of first metatarsal bone, r foot, init for opn fx
		S92.315B	Nondisp fx of first metatarsal bone, l foot, init for opn fx
		S92.316B	Nondisp fx of 1st metatarsal bone, unsp ft, init for opn fx
		S92.321B	Disp fx of second metatarsal bone, r foot, init for opn fx
		S92.322B	Disp fx of second metatarsal bone, l foot, init for opn fx
		S92.323B	Disp fx of 2nd metatarsal bone, unsp foot, init for opn fx
		S92.324B	Nondisp fx of 2nd metatarsal bone, r foot, init for opn fx
		S92.325B	Nondisp fx of 2nd metatarsal bone, l foot, init for opn fx
		S92.326B	Nondisp fx of 2nd metatarsal bone, unsp ft, init for opn fx
		S92.331B	Disp fx of third metatarsal bone, r foot, init for opn fx

(Continued on next page)

ICD-9-CM		ICD-10-CM	
825.35	OPEN FRACTURE OF METATARSAL BONE **(Continued on next page)**	**S92.332B**	Disp fx of third metatarsal bone, left foot, init for opn fx
		S92.333B	Disp fx of third metatarsal bone, unsp foot, init for opn fx
		S92.334B	Nondisp fx of third metatarsal bone, r foot, init for opn fx
		S92.335B	Nondisp fx of third metatarsal bone, l foot, init for opn fx
		S92.336B	Nondisp fx of 3rd metatarsal bone, unsp ft, init for opn fx
		S92.341B	Disp fx of fourth metatarsal bone, r foot, init for opn fx
		S92.342B	Disp fx of fourth metatarsal bone, l foot, init for opn fx
		S92.343B	Disp fx of 4th metatarsal bone, unsp foot, init for opn fx
		S92.344B	Nondisp fx of 4th metatarsal bone, r foot, init for opn fx
		S92.345B	Nondisp fx of 4th metatarsal bone, l foot, init for opn fx
		S92.346B	Nondisp fx of 4th metatarsal bone, unsp ft, init for opn fx
		S92.351B	Disp fx of fifth metatarsal bone, r foot, init for opn fx
		S92.352B	Disp fx of fifth metatarsal bone, left foot, init for opn fx
		S92.353B	Disp fx of fifth metatarsal bone, unsp foot, init for opn fx
		S92.354B	Nondisp fx of fifth metatarsal bone, r foot, init for opn fx
		S92.355B	Nondisp fx of fifth metatarsal bone, l foot, init for opn fx
		S92.356B	Nondisp fx of 5th metatarsal bone, unsp ft, init for opn fx
825.39	OTHER OPEN FRACTURES OF TARSAL&METATARSAL BONES	**S92.2Ø1B**	Fx unsp tarsal bone(s) of right foot, init for opn fx
		S92.2Ø2B	Fx unsp tarsal bone(s) of left foot, init for opn fx
		S92.2Ø9B	Fx unsp tarsal bone(s) of unsp foot, init for opn fx
		S92.3Ø9B	Fx unsp metatarsal bone(s), unsp foot, init for opn fx
826.Ø	CLOSED FRACTURE OF ONE OR MORE PHALANGES OF FOOT	**S92.4Ø1A**	Displaced unsp fracture of right great toe, init for clos fx
		S92.4Ø2A	Displaced unsp fracture of left great toe, init for clos fx
		S92.4Ø3A	Displaced unsp fracture of unsp great toe, init for clos fx
		S92.4Ø4A	Nondisplaced unsp fracture of right great toe, init
		S92.4Ø5A	Nondisplaced unsp fracture of left great toe, init
		S92.4Ø6A	Nondisplaced unsp fracture of unsp great toe, init
		S92.411A	Disp fx of proximal phalanx of right great toe, init
		S92.412A	Disp fx of proximal phalanx of left great toe, init
		S92.413A	Disp fx of proximal phalanx of unsp great toe, init
		S92.414A	Nondisp fx of proximal phalanx of right great toe, init
		S92.415A	Nondisp fx of proximal phalanx of left great toe, init
		S92.416A	Nondisp fx of proximal phalanx of unsp great toe, init
		S92.421A	Disp fx of distal phalanx of right great toe, init
		S92.422A	Disp fx of distal phalanx of left great toe, init
		S92.423A	Disp fx of distal phalanx of unsp great toe, init
		S92.424A	Nondisp fx of distal phalanx of right great toe, init
		S92.425A	Nondisp fx of distal phalanx of left great toe, init
		S92.426A	Nondisp fx of distal phalanx of unsp great toe, init
		S92.491A	Oth fracture of right great toe, init for clos fx
		S92.492A	Oth fracture of left great toe, init for clos fx
		S92.499A	Oth fracture of unsp great toe, init for clos fx
		S92.5Ø1A	Displaced unsp fracture of right lesser toe(s), init
		S92.5Ø2A	Displaced unsp fracture of left lesser toe(s), init
		S92.5Ø3A	Displaced unsp fracture of unsp lesser toe(s), init
		S92.5Ø4A	Nondisplaced unsp fracture of right lesser toe(s), init
		S92.5Ø5A	Nondisplaced unsp fracture of left lesser toe(s), init
		S92.5Ø6A	Nondisplaced unsp fracture of unsp lesser toe(s), init
		S92.511A	Disp fx of proximal phalanx of right lesser toe(s), init
		S92.512A	Disp fx of proximal phalanx of left lesser toe(s), init
		S92.513A	Disp fx of proximal phalanx of unsp lesser toe(s), init
		S92.514A	Nondisp fx of proximal phalanx of right lesser toe(s), init
		S92.515A	Nondisp fx of proximal phalanx of left lesser toe(s), init
		S92.516A	Nondisp fx of proximal phalanx of unsp lesser toe(s), init
		S92.521A	Disp fx of medial phalanx of right lesser toe(s), init
		S92.522A	Disp fx of medial phalanx of left lesser toe(s), init
		S92.523A	Disp fx of medial phalanx of unsp lesser toe(s), init
		S92.524A	Nondisp fx of medial phalanx of right lesser toe(s), init
		S92.525A	Nondisp fx of medial phalanx of left lesser toe(s), init
		S92.526A	Nondisp fx of medial phalanx of unsp lesser toe(s), init
		S92.531A	Disp fx of distal phalanx of right lesser toe(s), init
		S92.532A	Disp fx of distal phalanx of left lesser toe(s), init
		S92.533A	Disp fx of distal phalanx of unsp lesser toe(s), init
		S92.534A	Nondisp fx of distal phalanx of right lesser toe(s), init
		S92.535A	Nondisp fx of distal phalanx of left lesser toe(s), init
		S92.536A	Nondisp fx of distal phalanx of unsp lesser toe(s), init
		S92.591A	Oth fracture of right lesser toe(s), init for clos fx
		S92.592A	Oth fracture of left lesser toe(s), init for clos fx
		S92.599A	Oth fracture of unsp lesser toe(s), init for clos fx
		S92.911A	Unsp fracture of right toe(s), init for clos fx
		S92.912A	Unsp fracture of left toe(s), init for clos fx
		S92.919A	Unsp fracture of unsp toe(s), init for clos fx

ICD-9-CM		ICD-10-CM	
826.1	OPEN FRACTURE OF ONE OR MORE PHALANGES OF FOOT	**S92.4Ø1B**	Displaced unsp fracture of right great toe, init for opn fx
		S92.4Ø2B	Displaced unsp fracture of left great toe, init for opn fx
		S92.4Ø3B	Displaced unsp fracture of unsp great toe, init for opn fx
		S92.4Ø4B	Nondisp unsp fracture of right great toe, init for opn fx
		S92.4Ø5B	Nondisp unsp fracture of left great toe, init for opn fx
		S92.4Ø6B	Nondisp unsp fracture of unsp great toe, init for opn fx
		S92.411B	Disp fx of prox phalanx of right great toe, init for opn fx
		S92.412B	Disp fx of prox phalanx of left great toe, init for opn fx
		S92.413B	Disp fx of prox phalanx of unsp great toe, init for opn fx
		S92.414B	Nondisp fx of prox phalanx of r great toe, init for opn fx
		S92.415B	Nondisp fx of prox phalanx of l great toe, init for opn fx
		S92.416B	Nondisp fx of prox phalanx of unsp great toe, init op fx
		S92.421B	Disp fx of dist phalanx of right great toe, init for opn fx
		S92.422B	Disp fx of distal phalanx of left great toe, init for opn fx
		S92.423B	Disp fx of distal phalanx of unsp great toe, init for opn fx
		S92.424B	Nondisp fx of dist phalanx of r great toe, init for opn fx
		S92.425B	Nondisp fx of dist phalanx of l great toe, init for opn fx
		S92.426B	Nondisp fx of dist phalanx of unsp great toe, init op fx
		S92.491B	Oth fracture of right great toe, init for opn fx
		S92.492B	Oth fracture of left great toe, init for opn fx
		S92.499B	Oth fracture of unsp great toe, init for opn fx
		S92.5Ø1B	Displaced unsp fx right lesser toe(s), init for opn fx
		S92.5Ø2B	Displaced unsp fx left lesser toe(s), init for opn fx
		S92.5Ø3B	Displaced unsp fx unsp lesser toe(s), init for opn fx
		S92.5Ø4B	Nondisp unsp fx right lesser toe(s), init for opn fx
		S92.5Ø5B	Nondisp unsp fracture of left lesser toe(s), init for opn fx
		S92.5Ø6B	Nondisp unsp fracture of unsp lesser toe(s), init for opn fx
		S92.511B	Disp fx of prox phalanx of r less toe(s), init for opn fx
		S92.512B	Disp fx of prox phalanx of left less toe(s), init for opn fx
		S92.513B	Disp fx of prox phalanx of unsp less toe(s), init for opn fx
		S92.514B	Nondisp fx of prox phalanx of r less toe(s), init for opn fx
		S92.515B	Nondisp fx of prox phalanx of l less toe(s), init for opn fx
		S92.516B	Nondisp fx of prox phalanx of unsp less toe(s), init op fx
		S92.521B	Disp fx of med phalanx of right less toe(s), init for opn fx
		S92.522B	Disp fx of med phalanx of left less toe(s), init for opn fx
		S92.523B	Disp fx of med phalanx of unsp less toe(s), init for opn fx
		S92.524B	Nondisp fx of med phalanx of r less toe(s), init for opn fx
		S92.525B	Nondisp fx of med phalanx of l less toe(s), init for opn fx
		S92.526B	Nondisp fx of med phalanx of unsp less toe(s), init op fx
		S92.531B	Disp fx of dist phalanx of r less toe(s), init for opn fx
		S92.532B	Disp fx of dist phalanx of left less toe(s), init for opn fx
		S92.533B	Disp fx of dist phalanx of unsp less toe(s), init for opn fx
		S92.534B	Nondisp fx of dist phalanx of r less toe(s), init for opn fx
		S92.535B	Nondisp fx of dist phalanx of l less toe(s), init for opn fx
		S92.536B	Nondisp fx of dist phalanx of unsp less toe(s), init op fx
		S92.591B	Oth fracture of right lesser toe(s), init for opn fx
		S92.592B	Oth fracture of left lesser toe(s), init for opn fx
		S92.599B	Oth fracture of unsp lesser toe(s), init for opn fx
		S92.911B	Unsp fracture of right toe(s), init encntr for open fracture
		S92.912B	Unsp fracture of left toe(s), init encntr for open fracture
		S92.919B	Unsp fracture of unsp toe(s), init encntr for open fracture
827.Ø	OTH MULTIPLE&ILL-DEFINED CLOS FX LOWER LIMB	**S82.9ØXA**	Unsp fracture of unsp lower leg, init for clos fx
		S82.91XA	Unsp fracture of right lower leg, init for clos fx
		S82.92XA	Unsp fracture of left lower leg, init for clos fx
		T14.8	Other injury of unspecified body region
827.1	OTH MULTIPLE&ILL-DEFINED OPEN FX LOWER LIMB	**S82.9ØXB**	Unsp fracture of unsp lower leg, init for opn fx type I/2
		S82.9ØXC	Unsp fracture of unsp lower leg, init for opn fx type 3A/B/C
		S82.91XB	Unsp fracture of right lower leg, init for opn fx type I/2
		S82.91XC	Unsp fracture of r low leg, init for opn fx type 3A/B/C
		S82.92XB	Unsp fracture of left lower leg, init for opn fx type I/2
		S82.92XC	Unsp fracture of left lower leg, init for opn fx type 3A/B/C
		T14.8	Other injury of unspecified body region
828.Ø	MX CLOS FX LEGS LEGS W/ARM LEGS W/RIBS&STERNUM	**TØ7**	Unspecified multiple injuries
828.1	MX OPN FX LEGS LEGS W/ARM-LEGS W/RIBS&STERNUM	**TØ7**	Unspecified multiple injuries
829.Ø	CLOSED FRACTURE OF UNSPECIFIED BONE	**T14.8**	Other injury of unspecified body region
829.1	OPEN FRACTURE OF UNSPECIFIED BONE	**T14.8**	Other injury of unspecified body region
83Ø.Ø	CLOSED DISLOCATION OF JAW	**SØ3.ØXXA**	Dislocation of jaw, initial encounter
83Ø.1	OPEN DISLOCATION OF JAW	**SØ3.ØXXA**	Dislocation of jaw, initial encounter *and*
		SØ1.4Ø9A	Unsp open wound of unsp cheek and TMJ area, init
831.ØØ	CLOSED DISLOCATION OF SHOULDER UNSPECIFIED SITE	**S43.ØØ1A**	Unspecified subluxation of right shoulder joint, init encntr
		S43.ØØ2A	Unspecified subluxation of left shoulder joint, init encntr
		S43.ØØ3A	Unsp subluxation of unspecified shoulder joint, init encntr
		S43.ØØ4A	Unspecified dislocation of right shoulder joint, init encntr
		S43.ØØ5A	Unspecified dislocation of left shoulder joint, init encntr
		S43.ØØ6A	Unsp dislocation of unspecified shoulder joint, init encntr

ICD-9-CM		ICD-10-CM		
831.Ø1	CLOSED ANTERIOR DISLOCATION OF HUMERUS	**S43.Ø11A**	Anterior subluxation of right humerus, initial encounter	
		S43.Ø12A	Anterior subluxation of left humerus, initial encounter	
		S43.Ø13A	Anterior subluxation of unspecified humerus, init encntr	
		S43.Ø14A	Anterior dislocation of right humerus, initial encounter	
		S43.Ø15A	Anterior dislocation of left humerus, initial encounter	
		S43.Ø16A	Anterior dislocation of unspecified humerus, init encntr	
831.Ø2	CLOSED POSTERIOR DISLOCATION OF HUMERUS	**S43.Ø21A**	Posterior subluxation of right humerus, initial encounter	
		S43.Ø22A	Posterior subluxation of left humerus, initial encounter	
		S43.Ø23A	Posterior subluxation of unspecified humerus, init encntr	
		S43.Ø24A	Posterior dislocation of right humerus, initial encounter	
		S43.Ø25A	Posterior dislocation of left humerus, initial encounter	
		S43.Ø26A	Posterior dislocation of unspecified humerus, init encntr	
831.Ø3	CLOSED INFERIOR DISLOCATION OF HUMERUS	**S43.Ø31A**	Inferior subluxation of right humerus, initial encounter	
		S43.Ø32A	Inferior subluxation of left humerus, initial encounter	
		S43.Ø33A	Inferior subluxation of unspecified humerus, init encntr	
		S43.Ø34A	Inferior dislocation of right humerus, initial encounter	
		S43.Ø35A	Inferior dislocation of left humerus, initial encounter	
		S43.Ø36A	Inferior dislocation of unspecified humerus, init encntr	
831.Ø4	CLOSED DISLOCATION OF ACROMIOCLAVICULAR	**S43.1Ø1A**	Unsp dislocation of right acromioclavicular joint, init	
		S43.1Ø2A	Unsp dislocation of left acromioclavicular joint, init	
		S43.1Ø9A	Unsp dislocation of unsp acromioclavicular joint, init	
		S43.111A	Subluxation of right acromioclavicular joint, init encntr	
		S43.112A	Subluxation of left acromioclavicular joint, init encntr	
		S43.119A	Subluxation of unsp acromioclavicular joint, init encntr	
		S43.121A	Dislocation of r acromioclav jt, 100%-200% displacmnt, init	
		S43.122A	Dislocation of l acromioclav jt, 100%-200% displacmnt, init	
		S43.129A	Disloc of unsp acromioclav jt, 100%-200% displacmnt, init	
		S43.131A	Dislocation of r acromioclav jt, > 200% displacmnt, init	
		S43.132A	Dislocation of l acromioclav jt, > 200% displacmnt, init	
		S43.139A	Dislocation of unsp acromioclav jt, > 200% displacmnt, init	
		S43.141A	Inferior dislocation of right acromioclavicular joint, init	
		S43.142A	Inferior dislocation of left acromioclavicular joint, init	
		S43.149A	Inferior dislocation of unsp acromioclavicular joint, init	
		S43.151A	Posterior dislocation of right acromioclavicular joint, init	
		S43.152A	Posterior dislocation of left acromioclavicular joint, init	
		S43.159A	Posterior dislocation of unsp acromioclavicular joint, init	
831.Ø9	CLOSED DISLOCATION OF OTHER SITE OF SHOULDER	**S43.Ø81A**	Other subluxation of right shoulder joint, initial encounter	
		S43.Ø82A	Other subluxation of left shoulder joint, initial encounter	
		S43.Ø83A	Other subluxation of unspecified shoulder joint, init encntr	
		S43.Ø84A	Other dislocation of right shoulder joint, initial encounter	
		S43.Ø85A	Other dislocation of left shoulder joint, initial encounter	
		S43.Ø86A	Other dislocation of unspecified shoulder joint, init encntr	
		S43.3Ø1A	Subluxation of unsp parts of right shoulder girdle, init	
		S43.3Ø2A	Subluxation of unsp parts of left shoulder girdle, init	
		S43.3Ø3A	Subluxation of unsp parts of unsp shoulder girdle, init	
		S43.3Ø4A	Dislocation of unsp parts of right shoulder girdle, init	
		S43.3Ø5A	Dislocation of unsp parts of left shoulder girdle, init	
		S43.3Ø6A	Dislocation of unsp parts of unsp shoulder girdle, init	
		S43.311A	Subluxation of right scapula, initial encounter	
		S43.312A	Subluxation of left scapula, initial encounter	
		S43.313A	Subluxation of unspecified scapula, initial encounter	
		S43.314A	Dislocation of right scapula, initial encounter	
		S43.315A	Dislocation of left scapula, initial encounter	
		S43.316A	Dislocation of unspecified scapula, initial encounter	
		S43.391A	Subluxation of oth prt right shoulder girdle, init encntr	
		S43.392A	Subluxation of oth prt left shoulder girdle, init encntr	
		S43.393A	Subluxation of oth prt unsp shoulder girdle, init encntr	
		S43.394A	Dislocation of oth prt right shoulder girdle, init encntr	
		S43.395A	Dislocation of oth prt left shoulder girdle, init encntr	
		S43.396A	Dislocation of oth prt unsp shoulder girdle, init encntr	
831.1Ø	OPEN UNSPECIFIED DISLOCATION OF SHOULDER	**S43.ØØ6A**	Unsp dislocation of unspecified shoulder joint, init encntr	*and*
		S41.ØØ9A	Unspecified open wound of unspecified shoulder, init encntr	
831.11	OPEN ANTERIOR DISLOCATION OF HUMERUS	**S43.Ø16A**	Anterior dislocation of unspecified humerus, init encntr	*and*
		S41.1Ø9A	Unspecified open wound of unspecified upper arm, init encntr	
831.12	OPEN POSTERIOR DISLOCATION OF HUMERUS	**S43.Ø26A**	Posterior dislocation of unspecified humerus, init encntr	*and*
		S41.1Ø9A	Unspecified open wound of unspecified upper arm, init encntr	
831.13	OPEN INFERIOR DISLOCATION OF HUMERUS	**S43.Ø36A**	Inferior dislocation of unspecified humerus, init encntr	*and*
		S41.1Ø9A	Unspecified open wound of unspecified upper arm, init encntr	
831.14	OPEN DISLOCATION OF ACROMIOCLAVICULAR	**S43.1Ø9A**	Unsp dislocation of unsp acromioclavicular joint, init	*and*
		S41.ØØ9A	Unspecified open wound of unspecified shoulder, init encntr	
831.19	OPEN DISLOCATION OF OTHER SITE OF SHOULDER	**S43.Ø86A**	Other dislocation of unspecified shoulder joint, init encntr	*and*
		S41.ØØ9A	Unspecified open wound of unspecified shoulder, init encntr	

ICD-9-CM		ICD-10-CM		
832.00	CLOSED UNSPECIFIED DISLOCATION OF ELBOW	**S53.001A**	Unspecified subluxation of right radial head, init encntr	
		S53.002A	Unspecified subluxation of left radial head, init encntr	
		S53.003A	Unsp subluxation of unspecified radial head, init encntr	
		S53.004A	Unspecified dislocation of right radial head, init encntr	
		S53.005A	Unspecified dislocation of left radial head, init encntr	
		S53.006A	Unsp dislocation of unspecified radial head, init encntr	
		S53.101A	Unsp subluxation of right ulnohumeral joint, init encntr	
		S53.102A	Unsp subluxation of left ulnohumeral joint, init encntr	
		S53.103A	Unsp subluxation of unsp ulnohumeral joint, init encntr	
		S53.104A	Unsp dislocation of right ulnohumeral joint, init encntr	
		S53.105A	Unsp dislocation of left ulnohumeral joint, init encntr	
		S53.106A	Unsp dislocation of unsp ulnohumeral joint, init encntr	
832.01	CLOSED ANTERIOR DISLOCATION OF ELBOW	**S53.011A**	Anterior subluxation of right radial head, initial encounter	
		S53.012A	Anterior subluxation of left radial head, initial encounter	
		S53.013A	Anterior subluxation of unspecified radial head, init encntr	
		S53.014A	Anterior dislocation of right radial head, initial encounter	
		S53.015A	Anterior dislocation of left radial head, initial encounter	
		S53.016A	Anterior dislocation of unspecified radial head, init encntr	
		S53.111A	Anterior subluxation of right ulnohumeral joint, init encntr	
		S53.112A	Anterior subluxation of left ulnohumeral joint, init encntr	
		S53.113A	Anterior subluxation of unsp ulnohumeral joint, init encntr	
		S53.114A	Anterior dislocation of right ulnohumeral joint, init encntr	
		S53.115A	Anterior dislocation of left ulnohumeral joint, init encntr	
		S53.116A	Anterior dislocation of unsp ulnohumeral joint, init encntr	
832.02	CLOSED POSTERIOR DISLOCATION OF ELBOW	**S53.021A**	Posterior subluxation of right radial head, init encntr	
		S53.022A	Posterior subluxation of left radial head, initial encounter	
		S53.023A	Posterior subluxation of unsp radial head, init encntr	
		S53.024A	Posterior dislocation of right radial head, init encntr	
		S53.025A	Posterior dislocation of left radial head, initial encounter	
		S53.026A	Posterior dislocation of unsp radial head, init encntr	
		S53.121A	Posterior subluxation of right ulnohumeral joint, init	
		S53.122A	Posterior subluxation of left ulnohumeral joint, init encntr	
		S53.123A	Posterior subluxation of unsp ulnohumeral joint, init encntr	
		S53.124A	Posterior dislocation of right ulnohumeral joint, init	
		S53.125A	Posterior dislocation of left ulnohumeral joint, init encntr	
		S53.126A	Posterior dislocation of unsp ulnohumeral joint, init encntr	
832.03	CLOSED MEDIAL DISLOCATION OF ELBOW	**S53.131A**	Medial subluxation of right ulnohumeral joint, init encntr	
		S53.132A	Medial subluxation of left ulnohumeral joint, init encntr	
		S53.133A	Medial subluxation of unsp ulnohumeral joint, init encntr	
		S53.134A	Medial dislocation of right ulnohumeral joint, init encntr	
		S53.135A	Medial dislocation of left ulnohumeral joint, init encntr	
		S53.136A	Medial dislocation of unsp ulnohumeral joint, init encntr	
832.04	CLOSED LATERAL DISLOCATION OF ELBOW	**S53.141A**	Lateral subluxation of right ulnohumeral joint, init encntr	
		S53.142A	Lateral subluxation of left ulnohumeral joint, init encntr	
		S53.143A	Lateral subluxation of unsp ulnohumeral joint, init encntr	
		S53.144A	Lateral dislocation of right ulnohumeral joint, init encntr	
		S53.145A	Lateral dislocation of left ulnohumeral joint, init encntr	
		S53.146A	Lateral dislocation of unsp ulnohumeral joint, init encntr	
832.09	CLOSED DISLOCATION OF OTHER SITE OF ELBOW	**S53.091A**	Other subluxation of right radial head, initial encounter	
		S53.092A	Other subluxation of left radial head, initial encounter	
		S53.093A	Other subluxation of unspecified radial head, init encntr	
		S53.094A	Other dislocation of right radial head, initial encounter	
		S53.095A	Other dislocation of left radial head, initial encounter	
		S53.096A	Other dislocation of unspecified radial head, init encntr	
		S53.191A	Other subluxation of right ulnohumeral joint, init encntr	
		S53.192A	Other subluxation of left ulnohumeral joint, init encntr	
		S53.193A	Other subluxation of unsp ulnohumeral joint, init encntr	
		S53.194A	Other dislocation of right ulnohumeral joint, init encntr	
		S53.195A	Other dislocation of left ulnohumeral joint, init encntr	
		S53.196A	Other dislocation of unsp ulnohumeral joint, init encntr	
832.10	OPEN UNSPECIFIED DISLOCATION OF ELBOW	**S53.006A**	Unsp dislocation of unspecified radial head, init encntr	*and*
		S51.009A	Unspecified open wound of unspecified elbow, init encntr	
		S53.106A	Unsp dislocation of unsp ulnohumeral joint, init encntr	*and*
		S51.009A	Unspecified open wound of unspecified elbow, init encntr	
832.11	OPEN ANTERIOR DISLOCATION OF ELBOW	**S53.016A**	Anterior dislocation of unspecified radial head, init encntr	*and*
		S51.009A	Unspecified open wound of unspecified elbow, init encntr	
		S53.116A	Anterior dislocation of unsp ulnohumeral joint, init encntr	*and*
		S51.009A	Unspecified open wound of unspecified elbow, init encntr	
832.12	OPEN POSTERIOR DISLOCATION OF ELBOW	**S53.026A**	Posterior dislocation of unsp radial head, init encntr	*and*
		S51.009A	Unspecified open wound of unspecified elbow, init encntr	
832.13	OPEN MEDIAL DISLOCATION OF ELBOW	**S53.136A**	Medial dislocation of unsp ulnohumeral joint, init encntr	*and*
		S51.009A	Unspecified open wound of unspecified elbow, init encntr	
832.14	OPEN LATERAL DISLOCATION OF ELBOW	**S53.146A**	Lateral dislocation of unsp ulnohumeral joint, init encntr	*and*
		S51.009A	Unspecified open wound of unspecified elbow, init encntr	

ICD-9-CM		ICD-10-CM		
832.19	OPEN DISLOCATION OF OTHER SITE OF ELBOW	**S53.096A**	Other dislocation of unspecified radial head, init encntr	***and***
		S51.009A	Unspecified open wound of unspecified elbow, init encntr	
		S53.196A	Other dislocation of unsp ulnohumeral joint, init encntr	***and***
		S51.009A	Unspecified open wound of unspecified elbow, init encntr	
832.2	NURSEMAIDS ELBOW	**S53.031A**	Nursemaid's elbow, right elbow, initial encounter	
		S53.032A	Nursemaid's elbow, left elbow, initial encounter	
		S53.033A	Nursemaid's elbow, unspecified elbow, initial encounter	
833.00	CLOSED DISLOCATION OF WRIST UNSPECIFIED PART	**S63.001A**	Unspecified subluxation of right wrist and hand, init encntr	
		S63.002A	Unspecified subluxation of left wrist and hand, init encntr	
		S63.003A	Unsp subluxation of unspecified wrist and hand, init encntr	
		S63.004A	Unspecified dislocation of right wrist and hand, init encntr	
		S63.005A	Unspecified dislocation of left wrist and hand, init encntr	
		S63.006A	Unsp dislocation of unspecified wrist and hand, init encntr	
833.01	CLOSED DISLOCATION OF DISTAL RADIOULNAR	**S63.011A**	Subluxation of distal radioulnar joint of right wrist, init	
		S63.012A	Subluxation of distal radioulnar joint of left wrist, init	
		S63.013A	Subluxation of distal radioulnar joint of unsp wrist, init	
		S63.014A	Dislocation of distal radioulnar joint of right wrist, init	
		S63.015A	Dislocation of distal radioulnar joint of left wrist, init	
		S63.016A	Dislocation of distal radioulnar joint of unsp wrist, init	
833.02	CLOSED DISLOCATION OF RADIOCARPAL	**S63.021A**	Subluxation of radiocarpal joint of right wrist, init encntr	
		S63.022A	Subluxation of radiocarpal joint of left wrist, init encntr	
		S63.023A	Subluxation of radiocarpal joint of unsp wrist, init encntr	
		S63.024A	Dislocation of radiocarpal joint of right wrist, init encntr	
		S63.025A	Dislocation of radiocarpal joint of left wrist, init encntr	
		S63.026A	Dislocation of radiocarpal joint of unsp wrist, init encntr	
833.03	CLOSED DISLOCATION OF MIDCARPAL	**S63.031A**	Subluxation of midcarpal joint of right wrist, init encntr	
		S63.032A	Subluxation of midcarpal joint of left wrist, init encntr	
		S63.033A	Subluxation of midcarpal joint of unsp wrist, init encntr	
		S63.034A	Dislocation of midcarpal joint of right wrist, init encntr	
		S63.035A	Dislocation of midcarpal joint of left wrist, init encntr	
		S63.036A	Dislocation of midcarpal joint of unsp wrist, init encntr	
833.04	CLOSED DISLOCATION OF CARPOMETACARPAL	**S63.041A**	Subluxation of carpometacarpal joint of right thumb, init	
		S63.042A	Subluxation of carpometacarpal joint of left thumb, init	
		S63.043A	Subluxation of carpometacarpal joint of unsp thumb, init	
		S63.044A	Dislocation of carpometacarpal joint of right thumb, init	
		S63.045A	Dislocation of carpometacarpal joint of left thumb, init	
		S63.046A	Dislocation of carpometacarpal joint of unsp thumb, init	
		S63.051A	Subluxation of oth carpometacarpal joint of right hand, init	
		S63.052A	Subluxation of oth carpometacarpal joint of left hand, init	
		S63.053A	Subluxation of oth carpometacarpal joint of unsp hand, init	
		S63.054A	Dislocation of oth carpometacarpal joint of right hand, init	
		S63.055A	Dislocation of oth carpometacarpal joint of left hand, init	
		S63.056A	Dislocation of oth carpometacarpal joint of unsp hand, init	
833.05	CLOSED DISLOCATION OF PROXIMAL END OF METACARPAL	**S63.061A**	Sublux of MC (bone), proximal end of right hand, init	
		S63.062A	Sublux of metacarpal (bone), proximal end of left hand, init	
		S63.063A	Sublux of metacarpal (bone), proximal end of unsp hand, init	
		S63.064A	Disloc of MC (bone), proximal end of right hand, init	
		S63.065A	Disloc of metacarpal (bone), proximal end of left hand, init	
		S63.066A	Disloc of metacarpal (bone), proximal end of unsp hand, init	
833.09	CLOSED DISLOCATION OF OTHER PART OF WRIST	**S63.071A**	Subluxation of distal end of right ulna, initial encounter	
		S63.072A	Subluxation of distal end of left ulna, initial encounter	
		S63.073A	Subluxation of distal end of unspecified ulna, init encntr	
		S63.074A	Dislocation of distal end of right ulna, initial encounter	
		S63.075A	Dislocation of distal end of left ulna, initial encounter	
		S63.076A	Dislocation of distal end of unspecified ulna, init encntr	
		S63.091A	Other subluxation of right wrist and hand, initial encounter	
		S63.092A	Other subluxation of left wrist and hand, initial encounter	
		S63.093A	Other subluxation of unspecified wrist and hand, init encntr	
		S63.094A	Other dislocation of right wrist and hand, initial encounter	
		S63.095A	Other dislocation of left wrist and hand, initial encounter	
		S63.096A	Other dislocation of unspecified wrist and hand, init encntr	
833.10	OPEN DISLOCATION OF WRIST UNSPECIFIED PART	**S63.006A**	Unsp dislocation of unspecified wrist and hand, init encntr	***and***
		S61.509A	Unspecified open wound of unspecified wrist, init encntr	
833.11	OPEN DISLOCATION OF DISTAL RADIOULNAR	**S63.016A**	Dislocation of distal radioulnar joint of unsp wrist, init	***and***
		S61.509A	Unspecified open wound of unspecified wrist, init encntr	
833.12	OPEN DISLOCATION OF RADIOCARPAL	**S63.026A**	Dislocation of radiocarpal joint of unsp wrist, init encntr	***and***
		S61.509A	Unspecified open wound of unspecified wrist, init encntr	
833.13	OPEN DISLOCATION OF MIDCARPAL	**S63.036A**	Dislocation of midcarpal joint of unsp wrist, init encntr	***and***
		S61.509A	Unspecified open wound of unspecified wrist, init encntr	
833.14	OPEN DISLOCATION OF CARPOMETACARPAL	**S63.046A**	Dislocation of carpometacarpal joint of unsp thumb, init	***or***
		S63.056A	Dislocation of oth carpometacarpal joint of unsp hand, init	***and***
		S61.509A	Unspecified open wound of unspecified wrist, init encntr	
833.15	OPEN DISLOCATION OF PROXIMAL END OF METACARPAL	**S63.066A**	Disloc of metacarpal (bone), proximal end of unsp hand, init	***and***
		S61.509A	Unspecified open wound of unspecified wrist, init encntr	

ICD-9-CM		ICD-10-CM		
833.19	OPEN DISLOCATION OF OTHER PART OF WRIST	**S63.Ø76A**	Dislocation of distal end of unspecified ulna, init encntr	*or*
		S63.Ø96A	Other dislocation of unspecified wrist and hand, init encntr	*and*
		S61.5Ø9A	Unspecified open wound of unspecified wrist, init encntr	
834.ØØ	CLOSED DISLOCATION OF FINGER UNSPECIFIED PART	**S63.1Ø1A**	Unspecified subluxation of right thumb, initial encounter	
		S63.1Ø2A	Unspecified subluxation of left thumb, initial encounter	
		S63.1Ø3A	Unspecified subluxation of unspecified thumb, init encntr	
		S63.1Ø4A	Unspecified dislocation of right thumb, initial encounter	
		S63.1Ø5A	Unspecified dislocation of left thumb, initial encounter	
		S63.1Ø6A	Unspecified dislocation of unspecified thumb, init encntr	
		S63.2ØØA	Unspecified subluxation of right index finger, init encntr	
		S63.2Ø1A	Unspecified subluxation of left index finger, init encntr	
		S63.2Ø2A	Unspecified subluxation of right middle finger, init encntr	
		S63.2Ø3A	Unspecified subluxation of left middle finger, init encntr	
		S63.2Ø4A	Unspecified subluxation of right ring finger, init encntr	
		S63.2Ø5A	Unspecified subluxation of left ring finger, init encntr	
		S63.2Ø6A	Unspecified subluxation of right little finger, init encntr	
		S63.2Ø7A	Unspecified subluxation of left little finger, init encntr	
		S63.2Ø8A	Unspecified subluxation of other finger, initial encounter	
		S63.2Ø9A	Unspecified subluxation of unspecified finger, init encntr	
		S63.25ØA	Unspecified dislocation of right index finger, init encntr	
		S63.251A	Unspecified dislocation of left index finger, init encntr	
		S63.252A	Unspecified dislocation of right middle finger, init encntr	
		S63.253A	Unspecified dislocation of left middle finger, init encntr	
		S63.254A	Unspecified dislocation of right ring finger, init encntr	
		S63.255A	Unspecified dislocation of left ring finger, init encntr	
		S63.256A	Unspecified dislocation of right little finger, init encntr	
		S63.257A	Unspecified dislocation of left little finger, init encntr	
		S63.258A	Unspecified dislocation of other finger, initial encounter	
		S63.259A	Unspecified dislocation of unspecified finger, init encntr	
834.Ø1	CLOSED DISLOCATION OF METACARPOPHALANGEAL	**S63.111A**	Subluxation of MCP joint of right thumb, init	
		S63.112A	Subluxation of metacarpophalangeal joint of left thumb, init	
		S63.113A	Subluxation of metacarpophalangeal joint of unsp thumb, init	
		S63.114A	Dislocation of MCP joint of right thumb, init	
		S63.115A	Dislocation of metacarpophalangeal joint of left thumb, init	
		S63.116A	Dislocation of metacarpophalangeal joint of unsp thumb, init	
		S63.21ØA	Subluxation of MCP joint of right index finger, init	
		S63.211A	Subluxation of MCP joint of left index finger, init	
		S63.212A	Subluxation of MCP joint of right middle finger, init	
		S63.213A	Subluxation of MCP joint of left middle finger, init	
		S63.214A	Subluxation of MCP joint of right ring finger, init	
		S63.215A	Subluxation of MCP joint of left ring finger, init	
		S63.216A	Subluxation of MCP joint of right little finger, init	
		S63.217A	Subluxation of MCP joint of left little finger, init	
		S63.218A	Subluxation of metacarpophalangeal joint of oth finger, init	
		S63.219A	Subluxation of MCP joint of unsp finger, init	
		S63.26ØA	Dislocation of MCP joint of right index finger, init	
		S63.261A	Dislocation of MCP joint of left index finger, init	
		S63.262A	Dislocation of MCP joint of right middle finger, init	
		S63.263A	Dislocation of MCP joint of left middle finger, init	
		S63.264A	Dislocation of MCP joint of right ring finger, init	
		S63.265A	Dislocation of MCP joint of left ring finger, init	
		S63.266A	Dislocation of MCP joint of right little finger, init	
		S63.267A	Dislocation of MCP joint of left little finger, init	
		S63.268A	Dislocation of metacarpophalangeal joint of oth finger, init	
		S63.269A	Dislocation of MCP joint of unsp finger, init	
834.Ø2	CLOSED DISLOCATION OF INTERPHALANGEAL HAND	**S63.121A**	Subluxation of unsp interphaln joint of right thumb, init	
		S63.122A	Subluxation of unsp interphaln joint of left thumb, init	
		S63.123A	Subluxation of unsp interphalangeal joint of thmb, init	
		S63.124A	Dislocation of unsp interphaln joint of right thumb, init	
		S63.125A	Dislocation of unsp interphaln joint of left thumb, init	
		S63.126A	Dislocation of unsp interphalangeal joint of thmb, init	
		S63.131A	Subluxation of proximal interphaln joint of r thm, init	
		S63.132A	Subluxation of proximal interphaln joint of left thumb, init	
		S63.133A	Subluxation of proximal interphalangeal joint of thmb, init	
		S63.134A	Disloc of proximal interphaln joint of right thumb, init	
		S63.135A	Dislocation of proximal interphaln joint of left thumb, init	
		S63.136A	Dislocation of proximal interphalangeal joint of thmb, init	
		S63.141A	Subluxation of distal interphaln joint of right thumb, init	
		S63.142A	Subluxation of distal interphaln joint of left thumb, init	
		S63.143A	Subluxation of distal interphalangeal joint of thmb, init	
		S63.144A	Dislocation of distal interphaln joint of right thumb, init	
		S63.145A	Dislocation of distal interphaln joint of left thumb, init	
		S63.146A	Dislocation of distal interphalangeal joint of thmb, init	
		S63.22ØA	Subluxation of unsp interphaln joint of r idx fngr, init	
		S63.221A	Subluxation of unsp interphaln joint of l idx fngr, init	
		S63.222A	Subluxation of unsp interphaln joint of r mid finger, init	
		S63.223A	Subluxation of unsp interphaln joint of l mid finger, init	

(Continued on next page)

ICD-9-CM		ICD-10-CM		
834.Ø2	CLOSED DISLOCATION OF INTERPHALANGEAL HAND **(Continued)**	**S63.224A**	Subluxation of unsp interphaln joint of r rng fngr, init	
		S63.225A	Subluxation of unsp interphaln joint of l rng fngr, init	
		S63.226A	Sublux of unsp interphaln joint of r little finger, init	
		S63.227A	Sublux of unsp interphaln joint of l little finger, init	
		S63.228A	Subluxation of unsp interphalangeal joint of finger, init	
		S63.229A	Subluxation of unsp interphaln joint of unsp finger, init	
		S63.23ØA	Subluxation of proximal interphaln joint of r idx fngr, init	
		S63.231A	Subluxation of proximal interphaln joint of l idx fngr, init	
		S63.232A	Sublux of proximal interphaln joint of r mid finger, init	
		S63.233A	Sublux of proximal interphaln joint of l mid finger, init	
		S63.234A	Subluxation of proximal interphaln joint of r rng fngr, init	
		S63.235A	Subluxation of proximal interphaln joint of l rng fngr, init	
		S63.236A	Sublux of proximal interphaln joint of r little finger, init	
		S63.237A	Sublux of proximal interphaln joint of l little finger, init	
		S63.238A	Subluxation of proximal interphaln joint of finger, init	
		S63.239A	Sublux of proximal interphaln joint of unsp finger, init	
		S63.24ØA	Subluxation of distal interphaln joint of r idx fngr, init	
		S63.241A	Subluxation of distal interphaln joint of l idx fngr, init	
		S63.242A	Subluxation of distal interphaln joint of r mid finger, init	
		S63.243A	Subluxation of distal interphaln joint of l mid finger, init	
		S63.244A	Subluxation of distal interphaln joint of r rng fngr, init	
		S63.245A	Subluxation of distal interphaln joint of l rng fngr, init	
		S63.246A	Sublux of distal interphaln joint of r little finger, init	
		S63.247A	Sublux of distal interphaln joint of l little finger, init	
		S63.248A	Subluxation of distal interphalangeal joint of finger, init	
		S63.249A	Subluxation of distal interphaln joint of unsp finger, init	
		S63.27ØA	Dislocation of unsp interphaln joint of r idx fngr, init	
		S63.271A	Dislocation of unsp interphaln joint of l idx fngr, init	
		S63.272A	Dislocation of unsp interphaln joint of r mid finger, init	
		S63.273A	Dislocation of unsp interphaln joint of l mid finger, init	
		S63.274A	Dislocation of unsp interphaln joint of r rng fngr, init	
		S63.275A	Dislocation of unsp interphaln joint of l rng fngr, init	
		S63.276A	Disloc of unsp interphaln joint of r little finger, init	
		S63.277A	Disloc of unsp interphaln joint of l little finger, init	
		S63.278A	Dislocation of unsp interphalangeal joint of finger, init	
		S63.279A	Dislocation of unsp interphaln joint of unsp finger, init	
		S63.28ØA	Dislocation of proximal interphaln joint of r idx fngr, init	
		S63.281A	Dislocation of proximal interphaln joint of l idx fngr, init	
		S63.282A	Disloc of proximal interphaln joint of r mid finger, init	
		S63.283A	Disloc of proximal interphaln joint of l mid finger, init	
		S63.284A	Dislocation of proximal interphaln joint of r rng fngr, init	
		S63.285A	Dislocation of proximal interphaln joint of l rng fngr, init	
		S63.286A	Disloc of proximal interphaln joint of r little finger, init	
		S63.287A	Disloc of proximal interphaln joint of l little finger, init	
		S63.288A	Dislocation of proximal interphaln joint of finger, init	
		S63.289A	Disloc of proximal interphaln joint of unsp finger, init	
		S63.29ØA	Dislocation of distal interphaln joint of r idx fngr, init	
		S63.291A	Dislocation of distal interphaln joint of l idx fngr, init	
		S63.292A	Dislocation of distal interphaln joint of r mid finger, init	
		S63.293A	Dislocation of distal interphaln joint of l mid finger, init	
		S63.294A	Dislocation of distal interphaln joint of r rng fngr, init	
		S63.295A	Dislocation of distal interphaln joint of l rng fngr, init	
		S63.296A	Disloc of distal interphaln joint of r little finger, init	
		S63.297A	Disloc of distal interphaln joint of l little finger, init	
		S63.298A	Dislocation of distal interphalangeal joint of finger, init	
		S63.299A	Dislocation of distal interphaln joint of unsp finger, init	
834.1Ø	OPEN DISLOCATION OF FINGER UNSPECIFIED PART	**S63.1Ø6A**	Unspecified dislocation of unspecified thumb, init encntr	*and*
		S61.ØØ9A	Unsp open wound of unsp thumb w/o damage to nail, init	
		S63.259A	Unspecified dislocation of unspecified finger, init encntr	*and*
		S61.2Ø9A	Unsp open wound of unsp finger w/o damage to nail, init	
834.11	OPEN DISLOCATION OF METACARPOPHALANGEAL	**S63.116A**	Dislocation of metacarpophalangeal joint of unsp thumb, init	*or*
		S63.269A	Dislocation of MCP joint of unsp finger, init	*and*
		S61.4Ø9A	Unspecified open wound of unspecified hand, init encntr	
834.12	OPEN DISLOCATION INTERPHALANGEAL HAND	**S63.126A**	Dislocation of unsp interphalangeal joint of thmb, init	*and*
		S61.ØØ9A	Unsp open wound of unsp thumb w/o damage to nail, init	
		S63.279A	Dislocation of unsp interphaln joint of unsp finger, init	*and*
		S61.2Ø9A	Unsp open wound of unsp finger w/o damage to nail, init	
835.ØØ	CLOSED DISLOCATION OF HIP UNSPECIFIED SITE	**S73.ØØ1A**	Unspecified subluxation of right hip, initial encounter	
		S73.ØØ2A	Unspecified subluxation of left hip, initial encounter	
		S73.ØØ3A	Unspecified subluxation of unspecified hip, init encntr	
		S73.ØØ4A	Unspecified dislocation of right hip, initial encounter	
		S73.ØØ5A	Unspecified dislocation of left hip, initial encounter	
		S73.ØØ6A	Unspecified dislocation of unspecified hip, init encntr	
		S73.Ø41A	Central subluxation of right hip, initial encounter	
		S73.Ø42A	Central subluxation of left hip, initial encounter	
		S73.Ø43A	Central subluxation of unspecified hip, initial encounter	
		S73.Ø44A	Central dislocation of right hip, initial encounter	
		S73.Ø45A	Central dislocation of left hip, initial encounter	
		S73.Ø46A	Central dislocation of unspecified hip, initial encounter	

[Brackets] indicate valid character values for each code. Character value meanings provided for each code grouping.

ICD-9-CM		ICD-10-CM		
835.01	CLOSED POSTERIOR DISLOCATION OF HIP	**S73.011A**	Posterior subluxation of right hip, initial encounter	
		S73.012A	Posterior subluxation of left hip, initial encounter	
		S73.013A	Posterior subluxation of unspecified hip, initial encounter	
		S73.014A	Posterior dislocation of right hip, initial encounter	
		S73.015A	Posterior dislocation of left hip, initial encounter	
		S73.016A	Posterior dislocation of unspecified hip, initial encounter	
835.02	CLOSED OBTURATOR DISLOCATION OF HIP	**S73.021A**	Obturator subluxation of right hip, initial encounter	
		S73.022A	Obturator subluxation of left hip, initial encounter	
		S73.023A	Obturator subluxation of unspecified hip, initial encounter	
		S73.024A	Obturator dislocation of right hip, initial encounter	
		S73.025A	Obturator dislocation of left hip, initial encounter	
		S73.026A	Obturator dislocation of unspecified hip, initial encounter	
835.03	OTHER CLOSED ANTERIOR DISLOCATION OF HIP	**S73.031A**	Other anterior subluxation of right hip, initial encounter	
		S73.032A	Other anterior subluxation of left hip, initial encounter	
		S73.033A	Other anterior subluxation of unspecified hip, init encntr	
		S73.034A	Other anterior dislocation of right hip, initial encounter	
		S73.035A	Other anterior dislocation of left hip, initial encounter	
		S73.036A	Other anterior dislocation of unspecified hip, init encntr	
835.10	OPEN DISLOCATION OF HIP UNSPECIFIED SITE	**S73.006A**	Unspecified dislocation of unspecified hip, init encntr	*and*
		S71.009A	Unspecified open wound, unspecified hip, initial encounter	
835.11	OPEN POSTERIOR DISLOCATION OF HIP	**S73.016A**	Posterior dislocation of unspecified hip, initial encounter	*and*
		S71.009A	Unspecified open wound, unspecified hip, initial encounter	
835.12	OPEN OBTURATOR DISLOCATION OF HIP	**S73.026A**	Obturator dislocation of unspecified hip, initial encounter	*and*
		S71.009A	Unspecified open wound, unspecified hip, initial encounter	
835.13	OTHER OPEN ANTERIOR DISLOCATION OF HIP	**S73.036A**	Other anterior dislocation of unspecified hip, init encntr	*and*
		S71.009A	Unspecified open wound, unspecified hip, initial encounter	
836.0	TEAR MEDIAL CARTILAGE OR MENISCUS KNEE CURRENT	**S83.211A**	Bucket-hndl tear of medial mensc, crnt injury, r knee, init	
		S83.212A	Bucket-hndl tear of medial mensc, crnt injury, l knee, init	
		S83.219A	Bucket-hndl tear of medial mensc, crnt inj, unsp knee, init	
		S83.221A	Prph tear of medial meniscus, current injury, r knee, init	
		S83.222A	Prph tear of medial meniscus, current injury, l knee, init	
		S83.229A	Prph tear of medial mensc, current injury, unsp knee, init	
		S83.231A	Complex tear of medial mensc, current injury, r knee, init	
		S83.232A	Complex tear of medial mensc, current injury, l knee, init	
		S83.239A	Cmplx tear of medial mensc, current injury, unsp knee, init	
		S83.241A	Oth tear of medial meniscus, current injury, r knee, init	
		S83.242A	Oth tear of medial meniscus, current injury, left knee, init	
		S83.249A	Oth tear of medial meniscus, current injury, unsp knee, init	
836.1	TEAR LATERAL CARTILAGE OR MENISCUS KNEE CURRENT	**S83.251A**	Bucket-hndl tear of lat mensc, current injury, r knee, init	
		S83.252A	Bucket-hndl tear of lat mensc, current injury, l knee, init	
		S83.259A	Bucket-hndl tear of lat mensc, crnt injury, unsp knee, init	
		S83.261A	Prph tear of lat mensc, current injury, right knee, init	
		S83.262A	Prph tear of lat mensc, current injury, left knee, init	
		S83.269A	Prph tear of lat mensc, current injury, unsp knee, init	
		S83.271A	Complex tear of lat mensc, current injury, right knee, init	
		S83.272A	Complex tear of lat mensc, current injury, left knee, init	
		S83.279A	Complex tear of lat mensc, current injury, unsp knee, init	
		S83.281A	Oth tear of lat mensc, current injury, right knee, init	
		S83.282A	Oth tear of lat mensc, current injury, left knee, init	
		S83.289A	Oth tear of lat mensc, current injury, unsp knee, init	
836.2	OTHER TEAR CARTILAGE OR MENISCUS KNEE CURRENT	**S83.200A**	Bucket-hndl tear of unsp mensc, current injury, r knee, init	
		S83.201A	Bucket-hndl tear of unsp mensc, current injury, l knee, init	
		S83.202A	Bucket-hndl tear of unsp mensc, crnt injury, unsp knee, init	
		S83.203A	Oth tear of unsp meniscus, current injury, right knee, init	
		S83.204A	Oth tear of unsp meniscus, current injury, left knee, init	
		S83.205A	Oth tear of unsp meniscus, current injury, unsp knee, init	
		S83.206A	Unsp tear of unsp meniscus, current injury, right knee, init	
		S83.207A	Unsp tear of unsp meniscus, current injury, left knee, init	
		S83.209A	Unsp tear of unsp meniscus, current injury, unsp knee, init	
		S83.30XA	Tear of articular cartilage of unsp knee, current, init	
		S83.31XA	Tear of articular cartilage of right knee, current, init	
		S83.32XA	Tear of articular cartilage of left knee, current, init	
836.3	CLOSED DISLOCATION OF PATELLA	**S83.001A**	Unspecified subluxation of right patella, initial encounter	
		S83.002A	Unspecified subluxation of left patella, initial encounter	
		S83.003A	Unspecified subluxation of unspecified patella, init encntr	
		S83.004A	Unspecified dislocation of right patella, initial encounter	
		S83.005A	Unspecified dislocation of left patella, initial encounter	
		S83.006A	Unspecified dislocation of unspecified patella, init encntr	
		S83.011A	Lateral subluxation of right patella, initial encounter	
		S83.012A	Lateral subluxation of left patella, initial encounter	
		S83.013A	Lateral subluxation of unspecified patella, init encntr	
		S83.014A	Lateral dislocation of right patella, initial encounter	
		S83.015A	Lateral dislocation of left patella, initial encounter	
		S83.016A	Lateral dislocation of unspecified patella, init encntr	
		S83.091A	Other subluxation of right patella, initial encounter	
		S83.092A	Other subluxation of left patella, initial encounter	
		S83.093A	Other subluxation of unspecified patella, initial encounter	
		S83.094A	Other dislocation of right patella, initial encounter	

(Continued on next page)

ICD-9-CM		ICD-10-CM		
836.3	CLOSED DISLOCATION OF PATELLA **(Continued)**	**S83.Ø95A**	Other dislocation of left patella, initial encounter	
		S83.Ø96A	Other dislocation of unspecified patella, initial encounter	
836.4	OPEN DISLOCATION OF PATELLA	**S83.ØØ6A**	Unspecified dislocation of unspecified patella, init encntr	***and***
		S81.ØØ9A	Unspecified open wound, unspecified knee, initial encounter	
836.5Ø	CLOSED DISLOCATION OF KNEE UNSPECIFIED PART	**S83.1Ø1A**	Unspecified subluxation of right knee, initial encounter	
		S83.1Ø2A	Unspecified subluxation of left knee, initial encounter	
		S83.1Ø3A	Unspecified subluxation of unspecified knee, init encntr	
		S83.1Ø4A	Unspecified dislocation of right knee, initial encounter	
		S83.1Ø5A	Unspecified dislocation of left knee, initial encounter	
		S83.1Ø6A	Unspecified dislocation of unspecified knee, init encntr	
836.51	CLOSED ANTERIOR DISLOCATION TIBIA PROXIMAL END	**S83.111A**	Anterior sublux of proximal end of tibia, right knee, init	
		S83.112A	Anterior sublux of proximal end of tibia, left knee, init	
		S83.113A	Anterior sublux of proximal end of tibia, unsp knee, init	
		S83.114A	Anterior disloc of proximal end of tibia, right knee, init	
		S83.115A	Anterior disloc of proximal end of tibia, left knee, init	
		S83.116A	Anterior disloc of proximal end of tibia, unsp knee, init	
836.52	CLOSED POSTERIOR DISLOCATION TIBIA PROXIMAL END	**S83.121A**	Posterior sublux of proximal end of tibia, right knee, init	
		S83.122A	Posterior sublux of proximal end of tibia, left knee, init	
		S83.123A	Posterior sublux of proximal end of tibia, unsp knee, init	
		S83.124A	Posterior disloc of proximal end of tibia, right knee, init	
		S83.125A	Posterior disloc of proximal end of tibia, left knee, init	
		S83.126A	Posterior disloc of proximal end of tibia, unsp knee, init	
836.53	CLOSED MEDIAL DISLOCATION OF TIBIA PROXIMAL END	**S83.131A**	Medial sublux of proximal end of tibia, right knee, init	
		S83.132A	Medial subluxation of proximal end of tibia, left knee, init	
		S83.133A	Medial subluxation of proximal end of tibia, unsp knee, init	
		S83.134A	Medial disloc of proximal end of tibia, right knee, init	
		S83.135A	Medial dislocation of proximal end of tibia, left knee, init	
		S83.136A	Medial dislocation of proximal end of tibia, unsp knee, init	
836.54	CLOSED LATERAL DISLOCATION OF TIBIA PROXIMAL END	**S83.141A**	Lateral sublux of proximal end of tibia, right knee, init	
		S83.142A	Lateral sublux of proximal end of tibia, left knee, init	
		S83.143A	Lateral sublux of proximal end of tibia, unsp knee, init	
		S83.144A	Lateral disloc of proximal end of tibia, right knee, init	
		S83.145A	Lateral disloc of proximal end of tibia, left knee, init	
		S83.146A	Lateral disloc of proximal end of tibia, unsp knee, init	
836.59	OTHER DISLOCATION OF KNEE CLOSED OTHER	**S83.191A**	Other subluxation of right knee, initial encounter	
		S83.192A	Other subluxation of left knee, initial encounter	
		S83.193A	Other subluxation of unspecified knee, initial encounter	
		S83.194A	Other dislocation of right knee, initial encounter	
		S83.195A	Other dislocation of left knee, initial encounter	
		S83.196A	Other dislocation of unspecified knee, initial encounter	
836.6Ø	OPEN DISLOCATION OF KNEE UNSPECIFIED PART	**S83.1Ø6A**	Unspecified dislocation of unspecified knee, init encntr	***and***
		S81.ØØ9A	Unspecified open wound, unspecified knee, initial encounter	
836.61	OPEN ANTERIOR DISLOCATION OF TIBIA PROXIMAL END	**S83.116A**	Anterior disloc of proximal end of tibia, unsp knee, init	***and***
		S81.ØØ9A	Unspecified open wound, unspecified knee, initial encounter	
836.62	OPEN POSTERIOR DISLOCATION OF TIBIA PROXIMAL END	**S83.126A**	Posterior disloc of proximal end of tibia, unsp knee, init	***and***
		S81.ØØ9A	Unspecified open wound, unspecified knee, initial encounter	
836.63	OPEN MEDIAL DISLOCATION OF TIBIA PROXIMAL END	**S83.136A**	Medial dislocation of proximal end of tibia, unsp knee, init	***and***
		S81.ØØ9A	Unspecified open wound, unspecified knee, initial encounter	
836.64	OPEN LATERAL DISLOCATION OF TIBIA PROXIMAL END	**S83.146A**	Lateral disloc of proximal end of tibia, unsp knee, init	***and***
		S81.ØØ9A	Unspecified open wound, unspecified knee, initial encounter	
836.69	OTHER OPEN DISLOCATION OF KNEE	**S83.196A**	Other dislocation of unspecified knee, initial encounter	***and***
		S81.ØØ9A	Unspecified open wound, unspecified knee, initial encounter	
837.Ø	CLOSED DISLOCATION OF ANKLE	**S93.Ø1XA**	Subluxation of right ankle joint, initial encounter	
		S93.Ø2XA	Subluxation of left ankle joint, initial encounter	
		S93.Ø3XA	Subluxation of unspecified ankle joint, initial encounter	
		S93.Ø4XA	Dislocation of right ankle joint, initial encounter	
		S93.Ø5XA	Dislocation of left ankle joint, initial encounter	
		S93.Ø6XA	Dislocation of unspecified ankle joint, initial encounter	
837.1	OPEN DISLOCATION OF ANKLE	**S93.Ø6XA**	Dislocation of unspecified ankle joint, initial encounter	***and***
		S91.ØØ9A	Unspecified open wound, unspecified ankle, initial encounter	
838.ØØ	CLOSED DISLOCATION OF FOOT UNSPECIFIED PART	**S93.3Ø1A**	Unspecified subluxation of right foot, initial encounter	
		S93.3Ø2A	Unspecified subluxation of left foot, initial encounter	
		S93.3Ø3A	Unspecified subluxation of unspecified foot, init encntr	
		S93.3Ø4A	Unspecified dislocation of right foot, initial encounter	
		S93.3Ø5A	Unspecified dislocation of left foot, initial encounter	
		S93.3Ø6A	Unspecified dislocation of unspecified foot, init encntr	
838.Ø1	CLOSED DISLOCATION OF TARSAL JOINT UNSPECIFIED	**S93.316A**	Dislocation of tarsal joint of unspecified foot, init encntr	
838.Ø2	CLOSED DISLOCATION OF MIDTARSAL	**S93.311A**	Subluxation of tarsal joint of right foot, initial encounter	
		S93.312A	Subluxation of tarsal joint of left foot, initial encounter	
		S93.313A	Subluxation of tarsal joint of unspecified foot, init encntr	
		S93.314A	Dislocation of tarsal joint of right foot, initial encounter	
		S93.315A	Dislocation of tarsal joint of left foot, initial encounter	
		S93.316A	Dislocation of tarsal joint of unspecified foot, init encntr	

ICD-9-CM		ICD-10-CM		
838.Ø3	CLOSED DISLOCATION OF TARSOMETATARSAL	**S93.321A**	Subluxation of tarsometatarsal joint of right foot, init	
		S93.322A	Subluxation of tarsometatarsal joint of left foot, init	
		S93.323A	Subluxation of tarsometatarsal joint of unsp foot, init	
		S93.324A	Dislocation of tarsometatarsal joint of right foot, init	
		S93.325A	Dislocation of tarsometatarsal joint of left foot, init	
		S93.326A	Dislocation of tarsometatarsal joint of unsp foot, init	
838.Ø4	CLOSED DISLOCATION METATARSAL JOINT UNSPECIFIED	**S93.331A**	Other subluxation of right foot, initial encounter	
		S93.332A	Other subluxation of left foot, initial encounter	
		S93.333A	Other subluxation of unspecified foot, initial encounter	
		S93.334A	Other dislocation of right foot, initial encounter	
		S93.335A	Other dislocation of left foot, initial encounter	
		S93.336A	Other dislocation of unspecified foot, initial encounter	
838.Ø5	CLOSED DISLOCATION OF METATARSOPHALANGEAL	**S93.121A**	Dislocation of MTP joint of right great toe, init	
		S93.122A	Dislocation of MTP joint of left great toe, init	
		S93.123A	Dislocation of MTP joint of unsp great toe, init	
		S93.124A	Dislocation of MTP joint of right lesser toe(s), init	
		S93.125A	Dislocation of MTP joint of left lesser toe(s), init	
		S93.126A	Dislocation of MTP joint of unsp lesser toe(s), init	
		S93.129A	Dislocation of MTP joint of unsp toe(s), init	
		S93.141A	Subluxation of MTP joint of right great toe, init	
		S93.142A	Subluxation of MTP joint of left great toe, init	
		S93.143A	Subluxation of MTP joint of unsp great toe, init	
		S93.144A	Subluxation of MTP joint of right lesser toe(s), init	
		S93.145A	Subluxation of MTP joint of left lesser toe(s), init	
		S93.146A	Subluxation of MTP joint of unsp lesser toe(s), init	
		S93.149A	Subluxation of MTP joint of unsp toe(s), init	
838.Ø6	CLOSED DISLOCATION OF INTERPHALANGEAL FOOT	**S93.111A**	Dislocation of interphaln joint of right great toe, init	
		S93.112A	Dislocation of interphalangeal joint of left great toe, init	
		S93.113A	Dislocation of interphalangeal joint of unsp great toe, init	
		S93.114A	Dislocation of interphaln joint of right lesser toe(s), init	
		S93.115A	Dislocation of interphaln joint of left lesser toe(s), init	
		S93.116A	Dislocation of interphaln joint of unsp lesser toe(s), init	
		S93.119A	Dislocation of interphalangeal joint of unsp toe(s), init	
		S93.131A	Subluxation of interphaln joint of right great toe, init	
		S93.132A	Subluxation of interphalangeal joint of left great toe, init	
		S93.133A	Subluxation of interphalangeal joint of unsp great toe, init	
		S93.134A	Subluxation of interphaln joint of right lesser toe(s), init	
		S93.135A	Subluxation of interphaln joint of left lesser toe(s), init	
		S93.136A	Subluxation of interphaln joint of unsp lesser toe(s), init	
		S93.139A	Subluxation of interphalangeal joint of unsp toe(s), init	
838.Ø9	CLOSED DISLOCATION OF OTHER PART OF FOOT	**S93.1Ø1A**	Unspecified subluxation of right toe(s), initial encounter	
		S93.1Ø2A	Unspecified subluxation of left toe(s), initial encounter	
		S93.1Ø3A	Unspecified subluxation of unspecified toe(s), init encntr	
		S93.1Ø4A	Unspecified dislocation of right toe(s), initial encounter	
		S93.1Ø5A	Unspecified dislocation of left toe(s), initial encounter	
		S93.1Ø6A	Unspecified dislocation of unspecified toe(s), init encntr	
		S93.336A	Other dislocation of unspecified foot, initial encounter	
838.1Ø	OPEN DISLOCATION OF FOOT UNSPECIFIED PART	**S93.3Ø6A**	Unspecified dislocation of unspecified foot, init encntr	*and*
		S91.3Ø9A	Unspecified open wound, unspecified foot, initial encounter	
838.11	OPEN DISLOCATION OF TARSAL JOINT UNSPECIFIED	**S93.316A**	Dislocation of tarsal joint of unspecified foot, init encntr	*and*
		S91.3Ø9A	Unspecified open wound, unspecified foot, initial encounter	
838.12	OPEN DISLOCATION OF MIDTARSAL	**S93.316A**	Dislocation of tarsal joint of unspecified foot, init encntr	*and*
		S91.3Ø9A	Unspecified open wound, unspecified foot, initial encounter	
838.13	OPEN DISLOCATION OF TARSOMETATARSAL	**S93.326A**	Dislocation of tarsometatarsal joint of unsp foot, init	*and*
		S91.3Ø9A	Unspecified open wound, unspecified foot, initial encounter	
838.14	OPEN DISLOCATION OF METATARSAL JOINT UNSPECIFIED	**S93.336A**	Other dislocation of unspecified foot, initial encounter	*and*
		S91.3Ø9A	Unspecified open wound, unspecified foot, initial encounter	
838.15	OPEN DISLOCATION OF METATARSOPHALANGEAL	**S93.129A**	Dislocation of MTP joint of unsp toe(s), init	*and*
		S91.3Ø9A	Unspecified open wound, unspecified foot, initial encounter	
838.16	OPEN DISLOCATION OF INTERPHALANGEAL FOOT	**S93.119A**	Dislocation of interphalangeal joint of unsp toe(s), init	*and*
		S91.1Ø9A	Unsp open wound of unsp toe(s) w/o damage to nail, init	
838.19	OPEN DISLOCATION OF OTHER PART OF FOOT	**S93.336A**	Other dislocation of unspecified foot, initial encounter	*and*
		S91.1Ø9A	Unsp open wound of unsp toe(s) w/o damage to nail, init	
839.ØØ	CLOSED DISLOCATION UNSPECIFIED CERVICAL VERTEBRA	**M99.1Ø**	Subluxation complex (vertebral) of head region	
		M99.11	Subluxation complex (vertebral) of cervical region	
		S13.ØXXA	Traumatic rupture of cervical intervertebral disc, init	
		S13.1ØØA	Subluxation of unspecified cervical vertebrae, init encntr	
		S13.1Ø1A	Dislocation of unspecified cervical vertebrae, init encntr	
		S13.2ØXA	Dislocation of unspecified parts of neck, initial encounter	
		S13.29XA	Dislocation of other parts of neck, initial encounter	
839.Ø1	CLOSED DISLOCATION FIRST CERVICAL VERTEBRA	**S13.11ØA**	Subluxation of C0/C1 cervical vertebrae, initial encounter	
		S13.111A	Dislocation of C0/C1 cervical vertebrae, initial encounter	
839.Ø2	CLOSED DISLOCATION SECOND CERVICAL VERTEBRA	**S13.12ØA**	Subluxation of C1/C2 cervical vertebrae, initial encounter	
		S13.121A	Dislocation of C1/C2 cervical vertebrae, initial encounter	

ICD-9-CM		ICD-10-CM		
839.03	CLOSED DISLOCATION THIRD CERVICAL VERTEBRA	**S13.130A**	Subluxation of C2/C3 cervical vertebrae, initial encounter	
		S13.131A	Dislocation of C2/C3 cervical vertebrae, initial encounter	
839.04	CLOSED DISLOCATION FOURTH CERVICAL VERTEBRA	**S13.140A**	Subluxation of C3/C4 cervical vertebrae, initial encounter	
		S13.141A	Dislocation of C3/C4 cervical vertebrae, initial encounter	
839.05	CLOSED DISLOCATION FIFTH CERVICAL VERTEBRA	**S13.150A**	Subluxation of C4/C5 cervical vertebrae, initial encounter	
		S13.151A	Dislocation of C4/C5 cervical vertebrae, initial encounter	
839.06	CLOSED DISLOCATION SIXTH CERVICAL VERTEBRA	**S13.160A**	Subluxation of C5/C6 cervical vertebrae, initial encounter	
		S13.161A	Dislocation of C5/C6 cervical vertebrae, initial encounter	
839.07	CLOSED DISLOCATION SEVENTH CERVICAL VERTEBRA	**S13.170A**	Subluxation of C6/C7 cervical vertebrae, initial encounter	
		S13.171A	Dislocation of C6/C7 cervical vertebrae, initial encounter	
		S13.180A	Subluxation of C7/T1 cervical vertebrae, initial encounter	
		S13.181A	Dislocation of C7/T1 cervical vertebrae, initial encounter	
839.08	CLOSED DISLOCATION MULTIPLE CERVICAL VERTEBRAE	**S13.100A**	Subluxation of unspecified cervical vertebrae, init encntr	
		S13.101A	Dislocation of unspecified cervical vertebrae, init encntr	
839.10	OPEN DISLOCATION UNSPECIFIED CERVICAL VERTEBRA	**S13.101A**	Dislocation of unspecified cervical vertebrae, init encntr	*and*
		S11.90XA	Unsp open wound of unspecified part of neck, init encntr	
839.11	OPEN DISLOCATION FIRST CERVICAL VERTEBRA	**S13.111A**	Dislocation of C0/C1 cervical vertebrae, initial encounter	*and*
		S11.90XA	Unsp open wound of unspecified part of neck, init encntr	
839.12	OPEN DISLOCATION SECOND CERVICAL VERTEBRA	**S13.121A**	Dislocation of C1/C2 cervical vertebrae, initial encounter	*and*
		S11.90XA	Unsp open wound of unspecified part of neck, init encntr	
839.13	OPEN DISLOCATION THIRD CERVICAL VERTEBRA	**S13.131A**	Dislocation of C2/C3 cervical vertebrae, initial encounter	*and*
		S11.90XA	Unsp open wound of unspecified part of neck, init encntr	
839.14	OPEN DISLOCATION FOURTH CERVICAL VERTEBRA	**S13.141A**	Dislocation of C3/C4 cervical vertebrae, initial encounter	*and*
		S11.90XA	Unsp open wound of unspecified part of neck, init encntr	
839.15	OPEN DISLOCATION FIFTH CERVICAL VERTEBRA	**S13.151A**	Dislocation of C4/C5 cervical vertebrae, initial encounter	*and*
		S11.90XA	Unsp open wound of unspecified part of neck, init encntr	
839.16	OPEN DISLOCATION SIXTH CERVICAL VERTEBRA	**S13.161A**	Dislocation of C5/C6 cervical vertebrae, initial encounter	*and*
		S11.90XA	Unsp open wound of unspecified part of neck, init encntr	
839.17	OPEN DISLOCATION SEVENTH CERVICAL VERTEBRA	**S13.171A**	Dislocation of C6/C7 cervical vertebrae, initial encounter	*or*
		S13.181A	Dislocation of C7/T1 cervical vertebrae, initial encounter	*and*
		S11.90XA	Unsp open wound of unspecified part of neck, init encntr	
839.18	OPEN DISLOCATION MULTIPLE CERVICAL VERTEBRAE	**S13.101A**	Dislocation of unspecified cervical vertebrae, init encntr	*and*
		S11.90XA	Unsp open wound of unspecified part of neck, init encntr	
839.20	CLOSED DISLOCATION, LUMBAR VERTEBRA	**M99.13**	Subluxation complex (vertebral) of lumbar region	
		S33.0XXA	Traumatic rupture of lumbar intervertebral disc, init encntr	
		S33.100A	Subluxation of unspecified lumbar vertebra, init encntr	
		S33.101A	Dislocation of unspecified lumbar vertebra, init encntr	
		S33.110A	Subluxation of L1/L2 lumbar vertebra, initial encounter	
		S33.111A	Dislocation of L1/L2 lumbar vertebra, initial encounter	
		S33.120A	Subluxation of L2/L3 lumbar vertebra, initial encounter	
		S33.121A	Dislocation of L2/L3 lumbar vertebra, initial encounter	
		S33.130A	Subluxation of L3/L4 lumbar vertebra, initial encounter	
		S33.131A	Dislocation of L3/L4 lumbar vertebra, initial encounter	
		S33.140A	Subluxation of L4/L5 lumbar vertebra, initial encounter	
		S33.141A	Dislocation of L4/L5 lumbar vertebra, initial encounter	
839.21	CLOSED DISLOCATION THORACIC VERTEBRA	**M99.12**	Subluxation complex (vertebral) of thoracic region	
		S23.0XXA	Traumatic rupture of thoracic intervertebral disc, init	
		S23.100A	Subluxation of unspecified thoracic vertebra, init encntr	
		S23.101A	Dislocation of unspecified thoracic vertebra, init encntr	
		S23.110A	Subluxation of T1/T2 thoracic vertebra, initial encounter	
		S23.111A	Dislocation of T1/T2 thoracic vertebra, initial encounter	
		S23.120A	Subluxation of T2/T3 thoracic vertebra, initial encounter	
		S23.121A	Dislocation of T2/T3 thoracic vertebra, initial encounter	
		S23.122A	Subluxation of T3/T4 thoracic vertebra, initial encounter	
		S23.123A	Dislocation of T3/T4 thoracic vertebra, initial encounter	
		S23.130A	Subluxation of T4/T5 thoracic vertebra, initial encounter	
		S23.131A	Dislocation of T4/T5 thoracic vertebra, initial encounter	
		S23.132A	Subluxation of T5/T6 thoracic vertebra, initial encounter	
		S23.133A	Dislocation of T5/T6 thoracic vertebra, initial encounter	
		S23.140A	Subluxation of T6/T7 thoracic vertebra, initial encounter	
		S23.141A	Dislocation of T6/T7 thoracic vertebra, initial encounter	
		S23.142A	Subluxation of T7/T8 thoracic vertebra, initial encounter	
		S23.143A	Dislocation of T7/T8 thoracic vertebra, initial encounter	
		S23.150A	Subluxation of T8/T9 thoracic vertebra, initial encounter	
		S23.151A	Dislocation of T8/T9 thoracic vertebra, initial encounter	
		S23.152A	Subluxation of T9/T10 thoracic vertebra, initial encounter	
		S23.153A	Dislocation of T9/T10 thoracic vertebra, initial encounter	
		S23.160A	Subluxation of T10/T11 thoracic vertebra, initial encounter	
		S23.161A	Dislocation of T10/T11 thoracic vertebra, initial encounter	
		S23.162A	Subluxation of T11/T12 thoracic vertebra, initial encounter	
		S23.163A	Dislocation of T11/T12 thoracic vertebra, initial encounter	
		S23.170A	Subluxation of T12/L1 thoracic vertebra, initial encounter	
		S23.171A	Dislocation of T12/L1 thoracic vertebra, initial encounter	

[Brackets] indicate valid character values for each code. Character value meanings provided for each code grouping.

ICD-9-CM		ICD-10-CM		
839.30	OPEN DISLOCATION, LUMBAR VERTEBRA	**S33.101A**	Dislocation of unspecified lumbar vertebra, init encntr	*and*
		S31.000A	Unsp opn wnd low back and pelv w/o penet retroperiton, init	
839.31	OPEN DISLOCATION, THORACIC VERTEBRA	**S23.101A**	Dislocation of unspecified thoracic vertebra, init encntr	*and*
		S21.209A	Unsp opn wnd unsp bk wl of thorax w/o penet thor cav, init	
839.40	CLOSED DISLOCATION VERTEBRA UNSPECIFIED SITE	**S23.20XA**	Dislocation of unspecified part of thorax, initial encounter	
		S23.29XA	Dislocation of other parts of thorax, initial encounter	
839.41	CLOSED DISLOCATION, COCCYX	**S33.2XXA**	Dislocation of sacroiliac and sacrococcygeal joint, init	
839.42	CLOSED DISLOCATION, SACRUM	**M99.14**	Subluxation complex (vertebral) of sacral region	
		S33.2XXA	Dislocation of sacroiliac and sacrococcygeal joint, init	
839.49	CLOSED DISLOCATION OTHER VERTEBRA OTHER	**M99.15**	Subluxation complex (vertebral) of pelvic region	
		S33.39XA	Dislocation of oth prt lumbar spine and pelvis, init encntr	
839.50	OPEN DISLOCATION VERTEBRA UNSPECIFIED SITE	**S23.20XA**	Dislocation of unspecified part of thorax, initial encounter	*and*
		S31.000A	Unsp opn wnd low back and pelv w/o penet retroperiton, init	
839.51	OPEN DISLOCATION, COCCYX	**S33.2XXA**	Dislocation of sacroiliac and sacrococcygeal joint, init	*and*
		S31.000A	Unsp opn wnd low back and pelv w/o penet retroperiton, init	
839.52	OPEN DISLOCATION, SACRUM	**S33.2XXA**	Dislocation of sacroiliac and sacrococcygeal joint, init	*and*
		S31.000A	Unsp opn wnd low back and pelv w/o penet retroperiton, init	
839.59	OPEN DISLOCATION OTHER VERTEBRA OTHER	**S33.39XA**	Dislocation of oth prt lumbar spine and pelvis, init encntr	*and*
		S31.000A	Unsp opn wnd low back and pelv w/o penet retroperiton, init	
839.61	CLOSED DISLOCATION, STERNUM	**M99.18**	Subluxation complex (vertebral) of rib cage	
		S43.201A	Unsp subluxation of right sternoclavicular joint, init	
		S43.202A	Unsp subluxation of left sternoclavicular joint, init encntr	
		S43.203A	Unsp subluxation of unsp sternoclavicular joint, init encntr	
		S43.204A	Unsp dislocation of right sternoclavicular joint, init	
		S43.205A	Unsp dislocation of left sternoclavicular joint, init encntr	
		S43.206A	Unsp dislocation of unsp sternoclavicular joint, init encntr	
		S43.211A	Anterior subluxation of right sternoclavicular joint, init	
		S43.212A	Anterior subluxation of left sternoclavicular joint, init	
		S43.213A	Anterior subluxation of unsp sternoclavicular joint, init	
		S43.214A	Anterior dislocation of right sternoclavicular joint, init	
		S43.215A	Anterior dislocation of left sternoclavicular joint, init	
		S43.216A	Anterior dislocation of unsp sternoclavicular joint, init	
		S43.221A	Posterior subluxation of right sternoclavicular joint, init	
		S43.222A	Posterior subluxation of left sternoclavicular joint, init	
		S43.223A	Posterior subluxation of unsp sternoclavicular joint, init	
		S43.224A	Posterior dislocation of right sternoclavicular joint, init	
		S43.225A	Posterior dislocation of left sternoclavicular joint, init	
		S43.226A	Posterior dislocation of unsp sternoclavicular joint, init	
839.69	CLOSED DISLOCATION OTHER LOCATION OTHER	**M99.16**	Subluxation complex (vertebral) of lower extremity	
		M99.17	Subluxation complex (vertebral) of upper extremity	
		M99.19	Subluxation complex (vertebral) of abdomen and other regions	
		S03.1XXA	Dislocation of septal cartilage of nose, initial encounter	
		S33.30XA	Dislocation of unsp parts of lumbar spine and pelvis, init	
		S33.39XA	Dislocation of oth prt lumbar spine and pelvis, init encntr	
839.71	OPEN DISLOCATION, STERNUM	**S43.206A**	Unsp dislocation of unsp sternoclavicular joint, init encntr	*and*
		S21.109A	Unsp opn wnd unsp frnt wall of thrx w/o penet thor cav, init	
839.79	OPEN DISLOCATION OTHER LOCATION OTHER	**S33.39XA**	Dislocation of oth prt lumbar spine and pelvis, init encntr	*and*
		S31.000A	Unsp opn wnd low back and pelv w/o penet retroperiton, init	
839.8	CLOSED DISLOCATION MULTIPLE&ILL-DEFINED SITES	**T14.90**	Injury, unspecified	
839.9	OPEN DISLOCATION MULTIPLE AND ILL-DEFINED SITES	**T14.90**	Injury, unspecified	
840.0	ACROMIOCLAVICULAR SPRAIN AND STRAIN	**S43.50XA**	Sprain of unspecified acromioclavicular joint, init encntr	
		S43.51XA	Sprain of right acromioclavicular joint, initial encounter	
		S43.52XA	Sprain of left acromioclavicular joint, initial encounter	
840.1	CORACOCLAVICULAR SPRAIN AND STRAIN	**S43.80XA**	Sprain of oth parts of unsp shoulder girdle, init encntr	
		S43.81XA	Sprain of oth parts of right shoulder girdle, init encntr	
		S43.82XA	Sprain of oth parts of left shoulder girdle, init encntr	
840.2	CORACOHUMERAL SPRAIN AND STRAIN	**S43.411A**	Sprain of right coracohumeral (ligament), initial encounter	
		S43.412A	Sprain of left coracohumeral (ligament), initial encounter	
		S43.419A	Sprain of unspecified coracohumeral (ligament), init encntr	
840.3	INFRASPINATUS SPRAIN AND STRAIN	**S43.80XA**	Sprain of oth parts of unsp shoulder girdle, init encntr	
		S43.81XA	Sprain of oth parts of right shoulder girdle, init encntr	
		S43.82XA	Sprain of oth parts of left shoulder girdle, init encntr	
840.4	ROTATOR CUFF SPRAIN AND STRAIN	**S43.421A**	Sprain of right rotator cuff capsule, initial encounter	
		S43.422A	Sprain of left rotator cuff capsule, initial encounter	
		S43.429A	Sprain of unspecified rotator cuff capsule, init encntr	
840.5	SUBSCAPULARIS SPRAIN AND STRAIN	**S43.80XA**	Sprain of oth parts of unsp shoulder girdle, init encntr	
		S43.81XA	Sprain of oth parts of right shoulder girdle, init encntr	
		S43.82XA	Sprain of oth parts of left shoulder girdle, init encntr	
840.6	SUPRASPINATUS SPRAIN AND STRAIN	**S43.80XA**	Sprain of oth parts of unsp shoulder girdle, init encntr	
		S43.81XA	Sprain of oth parts of right shoulder girdle, init encntr	
		S43.82XA	Sprain of oth parts of left shoulder girdle, init encntr	

ICD-9-CM		ICD-10-CM	
840.7	SUPERIOR GLENOID LABRUM LESIONS	**S43.431A**	Superior glenoid labrum lesion of right shoulder, init
		S43.432A	Superior glenoid labrum lesion of left shoulder, init encntr
		S43.439A	Superior glenoid labrum lesion of unsp shoulder, init encntr
840.8	SPRAIN&STRAIN OTH SPEC SITES SHOULDER&UPPER ARM	**S43.491A**	Other sprain of right shoulder joint, initial encounter
		S43.492A	Other sprain of left shoulder joint, initial encounter
		S43.499A	Other sprain of unspecified shoulder joint, init encntr
		S43.60XA	Sprain of unspecified sternoclavicular joint, init encntr
		S43.61XA	Sprain of right sternoclavicular joint, initial encounter
		S43.62XA	Sprain of left sternoclavicular joint, initial encounter
		S46.011A	Strain of musc/tend the rotator cuff of right shoulder, init
		S46.012A	Strain of musc/tend the rotator cuff of left shoulder, init
		S46.019A	Strain of musc/tend the rotator cuff of unsp shoulder, init
		S46.111A	Strain of musc/fasc/tend long hd bicep, right arm, init
		S46.112A	Strain of musc/fasc/tend long head of biceps, left arm, init
		S46.119A	Strain of musc/fasc/tend long head of biceps, unsp arm, init
		S46.211A	Strain of musc/fasc/tend prt biceps, right arm, init
		S46.212A	Strain of musc/fasc/tend prt biceps, left arm, init
		S46.219A	Strain of musc/fasc/tend prt biceps, unsp arm, init
		S46.311A	Strain of musc/fasc/tend triceps, right arm, init
		S46.312A	Strain of musc/fasc/tend triceps, left arm, init
		S46.319A	Strain of musc/fasc/tend triceps, unsp arm, init
		S46.811A	Strain of musc/fasc/tend at shldr/up arm, right arm, init
		S46.812A	Strain of musc/fasc/tend at shldr/up arm, left arm, init
		S46.819A	Strain of musc/fasc/tend at shldr/up arm, unsp arm, init
840.9	SPRAIN&STRAIN UNSPEC SITE SHOULDER&UPPER ARM	**S43.401A**	Unspecified sprain of right shoulder joint, init encntr
		S43.402A	Unspecified sprain of left shoulder joint, initial encounter
		S43.409A	Unsp sprain of unspecified shoulder joint, init encntr
		S43.90XA	Sprain of unsp parts of unsp shoulder girdle, init encntr
		S43.91XA	Sprain of unsp parts of right shoulder girdle, init encntr
		S43.92XA	Sprain of unsp parts of left shoulder girdle, init encntr
		S46.911A	Strain unsp musc/fasc/tend at shldr/up arm, right arm, init
		S46.912A	Strain unsp musc/fasc/tend at shldr/up arm, left arm, init
		S46.919A	Strain unsp musc/fasc/tend at shldr/up arm, unsp arm, init
841.0	RADIAL COLLATERAL LIGAMENT SPRAIN AND STRAIN	**S53.20XA**	Traumatic rupture of unsp radial collateral ligament, init
		S53.21XA	Traumatic rupture of right radial collateral ligament, init
		S53.22XA	Traumatic rupture of left radial collateral ligament, init
		S53.431A	Radial collateral ligament sprain of right elbow, init
		S53.432A	Radial collateral ligament sprain of left elbow, init encntr
		S53.439A	Radial collateral ligament sprain of unsp elbow, init encntr
841.1	ULNAR COLLATERAL LIGAMENT SPRAIN AND STRAIN	**S53.30XA**	Traumatic rupture of unsp ulnar collateral ligament, init
		S53.31XA	Traumatic rupture of right ulnar collateral ligament, init
		S53.32XA	Traumatic rupture of left ulnar collateral ligament, init
		S53.441A	Ulnar collateral ligament sprain of right elbow, init encntr
		S53.442A	Ulnar collateral ligament sprain of left elbow, init encntr
		S53.449A	Ulnar collateral ligament sprain of unsp elbow, init encntr
841.2	RADIOHUMERAL SPRAIN AND STRAIN	**S53.411A**	Radiohumeral (joint) sprain of right elbow, init encntr
		S53.412A	Radiohumeral (joint) sprain of left elbow, initial encounter
		S53.419A	Radiohumeral (joint) sprain of unsp elbow, init encntr
841.3	ULNOHUMERAL SPRAIN AND STRAIN	**S53.421A**	Ulnohumeral (joint) sprain of right elbow, initial encounter
		S53.422A	Ulnohumeral (joint) sprain of left elbow, initial encounter
		S53.429A	Ulnohumeral (joint) sprain of unspecified elbow, init encntr
841.8	SPRAIN&STRAIN OTHER SPEC SITES ELBOW&FOREARM	**S53.401A**	Unspecified sprain of right elbow, initial encounter
		S53.402A	Unspecified sprain of left elbow, initial encounter
		S53.409A	Unspecified sprain of unspecified elbow, initial encounter
		S53.491A	Other sprain of right elbow, initial encounter
		S53.492A	Other sprain of left elbow, initial encounter
		S53.499A	Other sprain of unspecified elbow, initial encounter
841.9	SPRAIN&STRAIN UNSPECIFIED SITE ELBOW&FOREARM	**S53.401A**	Unspecified sprain of right elbow, initial encounter
		S53.402A	Unspecified sprain of left elbow, initial encounter
		S53.409A	Unspecified sprain of unspecified elbow, initial encounter
		S56.011A	Strain of flexor musc/fasc/tend r thm at forarm lv, init
		S56.012A	Strain of flexor musc/fasc/tend l thm at forarm lv, init
		S56.019A	Strain of flexor musc/fasc/tend thmb at forearm level, init
		S56.111A	Strain flexor musc/fasc/tend r idx fngr at forarm lv, init
		S56.112A	Strain flexor musc/fasc/tend l idx fngr at forarm lv, init
		S56.113A	Strain flexor musc/fasc/tend r mid finger at forarm lv, init
		S56.114A	Strain flexor musc/fasc/tend l mid finger at forarm lv, init
		S56.115A	Strain flexor musc/fasc/tend r rng fngr at forarm lv, init
		S56.116A	Strain flexor musc/fasc/tend l rng fngr at forarm lv, init
		S56.117A	Strain flxr musc/fasc/tend r little fngr at forarm lv, init
		S56.118A	Strain flxr musc/fasc/tend l little fngr at forarm lv, init
		S56.119A	Strain flexor musc/fasc/tend of unsp fngr at forarm lv, init
		S56.211A	Strain flexor musc/fasc/tend at forarm lv, right arm, init
		S56.212A	Strain of flexor musc/fasc/tend at forarm lv, left arm, init
		S56.219A	Strain of flexor musc/fasc/tend at forarm lv, unsp arm, init
		S56.311A	Strain extn/abdr musc/fasc/tend of r thm at forarm lv, init
		S56.312A	Strain extn/abdr musc/fasc/tend of l thm at forarm lv, init
		S56.319A	Strain extn/abdr musc/fasc/tend of thmb at forarm lv, init
		S56.411A	Strain extensor musc/fasc/tend r idx fngr at forarm lv, init
		S56.415A	Strain extensor musc/fasc/tend r rng fngr at forarm lv, init
		S56.416A	Strain extensor musc/fasc/tend l rng fngr at forarm lv, init

(Continued on next page)

ICD-9-CM		ICD-10-CM	
841.9	SPRAIN&STRAIN UNSPECIFIED SITE ELBOW&FOREARM (Continued)	**S56.417A**	Strain extn musc/fasc/tend r little fngr at forarm lv, init
		S56.418A	Strain extn musc/fasc/tend l little fngr at forarm lv, init
		S56.419A	Strain extn musc/fasc/tend fngr,unsp fngr at forarm lv, init
		S56.511A	Strain of extn musc/fasc/tend at forarm lv, right arm, init
		S56.512A	Strain of extn musc/fasc/tend at forarm lv, left arm, init
		S56.519A	Strain of extn musc/fasc/tend at forarm lv, unsp arm, init
		S56.811A	Strain of musc/fasc/tend at forearm level, right arm, init
		S56.812A	Strain of musc/fasc/tend at forearm level, left arm, init
		S56.819A	Strain of musc/fasc/tend at forearm level, unsp arm, init
		S56.911A	Strain of unsp musc/fasc/tend at forarm lv, right arm, init
		S56.912A	Strain of unsp musc/fasc/tend at forarm lv, left arm, init
		S56.919A	Strain of unsp musc/fasc/tend at forarm lv, unsp arm, init
842.ØØ	SPRAIN AND STRAIN OF UNSPECIFIED SITE OF WRIST	**S63.5Ø1A**	Unspecified sprain of right wrist, initial encounter
		S63.5Ø2A	Unspecified sprain of left wrist, initial encounter
		S63.5Ø9A	Unspecified sprain of unspecified wrist, initial encounter
		S66.911A	Strain of unsp musc/fasc/tend at wrs/hnd lv, r hand, init
		S66.912A	Strain of unsp musc/fasc/tend at wrs/hnd lv, left hand, init
		S66.919A	Strain of unsp musc/fasc/tend at wrs/hnd lv, unsp hand, init
842.Ø1	SPRAIN AND STRAIN OF CARPAL OF WRIST	**S63.511A**	Sprain of carpal joint of right wrist, initial encounter
		S63.512A	Sprain of carpal joint of left wrist, initial encounter
		S63.519A	Sprain of carpal joint of unspecified wrist, init encntr
842.Ø2	SPRAIN AND STRAIN OF RADIOCARPAL OF WRIST	**S63.321A**	Traumatic rupture of right radiocarpal ligament, init encntr
		S63.322A	Traumatic rupture of left radiocarpal ligament, init encntr
		S63.329A	Traumatic rupture of unsp radiocarpal ligament, init encntr
		S63.521A	Sprain of radiocarpal joint of right wrist, init encntr
		S63.522A	Sprain of radiocarpal joint of left wrist, initial encounter
		S63.529A	Sprain of radiocarpal joint of unsp wrist, init encntr
842.Ø9	OTHER WRIST SPRAIN AND STRAIN	**S63.3Ø1A**	Traumatic rupture of unsp ligament of right wrist, init
		S63.3Ø2A	Traumatic rupture of unsp ligament of left wrist, init
		S63.3Ø9A	Traumatic rupture of unsp ligament of unsp wrist, init
		S63.311A	Traumatic rupture of collateral ligament of r wrist, init
		S63.312A	Traumatic rupture of collateral ligament of left wrist, init
		S63.319A	Traumatic rupture of collateral ligament of unsp wrist, init
		S63.331A	Traum rupture of right ulnocarpal (palmar) ligament, init
		S63.332A	Traumatic rupture of left ulnocarpal (palmar) ligament, init
		S63.339A	Traumatic rupture of unsp ulnocarpal (palmar) ligament, init
		S63.391A	Traumatic rupture of oth ligament of right wrist, init
		S63.392A	Traumatic rupture of oth ligament of left wrist, init encntr
		S63.399A	Traumatic rupture of oth ligament of unsp wrist, init encntr
		S63.591A	Other specified sprain of right wrist, initial encounter
		S63.592A	Other specified sprain of left wrist, initial encounter
		S63.599A	Other specified sprain of unspecified wrist, init encntr
		S66.Ø11A	Strain long flexor musc/fasc/tend r thm at wrs/hnd lv, init
		S66.Ø12A	Strain long flexor musc/fasc/tend l thm at wrs/hnd lv, init
		S66.Ø19A	Strain long flexor musc/fasc/tend thmb at wrs/hnd lv, init
		S66.11ØA	Strain flexor musc/fasc/tend r idx fngr at wrs/hnd lv, init
		S66.111A	Strain flexor musc/fasc/tend l idx fngr at wrs/hnd lv, init
		S66.112A	Strain flexor musc/fasc/tend r mid fngr at wrs/hnd lv, init
		S66.113A	Strain flexor musc/fasc/tend l mid fngr at wrs/hnd lv, init
		S66.114A	Strain flexor musc/fasc/tend r rng fngr at wrs/hnd lv, init
		S66.115A	Strain flexor musc/fasc/tend l rng fngr at wrs/hnd lv, init
		S66.116A	Strain flxr musc/fasc/tend r little fngr at wrs/hnd lv, init
		S66.117A	Strain flxr musc/fasc/tend l little fngr at wrs/hnd lv, init
		S66.118A	Strain of flexor musc/fasc/tend finger at wrs/hnd lv, init
		S66.119A	Strain flexor musc/fasc/tend unsp finger at wrs/hnd lv, init
		S66.211A	Strain of extensor musc/fasc/tend r thm at wrs/hnd lv, init
		S66.212A	Strain of extensor musc/fasc/tend l thm at wrs/hnd lv, init
		S66.219A	Strain of extensor musc/fasc/tend thmb at wrs/hnd lv, init
		S66.31ØA	Strain extn musc/fasc/tend r idx fngr at wrs/hnd lv, init
		S66.311A	Strain extn musc/fasc/tend l idx fngr at wrs/hnd lv, init
		S66.312A	Strain extn musc/fasc/tend r mid finger at wrs/hnd lv, init
		S66.313A	Strain extn musc/fasc/tend l mid finger at wrs/hnd lv, init
		S66.314A	Strain extn musc/fasc/tend r rng fngr at wrs/hnd lv, init
		S66.315A	Strain extn musc/fasc/tend l rng fngr at wrs/hnd lv, init
		S66.316A	Strain extn musc/fasc/tend r little fngr at wrs/hnd lv, init
		S66.317A	Strain extn musc/fasc/tend l little fngr at wrs/hnd lv, init
		S66.318A	Strain of extensor musc/fasc/tend finger at wrs/hnd lv, init
		S66.319A	Strain extn musc/fasc/tend unsp finger at wrs/hnd lv, init
		S66.411A	Strain of intrinsic musc/fasc/tend r thm at wrs/hnd lv, init
		S66.412A	Strain of intrinsic musc/fasc/tend l thm at wrs/hnd lv, init
		S66.419A	Strain of intrinsic musc/fasc/tend thmb at wrs/hnd lv, init
		S66.51ØA	Strain intrns musc/fasc/tend r idx fngr at wrs/hnd lv, init
		S66.511A	Strain intrns musc/fasc/tend l idx fngr at wrs/hnd lv, init
		S66.512A	Strain intrns musc/fasc/tend r mid fngr at wrs/hnd lv, init
		S66.513A	Strain intrns musc/fasc/tend l mid fngr at wrs/hnd lv, init
		S66.514A	Strain intrns musc/fasc/tend r rng fngr at wrs/hnd lv, init
		S66.515A	Strain intrns musc/fasc/tend l rng fngr at wrs/hnd lv, init
		S66.516A	Strain intrns musc/fasc/tend r lit fngr at wrs/hnd lv, init
		S66.517A	Strain intrns musc/fasc/tend l lit fngr at wrs/hnd lv, init
		S66.518A	Strain of intrns musc/fasc/tend finger at wrs/hnd lv, init
	(Continued on next page)	**S66.519A**	Strain intrns musc/fasc/tend unsp finger at wrs/hnd lv, init

ICD-9-CM		ICD-10-CM	
842.Ø9	OTHER WRIST SPRAIN AND STRAIN **(Continued)**	**S66.811A**	Strain of musc/fasc/tend at wrs/hnd lv, right hand, init
		S66.812A	Strain of musc/fasc/tend at wrs/hnd lv, left hand, init
		S66.819A	Strain of musc/fasc/tend at wrs/hnd lv, unsp hand, init
842.1Ø	SPRAIN AND STRAIN OF UNSPECIFIED SITE OF HAND	**S63.9ØXA**	Sprain of unsp part of unsp wrist and hand, init encntr
		S63.91XA	Sprain of unsp part of right wrist and hand, init encntr
		S63.92XA	Sprain of unsp part of left wrist and hand, init encntr
		S66.911A	Strain of unsp musc/fasc/tend at wrs/hnd lv, r hand, init
		S66.912A	Strain of unsp musc/fasc/tend at wrs/hnd lv, left hand, init
		S66.919A	Strain of unsp musc/fasc/tend at wrs/hnd lv, unsp hand, init
842.11	SPRAIN AND STRAIN OF CARPOMETACARPAL OF HAND	**S63.8X9A**	Sprain of other part of unsp wrist and hand, init encntr
842.12	SPRAIN AND STRAIN OF METACARPOPHALANGEAL OF HAND	**S63.641A**	Sprain of metacarpophalangeal joint of right thumb, init
		S63.642A	Sprain of metacarpophalangeal joint of left thumb, init
		S63.649A	Sprain of metacarpophalangeal joint of unsp thumb, init
		S63.65ØA	Sprain of MCP joint of right index finger, init
		S63.651A	Sprain of MCP joint of left index finger, init
		S63.652A	Sprain of MCP joint of right middle finger, init
		S63.653A	Sprain of MCP joint of left middle finger, init
		S63.654A	Sprain of MCP joint of right ring finger, init
		S63.655A	Sprain of MCP joint of left ring finger, init
		S63.656A	Sprain of MCP joint of right little finger, init
		S63.657A	Sprain of MCP joint of left little finger, init
		S63.658A	Sprain of metacarpophalangeal joint of oth finger, init
		S63.659A	Sprain of metacarpophalangeal joint of unsp finger, init
842.13	SPRAIN AND STRAIN OF INTERPHALANGEAL OF HAND	**S63.621A**	Sprain of interphalangeal joint of right thumb, init encntr
		S63.622A	Sprain of interphalangeal joint of left thumb, init encntr
		S63.629A	Sprain of interphalangeal joint of unsp thumb, init encntr
		S63.63ØA	Sprain of interphalangeal joint of right index finger, init
		S63.631A	Sprain of interphalangeal joint of left index finger, init
		S63.632A	Sprain of interphalangeal joint of right middle finger, init
		S63.633A	Sprain of interphalangeal joint of left middle finger, init
		S63.634A	Sprain of interphalangeal joint of right ring finger, init
		S63.635A	Sprain of interphalangeal joint of left ring finger, init
		S63.636A	Sprain of interphalangeal joint of right little finger, init
		S63.637A	Sprain of interphalangeal joint of left little finger, init
		S63.638A	Sprain of interphalangeal joint of other finger, init encntr
		S63.639A	Sprain of interphalangeal joint of unsp finger, init encntr
842.19	OTHER HAND SPRAIN AND STRAIN	**S63.4ØØA**	Traum rupture of unsp ligmt of r idx fngr at MCP/IP jt, init
		S63.4Ø1A	Traum rupture of unsp ligmt of l idx fngr at MCP/IP jt, init
		S63.4Ø2A	Traum rupt of unsp ligmt of r mid finger at MCP/IP jt, init
		S63.4Ø3A	Traum rupt of unsp ligmt of l mid finger at MCP/IP jt, init
		S63.4Ø4A	Traum rupture of unsp ligmt of r rng fngr at MCP/IP jt, init
		S63.4Ø5A	Traum rupture of unsp ligmt of l rng fngr at MCP/IP jt, init
		S63.4Ø6A	Traum rupt of unsp ligmt of r little fngr at MCP/IP jt, init
		S63.4Ø7A	Traum rupt of unsp ligmt of l little fngr at MCP/IP jt, init
		S63.4Ø8A	Traum rupture of unsp ligament of finger at MCP/IP jt, init
		S63.4Ø9A	Traum rupt of unsp ligmt of unsp finger at MCP/IP jt, init
		S63.41ØA	Traum rupt of collat ligmt of r idx fngr at MCP/IP jt, init
		S63.411A	Traum rupt of collat ligmt of l idx fngr at MCP/IP jt, init
		S63.412A	Traum rupt of collat ligmt of r mid fngr at MCP/IP jt, init
		S63.413A	Traum rupt of collat ligmt of l mid fngr at MCP/IP jt, init
		S63.414A	Traum rupt of collat ligmt of r rng fngr at MCP/IP jt, init
		S63.415A	Traum rupt of collat ligmt of l rng fngr at MCP/IP jt, init
		S63.416A	Traum rupt of collat ligmt of r lit fngr at MCP/IP jt, init
		S63.417A	Traum rupt of collat ligmt of l lit fngr at MCP/IP jt, init
		S63.418A	Traum rupture of collat ligmt of finger at MCP/IP jt, init
		S63.419A	Traum rupt of collat ligmt of unsp finger at MCP/IP jt, init
		S63.42ØA	Traum rupt of palmar ligmt of r idx fngr at MCP/IP jt, init
		S63.421A	Traum rupt of palmar ligmt of l idx fngr at MCP/IP jt, init
		S63.422A	Traum rupt of palmar ligmt of r mid fngr at MCP/IP jt, init
		S63.423A	Traum rupt of palmar ligmt of l mid fngr at MCP/IP jt, init
		S63.424A	Traum rupt of palmar ligmt of r rng fngr at MCP/IP jt, init
		S63.425A	Traum rupt of palmar ligmt of l rng fngr at MCP/IP jt, init
		S63.426A	Traum rupt of palmar ligmt of r lit fngr at MCP/IP jt, init
		S63.427A	Traum rupt of palmar ligmt of l lit fngr at MCP/IP jt, init
		S63.428A	Traum rupture of palmar ligmt of finger at MCP/IP jt, init
		S63.429A	Traum rupt of palmar ligmt of unsp finger at MCP/IP jt, init
		S63.43ØA	Traum rupt of volar plate of r idx fngr at MCP/IP jt, init
		S63.431A	Traum rupt of volar plate of l idx fngr at MCP/IP jt, init
		S63.432A	Traum rupt of volar plate of r mid finger at MCP/IP jt, init
		S63.433A	Traum rupt of volar plate of l mid finger at MCP/IP jt, init
		S63.434A	Traum rupt of volar plate of r rng fngr at MCP/IP jt, init
		S63.435A	Traum rupt of volar plate of l rng fngr at MCP/IP jt, init
		S63.436A	Traum rupt of volar plate of r lit fngr at MCP/IP jt, init
		S63.437A	Traum rupt of volar plate of l lit fngr at MCP/IP jt, init
		S63.438A	Traum rupture of volar plate of finger at MCP/IP jt, init
		S63.439A	Traum rupt of volar plate of unsp finger at MCP/IP jt, init
		S63.49ØA	Traum rupture of ligament of r idx fngr at MCP/IP jt, init
		S63.491A	Traum rupture of ligament of l idx fngr at MCP/IP jt, init
		S63.492A	Traum rupture of ligament of r mid finger at MCP/IP jt, init
		S63.493A	Traum rupture of ligament of l mid finger at MCP/IP jt, init
	(Continued on next page)	**S63.494A**	Traum rupture of ligament of r rng fngr at MCP/IP jt, init

 [Brackets] indicate valid character values for each code. Character value meanings provided for each code grouping.

ICD-9-CM		ICD-10-CM	
842.19	OTHER HAND SPRAIN AND STRAIN **(Continued)**	**S63.495A**	Traum rupture of ligament of l rng fngr at MCP/IP jt, init
		S63.496A	Traum rupture of ligmt of r little finger at MCP/IP jt, init
		S63.497A	Traum rupture of ligmt of l little finger at MCP/IP jt, init
		S63.498A	Traumatic rupture of ligament of finger at MCP/IP jt, init
		S63.499A	Traum rupture of ligament of unsp finger at MCP/IP jt, init
		S63.6Ø1A	Unspecified sprain of right thumb, initial encounter
		S63.6Ø2A	Unspecified sprain of left thumb, initial encounter
		S63.6Ø9A	Unspecified sprain of unspecified thumb, initial encounter
		S63.61ØA	Unspecified sprain of right index finger, initial encounter
		S63.611A	Unspecified sprain of left index finger, initial encounter
		S63.612A	Unspecified sprain of right middle finger, initial encounter
		S63.613A	Unspecified sprain of left middle finger, initial encounter
		S63.614A	Unspecified sprain of right ring finger, initial encounter
		S63.615A	Unspecified sprain of left ring finger, initial encounter
		S63.616A	Unspecified sprain of right little finger, initial encounter
		S63.617A	Unspecified sprain of left little finger, initial encounter
		S63.618A	Unspecified sprain of other finger, initial encounter
		S63.619A	Unspecified sprain of unspecified finger, initial encounter
		S63.681A	Other sprain of right thumb, initial encounter
		S63.682A	Other sprain of left thumb, initial encounter
		S63.689A	Other sprain of unspecified thumb, initial encounter
		S63.69ØA	Other sprain of right index finger, initial encounter
		S63.691A	Other sprain of left index finger, initial encounter
		S63.692A	Other sprain of right middle finger, initial encounter
		S63.693A	Other sprain of left middle finger, initial encounter
		S63.694A	Other sprain of right ring finger, initial encounter
		S63.695A	Other sprain of left ring finger, initial encounter
		S63.696A	Other sprain of right little finger, initial encounter
		S63.697A	Other sprain of left little finger, initial encounter
		S63.698A	Other sprain of other finger, initial encounter
		S63.699A	Other sprain of unspecified finger, initial encounter
		S63.8X1A	Sprain of other part of right wrist and hand, init encntr
		S63.8X2A	Sprain of other part of left wrist and hand, init encntr
		S63.8X9A	Sprain of other part of unsp wrist and hand, init encntr
		S66.Ø11A	Strain long flexor musc/fasc/tend r thm at wrs/hnd lv, init
		S66.Ø12A	Strain long flexor musc/fasc/tend l thm at wrs/hnd lv, init
		S66.Ø19A	Strain long flexor musc/fasc/tend thmb at wrs/hnd lv, init
		S66.11ØA	Strain flexor musc/fasc/tend r idx fngr at wrs/hnd lv, init
		S66.111A	Strain flexor musc/fasc/tend l idx fngr at wrs/hnd lv, init
		S66.112A	Strain flexor musc/fasc/tend r mid fngr at wrs/hnd lv, init
		S66.113A	Strain flexor musc/fasc/tend l mid fngr at wrs/hnd lv, init
		S66.114A	Strain flexor musc/fasc/tend r rng fngr at wrs/hnd lv, init
		S66.115A	Strain flexor musc/fasc/tend l rng fngr at wrs/hnd lv, init
		S66.116A	Strain flxr musc/fasc/tend r little fngr at wrs/hnd lv, init
		S66.117A	Strain flxr musc/fasc/tend l little fngr at wrs/hnd lv, init
		S66.118A	Strain of flexor musc/fasc/tend finger at wrs/hnd lv, init
		S66.119A	Strain flexor musc/fasc/tend unsp finger at wrs/hnd lv, init
		S66.211A	Strain of extensor musc/fasc/tend r thm at wrs/hnd lv, init
		S66.212A	Strain of extensor musc/fasc/tend l thm at wrs/hnd lv, init
		S66.219A	Strain of extensor musc/fasc/tend thmb at wrs/hnd lv, init
		S66.31ØA	Strain extn musc/fasc/tend r idx fngr at wrs/hnd lv, init
		S66.311A	Strain extn musc/fasc/tend l idx fngr at wrs/hnd lv, init
		S66.312A	Strain extn musc/fasc/tend r mid finger at wrs/hnd lv, init
		S66.313A	Strain extn musc/fasc/tend l mid finger at wrs/hnd lv, init
		S66.314A	Strain extn musc/fasc/tend r rng fngr at wrs/hnd lv, init
		S66.315A	Strain extn musc/fasc/tend l rng fngr at wrs/hnd lv, init
		S66.316A	Strain extn musc/fasc/tend r little fngr at wrs/hnd lv, init
		S66.317A	Strain extn musc/fasc/tend l little fngr at wrs/hnd lv, init
		S66.318A	Strain of extensor musc/fasc/tend finger at wrs/hnd lv, init
		S66.319A	Strain extn musc/fasc/tend unsp finger at wrs/hnd lv, init
		S66.411A	Strain of intrinsic musc/fasc/tend r thm at wrs/hnd lv, init
		S66.412A	Strain of intrinsic musc/fasc/tend l thm at wrs/hnd lv, init
		S66.419A	Strain of intrinsic musc/fasc/tend thmb at wrs/hnd lv, init
		S66.51ØA	Strain intrns musc/fasc/tend r idx fngr at wrs/hnd lv, init
		S66.511A	Strain intrns musc/fasc/tend l idx fngr at wrs/hnd lv, init
		S66.512A	Strain intrns musc/fasc/tend r mid fngr at wrs/hnd lv, init
		S66.513A	Strain intrns musc/fasc/tend l mid fngr at wrs/hnd lv, init
		S66.514A	Strain intrns musc/fasc/tend r rng fngr at wrs/hnd lv, init
		S66.515A	Strain intrns musc/fasc/tend l rng fngr at wrs/hnd lv, init
		S66.516A	Strain intrns musc/fasc/tend r lit fngr at wrs/hnd lv, init
		S66.517A	Strain intrns musc/fasc/tend l lit fngr at wrs/hnd lv, init
		S66.518A	Strain of intrns musc/fasc/tend finger at wrs/hnd lv, init
		S66.519A	Strain intrns musc/fasc/tend unsp finger at wrs/hnd lv, init
		S66.811A	Strain of musc/fasc/tend at wrs/hnd lv, right hand, init
		S66.812A	Strain of musc/fasc/tend at wrs/hnd lv, left hand, init
		S66.819A	Strain of musc/fasc/tend at wrs/hnd lv, unsp hand, init
843.Ø	ILIOFEMORAL SPRAIN AND STRAIN	**S73.111A**	Iliofemoral ligament sprain of right hip, initial encounter
		S73.112A	Iliofemoral ligament sprain of left hip, initial encounter
		S73.119A	Iliofemoral ligament sprain of unspecified hip, init encntr
843.1	ISCHIOCAPSULAR SPRAIN AND STRAIN	**S73.121A**	Ischiocapsular ligament sprain of right hip, init encntr
		S73.122A	Ischiocapsular ligament sprain of left hip, init encntr
		S73.129A	Ischiocapsular ligament sprain of unsp hip, init encntr

ICD-9-CM		ICD-10-CM	
843.8	SPRAIN&STRAIN OTHER SPECIFIED SITES HIP&THIGH	**S73.191A**	Other sprain of right hip, initial encounter
		S73.192A	Other sprain of left hip, initial encounter
		S73.199A	Other sprain of unspecified hip, initial encounter
		S76.Ø11A	Strain of muscle, fascia and tendon of right hip, init
		S76.Ø12A	Strain of muscle, fascia and tendon of left hip, init encntr
		S76.Ø19A	Strain of muscle, fascia and tendon of unsp hip, init encntr
		S76.111A	Strain of right quadriceps muscle, fascia and tendon, init
		S76.112A	Strain of left quadriceps muscle, fascia and tendon, init
		S76.119A	Strain of unsp quadriceps muscle, fascia and tendon, init
		S76.211A	Strain of adductor musc/fasc/tend right thigh, init
		S76.212A	Strain of adductor musc/fasc/tend left thigh, init
		S76.219A	Strain of adductor musc/fasc/tend unsp thigh, init
		S76.311A	Strain msl/fasc/tnd post grp at thi lev, right thigh, init
		S76.312A	Strain of msl/fasc/tnd post grp at thi lev, left thigh, init
		S76.319A	Strain of msl/fasc/tnd post grp at thi lev, unsp thigh, init
		S76.811A	Strain of musc/fasc/tend at thigh level, right thigh, init
		S76.812A	Strain of musc/fasc/tend at thigh level, left thigh, init
		S76.819A	Strain of musc/fasc/tend at thigh level, unsp thigh, init
843.9	SPRAIN&STRAIN OF UNSPECIFIED SITE OF HIP&THIGH	**S73.1Ø1A**	Unspecified sprain of right hip, initial encounter
		S73.1Ø2A	Unspecified sprain of left hip, initial encounter
		S73.1Ø9A	Unspecified sprain of unspecified hip, initial encounter
		S76.911A	Strain of unsp musc/fasc/tend at thi lev, right thigh, init
		S76.912A	Strain of unsp musc/fasc/tend at thi lev, left thigh, init
		S76.919A	Strain of unsp musc/fasc/tend at thi lev, unsp thigh, init
844.Ø	SPRAIN&STRAIN LATERAL COLLATERAL LIGAMENT KNEE	**S83.421A**	Sprain of lateral collateral ligament of right knee, init
		S83.422A	Sprain of lateral collateral ligament of left knee, init
		S83.429A	Sprain of lateral collateral ligament of unsp knee, init
844.1	SPRAIN AND STRAIN OF MCL OF KNEE	**S83.411A**	Sprain of medial collateral ligament of right knee, init
		S83.412A	Sprain of medial collateral ligament of left knee, init
		S83.419A	Sprain of medial collateral ligament of unsp knee, init
844.2	SPRAIN AND STRAIN OF CRUCIATE LIGAMENT OF KNEE	**S83.5Ø1A**	Sprain of unsp cruciate ligament of right knee, init encntr
		S83.5Ø2A	Sprain of unsp cruciate ligament of left knee, init encntr
		S83.5Ø9A	Sprain of unsp cruciate ligament of unsp knee, init encntr
		S83.511A	Sprain of anterior cruciate ligament of right knee, init
		S83.512A	Sprain of anterior cruciate ligament of left knee, init
		S83.519A	Sprain of anterior cruciate ligament of unsp knee, init
		S83.521A	Sprain of posterior cruciate ligament of right knee, init
		S83.522A	Sprain of posterior cruciate ligament of left knee, init
		S83.529A	Sprain of posterior cruciate ligament of unsp knee, init
844.3	SPRAIN&STRAIN OF TIBIOFIBULAR SUPERIOR OF KNEE	**S83.6ØXA**	Sprain of super tibiofibul joint and ligmt, unsp knee, init
		S83.61XA	Sprain of the super tibiofibul joint and ligmt, r knee, init
		S83.62XA	Sprain of the super tibiofibul joint and ligmt, l knee, init
844.8	SPRAIN&STRAIN OTHER SPECIFIED SITES KNEE&LEG	**S83.4Ø1A**	Sprain of unsp collateral ligament of right knee, init
		S83.4Ø2A	Sprain of unsp collateral ligament of left knee, init encntr
		S83.4Ø9A	Sprain of unsp collateral ligament of unsp knee, init encntr
		S83.8X1A	Sprain of other specified parts of right knee, init encntr
		S83.8X2A	Sprain of other specified parts of left knee, init encntr
		S83.8X9A	Sprain of oth parts of unspecified knee, init encntr
		S86.111A	Strain musc/tend post grp at low leg level, right leg, init
		S86.112A	Strain musc/tend post grp at low leg level, left leg, init
		S86.119A	Strain musc/tend post grp at low leg level, unsp leg, init
		S86.211A	Strain musc/tend ant grp at low leg level, right leg, init
		S86.212A	Strain musc/tend ant grp at low leg level, left leg, init
		S86.219A	Strain musc/tend ant grp at low leg level, unsp leg, init
		S86.311A	Strain musc/tend peroneal grp at low leg lev, r leg, init
		S86.312A	Strain musc/tend peroneal grp at low leg lev, left leg, init
		S86.319A	Strain musc/tend peroneal grp at low leg lev, unsp leg, init
		S86.811A	Strain of musc/tend at lower leg level, right leg, init
		S86.812A	Strain of musc/tend at lower leg level, left leg, init
		S86.819A	Strain of musc/tend at lower leg level, unsp leg, init
844.9	SPRAIN&STRAIN OF UNSPECIFIED SITE OF KNEE&LEG	**S83.9ØXA**	Sprain of unspecified site of unspecified knee, init encntr
		S83.91XA	Sprain of unspecified site of right knee, initial encounter
		S83.92XA	Sprain of unspecified site of left knee, initial encounter
		S86.911A	Strain of unsp musc/tend at lower leg level, right leg, init
		S86.912A	Strain of unsp musc/tend at lower leg level, left leg, init
		S86.919A	Strain of unsp musc/tend at lower leg level, unsp leg, init
845.ØØ	UNSPECIFIED SITE OF ANKLE SPRAIN AND STRAIN	**S93.4Ø1A**	Sprain of unspecified ligament of right ankle, init encntr
		S93.4Ø2A	Sprain of unspecified ligament of left ankle, init encntr
		S93.4Ø9A	Sprain of unsp ligament of unspecified ankle, init encntr
		S96.919A	Strain of unsp msl/tnd at ank/ft level, unsp foot, init
845.Ø1	SPRAIN AND STRAIN OF DELTOID OF ANKLE	**S93.421A**	Sprain of deltoid ligament of right ankle, initial encounter
		S93.422A	Sprain of deltoid ligament of left ankle, initial encounter
		S93.429A	Sprain of deltoid ligament of unspecified ankle, init encntr
845.Ø2	SPRAIN AND STRAIN OF CALCANEOFIBULAR	**S93.411A**	Sprain of calcaneofibular ligament of right ankle, init
		S93.412A	Sprain of calcaneofibular ligament of left ankle, init
		S93.419A	Sprain of calcaneofibular ligament of unsp ankle, init
845.Ø3	SPRAIN AND STRAIN OF TIBIOFIBULAR	**S93.431A**	Sprain of tibiofibular ligament of right ankle, init encntr
		S93.432A	Sprain of tibiofibular ligament of left ankle, init encntr
		S93.439A	Sprain of tibiofibular ligament of unsp ankle, init encntr

ICD-9-CM		ICD-10-CM	
845.Ø9	OTHER ANKLE SPRAIN AND STRAIN	**S86.Ø11A**	Strain of right Achilles tendon, initial encounter
		S86.Ø12A	Strain of left Achilles tendon, initial encounter
		S86.Ø19A	Strain of unspecified Achilles tendon, initial encounter
		S93.491A	Sprain of other ligament of right ankle, initial encounter
		S93.492A	Sprain of other ligament of left ankle, initial encounter
		S93.499A	Sprain of other ligament of unspecified ankle, init encntr
		S96.Ø11A	Strain msl/tnd lng flxr msl toe at ank/ft lev, r foot, init
		S96.Ø12A	Strain msl/tnd lng flxr msl toe at ank/ft lev, l foot, init
		S96.Ø19A	Strain msl/tnd lng flxr msl toe at ank/ft lev, unsp ft, init
		S96.111A	Strain msl/tnd lng extn msl toe at ank/ft lev, r foot, init
		S96.112A	Strain msl/tnd lng extn msl toe at ank/ft lev, l foot, init
		S96.119A	Strain msl/tnd lng extn msl toe at ank/ft lev, unsp ft, init
		S96.211A	Strain of intrinsic msl/tnd at ank/ft level, r foot, init
		S96.212A	Strain of intrinsic msl/tnd at ank/ft level, left foot, init
		S96.219A	Strain of intrinsic msl/tnd at ank/ft level, unsp foot, init
		S96.811A	Strain of muscles and tendons at ank/ft level, r foot, init
		S96.812A	Strain of muscles and tendons at ank/ft level, l foot, init
		S96.819A	Strain muscles and tendons at ank/ft level, unsp foot, init
		S96.911A	Strain of unsp msl/tnd at ank/ft level, right foot, init
		S96.912A	Strain of unsp msl/tnd at ank/ft level, left foot, init
845.1Ø	SPRAIN AND STRAIN OF UNSPECIFIED SITE OF FOOT	**S93.6Ø1A**	Unspecified sprain of right foot, initial encounter
		S93.6Ø2A	Unspecified sprain of left foot, initial encounter
		S93.6Ø9A	Unspecified sprain of unspecified foot, initial encounter
		S96.919A	Strain of unsp msl/tnd at ank/ft level, unsp foot, init
845.11	SPRAIN AND STRAIN OF TARSOMETATARSAL	**S93.621A**	Sprain of tarsometatarsal ligament of right foot, init
		S93.622A	Sprain of tarsometatarsal ligament of left foot, init encntr
		S93.629A	Sprain of tarsometatarsal ligament of unsp foot, init encntr
845.12	SPRAIN AND STRAIN OF METATARSAOPHALANGEAL	**S93.521A**	Sprain of metatarsophalangeal joint of right great toe, init
		S93.522A	Sprain of metatarsophalangeal joint of left great toe, init
		S93.523A	Sprain of metatarsophalangeal joint of unsp great toe, init
		S93.524A	Sprain of MTP joint of right lesser toe(s), init
		S93.525A	Sprain of MTP joint of left lesser toe(s), init
		S93.526A	Sprain of MTP joint of unsp lesser toe(s), init
		S93.529A	Sprain of metatarsophalangeal joint of unsp toe(s), init
845.13	SPRAIN AND STRAIN OF INTERPHALANGEAL OF TOE	**S93.511A**	Sprain of interphalangeal joint of right great toe, init
		S93.512A	Sprain of interphalangeal joint of left great toe, init
		S93.513A	Sprain of interphalangeal joint of unsp great toe, init
		S93.514A	Sprain of interphalangeal joint of right lesser toe(s), init
		S93.515A	Sprain of interphalangeal joint of left lesser toe(s), init
		S93.516A	Sprain of interphalangeal joint of unsp lesser toe(s), init
		S93.519A	Sprain of interphalangeal joint of unsp toe(s), init encntr
845.19	OTHER FOOT SPRAIN AND STRAIN	**S93.5Ø1A**	Unspecified sprain of right great toe, initial encounter
		S93.5Ø2A	Unspecified sprain of left great toe, initial encounter
		S93.5Ø3A	Unspecified sprain of unspecified great toe, init encntr
		S93.5Ø4A	Unspecified sprain of right lesser toe(s), initial encounter
		S93.5Ø5A	Unspecified sprain of left lesser toe(s), initial encounter
		S93.5Ø6A	Unspecified sprain of unspecified lesser toe(s), init encntr
		S93.5Ø9A	Unspecified sprain of unspecified toe(s), initial encounter
		S93.611A	Sprain of tarsal ligament of right foot, initial encounter
		S93.612A	Sprain of tarsal ligament of left foot, initial encounter
		S93.619A	Sprain of tarsal ligament of unspecified foot, init encntr
		S93.691A	Other sprain of right foot, initial encounter
		S93.692A	Other sprain of left foot, initial encounter
		S93.699A	Other sprain of unspecified foot, initial encounter
		S96.Ø11A	Strain msl/tnd lng flxr msl toe at ank/ft lev, r foot, init
		S96.Ø12A	Strain msl/tnd lng flxr msl toe at ank/ft lev, l foot, init
		S96.Ø19A	Strain msl/tnd lng flxr msl toe at ank/ft lev, unsp ft, init
		S96.111A	Strain msl/tnd lng extn msl toe at ank/ft lev, r foot, init
		S96.112A	Strain msl/tnd lng extn msl toe at ank/ft lev, l foot, init
		S96.119A	Strain msl/tnd lng extn msl toe at ank/ft lev, unsp ft, init
		S96.211A	Strain of intrinsic msl/tnd at ank/ft level, r foot, init
		S96.212A	Strain of intrinsic msl/tnd at ank/ft level, left foot, init
		S96.219A	Strain of intrinsic msl/tnd at ank/ft level, unsp foot, init
		S96.811A	Strain of muscles and tendons at ank/ft level, r foot, init
		S96.812A	Strain of muscles and tendons at ank/ft level, l foot, init
		S96.819A	Strain muscles and tendons at ank/ft level, unsp foot, init
		S96.911A	Strain of unsp msl/tnd at ank/ft level, right foot, init
		S96.912A	Strain of unsp msl/tnd at ank/ft level, left foot, init
846.Ø	SPRAIN AND STRAIN OF LUMBOSACRAL	**S33.8XXA**	Sprain of oth parts of lumbar spine and pelvis, init encntr
846.1	SPRAIN AND STRAIN OF SACROILIAC	**S33.6XXA**	Sprain of sacroiliac joint, initial encounter
846.2	SPRAIN AND STRAIN OF SACROSPINATUS	**S33.8XXA**	Sprain of oth parts of lumbar spine and pelvis, init encntr
846.3	SPRAIN AND STRAIN OF SACROTUBEROUS	**S33.8XXA**	Sprain of oth parts of lumbar spine and pelvis, init encntr
846.8	OTHER SPEC SITES SACROILIAC REGION SPRAIN&STRAIN	**S33.8XXA**	Sprain of oth parts of lumbar spine and pelvis, init encntr
846.9	UNSPECIFIED SITE SACROILIAC REGION SPRAIN&STRAIN	**S33.9XXA**	Sprain of unsp parts of lumbar spine and pelvis, init encntr
847.Ø	NECK SPRAIN AND STRAIN	**S13.4XXA**	Sprain of ligaments of cervical spine, initial encounter
		S13.8XXA	Sprain of joints and ligaments of oth prt neck, init encntr
		S16.1XXA	Strain of muscle, fascia and tendon at neck level, init
847.1	THORACIC SPRAIN AND STRAIN	**S23.3XXA**	Sprain of ligaments of thoracic spine, initial encounter
		S23.8XXA	Sprain of other specified parts of thorax, initial encounter
847.2	LUMBAR SPRAIN AND STRAIN	**S33.5XXA**	Sprain of ligaments of lumbar spine, initial encounter

ICD-9-CM		ICD-10-CM		
847.3	SPRAIN AND STRAIN OF SACRUM	**S33.8XXA**	Sprain of oth parts of lumbar spine and pelvis, init encntr	
847.4	SPRAIN AND STRAIN OF COCCYX	**S33.8XXA**	Sprain of oth parts of lumbar spine and pelvis, init encntr	
847.9	SPRAIN AND STRAIN OF UNSPECIFIED SITE OF BACK	**S13.9XXA** **S23.9XXA** **S33.9XXA**	Sprain of joints and ligaments of unsp parts of neck, init Sprain of unspecified parts of thorax, initial encounter Sprain of unsp parts of lumbar spine and pelvis, init encntr	
848.0	SPRAIN AND STRAIN OF SEPTAL CARTILAGE OF NOSE	**S03.8XXA**	Sprain of joints and ligaments of oth prt head, init encntr	
848.1	SPRAIN AND STRAIN OF JAW	**S03.4XXA**	Sprain of jaw, initial encounter	
848.2	SPRAIN AND STRAIN OF THYROID REGION	**S13.5XXA**	Sprain of thyroid region, initial encounter	
848.3	SPRAIN AND STRAIN OF RIBS	**S23.41XA**	Sprain of ribs, initial encounter	
848.40	SPRAIN AND STRAIN OF STERNUM UNSPECIFIED PART	**S23.429A**	Unspecified sprain of sternum, initial encounter	
848.41	SPRAIN AND STRAIN OF STERNOCLAVICULAR	**S23.420A**	Sprain of sternoclavicular (joint) (ligament), init encntr	
848.42	SPRAIN AND STRAIN OF CHONDROSTERNAL	**S23.421A**	Sprain of chondrosternal joint, initial encounter	
848.49	OTHER SPRAIN AND STRAINS OF STERNUM	**S23.428A**	Other sprain of sternum, initial encounter	
848.5	PELVIC SPRAIN AND STRAINS	**S33.4XXA** **S33.8XXA** **S33.9XXA**	Traumatic rupture of symphysis pubis, initial encounter Sprain of oth parts of lumbar spine and pelvis, init encntr Sprain of unsp parts of lumbar spine and pelvis, init encntr	
848.8	OTHER SPECIFIED SITES OF SPRAINS AND STRAINS	**S03.8XXA** **S03.9XXA** **S29.011A** **S29.012A** **S29.019A** **S39.011A** **S39.012A** **S39.013A**	Sprain of joints and ligaments of oth prt head, init encntr Sprain of joints and ligaments of unsp parts of head, init Strain of muscle and tendon of front wall of thorax, init Strain of muscle and tendon of back wall of thorax, init Strain of muscle and tendon of unsp wall of thorax, init Strain of muscle, fascia and tendon of abdomen, init encntr Strain of muscle, fascia and tendon of lower back, init Strain of muscle, fascia and tendon of pelvis, init encntr	
848.9	UNSPECIFIED SITE OF SPRAIN AND STRAIN	**T14.90**	Injury, unspecified	
850.0	CONCUSSION WITH NO LOSS OF CONSCIOUSNESS	**S06.0X0A**	Concussion without loss of consciousness, initial encounter	
850.11	CONCUSSION WITH LOC OF 30 MINUTES OR LESS	**S06.0X1A**	Concussion w LOC of 30 minutes or less, init	
850.12	CONCUSSION WITH LOC FROM 31 TO 59 MINUTES	**S06.0X2A**	Concussion w loss of consciousness of 31-59 min, init	
850.2	CONCUSSION WITH MODERATE LOSS OF CONSCIOUSNESS	**S06.0X3A** **S06.0X4A**	Concussion w loss of consciousness of 1-5 hrs 59 min, init Concussion w LOC of 6 hours to 24 hours, init	
850.3	CONCUSS W/PROLNG LOC&RTN PRE-XST CONSCIOUS LEVL	**S06.0X5A**	Concussion w LOC >24 hr w ret consc lev, init	
850.4	CONCUS W/PROLNG LOC W/O RTN PRE-XST CONSC LEVL	**S06.0X6A**	Concussion w LOC >24 hr w/o ret consc w surv, init	
850.5	CONCUSSION WITH LOC OF UNSPECIFIED DURATION	**S06.0X7A** **S06.0X8A** **S06.0X9A**	Concussion w LOC w death due to brain injury bf consc, init Concussion w LOC w death due to oth cause bf consc, init Concussion w loss of consciousness of unsp duration, init	
850.9	UNSPECIFIED CONCUSSION	**S06.0X0A**	Concussion without loss of consciousness, initial encounter	
851.00	CORTX CONTUS W/O OPN ICW STATE CONSCIOUS UNS	**S06.330A**	Contus/lac cereb, w/o loss of consciousness, init	
851.01	CORTX CONTUS W/O MENTION OPN ICW NO LOC	**S06.339A**	Contus/lac cereb, w LOC of unsp duration, init	
851.02	CORTX CONTUS W/O MENTION OPN ICW BRF LOC	**S06.331A**	Contus/lac cereb, w LOC of 30 minutes or less, init	
851.03	CORTX CONTUS W/O MENTION OPN ICW MOD LOC	**S06.333A**	Contus/lac cereb, w LOC of 1-5 hrs 59 min, init	
851.04	CORTEX CONTUSION W/O OPN ICW LOC>24 HR&RETURN	**S06.335A**	Contus/lac cereb, w LOC >24 hr w ret consc lev, init	
851.05	CORTEX CONTUSION NO OPN ICW LOC >24 HR NO RTRN	**S06.336A**	Contus/lac cereb, w LOC >24 hr w/o ret consc w surv, init	
851.06	CORTX CONTUS W/O MENTION OPN ICW LOC UNS DUR	**S06.339A**	Contus/lac cereb, w LOC of unsp duration, init	
851.09	CORTX CONTUS W/O MENTION OPN ICW UNS CONCUS	**S06.330A** **S06.339A**	Contus/lac cereb, w/o loss of consciousness, init Contus/lac cereb, w LOC of unsp duration, init	
851.10	CORTX CONTUS W/OPEN ICW UNS STATE CONSCIOUS	**S06.330A** **S01.90XA**	Contus/lac cereb, w/o loss of consciousness, init Unsp open wound of unspecified part of head, init encntr	***and***
851.11	CORTEX CONTUS W/OPEN INTRACRANIAL WOUND NO LOC	**S06.330A** **S01.90XA**	Contus/lac cereb, w/o loss of consciousness, init Unsp open wound of unspecified part of head, init encntr	***and***
851.12	CORTEX CONTUS W/OPEN INTRACRANIAL WOUND BRF LOC	**S06.331A** **S06.332A** **S01.90XA**	Contus/lac cereb, w LOC of 30 minutes or less, init Contus/lac cereb, w loss of consciousness of 31-59 min, init Unsp open wound of unspecified part of head, init encntr	***or*** ***and***
851.13	CORTEX CONTUS W/OPEN INTRACRAN WOUND MOD LOC	**S06.333A** **S06.334A** **S01.90XA**	Contus/lac cereb, w LOC of 1-5 hrs 59 min, init Contus/lac cereb, w LOC of 6 hours to 24 hours, init Unsp open wound of unspecified part of head, init encntr	***or*** ***and***
851.14	CORTEX CONTUSION W/OPEN ICW LOC >24 HR&RETURN	**S06.335A** **S01.90XA**	Contus/lac cereb, w LOC >24 hr w ret consc lev, init Unsp open wound of unspecified part of head, init encntr	***and***
851.15	CORTEX CONTUSION W/OPN ICW LOC>24 HR NO RETURN	**S06.336A** **S06.337A** **S06.338A** **S01.90XA**	Contus/lac cereb, w LOC >24 hr w/o ret consc w surv, init Contus/lac cereb, w LOC w death d/t brain inj bf consc, init Contus/lac cereb, w LOC w death d/t oth cause bf consc, init Unsp open wound of unspecified part of head, init encntr	***or*** ***or*** ***and***
851.16	CORTX CONTUS W/OPEN INTRACRAN WND LOC UNS DURAT	**S06.339A** **S01.90XA**	Contus/lac cereb, w LOC of unsp duration, init Unsp open wound of unspecified part of head, init encntr	***and***
851.19	CORTX CONTUS W/OPEN INTRACRAN WOUND UNS CONCUSS	**S06.330A** **S06.339A** **S01.90XA**	Contus/lac cereb, w/o loss of consciousness, init Contus/lac cereb, w LOC of unsp duration, init Unsp open wound of unspecified part of head, init encntr	***or*** ***and***
851.20	CORTX LAC W/O OPN ICW UNS STATE CONSCIOUS	**S06.330A**	Contus/lac cereb, w/o loss of consciousness, init	
851.21	CORTX LAC W/O MENTION OPN INTRACRAN WOUND NO LOC	**S06.339A**	Contus/lac cereb, w LOC of unsp duration, init	
851.22	CORTX LAC W/O MENTION OPN INTRACRAN WND BRF LOC	**S06.331A**	Contus/lac cereb, w LOC of 30 minutes or less, init	

[Brackets] indicate valid character values for each code. Character value meanings provided for each code grouping.

ICD-9-CM		ICD-10-CM		
851.23	CORTX LAC W/O MENTION OPN INTRACRAN WND MOD LOC	**S06.333A**	Contus/lac cereb, w LOC of 1-5 hrs 59 min, init	
851.24	CORTEX LACERATION W/O OPN ICW LOC>24 HR&RTURN	**S06.335A**	Contus/lac cereb, w LOC >24 hr w ret consc lev, init	
851.25	CORTEX LACERATION W/O OPEN ICW LOC NO RTRN	**S06.336A**	Contus/lac cereb, w LOC >24 hr w/o ret consc w surv, init	
851.26	CORTX LAC W/O MENTION OPN ICW LOC UNS DUR	**S06.339A**	Contus/lac cereb, w LOC of unsp duration, init	
851.29	CORTX LAC W/O MENTION OPN ICW UNS CONCUS	**S06.330A**	Contus/lac cereb, w/o loss of consciousness, init	
		S06.339A	Contus/lac cereb, w LOC of unsp duration, init	
851.30	CORTX LAC W/OPEN ICW UNS STATE CONSCIOUS	**S06.330A**	Contus/lac cereb, w/o loss of consciousness, init	*and*
		S01.90XA	Unsp open wound of unspecified part of head, init encntr	
851.31	CORTEX LACERATION W/OPEN INTRACRAN WOUND NO LOC	**S06.330A**	Contus/lac cereb, w/o loss of consciousness, init	*and*
		S01.90XA	Unsp open wound of unspecified part of head, init encntr	
851.32	CORTEX LACERATION W/OPEN INTRACRAN WOUND BRF LOC	**S06.331A**	Contus/lac cereb, w LOC of 30 minutes or less, init	*or*
		S06.332A	Contus/lac cereb, w loss of consciousness of 31-59 min, init	*and*
		S01.90XA	Unsp open wound of unspecified part of head, init encntr	
851.33	CORTEX LACERATION W/OPEN INTRACRAN WOUND MOD LOC	**S06.333A**	Contus/lac cereb, w LOC of 1-5 hrs 59 min, init	*or*
		S06.334A	Contus/lac cereb, w LOC of 6 hours to 24 hours, init	*and*
		S01.90XA	Unsp open wound of unspecified part of head, init encntr	
851.34	CORTEX LACERATION W/OPN ICW LOC>24 HR&RETURN	**S06.335A**	Contus/lac cereb, w LOC >24 hr w ret consc lev, init	*and*
		S01.90XA	Unsp open wound of unspecified part of head, init encntr	
851.35	CORTEX LACERATION W/OPEN ICW LOC NO RTRN	**S06.336A**	Contus/lac cereb, w LOC >24 hr w/o ret consc w surv, init	*or*
		S06.337A	Contus/lac cereb, w LOC w death d/t brain inj bf consc, init	*or*
		S06.338A	Contus/lac cereb, w LOC w death d/t oth cause bf consc, init	*and*
		S01.90XA	Unsp open wound of unspecified part of head, init encntr	
851.36	CORTX LAC W/OPEN INTRACRAN WOUND LOC UNS DURAT	**S06.339A**	Contus/lac cereb, w LOC of unsp duration, init	*and*
		S01.90XA	Unsp open wound of unspecified part of head, init encntr	
851.39	CORTX LAC W/OPEN INTRACRAN WOUND UNSPEC CONCUSS	**S06.330A**	Contus/lac cereb, w/o loss of consciousness, init	*or*
		S06.339A	Contus/lac cereb, w LOC of unsp duration, init	*and*
		S01.90XA	Unsp open wound of unspecified part of head, init encntr	
851.40	CERBLLR/BRAIN STEM CONTUS W/O OPN ICW UNS SOC	**S06.370A**	Contus/lac/hem crblm w/o loss of consciousness, init	
		S06.380A	Contus/lac/hem brainstem w/o loss of consciousness, init	
851.41	CERBLLR/BRAIN STEM CONTUS W/O OPN ICW NO LOC	**S06.370A**	Contus/lac/hem crblm w/o loss of consciousness, init	
		S06.380A	Contus/lac/hem brainstem w/o loss of consciousness, init	
851.42	CERBLLR/BRAIN STEM CONTUS W/O OPN ICW BRIEF LOC	**S06.371A**	Contus/lac/hem crblm w LOC of 30 minutes or less, init	
		S06.372A	Contus/lac/hem crblm w LOC of 31-59 min, init	
		S06.381A	Contus/lac/hem brainstem w LOC of 30 minutes or less, init	
		S06.382A	Contus/lac/hem brainstem w LOC of 31-59 min, init	
851.43	CERBLLR/BRAIN STEM CONTUS W/O OPN ICW MOD LOC	**S06.373A**	Contus/lac/hem crblm w LOC of 1-5 hrs 59 min, init	
		S06.374A	Contus/lac/hem crblm w LOC of 6 hours to 24 hours, init	
		S06.383A	Contus/lac/hem brainstem w LOC of 1-5 hrs 59 min, init	
		S06.384A	Contus/lac/hem brainstem w LOC of 6 hours to 24 hours, init	
851.44	CERBLLR/BRAIN STEM CONTUS NO OPN ICW LOC>24&RTRN	**S06.375A**	Contus/lac/hem crblm w LOC >24 hr w ret consc lev, init	
		S06.385A	Contus/lac/hem brainstem w LOC >24 hr w ret consc lev, init	
851.45	CERBLLR/BRAIN STEM CONTUS NO OPN ICW LOC NO RTRN	**S06.376A**	Contus/lac/hem crblm w LOC >24 hr w/o ret consc w surv, init	
		S06.377A	Contus/lac/hem crblm w LOC w dth d/t brain inj bf consc,init	
		S06.378A	Contus/lac/hem crblm w LOC w dth d/t oth cause bf consc,init	
		S06.386A	Contus/lac/hem brnst w LOC >24 hr w/o ret consc w surv, init	
		S06.387A	Contus/lac/hem brnst w LOC w dth d/t brain inj bf consc,init	
		S06.388A	Contus/lac/hem brnst w LOC w dth d/t oth cause bf consc,init	
851.46	CERBLLR/BRAIN STEM CONTUS NO OPN ICW LOC UNS DUR	**S06.379A**	Contus/lac/hem crblm w LOC of unsp duration, init	
		S06.389A	Contus/lac/hem brainstem w LOC of unsp duration, init	
851.49	CERBLLR/BRAIN STEM CONTUS NO OPN ICW UNS CONCUSS	**S06.380A**	Contus/lac/hem brainstem w/o loss of consciousness, init	
		S06.389A	Contus/lac/hem brainstem w LOC of unsp duration, init	
851.50	CERBLLR/BRAIN STEM CONTUS W/OPN ICW UNS SOC	**S06.370A**	Contus/lac/hem crblm w/o loss of consciousness, init	*or*
		S06.380A	Contus/lac/hem brainstem w/o loss of consciousness, init	*and*
		S01.90XA	Unsp open wound of unspecified part of head, init encntr	
851.51	CERBLLR/BRAIN STEM CONTUS W/OPN ICW NO LOC	**S06.370A**	Contus/lac/hem crblm w/o loss of consciousness, init	*or*
		S06.380A	Contus/lac/hem brainstem w/o loss of consciousness, init	*and*
		S01.90XA	Unsp open wound of unspecified part of head, init encntr	
851.52	CERBLLR/BRAIN STEM CONTUS W/OPN ICW BRIEF LOC	**S06.371A**	Contus/lac/hem crblm w LOC of 30 minutes or less, init	*or*
		S06.372A	Contus/lac/hem crblm w LOC of 31-59 min, init	*or*
		S06.381A	Contus/lac/hem brainstem w LOC of 30 minutes or less, init	*or*
		S06.382A	Contus/lac/hem brainstem w LOC of 31-59 min, init	*and*
		S01.90XA	Unsp open wound of unspecified part of head, init encntr	
851.53	CERBLLR/BRAIN STEM CONTUS W/OPN ICW MOD LOC	**S06.373A**	Contus/lac/hem crblm w LOC of 1-5 hrs 59 min, init	*or*
		S06.374A	Contus/lac/hem crblm w LOC of 6 hours to 24 hours, init	*or*
		S06.383A	Contus/lac/hem brainstem w LOC of 1-5 hrs 59 min, init	*or*
		S06.384A	Contus/lac/hem brainstem w LOC of 6 hours to 24 hours, init	*and*
		S01.90XA	Unsp open wound of unspecified part of head, init encntr	
851.54	CERBLLR/BRAIN STEM CONTUS W/OPN ICW LOC>24&RETRN	**S06.375A**	Contus/lac/hem crblm w LOC >24 hr w ret consc lev, init	*or*
		S06.385A	Contus/lac/hem brainstem w LOC >24 hr w ret consc lev, init	*and*
		S01.90XA	Unsp open wound of unspecified part of head, init encntr	

ICD-9-CM		ICD-10-CM		
851.55	CERBLLR/BRAIN STEM CONTUS W/OPEN ICW LOC NO RTRN	**SØ6.376A**	Contus/lac/hem crblm w LOC >24 hr w/o ret consc w surv, init	*or*
		SØ6.377A	Contus/lac/hem crblm w LOC w dth d/t brain inj bf consc,init	*or*
		SØ6.378A	Contus/lac/hem crblm w LOC w dth d/t oth cause bf consc,init	*or*
		SØ6.386A	Contus/lac/hem brnst w LOC >24 hr w/o ret consc w surv, init	*or*
		SØ6.387A	Contus/lac/hem brnst w LOC w dth d/t brain inj bf consc,init	*or*
		SØ6.388A	Contus/lac/hem brnst w LOC w dth d/t oth cause bf consc,init	*and*
		SØ1.9ØXA	Unsp open wound of unspecified part of head, init encntr	
851.56	CERBLLR/BRAIN STEM CONTUS W/OPN ICW LOC UNS DUR	**SØ6.379A**	Contus/lac/hem crblm w LOC of unsp duration, init	*or*
		SØ6.389A	Contus/lac/hem brainstem w LOC of unsp duration, init	*and*
		SØ1.9ØXA	Unsp open wound of unspecified part of head, init encntr	
851.59	CERBLLR/BRAIN STEM CONTUS W/OPN ICW UNS CONCUSS	**SØ6.37ØA**	Contus/lac/hem crblm w/o loss of consciousness, init	*or*
		SØ6.379A	Contus/lac/hem crblm w LOC of unsp duration, init	*or*
		SØ6.38ØA	Contus/lac/hem brainstem w/o loss of consciousness, init	*or*
		SØ6.389A	Contus/lac/hem brainstem w LOC of unsp duration, init	*and*
		SØ1.9ØXA	Unsp open wound of unspecified part of head, init encntr	
851.6Ø	CERBLLR/BRAIN STEM LAC W/O OPN ICW UNS SOC	**SØ6.37ØA**	Contus/lac/hem crblm w/o loss of consciousness, init	
		SØ6.38ØA	Contus/lac/hem brainstem w/o loss of consciousness, init	
851.61	CERBLLR/BRAIN STEM LAC W/O MEN OPN ICW NO LOC	**SØ6.37ØA**	Contus/lac/hem crblm w/o loss of consciousness, init	
		SØ6.38ØA	Contus/lac/hem brainstem w/o loss of consciousness, init	
851.62	CERBLLR/BRAIN STEM LAC W/O OPN ICW BRIEF LOC	**SØ6.371A**	Contus/lac/hem crblm w LOC of 30 minutes or less, init	
		SØ6.372A	Contus/lac/hem crblm w LOC of 31-59 min, init	
		SØ6.381A	Contus/lac/hem brainstem w LOC of 30 minutes or less, init	
		SØ6.382A	Contus/lac/hem brainstem w LOC of 31-59 min, init	
851.63	CERBLLR/BRAIN STEM LAC W/O OPN ICW MOD LOC	**SØ6.373A**	Contus/lac/hem crblm w LOC of 1-5 hrs 59 min, init	
		SØ6.374A	Contus/lac/hem crblm w LOC of 6 hours to 24 hours, init	
		SØ6.383A	Contus/lac/hem brainstem w LOC of 1-5 hrs 59 min, init	
		SØ6.384A	Contus/lac/hem brainstem w LOC of 6 hours to 24 hours, init	
851.64	CEREBELLR/BRAIN STEM LAC W/O OPN ICW LOC>24&RTRN	**SØ6.375A**	Contus/lac/hem crblm w LOC >24 hr w ret consc lev, init	
		SØ6.385A	Contus/lac/hem brainstem w LOC >24 hr w ret consc lev, init	
851.65	CEREBELLR/BRAIN STEM LAC W/O OPN ICW LOC NO RTRN	**SØ6.376A**	Contus/lac/hem crblm w LOC >24 hr w/o ret consc w surv, init	
		SØ6.377A	Contus/lac/hem crblm w LOC w dth d/t brain inj bf consc,init	
		SØ6.378A	Contus/lac/hem crblm w LOC w dth d/t oth cause bf consc,init	
		SØ6.386A	Contus/lac/hem brnst w LOC >24 hr w/o ret consc w surv, init	
		SØ6.387A	Contus/lac/hem brnst w LOC w dth d/t brain inj bf consc,init	
		SØ6.388A	Contus/lac/hem brnst w LOC w dth d/t oth cause bf consc,init	
851.66	CERBLLR/BRAIN STEM LAC W/O OPN ICW LOC UNS DUR	**SØ6.379A**	Contus/lac/hem crblm w LOC of unsp duration, init	
		SØ6.389A	Contus/lac/hem brainstem w LOC of unsp duration, init	
851.69	CERBLLR/BRAIN STEM LAC W/O OPN ICW UNS CONCUSS	**SØ6.37ØA**	Contus/lac/hem crblm w/o loss of consciousness, init	
		SØ6.379A	Contus/lac/hem crblm w LOC of unsp duration, init	
		SØ6.38ØA	Contus/lac/hem brainstem w/o loss of consciousness, init	
		SØ6.389A	Contus/lac/hem brainstem w LOC of unsp duration, init	
851.7Ø	CERBLLR/BRAIN STEM LAC W/OPN ICW SOC UNS	**SØ6.37ØA**	Contus/lac/hem crblm w/o loss of consciousness, init	*or*
		SØ6.38ØA	Contus/lac/hem brainstem w/o loss of consciousness, init	*and*
		SØ1.9ØXA	Unsp open wound of unspecified part of head, init encntr	
851.71	CERBLLR/BRAIN STEM LAC W/OPN ICW NO LOC	**SØ6.37ØA**	Contus/lac/hem crblm w/o loss of consciousness, init	*or*
		SØ6.38ØA	Contus/lac/hem brainstem w/o loss of consciousness, init	*and*
		SØ1.9ØXA	Unsp open wound of unspecified part of head, init encntr	
851.72	CERBLLR/BRAIN STEM LAC W/OPN ICW BRIEF LOC	**SØ6.371A**	Contus/lac/hem crblm w LOC of 30 minutes or less, init	*or*
		SØ6.372A	Contus/lac/hem crblm w LOC of 31-59 min, init	*or*
		SØ6.381A	Contus/lac/hem brainstem w LOC of 30 minutes or less, init	*or*
		SØ6.382A	Contus/lac/hem brainstem w LOC of 31-59 min, init	*and*
		SØ1.9ØXA	Unsp open wound of unspecified part of head, init encntr	
851.73	CERBLLR/BRAIN STEM LAC W/OPN ICW MOD LOC	**SØ6.373A**	Contus/lac/hem crblm w LOC of 1-5 hrs 59 min, init	*or*
		SØ6.374A	Contus/lac/hem crblm w LOC of 6 hours to 24 hours, init	*or*
		SØ6.383A	Contus/lac/hem brainstem w LOC of 1-5 hrs 59 min, init	*or*
		SØ6.384A	Contus/lac/hem brainstem w LOC of 6 hours to 24 hours, init	*and*
		SØ1.9ØXA	Unsp open wound of unspecified part of head, init encntr	
851.74	CEREBELLR/BRAIN STEM LAC W/OPN ICW LOC>24&RETURN	**SØ6.375A**	Contus/lac/hem crblm w LOC >24 hr w ret consc lev, init	*or*
		SØ6.385A	Contus/lac/hem brainstem w LOC >24 hr w ret consc lev, init	*and*
		SØ1.9ØXA	Unsp open wound of unspecified part of head, init encntr	
851.75	CEREBELLR/BRAIN STEM LAC W/OPN ICW LOC NO RTRN	**SØ6.376A**	Contus/lac/hem crblm w LOC >24 hr w/o ret consc w surv, init	*or*
		SØ6.377A	Contus/lac/hem crblm w LOC w dth d/t brain inj bf consc,init	*or*
		SØ6.378A	Contus/lac/hem crblm w LOC w dth d/t oth cause bf consc,init	*or*
		SØ6.386A	Contus/lac/hem brnst w LOC >24 hr w/o ret consc w surv, init	*or*
		SØ6.387A	Contus/lac/hem brnst w LOC w dth d/t brain inj bf consc,init	*or*
		SØ6.388A	Contus/lac/hem brnst w LOC w dth d/t oth cause bf consc,init	*and*
		SØ1.9ØXA	Unsp open wound of unspecified part of head, init encntr	
851.76	CERBLLR/BRAIN STEM LAC W/OPN ICW LOC UNS DUR	**SØ6.379A**	Contus/lac/hem crblm w LOC of unsp duration, init	*or*
		SØ6.389A	Contus/lac/hem brainstem w LOC of unsp duration, init	*and*
		SØ1.9ØXA	Unsp open wound of unspecified part of head, init encntr	

ICD-9-CM		ICD-10-CM		
851.79	CERBLLR/BRAIN STEM LAC W/OPN ICW UNS CONCUS	**SØ6.37ØA**	Contus/lac/hem crblm w/o loss of consciousness, init	*or*
		SØ6.379A	Contus/lac/hem crblm w LOC of unsp duration, init	*or*
		SØ6.38ØA	Contus/lac/hem brainstem w/o loss of consciousness, init	*or*
		SØ6.389A	Contus/lac/hem brainstem w LOC of unsp duration, init	*and*
		SØ1.9ØXA	Unsp open wound of unspecified part of head, init encntr	
851.8Ø	OTH&UNS CERBRL LAC&CONTUS W/O OPN ICW UNS SOC	**SØ6.33ØA**	Contus/lac cereb, w/o loss of consciousness, init	
851.81	OTH&UNS CERBRL LAC&CONTUS W/O OPN ICW NO LOC	**SØ6.31ØA**	Contus/lac right cerebrum w/o loss of consciousness, init	
		SØ6.32ØA	Contus/lac left cerebrum w/o loss of consciousness, init	
		SØ6.33ØA	Contus/lac cereb, w/o loss of consciousness, init	
851.82	OTH&UNS CERBRL LAC&CONTUS W/O OPN ICW BRIEF LOC	**SØ6.311A**	Contus/lac right cerebrum w LOC of 30 minutes or less, init	
		SØ6.312A	Contus/lac right cerebrum w LOC of 31-59 min, init	
		SØ6.321A	Contus/lac left cerebrum w LOC of 30 minutes or less, init	
		SØ6.322A	Contus/lac left cerebrum w LOC of 31-59 min, init	
		SØ6.331A	Contus/lac cereb, w LOC of 30 minutes or less, init	
		SØ6.332A	Contus/lac cereb, w loss of consciousness of 31-59 min, init	
851.83	OTH&UNS CERBRL LAC&CONTUS W/O OPN ICW MOD LOC	**SØ6.313A**	Contus/lac right cerebrum w LOC of 1-5 hrs 59 min, init	
		SØ6.314A	Contus/lac right cerebrum w LOC of 6 hours to 24 hours, init	
		SØ6.323A	Contus/lac left cerebrum w LOC of 1-5 hrs 59 min, init	
		SØ6.324A	Contus/lac left cerebrum w LOC of 6 hours to 24 hours, init	
		SØ6.333A	Contus/lac cereb, w LOC of 1-5 hrs 59 min, init	
		SØ6.334A	Contus/lac cereb, w LOC of 6 hours to 24 hours, init	
851.84	OTH&UNS CERBRL LAC&CONTUS NO OPN ICW LOC>24&RTRN	**SØ6.315A**	Contus/lac right cerebrum w LOC >24 hr w ret consc lev, init	
		SØ6.325A	Contus/lac left cerebrum w LOC >24 hr w ret consc lev, init	
		SØ6.335A	Contus/lac cereb, w LOC >24 hr w ret consc lev, init	
851.85	OTH&UNS CERBRL LAC&CONTUS NO OPN ICW LOC NO RTRN	**SØ6.316A**	Contus/lac r cereb w LOC >24 hr w/o ret consc w surv, init	
		SØ6.317A	Contus/lac r cereb w LOC w dth d/t brain inj bf consc, init	
		SØ6.318A	Contus/lac r cereb w LOC w dth d/t oth cause bf consc, init	
		SØ6.326A	Contus/lac l cereb w LOC >24 hr w/o ret consc w surv, init	
		SØ6.327A	Contus/lac l cereb w LOC w dth d/t brain inj bf consc, init	
		SØ6.328A	Contus/lac l cereb w LOC w dth d/t oth cause bf consc, init	
		SØ6.336A	Contus/lac cereb, w LOC >24 hr w/o ret consc w surv, init	
		SØ6.337A	Contus/lac cereb, w LOC w death d/t brain inj bf consc, init	
		SØ6.338A	Contus/lac cereb, w LOC w death d/t oth cause bf consc, init	
851.86	OTH&UNS CERBRL LAC&CONTUS NO OPN ICW LOC UNS DUR	**SØ6.319A**	Contus/lac right cerebrum w LOC of unsp duration, init	
		SØ6.329A	Contus/lac left cerebrum w LOC of unsp duration, init	
		SØ6.339A	Contus/lac cereb, w LOC of unsp duration, init	
851.89	OTH&UNS CERBRL LAC&CONTUS NO OPN ICW UNS CONCUSS	**SØ6.33ØA**	Contus/lac cereb, w/o loss of consciousness, init	
		SØ6.339A	Contus/lac cereb, w LOC of unsp duration, init	
851.9Ø	OTH&UNS CERBRL LAC&CONTUS W/OPN ICW UNS SOC	**SØ6.33ØA**	Contus/lac cereb, w/o loss of consciousness, init	*and*
		SØ1.9ØXA	Unsp open wound of unspecified part of head, init encntr	
851.91	OTH&UNS CERBRL LAC&CONTUS W/OPN ICW NO LOC	**SØ6.33ØA**	Contus/lac cereb, w/o loss of consciousness, init	*and*
		SØ1.9ØXA	Unsp open wound of unspecified part of head, init encntr	
851.92	OTH&UNS CERBRL LAC&CONTUS W/OPN ICW BRIEF LOC	**SØ6.331A**	Contus/lac cereb, w LOC of 30 minutes or less, init	*or*
		SØ6.332A	Contus/lac cereb, w loss of consciousness of 31-59 min, init	*and*
		SØ1.9ØXA	Unsp open wound of unspecified part of head, init encntr	
851.93	OTH&UNS CERBRL LAC&CONTUS W/OPN ICW MOD LOC	**SØ6.333A**	Contus/lac cereb, w LOC of 1-5 hrs 59 min, init	*or*
		SØ6.334A	Contus/lac cereb, w LOC of 6 hours to 24 hours, init	*and*
		SØ1.9ØXA	Unsp open wound of unspecified part of head, init encntr	
851.94	OTH&UNS CERBRL LAC W/OPN ICW LOC>24&RETURN	**SØ6.335A**	Contus/lac cereb, w LOC >24 hr w ret consc lev, init	*and*
		SØ1.9ØXA	Unsp open wound of unspecified part of head, init encntr	
851.95	OTH&UNS CERBRL LAC&CONTUS W/OPEN ICW LOC NO RTRN	**SØ6.336A**	Contus/lac cereb, w LOC >24 hr w/o ret consc w surv, init	*or*
		SØ6.337A	Contus/lac cereb, w LOC w death d/t brain inj bf consc, init	*or*
		SØ6.338A	Contus/lac cereb, w LOC w death d/t oth cause bf consc, init	*and*
		SØ1.9ØXA	Unsp open wound of unspecified part of head, init encntr	
851.96	OTH&UNS CERBRL LAC&CONTUS W/OPN ICW LOC UNS DUR	**SØ6.339A**	Contus/lac cereb, w LOC of unsp duration, init	*and*
		SØ1.9ØXA	Unsp open wound of unspecified part of head, init encntr	
851.99	OTH&UNS CERBRL LAC&CONTUS W/OPN ICW UNS CONCUSS	**SØ6.33ØA**	Contus/lac cereb, w/o loss of consciousness, init	*or*
		SØ6.339A	Contus/lac cereb, w LOC of unsp duration, init	*and*
		SØ1.9ØXA	Unsp open wound of unspecified part of head, init encntr	
852.ØØ	SUBARACH HEMOR FLW INJR W/O OPN ICW UNS SOC	**SØ6.6XØA**	Traum subrac hem w/o loss of consciousness, init	
852.Ø1	SUBARACH HEMOR FLW INJR W/O OPN ICW NO LOC	**SØ6.6XØA**	Traum subrac hem w/o loss of consciousness, init	
852.Ø2	SUBARACH HEMOR FLW INJR W/O OPN ICW BRF LOC	**SØ6.6X1A**	Traum subrac hem w LOC of 30 minutes or less, init	
		SØ6.6X2A	Traum subrac hem w loss of consciousness of 31-59 min, init	
852.Ø3	SUBARACH HEMOR FLW INJR W/O OPN ICW MOD LOC	**SØ6.6X3A**	Traum subrac hem w LOC of 1-5 hrs 59 min, init	
		SØ6.6X4A	Traum subrac hem w LOC of 6 hours to 24 hours, init	
852.Ø4	SUBARACH HEMOR FLW INJR W/O OPN ICW LOC>24 RTRN	**SØ6.6X5A**	Traum subrac hem w LOC >24 hr w ret consc lev, init	
852.Ø5	SUBARAC HEMOR FLW INJR WO OPN ICW LOC>24 NO RTRN	**SØ6.6X6A**	Traum subrac hem w LOC >24 hr w/o ret consc w surv, init	
		SØ6.6X7A	Traum subrac hem w LOC w death d/t brain inj bf consc, init	
		SØ6.6X8A	Traum subrac hem w LOC w death d/t oth cause bf consc, init	
852.Ø6	SUBARACH HEMOR FLW INJR W/O OPN ICW LOC UNS DUR	**SØ6.6X9A**	Traum subrac hem w LOC of unsp duration, init	
852.Ø9	SUBARACH HEMOR FLW INJR W/O OPN ICW UNS CONCUS	**SØ6.6XØA**	Traum subrac hem w/o loss of consciousness, init	
		SØ6.6X9A	Traum subrac hem w LOC of unsp duration, init	

ICD-9-CM		ICD-10-CM		
852.1Ø	SUBARACH HEMOR FLW INJR W/OPEN ICW UNS SOC	**SØ6.6XØA**	Traum subrac hem w/o loss of consciousness, init	
852.11	SUBARACH HEMOR FLW INJR W/OPEN ICW NO LOC	**SØ6.6XØA**	Traum subrac hem w/o loss of consciousness, init	*and*
		SØ1.9ØXA	Unsp open wound of unspecified part of head, init encntr	
852.12	SUBARACH HEMOR FLW INJR W/OPEN ICW BRF LOC	**SØ6.6X1A**	Traum subrac hem w LOC of 30 minutes or less, init	*or*
		SØ6.6X2A	Traum subrac hem w loss of consciousness of 31-59 min, init	*and*
		SØ1.9ØXA	Unsp open wound of unspecified part of head, init encntr	
852.13	SUBARACH HEMOR FLW INJR W/OPEN ICW MOD LOC	**SØ6.6X3A**	Traum subrac hem w LOC of 1-5 hrs 59 min, init	*or*
		SØ6.6X4A	Traum subrac hem w LOC of 6 hours to 24 hours, init	*and*
		SØ1.9ØXA	Unsp open wound of unspecified part of head, init encntr	
852.14	SUBARACH HEMOR FLW INJR W/OPN ICW LOC>24 RTRN	**SØ6.6X5A**	Traum subrac hem w LOC >24 hr w ret consc lev, init	*and*
		SØ1.9ØXA	Unsp open wound of unspecified part of head, init encntr	
852.15	SUBARACH HEMOR FLW INJR W/OPN ICW LOC>24 NO RTRN	**SØ6.6X6A**	Traum subrac hem w LOC >24 hr w/o ret consc w surv, init	*or*
		SØ6.6X7A	Traum subrac hem w LOC w death d/t brain inj bf consc, init	*or*
		SØ6.6X8A	Traum subrac hem w LOC w death d/t oth cause bf consc, init	*and*
		SØ1.9ØXA	Unsp open wound of unspecified part of head, init encntr	
852.16	SUBARACH HEMOR FLW INJR W/OPEN ICW LOC UNS DUR	**SØ6.6X9A**	Traum subrac hem w LOC of unsp duration, init	*and*
		SØ1.9ØXA	Unsp open wound of unspecified part of head, init encntr	
852.19	SUBARACH HEMOR FLW INJR W/OPEN ICW UNS CONCUS	**SØ6.6XØA**	Traum subrac hem w/o loss of consciousness, init	*or*
		SØ6.6X9A	Traum subrac hem w LOC of unsp duration, init	*and*
		SØ1.9ØXA	Unsp open wound of unspecified part of head, init encntr	
852.2Ø	SUBDURAL HEMOR FLW INJR W/O OPN ICW UNS SOC	**SØ6.5XØA**	Traum subdr hem w/o loss of consciousness, init	
852.21	SUBDURAL HEMOR FLW INJR W/O OPN ICW NO LOC	**SØ6.5XØA**	Traum subdr hem w/o loss of consciousness, init	
852.22	SUBDURAL HEMOR FLW INJR W/O OPN ICW BRF LOC	**SØ6.5X1A**	Traum subdr hem w LOC of 30 minutes or less, init	
		SØ6.5X2A	Traum subdr hem w loss of consciousness of 31-59 min, init	
852.23	SUBDURAL HEMOR FLW INJR W/O OPN ICW MOD LOC	**SØ6.5X3A**	Traum subdr hem w LOC of 1-5 hrs 59 min, init	
		SØ6.5X4A	Traum subdr hem w LOC of 6 hours to 24 hours, init	
852.24	SUBDURL HEMOR FLW INJR W/O OPEN ICW LOC>24-RETRN	**SØ6.5X5A**	Traum subdr hem w LOC >24 hr w ret consc lev, init	
852.25	SUBDRL HEMOR FLW INJR W/O OPN ICW LOC>24 NO RTRN	**SØ6.5X6A**	Traum subdr hem w LOC >24 hr w/o ret consc w surv, init	
		SØ6.5X7A	Traum subdr hem w LOC w dth d/t brain inj bef reg consc,init	
		SØ6.5X8A	Traum subdr hem w LOC w dth d/t oth cause bef reg consc,init	
852.26	SUBDURAL HEMOR FLW INJR W/O OPN ICW LOC UNS DUR	**SØ6.5X9A**	Traum subdr hem w LOC of unsp duration, init	
852.29	SUBDURAL HEMOR FLW INJR W/O OPN ICW UNS CONCUS	**SØ6.5XØA**	Traum subdr hem w/o loss of consciousness, init	
		SØ6.5X9A	Traum subdr hem w LOC of unsp duration, init	
852.3Ø	SUBDURAL HEMOR FLW INJR W/OPEN ICW SOC UNS	**SØ6.5XØA**	Traum subdr hem w/o loss of consciousness, init	*and*
		SØ1.9ØXA	Unsp open wound of unspecified part of head, init encntr	
852.31	SUBDURAL HEMOR FLW INJR W/OPEN ICW NO LOC	**SØ6.5XØA**	Traum subdr hem w/o loss of consciousness, init	*and*
		SØ1.9ØXA	Unsp open wound of unspecified part of head, init encntr	
852.32	SUBDURAL HEMOR FLW INJR W/OPEN ICW BRF LOC	**SØ6.5X1A**	Traum subdr hem w LOC of 30 minutes or less, init	*or*
		SØ6.5X2A	Traum subdr hem w loss of consciousness of 31-59 min, init	*and*
		SØ1.9ØXA	Unsp open wound of unspecified part of head, init encntr	
852.33	SUBDURAL HEMOR FLW INJR W/OPEN ICW MOD LOC	**SØ6.5X3A**	Traum subdr hem w LOC of 1-5 hrs 59 min, init	*or*
		SØ6.5X4A	Traum subdr hem w LOC of 6 hours to 24 hours, init	*and*
		SØ1.9ØXA	Unsp open wound of unspecified part of head, init encntr	
852.34	SUBDURAL HEMORR FLW INJR W/OPEN ICW LOS>24 RTRN	**SØ6.5X5A**	Traum subdr hem w LOC >24 hr w ret consc lev, init	*and*
		SØ1.9ØXA	Unsp open wound of unspecified part of head, init encntr	
852.35	SUBDURAL HEMORR FLW INJR W/OPN ICW LOC>24 NO RTN	**SØ6.5X6A**	Traum subdr hem w LOC >24 hr w/o ret consc w surv, init	*or*
		SØ6.5X7A	Traum subdr hem w LOC w dth d/t brain inj bef reg consc,init	*or*
		SØ6.5X8A	Traum subdr hem w LOC w dth d/t oth cause bef reg consc,init	*and*
		SØ1.9ØXA	Unsp open wound of unspecified part of head, init encntr	
852.36	SUBDURAL HEMOR FLW INJR W/OPEN ICW LOC UNS DUR	**SØ6.5X9A**	Traum subdr hem w LOC of unsp duration, init	*and*
		SØ1.9ØXA	Unsp open wound of unspecified part of head, init encntr	
852.39	SUBDURAL HEMOR FLW INJR W/OPEN ICW UNS CONCUS	**SØ6.5XØA**	Traum subdr hem w/o loss of consciousness, init	*or*
		SØ6.5X9A	Traum subdr hem w LOC of unsp duration, init	*and*
		SØ1.9ØXA	Unsp open wound of unspecified part of head, init encntr	
852.4Ø	XTRADURL HEMOR FLW INJR W/O OPN ICW UNS SOC	**SØ6.4XØA**	Epidural hemorrhage w/o loss of consciousness, init encntr	
852.41	XTRADURL HEMOR FLW INJR W/O OPN ICW NO LOC	**SØ6.4XØA**	Epidural hemorrhage w/o loss of consciousness, init encntr	
852.42	XTRADURL HEMOR FLW INJR W/O OPN ICW BRF LOC	**SØ6.4X1A**	Epidural hemorrhage w LOC of 30 minutes or less, init	
		SØ6.4X2A	Epidural hemorrhage w LOC of 31-59 min, init	
852.43	XTRADURL HEMOR FLW INJR W/O OPN ICW MOD LOC	**SØ6.4X3A**	Epidural hemorrhage w LOC of 1-5 hrs 59 min, init	
		SØ6.4X4A	Epidural hemorrhage w LOC of 6 hours to 24 hours, init	
852.44	EXTRADUR HEMOR FLW INJR W/O OPN ICW LOC>24 RTRN	**SØ6.4X5A**	Epidural hemorrhage w LOC >24 hr w ret consc lev, init	
852.45	EXTRADUR HEMOR FLW INJR WO OP ICW LOC>24 NO RTRN	**SØ6.4X6A**	Epidural hemorrhage w LOC >24 hr w/o ret consc w surv, init	
		SØ6.4X7A	Epidur hemor w LOC w death d/t brain injury bf consc, init	
		SØ6.4X8A	Epidur hemor w LOC w death due to oth causes bf consc, init	
852.46	XTRADURL HEMOR FLW INJR W/O OPN ICW LOC UNS DUR	**SØ6.4X9A**	Epidural hemorrhage w LOC of unsp duration, init	
852.49	XTRADURL HEMOR FLW INJR W/O OPN ICW UNS CONCUS	**SØ6.4XØA**	Epidural hemorrhage w/o loss of consciousness, init encntr	
		SØ6.4X9A	Epidural hemorrhage w LOC of unsp duration, init	

[Brackets] indicate valid character values for each code. Character value meanings provided for each code grouping.

ICD-9-CM		ICD-10-CM		
852.5Ø	XTRADURL HEMOR FLW INJR W/OPEN ICW SOC UNS	S06.4X0A	Epidural hemorrhage w/o loss of consciousness, init encntr	and
		S01.90XA	Unsp open wound of unspecified part of head, init encntr	
852.51	XTRADURL HEMOR FLW INJR W/OPEN ICW NO LOC	S06.4X0A	Epidural hemorrhage w/o loss of consciousness, init encntr	and
		S01.90XA	Unsp open wound of unspecified part of head, init encntr	
852.52	XTRADURL HEMOR FLW INJR W/OPEN ICW BRF LOC	S06.4X1A	Epidural hemorrhage w LOC of 30 minutes or less, init	or
		S06.4X2A	Epidural hemorrhage w LOC of 31-59 min, init	and
		S01.90XA	Unsp open wound of unspecified part of head, init encntr	
852.53	XTRADURL HEMOR FLW INJR W/OPEN ICW MOD LOC	S06.4X3A	Epidural hemorrhage w LOC of 1-5 hrs 59 min, init	or
		S06.4X4A	Epidural hemorrhage w LOC of 6 hours to 24 hours, init	and
		S01.90XA	Unsp open wound of unspecified part of head, init encntr	
852.54	XTRADUR HEMOR FLW INJURY W/OPN ICW LOC>24 RETURN	S06.4X5A	Epidural hemorrhage w LOC >24 hr w ret consc lev, init	and
		S01.90XA	Unsp open wound of unspecified part of head, init encntr	
852.55	XTRADUR HEMOR FLW INJR W/OPN ICW LOC>24 NO RETRN	S06.4X6A	Epidural hemorrhage w LOC >24 hr w/o ret consc w surv, init	or
		S06.4X7A	Epidur hemor w LOC w death d/t brain injury bf consc, init	or
		S06.4X8A	Epidur hemor w LOC w death due to oth causes bf consc, init	and
		S01.90XA	Unsp open wound of unspecified part of head, init encntr	
852.56	XTRADURL HEMOR FLW INJR W/OPEN ICW LOC UNS DUR	S06.4X9A	Epidural hemorrhage w LOC of unsp duration, init	and
		S01.90XA	Unsp open wound of unspecified part of head, init encntr	
852.59	XTRADURL HEMOR FLW INJR W/OPEN ICW UNSCONCUS	S06.4X0A	Epidural hemorrhage w/o loss of consciousness, init encntr	or
		S06.4X9A	Epidural hemorrhage w LOC of unsp duration, init	and
		S01.90XA	Unsp open wound of unspecified part of head, init encntr	
853.00	OTH&UNS ICH FOLLOW INJR W/O OPEN ICW UNS SOC	S06.360A	Traum hemor cereb, w/o loss of consciousness, init	
853.01	OTH&UNS ICH FOLLOW INJR W/O OPN ICW NO LOC	S06.340A	Traum hemor right cerebrum w/o loss of consciousness, init	
		S06.350A	Traum hemor left cerebrum w/o loss of consciousness, init	
		S06.360A	Traum hemor cereb, w/o loss of consciousness, init	
853.02	UNS INTRACRAN HEMOR FLW INJR W/O OPN ICW BRF LOC	S06.341A	Traum hemor right cerebrum w LOC of 30 minutes or less, init	
		S06.342A	Traum hemor right cerebrum w LOC of 31-59 min, init	
		S06.351A	Traum hemor left cerebrum w LOC of 30 minutes or less, init	
		S06.352A	Traum hemor left cerebrum w LOC of 31-59 min, init	
		S06.361A	Traum hemor cereb, w LOC of 30 minutes or less, init	
		S06.362A	Traum hemor cereb, w LOC of 31-59 min, init	
853.03	OTH&UNS ICH FLW INJURY W/O OPEN ICW-MOD LOC	S06.343A	Traum hemor right cerebrum w LOC of 1-5 hrs 59 minutes, init	
		S06.344A	Traum hemor right cerebrum w LOC of 6-24 hrs, init	
		S06.353A	Traum hemor left cerebrum w LOC of 1-5 hrs 59 minutes, init	
		S06.354A	Traum hemor left cerebrum w LOC of 6 hours to 24 hours, init	
		S06.363A	Traum hemor cereb, w LOC of 1-5 hrs 59 minutes, init	
		S06.364A	Traum hemor cereb, w LOC of 6 hours to 24 hours, init	
853.04	OTH&UNS ICH FLW INJR W/O OPN ICW >24 LOC RTRN	S06.345A	Traum hemor r cereb w LOC >24 hr w ret consc lev, init	
		S06.355A	Traum hemor left cerebrum w LOC >24 hr w ret consc lev, init	
		S06.365A	Traum hemor cereb, w LOC >24 hr w ret consc lev, init	
853.05	OTH&UNS ICH FLW INJR W/O OPN ICW >24 LOC NO RTN	S06.346A	Traum hemor r cereb w LOC >24 hr w/o ret consc w surv, init	
		S06.347A	Traum hemor r cereb w LOC w dth d/t brain inj bf consc, init	
		S06.348A	Traum hemor r cereb w LOC w dth d/t oth cause bf consc, init	
		S06.356A	Traum hemor l cereb w LOC >24 hr w/o ret consc w surv, init	
		S06.357A	Traum hemor l cereb w LOC w dth d/t brain inj bf consc, init	
		S06.358A	Traum hemor l cereb w LOC w dth d/t oth cause bf consc, init	
		S06.366A	Traum hemor cereb, w LOC >24 hr w/o ret consc w surv, init	
		S06.367A	Traum hemor cereb, w LOC w dth d/t brain inj bf consc, init	
		S06.368A	Traum hemor cereb, w LOC w dth d/t oth cause bf consc, init	
853.06	OTH&UNS ICH FLW INJURY W/O OPN ICW-LOC UNS DUR	S06.349A	Traum hemor right cerebrum w LOC of unsp duration, init	
		S06.359A	Traum hemor left cerebrum w LOC of unsp duration, init	
		S06.369A	Traum hemor cereb, w LOC of unsp duration, init	
853.09	OTH&UNS ICH FLW INJURY W/O OPN ICW-UNS CONCUSS	S06.360A	Traum hemor cereb, w/o loss of consciousness, init	
		S06.369A	Traum hemor cereb, w LOC of unsp duration, init	
853.10	OTH&UNS ICH FOLLOW INJR W/OPEN ICW UNS SOC	S06.360A	Traum hemor cereb, w/o loss of consciousness, init	and
		S01.90XA	Unsp open wound of unspecified part of head, init encntr	
853.11	OTH&UNS ICH FOLLOW INJR W/OPEN ICW NO LOC	S06.360A	Traum hemor cereb, w/o loss of consciousness, init	and
		S01.90XA	Unsp open wound of unspecified part of head, init encntr	
853.12	UNS INTRACRAN HEMOR FLW INJR W/OPEN ICW BRF LOC	S06.361A	Traum hemor cereb, w LOC of 30 minutes or less, init	or
		S06.362A	Traum hemor cereb, w LOC of 31-59 min, init	and
		S01.90XA	Unsp open wound of unspecified part of head, init encntr	
853.13	OTH&UNS ICH FLW INJURY W/OPEN ICW-MOD LOC	S06.363A	Traum hemor cereb, w LOC of 1-5 hrs 59 minutes, in	or
		S06.364A	Traum hemor cereb, w LOC of 6 hours to 24 hours, init	and
		S01.90XA	Unsp open wound of unspecified part of head, init encntr	
853.14	OTH&UNS ICH FLW INJR W/OPEN ICW >24 LOC RTRN	S06.365A	Traum hemor cereb, w LOC >24 hr w ret consc lev, init	and
		S01.90XA	Unsp open wound of unspecified part of head, init encntr	
853.15	OTH&UNS ICH FLW INJR W/OPEN ICW >24 LOC NO RTN	S06.366A	Traum hemor cereb, w LOC >24 hr w/o ret consc w surv, init	or
		S06.367A	Traum hemor cereb, w LOC w dth d/t brain inj bf consc, init	or
		S06.368A	Traum hemor cereb, w LOC w dth d/t oth cause bf consc, init	and
		S01.90XA	Unsp open wound of unspecified part of head, init encntr	

ICD-9-CM		ICD-10-CM		
853.16	OTH&UNS ICH FLW INJURY W/OPEN ICW-LOC UNS DUR	**S06.369A**	Traum hemor cereb, w LOC of unsp duration, init	*and*
		S01.90XA	Unsp open wound of unspecified part of head, init encntr	
853.19	OTH&UNS ICH FLW INJURY W/OPEN ICW-UNS CONCUSS	**S06.360A**	Traum hemor cereb, w/o loss of consciousness, init	*or*
		S06.369A	Traum hemor cereb, w LOC of unsp duration, init	*and*
		S01.90XA	Unsp open wound of unspecified part of head, init encntr	
854.00	ICI OTH&UNS NATR W/O OPEN ICW UNS STATE CONSC	**S06.890A**	Intcran inj w/o loss of consciousness, init encntr	
854.01	INTRACRAN INJR OTH&UNS NATR W/O OPN ICW NO LOC	**S06.1X0A**	Traumatic cerebral edema w/o loss of consciousness, init	
		S06.2X0A	Diffuse TBI w/o loss of consciousness, init	
		S06.300A	Unsp focal TBI w/o loss of consciousness, init	
		S06.810A	Injury of r int carotid, intcr w/o LOC, init	
		S06.820A	Injury of l int carotid, intcr w/o LOC, init	
		S06.890A	Intcran inj w/o loss of consciousness, init encntr	
		S06.9X0A	Unsp intracranial injury w/o loss of consciousness, init	
854.02	ICI OTH&UNS NATURE W/O OPEN ICW BRIEF LOC	**S06.1X1A**	Traumatic cerebral edema w LOC of 30 minutes or less, init	
		S06.1X2A	Traumatic cerebral edema w LOC of 31-59 min, init	
		S06.2X1A	Diffuse TBI w LOC of 30 minutes or less, init	
		S06.2X2A	Diffuse TBI w loss of consciousness of 31-59 min, init	
		S06.301A	Unsp focal TBI w LOC of 30 minutes or less, init	
		S06.302A	Unsp focal TBI w loss of consciousness of 31-59 min, init	
		S06.811A	Inj r int carotid, intcr w LOC of 30 minutes or less, init	
		S06.812A	Injury of r int carotid, intcr w LOC of 31-59 min, init	
		S06.821A	Inj l int carotid, intcr w LOC of 30 minutes or less, init	
		S06.822A	Injury of l int carotid, intcr w LOC of 31-59 min, init	
		S06.891A	Intcran inj w LOC of 30 minutes or less, init	
		S06.892A	Intcran inj w loss of consciousness of 31-59 min, init	
		S06.9X1A	Unsp intracranial injury w LOC of 30 minutes or less, init	
		S06.9X2A	Unsp intracranial injury w LOC of 31-59 min, init	
854.03	INTRACRAN INJR OTH&UNS NATR W/O OPN ICW MOD LOC	**S06.1X3A**	Traumatic cerebral edema w LOC of 1-5 hrs 59 min, init	
		S06.1X4A	Traumatic cerebral edema w LOC of 6 hours to 24 hours, init	
		S06.2X3A	Diffuse TBI w loss of consciousness of 1-5 hrs 59 min, init	
		S06.2X4A	Diffuse TBI w LOC of 6 hours to 24 hours, init	
		S06.303A	Unsp focal TBI w LOC of 1-5 hrs 59 min, init	
		S06.304A	Unsp focal TBI w LOC of 6 hours to 24 hours, init	
		S06.813A	Injury of r int carotid, intcr w LOC of 1-5 hrs 59 min, init	
		S06.814A	Injury of r int carotid, intcr w LOC of 6-24 hrs, init	
		S06.823A	Injury of l int carotid, intcr w LOC of 1-5 hrs 59 min, init	
		S06.824A	Injury of l int carotid, intcr w LOC of 6-24 hrs, init	
		S06.893A	Intcran inj w loss of consciousness of 1-5 hrs 59 min, init	
		S06.894A	Intcran inj w LOC of 6 hours to 24 hours, init	
		S06.9X3A	Unsp intracranial injury w LOC of 1-5 hrs 59 min, init	
		S06.9X4A	Unsp intracranial injury w LOC of 6 hours to 24 hours, init	
854.04	ICI OTH&UNS NATR W/O OPEN ICW LOC>24 RETURN	**S06.1X5A**	Traumatic cerebral edema w LOC >24 hr w ret consc lev, init	
		S06.2X5A	Diffuse TBI w LOC >24 hr w return to conscious levels, init	
		S06.305A	Unsp focal TBI w LOC >24 hr w ret consc lev, init	
		S06.815A	Inj r int carotid, intcr w LOC >24 hr w ret consc lev, init	
		S06.825A	Inj l int carotid, intcr w LOC >24 hr w ret consc lev, init	
		S06.895A	Intcran inj w LOC >24 hr w ret consc lev, init	
		S06.9X5A	Unsp intracranial injury w LOC >24 hr w ret consc lev, init	
854.05	ICI OTH&UNS NATR W/O OPEN ICW LOC>24 NO RETURN	**S06.1X6A**	Traum cerebral edema w LOC >24 hr w/o ret consc w surv, init	
		S06.1X7A	Traum cereb edema w LOC w death d/t brain inj bf consc, init	
		S06.1X8A	Traum cereb edema w LOC w death d/t oth cause bf consc, init	
		S06.2X6A	Diffuse TBI w LOC >24 hr w/o ret consc w surv, init	
		S06.2X7A	Diffuse TBI w LOC w death due to brain injury bf consc, init	
		S06.2X8A	Diffuse TBI w LOC w death due to oth cause bf consc, init	
		S06.306A	Unsp focal TBI w LOC >24 hr w/o ret consc w surv, init	
		S06.307A	Unsp focal TBI w LOC w death d/t brain injury bf consc, init	
		S06.308A	Unsp focal TBI w LOC w death due to oth cause bf consc, init	
		S06.816A	Inj r int crtd,intcr w LOC >24 hr w/o ret consc w surv, init	
		S06.817A	Inj r int crtd,intcr w LOC w dth d/t brain inj bf consc,init	
		S06.818A	Inj r int crtd,intcr w LOC w dth d/t oth cause bf consc,init	
		S06.826A	Inj l int crtd,intcr w LOC >24 hr w/o ret consc w surv, init	
		S06.827A	Inj l int crtd,intcr w LOC w dth d/t brain inj bf consc,init	
		S06.828A	Inj l int crtd,intcr w LOC w dth d/t oth cause bf consc,init	
		S06.896A	Intcran inj w LOC >24 hr w/o ret consc w surv, init	
		S06.897A	Intcran inj w LOC w death due to brain injury bf consc, init	
		S06.898A	Intcran inj w LOC w death due to oth cause bf consc, init	
		S06.9X6A	Unsp intcrn injury w LOC >24 hr w/o ret consc w surv, init	
		S06.9X7A	Unsp intcrn inj w LOC w death d/t brain inj bf consc, init	
		S06.9X8A	Unsp intcrn inj w LOC w death d/t oth cause bf consc, init	
854.06	ICI OTH&UNS NATURE W/O OPEN ICW LOC UNS DUR	**S06.1X9A**	Traumatic cerebral edema w LOC of unsp duration, init	
		S06.2X9A	Diffuse TBI w loss of consciousness of unsp duration, init	
		S06.309A	Unsp focal TBI w LOC of unsp duration, init	
		S06.819A	Injury of r int carotid, intcr w LOC of unsp duration, init	
		S06.829A	Injury of l int carotid, intcr w LOC of unsp duration, init	
		S06.899A	Intcran inj w loss of consciousness of unsp duration, init	
		S06.9X9A	Unsp intracranial injury w LOC of unsp duration, init	
854.09	ICI OTH&UNS NATURE W/O OPEN ICW UNS CONCUSS	**S06.890A**	Intcran inj w/o loss of consciousness, init encntr	*and*
		S06.0X0A	Concussion without loss of consciousness, initial encounter	

ICD-9-CM		ICD-10-CM		
854.10	ICI OTH&UNS NATR W/OPEN ICW UNS STATE CONSC	S06.890A	Intcran inj w/o loss of consciousness, init encntr	and
		S01.90XA	Unsp open wound of unspecified part of head, init encntr	
854.11	INTRACRAN INJR OTH&UNS NATR W/OPEN ICW NO LOC	S06.890A	Intcran inj w/o loss of consciousness, init encntr	and
		S01.90XA	Unsp open wound of unspecified part of head, init encntr	
854.12	INTRACRAN INJR OTH&UNS NATR W/OPEN ICW BRF LOC	S06.891A	Intcran inj w LOC of 30 minutes or less, init	or
		S06.892A	Intcran inj w loss of consciousness of 31-59 min, init	and
		S01.90XA	Unsp open wound of unspecified part of head, init encntr	
854.13	INTRACRAN INJR OTH&UNS NATR W/OPEN ICW MOD LOC	S06.893A	Intcran inj w loss of consciousness of 1-5 hrs 59 min, init	or
		S06.894A	Intcran inj w LOC of 6 hours to 24 hours, init	and
		S01.90XA	Unsp open wound of unspecified part of head, init encntr	
854.14	ICI OTH&UNS NATR W/OPEN ICW LOC>24 RETURN	S06.895A	Intcran inj w LOC >24 hr w ret consc lev, init	and
		S01.90XA	Unsp open wound of unspecified part of head, init encntr	
854.15	ICI OTH&UNS NATR W/OPEN ICW LOC>24 NO RETURN	S06.896A	Intcran inj w LOC >24 hr w/o ret consc w surv, init	or
		S06.897A	Intcran inj w LOC w death due to brain injury bf consc, init	or
		S06.898A	Intcran inj w LOC w death due to oth cause bf consc, init	and
		S01.90XA	Unsp open wound of unspecified part of head, init encntr	
854.16	ICI OTH&UNS NATURE W/OPEN ICW LOC UNS DUR	S06.899A	Intcran inj w loss of consciousness of unsp duration, init	and
		S01.90XA	Unsp open wound of unspecified part of head, init encntr	
854.19	ICI OTH&UNS NATURE W/OPEN ICW UNS CONCUSS	S06.890A	Intcran inj w/o loss of consciousness, init encntr	or
		S06.899A	Intcran inj w loss of consciousness of unsp duration, init	and
		S01.90XA	Unsp open wound of unspecified part of head, init encntr	
860.0	TRAUMAT PNEUMO W/O MENTION OPEN WOUND INTO THOR	S27.0XXA	Traumatic pneumothorax, initial encounter	
860.1	TRAUMATIC PNEUMOTHORAX W/OPEN WOUND INTO THORAX	S27.0XXA	Traumatic pneumothorax, initial encounter	and
		S21.309A	Unsp opn wnd unsp front wall of thrx w penet thor cav, init	
860.2	TRAUMAT HEMOTHOR W/O MENTION OPEN WOUND IN THOR	S27.1XXA	Traumatic hemothorax, initial encounter	
860.3	TRAUMATIC HEMOTHORAX WITH OPEN WOUND INTO THORAX	S27.1XXA	Traumatic hemothorax, initial encounter	and
		S21.309A	Unsp opn wnd unsp front wall of thrx w penet thor cav, init	
860.4	TRAUMAT PNEUMOHEMOTHOR W/O OPN WND IN THOR	S27.2XXA	Traumatic hemopneumothorax, initial encounter	
860.5	TRAUMATIC PNEUMOHEMOTHOR W/OPEN WOUND INTO THOR	S27.2XXA	Traumatic hemopneumothorax, initial encounter	and
		S21.309A	Unsp opn wnd unsp front wall of thrx w penet thor cav, init	
861.00	UNSPEC INJURY HRT W/O MENTION OPEN WOUND IN THOR	S26.00XA	Unsp injury of heart with hemopericardium, init encntr	
		S26.09XA	Other injury of heart with hemopericardium, init encntr	
		S26.10XA	Unsp injury of heart without hemopericardium, init encntr	
		S26.19XA	Other injury of heart without hemopericardium, init encntr	
		S26.90XA	Unsp injury of heart, unsp w or w/o hemopericardium, init	
		S26.99XA	Inj heart, unsp w or w/o hemopericardium, init encntr	
861.01	HRT CONTUS WITHOUT MENTION OPEN WOUND INTO THOR	S26.01XA	Contusion of heart with hemopericardium, initial encounter	
		S26.11XA	Contusion of heart without hemopericardium, init encntr	
		S26.91XA	Contusion of heart, unsp w or w/o hemopericardium, init	
861.02	HRT LAC W/O PENETRAT HRT CHAMBS/ OPN WND IN THOR	S26.020A	Mild laceration of heart with hemopericardium, init encntr	
		S26.021A	Moderate laceration of heart w hemopericardium, init encntr	
		S26.12XA	Laceration of heart without hemopericardium, init encntr	
		S26.92XA	Laceration of heart, unsp w or w/o hemopericardium, init	
861.03	HEART LACERATION W/PENETRATION OF CHAMBERS	S26.022A	Major laceration of heart with hemopericardium, init encntr	
		S26.12XA	Laceration of heart without hemopericardium, init encntr	
		S26.92XA	Laceration of heart, unsp w or w/o hemopericardium, init	
861.10	UNSPEC INJURY HEART W/OPEN WOUND INTO THORAX	S26.90XA	Unsp injury of heart, unsp w or w/o hemopericardium, init	and
		S21.309A	Unsp opn wnd unsp front wall of thrx w penet thor cav, init	
861.11	HEART CONTUSION WITH OPEN WOUND INTO THORAX	S26.91XA	Contusion of heart, unsp w or w/o hemopericardium, init	and
		S21.309A	Unsp opn wnd unsp front wall of thrx w penet thor cav, init	
861.12	LACERATION OF HEART WO PENETRATION OF CHAMBERS	S26.020A	Mild laceration of heart with hemopericardium, init encntr	or
		S26.92XA	Laceration of heart, unsp w or w/o hemopericardium, init	and
		S21.309A	Unsp opn wnd unsp front wall of thrx w penet thor cav, init	
861.13	HRT LAC W/PENETRAT HRT CHAMBS&OPEN WOUND IN THOR	S26.021A	Moderate laceration of heart w hemopericardium, init encntr	or
		S26.022A	Major laceration of heart with hemopericardium, init encntr	and
		S21.309A	Unsp opn wnd unsp front wall of thrx w penet thor cav, init	
861.20	UNSPEC LUNG INJURY W/O MENTION OPN WOUND IN THOR	S27.301A	Unspecified injury of lung, unilateral, initial encounter	
		S27.302A	Unspecified injury of lung, bilateral, initial encounter	
		S27.309A	Unspecified injury of lung, unspecified, initial encounter	
		S27.311A	Primary blast injury of lung, unilateral, initial encounter	
		S27.312A	Primary blast injury of lung, bilateral, initial encounter	
		S27.319A	Primary blast injury of lung, unspecified, initial encounter	
		S27.391A	Other injuries of lung, unilateral, initial encounter	
		S27.392A	Other injuries of lung, bilateral, initial encounter	
		S27.399A	Other injuries of lung, unspecified, initial encounter	
861.21	LUNG CONTUS WITHOUT MENTION OPEN WOUND INTO THOR	S27.321A	Contusion of lung, unilateral, initial encounter	
		S27.322A	Contusion of lung, bilateral, initial encounter	
		S27.329A	Contusion of lung, unspecified, initial encounter	

ICD-9-CM		ICD-10-CM		
861.22	LUNG LACERATION W/O MENTION OPEN WOUND INTO THOR	**S27.331A**	Laceration of lung, unilateral, initial encounter	
		S27.332A	Laceration of lung, bilateral, initial encounter	
		S27.339A	Laceration of lung, unspecified, initial encounter	
861.30	UNSPECIFIED LUNG INJURY W/OPEN WOUND INTO THORAX	**S27.309A**	Unspecified injury of lung, unspecified, initial encounter	*and*
		S21.309A	Unsp opn wnd unsp front wall of thrx w penet thor cav, init	
861.31	LUNG CONTUSION WITH OPEN WOUND INTO THORAX	**S27.329A**	Contusion of lung, unspecified, initial encounter	*and*
		S21.309A	Unsp opn wnd unsp front wall of thrx w penet thor cav, init	
861.32	LUNG LACERATION WITH OPEN WOUND INTO THORAX	**S27.339A**	Laceration of lung, unspecified, initial encounter	*and*
		S21.309A	Unsp opn wnd unsp front wall of thrx w penet thor cav, init	
862.0	DIAPHRAGM INJURY W/O MENTION OPN WOUND IN CAVITY	**S27.802A**	Contusion of diaphragm, initial encounter	
		S27.803A	Laceration of diaphragm, initial encounter	
		S27.808A	Other injury of diaphragm, initial encounter	
		S27.809A	Unspecified injury of diaphragm, initial encounter	
862.1	DIAPHRAGM INJURY WITH OPEN WOUND INTO CAVITY	**S27.809A**	Unspecified injury of diaphragm, initial encounter	*and*
		S21.309A	Unsp opn wnd unsp front wall of thrx w penet thor cav, init	
862.21	BRONCHUS INJURY W/O MENTION OPEN WOUND IN CAVITY	**S27.401A**	Unspecified injury of bronchus, unilateral, init encntr	
		S27.402A	Unspecified injury of bronchus, bilateral, initial encounter	
		S27.409A	Unspecified injury of bronchus, unspecified, init encntr	
		S27.411A	Primary blast injury of bronchus, unilateral, init encntr	
		S27.412A	Primary blast injury of bronchus, bilateral, init encntr	
		S27.419A	Primary blast injury of bronchus, unspecified, init encntr	
		S27.421A	Contusion of bronchus, unilateral, initial encounter	
		S27.422A	Contusion of bronchus, bilateral, initial encounter	
		S27.429A	Contusion of bronchus, unspecified, initial encounter	
		S27.431A	Laceration of bronchus, unilateral, initial encounter	
		S27.432A	Laceration of bronchus, bilateral, initial encounter	
		S27.439A	Laceration of bronchus, unspecified, initial encounter	
		S27.491A	Other injury of bronchus, unilateral, initial encounter	
		S27.492A	Other injury of bronchus, bilateral, initial encounter	
		S27.499A	Other injury of bronchus, unspecified, initial encounter	
862.22	ESOPH INJURY W/O MENTION OPEN WOUND INTO CAVITY	**S27.812A**	Contusion of esophagus (thoracic part), initial encounter	
		S27.813A	Laceration of esophagus (thoracic part), initial encounter	
		S27.818A	Other injury of esophagus (thoracic part), initial encounter	
		S27.819A	Unspecified injury of esophagus (thoracic part), init encntr	
862.29	INJR OTH SPEC INTRATHR ORGN W/O OPN WND CAV OTH	**S27.50XA**	Unspecified injury of thoracic trachea, initial encounter	
		S27.51XA	Primary blast injury of thoracic trachea, initial encounter	
		S27.52XA	Contusion of thoracic trachea, initial encounter	
		S27.53XA	Laceration of thoracic trachea, initial encounter	
		S27.59XA	Other injury of thoracic trachea, initial encounter	
		S27.60XA	Unspecified injury of pleura, initial encounter	
		S27.63XA	Laceration of pleura, initial encounter	
		S27.69XA	Other injury of pleura, initial encounter	
		S27.892A	Contusion of oth intrathoracic organs, init encntr	
		S27.893A	Laceration of oth intrathoracic organs, init encntr	
		S27.898A	Other injury of oth intrathoracic organs, init encntr	
		S27.899A	Unspecified injury of oth intrathoracic organs, init encntr	
862.31	BRONCHUS INJURY WITH OPEN WOUND INTO CAVITY	**S27.409A**	Unspecified injury of bronchus, unspecified, init encntr	*and*
		S21.309A	Unsp opn wnd unsp front wall of thrx w penet thor cav, init	
862.32	ESOPHAGUS INJURY WITH OPEN WOUND INTO CAVITY	**S27.813A**	Laceration of esophagus (thoracic part), initial encounter	*and*
		S21.309A	Unsp opn wnd unsp front wall of thrx w penet thor cav, init	
862.39	INJR OTH SPEC INTRATHOR ORGN W/OPEN WND CAV OTH	**S27.893A**	Laceration of oth intrathoracic organs, init encntr	*and*
		S21.309A	Unsp opn wnd unsp front wall of thrx w penet thor cav, init	
862.8	INJR MX&UNS INTRATHR ORGN W/O OPN WND IN CAV	**S27.9XXA**	Injury of unspecified intrathoracic organ, initial encounter	
862.9	INJURY MX&UNS INTRATHOR ORGN W/OPEN WOUND IN CAV	**S27.9XXA**	Injury of unspecified intrathoracic organ, initial encounter	*and*
		S21.309A	Unsp opn wnd unsp front wall of thrx w penet thor cav, init	
		S21.301A	Unsp opn wnd r frnt wl of thorax w penet thor cavity, init	
		S21.302A	Unsp opn wnd l frnt wl of thorax w penet thor cavity, init	
		S21.311A	Lac w/o fb of r frnt wl of thorax w penet thor cavity, init	
		S21.312A	Lac w/o fb of l frnt wl of thorax w penet thor cavity, init	
		S21.319A	Lac w/o fb of unsp front wall of thrx w penet thor cav, init	
		S21.321A	Lac w fb of r frnt wl of thorax w penet thor cavity, init	
		S21.322A	Lac w fb of l frnt wl of thorax w penet thor cavity, init	
		S21.329A	Lac w fb of unsp front wall of thorax w penet thor cav, init	
		S21.331A	Pnctr w/o fb of r frnt wl of thorax w penet thor cav, init	
		S21.332A	Pnctr w/o fb of l frnt wl of thorax w penet thor cav, init	
		S21.339A	Pnctr w/o fb of unsp frnt wl of thrx w penet thor cav, init	
		S21.341A	Pnctr w fb of r frnt wl of thorax w penet thor cavity, init	
		S21.342A	Pnctr w fb of l frnt wl of thorax w penet thor cavity, init	
		S21.349A	Pnctr w fb of unsp front wall of thrx w penet thor cav, init	
		S21.351A	Open bite of r frnt wl of thorax w penet thor cavity, init	
		S21.352A	Open bite of l frnt wl of thorax w penet thor cavity, init	
		S21.359A	Open bite of unsp front wall of thrx w penet thor cav, init	
		S21.401A	Unsp opn wnd r bk wl of thorax w penet thoracic cavity, init	
		S21.402A	Unsp opn wnd l bk wl of thorax w penet thoracic cavity, init	
		S21.409A	Unsp opn wnd unsp bk wl of thorax w penet thor cavity, init	

(Continued on next page)

[Brackets] indicate valid character values for each code. Character value meanings provided for each code grouping.

ICD-9-CM		ICD-10-CM		
862.9	INJURY MX&UNS INTRATHOR ORGN W/OPEN WOUND IN CAV (Continued)	S21.411A	Lac w/o fb of r bk wl of thorax w penet thor cavity, init	
		S21.412A	Lac w/o fb of l bk wl of thorax w penet thor cavity, init	
		S21.419A	Lac w/o fb of unsp bk wl of thorax w penet thor cavity, init	
		S21.421A	Lac w fb of r bk wl of thorax w penet thoracic cavity, init	
		S21.422A	Lac w fb of l bk wl of thorax w penet thoracic cavity, init	
		S21.429A	Lac w fb of unsp bk wl of thorax w penet thor cavity, init	
		S21.431A	Pnctr w/o fb of r bk wl of thorax w penet thor cavity, init	
		S21.432A	Pnctr w/o fb of l bk wl of thorax w penet thor cavity, init	
		S21.439A	Pnctr w/o fb of unsp bk wl of thorax w penet thor cav, init	
		S21.441A	Pnctr w fb of r bk wl of thorax w penet thor cavity, init	
		S21.442A	Pnctr w fb of l bk wl of thorax w penet thor cavity, init	
		S21.449A	Pnctr w fb of unsp bk wl of thorax w penet thor cavity, init	
		S21.451A	Open bite of r bk wl of thorax w penet thoracic cavity, init	
		S21.452A	Open bite of l bk wl of thorax w penet thoracic cavity, init	
		S21.459A	Open bite of unsp bk wl of thorax w penet thor cavity, init	
863.0	STOMACH INJURY W/O MENTION OPEN WOUND IN CAVITY	S36.30XA	Unspecified injury of stomach, initial encounter	
		S36.32XA	Contusion of stomach, initial encounter	
		S36.33XA	Laceration of stomach, initial encounter	
		S36.39XA	Other injury of stomach, initial encounter	
863.1	STOMACH INJURY WITH OPEN WOUND INTO CAVITY	S36.30XA	Unspecified injury of stomach, initial encounter	and
		S31.609A	Unsp opn wnd abd wall, unsp quadrant w penet perit cav, init	
863.20	SM INTST INJR UNS SITE W/O OPN WND IN CAV	S36.409A	Unsp injury of unsp part of small intestine, init encntr	
		S36.419A	Primary blast injury of unsp part of small intestine, init	
		S36.429A	Contusion of unsp part of small intestine, init encntr	
		S36.439A	Laceration of unsp part of small intestine, init encntr	
		S36.499A	Other injury of unsp part of small intestine, init encntr	
863.21	DUODENUM INJURY W/O MENTION OPEN WOUND IN CAVITY	S36.400A	Unspecified injury of duodenum, initial encounter	
		S36.410A	Primary blast injury of duodenum, initial encounter	
		S36.420A	Contusion of duodenum, initial encounter	
		S36.430A	Laceration of duodenum, initial encounter	
		S36.490A	Other injury of duodenum, initial encounter	
863.29	OTH INJURY SM INTST W/O MENTION OPN WOUND IN CAV	S36.408A	Unsp injury of other part of small intestine, init encntr	
		S36.418A	Primary blast injury oth prt small intestine, init encntr	
		S36.428A	Contusion of other part of small intestine, init encntr	
		S36.438A	Laceration of other part of small intestine, init encntr	
		S36.498A	Other injury of other part of small intestine, init encntr	
863.30	SM INTEST INJURY UNSPEC SITE W/OPEN WOUND IN CAV	S36.409A	Unsp injury of unsp part of small intestine, init encntr	and
		S31.609A	Unsp opn wnd abd wall, unsp quadrant w penet perit cav, init	
863.31	DUODENUM INJURY WITH OPEN WOUND INTO CAVITY	S36.400A	Unspecified injury of duodenum, initial encounter	and
		S31.609A	Unsp opn wnd abd wall, unsp quadrant w penet perit cav, init	
863.39	OTH INJURY SM INTESTINE W/OPEN WOUND INTO CAVITY	S36.408A	Unsp injury of other part of small intestine, init encntr	and
		S31.609A	Unsp opn wnd abd wall, unsp quadrant w penet perit cav, init	
863.40	COLON INJURY UNS SITE W/O MENTION OPN WND IN CAV	S36.509A	Unspecified injury of unspecified part of colon, init encntr	
		S36.519A	Primary blast injury of unsp part of colon, init encntr	
		S36.529A	Contusion of unspecified part of colon, initial encounter	
		S36.539A	Laceration of unspecified part of colon, initial encounter	
		S36.599A	Other injury of unspecified part of colon, initial encounter	
863.41	ASCEND COLON INJURY W/O MENTION OPN WOUND IN CAV	S36.500A	Unspecified injury of ascending colon, initial encounter	
		S36.510A	Primary blast injury of ascending colon, initial encounter	
		S36.520A	Contusion of ascending [right] colon, initial encounter	
		S36.530A	Laceration of ascending [right] colon, initial encounter	
		S36.590A	Other injury of ascending [right] colon, initial encounter	
863.42	TRNS COLON INJURY W/O MENTION OPN WOUND IN CAV	S36.501A	Unspecified injury of transverse colon, initial encounter	
		S36.511A	Primary blast injury of transverse colon, initial encounter	
		S36.521A	Contusion of transverse colon, initial encounter	
		S36.531A	Laceration of transverse colon, initial encounter	
		S36.591A	Other injury of transverse colon, initial encounter	
863.43	DESCEND COLON INJURY W/O MENTION OPN WND IN CAV	S36.502A	Unspecified injury of descending colon, initial encounter	
		S36.512A	Primary blast injury of descending colon, initial encounter	
		S36.522A	Contusion of descending [left] colon, initial encounter	
		S36.532A	Laceration of descending [left] colon, initial encounter	
		S36.592A	Other injury of descending [left] colon, initial encounter	
863.44	SIGMOID COLON INJURY W/O MENTION OPN WND IN CAV	S36.503A	Unspecified injury of sigmoid colon, initial encounter	
		S36.513A	Primary blast injury of sigmoid colon, initial encounter	
		S36.523A	Contusion of sigmoid colon, initial encounter	
		S36.533A	Laceration of sigmoid colon, initial encounter	
		S36.593A	Other injury of sigmoid colon, initial encounter	
863.45	RECT INJURY W/O MENTION OPEN WOUND INTO CAVITY	S36.60XA	Unspecified injury of rectum, initial encounter	
		S36.61XA	Primary blast injury of rectum, initial encounter	
		S36.62XA	Contusion of rectum, initial encounter	
		S36.63XA	Laceration of rectum, initial encounter	
		S36.69XA	Other injury of rectum, initial encounter	
863.46	INJR MX SITE COLON&RECT W/O OPN WND IN CAV	S36.508A	Unspecified injury of other part of colon, initial encounter	
		S36.518A	Primary blast injury of other part of colon, init encntr	
		S36.528A	Contusion of other part of colon, initial encounter	
		S36.538A	Laceration of other part of colon, initial encounter	
		S36.598A	Other injury of other part of colon, initial encounter	

ICD-9-CM		ICD-10-CM		
863.49	OTH COLON&RECT INJURY W/O MENTION OPN WND IN CAV	**S36.508A**	Unspecified injury of other part of colon, initial encounter	
		S36.518A	Primary blast injury of other part of colon, init encntr	
		S36.528A	Contusion of other part of colon, initial encounter	
		S36.538A	Laceration of other part of colon, initial encounter	
		S36.598A	Other injury of other part of colon, initial encounter	
863.50	COLON INJURY UNSPEC SITE W/OPEN WOUND IN CAVITY	**S36.509A**	Unspecified injury of unspecified part of colon, init encntr	*and*
		S31.609A	Unsp opn wnd abd wall, unsp quadrant w penet perit cav, init	
863.51	ASCENDING COLON INJURY W/OPEN WOUND INTO CAVITY	**S36.500A**	Unspecified injury of ascending colon, initial encounter	*and*
		S31.609A	Unsp opn wnd abd wall, unsp quadrant w penet perit cav, init	
863.52	TRANSVERSE COLON INJURY W/OPEN WOUND INTO CAVITY	**S36.501A**	Unspecified injury of transverse colon, initial encounter	*and*
		S31.609A	Unsp opn wnd abd wall, unsp quadrant w penet perit cav, init	
863.53	DESCENDING COLON INJURY W/OPEN WOUND INTO CAVITY	**S36.502A**	Unspecified injury of descending colon, initial encounter	*and*
		S31.609A	Unsp opn wnd abd wall, unsp quadrant w penet perit cav, init	
863.54	SIGMOID COLON INJURY WITH OPEN WOUND INTO CAVITY	**S36.503A**	Unspecified injury of sigmoid colon, initial encounter	*and*
		S31.609A	Unsp opn wnd abd wall, unsp quadrant w penet perit cav, init	
863.55	RECTUM INJURY WITH OPEN WOUND INTO CAVITY	**S36.60XA**	Unspecified injury of rectum, initial encounter	*and*
		S31.609A	Unsp opn wnd abd wall, unsp quadrant w penet perit cav, init	
863.56	INJURY MX SITES COLON&RECT W/OPEN WOUND IN CAV	**S36.508A**	Unspecified injury of other part of colon, initial encounter	*and*
		S31.609A	Unsp opn wnd abd wall, unsp quadrant w penet perit cav, init	
863.59	OTH INJURY COLON&RECTUM W/OPEN WOUND INTO CAVITY	**S36.508A**	Unspecified injury of other part of colon, initial encounter	*and*
		S31.609A	Unsp opn wnd abd wall, unsp quadrant w penet perit cav, init	
863.80	GI TRACT INJR UNS SITE W/O OPN WND IN CAV	**S36.90XA**	Unsp injury of unsp intra-abdominal organ, init encntr	
863.81	PANC HEAD INJURY W/O MENTION OPN WOUND IN CAVITY	**S36.200A**	Unspecified injury of head of pancreas, initial encounter	
		S36.220A	Contusion of head of pancreas, initial encounter	
		S36.230A	Laceration of head of pancreas, unsp degree, init encntr	
		S36.240A	Minor laceration of head of pancreas, initial encounter	
		S36.250A	Moderate laceration of head of pancreas, initial encounter	
		S36.260A	Major laceration of head of pancreas, initial encounter	
		S36.290A	Other injury of head of pancreas, initial encounter	
863.82	PANC BODY INJURY W/O MENTION OPN WOUND IN CAVITY	**S36.201A**	Unspecified injury of body of pancreas, initial encounter	
		S36.221A	Contusion of body of pancreas, initial encounter	
		S36.231A	Laceration of body of pancreas, unsp degree, init encntr	
		S36.241A	Minor laceration of body of pancreas, initial encounter	
		S36.251A	Moderate laceration of body of pancreas, initial encounter	
		S36.261A	Major laceration of body of pancreas, initial encounter	
		S36.291A	Other injury of body of pancreas, initial encounter	
863.83	PANC TAIL INJURY W/O MENTION OPN WOUND IN CAVITY	**S36.202A**	Unspecified injury of tail of pancreas, initial encounter	
		S36.222A	Contusion of tail of pancreas, initial encounter	
		S36.232A	Laceration of tail of pancreas, unsp degree, init encntr	
		S36.242A	Minor laceration of tail of pancreas, initial encounter	
		S36.252A	Moderate laceration of tail of pancreas, initial encounter	
		S36.262A	Major laceration of tail of pancreas, initial encounter	
		S36.292A	Other injury of tail of pancreas, initial encounter	
863.84	PANC INJR MX&UNS SITE W/O MENTION OPN WND IN CAV	**S36.209A**	Unsp injury of unspecified part of pancreas, init encntr	
		S36.229A	Contusion of unspecified part of pancreas, initial encounter	
		S36.239A	Laceration of unsp part of pancreas, unsp degree, init	
		S36.249A	Minor laceration of unsp part of pancreas, init encntr	
		S36.259A	Moderate laceration of unsp part of pancreas, init encntr	
		S36.269A	Major laceration of unsp part of pancreas, init encntr	
		S36.299A	Other injury of unspecified part of pancreas, init encntr	
863.85	APPDX INJURY W/O MENTION OPEN WOUND INTO CAVITY	**S36.899A**	Unsp injury of other intra-abdominal organs, init encntr	
863.89	INJR OTH&UNS GI SITE W/O MEN OPN WND IN CAV OTH	**S36.899A**	Unsp injury of other intra-abdominal organs, init encntr	
863.90	GI TRACT INJURY UNSPEC SITE W/OPEN WOUND IN CAV	**S36.90XA**	Unsp injury of unsp intra-abdominal organ, init encntr	*and*
		S31.609A	Unsp opn wnd abd wall, unsp quadrant w penet perit cav, init	
863.91	PANCREAS HEAD INJURY WITH OPEN WOUND INTO CAVITY	**S36.200A**	Unspecified injury of head of pancreas, initial encounter	*and*
		S31.609A	Unsp opn wnd abd wall, unsp quadrant w penet perit cav, init	
863.92	PANCREAS BODY INJURY WITH OPEN WOUND INTO CAVITY	**S36.201A**	Unspecified injury of body of pancreas, initial encounter	*and*
		S31.609A	Unsp opn wnd abd wall, unsp quadrant w penet perit cav, init	
863.93	PANCREAS TAIL INJURY WITH OPEN WOUND INTO CAVITY	**S36.202A**	Unspecified injury of tail of pancreas, initial encounter	*and*
		S31.609A	Unsp opn wnd abd wall, unsp quadrant w penet perit cav, init	
863.94	PANC INJURY MX&UNSPEC SITES W/OPEN WOUND IN CAV	**S36.209A**	Unsp injury of unspecified part of pancreas, init encntr	*and*
		S31.609A	Unsp opn wnd abd wall, unsp quadrant w penet perit cav, init	
863.95	APPENDIX INJURY WITH OPEN WOUND INTO CAVITY	**S36.899A**	Unsp injury of other intra-abdominal organs, init encntr	*and*
		S31.609A	Unsp opn wnd abd wall, unsp quadrant w penet perit cav, init	
863.99	INJR OTH&UNSPEC GI SITES W/OPEN WOUND IN CAV OTH	**S36.899A**	Unsp injury of other intra-abdominal organs, init encntr	*and*
		S31.609A	Unsp opn wnd abd wall, unsp quadrant w penet perit cav, init	
864.00	UNSPEC INJURY LIVR W/O MENTION OPN WOUND IN CAV	**S36.119A**	Unspecified injury of liver, initial encounter	
864.01	LIVER HEMAT&CONTUS W/O MENTION OPN WOUND IN CAV	**S36.112A**	Contusion of liver, initial encounter	
864.02	LIVER LAC MINOR W/O MENTION OPN WOUND IN CAV	**S36.114A**	Minor laceration of liver, initial encounter	

[Brackets] indicate valid character values for each code. Character value meanings provided for each code grouping.

ICD-9-CM		ICD-10-CM		
864.Ø3	LIVER LAC MOD W/O MENTION OPN WOUND IN CAV	**S36.115A**	Moderate laceration of liver, initial encounter	
864.Ø4	LIVER LAC MAJ W/O MENTION OPN WOUND IN CAV	**S36.116A**	Major laceration of liver, initial encounter	
864.Ø5	LIVER INJURY W/O MENTION OPN WND IN CAV UNS LAC	**S36.113A**	Laceration of liver, unspecified degree, initial encounter	
864.Ø9	OTH LIVR INJURY W/O MENTION OPEN WOUND IN CAVITY	**S36.118A**	Other injury of liver, initial encounter	
864.1Ø	UNSPEC LIVER INJURY W/OPEN WOUND INTO CAVITY	**S36.119A**	Unspecified injury of liver, initial encounter	*and*
		S31.6Ø9A	Unsp opn wnd abd wall, unsp quadrant w penet perit cav, init	
864.11	LIVER HEMATOMA&CONTUS W/OPEN WOUND INTO CAVITY	**S36.112A**	Contusion of liver, initial encounter	*and*
		S31.6Ø9A	Unsp opn wnd abd wall, unsp quadrant w penet perit cav, init	
864.12	LIVER LACERATION MINOR W/OPEN WOUND INTO CAVITY	**S36.114A**	Minor laceration of liver, initial encounter	*and*
		S31.6Ø9A	Unsp opn wnd abd wall, unsp quadrant w penet perit cav, init	
864.13	LIVER LACERATION MOD W/OPEN WOUND INTO CAVITY	**S36.115A**	Moderate laceration of liver, initial encounter	*and*
		S31.6Ø9A	Unsp opn wnd abd wall, unsp quadrant w penet perit cav, init	
864.14	LIVER LACERATION MAJOR W/OPEN WOUND INTO CAVITY	**S36.116A**	Major laceration of liver, initial encounter	*and*
		S31.6Ø9A	Unsp opn wnd abd wall, unsp quadrant w penet perit cav, init	
864.15	LIVER INJURY W/OPEN WOUND IN CAV UNSPEC LAC	**S36.113A**	Laceration of liver, unspecified degree, initial encounter	*and*
		S31.6Ø9A	Unsp opn wnd abd wall, unsp quadrant w penet perit cav, init	
864.19	OTHER LIVER INJURY WITH OPEN WOUND INTO CAVITY	**S36.118A**	Other injury of liver, initial encounter	*and*
		S31.6Ø9A	Unsp opn wnd abd wall, unsp quadrant w penet perit cav, init	
865.ØØ	UNS SPLEEN INJURY W/O MENTION OPN WOUND IN CAV	**S36.ØØXA**	Unspecified injury of spleen, initial encounter	
865.Ø1	SPLEEN HEMAT W/O RUP CAP/MENTION OPN WND IN CAV	**S36.Ø2ØA**	Minor contusion of spleen, initial encounter	
		S36.Ø21A	Major contusion of spleen, initial encounter	
		S36.Ø29A	Unspecified contusion of spleen, initial encounter	
865.Ø2	SPLEEN INJR CAPSUL TEARS W/O MAJ DISRUP PARENCH	**S36.Ø3ØA**	Superficial (capsular) laceration of spleen, init encntr	
865.Ø3	SPLEEN LAC EXT IN PARENCHYMA W/O OPN WND IN CAV	**S36.Ø31A**	Moderate laceration of spleen, initial encounter	
865.Ø4	SPLEEN INJR MASSIV PARENCH DISRUP W/O OP WND CAV	**S36.Ø32A**	Major laceration of spleen, initial encounter	
865.Ø9	OTH SPLEEN INJURY W/O MENTION OPN WOUND IN CAV	**S36.Ø39A**	Unspecified laceration of spleen, initial encounter	
		S36.Ø9XA	Other injury of spleen, initial encounter	
865.1Ø	UNSPEC SPLEEN INJURY W/OPEN WOUND INTO CAVITY	**S36.ØØXA**	Unspecified injury of spleen, initial encounter	*and*
		S31.6Ø9A	Unsp opn wnd abd wall, unsp quadrant w penet perit cav, init	
865.11	SPLEEN HEMAT W/O RUPTURE CAP W/OPEN WOUND IN CAV	**S36.Ø2ØA**	Minor contusion of spleen, initial encounter	*or*
		S36.Ø21A	Major contusion of spleen, initial encounter	*or*
		S36.Ø29A	Unspecified contusion of spleen, initial encounter	*and*
		S31.6Ø9A	Unsp opn wnd abd wall, unsp quadrant w penet perit cav, init	
865.12	SPLEEN CAPSUL TEARS W/O DISRUP PARENCH W/WND CAV	**S36.Ø3ØA**	Superficial (capsular) laceration of spleen, init encntr	*and*
		S31.6Ø9A	Unsp opn wnd abd wall, unsp quadrant w penet perit cav, init	
865.13	SPLEEN LAC EXT IN PARENCHYMA W/OPEN WOUND IN CAV	**S36.Ø31A**	Moderate laceration of spleen, initial encounter	*and*
		S31.6Ø9A	Unsp opn wnd abd wall, unsp quadrant w penet perit cav, init	
865.14	SPLEEN MASSIVE PARENCHYMAL DISRUPT W/OPN WND CAV	**S36.Ø32A**	Major laceration of spleen, initial encounter	*and*
		S31.6Ø9A	Unsp opn wnd abd wall, unsp quadrant w penet perit cav, init	
865.19	OTHER SPLEEN INJURY WITH OPEN WOUND INTO CAVITY	**S36.Ø9XA**	Other injury of spleen, initial encounter	*and*
		S31.6Ø9A	Unsp opn wnd abd wall, unsp quadrant w penet perit cav, init	
866.ØØ	UNS KIDNEY INJURY W/O MENTION OPN WOUND IN CAV	**S37.ØØ1A**	Unspecified injury of right kidney, initial encounter	
		S37.ØØ2A	Unspecified injury of left kidney, initial encounter	
		S37.ØØ9A	Unspecified injury of unspecified kidney, initial encounter	
866.Ø1	KIDNEY HEMAT W/O RUP CAP/MENTION OPN WND IN CAV	**S37.Ø11A**	Minor contusion of right kidney, initial encounter	
		S37.Ø12A	Minor contusion of left kidney, initial encounter	
		S37.Ø19A	Minor contusion of unspecified kidney, initial encounter	
		S37.Ø21A	Major contusion of right kidney, initial encounter	
		S37.Ø22A	Major contusion of left kidney, initial encounter	
		S37.Ø29A	Major contusion of unspecified kidney, initial encounter	
866.Ø2	KIDNEY LACERATION W/O MENTION OPN WOUND IN CAV	**S37.Ø31A**	Laceration of right kidney, unspecified degree, init encntr	
		S37.Ø32A	Laceration of left kidney, unspecified degree, init encntr	
		S37.Ø39A	Laceration of unsp kidney, unspecified degree, init encntr	
		S37.Ø41A	Minor laceration of right kidney, initial encounter	
		S37.Ø42A	Minor laceration of left kidney, initial encounter	
		S37.Ø49A	Minor laceration of unspecified kidney, initial encounter	
		S37.Ø51A	Moderate laceration of right kidney, initial encounter	
		S37.Ø52A	Moderate laceration of left kidney, initial encounter	
		S37.Ø59A	Moderate laceration of unspecified kidney, initial encounter	
866.Ø3	CMPL DISRUPT KIDNEY PARENCHYMA W/O OP WND CAV	**S37.Ø61A**	Major laceration of right kidney, initial encounter	
		S37.Ø62A	Major laceration of left kidney, initial encounter	
		S37.Ø69A	Major laceration of unspecified kidney, initial encounter	
		S37.Ø91A	Other injury of right kidney, initial encounter	
		S37.Ø92A	Other injury of left kidney, initial encounter	
		S37.Ø99A	Other injury of unspecified kidney, initial encounter	
866.1Ø	UNSPEC IKIDNEY INJURY W/OPEN WOUND INTO CAVITY	**S37.ØØ9A**	Unspecified injury of unspecified kidney, initial encounter	*and*
		S31.ØØ1A	Unsp opn wnd low back and pelvis w penet retroperiton, init	

ICD-9-CM		ICD-10-CM		
866.11	KIDNEY HEMAT W/O RUPTURE CAP W/OPEN WOUND IN CAV	**S37.019A**	Minor contusion of unspecified kidney, initial encounter	*or*
		S37.029A	Major contusion of unspecified kidney, initial encounter	*and*
		S31.001A	Unsp opn wnd low back and pelvis w penet retroperiton, init	
866.12	KIDNEY LACERATION WITH OPEN WOUND INTO CAVITY	**S37.039A**	Laceration of unsp kidney, unspecified degree, init encntr	*or*
		S37.049A	Minor laceration of unspecified kidney, initial encounter	*or*
		S37.059A	Moderate laceration of unspecified kidney, initial encounter	*and*
		S31.001A	Unsp opn wnd low back and pelvis w penet retroperiton, init	
866.13	CMPL DISRUPT KIDNEY PARENCHYMA W/OPEN WND IN CAV	**S37.069A**	Major laceration of unspecified kidney, initial encounter	*and*
		S31.001A	Unsp opn wnd low back and pelvis w penet retroperiton, init	
867.0	BLADD&URETHRA INJURY W/O MENTION OPN WND IN CAV	**S37.20XA**	Unspecified injury of bladder, initial encounter	
		S37.22XA	Contusion of bladder, initial encounter	
		S37.23XA	Laceration of bladder, initial encounter	
		S37.29XA	Other injury of bladder, initial encounter	
		S37.30XA	Unspecified injury of urethra, initial encounter	
		S37.32XA	Contusion of urethra, initial encounter	
		S37.33XA	Laceration of urethra, initial encounter	
		S37.39XA	Other injury of urethra, initial encounter	
867.1	BLADDER&URETHRA INJURY W/OPEN WOUND INTO CAVITY	**S37.20XA**	Unspecified injury of bladder, initial encounter	*or*
		S37.30XA	Unspecified injury of urethra, initial encounter	*and*
		S31.001A	Unsp opn wnd low back and pelvis w penet retroperiton, init	
867.2	URETER INJURY W/O MENTION OPEN WOUND INTO CAVITY	**S37.10XA**	Unspecified injury of ureter, initial encounter	
		S37.12XA	Contusion of ureter, initial encounter	
		S37.13XA	Laceration of ureter, initial encounter	
		S37.19XA	Other injury of ureter, initial encounter	
867.3	URETER INJURY WITH OPEN WOUND INTO CAVITY	**S37.10XA**	Unspecified injury of ureter, initial encounter	*and*
		S31.001A	Unsp opn wnd low back and pelvis w penet retroperiton, init	
867.4	UTERUS INJURY W/O MENTION OPEN WOUND INTO CAVITY	**S37.60XA**	Unspecified injury of uterus, initial encounter	
		S37.62XA	Contusion of uterus, initial encounter	
		S37.63XA	Laceration of uterus, initial encounter	
		S37.69XA	Other injury of uterus, initial encounter	
867.5	UTERUS INJURY WITH OPEN WOUND INTO CAVITY	**S37.60XA**	Unspecified injury of uterus, initial encounter	*and*
		S31.001A	Unsp opn wnd low back and pelvis w penet retroperiton, init	
867.6	INJR OTH SPEC PELV ORGN W/O OPN WND IN CAV	**S37.401A**	Unspecified injury of ovary, unilateral, initial encounter	
		S37.402A	Unspecified injury of ovary, bilateral, initial encounter	
		S37.409A	Unspecified injury of ovary, unspecified, initial encounter	
		S37.421A	Contusion of ovary, unilateral, initial encounter	
		S37.422A	Contusion of ovary, bilateral, initial encounter	
		S37.429A	Contusion of ovary, unspecified, initial encounter	
		S37.431A	Laceration of ovary, unilateral, initial encounter	
		S37.432A	Laceration of ovary, bilateral, initial encounter	
		S37.439A	Laceration of ovary, unspecified, initial encounter	
		S37.491A	Other injury of ovary, unilateral, initial encounter	
		S37.492A	Other injury of ovary, bilateral, initial encounter	
		S37.499A	Other injury of ovary, unspecified, initial encounter	
		S37.501A	Unsp injury of fallopian tube, unilateral, init encntr	
		S37.502A	Unspecified injury of fallopian tube, bilateral, init encntr	
		S37.509A	Unsp injury of fallopian tube, unspecified, init encntr	
		S37.511A	Primary blast injury of fallopian tube, unilateral, init	
		S37.512A	Primary blast injury of fallopian tube, bilateral, init	
		S37.519A	Primary blast injury of fallopian tube, unsp, init encntr	
		S37.521A	Contusion of fallopian tube, unilateral, initial encounter	
		S37.522A	Contusion of fallopian tube, bilateral, initial encounter	
		S37.529A	Contusion of fallopian tube, unspecified, initial encounter	
		S37.531A	Laceration of fallopian tube, unilateral, initial encounter	
		S37.532A	Laceration of fallopian tube, bilateral, initial encounter	
		S37.539A	Laceration of fallopian tube, unspecified, initial encounter	
		S37.591A	Other injury of fallopian tube, unilateral, init encntr	
		S37.592A	Other injury of fallopian tube, bilateral, initial encounter	
		S37.599A	Other injury of fallopian tube, unspecified, init encntr	
		S37.822A	Contusion of prostate, initial encounter	
		S37.823A	Laceration of prostate, initial encounter	
		S37.828A	Other injury of prostate, initial encounter	
		S37.829A	Unspecified injury of prostate, initial encounter	
		S37.892A	Contusion of other urinary and pelvic organ, init encntr	
		S37.893A	Laceration of other urinary and pelvic organ, init encntr	
		S37.898A	Other injury of other urinary and pelvic organ, init encntr	
		S37.899A	Unsp injury of other urinary and pelvic organ, init encntr	
867.7	INJURY OTH SPEC PELV ORGN W/OPEN WOUND IN CAVITY	**S37.409A**	Unspecified injury of ovary, unspecified, initial encounter	*or*
		S37.509A	Unsp injury of fallopian tube, unspecified, init encntr	*or*
		S37.829A	Unspecified injury of prostate, initial encounter	*or*
		S37.899A	Unsp injury of other urinary and pelvic organ, init encntr	*and*
		S31.001A	Unsp opn wnd low back and pelvis w penet retroperiton, init	
867.8	INJURY UNS PELV ORGN W/O MENTION OPN WND IN CAV	**S37.90XA**	Unsp injury of unsp urinary and pelvic organ, init encntr	
		S37.92XA	Contusion of unsp urinary and pelvic organ, init encntr	
		S37.93XA	Laceration of unsp urinary and pelvic organ, init encntr	
		S37.99XA	Other injury of unsp urinary and pelvic organ, init encntr	

[Brackets] indicate valid character values for each code. Character value meanings provided for each code grouping.

ICD-9-CM		ICD-10-CM		
867.9	INJURY UNSPEC PELV ORGAN W/OPEN WOUND IN CAVITY	**S37.90XA**	Unsp injury of unsp urinary and pelvic organ, init encntr	*and*
		S31.001A	Unsp opn wnd low back and pelvis w penet retroperiton, init	
868.00	INJR UNS INTRA-ABD ORGN W/O OPN WND IN CAV	**S36.90XA**	Unsp injury of unsp intra-abdominal organ, init encntr	
		S36.92XA	Contusion of unspecified intra-abdominal organ, init encntr	
		S36.93XA	Laceration of unspecified intra-abdominal organ, init encntr	
		S36.99XA	Other injury of unsp intra-abdominal organ, init encntr	
868.01	ADRENL GLAND INJURY W/O MENTION OPN WOUND IN CAV	**S37.812A**	Contusion of adrenal gland, initial encounter	
		S37.813A	Laceration of adrenal gland, initial encounter	
		S37.818A	Other injury of adrenal gland, initial encounter	
		S37.819A	Unspecified injury of adrenal gland, initial encounter	
868.02	BD&GALLBLADD INJURY W/O MENTION OPN WOUND IN CAV	**S36.122A**	Contusion of gallbladder, initial encounter	
		S36.123A	Laceration of gallbladder, initial encounter	
		S36.128A	Other injury of gallbladder, initial encounter	
		S36.129A	Unspecified injury of gallbladder, initial encounter	
		S36.13XA	Injury of bile duct, initial encounter	
868.03	PERITON INJURY W/O MENTION OPEN WOUND IN CAVITY	**S36.81XA**	Injury of peritoneum, initial encounter	
868.04	RETROPERITON INJURY W/O MENTION OPN WOUND IN CAV	**S36.892A**	Contusion of other intra-abdominal organs, initial encounter	
		S36.893A	Laceration of other intra-abdominal organs, init encntr	
		S36.898A	Other injury of other intra-abdominal organs, init encntr	
		S36.899A	Unsp injury of other intra-abdominal organs, init encntr	
868.09	INJR OTH&MX INTRA-ABD ORGN W/O OPN WND IN CAV	**S36.892A**	Contusion of other intra-abdominal organs, initial encounter	
		S36.893A	Laceration of other intra-abdominal organs, init encntr	
		S36.898A	Other injury of other intra-abdominal organs, init encntr	
		S36.899A	Unsp injury of other intra-abdominal organs, init encntr	
868.10	INJURY UNSPEC INTRA-ABD ORGN W/OPEN WOUND IN CAV	**S36.90XA**	Unsp injury of unsp intra-abdominal organ, init encntr	*and*
		S31.001A	Unsp opn wnd low back and pelvis w penet retroperiton, init	
868.11	ADRENAL GLAND INJURY WITH OPEN WOUND INTO CAVITY	**S37.819A**	Unspecified injury of adrenal gland, initial encounter	*and*
		S31.001A	Unsp opn wnd low back and pelvis w penet retroperiton, init	
868.12	BD&GALLBLADDER INJURY W/OPEN WOUND INTO CAVITY	**S36.129A**	Unspecified injury of gallbladder, initial encounter	*or*
		S36.13XA	Injury of bile duct, initial encounter	*and*
		S31.001A	Unsp opn wnd low back and pelvis w penet retroperiton, init	
868.13	PERITONEUM INJURY WITH OPEN WOUND INTO CAVITY	**S31.600A**	Unsp opn wnd abd wall, right upper q w penet perit cav, init	
		S31.601A	Unsp open wound of abd wall, l upr q w penet perit cav, init	
		S31.602A	Unsp opn wnd abd wall, epigst rgn w penet perit cav, init	
		S31.603A	Unsp opn wnd abd wall, right lower q w penet perit cav, init	
		S31.604A	Unsp opn wnd abd wall, left lower q w penet perit cav, init	
		S31.605A	Unsp opn wnd abd wall, periumb rgn w penet perit cav, init	
		S31.609A	Unsp opn wnd abd wall, unsp quadrant w penet perit cav, init	
		S31.610A	Lac w/o fb of abd wall, r upper q w penet perit cav, init	
		S31.611A	Lac w/o fb of abd wall, l upr q w penet perit cav, init	
		S31.612A	Lac w/o fb of abd wall, epigst rgn w penet perit cav, init	
		S31.613A	Lac w/o fb of abd wall, right low q w penet perit cav, init	
		S31.614A	Lac w/o fb of abd wall, left lower q w penet perit cav, init	
		S31.615A	Lac w/o fb of abd wall, periumb rgn w penet perit cav, init	
		S31.619A	Lac w/o fb of abd wall, unsp q w penet perit cav, init	
		S31.620A	Lac w fb of abd wall, right upper q w penet perit cav, init	
		S31.621A	Laceration w fb of abd wall, l upr q w penet perit cav, init	
		S31.622A	Lac w fb of abd wall, epigst rgn w penet perit cav, init	
		S31.623A	Lac w fb of abd wall, right lower q w penet perit cav, init	
		S31.624A	Lac w fb of abd wall, left lower q w penet perit cav, init	
		S31.625A	Lac w fb of abd wall, periumb rgn w penet perit cav, init	
		S31.629A	Lac w fb of abd wall, unsp quadrant w penet perit cav, init	
		S31.630A	Pnctr w/o fb of abd wall, r upper q w penet perit cav, init	
		S31.631A	Pnctr w/o fb of abd wall, l upr q w penet perit cav, init	
		S31.632A	Pnctr w/o fb of abd wall, epigst rgn w penet perit cav, init	
		S31.633A	Pnctr w/o fb of abd wall, r low q w penet perit cav, init	
		S31.634A	Pnctr w/o fb of abd wall, left low q w penet perit cav, init	
		S31.635A	Pnctr w/o fb of abd wl, periumb rgn w penet perit cav, init	
		S31.639A	Pnctr w/o fb of abd wall, unsp q w penet perit cav, init	
		S31.640A	Pnctr w fb of abd wall, r upper q w penet perit cav, init	
		S31.641A	Pnctr w fb of abd wall, l upr q w penet perit cav, init	
		S31.642A	Pnctr w fb of abd wall, epigst rgn w penet perit cav, init	
		S31.643A	Pnctr w fb of abd wall, right low q w penet perit cav, init	
		S31.644A	Pnctr w fb of abd wall, left lower q w penet perit cav, init	
		S31.645A	Pnctr w fb of abd wall, periumb rgn w penet perit cav, init	
		S31.649A	Pnctr w fb of abd wall, unsp q w penet perit cav, init	
		S31.650A	Open bite of abd wall, right upper q w penet perit cav, init	
		S31.651A	Open bite of abdominal wall, l upr q w penet perit cav, init	
		S31.652A	Open bite of abd wall, epigst rgn w penet perit cav, init	
		S31.653A	Open bite of abd wall, right lower q w penet perit cav, init	
		S31.654A	Open bite of abd wall, left lower q w penet perit cav, init	
		S31.655A	Open bite of abd wall, periumb rgn w penet perit cav, init	
		S31.659A	Open bite of abd wall, unsp quadrant w penet perit cav, init	
		S36.81XA	Injury of peritoneum, initial encounter	

ICD-9-CM		ICD-10-CM		
868.14	RETROPERITONEUM INJURY W/OPEN WOUND INTO CAVITY	S36.899A	Unsp injury of other intra-abdominal organs, init encntr	and
		S31.001A	Unsp opn wnd low back and pelvis w penet retroperiton, init	
		S31.011A	Lac w/o fb of low back and pelvis w penet retroperiton, init	
		S31.021A	Lac w fb of lower back and pelvis w penet retroperiton, init	
		S31.031A	Pnctr w/o fb of low back and pelv w penet retroperiton, init	
		S31.041A	Pnctr w fb of low back and pelvis w penet retroperiton, init	
		S31.051A	Open bite of low back and pelvis w penet retroperiton, init	
868.19	INJURY OTH&MX INTRA-ABD ORGN W/OPEN WOUND IN CAV	S36.899A	Unsp injury of other intra-abdominal organs, init encntr	and
		S31.001A	Unsp opn wnd low back and pelvis w penet retroperiton, init	
869.0	INTRL INJURY UNS ORGANS W/O OPEN WND IN CAVITY	S36.90XA	Unsp injury of unsp intra-abdominal organ, init encntr	
		S36.92XA	Contusion of unspecified intra-abdominal organ, init encntr	
		S36.93XA	Laceration of unspecified intra-abdominal organ, init encntr	
		S36.99XA	Other injury of unsp intra-abdominal organ, init encntr	
		S37.90XA	Unsp injury of unsp urinary and pelvic organ, init encntr	
		S37.92XA	Contusion of unsp urinary and pelvic organ, init encntr	
		S37.93XA	Laceration of unsp urinary and pelvic organ, init encntr	
		S37.99XA	Other injury of unsp urinary and pelvic organ, init encntr	
869.1	INTRL INJR UNS/ILL-DEFIND ORGN W/OPEN WND IN CAV	S36.90XA	Unsp injury of unsp intra-abdominal organ, init encntr	and
		S31.001A	Unsp opn wnd low back and pelvis w penet retroperiton, init	
		S37.90XA	Unsp injury of unsp urinary and pelvic organ, init encntr	and
		S31.001A	Unsp opn wnd low back and pelvis w penet retroperiton, init	
870.0	LACERATION OF SKIN OF EYELID AND PERIOCULAR AREA	S01.111A	Laceration w/o fb of right eyelid and periocular area, init	
		S01.112A	Laceration w/o fb of left eyelid and periocular area, init	
		S01.119A	Laceration w/o fb of unsp eyelid and periocular area, init	
		S01.121A	Laceration w fb of right eyelid and periocular area, init	
		S01.122A	Laceration w fb of left eyelid and periocular area, init	
		S01.129A	Laceration w fb of unsp eyelid and periocular area, init	
		S01.131A	Pnctr w/o fb of right eyelid and periocular area, init	
		S01.132A	Pnctr w/o fb of left eyelid and periocular area, init	
		S01.139A	Pnctr w/o fb of unsp eyelid and periocular area, init	
		S01.141A	Pnctr w fb of right eyelid and periocular area, init	
		S01.142A	Pnctr w fb of left eyelid and periocular area, init	
		S01.149A	Pnctr w fb of unsp eyelid and periocular area, init	
		S01.151A	Open bite of right eyelid and periocular area, init encntr	
		S01.152A	Open bite of left eyelid and periocular area, init encntr	
		S01.159A	Open bite of unsp eyelid and periocular area, init encntr	
870.1	LAC EYELD FULL-THICK NOT INVLV LAC PASSAGES	S01.119A	Laceration w/o fb of unsp eyelid and periocular area, init	
		S01.129A	Laceration w fb of unsp eyelid and periocular area, init	
		S01.139A	Pnctr w/o fb of unsp eyelid and periocular area, init	
		S01.149A	Pnctr w fb of unsp eyelid and periocular area, init	
		S01.159A	Open bite of unsp eyelid and periocular area, init encntr	
870.2	LACERATION OF EYELID INVOLVING LACRIMAL PASSAGES	S01.111A	Laceration w/o fb of right eyelid and periocular area, init	
		S01.112A	Laceration w/o fb of left eyelid and periocular area, init	
		S01.119A	Laceration w/o fb of unsp eyelid and periocular area, init	
		S01.121A	Laceration w fb of right eyelid and periocular area, init	
		S01.122A	Laceration w fb of left eyelid and periocular area, init	
		S01.129A	Laceration w fb of unsp eyelid and periocular area, init	
		S01.131A	Pnctr w/o fb of right eyelid and periocular area, init	
		S01.132A	Pnctr w/o fb of left eyelid and periocular area, init	
		S01.139A	Pnctr w/o fb of unsp eyelid and periocular area, init	
		S01.141A	Pnctr w fb of right eyelid and periocular area, init	
		S01.142A	Pnctr w fb of left eyelid and periocular area, init	
		S01.149A	Pnctr w fb of unsp eyelid and periocular area, init	
		S01.151A	Open bite of right eyelid and periocular area, init encntr	
		S01.152A	Open bite of left eyelid and periocular area, init encntr	
		S01.159A	Open bite of unsp eyelid and periocular area, init encntr	
870.3	PENETRATING WOUND ORBIT WITHOUT MENTION FB	S05.40XA	Penetrating wound of orbit w or w/o fb, unsp eye, init	
		S05.41XA	Penetrating wound of orbit w or w/o fb, right eye, init	
		S05.42XA	Penetrating wound of orbit w or w/o fb, left eye, init	
870.4	PENETRATING WOUND OF ORBIT WITH FOREIGN BODY	S05.40XA	Penetrating wound of orbit w or w/o fb, unsp eye, init	
		S05.41XA	Penetrating wound of orbit w or w/o fb, right eye, init	
		S05.42XA	Penetrating wound of orbit w or w/o fb, left eye, init	
870.8	OTHER SPECIFIED OPEN WOUND OF OCULAR ADNEXA	S01.101A	Unsp open wound of right eyelid and periocular area, init	
		S01.102A	Unsp open wound of left eyelid and periocular area, init	
		S01.109A	Unsp open wound of unsp eyelid and periocular area, init	
870.9	UNSPECIFIED OPEN WOUND OF OCULAR ADNEXA	S01.101A	Unsp open wound of right eyelid and periocular area, init	
		S01.102A	Unsp open wound of left eyelid and periocular area, init	
		S01.109A	Unsp open wound of unsp eyelid and periocular area, init	
871.0	OCULR LACERATION W/O PROLAPSE INTRAOCULR TISSUE	S05.30XA	Oclr lac w/o prolaps/loss of intraoc tissue, unsp eye, init	
		S05.31XA	Ocular lac w/o prolaps/loss of intraoc tissue, r eye, init	
		S05.32XA	Ocular lac w/o prolaps/loss of intraoc tissue, l eye, init	
871.1	OCULR LAC WITH PROLAPSE/EXPOS INTRAOCULR TISSUE	S05.20XA	Oclr lac/rupt w prolaps/loss of intraoc tiss, unsp eye, init	
		S05.21XA	Oclr lac/rupt w prolaps/loss of intraoc tissue, r eye, init	
		S05.22XA	Oclr lac/rupt w prolaps/loss of intraoc tissue, l eye, init	
871.2	RUPTURE EYE W/PARTIAL LOSS INTRAOCULAR TISSUE	S05.20XA	Oclr lac/rupt w prolaps/loss of intraoc tiss, unsp eye, init	
		S05.21XA	Oclr lac/rupt w prolaps/loss of intraoc tissue, r eye, init	
		S05.22XA	Oclr lac/rupt w prolaps/loss of intraoc tissue, l eye, init	

ICD-9-CM		ICD-10-CM	
871.3	AVULSION OF EYE	**SØ5.7ØXA**	Avulsion of unspecified eye, initial encounter
		SØ5.71XA	Avulsion of right eye, initial encounter
		SØ5.72XA	Avulsion of left eye, initial encounter
871.4	UNSPECIFIED LACERATION OF EYE	**SØ5.3ØXA**	Oclr lac w/o prolaps/loss of intraoc tissue, unsp eye, init
871.5	PENETRATION OF EYEBALL W/MAGNETIC FOREIGN BODY	**SØ5.5ØXA**	Penetrating wound w foreign body of unsp eyeball, init
		SØ5.51XA	Penetrating wound w foreign body of right eyeball, init
		SØ5.52XA	Penetrating wound w foreign body of left eyeball, init
871.6	PENETRATION OF EYEBALL WITH FOREIGN BODY	**SØ5.5ØXA**	Penetrating wound w foreign body of unsp eyeball, init
		SØ5.51XA	Penetrating wound w foreign body of right eyeball, init
		SØ5.52XA	Penetrating wound w foreign body of left eyeball, init
871.7	UNSPECIFIED OCULAR PENETRATION	**SØ5.6ØXA**	Penetrating wound w/o foreign body of unsp eyeball, init
		SØ5.61XA	Penetrating wound w/o foreign body of right eyeball, init
		SØ5.62XA	Penetrating wound w/o foreign body of left eyeball, init
871.9	UNSPECIFIED OPEN WOUND OF EYEBALL	**SØ5.8X1A**	Other injuries of right eye and orbit, initial encounter
		SØ5.8X2A	Other injuries of left eye and orbit, initial encounter
		SØ5.8X9A	Other injuries of unspecified eye and orbit, init encntr
		SØ5.9ØXA	Unspecified injury of unspecified eye and orbit, init encntr
		SØ5.91XA	Unspecified injury of right eye and orbit, initial encounter
		SØ5.92XA	Unspecified injury of left eye and orbit, initial encounter
872.ØØ	OPEN WOUND EXT EAR UNSPEC SITE W/O MENTION COMP	**SØ1.3Ø1A**	Unspecified open wound of right ear, initial encounter
		SØ1.3Ø2A	Unspecified open wound of left ear, initial encounter
		SØ1.3Ø9A	Unspecified open wound of unspecified ear, initial encounter
872.Ø1	OPEN WOUND AURICLE WITHOUT MENTION COMPLICATION	**SØ1.3Ø2A**	Unspecified open wound of left ear, initial encounter
		SØ1.3Ø9A	Unspecified open wound of unspecified ear, initial encounter
		SØ1.311A	Laceration without foreign body of right ear, init encntr
		SØ1.312A	Laceration without foreign body of left ear, init encntr
		SØ1.319A	Laceration without foreign body of unsp ear, init encntr
		SØ1.331A	Puncture wound w/o foreign body of right ear, init encntr
		SØ1.332A	Puncture wound without foreign body of left ear, init encntr
		SØ1.339A	Puncture wound without foreign body of unsp ear, init encntr
		SØ1.351A	Open bite of right ear, initial encounter
		SØ1.352A	Open bite of left ear, initial encounter
		SØ1.359A	Open bite of unspecified ear, initial encounter
		SØ8.111A	Complete traumatic amputation of right ear, init encntr
		SØ8.112A	Complete traumatic amputation of left ear, initial encounter
		SØ8.119A	Complete traumatic amputation of unsp ear, init encntr
		SØ8.121A	Partial traumatic amputation of right ear, initial encounter
		SØ8.122A	Partial traumatic amputation of left ear, initial encounter
		SØ8.129A	Partial traumatic amputation of unspecified ear, init encntr
872.Ø2	OPEN WOUND AUDITRY CANAL WITHOUT MENTION COMP	**SØ1.3Ø1A**	Unspecified open wound of right ear, initial encounter
		SØ1.3Ø2A	Unspecified open wound of left ear, initial encounter
		SØ1.3Ø9A	Unspecified open wound of unspecified ear, initial encounter
		SØ1.311A	Laceration without foreign body of right ear, init encntr
		SØ1.312A	Laceration without foreign body of left ear, init encntr
		SØ1.319A	Laceration without foreign body of unsp ear, init encntr
		SØ1.331A	Puncture wound w/o foreign body of right ear, init encntr
		SØ1.332A	Puncture wound without foreign body of left ear, init encntr
		SØ1.339A	Puncture wound without foreign body of unsp ear, init encntr
		SØ1.351A	Open bite of right ear, initial encounter
		SØ1.352A	Open bite of left ear, initial encounter
		SØ1.359A	Open bite of unspecified ear, initial encounter
872.1Ø	OPEN WOUND EXTERNAL EAR UNSPEC SITE COMPLICATED	**SØ1.321A**	Laceration with foreign body of right ear, initial encounter
		SØ1.322A	Laceration with foreign body of left ear, initial encounter
		SØ1.329A	Laceration with foreign body of unspecified ear, init encntr
		SØ1.341A	Puncture wound with foreign body of right ear, init encntr
		SØ1.342A	Puncture wound with foreign body of left ear, init encntr
		SØ1.349A	Puncture wound with foreign body of unsp ear, init encntr
872.11	OPEN WOUND OF AURICLE, COMPLICATED	**SØ1.329A**	Laceration with foreign body of unspecified ear, init encntr
872.12	OPEN WOUND OF AUDITORY CANAL COMPLICATED	**SØ1.329A**	Laceration with foreign body of unspecified ear, init encntr
872.61	OPEN WOUND EAR DRUM WITHOUT MENTION COMPLICATION	**SØ9.2ØXA**	Traumatic rupture of unspecified ear drum, initial encounter
		SØ9.21XA	Traumatic rupture of right ear drum, initial encounter
		SØ9.22XA	Traumatic rupture of left ear drum, initial encounter
872.62	OPEN WOUND OSSICLES WITHOUT MENTION COMPLICATION	**SØ9.3Ø1A**	Unsp injury of right middle and inner ear, init encntr
		SØ9.3Ø2A	Unspecified injury of left middle and inner ear, init encntr
		SØ9.3Ø9A	Unsp injury of unspecified middle and inner ear, init encntr
		SØ9.311A	Primary blast injury of right ear, initial encounter
		SØ9.312A	Primary blast injury of left ear, initial encounter
		SØ9.313A	Primary blast injury of ear, bilateral, initial encounter
		SØ9.319A	Primary blast injury of unspecified ear, initial encounter
		SØ9.391A	Oth injury of right middle and inner ear, init encntr
		SØ9.392A	Oth injury of left middle and inner ear, init encntr
		SØ9.399A	Oth injury of unspecified middle and inner ear, init encntr

ICD-9-CM		ICD-10-CM	
872.63	OPEN WOUND EUSTACHIAN TUBE WITHOUT MENTION COMP	**S09.301A**	Unsp injury of right middle and inner ear, init encntr
		S09.302A	Unspecified injury of left middle and inner ear, init encntr
		S09.309A	Unsp injury of unspecified middle and inner ear, init encntr
		S09.311A	Primary blast injury of right ear, initial encounter
		S09.312A	Primary blast injury of left ear, initial encounter
		S09.313A	Primary blast injury of ear, bilateral, initial encounter
		S09.319A	Primary blast injury of unspecified ear, initial encounter
		S09.391A	Oth injury of right middle and inner ear, init encntr
		S09.392A	Oth injury of left middle and inner ear, init encntr
		S09.399A	Oth injury of unspecified middle and inner ear, init encntr
872.64	OPEN WOUND COCHLEA WITHOUT MENTION COMPLICATION	**S09.301A**	Unsp injury of right middle and inner ear, init encntr
		S09.302A	Unspecified injury of left middle and inner ear, init encntr
		S09.309A	Unsp injury of unspecified middle and inner ear, init encntr
		S09.311A	Primary blast injury of right ear, initial encounter
		S09.312A	Primary blast injury of left ear, initial encounter
		S09.313A	Primary blast injury of ear, bilateral, initial encounter
		S09.319A	Primary blast injury of unspecified ear, initial encounter
		S09.391A	Oth injury of right middle and inner ear, init encntr
		S09.392A	Oth injury of left middle and inner ear, init encntr
		S09.399A	Oth injury of unspecified middle and inner ear, init encntr
872.69	OPEN WOUND OTH&MX SITES WITHOUT MENTION COMP	**S09.391A**	Oth injury of right middle and inner ear, init encntr
		S09.392A	Oth injury of left middle and inner ear, init encntr
		S09.399A	Oth injury of unspecified middle and inner ear, init encntr
872.71	OPEN WOUND OF EAR DRUM, COMPLICATED	**S09.20XA**	Traumatic rupture of unspecified ear drum, initial encounter
		S09.21XA	Traumatic rupture of right ear drum, initial encounter
		S09.22XA	Traumatic rupture of left ear drum, initial encounter
872.72	OPEN WOUND OF OSSICLES, COMPLICATED	**S09.301A**	Unsp injury of right middle and inner ear, init encntr
		S09.302A	Unspecified injury of left middle and inner ear, init encntr
		S09.309A	Unsp injury of unspecified middle and inner ear, init encntr
		S09.311A	Primary blast injury of right ear, initial encounter
		S09.312A	Primary blast injury of left ear, initial encounter
		S09.313A	Primary blast injury of ear, bilateral, initial encounter
		S09.319A	Primary blast injury of unspecified ear, initial encounter
		S09.391A	Oth injury of right middle and inner ear, init encntr
		S09.392A	Oth injury of left middle and inner ear, init encntr
		S09.399A	Oth injury of unspecified middle and inner ear, init encntr
872.73	OPEN WOUND OF EUSTACHIAN TUBE COMPLICATED	**S09.301A**	Unsp injury of right middle and inner ear, init encntr
		S09.302A	Unspecified injury of left middle and inner ear, init encntr
		S09.309A	Unsp injury of unspecified middle and inner ear, init encntr
		S09.311A	Primary blast injury of right ear, initial encounter
		S09.312A	Primary blast injury of left ear, initial encounter
		S09.313A	Primary blast injury of ear, bilateral, initial encounter
		S09.319A	Primary blast injury of unspecified ear, initial encounter
		S09.391A	Oth injury of right middle and inner ear, init encntr
		S09.392A	Oth injury of left middle and inner ear, init encntr
		S09.399A	Oth injury of unspecified middle and inner ear, init encntr
872.74	OPEN WOUND OF COCHLEA, COMPLICATED	**S09.301A**	Unsp injury of right middle and inner ear, init encntr
		S09.302A	Unspecified injury of left middle and inner ear, init encntr
		S09.309A	Unsp injury of unspecified middle and inner ear, init encntr
		S09.311A	Primary blast injury of right ear, initial encounter
		S09.312A	Primary blast injury of left ear, initial encounter
		S09.313A	Primary blast injury of ear, bilateral, initial encounter
		S09.319A	Primary blast injury of unspecified ear, initial encounter
		S09.391A	Oth injury of right middle and inner ear, init encntr
		S09.392A	Oth injury of left middle and inner ear, init encntr
		S09.399A	Oth injury of unspecified middle and inner ear, init encntr
872.79	OPEN WOUND OF OTHER&MULTIPLE SITES COMPLICATED	**S09.8XXA**	Other specified injuries of head, initial encounter
872.8	OPEN WOUND EAR PART UNSPEC WITHOUT MENTION COMP	**S09.91XA**	Unspecified injury of ear, initial encounter
872.9	OPEN WOUND OF EAR PART UNSPECIFIED COMPLICATED	**S09.91XA**	Unspecified injury of ear, initial encounter
873.0	OPEN WOUND SCALP WITHOUT MENTION COMPLICATION	**S01.00XA**	Unspecified open wound of scalp, initial encounter
		S01.01XA	Laceration without foreign body of scalp, initial encounter
		S01.03XA	Puncture wound without foreign body of scalp, init encntr
		S01.05XA	Open bite of scalp, initial encounter
		S08.0XXA	Avulsion of scalp, initial encounter
873.1	OPEN WOUND OF SCALP, COMPLICATED	**S01.02XA**	Laceration with foreign body of scalp, initial encounter
		S01.04XA	Puncture wound with foreign body of scalp, initial encounter
873.20	OPEN WOUND NOSE UNSPEC SITE WITHOUT MENTION COMP	**S01.20XA**	Unspecified open wound of nose, initial encounter
		S01.21XA	Laceration without foreign body of nose, initial encounter
		S01.23XA	Puncture wound without foreign body of nose, init encntr
		S01.25XA	Open bite of nose, initial encounter
873.21	OPEN WOUND NASAL SEPTUM WITHOUT MENTION COMP	**S01.20XA**	Unspecified open wound of nose, initial encounter
		S01.21XA	Laceration without foreign body of nose, initial encounter
		S01.23XA	Puncture wound without foreign body of nose, init encntr
		S01.25XA	Open bite of nose, initial encounter
873.22	OPEN WOUND NASAL CAVITY WITHOUT MENTION COMP	**S01.20XA**	Unspecified open wound of nose, initial encounter
		S01.21XA	Laceration without foreign body of nose, initial encounter
		S01.23XA	Puncture wound without foreign body of nose, init encntr
		S01.25XA	Open bite of nose, initial encounter

ICD-9-CM		ICD-10-CM	
873.23	OPEN WOUND NASAL SINUS WITHOUT MENTION COMP	S01.20XA	Unspecified open wound of nose, initial encounter
		S01.21XA	Laceration without foreign body of nose, initial encounter
		S01.23XA	Puncture wound without foreign body of nose, init encntr
		S01.25XA	Open bite of nose, initial encounter
873.29	OPEN WOUND NOSE MX SITES WITHOUT MENTION COMP	S08.811A	Complete traumatic amputation of nose, initial encounter
		S08.812A	Partial traumatic amputation of nose, initial encounter
873.30	OPEN WOUND OF NOSE UNSPECIFIED SITE COMPLICATED	S01.22XA	Laceration with foreign body of nose, initial encounter
		S01.24XA	Puncture wound with foreign body of nose, initial encounter
873.31	OPEN WOUND OF NASAL SEPTUM COMPLICATED	S01.22XA	Laceration with foreign body of nose, initial encounter
		S01.24XA	Puncture wound with foreign body of nose, initial encounter
873.32	OPEN WOUND OF NASAL CAVITY COMPLICATED	S01.22XA	Laceration with foreign body of nose, initial encounter
		S01.24XA	Puncture wound with foreign body of nose, initial encounter
873.33	OPEN WOUND OF NASAL SINUS COMPLICATED	S01.22XA	Laceration with foreign body of nose, initial encounter
		S01.24XA	Puncture wound with foreign body of nose, initial encounter
873.39	OPEN WOUND OF NOSE MULTIPLE SITES COMPLICATED	S08.811A	Complete traumatic amputation of nose, initial encounter
873.40	OPEN WOUND FACE UNSPEC SITE WITHOUT MENTION COMP	S09.93XA	Unspecified injury of face, initial encounter
873.41	OPEN WOUND CHEEK WITHOUT MENTION COMPLICATION	S01.401A	Unsp open wound of right cheek and TMJ area, init
		S01.402A	Unsp open wound of left cheek and TMJ area, init
		S01.409A	Unsp open wound of unsp cheek and TMJ area, init
		S01.411A	Laceration w/o fb of right cheek and TMJ area, init
		S01.412A	Laceration w/o foreign body of left cheek and TMJ area, init
		S01.419A	Laceration w/o foreign body of unsp cheek and TMJ area, init
		S01.431A	Pnctr w/o foreign body of right cheek and TMJ area, init
		S01.432A	Pnctr w/o foreign body of left cheek and TMJ area, init
		S01.439A	Pnctr w/o foreign body of unsp cheek and TMJ area, init
		S01.451A	Open bite of right cheek and temporomandibular area, init
		S01.452A	Open bite of left cheek and temporomandibular area, init
		S01.459A	Open bite of unsp cheek and temporomandibular area, init
873.42	OPEN WOUND FOREHEAD WITHOUT MENTION COMPLICATION	S01.80XA	Unspecified open wound of other part of head, init encntr
		S01.81XA	Laceration w/o foreign body of oth part of head, init encntr
		S01.83XA	Puncture wound w/o foreign body oth prt head, init encntr
		S01.85XA	Open bite of other part of head, initial encounter
873.43	OPEN WOUND LIP WITHOUT MENTION COMPLICATION	S01.501A	Unspecified open wound of lip, initial encounter
		S01.511A	Laceration without foreign body of lip, initial encounter
		S01.531A	Puncture wound without foreign body of lip, init encntr
		S01.551A	Open bite of lip, initial encounter
873.44	OPEN WOUND JAW WITHOUT MENTION COMPLICATION	S01.401A	Unsp open wound of right cheek and TMJ area, init
		S01.402A	Unsp open wound of left cheek and TMJ area, init
		S01.409A	Unsp open wound of unsp cheek and TMJ area, init
		S01.411A	Laceration w/o fb of right cheek and TMJ area, init
		S01.412A	Laceration w/o foreign body of left cheek and TMJ area, init
		S01.419A	Laceration w/o foreign body of unsp cheek and TMJ area, init
		S01.431A	Pnctr w/o foreign body of right cheek and TMJ area, init
		S01.432A	Pnctr w/o foreign body of left cheek and TMJ area, init
		S01.439A	Pnctr w/o foreign body of unsp cheek and TMJ area, init
		S01.451A	Open bite of right cheek and temporomandibular area, init
		S01.452A	Open bite of left cheek and temporomandibular area, init
		S01.459A	Open bite of unsp cheek and temporomandibular area, init
		S01.80XA	Unspecified open wound of other part of head, init encntr
		S01.81XA	Laceration w/o foreign body of oth part of head, init encntr
		S01.83XA	Puncture wound w/o foreign body oth prt head, init encntr
		S01.85XA	Open bite of other part of head, initial encounter
873.49	OPEN WOUND FCE OTH&MX SITES WITHOUT MENTION COMP	S01.80XA	Unspecified open wound of other part of head, init encntr
		S01.81XA	Laceration w/o foreign body of oth part of head, init encntr
		S01.83XA	Puncture wound w/o foreign body oth prt head, init encntr
		S01.85XA	Open bite of other part of head, initial encounter
873.50	OPEN WOUND OF FACE UNSPECIFIED SITE COMPLICATED	S09.93XA	Unspecified injury of face, initial encounter
873.51	OPEN WOUND OF CHEEK, COMPLICATED	S01.421A	Laceration w foreign body of right cheek and TMJ area, init
		S01.422A	Laceration w foreign body of left cheek and TMJ area, init
		S01.429A	Laceration w foreign body of unsp cheek and TMJ area, init
		S01.441A	Pnctr w foreign body of right cheek and TMJ area, init
		S01.442A	Pnctr w foreign body of left cheek and TMJ area, init
		S01.449A	Pnctr w foreign body of unsp cheek and TMJ area, init
873.52	OPEN WOUND OF FOREHEAD, COMPLICATED	S01.82XA	Laceration w foreign body of oth part of head, init encntr
		S01.84XA	Puncture wound w foreign body oth prt head, init encntr
873.53	OPEN WOUND OF LIP, COMPLICATED	S01.521A	Laceration with foreign body of lip, initial encounter
		S01.541A	Puncture wound with foreign body of lip, initial encounter
873.54	OPEN WOUND OF JAW, COMPLICATED	S01.421A	Laceration w foreign body of right cheek and TMJ area, init
		S01.422A	Laceration w foreign body of left cheek and TMJ area, init
		S01.429A	Laceration w foreign body of unsp cheek and TMJ area, init
		S01.441A	Pnctr w foreign body of right cheek and TMJ area, init
		S01.442A	Pnctr w foreign body of left cheek and TMJ area, init
		S01.449A	Pnctr w foreign body of unsp cheek and TMJ area, init
873.59	OPEN WOUND FACE OTHER&MULTIPLE SITES COMPLICATED	S01.82XA	Laceration w foreign body of oth part of head, init encntr
		S01.84XA	Puncture wound w foreign body oth prt head, init encntr

ICD-9-CM		ICD-10-CM		
873.60	OPEN WOUND MOUTH UNSPEC SITE W/O MENTION COMP	**S01.502A**	Unspecified open wound of oral cavity, initial encounter	
		S01.512A	Laceration without foreign body of oral cavity, init encntr	
		S01.532A	Puncture wound w/o foreign body of oral cavity, init encntr	
		S01.552A	Open bite of oral cavity, initial encounter	
873.61	OPEN WOUND BUCCAL MUCOSA WITHOUT MENTION COMP	**S01.512A**	Laceration without foreign body of oral cavity, init encntr	
		S01.532A	Puncture wound w/o foreign body of oral cavity, init encntr	
		S01.552A	Open bite of oral cavity, initial encounter	
873.62	OPEN WOUND GUM WITHOUT MENTION COMPLICATION	**S01.512A**	Laceration without foreign body of oral cavity, init encntr	
		S01.532A	Puncture wound w/o foreign body of oral cavity, init encntr	
		S01.552A	Open bite of oral cavity, initial encounter	
873.63	TOOTH BROKEN FX DUE TO TRAUMA W/O MENTION COMP	**S02.5XXA**	Fracture of tooth (traumatic), init for clos fx	
		S02.5XXB	Fracture of tooth (traumatic), init encntr for open fracture	
		S03.2XXA	Dislocation of tooth, initial encounter	
873.64	OPEN WOUND TONGUE&FLR MOUTH WITHOUT MENTION COMP	**S01.512A**	Laceration without foreign body of oral cavity, init encntr	
		S01.532A	Puncture wound w/o foreign body of oral cavity, init encntr	
		S01.552A	Open bite of oral cavity, initial encounter	
873.65	OPEN WOUND PALATE WITHOUT MENTION COMPLICATION	**S01.512A**	Laceration without foreign body of oral cavity, init encntr	
		S01.532A	Puncture wound w/o foreign body of oral cavity, init encntr	
		S01.552A	Open bite of oral cavity, initial encounter	
873.69	OPEN WOUND MOUTH OTH&MX SITES W/O MENTION COMP	**S01.512A**	Laceration without foreign body of oral cavity, init encntr	
873.70	OPEN WOUND OF MOUTH UNSPECIFIED SITE COMPLICATED	**S01.522A**	Laceration with foreign body of oral cavity, init encntr	
		S01.542A	Puncture wound with foreign body of oral cavity, init encntr	
873.71	OPEN WOUND OF BUCCAL MUCOSA COMPLICATED	**S01.522A**	Laceration with foreign body of oral cavity, init encntr	
		S01.542A	Puncture wound with foreign body of oral cavity, init encntr	
873.72	OPEN WOUND OF GUM , COMPLICATED	**S01.522A**	Laceration with foreign body of oral cavity, init encntr	
		S01.542A	Puncture wound with foreign body of oral cavity, init encntr	
873.73	TOOTH BROKEN FRACTURE DUE TO TRAUMA COMPLICATED	**S02.5XXA**	Fracture of tooth (traumatic), init for clos fx	
		S02.5XXB	Fracture of tooth (traumatic), init encntr for open fracture	
873.74	OPEN WOUND OF TONGUE&FLOOR OF MOUTH COMPLICATED	**S01.522A**	Laceration with foreign body of oral cavity, init encntr	
		S01.542A	Puncture wound with foreign body of oral cavity, init encntr	
873.75	OPEN WOUND OF PALATE, COMPLICATED	**S01.522A**	Laceration with foreign body of oral cavity, init encntr	
		S01.542A	Puncture wound with foreign body of oral cavity, init encntr	
873.79	OPEN WOUND MOUTH OTH&MULTIPLE SITES COMPLICATED	**S01.522A**	Laceration with foreign body of oral cavity, init encntr	
873.8	OTH&UNSPEC OPEN WOUND HEAD WITHOUT MENTION COMP	**S01.90XA**	Unsp open wound of unspecified part of head, init encntr	
		S01.91XA	Laceration w/o foreign body of unsp part of head, init	
		S01.93XA	Puncture wound w/o foreign body of unsp part of head, init	
		S01.95XA	Open bite of unspecified part of head, initial encounter	
		S08.89XA	Traumatic amputation of other parts of head, init encntr	
		S09.12XA	Laceration of muscle and tendon of head, initial encounter	
		S09.8XXA	Other specified injuries of head, initial encounter	
		S09.90XA	Unspecified injury of head, initial encounter	
873.9	OTHER&UNSPECIFIED OPEN WOUND OF HEAD COMPLICATED	**S01.90XA**	Unsp open wound of unspecified part of head, init encntr	
		S01.92XA	Laceration w foreign body of unsp part of head, init encntr	
		S01.94XA	Puncture wound w foreign body of unsp part of head, init	
		S01.95XA	Open bite of unspecified part of head, initial encounter	
		S09.8XXA	Other specified injuries of head, initial encounter	
		S09.90XA	Unspecified injury of head, initial encounter	
874.00	OPEN WOUND LARYNX W/TRACHEA WITHOUT MENTION COMP	**S11.019A**	Unspecified open wound of larynx, initial encounter	*and*
		S11.029A	Unspecified open wound of trachea, initial encounter	
874.01	OPEN WOUND LARYNX WITHOUT MENTION COMPLICATION	**S11.011A**	Laceration without foreign body of larynx, initial encounter	
		S11.013A	Puncture wound without foreign body of larynx, init encntr	
		S11.015A	Open bite of larynx, initial encounter	
		S11.019A	Unspecified open wound of larynx, initial encounter	
		S11.031A	Laceration without foreign body of vocal cord, init encntr	
		S11.033A	Puncture wound w/o foreign body of vocal cord, init encntr	
		S11.035A	Open bite of vocal cord, initial encounter	
		S11.039A	Unspecified open wound of vocal cord, initial encounter	
874.02	OPEN WOUND TRACHEA WITHOUT MENTION COMPLICATION	**S11.021A**	Laceration without foreign body of trachea, init encntr	
		S11.023A	Puncture wound without foreign body of trachea, init encntr	
		S11.025A	Open bite of trachea, initial encounter	
		S11.029A	Unspecified open wound of trachea, initial encounter	
874.10	OPEN WOUND OF LARYNX WITH TRACHEA COMPLICATED	**S11.012A**	Laceration with foreign body of larynx, initial encounter	*and*
		S11.022A	Laceration with foreign body of trachea, initial encounter	
		S11.014A	Puncture wound with foreign body of larynx, init encntr	*and*
		S11.024A	Puncture wound with foreign body of trachea, init encntr	
874.11	OPEN WOUND OF LARYNX, COMPLICATED	**S11.012A**	Laceration with foreign body of larynx, initial encounter	
		S11.014A	Puncture wound with foreign body of larynx, init encntr	
		S11.032A	Laceration with foreign body of vocal cord, init encntr	
		S11.034A	Puncture wound with foreign body of vocal cord, init encntr	
874.12	OPEN WOUND OF TRACHEA, COMPLICATED	**S11.022A**	Laceration with foreign body of trachea, initial encounter	
		S11.024A	Puncture wound with foreign body of trachea, init encntr	
874.2	OPEN WOUND THYROID GLAND WITHOUT MENTION COMP	**S11.10XA**	Unspecified open wound of thyroid gland, initial encounter	
		S11.11XA	Laceration w/o foreign body of thyroid gland, init encntr	
		S11.13XA	Puncture wound w/o foreign body of thyroid gland, init	
		S11.15XA	Open bite of thyroid gland, initial encounter	

ICD-9-CM		ICD-10-CM	
874.3	OPEN WOUND OF THYROID GLAND COMPLICATED	**S11.12XA**	Laceration with foreign body of thyroid gland, init encntr
		S11.14XA	Puncture wound w foreign body of thyroid gland, init encntr
874.4	OPEN WOUND PHARYNX WITHOUT MENTION COMPLICATION	**S11.2ØXA**	Unsp open wound of pharynx and cervical esophagus, init
		S11.21XA	Laceration w/o fb of pharynx and cervical esophagus, init
		S11.23XA	Pnctr w/o fb of pharynx and cervical esophagus, init
		S11.25XA	Open bite of pharynx and cervical esophagus, init encntr
874.5	OPEN WOUND OF PHARYNX, COMPLICATED	**S11.22XA**	Laceration w fb of pharynx and cervical esophagus, init
		S11.24XA	Pnctr w foreign body of pharynx and cervical esophagus, init
874.8	OPEN WOUND OTH&UNSPEC PARTS NCK W/O MENTION COMP	**S11.8ØXA**	Unspecified open wound of oth part of neck, init encntr
		S11.81XA	Laceration w/o foreign body of oth part of neck, init encntr
		S11.83XA	Puncture wound w/o foreign body oth prt neck, init encntr
		S11.85XA	Open bite of other specified part of neck, initial encounter
		S11.89XA	Other open wound of oth part of neck, init encntr
		S11.9ØXA	Unsp open wound of unspecified part of neck, init encntr
		S11.91XA	Laceration w/o foreign body of unsp part of neck, init
		S11.93XA	Puncture wound w/o foreign body of unsp part of neck, init
		S11.95XA	Open bite of unspecified part of neck, initial encounter
		S16.2XXA	Laceration of muscle, fascia and tendon at neck level, init
874.9	OPEN WOUND OTHER&UNSPEC PARTS NECK COMPLICATED	**S11.82XA**	Laceration w foreign body of oth part of neck, init encntr
		S11.84XA	Puncture wound w foreign body oth prt neck, init encntr
		S11.92XA	Laceration w foreign body of unsp part of neck, init encntr
		S11.94XA	Puncture wound w foreign body of unsp part of neck, init
875.Ø	OPEN WOUND CHEST WITHOUT MENTION COMPLICATION	**S21.1Ø1A**	Unsp opn wnd r frnt wl of thorax w/o penet thor cavity, init
		S21.1Ø2A	Unsp opn wnd l frnt wl of thorax w/o penet thor cavity, init
		S21.1Ø9A	Unsp opn wnd unsp frnt wall of thrx w/o penet thor cav, init
		S21.111A	Lac w/o fb of r frnt wl of thorax w/o penet thor cav, init
		S21.112A	Lac w/o fb of l frnt wl of thorax w/o penet thor cav, init
		S21.119A	Lac w/o fb of unsp frnt wl of thrx w/o penet thor cav, init
		S21.131A	Pnctr w/o fb of r frnt wl of thorax w/o penet thor cav, init
		S21.132A	Pnctr w/o fb of l frnt wl of thorax w/o penet thor cav, init
		S21.139A	Pnctr w/o fb of unsp frnt wl of thrx w/o penet thor cav,init
		S21.151A	Open bite of r frnt wl of thorax w/o penet thor cavity, init
		S21.152A	Open bite of l frnt wl of thorax w/o penet thor cavity, init
		S21.159A	Open bite of unsp frnt wall of thrx w/o penet thor cav, init
		S21.9ØXA	Unsp open wound of unspecified part of thorax, init encntr
		S21.91XA	Laceration w/o foreign body of unsp part of thorax, init
		S21.93XA	Puncture wound w/o foreign body of unsp part of thorax, init
		S21.95XA	Open bite of unspecified part of thorax, initial encounter
		S28.1XXA	Traumatic amp of part of thorax, except breast, init
		S29.Ø21A	Laceration of msl/tnd of front wall of thorax, init
		S29.Ø29A	Laceration of muscle and tendon of unsp wall of thorax, init
875.1	OPEN WOUND OF CHEST , COMPLICATED	**S21.121A**	Lac w fb of r frnt wl of thorax w/o penet thor cavity, init
		S21.122A	Lac w fb of l frnt wl of thorax w/o penet thor cavity, init
		S21.129A	Lac w fb of unsp front wall of thrx w/o penet thor cav, init
		S21.141A	Pnctr w fb of r frnt wl of thorax w/o penet thor cav, init
		S21.142A	Pnctr w fb of l frnt wl of thorax w/o penet thor cav, init
		S21.149A	Pnctr w fb of unsp frnt wl of thrx w/o penet thor cav, init
		S21.92XA	Laceration w foreign body of unsp part of thorax, init
		S21.94XA	Puncture wound w foreign body of unsp part of thorax, init
876.Ø	OPEN WOUND BACK WITHOUT MENTION COMPLICATION	**S21.2Ø1A**	Unsp opn wnd r bk wl of thorax w/o penet thor cavity, init
		S21.2Ø2A	Unsp opn wnd l bk wl of thorax w/o penet thor cavity, init
		S21.2Ø9A	Unsp opn wnd unsp bk wl of thorax w/o penet thor cav, init
		S21.211A	Lac w/o fb of r bk wl of thorax w/o penet thor cavity, init
		S21.212A	Lac w/o fb of l bk wl of thorax w/o penet thor cavity, init
		S21.219A	Lac w/o fb of unsp bk wl of thorax w/o penet thor cav, init
		S21.231A	Pnctr w/o fb of r bk wl of thorax w/o penet thor cav, init
		S21.232A	Pnctr w/o fb of l bk wl of thorax w/o penet thor cav, init
		S21.239A	Pnctr w/o fb of unsp bk wl of thrx w/o penet thor cav, init
		S21.251A	Open bite of r bk wl of thorax w/o penet thor cavity, init
		S21.252A	Open bite of l bk wl of thorax w/o penet thor cavity, init
		S21.259A	Open bite of unsp bk wl of thorax w/o penet thor cav, init
		S29.Ø22A	Laceration of muscle and tendon of back wall of thorax, init
		S31.ØØØA	Unsp opn wnd low back and pelv w/o penet retroperiton, init
		S31.Ø1ØA	Lac w/o fb of low back and pelv w/o penet retroperiton, init
		S31.Ø3ØA	Pnctr w/o fb of low back & pelv w/o penet retroperiton, init
		S31.Ø5ØA	Open bite of low back and pelv w/o penet retroperiton, init
876.1	OPEN WOUND OF BACK, COMPLICATED	**S21.221A**	Lac w fb of r bk wl of thorax w/o penet thor cavity, init
		S21.222A	Lac w fb of l bk wl of thorax w/o penet thor cavity, init
		S21.229A	Lac w fb of unsp bk wl of thorax w/o penet thor cavity, init
		S21.241A	Pnctr w fb of r bk wl of thorax w/o penet thor cavity, init
		S21.242A	Pnctr w fb of l bk wl of thorax w/o penet thor cavity, init
		S21.249A	Pnctr w fb of unsp bk wl of thorax w/o penet thor cav, init
		S31.Ø2ØA	Lac w fb of low back and pelvis w/o penet retroperiton, init
		S31.Ø4ØA	Pnctr w fb of low back and pelv w/o penet retroperiton, init
877.Ø	OPEN WOUND BUTTOCK WITHOUT MENTION COMPLICATION	**S31.8Ø1A**	Laceration without foreign body of unsp buttock, init encntr
		S31.8Ø3A	Puncture wound w/o foreign body of unsp buttock, init encntr
		S31.8Ø5A	Open bite of unspecified buttock, initial encounter
		S31.8Ø9A	Unspecified open wound of unspecified buttock, init encntr
		S31.811A	Laceration w/o foreign body of right buttock, init encntr
	(Continued on next page)	**S31.813A**	Puncture wound w/o foreign body of right buttock, init

ICD-9-CM		ICD-10-CM	
877.Ø	OPEN WOUND BUTTOCK WITHOUT MENTION COMPLICATION **(Continued)**	**S31.815A**	Open bite of right buttock, initial encounter
		S31.819A	Unspecified open wound of right buttock, initial encounter
		S31.821A	Laceration without foreign body of left buttock, init encntr
		S31.823A	Puncture wound w/o foreign body of left buttock, init encntr
		S31.825A	Open bite of left buttock, initial encounter
		S31.829A	Unspecified open wound of left buttock, initial encounter
877.1	OPEN WOUND OF BUTTOCK, COMPLICATED	**S31.8Ø2A**	Laceration with foreign body of unsp buttock, init encntr
		S31.8Ø4A	Puncture wound w foreign body of unsp buttock, init encntr
		S31.812A	Laceration with foreign body of right buttock, init encntr
		S31.814A	Puncture wound w foreign body of right buttock, init encntr
		S31.822A	Laceration with foreign body of left buttock, init encntr
		S31.824A	Puncture wound w foreign body of left buttock, init encntr
878.Ø	OPEN WOUND PENIS WITHOUT MENTION COMPLICATION	**S31.2ØXA**	Unspecified open wound of penis, initial encounter
		S31.21XA	Laceration without foreign body of penis, initial encounter
		S31.23XA	Puncture wound without foreign body of penis, init encntr
		S31.25XA	Open bite of penis, initial encounter
		S38.221A	Complete traumatic amputation of penis, initial encounter
		S38.222A	Partial traumatic amputation of penis, initial encounter
878.1	OPEN WOUND OF PENIS, COMPLICATED	**S31.22XA**	Laceration with foreign body of penis, initial encounter
		S31.24XA	Puncture wound with foreign body of penis, initial encounter
878.2	OPEN WOUND SCROTUM&TESTES WITHOUT MENTION COMP	**S31.3ØXA**	Unspecified open wound of scrotum and testes, init encntr
		S31.31XA	Laceration w/o foreign body of scrotum and testes, init
		S31.33XA	Puncture wound w/o foreign body of scrotum and testes, init
		S31.35XA	Open bite of scrotum and testes, initial encounter
		S38.231A	Complete traumatic amputation of scrotum and testis, init
		S38.232A	Partial traumatic amputation of scrotum and testis, init
878.3	OPEN WOUND OF SCROTUM AND TESTES COMPLICATED	**S31.32XA**	Laceration w foreign body of scrotum and testes, init encntr
		S31.34XA	Puncture wound w foreign body of scrotum and testes, init
878.4	OPEN WOUND VULVA WITHOUT MENTION COMPLICATION	**S31.4ØXA**	Unspecified open wound of vagina and vulva, init encntr
		S31.41XA	Laceration w/o foreign body of vagina and vulva, init encntr
		S31.43XA	Puncture wound w/o foreign body of vagina and vulva, init
		S31.45XA	Open bite of vagina and vulva, initial encounter
878.5	OPEN WOUND OF VULVA, COMPLICATED	**S31.42XA**	Laceration w foreign body of vagina and vulva, init encntr
		S31.44XA	Puncture wound w foreign body of vagina and vulva, init
878.6	OPEN WOUND VAGINA WITHOUT MENTION COMPLICATION	**S31.4ØXA**	Unspecified open wound of vagina and vulva, init encntr
		S31.41XA	Laceration w/o foreign body of vagina and vulva, init encntr
		S31.43XA	Puncture wound w/o foreign body of vagina and vulva, init
		S31.45XA	Open bite of vagina and vulva, initial encounter
878.7	OPEN WOUND OF VAGINA, COMPLICATED	**S31.42XA**	Laceration w foreign body of vagina and vulva, init encntr
		S31.44XA	Puncture wound w foreign body of vagina and vulva, init
878.8	OPEN WND OTH&UNS PART GNT ORGN W/O MENTION COMP	**S31.5Ø1A**	Unsp open wound of unsp external genital organs, male, init
		S31.5Ø2A	Unsp opn wnd unsp external genital organs, female, init
		S31.511A	Lac w/o fb of unsp external genital organs, male, init
		S31.512A	Lac w/o fb of unsp external genital organs, female, init
		S31.531A	Pnctr w/o fb of unsp external genital organs, male, init
		S31.532A	Pnctr w/o fb of unsp external genital organs, female, init
		S31.551A	Open bite of unsp external genital organs, male, init encntr
		S31.552A	Open bite of unsp external genital organs, female, init
		S38.211A	Complete traum amp of female external genital organs, init
		S38.212A	Partial traum amp of female external genital organs, init
878.9	OPEN WOUND OTH&UNSPEC PARTS GENITAL ORGANS COMP	**S31.521A**	Laceration w fb of unsp external genital organs, male, init
		S31.522A	Lac w fb of unsp external genital organs, female, init
		S31.541A	Pnctr w fb of unsp external genital organs, male, init
		S31.542A	Pnctr w fb of unsp external genital organs, female, init
879.Ø	OPEN WOUND BREAST WITHOUT MENTION COMPLICATION	**S21.ØØ1A**	Unspecified open wound of right breast, initial encounter
		S21.ØØ2A	Unspecified open wound of left breast, initial encounter
		S21.ØØ9A	Unspecified open wound of unspecified breast, init encntr
		S21.Ø11A	Laceration without foreign body of right breast, init encntr
		S21.Ø12A	Laceration without foreign body of left breast, init encntr
		S21.Ø19A	Laceration without foreign body of unsp breast, init encntr
		S21.Ø31A	Puncture wound w/o foreign body of right breast, init encntr
		S21.Ø32A	Puncture wound w/o foreign body of left breast, init encntr
		S21.Ø39A	Puncture wound w/o foreign body of unsp breast, init encntr
		S21.Ø51A	Open bite of right breast, initial encounter
		S21.Ø52A	Open bite of left breast, initial encounter
		S21.Ø59A	Open bite of unspecified breast, initial encounter
		S28.211A	Complete traumatic amputation of right breast, init encntr
		S28.212A	Complete traumatic amputation of left breast, init encntr
		S28.219A	Complete traumatic amputation of unsp breast, init encntr
		S28.221A	Partial traumatic amputation of right breast, init encntr
		S28.222A	Partial traumatic amputation of left breast, init encntr
		S28.229A	Partial traumatic amputation of unsp breast, init encntr
879.1	OPEN WOUND OF BREAST, COMPLICATED	**S21.Ø21A**	Laceration with foreign body of right breast, init encntr
		S21.Ø22A	Laceration with foreign body of left breast, init encntr
		S21.Ø29A	Laceration with foreign body of unsp breast, init encntr
		S21.Ø41A	Puncture wound w foreign body of right breast, init encntr
		S21.Ø42A	Puncture wound with foreign body of left breast, init encntr
		S21.Ø49A	Puncture wound with foreign body of unsp breast, init encntr

ICD-9-CM		ICD-10-CM	
879.2	OPEN WOUND ABD WALL ANT WITHOUT MENTION COMP	S31.102A	Unsp opn wnd abd wall, epigst rgn w/o penet perit cav, init
		S31.105A	Unsp opn wnd abd wall, periumb rgn w/o penet perit cav, init
		S31.112A	Lac w/o fb of abd wall, epigst rgn w/o penet perit cav, init
		S31.115A	Lac w/o fb of abd wl, periumb rgn w/o penet perit cav, init
		S31.132A	Pnctr of abd wl w/o fb, epigst rgn w/o penet perit cav, init
		S31.135A	Pnctr of abd wl w/o fb,periumb rgn w/o penet perit cav, init
		S31.152A	Open bite of abd wall, epigst rgn w/o penet perit cav, init
		S31.155A	Open bite of abd wall, periumb rgn w/o penet perit cav, init
879.3	OPEN WOUND ABDOMINAL WALL ANTERIOR COMPLICATED	S31.122A	Lacerat abd wall w fb, epigst rgn w/o penet perit cav, init
		S31.125A	Lacerat abd wall w fb, periumb rgn w/o penet perit cav, init
		S31.142A	Pnctr of abd wall w fb, epigst rgn w/o penet perit cav, init
		S31.145A	Pnctr of abd wl w fb, periumb rgn w/o penet perit cav, init
879.4	OPEN WOUND ABD WALL LATERAL WITHOUT MENTION COMP	S31.100A	Unsp opn wnd abd wall, r upper q w/o penet perit cav, init
		S31.101A	Unsp opn wnd abd wall, l upr q w/o penet perit cav, init
		S31.103A	Unsp opn wnd abd wall, right low q w/o penet perit cav, init
		S31.104A	Unsp opn wnd abd wall, left low q w/o penet perit cav, init
		S31.109A	Unsp opn wnd abd wall, unsp q w/o penet perit cav, init
		S31.110A	Lac w/o fb of abd wall, r upper q w/o penet perit cav, init
		S31.111A	Lac w/o fb of abd wall, l upr q w/o penet perit cav, init
		S31.113A	Lac w/o fb of abd wall, r low q w/o penet perit cav, init
		S31.114A	Lac w/o fb of abd wall, left low q w/o penet perit cav, init
		S31.119A	Lac w/o fb of abd wall, unsp q w/o penet perit cav, init
		S31.130A	Pnctr of abd wall w/o fb, r upr q w/o penet perit cav, init
		S31.131A	Pnctr of abd wall w/o fb, l upr q w/o penet perit cav, init
		S31.133A	Pnctr of abd wall w/o fb, r low q w/o penet perit cav, init
		S31.134A	Pnctr of abd wall w/o fb, l low q w/o penet perit cav, init
		S31.139A	Pnctr of abd wall w/o fb, unsp q w/o penet perit cav, init
		S31.150A	Open bite of abd wall, r upper q w/o penet perit cav, init
		S31.151A	Open bite of abd wall, l upr q w/o penet perit cav, init
		S31.153A	Open bite of abd wall, right low q w/o penet perit cav, init
		S31.154A	Open bite of abd wall, left low q w/o penet perit cav, init
		S31.159A	Open bite of abd wall, unsp q w/o penet perit cav, init
879.5	OPEN WOUND OF ABDOMINAL WALL LATERAL COMPLICATED	S31.120A	Lacerat abd wall w fb, r upper q w/o penet perit cav, init
		S31.121A	Lacerat abd wall w fb, l upr q w/o penet perit cav, init
		S31.123A	Lacerat abd wall w fb, right low q w/o penet perit cav, init
		S31.124A	Lacerat abd wall w fb, left low q w/o penet perit cav, init
		S31.129A	Lacerat abd wall w fb, unsp q w/o penet perit cav, init
		S31.140A	Pnctr of abd wall w fb, r upper q w/o penet perit cav, init
		S31.141A	Pnctr of abd wall w fb, l upr q w/o penet perit cav, init
		S31.143A	Pnctr of abd wall w fb, r low q w/o penet perit cav, init
		S31.144A	Pnctr of abd wall w fb, left low q w/o penet perit cav, init
		S31.149A	Pnctr of abd wall w fb, unsp q w/o penet perit cav, init
879.6	OPEN WOUND OTH&UNSPEC PART TRNK W/O MENTION COMP	S31.000A	Unsp opn wnd low back and pelv w/o penet retroperiton, init
		S31.010A	Lac w/o fb of low back and pelv w/o penet retroperiton, init
		S31.030A	Pnctr w/o fb of low back & pelv w/o penet retroperiton, init
		S31.050A	Open bite of low back and pelv w/o penet retroperiton, init
		S31.831A	Laceration without foreign body of anus, initial encounter
		S31.833A	Puncture wound without foreign body of anus, init encntr
		S31.835A	Open bite of anus, initial encounter
		S31.839A	Unspecified open wound of anus, initial encounter
		S39.021A	Laceration of muscle, fascia and tendon of abdomen, init
		S39.022A	Laceration of muscle, fascia and tendon of lower back, init
		S39.023A	Laceration of muscle, fascia and tendon of pelvis, init
879.7	OPEN WOUND OTHER&UNSPEC PARTS TRUNK COMPLICATED	S31.020A	Lac w fb of low back and pelvis w/o penet retroperiton, init
		S31.040A	Pnctr w fb of low back and pelv w/o penet retroperiton, init
		S31.832A	Laceration with foreign body of anus, initial encounter
		S31.834A	Puncture wound with foreign body of anus, initial encounter
879.8	OPEN WOUND UNSPEC SITE WITHOUT MENTION COMP	S31.000A	Unsp opn wnd low back and pelv w/o penet retroperiton, init
		S31.010A	Lac w/o fb of low back and pelv w/o penet retroperiton, init
		S31.030A	Pnctr w/o fb of low back & pelv w/o penet retroperiton, init
		S31.050A	Open bite of low back and pelv w/o penet retroperiton, init
		S38.3XXA	Transection (partial) of abdomen, initial encounter
879.9	OPEN WOUND OF UNSPECIFIED SITE COMPLICATED	S31.020A	Lac w fb of low back and pelvis w/o penet retroperiton, init
		S31.040A	Pnctr w fb of low back and pelv w/o penet retroperiton, init
880.00	OPEN WOUND SHOULDER REGION WITHOUT MENTION COMP	S41.001A	Unspecified open wound of right shoulder, initial encounter
		S41.002A	Unspecified open wound of left shoulder, initial encounter
		S41.009A	Unspecified open wound of unspecified shoulder, init encntr
		S41.011A	Laceration w/o foreign body of right shoulder, init encntr
		S41.012A	Laceration w/o foreign body of left shoulder, init encntr
		S41.019A	Laceration w/o foreign body of unsp shoulder, init encntr
		S41.031A	Puncture wound w/o foreign body of right shoulder, init
		S41.032A	Puncture wound w/o foreign body of left shoulder, init
		S41.039A	Puncture wound w/o foreign body of unsp shoulder, init
		S41.051A	Open bite of right shoulder, initial encounter
		S41.052A	Open bite of left shoulder, initial encounter
		S41.059A	Open bite of unspecified shoulder, initial encounter

ICD-9-CM	ICD-10-CM	
880.01 OPEN WOUND SCAPULAR REGION WITHOUT MENTION COMP	**S41.001A**	Unspecified open wound of right shoulder, initial encounter
	S41.002A	Unspecified open wound of left shoulder, initial encounter
	S41.009A	Unspecified open wound of unspecified shoulder, init encntr
	S41.011A	Laceration w/o foreign body of right shoulder, init encntr
	S41.012A	Laceration w/o foreign body of left shoulder, init encntr
	S41.019A	Laceration w/o foreign body of unsp shoulder, init encntr
	S41.031A	Puncture wound w/o foreign body of right shoulder, init
	S41.032A	Puncture wound w/o foreign body of left shoulder, init
	S41.039A	Puncture wound w/o foreign body of unsp shoulder, init
	S41.051A	Open bite of right shoulder, initial encounter
	S41.052A	Open bite of left shoulder, initial encounter
	S41.059A	Open bite of unspecified shoulder, initial encounter
880.02 OPEN WOUND AX REGION WITHOUT MENTION COMP	**S41.001A**	Unspecified open wound of right shoulder, initial encounter
	S41.002A	Unspecified open wound of left shoulder, initial encounter
	S41.009A	Unspecified open wound of unspecified shoulder, init encntr
	S41.011A	Laceration w/o foreign body of right shoulder, init encntr
	S41.012A	Laceration w/o foreign body of left shoulder, init encntr
	S41.019A	Laceration w/o foreign body of unsp shoulder, init encntr
	S41.031A	Puncture wound w/o foreign body of right shoulder, init
	S41.032A	Puncture wound w/o foreign body of left shoulder, init
	S41.039A	Puncture wound w/o foreign body of unsp shoulder, init
	S41.051A	Open bite of right shoulder, initial encounter
	S41.052A	Open bite of left shoulder, initial encounter
	S41.059A	Open bite of unspecified shoulder, initial encounter
880.03 OPEN WOUND UPPER ARM WITHOUT MENTION COMP	**S41.101A**	Unspecified open wound of right upper arm, initial encounter
	S41.102A	Unspecified open wound of left upper arm, initial encounter
	S41.109A	Unspecified open wound of unspecified upper arm, init encntr
	S41.111A	Laceration w/o foreign body of right upper arm, init encntr
	S41.112A	Laceration w/o foreign body of left upper arm, init encntr
	S41.119A	Laceration w/o foreign body of unsp upper arm, init encntr
	S41.131A	Puncture wound w/o foreign body of right upper arm, init
	S41.132A	Puncture wound w/o foreign body of left upper arm, init
	S41.139A	Puncture wound w/o foreign body of unsp upper arm, init
	S41.151A	Open bite of right upper arm, initial encounter
	S41.152A	Open bite of left upper arm, initial encounter
	S41.159A	Open bite of unspecified upper arm, initial encounter
880.09 OPEN WOUND MX SITE SHLDR&UP ARM W/O MENTION COMP	**S41.101A**	Unspecified open wound of right upper arm, initial encounter
	S41.102A	Unspecified open wound of left upper arm, initial encounter
	S41.109A	Unspecified open wound of unspecified upper arm, init encntr
	S41.111A	Laceration w/o foreign body of right upper arm, init encntr
	S41.112A	Laceration w/o foreign body of left upper arm, init encntr
	S41.119A	Laceration w/o foreign body of unsp upper arm, init encntr
	S41.131A	Puncture wound w/o foreign body of right upper arm, init
	S41.132A	Puncture wound w/o foreign body of left upper arm, init
	S41.139A	Puncture wound w/o foreign body of unsp upper arm, init
	S41.151A	Open bite of right upper arm, initial encounter
	S41.152A	Open bite of left upper arm, initial encounter
	S41.159A	Open bite of unspecified upper arm, initial encounter
880.10 OPEN WOUND OF SHOULDER REGION COMPLICATED	**S41.021A**	Laceration with foreign body of right shoulder, init encntr
	S41.022A	Laceration with foreign body of left shoulder, init encntr
	S41.029A	Laceration with foreign body of unsp shoulder, init encntr
	S41.041A	Puncture wound w foreign body of right shoulder, init encntr
	S41.042A	Puncture wound w foreign body of left shoulder, init encntr
	S41.049A	Puncture wound w foreign body of unsp shoulder, init encntr
880.11 OPEN WOUND OF SCAPULAR REGION COMPLICATED	**S41.021A**	Laceration with foreign body of right shoulder, init encntr
	S41.022A	Laceration with foreign body of left shoulder, init encntr
	S41.029A	Laceration with foreign body of unsp shoulder, init encntr
	S41.041A	Puncture wound w foreign body of right shoulder, init encntr
	S41.042A	Puncture wound w foreign body of left shoulder, init encntr
	S41.049A	Puncture wound w foreign body of unsp shoulder, init encntr
880.12 OPEN WOUND OF AXILLARY REGION COMPLICATED	**S41.021A**	Laceration with foreign body of right shoulder, init encntr
	S41.022A	Laceration with foreign body of left shoulder, init encntr
	S41.029A	Laceration with foreign body of unsp shoulder, init encntr
	S41.041A	Puncture wound w foreign body of right shoulder, init encntr
	S41.042A	Puncture wound w foreign body of left shoulder, init encntr
	S41.049A	Puncture wound w foreign body of unsp shoulder, init encntr
880.13 OPEN WOUND OF UPPER ARM COMPLICATED	**S41.121A**	Laceration with foreign body of right upper arm, init encntr
	S41.122A	Laceration with foreign body of left upper arm, init encntr
	S41.129A	Laceration with foreign body of unsp upper arm, init encntr
	S41.141A	Puncture wound w foreign body of right upper arm, init
	S41.142A	Puncture wound w foreign body of left upper arm, init encntr
	S41.149A	Puncture wound w foreign body of unsp upper arm, init encntr
880.19 OPEN WOUND MX SITES SHOULDER&UPPER ARM COMP	**S41.121A**	Laceration with foreign body of right upper arm, init encntr
	S41.122A	Laceration with foreign body of left upper arm, init encntr
	S41.129A	Laceration with foreign body of unsp upper arm, init encntr
	S41.141A	Puncture wound w foreign body of right upper arm, init
	S41.142A	Puncture wound w foreign body of left upper arm, init encntr
	S41.149A	Puncture wound w foreign body of unsp upper arm, init encntr

ICD-9-CM		ICD-10-CM		
880.20	OPEN WOUND SHOULDER REGION W/TENDON INVOLVEMENT	**S46.929A**	Lacerat unsp musc/fasc/tend at shldr/up arm, unsp arm, init	*and*
		S41.009A	Unspecified open wound of unspecified shoulder, init encntr	
		S46.021A	Laceration of musc/tend the rotator cuff of r shoulder, init	
		S46.022A	Lacerat musc/tend the rotator cuff of left shoulder, init	
		S46.029A	Lacerat musc/tend the rotator cuff of unsp shoulder, init	
		S46.121A	Laceration of musc/fasc/tend long hd bicep, right arm, init	
		S46.122A	Laceration of musc/fasc/tend long hd bicep, left arm, init	
		S46.129A	Laceration of musc/fasc/tend long hd bicep, unsp arm, init	
		S46.221A	Laceration of musc/fasc/tend prt biceps, right arm, init	
		S46.222A	Laceration of musc/fasc/tend prt biceps, left arm, init	
		S46.229A	Laceration of musc/fasc/tend prt biceps, unsp arm, init	
		S46.321A	Laceration of musc/fasc/tend triceps, right arm, init	
		S46.322A	Laceration of musc/fasc/tend triceps, left arm, init	
		S46.329A	Laceration of musc/fasc/tend triceps, unsp arm, init	
		S46.821A	Lacerat musc/fasc/tend at shldr/up arm, right arm, init	
		S46.822A	Laceration of musc/fasc/tend at shldr/up arm, left arm, init	
		S46.829A	Laceration of musc/fasc/tend at shldr/up arm, unsp arm, init	
		S46.921A	Lacerat unsp musc/fasc/tend at shldr/up arm, right arm, init	
		S46.922A	Lacerat unsp musc/fasc/tend at shldr/up arm, left arm, init	
880.21	OPEN WOUND SCAPULAR REGION W/TENDON INVOLVEMENT	**S46.929A**	Lacerat unsp musc/fasc/tend at shldr/up arm, unsp arm, init	*and*
		S41.009A	Unspecified open wound of unspecified shoulder, init encntr	
880.22	OPEN WOUND AXILLARY REGION W/TENDON INVOLVEMENT	**S46.929A**	Lacerat unsp musc/fasc/tend at shldr/up arm, unsp arm, init	*and*
		S41.009A	Unspecified open wound of unspecified shoulder, init encntr	
880.23	OPEN WOUND OF UPPER ARM WITH TENDON INVOLVEMENT	**S46.929A**	Lacerat unsp musc/fasc/tend at shldr/up arm, unsp arm, init	*and*
		S41.109A	Unspecified open wound of unspecified upper arm, init encntr	
880.29	OPEN WOUND MX SITE SHLDR&UPPER ARM W/TEND INVLV	**S46.929A**	Lacerat unsp musc/fasc/tend at shldr/up arm, unsp arm, init	*and*
		S41.109A	Unspecified open wound of unspecified upper arm, init encntr	
881.00	OPEN WOUND FOREARM WITHOUT MENTION COMPLICATION	**S51.801A**	Unspecified open wound of right forearm, initial encounter	
		S51.802A	Unspecified open wound of left forearm, initial encounter	
		S51.809A	Unspecified open wound of unspecified forearm, init encntr	
		S51.811A	Laceration w/o foreign body of right forearm, init encntr	
		S51.812A	Laceration without foreign body of left forearm, init encntr	
		S51.819A	Laceration without foreign body of unsp forearm, init encntr	
		S51.831A	Puncture wound w/o foreign body of right forearm, init	
		S51.832A	Puncture wound w/o foreign body of left forearm, init encntr	
		S51.839A	Puncture wound w/o foreign body of unsp forearm, init encntr	
		S51.851A	Open bite of right forearm, initial encounter	
		S51.852A	Open bite of left forearm, initial encounter	
		S51.859A	Open bite of unspecified forearm, initial encounter	
881.01	OPEN WOUND ELBOW WITHOUT MENTION COMPLICATION	**S51.001A**	Unspecified open wound of right elbow, initial encounter	
		S51.002A	Unspecified open wound of left elbow, initial encounter	
		S51.009A	Unspecified open wound of unspecified elbow, init encntr	
		S51.011A	Laceration without foreign body of right elbow, init encntr	
		S51.012A	Laceration without foreign body of left elbow, init encntr	
		S51.019A	Laceration without foreign body of unsp elbow, init encntr	
		S51.031A	Puncture wound w/o foreign body of right elbow, init encntr	
		S51.032A	Puncture wound w/o foreign body of left elbow, init encntr	
		S51.039A	Puncture wound w/o foreign body of unsp elbow, init encntr	
		S51.051A	Open bite, right elbow, initial encounter	
		S51.052A	Open bite, left elbow, initial encounter	
		S51.059A	Open bite, unspecified elbow, initial encounter	
881.02	OPEN WOUND WRIST WITHOUT MENTION COMPLICATION	**S61.501A**	Unspecified open wound of right wrist, initial encounter	
		S61.502A	Unspecified open wound of left wrist, initial encounter	
		S61.509A	Unspecified open wound of unspecified wrist, init encntr	
		S61.511A	Laceration without foreign body of right wrist, init encntr	
		S61.512A	Laceration without foreign body of left wrist, init encntr	
		S61.519A	Laceration without foreign body of unsp wrist, init encntr	
		S61.531A	Puncture wound w/o foreign body of right wrist, init encntr	
		S61.532A	Puncture wound w/o foreign body of left wrist, init encntr	
		S61.539A	Puncture wound w/o foreign body of unsp wrist, init encntr	
		S61.551A	Open bite of right wrist, initial encounter	
		S61.552A	Open bite of left wrist, initial encounter	
		S61.559A	Open bite of unspecified wrist, initial encounter	
881.10	OPEN WOUND OF FOREARM, COMPLICATED	**S51.821A**	Laceration with foreign body of right forearm, init encntr	
		S51.822A	Laceration with foreign body of left forearm, init encntr	
		S51.829A	Laceration with foreign body of unsp forearm, init encntr	
		S51.841A	Puncture wound w foreign body of right forearm, init encntr	
		S51.842A	Puncture wound w foreign body of left forearm, init encntr	
		S51.849A	Puncture wound w foreign body of unsp forearm, init encntr	
881.11	OPEN WOUND OF ELBOW, COMPLICATED	**S51.021A**	Laceration with foreign body of right elbow, init encntr	
		S51.022A	Laceration with foreign body of left elbow, init encntr	
		S51.029A	Laceration with foreign body of unsp elbow, init encntr	
		S51.041A	Puncture wound with foreign body of right elbow, init encntr	
		S51.042A	Puncture wound with foreign body of left elbow, init encntr	
		S51.049A	Puncture wound with foreign body of unsp elbow, init encntr	

ICD-9-CM		ICD-10-CM		
881.12	OPEN WOUND OF WRIST, COMPLICATED	S61.521A	Laceration with foreign body of right wrist, init encntr	
		S61.522A	Laceration with foreign body of left wrist, init encntr	
		S61.529A	Laceration with foreign body of unsp wrist, init encntr	
		S61.541A	Puncture wound with foreign body of right wrist, init encntr	
		S61.542A	Puncture wound with foreign body of left wrist, init encntr	
		S61.549A	Puncture wound with foreign body of unsp wrist, init encntr	
881.2Ø	OPEN WOUND OF FOREARM WITH TENDON INVOLVEMENT	S56.929A	Lacerat unsp musc/fasc/tend at forarm lv, unsp arm, init	and
		S51.8Ø9A	Unspecified open wound of unspecified forearm, init encntr	
		S56.Ø21A	Lacerat flexor musc/fasc/tend right thumb at forarm lv, init	
		S56.Ø22A	Lacerat flexor musc/fasc/tend left thumb at forarm lv, init	
		S56.Ø29A	Laceration of flexor musc/fasc/tend thmb at forarm lv, init	
		S56.121A	Lacerat flexor musc/fasc/tend r idx fngr at forarm lv, init	
		S56.122A	Lacerat flexor musc/fasc/tend l idx fngr at forarm lv, init	
		S56.123A	Lacerat flexor musc/fasc/tend r mid fngr at forarm lv, init	
		S56.124A	Lacerat flexor musc/fasc/tend l mid fngr at forarm lv, init	
		S56.125A	Lacerat flexor musc/fasc/tend r rng fngr at forarm lv, init	
		S56.126A	Lacerat flexor musc/fasc/tend l rng fngr at forarm lv, init	
		S56.127A	Lacerat flxr musc/fasc/tend r little fngr at forarm lv, init	
		S56.128A	Lacerat flxr musc/fasc/tend l little fngr at forarm lv, init	
		S56.129A	Lacerat flexor musc/fasc/tend unsp finger at forarm lv, init	
		S56.221A	Lacerat flexor musc/fasc/tend at forarm lv, right arm, init	
		S56.222A	Lacerat flexor musc/fasc/tend at forarm lv, left arm, init	
		S56.229A	Lacerat flexor musc/fasc/tend at forarm lv, unsp arm, init	
		S56.321A	Lacerat extn/abdr musc/fasc/tend of r thm at forarm lv, init	
		S56.322A	Lacerat extn/abdr musc/fasc/tend of l thm at forarm lv, init	
		S56.329A	Lacerat extn/abdr musc/fasc/tend of thmb at forarm lv, init	
		S56.421A	Lacerat extn musc/fasc/tend r idx fngr at forarm lv, init	
		S56.422A	Lacerat extn musc/fasc/tend l idx fngr at forarm lv, init	
		S56.423A	Lacerat extn musc/fasc/tend r mid finger at forarm lv, init	
		S56.424A	Lacerat extn musc/fasc/tend l mid finger at forarm lv, init	
		S56.425A	Lacerat extn musc/fasc/tend r rng fngr at forarm lv, init	
		S56.426A	Lacerat extn musc/fasc/tend l rng fngr at forarm lv, init	
		S56.427A	Lacerat extn musc/fasc/tend r little fngr at forarm lv, init	
		S56.428A	Lacerat extn musc/fasc/tend l little fngr at forarm lv, init	
		S56.429A	Lacerat extn musc/fasc/tend unsp finger at forarm lv, init	
		S56.521A	Lacerat extn musc/fasc/tend at forarm lv, right arm, init	
		S56.522A	Lacerat extn musc/fasc/tend at forarm lv, left arm, init	
		S56.529A	Lacerat extn musc/fasc/tend at forarm lv, unsp arm, init	
		S56.821A	Laceration of musc/fasc/tend at forarm lv, right arm, init	
		S56.822A	Laceration of musc/fasc/tend at forarm lv, left arm, init	
		S56.829A	Laceration of musc/fasc/tend at forarm lv, unsp arm, init	
		S56.921A	Lacerat unsp musc/fasc/tend at forarm lv, right arm, init	
		S56.922A	Lacerat unsp musc/fasc/tend at forarm lv, left arm, init	
		S56.929A	Lacerat unsp musc/fasc/tend at forarm lv, unsp arm, init	
881.21	OPEN WOUND OF ELBOW WITH TENDON INVOLVEMENT	S56.929A	Lacerat unsp musc/fasc/tend at forarm lv, unsp arm, init	and
		S51.ØØ9A	Unspecified open wound of unspecified elbow, init encntr	
881.22	OPEN WOUND OF WRIST WITH TENDON INVOLVEMENT	S66.929A	Lacerat unsp musc/fasc/tend at wrs/hnd lv, unsp hand, init	and
		S61.5Ø9A	Unspecified open wound of unspecified wrist, init encntr	
		S66.Ø21A	Lacerat long flexor musc/fasc/tend r thm at wrs/hnd lv, init	
		S66.Ø22A	Lacerat long flexor musc/fasc/tend l thm at wrs/hnd lv, init	
		S66.Ø29A	Lacerat long flexor musc/fasc/tend thmb at wrs/hnd lv, init	
		S66.12ØA	Lacerat flexor musc/fasc/tend r idx fngr at wrs/hnd lv, init	
		S66.121A	Lacerat flexor musc/fasc/tend l idx fngr at wrs/hnd lv, init	
		S66.122A	Lacerat flexor musc/fasc/tend r mid fngr at wrs/hnd lv, init	
		S66.123A	Lacerat flexor musc/fasc/tend l mid fngr at wrs/hnd lv, init	
		S66.124A	Lacerat flexor musc/fasc/tend r rng fngr at wrs/hnd lv, init	
		S66.125A	Lacerat flexor musc/fasc/tend l rng fngr at wrs/hnd lv, init	
		S66.126A	Lacerat flxr musc/fasc/tend r lit fngr at wrs/hnd lv, init	
		S66.127A	Lacerat flxr musc/fasc/tend l lit fngr at wrs/hnd lv, init	
		S66.128A	Lacerat flexor musc/fasc/tend finger at wrs/hnd lv, init	
		S66.129A	Lacerat flexor musc/fasc/tend unsp fngr at wrs/hnd lv, init	
		S66.221A	Lacerat extensor musc/fasc/tend r thm at wrs/hnd lv, init	
		S66.222A	Lacerat extensor musc/fasc/tend l thm at wrs/hnd lv, init	
		S66.229A	Lacerat extensor musc/fasc/tend thmb at wrs/hnd lv, init	
		S66.32ØA	Lacerat extn musc/fasc/tend r idx fngr at wrs/hnd lv, init	
		S66.321A	Lacerat extn musc/fasc/tend l idx fngr at wrs/hnd lv, init	
		S66.322A	Lacerat extn musc/fasc/tend r mid finger at wrs/hnd lv, init	
		S66.323A	Lacerat extn musc/fasc/tend l mid finger at wrs/hnd lv, init	
		S66.324A	Lacerat extn musc/fasc/tend r rng fngr at wrs/hnd lv, init	
		S66.325A	Lacerat extn musc/fasc/tend l rng fngr at wrs/hnd lv, init	
		S66.326A	Lacerat extn musc/fasc/tend r lit fngr at wrs/hnd lv, init	
		S66.327A	Lacerat extn musc/fasc/tend l lit fngr at wrs/hnd lv, init	
		S66.328A	Lacerat extensor musc/fasc/tend finger at wrs/hnd lv, init	
		S66.329A	Lacerat extn musc/fasc/tend unsp finger at wrs/hnd lv, init	
		S66.421A	Lacerat intrinsic musc/fasc/tend r thm at wrs/hnd lv, init	
		S66.422A	Lacerat intrinsic musc/fasc/tend l thm at wrs/hnd lv, init	
		S66.429A	Lacerat intrinsic musc/fasc/tend thmb at wrs/hnd lv, init	

(Continued on next page)

[Brackets] indicate valid character values for each code. Character value meanings provided for each code grouping.

ICD-9-CM		ICD-10-CM	
881.22	OPEN WOUND OF WRIST WITH TENDON INVOLVEMENT (Continued)	**S66.52ØA**	Lacerat intrns musc/fasc/tend r idx fngr at wrs/hnd lv, init
		S66.521A	Lacerat intrns musc/fasc/tend l idx fngr at wrs/hnd lv, init
		S66.522A	Lacerat intrns musc/fasc/tend r mid fngr at wrs/hnd lv, init
		S66.523A	Lacerat intrns musc/fasc/tend l mid fngr at wrs/hnd lv, init
		S66.524A	Lacerat intrns musc/fasc/tend r rng fngr at wrs/hnd lv, init
		S66.525A	Lacerat intrns musc/fasc/tend l rng fngr at wrs/hnd lv, init
		S66.526A	Lacerat intrns musc/fasc/tend r lit fngr at wrs/hnd lv, init
		S66.527A	Lacerat intrns musc/fasc/tend l lit fngr at wrs/hnd lv, init
		S66.528A	Lacerat intrinsic musc/fasc/tend finger at wrs/hnd lv, init
		S66.529A	Lacerat intrns musc/fasc/tend unsp fngr at wrs/hnd lv, init
		S66.821A	Laceration of musc/fasc/tend at wrs/hnd lv, right hand, init
		S66.822A	Laceration of musc/fasc/tend at wrs/hnd lv, left hand, init
		S66.829A	Laceration of musc/fasc/tend at wrs/hnd lv, unsp hand, init
		S66.921A	Lacerat unsp musc/fasc/tend at wrs/hnd lv, right hand, init
		S66.922A	Lacerat unsp musc/fasc/tend at wrs/hnd lv, left hand, init
		S66.929A	Lacerat unsp musc/fasc/tend at wrs/hnd lv, unsp hand, init
882.Ø	OPEN WOUND HAND NO FINGER ALONE W/O MENTION COMP	**S61.4Ø1A**	Unspecified open wound of right hand, initial encounter
		S61.4Ø2A	Unspecified open wound of left hand, initial encounter
		S61.4Ø9A	Unspecified open wound of unspecified hand, init encntr
		S61.411A	Laceration without foreign body of right hand, init encntr
		S61.412A	Laceration without foreign body of left hand, init encntr
		S61.419A	Laceration without foreign body of unsp hand, init encntr
		S61.431A	Puncture wound w/o foreign body of right hand, init encntr
		S61.432A	Puncture wound w/o foreign body of left hand, init encntr
		S61.439A	Puncture wound w/o foreign body of unsp hand, init encntr
		S61.451A	Open bite of right hand, initial encounter
		S61.452A	Open bite of left hand, initial encounter
		S61.459A	Open bite of unspecified hand, initial encounter
882.1	OPEN WOUND HAND EXCEPT FINGER ALONE COMPLICATED	**S61.421A**	Laceration with foreign body of right hand, init encntr
		S61.422A	Laceration with foreign body of left hand, initial encounter
		S61.429A	Laceration with foreign body of unsp hand, init encntr
		S61.441A	Puncture wound with foreign body of right hand, init encntr
		S61.442A	Puncture wound with foreign body of left hand, init encntr
		S61.449A	Puncture wound with foreign body of unsp hand, init encntr
882.2	OPEN WOUND HAND NO FINGER ALONE W/TENDON INVLV	**S66.929A**	Lacerat unsp musc/fasc/tend at wrs/hnd lv, unsp hand, init *and*
		S61.4Ø9A	Unspecified open wound of unspecified hand, init encntr
		S66.Ø21A	Lacerat long flexor musc/fasc/tend r thm at wrs/hnd lv, init
		S66.Ø22A	Lacerat long flexor musc/fasc/tend l thm at wrs/hnd lv, init
		S66.Ø29A	Lacerat long flexor musc/fasc/tend thmb at wrs/hnd lv, init
		S66.12ØA	Lacerat flexor musc/fasc/tend r idx fngr at wrs/hnd lv, init
		S66.121A	Lacerat flexor musc/fasc/tend l idx fngr at wrs/hnd lv, init
		S66.122A	Lacerat flexor musc/fasc/tend r mid fngr at wrs/hnd lv, init
		S66.123A	Lacerat flexor musc/fasc/tend l mid fngr at wrs/hnd lv, init
		S66.124A	Lacerat flexor musc/fasc/tend r rng fngr at wrs/hnd lv, init
		S66.125A	Lacerat flexor musc/fasc/tend l rng fngr at wrs/hnd lv, init
		S66.126A	Lacerat flxr musc/fasc/tend r lit fngr at wrs/hnd lv, init
		S66.127A	Lacerat flxr musc/fasc/tend l lit fngr at wrs/hnd lv, init
		S66.128A	Lacerat flexor musc/fasc/tend finger at wrs/hnd lv, init
		S66.129A	Lacerat flexor musc/fasc/tend unsp fngr at wrs/hnd lv, init
		S66.221A	Lacerat extensor musc/fasc/tend r thm at wrs/hnd lv, init
		S66.222A	Lacerat extensor musc/fasc/tend l thm at wrs/hnd lv, init
		S66.229A	Lacerat extensor musc/fasc/tend thmb at wrs/hnd lv, init
		S66.32ØA	Lacerat extn musc/fasc/tend r idx fngr at wrs/hnd lv, init
		S66.321A	Lacerat extn musc/fasc/tend l idx fngr at wrs/hnd lv, init
		S66.322A	Lacerat extn musc/fasc/tend r mid finger at wrs/hnd lv, init
		S66.323A	Lacerat extn musc/fasc/tend l mid finger at wrs/hnd lv, init
		S66.324A	Lacerat extn musc/fasc/tend r rng fngr at wrs/hnd lv, init
		S66.325A	Lacerat extn musc/fasc/tend l rng fngr at wrs/hnd lv, init
		S66.326A	Lacerat extn musc/fasc/tend r lit fngr at wrs/hnd lv, init
		S66.327A	Lacerat extn musc/fasc/tend l lit fngr at wrs/hnd lv, init
		S66.328A	Lacerat extensor musc/fasc/tend finger at wrs/hnd lv, init
		S66.329A	Lacerat extn musc/fasc/tend unsp finger at wrs/hnd lv, init
		S66.421A	Lacerat intrinsic musc/fasc/tend r thm at wrs/hnd lv, init
		S66.422A	Lacerat intrinsic musc/fasc/tend l thm at wrs/hnd lv, init
		S66.429A	Lacerat intrinsic musc/fasc/tend thmb at wrs/hnd lv, init
		S66.52ØA	Lacerat intrns musc/fasc/tend r idx fngr at wrs/hnd lv, init
		S66.521A	Lacerat intrns musc/fasc/tend l idx fngr at wrs/hnd lv, init
		S66.522A	Lacerat intrns musc/fasc/tend r mid fngr at wrs/hnd lv, init
		S66.523A	Lacerat intrns musc/fasc/tend l mid fngr at wrs/hnd lv, init
		S66.524A	Lacerat intrns musc/fasc/tend r rng fngr at wrs/hnd lv, init
		S66.525A	Lacerat intrns musc/fasc/tend l rng fngr at wrs/hnd lv, init
		S66.526A	Lacerat intrns musc/fasc/tend r lit fngr at wrs/hnd lv, init
		S66.527A	Lacerat intrns musc/fasc/tend l lit fngr at wrs/hnd lv, init
		S66.528A	Lacerat intrinsic musc/fasc/tend finger at wrs/hnd lv, init
		S66.529A	Lacerat intrns musc/fasc/tend unsp fngr at wrs/hnd lv, init
		S66.821A	Laceration of musc/fasc/tend at wrs/hnd lv, right hand, init
		S66.822A	Laceration of musc/fasc/tend at wrs/hnd lv, left hand, init
		S66.829A	Laceration of musc/fasc/tend at wrs/hnd lv, unsp hand, init
		S66.921A	Lacerat unsp musc/fasc/tend at wrs/hnd lv, right hand, init
		S66.922A	Lacerat unsp musc/fasc/tend at wrs/hnd lv, left hand, init
		S66.929A	Lacerat unsp musc/fasc/tend at wrs/hnd lv, unsp hand, init

ICD-9-CM		ICD-10-CM	
883.0	OPEN WOUND FINGER WITHOUT MENTION COMPLICATION	**S61.001A**	Unsp open wound of right thumb w/o damage to nail, init
		S61.002A	Unsp open wound of left thumb w/o damage to nail, init
		S61.009A	Unsp open wound of unsp thumb w/o damage to nail, init
		S61.011A	Laceration w/o fb of right thumb w/o damage to nail, init
		S61.012A	Laceration w/o fb of left thumb w/o damage to nail, init
		S61.019A	Laceration w/o foreign body of thmb w/o damage to nail, init
		S61.031A	Pnctr w/o fb of right thumb w/o damage to nail, init
		S61.032A	Pnctr w/o fb of left thumb w/o damage to nail, init
		S61.039A	Pnctr w/o foreign body of thmb w/o damage to nail, init
		S61.051A	Open bite of right thumb without damage to nail, init encntr
		S61.052A	Open bite of left thumb without damage to nail, init encntr
		S61.059A	Open bite of unsp thumb without damage to nail, init encntr
		S61.101A	Unsp open wound of right thumb w damage to nail, init encntr
		S61.102A	Unsp open wound of left thumb w damage to nail, init encntr
		S61.109A	Unsp open wound of unsp thumb w damage to nail, init encntr
		S61.111A	Laceration w/o fb of right thumb w damage to nail, init
		S61.112A	Laceration w/o fb of left thumb w damage to nail, init
		S61.119A	Laceration w/o foreign body of thmb w damage to nail, init
		S61.131A	Pnctr w/o foreign body of right thumb w damage to nail, init
		S61.132A	Pnctr w/o foreign body of left thumb w damage to nail, init=
		S61.139A	Pnctr w/o foreign body of thmb w damage to nail, init
		S61.151A	Open bite of right thumb with damage to nail, init encntr
		S61.152A	Open bite of left thumb with damage to nail, init encntr
		S61.159A	Open bite of unsp thumb with damage to nail, init encntr
		S61.200A	Unsp open wound of r idx fngr w/o damage to nail, init
		S61.201A	Unsp open wound of l idx fngr w/o damage to nail, init
		S61.202A	Unsp open wound of r mid finger w/o damage to nail, init
		S61.203A	Unsp open wound of l mid finger w/o damage to nail, init
		S61.204A	Unsp open wound of r rng fngr w/o damage to nail, init
		S61.205A	Unsp open wound of left ring finger w/o damage to nail, init
		S61.206A	Unsp open wound of r little finger w/o damage to nail, init
		S61.207A	Unsp open wound of l little finger w/o damage to nail, init
		S61.208A	Unsp open wound of oth finger w/o damage to nail, init
		S61.209A	Unsp open wound of unsp finger w/o damage to nail, init
		S61.210A	Laceration w/o fb of r idx fngr w/o damage to nail, init
		S61.211A	Laceration w/o fb of l idx fngr w/o damage to nail, init
		S61.212A	Laceration w/o fb of r mid finger w/o damage to nail, init
		S61.213A	Laceration w/o fb of l mid finger w/o damage to nail, init
		S61.214A	Laceration w/o fb of r rng fngr w/o damage to nail, init
		S61.215A	Laceration w/o fb of l rng fngr w/o damage to nail, init
		S61.216A	Lac w/o fb of r little finger w/o damage to nail, init
		S61.217A	Lac w/o fb of l little finger w/o damage to nail, init
		S61.218A	Laceration w/o fb of finger w/o damage to nail, init
		S61.219A	Laceration w/o fb of unsp finger w/o damage to nail, init
		S61.230A	Pnctr w/o fb of r idx fngr w/o damage to nail, init
		S61.231A	Pnctr w/o fb of l idx fngr w/o damage to nail, init
		S61.232A	Pnctr w/o fb of r mid finger w/o damage to nail, init
		S61.233A	Pnctr w/o fb of l mid finger w/o damage to nail, init
		S61.234A	Pnctr w/o fb of r rng fngr w/o damage to nail, init
		S61.235A	Pnctr w/o fb of l rng fngr w/o damage to nail, init
		S61.236A	Pnctr w/o fb of r little finger w/o damage to nail, init
		S61.237A	Pnctr w/o fb of l little finger w/o damage to nail, init
		S61.238A	Pnctr w/o foreign body of finger w/o damage to nail, init
		S61.239A	Pnctr w/o fb of unsp finger w/o damage to nail, init
		S61.250A	Open bite of right index finger w/o damage to nail, init
		S61.251A	Open bite of left index finger w/o damage to nail, init
		S61.252A	Open bite of right middle finger w/o damage to nail, init
		S61.253A	Open bite of left middle finger w/o damage to nail, init
		S61.254A	Open bite of right ring finger w/o damage to nail, init
		S61.255A	Open bite of left ring finger w/o damage to nail, init
		S61.256A	Open bite of right little finger w/o damage to nail, init
		S61.257A	Open bite of left little finger w/o damage to nail, init
		S61.258A	Open bite of other finger w/o damage to nail, init encntr
		S61.259A	Open bite of unsp finger without damage to nail, init encntr
		S61.300A	Unsp open wound of right index finger w damage to nail, init
		S61.301A	Unsp open wound of left index finger w damage to nail, init
		S61.302A	Unsp open wound of r mid finger w damage to nail, init
		S61.303A	Unsp open wound of left middle finger w damage to nail, init
		S61.304A	Unsp open wound of right ring finger w damage to nail, init
		S61.305A	Unsp open wound of left ring finger w damage to nail, init
		S61.306A	Unsp open wound of r little finger w damage to nail, init
		S61.307A	Unsp open wound of left little finger w damage to nail, init
		S61.308A	Unsp open wound of oth finger w damage to nail, init encntr
		S61.309A	Unsp open wound of unsp finger w damage to nail, init encntr
		S61.310A	Laceration w/o fb of r idx fngr w damage to nail, init
		S61.311A	Laceration w/o fb of l idx fngr w damage to nail, init
		S61.312A	Laceration w/o fb of r mid finger w damage to nail, init
		S61.313A	Laceration w/o fb of l mid finger w damage to nail, init
		S61.314A	Laceration w/o fb of r rng fngr w damage to nail, init
		S61.315A	Laceration w/o fb of l rng fngr w damage to nail, init
		S61.316A	Laceration w/o fb of r little finger w damage to nail, init
		S61.317A	Laceration w/o fb of l little finger w damage to nail, init

(Continued on next page)

ICD-9-CM		ICD-10-CM		
883.Ø	OPEN WOUND FINGER WITHOUT MENTION COMPLICATION **(Continued)**	**S61.318A**	Laceration w/o foreign body of finger w damage to nail, init	
		S61.319A	Laceration w/o fb of unsp finger w damage to nail, init	
		S61.33ØA	Pnctr w/o foreign body of r idx fngr w damage to nail, init	
		S61.331A	Pnctr w/o foreign body of l idx fngr w damage to nail, init	
		S61.332A	Pnctr w/o fb of r mid finger w damage to nail, init	
		S61.333A	Pnctr w/o fb of l mid finger w damage to nail, init	
		S61.334A	Pnctr w/o foreign body of r rng fngr w damage to nail, init	
		S61.335A	Pnctr w/o foreign body of l rng fngr w damage to nail, init	
		S61.336A	Pnctr w/o fb of r little finger w damage to nail, init	
		S61.337A	Pnctr w/o fb of l little finger w damage to nail, init	
		S61.338A	Pnctr w/o foreign body of finger w damage to nail, init	
		S61.339A	Pnctr w/o foreign body of unsp finger w damage to nail, init	
		S61.35ØA	Open bite of right index finger w damage to nail, init	
		S61.351A	Open bite of left index finger w damage to nail, init encntr	
		S61.352A	Open bite of right middle finger w damage to nail, init	
		S61.353A	Open bite of left middle finger w damage to nail, init	
		S61.354A	Open bite of right ring finger w damage to nail, init encntr	
		S61.355A	Open bite of left ring finger w damage to nail, init encntr	
		S61.356A	Open bite of right little finger w damage to nail, init	
		S61.357A	Open bite of left little finger w damage to nail, init	
		S61.358A	Open bite of other finger with damage to nail, init encntr	
		S61.359A	Open bite of unsp finger with damage to nail, init encntr	
883.1	OPEN WOUND OF FINGER, COMPLICATED	**S61.Ø21A**	Laceration w fb of right thumb w/o damage to nail, init	
		S61.Ø22A	Laceration w fb of left thumb w/o damage to nail, init	
		S61.Ø29A	Laceration w foreign body of thmb w/o damage to nail, init	
		S61.Ø41A	Pnctr w foreign body of right thumb w/o damage to nail, init	
		S61.Ø42A	Pnctr w foreign body of left thumb w/o damage to nail, init	
		S61.Ø49A	Pnctr w foreign body of thmb w/o damage to nail, init	
		S61.121A	Laceration w fb of right thumb w damage to nail, init	
		S61.122A	Laceration w fb of left thumb w damage to nail, init	
		S61.129A	Laceration w foreign body of thmb w damage to nail, init	
		S61.141A	Pnctr w foreign body of right thumb w damage to nail, init	
		S61.142A	Pnctr w foreign body of left thumb w damage to nail, init	
		S61.149A	Puncture wound w foreign body of thmb w damage to nail, init	
		S61.22ØA	Laceration w fb of r idx fngr w/o damage to nail, init	
		S61.221A	Laceration w fb of l idx fngr w/o damage to nail, init	
		S61.222A	Laceration w fb of r mid finger w/o damage to nail, init	
		S61.223A	Laceration w fb of l mid finger w/o damage to nail, init	
		S61.224A	Laceration w fb of r rng fngr w/o damage to nail, init	
		S61.225A	Laceration w fb of l rng fngr w/o damage to nail, init	
		S61.226A	Laceration w fb of r little finger w/o damage to nail, init	
		S61.227A	Laceration w fb of l little finger w/o damage to nail, init	
		S61.228A	Laceration w foreign body of finger w/o damage to nail, init	
		S61.229A	Laceration w fb of unsp finger w/o damage to nail, init	
		S61.24ØA	Pnctr w foreign body of r idx fngr w/o damage to nail, init	
		S61.241A	Pnctr w foreign body of l idx fngr w/o damage to nail, init	
		S61.242A	Pnctr w fb of r mid finger w/o damage to nail, init	
		S61.243A	Pnctr w fb of l mid finger w/o damage to nail, init	
		S61.244A	Pnctr w foreign body of r rng fngr w/o damage to nail, init	
		S61.245A	Pnctr w foreign body of l rng fngr w/o damage to nail, init	
		S61.246A	Pnctr w fb of r little finger w/o damage to nail, init	
		S61.247A	Pnctr w fb of l little finger w/o damage to nail, init	
		S61.248A	Pnctr w foreign body of finger w/o damage to nail, init	
		S61.249A	Pnctr w foreign body of unsp finger w/o damage to nail, init	
		S61.32ØA	Laceration w fb of r idx fngr w damage to nail, init	
		S61.321A	Laceration w fb of l idx fngr w damage to nail, init	
		S61.322A	Laceration w fb of r mid finger w damage to nail, init	
		S61.323A	Laceration w fb of l mid finger w damage to nail, init	
		S61.324A	Laceration w fb of r rng fngr w damage to nail, init	
		S61.325A	Laceration w fb of l rng fngr w damage to nail, init	
		S61.326A	Laceration w fb of r little finger w damage to nail, init	
		S61.327A	Laceration w fb of l little finger w damage to nail, init	
		S61.328A	Laceration w foreign body of finger w damage to nail, init	
		S61.329A	Laceration w fb of unsp finger w damage to nail, init	
		S61.34ØA	Pnctr w foreign body of r idx fngr w damage to nail, init	
		S61.341A	Pnctr w foreign body of l idx fngr w damage to nail, init	
		S61.342A	Pnctr w foreign body of r mid finger w damage to nail, init	
		S61.343A	Pnctr w foreign body of l mid finger w damage to nail, init	
		S61.344A	Pnctr w foreign body of r rng fngr w damage to nail, init	
		S61.345A	Pnctr w foreign body of l rng fngr w damage to nail, init	
		S61.346A	Pnctr w fb of r little finger w damage to nail, init	
		S61.347A	Pnctr w fb of l little finger w damage to nail, init	
		S61.348A	Pnctr w foreign body of finger w damage to nail, init	
		S61.349A	Pnctr w foreign body of unsp finger w damage to nail, init	
883.2	OPEN WOUND OF FINGER WITH TENDON INVOLVEMENT	**S66.529A**	Lacerat intrns musc/fasc/tend unsp fngr at wrs/hnd lv, init	***and***
		S61.1Ø9A	Unsp open wound of unsp thumb w damage to nail, init encntr	***or***
		S61.2Ø9A	Unsp open wound of unsp finger w/o damage to nail, init	
884.Ø	MX&UNSPEC OPEN WOUND UPPER LIMB W/O MENTION COMP	**S41.ØØ9A**	Unspecified open wound of unspecified shoulder, init encntr	
884.1	MULTIPLE&UNSPEC OPEN WOUND UPPER LIMB COMP	**S41.Ø29A**	Laceration with foreign body of unsp shoulder, init encntr	
884.2	MX&UNSPEC OPEN WOUND UPPER LIMB W/TENDON INVLV	**S41.ØØ9A**	Unspecified open wound of unspecified shoulder, init encntr	

ICD-9-CM		ICD-10-CM	
885.Ø	TRAUMATIC AMP THUMB WITHOUT MENTION COMPLICATION	**S68.Ø11A**	Complete traumatic MCP amputation of right thumb, init
		S68.Ø12A	Complete traumatic MCP amputation of left thumb, init
		S68.Ø19A	Complete traumatic MCP amputation of thmb, init
		S68.Ø21A	Partial traumatic MCP amputation of right thumb, init
		S68.Ø22A	Partial traumatic MCP amputation of left thumb, init
		S68.Ø29A	Partial traumatic MCP amputation of thmb, init
		S68.511A	Complete traumatic trnsphal amputation of right thumb, init
		S68.512A	Complete traumatic trnsphal amputation of left thumb, init
		S68.519A	Complete traumatic transphalangeal amputation of thmb, init
		S68.521A	Partial traumatic trnsphal amputation of right thumb, init
		S68.522A	Partial traumatic trnsphal amputation of left thumb, init
		S68.529A	Partial traumatic transphalangeal amputation of thmb, init
885.1	TRAUMATIC AMPUTATION OF THUMB COMPLICATED	**S68.Ø19A**	Complete traumatic MCP amputation of thmb, init
		S68.Ø29A	Partial traumatic MCP amputation of thmb, init
		S68.519A	Complete traumatic transphalangeal amputation of thmb, init
		S68.529A	Partial traumatic transphalangeal amputation of thmb, init
886.Ø	TRAUMATIC AMP OTH FINGER WITHOUT MENTION COMP	**S68.11ØA**	Complete traumatic MCP amputation of r idx fngr, init
		S68.111A	Complete traumatic MCP amputation of left index finger, init
		S68.112A	Complete traumatic MCP amputation of r mid finger, init
		S68.113A	Complete traumatic MCP amputation of l mid finger, init
		S68.114A	Complete traumatic MCP amputation of right ring finger, init
		S68.115A	Complete traumatic MCP amputation of left ring finger, init
		S68.116A	Complete traumatic MCP amputation of r little finger, init
		S68.117A	Complete traumatic MCP amputation of l little finger, init
		S68.118A	Complete traumatic MCP amputation of finger, init
		S68.119A	Complete traumatic MCP amputation of unsp finger, init
		S68.12ØA	Partial traumatic MCP amputation of right index finger, init
		S68.121A	Partial traumatic MCP amputation of left index finger, init
		S68.122A	Partial traumatic MCP amputation of r mid finger, init
		S68.123A	Partial traumatic MCP amputation of left middle finger, init
		S68.124A	Partial traumatic MCP amputation of right ring finger, init
		S68.125A	Partial traumatic MCP amputation of left ring finger, init
		S68.126A	Partial traumatic MCP amputation of r little finger, init
		S68.127A	Partial traumatic MCP amputation of left little finger, init
		S68.128A	Partial traumatic MCP amputation of finger, init
		S68.129A	Partial traumatic MCP amputation of unsp finger, init
		S68.61ØA	Complete traumatic trnsphal amputation of r idx fngr, init
		S68.611A	Complete traumatic trnsphal amputation of l idx fngr, init
		S68.612A	Complete traumatic trnsphal amputation of r mid finger, init
		S68.613A	Complete traumatic trnsphal amputation of l mid finger, init
		S68.614A	Complete traumatic trnsphal amputation of r rng fngr, init
		S68.615A	Complete traumatic trnsphal amputation of l rng fngr, init
		S68.616A	Complete traumatic trnsphal amp of r little finger, init
		S68.617A	Complete traumatic trnsphal amp of l little finger, init
		S68.618A	Complete traumatic trnsphal amputation of finger, init
		S68.619A	Complete traumatic trnsphal amputation of unsp finger, init
		S68.62ØA	Partial traumatic trnsphal amputation of r idx fngr, init
		S68.621A	Partial traumatic trnsphal amputation of l idx fngr, init
		S68.622A	Partial traumatic trnsphal amputation of r mid finger, init
		S68.623A	Partial traumatic trnsphal amputation of l mid finger, init
		S68.624A	Partial traumatic trnsphal amputation of r rng fngr, init
		S68.625A	Partial traumatic trnsphal amputation of l rng fngr, init
		S68.626A	Partial traumatic trnsphal amp of r little finger, init
		S68.627A	Partial traumatic trnsphal amp of l little finger, init
		S68.628A	Partial traumatic transphalangeal amputation of finger, init
		S68.629A	Partial traumatic trnsphal amputation of unsp finger, init
886.1	TRAUMATIC AMPUTATION OF OTHER FINGER COMPLICATED	**S68.119A**	Complete traumatic MCP amputation of unsp finger, init
		S68.129A	Partial traumatic MCP amputation of unsp finger, init
		S68.619A	Complete traumatic trnsphal amputation of unsp finger, init
		S68.629A	Partial traumatic trnsphal amputation of unsp finger, init
887.Ø	TRAUMAT AMP ARM&HND UNILAT BELW ELB W/O COMP	**S58.111A**	Complete traum amp at lev betw elbow and wrist, r arm, init
		S58.112A	Complete traum amp at lev betw elbow and wrs, left arm, init
		S58.119A	Complete traum amp at lev betw elbow and wrs, unsp arm, init
		S58.121A	Part traum amp at lev betw elbow and wrist, right arm, init
		S58.122A	Part traum amp at level betw elbow and wrist, left arm, init
		S58.129A	Part traum amp at level betw elbow and wrist, unsp arm, init
		S58.911A	Complete traumatic amputation of r forearm, level unsp, init
		S58.912A	Complete traumatic amputation of l forearm, level unsp, init
		S58.919A	Complete traumatic amp of unsp forearm, level unsp, init
		S58.921A	Partial traumatic amputation of r forearm, level unsp, init
		S58.922A	Partial traumatic amputation of l forearm, level unsp, init
		S58.929A	Partial traumatic amp of unsp forearm, level unsp, init
		S68.411A	Complete traumatic amp of right hand at wrist level, init
		S68.412A	Complete traumatic amp of left hand at wrist level, init
		S68.419A	Complete traumatic amp of unsp hand at wrist level, init
		S68.421A	Partial traumatic amp of right hand at wrist level, init
		S68.422A	Partial traumatic amp of left hand at wrist level, init
		S68.429A	Partial traumatic amp of unsp hand at wrist level, init
	(Continued on next page)	**S68.711A**	Complete traumatic transmetcrpl amp of right hand, init

ICD-9-CM		ICD-10-CM		
887.Ø	TRAUMAT AMP ARM&HND UNILAT BELW ELB W/O COMP **(Continued)**	**S68.712A**	Complete traumatic transmetcrpl amp of left hand, init	
		S68.719A	Complete traumatic transmetcrpl amp of unsp hand, init	
		S68.721A	Partial traumatic transmetcrpl amp of right hand, init	
		S68.722A	Partial traumatic transmetcrpl amputation of left hand, init	
		S68.729A	Partial traumatic transmetcrpl amputation of unsp hand, init	
887.1	TRAUMATIC AMP ARM&HAND UNILATERAL BELOW ELB COMP	**S58.119A**	Complete traum amp at lev betw elbow and wrs, unsp arm, init	
		S58.129A	Part traum amp at level betw elbow and wrist, unsp arm, init	
		S58.919A	Complete traumatic amp of unsp forearm, level unsp, init	
		S58.929A	Partial traumatic amp of unsp forearm, level unsp, init	
		S68.419A	Complete traumatic amp of unsp hand at wrist level, init	
		S68.429A	Partial traumatic amp of unsp hand at wrist level, init	
		S68.719A	Complete traumatic transmetcrpl amp of unsp hand, init	
		S68.729A	Partial traumatic transmetcrpl amputation of unsp hand, init	
887.2	TRAUMAT AMP ARM&HND UNILAT@OR ABVE ELB W/O COMP	**S48.Ø11A**	Complete traumatic amputation at right shoulder joint, init	
		S48.Ø12A	Complete traumatic amputation at left shoulder joint, init	
		S48.Ø19A	Complete traumatic amputation at unsp shoulder joint, init	
		S48.Ø21A	Partial traumatic amputation at right shoulder joint, init	
		S48.Ø22A	Partial traumatic amputation at left shoulder joint, init	
		S48.Ø29A	Partial traumatic amputation at unsp shoulder joint, init	
		S48.111A	Complete traum amp at level betw r shoulder and elbow, init	
		S48.112A	Complete traum amp at level betw l shoulder and elbow, init	
		S48.119A	Complete traum amp at level betw unsp shldr and elbow, init	
		S48.121A	Partial traum amp at level betw r shoulder and elbow, init	
		S48.122A	Partial traum amp at level betw l shoulder and elbow, init	
		S48.129A	Partial traum amp at level betw unsp shldr and elbow, init	
		S58.Ø11A	Complete traumatic amp at elbow level, right arm, init	
		S58.Ø12A	Complete traumatic amputation at elbow level, left arm, init	
		S58.Ø19A	Complete traumatic amputation at elbow level, unsp arm, init	
		S58.Ø21A	Partial traumatic amputation at elbow level, right arm, init	
		S58.Ø22A	Partial traumatic amputation at elbow level, left arm, init	
		S58.Ø29A	Partial traumatic amputation at elbow level, unsp arm, init	
887.3	TRAUMATIC AMP ARM&HAND UNILAT@OR ABOVE ELB COMP	**S48.Ø19A**	Complete traumatic amputation at unsp shoulder joint, init	
		S48.Ø29A	Partial traumatic amputation at unsp shoulder joint, init	
		S48.119A	Complete traum amp at level betw unsp shldr and elbow, init	
		S48.129A	Partial traum amp at level betw unsp shldr and elbow, init	
		S58.Ø19A	Complete traumatic amputation at elbow level, unsp arm, init	
		S58.Ø29A	Partial traumatic amputation at elbow level, unsp arm, init	
887.4	TRAUMAT AMP ARM&HND UNILAT LEVL NOT W/O COMP	**S48.911A**	Complete traum amp of right shldr/up arm, level unsp, init	
		S48.912A	Complete traum amp of left shldr/up arm, level unsp, init	
		S48.919A	Complete traum amp of unsp shldr/up arm, level unsp, init	
		S48.921A	Partial traum amp of right shldr/up arm, level unsp, init	
		S48.922A	Partial traumatic amp of left shldr/up arm, level unsp, init	
		S48.929A	Partial traumatic amp of unsp shldr/up arm, level unsp, init	
887.5	TRAUMAT AMP ARM&HAND UNILAT LEVEL NOT SPEC COMP	**S48.919A**	Complete traum amp of unsp shldr/up arm, level unsp, init	
		S48.929A	Partial traumatic amp of unsp shldr/up arm, level unsp, init	
887.6	TRAUMAT AMP ARM&HAND BILAT WITHOUT MENTION COMP	**S48.911A**	Complete traum amp of right shldr/up arm, level unsp, init	***or***
		S48.921A	Partial traum amp of right shldr/up arm, level unsp, init	***and***
		S48.912A	Complete traum amp of left shldr/up arm, level unsp, init	***or***
		S48.922A	Partial traumatic amp of left shldr/up arm, level unsp, init	
887.7	TRAUMATIC AMP ARM&HAND BILATERAL COMPLICATED	**S48.911A**	Complete traum amp of right shldr/up arm, level unsp, init	***and***
		S48.912A	Complete traum amp of left shldr/up arm, level unsp, init	
89Ø.Ø	OPEN WOUND HIP&THIGH WITHOUT MENTION COMP	**S71.ØØ1A**	Unspecified open wound, right hip, initial encounter	
		S71.ØØ2A	Unspecified open wound, left hip, initial encounter	
		S71.ØØ9A	Unspecified open wound, unspecified hip, initial encounter	
		S71.Ø11A	Laceration without foreign body, right hip, init encntr	
		S71.Ø12A	Laceration without foreign body, left hip, initial encounter	
		S71.Ø19A	Laceration without foreign body, unsp hip, init encntr	
		S71.Ø31A	Puncture wound without foreign body, right hip, init encntr	
		S71.Ø32A	Puncture wound without foreign body, left hip, init encntr	
		S71.Ø39A	Puncture wound without foreign body, unsp hip, init encntr	
		S71.Ø51A	Open bite, right hip, initial encounter	
		S71.Ø52A	Open bite, left hip, initial encounter	
		S71.Ø59A	Open bite, unspecified hip, initial encounter	
		S71.1Ø1A	Unspecified open wound, right thigh, initial encounter	
		S71.1Ø2A	Unspecified open wound, left thigh, initial encounter	
		S71.1Ø9A	Unspecified open wound, unspecified thigh, initial encounter	
		S71.111A	Laceration without foreign body, right thigh, init encntr	
		S71.112A	Laceration without foreign body, left thigh, init encntr	
		S71.119A	Laceration without foreign body, unsp thigh, init encntr	
		S71.131A	Puncture wound w/o foreign body, right thigh, init encntr	
		S71.132A	Puncture wound without foreign body, left thigh, init encntr	
		S71.139A	Puncture wound without foreign body, unsp thigh, init encntr	
		S71.151A	Open bite, right thigh, initial encounter	
		S71.152A	Open bite, left thigh, initial encounter	
		S71.159A	Open bite, unspecified thigh, initial encounter	

ICD-9-CM		ICD-10-CM		
890.1	OPEN WOUND OF HIP AND THIGH COMPLICATED	**S71.021A**	Laceration with foreign body, right hip, initial encounter	
		S71.022A	Laceration with foreign body, left hip, initial encounter	
		S71.029A	Laceration with foreign body, unspecified hip, init encntr	
		S71.041A	Puncture wound with foreign body, right hip, init encntr	
		S71.042A	Puncture wound with foreign body, left hip, init encntr	
		S71.049A	Puncture wound with foreign body, unsp hip, init encntr	
		S71.121A	Laceration with foreign body, right thigh, initial encounter	
		S71.122A	Laceration with foreign body, left thigh, initial encounter	
		S71.129A	Laceration with foreign body, unspecified thigh, init encntr	
		S71.141A	Puncture wound with foreign body, right thigh, init encntr	
		S71.142A	Puncture wound with foreign body, left thigh, init encntr	
		S71.149A	Puncture wound with foreign body, unsp thigh, init encntr	
890.2	OPEN WOUND OF HIP AND THIGH W/TENDON INVOLVEMENT	**S76.929A**	Lacerat unsp musc/fasc/tend at thigh level, unsp thigh, init	***and***
		S71.009A	Unspecified open wound, unspecified hip, initial encounter	***or***
		S71.109A	Unspecified open wound, unspecified thigh, initial encounter	
		S76.021A	Laceration of muscle, fascia and tendon of right hip, init	
		S76.022A	Laceration of muscle, fascia and tendon of left hip, init	
		S76.029A	Laceration of muscle, fascia and tendon of unsp hip, init	
		S76.121A	Laceration of right quadriceps musc/fasc/tend, init	
		S76.122A	Laceration of left quadriceps musc/fasc/tend, init	
		S76.129A	Laceration of unsp quadriceps musc/fasc/tend, init	
		S76.221A	Laceration of adductor musc/fasc/tend right thigh, init	
		S76.222A	Laceration of adductor musc/fasc/tend left thigh, init	
		S76.229A	Laceration of adductor musc/fasc/tend unsp thigh, init	
		S76.321A	Lacerat msl/fasc/tnd post grp at thi lev, right thigh, init	
		S76.322A	Lacerat msl/fasc/tnd post grp at thi lev, left thigh, init	
		S76.329A	Lacerat msl/fasc/tnd post grp at thi lev, unsp thigh, init	
		S76.821A	Lacerat musc/fasc/tend at thigh level, right thigh, init	
		S76.822A	Lacerat musc/fasc/tend at thigh level, left thigh, init	
		S76.829A	Lacerat musc/fasc/tend at thigh level, unsp thigh, init	
		S76.921A	Lacerat unsp musc/fasc/tend at thi lev, right thigh, init	
		S76.922A	Lacerat unsp musc/fasc/tend at thigh level, left thigh, init	
		S76.929A	Lacerat unsp musc/fasc/tend at thigh level, unsp thigh, init	
891.0	OPEN WOUND KNEE LEG&ANK WITHOUT MENTION COMP	**S81.001A**	Unspecified open wound, right knee, initial encounter	
		S81.002A	Unspecified open wound, left knee, initial encounter	
		S81.009A	Unspecified open wound, unspecified knee, initial encounter	
		S81.011A	Laceration without foreign body, right knee, init encntr	
		S81.012A	Laceration without foreign body, left knee, init encntr	
		S81.019A	Laceration without foreign body, unsp knee, init encntr	
		S81.031A	Puncture wound without foreign body, right knee, init encntr	
		S81.032A	Puncture wound without foreign body, left knee, init encntr	
		S81.039A	Puncture wound without foreign body, unsp knee, init encntr	
		S81.051A	Open bite, right knee, initial encounter	
		S81.052A	Open bite, left knee, initial encounter	
		S81.059A	Open bite, unspecified knee, initial encounter	
		S81.801A	Unspecified open wound, right lower leg, initial encounter	
		S81.802A	Unspecified open wound, left lower leg, initial encounter	
		S81.809A	Unspecified open wound, unspecified lower leg, init encntr	
		S81.811A	Laceration w/o foreign body, right lower leg, init encntr	
		S81.812A	Laceration without foreign body, left lower leg, init encntr	
		S81.819A	Laceration without foreign body, unsp lower leg, init encntr	
		S81.831A	Puncture wound w/o foreign body, right lower leg, init	
		S81.832A	Puncture wound w/o foreign body, left lower leg, init encntr	
		S81.839A	Puncture wound w/o foreign body, unsp lower leg, init encntr	
		S81.851A	Open bite, right lower leg, initial encounter	
		S81.852A	Open bite, left lower leg, initial encounter	
		S81.859A	Open bite, unspecified lower leg, initial encounter	
		S91.001A	Unspecified open wound, right ankle, initial encounter	
		S91.002A	Unspecified open wound, left ankle, initial encounter	
		S91.009A	Unspecified open wound, unspecified ankle, initial encounter	
		S91.011A	Laceration without foreign body, right ankle, init encntr	
		S91.012A	Laceration without foreign body, left ankle, init encntr	
		S91.019A	Laceration without foreign body, unsp ankle, init encntr	
		S91.031A	Puncture wound w/o foreign body, right ankle, init encntr	
		S91.032A	Puncture wound without foreign body, left ankle, init encntr	
		S91.039A	Puncture wound without foreign body, unsp ankle, init encntr	
		S91.051A	Open bite, right ankle, initial encounter	
		S91.052A	Open bite, left ankle, initial encounter	
		S91.059A	Open bite, unspecified ankle, initial encounter	
891.1	OPEN WOUND OF KNEE LEG AND ANKLE COMPLICATED	**S81.021A**	Laceration with foreign body, right knee, initial encounter	
		S81.022A	Laceration with foreign body, left knee, initial encounter	
		S81.029A	Laceration with foreign body, unspecified knee, init encntr	
		S81.041A	Puncture wound with foreign body, right knee, init encntr	
		S81.042A	Puncture wound with foreign body, left knee, init encntr	
		S81.049A	Puncture wound with foreign body, unsp knee, init encntr	
		S81.821A	Laceration with foreign body, right lower leg, init encntr	
		S81.822A	Laceration with foreign body, left lower leg, init encntr	
		S81.829A	Laceration with foreign body, unsp lower leg, init encntr	
		S81.841A	Puncture wound w foreign body, right lower leg, init encntr	
		S81.842A	Puncture wound w foreign body, left lower leg, init encntr	

(Continued on next page)

[Brackets] indicate valid character values for each code. Character value meanings provided for each code grouping.

ICD-9-CM		ICD-10-CM		
891.1	OPEN WOUND OF KNEE LEG AND ANKLE COMPLICATED **(Continued)**	**S81.849A**	Puncture wound w foreign body, unsp lower leg, init encntr	
		S91.Ø21A	Laceration with foreign body, right ankle, initial encounter	
		S91.Ø22A	Laceration with foreign body, left ankle, initial encounter	
		S91.Ø29A	Laceration with foreign body, unspecified ankle, init encntr	
		S91.Ø41A	Puncture wound with foreign body, right ankle, init encntr	
		S91.Ø42A	Puncture wound with foreign body, left ankle, init encntr	
		S91.Ø49A	Puncture wound with foreign body, unsp ankle, init encntr	
891.2	OPEN WOUND KNEE LEG&ANKLE W/TENDON INVOLVEMENT	**S86.929A**	Lacerat unsp musc/tend at lower leg level, unsp leg, init	*and*
		S81.ØØ9A	Unspecified open wound, unspecified knee, initial encounter	*or*
		S81.8Ø9A	Unspecified open wound, unspecified lower leg, init encntr	
		S96.929A	Laceration of unsp msl/tnd at ank/ft level, unsp foot, init	*and*
		S91.ØØ9A	Unspecified open wound, unspecified ankle, initial encounter	
		S86.Ø21A	Laceration of right Achilles tendon, initial encounter	
		S86.Ø22A	Laceration of left Achilles tendon, initial encounter	
		S86.Ø29A	Laceration of unspecified Achilles tendon, initial encounter	
		S86.121A	Lacerat musc/tend post grp at low leg level, right leg, init	
		S86.122A	Lacerat musc/tend post grp at low leg level, left leg, init	
		S86.129A	Lacerat musc/tend post grp at low leg level, unsp leg, init	
		S86.221A	Lacerat musc/tend ant grp at low leg level, right leg, init	
		S86.222A	Lacerat musc/tend ant grp at low leg level, left leg, init	
		S86.229A	Lacerat musc/tend ant grp at low leg level, unsp leg, init	
		S86.321A	Lacerat musc/tend peroneal grp at low leg lev, r leg, init	
		S86.322A	Lacerat musc/tend peroneal grp at low leg lev, l leg, init	
		S86.329A	Lacerat musc/tend peroneal grp at low leg lev,unsp leg, init	
		S86.821A	Laceration of musc/tend at lower leg level, right leg, init	
		S86.822A	Laceration of musc/tend at lower leg level, left leg, init	
		S86.829A	Laceration of musc/tend at lower leg level, unsp leg, init	
		S86.921A	Lacerat unsp musc/tend at lower leg level, right leg, init	
		S86.922A	Lacerat unsp musc/tend at lower leg level, left leg, init	
		S86.929A	Lacerat unsp musc/tend at lower leg level, unsp leg, init	
		S96.Ø21A	Lacerat msl/tnd lng flxr msl toe at ank/ft lev, r foot, init	
		S96.Ø22A	Lacerat msl/tnd lng flxr msl toe at ank/ft lev, l foot, init	
		S96.Ø29A	Lacerat msl/tnd lng flxr msl toe at ank/ft lev,unsp ft, init	
		S96.121A	Lacerat msl/tnd lng extn msl toe at ank/ft lev, r foot, init	
		S96.122A	Lacerat msl/tnd lng extn msl toe at ank/ft lev, l foot, init	
		S96.129A	Lacerat msl/tnd lng extn msl toe at ank/ft lev,unsp ft, init	
		S96.221A	Lacerat intrinsic msl/tnd at ank/ft level, right foot, init	
		S96.222A	Lacerat intrinsic msl/tnd at ank/ft level, left foot, init	
		S96.229A	Lacerat intrinsic msl/tnd at ank/ft level, unsp foot, init	
		S96.821A	Lacerat muscles and tendons at ank/ft level, r foot, init	
		S96.822A	Lacerat muscles and tendons at ank/ft level, left foot, init	
		S96.829A	Lacerat muscles and tendons at ank/ft level, unsp foot, init	
		S96.921A	Laceration of unsp msl/tnd at ank/ft level, right foot, init	
		S96.922A	Laceration of unsp msl/tnd at ank/ft level, left foot, init	
		S96.929A	Lacerat unsp musc/tend at lower leg level, unsp leg, init	
		S96.929A	Laceration of unsp msl/tnd at ank/ft level, unsp foot, init	
892.Ø	OPEN WOUND FT NO TOE ALONE WITHOUT MENTION COMP	**S91.3Ø1A**	Unspecified open wound, right foot, initial encounter	
		S91.3Ø2A	Unspecified open wound, left foot, initial encounter	
		S91.3Ø9A	Unspecified open wound, unspecified foot, initial encounter	
		S91.311A	Laceration without foreign body, right foot, init encntr	
		S91.312A	Laceration without foreign body, left foot, init encntr	
		S91.319A	Laceration without foreign body, unsp foot, init encntr	
		S91.331A	Puncture wound without foreign body, right foot, init encntr	
		S91.332A	Puncture wound without foreign body, left foot, init encntr	
		S91.339A	Puncture wound without foreign body, unsp foot, init encntr	
		S91.351A	Open bite, right foot, initial encounter	
		S91.352A	Open bite, left foot, initial encounter	
		S91.359A	Open bite, unspecified foot, initial encounter	
892.1	OPEN WOUND OF FOOT EXCEPT TOE ALONE COMPLICATED	**S91.321A**	Laceration with foreign body, right foot, initial encounter	
		S91.322A	Laceration with foreign body, left foot, initial encounter	
		S91.329A	Laceration with foreign body, unspecified foot, init encntr	
		S91.341A	Puncture wound with foreign body, right foot, init encntr	
		S91.342A	Puncture wound with foreign body, left foot, init encntr	
		S91.349A	Puncture wound with foreign body, unsp foot, init encntr	
892.2	OPEN WOUND FT NO TOE ALONE W/TENDON INVOLVEMENT	**S96.929A**	Laceration of unsp msl/tnd at ank/ft level, unsp foot, init	*and*
		S91.3Ø9A	Unspecified open wound, unspecified foot, initial encounter	
893.Ø	OPEN WOUND TOE WITHOUT MENTION COMPLICATION	**S91.1Ø1A**	Unsp open wound of right great toe w/o damage to nail, init	
		S91.1Ø2A	Unsp open wound of left great toe w/o damage to nail, init	
		S91.1Ø3A	Unsp open wound of unsp great toe w/o damage to nail, init	
		S91.1Ø4A	Unsp opn wnd right lesser toe(s) w/o damage to nail, init	
		S91.1Ø5A	Unsp opn wnd left lesser toe(s) w/o damage to nail, init	
		S91.1Ø6A	Unsp opn wnd unsp lesser toe(s) w/o damage to nail, init	
		S91.1Ø9A	Unsp open wound of unsp toe(s) w/o damage to nail, init	
		S91.111A	Lac w/o fb of right great toe w/o damage to nail, init	
		S91.112A	Laceration w/o fb of left great toe w/o damage to nail, init	
		S91.113A	Laceration w/o fb of unsp great toe w/o damage to nail, init	
		S91.114A	Lac w/o fb of right lesser toe(s) w/o damage to nail, init	
		S91.115A	Lac w/o fb of left lesser toe(s) w/o damage to nail, init	
		S91.116A	Lac w/o fb of unsp lesser toe(s) w/o damage to nail, init	
		S91.119A	Laceration w/o fb of unsp toe w/o damage to nail, init	

(Continued on next page)

ICD-9-CM		ICD-10-CM		
893.Ø	OPEN WOUND TOE WITHOUT MENTION COMPLICATION **(Continued)**	**S91.131A**	Pnctr w/o fb of right great toe w/o damage to nail, init	
		S91.132A	Pnctr w/o fb of left great toe w/o damage to nail, init	
		S91.133A	Pnctr w/o fb of unsp great toe w/o damage to nail, init	
		S91.134A	Pnctr w/o fb of right lesser toe(s) w/o damage to nail, init	
		S91.135A	Pnctr w/o fb of left lesser toe(s) w/o damage to nail, init	
		S91.136A	Pnctr w/o fb of unsp lesser toe(s) w/o damage to nail, init	
		S91.139A	Pnctr w/o fb of unsp toe(s) w/o damage to nail, init	
		S91.151A	Open bite of right great toe w/o damage to nail, init encntr	
		S91.152A	Open bite of left great toe w/o damage to nail, init encntr	
		S91.153A	Open bite of unsp great toe w/o damage to nail, init encntr	
		S91.154A	Open bite of right lesser toe(s) w/o damage to nail, init	
		S91.155A	Open bite of left lesser toe(s) w/o damage to nail, init	
		S91.156A	Open bite of unsp lesser toe(s) w/o damage to nail, init	
		S91.159A	Open bite of unsp toe(s) without damage to nail, init encntr	
		S91.2Ø1A	Unsp open wound of right great toe w damage to nail, init	
		S91.2Ø2A	Unsp open wound of left great toe w damage to nail, init	
		S91.2Ø3A	Unsp open wound of unsp great toe w damage to nail, init	
		S91.2Ø4A	Unsp opn wnd right lesser toe(s) w damage to nail, init	
		S91.2Ø5A	Unsp open wound of left lesser toe(s) w damage to nail, init	
		S91.2Ø6A	Unsp open wound of unsp lesser toe(s) w damage to nail, init	
		S91.2Ø9A	Unsp open wound of unsp toe(s) w damage to nail, init encntr	
		S91.211A	Laceration w/o fb of right great toe w damage to nail, init	
		S91.212A	Laceration w/o fb of left great toe w damage to nail, init	
		S91.213A	Laceration w/o fb of unsp great toe w damage to nail, init	
		S91.214A	Lac w/o fb of right lesser toe(s) w damage to nail, init	
		S91.215A	Lac w/o fb of left lesser toe(s) w damage to nail, init	
		S91.216A	Lac w/o fb of unsp lesser toe(s) w damage to nail, init	
		S91.219A	Laceration w/o fb of unsp toe(s) w damage to nail, init	
		S91.231A	Pnctr w/o fb of right great toe w damage to nail, init	
		S91.232A	Pnctr w/o fb of left great toe w damage to nail, init	
		S91.233A	Pnctr w/o fb of unsp great toe w damage to nail, init	
		S91.234A	Pnctr w/o fb of right lesser toe(s) w damage to nail, init	
		S91.235A	Pnctr w/o fb of left lesser toe(s) w damage to nail, init	
		S91.236A	Pnctr w/o fb of unsp lesser toe(s) w damage to nail, init	
		S91.239A	Pnctr w/o foreign body of unsp toe(s) w damage to nail, init	
		S91.251A	Open bite of right great toe w damage to nail, init encntr	
		S91.252A	Open bite of left great toe with damage to nail, init encntr	
		S91.253A	Open bite of unsp great toe with damage to nail, init encntr	
		S91.254A	Open bite of right lesser toe(s) w damage to nail, init	
		S91.255A	Open bite of left lesser toe(s) w damage to nail, init	
		S91.256A	Open bite of unsp lesser toe(s) w damage to nail, init	
		S91.259A	Open bite of unsp toe(s) with damage to nail, init encntr	
893.1	OPEN WOUND OF TOE, COMPLICATED	**S91.121A**	Laceration w fb of right great toe w/o damage to nail, init	
		S91.122A	Laceration w fb of left great toe w/o damage to nail, init	
		S91.123A	Laceration w fb of unsp great toe w/o damage to nail, init	
		S91.124A	Lac w fb of right lesser toe(s) w/o damage to nail, init	
		S91.125A	Lac w fb of left lesser toe(s) w/o damage to nail, init	
		S91.126A	Lac w fb of unsp lesser toe(s) w/o damage to nail, init	
		S91.129A	Laceration w fb of unsp toe(s) w/o damage to nail, init	
		S91.141A	Pnctr w fb of right great toe w/o damage to nail, init	
		S91.142A	Pnctr w fb of left great toe w/o damage to nail, init	
		S91.143A	Pnctr w fb of unsp great toe w/o damage to nail, init	
		S91.144A	Pnctr w fb of right lesser toe(s) w/o damage to nail, init	
		S91.145A	Pnctr w fb of left lesser toe(s) w/o damage to nail, init	
		S91.146A	Pnctr w fb of unsp lesser toe(s) w/o damage to nail, init	
		S91.149A	Pnctr w foreign body of unsp toe(s) w/o damage to nail, init	
		S91.221A	Laceration w fb of right great toe w damage to nail, init	
		S91.222A	Laceration w fb of left great toe w damage to nail, init	
		S91.223A	Laceration w fb of unsp great toe w damage to nail, init	
		S91.224A	Lac w fb of right lesser toe(s) w damage to nail, init	
		S91.225A	Laceration w fb of left lesser toe(s) w damage to nail, init	
		S91.226A	Laceration w fb of unsp lesser toe(s) w damage to nail, init	
		S91.229A	Laceration w fb of unsp toe(s) w damage to nail, init	
		S91.241A	Pnctr w fb of right great toe w damage to nail, init	
		S91.242A	Pnctr w fb of left great toe w damage to nail, init	
		S91.243A	Pnctr w fb of unsp great toe w damage to nail, init	
		S91.244A	Pnctr w fb of right lesser toe(s) w damage to nail, init	
		S91.245A	Pnctr w fb of left lesser toe(s) w damage to nail, init	
		S91.246A	Pnctr w fb of unsp lesser toe(s) w damage to nail, init	
		S91.249A	Pnctr w foreign body of unsp toe(s) w damage to nail, init	
893.2	OPEN WOUND OF TOE WITH TENDON INVOLVEMENT	**S96.929A**	Laceration of unsp msl/tnd at ank/ft level, unsp foot, init	***and***
		S91.1Ø9A	Unsp open wound of unsp toe(s) w/o damage to nail, init	***or***
		S91.2Ø9A	Unsp open wound of unsp toe(s) w damage to nail, init encntr	
894.Ø	MX&UNSPEC OPEN WOUND LOW LIMB W/O MENTION COMP	**S71.ØØ9A**	Unspecified open wound, unspecified hip, initial encounter	
894.1	MULTIPLE&UNSPEC OPEN WOUND LOWER LIMB COMP	**S71.Ø29A**	Laceration with foreign body, unspecified hip, init encntr	
894.2	MX&UNSPEC OPEN WOUND LOWER LIMB W/TENDON INVLV	**S71.ØØ9A**	Unspecified open wound, unspecified hip, initial encounter	

[Brackets] indicate valid character values for each code. Character value meanings provided for each code grouping.

ICD-9-CM		ICD-10-CM		
895.Ø	TRAUMATIC AMP TOE WITHOUT MENTION COMPLICATION	**S98.111A**	Complete traumatic amputation of right great toe, init	
		S98.112A	Complete traumatic amputation of left great toe, init encntr	
		S98.119A	Complete traumatic amputation of unsp great toe, init encntr	
		S98.121A	Partial traumatic amputation of right great toe, init encntr	
		S98.122A	Partial traumatic amputation of left great toe, init encntr	
		S98.129A	Partial traumatic amputation of unsp great toe, init encntr	
		S98.131A	Complete traumatic amputation of one right lesser toe, init	
		S98.132A	Complete traumatic amputation of one left lesser toe, init	
		S98.139A	Complete traumatic amputation of one unsp lesser toe, init	
		S98.141A	Partial traumatic amputation of one right lesser toe, init	
		S98.142A	Partial traumatic amputation of one left lesser toe, init	
		S98.149A	Partial traumatic amputation of one unsp lesser toe, init	
		S98.211A	Complete traum amp of two or more right lesser toes, init	
		S98.212A	Complete traumatic amp of two or more left lesser toes, init	
		S98.219A	Complete traumatic amp of two or more unsp lesser toes, init	
		S98.221A	Partial traumatic amp of two or more right lesser toes, init	
		S98.222A	Partial traumatic amp of two or more left lesser toes, init	
		S98.229A	Partial traumatic amp of two or more unsp lesser toes, init	
895.1	TRAUMATIC AMPUTATION OF TOE COMPLICATED	**S98.119A**	Complete traumatic amputation of unsp great toe, init encntr	
		S98.129A	Partial traumatic amputation of unsp great toe, init encntr	
		S98.139A	Complete traumatic amputation of one unsp lesser toe, init	
		S98.149A	Partial traumatic amputation of one unsp lesser toe, init	
		S98.219A	Complete traumatic amp of two or more unsp lesser toes, init	
		S98.229A	Partial traumatic amp of two or more unsp lesser toes, init	
896.Ø	TRAUMATIC AMPUTATION FOOT UNI W/O MENTION COMP	**S98.Ø11A**	Complete traumatic amp of right foot at ankle level, init	
		S98.Ø12A	Complete traumatic amp of left foot at ankle level, init	
		S98.Ø19A	Complete traumatic amp of unsp foot at ankle level, init	
		S98.Ø21A	Partial traumatic amp of right foot at ankle level, init	
		S98.Ø22A	Partial traumatic amp of left foot at ankle level, init	
		S98.Ø29A	Partial traumatic amp of unsp foot at ankle level, init	
		S98.311A	Complete traumatic amputation of right midfoot, init encntr	
		S98.312A	Complete traumatic amputation of left midfoot, init encntr	
		S98.319A	Complete traumatic amputation of unsp midfoot, init encntr	
		S98.321A	Partial traumatic amputation of right midfoot, init encntr	
		S98.322A	Partial traumatic amputation of left midfoot, init encntr	
		S98.329A	Partial traumatic amputation of unsp midfoot, init encntr	
		S98.911A	Complete traumatic amp of right foot, level unsp, init	
		S98.912A	Complete traumatic amputation of left foot, level unsp, init	
		S98.919A	Complete traumatic amputation of unsp foot, level unsp, init	
		S98.921A	Partial traumatic amputation of right foot, level unsp, init	
		S98.922A	Partial traumatic amputation of left foot, level unsp, init	
		S98.929A	Partial traumatic amputation of unsp foot, level unsp, init	
896.1	TRAUMATIC AMPUTATION FOOT UNILATERAL COMPLICATED	**S98.Ø19A**	Complete traumatic amp of unsp foot at ankle level, init	
		S98.Ø29A	Partial traumatic amp of unsp foot at ankle level, init	
		S98.319A	Complete traumatic amputation of unsp midfoot, init encntr	
		S98.329A	Partial traumatic amputation of unsp midfoot, init encntr	
		S98.919A	Complete traumatic amputation of unsp foot, level unsp, init	
		S98.929A	Partial traumatic amputation of unsp foot, level unsp, init	
896.2	TRAUMATIC AMP FT BILATERAL WITHOUT MENTION COMP	**S98.911A**	Complete traumatic amp of right foot, level unsp, init	*or*
		S98.921A	Partial traumatic amputation of right foot, level unsp, init	*and*
		S98.912A	Complete traumatic amputation of left foot, level unsp, init	*or*
		S98.922A	Partial traumatic amputation of left foot, level unsp, init	
896.3	TRAUMATIC AMPUTATION FOOT BILATERAL COMPLICATED	**S98.911A**	Complete traumatic amp of right foot, level unsp, init	*and*
		S98.912A	Complete traumatic amputation of left foot, level unsp, init	
897.Ø	TRAUMAT AMP LEG UNILAT BELW KNEE W/O COMP	**S88.111A**	Complete traum amp at lev betw kn and ankl, r low leg, init	
		S88.112A	Complete traum amp at lev betw kn and ankl, l low leg, init	
		S88.119A	Complete traum amp at lev betw kn & ankl, unsp low leg, init	
		S88.121A	Part traum amp at level betw knee and ankle, r low leg, init	
		S88.122A	Part traum amp at level betw knee and ankle, l low leg, init	
		S88.129A	Part traum amp at lev betw knee and ankl, unsp low leg, init	
897.1	TRAUMATIC AMP LEG UNILATERAL BELOW KNEE COMP	**S88.119A**	Complete traum amp at lev betw kn & ankl, unsp low leg, init	
		S88.129A	Part traum amp at lev betw knee and ankl, unsp low leg, init	
897.2	TRAUMAT AMP LEG UNILAT@OR ABVE KNEE W/O COMP	**S78.Ø11A**	Complete traumatic amputation at right hip joint, init	
		S78.Ø12A	Complete traumatic amputation at left hip joint, init encntr	
		S78.Ø19A	Complete traumatic amputation at unsp hip joint, init encntr	
		S78.Ø21A	Partial traumatic amputation at right hip joint, init encntr	
		S78.Ø22A	Partial traumatic amputation at left hip joint, init encntr	
		S78.Ø29A	Partial traumatic amputation at unsp hip joint, init encntr	
		S78.111A	Complete traumatic amp at level betw r hip and knee, init	
		S78.112A	Complete traumatic amp at level betw left hip and knee, init	
		S78.119A	Complete traumatic amp at level betw unsp hip and knee, init	
		S78.121A	Partial traumatic amp at level betw right hip and knee, init	
		S78.122A	Partial traumatic amp at level betw left hip and knee, init	
		S78.129A	Partial traumatic amp at level betw unsp hip and knee, init	
		S78.919A	Complete traum amp of unsp hip and thigh, level unsp, init	
		S78.929A	Partial traum amp of unsp hip and thigh, level unsp, init	
		S88.Ø11A	Complete traumatic amputation at knee level, r low leg, init	
		S88.Ø12A	Complete traumatic amputation at knee level, l low leg, init	

(Continued on next page)

ICD-9-CM		ICD-10-CM		
897.2	TRAUMAT AMP LEG UNILAT@OR ABVE KNEE W/O COMP **(Continued)**	S88.019A	Complete traumatic amp at knee level, unsp lower leg, init	
		S88.021A	Partial traumatic amputation at knee level, r low leg, init	
		S88.022A	Partial traumatic amputation at knee level, l low leg, init	
		S88.029A	Partial traumatic amp at knee level, unsp lower leg, init	
897.3	TRAUMATIC AMP LEG UNILATERAL@OR ABOVE KNEE COMP	S78.019A	Complete traumatic amputation at unsp hip joint, init encntr	
		S78.029A	Partial traumatic amputation at unsp hip joint, init encntr	
		S78.119A	Complete traumatic amp at level betw unsp hip and knee, init	
		S78.129A	Partial traumatic amp at level betw unsp hip and knee, init	
		S88.019A	Complete traumatic amp at knee level, unsp lower leg, init	
		S88.029A	Partial traumatic amp at knee level, unsp lower leg, init	
897.4	TRAUMAT AMP LEG UNILAT LEVL NOT SPEC W/O COMP	S78.911A	Complete traumatic amp of r hip and thigh, level unsp, init	
		S78.912A	Complete traum amp of left hip and thigh, level unsp, init	
		S78.919A	Complete traum amp of unsp hip and thigh, level unsp, init	
		S78.921A	Partial traumatic amp of r hip and thigh, level unsp, init	
		S78.922A	Partial traum amp of left hip and thigh, level unsp, init	
		S78.929A	Partial traum amp of unsp hip and thigh, level unsp, init	
		S88.911A	Complete traumatic amputation of r low leg, level unsp, init	
		S88.912A	Complete traumatic amputation of l low leg, level unsp, init	
		S88.919A	Complete traumatic amp of unsp lower leg, level unsp, init	
		S88.921A	Partial traumatic amputation of r low leg, level unsp, init	
		S88.922A	Partial traumatic amputation of l low leg, level unsp, init	
		S88.929A	Partial traumatic amp of unsp lower leg, level unsp, init	
897.5	TRAUMATIC AMP LEG UNILATERAL LEVEL NOT SPEC COMP	S78.919A	Complete traum amp of unsp hip and thigh, level unsp, init	
		S78.929A	Partial traum amp of unsp hip and thigh, level unsp, init	
		S88.919A	Complete traumatic amp of unsp lower leg, level unsp, init	
		S88.929A	Partial traumatic amp of unsp lower leg, level unsp, init	
897.6	TRAUMATIC AMP LEG BILATERAL WITHOUT MENTION COMP	S88.911A	Complete traumatic amputation of r low leg, level unsp, init	*and*
		S88.912A	Complete traumatic amputation of l low leg, level unsp, init	
897.7	TRAUMATIC AMPUTATION LEG BILATERAL COMPLICATED	S88.911A	Complete traumatic amputation of r low leg, level unsp, init	*and*
		S88.912A	Complete traumatic amputation of l low leg, level unsp, init	
900.00	INJURY TO CAROTID ARTERY UNSPECIFIED	S15.009A	Unsp injury of unspecified carotid artery, init encntr	
		S15.019A	Minor laceration of unspecified carotid artery, init encntr	
		S15.029A	Major laceration of unspecified carotid artery, init encntr	
		S15.099A	Oth injury of unspecified carotid artery, init encntr	
900.01	COMMON CAROTID ARTERY INJURY	S15.001A	Unspecified injury of right carotid artery, init encntr	
		S15.002A	Unspecified injury of left carotid artery, initial encounter	
		S15.009A	Unsp injury of unspecified carotid artery, init encntr	
		S15.011A	Minor laceration of right carotid artery, initial encounter	
		S15.012A	Minor laceration of left carotid artery, initial encounter	
		S15.019A	Minor laceration of unspecified carotid artery, init encntr	
		S15.021A	Major laceration of right carotid artery, initial encounter	
		S15.022A	Major laceration of left carotid artery, initial encounter	
		S15.029A	Major laceration of unspecified carotid artery, init encntr	
		S15.091A	Other specified injury of right carotid artery, init encntr	
		S15.092A	Other specified injury of left carotid artery, init encntr	
		S15.099A	Oth injury of unspecified carotid artery, init encntr	
900.02	EXTERNAL CAROTID ARTERY INJURY	S15.001A	Unspecified injury of right carotid artery, init encntr	
		S15.002A	Unspecified injury of left carotid artery, initial encounter	
		S15.009A	Unsp injury of unspecified carotid artery, init encntr	
		S15.011A	Minor laceration of right carotid artery, initial encounter	
		S15.012A	Minor laceration of left carotid artery, initial encounter	
		S15.019A	Minor laceration of unspecified carotid artery, init encntr	
		S15.021A	Major laceration of right carotid artery, initial encounter	
		S15.022A	Major laceration of left carotid artery, initial encounter	
		S15.029A	Major laceration of unspecified carotid artery, init encntr	
		S15.091A	Other specified injury of right carotid artery, init encntr	
		S15.092A	Other specified injury of left carotid artery, init encntr	
		S15.099A	Oth injury of unspecified carotid artery, init encntr	
900.03	INTERNAL CAROTID ARTERY INJURY	S15.001A	Unspecified injury of right carotid artery, init encntr	
		S15.002A	Unspecified injury of left carotid artery, initial encounter	
		S15.009A	Unsp injury of unspecified carotid artery, init encntr	
		S15.011A	Minor laceration of right carotid artery, initial encounter	
		S15.012A	Minor laceration of left carotid artery, initial encounter	
		S15.019A	Minor laceration of unspecified carotid artery, init encntr	
		S15.021A	Major laceration of right carotid artery, initial encounter	
		S15.022A	Major laceration of left carotid artery, initial encounter	
		S15.029A	Major laceration of unspecified carotid artery, init encntr	
		S15.091A	Other specified injury of right carotid artery, init encntr	
		S15.092A	Other specified injury of left carotid artery, init encntr	
		S15.099A	Oth injury of unspecified carotid artery, init encntr	

ICD-9-CM		ICD-10-CM	
900.1	INTERNAL JUGULAR VEIN INJURY	**S15.301A**	Unsp injury of right internal jugular vein, init encntr
		S15.302A	Unsp injury of left internal jugular vein, init encntr
		S15.309A	Unsp injury of unsp internal jugular vein, init encntr
		S15.311A	Minor laceration of right internal jugular vein, init encntr
		S15.312A	Minor laceration of left internal jugular vein, init encntr
		S15.319A	Minor laceration of unsp internal jugular vein, init encntr
		S15.321A	Major laceration of right internal jugular vein, init encntr
		S15.322A	Major laceration of left internal jugular vein, init encntr
		S15.329A	Major laceration of unsp internal jugular vein, init encntr
		S15.391A	Oth injury of right internal jugular vein, init encntr
		S15.392A	Oth injury of left internal jugular vein, init encntr
		S15.399A	Oth injury of unspecified internal jugular vein, init encntr
900.81	EXTERNAL JUGULAR VEIN INJURY	**S15.201A**	Unsp injury of right external jugular vein, init encntr
		S15.202A	Unsp injury of left external jugular vein, init encntr
		S15.209A	Unsp injury of unsp external jugular vein, init encntr
		S15.211A	Minor laceration of right external jugular vein, init encntr
		S15.212A	Minor laceration of left external jugular vein, init encntr
		S15.219A	Minor laceration of unsp external jugular vein, init encntr
		S15.221A	Major laceration of right external jugular vein, init encntr
		S15.222A	Major laceration of left external jugular vein, init encntr
		S15.229A	Major laceration of unsp external jugular vein, init encntr
		S15.291A	Oth injury of right external jugular vein, init encntr
		S15.292A	Oth injury of left external jugular vein, init encntr
		S15.299A	Oth injury of unspecified external jugular vein, init encntr
900.82	INJURY TO MULTIPLE BLOOD VESSELS OF HEAD&NECK	**S15.8XXA**	Injury of oth blood vessels at neck level, init encntr
900.89	INJURY OTH SPECIFIED BLOOD VESSELS HEAD&NECK OTH	**S09.0XXA**	Injury of blood vessels of head, NEC, init
		S15.101A	Unspecified injury of right vertebral artery, init encntr
		S15.102A	Unspecified injury of left vertebral artery, init encntr
		S15.109A	Unsp injury of unspecified vertebral artery, init encntr
		S15.111A	Minor laceration of right vertebral artery, init encntr
		S15.112A	Minor laceration of left vertebral artery, initial encounter
		S15.119A	Minor laceration of unsp vertebral artery, init encntr
		S15.121A	Major laceration of right vertebral artery, init encntr
		S15.122A	Major laceration of left vertebral artery, initial encounter
		S15.129A	Major laceration of unsp vertebral artery, init encntr
		S15.191A	Oth injury of right vertebral artery, init encntr
		S15.192A	Other specified injury of left vertebral artery, init encntr
		S15.199A	Oth injury of unspecified vertebral artery, init encntr
		S15.8XXA	Injury of oth blood vessels at neck level, init encntr
900.9	INJURY TO UNSPECIFIED BLOOD VESSEL OF HEAD&NECK	**S15.9XXA**	Injury of unsp blood vessel at neck level, init encntr
901.0	THORACIC AORTA INJURY	**S25.00XA**	Unspecified injury of thoracic aorta, initial encounter
		S25.01XA	Minor laceration of thoracic aorta, initial encounter
		S25.02XA	Major laceration of thoracic aorta, initial encounter
		S25.09XA	Other specified injury of thoracic aorta, initial encounter
901.1	INNOMINATE AND SUBCLAVIAN ARTERY INJURY	**S25.101A**	Unsp injury of right innominate or subclavian artery, init
		S25.102A	Unsp injury of left innominate or subclavian artery, init
		S25.109A	Unsp injury of unsp innominate or subclavian artery, init
		S25.111A	Minor laceration of right innominate or subclav art, init
		S25.112A	Minor laceration of left innominate or subclav art, init
		S25.119A	Minor laceration of unsp innominate or subclav art, init
		S25.121A	Major laceration of right innominate or subclav art, init
		S25.122A	Major laceration of left innominate or subclav art, init
		S25.129A	Major laceration of unsp innominate or subclav art, init
		S25.191A	Inj right innominate or subclavian artery, init encntr
		S25.192A	Inj left innominate or subclavian artery, init encntr
		S25.199A	Inj unsp innominate or subclavian artery, init encntr
901.2	SUPERIOR VENA CAVA INJURY	**S25.20XA**	Unspecified injury of superior vena cava, initial encounter
		S25.21XA	Minor laceration of superior vena cava, initial encounter
		S25.22XA	Major laceration of superior vena cava, initial encounter
		S25.29XA	Other specified injury of superior vena cava, init encntr
901.3	INNOMINATE AND SUBCLAVIAN VEIN INJURY	**S25.301A**	Unsp injury of right innominate or subclavian vein, init
		S25.302A	Unsp injury of left innominate or subclavian vein, init
		S25.309A	Unsp injury of unsp innominate or subclavian vein, init
		S25.311A	Minor laceration of right innominate or subclav vein, init
		S25.312A	Minor laceration of left innominate or subclavian vein, init
		S25.319A	Minor laceration of unsp innominate or subclavian vein, init
		S25.321A	Major laceration of right innominate or subclav vein, init
		S25.322A	Major laceration of left innominate or subclavian vein, init
		S25.329A	Major laceration of unsp innominate or subclavian vein, init
		S25.391A	Inj right innominate or subclavian vein, init encntr
		S25.392A	Inj left innominate or subclavian vein, init encntr
		S25.399A	Inj unsp innominate or subclavian vein, init encntr
901.40	INJURY TO UNSPECIFIED PULMONARY VESSEL	**S25.409A**	Unsp injury of unsp pulmonary blood vessels, init encntr
		S25.419A	Minor laceration of unsp pulmonary blood vessels, init
		S25.429A	Major laceration of unsp pulmonary blood vessels, init
		S25.499A	Oth injury of unsp pulmonary blood vessels, init encntr

ICD-9-CM		ICD-10-CM	
901.41	PULMONARY ARTERY INJURY	**S25.401A**	Unsp injury of right pulmonary blood vessels, init encntr
		S25.402A	Unsp injury of left pulmonary blood vessels, init encntr
		S25.409A	Unsp injury of unsp pulmonary blood vessels, init encntr
		S25.411A	Minor laceration of right pulmonary blood vessels, init
		S25.412A	Minor laceration of left pulmonary blood vessels, init
		S25.419A	Minor laceration of unsp pulmonary blood vessels, init
		S25.421A	Major laceration of right pulmonary blood vessels, init
		S25.422A	Major laceration of left pulmonary blood vessels, init
		S25.429A	Major laceration of unsp pulmonary blood vessels, init
		S25.491A	Oth injury of right pulmonary blood vessels, init encntr
		S25.492A	Oth injury of left pulmonary blood vessels, init encntr
		S25.499A	Oth injury of unsp pulmonary blood vessels, init encntr
901.42	PULMONARY VEIN INJURY	**S25.401A**	Unsp injury of right pulmonary blood vessels, init encntr
		S25.402A	Unsp injury of left pulmonary blood vessels, init encntr
		S25.409A	Unsp injury of unsp pulmonary blood vessels, init encntr
		S25.411A	Minor laceration of right pulmonary blood vessels, init
		S25.412A	Minor laceration of left pulmonary blood vessels, init
		S25.419A	Minor laceration of unsp pulmonary blood vessels, init
		S25.421A	Major laceration of right pulmonary blood vessels, init
		S25.422A	Major laceration of left pulmonary blood vessels, init
		S25.429A	Major laceration of unsp pulmonary blood vessels, init
		S25.491A	Oth injury of right pulmonary blood vessels, init encntr
		S25.492A	Oth injury of left pulmonary blood vessels, init encntr
		S25.499A	Oth injury of unsp pulmonary blood vessels, init encntr
901.81	INTERCOSTAL ARTERY OR VEIN INJURY	**S25.501A**	Unsp injury of intercostal blood vessels, right side, init
		S25.502A	Unsp injury of intercostal blood vessels, left side, init
		S25.509A	Unsp injury of intercostal blood vessels, unsp side, init
		S25.511A	Laceration of intercostal blood vessels, right side, init
		S25.512A	Laceration of intercostal blood vessels, left side, init
		S25.519A	Laceration of intercostal blood vessels, unsp side, init
		S25.591A	Inj intercostal blood vessels, right side, init encntr
		S25.592A	Inj intercostal blood vessels, left side, init encntr
		S25.599A	Inj intercostal blood vessels, unsp side, init encntr
901.82	INTERNAL MAMMARY ARTERY OR VEIN INJURY	**S25.801A**	Unsp injury of oth blood vessels of thorax, right side, init
		S25.802A	Unsp injury of oth blood vessels of thorax, left side, init
		S25.809A	Unsp injury of oth blood vessels of thorax, unsp side, init
		S25.811A	Laceration of oth blood vessels of thorax, right side, init
		S25.812A	Laceration of oth blood vessels of thorax, left side, init
		S25.819A	Laceration of oth blood vessels of thorax, unsp side, init
		S25.891A	Inj oth blood vessels of thorax, right side, init encntr
		S25.892A	Inj oth blood vessels of thorax, left side, init encntr
		S25.899A	Inj oth blood vessels of thorax, unsp side, init encntr
901.83	INJURY TO MULTIPLE BLOOD VESSELS OF THORAX	**S25.809A**	Unsp injury of oth blood vessels of thorax, unsp side, init
901.89	INJURY TO SPECIFIED BLOOD VESSELS THORAX OTHER	**S25.801A**	Unsp injury of oth blood vessels of thorax, right side, init
		S25.802A	Unsp injury of oth blood vessels of thorax, left side, init
		S25.809A	Unsp injury of oth blood vessels of thorax, unsp side, init
		S25.811A	Laceration of oth blood vessels of thorax, right side, init
		S25.812A	Laceration of oth blood vessels of thorax, left side, init
		S25.819A	Laceration of oth blood vessels of thorax, unsp side, init
		S25.891A	Inj oth blood vessels of thorax, right side, init encntr
		S25.892A	Inj oth blood vessels of thorax, left side, init encntr
		S25.899A	Inj oth blood vessels of thorax, unsp side, init encntr
901.9	INJURY TO UNSPECIFIED BLOOD VESSEL OF THORAX	**S25.90XA**	Unsp injury of unsp blood vessel of thorax, init encntr
		S25.91XA	Laceration of unsp blood vessel of thorax, init encntr
		S25.99XA	Oth injury of unsp blood vessel of thorax, init encntr
902.0	ABDOMINAL AORTA INJURY	**S35.00XA**	Unspecified injury of abdominal aorta, initial encounter
		S35.01XA	Minor laceration of abdominal aorta, initial encounter
		S35.02XA	Major laceration of abdominal aorta, initial encounter
		S35.09XA	Other injury of abdominal aorta, initial encounter
902.10	UNSPECIFIED INFERIOR VENA CAVA INJURY	**S35.10XA**	Unspecified injury of inferior vena cava, initial encounter
		S35.11XA	Minor laceration of inferior vena cava, initial encounter
		S35.12XA	Major laceration of inferior vena cava, initial encounter
		S35.19XA	Other injury of inferior vena cava, initial encounter
902.11	HEPATIC VEIN INJURY	**S35.10XA**	Unspecified injury of inferior vena cava, initial encounter
		S35.11XA	Minor laceration of inferior vena cava, initial encounter
		S35.12XA	Major laceration of inferior vena cava, initial encounter
		S35.19XA	Other injury of inferior vena cava, initial encounter
902.19	INJURY SPEC BRANCHES INFERIOR VENA CAVA OTHER	**S35.10XA**	Unspecified injury of inferior vena cava, initial encounter
		S35.11XA	Minor laceration of inferior vena cava, initial encounter
		S35.12XA	Major laceration of inferior vena cava, initial encounter
		S35.19XA	Other injury of inferior vena cava, initial encounter
902.20	UNSPECIFIED CELIAC AND MESENTERIC ARTERY INJURY	**S35.291A**	Minor laceration of branches of celiac and mesent art, init
		S35.292A	Major laceration of branches of celiac and mesent art, init
		S35.298A	Inj branches of celiac and mesenteric artery, init encntr
		S35.299A	Unsp injury of branches of celiac and mesent art, init
902.21	GASTRIC ARTERY INJURY	**S35.291A**	Minor laceration of branches of celiac and mesent art, init
		S35.292A	Major laceration of branches of celiac and mesent art, init
		S35.298A	Inj branches of celiac and mesenteric artery, init encntr
		S35.299A	Unsp injury of branches of celiac and mesent art, init

ICD-9-CM		ICD-10-CM	
902.22	HEPATIC ARTERY INJURY	**S35.291A**	Minor laceration of branches of celiac and mesent art, init
		S35.292A	Major laceration of branches of celiac and mesent art, init
		S35.298A	Inj branches of celiac and mesenteric artery, init encntr
		S35.299A	Unsp injury of branches of celiac and mesent art, init
902.23	SPLENIC ARTERY INJURY	**S35.291A**	Minor laceration of branches of celiac and mesent art, init
		S35.292A	Major laceration of branches of celiac and mesent art, init
		S35.298A	Inj branches of celiac and mesenteric artery, init encntr
		S35.299A	Unsp injury of branches of celiac and mesent art, init
902.24	INJURY TO SPECIFIED BRANCHES CELIAC AXIS OTHER	**S35.211A**	Minor laceration of celiac artery, initial encounter
		S35.212A	Major laceration of celiac artery, initial encounter
		S35.218A	Other injury of celiac artery, initial encounter
		S35.219A	Unspecified injury of celiac artery, initial encounter
902.25	SUPERIOR MESENTERIC ARTERY INJURY	**S35.221A**	Minor laceration of superior mesenteric artery, init encntr
		S35.222A	Major laceration of superior mesenteric artery, init encntr
		S35.228A	Other injury of superior mesenteric artery, init encntr
		S35.229A	Unsp injury of superior mesenteric artery, init encntr
902.26	INJURY PRIMARY BRANCHES SUPERIOR MESENTERIC ART	**S35.221A**	Minor laceration of superior mesenteric artery, init encntr
		S35.222A	Major laceration of superior mesenteric artery, init encntr
		S35.228A	Other injury of superior mesenteric artery, init encntr
		S35.229A	Unsp injury of superior mesenteric artery, init encntr
902.27	INFERIOR MESENTERIC ARTERY INJURY	**S35.231A**	Minor laceration of inferior mesenteric artery, init encntr
		S35.232A	Major laceration of inferior mesenteric artery, init encntr
		S35.238A	Other injury of inferior mesenteric artery, init encntr
		S35.239A	Unsp injury of inferior mesenteric artery, init encntr
902.29	INJURY TO CELIAC AND MESENTERIC ARTERIES OTHER	**S35.291A**	Minor laceration of branches of celiac and mesent art, init
		S35.292A	Major laceration of branches of celiac and mesent art, init
		S35.298A	Inj branches of celiac and mesenteric artery, init encntr
		S35.299A	Unsp injury of branches of celiac and mesent art, init
902.31	INJURY SUPERIOR MESENTERIC VEIN&PRIMARY SUBDIVS	**S35.331A**	Laceration of superior mesenteric vein, initial encounter
		S35.338A	Oth injury of superior mesenteric vein, init encntr
		S35.339A	Unspecified injury of superior mesenteric vein, init encntr
902.32	INFERIOR MESENTERIC VEIN INJURY	**S35.341A**	Laceration of inferior mesenteric vein, initial encounter
		S35.348A	Oth injury of inferior mesenteric vein, init encntr
		S35.349A	Unspecified injury of inferior mesenteric vein, init encntr
902.33	PORTAL VEIN INJURY	**S35.311A**	Laceration of portal vein, initial encounter
		S35.318A	Other specified injury of portal vein, initial encounter
		S35.319A	Unspecified injury of portal vein, initial encounter
902.34	SPLENIC VEIN INJURY	**S35.321A**	Laceration of splenic vein, initial encounter
		S35.328A	Other specified injury of splenic vein, initial encounter
		S35.329A	Unspecified injury of splenic vein, initial encounter
902.39	INJURY TO PORTAL AND SPLENIC VEINS OTHER	**S35.8X9A**	Unsp inj blood vesls at abd, low back and pelvis level, init
902.40	RENAL VESSEL INJURY, UNSPECIFIED	**S35.403A**	Unspecified injury of unspecified renal artery, init encntr
		S35.406A	Unspecified injury of unspecified renal vein, init encntr
		S35.413A	Laceration of unspecified renal artery, initial encounter
		S35.416A	Laceration of unspecified renal vein, initial encounter
		S35.493A	Oth injury of unspecified renal artery, init encntr
		S35.496A	Oth injury of unspecified renal vein, init encntr
902.41	RENAL ARTERY INJURY	**S35.401A**	Unspecified injury of right renal artery, initial encounter
		S35.402A	Unspecified injury of left renal artery, initial encounter
		S35.403A	Unspecified injury of unspecified renal artery, init encntr
		S35.411A	Laceration of right renal artery, initial encounter
		S35.412A	Laceration of left renal artery, initial encounter
		S35.413A	Laceration of unspecified renal artery, initial encounter
		S35.491A	Other specified injury of right renal artery, init encntr
		S35.492A	Other specified injury of left renal artery, init encntr
		S35.493A	Oth injury of unspecified renal artery, init encntr
902.42	RENAL VEIN INJURY	**S35.404A**	Unspecified injury of right renal vein, initial encounter
		S35.405A	Unspecified injury of left renal vein, initial encounter
		S35.406A	Unspecified injury of unspecified renal vein, init encntr
		S35.414A	Laceration of right renal vein, initial encounter
		S35.415A	Laceration of left renal vein, initial encounter
		S35.416A	Laceration of unspecified renal vein, initial encounter
		S35.494A	Other specified injury of right renal vein, init encntr
		S35.495A	Other specified injury of left renal vein, initial encounter
		S35.496A	Oth injury of unspecified renal vein, init encntr
902.49	RENAL BLOOD VESSEL INJURY, OTHER	**S35.403A**	Unspecified injury of unspecified renal artery, init encntr
		S35.406A	Unspecified injury of unspecified renal vein, init encntr
		S35.413A	Laceration of unspecified renal artery, initial encounter
		S35.416A	Laceration of unspecified renal vein, initial encounter
		S35.493A	Oth injury of unspecified renal artery, init encntr
		S35.496A	Oth injury of unspecified renal vein, init encntr
902.50	UNSPECIFIED ILIAC VESSEL INJURY	**S35.513A**	Injury of unspecified iliac artery, initial encounter
902.51	HYPOGASTRIC ARTERY INJURY	**S35.511A**	Injury of right iliac artery, initial encounter
		S35.512A	Injury of left iliac artery, initial encounter
		S35.513A	Injury of unspecified iliac artery, initial encounter
902.52	HYPOGASTRIC VEIN INJURY	**S35.514A**	Injury of right iliac vein, initial encounter
		S35.515A	Injury of left iliac vein, initial encounter
		S35.516A	Injury of unspecified iliac vein, initial encounter

ICD-9-CM		ICD-10-CM	
9Ø2.53	ILIAC ARTERY INJURY	**S35.511A**	Injury of right iliac artery, initial encounter
		S35.512A	Injury of left iliac artery, initial encounter
		S35.513A	Injury of unspecified iliac artery, initial encounter
9Ø2.54	ILIAC VEIN INJURY	**S35.514A**	Injury of right iliac vein, initial encounter
		S35.515A	Injury of left iliac vein, initial encounter
		S35.516A	Injury of unspecified iliac vein, initial encounter
9Ø2.55	UTERINE ARTERY INJURY	**S35.531A**	Injury of right uterine artery, initial encounter
		S35.532A	Injury of left uterine artery, initial encounter
		S35.533A	Injury of unspecified uterine artery, initial encounter
9Ø2.56	UTERINE VEIN INJURY	**S35.534A**	Injury of right uterine vein, initial encounter
		S35.535A	Injury of left uterine vein, initial encounter
		S35.536A	Injury of unspecified uterine vein, initial encounter
9Ø2.59	INJURY TO ILIAC BLOOD VESSELS OTHER	**S35.5ØXA**	Injury of unspecified iliac blood vessel(s), init encntr
		S35.59XA	Injury of other iliac blood vessels, initial encounter
		S35.8X9A	Unsp inj blood vesls at abd, low back and pelvis level, init
9Ø2.81	OVARIAN ARTERY INJURY	**S35.8X1A**	Lacerat blood vesls at abd, low back and pelvis level, init
		S35.8X8A	Inj oth blood vesls at abd, low back and pelvis level, init
		S35.8X9A	Unsp inj blood vesls at abd, low back and pelvis level, init
9Ø2.82	OVARIAN VEIN INJURY	**S35.8X1A**	Lacerat blood vesls at abd, low back and pelvis level, init
		S35.8X8A	Inj oth blood vesls at abd, low back and pelvis level, init
		S35.8X9A	Unsp inj blood vesls at abd, low back and pelvis level, init
9Ø2.87	INJURY TO MULTIPLE BLOOD VESSELS ABDOMEN&PELVIS	**S35.8X9A**	Unsp inj blood vesls at abd, low back and pelvis level, init
9Ø2.89	INJR OTH SPEC BLOOD VES OF ABDOMEN & PELVIS OTH	**S35.8X1A**	Lacerat blood vesls at abd, low back and pelvis level, init
		S35.8X8A	Inj oth blood vesls at abd, low back and pelvis level, init
		S35.8X9A	Unsp inj blood vesls at abd, low back and pelvis level, init
9Ø2.9	INJURY BLOOD VESSEL ABDOMEN&PELVIS UNSPECIFIED	**S35.9ØXA**	Unsp inj unsp bld vess at abd, low back and pelv level, init
		S35.91XA	Lacerat unsp bld vess at abd, low back and pelv level, init
		S35.99XA	Inj unsp blood vess at abd, low back and pelvis level, init
9Ø3.ØØ	AXILLARY VESSEL INJURY, UNSPECIFIED	**S45.8Ø1A**	Unsp inj blood vessels at shldr/up arm, right arm, init
		S45.8Ø2A	Unsp injury of blood vessels at shldr/up arm, left arm, init
		S45.8Ø9A	Unsp injury of blood vessels at shldr/up arm, unsp arm, init
		S45.811A	Laceration of blood vessels at shldr/up arm, right arm, init
		S45.812A	Laceration of blood vessels at shldr/up arm, left arm, init
		S45.819A	Laceration of blood vessels at shldr/up arm, unsp arm, init
		S45.891A	Inj oth blood vessels at shldr/up arm, right arm, init
		S45.892A	Inj oth blood vessels at shldr/up arm, left arm, init
		S45.899A	Inj oth blood vessels at shldr/up arm, unsp arm, init
9Ø3.Ø1	AXILLARY ARTERY INJURY	**S45.ØØ1A**	Unsp injury of axillary artery, right side, init encntr
		S45.ØØ2A	Unsp injury of axillary artery, left side, init encntr
		S45.ØØ9A	Unsp injury of axillary artery, unsp side, init encntr
		S45.Ø11A	Laceration of axillary artery, right side, initial encounter
		S45.Ø12A	Laceration of axillary artery, left side, initial encounter
		S45.Ø19A	Laceration of axillary artery, unspecified side, init encntr
		S45.Ø91A	Oth injury of axillary artery, right side, init encntr
		S45.Ø92A	Oth injury of axillary artery, left side, init encntr
		S45.Ø99A	Oth injury of axillary artery, unspecified side, init encntr
9Ø3.Ø2	AXILLARY VEIN INJURY	**S45.2Ø1A**	Unsp injury of axillary or brachial vein, right side, init
		S45.2Ø2A	Unsp injury of axillary or brachial vein, left side, init
		S45.2Ø9A	Unsp injury of axillary or brachial vein, unsp side, init
		S45.211A	Laceration of axillary or brachial vein, right side, init
		S45.212A	Laceration of axillary or brachial vein, left side, init
		S45.219A	Laceration of axillary or brachial vein, unsp side, init
		S45.291A	Inj axillary or brachial vein, right side, init encntr
		S45.292A	Inj axillary or brachial vein, left side, init encntr
		S45.299A	Inj axillary or brachial vein, unsp side, init encntr
9Ø3.1	BRACHIAL BLOOD VESSELS INJURY	**S45.1Ø1A**	Unsp injury of brachial artery, right side, init encntr
		S45.1Ø2A	Unsp injury of brachial artery, left side, init encntr
		S45.1Ø9A	Unsp injury of brachial artery, unsp side, init encntr
		S45.111A	Laceration of brachial artery, right side, initial encounter
		S45.112A	Laceration of brachial artery, left side, initial encounter
		S45.119A	Laceration of brachial artery, unspecified side, init encntr
		S45.191A	Oth injury of brachial artery, right side, init encntr
		S45.192A	Oth injury of brachial artery, left side, init encntr
		S45.199A	Oth injury of brachial artery, unspecified side, init encntr
		S45.2Ø1A	Unsp injury of axillary or brachial vein, right side, init
		S45.2Ø2A	Unsp injury of axillary or brachial vein, left side, init
		S45.2Ø9A	Unsp injury of axillary or brachial vein, unsp side, init
		S45.211A	Laceration of axillary or brachial vein, right side, init
		S45.212A	Laceration of axillary or brachial vein, left side, init
		S45.219A	Laceration of axillary or brachial vein, unsp side, init
		S45.291A	Inj axillary or brachial vein, right side, init encntr
		S45.292A	Inj axillary or brachial vein, left side, init encntr
		S45.299A	Inj axillary or brachial vein, unsp side, init encntr

[Brackets] indicate valid character values for each code. Character value meanings provided for each code grouping.

ICD-9-CM		ICD-10-CM	
903.2	RADIAL BLOOD VESSELS INJURY	**S55.101A**	Unsp injury of radial artery at forarm lv, right arm, init
		S55.102A	Unsp injury of radial artery at forarm lv, left arm, init
		S55.109A	Unsp injury of radial artery at forarm lv, unsp arm, init
		S55.111A	Laceration of radial artery at forarm lv, right arm, init
		S55.112A	Laceration of radial artery at forearm level, left arm, init
		S55.119A	Laceration of radial artery at forearm level, unsp arm, init
		S55.191A	Inj radial artery at forearm level, right arm, init encntr
		S55.192A	Inj radial artery at forearm level, left arm, init encntr
		S55.199A	Inj radial artery at forearm level, unsp arm, init encntr
		S65.101A	Unsp injury of radial art at wrs/hnd lv of right arm, init
		S65.102A	Unsp injury of radial artery at wrs/hnd lv of left arm, init
		S65.109A	Unsp injury of radial artery at wrs/hnd lv of unsp arm, init
		S65.111A	Laceration of radial artery at wrs/hnd lv of right arm, init
		S65.112A	Laceration of radial artery at wrs/hnd lv of left arm, init
		S65.119A	Laceration of radial artery at wrs/hnd lv of unsp arm, init
		S65.191A	Inj radial artery at wrist and hand level of right arm, init
		S65.192A	Inj radial artery at wrist and hand level of left arm, init
		S65.199A	Inj radial artery at wrist and hand level of unsp arm, init
903.3	ULNAR BLOOD VESSELS INJURY	**S55.001A**	Unsp injury of ulnar artery at forarm lv, right arm, init
		S55.002A	Unsp injury of ulnar artery at forearm level, left arm, init
		S55.009A	Unsp injury of ulnar artery at forearm level, unsp arm, init
		S55.011A	Laceration of ulnar artery at forearm level, right arm, init
		S55.012A	Laceration of ulnar artery at forearm level, left arm, init
		S55.019A	Laceration of ulnar artery at forearm level, unsp arm, init
		S55.091A	Inj ulnar artery at forearm level, right arm, init encntr
		S55.092A	Inj ulnar artery at forearm level, left arm, init encntr
		S55.099A	Inj ulnar artery at forearm level, unsp arm, init encntr
		S65.001A	Unsp injury of ulnar artery at wrs/hnd lv of right arm, init
		S65.002A	Unsp injury of ulnar artery at wrs/hnd lv of left arm, init
		S65.009A	Unsp injury of ulnar artery at wrs/hnd lv of unsp arm, init
		S65.011A	Laceration of ulnar artery at wrs/hnd lv of right arm, init
		S65.012A	Laceration of ulnar artery at wrs/hnd lv of left arm, init
		S65.019A	Laceration of ulnar artery at wrs/hnd lv of unsp arm, init
		S65.091A	Inj ulnar artery at wrist and hand level of right arm, init
		S65.092A	Inj ulnar artery at wrist and hand level of left arm, init
		S65.099A	Inj ulnar artery at wrist and hand level of unsp arm, init
903.4	PALMAR ARTERY INJURY	**S65.201A**	Unsp injury of superficial palmar arch of right hand, init
		S65.202A	Unsp injury of superficial palmar arch of left hand, init
		S65.209A	Unsp injury of superficial palmar arch of unsp hand, init
		S65.211A	Laceration of superficial palmar arch of right hand, init
		S65.212A	Laceration of superficial palmar arch of left hand, init
		S65.219A	Laceration of superficial palmar arch of unsp hand, init
		S65.291A	Inj superficial palmar arch of right hand, init encntr
		S65.292A	Inj superficial palmar arch of left hand, init encntr
		S65.299A	Inj superficial palmar arch of unsp hand, init encntr
		S65.301A	Unsp injury of deep palmar arch of right hand, init encntr
		S65.302A	Unsp injury of deep palmar arch of left hand, init encntr
		S65.309A	Unsp injury of deep palmar arch of unsp hand, init encntr
		S65.311A	Laceration of deep palmar arch of right hand, init encntr
		S65.312A	Laceration of deep palmar arch of left hand, init encntr
		S65.319A	Laceration of deep palmar arch of unsp hand, init encntr
		S65.391A	Oth injury of deep palmar arch of right hand, init encntr
		S65.392A	Oth injury of deep palmar arch of left hand, init encntr
		S65.399A	Oth injury of deep palmar arch of unsp hand, init encntr
903.5	DIGITAL BLOOD VESSELS INJURY	**S65.401A**	Unsp injury of blood vessel of right thumb, init encntr
		S65.402A	Unsp injury of blood vessel of left thumb, init encntr
		S65.409A	Unsp injury of blood vessel of unsp thumb, init encntr
		S65.411A	Laceration of blood vessel of right thumb, initial encounter
		S65.412A	Laceration of blood vessel of left thumb, initial encounter
		S65.419A	Laceration of blood vessel of unspecified thumb, init encntr
		S65.491A	Oth injury of blood vessel of right thumb, init encntr
		S65.492A	Oth injury of blood vessel of left thumb, init encntr
		S65.499A	Oth injury of blood vessel of unspecified thumb, init encntr
		S65.500A	Unsp injury of blood vessel of right index finger, init
		S65.501A	Unsp injury of blood vessel of left index finger, init
		S65.502A	Unsp injury of blood vessel of right middle finger, init
		S65.503A	Unsp injury of blood vessel of left middle finger, init
		S65.504A	Unsp injury of blood vessel of right ring finger, init
		S65.505A	Unsp injury of blood vessel of left ring finger, init encntr
		S65.506A	Unsp injury of blood vessel of right little finger, init
		S65.507A	Unsp injury of blood vessel of left little finger, init
		S65.508A	Unsp injury of blood vessel of other finger, init encntr
		S65.509A	Unsp injury of blood vessel of unsp finger, init encntr
		S65.510A	Laceration of blood vessel of right index finger, init
		S65.511A	Laceration of blood vessel of left index finger, init encntr
		S65.512A	Laceration of blood vessel of right middle finger, init
		S65.513A	Laceration of blood vessel of left middle finger, init
		S65.514A	Laceration of blood vessel of right ring finger, init encntr
		S65.515A	Laceration of blood vessel of left ring finger, init encntr
		S65.516A	Laceration of blood vessel of right little finger, init
		S65.517A	Laceration of blood vessel of left little finger, init
		S65.518A	Laceration of blood vessel of other finger, init encntr

(Continued on next page)

ICD-9-CM		ICD-10-CM	
903.5	DIGITAL BLOOD VESSELS INJURY **(Continued)**	**S65.519A**	Laceration of blood vessel of unsp finger, init encntr
		S65.590A	Inj blood vessel of right index finger, init encntr
		S65.591A	Oth injury of blood vessel of left index finger, init encntr
		S65.592A	Inj blood vessel of right middle finger, init encntr
		S65.593A	Inj blood vessel of left middle finger, init encntr
		S65.594A	Oth injury of blood vessel of right ring finger, init encntr
		S65.595A	Oth injury of blood vessel of left ring finger, init encntr
		S65.596A	Inj blood vessel of right little finger, init encntr
		S65.597A	Inj blood vessel of left little finger, init encntr
		S65.598A	Oth injury of blood vessel of other finger, init encntr
		S65.599A	Oth injury of blood vessel of unsp finger, init encntr
903.8	INJURY SPEC BLOOD VESSELS UPPER EXTREMITY OTHER	**S45.301A**	Unsp injury of superfic vn at shldr/up arm, right arm, init
		S45.302A	Unsp injury of superfic vn at shldr/up arm, left arm, init
		S45.309A	Unsp injury of superfic vn at shldr/up arm, unsp arm, init
		S45.311A	Laceration of superfic vn at shldr/up arm, right arm, init
		S45.312A	Laceration of superfic vn at shldr/up arm, left arm, init
		S45.319A	Laceration of superfic vn at shldr/up arm, unsp arm, init
		S45.391A	Inj superficial vein at shldr/up arm, right arm, init
		S45.392A	Inj superficial vein at shldr/up arm, left arm, init
		S45.399A	Inj superficial vein at shldr/up arm, unsp arm, init
		S45.801A	Unsp inj blood vessels at shldr/up arm, right arm, init
		S45.802A	Unsp injury of blood vessels at shldr/up arm, left arm, init
		S45.809A	Unsp injury of blood vessels at shldr/up arm, unsp arm, init
		S45.811A	Laceration of blood vessels at shldr/up arm, right arm, init
		S45.812A	Laceration of blood vessels at shldr/up arm, left arm, init
		S45.819A	Laceration of blood vessels at shldr/up arm, unsp arm, init
		S45.891A	Inj oth blood vessels at shldr/up arm, right arm, init
		S45.892A	Inj oth blood vessels at shldr/up arm, left arm, init
		S45.899A	Inj oth blood vessels at shldr/up arm, unsp arm, init
		S55.201A	Unsp injury of vein at forearm level, right arm, init encntr
		S55.202A	Unsp injury of vein at forearm level, left arm, init encntr
		S55.209A	Unsp injury of vein at forearm level, unsp arm, init encntr
		S55.211A	Laceration of vein at forearm level, right arm, init encntr
		S55.212A	Laceration of vein at forearm level, left arm, init encntr
		S55.219A	Laceration of vein at forearm level, unsp arm, init encntr
		S55.291A	Oth injury of vein at forearm level, right arm, init encntr
		S55.292A	Oth injury of vein at forearm level, left arm, init encntr
		S55.299A	Oth injury of vein at forearm level, unsp arm, init encntr
		S55.801A	Unsp injury of blood vessels at forarm lv, right arm, init
		S55.802A	Unsp injury of blood vessels at forarm lv, left arm, init
		S55.809A	Unsp injury of blood vessels at forarm lv, unsp arm, init
		S55.811A	Laceration of blood vessels at forarm lv, right arm, init
		S55.812A	Laceration of blood vessels at forearm level, left arm, init
		S55.819A	Laceration of blood vessels at forearm level, unsp arm, init
		S55.891A	Inj oth blood vessels at forearm level, right arm, init
		S55.892A	Inj oth blood vessels at forearm level, left arm, init
		S55.899A	Inj oth blood vessels at forearm level, unsp arm, init
		S65.801A	Unsp inj blood vessels at wrs/hnd lv of right arm, init
		S65.802A	Unsp injury of blood vessels at wrs/hnd lv of left arm, init
		S65.809A	Unsp injury of blood vessels at wrs/hnd lv of unsp arm, init
		S65.811A	Laceration of blood vessels at wrs/hnd lv of right arm, init
		S65.812A	Laceration of blood vessels at wrs/hnd lv of left arm, init
		S65.819A	Laceration of blood vessels at wrs/hnd lv of unsp arm, init
		S65.891A	Inj oth blood vessels at wrs/hnd lv of right arm, init
		S65.892A	Inj oth blood vessels at wrs/hnd lv of left arm, init
		S65.899A	Inj oth blood vessels at wrs/hnd lv of unsp arm, init
903.9	INJURY UNSPECIFIED BLOOD VESSEL UPPER EXTREMITY	**S45.901A**	Unsp inj unsp blood vess at shldr/up arm, right arm, init
		S45.902A	Unsp inj unsp blood vess at shldr/up arm, left arm, init
		S45.909A	Unsp inj unsp blood vess at shldr/up arm, unsp arm, init
		S45.911A	Lacerat unsp blood vessel at shldr/up arm, right arm, init
		S45.912A	Lacerat unsp blood vessel at shldr/up arm, left arm, init
		S45.919A	Lacerat unsp blood vessel at shldr/up arm, unsp arm, init
		S45.991A	Inj unsp blood vessel at shldr/up arm, right arm, init
		S45.992A	Inj unsp blood vessel at shldr/up arm, left arm, init
		S45.999A	Inj unsp blood vessel at shldr/up arm, unsp arm, init
		S55.901A	Unsp injury of unsp blood vess at forarm lv, right arm, init
		S55.902A	Unsp injury of unsp blood vess at forarm lv, left arm, init
		S55.909A	Unsp injury of unsp blood vess at forarm lv, unsp arm, init
		S55.911A	Lacerat unsp blood vessel at forarm lv, right arm, init
		S55.912A	Laceration of unsp blood vessel at forarm lv, left arm, init
		S55.919A	Laceration of unsp blood vessel at forarm lv, unsp arm, init
		S55.991A	Inj unsp blood vessel at forearm level, right arm, init
		S55.992A	Inj unsp blood vessel at forearm level, left arm, init
		S55.999A	Inj unsp blood vessel at forearm level, unsp arm, init
		S65.901A	Unsp inj unsp blood vess at wrs/hnd lv of right arm, init
		S65.902A	Unsp inj unsp blood vess at wrs/hnd lv of left arm, init
		S65.909A	Unsp inj unsp blood vess at wrs/hnd lv of unsp arm, init
		S65.911A	Lacerat unsp blood vessel at wrs/hnd lv of right arm, init
		S65.912A	Lacerat unsp blood vessel at wrs/hnd lv of left arm, init
		S65.919A	Lacerat unsp blood vessel at wrs/hnd lv of unsp arm, init
		S65.991A	Inj unsp blood vessel at wrist and hand of right arm, init
		S65.992A	Inj unsp blood vessel at wrist and hand of left arm, init
		S65.999A	Inj unsp blood vessel at wrist and hand of unsp arm, init

ICD-9-CM		ICD-10-CM	
904.Ø	COMMON FEMORAL ARTERY INJURY	**S75.ØØ1A**	Unspecified injury of femoral artery, right leg, init encntr
		S75.ØØ2A	Unspecified injury of femoral artery, left leg, init encntr
		S75.ØØ9A	Unsp injury of femoral artery, unspecified leg, init encntr
		S75.Ø11A	Minor laceration of femoral artery, right leg, init encntr
		S75.Ø12A	Minor laceration of femoral artery, left leg, init encntr
		S75.Ø19A	Minor laceration of femoral artery, unsp leg, init encntr
		S75.Ø21A	Major laceration of femoral artery, right leg, init encntr
		S75.Ø22A	Major laceration of femoral artery, left leg, init encntr
		S75.Ø29A	Major laceration of femoral artery, unsp leg, init encntr
		S75.Ø91A	Oth injury of femoral artery, right leg, init encntr
		S75.Ø92A	Oth injury of femoral artery, left leg, init encntr
		S75.Ø99A	Oth injury of femoral artery, unspecified leg, init encntr
904.1	SUPERFICIAL FEMORAL ARTERY INJURY	**S75.ØØ1A**	Unspecified injury of femoral artery, right leg, init encntr
		S75.ØØ2A	Unspecified injury of femoral artery, left leg, init encntr
		S75.ØØ9A	Unsp injury of femoral artery, unspecified leg, init encntr
		S75.Ø11A	Minor laceration of femoral artery, right leg, init encntr
		S75.Ø12A	Minor laceration of femoral artery, left leg, init encntr
		S75.Ø19A	Minor laceration of femoral artery, unsp leg, init encntr
		S75.Ø21A	Major laceration of femoral artery, right leg, init encntr
		S75.Ø22A	Major laceration of femoral artery, left leg, init encntr
		S75.Ø29A	Major laceration of femoral artery, unsp leg, init encntr
		S75.Ø91A	Oth injury of femoral artery, right leg, init encntr
		S75.Ø92A	Oth injury of femoral artery, left leg, init encntr
		S75.Ø99A	Oth injury of femoral artery, unspecified leg, init encntr
904.2	FEMORAL VEIN INJURY	**S75.1Ø1A**	Unsp inj femor vein at hip and thi lev, right leg, init
		S75.1Ø2A	Unsp injury of femor vein at hip and thi lev, left leg, init
		S75.1Ø9A	Unsp injury of femor vein at hip and thi lev, unsp leg, init
		S75.111A	Minor lacerat femor vein at hip and thi lev, right leg, init
		S75.112A	Minor lacerat femor vein at hip and thi lev, left leg, init
		S75.119A	Minor lacerat femor vein at hip and thi lev, unsp leg, init
		S75.121A	Major lacerat femor vein at hip and thi lev, right leg, init
		S75.122A	Major lacerat femor vein at hip and thi lev, left leg, init
		S75.129A	Major lacerat femor vein at hip and thi lev, unsp leg, init
		S75.191A	Inj femoral vein at hip and thigh level, right leg, init
		S75.192A	Inj femoral vein at hip and thigh level, left leg, init
		S75.199A	Inj femoral vein at hip and thigh level, unsp leg, init
904.3	SAPHENOUS VEIN INJURY	**S75.2Ø1A**	Unsp inj great saphenous at hip and thi lev, right leg, init
		S75.2Ø2A	Unsp inj great saphenous at hip and thi lev, left leg, init
		S75.2Ø9A	Unsp inj great saphenous at hip and thi lev, unsp leg, init
		S75.211A	Minor lacerat great saph at hip and thi lev, right leg, init
		S75.212A	Minor lacerat great saph at hip and thi lev, left leg, init
		S75.219A	Minor lacerat great saph at hip and thi lev, unsp leg, init
		S75.221A	Major lacerat great saph at hip and thi lev, right leg, init
		S75.222A	Major lacerat great saph at hip and thi lev, left leg, init
		S75.229A	Major lacerat great saph at hip and thi lev, unsp leg, init
		S75.291A	Inj great saphenous at hip and thigh level, right leg, init
		S75.292A	Inj great saphenous at hip and thigh level, left leg, init
		S75.299A	Inj great saphenous at hip and thigh level, unsp leg, init
		S85.3Ø1A	Unsp inj great saphenous at lower leg level, right leg, init
		S85.3Ø2A	Unsp inj great saphenous at lower leg level, left leg, init
		S85.3Ø9A	Unsp inj great saphenous at lower leg level, unsp leg, init
		S85.311A	Lacerat great saphenous at lower leg level, right leg, init
		S85.312A	Lacerat great saphenous at lower leg level, left leg, init
		S85.319A	Lacerat great saphenous at lower leg level, unsp leg, init
		S85.391A	Inj great saphenous at lower leg level, right leg, init
		S85.392A	Inj great saphenous at lower leg level, left leg, init
		S85.399A	Inj great saphenous at lower leg level, unsp leg, init
		S85.4Ø1A	Unsp inj less saphenous at lower leg level, right leg, init
		S85.4Ø2A	Unsp inj less saphenous at lower leg level, left leg, init
		S85.4Ø9A	Unsp inj less saphenous at lower leg level, unsp leg, init
		S85.411A	Lacerat less saphenous at lower leg level, right leg, init
		S85.412A	Lacerat less saphenous at lower leg level, left leg, init
		S85.419A	Lacerat less saphenous at lower leg level, unsp leg, init
		S85.491A	Inj less saphenous at lower leg level, right leg, init
		S85.492A	Inj lesser saphenous vein at lower leg level, left leg, init
		S85.499A	Inj lesser saphenous vein at lower leg level, unsp leg, init
904.4Ø	UNSPECIFIED POPLITEAL VESSEL INJURY	**S85.ØØ9A**	Unsp injury of popliteal artery, unsp leg, init encntr
		S85.5Ø9A	Unsp injury of popliteal vein, unspecified leg, init encntr
904.41	POPLITEAL ARTERY INJURY	**S85.ØØ1A**	Unsp injury of popliteal artery, right leg, init encntr
		S85.ØØ2A	Unsp injury of popliteal artery, left leg, init encntr
		S85.ØØ9A	Unsp injury of popliteal artery, unsp leg, init encntr
		S85.Ø11A	Laceration of popliteal artery, right leg, initial encounter
		S85.Ø12A	Laceration of popliteal artery, left leg, initial encounter
		S85.Ø19A	Laceration of popliteal artery, unspecified leg, init encntr
		S85.Ø91A	Oth injury of popliteal artery, right leg, init encntr
		S85.Ø92A	Oth injury of popliteal artery, left leg, init encntr
		S85.Ø99A	Oth injury of popliteal artery, unspecified leg, init encntr

ICD-9-CM		ICD-10-CM	
9Ø4.42	POPLITEAL VEIN INJURY	**S85.5Ø1A**	Unspecified injury of popliteal vein, right leg, init encntr
		S85.5Ø2A	Unspecified injury of popliteal vein, left leg, init encntr
		S85.5Ø9A	Unsp injury of popliteal vein, unspecified leg, init encntr
		S85.511A	Laceration of popliteal vein, right leg, initial encounter
		S85.512A	Laceration of popliteal vein, left leg, initial encounter
		S85.519A	Laceration of popliteal vein, unspecified leg, init encntr
		S85.591A	Oth injury of popliteal vein, right leg, init encntr
		S85.592A	Oth injury of popliteal vein, left leg, init encntr
		S85.599A	Oth injury of popliteal vein, unspecified leg, init encntr
9Ø4.5Ø	UNSPECIFIED TIBIAL VESSEL INJURY	**S85.1Ø1A**	Unsp injury of unsp tibial artery, right leg, init encntr
		S85.1Ø2A	Unsp injury of unsp tibial artery, left leg, init encntr
		S85.1Ø9A	Unsp injury of unsp tibial artery, unsp leg, init encntr
		S85.111A	Laceration of unsp tibial artery, right leg, init encntr
		S85.112A	Laceration of unsp tibial artery, left leg, init encntr
		S85.119A	Laceration of unsp tibial artery, unsp leg, init encntr
		S85.121A	Oth injury of unsp tibial artery, right leg, init encntr
		S85.122A	Oth injury of unsp tibial artery, left leg, init encntr
		S85.129A	Oth injury of unsp tibial artery, unsp leg, init encntr
9Ø4.51	ANTERIOR TIBIAL ARTERY INJURY	**S85.131A**	Unsp injury of anterior tibial artery, right leg, init
		S85.132A	Unsp injury of anterior tibial artery, left leg, init encntr
		S85.139A	Unsp injury of anterior tibial artery, unsp leg, init encntr
		S85.141A	Laceration of anterior tibial artery, right leg, init encntr
		S85.142A	Laceration of anterior tibial artery, left leg, init encntr
		S85.149A	Laceration of anterior tibial artery, unsp leg, init encntr
		S85.151A	Oth injury of anterior tibial artery, right leg, init encntr
		S85.152A	Oth injury of anterior tibial artery, left leg, init encntr
		S85.159A	Oth injury of anterior tibial artery, unsp leg, init encntr
9Ø4.52	ANTERIOR TIBIAL VEIN INJURY	**S85.8Ø1A**	Unsp inj blood vessels at lower leg level, right leg, init
		S85.8Ø2A	Unsp inj blood vessels at lower leg level, left leg, init
		S85.8Ø9A	Unsp inj blood vessels at lower leg level, unsp leg, init
		S85.811A	Lacerat blood vessels at lower leg level, right leg, init
		S85.812A	Lacerat blood vessels at lower leg level, left leg, init
		S85.819A	Lacerat blood vessels at lower leg level, unsp leg, init
		S85.891A	Inj oth blood vessels at lower leg level, right leg, init
		S85.892A	Inj oth blood vessels at lower leg level, left leg, init
		S85.899A	Inj oth blood vessels at lower leg level, unsp leg, init
9Ø4.53	POSTERIOR TIBIAL ARTERY INJURY	**S85.161A**	Unsp injury of posterior tibial artery, right leg, init
		S85.162A	Unsp injury of posterior tibial artery, left leg, init
		S85.169A	Unsp injury of posterior tibial artery, unsp leg, init
		S85.171A	Laceration of posterior tibial artery, right leg, init
		S85.172A	Laceration of posterior tibial artery, left leg, init encntr
		S85.179A	Laceration of posterior tibial artery, unsp leg, init encntr
		S85.181A	Inj posterior tibial artery, right leg, init encntr
		S85.182A	Oth injury of posterior tibial artery, left leg, init encntr
		S85.189A	Oth injury of posterior tibial artery, unsp leg, init encntr
9Ø4.54	POSTERIOR TIBIAL VEIN INJURY	**S85.8Ø1A**	Unsp inj blood vessels at lower leg level, right leg, init
		S85.8Ø2A	Unsp inj blood vessels at lower leg level, left leg, init
		S85.8Ø9A	Unsp inj blood vessels at lower leg level, unsp leg, init
		S85.811A	Lacerat blood vessels at lower leg level, right leg, init
		S85.812A	Lacerat blood vessels at lower leg level, left leg, init
		S85.819A	Lacerat blood vessels at lower leg level, unsp leg, init
		S85.891A	Inj oth blood vessels at lower leg level, right leg, init
		S85.892A	Inj oth blood vessels at lower leg level, left leg, init
		S85.899A	Inj oth blood vessels at lower leg level, unsp leg, init
9Ø4.6	DEEP PLANTAR BLOOD VESSELS INJURY	**S95.1Ø1A**	Unsp injury of plantar artery of right foot, init encntr
		S95.1Ø2A	Unsp injury of plantar artery of left foot, init encntr
		S95.1Ø9A	Unsp injury of plantar artery of unsp foot, init encntr
		S95.111A	Laceration of plantar artery of right foot, init encntr
		S95.112A	Laceration of plantar artery of left foot, initial encounter
		S95.119A	Laceration of plantar artery of unsp foot, init encntr
		S95.191A	Oth injury of plantar artery of right foot, init encntr
		S95.192A	Oth injury of plantar artery of left foot, init encntr
		S95.199A	Oth injury of plantar artery of unsp foot, init encntr
9Ø4.7	INJURY SPEC BLOOD VESSELS LOWER EXTREMITY OTHER	**S75.8Ø1A**	Unsp inj blood vessels at hip and thi lev, right leg, init
		S75.8Ø2A	Unsp inj blood vessels at hip and thi lev, left leg, init
		S75.8Ø9A	Unsp inj blood vessels at hip and thi lev, unsp leg, init
		S75.811A	Lacerat blood vessels at hip and thi lev, right leg, init
		S75.812A	Lacerat blood vessels at hip and thigh level, left leg, init
		S75.819A	Lacerat blood vessels at hip and thigh level, unsp leg, init
		S75.891A	Inj oth blood vessels at hip and thi lev, right leg, init
		S75.892A	Inj oth blood vessels at hip and thigh level, left leg, init
		S75.899A	Inj oth blood vessels at hip and thigh level, unsp leg, init
		S85.2Ø1A	Unsp injury of peroneal artery, right leg, init encntr
		S85.2Ø2A	Unspecified injury of peroneal artery, left leg, init encntr
		S85.2Ø9A	Unsp injury of peroneal artery, unspecified leg, init encntr
		S85.211A	Laceration of peroneal artery, right leg, initial encounter
		S85.212A	Laceration of peroneal artery, left leg, initial encounter
		S85.219A	Laceration of peroneal artery, unspecified leg, init encntr
		S85.291A	Oth injury of peroneal artery, right leg, init encntr
		S85.292A	Oth injury of peroneal artery, left leg, init encntr

(Continued on next page)

ICD-9-CM		ICD-10-CM	
904.7	INJURY SPEC BLOOD VESSELS LOWER EXTREMITY OTHER **(Continued)**	**S85.299A**	Oth injury of peroneal artery, unspecified leg, init encntr
		S85.801A	Unsp inj blood vessels at lower leg level, right leg, init
		S85.802A	Unsp inj blood vessels at lower leg level, left leg, init
		S85.809A	Unsp inj blood vessels at lower leg level, unsp leg, init
		S85.811A	Lacerat blood vessels at lower leg level, right leg, init
		S85.812A	Lacerat blood vessels at lower leg level, left leg, init
		S85.819A	Lacerat blood vessels at lower leg level, unsp leg, init
		S85.891A	Inj oth blood vessels at lower leg level, right leg, init
		S85.892A	Inj oth blood vessels at lower leg level, left leg, init
		S85.899A	Inj oth blood vessels at lower leg level, unsp leg, init
		S95.001A	Unsp injury of dorsal artery of right foot, init encntr
		S95.002A	Unsp injury of dorsal artery of left foot, init encntr
		S95.009A	Unsp injury of dorsal artery of unsp foot, init encntr
		S95.011A	Laceration of dorsal artery of right foot, initial encounter
		S95.012A	Laceration of dorsal artery of left foot, initial encounter
		S95.019A	Laceration of dorsal artery of unspecified foot, init encntr
		S95.091A	Oth injury of dorsal artery of right foot, init encntr
		S95.092A	Oth injury of dorsal artery of left foot, init encntr
		S95.099A	Oth injury of dorsal artery of unspecified foot, init encntr
		S95.201A	Unspecified injury of dorsal vein of right foot, init encntr
		S95.202A	Unspecified injury of dorsal vein of left foot, init encntr
		S95.209A	Unsp injury of dorsal vein of unspecified foot, init encntr
		S95.211A	Laceration of dorsal vein of right foot, initial encounter
		S95.212A	Laceration of dorsal vein of left foot, initial encounter
		S95.219A	Laceration of dorsal vein of unspecified foot, init encntr
		S95.291A	Oth injury of dorsal vein of right foot, init encntr
		S95.292A	Oth injury of dorsal vein of left foot, init encntr
		S95.299A	Oth injury of dorsal vein of unspecified foot, init encntr
		S95.801A	Unsp inj blood vessels at ank/ft level, right leg, init
		S95.802A	Unsp injury of blood vessels at ank/ft level, left leg, init
		S95.809A	Unsp injury of blood vessels at ank/ft level, unsp leg, init
		S95.811A	Laceration of blood vessels at ank/ft level, right leg, init
		S95.812A	Laceration of blood vessels at ank/ft level, left leg, init
		S95.819A	Laceration of blood vessels at ank/ft level, unsp leg, init
		S95.891A	Inj oth blood vessels at ank/ft level, right leg, init
		S95.892A	Inj oth blood vessels at ank/ft level, left leg, init
		S95.899A	Inj oth blood vessels at ank/ft level, unsp leg, init
904.8	INJURY UNSPECIFIED BLOOD VESSEL LOWER EXTREMITY	**S75.901A**	Unsp inj unsp blood vess at hip and thi lev, right leg, init
		S75.902A	Unsp inj unsp blood vess at hip and thi lev, left leg, init
		S75.909A	Unsp inj unsp blood vess at hip and thi lev, unsp leg, init
		S75.911A	Lacerat unsp blood vess at hip and thi lev, right leg, init
		S75.912A	Lacerat unsp blood vess at hip and thi lev, left leg, init
		S75.919A	Lacerat unsp blood vess at hip and thi lev, unsp leg, init
		S75.991A	Inj unsp blood vess at hip and thigh level, right leg, init
		S75.992A	Inj unsp blood vessel at hip and thigh level, left leg, init
		S75.999A	Inj unsp blood vessel at hip and thigh level, unsp leg, init
		S85.901A	Unsp inj unsp blood vess at lower leg level, right leg, init
		S85.902A	Unsp inj unsp blood vess at lower leg level, left leg, init
		S85.909A	Unsp inj unsp blood vess at lower leg level, unsp leg, init
		S85.911A	Lacerat unsp blood vess at lower leg level, right leg, init
		S85.912A	Lacerat unsp blood vessel at lower leg level, left leg, init
		S85.919A	Lacerat unsp blood vessel at lower leg level, unsp leg, init
		S85.991A	Inj unsp blood vessel at lower leg level, right leg, init
		S85.992A	Inj unsp blood vessel at lower leg level, left leg, init
		S85.999A	Inj unsp blood vessel at lower leg level, unsp leg, init
		S95.901A	Unsp inj unsp blood vess at ank/ft level, right leg, init
		S95.902A	Unsp inj unsp blood vess at ank/ft level, left leg, init
		S95.909A	Unsp inj unsp blood vess at ank/ft level, unsp leg, init
		S95.911A	Lacerat unsp blood vessel at ank/ft level, right leg, init
		S95.912A	Lacerat unsp blood vessel at ank/ft level, left leg, init
		S95.919A	Lacerat unsp blood vessel at ank/ft level, unsp leg, init
		S95.991A	Inj unsp blood vessel at ank/ft level, right leg, init
		S95.992A	Inj unsp blood vessel at ank/ft level, left leg, init
		S95.999A	Inj unsp blood vessel at ank/ft level, unsp leg, init
904.9	INJURY TO BLOOD VESSELS UNSPECIFIED SITE	**T14.90**	Injury, unspecified
905.0	LATE EFFECT OF FRACTURE OF SKULL AND FACE BONES	**S02.0XXS**	Fracture of vault of skull, sequela
		S02.10XS	Unspecified fracture of base of skull, sequela
		S02.110S	Type I occipital condyle fracture, sequela
		S02.111S	Type II occipital condyle fracture, sequela
		S02.112S	Type III occipital condyle fracture, sequela
		S02.113S	Unspecified occipital condyle fracture, sequela
		S02.118S	Other fracture of occiput, sequela
		S02.119S	Unspecified fracture of occiput, sequela
		S02.19XS	Other fracture of base of skull, sequela
		S02.2XXS	Fracture of nasal bones, sequela
		S02.3XXS	Fracture of orbital floor, sequela
		S02.400S	Malar fracture unspecified, sequela
		S02.401S	Maxillary fracture, unspecified, sequela
		S02.402S	Zygomatic fracture, unspecified, sequela
		S02.411S	LeFort I fracture, sequela
		S02.412S	LeFort II fracture, sequela
	(Continued on next page)	**S02.413S**	LeFort III fracture, sequela

ICD-9-CM		ICD-10-CM	
905.Ø	LATE EFFECT OF FRACTURE OF SKULL AND FACE BONES **(Continued)**	**SØ2.42XS**	Fracture of alveolus of maxilla, sequela
		SØ2.5XXS	Fracture of tooth (traumatic), sequela
		SØ2.6ØØS	Fracture of unspecified part of body of mandible, sequela
		SØ2.6Ø9S	Fracture of mandible, unspecified, sequela
		SØ2.61XS	Fracture of condylar process of mandible, sequela
		SØ2.62XS	Fracture of subcondylar process of mandible, sequela
		SØ2.63XS	Fracture of coronoid process of mandible, sequela
		SØ2.64XS	Fracture of ramus of mandible, sequela
		SØ2.65XS	Fracture of angle of mandible, sequela
		SØ2.66XS	Fracture of symphysis of mandible, sequela
		SØ2.67XS	Fracture of alveolus of mandible, sequela
		SØ2.69XS	Fracture of mandible of other specified site, sequela
		SØ2.8XXS	Fractures of other specified skull and facial bones, sequela
		SØ2.91XS	Unspecified fracture of skull, sequela
		SØ2.92XS	Unspecified fracture of facial bones, sequela
9Ø5.1	LATE EFF FX SPN&TRNK W/O MENTION SPINAL CORD LES	**M48.4ØXS**	Fatigue fracture of vertebra, site unsp, sequela of fracture
		M48.41XS	Fatigue fracture of vertebra, occipt-atlan-ax region, sqla
		M48.42XS	Fatigue fracture of vertebra, cervical region, sqla
		M48.43XS	Fatigue fracture of vertebra, cervicothoracic region, sqla
		M48.44XS	Fatigue fracture of vertebra, thoracic region, sqla
		M48.45XS	Fatigue fracture of vertebra, thoracolumbar region, sqla
		M48.46XS	Fatigue fracture of vertebra, lumbar region, sqla
		M48.47XS	Fatigue fracture of vertebra, lumbosacral region, sqla
		M48.48XS	Fatigue fracture of vertebra, sacr/sacrocygl region, sqla
		M48.5ØXS	Collapsed vertebra, NEC, site unsp, sequela of fracture
		M48.51XS	Collapsed vertebra, NEC, occipt-atlan-ax region, sqla
		M48.52XS	Collapsed vertebra, NEC, cervical region, sqla
		M48.53XS	Collapsed vertebra, NEC, cervicothoracic region, sqla
		M48.54XS	Collapsed vertebra, NEC, thoracic region, sqla
		M48.55XS	Collapsed vertebra, NEC, thoracolumbar region, sqla
		M48.56XS	Collapsed vertebra, NEC, lumbar region, sequela of fracture
		M48.57XS	Collapsed vertebra, NEC, lumbosacral region, sqla
		M48.58XS	Collapsed vertebra, NEC, sacr/sacrocygl region, sqla
		M8Ø.Ø8XS	Age-rel osteopor w curr path fx, oth spec site, sequela
		M8Ø.88XS	Oth osteopor w current path fracture, vertebra(e), sequela
		M84.35ØS	Stress fracture, pelvis, sequela
		M84.454S	Pathological fracture, pelvis, sequela
		M84.55ØS	Pathological fracture in neoplastic disease, pelvis, sequela
		M84.58XS	Path fracture in neoplastic disease, vertebrae, sequela
		M84.65ØS	Pathological fracture in other disease, pelvis, sequela
		S12.ØØØS	Unspecified disp fx of first cervical vertebra, sequela
		S12.ØØ1S	Unspecified nondisp fx of first cervical vertebra, sequela
		S12.Ø1XS	Stable burst fracture of first cervical vertebra, sequela
		S12.Ø2XS	Unstable burst fracture of first cervical vertebra, sequela
		S12.Ø3ØS	Displaced posterior arch fx first cervcal vertebra, sequela
		S12.Ø31S	Nondisp posterior arch fx first cervcal vertebra, sequela
		S12.Ø4ØS	Displaced lateral mass fx first cervcal vertebra, sequela
		S12.Ø41S	Nondisp lateral mass fx first cervcal vertebra, sequela
		S12.Ø9ØS	Other displaced fracture of first cervical vertebra, sequela
		S12.Ø91S	Other nondisp fx of first cervical vertebra, sequela
		S12.1ØØS	Unspecified disp fx of second cervical vertebra, sequela
		S12.1Ø1S	Unspecified nondisp fx of second cervical vertebra, sequela
		S12.11ØS	Anterior displaced Type II dens fracture, sequela
		S12.111S	Posterior displaced Type II dens fracture, sequela
		S12.112S	Nondisplaced Type II dens fracture, sequela
		S12.12ØS	Other displaced dens fracture, sequela
		S12.121S	Other nondisplaced dens fracture, sequela
		S12.13ØS	Unsp traum displ spondylolysis of second cervcal vert, sqla
		S12.131S	Unsp traum nondisp spondylolysis of 2nd cervcal vert, sqla
		S12.14XS	Type III traum spondylolysis of second cervcal vert, sequela
		S12.15ØS	Oth traum displ spondylolysis of second cervcal vert, sqla
		S12.151S	Oth traum nondisp spondylolysis of second cervcal vert, sqla
		S12.19ØS	Other disp fx of second cervical vertebra, sequela
		S12.191S	Other nondisp fx of second cervical vertebra, sequela
		S12.2ØØS	Unspecified disp fx of third cervical vertebra, sequela
		S12.2Ø1S	Unspecified nondisp fx of third cervical vertebra, sequela
		S12.23ØS	Unsp traum displ spondylolysis of third cervcal vert, sqla
		S12.231S	Unsp traum nondisp spondylolysis of third cervcal vert, sqla
		S12.24XS	Type III traum spondylolysis of third cervcal vert, sequela
		S12.25ØS	Oth traum displ spondylolysis of third cervcal vert, sequela
		S12.251S	Oth traum nondisp spondylolysis of third cervcal vert, sqla
		S12.29ØS	Other displaced fracture of third cervical vertebra, sequela
		S12.291S	Other nondisp fx of third cervical vertebra, sequela
		S12.3ØØS	Unspecified disp fx of fourth cervical vertebra, sequela
		S12.3Ø1S	Unspecified nondisp fx of fourth cervical vertebra, sequela
		S12.33ØS	Unsp traum displ spondylolysis of fourth cervcal vert, sqla
		S12.331S	Unsp traum nondisp spondylolysis of 4th cervcal vert, sqla
		S12.34XS	Type III traum spondylolysis of fourth cervcal vert, sequela
		S12.35ØS	Oth traum displ spondylolysis of fourth cervcal vert, sqla
		S12.351S	Oth traum nondisp spondylolysis of fourth cervcal vert, sqla
		S12.39ØS	Other disp fx of fourth cervical vertebra, sequela
	(Continued on next page)	**S12.391S**	Other nondisp fx of fourth cervical vertebra, sequela

ICD-9-CM		ICD-10-CM	
9Ø5.1	LATE EFF FX SPN&TRNK W/O MENTION SPINAL CORD LES **(Continued)**	**S12.4ØØS**	Unspecified disp fx of fifth cervical vertebra, sequela
		S12.4Ø1S	Unspecified nondisp fx of fifth cervical vertebra, sequela
		S12.43ØS	Unsp traum displ spondylolysis of fifth cervcal vert, sqla
		S12.431S	Unsp traum nondisp spondylolysis of fifth cervcal vert, sqla
		S12.44XS	Type III traum spondylolysis of fifth cervcal vert, sequela
		S12.45ØS	Oth traum displ spondylolysis of fifth cervcal vert, sequela
		S12.451S	Oth traum nondisp spondylolysis of fifth cervcal vert, sqla
		S12.49ØS	Other displaced fracture of fifth cervical vertebra, sequela
		S12.491S	Other nondisp fx of fifth cervical vertebra, sequela
		S12.5ØØS	Unspecified disp fx of sixth cervical vertebra, sequela
		S12.5Ø1S	Unspecified nondisp fx of sixth cervical vertebra, sequela
		S12.53ØS	Unsp traum displ spondylolysis of sixth cervcal vert, sqla
		S12.531S	Unsp traum nondisp spondylolysis of sixth cervcal vert, sqla
		S12.54XS	Type III traum spondylolysis of sixth cervcal vert, sequela
		S12.55ØS	Oth traum displ spondylolysis of sixth cervcal vert, sequela
		S12.551S	Oth traum nondisp spondylolysis of sixth cervcal vert, sqla
		S12.59ØS	Other displaced fracture of sixth cervical vertebra, sequela
		S12.591S	Other nondisp fx of sixth cervical vertebra, sequela
		S12.6ØØS	Unspecified disp fx of seventh cervical vertebra, sequela
		S12.6Ø1S	Unspecified nondisp fx of seventh cervical vertebra, sequela
		S12.63ØS	Unsp traum displ spondylolysis of seventh cervcal vert, sqla
		S12.631S	Unsp traum nondisp spondylolysis of 7th cervcal vert, sqla
		S12.64XS	Type III traum spondylolysis of seventh cervcal vert, sqla
		S12.65ØS	Oth traum displ spondylolysis of seventh cervcal vert, sqla
		S12.651S	Oth traum nondisp spondylolysis of 7th cervcal vert, sqla
		S12.69ØS	Other disp fx of seventh cervical vertebra, sequela
		S12.691S	Other nondisp fx of seventh cervical vertebra, sequela
		S12.8XXS	Fracture of other parts of neck, sequela
		S12.9XXS	Fracture of neck, unspecified, sequela
		S22.ØØØS	Wedge compression fracture of unsp thor vertebra, sequela
		S22.ØØ1S	Stable burst fracture of unsp thoracic vertebra, sequela
		S22.ØØ2S	Unstable burst fracture of unsp thoracic vertebra, sequela
		S22.ØØ8S	Other fracture of unspecified thoracic vertebra, sequela
		S22.ØØ9S	Unsp fracture of unspecified thoracic vertebra, sequela
		S22.Ø1ØS	Wedge compression fracture of first thor vertebra, sequela
		S22.Ø11S	Stable burst fracture of first thoracic vertebra, sequela
		S22.Ø12S	Unstable burst fracture of first thoracic vertebra, sequela
		S22.Ø18S	Other fracture of first thoracic vertebra, sequela
		S22.Ø19S	Unspecified fracture of first thoracic vertebra, sequela
		S22.Ø2ØS	Wedge compression fracture of second thor vertebra, sequela
		S22.Ø21S	Stable burst fracture of second thoracic vertebra, sequela
		S22.Ø22S	Unstable burst fracture of second thoracic vertebra, sequela
		S22.Ø28S	Other fracture of second thoracic vertebra, sequela
		S22.Ø29S	Unspecified fracture of second thoracic vertebra, sequela
		S22.Ø3ØS	Wedge compression fracture of third thor vertebra, sequela
		S22.Ø31S	Stable burst fracture of third thoracic vertebra, sequela
		S22.Ø32S	Unstable burst fracture of third thoracic vertebra, sequela
		S22.Ø38S	Other fracture of third thoracic vertebra, sequela
		S22.Ø39S	Unspecified fracture of third thoracic vertebra, sequela
		S22.Ø4ØS	Wedge compression fracture of fourth thor vertebra, sequela
		S22.Ø41S	Stable burst fracture of fourth thoracic vertebra, sequela
		S22.Ø42S	Unstable burst fracture of fourth thoracic vertebra, sequela
		S22.Ø48S	Other fracture of fourth thoracic vertebra, sequela
		S22.Ø49S	Unspecified fracture of fourth thoracic vertebra, sequela
		S22.Ø5ØS	Wedge compression fracture of T5-T6 vertebra, sequela
		S22.Ø51S	Stable burst fracture of T5-T6 vertebra, sequela
		S22.Ø52S	Unstable burst fracture of T5-T6 vertebra, sequela
		S22.Ø58S	Other fracture of T5-T6 vertebra, sequela
		S22.Ø59S	Unspecified fracture of T5-T6 vertebra, sequela
		S22.Ø6ØS	Wedge compression fracture of T7-T8 vertebra, sequela
		S22.Ø61S	Stable burst fracture of T7-T8 vertebra, sequela
		S22.Ø62S	Unstable burst fracture of T7-T8 vertebra, sequela
		S22.Ø68S	Other fracture of T7-T8 thoracic vertebra, sequela
		S22.Ø69S	Unspecified fracture of T7-T8 vertebra, sequela
		S22.Ø7ØS	Wedge compression fracture of T9-T10 vertebra, sequela
		S22.Ø71S	Stable burst fracture of T9-T10 vertebra, sequela
		S22.Ø72S	Unstable burst fracture of T9-T10 vertebra, sequela
		S22.Ø78S	Other fracture of T9-T10 vertebra, sequela
		S22.Ø79S	Unspecified fracture of T9-T10 vertebra, sequela
		S22.Ø8ØS	Wedge compression fracture of T11-T12 vertebra, sequela
		S22.Ø81S	Stable burst fracture of T11-T12 vertebra, sequela
		S22.Ø82S	Unstable burst fracture of T11-T12 vertebra, sequela
		S22.Ø88S	Other fracture of T11-T12 vertebra, sequela
		S22.Ø89S	Unspecified fracture of T11-T12 vertebra, sequela
		S22.2ØXS	Unspecified fracture of sternum, sequela
		S22.21XS	Fracture of manubrium, sequela
		S22.22XS	Fracture of body of sternum, sequela
		S22.23XS	Sternal manubrial dissociation, sequela
		S22.24XS	Fracture of xiphoid process, sequela
		S22.31XS	Fracture of one rib, right side, sequela
	(Continued on next page)	**S22.32XS**	Fracture of one rib, left side, sequela

ICD-9-CM		ICD-10-CM	
9Ø5.1	LATE EFF FX SPN&TRNK W/O MENTION SPINAL CORD LES **(Continued)**	**S22.39XS**	Fracture of one rib, unspecified side, sequela
		S22.41XS	Multiple fractures of ribs, right side, sequela
		S22.42XS	Multiple fractures of ribs, left side, sequela
		S22.43XS	Multiple fractures of ribs, bilateral, sequela
		S22.49XS	Multiple fractures of ribs, unspecified side, sequela
		S22.5XXS	Flail chest, sequela
		S22.9XXS	Fracture of bony thorax, part unspecified, sequela
		S32.ØØØS	Wedge compression fracture of unsp lumbar vertebra, sequela
		S32.ØØ1S	Stable burst fracture of unsp lumbar vertebra, sequela
		S32.ØØ2S	Unstable burst fracture of unsp lumbar vertebra, sequela
		S32.ØØ8S	Other fracture of unspecified lumbar vertebra, sequela
		S32.ØØ9S	Unspecified fracture of unspecified lumbar vertebra, sequela
		S32.Ø1ØS	Wedge compression fracture of first lumbar vertebra, sequela
		S32.Ø11S	Stable burst fracture of first lumbar vertebra, sequela
		S32.Ø12S	Unstable burst fracture of first lumbar vertebra, sequela
		S32.Ø18S	Other fracture of first lumbar vertebra, sequela
		S32.Ø19S	Unspecified fracture of first lumbar vertebra, sequela
		S32.Ø2ØS	Wedge compression fracture of second lum vertebra, sequela
		S32.Ø21S	Stable burst fracture of second lumbar vertebra, sequela
		S32.Ø22S	Unstable burst fracture of second lumbar vertebra, sequela
		S32.Ø28S	Other fracture of second lumbar vertebra, sequela
		S32.Ø29S	Unspecified fracture of second lumbar vertebra, sequela
		S32.Ø3ØS	Wedge compression fracture of third lumbar vertebra, sequela
		S32.Ø31S	Stable burst fracture of third lumbar vertebra, sequela
		S32.Ø32S	Unstable burst fracture of third lumbar vertebra, sequela
		S32.Ø38S	Other fracture of third lumbar vertebra, sequela
		S32.Ø39S	Unspecified fracture of third lumbar vertebra, sequela
		S32.Ø4ØS	Wedge compression fracture of fourth lum vertebra, sequela
		S32.Ø41S	Stable burst fracture of fourth lumbar vertebra, sequela
		S32.Ø42S	Unstable burst fracture of fourth lumbar vertebra, sequela
		S32.Ø48S	Other fracture of fourth lumbar vertebra, sequela
		S32.Ø49S	Unspecified fracture of fourth lumbar vertebra, sequela
		S32.Ø5ØS	Wedge compression fracture of fifth lumbar vertebra, sequela
		S32.Ø51S	Stable burst fracture of fifth lumbar vertebra, sequela
		S32.Ø52S	Unstable burst fracture of fifth lumbar vertebra, sequela
		S32.Ø58S	Other fracture of fifth lumbar vertebra, sequela
		S32.Ø59S	Unspecified fracture of fifth lumbar vertebra, sequela
		S32.1ØXS	Unspecified fracture of sacrum, sequela
		S32.11ØS	Nondisplaced Zone I fracture of sacrum, sequela
		S32.111S	Minimally displaced Zone I fracture of sacrum, sequela
		S32.112S	Severely displaced Zone I fracture of sacrum, sequela
		S32.119S	Unspecified Zone I fracture of sacrum, sequela
		S32.12ØS	Nondisplaced Zone II fracture of sacrum, sequela
		S32.121S	Minimally displaced Zone II fracture of sacrum, sequela
		S32.122S	Severely displaced Zone II fracture of sacrum, sequela
		S32.129S	Unspecified Zone II fracture of sacrum, sequela
		S32.13ØS	Nondisplaced Zone III fracture of sacrum, sequela
		S32.131S	Minimally displaced Zone III fracture of sacrum, sequela
		S32.132S	Severely displaced Zone III fracture of sacrum, sequela
		S32.139S	Unspecified Zone III fracture of sacrum, sequela
		S32.14XS	Type 1 fracture of sacrum, sequela
		S32.15XS	Type 2 fracture of sacrum, sequela
		S32.16XS	Type 3 fracture of sacrum, sequela
		S32.17XS	Type 4 fracture of sacrum, sequela
		S32.19XS	Other fracture of sacrum, sequela
		S32.2XXS	Fracture of coccyx, sequela
		S32.3Ø1S	Unspecified fracture of right ilium, sequela
		S32.3Ø2S	Unspecified fracture of left ilium, sequela
		S32.3Ø9S	Unspecified fracture of unspecified ilium, sequela
		S32.311S	Displaced avulsion fracture of right ilium, sequela
		S32.312S	Displaced avulsion fracture of left ilium, sequela
		S32.313S	Displaced avulsion fracture of unspecified ilium, sequela
		S32.314S	Nondisplaced avulsion fracture of right ilium, sequela
		S32.315S	Nondisplaced avulsion fracture of left ilium, sequela
		S32.316S	Nondisplaced avulsion fracture of unspecified ilium, sequela
		S32.391S	Other fracture of right ilium, sequela
		S32.392S	Other fracture of left ilium, sequela
		S32.399S	Other fracture of unspecified ilium, sequela
		S32.4Ø1S	Unspecified fracture of right acetabulum, sequela
		S32.4Ø2S	Unspecified fracture of left acetabulum, sequela
		S32.4Ø9S	Unspecified fracture of unspecified acetabulum, sequela
		S32.411S	Disp fx of anterior wall of right acetabulum, sequela
		S32.412S	Disp fx of anterior wall of left acetabulum, sequela
		S32.413S	Disp fx of anterior wall of unspecified acetabulum, sequela
		S32.414S	Nondisp fx of anterior wall of right acetabulum, sequela
		S32.415S	Nondisp fx of anterior wall of left acetabulum, sequela
		S32.416S	Nondisp fx of anterior wall of unsp acetabulum, sequela
		S32.421S	Disp fx of posterior wall of right acetabulum, sequela
		S32.422S	Disp fx of posterior wall of left acetabulum, sequela
		S32.423S	Disp fx of posterior wall of unspecified acetabulum, sequela
		S32.424S	Nondisp fx of posterior wall of right acetabulum, sequela
		S32.425S	Nondisp fx of posterior wall of left acetabulum, sequela

(Continued on next page)

ICD-9-CM		ICD-10-CM	
905.1	LATE EFF FX SPN&TRNK W/O MENTION SPINAL CORD LES **(Continued)**	**S32.426S**	Nondisp fx of posterior wall of unsp acetabulum, sequela
		S32.431S	Disp fx of anterior column of right acetabulum, sequela
		S32.432S	Disp fx of anterior column of left acetabulum, sequela
		S32.433S	Disp fx of anterior column of unsp acetabulum, sequela
		S32.434S	Nondisp fx of anterior column of right acetabulum, sequela
		S32.435S	Nondisp fx of anterior column of left acetabulum, sequela
		S32.436S	Nondisp fx of anterior column of unsp acetabulum, sequela
		S32.441S	Disp fx of posterior column of right acetabulum, sequela
		S32.442S	Disp fx of posterior column of left acetabulum, sequela
		S32.443S	Disp fx of posterior column of unsp acetabulum, sequela
		S32.444S	Nondisp fx of posterior column of right acetabulum, sequela
		S32.445S	Nondisp fx of posterior column of left acetabulum, sequela
		S32.446S	Nondisp fx of posterior column of unsp acetabulum, sequela
		S32.451S	Displaced transverse fracture of right acetabulum, sequela
		S32.452S	Displaced transverse fracture of left acetabulum, sequela
		S32.453S	Displaced transverse fracture of unsp acetabulum, sequela
		S32.454S	Nondisp transverse fracture of right acetabulum, sequela
		S32.455S	Nondisplaced transverse fracture of left acetabulum, sequela
		S32.456S	Nondisplaced transverse fracture of unsp acetabulum, sequela
		S32.461S	Displaced associated transv/post fx right acetab, sequela
		S32.462S	Displaced associated transv/post fx left acetabulum, sequela
		S32.463S	Displaced associated transv/post fx unsp acetabulum, sequela
		S32.464S	Nondisp associated transv/post fx right acetabulum, sequela
		S32.465S	Nondisp associated transv/post fx left acetabulum, sequela
		S32.466S	Nondisp associated transv/post fx unsp acetabulum, sequela
		S32.471S	Disp fx of medial wall of right acetabulum, sequela
		S32.472S	Disp fx of medial wall of left acetabulum, sequela
		S32.473S	Disp fx of medial wall of unspecified acetabulum, sequela
		S32.474S	Nondisp fx of medial wall of right acetabulum, sequela
		S32.475S	Nondisp fx of medial wall of left acetabulum, sequela
		S32.476S	Nondisp fx of medial wall of unspecified acetabulum, sequela
		S32.481S	Displaced dome fracture of right acetabulum, sequela
		S32.482S	Displaced dome fracture of left acetabulum, sequela
		S32.483S	Displaced dome fracture of unspecified acetabulum, sequela
		S32.484S	Nondisplaced dome fracture of right acetabulum, sequela
		S32.485S	Nondisplaced dome fracture of left acetabulum, sequela
		S32.486S	Nondisplaced dome fracture of unsp acetabulum, sequela
		S32.491S	Other specified fracture of right acetabulum, sequela
		S32.492S	Other specified fracture of left acetabulum, sequela
		S32.499S	Other specified fracture of unspecified acetabulum, sequela
		S32.501S	Unspecified fracture of right pubis, sequela
		S32.502S	Unspecified fracture of left pubis, sequela
		S32.509S	Unspecified fracture of unspecified pubis, sequela
		S32.511S	Fracture of superior rim of right pubis, sequela
		S32.512S	Fracture of superior rim of left pubis, sequela
		S32.519S	Fracture of superior rim of unspecified pubis, sequela
		S32.591S	Other specified fracture of right pubis, sequela
		S32.592S	Other specified fracture of left pubis, sequela
		S32.599S	Other specified fracture of unspecified pubis, sequela
		S32.601S	Unspecified fracture of right ischium, sequela
		S32.602S	Unspecified fracture of left ischium, sequela
		S32.609S	Unspecified fracture of unspecified ischium, sequela
		S32.611S	Displaced avulsion fracture of right ischium, sequela
		S32.612S	Displaced avulsion fracture of left ischium, sequela
		S32.613S	Displaced avulsion fracture of unspecified ischium, sequela
		S32.614S	Nondisplaced avulsion fracture of right ischium, sequela
		S32.615S	Nondisplaced avulsion fracture of left ischium, sequela
		S32.616S	Nondisplaced avulsion fracture of unsp ischium, sequela
		S32.691S	Other specified fracture of right ischium, sequela
		S32.692S	Other specified fracture of left ischium, sequela
		S32.699S	Other specified fracture of unspecified ischium, sequela
		S32.810S	Mult fx of pelvis w stable disrupt of pelvic ring, sequela
		S32.811S	Mult fx of pelvis w unstable disrupt of pelvic ring, sequela
		S32.82XS	Multiple fx of pelvis w/o disrupt of pelvic ring, sequela
		S32.89XS	Fracture of other parts of pelvis, sequela
		S32.9XXS	Fx unsp parts of lumbosacral spine & pelvis, sequela
905.2	LATE EFFECT OF FRACTURE OF UPPER EXTREMITIES	**M80.011S**	Age-rel osteopor w current path fx, r shoulder, sequela
		M80.012S	Age-rel osteopor w current path fx, l shoulder, sequela
		M80.019S	Age-rel osteopor w current path fx, unsp shoulder, sequela
		M80.021S	Age-rel osteopor w current path fracture, r humerus, sequela
		M80.022S	Age-rel osteopor w current path fracture, l humerus, sequela
		M80.029S	Age-rel osteopor w current path fx, unsp humerus, sequela
		M80.031S	Age-rel osteopor w current path fracture, r forearm, sequela
		M80.032S	Age-rel osteopor w current path fracture, l forearm, sequela
		M80.039S	Age-rel osteopor w current path fx, unsp forearm, sequela
		M80.041S	Age-rel osteopor w current path fracture, r hand, sequela
		M80.042S	Age-rel osteopor w current path fracture, left hand, sequela
		M80.049S	Age-rel osteopor w current path fracture, unsp hand, sequela
		M80.811S	Oth osteopor w current path fracture, r shoulder, sequela
		M80.812S	Oth osteopor w current path fracture, l shoulder, sequela
		M80.819S	Oth osteopor w current path fracture, unsp shoulder, sequela
	(Continued on next page)	**M80.821S**	Oth osteopor w current path fracture, r humerus, sequela

ICD-9-CM		ICD-10-CM	
9Ø5.2	LATE EFFECT OF FRACTURE OF UPPER EXTREMITIES **(Continued)**	**M8Ø.822S**	Oth osteopor w current path fracture, l humerus, sequela
		M8Ø.829S	Oth osteopor w current path fracture, unsp humerus, sequela
		M8Ø.831S	Oth osteopor w current path fracture, r forearm, sequela
		M8Ø.832S	Oth osteopor w current path fracture, l forearm, sequela
		M8Ø.839S	Oth osteopor w current path fracture, unsp forearm, sequela
		M8Ø.841S	Oth osteopor w current path fracture, right hand, sequela
		M8Ø.842S	Oth osteopor w current path fracture, left hand, sequela
		M8Ø.849S	Oth osteopor w current path fracture, unsp hand, sequela
		M84.311S	Stress fracture, right shoulder, sequela
		M84.312S	Stress fracture, left shoulder, sequela
		M84.319S	Stress fracture, unspecified shoulder, sequela
		M84.321S	Stress fracture, right humerus, sequela
		M84.322S	Stress fracture, left humerus, sequela
		M84.329S	Stress fracture, unspecified humerus, sequela
		M84.331S	Stress fracture, right ulna, sequela
		M84.332S	Stress fracture, left ulna, sequela
		M84.333S	Stress fracture, right radius, sequela
		M84.334S	Stress fracture, left radius, sequela
		M84.339S	Stress fracture, unspecified ulna and radius, sequela
		M84.341S	Stress fracture, right hand, sequela
		M84.342S	Stress fracture, left hand, sequela
		M84.343S	Stress fracture, unspecified hand, sequela
		M84.344S	Stress fracture, right finger(s), sequela
		M84.345S	Stress fracture, left finger(s), sequela
		M84.346S	Stress fracture, unspecified finger(s), sequela
		M84.411S	Pathological fracture, right shoulder, sequela
		M84.412S	Pathological fracture, left shoulder, sequela
		M84.419S	Pathological fracture, unspecified shoulder, sequela
		M84.421S	Pathological fracture, right humerus, sequela
		M84.422S	Pathological fracture, left humerus, sequela
		M84.429S	Pathological fracture, unspecified humerus, sequela
		M84.431S	Pathological fracture, right ulna, sequela
		M84.432S	Pathological fracture, left ulna, sequela
		M84.433S	Pathological fracture, right radius, sequela
		M84.434S	Pathological fracture, left radius, sequela
		M84.439S	Pathological fracture, unspecified ulna and radius, sequela
		M84.441S	Pathological fracture, right hand, sequela
		M84.442S	Pathological fracture, left hand, sequela
		M84.443S	Pathological fracture, unspecified hand, sequela
		M84.444S	Pathological fracture, right finger(s), sequela
		M84.445S	Pathological fracture, left finger(s), sequela
		M84.446S	Pathological fracture, unspecified finger(s), sequela
		M84.511S	Path fracture in neoplastic disease, r shoulder, sequela
		M84.512S	Path fracture in neoplastic disease, l shoulder, sequela
		M84.519S	Path fracture in neoplastic disease, unsp shoulder, sequela
		M84.521S	Path fracture in neoplastic disease, r humerus, sequela
		M84.522S	Path fracture in neoplastic disease, l humerus, sequela
		M84.529S	Path fracture in neoplastic disease, unsp humerus, sequela
		M84.531S	Path fracture in neoplastic disease, right ulna, sequela
		M84.532S	Path fracture in neoplastic disease, left ulna, sequela
		M84.533S	Path fracture in neoplastic disease, right radius, sequela
		M84.534S	Path fracture in neoplastic disease, left radius, sequela
		M84.539S	Path fx in neopltc disease, unsp ulna and radius, sequela
		M84.541S	Path fracture in neoplastic disease, right hand, sequela
		M84.542S	Path fracture in neoplastic disease, left hand, sequela
		M84.549S	Path fracture in neoplastic disease, unsp hand, sequela
		M84.611S	Pathological fracture in oth disease, r shoulder, sequela
		M84.612S	Pathological fracture in oth disease, left shoulder, sequela
		M84.619S	Pathological fracture in oth disease, unsp shoulder, sequela
		M84.621S	Pathological fracture in oth disease, right humerus, sequela
		M84.622S	Pathological fracture in oth disease, left humerus, sequela
		M84.629S	Pathological fracture in oth disease, unsp humerus, sequela
		M84.631S	Pathological fracture in other disease, right ulna, sequela
		M84.632S	Pathological fracture in other disease, left ulna, sequela
		M84.633S	Pathological fracture in oth disease, right radius, sequela
		M84.634S	Pathological fracture in other disease, left radius, sequela
		M84.639S	Path fracture in oth disease, unsp ulna and radius, sequela
		M84.641S	Pathological fracture in other disease, right hand, sequela
		M84.642S	Pathological fracture in other disease, left hand, sequela
		M84.649S	Pathological fracture in other disease, unsp hand, sequela
		S42.ØØ1S	Fracture of unspecified part of right clavicle, sequela
		S42.ØØ2S	Fracture of unspecified part of left clavicle, sequela
		S42.ØØ9S	Fracture of unsp part of unspecified clavicle, sequela
		S42.Ø11S	Anterior disp fx of sternal end of right clavicle, sequela
		S42.Ø12S	Anterior disp fx of sternal end of left clavicle, sequela
		S42.Ø13S	Anterior disp fx of sternal end of unsp clavicle, sequela
		S42.Ø14S	Posterior disp fx of sternal end of right clavicle, sequela
		S42.Ø15S	Posterior disp fx of sternal end of left clavicle, sequela
		S42.Ø16S	Posterior disp fx of sternal end of unsp clavicle, sequela
		S42.Ø17S	Nondisp fx of sternal end of right clavicle, sequela
	(Continued on next page)	**S42.Ø18S**	Nondisp fx of sternal end of left clavicle, sequela

ICD-9-CM		ICD-10-CM	
9Ø5.2	LATE EFFECT OF FRACTURE OF UPPER EXTREMITIES **(Continued)**	**S42.Ø19S**	Nondisp fx of sternal end of unspecified clavicle, sequela
		S42.Ø21S	Displaced fracture of shaft of right clavicle, sequela
		S42.Ø22S	Displaced fracture of shaft of left clavicle, sequela
		S42.Ø23S	Displaced fracture of shaft of unspecified clavicle, sequela
		S42.Ø24S	Nondisplaced fracture of shaft of right clavicle, sequela
		S42.Ø25S	Nondisplaced fracture of shaft of left clavicle, sequela
		S42.Ø26S	Nondisp fx of shaft of unspecified clavicle, sequela
		S42.Ø31S	Displaced fracture of lateral end of right clavicle, sequela
		S42.Ø32S	Displaced fracture of lateral end of left clavicle, sequela
		S42.Ø33S	Disp fx of lateral end of unspecified clavicle, sequela
		S42.Ø34S	Nondisp fx of lateral end of right clavicle, sequela
		S42.Ø35S	Nondisp fx of lateral end of left clavicle, sequela
		S42.Ø36S	Nondisp fx of lateral end of unspecified clavicle, sequela
		S42.1Ø1S	Fracture of unsp part of scapula, right shoulder, sequela
		S42.1Ø2S	Fracture of unsp part of scapula, left shoulder, sequela
		S42.1Ø9S	Fracture of unsp part of scapula, unsp shoulder, sequela
		S42.111S	Disp fx of body of scapula, right shoulder, sequela
		S42.112S	Disp fx of body of scapula, left shoulder, sequela
		S42.113S	Disp fx of body of scapula, unspecified shoulder, sequela
		S42.114S	Nondisp fx of body of scapula, right shoulder, sequela
		S42.115S	Nondisp fx of body of scapula, left shoulder, sequela
		S42.116S	Nondisp fx of body of scapula, unspecified shoulder, sequela
		S42.121S	Disp fx of acromial process, right shoulder, sequela
		S42.122S	Disp fx of acromial process, left shoulder, sequela
		S42.123S	Disp fx of acromial process, unspecified shoulder, sequela
		S42.124S	Nondisp fx of acromial process, right shoulder, sequela
		S42.125S	Nondisp fx of acromial process, left shoulder, sequela
		S42.126S	Nondisp fx of acromial process, unsp shoulder, sequela
		S42.131S	Disp fx of coracoid process, right shoulder, sequela
		S42.132S	Disp fx of coracoid process, left shoulder, sequela
		S42.133S	Disp fx of coracoid process, unspecified shoulder, sequela
		S42.134S	Nondisp fx of coracoid process, right shoulder, sequela
		S42.135S	Nondisp fx of coracoid process, left shoulder, sequela
		S42.136S	Nondisp fx of coracoid process, unsp shoulder, sequela
		S42.141S	Disp fx of glenoid cav of scapula, right shoulder, sequela
		S42.142S	Disp fx of glenoid cavity of scapula, left shoulder, sequela
		S42.143S	Disp fx of glenoid cavity of scapula, unsp shoulder, sequela
		S42.144S	Nondisp fx of glenoid cav of scapula, r shoulder, sequela
		S42.145S	Nondisp fx of glenoid cav of scapula, left shoulder, sequela
		S42.146S	Nondisp fx of glenoid cav of scapula, unsp shoulder, sequela
		S42.151S	Disp fx of neck of scapula, right shoulder, sequela
		S42.152S	Disp fx of neck of scapula, left shoulder, sequela
		S42.153S	Disp fx of neck of scapula, unspecified shoulder, sequela
		S42.154S	Nondisp fx of neck of scapula, right shoulder, sequela
		S42.155S	Nondisp fx of neck of scapula, left shoulder, sequela
		S42.156S	Nondisp fx of neck of scapula, unspecified shoulder, sequela
		S42.191S	Fracture of other part of scapula, right shoulder, sequela
		S42.192S	Fracture of other part of scapula, left shoulder, sequela
		S42.199S	Fracture of other part of scapula, unsp shoulder, sequela
		S42.2Ø1S	Unspecified fracture of upper end of right humerus, sequela
		S42.2Ø2S	Unspecified fracture of upper end of left humerus, sequela
		S42.2Ø9S	Unsp fracture of upper end of unspecified humerus, sequela
		S42.211S	Unsp disp fx of surgical neck of right humerus, sequela
		S42.212S	Unsp disp fx of surgical neck of left humerus, sequela
		S42.213S	Unsp disp fx of surgical neck of unsp humerus, sequela
		S42.214S	Unsp nondisp fx of surgical neck of right humerus, sequela
		S42.215S	Unsp nondisp fx of surgical neck of left humerus, sequela
		S42.216S	Unsp nondisp fx of surgical neck of unsp humerus, sequela
		S42.221S	2-part disp fx of surgical neck of right humerus, sequela
		S42.222S	2-part disp fx of surgical neck of left humerus, sequela
		S42.223S	2-part disp fx of surgical neck of unsp humerus, sequela
		S42.224S	2-part nondisp fx of surgical neck of right humerus, sequela
		S42.225S	2-part nondisp fx of surgical neck of left humerus, sequela
		S42.226S	2-part nondisp fx of surgical neck of unsp humerus, sequela
		S42.231S	3-part fracture of surgical neck of right humerus, sequela
		S42.232S	3-part fracture of surgical neck of left humerus, sequela
		S42.239S	3-part fracture of surgical neck of unsp humerus, sequela
		S42.241S	4-part fracture of surgical neck of right humerus, sequela
		S42.242S	4-part fracture of surgical neck of left humerus, sequela
		S42.249S	4-part fracture of surgical neck of unsp humerus, sequela
		S42.251S	Disp fx of greater tuberosity of right humerus, sequela
		S42.252S	Disp fx of greater tuberosity of left humerus, sequela
		S42.253S	Disp fx of greater tuberosity of unsp humerus, sequela
		S42.254S	Nondisp fx of greater tuberosity of right humerus, sequela
		S42.255S	Nondisp fx of greater tuberosity of left humerus, sequela
		S42.256S	Nondisp fx of greater tuberosity of unsp humerus, sequela
		S42.261S	Disp fx of lesser tuberosity of right humerus, sequela
		S42.262S	Disp fx of lesser tuberosity of left humerus, sequela
		S42.263S	Disp fx of lesser tuberosity of unspecified humerus, sequela
		S42.264S	Nondisp fx of lesser tuberosity of right humerus, sequela
		S42.265S	Nondisp fx of lesser tuberosity of left humerus, sequela
		S42.266S	Nondisp fx of lesser tuberosity of unsp humerus, sequela
		S42.271S	Torus fracture of upper end of right humerus, sequela

(Continued on next page)

ICD-9-CM		ICD-10-CM	
905.2	LATE EFFECT OF FRACTURE OF UPPER EXTREMITIES **(Continued)**	**S42.272S**	Torus fracture of upper end of left humerus, sequela
		S42.279S	Torus fracture of upper end of unspecified humerus, sequela
		S42.291S	Other disp fx of upper end of right humerus, sequela
		S42.292S	Other disp fx of upper end of left humerus, sequela
		S42.293S	Other disp fx of upper end of unspecified humerus, sequela
		S42.294S	Other nondisp fx of upper end of right humerus, sequela
		S42.295S	Other nondisp fx of upper end of left humerus, sequela
		S42.296S	Other nondisp fx of upper end of unsp humerus, sequela
		S42.301S	Unspecified fracture of shaft of humerus, right arm, sequela
		S42.302S	Unspecified fracture of shaft of humerus, left arm, sequela
		S42.309S	Unsp fracture of shaft of humerus, unspecified arm, sequela
		S42.311S	Greenstick fracture of shaft of humerus, right arm, sequela
		S42.312S	Greenstick fracture of shaft of humerus, left arm, sequela
		S42.319S	Greenstick fracture of shaft of humerus, unsp arm, sequela
		S42.321S	Displaced transverse fx shaft of humerus, right arm, sequela
		S42.322S	Displaced transverse fx shaft of humerus, left arm, sequela
		S42.323S	Displaced transverse fx shaft of humerus, unsp arm, sequela
		S42.324S	Nondisp transverse fx shaft of humerus, right arm, sequela
		S42.325S	Nondisp transverse fx shaft of humerus, left arm, sequela
		S42.326S	Nondisp transverse fx shaft of humerus, unsp arm, sequela
		S42.331S	Displaced oblique fx shaft of humerus, right arm, sequela
		S42.332S	Displaced oblique fx shaft of humerus, left arm, sequela
		S42.333S	Displaced oblique fx shaft of humerus, unsp arm, sequela
		S42.334S	Nondisp oblique fx shaft of humerus, right arm, sequela
		S42.335S	Nondisp oblique fx shaft of humerus, left arm, sequela
		S42.336S	Nondisp oblique fx shaft of humerus, unsp arm, sequela
		S42.341S	Displaced spiral fx shaft of humerus, right arm, sequela
		S42.342S	Displaced spiral fx shaft of humerus, left arm, sequela
		S42.343S	Displaced spiral fx shaft of humerus, unsp arm, sequela
		S42.344S	Nondisp spiral fx shaft of humerus, right arm, sequela
		S42.345S	Nondisp spiral fx shaft of humerus, left arm, sequela
		S42.346S	Nondisp spiral fx shaft of humerus, unsp arm, sequela
		S42.351S	Displaced comminuted fx shaft of humerus, right arm, sequela
		S42.352S	Displaced comminuted fx shaft of humerus, left arm, sequela
		S42.353S	Displaced comminuted fx shaft of humerus, unsp arm, sequela
		S42.354S	Nondisp comminuted fx shaft of humerus, right arm, sequela
		S42.355S	Nondisp comminuted fx shaft of humerus, left arm, sequela
		S42.356S	Nondisp comminuted fx shaft of humerus, unsp arm, sequela
		S42.361S	Displaced segmental fx shaft of humerus, right arm, sequela
		S42.362S	Displaced segmental fx shaft of humerus, left arm, sequela
		S42.363S	Displaced segmental fx shaft of humerus, unsp arm, sequela
		S42.364S	Nondisp segmental fx shaft of humerus, right arm, sequela
		S42.365S	Nondisp segmental fx shaft of humerus, left arm, sequela
		S42.366S	Nondisp segmental fx shaft of humerus, unsp arm, sequela
		S42.391S	Other fracture of shaft of right humerus, sequela
		S42.392S	Other fracture of shaft of left humerus, sequela
		S42.399S	Other fracture of shaft of unspecified humerus, sequela
		S42.401S	Unspecified fracture of lower end of right humerus, sequela
		S42.402S	Unspecified fracture of lower end of left humerus, sequela
		S42.409S	Unsp fracture of lower end of unspecified humerus, sequela
		S42.411S	Displ simple suprcndl fx w/o intrcndl fx r humerus, sequela
		S42.412S	Displ simple suprcndl fx w/o intrcndl fx l humerus, sequela
		S42.413S	Displ simple suprcndl fx w/o intrcndl fx unsp humer, sequela
		S42.414S	Nondisp simple suprcndl fx w/o intrcndl fx r humer, sequela
		S42.415S	Nondisp simple suprcndl fx w/o intrcndl fx l humer, sequela
		S42.416S	Nondisp simple suprcndl fx w/o intrcndl fx unsp humer, sqla
		S42.421S	Displ commnt suprcndl fx w/o intrcndl fx r humerus, sequela
		S42.422S	Displ commnt suprcndl fx w/o intrcndl fx l humerus, sequela
		S42.423S	Displ commnt suprcndl fx w/o intrcndl fx unsp humer, sequela
		S42.424S	Nondisp commnt suprcndl fx w/o intrcndl fx r humer, sequela
		S42.425S	Nondisp commnt suprcndl fx w/o intrcndl fx l humer, sequela
		S42.426S	Nondisp commnt suprcndl fx w/o intrcndl fx unsp humer, sqla
		S42.431S	Disp fx of lateral epicondyle of r humerus, sequela
		S42.432S	Disp fx of lateral epicondyle of l humerus, sequela
		S42.433S	Disp fx of lateral epicondyle of unsp humerus, sequela
		S42.434S	Nondisp fx of lateral epicondyle of r humerus, sequela
		S42.435S	Nondisp fx of lateral epicondyle of l humerus, sequela
		S42.436S	Nondisp fx of lateral epicondyle of unsp humerus, sequela
		S42.441S	Disp fx of medial epicondyle of r humerus, sequela
		S42.442S	Disp fx of medial epicondyle of l humerus, sequela
		S42.443S	Disp fx of medial epicondyle of unsp humerus, sequela
		S42.444S	Nondisp fx of medial epicondyle of r humerus, sequela
		S42.445S	Nondisp fx of medial epicondyle of l humerus, sequela
		S42.446S	Nondisp fx of medial epicondyle of unsp humerus, sequela
		S42.447S	Incarcerated fx of medial epicondyl of r humerus, sequela
		S42.448S	Incarcerated fx of medial epicondyl of l humerus, sequela
		S42.449S	Incarcerated fx of medial epicondyl of unsp humerus, sequela
		S42.451S	Disp fx of lateral condyle of right humerus, sequela
		S42.452S	Disp fx of lateral condyle of left humerus, sequela
		S42.453S	Disp fx of lateral condyle of unspecified humerus, sequela
		S42.454S	Nondisp fx of lateral condyle of right humerus, sequela
	(Continued on next page)	**S42.455S**	Nondisp fx of lateral condyle of left humerus, sequela

ICD-9-CM		ICD-10-CM	
9Ø5.2	LATE EFFECT OF FRACTURE OF UPPER EXTREMITIES **(Continued)**	**S42.456S**	Nondisp fx of lateral condyle of unsp humerus, sequela
		S42.461S	Disp fx of medial condyle of right humerus, sequela
		S42.462S	Disp fx of medial condyle of left humerus, sequela
		S42.463S	Disp fx of medial condyle of unspecified humerus, sequela
		S42.464S	Nondisp fx of medial condyle of right humerus, sequela
		S42.465S	Nondisp fx of medial condyle of left humerus, sequela
		S42.466S	Nondisp fx of medial condyle of unspecified humerus, sequela
		S42.471S	Displaced transcondylar fracture of right humerus, sequela
		S42.472S	Displaced transcondylar fracture of left humerus, sequela
		S42.473S	Displaced transcondylar fracture of unsp humerus, sequela
		S42.474S	Nondisplaced transcondylar fracture of r humerus, sequela
		S42.475S	Nondisplaced transcondylar fracture of left humerus, sequela
		S42.476S	Nondisplaced transcondylar fracture of unsp humerus, sequela
		S42.481S	Torus fracture of lower end of right humerus, sequela
		S42.482S	Torus fracture of lower end of left humerus, sequela
		S42.489S	Torus fracture of lower end of unspecified humerus, sequela
		S42.491S	Other disp fx of lower end of right humerus, sequela
		S42.492S	Other disp fx of lower end of left humerus, sequela
		S42.493S	Other disp fx of lower end of unspecified humerus, sequela
		S42.494S	Other nondisp fx of lower end of right humerus, sequela
		S42.495S	Other nondisp fx of lower end of left humerus, sequela
		S42.496S	Other nondisp fx of lower end of unsp humerus, sequela
		S42.9ØXS	Fracture of unsp shoulder girdle, part unspecified, sequela
		S42.91XS	Fracture of right shoulder girdle, part unspecified, sequela
		S42.92XS	Fracture of left shoulder girdle, part unspecified, sequela
		S49.ØØ1S	Unsp physeal fx upper end of humerus, right arm, sequela
		S49.ØØ2S	Unsp physeal fx upper end of humerus, left arm, sequela
		S49.ØØ9S	Unsp physeal fx upper end of humerus, unsp arm, sequela
		S49.Ø11S	Sltr-haris Type I physl fx upper end humer, right arm, sqla
		S49.Ø12S	Sltr-haris Type I physl fx upper end humer, left arm, sqla
		S49.Ø19S	Sltr-haris Type I physl fx upper end humer, unsp arm, sqla
		S49.Ø21S	Sltr-haris Type II physl fx upper end humer, right arm, sqla
		S49.Ø22S	Sltr-haris Type II physl fx upper end humer, left arm, sqla
		S49.Ø29S	Sltr-haris Type II physl fx upper end humer, unsp arm, sqla
		S49.Ø31S	Sltr-haris Type III physl fx upper end humer, r arm, sqla
		S49.Ø32S	Sltr-haris Type III physl fx upper end humer, left arm, sqla
		S49.Ø39S	Sltr-haris Type III physl fx upper end humer, unsp arm, sqla
		S49.Ø41S	Sltr-haris Type IV physl fx upper end humer, right arm, sqla
		S49.Ø42S	Sltr-haris Type IV physl fx upper end humer, left arm, sqla
		S49.Ø49S	Sltr-haris Type IV physl fx upper end humer, unsp arm, sqla
		S49.Ø91S	Oth physeal fx upper end of humerus, right arm, sequela
		S49.Ø92S	Oth physeal fx upper end of humerus, left arm, sequela
		S49.Ø99S	Oth physeal fx upper end of humerus, unsp arm, sequela
		S49.1Ø1S	Unsp physeal fx lower end of humerus, right arm, sequela
		S49.1Ø2S	Unsp physeal fx lower end of humerus, left arm, sequela
		S49.1Ø9S	Unsp physeal fx lower end of humerus, unsp arm, sequela
		S49.111S	Sltr-haris Type I physl fx lower end humer, right arm, sqla
		S49.112S	Sltr-haris Type I physl fx lower end humer, left arm, sqla
		S49.119S	Sltr-haris Type I physl fx lower end humer, unsp arm, sqla
		S49.121S	Sltr-haris Type II physl fx lower end humer, right arm, sqla
		S49.122S	Sltr-haris Type II physl fx lower end humer, left arm, sqla
		S49.129S	Sltr-haris Type II physl fx lower end humer, unsp arm, sqla
		S49.131S	Sltr-haris Type III physl fx low end humer, right arm, sqla
		S49.132S	Sltr-haris Type III physl fx lower end humer, left arm, sqla
		S49.139S	Sltr-haris Type III physl fx lower end humer, unsp arm, sqla
		S49.141S	Sltr-haris Type IV physl fx lower end humer, right arm, sqla
		S49.142S	Sltr-haris Type IV physl fx lower end humer, left arm, sqla
		S49.149S	Sltr-haris Type IV physl fx lower end humer, unsp arm, sqla
		S49.191S	Oth physeal fx lower end of humerus, right arm, sequela
		S49.192S	Oth physeal fx lower end of humerus, left arm, sequela
		S49.199S	Oth physeal fx lower end of humerus, unsp arm, sequela
		S52.ØØ1S	Unspecified fracture of upper end of right ulna, sequela
		S52.ØØ2S	Unspecified fracture of upper end of left ulna, sequela
		S52.ØØ9S	Unsp fracture of upper end of unspecified ulna, sequela
		S52.Ø11S	Torus fracture of upper end of right ulna, sequela
		S52.Ø12S	Torus fracture of upper end of left ulna, sequela
		S52.Ø19S	Torus fracture of upper end of unspecified ulna, sequela
		S52.Ø21S	Disp fx of olecran pro w/o intartic extn right ulna, sequela
		S52.Ø22S	Disp fx of olecran pro w/o intartic extn left ulna, sequela
		S52.Ø23S	Disp fx of olecran pro w/o intartic extn unsp ulna, sequela
		S52.Ø24S	Nondisp fx of olecran pro w/o intartic extn r ulna, sequela
		S52.Ø25S	Nondisp fx of olecran pro w/o intartic extn l ulna, sequela
		S52.Ø26S	Nondisp fx of olecran pro w/o intartic extn unsp ulna, sqla
		S52.Ø31S	Disp fx of olecran pro w intartic extn right ulna, sequela
		S52.Ø32S	Disp fx of olecran pro w intartic extn left ulna, sequela
		S52.Ø33S	Disp fx of olecran pro w intartic extn unsp ulna, sequela
		S52.Ø34S	Nondisp fx of olecran pro w intartic extn r ulna, sequela
		S52.Ø35S	Nondisp fx of olecran pro w intartic extn left ulna, sequela
		S52.Ø36S	Nondisp fx of olecran pro w intartic extn unsp ulna, sequela
		S52.Ø41S	Disp fx of coronoid process of right ulna, sequela
		S52.Ø42S	Displaced fracture of coronoid process of left ulna, sequela
		S52.Ø43S	Disp fx of coronoid process of unspecified ulna, sequela
		S52.Ø44S	Nondisp fx of coronoid process of right ulna, sequela

(Continued on next page)

ICD-9-CM		ICD-10-CM	
9Ø5.2	LATE EFFECT OF FRACTURE OF UPPER EXTREMITIES **(Continued)**	**S52.Ø45S**	Nondisp fx of coronoid process of left ulna, sequela
		S52.Ø46S	Nondisp fx of coronoid process of unspecified ulna, sequela
		S52.Ø91S	Other fracture of upper end of right ulna, sequela
		S52.Ø92S	Other fracture of upper end of left ulna, sequela
		S52.Ø99S	Other fracture of upper end of unspecified ulna, sequela
		S52.1Ø1S	Unspecified fracture of upper end of right radius, sequela
		S52.1Ø2S	Unspecified fracture of upper end of left radius, sequela
		S52.1Ø9S	Unsp fracture of upper end of unspecified radius, sequela
		S52.111S	Torus fracture of upper end of right radius, sequela
		S52.112S	Torus fracture of upper end of left radius, sequela
		S52.119S	Torus fracture of upper end of unspecified radius, sequela
		S52.121S	Displaced fracture of head of right radius, sequela
		S52.122S	Displaced fracture of head of left radius, sequela
		S52.123S	Displaced fracture of head of unspecified radius, sequela
		S52.124S	Nondisplaced fracture of head of right radius, sequela
		S52.125S	Nondisplaced fracture of head of left radius, sequela
		S52.126S	Nondisplaced fracture of head of unspecified radius, sequela
		S52.131S	Displaced fracture of neck of right radius, sequela
		S52.132S	Displaced fracture of neck of left radius, sequela
		S52.133S	Displaced fracture of neck of unspecified radius, sequela
		S52.134S	Nondisplaced fracture of neck of right radius, sequela
		S52.135S	Nondisplaced fracture of neck of left radius, sequela
		S52.136S	Nondisplaced fracture of neck of unspecified radius, sequela
		S52.181S	Other fracture of upper end of right radius, sequela
		S52.182S	Other fracture of upper end of left radius, sequela
		S52.189S	Other fracture of upper end of unspecified radius, sequela
		S52.2Ø1S	Unspecified fracture of shaft of right ulna, sequela
		S52.2Ø2S	Unspecified fracture of shaft of left ulna, sequela
		S52.2Ø9S	Unspecified fracture of shaft of unspecified ulna, sequela
		S52.211S	Greenstick fracture of shaft of right ulna, sequela
		S52.212S	Greenstick fracture of shaft of left ulna, sequela
		S52.219S	Greenstick fracture of shaft of unspecified ulna, sequela
		S52.221S	Displaced transverse fx shaft of right ulna, sequela
		S52.222S	Displaced transverse fracture of shaft of left ulna, sequela
		S52.223S	Displaced transverse fracture of shaft of unsp ulna, sequela
		S52.224S	Nondisp transverse fracture of shaft of right ulna, sequela
		S52.225S	Nondisp transverse fracture of shaft of left ulna, sequela
		S52.226S	Nondisp transverse fracture of shaft of unsp ulna, sequela
		S52.231S	Displaced oblique fracture of shaft of right ulna, sequela
		S52.232S	Displaced oblique fracture of shaft of left ulna, sequela
		S52.233S	Displaced oblique fracture of shaft of unsp ulna, sequela
		S52.234S	Nondisp oblique fracture of shaft of right ulna, sequela
		S52.235S	Nondisplaced oblique fracture of shaft of left ulna, sequela
		S52.236S	Nondisplaced oblique fracture of shaft of unsp ulna, sequela
		S52.241S	Displaced spiral fx shaft of ulna, right arm, sequela
		S52.242S	Displaced spiral fx shaft of ulna, left arm, sequela
		S52.243S	Displaced spiral fx shaft of ulna, unsp arm, sequela
		S52.244S	Nondisp spiral fracture of shaft of ulna, right arm, sequela
		S52.245S	Nondisp spiral fracture of shaft of ulna, left arm, sequela
		S52.246S	Nondisp spiral fracture of shaft of ulna, unsp arm, sequela
		S52.251S	Displaced comminuted fx shaft of ulna, right arm, sequela
		S52.252S	Displaced comminuted fx shaft of ulna, left arm, sequela
		S52.253S	Displaced comminuted fx shaft of ulna, unsp arm, sequela
		S52.254S	Nondisp comminuted fx shaft of ulna, right arm, sequela
		S52.255S	Nondisp comminuted fx shaft of ulna, left arm, sequela
		S52.256S	Nondisp comminuted fx shaft of ulna, unsp arm, sequela
		S52.261S	Displaced segmental fx shaft of ulna, right arm, sequela
		S52.262S	Displaced segmental fx shaft of ulna, left arm, sequela
		S52.263S	Displaced segmental fx shaft of ulna, unsp arm, sequela
		S52.264S	Nondisp segmental fx shaft of ulna, right arm, sequela
		S52.265S	Nondisp segmental fx shaft of ulna, left arm, sequela
		S52.266S	Nondisp segmental fx shaft of ulna, unsp arm, sequela
		S52.271S	Monteggia's fracture of right ulna, sequela
		S52.272S	Monteggia's fracture of left ulna, sequela
		S52.279S	Monteggia's fracture of unspecified ulna, sequela
		S52.281S	Bent bone of right ulna, sequela
		S52.282S	Bent bone of left ulna, sequela
		S52.283S	Bent bone of unspecified ulna, sequela
		S52.291S	Other fracture of shaft of right ulna, sequela
		S52.292S	Other fracture of shaft of left ulna, sequela
		S52.299S	Other fracture of shaft of unspecified ulna, sequela
		S52.3Ø1S	Unspecified fracture of shaft of right radius, sequela
		S52.3Ø2S	Unspecified fracture of shaft of left radius, sequela
		S52.3Ø9S	Unspecified fracture of shaft of unspecified radius, sequela
		S52.311S	Greenstick fracture of shaft of radius, right arm, sequela
		S52.312S	Greenstick fracture of shaft of radius, left arm, sequela
		S52.319S	Greenstick fracture of shaft of radius, unsp arm, sequela
		S52.321S	Displaced transverse fracture of shaft of r radius, sequela
		S52.322S	Displaced transverse fx shaft of left radius, sequela
		S52.323S	Displaced transverse fx shaft of unsp radius, sequela
		S52.324S	Nondisp transverse fracture of shaft of r radius, sequela
		S52.325S	Nondisp transverse fracture of shaft of left radius, sequela
	(Continued on next page)	**S52.326S**	Nondisp transverse fracture of shaft of unsp radius, sequela

ICD-9-CM		ICD-10-CM	
9Ø5.2	LATE EFFECT OF FRACTURE OF UPPER EXTREMITIES **(Continued)**	**S52.331S**	Displaced oblique fracture of shaft of right radius, sequela
		S52.332S	Displaced oblique fracture of shaft of left radius, sequela
		S52.333S	Displaced oblique fracture of shaft of unsp radius, sequela
		S52.334S	Nondisp oblique fracture of shaft of right radius, sequela
		S52.335S	Nondisp oblique fracture of shaft of left radius, sequela
		S52.336S	Nondisp oblique fracture of shaft of unsp radius, sequela
		S52.341S	Displaced spiral fx shaft of radius, right arm, sequela
		S52.342S	Displaced spiral fx shaft of radius, left arm, sequela
		S52.343S	Displaced spiral fx shaft of radius, unsp arm, sequela
		S52.344S	Nondisp spiral fx shaft of radius, right arm, sequela
		S52.345S	Nondisp spiral fx shaft of radius, left arm, sequela
		S52.346S	Nondisp spiral fx shaft of radius, unsp arm, sequela
		S52.351S	Displaced comminuted fx shaft of radius, right arm, sequela
		S52.352S	Displaced comminuted fx shaft of radius, left arm, sequela
		S52.353S	Displaced comminuted fx shaft of radius, unsp arm, sequela
		S52.354S	Nondisp comminuted fx shaft of radius, right arm, sequela
		S52.355S	Nondisp comminuted fx shaft of radius, left arm, sequela
		S52.356S	Nondisp comminuted fx shaft of radius, unsp arm, sequela
		S52.361S	Displaced segmental fx shaft of radius, right arm, sequela
		S52.362S	Displaced segmental fx shaft of radius, left arm, sequela
		S52.363S	Displaced segmental fx shaft of radius, unsp arm, sequela
		S52.364S	Nondisp segmental fx shaft of radius, right arm, sequela
		S52.365S	Nondisp segmental fx shaft of radius, left arm, sequela
		S52.366S	Nondisp segmental fx shaft of radius, unsp arm, sequela
		S52.371S	Galeazzi's fracture of right radius, sequela
		S52.372S	Galeazzi's fracture of left radius, sequela
		S52.379S	Galeazzi's fracture of unspecified radius, sequela
		S52.381S	Bent bone of right radius, sequela
		S52.382S	Bent bone of left radius, sequela
		S52.389S	Bent bone of unspecified radius, sequela
		S52.391S	Other fracture of shaft of radius, right arm, sequela
		S52.392S	Other fracture of shaft of radius, left arm, sequela
		S52.399S	Other fracture of shaft of radius, unspecified arm, sequela
		S52.5Ø1S	Unsp fracture of the lower end of right radius, sequela
		S52.5Ø2S	Unsp fracture of the lower end of left radius, sequela
		S52.5Ø9S	Unsp fracture of the lower end of unsp radius, sequela
		S52.511S	Displaced fracture of right radial styloid process, sequela
		S52.512S	Displaced fracture of left radial styloid process, sequela
		S52.513S	Disp fx of unspecified radial styloid process, sequela
		S52.514S	Nondisp fx of right radial styloid process, sequela
		S52.515S	Nondisp fx of left radial styloid process, sequela
		S52.516S	Nondisp fx of unspecified radial styloid process, sequela
		S52.521S	Torus fracture of lower end of right radius, sequela
		S52.522S	Torus fracture of lower end of left radius, sequela
		S52.529S	Torus fracture of lower end of unspecified radius, sequela
		S52.531S	Colles' fracture of right radius, sequela
		S52.532S	Colles' fracture of left radius, sequela
		S52.539S	Colles' fracture of unspecified radius, sequela
		S52.541S	Smith's fracture of right radius, sequela
		S52.542S	Smith's fracture of left radius, sequela
		S52.549S	Smith's fracture of unspecified radius, sequela
		S52.551S	Oth extrartic fracture of lower end of right radius, sequela
		S52.552S	Oth extrartic fracture of lower end of left radius, sequela
		S52.559S	Oth extrartic fracture of lower end of unsp radius, sequela
		S52.561S	Barton's fracture of right radius, sequela
		S52.562S	Barton's fracture of left radius, sequela
		S52.569S	Barton's fracture of unspecified radius, sequela
		S52.571S	Oth intartic fracture of lower end of right radius, sequela
		S52.572S	Oth intartic fracture of lower end of left radius, sequela
		S52.579S	Oth intartic fracture of lower end of unsp radius, sequela
		S52.591S	Other fractures of lower end of right radius, sequela
		S52.592S	Other fractures of lower end of left radius, sequela
		S52.599S	Other fractures of lower end of unspecified radius, sequela
		S52.6Ø1S	Unspecified fracture of lower end of right ulna, sequela
		S52.6Ø2S	Unspecified fracture of lower end of left ulna, sequela
		S52.6Ø9S	Unsp fracture of lower end of unspecified ulna, sequela
		S52.611S	Displaced fracture of right ulna styloid process, sequela
		S52.612S	Displaced fracture of left ulna styloid process, sequela
		S52.613S	Disp fx of unspecified ulna styloid process, sequela
		S52.614S	Nondisplaced fracture of right ulna styloid process, sequela
		S52.615S	Nondisplaced fracture of left ulna styloid process, sequela
		S52.616S	Nondisp fx of unspecified ulna styloid process, sequela
		S52.621S	Torus fracture of lower end of right ulna, sequela
		S52.622S	Torus fracture of lower end of left ulna, sequela
		S52.629S	Torus fracture of lower end of unspecified ulna, sequela
		S52.691S	Other fracture of lower end of right ulna, sequela
		S52.692S	Other fracture of lower end of left ulna, sequela
		S52.699S	Other fracture of lower end of unspecified ulna, sequela
		S52.9ØXS	Unspecified fracture of unspecified forearm, sequela
		S52.91XS	Unspecified fracture of right forearm, sequela
		S52.92XS	Unspecified fracture of left forearm, sequela
		S59.ØØ1S	Unsp physeal fx lower end of ulna, right arm, sequela
	(Continued on next page)	**S59.ØØ2S**	Unsp physeal fx lower end of ulna, left arm, sequela

ICD-9-CM		ICD-10-CM	
905.2	LATE EFFECT OF FRACTURE OF UPPER EXTREMITIES **(Continued)**	**S59.009S**	Unsp physeal fx lower end of ulna, unsp arm, sequela
		S59.011S	Sltr-haris Type I physl fx lower end ulna, right arm, sqla
		S59.012S	Sltr-haris Type I physl fx lower end of ulna, left arm, sqla
		S59.019S	Sltr-haris Type I physl fx lower end of ulna, unsp arm, sqla
		S59.021S	Sltr-haris Type II physl fx lower end ulna, right arm, sqla
		S59.022S	Sltr-haris Type II physl fx lower end ulna, left arm, sqla
		S59.029S	Sltr-haris Type II physl fx lower end ulna, unsp arm, sqla
		S59.031S	Sltr-haris Type III physl fx lower end ulna, right arm, sqla
		S59.032S	Sltr-haris Type III physl fx lower end ulna, left arm, sqla
		S59.039S	Sltr-haris Type III physl fx lower end ulna, unsp arm, sqla
		S59.041S	Sltr-haris Type IV physl fx lower end ulna, right arm, sqla
		S59.042S	Sltr-haris Type IV physl fx lower end ulna, left arm, sqla
		S59.049S	Sltr-haris Type IV physl fx lower end ulna, unsp arm, sqla
		S59.091S	Oth physeal fx lower end of ulna, right arm, sequela
		S59.092S	Oth physeal fracture of lower end of ulna, left arm, sequela
		S59.099S	Oth physeal fracture of lower end of ulna, unsp arm, sequela
		S59.101S	Unsp physeal fx upper end radius, right arm, sequela
		S59.102S	Unsp physeal fracture of upper end radius, left arm, sequela
		S59.109S	Unsp physeal fracture of upper end radius, unsp arm, sequela
		S59.111S	Sltr-haris Type I physl fx upper end radius, right arm, sqla
		S59.112S	Sltr-haris Type I physl fx upper end radius, left arm, sqla
		S59.119S	Sltr-haris Type I physl fx upper end radius, unsp arm, sqla
		S59.121S	Sltr-haris Type II physl fx upper end rad, right arm, sqla
		S59.122S	Sltr-haris Type II physl fx upper end radius, left arm, sqla
		S59.129S	Sltr-haris Type II physl fx upper end radius, unsp arm, sqla
		S59.131S	Sltr-haris Type III physl fx upper end rad, right arm, sqla
		S59.132S	Sltr-haris Type III physl fx upper end rad, left arm, sqla
		S59.139S	Sltr-haris Type III physl fx upper end rad, unsp arm, sqla
		S59.141S	Sltr-haris Type IV physl fx upper end rad, right arm, sqla
		S59.142S	Sltr-haris Type IV physl fx upper end radius, left arm, sqla
		S59.149S	Sltr-haris Type IV physl fx upper end radius, unsp arm, sqla
		S59.191S	Oth physeal fracture of upper end radius, right arm, sequela
		S59.192S	Oth physeal fracture of upper end radius, left arm, sequela
		S59.199S	Oth physeal fracture of upper end radius, unsp arm, sequela
		S59.201S	Unsp physeal fx lower end radius, right arm, sequela
		S59.202S	Unsp physeal fracture of lower end radius, left arm, sequela
		S59.209S	Unsp physeal fracture of lower end radius, unsp arm, sequela
		S59.211S	Sltr-haris Type I physl fx lower end radius, right arm, sqla
		S59.212S	Sltr-haris Type I physl fx lower end radius, left arm, sqla
		S59.219S	Sltr-haris Type I physl fx lower end radius, unsp arm, sqla
		S59.221S	Sltr-haris Type II physl fx lower end rad, right arm, sqla
		S59.222S	Sltr-haris Type II physl fx lower end radius, left arm, sqla
		S59.229S	Sltr-haris Type II physl fx lower end radius, unsp arm, sqla
		S59.231S	Sltr-haris Type III physl fx lower end rad, right arm, sqla
		S59.232S	Sltr-haris Type III physl fx lower end rad, left arm, sqla
		S59.239S	Sltr-haris Type III physl fx lower end rad, unsp arm, sqla
		S59.241S	Sltr-haris Type IV physl fx lower end rad, right arm, sqla
		S59.242S	Sltr-haris Type IV physl fx lower end radius, left arm, sqla
		S59.249S	Sltr-haris Type IV physl fx lower end radius, unsp arm, sqla
		S59.291S	Oth physeal fracture of lower end radius, right arm, sequela
		S59.292S	Oth physeal fracture of lower end radius, left arm, sequela
		S59.299S	Oth physeal fracture of lower end radius, unsp arm, sequela
		S62.001S	Unsp fracture of navicular bone of right wrist, sequela
		S62.002S	Unsp fracture of navicular bone of left wrist, sequela
		S62.009S	Unsp fracture of navicular bone of unsp wrist, sequela
		S62.011S	Disp fx of distal pole of navicular bone of r wrist, sequela
		S62.012S	Disp fx of distal pole of navicular bone of l wrist, sequela
		S62.013S	Disp fx of distal pole of navic bone of unsp wrist, sequela
		S62.014S	Nondisp fx of distal pole of navic bone of r wrist, sequela
		S62.015S	Nondisp fx of distal pole of navic bone of l wrist, sequela
		S62.016S	Nondisp fx of distal pole of navic bone of unsp wrist, sqla
		S62.021S	Disp fx of middle third of navic bone of r wrist, sequela
		S62.022S	Disp fx of middle third of navic bone of l wrist, sequela
		S62.023S	Disp fx of middle third of navic bone of unsp wrist, sequela
		S62.024S	Nondisp fx of middle third of navic bone of r wrist, sequela
		S62.025S	Nondisp fx of middle third of navic bone of l wrist, sequela
		S62.026S	Nondisp fx of middle third of navic bone of unsp wrist, sqla
		S62.031S	Disp fx of proximal third of navic bone of r wrist, sequela
		S62.032S	Disp fx of proximal third of navic bone of l wrist, sequela
		S62.033S	Disp fx of prox third of navic bone of unsp wrist, sequela
		S62.034S	Nondisp fx of prox third of navic bone of r wrist, sequela
		S62.035S	Nondisp fx of prox third of navic bone of l wrist, sequela
		S62.036S	Nondisp fx of prox third of navic bone of unsp wrist, sqla
		S62.101S	Fracture of unspecified carpal bone, right wrist, sequela
		S62.102S	Fracture of unspecified carpal bone, left wrist, sequela
		S62.109S	Fracture of unsp carpal bone, unspecified wrist, sequela
		S62.111S	Displaced fracture of triquetrum bone, right wrist, sequela
		S62.112S	Displaced fracture of triquetrum bone, left wrist, sequela
		S62.113S	Disp fx of triquetrum bone, unspecified wrist, sequela
		S62.114S	Nondisp fx of triquetrum bone, right wrist, sequela
		S62.115S	Nondisp fx of triquetrum bone, left wrist, sequela
		S62.116S	Nondisp fx of triquetrum bone, unspecified wrist, sequela
	(Continued on next page)	**S62.121S**	Displaced fracture of lunate, right wrist, sequela

 [Brackets] indicate valid character values for each code. Character value meanings provided for each code grouping.

ICD-9-CM		ICD-10-CM	
905.2	LATE EFFECT OF FRACTURE OF UPPER EXTREMITIES **(Continued)**	**S62.122S**	Displaced fracture of lunate, left wrist, sequela
		S62.123S	Displaced fracture of lunate, unspecified wrist, sequela
		S62.124S	Nondisplaced fracture of lunate, right wrist, sequela
		S62.125S	Nondisplaced fracture of lunate, left wrist, sequela
		S62.126S	Nondisplaced fracture of lunate, unspecified wrist, sequela
		S62.131S	Displaced fracture of capitate bone, right wrist, sequela
		S62.132S	Displaced fracture of capitate bone, left wrist, sequela
		S62.133S	Disp fx of capitate bone, unspecified wrist, sequela
		S62.134S	Nondisplaced fracture of capitate bone, right wrist, sequela
		S62.135S	Nondisplaced fracture of capitate bone, left wrist, sequela
		S62.136S	Nondisp fx of capitate bone, unspecified wrist, sequela
		S62.141S	Disp fx of body of hamate bone, right wrist, sequela
		S62.142S	Disp fx of body of hamate bone, left wrist, sequela
		S62.143S	Disp fx of body of hamate bone, unspecified wrist, sequela
		S62.144S	Nondisp fx of body of hamate bone, right wrist, sequela
		S62.145S	Nondisp fx of body of hamate bone, left wrist, sequela
		S62.146S	Nondisp fx of body of hamate bone, unsp wrist, sequela
		S62.151S	Disp fx of hook process of hamate bone, right wrist, sequela
		S62.152S	Disp fx of hook process of hamate bone, left wrist, sequela
		S62.153S	Disp fx of hook process of hamate bone, unsp wrist, sequela
		S62.154S	Nondisp fx of hook process of hamate bone, r wrist, sequela
		S62.155S	Nondisp fx of hook process of hamate bone, l wrist, sequela
		S62.156S	Nondisp fx of hook pro of hamate bone, unsp wrist, sequela
		S62.161S	Displaced fracture of pisiform, right wrist, sequela
		S62.162S	Displaced fracture of pisiform, left wrist, sequela
		S62.163S	Displaced fracture of pisiform, unspecified wrist, sequela
		S62.164S	Nondisplaced fracture of pisiform, right wrist, sequela
		S62.165S	Nondisplaced fracture of pisiform, left wrist, sequela
		S62.166S	Nondisp fx of pisiform, unspecified wrist, sequela
		S62.171S	Displaced fracture of trapezium, right wrist, sequela
		S62.172S	Displaced fracture of trapezium, left wrist, sequela
		S62.173S	Displaced fracture of trapezium, unspecified wrist, sequela
		S62.174S	Nondisplaced fracture of trapezium, right wrist, sequela
		S62.175S	Nondisplaced fracture of trapezium, left wrist, sequela
		S62.176S	Nondisp fx of trapezium, unspecified wrist, sequela
		S62.181S	Displaced fracture of trapezoid, right wrist, sequela
		S62.182S	Displaced fracture of trapezoid, left wrist, sequela
		S62.183S	Displaced fracture of trapezoid, unspecified wrist, sequela
		S62.184S	Nondisplaced fracture of trapezoid, right wrist, sequela
		S62.185S	Nondisplaced fracture of trapezoid, left wrist, sequela
		S62.186S	Nondisp fx of trapezoid, unspecified wrist, sequela
		S62.201S	Unsp fracture of first metacarpal bone, right hand, sequela
		S62.202S	Unsp fracture of first metacarpal bone, left hand, sequela
		S62.209S	Unsp fracture of first metacarpal bone, unsp hand, sequela
		S62.211S	Bennett's fracture, right hand, sequela
		S62.212S	Bennett's fracture, left hand, sequela
		S62.213S	Bennett's fracture, unspecified hand, sequela
		S62.221S	Displaced Rolando's fracture, right hand, sequela
		S62.222S	Displaced Rolando's fracture, left hand, sequela
		S62.223S	Displaced Rolando's fracture, unspecified hand, sequela
		S62.224S	Nondisplaced Rolando's fracture, right hand, sequela
		S62.225S	Nondisplaced Rolando's fracture, left hand, sequela
		S62.226S	Nondisplaced Rolando's fracture, unspecified hand, sequela
		S62.231S	Oth disp fx of base of first MC bone, right hand, sequela
		S62.232S	Oth disp fx of base of first MC bone, left hand, sequela
		S62.233S	Oth disp fx of base of first MC bone, unsp hand, sequela
		S62.234S	Oth nondisp fx of base of first MC bone, right hand, sequela
		S62.235S	Oth nondisp fx of base of first MC bone, left hand, sequela
		S62.236S	Oth nondisp fx of base of first MC bone, unsp hand, sequela
		S62.241S	Disp fx of shaft of first MC bone, right hand, sequela
		S62.242S	Disp fx of shaft of first MC bone, left hand, sequela
		S62.243S	Disp fx of shaft of first MC bone, unsp hand, sequela
		S62.244S	Nondisp fx of shaft of first MC bone, right hand, sequela
		S62.245S	Nondisp fx of shaft of first MC bone, left hand, sequela
		S62.246S	Nondisp fx of shaft of first MC bone, unsp hand, sequela
		S62.251S	Disp fx of neck of first MC bone, right hand, sequela
		S62.252S	Disp fx of neck of first metacarpal bone, left hand, sequela
		S62.253S	Disp fx of neck of first metacarpal bone, unsp hand, sequela
		S62.254S	Nondisp fx of neck of first MC bone, right hand, sequela
		S62.255S	Nondisp fx of neck of first MC bone, left hand, sequela
		S62.256S	Nondisp fx of neck of first MC bone, unsp hand, sequela
		S62.291S	Other fracture of first metacarpal bone, right hand, sequela
		S62.292S	Other fracture of first metacarpal bone, left hand, sequela
		S62.299S	Other fracture of first metacarpal bone, unsp hand, sequela
		S62.300S	Unsp fracture of second metacarpal bone, right hand, sequela
		S62.301S	Unsp fracture of second metacarpal bone, left hand, sequela
		S62.302S	Unsp fracture of third metacarpal bone, right hand, sequela
		S62.303S	Unsp fracture of third metacarpal bone, left hand, sequela
		S62.304S	Unsp fracture of fourth metacarpal bone, right hand, sequela
		S62.305S	Unsp fracture of fourth metacarpal bone, left hand, sequela
		S62.306S	Unsp fracture of fifth metacarpal bone, right hand, sequela
		S62.307S	Unsp fracture of fifth metacarpal bone, left hand, sequela
	(Continued on next page)	**S62.308S**	Unspecified fracture of other metacarpal bone, sequela

ICD-9-CM		ICD-10-CM	
905.2	LATE EFFECT OF FRACTURE OF UPPER EXTREMITIES **(Continued)**	**S62.309S**	Unspecified fracture of unspecified metacarpal bone, sequela
		S62.310S	Disp fx of base of second MC bone, right hand, sequela
		S62.311S	Disp fx of base of second MC bone. left hand, sequela
		S62.312S	Disp fx of base of third MC bone, right hand, sequela
		S62.313S	Disp fx of base of third metacarpal bone, left hand, sequela
		S62.314S	Disp fx of base of fourth MC bone, right hand, sequela
		S62.315S	Disp fx of base of fourth MC bone, left hand, sequela
		S62.316S	Disp fx of base of fifth MC bone, right hand, sequela
		S62.317S	Disp fx of base of fifth metacarpal bone. left hand, sequela
		S62.318S	Displaced fracture of base of other metacarpal bone, sequela
		S62.319S	Disp fx of base of unspecified metacarpal bone, sequela
		S62.320S	Disp fx of shaft of second MC bone, right hand, sequela
		S62.321S	Disp fx of shaft of second MC bone, left hand, sequela
		S62.322S	Disp fx of shaft of third MC bone, right hand, sequela
		S62.323S	Disp fx of shaft of third MC bone, left hand, sequela
		S62.324S	Disp fx of shaft of fourth MC bone, right hand, sequela
		S62.325S	Disp fx of shaft of fourth MC bone, left hand, sequela
		S62.326S	Disp fx of shaft of fifth MC bone, right hand, sequela
		S62.327S	Disp fx of shaft of fifth MC bone, left hand, sequela
		S62.328S	Disp fx of shaft of other metacarpal bone, sequela
		S62.329S	Disp fx of shaft of unspecified metacarpal bone, sequela
		S62.330S	Disp fx of neck of second MC bone, right hand, sequela
		S62.331S	Disp fx of neck of second MC bone, left hand, sequela
		S62.332S	Disp fx of neck of third MC bone, right hand, sequela
		S62.333S	Disp fx of neck of third metacarpal bone, left hand, sequela
		S62.334S	Disp fx of neck of fourth MC bone, right hand, sequela
		S62.335S	Disp fx of neck of fourth MC bone, left hand, sequela
		S62.336S	Disp fx of neck of fifth MC bone, right hand, sequela
		S62.337S	Disp fx of neck of fifth metacarpal bone, left hand, sequela
		S62.338S	Displaced fracture of neck of other metacarpal bone, sequela
		S62.339S	Disp fx of neck of unspecified metacarpal bone, sequela
		S62.340S	Nondisp fx of base of second MC bone, right hand, sequela
		S62.341S	Nondisp fx of base of second MC bone. left hand, sequela
		S62.342S	Nondisp fx of base of third MC bone, right hand, sequela
		S62.343S	Nondisp fx of base of third MC bone, left hand, sequela
		S62.344S	Nondisp fx of base of fourth MC bone, right hand, sequela
		S62.345S	Nondisp fx of base of fourth MC bone, left hand, sequela
		S62.346S	Nondisp fx of base of fifth MC bone, right hand, sequela
		S62.347S	Nondisp fx of base of fifth MC bone. left hand, sequela
		S62.348S	Nondisp fx of base of other metacarpal bone, sequela
		S62.349S	Nondisp fx of base of unspecified metacarpal bone, sequela
		S62.350S	Nondisp fx of shaft of second MC bone, right hand, sequela
		S62.351S	Nondisp fx of shaft of second MC bone, left hand, sequela
		S62.352S	Nondisp fx of shaft of third MC bone, right hand, sequela
		S62.353S	Nondisp fx of shaft of third MC bone, left hand, sequela
		S62.354S	Nondisp fx of shaft of fourth MC bone, right hand, sequela
		S62.355S	Nondisp fx of shaft of fourth MC bone, left hand, sequela
		S62.356S	Nondisp fx of shaft of fifth MC bone, right hand, sequela
		S62.357S	Nondisp fx of shaft of fifth MC bone, left hand, sequela
		S62.358S	Nondisp fx of shaft of other metacarpal bone, sequela
		S62.359S	Nondisp fx of shaft of unspecified metacarpal bone, sequela
		S62.360S	Nondisp fx of neck of second MC bone, right hand, sequela
		S62.361S	Nondisp fx of neck of second MC bone, left hand, sequela
		S62.362S	Nondisp fx of neck of third MC bone, right hand, sequela
		S62.363S	Nondisp fx of neck of third MC bone, left hand, sequela
		S62.364S	Nondisp fx of neck of fourth MC bone, right hand, sequela
		S62.365S	Nondisp fx of neck of fourth MC bone, left hand, sequela
		S62.366S	Nondisp fx of neck of fifth MC bone, right hand, sequela
		S62.367S	Nondisp fx of neck of fifth MC bone, left hand, sequela
		S62.368S	Nondisp fx of neck of other metacarpal bone, sequela
		S62.369S	Nondisp fx of neck of unspecified metacarpal bone, sequela
		S62.390S	Oth fracture of second metacarpal bone, right hand, sequela
		S62.391S	Other fracture of second metacarpal bone, left hand, sequela
		S62.392S	Other fracture of third metacarpal bone, right hand, sequela
		S62.393S	Other fracture of third metacarpal bone, left hand, sequela
		S62.394S	Oth fracture of fourth metacarpal bone, right hand, sequela
		S62.395S	Other fracture of fourth metacarpal bone, left hand, sequela
		S62.396S	Other fracture of fifth metacarpal bone, right hand, sequela
		S62.397S	Other fracture of fifth metacarpal bone, left hand, sequela
		S62.398S	Other fracture of other metacarpal bone, sequela
		S62.399S	Other fracture of unspecified metacarpal bone, sequela
		S62.501S	Fracture of unspecified phalanx of right thumb, sequela
		S62.502S	Fracture of unspecified phalanx of left thumb, sequela
		S62.509S	Fracture of unsp phalanx of unspecified thumb, sequela
		S62.511S	Disp fx of proximal phalanx of right thumb, sequela
		S62.512S	Disp fx of proximal phalanx of left thumb, sequela
		S62.513S	Disp fx of proximal phalanx of unspecified thumb, sequela
		S62.514S	Nondisp fx of proximal phalanx of right thumb, sequela
		S62.515S	Nondisp fx of proximal phalanx of left thumb, sequela
		S62.516S	Nondisp fx of proximal phalanx of unspecified thumb, sequela
		S62.521S	Displaced fracture of distal phalanx of right thumb, sequela
		S62.522S	Displaced fracture of distal phalanx of left thumb, sequela
	(Continued on next page)	**S62.523S**	Disp fx of distal phalanx of unspecified thumb, sequela

[Brackets] indicate valid character values for each code. Character value meanings provided for each code grouping.

ICD-9-CM		ICD-10-CM	
905.2	LATE EFFECT OF FRACTURE OF UPPER EXTREMITIES **(Continued)**	**S62.524S**	Nondisp fx of distal phalanx of right thumb, sequela
		S62.525S	Nondisp fx of distal phalanx of left thumb, sequela
		S62.526S	Nondisp fx of distal phalanx of unspecified thumb, sequela
		S62.600S	Fracture of unsp phalanx of right index finger, sequela
		S62.601S	Fracture of unsp phalanx of left index finger, sequela
		S62.602S	Fracture of unsp phalanx of right middle finger, sequela
		S62.603S	Fracture of unsp phalanx of left middle finger, sequela
		S62.604S	Fracture of unsp phalanx of right ring finger, sequela
		S62.605S	Fracture of unspecified phalanx of left ring finger, sequela
		S62.606S	Fracture of unsp phalanx of right little finger, sequela
		S62.607S	Fracture of unsp phalanx of left little finger, sequela
		S62.608S	Fracture of unspecified phalanx of other finger, sequela
		S62.609S	Fracture of unsp phalanx of unspecified finger, sequela
		S62.610S	Disp fx of proximal phalanx of right index finger, sequela
		S62.611S	Disp fx of proximal phalanx of left index finger, sequela
		S62.612S	Disp fx of proximal phalanx of right middle finger, sequela
		S62.613S	Disp fx of proximal phalanx of left middle finger, sequela
		S62.614S	Disp fx of proximal phalanx of right ring finger, sequela
		S62.615S	Disp fx of proximal phalanx of left ring finger, sequela
		S62.616S	Disp fx of proximal phalanx of right little finger, sequela
		S62.617S	Disp fx of proximal phalanx of left little finger, sequela
		S62.618S	Disp fx of proximal phalanx of other finger, sequela
		S62.619S	Disp fx of proximal phalanx of unspecified finger, sequela
		S62.620S	Disp fx of medial phalanx of right index finger, sequela
		S62.621S	Disp fx of medial phalanx of left index finger, sequela
		S62.622S	Disp fx of medial phalanx of right middle finger, sequela
		S62.623S	Disp fx of medial phalanx of left middle finger, sequela
		S62.624S	Disp fx of medial phalanx of right ring finger, sequela
		S62.625S	Disp fx of medial phalanx of left ring finger, sequela
		S62.626S	Disp fx of medial phalanx of right little finger, sequela
		S62.627S	Disp fx of medial phalanx of left little finger, sequela
		S62.628S	Disp fx of medial phalanx of other finger, sequela
		S62.629S	Disp fx of medial phalanx of unspecified finger, sequela
		S62.630S	Disp fx of distal phalanx of right index finger, sequela
		S62.631S	Disp fx of distal phalanx of left index finger, sequela
		S62.632S	Disp fx of distal phalanx of right middle finger, sequela
		S62.633S	Disp fx of distal phalanx of left middle finger, sequela
		S62.634S	Disp fx of distal phalanx of right ring finger, sequela
		S62.635S	Disp fx of distal phalanx of left ring finger, sequela
		S62.636S	Disp fx of distal phalanx of right little finger, sequela
		S62.637S	Disp fx of distal phalanx of left little finger, sequela
		S62.638S	Disp fx of distal phalanx of other finger, sequela
		S62.639S	Disp fx of distal phalanx of unspecified finger, sequela
		S62.640S	Nondisp fx of proximal phalanx of r idx fngr, sequela
		S62.641S	Nondisp fx of proximal phalanx of left index finger, sequela
		S62.642S	Nondisp fx of proximal phalanx of r mid finger, sequela
		S62.643S	Nondisp fx of proximal phalanx of l mid finger, sequela
		S62.644S	Nondisp fx of proximal phalanx of right ring finger, sequela
		S62.645S	Nondisp fx of proximal phalanx of left ring finger, sequela
		S62.646S	Nondisp fx of proximal phalanx of r little finger, sequela
		S62.647S	Nondisp fx of proximal phalanx of l little finger, sequela
		S62.648S	Nondisp fx of proximal phalanx of other finger, sequela
		S62.649S	Nondisp fx of proximal phalanx of unsp finger, sequela
		S62.650S	Nondisp fx of medial phalanx of right index finger, sequela
		S62.651S	Nondisp fx of medial phalanx of left index finger, sequela
		S62.652S	Nondisp fx of medial phalanx of right middle finger, sequela
		S62.653S	Nondisp fx of medial phalanx of left middle finger, sequela
		S62.654S	Nondisp fx of medial phalanx of right ring finger, sequela
		S62.655S	Nondisp fx of medial phalanx of left ring finger, sequela
		S62.656S	Nondisp fx of medial phalanx of right little finger, sequela
		S62.657S	Nondisp fx of medial phalanx of left little finger, sequela
		S62.658S	Nondisp fx of medial phalanx of other finger, sequela
		S62.659S	Nondisp fx of medial phalanx of unspecified finger, sequela
		S62.660S	Nondisp fx of distal phalanx of right index finger, sequela
		S62.661S	Nondisp fx of distal phalanx of left index finger, sequela
		S62.662S	Nondisp fx of distal phalanx of right middle finger, sequela
		S62.663S	Nondisp fx of distal phalanx of left middle finger, sequela
		S62.664S	Nondisp fx of distal phalanx of right ring finger, sequela
		S62.665S	Nondisp fx of distal phalanx of left ring finger, sequela
		S62.666S	Nondisp fx of distal phalanx of right little finger, sequela
		S62.667S	Nondisp fx of distal phalanx of left little finger, sequela
		S62.668S	Nondisp fx of distal phalanx of other finger, sequela
		S62.669S	Nondisp fx of distal phalanx of unspecified finger, sequela
		S62.90XS	Unspecified fracture of unspecified wrist and hand, sequela
		S62.91XS	Unspecified fracture of right wrist and hand, sequela
		S62.92XS	Unspecified fracture of left wrist and hand, sequela
905.3	LATE EFFECT OF FRACTURE OF NECK OF FEMUR	**M80.051S**	Age-rel osteopor w current path fracture, r femur, sequela
		M80.052S	Age-rel osteopor w current path fracture, l femur, sequela
		M80.059S	Age-rel osteopor w current path fx, unsp femur, sequela
		M80.851S	Oth osteopor w current path fracture, right femur, sequela
		M80.852S	Oth osteopor w current path fracture, left femur, sequela
		M80.859S	Oth osteopor w current path fracture, unsp femur, sequela
	(Continued on next page)	**M84.359S**	Stress fracture, hip, unspecified, sequela

ICD-9-CM		ICD-10-CM	
9Ø5.3	LATE EFFECT OF FRACTURE OF NECK OF FEMUR **(Continued)**	**M84.451S**	Pathological fracture, right femur, sequela
		M84.452S	Pathological fracture, left femur, sequela
		M84.459S	Pathological fracture, hip, unspecified, sequela
		M84.551S	Path fracture in neoplastic disease, right femur, sequela
		M84.552S	Path fracture in neoplastic disease, left femur, sequela
		M84.553S	Path fracture in neoplastic disease, unsp femur, sequela
		M84.559S	Path fracture in neoplastic disease, hip, unsp, sequela
		M84.651S	Pathological fracture in other disease, right femur, sequela
		M84.652S	Pathological fracture in other disease, left femur, sequela
		M84.653S	Pathological fracture in other disease, unsp femur, sequela
		M84.659S	Pathological fracture in other disease, hip, unsp, sequela
		S72.ØØ1S	Fracture of unspecified part of neck of right femur, sequela
		S72.ØØ2S	Fracture of unspecified part of neck of left femur, sequela
		S72.ØØ9S	Fracture of unsp part of neck of unspecified femur, sequela
		S72.Ø11S	Unspecified intracapsular fracture of right femur, sequela
		S72.Ø12S	Unspecified intracapsular fracture of left femur, sequela
		S72.Ø19S	Unsp intracapsular fracture of unspecified femur, sequela
		S72.Ø21S	Disp fx of epiphy (separation) (upper) of r femur, sequela
		S72.Ø22S	Disp fx of epiphy (separation) (upper) of l femur, sequela
		S72.Ø23S	Disp fx of epiphy (separation) (upper) of unsp femur, sqla
		S72.Ø24S	Nondisp fx of epiphy (separation) (upper) of r femur, sqla
		S72.Ø25S	Nondisp fx of epiphy (separation) (upper) of l femur, sqla
		S72.Ø26S	Nondisp fx of epiphy (separation) (upper) of unsp femr, sqla
		S72.Ø31S	Displaced midcervical fracture of right femur, sequela
		S72.Ø32S	Displaced midcervical fracture of left femur, sequela
		S72.Ø33S	Displaced midcervical fracture of unspecified femur, sequela
		S72.Ø34S	Nondisplaced midcervical fracture of right femur, sequela
		S72.Ø35S	Nondisplaced midcervical fracture of left femur, sequela
		S72.Ø36S	Nondisplaced midcervical fracture of unsp femur, sequela
		S72.Ø41S	Displaced fracture of base of neck of right femur, sequela
		S72.Ø42S	Displaced fracture of base of neck of left femur, sequela
		S72.Ø43S	Disp fx of base of neck of unspecified femur, sequela
		S72.Ø44S	Nondisp fx of base of neck of right femur, sequela
		S72.Ø45S	Nondisplaced fracture of base of neck of left femur, sequela
		S72.Ø46S	Nondisp fx of base of neck of unspecified femur, sequela
		S72.Ø51S	Unspecified fracture of head of right femur, sequela
		S72.Ø52S	Unspecified fracture of head of left femur, sequela
		S72.Ø59S	Unspecified fracture of head of unspecified femur, sequela
		S72.Ø61S	Displaced articular fracture of head of right femur, sequela
		S72.Ø62S	Displaced articular fracture of head of left femur, sequela
		S72.Ø63S	Displaced articular fracture of head of unsp femur, sequela
		S72.Ø64S	Nondisp articular fracture of head of right femur, sequela
		S72.Ø65S	Nondisp articular fracture of head of left femur, sequela
		S72.Ø66S	Nondisp articular fracture of head of unsp femur, sequela
		S72.Ø91S	Other fracture of head and neck of right femur, sequela
		S72.Ø92S	Other fracture of head and neck of left femur, sequela
		S72.Ø99S	Other fracture of head and neck of unsp femur, sequela
		S72.1Ø1S	Unspecified trochanteric fracture of right femur, sequela
		S72.1Ø2S	Unspecified trochanteric fracture of left femur, sequela
		S72.1Ø9S	Unsp trochanteric fracture of unspecified femur, sequela
		S72.111S	Disp fx of greater trochanter of right femur, sequela
		S72.112S	Disp fx of greater trochanter of left femur, sequela
		S72.113S	Disp fx of greater trochanter of unspecified femur, sequela
		S72.114S	Nondisp fx of greater trochanter of right femur, sequela
		S72.115S	Nondisp fx of greater trochanter of left femur, sequela
		S72.116S	Nondisp fx of greater trochanter of unsp femur, sequela
		S72.121S	Disp fx of lesser trochanter of right femur, sequela
		S72.122S	Disp fx of lesser trochanter of left femur, sequela
		S72.123S	Disp fx of lesser trochanter of unspecified femur, sequela
		S72.124S	Nondisp fx of lesser trochanter of right femur, sequela
		S72.125S	Nondisp fx of lesser trochanter of left femur, sequela
		S72.126S	Nondisp fx of lesser trochanter of unsp femur, sequela
		S72.131S	Displaced apophyseal fracture of right femur, sequela
		S72.132S	Displaced apophyseal fracture of left femur, sequela
		S72.133S	Displaced apophyseal fracture of unspecified femur, sequela
		S72.134S	Nondisplaced apophyseal fracture of right femur, sequela
		S72.135S	Nondisplaced apophyseal fracture of left femur, sequela
		S72.136S	Nondisplaced apophyseal fracture of unsp femur, sequela
		S72.141S	Displaced intertrochanteric fracture of right femur, sequela
		S72.142S	Displaced intertrochanteric fracture of left femur, sequela
		S72.143S	Displaced intertrochanteric fracture of unsp femur, sequela
		S72.144S	Nondisplaced intertroch fracture of right femur, sequela
		S72.145S	Nondisplaced intertroch fracture of left femur, sequela
		S72.146S	Nondisplaced intertroch fracture of unsp femur, sequela
		S72.21XS	Displaced subtrochanteric fracture of right femur, sequela
		S72.22XS	Displaced subtrochanteric fracture of left femur, sequela
		S72.23XS	Displaced subtrochanteric fracture of unsp femur, sequela
		S72.24XS	Nondisplaced subtrochnt fracture of right femur, sequela
		S72.25XS	Nondisplaced subtrochanteric fracture of left femur, sequela
		S72.26XS	Nondisplaced subtrochanteric fracture of unsp femur, sequela

[Brackets] indicate valid character values for each code. Character value meanings provided for each code grouping.

ICD-9-CM		ICD-10-CM	
905.4	LATE EFFECT OF FRACTURE OF LOWER EXTREMITIES	**M80.061S**	Age-rel osteopor w current path fracture, r low leg, sequela
		M80.062S	Age-rel osteopor w current path fracture, l low leg, sequela
		M80.069S	Age-rel osteopor w current path fx, unsp low leg, sequela
		M80.071S	Age-rel osteopor w current path fx, right ank/ft, sequela
		M80.072S	Age-rel osteopor w current path fx, left ank/ft, sequela
		M80.079S	Age-rel osteopor w current path fx, unsp ank/ft, sequela
		M80.851S	Oth osteopor w current path fracture, right femur, sequela
		M80.852S	Oth osteopor w current path fracture, left femur, sequela
		M80.859S	Oth osteopor w current path fracture, unsp femur, sequela
		M80.861S	Oth osteopor w current path fracture, r low leg, sequela
		M80.862S	Oth osteopor w current path fracture, l low leg, sequela
		M80.869S	Oth osteopor w current path fracture, unsp low leg, sequela
		M80.871S	Oth osteopor w current path fracture, right ank/ft, sequela
		M80.872S	Oth osteopor w current path fracture, left ank/ft, sequela
		M80.879S	Oth osteopor w current path fracture, unsp ank/ft, sequela
		M84.351S	Stress fracture, right femur, sequela
		M84.352S	Stress fracture, left femur, sequela
		M84.353S	Stress fracture, unspecified femur, sequela
		M84.361S	Stress fracture, right tibia, sequela
		M84.362S	Stress fracture, left tibia, sequela
		M84.363S	Stress fracture, right fibula, sequela
		M84.364S	Stress fracture, left fibula, sequela
		M84.369S	Stress fracture, unspecified tibia and fibula, sequela
		M84.371S	Stress fracture, right ankle, sequela
		M84.372S	Stress fracture, left ankle, sequela
		M84.373S	Stress fracture, unspecified ankle, sequela
		M84.374S	Stress fracture, right foot, sequela
		M84.375S	Stress fracture, left foot, sequela
		M84.376S	Stress fracture, unspecified foot, sequela
		M84.377S	Stress fracture, right toe(s), sequela
		M84.378S	Stress fracture, left toe(s), sequela
		M84.379S	Stress fracture, unspecified toe(s), sequela
		M84.451S	Pathological fracture, right femur, sequela
		M84.452S	Pathological fracture, left femur, sequela
		M84.453S	Pathological fracture, unspecified femur, sequela
		M84.461S	Pathological fracture, right tibia, sequela
		M84.462S	Pathological fracture, left tibia, sequela
		M84.463S	Pathological fracture, right fibula, sequela
		M84.464S	Pathological fracture, left fibula, sequela
		M84.469S	Pathological fracture, unspecified tibia and fibula, sequela
		M84.471S	Pathological fracture, right ankle, sequela
		M84.472S	Pathological fracture, left ankle, sequela
		M84.473S	Pathological fracture, unspecified ankle, sequela
		M84.474S	Pathological fracture, right foot, sequela
		M84.475S	Pathological fracture, left foot, sequela
		M84.476S	Pathological fracture, unspecified foot, sequela
		M84.477S	Pathological fracture, right toe(s), sequela
		M84.478S	Pathological fracture, left toe(s), sequela
		M84.479S	Pathological fracture, unspecified toe(s), sequela
		M84.551S	Path fracture in neoplastic disease, right femur, sequela
		M84.552S	Path fracture in neoplastic disease, left femur, sequela
		M84.553S	Path fracture in neoplastic disease, unsp femur, sequela
		M84.561S	Path fracture in neoplastic disease, right tibia, sequela
		M84.562S	Path fracture in neoplastic disease, left tibia, sequela
		M84.563S	Path fracture in neoplastic disease, right fibula, sequela
		M84.564S	Path fracture in neoplastic disease, left fibula, sequela
		M84.569S	Path fx in neopltc disease, unsp tibia and fibula, sequela
		M84.571S	Path fracture in neoplastic disease, right ankle, sequela
		M84.572S	Path fracture in neoplastic disease, left ankle, sequela
		M84.573S	Path fracture in neoplastic disease, unsp ankle, sequela
		M84.574S	Path fracture in neoplastic disease, right foot, sequela
		M84.575S	Path fracture in neoplastic disease, left foot, sequela
		M84.576S	Path fracture in neoplastic disease, unsp foot, sequela
		M84.651S	Pathological fracture in other disease, right femur, sequela
		M84.652S	Pathological fracture in other disease, left femur, sequela
		M84.653S	Pathological fracture in other disease, unsp femur, sequela
		M84.661S	Pathological fracture in other disease, right tibia, sequela
		M84.662S	Pathological fracture in other disease, left tibia, sequela
		M84.663S	Pathological fracture in oth disease, right fibula, sequela
		M84.664S	Pathological fracture in other disease, left fibula, sequela
		M84.669S	Path fracture in oth disease, unsp tibia and fibula, sequela
		M84.671S	Pathological fracture in other disease, right ankle, sequela
		M84.672S	Pathological fracture in other disease, left ankle, sequela
		M84.673S	Pathological fracture in other disease, unsp ankle, sequela
		M84.674S	Pathological fracture in other disease, right foot, sequela
		M84.675S	Pathological fracture in other disease, left foot, sequela
		M84.676S	Pathological fracture in other disease, unsp foot, sequela
		S72.301S	Unspecified fracture of shaft of right femur, sequela
		S72.302S	Unspecified fracture of shaft of left femur, sequela
		S72.309S	Unspecified fracture of shaft of unspecified femur, sequela
		S72.321S	Displaced transverse fx shaft of right femur, sequela
		S72.322S	Displaced transverse fx shaft of left femur, sequela
	(Continued on next page)	**S72.323S**	Displaced transverse fx shaft of unsp femur, sequela

ICD-9-CM		ICD-10-CM	
905.4	LATE EFFECT OF FRACTURE OF LOWER EXTREMITIES **(Continued)**	**S72.324S**	Nondisp transverse fracture of shaft of right femur, sequela
		S72.325S	Nondisp transverse fracture of shaft of left femur, sequela
		S72.326S	Nondisp transverse fracture of shaft of unsp femur, sequela
		S72.331S	Displaced oblique fracture of shaft of right femur, sequela
		S72.332S	Displaced oblique fracture of shaft of left femur, sequela
		S72.333S	Displaced oblique fracture of shaft of unsp femur, sequela
		S72.334S	Nondisp oblique fracture of shaft of right femur, sequela
		S72.335S	Nondisp oblique fracture of shaft of left femur, sequela
		S72.336S	Nondisp oblique fracture of shaft of unsp femur, sequela
		S72.341S	Displaced spiral fracture of shaft of right femur, sequela
		S72.342S	Displaced spiral fracture of shaft of left femur, sequela
		S72.343S	Displaced spiral fracture of shaft of unsp femur, sequela
		S72.344S	Nondisp spiral fracture of shaft of right femur, sequela
		S72.345S	Nondisplaced spiral fracture of shaft of left femur, sequela
		S72.346S	Nondisplaced spiral fracture of shaft of unsp femur, sequela
		S72.351S	Displaced comminuted fx shaft of right femur, sequela
		S72.352S	Displaced comminuted fx shaft of left femur, sequela
		S72.353S	Displaced comminuted fx shaft of unsp femur, sequela
		S72.354S	Nondisp comminuted fracture of shaft of right femur, sequela
		S72.355S	Nondisp comminuted fracture of shaft of left femur, sequela
		S72.356S	Nondisp comminuted fracture of shaft of unsp femur, sequela
		S72.361S	Displaced segmental fx shaft of right femur, sequela
		S72.362S	Displaced segmental fracture of shaft of left femur, sequela
		S72.363S	Displaced segmental fracture of shaft of unsp femur, sequela
		S72.364S	Nondisp segmental fracture of shaft of right femur, sequela
		S72.365S	Nondisp segmental fracture of shaft of left femur, sequela
		S72.366S	Nondisp segmental fracture of shaft of unsp femur, sequela
		S72.391S	Other fracture of shaft of right femur, sequela
		S72.392S	Other fracture of shaft of left femur, sequela
		S72.399S	Other fracture of shaft of unspecified femur, sequela
		S72.401S	Unspecified fracture of lower end of right femur, sequela
		S72.402S	Unspecified fracture of lower end of left femur, sequela
		S72.409S	Unsp fracture of lower end of unspecified femur, sequela
		S72.411S	Displaced unsp condyle fx lower end of right femur, sequela
		S72.412S	Displaced unsp condyle fx lower end of left femur, sequela
		S72.413S	Displaced unsp condyle fx lower end of unsp femur, sequela
		S72.414S	Nondisp unsp condyle fx lower end of right femur, sequela
		S72.415S	Nondisp unsp condyle fx lower end of left femur, sequela
		S72.416S	Nondisp unsp condyle fx lower end of unsp femur, sequela
		S72.421S	Disp fx of lateral condyle of right femur, sequela
		S72.422S	Displaced fracture of lateral condyle of left femur, sequela
		S72.423S	Disp fx of lateral condyle of unspecified femur, sequela
		S72.424S	Nondisp fx of lateral condyle of right femur, sequela
		S72.425S	Nondisp fx of lateral condyle of left femur, sequela
		S72.426S	Nondisp fx of lateral condyle of unspecified femur, sequela
		S72.431S	Displaced fracture of medial condyle of right femur, sequela
		S72.432S	Displaced fracture of medial condyle of left femur, sequela
		S72.433S	Disp fx of medial condyle of unspecified femur, sequela
		S72.434S	Nondisp fx of medial condyle of right femur, sequela
		S72.435S	Nondisp fx of medial condyle of left femur, sequela
		S72.436S	Nondisp fx of medial condyle of unspecified femur, sequela
		S72.441S	Disp fx of lower epiphysis (separation) of r femur, sequela
		S72.442S	Disp fx of lower epiphysis (separation) of l femur, sequela
		S72.443S	Disp fx of lower epiphy (separation) of unsp femur, sequela
		S72.444S	Nondisp fx of lower epiphy (separation) of r femur, sequela
		S72.445S	Nondisp fx of lower epiphy (separation) of l femur, sequela
		S72.446S	Nondisp fx of lower epiphy (separation) of unsp femur, sqla
		S72.451S	Displ suprcndl fx w/o intrcndl extn lower end r femur, sqla
		S72.452S	Displ suprcndl fx w/o intrcndl extn lower end l femur, sqla
		S72.453S	Displ suprcndl fx w/o intrcndl extn low end unsp femr, sqla
		S72.454S	Nondisp suprcndl fx w/o intrcndl extn lower end r femr, sqla
		S72.455S	Nondisp suprcndl fx w/o intrcndl extn lower end l femr, sqla
		S72.456S	Nondisp suprcndl fx w/o intrcndl extn low end unsp femr,sqla
		S72.461S	Displ suprcndl fx w intrcndl extn lower end of r femur, sqla
		S72.462S	Displ suprcndl fx w intrcndl extn lower end of l femur, sqla
		S72.463S	Displ suprcndl fx w intrcndl extn lower end unsp femur, sqla
		S72.464S	Nondisp suprcndl fx w intrcndl extn lower end r femur, sqla
		S72.465S	Nondisp suprcndl fx w intrcndl extn lower end l femur, sqla
		S72.466S	Nondisp suprcndl fx w intrcndl extn low end unsp femr, sqla
		S72.471S	Torus fracture of lower end of right femur, sequela
		S72.472S	Torus fracture of lower end of left femur, sequela
		S72.479S	Torus fracture of lower end of unspecified femur, sequela
		S72.491S	Other fracture of lower end of right femur, sequela
		S72.492S	Other fracture of lower end of left femur, sequela
		S72.499S	Other fracture of lower end of unspecified femur, sequela
		S72.8X1S	Other fracture of right femur, sequela
		S72.8X2S	Other fracture of left femur, sequela
		S72.8X9S	Other fracture of unspecified femur, sequela
		S72.90XS	Unspecified fracture of unspecified femur, sequela
		S72.91XS	Unspecified fracture of right femur, sequela
		S72.92XS	Unspecified fracture of left femur, sequela
		S79.001S	Unsp physeal fracture of upper end of right femur, sequela
	(Continued on next page)	**S79.002S**	Unsp physeal fracture of upper end of left femur, sequela

ICD-9-CM		ICD-10-CM	
905.4	LATE EFFECT OF FRACTURE OF LOWER EXTREMITIES **(Continued)**	**S79.009S**	Unsp physeal fracture of upper end of unsp femur, sequela
		S79.011S	Sltr-haris Type I physeal fx upper end of r femur, sequela
		S79.012S	Sltr-haris Type I physeal fx upper end of l femur, sequela
		S79.019S	Sltr-haris Type I physl fx upper end of unsp femur, sequela
		S79.091S	Other physeal fracture of upper end of right femur, sequela
		S79.092S	Other physeal fracture of upper end of left femur, sequela
		S79.099S	Other physeal fracture of upper end of unsp femur, sequela
		S79.101S	Unsp physeal fracture of lower end of right femur, sequela
		S79.102S	Unsp physeal fracture of lower end of left femur, sequela
		S79.109S	Unsp physeal fracture of lower end of unsp femur, sequela
		S79.111S	Sltr-haris Type I physeal fx lower end of r femur, sequela
		S79.112S	Sltr-haris Type I physeal fx lower end of l femur, sequela
		S79.119S	Sltr-haris Type I physl fx lower end of unsp femur, sequela
		S79.121S	Sltr-haris Type II physeal fx lower end of r femur, sequela
		S79.122S	Sltr-haris Type II physeal fx lower end of l femur, sequela
		S79.129S	Sltr-haris Type II physl fx lower end of unsp femur, sequela
		S79.131S	Sltr-haris Type III physeal fx lower end of r femur, sequela
		S79.132S	Sltr-haris Type III physeal fx lower end of l femur, sequela
		S79.139S	Sltr-haris Type III physl fx lower end of unsp femur, sqla
		S79.141S	Sltr-haris Type IV physeal fx lower end of r femur, sequela
		S79.142S	Sltr-haris Type IV physeal fx lower end of l femur, sequela
		S79.149S	Sltr-haris Type IV physl fx lower end of unsp femur, sequela
		S79.191S	Other physeal fracture of lower end of right femur, sequela
		S79.192S	Other physeal fracture of lower end of left femur, sequela
		S79.199S	Other physeal fracture of lower end of unsp femur, sequela
		S82.001S	Unspecified fracture of right patella, sequela
		S82.002S	Unspecified fracture of left patella, sequela
		S82.009S	Unspecified fracture of unspecified patella, sequela
		S82.011S	Displaced osteochondral fracture of right patella, sequela
		S82.012S	Displaced osteochondral fracture of left patella, sequela
		S82.013S	Displaced osteochondral fracture of unsp patella, sequela
		S82.014S	Nondisplaced osteochon fracture of right patella, sequela
		S82.015S	Nondisplaced osteochondral fracture of left patella, sequela
		S82.016S	Nondisplaced osteochondral fracture of unsp patella, sequela
		S82.021S	Displaced longitudinal fracture of right patella, sequela
		S82.022S	Displaced longitudinal fracture of left patella, sequela
		S82.023S	Displaced longitudinal fracture of unsp patella, sequela
		S82.024S	Nondisplaced longitudinal fracture of right patella, sequela
		S82.025S	Nondisplaced longitudinal fracture of left patella, sequela
		S82.026S	Nondisplaced longitudinal fracture of unsp patella, sequela
		S82.031S	Displaced transverse fracture of right patella, sequela
		S82.032S	Displaced transverse fracture of left patella, sequela
		S82.033S	Displaced transverse fracture of unsp patella, sequela
		S82.034S	Nondisplaced transverse fracture of right patella, sequela
		S82.035S	Nondisplaced transverse fracture of left patella, sequela
		S82.036S	Nondisplaced transverse fracture of unsp patella, sequela
		S82.041S	Displaced comminuted fracture of right patella, sequela
		S82.042S	Displaced comminuted fracture of left patella, sequela
		S82.043S	Displaced comminuted fracture of unsp patella, sequela
		S82.044S	Nondisplaced comminuted fracture of right patella, sequela
		S82.045S	Nondisplaced comminuted fracture of left patella, sequela
		S82.046S	Nondisplaced comminuted fracture of unsp patella, sequela
		S82.091S	Other fracture of right patella, sequela
		S82.092S	Other fracture of left patella, sequela
		S82.099S	Other fracture of unspecified patella, sequela
		S82.101S	Unspecified fracture of upper end of right tibia, sequela
		S82.102S	Unspecified fracture of upper end of left tibia, sequela
		S82.109S	Unsp fracture of upper end of unspecified tibia, sequela
		S82.111S	Displaced fracture of right tibial spine, sequela
		S82.112S	Displaced fracture of left tibial spine, sequela
		S82.113S	Displaced fracture of unspecified tibial spine, sequela
		S82.114S	Nondisplaced fracture of right tibial spine, sequela
		S82.115S	Nondisplaced fracture of left tibial spine, sequela
		S82.116S	Nondisplaced fracture of unspecified tibial spine, sequela
		S82.121S	Disp fx of lateral condyle of right tibia, sequela
		S82.122S	Displaced fracture of lateral condyle of left tibia, sequela
		S82.123S	Disp fx of lateral condyle of unspecified tibia, sequela
		S82.124S	Nondisp fx of lateral condyle of right tibia, sequela
		S82.125S	Nondisp fx of lateral condyle of left tibia, sequela
		S82.126S	Nondisp fx of lateral condyle of unspecified tibia, sequela
		S82.131S	Displaced fracture of medial condyle of right tibia, sequela
		S82.132S	Displaced fracture of medial condyle of left tibia, sequela
		S82.133S	Disp fx of medial condyle of unspecified tibia, sequela
		S82.134S	Nondisp fx of medial condyle of right tibia, sequela
		S82.135S	Nondisp fx of medial condyle of left tibia, sequela
		S82.136S	Nondisp fx of medial condyle of unspecified tibia, sequela
		S82.141S	Displaced bicondylar fracture of right tibia, sequela
		S82.142S	Displaced bicondylar fracture of left tibia, sequela
		S82.143S	Displaced bicondylar fracture of unspecified tibia, sequela
		S82.144S	Nondisplaced bicondylar fracture of right tibia, sequela
		S82.145S	Nondisplaced bicondylar fracture of left tibia, sequela
		S82.146S	Nondisplaced bicondylar fracture of unsp tibia, sequela
	(Continued on next page)	**S82.151S**	Displaced fracture of right tibial tuberosity, sequela

ICD-9-CM		ICD-10-CM	
905.4	LATE EFFECT OF FRACTURE OF LOWER EXTREMITIES **(Continued)**	**S82.152S**	Displaced fracture of left tibial tuberosity, sequela
		S82.153S	Displaced fracture of unspecified tibial tuberosity, sequela
		S82.154S	Nondisplaced fracture of right tibial tuberosity, sequela
		S82.155S	Nondisplaced fracture of left tibial tuberosity, sequela
		S82.156S	Nondisp fx of unspecified tibial tuberosity, sequela
		S82.161S	Torus fracture of upper end of right tibia, sequela
		S82.162S	Torus fracture of upper end of left tibia, sequela
		S82.169S	Torus fracture of upper end of unspecified tibia, sequela
		S82.191S	Other fracture of upper end of right tibia, sequela
		S82.192S	Other fracture of upper end of left tibia, sequela
		S82.199S	Other fracture of upper end of unspecified tibia, sequela
		S82.201S	Unspecified fracture of shaft of right tibia, sequela
		S82.202S	Unspecified fracture of shaft of left tibia, sequela
		S82.209S	Unspecified fracture of shaft of unspecified tibia, sequela
		S82.221S	Displaced transverse fx shaft of right tibia, sequela
		S82.222S	Displaced transverse fx shaft of left tibia, sequela
		S82.223S	Displaced transverse fx shaft of unsp tibia, sequela
		S82.224S	Nondisp transverse fracture of shaft of right tibia, sequela
		S82.225S	Nondisp transverse fracture of shaft of left tibia, sequela
		S82.226S	Nondisp transverse fracture of shaft of unsp tibia, sequela
		S82.231S	Displaced oblique fracture of shaft of right tibia, sequela
		S82.232S	Displaced oblique fracture of shaft of left tibia, sequela
		S82.233S	Displaced oblique fracture of shaft of unsp tibia, sequela
		S82.234S	Nondisp oblique fracture of shaft of right tibia, sequela
		S82.235S	Nondisp oblique fracture of shaft of left tibia, sequela
		S82.236S	Nondisp oblique fracture of shaft of unsp tibia, sequela
		S82.241S	Displaced spiral fracture of shaft of right tibia, sequela
		S82.242S	Displaced spiral fracture of shaft of left tibia, sequela
		S82.243S	Displaced spiral fracture of shaft of unsp tibia, sequela
		S82.244S	Nondisp spiral fracture of shaft of right tibia, sequela
		S82.245S	Nondisplaced spiral fracture of shaft of left tibia, sequela
		S82.246S	Nondisplaced spiral fracture of shaft of unsp tibia, sequela
		S82.251S	Displaced comminuted fx shaft of right tibia, sequela
		S82.252S	Displaced comminuted fx shaft of left tibia, sequela
		S82.253S	Displaced comminuted fx shaft of unsp tibia, sequela
		S82.254S	Nondisp comminuted fracture of shaft of right tibia, sequela
		S82.255S	Nondisp comminuted fracture of shaft of left tibia, sequela
		S82.256S	Nondisp comminuted fracture of shaft of unsp tibia, sequela
		S82.261S	Displaced segmental fx shaft of right tibia, sequela
		S82.262S	Displaced segmental fracture of shaft of left tibia, sequela
		S82.263S	Displaced segmental fracture of shaft of unsp tibia, sequela
		S82.264S	Nondisp segmental fracture of shaft of right tibia, sequela
		S82.265S	Nondisp segmental fracture of shaft of left tibia, sequela
		S82.266S	Nondisp segmental fracture of shaft of unsp tibia, sequela
		S82.291S	Other fracture of shaft of right tibia, sequela
		S82.292S	Other fracture of shaft of left tibia, sequela
		S82.299S	Other fracture of shaft of unspecified tibia, sequela
		S82.301S	Unspecified fracture of lower end of right tibia, sequela
		S82.302S	Unspecified fracture of lower end of left tibia, sequela
		S82.309S	Unsp fracture of lower end of unspecified tibia, sequela
		S82.311S	Torus fracture of lower end of right tibia, sequela
		S82.312S	Torus fracture of lower end of left tibia, sequela
		S82.319S	Torus fracture of lower end of unspecified tibia, sequela
		S82.391S	Other fracture of lower end of right tibia, sequela
		S82.392S	Other fracture of lower end of left tibia, sequela
		S82.399S	Other fracture of lower end of unspecified tibia, sequela
		S82.401S	Unspecified fracture of shaft of right fibula, sequela
		S82.402S	Unspecified fracture of shaft of left fibula, sequela
		S82.409S	Unspecified fracture of shaft of unspecified fibula, sequela
		S82.421S	Displaced transverse fracture of shaft of r fibula, sequela
		S82.422S	Displaced transverse fx shaft of left fibula, sequela
		S82.423S	Displaced transverse fx shaft of unsp fibula, sequela
		S82.424S	Nondisp transverse fracture of shaft of r fibula, sequela
		S82.425S	Nondisp transverse fracture of shaft of left fibula, sequela
		S82.426S	Nondisp transverse fracture of shaft of unsp fibula, sequela
		S82.431S	Displaced oblique fracture of shaft of right fibula, sequela
		S82.432S	Displaced oblique fracture of shaft of left fibula, sequela
		S82.433S	Displaced oblique fracture of shaft of unsp fibula, sequela
		S82.434S	Nondisp oblique fracture of shaft of right fibula, sequela
		S82.435S	Nondisp oblique fracture of shaft of left fibula, sequela
		S82.436S	Nondisp oblique fracture of shaft of unsp fibula, sequela
		S82.441S	Displaced spiral fracture of shaft of right fibula, sequela
		S82.442S	Displaced spiral fracture of shaft of left fibula, sequela
		S82.443S	Displaced spiral fracture of shaft of unsp fibula, sequela
		S82.444S	Nondisp spiral fracture of shaft of right fibula, sequela
		S82.445S	Nondisp spiral fracture of shaft of left fibula, sequela
		S82.446S	Nondisp spiral fracture of shaft of unsp fibula, sequela
		S82.451S	Displaced comminuted fracture of shaft of r fibula, sequela
		S82.452S	Displaced comminuted fx shaft of left fibula, sequela
		S82.453S	Displaced comminuted fx shaft of unsp fibula, sequela
		S82.454S	Nondisp comminuted fracture of shaft of r fibula, sequela
	(Continued on next page)	**S82.455S**	Nondisp comminuted fracture of shaft of left fibula, sequela

[Brackets] indicate valid character values for each code. Character value meanings provided for each code grouping.

ICD-9-CM		ICD-10-CM	
9Ø5.4	LATE EFFECT OF FRACTURE OF LOWER EXTREMITIES **(Continued)**	**S82.456S**	Nondisp comminuted fracture of shaft of unsp fibula, sequela
		S82.461S	Displaced segmental fracture of shaft of r fibula, sequela
		S82.462S	Displaced segmental fx shaft of left fibula, sequela
		S82.463S	Displaced segmental fx shaft of unsp fibula, sequela
		S82.464S	Nondisp segmental fracture of shaft of right fibula, sequela
		S82.465S	Nondisp segmental fracture of shaft of left fibula, sequela
		S82.466S	Nondisp segmental fracture of shaft of unsp fibula, sequela
		S82.491S	Other fracture of shaft of right fibula, sequela
		S82.492S	Other fracture of shaft of left fibula, sequela
		S82.499S	Other fracture of shaft of unspecified fibula, sequela
		S82.51XS	Disp fx of medial malleolus of right tibia, sequela
		S82.52XS	Disp fx of medial malleolus of left tibia, sequela
		S82.53XS	Disp fx of medial malleolus of unspecified tibia, sequela
		S82.54XS	Nondisp fx of medial malleolus of right tibia, sequela
		S82.55XS	Nondisp fx of medial malleolus of left tibia, sequela
		S82.56XS	Nondisp fx of medial malleolus of unspecified tibia, sequela
		S82.61XS	Disp fx of lateral malleolus of right fibula, sequela
		S82.62XS	Disp fx of lateral malleolus of left fibula, sequela
		S82.63XS	Disp fx of lateral malleolus of unspecified fibula, sequela
		S82.64XS	Nondisp fx of lateral malleolus of right fibula, sequela
		S82.65XS	Nondisp fx of lateral malleolus of left fibula, sequela
		S82.66XS	Nondisp fx of lateral malleolus of unsp fibula, sequela
		S82.811S	Torus fracture of upper end of right fibula, sequela
		S82.812S	Torus fracture of upper end of left fibula, sequela
		S82.819S	Torus fracture of upper end of unspecified fibula, sequela
		S82.821S	Torus fracture of lower end of right fibula, sequela
		S82.822S	Torus fracture of lower end of left fibula, sequela
		S82.829S	Torus fracture of lower end of unspecified fibula, sequela
		S82.831S	Oth fracture of upper and lower end of right fibula, sequela
		S82.832S	Oth fracture of upper and lower end of left fibula, sequela
		S82.839S	Oth fracture of upper and lower end of unsp fibula, sequela
		S82.841S	Displaced bimalleolar fracture of right lower leg, sequela
		S82.842S	Displaced bimalleolar fracture of left lower leg, sequela
		S82.843S	Displaced bimalleolar fracture of unsp lower leg, sequela
		S82.844S	Nondisplaced bimalleolar fracture of r low leg, sequela
		S82.845S	Nondisplaced bimalleolar fracture of left lower leg, sequela
		S82.846S	Nondisplaced bimalleolar fracture of unsp lower leg, sequela
		S82.851S	Displaced trimalleolar fracture of right lower leg, sequela
		S82.852S	Displaced trimalleolar fracture of left lower leg, sequela
		S82.853S	Displaced trimalleolar fracture of unsp lower leg, sequela
		S82.854S	Nondisplaced trimalleolar fracture of r low leg, sequela
		S82.855S	Nondisplaced trimalleolar fracture of l low leg, sequela
		S82.856S	Nondisp trimalleolar fracture of unsp lower leg, sequela
		S82.861S	Displaced Maisonneuve's fracture of right leg, sequela
		S82.862S	Displaced Maisonneuve's fracture of left leg, sequela
		S82.863S	Displaced Maisonneuve's fracture of unspecified leg, sequela
		S82.864S	Nondisplaced Maisonneuve's fracture of right leg, sequela
		S82.865S	Nondisplaced Maisonneuve's fracture of left leg, sequela
		S82.866S	Nondisplaced Maisonneuve's fracture of unsp leg, sequela
		S82.871S	Displaced pilon fracture of right tibia, sequela
		S82.872S	Displaced pilon fracture of left tibia, sequela
		S82.873S	Displaced pilon fracture of unspecified tibia, sequela
		S82.874S	Nondisplaced pilon fracture of right tibia, sequela
		S82.875S	Nondisplaced pilon fracture of left tibia, sequela
		S82.876S	Nondisplaced pilon fracture of unspecified tibia, sequela
		S82.891S	Other fracture of right lower leg, sequela
		S82.892S	Other fracture of left lower leg, sequela
		S82.899S	Other fracture of unspecified lower leg, sequela
		S82.9ØXS	Unspecified fracture of unspecified lower leg, sequela
		S82.91XS	Unspecified fracture of right lower leg, sequela
		S82.92XS	Unspecified fracture of left lower leg, sequela
		S89.ØØ1S	Unsp physeal fracture of upper end of right tibia, sequela
		S89.ØØ2S	Unsp physeal fracture of upper end of left tibia, sequela
		S89.ØØ9S	Unsp physeal fracture of upper end of unsp tibia, sequela
		S89.Ø11S	Sltr-haris Type I physeal fx upper end of r tibia, sequela
		S89.Ø12S	Sltr-haris Type I physeal fx upper end of l tibia, sequela
		S89.Ø19S	Sltr-haris Type I physl fx upper end of unsp tibia, sequela
		S89.Ø21S	Sltr-haris Type II physeal fx upper end of r tibia, sequela
		S89.Ø22S	Sltr-haris Type II physeal fx upper end of l tibia, sequela
		S89.Ø29S	Sltr-haris Type II physl fx upper end of unsp tibia, sequela
		S89.Ø31S	Sltr-haris Type III physeal fx upper end of r tibia, sequela
		S89.Ø32S	Sltr-haris Type III physeal fx upper end of l tibia, sequela
		S89.Ø39S	Sltr-haris Type III physl fx upper end of unsp tibia, sqla
		S89.Ø41S	Sltr-haris Type IV physeal fx upper end of r tibia, sequela
		S89.Ø42S	Sltr-haris Type IV physeal fx upper end of l tibia, sequela
		S89.Ø49S	Sltr-haris Type IV physl fx upper end of unsp tibia, sequela
		S89.Ø91S	Other physeal fracture of upper end of right tibia, sequela
		S89.Ø92S	Other physeal fracture of upper end of left tibia, sequela
		S89.Ø99S	Other physeal fracture of upper end of unsp tibia, sequela
		S89.1Ø1S	Unsp physeal fracture of lower end of right tibia, sequela
		S89.1Ø2S	Unsp physeal fracture of lower end of left tibia, sequela
	(Continued on next page)	**S89.1Ø9S**	Unsp physeal fracture of lower end of unsp tibia, sequela

ICD-9-CM		ICD-10-CM	
905.4	LATE EFFECT OF FRACTURE OF LOWER EXTREMITIES **(Continued)**	**S89.111S**	Sltr-haris Type I physeal fx lower end of r tibia, sequela
		S89.112S	Sltr-haris Type I physeal fx lower end of l tibia, sequela
		S89.119S	Sltr-haris Type I physl fx lower end of unsp tibia, sequela
		S89.121S	Sltr-haris Type II physeal fx lower end of r tibia, sequela
		S89.122S	Sltr-haris Type II physeal fx lower end of l tibia, sequela
		S89.129S	Sltr-haris Type II physl fx lower end of unsp tibia, sequela
		S89.131S	Sltr-haris Type III physeal fx lower end of r tibia, sequela
		S89.132S	Sltr-haris Type III physeal fx lower end of l tibia, sequela
		S89.139S	Sltr-haris Type III physl fx lower end of unsp tibia, sqla
		S89.141S	Sltr-haris Type IV physeal fx lower end of r tibia, sequela
		S89.142S	Sltr-haris Type IV physeal fx lower end of l tibia, sequela
		S89.149S	Sltr-haris Type IV physl fx lower end of unsp tibia, sequela
		S89.191S	Other physeal fracture of lower end of right tibia, sequela
		S89.192S	Other physeal fracture of lower end of left tibia, sequela
		S89.199S	Other physeal fracture of lower end of unsp tibia, sequela
		S89.201S	Unsp physeal fracture of upper end of right fibula, sequela
		S89.202S	Unsp physeal fracture of upper end of left fibula, sequela
		S89.209S	Unsp physeal fracture of upper end of unsp fibula, sequela
		S89.211S	Sltr-haris Type I physeal fx upper end of r fibula, sequela
		S89.212S	Sltr-haris Type I physeal fx upper end of l fibula, sequela
		S89.219S	Sltr-haris Type I physl fx upper end of unsp fibula, sequela
		S89.221S	Sltr-haris Type II physeal fx upper end of r fibula, sequela
		S89.222S	Sltr-haris Type II physeal fx upper end of l fibula, sequela
		S89.229S	Sltr-haris Type II physl fx upper end of unsp fibula, sqla
		S89.291S	Other physeal fracture of upper end of right fibula, sequela
		S89.292S	Other physeal fracture of upper end of left fibula, sequela
		S89.299S	Other physeal fracture of upper end of unsp fibula, sequela
		S89.301S	Unsp physeal fracture of lower end of right fibula, sequela
		S89.302S	Unsp physeal fracture of lower end of left fibula, sequela
		S89.309S	Unsp physeal fracture of lower end of unsp fibula, sequela
		S89.311S	Sltr-haris Type I physeal fx lower end of r fibula, sequela
		S89.312S	Sltr-haris Type I physeal fx lower end of l fibula, sequela
		S89.319S	Sltr-haris Type I physl fx lower end of unsp fibula, sequela
		S89.321S	Sltr-haris Type II physeal fx lower end of r fibula, sequela
		S89.322S	Sltr-haris Type II physeal fx lower end of l fibula, sequela
		S89.329S	Sltr-haris Type II physl fx lower end of unsp fibula, sqla
		S89.391S	Other physeal fracture of lower end of right fibula, sequela
		S89.392S	Other physeal fracture of lower end of left fibula, sequela
		S89.399S	Other physeal fracture of lower end of unsp fibula, sequela
		S92.001S	Unspecified fracture of right calcaneus, sequela
		S92.002S	Unspecified fracture of left calcaneus, sequela
		S92.009S	Unspecified fracture of unspecified calcaneus, sequela
		S92.011S	Displaced fracture of body of right calcaneus, sequela
		S92.012S	Displaced fracture of body of left calcaneus, sequela
		S92.013S	Displaced fracture of body of unspecified calcaneus, sequela
		S92.014S	Nondisplaced fracture of body of right calcaneus, sequela
		S92.015S	Nondisplaced fracture of body of left calcaneus, sequela
		S92.016S	Nondisp fx of body of unspecified calcaneus, sequela
		S92.021S	Disp fx of anterior process of right calcaneus, sequela
		S92.022S	Disp fx of anterior process of left calcaneus, sequela
		S92.023S	Disp fx of anterior process of unsp calcaneus, sequela
		S92.024S	Nondisp fx of anterior process of right calcaneus, sequela
		S92.025S	Nondisp fx of anterior process of left calcaneus, sequela
		S92.026S	Nondisp fx of anterior process of unsp calcaneus, sequela
		S92.031S	Displaced avulsion fx tuberosity of r calcaneus, sequela
		S92.032S	Displaced avulsion fx tuberosity of l calcaneus, sequela
		S92.033S	Displaced avulsion fx tuberosity of unsp calcaneus, sequela
		S92.034S	Nondisp avulsion fx tuberosity of r calcaneus, sequela
		S92.035S	Nondisp avulsion fx tuberosity of l calcaneus, sequela
		S92.036S	Nondisp avulsion fx tuberosity of unsp calcaneus, sequela
		S92.041S	Displaced oth fracture of tuberosity of r calcaneus, sequela
		S92.042S	Displaced oth fracture of tuberosity of l calcaneus, sequela
		S92.043S	Displaced oth fx tuberosity of unsp calcaneus, sequela
		S92.044S	Nondisp oth fracture of tuberosity of r calcaneus, sequela
		S92.045S	Nondisp oth fracture of tuberosity of l calcaneus, sequela
		S92.046S	Nondisp oth fx tuberosity of unsp calcaneus, sequela
		S92.051S	Displaced oth extrartic fracture of r calcaneus, sequela
		S92.052S	Displaced oth extrartic fracture of left calcaneus, sequela
		S92.053S	Displaced oth extrartic fracture of unsp calcaneus, sequela
		S92.054S	Nondisplaced oth extrartic fracture of r calcaneus, sequela
		S92.055S	Nondisplaced oth extrartic fracture of l calcaneus, sequela
		S92.056S	Nondisp oth extrartic fracture of unsp calcaneus, sequela
		S92.061S	Displaced intraarticular fracture of r calcaneus, sequela
		S92.062S	Displaced intraarticular fracture of left calcaneus, sequela
		S92.063S	Displaced intraarticular fracture of unsp calcaneus, sequela
		S92.064S	Nondisplaced intraarticular fracture of r calcaneus, sequela
		S92.065S	Nondisplaced intartic fracture of left calcaneus, sequela
		S92.066S	Nondisplaced intartic fracture of unsp calcaneus, sequela
		S92.101S	Unspecified fracture of right talus, sequela
		S92.102S	Unspecified fracture of left talus, sequela
		S92.109S	Unspecified fracture of unspecified talus, sequela
	(Continued on next page)	**S92.111S**	Displaced fracture of neck of right talus, sequela

ICD-9-CM		ICD-10-CM	
905.4	LATE EFFECT OF FRACTURE OF LOWER EXTREMITIES **(Continued)**	**S92.112S**	Displaced fracture of neck of left talus, sequela
		S92.113S	Displaced fracture of neck of unspecified talus, sequela
		S92.114S	Nondisplaced fracture of neck of right talus, sequela
		S92.115S	Nondisplaced fracture of neck of left talus, sequela
		S92.116S	Nondisplaced fracture of neck of unspecified talus, sequela
		S92.121S	Displaced fracture of body of right talus, sequela
		S92.122S	Displaced fracture of body of left talus, sequela
		S92.123S	Displaced fracture of body of unspecified talus, sequela
		S92.124S	Nondisplaced fracture of body of right talus, sequela
		S92.125S	Nondisplaced fracture of body of left talus, sequela
		S92.126S	Nondisplaced fracture of body of unspecified talus, sequela
		S92.131S	Disp fx of posterior process of right talus, sequela
		S92.132S	Disp fx of posterior process of left talus, sequela
		S92.133S	Disp fx of posterior process of unspecified talus, sequela
		S92.134S	Nondisp fx of posterior process of right talus, sequela
		S92.135S	Nondisp fx of posterior process of left talus, sequela
		S92.136S	Nondisp fx of posterior process of unsp talus, sequela
		S92.141S	Displaced dome fracture of right talus, sequela
		S92.142S	Displaced dome fracture of left talus, sequela
		S92.143S	Displaced dome fracture of unspecified talus, sequela
		S92.144S	Nondisplaced dome fracture of right talus, sequela
		S92.145S	Nondisplaced dome fracture of left talus, sequela
		S92.146S	Nondisplaced dome fracture of unspecified talus, sequela
		S92.151S	Displ avuls fracture (chip fracture) of right talus, sequela
		S92.152S	Displ avuls fracture (chip fracture) of left talus, sequela
		S92.153S	Displ avuls fracture (chip fracture) of unsp talus, sequela
		S92.154S	Nondisp avuls fx (chip fracture) of right talus, sequela
		S92.155S	Nondisp avuls fx (chip fracture) of left talus, sequela
		S92.156S	Nondisp avuls fx (chip fracture) of unsp talus, sequela
		S92.191S	Other fracture of right talus, sequela
		S92.192S	Other fracture of left talus, sequela
		S92.199S	Other fracture of unspecified talus, sequela
		S92.201S	Fracture of unsp tarsal bone(s) of right foot, sequela
		S92.202S	Fracture of unspecified tarsal bone(s) of left foot, sequela
		S92.209S	Fracture of unsp tarsal bone(s) of unspecified foot, sequela
		S92.211S	Displaced fracture of cuboid bone of right foot, sequela
		S92.212S	Displaced fracture of cuboid bone of left foot, sequela
		S92.213S	Disp fx of cuboid bone of unspecified foot, sequela
		S92.214S	Nondisplaced fracture of cuboid bone of right foot, sequela
		S92.215S	Nondisplaced fracture of cuboid bone of left foot, sequela
		S92.216S	Nondisp fx of cuboid bone of unspecified foot, sequela
		S92.221S	Disp fx of lateral cuneiform of right foot, sequela
		S92.222S	Disp fx of lateral cuneiform of left foot, sequela
		S92.223S	Disp fx of lateral cuneiform of unspecified foot, sequela
		S92.224S	Nondisp fx of lateral cuneiform of right foot, sequela
		S92.225S	Nondisp fx of lateral cuneiform of left foot, sequela
		S92.226S	Nondisp fx of lateral cuneiform of unspecified foot, sequela
		S92.231S	Disp fx of intermediate cuneiform of right foot, sequela
		S92.232S	Disp fx of intermediate cuneiform of left foot, sequela
		S92.233S	Disp fx of intermediate cuneiform of unsp foot, sequela
		S92.234S	Nondisp fx of intermediate cuneiform of right foot, sequela
		S92.235S	Nondisp fx of intermediate cuneiform of left foot, sequela
		S92.236S	Nondisp fx of intermediate cuneiform of unsp foot, sequela
		S92.241S	Disp fx of medial cuneiform of right foot, sequela
		S92.242S	Displaced fracture of medial cuneiform of left foot, sequela
		S92.243S	Disp fx of medial cuneiform of unspecified foot, sequela
		S92.244S	Nondisp fx of medial cuneiform of right foot, sequela
		S92.245S	Nondisp fx of medial cuneiform of left foot, sequela
		S92.246S	Nondisp fx of medial cuneiform of unspecified foot, sequela
		S92.251S	Displaced fracture of navicular of right foot, sequela
		S92.252S	Displaced fracture of navicular of left foot, sequela
		S92.253S	Displaced fracture of navicular of unspecified foot, sequela
		S92.254S	Nondisplaced fracture of navicular of right foot, sequela
		S92.255S	Nondisplaced fracture of navicular of left foot, sequela
		S92.256S	Nondisp fx of navicular of unspecified foot, sequela
		S92.301S	Fracture of unsp metatarsal bone(s), right foot, sequela
		S92.302S	Fracture of unsp metatarsal bone(s), left foot, sequela
		S92.309S	Fracture of unsp metatarsal bone(s), unsp foot, sequela
		S92.311S	Disp fx of first metatarsal bone, right foot, sequela
		S92.312S	Disp fx of first metatarsal bone, left foot, sequela
		S92.313S	Disp fx of first metatarsal bone, unspecified foot, sequela
		S92.314S	Nondisp fx of first metatarsal bone, right foot, sequela
		S92.315S	Nondisp fx of first metatarsal bone, left foot, sequela
		S92.316S	Nondisp fx of first metatarsal bone, unsp foot, sequela
		S92.321S	Disp fx of second metatarsal bone, right foot, sequela
		S92.322S	Disp fx of second metatarsal bone, left foot, sequela
		S92.323S	Disp fx of second metatarsal bone, unspecified foot, sequela
		S92.324S	Nondisp fx of second metatarsal bone, right foot, sequela
		S92.325S	Nondisp fx of second metatarsal bone, left foot, sequela
		S92.326S	Nondisp fx of second metatarsal bone, unsp foot, sequela
		S92.331S	Disp fx of third metatarsal bone, right foot, sequela
905.4	**(Continued on next page)**	**S92.332S**	Disp fx of third metatarsal bone, left foot, sequela

ICD-9-CM		ICD-10-CM	
905.4	LATE EFFECT OF FRACTURE OF LOWER EXTREMITIES **(Continued)**	**S92.333S**	Disp fx of third metatarsal bone, unspecified foot, sequela
		S92.334S	Nondisp fx of third metatarsal bone, right foot, sequela
		S92.335S	Nondisp fx of third metatarsal bone, left foot, sequela
		S92.336S	Nondisp fx of third metatarsal bone, unsp foot, sequela
		S92.341S	Disp fx of fourth metatarsal bone, right foot, sequela
		S92.342S	Disp fx of fourth metatarsal bone, left foot, sequela
		S92.343S	Disp fx of fourth metatarsal bone, unspecified foot, sequela
		S92.344S	Nondisp fx of fourth metatarsal bone, right foot, sequela
		S92.345S	Nondisp fx of fourth metatarsal bone, left foot, sequela
		S92.346S	Nondisp fx of fourth metatarsal bone, unsp foot, sequela
		S92.351S	Disp fx of fifth metatarsal bone, right foot, sequela
		S92.352S	Disp fx of fifth metatarsal bone, left foot, sequela
		S92.353S	Disp fx of fifth metatarsal bone, unspecified foot, sequela
		S92.354S	Nondisp fx of fifth metatarsal bone, right foot, sequela
		S92.355S	Nondisp fx of fifth metatarsal bone, left foot, sequela
		S92.356S	Nondisp fx of fifth metatarsal bone, unsp foot, sequela
		S92.401S	Displaced unspecified fracture of right great toe, sequela
		S92.402S	Displaced unspecified fracture of left great toe, sequela
		S92.403S	Displaced unsp fracture of unspecified great toe, sequela
		S92.404S	Nondisplaced unsp fracture of right great toe, sequela
		S92.405S	Nondisplaced unspecified fracture of left great toe, sequela
		S92.406S	Nondisplaced unsp fracture of unspecified great toe, sequela
		S92.411S	Disp fx of proximal phalanx of right great toe, sequela
		S92.412S	Disp fx of proximal phalanx of left great toe, sequela
		S92.413S	Disp fx of proximal phalanx of unsp great toe, sequela
		S92.414S	Nondisp fx of proximal phalanx of right great toe, sequela
		S92.415S	Nondisp fx of proximal phalanx of left great toe, sequela
		S92.416S	Nondisp fx of proximal phalanx of unsp great toe, sequela
		S92.421S	Disp fx of distal phalanx of right great toe, sequela
		S92.422S	Disp fx of distal phalanx of left great toe, sequela
		S92.423S	Disp fx of distal phalanx of unspecified great toe, sequela
		S92.424S	Nondisp fx of distal phalanx of right great toe, sequela
		S92.425S	Nondisp fx of distal phalanx of left great toe, sequela
		S92.426S	Nondisp fx of distal phalanx of unsp great toe, sequela
		S92.491S	Other fracture of right great toe, sequela
		S92.492S	Other fracture of left great toe, sequela
		S92.499S	Other fracture of unspecified great toe, sequela
		S92.501S	Displaced unsp fracture of right lesser toe(s), sequela
		S92.502S	Displaced unsp fracture of left lesser toe(s), sequela
		S92.503S	Displaced unsp fracture of unsp lesser toe(s), sequela
		S92.504S	Nondisplaced unsp fracture of right lesser toe(s), sequela
		S92.505S	Nondisplaced unsp fracture of left lesser toe(s), sequela
		S92.506S	Nondisplaced unsp fracture of unsp lesser toe(s), sequela
		S92.511S	Disp fx of proximal phalanx of right lesser toe(s), sequela
		S92.512S	Disp fx of proximal phalanx of left lesser toe(s), sequela
		S92.513S	Disp fx of proximal phalanx of unsp lesser toe(s), sequela
		S92.514S	Nondisp fx of prox phalanx of right lesser toe(s), sequela
		S92.515S	Nondisp fx of prox phalanx of left lesser toe(s), sequela
		S92.516S	Nondisp fx of prox phalanx of unsp lesser toe(s), sequela
		S92.521S	Disp fx of medial phalanx of right lesser toe(s), sequela
		S92.522S	Disp fx of medial phalanx of left lesser toe(s), sequela
		S92.523S	Disp fx of medial phalanx of unsp lesser toe(s), sequela
		S92.524S	Nondisp fx of medial phalanx of right lesser toe(s), sequela
		S92.525S	Nondisp fx of medial phalanx of left lesser toe(s), sequela
		S92.526S	Nondisp fx of medial phalanx of unsp lesser toe(s), sequela
		S92.531S	Disp fx of distal phalanx of right lesser toe(s), sequela
		S92.532S	Disp fx of distal phalanx of left lesser toe(s), sequela
		S92.533S	Disp fx of distal phalanx of unsp lesser toe(s), sequela
		S92.534S	Nondisp fx of distal phalanx of right lesser toe(s), sequela
		S92.535S	Nondisp fx of distal phalanx of left lesser toe(s), sequela
		S92.536S	Nondisp fx of distal phalanx of unsp lesser toe(s), sequela
		S92.591S	Other fracture of right lesser toe(s), sequela
		S92.592S	Other fracture of left lesser toe(s), sequela
		S92.599S	Other fracture of unspecified lesser toe(s), sequela
		S92.901S	Unspecified fracture of right foot, sequela
		S92.902S	Unspecified fracture of left foot, sequela
		S92.909S	Unspecified fracture of unspecified foot, sequela
		S92.911S	Unspecified fracture of right toe(s), sequela
		S92.912S	Unspecified fracture of left toe(s), sequela
		S92.919S	Unspecified fracture of unspecified toe(s), sequela
905.5	LATE EFFECT FRACTURE MULTIPLE&UNSPECIFIED BONES	**M80.00XS**	Age-rel osteopor w current path fracture, unsp site, sequela
		M80.80XS	Oth osteopor w current path fracture, unsp site, sequela
		M84.30XS	Stress fracture, unspecified site, sequela
		M84.38XS	Stress fracture, other site, sequela
		M84.40XS	Pathological fracture, unspecified site, sequela
		M84.48XS	Pathological fracture, other site, sequela
		M84.50XS	Path fracture in neoplastic disease, unsp site, sequela
		M84.60XS	Pathological fracture in other disease, unsp site, sequela
		M84.68XS	Pathological fracture in other disease, other site, sequela

ICD-9-CM		ICD-10-CM	
905.6	LATE EFFECT OF DISLOCATION	**S03.0XXS**	Dislocation of jaw, sequela
		S03.1XXS	Dislocation of septal cartilage of nose, sequela
		S13.0XXS	Traumatic rupture of cervical intervertebral disc, sequela
		S13.100S	Subluxation of unspecified cervical vertebrae, sequela
		S13.101S	Dislocation of unspecified cervical vertebrae, sequela
		S13.110S	Subluxation of C0/C1 cervical vertebrae, sequela
		S13.111S	Dislocation of C0/C1 cervical vertebrae, sequela
		S13.120S	Subluxation of C1/C2 cervical vertebrae, sequela
		S13.121S	Dislocation of C1/C2 cervical vertebrae, sequela
		S13.130S	Subluxation of C2/C3 cervical vertebrae, sequela
		S13.131S	Dislocation of C2/C3 cervical vertebrae, sequela
		S13.140S	Subluxation of C3/C4 cervical vertebrae, sequela
		S13.141S	Dislocation of C3/C4 cervical vertebrae, sequela
		S13.150S	Subluxation of C4/C5 cervical vertebrae, sequela
		S13.151S	Dislocation of C4/C5 cervical vertebrae, sequela
		S13.160S	Subluxation of C5/C6 cervical vertebrae, sequela
		S13.161S	Dislocation of C5/C6 cervical vertebrae, sequela
		S13.170S	Subluxation of C6/C7 cervical vertebrae, sequela
		S13.171S	Dislocation of C6/C7 cervical vertebrae, sequela
		S13.180S	Subluxation of C7/T1 cervical vertebrae, sequela
		S13.181S	Dislocation of C7/T1 cervical vertebrae, sequela
		S13.20XS	Dislocation of unspecified parts of neck, sequela
		S13.29XS	Dislocation of other parts of neck, sequela
		S23.0XXS	Traumatic rupture of thoracic intervertebral disc, sequela
		S23.100S	Subluxation of unspecified thoracic vertebra, sequela
		S23.101S	Dislocation of unspecified thoracic vertebra, sequela
		S23.110S	Subluxation of T1/T2 thoracic vertebra, sequela
		S23.111S	Dislocation of T1/T2 thoracic vertebra, sequela
		S23.120S	Subluxation of T2/T3 thoracic vertebra, sequela
		S23.121S	Dislocation of T2/T3 thoracic vertebra, sequela
		S23.122S	Subluxation of T3/T4 thoracic vertebra, sequela
		S23.123S	Dislocation of T3/T4 thoracic vertebra, sequela
		S23.130S	Subluxation of T4/T5 thoracic vertebra, sequela
		S23.131S	Dislocation of T4/T5 thoracic vertebra, sequela
		S23.132S	Subluxation of T5/T6 thoracic vertebra, sequela
		S23.133S	Dislocation of T5/T6 thoracic vertebra, sequela
		S23.140S	Subluxation of T6/T7 thoracic vertebra, sequela
		S23.141S	Dislocation of T6/T7 thoracic vertebra, sequela
		S23.142S	Subluxation of T7/T8 thoracic vertebra, sequela
		S23.143S	Dislocation of T7/T8 thoracic vertebra, sequela
		S23.150S	Subluxation of T8/T9 thoracic vertebra, sequela
		S23.151S	Dislocation of T8/T9 thoracic vertebra, sequela
		S23.152S	Subluxation of T9/T10 thoracic vertebra, sequela
		S23.153S	Dislocation of T9/T10 thoracic vertebra, sequela
		S23.160S	Subluxation of T10/T11 thoracic vertebra, sequela
		S23.161S	Dislocation of T10/T11 thoracic vertebra, sequela
		S23.162S	Subluxation of T11/T12 thoracic vertebra, sequela
		S23.163S	Dislocation of T11/T12 thoracic vertebra, sequela
		S23.170S	Subluxation of T12/L1 thoracic vertebra, sequela
		S23.171S	Dislocation of T12/L1 thoracic vertebra, sequela
		S23.20XS	Dislocation of unspecified part of thorax, sequela
		S23.29XS	Dislocation of other parts of thorax, sequela
		S33.0XXS	Traumatic rupture of lumbar intervertebral disc, sequela
		S33.100S	Subluxation of unspecified lumbar vertebra, sequela
		S33.101S	Dislocation of unspecified lumbar vertebra, sequela
		S33.110S	Subluxation of L1/L2 lumbar vertebra, sequela
		S33.111S	Dislocation of L1/L2 lumbar vertebra, sequela
		S33.120S	Subluxation of L2/L3 lumbar vertebra, sequela
		S33.121S	Dislocation of L2/L3 lumbar vertebra, sequela
		S33.130S	Subluxation of L3/L4 lumbar vertebra, sequela
		S33.131S	Dislocation of L3/L4 lumbar vertebra, sequela
		S33.140S	Subluxation of L4/L5 lumbar vertebra, sequela
		S33.141S	Dislocation of L4/L5 lumbar vertebra, sequela
		S33.2XXS	Dislocation of sacroiliac and sacrococcygeal joint, sequela
		S33.30XS	Dislocation of unsp parts of lumbar spine & pelvis, sequela
		S33.39XS	Dislocation of oth parts of lumbar spine and pelvis, sequela
		S43.001S	Unspecified subluxation of right shoulder joint, sequela
		S43.002S	Unspecified subluxation of left shoulder joint, sequela
		S43.003S	Unsp subluxation of unspecified shoulder joint, sequela
		S43.004S	Unspecified dislocation of right shoulder joint, sequela
		S43.005S	Unspecified dislocation of left shoulder joint, sequela
		S43.006S	Unsp dislocation of unspecified shoulder joint, sequela
		S43.011S	Anterior subluxation of right humerus, sequela
		S43.012S	Anterior subluxation of left humerus, sequela
		S43.013S	Anterior subluxation of unspecified humerus, sequela
		S43.014S	Anterior dislocation of right humerus, sequela
		S43.015S	Anterior dislocation of left humerus, sequela
		S43.016S	Anterior dislocation of unspecified humerus, sequela
		S43.021S	Posterior subluxation of right humerus, sequela
		S43.022S	Posterior subluxation of left humerus, sequela
		S43.023S	Posterior subluxation of unspecified humerus, sequela
	(Continued on next page)	**S43.024S**	Posterior dislocation of right humerus, sequela

ICD-9-CM		ICD-10-CM	
905.6	LATE EFFECT OF DISLOCATION **(Continued)**	**S43.025S**	Posterior dislocation of left humerus, sequela
		S43.026S	Posterior dislocation of unspecified humerus, sequela
		S43.031S	Inferior subluxation of right humerus, sequela
		S43.032S	Inferior subluxation of left humerus, sequela
		S43.033S	Inferior subluxation of unspecified humerus, sequela
		S43.034S	Inferior dislocation of right humerus, sequela
		S43.035S	Inferior dislocation of left humerus, sequela
		S43.036S	Inferior dislocation of unspecified humerus, sequela
		S43.081S	Other subluxation of right shoulder joint, sequela
		S43.082S	Other subluxation of left shoulder joint, sequela
		S43.083S	Other subluxation of unspecified shoulder joint, sequela
		S43.084S	Other dislocation of right shoulder joint, sequela
		S43.085S	Other dislocation of left shoulder joint, sequela
		S43.086S	Other dislocation of unspecified shoulder joint, sequela
		S43.101S	Unsp dislocation of right acromioclavicular joint, sequela
		S43.102S	Unsp dislocation of left acromioclavicular joint, sequela
		S43.109S	Unsp dislocation of unsp acromioclavicular joint, sequela
		S43.111S	Subluxation of right acromioclavicular joint, sequela
		S43.112S	Subluxation of left acromioclavicular joint, sequela
		S43.119S	Subluxation of unspecified acromioclavicular joint, sequela
		S43.121S	Disloc of r acromioclav jt, 100%-200% displacmnt, sequela
		S43.122S	Disloc of l acromioclav jt, 100%-200% displacmnt, sequela
		S43.129S	Disloc of unsp acromioclav jt, 100%-200% displacmnt, sequela
		S43.131S	Dislocation of r acromioclav jt, > 200% displacmnt, sequela
		S43.132S	Dislocation of l acromioclav jt, > 200% displacmnt, sequela
		S43.139S	Disloc of unsp acromioclav jt, > 200% displacmnt, sequela
		S43.141S	Inferior dislocation of r acromioclav jt, sequela
		S43.142S	Inferior dislocation of l acromioclav jt, sequela
		S43.149S	Inferior dislocation of unsp acromioclav jt, sequela
		S43.151S	Posterior dislocation of r acromioclav jt, sequela
		S43.152S	Posterior dislocation of l acromioclav jt, sequela
		S43.159S	Posterior dislocation of unsp acromioclav jt, sequela
		S43.201S	Unsp subluxation of right sternoclavicular joint, sequela
		S43.202S	Unsp subluxation of left sternoclavicular joint, sequela
		S43.203S	Unsp subluxation of unsp sternoclavicular joint, sequela
		S43.204S	Unsp dislocation of right sternoclavicular joint, sequela
		S43.205S	Unsp dislocation of left sternoclavicular joint, sequela
		S43.206S	Unsp dislocation of unsp sternoclavicular joint, sequela
		S43.211S	Anterior subluxation of r sternoclav jt, sequela
		S43.212S	Anterior subluxation of left sternoclavicular joint, sequela
		S43.213S	Anterior subluxation of unsp sternoclavicular joint, sequela
		S43.214S	Anterior dislocation of r sternoclav jt, sequela
		S43.215S	Anterior dislocation of left sternoclavicular joint, sequela
		S43.216S	Anterior dislocation of unsp sternoclavicular joint, sequela
		S43.221S	Posterior subluxation of r sternoclav jt, sequela
		S43.222S	Posterior subluxation of l sternoclav jt, sequela
		S43.223S	Posterior subluxation of unsp sternoclav jt, sequela
		S43.224S	Posterior dislocation of r sternoclav jt, sequela
		S43.225S	Posterior dislocation of l sternoclav jt, sequela
		S43.226S	Posterior dislocation of unsp sternoclav jt, sequela
		S43.301S	Subluxation of unsp parts of right shoulder girdle, sequela
		S43.302S	Subluxation of unsp parts of left shoulder girdle, sequela
		S43.303S	Subluxation of unsp parts of unsp shoulder girdle, sequela
		S43.304S	Dislocation of unsp parts of right shoulder girdle, sequela
		S43.305S	Dislocation of unsp parts of left shoulder girdle, sequela
		S43.306S	Dislocation of unsp parts of unsp shoulder girdle, sequela
		S43.311S	Subluxation of right scapula, sequela
		S43.312S	Subluxation of left scapula, sequela
		S43.313S	Subluxation of unspecified scapula, sequela
		S43.314S	Dislocation of right scapula, sequela
		S43.315S	Dislocation of left scapula, sequela
		S43.316S	Dislocation of unspecified scapula, sequela
		S43.391S	Subluxation of other parts of right shoulder girdle, sequela
		S43.392S	Subluxation of other parts of left shoulder girdle, sequela
		S43.393S	Subluxation of other parts of unsp shoulder girdle, sequela
		S43.394S	Dislocation of other parts of right shoulder girdle, sequela
		S43.395S	Dislocation of other parts of left shoulder girdle, sequela
		S43.396S	Dislocation of other parts of unsp shoulder girdle, sequela
		S53.001S	Unspecified subluxation of right radial head, sequela
		S53.002S	Unspecified subluxation of left radial head, sequela
		S53.003S	Unspecified subluxation of unspecified radial head, sequela
		S53.004S	Unspecified dislocation of right radial head, sequela
		S53.005S	Unspecified dislocation of left radial head, sequela
		S53.006S	Unspecified dislocation of unspecified radial head, sequela
		S53.011S	Anterior subluxation of right radial head, sequela
		S53.012S	Anterior subluxation of left radial head, sequela
		S53.013S	Anterior subluxation of unspecified radial head, sequela
		S53.014S	Anterior dislocation of right radial head, sequela
		S53.015S	Anterior dislocation of left radial head, sequela
		S53.016S	Anterior dislocation of unspecified radial head, sequela
		S53.021S	Posterior subluxation of right radial head, sequela
905.6	**(Continued on next page)**	**S53.022S**	Posterior subluxation of left radial head, sequela

ICD-9-CM		ICD-10-CM	
905.6	LATE EFFECT OF DISLOCATION **(Continued)**	**S53.023S**	Posterior subluxation of unspecified radial head, sequela
		S53.024S	Posterior dislocation of right radial head, sequela
		S53.025S	Posterior dislocation of left radial head, sequela
		S53.026S	Posterior dislocation of unspecified radial head, sequela
		S53.031S	Nursemaid's elbow, right elbow, sequela
		S53.032S	Nursemaid's elbow, left elbow, sequela
		S53.033S	Nursemaid's elbow, unspecified elbow, sequela
		S53.091S	Other subluxation of right radial head, sequela
		S53.092S	Other subluxation of left radial head, sequela
		S53.093S	Other subluxation of unspecified radial head, sequela
		S53.094S	Other dislocation of right radial head, sequela
		S53.095S	Other dislocation of left radial head, sequela
		S53.096S	Other dislocation of unspecified radial head, sequela
		S53.101S	Unspecified subluxation of right ulnohumeral joint, sequela
		S53.102S	Unspecified subluxation of left ulnohumeral joint, sequela
		S53.103S	Unsp subluxation of unspecified ulnohumeral joint, sequela
		S53.104S	Unspecified dislocation of right ulnohumeral joint, sequela
		S53.105S	Unspecified dislocation of left ulnohumeral joint, sequela
		S53.106S	Unsp dislocation of unspecified ulnohumeral joint, sequela
		S53.111S	Anterior subluxation of right ulnohumeral joint, sequela
		S53.112S	Anterior subluxation of left ulnohumeral joint, sequela
		S53.113S	Anterior subluxation of unsp ulnohumeral joint, sequela
		S53.114S	Anterior dislocation of right ulnohumeral joint, sequela
		S53.115S	Anterior dislocation of left ulnohumeral joint, sequela
		S53.116S	Anterior dislocation of unsp ulnohumeral joint, sequela
		S53.121S	Posterior subluxation of right ulnohumeral joint, sequela
		S53.122S	Posterior subluxation of left ulnohumeral joint, sequela
		S53.123S	Posterior subluxation of unsp ulnohumeral joint, sequela
		S53.124S	Posterior dislocation of right ulnohumeral joint, sequela
		S53.125S	Posterior dislocation of left ulnohumeral joint, sequela
		S53.126S	Posterior dislocation of unsp ulnohumeral joint, sequela
		S53.131S	Medial subluxation of right ulnohumeral joint, sequela
		S53.132S	Medial subluxation of left ulnohumeral joint, sequela
		S53.133S	Medial subluxation of unspecified ulnohumeral joint, sequela
		S53.134S	Medial dislocation of right ulnohumeral joint, sequela
		S53.135S	Medial dislocation of left ulnohumeral joint, sequela
		S53.136S	Medial dislocation of unspecified ulnohumeral joint, sequela
		S53.141S	Lateral subluxation of right ulnohumeral joint, sequela
		S53.142S	Lateral subluxation of left ulnohumeral joint, sequela
		S53.143S	Lateral subluxation of unsp ulnohumeral joint, sequela
		S53.144S	Lateral dislocation of right ulnohumeral joint, sequela
		S53.145S	Lateral dislocation of left ulnohumeral joint, sequela
		S53.146S	Lateral dislocation of unsp ulnohumeral joint, sequela
		S53.191S	Other subluxation of right ulnohumeral joint, sequela
		S53.192S	Other subluxation of left ulnohumeral joint, sequela
		S53.193S	Other subluxation of unspecified ulnohumeral joint, sequela
		S53.194S	Other dislocation of right ulnohumeral joint, sequela
		S53.195S	Other dislocation of left ulnohumeral joint, sequela
		S53.196S	Other dislocation of unspecified ulnohumeral joint, sequela
		S63.001S	Unspecified subluxation of right wrist and hand, sequela
		S63.002S	Unspecified subluxation of left wrist and hand, sequela
		S63.003S	Unsp subluxation of unspecified wrist and hand, sequela
		S63.004S	Unspecified dislocation of right wrist and hand, sequela
		S63.005S	Unspecified dislocation of left wrist and hand, sequela
		S63.006S	Unsp dislocation of unspecified wrist and hand, sequela
		S63.011S	Subluxation of distal radioulnar joint of r wrist, sequela
		S63.012S	Sublux of distal radioulnar joint of left wrist, sequela
		S63.013S	Sublux of distal radioulnar joint of unsp wrist, sequela
		S63.014S	Disloc of distal radioulnar joint of right wrist, sequela
		S63.015S	Disloc of distal radioulnar joint of left wrist, sequela
		S63.016S	Disloc of distal radioulnar joint of unsp wrist, sequela
		S63.021S	Subluxation of radiocarpal joint of right wrist, sequela
		S63.022S	Subluxation of radiocarpal joint of left wrist, sequela
		S63.023S	Subluxation of radiocarpal joint of unsp wrist, sequela
		S63.024S	Dislocation of radiocarpal joint of right wrist, sequela
		S63.025S	Dislocation of radiocarpal joint of left wrist, sequela
		S63.026S	Dislocation of radiocarpal joint of unsp wrist, sequela
		S63.031S	Subluxation of midcarpal joint of right wrist, sequela
		S63.032S	Subluxation of midcarpal joint of left wrist, sequela
		S63.033S	Subluxation of midcarpal joint of unspecified wrist, sequela
		S63.034S	Dislocation of midcarpal joint of right wrist, sequela
		S63.035S	Dislocation of midcarpal joint of left wrist, sequela
		S63.036S	Dislocation of midcarpal joint of unspecified wrist, sequela
		S63.041S	Subluxation of carpometacarpal joint of right thumb, sequela
		S63.042S	Subluxation of carpometacarpal joint of left thumb, sequela
		S63.043S	Subluxation of carpometacarpal joint of unsp thumb, sequela
		S63.044S	Dislocation of carpometacarpal joint of right thumb, sequela
		S63.045S	Dislocation of carpometacarpal joint of left thumb, sequela
		S63.046S	Dislocation of carpometacarpal joint of unsp thumb, sequela
		S63.051S	Subluxation of carpometacarpal joint of right hand, sequela
		S63.052S	Subluxation of carpometacarpal joint of left hand, sequela
	(Continued on next page)	**S63.053S**	Subluxation of carpometacarpal joint of unsp hand, sequela

ICD-9-CM		ICD-10-CM	
905.6	LATE EFFECT OF DISLOCATION **(Continued)**	**S63.054S**	Dislocation of carpometacarpal joint of right hand, sequela
		S63.055S	Dislocation of carpometacarpal joint of left hand, sequela
		S63.056S	Dislocation of carpometacarpal joint of unsp hand, sequela
		S63.061S	Sublux of MC (bone), proximal end of right hand, sequela
		S63.062S	Sublux of MC (bone), proximal end of left hand, sequela
		S63.063S	Sublux of MC (bone), proximal end of unsp hand, sequela
		S63.064S	Disloc of MC (bone), proximal end of right hand, sequela
		S63.065S	Disloc of MC (bone), proximal end of left hand, sequela
		S63.066S	Disloc of MC (bone), proximal end of unsp hand, sequela
		S63.071S	Subluxation of distal end of right ulna, sequela
		S63.072S	Subluxation of distal end of left ulna, sequela
		S63.073S	Subluxation of distal end of unspecified ulna, sequela
		S63.074S	Dislocation of distal end of right ulna, sequela
		S63.075S	Dislocation of distal end of left ulna, sequela
		S63.076S	Dislocation of distal end of unspecified ulna, sequela
		S63.091S	Other subluxation of right wrist and hand, sequela
		S63.092S	Other subluxation of left wrist and hand, sequela
		S63.093S	Other subluxation of unspecified wrist and hand, sequela
		S63.094S	Other dislocation of right wrist and hand, sequela
		S63.095S	Other dislocation of left wrist and hand, sequela
		S63.096S	Other dislocation of unspecified wrist and hand, sequela
		S63.101S	Unspecified subluxation of right thumb, sequela
		S63.102S	Unspecified subluxation of left thumb, sequela
		S63.103S	Unspecified subluxation of unspecified thumb, sequela
		S63.104S	Unspecified dislocation of right thumb, sequela
		S63.105S	Unspecified dislocation of left thumb, sequela
		S63.106S	Unspecified dislocation of unspecified thumb, sequela
		S63.111S	Subluxation of MCP joint of right thumb, sequela
		S63.112S	Subluxation of MCP joint of left thumb, sequela
		S63.113S	Subluxation of metacarpophalangeal joint of thmb, sequela
		S63.114S	Dislocation of MCP joint of right thumb, sequela
		S63.115S	Dislocation of MCP joint of left thumb, sequela
		S63.116S	Dislocation of metacarpophalangeal joint of thmb, sequela
		S63.121S	Subluxation of unsp interphaln joint of right thumb, sequela
		S63.122S	Subluxation of unsp interphaln joint of left thumb, sequela
		S63.123S	Subluxation of unsp interphalangeal joint of thmb, sequela
		S63.124S	Dislocation of unsp interphaln joint of right thumb, sequela
		S63.125S	Dislocation of unsp interphaln joint of left thumb, sequela
		S63.126S	Dislocation of unsp interphalangeal joint of thmb, sequela
		S63.131S	Subluxation of proximal interphaln joint of r thm, sequela
		S63.132S	Sublux of proximal interphaln joint of left thumb, sequela
		S63.133S	Subluxation of proximal interphaln joint of thmb, sequela
		S63.134S	Disloc of proximal interphaln joint of right thumb, sequela
		S63.135S	Disloc of proximal interphaln joint of left thumb, sequela
		S63.136S	Dislocation of proximal interphaln joint of thmb, sequela
		S63.141S	Subluxation of distal interphaln joint of r thm, sequela
		S63.142S	Sublux of distal interphaln joint of left thumb, sequela
		S63.143S	Subluxation of distal interphalangeal joint of thmb, sequela
		S63.144S	Disloc of distal interphaln joint of right thumb, sequela
		S63.145S	Disloc of distal interphaln joint of left thumb, sequela
		S63.146S	Dislocation of distal interphalangeal joint of thmb, sequela
		S63.200S	Unspecified subluxation of right index finger, sequela
		S63.201S	Unspecified subluxation of left index finger, sequela
		S63.202S	Unspecified subluxation of right middle finger, sequela
		S63.203S	Unspecified subluxation of left middle finger, sequela
		S63.204S	Unspecified subluxation of right ring finger, sequela
		S63.205S	Unspecified subluxation of left ring finger, sequela
		S63.206S	Unspecified subluxation of right little finger, sequela
		S63.207S	Unspecified subluxation of left little finger, sequela
		S63.208S	Unspecified subluxation of other finger, sequela
		S63.209S	Unspecified subluxation of unspecified finger, sequela
		S63.210S	Subluxation of MCP joint of right index finger, sequela
		S63.211S	Subluxation of MCP joint of left index finger, sequela
		S63.212S	Subluxation of MCP joint of right middle finger, sequela
		S63.213S	Subluxation of MCP joint of left middle finger, sequela
		S63.214S	Subluxation of MCP joint of right ring finger, sequela
		S63.215S	Subluxation of MCP joint of left ring finger, sequela
		S63.216S	Subluxation of MCP joint of right little finger, sequela
		S63.217S	Subluxation of MCP joint of left little finger, sequela
		S63.218S	Subluxation of metacarpophalangeal joint of finger, sequela
		S63.219S	Subluxation of MCP joint of unsp finger, sequela
		S63.220S	Subluxation of unsp interphaln joint of r idx fngr, sequela
		S63.221S	Subluxation of unsp interphaln joint of l idx fngr, sequela
		S63.222S	Sublux of unsp interphaln joint of r mid finger, sequela
		S63.223S	Sublux of unsp interphaln joint of l mid finger, sequela
		S63.224S	Subluxation of unsp interphaln joint of r rng fngr, sequela
		S63.225S	Subluxation of unsp interphaln joint of l rng fngr, sequela
		S63.226S	Sublux of unsp interphaln joint of r little finger, sequela
		S63.227S	Sublux of unsp interphaln joint of l little finger, sequela
		S63.228S	Subluxation of unsp interphalangeal joint of finger, sequela
		S63.229S	Subluxation of unsp interphaln joint of unsp finger, sequela
	(Continued on next page)	**S63.230S**	Sublux of proximal interphaln joint of r idx fngr, sequela

ICD-9-CM		ICD-10-CM	
905.6	LATE EFFECT OF DISLOCATION **(Continued)**	**S63.231S**	Sublux of proximal interphaln joint of l idx fngr, sequela
		S63.232S	Sublux of proximal interphaln joint of r mid finger, sequela
		S63.233S	Sublux of proximal interphaln joint of l mid finger, sequela
		S63.234S	Sublux of proximal interphaln joint of r rng fngr, sequela
		S63.235S	Sublux of proximal interphaln joint of l rng fngr, sequela
		S63.236S	Sublux of prox interphaln joint of r little finger, sequela
		S63.237S	Sublux of prox interphaln joint of l little finger, sequela
		S63.238S	Subluxation of proximal interphaln joint of finger, sequela
		S63.239S	Sublux of proximal interphaln joint of unsp finger, sequela
		S63.240S	Sublux of distal interphaln joint of r idx fngr, sequela
		S63.241S	Sublux of distal interphaln joint of l idx fngr, sequela
		S63.242S	Sublux of distal interphaln joint of r mid finger, sequela
		S63.243S	Sublux of distal interphaln joint of l mid finger, sequela
		S63.244S	Sublux of distal interphaln joint of r rng fngr, sequela
		S63.245S	Sublux of distal interphaln joint of l rng fngr, sequela
		S63.246S	Sublux of distal interphaln joint of r little finger, sqla
		S63.247S	Sublux of distal interphaln joint of l little finger, sqla
		S63.248S	Subluxation of distal interphaln joint of finger, sequela
		S63.249S	Sublux of distal interphaln joint of unsp finger, sequela
		S63.250S	Unspecified dislocation of right index finger, sequela
		S63.251S	Unspecified dislocation of left index finger, sequela
		S63.252S	Unspecified dislocation of right middle finger, sequela
		S63.253S	Unspecified dislocation of left middle finger, sequela
		S63.254S	Unspecified dislocation of right ring finger, sequela
		S63.255S	Unspecified dislocation of left ring finger, sequela
		S63.256S	Unspecified dislocation of right little finger, sequela
		S63.257S	Unspecified dislocation of left little finger, sequela
		S63.258S	Unspecified dislocation of other finger, sequela
		S63.259S	Unspecified dislocation of unspecified finger, sequela
		S63.260S	Dislocation of MCP joint of right index finger, sequela
		S63.261S	Dislocation of MCP joint of left index finger, sequela
		S63.262S	Dislocation of MCP joint of right middle finger, sequela
		S63.263S	Dislocation of MCP joint of left middle finger, sequela
		S63.264S	Dislocation of MCP joint of right ring finger, sequela
		S63.265S	Dislocation of MCP joint of left ring finger, sequela
		S63.266S	Dislocation of MCP joint of right little finger, sequela
		S63.267S	Dislocation of MCP joint of left little finger, sequela
		S63.268S	Dislocation of metacarpophalangeal joint of finger, sequela
		S63.269S	Dislocation of MCP joint of unsp finger, sequela
		S63.270S	Dislocation of unsp interphaln joint of r idx fngr, sequela
		S63.271S	Dislocation of unsp interphaln joint of l idx fngr, sequela
		S63.272S	Disloc of unsp interphaln joint of r mid finger, sequela
		S63.273S	Disloc of unsp interphaln joint of l mid finger, sequela
		S63.274S	Dislocation of unsp interphaln joint of r rng fngr, sequela
		S63.275S	Dislocation of unsp interphaln joint of l rng fngr, sequela
		S63.276S	Disloc of unsp interphaln joint of r little finger, sequela
		S63.277S	Disloc of unsp interphaln joint of l little finger, sequela
		S63.278S	Dislocation of unsp interphalangeal joint of finger, sequela
		S63.279S	Dislocation of unsp interphaln joint of unsp finger, sequela
		S63.280S	Disloc of proximal interphaln joint of r idx fngr, sequela
		S63.281S	Disloc of proximal interphaln joint of l idx fngr, sequela
		S63.282S	Disloc of proximal interphaln joint of r mid finger, sequela
		S63.283S	Disloc of proximal interphaln joint of l mid finger, sequela
		S63.284S	Disloc of proximal interphaln joint of r rng fngr, sequela
		S63.285S	Disloc of proximal interphaln joint of l rng fngr, sequela
		S63.286S	Disloc of prox interphaln joint of r little finger, sequela
		S63.287S	Disloc of prox interphaln joint of l little finger, sequela
		S63.288S	Dislocation of proximal interphaln joint of finger, sequela
		S63.289S	Disloc of proximal interphaln joint of unsp finger, sequela
		S63.290S	Disloc of distal interphaln joint of r idx fngr, sequela
		S63.291S	Disloc of distal interphaln joint of l idx fngr, sequela
		S63.292S	Disloc of distal interphaln joint of r mid finger, sequela
		S63.293S	Disloc of distal interphaln joint of l mid finger, sequela
		S63.294S	Disloc of distal interphaln joint of r rng fngr, sequela
		S63.295S	Disloc of distal interphaln joint of l rng fngr, sequela
		S63.296S	Disloc of distal interphaln joint of r little finger, sqla
		S63.297S	Disloc of distal interphaln joint of l little finger, sqla
		S63.298S	Dislocation of distal interphaln joint of finger, sequela
		S63.299S	Disloc of distal interphaln joint of unsp finger, sequela
		S73.001S	Unspecified subluxation of right hip, sequela
		S73.002S	Unspecified subluxation of left hip, sequela
		S73.003S	Unspecified subluxation of unspecified hip, sequela
		S73.004S	Unspecified dislocation of right hip, sequela
		S73.005S	Unspecified dislocation of left hip, sequela
		S73.006S	Unspecified dislocation of unspecified hip, sequela
		S73.011S	Posterior subluxation of right hip, sequela
		S73.012S	Posterior subluxation of left hip, sequela
		S73.013S	Posterior subluxation of unspecified hip, sequela
		S73.014S	Posterior dislocation of right hip, sequela
		S73.015S	Posterior dislocation of left hip, sequela
		S73.016S	Posterior dislocation of unspecified hip, sequela
		S73.021S	Obturator subluxation of right hip, sequela

(Continued on next page)

ICD-9-CM		ICD-10-CM	
905.6	LATE EFFECT OF DISLOCATION **(Continued)**	**S73.022S**	Obturator subluxation of left hip, sequela
		S73.023S	Obturator subluxation of unspecified hip, sequela
		S73.024S	Obturator dislocation of right hip, sequela
		S73.025S	Obturator dislocation of left hip, sequela
		S73.026S	Obturator dislocation of unspecified hip, sequela
		S73.031S	Other anterior subluxation of right hip, sequela
		S73.032S	Other anterior subluxation of left hip, sequela
		S73.033S	Other anterior subluxation of unspecified hip, sequela
		S73.034S	Other anterior dislocation of right hip, sequela
		S73.035S	Other anterior dislocation of left hip, sequela
		S73.036S	Other anterior dislocation of unspecified hip, sequela
		S73.041S	Central subluxation of right hip, sequela
		S73.042S	Central subluxation of left hip, sequela
		S73.043S	Central subluxation of unspecified hip, sequela
		S73.044S	Central dislocation of right hip, sequela
		S73.045S	Central dislocation of left hip, sequela
		S73.046S	Central dislocation of unspecified hip, sequela
		S83.001S	Unspecified subluxation of right patella, sequela
		S83.002S	Unspecified subluxation of left patella, sequela
		S83.003S	Unspecified subluxation of unspecified patella, sequela
		S83.004S	Unspecified dislocation of right patella, sequela
		S83.005S	Unspecified dislocation of left patella, sequela
		S83.006S	Unspecified dislocation of unspecified patella, sequela
		S83.011S	Lateral subluxation of right patella, sequela
		S83.012S	Lateral subluxation of left patella, sequela
		S83.013S	Lateral subluxation of unspecified patella, sequela
		S83.014S	Lateral dislocation of right patella, sequela
		S83.015S	Lateral dislocation of left patella, sequela
		S83.016S	Lateral dislocation of unspecified patella, sequela
		S83.091S	Other subluxation of right patella, sequela
		S83.092S	Other subluxation of left patella, sequela
		S83.093S	Other subluxation of unspecified patella, sequela
		S83.094S	Other dislocation of right patella, sequela
		S83.095S	Other dislocation of left patella, sequela
		S83.096S	Other dislocation of unspecified patella, sequela
		S83.101S	Unspecified subluxation of right knee, sequela
		S83.102S	Unspecified subluxation of left knee, sequela
		S83.103S	Unspecified subluxation of unspecified knee, sequela
		S83.104S	Unspecified dislocation of right knee, sequela
		S83.105S	Unspecified dislocation of left knee, sequela
		S83.106S	Unspecified dislocation of unspecified knee, sequela
		S83.111S	Anterior sublux of proximal end of tibia, r knee, sequela
		S83.112S	Anterior sublux of proximal end of tibia, left knee, sequela
		S83.113S	Anterior sublux of proximal end of tibia, unsp knee, sequela
		S83.114S	Anterior disloc of proximal end of tibia, r knee, sequela
		S83.115S	Anterior disloc of proximal end of tibia, left knee, sequela
		S83.116S	Anterior disloc of proximal end of tibia, unsp knee, sequela
		S83.121S	Posterior sublux of proximal end of tibia, r knee, sequela
		S83.122S	Posterior sublux of proximal end of tibia, l knee, sequela
		S83.123S	Post sublux of proximal end of tibia, unsp knee, sequela
		S83.124S	Posterior disloc of proximal end of tibia, r knee, sequela
		S83.125S	Posterior disloc of proximal end of tibia, l knee, sequela
		S83.126S	Post disloc of proximal end of tibia, unsp knee, sequela
		S83.131S	Medial sublux of proximal end of tibia, right knee, sequela
		S83.132S	Medial sublux of proximal end of tibia, left knee, sequela
		S83.133S	Medial sublux of proximal end of tibia, unsp knee, sequela
		S83.134S	Medial disloc of proximal end of tibia, right knee, sequela
		S83.135S	Medial disloc of proximal end of tibia, left knee, sequela
		S83.136S	Medial disloc of proximal end of tibia, unsp knee, sequela
		S83.141S	Lateral sublux of proximal end of tibia, right knee, sequela
		S83.142S	Lateral sublux of proximal end of tibia, left knee, sequela
		S83.143S	Lateral sublux of proximal end of tibia, unsp knee, sequela
		S83.144S	Lateral disloc of proximal end of tibia, right knee, sequela
		S83.145S	Lateral disloc of proximal end of tibia, left knee, sequela
		S83.146S	Lateral disloc of proximal end of tibia, unsp knee, sequela
		S83.191S	Other subluxation of right knee, sequela
		S83.192S	Other subluxation of left knee, sequela
		S83.193S	Other subluxation of unspecified knee, sequela
		S83.194S	Other dislocation of right knee, sequela
		S83.195S	Other dislocation of left knee, sequela
		S83.196S	Other dislocation of unspecified knee, sequela
		S93.01XS	Subluxation of right ankle joint, sequela
		S93.02XS	Subluxation of left ankle joint, sequela
		S93.03XS	Subluxation of unspecified ankle joint, sequela
		S93.04XS	Dislocation of right ankle joint, sequela
		S93.05XS	Dislocation of left ankle joint, sequela
		S93.06XS	Dislocation of unspecified ankle joint, sequela
		S93.101S	Unspecified subluxation of right toe(s), sequela
		S93.102S	Unspecified subluxation of left toe(s), sequela
		S93.103S	Unspecified subluxation of unspecified toe(s), sequela
		S93.104S	Unspecified dislocation of right toe(s), sequela
	(Continued on next page)	**S93.105S**	Unspecified dislocation of left toe(s), sequela

[Brackets] indicate valid character values for each code. Character value meanings provided for each code grouping.

ICD-9-CM		ICD-10-CM	
9Ø5.6	LATE EFFECT OF DISLOCATION **(Continued)**	**S93.1Ø6S**	Unspecified dislocation of unspecified toe(s), sequela
		S93.111S	Dislocation of interphaln joint of right great toe, sequela
		S93.112S	Dislocation of interphaln joint of left great toe, sequela
		S93.113S	Dislocation of interphaln joint of unsp great toe, sequela
		S93.114S	Disloc of interphaln joint of right lesser toe(s), sequela
		S93.115S	Disloc of interphaln joint of left lesser toe(s), sequela
		S93.116S	Disloc of interphaln joint of unsp lesser toe(s), sequela
		S93.119S	Dislocation of interphalangeal joint of unsp toe(s), sequela
		S93.121S	Dislocation of MTP joint of right great toe, sequela
		S93.122S	Dislocation of MTP joint of left great toe, sequela
		S93.123S	Dislocation of MTP joint of unsp great toe, sequela
		S93.124S	Dislocation of MTP joint of right lesser toe(s), sequela
		S93.125S	Dislocation of MTP joint of left lesser toe(s), sequela
		S93.126S	Dislocation of MTP joint of unsp lesser toe(s), sequela
		S93.129S	Dislocation of MTP joint of unsp toe(s), sequela
		S93.131S	Subluxation of interphaln joint of right great toe, sequela
		S93.132S	Subluxation of interphaln joint of left great toe, sequela
		S93.133S	Subluxation of interphaln joint of unsp great toe, sequela
		S93.134S	Sublux of interphaln joint of right lesser toe(s), sequela
		S93.135S	Sublux of interphaln joint of left lesser toe(s), sequela
		S93.136S	Sublux of interphaln joint of unsp lesser toe(s), sequela
		S93.139S	Subluxation of interphalangeal joint of unsp toe(s), sequela
		S93.141S	Subluxation of MTP joint of right great toe, sequela
		S93.142S	Subluxation of MTP joint of left great toe, sequela
		S93.143S	Subluxation of MTP joint of unsp great toe, sequela
		S93.144S	Subluxation of MTP joint of right lesser toe(s), sequela
		S93.145S	Subluxation of MTP joint of left lesser toe(s), sequela
		S93.146S	Subluxation of MTP joint of unsp lesser toe(s), sequela
		S93.149S	Subluxation of MTP joint of unsp toe(s), sequela
		S93.3Ø1S	Unspecified subluxation of right foot, sequela
		S93.3Ø2S	Unspecified subluxation of left foot, sequela
		S93.3Ø3S	Unspecified subluxation of unspecified foot, sequela
		S93.3Ø4S	Unspecified dislocation of right foot, sequela
		S93.3Ø5S	Unspecified dislocation of left foot, sequela
		S93.3Ø6S	Unspecified dislocation of unspecified foot, sequela
		S93.311S	Subluxation of tarsal joint of right foot, sequela
		S93.312S	Subluxation of tarsal joint of left foot, sequela
		S93.313S	Subluxation of tarsal joint of unspecified foot, sequela
		S93.314S	Dislocation of tarsal joint of right foot, sequela
		S93.315S	Dislocation of tarsal joint of left foot, sequela
		S93.316S	Dislocation of tarsal joint of unspecified foot, sequela
		S93.321S	Subluxation of tarsometatarsal joint of right foot, sequela
		S93.322S	Subluxation of tarsometatarsal joint of left foot, sequela
		S93.323S	Subluxation of tarsometatarsal joint of unsp foot, sequela
		S93.324S	Dislocation of tarsometatarsal joint of right foot, sequela
		S93.325S	Dislocation of tarsometatarsal joint of left foot, sequela
		S93.326S	Dislocation of tarsometatarsal joint of unsp foot, sequela
		S93.331S	Other subluxation of right foot, sequela
		S93.332S	Other subluxation of left foot, sequela
		S93.333S	Other subluxation of unspecified foot, sequela
		S93.334S	Other dislocation of right foot, sequela
		S93.335S	Other dislocation of left foot, sequela
		S93.336S	Other dislocation of unspecified foot, sequela
9Ø5.7	LATE EFF SPRAIN&STRAIN W/O MENTION TENDON INJURY	**SØ3.4XXS**	Sprain of jaw, sequela
		SØ3.8XXS	Sprain of joints and ligaments of oth parts of head, sequela
		SØ3.9XXS	Sprain of joints and ligaments of unsp parts of head, sqla
		SØ9.11XS	Strain of muscle and tendon of head, sequela
		S13.4XXS	Sprain of ligaments of cervical spine, sequela
		S13.5XXS	Sprain of thyroid region, sequela
		S13.8XXS	Sprain of joints and ligaments of oth parts of neck, sequela
		S13.9XXS	Sprain of joints and ligaments of unsp parts of neck, sqla
		S16.1XXS	Strain of muscle, fascia and tendon at neck level, sequela
		S23.3XXS	Sprain of ligaments of thoracic spine, sequela
		S23.41XS	Sprain of ribs, sequela
		S23.42ØS	Sprain of sternoclavicular (joint) (ligament), sequela
		S23.421S	Sprain of chondrosternal joint, sequela
		S23.428S	Other sprain of sternum, sequela
		S23.429S	Unspecified sprain of sternum, sequela
		S23.8XXS	Sprain of other specified parts of thorax, sequela
		S23.9XXS	Sprain of unspecified parts of thorax, sequela
		S29.Ø11S	Strain of muscle and tendon of front wall of thorax, sequela
		S29.Ø12S	Strain of muscle and tendon of back wall of thorax, sequela
		S29.Ø19S	Strain of muscle and tendon of unsp wall of thorax, sequela
		S33.4XXS	Traumatic rupture of symphysis pubis, sequela
		S33.5XXS	Sprain of ligaments of lumbar spine, sequela
		S33.6XXS	Sprain of sacroiliac joint, sequela
		S33.8XXS	Sprain of other parts of lumbar spine and pelvis, sequela
		S33.9XXS	Sprain of unsp parts of lumbar spine and pelvis, sequela
		S39.Ø11S	Strain of muscle, fascia and tendon of abdomen, sequela
		S39.Ø12S	Strain of muscle, fascia and tendon of lower back, sequela
		S39.Ø13S	Strain of muscle, fascia and tendon of pelvis, sequela
	(Continued on next page)	**S43.4Ø1S**	Unspecified sprain of right shoulder joint, sequela

ICD-9-CM		ICD-10-CM	
9Ø5.7	LATE EFF SPRAIN&STRAIN W/O MENTION TENDON INJURY **(Continued)**	**S43.4Ø2S**	Unspecified sprain of left shoulder joint, sequela
		S43.4Ø9S	Unspecified sprain of unspecified shoulder joint, sequela
		S43.411S	Sprain of right coracohumeral (ligament), sequela
		S43.412S	Sprain of left coracohumeral (ligament), sequela
		S43.419S	Sprain of unspecified coracohumeral (ligament), sequela
		S43.421S	Sprain of right rotator cuff capsule, sequela
		S43.422S	Sprain of left rotator cuff capsule, sequela
		S43.429S	Sprain of unspecified rotator cuff capsule, sequela
		S43.431S	Superior glenoid labrum lesion of right shoulder, sequela
		S43.432S	Superior glenoid labrum lesion of left shoulder, sequela
		S43.439S	Superior glenoid labrum lesion of unsp shoulder, sequela
		S43.491S	Other sprain of right shoulder joint, sequela
		S43.492S	Other sprain of left shoulder joint, sequela
		S43.499S	Other sprain of unspecified shoulder joint, sequela
		S43.5ØXS	Sprain of unspecified acromioclavicular joint, sequela
		S43.51XS	Sprain of right acromioclavicular joint, sequela
		S43.52XS	Sprain of left acromioclavicular joint, sequela
		S43.6ØXS	Sprain of unspecified sternoclavicular joint, sequela
		S43.61XS	Sprain of right sternoclavicular joint, sequela
		S43.62XS	Sprain of left sternoclavicular joint, sequela
		S43.8ØXS	Sprain of oth parts of unspecified shoulder girdle, sequela
		S43.81XS	Sprain of oth parts of right shoulder girdle, sequela
		S43.82XS	Sprain of oth parts of left shoulder girdle, sequela
		S43.9ØXS	Sprain of unsp parts of unspecified shoulder girdle, sequela
		S43.91XS	Sprain of unsp parts of right shoulder girdle, sequela
		S43.92XS	Sprain of unspecified parts of left shoulder girdle, sequela
		S46.Ø11S	Strain of musc/tend the rotator cuff of r shoulder, sequela
		S46.Ø12S	Strain of musc/tend the rotator cuff of l shoulder, sequela
		S46.Ø19S	Strain musc/tend the rotator cuff of unsp shoulder, sequela
		S46.111S	Strain of musc/fasc/tend long hd bicep, right arm, sequela
		S46.112S	Strain of musc/fasc/tend long hd bicep, left arm, sequela
		S46.119S	Strain of musc/fasc/tend long hd bicep, unsp arm, sequela
		S46.211S	Strain of musc/fasc/tend prt biceps, right arm, sequela
		S46.212S	Strain of musc/fasc/tend prt biceps, left arm, sequela
		S46.219S	Strain of musc/fasc/tend prt biceps, unsp arm, sequela
		S46.311S	Strain of musc/fasc/tend triceps, right arm, sequela
		S46.312S	Strain of musc/fasc/tend triceps, left arm, sequela
		S46.319S	Strain of musc/fasc/tend triceps, unsp arm, sequela
		S46.811S	Strain of musc/fasc/tend at shldr/up arm, right arm, sequela
		S46.812S	Strain of musc/fasc/tend at shldr/up arm, left arm, sequela
		S46.819S	Strain of musc/fasc/tend at shldr/up arm, unsp arm, sequela
		S46.911S	Strain unsp musc/fasc/tend at shldr/up arm, right arm, sqla
		S46.912S	Strain unsp musc/fasc/tend at shldr/up arm, left arm, sqla
		S46.919S	Strain unsp musc/fasc/tend at shldr/up arm, unsp arm, sqla
		S53.2ØXS	Traumatic rupture of unsp radial collat ligament, sequela
		S53.21XS	Traumatic rupture of right radial collat ligament, sequela
		S53.22XS	Traumatic rupture of left radial collat ligament, sequela
		S53.3ØXS	Traumatic rupture of unsp ulnar collateral ligament, sequela
		S53.31XS	Traumatic rupture of right ulnar collat ligament, sequela
		S53.32XS	Traumatic rupture of left ulnar collateral ligament, sequela
		S53.4Ø1S	Unspecified sprain of right elbow, sequela
		S53.4Ø2S	Unspecified sprain of left elbow, sequela
		S53.4Ø9S	Unspecified sprain of unspecified elbow, sequela
		S53.411S	Radiohumeral (joint) sprain of right elbow, sequela
		S53.412S	Radiohumeral (joint) sprain of left elbow, sequela
		S53.419S	Radiohumeral (joint) sprain of unspecified elbow, sequela
		S53.421S	Ulnohumeral (joint) sprain of right elbow, sequela
		S53.422S	Ulnohumeral (joint) sprain of left elbow, sequela
		S53.429S	Ulnohumeral (joint) sprain of unspecified elbow, sequela
		S53.431S	Radial collateral ligament sprain of right elbow, sequela
		S53.432S	Radial collateral ligament sprain of left elbow, sequela
		S53.439S	Radial collateral ligament sprain of unsp elbow, sequela
		S53.441S	Ulnar collateral ligament sprain of right elbow, sequela
		S53.442S	Ulnar collateral ligament sprain of left elbow, sequela
		S53.449S	Ulnar collateral ligament sprain of unsp elbow, sequela
		S53.491S	Other sprain of right elbow, sequela
		S53.492S	Other sprain of left elbow, sequela
		S53.499S	Other sprain of unspecified elbow, sequela
		S56.Ø11S	Strain of flexor musc/fasc/tend r thm at forarm lv, sequela
		S56.Ø12S	Strain of flexor musc/fasc/tend l thm at forarm lv, sequela
		S56.Ø19S	Strain of flexor musc/fasc/tend thmb at forarm lv, sequela
		S56.111S	Strain flexor musc/fasc/tend r idx fngr at forarm lv, sqla
		S56.112S	Strain flexor musc/fasc/tend l idx fngr at forarm lv, sqla
		S56.113S	Strain flexor musc/fasc/tend r mid finger at forarm lv, sqla
		S56.114S	Strain flexor musc/fasc/tend l mid finger at forarm lv, sqla
		S56.115S	Strain flexor musc/fasc/tend r rng fngr at forarm lv, sqla
		S56.116S	Strain flexor musc/fasc/tend l rng fngr at forarm lv, sqla
		S56.117S	Strain flxr musc/fasc/tend r little fngr at forarm lv, sqla
		S56.118S	Strain flxr musc/fasc/tend l little fngr at forarm lv, sqla
		S56.119S	Strain flexor musc/fasc/tend of unsp fngr at forarm lv, sqla
		S56.211S	Strain flexor musc/fasc/tend at forarm lv, right arm, sqla
		S56.212S	Strain flexor musc/fasc/tend at forarm lv, left arm, sequela
	(Continued on next page)	**S56.219S**	Strain flexor musc/fasc/tend at forarm lv, unsp arm, sequela

ICD-9-CM		ICD-10-CM	
905.7	LATE EFF SPRAIN&STRAIN W/O MENTION TENDON INJURY **(Continued)**	**S56.311S**	Strain extn/abdr musc/fasc/tend of r thm at forarm lv, sqla
		S56.312S	Strain extn/abdr musc/fasc/tend of l thm at forarm lv, sqla
		S56.319S	Strain extn/abdr musc/fasc/tend of thmb at forarm lv, sqla
		S56.411S	Strain extn musc/fasc/tend r idx fngr at forarm lv, sequela
		S56.412S	Strain extn musc/fasc/tend l idx fngr at forarm lv, sequela
		S56.413S	Strain extn musc/fasc/tend r mid finger at forarm lv, sqla
		S56.414S	Strain extn musc/fasc/tend l mid finger at forarm lv, sqla
		S56.415S	Strain extn musc/fasc/tend r rng fngr at forarm lv, sequela
		S56.416S	Strain extn musc/fasc/tend l rng fngr at forarm lv, sequela
		S56.417S	Strain extn musc/fasc/tend r little fngr at forarm lv, sqla
		S56.418S	Strain extn musc/fasc/tend l little fngr at forarm lv, sqla
		S56.419S	Strain extn musc/fasc/tend fngr,unsp fngr at forarm lv, sqla
		S56.511S	Strain extn musc/fasc/tend at forarm lv, right arm, sequela
		S56.512S	Strain extn musc/fasc/tend at forarm lv, left arm, sequela
		S56.519S	Strain extn musc/fasc/tend at forarm lv, unsp arm, sequela
		S56.811S	Strain of musc/fasc/tend at forarm lv, right arm, sequela
		S56.812S	Strain of musc/fasc/tend at forearm level, left arm, sequela
		S56.819S	Strain of musc/fasc/tend at forearm level, unsp arm, sequela
		S56.911S	Strain unsp musc/fasc/tend at forarm lv, right arm, sequela
		S56.912S	Strain unsp musc/fasc/tend at forarm lv, left arm, sequela
		S56.919S	Strain unsp musc/fasc/tend at forarm lv, unsp arm, sequela
		S63.301S	Traumatic rupture of unsp ligament of right wrist, sequela
		S63.302S	Traumatic rupture of unsp ligament of left wrist, sequela
		S63.309S	Traumatic rupture of unsp ligament of unsp wrist, sequela
		S63.311S	Traumatic rupture of collateral ligament of r wrist, sequela
		S63.312S	Traumatic rupture of collat ligament of left wrist, sequela
		S63.319S	Traumatic rupture of collat ligament of unsp wrist, sequela
		S63.321S	Traumatic rupture of right radiocarpal ligament, sequela
		S63.322S	Traumatic rupture of left radiocarpal ligament, sequela
		S63.329S	Traumatic rupture of unsp radiocarpal ligament, sequela
		S63.331S	Traum rupture of right ulnocarpal (palmar) ligament, sequela
		S63.332S	Traum rupture of left ulnocarpal (palmar) ligament, sequela
		S63.339S	Traum rupture of unsp ulnocarpal (palmar) ligament, sequela
		S63.391S	Traumatic rupture of other ligament of right wrist, sequela
		S63.392S	Traumatic rupture of other ligament of left wrist, sequela
		S63.399S	Traumatic rupture of other ligament of unsp wrist, sequela
		S63.400S	Traum rupt of unsp ligmt of r idx fngr at MCP/IP jt, sequela
		S63.401S	Traum rupt of unsp ligmt of l idx fngr at MCP/IP jt, sequela
		S63.402S	Traum rupt of unsp ligmt of r mid finger at MCP/IP jt, sqla
		S63.403S	Traum rupt of unsp ligmt of l mid finger at MCP/IP jt, sqla
		S63.404S	Traum rupt of unsp ligmt of r rng fngr at MCP/IP jt, sequela
		S63.405S	Traum rupt of unsp ligmt of l rng fngr at MCP/IP jt, sequela
		S63.406S	Traum rupt of unsp ligmt of r little fngr at MCP/IP jt, sqla
		S63.407S	Traum rupt of unsp ligmt of l little fngr at MCP/IP jt, sqla
		S63.408S	Traum rupture of unsp ligmt of finger at MCP/IP jt, sequela
		S63.409S	Traum rupt of unsp ligmt of unsp finger at MCP/IP jt, sqla
		S63.410S	Traum rupt of collat ligmt of r idx fngr at MCP/IP jt, sqla
		S63.411S	Traum rupt of collat ligmt of l idx fngr at MCP/IP jt, sqla
		S63.412S	Traum rupt of collat ligmt of r mid fngr at MCP/IP jt, sqla
		S63.413S	Traum rupt of collat ligmt of l mid fngr at MCP/IP jt, sqla
		S63.414S	Traum rupt of collat ligmt of r rng fngr at MCP/IP jt, sqla
		S63.415S	Traum rupt of collat ligmt of l rng fngr at MCP/IP jt, sqla
		S63.416S	Traum rupt of collat ligmt of r lit fngr at MCP/IP jt, sqla
		S63.417S	Traum rupt of collat ligmt of l lit fngr at MCP/IP jt, sqla
		S63.418S	Traum rupt of collat ligmt of finger at MCP/IP jt, sequela
		S63.419S	Traum rupt of collat ligmt of unsp finger at MCP/IP jt, sqla
		S63.420S	Traum rupt of palmar ligmt of r idx fngr at MCP/IP jt, sqla
		S63.421S	Traum rupt of palmar ligmt of l idx fngr at MCP/IP jt, sqla
		S63.422S	Traum rupt of palmar ligmt of r mid fngr at MCP/IP jt, sqla
		S63.423S	Traum rupt of palmar ligmt of l mid fngr at MCP/IP jt, sqla
		S63.424S	Traum rupt of palmar ligmt of r rng fngr at MCP/IP jt, sqla
		S63.425S	Traum rupt of palmar ligmt of l rng fngr at MCP/IP jt, sqla
		S63.426S	Traum rupt of palmar ligmt of r lit fngr at MCP/IP jt, sqla
		S63.427S	Traum rupt of palmar ligmt of l lit fngr at MCP/IP jt, sqla
		S63.428S	Traum rupt of palmar ligmt of finger at MCP/IP jt, sequela
		S63.429S	Traum rupt of palmar ligmt of unsp finger at MCP/IP jt, sqla
		S63.430S	Traum rupt of volar plate of r idx fngr at MCP/IP jt, sqla
		S63.431S	Traum rupt of volar plate of l idx fngr at MCP/IP jt, sqla
		S63.432S	Traum rupt of volar plate of r mid finger at MCP/IP jt, sqla
		S63.433S	Traum rupt of volar plate of l mid finger at MCP/IP jt, sqla
		S63.434S	Traum rupt of volar plate of r rng fngr at MCP/IP jt, sqla
		S63.435S	Traum rupt of volar plate of l rng fngr at MCP/IP jt, sqla
		S63.436S	Traum rupt of volar plate of r lit fngr at MCP/IP jt, sqla
		S63.437S	Traum rupt of volar plate of l lit fngr at MCP/IP jt, sqla
		S63.438S	Traum rupture of volar plate of finger at MCP/IP jt, sequela
		S63.439S	Traum rupt of volar plate of unsp finger at MCP/IP jt, sqla
		S63.490S	Traum rupture of ligmt of r idx fngr at MCP/IP jt, sequela
		S63.491S	Traum rupture of ligmt of l idx fngr at MCP/IP jt, sequela
		S63.492S	Traum rupture of ligmt of r mid finger at MCP/IP jt, sequela
		S63.493S	Traum rupture of ligmt of l mid finger at MCP/IP jt, sequela
		S63.494S	Traum rupture of ligmt of r rng fngr at MCP/IP jt, sequela
		S63.495S	Traum rupture of ligmt of l rng fngr at MCP/IP jt, sequela
	(Continued on next page)	**S63.496S**	Traum rupt of ligmt of r little finger at MCP/IP jt, sequela

ICD-9-CM		ICD-10-CM	
905.7	LATE EFF SPRAIN&STRAIN W/O MENTION TENDON INJURY **(Continued)**	**S63.497S**	Traum rupt of ligmt of l little finger at MCP/IP jt, sequela
		S63.498S	Traum rupture of ligament of finger at MCP/IP jt, sequela
		S63.499S	Traum rupture of ligmt of unsp finger at MCP/IP jt, sequela
		S63.501S	Unspecified sprain of right wrist, sequela
		S63.502S	Unspecified sprain of left wrist, sequela
		S63.509S	Unspecified sprain of unspecified wrist, sequela
		S63.511S	Sprain of carpal joint of right wrist, sequela
		S63.512S	Sprain of carpal joint of left wrist, sequela
		S63.519S	Sprain of carpal joint of unspecified wrist, sequela
		S63.521S	Sprain of radiocarpal joint of right wrist, sequela
		S63.522S	Sprain of radiocarpal joint of left wrist, sequela
		S63.529S	Sprain of radiocarpal joint of unspecified wrist, sequela
		S63.591S	Other specified sprain of right wrist, sequela
		S63.592S	Other specified sprain of left wrist, sequela
		S63.599S	Other specified sprain of unspecified wrist, sequela
		S63.601S	Unspecified sprain of right thumb, sequela
		S63.602S	Unspecified sprain of left thumb, sequela
		S63.609S	Unspecified sprain of unspecified thumb, sequela
		S63.610S	Unspecified sprain of right index finger, sequela
		S63.611S	Unspecified sprain of left index finger, sequela
		S63.612S	Unspecified sprain of right middle finger, sequela
		S63.613S	Unspecified sprain of left middle finger, sequela
		S63.614S	Unspecified sprain of right ring finger, sequela
		S63.615S	Unspecified sprain of left ring finger, sequela
		S63.616S	Unspecified sprain of right little finger, sequela
		S63.617S	Unspecified sprain of left little finger, sequela
		S63.618S	Unspecified sprain of other finger, sequela
		S63.619S	Unspecified sprain of unspecified finger, sequela
		S63.621S	Sprain of interphalangeal joint of right thumb, sequela
		S63.622S	Sprain of interphalangeal joint of left thumb, sequela
		S63.629S	Sprain of interphalangeal joint of unsp thumb, sequela
		S63.630S	Sprain of interphalangeal joint of r idx fngr, sequela
		S63.631S	Sprain of interphalangeal joint of l idx fngr, sequela
		S63.632S	Sprain of interphalangeal joint of r mid finger, sequela
		S63.633S	Sprain of interphalangeal joint of l mid finger, sequela
		S63.634S	Sprain of interphalangeal joint of r rng fngr, sequela
		S63.635S	Sprain of interphalangeal joint of left ring finger, sequela
		S63.636S	Sprain of interphalangeal joint of r little finger, sequela
		S63.637S	Sprain of interphalangeal joint of l little finger, sequela
		S63.638S	Sprain of interphalangeal joint of other finger, sequela
		S63.639S	Sprain of interphalangeal joint of unsp finger, sequela
		S63.641S	Sprain of metacarpophalangeal joint of right thumb, sequela
		S63.642S	Sprain of metacarpophalangeal joint of left thumb, sequela
		S63.649S	Sprain of metacarpophalangeal joint of unsp thumb, sequela
		S63.650S	Sprain of MCP joint of right index finger, sequela
		S63.651S	Sprain of MCP joint of left index finger, sequela
		S63.652S	Sprain of MCP joint of right middle finger, sequela
		S63.653S	Sprain of MCP joint of left middle finger, sequela
		S63.654S	Sprain of MCP joint of right ring finger, sequela
		S63.655S	Sprain of MCP joint of left ring finger, sequela
		S63.656S	Sprain of MCP joint of right little finger, sequela
		S63.657S	Sprain of MCP joint of left little finger, sequela
		S63.658S	Sprain of metacarpophalangeal joint of other finger, sequela
		S63.659S	Sprain of metacarpophalangeal joint of unsp finger, sequela
		S63.681S	Other sprain of right thumb, sequela
		S63.682S	Other sprain of left thumb, sequela
		S63.689S	Other sprain of unspecified thumb, sequela
		S63.690S	Other sprain of right index finger, sequela
		S63.691S	Other sprain of left index finger, sequela
		S63.692S	Other sprain of right middle finger, sequela
		S63.693S	Other sprain of left middle finger, sequela
		S63.694S	Other sprain of right ring finger, sequela
		S63.695S	Other sprain of left ring finger, sequela
		S63.696S	Other sprain of right little finger, sequela
		S63.697S	Other sprain of left little finger, sequela
		S63.698S	Other sprain of other finger, sequela
		S63.699S	Other sprain of unspecified finger, sequela
		S63.8X1S	Sprain of other part of right wrist and hand, sequela
		S63.8X2S	Sprain of other part of left wrist and hand, sequela
		S63.8X9S	Sprain of other part of unspecified wrist and hand, sequela
		S63.90XS	Sprain of unsp part of unspecified wrist and hand, sequela
		S63.91XS	Sprain of unspecified part of right wrist and hand, sequela
		S63.92XS	Sprain of unspecified part of left wrist and hand, sequela
		S66.011S	Strain long flexor musc/fasc/tend r thm at wrs/hnd lv, sqla
		S66.012S	Strain long flexor musc/fasc/tend l thm at wrs/hnd lv, sqla
		S66.019S	Strain long flexor musc/fasc/tend thmb at wrs/hnd lv, sqla
		S66.110S	Strain flexor musc/fasc/tend r idx fngr at wrs/hnd lv, sqla
		S66.111S	Strain flexor musc/fasc/tend l idx fngr at wrs/hnd lv, sqla
		S66.112S	Strain flexor musc/fasc/tend r mid fngr at wrs/hnd lv, sqla
		S66.113S	Strain flexor musc/fasc/tend l mid fngr at wrs/hnd lv, sqla
		S66.114S	Strain flexor musc/fasc/tend r rng fngr at wrs/hnd lv, sqla
	(Continued on next page)	**S66.115S**	Strain flexor musc/fasc/tend l rng fngr at wrs/hnd lv, sqla

ICD-9-CM		ICD-10-CM	
905.7	LATE EFF SPRAIN&STRAIN W/O MENTION TENDON INJURY **(Continued)**	**S66.116S**	Strain flxr musc/fasc/tend r little fngr at wrs/hnd lv, sqla
		S66.117S	Strain flxr musc/fasc/tend l little fngr at wrs/hnd lv, sqla
		S66.118S	Strain flexor musc/fasc/tend finger at wrs/hnd lv, sequela
		S66.119S	Strain flexor musc/fasc/tend unsp finger at wrs/hnd lv, sqla
		S66.211S	Strain extensor musc/fasc/tend r thm at wrs/hnd lv, sequela
		S66.212S	Strain extensor musc/fasc/tend l thm at wrs/hnd lv, sequela
		S66.219S	Strain extensor musc/fasc/tend thmb at wrs/hnd lv, sequela
		S66.310S	Strain extn musc/fasc/tend r idx fngr at wrs/hnd lv, sequela
		S66.311S	Strain extn musc/fasc/tend l idx fngr at wrs/hnd lv, sequela
		S66.312S	Strain extn musc/fasc/tend r mid finger at wrs/hnd lv, sqla
		S66.313S	Strain extn musc/fasc/tend l mid finger at wrs/hnd lv, sqla
		S66.314S	Strain extn musc/fasc/tend r rng fngr at wrs/hnd lv, sequela
		S66.315S	Strain extn musc/fasc/tend l rng fngr at wrs/hnd lv, sequela
		S66.316S	Strain extn musc/fasc/tend r little fngr at wrs/hnd lv, sqla
		S66.317S	Strain extn musc/fasc/tend l little fngr at wrs/hnd lv, sqla
		S66.318S	Strain extensor musc/fasc/tend finger at wrs/hnd lv, sequela
		S66.319S	Strain extn musc/fasc/tend unsp finger at wrs/hnd lv, sqla
		S66.411S	Strain of intrns musc/fasc/tend r thm at wrs/hnd lv, sequela
		S66.412S	Strain of intrns musc/fasc/tend l thm at wrs/hnd lv, sequela
		S66.419S	Strain of intrns musc/fasc/tend thmb at wrs/hnd lv, sequela
		S66.510S	Strain intrns musc/fasc/tend r idx fngr at wrs/hnd lv, sqla
		S66.511S	Strain intrns musc/fasc/tend l idx fngr at wrs/hnd lv, sqla
		S66.512S	Strain intrns musc/fasc/tend r mid fngr at wrs/hnd lv, sqla
		S66.513S	Strain intrns musc/fasc/tend l mid fngr at wrs/hnd lv, sqla
		S66.514S	Strain intrns musc/fasc/tend r rng fngr at wrs/hnd lv, sqla
		S66.515S	Strain intrns musc/fasc/tend l rng fngr at wrs/hnd lv, sqla
		S66.516S	Strain intrns musc/fasc/tend r lit fngr at wrs/hnd lv, sqla
		S66.517S	Strain intrns musc/fasc/tend l lit fngr at wrs/hnd lv, sqla
		S66.518S	Strain intrns musc/fasc/tend finger at wrs/hnd lv, sequela
		S66.519S	Strain intrns musc/fasc/tend unsp finger at wrs/hnd lv, sqla
		S66.811S	Strain of musc/fasc/tend at wrs/hnd lv, right hand, sequela
		S66.812S	Strain of musc/fasc/tend at wrs/hnd lv, left hand, sequela
		S66.819S	Strain of musc/fasc/tend at wrs/hnd lv, unsp hand, sequela
		S66.911S	Strain of unsp musc/fasc/tend at wrs/hnd lv, r hand, sequela
		S66.912S	Strain of unsp musc/fasc/tend at wrs/hnd lv, l hand, sequela
		S66.919S	Strain unsp musc/fasc/tend at wrs/hnd lv, unsp hand, sequela
		S73.101S	Unspecified sprain of right hip, sequela
		S73.102S	Unspecified sprain of left hip, sequela
		S73.109S	Unspecified sprain of unspecified hip, sequela
		S73.111S	Iliofemoral ligament sprain of right hip, sequela
		S73.112S	Iliofemoral ligament sprain of left hip, sequela
		S73.119S	Iliofemoral ligament sprain of unspecified hip, sequela
		S73.121S	Ischiocapsular ligament sprain of right hip, sequela
		S73.122S	Ischiocapsular ligament sprain of left hip, sequela
		S73.129S	Ischiocapsular ligament sprain of unspecified hip, sequela
		S73.191S	Other sprain of right hip, sequela
		S73.192S	Other sprain of left hip, sequela
		S73.199S	Other sprain of unspecified hip, sequela
		S76.011S	Strain of muscle, fascia and tendon of right hip, sequela
		S76.012S	Strain of muscle, fascia and tendon of left hip, sequela
		S76.019S	Strain of muscle, fascia and tendon of unsp hip, sequela
		S76.111S	Strain of right quadriceps musc/fasc/tend, sequela
		S76.112S	Strain of left quadriceps muscle, fascia and tendon, sequela
		S76.119S	Strain of unsp quadriceps muscle, fascia and tendon, sequela
		S76.211S	Strain of adductor musc/fasc/tend right thigh, sequela
		S76.212S	Strain of adductor musc/fasc/tend left thigh, sequela
		S76.219S	Strain of adductor musc/fasc/tend unsp thigh, sequela
		S76.311S	Strain msl/fasc/tnd post grp at thi lev, right thigh, sqla
		S76.312S	Strain msl/fasc/tnd post grp at thi lev, left thigh, sequela
		S76.319S	Strain msl/fasc/tnd post grp at thi lev, unsp thigh, sequela
		S76.811S	Strain of musc/fasc/tend at thi lev, right thigh, sequela
		S76.812S	Strain of musc/fasc/tend at thigh level, left thigh, sequela
		S76.819S	Strain of musc/fasc/tend at thigh level, unsp thigh, sequela
		S76.911S	Strain unsp musc/fasc/tend at thi lev, right thigh, sequela
		S76.912S	Strain unsp musc/fasc/tend at thi lev, left thigh, sequela
		S76.919S	Strain unsp musc/fasc/tend at thi lev, unsp thigh, sequela
		S83.200S	Bucket-hndl tear of unsp mensc, crnt injury, r knee, sequela
		S83.201S	Bucket-hndl tear of unsp mensc, crnt injury, l knee, sequela
		S83.202S	Bucket-hndl tear of unsp mensc, crnt injury, unsp knee, sqla
		S83.203S	Oth tear of unsp meniscus, current injury, r knee, sequela
		S83.204S	Oth tear of unsp meniscus, current injury, l knee, sequela
		S83.205S	Oth tear of unsp mensc, current injury, unsp knee, sequela
		S83.206S	Unsp tear of unsp meniscus, current injury, r knee, sequela
		S83.207S	Unsp tear of unsp meniscus, current injury, l knee, sequela
		S83.209S	Unsp tear of unsp mensc, current injury, unsp knee, sequela
		S83.211S	Bucket-hndl tear of medial mensc, crnt injury, r knee, sqla
		S83.212S	Bucket-hndl tear of medial mensc, crnt injury, l knee, sqla
		S83.219S	Bucket-hndl tear of medial mensc, crnt inj, unsp knee, sqla
		S83.221S	Prph tear of medial mensc, current injury, r knee, sequela
		S83.222S	Prph tear of medial mensc, current injury, l knee, sequela
		S83.229S	Prph tear of medial mensc, crnt injury, unsp knee, sequela
	(Continued on next page)	**S83.231S**	Cmplx tear of medial mensc, current injury, r knee, sequela

ICD-9-CM		ICD-10-CM	
905.7	LATE EFF SPRAIN&STRAIN W/O MENTION TENDON INJURY **(Continued)**	**S83.232S**	Cmplx tear of medial mensc, current injury, l knee, sequela
		S83.239S	Cmplx tear of medial mensc, crnt injury, unsp knee, sequela
		S83.241S	Oth tear of medial meniscus, current injury, r knee, sequela
		S83.242S	Oth tear of medial meniscus, current injury, l knee, sequela
		S83.249S	Oth tear of medial mensc, current injury, unsp knee, sequela
		S83.251S	Bucket-hndl tear of lat mensc, crnt injury, r knee, sequela
		S83.252S	Bucket-hndl tear of lat mensc, crnt injury, l knee, sequela
		S83.259S	Bucket-hndl tear of lat mensc, crnt injury, unsp knee, sqla
		S83.261S	Prph tear of lat mensc, current injury, right knee, sequela
		S83.262S	Prph tear of lat mensc, current injury, left knee, sequela
		S83.269S	Prph tear of lat mensc, current injury, unsp knee, sequela
		S83.271S	Complex tear of lat mensc, current injury, r knee, sequela
		S83.272S	Complex tear of lat mensc, current injury, l knee, sequela
		S83.279S	Cmplx tear of lat mensc, current injury, unsp knee, sequela
		S83.281S	Oth tear of lat mensc, current injury, right knee, sequela
		S83.282S	Oth tear of lat mensc, current injury, left knee, sequela
		S83.289S	Oth tear of lat mensc, current injury, unsp knee, sequela
		S83.30XS	Tear of articular cartilage of unsp knee, current, sequela
		S83.31XS	Tear of articular cartilage of right knee, current, sequela
		S83.32XS	Tear of articular cartilage of left knee, current, sequela
		S83.401S	Sprain of unsp collateral ligament of right knee, sequela
		S83.402S	Sprain of unsp collateral ligament of left knee, sequela
		S83.409S	Sprain of unsp collateral ligament of unsp knee, sequela
		S83.411S	Sprain of medial collateral ligament of right knee, sequela
		S83.412S	Sprain of medial collateral ligament of left knee, sequela
		S83.419S	Sprain of medial collateral ligament of unsp knee, sequela
		S83.421S	Sprain of lateral collateral ligament of right knee, sequela
		S83.422S	Sprain of lateral collateral ligament of left knee, sequela
		S83.429S	Sprain of lateral collateral ligament of unsp knee, sequela
		S83.501S	Sprain of unsp cruciate ligament of right knee, sequela
		S83.502S	Sprain of unsp cruciate ligament of left knee, sequela
		S83.509S	Sprain of unsp cruciate ligament of unsp knee, sequela
		S83.511S	Sprain of anterior cruciate ligament of right knee, sequela
		S83.512S	Sprain of anterior cruciate ligament of left knee, sequela
		S83.519S	Sprain of anterior cruciate ligament of unsp knee, sequela
		S83.521S	Sprain of posterior cruciate ligament of right knee, sequela
		S83.522S	Sprain of posterior cruciate ligament of left knee, sequela
		S83.529S	Sprain of posterior cruciate ligament of unsp knee, sequela
		S83.60XS	Sprain of super tibiofibul joint and ligmt, unsp knee, sqla
		S83.61XS	Sprain of the super tibiofibul joint and ligmt, r knee, sqla
		S83.62XS	Sprain of the super tibiofibul joint and ligmt, l knee, sqla
		S83.8X1S	Sprain of other specified parts of right knee, sequela
		S83.8X2S	Sprain of other specified parts of left knee, sequela
		S83.8X9S	Sprain of other specified parts of unspecified knee, sequela
		S83.90XS	Sprain of unspecified site of unspecified knee, sequela
		S83.91XS	Sprain of unspecified site of right knee, sequela
		S83.92XS	Sprain of unspecified site of left knee, sequela
		S86.011S	Strain of right Achilles tendon, sequela
		S86.012S	Strain of left Achilles tendon, sequela
		S86.019S	Strain of unspecified Achilles tendon, sequela
		S86.111S	Strain musc/tend post grp at low leg level, right leg, sqla
		S86.112S	Strain musc/tend post grp at low leg level, left leg, sqla
		S86.119S	Strain musc/tend post grp at low leg level, unsp leg, sqla
		S86.211S	Strain musc/tend ant grp at low leg level, right leg, sqla
		S86.212S	Strain musc/tend ant grp at low leg level, left leg, sequela
		S86.219S	Strain musc/tend ant grp at low leg level, unsp leg, sequela
		S86.311S	Strain musc/tend peroneal grp at low leg lev, r leg, sqla
		S86.312S	Strain musc/tend peroneal grp at low leg lev, left leg, sqla
		S86.319S	Strain musc/tend peroneal grp at low leg lev, unsp leg, sqla
		S86.811S	Strain of musc/tend at lower leg level, right leg, sequela
		S86.812S	Strain of musc/tend at lower leg level, left leg, sequela
		S86.819S	Strain of musc/tend at lower leg level, unsp leg, sequela
		S86.911S	Strain unsp musc/tend at low leg level, right leg, sequela
		S86.912S	Strain of unsp musc/tend at low leg level, left leg, sequela
		S86.919S	Strain of unsp musc/tend at low leg level, unsp leg, sequela
		S93.401S	Sprain of unspecified ligament of right ankle, sequela
		S93.402S	Sprain of unspecified ligament of left ankle, sequela
		S93.409S	Sprain of unspecified ligament of unspecified ankle, sequela
		S93.411S	Sprain of calcaneofibular ligament of right ankle, sequela
		S93.412S	Sprain of calcaneofibular ligament of left ankle, sequela
		S93.419S	Sprain of calcaneofibular ligament of unsp ankle, sequela
		S93.421S	Sprain of deltoid ligament of right ankle, sequela
		S93.422S	Sprain of deltoid ligament of left ankle, sequela
		S93.429S	Sprain of deltoid ligament of unspecified ankle, sequela
		S93.431S	Sprain of tibiofibular ligament of right ankle, sequela
		S93.432S	Sprain of tibiofibular ligament of left ankle, sequela
		S93.439S	Sprain of tibiofibular ligament of unsp ankle, sequela
		S93.491S	Sprain of other ligament of right ankle, sequela
		S93.492S	Sprain of other ligament of left ankle, sequela
		S93.499S	Sprain of other ligament of unspecified ankle, sequela
		S93.501S	Unspecified sprain of right great toe, sequela
		S93.502S	Unspecified sprain of left great toe, sequela

(Continued on next page)

[Brackets] indicate valid character values for each code. Character value meanings provided for each code grouping.

ICD-9-CM		ICD-10-CM	
905.7	LATE EFF SPRAIN&STRAIN W/O MENTION TENDON INJURY **(Continued)**	**S93.503S**	Unspecified sprain of unspecified great toe, sequela
		S93.504S	Unspecified sprain of right lesser toe(s), sequela
		S93.505S	Unspecified sprain of left lesser toe(s), sequela
		S93.506S	Unspecified sprain of unspecified lesser toe(s), sequela
		S93.509S	Unspecified sprain of unspecified toe(s), sequela
		S93.511S	Sprain of interphalangeal joint of right great toe, sequela
		S93.512S	Sprain of interphalangeal joint of left great toe, sequela
		S93.513S	Sprain of interphalangeal joint of unsp great toe, sequela
		S93.514S	Sprain of interphaln joint of right lesser toe(s), sequela
		S93.515S	Sprain of interphaln joint of left lesser toe(s), sequela
		S93.516S	Sprain of interphaln joint of unsp lesser toe(s), sequela
		S93.519S	Sprain of interphalangeal joint of unsp toe(s), sequela
		S93.521S	Sprain of MTP joint of right great toe, sequela
		S93.522S	Sprain of MTP joint of left great toe, sequela
		S93.523S	Sprain of MTP joint of unsp great toe, sequela
		S93.524S	Sprain of MTP joint of right lesser toe(s), sequela
		S93.525S	Sprain of MTP joint of left lesser toe(s), sequela
		S93.526S	Sprain of MTP joint of unsp lesser toe(s), sequela
		S93.529S	Sprain of metatarsophalangeal joint of unsp toe(s), sequela
		S93.601S	Unspecified sprain of right foot, sequela
		S93.602S	Unspecified sprain of left foot, sequela
		S93.609S	Unspecified sprain of unspecified foot, sequela
		S93.611S	Sprain of tarsal ligament of right foot, sequela
		S93.612S	Sprain of tarsal ligament of left foot, sequela
		S93.619S	Sprain of tarsal ligament of unspecified foot, sequela
		S93.621S	Sprain of tarsometatarsal ligament of right foot, sequela
		S93.622S	Sprain of tarsometatarsal ligament of left foot, sequela
		S93.629S	Sprain of tarsometatarsal ligament of unsp foot, sequela
		S93.691S	Other sprain of right foot, sequela
		S93.692S	Other sprain of left foot, sequela
		S93.699S	Other sprain of unspecified foot, sequela
		S96.011S	Strain msl/tnd lng flxr msl toe at ank/ft lev, r foot, sqla
		S96.012S	Strain msl/tnd lng flxr msl toe at ank/ft lev, l foot, sqla
		S96.019S	Strain msl/tnd lng flxr msl toe at ank/ft lev, unsp ft, sqla
		S96.111S	Strain msl/tnd lng extn msl toe at ank/ft lev, r foot, sqla
		S96.112S	Strain msl/tnd lng extn msl toe at ank/ft lev, l foot, sqla
		S96.119S	Strain msl/tnd lng extn msl toe at ank/ft lev, unsp ft, sqla
		S96.211S	Strain of intrinsic msl/tnd at ank/ft level, r foot, sequela
		S96.212S	Strain of intrns msl/tnd at ank/ft level, left foot, sequela
		S96.219S	Strain of intrns msl/tnd at ank/ft level, unsp foot, sequela
		S96.811S	Strain muscles and tendons at ank/ft level, r foot, sequela
		S96.812S	Strain muscles and tendons at ank/ft level, l foot, sequela
		S96.819S	Strain musc and tendons at ank/ft level, unsp foot, sequela
		S96.911S	Strain of unsp msl/tnd at ank/ft level, right foot, sequela
		S96.912S	Strain of unsp msl/tnd at ank/ft level, left foot, sequela
		S96.919S	Strain of unsp msl/tnd at ank/ft level, unsp foot, sequela
905.8	LATE EFFECT OF TENDON INJURY	**M67.90**	Unsp disorder of synovium and tendon, unspecified site
905.9	LATE EFFECT OF TRAUMATIC AMPUTATION	**S48.011S**	Complete traumatic amputation at r shoulder jt, sequela
		S48.012S	Complete traumatic amputation at l shoulder jt, sequela
		S48.019S	Complete traumatic amputation at unsp shoulder jt, sequela
		S48.021S	Partial traumatic amputation at r shoulder jt, sequela
		S48.022S	Partial traumatic amputation at left shoulder joint, sequela
		S48.029S	Partial traumatic amputation at unsp shoulder joint, sequela
		S48.111S	Complete traum amp at level betw r shldr and elbow, sequela
		S48.112S	Complete traum amp at level betw l shldr and elbow, sequela
		S48.119S	Complete traum amp at level betw unsp shldr and elbow, sqla
		S48.121S	Partial traum amp at level betw r shldr and elbow, sequela
		S48.122S	Partial traum amp at level betw l shldr and elbow, sequela
		S48.129S	Part traum amp at level betw unsp shldr and elbow, sequela
		S48.911S	Complete traum amp of right shldr/up arm, level unsp, sqla
		S48.912S	Complete traum amp of left shldr/up arm, level unsp, sequela
		S48.919S	Complete traum amp of unsp shldr/up arm, level unsp, sequela
		S48.921S	Partial traum amp of right shldr/up arm, level unsp, sequela
		S48.922S	Partial traum amp of left shldr/up arm, level unsp, sequela
		S48.929S	Partial traum amp of unsp shldr/up arm, level unsp, sequela
		S58.011S	Complete traumatic amp at elbow level, right arm, sequela
		S58.012S	Complete traumatic amp at elbow level, left arm, sequela
		S58.019S	Complete traumatic amp at elbow level, unsp arm, sequela
		S58.021S	Partial traumatic amp at elbow level, right arm, sequela
		S58.022S	Partial traumatic amp at elbow level, left arm, sequela
		S58.029S	Partial traumatic amp at elbow level, unsp arm, sequela
		S58.111S	Complete traum amp at lev betw elbow and wrist, r arm, sqla
		S58.112S	Complete traum amp at lev betw elbow and wrs, left arm, sqla
		S58.119S	Complete traum amp at lev betw elbow and wrs, unsp arm, sqla
		S58.121S	Part traum amp at lev betw elbow and wrist, right arm, sqla
		S58.122S	Part traum amp at level betw elbow and wrist, left arm, sqla
		S58.129S	Part traum amp at level betw elbow and wrist, unsp arm, sqla
		S58.911S	Complete traumatic amp of r forearm, level unsp, sequela
		S58.912S	Complete traumatic amp of l forearm, level unsp, sequela
		S58.919S	Complete traumatic amp of unsp forearm, level unsp, sequela
		S58.921S	Partial traumatic amp of r forearm, level unsp, sequela
	(Continued on next page)	**S58.922S**	Partial traumatic amp of l forearm, level unsp, sequela

ICD-9-CM		ICD-10-CM	
905.9	LATE EFFECT OF TRAUMATIC AMPUTATION **(Continued)**	**S58.929S**	Partial traumatic amp of unsp forearm, level unsp, sequela
		S68.011S	Complete traumatic MCP amputation of right thumb, sequela
		S68.012S	Complete traumatic MCP amputation of left thumb, sequela
		S68.019S	Complete traumatic MCP amputation of thmb, sequela
		S68.021S	Partial traumatic MCP amputation of right thumb, sequela
		S68.022S	Partial traumatic MCP amputation of left thumb, sequela
		S68.029S	Partial traumatic MCP amputation of thmb, sequela
		S68.110S	Complete traumatic MCP amputation of r idx fngr, sequela
		S68.111S	Complete traumatic MCP amputation of l idx fngr, sequela
		S68.112S	Complete traumatic MCP amputation of r mid finger, sequela
		S68.113S	Complete traumatic MCP amputation of l mid finger, sequela
		S68.114S	Complete traumatic MCP amputation of r rng fngr, sequela
		S68.115S	Complete traumatic MCP amputation of l rng fngr, sequela
		S68.116S	Complete traumatic MCP amp of r little finger, sequela
		S68.117S	Complete traumatic MCP amp of l little finger, sequela
		S68.118S	Complete traumatic MCP amputation of finger, sequela
		S68.119S	Complete traumatic MCP amputation of unsp finger, sequela
		S68.120S	Partial traumatic MCP amputation of r idx fngr, sequela
		S68.121S	Partial traumatic MCP amputation of l idx fngr, sequela
		S68.122S	Partial traumatic MCP amputation of r mid finger, sequela
		S68.123S	Partial traumatic MCP amputation of l mid finger, sequela
		S68.124S	Partial traumatic MCP amputation of r rng fngr, sequela
		S68.125S	Partial traumatic MCP amputation of l rng fngr, sequela
		S68.126S	Partial traumatic MCP amputation of r little finger, sequela
		S68.127S	Partial traumatic MCP amputation of l little finger, sequela
		S68.128S	Partial traumatic MCP amputation of finger, sequela
		S68.129S	Partial traumatic MCP amputation of unsp finger, sequela
		S68.411S	Complete traumatic amp of right hand at wrist level, sequela
		S68.412S	Complete traumatic amp of left hand at wrist level, sequela
		S68.419S	Complete traumatic amp of unsp hand at wrist level, sequela
		S68.421S	Partial traumatic amp of right hand at wrist level, sequela
		S68.422S	Partial traumatic amp of left hand at wrist level, sequela
		S68.429S	Partial traumatic amp of unsp hand at wrist level, sequela
		S68.511S	Complete traumatic trnsphal amputation of r thm, sequela
		S68.512S	Complete traumatic trnsphal amp of left thumb, sequela
		S68.519S	Complete traumatic trnsphal amputation of thmb, sequela
		S68.521S	Partial traumatic trnsphal amputation of r thm, sequela
		S68.522S	Partial traumatic trnsphal amputation of left thumb, sequela
		S68.529S	Partial traumatic trnsphal amputation of thmb, sequela
		S68.610S	Complete traumatic trnsphal amp of r idx fngr, sequela
		S68.611S	Complete traumatic trnsphal amp of l idx fngr, sequela
		S68.612S	Complete traumatic trnsphal amp of r mid finger, sequela
		S68.613S	Complete traumatic trnsphal amp of l mid finger, sequela
		S68.614S	Complete traumatic trnsphal amp of r rng fngr, sequela
		S68.615S	Complete traumatic trnsphal amp of l rng fngr, sequela
		S68.616S	Complete traumatic trnsphal amp of r little finger, sequela
		S68.617S	Complete traumatic trnsphal amp of l little finger, sequela
		S68.618S	Complete traumatic trnsphal amputation of finger, sequela
		S68.619S	Complete traumatic trnsphal amp of unsp finger, sequela
		S68.620S	Partial traumatic trnsphal amputation of r idx fngr, sequela
		S68.621S	Partial traumatic trnsphal amputation of l idx fngr, sequela
		S68.622S	Partial traumatic trnsphal amp of r mid finger, sequela
		S68.623S	Partial traumatic trnsphal amp of l mid finger, sequela
		S68.624S	Partial traumatic trnsphal amputation of r rng fngr, sequela
		S68.625S	Partial traumatic trnsphal amputation of l rng fngr, sequela
		S68.626S	Partial traumatic trnsphal amp of r little finger, sequela
		S68.627S	Partial traumatic trnsphal amp of l little finger, sequela
		S68.628S	Partial traumatic trnsphal amputation of finger, sequela
		S68.629S	Partial traumatic trnsphal amp of unsp finger, sequela
		S68.711S	Complete traumatic transmetcrpl amp of right hand, sequela
		S68.712S	Complete traumatic transmetcrpl amp of left hand, sequela
		S68.719S	Complete traumatic transmetcrpl amp of unsp hand, sequela
		S68.721S	Partial traumatic transmetcrpl amp of right hand, sequela
		S68.722S	Partial traumatic transmetcrpl amp of left hand, sequela
		S68.729S	Partial traumatic transmetcrpl amp of unsp hand, sequela
		S78.011S	Complete traumatic amputation at right hip joint, sequela
		S78.012S	Complete traumatic amputation at left hip joint, sequela
		S78.019S	Complete traumatic amputation at unsp hip joint, sequela
		S78.021S	Partial traumatic amputation at right hip joint, sequela
		S78.022S	Partial traumatic amputation at left hip joint, sequela
		S78.029S	Partial traumatic amputation at unsp hip joint, sequela
		S78.111S	Complete traumatic amp at level betw r hip and knee, sequela
		S78.112S	Complete traum amp at level betw left hip and knee, sequela
		S78.119S	Complete traum amp at level betw unsp hip and knee, sequela
		S78.121S	Partial traumatic amp at level betw r hip and knee, sequela
		S78.122S	Partial traum amp at level betw left hip and knee, sequela
		S78.129S	Partial traum amp at level betw unsp hip and knee, sequela
		S78.911S	Complete traum amp of r hip and thigh, level unsp, sequela
		S78.912S	Complete traum amp of l hip and thigh, level unsp, sequela
		S78.919S	Complete traum amp of unsp hip and thigh, level unsp, sqla
		S78.921S	Partial traum amp of r hip and thigh, level unsp, sequela
		S78.922S	Partial traum amp of left hip and thigh, level unsp, sequela

(Continued on next page)

ICD-9-CM		ICD-10-CM	
905.9	LATE EFFECT OF TRAUMATIC AMPUTATION **(Continued)**	**S78.929S**	Partial traum amp of unsp hip and thigh, level unsp, sequela
		S88.011S	Complete traumatic amp at knee level, r low leg, sequela
		S88.012S	Complete traumatic amp at knee level, l low leg, sequela
		S88.019S	Complete traumatic amp at knee level, unsp low leg, sequela
		S88.021S	Partial traumatic amp at knee level, r low leg, sequela
		S88.022S	Partial traumatic amp at knee level, l low leg, sequela
		S88.029S	Partial traumatic amp at knee level, unsp lower leg, sequela
		S88.111S	Complete traum amp at lev betw kn and ankl, r low leg, sqla
		S88.112S	Complete traum amp at lev betw kn and ankl, l low leg, sqla
		S88.119S	Complete traum amp at lev betw kn & ankl, unsp low leg, sqla
		S88.121S	Part traum amp at level betw knee and ankle, r low leg, sqla
		S88.122S	Part traum amp at level betw knee and ankle, l low leg, sqla
		S88.129S	Part traum amp at lev betw knee and ankl, unsp low leg, sqla
		S88.911S	Complete traumatic amp of r low leg, level unsp, sequela
		S88.912S	Complete traumatic amp of l low leg, level unsp, sequela
		S88.919S	Complete traumatic amp of unsp low leg, level unsp, sequela
		S88.921S	Partial traumatic amp of r low leg, level unsp, sequela
		S88.922S	Partial traumatic amp of l low leg, level unsp, sequela
		S88.929S	Partial traumatic amp of unsp lower leg, level unsp, sequela
		S98.011S	Complete traumatic amp of right foot at ankle level, sequela
		S98.012S	Complete traumatic amp of left foot at ankle level, sequela
		S98.019S	Complete traumatic amp of unsp foot at ankle level, sequela
		S98.021S	Partial traumatic amp of right foot at ankle level, sequela
		S98.022S	Partial traumatic amp of left foot at ankle level, sequela
		S98.029S	Partial traumatic amp of unsp foot at ankle level, sequela
		S98.111S	Complete traumatic amputation of right great toe, sequela
		S98.112S	Complete traumatic amputation of left great toe, sequela
		S98.119S	Complete traumatic amputation of unsp great toe, sequela
		S98.121S	Partial traumatic amputation of right great toe, sequela
		S98.122S	Partial traumatic amputation of left great toe, sequela
		S98.129S	Partial traumatic amputation of unsp great toe, sequela
		S98.131S	Complete traumatic amp of one right lesser toe, sequela
		S98.132S	Complete traumatic amp of one left lesser toe, sequela
		S98.139S	Complete traumatic amp of one unsp lesser toe, sequela
		S98.141S	Partial traumatic amp of one right lesser toe, sequela
		S98.142S	Partial traumatic amputation of one left lesser toe, sequela
		S98.149S	Partial traumatic amputation of one unsp lesser toe, sequela
		S98.211S	Complete traum amp of two or more right lesser toes, sequela
		S98.212S	Complete traum amp of two or more left lesser toes, sequela
		S98.219S	Complete traum amp of two or more unsp lesser toes, sequela
		S98.221S	Partial traum amp of two or more right lesser toes, sequela
		S98.222S	Partial traum amp of two or more left lesser toes, sequela
		S98.229S	Partial traum amp of two or more unsp lesser toes, sequela
		S98.311S	Complete traumatic amputation of right midfoot, sequela
		S98.312S	Complete traumatic amputation of left midfoot, sequela
		S98.319S	Complete traumatic amputation of unsp midfoot, sequela
		S98.321S	Partial traumatic amputation of right midfoot, sequela
		S98.322S	Partial traumatic amputation of left midfoot, sequela
		S98.329S	Partial traumatic amputation of unspecified midfoot, sequela
		S98.911S	Complete traumatic amp of right foot, level unsp, sequela
		S98.912S	Complete traumatic amp of left foot, level unsp, sequela
		S98.919S	Complete traumatic amp of unsp foot, level unsp, sequela
		S98.921S	Partial traumatic amp of right foot, level unsp, sequela
		S98.922S	Partial traumatic amp of left foot, level unsp, sequela
		S98.929S	Partial traumatic amp of unsp foot, level unsp, sequela
906.0	LATE EFFECT OF OPEN WOUND OF HEAD NECK AND TRUNK	**S01.00XS**	Unspecified open wound of scalp, sequela
		S01.01XS	Laceration without foreign body of scalp, sequela
		S01.02XS	Laceration with foreign body of scalp, sequela
		S01.03XS	Puncture wound without foreign body of scalp, sequela
		S01.04XS	Puncture wound with foreign body of scalp, sequela
		S01.05XS	Open bite of scalp, sequela
		S01.101S	Unsp open wound of right eyelid and periocular area, sequela
		S01.102S	Unsp open wound of left eyelid and periocular area, sequela
		S01.109S	Unsp open wound of unsp eyelid and periocular area, sequela
		S01.111S	Lac w/o fb of right eyelid and periocular area, sequela
		S01.112S	Lac w/o fb of left eyelid and periocular area, sequela
		S01.119S	Lac w/o fb of unsp eyelid and periocular area, sequela
		S01.121S	Laceration w fb of right eyelid and periocular area, sequela
		S01.122S	Laceration w fb of left eyelid and periocular area, sequela
		S01.129S	Laceration w fb of unsp eyelid and periocular area, sequela
		S01.131S	Pnctr w/o fb of right eyelid and periocular area, sequela
		S01.132S	Pnctr w/o fb of left eyelid and periocular area, sequela
		S01.139S	Pnctr w/o fb of unsp eyelid and periocular area, sequela
		S01.141S	Pnctr w fb of right eyelid and periocular area, sequela
		S01.142S	Pnctr w fb of left eyelid and periocular area, sequela
		S01.149S	Pnctr w fb of unsp eyelid and periocular area, sequela
		S01.151S	Open bite of right eyelid and periocular area, sequela
		S01.152S	Open bite of left eyelid and periocular area, sequela
		S01.159S	Open bite of unspecified eyelid and periocular area, sequela
		S01.20XS	Unspecified open wound of nose, sequela
		S01.21XS	Laceration without foreign body of nose, sequela
	(Continued on next page)	**S01.22XS**	Laceration with foreign body of nose, sequela

ICD-9-CM		ICD-10-CM	
906.0	LATE EFFECT OF OPEN WOUND OF HEAD NECK AND TRUNK **(Continued)**	**S01.23XS**	Puncture wound without foreign body of nose, sequela
		S01.24XS	Puncture wound with foreign body of nose, sequela
		S01.25XS	Open bite of nose, sequela
		S01.301S	Unspecified open wound of right ear, sequela
		S01.302S	Unspecified open wound of left ear, sequela
		S01.309S	Unspecified open wound of unspecified ear, sequela
		S01.311S	Laceration without foreign body of right ear, sequela
		S01.312S	Laceration without foreign body of left ear, sequela
		S01.319S	Laceration without foreign body of unspecified ear, sequela
		S01.321S	Laceration with foreign body of right ear, sequela
		S01.322S	Laceration with foreign body of left ear, sequela
		S01.329S	Laceration with foreign body of unspecified ear, sequela
		S01.331S	Puncture wound without foreign body of right ear, sequela
		S01.332S	Puncture wound without foreign body of left ear, sequela
		S01.339S	Puncture wound without foreign body of unsp ear, sequela
		S01.341S	Puncture wound with foreign body of right ear, sequela
		S01.342S	Puncture wound with foreign body of left ear, sequela
		S01.349S	Puncture wound with foreign body of unspecified ear, sequela
		S01.351S	Open bite of right ear, sequela
		S01.352S	Open bite of left ear, sequela
		S01.359S	Open bite of unspecified ear, sequela
		S01.401S	Unsp open wound of right cheek and TMJ area, sequela
		S01.402S	Unsp open wound of left cheek and TMJ area, sequela
		S01.409S	Unsp open wound of unsp cheek and TMJ area, sequela
		S01.411S	Laceration w/o fb of right cheek and TMJ area, sequela
		S01.412S	Laceration w/o fb of left cheek and TMJ area, sequela
		S01.419S	Laceration w/o fb of unsp cheek and TMJ area, sequela
		S01.421S	Laceration w fb of right cheek and TMJ area, sequela
		S01.422S	Laceration w fb of left cheek and TMJ area, sequela
		S01.429S	Laceration w fb of unsp cheek and TMJ area, sequela
		S01.431S	Pnctr w/o foreign body of right cheek and TMJ area, sequela
		S01.432S	Pnctr w/o foreign body of left cheek and TMJ area, sequela
		S01.439S	Pnctr w/o foreign body of unsp cheek and TMJ area, sequela
		S01.441S	Pnctr w foreign body of right cheek and TMJ area, sequela
		S01.442S	Pnctr w foreign body of left cheek and TMJ area, sequela
		S01.449S	Pnctr w foreign body of unsp cheek and TMJ area, sequela
		S01.451S	Open bite of right cheek and temporomandibular area, sequela
		S01.452S	Open bite of left cheek and temporomandibular area, sequela
		S01.459S	Open bite of unsp cheek and temporomandibular area, sequela
		S01.501S	Unspecified open wound of lip, sequela
		S01.502S	Unspecified open wound of oral cavity, sequela
		S01.511S	Laceration without foreign body of lip, sequela
		S01.512S	Laceration without foreign body of oral cavity, sequela
		S01.521S	Laceration with foreign body of lip, sequela
		S01.522S	Laceration with foreign body of oral cavity, sequela
		S01.531S	Puncture wound without foreign body of lip, sequela
		S01.532S	Puncture wound without foreign body of oral cavity, sequela
		S01.541S	Puncture wound with foreign body of lip, sequela
		S01.542S	Puncture wound with foreign body of oral cavity, sequela
		S01.551S	Open bite of lip, sequela
		S01.552S	Open bite of oral cavity, sequela
		S01.80XS	Unspecified open wound of other part of head, sequela
		S01.81XS	Laceration w/o foreign body of other part of head, sequela
		S01.82XS	Laceration with foreign body of other part of head, sequela
		S01.83XS	Puncture wound w/o foreign body of oth part of head, sequela
		S01.84XS	Puncture wound w foreign body of oth part of head, sequela
		S01.85XS	Open bite of other part of head, sequela
		S01.90XS	Unspecified open wound of unspecified part of head, sequela
		S01.91XS	Laceration w/o foreign body of unsp part of head, sequela
		S01.92XS	Laceration with foreign body of unsp part of head, sequela
		S01.93XS	Pnctr w/o foreign body of unsp part of head, sequela
		S01.94XS	Puncture wound w foreign body of unsp part of head, sequela
		S01.95XS	Open bite of unspecified part of head, sequela
		S03.2XXS	Dislocation of tooth, sequela
		S05.20XS	Oclr lac/rupt w prolaps/loss of intraoc tiss, unsp eye, sqla
		S05.21XS	Oclr lac/rupt w prolaps/loss of intraoc tissue, r eye, sqla
		S05.22XS	Oclr lac/rupt w prolaps/loss of intraoc tissue, l eye, sqla
		S05.30XS	Oclr lac w/o prolaps/loss of intraoc tissue, unsp eye, sqla
		S05.31XS	Ocular lac w/o prolaps/loss of intraoc tissue, r eye, sqla
		S05.32XS	Ocular lac w/o prolaps/loss of intraoc tissue, l eye, sqla
		S05.40XS	Penetrating wound of orbit w or w/o fb, unsp eye, sequela
		S05.41XS	Penetrating wound of orbit w or w/o fb, right eye, sequela
		S05.42XS	Penetrating wound of orbit w or w/o fb, left eye, sequela
		S05.50XS	Penetrating wound with foreign body of unsp eyeball, sequela
		S05.51XS	Penetrating wound w foreign body of right eyeball, sequela
		S05.52XS	Penetrating wound with foreign body of left eyeball, sequela
		S05.60XS	Penetrating wound w/o foreign body of unsp eyeball, sequela
		S05.61XS	Penetrating wound w/o foreign body of right eyeball, sequela
		S05.62XS	Penetrating wound w/o foreign body of left eyeball, sequela
		S08.0XXS	Avulsion of scalp, sequela
		S08.111S	Complete traumatic amputation of right ear, sequela
	(Continued on next page)	**S08.112S**	Complete traumatic amputation of left ear, sequela

[Brackets] indicate valid character values for each code. Character value meanings provided for each code grouping.

ICD-9-CM		ICD-10-CM	
906.0	LATE EFFECT OF OPEN WOUND OF HEAD NECK AND TRUNK **(Continued)**	**S08.119S**	Complete traumatic amputation of unspecified ear, sequela
		S08.121S	Partial traumatic amputation of right ear, sequela
		S08.122S	Partial traumatic amputation of left ear, sequela
		S08.129S	Partial traumatic amputation of unspecified ear, sequela
		S08.811S	Complete traumatic amputation of nose, sequela
		S08.812S	Partial traumatic amputation of nose, sequela
		S08.89XS	Traumatic amputation of other parts of head, sequela
		S09.12XS	Laceration of muscle and tendon of head, sequela
		S09.21XS	Traumatic rupture of right ear drum, sequela
		S09.22XS	Traumatic rupture of left ear drum, sequela
		S09.311S	Primary blast injury of right ear, sequela
		S09.312S	Primary blast injury of left ear, sequela
		S09.313S	Primary blast injury of ear, bilateral, sequela
		S09.319S	Primary blast injury of unspecified ear, sequela
		S11.011S	Laceration without foreign body of larynx, sequela
		S11.012S	Laceration with foreign body of larynx, sequela
		S11.013S	Puncture wound without foreign body of larynx, sequela
		S11.014S	Puncture wound with foreign body of larynx, sequela
		S11.015S	Open bite of larynx, sequela
		S11.019S	Unspecified open wound of larynx, sequela
		S11.021S	Laceration without foreign body of trachea, sequela
		S11.022S	Laceration with foreign body of trachea, sequela
		S11.023S	Puncture wound without foreign body of trachea, sequela
		S11.024S	Puncture wound with foreign body of trachea, sequela
		S11.025S	Open bite of trachea, sequela
		S11.029S	Unspecified open wound of trachea, sequela
		S11.031S	Laceration without foreign body of vocal cord, sequela
		S11.032S	Laceration with foreign body of vocal cord, sequela
		S11.033S	Puncture wound without foreign body of vocal cord, sequela
		S11.034S	Puncture wound with foreign body of vocal cord, sequela
		S11.035S	Open bite of vocal cord, sequela
		S11.039S	Unspecified open wound of vocal cord, sequela
		S11.10XS	Unspecified open wound of thyroid gland, sequela
		S11.11XS	Laceration without foreign body of thyroid gland, sequela
		S11.12XS	Laceration with foreign body of thyroid gland, sequela
		S11.13XS	Puncture wound w/o foreign body of thyroid gland, sequela
		S11.14XS	Puncture wound with foreign body of thyroid gland, sequela
		S11.15XS	Open bite of thyroid gland, sequela
		S11.20XS	Unsp open wound of pharynx and cervical esophagus, sequela
		S11.21XS	Laceration w/o fb of pharynx and cervical esophagus, sequela
		S11.22XS	Laceration w fb of pharynx and cervical esophagus, sequela
		S11.23XS	Pnctr w/o fb of pharynx and cervical esophagus, sequela
		S11.24XS	Pnctr w fb of pharynx and cervical esophagus, sequela
		S11.25XS	Open bite of pharynx and cervical esophagus, sequela
		S11.80XS	Unspecified open wound of oth part of neck, sequela
		S11.81XS	Laceration without foreign body of oth part of neck, sequela
		S11.82XS	Laceration with foreign body of oth part of neck, sequela
		S11.83XS	Puncture wound w/o foreign body of oth part of neck, sequela
		S11.84XS	Puncture wound w foreign body of oth part of neck, sequela
		S11.85XS	Open bite of other specified part of neck, sequela
		S11.89XS	Other open wound of other specified part of neck, sequela
		S11.90XS	Unspecified open wound of unspecified part of neck, sequela
		S11.91XS	Laceration w/o foreign body of unsp part of neck, sequela
		S11.92XS	Laceration with foreign body of unsp part of neck, sequela
		S11.93XS	Pnctr w/o foreign body of unsp part of neck, sequela
		S11.94XS	Puncture wound w foreign body of unsp part of neck, sequela
		S11.95XS	Open bite of unspecified part of neck, sequela
		S16.2XXS	Laceration of musc/fasc/tend at neck level, sequela
		S21.001S	Unspecified open wound of right breast, sequela
		S21.002S	Unspecified open wound of left breast, sequela
		S21.009S	Unspecified open wound of unspecified breast, sequela
		S21.011S	Laceration without foreign body of right breast, sequela
		S21.012S	Laceration without foreign body of left breast, sequela
		S21.019S	Laceration without foreign body of unsp breast, sequela
		S21.021S	Laceration with foreign body of right breast, sequela
		S21.022S	Laceration with foreign body of left breast, sequela
		S21.029S	Laceration with foreign body of unspecified breast, sequela
		S21.031S	Puncture wound without foreign body of right breast, sequela
		S21.032S	Puncture wound without foreign body of left breast, sequela
		S21.039S	Puncture wound without foreign body of unsp breast, sequela
		S21.041S	Puncture wound with foreign body of right breast, sequela
		S21.042S	Puncture wound with foreign body of left breast, sequela
		S21.049S	Puncture wound with foreign body of unsp breast, sequela
		S21.051S	Open bite of right breast, sequela
		S21.052S	Open bite of left breast, sequela
		S21.059S	Open bite of unspecified breast, sequela
		S21.101S	Unsp opn wnd r frnt wl of thorax w/o penet thor cavity, sqla
		S21.102S	Unsp opn wnd l frnt wl of thorax w/o penet thor cavity, sqla
		S21.109S	Unsp opn wnd unsp frnt wall of thrx w/o penet thor cav, sqla
		S21.111S	Lac w/o fb of r frnt wl of thorax w/o penet thor cav, sqla
		S21.112S	Lac w/o fb of l frnt wl of thorax w/o penet thor cav, sqla
		S21.119S	Lac w/o fb of unsp frnt wl of thrx w/o penet thor cav, sqla

(Continued on next page)

ICD-9-CM		ICD-10-CM	
906.0	LATE EFFECT OF OPEN WOUND OF HEAD NECK AND TRUNK **(Continued)**	**S21.121S**	Lac w fb of r frnt wl of thorax w/o penet thor cavity, sqla
		S21.122S	Lac w fb of l frnt wl of thorax w/o penet thor cavity, sqla
		S21.129S	Lac w fb of unsp front wall of thrx w/o penet thor cav, sqla
		S21.131S	Pnctr w/o fb of r frnt wl of thorax w/o penet thor cav, sqla
		S21.132S	Pnctr w/o fb of l frnt wl of thorax w/o penet thor cav, sqla
		S21.139S	Pnctr w/o fb of unsp frnt wl of thrx w/o penet thor cav,sqla
		S21.141S	Pnctr w fb of r frnt wl of thorax w/o penet thor cav, sqla
		S21.142S	Pnctr w fb of l frnt wl of thorax w/o penet thor cav, sqla
		S21.149S	Pnctr w fb of unsp frnt wl of thrx w/o penet thor cav, sqla
		S21.151S	Open bite of r frnt wl of thorax w/o penet thor cavity, sqla
		S21.152S	Open bite of l frnt wl of thorax w/o penet thor cavity, sqla
		S21.159S	Open bite of unsp frnt wall of thrx w/o penet thor cav, sqla
		S21.201S	Unsp opn wnd r bk wl of thorax w/o penet thor cavity, sqla
		S21.202S	Unsp opn wnd l bk wl of thorax w/o penet thor cavity, sqla
		S21.209S	Unsp opn wnd unsp bk wl of thorax w/o penet thor cav, sqla
		S21.211S	Lac w/o fb of r bk wl of thorax w/o penet thor cavity, sqla
		S21.212S	Lac w/o fb of l bk wl of thorax w/o penet thor cavity, sqla
		S21.219S	Lac w/o fb of unsp bk wl of thorax w/o penet thor cav, sqla
		S21.221S	Lac w fb of r bk wl of thorax w/o penet thor cavity, sequela
		S21.222S	Lac w fb of l bk wl of thorax w/o penet thor cavity, sequela
		S21.229S	Lac w fb of unsp bk wl of thorax w/o penet thor cavity, sqla
		S21.231S	Pnctr w/o fb of r bk wl of thorax w/o penet thor cav, sqla
		S21.232S	Pnctr w/o fb of l bk wl of thorax w/o penet thor cav, sqla
		S21.239S	Pnctr w/o fb of unsp bk wl of thrx w/o penet thor cav, sqla
		S21.241S	Pnctr w fb of r bk wl of thorax w/o penet thor cavity, sqla
		S21.242S	Pnctr w fb of l bk wl of thorax w/o penet thor cavity, sqla
		S21.249S	Pnctr w fb of unsp bk wl of thorax w/o penet thor cav, sqla
		S21.251S	Open bite of r bk wl of thorax w/o penet thor cavity, sqla
		S21.252S	Open bite of l bk wl of thorax w/o penet thor cavity, sqla
		S21.259S	Open bite of unsp bk wl of thorax w/o penet thor cav, sqla
		S21.301S	Unsp opn wnd r frnt wl of thorax w penet thor cavity, sqla
		S21.302S	Unsp opn wnd l frnt wl of thorax w penet thor cavity, sqla
		S21.309S	Unsp opn wnd unsp front wall of thrx w penet thor cav, sqla
		S21.311S	Lac w/o fb of r frnt wl of thorax w penet thor cavity, sqla
		S21.312S	Lac w/o fb of l frnt wl of thorax w penet thor cavity, sqla
		S21.319S	Lac w/o fb of unsp front wall of thrx w penet thor cav, sqla
		S21.321S	Lac w fb of r frnt wl of thorax w penet thor cavity, sequela
		S21.322S	Lac w fb of l frnt wl of thorax w penet thor cavity, sequela
		S21.329S	Lac w fb of unsp front wall of thorax w penet thor cav, sqla
		S21.331S	Pnctr w/o fb of r frnt wl of thorax w penet thor cav, sqla
		S21.332S	Pnctr w/o fb of l frnt wl of thorax w penet thor cav, sqla
		S21.339S	Pnctr w/o fb of unsp frnt wl of thrx w penet thor cav, sqla
		S21.341S	Pnctr w fb of r frnt wl of thorax w penet thor cavity, sqla
		S21.342S	Pnctr w fb of l frnt wl of thorax w penet thor cavity, sqla
		S21.349S	Pnctr w fb of unsp front wall of thrx w penet thor cav, sqla
		S21.351S	Open bite of r frnt wl of thorax w penet thor cavity, sqla
		S21.352S	Open bite of l frnt wl of thorax w penet thor cavity, sqla
		S21.359S	Open bite of unsp front wall of thrx w penet thor cav, sqla
		S21.401S	Unsp opn wnd r bk wl of thorax w penet thor cavity, sequela
		S21.402S	Unsp opn wnd l bk wl of thorax w penet thor cavity, sequela
		S21.409S	Unsp opn wnd unsp bk wl of thorax w penet thor cavity, sqla
		S21.411S	Lac w/o fb of r bk wl of thorax w penet thor cavity, sequela
		S21.412S	Lac w/o fb of l bk wl of thorax w penet thor cavity, sequela
		S21.419S	Lac w/o fb of unsp bk wl of thorax w penet thor cavity, sqla
		S21.421S	Lac w fb of r bk wl of thorax w penet thor cavity, sequela
		S21.422S	Lac w fb of l bk wl of thorax w penet thor cavity, sequela
		S21.429S	Lac w fb of unsp bk wl of thorax w penet thor cavity, sqla
		S21.431S	Pnctr w/o fb of r bk wl of thorax w penet thor cavity, sqla
		S21.432S	Pnctr w/o fb of l bk wl of thorax w penet thor cavity, sqla
		S21.439S	Pnctr w/o fb of unsp bk wl of thorax w penet thor cav, sqla
		S21.441S	Pnctr w fb of r bk wl of thorax w penet thor cavity, sequela
		S21.442S	Pnctr w fb of l bk wl of thorax w penet thor cavity, sequela
		S21.449S	Pnctr w fb of unsp bk wl of thorax w penet thor cavity, sqla
		S21.451S	Open bite of r bk wl of thorax w penet thor cavity, sequela
		S21.452S	Open bite of l bk wl of thorax w penet thor cavity, sequela
		S21.459S	Open bite of unsp bk wl of thorax w penet thor cavity, sqla
		S21.90XS	Unsp open wound of unspecified part of thorax, sequela
		S21.91XS	Laceration w/o foreign body of unsp part of thorax, sequela
		S21.92XS	Laceration with foreign body of unsp part of thorax, sequela
		S21.93XS	Pnctr w/o foreign body of unsp part of thorax, sequela
		S21.94XS	Pnctr w foreign body of unsp part of thorax, sequela
		S21.95XS	Open bite of unspecified part of thorax, sequela
		S28.1XXS	Traumatic amp of part of thorax, except breast, sequela
		S28.211S	Complete traumatic amputation of right breast, sequela
		S28.212S	Complete traumatic amputation of left breast, sequela
		S28.219S	Complete traumatic amputation of unspecified breast, sequela
		S28.221S	Partial traumatic amputation of right breast, sequela
		S28.222S	Partial traumatic amputation of left breast, sequela
		S28.229S	Partial traumatic amputation of unspecified breast, sequela
		S29.021S	Laceration of msl/tnd of front wall of thorax, sequela
		S29.022S	Laceration of msl/tnd of back wall of thorax, sequela
	(Continued on next page)	**S29.029S**	Laceration of msl/tnd of unsp wall of thorax, sequela

ICD-9-CM		ICD-10-CM	
906.Ø	LATE EFFECT OF OPEN WOUND OF HEAD NECK AND TRUNK **(Continued)**	**S31.ØØØS**	Unsp opn wnd low back and pelv w/o penet retroperiton, sqla
		S31.ØØ1S	Unsp opn wnd low back and pelvis w penet retroperiton, sqla
		S31.Ø1ØS	Lac w/o fb of low back and pelv w/o penet retroperiton, sqla
		S31.Ø11S	Lac w/o fb of low back and pelvis w penet retroperiton, sqla
		S31.Ø2ØS	Lac w fb of low back and pelvis w/o penet retroperiton, sqla
		S31.Ø21S	Lac w fb of low back and pelvis w penet retroperiton, sqla
		S31.Ø3ØS	Pnctr w/o fb of low back & pelv w/o penet retroperiton, sqla
		S31.Ø31S	Pnctr w/o fb of low back and pelv w penet retroperiton, sqla
		S31.Ø4ØS	Pnctr w fb of low back and pelv w/o penet retroperiton, sqla
		S31.Ø41S	Pnctr w fb of low back and pelvis w penet retroperiton, sqla
		S31.Ø5ØS	Open bite of low back and pelv w/o penet retroperiton, sqla
		S31.Ø51S	Open bite of low back and pelvis w penet retroperiton, sqla
		S31.1ØØS	Unsp opn wnd abd wall, r upper q w/o penet perit cav, sqla
		S31.1Ø1S	Unsp opn wnd abd wall, l upr q w/o penet perit cav, sequela
		S31.1Ø2S	Unsp opn wnd abd wall, epigst rgn w/o penet perit cav, sqla
		S31.1Ø3S	Unsp opn wnd abd wall, right low q w/o penet perit cav, sqla
		S31.1Ø4S	Unsp opn wnd abd wall, left low q w/o penet perit cav, sqla
		S31.1Ø5S	Unsp opn wnd abd wall, periumb rgn w/o penet perit cav, sqla
		S31.1Ø9S	Unsp opn wnd abd wall, unsp q w/o penet perit cav, sequela
		S31.11ØS	Lac w/o fb of abd wall, r upper q w/o penet perit cav, sqla
		S31.111S	Lac w/o fb of abd wall, l upr q w/o penet perit cav, sequela
		S31.112S	Lac w/o fb of abd wall, epigst rgn w/o penet perit cav, sqla
		S31.113S	Lac w/o fb of abd wall, r low q w/o penet perit cav, sqla
		S31.114S	Lac w/o fb of abd wall, left low q w/o penet perit cav, sqla
		S31.115S	Lac w/o fb of abd wl, periumb rgn w/o penet perit cav, sqla
		S31.119S	Lac w/o fb of abd wall, unsp q w/o penet perit cav, sequela
		S31.12ØS	Lacerat abd wall w fb, r upper q w/o penet perit cav, sqla
		S31.121S	Lacerat abd wall w fb, l upr q w/o penet perit cav, sequela
		S31.122S	Lacerat abd wall w fb, epigst rgn w/o penet perit cav, sqla
		S31.123S	Lacerat abd wall w fb, right low q w/o penet perit cav, sqla
		S31.124S	Lacerat abd wall w fb, left low q w/o penet perit cav, sqla
		S31.125S	Lacerat abd wall w fb, periumb rgn w/o penet perit cav, sqla
		S31.129S	Lacerat abd wall w fb, unsp q w/o penet perit cav, sequela
		S31.13ØS	Pnctr of abd wall w/o fb, r upr q w/o penet perit cav, sqla
		S31.131S	Pnctr of abd wall w/o fb, l upr q w/o penet perit cav, sqla
		S31.132S	Pnctr of abd wl w/o fb, epigst rgn w/o penet perit cav, sqla
		S31.133S	Pnctr of abd wall w/o fb, r low q w/o penet perit cav, sqla
		S31.134S	Pnctr of abd wall w/o fb, l low q w/o penet perit cav, sqla
		S31.135S	Pnctr of abd wl w/o fb,periumb rgn w/o penet perit cav, sqla
		S31.139S	Pnctr of abd wall w/o fb, unsp q w/o penet perit cav, sqla
		S31.14ØS	Pnctr of abd wall w fb, r upper q w/o penet perit cav, sqla
		S31.141S	Pnctr of abd wall w fb, l upr q w/o penet perit cav, sequela
		S31.142S	Pnctr of abd wall w fb, epigst rgn w/o penet perit cav, sqla
		S31.143S	Pnctr of abd wall w fb, r low q w/o penet perit cav, sqla
		S31.144S	Pnctr of abd wall w fb, left low q w/o penet perit cav, sqla
		S31.145S	Pnctr of abd wl w fb, periumb rgn w/o penet perit cav, sqla
		S31.149S	Pnctr of abd wall w fb, unsp q w/o penet perit cav, sequela
		S31.15ØS	Open bite of abd wall, r upper q w/o penet perit cav, sqla
		S31.151S	Open bite of abd wall, l upr q w/o penet perit cav, sequela
		S31.152S	Open bite of abd wall, epigst rgn w/o penet perit cav, sqla
		S31.153S	Open bite of abd wall, right low q w/o penet perit cav, sqla
		S31.154S	Open bite of abd wall, left low q w/o penet perit cav, sqla
		S31.155S	Open bite of abd wall, periumb rgn w/o penet perit cav, sqla
		S31.159S	Open bite of abd wall, unsp q w/o penet perit cav, sequela
		S31.2ØXS	Unspecified open wound of penis, sequela
		S31.21XS	Laceration without foreign body of penis, sequela
		S31.22XS	Laceration with foreign body of penis, sequela
		S31.23XS	Puncture wound without foreign body of penis, sequela
		S31.24XS	Puncture wound with foreign body of penis, sequela
		S31.25XS	Open bite of penis, sequela
		S31.3ØXS	Unspecified open wound of scrotum and testes, sequela
		S31.31XS	Laceration w/o foreign body of scrotum and testes, sequela
		S31.32XS	Laceration with foreign body of scrotum and testes, sequela
		S31.33XS	Pnctr w/o foreign body of scrotum and testes, sequela
		S31.34XS	Puncture wound w foreign body of scrotum and testes, sequela
		S31.35XS	Open bite of scrotum and testes, sequela
		S31.4ØXS	Unspecified open wound of vagina and vulva, sequela
		S31.41XS	Laceration without foreign body of vagina and vulva, sequela
		S31.42XS	Laceration with foreign body of vagina and vulva, sequela
		S31.43XS	Puncture wound w/o foreign body of vagina and vulva, sequela
		S31.44XS	Puncture wound w foreign body of vagina and vulva, sequela
		S31.45XS	Open bite of vagina and vulva, sequela
		S31.6ØØS	Unsp opn wnd abd wall, right upper q w penet perit cav, sqla
		S31.6Ø1S	Unsp opn wnd abd wall, l upr q w penet perit cav, sequela
		S31.6Ø2S	Unsp opn wnd abd wall, epigst rgn w penet perit cav, sequela
		S31.6Ø3S	Unsp opn wnd abd wall, right lower q w penet perit cav, sqla
		S31.6Ø4S	Unsp opn wnd abd wall, left lower q w penet perit cav, sqla
		S31.6Ø5S	Unsp opn wnd abd wall, periumb rgn w penet perit cav, sqla
		S31.6Ø9S	Unsp opn wnd abd wall, unsp q w penet perit cav, sequela
		S31.61ØS	Lac w/o fb of abd wall, r upper q w penet perit cav, sqla
		S31.611S	Lac w/o fb of abd wall, l upr q w penet perit cav, sequela
		S31.612S	Lac w/o fb of abd wall, epigst rgn w penet perit cav, sqla

(Continued on next page)

ICD-9-CM		ICD-10-CM	
906.0	LATE EFFECT OF OPEN WOUND OF HEAD NECK AND TRUNK **(Continued)**	**S31.613S**	Lac w/o fb of abd wall, right low q w penet perit cav, sqla
		S31.614S	Lac w/o fb of abd wall, left lower q w penet perit cav, sqla
		S31.615S	Lac w/o fb of abd wall, periumb rgn w penet perit cav, sqla
		S31.619S	Lac w/o fb of abd wall, unsp q w penet perit cav, sequela
		S31.620S	Lac w fb of abd wall, right upper q w penet perit cav, sqla
		S31.621S	Lac w fb of abd wall, l upr q w penet perit cav, sequela
		S31.622S	Lac w fb of abd wall, epigst rgn w penet perit cav, sequela
		S31.623S	Lac w fb of abd wall, right lower q w penet perit cav, sqla
		S31.624S	Lac w fb of abd wall, left lower q w penet perit cav, sqla
		S31.625S	Lac w fb of abd wall, periumb rgn w penet perit cav, sequela
		S31.629S	Lac w fb of abd wall, unsp q w penet perit cav, sequela
		S31.630S	Pnctr w/o fb of abd wall, r upper q w penet perit cav, sqla
		S31.631S	Pnctr w/o fb of abd wall, l upr q w penet perit cav, sequela
		S31.632S	Pnctr w/o fb of abd wall, epigst rgn w penet perit cav, sqla
		S31.633S	Pnctr w/o fb of abd wall, r low q w penet perit cav, sqla
		S31.634S	Pnctr w/o fb of abd wall, left low q w penet perit cav, sqla
		S31.635S	Pnctr w/o fb of abd wl, periumb rgn w penet perit cav, sqla
		S31.639S	Pnctr w/o fb of abd wall, unsp q w penet perit cav, sequela
		S31.640S	Pnctr w fb of abd wall, r upper q w penet perit cav, sqla
		S31.641S	Pnctr w fb of abd wall, l upr q w penet perit cav, sequela
		S31.642S	Pnctr w fb of abd wall, epigst rgn w penet perit cav, sqla
		S31.643S	Pnctr w fb of abd wall, right low q w penet perit cav, sqla
		S31.644S	Pnctr w fb of abd wall, left lower q w penet perit cav, sqla
		S31.645S	Pnctr w fb of abd wall, periumb rgn w penet perit cav, sqla
		S31.649S	Pnctr w fb of abd wall, unsp q w penet perit cav, sequela
		S31.650S	Open bite of abd wall, right upper q w penet perit cav, sqla
		S31.651S	Open bite of abd wall, l upr q w penet perit cav, sequela
		S31.652S	Open bite of abd wall, epigst rgn w penet perit cav, sequela
		S31.653S	Open bite of abd wall, right lower q w penet perit cav, sqla
		S31.654S	Open bite of abd wall, left lower q w penet perit cav, sqla
		S31.655S	Open bite of abd wall, periumb rgn w penet perit cav, sqla
		S31.659S	Open bite of abd wall, unsp q w penet perit cav, sequela
		S31.801S	Laceration without foreign body of unsp buttock, sequela
		S31.802S	Laceration with foreign body of unspecified buttock, sequela
		S31.803S	Puncture wound without foreign body of unsp buttock, sequela
		S31.804S	Puncture wound with foreign body of unsp buttock, sequela
		S31.805S	Open bite of unspecified buttock, sequela
		S31.809S	Unspecified open wound of unspecified buttock, sequela
		S31.811S	Laceration without foreign body of right buttock, sequela
		S31.812S	Laceration with foreign body of right buttock, sequela
		S31.813S	Puncture wound w/o foreign body of right buttock, sequela
		S31.814S	Puncture wound with foreign body of right buttock, sequela
		S31.815S	Open bite of right buttock, sequela
		S31.819S	Unspecified open wound of right buttock, sequela
		S31.821S	Laceration without foreign body of left buttock, sequela
		S31.822S	Laceration with foreign body of left buttock, sequela
		S31.823S	Puncture wound without foreign body of left buttock, sequela
		S31.824S	Puncture wound with foreign body of left buttock, sequela
		S31.825S	Open bite of left buttock, sequela
		S31.829S	Unspecified open wound of left buttock, sequela
		S31.831S	Laceration without foreign body of anus, sequela
		S31.832S	Laceration with foreign body of anus, sequela
		S31.833S	Puncture wound without foreign body of anus, sequela
		S31.834S	Puncture wound with foreign body of anus, sequela
		S31.835S	Open bite of anus, sequela
		S31.839S	Unspecified open wound of anus, sequela
		S38.211S	Complete traum amp of female extrn genital organs, sequela
		S38.212S	Partial traum amp of female external genital organs, sequela
		S38.221S	Complete traumatic amputation of penis, sequela
		S38.222S	Partial traumatic amputation of penis, sequela
		S38.231S	Complete traumatic amputation of scrotum and testis, sequela
		S38.232S	Partial traumatic amputation of scrotum and testis, sequela
		S38.3XXS	Transection (partial) of abdomen, sequela
		S39.021S	Laceration of muscle, fascia and tendon of abdomen, sequela
		S39.022S	Laceration of musc/fasc/tend lower back, sequela
		S39.023S	Laceration of muscle, fascia and tendon of pelvis, sequela
906.1	LATE EFF OPN WND EXTREM W/O MENTION TEND INJURY	**S41.001S**	Unspecified open wound of right shoulder, sequela
		S41.002S	Unspecified open wound of left shoulder, sequela
		S41.009S	Unspecified open wound of unspecified shoulder, sequela
		S41.011S	Laceration without foreign body of right shoulder, sequela
		S41.012S	Laceration without foreign body of left shoulder, sequela
		S41.019S	Laceration without foreign body of unsp shoulder, sequela
		S41.021S	Laceration with foreign body of right shoulder, sequela
		S41.022S	Laceration with foreign body of left shoulder, sequela
		S41.029S	Laceration with foreign body of unsp shoulder, sequela
		S41.031S	Puncture wound w/o foreign body of right shoulder, sequela
		S41.032S	Puncture wound w/o foreign body of left shoulder, sequela
		S41.039S	Puncture wound w/o foreign body of unsp shoulder, sequela
		S41.041S	Puncture wound with foreign body of right shoulder, sequela
		S41.042S	Puncture wound with foreign body of left shoulder, sequela
		S41.049S	Puncture wound with foreign body of unsp shoulder, sequela
	(Continued on next page)	**S41.051S**	Open bite of right shoulder, sequela

ICD-9-CM		ICD-10-CM	
9Ø6.1	LATE EFF OPN WND EXTREM W/O MENTION TEND INJURY (Continued)	S41.Ø52S	Open bite of left shoulder, sequela
		S41.Ø59S	Open bite of unspecified shoulder, sequela
		S41.1Ø1S	Unspecified open wound of right upper arm, sequela
		S41.1Ø2S	Unspecified open wound of left upper arm, sequela
		S41.1Ø9S	Unspecified open wound of unspecified upper arm, sequela
		S41.111S	Laceration without foreign body of right upper arm, sequela
		S41.112S	Laceration without foreign body of left upper arm, sequela
		S41.119S	Laceration without foreign body of unsp upper arm, sequela
		S41.121S	Laceration with foreign body of right upper arm, sequela
		S41.122S	Laceration with foreign body of left upper arm, sequela
		S41.129S	Laceration with foreign body of unsp upper arm, sequela
		S41.131S	Puncture wound w/o foreign body of right upper arm, sequela
		S41.132S	Puncture wound w/o foreign body of left upper arm, sequela
		S41.139S	Puncture wound w/o foreign body of unsp upper arm, sequela
		S41.141S	Puncture wound with foreign body of right upper arm, sequela
		S41.142S	Puncture wound with foreign body of left upper arm, sequela
		S41.149S	Puncture wound with foreign body of unsp upper arm, sequela
		S41.151S	Open bite of right upper arm, sequela
		S41.152S	Open bite of left upper arm, sequela
		S41.159S	Open bite of unspecified upper arm, sequela
		S46.Ø21S	Lacerat musc/tend the rotator cuff of r shoulder, sequela
		S46.Ø22S	Lacerat musc/tend the rotator cuff of left shoulder, sequela
		S46.Ø29S	Lacerat musc/tend the rotator cuff of unsp shoulder, sequela
		S46.121S	Lacerat musc/fasc/tend long hd bicep, right arm, sequela
		S46.122S	Lacerat musc/fasc/tend long hd bicep, left arm, sequela
		S46.129S	Lacerat musc/fasc/tend long hd bicep, unsp arm, sequela
		S46.221S	Laceration of musc/fasc/tend prt biceps, right arm, sequela
		S46.222S	Laceration of musc/fasc/tend prt biceps, left arm, sequela
		S46.229S	Laceration of musc/fasc/tend prt biceps, unsp arm, sequela
		S46.321S	Laceration of musc/fasc/tend triceps, right arm, sequela
		S46.322S	Laceration of musc/fasc/tend triceps, left arm, sequela
		S46.329S	Laceration of musc/fasc/tend triceps, unsp arm, sequela
		S46.821S	Lacerat musc/fasc/tend at shldr/up arm, right arm, sequela
		S46.822S	Lacerat musc/fasc/tend at shldr/up arm, left arm, sequela
		S46.829S	Lacerat musc/fasc/tend at shldr/up arm, unsp arm, sequela
		S46.921S	Lacerat unsp musc/fasc/tend at shldr/up arm, right arm, sqla
		S46.922S	Lacerat unsp musc/fasc/tend at shldr/up arm, left arm, sqla
		S46.929S	Lacerat unsp musc/fasc/tend at shldr/up arm, unsp arm, sqla
		S51.ØØ1S	Unspecified open wound of right elbow, sequela
		S51.ØØ2S	Unspecified open wound of left elbow, sequela
		S51.ØØ9S	Unspecified open wound of unspecified elbow, sequela
		S51.Ø11S	Laceration without foreign body of right elbow, sequela
		S51.Ø12S	Laceration without foreign body of left elbow, sequela
		S51.Ø19S	Laceration without foreign body of unsp elbow, sequela
		S51.Ø21S	Laceration with foreign body of right elbow, sequela
		S51.Ø22S	Laceration with foreign body of left elbow, sequela
		S51.Ø29S	Laceration with foreign body of unspecified elbow, sequela
		S51.Ø31S	Puncture wound without foreign body of right elbow, sequela
		S51.Ø32S	Puncture wound without foreign body of left elbow, sequela
		S51.Ø39S	Puncture wound without foreign body of unsp elbow, sequela
		S51.Ø41S	Puncture wound with foreign body of right elbow, sequela
		S51.Ø42S	Puncture wound with foreign body of left elbow, sequela
		S51.Ø49S	Puncture wound with foreign body of unsp elbow, sequela
		S51.Ø51S	Open bite, right elbow, sequela
		S51.Ø52S	Open bite, left elbow, sequela
		S51.Ø59S	Open bite, unspecified elbow, sequela
		S51.8Ø1S	Unspecified open wound of right forearm, sequela
		S51.8Ø2S	Unspecified open wound of left forearm, sequela
		S51.8Ø9S	Unspecified open wound of unspecified forearm, sequela
		S51.811S	Laceration without foreign body of right forearm, sequela
		S51.812S	Laceration without foreign body of left forearm, sequela
		S51.819S	Laceration without foreign body of unsp forearm, sequela
		S51.821S	Laceration with foreign body of right forearm, sequela
		S51.822S	Laceration with foreign body of left forearm, sequela
		S51.829S	Laceration with foreign body of unspecified forearm, sequela
		S51.831S	Puncture wound w/o foreign body of right forearm, sequela
		S51.832S	Puncture wound without foreign body of left forearm, sequela
		S51.839S	Puncture wound without foreign body of unsp forearm, sequela
		S51.841S	Puncture wound with foreign body of right forearm, sequela
		S51.842S	Puncture wound with foreign body of left forearm, sequela
		S51.849S	Puncture wound with foreign body of unsp forearm, sequela
		S51.851S	Open bite of right forearm, sequela
		S51.852S	Open bite of left forearm, sequela
		S51.859S	Open bite of unspecified forearm, sequela
		S56.Ø21S	Lacerat flexor musc/fasc/tend r thm at forarm lv, sequela
		S56.Ø22S	Lacerat flexor musc/fasc/tend l thm at forarm lv, sequela
		S56.Ø29S	Lacerat flexor musc/fasc/tend thmb at forarm lv, sequela
		S56.121S	Lacerat flexor musc/fasc/tend r idx fngr at forarm lv, sqla
		S56.122S	Lacerat flexor musc/fasc/tend l idx fngr at forarm lv, sqla
		S56.123S	Lacerat flexor musc/fasc/tend r mid fngr at forarm lv, sqla
		S56.124S	Lacerat flexor musc/fasc/tend l mid fngr at forarm lv, sqla
9Ø6.1	(Continued on next page)	S56.125S	Lacerat flexor musc/fasc/tend r rng fngr at forarm lv, sqla

ICD-9-CM		ICD-10-CM	
9Ø6.1	LATE EFF OPN WND EXTREM W/O MENTION TEND INJURY **(Continued)**	**S56.126S**	Lacerat flexor musc/fasc/tend l rng fngr at forarm lv, sqla
		S56.127S	Lacerat flxr musc/fasc/tend r little fngr at forarm lv, sqla
		S56.128S	Lacerat flxr musc/fasc/tend l little fngr at forarm lv, sqla
		S56.129S	Lacerat flexor musc/fasc/tend unsp finger at forarm lv, sqla
		S56.221S	Lacerat flexor musc/fasc/tend at forarm lv, right arm, sqla
		S56.222S	Lacerat flexor musc/fasc/tend at forarm lv, left arm, sqla
		S56.229S	Lacerat flexor musc/fasc/tend at forarm lv, unsp arm, sqla
		S56.321S	Lacerat extn/abdr musc/fasc/tend of r thm at forarm lv, sqla
		S56.322S	Lacerat extn/abdr musc/fasc/tend of l thm at forarm lv, sqla
		S56.329S	Lacerat extn/abdr musc/fasc/tend of thmb at forarm lv, sqla
		S56.421S	Lacerat extn musc/fasc/tend r idx fngr at forarm lv, sequela
		S56.422S	Lacerat extn musc/fasc/tend l idx fngr at forarm lv, sequela
		S56.423S	Lacerat extn musc/fasc/tend r mid finger at forarm lv, sqla
		S56.424S	Lacerat extn musc/fasc/tend l mid finger at forarm lv, sqla
		S56.425S	Lacerat extn musc/fasc/tend r rng fngr at forarm lv, sequela
		S56.426S	Lacerat extn musc/fasc/tend l rng fngr at forarm lv, sequela
		S56.427S	Lacerat extn musc/fasc/tend r little fngr at forarm lv, sqla
		S56.428S	Lacerat extn musc/fasc/tend l little fngr at forarm lv, sqla
		S56.429S	Lacerat extn musc/fasc/tend unsp finger at forarm lv, sqla
		S56.521S	Lacerat extn musc/fasc/tend at forarm lv, right arm, sequela
		S56.522S	Lacerat extn musc/fasc/tend at forarm lv, left arm, sequela
		S56.529S	Lacerat extn musc/fasc/tend at forarm lv, unsp arm, sequela
		S56.821S	Lacerat musc/fasc/tend at forarm lv, right arm, sequela
		S56.822S	Laceration of musc/fasc/tend at forarm lv, left arm, sequela
		S56.829S	Laceration of musc/fasc/tend at forarm lv, unsp arm, sequela
		S56.921S	Lacerat unsp musc/fasc/tend at forarm lv, right arm, sequela
		S56.922S	Lacerat unsp musc/fasc/tend at forarm lv, left arm, sequela
		S56.929S	Lacerat unsp musc/fasc/tend at forarm lv, unsp arm, sequela
		S61.ØØ1S	Unsp open wound of right thumb w/o damage to nail, sequela
		S61.ØØ2S	Unsp open wound of left thumb w/o damage to nail, sequela
		S61.ØØ9S	Unsp open wound of unsp thumb w/o damage to nail, sequela
		S61.Ø11S	Laceration w/o fb of right thumb w/o damage to nail, sequela
		S61.Ø12S	Laceration w/o fb of left thumb w/o damage to nail, sequela
		S61.Ø19S	Laceration w/o fb of thmb w/o damage to nail, sequela
		S61.Ø21S	Laceration w fb of right thumb w/o damage to nail, sequela
		S61.Ø22S	Laceration w fb of left thumb w/o damage to nail, sequela
		S61.Ø29S	Laceration w fb of thmb w/o damage to nail, sequela
		S61.Ø31S	Pnctr w/o fb of right thumb w/o damage to nail, sequela
		S61.Ø32S	Pnctr w/o fb of left thumb w/o damage to nail, sequela
		S61.Ø39S	Pnctr w/o foreign body of thmb w/o damage to nail, sequela
		S61.Ø41S	Pnctr w fb of right thumb w/o damage to nail, sequela
		S61.Ø42S	Pnctr w fb of left thumb w/o damage to nail, sequela
		S61.Ø49S	Pnctr w foreign body of thmb w/o damage to nail, sequela
		S61.Ø51S	Open bite of right thumb without damage to nail, sequela
		S61.Ø52S	Open bite of left thumb without damage to nail, sequela
		S61.Ø59S	Open bite of unsp thumb without damage to nail, sequela
		S61.1Ø1S	Unsp open wound of right thumb with damage to nail, sequela
		S61.1Ø2S	Unsp open wound of left thumb with damage to nail, sequela
		S61.1Ø9S	Unsp open wound of unsp thumb with damage to nail, sequela
		S61.111S	Laceration w/o fb of right thumb w damage to nail, sequela
		S61.112S	Laceration w/o fb of left thumb w damage to nail, sequela
		S61.119S	Laceration w/o fb of thmb w damage to nail, sequela
		S61.121S	Laceration w fb of right thumb w damage to nail, sequela
		S61.122S	Laceration w fb of left thumb w damage to nail, sequela
		S61.129S	Laceration w foreign body of thmb w damage to nail, sequela
		S61.131S	Pnctr w/o fb of right thumb w damage to nail, sequela
		S61.132S	Pnctr w/o fb of left thumb w damage to nail, sequela
		S61.139S	Pnctr w/o foreign body of thmb w damage to nail, sequela
		S61.141S	Pnctr w fb of right thumb w damage to nail, sequela
		S61.142S	Pnctr w foreign body of left thumb w damage to nail, sequela
		S61.149S	Pnctr w foreign body of thmb w damage to nail, sequela
		S61.151S	Open bite of right thumb with damage to nail, sequela
		S61.152S	Open bite of left thumb with damage to nail, sequela
		S61.159S	Open bite of unspecified thumb with damage to nail, sequela
		S61.2ØØS	Unsp open wound of r idx fngr w/o damage to nail, sequela
		S61.2Ø1S	Unsp open wound of l idx fngr w/o damage to nail, sequela
		S61.2Ø2S	Unsp open wound of r mid finger w/o damage to nail, sequela
		S61.2Ø3S	Unsp open wound of l mid finger w/o damage to nail, sequela
		S61.2Ø4S	Unsp open wound of r rng fngr w/o damage to nail, sequela
		S61.2Ø5S	Unsp open wound of l rng fngr w/o damage to nail, sequela
		S61.2Ø6S	Unsp opn wnd r little finger w/o damage to nail, sequela
		S61.2Ø7S	Unsp opn wnd l little finger w/o damage to nail, sequela
		S61.2Ø8S	Unsp open wound of other finger w/o damage to nail, sequela
		S61.2Ø9S	Unsp open wound of unsp finger w/o damage to nail, sequela
		S61.21ØS	Laceration w/o fb of r idx fngr w/o damage to nail, sequela
		S61.211S	Laceration w/o fb of l idx fngr w/o damage to nail, sequela
		S61.212S	Lac w/o fb of r mid finger w/o damage to nail, sequela
		S61.213S	Lac w/o fb of l mid finger w/o damage to nail, sequela
		S61.214S	Laceration w/o fb of r rng fngr w/o damage to nail, sequela
		S61.215S	Laceration w/o fb of l rng fngr w/o damage to nail, sequela
		S61.216S	Lac w/o fb of r little finger w/o damage to nail, sequela
		S61.217S	Lac w/o fb of l little finger w/o damage to nail, sequela
	(Continued on next page)	**S61.218S**	Laceration w/o fb of finger w/o damage to nail, sequela

ICD-9-CM		ICD-10-CM	
906.1	LATE EFF OPN WND EXTREM W/O MENTION TEND INJURY **(Continued)**	**S61.219S**	Laceration w/o fb of unsp finger w/o damage to nail, sequela
		S61.220S	Laceration w fb of r idx fngr w/o damage to nail, sequela
		S61.221S	Laceration w fb of l idx fngr w/o damage to nail, sequela
		S61.222S	Laceration w fb of r mid finger w/o damage to nail, sequela
		S61.223S	Laceration w fb of l mid finger w/o damage to nail, sequela
		S61.224S	Laceration w fb of r rng fngr w/o damage to nail, sequela
		S61.225S	Laceration w fb of l rng fngr w/o damage to nail, sequela
		S61.226S	Lac w fb of r little finger w/o damage to nail, sequela
		S61.227S	Lac w fb of l little finger w/o damage to nail, sequela
		S61.228S	Laceration w fb of finger w/o damage to nail, sequela
		S61.229S	Laceration w fb of unsp finger w/o damage to nail, sequela
		S61.230S	Pnctr w/o fb of r idx fngr w/o damage to nail, sequela
		S61.231S	Pnctr w/o fb of l idx fngr w/o damage to nail, sequela
		S61.232S	Pnctr w/o fb of r mid finger w/o damage to nail, sequela
		S61.233S	Pnctr w/o fb of l mid finger w/o damage to nail, sequela
		S61.234S	Pnctr w/o fb of r rng fngr w/o damage to nail, sequela
		S61.235S	Pnctr w/o fb of l rng fngr w/o damage to nail, sequela
		S61.236S	Pnctr w/o fb of r little finger w/o damage to nail, sequela
		S61.237S	Pnctr w/o fb of l little finger w/o damage to nail, sequela
		S61.238S	Pnctr w/o foreign body of finger w/o damage to nail, sequela
		S61.239S	Pnctr w/o fb of unsp finger w/o damage to nail, sequela
		S61.240S	Pnctr w fb of r idx fngr w/o damage to nail, sequela
		S61.241S	Pnctr w fb of l idx fngr w/o damage to nail, sequela
		S61.242S	Pnctr w fb of r mid finger w/o damage to nail, sequela
		S61.243S	Pnctr w fb of l mid finger w/o damage to nail, sequela
		S61.244S	Pnctr w fb of r rng fngr w/o damage to nail, sequela
		S61.245S	Pnctr w fb of l rng fngr w/o damage to nail, sequela
		S61.246S	Pnctr w fb of r little finger w/o damage to nail, sequela
		S61.247S	Pnctr w fb of l little finger w/o damage to nail, sequela
		S61.248S	Pnctr w foreign body of finger w/o damage to nail, sequela
		S61.249S	Pnctr w fb of unsp finger w/o damage to nail, sequela
		S61.250S	Open bite of right index finger w/o damage to nail, sequela
		S61.251S	Open bite of left index finger w/o damage to nail, sequela
		S61.252S	Open bite of right middle finger w/o damage to nail, sequela
		S61.253S	Open bite of left middle finger w/o damage to nail, sequela
		S61.254S	Open bite of right ring finger w/o damage to nail, sequela
		S61.255S	Open bite of left ring finger w/o damage to nail, sequela
		S61.256S	Open bite of right little finger w/o damage to nail, sequela
		S61.257S	Open bite of left little finger w/o damage to nail, sequela
		S61.258S	Open bite of other finger without damage to nail, sequela
		S61.259S	Open bite of unsp finger without damage to nail, sequela
		S61.300S	Unsp open wound of r idx fngr w damage to nail, sequela
		S61.301S	Unsp open wound of l idx fngr w damage to nail, sequela
		S61.302S	Unsp open wound of r mid finger w damage to nail, sequela
		S61.303S	Unsp open wound of l mid finger w damage to nail, sequela
		S61.304S	Unsp open wound of r rng fngr w damage to nail, sequela
		S61.305S	Unsp open wound of l rng fngr w damage to nail, sequela
		S61.306S	Unsp open wound of r little finger w damage to nail, sequela
		S61.307S	Unsp open wound of l little finger w damage to nail, sequela
		S61.308S	Unsp open wound of other finger with damage to nail, sequela
		S61.309S	Unsp open wound of unsp finger with damage to nail, sequela
		S61.310S	Laceration w/o fb of r idx fngr w damage to nail, sequela
		S61.311S	Laceration w/o fb of l idx fngr w damage to nail, sequela
		S61.312S	Laceration w/o fb of r mid finger w damage to nail, sequela
		S61.313S	Laceration w/o fb of l mid finger w damage to nail, sequela
		S61.314S	Laceration w/o fb of r rng fngr w damage to nail, sequela
		S61.315S	Laceration w/o fb of l rng fngr w damage to nail, sequela
		S61.316S	Lac w/o fb of r little finger w damage to nail, sequela
		S61.317S	Lac w/o fb of l little finger w damage to nail, sequela
		S61.318S	Laceration w/o fb of finger w damage to nail, sequela
		S61.319S	Laceration w/o fb of unsp finger w damage to nail, sequela
		S61.320S	Laceration w fb of r idx fngr w damage to nail, sequela
		S61.321S	Laceration w fb of l idx fngr w damage to nail, sequela
		S61.322S	Laceration w fb of r mid finger w damage to nail, sequela
		S61.323S	Laceration w fb of l mid finger w damage to nail, sequela
		S61.324S	Laceration w fb of r rng fngr w damage to nail, sequela
		S61.325S	Laceration w fb of l rng fngr w damage to nail, sequela
		S61.326S	Laceration w fb of r little finger w damage to nail, sequela
		S61.327S	Laceration w fb of l little finger w damage to nail, sequela
		S61.328S	Laceration w fb of finger w damage to nail, sequela
		S61.329S	Laceration w fb of unsp finger w damage to nail, sequela
		S61.330S	Pnctr w/o fb of r idx fngr w damage to nail, sequela
		S61.331S	Pnctr w/o fb of l idx fngr w damage to nail, sequela
		S61.332S	Pnctr w/o fb of r mid finger w damage to nail, sequela
		S61.333S	Pnctr w/o fb of l mid finger w damage to nail, sequela
		S61.334S	Pnctr w/o fb of r rng fngr w damage to nail, sequela
		S61.335S	Pnctr w/o fb of l rng fngr w damage to nail, sequela
		S61.336S	Pnctr w/o fb of r little finger w damage to nail, sequela
		S61.337S	Pnctr w/o fb of l little finger w damage to nail, sequela
		S61.338S	Pnctr w/o foreign body of finger w damage to nail, sequela
		S61.339S	Pnctr w/o fb of unsp finger w damage to nail, sequela
	(Continued on next page)	**S61.340S**	Pnctr w foreign body of r idx fngr w damage to nail, sequela

ICD-9-CM		ICD-10-CM	
906.1	LATE EFF OPN WND EXTREM W/O MENTION TEND INJURY **(Continued)**	**S61.341S**	Pnctr w foreign body of l idx fngr w damage to nail, sequela
		S61.342S	Pnctr w fb of r mid finger w damage to nail, sequela
		S61.343S	Pnctr w fb of l mid finger w damage to nail, sequela
		S61.344S	Pnctr w foreign body of r rng fngr w damage to nail, sequela
		S61.345S	Pnctr w foreign body of l rng fngr w damage to nail, sequela
		S61.346S	Pnctr w fb of r little finger w damage to nail, sequela
		S61.347S	Pnctr w fb of l little finger w damage to nail, sequela
		S61.348S	Pnctr w foreign body of finger w damage to nail, sequela
		S61.349S	Pnctr w fb of unsp finger w damage to nail, sequela
		S61.350S	Open bite of right index finger with damage to nail, sequela
		S61.351S	Open bite of left index finger with damage to nail, sequela
		S61.352S	Open bite of right middle finger w damage to nail, sequela
		S61.353S	Open bite of left middle finger with damage to nail, sequela
		S61.354S	Open bite of right ring finger with damage to nail, sequela
		S61.355S	Open bite of left ring finger with damage to nail, sequela
		S61.356S	Open bite of right little finger w damage to nail, sequela
		S61.357S	Open bite of left little finger with damage to nail, sequela
		S61.358S	Open bite of other finger with damage to nail, sequela
		S61.359S	Open bite of unspecified finger with damage to nail, sequela
		S61.401S	Unspecified open wound of right hand, sequela
		S61.402S	Unspecified open wound of left hand, sequela
		S61.409S	Unspecified open wound of unspecified hand, sequela
		S61.411S	Laceration without foreign body of right hand, sequela
		S61.412S	Laceration without foreign body of left hand, sequela
		S61.419S	Laceration without foreign body of unspecified hand, sequela
		S61.421S	Laceration with foreign body of right hand, sequela
		S61.422S	Laceration with foreign body of left hand, sequela
		S61.429S	Laceration with foreign body of unspecified hand, sequela
		S61.431S	Puncture wound without foreign body of right hand, sequela
		S61.432S	Puncture wound without foreign body of left hand, sequela
		S61.439S	Puncture wound without foreign body of unsp hand, sequela
		S61.441S	Puncture wound with foreign body of right hand, sequela
		S61.442S	Puncture wound with foreign body of left hand, sequela
		S61.449S	Puncture wound with foreign body of unsp hand, sequela
		S61.451S	Open bite of right hand, sequela
		S61.452S	Open bite of left hand, sequela
		S61.459S	Open bite of unspecified hand, sequela
		S61.501S	Unspecified open wound of right wrist, sequela
		S61.502S	Unspecified open wound of left wrist, sequela
		S61.509S	Unspecified open wound of unspecified wrist, sequela
		S61.511S	Laceration without foreign body of right wrist, sequela
		S61.512S	Laceration without foreign body of left wrist, sequela
		S61.519S	Laceration without foreign body of unsp wrist, sequela
		S61.521S	Laceration with foreign body of right wrist, sequela
		S61.522S	Laceration with foreign body of left wrist, sequela
		S61.529S	Laceration with foreign body of unspecified wrist, sequela
		S61.531S	Puncture wound without foreign body of right wrist, sequela
		S61.532S	Puncture wound without foreign body of left wrist, sequela
		S61.539S	Puncture wound without foreign body of unsp wrist, sequela
		S61.541S	Puncture wound with foreign body of right wrist, sequela
		S61.542S	Puncture wound with foreign body of left wrist, sequela
		S61.549S	Puncture wound with foreign body of unsp wrist, sequela
		S61.551S	Open bite of right wrist, sequela
		S61.552S	Open bite of left wrist, sequela
		S61.559S	Open bite of unspecified wrist, sequela
		S66.021S	Lacerat long flexor musc/fasc/tend r thm at wrs/hnd lv, sqla
		S66.022S	Lacerat long flexor musc/fasc/tend l thm at wrs/hnd lv, sqla
		S66.029S	Lacerat long flexor musc/fasc/tend thmb at wrs/hnd lv, sqla
		S66.120S	Lacerat flexor musc/fasc/tend r idx fngr at wrs/hnd lv, sqla
		S66.121S	Lacerat flexor musc/fasc/tend l idx fngr at wrs/hnd lv, sqla
		S66.122S	Lacerat flexor musc/fasc/tend r mid fngr at wrs/hnd lv, sqla
		S66.123S	Lacerat flexor musc/fasc/tend l mid fngr at wrs/hnd lv, sqla
		S66.124S	Lacerat flexor musc/fasc/tend r rng fngr at wrs/hnd lv, sqla
		S66.125S	Lacerat flexor musc/fasc/tend l rng fngr at wrs/hnd lv, sqla
		S66.126S	Lacerat flxr musc/fasc/tend r lit fngr at wrs/hnd lv, sqla
		S66.127S	Lacerat flxr musc/fasc/tend l lit fngr at wrs/hnd lv, sqla
		S66.128S	Lacerat flexor musc/fasc/tend finger at wrs/hnd lv, sequela
		S66.129S	Lacerat flexor musc/fasc/tend unsp fngr at wrs/hnd lv, sqla
		S66.221S	Lacerat extensor musc/fasc/tend r thm at wrs/hnd lv, sequela
		S66.222S	Lacerat extensor musc/fasc/tend l thm at wrs/hnd lv, sequela
		S66.229S	Lacerat extensor musc/fasc/tend thmb at wrs/hnd lv, sequela
		S66.320S	Lacerat extn musc/fasc/tend r idx fngr at wrs/hnd lv, sqla
		S66.321S	Lacerat extn musc/fasc/tend l idx fngr at wrs/hnd lv, sqla
		S66.322S	Lacerat extn musc/fasc/tend r mid finger at wrs/hnd lv, sqla
		S66.323S	Lacerat extn musc/fasc/tend l mid finger at wrs/hnd lv, sqla
		S66.324S	Lacerat extn musc/fasc/tend r rng fngr at wrs/hnd lv, sqla
		S66.325S	Lacerat extn musc/fasc/tend l rng fngr at wrs/hnd lv, sqla
		S66.326S	Lacerat extn musc/fasc/tend r lit fngr at wrs/hnd lv, sqla
		S66.327S	Lacerat extn musc/fasc/tend l lit fngr at wrs/hnd lv, sqla
		S66.328S	Lacerat extn musc/fasc/tend finger at wrs/hnd lv, sequela
		S66.329S	Lacerat extn musc/fasc/tend unsp finger at wrs/hnd lv, sqla
	(Continued on next page)	**S66.421S**	Lacerat intrns musc/fasc/tend r thm at wrs/hnd lv, sequela

 [Brackets] indicate valid character values for each code. Character value meanings provided for each code grouping.

ICD-9-CM		ICD-10-CM	
9Ø6.1	LATE EFF OPN WND EXTREM W/O MENTION TEND INJURY **(Continued)**	**S66.422S**	Lacerat intrns musc/fasc/tend l thm at wrs/hnd lv, sequela
		S66.429S	Lacerat intrinsic musc/fasc/tend thmb at wrs/hnd lv, sequela
		S66.52ØS	Lacerat intrns musc/fasc/tend r idx fngr at wrs/hnd lv, sqla
		S66.521S	Lacerat intrns musc/fasc/tend l idx fngr at wrs/hnd lv, sqla
		S66.522S	Lacerat intrns musc/fasc/tend r mid fngr at wrs/hnd lv, sqla
		S66.523S	Lacerat intrns musc/fasc/tend l mid fngr at wrs/hnd lv, sqla
		S66.524S	Lacerat intrns musc/fasc/tend r rng fngr at wrs/hnd lv, sqla
		S66.525S	Lacerat intrns musc/fasc/tend l rng fngr at wrs/hnd lv, sqla
		S66.526S	Lacerat intrns musc/fasc/tend r lit fngr at wrs/hnd lv, sqla
		S66.527S	Lacerat intrns musc/fasc/tend l lit fngr at wrs/hnd lv, sqla
		S66.528S	Lacerat intrns musc/fasc/tend finger at wrs/hnd lv, sequela
		S66.529S	Lacerat intrns musc/fasc/tend unsp fngr at wrs/hnd lv, sqla
		S66.821S	Lacerat musc/fasc/tend at wrs/hnd lv, right hand, sequela
		S66.822S	Lacerat musc/fasc/tend at wrs/hnd lv, left hand, sequela
		S66.829S	Lacerat musc/fasc/tend at wrs/hnd lv, unsp hand, sequela
		S66.921S	Lacerat unsp musc/fasc/tend at wrs/hnd lv, r hand, sequela
		S66.922S	Lacerat unsp musc/fasc/tend at wrs/hnd lv, l hand, sequela
		S66.929S	Lacerat unsp musc/fasc/tend at wrs/hnd lv, unsp hand, sqla
		S71.ØØ1S	Unspecified open wound, right hip, sequela
		S71.ØØ2S	Unspecified open wound, left hip, sequela
		S71.ØØ9S	Unspecified open wound, unspecified hip, sequela
		S71.Ø11S	Laceration without foreign body, right hip, sequela
		S71.Ø12S	Laceration without foreign body, left hip, sequela
		S71.Ø19S	Laceration without foreign body, unspecified hip, sequela
		S71.Ø21S	Laceration with foreign body, right hip, sequela
		S71.Ø22S	Laceration with foreign body, left hip, sequela
		S71.Ø29S	Laceration with foreign body, unspecified hip, sequela
		S71.Ø31S	Puncture wound without foreign body, right hip, sequela
		S71.Ø32S	Puncture wound without foreign body, left hip, sequela
		S71.Ø39S	Puncture wound without foreign body, unsp hip, sequela
		S71.Ø41S	Puncture wound with foreign body, right hip, sequela
		S71.Ø42S	Puncture wound with foreign body, left hip, sequela
		S71.Ø49S	Puncture wound with foreign body, unspecified hip, sequela
		S71.Ø51S	Open bite, right hip, sequela
		S71.Ø52S	Open bite, left hip, sequela
		S71.Ø59S	Open bite, unspecified hip, sequela
		S71.1Ø1S	Unspecified open wound, right thigh, sequela
		S71.1Ø2S	Unspecified open wound, left thigh, sequela
		S71.1Ø9S	Unspecified open wound, unspecified thigh, sequela
		S71.111S	Laceration without foreign body, right thigh, sequela
		S71.112S	Laceration without foreign body, left thigh, sequela
		S71.119S	Laceration without foreign body, unspecified thigh, sequela
		S71.121S	Laceration with foreign body, right thigh, sequela
		S71.122S	Laceration with foreign body, left thigh, sequela
		S71.129S	Laceration with foreign body, unspecified thigh, sequela
		S71.131S	Puncture wound without foreign body, right thigh, sequela
		S71.132S	Puncture wound without foreign body, left thigh, sequela
		S71.139S	Puncture wound without foreign body, unsp thigh, sequela
		S71.141S	Puncture wound with foreign body, right thigh, sequela
		S71.142S	Puncture wound with foreign body, left thigh, sequela
		S71.149S	Puncture wound with foreign body, unspecified thigh, sequela
		S71.151S	Open bite, right thigh, sequela
		S71.152S	Open bite, left thigh, sequela
		S71.159S	Open bite, unspecified thigh, sequela
		S76.Ø21S	Laceration of musc/fasc/tend right hip, sequela
		S76.Ø22S	Laceration of muscle, fascia and tendon of left hip, sequela
		S76.Ø29S	Laceration of muscle, fascia and tendon of unsp hip, sequela
		S76.121S	Laceration of right quadriceps musc/fasc/tend, sequela
		S76.122S	Laceration of left quadriceps musc/fasc/tend, sequela
		S76.129S	Laceration of unsp quadriceps musc/fasc/tend, sequela
		S76.221S	Laceration of adductor musc/fasc/tend right thigh, sequela
		S76.222S	Laceration of adductor musc/fasc/tend left thigh, sequela
		S76.229S	Laceration of adductor musc/fasc/tend unsp thigh, sequela
		S76.321S	Lacerat msl/fasc/tnd post grp at thi lev, right thigh, sqla
		S76.322S	Lacerat msl/fasc/tnd post grp at thi lev, left thigh, sqla
		S76.329S	Lacerat msl/fasc/tnd post grp at thi lev, unsp thigh, sqla
		S76.821S	Lacerat musc/fasc/tend at thigh level, right thigh, sequela
		S76.822S	Lacerat musc/fasc/tend at thigh level, left thigh, sequela
		S76.829S	Lacerat musc/fasc/tend at thigh level, unsp thigh, sequela
		S76.921S	Lacerat unsp musc/fasc/tend at thi lev, right thigh, sequela
		S76.922S	Lacerat unsp musc/fasc/tend at thi lev, left thigh, sequela
		S76.929S	Lacerat unsp musc/fasc/tend at thi lev, unsp thigh, sequela
		S81.ØØ1S	Unspecified open wound, right knee, sequela
		S81.ØØ2S	Unspecified open wound, left knee, sequela
		S81.ØØ9S	Unspecified open wound, unspecified knee, sequela
		S81.Ø11S	Laceration without foreign body, right knee, sequela
		S81.Ø12S	Laceration without foreign body, left knee, sequela
		S81.Ø19S	Laceration without foreign body, unspecified knee, sequela
		S81.Ø21S	Laceration with foreign body, right knee, sequela
		S81.Ø22S	Laceration with foreign body, left knee, sequela
		S81.Ø29S	Laceration with foreign body, unspecified knee, sequela
	(Continued on next page)	**S81.Ø31S**	Puncture wound without foreign body, right knee, sequela

ICD-9-CM		ICD-10-CM	
906.1	LATE EFF OPN WND EXTREM W/O MENTION TEND INJURY **(Continued)**	**S81.032S**	Puncture wound without foreign body, left knee, sequela
		S81.039S	Puncture wound without foreign body, unsp knee, sequela
		S81.041S	Puncture wound with foreign body, right knee, sequela
		S81.042S	Puncture wound with foreign body, left knee, sequela
		S81.049S	Puncture wound with foreign body, unspecified knee, sequela
		S81.051S	Open bite, right knee, sequela
		S81.052S	Open bite, left knee, sequela
		S81.059S	Open bite, unspecified knee, sequela
		S81.801S	Unspecified open wound, right lower leg, sequela
		S81.802S	Unspecified open wound, left lower leg, sequela
		S81.809S	Unspecified open wound, unspecified lower leg, sequela
		S81.811S	Laceration without foreign body, right lower leg, sequela
		S81.812S	Laceration without foreign body, left lower leg, sequela
		S81.819S	Laceration without foreign body, unsp lower leg, sequela
		S81.821S	Laceration with foreign body, right lower leg, sequela
		S81.822S	Laceration with foreign body, left lower leg, sequela
		S81.829S	Laceration with foreign body, unspecified lower leg, sequela
		S81.831S	Puncture wound w/o foreign body, right lower leg, sequela
		S81.832S	Puncture wound without foreign body, left lower leg, sequela
		S81.839S	Puncture wound without foreign body, unsp lower leg, sequela
		S81.841S	Puncture wound with foreign body, right lower leg, sequela
		S81.842S	Puncture wound with foreign body, left lower leg, sequela
		S81.849S	Puncture wound with foreign body, unsp lower leg, sequela
		S81.851S	Open bite, right lower leg, sequela
		S81.852S	Open bite, left lower leg, sequela
		S81.859S	Open bite, unspecified lower leg, sequela
		S86.021S	Laceration of right Achilles tendon, sequela
		S86.022S	Laceration of left Achilles tendon, sequela
		S86.029S	Laceration of unspecified Achilles tendon, sequela
		S86.121S	Lacerat musc/tend post grp at low leg level, right leg, sqla
		S86.122S	Lacerat musc/tend post grp at low leg level, left leg, sqla
		S86.129S	Lacerat musc/tend post grp at low leg level, unsp leg, sqla
		S86.221S	Lacerat musc/tend ant grp at low leg level, right leg, sqla
		S86.222S	Lacerat musc/tend ant grp at low leg level, left leg, sqla
		S86.229S	Lacerat musc/tend ant grp at low leg level, unsp leg, sqla
		S86.321S	Lacerat musc/tend peroneal grp at low leg lev, r leg, sqla
		S86.322S	Lacerat musc/tend peroneal grp at low leg lev, l leg, sqla
		S86.329S	Lacerat musc/tend peroneal grp at low leg lev,unsp leg, sqla
		S86.821S	Lacerat musc/tend at lower leg level, right leg, sequela
		S86.822S	Lacerat musc/tend at lower leg level, left leg, sequela
		S86.829S	Lacerat musc/tend at lower leg level, unsp leg, sequela
		S86.921S	Lacerat unsp musc/tend at low leg level, right leg, sequela
		S86.922S	Lacerat unsp musc/tend at lower leg level, left leg, sequela
		S86.929S	Lacerat unsp musc/tend at lower leg level, unsp leg, sequela
		S91.001S	Unspecified open wound, right ankle, sequela
		S91.002S	Unspecified open wound, left ankle, sequela
		S91.009S	Unspecified open wound, unspecified ankle, sequela
		S91.011S	Laceration without foreign body, right ankle, sequela
		S91.012S	Laceration without foreign body, left ankle, sequela
		S91.019S	Laceration without foreign body, unspecified ankle, sequela
		S91.021S	Laceration with foreign body, right ankle, sequela
		S91.022S	Laceration with foreign body, left ankle, sequela
		S91.029S	Laceration with foreign body, unspecified ankle, sequela
		S91.031S	Puncture wound without foreign body, right ankle, sequela
		S91.032S	Puncture wound without foreign body, left ankle, sequela
		S91.039S	Puncture wound without foreign body, unsp ankle, sequela
		S91.041S	Puncture wound with foreign body, right ankle, sequela
		S91.042S	Puncture wound with foreign body, left ankle, sequela
		S91.049S	Puncture wound with foreign body, unspecified ankle, sequela
		S91.051S	Open bite, right ankle, sequela
		S91.052S	Open bite, left ankle, sequela
		S91.059S	Open bite, unspecified ankle, sequela
		S91.101S	Unsp opn wnd right great toe w/o damage to nail, sequela
		S91.102S	Unsp opn wnd left great toe w/o damage to nail, sequela
		S91.103S	Unsp opn wnd unsp great toe w/o damage to nail, sequela
		S91.104S	Unsp opn wnd right lesser toe(s) w/o damage to nail, sequela
		S91.105S	Unsp opn wnd left lesser toe(s) w/o damage to nail, sequela
		S91.106S	Unsp opn wnd unsp lesser toe(s) w/o damage to nail, sequela
		S91.109S	Unsp open wound of unsp toe(s) w/o damage to nail, sequela
		S91.111S	Lac w/o fb of right great toe w/o damage to nail, sequela
		S91.112S	Lac w/o fb of left great toe w/o damage to nail, sequela
		S91.113S	Lac w/o fb of unsp great toe w/o damage to nail, sequela
		S91.114S	Lac w/o fb of right lesser toe(s) w/o damage to nail, sqla
		S91.115S	Lac w/o fb of left lesser toe(s) w/o damage to nail, sequela
		S91.116S	Lac w/o fb of unsp lesser toe(s) w/o damage to nail, sequela
		S91.119S	Laceration w/o fb of unsp toe w/o damage to nail, sequela
		S91.121S	Lac w fb of right great toe w/o damage to nail, sequela
		S91.122S	Lac w fb of left great toe w/o damage to nail, sequela
		S91.123S	Lac w fb of unsp great toe w/o damage to nail, sequela
		S91.124S	Lac w fb of right lesser toe(s) w/o damage to nail, sequela
		S91.125S	Lac w fb of left lesser toe(s) w/o damage to nail, sequela
		S91.126S	Lac w fb of unsp lesser toe(s) w/o damage to nail, sequela

(Continued on next page)

ICD-9-CM		ICD-10-CM	
906.1	LATE EFF OPN WND EXTREM W/O MENTION TEND INJURY **(Continued)**	**S91.129S**	Laceration w fb of unsp toe(s) w/o damage to nail, sequela
		S91.131S	Pnctr w/o fb of right great toe w/o damage to nail, sequela
		S91.132S	Pnctr w/o fb of left great toe w/o damage to nail, sequela
		S91.133S	Pnctr w/o fb of unsp great toe w/o damage to nail, sequela
		S91.134S	Pnctr w/o fb of right lesser toe(s) w/o damage to nail, sqla
		S91.135S	Pnctr w/o fb of left lesser toe(s) w/o damage to nail, sqla
		S91.136S	Pnctr w/o fb of unsp lesser toe(s) w/o damage to nail, sqla
		S91.139S	Pnctr w/o fb of unsp toe(s) w/o damage to nail, sequela
		S91.141S	Pnctr w fb of right great toe w/o damage to nail, sequela
		S91.142S	Pnctr w fb of left great toe w/o damage to nail, sequela
		S91.143S	Pnctr w fb of unsp great toe w/o damage to nail, sequela
		S91.144S	Pnctr w fb of right lesser toe(s) w/o damage to nail, sqla
		S91.145S	Pnctr w fb of left lesser toe(s) w/o damage to nail, sequela
		S91.146S	Pnctr w fb of unsp lesser toe(s) w/o damage to nail, sequela
		S91.149S	Pnctr w fb of unsp toe(s) w/o damage to nail, sequela
		S91.151S	Open bite of right great toe without damage to nail, sequela
		S91.152S	Open bite of left great toe without damage to nail, sequela
		S91.153S	Open bite of unsp great toe without damage to nail, sequela
		S91.154S	Open bite of right lesser toe(s) w/o damage to nail, sequela
		S91.155S	Open bite of left lesser toe(s) w/o damage to nail, sequela
		S91.156S	Open bite of unsp lesser toe(s) w/o damage to nail, sequela
		S91.159S	Open bite of unsp toe(s) without damage to nail, sequela
		S91.201S	Unsp open wound of right great toe w damage to nail, sequela
		S91.202S	Unsp open wound of left great toe w damage to nail, sequela
		S91.203S	Unsp open wound of unsp great toe w damage to nail, sequela
		S91.204S	Unsp opn wnd right lesser toe(s) w damage to nail, sequela
		S91.205S	Unsp opn wnd left lesser toe(s) w damage to nail, sequela
		S91.206S	Unsp opn wnd unsp lesser toe(s) w damage to nail, sequela
		S91.209S	Unsp open wound of unsp toe(s) with damage to nail, sequela
		S91.211S	Lac w/o fb of right great toe w damage to nail, sequela
		S91.212S	Lac w/o fb of left great toe w damage to nail, sequela
		S91.213S	Lac w/o fb of unsp great toe w damage to nail, sequela
		S91.214S	Lac w/o fb of right lesser toe(s) w damage to nail, sequela
		S91.215S	Lac w/o fb of left lesser toe(s) w damage to nail, sequela
		S91.216S	Lac w/o fb of unsp lesser toe(s) w damage to nail, sequela
		S91.219S	Laceration w/o fb of unsp toe(s) w damage to nail, sequela
		S91.221S	Laceration w fb of right great toe w damage to nail, sequela
		S91.222S	Laceration w fb of left great toe w damage to nail, sequela
		S91.223S	Laceration w fb of unsp great toe w damage to nail, sequela
		S91.224S	Lac w fb of right lesser toe(s) w damage to nail, sequela
		S91.225S	Lac w fb of left lesser toe(s) w damage to nail, sequela
		S91.226S	Lac w fb of unsp lesser toe(s) w damage to nail, sequela
		S91.229S	Laceration w fb of unsp toe(s) w damage to nail, sequela
		S91.231S	Pnctr w/o fb of right great toe w damage to nail, sequela
		S91.232S	Pnctr w/o fb of left great toe w damage to nail, sequela
		S91.233S	Pnctr w/o fb of unsp great toe w damage to nail, sequela
		S91.234S	Pnctr w/o fb of right lesser toe(s) w damage to nail, sqla
		S91.235S	Pnctr w/o fb of left lesser toe(s) w damage to nail, sequela
		S91.236S	Pnctr w/o fb of unsp lesser toe(s) w damage to nail, sequela
		S91.239S	Pnctr w/o fb of unsp toe(s) w damage to nail, sequela
		S91.241S	Pnctr w fb of right great toe w damage to nail, sequela
		S91.242S	Pnctr w fb of left great toe w damage to nail, sequela
		S91.243S	Pnctr w fb of unsp great toe w damage to nail, sequela
		S91.244S	Pnctr w fb of right lesser toe(s) w damage to nail, sequela
		S91.245S	Pnctr w fb of left lesser toe(s) w damage to nail, sequela
		S91.246S	Pnctr w fb of unsp lesser toe(s) w damage to nail, sequela
		S91.249S	Pnctr w fb of unsp toe(s) w damage to nail, sequela
		S91.251S	Open bite of right great toe with damage to nail, sequela
		S91.252S	Open bite of left great toe with damage to nail, sequela
		S91.253S	Open bite of unsp great toe with damage to nail, sequela
		S91.254S	Open bite of right lesser toe(s) w damage to nail, sequela
		S91.255S	Open bite of left lesser toe(s) with damage to nail, sequela
		S91.256S	Open bite of unsp lesser toe(s) with damage to nail, sequela
		S91.259S	Open bite of unspecified toe(s) with damage to nail, sequela
		S91.301S	Unspecified open wound, right foot, sequela
		S91.302S	Unspecified open wound, left foot, sequela
		S91.309S	Unspecified open wound, unspecified foot, sequela
		S91.311S	Laceration without foreign body, right foot, sequela
		S91.312S	Laceration without foreign body, left foot, sequela
		S91.319S	Laceration without foreign body, unspecified foot, sequela
		S91.321S	Laceration with foreign body, right foot, sequela
		S91.322S	Laceration with foreign body, left foot, sequela
		S91.329S	Laceration with foreign body, unspecified foot, sequela
		S91.331S	Puncture wound without foreign body, right foot, sequela
		S91.332S	Puncture wound without foreign body, left foot, sequela
		S91.339S	Puncture wound without foreign body, unsp foot, sequela
		S91.341S	Puncture wound with foreign body, right foot, sequela
		S91.342S	Puncture wound with foreign body, left foot, sequela
		S91.349S	Puncture wound with foreign body, unspecified foot, sequela
		S91.351S	Open bite, right foot, sequela
		S91.352S	Open bite, left foot, sequela
	(Continued on next page)	**S91.359S**	Open bite, unspecified foot, sequela

ICD-9-CM		ICD-10-CM	
906.1	LATE EFF OPN WND EXTREM W/O MENTION TEND INJURY **(Continued)**	**S96.021S**	Lacerat msl/tnd lng flxr msl toe at ank/ft lev, r foot, sqla
		S96.022S	Lacerat msl/tnd lng flxr msl toe at ank/ft lev, l foot, sqla
		S96.029S	Lacerat msl/tnd lng flxr msl toe at ank/ft lev,unsp ft, sqla
		S96.121S	Lacerat msl/tnd lng extn msl toe at ank/ft lev, r foot, sqla
		S96.122S	Lacerat msl/tnd lng extn msl toe at ank/ft lev, l foot, sqla
		S96.129S	Lacerat msl/tnd lng extn msl toe at ank/ft lev,unsp ft, sqla
		S96.221S	Lacerat intrinsic msl/tnd at ank/ft level, r foot, sequela
		S96.222S	Lacerat intrns msl/tnd at ank/ft level, left foot, sequela
		S96.229S	Lacerat intrns msl/tnd at ank/ft level, unsp foot, sequela
		S96.821S	Lacerat muscles and tendons at ank/ft level, r foot, sequela
		S96.822S	Lacerat muscles and tendons at ank/ft level, l foot, sequela
		S96.829S	Lacerat musc and tendons at ank/ft level, unsp foot, sequela
		S96.921S	Lacerat unsp msl/tnd at ank/ft level, right foot, sequela
		S96.922S	Lacerat unsp msl/tnd at ank/ft level, left foot, sequela
		S96.929S	Lacerat unsp msl/tnd at ank/ft level, unsp foot, sequela
906.2	LATE EFFECT OF SUPERFICIAL INJURY	**S00.00XS**	Unspecified superficial injury of scalp, sequela
		S00.01XS	Abrasion of scalp, sequela
		S00.02XS	Blister (nonthermal) of scalp, sequela
		S00.04XS	External constriction of part of scalp, sequela
		S00.05XS	Superficial foreign body of scalp, sequela
		S00.06XS	Insect bite (nonvenomous) of scalp, sequela
		S00.07XS	Other superficial bite of scalp, sequela
		S00.201S	Unsp superfic inj right eyelid and periocular area, sequela
		S00.202S	Unsp superfic inj left eyelid and periocular area, sequela
		S00.209S	Unsp superfic inj unsp eyelid and periocular area, sequela
		S00.211S	Abrasion of right eyelid and periocular area, sequela
		S00.212S	Abrasion of left eyelid and periocular area, sequela
		S00.219S	Abrasion of unspecified eyelid and periocular area, sequela
		S00.221S	Blister of right eyelid and periocular area, sequela
		S00.222S	Blister of left eyelid and periocular area, sequela
		S00.229S	Blister of unsp eyelid and periocular area, sequela
		S00.241S	Extrn constrict of right eyelid and periocular area, sequela
		S00.242S	Extrn constrict of left eyelid and periocular area, sequela
		S00.249S	Extrn constrict of unsp eyelid and periocular area, sequela
		S00.251S	Superficial fb of right eyelid and periocular area, sequela
		S00.252S	Superficial fb of left eyelid and periocular area, sequela
		S00.259S	Superficial fb of unsp eyelid and periocular area, sequela
		S00.261S	Insect bite of right eyelid and periocular area, sequela
		S00.262S	Insect bite of left eyelid and periocular area, sequela
		S00.269S	Insect bite of unsp eyelid and periocular area, sequela
		S00.271S	Oth superfic bite of right eyelid and periocular area, sqla
		S00.272S	Oth superfic bite of left eyelid and periocular area, sequela
		S00.279S	Oth superfic bite of unsp eyelid and periocular area, sequela
		S00.30XS	Unspecified superficial injury of nose, sequela
		S00.31XS	Abrasion of nose, sequela
		S00.32XS	Blister (nonthermal) of nose, sequela
		S00.34XS	External constriction of nose, sequela
		S00.35XS	Superficial foreign body of nose, sequela
		S00.36XS	Insect bite (nonvenomous) of nose, sequela
		S00.37XS	Other superficial bite of nose, sequela
		S00.401S	Unspecified superficial injury of right ear, sequela
		S00.402S	Unspecified superficial injury of left ear, sequela
		S00.409S	Unspecified superficial injury of unspecified ear, sequela
		S00.411S	Abrasion of right ear, sequela
		S00.412S	Abrasion of left ear, sequela
		S00.419S	Abrasion of unspecified ear, sequela
		S00.421S	Blister (nonthermal) of right ear, sequela
		S00.422S	Blister (nonthermal) of left ear, sequela
		S00.429S	Blister (nonthermal) of unspecified ear, sequela
		S00.441S	External constriction of right ear, sequela
		S00.442S	External constriction of left ear, sequela
		S00.449S	External constriction of unspecified ear, sequela
		S00.451S	Superficial foreign body of right ear, sequela
		S00.452S	Superficial foreign body of left ear, sequela
		S00.459S	Superficial foreign body of unspecified ear, sequela
		S00.461S	Insect bite (nonvenomous) of right ear, sequela
		S00.462S	Insect bite (nonvenomous) of left ear, sequela
		S00.469S	Insect bite (nonvenomous) of unspecified ear, sequela
		S00.471S	Other superficial bite of right ear, sequela
		S00.472S	Other superficial bite of left ear, sequela
		S00.479S	Other superficial bite of unspecified ear, sequela
		S00.501S	Unspecified superficial injury of lip, sequela
		S00.502S	Unspecified superficial injury of oral cavity, sequela
		S00.511S	Abrasion of lip, sequela
		S00.512S	Abrasion of oral cavity, sequela
		S00.521S	Blister (nonthermal) of lip, sequela
		S00.522S	Blister (nonthermal) of oral cavity, sequela
		S00.541S	External constriction of lip, sequela
		S00.542S	External constriction of oral cavity, sequela
		S00.551S	Superficial foreign body of lip, sequela
		S00.552S	Superficial foreign body of oral cavity, sequela
		S00.561S	Insect bite (nonvenomous) of lip, sequela
	(Continued on next page)	**S00.562S**	Insect bite (nonvenomous) of oral cavity, sequela

ICD-9-CM		ICD-10-CM	
906.2	LATE EFFECT OF SUPERFICIAL INJURY **(Continued)**	**S00.571S**	Other superficial bite of lip, sequela
		S00.572S	Other superficial bite of oral cavity, sequela
		S00.80XS	Unsp superficial injury of other part of head, sequela
		S00.81XS	Abrasion of other part of head, sequela
		S00.82XS	Blister (nonthermal) of other part of head, sequela
		S00.84XS	External constriction of other part of head, sequela
		S00.85XS	Superficial foreign body of other part of head, sequela
		S00.86XS	Insect bite (nonvenomous) of other part of head, sequela
		S00.87XS	Other superficial bite of other part of head, sequela
		S00.90XS	Unsp superficial injury of unspecified part of head, sequela
		S00.91XS	Abrasion of unspecified part of head, sequela
		S00.92XS	Blister (nonthermal) of unspecified part of head, sequela
		S00.94XS	External constriction of unspecified part of head, sequela
		S00.95XS	Superficial foreign body of unsp part of head, sequela
		S00.96XS	Insect bite (nonvenomous) of unsp part of head, sequela
		S00.97XS	Other superficial bite of unspecified part of head, sequela
		S05.00XS	Inj conjunctiva and corneal abras w/o fb, unsp eye, sequela
		S05.01XS	Inj conjunctiva and corneal abrasion w/o fb, r eye, sequela
		S05.02XS	Inj conjunctiva and corneal abras w/o fb, left eye, sequela
		S10.10XS	Unspecified superficial injuries of throat, sequela
		S10.11XS	Abrasion of throat, sequela
		S10.12XS	Blister (nonthermal) of throat, sequela
		S10.14XS	External constriction of part of throat, sequela
		S10.15XS	Superficial foreign body of throat, sequela
		S10.16XS	Insect bite (nonvenomous) of throat, sequela
		S10.17XS	Other superficial bite of throat, sequela
		S10.80XS	Unspecified superficial injury of oth part of neck, sequela
		S10.81XS	Abrasion of other specified part of neck, sequela
		S10.82XS	Blister (nonthermal) of oth part of neck, sequela
		S10.84XS	External constriction of oth part of neck, sequela
		S10.85XS	Superficial foreign body of oth part of neck, sequela
		S10.86XS	Insect bite of other specified part of neck, sequela
		S10.87XS	Other superficial bite of oth part of neck, sequela
		S10.90XS	Unsp superficial injury of unspecified part of neck, sequela
		S10.91XS	Abrasion of unspecified part of neck, sequela
		S10.92XS	Blister (nonthermal) of unspecified part of neck, sequela
		S10.94XS	External constriction of unspecified part of neck, sequela
		S10.95XS	Superficial foreign body of unsp part of neck, sequela
		S10.96XS	Insect bite of unspecified part of neck, sequela
		S10.97XS	Other superficial bite of unspecified part of neck, sequela
		S20.101S	Unsp superficial injuries of breast, right breast, sequela
		S20.102S	Unsp superficial injuries of breast, left breast, sequela
		S20.109S	Unsp superficial injuries of breast, unsp breast, sequela
		S20.111S	Abrasion of breast, right breast, sequela
		S20.112S	Abrasion of breast, left breast, sequela
		S20.119S	Abrasion of breast, unspecified breast, sequela
		S20.121S	Blister (nonthermal) of breast, right breast, sequela
		S20.122S	Blister (nonthermal) of breast, left breast, sequela
		S20.129S	Blister (nonthermal) of breast, unspecified breast, sequela
		S20.141S	External constrict of part of breast, right breast, sequela
		S20.142S	External constrict of part of breast, left breast, sequela
		S20.149S	External constrict of part of breast, unsp breast, sequela
		S20.151S	Superficial foreign body of breast, right breast, sequela
		S20.152S	Superficial foreign body of breast, left breast, sequela
		S20.159S	Superficial foreign body of breast, unsp breast, sequela
		S20.161S	Insect bite (nonvenomous) of breast, right breast, sequela
		S20.162S	Insect bite (nonvenomous) of breast, left breast, sequela
		S20.169S	Insect bite (nonvenomous) of breast, unsp breast, sequela
		S20.171S	Other superficial bite of breast, right breast, sequela
		S20.172S	Other superficial bite of breast, left breast, sequela
		S20.179S	Other superficial bite of breast, unsp breast, sequela
		S20.301S	Unsp superficial injuries of r frnt wl of thorax, sequela
		S20.302S	Unsp superficial injuries of l frnt wl of thorax, sequela
		S20.309S	Unsp superfic injuries of unsp front wall of thorax, sequela
		S20.311S	Abrasion of right front wall of thorax, sequela
		S20.312S	Abrasion of left front wall of thorax, sequela
		S20.319S	Abrasion of unspecified front wall of thorax, sequela
		S20.321S	Blister (nonthermal) of right front wall of thorax, sequela
		S20.322S	Blister (nonthermal) of left front wall of thorax, sequela
		S20.329S	Blister (nonthermal) of unsp front wall of thorax, sequela
		S20.341S	External constriction of right front wall of thorax, sequela
		S20.342S	External constriction of left front wall of thorax, sequela
		S20.349S	External constriction of unsp front wall of thorax, sequela
		S20.351S	Superficial foreign body of r frnt wl of thorax, sequela
		S20.352S	Superficial foreign body of l frnt wl of thorax, sequela
		S20.359S	Superficial fb of unsp front wall of thorax, sequela
		S20.361S	Insect bite (nonvenomous) of r frnt wl of thorax, sequela
		S20.362S	Insect bite (nonvenomous) of l frnt wl of thorax, sequela
		S20.369S	Insect bite of unsp front wall of thorax, sequela
		S20.371S	Oth superficial bite of right front wall of thorax, sequela
		S20.372S	Other superficial bite of left front wall of thorax, sequela
		S20.379S	Other superficial bite of unsp front wall of thorax, sequela
	(Continued on next page)	**S20.401S**	Unsp superficial injuries of r bk wl of thorax, sequela

ICD-9-CM		ICD-10-CM	
9Ø6.2	LATE EFFECT OF SUPERFICIAL INJURY **(Continued)**	**S2Ø.4Ø2S**	Unsp superficial injuries of l bk wl of thorax, sequela
		S2Ø.4Ø9S	Unsp superfic injuries of unsp back wall of thorax, sequela
		S2Ø.411S	Abrasion of right back wall of thorax, sequela
		S2Ø.412S	Abrasion of left back wall of thorax, sequela
		S2Ø.419S	Abrasion of unspecified back wall of thorax, sequela
		S2Ø.421S	Blister (nonthermal) of right back wall of thorax, sequela
		S2Ø.422S	Blister (nonthermal) of left back wall of thorax, sequela
		S2Ø.429S	Blister (nonthermal) of unsp back wall of thorax, sequela
		S2Ø.441S	External constriction of right back wall of thorax, sequela
		S2Ø.442S	External constriction of left back wall of thorax, sequela
		S2Ø.449S	External constriction of unsp back wall of thorax, sequela
		S2Ø.451S	Superficial foreign body of r bk wl of thorax, sequela
		S2Ø.452S	Superficial foreign body of l bk wl of thorax, sequela
		S2Ø.459S	Superficial fb of unsp back wall of thorax, sequela
		S2Ø.461S	Insect bite (nonvenomous) of r bk wl of thorax, sequela
		S2Ø.462S	Insect bite (nonvenomous) of l bk wl of thorax, sequela
		S2Ø.469S	Insect bite of unsp back wall of thorax, sequela
		S2Ø.471S	Other superficial bite of right back wall of thorax, sequela
		S2Ø.472S	Other superficial bite of left back wall of thorax, sequela
		S2Ø.479S	Other superficial bite of unsp back wall of thorax, sequela
		S2Ø.9ØXS	Unsp superficial injury of unsp parts of thorax, sequela
		S2Ø.91XS	Abrasion of unspecified parts of thorax, sequela
		S2Ø.92XS	Blister (nonthermal) of unspecified parts of thorax, sequela
		S2Ø.94XS	External constriction of unsp parts of thorax, sequela
		S2Ø.95XS	Superficial foreign body of unsp parts of thorax, sequela
		S2Ø.96XS	Insect bite (nonvenomous) of unsp parts of thorax, sequela
		S2Ø.97XS	Other superficial bite of unsp parts of thorax, sequela
		S3Ø.81ØS	Abrasion of lower back and pelvis, sequela
		S3Ø.811S	Abrasion of abdominal wall, sequela
		S3Ø.812S	Abrasion of penis, sequela
		S3Ø.813S	Abrasion of scrotum and testes, sequela
		S3Ø.814S	Abrasion of vagina and vulva, sequela
		S3Ø.815S	Abrasion of unsp external genital organs, male, sequela
		S3Ø.816S	Abrasion of unsp external genital organs, female, sequela
		S3Ø.817S	Abrasion of anus, sequela
		S3Ø.82ØS	Blister (nonthermal) of lower back and pelvis, sequela
		S3Ø.821S	Blister (nonthermal) of abdominal wall, sequela
		S3Ø.822S	Blister (nonthermal) of penis, sequela
		S3Ø.823S	Blister (nonthermal) of scrotum and testes, sequela
		S3Ø.824S	Blister (nonthermal) of vagina and vulva, sequela
		S3Ø.825S	Blister of unsp external genital organs, male, sequela
		S3Ø.826S	Blister of unsp external genital organs, female, sequela
		S3Ø.827S	Blister (nonthermal) of anus, sequela
		S3Ø.84ØS	External constriction of lower back and pelvis, sequela
		S3Ø.841S	External constriction of abdominal wall, sequela
		S3Ø.842S	External constriction of penis, sequela
		S3Ø.843S	External constriction of scrotum and testes, sequela
		S3Ø.844S	External constriction of vagina and vulva, sequela
		S3Ø.845S	Extrn constrict of unsp extrn genital organs, male, sequela
		S3Ø.846S	Extrn constrict of unsp extrn gntl organs, female, sequela
		S3Ø.85ØS	Superficial foreign body of lower back and pelvis, sequela
		S3Ø.851S	Superficial foreign body of abdominal wall, sequela
		S3Ø.852S	Superficial foreign body of penis, sequela
		S3Ø.853S	Superficial foreign body of scrotum and testes, sequela
		S3Ø.854S	Superficial foreign body of vagina and vulva, sequela
		S3Ø.855S	Superfic fb of unsp external genital organs, male, sequela
		S3Ø.856S	Superfic fb of unsp external genital organs, female, sequela
		S3Ø.857S	Superficial foreign body of anus, sequela
		S3Ø.86ØS	Insect bite (nonvenomous) of lower back and pelvis, sequela
		S3Ø.861S	Insect bite (nonvenomous) of abdominal wall, sequela
		S3Ø.862S	Insect bite (nonvenomous) of penis, sequela
		S3Ø.863S	Insect bite (nonvenomous) of scrotum and testes, sequela
		S3Ø.864S	Insect bite (nonvenomous) of vagina and vulva, sequela
		S3Ø.865S	Insect bite of unsp external genital organs, male, sequela
		S3Ø.866S	Insect bite of unsp external genital organs, female, sequela
		S3Ø.867S	Insect bite (nonvenomous) of anus, sequela
		S3Ø.87ØS	Other superficial bite of lower back and pelvis, sequela
		S3Ø.871S	Other superficial bite of abdominal wall, sequela
		S3Ø.872S	Other superficial bite of penis, sequela
		S3Ø.873S	Other superficial bite of scrotum and testes, sequela
		S3Ø.874S	Other superficial bite of vagina and vulva, sequela
		S3Ø.875S	Oth superfic bite of unsp extrn gntl organs, male, sequela
		S3Ø.876S	Oth superfic bite of unsp extrn gntl organs, female, sequela
		S3Ø.877S	Other superficial bite of anus, sequela
		S3Ø.91XS	Unsp superficial injury of lower back and pelvis, sequela
		S3Ø.92XS	Unspecified superficial injury of abdominal wall, sequela
		S3Ø.93XS	Unspecified superficial injury of penis, sequela
		S3Ø.94XS	Unsp superficial injury of scrotum and testes, sequela
		S3Ø.95XS	Unspecified superficial injury of vagina and vulva, sequela
		S3Ø.96XS	Unsp superfic inj unsp extrn genital organs, male, sequela
		S3Ø.97XS	Unsp superfic inj unsp extrn genital organs, female, sequela
	(Continued on next page)	**S3Ø.98XS**	Unspecified superficial injury of anus, sequela

[Brackets] indicate valid character values for each code. Character value meanings provided for each code grouping.

ICD-9-CM		ICD-10-CM	
9Ø6.2	LATE EFFECT OF SUPERFICIAL INJURY **(Continued)**	**S4Ø.211S**	Abrasion of right shoulder, sequela
		S4Ø.212S	Abrasion of left shoulder, sequela
		S4Ø.219S	Abrasion of unspecified shoulder, sequela
		S4Ø.221S	Blister (nonthermal) of right shoulder, sequela
		S4Ø.222S	Blister (nonthermal) of left shoulder, sequela
		S4Ø.229S	Blister (nonthermal) of unspecified shoulder, sequela
		S4Ø.241S	External constriction of right shoulder, sequela
		S4Ø.242S	External constriction of left shoulder, sequela
		S4Ø.249S	External constriction of unspecified shoulder, sequela
		S4Ø.251S	Superficial foreign body of right shoulder, sequela
		S4Ø.252S	Superficial foreign body of left shoulder, sequela
		S4Ø.259S	Superficial foreign body of unspecified shoulder, sequela
		S4Ø.261S	Insect bite (nonvenomous) of right shoulder, sequela
		S4Ø.262S	Insect bite (nonvenomous) of left shoulder, sequela
		S4Ø.269S	Insect bite (nonvenomous) of unspecified shoulder, sequela
		S4Ø.271S	Other superficial bite of right shoulder, sequela
		S4Ø.272S	Other superficial bite of left shoulder, sequela
		S4Ø.279S	Other superficial bite of unspecified shoulder, sequela
		S4Ø.811S	Abrasion of right upper arm, sequela
		S4Ø.812S	Abrasion of left upper arm, sequela
		S4Ø.819S	Abrasion of unspecified upper arm, sequela
		S4Ø.821S	Blister (nonthermal) of right upper arm, sequela
		S4Ø.822S	Blister (nonthermal) of left upper arm, sequela
		S4Ø.829S	Blister (nonthermal) of unspecified upper arm, sequela
		S4Ø.841S	External constriction of right upper arm, sequela
		S4Ø.842S	External constriction of left upper arm, sequela
		S4Ø.849S	External constriction of unspecified upper arm, sequela
		S4Ø.851S	Superficial foreign body of right upper arm, sequela
		S4Ø.852S	Superficial foreign body of left upper arm, sequela
		S4Ø.859S	Superficial foreign body of unspecified upper arm, sequela
		S4Ø.861S	Insect bite (nonvenomous) of right upper arm, sequela
		S4Ø.862S	Insect bite (nonvenomous) of left upper arm, sequela
		S4Ø.869S	Insect bite (nonvenomous) of unspecified upper arm, sequela
		S4Ø.871S	Other superficial bite of right upper arm, sequela
		S4Ø.872S	Other superficial bite of left upper arm, sequela
		S4Ø.879S	Other superficial bite of unspecified upper arm, sequela
		S4Ø.911S	Unspecified superficial injury of right shoulder, sequela
		S4Ø.912S	Unspecified superficial injury of left shoulder, sequela
		S4Ø.919S	Unsp superficial injury of unspecified shoulder, sequela
		S4Ø.921S	Unspecified superficial injury of right upper arm, sequela
		S4Ø.922S	Unspecified superficial injury of left upper arm, sequela
		S4Ø.929S	Unsp superficial injury of unspecified upper arm, sequela
		S5Ø.311S	Abrasion of right elbow, sequela
		S5Ø.312S	Abrasion of left elbow, sequela
		S5Ø.319S	Abrasion of unspecified elbow, sequela
		S5Ø.321S	Blister (nonthermal) of right elbow, sequela
		S5Ø.322S	Blister (nonthermal) of left elbow, sequela
		S5Ø.329S	Blister (nonthermal) of unspecified elbow, sequela
		S5Ø.341S	External constriction of right elbow, sequela
		S5Ø.342S	External constriction of left elbow, sequela
		S5Ø.349S	External constriction of unspecified elbow, sequela
		S5Ø.351S	Superficial foreign body of right elbow, sequela
		S5Ø.352S	Superficial foreign body of left elbow, sequela
		S5Ø.359S	Superficial foreign body of unspecified elbow, sequela
		S5Ø.361S	Insect bite (nonvenomous) of right elbow, sequela
		S5Ø.362S	Insect bite (nonvenomous) of left elbow, sequela
		S5Ø.369S	Insect bite (nonvenomous) of unspecified elbow, sequela
		S5Ø.371S	Other superficial bite of right elbow, sequela
		S5Ø.372S	Other superficial bite of left elbow, sequela
		S5Ø.379S	Other superficial bite of unspecified elbow, sequela
		S5Ø.811S	Abrasion of right forearm, sequela
		S5Ø.812S	Abrasion of left forearm, sequela
		S5Ø.819S	Abrasion of unspecified forearm, sequela
		S5Ø.821S	Blister (nonthermal) of right forearm, sequela
		S5Ø.822S	Blister (nonthermal) of left forearm, sequela
		S5Ø.829S	Blister (nonthermal) of unspecified forearm, sequela
		S5Ø.841S	External constriction of right forearm, sequela
		S5Ø.842S	External constriction of left forearm, sequela
		S5Ø.849S	External constriction of unspecified forearm, sequela
		S5Ø.851S	Superficial foreign body of right forearm, sequela
		S5Ø.852S	Superficial foreign body of left forearm, sequela
		S5Ø.859S	Superficial foreign body of unspecified forearm, sequela
		S5Ø.861S	Insect bite (nonvenomous) of right forearm, sequela
		S5Ø.862S	Insect bite (nonvenomous) of left forearm, sequela
		S5Ø.869S	Insect bite (nonvenomous) of unspecified forearm, sequela
		S5Ø.871S	Other superficial bite of right forearm, sequela
		S5Ø.872S	Other superficial bite of left forearm, sequela
		S5Ø.879S	Other superficial bite of unspecified forearm, sequela
		S5Ø.9Ø1S	Unspecified superficial injury of right elbow, sequela
		S5Ø.9Ø2S	Unspecified superficial injury of left elbow, sequela
		S5Ø.9Ø9S	Unspecified superficial injury of unspecified elbow, sequela
	(Continued on next page)	**S5Ø.911S**	Unspecified superficial injury of right forearm, sequela

ICD-9-CM		ICD-10-CM	
906.2	LATE EFFECT OF SUPERFICIAL INJURY **(Continued)**	**S50.912S**	Unspecified superficial injury of left forearm, sequela
		S50.919S	Unsp superficial injury of unspecified forearm, sequela
		S60.311S	Abrasion of right thumb, sequela
		S60.312S	Abrasion of left thumb, sequela
		S60.319S	Abrasion of unspecified thumb, sequela
		S60.321S	Blister (nonthermal) of right thumb, sequela
		S60.322S	Blister (nonthermal) of left thumb, sequela
		S60.329S	Blister (nonthermal) of unspecified thumb, sequela
		S60.341S	External constriction of right thumb, sequela
		S60.342S	External constriction of left thumb, sequela
		S60.349S	External constriction of unspecified thumb, sequela
		S60.351S	Superficial foreign body of right thumb, sequela
		S60.352S	Superficial foreign body of left thumb, sequela
		S60.359S	Superficial foreign body of unspecified thumb, sequela
		S60.361S	Insect bite (nonvenomous) of right thumb, sequela
		S60.362S	Insect bite (nonvenomous) of left thumb, sequela
		S60.369S	Insect bite (nonvenomous) of unspecified thumb, sequela
		S60.371S	Other superficial bite of right thumb, sequela
		S60.372S	Other superficial bite of left thumb, sequela
		S60.379S	Other superficial bite of unspecified thumb, sequela
		S60.391S	Other superficial injuries of right thumb, sequela
		S60.392S	Other superficial injuries of left thumb, sequela
		S60.399S	Other superficial injuries of unspecified thumb, sequela
		S60.410S	Abrasion of right index finger, sequela
		S60.411S	Abrasion of left index finger, sequela
		S60.412S	Abrasion of right middle finger, sequela
		S60.413S	Abrasion of left middle finger, sequela
		S60.414S	Abrasion of right ring finger, sequela
		S60.415S	Abrasion of left ring finger, sequela
		S60.416S	Abrasion of right little finger, sequela
		S60.417S	Abrasion of left little finger, sequela
		S60.418S	Abrasion of other finger, sequela
		S60.419S	Abrasion of unspecified finger, sequela
		S60.420S	Blister (nonthermal) of right index finger, sequela
		S60.421S	Blister (nonthermal) of left index finger, sequela
		S60.422S	Blister (nonthermal) of right middle finger, sequela
		S60.423S	Blister (nonthermal) of left middle finger, sequela
		S60.424S	Blister (nonthermal) of right ring finger, sequela
		S60.425S	Blister (nonthermal) of left ring finger, sequela
		S60.426S	Blister (nonthermal) of right little finger, sequela
		S60.427S	Blister (nonthermal) of left little finger, sequela
		S60.428S	Blister (nonthermal) of other finger, sequela
		S60.429S	Blister (nonthermal) of unspecified finger, sequela
		S60.440S	External constriction of right index finger, sequela
		S60.441S	External constriction of left index finger, sequela
		S60.442S	External constriction of right middle finger, sequela
		S60.443S	External constriction of left middle finger, sequela
		S60.444S	External constriction of right ring finger, sequela
		S60.445S	External constriction of left ring finger, sequela
		S60.446S	External constriction of right little finger, sequela
		S60.447S	External constriction of left little finger, sequela
		S60.448S	External constriction of other finger, sequela
		S60.449S	External constriction of unspecified finger, sequela
		S60.450S	Superficial foreign body of right index finger, sequela
		S60.451S	Superficial foreign body of left index finger, sequela
		S60.452S	Superficial foreign body of right middle finger, sequela
		S60.453S	Superficial foreign body of left middle finger, sequela
		S60.454S	Superficial foreign body of right ring finger, sequela
		S60.455S	Superficial foreign body of left ring finger, sequela
		S60.456S	Superficial foreign body of right little finger, sequela
		S60.457S	Superficial foreign body of left little finger, sequela
		S60.458S	Superficial foreign body of other finger, sequela
		S60.459S	Superficial foreign body of unspecified finger, sequela
		S60.460S	Insect bite (nonvenomous) of right index finger, sequela
		S60.461S	Insect bite (nonvenomous) of left index finger, sequela
		S60.462S	Insect bite (nonvenomous) of right middle finger, sequela
		S60.463S	Insect bite (nonvenomous) of left middle finger, sequela
		S60.464S	Insect bite (nonvenomous) of right ring finger, sequela
		S60.465S	Insect bite (nonvenomous) of left ring finger, sequela
		S60.466S	Insect bite (nonvenomous) of right little finger, sequela
		S60.467S	Insect bite (nonvenomous) of left little finger, sequela
		S60.468S	Insect bite (nonvenomous) of other finger, sequela
		S60.469S	Insect bite (nonvenomous) of unspecified finger, sequela
		S60.470S	Other superficial bite of right index finger, sequela
		S60.471S	Other superficial bite of left index finger, sequela
		S60.472S	Other superficial bite of right middle finger, sequela
		S60.473S	Other superficial bite of left middle finger, sequela
		S60.474S	Other superficial bite of right ring finger, sequela
		S60.475S	Other superficial bite of left ring finger, sequela
		S60.476S	Other superficial bite of right little finger, sequela
		S60.477S	Other superficial bite of left little finger, sequela
	(Continued on next page)	**S60.478S**	Other superficial bite of other finger, sequela

 [Brackets] indicate valid character values for each code. Character value meanings provided for each code grouping.

ICD-9-CM		ICD-10-CM	
9Ø6.2	LATE EFFECT OF SUPERFICIAL INJURY **(Continued)**	**S6Ø.479S**	Other superficial bite of unspecified finger, sequela
		S6Ø.511S	Abrasion of right hand, sequela
		S6Ø.512S	Abrasion of left hand, sequela
		S6Ø.519S	Abrasion of unspecified hand, sequela
		S6Ø.521S	Blister (nonthermal) of right hand, sequela
		S6Ø.522S	Blister (nonthermal) of left hand, sequela
		S6Ø.529S	Blister (nonthermal) of unspecified hand, sequela
		S6Ø.541S	External constriction of right hand, sequela
		S6Ø.542S	External constriction of left hand, sequela
		S6Ø.549S	External constriction of unspecified hand, sequela
		S6Ø.551S	Superficial foreign body of right hand, sequela
		S6Ø.552S	Superficial foreign body of left hand, sequela
		S6Ø.559S	Superficial foreign body of unspecified hand, sequela
		S6Ø.561S	Insect bite (nonvenomous) of right hand, sequela
		S6Ø.562S	Insect bite (nonvenomous) of left hand, sequela
		S6Ø.569S	Insect bite (nonvenomous) of unspecified hand, sequela
		S6Ø.571S	Other superficial bite of hand of right hand, sequela
		S6Ø.572S	Other superficial bite of hand of left hand, sequela
		S6Ø.579S	Other superficial bite of hand of unspecified hand, sequela
		S6Ø.811S	Abrasion of right wrist, sequela
		S6Ø.812S	Abrasion of left wrist, sequela
		S6Ø.819S	Abrasion of unspecified wrist, sequela
		S6Ø.821S	Blister (nonthermal) of right wrist, sequela
		S6Ø.822S	Blister (nonthermal) of left wrist, sequela
		S6Ø.829S	Blister (nonthermal) of unspecified wrist, sequela
		S6Ø.841S	External constriction of right wrist, sequela
		S6Ø.842S	External constriction of left wrist, sequela
		S6Ø.849S	External constriction of unspecified wrist, sequela
		S6Ø.851S	Superficial foreign body of right wrist, sequela
		S6Ø.852S	Superficial foreign body of left wrist, sequela
		S6Ø.859S	Superficial foreign body of unspecified wrist, sequela
		S6Ø.861S	Insect bite (nonvenomous) of right wrist, sequela
		S6Ø.862S	Insect bite (nonvenomous) of left wrist, sequela
		S6Ø.869S	Insect bite (nonvenomous) of unspecified wrist, sequela
		S6Ø.871S	Other superficial bite of right wrist, sequela
		S6Ø.872S	Other superficial bite of left wrist, sequela
		S6Ø.879S	Other superficial bite of unspecified wrist, sequela
		S6Ø.911S	Unspecified superficial injury of right wrist, sequela
		S6Ø.912S	Unspecified superficial injury of left wrist, sequela
		S6Ø.919S	Unspecified superficial injury of unspecified wrist, sequela
		S6Ø.921S	Unspecified superficial injury of right hand, sequela
		S6Ø.922S	Unspecified superficial injury of left hand, sequela
		S6Ø.929S	Unspecified superficial injury of unspecified hand, sequela
		S6Ø.931S	Unspecified superficial injury of right thumb, sequela
		S6Ø.932S	Unspecified superficial injury of left thumb, sequela
		S6Ø.939S	Unspecified superficial injury of unspecified thumb, sequela
		S6Ø.94ØS	Unsp superficial injury of right index finger, sequela
		S6Ø.941S	Unspecified superficial injury of left index finger, sequela
		S6Ø.942S	Unsp superficial injury of right middle finger, sequela
		S6Ø.943S	Unsp superficial injury of left middle finger, sequela
		S6Ø.944S	Unspecified superficial injury of right ring finger, sequela
		S6Ø.945S	Unspecified superficial injury of left ring finger, sequela
		S6Ø.946S	Unsp superficial injury of right little finger, sequela
		S6Ø.947S	Unsp superficial injury of left little finger, sequela
		S6Ø.948S	Unspecified superficial injury of other finger, sequela
		S6Ø.949S	Unsp superficial injury of unspecified finger, sequela
		S7Ø.211S	Abrasion, right hip, sequela
		S7Ø.212S	Abrasion, left hip, sequela
		S7Ø.219S	Abrasion, unspecified hip, sequela
		S7Ø.221S	Blister (nonthermal), right hip, sequela
		S7Ø.222S	Blister (nonthermal), left hip, sequela
		S7Ø.229S	Blister (nonthermal), unspecified hip, sequela
		S7Ø.241S	External constriction, right hip, sequela
		S7Ø.242S	External constriction, left hip, sequela
		S7Ø.249S	External constriction, unspecified hip, sequela
		S7Ø.251S	Superficial foreign body, right hip, sequela
		S7Ø.252S	Superficial foreign body, left hip, sequela
		S7Ø.259S	Superficial foreign body, unspecified hip, sequela
		S7Ø.261S	Insect bite (nonvenomous), right hip, sequela
		S7Ø.262S	Insect bite (nonvenomous), left hip, sequela
		S7Ø.269S	Insect bite (nonvenomous), unspecified hip, sequela
		S7Ø.271S	Other superficial bite of hip, right hip, sequela
		S7Ø.272S	Other superficial bite of hip, left hip, sequela
		S7Ø.279S	Other superficial bite of hip, unspecified hip, sequela
		S7Ø.311S	Abrasion, right thigh, sequela
		S7Ø.312S	Abrasion, left thigh, sequela
		S7Ø.319S	Abrasion, unspecified thigh, sequela
		S7Ø.321S	Blister (nonthermal), right thigh, sequela
		S7Ø.322S	Blister (nonthermal), left thigh, sequela
		S7Ø.329S	Blister (nonthermal), unspecified thigh, sequela
		S7Ø.341S	External constriction, right thigh, sequela
	(Continued on next page)	**S7Ø.342S**	External constriction, left thigh, sequela

ICD-9-CM		ICD-10-CM	
9Ø6.2	LATE EFFECT OF SUPERFICIAL INJURY **(Continued)**	**S7Ø.349S**	External constriction, unspecified thigh, sequela
		S7Ø.351S	Superficial foreign body, right thigh, sequela
		S7Ø.352S	Superficial foreign body, left thigh, sequela
		S7Ø.359S	Superficial foreign body, unspecified thigh, sequela
		S7Ø.361S	Insect bite (nonvenomous), right thigh, sequela
		S7Ø.362S	Insect bite (nonvenomous), left thigh, sequela
		S7Ø.369S	Insect bite (nonvenomous), unspecified thigh, sequela
		S7Ø.371S	Other superficial bite of right thigh, sequela
		S7Ø.372S	Other superficial bite of left thigh, sequela
		S7Ø.379S	Other superficial bite of unspecified thigh, sequela
		S7Ø.911S	Unspecified superficial injury of right hip, sequela
		S7Ø.912S	Unspecified superficial injury of left hip, sequela
		S7Ø.919S	Unspecified superficial injury of unspecified hip, sequela
		S7Ø.921S	Unspecified superficial injury of right thigh, sequela
		S7Ø.922S	Unspecified superficial injury of left thigh, sequela
		S7Ø.929S	Unspecified superficial injury of unspecified thigh, sequela
		S8Ø.211S	Abrasion, right knee, sequela
		S8Ø.212S	Abrasion, left knee, sequela
		S8Ø.219S	Abrasion, unspecified knee, sequela
		S8Ø.221S	Blister (nonthermal), right knee, sequela
		S8Ø.222S	Blister (nonthermal), left knee, sequela
		S8Ø.229S	Blister (nonthermal), unspecified knee, sequela
		S8Ø.241S	External constriction, right knee, sequela
		S8Ø.242S	External constriction, left knee, sequela
		S8Ø.249S	External constriction, unspecified knee, sequela
		S8Ø.251S	Superficial foreign body, right knee, sequela
		S8Ø.252S	Superficial foreign body, left knee, sequela
		S8Ø.259S	Superficial foreign body, unspecified knee, sequela
		S8Ø.261S	Insect bite (nonvenomous), right knee, sequela
		S8Ø.262S	Insect bite (nonvenomous), left knee, sequela
		S8Ø.269S	Insect bite (nonvenomous), unspecified knee, sequela
		S8Ø.271S	Other superficial bite of right knee, sequela
		S8Ø.272S	Other superficial bite of left knee, sequela
		S8Ø.279S	Other superficial bite of unspecified knee, sequela
		S8Ø.811S	Abrasion, right lower leg, sequela
		S8Ø.812S	Abrasion, left lower leg, sequela
		S8Ø.819S	Abrasion, unspecified lower leg, sequela
		S8Ø.821S	Blister (nonthermal), right lower leg, sequela
		S8Ø.822S	Blister (nonthermal), left lower leg, sequela
		S8Ø.829S	Blister (nonthermal), unspecified lower leg, sequela
		S8Ø.841S	External constriction, right lower leg, sequela
		S8Ø.842S	External constriction, left lower leg, sequela
		S8Ø.849S	External constriction, unspecified lower leg, sequela
		S8Ø.851S	Superficial foreign body, right lower leg, sequela
		S8Ø.852S	Superficial foreign body, left lower leg, sequela
		S8Ø.859S	Superficial foreign body, unspecified lower leg, sequela
		S8Ø.861S	Insect bite (nonvenomous), right lower leg, sequela
		S8Ø.862S	Insect bite (nonvenomous), left lower leg, sequela
		S8Ø.869S	Insect bite (nonvenomous), unspecified lower leg, sequela
		S8Ø.871S	Other superficial bite, right lower leg, sequela
		S8Ø.872S	Other superficial bite, left lower leg, sequela
		S8Ø.879S	Other superficial bite, unspecified lower leg, sequela
		S8Ø.911S	Unspecified superficial injury of right knee, sequela
		S8Ø.912S	Unspecified superficial injury of left knee, sequela
		S8Ø.919S	Unspecified superficial injury of unspecified knee, sequela
		S8Ø.921S	Unspecified superficial injury of right lower leg, sequela
		S8Ø.922S	Unspecified superficial injury of left lower leg, sequela
		S8Ø.929S	Unsp superficial injury of unspecified lower leg, sequela
		S9Ø.411S	Abrasion, right great toe, sequela
		S9Ø.412S	Abrasion, left great toe, sequela
		S9Ø.413S	Abrasion, unspecified great toe, sequela
		S9Ø.414S	Abrasion, right lesser toe(s), sequela
		S9Ø.415S	Abrasion, left lesser toe(s), sequela
		S9Ø.416S	Abrasion, unspecified lesser toe(s), sequela
		S9Ø.421S	Blister (nonthermal), right great toe, sequela
		S9Ø.422S	Blister (nonthermal), left great toe, sequela
		S9Ø.423S	Blister (nonthermal), unspecified great toe, sequela
		S9Ø.424S	Blister (nonthermal), right lesser toe(s), sequela
		S9Ø.425S	Blister (nonthermal), left lesser toe(s), sequela
		S9Ø.426S	Blister (nonthermal), unspecified lesser toe(s), sequela
		S9Ø.441S	External constriction, right great toe, sequela
		S9Ø.442S	External constriction, left great toe, sequela
		S9Ø.443S	External constriction, unspecified great toe, sequela
		S9Ø.444S	External constriction, right lesser toe(s), sequela
		S9Ø.445S	External constriction, left lesser toe(s), sequela
		S9Ø.446S	External constriction, unspecified lesser toe(s), sequela
		S9Ø.451S	Superficial foreign body, right great toe, sequela
		S9Ø.452S	Superficial foreign body, left great toe, sequela
		S9Ø.453S	Superficial foreign body, unspecified great toe, sequela
		S9Ø.454S	Superficial foreign body, right lesser toe(s), sequela
		S9Ø.455S	Superficial foreign body, left lesser toe(s), sequela
	(Continued on next page)	**S9Ø.456S**	Superficial foreign body, unspecified lesser toe(s), sequela

ICD-9-CM		ICD-10-CM	
906.2	LATE EFFECT OF SUPERFICIAL INJURY **(Continued)**	**S90.461S**	Insect bite (nonvenomous), right great toe, sequela
		S90.462S	Insect bite (nonvenomous), left great toe, sequela
		S90.463S	Insect bite (nonvenomous), unspecified great toe, sequela
		S90.464S	Insect bite (nonvenomous), right lesser toe(s), sequela
		S90.465S	Insect bite (nonvenomous), left lesser toe(s), sequela
		S90.466S	Insect bite (nonvenomous), unsp lesser toe(s), sequela
		S90.471S	Other superficial bite of right great toe, sequela
		S90.472S	Other superficial bite of left great toe, sequela
		S90.473S	Other superficial bite of unspecified great toe, sequela
		S90.474S	Other superficial bite of right lesser toe(s), sequela
		S90.475S	Other superficial bite of left lesser toe(s), sequela
		S90.476S	Other superficial bite of unspecified lesser toe(s), sequela
		S90.511S	Abrasion, right ankle, sequela
		S90.512S	Abrasion, left ankle, sequela
		S90.519S	Abrasion, unspecified ankle, sequela
		S90.521S	Blister (nonthermal), right ankle, sequela
		S90.522S	Blister (nonthermal), left ankle, sequela
		S90.529S	Blister (nonthermal), unspecified ankle, sequela
		S90.541S	External constriction, right ankle, sequela
		S90.542S	External constriction, left ankle, sequela
		S90.549S	External constriction, unspecified ankle, sequela
		S90.551S	Superficial foreign body, right ankle, sequela
		S90.552S	Superficial foreign body, left ankle, sequela
		S90.559S	Superficial foreign body, unspecified ankle, sequela
		S90.561S	Insect bite (nonvenomous), right ankle, sequela
		S90.562S	Insect bite (nonvenomous), left ankle, sequela
		S90.569S	Insect bite (nonvenomous), unspecified ankle, sequela
		S90.571S	Other superficial bite of ankle, right ankle, sequela
		S90.572S	Other superficial bite of ankle, left ankle, sequela
		S90.579S	Other superficial bite of ankle, unspecified ankle, sequela
		S90.811S	Abrasion, right foot, sequela
		S90.812S	Abrasion, left foot, sequela
		S90.819S	Abrasion, unspecified foot, sequela
		S90.821S	Blister (nonthermal), right foot, sequela
		S90.822S	Blister (nonthermal), left foot, sequela
		S90.829S	Blister (nonthermal), unspecified foot, sequela
		S90.841S	External constriction, right foot, sequela
		S90.842S	External constriction, left foot, sequela
		S90.849S	External constriction, unspecified foot, sequela
		S90.851S	Superficial foreign body, right foot, sequela
		S90.852S	Superficial foreign body, left foot, sequela
		S90.859S	Superficial foreign body, unspecified foot, sequela
		S90.861S	Insect bite (nonvenomous), right foot, sequela
		S90.862S	Insect bite (nonvenomous), left foot, sequela
		S90.869S	Insect bite (nonvenomous), unspecified foot, sequela
		S90.871S	Other superficial bite of right foot, sequela
		S90.872S	Other superficial bite of left foot, sequela
		S90.879S	Other superficial bite of unspecified foot, sequela
		S90.911S	Unspecified superficial injury of right ankle, sequela
		S90.912S	Unspecified superficial injury of left ankle, sequela
		S90.919S	Unspecified superficial injury of unspecified ankle, sequela
		S90.921S	Unspecified superficial injury of right foot, sequela
		S90.922S	Unspecified superficial injury of left foot, sequela
		S90.929S	Unspecified superficial injury of unspecified foot, sequela
		S90.931S	Unspecified superficial injury of right great toe, sequela
		S90.932S	Unspecified superficial injury of left great toe, sequela
		S90.933S	Unsp superficial injury of unspecified great toe, sequela
		S90.934S	Unsp superficial injury of right lesser toe(s), sequela
		S90.935S	Unsp superficial injury of left lesser toe(s), sequela
		S90.936S	Unsp superficial injury of unsp lesser toe(s), sequela
906.3	LATE EFFECT OF CONTUSION	**S00.03XS**	Contusion of scalp, sequela
		S00.10XS	Contusion of unspecified eyelid and periocular area, sequela
		S00.11XS	Contusion of right eyelid and periocular area, sequela
		S00.12XS	Contusion of left eyelid and periocular area, sequela
		S00.33XS	Contusion of nose, sequela
		S00.431S	Contusion of right ear, sequela
		S00.432S	Contusion of left ear, sequela
		S00.439S	Contusion of unspecified ear, sequela
		S00.531S	Contusion of lip, sequela
		S00.532S	Contusion of oral cavity, sequela
		S00.83XS	Contusion of other part of head, sequela
		S00.93XS	Contusion of unspecified part of head, sequela
		S05.10XS	Contusion of eyeball and orbital tissues, unsp eye, sequela
		S05.11XS	Contusion of eyeball and orbital tissues, right eye, sequela
		S05.12XS	Contusion of eyeball and orbital tissues, left eye, sequela
		S10.0XXS	Contusion of throat, sequela
		S10.83XS	Contusion of other specified part of neck, sequela
		S10.93XS	Contusion of unspecified part of neck, sequela
		S20.00XS	Contusion of breast, unspecified breast, sequela
		S20.01XS	Contusion of right breast, sequela
		S20.02XS	Contusion of left breast, sequela
	(Continued on next page)	**S20.20XS**	Contusion of thorax, unspecified, sequela

ICD-9-CM		ICD-10-CM	
906.3	LATE EFFECT OF CONTUSION **(Continued)**	**S20.211S**	Contusion of right front wall of thorax, sequela
		S20.212S	Contusion of left front wall of thorax, sequela
		S20.219S	Contusion of unspecified front wall of thorax, sequela
		S20.221S	Contusion of right back wall of thorax, sequela
		S20.222S	Contusion of left back wall of thorax, sequela
		S20.229S	Contusion of unspecified back wall of thorax, sequela
		S30.0XXS	Contusion of lower back and pelvis, sequela
		S30.1XXS	Contusion of abdominal wall, sequela
		S30.201S	Contusion of unsp external genital organ, male, sequela
		S30.202S	Contusion of unsp external genital organ, female, sequela
		S30.21XS	Contusion of penis, sequela
		S30.22XS	Contusion of scrotum and testes, sequela
		S30.23XS	Contusion of vagina and vulva, sequela
		S30.3XXS	Contusion of anus, sequela
		S40.011S	Contusion of right shoulder, sequela
		S40.012S	Contusion of left shoulder, sequela
		S40.019S	Contusion of unspecified shoulder, sequela
		S40.021S	Contusion of right upper arm, sequela
		S40.022S	Contusion of left upper arm, sequela
		S40.029S	Contusion of unspecified upper arm, sequela
		S50.00XS	Contusion of unspecified elbow, sequela
		S50.01XS	Contusion of right elbow, sequela
		S50.02XS	Contusion of left elbow, sequela
		S50.10XS	Contusion of unspecified forearm, sequela
		S50.11XS	Contusion of right forearm, sequela
		S50.12XS	Contusion of left forearm, sequela
		S60.00XS	Contusion of unsp finger without damage to nail, sequela
		S60.011S	Contusion of right thumb without damage to nail, sequela
		S60.012S	Contusion of left thumb without damage to nail, sequela
		S60.019S	Contusion of unsp thumb without damage to nail, sequela
		S60.021S	Contusion of right index finger w/o damage to nail, sequela
		S60.022S	Contusion of left index finger w/o damage to nail, sequela
		S60.029S	Contusion of unsp index finger w/o damage to nail, sequela
		S60.031S	Contusion of right middle finger w/o damage to nail, sequela
		S60.032S	Contusion of left middle finger w/o damage to nail, sequela
		S60.039S	Contusion of unsp middle finger w/o damage to nail, sequela
		S60.041S	Contusion of right ring finger w/o damage to nail, sequela
		S60.042S	Contusion of left ring finger w/o damage to nail, sequela
		S60.049S	Contusion of unsp ring finger w/o damage to nail, sequela
		S60.051S	Contusion of right little finger w/o damage to nail, sequela
		S60.052S	Contusion of left little finger w/o damage to nail, sequela
		S60.059S	Contusion of unsp little finger w/o damage to nail, sequela
		S60.10XS	Contusion of unspecified finger with damage to nail, sequela
		S60.111S	Contusion of right thumb with damage to nail, sequela
		S60.112S	Contusion of left thumb with damage to nail, sequela
		S60.119S	Contusion of unspecified thumb with damage to nail, sequela
		S60.121S	Contusion of right index finger with damage to nail, sequela
		S60.122S	Contusion of left index finger with damage to nail, sequela
		S60.129S	Contusion of unsp index finger with damage to nail, sequela
		S60.131S	Contusion of right middle finger w damage to nail, sequela
		S60.132S	Contusion of left middle finger with damage to nail, sequela
		S60.139S	Contusion of unsp middle finger with damage to nail, sequela
		S60.141S	Contusion of right ring finger with damage to nail, sequela
		S60.142S	Contusion of left ring finger with damage to nail, sequela
		S60.149S	Contusion of unsp ring finger with damage to nail, sequela
		S60.151S	Contusion of right little finger w damage to nail, sequela
		S60.152S	Contusion of left little finger with damage to nail, sequela
		S60.159S	Contusion of unsp little finger with damage to nail, sequela
		S60.211S	Contusion of right wrist, sequela
		S60.212S	Contusion of left wrist, sequela
		S60.219S	Contusion of unspecified wrist, sequela
		S60.221S	Contusion of right hand, sequela
		S60.222S	Contusion of left hand, sequela
		S60.229S	Contusion of unspecified hand, sequela
		S70.00XS	Contusion of unspecified hip, sequela
		S70.01XS	Contusion of right hip, sequela
		S70.02XS	Contusion of left hip, sequela
		S70.10XS	Contusion of unspecified thigh, sequela
		S70.11XS	Contusion of right thigh, sequela
		S70.12XS	Contusion of left thigh, sequela
		S80.00XS	Contusion of unspecified knee, sequela
		S80.01XS	Contusion of right knee, sequela
		S80.02XS	Contusion of left knee, sequela
		S80.10XS	Contusion of unspecified lower leg, sequela
		S80.11XS	Contusion of right lower leg, sequela
		S80.12XS	Contusion of left lower leg, sequela
		S90.00XS	Contusion of unspecified ankle, sequela
		S90.01XS	Contusion of right ankle, sequela
		S90.02XS	Contusion of left ankle, sequela
		S90.111S	Contusion of right great toe without damage to nail, sequela
		S90.112S	Contusion of left great toe without damage to nail, sequela
		S90.119S	Contusion of unsp great toe without damage to nail, sequela
	(Continued on next page)	**S90.121S**	Contusion of right lesser toe(s) w/o damage to nail, sequela

 [Brackets] indicate valid character values for each code. Character value meanings provided for each code grouping.

ICD-9-CM		ICD-10-CM	
906.3	LATE EFFECT OF CONTUSION **(Continued)**	**S90.122S**	Contusion of left lesser toe(s) w/o damage to nail, sequela
		S90.129S	Contusion of unsp lesser toe(s) w/o damage to nail, sequela
		S90.211S	Contusion of right great toe with damage to nail, sequela
		S90.212S	Contusion of left great toe with damage to nail, sequela
		S90.219S	Contusion of unsp great toe with damage to nail, sequela
		S90.221S	Contusion of right lesser toe(s) w damage to nail, sequela
		S90.222S	Contusion of left lesser toe(s) with damage to nail, sequela
		S90.229S	Contusion of unsp lesser toe(s) with damage to nail, sequela
		S90.30XS	Contusion of unspecified foot, sequela
		S90.31XS	Contusion of right foot, sequela
		S90.32XS	Contusion of left foot, sequela
906.4	LATE EFFECT OF CRUSHING	**S07.0XXS**	Crushing injury of face, sequela
		S07.1XXS	Crushing injury of skull, sequela
		S07.8XXS	Crushing injury of other parts of head, sequela
		S07.9XXS	Crushing injury of head, part unspecified, sequela
		S17.0XXS	Crushing injury of larynx and trachea, sequela
		S17.8XXS	Crushing injury of other specified parts of neck, sequela
		S17.9XXS	Crushing injury of neck, part unspecified, sequela
		S28.0XXS	Crushed chest, sequela
		S38.001S	Crushing inj unsp external genital organs, male, sequela
		S38.002S	Crushing inj unsp external genital organs, female, sequela
		S38.01XS	Crushing injury of penis, sequela
		S38.02XS	Crushing injury of scrotum and testis, sequela
		S38.03XS	Crushing injury of vulva, sequela
		S38.1XXS	Crushing injury of abdomen, lower back, and pelvis, sequela
		S47.1XXS	Crushing injury of right shoulder and upper arm, sequela
		S47.2XXS	Crushing injury of left shoulder and upper arm, sequela
		S47.9XXS	Crushing injury of shoulder and upper arm, unsp arm, sequela
		S57.00XS	Crushing injury of unspecified elbow, sequela
		S57.01XS	Crushing injury of right elbow, sequela
		S57.02XS	Crushing injury of left elbow, sequela
		S57.80XS	Crushing injury of unspecified forearm, sequela
		S57.81XS	Crushing injury of right forearm, sequela
		S57.82XS	Crushing injury of left forearm, sequela
		S67.00XS	Crushing injury of unspecified thumb, sequela
		S67.01XS	Crushing injury of right thumb, sequela
		S67.02XS	Crushing injury of left thumb, sequela
		S67.10XS	Crushing injury of unspecified finger(s), sequela
		S67.190S	Crushing injury of right index finger, sequela
		S67.191S	Crushing injury of left index finger, sequela
		S67.192S	Crushing injury of right middle finger, sequela
		S67.193S	Crushing injury of left middle finger, sequela
		S67.194S	Crushing injury of right ring finger, sequela
		S67.195S	Crushing injury of left ring finger, sequela
		S67.196S	Crushing injury of right little finger, sequela
		S67.197S	Crushing injury of left little finger, sequela
		S67.198S	Crushing injury of other finger, sequela
		S67.20XS	Crushing injury of unspecified hand, sequela
		S67.21XS	Crushing injury of right hand, sequela
		S67.22XS	Crushing injury of left hand, sequela
		S67.30XS	Crushing injury of unspecified wrist, sequela
		S67.31XS	Crushing injury of right wrist, sequela
		S67.32XS	Crushing injury of left wrist, sequela
		S67.40XS	Crushing injury of unspecified wrist and hand, sequela
		S67.41XS	Crushing injury of right wrist and hand, sequela
		S67.42XS	Crushing injury of left wrist and hand, sequela
		S67.90XS	Crush inj unsp part(s) of unsp wrist, hand and fngr, sequela
		S67.91XS	Crush inj unsp part(s) of r wrist, hand and fingers, sequela
		S67.92XS	Crush inj unsp part(s) of l wrist, hand and fingers, sequela
		S77.00XS	Crushing injury of unspecified hip, sequela
		S77.01XS	Crushing injury of right hip, sequela
		S77.02XS	Crushing injury of left hip, sequela
		S77.10XS	Crushing injury of unspecified thigh, sequela
		S77.11XS	Crushing injury of right thigh, sequela
		S77.12XS	Crushing injury of left thigh, sequela
		S77.20XS	Crushing injury of unspecified hip with thigh, sequela
		S77.21XS	Crushing injury of right hip with thigh, sequela
		S77.22XS	Crushing injury of left hip with thigh, sequela
		S87.00XS	Crushing injury of unspecified knee, sequela
		S87.01XS	Crushing injury of right knee, sequela
		S87.02XS	Crushing injury of left knee, sequela
		S87.80XS	Crushing injury of unspecified lower leg, sequela
		S87.81XS	Crushing injury of right lower leg, sequela
		S87.82XS	Crushing injury of left lower leg, sequela
		S97.00XS	Crushing injury of unspecified ankle, sequela
		S97.01XS	Crushing injury of right ankle, sequela
		S97.02XS	Crushing injury of left ankle, sequela
		S97.101S	Crushing injury of unspecified right toe(s), sequela
		S97.102S	Crushing injury of unspecified left toe(s), sequela
		S97.109S	Crushing injury of unspecified toe(s), sequela
		S97.111S	Crushing injury of right great toe, sequela
	(Continued on next page)	**S97.112S**	Crushing injury of left great toe, sequela

ICD-9-CM		ICD-10-CM	
906.4	LATE EFFECT OF CRUSHING **(Continued)**	**S97.119S**	Crushing injury of unspecified great toe, sequela
		S97.121S	Crushing injury of right lesser toe(s), sequela
		S97.122S	Crushing injury of left lesser toe(s), sequela
		S97.129S	Crushing injury of unspecified lesser toe(s), sequela
		S97.80XS	Crushing injury of unspecified foot, sequela
		S97.81XS	Crushing injury of right foot, sequela
		S97.82XS	Crushing injury of left foot, sequela
906.5	LATE EFFECT OF BURN OF EYE FACE HEAD AND NECK	**T20.00XS**	Burn unsp degree of head, face, and neck, unsp site, sequela
		T20.011S	Burn of unspecified degree of right ear, sequela
		T20.012S	Burn of unspecified degree of left ear, sequela
		T20.019S	Burn of unspecified degree of unspecified ear, sequela
		T20.02XS	Burn of unspecified degree of lip(s), sequela
		T20.03XS	Burn of unspecified degree of chin, sequela
		T20.04XS	Burn of unspecified degree of nose (septum), sequela
		T20.05XS	Burn of unspecified degree of scalp [any part], sequela
		T20.06XS	Burn of unspecified degree of forehead and cheek, sequela
		T20.07XS	Burn of unspecified degree of neck, sequela
		T20.09XS	Burn of unsp deg mult sites of head, face, and neck, sequela
		T20.10XS	Burn first degree of head, face, and neck, unsp site, sqla
		T20.111S	Burn of first degree of right ear, sequela
		T20.112S	Burn of first degree of left ear, sequela
		T20.119S	Burn of first degree of unspecified ear, sequela
		T20.12XS	Burn of first degree of lip(s), sequela
		T20.13XS	Burn of first degree of chin, sequela
		T20.14XS	Burn of first degree of nose (septum), sequela
		T20.15XS	Burn of first degree of scalp [any part], sequela
		T20.16XS	Burn of first degree of forehead and cheek, sequela
		T20.17XS	Burn of first degree of neck, sequela
		T20.19XS	Burn first deg mult sites of head, face, and neck, sequela
		T20.20XS	Burn second degree of head, face, and neck, unsp site, sqla
		T20.211S	Burn of second degree of right ear, sequela
		T20.212S	Burn of second degree of left ear, sequela
		T20.219S	Burn of second degree of unspecified ear, sequela
		T20.22XS	Burn of second degree of lip(s), sequela
		T20.23XS	Burn of second degree of chin, sequela
		T20.24XS	Burn of second degree of nose (septum), sequela
		T20.25XS	Burn of second degree of scalp [any part], sequela
		T20.26XS	Burn of second degree of forehead and cheek, sequela
		T20.27XS	Burn of second degree of neck, sequela
		T20.29XS	Burn of 2nd deg mul sites of head, face, and neck, sequela
		T20.30XS	Burn third degree of head, face, and neck, unsp site, sqla
		T20.311S	Burn of third degree of right ear, sequela
		T20.312S	Burn of third degree of left ear, sequela
		T20.319S	Burn of third degree of unspecified ear, sequela
		T20.32XS	Burn of third degree of lip(s), sequela
		T20.33XS	Burn of third degree of chin, sequela
		T20.34XS	Burn of third degree of nose (septum), sequela
		T20.35XS	Burn of third degree of scalp [any part], sequela
		T20.36XS	Burn of third degree of forehead and cheek, sequela
		T20.37XS	Burn of third degree of neck, sequela
		T20.39XS	Burn of 3rd deg mu sites of head, face, and neck, sequela
		T20.40XS	Corros unsp degree of head, face, and neck, unsp site, sqla
		T20.411S	Corrosion of unspecified degree of right ear, sequela
		T20.412S	Corrosion of unspecified degree of left ear, sequela
		T20.419S	Corrosion of unspecified degree of unspecified ear, sequela
		T20.42XS	Corrosion of unspecified degree of lip(s), sequela
		T20.43XS	Corrosion of unspecified degree of chin, sequela
		T20.44XS	Corrosion of unspecified degree of nose (septum), sequela
		T20.45XS	Corrosion of unspecified degree of scalp [any part], sequela
		T20.46XS	Corrosion of unsp degree of forehead and cheek, sequela
		T20.47XS	Corrosion of unspecified degree of neck, sequela
		T20.49XS	Corros unsp deg mult sites of head, face, and neck, sequela
		T20.50XS	Corros first degree of head, face, and neck, unsp site, sqla
		T20.511S	Corrosion of first degree of right ear, sequela
		T20.512S	Corrosion of first degree of left ear, sequela
		T20.519S	Corrosion of first degree of unspecified ear, sequela
		T20.52XS	Corrosion of first degree of lip(s), sequela
		T20.53XS	Corrosion of first degree of chin, sequela
		T20.54XS	Corrosion of first degree of nose (septum), sequela
		T20.55XS	Corrosion of first degree of scalp [any part], sequela
		T20.56XS	Corrosion of first degree of forehead and cheek, sequela
		T20.57XS	Corrosion of first degree of neck, sequela
		T20.59XS	Corros first deg mult sites of head, face, and neck, sequela
		T20.60XS	Corros second deg of head, face, and neck, unsp site, sqla
		T20.611S	Corrosion of second degree of right ear, sequela
		T20.612S	Corrosion of second degree of left ear, sequela
		T20.619S	Corrosion of second degree of unspecified ear, sequela
		T20.62XS	Corrosion of second degree of lip(s), sequela
		T20.63XS	Corrosion of second degree of chin, sequela
		T20.64XS	Corrosion of second degree of nose (septum), sequela
		T20.65XS	Corrosion of second degree of scalp [any part], sequela
		T20.66XS	Corrosion of second degree of forehead and cheek, sequela

(Continued on next page)

ICD-9-CM		ICD-10-CM	
906.5	LATE EFFECT OF BURN OF EYE FACE HEAD AND NECK **(Continued)**	**T20.67XS**	Corrosion of second degree of neck, sequela
		T20.69XS	Corros 2nd deg mul sites of head, face, and neck, sequela
		T20.70XS	Corros third degree of head, face, and neck, unsp site, sqla
		T20.711S	Corrosion of third degree of right ear, sequela
		T20.712S	Corrosion of third degree of left ear, sequela
		T20.719S	Corrosion of third degree of unspecified ear, sequela
		T20.72XS	Corrosion of third degree of lip(s), sequela
		T20.73XS	Corrosion of third degree of chin, sequela
		T20.74XS	Corrosion of third degree of nose (septum), sequela
		T20.75XS	Corrosion of third degree of scalp [any part], sequela
		T20.76XS	Corrosion of third degree of forehead and cheek, sequela
		T20.77XS	Corrosion of third degree of neck, sequela
		T20.79XS	Corros 3rd deg mu sites of head, face, and neck, sequela
906.6	LATE EFFECT OF BURN OF WRIST AND HAND	**T23.001S**	Burn of unsp degree of right hand, unspecified site, sequela
		T23.002S	Burn of unsp degree of left hand, unspecified site, sequela
		T23.009S	Burn of unsp degree of unsp hand, unspecified site, sequela
		T23.011S	Burn of unspecified degree of right thumb (nail), sequela
		T23.012S	Burn of unspecified degree of left thumb (nail), sequela
		T23.019S	Burn of unsp degree of unspecified thumb (nail), sequela
		T23.021S	Burn unsp degree of single r finger except thumb, sqla
		T23.022S	Burn unsp degree of single l finger except thumb, sqla
		T23.029S	Burn unsp degree of unsp single finger except thumb, sqla
		T23.031S	Burn unsp deg mult right fngr (nail), not inc thumb, sequela
		T23.032S	Burn unsp deg mult left fngr (nail), not inc thumb, sequela
		T23.039S	Burn unsp degree of unsp mult fngr, not inc thumb, sqla
		T23.041S	Burn unsp deg mult right fingers (nail), inc thumb, sequela
		T23.042S	Burn unsp deg mult left fingers (nail), inc thumb, sequela
		T23.049S	Burn unsp degree of unsp mult fngr (nail), inc thumb, sqla
		T23.051S	Burn of unspecified degree of right palm, sequela
		T23.052S	Burn of unspecified degree of left palm, sequela
		T23.059S	Burn of unspecified degree of unspecified palm, sequela
		T23.061S	Burn of unspecified degree of back of right hand, sequela
		T23.062S	Burn of unspecified degree of back of left hand, sequela
		T23.069S	Burn of unsp degree of back of unspecified hand, sequela
		T23.071S	Burn of unspecified degree of right wrist, sequela
		T23.072S	Burn of unspecified degree of left wrist, sequela
		T23.079S	Burn of unspecified degree of unspecified wrist, sequela
		T23.091S	Burn of unsp deg mult sites of right wrist and hand, sequela
		T23.092S	Burn of unsp deg mult sites of left wrist and hand, sequela
		T23.099S	Burn of unsp deg mult sites of unsp wrist and hand, sequela
		T23.101S	Burn of first degree of right hand, unsp site, sequela
		T23.102S	Burn of first degree of left hand, unspecified site, sequela
		T23.109S	Burn of first degree of unsp hand, unspecified site, sequela
		T23.111S	Burn of first degree of right thumb (nail), sequela
		T23.112S	Burn of first degree of left thumb (nail), sequela
		T23.119S	Burn of first degree of unspecified thumb (nail), sequela
		T23.121S	Burn first degree of single r finger except thumb, sqla
		T23.122S	Burn first degree of single l finger except thumb, sqla
		T23.129S	Burn first degree of unsp single finger except thumb, sqla
		T23.131S	Burn first deg mult right fngr (nail), not inc thumb, sqla
		T23.132S	Burn first deg mult left fngr (nail), not inc thumb, sequela
		T23.139S	Burn first degree of unsp mult fngr, not inc thumb, sqla
		T23.141S	Burn first deg mult right fingers (nail), inc thumb, sequela
		T23.142S	Burn first deg mult left fingers (nail), inc thumb, sequela
		T23.149S	Burn first degree of unsp mult fngr (nail), inc thumb, sqla
		T23.151S	Burn of first degree of right palm, sequela
		T23.152S	Burn of first degree of left palm, sequela
		T23.159S	Burn of first degree of unspecified palm, sequela
		T23.161S	Burn of first degree of back of right hand, sequela
		T23.162S	Burn of first degree of back of left hand, sequela
		T23.169S	Burn of first degree of back of unspecified hand, sequela
		T23.171S	Burn of first degree of right wrist, sequela
		T23.172S	Burn of first degree of left wrist, sequela
		T23.179S	Burn of first degree of unspecified wrist, sequela
		T23.191S	Burn of first deg mult sites of right wrs/hnd, sequela
		T23.192S	Burn of first deg mult sites of left wrist and hand, sequela
		T23.199S	Burn of first deg mult sites of unsp wrist and hand, sequela
		T23.201S	Burn of second degree of right hand, unsp site, sequela
		T23.202S	Burn of second degree of left hand, unsp site, sequela
		T23.209S	Burn of second degree of unsp hand, unsp site, sequela
		T23.211S	Burn of second degree of right thumb (nail), sequela
		T23.212S	Burn of second degree of left thumb (nail), sequela
		T23.219S	Burn of second degree of unspecified thumb (nail), sequela
		T23.221S	Burn second degree of single r finger except thumb, sqla
		T23.222S	Burn second degree of single l finger except thumb, sqla
		T23.229S	Burn second degree of unsp single finger except thumb, sqla
		T23.231S	Burn 2nd deg mul right fngr (nail), not inc thumb, sequela
		T23.232S	Burn 2nd deg mul left fingers (nail), not inc thumb, sequela
		T23.239S	Burn second degree of unsp mult fngr, not inc thumb, sqla
		T23.241S	Burn of 2nd deg mul right fingers (nail), inc thumb, sequela
		T23.242S	Burn of 2nd deg mul left fingers (nail), inc thumb, sequela
	(Continued on next page)	**T23.249S**	Burn second degree of unsp mult fngr (nail), inc thumb, sqla

ICD-9-CM		ICD-10-CM	
906.6	LATE EFFECT OF BURN OF WRIST AND HAND **(Continued)**	**T23.251S**	Burn of second degree of right palm, sequela
		T23.252S	Burn of second degree of left palm, sequela
		T23.259S	Burn of second degree of unspecified palm, sequela
		T23.261S	Burn of second degree of back of right hand, sequela
		T23.262S	Burn of second degree of back of left hand, sequela
		T23.269S	Burn of second degree of back of unspecified hand, sequela
		T23.271S	Burn of second degree of right wrist, sequela
		T23.272S	Burn of second degree of left wrist, sequela
		T23.279S	Burn of second degree of unspecified wrist, sequela
		T23.291S	Burn of 2nd deg mul sites of right wrist and hand, sequela
		T23.292S	Burn of 2nd deg mul sites of left wrist and hand, sequela
		T23.299S	Burn of 2nd deg mul sites of unsp wrist and hand, sequela
		T23.301S	Burn of third degree of right hand, unsp site, sequela
		T23.302S	Burn of third degree of left hand, unspecified site, sequela
		T23.309S	Burn of third degree of unsp hand, unspecified site, sequela
		T23.311S	Burn of third degree of right thumb (nail), sequela
		T23.312S	Burn of third degree of left thumb (nail), sequela
		T23.319S	Burn of third degree of unspecified thumb (nail), sequela
		T23.321S	Burn third degree of single r finger except thumb, sqla
		T23.322S	Burn third degree of single l finger except thumb, sqla
		T23.329S	Burn third degree of unsp single finger except thumb, sqla
		T23.331S	Burn 3rd deg mu right fingers (nail), not inc thumb, sequela
		T23.332S	Burn 3rd deg mu left fingers (nail), not inc thumb, sequela
		T23.339S	Burn third degree of unsp mult fngr, not inc thumb, sqla
		T23.341S	Burn of 3rd deg mu right fingers (nail), inc thumb, sequela
		T23.342S	Burn of 3rd deg mu left fingers (nail), inc thumb, sequela
		T23.349S	Burn third degree of unsp mult fngr (nail), inc thumb, sqla
		T23.351S	Burn of third degree of right palm, sequela
		T23.352S	Burn of third degree of left palm, sequela
		T23.359S	Burn of third degree of unspecified palm, sequela
		T23.361S	Burn of third degree of back of right hand, sequela
		T23.362S	Burn of third degree of back of left hand, sequela
		T23.369S	Burn of third degree of back of unspecified hand, sequela
		T23.371S	Burn of third degree of right wrist, sequela
		T23.372S	Burn of third degree of left wrist, sequela
		T23.379S	Burn of third degree of unspecified wrist, sequela
		T23.391S	Burn of 3rd deg mu sites of right wrist and hand, sequela
		T23.392S	Burn of 3rd deg mu sites of left wrist and hand, sequela
		T23.399S	Burn of 3rd deg mu sites of unsp wrist and hand, sequela
		T23.401S	Corrosion of unsp degree of right hand, unsp site, sequela
		T23.402S	Corrosion of unsp degree of left hand, unsp site, sequela
		T23.409S	Corrosion of unsp degree of unsp hand, unsp site, sequela
		T23.411S	Corrosion of unsp degree of right thumb (nail), sequela
		T23.412S	Corrosion of unsp degree of left thumb (nail), sequela
		T23.419S	Corrosion of unsp degree of unsp thumb (nail), sequela
		T23.421S	Corros unsp degree of single r finger except thumb, sqla
		T23.422S	Corros unsp degree of single l finger except thumb, sqla
		T23.429S	Corros unsp degree of unsp single finger except thumb, sqla
		T23.431S	Corros unsp deg mult right fngr (nail), not inc thumb, sqla
		T23.432S	Corros unsp deg mult left fngr (nail), not inc thumb, sqla
		T23.439S	Corros unsp degree of unsp mult fngr, not inc thumb, sqla
		T23.441S	Corros unsp deg mult right fngr (nail), inc thumb, sequela
		T23.442S	Corros unsp deg mult left fingers (nail), inc thumb, sequela
		T23.449S	Corros unsp degree of unsp mult fngr (nail), inc thumb, sqla
		T23.451S	Corrosion of unspecified degree of right palm, sequela
		T23.452S	Corrosion of unspecified degree of left palm, sequela
		T23.459S	Corrosion of unspecified degree of unspecified palm, sequela
		T23.461S	Corrosion of unsp degree of back of right hand, sequela
		T23.462S	Corrosion of unsp degree of back of left hand, sequela
		T23.469S	Corrosion of unsp degree of back of unsp hand, sequela
		T23.471S	Corrosion of unspecified degree of right wrist, sequela
		T23.472S	Corrosion of unspecified degree of left wrist, sequela
		T23.479S	Corrosion of unsp degree of unspecified wrist, sequela
		T23.491S	Corrosion of unsp deg mult sites of right wrs/hnd, sequela
		T23.492S	Corrosion of unsp deg mult sites of left wrs/hnd, sequela
		T23.499S	Corrosion of unsp deg mult sites of unsp wrs/hnd, sequela
		T23.501S	Corrosion of first degree of right hand, unsp site, sequela
		T23.502S	Corrosion of first degree of left hand, unsp site, sequela
		T23.509S	Corrosion of first degree of unsp hand, unsp site, sequela
		T23.511S	Corrosion of first degree of right thumb (nail), sequela
		T23.512S	Corrosion of first degree of left thumb (nail), sequela
		T23.519S	Corrosion of first degree of unsp thumb (nail), sequela
		T23.521S	Corros first degree of single r finger except thumb, sqla
		T23.522S	Corros first degree of single l finger except thumb, sqla
		T23.529S	Corros first degree of unsp single finger except thumb, sqla
		T23.531S	Corros first deg mult right fngr (nail), not inc thumb, sqla
		T23.532S	Corros first deg mult left fngr (nail), not inc thumb, sqla
		T23.539S	Corros first degree of unsp mult fngr, not inc thumb, sqla
		T23.541S	Corros first deg mult right fngr (nail), inc thumb, sequela
		T23.542S	Corros first deg mult left fngr (nail), inc thumb, sequela
		T23.549S	Corros first degree of unsp mult fngr, inc thumb, sqla
	(Continued on next page)	**T23.551S**	Corrosion of first degree of right palm, sequela

ICD-9-CM		ICD-10-CM	
9Ø6.6	LATE EFFECT OF BURN OF WRIST AND HAND **(Continued)**	**T23.552S**	Corrosion of first degree of left palm, sequela
		T23.559S	Corrosion of first degree of unspecified palm, sequela
		T23.561S	Corrosion of first degree of back of right hand, sequela
		T23.562S	Corrosion of first degree of back of left hand, sequela
		T23.569S	Corrosion of first degree of back of unsp hand, sequela
		T23.571S	Corrosion of first degree of right wrist, sequela
		T23.572S	Corrosion of first degree of left wrist, sequela
		T23.579S	Corrosion of first degree of unspecified wrist, sequela
		T23.591S	Corrosion of first deg mult sites of right wrs/hnd, sequela
		T23.592S	Corrosion of first deg mult sites of left wrs/hnd, sequela
		T23.599S	Corrosion of first deg mult sites of unsp wrs/hnd, sequela
		T23.6Ø1S	Corrosion of second degree of right hand, unsp site, sequela
		T23.6Ø2S	Corrosion of second degree of left hand, unsp site, sequela
		T23.6Ø9S	Corrosion of second degree of unsp hand, unsp site, sequela
		T23.611S	Corrosion of second degree of right thumb (nail), sequela
		T23.612S	Corrosion of second degree of left thumb (nail), sequela
		T23.619S	Corrosion of second degree of unsp thumb (nail), sequela
		T23.621S	Corros second degree of single r finger except thumb, sqla
		T23.622S	Corros second degree of single l finger except thumb, sqla
		T23.629S	Corros second deg of unsp single finger except thumb, sqla
		T23.631S	Corros 2nd deg mul right fngr (nail), not inc thumb, sequela
		T23.632S	Corros 2nd deg mul left fngr (nail), not inc thumb, sequela
		T23.639S	Corros second degree of unsp mult fngr, not inc thumb, sqla
		T23.641S	Corros 2nd deg mul right fingers (nail), inc thumb, sequela
		T23.642S	Corros 2nd deg mul left fingers (nail), inc thumb, sequela
		T23.649S	Corros second degree of unsp mult fngr, inc thumb, sqla
		T23.651S	Corrosion of second degree of right palm, sequela
		T23.652S	Corrosion of second degree of left palm, sequela
		T23.659S	Corrosion of second degree of unspecified palm, sequela
		T23.661S	Corrosion of second degree back of right hand, sequela
		T23.662S	Corrosion of second degree back of left hand, sequela
		T23.669S	Corrosion of second degree back of unspecified hand, sequela
		T23.671S	Corrosion of second degree of right wrist, sequela
		T23.672S	Corrosion of second degree of left wrist, sequela
		T23.679S	Corrosion of second degree of unspecified wrist, sequela
		T23.691S	Corrosion of 2nd deg mul sites of right wrs/hnd, sequela
		T23.692S	Corrosion of 2nd deg mul sites of left wrs/hnd, sequela
		T23.699S	Corrosion of 2nd deg mul sites of unsp wrs/hnd, sequela
		T23.7Ø1S	Corrosion of third degree of right hand, unsp site, sequela
		T23.7Ø2S	Corrosion of third degree of left hand, unsp site, sequela
		T23.7Ø9S	Corrosion of third degree of unsp hand, unsp site, sequela
		T23.711S	Corrosion of third degree of right thumb (nail), sequela
		T23.712S	Corrosion of third degree of left thumb (nail), sequela
		T23.719S	Corrosion of third degree of unsp thumb (nail), sequela
		T23.721S	Corros third degree of single r finger except thumb, sqla
		T23.722S	Corros third degree of single l finger except thumb, sqla
		T23.729S	Corros third degree of unsp single finger except thumb, sqla
		T23.731S	Corros 3rd deg mu right fngr (nail), not inc thumb, sequela
		T23.732S	Corros 3rd deg mu left fngr (nail), not inc thumb, sequela
		T23.739S	Corros third degree of unsp mult fngr, not inc thumb, sqla
		T23.741S	Corros 3rd deg mu right fingers (nail), inc thumb, sequela
		T23.742S	Corros 3rd deg mu left fingers (nail), inc thumb, sequela
		T23.749S	Corros third degree of unsp mult fngr, inc thumb, sqla
		T23.751S	Corrosion of third degree of right palm, sequela
		T23.752S	Corrosion of third degree of left palm, sequela
		T23.759S	Corrosion of third degree of unspecified palm, sequela
		T23.761S	Corrosion of third degree of back of right hand, sequela
		T23.762S	Corrosion of third degree of back of left hand, sequela
		T23.769S	Corrosion of third degree back of unspecified hand, sequela
		T23.771S	Corrosion of third degree of right wrist, sequela
		T23.772S	Corrosion of third degree of left wrist, sequela
		T23.779S	Corrosion of third degree of unspecified wrist, sequela
		T23.791S	Corrosion of 3rd deg mu sites of right wrs/hnd, sequela
		T23.792S	Corrosion of 3rd deg mu sites of left wrs/hnd, sequela
		T23.799S	Corrosion of 3rd deg mu sites of unsp wrs/hnd, sequela
9Ø6.7	LATE EFFECT OF BURN OF OTHER EXTREMITIES	**T22.ØØXS**	Burn unsp deg of shldr/up lmb, ex wrs/hnd, unsp site, sqla
		T22.Ø11S	Burn of unspecified degree of right forearm, sequela
		T22.Ø12S	Burn of unspecified degree of left forearm, sequela
		T22.Ø19S	Burn of unspecified degree of unspecified forearm, sequela
		T22.Ø21S	Burn of unspecified degree of right elbow, sequela
		T22.Ø22S	Burn of unspecified degree of left elbow, sequela
		T22.Ø29S	Burn of unspecified degree of unspecified elbow, sequela
		T22.Ø31S	Burn of unspecified degree of right upper arm, sequela
		T22.Ø32S	Burn of unspecified degree of left upper arm, sequela
		T22.Ø39S	Burn of unspecified degree of unspecified upper arm, sequela
		T22.Ø41S	Burn of unspecified degree of right axilla, sequela
		T22.Ø42S	Burn of unspecified degree of left axilla, sequela
		T22.Ø49S	Burn of unspecified degree of unspecified axilla, sequela
		T22.Ø51S	Burn of unspecified degree of right shoulder, sequela
		T22.Ø52S	Burn of unspecified degree of left shoulder, sequela
		T22.Ø59S	Burn of unspecified degree of unspecified shoulder, sequela
	(Continued on next page)	**T22.Ø61S**	Burn of unspecified degree of right scapular region, sequela

ICD-9-CM		ICD-10-CM	
9Ø6.7	LATE EFFECT OF BURN OF OTHER EXTREMITIES **(Continued)**	**T22.Ø62S**	Burn of unspecified degree of left scapular region, sequela
		T22.Ø69S	Burn of unsp degree of unspecified scapular region, sequela
		T22.Ø91S	Burn unsp deg mult sites of r shldr/up lmb, ex wrs/hnd, sqla
		T22.Ø92S	Burn unsp deg mult site of l shldr/up lmb, ex wrs/hnd, sqla
		T22.Ø99S	Burn unsp deg mult sites of shldr/up lmb, ex wrs/hnd, sqla
		T22.1ØXS	Burn first deg of shldr/up lmb, ex wrs/hnd, unsp site, sqla
		T22.111S	Burn of first degree of right forearm, sequela
		T22.112S	Burn of first degree of left forearm, sequela
		T22.119S	Burn of first degree of unspecified forearm, sequela
		T22.121S	Burn of first degree of right elbow, sequela
		T22.122S	Burn of first degree of left elbow, sequela
		T22.129S	Burn of first degree of unspecified elbow, sequela
		T22.131S	Burn of first degree of right upper arm, sequela
		T22.132S	Burn of first degree of left upper arm, sequela
		T22.139S	Burn of first degree of unspecified upper arm, sequela
		T22.141S	Burn of first degree of right axilla, sequela
		T22.142S	Burn of first degree of left axilla, sequela
		T22.149S	Burn of first degree of unspecified axilla, sequela
		T22.151S	Burn of first degree of right shoulder, sequela
		T22.152S	Burn of first degree of left shoulder, sequela
		T22.159S	Burn of first degree of unspecified shoulder, sequela
		T22.161S	Burn of first degree of right scapular region, sequela
		T22.162S	Burn of first degree of left scapular region, sequela
		T22.169S	Burn of first degree of unspecified scapular region, sequela
		T22.191S	Burn 1st deg mult sites of r shldr/up lmb, ex wrs/hnd, sqla
		T22.192S	Burn 1st deg mult site of l shldr/up lmb, ex wrs/hnd, sqla
		T22.199S	Burn first deg mult sites of shldr/up lmb, ex wrs/hnd, sqla
		T22.2ØXS	Burn second deg of shldr/up lmb, ex wrs/hnd, unsp site, sqla
		T22.211S	Burn of second degree of right forearm, sequela
		T22.212S	Burn of second degree of left forearm, sequela
		T22.219S	Burn of second degree of unspecified forearm, sequela
		T22.221S	Burn of second degree of right elbow, sequela
		T22.222S	Burn of second degree of left elbow, sequela
		T22.229S	Burn of second degree of unspecified elbow, sequela
		T22.231S	Burn of second degree of right upper arm, sequela
		T22.232S	Burn of second degree of left upper arm, sequela
		T22.239S	Burn of second degree of unspecified upper arm, sequela
		T22.241S	Burn of second degree of right axilla, sequela
		T22.242S	Burn of second degree of left axilla, sequela
		T22.249S	Burn of second degree of unspecified axilla, sequela
		T22.251S	Burn of second degree of right shoulder, sequela
		T22.252S	Burn of second degree of left shoulder, sequela
		T22.259S	Burn of second degree of unspecified shoulder, sequela
		T22.261S	Burn of second degree of right scapular region, sequela
		T22.262S	Burn of second degree of left scapular region, sequela
		T22.269S	Burn of second degree of unsp scapular region, sequela
		T22.291S	Burn 2nd deg mul sites of r shldr/up lmb, ex wrs/hnd, sqla
		T22.292S	Burn 2nd deg mul site of left shldr/up lmb, ex wrs/hnd, sqla
		T22.299S	Burn 2nd deg mul sites of shldr/up lmb, except wrs/hnd, sqla
		T22.3ØXS	Burn third deg of shldr/up lmb, ex wrs/hnd, unsp site, sqla
		T22.311S	Burn of third degree of right forearm, sequela
		T22.312S	Burn of third degree of left forearm, sequela
		T22.319S	Burn of third degree of unspecified forearm, sequela
		T22.321S	Burn of third degree of right elbow, sequela
		T22.322S	Burn of third degree of left elbow, sequela
		T22.329S	Burn of third degree of unspecified elbow, sequela
		T22.331S	Burn of third degree of right upper arm, sequela
		T22.332S	Burn of third degree of left upper arm, sequela
		T22.339S	Burn of third degree of unspecified upper arm, sequela
		T22.341S	Burn of third degree of right axilla, sequela
		T22.342S	Burn of third degree of left axilla, sequela
		T22.349S	Burn of third degree of unspecified axilla, sequela
		T22.351S	Burn of third degree of right shoulder, sequela
		T22.352S	Burn of third degree of left shoulder, sequela
		T22.359S	Burn of third degree of unspecified shoulder, sequela
		T22.361S	Burn of third degree of right scapular region, sequela
		T22.362S	Burn of third degree of left scapular region, sequela
		T22.369S	Burn of third degree of unspecified scapular region, sequela
		T22.391S	Burn 3rd deg mu sites of r shldr/up lmb, ex wrs/hnd, sqla
		T22.392S	Burn 3rd deg mu sites of left shldr/up lmb, ex wrs/hnd, sqla
		T22.399S	Burn 3rd deg mu sites of shldr/up lmb, except wrs/hnd, sqla
		T22.4ØXS	Corros unsp deg of shldr/up lmb, ex wrs/hnd, unsp site, sqla
		T22.411S	Corrosion of unspecified degree of right forearm, sequela
		T22.412S	Corrosion of unspecified degree of left forearm, sequela
		T22.419S	Corrosion of unsp degree of unspecified forearm, sequela
		T22.421S	Corrosion of unspecified degree of right elbow, sequela
		T22.422S	Corrosion of unspecified degree of left elbow, sequela
		T22.429S	Corrosion of unsp degree of unspecified elbow, sequela
		T22.431S	Corrosion of unspecified degree of right upper arm, sequela
		T22.432S	Corrosion of unspecified degree of left upper arm, sequela
		T22.439S	Corrosion of unsp degree of unspecified upper arm, sequela
	(Continued on next page)	**T22.441S**	Corrosion of unspecified degree of right axilla, sequela

ICD-9-CM		ICD-10-CM	
906.7	LATE EFFECT OF BURN OF OTHER EXTREMITIES **(Continued)**	**T22.442S**	Corrosion of unspecified degree of left axilla, sequela
		T22.449S	Corrosion of unsp degree of unspecified axilla, sequela
		T22.451S	Corrosion of unspecified degree of right shoulder, sequela
		T22.452S	Corrosion of unspecified degree of left shoulder, sequela
		T22.459S	Corrosion of unsp degree of unspecified shoulder, sequela
		T22.461S	Corrosion of unsp degree of right scapular region, sequela
		T22.462S	Corrosion of unsp degree of left scapular region, sequela
		T22.469S	Corrosion of unsp degree of unsp scapular region, sequela
		T22.491S	Corros unsp deg mult site of r shldr/up lmb,ex wrs/hnd, sqla
		T22.492S	Corros unsp deg mult site of l shldr/up lmb,ex wrs/hnd, sqla
		T22.499S	Corros unsp deg mult sites of shldr/up lmb, ex wrs/hnd, sqla
		T22.50XS	Corros first deg of shldr/up lmb, ex wrs/hnd unsp site, sqla
		T22.511S	Corrosion of first degree of right forearm, sequela
		T22.512S	Corrosion of first degree of left forearm, sequela
		T22.519S	Corrosion of first degree of unspecified forearm, sequela
		T22.521S	Corrosion of first degree of right elbow, sequela
		T22.522S	Corrosion of first degree of left elbow, sequela
		T22.529S	Corrosion of first degree of unspecified elbow, sequela
		T22.531S	Corrosion of first degree of right upper arm, sequela
		T22.532S	Corrosion of first degree of left upper arm, sequela
		T22.539S	Corrosion of first degree of unspecified upper arm, sequela
		T22.541S	Corrosion of first degree of right axilla, sequela
		T22.542S	Corrosion of first degree of left axilla, sequela
		T22.549S	Corrosion of first degree of unspecified axilla, sequela
		T22.551S	Corrosion of first degree of right shoulder, sequela
		T22.552S	Corrosion of first degree of left shoulder, sequela
		T22.559S	Corrosion of first degree of unspecified shoulder, sequela
		T22.561S	Corrosion of first degree of right scapular region, sequela
		T22.562S	Corrosion of first degree of left scapular region, sequela
		T22.569S	Corrosion of first degree of unsp scapular region, sequela
		T22.591S	Corros 1st deg mult site of r shldr/up lmb, ex wrs/hnd, sqla
		T22.592S	Corros 1st deg mult site of l shldr/up lmb, ex wrs/hnd, sqla
		T22.599S	Corros 1st deg mult sites of shldr/up lmb, ex wrs/hnd, sqla
		T22.60XS	Corros 2nd deg of shldr/up lmb, ex wrs/hnd, unsp site, sqla
		T22.611S	Corrosion of second degree of right forearm, sequela
		T22.612S	Corrosion of second degree of left forearm, sequela
		T22.619S	Corrosion of second degree of unspecified forearm, sequela
		T22.621S	Corrosion of second degree of right elbow, sequela
		T22.622S	Corrosion of second degree of left elbow, sequela
		T22.629S	Corrosion of second degree of unspecified elbow, sequela
		T22.631S	Corrosion of second degree of right upper arm, sequela
		T22.632S	Corrosion of second degree of left upper arm, sequela
		T22.639S	Corrosion of second degree of unspecified upper arm, sequela
		T22.641S	Corrosion of second degree of right axilla, sequela
		T22.642S	Corrosion of second degree of left axilla, sequela
		T22.649S	Corrosion of second degree of unspecified axilla, sequela
		T22.651S	Corrosion of second degree of right shoulder, sequela
		T22.652S	Corrosion of second degree of left shoulder, sequela
		T22.659S	Corrosion of second degree of unspecified shoulder, sequela
		T22.661S	Corrosion of second degree of right scapular region, sequela
		T22.662S	Corrosion of second degree of left scapular region, sequela
		T22.669S	Corrosion of second degree of unsp scapular region, sequela
		T22.691S	Corros 2nd deg mul sites of r shldr/up lmb, ex wrs/hnd, sqla
		T22.692S	Corros 2nd deg mul site of l shldr/up lmb, ex wrs/hnd, sqla
		T22.699S	Corros 2nd deg mul sites of shldr/up lmb, ex wrs/hnd, sqla
		T22.70XS	Corros 3rd deg of shldr/up lmb, ex wrs/hnd, unsp site, sqla
		T22.711S	Corrosion of third degree of right forearm, sequela
		T22.712S	Corrosion of third degree of left forearm, sequela
		T22.719S	Corrosion of third degree of unspecified forearm, sequela
		T22.721S	Corrosion of third degree of right elbow, sequela
		T22.722S	Corrosion of third degree of left elbow, sequela
		T22.729S	Corrosion of third degree of unspecified elbow, sequela
		T22.731S	Corrosion of third degree of right upper arm, sequela
		T22.732S	Corrosion of third degree of left upper arm, sequela
		T22.739S	Corrosion of third degree of unspecified upper arm, sequela
		T22.741S	Corrosion of third degree of right axilla, sequela
		T22.742S	Corrosion of third degree of left axilla, sequela
		T22.749S	Corrosion of third degree of unspecified axilla, sequela
		T22.751S	Corrosion of third degree of right shoulder, sequela
		T22.752S	Corrosion of third degree of left shoulder, sequela
		T22.759S	Corrosion of third degree of unspecified shoulder, sequela
		T22.761S	Corrosion of third degree of right scapular region, sequela
		T22.762S	Corrosion of third degree of left scapular region, sequela
		T22.769S	Corrosion of third degree of unsp scapular region, sequela
		T22.791S	Corros 3rd deg mu sites of r shldr/up lmb, ex wrs/hnd, sqla
		T22.792S	Corros 3rd deg mu site of l shldr/up lmb, ex wrs/hnd, sqla
		T22.799S	Corros 3rd deg mu sites of shldr/up lmb, ex wrs/hnd, sqla
		T24.001S	Burn unsp deg of unsp site right lower limb, ex ank/ft, sqla
		T24.002S	Burn unsp deg of unsp site left lower limb, ex ank/ft, sqla
		T24.009S	Burn unsp deg of unsp site unsp lower limb, ex ank/ft, sqla
		T24.011S	Burn of unspecified degree of right thigh, sequela
	(Continued on next page)	**T24.012S**	Burn of unspecified degree of left thigh, sequela

ICD-9-CM		ICD-10-CM	
9Ø6.7	LATE EFFECT OF BURN OF OTHER EXTREMITIES **(Continued)**	**T24.Ø19S**	Burn of unspecified degree of unspecified thigh, sequela
		T24.Ø21S	Burn of unspecified degree of right knee, sequela
		T24.Ø22S	Burn of unspecified degree of left knee, sequela
		T24.Ø29S	Burn of unspecified degree of unspecified knee, sequela
		T24.Ø31S	Burn of unspecified degree of right lower leg, sequela
		T24.Ø32S	Burn of unspecified degree of left lower leg, sequela
		T24.Ø39S	Burn of unspecified degree of unspecified lower leg, sequela
		T24.Ø91S	Burn unsp deg mult sites of right low limb, ex ank/ft, sqla
		T24.Ø92S	Burn unsp deg mult sites of left lower limb, ex ank/ft, sqla
		T24.Ø99S	Burn unsp deg mult sites of unsp lower limb, ex ank/ft, sqla
		T24.1Ø1S	Burn 1st deg of unsp site right lower limb, ex ank/ft, sqla
		T24.1Ø2S	Burn first deg of unsp site left lower limb, ex ank/ft, sqla
		T24.1Ø9S	Burn first deg of unsp site unsp lower limb, ex ank/ft, sqla
		T24.111S	Burn of first degree of right thigh, sequela
		T24.112S	Burn of first degree of left thigh, sequela
		T24.119S	Burn of first degree of unspecified thigh, sequela
		T24.121S	Burn of first degree of right knee, sequela
		T24.122S	Burn of first degree of left knee, sequela
		T24.129S	Burn of first degree of unspecified knee, sequela
		T24.131S	Burn of first degree of right lower leg, sequela
		T24.132S	Burn of first degree of left lower leg, sequela
		T24.139S	Burn of first degree of unspecified lower leg, sequela
		T24.191S	Burn 1st deg mult sites of right lower limb, ex ank/ft, sqla
		T24.192S	Burn 1st deg mult sites of left lower limb, ex ank/ft, sqla
		T24.199S	Burn 1st deg mult sites of unsp lower limb, ex ank/ft, sqla
		T24.2Ø1S	Burn 2nd deg of unsp site right lower limb, ex ank/ft, sqla
		T24.2Ø2S	Burn 2nd deg of unsp site left lower limb, ex ank/ft, sqla
		T24.2Ø9S	Burn 2nd deg of unsp site unsp lower limb, ex ank/ft, sqla
		T24.211S	Burn of second degree of right thigh, sequela
		T24.212S	Burn of second degree of left thigh, sequela
		T24.219S	Burn of second degree of unspecified thigh, sequela
		T24.221S	Burn of second degree of right knee, sequela
		T24.222S	Burn of second degree of left knee, sequela
		T24.229S	Burn of second degree of unspecified knee, sequela
		T24.231S	Burn of second degree of right lower leg, sequela
		T24.232S	Burn of second degree of left lower leg, sequela
		T24.239S	Burn of second degree of unspecified lower leg, sequela
		T24.291S	Burn 2nd deg mul sites of right lower limb, ex ank/ft, sqla
		T24.292S	Burn 2nd deg mul sites of left lower limb, ex ank/ft, sqla
		T24.299S	Burn 2nd deg mul sites of unsp lower limb, ex ank/ft, sqla
		T24.3Ø1S	Burn third deg of unsp site right low limb, ex ank/ft, sqla
		T24.3Ø2S	Burn third deg of unsp site left lower limb, ex ank/ft, sqla
		T24.3Ø9S	Burn third deg of unsp site unsp lower limb, ex ank/ft, sqla
		T24.311S	Burn of third degree of right thigh, sequela
		T24.312S	Burn of third degree of left thigh, sequela
		T24.319S	Burn of third degree of unspecified thigh, sequela
		T24.321S	Burn of third degree of right knee, sequela
		T24.322S	Burn of third degree of left knee, sequela
		T24.329S	Burn of third degree of unspecified knee, sequela
		T24.331S	Burn of third degree of right lower leg, sequela
		T24.332S	Burn of third degree of left lower leg, sequela
		T24.339S	Burn of third degree of unspecified lower leg, sequela
		T24.391S	Burn 3rd deg mu sites of right lower limb, ex ank/ft, sqla
		T24.392S	Burn 3rd deg mu sites of left lower limb, ex ank/ft, sqla
		T24.399S	Burn 3rd deg mu sites of unsp lower limb, ex ank/ft, sqla
		T24.4Ø1S	Corros unsp deg of unsp site right low limb, ex ank/ft, sqla
		T24.4Ø2S	Corros unsp deg of unsp site left low limb, ex ank/ft, sqla
		T24.4Ø9S	Corros unsp deg of unsp site unsp low limb, ex ank/ft, sqla
		T24.411S	Corrosion of unspecified degree of right thigh, sequela
		T24.412S	Corrosion of unspecified degree of left thigh, sequela
		T24.419S	Corrosion of unsp degree of unspecified thigh, sequela
		T24.421S	Corrosion of unspecified degree of right knee, sequela
		T24.422S	Corrosion of unspecified degree of left knee, sequela
		T24.429S	Corrosion of unspecified degree of unspecified knee, sequela
		T24.431S	Corrosion of unspecified degree of right lower leg, sequela
		T24.432S	Corrosion of unspecified degree of left lower leg, sequela
		T24.439S	Corrosion of unsp degree of unspecified lower leg, sequela
		T24.491S	Corros unsp deg mult sites of r low limb, ex ank/ft, sqla
		T24.492S	Corros unsp deg mult sites of left low limb, ex ank/ft, sqla
		T24.499S	Corros unsp deg mult sites of unsp low limb, ex ank/ft, sqla
		T24.5Ø1S	Corros 1st deg of unsp site right low limb, ex ank/ft, sqla
		T24.5Ø2S	Corros 1st deg of unsp site left lower limb, ex ank/ft, sqla
		T24.5Ø9S	Corros 1st deg of unsp site unsp lower limb, ex ank/ft, sqla
		T24.511S	Corrosion of first degree of right thigh, sequela
		T24.512S	Corrosion of first degree of left thigh, sequela
		T24.519S	Corrosion of first degree of unspecified thigh, sequela
		T24.521S	Corrosion of first degree of right knee, sequela
		T24.522S	Corrosion of first degree of left knee, sequela
		T24.529S	Corrosion of first degree of unspecified knee, sequela
		T24.531S	Corrosion of first degree of right lower leg, sequela
		T24.532S	Corrosion of first degree of left lower leg, sequela
	(Continued on next page)	**T24.539S**	Corrosion of first degree of unspecified lower leg, sequela

[Brackets] indicate valid character values for each code. Character value meanings provided for each code grouping.

ICD-9-CM		ICD-10-CM	
906.7	LATE EFFECT OF BURN OF OTHER EXTREMITIES **(Continued)**	**T24.591S**	Corros 1st deg mult sites of right low limb, ex ank/ft, sqla
		T24.592S	Corros 1st deg mult sites of left low limb, ex ank/ft, sqla
		T24.599S	Corros 1st deg mult sites of unsp low limb, ex ank/ft, sqla
		T24.601S	Corros 2nd deg of unsp site right low limb, ex ank/ft, sqla
		T24.602S	Corros 2nd deg of unsp site left lower limb, ex ank/ft, sqla
		T24.609S	Corros 2nd deg of unsp site unsp lower limb, ex ank/ft, sqla
		T24.611S	Corrosion of second degree of right thigh, sequela
		T24.612S	Corrosion of second degree of left thigh, sequela
		T24.619S	Corrosion of second degree of unspecified thigh, sequela
		T24.621S	Corrosion of second degree of right knee, sequela
		T24.622S	Corrosion of second degree of left knee, sequela
		T24.629S	Corrosion of second degree of unspecified knee, sequela
		T24.631S	Corrosion of second degree of right lower leg, sequela
		T24.632S	Corrosion of second degree of left lower leg, sequela
		T24.639S	Corrosion of second degree of unspecified lower leg, sequela
		T24.691S	Corros 2nd deg mul sites of right low limb, ex ank/ft, sqla
		T24.692S	Corros 2nd deg mul sites of left lower limb, ex ank/ft, sqla
		T24.699S	Corros 2nd deg mul sites of unsp lower limb, ex ank/ft, sqla
		T24.701S	Corros third deg of unsp site r low limb, ex ank/ft, sqla
		T24.702S	Corros third deg of unsp site left low limb, ex ank/ft, sqla
		T24.709S	Corros third deg of unsp site unsp low limb, ex ank/ft, sqla
		T24.711S	Corrosion of third degree of right thigh, sequela
		T24.712S	Corrosion of third degree of left thigh, sequela
		T24.719S	Corrosion of third degree of unspecified thigh, sequela
		T24.721S	Corrosion of third degree of right knee, sequela
		T24.722S	Corrosion of third degree of left knee, sequela
		T24.729S	Corrosion of third degree of unspecified knee, sequela
		T24.731S	Corrosion of third degree of right lower leg, sequela
		T24.732S	Corrosion of third degree of left lower leg, sequela
		T24.739S	Corrosion of third degree of unspecified lower leg, sequela
		T24.791S	Corros 3rd deg mu sites of right lower limb, ex ank/ft, sqla
		T24.792S	Corros 3rd deg mu sites of left lower limb, ex ank/ft, sqla
		T24.799S	Corros 3rd deg mu sites of unsp lower limb, ex ank/ft, sqla
		T25.011S	Burn of unspecified degree of right ankle, sequela
		T25.012S	Burn of unspecified degree of left ankle, sequela
		T25.019S	Burn of unspecified degree of unspecified ankle, sequela
		T25.021S	Burn of unspecified degree of right foot, sequela
		T25.022S	Burn of unspecified degree of left foot, sequela
		T25.029S	Burn of unspecified degree of unspecified foot, sequela
		T25.031S	Burn of unspecified degree of right toe(s) (nail), sequela
		T25.032S	Burn of unspecified degree of left toe(s) (nail), sequela
		T25.039S	Burn of unsp degree of unspecified toe(s) (nail), sequela
		T25.091S	Burn of unsp deg mult sites of right ankle and foot, sequela
		T25.092S	Burn of unsp deg mult sites of left ankle and foot, sequela
		T25.099S	Burn of unsp deg mult sites of unsp ankle and foot, sequela
		T25.111S	Burn of first degree of right ankle, sequela
		T25.112S	Burn of first degree of left ankle, sequela
		T25.119S	Burn of first degree of unspecified ankle, sequela
		T25.121S	Burn of first degree of right foot, sequela
		T25.122S	Burn of first degree of left foot, sequela
		T25.129S	Burn of first degree of unspecified foot, sequela
		T25.131S	Burn of first degree of right toe(s) (nail), sequela
		T25.132S	Burn of first degree of left toe(s) (nail), sequela
		T25.139S	Burn of first degree of unspecified toe(s) (nail), sequela
		T25.191S	Burn of first deg mult sites of right ank/ft, sequela
		T25.192S	Burn of first deg mult sites of left ankle and foot, sequela
		T25.199S	Burn of first deg mult sites of unsp ankle and foot, sequela
		T25.211S	Burn of second degree of right ankle, sequela
		T25.212S	Burn of second degree of left ankle, sequela
		T25.219S	Burn of second degree of unspecified ankle, sequela
		T25.221S	Burn of second degree of right foot, sequela
		T25.222S	Burn of second degree of left foot, sequela
		T25.229S	Burn of second degree of unspecified foot, sequela
		T25.231S	Burn of second degree of right toe(s) (nail), sequela
		T25.232S	Burn of second degree of left toe(s) (nail), sequela
		T25.239S	Burn of second degree of unspecified toe(s) (nail), sequela
		T25.291S	Burn of 2nd deg mul sites of right ankle and foot, sequela
		T25.292S	Burn of 2nd deg mul sites of left ankle and foot, sequela
		T25.299S	Burn of 2nd deg mul sites of unsp ankle and foot, sequela
		T25.311S	Burn of third degree of right ankle, sequela
		T25.312S	Burn of third degree of left ankle, sequela
		T25.319S	Burn of third degree of unspecified ankle, sequela
		T25.321S	Burn of third degree of right foot, sequela
		T25.322S	Burn of third degree of left foot, sequela
		T25.329S	Burn of third degree of unspecified foot, sequela
		T25.331S	Burn of third degree of right toe(s) (nail), sequela
		T25.332S	Burn of third degree of left toe(s) (nail), sequela
		T25.339S	Burn of third degree of unspecified toe(s) (nail), sequela
		T25.391S	Burn of 3rd deg mu sites of right ankle and foot, sequela
		T25.392S	Burn of 3rd deg mu sites of left ankle and foot, sequela
		T25.399S	Burn of 3rd deg mu sites of unsp ankle and foot, sequela
	(Continued on next page)	**T25.411S**	Corrosion of unspecified degree of right ankle, sequela

ICD-9-CM		ICD-10-CM	
906.7	LATE EFFECT OF BURN OF OTHER EXTREMITIES **(Continued)**	**T25.412S**	Corrosion of unspecified degree of left ankle, sequela
		T25.419S	Corrosion of unsp degree of unspecified ankle, sequela
		T25.421S	Corrosion of unspecified degree of right foot, sequela
		T25.422S	Corrosion of unspecified degree of left foot, sequela
		T25.429S	Corrosion of unspecified degree of unspecified foot, sequela
		T25.431S	Corrosion of unsp degree of right toe(s) (nail), sequela
		T25.432S	Corrosion of unsp degree of left toe(s) (nail), sequela
		T25.439S	Corrosion of unsp degree of unsp toe(s) (nail), sequela
		T25.491S	Corrosion of unsp deg mult sites of right ank/ft, sequela
		T25.492S	Corrosion of unsp deg mult sites of left ank/ft, sequela
		T25.499S	Corrosion of unsp deg mult sites of unsp ank/ft, sequela
		T25.511S	Corrosion of first degree of right ankle, sequela
		T25.512S	Corrosion of first degree of left ankle, sequela
		T25.519S	Corrosion of first degree of unspecified ankle, sequela
		T25.521S	Corrosion of first degree of right foot, sequela
		T25.522S	Corrosion of first degree of left foot, sequela
		T25.529S	Corrosion of first degree of unspecified foot, sequela
		T25.531S	Corrosion of first degree of right toe(s) (nail), sequela
		T25.532S	Corrosion of first degree of left toe(s) (nail), sequela
		T25.539S	Corrosion of first degree of unsp toe(s) (nail), sequela
		T25.591S	Corrosion of first deg mult sites of right ank/ft, sequela
		T25.592S	Corrosion of first deg mult sites of left ank/ft, sequela
		T25.599S	Corrosion of first deg mult sites of unsp ank/ft, sequela
		T25.611S	Corrosion of second degree of right ankle, sequela
		T25.612S	Corrosion of second degree of left ankle, sequela
		T25.619S	Corrosion of second degree of unspecified ankle, sequela
		T25.621S	Corrosion of second degree of right foot, sequela
		T25.622S	Corrosion of second degree of left foot, sequela
		T25.629S	Corrosion of second degree of unspecified foot, sequela
		T25.631S	Corrosion of second degree of right toe(s) (nail), sequela
		T25.632S	Corrosion of second degree of left toe(s) (nail), sequela
		T25.639S	Corrosion of second degree of unsp toe(s) (nail), sequela
		T25.691S	Corrosion of second degree of right ankle and foot, sequela
		T25.692S	Corrosion of second degree of left ankle and foot, sequela
		T25.699S	Corrosion of second degree of unsp ankle and foot, sequela
		T25.711S	Corrosion of third degree of right ankle, sequela
		T25.712S	Corrosion of third degree of left ankle, sequela
		T25.719S	Corrosion of third degree of unspecified ankle, sequela
		T25.721S	Corrosion of third degree of right foot, sequela
		T25.722S	Corrosion of third degree of left foot, sequela
		T25.729S	Corrosion of third degree of unspecified foot, sequela
		T25.731S	Corrosion of third degree of right toe(s) (nail), sequela
		T25.732S	Corrosion of third degree of left toe(s) (nail), sequela
		T25.739S	Corrosion of third degree of unsp toe(s) (nail), sequela
		T25.791S	Corrosion of 3rd deg mu sites of right ank/ft, sequela
		T25.792S	Corrosion of 3rd deg mu sites of left ank/ft, sequela
		T25.799S	Corrosion of 3rd deg mu sites of unsp ank/ft, sequela
906.8	LATE EFFECT OF BURNS OF OTHER SPECIFIED SITES	**T21.00XS**	Burn of unsp degree of trunk, unspecified site, sequela
		T21.01XS	Burn of unspecified degree of chest wall, sequela
		T21.02XS	Burn of unspecified degree of abdominal wall, sequela
		T21.03XS	Burn of unspecified degree of upper back, sequela
		T21.04XS	Burn of unspecified degree of lower back, sequela
		T21.05XS	Burn of unspecified degree of buttock, sequela
		T21.06XS	Burn of unspecified degree of male genital region, sequela
		T21.07XS	Burn of unspecified degree of female genital region, sequela
		T21.09XS	Burn of unspecified degree of other site of trunk, sequela
		T21.10XS	Burn of first degree of trunk, unspecified site, sequela
		T21.11XS	Burn of first degree of chest wall, sequela
		T21.12XS	Burn of first degree of abdominal wall, sequela
		T21.13XS	Burn of first degree of upper back, sequela
		T21.14XS	Burn of first degree of lower back, sequela
		T21.15XS	Burn of first degree of buttock, sequela
		T21.16XS	Burn of first degree of male genital region, sequela
		T21.17XS	Burn of first degree of female genital region, sequela
		T21.19XS	Burn of first degree of other site of trunk, sequela
		T21.20XS	Burn of second degree of trunk, unspecified site, sequela
		T21.21XS	Burn of second degree of chest wall, sequela
		T21.22XS	Burn of second degree of abdominal wall, sequela
		T21.23XS	Burn of second degree of upper back, sequela
		T21.24XS	Burn of second degree of lower back, sequela
		T21.25XS	Burn of second degree of buttock, sequela
		T21.26XS	Burn of second degree of male genital region, sequela
		T21.27XS	Burn of second degree of female genital region, sequela
		T21.29XS	Burn of second degree of other site of trunk, sequela
		T21.30XS	Burn of third degree of trunk, unspecified site, sequela
		T21.31XS	Burn of third degree of chest wall, sequela
		T21.32XS	Burn of third degree of abdominal wall, sequela
		T21.33XS	Burn of third degree of upper back, sequela
		T21.34XS	Burn of third degree of lower back, sequela
		T21.35XS	Burn of third degree of buttock, sequela
		T21.36XS	Burn of third degree of male genital region, sequela
	(Continued on next page)	**T21.37XS**	Burn of third degree of female genital region, sequela

 [Brackets] indicate valid character values for each code. Character value meanings provided for each code grouping.

ICD-9-CM		ICD-10-CM	
9Ø6.8	LATE EFFECT OF BURNS OF OTHER SPECIFIED SITES **(Continued)**	**T21.39XS**	Burn of third degree of other site of trunk, sequela
		T21.4ØXS	Corrosion of unsp degree of trunk, unspecified site, sequela
		T21.41XS	Corrosion of unspecified degree of chest wall, sequela
		T21.42XS	Corrosion of unspecified degree of abdominal wall, sequela
		T21.43XS	Corrosion of unspecified degree of upper back, sequela
		T21.44XS	Corrosion of unspecified degree of lower back, sequela
		T21.45XS	Corrosion of unspecified degree of buttock, sequela
		T21.46XS	Corrosion of unsp degree of male genital region, sequela
		T21.47XS	Corrosion of unsp degree of female genital region, sequela
		T21.49XS	Corrosion of unsp degree of other site of trunk, sequela
		T21.5ØXS	Corrosion of first degree of trunk, unsp site, sequela
		T21.51XS	Corrosion of first degree of chest wall, sequela
		T21.52XS	Corrosion of first degree of abdominal wall, sequela
		T21.53XS	Corrosion of first degree of upper back, sequela
		T21.54XS	Corrosion of first degree of lower back, sequela
		T21.55XS	Corrosion of first degree of buttock, sequela
		T21.56XS	Corrosion of first degree of male genital region, sequela
		T21.57XS	Corrosion of first degree of female genital region, sequela
		T21.59XS	Corrosion of first degree of other site of trunk, sequela
		T21.6ØXS	Corrosion of second degree of trunk, unsp site, sequela
		T21.61XS	Corrosion of second degree of chest wall, sequela
		T21.62XS	Corrosion of second degree of abdominal wall, sequela
		T21.63XS	Corrosion of second degree of upper back, sequela
		T21.64XS	Corrosion of second degree of lower back, sequela
		T21.65XS	Corrosion of second degree of buttock, sequela
		T21.66XS	Corrosion of second degree of male genital region, sequela
		T21.67XS	Corrosion of second degree of female genital region, sequela
		T21.69XS	Corrosion of second degree of other site of trunk, sequela
		T21.7ØXS	Corrosion of third degree of trunk, unsp site, sequela
		T21.71XS	Corrosion of third degree of chest wall, sequela
		T21.72XS	Corrosion of third degree of abdominal wall, sequela
		T21.73XS	Corrosion of third degree of upper back, sequela
		T21.74XS	Corrosion of third degree of lower back, sequela
		T21.75XS	Corrosion of third degree of buttock, sequela
		T21.76XS	Corrosion of third degree of male genital region, sequela
		T21.77XS	Corrosion of third degree of female genital region, sequela
		T21.79XS	Corrosion of third degree of other site of trunk, sequela
		T26.ØØXS	Burn of unspecified eyelid and periocular area, sequela
		T26.Ø1XS	Burn of right eyelid and periocular area, sequela
		T26.Ø2XS	Burn of left eyelid and periocular area, sequela
		T26.1ØXS	Burn of cornea and conjunctival sac, unsp eye, sequela
		T26.11XS	Burn of cornea and conjunctival sac, right eye, sequela
		T26.12XS	Burn of cornea and conjunctival sac, left eye, sequela
		T26.2ØXS	Burn w resulting rupture and dest of unsp eyeball, sequela
		T26.21XS	Burn w resulting rupture and dest of right eyeball, sequela
		T26.22XS	Burn w resulting rupture and dest of left eyeball, sequela
		T26.3ØXS	Burns of oth parts of unspecified eye and adnexa, sequela
		T26.31XS	Burns of oth parts of right eye and adnexa, sequela
		T26.32XS	Burns of oth parts of left eye and adnexa, sequela
		T26.4ØXS	Burn of unsp eye and adnexa, part unspecified, sequela
		T26.41XS	Burn of right eye and adnexa, part unspecified, sequela
		T26.42XS	Burn of left eye and adnexa, part unspecified, sequela
		T26.5ØXS	Corrosion of unspecified eyelid and periocular area, sequela
		T26.51XS	Corrosion of right eyelid and periocular area, sequela
		T26.52XS	Corrosion of left eyelid and periocular area, sequela
		T26.6ØXS	Corrosion of cornea and conjunctival sac, unsp eye, sequela
		T26.61XS	Corrosion of cornea and conjunctival sac, right eye, sequela
		T26.62XS	Corrosion of cornea and conjunctival sac, left eye, sequela
		T26.7ØXS	Corros w resulting rupture and dest of unsp eyeball, sequela
		T26.71XS	Corros w rslt rupture and dest of right eyeball, sequela
		T26.72XS	Corros w resulting rupture and dest of left eyeball, sequela
		T26.8ØXS	Corrosions of oth parts of unsp eye and adnexa, sequela
		T26.81XS	Corrosions of oth parts of right eye and adnexa, sequela
		T26.82XS	Corrosions of oth parts of left eye and adnexa, sequela
		T26.9ØXS	Corrosion of unsp eye and adnexa, part unspecified, sequela
		T26.91XS	Corrosion of right eye and adnexa, part unspecified, sequela
		T26.92XS	Corrosion of left eye and adnexa, part unspecified, sequela
		T27.ØXXS	Burn of larynx and trachea, sequela
		T27.1XXS	Burn involving larynx and trachea with lung, sequela
		T27.2XXS	Burn of other parts of respiratory tract, sequela
		T27.3XXS	Burn of respiratory tract, part unspecified, sequela
		T27.4XXS	Corrosion of larynx and trachea, sequela
		T27.5XXS	Corrosion involving larynx and trachea with lung, sequela
		T27.6XXS	Corrosion of other parts of respiratory tract, sequela
		T27.7XXS	Corrosion of respiratory tract, part unspecified, sequela
		T28.ØXXS	Burn of mouth and pharynx, sequela
		T28.1XXS	Burn of esophagus, sequela
		T28.2XXS	Burn of other parts of alimentary tract, sequela
		T28.3XXS	Burn of internal genitourinary organs, sequela
		T28.4ØXS	Burn of unspecified internal organ, sequela
		T28.411S	Burn of right ear drum, sequela
		T28.412S	Burn of left ear drum, sequela
	(Continued on next page)	**T28.419S**	Burn of unspecified ear drum, sequela

ICD-9-CM		ICD-10-CM	
906.8	LATE EFFECT OF BURNS OF OTHER SPECIFIED SITES **(Continued)**	**T28.49XS**	Burn of other internal organ, sequela
		T28.5XXS	Corrosion of mouth and pharynx, sequela
		T28.6XXS	Corrosion of esophagus, sequela
		T28.7XXS	Corrosion of other parts of alimentary tract, sequela
		T28.8XXS	Corrosion of internal genitourinary organs, sequela
		T28.90XS	Corrosions of unspecified internal organs, sequela
		T28.911S	Corrosions of right ear drum, sequela
		T28.912S	Corrosions of left ear drum, sequela
		T28.919S	Corrosions of unspecified ear drum, sequela
		T28.99XS	Corrosions of other internal organs, sequela
906.9	LATE EFFECT OF BURN OF UNSPECIFIED SITE	**T20.00XS**	Burn unsp degree of head, face, and neck, unsp site, sequela
		T20.40XS	Corros unsp degree of head, face, and neck, unsp site, sqla
907.0	LATE EFF INTRACRAN INJURY W/O MENTION SKULL FX	**S06.0X0S**	Concussion without loss of consciousness, sequela
		S06.0X1S	Concussion w LOC of 30 minutes or less, sequela
		S06.0X2S	Concussion w loss of consciousness of 31-59 min, sequela
		S06.0X3S	Concussion w LOC of 1-5 hrs 59 min, sequela
		S06.0X4S	Concussion w LOC of 6 hours to 24 hours, sequela
		S06.0X5S	Concussion w LOC >24 hr w ret consc lev, sequela
		S06.0X6S	Concussion w LOC >24 hr w/o ret consc w surv, sequela
		S06.0X7S	Concuss w LOC w death due to brain injury bf consc, sequela
		S06.0X8S	Concussion w LOC w death due to oth cause bf consc, sequela
		S06.0X9S	Concussion w loss of consciousness of unsp duration, sequela
		S06.1X0S	Traumatic cerebral edema w/o loss of consciousness, sequela
		S06.1X1S	Traum cerebral edema w LOC of 30 minutes or less, sequela
		S06.1X2S	Traumatic cerebral edema w LOC of 31-59 min, sequela
		S06.1X3S	Traumatic cerebral edema w LOC of 1-5 hrs 59 min, sequela
		S06.1X4S	Traumatic cerebral edema w LOC of 6-24 hrs, sequela
		S06.1X5S	Traum cerebral edema w LOC >24 hr w ret consc lev, sequela
		S06.1X6S	Traum cereb edema w LOC >24 hr w/o ret consc w surv, sequela
		S06.1X7S	Traum cereb edema w LOC w death d/t brain inj bf consc, sqla
		S06.1X8S	Traum cereb edema w LOC w death d/t oth cause bf consc, sqla
		S06.1X9S	Traumatic cerebral edema w LOC of unsp duration, sequela
		S06.2X0S	Diffuse TBI w/o loss of consciousness, sequela
		S06.2X1S	Diffuse TBI w LOC of 30 minutes or less, sequela
		S06.2X2S	Diffuse TBI w loss of consciousness of 31-59 min, sequela
		S06.2X3S	Diffuse TBI w LOC of 1-5 hrs 59 min, sequela
		S06.2X4S	Diffuse TBI w LOC of 6 hours to 24 hours, sequela
		S06.2X5S	Diffuse TBI w LOC >24 hr w return to consc levels, sequela
		S06.2X6S	Diffuse TBI w LOC >24 hr w/o ret consc w surv, sequela
		S06.2X7S	Diffus TBI w LOC w death due to brain injury bf consc, sqla
		S06.2X8S	Diffuse TBI w LOC w death due to oth cause bf consc, sequela
		S06.2X9S	Diffuse TBI w LOC of unsp duration, sequela
		S06.300S	Unsp focal TBI w/o loss of consciousness, sequela
		S06.301S	Unsp focal TBI w LOC of 30 minutes or less, sequela
		S06.302S	Unsp focal TBI w loss of consciousness of 31-59 min, sequela
		S06.303S	Unsp focal TBI w LOC of 1-5 hrs 59 min, sequela
		S06.304S	Unsp focal TBI w LOC of 6 hours to 24 hours, sequela
		S06.305S	Unsp focal TBI w LOC >24 hr w ret consc lev, sequela
		S06.306S	Unsp focal TBI w LOC >24 hr w/o ret consc w surv, sequela
		S06.307S	Unsp focal TBI w LOC w death d/t brain injury bf consc, sqla
		S06.308S	Unsp focal TBI w LOC w death due to oth cause bf consc, sqla
		S06.309S	Unsp focal TBI w LOC of unsp duration, sequela
		S06.310S	Contus/lac right cerebrum w/o loss of consciousness, sequela
		S06.311S	Contus/lac r cereb w LOC of 30 minutes or less, sequela
		S06.312S	Contus/lac right cerebrum w LOC of 31-59 min, sequela
		S06.313S	Contus/lac right cerebrum w LOC of 1-5 hrs 59 min, sequela
		S06.314S	Contus/lac right cerebrum w LOC of 6-24 hrs, sequela
		S06.315S	Contus/lac r cereb w LOC >24 hr w ret consc lev, sequela
		S06.316S	Contus/lac r cereb w LOC >24 hr w/o ret consc w surv, sqla
		S06.317S	Contus/lac r cereb w LOC w dth d/t brain inj bf consc, sqla
		S06.318S	Contus/lac r cereb w LOC w dth d/t oth cause bf consc, sqla
		S06.319S	Contus/lac right cerebrum w LOC of unsp duration, sequela
		S06.320S	Contus/lac left cerebrum w/o loss of consciousness, sequela
		S06.321S	Contus/lac l cereb w LOC of 30 minutes or less, sequela
		S06.322S	Contus/lac left cerebrum w LOC of 31-59 min, sequela
		S06.323S	Contus/lac left cerebrum w LOC of 1-5 hrs 59 min, sequela
		S06.324S	Contus/lac left cerebrum w LOC of 6-24 hrs, sequela
		S06.325S	Contus/lac l cereb w LOC >24 hr w ret consc lev, sequela
		S06.326S	Contus/lac l cereb w LOC >24 hr w/o ret consc w surv, sqla
		S06.327S	Contus/lac l cereb w LOC w dth d/t brain inj bf consc, sqla
		S06.328S	Contus/lac l cereb w LOC w dth d/t oth cause bf consc, sqla
		S06.329S	Contus/lac left cerebrum w LOC of unsp duration, sequela
		S06.330S	Contus/lac cereb, w/o loss of consciousness, sequela
		S06.331S	Contus/lac cereb, w LOC of 30 minutes or less, sequela
		S06.332S	Contus/lac cereb, w LOC of 31-59 min, sequela
		S06.333S	Contus/lac cereb, w LOC of 1-5 hrs 59 min, sequela
		S06.334S	Contus/lac cereb, w LOC of 6 hours to 24 hours, sequela
		S06.335S	Contus/lac cereb, w LOC >24 hr w ret consc lev, sequela
		S06.336S	Contus/lac cereb, w LOC >24 hr w/o ret consc w surv, sequela
		S06.337S	Contus/lac cereb, w LOC w death d/t brain inj bf consc, sqla
		S06.338S	Contus/lac cereb, w LOC w death d/t oth cause bf consc, sqla
	(Continued on next page)	**S06.339S**	Contus/lac cereb, w LOC of unsp duration, sequela

ICD-9-CM		ICD-10-CM	
9Ø7.Ø	LATE EFF INTRACRAN INJURY W/O MENTION SKULL FX **(Continued)**	**SØ6.34ØS**	Traum hemor right cerebrum w/o LOC, sequela
		SØ6.341S	Traum hemor r cereb w LOC of 30 minutes or less, sequela
		SØ6.342S	Traum hemor right cerebrum w LOC of 31-59 min, sequela
		SØ6.343S	Traum hemor r cereb w LOC of 1-5 hrs 59 minutes, sequela
		SØ6.344S	Traum hemor right cerebrum w LOC of 6-24 hrs, sequela
		SØ6.345S	Traum hemor r cereb w LOC >24 hr w ret consc lev, sequela
		SØ6.346S	Traum hemor r cereb w LOC >24 hr w/o ret consc w surv, sqla
		SØ6.347S	Traum hemor r cereb w LOC w dth d/t brain inj bf consc, sqla
		SØ6.348S	Traum hemor r cereb w LOC w dth d/t oth cause bf consc, sqla
		SØ6.349S	Traum hemor right cerebrum w LOC of unsp duration, sequela
		SØ6.35ØS	Traum hemor left cerebrum w/o loss of consciousness, sequela
		SØ6.351S	Traum hemor l cereb w LOC of 30 minutes or less, sequela
		SØ6.352S	Traum hemor left cerebrum w LOC of 31-59 min, sequela
		SØ6.353S	Traum hemor l cereb w LOC of 1-5 hrs 59 minutes, sequela
		SØ6.354S	Traum hemor left cerebrum w LOC of 6-24 hrs, sequela
		SØ6.355S	Traum hemor l cereb w LOC >24 hr w ret consc lev, sequela
		SØ6.356S	Traum hemor l cereb w LOC >24 hr w/o ret consc w surv, sqla
		SØ6.357S	Traum hemor l cereb w LOC w dth d/t brain inj bf consc, sqla
		SØ6.358S	Traum hemor l cereb w LOC w dth d/t oth cause bf consc, sqla
		SØ6.359S	Traum hemor left cerebrum w LOC of unsp duration, sequela
		SØ6.36ØS	Traum hemor cereb, w/o loss of consciousness, sequela
		SØ6.361S	Traum hemor cereb, w LOC of 30 minutes or less, sequela
		SØ6.362S	Traum hemor cereb, w LOC of 31-59 min, sequela
		SØ6.363S	Traum hemor cereb, w LOC of 1-5 hrs 59 minutes, sequela
		SØ6.364S	Traum hemor cereb, w LOC of 6 hours to 24 hours, sequela
		SØ6.365S	Traum hemor cereb, w LOC >24 hr w ret consc lev, sequela
		SØ6.366S	Traum hemor cereb, w LOC >24 hr w/o ret consc w surv, sqla
		SØ6.367S	Traum hemor cereb, w LOC w dth d/t brain inj bf consc, sqla
		SØ6.368S	Traum hemor cereb, w LOC w dth d/t oth cause bf consc, sqla
		SØ6.369S	Traum hemor cereb, w LOC of unsp duration, sequela
		SØ6.37ØS	Contus/lac/hem crblm w/o loss of consciousness, sequela
		SØ6.371S	Contus/lac/hem crblm w LOC of 30 minutes or less, sequela
		SØ6.372S	Contus/lac/hem crblm w LOC of 31-59 min, sequela
		SØ6.373S	Contus/lac/hem crblm w LOC of 1-5 hrs 59 min, sequela
		SØ6.374S	Contus/lac/hem crblm w LOC of 6 hours to 24 hours, sequela
		SØ6.375S	Contus/lac/hem crblm w LOC >24 hr w ret consc lev, sequela
		SØ6.376S	Contus/lac/hem crblm w LOC >24 hr w/o ret consc w surv, sqla
		SØ6.377S	Contus/lac/hem crblm w LOC w dth d/t brain inj bf consc,sqla
		SØ6.378S	Contus/lac/hem crblm w LOC w dth d/t oth cause bf consc,sqla
		SØ6.379S	Contus/lac/hem crblm w LOC of unsp duration, sequela
		SØ6.38ØS	Contus/lac/hem brainstem w/o loss of consciousness, sequela
		SØ6.381S	Contus/lac/hem brnst w LOC of 30 minutes or less, sequela
		SØ6.382S	Contus/lac/hem brainstem w LOC of 31-59 min, sequela
		SØ6.383S	Contus/lac/hem brainstem w LOC of 1-5 hrs 59 min, sequela
		SØ6.384S	Contus/lac/hem brainstem w LOC of 6-24 hrs, sequela
		SØ6.385S	Contus/lac/hem brnst w LOC >24 hr w ret consc lev, sequela
		SØ6.386S	Contus/lac/hem brnst w LOC >24 hr w/o ret consc w surv, sqla
		SØ6.387S	Contus/lac/hem brnst w LOC w dth d/t brain inj bf consc,sqla
		SØ6.388S	Contus/lac/hem brnst w LOC w dth d/t oth cause bf consc,sqla
		SØ6.389S	Contus/lac/hem brainstem w LOC of unsp duration, sequela
		SØ6.4XØS	Epidural hemorrhage without loss of consciousness, sequela
		SØ6.4X1S	Epidural hemorrhage w LOC of 30 minutes or less, sequela
		SØ6.4X2S	Epidural hemorrhage w LOC of 31-59 min, sequela
		SØ6.4X3S	Epidural hemorrhage w LOC of 1-5 hrs 59 min, sequela
		SØ6.4X4S	Epidural hemorrhage w LOC of 6 hours to 24 hours, sequela
		SØ6.4X5S	Epidural hemorrhage w LOC >24 hr w ret consc lev, sequela
		SØ6.4X6S	Epidural hemor w LOC >24 hr w/o ret consc w surv, sequela
		SØ6.4X7S	Epidur hemor w LOC w death d/t brain injury bf consc, sqla
		SØ6.4X8S	Epidur hemor w LOC w death due to oth causes bf consc, sqla
		SØ6.4X9S	Epidural hemorrhage w LOC of unsp duration, sequela
		SØ6.5XØS	Traum subdr hem w/o loss of consciousness, sequela
		SØ6.5X1S	Traum subdr hem w LOC of 30 minutes or less, sequela
		SØ6.5X2S	Traum subdr hem w LOC of 31-59 min, sequela
		SØ6.5X3S	Traum subdr hem w LOC of 1-5 hrs 59 min, sequela
		SØ6.5X4S	Traum subdr hem w LOC of 6 hours to 24 hours, sequela
		SØ6.5X5S	Traum subdr hem w LOC >24 hr w ret consc lev, sequela
		SØ6.5X6S	Traum subdr hem w LOC >24 hr w/o ret consc w surv, sequela
		SØ6.5X7S	Traum subdr hem w LOC w dth d/t brain inj bef reg consc,sqla
		SØ6.5X8S	Traum subdr hem w LOC w dth d/t oth cause bef reg consc,sqla
		SØ6.5X9S	Traum subdr hem w LOC of unsp duration, sequela
		SØ6.6XØS	Traum subrac hem w/o loss of consciousness, sequela
		SØ6.6X1S	Traum subrac hem w LOC of 30 minutes or less, sequela
		SØ6.6X2S	Traum subrac hem w LOC of 31-59 min, sequela
		SØ6.6X3S	Traum subrac hem w LOC of 1-5 hrs 59 min, sequela
		SØ6.6X4S	Traum subrac hem w LOC of 6 hours to 24 hours, sequela
		SØ6.6X5S	Traum subrac hem w LOC >24 hr w ret consc lev, sequela
		SØ6.6X6S	Traum subrac hem w LOC >24 hr w/o ret consc w surv, sequela
		SØ6.6X7S	Traum subrac hem w LOC w death d/t brain inj bf consc, sqla
		SØ6.6X8S	Traum subrac hem w LOC w death d/t oth cause bf consc, sqla
		SØ6.6X9S	Traum subrac hem w LOC of unsp duration, sequela
		SØ6.81ØS	Injury of r int carotid, intcr w/o LOC, sequela
	(Continued on next page)	**SØ6.811S**	Inj r int crtd, intcr w LOC of 30 minutes or less, sequela

ICD-9-CM		ICD-10-CM	
907.0	LATE EFF INTRACRAN INJURY W/O MENTION SKULL FX **(Continued)**	**S06.812S**	Injury of r int carotid, intcr w LOC of 31-59 min, sequela
		S06.813S	Inj r int carotid, intcr w LOC of 1-5 hrs 59 min, sequela
		S06.814S	Injury of r int carotid, intcr w LOC of 6-24 hrs, sequela
		S06.815S	Inj r int crtd, intcr w LOC >24 hr w ret consc lev, sequela
		S06.816S	Inj r int crtd,intcr w LOC >24 hr w/o ret consc w surv, sqla
		S06.817S	Inj r int crtd,intcr w LOC w dth d/t brain inj bf consc,sqla
		S06.818S	Inj r int crtd,intcr w LOC w dth d/t oth cause bf consc,sqla
		S06.819S	Inj r int carotid, intcr w LOC of unsp duration, sequela
		S06.820S	Injury of l int carotid, intcr w/o LOC, sequela
		S06.821S	Inj l int crtd, intcr w LOC of 30 minutes or less, sequela
		S06.822S	Injury of l int carotid, intcr w LOC of 31-59 min, sequela
		S06.823S	Inj l int carotid, intcr w LOC of 1-5 hrs 59 min, sequela
		S06.824S	Injury of l int carotid, intcr w LOC of 6-24 hrs, sequela
		S06.825S	Inj l int crtd, intcr w LOC >24 hr w ret consc lev, sequela
		S06.826S	Inj l int crtd,intcr w LOC >24 hr w/o ret consc w surv, sqla
		S06.827S	Inj l int crtd,intcr w LOC w dth d/t brain inj bf consc,sqla
		S06.828S	Inj l int crtd,intcr w LOC w dth d/t oth cause bf consc,sqla
		S06.829S	Inj l int carotid, intcr w LOC of unsp duration, sequela
		S06.890S	Oth intracranial injury w/o loss of consciousness, sequela
		S06.891S	Intcran inj w LOC of 30 minutes or less, sequela
		S06.892S	Intcran inj w loss of consciousness of 31-59 min, sequela
		S06.893S	Intcran inj w LOC of 1-5 hrs 59 min, sequela
		S06.894S	Intcran inj w LOC of 6 hours to 24 hours, sequela
		S06.895S	Intcran inj w LOC >24 hr w ret consc lev, sequela
		S06.896S	Intcran inj w LOC >24 hr w/o ret consc w surv, sequela
		S06.897S	Intcran inj w LOC w death due to brain injury bf consc, sqla
		S06.898S	Intcran inj w LOC w death due to oth cause bf consc, sequela
		S06.899S	Intcran inj w LOC of unsp duration, sequela
		S06.9X0S	Unsp intracranial injury w/o loss of consciousness, sequela
		S06.9X1S	Unsp intcrn injury w LOC of 30 minutes or less, sequela
		S06.9X2S	Unsp intracranial injury w LOC of 31-59 min, sequela
		S06.9X3S	Unsp intracranial injury w LOC of 1-5 hrs 59 min, sequela
		S06.9X4S	Unsp intracranial injury w LOC of 6-24 hrs, sequela
		S06.9X5S	Unsp intcrn injury w LOC >24 hr w ret consc lev, sequela
		S06.9X6S	Unsp intcrn injury w LOC >24 hr w/o ret consc w surv, sqla
		S06.9X7S	Unsp intcrn inj w LOC w death d/t brain inj bf consc, sqla
		S06.9X8S	Unsp intcrn inj w LOC w death d/t oth cause bf consc, sqla
		S06.9X9S	Unsp intracranial injury w LOC of unsp duration, sequela
907.1	LATE EFFECT OF INJURY TO CRANIAL NERVE	**S04.011S**	Injury of optic nerve, right eye, sequela
		S04.012S	Injury of optic nerve, left eye, sequela
		S04.019S	Injury of optic nerve, unspecified eye, sequela
		S04.02XS	Injury of optic chiasm, sequela
		S04.031S	Injury of optic tract and pathways, right eye, sequela
		S04.032S	Injury of optic tract and pathways, left eye, sequela
		S04.039S	Injury of optic tract and pathways, unspecified eye, sequela
		S04.041S	Injury of visual cortex, right eye, sequela
		S04.042S	Injury of visual cortex, left eye, sequela
		S04.049S	Injury of visual cortex, unspecified eye, sequela
		S04.10XS	Injury of oculomotor nerve, unspecified side, sequela
		S04.11XS	Injury of oculomotor nerve, right side, sequela
		S04.12XS	Injury of oculomotor nerve, left side, sequela
		S04.20XS	Injury of trochlear nerve, unspecified side, sequela
		S04.21XS	Injury of trochlear nerve, right side, sequela
		S04.22XS	Injury of trochlear nerve, left side, sequela
		S04.30XS	Injury of trigeminal nerve, unspecified side, sequela
		S04.31XS	Injury of trigeminal nerve, right side, sequela
		S04.32XS	Injury of trigeminal nerve, left side, sequela
		S04.40XS	Injury of abducent nerve, unspecified side, sequela
		S04.41XS	Injury of abducent nerve, right side, sequela
		S04.42XS	Injury of abducent nerve, left side, sequela
		S04.50XS	Injury of facial nerve, unspecified side, sequela
		S04.51XS	Injury of facial nerve, right side, sequela
		S04.52XS	Injury of facial nerve, left side, sequela
		S04.60XS	Injury of acoustic nerve, unspecified side, sequela
		S04.61XS	Injury of acoustic nerve, right side, sequela
		S04.62XS	Injury of acoustic nerve, left side, sequela
		S04.70XS	Injury of accessory nerve, unspecified side, sequela
		S04.71XS	Injury of accessory nerve, right side, sequela
		S04.72XS	Injury of accessory nerve, left side, sequela
		S04.811S	Injury of olfactory [1st] nerve, right side, sequela
		S04.812S	Injury of olfactory [1st] nerve, left side, sequela
		S04.819S	Injury of olfactory [1st] nerve, unspecified side, sequela
		S04.891S	Injury of other cranial nerves, right side, sequela
		S04.892S	Injury of other cranial nerves, left side, sequela
		S04.899S	Injury of other cranial nerves, unspecified side, sequela
		S04.9XXS	Injury of unspecified cranial nerve, sequela

ICD-9-CM		ICD-10-CM	
9Ø7.2	LATE EFFECT OF SPINAL CORD INJURY	**S14.ØXXS**	Concussion and edema of cervical spinal cord, sequela
		S14.1Ø1S	Unsp injury at C1 level of cervical spinal cord, sequela
		S14.1Ø2S	Unsp injury at C2 level of cervical spinal cord, sequela
		S14.1Ø3S	Unsp injury at C3 level of cervical spinal cord, sequela
		S14.1Ø4S	Unsp injury at C4 level of cervical spinal cord, sequela
		S14.1Ø5S	Unsp injury at C5 level of cervical spinal cord, sequela
		S14.1Ø6S	Unsp injury at C6 level of cervical spinal cord, sequela
		S14.1Ø7S	Unsp injury at C7 level of cervical spinal cord, sequela
		S14.1Ø8S	Unsp injury at C8 level of cervical spinal cord, sequela
		S14.1Ø9S	Unsp injury at unsp level of cervical spinal cord, sequela
		S14.111S	Complete lesion at C1 level of cervical spinal cord, sequela
		S14.112S	Complete lesion at C2 level of cervical spinal cord, sequela
		S14.113S	Complete lesion at C3 level of cervical spinal cord, sequela
		S14.114S	Complete lesion at C4 level of cervical spinal cord, sequela
		S14.115S	Complete lesion at C5 level of cervical spinal cord, sequela
		S14.116S	Complete lesion at C6 level of cervical spinal cord, sequela
		S14.117S	Complete lesion at C7 level of cervical spinal cord, sequela
		S14.118S	Complete lesion at C8 level of cervical spinal cord, sequela
		S14.119S	Complete lesion at unsp level of cerv spinal cord, sequela
		S14.121S	Central cord syndrome at C1, sequela
		S14.122S	Central cord syndrome at C2, sequela
		S14.123S	Central cord syndrome at C3, sequela
		S14.124S	Central cord syndrome at C4, sequela
		S14.125S	Central cord syndrome at C5, sequela
		S14.126S	Central cord syndrome at C6, sequela
		S14.127S	Central cord syndrome at C7, sequela
		S14.128S	Central cord syndrome at C8, sequela
		S14.129S	Central cord synd at unsp level of cerv spinal cord, sequela
		S14.131S	Anterior cord syndrome at C1, sequela
		S14.132S	Anterior cord syndrome at C2, sequela
		S14.133S	Anterior cord syndrome at C3, sequela
		S14.134S	Anterior cord syndrome at C4, sequela
		S14.135S	Anterior cord syndrome at C5, sequela
		S14.136S	Anterior cord syndrome at C6, sequela
		S14.137S	Anterior cord syndrome at C7, sequela
		S14.138S	Anterior cord syndrome at C8, sequela
		S14.139S	Ant cord syndrome at unsp level of cerv spinal cord, sequela
		S14.141S	Brown-Sequard syndrome at C1, sequela
		S14.142S	Brown-Sequard syndrome at C2, sequela
		S14.143S	Brown-Sequard syndrome at C3, sequela
		S14.144S	Brown-Sequard syndrome at C4, sequela
		S14.145S	Brown-Sequard syndrome at C5, sequela
		S14.146S	Brown-Sequard syndrome at C6, sequela
		S14.147S	Brown-Sequard syndrome at C7, sequela
		S14.148S	Brown-Sequard syndrome at C8, sequela
		S14.149S	Brown-Sequard synd at unsp level of cerv spinal cord, sqla
		S14.151S	Oth incomplete lesion at C1, sequela
		S14.152S	Oth incomplete lesion at C2, sequela
		S14.153S	Oth incomplete lesion at C3, sequela
		S14.154S	Oth incomplete lesion at C4, sequela
		S14.155S	Oth incomplete lesion at C5, sequela
		S14.156S	Oth incomplete lesion at C6, sequela
		S14.157S	Oth incomplete lesion at C7, sequela
		S14.158S	Oth incomplete lesion at C8, sequela
		S14.159S	Oth incmpl lesion at unsp level of cerv spinal cord, sequela
		S24.ØXXS	Concussion and edema of thoracic spinal cord, sequela
		S24.1Ø1S	Unsp injury at T1 level of thoracic spinal cord, sequela
		S24.1Ø2S	Unsp injury at T2-T6 level of thoracic spinal cord, sequela
		S24.1Ø3S	Unsp injury at T7-T10 level of thoracic spinal cord, sequela
		S24.1Ø4S	Unsp injury at T11-T12, sequela
		S24.1Ø9S	Unsp injury at unsp level of thoracic spinal cord, sequela
		S24.111S	Complete lesion at T1 level of thoracic spinal cord, sequela
		S24.112S	Complete lesion at T2-T6, sequela
		S24.113S	Complete lesion at T7-T10, sequela
		S24.114S	Complete lesion at T11-T12, sequela
		S24.119S	Complete lesion at unsp level of thor spinal cord, sequela
		S24.131S	Anterior cord syndrome at T1, sequela
		S24.132S	Anterior cord syndrome at T2-T6, sequela
		S24.133S	Anterior cord syndrome at T7-T10, sequela
		S24.134S	Anterior cord syndrome at T11-T12, sequela
		S24.139S	Ant cord syndrome at unsp level of thor spinal cord, sequela
		S24.141S	Brown-Sequard syndrome at T1, sequela
		S24.142S	Brown-Sequard syndrome at T2-T6, sequela
		S24.143S	Brown-Sequard syndrome at T7-T10, sequela
		S24.144S	Brown-Sequard syndrome at T11-T12, sequela
		S24.149S	Brown-Sequard synd at unsp level of thor spinal cord, sqla
		S24.151S	Oth incomplete lesion at T1, sequela
		S24.152S	Oth incomplete lesion at T2-T6, sequela
		S24.153S	Oth incomplete lesion at T7-T10, sequela
		S24.154S	Oth incomplete lesion at T11-T12, sequela
		S24.159S	Oth incmpl lesion at unsp level of thor spinal cord, sequela
	(Continued on next page)	**S34.Ø1XS**	Concussion and edema of lumbar spinal cord, sequela

9Ø7.2–9Ø7.2

ICD-9-CM		ICD-10-CM	
907.2	LATE EFFECT OF SPINAL CORD INJURY **(Continued)**	**S34.02XS**	Concussion and edema of sacral spinal cord, sequela
		S34.101S	Unsp injury to L1 level of lumbar spinal cord, sequela
		S34.102S	Unsp injury to L2 level of lumbar spinal cord, sequela
		S34.103S	Unsp injury to L3 level of lumbar spinal cord, sequela
		S34.104S	Unsp injury to L4 level of lumbar spinal cord, sequela
		S34.105S	Unsp injury to L5 level of lumbar spinal cord, sequela
		S34.109S	Unsp injury to unsp level of lumbar spinal cord, sequela
		S34.111S	Complete lesion of L1 level of lumbar spinal cord, sequela
		S34.112S	Complete lesion of L2 level of lumbar spinal cord, sequela
		S34.113S	Complete lesion of L3 level of lumbar spinal cord, sequela
		S34.114S	Complete lesion of L4 level of lumbar spinal cord, sequela
		S34.115S	Complete lesion of L5 level of lumbar spinal cord, sequela
		S34.119S	Complete lesion of unsp level of lumbar spinal cord, sequela
		S34.121S	Incomplete lesion of L1 level of lumbar spinal cord, sequela
		S34.122S	Incomplete lesion of L2 level of lumbar spinal cord, sequela
		S34.123S	Incomplete lesion of L3 level of lumbar spinal cord, sequela
		S34.124S	Incomplete lesion of L4 level of lumbar spinal cord, sequela
		S34.125S	Incomplete lesion of L5 level of lumbar spinal cord, sequela
		S34.129S	Incomplete lesion of unsp level of lum spinal cord, sequela
		S34.131S	Complete lesion of sacral spinal cord, sequela
		S34.132S	Incomplete lesion of sacral spinal cord, sequela
		S34.139S	Unspecified injury to sacral spinal cord, sequela
907.3	LATE EFF INJR NERV ROOT SP PLEXUS&OTH NERV TRNK	**S14.2XXS**	Injury of nerve root of cervical spine, sequela
		S14.3XXS	Injury of brachial plexus, sequela
		S14.4XXS	Injury of peripheral nerves of neck, sequela
		S14.5XXS	Injury of cervical sympathetic nerves, sequela
		S14.8XXS	Injury of other specified nerves of neck, sequela
		S14.9XXS	Injury of unspecified nerves of neck, sequela
		S24.2XXS	Injury of nerve root of thoracic spine, sequela
		S24.3XXS	Injury of peripheral nerves of thorax, sequela
		S24.4XXS	Injury of thoracic sympathetic nervous system, sequela
		S24.8XXS	Injury of other specified nerves of thorax, sequela
		S24.9XXS	Injury of unspecified nerve of thorax, sequela
		S34.21XS	Injury of nerve root of lumbar spine, sequela
		S34.22XS	Injury of nerve root of sacral spine, sequela
		S34.3XXS	Injury of cauda equina, sequela
		S34.4XXS	Injury of lumbosacral plexus, sequela
		S34.5XXS	Inj lumbar, sacral and pelvic sympathetic nerves, sequela
		S34.6XXS	Inj prph nerve(s) at abd, low back and pelvis level, sequela
		S34.8XXS	Inj nerves at abdomen, low back and pelvis level, sequela
		S34.9XXS	Inj unsp nerves at abd, low back and pelvis level, sequela
907.4	LATE EFF INJURY PERIPH NERV SHLDR GIRDL&UP LIMB	**S44.00XS**	Injury of ulnar nerve at upper arm level, unsp arm, sequela
		S44.01XS	Injury of ulnar nerve at upper arm level, right arm, sequela
		S44.02XS	Injury of ulnar nerve at upper arm level, left arm, sequela
		S44.10XS	Injury of median nerve at upper arm level, unsp arm, sequela
		S44.11XS	Injury of median nrv at upper arm level, right arm, sequela
		S44.12XS	Injury of median nerve at upper arm level, left arm, sequela
		S44.20XS	Injury of radial nerve at upper arm level, unsp arm, sequela
		S44.21XS	Injury of radial nrv at upper arm level, right arm, sequela
		S44.22XS	Injury of radial nerve at upper arm level, left arm, sequela
		S44.30XS	Injury of axillary nerve, unspecified arm, sequela
		S44.31XS	Injury of axillary nerve, right arm, sequela
		S44.32XS	Injury of axillary nerve, left arm, sequela
		S44.40XS	Injury of musculocutaneous nerve, unspecified arm, sequela
		S44.41XS	Injury of musculocutaneous nerve, right arm, sequela
		S44.42XS	Injury of musculocutaneous nerve, left arm, sequela
		S44.50XS	Inj cutan sensory nerve at shldr/up arm, unsp arm, sequela
		S44.51XS	Inj cutan sensory nerve at shldr/up arm, right arm, sequela
		S44.52XS	Inj cutan sensory nerve at shldr/up arm, left arm, sequela
		S44.8X1S	Injury of nerves at shldr/up arm, right arm, sequela
		S44.8X2S	Injury of nerves at shldr/up arm, left arm, sequela
		S44.8X9S	Injury of nerves at shldr/up arm, unsp arm, sequela
		S44.90XS	Injury of unsp nerve at shldr/up arm, unsp arm, sequela
		S44.91XS	Injury of unsp nerve at shldr/up arm, right arm, sequela
		S44.92XS	Injury of unsp nerve at shldr/up arm, left arm, sequela
		S54.00XS	Injury of ulnar nerve at forearm level, unsp arm, sequela
		S54.01XS	Injury of ulnar nerve at forearm level, right arm, sequela
		S54.02XS	Injury of ulnar nerve at forearm level, left arm, sequela
		S54.10XS	Injury of median nerve at forearm level, unsp arm, sequela
		S54.11XS	Injury of median nerve at forearm level, right arm, sequela
		S54.12XS	Injury of median nerve at forearm level, left arm, sequela
		S54.20XS	Injury of radial nerve at forearm level, unsp arm, sequela
		S54.21XS	Injury of radial nerve at forearm level, right arm, sequela
		S54.22XS	Injury of radial nerve at forearm level, left arm, sequela
		S54.30XS	Inj cutan sensory nerve at forarm lv, unsp arm, sequela
		S54.31XS	Inj cutan sensory nerve at forarm lv, right arm, sequela
		S54.32XS	Inj cutan sensory nerve at forarm lv, left arm, sequela
		S54.8X1S	Unsp injury of nerves at forearm level, right arm, sequela
		S54.8X2S	Unsp injury of nerves at forearm level, left arm, sequela
		S54.8X9S	Unsp injury of nerves at forearm level, unsp arm, sequela
		S54.90XS	Injury of unsp nerve at forearm level, unsp arm, sequela
	(Continued on next page)	**S54.91XS**	Injury of unsp nerve at forearm level, right arm, sequela

[Brackets] indicate valid character values for each code. Character value meanings provided for each code grouping.

ICD-9-CM		ICD-10-CM	
907.4	LATE EFF INJURY PERIPH NERV SHLDR GIRDL&UP LIMB **(Continued)**	**S54.92XS**	Injury of unsp nerve at forearm level, left arm, sequela
		S64.00XS	Injury of ulnar nerve at wrs/hnd lv of unsp arm, sequela
		S64.01XS	Injury of ulnar nerve at wrs/hnd lv of right arm, sequela
		S64.02XS	Injury of ulnar nerve at wrs/hnd lv of left arm, sequela
		S64.10XS	Injury of median nerve at wrs/hnd lv of unsp arm, sequela
		S64.11XS	Injury of median nerve at wrs/hnd lv of right arm, sequela
		S64.12XS	Injury of median nerve at wrs/hnd lv of left arm, sequela
		S64.20XS	Injury of radial nerve at wrs/hnd lv of unsp arm, sequela
		S64.21XS	Injury of radial nerve at wrs/hnd lv of right arm, sequela
		S64.22XS	Injury of radial nerve at wrs/hnd lv of left arm, sequela
		S64.30XS	Injury of digital nerve of unspecified thumb, sequela
		S64.31XS	Injury of digital nerve of right thumb, sequela
		S64.32XS	Injury of digital nerve of left thumb, sequela
		S64.40XS	Injury of digital nerve of unspecified finger, sequela
		S64.490S	Injury of digital nerve of right index finger, sequela
		S64.491S	Injury of digital nerve of left index finger, sequela
		S64.492S	Injury of digital nerve of right middle finger, sequela
		S64.493S	Injury of digital nerve of left middle finger, sequela
		S64.494S	Injury of digital nerve of right ring finger, sequela
		S64.495S	Injury of digital nerve of left ring finger, sequela
		S64.496S	Injury of digital nerve of right little finger, sequela
		S64.497S	Injury of digital nerve of left little finger, sequela
		S64.498S	Injury of digital nerve of other finger, sequela
		S64.8X1S	Injury of nerves at wrs/hnd lv of right arm, sequela
		S64.8X2S	Injury of nerves at wrs/hnd lv of left arm, sequela
		S64.8X9S	Injury of nerves at wrs/hnd lv of unsp arm, sequela
		S64.90XS	Injury of unsp nerve at wrs/hnd lv of unsp arm, sequela
		S64.91XS	Injury of unsp nerve at wrs/hnd lv of right arm, sequela
		S64.92XS	Injury of unsp nerve at wrs/hnd lv of left arm, sequela
907.5	LATE EFF INJURY PERIPH NERVE PELV GIRDL&LOW LIMB	**S74.00XS**	Injury of sciatic nrv at hip and thi lev, unsp leg, sequela
		S74.01XS	Injury of sciatic nrv at hip and thi lev, right leg, sequela
		S74.02XS	Injury of sciatic nrv at hip and thi lev, left leg, sequela
		S74.10XS	Injury of femoral nrv at hip and thi lev, unsp leg, sequela
		S74.11XS	Injury of femoral nrv at hip and thi lev, right leg, sequela
		S74.12XS	Injury of femoral nrv at hip and thi lev, left leg, sequela
		S74.20XS	Inj cutan sens nerve at hip and thi lev, unsp leg, sequela
		S74.21XS	Inj cutan sens nerve at hip and high level, right leg, sqla
		S74.22XS	Inj cutan sens nerve at hip and thi lev, left leg, sequela
		S74.8X1S	Injury of nerves at hip and thigh level, right leg, sequela
		S74.8X2S	Injury of nerves at hip and thigh level, left leg, sequela
		S74.8X9S	Injury of nerves at hip and thigh level, unsp leg, sequela
		S74.90XS	Injury of unsp nerve at hip and thi lev, unsp leg, sequela
		S74.91XS	Injury of unsp nerve at hip and thi lev, right leg, sequela
		S74.92XS	Injury of unsp nerve at hip and thi lev, left leg, sequela
		S84.00XS	Injury of tibial nerve at lower leg level, unsp leg, sequela
		S84.01XS	Injury of tibial nrv at lower leg level, right leg, sequela
		S84.02XS	Injury of tibial nerve at lower leg level, left leg, sequela
		S84.10XS	Injury of peroneal nrv at lower leg level, unsp leg, sequela
		S84.11XS	Inj peroneal nrv at lower leg level, right leg, sequela
		S84.12XS	Injury of peroneal nrv at lower leg level, left leg, sequela
		S84.20XS	Inj cutan sensory nerve at low leg level, unsp leg, sequela
		S84.21XS	Inj cutan sensory nerve at low leg level, right leg, sequela
		S84.22XS	Inj cutan sensory nerve at low leg level, left leg, sequela
		S84.801S	Injury of oth nerves at lower leg level, right leg, sequela
		S84.802S	Injury of other nerves at lower leg level, left leg, sequela
		S84.809S	Injury of other nerves at lower leg level, unsp leg, sequela
		S84.90XS	Injury of unsp nerve at lower leg level, unsp leg, sequela
		S84.91XS	Injury of unsp nerve at lower leg level, right leg, sequela
		S84.92XS	Injury of unsp nerve at lower leg level, left leg, sequela
		S94.00XS	Injury of lateral plantar nerve, unspecified leg, sequela
		S94.01XS	Injury of lateral plantar nerve, right leg, sequela
		S94.02XS	Injury of lateral plantar nerve, left leg, sequela
		S94.10XS	Injury of medial plantar nerve, unspecified leg, sequela
		S94.11XS	Injury of medial plantar nerve, right leg, sequela
		S94.12XS	Injury of medial plantar nerve, left leg, sequela
		S94.20XS	Inj deep peroneal nrv at ank/ft level, unsp leg, sequela
		S94.21XS	Inj deep peroneal nrv at ank/ft level, right leg, sequela
		S94.22XS	Inj deep peroneal nrv at ank/ft level, left leg, sequela
		S94.30XS	Inj cutan sensory nerve at ank/ft level, unsp leg, sequela
		S94.31XS	Inj cutan sensory nerve at ank/ft level, right leg, sequela
		S94.32XS	Inj cutan sensory nerve at ank/ft level, left leg, sequela
		S94.8X1S	Injury of nerves at ankle and foot level, right leg, sequela
		S94.8X2S	Injury of nerves at ankle and foot level, left leg, sequela
		S94.8X9S	Injury of nerves at ankle and foot level, unsp leg, sequela
		S94.90XS	Injury of unsp nerve at ank/ft level, unsp leg, sequela
		S94.91XS	Injury of unsp nerve at ank/ft level, right leg, sequela
		S94.92XS	Injury of unsp nerve at ank/ft level, left leg, sequela

907.4–907.5

ICD-9-CM		ICD-10-CM	
907.9	LATE EFFECT OF INJURY TO OTHER&UNSPECIFIED NERVE	**S14.9XXS**	Injury of unspecified nerves of neck, sequela
		S24.9XXS	Injury of unspecified nerve of thorax, sequela
		S34.9XXS	Inj unsp nerves at abd, low back and pelvis level, sequela
		S44.90XS	Injury of unsp nerve at shldr/up arm, unsp arm, sequela
		S54.90XS	Injury of unsp nerve at forearm level, unsp arm, sequela
		S64.90XS	Injury of unsp nerve at wrs/hnd lv of unsp arm, sequela
		S74.90XS	Injury of unsp nerve at hip and thi lev, unsp leg, sequela
		S84.90XS	Injury of unsp nerve at lower leg level, unsp leg, sequela
		S94.90XS	Injury of unsp nerve at ank/ft level, unsp leg, sequela
908.0	LATE EFFECT OF INTERNAL INJURY TO CHEST	**S26.00XS**	Unspecified injury of heart with hemopericardium, sequela
		S26.01XS	Contusion of heart with hemopericardium, sequela
		S26.020S	Mild laceration of heart with hemopericardium, sequela
		S26.021S	Moderate laceration of heart with hemopericardium, sequela
		S26.022S	Major laceration of heart with hemopericardium, sequela
		S26.09XS	Other injury of heart with hemopericardium, sequela
		S26.10XS	Unspecified injury of heart without hemopericardium, sequela
		S26.11XS	Contusion of heart without hemopericardium, sequela
		S26.12XS	Laceration of heart without hemopericardium, sequela
		S26.19XS	Other injury of heart without hemopericardium, sequela
		S26.90XS	Unsp injury of heart, unsp w or w/o hemopericardium, sequela
		S26.91XS	Contusion of heart, unsp w or w/o hemopericardium, sequela
		S26.92XS	Laceration of heart, unsp w or w/o hemopericardium, sequela
		S26.99XS	Oth injury of heart, unsp w or w/o hemopericardium, sequela
		S27.0XXS	Traumatic pneumothorax, sequela
		S27.1XXS	Traumatic hemothorax, sequela
		S27.2XXS	Traumatic hemopneumothorax, sequela
		S27.301S	Unspecified injury of lung, unilateral, sequela
		S27.302S	Unspecified injury of lung, bilateral, sequela
		S27.309S	Unspecified injury of lung, unspecified, sequela
		S27.311S	Primary blast injury of lung, unilateral, sequela
		S27.312S	Primary blast injury of lung, bilateral, sequela
		S27.319S	Primary blast injury of lung, unspecified, sequela
		S27.321S	Contusion of lung, unilateral, sequela
		S27.322S	Contusion of lung, bilateral, sequela
		S27.329S	Contusion of lung, unspecified, sequela
		S27.331S	Laceration of lung, unilateral, sequela
		S27.332S	Laceration of lung, bilateral, sequela
		S27.339S	Laceration of lung, unspecified, sequela
		S27.391S	Other injuries of lung, unilateral, sequela
		S27.392S	Other injuries of lung, bilateral, sequela
		S27.399S	Other injuries of lung, unspecified, sequela
		S27.401S	Unspecified injury of bronchus, unilateral, sequela
		S27.402S	Unspecified injury of bronchus, bilateral, sequela
		S27.409S	Unspecified injury of bronchus, unspecified, sequela
		S27.411S	Primary blast injury of bronchus, unilateral, sequela
		S27.412S	Primary blast injury of bronchus, bilateral, sequela
		S27.419S	Primary blast injury of bronchus, unspecified, sequela
		S27.421S	Contusion of bronchus, unilateral, sequela
		S27.422S	Contusion of bronchus, bilateral, sequela
		S27.429S	Contusion of bronchus, unspecified, sequela
		S27.431S	Laceration of bronchus, unilateral, sequela
		S27.432S	Laceration of bronchus, bilateral, sequela
		S27.439S	Laceration of bronchus, unspecified, sequela
		S27.491S	Other injury of bronchus, unilateral, sequela
		S27.492S	Other injury of bronchus, bilateral, sequela
		S27.499S	Other injury of bronchus, unspecified, sequela
		S27.50XS	Unspecified injury of thoracic trachea, sequela
		S27.51XS	Primary blast injury of thoracic trachea, sequela
		S27.52XS	Contusion of thoracic trachea, sequela
		S27.53XS	Laceration of thoracic trachea, sequela
		S27.59XS	Other injury of thoracic trachea, sequela
		S27.60XS	Unspecified injury of pleura, sequela
		S27.63XS	Laceration of pleura, sequela
		S27.69XS	Other injury of pleura, sequela
		S27.802S	Contusion of diaphragm, sequela
		S27.803S	Laceration of diaphragm, sequela
		S27.808S	Other injury of diaphragm, sequela
		S27.809S	Unspecified injury of diaphragm, sequela
		S27.812S	Contusion of esophagus (thoracic part), sequela
		S27.813S	Laceration of esophagus (thoracic part), sequela
		S27.818S	Other injury of esophagus (thoracic part), sequela
		S27.819S	Unspecified injury of esophagus (thoracic part), sequela
		S27.892S	Contusion of other specified intrathoracic organs, sequela
		S27.893S	Laceration of other specified intrathoracic organs, sequela
		S27.898S	Other injury of oth intrathoracic organs, sequela
		S27.899S	Unspecified injury of oth intrathoracic organs, sequela
		S27.9XXS	Injury of unspecified intrathoracic organ, sequela

ICD-9-CM		ICD-10-CM	
9Ø8.1	LATE EFFECT INTERNAL INJURY INTRA-ABD ORGANS	**S36.ØØXS**	Unspecified injury of spleen, sequela
		S36.Ø2ØS	Minor contusion of spleen, sequela
		S36.Ø21S	Major contusion of spleen, sequela
		S36.Ø29S	Unspecified contusion of spleen, sequela
		S36.Ø3ØS	Superficial (capsular) laceration of spleen, sequela
		S36.Ø31S	Moderate laceration of spleen, sequela
		S36.Ø32S	Major laceration of spleen, sequela
		S36.Ø39S	Unspecified laceration of spleen, sequela
		S36.Ø9XS	Other injury of spleen, sequela
		S36.112S	Contusion of liver, sequela
		S36.113S	Laceration of liver, unspecified degree, sequela
		S36.114S	Minor laceration of liver, sequela
		S36.115S	Moderate laceration of liver, sequela
		S36.116S	Major laceration of liver, sequela
		S36.118S	Other injury of liver, sequela
		S36.119S	Unspecified injury of liver, sequela
		S36.122S	Contusion of gallbladder, sequela
		S36.123S	Laceration of gallbladder, sequela
		S36.128S	Other injury of gallbladder, sequela
		S36.129S	Unspecified injury of gallbladder, sequela
		S36.13XS	Injury of bile duct, sequela
		S36.2ØØS	Unspecified injury of head of pancreas, sequela
		S36.2Ø1S	Unspecified injury of body of pancreas, sequela
		S36.2Ø2S	Unspecified injury of tail of pancreas, sequela
		S36.2Ø9S	Unspecified injury of unspecified part of pancreas, sequela
		S36.22ØS	Contusion of head of pancreas, sequela
		S36.221S	Contusion of body of pancreas, sequela
		S36.222S	Contusion of tail of pancreas, sequela
		S36.229S	Contusion of unspecified part of pancreas, sequela
		S36.23ØS	Laceration of head of pancreas, unspecified degree, sequela
		S36.231S	Laceration of body of pancreas, unspecified degree, sequela
		S36.232S	Laceration of tail of pancreas, unspecified degree, sequela
		S36.239S	Laceration of unsp part of pancreas, unsp degree, sequela
		S36.24ØS	Minor laceration of head of pancreas, sequela
		S36.241S	Minor laceration of body of pancreas, sequela
		S36.242S	Minor laceration of tail of pancreas, sequela
		S36.249S	Minor laceration of unspecified part of pancreas, sequela
		S36.25ØS	Moderate laceration of head of pancreas, sequela
		S36.251S	Moderate laceration of body of pancreas, sequela
		S36.252S	Moderate laceration of tail of pancreas, sequela
		S36.259S	Moderate laceration of unspecified part of pancreas, sequela
		S36.26ØS	Major laceration of head of pancreas, sequela
		S36.261S	Major laceration of body of pancreas, sequela
		S36.262S	Major laceration of tail of pancreas, sequela
		S36.269S	Major laceration of unspecified part of pancreas, sequela
		S36.29ØS	Other injury of head of pancreas, sequela
		S36.291S	Other injury of body of pancreas, sequela
		S36.292S	Other injury of tail of pancreas, sequela
		S36.299S	Other injury of unspecified part of pancreas, sequela
		S36.3ØXS	Unspecified injury of stomach, sequela
		S36.32XS	Contusion of stomach, sequela
		S36.33XS	Laceration of stomach, sequela
		S36.39XS	Other injury of stomach, sequela
		S36.4ØØS	Unspecified injury of duodenum, sequela
		S36.4Ø8S	Unspecified injury of other part of small intestine, sequela
		S36.4Ø9S	Unsp injury of unspecified part of small intestine, sequela
		S36.41ØS	Primary blast injury of duodenum, sequela
		S36.418S	Primary blast injury of oth part of small intestine, sequela
		S36.419S	Primary blast injury of unsp part of sm int, sequela
		S36.42ØS	Contusion of duodenum, sequela
		S36.428S	Contusion of other part of small intestine, sequela
		S36.429S	Contusion of unspecified part of small intestine, sequela
		S36.43ØS	Laceration of duodenum, sequela
		S36.438S	Laceration of other part of small intestine, sequela
		S36.439S	Laceration of unspecified part of small intestine, sequela
		S36.49ØS	Other injury of duodenum, sequela
		S36.498S	Other injury of other part of small intestine, sequela
		S36.499S	Other injury of unspecified part of small intestine, sequela
		S36.5ØØS	Unspecified injury of ascending [right] colon, sequela
		S36.5Ø1S	Unspecified injury of transverse colon, sequela
		S36.5Ø2S	Unspecified injury of descending [left] colon, sequela
		S36.5Ø3S	Unspecified injury of sigmoid colon, sequela
		S36.5Ø8S	Unspecified injury of other part of colon, sequela
		S36.5Ø9S	Unspecified injury of unspecified part of colon, sequela
		S36.51ØS	Primary blast injury of ascending [right] colon, sequela
		S36.511S	Primary blast injury of transverse colon, sequela
		S36.512S	Primary blast injury of descending [left] colon, sequela
		S36.513S	Primary blast injury of sigmoid colon, sequela
		S36.518S	Primary blast injury of other part of colon, sequela
		S36.519S	Primary blast injury of unspecified part of colon, sequela
		S36.52ØS	Contusion of ascending [right] colon, sequela
	(Continued on next page)	**S36.521S**	Contusion of transverse colon, sequela

ICD-9-CM		ICD-10-CM	
9Ø8.1	LATE EFFECT INTERNAL INJURY INTRA-ABD ORGANS **(Continued)**	**S36.522S**	Contusion of descending [left] colon, sequela
		S36.523S	Contusion of sigmoid colon, sequela
		S36.528S	Contusion of other part of colon, sequela
		S36.529S	Contusion of unspecified part of colon, sequela
		S36.53ØS	Laceration of ascending [right] colon, sequela
		S36.531S	Laceration of transverse colon, sequela
		S36.532S	Laceration of descending [left] colon, sequela
		S36.533S	Laceration of sigmoid colon, sequela
		S36.538S	Laceration of other part of colon, sequela
		S36.539S	Laceration of unspecified part of colon, sequela
		S36.59ØS	Other injury of ascending [right] colon, sequela
		S36.591S	Other injury of transverse colon, sequela
		S36.592S	Other injury of descending [left] colon, sequela
		S36.593S	Other injury of sigmoid colon, sequela
		S36.598S	Other injury of other part of colon, sequela
		S36.599S	Other injury of unspecified part of colon, sequela
		S36.6ØXS	Unspecified injury of rectum, sequela
		S36.61XS	Primary blast injury of rectum, sequela
		S36.62XS	Contusion of rectum, sequela
		S36.63XS	Laceration of rectum, sequela
		S36.69XS	Other injury of rectum, sequela
		S36.81XS	Injury of peritoneum, sequela
		S36.892S	Contusion of other intra-abdominal organs, sequela
		S36.893S	Laceration of other intra-abdominal organs, sequela
		S36.898S	Other injury of other intra-abdominal organs, sequela
		S36.899S	Unspecified injury of other intra-abdominal organs, sequela
		S36.9ØXS	Unsp injury of unspecified intra-abdominal organ, sequela
		S36.92XS	Contusion of unspecified intra-abdominal organ, sequela
		S36.93XS	Laceration of unspecified intra-abdominal organ, sequela
		S36.99XS	Other injury of unspecified intra-abdominal organ, sequela
		S37.ØØ1S	Unspecified injury of right kidney, sequela
		S37.ØØ2S	Unspecified injury of left kidney, sequela
		S37.ØØ9S	Unspecified injury of unspecified kidney, sequela
		S37.Ø11S	Minor contusion of right kidney, sequela
		S37.Ø12S	Minor contusion of left kidney, sequela
		S37.Ø19S	Minor contusion of unspecified kidney, sequela
		S37.Ø21S	Major contusion of right kidney, sequela
		S37.Ø22S	Major contusion of left kidney, sequela
		S37.Ø29S	Major contusion of unspecified kidney, sequela
		S37.Ø31S	Laceration of right kidney, unspecified degree, sequela
		S37.Ø32S	Laceration of left kidney, unspecified degree, sequela
		S37.Ø39S	Laceration of unsp kidney, unspecified degree, sequela
		S37.Ø41S	Minor laceration of right kidney, sequela
		S37.Ø42S	Minor laceration of left kidney, sequela
		S37.Ø49S	Minor laceration of unspecified kidney, sequela
		S37.Ø51S	Moderate laceration of right kidney, sequela
		S37.Ø52S	Moderate laceration of left kidney, sequela
		S37.Ø59S	Moderate laceration of unspecified kidney, sequela
		S37.Ø61S	Major laceration of right kidney, sequela
		S37.Ø62S	Major laceration of left kidney, sequela
		S37.Ø69S	Major laceration of unspecified kidney, sequela
		S37.Ø91S	Other injury of right kidney, sequela
		S37.Ø92S	Other injury of left kidney, sequela
		S37.Ø99S	Other injury of unspecified kidney, sequela
9Ø8.2	LATE EFFECT INTERNAL INJURY OTH INTERNAL ORGANS	**S31.5Ø1S**	Unsp opn wnd unsp external genital organs, male, sequela
		S31.5Ø2S	Unsp opn wnd unsp external genital organs, female, sequela
		S31.511S	Lac w/o fb of unsp external genital organs, male, sequela
		S31.512S	Lac w/o fb of unsp external genital organs, female, sequela
		S31.521S	Lac w fb of unsp external genital organs, male, sequela
		S31.522S	Lac w fb of unsp external genital organs, female, sequela
		S31.531S	Pnctr w/o fb of unsp external genital organs, male, sequela
		S31.532S	Pnctr w/o fb of unsp extrn genital organs, female, sequela
		S31.541S	Pnctr w fb of unsp external genital organs, male, sequela
		S31.542S	Pnctr w fb of unsp external genital organs, female, sequela
		S31.551S	Open bite of unsp external genital organs, male, sequela
		S31.552S	Open bite of unsp external genital organs, female, sequela
		S37.1ØXS	Unspecified injury of ureter, sequela
		S37.12XS	Contusion of ureter, sequela
		S37.13XS	Laceration of ureter, sequela
		S37.19XS	Other injury of ureter, sequela
		S37.2ØXS	Unspecified injury of bladder, sequela
		S37.22XS	Contusion of bladder, sequela
		S37.23XS	Laceration of bladder, sequela
		S37.29XS	Other injury of bladder, sequela
		S37.3ØXS	Unspecified injury of urethra, sequela
		S37.32XS	Contusion of urethra, sequela
		S37.33XS	Laceration of urethra, sequela
		S37.39XS	Other injury of urethra, sequela
		S37.4Ø1S	Unspecified injury of ovary, unilateral, sequela
		S37.4Ø2S	Unspecified injury of ovary, bilateral, sequela
		S37.4Ø9S	Unspecified injury of ovary, unspecified, sequela
	(Continued on next page)	**S37.421S**	Contusion of ovary, unilateral, sequela

[Brackets] indicate valid character values for each code. Character value meanings provided for each code grouping.

ICD-9-CM		ICD-10-CM	
908.2	LATE EFFECT INTERNAL INJURY OTH INTERNAL ORGANS **(Continued)**	**S37.422S**	Contusion of ovary, bilateral, sequela
		S37.429S	Contusion of ovary, unspecified, sequela
		S37.431S	Laceration of ovary, unilateral, sequela
		S37.432S	Laceration of ovary, bilateral, sequela
		S37.439S	Laceration of ovary, unspecified, sequela
		S37.491S	Other injury of ovary, unilateral, sequela
		S37.492S	Other injury of ovary, bilateral, sequela
		S37.499S	Other injury of ovary, unspecified, sequela
		S37.501S	Unspecified injury of fallopian tube, unilateral, sequela
		S37.502S	Unspecified injury of fallopian tube, bilateral, sequela
		S37.509S	Unspecified injury of fallopian tube, unspecified, sequela
		S37.511S	Primary blast injury of fallopian tube, unilateral, sequela
		S37.512S	Primary blast injury of fallopian tube, bilateral, sequela
		S37.519S	Primary blast injury of fallopian tube, unspecified, sequela
		S37.521S	Contusion of fallopian tube, unilateral, sequela
		S37.522S	Contusion of fallopian tube, bilateral, sequela
		S37.529S	Contusion of fallopian tube, unspecified, sequela
		S37.531S	Laceration of fallopian tube, unilateral, sequela
		S37.532S	Laceration of fallopian tube, bilateral, sequela
		S37.539S	Laceration of fallopian tube, unspecified, sequela
		S37.591S	Other injury of fallopian tube, unilateral, sequela
		S37.592S	Other injury of fallopian tube, bilateral, sequela
		S37.599S	Other injury of fallopian tube, unspecified, sequela
		S37.60XS	Unspecified injury of uterus, sequela
		S37.62XS	Contusion of uterus, sequela
		S37.63XS	Laceration of uterus, sequela
		S37.69XS	Other injury of uterus, sequela
		S37.812S	Contusion of adrenal gland, sequela
		S37.813S	Laceration of adrenal gland, sequela
		S37.818S	Other injury of adrenal gland, sequela
		S37.819S	Unspecified injury of adrenal gland, sequela
		S37.822S	Contusion of prostate, sequela
		S37.823S	Laceration of prostate, sequela
		S37.828S	Other injury of prostate, sequela
		S37.829S	Unspecified injury of prostate, sequela
		S37.892S	Contusion of other urinary and pelvic organ, sequela
		S37.893S	Laceration of other urinary and pelvic organ, sequela
		S37.898S	Other injury of other urinary and pelvic organ, sequela
		S37.899S	Unsp injury of other urinary and pelvic organ, sequela
		S37.90XS	Unsp injury of unspecified urinary and pelvic organ, sequela
		S37.92XS	Contusion of unspecified urinary and pelvic organ, sequela
		S37.93XS	Laceration of unspecified urinary and pelvic organ, sequela
		S37.99XS	Other injury of unsp urinary and pelvic organ, sequela
908.3	LATE EFFECT INJURY BLD VESSEL HEAD NECK&EXTREM	**S09.0XXS**	Injury of blood vessels of head, NEC, sequela
		S15.001S	Unspecified injury of right carotid artery, sequela
		S15.002S	Unspecified injury of left carotid artery, sequela
		S15.009S	Unspecified injury of unspecified carotid artery, sequela
		S15.011S	Minor laceration of right carotid artery, sequela
		S15.012S	Minor laceration of left carotid artery, sequela
		S15.019S	Minor laceration of unspecified carotid artery, sequela
		S15.021S	Major laceration of right carotid artery, sequela
		S15.022S	Major laceration of left carotid artery, sequela
		S15.029S	Major laceration of unspecified carotid artery, sequela
		S15.091S	Other specified injury of right carotid artery, sequela
		S15.092S	Other specified injury of left carotid artery, sequela
		S15.099S	Oth injury of unspecified carotid artery, sequela
		S15.101S	Unspecified injury of right vertebral artery, sequela
		S15.102S	Unspecified injury of left vertebral artery, sequela
		S15.109S	Unspecified injury of unspecified vertebral artery, sequela
		S15.111S	Minor laceration of right vertebral artery, sequela
		S15.112S	Minor laceration of left vertebral artery, sequela
		S15.119S	Minor laceration of unspecified vertebral artery, sequela
		S15.121S	Major laceration of right vertebral artery, sequela
		S15.122S	Major laceration of left vertebral artery, sequela
		S15.129S	Major laceration of unspecified vertebral artery, sequela
		S15.191S	Other specified injury of right vertebral artery, sequela
		S15.192S	Other specified injury of left vertebral artery, sequela
		S15.199S	Oth injury of unspecified vertebral artery, sequela
		S15.201S	Unspecified injury of right external jugular vein, sequela
		S15.202S	Unspecified injury of left external jugular vein, sequela
		S15.209S	Unsp injury of unspecified external jugular vein, sequela
		S15.211S	Minor laceration of right external jugular vein, sequela
		S15.212S	Minor laceration of left external jugular vein, sequela
		S15.219S	Minor laceration of unsp external jugular vein, sequela
		S15.221S	Major laceration of right external jugular vein, sequela
		S15.222S	Major laceration of left external jugular vein, sequela
		S15.229S	Major laceration of unsp external jugular vein, sequela
		S15.291S	Oth injury of right external jugular vein, sequela
		S15.292S	Oth injury of left external jugular vein, sequela
		S15.299S	Oth injury of unspecified external jugular vein, sequela
		S15.301S	Unspecified injury of right internal jugular vein, sequela
	(Continued on next page)	**S15.302S**	Unspecified injury of left internal jugular vein, sequela

ICD-9-CM		ICD-10-CM	
908.3	LATE EFFECT INJURY BLD VESSEL HEAD NECK&EXTREM **(Continued)**	**S15.309S**	Unsp injury of unspecified internal jugular vein, sequela
		S15.311S	Minor laceration of right internal jugular vein, sequela
		S15.312S	Minor laceration of left internal jugular vein, sequela
		S15.319S	Minor laceration of unsp internal jugular vein, sequela
		S15.321S	Major laceration of right internal jugular vein, sequela
		S15.322S	Major laceration of left internal jugular vein, sequela
		S15.329S	Major laceration of unsp internal jugular vein, sequela
		S15.391S	Oth injury of right internal jugular vein, sequela
		S15.392S	Oth injury of left internal jugular vein, sequela
		S15.399S	Oth injury of unspecified internal jugular vein, sequela
		S15.8XXS	Injury of oth blood vessels at neck level, sequela
		S15.9XXS	Injury of unspecified blood vessel at neck level, sequela
		S45.001S	Unspecified injury of axillary artery, right side, sequela
		S45.002S	Unspecified injury of axillary artery, left side, sequela
		S45.009S	Unsp injury of axillary artery, unspecified side, sequela
		S45.011S	Laceration of axillary artery, right side, sequela
		S45.012S	Laceration of axillary artery, left side, sequela
		S45.019S	Laceration of axillary artery, unspecified side, sequela
		S45.091S	Oth injury of axillary artery, right side, sequela
		S45.092S	Oth injury of axillary artery, left side, sequela
		S45.099S	Oth injury of axillary artery, unspecified side, sequela
		S45.101S	Unspecified injury of brachial artery, right side, sequela
		S45.102S	Unspecified injury of brachial artery, left side, sequela
		S45.109S	Unsp injury of brachial artery, unspecified side, sequela
		S45.111S	Laceration of brachial artery, right side, sequela
		S45.112S	Laceration of brachial artery, left side, sequela
		S45.119S	Laceration of brachial artery, unspecified side, sequela
		S45.191S	Oth injury of brachial artery, right side, sequela
		S45.192S	Oth injury of brachial artery, left side, sequela
		S45.199S	Oth injury of brachial artery, unspecified side, sequela
		S45.201S	Unsp injury of axillary or brach vein, right side, sequela
		S45.202S	Unsp injury of axillary or brachial vein, left side, sequela
		S45.209S	Unsp injury of axillary or brachial vein, unsp side, sequela
		S45.211S	Laceration of axillary or brachial vein, right side, sequela
		S45.212S	Laceration of axillary or brachial vein, left side, sequela
		S45.219S	Laceration of axillary or brachial vein, unsp side, sequela
		S45.291S	Oth injury of axillary or brachial vein, right side, sequela
		S45.292S	Oth injury of axillary or brachial vein, left side, sequela
		S45.299S	Oth injury of axillary or brachial vein, unsp side, sequela
		S45.301S	Unsp inj superfic vn at shldr/up arm, right arm, sequela
		S45.302S	Unsp inj superfic vn at shldr/up arm, left arm, sequela
		S45.309S	Unsp inj superfic vn at shldr/up arm, unsp arm, sequela
		S45.311S	Lacerat superfic vn at shldr/up arm, right arm, sequela
		S45.312S	Laceration of superfic vn at shldr/up arm, left arm, sequela
		S45.319S	Laceration of superfic vn at shldr/up arm, unsp arm, sequela
		S45.391S	Inj superficial vein at shldr/up arm, right arm, sequela
		S45.392S	Inj superficial vein at shldr/up arm, left arm, sequela
		S45.399S	Inj superficial vein at shldr/up arm, unsp arm, sequela
		S45.801S	Unsp inj blood vessels at shldr/up arm, right arm, sequela
		S45.802S	Unsp inj blood vessels at shldr/up arm, left arm, sequela
		S45.809S	Unsp inj blood vessels at shldr/up arm, unsp arm, sequela
		S45.811S	Lacerat blood vessels at shldr/up arm, right arm, sequela
		S45.812S	Lacerat blood vessels at shldr/up arm, left arm, sequela
		S45.819S	Lacerat blood vessels at shldr/up arm, unsp arm, sequela
		S45.891S	Inj oth blood vessels at shldr/up arm, right arm, sequela
		S45.892S	Inj oth blood vessels at shldr/up arm, left arm, sequela
		S45.899S	Inj oth blood vessels at shldr/up arm, unsp arm, sequela
		S45.901S	Unsp inj unsp blood vess at shldr/up arm, right arm, sequela
		S45.902S	Unsp inj unsp blood vess at shldr/up arm, left arm, sequela
		S45.909S	Unsp inj unsp blood vess at shldr/up arm, unsp arm, sequela
		S45.911S	Lacerat unsp blood vess at shldr/up arm, right arm, sequela
		S45.912S	Lacerat unsp blood vessel at shldr/up arm, left arm, sequela
		S45.919S	Lacerat unsp blood vessel at shldr/up arm, unsp arm, sequela
		S45.991S	Inj unsp blood vessel at shldr/up arm, right arm, sequela
		S45.992S	Inj unsp blood vessel at shldr/up arm, left arm, sequela
		S45.999S	Inj unsp blood vessel at shldr/up arm, unsp arm, sequela
		S55.001S	Unsp injury of ulnar artery at forarm lv, right arm, sequela
		S55.002S	Unsp injury of ulnar artery at forarm lv, left arm, sequela
		S55.009S	Unsp injury of ulnar artery at forarm lv, unsp arm, sequela
		S55.011S	Laceration of ulnar artery at forarm lv, right arm, sequela
		S55.012S	Laceration of ulnar artery at forarm lv, left arm, sequela
		S55.019S	Laceration of ulnar artery at forarm lv, unsp arm, sequela
		S55.091S	Inj ulnar artery at forearm level, right arm, sequela
		S55.092S	Inj ulnar artery at forearm level, left arm, sequela
		S55.099S	Inj ulnar artery at forearm level, unsp arm, sequela
		S55.101S	Unsp injury of radial art at forarm lv, right arm, sequela
		S55.102S	Unsp injury of radial artery at forarm lv, left arm, sequela
		S55.109S	Unsp injury of radial artery at forarm lv, unsp arm, sequela
		S55.111S	Laceration of radial artery at forarm lv, right arm, sequela
		S55.112S	Laceration of radial artery at forarm lv, left arm, sequela
		S55.119S	Laceration of radial artery at forarm lv, unsp arm, sequela
		S55.191S	Inj radial artery at forearm level, right arm, sequela
	(Continued on next page)	**S55.192S**	Inj radial artery at forearm level, left arm, sequela

[Brackets] indicate valid character values for each code. Character value meanings provided for each code grouping.

ICD-9-CM		ICD-10-CM	
908.3	LATE EFFECT INJURY BLD VESSEL HEAD NECK&EXTREM **(Continued)**	S55.199S	Inj radial artery at forearm level, unsp arm, sequela
		S55.201S	Unsp injury of vein at forearm level, right arm, sequela
		S55.202S	Unsp injury of vein at forearm level, left arm, sequela
		S55.209S	Unsp injury of vein at forearm level, unsp arm, sequela
		S55.211S	Laceration of vein at forearm level, right arm, sequela
		S55.212S	Laceration of vein at forearm level, left arm, sequela
		S55.219S	Laceration of vein at forearm level, unsp arm, sequela
		S55.291S	Oth injury of vein at forearm level, right arm, sequela
		S55.292S	Oth injury of vein at forearm level, left arm, sequela
		S55.299S	Oth injury of vein at forearm level, unsp arm, sequela
		S55.801S	Unsp inj blood vessels at forarm lv, right arm, sequela
		S55.802S	Unsp injury of blood vessels at forarm lv, left arm, sequela
		S55.809S	Unsp injury of blood vessels at forarm lv, unsp arm, sequela
		S55.811S	Laceration of blood vessels at forarm lv, right arm, sequela
		S55.812S	Laceration of blood vessels at forarm lv, left arm, sequela
		S55.819S	Laceration of blood vessels at forarm lv, unsp arm, sequela
		S55.891S	Inj oth blood vessels at forearm level, right arm, sequela
		S55.892S	Inj oth blood vessels at forearm level, left arm, sequela
		S55.899S	Inj oth blood vessels at forearm level, unsp arm, sequela
		S55.901S	Unsp inj unsp blood vess at forarm lv, right arm, sequela
		S55.902S	Unsp inj unsp blood vess at forarm lv, left arm, sequela
		S55.909S	Unsp inj unsp blood vess at forarm lv, unsp arm, sequela
		S55.911S	Lacerat unsp blood vessel at forarm lv, right arm, sequela
		S55.912S	Lacerat unsp blood vessel at forarm lv, left arm, sequela
		S55.919S	Lacerat unsp blood vessel at forarm lv, unsp arm, sequela
		S55.991S	Inj unsp blood vessel at forearm level, right arm, sequela
		S55.992S	Inj unsp blood vessel at forearm level, left arm, sequela
		S55.999S	Inj unsp blood vessel at forearm level, unsp arm, sequela
		S65.001S	Unsp injury of ulnar art at wrs/hnd lv of right arm, sequela
		S65.002S	Unsp injury of ulnar art at wrs/hnd lv of left arm, sequela
		S65.009S	Unsp injury of ulnar art at wrs/hnd lv of unsp arm, sequela
		S65.011S	Lacerat ulnar artery at wrs/hnd lv of right arm, sequela
		S65.012S	Lacerat ulnar artery at wrs/hnd lv of left arm, sequela
		S65.019S	Lacerat ulnar artery at wrs/hnd lv of unsp arm, sequela
		S65.091S	Inj ulnar artery at wrs/hnd lv of right arm, sequela
		S65.092S	Inj ulnar artery at wrs/hnd lv of left arm, sequela
		S65.099S	Inj ulnar artery at wrs/hnd lv of unsp arm, sequela
		S65.101S	Unsp inj radial art at wrs/hnd lv of right arm, sequela
		S65.102S	Unsp injury of radial art at wrs/hnd lv of left arm, sequela
		S65.109S	Unsp injury of radial art at wrs/hnd lv of unsp arm, sequela
		S65.111S	Lacerat radial artery at wrs/hnd lv of right arm, sequela
		S65.112S	Lacerat radial artery at wrs/hnd lv of left arm, sequela
		S65.119S	Lacerat radial artery at wrs/hnd lv of unsp arm, sequela
		S65.191S	Inj radial artery at wrs/hnd lv of right arm, sequela
		S65.192S	Inj radial artery at wrs/hnd lv of left arm, sequela
		S65.199S	Inj radial artery at wrs/hnd lv of unsp arm, sequela
		S65.201S	Unsp injury of superfic palmar arch of right hand, sequela
		S65.202S	Unsp injury of superficial palmar arch of left hand, sequela
		S65.209S	Unsp injury of superficial palmar arch of unsp hand, sequela
		S65.211S	Laceration of superficial palmar arch of right hand, sequela
		S65.212S	Laceration of superficial palmar arch of left hand, sequela
		S65.219S	Laceration of superficial palmar arch of unsp hand, sequela
		S65.291S	Oth injury of superficial palmar arch of right hand, sequela
		S65.292S	Oth injury of superficial palmar arch of left hand, sequela
		S65.299S	Oth injury of superficial palmar arch of unsp hand, sequela
		S65.301S	Unsp injury of deep palmar arch of right hand, sequela
		S65.302S	Unspecified injury of deep palmar arch of left hand, sequela
		S65.309S	Unsp injury of deep palmar arch of unspecified hand, sequela
		S65.311S	Laceration of deep palmar arch of right hand, sequela
		S65.312S	Laceration of deep palmar arch of left hand, sequela
		S65.319S	Laceration of deep palmar arch of unspecified hand, sequela
		S65.391S	Oth injury of deep palmar arch of right hand, sequela
		S65.392S	Oth injury of deep palmar arch of left hand, sequela
		S65.399S	Oth injury of deep palmar arch of unspecified hand, sequela
		S65.401S	Unspecified injury of blood vessel of right thumb, sequela
		S65.402S	Unspecified injury of blood vessel of left thumb, sequela
		S65.409S	Unsp injury of blood vessel of unspecified thumb, sequela
		S65.411S	Laceration of blood vessel of right thumb, sequela
		S65.412S	Laceration of blood vessel of left thumb, sequela
		S65.419S	Laceration of blood vessel of unspecified thumb, sequela
		S65.491S	Oth injury of blood vessel of right thumb, sequela
		S65.492S	Oth injury of blood vessel of left thumb, sequela
		S65.499S	Oth injury of blood vessel of unspecified thumb, sequela
		S65.500S	Unsp injury of blood vessel of right index finger, sequela
		S65.501S	Unsp injury of blood vessel of left index finger, sequela
		S65.502S	Unsp injury of blood vessel of right middle finger, sequela
		S65.503S	Unsp injury of blood vessel of left middle finger, sequela
		S65.504S	Unsp injury of blood vessel of right ring finger, sequela
		S65.505S	Unsp injury of blood vessel of left ring finger, sequela
		S65.506S	Unsp injury of blood vessel of right little finger, sequela
		S65.507S	Unsp injury of blood vessel of left little finger, sequela
		S65.508S	Unspecified injury of blood vessel of other finger, sequela
	(Continued on next page)	S65.509S	Unsp injury of blood vessel of unspecified finger, sequela

ICD-9-CM		ICD-10-CM	
9Ø8.3	LATE EFFECT INJURY BLD VESSEL HEAD NECK&EXTREM **(Continued)**	**S65.51ØS**	Laceration of blood vessel of right index finger, sequela
		S65.511S	Laceration of blood vessel of left index finger, sequela
		S65.512S	Laceration of blood vessel of right middle finger, sequela
		S65.513S	Laceration of blood vessel of left middle finger, sequela
		S65.514S	Laceration of blood vessel of right ring finger, sequela
		S65.515S	Laceration of blood vessel of left ring finger, sequela
		S65.516S	Laceration of blood vessel of right little finger, sequela
		S65.517S	Laceration of blood vessel of left little finger, sequela
		S65.518S	Laceration of blood vessel of other finger, sequela
		S65.519S	Laceration of blood vessel of unspecified finger, sequela
		S65.59ØS	Oth injury of blood vessel of right index finger, sequela
		S65.591S	Oth injury of blood vessel of left index finger, sequela
		S65.592S	Oth injury of blood vessel of right middle finger, sequela
		S65.593S	Oth injury of blood vessel of left middle finger, sequela
		S65.594S	Oth injury of blood vessel of right ring finger, sequela
		S65.595S	Oth injury of blood vessel of left ring finger, sequela
		S65.596S	Oth injury of blood vessel of right little finger, sequela
		S65.597S	Oth injury of blood vessel of left little finger, sequela
		S65.598S	Oth injury of blood vessel of other finger, sequela
		S65.599S	Oth injury of blood vessel of unspecified finger, sequela
		S65.8Ø1S	Unsp inj blood vessels at wrs/hnd lv of right arm, sequela
		S65.8Ø2S	Unsp inj blood vessels at wrs/hnd lv of left arm, sequela
		S65.8Ø9S	Unsp inj blood vessels at wrs/hnd lv of unsp arm, sequela
		S65.811S	Lacerat blood vessels at wrs/hnd lv of right arm, sequela
		S65.812S	Lacerat blood vessels at wrs/hnd lv of left arm, sequela
		S65.819S	Lacerat blood vessels at wrs/hnd lv of unsp arm, sequela
		S65.891S	Inj oth blood vessels at wrs/hnd lv of right arm, sequela
		S65.892S	Inj oth blood vessels at wrs/hnd lv of left arm, sequela
		S65.899S	Inj oth blood vessels at wrs/hnd lv of unsp arm, sequela
		S65.9Ø1S	Unsp inj unsp blood vess at wrs/hnd lv of right arm, sequela
		S65.9Ø2S	Unsp inj unsp blood vess at wrs/hnd lv of left arm, sequela
		S65.9Ø9S	Unsp inj unsp blood vess at wrs/hnd lv of unsp arm, sequela
		S65.911S	Lacerat unsp blood vess at wrs/hnd lv of right arm, sequela
		S65.912S	Lacerat unsp blood vessel at wrs/hnd lv of left arm, sequela
		S65.919S	Lacerat unsp blood vessel at wrs/hnd lv of unsp arm, sequela
		S65.991S	Inj unsp blood vessel at wrs/hnd of right arm, sequela
		S65.992S	Inj unsp blood vessel at wrist and hand of left arm, sequela
		S65.999S	Inj unsp blood vessel at wrist and hand of unsp arm, sequela
		S75.ØØ1S	Unspecified injury of femoral artery, right leg, sequela
		S75.ØØ2S	Unspecified injury of femoral artery, left leg, sequela
		S75.ØØ9S	Unsp injury of femoral artery, unspecified leg, sequela
		S75.Ø11S	Minor laceration of femoral artery, right leg, sequela
		S75.Ø12S	Minor laceration of femoral artery, left leg, sequela
		S75.Ø19S	Minor laceration of femoral artery, unspecified leg, sequela
		S75.Ø21S	Major laceration of femoral artery, right leg, sequela
		S75.Ø22S	Major laceration of femoral artery, left leg, sequela
		S75.Ø29S	Major laceration of femoral artery, unspecified leg, sequela
		S75.Ø91S	Other specified injury of femoral artery, right leg, sequela
		S75.Ø92S	Other specified injury of femoral artery, left leg, sequela
		S75.Ø99S	Oth injury of femoral artery, unspecified leg, sequela
		S75.1Ø1S	Unsp inj femor vein at hip and thi lev, right leg, sequela
		S75.1Ø2S	Unsp inj femor vein at hip and thi lev, left leg, sequela
		S75.1Ø9S	Unsp inj femor vein at hip and thi lev, unsp leg, sequela
		S75.111S	Minor lacerat femor vein at hip and thi lev, right leg, sqla
		S75.112S	Minor lacerat femor vein at hip and thi lev, left leg, sqla
		S75.119S	Minor lacerat femor vein at hip and thi lev, unsp leg, sqla
		S75.121S	Major lacerat femor vein at hip and thi lev, right leg, sqla
		S75.122S	Major lacerat femor vein at hip and thi lev, left leg, sqla
		S75.129S	Major lacerat femor vein at hip and thi lev, unsp leg, sqla
		S75.191S	Inj femoral vein at hip and thigh level, right leg, sequela
		S75.192S	Inj femoral vein at hip and thigh level, left leg, sequela
		S75.199S	Inj femoral vein at hip and thigh level, unsp leg, sequela
		S75.2Ø1S	Unsp inj great saph at hip and thi lev, right leg, sequela
		S75.2Ø2S	Unsp inj great saph at hip and thi lev, left leg, sequela
		S75.2Ø9S	Unsp inj great saph at hip and thi lev, unsp leg, sequela
		S75.211S	Minor lacerat great saph at hip and thi lev, right leg, sqla
		S75.212S	Minor lacerat great saph at hip and thi lev, left leg, sqla
		S75.219S	Minor lacerat great saph at hip and thi lev, unsp leg, sqla
		S75.221S	Major lacerat great saph at hip and thi lev, right leg, sqla
		S75.222S	Major lacerat great saph at hip and thi lev, left leg, sqla
		S75.229S	Major lacerat great saph at hip and thi lev, unsp leg, sqla
		S75.291S	Inj great saphenous at hip and thi lev, right leg, sequela
		S75.292S	Inj great saphenous at hip and thi lev, left leg, sequela
		S75.299S	Inj great saphenous at hip and thi lev, unsp leg, sequela
		S75.8Ø1S	Unsp inj blood vessels at hip and thi lev, right leg, sqla
		S75.8Ø2S	Unsp inj blood vessels at hip and thi lev, left leg, sequela
		S75.8Ø9S	Unsp inj blood vessels at hip and thi lev, unsp leg, sequela
		S75.811S	Lacerat blood vessels at hip and thi lev, right leg, sequela
		S75.812S	Lacerat blood vessels at hip and thi lev, left leg, sequela
		S75.819S	Lacerat blood vessels at hip and thi lev, unsp leg, sequela
		S75.891S	Inj oth blood vessels at hip and thi lev, right leg, sequela
		S75.892S	Inj oth blood vessels at hip and thi lev, left leg, sequela
	(Continued on next page)	**S75.899S**	Inj oth blood vessels at hip and thi lev, unsp leg, sequela

[Brackets] indicate valid character values for each code. Character value meanings provided for each code grouping.

ICD-9-CM		ICD-10-CM	
9Ø8.3	LATE EFFECT INJURY BLD VESSEL HEAD NECK&EXTREM **(Continued)**	**S75.9Ø1S**	Unsp inj unsp blood vess at hip and thi lev, right leg, sqla
		S75.9Ø2S	Unsp inj unsp blood vess at hip and thi lev, left leg, sqla
		S75.9Ø9S	Unsp inj unsp blood vess at hip and thi lev, unsp leg, sqla
		S75.911S	Lacerat unsp blood vess at hip and thi lev, right leg, sqla
		S75.912S	Lacerat unsp blood vess at hip and thi lev, left leg, sqla
		S75.919S	Lacerat unsp blood vess at hip and thi lev, unsp leg, sqla
		S75.991S	Inj unsp blood vess at hip and thi lev, right leg, sequela
		S75.992S	Inj unsp blood vess at hip and thi lev, left leg, sequela
		S75.999S	Inj unsp blood vess at hip and thi lev, unsp leg, sequela
		S85.ØØ1S	Unspecified injury of popliteal artery, right leg, sequela
		S85.ØØ2S	Unspecified injury of popliteal artery, left leg, sequela
		S85.ØØ9S	Unsp injury of popliteal artery, unspecified leg, sequela
		S85.Ø11S	Laceration of popliteal artery, right leg, sequela
		S85.Ø12S	Laceration of popliteal artery, left leg, sequela
		S85.Ø19S	Laceration of popliteal artery, unspecified leg, sequela
		S85.Ø91S	Oth injury of popliteal artery, right leg, sequela
		S85.Ø92S	Oth injury of popliteal artery, left leg, sequela
		S85.Ø99S	Oth injury of popliteal artery, unspecified leg, sequela
		S85.1Ø1S	Unsp injury of unspecified tibial artery, right leg, sequela
		S85.1Ø2S	Unsp injury of unspecified tibial artery, left leg, sequela
		S85.1Ø9S	Unsp injury of unsp tibial artery, unspecified leg, sequela
		S85.111S	Laceration of unspecified tibial artery, right leg, sequela
		S85.112S	Laceration of unspecified tibial artery, left leg, sequela
		S85.119S	Laceration of unsp tibial artery, unspecified leg, sequela
		S85.121S	Oth injury of unspecified tibial artery, right leg, sequela
		S85.122S	Oth injury of unspecified tibial artery, left leg, sequela
		S85.129S	Oth injury of unsp tibial artery, unspecified leg, sequela
		S85.131S	Unsp injury of anterior tibial artery, right leg, sequela
		S85.132S	Unsp injury of anterior tibial artery, left leg, sequela
		S85.139S	Unsp injury of anterior tibial artery, unsp leg, sequela
		S85.141S	Laceration of anterior tibial artery, right leg, sequela
		S85.142S	Laceration of anterior tibial artery, left leg, sequela
		S85.149S	Laceration of anterior tibial artery, unsp leg, sequela
		S85.151S	Oth injury of anterior tibial artery, right leg, sequela
		S85.152S	Oth injury of anterior tibial artery, left leg, sequela
		S85.159S	Oth injury of anterior tibial artery, unsp leg, sequela
		S85.161S	Unsp injury of posterior tibial artery, right leg, sequela
		S85.162S	Unsp injury of posterior tibial artery, left leg, sequela
		S85.169S	Unsp injury of posterior tibial artery, unsp leg, sequela
		S85.171S	Laceration of posterior tibial artery, right leg, sequela
		S85.172S	Laceration of posterior tibial artery, left leg, sequela
		S85.179S	Laceration of posterior tibial artery, unsp leg, sequela
		S85.181S	Oth injury of posterior tibial artery, right leg, sequela
		S85.182S	Oth injury of posterior tibial artery, left leg, sequela
		S85.189S	Oth injury of posterior tibial artery, unsp leg, sequela
		S85.2Ø1S	Unspecified injury of peroneal artery, right leg, sequela
		S85.2Ø2S	Unspecified injury of peroneal artery, left leg, sequela
		S85.2Ø9S	Unsp injury of peroneal artery, unspecified leg, sequela
		S85.211S	Laceration of peroneal artery, right leg, sequela
		S85.212S	Laceration of peroneal artery, left leg, sequela
		S85.219S	Laceration of peroneal artery, unspecified leg, sequela
		S85.291S	Oth injury of peroneal artery, right leg, sequela
		S85.292S	Other specified injury of peroneal artery, left leg, sequela
		S85.299S	Oth injury of peroneal artery, unspecified leg, sequela
		S85.3Ø1S	Unsp inj great saph at low leg level, right leg, sequela
		S85.3Ø2S	Unsp inj great saphenous at low leg level, left leg, sequela
		S85.3Ø9S	Unsp inj great saphenous at low leg level, unsp leg, sequela
		S85.311S	Lacerat great saphenous at low leg level, right leg, sequela
		S85.312S	Lacerat great saphenous at low leg level, left leg, sequela
		S85.319S	Lacerat great saphenous at low leg level, unsp leg, sequela
		S85.391S	Inj great saphenous at lower leg level, right leg, sequela
		S85.392S	Inj great saphenous at lower leg level, left leg, sequela
		S85.399S	Inj great saphenous at lower leg level, unsp leg, sequela
		S85.4Ø1S	Unsp inj less saphenous at low leg level, right leg, sequela
		S85.4Ø2S	Unsp inj less saphenous at low leg level, left leg, sequela
		S85.4Ø9S	Unsp inj less saphenous at low leg level, unsp leg, sequela
		S85.411S	Lacerat less saphenous at low leg level, right leg, sequela
		S85.412S	Lacerat less saphenous at lower leg level, left leg, sequela
		S85.419S	Lacerat less saphenous at lower leg level, unsp leg, sequela
		S85.491S	Inj less saphenous at lower leg level, right leg, sequela
		S85.492S	Inj less saphenous at lower leg level, left leg, sequela
		S85.499S	Inj less saphenous at lower leg level, unsp leg, sequela
		S85.5Ø1S	Unspecified injury of popliteal vein, right leg, sequela
		S85.5Ø2S	Unspecified injury of popliteal vein, left leg, sequela
		S85.5Ø9S	Unsp injury of popliteal vein, unspecified leg, sequela
		S85.511S	Laceration of popliteal vein, right leg, sequela
		S85.512S	Laceration of popliteal vein, left leg, sequela
		S85.519S	Laceration of popliteal vein, unspecified leg, sequela
		S85.591S	Other specified injury of popliteal vein, right leg, sequela
		S85.592S	Other specified injury of popliteal vein, left leg, sequela
		S85.599S	Oth injury of popliteal vein, unspecified leg, sequela
		S85.8Ø1S	Unsp inj blood vessels at low leg level, right leg, sequela
	(Continued on next page)	**S85.8Ø2S**	Unsp inj blood vessels at lower leg level, left leg, sequela

ICD-9-CM		ICD-10-CM	
908.3	LATE EFFECT INJURY BLD VESSEL HEAD NECK&EXTREM **(Continued)**	**S85.809S**	Unsp inj blood vessels at lower leg level, unsp leg, sequela
		S85.811S	Lacerat blood vessels at lower leg level, right leg, sequela
		S85.812S	Lacerat blood vessels at lower leg level, left leg, sequela
		S85.819S	Lacerat blood vessels at lower leg level, unsp leg, sequela
		S85.891S	Inj oth blood vessels at lower leg level, right leg, sequela
		S85.892S	Inj oth blood vessels at lower leg level, left leg, sequela
		S85.899S	Inj oth blood vessels at lower leg level, unsp leg, sequela
		S85.901S	Unsp inj unsp blood vess at low leg level, right leg, sqla
		S85.902S	Unsp inj unsp blood vess at low leg level, left leg, sequela
		S85.909S	Unsp inj unsp blood vess at low leg level, unsp leg, sequela
		S85.911S	Lacerat unsp blood vess at low leg level, right leg, sequela
		S85.912S	Lacerat unsp blood vess at low leg level, left leg, sequela
		S85.919S	Lacerat unsp blood vess at low leg level, unsp leg, sequela
		S85.991S	Inj unsp blood vessel at lower leg level, right leg, sequela
		S85.992S	Inj unsp blood vessel at lower leg level, left leg, sequela
		S85.999S	Inj unsp blood vessel at lower leg level, unsp leg, sequela
		S95.001S	Unspecified injury of dorsal artery of right foot, sequela
		S95.002S	Unspecified injury of dorsal artery of left foot, sequela
		S95.009S	Unsp injury of dorsal artery of unspecified foot, sequela
		S95.011S	Laceration of dorsal artery of right foot, sequela
		S95.012S	Laceration of dorsal artery of left foot, sequela
		S95.019S	Laceration of dorsal artery of unspecified foot, sequela
		S95.091S	Oth injury of dorsal artery of right foot, sequela
		S95.092S	Oth injury of dorsal artery of left foot, sequela
		S95.099S	Oth injury of dorsal artery of unspecified foot, sequela
		S95.101S	Unspecified injury of plantar artery of right foot, sequela
		S95.102S	Unspecified injury of plantar artery of left foot, sequela
		S95.109S	Unsp injury of plantar artery of unspecified foot, sequela
		S95.111S	Laceration of plantar artery of right foot, sequela
		S95.112S	Laceration of plantar artery of left foot, sequela
		S95.119S	Laceration of plantar artery of unspecified foot, sequela
		S95.191S	Oth injury of plantar artery of right foot, sequela
		S95.192S	Oth injury of plantar artery of left foot, sequela
		S95.199S	Oth injury of plantar artery of unspecified foot, sequela
		S95.201S	Unspecified injury of dorsal vein of right foot, sequela
		S95.202S	Unspecified injury of dorsal vein of left foot, sequela
		S95.209S	Unsp injury of dorsal vein of unspecified foot, sequela
		S95.211S	Laceration of dorsal vein of right foot, sequela
		S95.212S	Laceration of dorsal vein of left foot, sequela
		S95.219S	Laceration of dorsal vein of unspecified foot, sequela
		S95.291S	Other specified injury of dorsal vein of right foot, sequela
		S95.292S	Other specified injury of dorsal vein of left foot, sequela
		S95.299S	Oth injury of dorsal vein of unspecified foot, sequela
		S95.801S	Unsp inj blood vessels at ank/ft level, right leg, sequela
		S95.802S	Unsp inj blood vessels at ank/ft level, left leg, sequela
		S95.809S	Unsp inj blood vessels at ank/ft level, unsp leg, sequela
		S95.811S	Lacerat blood vessels at ank/ft level, right leg, sequela
		S95.812S	Lacerat blood vessels at ank/ft level, left leg, sequela
		S95.819S	Lacerat blood vessels at ank/ft level, unsp leg, sequela
		S95.891S	Inj oth blood vessels at ank/ft level, right leg, sequela
		S95.892S	Inj oth blood vessels at ank/ft level, left leg, sequela
		S95.899S	Inj oth blood vessels at ank/ft level, unsp leg, sequela
		S95.901S	Unsp inj unsp blood vess at ank/ft level, right leg, sequela
		S95.902S	Unsp inj unsp blood vess at ank/ft level, left leg, sequela
		S95.909S	Unsp inj unsp blood vess at ank/ft level, unsp leg, sequela
		S95.911S	Lacerat unsp blood vess at ank/ft level, right leg, sequela
		S95.912S	Lacerat unsp blood vessel at ank/ft level, left leg, sequela
		S95.919S	Lacerat unsp blood vessel at ank/ft level, unsp leg, sequela
		S95.991S	Inj unsp blood vessel at ank/ft level, right leg, sequela
		S95.992S	Inj unsp blood vessel at ank/ft level, left leg, sequela
		S95.999S	Inj unsp blood vessel at ank/ft level, unsp leg, sequela
908.4	LATE EFFECT INJURY BLD VESSEL THORAX ABD&PELVIS	**S25.00XS**	Unspecified injury of thoracic aorta, sequela
		S25.01XS	Minor laceration of thoracic aorta, sequela
		S25.02XS	Major laceration of thoracic aorta, sequela
		S25.09XS	Other specified injury of thoracic aorta, sequela
		S25.101S	Unsp injury of right innominate or subclav art, sequela
		S25.102S	Unsp injury of left innominate or subclavian artery, sequela
		S25.109S	Unsp injury of unsp innominate or subclavian artery, sequela
		S25.111S	Minor laceration of right innominate or subclav art, sequela
		S25.112S	Minor laceration of left innominate or subclav art, sequela
		S25.119S	Minor laceration of unsp innominate or subclav art, sequela
		S25.121S	Major laceration of right innominate or subclav art, sequela
		S25.122S	Major laceration of left innominate or subclav art, sequela
		S25.129S	Major laceration of unsp innominate or subclav art, sequela
		S25.191S	Oth injury of right innominate or subclavian artery, sequela
		S25.192S	Oth injury of left innominate or subclavian artery, sequela
		S25.199S	Oth injury of unsp innominate or subclavian artery, sequela
		S25.20XS	Unspecified injury of superior vena cava, sequela
		S25.21XS	Minor laceration of superior vena cava, sequela
		S25.22XS	Major laceration of superior vena cava, sequela
		S25.29XS	Other specified injury of superior vena cava, sequela
	(Continued on next page)	**S25.301S**	Unsp injury of right innominate or subclavian vein, sequela

ICD-9-CM		ICD-10-CM	
9Ø8.4	LATE EFFECT INJURY BLD VESSEL THORAX ABD&PELVIS **(Continued)**	**S25.3Ø2S**	Unsp injury of left innominate or subclavian vein, sequela
		S25.3Ø9S	Unsp injury of unsp innominate or subclavian vein, sequela
		S25.311S	Minor lacerat right innominate or subclav vein, sequela
		S25.312S	Minor laceration of left innominate or subclav vein, sequela
		S25.319S	Minor laceration of unsp innominate or subclav vein, sequela
		S25.321S	Major lacerat right innominate or subclav vein, sequela
		S25.322S	Major laceration of left innominate or subclav vein, sequela
		S25.329S	Major laceration of unsp innominate or subclav vein, sequela
		S25.391S	Oth injury of right innominate or subclavian vein, sequela
		S25.392S	Oth injury of left innominate or subclavian vein, sequela
		S25.399S	Oth injury of unsp innominate or subclavian vein, sequela
		S25.4Ø1S	Unspecified injury of right pulmonary blood vessels, sequela
		S25.4Ø2S	Unspecified injury of left pulmonary blood vessels, sequela
		S25.4Ø9S	Unsp injury of unspecified pulmonary blood vessels, sequela
		S25.411S	Minor laceration of right pulmonary blood vessels, sequela
		S25.412S	Minor laceration of left pulmonary blood vessels, sequela
		S25.419S	Minor laceration of unsp pulmonary blood vessels, sequela
		S25.421S	Major laceration of right pulmonary blood vessels, sequela
		S25.422S	Major laceration of left pulmonary blood vessels, sequela
		S25.429S	Major laceration of unsp pulmonary blood vessels, sequela
		S25.491S	Oth injury of right pulmonary blood vessels, sequela
		S25.492S	Oth injury of left pulmonary blood vessels, sequela
		S25.499S	Oth injury of unspecified pulmonary blood vessels, sequela
		S25.5Ø1S	Unsp injury of intercostl blood vessels, right side, sequela
		S25.5Ø2S	Unsp injury of intercostal blood vessels, left side, sequela
		S25.5Ø9S	Unsp injury of intercostal blood vessels, unsp side, sequela
		S25.511S	Laceration of intercostal blood vessels, right side, sequela
		S25.512S	Laceration of intercostal blood vessels, left side, sequela
		S25.519S	Laceration of intercostal blood vessels, unsp side, sequela
		S25.591S	Oth injury of intercostal blood vessels, right side, sequela
		S25.592S	Oth injury of intercostal blood vessels, left side, sequela
		S25.599S	Oth injury of intercostal blood vessels, unsp side, sequela
		S25.8Ø1S	Unsp injury of blood vessels of thorax, right side, sequela
		S25.8Ø2S	Unsp injury of blood vessels of thorax, left side, sequela
		S25.8Ø9S	Unsp injury of blood vessels of thorax, unsp side, sequela
		S25.811S	Laceration of blood vessels of thorax, right side, sequela
		S25.812S	Laceration of blood vessels of thorax, left side, sequela
		S25.819S	Laceration of blood vessels of thorax, unsp side, sequela
		S25.891S	Inj oth blood vessels of thorax, right side, sequela
		S25.892S	Inj oth blood vessels of thorax, left side, sequela
		S25.899S	Inj oth blood vessels of thorax, unsp side, sequela
		S25.9ØXS	Unsp injury of unspecified blood vessel of thorax, sequela
		S25.91XS	Laceration of unspecified blood vessel of thorax, sequela
		S25.99XS	Oth injury of unspecified blood vessel of thorax, sequela
		S35.ØØXS	Unspecified injury of abdominal aorta, sequela
		S35.Ø1XS	Minor laceration of abdominal aorta, sequela
		S35.Ø2XS	Major laceration of abdominal aorta, sequela
		S35.Ø9XS	Other injury of abdominal aorta, sequela
		S35.1ØXS	Unspecified injury of inferior vena cava, sequela
		S35.11XS	Minor laceration of inferior vena cava, sequela
		S35.12XS	Major laceration of inferior vena cava, sequela
		S35.19XS	Other injury of inferior vena cava, sequela
		S35.211S	Minor laceration of celiac artery, sequela
		S35.212S	Major laceration of celiac artery, sequela
		S35.218S	Other injury of celiac artery, sequela
		S35.219S	Unspecified injury of celiac artery, sequela
		S35.221S	Minor laceration of superior mesenteric artery, sequela
		S35.222S	Major laceration of superior mesenteric artery, sequela
		S35.228S	Other injury of superior mesenteric artery, sequela
		S35.229S	Unspecified injury of superior mesenteric artery, sequela
		S35.231S	Minor laceration of inferior mesenteric artery, sequela
		S35.232S	Major laceration of inferior mesenteric artery, sequela
		S35.238S	Other injury of inferior mesenteric artery, sequela
		S35.239S	Unspecified injury of inferior mesenteric artery, sequela
		S35.291S	Minor lacerat branches of celiac and mesent art, sequela
		S35.292S	Major lacerat branches of celiac and mesent art, sequela
		S35.298S	Inj branches of celiac and mesenteric artery, sequela
		S35.299S	Unsp injury of branches of celiac and mesent art, sequela
		S35.311S	Laceration of portal vein, sequela
		S35.318S	Other specified injury of portal vein, sequela
		S35.319S	Unspecified injury of portal vein, sequela
		S35.321S	Laceration of splenic vein, sequela
		S35.328S	Other specified injury of splenic vein, sequela
		S35.329S	Unspecified injury of splenic vein, sequela
		S35.331S	Laceration of superior mesenteric vein, sequela
		S35.338S	Other specified injury of superior mesenteric vein, sequela
		S35.339S	Unspecified injury of superior mesenteric vein, sequela
		S35.341S	Laceration of inferior mesenteric vein, sequela
		S35.348S	Other specified injury of inferior mesenteric vein, sequela
		S35.349S	Unspecified injury of inferior mesenteric vein, sequela
		S35.4Ø1S	Unspecified injury of right renal artery, sequela
	(Continued on next page)	**S35.4Ø2S**	Unspecified injury of left renal artery, sequela

ICD-9-CM		ICD-10-CM	
908.4	LATE EFFECT INJURY BLD VESSEL THORAX ABD&PELVIS **(Continued)**	**S35.403S**	Unspecified injury of unspecified renal artery, sequela
		S35.404S	Unspecified injury of right renal vein, sequela
		S35.405S	Unspecified injury of left renal vein, sequela
		S35.406S	Unspecified injury of unspecified renal vein, sequela
		S35.411S	Laceration of right renal artery, sequela
		S35.412S	Laceration of left renal artery, sequela
		S35.413S	Laceration of unspecified renal artery, sequela
		S35.414S	Laceration of right renal vein, sequela
		S35.415S	Laceration of left renal vein, sequela
		S35.416S	Laceration of unspecified renal vein, sequela
		S35.491S	Other specified injury of right renal artery, sequela
		S35.492S	Other specified injury of left renal artery, sequela
		S35.493S	Other specified injury of unspecified renal artery, sequela
		S35.494S	Other specified injury of right renal vein, sequela
		S35.495S	Other specified injury of left renal vein, sequela
		S35.496S	Other specified injury of unspecified renal vein, sequela
		S35.50XS	Injury of unspecified iliac blood vessel(s), sequela
		S35.511S	Injury of right iliac artery, sequela
		S35.512S	Injury of left iliac artery, sequela
		S35.513S	Injury of unspecified iliac artery, sequela
		S35.514S	Injury of right iliac vein, sequela
		S35.515S	Injury of left iliac vein, sequela
		S35.516S	Injury of unspecified iliac vein, sequela
		S35.531S	Injury of right uterine artery, sequela
		S35.532S	Injury of left uterine artery, sequela
		S35.533S	Injury of unspecified uterine artery, sequela
		S35.534S	Injury of right uterine vein, sequela
		S35.535S	Injury of left uterine vein, sequela
		S35.536S	Injury of unspecified uterine vein, sequela
		S35.59XS	Injury of other iliac blood vessels, sequela
		S35.8X1S	Lacerat blood vesls at abd, low back and pelvis level, sqla
		S35.8X8S	Inj oth blood vesls at abd, low back and pelvis level, sqla
		S35.8X9S	Unsp inj blood vesls at abd, low back and pelvis level, sqla
		S35.90XS	Unsp inj unsp bld vess at abd, low back and pelv level, sqla
		S35.91XS	Lacerat unsp bld vess at abd, low back and pelv level, sqla
		S35.99XS	Inj unsp blood vess at abd, low back and pelvis level, sqla
908.5	LATE EFFECT OF FOREIGN BODY IN ORIFICE	**T15.00XS**	Foreign body in cornea, unspecified eye, sequela
		T15.01XS	Foreign body in cornea, right eye, sequela
		T15.02XS	Foreign body in cornea, left eye, sequela
		T15.10XS	Foreign body in conjunctival sac, unspecified eye, sequela
		T15.11XS	Foreign body in conjunctival sac, right eye, sequela
		T15.12XS	Foreign body in conjunctival sac, left eye, sequela
		T15.80XS	Fb in oth and multiple parts of extrn eye, unsp eye, sequela
		T15.81XS	Fb in oth and multiple parts of external eye, r eye, sequela
		T15.82XS	Fb in oth and multiple parts of extrn eye, left eye, sequela
		T15.90XS	Foreign body on external eye, part unsp, unsp eye, sequela
		T15.91XS	Foreign body on external eye, part unsp, right eye, sequela
		T15.92XS	Foreign body on external eye, part unsp, left eye, sequela
		T16.1XXS	Foreign body in right ear, sequela
		T16.2XXS	Foreign body in left ear, sequela
		T16.9XXS	Foreign body in ear, unspecified ear, sequela
		T17.0XXS	Foreign body in nasal sinus, sequela
		T17.1XXS	Foreign body in nostril, sequela
		T17.200S	Unsp foreign body in pharynx causing asphyxiation, sequela
		T17.208S	Unsp foreign body in pharynx causing other injury, sequela
		T17.210S	Gastric contents in pharynx causing asphyxiation, sequela
		T17.218S	Gastric contents in pharynx causing other injury, sequela
		T17.220S	Food in pharynx causing asphyxiation, sequela
		T17.228S	Food in pharynx causing other injury, sequela
		T17.290S	Oth foreign object in pharynx causing asphyxiation, sequela
		T17.298S	Oth foreign object in pharynx causing other injury, sequela
		T17.300S	Unsp foreign body in larynx causing asphyxiation, sequela
		T17.308S	Unsp foreign body in larynx causing other injury, sequela
		T17.310S	Gastric contents in larynx causing asphyxiation, sequela
		T17.318S	Gastric contents in larynx causing other injury, sequela
		T17.320S	Food in larynx causing asphyxiation, sequela
		T17.328S	Food in larynx causing other injury, sequela
		T17.390S	Other foreign object in larynx causing asphyxiation, sequela
		T17.398S	Other foreign object in larynx causing other injury, sequela
		T17.400S	Unsp foreign body in trachea causing asphyxiation, sequela
		T17.408S	Unsp foreign body in trachea causing other injury, sequela
		T17.410S	Gastric contents in trachea causing asphyxiation, sequela
		T17.418S	Gastric contents in trachea causing other injury, sequela
		T17.420S	Food in trachea causing asphyxiation, sequela
		T17.428S	Food in trachea causing other injury, sequela
		T17.490S	Oth foreign object in trachea causing asphyxiation, sequela
		T17.498S	Oth foreign object in trachea causing other injury, sequela
		T17.500S	Unsp foreign body in bronchus causing asphyxiation, sequela
		T17.508S	Unsp foreign body in bronchus causing other injury, sequela
		T17.510S	Gastric contents in bronchus causing asphyxiation, sequela
		T17.518S	Gastric contents in bronchus causing other injury, sequela
		T17.520S	Food in bronchus causing asphyxiation, sequela

(Continued on next page)

ICD-9-CM		ICD-10-CM	
9Ø8.5	LATE EFFECT OF FOREIGN BODY IN ORIFICE **(Continued)**	**T17.528S**	Food in bronchus causing other injury, sequela
		T17.59ØS	Oth foreign object in bronchus causing asphyxiation, sequela
		T17.598S	Oth foreign object in bronchus causing other injury, sequela
		T17.8ØØS	Unsp fb in oth prt resp tract causing asphyx, sequela
		T17.8Ø8S	Unsp fb in oth prt resp tract causing oth injury, sequela
		T17.81ØS	Gastric contents in oth prt resp tract cause asphyx, sequela
		T17.818S	Gastr contents in oth prt resp tract cause oth injury, sqla
		T17.82ØS	Food in oth prt resp tract causing asphyxiation, sequela
		T17.828S	Food in oth prt resp tract causing oth injury, sequela
		T17.89ØS	Oth forn object in oth prt resp tract cause asphyx, sequela
		T17.898S	Oth forn object in oth prt resp tract cause oth injury, sqla
		T17.9ØØS	Unsp fb in resp tract, part unsp causing asphyx, sequela
		T17.9Ø8S	Unsp fb in resp tract, part unsp causing oth injury, sequela
		T17.91ØS	Gastr contents in resp tract, part unsp cause asphyx, sqla
		T17.918S	Gastr contents in resp tract, part unsp cause oth inj, sqla
		T17.92ØS	Food in resp tract, part unsp causing asphyxiation, sequela
		T17.928S	Food in resp tract, part unsp causing oth injury, sequela
		T17.99ØS	Oth forn obj in resp tract, part unsp in cause asphyx, sqla
		T17.998S	Oth forn object in resp tract, part unsp cause oth inj, sqla
		T18.ØXXS	Foreign body in mouth, sequela
		T18.1ØØS	Unsp fb in esophagus causing compression of trachea, sequela
		T18.1Ø8S	Unsp foreign body in esophagus causing other injury, sequela
		T18.11ØS	Gastric contents in esoph cause comprsn of trachea, sequela
		T18.118S	Gastric contents in esophagus causing other injury, sequela
		T18.12ØS	Food in esophagus causing compression of trachea, sequela
		T18.128S	Food in esophagus causing other injury, sequela
		T18.19ØS	Oth forn object in esoph cause comprsn of trachea, sequela
		T18.198S	Oth foreign object in esophagus causing oth injury, sequela
		T18.2XXS	Foreign body in stomach, sequela
		T18.3XXS	Foreign body in small intestine, sequela
		T18.4XXS	Foreign body in colon, sequela
		T18.5XXS	Foreign body in anus and rectum, sequela
		T18.8XXS	Foreign body in other parts of alimentary tract, sequela
		T18.9XXS	Foreign body of alimentary tract, part unspecified, sequela
		T19.ØXXS	Foreign body in urethra, sequela
		T19.1XXS	Foreign body in bladder, sequela
		T19.2XXS	Foreign body in vulva and vagina, sequela
		T19.3XXS	Foreign body in uterus, sequela
		T19.4XXS	Foreign body in penis, sequela
		T19.8XXS	Foreign body in other parts of genitourinary tract, sequela
		T19.9XXS	Foreign body in genitourinary tract, part unsp, sequela
9Ø8.6	LATE EFFECT OF CERTAIN COMPLICATIONS OF TRAUMA	**T79.ØXXS**	Air embolism (traumatic), sequela
		T79.1XXS	Fat embolism (traumatic), sequela
		T79.2XXS	Traumatic secondary and recurrent hemor and seroma, sequela
		T79.4XXS	Traumatic shock, sequela
		T79.5XXS	Traumatic anuria, sequela
		T79.6XXS	Traumatic ischemia of muscle, sequela
		T79.7XXS	Traumatic subcutaneous emphysema, sequela
		T79.8XXS	Other early complications of trauma, sequela
		T79.9XXS	Unspecified early complication of trauma, sequela
		T79.AØXS	Compartment syndrome, unspecified, sequela
		T79.A11S	Traumatic compartment syndrome of r up extrem, sequela
		T79.A12S	Traumatic compartment syndrome of l up extrem, sequela
		T79.A19S	Traumatic compartment syndrome of unsp up extrem, sequela
		T79.A21S	Traumatic compartment syndrome of r low extrem, sequela
		T79.A22S	Traumatic compartment syndrome of l low extrem, sequela
		T79.A29S	Traumatic compartment syndrome of unsp low extrm, sequela
		T79.A3XS	Traumatic compartment syndrome of abdomen, sequela
		T79.A9XS	Traumatic compartment syndrome of other sites, sequela
9Ø8.9	LATE EFFECT OF UNSPECIFIED INJURY	**SØ5.7ØXS**	Avulsion of unspecified eye, sequela
		SØ5.71XS	Avulsion of right eye, sequela
		SØ5.72XS	Avulsion of left eye, sequela
		SØ5.8X1S	Other injuries of right eye and orbit, sequela
		SØ5.8X2S	Other injuries of left eye and orbit, sequela
		SØ5.8X9S	Other injuries of unspecified eye and orbit, sequela
		SØ5.9ØXS	Unspecified injury of unspecified eye and orbit, sequela
		SØ5.91XS	Unspecified injury of right eye and orbit, sequela
		SØ5.92XS	Unspecified injury of left eye and orbit, sequela
		SØ9.1ØXS	Unspecified injury of muscle and tendon of head, sequela
		SØ9.19XS	Other specified injury of muscle and tendon of head, sequela
		SØ9.2ØXS	Traumatic rupture of unspecified ear drum, sequela
		SØ9.3Ø1S	Unspecified injury of right middle and inner ear, sequela
		SØ9.3Ø2S	Unspecified injury of left middle and inner ear, sequela
		SØ9.3Ø9S	Unsp injury of unspecified middle and inner ear, sequela
		SØ9.391S	Oth injury of right middle and inner ear, sequela
		SØ9.392S	Other specified injury of left middle and inner ear, sequela
		SØ9.399S	Oth injury of unspecified middle and inner ear, sequela
		SØ9.8XXS	Other specified injuries of head, sequela
		SØ9.9ØXS	Unspecified injury of head, sequela
		SØ9.91XS	Unspecified injury of ear, sequela
		SØ9.92XS	Unspecified injury of nose, sequela
	(Continued on next page)	**SØ9.93XS**	Unspecified injury of face, sequela

ICD-9-CM		ICD-10-CM	
908.9	LATE EFFECT OF UNSPECIFIED INJURY **(Continued)**	**S16.8XXS**	Inj muscle, fascia and tendon at neck level, sequela
		S16.9XXS	Unsp injury of musc/fasc/tend at neck level, sequela
		S19.80XS	Oth injuries of unspecified part of neck, sequela
		S19.81XS	Other specified injuries of larynx, sequela
		S19.82XS	Other specified injuries of cervical trachea, sequela
		S19.83XS	Other specified injuries of vocal cord, sequela
		S19.84XS	Other specified injuries of thyroid gland, sequela
		S19.85XS	Oth injuries of pharynx and cervical esophagus, sequela
		S19.89XS	Oth injuries of other specified part of neck, sequela
		S19.9XXS	Unspecified injury of neck, sequela
		S29.001S	Unsp injury of msl/tnd of front wall of thorax, sequela
		S29.002S	Unsp injury of msl/tnd of back wall of thorax, sequela
		S29.009S	Unsp injury of msl/tnd of unsp wall of thorax, sequela
		S29.091S	Inj muscle and tendon of front wall of thorax, sequela
		S29.092S	Inj muscle and tendon of back wall of thorax, sequela
		S29.099S	Inj muscle and tendon of unsp wall of thorax, sequela
		S29.8XXS	Other specified injuries of thorax, sequela
		S29.9XXS	Unspecified injury of thorax, sequela
		S39.001S	Unsp injury of muscle, fascia and tendon of abdomen, sequela
		S39.002S	Unsp injury of musc/fasc/tend lower back, sequela
		S39.003S	Unsp injury of muscle, fascia and tendon of pelvis, sequela
		S39.091S	Oth injury of muscle, fascia and tendon of abdomen, sequela
		S39.092S	Inj muscle, fascia and tendon of lower back, sequela
		S39.093S	Other injury of muscle, fascia and tendon of pelvis, sequela
		S39.81XS	Other specified injuries of abdomen, sequela
		S39.82XS	Other specified injuries of lower back, sequela
		S39.83XS	Other specified injuries of pelvis, sequela
		S39.840S	Fracture of corpus cavernosum penis, sequela
		S39.848S	Other specified injuries of external genitals, sequela
		S39.91XS	Unspecified injury of abdomen, sequela
		S39.92XS	Unspecified injury of lower back, sequela
		S39.93XS	Unspecified injury of pelvis, sequela
		S39.94XS	Unspecified injury of external genitals, sequela
		S46.001S	Unsp inj musc/tend the rotator cuff of r shoulder, sequela
		S46.002S	Unsp inj musc/tend the rotator cuff of l shoulder, sequela
		S46.009S	Unsp inj musc/tend the rotator cuff of unsp shldr, sequela
		S46.091S	Inj musc/tend the rotator cuff of right shoulder, sequela
		S46.092S	Inj musc/tend the rotator cuff of left shoulder, sequela
		S46.099S	Inj musc/tend the rotator cuff of unsp shoulder, sequela
		S46.101S	Unsp inj musc/fasc/tend long hd bicep, right arm, sequela
		S46.102S	Unsp inj musc/fasc/tend long hd bicep, left arm, sequela
		S46.109S	Unsp inj musc/fasc/tend long hd bicep, unsp arm, sequela
		S46.191S	Inj musc/fasc/tend long head of biceps, right arm, sequela
		S46.192S	Inj musc/fasc/tend long head of biceps, left arm, sequela
		S46.199S	Inj musc/fasc/tend long head of biceps, unsp arm, sequela
		S46.201S	Unsp injury of musc/fasc/tend prt biceps, right arm, sequela
		S46.202S	Unsp injury of musc/fasc/tend prt biceps, left arm, sequela
		S46.209S	Unsp injury of musc/fasc/tend prt biceps, unsp arm, sequela
		S46.291S	Inj musc/fasc/tend prt biceps, right arm, sequela
		S46.292S	Inj musc/fasc/tend prt biceps, left arm, sequela
		S46.299S	Inj musc/fasc/tend prt biceps, unsp arm, sequela
		S46.301S	Unsp injury of musc/fasc/tend triceps, right arm, sequela
		S46.302S	Unsp injury of musc/fasc/tend triceps, left arm, sequela
		S46.309S	Unsp injury of musc/fasc/tend triceps, unsp arm, sequela
		S46.391S	Inj muscle, fascia and tendon of triceps, right arm, sequela
		S46.392S	Inj muscle, fascia and tendon of triceps, left arm, sequela
		S46.399S	Inj muscle, fascia and tendon of triceps, unsp arm, sequela
		S46.801S	Unsp inj musc/fasc/tend at shldr/up arm, right arm, sequela
		S46.802S	Unsp inj musc/fasc/tend at shldr/up arm, left arm, sequela
		S46.809S	Unsp inj musc/fasc/tend at shldr/up arm, unsp arm, sequela
		S46.891S	Inj musc/fasc/tend at shldr/up arm, right arm, sequela
		S46.892S	Inj musc/fasc/tend at shldr/up arm, left arm, sequela
		S46.899S	Inj musc/fasc/tend at shldr/up arm, unsp arm, sequela
		S46.901S	Unsp inj unsp musc/fasc/tend at shldr/up arm, r arm, sqla
		S46.902S	Unsp inj unsp musc/fasc/tend at shldr/up arm, left arm, sqla
		S46.909S	Unsp inj unsp musc/fasc/tend at shldr/up arm, unsp arm, sqla
		S46.991S	Inj unsp musc/fasc/tend at shldr/up arm, right arm, sequela
		S46.992S	Inj unsp musc/fasc/tend at shldr/up arm, left arm, sequela
		S46.999S	Inj unsp musc/fasc/tend at shldr/up arm, unsp arm, sequela
		S49.80XS	Oth injuries of shoulder and upper arm, unsp arm, sequela
		S49.81XS	Oth injuries of right shoulder and upper arm, sequela
		S49.82XS	Oth injuries of left shoulder and upper arm, sequela
		S49.90XS	Unsp injury of shoulder and upper arm, unsp arm, sequela
		S49.91XS	Unspecified injury of right shoulder and upper arm, sequela
		S49.92XS	Unspecified injury of left shoulder and upper arm, sequela
		S56.001S	Unsp inj flexor musc/fasc/tend r thm at forarm lv, sequela
		S56.002S	Unsp inj flexor musc/fasc/tend l thm at forarm lv, sequela
		S56.009S	Unsp inj flexor musc/fasc/tend thmb at forarm lv, sequela
		S56.091S	Inj flexor musc/fasc/tend right thumb at forarm lv, sequela
		S56.092S	Inj flexor musc/fasc/tend left thumb at forarm lv, sequela
		S56.099S	Inj flexor musc/fasc/tend thmb at forearm level, sequela
	(Continued on next page)	**S56.101S**	Unsp inj flexor musc/fasc/tend r idx fngr at forarm lv, sqla

ICD-9-CM		ICD-10-CM	
9Ø8.9	LATE EFFECT OF UNSPECIFIED INJURY **(Continued)**	**S56.1Ø2S**	Unsp inj flexor musc/fasc/tend l idx fngr at forarm lv, sqla
		S56.1Ø3S	Unsp inj flexor musc/fasc/tend r mid fngr at forarm lv, sqla
		S56.1Ø4S	Unsp inj flexor musc/fasc/tend l mid fngr at forarm lv, sqla
		S56.1Ø5S	Unsp inj flexor musc/fasc/tend r rng fngr at forarm lv, sqla
		S56.1Ø6S	Unsp inj flexor musc/fasc/tend l rng fngr at forarm lv, sqla
		S56.1Ø7S	Unsp inj flxr musc/fasc/tend r lit fngr at forarm lv, sqla
		S56.1Ø8S	Unsp inj flxr musc/fasc/tend l lit fngr at forarm lv, sqla
		S56.1Ø9S	Unsp inj flexor musc/fasc/tend unsp fngr at forarm lv, sqla
		S56.191S	Inj flexor musc/fasc/tend r idx fngr at forarm lv, sequela
		S56.192S	Inj flexor musc/fasc/tend l idx fngr at forarm lv, sequela
		S56.193S	Inj flexor musc/fasc/tend r mid finger at forarm lv, sequela
		S56.194S	Inj flexor musc/fasc/tend l mid finger at forarm lv, sequela
		S56.195S	Inj flexor musc/fasc/tend r rng fngr at forarm lv, sequela
		S56.196S	Inj flexor musc/fasc/tend l rng fngr at forarm lv, sequela
		S56.197S	Inj flexor musc/fasc/tend r little finger at forarm lv, sqla
		S56.198S	Inj flexor musc/fasc/tend l little finger at forarm lv, sqla
		S56.199S	Inj flexor musc/fasc/tend unsp finger at forarm lv, sequela
		S56.2Ø1S	Unsp inj flexor musc/fasc/tend at forarm lv, right arm, sqla
		S56.2Ø2S	Unsp inj flexor musc/fasc/tend at forarm lv, left arm, sqla
		S56.2Ø9S	Unsp inj flexor musc/fasc/tend at forarm lv, unsp arm, sqla
		S56.291S	Inj oth flexor musc/fasc/tend at forarm lv, right arm, sqla
		S56.292S	Inj oth flexor musc/fasc/tend at forarm lv, left arm, sqla
		S56.299S	Inj oth flexor musc/fasc/tend at forarm lv, unsp arm, sqla
		S56.3Ø1S	Unsp inj extn/abdr musc/fasc/tend of r thm at forarm lv,sqla
		S56.3Ø2S	Unsp inj extn/abdr musc/fasc/tend of l thm at forarm lv,sqla
		S56.3Ø9S	Unsp inj extn/abdr musc/fasc/tend of thmb at forarm lv, sqla
		S56.391S	Inj extn/abdr musc/fasc/tend of r thm at forarm lv, sequela
		S56.392S	Inj extn/abdr musc/fasc/tend of l thm at forarm lv, sequela
		S56.399S	Inj extn/abdr musc/fasc/tend of thmb at forarm lv, sequela
		S56.4Ø1S	Unsp inj extn musc/fasc/tend r idx fngr at forarm lv, sqla
		S56.4Ø2S	Unsp inj extn musc/fasc/tend l idx fngr at forarm lv, sqla
		S56.4Ø3S	Unsp inj extn musc/fasc/tend r mid finger at forarm lv, sqla
		S56.4Ø4S	Unsp inj extn musc/fasc/tend l mid finger at forarm lv, sqla
		S56.4Ø5S	Unsp inj extn musc/fasc/tend r rng fngr at forarm lv, sqla
		S56.4Ø6S	Unsp inj extn musc/fasc/tend l rng fngr at forarm lv, sqla
		S56.4Ø7S	Unsp inj extn musc/fasc/tend r lit fngr at forarm lv, sqla
		S56.4Ø8S	Unsp inj extn musc/fasc/tend l lit fngr at forarm lv, sqla
		S56.4Ø9S	Unsp inj extn musc/fasc/tend unsp finger at forarm lv, sqla
		S56.491S	Inj extensor musc/fasc/tend r idx fngr at forarm lv, sequela
		S56.492S	Inj extensor musc/fasc/tend l idx fngr at forarm lv, sequela
		S56.493S	Inj extn musc/fasc/tend r mid finger at forarm lv, sequela
		S56.494S	Inj extn musc/fasc/tend l mid finger at forarm lv, sequela
		S56.495S	Inj extensor musc/fasc/tend r rng fngr at forarm lv, sequela
		S56.496S	Inj extensor musc/fasc/tend l rng fngr at forarm lv, sequela
		S56.497S	Inj extn musc/fasc/tend r little finger at forarm lv, sqla
		S56.498S	Inj extn musc/fasc/tend l little finger at forarm lv, sqla
		S56.499S	Inj extn musc/fasc/tend unsp finger at forarm lv, sequela
		S56.5Ø1S	Unsp inj extn musc/fasc/tend at forarm lv, right arm, sqla
		S56.5Ø2S	Unsp inj extn musc/fasc/tend at forarm lv, left arm, sequela
		S56.5Ø9S	Unsp inj extn musc/fasc/tend at forarm lv, unsp arm, sequela
		S56.591S	Inj extn musc/fasc/tend at forearm level, right arm, sequela
		S56.592S	Inj extn musc/fasc/tend at forearm level, left arm, sequela
		S56.599S	Inj extn musc/fasc/tend at forearm level, unsp arm, sequela
		S56.8Ø1S	Unsp inj musc/fasc/tend at forarm lv, right arm, sequela
		S56.8Ø2S	Unsp inj musc/fasc/tend at forarm lv, left arm, sequela
		S56.8Ø9S	Unsp inj musc/fasc/tend at forarm lv, unsp arm, sequela
		S56.891S	Inj musc/fasc/tend at forearm level, right arm, sequela
		S56.892S	Inj musc/fasc/tend at forearm level, left arm, sequela
		S56.899S	Inj musc/fasc/tend at forearm level, unsp arm, sequela
		S56.9Ø1S	Unsp inj unsp musc/fasc/tend at forarm lv, right arm, sqla
		S56.9Ø2S	Unsp inj unsp musc/fasc/tend at forarm lv, left arm, sequela
		S56.9Ø9S	Unsp inj unsp musc/fasc/tend at forarm lv, unsp arm, sequela
		S56.991S	Inj unsp musc/fasc/tend at forearm level, right arm, sequela
		S56.992S	Inj unsp musc/fasc/tend at forearm level, left arm, sequela
		S56.999S	Inj unsp musc/fasc/tend at forearm level, unsp arm, sequela
		S59.8Ø1S	Other specified injuries of right elbow, sequela
		S59.8Ø2S	Other specified injuries of left elbow, sequela
		S59.8Ø9S	Other specified injuries of unspecified elbow, sequela
		S59.811S	Other specified injuries right forearm, sequela
		S59.812S	Other specified injuries left forearm, sequela
		S59.819S	Other specified injuries unspecified forearm, sequela
		S59.9Ø1S	Unspecified injury of right elbow, sequela
		S59.9Ø2S	Unspecified injury of left elbow, sequela
		S59.9Ø9S	Unspecified injury of unspecified elbow, sequela
		S59.911S	Unspecified injury of right forearm, sequela
		S59.912S	Unspecified injury of left forearm, sequela
		S59.919S	Unspecified injury of unspecified forearm, sequela
		S66.ØØ1S	Unsp inj long flxr musc/fasc/tend r thm at wrs/hnd lv, sqla
		S66.ØØ2S	Unsp inj long flxr musc/fasc/tend l thm at wrs/hnd lv, sqla
		S66.ØØ9S	Unsp inj long flexor musc/fasc/tend thmb at wrs/hnd lv, sqla
		S66.Ø91S	Inj long flexor musc/fasc/tend r thm at wrs/hnd lv, sequela
9Ø8.9	**(Continued on next page)**	**S66.Ø92S**	Inj long flexor musc/fasc/tend l thm at wrs/hnd lv, sequela

ICD-9-CM		ICD-10-CM	
908.9	LATE EFFECT OF UNSPECIFIED INJURY **(Continued)**	**S66.099S**	Inj long flexor musc/fasc/tend thmb at wrs/hnd lv, sequela
		S66.100S	Unsp inj flxr musc/fasc/tend r idx fngr at wrs/hnd lv, sqla
		S66.101S	Unsp inj flxr musc/fasc/tend l idx fngr at wrs/hnd lv, sqla
		S66.102S	Unsp inj flxr musc/fasc/tend r mid fngr at wrs/hnd lv, sqla
		S66.103S	Unsp inj flxr musc/fasc/tend l mid fngr at wrs/hnd lv, sqla
		S66.104S	Unsp inj flxr musc/fasc/tend r rng fngr at wrs/hnd lv, sqla
		S66.105S	Unsp inj flxr musc/fasc/tend l rng fngr at wrs/hnd lv, sqla
		S66.106S	Unsp inj flxr musc/fasc/tend r lit fngr at wrs/hnd lv, sqla
		S66.107S	Unsp inj flxr musc/fasc/tend l lit fngr at wrs/hnd lv, sqla
		S66.108S	Unsp inj flexor musc/fasc/tend finger at wrs/hnd lv, sequela
		S66.109S	Unsp inj flexor musc/fasc/tend unsp fngr at wrs/hnd lv, sqla
		S66.190S	Inj flexor musc/fasc/tend r idx fngr at wrs/hnd lv, sequela
		S66.191S	Inj flexor musc/fasc/tend l idx fngr at wrs/hnd lv, sequela
		S66.192S	Inj flexor musc/fasc/tend r mid finger at wrs/hnd lv, sqla
		S66.193S	Inj flexor musc/fasc/tend l mid finger at wrs/hnd lv, sqla
		S66.194S	Inj flexor musc/fasc/tend r rng fngr at wrs/hnd lv, sequela
		S66.195S	Inj flexor musc/fasc/tend l rng fngr at wrs/hnd lv, sequela
		S66.196S	Inj flexor musc/fasc/tend r little fngr at wrs/hnd lv, sqla
		S66.197S	Inj flexor musc/fasc/tend l little fngr at wrs/hnd lv, sqla
		S66.198S	Inj flexor musc/fasc/tend finger at wrs/hnd lv, sequela
		S66.199S	Inj flexor musc/fasc/tend unsp finger at wrs/hnd lv, sequela
		S66.201S	Unsp inj extn musc/fasc/tend r thm at wrs/hnd lv, sequela
		S66.202S	Unsp inj extn musc/fasc/tend l thm at wrs/hnd lv, sequela
		S66.209S	Unsp inj extensor musc/fasc/tend thmb at wrs/hnd lv, sequela
		S66.291S	Inj extensor musc/fasc/tend r thm at wrs/hnd lv, sequela
		S66.292S	Inj extensor musc/fasc/tend l thm at wrs/hnd lv, sequela
		S66.299S	Inj extensor musc/fasc/tend thmb at wrs/hnd lv, sequela
		S66.300S	Unsp inj extn musc/fasc/tend r idx fngr at wrs/hnd lv, sqla
		S66.301S	Unsp inj extn musc/fasc/tend l idx fngr at wrs/hnd lv, sqla
		S66.302S	Unsp inj extn musc/fasc/tend r mid fngr at wrs/hnd lv, sqla
		S66.303S	Unsp inj extn musc/fasc/tend l mid fngr at wrs/hnd lv, sqla
		S66.304S	Unsp inj extn musc/fasc/tend r rng fngr at wrs/hnd lv, sqla
		S66.305S	Unsp inj extn musc/fasc/tend l rng fngr at wrs/hnd lv, sqla
		S66.306S	Unsp inj extn musc/fasc/tend r lit fngr at wrs/hnd lv, sqla
		S66.307S	Unsp inj extn musc/fasc/tend l lit fngr at wrs/hnd lv, sqla
		S66.308S	Unsp inj extn musc/fasc/tend finger at wrs/hnd lv, sequela
		S66.309S	Unsp inj extn musc/fasc/tend unsp finger at wrs/hnd lv, sqla
		S66.390S	Inj extn musc/fasc/tend r idx fngr at wrs/hnd lv, sequela
		S66.391S	Inj extn musc/fasc/tend l idx fngr at wrs/hnd lv, sequela
		S66.392S	Inj extn musc/fasc/tend r mid finger at wrs/hnd lv, sequela
		S66.393S	Inj extn musc/fasc/tend l mid finger at wrs/hnd lv, sequela
		S66.394S	Inj extn musc/fasc/tend r rng fngr at wrs/hnd lv, sequela
		S66.395S	Inj extn musc/fasc/tend l rng fngr at wrs/hnd lv, sequela
		S66.396S	Inj extn musc/fasc/tend r little finger at wrs/hnd lv, sqla
		S66.397S	Inj extn musc/fasc/tend l little finger at wrs/hnd lv, sqla
		S66.398S	Inj extensor musc/fasc/tend finger at wrs/hnd lv, sequela
		S66.399S	Inj extn musc/fasc/tend unsp finger at wrs/hnd lv, sequela
		S66.401S	Unsp inj intrns musc/fasc/tend r thm at wrs/hnd lv, sequela
		S66.402S	Unsp inj intrns musc/fasc/tend l thm at wrs/hnd lv, sequela
		S66.409S	Unsp inj intrns musc/fasc/tend thmb at wrs/hnd lv, sequela
		S66.491S	Inj intrinsic musc/fasc/tend r thm at wrs/hnd lv, sequela
		S66.492S	Inj intrinsic musc/fasc/tend l thm at wrs/hnd lv, sequela
		S66.499S	Inj intrinsic musc/fasc/tend thmb at wrs/hnd lv, sequela
		S66.500S	Unsp inj intrns musc/fasc/tend r idx fngr at wrs/hnd lv,sqla
		S66.501S	Unsp inj intrns musc/fasc/tend l idx fngr at wrs/hnd lv,sqla
		S66.502S	Unsp inj intrns musc/fasc/tend r mid fngr at wrs/hnd lv,sqla
		S66.503S	Unsp inj intrns musc/fasc/tend l mid fngr at wrs/hnd lv,sqla
		S66.504S	Unsp inj intrns musc/fasc/tend r rng fngr at wrs/hnd lv,sqla
		S66.505S	Unsp inj intrns musc/fasc/tend l rng fngr at wrs/hnd lv,sqla
		S66.506S	Unsp inj intrns musc/fasc/tend r lit fngr at wrs/hnd lv,sqla
		S66.507S	Unsp inj intrns musc/fasc/tend l lit fngr at wrs/hnd lv,sqla
		S66.508S	Unsp inj intrns musc/fasc/tend finger at wrs/hnd lv, sequela
		S66.509S	Unsp inj intrns musc/fasc/tend unsp fngr at wrs/hnd lv, sqla
		S66.590S	Inj intrns musc/fasc/tend r idx fngr at wrs/hnd lv, sequela
		S66.591S	Inj intrns musc/fasc/tend l idx fngr at wrs/hnd lv, sequela
		S66.592S	Inj intrns musc/fasc/tend r mid finger at wrs/hnd lv, sqla
		S66.593S	Inj intrns musc/fasc/tend l mid finger at wrs/hnd lv, sqla
		S66.594S	Inj intrns musc/fasc/tend r rng fngr at wrs/hnd lv, sequela
		S66.595S	Inj intrns musc/fasc/tend l rng fngr at wrs/hnd lv, sequela
		S66.596S	Inj intrns musc/fasc/tend r little fngr at wrs/hnd lv, sqla
		S66.597S	Inj intrns musc/fasc/tend l little fngr at wrs/hnd lv, sqla
		S66.598S	Inj intrinsic musc/fasc/tend finger at wrs/hnd lv, sequela
		S66.599S	Inj intrns musc/fasc/tend unsp finger at wrs/hnd lv, sequela
		S66.801S	Unsp injury of musc/fasc/tend at wrs/hnd lv, r hand, sequela
		S66.802S	Unsp inj musc/fasc/tend at wrs/hnd lv, left hand, sequela
		S66.809S	Unsp inj musc/fasc/tend at wrs/hnd lv, unsp hand, sequela
		S66.891S	Inj musc/fasc/tend at wrs/hnd lv, right hand, sequela
		S66.892S	Inj musc/fasc/tend at wrs/hnd lv, left hand, sequela
		S66.899S	Inj musc/fasc/tend at wrs/hnd lv, unsp hand, sequela
		S66.901S	Unsp inj unsp musc/fasc/tend at wrs/hnd lv, r hand, sequela
		S66.902S	Unsp inj unsp musc/fasc/tend at wrs/hnd lv, l hand, sequela
		S66.909S	Unsp inj unsp musc/fasc/tend at wrs/hnd lv, unsp hand, sqla
	(Continued on next page)	**S66.991S**	Inj unsp musc/fasc/tend at wrs/hnd lv, right hand, sequela

ICD-9-CM		ICD-10-CM	
908.9	LATE EFFECT OF UNSPECIFIED INJURY **(Continued)**	**S66.992S**	Inj unsp musc/fasc/tend at wrs/hnd lv, left hand, sequela
		S66.999S	Inj unsp musc/fasc/tend at wrs/hnd lv, unsp hand, sequela
		S69.80XS	Oth injuries of unsp wrist, hand and finger(s), sequela
		S69.81XS	Oth injuries of right wrist, hand and finger(s), sequela
		S69.82XS	Oth injuries of left wrist, hand and finger(s), sequela
		S69.90XS	Unsp injury of unsp wrist, hand and finger(s), sequela
		S69.91XS	Unsp injury of right wrist, hand and finger(s), sequela
		S69.92XS	Unsp injury of left wrist, hand and finger(s), sequela
		S76.001S	Unsp injury of musc/fasc/tend right hip, sequela
		S76.002S	Unsp injury of musc/fasc/tend left hip, sequela
		S76.009S	Unsp injury of musc/fasc/tend unsp hip, sequela
		S76.091S	Inj muscle, fascia and tendon of right hip, sequela
		S76.092S	Oth injury of muscle, fascia and tendon of left hip, sequela
		S76.099S	Oth injury of muscle, fascia and tendon of unsp hip, sequela
		S76.101S	Unsp injury of right quadriceps musc/fasc/tend, sequela
		S76.102S	Unsp injury of left quadriceps musc/fasc/tend, sequela
		S76.109S	Unsp injury of unsp quadriceps musc/fasc/tend, sequela
		S76.191S	Inj right quadriceps muscle, fascia and tendon, sequela
		S76.192S	Inj left quadriceps muscle, fascia and tendon, sequela
		S76.199S	Inj unsp quadriceps muscle, fascia and tendon, sequela
		S76.201S	Unsp injury of adductor musc/fasc/tend right thigh, sequela
		S76.202S	Unsp injury of adductor musc/fasc/tend left thigh, sequela
		S76.209S	Unsp injury of adductor musc/fasc/tend unsp thigh, sequela
		S76.291S	Inj adductor musc/fasc/tend right thigh, sequela
		S76.292S	Inj adductor musc/fasc/tend left thigh, sequela
		S76.299S	Inj adductor musc/fasc/tend unsp thigh, sequela
		S76.301S	Unsp inj msl/fasc/tnd post grp at thi lev, right thigh, sqla
		S76.302S	Unsp inj msl/fasc/tnd post grp at thi lev, left thigh, sqla
		S76.309S	Unsp inj msl/fasc/tnd post grp at thi lev, unsp thigh, sqla
		S76.391S	Inj msl/fasc/tnd post grp at thi lev, right thigh, sequela
		S76.392S	Inj msl/fasc/tnd post grp at thi lev, left thigh, sequela
		S76.399S	Inj msl/fasc/tnd post grp at thi lev, unsp thigh, sequela
		S76.801S	Unsp inj musc/fasc/tend at thi lev, right thigh, sequela
		S76.802S	Unsp inj musc/fasc/tend at thi lev, left thigh, sequela
		S76.809S	Unsp inj musc/fasc/tend at thi lev, unsp thigh, sequela
		S76.891S	Inj musc/fasc/tend at thigh level, right thigh, sequela
		S76.892S	Inj musc/fasc/tend at thigh level, left thigh, sequela
		S76.899S	Inj musc/fasc/tend at thigh level, unsp thigh, sequela
		S76.901S	Unsp inj unsp musc/fasc/tend at thi lev, right thigh, sqla
		S76.902S	Unsp inj unsp musc/fasc/tend at thi lev, left thigh, sequela
		S76.909S	Unsp inj unsp musc/fasc/tend at thi lev, unsp thigh, sequela
		S76.991S	Inj unsp musc/fasc/tend at thigh level, right thigh, sequela
		S76.992S	Inj unsp musc/fasc/tend at thigh level, left thigh, sequela
		S76.999S	Inj unsp musc/fasc/tend at thigh level, unsp thigh, sequela
		S79.811S	Other specified injuries of right hip, sequela
		S79.812S	Other specified injuries of left hip, sequela
		S79.819S	Other specified injuries of unspecified hip, sequela
		S79.821S	Other specified injuries of right thigh, sequela
		S79.822S	Other specified injuries of left thigh, sequela
		S79.829S	Other specified injuries of unspecified thigh, sequela
		S79.911S	Unspecified injury of right hip, sequela
		S79.912S	Unspecified injury of left hip, sequela
		S79.919S	Unspecified injury of unspecified hip, sequela
		S79.921S	Unspecified injury of right thigh, sequela
		S79.922S	Unspecified injury of left thigh, sequela
		S79.929S	Unspecified injury of unspecified thigh, sequela
		S86.001S	Unspecified injury of right Achilles tendon, sequela
		S86.002S	Unspecified injury of left Achilles tendon, sequela
		S86.009S	Unspecified injury of unspecified Achilles tendon, sequela
		S86.091S	Other specified injury of right Achilles tendon, sequela
		S86.092S	Other specified injury of left Achilles tendon, sequela
		S86.099S	Oth injury of unspecified Achilles tendon, sequela
		S86.101S	Unsp inj musc/tend post grp at low leg lev, right leg, sqla
		S86.102S	Unsp inj musc/tend post grp at low leg level, left leg, sqla
		S86.109S	Unsp inj musc/tend post grp at low leg level, unsp leg, sqla
		S86.191S	Inj oth musc/tend post grp at low leg level, right leg, sqla
		S86.192S	Inj oth musc/tend post grp at low leg level, left leg, sqla
		S86.199S	Inj oth musc/tend post grp at low leg level, unsp leg, sqla
		S86.201S	Unsp inj musc/tend ant grp at low leg level, right leg, sqla
		S86.202S	Unsp inj musc/tend ant grp at low leg level, left leg, sqla
		S86.209S	Unsp inj musc/tend ant grp at low leg level, unsp leg, sqla
		S86.291S	Inj musc/tend ant grp at low leg level, right leg, sequela
		S86.292S	Inj musc/tend ant grp at low leg level, left leg, sequela
		S86.299S	Inj musc/tend ant grp at low leg level, unsp leg, sequela
		S86.301S	Unsp inj musc/tend peroneal grp at low leg lev, r leg, sqla
		S86.302S	Unsp inj musc/tend peroneal grp at low leg lev, l leg, sqla
		S86.309S	Unsp inj musc/tend peroneal grp at low leg lev,unsp leg,sqla
		S86.391S	Inj musc/tend peroneal grp at low leg level, right leg, sqla
		S86.392S	Inj musc/tend peroneal grp at low leg level, left leg, sqla
		S86.399S	Inj musc/tend peroneal grp at low leg level, unsp leg, sqla
		S86.801S	Unsp inj musc/tend at lower leg level, right leg, sequela
		S86.802S	Unsp inj musc/tend at lower leg level, left leg, sequela
	(Continued on next page)	**S86.809S**	Unsp inj musc/tend at lower leg level, unsp leg, sequela

ICD-9-CM		ICD-10-CM	
9Ø8.9	LATE EFFECT OF UNSPECIFIED INJURY **(Continued)**	**S86.891S**	Inj oth musc/tend at lower leg level, right leg, sequela
		S86.892S	Inj oth musc/tend at lower leg level, left leg, sequela
		S86.899S	Inj oth musc/tend at lower leg level, unsp leg, sequela
		S86.9Ø1S	Unsp inj unsp musc/tend at low leg level, right leg, sequela
		S86.9Ø2S	Unsp inj unsp musc/tend at low leg level, left leg, sequela
		S86.9Ø9S	Unsp inj unsp musc/tend at low leg level, unsp leg, sequela
		S86.991S	Inj unsp musc/tend at lower leg level, right leg, sequela
		S86.992S	Inj unsp musc/tend at lower leg level, left leg, sequela
		S86.999S	Inj unsp musc/tend at lower leg level, unsp leg, sequela
		S89.8ØXS	Other specified injuries of unspecified lower leg, sequela
		S89.81XS	Other specified injuries of right lower leg, sequela
		S89.82XS	Other specified injuries of left lower leg, sequela
		S89.9ØXS	Unspecified injury of unspecified lower leg, sequela
		S89.91XS	Unspecified injury of right lower leg, sequela
		S89.92XS	Unspecified injury of left lower leg, sequela
		S96.ØØ1S	Unsp inj msl/tnd lng flxr msl toe at ank/ft lev, r ft, sqla
		S96.ØØ2S	Unsp inj msl/tnd lng flxr msl toe at ank/ft lev, l ft, sqla
		S96.ØØ9S	Unsp inj msl/tnd lng flxr msl toe at ank/ft lev,unsp ft,sqla
		S96.Ø91S	Inj msl/tnd lng flxr msl toe at ank/ft level, r foot, sqla
		S96.Ø92S	Inj msl/tnd lng flxr msl toe at ank/ft level, l foot, sqla
		S96.Ø99S	Inj msl/tnd lng flxr msl toe at ank/ft lev, unsp foot, sqla
		S96.1Ø1S	Unsp inj msl/tnd lng extn msl toe at ank/ft lev, r ft, sqla
		S96.1Ø2S	Unsp inj msl/tnd lng extn msl toe at ank/ft lev, l ft, sqla
		S96.1Ø9S	Unsp inj msl/tnd lng extn msl toe at ank/ft lev,unsp ft,sqla
		S96.191S	Inj msl/tnd lng extn msl toe at ank/ft level, r foot, sqla
		S96.192S	Inj msl/tnd lng extn msl toe at ank/ft level, l foot, sqla
		S96.199S	Inj msl/tnd lng extn msl toe at ank/ft lev, unsp foot, sqla
		S96.2Ø1S	Unsp inj intrinsic msl/tnd at ank/ft level, r foot, sequela
		S96.2Ø2S	Unsp inj intrns msl/tnd at ank/ft level, left foot, sequela
		S96.2Ø9S	Unsp inj intrns msl/tnd at ank/ft level, unsp foot, sequela
		S96.291S	Inj intrinsic msl/tnd at ank/ft level, right foot, sequela
		S96.292S	Inj intrinsic msl/tnd at ank/ft level, left foot, sequela
		S96.299S	Inj intrinsic msl/tnd at ank/ft level, unsp foot, sequela
		S96.8Ø1S	Unsp inj musc and tendons at ank/ft level, r foot, sequela
		S96.8Ø2S	Unsp inj musc and tendons at ank/ft level, l foot, sequela
		S96.8Ø9S	Unsp inj musc and tendons at ank/ft level, unsp foot, sqla
		S96.891S	Inj oth muscles and tendons at ank/ft level, r foot, sequela
		S96.892S	Inj oth muscles and tendons at ank/ft level, l foot, sequela
		S96.899S	Inj oth musc and tendons at ank/ft level, unsp foot, sequela
		S96.9Ø1S	Unsp injury of unsp msl/tnd at ank/ft level, r foot, sequela
		S96.9Ø2S	Unsp inj unsp msl/tnd at ank/ft level, left foot, sequela
		S96.9Ø9S	Unsp inj unsp msl/tnd at ank/ft level, unsp foot, sequela
		S96.991S	Inj unsp msl/tnd at ank/ft level, right foot, sequela
		S96.992S	Inj unsp msl/tnd at ankle and foot level, left foot, sequela
		S96.999S	Inj unsp msl/tnd at ankle and foot level, unsp foot, sequela
		S99.811S	Other specified injuries of right ankle, sequela
		S99.812S	Other specified injuries of left ankle, sequela
		S99.819S	Other specified injuries of unspecified ankle, sequela
		S99.821S	Other specified injuries of right foot, sequela
		S99.822S	Other specified injuries of left foot, sequela
		S99.829S	Other specified injuries of unspecified foot, sequela
		S99.911S	Unspecified injury of right ankle, sequela
		S99.912S	Unspecified injury of left ankle, sequela
		S99.919S	Unspecified injury of unspecified ankle, sequela
		S99.921S	Unspecified injury of right foot, sequela
		S99.922S	Unspecified injury of left foot, sequela
		S99.929S	Unspecified injury of unspecified foot, sequela
9Ø9.Ø	LATE EFF POISN-RX MEDICINAL/BIOLOGICAL SUBSTANCE	**T36.ØX1S**	Poisoning by penicillins, accidental, sequela
		T36.ØX2S	Poisoning by penicillins, intentional self-harm, sequela
		T36.ØX3S	Poisoning by penicillins, assault, sequela
		T36.ØX4S	Poisoning by penicillins, undetermined, sequela
		T36.1X1S	Poisn by cephalospor/oth beta-lactm antibiot, acc, sequela
		T36.1X2S	Poisn by cephalospor/oth beta-lactm antibiot, slf-hrm, sqla
		T36.1X3S	Poisn by cephalospor/oth beta-lactm antibiot, asslt, sequela
		T36.1X4S	Poisn by cephalospor/oth beta-lactm antibiot, undet, sequela
		T36.2X1S	Poisoning by chloramphenicol group, accidental, sequela
		T36.2X2S	Poisoning by chloramphenicol group, self-harm, sequela
		T36.2X3S	Poisoning by chloramphenicol group, assault, sequela
		T36.2X4S	Poisoning by chloramphenicol group, undetermined, sequela
		T36.3X1S	Poisoning by macrolides, accidental (unintentional), sequela
		T36.3X2S	Poisoning by macrolides, intentional self-harm, sequela
		T36.3X3S	Poisoning by macrolides, assault, sequela
		T36.3X4S	Poisoning by macrolides, undetermined, sequela
		T36.4X1S	Poisoning by tetracyclines, accidental, sequela
		T36.4X2S	Poisoning by tetracyclines, intentional self-harm, sequela
		T36.4X3S	Poisoning by tetracyclines, assault, sequela
		T36.4X4S	Poisoning by tetracyclines, undetermined, sequela
		T36.5X1S	Poisoning by aminoglycosides, accidental, sequela
		T36.5X2S	Poisoning by aminoglycosides, intentional self-harm, sequela
		T36.5X3S	Poisoning by aminoglycosides, assault, sequela
	(Continued on next page)	**T36.5X4S**	Poisoning by aminoglycosides, undetermined, sequela

ICD-9-CM		ICD-10-CM	
909.0	LATE EFF POISN-RX MEDICINAL/BIOLOGICAL SUBSTANCE **(Continued)**	**T36.6X1S**	Poisoning by rifampicins, accidental, sequela
		T36.6X2S	Poisoning by rifampicins, intentional self-harm, sequela
		T36.6X3S	Poisoning by rifampicins, assault, sequela
		T36.6X4S	Poisoning by rifampicins, undetermined, sequela
		T36.7X1S	Poisoning by antifungal antibiot, sys used, acc, sequela
		T36.7X2S	Poisoning by antifung antibiot, sys used, self-harm, sequela
		T36.7X3S	Poisoning by antifungal antibiot, sys used, assault, sequela
		T36.7X4S	Poisoning by antifungal antibiot, sys used, undet, sequela
		T36.8X1S	Poisoning by oth systemic antibiotics, accidental, sequela
		T36.8X2S	Poisoning by oth systemic antibiotics, self-harm, sequela
		T36.8X3S	Poisoning by other systemic antibiotics, assault, sequela
		T36.8X4S	Poisoning by oth systemic antibiotics, undetermined, sequela
		T36.91XS	Poisoning by unsp systemic antibiotic, accidental, sequela
		T36.92XS	Poisoning by unsp systemic antibiotic, self-harm, sequela
		T36.93XS	Poisoning by unsp systemic antibiotic, assault, sequela
		T36.94XS	Poisoning by unsp systemic antibiotic, undetermined, sequela
		T37.0X1S	Poisoning by sulfonamides, accidental, sequela
		T37.0X2S	Poisoning by sulfonamides, intentional self-harm, sequela
		T37.0X3S	Poisoning by sulfonamides, assault, sequela
		T37.0X4S	Poisoning by sulfonamides, undetermined, sequela
		T37.1X1S	Poisoning by antimycobac drugs, accidental, sequela
		T37.1X2S	Poisoning by antimycobacterial drugs, self-harm, sequela
		T37.1X3S	Poisoning by antimycobacterial drugs, assault, sequela
		T37.1X4S	Poisoning by antimycobacterial drugs, undetermined, sequela
		T37.2X1S	Poisn by antimalari/drugs acting on bld protzoa, acc, sqla
		T37.2X2S	Poisn by antimalari/drugs act on bld protzoa, slf-hrm, sqla
		T37.2X3S	Poisn by antimalari/drugs acting on bld protzoa, asslt, sqla
		T37.2X4S	Poisn by antimalari/drugs acting on bld protzoa, undet, sqla
		T37.3X1S	Poisoning by oth antiprotozoal drugs, accidental, sequela
		T37.3X2S	Poisoning by oth antiprotozoal drugs, self-harm, sequela
		T37.3X3S	Poisoning by other antiprotozoal drugs, assault, sequela
		T37.3X4S	Poisoning by oth antiprotozoal drugs, undetermined, sequela
		T37.4X1S	Poisoning by anthelminthics, accidental, sequela
		T37.4X2S	Poisoning by anthelminthics, intentional self-harm, sequela
		T37.4X3S	Poisoning by anthelminthics, assault, sequela
		T37.4X4S	Poisoning by anthelminthics, undetermined, sequela
		T37.5X1S	Poisoning by antiviral drugs, accidental, sequela
		T37.5X2S	Poisoning by antiviral drugs, intentional self-harm, sequela
		T37.5X3S	Poisoning by antiviral drugs, assault, sequela
		T37.5X4S	Poisoning by antiviral drugs, undetermined, sequela
		T37.8X1S	Poisoning by oth systemic anti-infect/parasit, acc, sequela
		T37.8X2S	Poisn by oth systemic anti-infect/parasit, slf-hrm, sequela
		T37.8X3S	Poisn by oth systemic anti-infect/parasit, assault, sequela
		T37.8X4S	Poisn by oth systemic anti-infect/parasit, undet, sequela
		T37.91XS	Poisn by unsp sys anti-infect and antiparastc, acc, sequela
		T37.92XS	Poisn by unsp sys anti-infect and antiparastc, slf-hrm, sqla
		T37.93XS	Poisn by unsp sys anti-infect and antiparastc, asslt, sqla
		T37.94XS	Poisn by unsp sys anti-infect and antiparastc, undet, sqla
		T38.0X1S	Poisoning by glucocort/synth analog, accidental, sequela
		T38.0X2S	Poisoning by glucocort/synth analog, self-harm, sequela
		T38.0X3S	Poisoning by glucocort/synth analog, assault, sequela
		T38.0X4S	Poisoning by glucocort/synth analog, undetermined, sequela
		T38.1X1S	Poisoning by thyroid hormones and sub, accidental, sequela
		T38.1X2S	Poisoning by thyroid hormones and sub, self-harm, sequela
		T38.1X3S	Poisoning by thyroid hormones and sub, assault, sequela
		T38.1X4S	Poisoning by thyroid hormones and sub, undet, sequela
		T38.2X1S	Poisoning by antithyroid drugs, accidental, sequela
		T38.2X2S	Poisoning by antithyroid drugs, self-harm, sequela
		T38.2X3S	Poisoning by antithyroid drugs, assault, sequela
		T38.2X4S	Poisoning by antithyroid drugs, undetermined, sequela
		T38.3X1S	Poisn by insulin and oral hypoglycemic drugs, acc, sequela
		T38.3X2S	Poisn by insulin and oral hypoglycemic drugs, slf-hrm, sqla
		T38.3X3S	Poisn by insulin and oral hypoglycemic drugs, asslt, sequela
		T38.3X4S	Poisn by insulin and oral hypoglycemic drugs, undet, sequela
		T38.4X1S	Poisoning by oral contraceptives, accidental, sequela
		T38.4X2S	Poisoning by oral contraceptives, self-harm, sequela
		T38.4X3S	Poisoning by oral contraceptives, assault, sequela
		T38.4X4S	Poisoning by oral contraceptives, undetermined, sequela
		T38.5X1S	Poisoning by oth estrogens and progstrn, acc, sequela
		T38.5X2S	Poisoning by oth estrogens and progstrn, self-harm, sequela
		T38.5X3S	Poisoning by oth estrogens and progstrn, assault, sequela
		T38.5X4S	Poisoning by oth estrogens and progstrn, undet, sequela
		T38.6X1S	Poisn by antigonadtr/antiestr/antiandrg, NEC, acc, sequela
		T38.6X2S	Poisn by antigonadtr/antiestr/antiandrg, NEC, slf-hrm, sqla
		T38.6X3S	Poisn by antigonadtr/antiestr/antiandrg, NEC, asslt, sequela
		T38.6X4S	Poisn by antigonadtr/antiestr/antiandrg, NEC, undet, sequela
		T38.7X1S	Poisoning by androgens and anabolic congeners, acc, sequela
		T38.7X2S	Poisn by androgens and anabolic congeners, slf-hrm, sequela
	(Continued on next page)	**T38.7X3S**	Poisn by androgens and anabolic congeners, assault, sequela

ICD-9-CM		ICD-10-CM	
909.Ø	LATE EFF POISN-RX MEDICINAL/BIOLOGICAL SUBSTANCE **(Continued)**	**T38.7X4S**	Poisn by androgens and anabolic congeners, undet, sequela
		T38.8Ø1S	Poisoning by unsp hormones and synthetic sub, acc, sequela
		T38.8Ø2S	Poisn by unsp hormones and synthetic sub, self-harm, sequela
		T38.8Ø3S	Poisn by unsp hormones and synthetic sub, assault, sequela
		T38.8Ø4S	Poisoning by unsp hormones and synthetic sub, undet, sequela
		T38.811S	Poisoning by anterior pituitary hormones, acc, sequela
		T38.812S	Poisoning by anterior pituitary hormones, self-harm, sequela
		T38.813S	Poisoning by anterior pituitary hormones, assault, sequela
		T38.814S	Poisoning by anterior pituitary hormones, undet, sequela
		T38.891S	Poisoning by oth hormones and synthetic sub, acc, sequela
		T38.892S	Poisn by oth hormones and synthetic sub, self-harm, sequela
		T38.893S	Poisn by oth hormones and synthetic sub, assault, sequela
		T38.894S	Poisoning by oth hormones and synthetic sub, undet, sequela
		T38.9Ø1S	Poisoning by unsp hormone antagonists, accidental, sequela
		T38.9Ø2S	Poisoning by unsp hormone antagonists, self-harm, sequela
		T38.9Ø3S	Poisoning by unsp hormone antagonists, assault, sequela
		T38.9Ø4S	Poisoning by unsp hormone antagonists, undetermined, sequela
		T38.991S	Poisoning by oth hormone antagonists, accidental, sequela
		T38.992S	Poisoning by oth hormone antagonists, self-harm, sequela
		T38.993S	Poisoning by other hormone antagonists, assault, sequela
		T38.994S	Poisoning by oth hormone antagonists, undetermined, sequela
		T39.Ø11S	Poisoning by aspirin, accidental (unintentional), sequela
		T39.Ø12S	Poisoning by aspirin, intentional self-harm, sequela
		T39.Ø13S	Poisoning by aspirin, assault, sequela
		T39.Ø14S	Poisoning by aspirin, undetermined, sequela
		T39.Ø91S	Poisoning by salicylates, accidental, sequela
		T39.Ø92S	Poisoning by salicylates, intentional self-harm, sequela
		T39.Ø93S	Poisoning by salicylates, assault, sequela
		T39.Ø94S	Poisoning by salicylates, undetermined, sequela
		T39.1X1S	Poisoning by 4-Aminophenol derivatives, accidental, sequela
		T39.1X2S	Poisoning by 4-Aminophenol derivatives, self-harm, sequela
		T39.1X3S	Poisoning by 4-Aminophenol derivatives, assault, sequela
		T39.1X4S	Poisoning by 4-Aminophenol derivatives, undet, sequela
		T39.2X1S	Poisoning by pyrazolone derivatives, accidental, sequela
		T39.2X2S	Poisoning by pyrazolone derivatives, self-harm, sequela
		T39.2X3S	Poisoning by pyrazolone derivatives, assault, sequela
		T39.2X4S	Poisoning by pyrazolone derivatives, undetermined, sequela
		T39.311S	Poisoning by propionic acid deriv, accidental, sequela
		T39.312S	Poisoning by propionic acid derivatives, self-harm, sequela
		T39.313S	Poisoning by propionic acid derivatives, assault, sequela
		T39.314S	Poisoning by propionic acid derivatives, undet, sequela
		T39.391S	Poisoning by oth nonsteroid anti-inflam drugs, acc, sequela
		T39.392S	Poisn by oth nonsteroid anti-inflam drugs, slf-hrm, sequela
		T39.393S	Poisn by oth nonsteroid anti-inflam drugs, assault, sequela
		T39.394S	Poisn by oth nonsteroid anti-inflam drugs, undet, sequela
		T39.4X1S	Poisoning by antirheumatics, NEC, accidental, sequela
		T39.4X2S	Poisoning by antirheumatics, NEC, self-harm, sequela
		T39.4X3S	Poisoning by antirheumatics, NEC, assault, sequela
		T39.4X4S	Poisoning by antirheumatics, NEC, undetermined, sequela
		T39.8X1S	Poisn by oth nonopio analges/antipyret, NEC, acc, sequela
		T39.8X2S	Poisn by oth nonopio analges/antipyret, NEC, slf-hrm, sqla
		T39.8X3S	Poisn by oth nonopio analges/antipyret, NEC, asslt, sequela
		T39.8X4S	Poisn by oth nonopio analges/antipyret, NEC, undet, sequela
		T39.91XS	Poisn by unsp nonopi analgs/antipyr/antirheu, acc, sequela
		T39.92XS	Poisn by unsp nonopi analgs/antipyr/antirheu, slf-hrm, sqla
		T39.93XS	Poisn by unsp nonopi analgs/antipyr/antirheu, asslt, sequela
		T39.94XS	Poisn by unsp nonopi analgs/antipyr/antirheu, undet, sequela
		T4Ø.ØX1S	Poisoning by opium, accidental (unintentional), sequela
		T4Ø.ØX2S	Poisoning by opium, intentional self-harm, sequela
		T4Ø.ØX3S	Poisoning by opium, assault, sequela
		T4Ø.ØX4S	Poisoning by opium, undetermined, sequela
		T4Ø.1X1S	Poisoning by heroin, accidental (unintentional), sequela
		T4Ø.1X2S	Poisoning by heroin, intentional self-harm, sequela
		T4Ø.1X3S	Poisoning by heroin, assault, sequela
		T4Ø.1X4S	Poisoning by heroin, undetermined, sequela
		T4Ø.2X1S	Poisoning by oth opioids, accidental, sequela
		T4Ø.2X2S	Poisoning by other opioids, intentional self-harm, sequela
		T4Ø.2X3S	Poisoning by other opioids, assault, sequela
		T4Ø.2X4S	Poisoning by other opioids, undetermined, sequela
		T4Ø.3X1S	Poisoning by methadone, accidental (unintentional), sequela
		T4Ø.3X2S	Poisoning by methadone, intentional self-harm, sequela
		T4Ø.3X3S	Poisoning by methadone, assault, sequela
		T4Ø.3X4S	Poisoning by methadone, undetermined, sequela
		T4Ø.4X1S	Poisoning by oth synthetic narcotics, accidental, sequela
		T4Ø.4X2S	Poisoning by oth synthetic narcotics, self-harm, sequela
		T4Ø.4X3S	Poisoning by other synthetic narcotics, assault, sequela
		T4Ø.4X4S	Poisoning by oth synthetic narcotics, undetermined, sequela
		T4Ø.5X1S	Poisoning by cocaine, accidental (unintentional), sequela
	(Continued on next page)	**T4Ø.5X2S**	Poisoning by cocaine, intentional self-harm, sequela

ICD-9-CM		ICD-10-CM	
909.Ø	LATE EFF POISN-RX MEDICINAL/BIOLOGICAL SUBSTANCE **(Continued)**	**T40.5X3S**	Poisoning by cocaine, assault, sequela
		T40.5X4S	Poisoning by cocaine, undetermined, sequela
		T40.601S	Poisoning by unsp narcotics, accidental, sequela
		T40.602S	Poisoning by unsp narcotics, intentional self-harm, sequela
		T40.603S	Poisoning by unspecified narcotics, assault, sequela
		T40.604S	Poisoning by unspecified narcotics, undetermined, sequela
		T40.691S	Poisoning by oth narcotics, accidental, sequela
		T40.692S	Poisoning by other narcotics, intentional self-harm, sequela
		T40.693S	Poisoning by other narcotics, assault, sequela
		T40.694S	Poisoning by other narcotics, undetermined, sequela
		T40.7X1S	Poisoning by cannabis (derivatives), accidental, sequela
		T40.7X2S	Poisoning by cannabis (derivatives), self-harm, sequela
		T40.7X3S	Poisoning by cannabis (derivatives), assault, sequela
		T40.7X4S	Poisoning by cannabis (derivatives), undetermined, sequela
		T40.8X1S	Poisoning by lysergide, accidental (unintentional), sequela
		T40.8X2S	Poisoning by lysergide [LSD], intentional self-harm, sequela
		T40.8X3S	Poisoning by lysergide [LSD], assault, sequela
		T40.8X4S	Poisoning by lysergide [LSD], undetermined, sequela
		T40.901S	Poisoning by unsp psychodyslept, accidental, sequela
		T40.902S	Poisoning by unsp psychodysleptics, self-harm, sequela
		T40.903S	Poisoning by unspecified psychodysleptics, assault, sequela
		T40.904S	Poisoning by unsp psychodysleptics, undetermined, sequela
		T40.991S	Poisoning by oth psychodyslept, accidental, sequela
		T40.992S	Poisoning by oth psychodysleptics, self-harm, sequela
		T40.993S	Poisoning by other psychodysleptics, assault, sequela
		T40.994S	Poisoning by other psychodysleptics, undetermined, sequela
		T41.0X1S	Poisoning by inhaled anesthetics, accidental, sequela
		T41.0X2S	Poisoning by inhaled anesthetics, self-harm, sequela
		T41.0X3S	Poisoning by inhaled anesthetics, assault, sequela
		T41.0X4S	Poisoning by inhaled anesthetics, undetermined, sequela
		T41.1X1S	Poisoning by intravenous anesthetics, accidental, sequela
		T41.1X2S	Poisoning by intravenous anesthetics, self-harm, sequela
		T41.1X3S	Poisoning by intravenous anesthetics, assault, sequela
		T41.1X4S	Poisoning by intravenous anesthetics, undetermined, sequela
		T41.201S	Poisoning by unsp general anesthetics, accidental, sequela
		T41.202S	Poisoning by unsp general anesthetics, self-harm, sequela
		T41.203S	Poisoning by unsp general anesthetics, assault, sequela
		T41.204S	Poisoning by unsp general anesthetics, undetermined, sequela
		T41.291S	Poisoning by oth general anesthetics, accidental, sequela
		T41.292S	Poisoning by oth general anesthetics, self-harm, sequela
		T41.293S	Poisoning by other general anesthetics, assault, sequela
		T41.294S	Poisoning by oth general anesthetics, undetermined, sequela
		T41.3X1S	Poisoning by local anesthetics, accidental, sequela
		T41.3X2S	Poisoning by local anesthetics, self-harm, sequela
		T41.3X3S	Poisoning by local anesthetics, assault, sequela
		T41.3X4S	Poisoning by local anesthetics, undetermined, sequela
		T41.41XS	Poisoning by unsp anesthetic, accidental, sequela
		T41.42XS	Poisoning by unsp anesthetic, intentional self-harm, sequela
		T41.43XS	Poisoning by unspecified anesthetic, assault, sequela
		T41.44XS	Poisoning by unspecified anesthetic, undetermined, sequela
		T41.5X1S	Poisoning by therapeutic gases, accidental, sequela
		T41.5X2S	Poisoning by therapeutic gases, self-harm, sequela
		T41.5X3S	Poisoning by therapeutic gases, assault, sequela
		T41.5X4S	Poisoning by therapeutic gases, undetermined, sequela
		T42.0X1S	Poisoning by hydantoin derivatives, accidental, sequela
		T42.0X2S	Poisoning by hydantoin derivatives, self-harm, sequela
		T42.0X3S	Poisoning by hydantoin derivatives, assault, sequela
		T42.0X4S	Poisoning by hydantoin derivatives, undetermined, sequela
		T42.1X1S	Poisoning by iminostilbenes, accidental, sequela
		T42.1X2S	Poisoning by iminostilbenes, intentional self-harm, sequela
		T42.1X3S	Poisoning by iminostilbenes, assault, sequela
		T42.1X4S	Poisoning by iminostilbenes, undetermined, sequela
		T42.2X1S	Poisn by succinimides and oxazolidinediones, acc, sequela
		T42.2X2S	Poisn by succinimides and oxazolidinediones, slf-hrm, sqla
		T42.2X3S	Poisn by succinimides and oxazolidinediones, asslt, sequela
		T42.2X4S	Poisn by succinimides and oxazolidinediones, undet, sequela
		T42.3X1S	Poisoning by barbiturates, accidental, sequela
		T42.3X2S	Poisoning by barbiturates, intentional self-harm, sequela
		T42.3X3S	Poisoning by barbiturates, assault, sequela
		T42.3X4S	Poisoning by barbiturates, undetermined, sequela
		T42.4X1S	Poisoning by benzodiazepines, accidental, sequela
		T42.4X2S	Poisoning by benzodiazepines, intentional self-harm, sequela
		T42.4X3S	Poisoning by benzodiazepines, assault, sequela
		T42.4X4S	Poisoning by benzodiazepines, undetermined, sequela
		T42.5X1S	Poisoning by mixed antiepileptics, accidental, sequela
		T42.5X2S	Poisoning by mixed antiepileptics, self-harm, sequela
		T42.5X3S	Poisoning by mixed antiepileptics, assault, sequela
		T42.5X4S	Poisoning by mixed antiepileptics, undetermined, sequela
		T42.6X1S	Poisn by oth antieplptc and sed-hypntc drugs, acc, sequela

(Continued on next page)

ICD-9-CM		ICD-10-CM	
9Ø9.Ø	LATE EFF POISN-RX MEDICINAL/BIOLOGICAL SUBSTANCE **(Continued)**	**T42.6X2S**	Poisn by oth antieplptc and sed-hypntc drugs, slf-hrm, sqla
		T42.6X3S	Poisn by oth antieplptc and sed-hypntc drugs, asslt, sequela
		T42.6X4S	Poisn by oth antieplptc and sed-hypntc drugs, undet, sequela
		T42.71XS	Poisn by unsp antieplptc and sed-hypntc drugs, acc, sequela
		T42.72XS	Poisn by unsp antieplptc and sed-hypntc drugs, slf-hrm, sqla
		T42.73XS	Poisn by unsp antieplptc and sed-hypntc drugs, asslt, sqla
		T42.74XS	Poisn by unsp antieplptc and sed-hypntc drugs, undet, sqla
		T42.8X1S	Poisn by antiparkns drug/centr musc-tone depr, acc, sequela
		T42.8X2S	Poisn by antiparkns drug/centr musc-tone depr, slf-hrm, sqla
		T42.8X3S	Poisn by antiparkns drug/centr musc-tone depr, asslt, sqla
		T42.8X4S	Poisn by antiparkns drug/centr musc-tone depr, undet, sqla
		T43.Ø11S	Poisoning by tricyclic antidepressants, accidental, sequela
		T43.Ø12S	Poisoning by tricyclic antidepressants, self-harm, sequela
		T43.Ø13S	Poisoning by tricyclic antidepressants, assault, sequela
		T43.Ø14S	Poisoning by tricyclic antidepress, undetermined, sequela
		T43.Ø21S	Poisoning by tetracyclic antidepress, accidental, sequela
		T43.Ø22S	Poisoning by tetracyclic antidepressants, self-harm, sequela
		T43.Ø23S	Poisoning by tetracyclic antidepressants, assault, sequela
		T43.Ø24S	Poisoning by tetracyclic antidepress, undetermined, sequela
		T43.1X1S	Poisoning by MAO inhib antidepressants, accidental, sequela
		T43.1X2S	Poisoning by MAO inhib antidepressants, self-harm, sequela
		T43.1X3S	Poisoning by MAO inhib antidepressants, assault, sequela
		T43.1X4S	Poisoning by MAO inhib antidepress, undetermined, sequela
		T43.2Ø1S	Poisoning by unsp antidepressants, accidental, sequela
		T43.2Ø2S	Poisoning by unsp antidepressants, self-harm, sequela
		T43.2Ø3S	Poisoning by unspecified antidepressants, assault, sequela
		T43.2Ø4S	Poisoning by unsp antidepressants, undetermined, sequela
		T43.211S	Poisn by slctv seroton/norepineph reup inhibtr, acc, sqla
		T43.212S	Poisn by slctv seroton/norepineph reup inhibtr,slf-hrm, sqla
		T43.213S	Poisn by slctv seroton/norepineph reup inhibtr, asslt, sqla
		T43.214S	Poisn by slctv seroton/norepineph reup inhibtr, undet, sqla
		T43.221S	Poisn by selective serotonin reuptake inhibtr, acc, sequela
		T43.222S	Poisn by slctv serotonin reuptake inhibtr, slf-hrm, sequela
		T43.223S	Poisn by slctv serotonin reuptake inhibtr, assault, sequela
		T43.224S	Poisn by slctv serotonin reuptake inhibtr, undet, sequela
		T43.291S	Poisoning by oth antidepressants, accidental, sequela
		T43.292S	Poisoning by oth antidepressants, self-harm, sequela
		T43.293S	Poisoning by other antidepressants, assault, sequela
		T43.294S	Poisoning by other antidepressants, undetermined, sequela
		T43.3X1S	Poisoning by phenothiaz antipsychot/neurolept, acc, sequela
		T43.3X2S	Poisn by phenothiaz antipsychot/neurolept, slf-hrm, sequela
		T43.3X3S	Poisn by phenothiaz antipsychot/neurolept, assault, sequela
		T43.3X4S	Poisn by phenothiaz antipsychot/neurolept, undet, sequela
		T43.4X1S	Poisoning by butyrophen/thiothixen neuroleptc, acc, sequela
		T43.4X2S	Poisn by butyrophen/thiothixen neuroleptc, slf-hrm, sequela
		T43.4X3S	Poisn by butyrophen/thiothixen neuroleptc, assault, sequela
		T43.4X4S	Poisn by butyrophen/thiothixen neuroleptc, undet, sequela
		T43.5Ø1S	Poisoning by unsp antipsychot/neurolept, acc, sequela
		T43.5Ø2S	Poisoning by unsp antipsychot/neurolept, self-harm, sequela
		T43.5Ø3S	Poisoning by unsp antipsychot/neurolept, assault, sequela
		T43.5Ø4S	Poisoning by unsp antipsychot/neurolept, undet, sequela
		T43.591S	Poisoning by oth antipsychot/neurolept, accidental, sequela
		T43.592S	Poisoning by oth antipsychot/neurolept, self-harm, sequela
		T43.593S	Poisoning by oth antipsychot/neurolept, assault, sequela
		T43.594S	Poisoning by oth antipsychot/neurolept, undet, sequela
		T43.6Ø1S	Poisoning by unsp psychostim, accidental, sequela
		T43.6Ø2S	Poisoning by unsp psychostimulants, self-harm, sequela
		T43.6Ø3S	Poisoning by unspecified psychostimulants, assault, sequela
		T43.6Ø4S	Poisoning by unsp psychostimulants, undetermined, sequela
		T43.611S	Poisoning by caffeine, accidental (unintentional), sequela
		T43.612S	Poisoning by caffeine, intentional self-harm, sequela
		T43.613S	Poisoning by caffeine, assault, sequela
		T43.614S	Poisoning by caffeine, undetermined, sequela
		T43.621S	Poisoning by amphetamines, accidental, sequela
		T43.622S	Poisoning by amphetamines, intentional self-harm, sequela
		T43.623S	Poisoning by amphetamines, assault, sequela
		T43.624S	Poisoning by amphetamines, undetermined, sequela
		T43.631S	Poisoning by methylphenidate, accidental, sequela
		T43.632S	Poisoning by methylphenidate, intentional self-harm, sequela
		T43.633S	Poisoning by methylphenidate, assault, sequela
		T43.634S	Poisoning by methylphenidate, undetermined, sequela
		T43.691S	Poisoning by oth psychostim, accidental, sequela
		T43.692S	Poisoning by oth psychostimulants, self-harm, sequela
		T43.693S	Poisoning by other psychostimulants, assault, sequela
		T43.694S	Poisoning by other psychostimulants, undetermined, sequela
		T43.8X1S	Poisoning by oth psychotropic drugs, accidental, sequela
		T43.8X2S	Poisoning by oth psychotropic drugs, self-harm, sequela
		T43.8X3S	Poisoning by other psychotropic drugs, assault, sequela
	(Continued on next page)	**T43.8X4S**	Poisoning by other psychotropic drugs, undetermined, sequela

ICD-9-CM		ICD-10-CM	
909.Ø	LATE EFF POISN-RX MEDICINAL/BIOLOGICAL SUBSTANCE **(Continued)**	**T43.91XS**	Poisoning by unsp psychotropic drug, accidental, sequela
		T43.92XS	Poisoning by unsp psychotropic drug, self-harm, sequela
		T43.93XS	Poisoning by unspecified psychotropic drug, assault, sequela
		T43.94XS	Poisoning by unsp psychotropic drug, undetermined, sequela
		T44.ØX1S	Poisoning by anticholin agents, accidental, sequela
		T44.ØX2S	Poisoning by anticholinesterase agents, self-harm, sequela
		T44.ØX3S	Poisoning by anticholinesterase agents, assault, sequela
		T44.ØX4S	Poisoning by anticholin agents, undetermined, sequela
		T44.1X1S	Poisoning by oth parasympath, accidental, sequela
		T44.1X2S	Poisoning by oth parasympathomimetics, self-harm, sequela
		T44.1X3S	Poisoning by other parasympathomimetics, assault, sequela
		T44.1X4S	Poisoning by oth parasympathomimetics, undetermined, sequela
		T44.2X1S	Poisoning by ganglionic blocking drugs, accidental, sequela
		T44.2X2S	Poisoning by ganglionic blocking drugs, self-harm, sequela
		T44.2X3S	Poisoning by ganglionic blocking drugs, assault, sequela
		T44.2X4S	Poisoning by ganglionic blocking drugs, undet, sequela
		T44.3X1S	Poisoning by oth parasympath and spasmolytics, acc, sequela
		T44.3X2S	Poisn by oth parasympath and spasmolytics, slf-hrm, sequela
		T44.3X3S	Poisn by oth parasympath and spasmolytics, assault, sequela
		T44.3X4S	Poisn by oth parasympath and spasmolytics, undet, sequela
		T44.4X1S	Poisoning by predom alpha-adrenocpt agonists, acc, sequela
		T44.4X2S	Poisn by predom alpha-adrenocpt agonists, self-harm, sequela
		T44.4X3S	Poisn by predom alpha-adrenocpt agonists, assault, sequela
		T44.4X4S	Poisoning by predom alpha-adrenocpt agonists, undet, sequela
		T44.5X1S	Poisoning by predom beta-adrenocpt agonists, acc, sequela
		T44.5X2S	Poisn by predom beta-adrenocpt agonists, self-harm, sequela
		T44.5X3S	Poisn by predom beta-adrenocpt agonists, assault, sequela
		T44.5X4S	Poisoning by predom beta-adrenocpt agonists, undet, sequela
		T44.6X1S	Poisoning by alpha-adrenocpt antag, accidental, sequela
		T44.6X2S	Poisoning by alpha-adrenocpt antagonists, self-harm, sequela
		T44.6X3S	Poisoning by alpha-adrenocpt antagonists, assault, sequela
		T44.6X4S	Poisoning by alpha-adrenocpt antagonists, undet, sequela
		T44.7X1S	Poisoning by beta-adrenocpt antag, accidental, sequela
		T44.7X2S	Poisoning by beta-adrenocpt antagonists, self-harm, sequela
		T44.7X3S	Poisoning by beta-adrenocpt antagonists, assault, sequela
		T44.7X4S	Poisoning by beta-adrenocpt antagonists, undet, sequela
		T44.8X1S	Poisn by centr-acting/adren-neurn-block agnt, acc, sequela
		T44.8X2S	Poisn by centr-acting/adren-neurn-block agnt, slf-hrm, sqla
		T44.8X3S	Poisn by centr-acting/adren-neurn-block agnt, asslt, sequela
		T44.8X4S	Poisn by centr-acting/adren-neurn-block agnt, undet, sequela
		T44.9Ø1S	Poisn by unsp drugs aff the autonm nrv sys, acc, sequela
		T44.9Ø2S	Poisn by unsp drugs aff the autonm nrv sys, slf-hrm, sequela
		T44.9Ø3S	Poisn by unsp drugs aff the autonm nrv sys, asslt, sequela
		T44.9Ø4S	Poisn by unsp drugs aff the autonm nrv sys, undet, sequela
		T44.991S	Poisn by oth drug aff the autonm nervous sys, acc, sequela
		T44.992S	Poisn by oth drug aff the autonm nrv sys, slf-hrm, sequela
		T44.993S	Poisn by oth drug aff the autonm nervous sys, asslt, sequela
		T44.994S	Poisn by oth drug aff the autonm nervous sys, undet, sequela
		T45.ØX1S	Poisoning by antiallerg/antiemetic, accidental, sequela
		T45.ØX2S	Poisoning by antiallerg/antiemetic, self-harm, sequela
		T45.ØX3S	Poisoning by antiallerg/antiemetic, assault, sequela
		T45.ØX4S	Poisoning by antiallerg/antiemetic, undetermined, sequela
		T45.1X1S	Poisoning by antineopl and immunosup drugs, acc, sequela
		T45.1X2S	Poisn by antineopl and immunosup drugs, self-harm, sequela
		T45.1X3S	Poisoning by antineopl and immunosup drugs, assault, sequela
		T45.1X4S	Poisoning by antineopl and immunosup drugs, undet, sequela
		T45.2X1S	Poisoning by vitamins, accidental (unintentional), sequela
		T45.2X2S	Poisoning by vitamins, intentional self-harm, sequela
		T45.2X3S	Poisoning by vitamins, assault, sequela
		T45.2X4S	Poisoning by vitamins, undetermined, sequela
		T45.3X1S	Poisoning by enzymes, accidental (unintentional), sequela
		T45.3X2S	Poisoning by enzymes, intentional self-harm, sequela
		T45.3X3S	Poisoning by enzymes, assault, sequela
		T45.3X4S	Poisoning by enzymes, undetermined, sequela
		T45.4X1S	Poisoning by iron and its compounds, accidental, sequela
		T45.4X2S	Poisoning by iron and its compounds, self-harm, sequela
		T45.4X3S	Poisoning by iron and its compounds, assault, sequela
		T45.4X4S	Poisoning by iron and its compounds, undetermined, sequela
		T45.511S	Poisoning by anticoagulants, accidental, sequela
		T45.512S	Poisoning by anticoagulants, intentional self-harm, sequela
		T45.513S	Poisoning by anticoagulants, assault, sequela
		T45.514S	Poisoning by anticoagulants, undetermined, sequela
		T45.521S	Poisoning by antithrombotic drugs, accidental, sequela
		T45.522S	Poisoning by antithrombotic drugs, self-harm, sequela
		T45.523S	Poisoning by antithrombotic drugs, assault, sequela
		T45.524S	Poisoning by antithrombotic drugs, undetermined, sequela
		T45.6Ø1S	Poisoning by unsp fibrin-affct drugs, accidental, sequela
		T45.6Ø2S	Poisoning by unsp fibrin-affct drugs, self-harm, sequela
	(Continued on next page)	**T45.6Ø3S**	Poisoning by unsp fibrin-affct drugs, assault, sequela

ICD-9-CM		ICD-10-CM	
909.Ø	LATE EFF POISN-RX MEDICINAL/BIOLOGICAL SUBSTANCE **(Continued)**	**T45.6Ø4S**	Poisoning by unsp fibrin-affct drugs, undetermined, sequela
		T45.611S	Poisoning by thrombolytic drug, accidental, sequela
		T45.612S	Poisoning by thrombolytic drug, self-harm, sequela
		T45.613S	Poisoning by thrombolytic drug, assault, sequela
		T45.614S	Poisoning by thrombolytic drug, undetermined, sequela
		T45.621S	Poisoning by hemostatic drug, accidental, sequela
		T45.622S	Poisoning by hemostatic drug, intentional self-harm, sequela
		T45.623S	Poisoning by hemostatic drug, assault, sequela
		T45.624S	Poisoning by hemostatic drug, undetermined, sequela
		T45.691S	Poisoning by oth fibrin-affct drugs, accidental, sequela
		T45.692S	Poisoning by oth fibrin-affct drugs, self-harm, sequela
		T45.693S	Poisoning by oth fibrin-affct drugs, assault, sequela
		T45.694S	Poisoning by oth fibrin-affct drugs, undetermined, sequela
		T45.7X1S	Poisn by anticoag antag, vit K and oth coag, acc, sequela
		T45.7X2S	Poisn by anticoag antag, vit K and oth coag, slf-hrm, sqla
		T45.7X3S	Poisn by anticoag antag, vit K and oth coag, asslt, sequela
		T45.7X4S	Poisn by anticoag antag, vit K and oth coag, undet, sequela
		T45.8X1S	Poisn by oth prim sys and hematolog agents, acc, sequela
		T45.8X2S	Poisn by oth prim sys and hematolog agents, slf-hrm, sequela
		T45.8X3S	Poisn by oth prim sys and hematolog agents, assault, sequela
		T45.8X4S	Poisn by oth prim sys and hematolog agents, undet, sequela
		T45.91XS	Poisn by unsp prim sys and hematolog agent, acc, sequela
		T45.92XS	Poisn by unsp prim sys and hematolog agent, slf-hrm, sequela
		T45.93XS	Poisn by unsp prim sys and hematolog agent, assault, sequela
		T45.94XS	Poisn by unsp prim sys and hematolog agent, undet, sequela
		T46.ØX1S	Poisn by cardi-stim glycos/drug simlar act, acc, sequela
		T46.ØX2S	Poisn by cardi-stim glycos/drug simlar act, slf-hrm, sequela
		T46.ØX3S	Poisn by cardi-stim glycos/drug simlar act, assault, sequela
		T46.ØX4S	Poisn by cardi-stim glycos/drug simlar act, undet, sequela
		T46.1X1S	Poisoning by calcium-channel blockers, accidental, sequela
		T46.1X2S	Poisoning by calcium-channel blockers, self-harm, sequela
		T46.1X3S	Poisoning by calcium-channel blockers, assault, sequela
		T46.1X4S	Poisoning by calcium-channel blockers, undetermined, sequela
		T46.2X1S	Poisoning by oth antidysrhythmic drugs, accidental, sequela
		T46.2X2S	Poisoning by oth antidysrhythmic drugs, self-harm, sequela
		T46.2X3S	Poisoning by other antidysrhythmic drugs, assault, sequela
		T46.2X4S	Poisoning by oth antidysrhy drugs, undetermined, sequela
		T46.3X1S	Poisoning by coronary vasodilators, accidental, sequela
		T46.3X2S	Poisoning by coronary vasodilators, self-harm, sequela
		T46.3X3S	Poisoning by coronary vasodilators, assault, sequela
		T46.3X4S	Poisoning by coronary vasodilators, undetermined, sequela
		T46.4X1S	Poisoning by angiotens-convert-enzyme inhibtr, acc, sequela
		T46.4X2S	Poisn by angiotens-convert-enzyme inhibtr, slf-hrm, sequela
		T46.4X3S	Poisn by angiotens-convert-enzyme inhibtr, assault, sequela
		T46.4X4S	Poisn by angiotens-convert-enzyme inhibtr, undet, sequela
		T46.5X1S	Poisoning by oth antihypertn drugs, accidental, sequela
		T46.5X2S	Poisoning by oth antihypertensive drugs, self-harm, sequela
		T46.5X3S	Poisoning by other antihypertensive drugs, assault, sequela
		T46.5X4S	Poisoning by oth antihypertn drugs, undetermined, sequela
		T46.6X1S	Poisn by antihyperlip and antiarterio drugs, acc, sequela
		T46.6X2S	Poisn by antihyperlip and antiarterio drugs, slf-hrm, sqla
		T46.6X3S	Poisn by antihyperlip and antiarterio drugs, asslt, sequela
		T46.6X4S	Poisn by antihyperlip and antiarterio drugs, undet, sequela
		T46.7X1S	Poisoning by peripheral vasodilators, accidental, sequela
		T46.7X2S	Poisoning by peripheral vasodilators, self-harm, sequela
		T46.7X3S	Poisoning by peripheral vasodilators, assault, sequela
		T46.7X4S	Poisoning by peripheral vasodilators, undetermined, sequela
		T46.8X1S	Poisn by antivaric drugs, inc scler agents, acc, sequela
		T46.8X2S	Poisn by antivaric drugs, inc scler agents, slf-hrm, sequela
		T46.8X3S	Poisn by antivaric drugs, inc scler agents, assault, sequela
		T46.8X4S	Poisn by antivaric drugs, inc scler agents, undet, sequela
		T46.9Ø1S	Poisn by unsp agents aff the cardiovasc sys, acc, sequela
		T46.9Ø2S	Poisn by unsp agents aff the cardiovasc sys, slf-hrm, sqla
		T46.9Ø3S	Poisn by unsp agents aff the cardiovasc sys, asslt, sequela
		T46.9Ø4S	Poisn by unsp agents aff the cardiovasc sys, undet, sequela
		T46.991S	Poisn by oth agents aff the cardiovasc sys, acc, sequela
		T46.992S	Poisn by oth agents aff the cardiovasc sys, slf-hrm, sequela
		T46.993S	Poisn by oth agents aff the cardiovasc sys, assault, sequela
		T46.994S	Poisn by oth agents aff the cardiovasc sys, undet, sequela
		T47.ØX1S	Poisoning by histamine H2-receptor blockers, acc, sequela
		T47.ØX2S	Poisn by histamine H2-receptor blockers, self-harm, sequela
		T47.ØX3S	Poisn by histamine H2-receptor blockers, assault, sequela
		T47.ØX4S	Poisoning by histamine H2-receptor blockers, undet, sequela
		T47.1X1S	Poisn by oth antacids and anti-gstrc-sec drugs, acc, sqla
		T47.1X2S	Poisn by oth antacids & anti-gstrc-sec drugs, slf-hrm, sqla
		T47.1X3S	Poisn by oth antacids and anti-gstrc-sec drugs, asslt, sqla
		T47.1X4S	Poisn by oth antacids and anti-gstrc-sec drugs, undet, sqla
		T47.2X1S	Poisoning by stimulant laxatives, accidental, sequela
	(Continued on next page)	**T47.2X2S**	Poisoning by stimulant laxatives, self-harm, sequela

ICD-9-CM		ICD-10-CM	
9Ø9.Ø	LATE EFF POISN-RX MEDICINAL/BIOLOGICAL SUBSTANCE **(Continued)**	**T47.2X3S**	Poisoning by stimulant laxatives, assault, sequela
		T47.2X4S	Poisoning by stimulant laxatives, undetermined, sequela
		T47.3X1S	Poisoning by saline and osmotic laxatives, acc, sequela
		T47.3X2S	Poisoning by saline and osmotic laxtv, self-harm, sequela
		T47.3X3S	Poisoning by saline and osmotic laxatives, assault, sequela
		T47.3X4S	Poisoning by saline and osmotic laxatives, undet, sequela
		T47.4X1S	Poisoning by oth laxatives, accidental, sequela
		T47.4X2S	Poisoning by other laxatives, intentional self-harm, sequela
		T47.4X3S	Poisoning by other laxatives, assault, sequela
		T47.4X4S	Poisoning by other laxatives, undetermined, sequela
		T47.5X1S	Poisoning by digestants, accidental (unintentional), sequela
		T47.5X2S	Poisoning by digestants, intentional self-harm, sequela
		T47.5X3S	Poisoning by digestants, assault, sequela
		T47.5X4S	Poisoning by digestants, undetermined, sequela
		T47.6X1S	Poisoning by antidiarrheal drugs, accidental, sequela
		T47.6X2S	Poisoning by antidiarrheal drugs, self-harm, sequela
		T47.6X3S	Poisoning by antidiarrheal drugs, assault, sequela
		T47.6X4S	Poisoning by antidiarrheal drugs, undetermined, sequela
		T47.7X1S	Poisoning by emetics, accidental (unintentional), sequela
		T47.7X2S	Poisoning by emetics, intentional self-harm, sequela
		T47.7X3S	Poisoning by emetics, assault, sequela
		T47.7X4S	Poisoning by emetics, undetermined, sequela
		T47.8X1S	Poisoning by oth agents aff GI sys, accidental, sequela
		T47.8X2S	Poisoning by oth agents aff GI sys, self-harm, sequela
		T47.8X3S	Poisoning by oth agents aff GI sys, assault, sequela
		T47.8X4S	Poisoning by oth agents aff GI sys, undetermined, sequela
		T47.91XS	Poisoning by unsp agents aff the GI sys, acc, sequela
		T47.92XS	Poisoning by unsp agents aff the GI sys, self-harm, sequela
		T47.93XS	Poisoning by unsp agents aff the GI sys, assault, sequela
		T47.94XS	Poisoning by unsp agents aff the GI sys, undet, sequela
		T48.ØX1S	Poisoning by oxytocic drugs, accidental, sequela
		T48.ØX2S	Poisoning by oxytocic drugs, intentional self-harm, sequela
		T48.ØX3S	Poisoning by oxytocic drugs, assault, sequela
		T48.ØX4S	Poisoning by oxytocic drugs, undetermined, sequela
		T48.1X1S	Poisoning by skeletal muscle relaxants, accidental, sequela
		T48.1X2S	Poisoning by skeletal muscle relaxants, self-harm, sequela
		T48.1X3S	Poisoning by skeletal muscle relaxants, assault, sequela
		T48.1X4S	Poisoning by skeletal muscle relaxants, undet, sequela
		T48.2Ø1S	Poisoning by unsp drugs acting on muscles, acc, sequela
		T48.2Ø2S	Poisn by unsp drugs acting on muscles, self-harm, sequela
		T48.2Ø3S	Poisoning by unsp drugs acting on muscles, assault, sequela
		T48.2Ø4S	Poisoning by unsp drugs acting on muscles, undet, sequela
		T48.291S	Poisoning by oth drugs acting on muscles, acc, sequela
		T48.292S	Poisoning by oth drugs acting on muscles, self-harm, sequela
		T48.293S	Poisoning by other drugs acting on muscles, assault, sequela
		T48.294S	Poisoning by oth drugs acting on muscles, undet, sequela
		T48.3X1S	Poisoning by antitussives, accidental, sequela
		T48.3X2S	Poisoning by antitussives, intentional self-harm, sequela
		T48.3X3S	Poisoning by antitussives, assault, sequela
		T48.3X4S	Poisoning by antitussives, undetermined, sequela
		T48.4X1S	Poisoning by expectorants, accidental, sequela
		T48.4X2S	Poisoning by expectorants, intentional self-harm, sequela
		T48.4X3S	Poisoning by expectorants, assault, sequela
		T48.4X4S	Poisoning by expectorants, undetermined, sequela
		T48.5X1S	Poisoning by oth anti-cmn-cold drugs, accidental, sequela
		T48.5X2S	Poisoning by oth anti-common-cold drugs, self-harm, sequela
		T48.5X3S	Poisoning by other anti-common-cold drugs, assault, sequela
		T48.5X4S	Poisoning by oth anti-cmn-cold drugs, undetermined, sequela
		T48.6X1S	Poisoning by antiasthmatics, accidental, sequela
		T48.6X2S	Poisoning by antiasthmatics, intentional self-harm, sequela
		T48.6X3S	Poisoning by antiasthmatics, assault, sequela
		T48.6X4S	Poisoning by antiasthmatics, undetermined, sequela
		T48.9Ø1S	Poisn by unsp agents prim acting on the resp sys, acc, sqla
		T48.9Ø2S	Poisn by unsp agents prim act on the resp sys, slf-hrm, sqla
		T48.9Ø3S	Poisn by unsp agents prim act on the resp sys, asslt, sqla
		T48.9Ø4S	Poisn by unsp agents prim act on the resp sys, undet, sqla
		T48.991S	Poisn by oth agents prim acting on the resp sys, acc, sqla
		T48.992S	Poisn by oth agents prim act on the resp sys, slf-hrm, sqla
		T48.993S	Poisn by oth agents prim acting on the resp sys, asslt, sqla
		T48.994S	Poisn by oth agents prim acting on the resp sys, undet, sqla
		T49.ØX1S	Poisn by local antifung/infect/inflamm drugs, acc, sequela
		T49.ØX2S	Poisn by local antifung/infect/inflamm drugs, slf-hrm, sqla
		T49.ØX3S	Poisn by local antifung/infect/inflamm drugs, asslt, sequela
		T49.ØX4S	Poisn by local antifung/infect/inflamm drugs, undet, sequela
		T49.1X1S	Poisoning by antipruritics, accidental, sequela
		T49.1X2S	Poisoning by antipruritics, intentional self-harm, sequela
		T49.1X3S	Poisoning by antipruritics, assault, sequela
		T49.1X4S	Poisoning by antipruritics, undetermined, sequela
		T49.2X1S	Poisoning by local astringents/detergents, acc, sequela

(Continued on next page)

ICD-9-CM		ICD-10-CM	
909.0	LATE EFF POISN-RX MEDICINAL/BIOLOGICAL SUBSTANCE **(Continued)**	**T49.2X2S**	Poisn by local astringents/detergents, self-harm, sequela
		T49.2X3S	Poisoning by local astringents/detergents, assault, sequela
		T49.2X4S	Poisoning by local astringents/detergents, undet, sequela
		T49.3X1S	Poisn by emollients, demulcents and protect, acc, sequela
		T49.3X2S	Poisn by emollients, demulcents and protect, slf-hrm, sqla
		T49.3X3S	Poisn by emollients, demulcents and protect, asslt, sequela
		T49.3X4S	Poisn by emollients, demulcents and protect, undet, sequela
		T49.4X1S	Poisn by keratolyt/keratplst/hair trmt drug, acc, sequela
		T49.4X2S	Poisn by keratolyt/keratplst/hair trmt drug, slf-hrm, sqla
		T49.4X3S	Poisn by keratolyt/keratplst/hair trmt drug, asslt, sequela
		T49.4X4S	Poisn by keratolyt/keratplst/hair trmt drug, undet, sequela
		T49.5X1S	Poisoning by opth drugs and prep, accidental, sequela
		T49.5X2S	Poisoning by opth drugs and preparations, self-harm, sequela
		T49.5X3S	Poisoning by opth drugs and preparations, assault, sequela
		T49.5X4S	Poisoning by opth drugs and prep, undetermined, sequela
		T49.6X1S	Poisoning by otorhino drugs and prep, accidental, sequela
		T49.6X2S	Poisoning by otorhino drugs and prep, self-harm, sequela
		T49.6X3S	Poisoning by otorhino drugs and prep, assault, sequela
		T49.6X4S	Poisoning by otorhino drugs and prep, undetermined, sequela
		T49.7X1S	Poisoning by dental drugs, topically applied, acc, sequela
		T49.7X2S	Poisn by dental drugs, topically applied, self-harm, sequela
		T49.7X3S	Poisn by dental drugs, topically applied, assault, sequela
		T49.7X4S	Poisoning by dental drugs, topically applied, undet, sequela
		T49.8X1S	Poisoning by oth topical agents, accidental, sequela
		T49.8X2S	Poisoning by oth topical agents, self-harm, sequela
		T49.8X3S	Poisoning by other topical agents, assault, sequela
		T49.8X4S	Poisoning by other topical agents, undetermined, sequela
		T49.91XS	Poisoning by unsp topical agent, accidental, sequela
		T49.92XS	Poisoning by unsp topical agent, self-harm, sequela
		T49.93XS	Poisoning by unspecified topical agent, assault, sequela
		T49.94XS	Poisoning by unsp topical agent, undetermined, sequela
		T50.0X1S	Poisoning by mineralocorticoids and antag, acc, sequela
		T50.0X2S	Poisn by mineralocorticoids and antag, self-harm, sequela
		T50.0X3S	Poisoning by mineralocorticoids and antag, assault, sequela
		T50.0X4S	Poisoning by mineralocorticoids and antag, undet, sequela
		T50.1X1S	Poisoning by loop diuretics, accidental, sequela
		T50.1X2S	Poisoning by loop diuretics, intentional self-harm, sequela
		T50.1X3S	Poisoning by loop [high-ceiling] diuretics, assault, sequela
		T50.1X4S	Poisoning by loop diuretics, undetermined, sequela
		T50.2X1S	Poisn by crbnc-anhydr inhibtr, benzo/oth diuretc, acc, sqla
		T50.2X2S	Poisn by crbnc-anhydr inhibtr,benzo/oth diuretc,slf-hrm,sqla
		T50.2X3S	Poisn by crbnc-anhydr inhibtr,benzo/oth diuretc, asslt, sqla
		T50.2X4S	Poisn by crbnc-anhydr inhibtr,benzo/oth diuretc, undet, sqla
		T50.3X1S	Poisn by electrolytic/caloric/wtr-bal agnt, acc, sequela
		T50.3X2S	Poisn by electrolytic/caloric/wtr-bal agnt, slf-hrm, sequela
		T50.3X3S	Poisn by electrolytic/caloric/wtr-bal agnt, assault, sequela
		T50.3X4S	Poisn by electrolytic/caloric/wtr-bal agnt, undet, sequela
		T50.4X1S	Poisoning by drugs affecting uric acid metab, acc, sequela
		T50.4X2S	Poisoning by drugs aff uric acid metab, self-harm, sequela
		T50.4X3S	Poisoning by drugs aff uric acid metab, assault, sequela
		T50.4X4S	Poisoning by drugs affecting uric acid metab, undet, sequela
		T50.5X1S	Poisoning by appetite depressants, accidental, sequela
		T50.5X2S	Poisoning by appetite depressants, self-harm, sequela
		T50.5X3S	Poisoning by appetite depressants, assault, sequela
		T50.5X4S	Poisoning by appetite depressants, undetermined, sequela
		T50.6X1S	Poisoning by antidotes and chelating agents, acc, sequela
		T50.6X2S	Poisn by antidotes and chelating agents, self-harm, sequela
		T50.6X3S	Poisn by antidotes and chelating agents, assault, sequela
		T50.6X4S	Poisoning by antidotes and chelating agents, undet, sequela
		T50.7X1S	Poisn by analeptics and opioid receptor antag, acc, sequela
		T50.7X2S	Poisn by analeptics and opioid receptor antag, slf-hrm, sqla
		T50.7X3S	Poisn by analeptics and opioid receptor antag, asslt, sqla
		T50.7X4S	Poisn by analeptics and opioid receptor antag, undet, sqla
		T50.8X1S	Poisoning by diagnostic agents, accidental, sequela
		T50.8X2S	Poisoning by diagnostic agents, self-harm, sequela
		T50.8X3S	Poisoning by diagnostic agents, assault, sequela
		T50.8X4S	Poisoning by diagnostic agents, undetermined, sequela
		T50.901S	Poisoning by unsp drug/meds/biol subst, accidental, sequela
		T50.902S	Poisoning by unsp drug/meds/biol subst, self-harm, sequela
		T50.903S	Poisoning by unsp drug/meds/biol subst, assault, sequela
		T50.904S	Poisoning by unsp drug/meds/biol subst, undet, sequela
		T50.991S	Poisoning by oth drug/meds/biol subst, accidental, sequela
		T50.992S	Poisoning by oth drug/meds/biol subst, self-harm, sequela
		T50.993S	Poisoning by oth drug/meds/biol subst, assault, sequela
		T50.994S	Poisoning by oth drug/meds/biol subst, undetermined, sequela
		T50.A11S	Poisn by pertuss vaccine, inc combin w pertuss, acc, sqla
		T50.A12S	Poisn by pertuss vaccn, inc combin w pertuss, slf-hrm, sqla
		T50.A13S	Poisn by pertuss vaccine, inc combin w pertuss, asslt, sqla
	(Continued on next page)	**T50.A14S**	Poisn by pertuss vaccine, inc combin w pertuss, undet, sqla

ICD-9-CM		ICD-10-CM		
9Ø9.Ø	LATE EFF POISN-RX MEDICINAL/BIOLOGICAL SUBSTANCE **(Continued)**	◘	**T5Ø.A21S**	Poisn by mixed bact vaccines w/o a pertuss, acc, sequela
		◘	**T5Ø.A22S**	Poisn by mixed bact vaccines w/o a pertuss, slf-hrm, sequela
		◘	**T5Ø.A23S**	Poisn by mixed bact vaccines w/o a pertuss, assault, sequela
		◘	**T5Ø.A24S**	Poisn by mixed bact vaccines w/o a pertuss, undet, sequela
		◘	**T5Ø.A91S**	Poisoning by oth bacterial vaccines, accidental, sequela
		◘	**T5Ø.A92S**	Poisoning by oth bacterial vaccines, self-harm, sequela
		◘	**T5Ø.A93S**	Poisoning by other bacterial vaccines, assault, sequela
		◘	**T5Ø.A94S**	Poisoning by other bacterial vaccines, undetermined, sequela
		◘	**T5Ø.B11S**	Poisoning by smallpox vaccines, accidental, sequela
		◘	**T5Ø.B12S**	Poisoning by smallpox vaccines, self-harm, sequela
		◘	**T5Ø.B13S**	Poisoning by smallpox vaccines, assault, sequela
		◘	**T5Ø.B14S**	Poisoning by smallpox vaccines, undetermined, sequela
		◘	**T5Ø.B91S**	Poisoning by oth viral vaccines, accidental, sequela
		◘	**T5Ø.B92S**	Poisoning by oth viral vaccines, self-harm, sequela
		◘	**T5Ø.B93S**	Poisoning by other viral vaccines, assault, sequela
		◘	**T5Ø.B94S**	Poisoning by other viral vaccines, undetermined, sequela
		◘	**T5Ø.Z11S**	Poisoning by immunoglobulin, accidental, sequela
		◘	**T5Ø.Z12S**	Poisoning by immunoglobulin, intentional self-harm, sequela
		◘	**T5Ø.Z13S**	Poisoning by immunoglobulin, assault, sequela
		◘	**T5Ø.Z14S**	Poisoning by immunoglobulin, undetermined, sequela
		◘	**T5Ø.Z91S**	Poisoning by oth vaccines and biolg substnc, acc, sequela
		◘	**T5Ø.Z92S**	Poisn by oth vaccines and biolg substnc, self-harm, sequela
		◘	**T5Ø.Z93S**	Poisn by oth vaccines and biolg substnc, assault, sequela
		◘	**T5Ø.Z94S**	Poisoning by oth vaccines and biolg substnc, undet, sequela
9Ø9.1	LATE EFFECT TOXIC EFFECTS NONMEDICAL SUBSTANCES		**T51.ØX1S**	Toxic effect of ethanol, accidental (unintentional), sequela
			T51.ØX2S	Toxic effect of ethanol, intentional self-harm, sequela
			T51.ØX3S	Toxic effect of ethanol, assault, sequela
			T51.ØX4S	Toxic effect of ethanol, undetermined, sequela
			T51.1X1S	Toxic effect of methanol, accidental, sequela
			T51.1X2S	Toxic effect of methanol, intentional self-harm, sequela
			T51.1X3S	Toxic effect of methanol, assault, sequela
			T51.1X4S	Toxic effect of methanol, undetermined, sequela
			T51.2X1S	Toxic effect of 2-Propanol, accidental, sequela
			T51.2X2S	Toxic effect of 2-Propanol, intentional self-harm, sequela
			T51.2X3S	Toxic effect of 2-Propanol, assault, sequela
			T51.2X4S	Toxic effect of 2-Propanol, undetermined, sequela
			T51.3X1S	Toxic effect of fusel oil, accidental, sequela
			T51.3X2S	Toxic effect of fusel oil, intentional self-harm, sequela
			T51.3X3S	Toxic effect of fusel oil, assault, sequela
			T51.3X4S	Toxic effect of fusel oil, undetermined, sequela
			T51.8X1S	Toxic effect of alcohols, accidental, sequela
			T51.8X2S	Toxic effect of oth alcohols, intentional self-harm, sequela
			T51.8X3S	Toxic effect of other alcohols, assault, sequela
			T51.8X4S	Toxic effect of other alcohols, undetermined, sequela
			T51.91XS	Toxic effect of unsp alcohol, accidental, sequela
			T51.92XS	Toxic effect of unsp alcohol, intentional self-harm, sequela
			T51.93XS	Toxic effect of unspecified alcohol, assault, sequela
			T51.94XS	Toxic effect of unspecified alcohol, undetermined, sequela
			T52.ØX1S	Toxic effect of petroleum products, accidental, sequela
			T52.ØX2S	Toxic effect of petroleum products, self-harm, sequela
			T52.ØX3S	Toxic effect of petroleum products, assault, sequela
			T52.ØX4S	Toxic effect of petroleum products, undetermined, sequela
			T52.1X1S	Toxic effect of benzene, accidental (unintentional), sequela
			T52.1X2S	Toxic effect of benzene, intentional self-harm, sequela
			T52.1X3S	Toxic effect of benzene, assault, sequela
			T52.1X4S	Toxic effect of benzene, undetermined, sequela
			T52.2X1S	Toxic effect of homologues of benzene, accidental, sequela
			T52.2X2S	Toxic effect of homologues of benzene, self-harm, sequela
			T52.2X3S	Toxic effect of homologues of benzene, assault, sequela
			T52.2X4S	Toxic effect of homologues of benzene, undetermined, sequela
			T52.3X1S	Toxic effect of glycols, accidental (unintentional), sequela
			T52.3X2S	Toxic effect of glycols, intentional self-harm, sequela
			T52.3X3S	Toxic effect of glycols, assault, sequela
			T52.3X4S	Toxic effect of glycols, undetermined, sequela
			T52.4X1S	Toxic effect of ketones, accidental (unintentional), sequela
			T52.4X2S	Toxic effect of ketones, intentional self-harm, sequela
			T52.4X3S	Toxic effect of ketones, assault, sequela
			T52.4X4S	Toxic effect of ketones, undetermined, sequela
			T52.8X1S	Toxic effect of organic solvents, accidental, sequela
			T52.8X2S	Toxic effect of organic solvents, self-harm, sequela
			T52.8X3S	Toxic effect of other organic solvents, assault, sequela
			T52.8X4S	Toxic effect of oth organic solvents, undetermined, sequela
			T52.91XS	Toxic effect of unsp organic solvent, accidental, sequela
			T52.92XS	Toxic effect of unsp organic solvent, self-harm, sequela
			T52.93XS	Toxic effect of unsp organic solvent, assault, sequela
			T52.94XS	Toxic effect of unsp organic solvent, undetermined, sequela
			T53.ØX1S	Toxic effect of carbon tetrachloride, accidental, sequela
			T53.ØX2S	Toxic effect of carbon tetrachloride, self-harm, sequela
			T53.ØX3S	Toxic effect of carbon tetrachloride, assault, sequela
			T53.ØX4S	Toxic effect of carbon tetrachloride, undetermined, sequela
	(Continued on next page)		**T53.1X1S**	Toxic effect of chloroform, accidental, sequela

ICD-9-CM		ICD-10-CM	
909.1	LATE EFFECT TOXIC EFFECTS NONMEDICAL SUBSTANCES **(Continued)**	**T53.1X2S**	Toxic effect of chloroform, intentional self-harm, sequela
		T53.1X3S	Toxic effect of chloroform, assault, sequela
		T53.1X4S	Toxic effect of chloroform, undetermined, sequela
		T53.2X1S	Toxic effect of trichloroethylene, accidental, sequela
		T53.2X2S	Toxic effect of trichloroethylene, self-harm, sequela
		T53.2X3S	Toxic effect of trichloroethylene, assault, sequela
		T53.2X4S	Toxic effect of trichloroethylene, undetermined, sequela
		T53.3X1S	Toxic effect of tetrachloroethylene, accidental, sequela
		T53.3X2S	Toxic effect of tetrachloroethylene, self-harm, sequela
		T53.3X3S	Toxic effect of tetrachloroethylene, assault, sequela
		T53.3X4S	Toxic effect of tetrachloroethylene, undetermined, sequela
		T53.4X1S	Toxic effect of dichloromethane, accidental, sequela
		T53.4X2S	Toxic effect of dichloromethane, self-harm, sequela
		T53.4X3S	Toxic effect of dichloromethane, assault, sequela
		T53.4X4S	Toxic effect of dichloromethane, undetermined, sequela
		T53.5X1S	Toxic effect of chlorofluorocarbons, accidental, sequela
		T53.5X2S	Toxic effect of chlorofluorocarbons, self-harm, sequela
		T53.5X3S	Toxic effect of chlorofluorocarbons, assault, sequela
		T53.5X4S	Toxic effect of chlorofluorocarbons, undetermined, sequela
		T53.6X1S	Toxic eff of halgn deriv of aliphatic hydrocrb, acc, sqla
		T53.6X2S	Tox eff of halgn deriv of aliphatic hydrocrb, slf-hrm, sqla
		T53.6X3S	Toxic eff of halgn deriv of aliphatic hydrocrb, asslt, sqla
		T53.6X4S	Toxic eff of halgn deriv of aliphatic hydrocrb, undet, sqla
		T53.7X1S	Toxic effect of halgn deriv of aromatic hydrocrb, acc, sqla
		T53.7X2S	Toxic eff of halgn deriv of aromatic hydrocrb, slf-hrm, sqla
		T53.7X3S	Toxic eff of halgn deriv of aromatic hydrocrb, asslt, sqla
		T53.7X4S	Toxic eff of halgn deriv of aromatic hydrocrb, undet, sqla
		T53.91XS	Toxic eff of unsp halgn deriv of aromat hydrocrb, acc, sqla
		T53.92XS	Tox eff of unsp halgn deriv of aromat hydrocrb,slf-hrm, sqla
		T53.93XS	Tox eff of unsp halgn deriv of aromat hydrocrb, asslt, sqla
		T53.94XS	Tox eff of unsp halgn deriv of aromat hydrocrb, undet, sqla
		T54.ØX1S	Toxic effect of phenol and phenol homologues, acc, sequela
		T54.ØX2S	Toxic effect of phenol and phenol homolog, slf-hrm, sequela
		T54.ØX3S	Toxic effect of phenol and phenol homolog, assault, sequela
		T54.ØX4S	Toxic effect of phenol and phenol homologues, undet, sequela
		T54.1X1S	Toxic effect of corrosive organic compounds, acc, sequela
		T54.1X2S	Toxic effect of corrosive organic compnd, self-harm, sequela
		T54.1X3S	Toxic effect of corrosive organic compnd, assault, sequela
		T54.1X4S	Toxic effect of corrosive organic compounds, undet, sequela
		T54.2X1S	Toxic eff of corrosv acids and acid-like substnc, acc, sqla
		T54.2X2S	Tox eff of corrosv acids & acid-like substnc, slf-hrm, sqla
		T54.2X3S	Tox eff of corrosv acids and acid-like substnc, asslt, sqla
		T54.2X4S	Tox eff of corrosv acids and acid-like substnc, undet, sqla
		T54.3X1S	Tox eff of corrosv alkalis and alk-like substnc, acc, sqla
		T54.3X2S	Tox eff of corrosv alkalis & alk-like substnc, slf-hrm, sqla
		T54.3X3S	Tox eff of corrosv alkalis and alk-like substnc, asslt, sqla
		T54.3X4S	Tox eff of corrosv alkalis and alk-like substnc, undet, sqla
		T54.91XS	Toxic effect of unsp corrosive substance, acc, sequela
		T54.92XS	Toxic effect of unsp corrosive substance, self-harm, sequela
		T54.93XS	Toxic effect of unsp corrosive substance, assault, sequela
		T54.94XS	Toxic effect of unsp corrosive substance, undet, sequela
		T55.ØX1S	Toxic effect of soaps, accidental (unintentional), sequela
		T55.ØX2S	Toxic effect of soaps, intentional self-harm, sequela
		T55.ØX3S	Toxic effect of soaps, assault, sequela
		T55.ØX4S	Toxic effect of soaps, undetermined, sequela
		T55.1X1S	Toxic effect of detergents, accidental, sequela
		T55.1X2S	Toxic effect of detergents, intentional self-harm, sequela
		T55.1X3S	Toxic effect of detergents, assault, sequela
		T55.1X4S	Toxic effect of detergents, undetermined, sequela
		T56.ØX1S	Toxic effect of lead and its compounds, accidental, sequela
		T56.ØX2S	Toxic effect of lead and its compounds, self-harm, sequela
		T56.ØX3S	Toxic effect of lead and its compounds, assault, sequela
		T56.ØX4S	Toxic effect of lead and its compounds, undet, sequela
		T56.1X1S	Toxic effect of mercury and its compounds, acc, sequela
		T56.1X2S	Toxic effect of mercury and its compnd, self-harm, sequela
		T56.1X3S	Toxic effect of mercury and its compounds, assault, sequela
		T56.1X4S	Toxic effect of mercury and its compounds, undet, sequela
		T56.2X1S	Toxic effect of chromium and its compounds, acc, sequela
		T56.2X2S	Toxic effect of chromium and its compnd, self-harm, sequela
		T56.2X3S	Toxic effect of chromium and its compounds, assault, sequela
		T56.2X4S	Toxic effect of chromium and its compounds, undet, sequela
		T56.3X1S	Toxic effect of cadmium and its compounds, acc, sequela
		T56.3X2S	Toxic effect of cadmium and its compnd, self-harm, sequela
		T56.3X3S	Toxic effect of cadmium and its compounds, assault, sequela
		T56.3X4S	Toxic effect of cadmium and its compounds, undet, sequela
		T56.4X1S	Toxic effect of copper and its compounds, acc, sequela
		T56.4X2S	Toxic effect of copper and its compounds, self-harm, sequela
		T56.4X3S	Toxic effect of copper and its compounds, assault, sequela
		T56.4X4S	Toxic effect of copper and its compounds, undet, sequela
		T56.5X1S	Toxic effect of zinc and its compounds, accidental, sequela
		T56.5X2S	Toxic effect of zinc and its compounds, self-harm, sequela
		T56.5X3S	Toxic effect of zinc and its compounds, assault, sequela
	(Continued on next page)	**T56.5X4S**	Toxic effect of zinc and its compounds, undet, sequela

ICD-9-CM		ICD-10-CM	
9Ø9.1	LATE EFFECT TOXIC EFFECTS NONMEDICAL SUBSTANCES **(Continued)**	**T56.6X1S**	Toxic effect of tin and its compounds, accidental, sequela
		T56.6X2S	Toxic effect of tin and its compounds, self-harm, sequela
		T56.6X3S	Toxic effect of tin and its compounds, assault, sequela
		T56.6X4S	Toxic effect of tin and its compounds, undetermined, sequela
		T56.7X1S	Toxic effect of beryllium and its compounds, acc, sequela
		T56.7X2S	Toxic effect of beryllium and its compnd, self-harm, sequela
		T56.7X3S	Toxic effect of beryllium and its compnd, assault, sequela
		T56.7X4S	Toxic effect of beryllium and its compounds, undet, sequela
		T56.811S	Toxic effect of thallium, accidental, sequela
		T56.812S	Toxic effect of thallium, intentional self-harm, sequela
		T56.813S	Toxic effect of thallium, assault, sequela
		T56.814S	Toxic effect of thallium, undetermined, sequela
		T56.891S	Toxic effect of metals, accidental (unintentional), sequela
		T56.892S	Toxic effect of other metals, intentional self-harm, sequela
		T56.893S	Toxic effect of other metals, assault, sequela
		T56.894S	Toxic effect of other metals, undetermined, sequela
		T56.91XS	Toxic effect of unsp metal, accidental, sequela
		T56.92XS	Toxic effect of unsp metal, intentional self-harm, sequela
		T56.93XS	Toxic effect of unspecified metal, assault, sequela
		T56.94XS	Toxic effect of unspecified metal, undetermined, sequela
		T57.ØX1S	Toxic effect of arsenic and its compounds, acc, sequela
		T57.ØX2S	Toxic effect of arsenic and its compnd, self-harm, sequela
		T57.ØX3S	Toxic effect of arsenic and its compounds, assault, sequela
		T57.ØX4S	Toxic effect of arsenic and its compounds, undet, sequela
		T57.1X1S	Toxic effect of phosphorus and its compounds, acc, sequela
		T57.1X2S	Toxic effect of phosphorus and its compnd, slf-hrm, sequela
		T57.1X3S	Toxic effect of phosphorus and its compnd, assault, sequela
		T57.1X4S	Toxic effect of phosphorus and its compounds, undet, sequela
		T57.2X1S	Toxic effect of manganese and its compounds, acc, sequela
		T57.2X2S	Toxic effect of manganese and its compnd, self-harm, sequela
		T57.2X3S	Toxic effect of manganese and its compnd, assault, sequela
		T57.2X4S	Toxic effect of manganese and its compounds, undet, sequela
		T57.3X1S	Toxic effect of hydrogen cyanide, accidental, sequela
		T57.3X2S	Toxic effect of hydrogen cyanide, self-harm, sequela
		T57.3X3S	Toxic effect of hydrogen cyanide, assault, sequela
		T57.3X4S	Toxic effect of hydrogen cyanide, undetermined, sequela
		T57.8X1S	Toxic effect of inorganic substances, accidental, sequela
		T57.8X2S	Toxic effect of inorganic substances, self-harm, sequela
		T57.8X3S	Toxic effect of oth inorganic substances, assault, sequela
		T57.8X4S	Toxic effect of inorganic substances, undetermined, sequela
		T57.91XS	Toxic effect of unsp inorganic substance, acc, sequela
		T57.92XS	Toxic effect of unsp inorganic substance, self-harm, sequela
		T57.93XS	Toxic effect of unsp inorganic substance, assault, sequela
		T57.94XS	Toxic effect of unsp inorganic substance, undet, sequela
		T58.Ø1XS	Toxic effect of carb monx from mtr veh exhaust, acc, sqla
		T58.Ø2XS	Toxic eff of carb monx from mtr veh exhaust, slf-hrm, sqla
		T58.Ø3XS	Toxic effect of carb monx from mtr veh exhaust, asslt, sqla
		T58.Ø4XS	Toxic effect of carb monx from mtr veh exhaust, undet, sqla
		T58.11XS	Toxic effect of carb monx from utility gas, acc, sequela
		T58.12XS	Toxic effect of carb monx from utility gas, slf-hrm, sequela
		T58.13XS	Toxic effect of carb monx from utility gas, assault, sequela
		T58.14XS	Toxic effect of carb monx from utility gas, undet, sequela
		T58.2X1S	Tox eff of carb monx fr incmpl combst dmst fuel, acc, sqla
		T58.2X2S	Tox eff of carb monx fr incmpl combst dmst fuel,slf-hrm,sqla
		T58.2X3S	Tox eff of carb monx fr incmpl combst dmst fuel, asslt, sqla
		T58.2X4S	Tox eff of carb monx fr incmpl combst dmst fuel, undet, sqla
		T58.8X1S	Toxic effect of carb monx from oth source, acc, sequela
		T58.8X2S	Toxic effect of carb monx from oth source, slf-hrm, sequela
		T58.8X3S	Toxic effect of carb monx from oth source, assault, sequela
		T58.8X4S	Toxic effect of carb monx from oth source, undet, sequela
		T58.91XS	Toxic effect of carb monx from unsp source, acc, sequela
		T58.92XS	Toxic effect of carb monx from unsp source, slf-hrm, sequela
		T58.93XS	Toxic effect of carb monx from unsp source, assault, sequela
		T58.94XS	Toxic effect of carb monx from unsp source, undet, sequela
		T59.ØX1S	Toxic effect of nitrogen oxides, accidental, sequela
		T59.ØX2S	Toxic effect of nitrogen oxides, self-harm, sequela
		T59.ØX3S	Toxic effect of nitrogen oxides, assault, sequela
		T59.ØX4S	Toxic effect of nitrogen oxides, undetermined, sequela
		T59.1X1S	Toxic effect of sulfur dioxide, accidental, sequela
		T59.1X2S	Toxic effect of sulfur dioxide, self-harm, sequela
		T59.1X3S	Toxic effect of sulfur dioxide, assault, sequela
		T59.1X4S	Toxic effect of sulfur dioxide, undetermined, sequela
		T59.2X1S	Toxic effect of formaldehyde, accidental, sequela
		T59.2X2S	Toxic effect of formaldehyde, intentional self-harm, sequela
		T59.2X3S	Toxic effect of formaldehyde, assault, sequela
		T59.2X4S	Toxic effect of formaldehyde, undetermined, sequela
		T59.3X1S	Toxic effect of lacrimogenic gas, accidental, sequela
		T59.3X2S	Toxic effect of lacrimogenic gas, self-harm, sequela
		T59.3X3S	Toxic effect of lacrimogenic gas, assault, sequela
		T59.3X4S	Toxic effect of lacrimogenic gas, undetermined, sequela
		T59.4X1S	Toxic effect of chlorine gas, accidental, sequela
		T59.4X2S	Toxic effect of chlorine gas, intentional self-harm, sequela
	(Continued on next page)	**T59.4X3S**	Toxic effect of chlorine gas, assault, sequela

ICD-9-CM		ICD-10-CM	
9Ø9.1	LATE EFFECT TOXIC EFFECTS NONMEDICAL SUBSTANCES **(Continued)**	**T59.4X4S**	Toxic effect of chlorine gas, undetermined, sequela
		T59.5X1S	Toxic eff of fluorine gas and hydrogen fluoride, acc, sqla
		T59.5X2S	Tox eff of fluorine gas and hydrogen fluoride, slf-hrm, sqla
		T59.5X3S	Toxic eff of fluorine gas and hydrogen fluoride, asslt, sqla
		T59.5X4S	Toxic eff of fluorine gas and hydrogen fluoride, undet, sqla
		T59.6X1S	Toxic effect of hydrogen sulfide, accidental, sequela
		T59.6X2S	Toxic effect of hydrogen sulfide, self-harm, sequela
		T59.6X3S	Toxic effect of hydrogen sulfide, assault, sequela
		T59.6X4S	Toxic effect of hydrogen sulfide, undetermined, sequela
		T59.7X1S	Toxic effect of carbon dioxide, accidental, sequela
		T59.7X2S	Toxic effect of carbon dioxide, self-harm, sequela
		T59.7X3S	Toxic effect of carbon dioxide, assault, sequela
		T59.7X4S	Toxic effect of carbon dioxide, undetermined, sequela
		T59.811S	Toxic effect of smoke, accidental (unintentional), sequela
		T59.812S	Toxic effect of smoke, intentional self-harm, sequela
		T59.813S	Toxic effect of smoke, assault, sequela
		T59.814S	Toxic effect of smoke, undetermined, sequela
		T59.891S	Toxic effect of gases, fumes and vapors, acc, sequela
		T59.892S	Toxic effect of gases, fumes and vapors, self-harm, sequela
		T59.893S	Toxic effect of gases, fumes and vapors, assault, sequela
		T59.894S	Toxic effect of gases, fumes and vapors, undet, sequela
		T59.91XS	Toxic effect of unsp gases, fumes and vapors, acc, sequela
		T59.92XS	Toxic effect of unsp gases, fumes and vapors, slf-hrm, sqla
		T59.93XS	Toxic effect of unsp gases, fumes and vapors, asslt, sequela
		T59.94XS	Toxic effect of unsp gases, fumes and vapors, undet, sequela
		T6Ø.ØX1S	Toxic effect of organophos and carbamate insect, acc, sqla
		T6Ø.ØX2S	Toxic eff of organophos and carbamate insect, slf-hrm, sqla
		T6Ø.ØX3S	Toxic effect of organophos and carbamate insect, asslt, sqla
		T6Ø.ØX4S	Toxic effect of organophos and carbamate insect, undet, sqla
		T6Ø.1X1S	Toxic effect of halogenated insect, accidental, sequela
		T6Ø.1X2S	Toxic effect of halogenated insecticides, self-harm, sequela
		T6Ø.1X3S	Toxic effect of halogenated insecticides, assault, sequela
		T6Ø.1X4S	Toxic effect of halogenated insect, undetermined, sequela
		T6Ø.2X1S	Toxic effect of insecticides, accidental, sequela
		T6Ø.2X2S	Toxic effect of insecticides, intentional self-harm, sequela
		T6Ø.2X3S	Toxic effect of other insecticides, assault, sequela
		T6Ø.2X4S	Toxic effect of other insecticides, undetermined, sequela
		T6Ø.3X1S	Toxic effect of herbicides and fungicides, acc, sequela
		T6Ø.3X2S	Toxic effect of herbicides and fungicides, slf-hrm, sequela
		T6Ø.3X3S	Toxic effect of herbicides and fungicides, assault, sequela
		T6Ø.3X4S	Toxic effect of herbicides and fungicides, undet, sequela
		T6Ø.4X1S	Toxic effect of rodenticides, accidental, sequela
		T6Ø.4X2S	Toxic effect of rodenticides, intentional self-harm, sequela
		T6Ø.4X3S	Toxic effect of rodenticides, assault, sequela
		T6Ø.4X4S	Toxic effect of rodenticides, undetermined, sequela
		T6Ø.8X1S	Toxic effect of pesticides, accidental, sequela
		T6Ø.8X2S	Toxic effect of pesticides, intentional self-harm, sequela
		T6Ø.8X3S	Toxic effect of other pesticides, assault, sequela
		T6Ø.8X4S	Toxic effect of other pesticides, undetermined, sequela
		T6Ø.91XS	Toxic effect of unsp pesticide, accidental, sequela
		T6Ø.92XS	Toxic effect of unsp pesticide, self-harm, sequela
		T6Ø.93XS	Toxic effect of unspecified pesticide, assault, sequela
		T6Ø.94XS	Toxic effect of unspecified pesticide, undetermined, sequela
		T61.Ø1XS	Ciguatera fish poisoning, accidental, sequela
		T61.Ø2XS	Ciguatera fish poisoning, intentional self-harm, sequela
		T61.Ø3XS	Ciguatera fish poisoning, assault, sequela
		T61.Ø4XS	Ciguatera fish poisoning, undetermined, sequela
		T61.11XS	Scombroid fish poisoning, accidental, sequela
		T61.12XS	Scombroid fish poisoning, intentional self-harm, sequela
		T61.13XS	Scombroid fish poisoning, assault, sequela
		T61.14XS	Scombroid fish poisoning, undetermined, sequela
		T61.771S	Other fish poisoning, accidental (unintentional), sequela
		T61.772S	Other fish poisoning, intentional self-harm, sequela
		T61.773S	Other fish poisoning, assault, sequela
		T61.774S	Other fish poisoning, undetermined, sequela
		T61.781S	Oth shellfish poisoning, accidental (unintentional), sequela
		T61.782S	Other shellfish poisoning, intentional self-harm, sequela
		T61.783S	Other shellfish poisoning, assault, sequela
		T61.784S	Other shellfish poisoning, undetermined, sequela
		T61.8X1S	Toxic effect of seafood, accidental (unintentional), sequela
		T61.8X2S	Toxic effect of oth seafood, intentional self-harm, sequela
		T61.8X3S	Toxic effect of other seafood, assault, sequela
		T61.8X4S	Toxic effect of other seafood, undetermined, sequela
		T61.91XS	Toxic effect of unsp seafood, accidental, sequela
		T61.92XS	Toxic effect of unsp seafood, intentional self-harm, sequela
		T61.93XS	Toxic effect of unspecified seafood, assault, sequela
		T61.94XS	Toxic effect of unspecified seafood, undetermined, sequela
		T62.ØX1S	Toxic effect of ingested mushrooms, accidental, sequela
		T62.ØX2S	Toxic effect of ingested mushrooms, self-harm, sequela
		T62.ØX3S	Toxic effect of ingested mushrooms, assault, sequela

(Continued on next page)

ICD-9-CM		ICD-10-CM	
9Ø9.1	LATE EFFECT TOXIC EFFECTS NONMEDICAL SUBSTANCES **(Continued)**	**T62.ØX4S**	Toxic effect of ingested mushrooms, undetermined, sequela
		T62.1X1S	Toxic effect of ingested berries, accidental, sequela
		T62.1X2S	Toxic effect of ingested berries, self-harm, sequela
		T62.1X3S	Toxic effect of ingested berries, assault, sequela
		T62.1X4S	Toxic effect of ingested berries, undetermined, sequela
		T62.2X1S	Toxic effect of ingested (parts of) plant(s), acc, sequela
		T62.2X2S	Toxic effect of ingest (parts of) plant(s), slf-hrm, sequela
		T62.2X3S	Toxic effect of ingest (parts of) plant(s), assault, sequela
		T62.2X4S	Toxic effect of ingested (parts of) plant(s), undet, sequela
		T62.8X1S	Toxic effect of noxious substnc eaten as food, acc, sequela
		T62.8X2S	Toxic effect of noxious substnc eaten as food, slf-hrm, sqla
		T62.8X3S	Toxic effect of noxious substnc eaten as food, asslt, sqla
		T62.8X4S	Toxic effect of noxious substnc eaten as food, undet, sqla
		T62.91XS	Toxic effect of unsp noxious sub eaten as food, acc, sequela
		T62.92XS	Toxic eff of unsp noxious sub eaten as food, slf-hrm, sqla
		T62.93XS	Toxic effect of unsp noxious sub eaten as food, asslt, sqla
		T62.94XS	Toxic effect of unsp noxious sub eaten as food, undet, sqla
		T63.ØØ1S	Toxic effect of unsp snake venom, accidental, sequela
		T63.ØØ2S	Toxic effect of unsp snake venom, self-harm, sequela
		T63.ØØ3S	Toxic effect of unspecified snake venom, assault, sequela
		T63.ØØ4S	Toxic effect of unsp snake venom, undetermined, sequela
		T63.Ø11S	Toxic effect of rattlesnake venom, accidental, sequela
		T63.Ø12S	Toxic effect of rattlesnake venom, self-harm, sequela
		T63.Ø13S	Toxic effect of rattlesnake venom, assault, sequela
		T63.Ø14S	Toxic effect of rattlesnake venom, undetermined, sequela
		T63.Ø21S	Toxic effect of coral snake venom, accidental, sequela
		T63.Ø22S	Toxic effect of coral snake venom, self-harm, sequela
		T63.Ø23S	Toxic effect of coral snake venom, assault, sequela
		T63.Ø24S	Toxic effect of coral snake venom, undetermined, sequela
		T63.Ø31S	Toxic effect of taipan venom, accidental, sequela
		T63.Ø32S	Toxic effect of taipan venom, intentional self-harm, sequela
		T63.Ø33S	Toxic effect of taipan venom, assault, sequela
		T63.Ø34S	Toxic effect of taipan venom, undetermined, sequela
		T63.Ø41S	Toxic effect of cobra venom, accidental, sequela
		T63.Ø42S	Toxic effect of cobra venom, intentional self-harm, sequela
		T63.Ø43S	Toxic effect of cobra venom, assault, sequela
		T63.Ø44S	Toxic effect of cobra venom, undetermined, sequela
		T63.Ø61S	Toxic effect of venom of N & S American snake, acc, sequela
		T63.Ø62S	Toxic effect of venom of N & S American snake, slf-hrm, sqla
		T63.Ø63S	Toxic effect of venom of N & S American snake, asslt, sqla
		T63.Ø64S	Toxic effect of venom of N & S American snake, undet, sqla
		T63.Ø71S	Toxic effect of venom of Australian snake, acc, sequela
		T63.Ø72S	Toxic effect of venom of Australian snake, slf-hrm, sequela
		T63.Ø73S	Toxic effect of venom of Australian snake, assault, sequela
		T63.Ø74S	Toxic effect of venom of Australian snake, undet, sequela
		T63.Ø81S	Toxic effect of venom of African and Asian snake, acc, sqla
		T63.Ø82S	Toxic eff of venom of African and Asian snake, slf-hrm, sqla
		T63.Ø83S	Toxic eff of venom of African and Asian snake, asslt, sqla
		T63.Ø84S	Toxic eff of venom of African and Asian snake, undet, sqla
		T63.Ø91S	Toxic effect of venom of snake, accidental, sequela
		T63.Ø92S	Toxic effect of venom of snake, self-harm, sequela
		T63.Ø93S	Toxic effect of venom of other snake, assault, sequela
		T63.Ø94S	Toxic effect of venom of other snake, undetermined, sequela
		T63.111S	Toxic effect of venom of gila monster, accidental, sequela
		T63.112S	Toxic effect of venom of gila monster, self-harm, sequela
		T63.113S	Toxic effect of venom of gila monster, assault, sequela
		T63.114S	Toxic effect of venom of gila monster, undetermined, sequela
		T63.121S	Toxic effect of venom of venomous lizard, acc, sequela
		T63.122S	Toxic effect of venom of venomous lizard, self-harm, sequela
		T63.123S	Toxic effect of venom of venomous lizard, assault, sequela
		T63.124S	Toxic effect of venom of venomous lizard, undet, sequela
		T63.191S	Toxic effect of venom of reptiles, accidental, sequela
		T63.192S	Toxic effect of venom of reptiles, self-harm, sequela
		T63.193S	Toxic effect of venom of other reptiles, assault, sequela
		T63.194S	Toxic effect of venom of oth reptiles, undetermined, sequela
		T63.2X1S	Toxic effect of venom of scorpion, accidental, sequela
		T63.2X2S	Toxic effect of venom of scorpion, self-harm, sequela
		T63.2X3S	Toxic effect of venom of scorpion, assault, sequela
		T63.2X4S	Toxic effect of venom of scorpion, undetermined, sequela
		T63.3Ø1S	Toxic effect of unsp spider venom, accidental, sequela
		T63.3Ø2S	Toxic effect of unsp spider venom, self-harm, sequela
		T63.3Ø3S	Toxic effect of unspecified spider venom, assault, sequela
		T63.3Ø4S	Toxic effect of unsp spider venom, undetermined, sequela
		T63.311S	Toxic effect of venom of black widow spider, acc, sequela
		T63.312S	Toxic effect of venom of black widow spider, slf-hrm, sqla
		T63.313S	Toxic effect of venom of black widow spider, asslt, sequela
		T63.314S	Toxic effect of venom of black widow spider, undet, sequela
		T63.321S	Toxic effect of venom of tarantula, accidental, sequela
	(Continued on next page)	**T63.322S**	Toxic effect of venom of tarantula, self-harm, sequela

ICD-9-CM		ICD-10-CM	
909.1	LATE EFFECT TOXIC EFFECTS NONMEDICAL SUBSTANCES **(Continued)**	**T63.323S**	Toxic effect of venom of tarantula, assault, sequela
		T63.324S	Toxic effect of venom of tarantula, undetermined, sequela
		T63.331S	Toxic effect of venom of brown recluse spider, acc, sequela
		T63.332S	Toxic effect of venom of brown recluse spider, slf-hrm, sqla
		T63.333S	Toxic effect of venom of brown recluse spider, asslt, sqla
		T63.334S	Toxic effect of venom of brown recluse spider, undet, sqla
		T63.391S	Toxic effect of venom of spider, accidental, sequela
		T63.392S	Toxic effect of venom of spider, self-harm, sequela
		T63.393S	Toxic effect of venom of other spider, assault, sequela
		T63.394S	Toxic effect of venom of other spider, undetermined, sequela
		T63.411S	Toxic effect of venom of centipede/millipede, acc, sequela
		T63.412S	Toxic effect of venom of centipede/millipede, slf-hrm, sqla
		T63.413S	Toxic effect of venom of centipede/millipede, asslt, sequela
		T63.414S	Toxic effect of venom of centipede/millipede, undet, sequela
		T63.421S	Toxic effect of venom of ants, accidental, sequela
		T63.422S	Toxic effect of venom of ants, self-harm, sequela
		T63.423S	Toxic effect of venom of ants, assault, sequela
		T63.424S	Toxic effect of venom of ants, undetermined, sequela
		T63.431S	Toxic effect of venom of caterpillars, accidental, sequela
		T63.432S	Toxic effect of venom of caterpillars, self-harm, sequela
		T63.433S	Toxic effect of venom of caterpillars, assault, sequela
		T63.434S	Toxic effect of venom of caterpillars, undetermined, sequela
		T63.441S	Toxic effect of venom of bees, accidental, sequela
		T63.442S	Toxic effect of venom of bees, self-harm, sequela
		T63.443S	Toxic effect of venom of bees, assault, sequela
		T63.444S	Toxic effect of venom of bees, undetermined, sequela
		T63.451S	Toxic effect of venom of hornets, accidental, sequela
		T63.452S	Toxic effect of venom of hornets, self-harm, sequela
		T63.453S	Toxic effect of venom of hornets, assault, sequela
		T63.454S	Toxic effect of venom of hornets, undetermined, sequela
		T63.461S	Toxic effect of venom of wasps, accidental, sequela
		T63.462S	Toxic effect of venom of wasps, self-harm, sequela
		T63.463S	Toxic effect of venom of wasps, assault, sequela
		T63.464S	Toxic effect of venom of wasps, undetermined, sequela
		T63.481S	Toxic effect of venom of arthropod, accidental, sequela
		T63.482S	Toxic effect of venom of arthropod, self-harm, sequela
		T63.483S	Toxic effect of venom of other arthropod, assault, sequela
		T63.484S	Toxic effect of venom of arthropod, undetermined, sequela
		T63.511S	Toxic effect of contact w stingray, accidental, sequela
		T63.512S	Toxic effect of contact w stingray, self-harm, sequela
		T63.513S	Toxic effect of contact with stingray, assault, sequela
		T63.514S	Toxic effect of contact with stingray, undetermined, sequela
		T63.591S	Toxic effect of contact w oth venomous fish, acc, sequela
		T63.592S	Toxic effect of contact w oth venom fish, slf-hrm, sequela
		T63.593S	Toxic effect of contact w oth venom fish, assault, sequela
		T63.594S	Toxic effect of contact w oth venomous fish, undet, sequela
		T63.611S	Toxic effect of contact w Portugese Man-o-war, acc, sequela
		T63.612S	Toxic effect of cntct w Portugese Man-o-war, slf-hrm, sqla
		T63.613S	Toxic effect of cntct w Portugese Man-o-war, asslt, sequela
		T63.614S	Toxic effect of cntct w Portugese Man-o-war, undet, sequela
		T63.621S	Toxic effect of contact w oth jellyfish, acc, sequela
		T63.622S	Toxic effect of contact w oth jellyfish, self-harm, sequela
		T63.623S	Toxic effect of contact with oth jellyfish, assault, sequela
		T63.624S	Toxic effect of contact w oth jellyfish, undet, sequela
		T63.631S	Toxic effect of contact w sea anemone, accidental, sequela
		T63.632S	Toxic effect of contact w sea anemone, self-harm, sequela
		T63.633S	Toxic effect of contact with sea anemone, assault, sequela
		T63.634S	Toxic effect of contact w sea anemone, undetermined, sequela
		T63.691S	Toxic effect of cntct w oth venom marine animals, acc, sqla
		T63.692S	Toxic eff of cntct w oth venom marine animals, slf-hrm, sqla
		T63.693S	Toxic eff of cntct w oth venom marine animals, asslt, sqla
		T63.694S	Toxic eff of cntct w oth venom marine animals, undet, sqla
		T63.711S	Toxic effect of contact w venom marine plant, acc, sequela
		T63.712S	Toxic effect of cntct w venom marine plant, slf-hrm, sequela
		T63.713S	Toxic effect of contact w venom marine plant, asslt, sequela
		T63.714S	Toxic effect of contact w venom marine plant, undet, sequela
		T63.791S	Toxic effect of contact w oth venomous plant, acc, sequela
		T63.792S	Toxic effect of contact w oth venom plant, slf-hrm, sequela
		T63.793S	Toxic effect of contact w oth venom plant, assault, sequela
		T63.794S	Toxic effect of contact w oth venomous plant, undet, sequela
		T63.811S	Toxic effect of contact w venomous frog, acc, sequela
		T63.812S	Toxic effect of contact w venomous frog, self-harm, sequela
		T63.813S	Toxic effect of contact with venomous frog, assault, sequela
		T63.814S	Toxic effect of contact w venomous frog, undet, sequela
		T63.821S	Toxic effect of contact w venomous toad, acc, sequela
		T63.822S	Toxic effect of contact w venomous toad, self-harm, sequela
		T63.823S	Toxic effect of contact with venomous toad, assault, sequela
		T63.824S	Toxic effect of contact w venomous toad, undet, sequela
	(Continued on next page)	**T63.831S**	Toxic effect of contact w oth venomous amphib, acc, sequela

ICD-9-CM		ICD-10-CM		
9Ø9.1	LATE EFFECT TOXIC EFFECTS NONMEDICAL SUBSTANCES **(Continued)**	◘	**T63.832S**	Toxic effect of contact w oth venom amphib, slf-hrm, sequela
		◘	**T63.833S**	Toxic effect of contact w oth venom amphib, assault, sequela
		◘	**T63.834S**	Toxic effect of contact w oth venom amphib, undet, sequela
		◘	**T63.891S**	Toxic effect of contact w oth venom animals, acc, sequela
		◘	**T63.892S**	Toxic effect of cntct w oth venom animals, slf-hrm, sequela
		◘	**T63.893S**	Toxic effect of contact w oth venom animals, asslt, sequela
		◘	**T63.894S**	Toxic effect of contact w oth venom animals, undet, sequela
		◘	**T63.91XS**	Toxic effect of contact w unsp venom animal, acc, sequela
		◘	**T63.92XS**	Toxic effect of cntct w unsp venom animal, slf-hrm, sequela
		◘	**T63.93XS**	Toxic effect of contact w unsp venom animal, asslt, sequela
		◘	**T63.94XS**	Toxic effect of contact w unsp venom animal, undet, sequela
		◘	**T64.Ø1XS**	Toxic effect of aflatoxin, accidental, sequela
		◘	**T64.Ø2XS**	Toxic effect of aflatoxin, intentional self-harm, sequela
		◘	**T64.Ø3XS**	Toxic effect of aflatoxin, assault, sequela
		◘	**T64.Ø4XS**	Toxic effect of aflatoxin, undetermined, sequela
		◘	**T64.81XS**	Toxic effect of mycotoxin food contamnt, acc, sequela
		◘	**T64.82XS**	Toxic effect of mycotoxin food contamnt, self-harm, sequela
		◘	**T64.83XS**	Toxic effect of mycotoxin food contamnt, assault, sequela
		◘	**T64.84XS**	Toxic effect of mycotoxin food contamnt, undet, sequela
		◘	**T65.ØX1S**	Toxic effect of cyanides, accidental, sequela
		◘	**T65.ØX2S**	Toxic effect of cyanides, intentional self-harm, sequela
		◘	**T65.ØX3S**	Toxic effect of cyanides, assault, sequela
		◘	**T65.ØX4S**	Toxic effect of cyanides, undetermined, sequela
		◘	**T65.1X1S**	Toxic effect of strychnine and its salts, acc, sequela
		◘	**T65.1X2S**	Toxic effect of strychnine and its salts, self-harm, sequela
		◘	**T65.1X3S**	Toxic effect of strychnine and its salts, assault, sequela
		◘	**T65.1X4S**	Toxic effect of strychnine and its salts, undet, sequela
		◘	**T65.211S**	Toxic effect of chewing tobacco, accidental, sequela
		◘	**T65.212S**	Toxic effect of chewing tobacco, self-harm, sequela
		◘	**T65.213S**	Toxic effect of chewing tobacco, assault, sequela
		◘	**T65.214S**	Toxic effect of chewing tobacco, undetermined, sequela
		◘	**T65.221S**	Toxic effect of tobacco cigarettes, accidental, sequela
		◘	**T65.222S**	Toxic effect of tobacco cigarettes, self-harm, sequela
		◘	**T65.223S**	Toxic effect of tobacco cigarettes, assault, sequela
		◘	**T65.224S**	Toxic effect of tobacco cigarettes, undetermined, sequela
		◘	**T65.291S**	Toxic effect of tobacco and nicotine, accidental, sequela
		◘	**T65.292S**	Toxic effect of tobacco and nicotine, self-harm, sequela
		◘	**T65.293S**	Toxic effect of other tobacco and nicotine, assault, sequela
		◘	**T65.294S**	Toxic effect of tobacco and nicotine, undetermined, sequela
		◘	**T65.3X1S**	Toxic eff of nitrodrv/aminodrv of benzn/homolog, acc, sqla
		◘	**T65.3X2S**	Tox eff of nitrodrv/aminodrv of benzn/homolog, slf-hrm, sqla
		◘	**T65.3X3S**	Toxic eff of nitrodrv/aminodrv of benzn/homolog, asslt, sqla
		◘	**T65.3X4S**	Toxic eff of nitrodrv/aminodrv of benzn/homolog, undet, sqla
		◘	**T65.4X1S**	Toxic effect of carbon disulfide, accidental, sequela
		◘	**T65.4X2S**	Toxic effect of carbon disulfide, self-harm, sequela
		◘	**T65.4X3S**	Toxic effect of carbon disulfide, assault, sequela
		◘	**T65.4X4S**	Toxic effect of carbon disulfide, undetermined, sequela
		◘	**T65.5X1S**	Tox eff of nitro and oth nitric acids and esters, acc, sqla
		◘	**T65.5X2S**	Tox eff of nitro & oth nitric acids & esters, slf-hrm, sqla
		◘	**T65.5X3S**	Tox eff of nitro & oth nitric acids and esters, asslt, sqla
		◘	**T65.5X4S**	Tox eff of nitro & oth nitric acids and esters, undet, sqla
		◘	**T65.6X1S**	Toxic effect of paints and dyes, NEC, accidental, sequela
		◘	**T65.6X2S**	Toxic effect of paints and dyes, NEC, self-harm, sequela
		◘	**T65.6X3S**	Toxic effect of paints and dyes, NEC, assault, sequela
		◘	**T65.6X4S**	Toxic effect of paints and dyes, NEC, undetermined, sequela
		◘	**T65.811S**	Toxic effect of latex, accidental (unintentional), sequela
		◘	**T65.812S**	Toxic effect of latex, intentional self-harm, sequela
		◘	**T65.813S**	Toxic effect of latex, assault, sequela
		◘	**T65.814S**	Toxic effect of latex, undetermined, sequela
		◘	**T65.821S**	Toxic effect of harmful algae and algae toxins, acc, sqla
		◘	**T65.822S**	Toxic eff of harmful algae and algae toxins, slf-hrm, sqla
		◘	**T65.823S**	Toxic effect of harmful algae and algae toxins, asslt, sqla
		◘	**T65.824S**	Toxic effect of harmful algae and algae toxins, undet, sqla
		◘	**T65.831S**	Toxic effect of fiberglass, accidental, sequela
		◘	**T65.832S**	Toxic effect of fiberglass, intentional self-harm, sequela
		◘	**T65.833S**	Toxic effect of fiberglass, assault, sequela
		◘	**T65.834S**	Toxic effect of fiberglass, undetermined, sequela
		◘	**T65.891S**	Toxic effect of substances, accidental, sequela
		◘	**T65.892S**	Toxic effect of substances, intentional self-harm, sequela
		◘	**T65.893S**	Toxic effect of other specified substances, assault, sequela
		◘	**T65.894S**	Toxic effect of oth substances, undetermined, sequela
		◘	**T65.91XS**	Toxic effect of unsp substance, accidental, sequela
		◘	**T65.92XS**	Toxic effect of unsp substance, self-harm, sequela
		◘	**T65.93XS**	Toxic effect of unspecified substance, assault, sequela
		◘	**T65.94XS**	Toxic effect of unspecified substance, undetermined, sequela
9Ø9.2	LATE EFFECT OF RADIATION		**L59.9**	Disorder of the skin, subcu related to radiation, unsp

ICD-9-CM		ICD-10-CM	
909.3	LATE EFFECT COMPLICATIONS SURGICAL&MEDICAL CARE	**T80.0XXS**	Air emblsm fol infusn, tranfs and theraputc inject, sequela
		T80.1XXS	Vasc comp fol infusn, tranfs and theraputc inject, sequela
		T80.211S	Bloodstream infct due to central venous catheter, sequela
		T80.212S	Local infection due to central venous catheter, sequela
		T80.218S	Other infection due to central venous catheter, sequela
		T80.219S	Unsp infection due to central venous catheter, sequela
		T80.22XS	Acute infct fol tranfs,infusn,inject blood/products, sequela
		T80.29XS	Infct fol oth infusion, tranfs and theraputc inject, sequela
		T80.30XS	ABO incompat react due to tranfs of bld/bld prod, unsp, sqla
		T80.310S	ABO incompatibility w acute hemolytic transfs react, sequela
		T80.311S	ABO incompat w delayed hemolytic transfs react, sequela
		T80.319S	ABO incompatibility w hemolytic transfs react, unsp, sequela
		T80.39XS	Oth ABO incompat react due to tranfs of bld/bld prod, sqla
		T80.40XS	Rh incompat react due to tranfs of bld/bld prod, unsp, sqla
		T80.410S	Rh incompatibility w acute hemolytic transfs react, sequela
		T80.411S	Rh incompat w delayed hemolytic transfs react, sequela
		T80.419S	Rh incompatibility w hemolytic transfs react, unsp, sequela
		T80.49XS	Oth Rh incompat react due to tranfs of bld/bld prod, sequela
		T80.51XS	Anaphylactic reaction due to admin blood/products, sequela
		T80.52XS	Anaphylactic reaction due to vaccination, sequela
		T80.59XS	Anaphylactic reaction due to other serum, sequela
		T80.61XS	Oth serum reaction due to admin blood/products, sequela
		T80.62XS	Other serum reaction due to vaccination, sequela
		T80.69XS	Other serum reaction due to other serum, sequela
		T80.810S	Extravasation of vesicant antineopl chemotherapy, sequela
		T80.818S	Extravasation of other vesicant agent, sequela
		T80.89XS	Oth comp fol infusion, tranfs and theraputc inject, sequela
		T80.90XS	Unsp comp fol infusion and theraputc injection, sequela
		T80.910S	Acute hemolytic transfs react, unsp incompatibility, sequela
		T80.911S	Delayed hemolytic transfs react, unsp incompat, sequela
		T80.919S	Hemolytic transfs react, unsp incompat, unsp ac/delay, sqla
		T80.92XS	Unspecified transfusion reaction, sequela
		T80.A0XS	Non-ABO incompat react d/t tranfs of bld/bld prod,unsp, sqla
		T80.A10S	Non-ABO incompat w acute hemolytic transfs react, sequela
		T80.A11S	Non-ABO incompat w delayed hemolytic transfs react, sequela
		T80.A19S	Non-ABO incompat w hemolytic transfs react, unsp, sequela
		T80.A9XS	Oth non-ABO incompat react d/t tranfs of bld/bld prod, sqla
		T81.10XS	Postprocedural shock unspecified, sequela
		T81.11XS	Postprocedural cardiogenic shock, sequela
		T81.12XS	Postprocedural septic shock, sequela
		T81.19XS	Other postprocedural shock, sequela
		T81.30XS	Disruption of wound, unspecified, sequela
		T81.31XS	Disrupt of external operation (surgical) wound, NEC, sequela
		T81.32XS	Disrupt of internal operation (surgical) wound, NEC, sequela
		T81.33XS	Disruption of traumatic injury wound repair, sequela
		T81.4XXS	Infection following a procedure, sequela
		T81.500S	Unsp comp of fb acc left in body fol surgical op, sequela
		T81.501S	Unsp comp of fb acc left in body fol infusn/transfusn, sqla
		T81.502S	Unsp comp of fb acc left in body fol kidney dialysis, sqla
		T81.503S	Unsp comp of fb acc left in body fol inject or immuniz, sqla
		T81.504S	Unsp comp of fb acc left in body fol endo exam, sequela
		T81.505S	Unsp comp of fb acc left in body fol heart cath, sequela
		T81.506S	Unsp comp of fb acc left in body fol punctr/cath, sequela
		T81.507S	Unsp comp of fb acc left in body fol remov cath/pack, sqla
		T81.508S	Unsp comp of fb acc left in body fol oth procedure, sequela
		T81.509S	Unsp comp of fb acc left in body fol unsp procedure, sequela
		T81.510S	Adhes due to fb acc left in body fol surgical op, sequela
		T81.511S	Adhes due to fb acc left in body fol infusn/transfusn, sqla
		T81.512S	Adhes due to fb acc left in body fol kidney dialysis, sqla
		T81.513S	Adhes due to fb acc left in body fol inject or immuniz, sqla
		T81.514S	Adhes due to fb acc left in body fol endo exam, sequela
		T81.515S	Adhes due to fb acc left in body fol heart cath, sequela
		T81.516S	Adhes due to fb acc left in body fol punctr/cath, sequela
		T81.517S	Adhes due to fb acc left in body fol remov cath/pack, sqla
		T81.518S	Adhes due to fb acc left in body fol oth procedure, sequela
		T81.519S	Adhes due to fb acc left in body fol unsp procedure, sequela
		T81.520S	Obst due to fb acc left in body fol surgical op, sequela
		T81.521S	Obst due to fb acc left in body fol infusn/transfusn, sqla
		T81.522S	Obst due to fb acc left in body fol kidney dialysis, sequela
		T81.523S	Obst due to fb acc left in body fol inject or immuniz, sqla
		T81.524S	Obst due to fb acc left in body following endo exam, sequela
		T81.525S	Obst due to fb acc left in body fol heart cath, sequela
		T81.526S	Obst due to fb acc left in body fol punctr/cath, sequela
		T81.527S	Obst due to fb acc left in body fol remov cath/pack, sequela
		T81.528S	Obst due to fb acc left in body fol oth procedure, sequela
		T81.529S	Obst due to fb acc left in body fol unsp procedure, sequela
		T81.530S	Perf due to fb acc left in body fol surgical op, sequela
		T81.531S	Perf due to fb acc left in body fol infusn/transfusn, sqla
		T81.532S	Perf due to fb acc left in body fol kidney dialysis, sequela
		T81.533S	Perf due to fb acc left in body fol inject or immuniz, sqla
		T81.534S	Perf due to fb acc left in body following endo exam, sequela
		T81.535S	Perf due to fb acc left in body fol heart cath, sequela
	(Continued on next page)	**T81.536S**	Perf due to fb acc left in body fol punctr/cath, sequela

ICD-9-CM		ICD-10-CM	
9Ø9.3	LATE EFFECT COMPLICATIONS SURGICAL&MEDICAL CARE **(Continued)**	**T81.537S**	Perf due to fb acc left in body fol remov cath/pack, sequela
		T81.538S	Perf due to fb acc left in body fol oth procedure, sequela
		T81.539S	Perf due to fb acc left in body fol unsp procedure, sequela
		T81.59ØS	Oth comp of fb acc left in body fol surgical op, sequela
		T81.591S	Oth comp of fb acc left in body fol infusn/transfusn, sqla
		T81.592S	Oth comp of fb acc left in body fol kidney dialysis, sequela
		T81.593S	Oth comp of fb acc left in body fol inject or immuniz, sqla
		T81.594S	Oth comp of fb acc left in body following endo exam, sequela
		T81.595S	Oth comp of fb acc left in body fol heart cath, sequela
		T81.596S	Oth comp of fb acc left in body fol punctr/cath, sequela
		T81.597S	Oth comp of fb acc left in body fol remov cath/pack, sequela
		T81.598S	Oth comp of fb acc left in body fol oth procedure, sequela
		T81.599S	Oth comp of fb acc left in body fol unsp procedure, sequela
		T81.6ØXS	Unsp acute react to foreign sub acc left dur proc, sequela
		T81.61XS	Aseptic peritonitis due to forn sub acc left dur proc, sqla
		T81.69XS	Oth acute reaction to foreign sub acc left dur proc, sequela
		T81.71ØS	Comp of mesent art following a procedure, NEC, sequela
		T81.711S	Comp of renal artery following a procedure, NEC, sequela
		T81.718S	Complication of artery following a procedure, NEC, sequela
		T81.719S	Comp of unsp artery following a procedure, NEC, sequela
		T81.72XS	Complication of vein following a procedure, NEC, sequela
		T81.81XS	Complication of inhalation therapy, sequela
		T81.82XS	Emphysema (subcutaneous) resulting from a procedure, sequela
		T81.83XS	Persistent postprocedural fistula, sequela
		T81.89XS	Oth complications of procedures, NEC, sequela
		T81.9XXS	Unspecified complication of procedure, sequela
		T82.Ø1XS	Breakdown (mechanical) of heart valve prosthesis, sequela
		T82.Ø2XS	Displacement of heart valve prosthesis, sequela
		T82.Ø3XS	Leakage of heart valve prosthesis, sequela
		T82.Ø9XS	Mech compl of heart valve prosthesis, sequela
		T82.11ØS	Breakdown (mechanical) of cardiac electrode, sequela
		T82.111S	Breakdown of cardiac pulse generator (battery), sequela
		T82.118S	Breakdown (mechanical) of cardiac electronic device, sequela
		T82.119S	Breakdown of unsp cardiac electronic device, sequela
		T82.12ØS	Displacement of cardiac electrode, sequela
		T82.121S	Displacement of cardiac pulse generator (battery), sequela
		T82.128S	Displacement of other cardiac electronic device, sequela
		T82.129S	Displacement of unsp cardiac electronic device, sequela
		T82.19ØS	Other mechanical complication of cardiac electrode, sequela
		T82.191S	Mech compl of cardiac pulse generator (battery), sequela
		T82.198S	Mech compl of other cardiac electronic device, sequela
		T82.199S	Mech compl of unspecified cardiac device, sequela
		T82.211S	Breakdown (mechanical) of cor art bypass graft, sequela
		T82.212S	Displacement of coronary artery bypass graft, sequela
		T82.213S	Leakage of coronary artery bypass graft, sequela
		T82.218S	Mech compl of coronary artery bypass graft, sequela
		T82.221S	Breakdown of biological heart valve graft, sequela
		T82.222S	Displacement of biological heart valve graft, sequela
		T82.223S	Leakage of biological heart valve graft, sequela
		T82.228S	Mech compl of biological heart valve graft, sequela
		T82.31ØS	Breakdown of aortic (bifurcation) graft, sequela
		T82.311S	Breakdown of carotid arterial graft (bypass), sequela
		T82.312S	Breakdown of femoral arterial graft (bypass), sequela
		T82.318S	Breakdown (mechanical) of other vascular grafts, sequela
		T82.319S	Breakdown (mechanical) of unsp vascular grafts, sequela
		T82.32ØS	Displacement of aortic (bifurcation) graft, sequela
		T82.321S	Displacement of carotid arterial graft (bypass), sequela
		T82.322S	Displacement of femoral arterial graft (bypass), sequela
		T82.328S	Displacement of other vascular grafts, sequela
		T82.329S	Displacement of unspecified vascular grafts, sequela
		T82.33ØS	Leakage of aortic (bifurcation) graft (replacement), sequela
		T82.331S	Leakage of carotid arterial graft (bypass), sequela
		T82.332S	Leakage of femoral arterial graft (bypass), sequela
		T82.338S	Leakage of other vascular grafts, sequela
		T82.339S	Leakage of unspecified vascular graft, sequela
		T82.39ØS	Mech compl of aortic (bifurcation) graft, sequela
		T82.391S	Mech compl of carotid arterial graft (bypass), sequela
		T82.392S	Mech compl of femoral arterial graft (bypass), sequela
		T82.398S	Mech compl of other vascular grafts, sequela
		T82.399S	Mech compl of unspecified vascular grafts, sequela
		T82.41XS	Breakdown of vascular dialysis catheter, sequela
		T82.42XS	Displacement of vascular dialysis catheter, sequela
		T82.43XS	Leakage of vascular dialysis catheter, sequela
		T82.49XS	Other complication of vascular dialysis catheter, sequela
		T82.51ØS	Breakdown of surgically created AV fistula, sequela
		T82.511S	Breakdown of surgically created AV shunt, sequela
		T82.512S	Breakdown (mechanical) of artificial heart, sequela
		T82.513S	Breakdown of balloon (counterpulsation) device, sequela
		T82.514S	Breakdown (mechanical) of infusion catheter, sequela
		T82.515S	Breakdown (mechanical) of umbrella device, sequela
		T82.518S	Brkdwn cardiac and vascular devices and implants, sequela
		T82.519S	Brkdwn unsp cardiac and vascular devices and implnt, sequela
	(Continued on next page)	**T82.52ØS**	Displacement of surgically created AV fistula, sequela

ICD-9-CM		ICD-10-CM	
909.3	LATE EFFECT COMPLICATIONS SURGICAL&MEDICAL CARE **(Continued)**	**T82.521S**	Displacement of surgically created AV shunt, sequela
		T82.522S	Displacement of artificial heart, sequela
		T82.523S	Displacement of balloon (counterpulsation) device, sequela
		T82.524S	Displacement of infusion catheter, sequela
		T82.525S	Displacement of umbrella device, sequela
		T82.528S	Displacmnt of cardiac and vasc devices and implnt, sequela
		T82.529S	Displacmnt of unsp card and vasc devices and implnt, sequela
		T82.530S	Leakage of surgically created arteriovenous fistula, sequela
		T82.531S	Leakage of surgically created arteriovenous shunt, sequela
		T82.532S	Leakage of artificial heart, sequela
		T82.533S	Leakage of balloon (counterpulsation) device, sequela
		T82.534S	Leakage of infusion catheter, sequela
		T82.535S	Leakage of umbrella device, sequela
		T82.538S	Leakage of cardiac and vascular devices and implnt, sequela
		T82.539S	Leakage of unsp cardiac and vasc devices and implnt, sequela
		T82.590S	Mech compl of surgically created AV fistula, sequela
		T82.591S	Mech compl of surgically created AV shunt, sequela
		T82.592S	Other mechanical complication of artificial heart, sequela
		T82.593S	Mech compl of balloon (counterpulsation) device, sequela
		T82.594S	Other mechanical complication of infusion catheter, sequela
		T82.595S	Other mechanical complication of umbrella device, sequela
		T82.598S	Mech compl of cardiac and vasc devices and implnt, sequela
		T82.599S	Mech compl of unsp card and vasc devices and implnt, sequela
		T82.6XXS	Infect/inflm reaction due to cardiac valve prosth, sequela
		T82.7XXS	Infect/inflm react d/t oth cardi/vasc dev/implnt/grft, sqla
		T82.817S	Embolism of cardiac prosth dev/grft, sequela
		T82.818S	Embolism of vascular prosth dev/grft, sequela
		T82.827S	Fibrosis of cardiac prosth dev/grft, sequela
		T82.828S	Fibrosis of vascular prosth dev/grft, sequela
		T82.837S	Hemorrhage of cardiac prosth dev/grft, sequela
		T82.838S	Hemorrhage of vascular prosth dev/grft, sequela
		T82.847S	Pain from cardiac prosth dev/grft, sequela
		T82.848S	Pain from vascular prosth dev/grft, sequela
		T82.857S	Stenosis of cardiac prosth dev/grft, sequela
		T82.858S	Stenosis of vascular prosth dev/grft, sequela
		T82.867S	Thrombosis of cardiac prosth dev/grft, sequela
		T82.868S	Thrombosis of vascular prosth dev/grft, sequela
		T82.897S	Oth complication of cardiac prosth dev/grft, sequela
		T82.898S	Oth complication of vascular prosth dev/grft, sequela
		T82.9XXS	Unsp comp of cardiac and vascular prosth dev/grft, sequela
		T83.010S	Breakdown (mechanical) of cystostomy catheter, sequela
		T83.018S	Breakdown of indwelling urethral catheter, sequela
		T83.020S	Displacement of cystostomy catheter, sequela
		T83.028S	Displacement of other indwelling urethral catheter, sequela
		T83.030S	Leakage of cystostomy catheter, sequela
		T83.038S	Leakage of other indwelling urethral catheter, sequela
		T83.090S	Mech compl of cystostomy catheter, sequela
		T83.098S	Mech compl of other indwelling urethral catheter, sequela
		T83.110S	Breakdown of urinary electronic stimulator device, sequela
		T83.111S	Breakdown (mechanical) of urinary sphincter implant, sequela
		T83.112S	Breakdown (mechanical) of urinary stent, sequela
		T83.118S	Breakdown of urinary devices and implants, sequela
		T83.120S	Displacmnt of urinary electronic stimulator device, sequela
		T83.121S	Displacement of urinary sphincter implant, sequela
		T83.122S	Displacement of urinary stent, sequela
		T83.128S	Displacement of other urinary devices and implants, sequela
		T83.190S	Mech compl of urinary electronic stimulator device, sequela
		T83.191S	Mech compl of urinary sphincter implant, sequela
		T83.192S	Other mechanical complication of urinary stent, sequela
		T83.198S	Mech compl of other urinary devices and implants, sequela
		T83.21XS	Breakdown (mechanical) of graft of urinary organ, sequela
		T83.22XS	Displacement of graft of urinary organ, sequela
		T83.23XS	Leakage of graft of urinary organ, sequela
		T83.29XS	Mech compl of graft of urinary organ, sequela
		T83.31XS	Breakdown of intrauterine contracep dev, sequela
		T83.32XS	Displacement of intrauterine contraceptive device, sequela
		T83.39XS	Mech compl of intrauterine contraceptive device, sequela
		T83.410S	Breakdown of penile (implanted) prosthesis, sequela
		T83.418S	Breakdown of prosth dev/implnt/grft of genitl trct, sequela
		T83.420S	Displacement of penile (implanted) prosthesis, sequela
		T83.428S	Displacmnt of prosth dev/implnt/grft of genitl trct, sequela
		T83.490S	Mech compl of penile (implanted) prosthesis, sequela
		T83.498S	Mech compl of prosth dev/implnt/grft of genitl trct, sequela
		T83.51XS	Infect/inflm reaction due to indwell urinary cath, sequela
		T83.59XS	Infect/inflm react d/t prosth dev/grft in urinry sys, sqla
		T83.6XXS	Infect/inflm react d/t prosth dev/grft in genitl trct, sqla
		T83.711S	Erosion of implnt vag prstht mtrl to surrnd org/tiss, sqla
		T83.718S	Erosion of implanted prstht mtrl to surrnd org/tiss, sequela
		T83.721S	Exposure of implnt vag prstht mtrl into vagina, sequela
		T83.728S	Exposure of implnt prstht mtrl to surrnd org/tiss, sequela
		T83.81XS	Embolism of genitourinary prosth dev/grft, sequela
		T83.82XS	Fibrosis of genitourinary prosth dev/grft, sequela
	(Continued on next page)	**T83.83XS**	Hemorrhage of genitourinary prosth dev/grft, sequela

ICD-9-CM		ICD-10-CM	
909.3	LATE EFFECT COMPLICATIONS SURGICAL&MEDICAL CARE **(Continued)**	**T83.84XS**	Pain from genitourinary prosth dev/grft, sequela
		T83.85XS	Stenosis of genitourinary prosth dev/grft, sequela
		T83.86XS	Thrombosis of genitourinary prosth dev/grft, sequela
		T83.89XS	Oth complication of genitourinary prosth dev/grft, sequela
		T83.9XXS	Unsp complication of genitourinary prosth dev/grft, sequela
		T84.010S	Broken internal right hip prosthesis, sequela
		T84.011S	Broken internal left hip prosthesis, sequela
		T84.012S	Broken internal right knee prosthesis, sequela
		T84.013S	Broken internal left knee prosthesis, sequela
		T84.018S	Broken internal joint prosthesis, other site, sequela
		T84.019S	Broken internal joint prosthesis, unspecified site, sequela
		T84.020S	Dislocation of internal right hip prosthesis, sequela
		T84.021S	Dislocation of internal left hip prosthesis, sequela
		T84.022S	Instability of internal right knee prosthesis, sequela
		T84.023S	Instability of internal left knee prosthesis, sequela
		T84.028S	Dislocation of other internal joint prosthesis, sequela
		T84.029S	Dislocation of unsp internal joint prosthesis, sequela
		T84.030S	Mech loosening of internal right hip prosth joint, sequela
		T84.031S	Mech loosening of internal left hip prosth joint, sequela
		T84.032S	Mech loosening of internal right knee prosth joint, sequela
		T84.033S	Mech loosening of internal left knee prosth joint, sequela
		T84.038S	Mechanical loosening of internal prosthetic joint, sequela
		T84.039S	Mech loosening of unsp internal prosthetic joint, sequela
		T84.040S	Periprosth fracture around internal prosth r hip jt, sequela
		T84.041S	Periprosth fracture around internal prosth l hip jt, sequela
		T84.042S	Periprosth fx around internal prosth r knee jt, sequela
		T84.043S	Periprosth fx around internal prosth l knee jt, sequela
		T84.048S	Periprosth fx around oth internal prosth joint, sequela
		T84.049S	Periprosth fx around unsp internal prosth joint, sequela
		T84.050S	Periprosth osteolys of internal prosthetic r hip jt, sequela
		T84.051S	Periprosth osteolys of internal prosthetic l hip jt, sequela
		T84.052S	Periprosth osteolys of internal prosth r knee jt, sequela
		T84.053S	Periprosth osteolys of internal prosth l knee jt, sequela
		T84.058S	Periprosth osteolysis of internal prosthetic joint, sequela
		T84.059S	Periprosth osteolys of unsp internal prosth joint, sequela
		T84.060S	Wear of artic bearing surface of int prosth r hip jt, sqla
		T84.061S	Wear of artic bearing surface of int prosth l hip jt, sqla
		T84.062S	Wear of artic bearing surface of int prosth r knee jt, sqla
		T84.063S	Wear of artic bearing surface of int prosth l knee jt, sqla
		T84.068S	Wear of artic bearing surface of int prosth joint, sequela
		T84.069S	Wear of artic bearing surface of unsp int prosth joint, sqla
		T84.090S	Mech compl of internal right hip prosthesis, sequela
		T84.091S	Mech compl of internal left hip prosthesis, sequela
		T84.092S	Mech compl of internal right knee prosthesis, sequela
		T84.093S	Mech compl of internal left knee prosthesis, sequela
		T84.098S	Mech compl of other internal joint prosthesis, sequela
		T84.099S	Mech compl of unspecified internal joint prosthesis, sequela
		T84.110S	Breakdown (mechanical) of int fix of right humerus, sequela
		T84.111S	Breakdown (mechanical) of int fix of left humerus, sequela
		T84.112S	Breakdown of int fix of bone of r forearm, sequela
		T84.113S	Breakdown of int fix of bone of left forearm, sequela
		T84.114S	Breakdown (mechanical) of int fix of right femur, sequela
		T84.115S	Breakdown (mechanical) of int fix of left femur, sequela
		T84.116S	Breakdown of int fix of bone of r low leg, sequela
		T84.117S	Breakdown of int fix of bone of l low leg, sequela
		T84.119S	Breakdown of int fix of unsp bone of limb, sequela
		T84.120S	Displacement of int fix of right humerus, sequela
		T84.121S	Displacement of int fix of left humerus, sequela
		T84.122S	Displacement of int fix of bone of right forearm, sequela
		T84.123S	Displacement of int fix of bone of left forearm, sequela
		T84.124S	Displacement of int fix of right femur, sequela
		T84.125S	Displacement of int fix of left femur, sequela
		T84.126S	Displacement of int fix of bone of right lower leg, sequela
		T84.127S	Displacement of int fix of bone of left lower leg, sequela
		T84.129S	Displacement of int fix of unsp bone of limb, sequela
		T84.190S	Mech compl of int fix of right humerus, sequela
		T84.191S	Mech compl of int fix of left humerus, sequela
		T84.192S	Mech compl of int fix of bone of right forearm, sequela
		T84.193S	Mech compl of int fix of bone of left forearm, sequela
		T84.194S	Mech compl of int fix of right femur, sequela
		T84.195S	Mech compl of int fix of left femur, sequela
		T84.196S	Mech compl of int fix of bone of right lower leg, sequela
		T84.197S	Mech compl of int fix of bone of left lower leg, sequela
		T84.199S	Mech compl of int fix of unsp bone of limb, sequela
		T84.210S	Breakdown of int fix of bones of hand and fingers, sequela
		T84.213S	Breakdown of int fix of bones of foot and toes, sequela
		T84.216S	Breakdown (mechanical) of int fix of vertebrae, sequela
		T84.218S	Breakdown (mechanical) of int fix of bones, sequela
		T84.220S	Displacmnt of int fix of bones of hand and fingers, sequela
		T84.223S	Displacement of int fix of bones of foot and toes, sequela
		T84.226S	Displacement of int fix of vertebrae, sequela
	(Continued on next page)	**T84.228S**	Displacement of internal fixation device of bones, sequela

ICD-9-CM		ICD-10-CM	
909.3	LATE EFFECT COMPLICATIONS SURGICAL&MEDICAL CARE **(Continued)**	**T84.290S**	Mech compl of int fix of bones of hand and fingers, sequela
		T84.293S	Mech compl of int fix of bones of foot and toes, sequela
		T84.296S	Mech compl of internal fixation device of vertebrae, sequela
		T84.298S	Mech compl of internal fixation device of oth bones, sequela
		T84.310S	Breakdown of electronic bone stimulator, sequela
		T84.318S	Breakdown of bone devices, implants and grafts, sequela
		T84.320S	Displacement of electronic bone stimulator, sequela
		T84.328S	Displacement of bone devices, implants and grafts, sequela
		T84.390S	Mech compl of electronic bone stimulator, sequela
		T84.398S	Mech compl of oth bone devices, implants and grafts, sequela
		T84.410S	Breakdown (mechanical) of muscle and tendon graft, sequela
		T84.418S	Brkdwn internal orth devices, implants and grafts, sequela
		T84.420S	Displacement of muscle and tendon graft, sequela
		T84.428S	Displacmnt of int orth devices, implnt and grafts, sequela
		T84.490S	Mech compl of muscle and tendon graft, sequela
		T84.498S	Mech compl of int orth devices, implnt and grafts, sequela
		T84.50XS	Infect/inflm reaction due to unsp int joint prosth, sequela
		T84.51XS	Infect/inflm reaction due to internal r hip prosth, sequela
		T84.52XS	Infect/inflm reaction due to int left hip prosth, sequela
		T84.53XS	Infect/inflm reaction due to internal r knee prosth, sequela
		T84.54XS	Infect/inflm reaction due to internal l knee prosth, sequela
		T84.59XS	Infect/inflm reaction due to oth int joint prosth, sequela
		T84.60XS	Infect/inflm reaction due to int fix of unsp site, sequela
		T84.610S	Infect/inflm reaction due to int fix of r humerus, sequela
		T84.611S	Infect/inflm reaction due to int fix of l humerus, sequela
		T84.612S	Infect/inflm reaction due to int fix of r radius, sequela
		T84.613S	Infect/inflm reaction due to int fix of left radius, sequela
		T84.614S	Infect/inflm reaction due to int fix of right ulna, sequela
		T84.615S	Infect/inflm reaction due to int fix of left ulna, sequela
		T84.619S	Infect/inflm react due to int fix of unsp bone of arm, sqla
		T84.620S	Infect/inflm reaction due to int fix of right femur, sequela
		T84.621S	Infect/inflm reaction due to int fix of left femur, sequela
		T84.622S	Infect/inflm reaction due to int fix of right tibia, sequela
		T84.623S	Infect/inflm reaction due to int fix of left tibia, sequela
		T84.624S	Infect/inflm reaction due to int fix of r fibula, sequela
		T84.625S	Infect/inflm reaction due to int fix of left fibula, sequela
		T84.629S	Infect/inflm react due to int fix of unsp bone of leg, sqla
		T84.63XS	Infect/inflm reaction due to int fix of spine, sequela
		T84.69XS	Infect/inflm reaction due to int fix of site, sequela
		T84.7XXS	Infect/inflm react due to oth int orth prosth dev/grft, sqla
		T84.81XS	Embolism due to internal orthopedic prosth dev/grft, sequela
		T84.82XS	Fibrosis due to internal orthopedic prosth dev/grft, sequela
		T84.83XS	Hemor due to internal orthopedic prosth dev/grft, sequela
		T84.84XS	Pain due to internal orthopedic prosth dev/grft, sequela
		T84.85XS	Stenosis due to internal orthopedic prosth dev/grft, sequela
		T84.86XS	Thrombosis due to internal orth prosth dev/grft, sequela
		T84.89XS	Oth comp of internal orthopedic prosth dev/grft, sequela
		T84.9XXS	Unsp comp of internal orthopedic prosth dev/grft, sequela
		T85.01XS	Breakdown of ventricular intracranial shunt, sequela
		T85.02XS	Displacement of ventricular intracranial shunt, sequela
		T85.03XS	Leakage of ventricular intracranial shunt, sequela
		T85.09XS	Mech compl of ventricular intracranial shunt, sequela
		T85.110S	Brkdwn implanted electronic neurostim of brain, sequela
		T85.111S	Brkdwn implanted electronic neurostim of periph nrv, sequela
		T85.112S	Brkdwn implanted electrnc neurostim of spinal cord, sequela
		T85.118S	Brkdwn implanted electrnc stimulator of nervous sys, sequela
		T85.120S	Displacmnt of implanted electrnc neurostim of brain, sequela
		T85.121S	Displacmnt of implnt electrnc neurostim of periph nrv, sqla
		T85.122S	Displacmnt of implnt electrnc neurostim of spinal cord, sqla
		T85.128S	Displacmnt of implnt electrnc stimultr of nrv sys, sequela
		T85.190S	Mech compl of implanted electrnc neurostim of brain, sequela
		T85.191S	Mech compl of implnt electrnc neurostim of periph nrv, sqla
		T85.192S	Mech compl of implnt electrnc neurostim of spinal cord, sqla
		T85.199S	Mech compl of implnt electrnc stimultr of nrv sys, sequela
		T85.21XS	Breakdown (mechanical) of intraocular lens, sequela
		T85.22XS	Displacement of intraocular lens, sequela
		T85.29XS	Other mechanical complication of intraocular lens, sequela
		T85.310S	Breakdown of prosthetic orbit of right eye, sequela
		T85.311S	Breakdown of prosthetic orbit of left eye, sequela
		T85.318S	Breakdown (mechanical) of ocular prosth dev/grft, sequela
		T85.320S	Displacement of prosthetic orbit of right eye, sequela
		T85.321S	Displacement of prosthetic orbit of left eye, sequela
		T85.328S	Displacement of ocular prosth dev/grft, sequela
		T85.390S	Mech compl of prosthetic orbit of right eye, sequela
		T85.391S	Mech compl of prosthetic orbit of left eye, sequela
		T85.398S	Mech compl of ocular prosth dev/grft, sequela
		T85.41XS	Breakdown of breast prosthesis and implant, sequela
		T85.42XS	Displacement of breast prosthesis and implant, sequela
		T85.43XS	Leakage of breast prosthesis and implant, sequela
		T85.44XS	Capsular contracture of breast implant, sequela
		T85.49XS	Mech compl of breast prosthesis and implant, sequela
		T85.510S	Breakdown (mechanical) of bile duct prosthesis, sequela
	(Continued on next page)	**T85.511S**	Breakdown of esophageal anti-reflux device, sequela

ICD-9-CM		ICD-10-CM	
909.3	LATE EFFECT COMPLICATIONS SURGICAL&MEDICAL CARE **(Continued)**	**T85.518S**	Breakdown (mechanical) of GI prosth dev/grft, sequela
		T85.520S	Displacement of bile duct prosthesis, sequela
		T85.521S	Displacement of esophageal anti-reflux device, sequela
		T85.528S	Displacement of gastrointestinal prosth dev/grft, sequela
		T85.590S	Mech compl of bile duct prosthesis, sequela
		T85.591S	Mech compl of esophageal anti-reflux device, sequela
		T85.598S	Mech compl of gastrointestinal prosth dev/grft, sequela
		T85.610S	Brkdwn epidural and subdural infusion catheter, sequela
		T85.611S	Breakdown of intraperitoneal dialysis catheter, sequela
		T85.612S	Breakdown (mechanical) of permanent sutures, sequela
		T85.613S	Brkdwn artificial skin grft /decellular alloderm, sequela
		T85.614S	Breakdown (mechanical) of insulin pump, sequela
		T85.618S	Breakdown (mechanical) of internal prosth dev/grft, sequela
		T85.620S	Displacmnt of epidural and subdural infusion cath, sequela
		T85.621S	Displacement of intraperitoneal dialysis catheter, sequela
		T85.622S	Displacement of permanent sutures, sequela
		T85.623S	Displacmnt of artif skin grft /decellular alloderm, sequela
		T85.624S	Displacement of insulin pump, sequela
		T85.628S	Displacement of internal prosth dev/grft, sequela
		T85.630S	Leakage of epidural and subdural infusion catheter, sequela
		T85.631S	Leakage of intraperitoneal dialysis catheter, sequela
		T85.633S	Leakage of insulin pump, sequela
		T85.638S	Leakage of internal prosth dev/grft, sequela
		T85.690S	Mech compl of epidural and subdural infusion cath, sequela
		T85.691S	Mech compl of intraperitoneal dialysis catheter, sequela
		T85.692S	Other mechanical complication of permanent sutures, sequela
		T85.693S	Mech compl of artif skin grft /decellular alloderm, sequela
		T85.694S	Other mechanical complication of insulin pump, sequela
		T85.698S	Mech compl of internal prosth dev/grft, sequela
		T85.71XS	Infect/inflm reaction due to periton dialysis cath, sequela
		T85.72XS	Infect/inflm reaction due to insulin pump, sequela
		T85.79XS	Infect/inflm react due to oth int prosth dev/grft, sequela
		T85.81XS	Embolism due to internal prosth dev/grft, NEC, sequela
		T85.82XS	Fibrosis due to internal prosth dev/grft, NEC, sequela
		T85.83XS	Hemorrhage due to internal prosth dev/grft, NEC, sequela
		T85.84XS	Pain due to internal prosth dev/grft, NEC, sequela
		T85.85XS	Stenosis due to internal prosth dev/grft, NEC, sequela
		T85.86XS	Thrombosis due to internal prosth dev/grft, NEC, sequela
		T85.89XS	Oth complication of internal prosth dev/grft, NEC, sequela
		T85.9XXS	Unsp complication of internal prosth dev/grft, sequela
		T88.0XXS	Infection following immunization, sequela
		T88.1XXS	Oth complications following immunization, NEC, sequela
		T88.2XXS	Shock due to anesthesia, sequela
		T88.3XXS	Malignant hyperthermia due to anesthesia, sequela
		T88.4XXS	Failed or difficult intubation, sequela
		T88.51XS	Hypothermia following anesthesia, sequela
		T88.52XS	Failed moderate sedation during procedure, sequela
		T88.59XS	Other complications of anesthesia, sequela
		T88.8XXS	Oth complications of surgical and medical care, NEC, sequela
		T88.9XXS	Complication of surgical and medical care, unsp, sequela
909.4	LATE EFFECT OF CERTAIN OTHER EXTERNAL CAUSES	**T33.011S**	Superficial frostbite of right ear, sequela
		T33.012S	Superficial frostbite of left ear, sequela
		T33.019S	Superficial frostbite of unspecified ear, sequela
		T33.02XS	Superficial frostbite of nose, sequela
		T33.09XS	Superficial frostbite of other part of head, sequela
		T33.1XXS	Superficial frostbite of neck, sequela
		T33.2XXS	Superficial frostbite of thorax, sequela
		T33.3XXS	Superfic frostbite of abd wall, low back and pelvis, sequela
		T33.40XS	Superficial frostbite of unspecified arm, sequela
		T33.41XS	Superficial frostbite of right arm, sequela
		T33.42XS	Superficial frostbite of left arm, sequela
		T33.511S	Superficial frostbite of right wrist, sequela
		T33.512S	Superficial frostbite of left wrist, sequela
		T33.519S	Superficial frostbite of unspecified wrist, sequela
		T33.521S	Superficial frostbite of right hand, sequela
		T33.522S	Superficial frostbite of left hand, sequela
		T33.529S	Superficial frostbite of unspecified hand, sequela
		T33.531S	Superficial frostbite of right finger(s), sequela
		T33.532S	Superficial frostbite of left finger(s), sequela
		T33.539S	Superficial frostbite of unspecified finger(s), sequela
		T33.60XS	Superficial frostbite of unspecified hip and thigh, sequela
		T33.61XS	Superficial frostbite of right hip and thigh, sequela
		T33.62XS	Superficial frostbite of left hip and thigh, sequela
		T33.70XS	Superficial frostbite of unsp knee and lower leg, sequela
		T33.71XS	Superficial frostbite of right knee and lower leg, sequela
		T33.72XS	Superficial frostbite of left knee and lower leg, sequela
		T33.811S	Superficial frostbite of right ankle, sequela
		T33.812S	Superficial frostbite of left ankle, sequela
		T33.819S	Superficial frostbite of unspecified ankle, sequela
		T33.821S	Superficial frostbite of right foot, sequela
		T33.822S	Superficial frostbite of left foot, sequela
	(Continued on next page)	**T33.829S**	Superficial frostbite of unspecified foot, sequela

ICD-9-CM		ICD-10-CM	
909.4	LATE EFFECT OF CERTAIN OTHER EXTERNAL CAUSES **(Continued)**	**T33.831S**	Superficial frostbite of right toe(s), sequela
		T33.832S	Superficial frostbite of left toe(s), sequela
		T33.839S	Superficial frostbite of unspecified toe(s), sequela
		T33.90XS	Superficial frostbite of unspecified sites, sequela
		T33.99XS	Superficial frostbite of other sites, sequela
		T34.011S	Frostbite with tissue necrosis of right ear, sequela
		T34.012S	Frostbite with tissue necrosis of left ear, sequela
		T34.019S	Frostbite with tissue necrosis of unspecified ear, sequela
		T34.02XS	Frostbite with tissue necrosis of nose, sequela
		T34.09XS	Frostbite with tissue necrosis of oth part of head, sequela
		T34.1XXS	Frostbite with tissue necrosis of neck, sequela
		T34.2XXS	Frostbite with tissue necrosis of thorax, sequela
		T34.3XXS	Frstbte w tissue necros abd wall, low back and pelvis, sqla
		T34.40XS	Frostbite with tissue necrosis of unspecified arm, sequela
		T34.41XS	Frostbite with tissue necrosis of right arm, sequela
		T34.42XS	Frostbite with tissue necrosis of left arm, sequela
		T34.511S	Frostbite with tissue necrosis of right wrist, sequela
		T34.512S	Frostbite with tissue necrosis of left wrist, sequela
		T34.519S	Frostbite with tissue necrosis of unspecified wrist, sequela
		T34.521S	Frostbite with tissue necrosis of right hand, sequela
		T34.522S	Frostbite with tissue necrosis of left hand, sequela
		T34.529S	Frostbite with tissue necrosis of unspecified hand, sequela
		T34.531S	Frostbite with tissue necrosis of right finger(s), sequela
		T34.532S	Frostbite with tissue necrosis of left finger(s), sequela
		T34.539S	Frostbite with tissue necrosis of unsp finger(s), sequela
		T34.60XS	Frostbite w tissue necrosis of unsp hip and thigh, sequela
		T34.61XS	Frostbite w tissue necrosis of right hip and thigh, sequela
		T34.62XS	Frostbite w tissue necrosis of left hip and thigh, sequela
		T34.70XS	Frostbite w tissue necros unsp knee and lower leg, sequela
		T34.71XS	Frostbite w tissue necros right knee and lower leg, sequela
		T34.72XS	Frostbite w tissue necros left knee and lower leg, sequela
		T34.811S	Frostbite with tissue necrosis of right ankle, sequela
		T34.812S	Frostbite with tissue necrosis of left ankle, sequela
		T34.819S	Frostbite with tissue necrosis of unspecified ankle, sequela
		T34.821S	Frostbite with tissue necrosis of right foot, sequela
		T34.822S	Frostbite with tissue necrosis of left foot, sequela
		T34.829S	Frostbite with tissue necrosis of unspecified foot, sequela
		T34.831S	Frostbite with tissue necrosis of right toe(s), sequela
		T34.832S	Frostbite with tissue necrosis of left toe(s), sequela
		T34.839S	Frostbite with tissue necrosis of unsp toe(s), sequela
		T34.90XS	Frostbite with tissue necrosis of unspecified sites, sequela
		T34.99XS	Frostbite with tissue necrosis of other sites, sequela
		T66.XXXS	Radiation sickness, unspecified, sequela
		T67.0XXS	Heatstroke and sunstroke, sequela
		T67.1XXS	Heat syncope, sequela
		T67.2XXS	Heat cramp, sequela
		T67.3XXS	Heat exhaustion, anhydrotic, sequela
		T67.4XXS	Heat exhaustion due to salt depletion, sequela
		T67.5XXS	Heat exhaustion, unspecified, sequela
		T67.6XXS	Heat fatigue, transient, sequela
		T67.7XXS	Heat edema, sequela
		T67.8XXS	Other effects of heat and light, sequela
		T67.9XXS	Effect of heat and light, unspecified, sequela
		T68.XXXS	Hypothermia, sequela
		T69.011S	Immersion hand, right hand, sequela
		T69.012S	Immersion hand, left hand, sequela
		T69.019S	Immersion hand, unspecified hand, sequela
		T69.021S	Immersion foot, right foot, sequela
		T69.022S	Immersion foot, left foot, sequela
		T69.029S	Immersion foot, unspecified foot, sequela
		T69.1XXS	Chilblains, sequela
		T69.8XXS	Other specified effects of reduced temperature, sequela
		T69.9XXS	Effect of reduced temperature, unspecified, sequela
		T70.0XXS	Otitic barotrauma, sequela
		T70.1XXS	Sinus barotrauma, sequela
		T70.20XS	Unspecified effects of high altitude, sequela
		T70.29XS	Other effects of high altitude, sequela
		T70.3XXS	Caisson disease [decompression sickness], sequela
		T70.4XXS	Effects of high-pressure fluids, sequela
		T70.8XXS	Other effects of air pressure and water pressure, sequela
		T70.9XXS	Effect of air pressure and water pressure, unsp, sequela
		T71.111S	Asphyx due to smothering under pillow, accidental, sequela
		T71.112S	Asphyx due to smothering under pillow, self-harm, sequela
		T71.113S	Asphyx due to smothering under pillow, assault, sequela
		T71.114S	Asphyx due to smothering under pillow, undetermined, sequela
		T71.121S	Asphyxiation due to plastic bag, accidental, sequela
		T71.122S	Asphyxiation due to plastic bag, self-harm, sequela
		T71.123S	Asphyxiation due to plastic bag, assault, sequela
		T71.124S	Asphyxiation due to plastic bag, undetermined, sequela
		T71.131S	Asphyx due to being trapped in bed linens, acc, sequela
		T71.132S	Asphyx due to being trapped in bed linens, slf-hrm, sequela
	(Continued on next page)	**T71.133S**	Asphyx due to being trapped in bed linens, assault, sequela

ICD-9-CM		ICD-10-CM	
9Ø9.4	LATE EFFECT OF CERTAIN OTHER EXTERNAL CAUSES **(Continued)**	**T71.134S**	Asphyx due to being trapped in bed linens, undet, sequela
		T71.141S	Asphyx due to smothr under another person's body, acc, sqla
		T71.143S	Asphyx d/t smothr under another person's body, asslt, sqla
		T71.144S	Asphyx d/t smothr under another person's body, undet, sqla
		T71.151S	Asphyx due to smothering in furniture, accidental, sequela
		T71.152S	Asphyx due to smothering in furniture, self-harm, sequela
		T71.153S	Asphyx due to smothering in furniture, assault, sequela
		T71.154S	Asphyx due to smothering in furniture, undetermined, sequela
		T71.161S	Asphyxiation due to hanging, accidental, sequela
		T71.162S	Asphyxiation due to hanging, intentional self-harm, sequela
		T71.163S	Asphyxiation due to hanging, assault, sequela
		T71.164S	Asphyxiation due to hanging, undetermined, sequela
		T71.191S	Asphyx d/t mech threat to breathe d/t oth cause, acc, sqla
		T71.192S	Asphyx d/t mech thrt to breathe d/t oth cause, slf-hrm, sqla
		T71.193S	Asphyx d/t mech threat to breathe d/t oth cause, asslt, sqla
		T71.194S	Asphyx d/t mech threat to breathe d/t oth cause, undet, sqla
		T71.2ØXS	Asphyx d/t sys oxy defic d/t low oxy in air unsp cause, sqla
		T71.21XS	Asphyxiation due to cave-in or falling earth, sequela
		T71.221S	Asphyx due to being trapped in a car trunk, acc, sequela
		T71.222S	Asphyx due to being trapped in a car trunk, slf-hrm, sequela
		T71.223S	Asphyx due to being trapped in a car trunk, assault, sequela
		T71.224S	Asphyx due to being trapped in a car trunk, undet, sequela
		T71.231S	Asphyx due to being trap in a (discarded) refrig, acc, sqla
		T71.232S	Asphyx d/t being trap in a (discarded) refrig, slf-hrm, sqla
		T71.233S	Asphyx d/t being trap in a (discarded) refrig, asslt, sqla
		T71.234S	Asphyx d/t being trap in a (discarded) refrig, undet, sqla
		T71.29XS	Asphyx due to being trap in oth low oxygen environment, sqla
		T71.9XXS	Asphyxiation due to unspecified cause, sequela
		T73.ØXXS	Starvation, sequela
		T73.1XXS	Deprivation of water, sequela
		T73.2XXS	Exhaustion due to exposure, sequela
		T73.3XXS	Exhaustion due to excessive exertion, sequela
		T73.8XXS	Other effects of deprivation, sequela
		T73.9XXS	Effect of deprivation, unspecified, sequela
		T75.ØØXS	Unspecified effects of lightning, sequela
		T75.Ø1XS	Shock due to being struck by lightning, sequela
		T75.Ø9XS	Other effects of lightning, sequela
		T75.1XXS	Unsp effects of drowning and nonfatal submersion, sequela
		T75.2ØXS	Unspecified effects of vibration, sequela
		T75.21XS	Pneumatic hammer syndrome, sequela
		T75.22XS	Traumatic vasospastic syndrome, sequela
		T75.23XS	Vertigo from infrasound, sequela
		T75.29XS	Other effects of vibration, sequela
		T75.3XXS	Motion sickness, sequela
		T75.4XXS	Electrocution, sequela
		T75.81XS	Effects of abnormal gravitation [G] forces, sequela
		T75.82XS	Effects of weightlessness, sequela
		T75.89XS	Other specified effects of external causes, sequela
9Ø9.5	LATE EFF ADVRS EFF RX MED/BIOLOGICAL SUBSTANCE	**T36.ØX5S**	Adverse effect of penicillins, sequela
		T36.1X5S	Advrs effect of cephalospor/oth beta-lactm antibiot, sequela
		T36.2X5S	Adverse effect of chloramphenicol group, sequela
		T36.3X5S	Adverse effect of macrolides, sequela
		T36.4X5S	Adverse effect of tetracyclines, sequela
		T36.5X5S	Adverse effect of aminoglycosides, sequela
		T36.6X5S	Adverse effect of rifampicins, sequela
		T36.7X5S	Adverse effect of antifungal antibiotics, sys used, sequela
		T36.8X5S	Adverse effect of other systemic antibiotics, sequela
		T36.95XS	Adverse effect of unspecified systemic antibiotic, sequela
		T37.ØX5S	Adverse effect of sulfonamides, sequela
		T37.1X5S	Adverse effect of antimycobacterial drugs, sequela
		T37.2X5S	Advrs effect of antimalari/drugs acting on bld protzoa, sqla
		T37.3X5S	Adverse effect of other antiprotozoal drugs, sequela
		T37.4X5S	Adverse effect of anthelminthics, sequela
		T37.5X5S	Adverse effect of antiviral drugs, sequela
		T37.8X5S	Adverse effect of systemic anti-infect/parasit, sequela
		T37.95XS	Advrs effect of unsp sys anti-infect and antiparasitic, sqla
		T38.ØX5S	Adverse effect of glucocort/synth analog, sequela
		T38.1X5S	Adverse effect of thyroid hormones and substitutes, sequela
		T38.2X5S	Adverse effect of antithyroid drugs, sequela
		T38.3X5S	Advrs effect of insulin and oral hypoglycemic drugs, sequela
		T38.4X5S	Adverse effect of oral contraceptives, sequela
		T38.5X5S	Adverse effect of other estrogens and progestogens, sequela
		T38.6X5S	Advrs effect of antigonadtr/antiestr/antiandrg, NEC, sequela
		T38.7X5S	Adverse effect of androgens and anabolic congeners, sequela
		T38.8Ø5S	Adverse effect of unsp hormones and synthetic sub, sequela
		T38.815S	Adverse effect of anterior pituitary hormones, sequela
		T38.895S	Adverse effect of hormones and synthetic sub, sequela
		T38.9Ø5S	Adverse effect of unspecified hormone antagonists, sequela
		T38.995S	Adverse effect of other hormone antagonists, sequela
		T39.Ø15S	Adverse effect of aspirin, sequela
	(Continued on next page)	**T39.Ø95S**	Adverse effect of salicylates, sequela

ICD-9-CM		ICD-10-CM	
909.5	LATE EFF ADVRS EFF RX MED/BIOLOGICAL SUBSTANCE **(Continued)**	**T39.1X5S**	Adverse effect of 4-Aminophenol derivatives, sequela
		T39.2X5S	Adverse effect of pyrazolone derivatives, sequela
		T39.315S	Adverse effect of propionic acid derivatives, sequela
		T39.395S	Adverse effect of nonsteroidal anti-inflam drugs, sequela
		T39.4X5S	Adverse effect of antirheumatics, NEC, sequela
		T39.8X5S	Adverse effect of nonopioid analges/antipyret, NEC, sequela
		T39.95XS	Advrs effect of unsp nonopi analgs/antipyr/antirheu, sequela
		T40.0X5S	Adverse effect of opium, sequela
		T40.2X5S	Adverse effect of other opioids, sequela
		T40.3X5S	Adverse effect of methadone, sequela
		T40.4X5S	Adverse effect of other synthetic narcotics, sequela
		T40.5X5S	Adverse effect of cocaine, sequela
		T40.605S	Adverse effect of unspecified narcotics, sequela
		T40.695S	Adverse effect of other narcotics, sequela
		T40.7X5S	Adverse effect of cannabis (derivatives), sequela
		T40.905S	Adverse effect of unspecified psychodysleptics, sequela
		T40.995S	Adverse effect of other psychodysleptics, sequela
		T41.0X5S	Adverse effect of inhaled anesthetics, sequela
		T41.1X5S	Adverse effect of intravenous anesthetics, sequela
		T41.205S	Adverse effect of unspecified general anesthetics, sequela
		T41.295S	Adverse effect of other general anesthetics, sequela
		T41.3X5S	Adverse effect of local anesthetics, sequela
		T41.45XS	Adverse effect of unspecified anesthetic, sequela
		T41.5X5S	Adverse effect of therapeutic gases, sequela
		T42.0X5S	Adverse effect of hydantoin derivatives, sequela
		T42.1X5S	Adverse effect of iminostilbenes, sequela
		T42.2X5S	Advrs effect of succinimides and oxazolidinediones, sequela
		T42.3X5S	Adverse effect of barbiturates, sequela
		T42.4X5S	Adverse effect of benzodiazepines, sequela
		T42.5X5S	Adverse effect of mixed antiepileptics, sequela
		T42.6X5S	Adverse effect of antieplptc and sed-hypntc drugs, sequela
		T42.75XS	Advrs effect of unsp antieplptc and sed-hypntc drugs, sqla
		T42.8X5S	Advrs effect of antiparkns drug/centr musc-tone depr, sqla
		T43.015S	Adverse effect of tricyclic antidepressants, sequela
		T43.025S	Adverse effect of tetracyclic antidepressants, sequela
		T43.1X5S	Adverse effect of MAO inhib antidepressants, sequela
		T43.205S	Adverse effect of unspecified antidepressants, sequela
		T43.215S	Advrs effect of slctv seroton/norepineph reup inhibtr, sqla
		T43.225S	Adverse effect of slctv serotonin reuptake inhibtr, sequela
		T43.295S	Adverse effect of other antidepressants, sequela
		T43.3X5S	Adverse effect of phenothiaz antipsychot/neurolept, sequela
		T43.4X5S	Adverse effect of butyrophen/thiothixen neuroleptc, sequela
		T43.505S	Adverse effect of unsp antipsychot/neurolept, sequela
		T43.595S	Adverse effect of antipsychotics and neuroleptics, sequela
		T43.605S	Adverse effect of unspecified psychostimulants, sequela
		T43.615S	Adverse effect of caffeine, sequela
		T43.625S	Adverse effect of amphetamines, sequela
		T43.635S	Adverse effect of methylphenidate, sequela
		T43.695S	Adverse effect of other psychostimulants, sequela
		T43.8X5S	Adverse effect of other psychotropic drugs, sequela
		T43.95XS	Adverse effect of unspecified psychotropic drug, sequela
		T44.0X5S	Adverse effect of anticholinesterase agents, sequela
		T44.1X5S	Adverse effect of other parasympathomimetics, sequela
		T44.2X5S	Adverse effect of ganglionic blocking drugs, sequela
		T44.3X5S	Adverse effect of parasympath and spasmolytics, sequela
		T44.4X5S	Adverse effect of predom alpha-adrenocpt agonists, sequela
		T44.5X5S	Adverse effect of predom beta-adrenocpt agonists, sequela
		T44.6X5S	Adverse effect of alpha-adrenoreceptor antagonists, sequela
		T44.7X5S	Adverse effect of beta-adrenoreceptor antagonists, sequela
		T44.8X5S	Advrs effect of centr-acting/adren-neurn-block agnt, sequela
		T44.905S	Advrs effect of unsp drugs aff the autonm nrv sys, sequela
		T44.995S	Adverse effect of drug aff the autonm nervous sys, sequela
		T45.0X5S	Adverse effect of antiallergic and antiemetic drugs, sequela
		T45.1X5S	Adverse effect of antineopl and immunosup drugs, sequela
		T45.2X5S	Adverse effect of vitamins, sequela
		T45.3X5S	Adverse effect of enzymes, sequela
		T45.4X5S	Adverse effect of iron and its compounds, sequela
		T45.515S	Adverse effect of anticoagulants, sequela
		T45.525S	Adverse effect of antithrombotic drugs, sequela
		T45.605S	Adverse effect of unsp fibrinolysis-affecting drugs, sequela
		T45.615S	Adverse effect of thrombolytic drugs, sequela
		T45.625S	Adverse effect of hemostatic drug, sequela
		T45.695S	Adverse effect of oth fibrinolysis-affecting drugs, sequela
		T45.7X5S	Advrs effect of anticoag antag, vit K and oth coag, sequela
		T45.8X5S	Adverse effect of prim sys and hematolog agents, sequela
		T45.95XS	Adverse effect of unsp prim sys and hematolog agent, sequela
		T46.0X5S	Adverse effect of cardi-stim glycos/drug simlar act, sequela

(Continued on next page)

ICD-9-CM		ICD-10-CM	
9Ø9.5	LATE EFF ADVRS EFF RX MED/BIOLOGICAL SUBSTANCE **(Continued)**	**T46.1X5S**	Adverse effect of calcium-channel blockers, sequela
		T46.2X5S	Adverse effect of other antidysrhythmic drugs, sequela
		T46.3X5S	Adverse effect of coronary vasodilators, sequela
		T46.4X5S	Adverse effect of angiotens-convert-enzyme inhibtr, sequela
		T46.5X5S	Adverse effect of other antihypertensive drugs, sequela
		T46.6X5S	Advrs effect of antihyperlip and antiarterio drugs, sequela
		T46.7X5S	Adverse effect of peripheral vasodilators, sequela
		T46.8X5S	Adverse effect of antivaric drugs, inc scler agents, sequela
		T46.9Ø5S	Advrs effect of unsp agents aff the cardiovasc sys, sequela
		T46.995S	Adverse effect of agents aff the cardiovascular sys, sequela
		T47.ØX5S	Adverse effect of histamine H2-receptor blockers, sequela
		T47.1X5S	Adverse effect of antacids and anti-gstrc-sec drugs, sequela
		T47.2X5S	Adverse effect of stimulant laxatives, sequela
		T47.3X5S	Adverse effect of saline and osmotic laxatives, sequela
		T47.4X5S	Adverse effect of other laxatives, sequela
		T47.5X5S	Adverse effect of digestants, sequela
		T47.6X5S	Adverse effect of antidiarrheal drugs, sequela
		T47.7X5S	Adverse effect of emetics, sequela
		T47.8X5S	Adverse effect of agents primarily affecting GI sys, sequela
		T47.95XS	Adverse effect of unsp agents aff the GI sys, sequela
		T48.ØX5S	Adverse effect of oxytocic drugs, sequela
		T48.1X5S	Adverse effect of skeletal muscle relaxants, sequela
		T48.2Ø5S	Adverse effect of unsp drugs acting on muscles, sequela
		T48.295S	Adverse effect of other drugs acting on muscles, sequela
		T48.3X5S	Adverse effect of antitussives, sequela
		T48.4X5S	Adverse effect of expectorants, sequela
		T48.5X5S	Adverse effect of other anti-common-cold drugs, sequela
		T48.6X5S	Adverse effect of antiasthmatics, sequela
		T48.9Ø5S	Advrs effect of unsp agents prim act on the resp sys, sqla
		T48.995S	Advrs effect of agents prim acting on the resp sys, sequela
		T49.ØX5S	Advrs effect of local antifung/infect/inflamm drugs, sequela
		T49.1X5S	Adverse effect of antipruritics, sequela
		T49.2X5S	Adverse effect of local astringents/detergents, sequela
		T49.3X5S	Advrs effect of emollients, demulcents and protect, sequela
		T49.4X5S	Advrs effect of keratolyt/keratplst/hair trmt drug, sequela
		T49.5X5S	Adverse effect of opth drugs and preparations, sequela
		T49.6X5S	Adverse effect of otorhino drugs and preparations, sequela
		T49.7X5S	Adverse effect of dental drugs, topically applied, sequela
		T49.8X5S	Adverse effect of other topical agents, sequela
		T49.95XS	Adverse effect of unspecified topical agent, sequela
		T5Ø.ØX5S	Adverse effect of mineralocorticoids and antag, sequela
		T5Ø.1X5S	Adverse effect of loop [high-ceiling] diuretics, sequela
		T5Ø.2X5S	Advrs eff of crbnc-anhydr inhibtr, benzo/oth diuretc, sqla
		T5Ø.3X5S	Adverse effect of electrolytic/caloric/wtr-bal agnt, sequela
		T5Ø.4X5S	Adverse effect of drugs affecting uric acid metab, sequela
		T5Ø.5X5S	Adverse effect of appetite depressants, sequela
		T5Ø.6X5S	Adverse effect of antidotes and chelating agents, sequela
		T5Ø.7X5S	Advrs effect of analeptics and opioid receptor antag, sqla
		T5Ø.8X5S	Adverse effect of diagnostic agents, sequela
		T5Ø.9Ø5S	Adverse effect of unsp drug/meds/biol subst, sequela
		T5Ø.995S	Adverse effect of drug/meds/biol subst, sequela
		T5Ø.A15S	Advrs effect of pertuss vaccine, inc combin w pertuss, sqla
		T5Ø.A25S	Adverse effect of mixed bact vaccines w/o a pertuss, sequela
		T5Ø.A95S	Adverse effect of other bacterial vaccines, sequela
		T5Ø.B15S	Adverse effect of smallpox vaccines, sequela
		T5Ø.B95S	Adverse effect of other viral vaccines, sequela
		T5Ø.Z15S	Adverse effect of immunoglobulin, sequela
		T5Ø.Z95S	Adverse effect of vaccines and biolg substances, sequela
		T88.6XXS	Anaphyl react due to advrs eff drug/med prop admin, sequela
		T88.7XXS	Unspecified adverse effect of drug or medicament, sequela
9Ø9.9	LATE EFFECT OF OTHER&UNSPECIFIED EXTERNAL CAUSES	**T74.Ø1XS**	Adult neglect or abandonment, confirmed, sequela
		T74.Ø2XS	Child neglect or abandonment, confirmed, sequela
		T74.11XS	Adult physical abuse, confirmed, sequela
		T74.12XS	Child physical abuse, confirmed, sequela
		T74.21XS	Adult sexual abuse, confirmed, sequela
		T74.22XS	Child sexual abuse, confirmed, sequela
		T74.31XS	Adult psychological abuse, confirmed, sequela
		T74.32XS	Child psychological abuse, confirmed, sequela
		T74.4XXS	Shaken infant syndrome, sequela
		T74.91XS	Unspecified adult maltreatment, confirmed, sequela
		T74.92XS	Unspecified child maltreatment, confirmed, sequela
		T76.Ø1XS	Adult neglect or abandonment, suspected, sequela
		T76.Ø2XS	Child neglect or abandonment, suspected, sequela
		T76.11XS	Adult physical abuse, suspected, sequela
		T76.12XS	Child physical abuse, suspected, sequela
		T76.21XS	Adult sexual abuse, suspected, sequela
		T76.22XS	Child sexual abuse, suspected, sequela
		T76.31XS	Adult psychological abuse, suspected, sequela
		T76.32XS	Child psychological abuse, suspected, sequela
	(Continued on next page)	**T76.91XS**	Unspecified adult maltreatment, suspected, sequela

ICD-9-CM		ICD-10-CM		
909.9	LATE EFFECT OF OTHER&UNSPECIFIED EXTERNAL CAUSES **(Continued)**	**T76.92XS**	Unspecified child maltreatment, suspected, sequela	
		T78.00XS	Anaphylactic reaction due to unspecified food, sequela	
		T78.01XS	Anaphylactic reaction due to peanuts, sequela	
		T78.02XS	Anaphyl reaction due to shellfish (crustaceans), sequela	
		T78.03XS	Anaphylactic reaction due to other fish, sequela	
		T78.04XS	Anaphylactic reaction due to fruits and vegetables, sequela	
		T78.05XS	Anaphylactic reaction due to tree nuts and seeds, sequela	
		T78.06XS	Anaphylactic reaction due to food additives, sequela	
		T78.07XS	Anaphyl reaction due to milk and dairy products, sequela	
		T78.08XS	Anaphylactic reaction due to eggs, sequela	
		T78.09XS	Anaphylactic reaction due to other food products, sequela	
		T78.1XXS	Oth adverse food reactions, NEC, sequela	
		T78.2XXS	Anaphylactic shock, unspecified, sequela	
		T78.3XXS	Angioneurotic edema, sequela	
		T78.40XS	Allergy, unspecified, sequela	
		T78.41XS	Arthus phenomenon, sequela	
		T78.49XS	Other allergy, sequela	
		T78.8XXS	Other adverse effects, not elsewhere classified, sequela	
910.0	FCE NCK&SCLP NO EYE ABRAS/FRIC BURN W/O INF	**S00.01XA**	Abrasion of scalp, initial encounter	
		S00.31XA	Abrasion of nose, initial encounter	
		S00.411A	Abrasion of right ear, initial encounter	
		S00.412A	Abrasion of left ear, initial encounter	
		S00.419A	Abrasion of unspecified ear, initial encounter	
		S00.511A	Abrasion of lip, initial encounter	
		S00.512A	Abrasion of oral cavity, initial encounter	
		S00.81XA	Abrasion of other part of head, initial encounter	
		S00.91XA	Abrasion of unspecified part of head, initial encounter	
		S10.11XA	Abrasion of throat, initial encounter	
		S10.81XA	Abrasion of other specified part of neck, initial encounter	
		S10.91XA	Abrasion of unspecified part of neck, initial encounter	
910.1	FCE NECK&SCLP NO EYE ABRAS/FRIC BURN INFECTED	**S00.90XA**	Unsp superficial injury of unsp part of head, init encntr	***or***
		S10.91XA	Abrasion of unspecified part of neck, initial encounter	***and***
		L08.89	Oth local infections of the skin and subcutaneous tissue	
910.2	FCE NECK&SCLP NO EYE BLISTER WITHOUT MENTION INF	**S00.02XA**	Blister (nonthermal) of scalp, initial encounter	
		S00.32XA	Blister (nonthermal) of nose, initial encounter	
		S00.421A	Blister (nonthermal) of right ear, initial encounter	
		S00.422A	Blister (nonthermal) of left ear, initial encounter	
		S00.429A	Blister (nonthermal) of unspecified ear, initial encounter	
		S00.521A	Blister (nonthermal) of lip, initial encounter	
		S00.522A	Blister (nonthermal) of oral cavity, initial encounter	
		S00.82XA	Blister (nonthermal) of other part of head, init encntr	
		S00.92XA	Blister (nonthermal) of unsp part of head, init encntr	
		S10.12XA	Blister (nonthermal) of throat, initial encounter	
		S10.82XA	Blister (nonthermal) of oth part of neck, init encntr	
		S10.92XA	Blister (nonthermal) of unsp part of neck, init encntr	
910.3	FACE NECK AND SCALP EXCEPT EYE BLISTER INFECTED	**S00.92XA**	Blister (nonthermal) of unsp part of head, init encntr	***or***
		S10.92XA	Blister (nonthermal) of unsp part of neck, init encntr	***and***
		L08.89	Oth local infections of the skin and subcutaneous tissue	
910.4	FCE NCK&SCLP NO EYE INSECT BITE NONVNOM W/O INF	**S00.06XA**	Insect bite (nonvenomous) of scalp, initial encounter	
		S00.36XA	Insect bite (nonvenomous) of nose, initial encounter	
		S00.461A	Insect bite (nonvenomous) of right ear, initial encounter	
		S00.462A	Insect bite (nonvenomous) of left ear, initial encounter	
		S00.469A	Insect bite (nonvenomous) of unspecified ear, init encntr	
		S00.561A	Insect bite (nonvenomous) of lip, initial encounter	
		S00.562A	Insect bite (nonvenomous) of oral cavity, initial encounter	
		S00.86XA	Insect bite (nonvenomous) of other part of head, init encntr	
		S00.96XA	Insect bite (nonvenomous) of unsp part of head, init encntr	
		S10.16XA	Insect bite (nonvenomous) of throat, initial encounter	
		S10.86XA	Insect bite of other specified part of neck, init encntr	
		S10.96XA	Insect bite of unspecified part of neck, initial encounter	
910.5	FCE NECK&SCLP NO EYE INSECT BITE NONVENOM INF	**S00.96XA**	Insect bite (nonvenomous) of unsp part of head, init encntr	***or***
		S10.96XA	Insect bite of unspecified part of neck, initial encounter	***and***
		L08.89	Oth local infections of the skin and subcutaneous tissue	
910.6	FCE NCK&SCLP NO EYE SUP FB W/O MAJ OPN WND/INF	**S00.05XA**	Superficial foreign body of scalp, initial encounter	
		S00.35XA	Superficial foreign body of nose, initial encounter	
		S00.451A	Superficial foreign body of right ear, initial encounter	
		S00.452A	Superficial foreign body of left ear, initial encounter	
		S00.459A	Superficial foreign body of unspecified ear, init encntr	
		S00.551A	Superficial foreign body of lip, initial encounter	
		S00.552A	Superficial foreign body of oral cavity, initial encounter	
		S00.85XA	Superficial foreign body of other part of head, init encntr	
		S00.95XA	Superficial foreign body of unsp part of head, init encntr	
		S10.15XA	Superficial foreign body of throat, initial encounter	
		S10.85XA	Superficial foreign body of oth part of neck, init encntr	
		S10.95XA	Superficial foreign body of unsp part of neck, init encntr	
910.7	FCE NCK&SCLP NO EYE SUP FB NO MAJ OPN WND-INF	**S00.95XA**	Superficial foreign body of unsp part of head, init encntr	***or***
		S10.95XA	Superficial foreign body of unsp part of neck, init encntr	***and***
		L08.89	Oth local infections of the skin and subcutaneous tissue	

ICD-9-CM		ICD-10-CM		
910.8	OTH&UNS SUP INJURY FCE NCK&SCLP W/O MENTION INF	**S00.00XA**	Unspecified superficial injury of scalp, initial encounter	
		S00.04XA	External constriction of part of scalp, initial encounter	
		S00.07XA	Other superficial bite of scalp, initial encounter	
		S00.30XA	Unspecified superficial injury of nose, initial encounter	
		S00.34XA	External constriction of nose, initial encounter	
		S00.37XA	Other superficial bite of nose, initial encounter	
		S00.401A	Unspecified superficial injury of right ear, init encntr	
		S00.402A	Unspecified superficial injury of left ear, init encntr	
		S00.409A	Unsp superficial injury of unspecified ear, init encntr	
		S00.441A	External constriction of right ear, initial encounter	
		S00.442A	External constriction of left ear, initial encounter	
		S00.449A	External constriction of unspecified ear, initial encounter	
		S00.471A	Other superficial bite of right ear, initial encounter	
		S00.472A	Other superficial bite of left ear, initial encounter	
		S00.479A	Other superficial bite of unspecified ear, initial encounter	
		S00.501A	Unspecified superficial injury of lip, initial encounter	
		S00.502A	Unspecified superficial injury of oral cavity, init encntr	
		S00.541A	External constriction of lip, initial encounter	
		S00.542A	External constriction of oral cavity, initial encounter	
		S00.571A	Other superficial bite of lip, initial encounter	
		S00.572A	Other superficial bite of oral cavity, initial encounter	
		S00.80XA	Unsp superficial injury of other part of head, init encntr	
		S00.84XA	External constriction of other part of head, init encntr	
		S00.87XA	Other superficial bite of other part of head, init encntr	
		S00.90XA	Unsp superficial injury of unsp part of head, init encntr	
		S00.94XA	External constriction of unsp part of head, init encntr	
		S00.97XA	Other superficial bite of unsp part of head, init encntr	
		S10.10XA	Unspecified superficial injuries of throat, init encntr	
		S10.14XA	External constriction of part of throat, initial encounter	
		S10.17XA	Other superficial bite of throat, initial encounter	
		S10.80XA	Unsp superficial injury of oth part of neck, init encntr	
		S10.84XA	External constriction of oth part of neck, init encntr	
		S10.87XA	Other superficial bite of oth part of neck, init encntr	
		S10.90XA	Unsp superficial injury of unsp part of neck, init encntr	
		S10.94XA	External constriction of unsp part of neck, init encntr	
		S10.97XA	Other superficial bite of unsp part of neck, init encntr	
910.9	OTH&UNSPEC SUPERFICIAL INJURY FACE NECK&SCLP INF	**S00.90XA**	Unsp superficial injury of unsp part of head, init encntr	*or*
		S10.90XA	Unsp superficial injury of unsp part of neck, init encntr	*and*
		L08.89	Oth local infections of the skin and subcutaneous tissue	
911.0	TRUNK ABRASION/FRICTION BURN WITHOUT MENTION INF	**S20.111A**	Abrasion of breast, right breast, initial encounter	
		S20.112A	Abrasion of breast, left breast, initial encounter	
		S20.119A	Abrasion of breast, unspecified breast, initial encounter	
		S20.311A	Abrasion of right front wall of thorax, initial encounter	
		S20.312A	Abrasion of left front wall of thorax, initial encounter	
		S20.319A	Abrasion of unspecified front wall of thorax, init encntr	
		S20.411A	Abrasion of right back wall of thorax, initial encounter	
		S20.412A	Abrasion of left back wall of thorax, initial encounter	
		S20.419A	Abrasion of unspecified back wall of thorax, init encntr	
		S20.91XA	Abrasion of unspecified parts of thorax, initial encounter	
		S30.810A	Abrasion of lower back and pelvis, initial encounter	
		S30.811A	Abrasion of abdominal wall, initial encounter	
		S30.812A	Abrasion of penis, initial encounter	
		S30.813A	Abrasion of scrotum and testes, initial encounter	
		S30.814A	Abrasion of vagina and vulva, initial encounter	
		S30.815A	Abrasion of unsp external genital organs, male, init encntr	
		S30.816A	Abrasion of unsp external genital organs, female, init	
		S30.817A	Abrasion of anus, initial encounter	
911.1	TRUNK ABRASION OR FRICTION BURN INFECTED	**S20.91XA**	Abrasion of unspecified parts of thorax, initial encounter	*and*
		L08.89	Oth local infections of the skin and subcutaneous tissue	
911.2	TRUNK BLISTER WITHOUT MENTION OF INFECTION	**S20.121A**	Blister (nonthermal) of breast, right breast, init encntr	
		S20.122A	Blister (nonthermal) of breast, left breast, init encntr	
		S20.129A	Blister (nonthermal) of breast, unsp breast, init encntr	
		S20.321A	Blister (nonthermal) of right front wall of thorax, init	
		S20.322A	Blister (nonthermal) of left front wall of thorax, init	
		S20.329A	Blister (nonthermal) of unsp front wall of thorax, init	
		S20.421A	Blister (nonthermal) of right back wall of thorax, init	
		S20.422A	Blister (nonthermal) of left back wall of thorax, init	
		S20.429A	Blister (nonthermal) of unsp back wall of thorax, init	
		S20.92XA	Blister (nonthermal) of unsp parts of thorax, init encntr	
		S30.820A	Blister (nonthermal) of lower back and pelvis, init encntr	
		S30.821A	Blister (nonthermal) of abdominal wall, initial encounter	
		S30.822A	Blister (nonthermal) of penis, initial encounter	
		S30.823A	Blister (nonthermal) of scrotum and testes, init encntr	
		S30.824A	Blister (nonthermal) of vagina and vulva, initial encounter	
		S30.825A	Blister of unsp external genital organs, male, init	
		S30.826A	Blister of unsp external genital organs, female, init	
		S30.827A	Blister (nonthermal) of anus, initial encounter	
911.3	TRUNK BLISTER, INFECTED	**S20.92XA**	Blister (nonthermal) of unsp parts of thorax, init encntr	*and*
		L08.89	Oth local infections of the skin and subcutaneous tissue	

ICD-9-CM		ICD-10-CM		
911.4	TRNK INSECT BITE NONVENOMOUS WITHOUT MENTION INF	**S2Ø.161A**	Insect bite (nonvenomous) of breast, right breast, init	
		S2Ø.162A	Insect bite (nonvenomous) of breast, left breast, init	
		S2Ø.169A	Insect bite (nonvenomous) of breast, unsp breast, init	
		S2Ø.361A	Insect bite (nonvenomous) of r frnt wl of thorax, init	
		S2Ø.362A	Insect bite (nonvenomous) of left front wall of thorax, init	
		S2Ø.369A	Insect bite (nonvenomous) of unsp front wall of thorax, init	
		S2Ø.461A	Insect bite (nonvenomous) of right back wall of thorax, init	
		S2Ø.462A	Insect bite (nonvenomous) of left back wall of thorax, init	
		S2Ø.469A	Insect bite (nonvenomous) of unsp back wall of thorax, init	
		S2Ø.96XA	Insect bite (nonvenomous) of unsp parts of thorax, init	
		S3Ø.86ØA	Insect bite (nonvenomous) of lower back and pelvis, init	
		S3Ø.861A	Insect bite (nonvenomous) of abdominal wall, init encntr	
		S3Ø.862A	Insect bite (nonvenomous) of penis, initial encounter	
		S3Ø.863A	Insect bite (nonvenomous) of scrotum and testes, init encntr	
		S3Ø.864A	Insect bite (nonvenomous) of vagina and vulva, init encntr	
		S3Ø.865A	Insect bite of unsp external genital organs, male, init	
		S3Ø.866A	Insect bite of unsp external genital organs, female, init	
		S3Ø.867A	Insect bite (nonvenomous) of anus, initial encounter	
911.5	TRUNK INSECT BITE NONVENOMOUS INFECTED	**S2Ø.96XA**	Insect bite (nonvenomous) of unsp parts of thorax, init	*and*
		LØ8.89	Oth local infections of the skin and subcutaneous tissue	
911.6	TRNK SUP FB W/O MAJ OPEN WOUND&W/O MENTION INF	**S2Ø.151A**	Superficial foreign body of breast, right breast, init	
		S2Ø.152A	Superficial foreign body of breast, left breast, init encntr	
		S2Ø.159A	Superficial foreign body of breast, unsp breast, init encntr	
		S2Ø.351A	Superficial foreign body of right front wall of thorax, init	
		S2Ø.352A	Superficial foreign body of left front wall of thorax, init	
		S2Ø.359A	Superficial foreign body of unsp front wall of thorax, init	
		S2Ø.451A	Superficial foreign body of right back wall of thorax, init	
		S2Ø.452A	Superficial foreign body of left back wall of thorax, init	
		S2Ø.459A	Superficial foreign body of unsp back wall of thorax, init	
		S2Ø.95XA	Superficial foreign body of unsp parts of thorax, init	
		S3Ø.85ØA	Superficial foreign body of lower back and pelvis, init	
		S3Ø.851A	Superficial foreign body of abdominal wall, init encntr	
		S3Ø.852A	Superficial foreign body of penis, initial encounter	
		S3Ø.853A	Superficial foreign body of scrotum and testes, init encntr	
		S3Ø.854A	Superficial foreign body of vagina and vulva, init encntr	
		S3Ø.855A	Superficial fb of unsp external genital organs, male, init	
		S3Ø.856A	Superficial fb of unsp external genital organs, female, init	
		S3Ø.857A	Superficial foreign body of anus, initial encounter	
911.7	TRUNK SUP FB WITHOUT MAJOR OPEN WOUND INF	**S2Ø.95XA**	Superficial foreign body of unsp parts of thorax, init	*and*
		LØ8.89	Oth local infections of the skin and subcutaneous tissue	
911.8	OTH&UNSPEC SUP INJURY TRUNK WITHOUT MENTION INF	**S2Ø.1Ø1A**	Unsp superficial injuries of breast, right breast, init	
		S2Ø.1Ø2A	Unsp superficial injuries of breast, left breast, init	
		S2Ø.1Ø9A	Unsp superficial injuries of breast, unsp breast, init	
		S2Ø.141A	External constriction of part of breast, right breast, init	
		S2Ø.142A	External constriction of part of breast, left breast, init	
		S2Ø.149A	External constriction of part of breast, unsp breast, init	
		S2Ø.171A	Other superficial bite of breast, right breast, init encntr	
		S2Ø.172A	Other superficial bite of breast, left breast, init encntr	
		S2Ø.179A	Other superficial bite of breast, unsp breast, init encntr	
		S2Ø.3Ø1A	Unsp superficial injuries of r frnt wl of thorax, init	
		S2Ø.3Ø2A	Unsp superficial injuries of left front wall of thorax, init	
		S2Ø.3Ø9A	Unsp superficial injuries of unsp front wall of thorax, init	
		S2Ø.341A	External constriction of right front wall of thorax, init	
		S2Ø.342A	External constriction of left front wall of thorax, init	
		S2Ø.349A	External constriction of unsp front wall of thorax, init	
		S2Ø.371A	Oth superficial bite of right front wall of thorax, init	
		S2Ø.372A	Oth superficial bite of left front wall of thorax, init	
		S2Ø.379A	Oth superficial bite of unsp front wall of thorax, init	
		S2Ø.4Ø1A	Unsp superficial injuries of right back wall of thorax, init	
		S2Ø.4Ø2A	Unsp superficial injuries of left back wall of thorax, init	
		S2Ø.4Ø9A	Unsp superficial injuries of unsp back wall of thorax, init	
		S2Ø.441A	External constriction of right back wall of thorax, init	
		S2Ø.442A	External constriction of left back wall of thorax, init	
		S2Ø.449A	External constriction of unsp back wall of thorax, init	
		S2Ø.471A	Oth superficial bite of right back wall of thorax, init	
		S2Ø.472A	Oth superficial bite of left back wall of thorax, init	
		S2Ø.479A	Oth superficial bite of unsp back wall of thorax, init	
		S2Ø.9ØXA	Unsp superficial injury of unsp parts of thorax, init encntr	
		S2Ø.94XA	External constriction of unsp parts of thorax, init encntr	
		S2Ø.97XA	Other superficial bite of unsp parts of thorax, init encntr	
		S3Ø.81ØA	Abrasion of lower back and pelvis, initial encounter	
		S3Ø.84ØA	External constriction of lower back and pelvis, init encntr	
		S3Ø.841A	External constriction of abdominal wall, initial encounter	
		S3Ø.842A	External constriction of penis, initial encounter	
		S3Ø.843A	External constriction of scrotum and testes, init encntr	
		S3Ø.844A	External constriction of vagina and vulva, initial encounter	
		S3Ø.845A	Extrn constrict of unsp external genital organs, male, init	
		S3Ø.846A	Extrn constrict of unsp extrn genital organs, female, init	
		S3Ø.87ØA	Other superficial bite of lower back and pelvis, init encntr	
		S3Ø.871A	Other superficial bite of abdominal wall, initial encounter	
		S3Ø.872A	Other superficial bite of penis, initial encounter	

(Continued on next page)

ICD-9-CM		ICD-10-CM		
911.8	OTH&UNSPEC SUP INJURY TRUNK WITHOUT MENTION INF **(Continued)**	**S3Ø.873A**	Other superficial bite of scrotum and testes, init encntr	
		S3Ø.874A	Other superficial bite of vagina and vulva, init encntr	
		S3Ø.875A	Oth superfic bite of unsp extrn genital organs, male, init	
		S3Ø.876A	Oth superfic bite of unsp extrn genital organs, female, init	
		S3Ø.877A	Other superficial bite of anus, initial encounter	
		S3Ø.91XA	Unsp superficial injury of lower back and pelvis, init	
		S3Ø.92XA	Unsp superficial injury of abdominal wall, init encntr	
		S3Ø.93XA	Unspecified superficial injury of penis, initial encounter	
		S3Ø.94XA	Unsp superficial injury of scrotum and testes, init encntr	
		S3Ø.95XA	Unsp superficial injury of vagina and vulva, init encntr	
		S3Ø.96XA	Unsp superfic inj unsp external genital organs, male, init	
		S3Ø.97XA	Unsp superfic inj unsp external genital organs, female, init	
		S3Ø.98XA	Unspecified superficial injury of anus, initial encounter	
911.9	OTHER&UNSPEC SUPERFICIAL INJURY TRUNK INFECTED	**S2Ø.9ØXA**	Unsp superficial injury of unsp parts of thorax, init encntr	*and*
		LØ8.89	Oth local infections of the skin and subcutaneous tissue	
912.Ø	SHLDR&UP ARM ABRASION/FRICION BURN W/O INF	**S4Ø.211A**	Abrasion of right shoulder, initial encounter	
		S4Ø.212A	Abrasion of left shoulder, initial encounter	
		S4Ø.219A	Abrasion of unspecified shoulder, initial encounter	
		S4Ø.811A	Abrasion of right upper arm, initial encounter	
		S4Ø.812A	Abrasion of left upper arm, initial encounter	
		S4Ø.819A	Abrasion of unspecified upper arm, initial encounter	
912.1	SHOULDR&UPPR ARM ABRASION/FRICTION BURN INFECTED	**S4Ø.219A**	Abrasion of unspecified shoulder, initial encounter	*or*
		S4Ø.819A	Abrasion of unspecified upper arm, initial encounter	*and*
		LØ8.89	Oth local infections of the skin and subcutaneous tissue	
912.2	SHOULDER&UPPER ARM BLISTER WITHOUT MENTION INF	**S4Ø.221A**	Blister (nonthermal) of right shoulder, initial encounter	
		S4Ø.222A	Blister (nonthermal) of left shoulder, initial encounter	
		S4Ø.229A	Blister (nonthermal) of unspecified shoulder, init encntr	
		S4Ø.821A	Blister (nonthermal) of right upper arm, initial encounter	
		S4Ø.822A	Blister (nonthermal) of left upper arm, initial encounter	
		S4Ø.829A	Blister (nonthermal) of unspecified upper arm, init encntr	
912.3	SHOULDER AND UPPER ARM BLISTER INFECTED	**S4Ø.229A**	Blister (nonthermal) of unspecified shoulder, init encntr	*or*
		S4Ø.829A	Blister (nonthermal) of unspecified upper arm, init encntr	*and*
		LØ8.89	Oth local infections of the skin and subcutaneous tissue	
912.4	SHLDR&UP ARM INSECT BITE NONVENOMOUS W/O INF	**S4Ø.261A**	Insect bite (nonvenomous) of right shoulder, init encntr	
		S4Ø.262A	Insect bite (nonvenomous) of left shoulder, init encntr	
		S4Ø.269A	Insect bite (nonvenomous) of unsp shoulder, init encntr	
		S4Ø.861A	Insect bite (nonvenomous) of right upper arm, init encntr	
		S4Ø.862A	Insect bite (nonvenomous) of left upper arm, init encntr	
		S4Ø.869A	Insect bite (nonvenomous) of unsp upper arm, init encntr	
912.5	SHOULDER&UPPER ARM INSECT BITE NONVEN INFECTD	**S4Ø.269A**	Insect bite (nonvenomous) of unsp shoulder, init encntr	*or*
		S4Ø.869A	Insect bite (nonvenomous) of unsp upper arm, init encntr	*and*
		LØ8.89	Oth local infections of the skin and subcutaneous tissue	
912.6	SHLDR&UP ARM SUP FB W/O MAJ OPN WND&W/O INF	**S4Ø.251A**	Superficial foreign body of right shoulder, init encntr	
		S4Ø.252A	Superficial foreign body of left shoulder, initial encounter	
		S4Ø.259A	Superficial foreign body of unsp shoulder, init encntr	
		S4Ø.851A	Superficial foreign body of right upper arm, init encntr	
		S4Ø.852A	Superficial foreign body of left upper arm, init encntr	
		S4Ø.859A	Superficial foreign body of unsp upper arm, init encntr	
912.7	SHLDR&UPPER ARM SUP FB NO MAJ OPN WOUND INFECTED	**S4Ø.259A**	Superficial foreign body of unsp shoulder, init encntr	*or*
		S4Ø.859A	Superficial foreign body of unsp upper arm, init encntr	*and*
		LØ8.89	Oth local infections of the skin and subcutaneous tissue	
912.8	OTH&UNS SUP INJURY SHLDR&UP ARM W/O MENTION INF	**S4Ø.241A**	External constriction of right shoulder, initial encounter	
		S4Ø.242A	External constriction of left shoulder, initial encounter	
		S4Ø.249A	External constriction of unspecified shoulder, init encntr	
		S4Ø.271A	Other superficial bite of right shoulder, initial encounter	
		S4Ø.272A	Other superficial bite of left shoulder, initial encounter	
		S4Ø.279A	Other superficial bite of unspecified shoulder, init encntr	
		S4Ø.841A	External constriction of right upper arm, initial encounter	
		S4Ø.842A	External constriction of left upper arm, initial encounter	
		S4Ø.849A	External constriction of unspecified upper arm, init encntr	
		S4Ø.871A	Other superficial bite of right upper arm, initial encounter	
		S4Ø.872A	Other superficial bite of left upper arm, initial encounter	
		S4Ø.879A	Other superficial bite of unspecified upper arm, init encntr	
		S4Ø.911A	Unsp superficial injury of right shoulder, init encntr	
		S4Ø.912A	Unspecified superficial injury of left shoulder, init encntr	
		S4Ø.919A	Unsp superficial injury of unspecified shoulder, init encntr	
		S4Ø.921A	Unsp superficial injury of right upper arm, init encntr	
		S4Ø.922A	Unsp superficial injury of left upper arm, init encntr	
		S4Ø.929A	Unsp superficial injury of unsp upper arm, init encntr	
912.9	OTH&UNSPEC SUP INJURY SHLDR&UPPER ARM INF	**S4Ø.919A**	Unsp superficial injury of unspecified shoulder, init encntr	*or*
		S4Ø.929A	Unsp superficial injury of unsp upper arm, init encntr	*and*
		LØ8.89	Oth local infections of the skin and subcutaneous tissue	

ICD-9-CM		ICD-10-CM		
913.Ø	ELB FORARM&WRST ABRASION/FRICION BURN W/O INF	S5Ø.311A	Abrasion of right elbow, initial encounter	
		S5Ø.312A	Abrasion of left elbow, initial encounter	
		S5Ø.319A	Abrasion of unspecified elbow, initial encounter	
		S5Ø.811A	Abrasion of right forearm, initial encounter	
		S5Ø.812A	Abrasion of left forearm, initial encounter	
		S5Ø.819A	Abrasion of unspecified forearm, initial encounter	
		S6Ø.811A	Abrasion of right wrist, initial encounter	
		S6Ø.812A	Abrasion of left wrist, initial encounter	
		S6Ø.819A	Abrasion of unspecified wrist, initial encounter	
913.1	ELB FOREARM&WRIST ABRASION/FRICTION BURN INF	S5Ø.319A	Abrasion of unspecified elbow, initial encounter	*or*
		S5Ø.819A	Abrasion of unspecified forearm, initial encounter	*or*
		S6Ø.819A	Abrasion of unspecified wrist, initial encounter	*and*
		LØ8.89	Oth local infections of the skin and subcutaneous tissue	
913.2	ELB FOREARM&WRIST BLISTER WITHOUT MENTION INF	S5Ø.321A	Blister (nonthermal) of right elbow, initial encounter	
		S5Ø.322A	Blister (nonthermal) of left elbow, initial encounter	
		S5Ø.329A	Blister (nonthermal) of unspecified elbow, initial encounter	
		S5Ø.821A	Blister (nonthermal) of right forearm, initial encounter	
		S5Ø.822A	Blister (nonthermal) of left forearm, initial encounter	
		S5Ø.829A	Blister (nonthermal) of unspecified forearm, init encntr	
		S6Ø.821A	Blister (nonthermal) of right wrist, initial encounter	
		S6Ø.822A	Blister (nonthermal) of left wrist, initial encounter	
		S6Ø.829A	Blister (nonthermal) of unspecified wrist, initial encounter	
913.3	ELBOW FOREARM AND WRIST BLISTER INFECTED	S5Ø.329A	Blister (nonthermal) of unspecified elbow, initial encounter	*or*
		S5Ø.829A	Blister (nonthermal) of unspecified forearm, init encntr	*or*
		S6Ø.829A	Blister (nonthermal) of unspecified wrist, initial encounter	*and*
		LØ8.89	Oth local infections of the skin and subcutaneous tissue	
913.4	ELB FORARM&WRST INSECT BITE NONVENOMOUS W/O INF	S5Ø.361A	Insect bite (nonvenomous) of right elbow, initial encounter	
		S5Ø.362A	Insect bite (nonvenomous) of left elbow, initial encounter	
		S5Ø.369A	Insect bite (nonvenomous) of unspecified elbow, init encntr	
		S5Ø.861A	Insect bite (nonvenomous) of right forearm, init encntr	
		S5Ø.862A	Insect bite (nonvenomous) of left forearm, initial encounter	
		S5Ø.869A	Insect bite (nonvenomous) of unsp forearm, init encntr	
		S6Ø.861A	Insect bite (nonvenomous) of right wrist, initial encounter	
		S6Ø.862A	Insect bite (nonvenomous) of left wrist, initial encounter	
		S6Ø.869A	Insect bite (nonvenomous) of unspecified wrist, init encntr	
913.5	ELB FOREARM&WRIST INSECT BITE NONVENOMOUS INF	S5Ø.369A	Insect bite (nonvenomous) of unspecified elbow, init encntr	*or*
		S5Ø.869A	Insect bite (nonvenomous) of unsp forearm, init encntr	*or*
		S6Ø.869A	Insect bite (nonvenomous) of unspecified wrist, init encntr	*and*
		LØ8.89	Oth local infections of the skin and subcutaneous tissue	
913.6	ELB FORARM&WRST SUP FB W/O MAJ OPN WND&W/O INF	S5Ø.351A	Superficial foreign body of right elbow, initial encounter	
		S5Ø.352A	Superficial foreign body of left elbow, initial encounter	
		S5Ø.359A	Superficial foreign body of unspecified elbow, init encntr	
		S5Ø.851A	Superficial foreign body of right forearm, initial encounter	
		S5Ø.852A	Superficial foreign body of left forearm, initial encounter	
		S5Ø.859A	Superficial foreign body of unspecified forearm, init encntr	
		S6Ø.851A	Superficial foreign body of right wrist, initial encounter	
		S6Ø.852A	Superficial foreign body of left wrist, initial encounter	
		S6Ø.859A	Superficial foreign body of unspecified wrist, init encntr	
913.7	ELB FOREARM&WRST SUP FB WITHOUT MAJ OPN WND INF	S5Ø.359A	Superficial foreign body of unspecified elbow, init encntr	*or*
		S5Ø.859A	Superficial foreign body of unspecified forearm, init encntr	*or*
		S6Ø.859A	Superficial foreign body of unspecified wrist, init encntr	*and*
		LØ8.89	Oth local infections of the skin and subcutaneous tissue	
913.8	OTH&UNS SUP INJR ELB FORARM&WRST W/O MENTION INF	S5Ø.341A	External constriction of right elbow, initial encounter	
		S5Ø.342A	External constriction of left elbow, initial encounter	
		S5Ø.349A	External constriction of unspecified elbow, init encntr	
		S5Ø.371A	Other superficial bite of right elbow, initial encounter	
		S5Ø.372A	Other superficial bite of left elbow, initial encounter	
		S5Ø.379A	Other superficial bite of unspecified elbow, init encntr	
		S5Ø.841A	External constriction of right forearm, initial encounter	
		S5Ø.842A	External constriction of left forearm, initial encounter	
		S5Ø.849A	External constriction of unspecified forearm, init encntr	
		S5Ø.871A	Other superficial bite of right forearm, initial encounter	
		S5Ø.872A	Other superficial bite of left forearm, initial encounter	
		S5Ø.879A	Other superficial bite of unspecified forearm, init encntr	
		S5Ø.9Ø1A	Unspecified superficial injury of right elbow, init encntr	
		S5Ø.9Ø2A	Unspecified superficial injury of left elbow, init encntr	
		S5Ø.9Ø9A	Unsp superficial injury of unspecified elbow, init encntr	
		S5Ø.911A	Unspecified superficial injury of right forearm, init encntr	
		S5Ø.912A	Unspecified superficial injury of left forearm, init encntr	
		S5Ø.919A	Unsp superficial injury of unspecified forearm, init encntr	
		S6Ø.841A	External constriction of right wrist, initial encounter	
		S6Ø.842A	External constriction of left wrist, initial encounter	
		S6Ø.849A	External constriction of unspecified wrist, init encntr	
		S6Ø.871A	Other superficial bite of right wrist, initial encounter	
		S6Ø.872A	Other superficial bite of left wrist, initial encounter	
		S6Ø.879A	Other superficial bite of unspecified wrist, init encntr	
		S6Ø.911A	Unspecified superficial injury of right wrist, init encntr	
		S6Ø.912A	Unspecified superficial injury of left wrist, init encntr	
		S6Ø.919A	Unsp superficial injury of unspecified wrist, init encntr	

ICD-9-CM		ICD-10-CM		
913.9	OTH&UNSPEC SUP INJURY ELB FOREARM&WRIST INF	S5Ø.9Ø9A	Unsp superficial injury of unspecified elbow, init encntr	or
		S5Ø.919A	Unsp superficial injury of unspecified forearm, init encntr	or
		S6Ø.919A	Unsp superficial injury of unspecified wrist, init encntr	and
		LØ8.89	Oth local infections of the skin and subcutaneous tissue	
914.Ø	HAND NO FINGER ALONE ABRAS/FRIC BURN W/O INF	S6Ø.511A	Abrasion of right hand, initial encounter	
		S6Ø.512A	Abrasion of left hand, initial encounter	
		S6Ø.519A	Abrasion of unspecified hand, initial encounter	
914.1	HAND NO FINGER ALONE ABRASION/FRICTION BURN INF	S6Ø.519A	Abrasion of unspecified hand, initial encounter	and
		LØ8.89	Oth local infections of the skin and subcutaneous tissue	
914.2	HAND NO FINGER ALONE BLISTER WITHOUT MENTION INF	S6Ø.521A	Blister (nonthermal) of right hand, initial encounter	
		S6Ø.522A	Blister (nonthermal) of left hand, initial encounter	
		S6Ø.529A	Blister (nonthermal) of unspecified hand, initial encounter	
914.3	HAND EXCEPT FINGER ALONE BLISTER INFECTED	S6Ø.529A	Blister (nonthermal) of unspecified hand, initial encounter	and
		LØ8.89	Oth local infections of the skin and subcutaneous tissue	
914.4	HND NO FNGR ALONE INSECT BITE NONVNOM W/O INF	S6Ø.561A	Insect bite (nonvenomous) of right hand, initial encounter	
		S6Ø.562A	Insect bite (nonvenomous) of left hand, initial encounter	
		S6Ø.569A	Insect bite (nonvenomous) of unspecified hand, init encntr	
914.5	HAND NO FINGER ALONE INSECT BITE NONVENOMOUS INF	S6Ø.569A	Insect bite (nonvenomous) of unspecified hand, init encntr	and
		LØ8.89	Oth local infections of the skin and subcutaneous tissue	
914.6	HND NO FINGR SUP FB W/O MAJ OPN WND&W/O INF	S6Ø.551A	Superficial foreign body of right hand, initial encounter	
		S6Ø.552A	Superficial foreign body of left hand, initial encounter	
		S6Ø.559A	Superficial foreign body of unspecified hand, init encntr	
914.7	HAND NO FINGR ALONE SUP FB W/O MAJ OPN WOUND INF	S6Ø.559A	Superficial foreign body of unspecified hand, init encntr	and
		LØ8.89	Oth local infections of the skin and subcutaneous tissue	
914.8	OTH&UNS SUP INJURY HND NO FINGR ALONE W/O INF	S6Ø.541A	External constriction of right hand, initial encounter	
		S6Ø.542A	External constriction of left hand, initial encounter	
		S6Ø.549A	External constriction of unspecified hand, initial encounter	
		S6Ø.571A	Other superficial bite of hand of right hand, init encntr	
		S6Ø.572A	Other superficial bite of hand of left hand, init encntr	
		S6Ø.579A	Other superficial bite of hand of unsp hand, init encntr	
		S6Ø.921A	Unspecified superficial injury of right hand, init encntr	
		S6Ø.922A	Unspecified superficial injury of left hand, init encntr	
		S6Ø.929A	Unsp superficial injury of unspecified hand, init encntr	
914.9	OTH&UNSPEC SUP INJURY HAND NO FINGR ALONE INF	S6Ø.929A	Unsp superficial injury of unspecified hand, init encntr	and
		LØ8.89	Oth local infections of the skin and subcutaneous tissue	
915.Ø	ABRASION/FRICTION BURN FINGER W/O MENTION INF	S6Ø.311A	Abrasion of right thumb, initial encounter	
		S6Ø.312A	Abrasion of left thumb, initial encounter	
		S6Ø.319A	Abrasion of unspecified thumb, initial encounter	
		S6Ø.41ØA	Abrasion of right index finger, initial encounter	
		S6Ø.411A	Abrasion of left index finger, initial encounter	
		S6Ø.412A	Abrasion of right middle finger, initial encounter	
		S6Ø.413A	Abrasion of left middle finger, initial encounter	
		S6Ø.414A	Abrasion of right ring finger, initial encounter	
		S6Ø.415A	Abrasion of left ring finger, initial encounter	
		S6Ø.416A	Abrasion of right little finger, initial encounter	
		S6Ø.417A	Abrasion of left little finger, initial encounter	
		S6Ø.418A	Abrasion of other finger, initial encounter	
		S6Ø.419A	Abrasion of unspecified finger, initial encounter	
915.1	FINGER ABRASION OR FRICTION BURN INFECTED	S6Ø.319A	Abrasion of unspecified thumb, initial encounter	or
		S6Ø.419A	Abrasion of unspecified finger, initial encounter	and
		LØ8.89	Oth local infections of the skin and subcutaneous tissue	
915.2	FINGER BLISTER WITHOUT MENTION OF INFECTION	S6Ø.321A	Blister (nonthermal) of right thumb, initial encounter	
		S6Ø.322A	Blister (nonthermal) of left thumb, initial encounter	
		S6Ø.329A	Blister (nonthermal) of unspecified thumb, initial encounter	
		S6Ø.42ØA	Blister (nonthermal) of right index finger, init encntr	
		S6Ø.421A	Blister (nonthermal) of left index finger, initial encounter	
		S6Ø.422A	Blister (nonthermal) of right middle finger, init encntr	
		S6Ø.423A	Blister (nonthermal) of left middle finger, init encntr	
		S6Ø.424A	Blister (nonthermal) of right ring finger, initial encounter	
		S6Ø.425A	Blister (nonthermal) of left ring finger, initial encounter	
		S6Ø.426A	Blister (nonthermal) of right little finger, init encntr	
		S6Ø.427A	Blister (nonthermal) of left little finger, init encntr	
		S6Ø.428A	Blister (nonthermal) of other finger, initial encounter	
		S6Ø.429A	Blister (nonthermal) of unspecified finger, init encntr	
915.3	FINGER, BLISTER, INFECTED	S6Ø.329A	Blister (nonthermal) of unspecified thumb, initial encounter	or
		S6Ø.429A	Blister (nonthermal) of unspecified finger, init encntr	and
		LØ8.89	Oth local infections of the skin and subcutaneous tissue	

ICD-9-CM		ICD-10-CM		
915.4	FINGER INSECT BITE NONVENOMOUS W/O MENTION INF	**S6Ø.361A**	Insect bite (nonvenomous) of right thumb, initial encounter	
		S6Ø.362A	Insect bite (nonvenomous) of left thumb, initial encounter	
		S6Ø.369A	Insect bite (nonvenomous) of unspecified thumb, init encntr	
		S6Ø.46ØA	Insect bite (nonvenomous) of right index finger, init encntr	
		S6Ø.461A	Insect bite (nonvenomous) of left index finger, init encntr	
		S6Ø.462A	Insect bite (nonvenomous) of right middle finger, init	
		S6Ø.463A	Insect bite (nonvenomous) of left middle finger, init encntr	
		S6Ø.464A	Insect bite (nonvenomous) of right ring finger, init encntr	
		S6Ø.465A	Insect bite (nonvenomous) of left ring finger, init encntr	
		S6Ø.466A	Insect bite (nonvenomous) of right little finger, init	
		S6Ø.467A	Insect bite (nonvenomous) of left little finger, init encntr	
		S6Ø.468A	Insect bite (nonvenomous) of other finger, initial encounter	
		S6Ø.469A	Insect bite (nonvenomous) of unspecified finger, init encntr	
915.5	FINGER INSECT BITE NONVENOMOUS INFECTED	**S6Ø.369A**	Insect bite (nonvenomous) of unspecified thumb, init encntr	***or***
		S6Ø.469A	Insect bite (nonvenomous) of unspecified finger, init encntr	***and***
		LØ8.89	Oth local infections of the skin and subcutaneous tissue	
915.6	FINGER SUP FB W/O MAJ OPEN WOUND&W/O MENTION INF	**S6Ø.351A**	Superficial foreign body of right thumb, initial encounter	
		S6Ø.352A	Superficial foreign body of left thumb, initial encounter	
		S6Ø.359A	Superficial foreign body of unspecified thumb, init encntr	
		S6Ø.45ØA	Superficial foreign body of right index finger, init encntr	
		S6Ø.451A	Superficial foreign body of left index finger, init encntr	
		S6Ø.452A	Superficial foreign body of right middle finger, init encntr	
		S6Ø.453A	Superficial foreign body of left middle finger, init encntr	
		S6Ø.454A	Superficial foreign body of right ring finger, init encntr	
		S6Ø.455A	Superficial foreign body of left ring finger, init encntr	
		S6Ø.456A	Superficial foreign body of right little finger, init encntr	
		S6Ø.457A	Superficial foreign body of left little finger, init encntr	
		S6Ø.458A	Superficial foreign body of other finger, initial encounter	
		S6Ø.459A	Superficial foreign body of unspecified finger, init encntr	
915.7	FINGER SUP FB WITHOUT MAJOR OPEN WOUND INF	**S6Ø.359A**	Superficial foreign body of unspecified thumb, init encntr	***or***
		S6Ø.459A	Superficial foreign body of unspecified finger, init encntr	***and***
		LØ8.89	Oth local infections of the skin and subcutaneous tissue	
915.8	OTH&UNSPEC SUP INJURY FINGER WITHOUT MENTION INF	**S6Ø.449A**	External constriction of unspecified finger, init encntr	
		S6Ø.47ØA	Other superficial bite of right index finger, init encntr	
		S6Ø.471A	Other superficial bite of left index finger, init encntr	
		S6Ø.472A	Other superficial bite of right middle finger, init encntr	
		S6Ø.473A	Other superficial bite of left middle finger, init encntr	
		S6Ø.474A	Other superficial bite of right ring finger, init encntr	
		S6Ø.475A	Other superficial bite of left ring finger, init encntr	
		S6Ø.476A	Other superficial bite of right little finger, init encntr	
		S6Ø.477A	Other superficial bite of left little finger, init encntr	
		S6Ø.478A	Other superficial bite of other finger, initial encounter	
		S6Ø.479A	Other superficial bite of unspecified finger, init encntr	
		S6Ø.931A	Unspecified superficial injury of right thumb, init encntr	
		S6Ø.932A	Unspecified superficial injury of left thumb, init encntr	
		S6Ø.939A	Unsp superficial injury of unspecified thumb, init encntr	
		S6Ø.94ØA	Unsp superficial injury of right index finger, init encntr	
		S6Ø.941A	Unsp superficial injury of left index finger, init encntr	
		S6Ø.942A	Unsp superficial injury of right middle finger, init encntr	
		S6Ø.943A	Unsp superficial injury of left middle finger, init encntr	
		S6Ø.944A	Unsp superficial injury of right ring finger, init encntr	
		S6Ø.945A	Unsp superficial injury of left ring finger, init encntr	
		S6Ø.946A	Unsp superficial injury of right little finger, init encntr	
		S6Ø.947A	Unsp superficial injury of left little finger, init encntr	
		S6Ø.948A	Unspecified superficial injury of other finger, init encntr	
		S6Ø.949A	Unsp superficial injury of unspecified finger, init encntr	
915.9	OTHER&UNSPEC SUPERFICIAL INJURY FINGER INFECTED	**S6Ø.939A**	Unsp superficial injury of unspecified thumb, init encntr	***or***
		S6Ø.949A	Unsp superficial injury of unspecified finger, init encntr	***and***
		LØ8.89	Oth local infections of the skin and subcutaneous tissue	
916.Ø	HIP THI LEG&ANK ABRASION/FRICION BURN W/O INF	**S7Ø.211A**	Abrasion, right hip, initial encounter	
		S7Ø.212A	Abrasion, left hip, initial encounter	
		S7Ø.219A	Abrasion, unspecified hip, initial encounter	
		S7Ø.311A	Abrasion, right thigh, initial encounter	
		S7Ø.312A	Abrasion, left thigh, initial encounter	
		S7Ø.319A	Abrasion, unspecified thigh, initial encounter	
		S8Ø.211A	Abrasion, right knee, initial encounter	
		S8Ø.212A	Abrasion, left knee, initial encounter	
		S8Ø.219A	Abrasion, unspecified knee, initial encounter	
		S8Ø.811A	Abrasion, right lower leg, initial encounter	
		S8Ø.812A	Abrasion, left lower leg, initial encounter	
		S8Ø.819A	Abrasion, unspecified lower leg, initial encounter	
		S9Ø.511A	Abrasion, right ankle, initial encounter	
		S9Ø.512A	Abrasion, left ankle, initial encounter	
		S9Ø.519A	Abrasion, unspecified ankle, initial encounter	

ICD-9-CM		ICD-10-CM		
916.1	HIP THIGH LEG&ANK ABRASION/FRICTION BURN INF	**S7Ø.219A**	Abrasion, unspecified hip, initial encounter	*or*
		S7Ø.319A	Abrasion, unspecified thigh, initial encounter	*or*
		S8Ø.219A	Abrasion, unspecified knee, initial encounter	*or*
		S8Ø.819A	Abrasion, unspecified lower leg, initial encounter	*or*
		S9Ø.519A	Abrasion, unspecified ankle, initial encounter	*and*
		LØ8.89	Oth local infections of the skin and subcutaneous tissue	
916.2	HIP THIGH LEG&ANK BLISTER WITHOUT MENTION INF	**S7Ø.221A**	Blister (nonthermal), right hip, initial encounter	
		S7Ø.222A	Blister (nonthermal), left hip, initial encounter	
		S7Ø.229A	Blister (nonthermal), unspecified hip, initial encounter	
		S7Ø.321A	Blister (nonthermal), right thigh, initial encounter	
		S7Ø.322A	Blister (nonthermal), left thigh, initial encounter	
		S7Ø.329A	Blister (nonthermal), unspecified thigh, initial encounter	
		S8Ø.221A	Blister (nonthermal), right knee, initial encounter	
		S8Ø.222A	Blister (nonthermal), left knee, initial encounter	
		S8Ø.229A	Blister (nonthermal), unspecified knee, initial encounter	
		S8Ø.821A	Blister (nonthermal), right lower leg, initial encounter	
		S8Ø.822A	Blister (nonthermal), left lower leg, initial encounter	
		S8Ø.829A	Blister (nonthermal), unspecified lower leg, init encntr	
		S9Ø.521A	Blister (nonthermal), right ankle, initial encounter	
		S9Ø.522A	Blister (nonthermal), left ankle, initial encounter	
		S9Ø.529A	Blister (nonthermal), unspecified ankle, initial encounter	
916.3	HIP THIGH LEG AND ANKLE BLISTER INFECTED	**S7Ø.229A**	Blister (nonthermal), unspecified hip, initial encounter	*or*
		S7Ø.329A	Blister (nonthermal), unspecified thigh, initial encounter	*or*
		S8Ø.229A	Blister (nonthermal), unspecified knee, initial encounter	*or*
		S8Ø.829A	Blister (nonthermal), unspecified lower leg, init encntr	*or*
		S9Ø.529A	Blister (nonthermal), unspecified ankle, initial encounter	*and*
		LØ8.89	Oth local infections of the skin and subcutaneous tissue	
916.4	HIP THI LEG&ANK INSECT BITE NONVENOMOUS W/O INF	**S7Ø.261A**	Insect bite (nonvenomous), right hip, initial encounter	
		S7Ø.262A	Insect bite (nonvenomous), left hip, initial encounter	
		S7Ø.269A	Insect bite (nonvenomous), unspecified hip, init encntr	
		S7Ø.361A	Insect bite (nonvenomous), right thigh, initial encounter	
		S7Ø.362A	Insect bite (nonvenomous), left thigh, initial encounter	
		S7Ø.369A	Insect bite (nonvenomous), unspecified thigh, init encntr	
		S8Ø.261A	Insect bite (nonvenomous), right knee, initial encounter	
		S8Ø.262A	Insect bite (nonvenomous), left knee, initial encounter	
		S8Ø.269A	Insect bite (nonvenomous), unspecified knee, init encntr	
		S8Ø.861A	Insect bite (nonvenomous), right lower leg, init encntr	
		S8Ø.862A	Insect bite (nonvenomous), left lower leg, initial encounter	
		S8Ø.869A	Insect bite (nonvenomous), unsp lower leg, init encntr	
		S9Ø.561A	Insect bite (nonvenomous), right ankle, initial encounter	
		S9Ø.562A	Insect bite (nonvenomous), left ankle, initial encounter	
		S9Ø.569A	Insect bite (nonvenomous), unspecified ankle, init encntr	
916.5	HIP THIGH LEG&ANK INSECT BITE NONVENOMOUS INF	**S7Ø.269A**	Insect bite (nonvenomous), unspecified hip, init encntr	*or*
		S7Ø.369A	Insect bite (nonvenomous), unspecified thigh, init encntr	*or*
		S8Ø.269A	Insect bite (nonvenomous), unspecified knee, init encntr	*or*
		S8Ø.869A	Insect bite (nonvenomous), unsp lower leg, init encntr	*or*
		S9Ø.569A	Insect bite (nonvenomous), unspecified ankle, init encntr	*and*
		LØ8.89	Oth local infections of the skin and subcutaneous tissue	
916.6	HIP THI LEG&ANK SUP FB W/O MAJ OPN WND&W/O INF	**S7Ø.251A**	Superficial foreign body, right hip, initial encounter	
		S7Ø.252A	Superficial foreign body, left hip, initial encounter	
		S7Ø.259A	Superficial foreign body, unspecified hip, initial encounter	
		S7Ø.351A	Superficial foreign body, right thigh, initial encounter	
		S7Ø.352A	Superficial foreign body, left thigh, initial encounter	
		S7Ø.359A	Superficial foreign body, unspecified thigh, init encntr	
		S8Ø.251A	Superficial foreign body, right knee, initial encounter	
		S8Ø.252A	Superficial foreign body, left knee, initial encounter	
		S8Ø.259A	Superficial foreign body, unspecified knee, init encntr	
		S8Ø.851A	Superficial foreign body, right lower leg, initial encounter	
		S8Ø.852A	Superficial foreign body, left lower leg, initial encounter	
		S8Ø.859A	Superficial foreign body, unspecified lower leg, init encntr	
		S9Ø.551A	Superficial foreign body, right ankle, initial encounter	
		S9Ø.552A	Superficial foreign body, left ankle, initial encounter	
		S9Ø.559A	Superficial foreign body, unspecified ankle, init encntr	
916.7	HIP THIGH LEG&ANK SUP FB W/O MAJ OPN WOUND INF	**S7Ø.259A**	Superficial foreign body, unspecified hip, initial encounter	*or*
		S7Ø.359A	Superficial foreign body, unspecified thigh, init encntr	*or*
		S8Ø.259A	Superficial foreign body, unspecified knee, init encntr	*or*
		S8Ø.859A	Superficial foreign body, unspecified lower leg, init encntr	*or*
		S9Ø.559A	Superficial foreign body, unspecified ankle, init encntr	*and*
		LØ8.89	Oth local infections of the skin and subcutaneous tissue	

ICD-9-CM		ICD-10-CM		
916.8	OTH&UNS SUP INJR HIP THI LEG&ANK W/O MENTION INF	**S7Ø.241A**	External constriction, right hip, initial encounter	
		S7Ø.242A	External constriction, left hip, initial encounter	
		S7Ø.249A	External constriction, unspecified hip, initial encounter	
		S7Ø.271A	Other superficial bite of hip, right hip, initial encounter	
		S7Ø.272A	Other superficial bite of hip, left hip, initial encounter	
		S7Ø.279A	Other superficial bite of hip, unspecified hip, init encntr	
		S7Ø.341A	External constriction, right thigh, initial encounter	
		S7Ø.342A	External constriction, left thigh, initial encounter	
		S7Ø.349A	External constriction, unspecified thigh, initial encounter	
		S7Ø.371A	Other superficial bite of right thigh, initial encounter	
		S7Ø.372A	Other superficial bite of left thigh, initial encounter	
		S7Ø.379A	Other superficial bite of unspecified thigh, init encntr	
		S7Ø.911A	Unspecified superficial injury of right hip, init encntr	
		S7Ø.912A	Unspecified superficial injury of left hip, init encntr	
		S7Ø.919A	Unsp superficial injury of unspecified hip, init encntr	
		S7Ø.921A	Unspecified superficial injury of right thigh, init encntr	
		S7Ø.922A	Unspecified superficial injury of left thigh, init encntr	
		S7Ø.929A	Unsp superficial injury of unspecified thigh, init encntr	
		S8Ø.241A	External constriction, right knee, initial encounter	
		S8Ø.242A	External constriction, left knee, initial encounter	
		S8Ø.249A	External constriction, unspecified knee, initial encounter	
		S8Ø.271A	Other superficial bite of right knee, initial encounter	
		S8Ø.272A	Other superficial bite of left knee, initial encounter	
		S8Ø.279A	Other superficial bite of unspecified knee, init encntr	
		S8Ø.841A	External constriction, right lower leg, initial encounter	
		S8Ø.842A	External constriction, left lower leg, initial encounter	
		S8Ø.849A	External constriction, unspecified lower leg, init encntr	
		S8Ø.871A	Other superficial bite, right lower leg, initial encounter	
		S8Ø.872A	Other superficial bite, left lower leg, initial encounter	
		S8Ø.879A	Other superficial bite, unspecified lower leg, init encntr	
		S8Ø.911A	Unspecified superficial injury of right knee, init encntr	
		S8Ø.912A	Unspecified superficial injury of left knee, init encntr	
		S8Ø.919A	Unsp superficial injury of unspecified knee, init encntr	
		S8Ø.921A	Unsp superficial injury of right lower leg, init encntr	
		S8Ø.922A	Unsp superficial injury of left lower leg, init encntr	
		S8Ø.929A	Unsp superficial injury of unsp lower leg, init encntr	
		S9Ø.541A	External constriction, right ankle, initial encounter	
		S9Ø.542A	External constriction, left ankle, initial encounter	
		S9Ø.549A	External constriction, unspecified ankle, initial encounter	
		S9Ø.571A	Other superficial bite of ankle, right ankle, init encntr	
		S9Ø.572A	Other superficial bite of ankle, left ankle, init encntr	
		S9Ø.579A	Other superficial bite of ankle, unsp ankle, init encntr	
		S9Ø.911A	Unspecified superficial injury of right ankle, init encntr	
		S9Ø.912A	Unspecified superficial injury of left ankle, init encntr	
		S9Ø.919A	Unsp superficial injury of unspecified ankle, init encntr	
916.9	OTH&UNSPEC SUP INJURY HIP THIGH LEG&ANK INF	**S7Ø.919A**	Unsp superficial injury of unspecified hip, init encntr	*or*
		S7Ø.929A	Unsp superficial injury of unspecified thigh, init encntr	*or*
		S8Ø.919A	Unsp superficial injury of unspecified knee, init encntr	*or*
		S8Ø.929A	Unsp superficial injury of unsp lower leg, init encntr	*or*
		S9Ø.919A	Unsp superficial injury of unspecified ankle, init encntr	*and*
		LØ8.89	Oth local infections of the skin and subcutaneous tissue	
917.Ø	ABRASION/FRICTION BURN FOOT&TOE W/O MENTION INF	**S9Ø.411A**	Abrasion, right great toe, initial encounter	
		S9Ø.412A	Abrasion, left great toe, initial encounter	
		S9Ø.413A	Abrasion, unspecified great toe, initial encounter	
		S9Ø.414A	Abrasion, right lesser toe(s), initial encounter	
		S9Ø.415A	Abrasion, left lesser toe(s), initial encounter	
		S9Ø.416A	Abrasion, unspecified lesser toe(s), initial encounter	
		S9Ø.811A	Abrasion, right foot, initial encounter	
		S9Ø.812A	Abrasion, left foot, initial encounter	
		S9Ø.819A	Abrasion, unspecified foot, initial encounter	
917.1	FOOT AND TOE ABRASION OR FRICTION BURN INFECTED	**S9Ø.413A**	Abrasion, unspecified great toe, initial encounter	*or*
		S9Ø.416A	Abrasion, unspecified lesser toe(s), initial encounter	*or*
		S9Ø.819A	Abrasion, unspecified foot, initial encounter	*and*
		LØ8.89	Oth local infections of the skin and subcutaneous tissu	
917.2	FOOT&TOE BLISTER WITHOUT MENTION OF INFECTION	**S9Ø.421A**	Blister (nonthermal), right great toe, initial encounter	
		S9Ø.422A	Blister (nonthermal), left great toe, initial encounter	
		S9Ø.423A	Blister (nonthermal), unspecified great toe, init encntr	
		S9Ø.424A	Blister (nonthermal), right lesser toe(s), initial encounter	
		S9Ø.425A	Blister (nonthermal), left lesser toe(s), initial encounter	
		S9Ø.426A	Blister (nonthermal), unspecified lesser toe(s), init encntr	
		S9Ø.821A	Blister (nonthermal), right foot, initial encounter	
		S9Ø.822A	Blister (nonthermal), left foot, initial encounter	
		S9Ø.829A	Blister (nonthermal), unspecified foot, initial encounter	
917.3	FOOT AND TOE, BLISTER, INFECTED	**S9Ø.423A**	Blister (nonthermal), unspecified great toe, init encntr	*or*
		S9Ø.426A	Blister (nonthermal), unspecified lesser toe(s), init encntr	*or*
		S9Ø.829A	Blister (nonthermal), unspecified foot, initial encounter	*and*
		LØ8.89	Oth local infections of the skin and subcutaneous tissue	

ICD-9-CM		ICD-10-CM		
917.4	FOOT&TOE INSECT BITE NONVENOMOUS W/O MENTION INF	S9Ø.461A	Insect bite (nonvenomous), right great toe, init encntr	
		S9Ø.462A	Insect bite (nonvenomous), left great toe, initial encounter	
		S9Ø.463A	Insect bite (nonvenomous), unsp great toe, init encntr	
		S9Ø.464A	Insect bite (nonvenomous), right lesser toe(s), init encntr	
		S9Ø.465A	Insect bite (nonvenomous), left lesser toe(s), init encntr	
		S9Ø.466A	Insect bite (nonvenomous), unsp lesser toe(s), init encntr	
		S9Ø.861A	Insect bite (nonvenomous), right foot, initial encounter	
		S9Ø.862A	Insect bite (nonvenomous), left foot, initial encounter	
		S9Ø.869A	Insect bite (nonvenomous), unspecified foot, init encntr	
917.5	FOOT AND TOE INSECT BITE NONVENOMOUS INFECTED	S9Ø.463A	Insect bite (nonvenomous), unsp great toe, init encntr	*or*
		S9Ø.466A	Insect bite (nonvenomous), unsp lesser toe(s), init encntr	*or*
		S9Ø.869A	Insect bite (nonvenomous), unspecified foot, init encntr	*and*
		LØ8.89	Oth local infections of the skin and subcutaneous tissue	
917.6	FOOT&TOE SUP FB W/O MAJ OPN WND&W/O MENTION INF	S9Ø.451A	Superficial foreign body, right great toe, initial encounter	
		S9Ø.452A	Superficial foreign body, left great toe, initial encounter	
		S9Ø.453A	Superficial foreign body, unspecified great toe, init encntr	
		S9Ø.454A	Superficial foreign body, right lesser toe(s), init encntr	
		S9Ø.455A	Superficial foreign body, left lesser toe(s), init encntr	
		S9Ø.456A	Superficial foreign body, unsp lesser toe(s), init encntr	
		S9Ø.851A	Superficial foreign body, right foot, initial encounter	
		S9Ø.852A	Superficial foreign body, left foot, initial encounter	
		S9Ø.859A	Superficial foreign body, unspecified foot, init encntr	
917.7	FOOT&TOE SUP FB WITHOUT MAJOR OPEN WOUND INF	S9Ø.453A	Superficial foreign body, unspecified great toe, init encntr	*or*
		S9Ø.456A	Superficial foreign body, unsp lesser toe(s), init encntr	*or*
		S9Ø.859A	Superficial foreign body, unspecified foot, init encntr	*and*
		LØ8.89	Oth local infections of the skin and subcutaneous tissue	
917.8	OTH&UNSPEC SUP INJURY FOOT&TOES W/O MENTION INF	S9Ø.441A	External constriction, right great toe, initial encounter	
		S9Ø.442A	External constriction, left great toe, initial encounter	
		S9Ø.443A	External constriction, unspecified great toe, init encntr	
		S9Ø.444A	External constriction, right lesser toe(s), init encntr	
		S9Ø.445A	External constriction, left lesser toe(s), initial encounter	
		S9Ø.446A	External constriction, unsp lesser toe(s), init encntr	
		S9Ø.471A	Other superficial bite of right great toe, initial encounter	
		S9Ø.472A	Other superficial bite of left great toe, initial encounter	
		S9Ø.473A	Other superficial bite of unspecified great toe, init encntr	
		S9Ø.474A	Other superficial bite of right lesser toe(s), init encntr	
		S9Ø.475A	Other superficial bite of left lesser toe(s), init encntr	
		S9Ø.476A	Other superficial bite of unsp lesser toe(s), init encntr	
		S9Ø.841A	External constriction, right foot, initial encounter	
		S9Ø.842A	External constriction, left foot, initial encounter	
		S9Ø.849A	External constriction, unspecified foot, initial encounter	
		S9Ø.871A	Other superficial bite of right foot, initial encounter	
		S9Ø.872A	Other superficial bite of left foot, initial encounter	
		S9Ø.879A	Other superficial bite of unspecified foot, init encntr	
		S9Ø.921A	Unspecified superficial injury of right foot, init encntr	
		S9Ø.922A	Unspecified superficial injury of left foot, init encntr	
		S9Ø.929A	Unsp superficial injury of unspecified foot, init encntr	
		S9Ø.931A	Unsp superficial injury of right great toe, init encntr	
		S9Ø.932A	Unsp superficial injury of left great toe, init encntr	
		S9Ø.933A	Unsp superficial injury of unsp great toe, init encntr	
		S9Ø.934A	Unsp superficial injury of right lesser toe(s), init encntr	
		S9Ø.935A	Unsp superficial injury of left lesser toe(s), init encntr	
		S9Ø.936A	Unsp superficial injury of unsp lesser toe(s), init encntr	
917.9	OTH&UNSPEC SUPERFICIAL INJURY FOOT&TOES INFECTED	S9Ø.929A	Unsp superficial injury of unspecified foot, init encntr	*or*
		S9Ø.933A	Unsp superficial injury of unsp great toe, init encntr	*or*
		S9Ø.936A	Unsp superficial injury of unsp lesser toe(s), init encntr	*and*
		LØ8.89	Oth local infections of the skin and subcutaneous tissue	
918.Ø	SUPERFICIAL INJURY OF EYELIDS&PERIOCULAR AREA	SØØ.2Ø1A	Unsp superfic inj right eyelid and periocular area, init	
		SØØ.2Ø2A	Unsp superfic injury of left eyelid and periocular area, init	
		SØØ.2Ø9A	Unsp superfic injury of unsp eyelid and periocular area, init	
		SØØ.211A	Abrasion of right eyelid and periocular area, init encntr	
		SØØ.212A	Abrasion of left eyelid and periocular area, init encntr	
		SØØ.219A	Abrasion of unsp eyelid and periocular area, init encntr	
		SØØ.221A	Blister of right eyelid and periocular area, init	
		SØØ.222A	Blister of left eyelid and periocular area, init	
		SØØ.229A	Blister of unsp eyelid and periocular area, init	
		SØØ.241A	External constrict of right eyelid and periocular area, init	
		SØØ.242A	External constrict of left eyelid and periocular area, init	
		SØØ.249A	External constrict of unsp eyelid and periocular area, init	
		SØØ.251A	Superficial fb of right eyelid and periocular area, init	
		SØØ.252A	Superficial fb of left eyelid and periocular area, Init	
		SØØ.259A	Superficial fb of unsp eyelid and periocular area, init	
		SØØ.261A	Insect bite of right eyelid and periocular area, init	
		SØØ.262A	Insect bite of left eyelid and periocular area, init	
		SØØ.269A	Insect bite of unsp eyelid and periocular area, init	
		SØØ.271A	Oth superfic bite of right eyelid and periocular area, init	
		SØØ.272A	Oth superfic bite of left eyelid and periocular area, init	
		SØØ.279A	Oth superfic bite of unsp eyelid and periocular area, init	

ICD-9-CM		ICD-10-CM		
918.1	SUPERFICIAL INJURY OF CORNEA	**SØ5.ØØXA**	Inj conjunctiva and corneal abrasion w/o fb, unsp eye, init	
		SØ5.Ø1XA	Inj conjunctiva and corneal abrasion w/o fb, right eye, init	
		SØ5.Ø2XA	Inj conjunctiva and corneal abrasion w/o fb, left eye, init	
918.2	SUPERFICIAL INJURY OF CONJUNCTIVA	**SØ5.ØØXA**	Inj conjunctiva and corneal abrasion w/o fb, unsp eye, init	
		SØ5.Ø1XA	Inj conjunctiva and corneal abrasion w/o fb, right eye, init	
		SØ5.Ø2XA	Inj conjunctiva and corneal abrasion w/o fb, left eye, init	
918.9	OTHER&UNSPECIFIED SUPERFICIAL INJURIES OF EYE	**SØ5.9ØXA**	Unspecified injury of unspecified eye and orbit, init encntr	
919.Ø	ABRASION/FRICION BURN OTH MX&UNS SITE W/O INF	**TØ7**	Unspecified multiple injuries	
919.1	OTH MX&UNSPEC SITES ABRASION/FRICTION BURN INF	**TØ7**	Unspecified multiple injuries	*and*
		LØ8.89	Oth local infections of the skin and subcutaneous tissue	
919.2	OTH MX&UNSPEC SITES BLISTER WITHOUT MENTION INF	**TØ7**	Unspecified multiple injuries	
919.3	OTHER MULTIPLE&UNSPEC SITES BLISTER INFECTED	**TØ7**	Unspecified multiple injuries	*and*
		LØ8.89	Oth local infections of the skin and subcutaneous tissue	
919.4	OTH MX&UNS SITE INSECT BITE NONVENOMOUS W/O INF	**TØ7**	Unspecified multiple injuries	
919.5	OTH MX&UNSPEC SITES INSECT BITE NONVENOMOUS INF	**TØ7**	Unspecified multiple injuries	*and*
		LØ8.89	Oth local infections of the skin and subcutaneous tissue	
919.6	OTH MULT&UNS SITE SUP FB W/O MAJ OPN WND&W/O INF	**TØ7**	Unspecified multiple injuries	
919.7	OTH MX&UNSPEC SITES SUP FB W/O MAJ OPN WOUND INF	**TØ7**	Unspecified multiple injuries	*and*
		LØ8.89	Oth local infections of the skin and subcutaneous tissue	
919.8	OTH&UNS SUP INJR OTH MX&UNS SITE W/O MENTION INF	**TØ7**	Unspecified multiple injuries	
919.9	OTH&UNSPEC SUP INJURY OTH MX&UNSPEC SITES INF	**TØ7**	Unspecified multiple injuries	*and*
		LØ8.89	Oth local infections of the skin and subcutaneous tissue	
92Ø	CONTUSION OF FACE SCALP AND NECK EXCEPT EYE	**SØØ.Ø3XA**	Contusion of scalp, initial encounter	
		SØØ.33XA	Contusion of nose, initial encounter	
		SØØ.431A	Contusion of right ear, initial encounter	
		SØØ.432A	Contusion of left ear, initial encounter	
		SØØ.439A	Contusion of unspecified ear, initial encounter	
		SØØ.531A	Contusion of lip, initial encounter	
		SØØ.532A	Contusion of oral cavity, initial encounter	
		SØØ.83XA	Contusion of other part of head, initial encounter	
		SØØ.93XA	Contusion of unspecified part of head, initial encounter	
		S1Ø.ØXXA	Contusion of throat, initial encounter	
		S1Ø.83XA	Contusion of other specified part of neck, initial encounter	
		S1Ø.93XA	Contusion of unspecified part of neck, initial encounter	
921.Ø	BLACK EYE, NOT OTHERWISE SPECIFIED	**SØØ.1ØXA**	Contusion of unsp eyelid and periocular area, init encntr	
		SØØ.11XA	Contusion of right eyelid and periocular area, init encntr	
		SØØ.12XA	Contusion of left eyelid and periocular area, init encntr	
921.1	CONTUSION OF EYELIDS AND PERIOCULAR AREA	**SØØ.1ØXA**	Contusion of unsp eyelid and periocular area, init encntr	
		SØØ.11XA	Contusion of right eyelid and periocular area, init encntr	
		SØØ.12XA	Contusion of left eyelid and periocular area, init encntr	
921.2	CONTUSION OF ORBITAL TISSUES	**SØ5.1ØXA**	Contusion of eyeball and orbital tissues, unsp eye, init	
		SØ5.11XA	Contusion of eyeball and orbital tissues, right eye, init	
		SØ5.12XA	Contusion of eyeball and orbital tissues, left eye, init	
921.3	CONTUSION OF EYEBALL	**SØ5.1ØXA**	Contusion of eyeball and orbital tissues, unsp eye, init	
		SØ5.11XA	Contusion of eyeball and orbital tissues, right eye, init	
		SØ5.12XA	Contusion of eyeball and orbital tissues, left eye, init	
921.9	UNSPECIFIED CONTUSION OF EYE	**SØ5.9ØXA**	Unspecified injury of unspecified eye and orbit, init encntr	
922.Ø	CONTUSION OF BREAST	**S2Ø.ØØXA**	Contusion of breast, unspecified breast, initial encounter	
		S2Ø.Ø1XA	Contusion of right breast, initial encounter	
		S2Ø.Ø2XA	Contusion of left breast, initial encounter	
922.1	CONTUSION OF CHEST WALL	**S2Ø.211A**	Contusion of right front wall of thorax, initial encounter	
		S2Ø.212A	Contusion of left front wall of thorax, initial encounter	
		S2Ø.219A	Contusion of unspecified front wall of thorax, init encntr	
922.2	CONTUSION OF ABDOMINAL WALL	**S3Ø.1XXA**	Contusion of abdominal wall, initial encounter	
922.31	CONTUSION OF BACK	**S3Ø.ØXXA**	Contusion of lower back and pelvis, initial encounter	
922.32	CONTUSION OF BUTTOCK	**S3Ø.ØXXA**	Contusion of lower back and pelvis, initial encounter	
		S3Ø.3XXA	Contusion of anus, initial encounter	
922.33	CONTUSION OF INTERSCAPULAR REGION	**S2Ø.221A**	Contusion of right back wall of thorax, initial encounter	
		S2Ø.222A	Contusion of left back wall of thorax, initial encounter	
		S2Ø.229A	Contusion of unspecified back wall of thorax, init encntr	
922.4	CONTUSION OF GENITAL ORGANS	**S3Ø.2Ø1A**	Contusion of unsp external genital organ, male, init encntr	
		S3Ø.2Ø2A	Contusion of unsp external genital organ, female, init	
		S3Ø.21XA	Contusion of penis, initial encounter	
		S3Ø.22XA	Contusion of scrotum and testes, initial encounter	
		S3Ø.23XA	Contusion of vagina and vulva, initial encounter	
922.8	CONTUSION OF MULTIPLE SITES OF TRUNK	**T14.8**	Other injury of unspecified body region	
922.9	CONTUSION OF UNSPECIFIED PART OF TRUNK	**S2Ø.2ØXA**	Contusion of thorax, unspecified, initial encounter	
923.ØØ	CONTUSION OF SHOULDER REGION	**S4Ø.Ø11A**	Contusion of right shoulder, initial encounter	
		S4Ø.Ø12A	Contusion of left shoulder, initial encounter	
		S4Ø.Ø19A	Contusion of unspecified shoulder, initial encounter	
923.Ø1	CONTUSION OF SCAPULAR REGION	**S4Ø.Ø11A**	Contusion of right shoulder, initial encounter	
		S4Ø.Ø12A	Contusion of left shoulder, initial encounter	
		S4Ø.Ø19A	Contusion of unspecified shoulder, initial encounter	

[Brackets] indicate valid character values for each code. Character value meanings provided for each code grouping.

ICD-9-CM		ICD-10-CM	
923.02	CONTUSION OF AXILLARY REGION	**S40.011A**	Contusion of right shoulder, initial encounter
		S40.012A	Contusion of left shoulder, initial encounter
		S40.019A	Contusion of unspecified shoulder, initial encounter
923.03	CONTUSION OF UPPER ARM	**S40.021A**	Contusion of right upper arm, initial encounter
		S40.022A	Contusion of left upper arm, initial encounter
		S40.029A	Contusion of unspecified upper arm, initial encounter
923.09	CONTUSION MULTIPLE SITES SHOULDER&UPPER ARM	**S40.019A**	Contusion of unspecified shoulder, initial encounter
923.10	CONTUSION OF FOREARM	**S50.10XA**	Contusion of unspecified forearm, initial encounter
		S50.11XA	Contusion of right forearm, initial encounter
		S50.12XA	Contusion of left forearm, initial encounter
923.11	CONTUSION OF ELBOW	**S50.00XA**	Contusion of unspecified elbow, initial encounter
		S50.01XA	Contusion of right elbow, initial encounter
		S50.02XA	Contusion of left elbow, initial encounter
923.20	CONTUSION OF HAND	**S60.221A**	Contusion of right hand, initial encounter
		S60.222A	Contusion of left hand, initial encounter
		S60.229A	Contusion of unspecified hand, initial encounter
923.21	CONTUSION OF WRIST	**S60.211A**	Contusion of right wrist, initial encounter
		S60.212A	Contusion of left wrist, initial encounter
		S60.219A	Contusion of unspecified wrist, initial encounter
923.3	CONTUSION OF FINGER	**S60.00XA**	Contusion of unsp finger without damage to nail, init encntr
		S60.011A	Contusion of right thumb without damage to nail, init encntr
		S60.012A	Contusion of left thumb without damage to nail, init encntr
		S60.019A	Contusion of unsp thumb without damage to nail, init encntr
		S60.021A	Contusion of right index finger w/o damage to nail, init
		S60.022A	Contusion of left index finger w/o damage to nail, init
		S60.029A	Contusion of unsp index finger w/o damage to nail, init
		S60.031A	Contusion of right middle finger w/o damage to nail, init
		S60.032A	Contusion of left middle finger w/o damage to nail, init
		S60.039A	Contusion of unsp middle finger w/o damage to nail, init
		S60.041A	Contusion of right ring finger w/o damage to nail, init
		S60.042A	Contusion of left ring finger w/o damage to nail, init
		S60.049A	Contusion of unsp ring finger w/o damage to nail, init
		S60.051A	Contusion of right little finger w/o damage to nail, init
		S60.052A	Contusion of left little finger w/o damage to nail, init
		S60.059A	Contusion of unsp little finger w/o damage to nail, init
		S60.10XA	Contusion of unsp finger with damage to nail, init encntr
		S60.111A	Contusion of right thumb with damage to nail, init encntr
		S60.112A	Contusion of left thumb with damage to nail, init encntr
		S60.119A	Contusion of unsp thumb with damage to nail, init encntr
		S60.121A	Contusion of right index finger w damage to nail, init
		S60.122A	Contusion of left index finger w damage to nail, init encntr
		S60.129A	Contusion of unsp index finger w damage to nail, init encntr
		S60.131A	Contusion of right middle finger w damage to nail, init
		S60.132A	Contusion of left middle finger w damage to nail, init
		S60.139A	Contusion of unsp middle finger w damage to nail, init
		S60.141A	Contusion of right ring finger w damage to nail, init encntr
		S60.142A	Contusion of left ring finger w damage to nail, init encntr
		S60.149A	Contusion of unsp ring finger w damage to nail, init encntr
		S60.151A	Contusion of right little finger w damage to nail, init
		S60.152A	Contusion of left little finger w damage to nail, init
		S60.159A	Contusion of unsp little finger w damage to nail, init
923.8	CONTUSION OF MULTIPLE SITES OF UPPER LIMB	**S40.019A**	Contusion of unspecified shoulder, initial encounter
923.9	CONTUSION OF UNSPECIFIED PART OF UPPER LIMB	**S40.019A**	Contusion of unspecified shoulder, initial encounter
924.00	CONTUSION OF THIGH	**S70.10XA**	Contusion of unspecified thigh, initial encounter
		S70.11XA	Contusion of right thigh, initial encounter
		S70.12XA	Contusion of left thigh, initial encounter
924.01	CONTUSION OF HIP	**S70.00XA**	Contusion of unspecified hip, initial encounter
		S70.01XA	Contusion of right hip, initial encounter
		S70.02XA	Contusion of left hip, initial encounter
924.10	CONTUSION OF LOWER LEG	**S80.10XA**	Contusion of unspecified lower leg, initial encounter
		S80.11XA	Contusion of right lower leg, initial encounter
		S80.12XA	Contusion of left lower leg, initial encounter
924.11	CONTUSION OF KNEE	**S80.00XA**	Contusion of unspecified knee, initial encounter
		S80.01XA	Contusion of right knee, initial encounter
		S80.02XA	Contusion of left knee, initial encounter
924.20	CONTUSION OF FOOT	**S90.30XA**	Contusion of unspecified foot, initial encounter
		S90.31XA	Contusion of right foot, initial encounter
		S90.32XA	Contusion of left foot, initial encounter
924.21	CONTUSION OF ANKLE	**S90.00XA**	Contusion of unspecified ankle, initial encounter
		S90.01XA	Contusion of right ankle, initial encounter
		S90.02XA	Contusion of left ankle, initial encounter

ICD-9-CM		ICD-10-CM	
924.3	CONTUSION OF TOE	**S9Ø.111A**	Contusion of right great toe w/o damage to nail, init encntr
		S9Ø.112A	Contusion of left great toe w/o damage to nail, init encntr
		S9Ø.119A	Contusion of unsp great toe w/o damage to nail, init encntr
		S9Ø.121A	Contusion of right lesser toe(s) w/o damage to nail, init
		S9Ø.122A	Contusion of left lesser toe(s) w/o damage to nail, init
		S9Ø.129A	Contusion of unsp lesser toe(s) w/o damage to nail, init
		S9Ø.211A	Contusion of right great toe w damage to nail, init encntr
		S9Ø.212A	Contusion of left great toe with damage to nail, init encntr
		S9Ø.219A	Contusion of unsp great toe with damage to nail, init encntr
		S9Ø.221A	Contusion of right lesser toe(s) w damage to nail, init
		S9Ø.222A	Contusion of left lesser toe(s) w damage to nail, init
		S9Ø.229A	Contusion of unsp lesser toe(s) w damage to nail, init
924.4	CONTUSION OF MULTIPLE SITES OF LOWER LIMB	**S7Ø.1ØXA**	Contusion of unspecified thigh, initial encounter
924.5	CONTUSION OF UNSPECIFIED PART OF LOWER LIMB	**S7Ø.1ØXA**	Contusion of unspecified thigh, initial encounter
924.8	CONTUSION OF MULTIPLE SITES NEC	**T14.8**	Other injury of unspecified body region
924.9	CONTUSION OF UNSPECIFIED SITE	**T14.9Ø**	Injury, unspecified
925.1	CRUSHING INJURY OF FACE AND SCALP	**SØ7.ØXXA**	Crushing injury of face, initial encounter
		SØ7.1XXA	Crushing injury of skull, initial encounter
		SØ7.8XXA	Crushing injury of other parts of head, initial encounter
		SØ7.9XXA	Crushing injury of head, part unspecified, initial encounter
925.2	CRUSHING INJURY OF NECK	**S17.ØXXA**	Crushing injury of larynx and trachea, initial encounter
		S17.8XXA	Crushing injury of oth parts of neck, init encntr
		S17.9XXA	Crushing injury of neck, part unspecified, initial encounter
926.Ø	CRUSHING INJURY OF EXTERNAL GENITALIA	**S38.ØØ1A**	Crushing injury of unsp external genital organs, male, init
		S38.ØØ2A	Crushing inj unsp external genital organs, female, init
		S38.Ø1XA	Crushing injury of penis, initial encounter
		S38.Ø2XA	Crushing injury of scrotum and testis, initial encounter
		S38.Ø3XA	Crushing injury of vulva, initial encounter
926.11	CRUSHING INJURY OF BACK	**S38.1XXA**	Crushing injury of abdomen, lower back, and pelvis, init
926.12	CRUSHING INJURY OF BUTTOCK	**S38.1XXA**	Crushing injury of abdomen, lower back, and pelvis, init
926.19	CRUSHING INJURY OTHER SPECIFIED SITES TRUNK OTH	**S28.ØXXA**	Crushed chest, initial encounter
926.8	CRUSHING INJURY OF MULTIPLE SITES OF TRUNK	**S28.ØXXA**	Crushed chest, initial encounter
926.9	CRUSHING INJURY OF UNSPECIFIED SITE OF TRUNK	**S28.ØXXA**	Crushed chest, initial encounter
927.ØØ	CRUSHING INJURY OF SHOULDER REGION	**S47.1XXA**	Crushing injury of right shoulder and upper arm, init encntr
		S47.2XXA	Crushing injury of left shoulder and upper arm, init encntr
		S47.9XXA	Crushing injury of shoulder and upper arm, unsp arm, init
927.Ø1	CRUSHING INJURY OF SCAPULAR REGION	**S47.1XXA**	Crushing injury of right shoulder and upper arm, init encntr
		S47.2XXA	Crushing injury of left shoulder and upper arm, init encntr
		S47.9XXA	Crushing injury of shoulder and upper arm, unsp arm, init
927.Ø2	CRUSHING INJURY OF AXILLARY REGION	**S47.1XXA**	Crushing injury of right shoulder and upper arm, init encntr
		S47.2XXA	Crushing injury of left shoulder and upper arm, init encntr
		S47.9XXA	Crushing injury of shoulder and upper arm, unsp arm, init
927.Ø3	CRUSHING INJURY OF UPPER ARM	**S47.1XXA**	Crushing injury of right shoulder and upper arm, init encntr
		S47.2XXA	Crushing injury of left shoulder and upper arm, init encntr
		S47.9XXA	Crushing injury of shoulder and upper arm, unsp arm, init
927.Ø9	CRUSHING INJURY OF MULTIPLE SITES OF UPPER ARM	**S47.9XXA**	Crushing injury of shoulder and upper arm, unsp arm, init
927.1Ø	CRUSHING INJURY OF FOREARM	**S57.8ØXA**	Crushing injury of unspecified forearm, initial encounter
		S57.81XA	Crushing injury of right forearm, initial encounter
		S57.82XA	Crushing injury of left forearm, initial encounter
927.11	CRUSHING INJURY OF ELBOW	**S57.ØØXA**	Crushing injury of unspecified elbow, initial encounter
		S57.Ø1XA	Crushing injury of right elbow, initial encounter
		S57.Ø2XA	Crushing injury of left elbow, initial encounter
927.2Ø	CRUSHING INJURY OF HAND	**S67.2ØXA**	Crushing injury of unspecified hand, initial encounter
		S67.21XA	Crushing injury of right hand, initial encounter
		S67.22XA	Crushing injury of left hand, initial encounter
927.21	CRUSHING INJURY OF WRIST	**S67.3ØXA**	Crushing injury of unspecified wrist, initial encounter
		S67.31XA	Crushing injury of right wrist, initial encounter
		S67.32XA	Crushing injury of left wrist, initial encounter
		S67.4ØXA	Crushing injury of unspecified wrist and hand, init encntr
		S67.41XA	Crushing injury of right wrist and hand, initial encounter
		S67.42XA	Crushing injury of left wrist and hand, initial encounter
		S67.9ØXA	Crush inj unsp part(s) of unsp wrist, hand and fingers, init
		S67.91XA	Crushing inj unsp part(s) of r wrist, hand and fingers, init
		S67.92XA	Crushing inj unsp part(s) of l wrist, hand and fingers, init
927.3	CRUSHING INJURY OF FINGER	**S67.ØØXA**	Crushing injury of unspecified thumb, initial encounter
		S67.Ø1XA	Crushing injury of right thumb, initial encounter
		S67.Ø2XA	Crushing injury of left thumb, initial encounter
		S67.1ØXA	Crushing injury of unspecified finger(s), initial encounter
		S67.19ØA	Crushing injury of right index finger, initial encounter
		S67.191A	Crushing injury of left index finger, initial encounter
		S67.192A	Crushing injury of right middle finger, initial encounter
		S67.193A	Crushing injury of left middle finger, initial encounter
		S67.194A	Crushing injury of right ring finger, initial encounter
		S67.195A	Crushing injury of left ring finger, initial encounter
		S67.196A	Crushing injury of right little finger, initial encounter
		S67.197A	Crushing injury of left little finger, initial encounter
		S67.198A	Crushing injury of other finger, initial encounter

[Brackets] indicate valid character values for each code. Character value meanings provided for each code grouping.

ICD-9-CM		ICD-10-CM	
927.8	CRUSHING INJURY OF MULTIPLE SITES OF UPPER LIMB	S47.1XXA	Crushing injury of right shoulder and upper arm, init encntr
		S47.2XXA	Crushing injury of left shoulder and upper arm, init encntr
		S47.9XXA	Crushing injury of shoulder and upper arm, unsp arm, init
927.9	CRUSHING INJURY UNSPECIFIED SITE UPPER LIMB	S47.1XXA	Crushing injury of right shoulder and upper arm, init encntr
		S47.2XXA	Crushing injury of left shoulder and upper arm, init encntr
		S47.9XXA	Crushing injury of shoulder and upper arm, unsp arm, init
928.ØØ	CRUSHING INJURY OF THIGH	S77.1ØXA	Crushing injury of unspecified thigh, initial encounter
		S77.11XA	Crushing injury of right thigh, initial encounter
		S77.12XA	Crushing injury of left thigh, initial encounter
928.Ø1	CRUSHING INJURY OF HIP	S77.ØØXA	Crushing injury of unspecified hip, initial encounter
		S77.Ø1XA	Crushing injury of right hip, initial encounter
		S77.Ø2XA	Crushing injury of left hip, initial encounter
928.1Ø	CRUSHING INJURY OF LOWER LEG	S87.8ØXA	Crushing injury of unspecified lower leg, initial encounter
		S87.81XA	Crushing injury of right lower leg, initial encounter
		S87.82XA	Crushing injury of left lower leg, initial encounter
928.11	CRUSHING INJURY OF KNEE	S87.ØØXA	Crushing injury of unspecified knee, initial encounter
		S87.Ø1XA	Crushing injury of right knee, initial encounter
		S87.Ø2XA	Crushing injury of left knee, initial encounter
928.2Ø	CRUSHING INJURY OF FOOT	S97.8ØXA	Crushing injury of unspecified foot, initial encounter
		S97.81XA	Crushing injury of right foot, initial encounter
		S97.82XA	Crushing injury of left foot, initial encounter
928.21	CRUSHING INJURY OF ANKLE	S97.ØØXA	Crushing injury of unspecified ankle, initial encounter
		S97.Ø1XA	Crushing injury of right ankle, initial encounter
		S97.Ø2XA	Crushing injury of left ankle, initial encounter
928.3	CRUSHING INJURY OF TOE	S97.1Ø1A	Crushing injury of unspecified right toe(s), init encntr
		S97.1Ø2A	Crushing injury of unspecified left toe(s), init encntr
		S97.1Ø9A	Crushing injury of unspecified toe(s), initial encounter
		S97.111A	Crushing injury of right great toe, initial encounter
		S97.112A	Crushing injury of left great toe, initial encounter
		S97.119A	Crushing injury of unspecified great toe, initial encounter
		S97.121A	Crushing injury of right lesser toe(s), initial encounter
		S97.122A	Crushing injury of left lesser toe(s), initial encounter
		S97.129A	Crushing injury of unspecified lesser toe(s), init encntr
928.8	CRUSHING INJURY OF MULTIPLE SITES OF LOWER LIMB	S77.2ØXA	Crushing injury of unspecified hip with thigh, init encntr
		S77.21XA	Crushing injury of right hip with thigh, initial encounter
		S77.22XA	Crushing injury of left hip with thigh, initial encounter
928.9	CRUSHING INJURY UNSPECIFIED SITE LOWER LIMB	S77.2ØXA	Crushing injury of unspecified hip with thigh, init encntr
929.Ø	CRUSHING INJURY OF MULTIPLE SITES NEC	S77.2ØXA	Crushing injury of unspecified hip with thigh, init encntr
929.9	CRUSHING INJURY OF UNSPECIFIED SITE	S77.2ØXA	Crushing injury of unspecified hip with thigh, init encntr
93Ø.Ø	FOREIGN BODY IN CORNEA	T15.ØØXA	Foreign body in cornea, unspecified eye, initial encounter
		T15.Ø1XA	Foreign body in cornea, right eye, initial encounter
		T15.Ø2XA	Foreign body in cornea, left eye, initial encounter
93Ø.1	FOREIGN BODY IN CONJUNCTIVAL SAC	T15.1ØXA	Foreign body in conjunctival sac, unsp eye, init encntr
		T15.11XA	Foreign body in conjunctival sac, right eye, init encntr
		T15.12XA	Foreign body in conjunctival sac, left eye, init encntr
93Ø.2	FOREIGN BODY IN LACRIMAL PUNCTUM	T15.8ØXA	Fb in oth and multiple parts of external eye, unsp eye, init
		T15.81XA	Fb in oth and multiple parts of external eye, r eye, init
		T15.82XA	Fb in oth and multiple parts of external eye, left eye, init
93Ø.8	FOREIGN BODY OTHER&COMBINED SITES EXTERNAL EYE	T15.8ØXA	Fb in oth and multiple parts of external eye, unsp eye, init
		T15.81XA	Fb in oth and multiple parts of external eye, r eye, init
		T15.82XA	Fb in oth and multiple parts of external eye, left eye, init
93Ø.9	FOREIGN BODY IN UNSPECIFIED SITE ON EXTERNAL EYE	T15.9ØXA	Foreign body on external eye, part unsp, unsp eye, init
		T15.91XA	Foreign body on external eye, part unsp, right eye, init
		T15.92XA	Foreign body on external eye, part unsp, left eye, init
931	FOREIGN BODY IN EAR	T16.1XXA	Foreign body in right ear, initial encounter
		T16.2XXA	Foreign body in left ear, initial encounter
		T16.9XXA	Foreign body in ear, unspecified ear, initial encounter
932	FOREIGN BODY IN NOSE	T17.ØXXA	Foreign body in nasal sinus, initial encounter
		T17.1XXA	Foreign body in nostril, initial encounter
933.Ø	FOREIGN BODY IN PHARYNX	T17.2ØØA	Unsp foreign body in pharynx causing asphyxiation, init
		T17.2Ø8A	Unsp foreign body in pharynx causing oth injury, init encntr
		T17.21ØA	Gastric contents in pharynx causing asphyxiation, init
		T17.218A	Gastric contents in pharynx causing oth injury, init encntr
		T17.22ØA	Food in pharynx causing asphyxiation, initial encounter
		T17.228A	Food in pharynx causing other injury, initial encounter
		T17.29ØA	Oth foreign object in pharynx causing asphyxiation, init
		T17.298A	Oth foreign object in pharynx causing oth injury, init
933.1	FOREIGN BODY IN LARYNX	T17.3ØØA	Unsp foreign body in larynx causing asphyxiation, init
		T17.3Ø8A	Unsp foreign body in larynx causing oth injury, init encntr
		T17.31ØA	Gastric contents in larynx causing asphyxiation, init encntr
		T17.318A	Gastric contents in larynx causing other injury, init encntr
		T17.32ØA	Food in larynx causing asphyxiation, initial encounter
		T17.328A	Food in larynx causing other injury, initial encounter
		T17.39ØA	Oth foreign object in larynx causing asphyxiation, init
		T17.398A	Oth foreign object in larynx causing oth injury, init encntr

ICD-9-CM		ICD-10-CM	
934.Ø	FOREIGN BODY IN TRACHEA	**T17.4ØØA**	Unsp foreign body in trachea causing asphyxiation, init
		T17.4Ø8A	Unsp foreign body in trachea causing oth injury, init encntr
		T17.41ØA	Gastric contents in trachea causing asphyxiation, init
		T17.418A	Gastric contents in trachea causing oth injury, init encntr
		T17.42ØA	Food in trachea causing asphyxiation, initial encounter
		T17.428A	Food in trachea causing other injury, initial encounter
		T17.49ØA	Oth foreign object in trachea causing asphyxiation, init
		T17.498A	Oth foreign object in trachea causing oth injury, init
934.1	FOREIGN BODY IN MAIN BRONCHUS	**T17.5ØØA**	Unsp foreign body in bronchus causing asphyxiation, init
		T17.5Ø8A	Unsp foreign body in bronchus causing oth injury, init
		T17.51ØA	Gastric contents in bronchus causing asphyxiation, init
		T17.518A	Gastric contents in bronchus causing oth injury, init encntr
		T17.52ØA	Food in bronchus causing asphyxiation, initial encounter
		T17.528A	Food in bronchus causing other injury, initial encounter
		T17.59ØA	Oth foreign object in bronchus causing asphyxiation, init
		T17.598A	Oth foreign object in bronchus causing oth injury, init
934.8	FB OTH SPEC PARTS TRACHEA BRONCHUS&LUNG	**T17.8ØØA**	Unsp foreign body in oth prt resp tract causing asphyx, init
		T17.8Ø8A	Unsp fb in oth prt resp tract causing oth injury, init
		T17.81ØA	Gastric contents in oth prt resp tract causing asphyx, init
		T17.818A	Gastr contents in oth prt resp tract cause oth injury, init
		T17.82ØA	Food in oth prt respiratory tract causing asphyxiation, init
		T17.828A	Food in oth prt respiratory tract causing oth injury, init
		T17.89ØA	Oth foreign object in oth prt resp tract cause asphyx, init
		T17.898A	Oth forn object in oth prt resp tract cause oth injury, init
934.9	FOREIGN BODY IN RESPIRATORY TREE UNSPECIFIED	**T17.9ØØA**	Unsp fb in resp tract, part unsp causing asphyx, init
		T17.9Ø8A	Unsp fb in resp tract, part unsp causing oth injury, init
		T17.91ØA	Gastric contents in resp tract, part unsp cause asphyx, init
		T17.918A	Gastr contents in resp tract, part unsp cause oth inj, init
		T17.92ØA	Food in resp tract, part unsp causing asphyxiation, init
		T17.928A	Food in resp tract, part unsp causing oth injury, init
		T17.99ØA	Oth forn obj in resp tract, part unsp in cause asphyx, init
		T17.998A	Oth forn object in resp tract, part unsp cause oth inj, init
935.Ø	FOREIGN BODY IN MOUTH	**T18.ØXXA**	Foreign body in mouth, initial encounter
935.1	FOREIGN BODY IN ESOPHAGUS	**T18.1ØØA**	Unsp fb in esophagus causing compression of trachea, init
		T18.1Ø8A	Unsp foreign body in esophagus causing oth injury, init
		T18.11ØA	Gastric contents in esoph causing comprsn of trachea, init
		T18.118A	Gastric contents in esophagus causing oth injury, init
		T18.12ØA	Food in esophagus causing compression of trachea, init
		T18.128A	Food in esophagus causing other injury, initial encounter
		T18.19ØA	Oth foreign object in esoph causing comprsn of trachea, init
		T18.198A	Oth foreign object in esophagus causing oth injury, init
935.2	FOREIGN BODY IN STOMACH	**T18.2XXA**	Foreign body in stomach, initial encounter
936	FOREIGN BODY IN INTESTINE AND COLON	**T18.3XXA**	Foreign body in small intestine, initial encounter
		T18.4XXA	Foreign body in colon, initial encounter
937	FOREIGN BODY IN ANUS AND RECTUM	**T18.5XXA**	Foreign body in anus and rectum, initial encounter
938	FOREIGN BODY IN DIGESTIVE SYSTEM UNSPECIFIED	**T18.8XXA**	Foreign body in other parts of alimentary tract, init encntr
		T18.9XXA	Foreign body of alimentary tract, part unsp, init encntr
939.Ø	FOREIGN BODY IN BLADDER AND URETHRA	**T19.ØXXA**	Foreign body in urethra, initial encounter
		T19.1XXA	Foreign body in bladder, initial encounter
939.1	FOREIGN BODY IN UTERUS, ANY PART	**T19.3XXA**	Foreign body in uterus, initial encounter
939.2	FOREIGN BODY IN VULVA AND VAGINA	**T19.2XXA**	Foreign body in vulva and vagina, initial encounter
939.3	FOREIGN BODY IN PENIS	**T19.4XXA**	Foreign body in penis, initial encounter
939.9	FOREIGN BODY UNSPEC SITE GENITOURINARY TRACT	**T19.8XXA**	Foreign body in oth prt genitourinary tract, init encntr
		T19.9XXA	Foreign body in genitourinary tract, part unsp, init encntr
94Ø.Ø	CHEMICAL BURN OF EYELIDS AND PERIOCULAR AREA	**T26.5ØXA**	Corrosion of unsp eyelid and periocular area, init encntr
		T26.51XA	Corrosion of right eyelid and periocular area, init encntr
		T26.52XA	Corrosion of left eyelid and periocular area, init encntr
94Ø.1	OTHER BURNS OF EYELIDS AND PERIOCULAR AREA	**T26.ØØXA**	Burn of unspecified eyelid and periocular area, init encntr
		T26.Ø1XA	Burn of right eyelid and periocular area, initial encounter
		T26.Ø2XA	Burn of left eyelid and periocular area, initial encounter
94Ø.2	ALKALINE CHEMICAL BURN CORNEA&CONJUNCTIVAL SAC	**T26.6ØXA**	Corrosion of cornea and conjunctival sac, unsp eye, init
		T26.61XA	Corrosion of cornea and conjunctival sac, right eye, init
		T26.62XA	Corrosion of cornea and conjunctival sac, left eye, init
94Ø.3	ACID CHEMICAL BURN OF CORNEA&CONJUNCTIVAL SAC	**T26.6ØXA**	Corrosion of cornea and conjunctival sac, unsp eye, init
		T26.61XA	Corrosion of cornea and conjunctival sac, right eye, init
		T26.62XA	Corrosion of cornea and conjunctival sac, left eye, init
94Ø.4	OTHER BURN OF CORNEA AND CONJUNCTIVAL SAC	**T26.1ØXA**	Burn of cornea and conjunctival sac, unsp eye, init encntr
		T26.11XA	Burn of cornea and conjunctival sac, right eye, init encntr
		T26.12XA	Burn of cornea and conjunctival sac, left eye, init encntr
94Ø.5	BURN W/RESULTING RUPTURE&DESTRUCTION OF EYEBALL	**T26.2ØXA**	Burn w resulting rupture and dest of unsp eyeball, init
		T26.21XA	Burn w resulting rupture and dest of right eyeball, init
		T26.22XA	Burn w resulting rupture and dest of left eyeball, init
		T26.7ØXA	Corrosion w resulting rupture and dest of unsp eyeball, init
		T26.71XA	Corros w resulting rupture and dest of right eyeball, init
		T26.72XA	Corrosion w resulting rupture and dest of left eyeball, init

 [Brackets] indicate valid character values for each code. Character value meanings provided for each code grouping.

ICD-9-CM		ICD-10-CM	
940.9	UNSPECIFIED BURN OF EYE AND ADNEXA	**T26.30XA**	Burns of oth parts of unsp eye and adnexa, init encntr
		T26.31XA	Burns of oth parts of right eye and adnexa, init encntr
		T26.32XA	Burns of oth parts of left eye and adnexa, init encntr
		T26.40XA	Burn of unsp eye and adnexa, part unspecified, init encntr
		T26.41XA	Burn of right eye and adnexa, part unspecified, init encntr
		T26.42XA	Burn of left eye and adnexa, part unspecified, init encntr
		T26.80XA	Corrosions of oth parts of unsp eye and adnexa, init encntr
		T26.81XA	Corrosions of oth parts of right eye and adnexa, init encntr
		T26.82XA	Corrosions of oth parts of left eye and adnexa, init encntr
		T26.90XA	Corrosion of unsp eye and adnexa, part unsp, init encntr
		T26.91XA	Corrosion of right eye and adnexa, part unsp, init encntr
		T26.92XA	Corrosion of left eye and adnexa, part unsp, init encntr
941.00	BURN UNSPEC DEGREE UNSPEC SITE FACE&HEAD	**T20.00XA**	Burn of unsp degree of head, face, and neck, unsp site, init
		T20.40XA	Corros unsp degree of head, face, and neck, unsp site, init
941.01	BURN OF UNSPECIFIED DEGREE OF EAR	**T20.011A**	Burn of unspecified degree of right ear, initial encounter
		T20.012A	Burn of unspecified degree of left ear, initial encounter
		T20.019A	Burn of unspecified degree of unspecified ear, init encntr
		T20.411A	Corrosion of unspecified degree of right ear, init encntr
		T20.412A	Corrosion of unspecified degree of left ear, init encntr
		T20.419A	Corrosion of unsp degree of unspecified ear, init encntr
941.02	BURN OF UNSPECIFIED DEGREE OF EYE	**T26.40XA**	Burn of unsp eye and adnexa, part unspecified, init encntr
		T26.41XA	Burn of right eye and adnexa, part unspecified, init encntr
		T26.42XA	Burn of left eye and adnexa, part unspecified, init encntr
941.03	BURN OF UNSPECIFIED DEGREE OF LIP	**T20.02XA**	Burn of unspecified degree of lip(s), initial encounter
		T20.42XA	Corrosion of unspecified degree of lip(s), initial encounter
941.04	BURN OF UNSPECIFIED DEGREE OF CHIN	**T20.03XA**	Burn of unspecified degree of chin, initial encounter
		T20.43XA	Corrosion of unspecified degree of chin, initial encounter
941.05	BURN OF UNSPECIFIED DEGREE OF NOSE	**T20.04XA**	Burn of unspecified degree of nose (septum), init encntr
		T20.44XA	Corrosion of unsp degree of nose (septum), init encntr
941.06	BURN OF UNSPECIFIED DEGREE OF SCALP	**T20.05XA**	Burn of unspecified degree of scalp, initial encounter
		T20.45XA	Corrosion of unspecified degree of scalp, initial encounter
941.07	BURN OF UNSPECIFIED DEGREE OF FOREHEAD AND CHEEK	**T20.06XA**	Burn of unsp degree of forehead and cheek, init encntr
		T20.46XA	Corrosion of unsp degree of forehead and cheek, init encntr
941.08	BURN OF UNSPECIFIED DEGREE OF NECK	**T20.07XA**	Burn of unspecified degree of neck, initial encounter
		T20.47XA	Corrosion of unspecified degree of neck, initial encounter
941.09	BURN UNSPEC DEGREE MULTIPLE SITES FACE HEAD&NECK	**T20.09XA**	Burn of unsp deg mult sites of head, face, and neck, init
		T20.49XA	Corros unsp deg mult sites of head, face, and neck, init
941.10	ERYTHEMA DUE TO BURN UNSPECIFIED SITE FACE&HEAD	**T20.10XA**	Burn first degree of head, face, and neck, unsp site, init
		T20.50XA	Corros first degree of head, face, and neck, unsp site, init
941.11	ERYTHEMA DUE TO BURN OF EAR	**T20.111A**	Burn of first degree of right ear, initial encounter
		T20.112A	Burn of first degree of left ear, initial encounter
		T20.119A	Burn of first degree of unspecified ear, initial encounter
		T20.511A	Corrosion of first degree of right ear, initial encounter
		T20.512A	Corrosion of first degree of left ear, initial encounter
		T20.519A	Corrosion of first degree of unspecified ear, init encntr
941.12	ERYTHEMA DUE TO BURN OF EYE	**T26.40XA**	Burn of unsp eye and adnexa, part unspecified, init encntr
		T26.41XA	Burn of right eye and adnexa, part unspecified, init encntr
		T26.42XA	Burn of left eye and adnexa, part unspecified, init encntr
941.13	ERYTHEMA DUE TO BURN OF LIP	**T20.12XA**	Burn of first degree of lip(s), initial encounter
		T20.52XA	Corrosion of first degree of lip(s), initial encounter
941.14	ERYTHEMA DUE TO BURN OF CHIN	**T20.13XA**	Burn of first degree of chin, initial encounter
		T20.53XA	Corrosion of first degree of chin, initial encounter
941.15	ERYTHEMA DUE TO BURN OF NOSE	**T20.14XA**	Burn of first degree of nose (septum), initial encounter
		T20.54XA	Corrosion of first degree of nose (septum), init encntr
941.16	ERYTHEMA DUE TO BURN OF SCALP	**T20.15XA**	Burn of first degree of scalp [any part], initial encounter
		T20.55XA	Corrosion of first degree of scalp, initial encounter
941.17	ERYTHEMA DUE TO BURN OF FOREHEAD AND CHEEK	**T20.16XA**	Burn of first degree of forehead and cheek, init encntr
		T20.56XA	Corrosion of first degree of forehead and cheek, initial encounter
941.18	ERYTHEMA DUE TO BURN OF NECK	**T20.17XA**	Burn of first degree of neck, initial encounter
		T20.57XA	Corrosion of first degree of neck, initial encounter
941.19	ERYTHEMA DUE BURN MULTIPLE SITES FACE HEAD&NECK	**T20.19XA**	Burn of first deg mult sites of head, face, and neck, init
		T20.59XA	Corros first deg mult sites of head, face, and neck, init
941.20	BLISTR W/EPID LOSS DUE BURN FCE&HEAD UNSPEC SITE	**T20.20XA**	Burn second degree of head, face, and neck, unsp site, init
		T20.60XA	Corros second deg of head, face, and neck, unsp site, init
941.21	BLISTERS WITH EPIDERMAL LOSS DUE TO BURN OF EAR	**T20.211A**	Burn of second degree of right ear, initial encounter
		T20.212A	Burn of second degree of left ear, initial encounter
		T20.219A	Burn of second degree of unspecified ear, initial encounter
		T20.611A	Corrosion of second degree of right ear, initial encounter
		T20.612A	Corrosion of second degree of left ear, initial encounter
		T20.619A	Corrosion of second degree of unspecified ear, init encntr
941.22	BLISTERS WITH EPIDERMAL LOSS DUE TO BURN OF EYE	**T26.40XA**	Burn of unsp eye and adnexa, part unspecified, init encntr
		T26.41XA	Burn of right eye and adnexa, part unspecified, init encntr
		T26.42XA	Burn of left eye and adnexa, part unspecified, init encntr
941.23	BLISTERS WITH EPIDERMAL LOSS DUE TO BURN OF LIP	**T20.22XA**	Burn of second degree of lip(s), initial encounter
		T20.62XA	Corrosion of second degree of lip(s), initial encounter
941.24	BLISTERS W/EPID LOSS D/T BURN-2ND DEG-CHIN	**T20.23XA**	Burn of second degree of chin, initial encounter
		T20.63XA	Corrosion of second degree of chin, initial encounter

ICD-9-CM		ICD-10-CM	
941.25	BLISTERS WITH EPIDERMAL LOSS DUE TO BURN OF NOSE	**T2Ø.24XA** **T2Ø.64XA**	Burn of second degree of nose (septum), initial encounter Corrosion of second degree of nose (septum), init encntr
941.26	BLISTERS W/EPIDERMAL LOSS DUE TO BURN OF SCALP	**T2Ø.25XA** **T2Ø.65XA**	Burn of second degree of scalp [any part], initial encounter Corrosion of second degree of scalp, initial encounter
941.27	BLISTERS-EPID LOSS D/T BURN-2ND DEG-FORHED&CHEEK	**T2Ø.26XA** **T2Ø.66XA**	Burn of second degree of forehead and cheek, init encntr Corrosion of second degree of forehead and cheek, init
941.28	BLISTERS WITH EPIDERMAL LOSS DUE TO BURN OF NECK	**T2Ø.27XA** **T2Ø.67XA**	Burn of second degree of neck, initial encounter Corrosion of second degree of neck, initial encounter
941.29	BLISTERS W/2ND DEG BURN-MX SITE FACE HEAD&NECK	**T2Ø.29XA** **T2Ø.69XA**	Burn of 2nd deg mul sites of head, face, and neck, init Corrosion of 2nd deg mul sites of head, face, and neck, init
941.3Ø	FULL-THICK SKN LOSS DUE BURN UNS SITE FCE&HEAD	**T2Ø.3ØXA** **T2Ø.7ØXA**	Burn third degree of head, face, and neck, unsp site, init Corros third degree of head, face, and neck, unsp site, init
941.31	FULL-THICKNESS SKIN LOSS DUE TO BURN OF EAR	**T2Ø.311A** **T2Ø.312A** **T2Ø.319A** **T2Ø.711A** **T2Ø.712A** **T2Ø.719A**	Burn of third degree of right ear, initial encounter Burn of third degree of left ear, initial encounter Burn of third degree of unspecified ear, initial encounter Corrosion of third degree of right ear, initial encounter Corrosion of third degree of left ear, initial encounter Corrosion of third degree of unspecified ear, init encntr
941.32	FULL-THICKNESS SKIN LOSS DUE TO BURN OF EYE	**T26.4ØXA** **T26.41XA** **T26.42XA**	Burn of unsp eye and adnexa, part unspecified, init encntr Burn of right eye and adnexa, part unspecified, init encntr Burn of left eye and adnexa, part unspecified, init encntr
941.33	FULL-THICKNESS SKIN LOSS DUE TO BURN OF LIP	**T2Ø.32XA** **T2Ø.72XA**	Burn of third degree of lip(s), initial encounter Corrosion of third degree of lip(s), initial encounter
941.34	FULL-THICKNESS SKIN LOSS DUE TO BURN OF CHIN	**T2Ø.33XA** **T2Ø.73XA**	Burn of third degree of chin, initial encounter Corrosion of third degree of chin, initial encounter
941.35	FULL-THICKNESS SKIN LOSS DUE TO BURN OF NOSE	**T2Ø.34XA** **T2Ø.74XA**	Burn of third degree of nose (septum), initial encounter Corrosion of third degree of nose (septum), init encntr
941.36	FULL-THICKNESS SKIN LOSS DUE TO BURN OF SCALP	**T2Ø.35XA** **T2Ø.75XA**	Burn of third degree of scalp [any part], initial encounter Corrosion of third degree of scalp, initial encounter
941.37	FULL-THICKNESS SKIN LOSS DUE BURN FOREHEAD&CHEEK	**T2Ø.36XA** **T2Ø.76XA**	Burn of third degree of forehead and cheek, init encntr Corrosion of third degree of forehead and cheek, init encntr
941.38	FULL-THICKNESS SKIN LOSS DUE TO BURN OF NECK	**T2Ø.37XA** **T2Ø.77XA**	Burn of third degree of neck, initial encounter Corrosion of third degree of neck, initial encounter
941.39	FULL-THICK SKN LOSS-BURN-MX SITE FACE HEAD&NECK	**T2Ø.39XA** **T2Ø.79XA**	Burn of 3rd deg mu sites of head, face, and neck, init Corrosion of 3rd deg mu sites of head, face, and neck, init
941.4Ø	DEEP 3RD DEG BURN-UNS SITE FACE&HEAD W/O LOBP	**T2Ø.3ØXA** **T2Ø.7ØXA**	Burn third degree of head, face, and neck, unsp site, init Corros third degree of head, face, and neck, unsp site, init
941.41	DEEP 3RD DEG BURN-NECROS-EAR W/O LOBP	**T2Ø.311A** **T2Ø.312A** **T2Ø.319A** **T2Ø.711A** **T2Ø.712A** **T2Ø.719A**	Burn of third degree of right ear, initial encounter Burn of third degree of left ear, initial encounter Burn of third degree of unspecified ear, initial encounter Corrosion of third degree of right ear, initial encounter Corrosion of third degree of left ear, initial encounter Corrosion of third degree of unspecified ear, init encntr
941.42	DEEP 3RD DEG BURN-NECROSIS-EYE W/O LOBP	**T26.4ØXA** **T26.41XA** **T26.42XA**	Burn of unsp eye and adnexa, part unspecified, init encntr Burn of right eye and adnexa, part unspecified, init encntr Burn of left eye and adnexa, part unspecified, init encntr
941.43	DEEP 3RD DEG BURN-NECROSIS-LIP W/O LOBP	**T2Ø.32XA** **T2Ø.72XA**	Burn of third degree of lip(s), initial encounter Corrosion of third degree of lip(s), initial encounter
941.44	DEEP 3RD DEG BURN-NECROSIS-CHIN W/O LOBP	**T2Ø.33XA** **T2Ø.73XA**	Burn of third degree of chin, initial encounter Corrosion of third degree of chin, initial encounter
941.45	DEEP 3RD DEG BURN-NECROSIS-NOSE W/O LOBP	**T2Ø.34XA** **T2Ø.74XA**	Burn of third degree of nose (septum), initial encounter Corrosion of third degree of nose (septum), init encntr
941.46	DEEP 3RD DEG BURN-NECROSIS-SCALP W/O LOBP	**T2Ø.35XA** **T2Ø.75XA**	Burn of third degree of scalp [any part], initial encounter Corrosion of third degree of scalp, initial encounter
941.47	DEEP 3RD DEG BURN-NECROS-FOREHEAD-CHEEK W/O LOBP	**T2Ø.36XA** **T2Ø.76XA**	Burn of third degree of forehead and cheek, init encntr Corrosion of third degree of forehead and cheek, init encntr
941.48	DEEP 3RD DEG BURN-NECROSIS-NECK W/O LOBP	**T2Ø.37XA** **T2Ø.77XA**	Burn of third degree of neck, initial encounter Corrosion of third degree of neck, initial encounter
941.49	DEEP 3RD DEG BURN-MX SITE FACE HEAD&NCK W/O LOBP	**T2Ø.39XA** **T2Ø.79XA**	Burn of 3rd deg mu sites of head, face, and neck, init Corrosion of 3rd deg mu sites of head, face, and neck, init
941.5Ø	DEEP 3RD DEG BURN-FACE&HEAD UNS SITE W/LOBP	**T2Ø.3ØXA** **T2Ø.7ØXA**	Burn third degree of head, face, and neck, unsp site, init Corros third degree of head, face, and neck, unsp site, init
941.51	DP 3RD DEG UNDLYING TISS-BRN EAR W/LOSS BDY PART	**T2Ø.319A** **T2Ø.719A**	Burn of third degree of unspecified ear, initial encounter Corrosion of third degree of unspecified ear, init encntr
941.52	DP 3RD DEG UNDLYING TISS-BRN EYE W/LOSS BDY PART	**T26.2ØXA** **T26.21XA** **T26.22XA**	Burn w resulting rupture and dest of unsp eyeball, init Burn w resulting rupture and dest of right eyeball, init Burn w resulting rupture and dest of left eyeball, init
941.53	DP 3RD DEG UNDLYING TISS-BRN LIP W/LOSS BDY PART	**T2Ø.32XA** **T2Ø.72XA**	Burn of third degree of lip(s), initial encounter Corrosion of third degree of lip(s), initial encounter
941.54	DP 3RD DEG UNDLY TISS-BRN CHIN W/LOSS BDY PART	**T2Ø.33XA** **T2Ø.73XA**	Burn of third degree of chin, initial encounter Corrosion of third degree of chin, initial encounter
941.55	DP 3RD DEG UNDLYING TISS-BRN NSE W/LOSS BDY PART	**T2Ø.34XA** **T2Ø.74XA**	Burn of third degree of nose (septum), initial encounter Corrosion of third degree of nose (septum), init encntr
941.56	DP 3RD DEG UNDLY TISS-BRN SCLP W/LOSS BDY PART	**T2Ø.35XA** **T2Ø.75XA**	Burn of third degree of scalp [any part], initial encounter Corrosion of third degree of scalp, initial encounter

ICD-9-CM		ICD-10-CM	
941.57	DEEP 3RD DGR BURN-NECROSIS-FOREHEAD&CHEEK W/LOBP	**T20.36XA** **T20.76XA**	Burn of third degree of forehead and cheek, init encntr Corrosion of third degree of forehead and cheek, init encntr
941.58	DP 3RD DEG UNDLYING TISS-BRN NCK W/LOSS BDY PART	**T20.37XA** **T20.77XA**	Burn of third degree of neck, initial encounter Corrosion of third degree of neck, initial encounter
941.59	DEEP 3RD DGR BURN-MULT-FACE-HEAD&NECK W/LOBP	**T20.39XA** **T20.79XA**	Burn of 3rd deg mu sites of head, face, and neck, init Corrosion of 3rd deg mu sites of head, face, and neck, init
942.00	BURN UNSPECIFIED DEGREE TRUNK UNSPECIFIED SITE	**T21.00XA** **T21.40XA**	Burn of unsp degree of trunk, unspecified site, init encntr Corrosion of unsp degree of trunk, unsp site, init encntr
942.01	BURN OF TRUNK UNSPECIFIED DEGREE OF BREAST	**T21.01XA** **T21.41XA**	Burn of unspecified degree of chest wall, initial encounter Corrosion of unspecified degree of chest wall, init encntr
942.02	BURN-TRNK UNS DEG CHEST WALL NOT BREAST&NIPPLE	**T21.01XA** **T21.41XA**	Burn of unspecified degree of chest wall, initial encounter Corrosion of unspecified degree of chest wall, init encntr
942.03	BURN TRUNK UNSPECIFIED DEGREE ABDOMINAL WALL	**T21.02XA** **T21.42XA**	Burn of unspecified degree of abdominal wall, init encntr Corrosion of unsp degree of abdominal wall, init encntr
942.04	BURN OF TRUNK UNSPECIFIED DEGREE OF BACK	**T21.03XA** **T21.04XA** **T21.05XA** **T21.43XA** **T21.44XA** **T21.45XA**	Burn of unspecified degree of upper back, initial encounter Burn of unspecified degree of lower back, initial encounter Burn of unspecified degree of buttock, initial encounter Corrosion of unspecified degree of upper back, init encntr Corrosion of unspecified degree of lower back, init encntr Corrosion of unspecified degree of buttock, init encntr
942.05	BURN OF TRUNK UNSPECIFIED DEGREE OF GENITALIA	**T21.06XA** **T21.07XA** **T21.46XA** **T21.47XA**	Burn of unsp degree of male genital region, init encntr Burn of unsp degree of female genital region, init encntr Corrosion of unsp degree of male genital region, init encntr Corrosion of unsp degree of female genital region, init
942.09	BURN TRUNK UNSPEC DEGREE OTHER&MULTIPLE SITES	**T21.09XA** **T21.49XA**	Burn of unsp degree of other site of trunk, init encntr Corrosion of unsp degree of other site of trunk, init encntr
942.10	ERYTHEMA DUE TO BURN UNSPECIFIED SITE TRUNK	**T21.10XA** **T21.50XA**	Burn of first degree of trunk, unspecified site, init encntr Corrosion of first degree of trunk, unsp site, init encntr
942.11	ERYTHEMA DUE TO BURN OF BREAST	**T21.11XA** **T21.51XA**	Burn of first degree of chest wall, initial encounter Corrosion of first degree of chest wall, initial encounter
942.12	ERYTHMA DUE BURN CHST WALL EXCLD BREAST&NIPPLE	**T21.11XA** **T21.51XA**	Burn of first degree of chest wall, initial encounter Corrosion of first degree of chest wall, initial encounter
942.13	ERYTHEMA DUE TO BURN OF ABDOMINAL WALL	**T21.12XA** **T21.52XA**	Burn of first degree of abdominal wall, initial encounter Corrosion of first degree of abdominal wall, init encntr
942.14	ERYTHEMA DUE TO BURN OF BACK	**T21.13XA** **T21.14XA** **T21.15XA** **T21.53XA** **T21.54XA** **T21.55XA**	Burn of first degree of upper back, initial encounter Burn of first degree of lower back, initial encounter Burn of first degree of buttock, initial encounter Corrosion of first degree of upper back, initial encounter Corrosion of first degree of lower back, initial encounter Corrosion of first degree of buttock, initial encounter
942.15	ERYTHEMA DUE TO BURN OF GENITALIA	**T21.16XA** **T21.17XA** **T21.56XA** **T21.57XA**	Burn of first degree of male genital region, init encntr Burn of first degree of female genital region, init encntr Corrosion of first degree of male genital region, init Corrosion of first degree of female genital region, init
942.19	ERYTHEMA DUE TO BURN OTHER&MULTIPLE SITES TRUNK	**T21.19XA** **T21.59XA**	Burn of first degree of other site of trunk, init encntr Corrosion of first degree of oth site of trunk, init encntr
942.20	BLISTERS W/EPID LOSS DUE BURN UNSPEC SITE-TRUNK	**T21.20XA** **T21.60XA**	Burn of second degree of trunk, unsp site, init encntr Corrosion of second degree of trunk, unsp site, init encntr
942.21	BLISTERS WITH EPIDERMAL LOSS DUE TO BURN-BREAST	**T21.21XA** **T21.61XA**	Burn of second degree of chest wall, initial encounter Corrosion of second degree of chest wall, initial encounter
942.22	BLISTRS-2ND DEG BURN-CHEST WALL NOT BREAST&NIPPL	**T21.21XA** **T21.61XA**	Burn of second degree of chest wall, initial encounter Corrosion of second degree of chest wall, initial encounter
942.23	BLISTERS W/EPIDERMAL LOSS DUE BURN ABD WALL	**T21.22XA** **T21.62XA**	Burn of second degree of abdominal wall, initial encounter Corrosion of second degree of abdominal wall, init encntr
942.24	BLISTERS WITH EPIDERMAL LOSS DUE TO BURN OF BACK	**T21.23XA** **T21.24XA** **T21.25XA** **T21.63XA** **T21.64XA** **T21.65XA**	Burn of second degree of upper back, initial encounter Burn of second degree of lower back, initial encounter Burn of second degree of buttock, initial encounter Corrosion of second degree of upper back, initial encounter Corrosion of second degree of lower back, initial encounter Corrosion of second degree of buttock, initial encounter
942.25	BLISTERS W/EPIDERMAL LOSS DUE TO BURN GENITALIA	**T21.26XA** **T21.27XA** **T21.66XA** **T21.67XA**	Burn of second degree of male genital region, init encntr Burn of second degree of female genital region, init encntr Corrosion of second degree of male genital region, init Corrosion of second degree of female genital region, init
942.29	BLISTERS W/EPID LOSS DUE BURN-OTH&MULT SITE TRNK	**T21.29XA** **T21.69XA**	Burn of second degree of other site of trunk, init encntr Corrosion of second degree of oth site of trunk, init encntr
942.30	FULL-THICK SKIN LOSS DUE BURN UNSPEC SITE TRUNK	**T21.30XA** **T21.70XA**	Burn of third degree of trunk, unspecified site, init encntr Corrosion of third degree of trunk, unsp site, init encntr
942.31	FULL-THICKNESS SKIN LOSS DUE TO BURN OF BREAST	**T21.31XA** **T21.71XA**	Burn of third degree of chest wall, initial encounter Corrosion of third degree of chest wall, initial encounter
942.32	FULL-THICK SKIN LOSS-BURN-CHEST WALL NOT BREST	**T21.31XA** **T21.71XA**	Burn of third degree of chest wall, initial encounter Corrosion of third degree of chest wall, initial encounter
942.33	FULL-THICKNESS SKIN LOSS DUE BURN ABDOMINAL WALL	**T21.32XA** **T21.72XA**	Burn of third degree of abdominal wall, initial encounter Corrosion of third degree of abdominal wall, init encntr

ICD-9-CM		ICD-10-CM	
942.34	FULL-THICKNESS SKIN LOSS DUE TO BURN OF BACK	**T21.33XA**	Burn of third degree of upper back, initial encounter
		T21.34XA	Burn of third degree of lower back, initial encounter
		T21.35XA	Burn of third degree of buttock, initial encounter
		T21.73XA	Corrosion of third degree of upper back, initial encounter
		T21.74XA	Corrosion of third degree of lower back, initial encounter
		T21.75XA	Corrosion of third degree of buttock, initial encounter
942.35	FULL-THICKNESS SKIN LOSS DUE TO BURN GENITALIA	**T21.36XA**	Burn of third degree of male genital region, init encntr
		T21.37XA	Burn of third degree of female genital region, init encntr
		T21.76XA	Corrosion of third degree of male genital region, init
		T21.77XA	Corrosion of third degree of female genital region, init
942.39	FULL-THICK SKIN LOSS DUE BURN-OTH&MULT SITE TRNK	**T21.39XA**	Burn of third degree of other site of trunk, init encntr
		T21.79XA	Corrosion of third degree of oth site of trunk, init encntr
942.4Ø	DEEP 3RD DEG BURN-NECROS-TRUNK-UNS SITE W/O LOBP	**T21.3ØXA**	Burn of third degree of trunk, unspecified site, init encntr
		T21.7ØXA	Corrosion of third degree of trunk, unsp site, init encntr
942.41	DEEP 3RD DEG BURN-NECROSIS-BREAST W/O LOBP	**T21.31XA**	Burn of third degree of chest wall, initial encounter
		T21.71XA	Corrosion of third degree of chest wall, initial encounter
942.42	DEEP 3RD DEG BURN-NECROSIS-CHEST WALL W/O LOBP	**T21.31XA**	Burn of third degree of chest wall, initial encounter
		T21.71XA	Corrosion of third degree of chest wall, initial encounter
942.43	DEEP 3RD DEG BURN-NECROSIS-ABD WALL W/O LOBP	**T21.32XA**	Burn of third degree of abdominal wall, initial encounter
		T21.72XA	Corrosion of third degree of abdominal wall, init encntr
942.44	DEEP 3RD DEG BURN-NECROS-BACK W/O LOBP	**T21.33XA**	Burn of third degree of upper back, initial encounter
		T21.34XA	Burn of third degree of lower back, initial encounter
		T21.35XA	Burn of third degree of buttock, initial encounter
		T21.73XA	Corrosion of third degree of upper back, initial encounter
		T21.74XA	Corrosion of third degree of lower back, initial encounter
		T21.75XA	Corrosion of third degree of buttock, initial encounter
942.45	DEEP 3RD DEG BURN-NECROSIS-GENITALIA W/O LOBP	**T21.36XA**	Burn of third degree of male genital region, init encntr
		T21.37XA	Burn of third degree of female genital region, init encntr
		T21.76XA	Corrosion of third degree of male genital region, init
		T21.77XA	Corrosion of third degree of female genital region, init
942.49	DEEP 3RD DEG BURN-NECROS-OTH&MULT-TRUNK W/O LOBP	**T21.39XA**	Burn of third degree of other site of trunk, init encntr
		T21.79XA	Corrosion of third degree of oth site of trunk, init encntr
942.5Ø	DEEP 3RD DEG BURN-NECROSIS-TRUNK-UNS SITE W/LOBP	**T21.3ØXA**	Burn of third degree of trunk, unspecified site, init encntr
		T21.7ØXA	Corrosion of third degree of trunk, unsp site, init encntr
942.51	DEEP 3RD DEG UNDLY TISS-BRN BRST W/LOSS BDY PART	**T21.31XA**	Burn of third degree of chest wall, initial encounter
		T21.71XA	Corrosion of third degree of chest wall, initial encounter
942.52	DEEP 3RD DEG BURN-NECROSIS-CHEST WALL W/LOBP	**T21.31XA**	Burn of third degree of chest wall, initial encounter
		T21.71XA	Corrosion of third degree of chest wall, initial encounter
942.53	DEEP 3RD DEG BURN-NECROSIS-ABD WALL W/LOBP	**T21.32XA**	Burn of third degree of abdominal wall, initial encounter
		T21.72XA	Corrosion of third degree of abdominal wall, init encntr
942.54	DEEP 3RD DEG UNDLY TISS-BRN BACK W/LOSS BDY PART	**T21.33XA**	Burn of third degree of upper back, initial encounter
		T21.73XA	Corrosion of third degree of upper back, initial encounter
942.55	DEEP 3RD DEG UNDLY TISS-BURN GNT W/LOSS BDY PART	**T21.36XA**	Burn of third degree of male genital region, init encntr
		T21.37XA	Burn of third degree of female genital region, init encntr
		T21.76XA	Corrosion of third degree of male genital region, init
		T21.77XA	Corrosion of third degree of female genital region, init
942.59	DEEP 3RD DEG BURN-NECROSIS-OTH&MULT-TRUNK W/LOBP	**T21.39XA**	Burn of third degree of other site of trunk, init encntr
		T21.79XA	Corrosion of third degree of oth site of trunk, init encntr
943.ØØ	BURN UNSPEC DEGREE UNSPEC SITE UPPER LIMB	**T22.ØØXA**	Burn unsp deg of shldr/up lmb, ex wrs/hnd, unsp site, init
		T22.4ØXA	Corros unsp deg of shldr/up lmb, ex wrs/hnd, unsp site, init
943.Ø1	BURN OF UNSPECIFIED DEGREE OF FOREARM	**T22.Ø11A**	Burn of unspecified degree of right forearm, init encntr
		T22.Ø12A	Burn of unspecified degree of left forearm, init encntr
		T22.Ø19A	Burn of unsp degree of unspecified forearm, init encntr
		T22.411A	Corrosion of unsp degree of right forearm, init encntr
		T22.412A	Corrosion of unspecified degree of left forearm, init encntr
		T22.419A	Corrosion of unsp degree of unspecified forearm, init encntr
943.Ø2	BURN OF UNSPECIFIED DEGREE OF ELBOW	**T22.Ø21A**	Burn of unspecified degree of right elbow, initial encounter
		T22.Ø22A	Burn of unspecified degree of left elbow, initial encounter
		T22.Ø29A	Burn of unspecified degree of unspecified elbow, init encntr
		T22.421A	Corrosion of unspecified degree of right elbow, init encntr
		T22.422A	Corrosion of unspecified degree of left elbow, init encntr
		T22.429A	Corrosion of unsp degree of unspecified elbow, init encntr
943.Ø3	BURN OF UNSPECIFIED DEGREE OF UPPER ARM	**T22.Ø31A**	Burn of unspecified degree of right upper arm, init encntr
		T22.Ø32A	Burn of unspecified degree of left upper arm, init encntr
		T22.Ø39A	Burn of unsp degree of unspecified upper arm, init encntr
		T22.431A	Corrosion of unsp degree of right upper arm, init encntr
		T22.432A	Corrosion of unsp degree of left upper arm, init encntr
		T22.439A	Corrosion of unsp degree of unsp upper arm, init encntr
943.Ø4	BURN OF UNSPECIFIED DEGREE OF AXILLA	**T22.Ø41A**	Burn of unspecified degree of right axilla, init encntr
		T22.Ø42A	Burn of unspecified degree of left axilla, initial encounter
		T22.Ø49A	Burn of unsp degree of unspecified axilla, init encntr
		T22.441A	Corrosion of unspecified degree of right axilla, init encntr
		T22.442A	Corrosion of unspecified degree of left axilla, init encntr
		T22.449A	Corrosion of unsp degree of unspecified axilla, init encntr

 [Brackets] indicate valid character values for each code. Character value meanings provided for each code grouping.

ICD-9-CM		ICD-10-CM	
943.Ø5	BURN OF UNSPECIFIED DEGREE OF SHOULDER	**T22.Ø51A**	Burn of unspecified degree of right shoulder, init encntr
		T22.Ø52A	Burn of unspecified degree of left shoulder, init encntr
		T22.Ø59A	Burn of unsp degree of unspecified shoulder, init encntr
		T22.451A	Corrosion of unsp degree of right shoulder, init encntr
		T22.452A	Corrosion of unsp degree of left shoulder, init encntr
		T22.459A	Corrosion of unsp degree of unsp shoulder, init encntr
943.Ø6	BURN OF UNSPECIFIED DEGREE OF SCAPULAR REGION	**T22.Ø61A**	Burn of unsp degree of right scapular region, init encntr
		T22.Ø62A	Burn of unsp degree of left scapular region, init encntr
		T22.Ø69A	Burn of unsp degree of unsp scapular region, init encntr
		T22.461A	Corrosion of unsp degree of right scapular region, init
		T22.462A	Corrosion of unsp degree of left scapular region, init
		T22.469A	Corrosion of unsp degree of unsp scapular region, init
943.Ø9	BURN UNSPEC DEG MX SITES UPPER LIMB NO WRST&HAND	**T22.Ø91A**	Burn unsp deg mult sites of r shldr/up lmb, ex wrs/hnd, init
		T22.Ø92A	Burn unsp deg mult site of l shldr/up lmb, ex wrs/hnd, init
		T22.Ø99A	Burn unsp deg mult sites of shldr/up lmb, ex wrs/hnd, init
		T22.491A	Corros unsp deg mult site of r shldr/up lmb,ex wrs/hnd, init
		T22.492A	Corros unsp deg mult site of l shldr/up lmb,ex wrs/hnd, init
		T22.499A	Corros unsp deg mult sites of shldr/up lmb, ex wrs/hnd, init
943.1Ø	ERYTHEMA DUE TO BURN UNSPECIFIED SITE UPPER LIMB	**T22.1ØXA**	Burn first deg of shldr/up lmb, ex wrs/hnd, unsp site, init
		T22.5ØXA	Corros first deg of shldr/up lmb, ex wrs/hnd unsp site, init
943.11	ERYTHEMA DUE TO BURN OF FOREARM	**T22.111A**	Burn of first degree of right forearm, initial encounter
		T22.112A	Burn of first degree of left forearm, initial encounter
		T22.119A	Burn of first degree of unspecified forearm, init encntr
		T22.511A	Corrosion of first degree of right forearm, init encntr
		T22.512A	Corrosion of first degree of left forearm, initial encounter
		T22.519A	Corrosion of first degree of unsp forearm, init encntr
943.12	ERYTHEMA DUE TO BURN OF ELBOW	**T22.121A**	Burn of first degree of right elbow, initial encounter
		T22.122A	Burn of first degree of left elbow, initial encounter
		T22.129A	Burn of first degree of unspecified elbow, initial encounter
		T22.521A	Corrosion of first degree of right elbow, initial encounter
		T22.522A	Corrosion of first degree of left elbow, initial encounter
		T22.529A	Corrosion of first degree of unspecified elbow, init encntr
943.13	ERYTHEMA DUE TO BURN OF UPPER ARM	**T22.131A**	Burn of first degree of right upper arm, initial encounter
		T22.132A	Burn of first degree of left upper arm, initial encounter
		T22.139A	Burn of first degree of unspecified upper arm, init encntr
		T22.531A	Corrosion of first degree of right upper arm, init encntr
		T22.532A	Corrosion of first degree of left upper arm, init encntr
		T22.539A	Corrosion of first degree of unsp upper arm, init encntr
943.14	ERYTHEMA DUE TO BURN OF AXILLA	**T22.141A**	Burn of first degree of right axilla, initial encounter
		T22.142A	Burn of first degree of left axilla, initial encounter
		T22.149A	Burn of first degree of unspecified axilla, init encntr
		T22.541A	Corrosion of first degree of right axilla, initial encounter
		T22.542A	Corrosion of first degree of left axilla, initial encounter
		T22.549A	Corrosion of first degree of unspecified axilla, init encntr
943.15	ERYTHEMA DUE TO BURN OF SHOULDER	**T22.151A**	Burn of first degree of right shoulder, initial encounter
		T22.152A	Burn of first degree of left shoulder, initial encounter
		T22.159A	Burn of first degree of unspecified shoulder, init encntr
		T22.551A	Corrosion of first degree of right shoulder, init encntr
		T22.552A	Corrosion of first degree of left shoulder, init encntr
		T22.559A	Corrosion of first degree of unsp shoulder, init encntr
943.16	ERYTHEMA DUE TO BURN OF SCAPULAR REGION	**T22.161A**	Burn of first degree of right scapular region, init encntr
		T22.162A	Burn of first degree of left scapular region, init encntr
		T22.169A	Burn of first degree of unsp scapular region, init encntr
		T22.561A	Corrosion of first degree of right scapular region, init
		T22.562A	Corrosion of first degree of left scapular region, init
		T22.569A	Corrosion of first degree of unsp scapular region, init
943.19	ERYTHMA DUE BURN-MULT SITE UP LIMB EXP WRST&HND	**T22.191A**	Burn 1st deg mult sites of r shldr/up lmb, ex wrs/hnd, init
		T22.192A	Burn 1st deg mult site of l shldr/up lmb, ex wrs/hnd, init
		T22.199A	Burn first deg mult sites of shldr/up lmb, ex wrs/hnd, init
		T22.591A	Corros 1st deg mult site of r shldr/up lmb, ex wrs/hnd, init
		T22.592A	Corros 1st deg mult site of l shldr/up lmb, ex wrs/hnd, init
		T22.599A	Corros 1st deg mult sites of shldr/up lmb, ex wrs/hnd, init
943.2Ø	BLISTR W/EPID LOSS DUE BURN UNS SITE UPPER LIMB	**T22.2ØXA**	Burn second deg of shldr/up lmb, ex wrs/hnd, unsp site, init
		T22.6ØXA	Corros 2nd deg of shldr/up lmb, ex wrs/hnd, unsp site, init
943.21	BLISTERS W/EPIDERMAL LOSS DUE TO BURN OF FOREARM	**T22.211A**	Burn of second degree of right forearm, initial encounter
		T22.212A	Burn of second degree of left forearm, initial encounter
		T22.219A	Burn of second degree of unspecified forearm, init encntr
		T22.611A	Corrosion of second degree of right forearm, init encntr
		T22.612A	Corrosion of second degree of left forearm, init encntr
		T22.619A	Corrosion of second degree of unsp forearm, Init encntr
943.22	BLISTERS W/EPIDERMAL LOSS DUE TO BURN OF ELBOW	**T22.221A**	Burn of second degree of right elbow, initial encounter
		T22.222A	Burn of second degree of left elbow, initial encounter
		T22.229A	Burn of second degree of unspecified elbow, init encntr
		T22.621A	Corrosion of second degree of right elbow, initial encounter
		T22.622A	Corrosion of second degree of left elbow, initial encounter
		T22.629A	Corrosion of second degree of unspecified elbow, init encntr

ICD-9-CM		ICD-10-CM	
943.23	BLISTERS W/EPIDERMAL LOSS DUE TO BURN UPPER ARM	**T22.231A**	Burn of second degree of right upper arm, initial encounter
		T22.232A	Burn of second degree of left upper arm, initial encounter
		T22.239A	Burn of second degree of unspecified upper arm, init encntr
		T22.631A	Corrosion of second degree of right upper arm, init encntr
		T22.632A	Corrosion of second degree of left upper arm, init encntr
		T22.639A	Corrosion of second degree of unsp upper arm, init encntr
943.24	BLISTERS W/EPIDERMAL LOSS DUE TO BURN OF AXILLA	**T22.241A**	Burn of second degree of right axilla, initial encounter
		T22.242A	Burn of second degree of left axilla, initial encounter
		T22.249A	Burn of second degree of unspecified axilla, init encntr
		T22.641A	Corrosion of second degree of right axilla, init encntr
		T22.642A	Corrosion of second degree of left axilla, initial encounter
		T22.649A	Corrosion of second degree of unsp axilla, init encntr
943.25	BLISTERS W/EPIDERMAL LOSS DUE TO BURN SHOULDER	**T22.251A**	Burn of second degree of right shoulder, initial encounter
		T22.252A	Burn of second degree of left shoulder, initial encounter
		T22.259A	Burn of second degree of unspecified shoulder, init encntr
		T22.651A	Corrosion of second degree of right shoulder, init encntr
		T22.652A	Corrosion of second degree of left shoulder, init encntr
		T22.659A	Corrosion of second degree of unsp shoulder, init encntr
943.26	BLISTR W/EPIDERMAL LOSS DUE BURN SCAPULAR REGION	**T22.261A**	Burn of second degree of right scapular region, init encntr
		T22.262A	Burn of second degree of left scapular region, init encntr
		T22.269A	Burn of second degree of unsp scapular region, init encntr
		T22.661A	Corrosion of second degree of right scapular region, init
		T22.662A	Corrosion of second degree of left scapular region, init
		T22.669A	Corrosion of second degree of unsp scapular region, init
943.29	BLISTERS-EPID LOSS-BURN-MX SITE-UPPER LIMB	**T22.291A**	Burn 2nd deg mul sites of r shldr/up lmb, ex wrs/hnd, init
		T22.292A	Burn 2nd deg mul site of left shldr/up lmb, ex wrs/hnd, init
		T22.299A	Burn 2nd deg mul sites of shldr/up lmb, except wrs/hnd, init
		T22.691A	Corros 2nd deg mul sites of r shldr/up lmb, ex wrs/hnd, init
		T22.692A	Corros 2nd deg mul site of l shldr/up lmb, ex wrs/hnd, init
		T22.699A	Corros 2nd deg mul sites of shldr/up lmb, ex wrs/hnd, init
943.3Ø	FULL-THICK SKN LOSS DUE BURN UNS SITE UPPER LIMB	**T22.3ØXA**	Burn third deg of shldr/up lmb, ex wrs/hnd, unsp site, init
		T22.7ØXA	Corros 3rd deg of shldr/up lmb, ex wrs/hnd, unsp site, init
943.31	FULL-THICKNESS SKIN LOSS DUE TO BURN OF FOREARM	**T22.311A**	Burn of third degree of right forearm, initial encounter
		T22.312A	Burn of third degree of left forearm, initial encounter
		T22.319A	Burn of third degree of unspecified forearm, init encntr
		T22.711A	Corrosion of third degree of right forearm, init encntr
		T22.712A	Corrosion of third degree of left forearm, initial encounter
		T22.719A	Corrosion of third degree of unsp forearm, init encntr
943.32	FULL-THICKNESS SKIN LOSS DUE TO BURN OF ELBOW	**T22.321A**	Burn of third degree of right elbow, initial encounter
		T22.322A	Burn of third degree of left elbow, initial encounter
		T22.329A	Burn of third degree of unspecified elbow, initial encounter
		T22.721A	Corrosion of third degree of right elbow, initial encounter
		T22.722A	Corrosion of third degree of left elbow, initial encounter
		T22.729A	Corrosion of third degree of unspecified elbow, init encntr
943.33	FULL-THICKNESS SKIN LOSS DUE TO BURN UPPER ARM	**T22.331A**	Burn of third degree of right upper arm, initial encounter
		T22.332A	Burn of third degree of left upper arm, initial encounter
		T22.339A	Burn of third degree of unspecified upper arm, init encntr
		T22.731A	Corrosion of third degree of right upper arm, init encntr
		T22.732A	Corrosion of third degree of left upper arm, init encntr
		T22.739A	Corrosion of third degree of unsp upper arm, init encntr
943.34	FULL-THICKNESS SKIN LOSS DUE TO BURN OF AXILLA	**T22.341A**	Burn of third degree of right axilla, initial encounter
		T22.342A	Burn of third degree of left axilla, initial encounter
		T22.349A	Burn of third degree of unspecified axilla, init encntr
		T22.741A	Corrosion of third degree of right axilla, initial encounter
		T22.742A	Corrosion of third degree of left axilla, initial encounter
		T22.749A	Corrosion of third degree of unspecified axilla, init encntr
943.35	FULL-THICKNESS SKIN LOSS DUE TO BURN OF SHOULDER	**T22.351A**	Burn of third degree of right shoulder, initial encounter
		T22.352A	Burn of third degree of left shoulder, initial encounter
		T22.359A	Burn of third degree of unspecified shoulder, init encntr
		T22.751A	Corrosion of third degree of right shoulder, init encntr
		T22.752A	Corrosion of third degree of left shoulder, init encntr
		T22.759A	Corrosion of third degree of unsp shoulder, init encntr
943.36	FULL-THICKNESS SKIN LOSS DUE BURN SCAP REGION	**T22.361A**	Burn of third degree of right scapular region, init encntr
		T22.362A	Burn of third degree of left scapular region, init encntr
		T22.369A	Burn of third degree of unsp scapular region, init encntr
		T22.761A	Corrosion of third degree of right scapular region, init
		T22.762A	Corrosion of third degree of left scapular region, init
		T22.769A	Corrosion of third degree of unsp scapular region, init
943.39	FULL-THICK SKIN LOSS-BURN-MX SITES UPPER LIMB	**T22.391A**	Burn 3rd deg mu sites of r shldr/up lmb, ex wrs/hnd, init
		T22.392A	Burn 3rd deg mu sites of left shldr/up lmb, ex wrs/hnd, init
		T22.399A	Burn 3rd deg mu sites of shldr/up lmb, except wrs/hnd, init
		T22.791A	Corros 3rd deg mu sites of r shldr/up lmb, ex wrs/hnd, init
		T22.792A	Corros 3rd deg mu site of l shldr/up lmb, ex wrs/hnd, init
		T22.799A	Corros 3rd deg mu sites of shldr/up lmb, ex wrs/hnd, init
943.4Ø	DEEP 3RD DEG BURN-UPPER LIMB-UNS SITE W/O LOBP	**T22.3ØXA**	Burn third deg of shldr/up lmb, ex wrs/hnd, unsp site, init
		T22.7ØXA	Corros 3rd deg of shldr/up lmb, ex wrs/hnd, unsp site, init

ICD-9-CM		ICD-10-CM	
943.41	DEEP 3RD DEG BURN-NECROSIS-FOREARM W/O LOBP	**T22.311A**	Burn of third degree of right forearm, initial encounter
		T22.312A	Burn of third degree of left forearm, initial encounter
		T22.319A	Burn of third degree of unspecified forearm, init encntr
		T22.711A	Corrosion of third degree of right forearm, init encntr
		T22.712A	Corrosion of third degree of left forearm, initial encounter
		T22.719A	Corrosion of third degree of unsp forearm, init encntr
943.42	DEEP 3RD DEG BURN-NECROSIS-ELBOW W/O LOBP	**T22.321A**	Burn of third degree of right elbow, initial encounter
		T22.322A	Burn of third degree of left elbow, initial encounter
		T22.329A	Burn of third degree of unspecified elbow, initial encounter
		T22.721A	Corrosion of third degree of right elbow, initial encounter
		T22.722A	Corrosion of third degree of left elbow, initial encounter
		T22.729A	Corrosion of third degree of unspecified elbow, init encntr
943.43	DEEP 3RD DEG BURN-NECROSIS-UPPER ARM W/O LOBP	**T22.331A**	Burn of third degree of right upper arm, initial encounter
		T22.332A	Burn of third degree of left upper arm, initial encounter
		T22.339A	Burn of third degree of unspecified upper arm, init encntr
		T22.731A	Corrosion of third degree of right upper arm, init encntr
		T22.732A	Corrosion of third degree of left upper arm, init encntr
		T22.739A	Corrosion of third degree of unsp upper arm, init encntr
943.44	DEEP 3RD DEG UNDLY TISS-BRN AX W/O LOSS BDY PART	**T22.341A**	Burn of third degree of right axilla, initial encounter
		T22.342A	Burn of third degree of left axilla, initial encounter
		T22.349A	Burn of third degree of unspecified axilla, init encntr
		T22.741A	Corrosion of third degree of right axilla, initial encounter
		T22.742A	Corrosion of third degree of left axilla, initial encounter
		T22.749A	Corrosion of third degree of unspecified axilla, init encntr
943.45	DEEP 3RD DEG BURN-NECROSIS-SHOULDER W/O LOBP	**T22.351A**	Burn of third degree of right shoulder, initial encounter
		T22.352A	Burn of third degree of left shoulder, initial encounter
		T22.359A	Burn of third degree of unspecified shoulder, init encntr
		T22.751A	Corrosion of third degree of right shoulder, init encntr
		T22.752A	Corrosion of third degree of left shoulder, init encntr
		T22.759A	Corrosion of third degree of unsp shoulder, init encntr
943.46	DEEP 3RD DEG BURN-SCAPULA W/O LOBP	**T22.361A**	Burn of third degree of right scapular region, init encntr
		T22.362A	Burn of third degree of left scapular region, init encntr
		T22.369A	Burn of third degree of unsp scapular region, init encntr
		T22.761A	Corrosion of third degree of right scapular region, init
		T22.762A	Corrosion of third degree of left scapular region, init
		T22.769A	Corrosion of third degree of unsp scapular region, init
943.49	DEEP 3RD DEG BURN-MX SITES-UP LIMB W/O LOBP	**T22.391A**	Burn 3rd deg mu sites of r shldr/up lmb, ex wrs/hnd, init
		T22.392A	Burn 3rd deg mu sites of left shldr/up lmb, ex wrs/hnd, init
		T22.399A	Burn 3rd deg mu sites of shldr/up lmb, except wrs/hnd, init
		T22.791A	Corros 3rd deg mu sites of r shldr/up lmb, ex wrs/hnd, init
		T22.792A	Corros 3rd deg mu site of l shldr/up lmb, ex wrs/hnd, init
		T22.799A	Corros 3rd deg mu sites of shldr/up lmb, ex wrs/hnd, init
943.5Ø	DEEP 3RD DEG BURN-UNS SITE-UPPR LIMB W/LOBP	**T22.3ØXA**	Burn third deg of shldr/up lmb, ex wrs/hnd, unsp site, init
		T22.7ØXA	Corros 3rd deg of shldr/up lmb, ex wrs/hnd, unsp site, init
943.51	DEEP 3RD DEG BURN-NECROSIS-FOREARM W/LOBP	**T22.311A**	Burn of third degree of right forearm, initial encounter
		T22.312A	Burn of third degree of left forearm, initial encounter
		T22.319A	Burn of third degree of unspecified forearm, init encntr
		T22.711A	Corrosion of third degree of right forearm, init encntr
		T22.712A	Corrosion of third degree of left forearm, initial encounter
		T22.719A	Corrosion of third degree of unsp forearm, init encntr
943.52	DP 3RD DEG UNDLYING TISS-BRN ELB W/LOSS BDY PART	**T22.321A**	Burn of third degree of right elbow, initial encounter
		T22.322A	Burn of third degree of left elbow, initial encounter
		T22.329A	Burn of third degree of unspecified elbow, initial encounter
		T22.721A	Corrosion of third degree of right elbow, initial encounter
		T22.722A	Corrosion of third degree of left elbow, initial encounter
		T22.729A	Corrosion of third degree of unspecified elbow, init encntr
943.53	DEEP 3RD DEG BURN-NECROSIS-UPPER ARM W/LOBP	**T22.331A**	Burn of third degree of right upper arm, initial encounter
		T22.332A	Burn of third degree of left upper arm, initial encounter
		T22.339A	Burn of third degree of unspecified upper arm, init encntr
		T22.731A	Corrosion of third degree of right upper arm, init encntr
		T22.732A	Corrosion of third degree of left upper arm, init encntr
		T22.739A	Corrosion of third degree of unsp upper arm, init encntr
943.54	DP 3RD DEG UNDLYING TISS-BURN AX W/LOSS BDY PART	**T22.341A**	Burn of third degree of right axilla, initial encounter
		T22.342A	Burn of third degree of left axilla, initial encounter
		T22.349A	Burn of third degree of unspecified axilla, init encntr
		T22.741A	Corrosion of third degree of right axilla, initial encounter
		T22.742A	Corrosion of third degree of left axilla, initial encounter
		T22.749A	Corrosion of third degree of unspecified axilla, init encntr
943.55	DEEP 3RD DEG BURN-NECROSIS-SHOULDER W/LOBP	**T22.351A**	Burn of third degree of right shoulder, initial encounter
		T22.352A	Burn of third degree of left shoulder, initial encounter
		T22.359A	Burn of third degree of unspecified shoulder, init encntr
		T22.751A	Corrosion of third degree of right shoulder, init encntr
		T22.752A	Corrosion of third degree of left shoulder, init encntr
		T22.759A	Corrosion of third degree of unsp shoulder, init encntr
943.56	DEEP 3RD DEG BURN-NECROSIS-SCAPULA W/LOBP	**T22.361A**	Burn of third degree of right scapular region, init encntr
		T22.362A	Burn of third degree of left scapular region, init encntr
		T22.369A	Burn of third degree of unsp scapular region, init encntr
		T22.761A	Corrosion of third degree of right scapular region, init
		T22.762A	Corrosion of third degree of left scapular region, init
		T22.769A	Corrosion of third degree of unsp scapular region, init

Injury and Poisoning

ICD-9-CM		ICD-10-CM	
943.59	DEEP 3RD DEG BURN-MX SITES-UPPER LIMB W/LOBP	**T22.391A**	Burn 3rd deg mu sites of r shldr/up lmb, ex wrs/hnd, init
		T22.392A	Burn 3rd deg mu sites of left shldr/up lmb, ex wrs/hnd, init
		T22.399A	Burn 3rd deg mu sites of shldr/up lmb, except wrs/hnd, init
		T22.791A	Corros 3rd deg mu sites of r shldr/up lmb, ex wrs/hnd, init
		T22.792A	Corros 3rd deg mu site of l shldr/up lmb, ex wrs/hnd, init
		T22.799A	Corros 3rd deg mu sites of shldr/up lmb, ex wrs/hnd, init
944.00	BURN UNSPECIFIED DEGREE UNSPECIFIED SITE HAND	**T23.001A**	Burn of unsp degree of right hand, unsp site, init encntr
		T23.002A	Burn of unsp degree of left hand, unsp site, init encntr
		T23.009A	Burn of unsp degree of unsp hand, unsp site, init encntr
		T23.401A	Corrosion of unsp degree of right hand, unsp site, init
		T23.402A	Corrosion of unsp degree of left hand, unsp site, init
		T23.409A	Corrosion of unsp degree of unsp hand, unsp site, init
944.01	BURN-UNS DEGREE-1 FINGER OTH THAN THUMB	**T23.021A**	Burn unsp degree of single r finger except thumb, init
		T23.022A	Burn unsp degree of single l finger except thumb, init
		T23.029A	Burn unsp degree of unsp single finger except thumb, init
		T23.421A	Corros unsp degree of single r finger except thumb, init
		T23.422A	Corros unsp degree of single l finger except thumb, init
		T23.429A	Corros unsp degree of unsp single finger except thumb, init
944.02	BURN OF UNSPECIFIED DEGREE OF THUMB	**T23.011A**	Burn of unsp degree of right thumb (nail), init encntr
		T23.012A	Burn of unspecified degree of left thumb (nail), init encntr
		T23.019A	Burn of unsp degree of unspecified thumb (nail), init encntr
		T23.411A	Corrosion of unsp degree of right thumb (nail), init encntr
		T23.412A	Corrosion of unsp degree of left thumb (nail), init encntr
		T23.419A	Corrosion of unsp degree of unsp thumb (nail), init encntr
944.03	BURN-UNS DEG-2/MORE DIGITS OF HAND NOT THUMB	**T23.031A**	Burn unsp deg mult right fingers (nail), not inc thumb, init
		T23.032A	Burn unsp deg mult left fingers (nail), not inc thumb, init
		T23.039A	Burn unsp degree of unsp mult fngr, not inc thumb, init
		T23.431A	Corros unsp deg mult right fngr (nail), not inc thumb, init
		T23.432A	Corros unsp deg mult left fngr (nail), not inc thumb, init
		T23.439A	Corros unsp degree of unsp mult fngr, not inc thumb, init
944.04	BURN-UNS DEG-2/MORE DIGITS OF HAND W/THUMB	**T23.041A**	Burn of unsp deg mult right fingers (nail), inc thumb, init
		T23.042A	Burn of unsp deg mult left fingers (nail), inc thumb, init
		T23.049A	Burn unsp degree of unsp mult fngr (nail), inc thumb, init
		T23.441A	Corros unsp deg mult right fingers (nail), inc thumb, init
		T23.442A	Corros unsp deg mult left fingers (nail), inc thumb, init
		T23.449A	Corros unsp degree of unsp mult fngr (nail), inc thumb, init
944.05	BURN OF UNSPECIFIED DEGREE OF PALM OF HAND	**T23.051A**	Burn of unspecified degree of right palm, initial encounter
		T23.052A	Burn of unspecified degree of left palm, initial encounter
		T23.059A	Burn of unspecified degree of unspecified palm, init encntr
		T23.451A	Corrosion of unspecified degree of right palm, init encntr
		T23.452A	Corrosion of unspecified degree of left palm, init encntr
		T23.459A	Corrosion of unsp degree of unspecified palm, init encntr
944.06	BURN OF UNSPECIFIED DEGREE OF BACK OF HAND	**T23.061A**	Burn of unsp degree of back of right hand, init encntr
		T23.062A	Burn of unspecified degree of back of left hand, init encntr
		T23.069A	Burn of unsp degree of back of unspecified hand, init encntr
		T23.461A	Corrosion of unsp degree of back of right hand, init encntr
		T23.462A	Corrosion of unsp degree of back of left hand, init encntr
		T23.469A	Corrosion of unsp degree of back of unsp hand, init encntr
944.07	BURN OF UNSPECIFIED DEGREE OF WRIST	**T23.071A**	Burn of unspecified degree of right wrist, initial encounter
		T23.072A	Burn of unspecified degree of left wrist, initial encounter
		T23.079A	Burn of unspecified degree of unspecified wrist, init encntr
		T23.471A	Corrosion of unspecified degree of right wrist, init encntr
		T23.472A	Corrosion of unspecified degree of left wrist, init encntr
		T23.479A	Corrosion of unsp degree of unspecified wrist, init encntr
944.08	BURN UNSPEC DEGREE MULTIPLE SITES WRIST&HAND	**T23.091A**	Burn of unsp deg mult sites of right wrist and hand, init
		T23.092A	Burn of unsp deg mult sites of left wrist and hand, init
		T23.099A	Burn of unsp deg mult sites of unsp wrist and hand, init
		T23.491A	Corrosion of unsp deg mult sites of right wrs/hnd, init
		T23.492A	Corrosion of unsp deg mult sites of left wrs/hnd, init
		T23.499A	Corrosion of unsp deg mult sites of unsp wrs/hnd, init
944.10	ERYTHEMA DUE TO BURN OF UNSPECIFIED SITE OF HAND	**T23.101A**	Burn of first degree of right hand, unsp site, init encntr
		T23.102A	Burn of first degree of left hand, unsp site, init encntr
		T23.109A	Burn of first degree of unsp hand, unsp site, init encntr
		T23.501A	Corrosion of first degree of right hand, unsp site, init
		T23.502A	Corrosion of first degree of left hand, unsp site, init
		T23.509A	Corrosion of first degree of unsp hand, unsp site, init
944.11	ERYTHEMA DUE BURN-SINGLE DIGIT OTH THAN THUMB	**T23.121A**	Burn first degree of single r finger except thumb, init
		T23.122A	Burn first degree of single l finger except thumb, init
		T23.129A	Burn first degree of unsp single finger except thumb, init
		T23.521A	Corros first degree of single r finger except thumb, init
		T23.522A	Corros first degree of single l finger except thumb, init
		T23.529A	Corros first degree of unsp single finger except thumb, init
944.12	ERYTHEMA DUE TO BURN OF THUMB	**T23.111A**	Burn of first degree of right thumb (nail), init encntr
		T23.112A	Burn of first degree of left thumb (nail), initial encounter
		T23.119A	Burn of first degree of unsp thumb (nail), init encntr
		T23.511A	Corrosion of first degree of right thumb (nail), init encntr
		T23.512A	Corrosion of first degree of left thumb (nail), init encntr
		T23.519A	Corrosion of first degree of unsp thumb (nail), init encntr

943.59–944.12

[Brackets] indicate valid character values for each code. Character value meanings provided for each code grouping.

ICD-9-CM		ICD-10-CM	
944.13	ERYTHEMA DUE BURN-2/MORE DIGITS HAND NOT THUMB	**T23.131A**	Burn first deg mult right fngr (nail), not inc thumb, init
		T23.132A	Burn first deg mult left fingers (nail), not inc thumb, init
		T23.139A	Burn first degree of unsp mult fngr, not inc thumb, init
		T23.531A	Corros first deg mult right fngr (nail), not inc thumb, init
		T23.532A	Corros first deg mult left fngr (nail), not inc thumb, init
		T23.539A	Corros first degree of unsp mult fngr, not inc thumb, init
944.14	ERYTHEMA DUE BURN-2/MORE DIGITS HAND INCL THUMB	**T23.141A**	Burn of first deg mult right fingers (nail), inc thumb, init
		T23.142A	Burn of first deg mult left fingers (nail), inc thumb, init
		T23.149A	Burn first degree of unsp mult fngr (nail), inc thumb, init
		T23.541A	Corros first deg mult right fingers (nail), inc thumb, init
		T23.542A	Corros first deg mult left fingers (nail), inc thumb, init
		T23.549A	Corros first degree of unsp mult fngr, inc thumb, init
944.15	ERYTHEMA DUE TO BURN OF PALM OF HAND	**T23.151A**	Burn of first degree of right palm, initial encounter
		T23.152A	Burn of first degree of left palm, initial encounter
		T23.159A	Burn of first degree of unspecified palm, initial encounter
		T23.551A	Corrosion of first degree of right palm, initial encounter
		T23.552A	Corrosion of first degree of left palm, initial encounter
		T23.559A	Corrosion of first degree of unspecified palm, init encntr
944.16	ERYTHEMA DUE TO BURN OF BACK OF HAND	**T23.161A**	Burn of first degree of back of right hand, init encntr
		T23.162A	Burn of first degree of back of left hand, initial encounter
		T23.169A	Burn of first degree of back of unsp hand, init encntr
		T23.561A	Corrosion of first degree of back of right hand, init encntr
		T23.562A	Corrosion of first degree of back of left hand, init encntr
		T23.569A	Corrosion of first degree of back of unsp hand, init encntr
944.17	ERYTHEMA DUE TO BURN OF WRIST	**T23.171A**	Burn of first degree of right wrist, initial encounter
		T23.172A	Burn of first degree of left wrist, initial encounter
		T23.179A	Burn of first degree of unspecified wrist, initial encounter
		T23.571A	Corrosion of first degree of right wrist, initial encounter
		T23.572A	Corrosion of first degree of left wrist, initial encounter
		T23.579A	Corrosion of first degree of unspecified wrist, init encntr
944.18	ERYTHEMA DUE TO BURN MULTIPLE SITES WRIST&HAND	**T23.191A**	Burn of first deg mult sites of right wrist and hand, init
		T23.192A	Burn of first deg mult sites of left wrist and hand, init
		T23.199A	Burn of first deg mult sites of unsp wrist and hand, init
		T23.591A	Corrosion of first deg mult sites of right wrs/hnd, init
		T23.592A	Corrosion of first deg mult sites of left wrs/hnd, init
		T23.599A	Corrosion of first deg mult sites of unsp wrs/hnd, init
944.2Ø	BLISTR W/EPID LOSS DUE BURN UNSPEC SITE HAND	**T23.2Ø1A**	Burn of second degree of right hand, unsp site, init encntr
		T23.2Ø2A	Burn of second degree of left hand, unsp site, init encntr
		T23.2Ø9A	Burn of second degree of unsp hand, unsp site, init encntr
		T23.6Ø1A	Corrosion of second degree of right hand, unsp site, init
		T23.6Ø2A	Corrosion of second degree of left hand, unsp site, init
		T23.6Ø9A	Corrosion of second degree of unsp hand, unsp site, init
944.21	BLISTERS W/EPID LOSS-BURN-SINGLE DIGIT NOT THUMB	**T23.221A**	Burn second degree of single r finger except thumb, init
		T23.222A	Burn second degree of single l finger except thumb, init
		T23.229A	Burn second degree of unsp single finger except thumb, init
		T23.621A	Corros second degree of single r finger except thumb, init
		T23.622A	Corros second degree of single l finger except thumb, init
		T23.629A	Corros second deg of unsp single finger except thumb, init
944.22	BLISTERS W/EPIDERMAL LOSS DUE TO BURN OF THUMB	**T23.211A**	Burn of second degree of right thumb (nail), init encntr
		T23.212A	Burn of second degree of left thumb (nail), init encntr
		T23.219A	Burn of second degree of unsp thumb (nail), init encntr
		T23.611A	Corrosion of second degree of right thumb (nail), init
		T23.612A	Corrosion of second degree of left thumb (nail), init encntr
		T23.619A	Corrosion of second degree of unsp thumb (nail), init encntr
944.23	BLISTRS W/EPID LOSS-BURN-2/MORE DIGITS NOT THUMB	**T23.231A**	Burn 2nd deg mul right fingers (nail), not inc thumb, init
		T23.232A	Burn of 2nd deg mul left fingers (nail), not inc thumb, init
		T23.239A	Burn second degree of unsp mult fngr, not inc thumb, init
		T23.631A	Corros 2nd deg mul right fingers (nail), not inc thumb, init
		T23.632A	Corros 2nd deg mul left fingers (nail), not inc thumb, init
		T23.639A	Corros second degree of unsp mult fngr, not inc thumb, init
944.24	BLISTERS W/EPID LOSS-BURN-2/MORE DIGITS W/THUMB	**T23.241A**	Burn of 2nd deg mul right fingers (nail), inc thumb, init
		T23.242A	Burn of 2nd deg mul left fingers (nail), inc thumb, init
		T23.249A	Burn second degree of unsp mult fngr (nail), inc thumb, init
		T23.641A	Corros 2nd deg mul right fingers (nail), inc thumb, init
		T23.642A	Corros 2nd deg mul left fingers (nail), inc thumb, init
		T23.649A	Corros second degree of unsp mult fngr, inc thumb, init
944.25	BLISTERS W/EPIDERMAL LOSS-BURN-PALM HAND	**T23.251A**	Burn of second degree of right palm, initial encounter
		T23.252A	Burn of second degree of left palm, initial encounter
		T23.259A	Burn of second degree of unspecified palm, initial encounter
		T23.651A	Corrosion of second degree of right palm, initial encounter
		T23.652A	Corrosion of second degree of left palm, initial encounter
		T23.659A	Corrosion of second degree of unspecified palm, init encntr
944.26	BLISTERS W/EPIDERMAL LOSS DUE TO BURN BACK HAND	**T23.261A**	Burn of second degree of back of right hand, init encntr
		T23.262A	Burn of second degree of back of left hand, init encntr
		T23.269A	Burn of second degree of back of unsp hand, init encntr
		T23.661A	Corrosion of second degree back of right hand, init encntr
		T23.662A	Corrosion of second degree back of left hand, init encntr
		T23.669A	Corrosion of second degree back of unsp hand, init encntr

ICD-9-CM		ICD-10-CM	
944.27	BLISTERS W/EPIDERMAL LOSS DUE TO BURN OF WRIST	**T23.271A**	Burn of second degree of right wrist, initial encounter
		T23.272A	Burn of second degree of left wrist, initial encounter
		T23.279A	Burn of second degree of unspecified wrist, init encntr
		T23.671A	Corrosion of second degree of right wrist, initial encounter
		T23.672A	Corrosion of second degree of left wrist, initial encounter
		T23.679A	Corrosion of second degree of unspecified wrist, init encntr
944.28	BLISTERS W/EPID LOSS-BURN-MULT SITE-WRIST&HAND	**T23.291A**	Burn of 2nd deg mul sites of right wrist and hand, init
		T23.292A	Burn of 2nd deg mul sites of left wrist and hand, init
		T23.299A	Burn of 2nd deg mul sites of unsp wrist and hand, init
		T23.691A	Corrosion of 2nd deg mul sites of right wrist and hand, init
		T23.692A	Corrosion of 2nd deg mul sites of left wrist and hand, init
		T23.699A	Corrosion of 2nd deg mul sites of unsp wrist and hand, init
944.30	FULL-THICK SKIN LOSS DUE BURN UNSPEC SITE HAND	**T23.301A**	Burn of third degree of right hand, unsp site, init encntr
		T23.302A	Burn of third degree of left hand, unsp site, init encntr
		T23.309A	Burn of third degree of unsp hand, unsp site, init encntr
		T23.701A	Corrosion of third degree of right hand, unsp site, init
		T23.702A	Corrosion of third degree of left hand, unsp site, init
		T23.709A	Corrosion of third degree of unsp hand, unsp site, init
944.31	FULL-THICK SKIN LOSS-BURN-SINGLE DIGIT NOT THUMB	**T23.321A**	Burn third degree of single r finger except thumb, init
		T23.322A	Burn third degree of single l finger except thumb, init
		T23.329A	Burn third degree of unsp single finger except thumb, init
		T23.721A	Corros third degree of single r finger except thumb, init
		T23.722A	Corros third degree of single l finger except thumb, init
		T23.729A	Corros third degree of unsp single finger except thumb, init
944.32	FULL-THICKNESS SKIN LOSS DUE TO BURN OF THUMB	**T23.311A**	Burn of third degree of right thumb (nail), init encntr
		T23.312A	Burn of third degree of left thumb (nail), initial encounter
		T23.319A	Burn of third degree of unsp thumb (nail), init encntr
		T23.711A	Corrosion of third degree of right thumb (nail), init encntr
		T23.712A	Corrosion of third degree of left thumb (nail), init encntr
		T23.719A	Corrosion of third degree of unsp thumb (nail), init encntr
944.33	FULL-THICK SKIN LOSS-BURN-2/MORE DIGTS NOT THUMB	**T23.331A**	Burn of 3rd deg mu right fingers (nail), not inc thumb, init
		T23.332A	Burn of 3rd deg mu left fingers (nail), not inc thumb, init
		T23.339A	Burn third degree of unsp mult fngr, not inc thumb, init
		T23.731A	Corros 3rd deg mu right fingers (nail), not inc thumb, init
		T23.732A	Corros 3rd deg mu left fingers (nail), not inc thumb, init
		T23.739A	Corros third degree of unsp mult fngr, not inc thumb, init
944.34	FULL-THICK SKIN LOSS-BURN-2/MORE DIGTS W/THUMB	**T23.341A**	Burn of 3rd deg mu right fingers (nail), inc thumb, init
		T23.342A	Burn of 3rd deg mu left fingers (nail), inc thumb, init
		T23.349A	Burn third degree of unsp mult fngr (nail), inc thumb, init
		T23.741A	Corros 3rd deg mu right fingers (nail), inc thumb, init
		T23.742A	Corros 3rd deg mu left fingers (nail), including thumb, init
		T23.749A	Corros third degree of unsp mult fngr, inc thumb, init
944.35	FULL-THICKNESS SKIN LOSS DUE TO BURN PALM HAND	**T23.351A**	Burn of third degree of right palm, initial encounter
		T23.352A	Burn of third degree of left palm, initial encounter
		T23.359A	Burn of third degree of unspecified palm, initial encounter
		T23.751A	Corrosion of third degree of right palm, initial encounter
		T23.752A	Corrosion of third degree of left palm, initial encounter
		T23.759A	Corrosion of third degree of unspecified palm, init encntr
944.36	FULL-THICKNESS SKIN LOSS DUE TO BURN BACK HAND	**T23.361A**	Burn of third degree of back of right hand, init encntr
		T23.362A	Burn of third degree of back of left hand, initial encounter
		T23.369A	Burn of third degree of back of unsp hand, init encntr
		T23.761A	Corrosion of third degree of back of right hand, init encntr
		T23.762A	Corrosion of third degree of back of left hand, init encntr
		T23.769A	Corrosion of third degree back of unsp hand, init encntr
944.37	FULL-THICKNESS SKIN LOSS DUE TO BURN OF WRIST	**T23.371A**	Burn of third degree of right wrist, initial encounter
		T23.372A	Burn of third degree of left wrist, initial encounter
		T23.379A	Burn of third degree of unspecified wrist, initial encounter
		T23.771A	Corrosion of third degree of right wrist, initial encounter
		T23.772A	Corrosion of third degree of left wrist, initial encounter
		T23.779A	Corrosion of third degree of unspecified wrist, init encntr
944.38	FULL-THICK SKIN LOSS-BURN-MULT SITE-WRIST&HAND	**T23.391A**	Burn of 3rd deg mu sites of right wrist and hand, init
		T23.392A	Burn of 3rd deg mu sites of left wrist and hand, init
		T23.399A	Burn of 3rd deg mu sites of unsp wrist and hand, init
		T23.791A	Corrosion of 3rd deg mu sites of right wrist and hand, init
		T23.792A	Corrosion of 3rd deg mu sites of left wrist and hand, init
		T23.799A	Corrosion of 3rd deg mu sites of unsp wrist and hand, init
944.40	DEEP 3RD DEG BURN-NECROS-UNS SITE-HAND W/O LOBP	**T23.301A**	Burn of third degree of right hand, unsp site, init encntr
		T23.302A	Burn of third degree of left hand, unsp site, init encntr
		T23.309A	Burn of third degree of unsp hand, unsp site, init encntr
		T23.701A	Corrosion of third degree of right hand, unsp site, init
		T23.702A	Corrosion of third degree of left hand, unsp site, init
		T23.709A	Corrosion of third degree of unsp hand, unsp site, init
944.41	DEEP 3RD DEG BURN OF 1 DIGIT-NOT THUMB W/O LOBP	**T23.321A**	Burn third degree of single r finger except thumb, init
		T23.322A	Burn third degree of single l finger except thumb, init
		T23.329A	Burn third degree of unsp single finger except thumb, init
		T23.721A	Corros third degree of single r finger except thumb, init
		T23.722A	Corros third degree of single l finger except thumb, init
		T23.729A	Corros third degree of unsp single finger except thumb, init

ICD-9-CM		ICD-10-CM	
944.42	DEEP 3RD DEG BURN-NECROSIS-THUMB W/O LOBP	**T23.311A**	Burn of third degree of right thumb (nail), init encntr
		T23.312A	Burn of third degree of left thumb (nail), initial encounter
		T23.319A	Burn of third degree of unsp thumb (nail), init encntr
		T23.711A	Corrosion of third degree of right thumb (nail), init encntr
		T23.712A	Corrosion of third degree of left thumb (nail), init encntr
		T23.719A	Corrosion of third degree of unsp thumb (nail), init encntr
944.43	DEEP 3RD DEG BURN-2/MORE DIGTS-NO THUMB W/O LOBP	**T23.331A**	Burn of 3rd deg mu right fingers (nail), not inc thumb, init
		T23.332A	Burn of 3rd deg mu left fingers (nail), not inc thumb, init
		T23.339A	Burn third degree of unsp mult fngr, not inc thumb, init
		T23.731A	Corros 3rd deg mu right fingers (nail), not inc thumb, init
		T23.732A	Corros 3rd deg mu left fingers (nail), not inc thumb, init
		T23.739A	Corros third degree of unsp mult fngr, not inc thumb, init
944.44	DEEP 3RD DEG BURN-2/MORE DIGITS W/THUMB W/O LOBP	**T23.341A**	Burn of 3rd deg mu right fingers (nail), inc thumb, init
		T23.342A	Burn of 3rd deg mu left fingers (nail), inc thumb, init
		T23.349A	Burn third degree of unsp mult fngr (nail), inc thumb, init
		T23.741A	Corros 3rd deg mu right fingers (nail), inc thumb, init
		T23.742A	Corros 3rd deg mu left fingers (nail), including thumb, init
		T23.749A	Corros third degree of unsp mult fngr, inc thumb, init
944.45	DEEP 3RD DEG BURN-NECROSIS-PALM W/O LOBP	**T23.351A**	Burn of third degree of right palm, initial encounter
		T23.352A	Burn of third degree of left palm, initial encounter
		T23.359A	Burn of third degree of unspecified palm, initial encounter
		T23.751A	Corrosion of third degree of right palm, initial encounter
		T23.752A	Corrosion of third degree of left palm, initial encounter
		T23.759A	Corrosion of third degree of unspecified palm, init encntr
944.46	DEEP 3RD DEG BURN-NECROSIS-BACK OF HAND W/O LOBP	**T23.361A**	Burn of third degree of back of right hand, init encntr
		T23.362A	Burn of third degree of back of left hand, initial encounter
		T23.369A	Burn of third degree of back of unsp hand, init encntr
		T23.761A	Corrosion of third degree of back of right hand, init encntr
		T23.762A	Corrosion of third degree of back of left hand, init encntr
		T23.769A	Corrosion of third degree back of unsp hand, init encntr
944.47	DEEP 3RD DEG BURN-NECROSIS OF WRIST W/O LOBP	**T23.371A**	Burn of third degree of right wrist, initial encounter
		T23.372A	Burn of third degree of left wrist, initial encounter
		T23.379A	Burn of third degree of unspecified wrist, initial encounter
		T23.771A	Corrosion of third degree of right wrist, initial encounter
		T23.772A	Corrosion of third degree of left wrist, initial encounter
		T23.779A	Corrosion of third degree of unspecified wrist, init encntr
944.48	DEEP 3RD DEG BURN-MX SITES WRIST-HAND W/O LOBP	**T23.391A**	Burn of 3rd deg mu sites of right wrist and hand, init
		T23.392A	Burn of 3rd deg mu sites of left wrist and hand, init
		T23.399A	Burn of 3rd deg mu sites of unsp wrist and hand, init
		T23.791A	Corrosion of 3rd deg mu sites of right wrist and hand, init
		T23.792A	Corrosion of 3rd deg mu sites of left wrist and hand, init
		T23.799A	Corrosion of 3rd deg mu sites of unsp wrist and hand, init
944.50	DP 3RD DEF UNDLYING TISS-BRN HND W/LOSS BDY PART	**T23.301A**	Burn of third degree of right hand, unsp site, init encntr
		T23.302A	Burn of third degree of left hand, unsp site, init encntr
		T23.309A	Burn of third degree of unsp hand, unsp site, init encntr
		T23.701A	Corrosion of third degree of right hand, unsp site, init
		T23.702A	Corrosion of third degree of left hand, unsp site, init
		T23.709A	Corrosion of third degree of unsp hand, unsp site, init
944.51	DEEP 3RD DEGR BURN-SINGLE DIGIT-NOT THUMB W/LOBP	**T23.321A**	Burn third degree of single r finger except thumb, init
		T23.322A	Burn third degree of single l finger except thumb, init
		T23.329A	Burn third degree of unsp single finger except thumb, init
		T23.721A	Corros third degree of single r finger except thumb, init
		T23.722A	Corros third degree of single l finger except thumb, init
		T23.729A	Corros third degree of unsp single finger except thumb, init
944.52	DEEP 3RD DEG BURN-NECROSIS-THUMB W/LOBP	**T23.311A**	Burn of third degree of right thumb (nail), init encntr
		T23.312A	Burn of third degree of left thumb (nail), initial encounter
		T23.319A	Burn of third degree of unsp thumb (nail), init encntr
		T23.711A	Corrosion of third degree of right thumb (nail), init encntr
		T23.712A	Corrosion of third degree of left thumb (nail), init encntr
		T23.719A	Corrosion of third degree of unsp thumb (nail), init encntr
944.53	DEEP 3RD DGR BURN-2/MORE DIGITS-NO THUMB W/LOBP	**T23.331A**	Burn of 3rd deg mu right fingers (nail), not inc thumb, init
		T23.332A	Burn of 3rd deg mu left fingers (nail), not inc thumb, init
		T23.339A	Burn third degree of unsp mult fngr, not inc thumb, init
		T23.731A	Corros 3rd deg mu right fingers (nail), not inc thumb, init
		T23.732A	Corros 3rd deg mu left fingers (nail), not inc thumb, init
		T23.739A	Corros third degree of unsp mult fngr, not inc thumb, init
944.54	DEEP 3RD DEG BURN-2/MORE DIGITS W/THUMB W/LOBP	**T23.341A**	Burn of 3rd deg mu right fingers (nail), inc thumb, init
		T23.342A	Burn of 3rd deg mu left fingers (nail), inc thumb, init
		T23.349A	Burn third degree of unsp mult fngr (nail), inc thumb, init
		T23.741A	Corros 3rd deg mu right fingers (nail), inc thumb, init
		T23.742A	Corros 3rd deg mu left fingers (nail), including thumb, init
		T23.749A	Corros third degree of unsp mult fngr, inc thumb, init
944.55	DEEP 3RD DEG BURN-NECROSIS-PALM W/LOBP	**T23.351A**	Burn of third degree of right palm, initial encounter
		T23.352A	Burn of third degree of left palm, initial encounter
		T23.359A	Burn of third degree of unspecified palm, initial encounter
		T23.751A	Corrosion of third degree of right palm, initial encounter
		T23.752A	Corrosion of third degree of left palm, initial encounter
		T23.759A	Corrosion of third degree of unspecified palm, init encntr

ICD-9-CM		ICD-10-CM	
944.56	DEEP 3RD DEG BURN-NECROSIS-BACK OF HAND W/LOBP	**T23.361A**	Burn of third degree of back of right hand, init encntr
		T23.362A	Burn of third degree of back of left hand, initial encounter
		T23.369A	Burn of third degree of back of unsp hand, init encntr
		T23.761A	Corrosion of third degree of back of right hand, init encntr
		T23.762A	Corrosion of third degree of back of left hand, init encntr
		T23.769A	Corrosion of third degree back of unsp hand, init encntr
944.57	DEEP 3RD DEG UNDLY TISS-BRN WRST W/LOSS BDY PART	**T23.371A**	Burn of third degree of right wrist, initial encounter
		T23.372A	Burn of third degree of left wrist, initial encounter
		T23.379A	Burn of third degree of unspecified wrist, initial encounter
		T23.771A	Corrosion of third degree of right wrist, initial encounter
		T23.772A	Corrosion of third degree of left wrist, initial encounter
		T23.779A	Corrosion of third degree of unspecified wrist, init encntr
944.58	DEEP 3RD DEG BURN-MX SITES-WRIST&HAND W/LOBP	**T23.391A**	Burn of 3rd deg mu sites of right wrist and hand, init
		T23.392A	Burn of 3rd deg mu sites of left wrist and hand, init
		T23.399A	Burn of 3rd deg mu sites of unsp wrist and hand, init
		T23.791A	Corrosion of 3rd deg mu sites of right wrist and hand, init
		T23.792A	Corrosion of 3rd deg mu sites of left wrist and hand, init
		T23.799A	Corrosion of 3rd deg mu sites of unsp wrist and hand, init
945.ØØ	BURN UNSPEC DEGREE UNSPEC SITE LOWER LIMB	**T24.ØØ1A**	Burn unsp deg of unsp site right lower limb, ex ank/ft, init
		T24.ØØ2A	Burn unsp deg of unsp site left lower limb, ex ank/ft, init
		T24.ØØ9A	Burn unsp deg of unsp site unsp lower limb, ex ank/ft, init
		T24.4Ø1A	Corros unsp deg of unsp site right low limb, ex ank/ft, init
		T24.4Ø2A	Corros unsp deg of unsp site left low limb, ex ank/ft, init
		T24.4Ø9A	Corros unsp deg of unsp site unsp low limb, ex ank/ft, init
945.Ø1	BURN OF UNSPECIFIED DEGREE OF TOE	**T25.Ø31A**	Burn of unsp degree of right toe(s) (nail), init encntr
		T25.Ø32A	Burn of unsp degree of left toe(s) (nail), init encntr
		T25.Ø39A	Burn of unsp degree of unsp toe(s) (nail), init encntr
		T25.431A	Corrosion of unsp degree of right toe(s) (nail), init encntr
		T25.432A	Corrosion of unsp degree of left toe(s) (nail), init encntr
		T25.439A	Corrosion of unsp degree of unsp toe(s) (nail), init encntr
945.Ø2	BURN OF UNSPECIFIED DEGREE OF FOOT	**T25.Ø21A**	Burn of unspecified degree of right foot, initial encounter
		T25.Ø22A	Burn of unspecified degree of left foot, initial encounter
		T25.Ø29A	Burn of unspecified degree of unspecified foot, init encntr
		T25.421A	Corrosion of unspecified degree of right foot, init encntr
		T25.422A	Corrosion of unspecified degree of left foot, init encntr
		T25.429A	Corrosion of unsp degree of unspecified foot, init encntr
945.Ø3	BURN OF UNSPECIFIED DEGREE OF ANKLE	**T25.Ø11A**	Burn of unspecified degree of right ankle, initial encounter
		T25.Ø12A	Burn of unspecified degree of left ankle, initial encounter
		T25.Ø19A	Burn of unspecified degree of unspecified ankle, init encntr
		T25.411A	Corrosion of unspecified degree of right ankle, init encntr
		T25.412A	Corrosion of unspecified degree of left ankle, init encntr
		T25.419A	Corrosion of unsp degree of unspecified ankle, init encntr
945.Ø4	BURN OF UNSPECIFIED DEGREE OF LOWER LEG	**T24.Ø31A**	Burn of unspecified degree of right lower leg, init encntr
		T24.Ø32A	Burn of unspecified degree of left lower leg, init encntr
		T24.Ø39A	Burn of unsp degree of unspecified lower leg, init encntr
		T24.431A	Corrosion of unsp degree of right lower leg, init encntr
		T24.432A	Corrosion of unsp degree of left lower leg, init encntr
		T24.439A	Corrosion of unsp degree of unsp lower leg, init encntr
945.Ø5	BURN OF UNSPECIFIED DEGREE OF KNEE	**T24.Ø21A**	Burn of unspecified degree of right knee, initial encounter
		T24.Ø22A	Burn of unspecified degree of left knee, initial encounter
		T24.Ø29A	Burn of unspecified degree of unspecified knee, init encntr
		T24.421A	Corrosion of unspecified degree of right knee, init encntr
		T24.422A	Corrosion of unspecified degree of left knee, init encntr
		T24.429A	Corrosion of unsp degree of unspecified knee, init encntr
945.Ø6	BURN OF UNSPECIFIED DEGREE OF THIGH	**T24.Ø11A**	Burn of unspecified degree of right thigh, initial encounter
		T24.Ø12A	Burn of unspecified degree of left thigh, initial encounter
		T24.Ø19A	Burn of unspecified degree of unspecified thigh, init encntr
		T24.411A	Corrosion of unspecified degree of right thigh, init encntr
		T24.412A	Corrosion of unspecified degree of left thigh, init encntr
		T24.419A	Corrosion of unsp degree of unspecified thigh, init encntr
945.Ø9	BURN UNSPEC DEGREE MULTIPLE SITES LOWER LIMB	**T24.Ø91A**	Burn unsp deg mult sites of right low limb, ex ank/ft, init
		T24.Ø92A	Burn unsp deg mult sites of left lower limb, ex ank/ft, init
		T24.Ø99A	Burn unsp deg mult sites of unsp lower limb, ex ank/ft, init
		T24.491A	Corros unsp deg mult sites of r low limb, ex ank/ft, init
		T24.492A	Corros unsp deg mult sites of left low limb, ex ank/ft, init
		T24.499A	Corros unsp deg mult sites of unsp low limb, ex ank/ft, init
		T25.Ø91A	Burn of unsp deg mult sites of right ankle and foot, init
		T25.Ø92A	Burn of unsp deg mult sites of left ankle and foot, init
		T25.Ø99A	Burn of unsp deg mult sites of unsp ankle and foot, init
		T25.491A	Corrosion of unsp deg mult sites of right ank/ft, init
		T25.492A	Corrosion of unsp deg mult sites of left ank/ft, init
		T25.499A	Corrosion of unsp deg mult sites of unsp ank/ft, init
945.1Ø	ERYTHEMA DUE TO BURN UNSPECIFIED SITE LOWER LIMB	**T24.1Ø1A**	Burn 1st deg of unsp site right lower limb, ex ank/ft, init
		T24.1Ø2A	Burn first deg of unsp site left lower limb, ex ank/ft, init
		T24.1Ø9A	Burn first deg of unsp site unsp lower limb, ex ank/ft, init
		T24.5Ø1A	Corros 1st deg of unsp site right low limb, ex ank/ft, init
		T24.5Ø2A	Corros 1st deg of unsp site left lower limb, ex ank/ft, init
		T24.5Ø9A	Corros 1st deg of unsp site unsp lower limb, ex ank/ft, init

ICD-9-CM		ICD-10-CM	
945.11	ERYTHEMA DUE TO BURN OF TOE	**T25.131A**	Burn of first degree of right toe(s) (nail), init encntr
		T25.132A	Burn of first degree of left toe(s) (nail), init encntr
		T25.139A	Burn of first degree of unsp toe(s) (nail), init encntr
		T25.531A	Corrosion of first degree of right toe(s) (nail), init
		T25.532A	Corrosion of first degree of left toe(s) (nail), init encntr
		T25.539A	Corrosion of first degree of unsp toe(s) (nail), init encntr
945.12	ERYTHEMA DUE TO BURN OF FOOT	**T25.121A**	Burn of first degree of right foot, initial encounter
		T25.122A	Burn of first degree of left foot, initial encounter
		T25.129A	Burn of first degree of unspecified foot, initial encounter
		T25.521A	Corrosion of first degree of right foot, initial encounter
		T25.522A	Corrosion of first degree of left foot, initial encounter
		T25.529A	Corrosion of first degree of unspecified foot, init encntr
945.13	ERYTHEMA DUE TO BURN OF ANKLE	**T25.111A**	Burn of first degree of right ankle, initial encounter
		T25.112A	Burn of first degree of left ankle, initial encounter
		T25.119A	Burn of first degree of unspecified ankle, initial encounter
		T25.511A	Corrosion of first degree of right ankle, initial encounter
		T25.512A	Corrosion of first degree of left ankle, initial encounter
		T25.519A	Corrosion of first degree of unspecified ankle, init encntr
945.14	ERYTHEMA DUE TO BURN OF LOWER LEG	**T24.131A**	Burn of first degree of right lower leg, initial encounter
		T24.132A	Burn of first degree of left lower leg, initial encounter
		T24.139A	Burn of first degree of unspecified lower leg, init encntr
		T24.531A	Corrosion of first degree of right lower leg, init encntr
		T24.532A	Corrosion of first degree of left lower leg, init encntr
		T24.539A	Corrosion of first degree of unsp lower leg, init encntr
945.15	ERYTHEMA DUE TO BURN OF KNEE	**T24.121A**	Burn of first degree of right knee, initial encounter
		T24.122A	Burn of first degree of left knee, initial encounter
		T24.129A	Burn of first degree of unspecified knee, initial encounter
		T24.521A	Corrosion of first degree of right knee, initial encounter
		T24.522A	Corrosion of first degree of left knee, initial encounter
		T24.529A	Corrosion of first degree of unspecified knee, init encntr
945.16	ERYTHEMA DUE TO BURN OF THIGH	**T24.111A**	Burn of first degree of right thigh, initial encounter
		T24.112A	Burn of first degree of left thigh, initial encounter
		T24.119A	Burn of first degree of unspecified thigh, initial encounter
		T24.511A	Corrosion of first degree of right thigh, initial encounter
		T24.512A	Corrosion of first degree of left thigh, initial encounter
		T24.519A	Corrosion of first degree of unspecified thigh, init encntr
945.19	ERYTHEMA DUE TO BURN MULTIPLE SITES LOWER LIMB	**T24.191A**	Burn 1st deg mult sites of right lower limb, ex ank/ft, init
		T24.192A	Burn 1st deg mult sites of left lower limb, ex ank/ft, init
		T24.199A	Burn 1st deg mult sites of unsp lower limb, ex ank/ft, init
		T24.591A	Corros 1st deg mult sites of right low limb, ex ank/ft, init
		T24.592A	Corros 1st deg mult sites of left low limb, ex ank/ft, init
		T24.599A	Corros 1st deg mult sites of unsp low limb, ex ank/ft, init
		T25.191A	Burn of first deg mult sites of right ankle and foot, init
		T25.192A	Burn of first deg mult sites of left ankle and foot, init
		T25.199A	Burn of first deg mult sites of unsp ankle and foot, init
		T25.591A	Corrosion of first deg mult sites of right ank/ft, init
		T25.592A	Corrosion of first deg mult sites of left ank/ft, init
		T25.599A	Corrosion of first deg mult sites of unsp ank/ft, init
945.20	BLISTR W/EPID LOSS DUE BURN UNSPEC SITE LOW LIMB	**T24.201A**	Burn 2nd deg of unsp site right lower limb, ex ank/ft, init
		T24.202A	Burn 2nd deg of unsp site left lower limb, ex ank/ft, init
		T24.209A	Burn 2nd deg of unsp site unsp lower limb, ex ank/ft, init
		T24.601A	Corros 2nd deg of unsp site right low limb, ex ank/ft, init
		T24.602A	Corros 2nd deg of unsp site left lower limb, ex ank/ft, init
		T24.609A	Corros 2nd deg of unsp site unsp lower limb, ex ank/ft, init
945.21	BLISTERS WITH EPIDERMAL LOSS DUE TO BURN OF TOE	**T25.231A**	Burn of second degree of right toe(s) (nail), init encntr
		T25.232A	Burn of second degree of left toe(s) (nail), init encntr
		T25.239A	Burn of second degree of unsp toe(s) (nail), init encntr
		T25.631A	Corrosion of second degree of right toe(s) (nail), init
		T25.632A	Corrosion of second degree of left toe(s) (nail), init
		T25.639A	Corrosion of second degree of unsp toe(s) (nail), init
945.22	BLISTERS WITH EPIDERMAL LOSS DUE TO BURN OF FOOT	**T25.221A**	Burn of second degree of right foot, initial encounter
		T25.222A	Burn of second degree of left foot, initial encounter
		T25.229A	Burn of second degree of unspecified foot, initial encounter
		T25.621A	Corrosion of second degree of right foot, initial encounter
		T25.622A	Corrosion of second degree of left foot, initial encounter
		T25.629A	Corrosion of second degree of unspecified foot, init encntr
945.23	BLISTERS W/EPIDERMAL LOSS DUE TO BURN OF ANKLE	**T25.211A**	Burn of second degree of right ankle, initial encounter
		T25.212A	Burn of second degree of left ankle, initial encounter
		T25.219A	Burn of second degree of unspecified ankle, init encntr
		T25.611A	Corrosion of second degree of right ankle, initial encounter
		T25.612A	Corrosion of second degree of left ankle, initial encounter
		T25.619A	Corrosion of second degree of unspecified ankle, init encntr
945.24	BLISTERS W/EPIDERMAL LOSS DUE TO BURN LOWER LEG	**T24.231A**	Burn of second degree of right lower leg, initial encounter
		T24.232A	Burn of second degree of left lower leg, initial encounter
		T24.239A	Burn of second degree of unspecified lower leg, init encntr
		T24.631A	Corrosion of second degree of right lower leg, init encntr
		T24.632A	Corrosion of second degree of left lower leg, init encntr
		T24.639A	Corrosion of second degree of unsp lower leg, init encntr

ICD-9-CM		ICD-10-CM	
945.25	BLISTERS WITH EPIDERMAL LOSS DUE TO BURN OF KNEE	**T24.221A**	Burn of second degree of right knee, initial encounter
		T24.222A	Burn of second degree of left knee, initial encounter
		T24.229A	Burn of second degree of unspecified knee, initial encounter
		T24.621A	Corrosion of second degree of right knee, initial encounter
		T24.622A	Corrosion of second degree of left knee, initial encounter
		T24.629A	Corrosion of second degree of unspecified knee, init encntr
945.26	BLISTERS W/EPIDERMAL LOSS DUE TO BURN OF THIGH	**T24.211A**	Burn of second degree of right thigh, initial encounter
		T24.212A	Burn of second degree of left thigh, initial encounter
		T24.219A	Burn of second degree of unspecified thigh, init encntr
		T24.611A	Corrosion of second degree of right thigh, initial encounter
		T24.612A	Corrosion of second degree of left thigh, initial encounter
		T24.619A	Corrosion of second degree of unspecified thigh, init encntr
945.29	BLISTERS W/EPID LOSS DUE BURN MULT SITE LW LIMB	**T24.291A**	Burn 2nd deg mul sites of right lower limb, ex ank/ft, init
		T24.292A	Burn 2nd deg mul sites of left lower limb, ex ank/ft, init
		T24.299A	Burn 2nd deg mul sites of unsp lower limb, ex ank/ft, init
		T24.691A	Corros 2nd deg mul sites of right low limb, ex ank/ft, init
		T24.692A	Corros 2nd deg mul sites of left lower limb, ex ank/ft, init
		T24.699A	Corros 2nd deg mul sites of unsp lower limb, ex ank/ft, init
		T25.291A	Burn of 2nd deg mul sites of right ankle and foot, init
		T25.292A	Burn of 2nd deg mul sites of left ankle and foot, init
		T25.299A	Burn of 2nd deg mul sites of unsp ankle and foot, init
		T25.691A	Corrosion of second degree of right ankle and foot, init
		T25.692A	Corrosion of second degree of left ankle and foot, init
		T25.699A	Corrosion of second degree of unsp ankle and foot, init
945.30	FULL-THICK SKN LOSS DUE BURN UNS SITE LOW LIMB	**T24.301A**	Burn third deg of unsp site right low limb, ex ank/ft, init
		T24.302A	Burn third deg of unsp site left lower limb, ex ank/ft, init
		T24.309A	Burn third deg of unsp site unsp lower limb, ex ank/ft, init
		T24.701A	Corros third deg of unsp site r low limb, ex ank/ft, init
		T24.702A	Corros third deg of unsp site left low limb, ex ank/ft, init
		T24.709A	Corros third deg of unsp site unsp low limb, ex ank/ft, init
945.31	FULL-THICKNESS SKIN LOSS DUE TO BURN OF TOE	**T25.331A**	Burn of third degree of right toe(s) (nail), init encntr
		T25.332A	Burn of third degree of left toe(s) (nail), init encntr
		T25.339A	Burn of third degree of unsp toe(s) (nail), init encntr
		T25.731A	Corrosion of third degree of right toe(s) (nail), init
		T25.732A	Corrosion of third degree of left toe(s) (nail), init encntr
		T25.739A	Corrosion of third degree of unsp toe(s) (nail), init encntr
945.32	FULL-THICKNESS SKIN LOSS DUE TO BURN OF FOOT	**T25.321A**	Burn of third degree of right foot, initial encounter
		T25.322A	Burn of third degree of left foot, initial encounter
		T25.329A	Burn of third degree of unspecified foot, initial encounter
		T25.721A	Corrosion of third degree of right foot, initial encounter
		T25.722A	Corrosion of third degree of left foot, initial encounter
		T25.729A	Corrosion of third degree of unspecified foot, init encntr
945.33	FULL-THICKNESS SKIN LOSS DUE TO BURN OF ANKLE	**T25.311A**	Burn of third degree of right ankle, initial encounter
		T25.312A	Burn of third degree of left ankle, initial encounter
		T25.319A	Burn of third degree of unspecified ankle, initial encounter
		T25.711A	Corrosion of third degree of right ankle, initial encounter
		T25.712A	Corrosion of third degree of left ankle, initial encounter
		T25.719A	Corrosion of third degree of unspecified ankle, init encntr
945.34	FULL-THICKNESS SKIN LOSS DUE TO BURN LOWER LEG	**T24.331A**	Burn of third degree of right lower leg, initial encounter
		T24.332A	Burn of third degree of left lower leg, initial encounter
		T24.339A	Burn of third degree of unspecified lower leg, init encntr
		T24.731A	Corrosion of third degree of right lower leg, init encntr
		T24.732A	Corrosion of third degree of left lower leg, init encntr
		T24.739A	Corrosion of third degree of unsp lower leg, init encntr
945.35	FULL-THICKNESS SKIN LOSS DUE TO BURN OF KNEE	**T24.321A**	Burn of third degree of right knee, initial encounter
		T24.322A	Burn of third degree of left knee, initial encounter
		T24.329A	Burn of third degree of unspecified knee, initial encounter
		T24.721A	Corrosion of third degree of right knee, initial encounter
		T24.722A	Corrosion of third degree of left knee, initial encounter
		T24.729A	Corrosion of third degree of unspecified knee, init encntr
945.36	FULL-THICKNESS SKIN LOSS DUE TO BURN OF THIGH	**T24.311A**	Burn of third degree of right thigh, initial encounter
		T24.312A	Burn of third degree of left thigh, initial encounter
		T24.319A	Burn of third degree of unspecified thigh, initial encounter
		T24.711A	Corrosion of third degree of right thigh, initial encounter
		T24.712A	Corrosion of third degree of left thigh, initial encounter
		T24.719A	Corrosion of third degree of unspecified thigh, init encntr
945.39	FULL-THICK SKIN LOSS DUE BURN MX SITES LOW LIMB	**T24.391A**	Burn 3rd deg mu sites of right lower limb, ex ank/ft, init
		T24.392A	Burn 3rd deg mu sites of left lower limb, ex ank/ft, init
		T24.399A	Burn 3rd deg mu sites of unsp lower limb, ex ank/ft, init
		T24.791A	Corros 3rd deg mu sites of right lower limb, ex ank/ft, init
		T24.792A	Corros 3rd deg mu sites of left lower limb, ex ank/ft, init
		T24.799A	Corros 3rd deg mu sites of unsp lower limb, ex ank/ft, init
		T25.391A	Burn of 3rd deg mu sites of right ankle and foot, init
		T25.392A	Burn of 3rd deg mu sites of left ankle and foot, init
		T25.399A	Burn of 3rd deg mu sites of unsp ankle and foot, init
		T25.791A	Corrosion of 3rd deg mu sites of right ankle and foot, init
		T25.792A	Corrosion of 3rd deg mu sites of left ankle and foot, init
		T25.799A	Corrosion of 3rd deg mu sites of unsp ankle and foot, init

ICD-9-CM		ICD-10-CM	
945.40	DEEP 3RD DEG BURN-UNS SITE-LW LIMB W/O LOBP	T24.301A	Burn third deg of unsp site right low limb, ex ank/ft, init
		T24.302A	Burn third deg of unsp site left lower limb, ex ank/ft, init
		T24.309A	Burn third deg of unsp site unsp lower limb, ex ank/ft, init
		T24.701A	Corros third deg of unsp site r low limb, ex ank/ft, init
		T24.702A	Corros third deg of unsp site left low limb, ex ank/ft, init
		T24.709A	Corros third deg of unsp site unsp low limb, ex ank/ft, init
945.41	DEEP 3RD DEG BURN-NECROSIS-TOE W/O LOBP	T25.331A	Burn of third degree of right toe(s) (nail), init encntr
		T25.332A	Burn of third degree of left toe(s) (nail), init encntr
		T25.339A	Burn of third degree of unsp toe(s) (nail), init encntr
		T25.731A	Corrosion of third degree of right toe(s) (nail), init
		T25.732A	Corrosion of third degree of left toe(s) (nail), init encntr
		T25.739A	Corrosion of third degree of unsp toe(s) (nail), init encntr
945.42	DEEP 3RD DEG UNDLY TISS-BRN FT W/O LOSS BDY PART	T25.321A	Burn of third degree of right foot, initial encounter
		T25.322A	Burn of third degree of left foot, initial encounter
		T25.329A	Burn of third degree of unspecified foot, initial encounter
		T25.721A	Corrosion of third degree of right foot, initial encounter
		T25.722A	Corrosion of third degree of left foot, initial encounter
		T25.729A	Corrosion of third degree of unspecified foot, init encntr
945.43	DEEP 3RD DEG BURN-NECROSIS OF ANKLE W/O LOBP	T25.311A	Burn of third degree of right ankle, initial encounter
		T25.312A	Burn of third degree of left ankle, initial encounter
		T25.319A	Burn of third degree of unspecified ankle, initial encounter
		T25.711A	Corrosion of third degree of right ankle, initial encounter
		T25.712A	Corrosion of third degree of left ankle, initial encounter
		T25.719A	Corrosion of third degree of unspecified ankle, init encntr
945.44	DEEP 3RD DEG BURN-NECROSIS OF LW LEG W/O LOBP	T24.331A	Burn of third degree of right lower leg, initial encounter
		T24.332A	Burn of third degree of left lower leg, initial encounter
		T24.339A	Burn of third degree of unspecified lower leg, init encntr
		T24.731A	Corrosion of third degree of right lower leg, init encntr
		T24.732A	Corrosion of third degree of left lower leg, init encntr
		T24.739A	Corrosion of third degree of unsp lower leg, init encntr
945.45	DEEP 3RD DG BURN-NECROSIS OF KNEE W/O LOBP	T24.321A	Burn of third degree of right knee, initial encounter
		T24.322A	Burn of third degree of left knee, initial encounter
		T24.329A	Burn of third degree of unspecified knee, initial encounter
		T24.721A	Corrosion of third degree of right knee, initial encounter
		T24.722A	Corrosion of third degree of left knee, initial encounter
		T24.729A	Corrosion of third degree of unspecified knee, init encntr
945.46	DEEP 3RD DEG BURN OF THIGH W/O LOBP	T24.311A	Burn of third degree of right thigh, initial encounter
		T24.312A	Burn of third degree of left thigh, initial encounter
		T24.319A	Burn of third degree of unspecified thigh, initial encounter
		T24.711A	Corrosion of third degree of right thigh, initial encounter
		T24.712A	Corrosion of third degree of left thigh, initial encounter
		T24.719A	Corrosion of third degree of unspecified thigh, init encntr
945.49	DEEP 3RD DEG BURN-MULT SITES-LOWER LIMB W/O LOBP	T24.391A	Burn 3rd deg mu sites of right lower limb, ex ank/ft, init
		T24.392A	Burn 3rd deg mu sites of left lower limb, ex ank/ft, init
		T24.399A	Burn 3rd deg mu sites of unsp lower limb, ex ank/ft, init
		T24.791A	Corros 3rd deg mu sites of right lower limb, ex ank/ft, init
		T24.792A	Corros 3rd deg mu sites of left lower limb, ex ank/ft, init
		T24.799A	Corros 3rd deg mu sites of unsp lower limb, ex ank/ft, init
		T25.391A	Burn of 3rd deg mu sites of right ankle and foot, init
		T25.392A	Burn of 3rd deg mu sites of left ankle and foot, init
		T25.399A	Burn of 3rd deg mu sites of unsp ankle and foot, init
		T25.791A	Corrosion of 3rd deg mu sites of right ankle and foot, init
		T25.792A	Corrosion of 3rd deg mu sites of left ankle and foot, init
		T25.799A	Corrosion of 3rd deg mu sites of unsp ankle and foot, init
945.50	DEEP 3RD DEG BURN-UNS SITE-LOWER LIMB W/LOBP	T24.301A	Burn third deg of unsp site right low limb, ex ank/ft, init
		T24.302A	Burn third deg of unsp site left lower limb, ex ank/ft, init
		T24.309A	Burn third deg of unsp site unsp lower limb, ex ank/ft, init
		T24.701A	Corros third deg of unsp site r low limb, ex ank/ft, init
		T24.702A	Corros third deg of unsp site left low limb, ex ank/ft, init
		T24.709A	Corros third deg of unsp site unsp low limb, ex ank/ft, init
945.51	DP 3RD DEG UNDLYING TISS-BRN TOE W/LOSS BDY PART	T25.331A	Burn of third degree of right toe(s) (nail), init encntr
		T25.332A	Burn of third degree of left toe(s) (nail), init encntr
		T25.339A	Burn of third degree of unsp toe(s) (nail), init encntr
		T25.731A	Corrosion of third degree of right toe(s) (nail), init
		T25.732A	Corrosion of third degree of left toe(s) (nail), init encntr
		T25.739A	Corrosion of third degree of unsp toe(s) (nail), init encntr
945.52	DP 3RD DEG UNDLYING TISS-BURN FT W/LOSS BDY PART	T25.321A	Burn of third degree of right foot, initial encounter
		T25.322A	Burn of third degree of left foot, initial encounter
		T25.329A	Burn of third degree of unspecified foot, initial encounter
		T25.721A	Corrosion of third degree of right foot, initial encounter
		T25.722A	Corrosion of third degree of left foot, initial encounter
		T25.729A	Corrosion of third degree of unspecified foot, init encntr
945.53	DP 3RD DEG UNDLYING TISS-BRN ANK W/LOSS BDY PART	T25.311A	Burn of third degree of right ankle, initial encounter
		T25.312A	Burn of third degree of left ankle, initial encounter
		T25.319A	Burn of third degree of unspecified ankle, initial encounter
		T25.711A	Corrosion of third degree of right ankle, initial encounter
		T25.712A	Corrosion of third degree of left ankle, initial encounter
		T25.719A	Corrosion of third degree of unspecified ankle, init encntr

ICD-9-CM		ICD-10-CM	
945.54	DEEP 3RD DEG BURN-NECROSIS OF LOWER LEG W/LOBP	**T24.331A**	Burn of third degree of right lower leg, initial encounter
		T24.332A	Burn of third degree of left lower leg, initial encounter
		T24.339A	Burn of third degree of unspecified lower leg, init encntr
		T24.731A	Corrosion of third degree of right lower leg, init encntr
		T24.732A	Corrosion of third degree of left lower leg, init encntr
		T24.739A	Corrosion of third degree of unsp lower leg, init encntr
945.55	DEEP 3RD DEG UNDLY TISS-BRN KNEE W/LOSS BDY PART	**T24.321A**	Burn of third degree of right knee, initial encounter
		T24.322A	Burn of third degree of left knee, initial encounter
		T24.329A	Burn of third degree of unspecified knee, initial encounter
		T24.721A	Corrosion of third degree of right knee, initial encounter
		T24.722A	Corrosion of third degree of left knee, initial encounter
		T24.729A	Corrosion of third degree of unspecified knee, init encntr
945.56	DP 3RD DEG UNDLYING TISS-BRN THI W/LOSS BDY PART	**T24.311A**	Burn of third degree of right thigh, initial encounter
		T24.312A	Burn of third degree of left thigh, initial encounter
		T24.319A	Burn of third degree of unspecified thigh, initial encounter
		T24.711A	Corrosion of third degree of right thigh, initial encounter
		T24.712A	Corrosion of third degree of left thigh, initial encounter
		T24.719A	Corrosion of third degree of unspecified thigh, init encntr
945.59	DEEP 3RD DEG BURN-MX SITE-LW LIMB W/LOBP	**T24.391A**	Burn 3rd deg mu sites of right lower limb, ex ank/ft, init
		T24.392A	Burn 3rd deg mu sites of left lower limb, ex ank/ft, init
		T24.399A	Burn 3rd deg mu sites of unsp lower limb, ex ank/ft, init
		T24.791A	Corros 3rd deg mu sites of right lower limb, ex ank/ft, init
		T24.792A	Corros 3rd deg mu sites of left lower limb, ex ank/ft, init
		T24.799A	Corros 3rd deg mu sites of unsp lower limb, ex ank/ft, init
		T25.391A	Burn of 3rd deg mu sites of right ankle and foot, init
		T25.392A	Burn of 3rd deg mu sites of left ankle and foot, init
		T25.399A	Burn of 3rd deg mu sites of unsp ankle and foot, init
		T25.791A	Corrosion of 3rd deg mu sites of right ankle and foot, init
		T25.792A	Corrosion of 3rd deg mu sites of left ankle and foot, init
		T25.799A	Corrosion of 3rd deg mu sites of unsp ankle and foot, init
946.Ø	BURNS MULTIPLE SPEC SITES UNSPEC DEGREE	**T3Ø.Ø**	Burn of unspecified body region, unspecified degree
		T3Ø.4	Corrosion of unspecified body region, unspecified degree
946.1	ERYTHEMA DUE TO BURN OF MULTIPLE SPECIFIED SITES	**T3Ø.Ø**	Burn of unspecified body region, unspecified degree
		T3Ø.4	Corrosion of unspecified body region, unspecified degree
946.2	BLISTR W/EPID LOSS DUE BURN MULTIPLE SPEC SITES	**T3Ø.Ø**	Burn of unspecified body region, unspecified degree
		T3Ø.4	Corrosion of unspecified body region, unspecified degree
946.3	FULL-THICKNESS SKIN LOSS DUE BURN MX SPEC SITES	**T3Ø.Ø**	Burn of unspecified body region, unspecified degree
		T3Ø.4	Corrosion of unspecified body region, unspecified degree
946.4	DEEP 3RD DEG BURN-NECROS-MX SPEC SITES W/O LOBP	**T3Ø.Ø**	Burn of unspecified body region, unspecified degree
946.5	DEEP 3RD DEG BURN-NECROS-MULT SPEC SITES W/LOBP	**T3Ø.Ø**	Burn of unspecified body region, unspecified degree
		T3Ø.4	Corrosion of unspecified body region, unspecified degree
947.Ø	BURN OF MOUTH AND PHARYNX	**T28.ØXXA**	Burn of mouth and pharynx, initial encounter
		T28.5XXA	Corrosion of mouth and pharynx, initial encounter
947.1	BURN OF LARYNX, TRACHEA, AND LUNG	**T27.ØXXA**	Burn of larynx and trachea, initial encounter
		T27.1XXA	Burn involving larynx and trachea with lung, init encntr
		T27.2XXA	Burn of other parts of respiratory tract, initial encounter
		T27.3XXA	Burn of respiratory tract, part unspecified, init encntr
		T27.4XXA	Corrosion of larynx and trachea, initial encounter
		T27.5XXA	Corrosion involving larynx and trachea w lung, init encntr
		T27.6XXA	Corrosion of other parts of respiratory tract, init encntr
		T27.7XXA	Corrosion of respiratory tract, part unsp, init encntr
947.2	BURN OF ESOPHAGUS	**T28.1XXA**	Burn of esophagus, initial encounter
		T28.6XXA	Corrosion of esophagus, initial encounter
947.3	BURN OF GASTROINTESTINAL TRACT	**T28.2XXA**	Burn of other parts of alimentary tract, initial encounter
		T28.7XXA	Corrosion of other parts of alimentary tract, init encntr
947.4	BURN OF VAGINA AND UTERUS	**T28.3XXA**	Burn of internal genitourinary organs, initial encounter
		T28.8XXA	Corrosion of internal genitourinary organs, init encntr
947.8	BURN OF OTHER SPECIFIED SITES OF INTERNAL ORGANS	**T28.3XXA**	Burn of internal genitourinary organs, initial encounter
		T28.411A	Burn of right ear drum, initial encounter
		T28.412A	Burn of left ear drum, initial encounter
		T28.419A	Burn of unspecified ear drum, initial encounter
		T28.49XA	Burn of other internal organ, initial encounter
		T28.8XXA	Corrosion of internal genitourinary organs, init encntr
		T28.911A	Corrosions of right ear drum, initial encounter
		T28.912A	Corrosions of left ear drum, initial encounter
		T28.919A	Corrosions of unspecified ear drum, initial encounter
		T28.99XA	Corrosions of other internal organs, initial encounter
947.9	BURN OF INTERNAL ORGANS UNSPECIFIED SITE	**T28.4ØXA**	Burn of unspecified internal organ, initial encounter
		T28.9ØXA	Corrosions of unspecified internal organs, initial encounter
948.ØØ	BURN <10% BODY SURF W/3RD DEG BURN<10%/UNS AMT	**T31.Ø**	Burns involving less than 10% of body surface
		T32.Ø	Corrosions involving less than 10% of body surface
948.1Ø	BURN 10-19% BODY SURF W/3RD DEG BURN<10%/UNS AMT	**T31.1Ø**	Burns of 10-19% of body surfc w 0% to 9% third degree burns
		T32.1Ø	Corros 10-19% of body surface w 0% to 9% third degree corros
948.11	BURN 10-19% BODY SURF W/3RD DEG BURN 10-19%	**T31.11**	Burns of 10-19% of body surface w 10-19% third degree burns
		T32.11	Corros 10-19% of body surface w 10-19% third degree corros
948.2Ø	BURN 20-29% BODY SURF W/3RD DEG BURN<10%/UNS AMT	**T31.2Ø**	Burns of 20-29% of body surfc w 0% to 9% third degree burns
		T32.2Ø	Corros 20-29% of body surface w 0% to 9% third degree corros

[Brackets] indicate valid character values for each code. Character value meanings provided for each code grouping.

ICD-9-CM		ICD-10-CM	
948.21	BURN 20-29% BODY SURF W/3RD DEG BURN 10-19%	**T31.21** **T32.21**	Burns of 20-29% of body surface w 10-19% third degree burns Corros 20-29% of body surface w 10-19% third degree corros
948.22	BURN 20-29% BODY SURF W/3RD DEG BURN 20-29%	**T31.22** **T32.22**	Burns of 20-29% of body surface w 20-29% third degree burns Corros 20-29% of body surface w 20-29% third degree corros
948.30	BURN 30-39% BODY SURF W/3RD DEG BURN<10%/UNS AMT	**T31.30** **T32.30**	Burns of 30-39% of body surfc w 0% to 9% third degree burns Corros 30-39% of body surface w 0% to 9% third degree corros
948.31	BURN 30-39% BODY SURFACE W/3RD DEG BURN 10-19%	**T31.31** **T32.31**	Burns of 30-39% of body surface w 10-19% third degree burns Corros 30-39% of body surface w 10-19% third degree corros
948.32	BURN 30-39% BODY SURFACE W/3RD DEG BURN 20-29%	**T31.32** **T32.32**	Burns of 30-39% of body surface w 20-29% third degree burns Corros 30-39% of body surface w 20-29% third degree corros
948.33	BURN 30-39% BODY SURFACE W/3RD DEG BURN 30-39%	**T31.33** **T32.33**	Burns of 30-39% of body surface w 30-39% third degree burns Corros 30-39% of body surface w 30-39% third degree corros
948.40	BURN 40-49% BODY SURF W/3RD DEG BURN<10%/UNS AMT	**T31.40** **T32.40**	Burns of 40-49% of body surfc w 0% to 9% third degree burns Corros 40-49% of body surface w 0% to 9% third degree corros
948.41	BURN 40-49% BODY SURFACE W/3RD DEG BURN 10-19%	**T31.41** **T32.41**	Burns of 40-49% of body surface w 10-19% third degree burns Corros 40-49% of body surface w 10-19% third degree corros
948.42	BURN 40-49% BODY SURFACE W/3RD DEG BURN 20-29%	**T31.42** **T32.42**	Burns of 40-49% of body surface w 20-29% third degree burns Corros 40-49% of body surface w 20-29% third degree corros
948.43	BURN 40-49% BODY SURFACE W/3RD DEG BURN 30-39%	**T31.43** **T32.43**	Burns of 40-49% of body surface w 30-39% third degree burns Corros 40-49% of body surface w 30-39% third degree corros
948.44	BURN 40-49% BODY SURFACE W/3RD DEG BURN 40-49%	**T31.44** **T32.44**	Burns of 40-49% of body surface w 40-49% third degree burns Corros 40-49% of body surface w 40-49% third degree corros
948.50	BURN 50-59% BODY SURF W/3RD DEG BURN<10%/UNS AMT	**T31.50** **T32.50**	Burns of 50-59% of body surfc w 0% to 9% third degree burns Corros 50-59% of body surface w 0% to 9% third degree corros
948.51	BURN 50-59% BODY SURFACE W/3RD DEG BURN 10-19%	**T31.51** **T32.51**	Burns of 50-59% of body surface w 10-19% third degree burns Corros 50-59% of body surface w 10-19% third degree corros
948.52	BURN 50-59% BODY SURFACE W/3RD DEG BURN 20-29%	**T31.52** **T32.52**	Burns of 50-59% of body surface w 20-29% third degree burns Corros 50-59% of body surface w 20-29% third degree corros
948.53	BURN 50-59% BODY SURFACE W/3RD DEG BURN 30-39%	**T31.53** **T32.53**	Burns of 50-59% of body surface w 30-39% third degree burns Corros 50-59% of body surface w 30-39% third degree corros
948.54	BURN 50-59% BODY SURFACE W/3RD DEG BURN 40-49%	**T31.54** **T32.54**	Burns of 50-59% of body surface w 40-49% third degree burns Corros 50-59% of body surface w 40-49% third degree corros
948.55	BURN 50-59% BODY SURFACE W/3RD DEG BURN 50-59%	**T31.55** **T32.55**	Burns of 50-59% of body surface w 50-59% third degree burns Corros 50-59% of body surface w 50-59% third degree corros
948.60	BURN 60-69% BODY SURF W/3RD DEG BURN<10%/UNS AMT	**T31.60** **T32.60**	Burns of 60-69% of body surfc w 0% to 9% third degree burns Corros 60-69% of body surface w 0% to 9% third degree corros
948.61	BURN 60-69% BODY SURFACE W/3RD DEG BURN 10-19%	**T31.61** **T32.61**	Burns of 60-69% of body surface w 10-19% third degree burns Corros 60-69% of body surface w 10-19% third degree corros
948.62	BURN 60-69% BODY SURFACE W/3RD DEG BURN 20-29%	**T31.62** **T32.62**	Burns of 60-69% of body surface w 20-29% third degree burns Corros 60-69% of body surface w 20-29% third degree corros
948.63	BURN 60-69% BODY SURFACE W/3RD DEG BURN 30-39%	**T31.63** **T32.63**	Burns of 60-69% of body surface w 30-39% third degree burns Corros 60-69% of body surface w 30-39% third degree corros
948.64	BURN 60-69% BODY SURFACE W/3RD DEG BURN 40-49%	**T31.64** **T32.64**	Burns of 60-69% of body surface w 40-49% third degree burns Corros 60-69% of body surface w 40-49% third degree corros
948.65	BURN 60-69% BODY SURFACE W/3RD DEG BURN 50-59%	**T31.65** **T32.65**	Burns of 60-69% of body surface w 50-59% third degree burns Corros 60-69% of body surface w 50-59% third degree corros
948.66	BURN 60-69% BODY SURFACE W/3RD DEG BURN 60-69%	**T31.66** **T32.66**	Burns of 60-69% of body surface w 60-69% third degree burns Corros 60-69% of body surface w 60-69% third degree corros
948.70	BURN 70-79% BODY SURF W/3RD DEG BURN<10%/UNS AMT	**T31.70** **T32.70**	Burns of 70-79% of body surfc w 0% to 9% third degree burns Corros 70-79% of body surface w 0% to 9% third degree corros
948.71	BURN 70-79% BODY SURFACE W/3RD DEG BURN 10-19%	**T31.71** **T32.71**	Burns of 70-79% of body surface w 10-19% third degree burns Corros 70-79% of body surface w 10-19% third degree corros
948.72	BURN 70-79% BODY SURFACE W/3RD DEG BURN 20-29%	**T31.72** **T32.72**	Burns of 70-79% of body surface w 20-29% third degree burns Corros 70-79% of body surface w 20-29% third degree corros
948.73	BURN 70-79% BODY SURFACE W/3RD DEG BURN 30-39%	**T31.73** **T32.73**	Burns of 70-79% of body surface w 30-39% third degree burns Corros 70-79% of body surface w 30-39% third degree corros
948.74	BURN 70-79% BODY SURFACE W/3RD DEG BURN 40-49%	**T31.74** **T32.74**	Burns of 70-79% of body surface w 40-49% third degree burns Corros 70-79% of body surface w 40-49% third degree corros
948.75	BURN 70-79% BODY SURFACE W/3RD DEG BURN 50-59%	**T31.75** **T32.75**	Burns of 70-79% of body surface w 50-59% third degree burns Corros 70-79% of body surface w 50-59% third degree corros
948.76	BURN 70-79% BODY SURFACE W/3RD DEG BURN 60-69%	**T31.76** **T32.76**	Burns of 70-79% of body surface w 60-69% third degree burns Corros 70-79% of body surface w 60-69% third degree corros
948.77	BURN 70-79% BODY SURFACE W/3RD DEG BURN 70-79%	**T31.77** **T32.77**	Burns of 70-79% of body surface w 70-79% third degree burns Corros 70-79% of body surface w 70-79% third degree corros
948.80	BURN 80-89% BODY SURF W/3RD DEG BURN<10%/UNS AMT	**T31.80** **T32.80**	Burns of 80-89% of body surfc w 0% to 9% third degree burns Corros 80-89% of body surface w 0% to 9% third degree corros
948.81	BURN 80-89% BODY SURFACE W/3RD DEG BURN 10-19%	**T31.81** **T32.81**	Burns of 80-89% of body surface w 10-19% third degree burns Corros 80-89% of body surface w 10-19% third degree corros
948.82	BURN 80-89% BODY SURFACE W/3RD DEG BURN 20-29%	**T31.82** **T32.82**	Burns of 80-89% of body surface w 20-29% third degree burns Corros 80-89% of body surface w 20-29% third degree corros
948.83	BURN 80-89% BODY SURFACE W/3RD DEG BURN 30-39%	**T31.83** **T32.83**	Burns of 80-89% of body surface w 30-39% third degree burns Corros 80-89% of body surface w 30-39% third degree corros
948.84	BURN 80-89% BODY SURFACE W/3RD DEG BURN 40-49%	**T31.84** **T32.84**	Burns of 80-89% of body surface w 40-49% third degree burns Corros 80-89% of body surface w 40-49% third degree corros

ICD-9-CM		ICD-10-CM	
948.85	BURN 80-89% BODY SURFACE W/3RD DEG BURN 50-59%	**T31.85**	Burns of 80-89% of body surface w 50-59% third degree burns
		T32.85	Corros 80-89% of body surface w 50-59% third degree corros
948.86	BURN 80-89% BODY SURFACE W/3RD DEG BURN 60-69%	**T31.86**	Burns of 80-89% of body surface w 60-69% third degree burns
		T32.86	Corros 80-89% of body surface w 60-69% third degree corros
948.87	BURN 80-89% BODY SURFACE W/3RD DEG BURN 70-79%	**T31.87**	Burns of 80-89% of body surface w 70-79% third degree burns
		T32.87	Corros 80-89% of body surface w 70-79% third degree corros
948.88	BURN 80-89% BODY SURFACE W/3RD DEG BURN 80-89%	**T31.88**	Burns of 80-89% of body surface w 80-89% third degree burns
		T32.88	Corros 80-89% of body surface w 80-89% third degree corros
948.90	BURN 90%/MORE BDY SURF W/3RD DEG<10%/UNS AMT	**T31.90**	Burns of 90%/more of body surfc w 0% to 9% third deg burns
		T32.90	Corros 90%/more of body surfc w 0% to 9% third degree corros
948.91	BURN 90%/MORE BODY SURFACE W/3RD DEG BURN 10-19%	**T31.91**	Burns of 90%/more of body surfc w 10-19% third degree burns
		T32.91	Corros 90%/more of body surface w 10-19% third degree corros
948.92	BURN 90%/MORE BODY SURFACE W/3RD DEG BURN 20-29%	**T31.92**	Burns of 90%/more of body surfc w 20-29% third degree burns
		T32.92	Corros 90%/more of body surface w 20-29% third degree corros
948.93	BURN 90%/MORE BODY SURFACE W/3RD DEG BURN 30-39%	**T31.93**	Burns of 90%/more of body surfc w 30-39% third degree burns
		T32.93	Corros 90%/more of body surface w 30-39% third degree corros
948.94	BURN 90%/MORE BODY SURFACE W/3RD DEG BURN 40-49%	**T31.94**	Burns of 90%/more of body surfc w 40-49% third degree burns
		T32.94	Corros 90%/more of body surface w 40-49% third degree corros
948.95	BURN 90%/MORE BODY SURFACE W/3RD DEG BURN 50-59%	**T31.95**	Burns of 90%/more of body surfc w 50-59% third degree burns
		T32.95	Corros 90%/more of body surface w 50-59% third degree corros
948.96	BURN 90%/MORE BODY SURFACE W/3RD DEG BURN 60-69%	**T31.96**	Burns of 90%/more of body surfc w 60-69% third degree burns
		T32.96	Corros 90%/more of body surface w 60-69% third degree corros
948.97	BURN 90%/MORE BODY SURFACE W/3RD DEG BURN 70-79%	**T31.97**	Burns of 90%/more of body surfc w 70-79% third degree burns
		T32.97	Corros 90%/more of body surface w 70-79% third degree corros
948.98	BURN 90%/MORE BODY SURFACE W/3RD DEG BURN 80-89%	**T31.98**	Burns of 90%/more of body surfc w 80-89% third degree burns
		T32.98	Corros 90%/more of body surface w 80-89% third degree corros
948.99	BURN 90%/MORE BODY SURF W/3RD DEG 90%/MORE SURF	**T31.99**	Burns of 90%/more of body surfc w 90%/more third deg burns
		T32.99	Corros 90%/more of body surfc w 90%/more third degree corros
949.0	BURN OF UNSPECIFIED SITE UNSPECIFIED DEGREE	**T30.0**	Burn of unspecified body region, unspecified degree
		T30.4	Corrosion of unspecified body region, unspecified degree
949.1	ERYTHEMA DUE TO BURN UNSPECIFIED SITE	**T30.0**	Burn of unspecified body region, unspecified degree
949.2	BLISTERS W/EPIDERMAL LOSS DUE BURN UNSPEC SITE	**T30.0**	Burn of unspecified body region, unspecified degree
949.3	FULL-THICKNESS SKIN LOSS DUE BURN UNSPEC SITE	**T30.0**	Burn of unspecified body region, unspecified degree
949.4	DEEP 3RD DEGREE BURN-NECROSIS-UNS SITE-W/O LOBP	**T30.0**	Burn of unspecified body region, unspecified degree
949.5	DEEP 3RD DEGREE BURN-NECROSIS-UNS SITE-W/LOBP	**T30.0**	Burn of unspecified body region, unspecified degree
		T30.4	Corrosion of unspecified body region, unspecified degree
950.0	OPTIC NERVE INJURY	**S04.011A**	Injury of optic nerve, right eye, initial encounter
		S04.012A	Injury of optic nerve, left eye, initial encounter
		S04.019A	Injury of optic nerve, unspecified eye, initial encounter
950.1	INJURY TO OPTIC CHIASM	**S04.02XA**	Injury of optic chiasm, initial encounter
950.2	INJURY TO OPTIC PATHWAYS	**S04.031A**	Injury of optic tract and pathways, right eye, init encntr
		S04.032A	Injury of optic tract and pathways, left eye, init encntr
		S04.039A	Injury of optic tract and pathways, unsp eye, init encntr
950.3	INJURY TO VISUAL CORTEX	**S04.041A**	Injury of visual cortex, right eye, initial encounter
		S04.042A	Injury of visual cortex, left eye, initial encounter
		S04.049A	Injury of visual cortex, unspecified eye, initial encounter
950.9	INJURY TO UNSPECIFIED OPTIC NERVE AND PATHWAYS	**S04.019A**	Injury of optic nerve, unspecified eye, initial encounter
951.0	INJURY TO OCULOMOTOR NERVE	**S04.10XA**	Injury of oculomotor nerve, unspecified side, init encntr
		S04.11XA	Injury of oculomotor nerve, right side, initial encounter
		S04.12XA	Injury of oculomotor nerve, left side, initial encounter
951.1	INJURY TO TROCHLEAR NERVE	**S04.20XA**	Injury of trochlear nerve, unspecified side, init encntr
		S04.21XA	Injury of trochlear nerve, right side, initial encounter
		S04.22XA	Injury of trochlear nerve, left side, initial encounter
951.2	INJURY TO TRIGEMINAL NERVE	**S04.30XA**	Injury of trigeminal nerve, unspecified side, init encntr
		S04.31XA	Injury of trigeminal nerve, right side, initial encounter
		S04.32XA	Injury of trigeminal nerve, left side, initial encounter
951.3	INJURY TO ABDUCENS NERVE	**S04.40XA**	Injury of abducent nerve, unspecified side, init encntr
		S04.41XA	Injury of abducent nerve, right side, initial encounter
		S04.42XA	Injury of abducent nerve, left side, initial encounter
951.4	INJURY TO FACIAL NERVE	**S04.50XA**	Injury of facial nerve, unspecified side, initial encounter
		S04.51XA	Injury of facial nerve, right side, initial encounter
		S04.52XA	Injury of facial nerve, left side, initial encounter
951.5	INJURY TO ACOUSTIC NERVE	**S04.60XA**	Injury of acoustic nerve, unspecified side, init encntr
		S04.61XA	Injury of acoustic nerve, right side, initial encounter
		S04.62XA	Injury of acoustic nerve, left side, initial encounter
951.6	INJURY TO ACCESSORY NERVE	**S04.70XA**	Injury of accessory nerve, unspecified side, init encntr
		S04.71XA	Injury of accessory nerve, right side, initial encounter
		S04.72XA	Injury of accessory nerve, left side, initial encounter
951.7	INJURY TO HYPOGLOSSAL NERVE	**S04.891A**	Injury of other cranial nerves, right side, init encntr
		S04.892A	Injury of other cranial nerves, left side, initial encounter
		S04.899A	Injury of other cranial nerves, unsp side, init encntr

[Brackets] indicate valid character values for each code. Character value meanings provided for each code grouping.

ICD-9-CM		ICD-10-CM	
951.8	INJURY TO OTHER SPECIFIED CRANIAL NERVES	**S04.811A**	Injury of olfactory nerve, right side, initial encounter
		S04.812A	Injury of olfactory nerve, left side, initial encounter
		S04.819A	Injury of olfactory nerve, unspecified side, init encntr
		S04.891A	Injury of other cranial nerves, right side, init encntr
		S04.892A	Injury of other cranial nerves, left side, initial encounter
		S04.899A	Injury of other cranial nerves, unsp side, init encntr
951.9	INJURY TO UNSPECIFIED CRANIAL NERVE	**S04.9XXA**	Injury of unspecified cranial nerve, initial encounter
952.00	C1-C4 LEVEL SPINAL CORD INJURY UNSPECIFIED	**S14.101A**	Unsp injury at C1 level of cervical spinal cord, init encntr
		S14.102A	Unsp injury at C2 level of cervical spinal cord, init encntr
		S14.103A	Unsp injury at C3 level of cervical spinal cord, init encntr
		S14.104A	Unsp injury at C4 level of cervical spinal cord, init encntr
952.01	C1-C4 LEVEL WITH COMPLETE LESION OF SPINAL CORD	**S14.111A**	Complete lesion at C1 level of cervical spinal cord, init
		S14.112A	Complete lesion at C2 level of cervical spinal cord, init
		S14.113A	Complete lesion at C3 level of cervical spinal cord, init
		S14.114A	Complete lesion at C4 level of cervical spinal cord, init
952.02	C1-C4 LEVEL WITH ANTERIOR CORD SYNDROME	**S14.131A**	Anterior cord syndrome at C1, init
		S14.132A	Anterior cord syndrome at C2, init
		S14.133A	Anterior cord syndrome at C3, init
		S14.134A	Anterior cord syndrome at C4, init
952.03	C1-C4 LEVEL WITH CENTRAL CORD SYNDROME	**S14.121A**	Central cord syndrome at C1, init
		S14.122A	Central cord syndrome at C2, init
		S14.123A	Central cord syndrome at C3, init
		S14.124A	Central cord syndrome at C4, init
952.04	C1-C4 LEVEL W/OTHER SPECIFIED SPINAL CORD INJURY	**S14.0XXA**	Concussion and edema of cervical spinal cord, init encntr
		S14.141A	Brown-Sequard syndrome at C1, init
		S14.142A	Brown-Sequard syndrome at C2, init
		S14.143A	Brown-Sequard syndrome at C3, init
		S14.144A	Brown-Sequard syndrome at C4, init
		S14.151A	Oth incomplete lesion at C1, init
		S14.152A	Oth incomplete lesion at C2, init
		S14.153A	Oth incomplete lesion at C3, init
		S14.154A	Oth incomplete lesion at C4, init
952.05	C5-C7 LEVEL SPINAL CORD INJURY UNSPECIFIED	**S14.105A**	Unsp injury at C5 level of cervical spinal cord, init encntr
		S14.106A	Unsp injury at C6 level of cervical spinal cord, init encntr
		S14.107A	Unsp injury at C7 level of cervical spinal cord, init encntr
		S14.108A	Unsp injury at C8 level of cervical spinal cord, init encntr
952.06	C5-C7 LEVEL WITH COMPLETE LESION OF SPINAL CORD	**S14.115A**	Complete lesion at C5 level of cervical spinal cord, init
		S14.116A	Complete lesion at C6 level of cervical spinal cord, init
		S14.117A	Complete lesion at C7 level of cervical spinal cord, init
		S14.118A	Complete lesion at C8 level of cervical spinal cord, init
952.07	C5-C7 LEVEL WITH ANTERIOR CORD SYNDROME	**S14.135A**	Anterior cord syndrome at C5, init
		S14.136A	Anterior cord syndrome at C6, init
		S14.137A	Anterior cord syndrome at C7, init
		S14.138A	Anterior cord syndrome at C8, init
952.08	C5-C7 LEVEL WITH CENTRAL CORD SYNDROME	**S14.125A**	Central cord syndrome at C5, init
		S14.126A	Central cord syndrome at C6, init
		S14.127A	Central cord syndrome at C7, init
		S14.128A	Central cord syndrome at C8, init
952.09	C5-C7 LEVEL W/OTHER SPECIFIED SPINAL CORD INJURY	**S14.0XXA**	Concussion and edema of cervical spinal cord, init encntr
		S14.145A	Brown-Sequard syndrome at C5, init
		S14.146A	Brown-Sequard syndrome at C6, init
		S14.147A	Brown-Sequard syndrome at C7, init
		S14.148A	Brown-Sequard syndrome at C8, init
		S14.155A	Oth incomplete lesion at C5, init
		S14.156A	Oth incomplete lesion at C6, init
		S14.157A	Oth incomplete lesion at C7, init
		S14.158A	Oth incomplete lesion at C8, init
952.10	T1-T6 LEVEL SPINAL CORD INJURY UNSPECIFIED	**S24.101A**	Unsp injury at T1 level of thoracic spinal cord, init encntr
		S24.102A	Unsp injury at T2-T6 level of thoracic spinal cord, init
952.11	T1-T6 LEVEL WITH COMPLETE LESION OF SPINAL CORD	**S24.111A**	Complete lesion at T1 level of thoracic spinal cord, init
		S24.112A	Complete lesion at T2-T6 level of thoracic spinal cord, init
952.12	T1-T6 LEVEL WITH ANTERIOR CORD SYNDROME	**S24.131A**	Anterior cord syndrome at T1, init
		S24.132A	Anterior cord syndrome at T2-T6, init
952.13	T1-T6 LEVEL WITH CENTRAL CORD SYNDROME	**S24.151A**	Oth incomplete lesion at T1, init
		S24.152A	Oth incomplete lesion at T2-T6, init
952.14	T1-T6 LEVEL W/OTHER SPECIFIED SPINAL CORD INJURY	**S24.0XXA**	Concussion and edema of thoracic spinal cord, init encntr
		S24.141A	Brown-Sequard syndrome at T1, init
		S24.142A	Brown-Sequard syndrome at T2-T6, init
		S24.151A	Oth incomplete lesion at T1, init
		S24.152A	Oth incomplete lesion at T2-T6, init
952.15	T7-T12 LEVEL SPINAL CORD INJURY UNSPECIFIED	**S24.103A**	Unsp injury at T7-T10 level of thoracic spinal cord, init
		S24.104A	Unsp injury at T11-T12 level of thoracic spinal cord, init
952.16	T7-T12 LEVEL WITH COMPLETE LESION OF SPINAL CORD	**S24.113A**	Complete lesion at T7-T10, init
		S24.114A	Complete lesion at T11-T12, init
952.17	T7-T12 LEVEL WITH ANTERIOR CORD SYNDROME	**S24.133A**	Anterior cord syndrome at T7-T10, init
		S24.134A	Anterior cord syndrome at T11-T12, init
952.18	T7-T12 LEVEL WITH CENTRAL CORD SYNDROME	**S24.153A**	Oth incomplete lesion at T7-T10, init
		S24.154A	Oth incomplete lesion at T11-T12, init

ICD-9-CM		ICD-10-CM	
952.19	T7-T12 LEVEL W/OTHER SPEC SPINAL CORD INJURY	**S24.ØXXA**	Concussion and edema of thoracic spinal cord, init encntr
		S24.143A	Brown-Sequard syndrome at T7-T10, init
		S24.144A	Brown-Sequard syndrome at T11-T12, init
		S24.153A	Oth incomplete lesion at T7-T10, init
		S24.154A	Oth incomplete lesion at T11-T12, init
952.2	LUMBAR SPINAL CORD INJURY W/O SPINAL BONE INJURY	**S34.Ø1XA**	Concussion and edema of lumbar spinal cord, init encntr
		S34.1Ø1A	Unsp injury to L1 level of lumbar spinal cord, init encntr
		S34.1Ø2A	Unsp injury to L2 level of lumbar spinal cord, init encntr
		S34.1Ø3A	Unsp injury to L3 level of lumbar spinal cord, init encntr
		S34.1Ø4A	Unsp injury to L4 level of lumbar spinal cord, init encntr
		S34.1Ø5A	Unsp injury to L5 level of lumbar spinal cord, init encntr
		S34.1Ø9A	Unsp injury to unsp level of lumbar spinal cord, init encntr
		S34.111A	Complete lesion of L1 level of lumbar spinal cord, init
		S34.112A	Complete lesion of L2 level of lumbar spinal cord, init
		S34.113A	Complete lesion of L3 level of lumbar spinal cord, init
		S34.114A	Complete lesion of L4 level of lumbar spinal cord, init
		S34.115A	Complete lesion of L5 level of lumbar spinal cord, init
		S34.119A	Complete lesion of unsp level of lumbar spinal cord, init
		S34.121A	Incomplete lesion of L1 level of lumbar spinal cord, init
		S34.122A	Incomplete lesion of L2 level of lumbar spinal cord, init
		S34.123A	Incomplete lesion of L3 level of lumbar spinal cord, init
		S34.124A	Incomplete lesion of L4 level of lumbar spinal cord, init
		S34.125A	Incomplete lesion of L5 level of lumbar spinal cord, init
		S34.129A	Incomplete lesion of unsp level of lumbar spinal cord, init
952.3	SAC SPINAL CORD INJURY W/O SPINAL BONE INJURY	**S34.Ø2XA**	Concussion and edema of sacral spinal cord, init encntr
		S34.131A	Complete lesion of sacral spinal cord, initial encounter
		S34.132A	Incomplete lesion of sacral spinal cord, initial encounter
		S34.139A	Unspecified injury to sacral spinal cord, initial encounter
952.4	CAUDA EQUINA SPINL CORD INJURY W/O SP BN INJURY	**S34.3XXA**	Injury of cauda equina, initial encounter
952.8	MX SITES SPINAL CORD INJURY W/O SPINAL BN INJURY	**S34.139A**	Unspecified injury to sacral spinal cord, initial encounter
952.9	UNSPEC SITE SP CORD INJURY W/O SP BN INJURY	**S14.1Ø9A**	Unsp injury at unsp level of cervical spinal cord, init
		S14.119A	Complete lesion at unsp level of cervical spinal cord, init
		S14.129A	Central cord synd at unsp level of cerv spinal cord, init
		S14.139A	Ant cord syndrome at unsp level of cerv spinal cord, init
		S14.149A	Brown-Sequard synd at unsp level of cerv spinal cord, init
		S14.159A	Oth incmpl lesion at unsp level of cerv spinal cord, init
		S24.1Ø9A	Unsp injury at unsp level of thoracic spinal cord, init
		S24.119A	Complete lesion at unsp level of thoracic spinal cord, init
		S24.139A	Ant cord syndrome at unsp level of thor spinal cord, init
		S24.149A	Brown-Sequard synd at unsp level of thor spinal cord, init
		S24.159A	Oth incmpl lesion at unsp level of thor spinal cord, init
		S34.1Ø9A	Unsp injury to unsp level of lumbar spinal cord, init encntr
		S34.139A	Unspecified injury to sacral spinal cord, initial encounter
953.Ø	INJURY TO CERVICAL NERVE ROOT	**S14.2XXA**	Injury of nerve root of cervical spine, initial encounter
953.1	INJURY TO DORSAL NERVE ROOT	**S24.2XXA**	Injury of nerve root of thoracic spine, initial encounter
953.2	INJURY TO LUMBAR NERVE ROOT	**S34.21XA**	Injury of nerve root of lumbar spine, initial encounter
953.3	INJURY TO SACRAL NERVE ROOT	**S34.22XA**	Injury of nerve root of sacral spine, initial encounter
953.4	INJURY TO BRACHIAL PLEXUS	**S14.3XXA**	Injury of brachial plexus, initial encounter
953.5	INJURY TO LUMBOSACRAL PLEXUS	**S34.4XXA**	Injury of lumbosacral plexus, initial encounter
953.8	INJURY MULTIPLE SITES NERVE ROOTS&SPINAL PLEXUS	**S14.2XXA**	Injury of nerve root of cervical spine, initial encounter
		S24.2XXA	Injury of nerve root of thoracic spine, initial encounter
		S34.21XA	Injury of nerve root of lumbar spine, initial encounter
		S34.22XA	Injury of nerve root of sacral spine, initial encounter
		S34.4XXA	Injury of lumbosacral plexus, initial encounter
953.9	INJURY UNSPEC SITE NERVE ROOTS&SPINAL PLEXUS	**S14.2XXA**	Injury of nerve root of cervical spine, initial encounter
		S24.2XXA	Injury of nerve root of thoracic spine, initial encounter
		S34.21XA	Injury of nerve root of lumbar spine, initial encounter
		S34.22XA	Injury of nerve root of sacral spine, initial encounter
		S34.4XXA	Injury of lumbosacral plexus, initial encounter
954.Ø	INJR CERV SYMPATHET NERV EXCLD SHLDR&PELV GIRDLS	**S14.5XXA**	Injury of cervical sympathetic nerves, initial encounter
954.1	INJR OTH SYMPATHET NERV EXCLD SHLDR&PELV GIRDLS	**S24.4XXA**	Injury of thoracic sympathetic nervous system, init encntr
		S34.5XXA	Injury of lumbar, sacral and pelvic sympathetic nerves, init
954.8	INJR OTH SPEC NERV TRNK EXCLD SHLDR&PELV GIRDLS	**S24.3XXA**	Injury of peripheral nerves of thorax, initial encounter
		S24.8XXA	Injury of other specified nerves of thorax, init encntr
		S34.6XXA	Inj prph nerve(s) at abd, low back and pelvis level, init
		S34.8XXA	Injury of nerves at abdomen, low back and pelvis level, init
954.9	INJURY UNSPEC NERVE TRUNK NOT SHLDR&PELV GIRDLS	**S24.9XXA**	Injury of unspecified nerve of thorax, initial encounter
		S34.9XXA	Inj unsp nerves at abdomen, low back and pelvis level, init
955.Ø	INJURY TO AXILLARY NERVE	**S44.3ØXA**	Injury of axillary nerve, unspecified arm, initial encounter
		S44.31XA	Injury of axillary nerve, right arm, initial encounter
		S44.32XA	Injury of axillary nerve, left arm, initial encounter

ICD-9-CM		ICD-10-CM	
955.1	INJURY TO MEDIAN NERVE	**S44.1ØXA**	Injury of median nerve at upper arm level, unsp arm, init
		S44.11XA	Injury of median nerve at upper arm level, right arm, init
		S44.12XA	Injury of median nerve at upper arm level, left arm, init
		S54.1ØXA	Injury of median nerve at forearm level, unsp arm, init
		S54.11XA	Injury of median nerve at forearm level, right arm, init
		S54.12XA	Injury of median nerve at forearm level, left arm, init
		S64.1ØXA	Injury of median nerve at wrs/hnd lv of unsp arm, init
		S64.11XA	Injury of median nerve at wrs/hnd lv of right arm, init
		S64.12XA	Injury of median nerve at wrs/hnd lv of left arm, init
955.2	INJURY TO ULNAR NERVE	**S44.ØØXA**	Injury of ulnar nerve at upper arm level, unsp arm, init
		S44.Ø1XA	Injury of ulnar nerve at upper arm level, right arm, init
		S44.Ø2XA	Injury of ulnar nerve at upper arm level, left arm, init
		S54.ØØXA	Injury of ulnar nerve at forearm level, unsp arm, init
		S54.Ø1XA	Injury of ulnar nerve at forearm level, right arm, init
		S54.Ø2XA	Injury of ulnar nerve at forearm level, left arm, init
		S64.ØØXA	Injury of ulnar nerve at wrs/hnd lv of unsp arm, init
		S64.Ø1XA	Injury of ulnar nerve at wrs/hnd lv of right arm, init
		S64.Ø2XA	Injury of ulnar nerve at wrs/hnd lv of left arm, init
955.3	INJURY TO RADIAL NERVE	**S44.2ØXA**	Injury of radial nerve at upper arm level, unsp arm, init
		S44.21XA	Injury of radial nerve at upper arm level, right arm, init
		S44.22XA	Injury of radial nerve at upper arm level, left arm, init
		S54.2ØXA	Injury of radial nerve at forearm level, unsp arm, init
		S54.21XA	Injury of radial nerve at forearm level, right arm, init
		S54.22XA	Injury of radial nerve at forearm level, left arm, init
		S64.2ØXA	Injury of radial nerve at wrs/hnd lv of unsp arm, init
		S64.21XA	Injury of radial nerve at wrs/hnd lv of right arm, init
		S64.22XA	Injury of radial nerve at wrs/hnd lv of left arm, init
955.4	INJURY TO MUSCULOCUTANEOUS NERVE	**S44.4ØXA**	Injury of musculocutaneous nerve, unsp arm, init encntr
		S44.41XA	Injury of musculocutaneous nerve, right arm, init encntr
		S44.42XA	Injury of musculocutaneous nerve, left arm, init encntr
955.5	INJURY TO CUTANEOUS SENSORY NERVE UPPER LIMB	**S44.5ØXA**	Inj cutan sensory nerve at shldr/up arm, unsp arm, init
		S44.51XA	Inj cutan sensory nerve at shldr/up arm, right arm, init
		S44.52XA	Inj cutan sensory nerve at shldr/up arm, left arm, init
		S54.3ØXA	Injury of cutan sensory nerve at forarm lv, unsp arm, init
		S54.31XA	Injury of cutan sensory nerve at forarm lv, right arm, init
		S54.32XA	Injury of cutan sensory nerve at forarm lv, left arm, init
955.6	INJURY TO DIGITAL NERVE, UPPER LIMB	**S64.3ØXA**	Injury of digital nerve of unspecified thumb, init encntr
		S64.31XA	Injury of digital nerve of right thumb, initial encounter
		S64.32XA	Injury of digital nerve of left thumb, initial encounter
		S64.4ØXA	Injury of digital nerve of unspecified finger, init encntr
		S64.49ØA	Injury of digital nerve of right index finger, init encntr
		S64.491A	Injury of digital nerve of left index finger, init encntr
		S64.492A	Injury of digital nerve of right middle finger, init encntr
		S64.493A	Injury of digital nerve of left middle finger, init encntr
		S64.494A	Injury of digital nerve of right ring finger, init encntr
		S64.495A	Injury of digital nerve of left ring finger, init encntr
		S64.496A	Injury of digital nerve of right little finger, init encntr
		S64.497A	Injury of digital nerve of left little finger, init encntr
		S64.498A	Injury of digital nerve of other finger, initial encounter
955.7	INJURY OTH SPEC NERVE SHOULDER GIRDLE&UPPER LIMB	**S44.8X1A**	Injury of nerves at shldr/up arm, right arm, init
		S44.8X2A	Injury of nerves at shldr/up arm, left arm, init
		S44.8X9A	Injury of nerves at shldr/up arm, unsp arm, init
		S54.8X1A	Unsp injury of oth nerves at forearm level, right arm, init
		S54.8X2A	Unsp injury of oth nerves at forearm level, left arm, init
		S54.8X9A	Unsp injury of oth nerves at forearm level, unsp arm, init
		S64.8X1A	Injury of nerves at wrist and hand level of right arm, init
		S64.8X2A	Injury of nerves at wrist and hand level of left arm, init
		S64.8X9A	Injury of nerves at wrist and hand level of unsp arm, init
955.8	INJURY MULTIPLE NERVES SHOULDER GIRDL&UPPER LIMB	**S44.8X1A**	Injury of nerves at shldr/up arm, right arm, init
		S44.8X2A	Injury of nerves at shldr/up arm, left arm, init
		S44.8X9A	Injury of nerves at shldr/up arm, unsp arm, init
		S54.8X1A	Unsp injury of oth nerves at forearm level, right arm, init
		S54.8X2A	Unsp injury of oth nerves at forearm level, left arm, init
		S54.8X9A	Unsp injury of oth nerves at forearm level, unsp arm, init
		S64.8X1A	Injury of nerves at wrist and hand level of right arm, init
		S64.8X2A	Injury of nerves at wrist and hand level of left arm, init
		S64.8X9A	Injury of nerves at wrist and hand level of unsp arm, init
955.9	INJURY UNSPEC NERVE SHOULDER GIRDLE&UPPER LIMB	**S44.9ØXA**	Injury of unsp nerve at shldr/up arm, unsp arm, init
		S44.91XA	Injury of unsp nerve at shldr/up arm, right arm, init
		S44.92XA	Injury of unsp nerve at shldr/up arm, left arm, init
		S54.9ØXA	Injury of unsp nerve at forearm level, unsp arm, init encntr
		S54.91XA	Injury of unsp nerve at forearm level, right arm, init
		S54.92XA	Injury of unsp nerve at forearm level, left arm, init encntr
		S64.9ØXA	Injury of unsp nerve at wrs/hnd lv of unsp arm, init
		S64.91XA	Injury of unsp nerve at wrs/hnd lv of right arm, init
		S64.92XA	Injury of unsp nerve at wrs/hnd lv of left arm, init
956.Ø	INJURY TO SCIATIC NERVE	**S74.ØØXA**	Injury of sciatic nrv at hip and thigh level, unsp leg, init
		S74.Ø1XA	Injury of sciatic nrv at hip and thi lev, right leg, init
		S74.Ø2XA	Injury of sciatic nrv at hip and thigh level, left leg, init

ICD-9-CM		ICD-10-CM	
956.1	INJURY TO FEMORAL NERVE	**S74.1ØXA**	Injury of femoral nrv at hip and thigh level, unsp leg, init
		S74.11XA	Injury of femoral nrv at hip and thi lev, right leg, init
		S74.12XA	Injury of femoral nrv at hip and thigh level, left leg, init
956.2	INJURY TO POSTERIOR TIBIAL NERVE	**S84.ØØXA**	Injury of tibial nerve at lower leg level, unsp leg, init
		S84.Ø1XA	Injury of tibial nerve at lower leg level, right leg, init
		S84.Ø2XA	Injury of tibial nerve at lower leg level, left leg, init
956.3	INJURY TO PERONEAL NERVE	**S84.1ØXA**	Injury of peroneal nerve at lower leg level, unsp leg, init
		S84.11XA	Injury of peroneal nerve at lower leg level, right leg, init
		S84.12XA	Injury of peroneal nerve at lower leg level, left leg, init
		S94.2ØXA	Injury of deep peroneal nrv at ank/ft level, unsp leg, init
		S94.21XA	Injury of deep peroneal nrv at ank/ft level, right leg, init
		S94.22XA	Injury of deep peroneal nrv at ank/ft level, left leg, init
956.4	INJURY TO CUTANEOUS SENSORY NERVE LOWER LIMB	**S74.2ØXA**	Inj cutan sensory nerve at hip and thi lev, unsp leg, init
		S74.21XA	Inj cutan sens nerve at hip and high level, right leg, init
		S74.22XA	Inj cutan sensory nerve at hip and thi lev, left leg, init
		S84.2ØXA	Inj cutan sensory nerve at lower leg level, unsp leg, init
		S84.21XA	Inj cutan sensory nerve at lower leg level, right leg, init
		S84.22XA	Inj cutan sensory nerve at lower leg level, left leg, init
		S94.3ØXA	Inj cutan sensory nerve at ank/ft level, unsp leg, init
		S94.31XA	Inj cutan sensory nerve at ank/ft level, right leg, init
		S94.32XA	Inj cutan sensory nerve at ank/ft level, left leg, init
956.5	INJURY OTHER SPEC NERVE PELVIC GIRDLE&LOWER LIMB	**S74.8X1A**	Injury of oth nerves at hip and thigh level, right leg, init
		S74.8X2A	Injury of oth nerves at hip and thigh level, left leg, init
		S74.8X9A	Injury of oth nerves at hip and thigh level, unsp leg, init
		S84.8Ø1A	Injury of oth nerves at lower leg level, right leg, init
		S84.8Ø2A	Injury of oth nerves at lower leg level, left leg, init
		S84.8Ø9A	Injury of oth nerves at lower leg level, unsp leg, init
		S94.ØØXA	Injury of lateral plantar nerve, unsp leg, init encntr
		S94.Ø1XA	Injury of lateral plantar nerve, right leg, init encntr
		S94.Ø2XA	Injury of lateral plantar nerve, left leg, initial encounter
		S94.1ØXA	Injury of medial plantar nerve, unspecified leg, init encntr
		S94.11XA	Injury of medial plantar nerve, right leg, initial encounter
		S94.12XA	Injury of medial plantar nerve, left leg, initial encounter
		S94.8X1A	Injury of nerves at ankle and foot level, right leg, init
		S94.8X2A	Injury of oth nerves at ankle and foot level, left leg, init
		S94.8X9A	Injury of oth nerves at ankle and foot level, unsp leg, init
956.8	INJURY MULTIPLE NERVES PELVIC GIRDLE&LOWER LIMB	**S74.8X1A**	Injury of oth nerves at hip and thigh level, right leg, init
		S74.8X2A	Injury of oth nerves at hip and thigh level, left leg, init
		S74.8X9A	Injury of oth nerves at hip and thigh level, unsp leg, init
		S84.8Ø1A	Injury of oth nerves at lower leg level, right leg, init
		S84.8Ø2A	Injury of oth nerves at lower leg level, left leg, init
		S84.8Ø9A	Injury of oth nerves at lower leg level, unsp leg, init
		S94.8X1A	Injury of nerves at ankle and foot level, right leg, init
		S94.8X2A	Injury of oth nerves at ankle and foot level, left leg, init
		S94.8X9A	Injury of oth nerves at ankle and foot level, unsp leg, init
956.9	INJURY UNSPEC NERVE PELVIC GIRDLE&LOWER LIMB	**S74.9ØXA**	Injury of unsp nerve at hip and thigh level, unsp leg, init
		S74.91XA	Injury of unsp nerve at hip and thigh level, right leg, init
		S74.92XA	Injury of unsp nerve at hip and thigh level, left leg, init
		S84.9ØXA	Injury of unsp nerve at lower leg level, unsp leg, init
		S84.91XA	Injury of unsp nerve at lower leg level, right leg, init
		S84.92XA	Injury of unsp nerve at lower leg level, left leg, init
		S94.9ØXA	Injury of unsp nerve at ankle and foot level, unsp leg, init
		S94.91XA	Injury of unsp nerve at ank/ft level, right leg, init
		S94.92XA	Injury of unsp nerve at ankle and foot level, left leg, init
957.Ø	INJURY TO SUPERFICIAL NERVES OF HEAD AND NECK	**S14.4XXA**	Injury of peripheral nerves of neck, initial encounter
		S14.8XXA	Injury of other specified nerves of neck, initial encounter
957.1	INJURY TO OTHER SPECIFIED NERVE	**S14.9XXA**	Injury of unspecified nerves of neck, initial encounter
957.8	INJURY TO MULTIPLE NERVES IN SEVERAL PARTS	**S14.9XXA**	Injury of unspecified nerves of neck, initial encounter
957.9	INJURY TO NERVES UNSPECIFIED SITE	**S14.9XXA**	Injury of unspecified nerves of neck, initial encounter
		S24.9XXA	Injury of unspecified nerve of thorax, initial encounter
		S34.9XXA	Inj unsp nerves at abdomen, low back and pelvis level, init
		S44.9ØXA	Injury of unsp nerve at shldr/up arm, unsp arm, init
		S44.91XA	Injury of unsp nerve at shldr/up arm, right arm, init
		S44.92XA	Injury of unsp nerve at shldr/up arm, left arm, init
		S54.9ØXA	Injury of unsp nerve at forearm level, unsp arm, init encntr
		S54.91XA	Injury of unsp nerve at forearm level, right arm, init
		S54.92XA	Injury of unsp nerve at forearm level, left arm, init encntr
		S64.9ØXA	Injury of unsp nerve at wrs/hnd lv of unsp arm, init
		S64.91XA	Injury of unsp nerve at wrs/hnd lv of right arm, init
		S64.92XA	Injury of unsp nerve at wrs/hnd lv of left arm, init
		S74.9ØXA	Injury of unsp nerve at hip and thigh level, unsp leg, init
		S74.91XA	Injury of unsp nerve at hip and thigh level, right leg, init
		S74.92XA	Injury of unsp nerve at hip and thigh level, left leg, init
		S84.9ØXA	Injury of unsp nerve at lower leg level, unsp leg, init
		S84.91XA	Injury of unsp nerve at lower leg level, right leg, init
		S84.92XA	Injury of unsp nerve at lower leg level, left leg, init
		S94.9ØXA	Injury of unsp nerve at ankle and foot level, unsp leg, init
		S94.91XA	Injury of unsp nerve at ank/ft level, right leg, init
		S94.92XA	Injury of unsp nerve at ankle and foot level, left leg, init
958.Ø	AIR EMBOLISM AS AN EARLY COMPLICATION OF TRAUMA	**T79.ØXXA**	Air embolism (traumatic), initial encounter

[Brackets] indicate valid character values for each code. Character value meanings provided for each code grouping.

ICD-9-CM		ICD-10-CM	
958.1	FAT EMBOLISM AS AN EARLY COMPLICATION OF TRAUMA	**T79.1XXA**	Fat embolism (traumatic), initial encounter
958.2	SEC&RECURRENT HEMORRHAGE AS AN EARLY COMP TRAUMA	**T79.2XXA**	Traumatic secondary and recurrent hemor and seroma, init
958.3	POSTTRAUMATIC WOUND INFECTION NEC	**T79.8XXA**	Other early complications of trauma, initial encounter
958.4	TRAUMATIC SHOCK	**T79.4XXA**	Traumatic shock, initial encounter
958.5	TRAUMATIC ANURIA	**T79.5XXA**	Traumatic anuria, initial encounter
958.6	VOLKMANNS ISCHEMIC CONTRACTURE	**T79.6XXA**	Traumatic ischemia of muscle, initial encounter
958.7	TRAUMATIC SUBCUTANEOUS EMPHYSEMA	**T79.7XXA**	Traumatic subcutaneous emphysema, initial encounter
958.8	OTHER EARLY COMPLICATIONS OF TRAUMA	**T79.8XXA**	Other early complications of trauma, initial encounter
		T79.9XXA	Unspecified early complication of trauma, initial encounter
958.90	COMPARTMENT SYNDROME UNSPECIFIED	**T79.A0XA**	Compartment syndrome, unspecified, initial encounter
958.91	TRAUMATIC COMPARTMENT SYNDROME UPPER EXTREMITY	**T79.A11A**	Traumatic compartment syndrome of r up extrem, init
		T79.A12A	Traumatic compartment syndrome of left upper extremity, init
		T79.A19A	Traumatic compartment syndrome of unsp upper extremity, init
958.92	TRAUMATIC COMPARTMENT SYNDROME LOWER EXTREMITY	**T79.A21A**	Traumatic compartment syndrome of r low extrem, init
		T79.A22A	Traumatic compartment syndrome of left lower extremity, init
		T79.A29A	Traumatic compartment syndrome of unsp lower extremity, init
958.93	TRAUMATIC COMPARTMENT SYNDROME OF ABDOMEN	**T79.A3XA**	Traumatic compartment syndrome of abdomen, initial encounter
958.99	TRAUMATIC COMPARTMENT SYNDROME OF OTHER SITES	**T79.A9XA**	Traumatic compartment syndrome of other sites, init encntr
959.01	HEAD INJURY, UNSPECIFIED	**S09.10XA**	Unspecified injury of muscle and tendon of head, init encntr
		S09.11XA	Strain of muscle and tendon of head, initial encounter
		S09.19XA	Oth injury of muscle and tendon of head, init encntr
		S09.8XXA	Other specified injuries of head, initial encounter
		S09.90XA	Unspecified injury of head, initial encounter
959.09	INJURY OF FACE AND NECK OTHER AND UNSPECIFIED	**S09.92XA**	Unspecified injury of nose, initial encounter
		S09.93XA	Unspecified injury of face, initial encounter
		S16.8XXA	Inj muscle, fascia and tendon at neck level, init encntr
		S16.9XXA	Unsp injury of muscle, fascia and tendon at neck level, init
		S19.80XA	Oth injuries of unspecified part of neck, init encntr
		S19.81XA	Other specified injuries of larynx, initial encounter
		S19.82XA	Other specified injuries of cervical trachea, init encntr
		S19.83XA	Other specified injuries of vocal cord, initial encounter
		S19.84XA	Other specified injuries of thyroid gland, initial encounter
		S19.85XA	Oth injuries of pharynx and cervical esophagus, init encntr
		S19.89XA	Oth injuries of other specified part of neck, init encntr
		S19.9XXA	Unspecified injury of neck, initial encounter
959.11	OTHER INJURY OF CHEST WALL	**S29.001A**	Unsp injury of msl/tnd of front wall of thorax, init
		S29.002A	Unsp injury of msl/tnd of back wall of thorax, init
		S29.009A	Unsp injury of msl/tnd of unsp wall of thorax, init
		S29.091A	Inj muscle and tendon of front wall of thorax, init encntr
		S29.092A	Inj muscle and tendon of back wall of thorax, init encntr
		S29.099A	Inj muscle and tendon of unsp wall of thorax, init encntr
		S29.8XXA	Other specified injuries of thorax, initial encounter
		S29.9XXA	Unspecified injury of thorax, initial encounter
959.12	OTHER INJURY OF ABDOMEN	**S39.001A**	Unsp injury of muscle, fascia and tendon of abdomen, init
		S39.091A	Inj muscle, fascia and tendon of abdomen, init encntr
		S39.81XA	Other specified injuries of abdomen, initial encounter
		S39.91XA	Unspecified injury of abdomen, initial encounter
959.13	FRACTURE OF CORPUS CAVERNOSUM PENIS	**S39.840A**	Fracture of corpus cavernosum penis, initial encounter
959.14	OTHER INJURY OF EXTERNAL GENITALS	**S39.848A**	Other specified injuries of external genitals, init encntr
		S39.94XA	Unspecified injury of external genitals, initial encounter
959.19	OTHER INJURY OF OTHER SITES OF TRUNK	**S39.002A**	Unsp injury of muscle, fascia and tendon of lower back, init
		S39.003A	Unsp injury of muscle, fascia and tendon of pelvis, init
		S39.092A	Inj muscle, fascia and tendon of lower back, init encntr
		S39.093A	Inj muscle, fascia and tendon of pelvis, init encntr
		S39.82XA	Other specified injuries of lower back, initial encounter
		S39.83XA	Other specified injuries of pelvis, initial encounter
		S39.92XA	Unspecified injury of lower back, initial encounter
		S39.93XA	Unspecified injury of pelvis, initial encounter
959.2	INJURY OTHER&UNSPECIFIED SHOULDER&UPPER ARM	**S46.001A**	Unsp inj musc/tend the rotator cuff of r shoulder, init
		S46.002A	Unsp inj musc/tend the rotator cuff of l shoulder, init
		S46.009A	Unsp inj musc/tend the rotator cuff of unsp shoulder, init
		S46.091A	Inj musc/tend the rotator cuff of right shoulder, init
		S46.092A	Inj musc/tend the rotator cuff of left shoulder, init
		S46.099A	Inj musc/tend the rotator cuff of unsp shoulder, init
		S46.101A	Unsp injury of musc/fasc/tend long hd bicep, right arm, init
		S46.102A	Unsp injury of musc/fasc/tend long hd bicep, left arm, init
		S46.109A	Unsp injury of musc/fasc/tend long hd bicep, unsp arm, init
		S46.191A	Inj musc/fasc/tend long head of biceps, right arm, init
		S46.192A	Inj musc/fasc/tend long head of biceps, left arm, init
		S46.199A	Inj musc/fasc/tend long head of biceps, unsp arm, init
		S46.201A	Unsp injury of musc/fasc/tend prt biceps, right arm, init
		S46.202A	Unsp injury of musc/fasc/tend prt biceps, left arm, init
		S46.209A	Unsp injury of musc/fasc/tend prt biceps, unsp arm, init
		S46.291A	Inj muscle, fascia and tendon of prt biceps, right arm, init
		S46.292A	Inj muscle, fascia and tendon of prt biceps, left arm, init
		S46.299A	Inj muscle, fascia and tendon of prt biceps, unsp arm, init
		S46.301A	Unsp injury of musc/fasc/tend triceps, right arm, init
	(Continued on next page)	**S46.302A**	Unsp injury of musc/fasc/tend triceps, left arm, init

ICD-9-CM		ICD-10-CM	
959.2	INJURY OTHER&UNSPECIFIED SHOULDER&UPPER ARM **(Continued)**	**S46.309A**	Unsp injury of musc/fasc/tend triceps, unsp arm, init
		S46.391A	Inj muscle, fascia and tendon of triceps, right arm, init
		S46.392A	Inj muscle, fascia and tendon of triceps, left arm, init
		S46.399A	Inj muscle, fascia and tendon of triceps, unsp arm, init
		S46.801A	Unsp inj musc/fasc/tend at shldr/up arm, right arm, init
		S46.802A	Unsp inj musc/fasc/tend at shldr/up arm, left arm, init
		S46.809A	Unsp inj musc/fasc/tend at shldr/up arm, unsp arm, init
		S46.891A	Inj musc/fasc/tend at shldr/up arm, right arm, init
		S46.892A	Inj musc/fasc/tend at shldr/up arm, left arm, init
		S46.899A	Inj musc/fasc/tend at shldr/up arm, unsp arm, init
		S46.901A	Unsp inj unsp musc/fasc/tend at shldr/up arm, r arm, init
		S46.902A	Unsp inj unsp musc/fasc/tend at shldr/up arm, left arm, init
		S46.909A	Unsp inj unsp musc/fasc/tend at shldr/up arm, unsp arm, init
		S46.991A	Inj unsp musc/fasc/tend at shldr/up arm, right arm, init
		S46.992A	Inj unsp musc/fasc/tend at shldr/up arm, left arm, init
		S46.999A	Inj unsp musc/fasc/tend at shldr/up arm, unsp arm, init
		S49.80XA	Oth injuries of shoulder and upper arm, unsp arm, init
		S49.81XA	Oth injuries of right shoulder and upper arm, init encntr
		S49.82XA	Oth injuries of left shoulder and upper arm, init encntr
		S49.90XA	Unsp injury of shoulder and upper arm, unsp arm, init encntr
		S49.91XA	Unsp injury of right shoulder and upper arm, init encntr
		S49.92XA	Unsp injury of left shoulder and upper arm, init encntr
959.3	INJURY OTHER&UNSPECIFIED ELBOW FOREARM&WRIST	**S56.001A**	Unsp inj flexor musc/fasc/tend r thm at forarm lv, init
		S56.002A	Unsp inj flexor musc/fasc/tend l thm at forarm lv, init
		S56.009A	Unsp injury of flexor musc/fasc/tend thmb at forarm lv, init
		S56.091A	Inj flexor musc/fasc/tend right thumb at forearm level, init
		S56.092A	Inj flexor musc/fasc/tend left thumb at forearm level, init
		S56.099A	Inj flexor musc/fasc/tend thmb at forearm level, init
		S56.101A	Unsp inj flexor musc/fasc/tend r idx fngr at forarm lv, init
		S56.102A	Unsp inj flexor musc/fasc/tend l idx fngr at forarm lv, init
		S56.103A	Unsp inj flexor musc/fasc/tend r mid fngr at forarm lv, init
		S56.104A	Unsp inj flexor musc/fasc/tend l mid fngr at forarm lv, init
		S56.105A	Unsp inj flexor musc/fasc/tend r rng fngr at forarm lv, init
		S56.106A	Unsp inj flexor musc/fasc/tend l rng fngr at forarm lv, init
		S56.107A	Unsp inj flxr musc/fasc/tend r lit fngr at forarm lv, init
		S56.108A	Unsp inj flxr musc/fasc/tend l lit fngr at forarm lv, init
		S56.109A	Unsp inj flexor musc/fasc/tend unsp fngr at forarm lv, init
		S56.191A	Inj flexor musc/fasc/tend r idx fngr at forearm level, init
		S56.192A	Inj flexor musc/fasc/tend l idx fngr at forearm level, init
		S56.193A	Inj flexor musc/fasc/tend r mid finger at forarm lv, init
		S56.194A	Inj flexor musc/fasc/tend l mid finger at forarm lv, init
		S56.195A	Inj flexor musc/fasc/tend r rng fngr at forearm level, init
		S56.196A	Inj flexor musc/fasc/tend l rng fngr at forearm level, init
		S56.197A	Inj flexor musc/fasc/tend r little finger at forarm lv, init
		S56.198A	Inj flexor musc/fasc/tend l little finger at forarm lv, init
		S56.199A	Inj flexor musc/fasc/tend unsp finger at forearm level, init
		S56.201A	Unsp inj flexor musc/fasc/tend at forarm lv, right arm, init
		S56.202A	Unsp inj flexor musc/fasc/tend at forarm lv, left arm, init
		S56.209A	Unsp inj flexor musc/fasc/tend at forarm lv, unsp arm, init
		S56.291A	Inj oth flexor musc/fasc/tend at forarm lv, right arm, init
		S56.292A	Inj oth flexor musc/fasc/tend at forarm lv, left arm, init
		S56.299A	Inj oth flexor musc/fasc/tend at forarm lv, unsp arm, init
		S56.301A	Unsp inj extn/abdr musc/fasc/tend of r thm at forarm lv,init
		S56.302A	Unsp inj extn/abdr musc/fasc/tend of l thm at forarm lv,init
		S56.309A	Unsp inj extn/abdr musc/fasc/tend of thmb at forarm lv, init
		S56.391A	Inj extn/abdr musc/fasc/tend of r thm at forarm lv, init
		S56.392A	Inj extn/abdr musc/fasc/tend of l thm at forarm lv, init
		S56.399A	Inj extn/abdr musc/fasc/tend of thmb at forearm level, init
		S56.401A	Unsp inj extn musc/fasc/tend r idx fngr at forarm lv, init
		S56.402A	Unsp inj extn musc/fasc/tend l idx fngr at forarm lv, init
		S56.403A	Unsp inj extn musc/fasc/tend r mid finger at forarm lv, init
		S56.404A	Unsp inj extn musc/fasc/tend l mid finger at forarm lv, init
		S56.405A	Unsp inj extn musc/fasc/tend r rng fngr at forarm lv, init
		S56.406A	Unsp inj extn musc/fasc/tend l rng fngr at forarm lv, init
		S56.407A	Unsp inj extn musc/fasc/tend r lit fngr at forarm lv, init
		S56.408A	Unsp inj extn musc/fasc/tend l lit fngr at forarm lv, init
		S56.409A	Unsp inj extn musc/fasc/tend unsp finger at forarm lv, init
		S56.491A	Inj extensor musc/fasc/tend r idx fngr at forarm lv, init
		S56.492A	Inj extensor musc/fasc/tend l idx fngr at forarm lv, init
		S56.493A	Inj extensor musc/fasc/tend r mid finger at forarm lv, init
		S56.494A	Inj extensor musc/fasc/tend l mid finger at forarm lv, init
		S56.495A	Inj extensor musc/fasc/tend r rng fngr at forarm lv, init
		S56.496A	Inj extensor musc/fasc/tend l rng fngr at forarm lv, init
		S56.497A	Inj extn musc/fasc/tend r little finger at forarm lv, init
		S56.498A	Inj extn musc/fasc/tend l little finger at forarm lv, init
		S56.499A	Inj extensor musc/fasc/tend unsp finger at forarm lv, init
		S56.501A	Unsp inj extn musc/fasc/tend at forarm lv, right arm, init
		S56.502A	Unsp inj extn musc/fasc/tend at forarm lv, left arm, init
		S56.509A	Unsp inj extn musc/fasc/tend at forarm lv, unsp arm, init
		S56.591A	Inj extn musc/fasc/tend at forearm level, right arm, init
		S56.592A	Inj extn musc/fasc/tend at forearm level, left arm, init
	(Continued on next page)	**S56.599A**	Inj extn musc/fasc/tend at forearm level, unsp arm, init

ICD-9-CM		ICD-10-CM	
959.3	INJURY OTHER&UNSPECIFIED ELBOW FOREARM&WRIST **(Continued)**	**S56.801A**	Unsp injury of musc/fasc/tend at forarm lv, right arm, init
		S56.802A	Unsp injury of musc/fasc/tend at forarm lv, left arm, init
		S56.809A	Unsp injury of musc/fasc/tend at forarm lv, unsp arm, init
		S56.891A	Inj musc/fasc/tend at forearm level, right arm, init encntr
		S56.892A	Inj musc/fasc/tend at forearm level, left arm, init encntr
		S56.899A	Inj musc/fasc/tend at forearm level, unsp arm, init encntr
		S56.901A	Unsp inj unsp musc/fasc/tend at forarm lv, right arm, init
		S56.902A	Unsp inj unsp musc/fasc/tend at forarm lv, left arm, init
		S56.909A	Unsp inj unsp musc/fasc/tend at forarm lv, unsp arm, init
		S56.991A	Inj unsp musc/fasc/tend at forearm level, right arm, init
		S56.992A	Inj unsp musc/fasc/tend at forearm level, left arm, init
		S56.999A	Inj unsp musc/fasc/tend at forearm level, unsp arm, init
		S59.801A	Other specified injuries of right elbow, initial encounter
		S59.802A	Other specified injuries of left elbow, initial encounter
		S59.809A	Other specified injuries of unspecified elbow, init encntr
		S59.811A	Other specified injuries right forearm, initial encounter
		S59.812A	Other specified injuries left forearm, initial encounter
		S59.819A	Other specified injuries unspecified forearm, init encntr
		S59.901A	Unspecified injury of right elbow, initial encounter
		S59.902A	Unspecified injury of left elbow, initial encounter
		S59.909A	Unspecified injury of unspecified elbow, initial encounter
		S59.911A	Unspecified injury of right forearm, initial encounter
		S59.912A	Unspecified injury of left forearm, initial encounter
		S59.919A	Unspecified injury of unspecified forearm, initial encounter
		S66.001A	Unsp inj long flxr musc/fasc/tend r thm at wrs/hnd lv, init
		S66.002A	Unsp inj long flxr musc/fasc/tend l thm at wrs/hnd lv, init
		S66.009A	Unsp inj long flexor musc/fasc/tend thmb at wrs/hnd lv, init
		S66.091A	Inj long flexor musc/fasc/tend r thm at wrs/hnd lv, init
		S66.092A	Inj long flexor musc/fasc/tend l thm at wrs/hnd lv, init
		S66.099A	Inj long flexor musc/fasc/tend thmb at wrs/hnd lv, init
		S66.100A	Unsp inj flxr musc/fasc/tend r idx fngr at wrs/hnd lv, init
		S66.101A	Unsp inj flxr musc/fasc/tend l idx fngr at wrs/hnd lv, init
		S66.102A	Unsp inj flxr musc/fasc/tend r mid fngr at wrs/hnd lv, init
		S66.103A	Unsp inj flxr musc/fasc/tend l mid fngr at wrs/hnd lv, init
		S66.104A	Unsp inj flxr musc/fasc/tend r rng fngr at wrs/hnd lv, init
		S66.105A	Unsp inj flxr musc/fasc/tend l rng fngr at wrs/hnd lv, init
		S66.106A	Unsp inj flxr musc/fasc/tend r lit fngr at wrs/hnd lv, init
		S66.107A	Unsp inj flxr musc/fasc/tend l lit fngr at wrs/hnd lv, init
		S66.108A	Unsp inj flexor musc/fasc/tend finger at wrs/hnd lv, init
		S66.109A	Unsp inj flexor musc/fasc/tend unsp fngr at wrs/hnd lv, init
		S66.190A	Inj flexor musc/fasc/tend r idx fngr at wrs/hnd lv, init
		S66.191A	Inj flexor musc/fasc/tend l idx fngr at wrs/hnd lv, init
		S66.192A	Inj flexor musc/fasc/tend r mid finger at wrs/hnd lv, init
		S66.193A	Inj flexor musc/fasc/tend l mid finger at wrs/hnd lv, init
		S66.194A	Inj flexor musc/fasc/tend r rng fngr at wrs/hnd lv, init
		S66.195A	Inj flexor musc/fasc/tend l rng fngr at wrs/hnd lv, init
		S66.196A	Inj flexor musc/fasc/tend r little fngr at wrs/hnd lv, init
		S66.197A	Inj flexor musc/fasc/tend l little fngr at wrs/hnd lv, init
		S66.198A	Inj flexor musc/fasc/tend finger at wrs/hnd lv, init
		S66.199A	Inj flexor musc/fasc/tend unsp finger at wrs/hnd lv, init
		S66.201A	Unsp inj extensor musc/fasc/tend r thm at wrs/hnd lv, init
		S66.202A	Unsp inj extensor musc/fasc/tend l thm at wrs/hnd lv, init
		S66.291A	Inj extensor musc/fasc/tend right thumb at wrs/hnd lv, init
		S66.292A	Inj extensor musc/fasc/tend left thumb at wrs/hnd lv, init
		S66.299A	Inj extensor musc/fasc/tend thmb at wrs/hnd lv, init
		S66.300A	Unsp inj extn musc/fasc/tend r idx fngr at wrs/hnd lv, init
		S66.301A	Unsp inj extn musc/fasc/tend l idx fngr at wrs/hnd lv, init
		S66.302A	Unsp inj extn musc/fasc/tend r mid fngr at wrs/hnd lv, init
		S66.303A	Unsp inj extn musc/fasc/tend l mid fngr at wrs/hnd lv, init
		S66.304A	Unsp inj extn musc/fasc/tend r rng fngr at wrs/hnd lv, init
		S66.305A	Unsp inj extn musc/fasc/tend l rng fngr at wrs/hnd lv, init
		S66.306A	Unsp inj extn musc/fasc/tend r lit fngr at wrs/hnd lv, init
		S66.307A	Unsp inj extn musc/fasc/tend l lit fngr at wrs/hnd lv, init
		S66.308A	Unsp inj extensor musc/fasc/tend finger at wrs/hnd lv, init
		S66.309A	Unsp inj extn musc/fasc/tend unsp finger at wrs/hnd lv, init
		S66.390A	Inj extensor musc/fasc/tend r idx fngr at wrs/hnd lv, init
		S66.391A	Inj extensor musc/fasc/tend l idx fngr at wrs/hnd lv, init
		S66.392A	Inj extensor musc/fasc/tend r mid finger at wrs/hnd lv, init
		S66.393A	Inj extensor musc/fasc/tend l mid finger at wrs/hnd lv, init
		S66.394A	Inj extensor musc/fasc/tend r rng fngr at wrs/hnd lv, init
		S66.395A	Inj extensor musc/fasc/tend l rng fngr at wrs/hnd lv, init
		S66.396A	Inj extn musc/fasc/tend r little finger at wrs/hnd lv, init
		S66.397A	Inj extn musc/fasc/tend l little finger at wrs/hnd lv, init
		S66.398A	Inj extensor musc/fasc/tend finger at wrs/hnd lv, init
		S66.399A	Inj extensor musc/fasc/tend unsp finger at wrs/hnd lv, init
		S66.401A	Unsp inj intrinsic musc/fasc/tend r thm at wrs/hnd lv, init
		S66.402A	Unsp inj intrinsic musc/fasc/tend l thm at wrs/hnd lv, init
		S66.409A	Unsp inj intrinsic musc/fasc/tend thmb at wrs/hnd lv, init
		S66.491A	Inj intrinsic musc/fasc/tend right thumb at wrs/hnd lv, init
		S66.492A	Inj intrinsic musc/fasc/tend left thumb at wrs/hnd lv, init
		S66.499A	Inj intrinsic musc/fasc/tend thmb at wrs/hnd lv, init
		S66.500A	Unsp inj intrns musc/fasc/tend r idx fngr at wrs/hnd lv,init
	(Continued on next page)	**S66.501A**	Unsp inj intrns musc/fasc/tend l idx fngr at wrs/hnd lv,init

ICD-9-CM		ICD-10-CM	
959.3	INJURY OTHER&UNSPECIFIED ELBOW FOREARM&WRIST **(Continued)**	**S66.502A**	Unsp inj intrns musc/fasc/tend r mid fngr at wrs/hnd lv,init
		S66.503A	Unsp inj intrns musc/fasc/tend l mid fngr at wrs/hnd lv,init
		S66.504A	Unsp inj intrns musc/fasc/tend r rng fngr at wrs/hnd lv,init
		S66.505A	Unsp inj intrns musc/fasc/tend l rng fngr at wrs/hnd lv,init
		S66.506A	Unsp inj intrns musc/fasc/tend r lit fngr at wrs/hnd lv,init
		S66.507A	Unsp inj intrns musc/fasc/tend l lit fngr at wrs/hnd lv,init
		S66.508A	Unsp inj intrinsic musc/fasc/tend finger at wrs/hnd lv, init
		S66.509A	Unsp inj intrns musc/fasc/tend unsp fngr at wrs/hnd lv, init
		S66.590A	Inj intrinsic musc/fasc/tend r idx fngr at wrs/hnd lv, init
		S66.591A	Inj intrinsic musc/fasc/tend l idx fngr at wrs/hnd lv, init
		S66.592A	Inj intrns musc/fasc/tend r mid finger at wrs/hnd lv, init
		S66.593A	Inj intrns musc/fasc/tend l mid finger at wrs/hnd lv, init
		S66.594A	Inj intrinsic musc/fasc/tend r rng fngr at wrs/hnd lv, init
		S66.595A	Inj intrinsic musc/fasc/tend l rng fngr at wrs/hnd lv, init
		S66.596A	Inj intrns musc/fasc/tend r little fngr at wrs/hnd lv, init
		S66.597A	Inj intrns musc/fasc/tend l little fngr at wrs/hnd lv, init
		S66.598A	Inj intrinsic musc/fasc/tend finger at wrs/hnd lv, init
		S66.599A	Inj intrinsic musc/fasc/tend unsp finger at wrs/hnd lv, init
		S66.801A	Unsp injury of musc/fasc/tend at wrs/hnd lv, r hand, init
		S66.802A	Unsp injury of musc/fasc/tend at wrs/hnd lv, left hand, init
		S66.809A	Unsp injury of musc/fasc/tend at wrs/hnd lv, unsp hand, init
		S66.891A	Inj musc/fasc/tend at wrist and hand level, right hand, init
		S66.892A	Inj musc/fasc/tend at wrist and hand level, left hand, init
		S66.899A	Inj musc/fasc/tend at wrist and hand level, unsp hand, init
		S66.901A	Unsp inj unsp musc/fasc/tend at wrs/hnd lv, r hand, init
		S66.902A	Unsp inj unsp musc/fasc/tend at wrs/hnd lv, left hand, init
		S66.909A	Unsp inj unsp musc/fasc/tend at wrs/hnd lv, unsp hand, init
		S66.991A	Inj unsp musc/fasc/tend at wrs/hnd lv, right hand, init
		S66.992A	Inj unsp musc/fasc/tend at wrs/hnd lv, left hand, init
		S66.999A	Inj unsp musc/fasc/tend at wrs/hnd lv, unsp hand, init
		S69.80XA	Oth injuries of unsp wrist, hand and finger(s), init encntr
		S69.81XA	Oth injuries of right wrist, hand and finger(s), init encntr
		S69.82XA	Oth injuries of left wrist, hand and finger(s), init encntr
		S69.90XA	Unsp injury of unsp wrist, hand and finger(s), init encntr
		S69.91XA	Unsp injury of right wrist, hand and finger(s), init encntr
		S69.92XA	Unsp injury of left wrist, hand and finger(s), init encntr
959.4	INJURY OTHER AND UNSPECIFIED HAND EXCEPT FINGER	**S66.001A**	Unsp inj long flxr musc/fasc/tend r thm at wrs/hnd lv, init
		S66.002A	Unsp inj long flxr musc/fasc/tend l thm at wrs/hnd lv, init
		S66.009A	Unsp inj long flexor musc/fasc/tend thmb at wrs/hnd lv, init
		S66.092A	Inj long flexor musc/fasc/tend l thm at wrs/hnd lv, init
		S66.099A	Inj long flexor musc/fasc/tend thmb at wrs/hnd lv, init
		S66.100A	Unsp inj flxr musc/fasc/tend r idx fngr at wrs/hnd lv, init
		S66.101A	Unsp inj flxr musc/fasc/tend l idx fngr at wrs/hnd lv, init
		S66.102A	Unsp inj flxr musc/fasc/tend r mid fngr at wrs/hnd lv, init
		S66.103A	Unsp inj flxr musc/fasc/tend l mid fngr at wrs/hnd lv, init
		S66.104A	Unsp inj flxr musc/fasc/tend r rng fngr at wrs/hnd lv, init
		S66.105A	Unsp inj flxr musc/fasc/tend l rng fngr at wrs/hnd lv, init
		S66.106A	Unsp inj flxr musc/fasc/tend r lit fngr at wrs/hnd lv, init
		S66.107A	Unsp inj flxr musc/fasc/tend l lit fngr at wrs/hnd lv, init
		S66.108A	Unsp inj flexor musc/fasc/tend finger at wrs/hnd lv, init
		S66.109A	Unsp inj flexor musc/fasc/tend unsp fngr at wrs/hnd lv, init
		S66.190A	Inj flexor musc/fasc/tend r idx fngr at wrs/hnd lv, init
		S66.191A	Inj flexor musc/fasc/tend l idx fngr at wrs/hnd lv, init
		S66.192A	Inj flexor musc/fasc/tend r mid finger at wrs/hnd lv, init
		S66.193A	Inj flexor musc/fasc/tend l mid finger at wrs/hnd lv, init
		S66.194A	Inj flexor musc/fasc/tend r rng fngr at wrs/hnd lv, init
		S66.195A	Inj flexor musc/fasc/tend l rng fngr at wrs/hnd lv, init
		S66.196A	Inj flexor musc/fasc/tend r little fngr at wrs/hnd lv, init
		S66.197A	Inj flexor musc/fasc/tend l little fngr at wrs/hnd lv, init
		S66.198A	Inj flexor musc/fasc/tend finger at wrs/hnd lv, init
		S66.199A	Inj flexor musc/fasc/tend unsp finger at wrs/hnd lv, init
		S66.201A	Unsp inj extensor musc/fasc/tend r thm at wrs/hnd lv, init
		S66.202A	Unsp inj extensor musc/fasc/tend l thm at wrs/hnd lv, init
		S66.209A	Unsp inj extensor musc/fasc/tend thmb at wrs/hnd lv, init
		S66.291A	Inj extensor musc/fasc/tend right thumb at wrs/hnd lv, init
		S66.292A	Inj extensor musc/fasc/tend left thumb at wrs/hnd lv, init
		S66.299A	Inj extensor musc/fasc/tend thmb at wrs/hnd lv, init
		S66.300A	Unsp inj extn musc/fasc/tend r idx fngr at wrs/hnd lv, init
		S66.301A	Unsp inj extn musc/fasc/tend l idx fngr at wrs/hnd lv, init
		S66.302A	Unsp inj extn musc/fasc/tend r mid fngr at wrs/hnd lv, init
		S66.303A	Unsp inj extn musc/fasc/tend l mid fngr at wrs/hnd lv, init
		S66.304A	Unsp inj extn musc/fasc/tend r rng fngr at wrs/hnd lv, init
		S66.305A	Unsp inj extn musc/fasc/tend l rng fngr at wrs/hnd lv, init
		S66.306A	Unsp inj extn musc/fasc/tend r lit fngr at wrs/hnd lv, init
		S66.307A	Unsp inj extn musc/fasc/tend l lit fngr at wrs/hnd lv, init
		S66.308A	Unsp inj extensor musc/fasc/tend finger at wrs/hnd lv, init
		S66.309A	Unsp inj extn musc/fasc/tend unsp finger at wrs/hnd lv, init
		S66.390A	Inj extensor musc/fasc/tend r idx fngr at wrs/hnd lv, init
		S66.391A	Inj extensor musc/fasc/tend l idx fngr at wrs/hnd lv, init
		S66.392A	Inj extensor musc/fasc/tend r mid finger at wrs/hnd lv, init
		S66.393A	Inj extensor musc/fasc/tend l mid finger at wrs/hnd lv, init
		S66.394A	Inj extensor musc/fasc/tend r rng fngr at wrs/hnd lv, init
	(Continued on next page)	**S66.395A**	Inj extensor musc/fasc/tend l rng fngr at wrs/hnd lv, init

ICD-9-CM		ICD-10-CM	
959.4	INJURY OTHER AND UNSPECIFIED HAND EXCEPT FINGER **(Continued)**	**S66.396A**	Inj extn musc/fasc/tend r little finger at wrs/hnd lv, init
		S66.397A	Inj extn musc/fasc/tend l little finger at wrs/hnd lv, init
		S66.398A	Inj extensor musc/fasc/tend finger at wrs/hnd lv, init
		S66.399A	Inj extensor musc/fasc/tend unsp finger at wrs/hnd lv, init
		S66.401A	Unsp inj intrinsic musc/fasc/tend r thm at wrs/hnd lv, init
		S66.402A	Unsp inj intrinsic musc/fasc/tend l thm at wrs/hnd lv, init
		S66.409A	Unsp inj intrinsic musc/fasc/tend thmb at wrs/hnd lv, init
		S66.491A	Inj intrinsic musc/fasc/tend right thumb at wrs/hnd lv, init
		S66.492A	Inj intrinsic musc/fasc/tend left thumb at wrs/hnd lv, init
		S66.499A	Inj intrinsic musc/fasc/tend thmb at wrs/hnd lv, init
		S66.500A	Unsp inj intrns musc/fasc/tend r idx fngr at wrs/hnd lv,init
		S66.501A	Unsp inj intrns musc/fasc/tend l idx fngr at wrs/hnd lv,init
		S66.502A	Unsp inj intrns musc/fasc/tend r mid fngr at wrs/hnd lv,init
		S66.503A	Unsp inj intrns musc/fasc/tend l mid fngr at wrs/hnd lv,init
		S66.504A	Unsp inj intrns musc/fasc/tend r rng fngr at wrs/hnd lv,init
		S66.505A	Unsp inj intrns musc/fasc/tend l rng fngr at wrs/hnd lv,init
		S66.506A	Unsp inj intrns musc/fasc/tend r lit fngr at wrs/hnd lv,init
		S66.507A	Unsp inj intrns musc/fasc/tend l lit fngr at wrs/hnd lv,init
		S66.508A	Unsp inj intrinsic musc/fasc/tend finger at wrs/hnd lv, init
		S66.509A	Unsp inj intrns musc/fasc/tend unsp fngr at wrs/hnd lv, init
		S66.590A	Inj intrinsic musc/fasc/tend r idx fngr at wrs/hnd lv, init
		S66.591A	Inj intrinsic musc/fasc/tend l idx fngr at wrs/hnd lv, init
		S66.592A	Inj intrns musc/fasc/tend r mid finger at wrs/hnd lv, init
		S66.593A	Inj intrns musc/fasc/tend l mid finger at wrs/hnd lv, init
		S66.594A	Inj intrinsic musc/fasc/tend r rng fngr at wrs/hnd lv, init
		S66.595A	Inj intrinsic musc/fasc/tend l rng fngr at wrs/hnd lv, init
		S66.596A	Inj intrns musc/fasc/tend r little fngr at wrs/hnd lv, init
		S66.597A	Inj intrns musc/fasc/tend l little fngr at wrs/hnd lv, init
		S66.598A	Inj intrinsic musc/fasc/tend finger at wrs/hnd lv, init
		S66.599A	Inj intrinsic musc/fasc/tend unsp finger at wrs/hnd lv, init
		S66.801A	Unsp injury of musc/fasc/tend at wrs/hnd lv, r hand, init
		S66.802A	Unsp injury of musc/fasc/tend at wrs/hnd lv, left hand, init
		S66.809A	Unsp injury of musc/fasc/tend at wrs/hnd lv, unsp hand, init
		S66.891A	Inj musc/fasc/tend at wrist and hand level, right hand, init
		S66.892A	Inj musc/fasc/tend at wrist and hand level, left hand, init
		S66.899A	Inj musc/fasc/tend at wrist and hand level, unsp hand, init
		S66.901A	Unsp inj unsp musc/fasc/tend at wrs/hnd lv, r hand, init
		S66.902A	Unsp inj unsp musc/fasc/tend at wrs/hnd lv, left hand, init
		S66.909A	Unsp inj unsp musc/fasc/tend at wrs/hnd lv, unsp hand, init
		S66.991A	Inj unsp musc/fasc/tend at wrs/hnd lv, right hand, init
		S66.992A	Inj unsp musc/fasc/tend at wrs/hnd lv, left hand, init
		S66.999A	Inj unsp musc/fasc/tend at wrs/hnd lv, unsp hand, init
		S69.80XA	Oth injuries of unsp wrist, hand and finger(s), init encntr
		S69.81XA	Oth injuries of right wrist, hand and finger(s), init encntr
		S69.82XA	Oth injuries of left wrist, hand and finger(s), init encntr
		S69.90XA	Unsp injury of unsp wrist, hand and finger(s), init encntr
		S69.91XA	Unsp injury of right wrist, hand and finger(s), init encntr
		S69.92XA	Unsp injury of left wrist, hand and finger(s), init encntr
959.5	INJURY OTHER AND UNSPECIFIED FINGER	**S69.80XA**	Oth injuries of unsp wrist, hand and finger(s), init encntr
		S69.81XA	Oth injuries of right wrist, hand and finger(s), init encntr
		S69.82XA	Oth injuries of left wrist, hand and finger(s), init encntr
		S69.90XA	Unsp injury of unsp wrist, hand and finger(s), init encntr
		S69.91XA	Unsp injury of right wrist, hand and finger(s), init encntr
		S69.92XA	Unsp injury of left wrist, hand and finger(s), init encntr
959.6	INJURY OTHER AND UNSPECIFIED HIP AND THIGH	**S76.001A**	Unsp injury of muscle, fascia and tendon of right hip, init
		S76.002A	Unsp injury of muscle, fascia and tendon of left hip, init
		S76.009A	Unsp injury of muscle, fascia and tendon of unsp hip, init
		S76.091A	Inj muscle, fascia and tendon of right hip, init encntr
		S76.092A	Inj muscle, fascia and tendon of left hip, init encntr
		S76.099A	Inj muscle, fascia and tendon of unsp hip, init encntr
		S76.101A	Unsp injury of right quadriceps musc/fasc/tend, init
		S76.102A	Unsp injury of left quadriceps musc/fasc/tend, init
		S76.109A	Unsp injury of unsp quadriceps musc/fasc/tend, init
		S76.191A	Inj right quadriceps muscle, fascia and tendon, init encntr
		S76.192A	Inj left quadriceps muscle, fascia and tendon, init encntr
		S76.199A	Inj unsp quadriceps muscle, fascia and tendon, init encntr
		S76.201A	Unsp injury of adductor musc/fasc/tend right thigh, init
		S76.202A	Unsp injury of adductor musc/fasc/tend left thigh, init
		S76.209A	Unsp injury of adductor musc/fasc/tend unsp thigh, init
		S76.291A	Inj adductor muscle, fascia and tendon of right thigh, init
		S76.292A	Inj adductor muscle, fascia and tendon of left thigh, init
		S76.299A	Inj adductor muscle, fascia and tendon of unsp thigh, init
		S76.301A	Unsp inj msl/fasc/tnd post grp at thi lev, right thigh, init
		S76.302A	Unsp inj msl/fasc/tnd post grp at thi lev, left thigh, init
		S76.309A	Unsp inj msl/fasc/tnd post grp at thi lev, unsp thigh, init
		S76.391A	Inj msl/fasc/tnd posterior grp at thi lev, right thigh, init
		S76.392A	Inj msl/fasc/tnd posterior grp at thi lev, left thigh, init
		S76.399A	Inj msl/fasc/tnd posterior grp at thi lev, unsp thigh, init
		S76.801A	Unsp injury of musc/fasc/tend at thi lev, right thigh, init
		S76.802A	Unsp injury of musc/fasc/tend at thi lev, left thigh, init
		S76.809A	Unsp injury of musc/fasc/tend at thi lev, unsp thigh, init
	(Continued on next page)	**S76.891A**	Inj musc/fasc/tend at thigh level, right thigh, init encntr

ICD-9-CM		ICD-10-CM	
959.6	INJURY OTHER AND UNSPECIFIED HIP AND THIGH **(Continued)**	**S76.892A**	Inj musc/fasc/tend at thigh level, left thigh, init encntr
		S76.899A	Inj musc/fasc/tend at thigh level, unsp thigh, init encntr
		S76.901A	Unsp inj unsp musc/fasc/tend at thi lev, right thigh, init
		S76.902A	Unsp inj unsp musc/fasc/tend at thi lev, left thigh, init
		S76.909A	Unsp inj unsp musc/fasc/tend at thi lev, unsp thigh, init
		S76.991A	Inj unsp musc/fasc/tend at thigh level, right thigh, init
		S76.992A	Inj unsp musc/fasc/tend at thigh level, left thigh, init
		S76.999A	Inj unsp musc/fasc/tend at thigh level, unsp thigh, init
		S79.811A	Other specified injuries of right hip, initial encounter
		S79.812A	Other specified injuries of left hip, initial encounter
		S79.819A	Other specified injuries of unspecified hip, init encntr
		S79.821A	Other specified injuries of right thigh, initial encounter
		S79.822A	Other specified injuries of left thigh, initial encounter
		S79.829A	Other specified injuries of unspecified thigh, init encntr
		S79.911A	Unspecified injury of right hip, initial encounter
		S79.912A	Unspecified injury of left hip, initial encounter
		S79.919A	Unspecified injury of unspecified hip, initial encounter
		S79.921A	Unspecified injury of right thigh, initial encounter
		S79.922A	Unspecified injury of left thigh, initial encounter
		S79.929A	Unspecified injury of unspecified thigh, initial encounter
959.7	INJURY OTHER&UNSPECIFIED KNEE LEG ANKLE&FOOT	**S86.001A**	Unspecified injury of right Achilles tendon, init encntr
		S86.002A	Unspecified injury of left Achilles tendon, init encntr
		S86.009A	Unsp injury of unspecified Achilles tendon, init encntr
		S86.091A	Other specified injury of right Achilles tendon, init encntr
		S86.092A	Other specified injury of left Achilles tendon, init encntr
		S86.099A	Oth injury of unspecified Achilles tendon, init encntr
		S86.101A	Unsp inj musc/tend post grp at low leg lev, right leg, init
		S86.102A	Unsp inj musc/tend post grp at low leg level, left leg, init
		S86.109A	Unsp inj musc/tend post grp at low leg level, unsp leg, init
		S86.191A	Inj oth musc/tend post grp at low leg level, right leg, init
		S86.192A	Inj oth musc/tend post grp at low leg level, left leg, init
		S86.199A	Inj oth musc/tend post grp at low leg level, unsp leg, init
		S86.201A	Unsp inj musc/tend ant grp at low leg level, right leg, init
		S86.202A	Unsp inj musc/tend ant grp at low leg level, left leg, init
		S86.209A	Unsp inj musc/tend ant grp at low leg level, unsp leg, init
		S86.291A	Inj musc/tend anterior grp at low leg level, right leg, init
		S86.292A	Inj musc/tend anterior grp at low leg level, left leg, init
		S86.299A	Inj musc/tend anterior grp at low leg level, unsp leg, init
		S86.301A	Unsp inj musc/tend peroneal grp at low leg lev, r leg, init
		S86.302A	Unsp inj musc/tend peroneal grp at low leg lev, l leg, init
		S86.309A	Unsp inj musc/tend peroneal grp at low leg lev,unsp leg,init
		S86.391A	Inj musc/tend peroneal grp at low leg level, right leg, init
		S86.392A	Inj musc/tend peroneal grp at low leg level, left leg, init
		S86.399A	Inj musc/tend peroneal grp at low leg level, unsp leg, init
		S86.801A	Unsp injury of musc/tend at lower leg level, right leg, init
		S86.802A	Unsp injury of musc/tend at lower leg level, left leg, init
		S86.809A	Unsp injury of musc/tend at lower leg level, unsp leg, init
		S86.891A	Inj oth musc/tend at lower leg level, right leg, init
		S86.892A	Inj oth musc/tend at lower leg level, left leg, init
		S86.899A	Inj oth musc/tend at lower leg level, unsp leg, init
		S86.901A	Unsp inj unsp musc/tend at lower leg level, right leg, init
		S86.902A	Unsp inj unsp musc/tend at lower leg level, left leg, init
		S86.909A	Unsp inj unsp musc/tend at lower leg level, unsp leg, init
		S86.991A	Inj unsp musc/tend at lower leg level, right leg, init
		S86.992A	Inj unsp musc/tend at lower leg level, left leg, init
		S86.999A	Inj unsp musc/tend at lower leg level, unsp leg, init
		S89.80XA	Oth injuries of unspecified lower leg, init encntr
		S89.81XA	Other specified injuries of right lower leg, init encntr
		S89.82XA	Other specified injuries of left lower leg, init encntr
		S89.90XA	Unspecified injury of unspecified lower leg, init encntr
		S89.91XA	Unspecified injury of right lower leg, initial encounter
		S89.92XA	Unspecified injury of left lower leg, initial encounter
		S96.001A	Unsp inj msl/tnd lng flxr msl toe at ank/ft lev, r ft, init
		S96.002A	Unsp inj msl/tnd lng flxr msl toe at ank/ft lev, l ft, init
		S96.009A	Unsp inj msl/tnd lng flxr msl toe at ank/ft lev,unsp ft,init
		S96.091A	Inj msl/tnd lng flxr msl toe at ank/ft level, r foot, init
		S96.092A	Inj msl/tnd lng flxr msl toe at ank/ft level, l foot, init
		S96.099A	Inj msl/tnd lng flxr msl toe at ank/ft lev, unsp foot, init
		S96.101A	Unsp inj msl/tnd lng extn msl toe at ank/ft lev, r ft, init
		S96.102A	Unsp inj msl/tnd lng extn msl toe at ank/ft lev, l ft, init
		S96.109A	Unsp inj msl/tnd lng extn msl toe at ank/ft lev,unsp ft,init
		S96.191A	Inj msl/tnd lng extn msl toe at ank/ft level, r foot, init
		S96.192A	Inj msl/tnd lng extn msl toe at ank/ft level, l foot, init
		S96.199A	Inj msl/tnd lng extn msl toe at ank/ft lev, unsp foot, init
		S96.201A	Unsp inj intrinsic msl/tnd at ank/ft level, r foot, init
		S96.202A	Unsp inj intrinsic msl/tnd at ank/ft level, left foot, init
		S96.209A	Unsp inj intrinsic msl/tnd at ank/ft level, unsp foot, init
		S96.291A	Inj intrinsic msl/tnd at ank/ft level, right foot, init
		S96.292A	Inj intrinsic msl/tnd at ank/ft level, left foot, init
		S96.299A	Inj intrinsic msl/tnd at ank/ft level, unsp foot, init
		S96.801A	Unsp inj muscles and tendons at ank/ft level, r foot, init
	(Continued on next page)	**S96.802A**	Unsp inj muscles and tendons at ank/ft level, l foot, init

ICD-9-CM		ICD-10-CM	
959.7	INJURY OTHER&UNSPECIFIED KNEE LEG ANKLE&FOOT **(Continued)**	**S96.8Ø9A**	Unsp inj musc and tendons at ank/ft level, unsp foot, init
		S96.891A	Inj oth muscles and tendons at ank/ft level, r foot, init
		S96.892A	Inj oth muscles and tendons at ank/ft level, left foot, init
		S96.899A	Inj oth muscles and tendons at ank/ft level, unsp foot, init
		S96.9Ø1A	Unsp injury of unsp msl/tnd at ank/ft level, r foot, init
		S96.9Ø2A	Unsp injury of unsp msl/tnd at ank/ft level, left foot, init
		S96.9Ø9A	Unsp injury of unsp msl/tnd at ank/ft level, unsp foot, init
		S96.991A	Inj unsp msl/tnd at ankle and foot level, right foot, init
		S96.992A	Inj unsp msl/tnd at ankle and foot level, left foot, init
		S96.999A	Inj unsp msl/tnd at ankle and foot level, unsp foot, init
		S99.811A	Other specified injuries of right ankle, initial encounter
		S99.812A	Other specified injuries of left ankle, initial encounter
		S99.819A	Other specified injuries of unspecified ankle, init encntr
"CONTINUED"		**S99.821A**	Other specified injuries of right foot, initial encounter
		S99.822A	Other specified injuries of left foot, initial encounter
		S99.829A	Other specified injuries of unspecified foot, init encntr
		S99.911A	Unspecified injury of right ankle, initial encounter
		S99.912A	Unspecified injury of left ankle, initial encounter
		S99.919A	Unspecified injury of unspecified ankle, initial encounter
		S99.921A	Unspecified injury of right foot, initial encounter
		S99.922A	Unspecified injury of left foot, initial encounter
		S99.929A	Unspecified injury of unspecified foot, initial encounter
959.8	INJURY OTH&UNSPEC OTH SPEC SITES INCL MULTIPLE	**TØ7**	Unspecified multiple injuries
959.9	INJURY OTHER AND UNSPECIFIED UNSPECIFIED SITE	**T14.8**	Other injury of unspecified body region
		T14.9Ø	Injury, unspecified
		T14.91	Suicide attempt
96Ø.Ø	POISONING BY PENICILLINS	**T36.ØX1A**	Poisoning by penicillins, accidental (unintentional), init
		T36.ØX2A	Poisoning by penicillins, intentional self-harm, init encntr
		T36.ØX3A	Poisoning by penicillins, assault, initial encounter
		T36.ØX4A	Poisoning by penicillins, undetermined, initial encounter
96Ø.1	POISONING BY ANTIFUNGAL ANTIBIOTICS	**T36.7X1A**	Poisoning by antifungal antibiot, sys used, acc, init
		T36.7X2A	Poisoning by antifungal antibiot, sys used, self-harm, init
		T36.7X3A	Poisoning by antifungal antibiotics, sys used, assault, init
		T36.7X4A	Poisoning by antifungal antibiotics, sys used, undet, init
96Ø.2	POISONING BY CHLORAMPHENICOL GROUP	**T36.2X1A**	Poisoning by chloramphenicol group, accidental, init
		T36.2X2A	Poisoning by chloramphenicol group, self-harm, init
		T36.2X3A	Poisoning by chloramphenicol group, assault, init encntr
		T36.2X4A	Poisoning by chloramphenicol group, undetermined, init
96Ø.3	POISONING BY ERYTHROMYCIN AND OTHER MACROLIDES	**T36.3X1A**	Poisoning by macrolides, accidental (unintentional), init
		T36.3X2A	Poisoning by macrolides, intentional self-harm, init encntr
		T36.3X3A	Poisoning by macrolides, assault, initial encounter
		T36.3X4A	Poisoning by macrolides, undetermined, initial encounter
96Ø.4	POISONING BY TETRACYCLINE GROUP	**T36.4X1A**	Poisoning by tetracyclines, accidental (unintentional), init
		T36.4X2A	Poisoning by tetracyclines, intentional self-harm, init
		T36.4X3A	Poisoning by tetracyclines, assault, initial encounter
		T36.4X4A	Poisoning by tetracyclines, undetermined, initial encounter
96Ø.5	POISONING OF CEPHALOSPORIN GROUP	**T36.1X1A**	Poisoning by cephalospor/oth beta-lactm antibiot, acc, init
		T36.1X2A	Poisn by cephalospor/oth beta-lactm antibiot, slf-hrm, init
		T36.1X3A	Poisn by cephalospor/oth beta-lactm antibiot, assault, init
		T36.1X4A	Poisn by cephalospor/oth beta-lactm antibiot, undet, init
96Ø.6	POISONING OF ANTIMYCOBACTERIAL ANTIBIOTICS	**T36.6X1A**	Poisoning by rifampicins, accidental (unintentional), init
		T36.6X2A	Poisoning by rifampicins, intentional self-harm, init encntr
		T36.6X3A	Poisoning by rifampicins, assault, initial encounter
		T36.6X4A	Poisoning by rifampicins, undetermined, initial encounter
96Ø.7	POISONING BY ANTINEOPLASTIC ANTIBIOTICS	**T45.1X1A**	Poisoning by antineopl and immunosup drugs, acc, init
96Ø.8	POISONING BY OTHER SPECIFIED ANTIBIOTICS	**T36.5X1A**	Poisoning by aminoglycosides, accidental, init
		T36.5X2A	Poisoning by aminoglycosides, intentional self-harm, init
		T36.5X3A	Poisoning by aminoglycosides, assault, initial encounter
		T36.5X4A	Poisoning by aminoglycosides, undetermined, init encntr
		T36.8X1A	Poisoning by oth systemic antibiotics, accidental, init
		T36.8X2A	Poisoning by oth systemic antibiotics, self-harm, init
		T36.8X3A	Poisoning by oth systemic antibiotics, assault, init encntr
		T36.8X4A	Poisoning by oth systemic antibiotics, undetermined, init
96Ø.9	POISONING BY UNSPECIFIED ANTIBIOTIC	**T36.91XA**	Poisoning by unsp systemic antibiotic, accidental, init
		T36.92XA	Poisoning by unsp systemic antibiotic, self-harm, init
		T36.93XA	Poisoning by unsp systemic antibiotic, assault, init encntr
		T36.94XA	Poisoning by unsp systemic antibiotic, undetermined, init
961.Ø	POISONING BY SULFONAMIDES	**T37.ØX1A**	Poisoning by sulfonamides, accidental (unintentional), init
		T37.ØX2A	Poisoning by sulfonamides, intentional self-harm, init
		T37.ØX3A	Poisoning by sulfonamides, assault, initial encounter
		T37.ØX4A	Poisoning by sulfonamides, undetermined, initial encounter
961.1	POISONING BY ARSENICAL ANTI-INFECTIVES	**T37.8X1A**	Poisoning by oth systemic anti-infect/parasit, acc, init
961.2	POISONING BY HEAVY METAL ANTI-INFECTIVES	**T37.8X1A**	Poisoning by oth systemic anti-infect/parasit, acc, init
961.3	POISONING QUINOLINE&HYDROXYQUINOLINE DERIVATIVES	**T37.8X1A**	Poisoning by oth systemic anti-infect/parasit, acc, init

ICD-9-CM		ICD-10-CM	
961.4	POISN ANTIMALARIALS&RX ACTING OTH BLD PROTOZOA	**T37.2X1A**	Poisn by antimalari/drugs acting on bld protzoa, acc, init
		T37.2X2A	Poisn by antimalari/drugs act on bld protzoa, slf-hrm, init
		T37.2X3A	Poisn by antimalari/drugs acting on bld protzoa, asslt, init
		T37.2X4A	Poisn by antimalari/drugs acting on bld protzoa, undet, init
961.5	POISONING BY OTHER ANTIPROTOZOAL DRUGS	**T37.3X1A**	Poisoning by oth antiprotozoal drugs, accidental, init
		T37.3X2A	Poisoning by oth antiprotozoal drugs, self-harm, init
		T37.3X3A	Poisoning by other antiprotozoal drugs, assault, init encntr
		T37.3X4A	Poisoning by oth antiprotozoal drugs, undetermined, init
961.6	POISONING BY ANTHELMINTICS	**T37.4X1A**	Poisoning by anthelminthics, accidental, init
		T37.4X2A	Poisoning by anthelminthics, intentional self-harm, init
		T37.4X3A	Poisoning by anthelminthics, assault, initial encounter
		T37.4X4A	Poisoning by anthelminthics, undetermined, initial encounter
961.7	POISONING BY ANTIVIRAL DRUGS	**T37.5X1A**	Poisoning by antiviral drugs, accidental, init
		T37.5X2A	Poisoning by antiviral drugs, intentional self-harm, init
		T37.5X3A	Poisoning by antiviral drugs, assault, initial encounter
		T37.5X4A	Poisoning by antiviral drugs, undetermined, init encntr
961.8	POISONING BY OTHER ANTIMYCOBACTERIAL DRUGS	**T37.1X1A**	Poisoning by antimycobac drugs, accidental, init
		T37.1X2A	Poisoning by antimycobacterial drugs, self-harm, init
		T37.1X3A	Poisoning by antimycobacterial drugs, assault, init encntr
		T37.1X4A	Poisoning by antimycobacterial drugs, undetermined, init
961.9	POISONING OTHER AND UNSPECIFIED ANTI-INFECTIVES	**T37.8X1A**	Poisoning by oth systemic anti-infect/parasit, acc, init
		T37.8X2A	Poisn by oth systemic anti-infect/parasit, self-harm, init
		T37.8X3A	Poisoning by oth systemic anti-infect/parasit, assault, init
		T37.8X4A	Poisoning by oth systemic anti-infect/parasit, undet, init
		T37.91XA	Poisn by unsp sys anti-infect and antiparastc, acc, init
		T37.92XA	Poisn by unsp sys anti-infect and antiparastc, slf-hrm, init
		T37.93XA	Poisn by unsp sys anti-infect and antiparastc, assault, init
		T37.94XA	Poisn by unsp sys anti-infect and antiparastc, undet, init
962.Ø	POISONING BY ADRENAL CORTICAL STEROIDS	**T38.ØX1A**	Poisoning by glucocort/synth analog, accidental, init
		T38.ØX2A	Poisoning by glucocort/synth analog, self-harm, init
		T38.ØX3A	Poisoning by glucocort/synth analog, assault, init
		T38.ØX4A	Poisoning by glucocort/synth analog, undetermined, init
		T5Ø.ØX1A	Poisoning by mineralocorticoids and their antag, acc, init
		T5Ø.ØX2A	Poisoning by mineralocorticoids and antag, self-harm, init
		T5Ø.ØX3A	Poisoning by mineralocorticoids and antag, assault, init
		T5Ø.ØX4A	Poisoning by mineralocorticoids and their antag, undet, init
962.1	POISONING BY ANDROGENS AND ANABOLIC CONGENERS	**T38.6X1A**	Poisoning by antigonadtr/antiestr/antiandrg, NEC, acc, init
		T38.6X2A	Poisn by antigonadtr/antiestr/antiandrg, NEC, slf-hrm, init
		T38.6X3A	Poisn by antigonadtr/antiestr/antiandrg, NEC, assault, init
		T38.6X4A	Poisn by antigonadtr/antiestr/antiandrg, NEC, undet, init
		T38.7X1A	Poisoning by androgens and anabolic congeners, acc, init
		T38.7X2A	Poisn by androgens and anabolic congeners, self-harm, init
		T38.7X3A	Poisoning by androgens and anabolic congeners, assault, init
		T38.7X4A	Poisoning by androgens and anabolic congeners, undet, init
962.2	POISONING OVARIAN HORMONES&SYNTHETIC SUBSTITUTES	**T38.4X1A**	Poisoning by oral contraceptives, accidental, init
		T38.4X2A	Poisoning by oral contraceptives, self-harm, init
		T38.4X3A	Poisoning by oral contraceptives, assault, initial encounter
		T38.4X4A	Poisoning by oral contraceptives, undetermined, init encntr
		T38.5X1A	Poisoning by oth estrogens and progstrn, accidental, init
		T38.5X2A	Poisoning by oth estrogens and progestogens, self-harm, init
		T38.5X3A	Poisoning by oth estrogens and progestogens, assault, init
		T38.5X4A	Poisoning by oth estrogens and progstrn, undetermined, init
962.3	POISONING BY INSULINS AND ANTIDIABETIC AGENTS	**T38.3X1A**	Poisoning by insulin and oral hypoglycemic drugs, acc, init
		T38.3X2A	Poisn by insulin and oral hypoglycemic drugs, slf-hrm, init
		T38.3X3A	Poisn by insulin and oral hypoglycemic drugs, assault, init
		T38.3X4A	Poisn by insulin and oral hypoglycemic drugs, undet, init
962.4	POISONING BY ANTERIOR PITUITARY HORMONES	**T38.811A**	Poisoning by anterior pituitary hormones, accidental, init
		T38.812A	Poisoning by anterior pituitary hormones, self-harm, init
		T38.813A	Poisoning by anterior pituitary hormones, assault, init
		T38.814A	Poisoning by anterior pituitary hormones, undetermined, init
962.5	POISONING BY POSTERIOR PITUITARY HORMONES	**T38.891A**	Poisoning by oth hormones and synthetic sub, acc, init
962.6	POISONING PARATHYROID&PARATHYROID DERIVATIVES	**T38.891A**	Poisoning by oth hormones and synthetic sub, acc, init
962.7	POISONING BY THYROID AND THYROID DERIVATIVES	**T38.1X1A**	Poisoning by thyroid hormones and sub, accidental, init
		T38.1X2A	Poisoning by thyroid hormones and sub, self-harm, init
		T38.1X3A	Poisoning by thyroid hormones and substitutes, assault, init
		T38.1X4A	Poisoning by thyroid hormones and substitutes, undet, init
962.8	POISONING BY ANTITHYROID AGENTS	**T38.2X1A**	Poisoning by antithyroid drugs, accidental, init
		T38.2X2A	Poisoning by antithyroid drugs, intentional self-harm, init
		T38.2X3A	Poisoning by antithyroid drugs, assault, initial encounter
		T38.2X4A	Poisoning by antithyroid drugs, undetermined, init encntr

ICD-9-CM		ICD-10-CM	
962.9	POISN OTH&UNSPEC HORMONES&SYNTHETIC SUBSTITUTES	**T38.8Ø1A**	Poisoning by unsp hormones and synthetic sub, acc, init
		T38.8Ø2A	Poisn by unsp hormones and synthetic sub, self-harm, init
		T38.8Ø3A	Poisoning by unsp hormones and synthetic sub, assault, init
		T38.8Ø4A	Poisoning by unsp hormones and synthetic sub, undet, init
		T38.891A	Poisoning by oth hormones and synthetic sub, acc, init
		T38.892A	Poisoning by oth hormones and synthetic sub, self-harm, init
		T38.893A	Poisoning by oth hormones and synthetic sub, assault, init
		T38.894A	Poisoning by oth hormones and synthetic sub, undet, init
		T38.9Ø1A	Poisoning by unsp hormone antagonists, accidental, init
		T38.9Ø2A	Poisoning by unsp hormone antagonists, self-harm, init
		T38.9Ø3A	Poisoning by unsp hormone antagonists, assault, init encntr
		T38.9Ø4A	Poisoning by unsp hormone antagonists, undetermined, init
		T38.991A	Poisoning by oth hormone antagonists, accidental, init
		T38.992A	Poisoning by oth hormone antagonists, self-harm, init
		T38.993A	Poisoning by other hormone antagonists, assault, init encntr
		T38.994A	Poisoning by oth hormone antagonists, undetermined, init
963.Ø	POISONING BY ANTIALLERGIC AND ANTIEMETIC DRUGS	**T45.ØX1A**	Poisoning by antiallerg/antiemetic, accidental, init
		T45.ØX2A	Poisoning by antiallerg/antiemetic, self-harm, init
		T45.ØX3A	Poisoning by antiallerg/antiemetic, assault, init
		T45.ØX4A	Poisoning by antiallerg/antiemetic, undetermined, init
963.1	POISONING ANTINEOPLASTIC&IMMUNOSUPPRESSIVE DRUGS	**T45.1X1A**	Poisoning by antineopl and immunosup drugs, acc, init
		T45.1X2A	Poisoning by antineopl and immunosup drugs, self-harm, init
		T45.1X3A	Poisoning by antineopl and immunosup drugs, assault, init
		T45.1X4A	Poisoning by antineopl and immunosup drugs, undet, init
963.2	POISONING BY ACIDIFYING AGENTS	**T45.8X1A**	Poisn by oth prim systemic and hematolog agents, acc, init
963.3	POISONING BY ALKALIZING AGENTS	**T45.8X1A**	Poisn by oth prim systemic and hematolog agents, acc, init
963.4	POISONING BY ENZYMES NOT ELSEWHERE CLASSIFIED	**T45.3X1A**	Poisoning by enzymes, accidental (unintentional), init
		T45.3X2A	Poisoning by enzymes, intentional self-harm, init encntr
		T45.3X3A	Poisoning by enzymes, assault, initial encounter
		T45.3X4A	Poisoning by enzymes, undetermined, initial encounter
963.5	POISONING BY VITAMINS NOT ELSEWHERE CLASSIFIED	**T45.2X1A**	Poisoning by vitamins, accidental (unintentional), init
		T45.2X2A	Poisoning by vitamins, intentional self-harm, init encntr
		T45.2X3A	Poisoning by vitamins, assault, initial encounter
		T45.2X4A	Poisoning by vitamins, undetermined, initial encounter
963.8	POISONING BY OTHER SPECIFIED SYSTEMIC AGENTS	**T45.8X1A**	Poisn by oth prim systemic and hematolog agents, acc, init
		T45.8X2A	Poisn by oth prim sys and hematolog agents, slf-hrm, init
		T45.8X3A	Poisn by oth prim sys and hematolog agents, assault, init
		T45.8X4A	Poisn by oth prim systemic and hematolog agents, undet, init
963.9	POISONING BY UNSPECIFIED SYSTEMIC AGENT	**T45.91XA**	Poisn by unsp prim systemic and hematolog agent, acc, init
		T45.92XA	Poisn by unsp prim sys and hematolog agent, slf-hrm, init
		T45.93XA	Poisn by unsp prim sys and hematolog agent, assault, init
		T45.94XA	Poisn by unsp prim systemic and hematolog agent, undet, init
964.Ø	POISONING BY IRON AND ITS COMPOUNDS	**T45.4X1A**	Poisoning by iron and its compounds, accidental, init
		T45.4X2A	Poisoning by iron and its compounds, self-harm, init
		T45.4X3A	Poisoning by iron and its compounds, assault, init encntr
		T45.4X4A	Poisoning by iron and its compounds, undetermined, init
964.1	POISONING LIVER PREPARATIONS&OTH ANTIANEMIC AGTS	**T45.8X1A**	Poisn by oth prim systemic and hematolog agents, acc, init
964.2	POISONING BY ANTICOAGULANTS	**T45.511A**	Poisoning by anticoagulants, accidental, init
		T45.512A	Poisoning by anticoagulants, intentional self-harm, init
		T45.513A	Poisoning by anticoagulants, assault, initial encounter
		T45.514A	Poisoning by anticoagulants, undetermined, initial encounter
		T45.521A	Poisoning by antithrombotic drugs, accidental, init
		T45.522A	Poisoning by antithrombotic drugs, self-harm, init
		T45.523A	Poisoning by antithrombotic drugs, assault, init encntr
		T45.524A	Poisoning by antithrombotic drugs, undetermined, init encntr
964.3	POISONING BY VITAMIN K	**T45.7X1A**	Poisn by anticoag antag, vitamin K and oth coag, acc, init
		T45.7X2A	Poisn by anticoag antag, vit K and oth coag, slf-hrm, init
		T45.7X3A	Poisn by anticoag antag, vit K and oth coag, assault, init
964.4	POISONING BY FIBRINOLYSIS-AFFECTING DRUGS	**T45.6Ø1A**	Poisoning by unsp fibrin-affct drugs, accidental, init
		T45.6Ø2A	Poisoning by unsp fibrin-affct drugs, self-harm, init
		T45.6Ø3A	Poisoning by unsp fibrin-affct drugs, assault, init
		T45.6Ø4A	Poisoning by unsp fibrin-affct drugs, undetermined, init
		T45.611A	Poisoning by thrombolytic drug, accidental, init
		T45.612A	Poisoning by thrombolytic drug, intentional self-harm, init
		T45.613A	Poisoning by thrombolytic drug, assault, initial encounter
		T45.614A	Poisoning by thrombolytic drug, undetermined, init encntr
		T45.691A	Poisoning by oth fibrin-affct drugs, accidental, init
		T45.692A	Poisoning by oth fibrin-affct drugs, self-harm, init
		T45.693A	Poisoning by oth fibrinolysis-affecting drugs, assault, init
		T45.694A	Poisoning by oth fibrin-affct drugs, undetermined, init
964.5	POISN ANTICOAGULANT ANTAGONISTS&OTH COAGULANTS	**T45.7X1A**	Poisn by anticoag antag, vitamin K and oth coag, acc, init
		T45.7X2A	Poisn by anticoag antag, vit K and oth coag, slf-hrm, init
		T45.7X3A	Poisn by anticoag antag, vit K and oth coag, assault, init
		T45.7X4A	Poisn by anticoag antag, vitamin K and oth coag, undet, init

ICD-9-CM		ICD-10-CM	
964.6	POISONING BY GAMMA GLOBULIN	**T45.8X1A**	Poisn by oth prim systemic and hematolog agents, acc, init
		T5Ø.Z11A	Poisoning by immunoglobulin, accidental, init
		T5Ø.Z12A	Poisoning by immunoglobulin, intentional self-harm, init
		T5Ø.Z13A	Poisoning by immunoglobulin, assault, initial encounter
		T5Ø.Z14A	Poisoning by immunoglobulin, undetermined, initial encounter
964.7	POISONING BY NATURAL BLOOD AND BLOOD PRODUCTS	**T45.8X1A**	Poisn by oth prim systemic and hematolog agents, acc, init
964.8	POISONING OTH SPEC AGTS AFFECT BLD CONSTITUENTS	**T45.621A**	Poisoning by hemostatic drug, accidental, init
		T45.622A	Poisoning by hemostatic drug, intentional self-harm, init
		T45.623A	Poisoning by hemostatic drug, assault, initial encounter
		T45.624A	Poisoning by hemostatic drug, undetermined, init encntr
		T45.8X1A	Poisn by oth prim systemic and hematolog agents, acc, init
		T45.8X2A	Poisn by oth prim sys and hematolog agents, slf-hrm, init
		T45.8X3A	Poisn by oth prim sys and hematolog agents, assault, init
		T45.8X4A	Poisn by oth prim systemic and hematolog agents, undet, init
964.9	POISONING UNSPEC AGENT AFFECT BLOOD CONSTITUENTS	**T45.91XA**	Poisn by unsp prim systemic and hematolog agent, acc, init
		T45.92XA	Poisn by unsp prim sys and hematolog agent, slf-hrm, init
		T45.93XA	Poisn by unsp prim sys and hematolog agent, assault, init
		T45.94XA	Poisn by unsp prim systemic and hematolog agent, undet, init
965.ØØ	POISONING BY OPIUM , UNSPECIFIED	**T4Ø.ØX1A**	Poisoning by opium, accidental (unintentional), init encntr
		T4Ø.ØX2A	Poisoning by opium, intentional self-harm, initial encounter
		T4Ø.ØX3A	Poisoning by opium, assault, initial encounter
		T4Ø.ØX4A	Poisoning by opium, undetermined, initial encounter
965.Ø1	POISONING BY HEROIN	**T4Ø.1X1A**	Poisoning by heroin, accidental (unintentional), init encntr
		T4Ø.1X2A	Poisoning by heroin, intentional self-harm, init encntr
		T4Ø.1X3A	Poisoning by heroin, assault, initial encounter
		T4Ø.1X4A	Poisoning by heroin, undetermined, initial encounter
965.Ø2	POISONING BY METHADONE	**T4Ø.3X1A**	Poisoning by methadone, accidental (unintentional), init
		T4Ø.3X2A	Poisoning by methadone, intentional self-harm, init encntr
		T4Ø.3X3A	Poisoning by methadone, assault, initial encounter
		T4Ø.3X4A	Poisoning by methadone, undetermined, initial encounter
965.Ø9	POISONING BY OPIATES AND RELATED NARCOTICS OTHER	**T4Ø.2X1A**	Poisoning by oth opioids, accidental (unintentional), init
		T4Ø.2X2A	Poisoning by oth opioids, intentional self-harm, init encntr
		T4Ø.2X3A	Poisoning by other opioids, assault, initial encounter
		T4Ø.2X4A	Poisoning by other opioids, undetermined, initial encounter
		T4Ø.4X1A	Poisoning by oth synthetic narcotics, accidental, init
		T4Ø.4X2A	Poisoning by oth synthetic narcotics, self-harm, init
		T4Ø.4X3A	Poisoning by other synthetic narcotics, assault, init encntr
		T4Ø.4X4A	Poisoning by oth synthetic narcotics, undetermined, init
		T4Ø.6Ø1A	Poisoning by unsp narcotics, accidental, init
		T4Ø.6Ø2A	Poisoning by unsp narcotics, intentional self-harm, init
		T4Ø.6Ø3A	Poisoning by unspecified narcotics, assault, init encntr
		T4Ø.6Ø4A	Poisoning by unsp narcotics, undetermined, init encntr
		T4Ø.691A	Poisoning by oth narcotics, accidental (unintentional), init
		T4Ø.692A	Poisoning by oth narcotics, intentional self-harm, init
		T4Ø.693A	Poisoning by other narcotics, assault, initial encounter
		T4Ø.694A	Poisoning by other narcotics, undetermined, init encntr
965.1	POISONING BY SALICYLATES	**T39.Ø11A**	Poisoning by aspirin, accidental (unintentional), init
		T39.Ø12A	Poisoning by aspirin, intentional self-harm, init encntr
		T39.Ø13A	Poisoning by aspirin, assault, initial encounter
		T39.Ø14A	Poisoning by aspirin, undetermined, initial encounter
		T39.Ø91A	Poisoning by salicylates, accidental (unintentional), init
		T39.Ø92A	Poisoning by salicylates, intentional self-harm, init encntr
		T39.Ø93A	Poisoning by salicylates, assault, initial encounter
		T39.Ø94A	Poisoning by salicylates, undetermined, initial encounter
		T39.314A	Poisoning by propionic acid derivatives, undetermined, init
965.4	POISONING BY AROMATIC ANALGESICS NEC	**T39.1X1A**	Poisoning by 4-Aminophenol derivatives, accidental, init
		T39.1X2A	Poisoning by 4-Aminophenol derivatives, self-harm, init
		T39.1X3A	Poisoning by 4-Aminophenol derivatives, assault, init encntr
		T39.1X4A	Poisoning by 4-Aminophenol derivatives, undetermined, init
965.5	POISONING BY PYRAZOLE DERIVATIVES	**T39.2X1A**	Poisoning by pyrazolone derivatives, accidental, init
		T39.2X2A	Poisoning by pyrazolone derivatives, self-harm, init
		T39.2X3A	Poisoning by pyrazolone derivatives, assault, init encntr
		T39.2X4A	Poisoning by pyrazolone derivatives, undetermined, init
965.61	POISONING BY PROPIONIC ACID DERIVATIVES	**T39.311A**	Poisoning by propionic acid derivatives, accidental, init
		T39.312A	Poisoning by propionic acid derivatives, self-harm, init
		T39.313A	Poisoning by propionic acid derivatives, assault, init
		T39.391A	Poisoning by oth nonsteroid anti-inflam drugs, acc, init
		T39.392A	Poisn by oth nonsteroid anti-inflam drugs, self-harm, init
		T39.393A	Poisoning by oth nonsteroid anti-inflam drugs, assault, init
		T39.394A	Poisoning by oth nonsteroid anti-inflam drugs, undet, init
965.69	POISONING BY OTHER ANTIRHEUMATICS	**T39.4X1A**	Poisoning by antirheumatics, NEC, accidental, init
		T39.4X2A	Poisoning by antirheumatics, NEC, self-harm, init
		T39.4X3A	Poisoning by antirheumatics, NEC, assault, init
		T39.4X4A	Poisoning by antirheumatics, NEC, undetermined, init

ICD-9-CM		ICD-10-CM	
965.7	POISONING BY OTHER NON-NARCOTIC ANALGESICS	T39.8X1A	Poisoning by oth nonopio analges/antipyret, NEC, acc, init
		T39.8X2A	Poisn by oth nonopio analges/antipyret, NEC, self-harm, init
		T39.8X3A	Poisn by oth nonopio analges/antipyret, NEC, assault, init
		T39.8X4A	Poisoning by oth nonopio analges/antipyret, NEC, undet, init
965.8	POISONING OTHER SPEC ANALGESICS&ANTIPYRETICS	T39.8X1A	Poisoning by oth nonopio analges/antipyret, NEC, acc, init
		T39.8X2A	Poisn by oth nonopio analges/antipyret, NEC, self-harm, init
		T39.8X3A	Poisn by oth nonopio analges/antipyret, NEC, assault, init
		T39.8X4A	Poisoning by oth nonopio analges/antipyret, NEC, undet, init
965.9	POISONING UNSPECIFIED ANALGESIC AND ANTIPYRETIC	T39.91XA	Poisoning by unsp nonopi analgs/antipyr/antirheu, acc, init
		T39.92XA	Poisn by unsp nonopi analgs/antipyr/antirheu, slf-hrm, init
		T39.93XA	Poisn by unsp nonopi analgs/antipyr/antirheu, assault, init
		T39.94XA	Poisn by unsp nonopi analgs/antipyr/antirheu, undet, init
966.Ø	POISONING BY OXAZOLIDINE DERIVATIVES	T42.2X1A	Poisoning by succinimides and oxazolidinediones, acc, init
		T42.2X2A	Poisn by succinimides and oxazolidinediones, self-harm, init
		T42.2X3A	Poisn by succinimides and oxazolidinediones, assault, init
		T42.2X4A	Poisoning by succinimides and oxazolidinediones, undet, init
966.1	POISONING BY HYDANTOIN DERIVATIVES	T42.ØX1A	Poisoning by hydantoin derivatives, accidental, init
		T42.ØX2A	Poisoning by hydantoin derivatives, self-harm, init
		T42.ØX3A	Poisoning by hydantoin derivatives, assault, init encntr
		T42.ØX4A	Poisoning by hydantoin derivatives, undetermined, init
966.2	POISONING BY SUCCINIMIDES	T42.2X1A	Poisoning by succinimides and oxazolidinediones, acc, init
		T42.2X2A	Poisn by succinimides and oxazolidinediones, self-harm, init
		T42.2X3A	Poisn by succinimides and oxazolidinediones, assault, init
		T42.2X4A	Poisoning by succinimides and oxazolidinediones, undet, init
966.3	POISONING OTHER AND UNSPECIFIED ANTICONVULSANTS	T42.1X1A	Poisoning by iminostilbenes, accidental, init
		T42.1X2A	Poisoning by iminostilbenes, intentional self-harm, init
		T42.1X3A	Poisoning by iminostilbenes, assault, initial encounter
		T42.1X4A	Poisoning by iminostilbenes, undetermined, initial encounter
		T42.5X1A	Poisoning by mixed antiepileptics, accidental, init
		T42.5X2A	Poisoning by mixed antiepileptics, self-harm, init
		T42.5X3A	Poisoning by mixed antiepileptics, assault, init encntr
		T42.5X4A	Poisoning by mixed antiepileptics, undetermined, init encntr
		T42.6X1A	Poisoning by oth antieplptc and sed-hypntc drugs, acc, init
		T42.6X2A	Poisn by oth antieplptc and sed-hypntc drugs, slf-hrm, init
		T42.6X3A	Poisn by oth antieplptc and sed-hypntc drugs, assault, init
		T42.6X4A	Poisn by oth antieplptc and sed-hypntc drugs, undet, init
		T42.71XA	Poisn by unsp antieplptc and sed-hypntc drugs, acc, init
		T42.72XA	Poisn by unsp antieplptc and sed-hypntc drugs, slf-hrm, init
		T42.73XA	Poisn by unsp antieplptc and sed-hypntc drugs, assault, init
		T42.74XA	Poisn by unsp antieplptc and sed-hypntc drugs, undet, init
966.4	POISONING BY ANTI-PARKINSONISM DRUGS	T42.8X1A	Poisn by antiparkns drug/centr musc-tone depr, acc, init
		T42.8X2A	Poisn by antiparkns drug/centr musc-tone depr, slf-hrm, init
		T42.8X3A	Poisn by antiparkns drug/centr musc-tone depr, assault, init
		T42.8X4A	Poisn by antiparkns drug/centr musc-tone depr, undet, init
967.Ø	POISONING BY BARBITURATES	T42.3X1A	Poisoning by barbiturates, accidental (unintentional), init
		T42.3X2A	Poisoning by barbiturates, intentional self-harm, init
		T42.3X3A	Poisoning by barbiturates, assault, initial encounter
		T42.3X4A	Poisoning by barbiturates, undetermined, initial encounter
967.1	POISONING BY CHLORAL HYDRATE GROUP	T42.6X1A	Poisoning by oth antieplptc and sed-hypntc drugs, acc, init
		T42.6X2A	Poisn by oth antieplptc and sed-hypntc drugs, slf-hrm, init
		T42.6X3A	Poisn by oth antieplptc and sed-hypntc drugs, assault, init
		T42.6X4A	Poisn by oth antieplptc and sed-hypntc drugs, undet, init
967.2	POISONING BY PARALDEHYDE	T42.6X1A	Poisoning by oth antieplptc and sed-hypntc drugs, acc, init
		T42.6X2A	Poisn by oth antieplptc and sed-hypntc drugs, slf-hrm, init
		T42.6X3A	Poisn by oth antieplptc and sed-hypntc drugs, assault, init
		T42.6X4A	Poisn by oth antieplptc and sed-hypntc drugs, undet, init
967.3	POISONING BY BROMINE COMPOUNDS	T42.6X1A	Poisoning by oth antieplptc and sed-hypntc drugs, acc, init
		T42.6X2A	Poisn by oth antieplptc and sed-hypntc drugs, slf-hrm, init
		T42.6X3A	Poisn by oth antieplptc and sed-hypntc drugs, assault, init
		T42.6X4A	Poisn by oth antieplptc and sed-hypntc drugs, undet, init
967.4	POISONING BY METHAQUALONE COMPOUNDS	T42.6X1A	Poisoning by oth antieplptc and sed-hypntc drugs, acc, init
		T42.6X2A	Poisn by oth antieplptc and sed-hypntc drugs, slf-hrm, init
		T42.6X3A	Poisn by oth antieplptc and sed-hypntc drugs, assault, init
		T42.6X4A	Poisn by oth antieplptc and sed-hypntc drugs, undet, init
967.5	POISONING BY GLUTETHIMIDE GROUP	T42.6X1A	Poisoning by oth antieplptc and sed-hypntc drugs, acc, init
		T42.6X2A	Poisn by oth antieplptc and sed-hypntc drugs, slf-hrm, init
		T42.6X3A	Poisn by oth antieplptc and sed-hypntc drugs, assault, init
		T42.6X4A	Poisn by oth antieplptc and sed-hypntc drugs, undet, init
967.6	POISONING BY MIXED SEDATIVES NEC	T42.6X1A	Poisoning by oth antieplptc and sed-hypntc drugs, acc, init
		T42.6X2A	Poisn by oth antieplptc and sed-hypntc drugs, slf-hrm, init
		T42.6X3A	Poisn by oth antieplptc and sed-hypntc drugs, assault, init
		T42.6X4A	Poisn by oth antieplptc and sed-hypntc drugs, undet, init
967.8	POISONING BY OTHER SEDATIVES AND HYPNOTICS	T42.6X1A	Poisoning by oth antieplptc and sed-hypntc drugs, acc, init
		T42.6X2A	Poisn by oth antieplptc and sed-hypntc drugs, slf-hrm, init
		T42.6X3A	Poisn by oth antieplptc and sed-hypntc drugs, assault, init
		T42.6X4A	Poisn by oth antieplptc and sed-hypntc drugs, undet, init

ICD-9-CM		ICD-10-CM	
967.9	POISONING BY UNSPECIFIED SEDATIVE OR HYPNOTIC	**T42.71XA**	Poisn by unsp antieplptc and sed-hypntc drugs, acc, init
		T42.72XA	Poisn by unsp antieplptc and sed-hypntc drugs, slf-hrm, init
		T42.73XA	Poisn by unsp antieplptc and sed-hypntc drugs, assault, init
		T42.74XA	Poisn by unsp antieplptc and sed-hypntc drugs, undet, init
968.0	POISONING CNTRL NERV SYS MUSCLE-TONE DEPRESSANTS	**T42.8X1A**	Poisn by antiparkns drug/centr musc-tone depr, acc, init
		T42.8X2A	Poisn by antiparkns drug/centr musc-tone depr, slf-hrm, init
		T42.8X3A	Poisn by antiparkns drug/centr musc-tone depr, assault, init
		T42.8X4A	Poisn by antiparkns drug/centr musc-tone depr, undet, init
968.1	POISONING BY HALOTHANE	**T41.0X1A**	Poisoning by inhaled anesthetics, accidental, init
		T41.0X2A	Poisoning by inhaled anesthetics, self-harm, init
		T41.0X3A	Poisoning by inhaled anesthetics, assault, initial encounter
		T41.0X4A	Poisoning by inhaled anesthetics, undetermined, init encntr
968.2	POISONING BY OTHER GASEOUS ANESTHETICS	**T41.0X1A**	Poisoning by inhaled anesthetics, accidental, init
		T41.0X2A	Poisoning by inhaled anesthetics, self-harm, init
		T41.0X3A	Poisoning by inhaled anesthetics, assault, initial encounter
		T41.0X4A	Poisoning by inhaled anesthetics, undetermined, init encntr
968.3	POISONING BY INTRAVENOUS ANESTHETICS	**T41.1X1A**	Poisoning by intravenous anesthetics, accidental, init
		T41.1X2A	Poisoning by intravenous anesthetics, self-harm, init
		T41.1X3A	Poisoning by intravenous anesthetics, assault, init encntr
		T41.1X4A	Poisoning by intravenous anesthetics, undetermined, init
968.4	POISONING OTHER&UNSPECIFIED GENERAL ANESTHETICS	**T41.201A**	Poisoning by unsp general anesthetics, accidental, init
		T41.202A	Poisoning by unsp general anesthetics, self-harm, init
		T41.203A	Poisoning by unsp general anesthetics, assault, init encntr
		T41.204A	Poisoning by unsp general anesthetics, undetermined, init
		T41.291A	Poisoning by oth general anesthetics, accidental, init
		T41.292A	Poisoning by oth general anesthetics, self-harm, init
		T41.293A	Poisoning by other general anesthetics, assault, init encntr
		T41.294A	Poisoning by oth general anesthetics, undetermined, init
968.5	POISN OTH CNS DEPRESSNT ANES SURF INFILTRAT ANES	**T41.3X1A**	Poisoning by local anesthetics, accidental, init
		T41.3X2A	Poisoning by local anesthetics, intentional self-harm, init
		T41.3X3A	Poisoning by local anesthetics, assault, initial encounter
		T41.3X4A	Poisoning by local anesthetics, undetermined, init encntr
968.6	POISONING PERIPHERAL NERVE-&PLEXUS-BLOCKING ANES	**T41.3X1A**	Poisoning by local anesthetics, accidental, init
968.7	POISONING BY SPINAL ANESTHETICS	**T41.3X1A**	Poisoning by local anesthetics, accidental, init
968.9	POISONING OTHER&UNSPECIFIED LOCAL ANESTHETICS	**T41.3X1A**	Poisoning by local anesthetics, accidental, init
		T41.3X2A	Poisoning by local anesthetics, intentional self-harm, init
		T41.3X3A	Poisoning by local anesthetics, assault, initial encounter
		T41.3X4A	Poisoning by local anesthetics, undetermined, init encntr
		T41.41XA	Poisoning by unsp anesthetic, accidental, init
		T41.42XA	Poisoning by unsp anesthetic, intentional self-harm, init
		T41.43XA	Poisoning by unspecified anesthetic, assault, init encntr
		T41.44XA	Poisoning by unsp anesthetic, undetermined, init encntr
969.00	POISONING BY ANTIDEPRESSANT UNSPECIFIED	**T43.201A**	Poisoning by unsp antidepressants, accidental, init
		T43.202A	Poisoning by unsp antidepressants, self-harm, init
		T43.203A	Poisoning by unsp antidepressants, assault, init encntr
		T43.204A	Poisoning by unsp antidepressants, undetermined, init encntr
969.01	POISONING BY MONOAMINE OXIDASE INHIBITORS	**T43.1X1A**	Poisoning by MAO inhib antidepressants, accidental, init
		T43.1X2A	Poisoning by MAO inhib antidepressants, self-harm, init
		T43.1X3A	Poisoning by MAO inhib antidepressants, assault, init
		T43.1X4A	Poisoning by MAO inhib antidepressants, undetermined, init
969.02	POISONING BY SSRI AND NRI	**T43.211A**	Poisn by slctv seroton/norepineph reup inhibtr, acc, init
		T43.212A	Poisn by slctv seroton/norepineph reup inhibtr,slf-hrm, init
		T43.213A	Poisn by slctv seroton/norepineph reup inhibtr, asslt, init
		T43.214A	Poisn by slctv seroton/norepineph reup inhibtr, undet, init
969.03	POISONING SELECTIVE SEROTONIN REUPTAKE INHIBITOR	**T43.221A**	Poisn by selective serotonin reuptake inhibtr, acc, init
		T43.222A	Poisn by slctv serotonin reuptake inhibtr, self-harm, init
		T43.223A	Poisn by selective serotonin reuptake inhibtr, assault, init
		T43.224A	Poisn by selective serotonin reuptake inhibtr, undet, init
969.04	POISONING BY TETRACYCLIC ANTIDEPRESSANTS	**T43.021A**	Poisoning by tetracyclic antidepressants, accidental, init
		T43.022A	Poisoning by tetracyclic antidepressants, self-harm, init
		T43.023A	Poisoning by tetracyclic antidepressants, assault, init
		T43.024A	Poisoning by tetracyclic antidepressants, undetermined, init
969.05	POISONING BY TRICYCLIC ANTIDEPRESSANTS	**T43.011A**	Poisoning by tricyclic antidepressants, accidental, init
		T43.012A	Poisoning by tricyclic antidepressants, self-harm, init
		T43.013A	Poisoning by tricyclic antidepressants, assault, init encntr
		T43.014A	Poisoning by tricyclic antidepressants, undetermined, init
969.09	POISONING BY OTHER ANTIDEPRESSANTS	**T43.291A**	Poisoning by oth antidepressants, accidental, init
		T43.292A	Poisoning by oth antidepressants, self-harm, init
		T43.293A	Poisoning by other antidepressants, assault, init encntr
		T43.294A	Poisoning by oth antidepressants, undetermined, init encntr
969.1	POISONING BY PHENOTHIAZINE-BASED TRANQUILIZERS	**T43.3X1A**	Poisoning by phenothiaz antipsychot/neurolept, acc, init
		T43.3X2A	Poisn by phenothiaz antipsychot/neurolept, self-harm, init
		T43.3X3A	Poisoning by phenothiaz antipsychot/neurolept, assault, init
		T43.3X4A	Poisoning by phenothiaz antipsychot/neurolept, undet, init

[Brackets] indicate valid character values for each code. Character value meanings provided for each code grouping.

ICD-9-CM			ICD-10-CM	
969.2	POISONING BY BUTYROPHENONE-BASED TRANQUILIZERS	🗔	T43.4X1A	Poisoning by butyrophen/thiothixen neuroleptc, acc, init
		🗔	T43.4X2A	Poisn by butyrophen/thiothixen neuroleptc, self-harm, init
		🗔	T43.4X3A	Poisoning by butyrophen/thiothixen neuroleptc, assault, init
		🗔	T43.4X4A	Poisoning by butyrophen/thiothixen neuroleptc, undet, init
969.3	POISN OTH ANTIPSYCHOTS NEUROLEPTICS&MAJOR TRANQ	🗔	T43.501A	Poisoning by unsp antipsychot/neurolept, accidental, init
		🗔	T43.502A	Poisoning by unsp antipsychot/neurolept, self-harm, init
		🗔	T43.503A	Poisoning by unsp antipsychot/neurolept, assault, init
		🗔	T43.504A	Poisoning by unsp antipsychot/neurolept, undetermined, init
		🗔	T43.591A	Poisoning by oth antipsychot/neurolept, accidental, init
		🗔	T43.592A	Poisoning by oth antipsychot/neurolept, self-harm, init
		🗔	T43.593A	Poisoning by oth antipsychot/neurolept, assault, init
		🗔	T43.594A	Poisoning by oth antipsychot/neurolept, undetermined, init
969.4	POISONING BY BENZODIAZEPINE-BASED TRANQUILIZERS	🗔	T42.4X1A	Poisoning by benzodiazepines, accidental, init
		🗔	T42.4X2A	Poisoning by benzodiazepines, intentional self-harm, init
		🗔	T42.4X3A	Poisoning by benzodiazepines, assault, initial encounter
		🗔	T42.4X4A	Poisoning by benzodiazepines, undetermined, init encntr
969.5	POISONING BY OTHER TRANQUILIZERS		T43.591A	Poisoning by oth antipsychot/neurolept, accidental, init
969.6	POISONING BY PSYCHODYSLEPTICS	🗔	T40.7X1A	Poisoning by cannabis (derivatives), accidental, init
		🗔	T40.7X2A	Poisoning by cannabis (derivatives), self-harm, init
		🗔	T40.7X3A	Poisoning by cannabis (derivatives), assault, init encntr
		🗔	T40.7X4A	Poisoning by cannabis (derivatives), undetermined, init
		🗔	T40.8X1A	Poisoning by lysergide, accidental (unintentional), init
		🗔	T40.8X2A	Poisoning by lysergide, intentional self-harm, init encntr
		🗔	T40.8X3A	Poisoning by lysergide [LSD], assault, initial encounter
		🗔	T40.8X4A	Poisoning by lysergide, undetermined, initial encounter
		🗔	T40.901A	Poisoning by unsp psychodyslept, accidental, init
		🗔	T40.902A	Poisoning by unsp psychodysleptics, self-harm, init
		🗔	T40.903A	Poisoning by unsp psychodysleptics, assault, init encntr
		🗔	T40.904A	Poisoning by unsp psychodysleptics, undetermined, init
		🗔	T40.991A	Poisoning by oth psychodyslept, accidental, init
		🗔	T40.992A	Poisoning by oth psychodysleptics, self-harm, init
		🗔	T40.993A	Poisoning by other psychodysleptics, assault, init encntr
		🗔	T40.994A	Poisoning by oth psychodysleptics, undetermined, init encntr
969.70	POISONING BY PSYCHOSTIMULANT UNSPECIFIED	🗔	T43.601A	Poisoning by unsp psychostim, accidental, init
		🗔	T43.602A	Poisoning by unsp psychostimulants, self-harm, init
		🗔	T43.603A	Poisoning by unsp psychostimulants, assault, init encntr
		🗔	T43.604A	Poisoning by unsp psychostimulants, undetermined, init
969.71	POISONING BY CAFFEINE	🗔	T43.611A	Poisoning by caffeine, accidental (unintentional), init
		🗔	T43.612A	Poisoning by caffeine, intentional self-harm, init encntr
		🗔	T43.613A	Poisoning by caffeine, assault, initial encounter
		🗔	T43.614A	Poisoning by caffeine, undetermined, initial encounter
969.72	POISONING BY AMPHETAMINES	🗔	T43.621A	Poisoning by amphetamines, accidental (unintentional), init
		🗔	T43.622A	Poisoning by amphetamines, intentional self-harm, init
		🗔	T43.623A	Poisoning by amphetamines, assault, initial encounter
		🗔	T43.624A	Poisoning by amphetamines, undetermined, initial encounter
969.73	POISONING BY METHYLPHENIDATE	🗔	T43.631A	Poisoning by methylphenidate, accidental, init
		🗔	T43.632A	Poisoning by methylphenidate, intentional self-harm, init
		🗔	T43.633A	Poisoning by methylphenidate, assault, initial encounter
		🗔	T43.634A	Poisoning by methylphenidate, undetermined, init encntr
969.79	POISONING BY OTHER PSYCHOSTIMULANTS	🗔	T43.691A	Poisoning by oth psychostim, accidental, init
		🗔	T43.692A	Poisoning by oth psychostimulants, self-harm, init
		🗔	T43.693A	Poisoning by other psychostimulants, assault, init encntr
		🗔	T43.694A	Poisoning by oth psychostimulants, undetermined, init encntr
969.8	POISONING BY OTHER SPECIFIED PSYCHOTROPIC AGENTS	🗔	T43.8X1A	Poisoning by oth psychotropic drugs, accidental, init
		🗔	T43.8X2A	Poisoning by oth psychotropic drugs, self-harm, init
		🗔	T43.8X3A	Poisoning by other psychotropic drugs, assault, init encntr
		🗔	T43.8X4A	Poisoning by oth psychotropic drugs, undetermined, init
969.9	POISONING BY UNSPECIFIED PSYCHOTROPIC AGENT	🗔	T43.91XA	Poisoning by unsp psychotropic drug, accidental, init
		🗔	T43.92XA	Poisoning by unsp psychotropic drug, self-harm, init
		🗔	T43.93XA	Poisoning by unsp psychotropic drug, assault, init encntr
		🗔	T43.94XA	Poisoning by unsp psychotropic drug, undetermined, init
970.0	POISONING BY ANALEPTICS	🗔	T50.7X1A	Poisn by analeptics and opioid receptor antag, acc, init
		🗔	T50.7X2A	Poisn by analeptics and opioid receptor antag, slf-hrm, init
		🗔	T50.7X3A	Poisn by analeptics and opioid receptor antag, assault, init
		🗔	T50.7X4A	Poisn by analeptics and opioid receptor antag, undet, init
970.1	POISONING BY OPIATE ANTAGONISTS	🗔	T50.7X1A	Poisn by analeptics and opioid receptor antag, acc, init
		🗔	T50.7X2A	Poisn by analeptics and opioid receptor antag, slf-hrm, init
		🗔	T50.7X3A	Poisn by analeptics and opioid receptor antag, assault, init
		🗔	T50.7X4A	Poisn by analeptics and opioid receptor antag, undet, init
970.81	POISONING BY COCAINE	🗔	T40.5X1A	Poisoning by cocaine, accidental (unintentional), init
		🗔	T40.5X2A	Poisoning by cocaine, intentional self-harm, init encntr
		🗔	T40.5X3A	Poisoning by cocaine, assault, initial encounter
		🗔	T40.5X4A	Poisoning by cocaine, undetermined, initial encounter
970.89	POISONING BY OTHER CENTRAL NERV SYS STIMULANTS		T50.991A	Poisoning by oth drug/meds/biol subst, accidental, init
970.9	POISONING UNSPECIFIED CNTRL NERV SYS STIMULANT		T50.991A	Poisoning by oth drug/meds/biol subst, accidental, init

ICD-9-CM		ICD-10-CM	
971.Ø	POISONING BY PARASYMPATHOMIMETICS	**T44.ØX1A**	Poisoning by anticholin agents, accidental, init
		T44.ØX2A	Poisoning by anticholinesterase agents, self-harm, init
		T44.ØX3A	Poisoning by anticholinesterase agents, assault, init encntr
		T44.ØX4A	Poisoning by anticholinesterase agents, undetermined, init
		T44.1X1A	Poisoning by oth parasympath, accidental, init
		T44.1X2A	Poisoning by oth parasympathomimetics, self-harm, init
		T44.1X3A	Poisoning by oth parasympathomimetics, assault, init encntr
		T44.1X4A	Poisoning by oth parasympathomimetics, undetermined, init
971.1	POISONING BY PARASYMPATHOLYTICS AND SPASMOLYTICS	**T44.3X1A**	Poisoning by oth parasympath and spasmolytics, acc, init
		T44.3X2A	Poisn by oth parasympath and spasmolytics, self-harm, init
		T44.3X3A	Poisoning by oth parasympath and spasmolytics, assault, init
		T44.3X4A	Poisoning by oth parasympath and spasmolytics, undet, init
971.2	POISONING BY SYMPATHOMIMETICS	**T44.4X1A**	Poisoning by predom alpha-adrenocpt agonists, acc, init
		T44.4X2A	Poisn by predom alpha-adrenocpt agonists, self-harm, init
		T44.4X3A	Poisoning by predom alpha-adrenocpt agonists, assault, init
		T44.4X4A	Poisoning by predom alpha-adrenocpt agonists, undet, init
		T44.5X1A	Poisoning by predom beta-adrenocpt agonists, acc, init
		T44.5X2A	Poisoning by predom beta-adrenocpt agonists, self-harm, init
		T44.5X3A	Poisoning by predom beta-adrenocpt agonists, assault, init
		T44.5X4A	Poisoning by predom beta-adrenocpt agonists, undet, init
971.3	POISONING BY SYMPATHOLYTICS	**T44.6X1A**	Poisoning by alpha-adrenocpt antagonists, accidental, init
		T44.6X2A	Poisoning by alpha-adrenocpt antagonists, self-harm, init
		T44.6X3A	Poisoning by alpha-adrenoreceptor antagonists, assault, init
		T44.6X4A	Poisoning by alpha-adrenocpt antagonists, undetermined, init
		T44.7X1A	Poisoning by beta-adrenocpt antagonists, accidental, init
		T44.7X2A	Poisoning by beta-adrenocpt antagonists, self-harm, init
		T44.7X3A	Poisoning by beta-adrenoreceptor antagonists, assault, init
		T44.7X4A	Poisoning by beta-adrenocpt antagonists, undetermined, init
		T44.8X1A	Poisoning by centr-acting/adren-neurn-block agnt, acc, init
		T44.8X2A	Poisn by centr-acting/adren-neurn-block agnt, slf-hrm, init
		T44.8X3A	Poisn by centr-acting/adren-neurn-block agnt, assault, init
		T44.8X4A	Poisn by centr-acting/adren-neurn-block agnt, undet, init
971.9	POISN UNSPEC DRUG PRIM AFFCT AUTONOM NERV SYSTEM	**T44.9Ø1A**	Poisn by unsp drugs aff the autonm nervous sys, acc, init
		T44.9Ø2A	Poisn by unsp drugs aff the autonm nrv sys, slf-hrm, init
		T44.9Ø3A	Poisn by unsp drugs aff the autonm nervous sys, asslt, init
		T44.9Ø4A	Poisn by unsp drugs aff the autonm nervous sys, undet, init
		T44.991A	Poisoning by oth drug aff the autonm nervous sys, acc, init
		T44.992A	Poisn by oth drug aff the autonm nervous sys, slf-hrm, init
		T44.993A	Poisn by oth drug aff the autonm nervous sys, assault, init
		T44.994A	Poisn by oth drug aff the autonm nervous sys, undet, init
972.Ø	POISONING BY CARDIAC RHYTHM REGULATORS	**T46.2X1A**	Poisoning by oth antidysrhythmic drugs, accidental, init
		T46.2X2A	Poisoning by oth antidysrhythmic drugs, self-harm, init
		T46.2X3A	Poisoning by oth antidysrhythmic drugs, assault, init encntr
		T46.2X4A	Poisoning by oth antidysrhythmic drugs, undetermined, init
972.1	POISN CARDIOTONIC GLYCOSIDES&RX SIMILAR ACTION	**T46.ØX1A**	Poisoning by cardi-stim glycos/drug simlar act, acc, init
		T46.ØX2A	Poisn by cardi-stim glycos/drug simlar act, self-harm, init
		T46.ØX3A	Poisn by cardi-stim glycos/drug simlar act, assault, init
		T46.ØX4A	Poisoning by cardi-stim glycos/drug simlar act, undet, init
972.2	POISONING ANTILIPEMIC&ANTIARTERIOSCLEROTIC DRUGS	**T46.6X1A**	Poisoning by antihyperlip and antiarterio drugs, acc, init
		T46.6X2A	Poisn by antihyperlip and antiarterio drugs, self-harm, init
		T46.6X3A	Poisn by antihyperlip and antiarterio drugs, assault, init
		T46.6X4A	Poisoning by antihyperlip and antiarterio drugs, undet, init
972.3	POISONING BY GANGLION-BLOCKING AGENTS	**T44.2X1A**	Poisoning by ganglionic blocking drugs, accidental, init
		T44.2X2A	Poisoning by ganglionic blocking drugs, self-harm, init
		T44.2X3A	Poisoning by ganglionic blocking drugs, assault, init encntr
		T44.2X4A	Poisoning by ganglionic blocking drugs, undetermined, init
972.4	POISONING BY CORONARY VASODILATORS	**T46.3X1A**	Poisoning by coronary vasodilators, accidental, init
		T46.3X2A	Poisoning by coronary vasodilators, self-harm, init
		T46.3X3A	Poisoning by coronary vasodilators, assault, init encntr
		T46.3X4A	Poisoning by coronary vasodilators, undetermined, init
972.5	POISONING BY OTHER VASODILATORS	**T46.7X1A**	Poisoning by peripheral vasodilators, accidental, init
		T46.7X2A	Poisoning by peripheral vasodilators, self-harm, init
		T46.7X3A	Poisoning by peripheral vasodilators, assault, init encntr
		T46.7X4A	Poisoning by peripheral vasodilators, undetermined, init
972.6	POISONING BY OTHER ANTIHYPERTENSIVE AGENTS	**T46.4X1A**	Poisoning by angiotens-convert-enzyme inhibitors, acc, init
		T46.4X2A	Poisn by angiotens-convert-enzyme inhibtr, self-harm, init
		T46.4X3A	Poisoning by angiotens-convert-enzyme inhibtr, assault, init
		T46.4X4A	Poisoning by angiotens-convert-enzyme inhibtr, undet, init
		T46.5X1A	Poisoning by oth antihypertn drugs, accidental, init
		T46.5X2A	Poisoning by oth antihypertensive drugs, self-harm, init
		T46.5X3A	Poisoning by oth antihypertensive drugs, assault, init
		T46.5X4A	Poisoning by oth antihypertensive drugs, undetermined, init
972.7	POISONING ANTIVARICOSE RX INCL SCLEROSING AGTS	**T46.8X1A**	Poisoning by antivaric drugs, inc scler agents, acc, init
		T46.8X2A	Poisn by antivaric drugs, inc scler agents, self-harm, init
		T46.8X3A	Poisn by antivaric drugs, inc scler agents, assault, init
		T46.8X4A	Poisoning by antivaric drugs, inc scler agents, undet, init
972.8	POISONING BY CAPILLARY-ACTIVE DRUGS	**T46.991A**	Poisoning by oth agents aff the cardiovasc sys, acc, init

 [Brackets] indicate valid character values for each code. Character value meanings provided for each code grouping.

ICD-9-CM		ICD-10-CM	
972.9	POISN OTH&UNSPEC AGTS PRIMARILY AFFECT CV SYSTEM	T46.1X1A	Poisoning by calcium-channel blockers, accidental, init
		T46.1X2A	Poisoning by calcium-channel blockers, self-harm, init
		T46.1X3A	Poisoning by calcium-channel blockers, assault, init encntr
		T46.1X4A	Poisoning by calcium-channel blockers, undetermined, init
		T46.901A	Poisoning by unsp agents aff the cardiovasc sys, acc, init
		T46.902A	Poisn by unsp agents aff the cardiovasc sys, self-harm, init
		T46.903A	Poisn by unsp agents aff the cardiovasc sys, assault, init
		T46.904A	Poisoning by unsp agents aff the cardiovasc sys, undet, init
		T46.991A	Poisoning by oth agents aff the cardiovasc sys, acc, init
		T46.992A	Poisn by oth agents aff the cardiovasc sys, self-harm, init
		T46.993A	Poisn by oth agents aff the cardiovasc sys, assault, init
		T46.994A	Poisoning by oth agents aff the cardiovasc sys, undet, init
973.0	POISONING ANTACIDS&ANTIGASTRIC SECRETION DRUGS	T47.0X1A	Poisoning by histamine H2-receptor blockers, acc, init
		T47.0X2A	Poisoning by histamine H2-receptor blockers, self-harm, init
		T47.0X3A	Poisoning by histamine H2-receptor blockers, assault, init
		T47.0X4A	Poisoning by histamine H2-receptor blockers, undet, init
		T47.1X1A	Poisn by oth antacids and anti-gstrc-sec drugs, acc, init
		T47.1X2A	Poisn by oth antacids & anti-gstrc-sec drugs, slf-hrm, init
		T47.1X3A	Poisn by oth antacids and anti-gstrc-sec drugs, asslt, init
		T47.1X4A	Poisn by oth antacids and anti-gstrc-sec drugs, undet, init
973.1	POISONING BY IRRITANT CATHARTICS	T47.2X1A	Poisoning by stimulant laxatives, accidental, init
		T47.2X2A	Poisoning by stimulant laxatives, self-harm, init
		T47.2X3A	Poisoning by stimulant laxatives, assault, initial encounter
		T47.2X4A	Poisoning by stimulant laxatives, undetermined, init encntr
973.2	POISONING BY EMOLLIENT CATHARTICS	T47.3X1A	Poisoning by saline and osmotic laxatives, accidental, init
		T47.3X2A	Poisoning by saline and osmotic laxatives, self-harm, init
		T47.3X3A	Poisoning by saline and osmotic laxatives, assault, init
		T47.3X4A	Poisoning by saline and osmotic laxatives, undet, init
973.3	POISONING OTH CATHRT INCL INTESTINAL ATONIA RX	T47.4X1A	Poisoning by oth laxatives, accidental (unintentional), init
		T47.4X2A	Poisoning by oth laxatives, intentional self-harm, init
		T47.4X3A	Poisoning by other laxatives, assault, initial encounter
		T47.4X4A	Poisoning by other laxatives, undetermined, init encntr
973.4	POISONING BY DIGESTANTS	T47.5X1A	Poisoning by digestants, accidental (unintentional), init
		T47.5X2A	Poisoning by digestants, intentional self-harm, init encntr
		T47.5X3A	Poisoning by digestants, assault, initial encounter
		T47.5X4A	Poisoning by digestants, undetermined, initial encounter
973.5	POISONING BY ANTIDIARRHEAL DRUGS	T47.6X1A	Poisoning by antidiarrheal drugs, accidental, init
		T47.6X2A	Poisoning by antidiarrheal drugs, self-harm, init
		T47.6X3A	Poisoning by antidiarrheal drugs, assault, initial encounter
		T47.6X4A	Poisoning by antidiarrheal drugs, undetermined, init encntr
973.6	POISONING BY EMETICS	T47.7X1A	Poisoning by emetics, accidental (unintentional), init
		T47.7X2A	Poisoning by emetics, intentional self-harm, init encntr
		T47.7X3A	Poisoning by emetics, assault, initial encounter
		T47.7X4A	Poisoning by emetics, undetermined, initial encounter
973.8	POISN OTH SPEC AGTS PRIMARILY AFFECT GI SYSTEM	T47.8X1A	Poisoning by oth agents aff GI sys, accidental, init
		T47.8X2A	Poisoning by oth agents aff GI sys, self-harm, init
		T47.8X3A	Poisoning by oth agents aff GI sys, assault, init
		T47.8X4A	Poisoning by oth agents aff GI sys, undetermined, init
973.9	POISONING UNSPEC AGT PRIMARILY AFFECT GI SYSTEM	T47.91XA	Poisoning by unsp agents aff the GI sys, accidental, init
		T47.92XA	Poisoning by unsp agents aff the GI sys, self-harm, init
		T47.93XA	Poisoning by unsp agents aff the GI sys, assault, init
		T47.94XA	Poisoning by unsp agents aff the GI sys, undetermined, init
974.0	POISONING BY MERCURIAL DIURETICS	T50.2X1A	Poisn by crbnc-anhydr inhibtr, benzo/oth diuretc, acc, init
974.1	POISONING BY PURINE DERIVATIVE DIURETICS	T50.2X1A	Poisn by crbnc-anhydr inhibtr, benzo/oth diuretc, acc, init
974.2	POISONING BY CARBONIC ACID ANHYDRASE INHIBITORS	T50.2X1A	Poisn by crbnc-anhydr inhibtr, benzo/oth diuretc, acc, init
		T50.2X2A	Poisn by crbnc-anhydr inhibtr,benzo/oth diuretc,slf-hrm,init
		T50.2X3A	Poisn by crbnc-anhydr inhibtr,benzo/oth diuretc, asslt, init
		T50.2X4A	Poisn by crbnc-anhydr inhibtr,benzo/oth diuretc, undet, init
974.3	POISONING BY SALURETICS	T50.2X1A	Poisn by crbnc-anhydr inhibtr, benzo/oth diuretc, acc, init
974.4	POISONING BY OTHER DIURETICS	T50.1X1A	Poisoning by loop diuretics, accidental, init
		T50.1X2A	Poisoning by loop diuretics, intentional self-harm, init
		T50.1X3A	Poisoning by loop diuretics, assault, initial encounter
		T50.1X4A	Poisoning by loop diuretics, undetermined, initial encounter
		T50.2X1A	Poisn by crbnc-anhydr inhibtr, benzo/oth diuretc, acc, init
		T50.2X2A	Poisn by crbnc-anhydr inhibtr,benzo/oth diuretc,slf-hrm,init
		T50.2X3A	Poisn by crbnc-anhydr inhibtr,benzo/oth diuretc, asslt, init
		T50.2X4A	Poisn by crbnc-anhydr inhibtr,benzo/oth diuretc, undet, init
974.5	POISN ELECTROLYTIC CALORIC&WATER-BALANCE AGTS	T50.3X1A	Poisoning by electrolytic/caloric/wtr-bal agnt, acc, init
		T50.3X2A	Poisn by electrolytic/caloric/wtr-bal agnt, self-harm, init
		T50.3X3A	Poisn by electrolytic/caloric/wtr-bal agnt, assault, init
		T50.3X4A	Poisoning by electrolytic/caloric/wtr-bal agnt, undet, init
974.6	POISONING BY OTHER MINERAL SALTS NEC	T50.3X1A	Poisoning by electrolytic/caloric/wtr-bal agnt, acc, init
974.7	POISONING BY URIC ACID METABOLISM DRUGS	T50.4X1A	Poisoning by drugs affecting uric acid metab, acc, init
		T50.4X2A	Poisoning by drugs aff uric acid metab, self-harm, init
		T50.4X3A	Poisoning by drugs affecting uric acid metab, assault, init
		T50.4X4A	Poisoning by drugs affecting uric acid metab, undet, init

ICD-9-CM		ICD-10-CM	
975.Ø	POISONING BY OXYTOCIC AGENTS	T48.ØX1A	Poisoning by oxytocic drugs, accidental, init
		T48.ØX2A	Poisoning by oxytocic drugs, intentional self-harm, init
		T48.ØX3A	Poisoning by oxytocic drugs, assault, initial encounter
		T48.ØX4A	Poisoning by oxytocic drugs, undetermined, initial encounter
975.1	POISONING BY SMOOTH MUSCLE RELAXANTS	T48.2Ø1A	Poisoning by unsp drugs acting on muscles, accidental, init
		T48.291A	Poisoning by oth drugs acting on muscles, accidental, init
		T48.294A	Poisoning by oth drugs acting on muscles, undetermined, init
975.2	POISONING BY SKELETAL MUSCLE RELAXANTS	T48.1X1A	Poisoning by skeletal muscle relaxants, accidental, init
		T48.1X2A	Poisoning by skeletal muscle relaxants, self-harm, init
		T48.1X3A	Poisoning by skeletal muscle relaxants, assault, init encntr
		T48.1X4A	Poisoning by skeletal muscle relaxants, undetermined, init
975.3	POISONING OTHER&UNSPECIFIED DRUGS ACTING MUSCLES	T48.2Ø1A	Poisoning by unsp drugs acting on muscles, accidental, init
		T48.2Ø2A	Poisoning by unsp drugs acting on muscles, self-harm, init
		T48.2Ø3A	Poisoning by unsp drugs acting on muscles, assault, init
		T48.2Ø4A	Poisoning by unsp drugs acting on muscles, undet, init
		T48.291A	Poisoning by oth drugs acting on muscles, accidental, init
		T48.292A	Poisoning by oth drugs acting on muscles, self-harm, init
		T48.293A	Poisoning by oth drugs acting on muscles, assault, init
		T48.294A	Poisoning by oth drugs acting on muscles, undetermined, init
975.4	POISONING BY ANTITUSSIVES	T48.3X1A	Poisoning by antitussives, accidental (unintentional), init
		T48.3X2A	Poisoning by antitussives, intentional self-harm, init
		T48.3X3A	Poisoning by antitussives, assault, initial encounter
		T48.3X4A	Poisoning by antitussives, undetermined, initial encounter
975.5	POISONING BY EXPECTORANTS	T48.4X1A	Poisoning by expectorants, accidental (unintentional), init
		T48.4X2A	Poisoning by expectorants, intentional self-harm, init
		T48.4X3A	Poisoning by expectorants, assault, initial encounter
		T48.4X4A	Poisoning by expectorants, undetermined, initial encounter
975.6	POISONING BY ANTI-COMMON COLD DRUGS	T48.5X1A	Poisoning by oth anti-cmn-cold drugs, accidental, init
		T48.5X2A	Poisoning by oth anti-common-cold drugs, self-harm, init
		T48.5X3A	Poisoning by oth anti-common-cold drugs, assault, init
		T48.5X4A	Poisoning by oth anti-common-cold drugs, undetermined, init
975.7	POISONING BY ANTIASTHMATICS	T48.6X1A	Poisoning by antiasthmatics, accidental, init
		T48.6X2A	Poisoning by antiasthmatics, intentional self-harm, init
		T48.6X3A	Poisoning by antiasthmatics, assault, initial encounter
		T48.6X4A	Poisoning by antiasthmatics, undetermined, initial encounter
975.8	POISONING OTHER&UNSPECIFIED RESPIRATORY DRUGS	T41.5X1A	Poisoning by therapeutic gases, accidental, init
		T41.5X2A	Poisoning by therapeutic gases, intentional self-harm, init
		T41.5X3A	Poisoning by therapeutic gases, assault, initial encounter
		T41.5X4A	Poisoning by therapeutic gases, undetermined, init encntr
		T48.9Ø1A	Poisn by unsp agents prim acting on the resp sys, acc, init
		T48.9Ø2A	Poisn by unsp agents prim act on the resp sys, slf-hrm, init
		T48.9Ø3A	Poisn by unsp agents prim act on the resp sys, asslt, init
		T48.9Ø4A	Poisn by unsp agents prim act on the resp sys, undet, init
		T48.991A	Poisn by oth agents prim acting on the resp sys, acc, init
		T48.992A	Poisn by oth agents prim act on the resp sys, slf-hrm, init
		T48.993A	Poisn by oth agents prim acting on the resp sys, asslt, init
		T48.994A	Poisn by oth agents prim acting on the resp sys, undet, init
976.Ø	POISONING LOCAL ANTI-INFECTIVES&ANTI-INFLAM RX	T49.ØX1A	Poisoning by local antifung/infect/inflamm drugs, acc, init
		T49.ØX2A	Poisn by local antifung/infect/inflamm drugs, slf-hrm, init
		T49.ØX3A	Poisn by local antifung/infect/inflamm drugs, assault, init
		T49.ØX4A	Poisn by local antifung/infect/inflamm drugs, undet, init
976.1	POISONING BY ANTIPRURITICS	T49.1X1A	Poisoning by antipruritics, accidental (unintentional), init
		T49.1X2A	Poisoning by antipruritics, intentional self-harm, init
		T49.1X3A	Poisoning by antipruritics, assault, initial encounter
		T49.1X4A	Poisoning by antipruritics, undetermined, initial encounter
976.2	POISONING LOCAL ASTRINGENTS AND LOCAL DETERGENTS	T49.2X1A	Poisoning by local astringents/detergents, accidental, init
		T49.2X2A	Poisoning by local astringents/detergents, self-harm, init
		T49.2X3A	Poisoning by local astringents/detergents, assault, init
		T49.2X4A	Poisoning by local astringents/detergents, undet, init
976.3	POISONING EMOLLIENTS DEMULCENTS AND PROTECTANTS	T49.3X1A	Poisoning by emollients, demulcents and protect, acc, init
		T49.3X2A	Poisn by emollients, demulcents and protect, self-harm, init
		T49.3X3A	Poisn by emollients, demulcents and protect, assault, init
		T49.3X4A	Poisoning by emollients, demulcents and protect, undet, init
976.4	POISON-KERATOLYTICS-KERATOPLASTICS-OTH HAIR RX	T49.4X1A	Poisoning by keratolyt/keratplst/hair trmt drug, acc, init
		T49.4X2A	Poisn by keratolyt/keratplst/hair trmt drug, self-harm, init
		T49.4X3A	Poisn by keratolyt/keratplst/hair trmt drug, assault, init
		T49.4X4A	Poisoning by keratolyt/keratplst/hair trmt drug, undet, init
976.5	POISONING EYE ANTI-INFECTIVES&OTHER EYE DRUGS	T49.5X1A	Poisoning by opth drugs and preparations, accidental, init
		T49.5X2A	Poisoning by opth drugs and preparations, self-harm, init
		T49.5X3A	Poisoning by opth drugs and preparations, assault, init
		T49.5X4A	Poisoning by opth drugs and preparations, undetermined, init
976.6	POISN ANTI-INFECTIVES&OTH RX&PREP EAR NSE&THROAT	T49.6X1A	Poisoning by otorhino drugs and prep, accidental, init
		T49.6X2A	Poisoning by otorhino drugs and prep, self-harm, init
		T49.6X3A	Poisoning by otorhino drugs and preparations, assault, init
		T49.6X4A	Poisoning by otorhino drugs and prep, undetermined, init

ICD-9-CM		ICD-10-CM	
976.7	POISONING BY DENTAL DRUGS TOPICALLY APPLIED	T49.7X1A	Poisoning by dental drugs, topically applied, acc, init
		T49.7X2A	Poisn by dental drugs, topically applied, self-harm, init
		T49.7X3A	Poisoning by dental drugs, topically applied, assault, init
		T49.7X4A	Poisoning by dental drugs, topically applied, undet, init
976.8	POISN OTH AGTS PRIM AFFECT SKIN&MUCOS MEMBRANE	T49.8X1A	Poisoning by oth topical agents, accidental, init
		T49.8X2A	Poisoning by oth topical agents, intentional self-harm, init
		T49.8X3A	Poisoning by other topical agents, assault, init encntr
		T49.8X4A	Poisoning by other topical agents, undetermined, init encntr
976.9	POISN UNSPEC AGT PRIM AFFECT SKIN&MUCOS MEMBRANE	T49.91XA	Poisoning by unsp topical agent, accidental, init
		T49.92XA	Poisoning by unsp topical agent, intentional self-harm, init
		T49.93XA	Poisoning by unspecified topical agent, assault, init encntr
		T49.94XA	Poisoning by unsp topical agent, undetermined, init encntr
977.Ø	POISONING BY DIETETICS	T5Ø.5X1A	Poisoning by appetite depressants, accidental, init
		T5Ø.5X2A	Poisoning by appetite depressants, self-harm, init
		T5Ø.5X3A	Poisoning by appetite depressants, assault, init encntr
		T5Ø.5X4A	Poisoning by appetite depressants, undetermined, init encntr
977.1	POISONING BY LIPOTROPIC DRUGS	T5Ø.991A	Poisoning by oth drug/meds/biol subst, accidental, init
977.2	POISONING BY ANTIDOTES AND CHELATING AGENTS NEC	T5Ø.6X1A	Poisoning by antidotes and chelating agents, acc, init
		T5Ø.6X2A	Poisoning by antidotes and chelating agents, self-harm, init
		T5Ø.6X3A	Poisoning by antidotes and chelating agents, assault, init
		T5Ø.6X4A	Poisoning by antidotes and chelating agents, undet, init
977.3	POISONING BY ALCOHOL DETERRENTS	T5Ø.991A	Poisoning by oth drug/meds/biol subst, accidental, init
977.4	POISONING BY PHARMACEUTICAL EXCIPIENTS	T5Ø.991A	Poisoning by oth drug/meds/biol subst, accidental, init
977.8	POISONING OTHER SPEC DRUGS&MEDICINAL SUBSTANCES	T5Ø.8X1A	Poisoning by diagnostic agents, accidental, init
		T5Ø.8X2A	Poisoning by diagnostic agents, intentional self-harm, init
		T5Ø.8X3A	Poisoning by diagnostic agents, assault, initial encounter
		T5Ø.8X4A	Poisoning by diagnostic agents, undetermined, init encntr
977.9	POISONING UNSPECIFIED DRUG/MEDICINAL SUBSTANCE	T5Ø.9Ø1A	Poisoning by unsp drug/meds/biol subst, accidental, init
		T5Ø.9Ø2A	Poisoning by unsp drug/meds/biol subst, self-harm, init
		T5Ø.9Ø3A	Poisoning by unsp drug/meds/biol subst, assault, init
		T5Ø.9Ø4A	Poisoning by unsp drug/meds/biol subst, undetermined, init
978.Ø	POISONING BY BCG VACCINE	T5Ø.A91A	Poisoning by oth bacterial vaccines, accidental, init
978.1	POISONING BY TYPHOID AND PARATYPHOID VACCINE	T5Ø.A92A	Poisoning by oth bacterial vaccines, self-harm, init
978.2	POISONING BY CHOLERA VACCINE	T5Ø.A92A	Poisoning by oth bacterial vaccines, self-harm, init
978.3	POISONING BY PLAGUE VACCINE	T5Ø.A92A	Poisoning by oth bacterial vaccines, self-harm, init
978.4	POISONING BY TETANUS VACCINE	T5Ø.A92A	Poisoning by oth bacterial vaccines, self-harm, init
978.5	POISONING BY DIPHTHERIA VACCINE	T5Ø.A92A	Poisoning by oth bacterial vaccines, self-harm, init
978.6	POISN PERTUSS VACCINE INCL COMB W/PERTUSS CMPNT	T5Ø.A11A	Poisn by pertuss vaccine, inc combin w pertuss, acc, init
		T5Ø.A12A	Poisn by pertuss vaccn, inc combin w pertuss, slf-hrm, init
		T5Ø.A13A	Poisn by pertuss vaccine, inc combin w pertuss, asslt, init
		T5Ø.A14A	Poisn by pertuss vaccine, inc combin w pertuss, undet, init
978.8	POISONING OTHER&UNSPECIFIED BACTERIAL VACCINES	T5Ø.A91A	Poisoning by oth bacterial vaccines, accidental, init
		T5Ø.A92A	Poisoning by oth bacterial vaccines, self-harm, init
		T5Ø.A93A	Poisoning by other bacterial vaccines, assault, init encntr
		T5Ø.A94A	Poisoning by oth bacterial vaccines, undetermined, init
978.9	POISN MIX BACTERL VACCS NO COMB W/PERTUSS CMPNT	T5Ø.A21A	Poisoning by mixed bact vaccines w/o a pertuss, acc, init
		T5Ø.A22A	Poisn by mixed bact vaccines w/o a pertuss, self-harm, init
		T5Ø.A23A	Poisn by mixed bact vaccines w/o a pertuss, assault, init
		T5Ø.A24A	Poisoning by mixed bact vaccines w/o a pertuss, undet, init
979.Ø	POISONING BY SMALLPOX VACCINE	T5Ø.B11A	Poisoning by smallpox vaccines, accidental, init
		T5Ø.B12A	Poisoning by smallpox vaccines, intentional self-harm, init
		T5Ø.B13A	Poisoning by smallpox vaccines, assault, initial encounter
		T5Ø.B14A	Poisoning by smallpox vaccines, undetermined, init encntr
979.1	POISONING BY RABIES VACCINE	T5Ø.B91A	Poisoning by oth viral vaccines, accidental, init
979.2	POISONING BY TYPHUS VACCINE	T5Ø.B91A	Poisoning by oth viral vaccines, accidental, init
979.3	POISONING BY YELLOW FEVER VACCINE	T5Ø.B91A	Poisoning by oth viral vaccines, accidental, init
979.4	POISONING BY MEASLES VACCINE	T5Ø.B91A	Poisoning by oth viral vaccines, accidental, init
979.5	POISONING BY POLIOMYELITIS VACCINE	T5Ø.B91A	Poisoning by oth viral vaccines, accidental, init
979.6	POISONING OTH&UNSPEC VIRAL&RICKETTSIAL VACCINES	T5Ø.B91A	Poisoning by oth viral vaccines, accidental, init
		T5Ø.B92A	Poisoning by oth viral vaccines, intentional self-harm, init
		T5Ø.B93A	Poisoning by other viral vaccines, assault, init encntr
		T5Ø.B94A	Poisoning by other viral vaccines, undetermined, init encntr
979.7	POISON-VIRAL-RICKETTSIAL-BACT VACCINE NO PERTUSS	T5Ø.Z91A	Poisoning by oth vaccines and biolg substances, acc, init
979.9	POISN OTH&UNSPEC VACCINES&BIOLOGICAL SUBSTANCES	T5Ø.9Ø1A	Poisoning by unsp drug/meds/biol subst, accidental, init
		T5Ø.991A	Poisoning by oth drug/meds/biol subst, accidental, init
		T5Ø.992A	Poisoning by oth drug/meds/biol subst, self-harm, init
		T5Ø.993A	Poisoning by oth drug/meds/biol subst, assault, init
		T5Ø.994A	Poisoning by oth drug/meds/biol subst, undetermined, init
		T5Ø.Z91A	Poisoning by oth vaccines and biolg substances, acc, init
		T5Ø.Z92A	Poisoning by oth vaccines and biolg substnc, self-harm, init
		T5Ø.Z93A	Poisoning by oth vaccines and biolg substnc, assault, init
		T5Ø.Z94A	Poisoning by oth vaccines and biolg substances, undet, init

ICD-9-CM		ICD-10-CM	
980.Ø	TOXIC EFFECT OF ETHYL ALCOHOL	T51.ØX1A	Toxic effect of ethanol, accidental (unintentional), init
		T51.ØX2A	Toxic effect of ethanol, intentional self-harm, init encntr
		T51.ØX3A	Toxic effect of ethanol, assault, initial encounter
		T51.ØX4A	Toxic effect of ethanol, undetermined, initial encounter
980.1	TOXIC EFFECT OF METHYL ALCOHOL	T51.1X1A	Toxic effect of methanol, accidental (unintentional), init
		T51.1X2A	Toxic effect of methanol, intentional self-harm, init encntr
		T51.1X3A	Toxic effect of methanol, assault, initial encounter
		T51.1X4A	Toxic effect of methanol, undetermined, initial encounter
980.2	TOXIC EFFECT OF ISOPROPYL ALCOHOL	T51.2X1A	Toxic effect of 2-Propanol, accidental (unintentional), init
		T51.2X2A	Toxic effect of 2-Propanol, intentional self-harm, init
		T51.2X3A	Toxic effect of 2-Propanol, assault, initial encounter
		T51.2X4A	Toxic effect of 2-Propanol, undetermined, initial encounter
980.3	TOXIC EFFECT OF FUSEL OIL	T51.3X1A	Toxic effect of fusel oil, accidental (unintentional), init
		T51.3X2A	Toxic effect of fusel oil, intentional self-harm, init
		T51.3X3A	Toxic effect of fusel oil, assault, initial encounter
		T51.3X4A	Toxic effect of fusel oil, undetermined, initial encounter
980.8	TOXIC EFFECT OF OTHER SPECIFIED ALCOHOLS	T51.8X1A	Toxic effect of alcohols, accidental (unintentional), init
		T51.8X2A	Toxic effect of oth alcohols, intentional self-harm, init
		T51.8X3A	Toxic effect of other alcohols, assault, initial encounter
		T51.8X4A	Toxic effect of other alcohols, undetermined, init encntr
980.9	TOXIC EFFECT OF UNSPECIFIED ALCOHOL	T51.91XA	Toxic effect of unsp alcohol, accidental, init
		T51.92XA	Toxic effect of unsp alcohol, intentional self-harm, init
		T51.93XA	Toxic effect of unspecified alcohol, assault, init encntr
		T51.94XA	Toxic effect of unsp alcohol, undetermined, init encntr
981	TOXIC EFFECT OF PETROLEUM PRODUCTS	T52.ØX1A	Toxic effect of petroleum products, accidental, init
		T52.ØX2A	Toxic effect of petroleum products, self-harm, init
		T52.ØX3A	Toxic effect of petroleum products, assault, init encntr
		T52.ØX4A	Toxic effect of petroleum products, undetermined, init
982.Ø	TOXIC EFFECT OF BENZENE AND HOMOLOGUES	T52.1X1A	Toxic effect of benzene, accidental (unintentional), init
		T52.1X2A	Toxic effect of benzene, intentional self-harm, init encntr
		T52.1X3A	Toxic effect of benzene, assault, initial encounter
		T52.1X4A	Toxic effect of benzene, undetermined, initial encounter
		T52.2X1A	Toxic effect of homologues of benzene, accidental, init
		T52.2X2A	Toxic effect of homologues of benzene, self-harm, init
		T52.2X3A	Toxic effect of homologues of benzene, assault, init encntr
		T52.2X4A	Toxic effect of homologues of benzene, undetermined, init
		T65.3X1A	Toxic eff of nitrodrv/aminodrv of benzn/homolog, acc, init
		T65.3X2A	Tox eff of nitrodrv/aminodrv of benzn/homolog, slf-hrm, init
		T65.3X3A	Toxic eff of nitrodrv/aminodrv of benzn/homolog, asslt, init
		T65.3X4A	Toxic eff of nitrodrv/aminodrv of benzn/homolog, undet, init
982.1	TOXIC EFFECT OF CARBON TETRACHLORIDE	T53.ØX1A	Toxic effect of carbon tetrachloride, accidental, init
		T53.ØX2A	Toxic effect of carbon tetrachloride, self-harm, init
		T53.ØX3A	Toxic effect of carbon tetrachloride, assault, init encntr
		T53.ØX4A	Toxic effect of carbon tetrachloride, undetermined, init
982.2	TOXIC EFFECT OF CARBON DISULFIDE	T65.4X1A	Toxic effect of carbon disulfide, accidental, init
		T65.4X2A	Toxic effect of carbon disulfide, self-harm, init
		T65.4X3A	Toxic effect of carbon disulfide, assault, initial encounter
		T65.4X4A	Toxic effect of carbon disulfide, undetermined, init encntr
982.3	TOXIC EFFECT OTH CHLORINATED HYDROCARBON SOLVNTS	T53.1X1A	Toxic effect of chloroform, accidental (unintentional), init
		T53.1X2A	Toxic effect of chloroform, intentional self-harm, init
		T53.1X3A	Toxic effect of chloroform, assault, initial encounter
		T53.1X4A	Toxic effect of chloroform, undetermined, initial encounter
		T53.2X1A	Toxic effect of trichloroethylene, accidental, init
		T53.2X2A	Toxic effect of trichloroethylene, self-harm, init
		T53.2X3A	Toxic effect of trichloroethylene, assault, init encntr
		T53.2X4A	Toxic effect of trichloroethylene, undetermined, init encntr
		T53.3X1A	Toxic effect of tetrachloroethylene, accidental, init
		T53.3X2A	Toxic effect of tetrachloroethylene, self-harm, init
		T53.3X3A	Toxic effect of tetrachloroethylene, assault, init encntr
		T53.3X4A	Toxic effect of tetrachloroethylene, undetermined, init
		T53.4X1A	Toxic effect of dichloromethane, accidental, init
		T53.4X2A	Toxic effect of dichloromethane, intentional self-harm, init
		T53.4X3A	Toxic effect of dichloromethane, assault, initial encounter
		T53.4X4A	Toxic effect of dichloromethane, undetermined, init encntr
		T53.6X1A	Toxic eff of halgn deriv of aliphatic hydrocrb, acc, init
		T53.6X2A	Tox eff of halgn deriv of aliphatic hydrocrb, slf-hrm, init
		T53.6X3A	Toxic eff of halgn deriv of aliphatic hydrocrb, asslt, init
		T53.6X4A	Toxic eff of halgn deriv of aliphatic hydrocrb, undet, init
		T53.7X1A	Toxic effect of halgn deriv of aromatic hydrocrb, acc, init
		T53.7X2A	Toxic eff of halgn deriv of aromatic hydrocrb, slf-hrm, init
		T53.7X3A	Toxic eff of halgn deriv of aromatic hydrocrb, asslt, init
		T53.7X4A	Toxic eff of halgn deriv of aromatic hydrocrb, undet, init
		T53.91XA	Toxic eff of unsp halgn deriv of aromat hydrocrb, acc, init
		T53.92XA	Tox eff of unsp halgn deriv of aromat hydrocrb,slf-hrm, init
		T53.93XA	Tox eff of unsp halgn deriv of aromat hydrocrb, asslt, init
		T53.94XA	Tox eff of unsp halgn deriv of aromat hydrocrb, undet, init

[Brackets] indicate valid character values for each code. Character value meanings provided for each code grouping.

ICD-9-CM		ICD-10-CM	
982.4	TOXIC EFFECT OF NITROGLYCOL	**T52.3X1A**	Toxic effect of glycols, accidental (unintentional), init
		T52.3X2A	Toxic effect of glycols, intentional self-harm, init encntr
		T52.3X3A	Toxic effect of glycols, assault, initial encounter
		T52.3X4A	Toxic effect of glycols, undetermined, initial encounter
982.8	TOXIC EFFECT OTHER NONPETROLEUM-BASED SOLVENTS	**T52.4X1A**	Toxic effect of ketones, accidental (unintentional), init
		T52.4X2A	Toxic effect of ketones, intentional self-harm, init encntr
		T52.4X3A	Toxic effect of ketones, assault, initial encounter
		T52.4X4A	Toxic effect of ketones, undetermined, initial encounter
		T52.8X1A	Toxic effect of organic solvents, accidental, init
		T52.8X2A	Toxic effect of organic solvents, self-harm, init
		T52.8X3A	Toxic effect of other organic solvents, assault, init encntr
		T52.8X4A	Toxic effect of oth organic solvents, undetermined, init
		T52.91XA	Toxic effect of unsp organic solvent, accidental, init
		T52.92XA	Toxic effect of unsp organic solvent, self-harm, init
		T52.93XA	Toxic effect of unsp organic solvent, assault, init encntr
		T52.94XA	Toxic effect of unsp organic solvent, undetermined, init
983.Ø	TOXIC EFFECT OF CORROSIVE AROMATICS	**T54.ØX1A**	Toxic effect of phenol and phenol homologues, acc, init
		T54.ØX2A	Toxic effect of phenol and phenol homolog, self-harm, init
		T54.ØX3A	Toxic effect of phenol and phenol homologues, assault, init
		T54.ØX4A	Toxic effect of phenol and phenol homologues, undet, init
983.1	TOXIC EFFECT OF ACIDS	**T54.2X1A**	Toxic eff of corrosv acids and acid-like substnc, acc, init
		T54.2X2A	Tox eff of corrosv acids & acid-like substnc, slf-hrm, init
		T54.2X3A	Tox eff of corrosv acids and acid-like substnc, asslt, init
		T54.2X4A	Tox eff of corrosv acids and acid-like substnc, undet, init
983.2	TOXIC EFFECT OF CAUSTIC ALKALIS	**T54.3X1A**	Tox eff of corrosv alkalis and alk-like substnc, acc, init
		T54.3X2A	Tox eff of corrosv alkalis & alk-like substnc, slf-hrm, init
		T54.3X3A	Tox eff of corrosv alkalis and alk-like substnc, asslt, init
		T54.3X4A	Tox eff of corrosv alkalis and alk-like substnc, undet, init
983.9	TOXIC EFFECT OF CAUSTIC UNSPECIFIED	**T54.1X1A**	Toxic effect of corrosive organic compounds, acc, init
		T54.1X2A	Toxic effect of corrosive organic compounds, self-harm, init
		T54.1X3A	Toxic effect of corrosive organic compounds, assault, init
		T54.1X4A	Toxic effect of corrosive organic compounds, undet, init
		T54.91XA	Toxic effect of unsp corrosive substance, accidental, init
		T54.92XA	Toxic effect of unsp corrosive substance, self-harm, init
		T54.93XA	Toxic effect of unsp corrosive substance, assault, init
		T54.94XA	Toxic effect of unsp corrosive substance, undetermined, init
		T57.1X1A	Toxic effect of phosphorus and its compounds, acc, init
		T57.1X2A	Toxic effect of phosphorus and its compnd, self-harm, init
		T57.1X3A	Toxic effect of phosphorus and its compounds, assault, init
		T57.1X4A	Toxic effect of phosphorus and its compounds, undet, init
984.Ø	TOXIC EFFECT OF INORGANIC LEAD COMPOUNDS	**T56.ØX1A**	Toxic effect of lead and its compounds, accidental, init
		T56.ØX2A	Toxic effect of lead and its compounds, self-harm, init
		T56.ØX3A	Toxic effect of lead and its compounds, assault, init encntr
		T56.ØX4A	Toxic effect of lead and its compounds, undetermined, init
984.1	TOXIC EFFECT OF ORGANIC LEAD COMPOUNDS	**T56.ØX1A**	Toxic effect of lead and its compounds, accidental, init
		T56.ØX2A	Toxic effect of lead and its compounds, self-harm, init
		T56.ØX3A	Toxic effect of lead and its compounds, assault, init encntr
		T56.ØX4A	Toxic effect of lead and its compounds, undetermined, init
984.8	TOXIC EFFECT OF OTHER LEAD COMPOUNDS	**T56.ØX1A**	Toxic effect of lead and its compounds, accidental, init
		T56.ØX2A	Toxic effect of lead and its compounds, self-harm, init
		T56.ØX3A	Toxic effect of lead and its compounds, assault, init encntr
		T56.ØX4A	Toxic effect of lead and its compounds, undetermined, init
984.9	TOXIC EFFECT OF UNSPECIFIED LEAD COMPOUND	**M1A.1ØXØ**	Lead-induced chronic gout, unspecified site, without tophus
		M1A.1ØX1	Lead-induced chronic gout, unspecified site, with tophus
		M1A.111Ø	Lead-induced chronic gout, right shoulder, without tophus
		M1A.1111	Lead-induced chronic gout, right shoulder, with tophus
		M1A.112Ø	Lead-induced chronic gout, left shoulder, without tophus
		M1A.1121	Lead-induced chronic gout, left shoulder, with tophus
		M1A.119Ø	Lead-induced chronic gout, unsp shoulder, without tophus
		M1A.1191	Lead-induced chronic gout, unspecified shoulder, with tophus
		M1A.121Ø	Lead-induced chronic gout, right elbow, without tophus
		M1A.1211	Lead-induced chronic gout, right elbow, with tophus (tophi)
		M1A.122Ø	Lead-induced chronic gout, left elbow, without tophus
		M1A.1221	Lead-induced chronic gout, left elbow, with tophus (tophi)
		M1A.129Ø	Lead-induced chronic gout, unspecified elbow, without tophus
		M1A.1291	Lead-induced chronic gout, unspecified elbow, with tophus
		M1A.131Ø	Lead-induced chronic gout, right wrist, without tophus
		M1A.1311	Lead-induced chronic gout, right wrist, with tophus (tophi)
		M1A.132Ø	Lead-induced chronic gout, left wrist, without tophus
		M1A.1321	Lead-induced chronic gout, left wrist, with tophus (tophi)
		M1A.139Ø	Lead-induced chronic gout, unspecified wrist, without tophus
		M1A.1391	Lead-induced chronic gout, unspecified wrist, with tophus
		M1A.141Ø	Lead-induced chronic gout, right hand, without tophus
		M1A.1411	Lead-induced chronic gout, right hand, with tophus (tophi)
		M1A.142Ø	Lead-induced chronic gout, left hand, without tophus (tophi)
		M1A.1421	Lead-induced chronic gout, left hand, with tophus (tophi)
		M1A.149Ø	Lead-induced chronic gout, unspecified hand, without tophus
		M1A.1491	Lead-induced chronic gout, unspecified hand, with tophus
		M1A.151Ø	Lead-induced chronic gout, right hip, without tophus (tophi)

(Continued on next page)

See Appendix A ➡ Equivalent Mapping Scenario Scenario

ICD-9-CM		ICD-10-CM	
984.9	TOXIC EFFECT OF UNSPECIFIED LEAD COMPOUND **(Continued)**	M1A.1511	Lead-induced chronic gout, right hip, with tophus (tophi)
		M1A.152Ø	Lead-induced chronic gout, left hip, without tophus (tophi)
		M1A.1521	Lead-induced chronic gout, left hip, with tophus (tophi)
		M1A.159Ø	Lead-induced chronic gout, unspecified hip, without tophus
		M1A.1591	Lead-induced chronic gout, unspecified hip, with tophus
		M1A.161Ø	Lead-induced chronic gout, right knee, without tophus
		M1A.1611	Lead-induced chronic gout, right knee, with tophus (tophi)
		M1A.162Ø	Lead-induced chronic gout, left knee, without tophus (tophi)
		M1A.1621	Lead-induced chronic gout, left knee, with tophus (tophi)
		M1A.169Ø	Lead-induced chronic gout, unspecified knee, without tophus
		M1A.1691	Lead-induced chronic gout, unspecified knee, with tophus
		M1A.171Ø	Lead-induced chronic gout, right ankle and foot, w/o tophus
		M1A.1711	Lead-induced chronic gout, right ankle and foot, with tophus
		M1A.172Ø	Lead-induced chronic gout, left ankle and foot, w/o tophus
		M1A.1721	Lead-induced chronic gout, left ankle and foot, with tophus
		M1A.179Ø	Lead-induced chronic gout, unsp ankle and foot, w/o tophus
		M1A.1791	Lead-induced chronic gout, unsp ankle and foot, with tophus
		M1A.18XØ	Lead-induced chronic gout, vertebrae, without tophus (tophi)
		M1A.18X1	Lead-induced chronic gout, vertebrae, with tophus (tophi)
		M1A.19XØ	Lead-induced chronic gout, multiple sites, without tophus
		M1A.19X1	Lead-induced chronic gout, multiple sites, with tophus
		T56.ØX1A	Toxic effect of lead and its compounds, accidental, init
		T56.ØX2A	Toxic effect of lead and its compounds, self-harm, init
		T56.ØX3A	Toxic effect of lead and its compounds, assault, init encntr
		T56.ØX4A	Toxic effect of lead and its compounds, undetermined, init
985.Ø	TOXIC EFFECT OF MERCURY AND ITS COMPOUNDS	T56.1X1A	Toxic effect of mercury and its compounds, accidental, init
		T56.1X2A	Toxic effect of mercury and its compounds, self-harm, init
		T56.1X3A	Toxic effect of mercury and its compounds, assault, init
		T56.1X4A	Toxic effect of mercury and its compounds, undet, init
985.1	TOXIC EFFECT OF ARSENIC AND ITS COMPOUNDS	T57.ØX1A	Toxic effect of arsenic and its compounds, accidental, init
		T57.ØX2A	Toxic effect of arsenic and its compounds, self-harm, init
		T57.ØX3A	Toxic effect of arsenic and its compounds, assault, init
		T57.ØX4A	Toxic effect of arsenic and its compounds, undet, init
985.2	TOXIC EFFECT OF MANGANESE AND ITS COMPOUNDS	T57.2X1A	Toxic effect of manganese and its compounds, acc, init
		T57.2X2A	Toxic effect of manganese and its compounds, self-harm, init
		T57.2X3A	Toxic effect of manganese and its compounds, assault, init
		T57.2X4A	Toxic effect of manganese and its compounds, undet, init
985.3	TOXIC EFFECT OF BERYLLIUM AND ITS COMPOUNDS	T56.7X1A	Toxic effect of beryllium and its compounds, acc, init
		T56.7X2A	Toxic effect of beryllium and its compounds, self-harm, init
		T56.7X3A	Toxic effect of beryllium and its compounds, assault, init
		T56.7X4A	Toxic effect of beryllium and its compounds, undet, init
985.4	TOXIC EFFECT OF ANTIMONY AND ITS COMPOUNDS	T56.891A	Toxic effect of oth metals, accidental (unintentional), init
985.5	TOXIC EFFECT OF CADMIUM AND ITS COMPOUNDS	T56.3X1A	Toxic effect of cadmium and its compounds, accidental, init
		T56.3X2A	Toxic effect of cadmium and its compounds, self-harm, init
		T56.3X3A	Toxic effect of cadmium and its compounds, assault, init
		T56.3X4A	Toxic effect of cadmium and its compounds, undet, init
985.6	TOXIC EFFECT OF CHROMIUM	T56.2X1A	Toxic effect of chromium and its compounds, acc, init
		T56.2X2A	Toxic effect of chromium and its compounds, self-harm, init
		T56.2X3A	Toxic effect of chromium and its compounds, assault, init
		T56.2X4A	Toxic effect of chromium and its compounds, undet, init
985.8	TOXIC EFFECT OF OTHER SPECIFIED METALS	T56.4X1A	Toxic effect of copper and its compounds, accidental, init
		T56.4X2A	Toxic effect of copper and its compounds, self-harm, init
		T56.4X3A	Toxic effect of copper and its compounds, assault, init
		T56.4X4A	Toxic effect of copper and its compounds, undetermined, init
		T56.5X1A	Toxic effect of zinc and its compounds, accidental, init
		T56.5X2A	Toxic effect of zinc and its compounds, self-harm, init
		T56.5X3A	Toxic effect of zinc and its compounds, assault, init encntr
		T56.5X4A	Toxic effect of zinc and its compounds, undetermined, init
		T56.6X1A	Toxic effect of tin and its compounds, accidental, init
		T56.6X2A	Toxic effect of tin and its compounds, self-harm, init
		T56.6X3A	Toxic effect of tin and its compounds, assault, init encntr
		T56.6X4A	Toxic effect of tin and its compounds, undetermined, init
		T56.811A	Toxic effect of thallium, accidental (unintentional), init
		T56.812A	Toxic effect of thallium, intentional self-harm, init encntr
		T56.813A	Toxic effect of thallium, assault, initial encounter
		T56.814A	Toxic effect of thallium, undetermined, initial encounter
		T56.891A	Toxic effect of oth metals, accidental (unintentional), init
		T56.892A	Toxic effect of oth metals, intentional self-harm, init
		T56.893A	Toxic effect of other metals, assault, initial encounter
		T56.894A	Toxic effect of other metals, undetermined, init encntr
985.9	TOXIC EFFECT OF UNSPECIFIED METAL	T56.91XA	Toxic effect of unsp metal, accidental (unintentional), init
		T56.92XA	Toxic effect of unsp metal, intentional self-harm, init
		T56.93XA	Toxic effect of unspecified metal, assault, init encntr
		T56.94XA	Toxic effect of unspecified metal, undetermined, init encntr

ICD-9-CM		ICD-10-CM	
986	TOXIC EFFECT OF CARBON MONOXIDE	**T58.Ø1XA**	Toxic effect of carb monx from mtr veh exhaust, acc, init
		T58.Ø2XA	Toxic eff of carb monx from mtr veh exhaust, slf-hrm, init
		T58.Ø3XA	Toxic effect of carb monx from mtr veh exhaust, asslt, init
		T58.Ø4XA	Toxic effect of carb monx from mtr veh exhaust, undet, init
		T58.11XA	Toxic effect of carb monx from utility gas, acc, init
		T58.12XA	Toxic effect of carb monx from utility gas, self-harm, init
		T58.13XA	Toxic effect of carb monx from utility gas, assault, init
		T58.14XA	Toxic effect of carb monx from utility gas, undet, init
		T58.2X1A	Tox eff of carb monx fr incmpl combst dmst fuel, acc, init
		T58.2X2A	Tox eff of carb monx fr incmpl combst dmst fuel,slf-hrm,init
		T58.2X3A	Tox eff of carb monx fr incmpl combst dmst fuel, asslt, init
		T58.2X4A	Tox eff of carb monx fr incmpl combst dmst fuel, undet, init
		T58.8X1A	Toxic effect of carb monx from oth source, accidental, init
		T58.8X2A	Toxic effect of carb monx from oth source, self-harm, init
		T58.8X3A	Toxic effect of carb monx from oth source, assault, init
		T58.8X4A	Toxic effect of carb monx from oth source, undet, init
		T58.91XA	Toxic effect of carb monx from unsp source, acc, init
		T58.92XA	Toxic effect of carb monx from unsp source, self-harm, init
		T58.93XA	Toxic effect of carb monx from unsp source, assault, init
		T58.94XA	Toxic effect of carb monx from unsp source, undet, init
987.Ø	TOXIC EFFECT OF LIQUEFIED PETROLEUM GASES	**T59.891A**	Toxic effect of gases, fumes and vapors, accidental, init
987.1	TOXIC EFFECT OF OTHER HYDROCARBON GAS	**T59.2X1A**	Toxic effect of formaldehyde, accidental, init
		T59.2X2A	Toxic effect of formaldehyde, intentional self-harm, init
		T59.2X3A	Toxic effect of formaldehyde, assault, initial encounter
		T59.2X4A	Toxic effect of formaldehyde, undetermined, init encntr
987.2	TOXIC EFFECT OF NITROGEN OXIDES	**T59.ØX1A**	Toxic effect of nitrogen oxides, accidental, init
		T59.ØX2A	Toxic effect of nitrogen oxides, intentional self-harm, init
		T59.ØX3A	Toxic effect of nitrogen oxides, assault, initial encounter
		T59.ØX4A	Toxic effect of nitrogen oxides, undetermined, init encntr
987.3	TOXIC EFFECT OF SULFUR DIOXIDE	**T59.1X1A**	Toxic effect of sulfur dioxide, accidental, init
		T59.1X2A	Toxic effect of sulfur dioxide, intentional self-harm, init
		T59.1X3A	Toxic effect of sulfur dioxide, assault, initial encounter
		T59.1X4A	Toxic effect of sulfur dioxide, undetermined, init encntr
987.4	TOXIC EFFECT OF FREON	**T53.5X1A**	Toxic effect of chlorofluorocarbons, accidental, init
		T53.5X2A	Toxic effect of chlorofluorocarbons, self-harm, init
		T53.5X3A	Toxic effect of chlorofluorocarbons, assault, init encntr
		T53.5X4A	Toxic effect of chlorofluorocarbons, undetermined, init
987.5	TOXIC EFFECT OF LACRIMOGENIC GAS	**T59.3X1A**	Toxic effect of lacrimogenic gas, accidental, init
		T59.3X2A	Toxic effect of lacrimogenic gas, self-harm, init
		T59.3X3A	Toxic effect of lacrimogenic gas, assault, initial encounter
		T59.3X4A	Toxic effect of lacrimogenic gas, undetermined, init encntr
987.6	TOXIC EFFECT OF CHLORINE GAS	**T59.4X1A**	Toxic effect of chlorine gas, accidental, init
		T59.4X2A	Toxic effect of chlorine gas, intentional self-harm, init
		T59.4X3A	Toxic effect of chlorine gas, assault, initial encounter
		T59.4X4A	Toxic effect of chlorine gas, undetermined, init encntr
987.7	TOXIC EFFECT OF HYDROCYANIC ACID GAS	**T57.3X1A**	Toxic effect of hydrogen cyanide, accidental, init
		T57.3X2A	Toxic effect of hydrogen cyanide, self-harm, init
		T57.3X3A	Toxic effect of hydrogen cyanide, assault, initial encounter
		T57.3X4A	Toxic effect of hydrogen cyanide, undetermined, init encntr
987.8	TOXIC EFFECT OTHER SPECIFIED GASES FUMES/VAPORS	**T59.5X1A**	Toxic eff of fluorine gas and hydrogen fluoride, acc, init
		T59.5X2A	Tox eff of fluorine gas and hydrogen fluoride, slf-hrm, init
		T59.5X3A	Toxic eff of fluorine gas and hydrogen fluoride, asslt, init
		T59.5X4A	Toxic eff of fluorine gas and hydrogen fluoride, undet, init
		T59.6X1A	Toxic effect of hydrogen sulfide, accidental, init
		T59.6X2A	Toxic effect of hydrogen sulfide, self-harm, init
		T59.6X3A	Toxic effect of hydrogen sulfide, assault, initial encounter
		T59.6X4A	Toxic effect of hydrogen sulfide, undetermined, init encntr
		T59.7X1A	Toxic effect of carbon dioxide, accidental, init
		T59.7X2A	Toxic effect of carbon dioxide, intentional self-harm, init
		T59.7X3A	Toxic effect of carbon dioxide, assault, initial encounter
		T59.7X4A	Toxic effect of carbon dioxide, undetermined, init encntr
		T59.811A	Toxic effect of smoke, accidental (unintentional), init
		T59.812A	Toxic effect of smoke, intentional self-harm, init encntr
		T59.813A	Toxic effect of smoke, assault, initial encounter
		T59.814A	Toxic effect of smoke, undetermined, initial encounter
		T59.891A	Toxic effect of gases, fumes and vapors, accidental, init
		T59.892A	Toxic effect of gases, fumes and vapors, self-harm, init
		T59.893A	Toxic effect of oth gases, fumes and vapors, assault, init
		T59.894A	Toxic effect of gases, fumes and vapors, undetermined, init

ICD-9-CM		ICD-10-CM	
987.9	TOXIC EFFECT OF UNSPECIFIED GAS FUME OR VAPOR	T59.811A	Toxic effect of smoke, accidental (unintentional), init
		T59.812A	Toxic effect of smoke, intentional self-harm, init encntr
		T59.813A	Toxic effect of smoke, assault, initial encounter
		T59.814A	Toxic effect of smoke, undetermined, initial encounter
		T59.891A	Toxic effect of gases, fumes and vapors, accidental, init
		T59.892A	Toxic effect of gases, fumes and vapors, self-harm, init
		T59.893A	Toxic effect of oth gases, fumes and vapors, assault, init
		T59.894A	Toxic effect of gases, fumes and vapors, undetermined, init
		T59.91XA	Toxic effect of unsp gases, fumes and vapors, acc, init
		T59.92XA	Toxic effect of unsp gases, fumes and vapors, slf-hrm, init
		T59.93XA	Toxic effect of unsp gases, fumes and vapors, assault, init
		T59.94XA	Toxic effect of unsp gases, fumes and vapors, undet, init
988.Ø	TOXIC EFFECT OF FISH AND SHELLFISH	T61.Ø1XA	Ciguatera fish poisoning, accidental (unintentional), init
		T61.Ø2XA	Ciguatera fish poisoning, intentional self-harm, init encntr
		T61.Ø3XA	Ciguatera fish poisoning, assault, initial encounter
		T61.Ø4XA	Ciguatera fish poisoning, undetermined, initial encounter
		T61.11XA	Scombroid fish poisoning, accidental (unintentional), init
		T61.12XA	Scombroid fish poisoning, intentional self-harm, init encntr
		T61.13XA	Scombroid fish poisoning, assault, initial encounter
		T61.14XA	Scombroid fish poisoning, undetermined, initial encounter
		T61.771A	Oth fish poisoning, accidental (unintentional), init encntr
		T61.772A	Other fish poisoning, intentional self-harm, init encntr
		T61.773A	Other fish poisoning, assault, initial encounter
		T61.774A	Other fish poisoning, undetermined, initial encounter
		T61.781A	Oth shellfish poisoning, accidental (unintentional), init
		T61.782A	Oth shellfish poisoning, intentional self-harm, init encntr
		T61.783A	Other shellfish poisoning, assault, initial encounter
		T61.784A	Other shellfish poisoning, undetermined, initial encounter
		T61.8X1A	Toxic effect of seafood, accidental (unintentional), init
		T61.8X2A	Toxic effect of oth seafood, intentional self-harm, init
		T61.8X3A	Toxic effect of other seafood, assault, initial encounter
		T61.8X4A	Toxic effect of other seafood, undetermined, init encntr
		T61.91XA	Toxic effect of unsp seafood, accidental, init
		T61.92XA	Toxic effect of unsp seafood, intentional self-harm, init
		T61.93XA	Toxic effect of unspecified seafood, assault, init encntr
		T61.94XA	Toxic effect of unsp seafood, undetermined, init encntr
988.1	TOXIC EFFECT OF MUSHROOMS	T62.ØX1A	Toxic effect of ingested mushrooms, accidental, init
		T62.ØX2A	Toxic effect of ingested mushrooms, self-harm, init
		T62.ØX3A	Toxic effect of ingested mushrooms, assault, init encntr
		T62.ØX4A	Toxic effect of ingested mushrooms, undetermined, init
988.2	TOXIC EFFECT OF BERRIES AND OTHER PLANTS	T62.1X1A	Toxic effect of ingested berries, accidental, init
		T62.1X2A	Toxic effect of ingested berries, self-harm, init
		T62.1X3A	Toxic effect of ingested berries, assault, initial encounter
		T62.1X4A	Toxic effect of ingested berries, undetermined, init encntr
		T62.2X1A	Toxic effect of ingested (parts of) plant(s), acc, init
		T62.2X2A	Toxic effect of ingested (parts of) plant(s), slf-hrm, init
		T62.2X3A	Toxic effect of ingested (parts of) plant(s), assault, init
		T62.2X4A	Toxic effect of ingested (parts of) plant(s), undet, init
988.8	TOXIC EFFECT OTHER SPECIFIED NOXIOUS SUBSTANCES	T62.8X1A	Toxic effect of noxious substances eaten as food, acc, init
		T62.8X2A	Toxic effect of noxious substnc eaten as food, slf-hrm, init
		T62.8X3A	Toxic effect of noxious substnc eaten as food, assault, init
		T62.8X4A	Toxic effect of noxious substnc eaten as food, undet, init
988.9	TOXIC EFFECT OF UNSPECIFIED NOXIOUS SUBSTANCE	T62.91XA	Toxic effect of unsp noxious sub eaten as food, acc, init
		T62.92XA	Toxic eff of unsp noxious sub eaten as food, slf-hrm, init
		T62.93XA	Toxic effect of unsp noxious sub eaten as food, asslt, init
		T62.94XA	Toxic effect of unsp noxious sub eaten as food, undet, init
		T78.1XXA	Oth adverse food reactions, not elsewhere classified, init
989.Ø	TOXIC EFFECT OF HYDROCYANIC ACID AND CYANIDES	T65.ØX1A	Toxic effect of cyanides, accidental (unintentional), init
		T65.ØX2A	Toxic effect of cyanides, intentional self-harm, init encntr
		T65.ØX3A	Toxic effect of cyanides, assault, initial encounter
		T65.ØX4A	Toxic effect of cyanides, undetermined, initial encounter
989.1	TOXIC EFFECT OF STRYCHNINE AND SALTS	T65.1X1A	Toxic effect of strychnine and its salts, accidental, init
		T65.1X2A	Toxic effect of strychnine and its salts, self-harm, init
		T65.1X3A	Toxic effect of strychnine and its salts, assault, init
		T65.1X4A	Toxic effect of strychnine and its salts, undetermined, init
989.2	TOXIC EFFECT OF CHLORINATED HYDROCARBONS	T53.91XA	Toxic eff of unsp halgn deriv of aromat hydrocrb, acc, init
		T53.92XA	Tox eff of unsp halgn deriv of aromat hydrocrb,slf-hrm, init
		T53.93XA	Tox eff of unsp halgn deriv of aromat hydrocrb, asslt, init
		T53.94XA	Tox eff of unsp halgn deriv of aromat hydrocrb, undet, init
989.3	TOXIC EFFECT OF ORGANOPHOSPHATE AND CARBAMATE	T6Ø.ØX1A	Toxic effect of organophos and carbamate insect, acc, init
		T6Ø.ØX2A	Toxic eff of organophos and carbamate insect, slf-hrm, init
		T6Ø.ØX3A	Toxic effect of organophos and carbamate insect, asslt, init
		T6Ø.ØX4A	Toxic effect of organophos and carbamate insect, undet, init

ICD-9-CM		ICD-10-CM	
989.4	TOXIC EFFECT OF OTHER PESTICIDES NEC	**T6Ø.1X1A**	Toxic effect of halogenated insecticides, accidental, init
		T6Ø.1X2A	Toxic effect of halogenated insecticides, self-harm, init
		T6Ø.1X3A	Toxic effect of halogenated insecticides, assault, init
		T6Ø.1X4A	Toxic effect of halogenated insecticides, undetermined, init
		T6Ø.2X1A	Toxic effect of insecticides, accidental, init
		T6Ø.2X2A	Toxic effect of insecticides, intentional self-harm, init
		T6Ø.2X3A	Toxic effect of other insecticides, assault, init encntr
		T6Ø.2X4A	Toxic effect of oth insecticides, undetermined, init encntr
		T6Ø.4X1A	Toxic effect of rodenticides, accidental, init
		T6Ø.4X2A	Toxic effect of rodenticides, intentional self-harm, init
		T6Ø.4X3A	Toxic effect of rodenticides, assault, initial encounter
		T6Ø.4X4A	Toxic effect of rodenticides, undetermined, init encntr
		T6Ø.8X1A	Toxic effect of pesticides, accidental (unintentional), init
		T6Ø.8X2A	Toxic effect of oth pesticides, intentional self-harm, init
		T6Ø.8X3A	Toxic effect of other pesticides, assault, initial encounter
		T6Ø.8X4A	Toxic effect of other pesticides, undetermined, init encntr
		T6Ø.91XA	Toxic effect of unsp pesticide, accidental, init
		T6Ø.92XA	Toxic effect of unsp pesticide, intentional self-harm, init
		T6Ø.93XA	Toxic effect of unspecified pesticide, assault, init encntr
		T6Ø.94XA	Toxic effect of unsp pesticide, undetermined, init encntr
989.5	TOXIC EFFECT OF VENOM	**T63.ØØ1A**	Toxic effect of unsp snake venom, accidental, init
		T63.ØØ2A	Toxic effect of unsp snake venom, self-harm, init
		T63.ØØ3A	Toxic effect of unsp snake venom, assault, init encntr
		T63.ØØ4A	Toxic effect of unsp snake venom, undetermined, init encntr
		T63.Ø11A	Toxic effect of rattlesnake venom, accidental, init
		T63.Ø12A	Toxic effect of rattlesnake venom, self-harm, init
		T63.Ø13A	Toxic effect of rattlesnake venom, assault, init encntr
		T63.Ø14A	Toxic effect of rattlesnake venom, undetermined, init encntr
		T63.Ø21A	Toxic effect of coral snake venom, accidental, init
		T63.Ø22A	Toxic effect of coral snake venom, self-harm, init
		T63.Ø23A	Toxic effect of coral snake venom, assault, init encntr
		T63.Ø24A	Toxic effect of coral snake venom, undetermined, init encntr
		T63.Ø31A	Toxic effect of taipan venom, accidental, init
		T63.Ø32A	Toxic effect of taipan venom, intentional self-harm, init
		T63.Ø33A	Toxic effect of taipan venom, assault, initial encounter
		T63.Ø34A	Toxic effect of taipan venom, undetermined, init encntr
		T63.Ø41A	Toxic effect of cobra venom, accidental, init
		T63.Ø42A	Toxic effect of cobra venom, intentional self-harm, init
		T63.Ø43A	Toxic effect of cobra venom, assault, initial encounter
		T63.Ø44A	Toxic effect of cobra venom, undetermined, initial encounter
		T63.Ø61A	Toxic effect of venom of N & S American snake, acc, init
		T63.Ø62A	Toxic effect of venom of N & S American snake, slf-hrm, init
		T63.Ø63A	Toxic effect of venom of N & S American snake, assault, init
		T63.Ø64A	Toxic effect of venom of N & S American snake, undet, init
		T63.Ø71A	Toxic effect of venom of Australian snake, accidental, init
		T63.Ø72A	Toxic effect of venom of Australian snake, self-harm, init
		T63.Ø73A	Toxic effect of venom of oth Australian snake, assault, init
		T63.Ø74A	Toxic effect of venom of Australian snake, undet, init
		T63.Ø81A	Toxic effect of venom of African and Asian snake, acc, init
		T63.Ø82A	Toxic eff of venom of African and Asian snake, slf-hrm, init
		T63.Ø83A	Toxic eff of venom of African and Asian snake, asslt, init
		T63.Ø84A	Toxic eff of venom of African and Asian snake, undet, init
		T63.Ø91A	Toxic effect of venom of snake, accidental, init
		T63.Ø92A	Toxic effect of venom of snake, intentional self-harm, init
		T63.Ø93A	Toxic effect of venom of other snake, assault, init encntr
		T63.Ø94A	Toxic effect of venom of oth snake, undetermined, init
		T63.111A	Toxic effect of venom of gila monster, accidental, init
		T63.112A	Toxic effect of venom of gila monster, self-harm, init
		T63.113A	Toxic effect of venom of gila monster, assault, init encntr
		T63.114A	Toxic effect of venom of gila monster, undetermined, init
		T63.121A	Toxic effect of venom of venomous lizard, accidental, init
		T63.122A	Toxic effect of venom of venomous lizard, self-harm, init
		T63.123A	Toxic effect of venom of oth venomous lizard, assault, init
		T63.124A	Toxic effect of venom of venomous lizard, undetermined, init
		T63.191A	Toxic effect of venom of reptiles, accidental, init
		T63.192A	Toxic effect of venom of reptiles, self-harm, init
		T63.193A	Toxic effect of venom of oth reptiles, assault, init encntr
		T63.194A	Toxic effect of venom of oth reptiles, undetermined, init
		T63.2X1A	Toxic effect of venom of scorpion, accidental, init
		T63.2X2A	Toxic effect of venom of scorpion, self-harm, init
		T63.2X3A	Toxic effect of venom of scorpion, assault, init encntr
		T63.2X4A	Toxic effect of venom of scorpion, undetermined, init encntr
		T63.3Ø1A	Toxic effect of unsp spider venom, accidental, init
		T63.3Ø2A	Toxic effect of unsp spider venom, self-harm, init
		T63.3Ø3A	Toxic effect of unsp spider venom, assault, init encntr
		T63.3Ø4A	Toxic effect of unsp spider venom, undetermined, init encntr
		T63.311A	Toxic effect of venom of black widow spider, acc, init
		T63.312A	Toxic effect of venom of black widow spider, self-harm, init
	(Continued on next page)	**T63.313A**	Toxic effect of venom of black widow spider, assault, init

ICD-9-CM		ICD-10-CM	
989.5	TOXIC EFFECT OF VENOM **(Continued)**	**T63.314A**	Toxic effect of venom of black widow spider, undet, init
		T63.321A	Toxic effect of venom of tarantula, accidental, init
		T63.322A	Toxic effect of venom of tarantula, self-harm, init
		T63.323A	Toxic effect of venom of tarantula, assault, init encntr
		T63.324A	Toxic effect of venom of tarantula, undetermined, init
		T63.331A	Toxic effect of venom of brown recluse spider, acc, init
		T63.332A	Toxic effect of venom of brown recluse spider, slf-hrm, init
		T63.333A	Toxic effect of venom of brown recluse spider, assault, init
		T63.334A	Toxic effect of venom of brown recluse spider, undet, init
		T63.391A	Toxic effect of venom of spider, accidental, init
		T63.392A	Toxic effect of venom of spider, intentional self-harm, init
		T63.393A	Toxic effect of venom of other spider, assault, init encntr
		T63.394A	Toxic effect of venom of oth spider, undetermined, init
		T63.411A	Toxic effect of venom of centipede/millipede, acc, init
		T63.412A	Toxic effect of venom of centipede/millipede, slf-hrm, init
		T63.413A	Toxic effect of venom of centipede/millipede, assault, init
		T63.414A	Toxic effect of venom of centipede/millipede, undet, init
		T63.421A	Toxic effect of venom of ants, accidental, init
		T63.422A	Toxic effect of venom of ants, intentional self-harm, init
		T63.423A	Toxic effect of venom of ants, assault, initial encounter
		T63.424A	Toxic effect of venom of ants, undetermined, init encntr
		T63.431A	Toxic effect of venom of caterpillars, accidental, init
		T63.432A	Toxic effect of venom of caterpillars, self-harm, init
		T63.433A	Toxic effect of venom of caterpillars, assault, init encntr
		T63.434A	Toxic effect of venom of caterpillars, undetermined, init
		T63.441A	Toxic effect of venom of bees, accidental, init
		T63.442A	Toxic effect of venom of bees, intentional self-harm, init
		T63.443A	Toxic effect of venom of bees, assault, initial encounter
		T63.444A	Toxic effect of venom of bees, undetermined, init encntr
		T63.451A	Toxic effect of venom of hornets, accidental, init
		T63.452A	Toxic effect of venom of hornets, self-harm, init
		T63.453A	Toxic effect of venom of hornets, assault, initial encounter
		T63.454A	Toxic effect of venom of hornets, undetermined, init encntr
		T63.461A	Toxic effect of venom of wasps, accidental, init
		T63.462A	Toxic effect of venom of wasps, intentional self-harm, init
		T63.463A	Toxic effect of venom of wasps, assault, initial encounter
		T63.464A	Toxic effect of venom of wasps, undetermined, init encntr
		T63.481A	Toxic effect of venom of arthropod, accidental, init
		T63.482A	Toxic effect of venom of arthropod, self-harm, init
		T63.483A	Toxic effect of venom of oth arthropod, assault, init encntr
		T63.484A	Toxic effect of venom of oth arthropod, undetermined, init
		T63.511A	Toxic effect of contact w stingray, accidental, init
		T63.512A	Toxic effect of contact w stingray, self-harm, init
		T63.513A	Toxic effect of contact with stingray, assault, init encntr
		T63.514A	Toxic effect of contact w stingray, undetermined, init
		T63.591A	Toxic effect of contact w oth venomous fish, acc, init
		T63.592A	Toxic effect of contact w oth venomous fish, self-harm, init
		T63.593A	Toxic effect of contact w oth venomous fish, assault, init
		T63.594A	Toxic effect of contact w oth venomous fish, undet, init
		T63.611A	Toxic effect of contact w Portugese Man-o-war, acc, init
		T63.612A	Toxic effect of contact w Portugese Man-o-war, slf-hrm, init
		T63.613A	Toxic effect of contact w Portugese Man-o-war, assault, init
		T63.614A	Toxic effect of contact w Portugese Man-o-war, undet, init
		T63.621A	Toxic effect of contact w oth jellyfish, accidental, init
		T63.622A	Toxic effect of contact w oth jellyfish, self-harm, init
		T63.623A	Toxic effect of contact w oth jellyfish, assault, init
		T63.624A	Toxic effect of contact w oth jellyfish, undetermined, init
		T63.631A	Toxic effect of contact w sea anemone, accidental, init
		T63.632A	Toxic effect of contact w sea anemone, self-harm, init
		T63.633A	Toxic effect of contact w sea anemone, assault, init encntr
		T63.634A	Toxic effect of contact w sea anemone, undetermined, init
		T63.691A	Toxic effect of cntct w oth venom marine animals, acc, init
		T63.692A	Toxic eff of cntct w oth venom marine animals, slf-hrm, init
		T63.693A	Toxic eff of cntct w oth venom marine animals, asslt, init
		T63.694A	Toxic eff of cntct w oth venom marine animals, undet, init
		T63.711A	Toxic effect of contact w venomous marine plant, acc, init
		T63.712A	Toxic effect of contact w venom marine plant, slf-hrm, init
		T63.713A	Toxic effect of contact w venom marine plant, assault, init
		T63.714A	Toxic effect of contact w venomous marine plant, undet, init
		T63.791A	Toxic effect of contact w oth venomous plant, acc, init
		T63.792A	Toxic effect of contact w oth venomous plant, slf-hrm, init
		T63.793A	Toxic effect of contact w oth venomous plant, assault, init
		T63.794A	Toxic effect of contact w oth venomous plant, undet, init
		T63.811A	Toxic effect of contact w venomous frog, accidental, init
		T63.812A	Toxic effect of contact w venomous frog, self-harm, init
		T63.813A	Toxic effect of contact w venomous frog, assault, init
		T63.814A	Toxic effect of contact w venomous frog, undetermined, init
		T63.821A	Toxic effect of contact w venomous toad, accidental, init
	(Continued on next page)	**T63.822A**	Toxic effect of contact w venomous toad, self-harm, init

ICD-9-CM		ICD-10-CM	
989.5	TOXIC EFFECT OF VENOM **(Continued)**	**T63.891A**	Toxic effect of contact w oth venomous animals, acc, init
		T63.892A	Toxic effect of contact w oth venom animals, slf-hrm, init
		T63.823A	Toxic effect of contact w venomous toad, assault, init
		T63.824A	Toxic effect of contact w venomous toad, undetermined, init
		T63.831A	Toxic effect of contact w oth venomous amphibian, acc, init
		T63.832A	Toxic effect of contact w oth venomous amphib, slf-hrm, init
		T63.833A	Toxic effect of contact w oth venomous amphib, assault, init
		T63.834A	Toxic effect of contact w oth venomous amphib, undet, init
		T63.893A	Toxic effect of contact w oth venom animals, assault, init
		T63.894A	Toxic effect of contact w oth venomous animals, undet, init
		T63.91XA	Toxic effect of contact w unsp venomous animal, acc, init
		T63.92XA	Toxic effect of contact w unsp venom animal, slf-hrm, init
		T63.93XA	Toxic effect of contact w unsp venom animal, assault, init
		T63.94XA	Toxic effect of contact w unsp venomous animal, undet, init
989.6	TOXIC EFFECT OF SOAPS AND DETERGENTS	**T55.ØX1A**	Toxic effect of soaps, accidental (unintentional), init
		T55.ØX2A	Toxic effect of soaps, intentional self-harm, init encntr
		T55.ØX3A	Toxic effect of soaps, assault, initial encounter
		T55.ØX4A	Toxic effect of soaps, undetermined, initial encounter
		T55.1X1A	Toxic effect of detergents, accidental (unintentional), init
		T55.1X2A	Toxic effect of detergents, intentional self-harm, init
		T55.1X3A	Toxic effect of detergents, assault, initial encounter
		T55.1X4A	Toxic effect of detergents, undetermined, initial encounter
989.7	TOXIC EFFECT OF AFLATOXIN AND OTHER MYCOTOXIN	**T64.Ø1XA**	Toxic effect of aflatoxin, accidental (unintentional), init
		T64.Ø2XA	Toxic effect of aflatoxin, intentional self-harm, init
		T64.Ø3XA	Toxic effect of aflatoxin, assault, initial encounter
		T64.Ø4XA	Toxic effect of aflatoxin, undetermined, initial encounter
		T64.81XA	Toxic effect of mycotoxin food contamnt, accidental, init
		T64.82XA	Toxic effect of mycotoxin food contaminants, self-harm, init
		T64.83XA	Toxic effect of mycotoxin food contaminants, assault, init
		T64.84XA	Toxic effect of mycotoxin food contamnt, undetermined, init
989.81	TOXIC EFFECT OF ASBESTOS	**T65.894A**	Toxic effect of oth substances, undetermined, init encntr
989.82	TOXIC EFFECT OF LATEX	**T65.811A**	Toxic effect of latex, accidental (unintentional), init
		T65.812A	Toxic effect of latex, intentional self-harm, init encntr
		T65.813A	Toxic effect of latex, assault, initial encounter
		T65.814A	Toxic effect of latex, undetermined, initial encounter
989.83	TOXIC EFFECT OF SILICONE	**T65.894A**	Toxic effect of oth substances, undetermined, init encntr
989.84	TOXIC EFFECT OF TOBACCO	**T65.211A**	Toxic effect of chewing tobacco, accidental, init
		T65.212A	Toxic effect of chewing tobacco, intentional self-harm, init
		T65.213A	Toxic effect of chewing tobacco, assault, initial encounter
		T65.214A	Toxic effect of chewing tobacco, undetermined, init encntr
		T65.221A	Toxic effect of tobacco cigarettes, accidental, init
		T65.222A	Toxic effect of tobacco cigarettes, self-harm, init
		T65.223A	Toxic effect of tobacco cigarettes, assault, init encntr
		T65.224A	Toxic effect of tobacco cigarettes, undetermined, init
		T65.291A	Toxic effect of tobacco and nicotine, accidental, init
		T65.292A	Toxic effect of tobacco and nicotine, self-harm, init
		T65.293A	Toxic effect of oth tobacco and nicotine, assault, init
		T65.294A	Toxic effect of oth tobacco and nicotine, undetermined, init
989.89	TOXIC EFFECT OF OTHER SUBSTANCES	**T57.8X1A**	Toxic effect of inorganic substances, accidental, init
		T57.8X2A	Toxic effect of inorganic substances, self-harm, init
		T57.8X3A	Toxic effect of oth inorganic substances, assault, init
		T57.8X4A	Toxic effect of oth inorganic substances, undetermined, init
		T6Ø.3X1A	Toxic effect of herbicides and fungicides, accidental, init
		T6Ø.3X2A	Toxic effect of herbicides and fungicides, self-harm, init
		T6Ø.3X3A	Toxic effect of herbicides and fungicides, assault, init
		T6Ø.3X4A	Toxic effect of herbicides and fungicides, undet, init
		T65.5X1A	Tox eff of nitro and oth nitric acids and esters, acc, init
		T65.5X2A	Tox eff of nitro & oth nitric acids & esters, slf-hrm, init
		T65.5X3A	Tox eff of nitro & oth nitric acids and esters, asslt, init
		T65.5X4A	Tox eff of nitro & oth nitric acids and esters, undet, init
		T65.6X1A	Toxic effect of paints and dyes, NEC, accidental, init
		T65.6X2A	Toxic effect of paints and dyes, NEC, self-harm, init
		T65.6X3A	Toxic effect of paints and dyes, NEC, assault, init
		T65.6X4A	Toxic effect of paints and dyes, NEC, undetermined, init
		T65.821A	Toxic effect of harmful algae and algae toxins, acc, init
		T65.822A	Toxic eff of harmful algae and algae toxins, slf-hrm, init
		T65.823A	Toxic effect of harmful algae and algae toxins, asslt, init
		T65.824A	Toxic effect of harmful algae and algae toxins, undet, init
		T65.831A	Toxic effect of fiberglass, accidental (unintentional), init
		T65.832A	Toxic effect of fiberglass, intentional self-harm, init
		T65.833A	Toxic effect of fiberglass, assault, initial encounter
		T65.834A	Toxic effect of fiberglass, undetermined, initial encounter
		T65.891A	Toxic effect of substances, accidental (unintentional), init
		T65.892A	Toxic effect of oth substances, intentional self-harm, init
		T65.893A	Toxic effect of oth substances, assault, init encntr
		T65.894A	Toxic effect of oth substances, undetermined, init encntr

ICD-9-CM		ICD-10-CM	
989.9	TOX EFF UNS SBSTNC CHIEFLY NONMEDICINAL AS SRC	T57.91XA	Toxic effect of unsp inorganic substance, accidental, init
		T57.92XA	Toxic effect of unsp inorganic substance, self-harm, init
		T57.93XA	Toxic effect of unsp inorganic substance, assault, init
		T57.94XA	Toxic effect of unsp inorganic substance, undetermined, init
		T65.91XA	Toxic effect of unsp substance, accidental, init
		T65.92XA	Toxic effect of unsp substance, intentional self-harm, init
		T65.93XA	Toxic effect of unspecified substance, assault, init encntr
		T65.94XA	Toxic effect of unsp substance, undetermined, init encntr
990	EFFECTS OF RADIATION, UNSPECIFIED	T66.XXXA	Radiation sickness, unspecified, initial encounter
991.0	FROSTBITE OF FACE	T33.011A	Superficial frostbite of right ear, initial encounter
		T33.012A	Superficial frostbite of left ear, initial encounter
		T33.019A	Superficial frostbite of unspecified ear, initial encounter
		T33.02XA	Superficial frostbite of nose, initial encounter
		T33.09XA	Superficial frostbite of other part of head, init encntr
		T33.1XXA	Superficial frostbite of neck, initial encounter
		T34.011A	Frostbite with tissue necrosis of right ear, init encntr
		T34.012A	Frostbite with tissue necrosis of left ear, init encntr
		T34.019A	Frostbite with tissue necrosis of unsp ear, init encntr
		T34.02XA	Frostbite with tissue necrosis of nose, initial encounter
		T34.09XA	Frostbite w tissue necrosis of oth part of head, init encntr
		T34.1XXA	Frostbite with tissue necrosis of neck, initial encounter
991.1	FROSTBITE OF HAND	T33.511A	Superficial frostbite of right wrist, initial encounter
		T33.512A	Superficial frostbite of left wrist, initial encounter
		T33.519A	Superficial frostbite of unspecified wrist, init encntr
		T33.521A	Superficial frostbite of right hand, initial encounter
		T33.522A	Superficial frostbite of left hand, initial encounter
		T33.529A	Superficial frostbite of unspecified hand, initial encounter
		T33.531A	Superficial frostbite of right finger(s), initial encounter
		T33.532A	Superficial frostbite of left finger(s), initial encounter
		T33.539A	Superficial frostbite of unspecified finger(s), init encntr
		T34.511A	Frostbite with tissue necrosis of right wrist, init encntr
		T34.512A	Frostbite with tissue necrosis of left wrist, init encntr
		T34.519A	Frostbite with tissue necrosis of unsp wrist, init encntr
		T34.521A	Frostbite with tissue necrosis of right hand, init encntr
		T34.522A	Frostbite with tissue necrosis of left hand, init encntr
		T34.529A	Frostbite with tissue necrosis of unsp hand, init encntr
		T34.531A	Frostbite w tissue necrosis of right finger(s), init encntr
		T34.532A	Frostbite w tissue necrosis of left finger(s), init encntr
		T34.539A	Frostbite w tissue necrosis of unsp finger(s), init encntr
991.2	FROSTBITE OF FOOT	T33.811A	Superficial frostbite of right ankle, initial encounter
		T33.812A	Superficial frostbite of left ankle, initial encounter
		T33.819A	Superficial frostbite of unspecified ankle, init encntr
		T33.821A	Superficial frostbite of right foot, initial encounter
		T33.822A	Superficial frostbite of left foot, initial encounter
		T33.829A	Superficial frostbite of unspecified foot, initial encounter
		T33.831A	Superficial frostbite of right toe(s), initial encounter
		T33.832A	Superficial frostbite of left toe(s), initial encounter
		T33.839A	Superficial frostbite of unspecified toe(s), init encntr
		T34.811A	Frostbite with tissue necrosis of right ankle, init encntr
		T34.812A	Frostbite with tissue necrosis of left ankle, init encntr
		T34.819A	Frostbite with tissue necrosis of unsp ankle, init encntr
		T34.821A	Frostbite with tissue necrosis of right foot, init encntr
		T34.822A	Frostbite with tissue necrosis of left foot, init encntr
		T34.829A	Frostbite with tissue necrosis of unsp foot, init encntr
		T34.831A	Frostbite with tissue necrosis of right toe(s), init encntr
		T34.832A	Frostbite with tissue necrosis of left toe(s), init encntr
		T34.839A	Frostbite with tissue necrosis of unsp toe(s), init encntr

ICD-9-CM		ICD-10-CM	
991.3	FROSTBITE OF OTHER AND UNSPECIFIED SITES	**T33.2XXA**	Superficial frostbite of thorax, initial encounter
		T33.3XXA	Superfic frostbite of abd wall, lower back and pelvis, init
		T33.40XA	Superficial frostbite of unspecified arm, initial encounter
		T33.41XA	Superficial frostbite of right arm, initial encounter
		T33.42XA	Superficial frostbite of left arm, initial encounter
		T33.60XA	Superficial frostbite of unsp hip and thigh, init encntr
		T33.61XA	Superficial frostbite of right hip and thigh, init encntr
		T33.62XA	Superficial frostbite of left hip and thigh, init encntr
		T33.70XA	Superficial frostbite of unsp knee and lower leg, init
		T33.71XA	Superficial frostbite of right knee and lower leg, init
		T33.72XA	Superficial frostbite of left knee and lower leg, init
		T33.90XA	Superficial frostbite of unspecified sites, init encntr
		T33.99XA	Superficial frostbite of other sites, initial encounter
		T34.2XXA	Frostbite with tissue necrosis of thorax, initial encounter
		T34.3XXA	Frstbte w tissue necros abd wall, low back and pelvis, init
		T34.40XA	Frostbite with tissue necrosis of unsp arm, init encntr
		T34.41XA	Frostbite with tissue necrosis of right arm, init encntr
		T34.42XA	Frostbite with tissue necrosis of left arm, init encntr
		T34.60XA	Frostbite w tissue necrosis of unsp hip and thigh, init
		T34.61XA	Frostbite w tissue necrosis of right hip and thigh, init
		T34.62XA	Frostbite w tissue necrosis of left hip and thigh, init
		T34.70XA	Frostbite w tissue necrosis of unsp knee and lower leg, init
		T34.71XA	Frostbite w tissue necros right knee and lower leg, init
		T34.72XA	Frostbite w tissue necrosis of left knee and lower leg, init
		T34.90XA	Frostbite with tissue necrosis of unsp sites, init encntr
		T34.99XA	Frostbite with tissue necrosis of other sites, init encntr
991.4	EFFECTS OF IMMERSION OF FOOT	**T69.021A**	Immersion foot, right foot, initial encounter
		T69.022A	Immersion foot, left foot, initial encounter
		T69.029A	Immersion foot, unspecified foot, initial encounter
991.5	EFFECTS OF CHILBLAINS	**T69.1XXA**	Chilblains, initial encounter
991.6	EFFECTS OF HYPOTHERMIA	**T68.XXXA**	Hypothermia, initial encounter
991.8	OTHER SPECIFIED EFFECTS OF REDUCED TEMPERATURE	**T69.011A**	Immersion hand, right hand, initial encounter
		T69.012A	Immersion hand, left hand, initial encounter
		T69.019A	Immersion hand, unspecified hand, initial encounter
		T69.8XXA	Other specified effects of reduced temperature, init encntr
991.9	UNSPECIFIED EFFECT OF REDUCED TEMPERATURE	**T69.9XXA**	Effect of reduced temperature, unspecified, init encntr
992.0	HEAT STROKE AND SUNSTROKE	**T67.0XXA**	Heatstroke and sunstroke, initial encounter
992.1	HEAT SYNCOPE	**T67.1XXA**	Heat syncope, initial encounter
992.2	HEAT CRAMPS	**T67.2XXA**	Heat cramp, initial encounter
992.3	HEAT EXHAUSTION, ANHYDROTIC	**T67.3XXA**	Heat exhaustion, anhydrotic, initial encounter
992.4	HEAT EXHAUSTION DUE TO SALT DEPLETION	**T67.4XXA**	Heat exhaustion due to salt depletion, initial encounter
992.5	HEAT EXHAUSTION, UNSPECIFIED	**T67.5XXA**	Heat exhaustion, unspecified, initial encounter
992.6	HEAT FATIGUE, TRANSIENT	**T67.6XXA**	Heat fatigue, transient, initial encounter
992.7	HEAT EDEMA	**T67.7XXA**	Heat edema, initial encounter
992.8	OTHER SPECIFIED HEAT EFFECTS	**T67.8XXA**	Other effects of heat and light, initial encounter
992.9	UNSPECIFIED EFFECTS OF HEAT AND LIGHT	**T67.9XXA**	Effect of heat and light, unspecified, initial encounter
993.0	BAROTRAUMA, OTITIC	**T70.0XXA**	Otitic barotrauma, initial encounter
993.1	BAROTRAUMA, SINUS	**T70.1XXA**	Sinus barotrauma, initial encounter
993.2	OTHER AND UNSPECIFIED EFFECTS OF HIGH ALTITUDE	**T70.20XA**	Unspecified effects of high altitude, initial encounter
		T70.29XA	Other effects of high altitude, initial encounter
993.3	CAISSON DISEASE	**T70.3XXA**	Caisson disease [decompression sickness], initial encounter
993.4	EFFECTS OF AIR PRESSURE CAUSED BY EXPLOSION	**T70.4XXA**	Effects of high-pressure fluids, initial encounter
993.8	OTHER SPECIFIED EFFECTS OF AIR PRESSURE	**T70.8XXA**	Oth effects of air pressure and water pressure, init encntr
993.9	UNSPECIFIED EFFECT OF AIR PRESSURE	**T70.9XXA**	Effect of air pressure and water pressure, unsp, init encntr
994.0	EFFECTS OF LIGHTNING	**T75.00XA**	Unspecified effects of lightning, initial encounter
		T75.01XA	Shock due to being struck by lightning, initial encounter
		T75.09XA	Other effects of lightning, initial encounter
994.1	DROWNING AND NONFATAL SUBMERSION	**T75.1XXA**	Unsp effects of drowning and nonfatal submersion, init
994.2	EFFECTS OF HUNGER	◘ **T73.0XXA**	Starvation, initial encounter
994.3	EFFECTS OF THIRST	◘ **T73.1XXA**	Deprivation of water, initial encounter
994.4	EXHAUSTION DUE TO EXPOSURE	◘ **T73.2XXA**	Exhaustion due to exposure, initial encounter
994.5	EXHAUSTION DUE TO EXCESSIVE EXERTION	◘ **T73.3XXA**	Exhaustion due to excessive exertion, initial encounter
994.6	MOTION SICKNESS	◘ **T75.3XXA**	Motion sickness, initial encounter

ICD-9-CM		ICD-10-CM	
994.7	ASPHYXIATION AND STRANGULATION	T71.111A	Asphyx due to smothering under pillow, accidental, init
		T71.112A	Asphyxiation due to smothering under pillow, self-harm, init
		T71.113A	Asphyxiation due to smothering under pillow, assault, init
		T71.114A	Asphyx due to smothering under pillow, undetermined, init
		T71.121A	Asphyxiation due to plastic bag, accidental, init encntr
		T71.122A	Asphyxiation due to plastic bag, intentional self-harm, init
		T71.123A	Asphyxiation due to plastic bag, assault, initial encounter
		T71.124A	Asphyxiation due to plastic bag, undetermined, init encntr
		T71.131A	Asphyx due to being trapped in bed linens, accidental, init
		T71.132A	Asphyx due to being trapped in bed linens, self-harm, init
		T71.133A	Asphyx due to being trapped in bed linens, assault, init
		T71.134A	Asphyx due to being trapped in bed linens, undet, init
		T71.141A	Asphyx due to smothr under another person's body, acc, init
		T71.143A	Asphyx d/t smothr under another person's body, asslt, init
		T71.144A	Asphyx d/t smothr under another person's body, undet, init
		T71.151A	Asphyx due to smothering in furniture, accidental, init
		T71.152A	Asphyxiation due to smothering in furniture, self-harm, init
		T71.153A	Asphyxiation due to smothering in furniture, assault, init
		T71.154A	Asphyx due to smothering in furniture, undetermined, init
		T71.161A	Asphyxiation due to hanging, accidental, initial encounter
		T71.162A	Asphyxiation due to hanging, intentional self-harm, init
		T71.163A	Asphyxiation due to hanging, assault, initial encounter
		T71.164A	Asphyxiation due to hanging, undetermined, initial encounter
		T71.191A	Asphyx d/t mech threat to breathe d/t oth cause, acc, init
		T71.192A	Asphyx d/t mech thrt to breathe d/t oth cause, slf-hrm, init
		T71.193A	Asphyx d/t mech threat to breathe d/t oth cause, asslt, init
		T71.194A	Asphyx d/t mech threat to breathe d/t oth cause, undet, init
		T71.2ØXA	Asphyx d/t sys oxy defic d/t low oxy in air unsp cause, init
		T71.21XA	Asphyxiation due to cave-in or falling earth, init encntr
		T71.221A	Asphyx due to being trapped in a car trunk, accidental, init
		T71.222A	Asphyx due to being trapped in a car trunk, self-harm, init
		T71.223A	Asphyx due to being trapped in a car trunk, assault, init
		T71.224A	Asphyx due to being trapped in a car trunk, undet, init
		T71.231A	Asphyx due to being trap in a (discarded) refrig, acc, init
		T71.232A	Asphyx d/t being trap in a (discarded) refrig, slf-hrm, init
		T71.233A	Asphyx d/t being trap in a (discarded) refrig, asslt, init
		T71.234A	Asphyx d/t being trap in a (discarded) refrig, undet, init
		T71.29XA	Asphyx due to being trap in oth low oxygen environment, init
		T71.9XXA	Asphyxiation due to unspecified cause, initial encounter
994.8	ELECTROCUTION&NONFATAL EFFECTS ELECTRIC CURRENT	T75.4XXA	Electrocution, initial encounter
994.9	OTHER EFFECTS OF EXTERNAL CAUSES	T73.8XXA	Other effects of deprivation, initial encounter
		T73.9XXA	Effect of deprivation, unspecified, initial encounter
		T75.2ØXA	Unspecified effects of vibration, initial encounter
		T75.21XA	Pneumatic hammer syndrome, initial encounter
		T75.22XA	Traumatic vasospastic syndrome, initial encounter
		T75.23XA	Vertigo from infrasound, initial encounter
		T75.29XA	Other effects of vibration, initial encounter
		T75.81XA	Effects of abnormal gravitation forces, initial encounter
		T75.82XA	Effects of weightlessness, initial encounter
		T75.89XA	Other specified effects of external causes, init encntr
995.Ø	OTHER ANAPHYLACTIC REACTION	T78.2XXA	Anaphylactic shock, unspecified, initial encounter
		T88.6XXA	Anaphyl reaction due to advrs eff drug/med prop admin, init
995.1	ANGIONEUROTIC EDEMA NOT ELSEWHERE CLASSIFIED	T78.3XXA	Angioneurotic edema, initial encounter
995.2Ø	UNS ADVRS EFF UNS RX MEDICINAL&BIOLOGICAL SBSTNC	T5Ø.9Ø5A	Adverse effect of unsp drug/meds/biol subst, init
995.21	ARTHUS PHENOMENON	T78.41XA	Arthus phenomenon, initial encounter
995.22	UNSPECIFIED ADVERSE EFFECT OF ANESTHESIA	T41.ØX5A	Adverse effect of inhaled anesthetics, initial encounter
		T41.1X5A	Adverse effect of intravenous anesthetics, initial encounter
		T41.2Ø5A	Adverse effect of unsp general anesthetics, init encntr
		T41.295A	Adverse effect of other general anesthetics, init encntr
		T41.3X5A	Adverse effect of local anesthetics, initial encounter
		T41.45XA	Adverse effect of unspecified anesthetic, initial encounter
		T88.59XA	Other complications of anesthesia, initial encounter
995.23	UNSPECIFIED ADVERSE EFFECT OF INSULIN	T38.3X5A	Adverse effect of insulin and oral hypoglycemic drugs, init
995.24	FAILED MODERATE SEDATION DURING PROCEDURE	T88.52XA	Failed moderate sedation during procedure, initial encounter
995.27	OTHER DRUG ALLERGY	T5Ø.995A	Adverse effect of drug/meds/biol subst, init

ICD-9-CM		ICD-10-CM	
995.29	UNS ADVRS EFF OTH RX MEDICINAL&BIOLOGICAL SBSTNC	**T36.ØX5A**	Adverse effect of penicillins, initial encounter
		T36.1X5A	Adverse effect of cephalospor/oth beta-lactm antibiot, init
		T36.2X5A	Adverse effect of chloramphenicol group, initial encounter
		T36.3X5A	Adverse effect of macrolides, initial encounter
		T36.4X5A	Adverse effect of tetracyclines, initial encounter
		T36.5X5A	Adverse effect of aminoglycosides, initial encounter
		T36.6X5A	Adverse effect of rifampicins, initial encounter
		T36.7X5A	Adverse effect of antifungal antibiotics, sys used, init
		T36.8X5A	Adverse effect of other systemic antibiotics, init encntr
		T36.95XA	Adverse effect of unsp systemic antibiotic, init encntr
		T37.ØX5A	Adverse effect of sulfonamides, initial encounter
		T37.1X5A	Adverse effect of antimycobacterial drugs, initial encounter
		T37.2X5A	Advrs effect of antimalari/drugs acting on bld protzoa, init
		T37.3X5A	Adverse effect of other antiprotozoal drugs, init encntr
		T37.4X5A	Adverse effect of anthelminthics, initial encounter
		T37.5X5A	Adverse effect of antiviral drugs, initial encounter
		T37.8X5A	Adverse effect of systemic anti-infect/parasit, init
		T37.95XA	Advrs effect of unsp sys anti-infect and antiparasitic, init
		T38.ØX5A	Adverse effect of glucocort/synth analog, init
		T38.1X5A	Adverse effect of thyroid hormones and substitutes, init
		T38.2X5A	Adverse effect of antithyroid drugs, initial encounter
		T38.4X5A	Adverse effect of oral contraceptives, initial encounter
		T38.5X5A	Adverse effect of oth estrogens and progestogens, init
		T38.6X5A	Adverse effect of antigonadtr/antiestr/antiandrg, NEC, init
		T38.7X5A	Adverse effect of androgens and anabolic congeners, init
		T38.8Ø5A	Adverse effect of unsp hormones and synthetic sub, init
		T38.815A	Adverse effect of anterior pituitary hormones, init encntr
		T38.895A	Adverse effect of hormones and synthetic substitutes, init
		T38.9Ø5A	Adverse effect of unsp hormone antagonists, init encntr
		T38.995A	Adverse effect of other hormone antagonists, init encntr
		T39.Ø15A	Adverse effect of aspirin, initial encounter
		T39.Ø95A	Adverse effect of salicylates, initial encounter
		T39.1X5A	Adverse effect of 4-Aminophenol derivatives, init encntr
		T39.2X5A	Adverse effect of pyrazolone derivatives, initial encounter
		T39.315A	Adverse effect of propionic acid derivatives, init encntr
		T39.395A	Adverse effect of nonsteroidal anti-inflammatory drugs, init
		T39.4X5A	Adverse effect of antirheumatics, NEC, init
		T39.8X5A	Adverse effect of nonopioid analges/antipyret, NEC, init
		T39.95XA	Adverse effect of unsp nonopi analgs/antipyr/antirheu, init
		T4Ø.ØX5A	Adverse effect of opium, initial encounter
		T4Ø.2X5A	Adverse effect of other opioids, initial encounter
		T4Ø.3X5A	Adverse effect of methadone, initial encounter
		T4Ø.4X5A	Adverse effect of other synthetic narcotics, init encntr
		T4Ø.5X5A	Adverse effect of cocaine, initial encounter
		T4Ø.6Ø5A	Adverse effect of unspecified narcotics, initial encounter
		T4Ø.695A	Adverse effect of other narcotics, initial encounter
		T4Ø.7X5A	Adverse effect of cannabis (derivatives), initial encounter
		T4Ø.9Ø5A	Adverse effect of unspecified psychodysleptics, init encntr
		T4Ø.995A	Adverse effect of other psychodysleptics, initial encounter
		T41.5X5A	Adverse effect of therapeutic gases, initial encounter
		T42.ØX5A	Adverse effect of hydantoin derivatives, initial encounter
		T42.1X5A	Adverse effect of iminostilbenes, initial encounter
		T42.2X5A	Adverse effect of succinimides and oxazolidinediones, init
		T42.3X5A	Adverse effect of barbiturates, initial encounter
		T42.4X5A	Adverse effect of benzodiazepines, initial encounter
		T42.5X5A	Adverse effect of mixed antiepileptics, initial encounter
		T42.6X5A	Adverse effect of antiepileptic and sed-hypntc drugs, init
		T42.75XA	Adverse effect of unsp antieplptc and sed-hypntc drugs, init
		T42.8X5A	Adverse effect of antiparkns drug/centr musc-tone depr, init
		T43.Ø15A	Adverse effect of tricyclic antidepressants, init encntr
		T43.Ø25A	Adverse effect of tetracyclic antidepressants, init encntr
		T43.1X5A	Adverse effect of MAO inhib antidepressants, init
		T43.2Ø5A	Adverse effect of unspecified antidepressants, init encntr
		T43.215A	Advrs effect of slctv seroton/norepineph reup inhibtr, init
		T43.225A	Adverse effect of selective serotonin reuptake inhibtr, init
		T43.295A	Adverse effect of other antidepressants, initial encounter
		T43.3X5A	Adverse effect of phenothiazine antipsychot/neurolept, init
		T43.4X5A	Adverse effect of butyrophen/thiothixen neuroleptics, init
		T43.5Ø5A	Adverse effect of unsp antipsychotics and neuroleptics, init
		T43.595A	Adverse effect of oth antipsychotics and neuroleptics, init
		T43.6Ø5A	Adverse effect of unspecified psychostimulants, init encntr
		T43.615A	Adverse effect of caffeine, initial encounter
		T43.625A	Adverse effect of amphetamines, initial encounter
		T43.635A	Adverse effect of methylphenidate, initial encounter
		T43.695A	Adverse effect of other psychostimulants, initial encounter
		T43.8X5A	Adverse effect of other psychotropic drugs, init encntr
		T43.95XA	Adverse effect of unspecified psychotropic drug, init encntr
		T44.ØX5A	Adverse effect of anticholinesterase agents, init encntr
		T44.1X5A	Adverse effect of other parasympathomimetics, init encntr
		T44.2X5A	Adverse effect of ganglionic blocking drugs, init encntr

(Continued on next page)

ICD-9-CM		ICD-10-CM	
995.29	UNS ADVRS EFF OTH RX MEDICINAL&BIOLOGICAL SBSTNC **(Continued)**	T44.3X5A	Adverse effect of parasympatholytics and spasmolytics, init
		T44.4X5A	Adverse effect of predom alpha-adrenocpt agonists, init
		T44.5X5A	Adverse effect of predom beta-adrenocpt agonists, init
		T44.6X5A	Adverse effect of alpha-adrenoreceptor antagonists, init
		T44.7X5A	Adverse effect of beta-adrenoreceptor antagonists, init
		T44.8X5A	Adverse effect of centr-acting/adren-neurn-block agnt, init
		T44.9Ø5A	Adverse effect of unsp drugs aff the autonm nervous sys, init
		T44.995A	Adverse effect of drug aff the autonomic nervous sys, init
		T45.ØX5A	Adverse effect of antiallergic and antiemetic drugs, init
		T45.1X5A	Adverse effect of antineoplastic and immunosup drugs, init
		T45.2X5A	Adverse effect of vitamins, initial encounter
		T45.3X5A	Adverse effect of enzymes, initial encounter
		T45.4X5A	Adverse effect of iron and its compounds, initial encounter
		T45.515A	Adverse effect of anticoagulants, initial encounter
		T45.525A	Adverse effect of antithrombotic drugs, initial encounter
		T45.6Ø5A	Adverse effect of unsp fibrinolysis-affecting drugs, init
		T45.615A	Adverse effect of thrombolytic drugs, initial encounter
		T45.625A	Adverse effect of hemostatic drug, initial encounter
		T45.695A	Adverse effect of oth fibrinolysis-affecting drugs, init
		T45.7X5A	Adverse effect of anticoag antag, vit K and oth coag, init
		T45.8X5A	Adverse effect of prim systemic and hematolog agents, init
		T45.95XA	Adverse effect of unsp prim sys and hematolog agent, init
		T46.ØX5A	Adverse effect of cardi-stim glycos/drug simlar act, init
		T46.1X5A	Adverse effect of calcium-channel blockers, init encntr
		T46.2X5A	Adverse effect of other antidysrhythmic drugs, init encntr
		T46.3X5A	Adverse effect of coronary vasodilators, initial encounter
		T46.4X5A	Adverse effect of angiotens-convert-enzyme inhibitors, init
		T46.5X5A	Adverse effect of other antihypertensive drugs, init encntr
		T46.6X5A	Adverse effect of antihyperlip and antiarterio drugs, init
		T46.7X5A	Adverse effect of peripheral vasodilators, initial encounter
		T46.8X5A	Adverse effect of antivaric drugs, inc scler agents, init
		T46.9Ø5A	Adverse effect of unsp agents aff the cardiovasc sys, init
		T46.995A	Adverse effect of agents aff the cardiovascular sys, init
		T47.ØX5A	Adverse effect of histamine H2-receptor blockers, init
		T47.1X5A	Adverse effect of antacids and anti-gstrc-sec drugs, init
		T47.2X5A	Adverse effect of stimulant laxatives, initial encounter
		T47.3X5A	Adverse effect of saline and osmotic laxatives, init encntr
		T47.4X5A	Adverse effect of other laxatives, initial encounter
		T47.5X5A	Adverse effect of digestants, initial encounter
		T47.6X5A	Adverse effect of antidiarrheal drugs, initial encounter
		T47.7X5A	Adverse effect of emetics, initial encounter
		T47.8X5A	Adverse effect of agents primarily affecting GI sys, init
		T47.95XA	Adverse effect of unsp agents aff the GI sys, init
		T48.ØX5A	Adverse effect of oxytocic drugs, initial encounter
		T48.1X5A	Adverse effect of skeletal muscle relaxants, init encntr
		T48.2Ø5A	Adverse effect of unsp drugs acting on muscles, init encntr
		T48.295A	Adverse effect of other drugs acting on muscles, init encntr
		T48.3X5A	Adverse effect of antitussives, initial encounter
		T48.4X5A	Adverse effect of expectorants, initial encounter
		T48.5X5A	Adverse effect of other anti-common-cold drugs, init encntr
		T48.6X5A	Adverse effect of antiasthmatics, initial encounter
		T48.9Ø5A	Advrs effect of unsp agents prim act on the resp sys, init
		T48.995A	Adverse effect of agents prim acting on the resp sys, init
		T49.ØX5A	Adverse effect of local antifung/infect/inflamm drugs, init
		T49.1X5A	Adverse effect of antipruritics, initial encounter
		T49.2X5A	Adverse effect of local astringents/detergents, init
		T49.3X5A	Adverse effect of emollients, demulcents and protect, init
		T49.4X5A	Adverse effect of keratolyt/keratplst/hair trmt drug, init
		T49.5X5A	Adverse effect of opth drugs and preparations, init
		T49.6X5A	Adverse effect of otorhino drugs and preparations, init
		T49.7X5A	Adverse effect of dental drugs, topically applied, init
		T49.8X5A	Adverse effect of other topical agents, initial encounter
		T49.95XA	Adverse effect of unspecified topical agent, init encntr
		T5Ø.ØX5A	Adverse effect of mineralocorticoids and their antag, init
		T5Ø.1X5A	Adverse effect of loop diuretics, initial encounter
		T5Ø.2X5A	Advrs eff of crbnc-anhydr inhibtr, benzo/oth diuretc, init
		T5Ø.3X5A	Adverse effect of electrolytic/caloric/wtr-bal agnt, init
		T5Ø.4X5A	Adverse effect of drugs affecting uric acid metabolism, init
		T5Ø.5X5A	Adverse effect of appetite depressants, initial encounter
		T5Ø.6X5A	Adverse effect of antidotes and chelating agents, init
		T5Ø.7X5A	Adverse effect of analeptics and opioid receptor antag, init
		T5Ø.8X5A	Adverse effect of diagnostic agents, initial encounter
		T5Ø.995A	Adverse effect of drug/meds/biol subst, init
		T5Ø.A15A	Advrs effect of pertuss vaccine, inc combin w pertuss, init
		T5Ø.A25A	Adverse effect of mixed bact vaccines w/o a pertuss, init
		T5Ø.A95A	Adverse effect of other bacterial vaccines, init encntr
		T5Ø.B15A	Adverse effect of smallpox vaccines, initial encounter
		T5Ø.B95A	Adverse effect of other viral vaccines, initial encounter
		T5Ø.Z15A	Adverse effect of immunoglobulin, initial encounter
		T5Ø.Z95A	Adverse effect of vaccines and biological substances, init

 [Brackets] indicate valid character values for each code. Character value meanings provided for each code grouping.

ICD-9-CM		ICD-10-CM	
995.3	ALLERGY UNSPECIFIED NOT ELSEWHERE CLASSIFIED	T78.4ØXA	Allergy, unspecified, initial encounter
		T78.49XA	Other allergy, initial encounter
995.4	SHOCK DUE TO ANESTHESIA NOT ELSEWHERE CLASSIFIED	T88.2XXA	Shock due to anesthesia, initial encounter
995.5Ø	CHILD ABUSE, UNSPECIFIED	T74.92XA	Unspecified child maltreatment, confirmed, initial encounter
		T76.92XA	Unspecified child maltreatment, suspected, initial encounter
995.51	CHILD EMOTIONAL/PSYCHOLOGICAL ABUSE	T74.32XA	Child psychological abuse, confirmed, initial encounter
		T76.32XA	Child psychological abuse, suspected, initial encounter
995.52	CHILD NEGLECT	▣ T74.Ø2XA	Child neglect or abandonment, confirmed, initial encounter
		T76.Ø2XA	Child neglect or abandonment, suspected, initial encounter
995.53	CHILD SEXUAL ABUSE	T74.22XA	Child sexual abuse, confirmed, initial encounter
		T76.22XA	Child sexual abuse, suspected, initial encounter
995.54	CHILD PHYSICAL ABUSE	T74.12XA	Child physical abuse, confirmed, initial encounter
		T76.12XA	Child physical abuse, suspected, initial encounter
995.55	SHAKEN INFANT SYNDROME	T74.4XXA	Shaken infant syndrome, initial encounter
995.59	OTHER CHILD ABUSE AND NEGLECT	T74.92XA	Unspecified child maltreatment, confirmed, initial encounter
		T76.92XA	Unspecified child maltreatment, suspected, initial encounter
995.6Ø	ANAPHYLACTIC REACTION DUE TO UNSPECIFIED FOOD	T78.ØØXA	Anaphylactic reaction due to unspecified food, init encntr
995.61	ANAPHYLACTIC REACTION DUE TO PEANUTS	T78.Ø1XA	Anaphylactic reaction due to peanuts, initial encounter
995.62	ANAPHYLACTIC REACTION DUE TO CRUSTACEANS	T78.Ø2XA	Anaphylactic reaction due to shellfish (crustaceans), init
995.63	ANAPHYLACTIC REACTION DUE TO FRUITS & VEGETABLES	T78.Ø4XA	Anaphylactic reaction due to fruits and vegetables, init
995.64	ANAPHYLACTIC REACTION DUE TO TREE NUTS AND SEEDS	T78.Ø5XA	Anaphylactic reaction due to tree nuts and seeds, init
995.65	ANAPHYLACTIC REACTION DUE TO FISH	T78.Ø3XA	Anaphylactic reaction due to other fish, initial encounter
995.66	ANAPHYLACTIC REACTION DUE TO FOOD ADDITIVES	T78.Ø6XA	Anaphylactic reaction due to food additives, init encntr
995.67	ANAPHYLACTIC REACTION DUE TO MILK PRODUCTS	T78.Ø7XA	Anaphylactic reaction due to milk and dairy products, init
995.68	ANAPHYLACTIC REACTION DUE TO EGGS	T78.Ø8XA	Anaphylactic reaction due to eggs, initial encounter
995.69	ANAPHYLACTIC REACTION DUE TO OTH SPECIFIED FOOD	T78.Ø9XA	Anaphylactic reaction due to oth food products, init encntr
995.7	OTHER ADVERSE FOOD REACTIONS NEC	T78.1XXA	Oth adverse food reactions, not elsewhere classified, init
995.8Ø	ADULT MALTREATMENT UNSPECIFIED NEC	T74.91XA	Unspecified adult maltreatment, confirmed, initial encounter
		T76.91XA	Unspecified adult maltreatment, suspected, initial encounter
995.81	ADULT PHYSICAL ABUSE NEC	T74.11XA	Adult physical abuse, confirmed, initial encounter
		T76.11XA	Adult physical abuse, suspected, initial encounter
995.82	ADULT EMOTIONAL/PSYCHOLOGICAL ABUSE NEC	T74.31XA	Adult psychological abuse, confirmed, initial encounter
		T76.31XA	Adult psychological abuse, suspected, initial encounter
995.83	ADULT SEXUAL ABUSE NEC	T74.21XA	Adult sexual abuse, confirmed, initial encounter
		T76.21XA	Adult sexual abuse, suspected, initial encounter
995.84	ADULT NEGLECT NEC	▣ T74.Ø1XA	Adult neglect or abandonment, confirmed, initial encounter
		T76.Ø1XA	Adult neglect or abandonment, suspected, initial encounter
995.85	OTHER ADULT ABUSE AND NEGLECT NEC	T74.91XA	Unspecified adult maltreatment, confirmed, initial encounter
		T76.91XA	Unspecified adult maltreatment, suspected, initial encounter
995.86	MALIGNANT HYPERTHERMIA NEC	T88.3XXA	Malignant hyperthermia due to anesthesia, initial encounter
995.89	CERTAIN ADVERSE EFFECTS NEC OTHER	T78.8XXA	Other adverse effects, not elsewhere classified, init encntr
		T88.51XA	Hypothermia following anesthesia, initial encounter
995.9Ø	SYSTEMIC INFLAMMATORY RESPONSE SYNDROME UNSPEC	R65.1Ø	SIRS of non-infectious origin w/o acute organ dysfunction
995.91	SEPSIS	▣ AØ2.1	Salmonella sepsis
		▣ A22.7	Anthrax sepsis
		▣ A26.7	Erysipelothrix sepsis
		▣ A32.7	Listerial sepsis
		▣ A4Ø.Ø	Sepsis due to streptococcus, group A
		▣ A4Ø.1	Sepsis due to streptococcus, group B
		▣ A4Ø.3	Sepsis due to Streptococcus pneumoniae
		▣ A4Ø.8	Other streptococcal sepsis
		▣ A4Ø.9	Streptococcal sepsis, unspecified
		▣ A41.Ø1	Sepsis due to Methicillin susceptible Staphylococcus aureus
		▣ A41.Ø2	Sepsis due to Methicillin resistant Staphylococcus aureus
		▣ A41.1	Sepsis due to other specified staphylococcus
		▣ A41.2	Sepsis due to unspecified staphylococcus
		▣ A41.3	Sepsis due to Hemophilus influenzae
		▣ A41.4	Sepsis due to anaerobes
		▣ A41.5Ø	Gram-negative sepsis, unspecified
		▣ A41.51	Sepsis due to Escherichia coli [E. coli]
		▣ A41.52	Sepsis due to Pseudomonas
		▣ A41.53	Sepsis due to Serratia
		▣ A41.59	Other Gram-negative sepsis
		▣ A41.81	Sepsis due to Enterococcus
		▣ A41.89	Other specified sepsis
		▣ A41.9	Sepsis, unspecified organism
		▣ A42.7	Actinomycotic sepsis
		▣ A54.86	Gonococcal sepsis
		▣ B37.7	Candidal sepsis
995.92	SEVERE SEPSIS	R65.2Ø	Severe sepsis without septic shock
		▣ R65.21	Severe sepsis with septic shock
995.93	SYS INFLAM RSPN SYND-NON-INF W/O ACUTE ORGN DYSF	R65.1Ø	SIRS of non-infectious origin w/o acute organ dysfunction
995.94	SYS INFLAM RSPN SYND NON-INF W/ACUTE ORGN DYSF	➡ R65.11	SIRS of non-infectious origin w acute organ dysfunction

995.3–995.94

ICD-9-CM		ICD-10-CM	
996.00	MECH COMP UNSPEC CARD DEVICE IMPLANT&GRAFT	**T82.519A**	Brkdwn unsp cardiac and vascular devices and implants, init
		T82.529A	Displacmnt of unsp cardiac and vasc devices and implnt, init
		T82.539A	Leakage of unsp cardiac and vasc devices and implnt, init
		T82.599A	Mech compl of unsp cardiac and vasc devices and implnt, init
996.00	MECH COMP UNSPEC CARD DEVICE IMPLANT&GRAFT	**T82.119A**	Breakdown of unsp cardiac electronic device, init
		T82.129A	Displacement of unsp cardiac electronic device, init encntr
		T82.199A	Mech compl of unspecified cardiac device, initial encounter
		T82.519A	Brkdwn unsp cardiac and vascular devices and implants, init
		T82.529A	Displacmnt of unsp cardiac and vasc devices and implnt, init
		T82.539A	Leakage of unsp cardiac and vasc devices and implnt, init
		T82.599A	Mech compl of unsp cardiac and vasc devices and implnt, init
996.01	MECHANICAL COMPLICATION DUE TO CARDIAC PACEMAKER	**T82.110A**	Breakdown (mechanical) of cardiac electrode, init encntr
		T82.111A	Breakdown of cardiac pulse generator (battery), init
		T82.120A	Displacement of cardiac electrode, initial encounter
		T82.121A	Displacement of cardiac pulse generator (battery), init
		T82.190A	Mech compl of cardiac electrode, initial encounter
		T82.191A	Mech compl of cardiac pulse generator (battery), init encntr
996.02	MECH COMPLICATION DUE HEART VALVE PROSTHESIS	**T82.01XA**	Breakdown (mechanical) of heart valve prosthesis, init
		T82.02XA	Displacement of heart valve prosthesis, initial encounter
		T82.03XA	Leakage of heart valve prosthesis, initial encounter
		T82.09XA	Mech compl of heart valve prosthesis, initial encounter
996.03	MECH COMPLICATION DUE CORONARY BYPASS GRAFT	**T82.211A**	Breakdown (mechanical) of coronary artery bypass graft, init
		T82.212A	Displacement of coronary artery bypass graft, init encntr
		T82.213A	Leakage of coronary artery bypass graft, initial encounter
		T82.218A	Mech compl of coronary artery bypass graft, init encntr
996.04	MECH COMP DUE AUTO IMPLANTABLE CARD DEFIB	**T82.110A**	Breakdown (mechanical) of cardiac electrode, init encntr
		T82.111A	Breakdown of cardiac pulse generator (battery), init
		T82.120A	Displacement of cardiac electrode, initial encounter
		T82.121A	Displacement of cardiac pulse generator (battery), init
		T82.190A	Mech compl of cardiac electrode, initial encounter
		T82.191A	Mech compl of cardiac pulse generator (battery), init encntr
996.09	MECH COMPLICATION CARD DEVICE IMPLANT&GRAFT OTH	**T82.118A**	Breakdown (mechanical) of cardiac electronic device, init
		T82.128A	Displacement of other cardiac electronic device, init encntr
		T82.198A	Mech compl of other cardiac electronic device, init encntr
		T82.221A	Breakdown (mechanical) of biological heart valve graft, init
		T82.222A	Displacement of biological heart valve graft, init encntr
		T82.223A	Leakage of biological heart valve graft, initial encounter
		T82.228A	Mech compl of biological heart valve graft, init encntr
		T82.512A	Breakdown (mechanical) of artificial heart, init encntr
		T82.514A	Breakdown (mechanical) of infusion catheter, init encntr
		T82.518A	Breakdown of cardiac and vascular devices and implants, init
		T82.522A	Displacement of artificial heart, initial encounter
		T82.524A	Displacement of infusion catheter, initial encounter
		T82.528A	Displacmnt of cardiac and vascular devices and implnt, init
		T82.529A	Displacmnt of unsp cardiac and vasc devices and implnt, init
		T82.532A	Leakage of artificial heart, initial encounter
		T82.534A	Leakage of infusion catheter, initial encounter
		T82.538A	Leakage of cardiac and vascular devices and implants, init
		T82.592A	Mech compl of artificial heart, initial encounter
		T82.594A	Mech compl of infusion catheter, initial encounter
		T82.598A	Mech compl of cardiac and vascular devices and implnt, init
996.1	MECH COMP OTH VASCULAR DEVICE IMPLANT&GRAFT	**T82.310A**	Breakdown (mechanical) of aortic (bifurcation) graft, init
		T82.311A	Breakdown of carotid arterial graft (bypass), init
		T82.312A	Breakdown of femoral arterial graft (bypass), init
		T82.318A	Breakdown (mechanical) of other vascular grafts, init encntr
		T82.319A	Breakdown (mechanical) of unsp vascular grafts, init encntr
		T82.320A	Displacement of aortic (bifurcation) graft, init
		T82.321A	Displacement of carotid arterial graft (bypass), init encntr
		T82.322A	Displacement of femoral arterial graft (bypass), init encntr
		T82.328A	Displacement of other vascular grafts, initial encounter
		T82.329A	Displacement of unspecified vascular grafts, init encntr
		T82.330A	Leakage of aortic (bifurcation) graft (replacement), init
		T82.331A	Leakage of carotid arterial graft (bypass), init encntr
		T82.332A	Leakage of femoral arterial graft (bypass), init encntr
		T82.338A	Leakage of other vascular grafts, initial encounter
		T82.339A	Leakage of unspecified vascular graft, initial encounter
		T82.390A	Mech compl of aortic (bifurcation) graft (replacement), init
		T82.391A	Mech compl of carotid arterial graft (bypass), init encntr
		T82.392A	Mech compl of femoral arterial graft (bypass), init encntr
		T82.398A	Mech compl of other vascular grafts, initial encounter
		T82.399A	Mech compl of unspecified vascular grafts, initial encounter
		T82.41XA	Breakdown (mechanical) of vascular dialysis catheter, init
		T82.42XA	Displacement of vascular dialysis catheter, init encntr
		T82.43XA	Leakage of vascular dialysis catheter, initial encounter
		T82.49XA	Oth complication of vascular dialysis catheter, init encntr
		T82.510A	Breakdown of surgically created AV fistula, init
		T82.511A	Breakdown (mechanical) of surgically created AV shunt, init
		T82.513A	Breakdown of balloon (counterpulsation) device, init
		T82.514A	Breakdown (mechanical) of infusion catheter, init encntr
		T82.515A	Breakdown (mechanical) of umbrella device, initial encounter
	(Continued on next page)	**T82.518A**	Breakdown of cardiac and vascular devices and implants, init

ICD-9-CM		ICD-10-CM	
996.1	MECH COMP OTH VASCULAR DEVICE IMPLANT&GRAFT **(Continued)**	**T82.520A**	Displacement of surgically created AV fistula, init
		T82.521A	Displacement of surgically created arteriovenous shunt, init
		T82.523A	Displacement of balloon (counterpulsation) device, init
		T82.524A	Displacement of infusion catheter, initial encounter
		T82.525A	Displacement of umbrella device, initial encounter
		T82.528A	Displacmnt of cardiac and vascular devices and implnt, init
		T82.529A	Displacmnt of unsp cardiac and vasc devices and implnt, init
		T82.530A	Leakage of surgically created arteriovenous fistula, init
		T82.531A	Leakage of surgically created arteriovenous shunt, init
		T82.533A	Leakage of balloon (counterpulsation) device, init encntr
		T82.534A	Leakage of infusion catheter, initial encounter
		T82.535A	Leakage of umbrella device, initial encounter
		T82.538A	Leakage of cardiac and vascular devices and implants, init
		T82.590A	Mech compl of surgically created arteriovenous fistula, init
		T82.591A	Mech compl of surgically created arteriovenous shunt, init
		T82.593A	Mech compl of balloon (counterpulsation) device, init encntr
		T82.594A	Mech compl of infusion catheter, initial encounter
		T82.595A	Mech compl of umbrella device, initial encounter
		T82.598A	Mech compl of cardiac and vascular devices and implnt, init
996.2	MECH COMP NERVOUS SYSTEM DEVICE IMPLANT&GRAFT	**T85.01XA**	Breakdown of ventricular intracranial shunt, init
		T85.02XA	Displacement of ventricular intracranial shunt, init
		T85.03XA	Leakage of ventricular intracranial shunt, init
		T85.09XA	Mech compl of ventricular intracranial shunt, init
		T85.110A	Brkdwn implanted electronic neurostim of brain, init
		T85.111A	Brkdwn implanted electronic neurostim of periph nrv, init
		T85.112A	Brkdwn implanted electronic neurostim of spinal cord, init
		T85.118A	Brkdwn implanted electronic stimulator of nervous sys, init
		T85.120A	Displacmnt of implanted electronic neurostim of brain, init
		T85.121A	Displacmnt of implnt electrnc neurostim of periph nrv, init
		T85.122A	Displacmnt of implnt electrnc neurostim of spinal cord, init
		T85.128A	Displacmnt of implnt electrnc stimultr of nervous sys, init
		T85.190A	Mech compl of implanted electronic neurostim of brain, init
		T85.191A	Mech compl of implnt electrnc neurostim of periph nrv, init
		T85.192A	Mech compl of implnt electrnc neurostim of spinal cord, init
		T85.199A	Mech compl of implnt electrnc stimultr of nervous sys, init
996.30	MECH COMP UNSPEC GU DEVICE IMPLANT&GRAFT	**T83.498A**	Mech compl of prosth dev/implnt/grft of genital tract, init
996.31	MECHANICAL COMPLICATION DUE TO URETHRAL CATHETER	**T83.018A**	Breakdown (mechanical) of indwelling urethral catheter, init
		T83.028A	Displacement of oth indwelling urethral catheter, init
		T83.038A	Leakage of other indwelling urethral catheter, init encntr
		T83.098A	Mech compl of oth indwelling urethral catheter, init encntr
996.32	MECH COMP DUE INTRAUTERINE CONTRACEPTIVE DEVICE	**T83.31XA**	Breakdown (mechanical) of intrauterine contracep dev, init
		T83.32XA	Displacement of intrauterine contraceptive device, init
		T83.39XA	Mech compl of intrauterine contraceptive device, init encntr
996.39	MECH COMP GENITOURINARY DEVICE IMPLANT&GRAFT OTH	**T83.010A**	Breakdown (mechanical) of cystostomy catheter, init encntr
		T83.020A	Displacement of cystostomy catheter, initial encounter
		T83.030A	Leakage of cystostomy catheter, initial encounter
		T83.090A	Mech compl of cystostomy catheter, initial encounter
		T83.110A	Breakdown of urinary electronic stimulator device, init
		T83.111A	Breakdown (mechanical) of urinary sphincter implant, init
		T83.112A	Breakdown (mechanical) of urinary stent, initial encounter
		T83.118A	Breakdown (mechanical) of urinary devices and implants, init
		T83.120A	Displacement of urinary electronic stimulator device, init
		T83.121A	Displacement of urinary sphincter implant, initial encounter
		T83.122A	Displacement of urinary stent, initial encounter
		T83.128A	Displacement of oth urinary devices and implants, init
		T83.190A	Mech compl of urinary electronic stimulator device, init
		T83.191A	Mech compl of urinary sphincter implant, initial encounter
		T83.192A	Mech compl of urinary stent, initial encounter
		T83.198A	Mech compl of oth urinary devices and implants, init encntr
		T83.21XA	Breakdown (mechanical) of graft of urinary organ, init
		T83.22XA	Displacement of graft of urinary organ, initial encounter
		T83.23XA	Leakage of graft of urinary organ, initial encounter
		T83.29XA	Mech compl of graft of urinary organ, initial encounter
		T83.410A	Breakdown of penile (implanted) prosthesis, init
		T83.418A	Breakdown of prosth dev/implnt/grft of genitl trct, init
		T83.420A	Displacement of penile (implanted) prosthesis, init encntr
		T83.428A	Displacement of prosth dev/implnt/grft of genitl trct, init
		T83.490A	Mech compl of penile (implanted) prosthesis, init encntr
		T83.498A	Mech compl of prosth dev/implnt/grft of genital tract, init
		T83.718A	Erosion of implanted prstht mtrl to surrnd org/tiss, init
		T83.728A	Exposure of implanted prstht mtrl to surrnd org/tiss, init
996.40	UNS MECH COMPL INT ORTHOPEDIC DEVC IMPLANT&GRAFT	**T84.498A**	Mech compl of internal orth devices, implnt and grafts, init
996.41	MECHANICAL LOOSENING OF PROSTHETIC JOINT	**T84.030A**	Mech loosening of internal right hip prosthetic joint, init
		T84.031A	Mech loosening of internal left hip prosthetic joint, init
		T84.032A	Mech loosening of internal right knee prosthetic joint, init
		T84.033A	Mech loosening of internal left knee prosthetic joint, init
		T84.038A	Mechanical loosening of oth internal prosthetic joint, init
		T84.039A	Mechanical loosening of unsp internal prosthetic joint, init

ICD-9-CM		ICD-10-CM	
996.42	DISLOCATION OF PROSTHETIC JOINT	**T84.Ø2ØA**	Dislocation of internal right hip prosthesis, init encntr
		T84.Ø21A	Dislocation of internal left hip prosthesis, init encntr
		T84.Ø22A	Instability of internal right knee prosthesis, init encntr
		T84.Ø23A	Instability of internal left knee prosthesis, init encntr
		T84.Ø28A	Dislocation of other internal joint prosthesis, init encntr
		T84.Ø29A	Dislocation of unsp internal joint prosthesis, init encntr
996.43	BROKEN PROSTHETIC JOINT IMPLANT	**T84.Ø1ØA**	Broken internal right hip prosthesis, initial encounter
		T84.Ø11A	Broken internal left hip prosthesis, initial encounter
		T84.Ø12A	Broken internal right knee prosthesis, initial encounter
		T84.Ø13A	Broken internal left knee prosthesis, initial encounter
		T84.Ø18A	Broken internal joint prosthesis, other site, init encntr
		T84.Ø19A	Broken internal joint prosthesis, unsp site, init encntr
996.44	PERIPROSTHETIC FRACTURE AROUND PROSTHETIC JOINT	**T84.Ø4ØA**	Periprosth fracture around internal prosth r hip jt, init
		T84.Ø41A	Periprosth fracture around internal prosth l hip jt, init
		T84.Ø42A	Periprosth fracture around internal prosth r knee jt, init
		T84.Ø43A	Periprosth fracture around internal prosth l knee jt, init
		T84.Ø48A	Periprosth fracture around oth internal prosth joint, init
		T84.Ø49A	Periprosth fracture around unsp internal prosth joint, init
996.45	PERIPROSTHETIC OSTEOLYSIS	**T84.Ø5ØA**	Periprosth osteolysis of internal prosthetic r hip jt, init
		T84.Ø51A	Periprosth osteolysis of internal prosthetic l hip jt, init
		T84.Ø52A	Periprosth osteolysis of internal prosthetic r knee jt, init
		T84.Ø53A	Periprosth osteolysis of internal prosthetic l knee jt, init
		T84.Ø58A	Periprosthetic osteolysis of internal prosthetic joint, init
		T84.Ø59A	Periprosth osteolys of unsp internal prosthetic joint, init
996.46	ARTICULAR BEARING SURFACE WEAR PROSTHETIC JOINT	**T84.Ø6ØA**	Wear of artic bearing surface of int prosth r hip jt, init
		T84.Ø61A	Wear of artic bearing surface of int prosth l hip jt, init
		T84.Ø62A	Wear of artic bearing surface of int prosth r knee jt, init
		T84.Ø63A	Wear of artic bearing surface of int prosth l knee jt, init
		T84.Ø68A	Wear of artic bearing surface of internal prosth joint, init
		T84.Ø69A	Wear of artic bearing surface of unsp int prosth joint, init
996.47	OTHER MECH COMPLICATION PROSTHETIC JOINT IMPLANT	**T84.Ø9ØA**	Mech compl of internal right hip prosthesis, init encntr
		T84.Ø91A	Mech compl of internal left hip prosthesis, init encntr
		T84.Ø92A	Mech compl of internal right knee prosthesis, init encntr
		T84.Ø93A	Mech compl of internal left knee prosthesis, init encntr
		T84.Ø98A	Mech compl of other internal joint prosthesis, init encntr
		T84.Ø99A	Mech compl of unsp internal joint prosthesis, init encntr
996.49	OTH MECH COMPL OTH INT ORTHOPEDIC DEVC IMPL&GFT	**M96.Ø**	Pseudarthrosis after fusion or arthrodesis
		M96.621	Fx humerus fol insrt ortho implnt/prosth/bone plt, right arm
		M96.622	Fx humerus fol insrt ortho implnt/prosth/bone plt, left arm
		M96.629	Fx humerus fol insrt ortho implnt/prosth/bone plt, unsp arm
		M96.631	Fx rad/ulna fol insrt ortho implnt/prosth/bone plt, r arm
		M96.632	Fx rad/ulna fol insrt ortho implnt/prosth/bone plt, left arm
		M96.639	Fx rad/ulna fol insrt ortho implnt/prosth/bone plt, unsp arm
		M96.65	Fx pelvis following insrt ortho implnt/prosth/bone plt
		M96.661	Fx femur fol insrt ortho implnt/prosth/bone plt, right leg
		M96.662	Fx femur fol insrt ortho implnt/prosth/bone plt, left leg
		M96.669	Fx femur fol insrt ortho implnt/prosth/bone plt, unsp leg
		M96.671	Fx tib/fib fol insrt ortho implnt/prosth/bone plt, right leg
		M96.672	Fx tib/fib fol insrt ortho implnt/prosth/bone plt, left leg
		M96.679	Fx tib/fib fol insrt ortho implnt/prosth/bone plt, unsp leg
		M96.69	Fx bone following insrt ortho implnt/prosth/bone plt
		T84.11ØA	Breakdown (mechanical) of int fix of right humerus, init
		T84.111A	Breakdown (mechanical) of int fix of left humerus, init
		T84.112A	Breakdown (mechanical) of int fix of bone of r forearm, init
		T84.113A	Breakdown of int fix of bone of left forearm, init
		T84.114A	Breakdown (mechanical) of int fix of right femur, init
		T84.115A	Breakdown (mechanical) of int fix of left femur, init
		T84.116A	Breakdown (mechanical) of int fix of bone of r low leg, init
		T84.117A	Breakdown (mechanical) of int fix of bone of l low leg, init
		T84.119A	Breakdown (mechanical) of int fix of unsp bone of limb, init
		T84.12ØA	Displacement of int fix of right humerus, init
		T84.121A	Displacement of int fix of left humerus, init
		T84.122A	Displacement of int fix of bone of right forearm, init
		T84.123A	Displacement of int fix of bone of left forearm, init
		T84.124A	Displacement of int fix of right femur, init
		T84.125A	Displacement of internal fixation device of left femur, init
		T84.126A	Displacement of int fix of bone of right lower leg, init
		T84.127A	Displacement of int fix of bone of left lower leg, init
		T84.129A	Displacement of int fix of unsp bone of limb, init
		T84.19ØA	Mech compl of int fix of right humerus, init
		T84.191A	Mech compl of internal fixation device of left humerus, init
		T84.192A	Mech compl of int fix of bone of right forearm, init
		T84.193A	Mech compl of int fix of bone of left forearm, init
		T84.194A	Mech compl of internal fixation device of right femur, init
		T84.195A	Mech compl of internal fixation device of left femur, init
		T84.196A	Mech compl of int fix of bone of right lower leg, init
		T84.197A	Mech compl of int fix of bone of left lower leg, init
		T84.199A	Mech compl of int fix of unsp bone of limb, init
		T84.21ØA	Breakdown of int fix of bones of hand and fingers, init
		T84.213A	Breakdown of int fix of bones of foot and toes, init
		T84.216A	Breakdown (mechanical) of int fix of vertebrae, init
		T84.218A	Breakdown (mechanical) of int fix of bones, init

(Continued on next page)

[Brackets] indicate valid character values for each code. Character value meanings provided for each code grouping.

ICD-9-CM		ICD-10-CM	
996.49	OTH MECH COMPL OTH INT ORTHOPEDIC DEVC IMPL&GFT **(Continued)**	**T84.22ØA**	Displacement of int fix of bones of hand and fingers, init
		T84.223A	Displacement of int fix of bones of foot and toes, init
		T84.226A	Displacement of internal fixation device of vertebrae, init
		T84.228A	Displacement of internal fixation device of oth bones, init
		T84.29ØA	Mech compl of int fix of bones of hand and fingers, init
		T84.293A	Mech compl of int fix of bones of foot and toes, init
		T84.296A	Mech compl of internal fixation device of vertebrae, init
		T84.298A	Mech compl of internal fixation device of oth bones, init
		T84.31ØA	Breakdown (mechanical) of electronic bone stimulator, init
		T84.318A	Breakdown of bone devices, implants and grafts, init
		T84.32ØA	Displacement of electronic bone stimulator, init encntr
		T84.328A	Displacement of oth bone devices, implants and grafts, init
		T84.39ØA	Mech compl of electronic bone stimulator, initial encounter
		T84.398A	Mech compl of oth bone devices, implants and grafts, init
		T84.41ØA	Breakdown (mechanical) of muscle and tendon graft, init
		T84.418A	Brkdwn internal orth devices, implants and grafts, init
		T84.42ØA	Displacement of muscle and tendon graft, initial encounter
		T84.428A	Displacmnt of internal orth devices, implnt and grafts, init
		T84.49ØA	Mech compl of muscle and tendon graft, initial encounter
		T84.498A	Mech compl of internal orth devices, implnt and grafts, init
996.51	MECHANICAL COMPLICATION DUE TO CORNEAL GRAFT	**T85.318A**	Breakdown (mechanical) of ocular prosth dev/grft, init
		T85.328A	Displacement of ocular prosth dev/grft, init
		T85.398A	Mech compl of ocular prosth dev/grft, init
		T86.84Ø	Corneal transplant rejection
		T86.841	Corneal transplant failure
996.52	MECH COMPLICATION DUE OTHER TISSUE GRAFT NEC	**T86.82Ø**	Skin graft (allograft) rejection
		T86.821	Skin graft (allograft) (autograft) failure
		T86.822	Skin graft (allograft) (autograft) infection
		T86.828	Other complications of skin graft (allograft) (autograft)
		T86.829	Unsp complication of skin graft (allograft) (autograft)
996.53	MECH COMPLICATION DUE OCULAR LENS PROSTHESIS	**T85.21XA**	Breakdown (mechanical) of intraocular lens, init encntr
		T85.22XA	Displacement of intraocular lens, initial encounter
		T85.29XA	Mech compl of intraocular lens, initial encounter
996.54	MECHANICAL COMPLICATION DUE TO BREAST PROSTHESIS	**T85.41XA**	Breakdown of breast prosthesis and implant, init
		T85.42XA	Displacement of breast prosthesis and implant, init encntr
		T85.43XA	Leakage of breast prosthesis and implant, initial encounter
		T85.44XA	Capsular contracture of breast implant, initial encounter
		T85.49XA	Mech compl of breast prosthesis and implant, init encntr
996.55	MECHANICAL COMPLICATION DUE ARTIFICIAL SKIN GRAF	**T85.613A**	Breakdown of artificial skin grft /decellular alloderm, init
		T85.623A	Displacmnt of artif skin grft /decellular alloderm, init
		T85.693A	Mech compl of artif skin grft /decellular alloderm, init
996.56	MECH COMPS DUE PERITONEAL DIALYSIS CATHETER	**T85.611A**	Breakdown of intraperitoneal dialysis catheter, init
		T85.621A	Displacement of intraperitoneal dialysis catheter, init
		T85.631A	Leakage of intraperitoneal dialysis catheter, init encntr
		T85.691A	Mech compl of intraperitoneal dialysis catheter, init encntr
996.57	COMPLICATION, DUE TO INSULIN PUMP	**T85.614A**	Breakdown (mechanical) of insulin pump, initial encounter
		T85.624A	Displacement of insulin pump, initial encounter
		T85.633A	Leakage of insulin pump, initial encounter
		T85.694A	Mech compl of insulin pump, initial encounter
996.59	MECH COMP DUE OTH IMPLANT&INTERNAL DEVICE NEC	**T85.31ØA**	Breakdown of prosthetic orbit of right eye, init
		T85.311A	Breakdown (mechanical) of prosthetic orbit of left eye, init
		T85.318A	Breakdown (mechanical) of ocular prosth dev/grft, init
		T85.32ØA	Displacement of prosthetic orbit of right eye, init encntr
		T85.321A	Displacement of prosthetic orbit of left eye, init encntr
		T85.328A	Displacement of ocular prosth dev/grft, init
		T85.39ØA	Mech compl of prosthetic orbit of right eye, init encntr
		T85.391A	Mech compl of prosthetic orbit of left eye, init encntr
		T85.398A	Mech compl of ocular prosth dev/grft, init
		T85.51ØA	Breakdown (mechanical) of bile duct prosthesis, init encntr
		T85.511A	Breakdown of esophageal anti-reflux device, init
		T85.518A	Breakdown (mechanical) of GI prosth dev/grft, init
		T85.52ØA	Displacement of bile duct prosthesis, initial encounter
		T85.521A	Displacement of esophageal anti-reflux device, init encntr
		T85.528A	Displacement of gastrointestinal prosth dev/grft, init
		T85.59ØA	Mech compl of bile duct prosthesis, initial encounter
		T85.591A	Mech compl of esophageal anti-reflux device, init encntr
		T85.598A	Mech compl of gastrointestinal prosth dev/grft, init
		T85.61ØA	Breakdown of epidural and subdural infusion catheter, init
		T85.612A	Breakdown (mechanical) of permanent sutures, init encntr
		T85.618A	Breakdown (mechanical) of internal prosth dev/grft, init
		T85.62ØA	Displacmnt of epidural and subdural infusion catheter, init
		T85.622A	Displacement of permanent sutures, initial encounter
		T85.628A	Displacement of internal prosth dev/grft, init
		T85.63ØA	Leakage of epidural and subdural infusion catheter, init
		T85.638A	Leakage of internal prosth dev/grft, init
		T85.69ØA	Mech compl of epidural and subdural infusion catheter, init
		T85.692A	Mech compl of permanent sutures, initial encounter
		T85.698A	Mech compl of internal prosth dev/grft, init
996.6Ø	INF&INFLAM REACT DUE UNSPEC DEVICE IMPLANT&GRAFT	**T85.79XA**	Infect/inflm reaction due to oth int prosth dev/grft, init
996.61	INF&INFLAM REACT DUE CARD DEVICE IMPLANT&GRAFT	**T82.6XXA**	Infect/inflm reaction due to cardiac valve prosthesis, init
		T82.7XXA	Infect/inflm react d/t oth cardi/vasc dev/implnt/grft, init

ICD-9-CM		ICD-10-CM	
996.62	INF&INFLAM REACT DUE OTH VASC DEVICE IMPLANT&GFT	**T82.7XXA**	Infect/inflm react d/t oth cardi/vasc dev/implnt/grft, init
996.63	INF&INFLAM REACT DUE NERV SYSTEM DEVICE IMPL&GFT	**T85.79XA**	Infect/inflm reaction due to oth int prosth dev/grft, init
996.64	INF&INFLAM REACTION DUE INDWELL URINARY CATHETER	**T83.51XA**	Infect/inflm reaction due to indwell urinary catheter, init
996.65	INF&INFLAM REACT DUE OTH GU DEVICE IMPLANT&GRAFT	**T83.59XA**	Infect/inflm react d/t prosth dev/grft in urinry sys, init
		T83.6XXA	Infect/inflm react d/t prosth dev/grft in genitl trct, init
996.66	INF&INFLAM REACTION DUE INTRL JOINT PROSTHESIS	**T84.5ØXA**	Infect/inflm reaction due to unsp int joint prosth, init
		T84.51XA	Infect/inflm reaction due to internal right hip prosth, init
		T84.52XA	Infect/inflm reaction due to internal left hip prosth, init
		T84.53XA	Infect/inflm reaction due to internal r knee prosth, init
		T84.54XA	Infect/inflm reaction due to internal left knee prosth, init
		T84.59XA	Infect/inflm reaction due to oth internal joint prosth, init
996.67	INF&INFLAM-OTH INTRL ORTH DEVICE IMPLANT&GRAFT	**T84.6ØXA**	Infect/inflm reaction due to int fix of unsp site, init
		T84.61ØA	Infect/inflm reaction due to int fix of right humerus, init
		T84.611A	Infect/inflm reaction due to int fix of left humerus, init
		T84.612A	Infect/inflm reaction due to int fix of right radius, init
		T84.613A	Infect/inflm reaction due to int fix of left radius, init
		T84.614A	Infect/inflm reaction due to int fix of right ulna, init
		T84.615A	Infect/inflm reaction due to int fix of left ulna, init
		T84.619A	Infect/inflm react due to int fix of unsp bone of arm, init
		T84.62ØA	Infect/inflm reaction due to int fix of right femur, init
		T84.621A	Infect/inflm reaction due to int fix of left femur, init
		T84.622A	Infect/inflm reaction due to int fix of right tibia, init
		T84.623A	Infect/inflm reaction due to int fix of left tibia, init
		T84.624A	Infect/inflm reaction due to int fix of right fibula, init
		T84.625A	Infect/inflm reaction due to int fix of left fibula, init
		T84.629A	Infect/inflm react due to int fix of unsp bone of leg, init
		T84.63XA	Infect/inflm reaction due to int fix of spine, init
		T84.69XA	Infect/inflm reaction due to int fix of site, init
		T84.7XXA	Infect/inflm react due to oth int orth prosth dev/grft, init
996.68	INF&INFLAM REACT DUE PERITON DIALYSIS CATHETER	**T85.71XA**	Infect/inflm reaction due to periton dialysis catheter, init
996.69	INF&INFLAM REACT-OTH INTRL PROSTH DEVC IMPL&GFT	**T85.72XA**	Infect/inflm reaction due to insulin pump, init
		T85.79XA	Infect/inflm reaction due to oth int prosth dev/grft, init
		T86.842	Corneal transplant infection
996.7Ø	OTH COMPS DUE UNSPEC DEVICE IMPLANT&GRAFT	**T85.9XXA**	Unsp complication of internal prosth dev/grft, init
996.71	OTHER COMPLICATIONS DUE HEART VALVE PROSTHESIS	**T82.817A**	Embolism of cardiac prosth dev/grft, init
		T82.827A	Fibrosis of cardiac prosth dev/grft, init
		T82.837A	Hemorrhage of cardiac prosth dev/grft, init
		T82.847A	Pain from cardiac prosth dev/grft, init
		T82.857A	Stenosis of cardiac prosth dev/grft, init
		T82.867A	Thrombosis of cardiac prosth dev/grft, init
		T82.897A	Oth complication of cardiac prosth dev/grft, init
		T82.9XXA	Unsp comp of cardiac and vascular prosth dev/grft, init
996.72	OTH COMPS DUE OTH CARD DEVICE IMPLANT&GRAFT	**T82.817A**	Embolism of cardiac prosth dev/grft, init
		T82.827A	Fibrosis of cardiac prosth dev/grft, init
		T82.837A	Hemorrhage of cardiac prosth dev/grft, init
		T82.847A	Pain from cardiac prosth dev/grft, init
		T82.857A	Stenosis of cardiac prosth dev/grft, init
		T82.867A	Thrombosis of cardiac prosth dev/grft, init
		T82.897A	Oth complication of cardiac prosth dev/grft, init
		T82.9XXA	Unsp comp of cardiac and vascular prosth dev/grft, init
996.73	OTH COMPS DUE RENAL DIALYSIS DEVICE IMPLANT&GFT	**T82.818A**	Embolism of vascular prosth dev/grft, init
		T82.828A	Fibrosis of vascular prosth dev/grft, init
		T82.838A	Hemorrhage of vascular prosth dev/grft, init
		T82.848A	Pain from vascular prosth dev/grft, init
		T82.858A	Stenosis of vascular prosth dev/grft, init
		T82.868A	Thrombosis of vascular prosth dev/grft, init
		T82.898A	Oth complication of vascular prosth dev/grft, init
996.74	OTH COMPS DUE OTH VASCULAR DEVICE IMPLANT&GRAFT	**T82.818A**	Embolism of vascular prosth dev/grft, init
		T82.828A	Fibrosis of vascular prosth dev/grft, init
		T82.838A	Hemorrhage of vascular prosth dev/grft, init
		T82.848A	Pain from vascular prosth dev/grft, init
		T82.858A	Stenosis of vascular prosth dev/grft, init
		T82.868A	Thrombosis of vascular prosth dev/grft, init
		T82.898A	Oth complication of vascular prosth dev/grft, init
		T82.9XXA	Unsp comp of cardiac and vascular prosth dev/grft, init
996.75	OTH COMPS DUE NERV SYSTEM DEVICE IMPLANT&GRAFT	**T85.81XA**	Embolism due to internal prosth dev/grft, NEC, init
		T85.82XA	Fibrosis due to internal prosth dev/grft, NEC, init
		T85.83XA	Hemorrhage due to internal prosth dev/grft, NEC, init
		T85.84XA	Pain due to internal prosth dev/grft, NEC, init
		T85.85XA	Stenosis due to internal prosth dev/grft, NEC, init
		T85.86XA	Thrombosis due to internal prosth dev/grft, NEC, init
		T85.89XA	Oth complication of internal prosth dev/grft, NEC, init
996.76	OTH COMPS DUE GENITOURINARY DEVICE IMPLANT&GRAFT	**T83.81XA**	Embolism of genitourinary prosth dev/grft, init
		T83.82XA	Fibrosis of genitourinary prosth dev/grft, init
		T83.83XA	Hemorrhage of genitourinary prosth dev/grft, init
		T83.84XA	Pain from genitourinary prosth dev/grft, init
		T83.85XA	Stenosis of genitourinary prosth dev/grft, init
		T83.86XA	Thrombosis of genitourinary prosth dev/grft, init
		T83.89XA	Oth complication of genitourinary prosth dev/grft, init
		T83.9XXA	Unsp complication of genitourinary prosth dev/grft, init

ICD-9-CM			ICD-10-CM	
996.77	OTH COMPLICATIONS DUE INTERNAL JOINT PROSTHESIS		**T84.81XA**	Embolism due to internal orthopedic prosth dev/grft, init
			T84.82XA	Fibrosis due to internal orthopedic prosth dev/grft, init
			T84.83XA	Hemorrhage due to internal orthopedic prosth dev/grft, init
			T84.84XA	Pain due to internal orthopedic prosth dev/grft, init
			T84.85XA	Stenosis due to internal orthopedic prosth dev/grft, init
			T84.86XA	Thrombosis due to internal orthopedic prosth dev/grft, init
			T84.89XA	Oth comp of internal orthopedic prosth dev/grft, init
			T84.9XXA	Unsp comp of internal orthopedic prosth dev/grft, init
996.78	OTH COMPS DUE OTH INTRL ORTHOPED DEVICE IMPL&GFT		**T84.81XA**	Embolism due to internal orthopedic prosth dev/grft, init
			T84.82XA	Fibrosis due to internal orthopedic prosth dev/grft, init
			T84.83XA	Hemorrhage due to internal orthopedic prosth dev/grft, init
			T84.84XA	Pain due to internal orthopedic prosth dev/grft, init
			T84.85XA	Stenosis due to internal orthopedic prosth dev/grft, init
			T84.86XA	Thrombosis due to internal orthopedic prosth dev/grft, init
			T84.89XA	Oth comp of internal orthopedic prosth dev/grft, init
			T84.9XXA	Unsp comp of internal orthopedic prosth dev/grft, init
996.79	OTH COMPS DUE OTH INTRL PROSTH DEVICE IMPL&GFT		**T85.81XA**	Embolism due to internal prosth dev/grft, NEC, init
			T85.82XA	Fibrosis due to internal prosth dev/grft, NEC, init
			T85.83XA	Hemorrhage due to internal prosth dev/grft, NEC, init
			T85.84XA	Pain due to internal prosth dev/grft, NEC, init
			T85.85XA	Stenosis due to internal prosth dev/grft, NEC, init
			T85.86XA	Thrombosis due to internal prosth dev/grft, NEC, init
			T85.89XA	Oth complication of internal prosth dev/grft, NEC, init
			T86.848	Other complications of corneal transplant
			T86.849	Unspecified complication of corneal transplant
996.8Ø	COMPLICATIONS TRANSPLANTED ORGAN UNSPEC SITE		**T86.9Ø**	Unsp complication of unsp transplanted organ and tissue
			T86.91	Unspecified transplanted organ and tissue rejection
			T86.92	Unspecified transplanted organ and tissue failure
			T86.93	Unspecified transplanted organ and tissue infection
			T86.99	Other complications of unsp transplanted organ and tissue
996.81	COMPLICATIONS OF TRANSPLANTED KIDNEY		**T86.1Ø**	Unspecified complication of kidney transplant
			T86.11	Kidney transplant rejection
			T86.12	Kidney transplant failure
			T86.13	Kidney transplant infection
			T86.19	Other complication of kidney transplant
996.82	COMPLICATIONS OF TRANSPLANTED LIVER		**T86.4Ø**	Unspecified complication of liver transplant
			T86.41	Liver transplant rejection
			T86.42	Liver transplant failure
			T86.43	Liver transplant infection
			T86.49	Other complications of liver transplant
996.83	COMPLICATIONS OF TRANSPLANTED HEART		**T86.2Ø**	Unspecified complication of heart transplant
			T86.21	Heart transplant rejection
			T86.22	Heart transplant failure
			T86.23	Heart transplant infection
			T86.29Ø	Cardiac allograft vasculopathy
			T86.298	Other complications of heart transplant
		◘	**T86.3Ø**	Unspecified complication of heart-lung transplant
		◘	**T86.31**	Heart-lung transplant rejection
		◘	**T86.32**	Heart-lung transplant failure
		◘	**T86.33**	Heart-lung transplant infection
		◘	**T86.39**	Other complications of heart-lung transplant
996.84	COMPLICATIONS OF TRANSPLANTED LUNG	◘	**T86.3Ø**	Unspecified complication of heart-lung transplant
		◘	**T86.31**	Heart-lung transplant rejection
		◘	**T86.32**	Heart-lung transplant failure
		◘	**T86.33**	Heart-lung transplant infection
		◘	**T86.39**	Other complications of heart-lung transplant
			T86.81Ø	Lung transplant rejection
			T86.811	Lung transplant failure
			T86.812	Lung transplant infection
			T86.818	Other complications of lung transplant
			T86.819	Unspecified complication of lung transplant
996.85	COMPLICATIONS OF BONE MARROW TRANSPLANT		**T86.ØØ**	Unspecified complication of bone marrow transplant
			T86.Ø1	Bone marrow transplant rejection
			T86.Ø2	Bone marrow transplant failure
			T86.Ø3	Bone marrow transplant infection
			T86.Ø9	Other complications of bone marrow transplant
996.86	COMPLICATIONS OF TRANSPLANTED PANCREAS		**T86.89Ø**	Other transplanted tissue rejection
			T86.891	Other transplanted tissue failure
			T86.892	Other transplanted tissue infection
			T86.898	Other complications of other transplanted tissue
			T86.899	Unspecified complication of other transplanted tissue
996.87	COMPLICATIONS OF TRANSPLANTED ORGAN INTESTINE		**T86.85Ø**	Intestine transplant rejection
			T86.851	Intestine transplant failure
			T86.852	Intestine transplant infection
			T86.858	Other complications of intestine transplant
			T86.859	Unspecified complication of intestine transplant
996.88	COMPLICATIONS OF TRANSPLANTED ORGAN STEM CELL		**T86.5**	Complications of stem cell transplant

ICD-9-CM		ICD-10-CM	
996.89	COMPLICATIONS OF OTHER TRANSPLANTED ORGAN	**T86.83Ø**	Bone graft rejection
		T86.831	Bone graft failure
		T86.832	Bone graft infection
		T86.838	Other complications of bone graft
		T86.839	Unspecified complication of bone graft
		T86.89Ø	Other transplanted tissue rejection
		T86.891	Other transplanted tissue failure
		T86.892	Other transplanted tissue infection
		T86.898	Other complications of other transplanted tissue
		T86.899	Unspecified complication of other transplanted tissue
996.9Ø	COMPLICATIONS UNSPECIFIED REATTACHED EXTREMITY	**T87.ØX9**	Complications of reattached (part of) unsp upper extremity
		T87.1X9	Complications of reattached (part of) unsp lower extremity
996.91	COMPLICATIONS OF REATTACHED FOREARM	**T87.ØX9**	Complications of reattached (part of) unsp upper extremity
996.92	COMPLICATIONS OF REATTACHED HAND	**T87.ØX9**	Complications of reattached (part of) unsp upper extremity
996.93	COMPLICATIONS OF REATTACHED FINGER	**T87.ØX9**	Complications of reattached (part of) unsp upper extremity
996.94	COMPLICATIONS REATTCH UPPER EXTREMITY OTH&UNSPEC	**T87.ØX1**	Complications of reattached (part of) right upper extremity
		T87.ØX2	Complications of reattached (part of) left upper extremity
		T87.ØX9	Complications of reattached (part of) unsp upper extremity
996.95	COMPLICATIONS OF REATTACHED FOOT AND TOE	**T87.1X9**	Complications of reattached (part of) unsp lower extremity
996.96	COMPLICATIONS REATTCH LOWER EXTREMITY OTH&UNSPEC	**T87.1X1**	Complications of reattached (part of) right lower extremity
		T87.1X2	Complications of reattached (part of) left lower extremity
		T87.1X9	Complications of reattached (part of) unsp lower extremity
996.99	COMPLICATIONS OTHER SPEC REATTACHED BODY PART	**T87.1X9**	Complications of reattached (part of) unsp lower extremity
		T87.2	Complications of other reattached body part
997.ØØ	UNSPECIFIED NERVOUS SYSTEM COMPLICATION NEC	**G97.81**	Other intraoperative complications of nervous system
997.Ø1	CENTRAL NERVOUS SYSTEM COMPLICATION NEC	**G97.2**	Intracranial hypotension following ventricular shunting
		G97.81	Other intraoperative complications of nervous system
		G97.82	Oth postproc complications and disorders of nervous sys
997.Ø2	IATROGENIC CEREBROVASCULAR INFARCT/HEMORRHAGE NE	**G97.31**	Intraop hemor/hemtom of a nervous sys org comp nrv sys proc
		G97.32	Intraop hemor/hemtom of a nervous sys org comp oth procedure
		I97.81Ø	Intraoperative cerebvasc infarction during cardiac surgery
		I97.811	Intraoperative cerebrovascular infarction during oth surgery
		I97.82Ø	Postprocedural cerebvasc infarction during cardiac surgery
		I97.821	Postprocedural cerebrovascular infarction during oth surgery
997.Ø9	OTHER NERVOUS SYSTEM COMPLICATIONS NEC	**GØ3.8**	Meningitis due to other specified causes
		G97.Ø	Cerebrospinal fluid leak from spinal puncture
		G97.81	Other intraoperative complications of nervous system
		G97.82	Oth postproc complications and disorders of nervous sys
997.1	CARDIAC COMPLICATIONS NEC	**I97.11Ø**	Postproc cardiac insufficiency following cardiac surgery
		I97.111	Postprocedural cardiac insufficiency following other surgery
		I97.12Ø	Postprocedural cardiac arrest following cardiac surgery
		I97.121	Postprocedural cardiac arrest following other surgery
		I97.13Ø	Postprocedural heart failure following cardiac surgery
		I97.131	Postprocedural heart failure following other surgery
		I97.19Ø	Oth postproc cardiac functn disturb fol cardiac surgery
		I97.191	Oth postproc cardiac functn disturb following oth surgery
		I97.71Ø	Intraoperative cardiac arrest during cardiac surgery
		I97.711	Intraoperative cardiac arrest during other surgery
		I97.79Ø	Oth intraop cardiac functn disturb during cardiac surgery
		I97.791	Oth intraop cardiac functional disturb during oth surgery
		I97.88	Oth intraoperative complications of the circ sys, NEC
		I97.89	Oth postproc comp and disorders of the circ sys, NEC
997.2	PERIPHERAL VASCULAR COMPLICATIONS NEC	**T81.718A**	Complication of artery following a procedure, NEC, init
		T81.719A	Complication of unsp artery following a procedure, NEC, init
		T81.72XA	Complication of vein following a procedure, NEC, init
997.31	VENTILATOR ASSOCIATED PNEUMONIA	**J95.851**	Ventilator associated pneumonia
997.32	POSTPROCEDURAL ASPIRATION PNEUMONIA	**J95.89**	Oth postproc complications and disorders of resp sys, NEC
997.39	OTHER RESPIRATORY COMPLICATIONS	**J95.4**	Chemical pneumonitis due to anesthesia
		J95.5	Postprocedural subglottic stenosis
		J95.859	Other complication of respirator [ventilator]
		J95.88	Oth intraoperative complications of respiratory system, NEC
		J95.89	Oth postproc complications and disorders of resp sys, NEC
997.41	RETAINED CHOLELITHIASIS FOLLOW CHOLECYSTECTOMY	**K91.86**	Retained cholelithiasis following cholecystectomy
997.49	OTHER DIGESTIVE SYSTEM COMPLICATIONS	**K91.3**	Postprocedural intestinal obstruction
		K91.81	Other intraoperative complications of digestive system
		K91.82	Postprocedural hepatic failure
		K91.83	Postprocedural hepatorenal syndrome
		K91.89	Oth postprocedural complications and disorders of dgstv sys

[Brackets] indicate valid character values for each code. Character value meanings provided for each code grouping.

ICD-9-CM		ICD-10-CM	
997.5	URINARY COMPLICATIONS NEC	**N99.Ø**	Postprocedural (acute) (chronic) kidney failure
		N99.52Ø	Hemorrhage of other external stoma of urinary tract
		N99.521	Infection of other external stoma of urinary tract
		N99.522	Malfunction of other external stoma of urinary tract
		N99.528	Other complication of other external stoma of urinary tract
		N99.53Ø	Hemorrhage of other stoma of urinary tract
		N99.531	Infection of other stoma of urinary tract
		N99.532	Malfunction of other stoma of urinary tract
		N99.538	Other complication of other stoma of urinary tract
		N99.81	Other intraoperative complications of genitourinary system
		N99.89	Oth postprocedural complications and disorders of GU sys
997.6Ø	LATE COMPLICATIONS AMPUTATION STUMP UNS NEC	**T87.9**	Unspecified complications of amputation stump
997.61	NEUROMA OF AMPUTATION STUMP NEC	**T87.3Ø**	Neuroma of amputation stump, unspecified extremity
		T87.31	Neuroma of amputation stump, right upper extremity
		T87.32	Neuroma of amputation stump, left upper extremity
		T87.33	Neuroma of amputation stump, right lower extremity
		T87.34	Neuroma of amputation stump, left lower extremity
997.62	INFECTION OF AMPUTATION STUMP NEC	**T87.4Ø**	Infection of amputation stump, unspecified extremity
		T87.41	Infection of amputation stump, right upper extremity
		T87.42	Infection of amputation stump, left upper extremity
		T87.43	Infection of amputation stump, right lower extremity
		T87.44	Infection of amputation stump, left lower extremity
997.69	OTHER LATE AMPUTATION STUMP COMPLICATION NEC	**T87.5Ø**	Necrosis of amputation stump, unspecified extremity
		T87.51	Necrosis of amputation stump, right upper extremity
		T87.52	Necrosis of amputation stump, left upper extremity
		T87.53	Necrosis of amputation stump, right lower extremity
		T87.54	Necrosis of amputation stump, left lower extremity
		T87.81	Dehiscence of amputation stump
		T87.89	Other complications of amputation stump
997.71	VASCULAR COMPLICATIONS OF MESENTERIC ARTERY	**T81.71ØA**	Complication of mesent art following a procedure, NEC, init
997.72	VASCULAR COMPLICATIONS OF RENAL ARTERY	**T81.711A**	Comp of renal artery following a procedure, NEC, init
997.79	VASCULAR COMPLICATIONS OF OTHER VESSELS	**T81.718A**	Complication of artery following a procedure, NEC, init
		T81.719A	Complication of unsp artery following a procedure, NEC, init
		T81.72XA	Complication of vein following a procedure, NEC, init
997.91	HYPERTENSION NEC	➡ **I97.3**	Postprocedural hypertension
997.99	OTH COMPS AFFECT OTH SPEC BODY SYSTEMS NEC	**D78.81**	Other intraoperative complications of the spleen
		D78.89	Other postprocedural complications of the spleen
		E89.81Ø	Postproc hemor/hemtom of endo sys org fol an endo sys proc
		E89.811	Postproc hemor/hemtom of an endo sys org fol oth procedure
		E89.89	Oth postproc endocrine and metabolic comp and disorders
		H59.Ø11	Keratopathy (bullous aphakic) fol cataract surgery, r eye
		H59.Ø12	Keratopathy (bullous aphakic) fol cataract surgery, left eye
		H59.Ø13	Keratopathy (bullous aphakic) following cataract surgery, bi
		H59.Ø19	Keratopathy (bullous aphakic) fol cataract surgery, unsp eye
		H59.Ø31	Cystoid macular edema following cataract surgery, right eye
		H59.Ø32	Cystoid macular edema following cataract surgery, left eye
		H59.Ø33	Cystoid macular edema following cataract surgery, bilateral
		H59.Ø39	Cystoid macular edema following cataract surgery, unsp eye
		H59.Ø91	Other disorders of the right eye following cataract surgery
		H59.Ø92	Other disorders of the left eye following cataract surgery
		H59.Ø93	Oth disorders of the eye following cataract surgery, bi
		H59.Ø99	Other disorders of unsp eye following cataract surgery
		H59.811	Chorioretinal scars after surgery for detachment, right eye
		H59.812	Chorioretinal scars after surgery for detachment, left eye
		H59.813	Chorioretinal scars after surgery for detachment, bilateral
		H59.819	Chorioretinal scars after surgery for detachment, unsp eye
		H59.88	Oth intraoperative complications of eye and adnexa, NEC
		H59.89	Oth postproc comp and disorders of eye and adnexa, NEC
		H95.811	Postprocedural stenosis of right external ear canal
		H95.812	Postprocedural stenosis of left external ear canal
		H95.813	Postprocedural stenosis of external ear canal, bilateral
		H95.819	Postprocedural stenosis of unspecified external ear canal
		H95.88	Oth intraop comp and disorders of the ear/mastd, NEC
		H95.89	Oth postproc comp and disorders of the ear/mastd, NEC
		M96.89	Oth intraop and postproc comp and disorders of the ms sys
		N98.1	Hyperstimulation of ovaries
		N98.2	Comp of attempt introduce of fertilized ovum fol in vitro
		N98.3	Comp of attempted introduction of embryo in embryo transfer
		N98.8	Other complications associated with artificial fertilization
		N98.9	Complication associated with artificial fertilization, unsp
998.ØØ	POSTOPERATIVE SHOCK UNSPECIFIED	**T81.1ØXA**	Postprocedural shock unspecified, initial encounter
998.Ø1	POSTOPERATIVE SHOCK CARDIOGENIC	**T81.11XA**	Postprocedural cardiogenic shock, initial encounter
998.Ø2	POSTOPERATIVE SHOCK SEPTIC	**T81.12XA**	Postprocedural septic shock, initial encounter
998.Ø9	POSTOPERATIVE SHOCK OTHER	**T81.19XA**	Other postprocedural shock, initial encounter

ICD-9-CM	ICD-10-CM	
998.11 HEMORRHAGE COMPLICATING A PROCEDURE NEC	**D78.Ø1**	Intraop hemor/hemtom of the spleen comp a proc on the spleen
	D78.Ø2	Intraop hemor/hemtom of the spleen comp oth procedure
	D78.21	Postprocedural hemor/hemtom of the spleen fol proc on spleen
	D78.22	Postproc hemor/hemtom of the spleen following oth procedure
	E36.Ø1	Intraop hemor/hemtom of endo sys org comp an endo sys proc
	E36.Ø2	Intraop hemor/hemtom of an endo sys org comp oth procedure
	G97.31	Intraop hemor/hemtom of a nervous sys org comp nrv sys proc
	G97.32	Intraop hemor/hemtom of a nervous sys org comp oth procedure
	G97.51	Postproc hemor/hemtom of a nrv sys org fol a nrv sys proc
	G97.52	Postproc hemor/hemtom of a nervous sys org fol oth procedure
	H59.111	Intraop hemor/hemtom of r eye and adnexa comp an opth proc
	H59.112	Intraop hemor/hemtom of l eye and adnexa comp an opth proc
	H59.113	Intraop hemor/hemtom of eye and adnexa comp an opth proc, bi
	H59.119	Intraop hemor/hemtom of unsp eye and adnx comp an opth proc
	H59.121	Intraop hemor/hemtom of right eye and adnexa comp oth proc
	H59.122	Intraop hemor/hemtom of left eye and adnexa comp oth proc
	H59.123	Intraop hemor/hemtom of eye and adnexa comp oth proc, bi
	H59.129	Intraop hemor/hemtom of unsp eye and adnexa comp oth proc
	H59.311	Postproc hemor/hemtom of r eye and adnexa fol an opth proc
	H59.312	Postproc hemor/hemtom of l eye and adnexa fol an opth proc
	H59.313	Postproc hemor/hemtom of eye and adnexa fol an opth proc, bi
	H59.319	Postproc hemor/hemtom of unsp eye and adnx fol an opth proc
	H59.321	Postproc hemor/hemtom of right eye and adnexa fol oth proc
	H59.322	Postproc hemor/hemtom of left eye and adnexa fol oth proc
	H59.323	Postproc hemor/hemtom of eye and adnexa fol oth proc, bi
	H59.329	Postproc hemor/hemtom of unsp eye and adnexa fol oth proc
	H95.21	Intraop hemor/hemtom of ear/mastd comp a proc on ear/mastd
	H95.22	Intraop hemor/hemtom of ear/mastd complicating oth procedure
	H95.41	Postproc hemor/hemtom of ear/mastd fol proc on ear/mastd
	H95.42	Postproc hemor/hemtom of ear/mastd following oth procedure
	I97.41Ø	Intraoperative hemor/hemtom of a circ sys org comp card cath
	I97.411	Intraop hemor/hemtom of a circ sys org comp card bypass
	I97.418	Intraop hemor/hemtom of circ sys org comp oth circ sys proc
	I97.42	Intraop hemor/hemtom of a circ sys org comp oth procedure
	I97.61Ø	Postproc hemor/hemtom of a circ sys org fol a cardiac cath
	I97.611	Postproc hemor/hemtom of a circ sys org fol cardiac bypass
	I97.618	Postproc hemor/hemtom of circ sys org fol oth circ sys proc
	I97.62	Postproc hemor/hemtom of a circ sys org fol oth procedure
	J95.61	Intraop hemor/hemtom of a resp sys org comp resp sys proc
	J95.62	Intraop hemor/hemtom of a resp sys org comp oth procedure
	J95.83Ø	Postproc hemor/hemtom of a resp sys org fol a resp sys proc
	J95.831	Postproc hemor/hemtom of a resp sys org fol oth procedure
	K91.61	Intraop hemor/hemtom of dgstv sys org comp a dgstv sys proc
	K91.62	Intraop hemor/hemtom of a dgstv sys org comp oth procedure
	K91.84Ø	Postproc hemor/hemtom of dgstv sys org fol a dgstv sys proc
	K91.841	Postproc hemor/hemtom of a dgstv sys org fol oth procedure
	L76.Ø1	Intraop hemor/hemtom of skin, subcu comp a dermatologic proc
	L76.Ø2	Intraop hemor/hemtom of skin, subcu comp oth procedure
	L76.21	Postproc hemor/hemtom of skin, subcu fol a dermatologic proc
	L76.22	Postproc hemor/hemtom of skin, subcu following oth procedure
	M96.81Ø	Intraop hemor/hemtom of a ms structure comp a ms sys proc
	M96.811	Intraop hemor/hemtom of a ms structure comp oth procedure
	M96.83Ø	Postproc hemor/hemtom of a ms structure fol a ms sys proc
	M96.831	Postproc hemor/hemtom of a ms structure fol oth procedure
	N99.61	Intraop hemor/hemtom of a GU sys org comp a GU sys procedure
	N99.62	Intraop hemor/hemtom of a GU sys org comp oth procedure
	N99.82Ø	Postproc hemor/hemtom of a GU sys org fol a GU sys procedure
	N99.821	Postproc hemor/hemtom of a GU sys org fol oth procedure
998.12 HEMATOMA COMPLICATING A PROCEDURE NEC	**D78.Ø1**	Intraop hemor/hemtom of the spleen comp a proc on the spleen
	D78.Ø2	Intraop hemor/hemtom of the spleen comp oth procedure
	D78.21	Postprocedural hemor/hemtom of the spleen fol proc on spleen
	D78.22	Postproc hemor/hemtom of the spleen following oth procedure
	E36.Ø1	Intraop hemor/hemtom of endo sys org comp an endo sys proc
	E36.Ø2	Intraop hemor/hemtom of an endo sys org comp oth procedure
	G97.31	Intraop hemor/hemtom of a nervous sys org comp nrv sys proc
	G97.32	Intraop hemor/hemtom of a nervous sys org comp oth procedure
	G97.51	Postproc hemor/hemtom of a nrv sys org fol a nrv sys proc
	G97.52	Postproc hemor/hemtom of a nervous sys org fol oth procedure
	H59.111	Intraop hemor/hemtom of r eye and adnexa comp an opth proc
	H59.112	Intraop hemor/hemtom of l eye and adnexa comp an opth proc
	H59.113	Intraop hemor/hemtom of eye and adnexa comp an opth proc, bi
	H59.119	Intraop hemor/hemtom of unsp eye and adnx comp an opth proc
	H59.121	Intraop hemor/hemtom of right eye and adnexa comp oth proc
	H59.122	Intraop hemor/hemtom of left eye and adnexa comp oth proc
	H59.123	Intraop hemor/hemtom of eye and adnexa comp oth proc, bi
	H59.129	Intraop hemor/hemtom of unsp eye and adnexa comp oth proc
	H59.311	Postproc hemor/hemtom of r eye and adnexa fol an opth proc
	H59.312	Postproc hemor/hemtom of l eye and adnexa fol an opth proc
	H59.313	Postproc hemor/hemtom of eye and adnexa fol an opth proc, bi
	H59.319	Postproc hemor/hemtom of unsp eye and adnx fol an opth proc
	H59.321	Postproc hemor/hemtom of right eye and adnexa fol oth proc
(Continued on next page)	**H59.322**	Postproc hemor/hemtom of left eye and adnexa fol oth proc

[Brackets] indicate valid character values for each code. Character value meanings provided for each code grouping.

ICD-9-CM		ICD-10-CM	
998.12	HEMATOMA COMPLICATING A PROCEDURE NEC **(Continued)**	**H59.323**	Postproc hemor/hemtom of eye and adnexa fol oth proc, bi
		H59.329	Postproc hemor/hemtom of unsp eye and adnexa fol oth proc
		H95.21	Intraop hemor/hemtom of ear/mastd comp a proc on ear/mastd
		H95.22	Intraop hemor/hemtom of ear/mastd complicating oth procedure
		H95.41	Postproc hemor/hemtom of ear/mastd fol proc on ear/mastd
		H95.42	Postproc hemor/hemtom of ear/mastd following oth procedure
		I97.41Ø	Intraoperative hemor/hemtom of a circ sys org comp card cath
		I97.411	Intraop hemor/hemtom of a circ sys org comp card bypass
		I97.418	Intraop hemor/hemtom of circ sys org comp oth circ sys proc
		I97.42	Intraop hemor/hemtom of a circ sys org comp oth procedure
		I97.61Ø	Postproc hemor/hemtom of a circ sys org fol a cardiac cath
		I97.611	Postproc hemor/hemtom of a circ sys org fol cardiac bypass
		I97.618	Postproc hemor/hemtom of circ sys org fol oth circ sys proc
		I97.62	Postproc hemor/hemtom of a circ sys org fol oth procedure
		J95.61	Intraop hemor/hemtom of a resp sys org comp resp sys proc
		J95.62	Intraop hemor/hemtom of a resp sys org comp oth procedure
		J95.83Ø	Postproc hemor/hemtom of a resp sys org fol a resp sys proc
		J95.831	Postproc hemor/hemtom of a resp sys org fol oth procedure
		K91.61	Intraop hemor/hemtom of dgstv sys org comp a dgstv sys proc
		K91.62	Intraop hemor/hemtom of a dgstv sys org comp oth procedure
		K91.84Ø	Postproc hemor/hemtom of dgstv sys org fol a dgstv sys proc
		K91.841	Postproc hemor/hemtom of a dgstv sys org fol oth procedure
		L76.Ø1	Intraop hemor/hemtom of skin, subcu comp a dermatologic proc
		L76.Ø2	Intraop hemor/hemtom of skin, subcu comp oth procedure
		L76.21	Postproc hemor/hemtom of skin, subcu fol a dermatologic proc
		L76.22	Postproc hemor/hemtom of skin, subcu following oth procedure
		M96.81Ø	Intraop hemor/hemtom of a ms structure comp a ms sys proc
		M96.811	Intraop hemor/hemtom of a ms structure comp oth procedure
		M96.83Ø	Postproc hemor/hemtom of a ms structure fol a ms sys proc
		M96.831	Postproc hemor/hemtom of a ms structure fol oth procedure
		N99.61	Intraop hemor/hemtom of a GU sys org comp a GU sys procedure
		N99.62	Intraop hemor/hemtom of a GU sys org comp oth procedure
		N99.82Ø	Postproc hemor/hemtom of a GU sys org fol a GU sys procedure
		N99.821	Postproc hemor/hemtom of a GU sys org fol oth procedure
998.13	SEROMA COMPLICATING A PROCEDURE NEC	**T88.8XXA**	Oth complications of surgical and medical care, NEC, init
998.2	ACCIDENTAL PUNCTURE/LACERATION DURING PROC NEC	**D78.11**	Accidental pnctr & lac of the spleen dur proc on the spleen
		D78.12	Accidental pnctr & lac of the spleen during oth procedure
		E36.11	Acc pnctr & lac of an endo sys org during an endo sys proc
		E36.12	Acc pnctr & lac of an endo sys org during oth procedure
		G97.48	Acc pnctr & lac of nervous sys org during a nervous sys proc
		G97.49	Acc pnctr & lac of nervous sys org during oth procedure
		H59.211	Acc pnctr & lac of right eye and adnexa during an opth proc
		H59.212	Acc pnctr & lac of left eye and adnexa during an opth proc
		H59.213	Acc pnctr & lac of eye and adnexa during an opth proc, bi
		H59.219	Acc pnctr & lac of unsp eye and adnexa during an opth proc
		H59.221	Acc pnctr & lac of right eye and adnexa during oth procedure
		H59.222	Acc pnctr & lac of left eye and adnexa during oth procedure
		H59.223	Acc pnctr & lac of eye and adnexa during oth procedure, bi
		H59.229	Acc pnctr & lac of unsp eye and adnexa during oth procedure
		H95.31	Acc pnctr & lac of the ear/mastd dur proc on the ear/mastd
		H95.32	Accidental pnctr & lac of the ear/mastd during oth procedure
		I97.51	Acc pnctr & lac of a circ sys org during a circ sys proc
		I97.52	Acc pnctr & lac of a circ sys org during oth procedure
		J95.71	Accidental pnctr & lac of a resp sys org dur resp sys proc
		J95.72	Acc pnctr & lac of a resp sys org during oth procedure
		K91.71	Accidental pnctr & lac of a dgstv sys org dur dgstv sys proc
		K91.72	Acc pnctr & lac of a dgstv sys org during oth procedure
		L76.11	Acc pnctr & lac of skin, subcu during a dermatologic proc
		L76.12	Accidental pnctr & lac of skin, subcu during oth procedure
		M96.82Ø	Acc pnctr & lac of a ms structure during a ms sys procedure
		M96.821	Acc pnctr & lac of a ms structure during oth procedure
		N99.71	Acc pnctr & lac of a GU sys org during a GU sys procedure
		N99.72	Accidental pnctr & lac of a GU sys org during oth procedure
		T88.8XXA	Oth complications of surgical and medical care, NEC, init
998.3Ø	DISRUPTION OF WOUND UNSPECIFIED	**T81.3ØXA**	Disruption of wound, unspecified, initial encounter
998.31	DISRUPTION OF INTERNAL OPERATION SURGICAL WOUND	**T81.32XA**	Disruption of internal operation (surgical) wound, NEC, init
998.32	DISRUPTION OF EXTERNAL OPERATION SURGICAL WOUND	**T81.31XA**	Disruption of external operation (surgical) wound, NEC, init
998.33	DISRUPTION OF TRAUMATIC INJURY WOUND REPAIR	**T81.33XA**	Disruption of traumatic injury wound repair, init encntr

ICD-9-CM		ICD-10-CM	
998.4	FOREIGN BODY ACCIDENTALLY LEFT DURING PROC NEC	**T81.500A**	Unsp comp of fb acc left in body fol surgical op, init
		T81.501A	Unsp comp of fb acc left in body fol infusn/transfusn, init
		T81.502A	Unsp comp of fb acc left in body fol kidney dialysis, init
		T81.503A	Unsp comp of fb acc left in body fol inject or immuniz, init
		T81.504A	Unsp comp of fb acc left in body following endo exam, init
		T81.505A	Unsp comp of fb acc left in body following heart cath, init
		T81.506A	Unsp comp of fb acc left in body following punctr/cath, init
		T81.507A	Unsp comp of fb acc left in body fol remov cath/pack, init
		T81.508A	Unsp comp of fb acc left in body fol oth procedure, init
		T81.509A	Unsp comp of fb acc left in body fol unsp procedure, init
		T81.510A	Adhes due to fb acc left in body fol surgical op, init
		T81.511A	Adhes due to fb acc left in body fol infusn/transfusn, init
		T81.512A	Adhes due to fb acc left in body fol kidney dialysis, init
		T81.513A	Adhes due to fb acc left in body fol inject or immuniz, init
		T81.514A	Adhes due to fb acc left in body following endo exam, init
		T81.515A	Adhes due to fb acc left in body following heart cath, init
		T81.516A	Adhes due to fb acc left in body following punctr/cath, init
		T81.517A	Adhes due to fb acc left in body fol remov cath/pack, init
		T81.518A	Adhes due to fb acc left in body fol oth procedure, init
		T81.519A	Adhes due to fb acc left in body fol unsp procedure, init
		T81.520A	Obst due to fb acc left in body fol surgical operation, init
		T81.521A	Obst due to fb acc left in body fol infusn/transfusn, init
		T81.522A	Obst due to fb acc left in body fol kidney dialysis, init
		T81.523A	Obst due to fb acc left in body fol inject or immuniz, init
		T81.524A	Obst due to fb acc left in body following endo exam, init
		T81.525A	Obst due to fb acc left in body following heart cath, init
		T81.526A	Obst due to fb acc left in body following punctr/cath, init
		T81.527A	Obst due to fb acc left in body fol remov cath/pack, init
		T81.528A	Obst due to fb acc left in body fol oth procedure, init
		T81.529A	Obst due to fb acc left in body fol unsp procedure, init
		T81.530A	Perf due to fb acc left in body fol surgical operation, init
		T81.531A	Perf due to fb acc left in body fol infusn/transfusn, init
		T81.532A	Perf due to fb acc left in body fol kidney dialysis, init
		T81.533A	Perf due to fb acc left in body fol inject or immuniz, init
		T81.534A	Perf due to fb acc left in body following endo exam, init
		T81.535A	Perf due to fb acc left in body following heart cath, init
		T81.536A	Perf due to fb acc left in body following punctr/cath, init
		T81.537A	Perf due to fb acc left in body fol remov cath/pack, init
		T81.538A	Perf due to fb acc left in body fol oth procedure, init
		T81.539A	Perf due to fb acc left in body fol unsp procedure, init
		T81.590A	Oth comp of fb acc left in body fol surgical operation, init
		T81.591A	Oth comp of fb acc left in body fol infusn/transfusn, init
		T81.592A	Oth comp of fb acc left in body fol kidney dialysis, init
		T81.593A	Oth comp of fb acc left in body fol inject or immuniz, init
		T81.594A	Oth comp of fb acc left in body following endo exam, init
		T81.595A	Oth comp of fb acc left in body following heart cath, init
		T81.596A	Oth comp of fb acc left in body following punctr/cath, init
		T81.597A	Oth comp of fb acc left in body fol remov cath/pack, init
		T81.598A	Oth comp of fb acc left in body fol oth procedure, init
		T81.599A	Oth comp of fb acc left in body fol unsp procedure, init
998.51	INFECTED POSTOPERATIVE SEROMA NEC	**T81.4XXA**	Infection following a procedure, initial encounter
998.59	OTHER POSTOPERATIVE INFECTION NEC	**K68.11**	Postprocedural retroperitoneal abscess
		T81.4XXA	Infection following a procedure, initial encounter
998.6	PERSISTENT POSTOPERATIVE FISTULA NEC	**T81.83XA**	Persistent postprocedural fistula, initial encounter
998.7	ACUT REACT FOREIGN SUBSTANCE ACC LT DUR PROC NEC	**T81.60XA**	Unsp acute reaction to foreign sub acc left dur proc, init
		T81.61XA	Aseptic peritonitis due to forn sub acc left dur proc, init
		T81.69XA	Oth acute reaction to foreign sub acc left dur proc, init
998.81	EMPHYSEMA RESULTING FROM A PROCEDURE NEC	**T81.82XA**	Emphysema (subcutaneous) resulting from a procedure, init
998.82	CATARACT FRAGMENTS IN EYE FOLLOWING SURG NEC	**H59.021**	Cataract (lens) fragmt in eye fol cataract surgery, r eye
		H59.022	Cataract (lens) fragmt in eye fol cataract surgery, left eye
		H59.023	Cataract (lens) fragments in eye fol cataract surgery, bi
		H59.029	Cataract (lens) fragmt in eye fol cataract surgery, unsp eye
998.83	NON-HEALING SURGICAL WOUND NEC	**T81.89XA**	Oth complications of procedures, NEC, init
998.89	OTHER SPECIFIED COMPLICATIONS NEC	**E36.8**	Other intraoperative complications of endocrine system
		L76.81	Oth intraoperative complications of skin, subcu
		L76.82	Oth postprocedural complications of skin, subcu
		T81.89XA	Oth complications of procedures, NEC, init
998.9	UNSPECIFIED COMPLICATION OF PROCEDURE NEC	**T81.9XXA**	Unspecified complication of procedure, initial encounter
999.0	GENERALIZED VACCINIA AS COMP MEDICAL CARE NEC	**T88.1XXA**	Oth complications following immunization, NEC, init
999.1	AIR EMBOLISM AS COMPLICATION OF MEDICAL CARE NEC	**T80.0XXA**	Air embolism fol infusion, tranfs and theraputc inject, init
999.2	OTHER VASCULAR COMPLICATIONS OF MEDICAL CARE NEC	**T80.1XXA**	Vascular comp fol infusn, tranfs and theraputc inject, init
999.31	OTHER & UNS INFECTION D/T CENTRAL VENOUS CATH	**T80.218A**	Other infection due to central venous catheter, init encntr
		T80.219A	Unsp infection due to central venous catheter, init encntr
999.32	BLOODSTREAM INFECT D/T CENTRAL VENOUS CATHETER	**T80.211A**	Bloodstream infection due to central venous catheter, init
999.33	LOCAL INFECTION DUE TO CENTRAL VENOUS CATHETER	**T80.212A**	Local infection due to central venous catheter, init encntr
999.34	ACUTE INFECT FLW TRAN INF/INJ BLOOD & BLOOD PROD	**T80.22XA**	Acute infct fol tranfs,infusn,inject blood/products, init
999.39	COMP MED CARE NEC INF FLW INFUS INJ TRANSFUS/VAC	**N98.0**	Infection associated with artificial insemination
		T80.29XA	Infct fol oth infusion, transfuse and theraputc inject, init
		T88.0XXA	Infection following immunization, initial encounter

ICD-9-CM		ICD-10-CM		
999.41	ANAPHYLACT REACTION D/T ADMIN BLOOD & BLOOD PROD		T80.51XA	Anaphylactic reaction due to admin blood/products, init
999.42	ANAPHYLACTIC REACTION DUE TO VACCINATION		T80.52XA	Anaphylactic reaction due to vaccination, initial encounter
999.49	ANAPHYLACTIC REACTION DUE TO OTHER SERUM		T80.59XA	Anaphylactic reaction due to other serum, initial encounter
999.51	OTH SERUM REACTION D/T ADMIN BLD BLOOD PRODUCTS		T80.61XA	Oth serum reaction due to admin blood/products, init
999.52	OTHER SERUM REACTION DUE TO VACCINATION	▣	M02.211	Postimmunization arthropathy, right shoulder
		▣	M02.212	Postimmunization arthropathy, left shoulder
		▣	M02.219	Postimmunization arthropathy, unspecified shoulder
		▣	M02.221	Postimmunization arthropathy, right elbow
		▣	M02.222	Postimmunization arthropathy, left elbow
		▣	M02.229	Postimmunization arthropathy, unspecified elbow
		▣	M02.231	Postimmunization arthropathy, right wrist
		▣	M02.232	Postimmunization arthropathy, left wrist
		▣	M02.239	Postimmunization arthropathy, unspecified wrist
		▣	M02.241	Postimmunization arthropathy, right hand
		▣	M02.242	Postimmunization arthropathy, left hand
		▣	M02.249	Postimmunization arthropathy, unspecified hand
		▣	M02.251	Postimmunization arthropathy, right hip
		▣	M02.252	Postimmunization arthropathy, left hip
		▣	M02.259	Postimmunization arthropathy, unspecified hip
		▣	M02.261	Postimmunization arthropathy, right knee
		▣	M02.262	Postimmunization arthropathy, left knee
		▣	M02.269	Postimmunization arthropathy, unspecified knee
		▣	M02.271	Postimmunization arthropathy, right ankle and foot
		▣	M02.272	Postimmunization arthropathy, left ankle and foot
		▣	M02.279	Postimmunization arthropathy, unspecified ankle and foot
		▣	M02.28	Postimmunization arthropathy, vertebrae
		▣	M02.29	Postimmunization arthropathy, multiple sites
			T80.62XA	Other serum reaction due to vaccination, initial encounter
999.59	OTHER SERUM REACTION		T80.69XA	Other serum reaction due to other serum, initial encounter
999.60	ABO INCOMPATIBILITY REACTION UNSPECIFIED		T80.30XA	ABO incompat react due to tranfs of bld/bld prod, unsp, init
999.61	ABO INCOMPAT HEMOLYT TRAN REACT NOT ACUT/DELAY		T80.319A	ABO incompatibility w hemolytic transfs react, unsp, init
999.62	ABO INCOMPAT ACUTE HEMOLYT TRANSFUSION REACTION		T80.310A	ABO incompatibility w acute hemolytic transfs react, init
999.63	ABO INCOMPAT DELAYD HEMOLYT TRANSFUSION REACTION		T80.311A	ABO incompatibility w delayed hemolytic transfs react, init
999.69	OTHER ABO INCOMPATIBILITY REACTION		T80.39XA	Oth ABO incompat react due to tranfs of bld/bld prod, init
999.70	RH INCOMPATIBILITY REACTION UNSPECIFIED		T80.40XA	Rh incompat react due to tranfs of bld/bld prod, unsp, init
999.71	RH INCOMPATIBILITY W/HTR NOT SPEC ACUTE/DELAY		T80.419A	Rh incompatibility w hemolytic transfs react, unsp, init
999.72	RH INCOMPAT ACUTE HEMOLYTIC TRANSFUSION REACTION		T80.410A	Rh incompatibility w acute hemolytic transfs react, init
999.73	RH INCOMPAT DELAY HEMOLYTIC TRANSFUSION REACTION		T80.411A	Rh incompatibility w delayed hemolytic transfs react, init
999.74	OTHER RH INCOMPATIBILITY REACTION		T80.49XA	Oth Rh incompat reaction due to tranfs of bld/bld prod, init
999.75	NON-ABO INCOMPATIBILITY REACTION UNSPECIFIED		T80.A0XA	Non-ABO incompat react d/t tranfs of bld/bld prod,unsp, init
999.76	NON-ABO INCOMPATIBILITY W/HTR NOT SPEC AC/DELAY		T80.A19A	Non-ABO incompat w hemolytic transfs react, unsp, init
999.77	NON-ABO INCOMPATIBILITY W/ACUTE HTR		T80.A10A	Non-ABO incompat w acute hemolytic transfs react, init
999.78	NON-ABO INCOMPAT DELAYED HEMOLYTIC TRAN REACTION		T80.A11A	Non-ABO incompat w delayed hemolytic transfs react, init
999.79	OTHER NON-ABO INCOMPATIBILITY REACTION		T80.A9XA	Oth non-ABO incompat react d/t tranfs of bld/bld prod, init
999.80	TRANSFUSION REACTION UNSPECIFIED		T80.92XA	Unspecified transfusion reaction, initial encounter
999.81	EXTRAVASATION OF VESICANT CHEMOTHERAPY		T80.810A	Extravasation of vesicant antineoplastic chemotherapy, init
999.82	EXTRAVASATION OF OTHER VESICANT AGENT		T80.818A	Extravasation of other vesicant agent, initial encounter
999.83	HEMOLYTIC TRANSFUSION REACT INCOMPATIBILITY UNS		T80.919A	Hemolytic transfs react, unsp incompat, unsp ac/delay, init
999.84	AC HEMOLYT TRANSFUSION REACT INCOMPATIBILITY UNS		T80.910A	Acute hemolytic transfs react, unsp incompatibility, init
999.85	DELAYED HEMOLYT TRANSFUSION REACT INCOMPAT UNS		T80.911A	Delayed hemolytic transfs react, unsp incompatibility, init
999.88	OTHER INFUSION REACTION		T80.89XA	Oth comp fol infusion, transfuse and theraputc inject, init
			T80.90XA	Unsp comp following infusion and therapeutic injection, init
999.89	OTHER TRANSFUSION REACTION		T80.89XA	Oth comp fol infusion, transfuse and theraputc inject, init
999.9	OTHER&UNSPECIFIED COMPLICATIONS MEDICAL CARE NEC		T81.81XA	Complication of inhalation therapy, initial encounter
			T88.4XXA	Failed or difficult intubation, initial encounter
			T88.7XXA	Unsp adverse effect of drug or medicament, init encntr
			T88.8XXA	Oth complications of surgical and medical care, NEC, init
			T88.9XXA	Complication of surgical and medical care, unsp, init encntr

V Codes

ICD-9-CM			ICD-10-CM	
V01.0	CONTACT WITH OR EXPOSURE TO CHOLERA		**Z20.09**	Contact w and exposure to oth intestinal infectious diseases
V01.1	CONTACT WITH OR EXPOSURE TO TUBERCULOSIS	➡	**Z20.1**	Contact with and (suspected) exposure to tuberculosis
V01.2	CONTACT WITH OR EXPOSURE TO POLIOMYELITIS		**Z20.89**	Contact w and exposure to oth communicable diseases
V01.3	CONTACT WITH OR EXPOSURE TO SMALLPOX		**Z20.89**	Contact w and exposure to oth communicable diseases
V01.4	CONTACT WITH OR EXPOSURE TO RUBELLA	➡	**Z20.4**	Contact with and (suspected) exposure to rubella
V01.5	CONTACT WITH OR EXPOSURE TO RABIES	➡	**Z20.3**	Contact with and (suspected) exposure to rabies
V01.6	CONTACT WITH OR EXPOSURE TO VENEREAL DISEASES	➡	**Z20.2**	Contact w and exposure to infect w a sexl mode of transmiss
V01.71	CONTACT OR EXPOSURE TO VARICELLA	➡	**Z20.820**	Contact with and (suspected) exposure to varicella
V01.79	CONTACT OR EXPOSURE TO OTHER VIRAL DISEASES		**Z20.5** **Z20.6** **Z20.828**	Contact with and (suspected) exposure to viral hepatitis Contact w and (suspected) exposure to human immunodef virus Contact w and exposure to oth viral communicable diseases
V01.81	CONTACT WITH OR EXPOSURE TO ANTHRAX	➡	**Z20.810**	Contact with and (suspected) exposure to anthrax
V01.82	EXPOSURE TO SARS-ASSOCIATED CORONAVIRUS		**Z20.89**	Contact w and exposure to oth communicable diseases
V01.83	CONTACT OR EXPOSURE TO ESCHERICHIA COLI	➡	**Z20.01**	Cntct w and expsr to intestnl infct dis d/t E coli (E. coli)
V01.84	CONTACT OR EXPOSURE TO MENINGOCOCCUS	➡	**Z20.811**	Contact with and (suspected) exposure to meningococcus
V01.89	CONTACT/EXPOSURE TO OTHER COMMUNICABLE DISEASES		**Z20.09** **Z20.7** **Z20.818** **Z20.89**	Contact w and exposure to oth intestinal infectious diseases Cntct w & expsr to pediculosis, acariasis & oth infestations Contact w and exposure to oth bact communicable diseases Contact w and exposure to oth communicable diseases
V01.9	CNTC W/OR EXPOSURE UNSPEC COMMUNICABLE DISEASE	➡	**Z20.9**	Contact w and exposure to unsp communicable disease
V02.0	CARRIER OR SUSPECTED CARRIER OF CHOLERA		**Z22.1**	Carrier of other intestinal infectious diseases
V02.1	CARRIER OR SUSPECTED CARRIER OF TYPHOID	➡	**Z22.0**	Carrier of typhoid
V02.2	CARRIER OR SUSPECTED CARRIER OF AMEBIASIS		**Z22.1**	Carrier of other intestinal infectious diseases
V02.3	CARR/SUSPECTED CARR OTH GI PATHOGENS		**Z22.1**	Carrier of other intestinal infectious diseases
V02.4	CARRIER OR SUSPECTED CARRIER OF DIPHTHERIA	➡	**Z22.2**	Carrier of diphtheria
V02.51	CARRIER/SUSPECTED CARRIER GROUP B STREPTOCOCCUS	▣ ▣ ▣	**O99.820** **O99.824** **O99.825** **Z22.330**	Streptococcus B carrier state complicating pregnancy Streptococcus B carrier state complicating childbirth Streptococcus B carrier state complicating the puerperium Carrier of Group B streptococcus
V02.52	CARRIER OR SUSPECTED CARRIER OTHER STREPTOCOCCUS	➡	**Z22.338**	Carrier of other streptococcus
V02.53	CARRIER OR SUSPECTED CARRIER OF MSSA		**Z22.321**	Carrier or suspected carrier of methicillin suscep staph
V02.54	CARR/SPCT CARRIER METHICILLIN RSIST STAPH AUREUS		**Z22.322**	Carrier or suspected carrier of methicillin resis staph
V02.59	CARR/SUSPECTED CARR OTH SPEC BACTERL DISEASES		**Z22.31** **Z22.39**	Carrier of bacterial disease due to meningococci Carrier of other specified bacterial diseases
V02.60	UNSPECIFIED VIRAL HEPATITIS CARRIER	➡	**Z22.50**	Carrier of unspecified viral hepatitis
V02.61	HEPATITIS B CARRIER	➡	**Z22.51**	Carrier of viral hepatitis B
V02.62	HEPATITIS C CARRIER	➡	**Z22.52**	Carrier of viral hepatitis C
V02.69	OTHER VIRAL HEPATITIS CARRIER	➡	**Z22.59**	Carrier of other viral hepatitis
V02.7	CARRIER OR SUSPECTED CARRIER OF GONORRHEA		**Z22.4**	Carrier of infections w sexl mode of transmiss
V02.8	CARRIER/SUSPECTED CARRIER OTH VENEREAL DISEASES		**Z22.4**	Carrier of infections w sexl mode of transmiss
V02.9	CARR/SUSPECTED CARR OTH SPEC INFECTIOUS ORGANISM		**Z22.6** **Z22.8** **Z22.9**	Carrier of human T-lymphotropic virus type-1 infection Carrier of other infectious diseases Carrier of infectious disease, unspecified
V03.0	NEED PROPH VACC&INOCULAT AGAINST CHOLERA ALONE		**Z23**	Encounter for immunization
V03.1	NEED PROPH VACC W/TYPHOID-PARATYPHIOD ALONE		**Z23**	Encounter for immunization
V03.2	NEED PROPH VACCINATION W/TUBERCULOSIS VACCINE		**Z23**	Encounter for immunization
V03.3	NEED PROPH VACCINATION&INOCULAT AGAINST PLAGUE		**Z23**	Encounter for immunization
V03.4	NEED PROPH VACC&INOCULAT AGAINST TULAREMIA		**Z23**	Encounter for immunization
V03.5	NEED PROPH VACC&INOCULAT AGAINST DIPHTH ALONE		**Z23**	Encounter for immunization
V03.6	NEED PROPH VACC&INOCULAT AGAINST PERTUSS ALONE		**Z23**	Encounter for immunization
V03.7	NEED PROPH VACCINATION W/TETANUS TOXOID ALONE		**Z23**	Encounter for immunization
V03.81	NEED PROPH VACC AGAINST HEMOPHILUS FLU TYPE B		**Z23**	Encounter for immunization
V03.82	NEED PROPH VACCINATION AGAINST STREP PNEUMONE		**Z23**	Encounter for immunization
V03.89	NEED PROPH VACC AGAINST OTH SPEC VACC		**Z23**	Encounter for immunization
V03.9	NEED PROPH VACC&INOCULAT AGNST UNS 1 BACTERL DZ		**Z23**	Encounter for immunization
V04.0	NEED PROPH VACC&INOCULAT AGAINST POLIOMYEL		**Z23**	Encounter for immunization
V04.1	NEED PROPH VACCINATION&INOCULAT AGAINST SMALLPOX		**Z23**	Encounter for immunization
V04.2	NEED PROPH VACC&INOCULAT AGAINST MEASLES ALONE		**Z23**	Encounter for immunization
V04.3	NEED PROPH VACC&INOCULAT AGAINST RUBELLA ALONE		**Z23**	Encounter for immunization
V04.4	NEED PROPH VACC&INOCULAT AGAINST YELLOW FEVER		**Z23**	Encounter for immunization
V04.5	NEED PROPH VACCINATION&INOCULAT AGAINST RABIES		**Z23**	Encounter for immunization
V04.6	NEED PROPH VACC&INOCULAT AGAINST MUMPS ALONE		**Z23**	Encounter for immunization
V04.7	NEED PROPH VACC&INOCULAT AGAINST COMMON COLD		**Z23**	Encounter for immunization
V04.81	NEED PROPHYLACTIC VACCINATION&INOCULATION FLU		**Z23**	Encounter for immunization
V04.82	NEED PROPH VACC&INOCULAT RESP SYNCTIAL VIRUS		**Z23**	Encounter for immunization
V04.89	NEED PROPH VACCINATION&INOCULAT OTH VIRAL DZ		**Z23**	Encounter for immunization
V05.0	NEED PROPH VACC ARTHROPOD-BORN VIRL ENCEPHALITIS		**Z23**	Encounter for immunization
V05.1	NEED PROPH VACC OTH ARTHROPOD-BORNE VIRAL DZ		**Z23**	Encounter for immunization
V05.2	NEED PROPH VACC&INOCULAT AGAINST LEISHMANIASIS		**Z23**	Encounter for immunization

ICD-9-CM			ICD-10-CM	
V05.3	NEED PROPH VACC&INOCULAT AGAINST VIRAL HEP		Z23	Encounter for immunization
V05.4	NEED PROPH VACC&INOCULAT AGAINST VARICELLA		Z23	Encounter for immunization
V05.8	NEED PROPH VACC&INOCULAT AGNST OTH SPEC DISEASE		Z23	Encounter for immunization
V05.9	NEED PROPH VACC&INOCULAT AGNST UNSPEC SINGLE DZ		Z23	Encounter for immunization
V06.0	NEED PROPH VACCINATE AGAINST CHOLERA+TAB VACCINE		Z23	Encounter for immunization
V06.1	NEED PROPH VAC W/COMB DIPHTH-TETANUS-PERTUSS VAC		Z23	Encounter for immunization
V06.2	NEED PROPH VACCINATION W/DTP + TAB VACCINE		Z23	Encounter for immunization
V06.3	NEED PROPH VACCINATION W/DTP + POLIO VACCINE		Z23	Encounter for immunization
V06.4	NEED PROPH VACC W/MEASLES-MUMPS-RUBELLA VACCINE		Z23	Encounter for immunization
V06.5	NEED PROPHYLACTIC VACCINATION W/TETANUS-DIPHTH		Z23	Encounter for immunization
V06.6	NEED PROPH VACCINATION W/STREP PNEUMONE&FLU		Z23	Encounter for immunization
V06.8	NEED PROPH VACC&INOCULAT AGAINST OTH COMB DZ		Z23	Encounter for immunization
V06.9	NEED PROPH VACCINATION W/UNSPEC COMB VACCINE		Z23	Encounter for immunization
V07.0	NEED FOR ISOLATION		Z51.89	Encounter for other specified aftercare
V07.1	NEED FOR DESENSITIZATION TO ALLERGENS		Z51.89	Encounter for other specified aftercare
V07.2	NEED FOR PROPHYLACTIC IMMUNOTHERAPY		Z41.8	Encntr for oth proc for purpose oth than remedy health state
V07.31	NEED FOR PROPHYLACTIC FLUORIDE ADMINISTRATION		Z41.8	Encntr for oth proc for purpose oth than remedy health state
V07.39	NEED FOR OTHER PROPHYLACTIC CHEMOTHERAPY		Z41.8	Encntr for oth proc for purpose oth than remedy health state
V07.4	HORMONE REPLACEMENT THERAPY	➡	Z79.890	Hormone replacement therapy (postmenopausal)
V07.51	USE OF SELECTIVE ESTROGEN RECEPTOR MODULATORS	➡	Z79.810	Lng trm (crnt) use of slctv estrog receptor modulators
V07.52	USE OF AROMATASE INHIBITORS	➡	Z79.811	Long term (current) use of aromatase inhibitors
V07.59	USE OTH AGENTS AFFECT ESTROGEN RECEPTOR & LEVELS	➡	Z79.818	Lng trm (crnt) use of agnt aff estrog recpt & estrog levels
V07.8	NEED FOR OTHER SPEC PROPHYLACTIC OR TX MEASURE		Z41.8	Encntr for oth proc for purpose oth than remedy health state
V07.9	NEED FOR UNSPECIFIED PROPHYLACTIC OR TX MEASURE		Z41.8	Encntr for oth proc for purpose oth than remedy health state
V08	ASYMPTOMATIC HIV INFECTION STATUS	➡	Z21	Asymptomatic human immunodeficiency virus infection status
V09.0	INFECTION W/MICROORGANISMS RESISTANT PENICILLINS		Z16.11	Resistance to penicillins
V09.1	CEPHALOSPORINS-OTH B-LACTAM RESIST MICROORGAN		Z16.10 Z16.12 Z16.19	Resistance to unspecified beta lactam antibiotics Extended spectrum beta lactamase (ESBL) resistance Resistance to other specified beta lactam antibiotics
V09.2	INFECTION W/MICROORGANISMS RESISTANT MACROLIDES		Z16.29	Resistance to other single specified antibiotic
V09.3	INF W/MICROORGANISMS RESISTANT TETRACYCLINES		Z16.29	Resistance to other single specified antibiotic
V09.4	INF W/MICROORGANISMS RESISTANT AMINOGLYCOSIDES		Z16.29	Resistance to other single specified antibiotic
V09.50	QUINOLONE-FLUOROQUINOLE-NON-MULT RESIST MICROORG		Z16.23	Resistance to quinolones and fluoroquinolones
V09.51	QUINOLONES-FUOROQUINOLE-MULT RESIST MICROORGAN		Z16.23	Resistance to quinolones and fluoroquinolones
V09.6	INF W/MICROORGANISMS RESIST TO SULFONAMIDES		Z16.29	Resistance to other single specified antibiotic
V09.70	OTH ANTIMYCOBACTER-NON MULT RESIST MICROORGANISM		Z16.341	Resistance to single antimycobacterial drug
V09.71	OTH ANTIMYCOBACTER-MULT RESIST MICROORGANISMS		Z16.342	Resistance to multiple antimycobacterial drugs
V09.80	INF MICROORG RESIST-OTH SPEC RX NO RESIST MX RX		Z16.20 Z16.21 Z16.22 Z16.31 Z16.32 Z16.33 Z16.39	Resistance to unspecified antibiotic Resistance to vancomycin Resistance to vancomycin related antibiotics Resistance to antiparasitic drug(s) Resistance to antifungal drug(s) Resistance to antiviral drug(s) Resistance to other specified antimicrobial drug
V09.81	INF W/MICROORG RESIST-OTH SPEC RX W/RESIST MX RX		Z16.35	Resistance to multiple antimicrobial drugs
V09.90	UNS NON-MULT DRUG-RESISTANT MICROORGANISMS		Z16.30	Resistance to unspecified antimicrobial drugs
V09.91	INF W/UNS RX-RSISTANT MICROORGNSMS W/MX RX RSIST		Z16.24	Resistance to multiple antibiotics
V10.00	PERSONAL HX MALIG NEOPLASM UNSPEC SITE GI TRACT	➡	Z85.00	Personal history of malignant neoplasm of unsp dgstv org
V10.01	PERSONAL HISTORY OF MALIGNANT NEOPLASM OF TONGUE	➡	Z85.810	Personal history of malignant neoplasm of tongue
V10.02	PERS HX MAL NEOPLSM OTH&UNS PART ORL CAV&PHARYNX		Z85.818 Z85.819	Prsnl hx of malig neoplm of site of lip, oral cav, & pharynx Prsnl hx of malig neoplm of unsp site lip,oral cav,& pharynx
V10.03	PERSONAL HISTORY MALIGNANT NEOPLASM ESOPHAGUS	➡	Z85.01	Personal history of malignant neoplasm of esophagus
V10.04	PERSONAL HISTORY MALIGNANT NEOPLASM STOMACH		Z85.028	Personal history of other malignant neoplasm of stomach
V10.05	PERSONAL HISTORY MALIG NEOPLASM LARGE INTESTINE		Z85.038	Personal history of malignant neoplasm of large intestine
V10.06	PERS HX MAL NEOPLSM RECT RECTOSIGMOID JUNC&ANUS		Z85.048	Prsnl hx of malig neoplm of rectum, rectosig junct, and anus
V10.07	PERSONAL HISTORY OF MALIGNANT NEOPLASM OF LIVER	➡	Z85.05	Personal history of malignant neoplasm of liver
V10.09	PERSONAL HX MALIG NEOPLASM OTH SITE GI TRACT		Z85.068 Z85.07 Z85.09	Personal history of malignant neoplasm of small intestine Personal history of malignant neoplasm of pancreas Personal history of malignant neoplasm of digestive organs
V10.11	PERSONAL HISTORY MALIG NEOPLASM BRONCHUS&LUNG		Z85.118	Personal history of malignant neoplasm of bronchus and lung
V10.12	PERSONAL HISTORY MALIGNANT NEOPLASM TRACHEA	➡	Z85.12	Personal history of malignant neoplasm of trachea
V10.20	PERS HX MALIG NEOPLASM UNSPEC RESPIRATORY ORGAN	➡	Z85.20	Personal history of malignant neoplasm of unsp resp organ
V10.21	PERSONAL HISTORY OF MALIGNANT NEOPLASM OF LARYNX	➡	Z85.21	Personal history of malignant neoplasm of larynx
V10.22	PHO MALIG NEO OF NASAL CAVITY-MIDDLE EAR-SINUSES	➡	Z85.22	Prsnl hx of malig neoplm of nasl cav, mid ear, & acces sinus
V10.29	PERS HX MAL NEOPLSM OTH RESP&INTRATHOR ORGN OTH		Z85.238 Z85.29	Personal history of other malignant neoplasm of thymus Prsnl history of malig neoplm of resp and intrathorac organs
V10.3	PERSONAL HISTORY OF MALIGNANT NEOPLASM OF BREAST	➡	Z85.3	Personal history of malignant neoplasm of breast
V10.40	PERS HX MALIG NEOPLASM UNSPEC FE GENITAL ORGAN	➡	Z85.40	Prsnl history of malig neoplm of unsp female genital organ
V10.41	PERSONAL HISTORY MALIGNANT NEOPLASM CERVIX UTERI	➡	Z85.41	Personal history of malignant neoplasm of cervix uteri

[Brackets] indicate valid character values for each code. Character value meanings provided for each code grouping.

ICD-9-CM			ICD-10-CM	
V10.42	PERSONAL HISTORY MALIG NEOPLASM OTH PARTS UTERUS	➡	**Z85.42**	Personal history of malignant neoplasm of oth prt uterus
V10.43	PERSONAL HISTORY OF MALIGNANT NEOPLASM OF OVARY	➡	**Z85.43**	Personal history of malignant neoplasm of ovary
V10.44	PERSONAL HX MALIG NEOPLASM OTH FE GENITAL ORGANS	➡	**Z85.44**	Personal history of malig neoplasm of female genital organs
V10.45	PERS HX MALIG NEOPLASM UNSPEC MALE GENITAL ORGAN	➡	**Z85.45**	Personal history of malig neoplm of unsp male genital organ
V10.46	PERSONAL HISTORY MALIGNANT NEOPLASM PROSTATE	➡	**Z85.46**	Personal history of malignant neoplasm of prostate
V10.47	PERSONAL HISTORY OF MALIGNANT NEOPLASM OF TESTIS	➡	**Z85.47**	Personal history of malignant neoplasm of testis
V10.48	PERSONAL HISTORY MALIGNANT NEOPLASM EPIDIDYMIS	➡	**Z85.48**	Personal history of malignant neoplasm of epididymis
V10.49	PERSONAL HX MALIG NEOPLASM OTH MALE GENITAL ORGN	➡	**Z85.49**	Personal history of malig neoplasm of male genital organs
V10.50	PERSONAL HX MALIG NEOPLASM UNSPEC URINARY ORGAN	➡	**Z85.50**	Personal history of malig neoplm of unsp urinary tract organ
V10.51	PERSONAL HISTORY MALIGNANT NEOPLASM BLADDER	➡	**Z85.51**	Personal history of malignant neoplasm of bladder
V10.52	PERSONAL HISTORY OF MALIGNANT NEOPLASM OF KIDNEY		**Z85.528**	Personal history of other malignant neoplasm of kidney
V10.53	PERSONAL HISTORY MALIGNANT NEOPLASM RENAL PELVIS	➡	**Z85.53**	Personal history of malignant neoplasm of renal pelvis
V10.59	PERSONAL HX MALIG NEOPLASM OTH URINARY ORGAN		**Z85.54** **Z85.59**	Personal history of malignant neoplasm of ureter Personal history of malig neoplasm of urinary tract organ
V10.60	PERSONAL HISTORY OF UNSPECIFIED LEUKEMIA		**Z85.6**	Personal history of leukemia
V10.61	PERSONAL HISTORY OF LYMPHOID LEUKEMIA		**Z85.6**	Personal history of leukemia
V10.62	PERSONAL HISTORY OF MYELOID LEUKEMIA		**Z85.6**	Personal history of leukemia
V10.63	PERSONAL HISTORY OF MONOCYTIC LEUKEMIA		**Z85.6**	Personal history of leukemia
V10.69	PERSONAL HISTORY OF OTHER LEUKEMIA		**Z85.6**	Personal history of leukemia
V10.71	PERSONAL HISTORY LYMPHOSARCOMA&RETICULOSARCOMA		**Z85.79** **Z85.831**	Prsnl hx of malig neoplm of lymphoid, hematpoetc & rel tiss Personal history of malignant neoplasm of soft tissue
V10.72	PERSONAL HISTORY OF HODGKINS DISEASE	➡	**Z85.71**	Personal history of Hodgkin lymphoma
V10.79	PERSONAL HX OTH LYMPHATIC&HEMATOPOIETIC NEOPLASM		**Z85.72** **Z85.79**	Personal history of non-Hodgkin lymphomas Prsnl hx of malig neoplm of lymphoid, hematpoetc & rel tiss
V10.81	PERSONAL HISTORY OF MALIGNANT NEOPLASM OF BONE	➡	**Z85.830**	Personal history of malignant neoplasm of bone
V10.82	PERSONAL HISTORY OF MALIGNANT MELANOMA OF SKIN	➡	**Z85.820**	Personal history of malignant melanoma of skin
V10.83	PERSONAL HISTORY OTHER MALIGNANT NEOPLASM SKIN		**Z85.828**	Personal history of other malignant neoplasm of skin
V10.84	PERSONAL HISTORY OF MALIGNANT NEOPLASM OF EYE	➡	**Z85.840**	Personal history of malignant neoplasm of eye
V10.85	PERSONAL HISTORY OF MALIGNANT NEOPLASM OF BRAIN	➡	**Z85.841**	Personal history of malignant neoplasm of brain
V10.86	PERSONAL HX MALIG NEOPLASM OTH PARTS NERV SYSTEM	➡	**Z85.848**	Personal history of malignant neoplasm of prt nervous tissue
V10.87	PERSONAL HISTORY MALIGNANT NEOPLASM THYROID	➡	**Z85.850**	Personal history of malignant neoplasm of thyroid
V10.88	PERS HX MALIG NEOPLSM OTH ENDOCRN GLND&REL STRCT	➡	**Z85.858**	Personal history of malignant neoplasm of endocrine glands
V10.89	PERSONAL HISTORY MALIGNANT NEOPLASM OTHER SITE		**Z85.831** **Z85.89**	Personal history of malignant neoplasm of soft tissue Personal history of malignant neoplasm of organs and systems
V10.90	PERSONAL HISTORY UNSPECIFIED MALIGNANT NEOPLASM	➡	**Z85.9**	Personal history of malignant neoplasm, unspecified
V10.91	PERSONAL HISTORY MALIGNANT NEUROENDOCRINE TUMOR		**Z85.020** **Z85.030** **Z85.040** **Z85.060** **Z85.110** **Z85.230** **Z85.520** **Z85.821**	Personal history of malignant carcinoid tumor of stomach Personal history of malignant carcinoid tumor of lg int Personal history of malignant carcinoid tumor of rectum Personal history of malignant carcinoid tumor of sm int Personal history of malig carcinoid tumor of bronc and lung Personal history of malignant carcinoid tumor of thymus Personal history of malignant carcinoid tumor of kidney Personal history of Merkel cell carcinoma
V11.0	PERSONAL HISTORY OF SCHIZOPHRENIA		**Z65.8**	Oth problems related to psychosocial circumstances
V11.1	PERSONAL HISTORY OF AFFECTIVE DISORDER		**Z65.8**	Oth problems related to psychosocial circumstances
V11.2	PERSONAL HISTORY OF NEUROSIS		**Z65.8**	Oth problems related to psychosocial circumstances
V11.3	PERSONAL HISTORY OF ALCOHOLISM		**Z65.8**	Oth problems related to psychosocial circumstances
V11.4	PERSONAL HX COMBAT OPERATIONAL STRESS REACTION	➡	**Z86.51**	Personal history of combat and operational stress reaction
V11.8	PERSONAL HISTORY OF OTHER MENTAL DISORDER		**Z86.59**	Personal history of other mental and behavioral disorders
V11.9	PERSONAL HISTORY OF UNSPECIFIED MENTAL DISORDER		**Z86.59**	Personal history of other mental and behavioral disorders
V12.00	PERSONAL HX UNSPEC INFECTIOUS&PARASITIC DISEASE		**Z86.19**	Personal history of other infectious and parasitic diseases
V12.01	PERSONAL HISTORY OF TUBERCULOSIS	➡	**Z86.11**	Personal history of tuberculosis
V12.02	PERSONAL HISTORY OF POLIOMYELITIS	➡	**Z86.12**	Personal history of poliomyelitis
V12.03	PERSONAL HISTORY OF MALARIA	➡	**Z86.13**	Personal history of malaria
V12.04	PERSONAL HX OF METHICILLIN RESIST STAPH AUREUS		**Z86.14**	Personal history of methicillin resis staph infection
V12.09	PERSONAL HX OTH INFECTIOUS&PARASITIC DISEASE		**Z86.19**	Personal history of other infectious and parasitic diseases
V12.1	PERSONAL HISTORY OF NUTRITIONAL DEFICIENCY		**Z86.39**	Personal history of endo, nutritional and metabolic disease
V12.21	PERSONAL HISTORY OF GESTATIONAL DIABETES	➡	**Z86.32**	Personal history of gestational diabetes
V12.29	PERSONAL HX OTH ENDOCRN METABOLIC IMMUNITY D/O		**Z86.2** **Z86.31** **Z86.39**	Prsnl history of dis of the bld/bld-form org/immun mechnsm Personal history of diabetic foot ulcer Personal history of endo, nutritional and metabolic disease
V12.3	PERSONAL HISTORY DISEASES BLD&BLD-FORMING ORGANS		**Z86.2**	Prsnl history of dis of the bld/bld-form org/immun mechnsm
V12.40	UNSPECIFIED DISORER NERVOUS SYSTEM&SENSE ORGANS		**Z86.69**	Personal history of dis of the nervous sys and sense organs
V12.41	BENIGN NEOPLASM OF THE BRAIN	➡	**Z86.011**	Personal history of benign neoplasm of the brain
V12.42	PERSONAL HISTORY INFECTIONS CENTRAL NERVOUS SYS	➡	**Z86.61**	Personal history of infections of the central nervous system
V12.49	OTHER DISORDERS OF NERVOUS SYSTEM&SENSE ORGANS		**Z86.69**	Personal history of dis of the nervous sys and sense organs
V12.50	UNSPECIFIED CIRCULATORY DISEASE		**Z86.79**	Personal history of other diseases of the circulatory system
V12.51	PERSONAL HISTORY, VENOUS THROMBOSIS AND EMBOLISM	➡	**Z86.718**	Personal history of other venous thrombosis and embolism
V12.52	PERSONAL HISTORY OF THROMBOPHLEBITIS	➡	**Z86.72**	Personal history of thrombophlebitis

ICD-9-CM			ICD-10-CM	
V12.53	PERSONAL HISTORY OF SUDDEN CARDIAC ARREST	➡	**Z86.74**	Personal history of sudden cardiac arrest
V12.54	PERSONAL HX TIA & CI W/O RESIDUAL DEFICITS	➡	**Z86.73**	Prsnl hx of TIA (TIA), and cereb infrc w/o resid deficits
V12.55	PERSONAL HISTORY OF PULMONARY EMBOLISM	➡	**Z86.711**	Personal history of pulmonary embolism
V12.59	PERS HX, OTHER DISEASES OF CIRCULATORY SYSTEM		**Z86.79**	Personal history of other diseases of the circulatory system
V12.60	PERSONAL HISTORY UNS DISEASE RESPIRATORY SYS		**Z87.09**	Personal history of other diseases of the respiratory system
V12.61	PERSONAL HISTORY PNEUMONIA RECURRENT	➡	**Z87.01**	Personal history of pneumonia (recurrent)
V12.69	PERSONAL HISTORY OTHER DISEASES RESPIRATORY SYS		**Z87.09**	Personal history of other diseases of the respiratory system
V12.70	PERSONAL HISTORY UNSPECIFIED DIGESTIVE DISEASE		**Z87.19**	Personal history of other diseases of the digestive system
V12.71	PERSONAL HISTORY OF PEPTIC ULCER DISEASE	➡	**Z87.11**	Personal history of peptic ulcer disease
V12.72	PERSONAL HISTORY OF COLONIC POLYPS	➡	**Z86.010**	Personal history of colonic polyps
V12.79	PERSONAL HISTORY OTH DISEASES DIGESTIVE DISEASE		**Z87.19**	Personal history of other diseases of the digestive system
V13.00	PERSONAL HISTORY OF UNSPECIFIED URINARY DISORDER		**Z87.448**	Personal history of other diseases of urinary system
V13.01	PERSONAL HISTORY OF URINARY CALCULI	➡	**Z87.442**	Personal history of urinary calculi
V13.02	PERSONAL HISTORY OF URINARY TRACT INFECTION	➡	**Z87.440**	Personal history of urinary (tract) infections
V13.03	PERSONAL HISTORY OF NEPHROTIC SYNDROME	➡	**Z87.441**	Personal history of nephrotic syndrome
V13.09	PERSONAL HISTORY OTHER DISORDER URINARY SYSTEM		**Z87.448**	Personal history of other diseases of urinary system
V13.1	PERSONAL HISTORY OF TROPHOBLASTIC DISEASE		**Z87.59**	Personal history of comp of preg, chldbrth and the puerp
V13.21	PERSONAL HISTORY OF PRE-TERM LABOR	➡	**Z87.51**	Personal history of pre-term labor
V13.22	PERSONAL HISTORY OF CERVICAL DYSPLASIA	➡	**Z87.410**	Personal history of cervical dysplasia
V13.23	PERSONAL HISTORY OF VAGINAL DYSPLASIA	➡	**Z87.411**	Personal history of vaginal dysplasia
V13.24	PERSONAL HISTORY OF VULVAR DYSPLASIA	➡	**Z87.412**	Personal history of vulvar dysplasia
V13.29	PERSONAL HX OTH GENITAL SYSTEM&OBSTETRIC D/O		**Z87.42**	Personal history of oth diseases of the female genital tract
			Z87.59	Personal history of comp of preg, chldbrth and the puerp
V13.3	PERSONAL HISTORY DISEASES SKIN&SUBCUT TISSUE	➡	**Z87.2**	Personal history of diseases of the skin, subcu
V13.4	PERSONAL HISTORY OF ARTHRITIS		**Z87.39**	Personal history of diseases of the ms sys and conn tiss
V13.51	PERSONAL HISTORY OF PATHOLOGIC FRACTURE		**Z87.310**	Personal history of (healed) osteoporosis fracture
			Z87.311	Personal history of (healed) other pathological fracture
V13.52	PERSONAL HISTORY OF STRESS FRACTURE	➡	**Z87.312**	Personal history of (healed) stress fracture
V13.59	PERSONAL HISTORY OF OTH MUSCULOSKELETAL D/O		**Z87.39**	Personal history of diseases of the ms sys and conn tiss
V13.61	PERSONAL HISTORY OF CORRECTED HYPOSPADIAS	➡	**Z87.710**	Personal history of (corrected) hypospadias
V13.62	PERSONAL HX OTH CORRECTED CONGEN MALF GU SYSTEM	➡	**Z87.718**	Personal history of (corrected) congenital malform of GU sys
V13.63	PERSONAL HX CORRECTED CONGEN MALFORM NERV SYS		**Z87.728**	Prsnl hx of congen malform of nervous sys and sense organs
V13.64	PERS HX CORRECTED CONGEN MALF EYE EAR FACE NECK		**Z87.720**	Personal history of (corrected) congenital malform of eye
			Z87.721	Personal history of (corrected) congenital malform of ear
			Z87.730	Personal history of (corrected) cleft lip and palate
			Z87.790	Personal history of congenital malform of face and neck
V13.65	PERS HX CORRECTED CONGEN MALF HEART CIRC SYSTEM	➡	**Z87.74**	Personal history of congenital malform of heart and circ sys
V13.66	PERS HX CORRECTED CONGEN MALF RESPIRATORY SYSTEM	➡	**Z87.75**	Personal history of congenital malform of resp sys
V13.67	PERS HX CORRECTED CONGEN MALF DIGESTIVE SYSTEM		**Z87.738**	Personal history of congenital malform of dgstv sys
V13.68	PERS HX CORRECTED CONGN MALF INTEG LIMBS MSK SYS	➡	**Z87.76**	Prsnl hx of congen malform of integument, limbs and ms sys
V13.69	PERSONL HX OTH CORRECTED CONGENITAL MALFORMATION	➡	**Z87.798**	Personal history of oth (corrected) congenital malformations
V13.7	PERSONAL HISTORY OF PERINATAL PROBLEMS		**Z87.898**	Personal history of other specified conditions
V13.81	PERSONAL HISTORY OF ANAPHYLAXIS	➡	**Z87.892**	Personal history of anaphylaxis
V13.89	PERSONAL HISTORY OF OTHER SPECIFIED DISEASES		**Z86.000**	Personal history of in-situ neoplasm of breast
			Z86.001	Personal history of in-situ neoplasm of cervix uteri
			Z86.008	Personal history of in-situ neoplasm of other site
			Z86.012	Personal history of benign carcinoid tumor
			Z86.018	Personal history of other benign neoplasm
			Z86.03	Personal history of neoplasm of uncertain behavior
			Z87.430	Personal history of prostatic dysplasia
			Z87.438	Personal history of other diseases of male genital organs
			Z87.898	Personal history of other specified conditions
V13.9	PERSONAL HISTORY OF UNSPECIFIED DISEASE		**Z87.898**	Personal history of other specified conditions
V14.0	PERSONAL HISTORY OF ALLERGY TO PENICILLIN	➡	**Z88.0**	Allergy status to penicillin
V14.1	PERSONAL HISTORY ALLERGY OTHER ANTIBIOTIC AGENT	➡	**Z88.1**	Allergy status to other antibiotic agents status
V14.2	PERSONAL HISTORY OF ALLERGY TO SULFONAMIDES	➡	**Z88.2**	Allergy status to sulfonamides status
V14.3	PERSONAL HISTORY ALLERGY OTH ANTI-INFECTIVE AGT	➡	**Z88.3**	Allergy status to other anti-infective agents status
V14.4	PERSONAL HISTORY OF ALLERGY TO ANESTHETIC AGENT	➡	**Z88.4**	Allergy status to anesthetic agent status
V14.5	PERSONAL HISTORY OF ALLERGY TO NARCOTIC AGENT	➡	**Z88.5**	Allergy status to narcotic agent status
V14.6	PERSONAL HISTORY OF ALLERGY TO ANALGESIC AGENT	➡	**Z88.6**	Allergy status to analgesic agent status
V14.7	PERSONAL HISTORY OF ALLERGY TO SERUM OR VACCINE	➡	**Z88.7**	Allergy status to serum and vaccine status
V14.8	PERSONAL HISTORY ALLERGY OTH SPEC MEDICINAL AGTS	➡	**Z88.8**	Allergy status to oth drug/meds/biol subst status
V14.9	PERSONAL HISTORY ALLERGY UNSPEC MEDICINAL AGENT	➡	**Z88.9**	Allergy status to unsp drug/meds/biol subst status
V15.01	PERSONAL HISTORY OF ALLERGY TO PEANUTS	➡	**Z91.010**	Allergy to peanuts
V15.02	PERSONAL HISTORY OF ALLERGY TO MILK PRODUCTS	➡	**Z91.011**	Allergy to milk products
V15.03	PERSONAL HISTORY OF ALLERGY TO EGGS	➡	**Z91.012**	Allergy to eggs
V15.04	PERSONAL HISTORY OF ALLERGY TO SEAFOOD	➡	**Z91.013**	Allergy to seafood
V15.05	PERSONAL HISTORY OF ALLERGY TO OTHER FOODS		**Z91.018**	Allergy to other foods
			Z91.02	Food additives allergy status

ICD-9-CM			ICD-10-CM	
V15.06	ALLERGY TO INSECTS AND ARACHNIDS		**Z91.030** **Z91.038**	Bee allergy status Other insect allergy status
V15.07	PERSONAL HISTORY OF ALLERGY TO LATEX	➡	**Z91.040**	Latex allergy status
V15.08	PERSONAL HISTORY OF ALLERGY TO RADIOGRAPHIC DYE	➡	**Z91.041**	Radiographic dye allergy status
V15.09	PERSONAL HX OTH ALLERG OTH THAN MEDICINAL AGTS		**Z91.048** **Z91.09**	Other nonmedicinal substance allergy status Oth allergy status, oth than to drugs and biolg substances
V15.1	PERS HX SURG HRT&GREAT VES PRS HAZARDS HEALTH		**Z98.89**	Other specified postprocedural states
V15.21	PERSONAL HX OF UNDERGOING IN UTERO PROC DUR PG	➡	**Z98.870**	Personal history of in utero procedure during pregnancy
V15.22	PERSONAL HX OF UNDERGOING IN UTERO PROC FETUS	➡	**Z98.871**	Personal history of in utero procedure while a fetus
V15.29	PERSONAL HISTORY OF SURGERY TO OTHER ORGANS		**Z98.89**	Other specified postprocedural states
V15.3	PERS HX IRRADIATION PRESENTING HAZARDS HEALTH	➡	**Z92.3**	Personal history of irradiation
V15.41	PERS HX PHYSICAL ABS PRESENTING HAZARDS HEALTH		**Z91.410**	Personal history of adult physical and sexual abuse
V15.42	PERS HX EMOTIONAL ABS PRESENTING HAZARDS HEALTH		**Z91.411** **Z91.412**	Personal history of adult psychological abuse Personal history of adult neglect
V15.49	OTH PERS HX PSYCHOLOGICAL TRAUMA PRS HAZS HLTH		**Z91.419** **Z91.49**	Personal history of unspecified adult abuse Oth personal history of psychological trauma, NEC
V15.51	PERSONAL HISTORY OF TRAUMATIC FRACTURE	➡	**Z87.81**	Personal history of (healed) traumatic fracture
V15.52	PERSONAL HISTORY OF TRAUMATIC BRAIN INJURY	➡	**Z87.820**	Personal history of traumatic brain injury
V15.53	PERSONAL HISTORY RETAINED FB FULLY REMOVED	➡	**Z87.821**	Personal history of retained foreign body fully removed
V15.59	PERSONAL HISTORY OF OTHER INJURY		**Z87.828** **Z91.5**	Personal history of oth (healed) physical injury and trauma Personal history of self-harm
V15.6	PERSONAL HX POISONING PRESENTING HAZARDS HEALTH		**Z91.89**	Oth personal risk factors, not elsewhere classified
V15.7	PERS HX CONTRACEPTION PRESENTING HAZARDS HEALTH	➡	**Z92.0**	Personal history of contraception
V15.80	PERSONAL HISTORY OF FAILED MODERATE SEDATION	➡	**Z92.83**	Personal history of failed moderate sedation
V15.81	PERS HX NONCOMPLIANCE W/MED TX PRS HAZARDS HLTH		**Z91.11** **Z91.120** **Z91.128** **Z91.130** **Z91.138** **Z91.14** **Z91.19**	Patient's noncompliance with dietary regimen Pt intentl undrdose of meds regimen due to financl hardship Patient's intentl undrdose of meds regimen for oth reason Pt unintent undrdose of meds regimen due to age-rel debility Patient's unintent undrdose of meds regimen for oth reason Patient's other noncompliance with medication regimen Patient's noncompliance w oth medical treatment and regimen
V15.82	PERS HX TOBACCO USE PRESENTING HAZARDS HEALTH		**Z87.891**	Personal history of nicotine dependence
V15.83	PERSONAL HISTORY OF UNDERIMMUNIZATION STATUS	➡	**Z28.3**	Underimmunization status
V15.84	PERSONAL HX CONTACT WITH AND EXPOSURE ASBESTOS	➡	**Z77.090**	Contact with and (suspected) exposure to asbestos
V15.85	PERSONAL HX CONTACT & EXPOSUR HAZARDOUS BODY FLD		**Z57.8**	Occupational exposure to other risk factors
V15.86	PERSONAL HISTORY CONTACT WITH & EXPOSURE TO LEAD	➡	**Z77.011**	Contact with and (suspected) exposure to lead
V15.87	HISTORY OF EXTRACORPOREAL MEMBRANE OXYGENATION	➡	**Z92.81**	Prsnl history of extracorporeal membrane oxygenation (ECMO)
V15.88	PERSONAL HISTORY OF FALL	➡	**Z91.81**	History of falling
V15.89	OTH SPEC PERS HX PRESENTING HAZARDS HEALTH OTH		**Z77.110** **Z77.111** **Z77.112** **Z77.118** **Z77.122** **Z77.123** **Z77.128** **Z77.21** **Z77.22** **Z77.9** **Z91.82** **Z91.89** **Z92.89**	Contact with and (suspected) exposure to air pollution Contact with and (suspected) exposure to water pollution Contact with and (suspected) exposure to soil pollution Contact w and (suspected) exposure to oth environ pollution Contact with and (suspected) exposure to noise Cntct w & expsr to radon & oth naturally occuring radiation Contact w and expsr to oth hazards in the physcl environment Contact w and exposure to potentially hazardous body fluids Cntct w and expsr to environ tobacco smoke (acute) (chronic) Oth contact w and (suspected) exposures hazardous to health Personal history of military deployment Oth personal risk factors, not elsewhere classified Personal history of other medical treatment
V15.9	UNSPEC PERSONAL HX PRESENTING HAZARDS HEALTH		**Z91.89**	Oth personal risk factors, not elsewhere classified
V16.0	FM HX MALIGNANT NEOPLASM GASTROINTESTINAL TRACT	➡	**Z80.0**	Family history of malignant neoplasm of digestive organs
V16.1	FM HX MALIGNANT NEOPLASM TRACHEA BRONCHUS&LUNG	➡	**Z80.1**	Family history of malig neoplasm of trachea, bronc and lung
V16.2	FM HX MALIG NEOPLASM OTH RESP&INTRATHORACIC ORGN	➡	**Z80.2**	Family hx of malig neoplm of resp and intrathorac organs
V16.3	FAMILY HISTORY OF MALIGNANT NEOPLASM OF BREAST	➡	**Z80.3**	Family history of malignant neoplasm of breast
V16.40	FM HX MALIGNANT NEOPLASM UNSPEC GENITAL ORGAN		**Z80.49**	Family history of malignant neoplasm of other genital organs
V16.41	FAMILY HISTORY OF MALIGNANT NEOPLASM OVARY	➡	**Z80.41**	Family history of malignant neoplasm of ovary
V16.42	FAMILY HISTORY OF MALIGNANT NEOPLASM PROSTATE	➡	**Z80.42**	Family history of malignant neoplasm of prostate
V16.43	FAMILY HISTORY OF MALIGNANT NEOPLASM TESTIS	➡	**Z80.43**	Family history of malignant neoplasm of testis
V16.49	FAMILY HISTORY OF OTHER MALIGNANT NEOPLASM		**Z80.49**	Family history of malignant neoplasm of other genital organs
V16.51	FAMILY HISTORY OF MALIGNANT NEOPLASM OF KIDNEY	➡	**Z80.51**	Family history of malignant neoplasm of kidney
V16.52	FAMILY HISTORY OF MALIGNANT NEOPLASM BLADDER	➡	**Z80.52**	Family history of malignant neoplasm of bladder
V16.59	FAMILIY HX MALIG NEOPLASM OTH URINARY ORGANS	➡	**Z80.59**	Family history of malignant neoplasm of urinary tract organ
V16.6	FAMILY HISTORY OF LEUKEMIA	➡	**Z80.6**	Family history of leukemia
V16.7	FM HX OF OTHER LYMPHATIC&HEMATOPOIETIC NEOPLASMS	➡	**Z80.7**	Fam hx of malig neoplm of lymphoid, hematpoetc and rel tiss
V16.8	FM HX OF OTHER SPECIFIED MALIGNANT NEOPLASM	➡	**Z80.8**	Family history of malignant neoplasm of organs or systems
V16.9	FAMILY HISTORY OF UNSPECIFIED MALIGNANT NEOPLASM	➡	**Z80.9**	Family history of malignant neoplasm, unspecified
V17.0	FAMILY HISTORY OF PSYCHIATRIC CONDITION	➡	**Z81.8**	Family history of other mental and behavioral disorders
V17.1	FAMILY HISTORY OF STROKE	➡	**Z82.3**	Family history of stroke
V17.2	FAMILY HISTORY OF OTHER NEUROLOGICAL DISEASES	➡	**Z82.0**	Family history of epilepsy and oth dis of the nervous sys

See Appendix A ➡ Equivalent Mapping Scenario Scenario

ICD-9-CM		ICD-10-CM	
V17.3	FAMILY HISTORY OF ISCHEMIC HEART DISEASE	**Z82.49**	Family hx of ischem heart dis and oth dis of the circ sys
V17.41	FAMILY HISTORY OF SUDDEN CARDIAC DEATH	➡ **Z82.41**	Family history of sudden cardiac death
V17.49	FAMILY HISTORY OF OTHER CARDIOVASCULAR DISEASES	**Z82.49**	Family hx of ischem heart dis and oth dis of the circ sys
V17.5	FAMILY HISTORY OF ASTHMA	**Z82.5**	Family history of asthma and oth chronic lower resp diseases
V17.6	FM HX OF OTHER CHRONIC RESPIRATORY CONDITIONS	**Z83.6**	Family history of other diseases of the respiratory system
V17.7	FAMILY HISTORY OF ARTHRITIS	➡ **Z82.61**	Family history of arthritis
V17.81	FAMILY HISTORY OSTEOPOROSIS	➡ **Z82.62**	Family history of osteoporosis
V17.89	FAMILY HISTORY OTHER MUSCULOSKELETAL DISEASES	➡ **Z82.69**	Family history of diseases of the ms sys and connective tiss
V18.0	FAMILY HISTORY OF DIABETES MELLITUS	➡ **Z83.3**	Family history of diabetes mellitus
V18.11	FAM HX OF MULTIPLE ENDOCRINE NEOPLASIA SYNDROME	➡ **Z83.41**	Family history of multiple endocrine neoplasia syndrome
V18.19	FAMILY HX OF OTHER ENDOCRINE & METABOLIC DX	➡ **Z83.49**	Family history of endo, nutritional and metabolic diseases
V18.2	FAMILY HISTORY OF ANEMIA	**Z83.2**	Family history of dis of the bld/bld-form org/immun mechnsm
V18.3	FAMILY HISTORY OF OTHER BLOOD DISORDERS	**Z83.2**	Family history of dis of the bld/bld-form org/immun mechnsm
V18.4	FAMILY HISTORY OF INTELLECTUAL DISABILITIES	➡ **Z81.0**	Family history of intellectual disabilities
V18.51	FAMILY HISTORY COLONIC POLYPS	➡ **Z83.71**	Family history of colonic polyps
V18.59	FAMILY HISTORY OTHER DIGESTIVE DISORDERS	➡ **Z83.79**	Family history of other diseases of the digestive system
V18.61	FAMILY HISTORY OF POLYCYSTIC KIDNEY	➡ **Z82.71**	Family history of polycystic kidney
V18.69	FAMILY HISTORY OF OTHER KIDNEY DISEASES	**Z84.1**	Family history of disorders of kidney and ureter
V18.7	FAMILY HISTORY OF OTHER GENITOURINARY DISEASES	➡ **Z84.2**	Family history of other diseases of the genitourinary system
V18.8	FM HX OF INFECTIOUS AND PARASITIC DISEASES	➡ **Z83.1**	Family history of other infectious and parasitic diseases
V18.9	FAMILY HISTORY GENETIC DISEASE CARRIER	**Z84.81**	Family history of carrier of genetic disease
V19.0	FAMILY HISTORY OF BLINDNESS OR VISUAL LOSS	➡ **Z82.1**	Family history of blindness and visual loss
V19.11	FAMILY HISTORY OF GLAUCOMA	➡ **Z83.511**	Family history of glaucoma
V19.19	FAMILY HISTORY OF OTHER SPECIFIED EYE DISORDER	➡ **Z83.518**	Family history of other specified eye disorder
V19.2	FAMILY HISTORY OF DEAFNESS OR HEARING LOSS	➡ **Z82.2**	Family history of deafness and hearing loss
V19.3	FAMILY HISTORY OF OTHER EAR DISORDERS	**Z83.52**	Family history of ear disorders
V19.4	FAMILY HISTORY OF SKIN CONDITIONS	**Z84.0**	Family history of diseases of the skin, subcu
V19.5	FAMILY HISTORY OF CONGENITAL ANOMALIES	➡ **Z82.79**	Fam hx of congen malform, deformations and chromsoml abnlt
V19.6	FAMILY HISTORY OF ALLERGIC DISORDERS	**Z84.89**	Family history of other specified conditions
V19.7	FAMILY HISTORY OF CONSANGUINITY	➡ **Z84.3**	Family history of consanguinity
V19.8	FAMILY HISTORY OF OTHER CONDITION	**Z81.1** **Z81.2** **Z81.3** **Z81.4** **Z82.8** **Z83.0** **Z84.89**	Family history of alcohol abuse and dependence Family history of tobacco abuse and dependence Family history of psychoactv substance abuse and dependence Family history of other substance abuse and dependence Family hx of disabil and chr dis leading to disablement, NEC Family history of human immunodeficiency virus [HIV] disease Family history of other specified conditions
V20.0	HEALTH SUPERVISION OF FOUNDLING	➡ **Z76.1**	Encounter for health supervision and care of foundling
V20.1	HEALTH SUP-OTH HEALTHY INFNT/CHLD RECEIVING CARE	➡ **Z76.2**	Encntr for hlth suprvsn and care of healthy infant and child
V20.2	ROUTINE INFANT OR CHILD HEALTH CHECK	**Z00.121** **Z00.129**	Encounter for routine child health exam w abnormal findings Encntr for routine child health exam w/o abnormal findings
V20.31	HEALTH SUPERVISION FOR NEWBORN UNDER 8 DAYS OLD	➡ **Z00.110**	Health examination for newborn under 8 days old
V20.32	HEALTH SUPERVISION FOR NEWBORN 8 TO 28 DAYS OLD	➡ **Z00.111**	Health examination for newborn 8 to 28 days old
V21.0	PERIOD OF RAPID GROWTH IN CHILDHOOD	**Z00.2**	Encounter for exam for period of rapid growth in childhood
V21.1	PUBERTY	**Z00.3**	Encounter for examination for adolescent development state
V21.2	OTHER DEVELOPMENT OF ADOLESCENCE	**Z00.3**	Encounter for examination for adolescent development state
V21.30	LOW BIRTH WEIGHT STATUS UNSPECIFIED	**P07.10**	Other low birth weight newborn, unspecified weight
V21.31	LOW BIRTH WEIGHT STATUS LESS THAN 500 GRAMS	**P07.01**	Extremely low birth weight newborn, less than 500 grams
V21.32	LOW BIRTH WEIGHT STATUS 500-999 GRAMS	**P07.02** **P07.03**	Extremely low birth weight newborn, 500-749 grams Extremely low birth weight newborn, 750-999 grams
V21.33	LOW BIRTH WEIGHT STATUS 1000-1499 GRAMS	**P07.14** **P07.15**	Other low birth weight newborn, 1000-1249 grams Other low birth weight newborn, 1250-1499 grams
V21.34	LOW BIRTH WEIGHT STATUS 1500-1999 GRAMS	**P07.16** **P07.17**	Other low birth weight newborn, 1500-1749 grams Other low birth weight newborn, 1750-1999 grams
V21.35	LOW BIRTH WEIGHT STATUS 2000-2500 GRAMS	**P07.18**	Other low birth weight newborn, 2000-2499 grams
V21.8	OTHER SPEC CONSTITUTIONAL STATES DEVELOPMENT	**Z00.2** **Z00.3**	Encounter for exam for period of rapid growth in childhood Encounter for examination for adolescent development state
V21.9	UNSPECIFIED CONSTITUTIONAL STATE IN DEVELOPMENT	**Z87.898**	Personal history of other specified conditions
V22.0	SUPERVISION OF NORMAL FIRST PREGNANCY	**Z34.00** **Z34.01** **Z34.02** **Z34.03**	Encntr for suprvsn of normal first pregnancy, unsp trimester Encntr for suprvsn of normal first preg, first trimester Encntr for suprvsn of normal first preg, second trimester Encntr for suprvsn of normal first preg, third trimester
V22.1	SUPERVISION OF OTHER NORMAL PREGNANCY	**Z34.80** **Z34.81** **Z34.82** **Z34.83** **Z34.90** **Z34.91** **Z34.92** **Z34.93**	Encounter for suprvsn of normal pregnancy, unsp trimester Encounter for suprvsn of normal pregnancy, first trimester Encounter for suprvsn of normal pregnancy, second trimester Encounter for suprvsn of normal pregnancy, third trimester Encntr for suprvsn of normal pregnancy, unsp, unsp trimester Encntr for suprvsn of normal preg, unsp, first trimester Encntr for suprvsn of normal preg, unsp, second trimester Encntr for suprvsn of normal preg, unsp, third trimester
V22.2	PREGNANT STATE, INCIDENTAL	➡ **Z33.1**	Pregnant state, incidental

ICD-9-CM		ICD-10-CM	
V23.Ø	PREGNANCY WITH HISTORY OF INFERTILITY	**O09.00**	Suprvsn of preg w history of infertility, unsp trimester
		O09.01	Suprvsn of preg w history of infertility, first trimester
		O09.02	Suprvsn of preg w history of infertility, second trimester
		O09.03	Suprvsn of preg w history of infertility, third trimester
V23.1	PREGNANCY WITH HISTORY OF TROPHOBLASTIC DISEASE	**O09.10**	Suprvsn of preg w history of ectopic or molar preg, unsp tri
		O09.11	Suprvsn of preg w history of ect or molar preg, first tri
		O09.12	Suprvsn of preg w history of ect or molar preg, second tri
		O09.13	Suprvsn of preg w history of ect or molar preg, third tri
V23.2	PREGNANCY WITH HISTORY OF ABORTION	**O09.291**	Suprvsn of preg w poor reprodctv or obstet hx, first tri
V23.3	PREGNANCY WITH GRAND MULTIPARITY	**O09.40**	Supervision of pregnancy w grand multiparity, unsp trimester
		O09.41	Suprvsn of pregnancy w grand multiparity, first trimester
		O09.42	Suprvsn of pregnancy w grand multiparity, second trimester
		O09.43	Suprvsn of pregnancy w grand multiparity, third trimester
V23.41	SUPERVISION PREGNANCY W/HISTORY PRE-TERM LABOR	**O09.211**	Suprvsn of preg w history of pre-term labor, first trimester
		O09.212	Suprvsn of preg w history of pre-term labor, second tri
		O09.213	Suprvsn of preg w history of pre-term labor, third trimester
		O09.219	Suprvsn of preg w history of pre-term labor, unsp trimester
V23.42	PREGNANCY WITH HISTORY OF ECTOPIC PREGNANCY	**O09.10**	Suprvsn of preg w history of ectopic or molar preg, unsp tri
		O09.11	Suprvsn of preg w history of ect or molar preg, first tri
		O09.12	Suprvsn of preg w history of ect or molar preg, second tri
		O09.13	Suprvsn of preg w history of ect or molar preg, third tri
V23.49	SUPERVISION PREGNANCY W/OTH POOR OBSTETRIC HX	**O09.291**	Suprvsn of preg w poor reprodctv or obstet hx, first tri
		O09.292	Suprvsn of preg w poor reprodctv or obstet hx, second tri
		O09.293	Suprvsn of preg w poor reprodctv or obstet hx, third tri
		O09.299	Suprvsn of preg w poor reprodctv or obstet history, unsp tri
V23.5	PREGNANCY WITH OTHER POOR REPRODUCTIVE HISTORY	**O09.291**	Suprvsn of preg w poor reprodctv or obstet hx, first tri
		O09.292	Suprvsn of preg w poor reprodctv or obstet hx, second tri
		O09.293	Suprvsn of preg w poor reprodctv or obstet hx, third tri
		O09.299	Suprvsn of preg w poor reprodctv or obstet history, unsp tri
V23.7	INSUFFICIENT PRENATAL CARE	**O09.30**	Suprvsn of preg w insufficient antenat care, unsp trimester
		O09.31	Suprvsn of preg w insufficient antenat care, first trimester
		O09.32	Suprvsn of preg w insufficient antenat care, second tri
		O09.33	Suprvsn of preg w insufficient antenat care, third trimester
V23.81	SUPERVISION HIGH-RISK PG ELDER PRIMIGRAVIDA	**O09.511**	Supervision of elderly primigravida, first trimester
		O09.512	Supervision of elderly primigravida, second trimester
		O09.513	Supervision of elderly primigravida, third trimester
		O09.519	Supervision of elderly primigravida, unspecified trimester
V23.82	SUPERVISION HIGH-RISK PG ELDER MULTIGRAVIDA	**O09.521**	Supervision of elderly multigravida, first trimester
		O09.522	Supervision of elderly multigravida, second trimester
		O09.523	Supervision of elderly multigravida, third trimester
		O09.529	Supervision of elderly multigravida, unspecified trimester
V23.83	SUPERVISION HIGH-RISK PG YOUNG PRIMIGRAVIDA	**O09.611**	Supervision of young primigravida, first trimester
		O09.612	Supervision of young primigravida, second trimester
		O09.613	Supervision of young primigravida, third trimester
		O09.619	Supervision of young primigravida, unspecified trimester
V23.84	SUPERVISION HIGH-RISK PG YOUNG MULTIGRAVIDA	**O09.621**	Supervision of young multigravida, first trimester
		O09.622	Supervision of young multigravida, second trimester
		O09.623	Supervision of young multigravida, third trimester
		O09.629	Supervision of young multigravida, unspecified trimester
V23.85	SUPERVISION OF HIGH RISK PG PG RESULT FROM ART	**O09.811**	Suprvsn of preg rslt from assisted reprodctv tech, first tri
		O09.812	Suprvsn of preg rslt from assist reprodctv tech, second tri
		O09.813	Suprvsn of preg rslt from assisted reprodctv tech, third tri
		O09.819	Suprvsn of preg rslt from assisted reprodctv tech, unsp tri
V23.86	SUPERVISION OF HRP PG HX OF IU PROC DUR PREV PG	**O09.821**	Suprvsn of preg w hx of in utero proc dur prev preg, 1st tri
		O09.822	Suprvsn of preg w hx of in utero proc dur prev preg, 2nd tri
		O09.823	Suprvsn of preg w hx of in utero proc dur prev preg, 3rd tri
		O09.829	Suprvsn of preg w hx of in utero proc dur prev preg,unsp tri
V23.87	PREGNANCY WITH INCONCLUSIVE FETAL VIABILITY	**O36.80X0**	Pregnancy w inconclusive fetal viability, unsp
		O36.80X1	Pregnancy with inconclusive fetal viability, fetus 1
		O36.80X2	Pregnancy with inconclusive fetal viability, fetus 2
		O36.80X3	Pregnancy with inconclusive fetal viability, fetus 3
		O36.80X4	Pregnancy with inconclusive fetal viability, fetus 4
		O36.80X5	Pregnancy with inconclusive fetal viability, fetus 5
		O36.80X9	Pregnancy with inconclusive fetal viability, other fetus
V23.89	SUPERVISION OF OTHER HIGH-RISK PREGNANCY	**O09.70**	Suprvsn of high risk preg due to social problems, unsp tri
		O09.71	Suprvsn of high risk preg due to social problems, first tri
		O09.72	Suprvsn of high risk preg due to social problems, second tri
		O09.73	Suprvsn of high risk preg due to social problems, third tri
		O09.891	Supervision of other high risk pregnancies, first trimester
		O09.892	Supervision of other high risk pregnancies, second trimester
		O09.893	Supervision of other high risk pregnancies, third trimester
		O09.899	Supervision of other high risk pregnancies, unsp trimester
V23.9	UNSPECIFIED HIGH-RISK PREGNANCY	**O09.90**	Supervision of high risk pregnancy, unsp, unsp trimester
		O09.91	Supervision of high risk pregnancy, unsp, first trimester
		O09.92	Supervision of high risk pregnancy, unsp, second trimester
		O09.93	Supervision of high risk pregnancy, unsp, third trimester
V24.Ø	POSTPARTUM CARE&EXAMINATION IMMED AFTER DELIV	➡ **Z39.0**	Encntr for care and exam of mother immediately after del
V24.1	POSTPARTUM CARE&EXAMINATION OF LACTATING MOTHER	➡ **Z39.1**	Encounter for care and examination of lactating mother

ICD-9-CM			ICD-10-CM	
V24.2	ROUTINE POSTPARTUM FOLLOW-UP	➡	**Z39.2**	Encounter for routine postpartum follow-up
V25.Ø1	GENERAL COUNSELING PRESCRIPTION ORAL CONTRACEPTS	➡	**Z3Ø.Ø11**	Encounter for initial prescription of contraceptive pills
V25.Ø2	GENERAL CNSL INITIATION OTH CONTRACEPT MEASURES		**Z3Ø.Ø13** **Z3Ø.Ø14** **Z3Ø.Ø18** **Z3Ø.Ø19**	Encounter for initial prescription of injectable contracep Encounter for initial prescription of uterin contracep dev Encounter for initial prescription of other contraceptives Encounter for initial prescription of contraceptives, unsp
V25.Ø3	ENCOUNTER EMERGENCY CONTRACEPT CNSL&PRESCRIPTION	➡	**Z3Ø.Ø12**	Encounter for prescription of emergency contraception
V25.Ø4	CNSL&INSTRCTION NATURAL FAM PLANNG AVOID PREG	➡	**Z3Ø.Ø2**	Cnsl and instruction in natrl family planning to avoid preg
V25.Ø9	OTH GENERAL CNSL&ADVICE CONTRACEPT MANAGEMENT	➡	**Z3Ø.Ø9**	Encounter for oth general cnsl and advice on contraception
V25.11	ENC FOR INSERTION INTRAUTERINE CONTRACEPT DEVICE	➡	**Z3Ø.43Ø**	Encounter for insertion of intrauterine contraceptive device
V25.12	ENCOUNTER FOR REMOVAL IU CONTRACEPT DEVICE	➡	**Z3Ø.432**	Encounter for removal of intrauterine contraceptive device
V25.13	ENC REMOVAL REINSERTION IU CONTRACEPT DEVICE	➡	**Z3Ø.433**	Encntr for removal and reinsertion of uterin contracep dev
V25.2	STERILIZATION	➡	**Z3Ø.2**	Encounter for sterilization
V25.3	MENSTRUAL EXTRACTION		**Z3Ø.8**	Encounter for other contraceptive management
V25.4Ø	UNSPECIFIED CONTRACEPTIVE SURVEILLANCE	➡	**Z3Ø.4Ø**	Encounter for surveillance of contraceptives, unspecified
V25.41	SURVEILLANCE PREV PRESCRIBED CONTRACEPT PILL	➡	**Z3Ø.41**	Encounter for surveillance of contraceptive pills
V25.42	SURVEILLANCE PREV PRSC INTRAUTERN CNTRACPT DEVC	➡	**Z3Ø.431**	Encounter for routine checking of intrauterine contracep dev
V25.43	SURVEILLANCE PREV PRSC IMPL SUBDERMAL CONTRACEPT		**Z3Ø.49**	Encounter for surveillance of other contraceptives
V25.49	SURVEILLANCE OTH PREV PRSC CONTRACEPT METHOD		**Z3Ø.42** **Z3Ø.49**	Encounter for surveillance of injectable contraceptive Encounter for surveillance of other contraceptives
V25.5	INSERTION OF IMPLANTABLE SUBDERMAL CONTRACEPTIVE		**Z3Ø.49**	Encounter for surveillance of other contraceptives
V25.8	OTHER SPECIFIED CONTRACEPTIVE MANAGEMENT		**Z3Ø.8**	Encounter for other contraceptive management
V25.9	UNSPECIFIED CONTRACEPTIVE MANAGEMENT	➡	**Z3Ø.9**	Encounter for contraceptive management, unspecified
V26.Ø	TUBOPLASTY/VASOPLASTY AFTER PREVIOUS STERILIZ	➡	**Z31.Ø**	Encounter for reversal of previous sterilization
V26.1	ARTIFICIAL INSEMINATION		**Z31.89**	Encounter for other procreative management
V26.21	FERTILITY TESTING	➡	**Z31.41**	Encounter for fertility testing
V26.22	AFTERCARE FOLLOWING STERILIZATION REVERSAL	➡	**Z31.42**	Aftercare following sterilization reversal
V26.29	OTHER INVESTIGATION AND TESTING	➡	**Z31.49**	Encounter for other procreative investigation and testing
V26.31	TESTING FEMALE GENETIC DISEASE CARRIER STATUS	➡	**Z31.43Ø**	Encntr fem for test for genetc dis carrier stat for pro mgmt
V26.32	OTHER GENETIC TESTING OF FEMALE		**Z31.438**	Encounter for oth genetic testing of female for pro mgmt
V26.33	GENETIC COUNSELING		**Z31.5**	Encounter for genetic counseling
V26.34	TESTING OF MALE GENETIC DISEASE CARRIER STATUS	➡	**Z31.44Ø**	Encntr male test for genetic dis carrier status for pro mgmt
V26.35	ENCOUNTER TEST MALE PARTNER FEM RECUR PREG LOSS	➡	**Z31.441**	Encntr for testing of male prtnr of pt w recur preg loss
V26.39	OTHER GENETIC TESTING OF MALE		**Z31.448**	Encounter for oth genetic testing of male for pro mgmt
V26.41	PROCREATIVE COUNSELING & ADVICE NATURAL FAM PLAN	➡	**Z31.61**	Procreat counseling and advice using natural family planning
V26.42	ENCOUNTER FOR FERTILITY PRESERVATION COUNSELING	➡	**Z31.62**	Encounter for fertility preservation counseling
V26.49	OTHER PROCREATIVE MANAGEMENT COUNSELING&ADVICE	➡	**Z31.69**	Encounter for oth general cnsl and advice on procreation
V26.51	TUBAL LIGATION STERILIZATION STATUS	➡	**Z98.51**	Tubal ligation status
V26.52	VASECTOMY STERILIZATION STATUS	➡	**Z98.52**	Vasectomy status
V26.81	ENCOUNTER ASSTD REPRODIVE FERTILITY PROC CYCL	➡	**Z31.83**	Encounter for assisted reprodctv fertility procedure cycle
V26.82	ENCOUNTER FOR FERTILITY PRESERVATION PROCEDURE	➡	**Z31.84**	Encounter for fertility preservation procedure
V26.89	OTHER SPECIFIED PROCREATIVE MANAGEMENT		**Z31.81** **Z31.82** **Z31.89**	Encounter for male factor infertility in female patient Encounter for Rh incompatibility status Encounter for other procreative management
V26.9	UNSPECIFIED PROCREATIVE MANAGEMENT	➡	**Z31.9**	Encounter for procreative management, unspecified
V27.Ø	OUTCOME OF DELIVERY SINGLE LIVEBORN	➡	**Z37.Ø**	Single live birth
V27.1	OUTCOME OF DELIVERY SINGLE STILLBORN	➡	**Z37.1**	Single stillbirth
V27.2	OUTCOME OF DELIVERY TWINS BOTH LIVEBORN	➡	**Z37.2**	Twins, both liveborn
V27.3	OUTCOME DELIVERY TWINS 1 LIVEBORN& 1 STILLBORN	➡	**Z37.3**	Twins, one liveborn and one stillborn
V27.4	OUTCOME OF DELIVERY TWINS BOTH STILLBORN	➡	**Z37.4**	Twins, both stillborn
V27.5	OUTCOME DELIVERY OTH MULTIPLE BIRTH ALL LIVEBORN		**Z37.5Ø** **Z37.51** **Z37.52** **Z37.53** **Z37.54** **Z37.59**	Multiple births, unspecified, all liveborn Triplets, all liveborn Quadruplets, all liveborn Quintuplets, all liveborn Sextuplets, all liveborn Other multiple births, all liveborn
V27.6	OUTCOME DELIV OTH MULTIPLE BIRTH SOME LIVEBORN		**Z37.6Ø** **Z37.61** **Z37.62** **Z37.63** **Z37.64** **Z37.69**	Multiple births, unspecified, some liveborn Triplets, some liveborn Quadruplets, some liveborn Quintuplets, some liveborn Sextuplets, some liveborn Other multiple births, some liveborn
V27.7	OUTCOME DELIV OTH MULTIPLE BIRTH ALL STILLBORN	➡	**Z37.7**	Other multiple births, all stillborn
V27.9	OUTCOME OF DELIVERY, UNSPECIFIED	➡	**Z37.9**	Outcome of delivery, unspecified
V28.Ø	SCREENING CHROMOSOMAL ANOMALIES AMNIOCENTESIS		**Z36**	Encounter for antenatal screening of mother
V28.1	SCREEN RAISED ALPHAFETOPROTEIN LEVEL AMNIOTIC FL		**Z36**	Encounter for antenatal screening of mother
V28.2	OTHER ANTENATAL SCREENING BASED ON AMNIOCENTESIS		**Z36**	Encounter for antenatal screening of mother
V28.3	ENCOUNTER ROUTINE SCREEN MALFORMATION ULTRASONIC		**Z36**	Encounter for antenatal screening of mother
V28.4	ANTENATAL SCR FETAL GROWTH RETARDATION USING US		**Z36**	Encounter for antenatal screening of mother
V28.5	ANTENATAL SCREENING FOR ISOIMMUNIZATION		**Z36**	Encounter for antenatal screening of mother

ICD-9-CM		ICD-10-CM	
V28.6	SCREENING OF STREPTOCOCCUS B	**Z36**	Encounter for antenatal screening of mother
V28.81	ENCOUNTER FOR FETAL ANATOMIC SURVEY	**Z36**	Encounter for antenatal screening of mother
V28.82	ENCOUNTER SCREENING FOR RISK OF PRE-TERM LABOR	**Z36**	Encounter for antenatal screening of mother
V28.89	OTHER SPECIFIED ANTENATAL SCREENING	**Z36**	Encounter for antenatal screening of mother
V28.9	UNSPECIFIED ANTENATAL SCREENING	**Z36**	Encounter for antenatal screening of mother
V29.Ø	OBS&EVAL NBS&INFNTS SPCT INF COND NOT FOUND	**PØØ.2**	Newborn affected by maternal infec/parastc diseases
V29.1	OBS&EVAL NBS&INFNTS SPCT NEURO COND NOT FOUND	**PØØ.89**	Newborn affected by oth maternal conditions
V29.2	OBS&EVAL NBS&INFNTS SPCT RESP COND NOT FOUND	**PØØ.3**	Newborn affected by oth maternal circ and resp diseases
V29.3	OBSERVATION SUSPECTED GENETIC/METABOLIC COND	**PØØ.89**	Newborn affected by oth maternal conditions
V29.8	OBS&EVAL NBS&INFNTS OTH SPEC SPCT COND NOT FOUND	**PØØ.89**	Newborn affected by oth maternal conditions
V29.9	OBS&EVAL NBS&INFNTS UNSPEC SPCT COND NOT FOUND	**PØØ.9**	Newborn affected by unsp maternal condition
V3Ø.ØØ	SINGLE LIVEBORN HOSPITAL W/O C-SECTION	**Z38.ØØ** **Z38.2**	Single liveborn infant, delivered vaginally Single liveborn infant, unspecified as to place of birth
V3Ø.Ø1	SINGLE LIVEBORN HOSPITAL DELIV BY C-SECTION	**Z38.Ø1**	Single liveborn infant, delivered by cesarean
V3Ø.1	SINGLE LIVEBORN BORN BEFORE ADMISSION HOSPITAL	**Z38.1**	Single liveborn infant, born outside hospital
V3Ø.2	SINGLE LIVEBORN BORN OUTSIDE HOSPITAL&NOT HOSP	**Z38.1**	Single liveborn infant, born outside hospital
V31.ØØ	LIVEBORN TWIN-MATE LIVEBORN HOSP W/O C-SEC	**Z38.3Ø** **Z38.5**	Twin liveborn infant, delivered vaginally Twin liveborn infant, unspecified as to place of birth
V31.Ø1	LIVEBORN TWIN-MATE LIVEBORN HOSP C-SEC	**Z38.31**	Twin liveborn infant, delivered by cesarean
V31.1	LIVEBORN TWIN-MATE LIVEBORN BEFORE ADMISS	**Z38.4**	Twin liveborn infant, born outside hospital
V31.2	LIVEBORN TWIN-MATE LIVEBORN OUTSIDE HOSP	**Z38.4**	Twin liveborn infant, born outside hospital
V32.ØØ	LIVEBORN TWIN-MATE STILLBORN HOSP W/O C-SEC	**Z38.3Ø**	Twin liveborn infant, delivered vaginally
V32.Ø1	LIVEBORN TWIN-MATE STILLBORN HOSPITAL C-SEC	**Z38.31**	Twin liveborn infant, delivered by cesarean
V32.1	LIVEBORN TWIN-MATE STILLBORN BEFORE ADMISS	**Z38.4**	Twin liveborn infant, born outside hospital
V32.2	LIVEBORN TWIN-MATE STILLB OUTSIDE HOSP&NOT HOSP	**Z38.4**	Twin liveborn infant, born outside hospital
V33.ØØ	LIVEB TWIN-UNS MATE LIVEB/STILLB-HOSP W/O C-SEC	**Z38.3Ø**	Twin liveborn infant, delivered vaginally
V33.Ø1	TWIN UNS MATE STILLB/LIVEB BORN HOS DEL C/S DEL	**Z38.31**	Twin liveborn infant, delivered by cesarean
V33.1	LIVB TWIN-UNS MATE LIVEB/STILLB-BEFORE ADMISS	**Z38.4**	Twin liveborn infant, born outside hospital
V33.2	LIVEB TWIN-UNS MATE LIVEB/STILLB OUTSIDE HOSP	**Z38.4**	Twin liveborn infant, born outside hospital
V34.ØØ	OTH MX MATES ALL LIVEB BORN HOS DEL W/O C/S DEL	**Z38.61** **Z38.63** **Z38.65** **Z38.68** **Z38.8**	Triplet liveborn infant, delivered vaginally Quadruplet liveborn infant, delivered vaginally Quintuplet liveborn infant, delivered vaginally Other multiple liveborn infant, delivered vaginally Other multiple liveborn infant, unsp as to place of birth
V34.Ø1	LIVEBORN OTH MX-MATES LIVEBORN HOSP C-SEC	**Z38.62** **Z38.64** **Z38.66** **Z38.69**	Triplet liveborn infant, delivered by cesarean Quadruplet liveborn infant, delivered by cesarean Quintuplet liveborn infant, delivered by cesarean Other multiple liveborn infant, delivered by cesarean
V34.1	LIVEBORN OTH MX-MATES LIVEBORN BEFOR ADMISSION	**Z38.7**	Other multiple liveborn infant, born outside hospital
V34.2	LIVEBORN OTH MX-MATES LIVEBORN OUTSIDE HOSP	**Z38.7**	Other multiple liveborn infant, born outside hospital
V35.ØØ	LIVEBORN OTH MX-MATES STILLB HOSP W/O C-SEC	**Z38.61** **Z38.63** **Z38.65** **Z38.68** **Z38.8**	Triplet liveborn infant, delivered vaginally Quadruplet liveborn infant, delivered vaginally Quintuplet liveborn infant, delivered vaginally Other multiple liveborn infant, delivered vaginally Other multiple liveborn infant, unsp as to place of birth
V35.Ø1	LIVEBORN OTH MX-MATES STILLBORN HOSP C-SEC	**Z38.62** **Z38.64** **Z38.66** **Z38.69** **Z38.8**	Triplet liveborn infant, delivered by cesarean Quadruplet liveborn infant, delivered by cesarean Quintuplet liveborn infant, delivered by cesarean Other multiple liveborn infant, delivered by cesarean Other multiple liveborn infant, unsp as to place of birth
V35.1	LIVEBORN OTH MX-MATES STILLB BEFORE ADMISSION	**Z38.7**	Other multiple liveborn infant, born outside hospital
V35.2	LIVEBORN OTH MX-MATES STILLB OUTSIDE HOSP	**Z38.7**	Other multiple liveborn infant, born outside hospital
V36.ØØ	LIVEB OTH MX-MATES LIVEB&STILLB HOSP W/O C-SEC	**Z38.61** **Z38.63** **Z38.65** **Z38.68** **Z38.8**	Triplet liveborn infant, delivered vaginally Quadruplet liveborn infant, delivered vaginally Quintuplet liveborn infant, delivered vaginally Other multiple liveborn infant, delivered vaginally Other multiple liveborn infant, unsp as to place of birth
V36.Ø1	LIVEBORN OTH MX-MATES LIVEB&STILLB HOSP C-SEC	**Z38.62** **Z38.64** **Z38.66** **Z38.69** **Z38.8**	Triplet liveborn infant, delivered by cesarean Quadruplet liveborn infant, delivered by cesarean Quintuplet liveborn infant, delivered by cesarean Other multiple liveborn infant, delivered by cesarean Other multiple liveborn infant, unsp as to place of birth
V36.1	LIVEB OTH MX-MATES LIVEB&STILLB BEFORE ADMISS	**Z38.7**	Other multiple liveborn infant, born outside hospital
V36.2	LIVEB OTH MX-MATES LIVEB&STILLB OUTSIDE HOSP	**Z38.7**	Other multiple liveborn infant, born outside hospital
V37.ØØ	LIVEB OTH MX-UNS MATE LIVEB/STILLB-HOSP WO C-SEC	**Z38.61** **Z38.63** **Z38.65** **Z38.68** **Z38.8**	Triplet liveborn infant, delivered vaginally Quadruplet liveborn infant, delivered vaginally Quintuplet liveborn infant, delivered vaginally Other multiple liveborn infant, delivered vaginally Other multiple liveborn infant, unsp as to place of birth

ICD-9-CM		ICD-10-CM	
V37.01	LIVEB OTH MX-UNS MATES LIVEB/STILLB HOSP C-SEC	**Z38.62** **Z38.64** **Z38.66** **Z38.69** **Z38.8**	Triplet liveborn infant, delivered by cesarean Quadruplet liveborn infant, delivered by cesarean Quintuplet liveborn infant, delivered by cesarean Other multiple liveborn infant, delivered by cesarean Other multiple liveborn infant, unsp as to place of birth
V37.1	LIVEB OTH MX-UNS MATES LIVEB/STILLB BEFOR ADMISS	**Z38.7**	Other multiple liveborn infant, born outside hospital
V37.2	LIVEB OTH MX-UNS MATES LIVEB/STILLB OUTSIDE HOSP	**Z38.7**	Other multiple liveborn infant, born outside hospital
V39.00	LIVEBORN UNS SINGLE TWIN/MX IN HOSP W/O C-SEC	**Z38.00** **Z38.2**	Single liveborn infant, delivered vaginally Single liveborn infant, unspecified as to place of birth
V39.01	LIVEBORN UNS SINGLE TWIN/MX IN HOSP C-SEC	**Z38.01**	Single liveborn infant, delivered by cesarean
V39.1	LIVEBORN UNS SINGLE TWIN/MX BEFORE ADMISSION	**Z38.1**	Single liveborn infant, born outside hospital
V39.2	LIVEBORN UNS SINGLE TWIN/MX OUTSIDE HOSP	**Z38.1**	Single liveborn infant, born outside hospital
V40.0	PROBLEMS WITH LEARNING	**F81.9**	Developmental disorder of scholastic skills, unspecified
V40.1	PROBLEMS WITH COMMUNICATION	**Z86.59**	Personal history of other mental and behavioral disorders
V40.2	OTHER MENTAL PROBLEMS	**F48.9**	Nonpsychotic mental disorder, unspecified
V40.31	WANDERING IN DISEASES CLASSIFIED ELSEWHERE	**Z91.83**	Wandering in diseases classified elsewhere
V40.39	OTHER SPECIFIED BEHAVIORAL PROBLEM	**F69** **R46.81** **R46.89**	Unspecified disorder of adult personality and behavior Obsessive-compulsive behavior Other symptoms and signs involving appearance and behavior
V40.9	UNSPECIFIED MENTAL OR BEHAVIORAL PROBLEM	**F48.9** **F69**	Nonpsychotic mental disorder, unspecified Unspecified disorder of adult personality and behavior
V41.0	PROBLEMS WITH SIGHT	**H54.7** **Z97.3**	Unspecified visual loss Presence of spectacles and contact lenses
V41.1	OTHER EYE PROBLEMS	**H57.9**	Unspecified disorder of eye and adnexa
V41.2	PROBLEMS WITH HEARING	**R68.89**	Other general symptoms and signs
V41.3	OTHER EAR PROBLEMS	**H93.90** **H93.91** **H93.92** **H93.93**	Unspecified disorder of ear, unspecified ear Unspecified disorder of right ear Unspecified disorder of left ear Unspecified disorder of ear, bilateral
V41.4	PROBLEMS WITH VOICE PRODUCTION	**R47.89**	Other speech disturbances
V41.5	PROBLEMS WITH SMELL AND TASTE	**R43.9**	Unspecified disturbances of smell and taste
V41.6	PROBLEMS WITH SWALLOWING AND MASTICATION	**R13.10**	Dysphagia, unspecified
V41.7	PROBLEMS WITH SEXUAL FUNCTION	**F52.9**	Unsp sexual dysfnct not due to a sub or known physiol cond
V41.8	OTHER PROBLEMS WITH SPECIAL FUNCTIONS	**R68.89**	Other general symptoms and signs
V41.9	UNSPECIFIED PROBLEM WITH SPECIAL FUNCTIONS	**R69**	Illness, unspecified
V42.0	KIDNEY REPLACED BY TRANSPLANT	**Z48.22** **Z94.0**	Encounter for aftercare following kidney transplant Kidney transplant status
V42.1	HEART REPLACED BY TRANSPLANT	**Z48.21** **Z48.280** **Z94.1** **Z94.3**	Encounter for aftercare following heart transplant Encounter for aftercare following heart-lung transplant Heart transplant status Heart and lungs transplant status
V42.2	HEART VALVE REPLACED BY TRANSPLANT	**Z95.3** **Z95.4**	Presence of xenogenic heart valve Presence of other heart-valve replacement
V42.3	SKIN REPLACED BY TRANSPLANT	**Z94.5**	Skin transplant status
V42.4	BONE REPLACED BY TRANSPLANT	**Z94.6**	Bone transplant status
V42.5	CORNEA REPLACED BY TRANSPLANT	**Z94.7**	Corneal transplant status
V42.6	LUNG REPLACED BY TRANSPLANT	**Z48.24** **Z48.280** **Z94.2** **Z94.3**	Encounter for aftercare following lung transplant Encounter for aftercare following heart-lung transplant Lung transplant status Heart and lungs transplant status
V42.7	LIVER REPLACED BY TRANSPLANT	**Z48.23** **Z94.4**	Encounter for aftercare following liver transplant Liver transplant status
V42.81	BONE MARROW REPLACED BY TRANSPLANT	**Z48.290** **Z94.81**	Encounter for aftercare following bone marrow transplant Bone marrow transplant status
V42.82	PERIPHERAL STEM CELLS REPLACED BY TRANSPLANT	**Z94.84**	Stem cells transplant status
V42.83	PANCREAS REPLACED BY TRANSPLANT	**Z94.83**	Pancreas transplant status
V42.84	ORGAN OR TISSUE REPLACED TRANSPLANT INTESTINES	**Z94.82**	Intestine transplant status
V42.89	OTHER ORGAN OR TISSUE REPLACED BY TRANSPLANT	**Z48.298** **Z94.89**	Encounter for aftercare following other organ transplant Other transplanted organ and tissue status
V42.9	UNSPECIFIED ORGAN OR TISSUE REPLACED TRANSPLANT	**Z48.288** **Z94.9**	Encounter for aftercare following multiple organ transplant Transplanted organ and tissue status, unspecified
V43.0	EYE GLOBE REPLACED BY OTHER MEANS	**Z97.0**	Presence of artificial eye
V43.1	LENS REPLACED BY OTHER MEANS	**Z96.1**	Presence of intraocular lens
V43.21	ORGAN/TISSUE REPL OTH MEANS HRT ASSIST DEVICE	**Z95.811**	Presence of heart assist device
V43.22	ORGAN/TISS REPL OTH MEANS FULL IMPL ARTFICL HRT	**Z95.812**	Presence of fully implantable artificial heart
V43.3	HEART VALVE REPLACED BY OTHER MEANS	**Z95.2**	Presence of prosthetic heart valve
V43.4	BLOOD VESSEL REPLACED BY OTHER MEANS	**Z95.820** **Z95.828**	Peripheral vascular angioplasty status w implants and grafts Presence of other vascular implants and grafts
V43.5	BLADDER REPLACED BY OTHER MEANS	**Z96.0**	Presence of urogenital implants
V43.60	UNSPECIFIED JOINT REPLACEMENT BY OTHER MEANS	**Z96.60**	Presence of unspecified orthopedic joint implant

[Brackets] indicate valid character values for each code. Character value meanings provided for each code grouping.

ICD-9-CM			ICD-10-CM	
V43.61	SHOULDER JOINT REPLACEMENT BY OTHER MEANS		**Z96.611**	Presence of right artificial shoulder joint
			Z96.612	Presence of left artificial shoulder joint
			Z96.619	Presence of unspecified artificial shoulder joint
V43.62	ELBOW JOINT REPLACEMENT BY OTHER MEANS		**Z96.621**	Presence of right artificial elbow joint
			Z96.622	Presence of left artificial elbow joint
			Z96.629	Presence of unspecified artificial elbow joint
V43.63	WRIST JOINT REPLACEMENT BY OTHER MEANS		**Z96.631**	Presence of right artificial wrist joint
			Z96.632	Presence of left artificial wrist joint
			Z96.639	Presence of unspecified artificial wrist joint
V43.64	HIP JOINT REPLACEMENT BY OTHER MEANS		**Z96.641**	Presence of right artificial hip joint
			Z96.642	Presence of left artificial hip joint
			Z96.643	Presence of artificial hip joint, bilateral
			Z96.649	Presence of unspecified artificial hip joint
V43.65	KNEE JOINT REPLACEMENT BY OTHER MEANS		**Z96.651**	Presence of right artificial knee joint
			Z96.652	Presence of left artificial knee joint
			Z96.653	Presence of artificial knee joint, bilateral
			Z96.659	Presence of unspecified artificial knee joint
V43.66	ANKLE JOINT REPLACEMENT BY OTHER MEANS		**Z96.661**	Presence of right artificial ankle joint
			Z96.662	Presence of left artificial ankle joint
			Z96.669	Presence of unspecified artificial ankle joint
V43.69	OTHER JOINT REPLACEMENT BY OTHER MEANS		**Z96.691**	Finger-joint replacement of right hand
			Z96.692	Finger-joint replacement of left hand
			Z96.693	Finger-joint replacement, bilateral
			Z96.698	Presence of other orthopedic joint implants
			Z96.7	Presence of other bone and tendon implants
V43.7	LIMB REPLACED BY OTHER MEANS		**Z97.10**	Presence of artificial limb (complete) (partial), unsp
			Z97.11	Presence of artificial right arm (complete) (partial)
			Z97.12	Presence of artificial left arm (complete) (partial)
			Z97.13	Presence of artificial right leg (complete) (partial)
			Z97.14	Presence of artificial left leg (complete) (partial)
			Z97.15	Presence of artificial arms, bilateral (complete) (partial)
			Z97.16	Presence of artificial legs, bilateral (complete) (partial)
V43.81	LARYNX REPLACED BY OTHER MEANS	➡	**Z96.3**	Presence of artificial larynx
V43.82	BREAST REPLACED BY OTHER MEANS		**Z98.82**	Breast implant status
V43.83	ORGAN OR TISSUE REPLACED BY ARTIFICIAL SKIN	➡	**Z96.81**	Presence of artificial skin
V43.89	OTHER ORGAN/TISSUE REPLACED BY OTHER MEANS OTHER		**Z96.20**	Presence of otological and audiological implant, unspecified
			Z96.29	Presence of other otological and audiological implants
			Z96.49	Presence of other endocrine implants
			Z96.5	Presence of tooth-root and mandibular implants
			Z96.89	Presence of other specified functional implants
			Z96.9	Presence of functional implant, unspecified
V44.0	TRACHEOSTOMY STATUS	➡	**Z93.0**	Tracheostomy status
V44.1	GASTROSTOMY STATUS	➡	**Z93.1**	Gastrostomy status
V44.2	ILEOSTOMY STATUS	➡	**Z93.2**	Ileostomy status
V44.3	COLOSTOMY STATUS	➡	**Z93.3**	Colostomy status
V44.4	STATUS OTH ARTFICL OPENING GI TRACT	➡	**Z93.4**	Other artificial openings of gastrointestinal tract status
V44.50	UNSPECIFIED CYSTOSTOMY STATUS	➡	**Z93.50**	Unspecified cystostomy status
V44.51	CUTANEOUS-VESICOSTOMY STATUS	➡	**Z93.51**	Cutaneous-vesicostomy status
V44.52	APPENDICO-VESICOSTOMY STATUS	➡	**Z93.52**	Appendico-vesicostomy status
V44.59	OTHER CYSTOSTOMY STATUS	➡	**Z93.59**	Other cystostomy status
V44.6	STATUS OTHER ARTIFICIAL OPENING URINARY TRACT	➡	**Z93.6**	Other artificial openings of urinary tract status
V44.7	ARTIFICIAL VAGINA STATUS		**Z93.8**	Other artificial opening status
V44.8	OTHER ARTIFICIAL OPENING STATUS		**Z93.8**	Other artificial opening status
V44.9	UNSPECIFIED ARTIFICIAL OPENING STATUS	➡	**Z93.9**	Artificial opening status, unspecified
V45.00	UNSPECIFIED CARDIAC DEVICE IN SITU		**Z95.9**	Presence of cardiac and vascular implant and graft, unsp
V45.01	CARDIAC PACEMAKER IN SITU	➡	**Z95.0**	Presence of cardiac pacemaker
V45.02	AUTOMATIC IMPLANTABLE CARDIAC DEFIBRILLATOR SITU	➡	**Z95.810**	Presence of automatic (implantable) cardiac defibrillator
V45.09	OTHER SPECIFIED CARDIAC DEVICE IN SITU		**Z95.818**	Presence of other cardiac implants and grafts
V45.11	RENAL DIALYSIS STATUS	➡	**Z99.2**	Dependence on renal dialysis
V45.12	NONCOMPLIANCE WITH RENAL DIALYSIS	➡	**Z91.15**	Patient's noncompliance with renal dialysis
V45.2	PRESENCE OF CEREBROSPINAL FLUID DRAINAGE DEVICE	➡	**Z98.2**	Presence of cerebrospinal fluid drainage device
V45.3	INTESTINAL BYPASS OR ANASTOMOSIS STATUS	➡	**Z98.0**	Intestinal bypass and anastomosis status
V45.4	ARTHRODESIS STATUS		**M96.0**	Pseudarthrosis after fusion or arthrodesis
			Z98.1	Arthrodesis status
V45.51	PRESENCE OF INTRAUTERINE CONTRACEPTIVE DEVICE		**Z97.5**	Presence of (intrauterine) contraceptive device
V45.52	PRESENCE OF SUBDERMAL CONTRACEPTIVE DEVICE		**Z97.5**	Presence of (intrauterine) contraceptive device
V45.59	PRESENCE OF OTHER CONTRACEPTIVE DEVICE		**Z97.5**	Presence of (intrauterine) contraceptive device
V45.61	CATARACT EXTRACTION STATUS		**Z98.41**	Cataract extraction status, right eye
			Z98.42	Cataract extraction status, left eye
			Z98.49	Cataract extraction status, unspecified eye
V45.69	OTHER STATES FOLLOWING SURGERY OF EYE AND ADNEXA		**Z98.83**	Filtering (vitreous) bleb after glaucoma surgery status

ICD-9-CM			ICD-10-CM	
V45.71	ACQUIRED ABSENCE OF BREAST AND NIPPLE		**Z9Ø.1Ø** **Z9Ø.11** **Z9Ø.12** **Z9Ø.13**	Acquired absence of unspecified breast and nipple Acquired absence of right breast and nipple Acquired absence of left breast and nipple Acquired absence of bilateral breasts and nipples
V45.72	ACQUIRED ABSENCE OF INTESTINE		**Z9Ø.49**	Acquired absence of other specified parts of digestive tract
V45.73	ACQUIRED ABSENCE OF KIDNEY	➡	**Z9Ø.5**	Acquired absence of kidney
V45.74	ACQUIRED ABSENCE ORGAN OTHER PARTS URINARY TRACT	➡	**Z9Ø.6**	Acquired absence of other parts of urinary tract
V45.75	ACQUIRED ABSENCE OF ORGAN, STOMACH	➡	**Z9Ø.3**	Acquired absence of stomach [part of]
V45.76	ACQUIRED ABSENCE OF ORGAN, LUNG	➡	**Z9Ø.2**	Acquired absence of lung [part of]
V45.77	ACQUIRED ABSENCE OF ORGAN GENITAL ORGANS		**Z9Ø.721** **Z9Ø.722** **Z9Ø.79**	Acquired absence of ovaries, unilateral Acquired absence of ovaries, bilateral Acquired absence of other genital organ(s)
V45.78	ACQUIRED ABSENCE OF ORGAN, EYE	➡	**Z9Ø.Ø1**	Acquired absence of eye
V45.79	OTHER ACQUIRED ABSENCE OF ORGAN		**Z9Ø.Ø2** **Z9Ø.Ø9** **Z9Ø.81** **Z9Ø.89**	Acquired absence of larynx Acquired absence of other part of head and neck Acquired absence of spleen Acquired absence of other organs
V45.81	POSTSURGICAL AORTOCORONARY BYPASS STATUS	➡	**Z95.1**	Presence of aortocoronary bypass graft
V45.82	POSTSURG PERCUT TRANSLUMINAL COR ANGPLSTY STS		**Z95.5** **Z98.61**	Presence of coronary angioplasty implant and graft Coronary angioplasty status
V45.83	BREAST IMPLANT REMOVAL STATUS	➡	**Z98.86**	Personal history of breast implant removal
V45.84	DENTAL RESTORATION STATUS		**Z97.2** **Z98.811** **Z98.818**	Presence of dental prosthetic device (complete) (partial) Dental restoration status Other dental procedure status
V45.85	INSULIN PUMP STATUS	➡	**Z96.41**	Presence of insulin pump (external) (internal)
V45.86	BARIATRIC SURGERY STATUS	➡	**Z98.84**	Bariatric surgery status
V45.87	TRANSPLANTED ORGAN REMOVAL STATUS	➡	**Z98.85**	Transplanted organ removal status
V45.88	S/P ADM TPA DIF FACILTY LAST 24H PTA CUR FACILTY	➡	**Z92.82**	S/p admn tPA in diff fac w/n last 24 hr bef adm to crnt fac
V45.89	OTHER POSTSURGICAL STATUS OTHER		**Z96.21** **Z96.22** **Z97.4** **Z97.8** **Z98.3** **Z98.62** **Z98.89**	Cochlear implant status Myringotomy tube(s) status Presence of external hearing-aid Presence of other specified devices Post therapeutic collapse of lung status Peripheral vascular angioplasty status Other specified postprocedural states
V46.Ø	DEPENDENCE ON ASPIRATOR	➡	**Z99.Ø**	Dependence on aspirator
V46.11	DEPENDENCE ON RESPIRATOR STATUS		**Z99.11**	Dependence on respirator [ventilator] status
V46.12	ENCOUNTER RESPIRATOR DEPEND DURING POWER FAILURE	➡	**Z99.12**	Encounter for respirator dependence during power failure
V46.13	ENCOUNTER FOR WEANING FROM RESPIRATOR VENTILATOR		**Z99.11**	Dependence on respirator [ventilator] status
V46.14	MECHANICAL COMPLICATION OF RESPIRATOR VENTILATOR	➡	**J95.85Ø**	Mechanical complication of respirator
V46.2	DEPENDENCE ON MACHINE FOR SUPPLEMENTAL OXYGEN	➡	**Z99.81**	Dependence on supplemental oxygen
V46.3	WHEELCHAIR DEPENDENCE	➡	**Z99.3**	Dependence on wheelchair
V46.8	DEPENDENCE ON OTHER ENABLING MACHINE		**Z99.89**	Dependence on other enabling machines and devices
V46.9	UNSPECIFIED MACHINE DEPENDENCE		**Z99.89**	Dependence on other enabling machines and devices
V47.Ø	DEFICIENCIES OF INTERNAL ORGANS		**Z87.898**	Personal history of other specified conditions
V47.1	MECHANICAL AND MOTOR PROBLEMS W/INTERNAL ORGANS		**R68.89**	Other general symptoms and signs
V47.2	OTHER CARDIORESPIRATORY PROBLEMS		**R68.89**	Other general symptoms and signs
V47.3	OTHER DIGESTIVE PROBLEMS		**R68.89**	Other general symptoms and signs
V47.4	OTHER URINARY PROBLEMS		**R68.89**	Other general symptoms and signs
V47.5	OTHER GENITAL PROBLEMS		**R68.89**	Other general symptoms and signs
V47.9	UNSPECIFIED PROBLEMS WITH INTERNAL ORGANS		**R68.89**	Other general symptoms and signs
V48.Ø	DEFICIENCIES OF HEAD		**R68.89**	Other general symptoms and signs
V48.1	DEFICIENCIES OF NECK AND TRUNK		**R68.89**	Other general symptoms and signs
V48.2	MECHANICAL AND MOTOR PROBLEMS WITH HEAD		**R68.89**	Other general symptoms and signs
V48.3	MECHANICAL AND MOTOR PROBLEMS W/NECK AND TRUNK		**R68.89**	Other general symptoms and signs
V48.4	SENSORY PROBLEM WITH HEAD		**R68.89**	Other general symptoms and signs
V48.5	SENSORY PROBLEM WITH NECK AND TRUNK		**R68.89**	Other general symptoms and signs
V48.6	DISFIGUREMENTS OF HEAD		**R68.89**	Other general symptoms and signs
V48.7	DISFIGUREMENTS OF NECK AND TRUNK		**R68.89**	Other general symptoms and signs
V48.8	OTHER PROBLEMS WITH HEAD NECK AND TRUNK		**R68.89**	Other general symptoms and signs
V48.9	UNSPECIFIED PROBLEM WITH HEAD NECK OR TRUNK		**R68.89**	Other general symptoms and signs
V49.Ø	DEFICIENCIES OF LIMBS		**R68.89**	Other general symptoms and signs
V49.1	MECHANICAL PROBLEMS WITH LIMBS		**R68.89**	Other general symptoms and signs
V49.2	MOTOR PROBLEMS WITH LIMBS		**R68.89**	Other general symptoms and signs
V49.3	SENSORY PROBLEMS WITH LIMBS		**R68.89**	Other general symptoms and signs
V49.4	DISFIGUREMENTS OF LIMBS		**R68.89**	Other general symptoms and signs
V49.5	OTHER PROBLEMS OF LIMBS		**R68.89**	Other general symptoms and signs
V49.6Ø	UPPER LIMB AMPUTATION STATUS UNSPEC LEVEL **(Continued on next page)**		**Z89.2Ø1** **Z89.2Ø2**	Acquired absence of right upper limb, unspecified level Acquired absence of left upper limb, unspecified level

ICD-9-CM		ICD-10-CM	
V49.6Ø	UPPER LIMB AMPUTATION STATUS UNSPEC LEVEL **(Continued)**	**Z89.2Ø9** **Z89.9**	Acquired absence of unsp upper limb, unspecified level Acquired absence of limb, unspecified
V49.61	UPPER LIMB AMPUTATION, THUMB	**Z89.Ø11** **Z89.Ø12** **Z89.Ø19**	Acquired absence of right thumb Acquired absence of left thumb Acquired absence of unspecified thumb
V49.62	UPPER LIMB AMPUTATION, OTHER FINGER	**Z89.Ø21** **Z89.Ø22** **Z89.Ø29**	Acquired absence of right finger(s) Acquired absence of left finger(s) Acquired absence of unspecified finger(s)
V49.63	UPPER LIMB AMPUTATION, HAND	**Z89.111** **Z89.112** **Z89.119**	Acquired absence of right hand Acquired absence of left hand Acquired absence of unspecified hand
V49.64	UPPER LIMB AMPUTATION, WRIST	**Z89.121** **Z89.122** **Z89.129**	Acquired absence of right wrist Acquired absence of left wrist Acquired absence of unspecified wrist
V49.65	UPPER LIMB AMPUTATION, BELOW ELBOW	**Z89.211** **Z89.212** **Z89.219**	Acquired absence of right upper limb below elbow Acquired absence of left upper limb below elbow Acquired absence of unspecified upper limb below elbow
V49.66	UPPER LIMB AMPUTATION, ABOVE ELBOW	**Z89.221** **Z89.222** **Z89.229**	Acquired absence of right upper limb above elbow Acquired absence of left upper limb above elbow Acquired absence of unspecified upper limb above elbow
V49.67	UPPER LIMB AMPUTATION, SHOULDER	**Z89.231** **Z89.232** **Z89.239**	Acquired absence of right shoulder Acquired absence of left shoulder Acquired absence of unspecified shoulder
V49.7Ø	LOWER LIMB AMPUTATION STATUS UNSPEC LEVEL	**Z89.9**	Acquired absence of limb, unspecified
V49.71	LOWER LIMB AMPUTATION, GREAT TOE	**Z89.411** **Z89.412** **Z89.419**	Acquired absence of right great toe Acquired absence of left great toe Acquired absence of unspecified great toe
V49.72	LOWER LIMB AMPUTATION, OTHER TOE	**Z89.421** **Z89.422** **Z89.429**	Acquired absence of other right toe(s) Acquired absence of other left toe(s) Acquired absence of other toe(s), unspecified side
V49.73	LOWER LIMB AMPUTATION, FOOT	**Z89.431** **Z89.432** **Z89.439**	Acquired absence of right foot Acquired absence of left foot Acquired absence of unspecified foot
V49.74	LOWER LIMB AMPUTATION, ANKLE	**Z89.441** **Z89.442** **Z89.449**	Acquired absence of right ankle Acquired absence of left ankle Acquired absence of unspecified ankle
V49.75	LOWER LIMB AMPUTATION, BELOW KNEE	**Z89.511** **Z89.512** **Z89.519**	Acquired absence of right leg below knee Acquired absence of left leg below knee Acquired absence of unspecified leg below knee
V49.76	LOWER LIMB AMPUTATION, ABOVE KNEE	**Z89.611** **Z89.612** **Z89.619**	Acquired absence of right leg above knee Acquired absence of left leg above knee Acquired absence of unspecified leg above knee
V49.77	LOWER LIMB AMPUTATION, HIP	**Z89.621** **Z89.622** **Z89.629**	Acquired absence of right hip joint Acquired absence of left hip joint Acquired absence of unspecified hip joint
V49.81	ASYMPTOMATIC POSTMENOPAUSAL STATUS	**Z78.Ø**	Asymptomatic menopausal state
V49.82	DENTAL SEALANT STATUS	➡ **Z98.81Ø**	Dental sealant status
V49.83	AWAITING ORGAN TRANSPLANT STATUS	➡ **Z76.82**	Awaiting organ transplant status
V49.84	BED CONFINEMENT STATUS	➡ **Z74.Ø1**	Bed confinement status
V49.85	DUAL SENSORY IMPAIRMENT	➡ **Z73.82**	Dual sensory impairment
V49.86	DO NOT RESUSCITATE STATUS	➡ **Z66**	Do not resuscitate
V49.87	PHYSICAL RESTRAINTS STATUS	➡ **Z78.1**	Physical restraint status
V49.89	OTHER SPEC CONDITIONS INFLUENCING HEALTH STATUS	**Z74.Ø9** **Z78.9**	Other reduced mobility Other specified health status
V49.9	UNSPECIFIED PROBLEMS W/LIMBS AND OTHER PROBLEMS	**Z87.898**	Personal history of other specified conditions
V5Ø.Ø	ELCTV HAIR TPLNT PRPSS OTH THAN REMEDYING HLTH	**Z41.1**	Encounter for cosmetic surgery
V5Ø.1	OTH PLASTIC SURGERY UNACCEPTABLE COSMETIC APPEAR	**Z41.1**	Encounter for cosmetic surgery
V5Ø.2	ROUTINE OR RITUAL CIRCUMCISION	➡ **Z41.2**	Encounter for routine and ritual male circumcision
V5Ø.3	EAR PIERCING	➡ **Z41.3**	Encounter for ear piercing
V5Ø.41	PROPHYLACTIC BREAST REMOVAL	➡ **Z4Ø.Ø1**	Encounter for prophylactic removal of breast
V5Ø.42	PROPHYLACTIC OVARY REMOVAL	➡ **Z4Ø.Ø2**	Encounter for prophylactic removal of ovary
V5Ø.49	OTHER PROPHYLACTIC ORGAN REMOVAL	**Z4Ø.ØØ** **Z4Ø.Ø9**	Encounter for prophylactic removal of unspecified organ Encounter for prophylactic removal of other organ
V5Ø.8	OTH ELCTV SURG PRPSS OTH THAN REMEDYING HLTH	**Z4Ø.8** **Z4Ø.9** **Z41.8**	Encounter for other prophylactic surgery Encounter for prophylactic surgery, unspecified Encntr for oth proc for purpose oth than remedy health state
V5Ø.9	UNS ELCTV SURG PRPSS OTH THAN REMEDYING HLTH	➡ **Z41.9**	Encntr for proc for purpose oth than remedy hlth state, unsp
V51.Ø	ENCOUNTER BREAST RECONSTRUCTION FLW MASTECTOMY	➡ **Z42.1**	Encounter for breast reconstruction following mastectomy
V51.8	OTHER AFTERCARE INVLV THE USE OF PLASTIC SURGERY	**Z42.8**	Encntr for oth plast/recnst surg fol med proc or heal injury
V52.Ø	FITTING AND ADJUSTMENT OF ARTIFICIAL ARM **(Continued on next page)**	**Z44.ØØ1** **Z44.ØØ2** **Z44.ØØ9** **Z44.Ø11** **Z44.Ø12**	Encounter for fit/adjst of unsp right artificial arm Encounter for fit/adjst of unsp left artificial arm Encounter for fit/adjst of unsp artificial arm, unsp arm Encounter for fit/adjst of complete right artificial arm Encounter for fit/adjst of complete left artificial arm

ICD-9-CM			ICD-10-CM	
V52.Ø	FITTING AND ADJUSTMENT OF ARTIFICIAL ARM **(Continued)**		**Z44.Ø19**	Encounter for fit/adjst of complete artificial arm, unsp arm
			Z44.Ø21	Encounter for fit/adjst of partial artificial right arm
			Z44.Ø22	Encounter for fit/adjst of partial artificial left arm
			Z44.Ø29	Encounter for fit/adjst of partial artificial arm, unsp arm
V52.1	FITTING AND ADJUSTMENT OF ARTIFICIAL LEG		**Z44.1Ø1**	Encounter for fit/adjst of unsp right artificial leg
			Z44.1Ø2	Encounter for fit/adjst of unsp left artificial leg
			Z44.1Ø9	Encounter for fit/adjst of unsp artificial leg, unsp leg
			Z44.111	Encounter for fit/adjst of complete right artificial leg
			Z44.112	Encounter for fit/adjst of complete left artificial leg
			Z44.119	Encounter for fit/adjst of complete artificial leg, unsp leg
			Z44.121	Encounter for fit/adjst of partial artificial right leg
			Z44.122	Encounter for fit/adjst of partial artificial left leg
			Z44.129	Encounter for fit/adjst of partial artificial leg, unsp leg
V52.2	FITTING AND ADJUSTMENT OF ARTIFICIAL EYE		**Z44.2Ø**	Encounter for fitting and adjustment of artificial eye, unsp
			Z44.21	Encounter for fitting and adjustment of artificial right eye
			Z44.22	Encounter for fitting and adjustment of artificial left eye
V52.3	FITTING&ADJUSTMENT OF DENTAL PROSTHETIC DEVICE	➡	**Z46.3**	Encounter for fit/adjst of dental prosthetic device
V52.4	FITTING&ADJUSTMENT OF BREAST PROSTHESIS&IMPLANT		**Z44.3Ø**	Encntr for fit/adjst of external breast prosth, unsp breast
			Z44.31	Encounter for fit/adjst of external right breast prosthesis
			Z44.32	Encounter for fit/adjst of external left breast prosthesis
			Z45.811	Encounter for adjustment or removal of right breast implant
			Z45.812	Encounter for adjustment or removal of left breast implant
			Z45.819	Encounter for adjustment or removal of unsp breast implant
V52.8	FITTING&ADJUSTMENT OTHER SPEC PROSTHETIC DEVICE		**Z44.8**	Encounter for fit/adjst of external prosthetic devices
V52.9	FITTING&ADJUSTMENT UNSPECIFIED PROSTHETIC DEVICE	➡	**Z44.9**	Encounter for fit/adjst of unsp external prosthetic device
V53.Ø1	FITTING&ADJUSTMENT OF CEREBRAL VENTRICULAR SHUNT	➡	**Z45.41**	Encounter for adjustment and management of CSF drain dev
V53.Ø2	NEUROPACEMAKER	➡	**Z45.42**	Encounter for adjust and mgmt of neuropacemaker (brain)
V53.Ø9	FIT&ADJ OTH DEVC RELATED NERV SYSTEM&SPCL SENSES		**Z45.31**	Encntr for adjust and mgmt of implnt visual substitution dev
			Z45.32Ø	Encounter for adjust and mgmt of bone conduction device
			Z45.321	Encounter for adjustment and management of cochlear device
			Z45.328	Encounter for adjust and management of implanted hear dev
			Z45.49	Encntr for adjust and mgmt of implanted nervous sys device
			Z46.2	Encntr for fit/adjst of dev rel to nrv sys and specl senses
V53.1	FITTING&ADJUSTMENT OF SPECTACLES&CONTACT LENSES	➡	**Z46.Ø**	Encounter for fit/adjst of spectacles and contact lenses
V53.2	FITTING AND ADJUSTMENT OF HEARING AID	➡	**Z46.1**	Encounter for fitting and adjustment of hearing aid
V53.31	FITTING AND ADJUSTMENT OF CARDIAC PACEMAKER		**Z45.Ø1Ø**	Encntr for checking and test of card pacemaker pulse gnrtr
			Z45.Ø18	Encounter for adjust and mgmt oth prt cardiac pacemaker
V53.32	FITTING&ADJ AUTO IMPLANTABLE CARD DEFIBRILLATOR	➡	**Z45.Ø2**	Encntr for adjust and mgmt of automatic implntbl card defib
V53.39	FITTING AND ADJUSTMENT OF OTHER CARDIAC DEVICE	➡	**Z45.Ø9**	Encounter for adjustment and management of cardiac device
V53.4	FITTING AND ADJUSTMENT OF ORTHODONTIC DEVICES		**Z46.4**	Encounter for fitting and adjustment of orthodontic device
V53.5Ø	FITTING & ADJUSTMENT INTESTINAL APPLIANCE&DEVICE		**Z46.59**	Encounter for fit/adjst of GI appliance and device
V53.51	FITTING & ADJUSTMENT OF GASTRIC LAP BAND	➡	**Z46.51**	Encounter for fitting and adjustment of gastric lap band
V53.59	FITTING & ADJUSTMENT OTHER GI APPLIANCE & DEVICE		**Z46.59**	Encounter for fit/adjst of GI appliance and device
V53.6	FITTING AND ADJUSTMENT OF URINARY DEVICE	➡	**Z46.6**	Encounter for fitting and adjustment of urinary device
V53.7	FITTING AND ADJUSTMENT OF ORTHOPEDIC DEVICE		**Z46.89**	Encounter for fitting and adjustment of oth devices
V53.8	FITTING AND ADJUSTMENT OF WHEELCHAIR		**Z46.89**	Encounter for fitting and adjustment of oth devices
V53.9Ø	FITTING AND ADJUSTMENT UNSPECIFIED DEVICE		**Z45.9**	Encounter for adjust and management of unsp implanted device
			Z46.9	Encounter for fitting and adjustment of unspecified device
V53.91	FITTING AND ADJUSTMENT OF INSULIN PUMP		**Z46.81**	Encounter for fitting and adjustment of insulin pump
V53.99	FITTING AND ADJUSTMENT OTHER DEVICE		**Z45.82**	Encntr for adjust or removal of myringotomy device (tube)
			Z45.89	Encounter for adjustment and management of implanted devices
			Z46.89	Encounter for fitting and adjustment of oth devices
V54.Ø1	ENCOUNTER REMOVAL OF INTERNAL FIXATION DEVICE	➡	**Z47.2**	Encounter for removal of internal fixation device
V54.Ø2	ENCOUNTER LENGTHENING/ADJUSTMENT OF GROWTH ROD		**Z51.89**	Encounter for other specified aftercare
V54.Ø9	OTH AFTERCARE INVOLVING INTERNAL FIXATION DEVICE		**Z51.89**	Encounter for other specified aftercare
V54.1Ø	AFTERCARE HEALING TRAUMATIC FRACTURE ARM UNSPEC		**S52.9ØXD**	Unsp fracture of unsp forearm, subs for clos fx w routn heal
			S52.9ØXE	Unsp fx unsp forearm, subs for opn fx type I/2 w routn heal
			S52.9ØXF	Unsp fx unsp forearm, sub op fx typ 3 A/B/C w rout heal
			S52.9ØXG	Unsp fracture of unsp forearm, subs for clos fx w delay heal
			S52.9ØXH	Unsp fx unsp forearm, subs for opn fx type I/2 w delay heal
			S52.9ØXJ	Unsp fx unsp forearm, sub op fx typ 3 A/B/C w delay heal
V54.11	AFTERCARE HEALING TRAUMATIC FRACTURE UPPER ARM		**S42.1Ø1D**	Fx unsp part of scapula, r shldr, subs for fx w routn heal
			S42.1Ø1G	Fx unsp part of scapula, r shldr, subs for fx w delay heal
			S42.1Ø2D	Fx unsp part of scapula, l shldr, subs for fx w routn heal
			S42.1Ø2G	Fx unsp part of scapula, l shldr, subs for fx w delay heal
			S42.1Ø9D	Fx unsp prt of scapula, unsp shldr, subs for fx w routn heal
			S42.1Ø9G	Fx unsp prt of scapula, unsp shldr, subs for fx w delay heal
			S42.111D	Disp fx of body of scapula, r shldr, sub for fx w rout heal
			S42.111G	Disp fx of body of scapula, r shldr, sub for fx w delay heal
			S42.112D	Disp fx of body of scapula, l shldr, sub for fx w rout heal
			S42.112G	Disp fx of body of scapula, l shldr, sub for fx w delay heal
			S42.113D	Disp fx of body of scapula, unsp shldr, sub for fx w rout heal
			S42.113G	Disp fx of body of scapula, unsp shldr, sub for fx w delay heal
			S42.114D	Nondisp fx of body of scapula, r shldr, sub for fx w rout heal
			S42.114G	Nondisp fx of body of scapula, r shldr, sub for fx w delay heal
	(Continued on next page)		**S42.115D**	Nondisp fx of body of scapula, l shldr, sub for fx w rout heal

ICD-9-CM		ICD-10-CM	
V54.11	AFTERCARE HEALING TRAUMATIC FRACTURE UPPER ARM **(Continued)**	**S42.115G**	Nondisp fx of body of scapula, l shldr, sub for fx w delay heal
		S42.116D	Nondisp fx of body of scapula, unsp shldr, sub for fx w rout heal
		S42.116G	Nondisp fx of body of scapula, unsp shldr, sub for fx w delay heal
		S42.121D	Disp fx of acromial pro, r shldr, subs for fx w routn heal
		S42.121G	Disp fx of acromial pro, r shldr, subs for fx w delay heal
		S42.122D	Disp fx of acromial pro, l shldr, subs for fx w routn heal
		S42.122G	Disp fx of acromial pro, l shldr, subs for fx w delay heal
		S42.123D	Disp fx of acromial pro, unsp shldr, sub for fx w rout heal
		S42.123G	Disp fx of acromial pro, unsp shldr, sub for fx w delay heal
		S42.124D	Nondisp fx of acromial pro, r shldr, sub for fx w rout heal
		S42.124G	Nondisp fx of acromial pro, r shldr, sub for fx w delay heal
		S42.125D	Nondisp fx of acromial pro, l shldr, sub for fx w rout heal
		S42.125G	Nondisp fx of acromial pro, l shldr, sub for fx w delay heal
		S42.126D	Nondisp fx of acromial pro, unsp shldr, sub for fx w rout heal
		S42.126G	Nondisp fx of acromial pro, unsp shldr, sub for fx w delay heal
		S42.131D	Disp fx of coracoid pro, r shldr, subs for fx w routn heal
		S42.131G	Disp fx of coracoid pro, r shldr, subs for fx w delay heal
		S42.132D	Disp fx of coracoid pro, l shldr, subs for fx w routn heal
		S42.132G	Disp fx of coracoid pro, l shldr, subs for fx w delay heal
		S42.133D	Disp fx of coracoid pro, unsp shldr, sub for fx w rout heal
		S42.133G	Disp fx of coracoid pro, unsp shldr, sub for fx w delay heal
		S42.134D	Nondisp fx of coracoid pro, r shldr, sub for fx w rout heal
		S42.134G	Nondisp fx of coracoid pro, r shldr, sub for fx w delay heal
		S42.135D	Nondisp fx of coracoid pro, l shldr, sub for fx w rout heal
		S42.135G	Nondisp fx of coracoid pro, l shldr, sub for fx w delay heal
		S42.136D	Nondisp fx of coracoid pro, unsp shldr, sub for fx w rout heal
		S42.136G	Nondisp fx of coracoid pro, unsp shldr, sub for fx w delay heal
		S42.141D	Disp fx of glenoid cav of scapula, r shldr, sub for fx w rout heal
		S42.141G	Disp fx of glenoid cav of scapula, r shldr, sub for fx w delay heal
		S42.142D	Disp fx of glenoid cav of scapula, l shldr, sub for fx w rout heal
		S42.142G	Disp fx of glenoid cav of scapula, l shldr, sub for fx w delay heal
		S42.143D	Disp fx of glenoid cav of scapula, unsp shldr, sub for fx w rout heal
		S42.143G	Disp fx of glenoid cav of scapula, unsp shldr, sub for fx w delay heal
		S42.144D	Nondisp fx of glenoid cav of scapula, r shldr, sub for fx w rout heal
		S42.144G	Nondisp fx of glenoid cav of scapula, r shldr, sub for fx w delay heal
		S42.145D	Nondisp fx of glenoid cav of scapula, l shldr, sub for fx w rout heal
		S42.145G	Nondisp fx of glenoid cav of scapula, l shldr, sub for fx w delay heal
		S42.146D	Nondisp fx of glenoid cav of scapula, unsp shldr, sub for fx w rout heal
		S42.146G	Nondisp fx of glenoid cav of scapula, unsp shldr, sub for fx w delay heal
		S42.151D	Disp fx of nk of scapula, r shldr, subs for fx w routn heal
		S42.151G	Disp fx of nk of scapula, r shldr, subs for fx w delay heal
		S42.152D	Disp fx of nk of scapula, l shldr, subs for fx w routn heal
		S42.152G	Disp fx of nk of scapula, l shldr, subs for fx w delay heal
		S42.153D	Disp fx of nk of scapula, unsp shldr, sub for fx w rout heal
		S42.153G	Disp fx of nk of scapula, unsp shldr, sub for fx w delay heal
		S42.154D	Nondisp fx of nk of scapula, r shldr, sub for fx w rout heal
		S42.154G	Nondisp fx of nk of scapula, r shldr, sub for fx w delay heal
		S42.155D	Nondisp fx of nk of scapula, l shldr, sub for fx w rout heal
		S42.155G	Nondisp fx of nk of scapula, l shldr, sub for fx w delay heal
		S42.156D	Nondisp fx of nk of scapula, unsp shldr, sub for fx w rout heal
		S42.156G	Nondisp fx of nk of scapula, unsp shldr, sub for fx w delay heal
		S42.191D	Fx oth prt scapula, r shoulder, subs for fx w routn heal
		S42.191G	Fx oth prt scapula, r shoulder, subs for fx w delay heal
		S42.192D	Fx oth prt scapula, l shoulder, subs for fx w routn heal
		S42.192G	Fx oth prt scapula, l shoulder, subs for fx w delay heal
		S42.199D	Fx oth prt scapula, unsp shoulder, subs for fx w routn heal
		S42.199G	Fx oth prt scapula, unsp shoulder, subs for fx w delay heal
		S42.201D	Unsp fx upper end of r humerus, subs for fx w routn heal
		S42.201G	Unsp fx upper end of r humerus, subs for fx w delay heal
		S42.202D	Unsp fx upper end of l humerus, subs for fx w routn heal
		S42.202G	Unsp fx upper end of l humerus, subs for fx w delay heal
		S42.209D	Unsp fx upper end of unsp humerus, subs for fx w routn heal
		S42.209G	Unsp fx upper end of unsp humerus, subs for fx w delay heal
		S42.211D	Unsp disp fx of surg nk of r humer, subs for fx w routn heal
		S42.211G	Unsp disp fx of surg nk of r humer, subs for fx w delay heal
		S42.212D	Unsp disp fx of surg nk of l humer, subs for fx w routn heal
		S42.212G	Unsp disp fx of surg nk of l humer, subs for fx w delay heal
		S42.213D	Unsp disp fx of surg nk of unsp humer, sub for fx w rout heal
		S42.213G	Unsp disp fx of surg nk of unsp humer, sub for fx w delay heal
		S42.214D	Unsp nondisp fx of surg nk of r humer, sub for fx w rout heal
		S42.214G	Unsp nondisp fx of surg nk of r humer, sub for fx w delay heal
		S42.215D	Unsp nondisp fx of surg nk of l humer, sub for fx w rout heal
		S42.215G	Unsp nondisp fx of surg nk of l humer, sub for fx w delay heal
		S42.216D	Unsp nondisp fx of surg nk of unsp humer, sub for fx w rout heal
		S42.216G	Unsp nondisp fx of surg nk of unsp humer, sub for fx w delay heal
		S42.221D	2-part disp fx of surg nk of r humer, sub for fx w rout heal
		S42.221G	2-part disp fx of surg nk of r humer, sub for fx w delay heal
		S42.222D	2-part disp fx of surg nk of l humer, sub for fx w rout heal
		S42.222G	2-part disp fx of surg nk of l humer, sub for fx w delay heal
		S42.223D	2-part disp fx of surg nk of unsp humer, sub for fx w rout heal
		S42.223G	2-part disp fx of surg nk of unsp humer, sub for fx w delay heal
	(Continued on next page)	**S42.224D**	2-part nondisp fx of surg nk of r humer, sub for fx w rout heal

ICD-9-CM		ICD-10-CM	
V54.11	AFTERCARE HEALING TRAUMATIC FRACTURE UPPER ARM **(Continued)**	**S42.224G**	2-part nondisp fx of surg nk of r humer, sub for fx w delay heal
		S42.225D	2-part nondisp fx of surg nk of l humer, sub for fx w rout heal
		S42.225G	2-part nondisp fx of surg nk of l humer, sub for fx w delay heal
		S42.226D	2-part nondisp fx of surg nk of unsp humer, sub for fx w rout heal
		S42.226G	2-part nondisp fx of surg nk of unsp humer, sub for fx w delay heal
		S42.231D	3-part fx surg neck of r humerus, subs for fx w routn heal
		S42.231G	3-part fx surg neck of r humerus, subs for fx w delay heal
		S42.232D	3-part fx surg neck of l humerus, subs for fx w routn heal
		S42.232G	3-part fx surg neck of l humerus, subs for fx w delay heal
		S42.239D	3-part fx surg neck of unsp humer, subs for fx w routn heal
		S42.239G	3-part fx surg neck of unsp humer, subs for fx w delay heal
		S42.241D	4-part fx surg neck of r humerus, subs for fx w routn heal
		S42.241G	4-part fx surg neck of r humerus, subs for fx w delay heal
		S42.242D	4-part fx surg neck of l humerus, subs for fx w routn heal
		S42.242G	4-part fx surg neck of l humerus, subs for fx w delay heal
		S42.249D	4-part fx surg neck of unsp humer, subs for fx w routn heal
		S42.249G	4-part fx surg neck of unsp humer, subs for fx w delay heal
		S42.251D	Disp fx of greater tuberosity of r humer, sub for fx w rout heal
		S42.251G	Disp fx of greater tuberosity of r humer, sub for fx w delay heal
		S42.252D	Disp fx of greater tuberosity of l humer, sub for fx w rout heal
		S42.252G	Disp fx of greater tuberosity of l humer, sub for fx w delay heal
		S42.253D	Disp fx of greater tuberosity of unsp humer, sub for fx w rout heal
		S42.253G	Disp fx of greater tuberosity of unsp humer, sub for fx w delay heal
		S42.254D	Nondisp fx of greater tuberosity of r humer, sub for fx w rout heal
		S42.254G	Nondisp fx of greater tuberosity of r humer, sub for fx w delay heal
		S42.255D	Nondisp fx of greater tuberosity of l humer, sub for fx w rout heal
		S42.255G	Nondisp fx of greater tuberosity of l humer, sub for fx w delay heal
		S42.256D	Nondisp fx of greater tuberosity of unsp humer, sub for fx w rout heal
		S42.256G	Nondisp fx of greater tuberosity of unsp humer, sub for fx w delay heal
		S42.261D	Disp fx of less tuberosity of r humer, sub for fx w rout heal
		S42.261G	Disp fx of less tuberosity of r humer, sub for fx w delay heal
		S42.262D	Disp fx of less tuberosity of l humer, sub for fx w rout heal
		S42.262G	Disp fx of less tuberosity of l humer, sub for fx w delay heal
		S42.263D	Disp fx of less tuberosity of unsp humer, sub for fx w rout heal
		S42.263G	Disp fx of less tuberosity of unsp humer, sub for fx w delay heal
		S42.264D	Nondisp fx of less tuberosity of r humer, sub for fx w rout heal
		S42.264G	Nondisp fx of less tuberosity of r humer, sub for fx w delay heal
		S42.265D	Nondisp fx of less tuberosity of l humer, sub for fx w rout heal
		S42.265G	Nondisp fx of less tuberosity of l humer, sub for fx w delay heal
		S42.266D	Nondisp fx of less tuberosity of unsp humer, sub for fx w rout heal
		S42.266G	Nondisp fx of less tuberosity of unsp humer, sub for fx w delay heal
		S42.271D	Torus fx upper end of r humerus, subs for fx w routn heal
		S42.271G	Torus fx upper end of r humerus, subs for fx w delay heal
		S42.272D	Torus fx upper end of l humerus, subs for fx w routn heal
		S42.272G	Torus fx upper end of l humerus, subs for fx w delay heal
		S42.279D	Torus fx upper end of unsp humerus, subs for fx w routn heal
		S42.279G	Torus fx upper end of unsp humerus, subs for fx w delay heal
		S42.291D	Oth disp fx of upper end r humer, subs for fx w routn heal
		S42.291G	Oth disp fx of upper end r humer, subs for fx w delay heal
		S42.292D	Oth disp fx of upper end l humer, subs for fx w routn heal
		S42.292G	Oth disp fx of upper end l humer, subs for fx w delay heal
		S42.293D	Oth disp fx of upr end unsp humer, subs for fx w routn heal
		S42.293G	Oth disp fx of upr end unsp humer, subs for fx w delay heal
		S42.294D	Oth nondisp fx of upr end r humer, subs for fx w routn heal
		S42.294G	Oth nondisp fx of upr end r humer, subs for fx w delay heal
		S42.295D	Oth nondisp fx of upr end l humer, subs for fx w routn heal
		S42.295G	Oth nondisp fx of upr end l humer, subs for fx w delay heal
		S42.296D	Oth nondisp fx of upr end unsp humer, sub for fx w rout heal
		S42.296G	Oth nondisp fx of upr end unsp humer, sub for fx w delay heal
		S42.301D	Unsp fx shaft of humer, right arm, subs for fx w routn heal
		S42.301G	Unsp fx shaft of humer, right arm, subs for fx w delay heal
		S42.302D	Unsp fx shaft of humerus, left arm, subs for fx w routn heal
		S42.302G	Unsp fx shaft of humerus, left arm, subs for fx w delay heal
		S42.309D	Unsp fx shaft of humerus, unsp arm, subs for fx w routn heal
		S42.309G	Unsp fx shaft of humerus, unsp arm, subs for fx w delay heal
		S42.311D	Greenstick fx shaft of humer, r arm, sub for fx w rout heal
		S42.311G	Greenstick fx shaft of humer, r arm, sub for fx w delay heal
		S42.312D	Greenstick fx shaft of humer, l arm, sub for fx w rout heal
		S42.312G	Greenstick fx shaft of humer, l arm, sub for fx w delay heal
		S42.319D	Greenstick fx shaft of humer, unsp arm, sub for fx w rout heal
		S42.319G	Greenstick fx shaft of humer, unsp arm, sub for fx w delay heal
		S42.321D	Displ transverse fx shaft of humer, r arm, sub for fx w rout heal
		S42.321G	Displ transverse fx shaft of humer, r arm, sub for fx w delay heal
		S42.322D	Displ transverse fx shaft of humer, l arm, sub for fx w rout heal
		S42.322G	Displ transverse fx shaft of humer, l arm, sub for fx w delay heal
		S42.323D	Displ transverse fx shaft of humer, unsp arm, sub for fx w rout heal
		S42.323G	Displ transverse fx shaft of humer, unsp arm, sub for fx w delay heal
		S42.324D	Nondisp transverse fx shaft of humer, r arm, sub for fx w rout heal
		S42.324G	Nondisp transverse fx shaft of humer, r arm, sub for fx w delay heal
		S42.325D	Nondisp transverse fx shaft of humer, l arm, sub for fx w rout heal
	(Continued on next page)	**S42.325G**	Nondisp transverse fx shaft of humer, l arm, sub for fx w delay heal

ICD-9-CM		ICD-10-CM	
V54.11	AFTERCARE HEALING TRAUMATIC FRACTURE UPPER ARM **(Continued)**	**S42.326D**	Nondisp transverse fx shaft of humer, unsp arm, sub for fx w rout heal
		S42.326G	Nondisp transverse fx shaft of humer, unsp arm, sub for fx w delay heal
		S42.331D	Displ oblique fx shaft of humer, r arm, sub for fx w rout heal
		S42.331G	Displ oblique fx shaft of humer, r arm, sub for fx w delay heal
		S42.332D	Displ oblique fx shaft of humer, l arm, sub for fx w rout heal
		S42.332G	Displ oblique fx shaft of humer, l arm, sub for fx w delay heal
		S42.333D	Displ oblique fx shaft of humer, unsp arm, sub for fx w rout heal
		S42.333G	Displ oblique fx shaft of humer, unsp arm, sub for fx w delay heal
		S42.334D	Nondisp oblique fx shaft of humer, r arm, sub for fx w rout heal
		S42.334G	Nondisp oblique fx shaft of humer, r arm, sub for fx w delay heal
		S42.335D	Nondisp oblique fx shaft of humer, l arm, sub for fx w rout heal
		S42.335G	Nondisp oblique fx shaft of humer, l arm, sub for fx w delay heal
		S42.336D	Nondisp oblique fx shaft of humer, unsp arm, sub for fx w rout heal
		S42.336G	Nondisp oblique fx shaft of humer, unsp arm, sub for fx w delay heal
		S42.341D	Displ spiral fx shaft of humer, r arm, sub for fx w rout heal
		S42.341G	Displ spiral fx shaft of humer, r arm, sub for fx w delay heal
		S42.342D	Displ spiral fx shaft of humer, l arm, sub for fx w rout heal
		S42.342G	Displ spiral fx shaft of humer, l arm, sub for fx w delay heal
		S42.343D	Displ spiral fx shaft of humer, unsp arm, sub for fx w rout heal
		S42.343G	Displ spiral fx shaft of humer, unsp arm, sub for fx w delay heal
		S42.344D	Nondisp spiral fx shaft of humer, r arm, sub for fx w rout heal
		S42.344G	Nondisp spiral fx shaft of humer, r arm, sub for fx w delay heal
		S42.345D	Nondisp spiral fx shaft of humer, l arm, sub for fx w rout heal
		S42.345G	Nondisp spiral fx shaft of humer, l arm, sub for fx w delay heal
		S42.346D	Nondisp spiral fx shaft of humer, unsp arm, sub for fx w rout heal
		S42.346G	Nondisp spiral fx shaft of humer, unsp arm, sub for fx w delay heal
		S42.351D	Displ commnt fx shaft of humer, r arm, sub for fx w rout heal
		S42.351G	Displ commnt fx shaft of humer, r arm, sub for fx w delay heal
		S42.352D	Displ commnt fx shaft of humer, l arm, sub for fx w rout heal
		S42.352G	Displ commnt fx shaft of humer, l arm, sub for fx w delay heal
		S42.353D	Displ commnt fx shaft of humer, unsp arm, sub for fx w rout heal
		S42.353G	Displ commnt fx shaft of humer, unsp arm, sub for fx w delay heal
		S42.354D	Nondisp commnt fx shaft of humer, r arm, sub for fx w rout heal
		S42.354G	Nondisp commnt fx shaft of humer, r arm, sub for fx w delay heal
		S42.355D	Nondisp commnt fx shaft of humer, l arm, sub for fx w rout heal
		S42.355G	Nondisp commnt fx shaft of humer, l arm, sub for fx w delay heal
		S42.356D	Nondisp commnt fx shaft of humer, unsp arm, sub for fx w rout heal
		S42.356G	Nondisp commnt fx shaft of humer, unsp arm, sub for fx w delay heal
		S42.361D	Displ seg fx shaft of humer, r arm, subs for fx w routn heal
		S42.361G	Displ seg fx shaft of humer, r arm, subs for fx w delay heal
		S42.362D	Displ seg fx shaft of humer, l arm, subs for fx w routn heal
		S42.362G	Displ seg fx shaft of humer, l arm, subs for fx w delay heal
		S42.363D	Displ seg fx shaft of humer, unsp arm, sub for fx w rout heal
		S42.363G	Displ seg fx shaft of humer, unsp arm, sub for fx w delay heal
		S42.364D	Nondisp seg fx shaft of humer, r arm, sub for fx w rout heal
		S42.364G	Nondisp seg fx shaft of humer, r arm, sub for fx w delay heal
		S42.365D	Nondisp seg fx shaft of humer, l arm, sub for fx w rout heal
		S42.365G	Nondisp seg fx shaft of humer, l arm, sub for fx w delay heal
		S42.366D	Nondisp seg fx shaft of humer, unsp arm, sub for fx w rout heal
		S42.366G	Nondisp seg fx shaft of humer, unsp arm, sub for fx w delay heal
		S42.391D	Oth fracture of shaft of r humerus, subs for fx w routn heal
		S42.391G	Oth fracture of shaft of r humerus, subs for fx w delay heal
		S42.392D	Oth fracture of shaft of l humerus, subs for fx w routn heal
		S42.392G	Oth fracture of shaft of l humerus, subs for fx w delay heal
		S42.399D	Oth fx shaft of unsp humerus, subs for fx w routn heal
		S42.399G	Oth fx shaft of unsp humerus, subs for fx w delay heal
		S42.401D	Unsp fx lower end of r humerus, subs for fx w routn heal
		S42.401G	Unsp fx lower end of r humerus, subs for fx w delay heal
		S42.402D	Unsp fx lower end of l humerus, subs for fx w routn heal
		S42.402G	Unsp fx lower end of l humerus, subs for fx w delay heal
		S42.409D	Unsp fx lower end of unsp humerus, subs for fx w routn heal
		S42.409G	Unsp fx lower end of unsp humerus, subs for fx w delay heal
		S42.411D	Displ simp suprcndl fx w/o intrcndl fx r humer, sub for fx w rout heal
		S42.411G	Displ simp suprcndl fx w/o intrcndl fx r humer, sub for fx w delay heal
		S42.412D	Displ simp suprcndl fx w/o intrcndl fx l humer, sub for fx w rout heal
		S42.412G	Displ simp suprcndl fx w/o intrcndl fx l humer, sub for fx w delay heal
		S42.413D	Displ simp suprcndl fx w/o intrcndl fx unsp humer, sub for fx w rout heal
		S42.413G	Displ simp suprcndl fx w/o intrcndl fx unsp humer, sub for fx w delay heal
		S42.414D	Nondisp simp suprcndl fx w/o intrcndl fx r humer, sub for fx w rout heal
		S42.414G	Nondisp simp suprcndl fx w/o intrcndl fx r humer, sub for fx w delay heal
		S42.415D	Nondisp simp suprcndl fx w/o intrcndl fx l humer, sub for fx w rout heal
		S42.415G	Nondisp simp suprcndl fx w/o intrcndl fx l humer, sub for fx w delay heal
		S42.416D	Nondisp simp suprcndl fx w/o intrcndl fx unsp humer, sub for fx w rout heal
		S42.416G	Nondisp simp suprcndl fx w/o intrcndl fx unsp humer, sub fx w delay heal
		S42.421D	Displ commnt suprcndl fx w/o intrcndl fx r humer, sub for fx w rout heal
		S42.421G	Displ commnt suprcndl fx w/o intrcndl fx r humer, sub for fx w delay heal
		S42.422D	Displ commnt suprcndl fx w/o intrcndl fx l humer, sub for fx w rout heal
		S42.422G	Displ commnt suprcndl fx w/o intrcndl fx l humer, sub for fx w delay heal
		S42.423D	Displ commnt suprcndl fx w/o intrcndl fx unsp humer, sub for fx w rout heal
		S42.423G	Displ commnt suprcndl fx w/o intrcndl fx unsp humer, sub fx w delay heal
		S42.424D	Nondisp commnt suprcndl fx w/o intrcndl fx r humer, sub for fx w rout heal
	(Continued on next page)	**S42.424G**	Nondisp commnt suprcndl fx w/o intrcndl fx r humer, sub fx w delay heal

ICD-9-CM		ICD-10-CM	
V54.11	AFTERCARE HEALING TRAUMATIC FRACTURE UPPER ARM **(Continued)**	**S42.425D**	Nondisp commnt suprcndl fx w/o intrcndl fx l humer, sub for fx w rout heal
		S42.425G	Nondisp commnt suprcndl fx w/o intrcndl fx l humer, sub for fx w delay heal
		S42.426D	Nondisp commnt suprcndl fx w/o intrcndl fx unsp humer, sub for fx w rout heal
		S42.426G	Nondisp commnt suprcndl fx w/o intrcndl fx unsp humer, sub fx w delay heal
		S42.431D	Disp fx of lateral epicondyl of r humer, sub for fx w rout heal
		S42.431G	Disp fx of lateral epicondyl of r humer, sub for fx w delay heal
		S42.432D	Disp fx of lateral epicondyl of l humer, sub for fx w rout heal
		S42.432G	Disp fx of lateral epicondyl of l humer, sub for fx w delay heal
		S42.433D	Disp fx of lateral epicondyl of unsp humer, sub for fx w rout heal
		S42.433G	Disp fx of lateral epicondyl of unsp humer, sub for fx w delay heal
		S42.434D	Nondisp fx of lateral epicondyl of r humer, sub for fx w rout heal
		S42.434G	Nondisp fx of lateral epicondyl of r humer, sub for fx w delay heal
		S42.435D	Nondisp fx of lateral epicondyl of l humer, sub for fx w rout heal
		S42.435G	Nondisp fx of lateral epicondyl of l humer, sub for fx w delay heal
		S42.436D	Nondisp fx of lateral epicondyl of unsp humer, sub for fx w rout heal
		S42.436G	Nondisp fx of lateral epicondyl of unsp humer, sub for fx w delay heal
		S42.441D	Disp fx of med epicondyl of r humer, sub for fx w rout heal
		S42.441G	Disp fx of med epicondyl of r humer, sub for fx w delay heal
		S42.442D	Disp fx of med epicondyl of l humer, sub for fx w rout heal
		S42.442G	Disp fx of med epicondyl of l humer, sub for fx w delay heal
		S42.443D	Disp fx of med epicondyl of unsp humer, sub for fx w rout heal
		S42.443G	Disp fx of med epicondyl of unsp humer, sub for fx w delay heal
		S42.444D	Nondisp fx of med epicondyl of r humer, sub for fx w rout heal
		S42.444G	Nondisp fx of med epicondyl of r humer, sub for fx w delay heal
		S42.445D	Nondisp fx of med epicondyl of l humer, sub for fx w rout heal
		S42.445G	Nondisp fx of med epicondyl of l humer, sub for fx w delay heal
		S42.446D	Nondisp fx of med epicondyl of unsp humer, sub for fx w rout heal
		S42.446G	Nondisp fx of med epicondyl of unsp humer, sub for fx w delay heal
		S42.447D	Incarcerated fx of med epicondyl of r humer, sub for fx w rout heal
		S42.447G	Incarcerated fx of med epicondyl of r humer, sub for fx w delay heal
		S42.448D	Incarcerated fx of med epicondyl of l humer, sub for fx w rout heal
		S42.448G	Incarcerated fx of med epicondyl of l humer, sub for fx w delay heal
		S42.449D	Incarcerated fx of med epicondyl of unsp humer, sub for fx w rout heal
		S42.449G	Incarcerated fx of med epicondyl of unsp humer, sub for fx w delay heal
		S42.451D	Disp fx of lateral condyle of r humer, sub for fx w rout heal
		S42.451G	Disp fx of lateral condyle of r humer, sub for fx w delay heal
		S42.452D	Disp fx of lateral condyle of l humer, sub for fx w rout heal
		S42.452G	Disp fx of lateral condyle of l humer, sub for fx w delay heal
		S42.453D	Disp fx of lateral condyle of unsp humer, sub for fx w rout heal
		S42.453G	Disp fx of lateral condyle of unsp humer, sub for fx w delay heal
		S42.454D	Nondisp fx of lateral condyle of r humer, sub for fx w rout heal
		S42.454G	Nondisp fx of lateral condyle of r humer, sub for fx w delay heal
		S42.455D	Nondisp fx of lateral condyle of l humer, sub for fx w rout heal
		S42.455G	Nondisp fx of lateral condyle of l humer, sub for fx w delay heal
		S42.456D	Nondisp fx of lateral condyle of unsp humer, sub for fx w rout heal
		S42.456G	Nondisp fx of lateral condyle of unsp humer, sub for fx w delay heal
		S42.461D	Disp fx of med condyle of r humer, subs for fx w routn heal
		S42.461G	Disp fx of med condyle of r humer, subs for fx w delay heal
		S42.462D	Disp fx of med condyle of l humer, subs for fx w routn heal
		S42.462G	Disp fx of med condyle of l humer, subs for fx w delay heal
		S42.463D	Disp fx of med condyle of unsp humer, sub for fx w rout heal
		S42.463G	Disp fx of med condyle of unsp humer, sub for fx w delay heal
		S42.464D	Nondisp fx of med condyle of r humer, sub for fx w rout heal
		S42.464G	Nondisp fx of med condyle of r humer, sub for fx w delay heal
		S42.465D	Nondisp fx of med condyle of l humer, sub for fx w rout heal
		S42.465G	Nondisp fx of med condyle of l humer, sub for fx w delay heal
		S42.466D	Nondisp fx of med condyle of unsp humer, sub for fx w rout heal
		S42.466G	Nondisp fx of med condyle of unsp humer, sub for fx w delay heal
		S42.471D	Displaced transcondy fx r humerus, subs for fx w routn heal
		S42.471G	Displaced transcondy fx r humerus, subs for fx w delay heal
		S42.472D	Displaced transcondy fx l humerus, subs for fx w routn heal
		S42.472G	Displaced transcondy fx l humerus, subs for fx w delay heal
		S42.473D	Displ transcondy fx unsp humerus, subs for fx w routn heal
		S42.473G	Displ transcondy fx unsp humerus, subs for fx w delay heal
		S42.474D	Nondisp transcondy fx r humerus, subs for fx w routn heal
		S42.474G	Nondisp transcondy fx r humerus, subs for fx w delay heal
		S42.475D	Nondisp transcondy fx l humerus, subs for fx w routn heal
		S42.475G	Nondisp transcondy fx l humerus, subs for fx w delay heal
		S42.476D	Nondisp transcondy fx unsp humerus, subs for fx w routn heal
		S42.476G	Nondisp transcondy fx unsp humerus, subs for fx w delay heal
		S42.481D	Torus fx lower end of r humerus, subs for fx w routn heal
		S42.481G	Torus fx lower end of r humerus, subs for fx w delay heal
		S42.482D	Torus fx lower end of l humerus, subs for fx w routn heal
		S42.482G	Torus fx lower end of l humerus, subs for fx w delay heal
		S42.489D	Torus fx lower end of unsp humerus, subs for fx w routn heal
		S42.489G	Torus fx lower end of unsp humerus, subs for fx w delay heal
		S42.491D	Oth disp fx of lower end r humer, subs for fx w routn heal
		S42.491G	Oth disp fx of lower end r humer, subs for fx w delay heal
		S42.492D	Oth disp fx of lower end l humer, subs for fx w routn heal
		S42.492G	Oth disp fx of lower end l humer, subs for fx w delay heal
		S42.493D	Oth disp fx of low end unsp humer, subs for fx w routn heal
		S42.493G	Oth disp fx of low end unsp humer, subs for fx w delay heal
	(Continued on next page)	**S42.494D**	Oth nondisp fx of low end r humer, subs for fx w routn heal

ICD-9-CM		ICD-10-CM	
V54.11	AFTERCARE HEALING TRAUMATIC FRACTURE UPPER ARM **(Continued)**	**S42.494G**	Oth nondisp fx of low end r humer, subs for fx w delay heal
		S42.495D	Oth nondisp fx of low end l humer, subs for fx w routn heal
		S42.495G	Oth nondisp fx of low end l humer, subs for fx w delay heal
		S42.496D	Oth nondisp fx of low end unsp humer, sub for fx w rout heal
		S42.496G	Oth nondisp fx of low end unsp humer, sub for fx w delay heal
		S42.9ØXD	Fx unsp shoulder girdle, part unsp, subs for fx w routn heal
		S42.9ØXG	Fx unsp shoulder girdle, part unsp, subs for fx w delay heal
		S42.91XD	Fx r shoulder girdle, part unsp, subs for fx w routn heal
		S42.91XG	Fx r shoulder girdle, part unsp, subs for fx w delay heal
		S42.92XD	Fx l shoulder girdle, part unsp, subs for fx w routn heal
		S42.92XG	Fx l shoulder girdle, part unsp, subs for fx w delay heal
		S49.ØØ1D	Unsp physl fx upr end humer, r arm, subs for fx w routn heal
		S49.ØØ1G	Unsp physl fx upr end humer, r arm, subs for fx w delay heal
		S49.ØØ2D	Unsp physl fx upr end humer, l arm, subs for fx w routn heal
		S49.ØØ2G	Unsp physl fx upr end humer, l arm, subs for fx w delay heal
		S49.ØØ9D	Unsp physl fx upr end humer, unsp arm, sub for fx w rout heal
		S49.ØØ9G	Unsp physl fx upr end humer, unsp arm, sub for fx w delay heal
		S49.Ø11D	Sltr-haris Type I physl fx upr end humer, r arm, sub for fx w rout heal
		S49.Ø11G	Sltr-haris Type I physl fx upr end humer, r arm, sub for fx w delay heal
		S49.Ø12D	Sltr-haris Type I physl fx upr end humer, l arm, sub for fx w rout heal
		S49.Ø12G	Sltr-haris Type I physl fx upr end humer, l arm, sub for fx w delay heal
		S49.Ø19D	Sltr-haris Type I physl fx upr end humer, unsp arm, sub for fx w rout heal
		S49.Ø19G	Sltr-haris Type I physl fx upr end humer, unsp arm, sub for fx w delay heal
		S49.Ø21D	Sltr-haris Type II physl fx upr end humer, r arm, sub for fx w rout heal
		S49.Ø21G	Sltr-haris Type II physl fx upr end humer, r arm, sub for fx w delay heal
		S49.Ø22D	Sltr-haris Type II physl fx upr end humer, l arm, sub for fx w rout heal
		S49.Ø22G	Sltr-haris Type II physl fx upr end humer, l arm, sub for fx w delay heal
		S49.Ø29D	Sltr-haris Type II physl fx upr end humer, unsp arm, sub for fx w rout heal
		S49.Ø29G	Sltr-haris Type II physl fx upr end humer, unsp arm, sub for fx w delay heal
		S49.Ø31D	Sltr-haris Type III physl fx upr end humer, r arm, sub for fx w rout heal
		S49.Ø31G	Sltr-haris Type III physl fx upr end humer, r arm, sub for fx w delay heal
		S49.Ø32D	Sltr-haris Type III physl fx upr end humer, l arm, sub for fx w rout heal
		S49.Ø32G	Sltr-haris Type III physl fx upr end humer, l arm, sub for fx w delay heal
		S49.Ø39D	Sltr-haris Type III physl fx upr end humer, unsp arm, sub for fx w rout heal
		S49.Ø39G	Sltr-haris Type III physl fx upr end humer, unsp arm, sub for fx w delay heal
		S49.Ø41D	Sltr-haris Type IV physl fx upr end humer, r arm, sub for fx w rout heal
		S49.Ø41G	Sltr-haris Type IV physl fx upr end humer, r arm, sub for fx w delay heal
		S49.Ø42D	Sltr-haris Type IV physl fx upr end humer, l arm, sub for fx w rout heal
		S49.Ø42G	Sltr-haris Type IV physl fx upr end humer, l arm, sub for fx w delay heal
		S49.Ø49D	Sltr-haris Type IV physl fx upr end humer, unsp arm, sub for fx w rout heal
		S49.Ø49G	Sltr-haris Type IV physl fx upr end humer, unsp arm, sub for fx w delay heal
		S49.Ø91D	Oth physl fx upr end humer, r arm, subs for fx w routn heal
		S49.Ø91G	Oth physl fx upr end humer, r arm, subs for fx w delay heal
		S49.Ø92D	Oth physl fx upr end humer, l arm, subs for fx w routn heal
		S49.Ø92G	Oth physl fx upr end humer, l arm, subs for fx w delay heal
		S49.Ø99D	Oth physl fx upr end humer, unsp arm, sub for fx w rout heal
		S49.Ø99G	Oth physl fx upr end humer, unsp arm, sub for fx w delay heal
		S49.1Ø1D	Unsp physl fx low end humer, r arm, subs for fx w routn heal
		S49.1Ø1G	Unsp physl fx low end humer, r arm, subs for fx w delay heal
		S49.1Ø2D	Unsp physl fx low end humer, l arm, subs for fx w routn heal
		S49.1Ø2G	Unsp physl fx low end humer, l arm, subs for fx w delay heal
		S49.1Ø9D	Unsp physl fx low end humer, unsp arm, sub for fx w rout heal
		S49.1Ø9G	Unsp physl fx low end humer, unsp arm, sub for fx w delay heal
		S49.111D	Sltr-haris Type I physl fx low end humer, r arm, sub for fx w rout heal
		S49.111G	Sltr-haris Type I physl fx low end humer, r arm, sub for fx w delay heal
		S49.112D	Sltr-haris Type I physl fx low end humer, l arm, sub for fx w rout heal
		S49.112G	Sltr-haris Type I physl fx low end humer, l arm, sub for fx w delay heal
		S49.119D	Sltr-haris Type I physl fx low end humer, unsp arm, sub for fx w rout heal
		S49.119G	Sltr-haris Type I physl fx low end humer, unsp arm, sub for fx w delay heal
		S49.121D	Sltr-haris Type II physl fx low end humer, r arm, sub for fx w rout heal
		S49.121G	Sltr-haris Type II physl fx low end humer, r arm, sub for fx w delay heal
		S49.122D	Sltr-haris Type II physl fx low end humer, l arm, sub for fx w rout heal
		S49.122G	Sltr-haris Type II physl fx low end humer, l arm, sub for fx w delay heal
		S49.129D	Sltr-haris Type II physl fx low end humer, unsp arm, sub for fx w rout heal
		S49.129G	Sltr-haris Type II physl fx low end humer, unsp arm, sub for fx w delay heal
		S49.131D	Sltr-haris Type III physl fx low end humer, r arm, sub for fx w rout heal
		S49.131G	Sltr-haris Type III physl fx low end humer, r arm, sub for fx w delay heal
		S49.132D	Sltr-haris Type III physl fx low end humer, l arm, sub for fx w rout heal
		S49.132G	Sltr-haris Type III physl fx low end humer, l arm, sub for fx w delay heal
		S49.139D	Sltr-haris Type III physl fx low end humer, unsp arm, sub for fx w rout heal
		S49.139G	Sltr-haris Type III physl fx low end humer, unsp arm, sub for fx w delay heal
		S49.141D	Sltr-haris Type IV physl fx low end humer, r arm, sub for fx w rout heal
		S49.141G	Sltr-haris Type IV physl fx low end humer, r arm, sub for fx w delay heal
		S49.142D	Sltr-haris Type IV physl fx low end humer, l arm, sub for fx w rout heal
		S49.142G	Sltr-haris Type IV physl fx low end humer, l arm, sub for fx w delay heal
		S49.149D	Sltr-haris Type IV physl fx low end humer, unsp arm, sub for fx w rout heal
		S49.149G	Sltr-haris Type IV physl fx low end humer, unsp arm, sub for fx w delay heal
		S49.191D	Oth physl fx low end humer, r arm, subs for fx w routn heal
		S49.191G	Oth physl fx low end humer, r arm, subs for fx w delay heal
		S49.192D	Oth physl fx low end humer, l arm, subs for fx w routn heal
		S49.192G	Oth physl fx low end humer, l arm, subs for fx w delay heal
		S49.199D	Oth physl fx low end humer, unsp arm, sub for fx w rout heal
		S49.199G	Oth physl fx low end humer, unsp arm, sub for fx w delay heal

ICD-9-CM		ICD-10-CM	
V54.12	AFTERCARE HEALING TRAUMATIC FRACTURE LOWER ARM	**S52.ØØ1**[D,E,F,G,H,J]	Unsp fx upper end of r ulna
		S52.ØØ2[D,E,F,G,H,J]	Unsp fx upper end of l ulna
		S52.ØØ9[D,E,F,G,H,J]	Unsp fx upper end unsp ulna
		S52.Ø11D	Torus fx upper end of right ulna, subs for fx w rout heal
		S52.Ø11G	Torus fx upper end of right ulna, subs for fx w delay heal
		S52.Ø12D	Torus fx upper end of left ulna, subs for fx w rout heal
		S52.Ø12G	Torus fx upper end of left ulna, subs for fx w delay heal
		S52.Ø19D	Torus fx upper end of unsp ulna, subs for fx w rout heal
		S52.Ø19G	Torus fx upper end of unsp ulna, subs for fx w delay heal
		S52.Ø21[D,E,F,G,H,J]	Disp fx olcrn pro w/o intartic extn r ulna
		S52.Ø22[D,E,F,G,H,J]	Disp fx olcrn pro w/o intartic extn l ulna
		S52.Ø23[D,E,F,G,H,J]	Disp fx olcrn pro w/o intartic extn unsp ulna,
		S52.Ø24[D,E,F,G,H,J]	Ndsplc fx olcrn pro w/o intartic extn r ulna
		S52.Ø25[D,E,F,G,H,J]	Ndsplc fx olcrn pro w/o intartic extn l ulna
		S52.Ø26[D,E,F,G,H,J]	Ndsplc fx olcrn pro w/o intartic extn unsp ulna
		S52.Ø31[D,E,F,G,H,J]	Disp fx olcrn pro w intartic extn r ulna
		S52.Ø32[D,E,F,G,H,J]	Disp fx olcrn pro w intartic extn l ulna
		S52.Ø33[D,E,F,G,H,J]	Disp fx olcrn pro w intartic extn unsp ulna
		S52.Ø34[D,E,F,G,H,J]	Nondisp fx olcrn pro w intartic extn r ulna
		S52.Ø35[D,E,F,G,H,J]	Nondisp fx olcrn pro w intartic extn l ulna,
		S52.Ø36[D,E,F,G,H,J]	Nondisp fx olcrn pro w intartic extn unsp ulna
		S52.Ø41[D,E,F,G,H,J]	Disp fx coronoid pro of r ulna
		S52.Ø42[D,E,F,G,H,J]	Disp fx coronoid pro of l ulna
		S52.Ø43[D,E,F,G,H,J]	Disp fx coronoid pro of unsp ulna
		S52.Ø44[D,E,F,G,H,J]	Nondisp fx coronoid pro of r ulna
		S52.Ø45[D,E,F,G,H,J]	Nondisp fx coronoid pro of l ulna
		S52.Ø46[D,E,F,G,H,J]	Nondisp fx coronoid pro of unsp ulna
		S52.Ø91[D,E,F,G,H,J]	Oth fx upper end of r ulna
		S52.Ø92[D,E,F,G,H,J]	Oth fx upper end of left ulna
		S52.Ø99[D,E,F,G,H,J]	Oth fx upper end of unsp ulna
		S52.1Ø1[D,E,F,G,H,J]	Unsp fx upper end of r radius
		S52.1Ø2[D,E,F,G,H,J]	Unsp fx upper end left radius
		S52.1Ø9[D,E,F,G,H,J]	Unsp fx upper end unsp radius
		S52.111D	Torus fx upper end of r radius, subs for fx w rout heal
		S52.111G	Torus fx upper end of r radius, subs for fx w delay heal
		S52.112D	Torus fx upper end of left radius, subs for fx w rout heal
		S52.112G	Torus fx upper end of left radius, subs for fx w delay heal
		S52.119D	Torus fx upper end of unsp radius, subs for fx w rout heal
		S52.119G	Torus fx upper end of unsp radius, subs for fx w delay heal
		S52.121[D,E,F,G,H,J]	Disp fx head of r radius
		S52.122[D,E,F,G,H,J]	Disp fx head of left rad
		S52.123[D,E,F,G,H,J]	Disp fx head of unsp rad
		S52.124[D,E,F,G,H,J]	Nondisp fx head of r rad
		S52.125[D,E,F,G,H,J]	Nondisp fx head of l rad
		S52.126[D,E,F,G,H,J]	Nondisp fx head of unsp rad
		S52.131[D,E,F,G,H,J]	Disp fx neck of r radius
		S52.132[D,E,F,G,H,J]	Disp fx neck of left rad
		S52.133[D,E,F,G,H,J]	Disp fx neck of unsp rad
		S52.134[D,E,F,G,H,J]	Nondisp fx neck of r rad
		S52.135[D,E,F,G,H,J]	Nondisp fx neck of l rad
		S52.136[D,E,F,G,H,J]	Nondisp fx nk of unsp rad
		S52.181[D,E,F,G,H,J]	Oth fx upper end of r radius
		S52.182[D,E,F,G,H,J]	Oth fx upper end left radius
		S52.189[D,E,F,G,H,J]	Oth fx upper end unsp radius
		S52.2Ø1[D,E,F,G,H,J]	Unsp fx shaft of right ulna
		S52.2Ø2[D,E,F,G,H,J]	Unsp fx shaft of left ulna
		S52.2Ø9[D,E,F,G,H,J]	Unsp fx shaft of unsp ulna
		S52.211D	Greenstick fx shaft of right ulna, subs for fx w rout heal
		S52.211G	Greenstick fx shaft of right ulna, subs for fx w delay heal
		S52.212D	Greenstick fx shaft of left ulna, subs for fx w rout heal
		S52.212G	Greenstick fx shaft of left ulna, subs for fx w delay heal
		S52.219D	Greenstick fx shaft of unsp ulna, subs for fx w rout heal
		S52.219G	Greenstick fx shaft of unsp ulna, subs for fx w delay heal
		S52.221[D,E,F,G,H,J]	Displ transvs fx shaft of r ulna
		S52.222[D,E,F,G,H,J]	Displ transvs fx shaft of l ulna
		S52.223[D,E,F,G,H,J]	Displ transvs fx shaft of unsp ulna
		S52.224[D,E,F,G,H,J]	Nondisp transvs fx shaft of r ulna
		S52.225[D,E,F,G,H,J]	Nondisp transvs fx shaft of l ulna
		S52.226[D,E,F,G,H,J]	Nondisp transvs fx shaft of unsp ulna
		S52.231[D,E,F,G,H,J]	Displ oblique fx shaft r ulna
		S52.232[D,E,F,G,H,J]	Displ oblique fx shaft l ulna
		S52.233[D,E,F,G,H,J]	Displ oblique fx shaft unsp ulna
		S52.234[D,E,F,G,H,J]	Nondisp oblique fx shaft r ulna
		S52.235[D,E,F,G,H,J]	Nondisp oblique fx shaft l ulna
		S52.236[D,E,F,G,H,J]	Nondisp oblique fx shaft unsp ulna
		S52.241[D,E,F,G,H,J]	Displ spiral fx shaft ulna, r arm

7th Character meanings for code S52.-

D subs enc for clos fx w rout heal
E subs enc for op fx typ 1/2 w rout heal
F subs enc
G subs enc for op fx typ 3 A/B/C w rout heal
H subs enc for op fx typ 1/2 w del heal
J subs enc for op fx typ 3 A/B/C w del heal

(Continued on next page)

ICD-9-CM		ICD-10-CM	
V54.12	AFTERCARE HEALING TRAUMATIC FRACTURE LOWER ARM **(Continued)**	**S52.242**[D,E,F,G,H,J]	Displ spiral fx shaft ulna, l arm
		S52.243[D,E,F,G,H,J]	Displ spiral fx shaft ulna, unsp arm
		S52.244[D,E,F,G,H,J]	Nondisp spiral fx shaft ulna, r arm
		S52.245[D,E,F,G,H,J]	Nondisp spiral fx shaft ulna, l arm
		S52.246[D,E,F,G,H,J]	Nondisp spiral fx shaft ulna, unsp arm
		S52.251[D,E,F,G,H,J]	Displ commnt fx shaft ulna, r arm
		S52.252[D,E,F,G,H,J]	Displ commnt fx shaft ulna, l arm
		S52.253[D,E,F,G,H,J]	Displ commnt fx shaft ulna, unsp arm
		S52.254[D,E,F,G,H,J]	Nondisp commnt fx shaft ulna, r arm
		S52.255[D,E,F,G,H,J]	Nondisp commnt fx shaft ulna, l arm
		S52.256[D,E,F,G,H,J]	Nondisp commnt fx shaft ulna, unsp arm
		S52.261[D,E,F,G,H,J]	Displ seg fx shaft ulna, r arm
		S52.262[D,E,F,G,H,J]	Displ seg fx shaft ulna, l arm
		S52.263[D,E,F,G,H,J]	Displ seg fx shaft ulna, unsp arm
		S52.264[D,E,F,G,H,J]	Nondisp seg fx shaft ulna, r arm
		S52.265[D,E,F,G,H,J]	Nondisp seg fx shaft ulna, l arm
		S52.266[D,E,F,G,H,J]	Nondisp seg fx shaft ulna, unsp arm
		S52.271[D,E,F,G,H,J]	Monteggia's fx right ulna
		S52.272[D,E,F,G,H,J]	Monteggia's fx left ulna
		S52.279[D,E,F,G,H,J]	Monteggia's fx unsp ulna
		S52.281[D,E,F,G,H,J]	Bent bone right ulna
		S52.282[D,E,F,G,H,J]	Bent bone left ulna
		S52.283[D,E,F,G,H,J]	Bent bone unsp ulna
		S52.291[D,E,F,G,H,J]	Oth fx shaft right ulna
		S52.292[D,E,F,G,H,J]	Oth fx shaft left ulna
		S52.299[D,E,F,G,H,J]	Oth fx shaft unsp ulna
		S52.301[D,E,F,G,H,J]	Unsp fx shaft r radius
		S52.302[D,E,F,G,H,J]	Unsp fx shaft left radius
		S52.309[D,E,F,G,H,J]	Unsp fx shaft unsp radius
		S52.311D	Greenstick fx shaft rad, r arm, subs for fx w rout heal
		S52.311G	Greenstick fx shaft rad, r arm, subs for fx w delay heal
		S52.312D	Greenstick fx shaft rad, l arm, subs for fx w rout heal
		S52.312G	Greenstick fx shaft rad, l arm, subs for fx w delay heal
		S52.319D	Greenstick fx shaft rad, unsp arm
		S52.319G	Greenstick fx shaft rad, unsp arm, sub for clsd fx w delay heal
		S52.321[D,E,F,G,H,J]	Displ transvs fx shaft r rad
		S52.322[D,E,F,G,H,J]	Displ transvs fx shaft l rad
		S52.323[D,E,F,G,H,J]	Displ transvs fx shaft unsp rad
		S52.324[D,E,F,G,H,J]	Nondisp transvs fx shaft r rad
		S52.325[D,E,F,G,H,J]	Nondisp transvs fx shaft l rad
		S52.326[D,E,F,G,H,J]	Nondisp transvs fx shaft unsp rad
		S52.331[D,E,F,G,H,J]	Displ oblique fx shaft r rad
		S52.332[D,E,F,G,H,J]	Displ oblique fx shaft l rad
		S52.333[D,E,F,G,H,J]	Displ oblique fx shaft unsp rad
		S52.334[D,E,F,G,H,J]	Nondisp oblique fx shaft r rad
		S52.335[D,E,F,G,H,J]	Nondisp oblique fx shaft l rad
		S52.336[D,E,F,G,H,J]	Nondisp oblique fx shaft unsp rad
		S52.341[D,E,F,G,H,J]	Displ spiral fx shaft rad, r arm
		S52.342[D,E,F,G,H,J]	Displ spiral fx shaft rad, l arm
		S52.343[D,E,F,G,H,J]	Displ spiral fx shaft rad, unsp arm
		S52.344[D,E,F,G,H,J]	Nondisp spiral fx shaft rad, r arm
		S52.345[D,E,F,G,H,J]	Nondisp spiral fx shaft rad, l arm
		S52.346[D,E,F,G,H,J]	Nondisp spiral fx shaft rad, unsp arm
		S52.351[D,E,F,G,H,J]	Displ commnt fx shaft rad, r arm
		S52.352[D,E,F,G,H,J]	Displ commnt fx shaft rad, l arm
		S52.353[D,E,F,G,H,J]	Displ commnt fx shaft rad, unsp arm
		S52.354[D,E,F,G,H,J]	Nondisp commnt fx shaft rad, r arm
		S52.355[D,E,F,G,H,J]	Nondisp commnt fx shaft rad, l arm
		S52.356[D,E,F,G,H,J]	Nondisp commnt fx shaft rad, unsp arm
		S52.361[D,E,F,G,H,J]	Displ seg fx shaft rad, r arm
		S52.362[D,E,F,G,H,J]	Displ seg fx shaft rad, l arm
		S52.363[D,E,F,G,H,J]	Displ seg fx shaft rad, unsp arm
		S52.364[D,E,F,G,H,J]	Nondisp seg fx shaft rad, r arm
		S52.365[D,E,F,G,H,J]	Nondisp seg fx shaft rad, l arm
		S52.366[D,E,F,G,H,J]	Nondisp seg fx shaft rad, unsp arm
		S52.371[D,E,F,G,H,J]	Galeazzi's fx r radius
		S52.372[D,E,F,G,H,J]	Galeazzi's fx left radius
		S52.379[D,E,F,G,H,J]	Galeazzi's fx unsp radius
		S52.381[D,E,F,G,H,J]	Bent bone right radius
		S52.382[D,E,F,G,H,J]	Bent bone left radius
		S52.389[D,E,F,G,H,J]	Bent bone unsp radius
		S52.391[D,E,F,G,H,J]	Oth fx shaft rad, r arm
		S52.392[D,E,F,G,H,J]	Oth fx shaft rad, left arm
		S52.399[D,E,F,G,H,J]	Oth fx shaft rad, unsp arm
		S52.501[D,E,F,G,H,J]	Unsp fx the lower end r rad

7th Character meanings for code S52.-
- ***D** subs enc for clos fx w rout heal*
- ***E** subs enc for op fx typ 1/2 w rout heal*
- ***F** subs enc*
- ***G** subs enc for op fx typ 3 A/B/C w rout heal*
- ***H** subs enc for op fx typ 1/2 w del heal*
- ***J** subs enc for op fx typ 3 A/B/C w del heal*

(Continued on next page)

ICD-9-CM		ICD-10-CM	
V54.12	AFTERCARE HEALING TRAUMATIC FRACTURE LOWER ARM **(Continued)**	**S52.502**[D,E,F,G,H,J]	Unsp fx the low end left rad
		S52.509[D,E,F,G,H,J]	Unsp fx the low end unsp rad
		S52.511[D,E,F,G,H,J]	Disp fx r radial styloid pro
		S52.512[D,E,F,G,H,J]	Disp fx l radial styloid pro
		S52.513[D,E,F,G,H,J]	Disp fx unsp radial styloid pro
		S52.514[D,E,F,G,H,J]	Nondisp fx r radial styloid pro
		S52.515[D,E,F,G,H,J]	Nondisp fx l radial styloid pro
		S52.516[D,E,F,G,H,J]	Nondisp fx unsp radial styloid pro
		S52.521D	Torus fx lower end r radius, subs for fx w rout heal
		S52.521G	Torus fx lower end r radius, subs for fx w delay heal
		S52.522D	Torus fx lower end left radius, subs for fx w rout heal
		S52.522G	Torus fx lower end left radius, subs for fx w delay heal
		S52.529D	Torus fx lower end unsp radius, subs for fx w rout heal
		S52.529G	Torus fx lower end unsp radius, subs for fx w delay heal
		S52.531[D,E,F,G,H,J]	Colles' fracture r radius
		S52.532[D,E,F,G,H,J]	Colles' fx left radius
		S52.539[D,E,F,G,H,J]	Colles' fx unsp radius
		S52.541[D,E,F,G,H,J]	Smith's fracture r radius
		S52.542[D,E,F,G,H,J]	Smith's fx left radius
		S52.549[D,E,F,G,H,J]	Smith's fx unsp radius
		S52.551[D,E,F,G,H,J]	Oth extrartic fx low end r rad
		S52.552[D,E,F,G,H,J]	Oth extrartic fx low end l rad
		S52.559[D,E,F,G,H,J]	Oth extrartic fx low end unsp rad
		S52.561[D,E,F,G,H,J]	Barton's fracture r radius
		S52.562[D,E,F,G,H,J]	Barton's fx left radius
		S52.569[D,E,F,G,H,J]	Barton's fx unsp radius
		S52.571[D,E,F,G,H,J]	Oth intartic fx low end r rad
		S52.572[D,E,F,G,H,J]	Oth intartic fx low end l rad
		S52.579[D,E,F,G,H,J]	Oth intartic fx low end unsp rad
		S52.591[D,E,F,G,H,J]	Oth fx lower end r radius
		S52.592[D,E,F,G,H,J]	Oth fx lower end left rad
		S52.599[D,E,F,G,H,J]	Oth fx lower end unsp rad
		S52.601[D,E,F,G,H,J]	Unsp fx lower end r ulna
		S52.602[D,E,F,G,H,J]	Unsp fx lower end l ulna
		S52.609[D,E,F,G,H,J]	Unsp fx lower end unsp ulna
		S52.611[D,E,F,G,H,J]	Disp fx r ulna styloid pro
		S52.612[D,E,F,G,H,J]	Disp fx l ulna styloid pro
		S52.613[D,E,F,G,H,J]	Disp fx unsp ulna styloid pro
		S52.614[D,E,F,G,H,J]	Nondisp fx r ulna styloid pro
		S52.615[D,E,F,G,H,J]	Nondisp fx l ulna styloid pro
		S52.616[D,E,F,G,H,J]	Nondisp fx unsp ulna styloid pro
		S52.621D	Torus fx lower end right ulna, subs for fx w rout heal
		S52.621G	Torus fx lower end right ulna, subs for fx w delay heal
		S52.622D	Torus fx lower end left ulna, subs for fx w rout heal
		S52.622G	Torus fx lower end left ulna, subs for fx w delay heal
		S52.629D	Torus fx lower end unsp ulna, subs for fx w rout heal
		S52.629G	Torus fx lower end unsp ulna, subs for fx w delay heal
		S52.691[D,E,F,G,H,J]	Oth fx lower end r ulna
		S52.692[D,E,F,G,H,J]	Oth fx lower end left ulna
		S52.699[D,E,F,G,H,J]	Oth fx lower end unsp ulna
		S52.91X[D,E,F,G,H,J]	Unsp fracture r forearm
		S52.92X[D,E,F,G,H,J]	Unsp fracture left forearm
		S59.001D	Unsp fx low end ulna, r arm, sub for fx w rout heal
		S59.001G	Unsp fx low end ulna, r arm, subs for fx w delay heal
		S59.002D	Unsp fx low end ulna, l arm, sub for fx w rout heal
		S59.002G	Unsp fx low end ulna, l arm, sub for fx w delay heal
		S59.009D	Unsp fx low end ulna, unsp arm, sub for fx w rout heal
		S59.009G	Unsp fx low end ulna, unsp arm, sub for clsd fx w delay heal
		S59.011D	Sltr-haris Type I fx low end ulna, r arm, sub for fx w rout heal
		S59.011G	Sltr-haris Type I fx low end ulna, r arm, sub for fx w delay heal
		S59.012D	Sltr-haris Type I fx low end ulna, l arm, sub for fx w rout heal
		S59.012G	Sltr-haris Type I fx low end ulna, l arm, sub for fx w delay heal
		S59.019D	Sltr-haris Type I fx low end ulna, unsp arm, sub for fx w rout heal
		S59.019G	Sltr-haris Type I fx low end ulna, unsp arm, sub for fx w del heal
		S59.021D	Sltr-haris Type II fx low end ulna, r arm, sub for fx w rout heal
		S59.021G	Sltr-haris Type II fx low end ulna, r arm, sub for fx w delay heal
		S59.022D	Sltr-haris Type II fx low end ulna, l arm, sub for fx w rout heal
		S59.022G	Sltr-haris Type II fx low end ulna, l arm, sub for fx w delay heal
		S59.029D	Sltr-haris Type II fx low end ulna, unsp arm, sub for fx w rout heal
		S59.029G	Sltr-haris Type II fx low end ulna, unsp arm, sub for fx w del heal
		S59.031D	Sltr-haris Type III fx low end ulna, r arm, sub for fx w rout heal
		S59.031G	Sltr-haris Type III fx low end ulna, r arm, sub for fx w delay heal
		S59.032D	Sltr-haris Type III fx low end ulna, l arm, sub for fx w rout heal
		S59.032G	Sltr-haris Type III fx low end ulna, l arm, sub for fx w delay heal
		S59.039D	Sltr-haris Type III fx low end ulna, unsp arm, sub for fx w rout heal
		S59.039G	Sltr-haris Type III fx low end ulna, unsp arm, sub for fx w del heal

7th Character meanings for code S52.-
D subs enc for clos fx w rout heal
E subs enc for op fx typ 1/2 w rout heal
F subs enc
G subs enc for op fx typ 3 A/B/C w rout heal
H subs enc for op fx typ 1/2 w del heal
J subs enc for op fx typ 3 A/B/C w del heal

(Continued on next page)

ICD-9-CM		ICD-10-CM	
V54.12	AFTERCARE HEALING TRAUMATIC FRACTURE LOWER ARM **(Continued)**	**S59.041D**	Sltr-haris Type IV fx low end ulna, r arm, sub for fx w rout heal
		S59.041G	Sltr-haris Type IV fx low end ulna, r arm, sub for fx w delay heal
		S59.042D	Sltr-haris Type IV fx low end ulna, l arm, sub for fx w rout heal
		S59.042G	Sltr-haris Type IV fx low end ulna, l arm, sub for fx w delay heal
		S59.049D	Sltr-haris Type IV fx low end ulna, unsp arm, sub for fx w rout heal
		S59.049G	Sltr-haris Type IV fx low end ulna, unsp arm, sub for fx w delay heal
		S59.091D	Oth fx low end ulna, r arm, sub for fx w rout heal
		S59.091G	Oth fx low end ulna, r arm, sub for fx w delay heal
		S59.092D	Oth fx low end ulna, l arm, sub for fx w rout heal
		S59.092G	Oth fx low end ulna, l arm, sub for fx w delay heal
		S59.099D	Oth fx low end ulna, unsp arm, sub for fx w rout heal
		S59.099G	Oth fx low end ulna, unsp arm, sub for fx w delay heal
		S59.101D	Unsp fx upper end rad, r arm, sub for fx w rout heal
		S59.101G	Unsp fx upper end rad, r arm, sub for fx w delay heal
		S59.102D	Unsp fx upr end rad, l arm, sub for fx w rout heal
		S59.102G	Unsp fx upr end rad, l arm, sub for fx w delay heal
		S59.109D	Unsp fx upr end rad, unsp arm, sub for fx w rout heal
		S59.109G	Unsp fx upr end rad, unsp arm, sub for fx w delay heal
		S59.111D	Sltr-haris Type I fx upr end rad, r arm, sub for fx w rout heal
		S59.111G	Sltr-haris Type I fx upr end rad, r arm, sub for fx w delay heal
		S59.112D	Sltr-haris Type I fx upr end rad, l arm, sub for fx w rout heal
		S59.112G	Sltr-haris Type I fx upr end rad, l arm, sub for fx w delay heal
		S59.119D	Sltr-haris Type I fx upr end rad, unsp arm, sub for fx w rout heal
		S59.119G	Sltr-haris Type I fx upr end rad, unsp arm, sub for fx w delay heal
		S59.121D	Sltr-haris Type II fx upr end rad, r arm, sub for fx w rout heal
		S59.121G	Sltr-haris Type II fx upr end rad, r arm, sub for fx w delay heal
		S59.122D	Sltr-haris Type II fx upr end rad, l arm, sub for fx w rout heal
		S59.122G	Sltr-haris Type II fx upr end rad, l arm, sub for fx w delay heal
		S59.129D	Sltr-haris Type II fx upr end rad, unsp arm, sub for fx w rout heal
		S59.129G	Sltr-haris Type II fx upr end rad, unsp arm, sub for fx w delay heal
		S59.131D	Sltr-haris Type III fx upr end rad, r arm, sub for fx w rout heal
		S59.131G	Sltr-haris Type III fx upr end rad, r arm, sub for fx w delay heal
		S59.132D	Sltr-haris Type III fx upr end rad, l arm, sub for fx w rout heal
		S59.132G	Sltr-haris Type III fx upr end rad, l arm, sub for fx w delay heal
		S59.139D	Sltr-haris Type III fx upr end rad, unsp arm, sub for fx w rout heal
		S59.139G	Sltr-haris Type III fx upr end rad, unsp arm, sub for fx w delay heal
		S59.141D	Sltr-haris Type IV fx upr end rad, r arm, sub for fx w rout heal
		S59.141G	Sltr-haris Type IV fx upr end rad, r arm, sub for fx w delay heal
		S59.142D	Sltr-haris Type IV fx upr end rad, l arm, sub for fx w rout heal
		S59.142G	Sltr-haris Type IV fx upr end rad, l arm, sub for fx w delay heal
		S59.149D	Sltr-haris Type IV fx upr end rad, unsp arm, sub for fx w rout heal
		S59.149G	Sltr-haris Type IV fx upr end rad, unsp arm, sub for fx w delay heal
		S59.191D	Oth fx upper end rad, r arm, sub for fx w rout heal
		S59.191G	Oth fx upper end rad, r arm, sub for fx w delay heal
		S59.192D	Oth fx upr end rad, left arm, sub for fx w rout heal
		S59.192G	Oth fx upr end rad, left arm, sub for fx w delay heal
		S59.199D	Oth fx upr end rad, unsp arm, sub for fx w rout heal
		S59.199G	Oth fx upr end rad, unsp arm, sub for fx w delay heal
		S59.201D	Unsp fx low end rad, r arm, sub for fx w rout heal
		S59.201G	Unsp fx low end rad, r arm, sub for fx w delay heal
		S59.202D	Unsp fx low end rad, l arm, sub for fx w rout heal
		S59.202G	Unsp fx low end rad, l arm, sub for fx w delay heal
		S59.209D	Unsp fx low end rad, unsp arm, sub for fx w rout heal
		S59.209G	Unsp fx low end rad, unsp arm, sub for fx w delay heal
		S59.211D	Sltr-haris Type I fx low end rad, r arm, sub for fx w rout heal
		S59.211G	Sltr-haris Type I fx low end rad, r arm, sub for fx w delay heal
		S59.212D	Sltr-haris Type I fx low end rad, l arm, sub for fx w rout heal
		S59.212G	Sltr-haris Type I fx low end rad, l arm, sub for fx w delay heal
		S59.219D	Sltr-haris Type I fx low end rad, unsp arm, sub for fx w rout heal
		S59.219G	Sltr-haris Type I fx low end rad, unsp arm, sub for fx w delay heal
		S59.221D	Sltr-haris Type II fx low end rad, r arm, sub for fx w rout heal
		S59.221G	Sltr-haris Type II fx low end rad, r arm, sub for fx w delay heal
		S59.222D	Sltr-haris Type II fx low end rad, l arm, sub for fx w rout heal
		S59.222G	Sltr-haris Type II fx low end rad, l arm, sub for fx w delay heal
		S59.229D	Sltr-haris Type II fx low end rad, unsp arm, sub for fx w rout heal
		S59.229G	Sltr-haris Type II fx low end rad, unsp arm, sub for fx w delay heal
		S59.231D	Sltr-haris Type III fx low end rad, r arm, sub for fx w rout heal
		S59.231G	Sltr-haris Type III fx low end rad, r arm, sub for fx w delay heal
		S59.232D	Sltr-haris Type III fx low end rad, l arm, sub for fx w rout heal
		S59.232G	Sltr-haris Type III fx low end rad, l arm, sub for fx w delay heal
		S59.239D	Sltr-haris Type III fx low end rad, unsp arm, sub for fx w rout heal
		S59.239G	Sltr-haris Type III fx low end rad, unsp arm, sub for fx w delay heal
		S59.241D	Sltr-haris Type IV fx low end rad, r arm, sub for fx w rout heal
		S59.241G	Sltr-haris Type IV fx low end rad, r arm, sub for fx w delay heal
		S59.242D	Sltr-haris Type IV fx low end rad, l arm, sub for fx w rout heal
		S59.242G	Sltr-haris Type IV fx low end rad, l arm, sub for fx w delay heal
		S59.249D	Sltr-haris Type IV fx low end rad, unsp arm, sub for fx w rout heal
		S59.249G	Sltr-haris Type IV fx low end rad, unsp arm, sub for fx w delay heal
		S59.291D	Oth fx low end rad, r arm, sub for fx w rout heal
		S59.291G	Oth fx low end rad, r arm, sub for fx w delay heal
		S59.292D	Oth fx low end rad, left arm, sub for fx w rout heal
		S59.292G	Oth fx low end rad, left arm, sub for fx w delay heal
	(Continued on next page)	**S59.299D**	Oth fx low end rad, unsp arm, sub for fx w rout heal

ICD-9-CM		ICD-10-CM	
V54.12	AFTERCARE HEALING TRAUMATIC FRACTURE LOWER ARM **(Continued)**	**S59.299G**	Oth fx low end rad, unsp arm, sub for fx w delay heal
		S62.001D	Unsp fx navicular bone r wrist, sub for fx w rout heal
		S62.001G	Unsp fx navicular bone r wrist, subs for fx w delay heal
		S62.002D	Unsp fx navicular bone l wrist, sub for fx w rout heal
		S62.002G	Unsp fx navicular bone l wrist, subs for fx w delay heal
		S62.009D	Unsp fx navic bone unsp wrist, sub for fx w rout heal
		S62.009G	Unsp fx navic bone unsp wrist, subs for fx w delay heal
		S62.011D	Disp fx dist pole navic bone r of wrs, sub for fx w rout heal
		S62.011G	Disp fx dist pole navic bone of r wrs, sub for fx w delay heal
		S62.012D	Disp fx dist pole navic bone of l wrs, sub for fx w rout heal
		S62.012G	Disp fx dist pole navic bone of l wrs, sub for fx w delay heal
		S62.013D	Disp fx dist pole navic bone of unsp wrs, sub for fx w rout heal
		S62.013G	Disp fx dist pole navic bone of unsp wrs, sub for fx w delay heal
		S62.014D	Nondisp fx dist pole of navic bone of r wrs, sub for fx w rout heal
		S62.014G	Nondisp fx dist pole of navic bone of r wrs, sub for fx w delay heal
		S62.015D	Nondisp fx dist pole of navic bone of l wrs, sub for fx w rout heal
		S62.015G	Nondisp fx dist pole of navic bone of l wrs, sub for fx w delay heal
		S62.016D	Nondisp fx dist pole of navic bone of unsp wrs, sub for fx w rout heal
		S62.016G	Nondisp fx dist pole of navic bone of unsp wrs, sub for fx w delay heal
		S62.021D	Disp fx mid 3rd of navic bone of r wrs, sub for fx w rout heal
		S62.021G	Disp fx mid 3rd of navic bone of r wrs, sub for fx w delay heal
		S62.022D	Disp fx mid 3rd of navic bone of l wrs, sub for fx w rout heal
		S62.022G	Disp fx mid 3rd of navic bone of l wrs, sub for fx w delay heal
		S62.023D	Disp fx mid 3rd of navic bone of unsp wrs, sub for fx w rout heal
		S62.023G	Disp fx mid 3rd of navic bone of unsp wrs, sub for fx w delay heal
		S62.024D	Nondisp fx mid 3rd of navic bone of r wrs, sub for fx w rout heal
		S62.024G	Nondisp fx mid 3rd of navic bone of r wrs, sub for fx w delay heal
		S62.025D	Nondisp fx mid 3rd of navic bone of l wrs, sub for fx w rout heal
		S62.025G	Nondisp fx mid 3rd of navic bone of l wrs, sub for fx w delay heal
		S62.026D	Nondisp fx mid 3rd of navic bone of unsp wrs, sub for fx w rout heal
		S62.026G	Nondisp fx mid 3rd of navic bone of unsp wrs, sub for fx w delay heal
		S62.031D	Disp fx prox 3rd of navic bone of r wrs, sub for fx w rout heal
		S62.031G	Disp fx prox 3rd of navic bone of r wrs, sub for fx w delay heal
		S62.032D	Disp fx prox 3rd of navic bone of l wrs, sub for fx w rout heal
		S62.032G	Disp fx prox 3rd of navic bone of l wrs, sub for fx w delay heal
		S62.033D	Disp fx prox 3rd of navic bone of unsp wrs, sub for fx w rout heal
		S62.033G	Disp fx prox 3rd of navic bone of unsp wrs, sub for fx w delay heal
		S62.034D	Nondisp fx prox 3rd of navic bone of r wrs, sub for fx w rout heal
		S62.034G	Nondisp fx prox 3rd of navic bone of r wrs, sub for fx w delay heal
		S62.035D	Nondisp fx prox 3rd of navic bone of l wrs, sub for fx w rout heal
		S62.035G	Nondisp fx prox 3rd of navic bone of l wrs, sub for fx w delay heal
		S62.036D	Nondisp fx prox 3rd of navic bone of unsp wrs, sub for fx w rout heal
		S62.036G	Nondisp fx prox 3rd of navic bone of unsp wrs, sub for fx w delay heal
		S62.101D	Fx unsp carpal bone, right wrist, sub for fx w rout heal
		S62.101G	Fx unsp carpal bone, right wrist, subs for fx w delay heal
		S62.102D	Fx unsp carpal bone, left wrist, subs for fx w rout heal
		S62.102G	Fx unsp carpal bone, left wrist, subs for fx w delay heal
		S62.109D	Fx unsp carpal bone, unsp wrist, subs for fx w rout heal
		S62.109G	Fx unsp carpal bone, unsp wrist, subs for fx w delay heal
		S62.111D	Disp fx triquetrum bone, r wrs, subs for fx w rout heal
		S62.111G	Disp fx triquetrum bone, r wrs, subs for fx w delay heal
		S62.112D	Disp fx triquetrum bone, l wrs, subs for fx w rout heal
		S62.112G	Disp fx triquetrum bone, l wrs, subs for fx w delay heal
		S62.113D	Disp fx triquetrum bone, unsp wrs, sub for fx w rout heal
		S62.113G	Disp fx triquetrum bone, unsp wrs, sub for fx w delay heal
		S62.114D	Nondisp fx triquetrum bone, r wrs, sub for fx w rout heal
		S62.114G	Nondisp fx triquetrum bone, r wrs, sub for fx w delay heal
		S62.115D	Nondisp fx triquetrum bone, l wrs, sub for fx w rout heal
		S62.115G	Nondisp fx triquetrum bone, l wrs, sub for fx w delay heal
		S62.116D	Nondisp fx triquetrum bone, unsp wrs, sub for fx w rout heal
		S62.116G	Nondisp fx triquetrum bone, unsp wrs, sub for fx w delay heal
		S62.121D	Disp fx lunate, right wrist, subs for fx w rout heal
		S62.121G	Disp fx lunate, right wrist, subs for fx w delay heal
		S62.122D	Disp fx lunate, left wrist, subs for fx w rout heal
		S62.122G	Disp fx lunate, left wrist, subs for fx w delay heal
		S62.123D	Disp fx lunate, unsp wrist, subs for fx w rout heal
		S62.123G	Disp fx lunate, unsp wrist, subs for fx w delay heal
		S62.124D	Nondisp fx lunate, right wrist, subs for fx w rout heal
		S62.124G	Nondisp fx lunate, right wrist, subs for fx w delay heal
		S62.125D	Nondisp fx lunate, left wrist, subs for fx w rout heal
		S62.125G	Nondisp fx lunate, left wrist, subs for fx w delay heal
		S62.126D	Nondisp fx lunate, unsp wrist, subs for fx w rout heal
		S62.126G	Nondisp fx lunate, unsp wrist, subs for fx w delay heal
		S62.131D	Disp fx capitate bone, r wrist, subs for fx w rout heal
		S62.131G	Disp fx capitate bone, r wrist, subs for fx w delay heal
		S62.132D	Disp fx capitate bone, l wrist, subs for fx w rout heal
		S62.132G	Disp fx capitate bone, l wrist, subs for fx w delay heal
		S62.133D	Disp fx capitate bone, unsp wrs, subs for fx w rout heal
		S62.133G	Disp fx capitate bone, unsp wrs, subs for fx w delay heal
		S62.134D	Nondisp fx capitate bone, r wrs, subs for fx w rout heal
		S62.134G	Nondisp fx capitate bone, r wrs, subs for fx w delay heal
		S62.135D	Nondisp fx capitate bone, l wrs, subs for fx w rout heal
	(Continued on next page)	**S62.135G**	Nondisp fx capitate bone, l wrs, subs for fx w delay heal

ICD-9-CM		ICD-10-CM	
V54.12	AFTERCARE HEALING TRAUMATIC FRACTURE LOWER ARM **(Continued)**	**S62.136D**	Nondisp fx capitate bone, unsp wrs, sub for fx w rout heal
		S62.136G	Nondisp fx capitate bone, unsp wrs, sub for fx w delay heal
		S62.141D	Disp fx body of hamate bone, r wrs, sub for fx w rout heal
		S62.141G	Disp fx body of hamate bone, r wrs, sub for fx w delay heal
		S62.142D	Disp fx body of hamate bone, l wrs, sub for fx w rout heal
		S62.142G	Disp fx body of hamate bone, l wrs, sub for fx w delay heal
		S62.143D	Disp fx body of hamate bone, unsp wrs, sub for fx w rout heal
		S62.143G	Disp fx body of hamate bone, unsp wrs, sub for fx w delay heal
		S62.144D	Nondisp fx body of hamate bone, r wrs, sub for fx w rout heal
		S62.144G	Nondisp fx body of hamate bone, r wrs, sub for fx w delay heal
		S62.145D	Nondisp fx body of hamate bone, l wrs, sub for fx w rout heal
		S62.145G	Nondisp fx body of hamate bone, l wrs, sub for fx w delay heal
		S62.146D	Nondisp fx body of hamate bone, unsp wrs, sub for fx w rout heal
		S62.146G	Nondisp fx body of hamate bone, unsp wrs, sub for fx w delay heal
		S62.151D	Disp fx hook pro of hamate bone, r wrs, sub for fx w rout heal
		S62.151G	Disp fx hook pro of hamate bone, r wrs, sub for fx w delay heal
		S62.152D	Disp fx hook pro of hamate bone, l wrs, sub for fx w rout heal
		S62.152G	Disp fx hook pro of hamate bone, l wrs, sub for fx w delay heal
		S62.153D	Disp fx hook pro of hamate bone, unsp wrs, sub for fx w rout heal
		S62.153G	Disp fx hook pro of hamate bone, unsp wrs, sub for fx w delay heal
		S62.154D	Nondisp fx hook pro of hamate bone, r wrs, sub for fx w rout heal
		S62.154G	Nondisp fx hook pro of hamate bone, r wrs, sub for fx w delay heal
		S62.155D	Nondisp fx hook pro of hamate bone, l wrs, sub for fx w rout heal
		S62.155G	Nondisp fx hook pro of hamate bone, l wrs, sub for fx w delay heal
		S62.156D	Nondisp fx hook pro of hamate bone, unsp wrs, sub for fx w rout heal
		S62.156G	Nondisp fx hook pro of hamate bone, unsp wrs, sub for fx w delay heal
		S62.161D	Disp fx pisiform, right wrist, subs for fx w rout heal
		S62.161G	Disp fx pisiform, right wrist, subs for fx w delay heal
		S62.162D	Disp fx pisiform, left wrist, subs for fx w rout heal
		S62.162G	Disp fx pisiform, left wrist, subs for fx w delay heal
		S62.163D	Disp fx pisiform, unsp wrist, subs for fx w rout heal
		S62.163G	Disp fx pisiform, unsp wrist, subs for fx w delay heal
		S62.164D	Nondisp fx pisiform, r wrist, subs for fx w rout heal
		S62.164G	Nondisp fx pisiform, r wrist, subs for fx w delay heal
		S62.165D	Nondisp fx pisiform, left wrist, subs for fx w rout heal
		S62.165G	Nondisp fx pisiform, left wrist, subs for fx w delay heal
		S62.166D	Nondisp fx pisiform, unsp wrist, subs for fx w rout heal
		S62.166G	Nondisp fx pisiform, unsp wrist, subs for fx w delay heal
		S62.171D	Disp fx trapezium, right wrist, subs for fx w rout heal
		S62.171G	Disp fx trapezium, right wrist, subs for fx w delay heal
		S62.172D	Disp fx trapezium, left wrist, subs for fx w rout heal
		S62.172G	Disp fx trapezium, left wrist, subs for fx w delay heal
		S62.173D	Disp fx trapezium, unsp wrist, subs for fx w rout heal
		S62.173G	Disp fx trapezium, unsp wrist, subs for fx w delay heal
		S62.174D	Nondisp fx trapezium, r wrist, subs for fx w rout heal
		S62.174G	Nondisp fx trapezium, r wrist, subs for fx w delay heal
		S62.175D	Nondisp fx trapezium, l wrist, subs for fx w rout heal
		S62.175G	Nondisp fx trapezium, l wrist, subs for fx w delay heal
		S62.176D	Nondisp fx trapezm, unsp wrist, subs for fx w rout heal
		S62.176G	Nondisp fx trapezm, unsp wrist, subs for fx w delay heal
		S62.181D	Disp fx trapezoid, right wrist, subs for fx w rout heal
		S62.181G	Disp fx trapezoid, right wrist, subs for fx w delay heal
		S62.182D	Disp fx trapezoid, left wrist, subs for fx w rout heal
		S62.182G	Disp fx trapezoid, left wrist, subs for fx w delay heal
		S62.183D	Disp fx trapezoid, unsp wrist, subs for fx w rout heal
		S62.183G	Disp fx trapezoid, unsp wrist, subs for fx w delay heal
		S62.184D	Nondisp fx trapezoid, r wrist, subs for fx w rout heal
		S62.184G	Nondisp fx trapezoid, r wrist, subs for fx w delay heal
		S62.185D	Nondisp fx trapezoid, l wrist, subs for fx w rout heal
		S62.185G	Nondisp fx trapezoid, l wrist, subs for fx w delay heal
		S62.186D	Nondisp fx trapezd, unsp wrist, subs for fx w rout heal
		S62.186G	Nondisp fx trapezd, unsp wrist, subs for fx w delay heal
		S62.201D	Unsp fx first MC bone, right hand, subs for fx w rout heal
		S62.201G	Unsp fx first MC bone, right hand, subs for fx w delay heal
		S62.202D	Unsp fx first MC bone, left hand, subs for fx w rout heal
		S62.202G	Unsp fx first MC bone, left hand, subs for fx w delay heal
		S62.209D	Unsp fx first MC bone, unsp hand, subs for fx w rout heal
		S62.209G	Unsp fx first MC bone, unsp hand, subs for fx w delay heal
		S62.211D	Bennett's fracture, right hand, subs for fx w rout heal
		S62.211G	Bennett's fracture, right hand, subs for fx w delay heal
		S62.212D	Bennett's fracture, left hand, subs for fx w rout heal
		S62.212G	Bennett's fracture, left hand, subs for fx w delay heal
		S62.213D	Bennett's fracture, unsp hand, subs for fx w rout heal
		S62.213G	Bennett's fracture, unsp hand, subs for fx w delay heal
		S62.221D	Displ Rolando's fracture, r hand, subs for fx w rout heal
		S62.221G	Displ Rolando's fracture, r hand, subs for fx w delay heal
		S62.222D	Displ Rolando's fracture, l hand, subs for fx w rout heal
		S62.222G	Displ Rolando's fracture, l hand, subs for fx w delay heal
		S62.223D	Displ Rolando's fx, unsp hand, subs for fx w rout heal
		S62.223G	Displ Rolando's fx, unsp hand, subs for fx w delay heal
		S62.224D	Nondisp Rolando's fracture, r hand, subs for fx w rout heal
		S62.224G	Nondisp Rolando's fracture, r hand, subs for fx w delay heal
	(Continued on next page)	**S62.225D**	Nondisp Rolando's fracture, l hand, subs for fx w rout heal

ICD-9-CM	ICD-10-CM	
V54.12 AFTERCARE HEALING TRAUMATIC FRACTURE LOWER ARM **(Continued)**	**S62.225G**	Nondisp Rolando's fracture, l hand, subs for fx w delay heal
	S62.226D	Nondisp Rolando's fx, unsp hand, subs for fx w rout heal
	S62.226G	Nondisp Rolando's fx, unsp hand, subs for fx w delay heal
	S62.231D	Oth Disp fx base of 1st MC bone, r hand, sub for fx w rout heal
	S62.231G	Oth Disp fx base of 1st MC bone, r hand, sub for fx w delay heal
	S62.232D	Oth Disp fx base of 1st MC bone, l hand, sub for fx w rout heal
	S62.232G	Oth Disp fx base of 1st MC bone, l hand, sub for fx w delay heal
	S62.233D	Oth Disp fx base of 1st MC bone, unsp hand, sub for fx w rout heal
	S62.233G	Oth Disp fx base of 1st MC bone, unsp hand, sub for fx w delay heal
	S62.234D	Oth Nondisp fx base of 1st MC bone, r hand, sub for fx w rout heal
	S62.234G	Oth Nondisp fx base of 1st MC bone, r hand, sub for fx w delay heal
	S62.235D	Oth Nondisp fx base of 1st MC bone, l hand, sub for fx w rout heal
	S62.235G	Oth Nondisp fx base of 1st MC bone, l hand, sub for fx w delay heal
	S62.236D	Oth Nondisp fx base of 1st MC bone, unsp hand, sub for fx w rout heal
	S62.236G	Oth Nondisp fx base of 1st MC bone, unsp hand, sub for fx w delay heal
	S62.241D	Disp fx shaft of 1st MC bone, r hand, sub for fx w rout heal
	S62.241G	Disp fx shaft of 1st MC bone, r hand, sub for fx w delay heal
	S62.242D	Disp fx shaft of 1st MC bone, l hand, sub for fx w rout heal
	S62.242G	Disp fx shaft of 1st MC bone, l hand, sub for fx w delay heal
	S62.243D	Disp fx shaft of 1st MC bone, unsp hand, sub for fx w rout heal
	S62.243G	Disp fx shaft of 1st MC bone, unsp hand, sub for fx w delay heal
	S62.244D	Nondisp fx shaft of 1st MC bone, r hand, sub for fx w rout heal
	S62.244G	Nondisp fx shaft of 1st MC bone, r hand, sub for fx w delay heal
	S62.245D	Nondisp fx shaft of 1st MC bone, l hand, sub for fx w rout heal
	S62.245G	Nondisp fx shaft of 1st MC bone, l hand, sub for fx w delay heal
	S62.246D	Nondisp fx shaft of 1st MC bone, unsp hand, sub for fx w rout heal
	S62.246G	Nondisp fx shaft of 1st MC bone, unsp hand, sub for fx w delay heal
	S62.251D	Disp fx nk of 1st MC bone, r hand, sub for fx w rout heal
	S62.251G	Disp fx nk of 1st MC bone, r hand, sub for fx w delay heal
	S62.252D	Disp fx nk of 1st MC bone, l hand, sub for fx w rout heal
	S62.252G	Disp fx nk of 1st MC bone, l hand, sub for fx w delay heal
	S62.253D	Disp fx nk of 1st MC bone, unsp hand, sub for fx w rout heal
	S62.253G	Disp fx nk of 1st MC bone, unsp hand, sub for fx w delay heal
	S62.254D	Nondisp fx nk of 1st MC bone, r hand, sub for fx w rout heal
	S62.254G	Nondisp fx nk of 1st MC bone, r hand, sub for fx w delay heal
	S62.255D	Nondisp fx nk of 1st MC bone, l hand, sub for fx w rout heal
	S62.255G	Nondisp fx nk of 1st MC bone, l hand, sub for fx w delay heal
	S62.256D	Nondisp fx nk of 1st MC bone, unsp hand, sub for fx w rout heal
	S62.256G	Nondisp fx nk of 1st MC bone, unsp hand, sub for fx w delay heal
	S62.291D	Oth fx first MC bone, right hand, subs for fx w rout heal
	S62.291G	Oth fx first MC bone, right hand, subs for fx w delay heal
	S62.292D	Oth fx first MC bone, left hand, subs for fx w rout heal
	S62.292G	Oth fx first MC bone, left hand, subs for fx w delay heal
	S62.299D	Oth fx first MC bone, unsp hand, subs for fx w rout heal
	S62.299G	Oth fx first MC bone, unsp hand, subs for fx w delay heal
	S62.300D	Unsp fx second MC bone, right hand, subs for fx w rout heal
	S62.300G	Unsp fx second MC bone, right hand, subs for fx w delay heal
	S62.301D	Unsp fx second MC bone, left hand, subs for fx w rout heal
	S62.301G	Unsp fx second MC bone, left hand, subs for fx w delay heal
	S62.302D	Unsp fx third MC bone, right hand, subs for fx w rout heal
	S62.302G	Unsp fx third MC bone, right hand, subs for fx w delay heal
	S62.303D	Unsp fx third MC bone, left hand, subs for fx w rout heal
	S62.303G	Unsp fx third MC bone, left hand, subs for fx w delay heal
	S62.304D	Unsp fx fourth MC bone, right hand, subs for fx w rout heal
	S62.304G	Unsp fx fourth MC bone, right hand, subs for fx w delay heal
	S62.305D	Unsp fx fourth MC bone, left hand, subs for fx w rout heal
	S62.305G	Unsp fx fourth MC bone, left hand, subs for fx w delay heal
	S62.306D	Unsp fx fifth MC bone, right hand, subs for fx w rout heal
	S62.306G	Unsp fx fifth MC bone, right hand, subs for fx w delay heal
	S62.307D	Unsp fx fifth MC bone, left hand, subs for fx w rout heal
	S62.307G	Unsp fx fifth MC bone, left hand, subs for fx w delay heal
	S62.308D	Unsp fracture of metacarpal bone, subs for fx w rout heal
	S62.308G	Unsp fracture of metacarpal bone, subs for fx w delay heal
	S62.309D	Unsp fx unsp metacarpal bone, subs for fx w rout heal
	S62.309G	Unsp fx unsp metacarpal bone, subs for fx w delay heal
	S62.310D	Disp fx base of 2nd MC bone, r hand, sub for fx w rout heal
	S62.310G	Disp fx base of 2nd MC bone, r hand, sub for fx w delay heal
	S62.311D	Disp fx base of 2nd MC bone. l hand, sub for fx w rout heal
	S62.311G	Disp fx base of 2nd MC bone. l hand, sub for fx w delay heal
	S62.312D	Disp fx base of 3rd MC bone, r hand, sub for fx w rout heal
	S62.312G	Disp fx base of 3rd MC bone, r hand, sub for fx w delay heal
	S62.313D	Disp fx base of 3rd MC bone, l hand, sub for fx w rout heal
	S62.313G	Disp fx base of 3rd MC bone, l hand, sub for fx w delay heal
	S62.314D	Disp fx base of 4th MC bone, r hand, sub for fx w rout heal
	S62.314G	Disp fx base of 4th MC bone, r hand, sub for fx w delay heal
	S62.315D	Disp fx base of 4th MC bone, l hand, sub for fx w rout heal
	S62.315G	Disp fx base of 4th MC bone, l hand, sub for fx w delay heal
	S62.316D	Disp fx base of 5th MC bone, r hand, sub for fx w rout heal
	S62.316G	Disp fx base of 5th MC bone, r hand, sub for fx w delay heal
	S62.317D	Disp fx base of 5th MC bone. l hand, sub for fx w rout heal
	S62.317G	Disp fx base of 5th MC bone. l hand, sub for fx w delay heal
	S62.318D	Disp fx base of metacarpal bone, subs for fx w rout heal
(Continued on next page)	**S62.318G**	Disp fx base of metacarpal bone, subs for fx w delay heal

ICD-9-CM		ICD-10-CM	
V54.12	AFTERCARE HEALING TRAUMATIC FRACTURE LOWER ARM **(Continued)**	**S62.319D**	Disp fx base of unsp MC bone, subs for fx w rout heal
		S62.319G	Disp fx base of unsp MC bone, subs for fx w delay heal
		S62.32ØD	Disp fx shaft of 2nd MC bone, r hand, sub for fx w rout heal
		S62.32ØG	Disp fx shaft of 2nd MC bone, r hand, sub for fx w delay heal
		S62.321D	Disp fx shaft of 2nd MC bone, l hand, sub for fx w rout heal
		S62.321G	Disp fx shaft of 2nd MC bone, l hand, sub for fx w delay heal
		S62.322D	Disp fx shaft of 3rd MC bone, r hand, sub for fx w rout heal
		S62.322G	Disp fx shaft of 3rd MC bone, r hand, sub for fx w delay heal
		S62.323D	Disp fx shaft of 3rd MC bone, l hand, sub for fx w rout heal
		S62.323G	Disp fx shaft of 3rd MC bone, l hand, sub for fx w delay heal
		S62.324D	Disp fx shaft of 4th MC bone, r hand, sub for fx w rout heal
		S62.324G	Disp fx shaft of 4th MC bone, r hand, sub for fx w delay heal
		S62.325D	Disp fx shaft of 4th MC bone, l hand, sub for fx w rout heal
		S62.325G	Disp fx shaft of 4th MC bone, l hand, sub for fx w delay heal
		S62.326D	Disp fx shaft of 5th MC bone, r hand, sub for fx w rout heal
		S62.326G	Disp fx shaft of 5th MC bone, r hand, sub for fx w delay heal
		S62.327D	Disp fx shaft of 5th MC bone, l hand, sub for fx w rout heal
		S62.327G	Disp fx shaft of 5th MC bone, l hand, sub for fx w delay heal
		S62.328D	Disp fx shaft of MC bone, subs for fx w rout heal
		S62.328G	Disp fx shaft of MC bone, subs for fx w delay heal
		S62.329D	Disp fx shaft of unsp MC bone, subs for fx w rout heal
		S62.329G	Disp fx shaft of unsp MC bone, subs for fx w delay heal
		S62.33ØD	Disp fx nk of 2nd MC bone, r hand, sub for fx w rout heal
		S62.33ØG	Disp fx nk of 2nd MC bone, r hand, sub for fx w delay heal
		S62.331D	Disp fx nk of 2nd MC bone, l hand, sub for fx w rout heal
		S62.331G	Disp fx nk of 2nd MC bone, l hand, sub for fx w delay heal
		S62.332D	Disp fx nk of 3rd MC bone, r hand, sub for fx w rout heal
		S62.332G	Disp fx nk of 3rd MC bone, r hand, sub for fx w delay heal
		S62.333D	Disp fx nk of 3rd MC bone, l hand, sub for fx w rout heal
		S62.333G	Disp fx nk of 3rd MC bone, l hand, sub for fx w delay heal
		S62.334D	Disp fx nk of 4th MC bone, r hand, sub for fx w rout heal
		S62.334G	Disp fx nk of 4th MC bone, r hand, sub for fx w delay heal
		S62.335D	Disp fx nk of 4th MC bone, l hand, sub for fx w rout heal
		S62.335G	Disp fx nk of 4th MC bone, l hand, sub for fx w delay heal
		S62.336D	Disp fx nk of 5th MC bone, r hand, sub for fx w rout heal
		S62.336G	Disp fx nk of 5th MC bone, r hand, sub for fx w delay heal
		S62.337D	Disp fx nk of 5th MC bone, l hand, sub for fx w rout heal
		S62.337G	Disp fx nk of 5th MC bone, l hand, sub for fx w delay heal
		S62.338D	Disp fx neck of metacarpal bone, subs for fx w rout heal
		S62.338G	Disp fx neck of metacarpal bone, subs for fx w delay heal
		S62.339D	Disp fx neck of unsp MC bone, subs for fx w rout heal
		S62.339G	Disp fx neck of unsp MC bone, subs for fx w delay heal
		S62.34ØD	Nondisp fx base of 2nd MC bone, r hand, sub for fx w rout heal
		S62.34ØG	Nondisp fx base of 2nd MC bone, r hand, sub for fx w delay heal
		S62.341D	Nondisp fx base of 2nd MC bone. l hand, sub for fx w rout heal
		S62.341G	Nondisp fx base of 2nd MC bone. l hand, sub for fx w delay heal
		S62.342D	Nondisp fx base of 3rd MC bone, r hand, sub for fx w rout heal
		S62.342G	Nondisp fx base of 3rd MC bone, r hand, sub for fx w delay heal
		S62.343D	Nondisp fx base of 3rd MC bone, l hand, sub for fx w rout heal
		S62.343G	Nondisp fx base of 3rd MC bone, l hand, sub for fx w delay heal
		S62.344D	Nondisp fx base of 4th MC bone, r hand, sub for fx w rout heal
		S62.344G	Nondisp fx base of 4th MC bone, r hand, sub for fx w delay heal
		S62.345D	Nondisp fx base of 4th MC bone, l hand, sub for fx w rout heal
		S62.345G	Nondisp fx base of 4th MC bone, l hand, sub for fx w delay heal
		S62.346D	Nondisp fx base of 5th MC bone, r hand, sub for fx w rout heal
		S62.346G	Nondisp fx base of 5th MC bone, r hand, sub for fx w delay heal
		S62.347D	Nondisp fx base of 5th MC bone. l hand, sub for fx w rout heal
		S62.347G	Nondisp fx base of 5th MC bone. l hand, sub for fx w delay heal
		S62.348D	Nondisp fx base of MC bone, subs for fx w rout heal
		S62.348G	Nondisp fx base of MC bone, subs for fx w delay heal
		S62.349D	Nondisp fx base of unsp MC bone, subs for fx w rout heal
		S62.349G	Nondisp fx base of unsp MC bone, subs for fx w delay heal
		S62.35ØD	Nondisp fx shaft of 2nd MC bone, r hand, sub for fx w rout heal
		S62.35ØG	Nondisp fx shaft of 2nd MC bone, r hand, sub for fx w delay heal
		S62.351D	Nondisp fx shaft of 2nd MC bone, l hand, sub for fx w rout heal
		S62.351G	Nondisp fx shaft of 2nd MC bone, l hand, sub for fx w delay heal
		S62.352D	Nondisp fx shaft of 3rd MC bone, r hand, sub for fx w rout heal
		S62.352G	Nondisp fx shaft of 3rd MC bone, r hand, sub for fx w delay heal
		S62.353D	Nondisp fx shaft of 3rd MC bone, l hand, sub for fx w rout heal
		S62.353G	Nondisp fx shaft of 3rd MC bone, l hand, sub for fx w delay heal
		S62.354D	Nondisp fx shaft of 4th MC bone, r hand, sub for fx w rout heal
		S62.354G	Nondisp fx shaft of 4th MC bone, r hand, sub for fx w delay heal
		S62.355D	Nondisp fx shaft of 4th MC bone, l hand, sub for fx w rout heal
		S62.355G	Nondisp fx shaft of 4th MC bone, l hand, sub for fx w delay heal
		S62.356D	Nondisp fx shaft of 5th MC bone, r hand, sub for fx w rout heal
		S62.356G	Nondisp fx shaft of 5th MC bone, r hand, sub for fx w delay heal
		S62.357D	Nondisp fx shaft of 5th MC bone, l hand, sub for fx w rout heal
		S62.357G	Nondisp fx shaft of 5th MC bone, l hand, sub for fx w delay heal
		S62.358D	Nondisp fx shaft of MC bone, subs for fx w rout heal
		S62.358G	Nondisp fx shaft of MC bone, subs for fx w delay heal
		S62.359D	Nondisp fx shaft of unsp MC bone, sub for fx w rout heal
		S62.359G	Nondisp fx shaft of unsp MC bone, sub for fx w delay heal
		S62.36ØD	Nondisp fx nk of 2nd MC bone, r hand, sub for fx w rout heal

(Continued on next page)

ICD-9-CM		ICD-10-CM	
V54.12	AFTERCARE HEALING TRAUMATIC FRACTURE LOWER ARM **(Continued)**	**S62.360G**	Nondisp fx nk of 2nd MC bone, r hand, sub for fx w delay heal
		S62.361D	Nondisp fx nk of 2nd MC bone, l hand, sub for fx w rout heal
		S62.361G	Nondisp fx nk of 2nd MC bone, l hand, sub for fx w delay heal
		S62.362D	Nondisp fx nk of 3rd MC bone, r hand, sub for fx w rout heal
		S62.362G	Nondisp fx nk of 3rd MC bone, r hand, sub for fx w delay heal
		S62.363D	Nondisp fx nk of 3rd MC bone, l hand, sub for fx w rout heal
		S62.363G	Nondisp fx nk of 3rd MC bone, l hand, sub for fx w delay heal
		S62.364D	Nondisp fx nk of 4th MC bone, r hand, sub for fx w rout heal
		S62.364G	Nondisp fx nk of 4th MC bone, r hand, sub for fx w delay heal
		S62.365D	Nondisp fx nk of 4th MC bone, l hand, sub for fx w rout heal
		S62.365G	Nondisp fx nk of 4th MC bone, l hand, sub for fx w delay heal
		S62.366D	Nondisp fx nk of 5th MC bone, r hand, sub for fx w rout heal
		S62.366G	Nondisp fx nk of 5th MC bone, r hand, sub for fx w delay heal
		S62.367D	Nondisp fx nk of 5th MC bone, l hand, sub for fx w rout heal
		S62.367G	Nondisp fx nk of 5th MC bone, l hand, sub for fx w delay heal
		S62.368D	Nondisp fx neck of MC bone, subs for fx w rout heal
		S62.368G	Nondisp fx neck of MC bone, subs for fx w delay heal
		S62.369D	Nondisp fx neck of unsp MC bone, subs for fx w rout heal
		S62.369G	Nondisp fx neck of unsp MC bone, subs for fx w delay heal
		S62.390D	Oth fx second MC bone, right hand, subs for fx w rout heal
		S62.390G	Oth fx second MC bone, right hand, subs for fx w delay heal
		S62.391D	Oth fx second MC bone, left hand, subs for fx w rout heal
		S62.391G	Oth fx second MC bone, left hand, subs for fx w delay heal
		S62.392D	Oth fx third MC bone, right hand, subs for fx w rout heal
		S62.392G	Oth fx third MC bone, right hand, subs for fx w delay heal
		S62.393D	Oth fx third MC bone, left hand, subs for fx w rout heal
		S62.393G	Oth fx third MC bone, left hand, subs for fx w delay heal
		S62.394D	Oth fx fourth MC bone, right hand, subs for fx w rout heal
		S62.394G	Oth fx fourth MC bone, right hand, subs for fx w delay heal
		S62.395D	Oth fx fourth MC bone, left hand, subs for fx w rout heal
		S62.395G	Oth fx fourth MC bone, left hand, subs for fx w delay heal
		S62.396D	Oth fx fifth MC bone, right hand, subs for fx w rout heal
		S62.396G	Oth fx fifth MC bone, right hand, subs for fx w delay heal
		S62.397D	Oth fx fifth MC bone, left hand, subs for fx w rout heal
		S62.397G	Oth fx fifth MC bone, left hand, subs for fx w delay heal
		S62.398D	Oth fracture of metacarpal bone, subs for fx w rout heal
		S62.398G	Oth fracture of metacarpal bone, subs for fx w delay heal
		S62.399D	Oth fx unsp metacarpal bone, subs for fx w rout heal
		S62.399G	Oth fx unsp metacarpal bone, subs for fx w delay heal
		S62.501D	Fx unsp phalanx of right thumb, subs for fx w rout heal
		S62.501G	Fx unsp phalanx of right thumb, subs for fx w delay heal
		S62.502D	Fx unsp phalanx of left thumb, subs for fx w rout heal
		S62.502G	Fx unsp phalanx of left thumb, subs for fx w delay heal
		S62.509D	Fracture of unsp phalanx of thmb, subs for fx w rout heal
		S62.509G	Fracture of unsp phalanx of thmb, subs for fx w delay heal
		S62.511D	Disp fx prox phalanx of r thm, subs for fx w rout heal
		S62.511G	Disp fx prox phalanx of r thm, subs for fx w delay heal
		S62.512D	Disp fx prox phalanx of l thm, subs for fx w rout heal
		S62.512G	Disp fx prox phalanx of l thm, subs for fx w delay heal
		S62.513D	Disp fx prox phalanx of thmb, subs for fx w rout heal
		S62.513G	Disp fx prox phalanx of thmb, subs for fx w delay heal
		S62.514D	Nondisp fx prox phalanx of r thm, sub for fx w rout heal
		S62.514G	Nondisp fx prox phalanx of r thm, sub for fx w delay heal
		S62.515D	Nondisp fx prox phalanx of l thm, sub for fx w rout heal
		S62.515G	Nondisp fx prox phalanx of l thm, sub for fx w delay heal
		S62.516D	Nondisp fx prox phalanx of thmb, subs for fx w rout heal
		S62.516G	Nondisp fx prox phalanx of thmb, subs for fx w delay heal
		S62.521D	Disp fx distal phalanx of r thm, subs for fx w rout heal
		S62.521G	Disp fx distal phalanx of r thm, subs for fx w delay heal
		S62.522D	Disp fx distal phalanx of l thm, subs for fx w rout heal
		S62.522G	Disp fx distal phalanx of l thm, subs for fx w delay heal
		S62.523D	Disp fx distal phalanx of thmb, subs for fx w rout heal
		S62.523G	Disp fx distal phalanx of thmb, subs for fx w delay heal
		S62.524D	Nondisp fx dist phalanx of r thm, sub for fx w rout heal
		S62.524G	Nondisp fx dist phalanx of r thm, sub for fx w delay heal
		S62.525D	Nondisp fx dist phalanx of l thm, sub for fx w rout heal
		S62.525G	Nondisp fx dist phalanx of l thm, sub for fx w delay heal
		S62.526D	Nondisp fx dist phalanx of thmb, sub for fx w rout heal
		S62.526G	Nondisp fx dist phalanx of thmb, sub for fx w delay heal
		S62.600D	Fx unsp phalanx of r idx fngr, subs for fx w rout heal
		S62.600G	Fx unsp phalanx of r idx fngr, subs for fx w delay heal
		S62.601D	Fx unsp phalanx of l idx fngr, subs for fx w rout heal
		S62.601G	Fx unsp phalanx of l idx fngr, subs for fx w delay heal
		S62.602D	Fx unsp phalanx of r mid finger, subs for fx w rout heal
		S62.602G	Fx unsp phalanx of r mid finger, subs for fx w delay heal
		S62.603D	Fx unsp phalanx of l mid finger, subs for fx w rout heal
		S62.603G	Fx unsp phalanx of l mid finger, subs for fx w delay heal
		S62.604D	Fx unsp phalanx of r rng fngr, subs for fx w rout heal
		S62.604G	Fx unsp phalanx of r rng fngr, subs for fx w delay heal
		S62.605D	Fx unsp phalanx of l rng fngr, subs for fx w rout heal
		S62.605G	Fx unsp phalanx of l rng fngr, subs for fx w delay heal
		S62.606D	Fx unsp phalanx of r little finger, subs for fx w rout heal
		S62.606G	Fx unsp phalanx of r little finger, subs for fx w delay heal
		S62.607D	Fx unsp phalanx of l little finger, subs for fx w rout heal

(Continued on next page)

ICD-9-CM		ICD-10-CM	
V54.12	AFTERCARE HEALING TRAUMATIC FRACTURE LOWER ARM **(Continued)**	**S62.6Ø7G**	Fx unsp phalanx of l little finger, subs for fx w delay heal
		S62.6Ø8D	Fracture of unsp phalanx of finger, subs for fx w rout heal
		S62.6Ø8G	Fracture of unsp phalanx of finger, subs for fx w delay heal
		S62.6Ø9D	Fx unsp phalanx of unsp finger, subs for fx w rout heal
		S62.6Ø9G	Fx unsp phalanx of unsp finger, subs for fx w delay heal
		S62.61ØD	Disp fx prox phalanx of r idx fngr, sub for fx w rout heal
		S62.61ØG	Disp fx prox phalanx of r idx fngr, sub for fx w delay heal
		S62.611D	Disp fx prox phalanx of l idx fngr, sub for fx w rout heal
		S62.611G	Disp fx prox phalanx of l idx fngr, sub for fx w delay heal
		S62.612D	Disp fx prox phalanx of r mid fngr, sub for fx w rout heal
		S62.612G	Disp fx prox phalanx of r mid fngr, sub for fx w delay heal
		S62.613D	Disp fx prox phalanx of l mid fngr, sub for fx w rout heal
		S62.613G	Disp fx prox phalanx of l mid fngr, sub for fx w delay heal
		S62.614D	Disp fx prox phalanx of r rng fngr, sub for fx w rout heal
		S62.614G	Disp fx prox phalanx of r rng fngr, sub for fx w delay heal
		S62.615D	Disp fx prox phalanx of l rng fngr, sub for fx w rout heal
		S62.615G	Disp fx prox phalanx of l rng fngr, sub for fx w delay heal
		S62.616D	Disp fx prox phalanx of r lit fngr, sub for fx w rout heal
		S62.616G	Disp fx prox phalanx of r lit fngr, sub for fx w delay heal
		S62.617D	Disp fx prox phalanx of l lit fngr, sub for fx w rout heal
		S62.617G	Disp fx prox phalanx of l lit fngr, sub for fx w delay heal
		S62.618D	Disp fx prox phalanx of finger, subs for fx w rout heal
		S62.618G	Disp fx prox phalanx of finger, subs for fx w delay heal
		S62.619D	Disp fx prox phalanx of unsp fngr, sub for fx w rout heal
		S62.619G	Disp fx prox phalanx of unsp fngr, sub for fx w delay heal
		S62.62ØD	Disp fx med phalanx of r idx fngr, sub for fx w rout heal
		S62.62ØG	Disp fx med phalanx of r idx fngr, sub for fx w delay heal
		S62.621D	Disp fx med phalanx of l idx fngr, sub for fx w rout heal
		S62.621G	Disp fx med phalanx of l idx fngr, sub for fx w delay heal
		S62.622D	Disp fx med phalanx of r mid fngr, sub for fx w rout heal
		S62.622G	Disp fx med phalanx of r mid fngr, sub for fx w delay heal
		S62.623D	Disp fx med phalanx of l mid fngr, sub for fx w rout heal
		S62.623G	Disp fx med phalanx of l mid fngr, sub for fx w delay heal
		S62.624D	Disp fx med phalanx of r rng fngr, sub for fx w rout heal
		S62.624G	Disp fx med phalanx of r rng fngr, sub for fx w delay heal
		S62.625D	Disp fx med phalanx of l rng fngr, sub for fx w rout heal
		S62.625G	Disp fx med phalanx of l rng fngr, sub for fx w delay heal
		S62.626D	Disp fx med phalanx of r lit fngr, sub for fx w rout heal
		S62.626G	Disp fx med phalanx of r lit fngr, sub for fx w delay heal
		S62.627D	Disp fx med phalanx of l lit fngr, sub for fx w rout heal
		S62.627G	Disp fx med phalanx of l lit fngr, sub for fx w delay heal
		S62.628D	Disp fx medial phalanx of fngr, subs for fx w rout heal
		S62.628G	Disp fx medial phalanx of fngr, subs for fx w delay heal
		S62.629D	Disp fx med phalanx of unsp fngr, sub for fx w rout heal
		S62.629G	Disp fx med phalanx of unsp fngr, sub for fx w delay heal
		S62.63ØD	Disp fx dist phalanx of r idx fngr, sub for fx w rout heal
		S62.63ØG	Disp fx dist phalanx of r idx fngr, sub for fx w delay heal
		S62.631D	Disp fx dist phalanx of l idx fngr, sub for fx w rout heal
		S62.631G	Disp fx dist phalanx of l idx fngr, sub for fx w delay heal
		S62.632D	Disp fx dist phalanx of r mid fngr, sub for fx w rout heal
		S62.632G	Disp fx dist phalanx of r mid fngr, sub for fx w delay heal
		S62.633D	Disp fx dist phalanx of l mid fngr, sub for fx w rout heal
		S62.633G	Disp fx dist phalanx of l mid fngr, sub for fx w delay heal
		S62.634D	Disp fx dist phalanx of r rng fngr, sub for fx w rout heal
		S62.634G	Disp fx dist phalanx of r rng fngr, sub for fx w delay heal
		S62.635D	Disp fx dist phalanx of l rng fngr, sub for fx w rout heal
		S62.635G	Disp fx dist phalanx of l rng fngr, sub for fx w delay heal
		S62.636D	Disp fx dist phalanx of r lit fngr, sub for fx w rout heal
		S62.636G	Disp fx dist phalanx of r lit fngr, sub for fx w delay heal
		S62.637D	Disp fx dist phalanx of l lit fngr, sub for fx w rout heal
		S62.637G	Disp fx dist phalanx of l lit fngr, sub for fx w delay heal
		S62.638D	Disp fx dist phalanx of finger, subs for fx w rout heal
		S62.638G	Disp fx dist phalanx of finger, subs for fx w delay heal
		S62.639D	Disp fx dist phalanx of unsp fngr, sub for fx w rout heal
		S62.639G	Disp fx dist phalanx of unsp fngr, sub for fx w delay heal
		S62.64ØD	Nondisp fx prox phalanx of r idx fngr, sub for fx w rout heal
		S62.64ØG	Nondisp fx prox phalanx of r idx fngr, sub for fx w delay heal
		S62.641D	Nondisp fx prox phalanx of l idx fngr, sub for fx w rout heal
		S62.641G	Nondisp fx prox phalanx of l idx fngr, sub for fx w delay heal
		S62.642D	Nondisp fx prox phalanx of r mid fngr, sub for fx w rout heal
		S62.642G	Nondisp fx prox phalanx of r mid fngr, sub for fx w delay heal
		S62.643D	Nondisp fx prox phalanx of l mid fngr, sub for fx w rout heal
		S62.643G	Nondisp fx prox phalanx of l mid fngr, sub for fx w delay heal
		S62.644D	Nondisp fx prox phalanx of r rng fngr, sub for fx w rout heal
		S62.644G	Nondisp fx prox phalanx of r rng fngr, sub for fx w delay heal
		S62.645D	Nondisp fx prox phalanx of l rng fngr, sub for fx w rout heal
		S62.645G	Nondisp fx prox phalanx of l rng fngr, sub for fx w delay heal
		S62.646D	Nondisp fx prox phalanx of r lit fngr, sub for fx w rout heal
		S62.646G	Nondisp fx prox phalanx of r lit fngr, sub for fx w delay heal
		S62.647D	Nondisp fx prox phalanx of l lit fngr, sub for fx w rout heal
		S62.647G	Nondisp fx prox phalanx of l lit fngr, sub for fx w delay heal
		S62.648D	Nondisp fx prox phalanx of fngr, subs for fx w rout heal
		S62.648G	Nondisp fx prox phalanx of fngr, subs for fx w delay heal
	(Continued on next page)	**S62.649D**	Nondisp fx prox phalanx of unsp fngr, sub for fx w rout heal

ICD-9-CM		ICD-10-CM	
V54.12	AFTERCARE HEALING TRAUMATIC FRACTURE LOWER ARM **(Continued)**	**S62.649G**	Nondisp fx prox phalanx of unsp fngr, sub for fx w delay heal
		S62.65ØD	Nondisp fx med phalanx of r idx fngr, sub for fx w rout heal
		S62.65ØG	Nondisp fx med phalanx of r idx fngr, sub for fx w delay heal
		S62.651D	Nondisp fx med phalanx of l idx fngr, sub for fx w rout heal
		S62.651G	Nondisp fx med phalanx of l idx fngr, sub for fx w delay heal
		S62.652D	Nondisp fx med phalanx of r mid fngr, sub for fx w rout heal
		S62.652G	Nondisp fx med phalanx of r mid fngr, sub for fx w delay heal
		S62.653D	Nondisp fx med phalanx of l mid fngr, sub for fx w rout heal
		S62.653G	Nondisp fx med phalanx of l mid fngr, sub for fx w delay heal
		S62.654D	Nondisp fx med phalanx of r rng fngr, sub for fx w rout heal
		S62.654G	Nondisp fx med phalanx of r rng fngr, sub for fx w delay heal
		S62.655D	Nondisp fx med phalanx of l rng fngr, sub for fx w rout heal
		S62.655G	Nondisp fx med phalanx of l rng fngr, sub for fx w delay heal
		S62.656D	Nondisp fx med phalanx of r lit fngr, sub for fx w rout heal
		S62.656G	Nondisp fx med phalanx of r lit fngr, sub for fx w delay heal
		S62.657D	Nondisp fx med phalanx of l lit fngr, sub for fx w rout heal
		S62.657G	Nondisp fx med phalanx of l lit fngr, sub for fx w delay heal
		S62.658D	Nondisp fx med phalanx of fngr, subs for fx w rout heal
		S62.658G	Nondisp fx med phalanx of fngr, subs for fx w delay heal
		S62.659D	Nondisp fx med phalanx of unsp fngr, sub for fx w rout heal
		S62.659G	Nondisp fx med phalanx of unsp fngr, sub for fx w delay heal
		S62.66ØD	Nondisp fx dist phalanx of r idx fngr, sub for fx w rout heal
		S62.66ØG	Nondisp fx dist phalanx of r idx fngr, sub for fx w delay heal
		S62.661D	Nondisp fx dist phalanx of l idx fngr, sub for fx w rout heal
		S62.661G	Nondisp fx dist phalanx of l idx fngr, sub for fx w delay heal
		S62.662D	Nondisp fx dist phalanx of r mid fngr, sub for fx w rout heal
		S62.662G	Nondisp fx dist phalanx of r mid fngr, sub for fx w delay heal
		S62.663D	Nondisp fx dist phalanx of l mid fngr, sub for fx w rout heal
		S62.663G	Nondisp fx dist phalanx of l mid fngr, sub for fx w delay heal
		S62.664D	Nondisp fx dist phalanx of r rng fngr, sub for fx w rout heal
		S62.664G	Nondisp fx dist phalanx of r rng fngr, sub for fx w delay heal
		S62.665D	Nondisp fx dist phalanx of l rng fngr, sub for fx w rout heal
		S62.665G	Nondisp fx dist phalanx of l rng fngr, sub for fx w delay heal
		S62.666D	Nondisp fx dist phalanx of r lit fngr, sub for fx w rout heal
		S62.666G	Nondisp fx dist phalanx of r lit fngr, sub for fx w delay heal
		S62.667D	Nondisp fx dist phalanx of l lit fngr, sub for fx w rout heal
		S62.667G	Nondisp fx dist phalanx of l lit fngr, sub for fx w delay heal
		S62.668D	Nondisp fx dist phalanx of fngr, subs for fx w rout heal
		S62.668G	Nondisp fx dist phalanx of fngr, subs for fx w delay heal
		S62.669D	Nondisp fx dist phalanx of unsp fngr, sub for fx w rout heal
		S62.669G	Nondisp fx dist phalanx of unsp fngr, sub for fx w delay heal
		S62.9ØXD	Unsp fracture of unsp wrs/hnd, subs for fx w rout heal
		S62.9ØXG	Unsp fracture of unsp wrs/hnd, subs for fx w delay heal
		S62.91XD	Unsp fracture of right wrs/hnd, subs for fx w rout heal
		S62.91XG	Unsp fracture of right wrs/hnd, subs for fx w delay heal
		S62.92XD	Unsp fracture of left wrs/hnd, subs for fx w rout heal
		S62.92XG	Unsp fracture of left wrs/hnd, subs for fx w delay heal
V54.13	AFTERCARE FOR HEALING TRAUMATIC FRACTURE OF HIP	**S32.3Ø1D**	Unsp fracture of right ilium, subs for fx w routn heal
		S32.3Ø1G	Unsp fracture of right ilium, subs for fx w delay heal
		S32.3Ø2D	Unsp fracture of left ilium, subs for fx w routn heal
		S32.3Ø2G	Unsp fracture of left ilium, subs for fx w delay heal
		S32.3Ø9D	Unsp fracture of unsp ilium, subs for fx w routn heal
		S32.3Ø9G	Unsp fracture of unsp ilium, subs for fx w delay heal
		S32.311D	Displaced avulsion fx right ilium, subs for fx w routn heal
		S32.311G	Displaced avulsion fx right ilium, subs for fx w delay heal
		S32.312D	Displaced avulsion fx left ilium, subs for fx w routn heal
		S32.312G	Displaced avulsion fx left ilium, subs for fx w delay heal
		S32.313D	Displaced avulsion fx unsp ilium, subs for fx w routn heal
		S32.313G	Displaced avulsion fx unsp ilium, subs for fx w delay heal
		S32.314D	Nondisp avulsion fx right ilium, subs for fx w routn heal
		S32.314G	Nondisp avulsion fx right ilium, subs for fx w delay heal
		S32.315D	Nondisp avulsion fx left ilium, subs for fx w routn heal
		S32.315G	Nondisp avulsion fx left ilium, subs for fx w delay heal
		S32.316D	Nondisp avulsion fx unsp ilium, subs for fx w routn heal
		S32.316G	Nondisp avulsion fx unsp ilium, subs for fx w delay heal
		S32.391D	Oth fracture of right ilium, subs for fx w routn heal
		S32.391G	Oth fracture of right ilium, subs for fx w delay heal
		S32.392D	Oth fracture of left ilium, subs for fx w routn heal
		S32.392G	Oth fracture of left ilium, subs for fx w delay heal
		S32.399D	Oth fracture of unsp ilium, subs for fx w routn heal
		S32.399G	Oth fracture of unsp ilium, subs for fx w delay heal
		S32.4Ø1D	Unsp fracture of right acetabulum, subs for fx w routn heal
		S32.4Ø1G	Unsp fracture of right acetabulum, subs for fx w delay heal
		S32.4Ø2D	Unsp fracture of left acetabulum, subs for fx w routn heal
		S32.4Ø2G	Unsp fracture of left acetabulum, subs for fx w delay heal
		S32.4Ø9D	Unsp fracture of unsp acetabulum, subs for fx w routn heal
		S32.4Ø9G	Unsp fracture of unsp acetabulum, subs for fx w delay heal
		S32.411D	Disp fx of ant wall of r acetab, subs for fx w routn heal
		S32.411G	Disp fx of ant wall of r acetab, subs for fx w delay heal
		S32.412D	Disp fx of ant wall of left acetab, subs for fx w routn heal
		S32.412G	Disp fx of ant wall of left acetab, subs for fx w delay heal
		S32.413D	Disp fx of ant wall of unsp acetab, subs for fx w routn heal
	(Continued on next page)	**S32.413G**	Disp fx of ant wall of unsp acetab, subs for fx w delay heal

ICD-9-CM		ICD-10-CM	
V54.13	AFTERCARE FOR HEALING TRAUMATIC FRACTURE OF HIP **(Continued)**	**S32.414D**	Nondisp fx of ant wall of r acetab, subs for fx w routn heal
		S32.414G	Nondisp fx of ant wall of r acetab, subs for fx w delay heal
		S32.415D	Nondisp fx of ant wall of l acetab, subs for fx w routn heal
		S32.415G	Nondisp fx of ant wall of l acetab, subs for fx w delay heal
		S32.416D	Nondisp fx of ant wl of unsp acetab, sub for fx w rout heal
		S32.416G	Nondisp fx of ant wl of unsp acetab, sub for fx w delay heal
		S32.421D	Disp fx of post wall of r acetab, subs for fx w routn heal
		S32.421G	Disp fx of post wall of r acetab, subs for fx w delay heal
		S32.422D	Disp fx of post wall of l acetab, subs for fx w routn heal
		S32.422G	Disp fx of post wall of l acetab, subs for fx w delay heal
		S32.423D	Disp fx of post wl of unsp acetab, subs for fx w routn heal
		S32.423G	Disp fx of post wl of unsp acetab, subs for fx w delay heal
		S32.424D	Nondisp fx of post wl of r acetab, subs for fx w routn heal
		S32.424G	Nondisp fx of post wl of r acetab, subs for fx w delay heal
		S32.425D	Nondisp fx of post wl of l acetab, subs for fx w routn heal
		S32.425G	Nondisp fx of post wl of l acetab, subs for fx w delay heal
		S32.426D	Nondisp fx of post wl of unsp acetab, sub for fx w rout heal
		S32.426G	Nondisp fx of post wl of unsp acetab, sub for fx w delay heal
		S32.431D	Disp fx of ant column of r acetab, subs for fx w routn heal
		S32.431G	Disp fx of ant column of r acetab, subs for fx w delay heal
		S32.432D	Disp fx of ant column of l acetab, subs for fx w routn heal
		S32.432G	Disp fx of ant column of l acetab, subs for fx w delay heal
		S32.433D	Disp fx of ant column of unsp acetab, sub for fx w rout heal
		S32.433G	Disp fx of ant column of unsp acetab, sub for fx w delay heal
		S32.434D	Nondisp fx of ant column of r acetab, sub for fx w rout heal
		S32.434G	Nondisp fx of ant column of r acetab, sub for fx w delay heal
		S32.435D	Nondisp fx of ant column of l acetab, sub for fx w rout heal
		S32.435G	Nondisp fx of ant column of l acetab, sub for fx w delay heal
		S32.436D	Nondisp fx of ant column of unsp acetab, sub for fx w rout heal
		S32.436G	Nondisp fx of ant column of unsp acetab, sub for fx w delay heal
		S32.441D	Disp fx of post column of r acetab, subs for fx w routn heal
		S32.441G	Disp fx of post column of r acetab, subs for fx w delay heal
		S32.442D	Disp fx of post column of l acetab, subs for fx w routn heal
		S32.442G	Disp fx of post column of l acetab, subs for fx w delay heal
		S32.443D	Disp fx of post column of unsp acetab, sub for fx w rout heal
		S32.443G	Disp fx of post column of unsp acetab, sub for fx w delay heal
		S32.444D	Nondisp fx of post column of r acetab, sub for fx w rout heal
		S32.444G	Nondisp fx of post column of r acetab, sub for fx w delay heal
		S32.445D	Nondisp fx of post column of l acetab, sub for fx w rout heal
		S32.445G	Nondisp fx of post column of l acetab, sub for fx w delay heal
		S32.446D	Nondisp fx of post column of unsp acetab, sub for fx w rout heal
		S32.446G	Nondisp fx of post column of unsp acetab, sub for fx w delay heal
		S32.451D	Displ transverse fx right acetab, subs for fx w routn heal
		S32.451G	Displ transverse fx right acetab, subs for fx w delay heal
		S32.452D	Displ transverse fx left acetab, subs for fx w routn heal
		S32.452G	Displ transverse fx left acetab, subs for fx w delay heal
		S32.453D	Displ transverse fx unsp acetab, subs for fx w routn heal
		S32.453G	Displ transverse fx unsp acetab, subs for fx w delay heal
		S32.454D	Nondisp transverse fx right acetab, subs for fx w routn heal
		S32.454G	Nondisp transverse fx right acetab, subs for fx w delay heal
		S32.455D	Nondisp transverse fx left acetab, subs for fx w routn heal
		S32.455G	Nondisp transverse fx left acetab, subs for fx w delay heal
		S32.456D	Nondisp transverse fx unsp acetab, subs for fx w routn heal
		S32.456G	Nondisp transverse fx unsp acetab, subs for fx w delay heal
		S32.461D	Displ assoc transv/post fx r acetab, sub for fx w rout heal
		S32.461G	Displ assoc transv/post fx r acetab, sub for fx w delay heal
		S32.462D	Displ assoc transv/post fx l acetab, sub for fx w rout heal
		S32.462G	Displ assoc transv/post fx l acetab, sub for fx w delay heal
		S32.463D	Displ assoc transv/post fx unsp acetab, sub for fx w rout heal
		S32.463G	Displ assoc transv/post fx unsp acetab, sub for fx w delay heal
		S32.464D	Nondisp assoc transv/post fx r acetab, sub for fx w rout heal
		S32.464G	Nondisp assoc transv/post fx r acetab, sub for fx w delay heal
		S32.465D	Nondisp assoc transv/post fx l acetab, sub for fx w rout heal
		S32.465G	Nondisp assoc transv/post fx l acetab, sub for fx w delay heal
		S32.466D	Nondisp assoc transv/post fx unsp acetab, sub for fx w rout heal
		S32.466G	Nondisp assoc transv/post fx unsp acetab, sub for fx w delay heal
		S32.471D	Disp fx of med wall of r acetab, subs for fx w routn heal
		S32.471G	Disp fx of med wall of r acetab, subs for fx w delay heal
		S32.472D	Disp fx of med wall of left acetab, subs for fx w routn heal
		S32.472G	Disp fx of med wall of left acetab, subs for fx w delay heal
		S32.473D	Disp fx of med wall of unsp acetab, subs for fx w routn heal
		S32.473G	Disp fx of med wall of unsp acetab, subs for fx w delay heal
		S32.474D	Nondisp fx of med wall of r acetab, subs for fx w routn heal
		S32.474G	Nondisp fx of med wall of r acetab, subs for fx w delay heal
		S32.475D	Nondisp fx of med wall of l acetab, subs for fx w routn heal
		S32.475G	Nondisp fx of med wall of l acetab, subs for fx w delay heal
		S32.476D	Nondisp fx of med wl of unsp acetab, sub for fx w rout heal
		S32.476G	Nondisp fx of med wl of unsp acetab, sub for fx w delay heal
		S32.481D	Displaced dome fx right acetabulum, subs for fx w routn heal
		S32.481G	Displaced dome fx right acetabulum, subs for fx w delay heal
		S32.482D	Displaced dome fx left acetabulum, subs for fx w routn heal
		S32.482G	Displaced dome fx left acetabulum, subs for fx w delay heal
		S32.483D	Displaced dome fx unsp acetabulum, subs for fx w routn heal
	(Continued on next page)	**S32.483G**	Displaced dome fx unsp acetabulum, subs for fx w delay heal

ICD-9-CM		ICD-10-CM	
V54.13	AFTERCARE FOR HEALING TRAUMATIC FRACTURE OF HIP **(Continued)**	**S32.484D**	Nondisp dome fx right acetabulum, subs for fx w routn heal
		S32.484G	Nondisp dome fx right acetabulum, subs for fx w delay heal
		S32.485D	Nondisp dome fx left acetabulum, subs for fx w routn heal
		S32.485G	Nondisp dome fx left acetabulum, subs for fx w delay heal
		S32.486D	Nondisp dome fx unsp acetabulum, subs for fx w routn heal
		S32.486G	Nondisp dome fx unsp acetabulum, subs for fx w delay heal
		S32.491D	Oth fracture of right acetabulum, subs for fx w routn heal
		S32.491G	Oth fracture of right acetabulum, subs for fx w delay heal
		S32.492D	Oth fracture of left acetabulum, subs for fx w routn heal
		S32.492G	Oth fracture of left acetabulum, subs for fx w delay heal
		S32.499D	Oth fracture of unsp acetabulum, subs for fx w routn heal
		S32.499G	Oth fracture of unsp acetabulum, subs for fx w delay heal
		S32.5Ø1D	Unsp fracture of right pubis, subs for fx w routn heal
		S32.5Ø1G	Unsp fracture of right pubis, subs for fx w delay heal
		S32.5Ø2D	Unsp fracture of left pubis, subs for fx w routn heal
		S32.5Ø2G	Unsp fracture of left pubis, subs for fx w delay heal
		S32.5Ø9D	Unsp fracture of unsp pubis, subs for fx w routn heal
		S32.5Ø9G	Unsp fracture of unsp pubis, subs for fx w delay heal
		S32.511D	Fx superior rim of right pubis, subs for fx w routn heal
		S32.511G	Fx superior rim of right pubis, subs for fx w delay heal
		S32.512D	Fx superior rim of left pubis, subs for fx w routn heal
		S32.512G	Fx superior rim of left pubis, subs for fx w delay heal
		S32.519D	Fx superior rim of unsp pubis, subs for fx w routn heal
		S32.519G	Fx superior rim of unsp pubis, subs for fx w delay heal
		S32.591D	Oth fracture of right pubis, subs for fx w routn heal
		S32.591G	Oth fracture of right pubis, subs for fx w delay heal
		S32.592D	Oth fracture of left pubis, subs for fx w routn heal
		S32.592G	Oth fracture of left pubis, subs for fx w delay heal
		S32.599D	Oth fracture of unsp pubis, subs for fx w routn heal
		S32.599G	Oth fracture of unsp pubis, subs for fx w delay heal
		S32.6Ø1D	Unsp fracture of right ischium, subs for fx w routn heal
		S32.6Ø1G	Unsp fracture of right ischium, subs for fx w delay heal
		S32.6Ø2D	Unsp fracture of left ischium, subs for fx w routn heal
		S32.6Ø2G	Unsp fracture of left ischium, subs for fx w delay heal
		S32.6Ø9D	Unsp fracture of unsp ischium, subs for fx w routn heal
		S32.6Ø9G	Unsp fracture of unsp ischium, subs for fx w delay heal
		S32.611D	Displ avulsion fx right ischium, subs for fx w routn heal
		S32.611G	Displ avulsion fx right ischium, subs for fx w delay heal
		S32.612D	Displaced avulsion fx left ischium, subs for fx w routn heal
		S32.612G	Displaced avulsion fx left ischium, subs for fx w delay heal
		S32.613D	Displaced avulsion fx unsp ischium, subs for fx w routn heal
		S32.613G	Displaced avulsion fx unsp ischium, subs for fx w delay heal
		S32.614D	Nondisp avulsion fx right ischium, subs for fx w routn heal
		S32.614G	Nondisp avulsion fx right ischium, subs for fx w delay heal
		S32.615D	Nondisp avulsion fx left ischium, subs for fx w routn heal
		S32.615G	Nondisp avulsion fx left ischium, subs for fx w delay heal
		S32.616D	Nondisp avulsion fx unsp ischium, subs for fx w routn heal
		S32.616G	Nondisp avulsion fx unsp ischium, subs for fx w delay heal
		S32.691D	Oth fracture of right ischium, subs for fx w routn heal
		S32.691G	Oth fracture of right ischium, subs for fx w delay heal
		S32.692D	Oth fracture of left ischium, subs for fx w routn heal
		S32.692G	Oth fracture of left ischium, subs for fx w delay heal
		S32.699D	Oth fracture of unsp ischium, subs for fx w routn heal
		S32.699G	Oth fracture of unsp ischium, subs for fx w delay heal
		S72.ØØ1[D,E,F,G,H,J]	Fx unsp part of nk of r femr
		S72.ØØ2[D,E,F,G,H,J]	Fx unsp part of nk of l femr
		S72.ØØ9[D,E,F,G,H,J]	Fx unsp prt of nk of unsp femr
		S72.Ø11[D,E,F,G,H,J]	Unsp intracap fx right femur
		S72.Ø12[D,E,F,G,H,J]	Unsp intracap fx left femur
		S72.Ø19[D,E,F,G,H,J]	Unsp intracap fx unsp femur
		S72.Ø21[D,E,F,G,H,J]	Disp fx epiphy (sep) (up) r femr
		S72.Ø22[D,E,F,G,H,J]	Disp fx epiphy (sep) (up) l femr
		S72.Ø23[D,E,F,G,H,J]	Disp fx epiphy (sep) (up) unsp femr
		S72.Ø24[D,E,F,G,H,J]	Nondisp fx epiphy (sep) (up) r femr
		S72.Ø25[D,E,F,G,H,J]	Nondisp fx epiphy (sep) (up) l femr
		S72.Ø26[D,E,F,G,H,J]	Nondisp fx epiphy (sep) (up) unsp femr
		S72.Ø31[D,E,F,G,H,J]	Displ midcervical fx r femur
		S72.Ø32[D,E,F,G,H,J]	Displ midcervical fx l femur
		S72.Ø33[D,E,F,G,H,J]	Displ midcervical fx unsp femr
		S72.Ø34[D,E,F,G,H,J]	Nondisp midcervical fx r femr
		S72.Ø35[D,E,F,G,H,J]	Nondisp midcervical fx l femr
		S72.Ø36[D,E,F,G,H,J]	Nondisp midcervical fx unsp femr
		S72.Ø41[D,E,F,G,H,J]	Disp fx of base of nk of r femr
		S72.Ø42[D,E,F,G,H,J]	Disp fx of base of nk of l femr
		S72.Ø43[D,E,F,G,H,J]	Disp fx of base of nk of unsp femr
		S72.Ø44[D,E,F,G,H,J]	Nondisp fx of base of nk of r femr

7th Character meanings for code S72.-
***D** subs enc for clos fx w rout heal*
***E** subs enc for op fx typ 1/2 w rout heal*
***F** subs enc*
***G** subs enc for op fx typ 3 A/B/C w rout heal*
***H** subs enc for op fx typ 1/2 w del heal*
***J** subs enc for op fx typ 3 A/B/C w del heal*

(Continued on next page)

ICD-9-CM		ICD-10-CM	
V54.13	AFTERCARE FOR HEALING TRAUMATIC FRACTURE OF HIP **(Continued)**	**S72.Ø45**[D,E,F,G,H,J]	Nondisp fx of base of nk of l femr
		S72.Ø46[D,E,F,G,H,J]	Nondisp fx of base of nk of unsp femr
		S72.Ø51[D,E,F,G,H,J]	Unsp fx head of right femur
		S72.Ø52[D,E,F,G,H,J]	Unsp fx head of left femur
		S72.Ø59[D,E,F,G,H,J]	Unsp fx head of unsp femur
		S72.Ø61[D,E,F,G,H,J]	Displ artic fx head of r femr
		S72.Ø62[D,E,F,G,H,J]	Displ artic fx head of l femr
		S72.Ø63[D,E,F,G,H,J]	Displ artic fx head of unsp femr
		S72.Ø64[D,E,F,G,H,J]	Nondisp artic fx head of r femr
		S72.Ø65[D,E,F,G,H,J]	Nondisp artic fx head of l femr
		S72.Ø66[D,E,F,G,H,J]	Nondisp artic fx head of unsp femr
		S72.Ø91[D,E,F,G,H,J]	Oth fx head/neck of r femur
		S72.Ø92[D,E,F,G,H,J]	Oth fx head/neck of l femur
		S72.Ø99[D,E,F,G,H,J]	Oth fx head/neck of unsp femr
		S72.1Ø1[D,E,F,G,H,J]	Unsp trochan fx right femur
		S72.1Ø2[D,E,F,G,H,J]	Unsp trochan fx left femur
		S72.1Ø9[D,E,F,G,H,J]	Unsp trochan fx unsp femur
		S72.111[D,E,F,G,H,J]	Disp fx greater trochanter r femr
		S72.112[D,E,F,G,H,J]	Disp fx greater trochanter l femr
		S72.113[D,E,F,G,H,J]	Disp fx greater trochanter unsp femr
		S72.114[D,E,F,G,H,J]	Nondisp fx greater trochanter r femr
		S72.115[D,E,F,G,H,J]	Nondisp fx greater trochanter l femr
		S72.116[D,E,F,G,H,J]	Nondisp fx greater trochanter unsp femr
		S72.121[D,E,F,G,H,J]	Disp fx less trochanter r femr
		S72.122[D,E,F,G,H,J]	Disp fx less trochanter l femr
		S72.123[D,E,F,G,H,J]	Disp fx less trochanter unsp femr
		S72.124[D,E,F,G,H,J]	Nondisp fx less trochanter r femr
		S72.125[D,E,F,G,H,J]	Nondisp fx less trochanter l femr
		S72.126[D,E,F,G,H,J]	Nondisp fx less trochanter unsp femr
		S72.131[D,E,F,G,H,J]	Displ apophyseal fx r femur
		S72.132[D,E,F,G,H,J]	Displ apophyseal fx l femur
		S72.133[D,E,F,G,H,J]	Displ apophyseal fx unsp femr
		S72.134[D,E,F,G,H,J]	Nondisp apophyseal fx r femur
		S72.135[D,E,F,G,H,J]	Nondisp apophyseal fx l femur
		S72.136[D,E,F,G,H,J]	Nondisp apophyseal fx unsp femr
		S72.141[D,E,F,G,H,J]	Displ intertroch fx r femur
		S72.142[D,E,F,G,H,J]	Displ intertroch fx l femur
		S72.143[D,E,F,G,H,J]	Displ intertroch fx unsp femr
		S72.144[D,E,F,G,H,J]	Nondisp intertroch fx r femur
		S72.145[D,E,F,G,H,J]	Nondisp intertroch fx l femur
		S72.146[D,E,F,G,H,J]	Nondisp intertroch fx unsp femr
			7th Character meanings for code S72.- ***D subs enc for clos fx w rout heal*** ***E subs enc for op fx typ 1/2 w rout heal*** ***F subs enc*** ***G subs enc for op fx typ 3 A/B/C w rout heal*** ***H subs enc for op fx typ 1/2 w del heal*** ***J subs enc for op fx typ 3 A/B/C w del heal***
V54.14	AFTERCARE HEALING TRAUMATIC FRACTURE LEG UNSPEC	**S82.9ØXD**	Unsp fx unsp lower leg, subs for clos fx w routn heal
		S82.9ØXE	Unsp fx unsp low leg, subs for opn fx type I/2 w routn heal
		S82.9ØXF	Unsp fx unsp low leg, 7thF
V54.15	AFTERCARE HEALING TRAUMATIC FRACTURE UPPER LEG	**S72.21X**[D,E,F,G,H,J]	Displ subtrochnt fx r femur
		S72.22X[D,E,F,G,H,J]	Displ subtrochnt fx l femur
		S72.23X[D,E,F,G,H,J]	Displ subtrochnt fx unsp femr
		S72.24X[D,E,F,G,H,J]	Nondisp subtrochnt fx r femur
		S72.25X[D,E,F,G,H,J]	Nondisp subtrochnt fx l femur
		S72.26X[D,E,F,G,H,J]	Nondisp subtrochnt fx unsp femr
		S72.3Ø1[D,E,F,G,H,J]	Unsp fx shaft right femur
		S72.3Ø2[D,E,F,G,H,J]	Unsp fx shaft left femur
		S72.3Ø9[D,E,F,G,H,J]	Unsp fx shaft unsp femur
		S72.321[D,E,F,G,H,J]	Displ transverse fx shaft of r femr
		S72.322[D,E,F,G,H,J]	Displ transverse fx shaft of l femr
		S72.323[D,E,F,G,H,J]	Displ transverse fx shaft of unsp femr
		S72.324[D,E,F,G,H,J]	Nondisp transvrs fx shaft of r femr
		S72.325[D,E,F,G,H,J]	Nondisp transvrs fx shaft of l femr
		S72.326[D,E,F,G,H,J]	Nondisp transvrs fx shaft of unsp femr
		S72.331[D,E,F,G,H,J]	Displ oblique fx shaft of r femr
		S72.332[D,E,F,G,H,J]	Displ oblique fx shaft of l femr
		S72.333[D,E,F,G,H,J]	Displ oblique fx shaft of unsp femr
		S72.334[D,E,F,G,H,J]	Nondisp oblique fx shaft of r femr
		S72.335[D,E,F,G,H,J]	Nondisp oblique fx shaft of l femr
		S72.336[D,E,F,G,H,J]	Nondisp oblique fx shaft of unsp femr
		S72.341[D,E,F,G,H,J]	Displ spiral fx shaft of r femr
		S72.342[D,E,F,G,H,J]	Displ spiral fx shaft of l femr
			7th Character meanings for code S72.- ***D subs enc for clos fx w rout heal*** ***E subs enc for op fx typ 1/2 w rout heal*** ***F subs enc*** ***G subs enc for op fx typ 3 A/B/C w rout heal*** ***H subs enc for op fx typ 1/2 w del heal*** ***J subs enc for op fx typ 3 A/B/C w del heal***
	(Continued on next page)		

ICD-9-CM		ICD-10-CM	
V54.15	AFTERCARE HEALING TRAUMATIC FRACTURE UPPER LEG **(Continued)**	**S72.343**[D,E,F,G,H,J]	Displ spiral fx shaft of unsp femr
		S72.344[D,E,F,G,H,J]	Nondisp spiral fx shaft r femr
		S72.345[D,E,F,G,H,J]	Nondisp spiral fx shaft l femr
		S72.346[D,E,F,G,H,J]	Nondisp spiral fx shaft unsp femr
		S72.351[D,E,F,G,H,J]	Displ commnt fx shaft of r femr
		S72.352[D,E,F,G,H,J]	Displ commnt fx shaft of l femr
		S72.353[D,E,F,G,H,J]	Displ commnt fx shaft of unsp femr
		S72.354[D,E,F,G,H,J]	Nondisp commnt fx shaft r femr
		S72.355[D,E,F,G,H,J]	Nondisp commnt fx shaft l femr
		S72.356[D,E,F,G,H,J]	Nondisp commnt fx shaft unsp femr
		S72.361[D,E,F,G,H,J]	Displ seg fx shaft of r femur
		S72.362[D,E,F,G,H,J]	Displ seg fx shaft of l femur
		S72.363[D,E,F,G,H,J]	Displ seg fx shaft of unsp femr
		S72.364[D,E,F,G,H,J]	Nondisp seg fx shaft of r femr
		S72.365[D,E,F,G,H,J]	Nondisp seg fx shaft of l femr
		S72.366[D,E,F,G,H,J]	Nondisp seg fx shaft of unsp femr
		S72.391[D,E,F,G,H,J]	Oth fx shaft of right femur
		S72.392[D,E,F,G,H,J]	Oth fx shaft of left femur
		S72.399[D,E,F,G,H,J]	Oth fx shaft of unsp femur
		S72.4Ø1[D,E,F,G,H,J]	Unsp fx lower end r femur
		S72.4Ø2[D,E,F,G,H,J]	Unsp fx lower end l femur
		S72.4Ø9[D,E,F,G,H,J]	Unsp fx lower end unsp femur
		S72.411[D,E,F,G,H,J]	Displ unsp condyle fx low end r femr
		S72.412[D,E,F,G,H,J]	Displ unsp condyle fx low end l femr
		S72.413[D,E,F,G,H,J]	Displ unsp condyle fx low end unsp femr
		S72.414[D,E,F,G,H,J]	Nondisp unsp condyle fx low end r femr
		S72.415[D,E,F,G,H,J]	Nondisp unsp condyle fx low end l femr
		S72.416[D,E,F,G,H,J]	Nondisp unsp condyle fx low end unsp femr
		S72.421[D,E,F,G,H,J]	Disp fx lateral condyle r femr
		S72.422[D,E,F,G,H,J]	Disp fx lateral condyle l femr
		S72.423[D,E,F,G,H,J]	Disp fx lateral condyle unsp femr
		S72.424[D,E,F,G,H,J]	Nondisp fx lateral condyle r femr
		S72.425[D,E,F,G,H,J]	Nondisp fx lateral condyle l femr
		S72.426[D,E,F,G,H,J]	Nondisp fx lateral condyle unsp femr
		S72.431[D,E,F,G,H,J]	Disp fx med condyle r femr
		S72.432[D,E,F,G,H,J]	Disp fx med condyle l femr
		S72.433[D,E,F,G,H,J]	Disp fx med condyle unsp femr
		S72.434[D,E,F,G,H,J]	Nondisp fx med condyle r femr
		S72.435[D,E,F,G,H,J]	Nondisp fx med condyle l femr
		S72.436[D,E,F,G,H,J]	Nondisp fx med condyle unsp femr
		S72.441[D,E,F,G,H,J]	Disp fx low epiphy (sep) r femr
		S72.442[D,E,F,G,H,J]	Disp fx low epiphy (sep) l femr
		S72.443[D,E,F,G,H,J]	Disp fx low epiphy (sep) unsp femr
		S72.444[D,E,F,G,H,J]	Nondisp fx low epiphy (sep) r femr
		S72.445[D,E,F,G,H,J]	Nondisp fx low epiphy (sep) l femr
		S72.446[D,E,F,G,H,J]	Nondisp fx low epiphy (sep) unsp femr
		S72.451[D,E,F,G,H,J]	Dspl sprcond fx w/o intrcndl extn low end r femr
		S72.452[D,E,F,G,H,J]	Dspl sprcond fx w/o intrcndl extn low end l femr
		S72.453[D,E,F,G,H,J]	Dspl sprcond fx w/o intrcndl extn low end unsp femr
		S72.454[D,E,F,G,H,J]	Ndsplc sprcond fx w/o intrcndl extn low end r femr
		S72.455[D,E,F,G,H,J]	Ndsplc sprcond fx w/o intrcndl extn low end l femr
		S72.456[D,E,F,G,H,J]	Ndsplc sprcond fx w/o intrcndl extn low end unsp femr
		S72.461[D,E,F,G,H,J]	Dspl sprcond fx w intrcndl extn low end r femr
		S72.462[D,E,F,G,H,J]	Dspl sprcnd fx w intrcndl extn low end l femr
		S72.463[D,E,F,G,H,J]	Dspl sprcnd fx w intrcndl extn lw end unsp fmr
		S72.464[D,E,F,G,H,J]	Ndsplc sprcnd fx w intrcndl extn low end r femr
		S72.465[D,E,F,G,H,J]	Ndsplc sprcnd fx w intrcndl extn low end l femr
		S72.466[D,E,F,G,H,J]	Ndsplc sprcnd fx w intrcndl extn low end unsp femr
		S72.471D	Torus fx lower end right femur, subs for fx w routn heal
		S72.471G	Torus fx lower end right femur, subs for fx w delay heal
		S72.472D	Torus fx lower end left femur, subs for fx w routn heal
		S72.472G	Torus fx lower end left femur, subs for fx w delay heal
		S72.479D	Torus fx lower end unsp femur, subs for fx w routn heal
		S72.479G	Torus fx lower end unsp femur, subs for fx w delay heal
		S72.491[D,E,F,G,H,J]	Oth fx lower end r femur
		S72.492[D,E,F,G,H,J]	Oth fx lower end l femur
		S72.499[D,E,F,G,H,J]	Oth fx lower end unsp femur
		S72.8X1[D,E,F,G,H,J]	Oth fracture right femur
		S72.8X2[D,E,F,G,H,J]	Oth fracture left femur
		S72.8X9[D,E,F,G,H,J]	Oth fracture unsp femur
		S72.9ØX[D,E,F,G,H,J]	Unsp fracture unsp femur
		S72.91X[D,E,F,G,H,J]	Unsp fracture right femur
		S72.92X[D,E,F,G,H,J]	Unsp fracture left femur
		S79.ØØ1D	Unsp physl fx upper end r femur, subs for fx w routn heal
		S79.ØØ1G	Unsp physl fx upper end r femur, subs for fx w delay heal

7th Character meanings for code S72.-
- ***D** subs enc for clos fx w rout heal*
- ***E** subs enc for op fx typ 1/2 w rout heal*
- ***F** subs enc*
- ***G** subs enc for op fx typ 3 A/B/C w rout heal*
- ***H** subs enc for op fx typ 1/2 w del heal*
- ***J** subs enc for op fx typ 3 A/B/C w del heal*

(Continued on next page)

ICD-9-CM		ICD-10-CM	
V54.15	AFTERCARE HEALING TRAUMATIC FRACTURE UPPER LEG **(Continued)**	**S79.002D**	Unsp physl fx upper end l femur, subs for fx w routn heal
		S79.002G	Unsp physl fx upper end l femur, subs for fx w delay heal
		S79.009D	Unsp physl fx upper end unsp femur, subs for fx w routn heal
		S79.009G	Unsp physl fx upper end unsp femur, subs for fx w delay heal
		S79.011D	Sltr-haris Type I physl fx upr end r femr, sub for clos fx w rout heal
		S79.011G	Sltr-haris Type I physl fx upr end r femr, sub for fx w delay heal
		S79.012D	Sltr-haris Type I physl fx upr end l femr, sub for fx w rout heal
		S79.012G	Sltr-haris Type I physl fx upr end l femr, sub for fx w delay heal
		S79.019D	Sltr-haris Type I physl fx upr end unsp femr, sub for fx w rout heal
		S79.019G	Sltr-haris Type I physl fx upr end unsp femr, sub for fx w delay heal
		S79.091D	Oth physl fx upper end r femur, subs for fx w routn heal
		S79.091G	Oth physl fx upper end r femur, subs for fx w delay heal
		S79.092D	Oth physl fx upper end l femur, subs for fx w routn heal
		S79.092G	Oth physl fx upper end l femur, subs for fx w delay heal
		S79.099D	Oth physl fx upper end unsp femur, subs for fx w routn heal
		S79.099G	Oth physl fx upper end unsp femur, subs for fx w delay heal
		S79.101D	Unsp physl fx lower end r femur, subs for fx w routn heal
		S79.101G	Unsp physl fx lower end r femur, subs for fx w delay heal
		S79.102D	Unsp physl fx lower end l femur, subs for fx w routn heal
		S79.102G	Unsp physl fx lower end l femur, subs for fx w delay heal
		S79.109D	Unsp physl fx lower end unsp femur, subs for fx w routn heal
		S79.109G	Unsp physl fx lower end unsp femur, subs for fx w delay heal
		S79.111D	Sltr-haris Type I physl fx low end r femr, sub for fx w rout heal
		S79.111G	Sltr-haris Type I physl fx low end r femr, sub for fx w delay heal
		S79.112D	Sltr-haris Type I physl fx low end l femr, sub for fx w rout heal
		S79.112G	Sltr-haris Type I physl fx low end l femr, sub for fx w delay heal
		S79.119D	Sltr-haris Type I physl fx low end unsp femr, sub for fx w rout heal
		S79.119G	Sltr-haris Type I physl fx low end unsp femr, sub for fx w delay heal
		S79.121D	Sltr-haris Type II physl fx low end r femr, sub for fx w rout heal
		S79.121G	Sltr-haris Type II physl fx low end r femr, sub for fx w delay heal
		S79.122D	Sltr-haris Type II physl fx low end l femr, sub for fx w rout heal
		S79.122G	Sltr-haris Type II physl fx low end l femr, sub for fx w delay heal
		S79.129D	Sltr-haris Type II physl fx low end unsp femr, sub for fx w rout heal
		S79.129G	Sltr-haris Type II physl fx low end unsp femr, sub for fx w delay heal
		S79.131D	Sltr-haris Type III physl fx low end r femr, sub for fx w rout heal
		S79.131G	Sltr-haris Type III physl fx low end r femr, sub for fx w delay heal
		S79.132D	Sltr-haris Type III physl fx low end l femr, sub for fx w rout heal
		S79.132G	Sltr-haris Type III physl fx low end l femr, sub for fx w delay heal
		S79.139D	Sltr-haris Type III physl fx low end unsp femr, sub for fx w rout heal
		S79.139G	Sltr-haris Type III physl fx low end unsp femr, sub for fx w delay heal
		S79.141D	Sltr-haris Type IV physl fx low end r femr, sub for fx w rout heal
		S79.141G	Sltr-haris Type IV physl fx low end r femr, sub for fx w delay heal
		S79.142D	Sltr-haris Type IV physl fx low end l femr, sub for fx w rout heal
		S79.142G	Sltr-haris Type IV physl fx low end l femr, sub for fx w delay heal
		S79.149D	Sltr-haris Type IV physl fx low end unsp femr, sub for fx w rout heal
		S79.149G	Sltr-haris Type IV physl fx low end unsp femr, sub for fx w delay heal
		S79.191D	Oth physl fx lower end r femur, subs for fx w routn heal
		S79.191G	Oth physl fx lower end r femur, subs for fx w delay heal
		S79.192D	Oth physl fx lower end l femur, subs for fx w routn heal
		S79.192G	Oth physl fx lower end l femur, subs for fx w delay heal
		S79.199D	Oth physl fx lower end unsp femur, subs for fx w routn heal
		S79.199G	Oth physl fx lower end unsp femur, subs for fx w delay heal
V54.16	AFTERCARE HEALING TRAUMATIC FRACTURE LOWER LEG	**S82.001**[D,E,F,G,H,J]	Unsp fx right patella
		S82.002[D,E,F,G,H,J]	Unsp fracture of left patella
		S82.009[D,E,F,G,H,J]	Unsp fracture of unsp patella
		S82.011[D,E,F,G,H,J]	Displ osteochon fx r patella
		S82.012[D,E,F,G,H,J]	Displ osteochon fx l patella
		S82.013[D,E,F,G,H,J]	Displ osteochon fx unsp patella
		S82.014[D,E,F,G,H,J]	Nondisp osteochon fx r patella
		S82.015[D,E,F,G,H,J]	Nondisp osteochon fx l patella
		S82.016[D,E,F,G,H,J]	Nondisp osteochon fx unsp patella
		S82.021[D,E,F,G,H,J]	Displ longitud fx r patella
		S82.022[D,E,F,G,H,J]	Displ longitud fx l patella
		S82.023[D,E,F,G,H,J]	Displ longitud fx unsp patella
		S82.024[D,E,F,G,H,J]	Nondisp longitud fx r patella
		S82.025[D,E,F,G,H,J]	Nondisp longitud fx l patella
		S82.026[D,E,F,G,H,J]	Nondisp longitud fx unsp patella
		S82.031[D,E,F,G,H,J]	Displ transverse fx r patella
		S82.032[D,E,F,G,H,J]	Displ transverse fx l patella
		S82.033[D,E,F,G,H,J]	Displ transverse fx unsp patella
		S82.034[D,E,F,G,H,J]	Nondisp transverse fx r patella
		S82.035[D,E,F,G,H,J]	Nondisp transverse fx l patella
		S82.036[D,E,F,G,H,J]	Nondisp transverse fx unsp patella
		S82.041[D,E,F,G,H,J]	Displ commnt fx right patella

7th Character meanings for code S82.-
***D** subs enc for clos fx w rout heal*
***E** subs enc for op fx typ 1/2 w rout heal*
***F** subs enc*
***G** subs enc for op fx typ 3 A/B/C w rout heal*
***H** subs enc for op fx typ 1/2 w del heal*
***J** subs enc for op fx typ 3 A/B/C w del heal*

(Continued on next page)

ICD-9-CM		ICD-10-CM	
V54.16	AFTERCARE HEALING TRAUMATIC FRACTURE LOWER LEG **(Continued)**	**S82.Ø42**[D,E,F,G,H,J]	Displ commnt fx left patella
		S82.Ø43[D,E,F,G,H,J]	Displ commnt fx unsp patella
		S82.Ø44[D,E,F,G,H,J]	Nondisp commnt fx r patella
		S82.Ø45[D,E,F,G,H,J]	Nondisp commnt fx l patella
		S82.Ø46[D,E,F,G,H,J]	Nondisp commnt fx unsp patella
		S82.Ø91[D,E,F,G,H,J]	Oth fracture of right patella
		S82.Ø92[D,E,F,G,H,J]	Oth fracture of left patella
		S82.Ø99[D,E,F,G,H,J]	Oth fracture of unsp patella
		S82.1Ø1[D,E,F,G,H,J]	Unsp fx upper end of r tibia
		S82.1Ø2[D,E,F,G,H,J]	Unsp fx upper end of l tibia
		S82.1Ø9[D,E,F,G,H,J]	Unsp fx upper end unsp tibia
		S82.111[D,E,F,G,H,J]	Disp fx of right tibial spine
		S82.112[D,E,F,G,H,J]	Disp fx of left tibial spine
		S82.113[D,E,F,G,H,J]	Disp fx of unsp tibial spine
		S82.114[D,E,F,G,H,J]	Nondisp fx of r tibial spine
		S82.115[D,E,F,G,H,J]	Nondisp fx of l tibial spin
		S82.116[D,E,F,G,H,J]	Nondisp fx of unsp tibial spin
		S82.121[D,E,F,G,H,J]	Disp fx of lateral condyle of r tibia
		S82.122[D,E,F,G,H,J]	Disp fx of lateral condyle of l tibia
		S82.123[D,E,F,G,H,J]	Disp fx of lateral condyle of unsp tibia
		S82.124[D,E,F,G,H,J]	Nondisp fx of lateral condyle of r tibia
		S82.125[D,E,F,G,H,J]	Nondisp fx of lateral condyle of l tibia
		S82.126[D,E,F,G,H,J]	Nondisp fx of lateral condyle of unsp tibia
		S82.131[D,E,F,G,H,J]	Disp fx of med condyle of r tibia
		S82.132[D,E,F,G,H,J]	Disp fx of med condyle of l tibia
		S82.133[D,E,F,G,H,J]	Disp fx of med condyle of unsp tibia
		S82.134[D,E,F,G,H,J]	Nondisp fx of med condyle of r tibia
		S82.135[D,E,F,G,H,J]	Nondisp fx of med condyle of l tibia
		S82.136[D,E,F,G,H,J]	Nondisp fx of med condyle of unsp tibia
		S82.141[D,E,F,G,H,J]	Displ bicondylar fx r tibia
		S82.142[D,E,F,G,H,J]	Displ bicondylar fx l tibia
		S82.143[D,E,F,G,H,J]	Displ bicondylar fx unsp tibia
		S82.144[D,E,F,G,H,J]	Nondisp bicondylar fx r tibia
		S82.145[D,E,F,G,H,J]	Nondisp bicondylar fx l tibia
		S82.146[D,E,F,G,H,J]	Nondisp bicondylar fx unsp tibia
		S82.151[D,E,F,G,H,J]	Disp fx of r tibial tuberosity
		S82.152[D,E,F,G,H,J]	Disp fx of l tibial tuberosity
		S82.153[D,E,F,G,H,J]	Disp fx of unsp tibial tuberosity
		S82.154[D,E,F,G,H,J]	Nondisp fx of r tibial tuberosity
		S82.155[D,E,F,G,H,J]	Nondisp fx of l tibial tuberosity
		S82.156[D,E,F,G,H,J]	Nondisp fx of unsp tibial tuberosity
		S82.161D	Torus fx upper end of right tibia, subs for fx w routn heal
		S82.161G	Torus fx upper end of right tibia, subs for fx w delay heal
		S82.162D	Torus fx upper end of left tibia, subs for fx w routn heal
		S82.162G	Torus fx upper end of left tibia, subs for fx w delay heal
		S82.169D	Torus fx upper end of unsp tibia, subs for fx w routn heal
		S82.169G	Torus fx upper end of unsp tibia, subs for fx w delay heal
		S82.191[D,E,F,G,H,J]	Oth fx upper end of r tibia
		S82.192[D,E,F,G,H,J]	Oth fx upper end of l tibia
		S82.199[D,E,F,G,H,J]	Oth fx upper end unsp tibia
		S82.2Ø1[D,E,F,G,H,J]	Unsp fx shaft of right tibia
		S82.2Ø2[D,E,F,G,H,J]	Unsp fx shaft of left tibia
		S82.2Ø9[D,E,F,G,H,J]	Unsp fx shaft of unsp tibia
		S82.221[D,E,F,G,H,J]	Displ transverse fx shaft of r tibia
		S82.222[D,E,F,G,H,J]	Displ transverse fx shaft of l tibia
		S82.223[D,E,F,G,H,J]	Displ transverse fx shaft of unsp tibia
		S82.224[D,E,F,G,H,J]	Nondisp transvs fx shaft of r tibia
		S82.225[D,E,F,G,H,J]	Nondisp transvs fx shaft of l tibia
		S82.226[D,E,F,G,H,J]	Nondisp transvs fx shaft of unsp tibia
		S82.231[D,E,F,G,H,J]	Displ oblique fx shaft of r tibia
		S82.232[D,E,F,G,H,J]	Displ oblique fx shaft of l tibia
		S82.233[D,E,F,G,H,J]	Displ oblique fx shaft of unsp tibia
		S82.234[D,E,F,G,H,J]	Nondisp oblique fx shaft of r tibia
		S82.235[D,E,F,G,H,J]	Nondisp oblique fx shaft of l tibia
		S82.236[D,E,F,G,H,J]	Nondisp oblique fx shaft of unsp tibia
		S82.241[D,E,F,G,H,J]	Displ spiral fx shaft of r tibia
		S82.242[D,E,F,G,H,J]	Displ spiral fx shaft of l tibia
		S82.243[D,E,F,G,H,J]	Displ spiral fx shaft of unsp tibia
		S82.244[D,E,F,G,H,J]	Nondisp spiral fx shaft of r tibia
		S82.245[D,E,F,G,H,J]	Nondisp spiral fx shaft of l tibia
		S82.246[D,E,F,G,H,J]	Nondisp spiral fx shaft of unsp tibia
		S82.251[D,E,F,G,H,J]	Displ commnt fx shaft of r tibia
		S82.252[D,E,F,G,H,J]	Displ commnt fx shaft of l tibia
		S82.253[D,E,F,G,H,J]	Displ commnt fx shaft of unsp tibia

7th Character meanings for code S82.-
D subs enc for clos fx w rout heal
E subs enc for op fx typ 1/2 w rout heal
F subs enc
G subs enc for op fx typ 3 A/B/C w rout heal
H subs enc for op fx typ 1/2 w del heal
J subs enc for op fx typ 3 A/B/C w del heal

(Continued on next page)

[Brackets] indicate valid character values for each code. Character value meanings provided for each code grouping.

ICD-9-CM		ICD-10-CM	
V54.16	AFTERCARE HEALING TRAUMATIC FRACTURE LOWER LEG **(Continued)**	**S82.254**[D,E,F,G,H,J]	Nondisp commnt fx shaft of r tibia
		S82.255[D,E,F,G,H,J]	Nondisp commnt fx shaft of l tibia
		S82.256[D,E,F,G,H,J]	Nondisp commnt fx shaft of unsp tibia
		S82.261[D,E,F,G,H,J]	Displ seg fx shaft of r tibia
		S82.262[D,E,F,G,H,J]	Displ seg fx shaft of l tibia
		S82.263[D,E,F,G,H,J]	Displ seg fx shaft of unsp tibia
		S82.264[D,E,F,G,H,J]	Nondisp seg fx shaft of r tibia
		S82.265[D,E,F,G,H,J]	Nondisp seg fx shaft of l tibia
		S82.266[D,E,F,G,H,J]	Nondisp seg fx shaft of unsp tibia
		S82.291[D,E,F,G,H,J]	Oth fx shaft of right tibia
		S82.292[D,E,F,G,H,J]	Oth fx shaft of left tibia
		S82.299[D,E,F,G,H,J]	Oth fx shaft of unsp tibia
		S82.3Ø1[D,E,F,G,H,J]	Unsp fx lower end of r tibia
		S82.3Ø2[D,E,F,G,H,J]	Unsp fx lower end of l tibia
		S82.3Ø9[D,E,F,G,H,J]	Unsp fx lower end unsp tibia
		S82.311D	Torus fx lower end of right tibia, subs for fx w routn heal
		S82.311G	Torus fx lower end of right tibia, subs for fx w delay heal
		S82.312D	Torus fx lower end of left tibia, subs for fx w routn heal
		S82.312G	Torus fx lower end of left tibia, subs for fx w delay heal
		S82.319D	Torus fx lower end of unsp tibia, subs for fx w routn heal
		S82.319G	Torus fx lower end of unsp tibia, subs for fx w delay heal
		S82.391[D,E,F,G,H,J]	Oth fx lower end of r tibia
		S82.392[D,E,F,G,H,J]	Oth fx lower end of l tibia
		S82.399[D,E,F,G,H,J]	Oth fx lower end unsp tibia
		S82.4Ø1[D,E,F,G,H,J]	Unsp fx shaft of r fibula
		S82.4Ø2[D,E,F,G,H,J]	Unsp fx shaft of left fibula
		S82.4Ø9[D,E,F,G,H,J]	Unsp fx shaft of unsp fibula
		S82.421[D,E,F,G,H,J]	Displ transverse fx shaft of r fibula
		S82.422[D,E,F,G,H,J]	Displ transverse fx shaft of l fibula
		S82.423[D,E,F,G,H,J]	Displ transverse fx shaft of unsp fibula
		S82.424[D,E,F,G,H,J]	Nondisp transverse fx shaft of r fibula
		S82.425[D,E,F,G,H,J]	Nondisp transverse fx shaft of l fibula
		S82.426[D,E,F,G,H,J]	Nondisp transverse fx shaft of unsp fibula
		S82.431[D,E,F,G,H,J]	Displ oblique fx shaft of r fibula
		S82.432[D,E,F,G,H,J]	Displ oblique fx shaft of l fibula
		S82.433[D,E,F,G,H,J]	Displ oblique fx shaft of unsp fibula
		S82.434[D,E,F,G,H,J]	Nondisp oblique fx shaft of r fibula
		S82.435[D,E,F,G,H,J]	Nondisp oblique fx shaft of l fibula
		S82.436[D,E,F,G,H,J]	Nondisp oblique fx shaft of unsp fibula
		S82.441[D,E,F,G,H,J]	Displ spiral fx shaft of r fibula
		S82.442[D,E,F,G,H,J]	Displ spiral fx shaft of l fibula
		S82.443[D,E,F,G,H,J]	Displ spiral fx shaft of unsp fibula
		S82.444[D,E,F,G,H,J]	Nondisp spiral fx shaft of r fibula
		S82.445[D,E,F,G,H,J]	Nondisp spiral fx shaft of l fibula
		S82.446[D,E,F,G,H,J]	Nondisp spiral fx shaft of unsp fibula
		S82.451[D,E,F,G,H,J]	Displ commnt fx shaft of r fibula
		S82.452[D,E,F,G,H,J]	Displ commnt fx shaft of l fibula
		S82.453[D,E,F,G,H,J]	Displ commnt fx shaft of unsp fibula
		S82.454[D,E,F,G,H,J]	Nondisp commnt fx shaft of r fibula
		S82.455[D,E,F,G,H,J]	Nondisp commnt fx shaft of l fibula
		S82.456[D,E,F,G,H,J]	Nondisp commnt fx shaft of unsp fibula
		S82.461[D,E,F,G,H,J]	Displ seg fx shaft of r fibula
		S82.462[D,E,F,G,H,J]	Displ seg fx shaft of l fibula
		S82.463[D,E,F,G,H,J]	Displ seg fx shaft of unsp fibula
		S82.464[D,E,F,G,H,J]	Nondisp seg fx shaft of r fibula
		S82.465[D,E,F,G,H,J]	Nondisp seg fx shaft of l fibula
		S82.466[D,E,F,G,H,J]	Nondisp seg fx shaft of unsp fibula
		S82.491[D,E,F,G,H,J]	Oth fx shaft of r fibula
		S82.492[D,E,F,G,H,J]	Oth fx shaft of left fibula
		S82.499[D,E,F,G,H,J]	Oth fx shaft of unsp fibula
		S82.51X[D,E,F,G,H,J]	Disp fx of med malleolus of r tibia
		S82.52X[D,E,F,G,H,J]	Disp fx of med malleolus of l tibia
		S82.53X[D,E,F,G,H,J]	Disp fx of med malleolus of unsp tibia
		S82.54X[D,E,F,G,H,J]	Nondisp fx of med malleolus of r tibia
		S82.55X[D,E,F,G,H,J]	Nondisp fx of med malleolus of l tibia
		S82.56X[D,E,F,G,H,J]	Nondisp fx of med malleolus of unsp tibia
		S82.61X[D,E,F,G,H,J]	Disp fx of lateral malleolus of r fibula
		S82.62X[D,E,F,G,H,J]	Disp fx of lateral malleolus of l fibula
		S82.63X[D,E,F,G,H,J]	Disp fx of lateral malleolus of unsp fibula
		S82.64X[D,E,F,G,H,J]	Nondisp fx lateral malleolus r fibula
		S82.65X[D,E,F,G,H,J]	Nondisp fx lateral malleolus l fibula
		S82.66X[D,E,F,G,H,J]	Nondisp fx lateral malleolus unsp fibula
		S82.811D	Torus fx upper end of r fibula, subs for fx w routn heal
		S82.811G	Torus fx upper end of r fibula, subs for fx w delay heal

7th Character meanings for code S82.-
D subs enc for clos fx w rout heal
E subs enc for op fx typ 1/2 w rout heal
F subs enc
G subs enc for op fx typ 3 A/B/C w rout heal
H subs enc for op fx typ 1/2 w del heal
J subs enc for op fx typ 3 A/B/C w del heal

(Continued on next page)

ICD-9-CM	ICD-10-CM	
V54.16 AFTERCARE HEALING TRAUMATIC FRACTURE LOWER LEG **(Continued)**	**S82.812D**	Torus fx upper end of left fibula, subs for fx w routn heal
	S82.812G	Torus fx upper end of left fibula, subs for fx w delay heal
	S82.819D	Torus fx upper end of unsp fibula, subs for fx w routn heal
	S82.819G	Torus fx upper end of unsp fibula, subs for fx w delay heal
	S82.821D	Torus fx lower end of r fibula, subs for fx w routn heal
	S82.821G	Torus fx lower end of r fibula, subs for fx w delay heal
	S82.822D	Torus fx lower end of left fibula, subs for fx w routn heal
	S82.822G	Torus fx lower end of left fibula, subs for fx w delay heal
	S82.829D	Torus fx lower end of unsp fibula, subs for fx w routn heal
	S82.829G	Torus fx lower end of unsp fibula, subs for fx w delay heal
	S82.831[D,E,F,G,H,J]	Oth fx upr & low end r fibula
	S82.832[D,E,F,G,H,J]	Oth fx upr & low end l fibula
	S82.839[D,E,F,G,H,J]	Oth fx upr & low end unsp fibula
	S82.841[D,E,F,G,H,J]	Displ bimalleol fx r low leg
	S82.842[D,E,F,G,H,J]	Displ bimalleol fx l low leg
	S82.843[D,E,F,G,H,J]	Displ bimalleol fx unsp low leg
	S82.844[D,E,F,G,H,J]	Nondisp bimalleol fx r low leg
	S82.845[D,E,F,G,H,J]	Nondisp bimalleol fx l low leg
	S82.846[D,E,F,G,H,J]	Nondisp bimalleol fx unsp low leg
	S82.851[D,E,F,G,H,J]	Displ trimalleol fx r low leg
	S82.852[D,E,F,G,H,J]	Displ trimalleol fx l low leg
	S82.853[D,E,F,G,H,J]	Displ trimalleol fx unsp low leg
	S82.854[D,E,F,G,H,J]	Nondisp trimalleol fx r low leg
	S82.855[D,E,F,G,H,J]	Nondisp trimalleol fx l low leg
	S82.856[D,E,F,G,H,J]	Nondisp trimalleol fx unsp low leg
	S82.861[D,E,F,G,H,J]	Displ Maisonneuve's fx r leg
	S82.862[D,E,F,G,H,J]	Displ Maisonneuve's fx l leg
	S82.863[D,E,F,G,H,J]	Displ Maisonneuve's fx unsp leg
	S82.864[D,E,F,G,H,J]	Nondisp Maisonneuve's fx r leg
	S82.865[D,E,F,G,H,J]	Nondisp Maisonneuve's fx l leg
	S82.866[D,E,F,G,H,J]	Nondisp Maisonneuve's fx unsp leg
	S82.871[D,E,F,G,H,J]	Displaced pilon fx r tibia
	S82.872[D,E,F,G,H,J]	Displaced pilon fx left tibia
	S82.873[D,E,F,G,H,J]	Displaced pilon fx unsp tibia
	S82.874[D,E,F,G,H,J]	Nondisp pilon fx right tibia
	S82.875[D,E,F,G,H,J]	Nondisp pilon fx left tibia
	S82.876[D,E,F,G,H,J]	Nondisp pilon fx unsp tibia
	S82.891[D,E,F,G,H,J]	Oth fracture of r low leg
	S82.892[D,E,F,G,H,J]	Oth fracture of l low leg
	S82.899[D,E,F,G,H,J]	Oth fx unsp lower leg
	S82.9ØX[D,E,F,G,H,J]	Unsp fx unsp lower leg
	S82.91X[D,E,F,G,H,J]	Unsp fracture of r low leg
	S82.92X[D,E,F,G,H,J]	Unsp fracture of l low leg
	S89.ØØ1D	Unsp physl fx upper end of r tibia, subs for fx w routn heal
	S89.ØØ1G	Unsp physl fx upper end of r tibia, subs for fx w delay heal
	S89.ØØ2D	Unsp physl fx upper end of l tibia, subs for fx w routn heal
	S89.ØØ2G	Unsp physl fx upper end of l tibia, subs for fx w delay heal
	S89.ØØ9D	Unsp physl fx upper end unsp tibia, subs for fx w routn heal
	S89.ØØ9G	Unsp physl fx upper end unsp tibia, subs for fx w delay heal
	S89.Ø11D	Sltr-haris Type I physl fx upr end r tibia, sub for fx w rout heal
	S89.Ø11G	Sltr-haris Type I physl fx upr end r tibia,sub for fx w delay heal
	S89.Ø12D	Sltr-haris Type I physl fx upr end l tibia, sub for fx w rout heal
	S89.Ø12G	Sltr-haris Type I physl fx upr end l tibia, sub for fx w delay heal
	S89.Ø19D	Sltr-haris Type I physl fx upr end unsp tibia, sub for fx w rout heal
	S89.Ø19G	Sltr-haris Type I physl fx upr end unsp tibia, sub for fx w del heal
	S89.Ø21D	Sltr-haris Type II physl fx upr end r tibia, sub for fx w rout heal
	S89.Ø21G	Sltr-haris Type II physl fx upr end r tibia, sub for fx w delay heal
	S89.Ø22D	Sltr-haris Type II physl fx upr end l tibia, sub for fx w rout heal
	S89.Ø22G	Sltr-haris Type II physl fx upr end l tibia, sub for fx w delay heal
	S89.Ø29D	Sltr-haris Type II physl fx upr end unsp tibia, sub for fx w rout heal
	S89.Ø29G	Sltr-haris Type II physl fx upr end unsp tibia, sub for fx w del heal
	S89.Ø31D	Sltr-haris Type III physl fx upr end r tibia, sub for fx w rout heal
	S89.Ø31G	Sltr-haris Type III physl fx upr end r tibia, sub for fx w delay heal
	S89.Ø32D	Sltr-haris Type III physl fx upr end l tibia, sub for fx w rout heal
	S89.Ø32G	Sltr-haris Type III physl fx upr end l tibia, sub for fx w delay heal
	S89.Ø39D	Sltr-haris Type III physl fx upr end unsp tibia, sub for fx w rout heal
	S89.Ø39G	Sltr-haris Type III physl fx upr end unsp tibia, sub for fx w del heal
	S89.Ø41D	Sltr-haris Type IV physl fx upr end r tibia, sub for fx w rout heal
	S89.Ø41G	Sltr-haris Type IV physl fx upr end r tibia, sub for fx w delay heal
	S89.Ø42D	Sltr-haris Type IV physl fx upr end l tibia, sub for fx w rout heal
	S89.Ø42G	Sltr-haris Type IV physl fx upr end l tibia, sub for fx w delay heal
	S89.Ø49D	Sltr-haris Type IV physl fx upr end unsp tibia, sub for fx w rout heal
	S89.Ø49G	Sltr-haris Type IV physl fx upr end unsp tibia, sub for fx w del heal

7th Character meanings for code S82.-
- ***D** subs enc for clos fx w rout heal*
- ***E** subs enc for op fx typ 1/2 w rout heal*
- ***F** subs enc*
- ***G** subs enc for op fx typ 3 A/B/C w rout heal*
- ***H** subs enc for op fx typ 1/2 w del heal*
- ***J** subs enc for op fx typ 3 A/B/C w del heal*

(Continued on next page)

[Brackets] indicate valid character values for each code. Character value meanings provided for each code grouping.

ICD-9-CM		ICD-10-CM	
V54.16	AFTERCARE HEALING TRAUMATIC FRACTURE LOWER LEG **(Continued)**	**S89.091D**	Oth physl fx upper end of r tibia, subs for fx w routn heal
		S89.091G	Oth physl fx upper end of r tibia, subs for fx w delay heal
		S89.092D	Oth physl fx upper end of l tibia, subs for fx w routn heal
		S89.092G	Oth physl fx upper end of l tibia, subs for fx w delay heal
		S89.099D	Oth physl fx upper end unsp tibia, subs for fx w routn heal
		S89.099G	Oth physl fx upper end unsp tibia, subs for fx w delay heal
		S89.101D	Unsp physl fx lower end of r tibia, subs for fx w routn heal
		S89.101G	Unsp physl fx lower end of r tibia, subs for fx w delay heal
		S89.102D	Unsp physl fx lower end of l tibia, subs for fx w routn heal
		S89.102G	Unsp physl fx lower end of l tibia, subs for fx w delay heal
		S89.109D	Unsp physl fx lower end unsp tibia, subs for fx w routn heal
		S89.109G	Unsp physl fx lower end unsp tibia, subs for fx w delay heal
		S89.111D	Sltr-haris Type I physl fx low end r tibia, sub for fx w rout heal
		S89.111G	Sltr-haris Type I physl fx low end r tibia, sub for fx w delay heal
		S89.112D	Sltr-haris Type I physl fx low end l tibia, sub for fx w rout heal
		S89.112G	Sltr-haris Type I physl fx low end l tibia, sub for fx w delay heal
		S89.119D	Sltr-haris Type I physl fx low end unsp tibia, sub for fx w rout heal
		S89.119G	Sltr-haris Type I physl fx low end unsp tibia, sub for fx w del heal
		S89.121D	Sltr-haris Type II physl fx low end r tibia, sub for fx w rout heal
		S89.121G	Sltr-haris Type II physl fx low end r tibia, sub for fx w delay heal
		S89.122D	Sltr-haris Type II physl fx low end l tibia, sub for fx w rout heal
		S89.122G	Sltr-haris Type II physl fx low end l tibia, sub for fx w delay heal
		S89.129D	Sltr-haris Type II physl fx low end unsp tibia, sub for fx w rout heal
		S89.129G	Sltr-haris Type II physl fx low end unsp tibia, sub for fx w delay heal
		S89.131D	Sltr-haris Type III physl fx low end r tibia, sub for fx w rout heal
		S89.131G	Sltr-haris Type III physl fx low end r tibia, sub for fx w delay heal
		S89.132D	Sltr-haris Type III physl fx low end l tibia, sub for fx w rout heal
		S89.132G	Sltr-haris Type III physl fx low end l tibia, sub for fx w delay heal
		S89.139D	Sltr-haris Type III physl fx low end unsp tibia, sub for fx w rout heal
		S89.139G	Sltr-haris Type III physl fx low end unsp tibia, sub for fx w delay heal
		S89.141D	Sltr-haris Type IV physl fx low end r tibia, sub for fx w rout heal
		S89.141G	Sltr-haris Type IV physl fx low end r tibia, sub for fx w delay heal
		S89.142D	Sltr-haris Type IV physl fx low end l tibia, sub for fx w rout heal
		S89.142G	Sltr-haris Type IV physl fx low end l tibia, sub for fx w delay heal
		S89.149D	Sltr-haris Type IV physl fx low end unsp tibia, sub for fx w rout heal
		S89.149G	Sltr-haris Type IV physl fx low end unsp tibia, sub for fx w delay heal
		S89.191D	Oth physl fx lower end of r tibia, subs for fx w routn heal
		S89.191G	Oth physl fx lower end of r tibia, subs for fx w delay heal
		S89.192D	Oth physl fx lower end of l tibia, subs for fx w routn heal
		S89.192G	Oth physl fx lower end of l tibia, subs for fx w delay heal
		S89.199D	Oth physl fx lower end unsp tibia, subs for fx w routn heal
		S89.199G	Oth physl fx lower end unsp tibia, subs for fx w delay heal
		S89.201D	Unsp physl fx upper end r fibula, subs for fx w routn heal
		S89.201G	Unsp physl fx upper end r fibula, subs for fx w delay heal
		S89.202D	Unsp physl fx upper end l fibula, subs for fx w routn heal
		S89.202G	Unsp physl fx upper end l fibula, subs for fx w delay heal
		S89.209D	Unsp physl fx upr end unsp fibula, subs for fx w routn heal
		S89.209G	Unsp physl fx upr end unsp fibula, subs for fx w delay heal
		S89.211D	Sltr-haris Type I physl fx upr end r fibula, sub for fx w rout heal
		S89.211G	Sltr-haris Type I physl fx upr end r fibula, sub for fx w delay heal
		S89.212D	Sltr-haris Type I physl fx upr end l fibula, sub for fx w rout heal
		S89.212G	Sltr-haris Type I physl fx upr end l fibula, sub for fx w delay heal
		S89.219D	Sltr-haris Type I physl fx upr end unsp fibula, sub for fx w rout heal
		S89.219G	Sltr-haris Type I physl fx upr end unsp fibula, sub for fx w delay heal
		S89.221D	Sltr-haris Type II physl fx upr end r fibula, sub for fx w rout heal
		S89.221G	Sltr-haris Type II physl fx upr end r fibula, sub for fx w delay heal
		S89.222D	Sltr-haris Type II physl fx upr end l fibula, sub for fx w rout heal
		S89.222G	Sltr-haris Type II physl fx upr end l fibula, sub for fx w delay heal
		S89.229D	Sltr-haris Type II physl fx upr end unsp fibula, sub for fx w rout heal
		S89.229G	Sltr-haris Type II physl fx upr end unsp fibula, sub for fx w delay heal
		S89.291D	Oth physl fx upper end of r fibula, subs for fx w routn heal
		S89.291G	Oth physl fx upper end of r fibula, subs for fx w delay heal
		S89.292D	Oth physl fx upper end of l fibula, subs for fx w routn heal
		S89.292G	Oth physl fx upper end of l fibula, subs for fx w delay heal
		S89.299D	Oth physl fx upper end unsp fibula, subs for fx w routn heal
		S89.299G	Oth physl fx upper end unsp fibula, subs for fx w delay heal
		S89.301D	Unsp physl fx lower end r fibula, subs for fx w routn heal
		S89.301G	Unsp physl fx lower end r fibula, subs for fx w delay heal
		S89.302D	Unsp physl fx lower end l fibula, subs for fx w routn heal
		S89.302G	Unsp physl fx lower end l fibula, subs for fx w delay heal
		S89.309D	Unsp physl fx low end unsp fibula, subs for fx w routn heal
		S89.309G	Unsp physl fx low end unsp fibula, subs for fx w delay heal
		S89.311D	Sltr-haris Type I physl fx low end r fibula, sub for fx w rout heal
		S89.311G	Sltr-haris Type I physl fx low end r fibula, sub for fx w delay heal
		S89.312D	Sltr-haris Type I physl fx low end l fibula, sub for fx w rout heal
		S89.312G	Sltr-haris Type I physl fx low end l fibula, sub for fx w delay heal
		S89.319D	Sltr-haris Type I physl fx low end unsp fibula, sub for fx w rout heal
		S89.319G	Sltr-haris Type I physl fx low end unsp fibula, sub for fx w delay heal
		S89.321D	Sltr-haris Type II physl fx low end r fibula, sub for fx w rout heal
		S89.321G	Sltr-haris Type II physl fx low end r fibula, sub for fx w delay heal
		S89.322D	Sltr-haris Type II physl fx low end l fibula, sub for fx w rout heal
	(Continued on next page)	**S89.322G**	Sltr-haris Type II physl fx low end l fibula, sub for fx w delay heal

ICD-9-CM		ICD-10-CM	
V54.16	AFTERCARE HEALING TRAUMATIC FRACTURE LOWER LEG **(Continued)**	**S89.329D**	Sltr-haris Type II physl fx low end unsp fibula, sub for fx w rout heal
		S89.329G	Sltr-haris Type II physl fx low end unsp fibula, sub for fx w delay heal
		S89.391D	Oth physl fx lower end of r fibula, subs for fx w routn heal
		S89.391G	Oth physl fx lower end of r fibula, subs for fx w delay heal
		S89.392D	Oth physl fx lower end of l fibula, subs for fx w routn heal
		S89.392G	Oth physl fx lower end of l fibula, subs for fx w delay heal
		S89.399D	Oth physl fx lower end unsp fibula, subs for fx w routn heal
		S89.399G	Oth physl fx lower end unsp fibula, subs for fx w delay heal
		S92.001D	Unsp fracture of right calcaneus, subs for fx w routn heal
		S92.001G	Unsp fracture of right calcaneus, subs for fx w delay heal
		S92.002D	Unsp fracture of left calcaneus, subs for fx w routn heal
		S92.002G	Unsp fracture of left calcaneus, subs for fx w delay heal
		S92.009D	Unsp fracture of unsp calcaneus, subs for fx w routn heal
		S92.009G	Unsp fracture of unsp calcaneus, subs for fx w delay heal
		S92.011D	Disp fx of body of right calcaneus, subs for fx w routn heal
		S92.011G	Disp fx of body of right calcaneus, subs for fx w delay heal
		S92.012D	Disp fx of body of left calcaneus, subs for fx w routn heal
		S92.012G	Disp fx of body of left calcaneus, subs for fx w delay heal
		S92.013D	Disp fx of body of unsp calcaneus, subs for fx w routn heal
		S92.013G	Disp fx of body of unsp calcaneus, subs for fx w delay heal
		S92.014D	Nondisp fx of body of r calcaneus, subs for fx w routn heal
		S92.014G	Nondisp fx of body of r calcaneus, subs for fx w delay heal
		S92.015D	Nondisp fx of body of l calcaneus, subs for fx w routn heal
		S92.015G	Nondisp fx of body of l calcaneus, subs for fx w delay heal
		S92.016D	Nondisp fx of body of unsp calcaneus, sub for fx w rout heal
		S92.016G	Nondisp fx of body of unsp calcaneus, sub for fx w delay heal
		S92.021D	Disp fx of ant pro of r calcaneus, subs for fx w routn heal
		S92.021G	Disp fx of ant pro of r calcaneus, subs for fx w delay heal
		S92.022D	Disp fx of ant pro of l calcaneus, subs for fx w routn heal
		S92.022G	Disp fx of ant pro of l calcaneus, subs for fx w delay heal
		S92.023D	Disp fx of ant pro of unsp calcaneus, sub for fx w rout heal
		S92.023G	Disp fx of ant pro of unsp calcaneus, sub for fx w delay heal
		S92.024D	Nondisp fx of ant pro of r calcaneus, sub for fx w rout heal
		S92.024G	Nondisp fx of ant pro of r calcaneus, sub for fx w delay heal
		S92.025D	Nondisp fx of ant pro of l calcaneus, sub for fx w rout heal
		S92.025G	Nondisp fx of ant pro of l calcaneus, sub for fx w delay heal
		S92.026D	Nondisp fx of ant pro of unsp calcaneus, sub for fx w rout heal
		S92.026G	Nondisp fx of ant pro of unsp calcaneus, sub for fx w delay heal
		S92.031D	Displ avuls fx tuberosity of r calcaneus, sub for fx w rout heal
		S92.031G	Displ avuls fx tuberosity of r calcaneus, sub for fx w delay heal
		S92.032D	Displ avuls fx tuberosity of l calcaneus, sub for fx w rout heal
		S92.032G	Displ avuls fx tuberosity of l calcaneus, sub for fx w delay heal
		S92.033D	Displ avuls fx tuberosity of unsp calcaneus, sub for fx w rout heal
		S92.033G	Displ avuls fx tuberosity of unsp calcaneus, sub for fx w delay heal
		S92.034D	Nondisp avuls fx tuberosity of r calcaneus, sub for fx w rout heal
		S92.034G	Nondisp avuls fx tuberosity of r calcaneus, sub for fx w delay heal
		S92.035D	Nondisp avuls fx tuberosity of l calcaneus, sub for fx w rout heal
		S92.035G	Nondisp avuls fx tuberosity of l calcaneus, sub for fx w delay heal
		S92.036D	Nondisp avuls fx tuberosity of unsp calcaneus, sub for fx w rout heal
		S92.036G	Nondisp avuls fx tuberosity of unsp calcaneus, sub for fx w delay heal
		S92.041D	Displ oth fx tuberosity of r calcaneus, sub for fx w rout heal
		S92.041G	Displ oth fx tuberosity of r calcaneus, sub for fx w delay heal
		S92.042D	Displ oth fx tuberosity of l calcaneus, sub for fx w rout heal
		S92.042G	Displ oth fx tuberosity of l calcaneus, sub for fx w delay heal
		S92.043D	Displ oth fx tuberosity of unsp calcaneus, sub for fx w rout heal
		S92.043G	Displ oth fx tuberosity of unsp calcaneus, sub for fx w delay heal
		S92.044D	Nondisp oth fx tuberosity of r calcaneus, sub for fx w rout heal
		S92.044G	Nondisp oth fx tuberosity of r calcaneus, sub for fx w delay heal
		S92.045D	Nondisp oth fx tuberosity of l calcaneus, sub for fx w rout heal
		S92.045G	Nondisp oth fx tuberosity of l calcaneus, sub for fx w delay heal
		S92.046D	Nondisp oth fx tuberosity of unsp calcaneus, sub for fx w rout heal
		S92.046G	Nondisp oth fx tuberosity of unsp calcaneus, sub for fx w delay heal
		S92.051D	Displ oth extrartic fx r calcaneus, subs for fx w routn heal
		S92.051G	Displ oth extrartic fx r calcaneus, subs for fx w delay heal
		S92.052D	Displ oth extrartic fx l calcaneus, subs for fx w routn heal
		S92.052G	Displ oth extrartic fx l calcaneus, subs for fx w delay heal
		S92.053D	Displ oth extrartic fx unsp calcaneus, sub for fx w rout heal
		S92.053G	Displ oth extrartic fx unsp calcaneus, sub for fx w delay heal
		S92.054D	Nondisp oth extrartic fx r calcaneus, sub for fx w rout heal
		S92.054G	Nondisp oth extrartic fx r calcaneus, sub for fx w delay heal
		S92.055D	Nondisp oth extrartic fx l calcaneus, sub for fx w rout heal
		S92.055G	Nondisp oth extrartic fx l calcaneus, sub for fx w delay heal
		S92.056D	Nondisp oth extrartic fx unsp calcaneus, sub for fx w rout heal
		S92.056G	Nondisp oth extrartic fx unsp calcaneus, sub for fx w delay heal
		S92.061D	Displaced intartic fx r calcaneus, subs for fx w routn heal
		S92.061G	Displaced intartic fx r calcaneus, subs for fx w delay heal
		S92.062D	Displaced intartic fx l calcaneus, subs for fx w routn heal
		S92.062G	Displaced intartic fx l calcaneus, subs for fx w delay heal
		S92.063D	Displ intartic fx unsp calcaneus, subs for fx w routn heal
		S92.063G	Displ intartic fx unsp calcaneus, subs for fx w delay heal
		S92.064D	Nondisp intartic fx r calcaneus, subs for fx w routn heal
		S92.064G	Nondisp intartic fx r calcaneus, subs for fx w delay heal
	(Continued on next page)	**S92.065D**	Nondisp intartic fx l calcaneus, subs for fx w routn heal

ICD-9-CM		ICD-10-CM	
V54.16	AFTERCARE HEALING TRAUMATIC FRACTURE LOWER LEG **(Continued)**	**S92.Ø65G**	Nondisp intartic fx l calcaneus, subs for fx w delay heal
		S92.Ø66D	Nondisp intartic fx unsp calcaneus, subs for fx w routn heal
		S92.Ø66G	Nondisp intartic fx unsp calcaneus, subs for fx w delay heal
		S92.1Ø1D	Unsp fracture of right talus, subs for fx w routn heal
		S92.1Ø1G	Unsp fracture of right talus, subs for fx w delay heal
		S92.1Ø2D	Unsp fracture of left talus, subs for fx w routn heal
		S92.1Ø2G	Unsp fracture of left talus, subs for fx w delay heal
		S92.1Ø9D	Unsp fracture of unsp talus, subs for fx w routn heal
		S92.1Ø9G	Unsp fracture of unsp talus, subs for fx w delay heal
		S92.111D	Disp fx of neck of right talus, subs for fx w routn heal
		S92.111G	Disp fx of neck of right talus, subs for fx w delay heal
		S92.112D	Disp fx of neck of left talus, subs for fx w routn heal
		S92.112G	Disp fx of neck of left talus, subs for fx w delay heal
		S92.113D	Disp fx of neck of unsp talus, subs for fx w routn heal
		S92.113G	Disp fx of neck of unsp talus, subs for fx w delay heal
		S92.114D	Nondisp fx of neck of right talus, subs for fx w routn heal
		S92.114G	Nondisp fx of neck of right talus, subs for fx w delay heal
		S92.115D	Nondisp fx of neck of left talus, subs for fx w routn heal
		S92.115G	Nondisp fx of neck of left talus, subs for fx w delay heal
		S92.116D	Nondisp fx of neck of unsp talus, subs for fx w routn heal
		S92.116G	Nondisp fx of neck of unsp talus, subs for fx w delay heal
		S92.121D	Disp fx of body of right talus, subs for fx w routn heal
		S92.121G	Disp fx of body of right talus, subs for fx w delay heal
		S92.122D	Disp fx of body of left talus, subs for fx w routn heal
		S92.122G	Disp fx of body of left talus, subs for fx w delay heal
		S92.123D	Disp fx of body of unsp talus, subs for fx w routn heal
		S92.123G	Disp fx of body of unsp talus, subs for fx w delay heal
		S92.124D	Nondisp fx of body of right talus, subs for fx w routn heal
		S92.124G	Nondisp fx of body of right talus, subs for fx w delay heal
		S92.125D	Nondisp fx of body of left talus, subs for fx w routn heal
		S92.125G	Nondisp fx of body of left talus, subs for fx w delay heal
		S92.126D	Nondisp fx of body of unsp talus, subs for fx w routn heal
		S92.126G	Nondisp fx of body of unsp talus, subs for fx w delay heal
		S92.131D	Disp fx of post pro of right talus, subs for fx w routn heal
		S92.131G	Disp fx of post pro of right talus, subs for fx w delay heal
		S92.132D	Disp fx of post pro of left talus, subs for fx w routn heal
		S92.132G	Disp fx of post pro of left talus, subs for fx w delay heal
		S92.133D	Disp fx of post pro of unsp talus, subs for fx w routn heal
		S92.133G	Disp fx of post pro of unsp talus, subs for fx w delay heal
		S92.134D	Nondisp fx of post pro of r talus, subs for fx w routn heal
		S92.134G	Nondisp fx of post pro of r talus, subs for fx w delay heal
		S92.135D	Nondisp fx of post pro of l talus, subs for fx w routn heal
		S92.135G	Nondisp fx of post pro of l talus, subs for fx w delay heal
		S92.136D	Nondisp fx of post pro of unsp talus, sub for fx w rout heal
		S92.136G	Nondisp fx of post pro of unsp talus, sub for fx w delay heal
		S92.141D	Displaced dome fx right talus, subs for fx w routn heal
		S92.141G	Displaced dome fx right talus, subs for fx w delay heal
		S92.142D	Displaced dome fx left talus, subs for fx w routn heal
		S92.142G	Displaced dome fx left talus, subs for fx w delay heal
		S92.143D	Displaced dome fx unsp talus, subs for fx w routn heal
		S92.143G	Displaced dome fx unsp talus, subs for fx w delay heal
		S92.144D	Nondisp dome fx right talus, subs for fx w routn heal
		S92.144G	Nondisp dome fx right talus, subs for fx w delay heal
		S92.145D	Nondisp dome fx left talus, subs for fx w routn heal
		S92.145G	Nondisp dome fx left talus, subs for fx w delay heal
		S92.146D	Nondisp dome fx unsp talus, subs for fx w routn heal
		S92.146G	Nondisp dome fx unsp talus, subs for fx w delay heal
		S92.151D	Displ avuls fx (chip fracture) of r talus, sub for fx w rout heal
		S92.151G	Displ avuls fx (chip fracture) of r talus, sub for fx w delay heal
		S92.152D	Displ avuls fx (chip fracture) of l talus, sub for fx w rout heal
		S92.152G	Displ avuls fx (chip fracture) of l talus, sub for fx w delay heal
		S92.153D	Displ avuls fx (chip fracture) of unsp talus, sub for fx w rout heal
		S92.153G	Displ avuls fx (chip fracture) of unsp talus, sub for fx w delay heal
		S92.154D	Nondisp avuls fx (chip fracture) of r talus, sub for fx w rout heal
		S92.154G	Nondisp avuls fx (chip fracture) of r talus, sub for fx w delay heal
		S92.155D	Nondisp avuls fx (chip fracture) of l talus, sub for fx w rout heal
		S92.155G	Nondisp avuls fx (chip fracture) of l talus, sub for fx w delay heal
		S92.156D	Nondisp avuls fx (chip fracture) of unsp talus, sub for fx w rout heal
		S92.156G	Nondisp avuls fx (chip fracture) of unsp talus, sub for fx w delay heal
		S92.191D	Oth fracture of right talus, subs for fx w routn heal
		S92.191G	Oth fracture of right talus, subs for fx w delay heal
		S92.192D	Oth fracture of left talus, subs for fx w routn heal
		S92.192G	Oth fracture of left talus, subs for fx w delay heal
		S92.199D	Oth fracture of unsp talus, subs for fx w routn heal
		S92.199G	Oth fracture of unsp talus, subs for fx w delay heal
		S92.2Ø1D	Fx unsp tarsal bone(s) of r foot, subs for fx w routn heal
		S92.2Ø1G	Fx unsp tarsal bone(s) of r foot, subs for fx w delay heal
		S92.2Ø2D	Fx unsp tarsal bone(s) of l foot, subs for fx w routn heal
		S92.2Ø2G	Fx unsp tarsal bone(s) of l foot, subs for fx w delay heal
		S92.2Ø9D	Fx unsp tarsal bone(s) of unsp ft, subs for fx w routn heal
		S92.2Ø9G	Fx unsp tarsal bone(s) of unsp ft, subs for fx w delay heal
		S92.211D	Disp fx of cuboid bone of r foot, subs for fx w routn heal
		S92.211G	Disp fx of cuboid bone of r foot, subs for fx w delay heal

(Continued on next page)

ICD-9-CM		ICD-10-CM	
V54.16	AFTERCARE HEALING TRAUMATIC FRACTURE LOWER LEG **(Continued)**	**S92.212D**	Disp fx of cuboid bone of l foot, subs for fx w routn heal
		S92.212G	Disp fx of cuboid bone of l foot, subs for fx w delay heal
		S92.213D	Disp fx of cuboid bone of unsp ft, subs for fx w routn heal
		S92.213G	Disp fx of cuboid bone of unsp ft, subs for fx w delay heal
		S92.214D	Nondisp fx of cuboid bone of r ft, subs for fx w routn heal
		S92.214G	Nondisp fx of cuboid bone of r ft, subs for fx w delay heal
		S92.215D	Nondisp fx of cuboid bone of l ft, subs for fx w routn heal
		S92.215G	Nondisp fx of cuboid bone of l ft, subs for fx w delay heal
		S92.216D	Nondisp fx of cuboid bone of unsp ft, sub for fx w rout heal
		S92.216G	Nondisp fx of cuboid bone of unsp ft, sub for fx w delay heal
		S92.221D	Disp fx of lateral cuneiform of r ft, sub for fx w rout heal
		S92.221G	Disp fx of lateral cuneiform of r ft, sub for fx w delay heal
		S92.222D	Disp fx of lateral cuneiform of l ft, sub for fx w rout heal
		S92.222G	Disp fx of lateral cuneiform of l ft, sub for fx w delay heal
		S92.223D	Disp fx of lateral cuneiform of unsp ft, sub for fx w rout heal
		S92.223G	Disp fx of lateral cuneiform of unsp ft, sub for fx w delay heal
		S92.224D	Nondisp fx of lateral cuneiform of r ft, sub for fx w rout heal
		S92.224G	Nondisp fx of lateral cuneiform of r ft, sub for fx w delay heal
		S92.225D	Nondisp fx of lateral cuneiform of l ft, sub for fx w rout heal
		S92.225G	Nondisp fx of lateral cuneiform of l ft, sub for fx w delay heal
		S92.226D	Nondisp fx of lateral cuneiform of unsp ft, sub for fx w rout heal
		S92.226G	Nondisp fx of lateral cuneiform of unsp ft, sub for fx w delay heal
		S92.231D	Disp fx of intermed cuneiform of r ft, sub for fx w rout heal
		S92.231G	Disp fx of intermed cuneiform of r ft, sub for fx w delay heal
		S92.232D	Disp fx of intermed cuneiform of l ft, sub for fx w rout heal
		S92.232G	Disp fx of intermed cuneiform of l ft, sub for fx w delay heal
		S92.233D	Disp fx of intermed cuneiform of unsp ft, sub for fx w rout heal
		S92.233G	Disp fx of intermed cuneiform of unsp ft, sub for fx w delay heal
		S92.234D	Nondisp fx of intermed cuneiform of r ft, sub for fx w rout heal
		S92.234G	Nondisp fx of intermed cuneiform of r ft, sub for fx w delay heal
		S92.235D	Nondisp fx of intermed cuneiform of l ft, sub for fx w rout heal
		S92.235G	Nondisp fx of intermed cuneiform of l ft, sub for fx w delay heal
		S92.236D	Nondisp fx of intermed cuneiform of unsp ft, sub for fx w rout heal
		S92.236G	Nondisp fx of intermed cuneiform of unsp ft, sub for fx w delay heal
		S92.241D	Disp fx of med cuneiform of r foot, subs for fx w routn heal
		S92.241G	Disp fx of med cuneiform of r foot, subs for fx w delay heal
		S92.242D	Disp fx of med cuneiform of l foot, subs for fx w routn heal
		S92.242G	Disp fx of med cuneiform of l foot, subs for fx w delay heal
		S92.243D	Disp fx of med cuneiform of unsp ft, sub for fx w rout heal
		S92.243G	Disp fx of med cuneiform of unsp ft, sub for fx w delay heal
		S92.244D	Nondisp fx of med cuneiform of r ft, sub for fx w rout heal
		S92.244G	Nondisp fx of med cuneiform of r ft, sub for fx w delay heal
		S92.245D	Nondisp fx of med cuneiform of l ft, sub for fx w rout heal
		S92.245G	Nondisp fx of med cuneiform of l ft, sub for fx w delay heal
		S92.246D	Nondisp fx of med cuneiform of unsp ft, sub for fx w rout heal
		S92.246G	Nondisp fx of med cuneiform of unsp ft, sub for fx w delay heal
		S92.251D	Disp fx of navicular of right foot, subs for fx w routn heal
		S92.251G	Disp fx of navicular of right foot, subs for fx w delay heal
		S92.252D	Disp fx of navicular of left foot, subs for fx w routn heal
		S92.252G	Disp fx of navicular of left foot, subs for fx w delay heal
		S92.253D	Disp fx of navicular of unsp foot, subs for fx w routn heal
		S92.253G	Disp fx of navicular of unsp foot, subs for fx w delay heal
		S92.254D	Nondisp fx of navicular of r foot, subs for fx w routn heal
		S92.254G	Nondisp fx of navicular of r foot, subs for fx w delay heal
		S92.255D	Nondisp fx of navicular of l foot, subs for fx w routn heal
		S92.255G	Nondisp fx of navicular of l foot, subs for fx w delay heal
		S92.256D	Nondisp fx of navic of unsp foot, subs for fx w routn heal
		S92.256G	Nondisp fx of navic of unsp foot, subs for fx w delay heal
		S92.3Ø1D	Fx unsp metatarsal bone(s), r foot, subs for fx w routn heal
		S92.3Ø1G	Fx unsp metatarsal bone(s), r foot, subs for fx w delay heal
		S92.3Ø2D	Fx unsp metatarsal bone(s), l foot, subs for fx w routn heal
		S92.3Ø2G	Fx unsp metatarsal bone(s), l foot, subs for fx w delay heal
		S92.3Ø9D	Fx unsp metatarsal bone(s), unsp ft, sub for fx w rout heal
		S92.3Ø9G	Fx unsp metatarsal bone(s), unsp ft, sub for fx w delay heal
		S92.311D	Disp fx of 1st metatarsal bone, r ft, sub for fx w rout heal
		S92.311G	Disp fx of 1st metatarsal bone, r ft, sub for fx w delay heal
		S92.312D	Disp fx of 1st metatarsal bone, l ft, sub for fx w rout heal
		S92.312G	Disp fx of 1st metatarsal bone, l ft, sub for fx w delay heal
		S92.313D	Disp fx of 1st metatarsal bone, unsp ft, sub for fx w rout heal
		S92.313G	Disp fx of 1st metatarsal bone, unsp ft, sub for fx w delay heal
		S92.314D	Nondisp fx of 1st metatarsal bone, r ft, sub for fx w rout heal
		S92.314G	Nondisp fx of 1st metatarsal bone, r ft, sub for fx w delay heal
		S92.315D	Nondisp fx of 1st metatarsal bone, l ft, sub for fx w rout heal
		S92.315G	Nondisp fx of 1st metatarsal bone, l ft, sub for fx w delay heal
		S92.316D	Nondisp fx of 1st metatarsal bone, unsp ft, sub for fx w rout heal
		S92.316G	Nondisp fx of 1st metatarsal bone, unsp ft, sub for fx w delay heal
		S92.321D	Disp fx of 2nd metatarsal bone, r ft, sub for fx w rout heal
		S92.321G	Disp fx of 2nd metatarsal bone, r ft, sub for fx w delay heal
		S92.322D	Disp fx of 2nd metatarsal bone, l ft, sub for fx w rout heal
		S92.322G	Disp fx of 2nd metatarsal bone, l ft, sub for fx w delay heal
		S92.323D	Disp fx of 2nd metatarsal bone, unsp ft, sub for fx w rout heal
		S92.323G	Disp fx of 2nd metatarsal bone, unsp ft, sub for fx w delay heal
	(Continued on next page)	**S92.324D**	Nondisp fx of 2nd metatarsal bone, r ft, sub for fx w rout heal

ICD-9-CM		ICD-10-CM	
V54.16	AFTERCARE HEALING TRAUMATIC FRACTURE LOWER LEG **(Continued)**	**S92.324G**	Nondisp fx of 2nd metatarsal bone, r ft, sub for fx w delay heal
		S92.325D	Nondisp fx of 2nd metatarsal bone, l ft, sub for fx w rout heal
		S92.325G	Nondisp fx of 2nd metatarsal bone, l ft, sub for fx w delay heal
		S92.326D	Nondisp fx of 2nd metatarsal bone, unsp ft, sub for fx w rout heal
		S92.326G	Nondisp fx of 2nd metatarsal bone, unsp ft, sub for fx w delay heal
		S92.331D	Disp fx of 3rd metatarsal bone, r ft, sub for fx w rout heal
		S92.331G	Disp fx of 3rd metatarsal bone, r ft, sub for fx w delay heal
		S92.332D	Disp fx of 3rd metatarsal bone, l ft, sub for fx w rout heal
		S92.332G	Disp fx of 3rd metatarsal bone, l ft, sub for fx w delay heal
		S92.333D	Disp fx of 3rd metatarsal bone, unsp ft, sub for fx w rout heal
		S92.333G	Disp fx of 3rd metatarsal bone, unsp ft, sub for fx w delay heal
		S92.334D	Nondisp fx of 3rd metatarsal bone, r ft, sub for fx w rout heal
		S92.334G	Nondisp fx of 3rd metatarsal bone, r ft, sub for fx w delay heal
		S92.335D	Nondisp fx of 3rd metatarsal bone, l ft, sub for fx w rout heal
		S92.335G	Nondisp fx of 3rd metatarsal bone, l ft, sub for fx w delay heal
		S92.336D	Nondisp fx of 3rd metatarsal bone, unsp ft, sub for fx w rout heal
		S92.336G	Nondisp fx of 3rd metatarsal bone, unsp ft, sub for fx w delay heal
		S92.341D	Disp fx of 4th metatarsal bone, r ft, sub for fx w rout heal
		S92.341G	Disp fx of 4th metatarsal bone, r ft, sub for fx w delay heal
		S92.342D	Disp fx of 4th metatarsal bone, l ft, sub for fx w rout heal
		S92.342G	Disp fx of 4th metatarsal bone, l ft, sub for fx w delay heal
		S92.343D	Disp fx of 4th metatarsal bone, unsp ft, sub for fx w rout heal
		S92.343G	Disp fx of 4th metatarsal bone, unsp ft, sub for fx w delay heal
		S92.344D	Nondisp fx of 4th metatarsal bone, r ft, sub for fx w rout heal
		S92.344G	Nondisp fx of 4th metatarsal bone, r ft, sub for fx w delay heal
		S92.345D	Nondisp fx of 4th metatarsal bone, l ft, sub for fx w rout heal
		S92.345G	Nondisp fx of 4th metatarsal bone, l ft, sub for fx w delay heal
		S92.346D	Nondisp fx of 4th metatarsal bone, unsp ft, sub for fx w rout heal
		S92.346G	Nondisp fx of 4th metatarsal bone, unsp ft, sub for fx w delay heal
		S92.351D	Disp fx of 5th metatarsal bone, r ft, sub for fx w rout heal
		S92.351G	Disp fx of 5th metatarsal bone, r ft, sub for fx w delay heal
		S92.352D	Disp fx of 5th metatarsal bone, l ft, sub for fx w rout heal
		S92.352G	Disp fx of 5th metatarsal bone, l ft, sub for fx w delay heal
		S92.353D	Disp fx of 5th metatarsal bone, unsp ft, sub for fx w rout heal
		S92.353G	Disp fx of 5th metatarsal bone, unsp ft, sub for fx w delay heal
		S92.354D	Nondisp fx of 5th metatarsal bone, r ft, sub for fx w rout heal
		S92.354G	Nondisp fx of 5th metatarsal bone, r ft, sub for fx w delay heal
		S92.355D	Nondisp fx of 5th metatarsal bone, l ft, sub for fx w rout heal
		S92.355G	Nondisp fx of 5th metatarsal bone, l ft, sub for fx w delay heal
		S92.356D	Nondisp fx of 5th metatarsal bone, unsp ft, sub for fx w rout heal
		S92.356G	Nondisp fx of 5th metatarsal bone, unsp ft, sub for fx w delay heal
		S92.401D	Displaced unsp fx right great toe, subs for fx w routn heal
		S92.401G	Displaced unsp fx right great toe, subs for fx w delay heal
		S92.402D	Displaced unsp fx left great toe, subs for fx w routn heal
		S92.402G	Displaced unsp fx left great toe, subs for fx w delay heal
		S92.403D	Displaced unsp fx unsp great toe, subs for fx w routn heal
		S92.403G	Displaced unsp fx unsp great toe, subs for fx w delay heal
		S92.404D	Nondisp unsp fx right great toe, subs for fx w routn heal
		S92.404G	Nondisp unsp fx right great toe, subs for fx w delay heal
		S92.405D	Nondisp unsp fx left great toe, subs for fx w routn heal
		S92.405G	Nondisp unsp fx left great toe, subs for fx w delay heal
		S92.406D	Nondisp unsp fx unsp great toe, subs for fx w routn heal
		S92.406G	Nondisp unsp fx unsp great toe, subs for fx w delay heal
		S92.411D	Disp fx of prox phalanx of r great toe, sub for fx w rout heal
		S92.411G	Disp fx of prox phalanx of r great toe, sub for fx w delay heal
		S92.412D	Disp fx of prox phalanx of l great toe, sub for fx w rout heal
		S92.412G	Disp fx of prox phalanx of l great toe, sub for fx w delay heal
		S92.413D	Disp fx of prox phalanx of unsp great toe, sub for fx w rout heal
		S92.413G	Disp fx of prox phalanx of unsp great toe, sub for fx w delay heal
		S92.414D	Nondisp fx of prox phalanx of r great toe, sub for fx w rout heal
		S92.414G	Nondisp fx of prox phalanx of r great toe, sub for fx w delay heal
		S92.415D	Nondisp fx of prox phalanx of l great toe, sub for fx w rout heal
		S92.415G	Nondisp fx of prox phalanx of l great toe, sub for fx w delay heal
		S92.416D	Nondisp fx of prox phalanx of unsp great toe, sub for fx w rout heal
		S92.416G	Nondisp fx of prox phalanx of unsp great toe, sub for fx w delay heal
		S92.421D	Disp fx of dist phalanx of r great toe, sub for fx w rout heal
		S92.421G	Disp fx of dist phalanx of r great toe, sub for fx w delay heal
		S92.422D	Disp fx of dist phalanx of l great toe, sub for fx w rout heal
		S92.422G	Disp fx of dist phalanx of l great toe, sub for fx w delay heal
		S92.423D	Disp fx of dist phalanx of unsp great toe, sub for fx w rout heal
		S92.423G	Disp fx of dist phalanx of unsp great toe, sub for fx w delay heal
		S92.424D	Nondisp fx of dist phalanx of r great toe, sub for fx w rout heal
		S92.424G	Nondisp fx of dist phalanx of r great toe, sub for fx w delay heal
		S92.425D	Nondisp fx of dist phalanx of l great toe, sub for fx w rout heal
		S92.425G	Nondisp fx of dist phalanx of l great toe, sub for fx w delay heal
		S92.426D	Nondisp fx of dist phalanx of unsp great toe, sub for fx w rout heal
		S92.426G	Nondisp fx of dist phalanx of unsp great toe, sub for fx w delay heal
		S92.491D	Oth fracture of right great toe, subs for fx w routn heal
		S92.491G	Oth fracture of right great toe, subs for fx w delay heal
		S92.492D	Oth fracture of left great toe, subs for fx w routn heal
		S92.492G	Oth fracture of left great toe, subs for fx w delay heal
		S92.499D	Oth fracture of unsp great toe, subs for fx w routn heal
	(Continued on next page)	**S92.499G**	Oth fracture of unsp great toe, subs for fx w delay heal

ICD-9-CM		ICD-10-CM	
V54.16	AFTERCARE HEALING TRAUMATIC FRACTURE LOWER LEG **(Continued)**	**S92.501D**	Displ unsp fx right lesser toe(s), subs for fx w routn heal
		S92.501G	Displ unsp fx right lesser toe(s), subs for fx w delay heal
		S92.502D	Displ unsp fx left lesser toe(s), subs for fx w routn heal
		S92.502G	Displ unsp fx left lesser toe(s), subs for fx w delay heal
		S92.503D	Displ unsp fx unsp lesser toe(s), subs for fx w routn heal
		S92.503G	Displ unsp fx unsp lesser toe(s), subs for fx w delay heal
		S92.504D	Nondisp unsp fx right less toe(s), subs for fx w routn heal
		S92.504G	Nondisp unsp fx right less toe(s), subs for fx w delay heal
		S92.505D	Nondisp unsp fx left lesser toe(s), subs for fx w routn heal
		S92.505G	Nondisp unsp fx left lesser toe(s), subs for fx w delay heal
		S92.506D	Nondisp unsp fx unsp lesser toe(s), subs for fx w routn heal
		S92.506G	Nondisp unsp fx unsp lesser toe(s), subs for fx w delay heal
		S92.511D	Disp fx of prox phalanx of r less toe(s), sub for fx w rout heal
		S92.511G	Disp fx of prox phalanx of r less toe(s), sub for fx w delay heal
		S92.512D	Disp fx of prox phalanx of l less toe(s), sub for fx w rout heal
		S92.512G	Disp fx of prox phalanx of l less toe(s), sub for fx w delay heal
		S92.513D	Disp fx of prox phalanx of unsp less toe(s), sub for fx w rout heal
		S92.513G	Disp fx of prox phalanx of unsp less toe(s), sub for fx w delay heal
		S92.514D	Nondisp fx of prox phalanx of r less toe(s), sub for fx w rout heal
		S92.514G	Nondisp fx of prox phalanx of r less toe(s), sub for fx w delay heal
		S92.515D	Nondisp fx of prox phalanx of l less toe(s), sub for fx w rout heal
		S92.515G	Nondisp fx of prox phalanx of l less toe(s), sub for fx w delay heal
		S92.516D	Nondisp fx of prox phalanx of unsp less toe(s), sub for fx w rout heal
		S92.516G	Nondisp fx of prox phalanx of unsp less toe(s), sub for fx w delay heal
		S92.521D	Disp fx of med phalanx of r less toe(s), sub for fx w rout heal
		S92.521G	Disp fx of med phalanx of r less toe(s), sub for fx w delay heal
		S92.522D	Disp fx of med phalanx of l less toe(s), sub for fx w rout heal
		S92.522G	Disp fx of med phalanx of l less toe(s), sub for fx w delay heal
		S92.523D	Disp fx of med phalanx of unsp less toe(s), sub for fx w rout heal
		S92.523G	Disp fx of med phalanx of unsp less toe(s), sub for fx w delay heal
		S92.524D	Nondisp fx of med phalanx of r less toe(s), sub for fx w rout heal
		S92.524G	Nondisp fx of med phalanx of r less toe(s), sub for fx w delay heal
		S92.525D	Nondisp fx of med phalanx of l less toe(s), sub for fx w rout heal
		S92.525G	Nondisp fx of med phalanx of l less toe(s), sub for fx w delay heal
		S92.526D	Nondisp fx of med phalanx of unsp less toe(s), sub for fx w rout heal
		S92.526G	Nondisp fx of med phalanx of unsp less toe(s), sub for fx w delay heal
		S92.531D	Disp fx of dist phalanx of r less toe(s), sub for fx w rout heal
		S92.531G	Disp fx of dist phalanx of r less toe(s), sub for fx w delay heal
		S92.532D	Disp fx of dist phalanx of l less toe(s), sub for fx w rout heal
		S92.532G	Disp fx of dist phalanx of l less toe(s), sub for fx w delay heal
		S92.533D	Disp fx of dist phalanx of unsp less toe(s), sub for fx w rout heal
		S92.533G	Disp fx of dist phalanx of unsp less toe(s), sub for fx w delay heal
		S92.534D	Nondisp fx of dist phalanx of r less toe(s), sub for fx w rout heal
		S92.534G	Nondisp fx of dist phalanx of r less toe(s), sub for fx w delay heal
		S92.535D	Nondisp fx of dist phalanx of l less toe(s), sub for fx w rout heal
		S92.535G	Nondisp fx of dist phalanx of l less toe(s), sub for fx w delay heal
		S92.536D	Nondisp fx of dist phalanx of unsp less toe(s), sub for fx w rout heal
		S92.536G	Nondisp fx of dist phalanx of unsp less toe(s), sub for fx w delay heal
		S92.591D	Oth fx right lesser toe(s), subs for fx w routn heal
		S92.591G	Oth fx right lesser toe(s), subs for fx w delay heal
		S92.592D	Oth fracture of left lesser toe(s), subs for fx w routn heal
		S92.592G	Oth fracture of left lesser toe(s), subs for fx w delay heal
		S92.599D	Oth fracture of unsp lesser toe(s), subs for fx w routn heal
		S92.599G	Oth fracture of unsp lesser toe(s), subs for fx w delay heal
		S92.901D	Unsp fracture of right foot, subs for fx w routn heal
		S92.901G	Unsp fracture of right foot, subs for fx w delay heal
		S92.902D	Unsp fracture of left foot, subs for fx w routn heal
		S92.902G	Unsp fracture of left foot, subs for fx w delay heal
		S92.909D	Unsp fracture of unsp foot, subs for fx w routn heal
		S92.909G	Unsp fracture of unsp foot, subs for fx w delay heal
		S92.911D	Unsp fracture of right toe(s), subs for fx w routn heal
		S92.911G	Unsp fracture of right toe(s), subs for fx w delay heal
		S92.912D	Unsp fracture of left toe(s), subs for fx w routn heal
		S92.912G	Unsp fracture of left toe(s), subs for fx w delay heal
		S92.919D	Unsp fracture of unsp toe(s), subs for fx w routn heal
		S92.919G	Unsp fracture of unsp toe(s), subs for fx w delay heal
V54.17	AFTERCARE HEALING TRAUMATIC FRACTURE VERTEBRAE	**S12.000D**	Unsp disp fx of first cervcal vert, subs for fx w routn heal
		S12.000G	Unsp disp fx of first cervcal vert, subs for fx w delay heal
		S12.001D	Unsp nondisp fx of 1st cervcal vert, sub for fx w rout heal
		S12.001G	Unsp nondisp fx of 1st cervcal vert, sub for fx w delay heal
		S12.01XD	Stable burst fx first cervcal vert, subs for fx w routn heal
		S12.01XG	Stable burst fx first cervcal vert, subs for fx w delay heal
		S12.02XD	Unstbl burst fx first cervcal vert, subs for fx w routn heal
		S12.02XG	Unstbl burst fx first cervcal vert, subs for fx w delay heal
		S12.030D	Displ post arch fx 1st cervcal vert, sub for fx w rout heal
		S12.030G	Displ post arch fx 1st cervcal vert, sub for fx w delay heal
		S12.031D	Nondisp post arch fx 1st cervcal vert, sub for fx w rout heal
		S12.031G	Nondisp post arch fx 1st cervcal vert, sub for fx w delay heal
		S12.040D	Displ lateral mass fx 1st cervcal vert, sub for fx w rout heal
		S12.040G	Displ lateral mass fx 1st cervcal vert, sub for fx w delay heal
		S12.041D	Nondisp lateral mass fx 1st cervcal vert, sub for fx w rout heal
		S12.041G	Nondisp lateral mass fx 1st cervcal vert, sub for fx w delay heal
	(Continued on next page)	**S12.090D**	Oth disp fx of first cervcal vert, subs for fx w routn heal

ICD-9-CM		ICD-10-CM	
V54.17	AFTERCARE HEALING TRAUMATIC FRACTURE VERTEBRAE **(Continued)**	**S12.090G**	Oth disp fx of first cervcal vert, subs for fx w delay heal
		S12.091D	Oth nondisp fx of 1st cervcal vert, subs for fx w routn heal
		S12.091G	Oth nondisp fx of 1st cervcal vert, subs for fx w delay heal
		S12.100D	Unsp disp fx of 2nd cervcal vert, subs for fx w routn heal
		S12.100G	Unsp disp fx of 2nd cervcal vert, subs for fx w delay heal
		S12.101D	Unsp nondisp fx of 2nd cervcal vert, sub for fx w rout heal
		S12.101G	Unsp nondisp fx of 2nd cervcal vert, sub for fx w delay heal
		S12.110D	Ant displ Type II dens fracture, subs for fx w routn heal
		S12.110G	Ant displ Type II dens fracture, subs for fx w delay heal
		S12.111D	Post displ Type II dens fracture, subs for fx w routn heal
		S12.111G	Post displ Type II dens fracture, subs for fx w delay heal
		S12.112D	Nondisplaced Type II dens fracture, subs for fx w routn heal
		S12.112G	Nondisplaced Type II dens fracture, subs for fx w delay heal
		S12.120D	Oth displaced dens fracture, subs for fx w routn heal
		S12.120G	Oth displaced dens fracture, subs for fx w delay heal
		S12.121D	Oth nondisplaced dens fracture, subs for fx w routn heal
		S12.121G	Oth nondisplaced dens fracture, subs for fx w delay heal
		S12.130D	Unsp traum displ spondylolysis of 2nd cervcal vert, sub for fx w rout heal
		S12.130G	Unsp traum displ spondylolysis of 2nd cervcal vert, sub for fx w delay heal
		S12.131D	Unsp traum nondisp spondylolysis of 2nd cervcal vert, sub for fx w rout heal
		S12.131G	Unsp traum nondisp spondylolysis of 2nd cervcal vert, sub for fx w delay heal
		S12.14XD	Type III traum spondylolysis of 2nd cervcal vert, sub for fx w rout heal
		S12.14XG	Type III traum spondylolysis of 2nd cervcal vert, sub for fx w delay heal
		S12.150D	Oth traum displ spondylolysis of 2nd cervcal vert, sub for fx w rout heal
		S12.150G	Oth traum displ spondylolysis of 2nd cervcal vert, sub for fx w delay heal
		S12.151D	Oth traum nondisp spondylolysis of 2nd cervcal vert, sub for fx w rout heal
		S12.151G	Oth traum nondisp spondylolysis of 2nd cervcal vert, sub for fx w delay heal
		S12.190D	Oth disp fx of second cervcal vert, subs for fx w routn heal
		S12.190G	Oth disp fx of second cervcal vert, subs for fx w delay heal
		S12.191D	Oth nondisp fx of 2nd cervcal vert, subs for fx w routn heal
		S12.191G	Oth nondisp fx of 2nd cervcal vert, subs for fx w delay heal
		S12.200D	Unsp disp fx of third cervcal vert, subs for fx w routn heal
		S12.200G	Unsp disp fx of third cervcal vert, subs for fx w delay heal
		S12.201D	Unsp nondisp fx of 3rd cervcal vert, sub for fx w rout heal
		S12.201G	Unsp nondisp fx of 3rd cervcal vert, sub for fx w delay heal
		S12.230D	Unsp traum displ spondylolysis of 3rd cervcal vert, sub for fx w rout heal
		S12.230G	Unsp traum displ spondylolysis of 3rd cervcal vert, sub for fx w delay heal
		S12.231D	Unsp traum nondisp spondylolysis of 3rd cervcal vert, sub for fx w rout heal
		S12.231G	Unsp traum nondisp spondylolysis of 3rd cervcal vert, sub for fx w delay heal
		S12.24XD	Type III traum spondylolysis of 3rd cervcal vert, sub for fx w rout heal
		S12.24XG	Type III traum spondylolysis of 3rd cervcal vert, sub for fx w delay heal
		S12.250D	Oth traum displ spondylolysis of 3rd cervcal vert, sub for fx w rout heal
		S12.250G	Oth traum displ spondylolysis of 3rd cervcal vert, sub for fx w delay heal
		S12.251D	Oth traum nondisp spondylolysis of 3rd cervcal vert, sub for fx w rout heal
		S12.251G	Oth traum nondisp spondylolysis of 3rd cervcal vert, sub for fx w delay heal
		S12.290D	Oth disp fx of third cervcal vert, subs for fx w routn heal
		S12.290G	Oth disp fx of third cervcal vert, subs for fx w delay heal
		S12.291D	Oth nondisp fx of 3rd cervcal vert, subs for fx w routn heal
		S12.291G	Oth nondisp fx of 3rd cervcal vert, subs for fx w delay heal
		S12.300D	Unsp disp fx of 4th cervcal vert, subs for fx w routn heal
		S12.300G	Unsp disp fx of 4th cervcal vert, subs for fx w delay heal
		S12.301D	Unsp nondisp fx of 4th cervcal vert, sub for fx w rout heal
		S12.301G	Unsp nondisp fx of 4th cervcal vert, sub for fx w delay heal
		S12.330D	Unsp traum displ spondylolysis of 4th cervcal vert, sub for fx w rout heal
		S12.330G	Unsp traum displ spondylolysis of 4th cervcal vert, sub for fx w delay heal
		S12.331D	Unsp traum nondisp spondylolysis of 4th cervcal vert, sub for fx w rout heal
		S12.331G	Unsp traum nondisp spondylolysis of 4th cervcal vert, sub for fx w delay heal
		S12.34XD	Type III traum spondylolysis of 4th cervcal vert, sub for fx w rout heal
		S12.34XG	Type III traum spondylolysis of 4th cervcal vert, sub for fx w delay heal
		S12.350D	Oth traum displ spondylolysis of 4th cervcal vert, sub for fx w rout heal
		S12.350G	Oth traum displ spondylolysis of 4th cervcal vert, sub for fx w delay heal
		S12.351D	Oth traum nondisp spondylolysis of 4th cervcal vert, sub for fx w rout heal
		S12.351G	Oth traum nondisp spondylolysis of 4th cervcal vert, sub for fx w delay heal
		S12.390D	Oth disp fx of fourth cervcal vert, subs for fx w routn heal
		S12.390G	Oth disp fx of fourth cervcal vert, subs for fx w delay heal
		S12.391D	Oth nondisp fx of 4th cervcal vert, subs for fx w routn heal
		S12.391G	Oth nondisp fx of 4th cervcal vert, subs for fx w delay heal
		S12.400D	Unsp disp fx of fifth cervcal vert, subs for fx w routn heal
		S12.400G	Unsp disp fx of fifth cervcal vert, subs for fx w delay heal
		S12.401D	Unsp nondisp fx of 5th cervcal vert, sub for fx w rout heal
		S12.401G	Unsp nondisp fx of 5th cervcal vert, sub for fx w delay heal
		S12.430D	Unsp traum displ spondylolysis of 5th cervcal vert, sub for fx w rout heal
		S12.430G	Unsp traum displ spondylolysis of 5th cervcal vert, sub for fx w delay heal
		S12.431D	Unsp traum nondisp spondylolysis of 5th cervcal vert, sub for fx w rout heal
		S12.431G	Unsp traum nondisp spondylolysis of 5th cervcal vert, sub for fx w delay heal
		S12.44XD	Type III traum spondylolysis of 5th cervcal vert, sub for fx w rout heal
		S12.44XG	Type III traum spondylolysis of 5th cervcal vert, sub for fx w delay heal
		S12.450D	Oth traum displ spondylolysis of 5th cervcal vert, sub for fx w rout heal
		S12.450G	Oth traum displ spondylolysis of 5th cervcal vert, sub for fx w delay heal
		S12.451D	Oth traum nondisp spondylolysis of 5th cervcal vert, sub for fx w rout heal
		S12.451G	Oth traum nondisp spondylolysis of 5th cervcal vert, sub for fx w delay heal
		S12.490D	Oth disp fx of fifth cervcal vert, subs for fx w routn heal
	(Continued on next page)	**S12.490G**	Oth disp fx of fifth cervcal vert, subs for fx w delay heal

ICD-9-CM		ICD-10-CM	
V54.17	AFTERCARE HEALING TRAUMATIC FRACTURE VERTEBRAE **(Continued)**	**S12.491D**	Oth nondisp fx of 5th cervcal vert, subs for fx w routn heal
		S12.491G	Oth nondisp fx of 5th cervcal vert, subs for fx w delay heal
		S12.500D	Unsp disp fx of sixth cervcal vert, subs for fx w routn heal
		S12.500G	Unsp disp fx of sixth cervcal vert, subs for fx w delay heal
		S12.501D	Unsp nondisp fx of sixth cervcal vert, sub for fx w rout heal
		S12.501G	Unsp nondisp fx of sixth cervcal vert, sub for fx w delay heal
		S12.530D	Unsp traum displ spondylolysis of sixth cervcal vert, sub for fx w rout heal
		S12.530G	Unsp traum displ spondylolysis of sixth cervcal vert, sub for fx w delay heal
		S12.531D	Unsp traum nondisp spondylolysis of sixth cervcal vert, sub for fx w rout heal
		S12.531G	Unsp traum nondisp spondylolysis of sixth cervcal vert, sub for fx w del heal
		S12.54XD	Type III traum spondylolysis of sixth cervcal vert, sub for fx w rout heal
		S12.54XG	Type III traum spondylolysis of sixth cervcal vert, sub for fx w delay heal
		S12.550D	Oth traum displ spondylolysis of sixth cervcal vert, sub for fx w rout heal
		S12.550G	Oth traum displ spondylolysis of sixth cervcal vert, sub for fx w delay heal
		S12.551D	Oth traum nondisp spondylolysis of sixth cervcal vert, sub for fx w rout heal
		S12.551G	Oth traum nondisp spondylolysis of sixth cervcal vert, sub for fx w delay heal
		S12.590D	Oth disp fx of sixth cervcal vert, subs for fx w routn heal
		S12.590G	Oth disp fx of sixth cervcal vert, subs for fx w delay heal
		S12.591D	Oth nondisp fx of sixth cervcal vert, sub for fx w rout heal
		S12.591G	Oth nondisp fx of sixth cervcal vert, sub for fx w delay heal
		S12.600D	Unsp disp fx of 7th cervcal vert, subs for fx w routn heal
		S12.600G	Unsp disp fx of 7th cervcal vert, subs for fx w delay heal
		S12.601D	Unsp nondisp fx of 7th cervcal vert, sub for fx w rout heal
		S12.601G	Unsp nondisp fx of 7th cervcal vert, sub for fx w delay heal
		S12.630D	Unsp traum displ spondylolysis of 7th cervcal vert, sub for fx w rout heal
		S12.630G	Unsp traum displ spondylolysis of 7th cervcal vert, sub for fx w delay heal
		S12.631D	Unsp traum nondisp spondylolysis of 7th cervcal vert, sub for fx w rout heal
		S12.631G	Unsp traum nondisp spondylolysis of 7th cervcal vert, sub for fx w delay heal
		S12.64XD	Type III traum spondylolysis of 7th cervcal vert, sub for fx w rout heal
		S12.64XG	Type III traum spondylolysis of 7th cervcal vert, sub for fx w delay heal
		S12.650D	Oth traum displ spondylolysis of 7th cervcal vert, sub for fx w rout heal
		S12.650G	Oth traum displ spondylolysis of 7th cervcal vert, sub for fx w delay heal
		S12.651D	Oth traum nondisp spondylolysis of 7th cervcal vert, sub for fx w rout heal
		S12.651G	Oth traum nondisp spondylolysis of 7th cervcal vert, sub for fx w delay heal
		S12.690D	Oth disp fx of 7th cervcal vert, subs for fx w routn heal
		S12.690G	Oth disp fx of 7th cervcal vert, subs for fx w delay heal
		S12.691D	Oth nondisp fx of 7th cervcal vert, subs for fx w routn heal
		S12.691G	Oth nondisp fx of 7th cervcal vert, subs for fx w delay heal
		S12.9XXD	Fracture of neck, unspecified, subsequent encounter
		S22.000D	Wedge comprsn fx unsp thor vert, subs for fx w routn heal
		S22.000G	Wedge comprsn fx unsp thor vert, subs for fx w delay heal
		S22.001D	Stable burst fx unsp thor vertebra, subs for fx w routn heal
		S22.001G	Stable burst fx unsp thor vertebra, subs for fx w delay heal
		S22.002D	Unstbl burst fx unsp thor vertebra, subs for fx w routn heal
		S22.002G	Unstbl burst fx unsp thor vertebra, subs for fx w delay heal
		S22.008D	Oth fracture of unsp thor vertebra, subs for fx w routn heal
		S22.008G	Oth fracture of unsp thor vertebra, subs for fx w delay heal
		S22.009D	Unsp fx unsp thor vertebra, subs for fx w routn heal
		S22.009G	Unsp fx unsp thor vertebra, subs for fx w delay heal
		S22.010D	Wedge comprsn fx first thor vert, subs for fx w routn heal
		S22.010G	Wedge comprsn fx first thor vert, subs for fx w delay heal
		S22.011D	Stable burst fx first thor vert, subs for fx w routn heal
		S22.011G	Stable burst fx first thor vert, subs for fx w delay heal
		S22.012D	Unstbl burst fx first thor vert, subs for fx w routn heal
		S22.012G	Unstbl burst fx first thor vert, subs for fx w delay heal
		S22.018D	Oth fx first thor vertebra, subs for fx w routn heal
		S22.018G	Oth fx first thor vertebra, subs for fx w delay heal
		S22.019D	Unsp fx first thor vertebra, subs for fx w routn heal
		S22.019G	Unsp fx first thor vertebra, subs for fx w delay heal
		S22.020D	Wedge comprsn fx second thor vert, subs for fx w routn heal
		S22.020G	Wedge comprsn fx second thor vert, subs for fx w delay heal
		S22.021D	Stable burst fx second thor vert, subs for fx w routn heal
		S22.021G	Stable burst fx second thor vert, subs for fx w delay heal
		S22.022D	Unstbl burst fx second thor vert, subs for fx w routn heal
		S22.022G	Unstbl burst fx second thor vert, subs for fx w delay heal
		S22.028D	Oth fx second thor vertebra, subs for fx w routn heal
		S22.028G	Oth fx second thor vertebra, subs for fx w delay heal
		S22.029D	Unsp fx second thor vertebra, subs for fx w routn heal
		S22.029G	Unsp fx second thor vertebra, subs for fx w delay heal
		S22.030D	Wedge comprsn fx third thor vert, subs for fx w routn heal
		S22.030G	Wedge comprsn fx third thor vert, subs for fx w delay heal
		S22.031D	Stable burst fx third thor vert, subs for fx w routn heal
		S22.031G	Stable burst fx third thor vert, subs for fx w delay heal
		S22.032D	Unstbl burst fx third thor vert, subs for fx w routn heal
		S22.032G	Unstbl burst fx third thor vert, subs for fx w delay heal
		S22.038D	Oth fx third thor vertebra, subs for fx w routn heal
		S22.038G	Oth fx third thor vertebra, subs for fx w delay heal
		S22.039D	Unsp fx third thor vertebra, subs for fx w routn heal
		S22.039G	Unsp fx third thor vertebra, subs for fx w delay heal
		S22.040D	Wedge comprsn fx fourth thor vert, subs for fx w routn heal
		S22.040G	Wedge comprsn fx fourth thor vert, subs for fx w delay heal
		S22.041D	Stable burst fx fourth thor vert, subs for fx w routn heal
	(Continued on next page)	**S22.041G**	Stable burst fx fourth thor vert, subs for fx w delay heal

ICD-9-CM		ICD-10-CM	
V54.17	AFTERCARE HEALING TRAUMATIC FRACTURE VERTEBRAE **(Continued)**	**S22.Ø42D**	Unstbl burst fx fourth thor vert, subs for fx w routn heal
		S22.Ø42G	Unstbl burst fx fourth thor vert, subs for fx w delay heal
		S22.Ø48D	Oth fx fourth thor vertebra, subs for fx w routn heal
		S22.Ø48G	Oth fx fourth thor vertebra, subs for fx w delay heal
		S22.Ø49D	Unsp fx fourth thor vertebra, subs for fx w routn heal
		S22.Ø49G	Unsp fx fourth thor vertebra, subs for fx w delay heal
		S22.Ø5ØD	Wedge comprsn fx T5-T6 vertebra, subs for fx w routn heal
		S22.Ø5ØG	Wedge comprsn fx T5-T6 vertebra, subs for fx w delay heal
		S22.Ø51D	Stable burst fx T5-T6 vertebra, subs for fx w routn heal
		S22.Ø51G	Stable burst fx T5-T6 vertebra, subs for fx w delay heal
		S22.Ø52D	Unstable burst fx T5-T6 vertebra, subs for fx w routn heal
		S22.Ø52G	Unstable burst fx T5-T6 vertebra, subs for fx w delay heal
		S22.Ø58D	Oth fracture of T5-T6 vertebra, subs for fx w routn heal
		S22.Ø58G	Oth fracture of T5-T6 vertebra, subs for fx w delay heal
		S22.Ø59D	Unsp fracture of T5-T6 vertebra, subs for fx w routn heal
		S22.Ø59G	Unsp fracture of T5-T6 vertebra, subs for fx w delay heal
		S22.Ø6ØD	Wedge comprsn fx T7-T8 vertebra, subs for fx w routn heal
		S22.Ø6ØG	Wedge comprsn fx T7-T8 vertebra, subs for fx w delay heal
		S22.Ø61D	Stable burst fx T7-T8 vertebra, subs for fx w routn heal
		S22.Ø61G	Stable burst fx T7-T8 vertebra, subs for fx w delay heal
		S22.Ø62D	Unstable burst fx T7-T8 vertebra, subs for fx w routn heal
		S22.Ø62G	Unstable burst fx T7-T8 vertebra, subs for fx w delay heal
		S22.Ø68D	Oth fx T7-T8 thor vertebra, subs for fx w routn heal
		S22.Ø68G	Oth fx T7-T8 thor vertebra, subs for fx w delay heal
		S22.Ø69D	Unsp fracture of T7-T8 vertebra, subs for fx w routn heal
		S22.Ø69G	Unsp fracture of T7-T8 vertebra, subs for fx w delay heal
		S22.Ø7ØD	Wedge comprsn fx T9-T10 vertebra, subs for fx w routn heal
		S22.Ø7ØG	Wedge comprsn fx T9-T10 vertebra, subs for fx w delay heal
		S22.Ø71D	Stable burst fx T9-T10 vertebra, subs for fx w routn heal
		S22.Ø71G	Stable burst fx T9-T10 vertebra, subs for fx w delay heal
		S22.Ø72D	Unstable burst fx T9-T10 vertebra, subs for fx w routn heal
		S22.Ø72G	Unstable burst fx T9-T10 vertebra, subs for fx w delay heal
		S22.Ø78D	Oth fracture of T9-T10 vertebra, subs for fx w routn heal
		S22.Ø78G	Oth fracture of T9-T10 vertebra, subs for fx w delay heal
		S22.Ø79D	Unsp fracture of T9-T10 vertebra, subs for fx w routn heal
		S22.Ø79G	Unsp fracture of T9-T10 vertebra, subs for fx w delay heal
		S22.Ø8ØD	Wedge comprsn fx T11-T12 vertebra, subs for fx w routn heal
		S22.Ø8ØG	Wedge comprsn fx T11-T12 vertebra, subs for fx w delay heal
		S22.Ø81D	Stable burst fx T11-T12 vertebra, subs for fx w routn heal
		S22.Ø81G	Stable burst fx T11-T12 vertebra, subs for fx w delay heal
		S22.Ø82D	Unstable burst fx T11-T12 vertebra, subs for fx w routn heal
		S22.Ø82G	Unstable burst fx T11-T12 vertebra, subs for fx w delay heal
		S22.Ø88D	Oth fracture of T11-T12 vertebra, subs for fx w routn heal
		S22.Ø88G	Oth fracture of T11-T12 vertebra, subs for fx w delay heal
		S22.Ø89D	Unsp fracture of T11-T12 vertebra, subs for fx w routn heal
		S22.Ø89G	Unsp fracture of T11-T12 vertebra, subs for fx w delay heal
		S32.ØØØD	Wedge comprsn fx unsp lum vertebra, subs for fx w routn heal
		S32.ØØØG	Wedge comprsn fx unsp lum vertebra, subs for fx w delay heal
		S32.ØØ1D	Stable burst fx unsp lum vertebra, subs for fx w routn heal
		S32.ØØ1G	Stable burst fx unsp lum vertebra, subs for fx w delay heal
		S32.ØØ2D	Unstbl burst fx unsp lum vertebra, subs for fx w routn heal
		S32.ØØ2G	Unstbl burst fx unsp lum vertebra, subs for fx w delay heal
		S32.ØØ8D	Oth fracture of unsp lum vertebra, subs for fx w routn heal
		S32.ØØ8G	Oth fracture of unsp lum vertebra, subs for fx w delay heal
		S32.ØØ9D	Unsp fracture of unsp lum vertebra, subs for fx w routn heal
		S32.ØØ9G	Unsp fracture of unsp lum vertebra, subs for fx w delay heal
		S32.Ø1ØD	Wedge comprsn fx first lum vert, subs for fx w routn heal
		S32.Ø1ØG	Wedge comprsn fx first lum vert, subs for fx w delay heal
		S32.Ø11D	Stable burst fx first lum vertebra, subs for fx w routn heal
		S32.Ø11G	Stable burst fx first lum vertebra, subs for fx w delay heal
		S32.Ø12D	Unstbl burst fx first lum vertebra, subs for fx w routn heal
		S32.Ø12G	Unstbl burst fx first lum vertebra, subs for fx w delay heal
		S32.Ø18D	Oth fracture of first lum vertebra, subs for fx w routn heal
		S32.Ø18G	Oth fracture of first lum vertebra, subs for fx w delay heal
		S32.Ø19D	Unsp fx first lum vertebra, subs for fx w routn heal
		S32.Ø19G	Unsp fx first lum vertebra, subs for fx w delay heal
		S32.Ø2ØD	Wedge comprsn fx second lum vert, subs for fx w routn heal
		S32.Ø2ØG	Wedge comprsn fx second lum vert, subs for fx w delay heal
		S32.Ø21D	Stable burst fx second lum vert, subs for fx w routn heal
		S32.Ø21G	Stable burst fx second lum vert, subs for fx w delay heal
		S32.Ø22D	Unstbl burst fx second lum vert, subs for fx w routn heal
		S32.Ø22G	Unstbl burst fx second lum vert, subs for fx w delay heal
		S32.Ø28D	Oth fx second lum vertebra, subs for fx w routn heal
		S32.Ø28G	Oth fx second lum vertebra, subs for fx w delay heal
		S32.Ø29D	Unsp fx second lum vertebra, subs for fx w routn heal
		S32.Ø29G	Unsp fx second lum vertebra, subs for fx w delay heal
		S32.Ø3ØD	Wedge comprsn fx third lum vert, subs for fx w routn heal
		S32.Ø3ØG	Wedge comprsn fx third lum vert, subs for fx w delay heal
		S32.Ø31D	Stable burst fx third lum vertebra, subs for fx w routn heal
		S32.Ø31G	Stable burst fx third lum vertebra, subs for fx w delay heal
		S32.Ø32D	Unstbl burst fx third lum vertebra, subs for fx w routn heal
		S32.Ø32G	Unstbl burst fx third lum vertebra, subs for fx w delay heal

(Continued on next page)

ICD-9-CM		ICD-10-CM	
V54.17	AFTERCARE HEALING TRAUMATIC FRACTURE VERTEBRAE **(Continued)**	**S32.038D**	Oth fracture of third lum vertebra, subs for fx w routn heal
		S32.038G	Oth fracture of third lum vertebra, subs for fx w delay heal
		S32.039D	Unsp fx third lum vertebra, subs for fx w routn heal
		S32.039G	Unsp fx third lum vertebra, subs for fx w delay heal
		S32.040D	Wedge comprsn fx fourth lum vert, subs for fx w routn heal
		S32.040G	Wedge comprsn fx fourth lum vert, subs for fx w delay heal
		S32.041D	Stable burst fx fourth lum vert, subs for fx w routn heal
		S32.041G	Stable burst fx fourth lum vert, subs for fx w delay heal
		S32.042D	Unstbl burst fx fourth lum vert, subs for fx w routn heal
		S32.042G	Unstbl burst fx fourth lum vert, subs for fx w delay heal
		S32.048D	Oth fx fourth lum vertebra, subs for fx w routn heal
		S32.048G	Oth fx fourth lum vertebra, subs for fx w delay heal
		S32.049D	Unsp fx fourth lum vertebra, subs for fx w routn heal
		S32.049G	Unsp fx fourth lum vertebra, subs for fx w delay heal
		S32.050D	Wedge comprsn fx fifth lum vert, subs for fx w routn heal
		S32.050G	Wedge comprsn fx fifth lum vert, subs for fx w delay heal
		S32.051D	Stable burst fx fifth lum vertebra, subs for fx w routn heal
		S32.051G	Stable burst fx fifth lum vertebra, subs for fx w delay heal
		S32.052D	Unstbl burst fx fifth lum vertebra, subs for fx w routn heal
		S32.052G	Unstbl burst fx fifth lum vertebra, subs for fx w delay heal
		S32.058D	Oth fracture of fifth lum vertebra, subs for fx w routn heal
		S32.058G	Oth fracture of fifth lum vertebra, subs for fx w delay heal
		S32.059D	Unsp fx fifth lum vertebra, subs for fx w routn heal
		S32.059G	Unsp fx fifth lum vertebra, subs for fx w delay heal
V54.19	AFTERCARE HEALING TRAUMATIC FRACTURE OTHER BONE	**S02.0XXD**	Fracture of vault of skull, subs for fx w routn heal
		S02.0XXG	Fracture of vault of skull, subs for fx w delay heal
		S02.10XD	Unsp fracture of base of skull, subs for fx w routn heal
		S02.10XG	Unsp fracture of base of skull, subs for fx w delay heal
		S02.110D	Type I occipital condyle fracture, subs for fx w routn heal
		S02.110G	Type I occipital condyle fracture, subs for fx w delay heal
		S02.111D	Type II occipital condyle fracture, subs for fx w routn heal
		S02.111G	Type II occipital condyle fracture, subs for fx w delay heal
		S02.112D	Type III occipital condyle fx, subs for fx w routn heal
		S02.112G	Type III occipital condyle fx, subs for fx w delay heal
		S02.113D	Unsp occipital condyle fracture, subs for fx w routn heal
		S02.113G	Unsp occipital condyle fracture, subs for fx w delay heal
		S02.118D	Oth fracture of occiput, subs for fx w routn heal
		S02.118G	Oth fracture of occiput, subs for fx w delay heal
		S02.119D	Unsp fracture of occiput, subs for fx w routn heal
		S02.119G	Unsp fracture of occiput, subs for fx w delay heal
		S02.19XD	Oth fracture of base of skull, subs for fx w routn heal
		S02.19XG	Oth fracture of base of skull, subs for fx w delay heal
		S02.2XXD	Fracture of nasal bones, subs for fx w routn heal
		S02.2XXG	Fracture of nasal bones, subs for fx w delay heal
		S02.3XXD	Fracture of orbital floor, subs for fx w routn heal
		S02.3XXG	Fracture of orbital floor, subs for fx w delay heal
		S02.400D	Malar fracture unsp, subs for fx w routn heal
		S02.400G	Malar fracture unsp, subs for fx w delay heal
		S02.401D	Maxillary fracture, unsp, subs for fx w routn heal
		S02.401G	Maxillary fracture, unsp, subs for fx w delay heal
		S02.402D	Zygomatic fracture, unsp, subs for fx w routn heal
		S02.402G	Zygomatic fracture, unsp, subs for fx w delay heal
		S02.411D	LeFort I fracture, subs for fx w routn heal
		S02.411G	LeFort I fracture, subs for fx w delay heal
		S02.412D	LeFort II fracture, subs for fx w routn heal
		S02.412G	LeFort II fracture, subs for fx w delay heal
		S02.413D	LeFort III fracture, subs for fx w routn heal
		S02.413G	LeFort III fracture, subs for fx w delay heal
		S02.42XD	Fracture of alveolus of maxilla, subs for fx w routn heal
		S02.42XG	Fracture of alveolus of maxilla, subs for fx w delay heal
		S02.5XXD	Fracture of tooth (traumatic), subs for fx w routn heal
		S02.5XXG	Fracture of tooth (traumatic), subs for fx w delay heal
		S02.600D	Fx unsp part of body of mandible, subs for fx w routn heal
		S02.600G	Fx unsp part of body of mandible, subs for fx w delay heal
		S02.609D	Fracture of mandible, unsp, subs for fx w routn heal
		S02.609G	Fracture of mandible, unsp, subs for fx w delay heal
		S02.61XD	Fx condylar process of mandible, subs for fx w routn heal
		S02.61XG	Fx condylar process of mandible, subs for fx w delay heal
		S02.62XD	Fx subcondylar process of mandible, subs for fx w routn heal
		S02.62XG	Fx subcondylar process of mandible, subs for fx w delay heal
		S02.63XD	Fx coronoid process of mandible, subs for fx w routn heal
		S02.63XG	Fx coronoid process of mandible, subs for fx w delay heal
		S02.64XD	Fracture of ramus of mandible, subs for fx w routn heal
		S02.64XG	Fracture of ramus of mandible, subs for fx w delay heal
		S02.65XD	Fracture of angle of mandible, subs for fx w routn heal
		S02.65XG	Fracture of angle of mandible, subs for fx w delay heal
		S02.66XD	Fracture of symphysis of mandible, subs for fx w routn heal
		S02.66XG	Fracture of symphysis of mandible, subs for fx w delay heal
		S02.67XD	Fracture of alveolus of mandible, subs for fx w routn heal
		S02.67XG	Fracture of alveolus of mandible, subs for fx w delay heal
		S02.69XD	Fracture of mandible of oth site, subs for fx w routn heal
		S02.69XG	Fracture of mandible of oth site, subs for fx w delay heal
	(Continued on next page)	**S02.8XXD**	Fx of skull and facial bones, subs for fx w routn heal

ICD-9-CM		ICD-10-CM	
V54.19	AFTERCARE HEALING TRAUMATIC FRACTURE OTHER BONE **(Continued)**	**SØ2.8XXG**	Fx of skull and facial bones, subs for fx w delay heal
		SØ2.91XD	Unsp fracture of skull, subs for fx w routn heal
		SØ2.91XG	Unsp fracture of skull, subs for fx w delay heal
		SØ2.92XD	Unsp fracture of facial bones, subs for fx w routn heal
		SØ2.92XG	Unsp fracture of facial bones, subs for fx w delay heal
		S12.8XXD	Fracture of other parts of neck, subsequent encounter
		S22.2ØXD	Unsp fracture of sternum, subs for fx w routn heal
		S22.2ØXG	Unsp fracture of sternum, subs for fx w delay heal
		S22.21XD	Fracture of manubrium, subs for fx w routn heal
		S22.21XG	Fracture of manubrium, subs for fx w delay heal
		S22.22XD	Fracture of body of sternum, subs for fx w routn heal
		S22.22XG	Fracture of body of sternum, subs for fx w delay heal
		S22.23XD	Sternal manubrial dissociation, subs for fx w routn heal
		S22.23XG	Sternal manubrial dissociation, subs for fx w delay heal
		S22.24XD	Fracture of xiphoid process, subs for fx w routn heal
		S22.24XG	Fracture of xiphoid process, subs for fx w delay heal
		S22.31XD	Fracture of one rib, right side, subs for fx w routn heal
		S22.31XG	Fracture of one rib, right side, subs for fx w delay heal
		S22.32XD	Fracture of one rib, left side, subs for fx w routn heal
		S22.32XG	Fracture of one rib, left side, subs for fx w delay heal
		S22.39XD	Fracture of one rib, unsp side, subs for fx w routn heal
		S22.39XG	Fracture of one rib, unsp side, subs for fx w delay heal
		S22.41XD	Multiple fx of ribs, right side, subs for fx w routn heal
		S22.41XG	Multiple fx of ribs, right side, subs for fx w delay heal
		S22.42XD	Multiple fx of ribs, left side, subs for fx w routn heal
		S22.42XG	Multiple fx of ribs, left side, subs for fx w delay heal
		S22.43XD	Multiple fractures of ribs, bi, subs for fx w routn heal
		S22.43XG	Multiple fractures of ribs, bi, subs for fx w delay heal
		S22.49XD	Multiple fx of ribs, unsp side, subs for fx w routn heal
		S22.49XG	Multiple fx of ribs, unsp side, subs for fx w delay heal
		S22.5XXD	Flail chest, subs encntr for fracture with routine healing
		S22.5XXG	Flail chest, subs encntr for fracture with delayed healing
		S22.9XXD	Fracture of bony thorax, part unsp, subs for fx w routn heal
		S22.9XXG	Fracture of bony thorax, part unsp, subs for fx w delay heal
		S32.1ØXD	Unsp fracture of sacrum, subs for fx w routn heal
		S32.1ØXG	Unsp fracture of sacrum, subs for fx w delay heal
		S32.11ØD	Nondisp Zone I fracture of sacrum, subs for fx w routn heal
		S32.11ØG	Nondisp Zone I fracture of sacrum, subs for fx w delay heal
		S32.111D	Minimally displ Zone I fx sacrum, subs for fx w routn heal
		S32.111G	Minimally displ Zone I fx sacrum, subs for fx w delay heal
		S32.112D	Severely displ Zone I fx sacrum, subs for fx w routn heal
		S32.112G	Severely displ Zone I fx sacrum, subs for fx w delay heal
		S32.119D	Unsp Zone I fracture of sacrum, subs for fx w routn heal
		S32.119G	Unsp Zone I fracture of sacrum, subs for fx w delay heal
		S32.12ØD	Nondisp Zone II fracture of sacrum, subs for fx w routn heal
		S32.12ØG	Nondisp Zone II fracture of sacrum, subs for fx w delay heal
		S32.121D	Minimally displ Zone II fx sacrum, subs for fx w routn heal
		S32.121G	Minimally displ Zone II fx sacrum, subs for fx w delay heal
		S32.122D	Severely displ Zone II fx sacrum, subs for fx w routn heal
		S32.122G	Severely displ Zone II fx sacrum, subs for fx w delay heal
		S32.129D	Unsp Zone II fracture of sacrum, subs for fx w routn heal
		S32.129G	Unsp Zone II fracture of sacrum, subs for fx w delay heal
		S32.13ØD	Nondisp Zone III fx sacrum, subs for fx w routn heal
		S32.13ØG	Nondisp Zone III fx sacrum, subs for fx w delay heal
		S32.131D	Minimally displ Zone III fx sacrum, subs for fx w routn heal
		S32.131G	Minimally displ Zone III fx sacrum, subs for fx w delay heal
		S32.132D	Severely displ Zone III fx sacrum, subs for fx w routn heal
		S32.132G	Severely displ Zone III fx sacrum, subs for fx w delay heal
		S32.139D	Unsp Zone III fracture of sacrum, subs for fx w routn heal
		S32.139G	Unsp Zone III fracture of sacrum, subs for fx w delay heal
		S32.14XD	Type 1 fracture of sacrum, subs for fx w routn heal
		S32.14XG	Type 1 fracture of sacrum, subs for fx w delay heal
		S32.15XD	Type 2 fracture of sacrum, subs for fx w routn heal
		S32.15XG	Type 2 fracture of sacrum, subs for fx w delay heal
		S32.16XD	Type 3 fracture of sacrum, subs for fx w routn heal
		S32.16XG	Type 3 fracture of sacrum, subs for fx w delay heal
		S32.17XD	Type 4 fracture of sacrum, subs for fx w routn heal
		S32.17XG	Type 4 fracture of sacrum, subs for fx w delay heal
		S32.19XD	Oth fracture of sacrum, subs for fx w routn heal
		S32.19XG	Oth fracture of sacrum, subs for fx w delay heal
		S32.2XXD	Fracture of coccyx, subs for fx w routn heal
		S32.2XXG	Fracture of coccyx, subs for fx w delay heal
		S32.81ØD	Mult fx of pelv w stable disrupt of pelv ring, sub for fx w rout heal
		S32.81ØG	Mult fx of pelv w stable disrupt of pelv ring, sub for fx w delay heal
		S32.811D	Mult fx of pelv w unstbl disrupt of pelv ring, sub for fx w rout heal
		S32.811G	Mult fx of pelv w unstbl disrupt of pelv ring, sub for fx w delay heal
		S32.82XD	Mult fx of pelv w/o disrupt of pelv ring, sub for fx w rout heal
		S32.82XG	Mult fx of pelv w/o disrupt of pelv ring, sub for fx w delay heal
		S32.89XD	Fracture of oth parts of pelvis, subs for fx w routn heal
		S32.89XG	Fracture of oth parts of pelvis, subs for fx w delay heal
		S32.9XXD	Fx unsp parts of lumbosacr spin & pelv, sub for fx w rout heal
		S32.9XXG	Fx unsp parts of lumbosacr spin & pelv, sub for fx w delay heal
	(Continued on next page)	**S42.ØØ1D**	Fx unsp part of r clavicle, subs for fx w routn heal

ICD-9-CM		ICD-10-CM	
V54.19	AFTERCARE HEALING TRAUMATIC FRACTURE OTHER BONE **(Continued)**	**S42.001G**	Fx unsp part of r clavicle, subs for fx w delay heal
		S42.002D	Fx unsp part of l clavicle, subs for fx w routn heal
		S42.002G	Fx unsp part of l clavicle, subs for fx w delay heal
		S42.009D	Fx unsp part of unsp clavicle, subs for fx w routn heal
		S42.009G	Fx unsp part of unsp clavicle, subs for fx w delay heal
		S42.011D	Ant disp fx of sternal end r clavicle, sub for fx w rout heal
		S42.011G	Ant disp fx of sternal end r clavicle, sub for fx w delay heal
		S42.012D	Ant disp fx of sternal end l clavicle, sub for fx w rout heal
		S42.012G	Ant disp fx of sternal end l clavicle, sub for fx w delay heal
		S42.013D	Ant disp fx of sternal end unsp clavicle, sub for fx w rout heal
		S42.013G	Ant disp fx of sternal end unsp clavicle, sub for fx w delay heal
		S42.014D	Post disp fx of sternal end r clavicle, sub for fx w rout heal
		S42.014G	Post disp fx of sternal end r clavicle, sub for fx w delay heal
		S42.015D	Post disp fx of sternal end l clavicle, sub for fx w rout heal
		S42.015G	Post disp fx of sternal end l clavicle, sub for fx w delay heal
		S42.016D	Post disp fx of sternal end unsp clavicle, sub for fx w rout heal
		S42.016G	Post disp fx of sternal end unsp clavicle, sub for fx w delay heal
		S42.017D	Nondisp fx of sternal end r clavicle, sub for fx w rout heal
		S42.017G	Nondisp fx of sternal end r clavicle, sub for fx w delay heal
		S42.018D	Nondisp fx of sternal end l clavicle, sub for fx w rout heal
		S42.018G	Nondisp fx of sternal end l clavicle, sub for fx w delay heal
		S42.019D	Nondisp fx of sternal end unsp clavicle, sub for fx w rout heal
		S42.019G	Nondisp fx of sternal end unsp clavicle, sub for fx w delay heal
		S42.021D	Disp fx of shaft of right clavicle, subs for fx w routn heal
		S42.021G	Disp fx of shaft of right clavicle, subs for fx w delay heal
		S42.022D	Disp fx of shaft of left clavicle, subs for fx w routn heal
		S42.022G	Disp fx of shaft of left clavicle, subs for fx w delay heal
		S42.023D	Disp fx of shaft of unsp clavicle, subs for fx w routn heal
		S42.023G	Disp fx of shaft of unsp clavicle, subs for fx w delay heal
		S42.024D	Nondisp fx of shaft of r clavicle, subs for fx w routn heal
		S42.024G	Nondisp fx of shaft of r clavicle, subs for fx w delay heal
		S42.025D	Nondisp fx of shaft of l clavicle, subs for fx w routn heal
		S42.025G	Nondisp fx of shaft of l clavicle, subs for fx w delay heal
		S42.026D	Nondisp fx of shaft of unsp clavicle, sub for fx w rout heal
		S42.026G	Nondisp fx of shaft of unsp clavicle, sub for fx w delay heal
		S42.031D	Disp fx of lateral end r clavicle, subs for fx w routn heal
		S42.031G	Disp fx of lateral end r clavicle, subs for fx w delay heal
		S42.032D	Disp fx of lateral end l clavicle, subs for fx w routn heal
		S42.032G	Disp fx of lateral end l clavicle, subs for fx w delay heal
		S42.033D	Disp fx of lateral end unsp clavicle, sub for fx w rout heal
		S42.033G	Disp fx of lateral end unsp clavicle, sub for fx w delay heal
		S42.034D	Nondisp fx of lateral end r clavicle, sub for fx w rout heal
		S42.034G	Nondisp fx of lateral end r clavicle, sub for fx w delay heal
		S42.035D	Nondisp fx of lateral end l clavicle, sub for fx w rout heal
		S42.035G	Nondisp fx of lateral end l clavicle, sub for fx w delay heal
		S42.036D	Nondisp fx of lateral end unsp clavicle, sub for fx w rout heal
		S42.036G	Nondisp fx of lateral end unsp clavicle, sub for fx w delay heal
V54.20	AFTERCARE HEALING PATHOLOGIC FRACTURE ARM UNSPEC	**M84.40XD**	Pathological fracture, unsp site, subs for fx w routn heal
V54.21	AFTERCARE HEALING PATHOLOGIC FRACTURE UPPER ARM	**M80.011D**	Age-rel osteopor w crnt path fx, r shldr, sub for fx w rout heal
		M80.011G	Age-rel osteopor w crnt path fx, r shldr, sub for fx w delay heal
		M80.012D	Age-rel osteopor w crnt path fx, l shldr, sub for fx w rout heal
		M80.012G	Age-rel osteopor w crnt path fx, l shldr, sub for fx w delay heal
		M80.019D	Age-rel osteopor w crnt path fx, unsp shldr, sub for fx w rout heal
		M80.019G	Age-rel osteopor w crnt path fx, unsp shldr, sub for fx w delay heal
		M80.021D	Age-rel osteopor w crnt path fx, r humer, sub for fx w rout heal
		M80.021G	Age-rel osteopor w crnt path fx, r humer, sub for fx w delay heal
		M80.022D	Age-rel osteopor w crnt path fx, l humer, sub for fx w rout heal
		M80.022G	Age-rel osteopor w crnt path fx, l humer, sub for fx w delay heal
		M80.029D	Age-rel osteopor w crnt path fx, unsp humer, sub for fx w rout heal
		M80.029G	Age-rel osteopor w crnt path fx, unsp humer, sub for fx w delay heal
		M80.811D	Oth osteopor w crnt path fx, r shldr, sub for fx w rout heal
		M80.811G	Oth osteopor w crnt path fx, r shldr, sub for fx w delay heal
		M80.812D	Oth osteopor w crnt path fx, l shldr, sub for fx w rout heal
		M80.812G	Oth osteopor w crnt path fx, l shldr, sub for fx w delay heal
		M80.819D	Oth osteopor w crnt path fx, unsp shldr, sub for fx w rout heal
		M80.819G	Oth osteopor w crnt path fx, unsp shldr, sub for fx w delay heal
		M80.821D	Oth osteopor w crnt path fx, r humer, sub for fx w rout heal
		M80.821G	Oth osteopor w crnt path fx, r humer, sub for fx w delay heal
		M80.822D	Oth osteopor w crnt path fx, l humer, sub for fx w rout heal
		M80.822G	Oth osteopor w crnt path fx, l humer, sub for fx w delay heal
		M80.829D	Oth osteopor w crnt path fx, unsp humer, sub for fx w rout heal
		M80.829G	Oth osteopor w crnt path fx, unsp humer, sub for fx w delay heal
		M84.311D	Stress fracture, right shoulder, subs for fx w routn heal
		M84.311G	Stress fracture, right shoulder, subs for fx w delay heal
		M84.312D	Stress fracture, left shoulder, subs for fx w routn heal
		M84.312G	Stress fracture, left shoulder, subs for fx w delay heal
		M84.319D	Stress fracture, unsp shoulder, subs for fx w routn heal
		M84.319G	Stress fracture, unsp shoulder, subs for fx w delay heal
		M84.321D	Stress fracture, right humerus, subs for fx w routn heal
		M84.321G	Stress fracture, right humerus, subs for fx w delay heal
	(Continued on next page)	**M84.322D**	Stress fracture, left humerus, subs for fx w routn heal

ICD-9-CM		ICD-10-CM	
V54.21	AFTERCARE HEALING PATHOLOGIC FRACTURE UPPER ARM **(Continued)**	**M84.322G**	Stress fracture, left humerus, subs for fx w delay heal
		M84.329D	Stress fracture, unsp humerus, subs for fx w routn heal
		M84.329G	Stress fracture, unsp humerus, subs for fx w delay heal
		M84.411D	Pathological fracture, r shoulder, subs for fx w routn heal
		M84.411G	Pathological fracture, r shoulder, subs for fx w delay heal
		M84.412D	Pathological fracture, l shoulder, subs for fx w routn heal
		M84.412G	Pathological fracture, l shoulder, subs for fx w delay heal
		M84.419D	Path fracture, unsp shoulder, subs for fx w routn heal
		M84.419G	Path fracture, unsp shoulder, subs for fx w delay heal
		M84.421D	Pathological fracture, r humerus, subs for fx w routn heal
		M84.421G	Pathological fracture, r humerus, subs for fx w delay heal
		M84.422D	Pathological fracture, l humerus, subs for fx w routn heal
		M84.422G	Pathological fracture, l humerus, subs for fx w delay heal
		M84.429D	Path fracture, unsp humerus, subs for fx w routn heal
		M84.429G	Path fracture, unsp humerus, subs for fx w delay heal
		M84.511D	Path fx in neopltc dis, r shldr, subs for fx w routn heal
		M84.511G	Path fx in neopltc dis, r shldr, subs for fx w delay heal
		M84.512D	Path fx in neopltc dis, l shldr, subs for fx w routn heal
		M84.512G	Path fx in neopltc dis, l shldr, subs for fx w delay heal
		M84.519D	Path fx in neopltc dis, unsp shldr, subs for fx w routn heal
		M84.519G	Path fx in neopltc dis, unsp shldr, subs for fx w delay heal
		M84.521D	Path fx in neopltc dis, r humerus, subs for fx w routn heal
		M84.521G	Path fx in neopltc dis, r humerus, subs for fx w delay heal
		M84.522D	Path fx in neopltc dis, l humerus, subs for fx w routn heal
		M84.522G	Path fx in neopltc dis, l humerus, subs for fx w delay heal
		M84.529D	Path fx in neopltc dis, unsp humer, subs for fx w routn heal
		M84.529G	Path fx in neopltc dis, unsp humer, subs for fx w delay heal
		M84.611D	Path fx in oth disease, r shoulder, subs for fx w routn heal
		M84.611G	Path fx in oth disease, r shoulder, subs for fx w delay heal
		M84.612D	Path fx in oth disease, l shoulder, subs for fx w routn heal
		M84.612G	Path fx in oth disease, l shoulder, subs for fx w delay heal
		M84.619D	Path fx in oth disease, unsp shldr, subs for fx w routn heal
		M84.619G	Path fx in oth disease, unsp shldr, subs for fx w delay heal
		M84.621D	Path fx in oth disease, r humerus, subs for fx w routn heal
		M84.621G	Path fx in oth disease, r humerus, subs for fx w delay heal
		M84.622D	Path fx in oth disease, l humerus, subs for fx w routn heal
		M84.622G	Path fx in oth disease, l humerus, subs for fx w delay heal
		M84.629D	Path fx in oth dis, unsp humerus, subs for fx w routn heal
		M84.629G	Path fx in oth dis, unsp humerus, subs for fx w delay heal
V54.22	AFTERCARE HEALING PATHOLOGIC FRACTURE LOWER ARM	**M80.031D**	Age-rel osteopor w crnt path fx, r forearm, sub for fx w rout heal
		M80.031G	Age-rel osteopor w crnt path fx, r forearm, sub for fx w delay heal
		M80.032D	Age-rel osteopor w crnt path fx, l forearm, sub for fx w rout heal
		M80.032G	Age-rel osteopor w crnt path fx, l forearm, sub for fx w delay heal
		M80.039D	Age-rel osteopor w crnt path fx, unsp forearm, sub for fx w rout heal
		M80.039G	Age-rel osteopor w crnt path fx, unsp forearm, sub for fx w delay heal
		M80.041D	Age-rel osteopor w crnt path fx, r hand, sub for fx w rout heal
		M80.041G	Age-rel osteopor w crnt path fx, r hand, sub for fx w delay heal
		M80.042D	Age-rel osteopor w crnt path fx, l hand, sub for fx w rout heal
		M80.042G	Age-rel osteopor w crnt path fx, l hand, sub for fx w delay heal
		M80.049D	Age-rel osteopor w crnt path fx, unsp hand, sub for fx w rout heal
		M80.049G	Age-rel osteopor w crnt path fx, unsp hand, sub for fx w delay heal
		M80.831D	Oth osteopor w crnt path fx, r forearm, sub for fx w rout heal
		M80.831G	Oth osteopor w crnt path fx, r forearm, sub for fx w delay heal
		M80.832D	Oth osteopor w crnt path fx, l forearm, sub for fx w rout heal
		M80.832G	Oth osteopor w crnt path fx, l forearm, sub for fx w delay heal
		M80.839D	Oth osteopor w crnt path fx, unsp forearm, sub for fx w rout heal
		M80.839G	Oth osteopor w crnt path fx, unsp forearm, sub for fx w delay heal
		M80.841D	Oth osteopor w crnt path fx, r hand, sub for fx w rout heal
		M80.841G	Oth osteopor w crnt path fx, r hand, sub for fx w delay heal
		M80.842D	Oth osteopor w crnt path fx, l hand, sub for fx w rout heal
		M80.842G	Oth osteopor w crnt path fx, l hand, sub for fx w delay heal
		M80.849D	Oth osteopor w crnt path fx, unsp hand, sub for fx w rout heal
		M80.849G	Oth osteopor w crnt path fx, unsp hand, sub for fx w delay heal
		M84.331D	Stress fracture, right ulna, subs for fx w routn heal
		M84.331G	Stress fracture, right ulna, subs for fx w delay heal
		M84.332D	Stress fracture, left ulna, subs for fx w routn heal
		M84.332G	Stress fracture, left ulna, subs for fx w delay heal
		M84.333D	Stress fracture, right radius, subs for fx w routn heal
		M84.333G	Stress fracture, right radius, subs for fx w delay heal
		M84.334D	Stress fracture, left radius, subs for fx w routn heal
		M84.334G	Stress fracture, left radius, subs for fx w delay heal
		M84.339D	Stress fx, unsp ulna and radius, subs for fx w routn heal
		M84.339G	Stress fx, unsp ulna and radius, subs for fx w delay heal
		M84.341D	Stress fracture, right hand, subs for fx w routn heal
		M84.341G	Stress fracture, right hand, subs for fx w delay heal
		M84.342D	Stress fracture, left hand, subs for fx w routn heal
		M84.342G	Stress fracture, left hand, subs for fx w delay heal
		M84.343D	Stress fracture, unsp hand, subs for fx w routn heal
		M84.343G	Stress fracture, unsp hand, subs for fx w delay heal
		M84.344D	Stress fracture, right finger(s), subs for fx w routn heal
		M84.344G	Stress fracture, right finger(s), subs for fx w delay heal
		M84.345D	Stress fracture, left finger(s), subs for fx w routn heal
	(Continued on next page)	**M84.345G**	Stress fracture, left finger(s), subs for fx w delay heal

ICD-9-CM		ICD-10-CM	
V54.22	AFTERCARE HEALING PATHOLOGIC FRACTURE LOWER ARM **(Continued)**	**M84.346D**	Stress fracture, unsp finger(s), subs for fx w routn heal
		M84.346G	Stress fracture, unsp finger(s), subs for fx w delay heal
		M84.431D	Pathological fracture, right ulna, subs for fx w routn heal
		M84.431G	Pathological fracture, right ulna, subs for fx w delay heal
		M84.432D	Pathological fracture, left ulna, subs for fx w routn heal
		M84.432G	Pathological fracture, left ulna, subs for fx w delay heal
		M84.433D	Path fracture, right radius, subs for fx w routn heal
		M84.433G	Path fracture, right radius, subs for fx w delay heal
		M84.434D	Pathological fracture, left radius, subs for fx w routn heal
		M84.434G	Pathological fracture, left radius, subs for fx w delay heal
		M84.439D	Path fx, unsp ulna and radius, subs for fx w routn heal
		M84.439G	Path fx, unsp ulna and radius, subs for fx w delay heal
		M84.441D	Pathological fracture, right hand, subs for fx w routn heal
		M84.441G	Pathological fracture, right hand, subs for fx w delay heal
		M84.442D	Pathological fracture, left hand, subs for fx w routn heal
		M84.442G	Pathological fracture, left hand, subs for fx w delay heal
		M84.443D	Pathological fracture, unsp hand, subs for fx w routn heal
		M84.443G	Pathological fracture, unsp hand, subs for fx w delay heal
		M84.444D	Path fracture, right finger(s), subs for fx w routn heal
		M84.444G	Path fracture, right finger(s), subs for fx w delay heal
		M84.445D	Path fracture, left finger(s), subs for fx w routn heal
		M84.445G	Path fracture, left finger(s), subs for fx w delay heal
		M84.446D	Path fracture, unsp finger(s), subs for fx w routn heal
		M84.446G	Path fracture, unsp finger(s), subs for fx w delay heal
		M84.531D	Path fx in neopltc disease, r ulna, subs for fx w routn heal
		M84.531G	Path fx in neopltc disease, r ulna, subs for fx w delay heal
		M84.532D	Path fx in neopltc disease, l ulna, subs for fx w routn heal
		M84.532G	Path fx in neopltc disease, l ulna, subs for fx w delay heal
		M84.533D	Path fx in neopltc dis, r radius, subs for fx w routn heal
		M84.533G	Path fx in neopltc dis, r radius, subs for fx w delay heal
		M84.534D	Path fx in neopltc dis, left rad, subs for fx w routn heal
		M84.534G	Path fx in neopltc dis, left rad, subs for fx w delay heal
		M84.539D	Path fx in neopltc dis, unsp ulna & rad, sub for fx w rout heal
		M84.539G	Path fx in neopltc dis, unsp ulna & rad, sub for fx w delay heal
		M84.541D	Path fx in neopltc disease, r hand, subs for fx w routn heal
		M84.541G	Path fx in neopltc disease, r hand, subs for fx w delay heal
		M84.542D	Path fx in neopltc disease, l hand, subs for fx w routn heal
		M84.542G	Path fx in neopltc disease, l hand, subs for fx w delay heal
		M84.549D	Path fx in neopltc dis, unsp hand, subs for fx w routn heal
		M84.549G	Path fx in neopltc dis, unsp hand, subs for fx w delay heal
		M84.631D	Path fx in oth disease, r ulna, subs for fx w routn heal
		M84.631G	Path fx in oth disease, r ulna, subs for fx w delay heal
		M84.632D	Path fx in oth disease, l ulna, subs for fx w routn heal
		M84.632G	Path fx in oth disease, l ulna, subs for fx w delay heal
		M84.633D	Path fx in oth disease, r radius, subs for fx w routn heal
		M84.633G	Path fx in oth disease, r radius, subs for fx w delay heal
		M84.634D	Path fx in oth dis, left radius, subs for fx w routn heal
		M84.634G	Path fx in oth dis, left radius, subs for fx w delay heal
		M84.639D	Path fx in oth dis, unsp ulna & rad, sub for fx w rout heal
		M84.639G	Path fx in oth dis, unsp ulna & rad, sub for fx w delay heal
		M84.641D	Path fx in oth disease, r hand, subs for fx w routn heal
		M84.641G	Path fx in oth disease, r hand, subs for fx w delay heal
		M84.642D	Path fx in oth disease, l hand, subs for fx w routn heal
		M84.642G	Path fx in oth disease, l hand, subs for fx w delay heal
		M84.649D	Path fx in oth disease, unsp hand, subs for fx w routn heal
		M84.649G	Path fx in oth disease, unsp hand, subs for fx w delay heal
V54.23	AFTERCARE FOR HEALING PATHOLOGIC FRACTURE OF HIP	**M8Ø.Ø51D**	Age-rel osteopor w crnt path fx, r femr, sub for fx w rout heal
		M8Ø.Ø51G	Age-rel osteopor w crnt path fx, r femr, sub for fx w delay heal
		M8Ø.Ø52D	Age-rel osteopor w crnt path fx, l femr, sub for fx w rout heal
		M8Ø.Ø52G	Age-rel osteopor w crnt path fx, l femr, sub for fx w delay heal
		M8Ø.Ø59D	Age-rel osteopor w crnt path fx, unsp femr, sub for fx w rout heal
		M8Ø.Ø59G	Age-rel osteopor w crnt path fx, unsp femr, sub for fx w delay heal
		M8Ø.851D	Oth osteopor w crnt path fx, r femr, sub for fx w rout heal
		M8Ø.851G	Oth osteopor w crnt path fx, r femr, sub for fx w delay heal
		M8Ø.852D	Oth osteopor w crnt path fx, l femr, sub for fx w rout heal
		M8Ø.852G	Oth osteopor w crnt path fx, l femr, sub for fx w delay heal
		M8Ø.859D	Oth osteopor w crnt path fx, unsp femr, sub for fx w rout heal
		M8Ø.859G	Oth osteopor w crnt path fx, unsp femr, sub for fx w delay heal
		M84.359D	Stress fracture, hip, unsp, subs for fx w routn heal
		M84.359G	Stress fracture, hip, unsp, subs for fx w delay heal
		M84.459D	Pathological fracture, hip, unsp, subs for fx w routn heal
		M84.459G	Pathological fracture, hip, unsp, subs for fx w delay heal
		M84.551D	Path fx in neopltc dis, r femur, subs for fx w routn heal
		M84.551G	Path fx in neopltc dis, r femur, subs for fx w delay heal
		M84.552D	Path fx in neopltc dis, l femur, subs for fx w routn heal
		M84.552G	Path fx in neopltc dis, l femur, subs for fx w delay heal
		M84.553D	Path fx in neopltc dis, unsp femur, subs for fx w routn heal
		M84.553G	Path fx in neopltc dis, unsp femur, subs for fx w delay heal
		M84.559D	Path fx in neopltc dis, hip, unsp, subs for fx w routn heal
		M84.559G	Path fx in neopltc dis, hip, unsp, subs for fx w delay heal
		M84.651D	Path fx in oth disease, r femur, subs for fx w routn heal
		M84.651G	Path fx in oth disease, r femur, subs for fx w delay heal
	(Continued on next page)		

ICD-9-CM		ICD-10-CM	
V54.23	AFTERCARE FOR HEALING PATHOLOGIC FRACTURE OF HIP **(Continued)**	**M84.652D**	Path fx in oth disease, l femur, subs for fx w routn heal
		M84.652G	Path fx in oth disease, l femur, subs for fx w delay heal
		M84.653D	Path fx in oth disease, unsp femur, subs for fx w routn heal
		M84.653G	Path fx in oth disease, unsp femur, subs for fx w delay heal
		M84.659D	Path fx in oth disease, hip, unsp, subs for fx w routn heal
		M84.659G	Path fx in oth disease, hip, unsp, subs for fx w delay heal
		T84.Ø4ØD	Periprosth fracture around internal prosth r hip jt, subs
		T84.Ø41D	Periprosth fracture around internal prosth l hip jt, subs
V54.24	AFTERCARE HEALING PATHOLOGIC FRACTURE LEG UNSPEC	**M84.4ØXD**	Pathological fracture, unsp site, subs for fx w routn heal
V54.25	AFTERCARE HEALING PATHOLOGIC FRACTURE UPPER LEG	**M84.351D**	Stress fracture, right femur, subs for fx w routn heal
		M84.351G	Stress fracture, right femur, subs for fx w delay heal
		M84.352D	Stress fracture, left femur, subs for fx w routn heal
		M84.352G	Stress fracture, left femur, subs for fx w delay heal
		M84.353D	Stress fracture, unsp femur, subs for fx w routn heal
		M84.353G	Stress fracture, unsp femur, subs for fx w delay heal
		M84.451D	Pathological fracture, right femur, subs for fx w routn heal
		M84.451G	Pathological fracture, right femur, subs for fx w delay heal
		M84.452D	Pathological fracture, left femur, subs for fx w routn heal
		M84.452G	Pathological fracture, left femur, subs for fx w delay heal
		M84.453D	Pathological fracture, unsp femur, subs for fx w routn heal
		M84.453G	Pathological fracture, unsp femur, subs for fx w delay heal
V54.26	AFTERCARE HEALING PATHOLOGIC FRACTURE LOWER LEG	**M8Ø.Ø61D**	Age-rel osteopor w crnt path fx, r low leg, sub for fx w rout heal
		M8Ø.Ø61G	Age-rel osteopor w crnt path fx, r low leg, sub for fx w delay heal
		M8Ø.Ø62D	Age-rel osteopor w crnt path fx, l low leg, sub for fx w rout heal
		M8Ø.Ø62G	Age-rel osteopor w crnt path fx, l low leg, sub for fx w delay heal
		M8Ø.Ø69D	Age-rel osteopor w crnt path fx, unsp low leg, sub for fx w rout heal
		M8Ø.Ø69G	Age-rel osteopor w crnt path fx, unsp low leg, sub for fx w delay heal
		M8Ø.Ø71D	Age-rel osteopor w crnt path fx, r ank/ft, sub for fx w rout heal
		M8Ø.Ø71G	Age-rel osteopor w crnt path fx, r ank/ft, sub for fx w delay heal
		M8Ø.Ø72D	Age-rel osteopor w crnt path fx, l ank/ft, sub for fx w rout heal
		M8Ø.Ø72G	Age-rel osteopor w crnt path fx, l ank/ft, sub for fx w delay heal
		M8Ø.Ø79D	Age-rel osteopor w crnt path fx, unsp ank/ft, sub for fx w rout heal
		M8Ø.Ø79G	Age-rel osteopor w crnt path fx, unsp ank/ft, sub for fx w delay heal
		M8Ø.861D	Oth osteopor w crnt path fx, r low leg, sub for fx w rout heal
		M8Ø.861G	Oth osteopor w crnt path fx, r low leg, sub for fx w delay heal
		M8Ø.862D	Oth osteopor w crnt path fx, l low leg, sub for fx w rout heal
		M8Ø.862G	Oth osteopor w crnt path fx, l low leg, sub for fx w delay heal
		M8Ø.869D	Oth osteopor w crnt path fx, unsp low leg, sub for fx w rout heal
		M8Ø.869G	Oth osteopor w crnt path fx, unsp low leg, sub for fx w delay heal
		M8Ø.871D	Oth osteopor w crnt path fx, r ank/ft, sub for fx w rout heal
		M8Ø.871G	Oth osteopor w crnt path fx, r ank/ft, sub for fx w delay heal
		M8Ø.872D	Oth osteopor w crnt path fx, l ank/ft, sub for fx w rout heal
		M8Ø.872G	Oth osteopor w crnt path fx, l ank/ft, sub for fx w delay heal
		M8Ø.879D	Oth osteopor w crnt path fx, unsp ank/ft, sub for fx w rout heal
		M8Ø.879G	Oth osteopor w crnt path fx, unsp ank/ft, sub for fx w delay heal
		M84.361D	Stress fracture, right tibia, subs for fx w routn heal
		M84.361G	Stress fracture, right tibia, subs for fx w delay heal
		M84.362D	Stress fracture, left tibia, subs for fx w routn heal
		M84.362G	Stress fracture, left tibia, subs for fx w delay heal
		M84.363D	Stress fracture, right fibula, subs for fx w routn heal
		M84.363G	Stress fracture, right fibula, subs for fx w delay heal
		M84.364D	Stress fracture, left fibula, subs for fx w routn heal
		M84.364G	Stress fracture, left fibula, subs for fx w delay heal
		M84.369D	Stress fx, unsp tibia and fibula, subs for fx w routn heal
		M84.369G	Stress fx, unsp tibia and fibula, subs for fx w delay heal
		M84.371D	Stress fracture, right ankle, subs for fx w routn heal
		M84.371G	Stress fracture, right ankle, subs for fx w delay heal
		M84.372D	Stress fracture, left ankle, subs for fx w routn heal
		M84.372G	Stress fracture, left ankle, subs for fx w delay heal
		M84.373D	Stress fracture, unsp ankle, subs for fx w routn heal
		M84.373G	Stress fracture, unsp ankle, subs for fx w delay heal
		M84.374D	Stress fracture, right foot, subs for fx w routn heal
		M84.374G	Stress fracture, right foot, subs for fx w delay heal
		M84.375D	Stress fracture, left foot, subs for fx w routn heal
		M84.375G	Stress fracture, left foot, subs for fx w delay heal
		M84.376D	Stress fracture, unsp foot, subs for fx w routn heal
		M84.376G	Stress fracture, unsp foot, subs for fx w delay heal
		M84.377D	Stress fracture, right toe(s), subs for fx w routn heal
		M84.377G	Stress fracture, right toe(s), subs for fx w delay heal
		M84.378D	Stress fracture, left toe(s), subs for fx w routn heal
		M84.378G	Stress fracture, left toe(s), subs for fx w delay heal
		M84.379D	Stress fracture, unsp toe(s), subs for fx w routn heal
		M84.379G	Stress fracture, unsp toe(s), subs for fx w delay heal
		M84.461D	Pathological fracture, right tibia, subs for fx w routn heal
		M84.461G	Pathological fracture, right tibia, subs for fx w delay heal
		M84.462D	Pathological fracture, left tibia, subs for fx w routn heal
		M84.462G	Pathological fracture, left tibia, subs for fx w delay heal
		M84.463D	Path fracture, right fibula, subs for fx w routn heal
		M84.463G	Path fracture, right fibula, subs for fx w delay heal
		M84.464D	Pathological fracture, left fibula, subs for fx w routn heal
		M84.464G	Pathological fracture, left fibula, subs for fx w delay heal
	(Continued on next page)	**M84.469D**	Path fx, unsp tibia and fibula, subs for fx w routn heal

ICD-9-CM		ICD-10-CM	
V54.26	AFTERCARE HEALING PATHOLOGIC FRACTURE LOWER LEG **(Continued)**	**M84.469G**	Path fx, unsp tibia and fibula, subs for fx w delay heal
		M84.471D	Pathological fracture, right ankle, subs for fx w routn heal
		M84.471G	Pathological fracture, right ankle, subs for fx w delay heal
		M84.472D	Pathological fracture, left ankle, subs for fx w routn heal
		M84.472G	Pathological fracture, left ankle, subs for fx w delay heal
		M84.473D	Pathological fracture, unsp ankle, subs for fx w routn heal
		M84.473G	Pathological fracture, unsp ankle, subs for fx w delay heal
		M84.474D	Pathological fracture, right foot, subs for fx w routn heal
		M84.474G	Pathological fracture, right foot, subs for fx w delay heal
		M84.475D	Pathological fracture, left foot, subs for fx w routn heal
		M84.475G	Pathological fracture, left foot, subs for fx w delay heal
		M84.476D	Pathological fracture, unsp foot, subs for fx w routn heal
		M84.476G	Pathological fracture, unsp foot, subs for fx w delay heal
		M84.477D	Path fracture, right toe(s), subs for fx w routn heal
		M84.477G	Path fracture, right toe(s), subs for fx w delay heal
		M84.478D	Pathological fracture, left toe(s), subs for fx w routn heal
		M84.478G	Pathological fracture, left toe(s), subs for fx w delay heal
		M84.479D	Pathological fracture, unsp toe(s), subs for fx w routn heal
		M84.479G	Pathological fracture, unsp toe(s), subs for fx w delay heal
		M84.561D	Path fx in neopltc dis, r tibia, subs for fx w routn heal
		M84.561G	Path fx in neopltc dis, r tibia, subs for fx w delay heal
		M84.562D	Path fx in neopltc dis, l tibia, subs for fx w routn heal
		M84.562G	Path fx in neopltc dis, l tibia, subs for fx w delay heal
		M84.563D	Path fx in neopltc dis, r fibula, subs for fx w routn heal
		M84.563G	Path fx in neopltc dis, r fibula, subs for fx w delay heal
		M84.564D	Path fx in neopltc dis, l fibula, subs for fx w routn heal
		M84.564G	Path fx in neopltc dis, l fibula, subs for fx w delay heal
		M84.569D	Path fx in neopltc dis, unsp tibia & fibula, sub for fx w rout heal
		M84.569G	Path fx in neopltc dis, unsp tibia & fibula, sub for fx w delay heal
		M84.571D	Path fx in neopltc dis, r ankle, subs for fx w routn heal
		M84.571G	Path fx in neopltc dis, r ankle, subs for fx w delay heal
		M84.572D	Path fx in neopltc dis, l ankle, subs for fx w routn heal
		M84.572G	Path fx in neopltc dis, l ankle, subs for fx w delay heal
		M84.573D	Path fx in neopltc dis, unsp ankle, subs for fx w routn heal
		M84.573G	Path fx in neopltc dis, unsp ankle, subs for fx w delay heal
		M84.574D	Path fx in neopltc disease, r foot, subs for fx w routn heal
		M84.574G	Path fx in neopltc disease, r foot, subs for fx w delay heal
		M84.575D	Path fx in neopltc disease, l foot, subs for fx w routn heal
		M84.575G	Path fx in neopltc disease, l foot, subs for fx w delay heal
		M84.576D	Path fx in neopltc dis, unsp foot, subs for fx w routn heal
		M84.576G	Path fx in neopltc dis, unsp foot, subs for fx w delay heal
		M84.661D	Path fx in oth disease, r tibia, subs for fx w routn heal
		M84.661G	Path fx in oth disease, r tibia, subs for fx w delay heal
		M84.662D	Path fx in oth disease, l tibia, subs for fx w routn heal
		M84.662G	Path fx in oth disease, l tibia, subs for fx w delay heal
		M84.663D	Path fx in oth disease, r fibula, subs for fx w routn heal
		M84.663G	Path fx in oth disease, r fibula, subs for fx w delay heal
		M84.664D	Path fx in oth disease, l fibula, subs for fx w routn heal
		M84.664G	Path fx in oth disease, l fibula, subs for fx w delay heal
		M84.669D	Path fx in oth dis, unsp tibia & fibula, sub for fx w rout heal
		M84.669G	Path fx in oth dis, unsp tibia & fibula, sub for fx w delay heal
		M84.671D	Path fx in oth disease, r ankle, subs for fx w routn heal
		M84.671G	Path fx in oth disease, r ankle, subs for fx w delay heal
		M84.672D	Path fx in oth disease, l ankle, subs for fx w routn heal
		M84.672G	Path fx in oth disease, l ankle, subs for fx w delay heal
		M84.673D	Path fx in oth disease, unsp ankle, subs for fx w routn heal
		M84.673G	Path fx in oth disease, unsp ankle, subs for fx w delay heal
		M84.674D	Path fx in oth disease, r foot, subs for fx w routn heal
		M84.674G	Path fx in oth disease, r foot, subs for fx w delay heal
		M84.675D	Path fx in oth disease, l foot, subs for fx w routn heal
		M84.675G	Path fx in oth disease, l foot, subs for fx w delay heal
		M84.676D	Path fx in oth disease, unsp foot, subs for fx w routn heal
		M84.676G	Path fx in oth disease, unsp foot, subs for fx w delay heal
		T84.Ø42D	Periprosth fracture around internal prosth r knee jt, subs
		T84.Ø43D	Periprosth fracture around internal prosth l knee jt, subs
V54.27	AFTERCARE HEALING PATHOLOGIC FRACTURE VERTEBRAE	**M48.4ØXD**	Fatigue fx vertebra, site unsp, subs for fx w routn heal
		M48.4ØXG	Fatigue fx vertebra, site unsp, subs for fx w delay heal
		M48.41XD	Fatigue fx vert, occipt-atlan-ax rgn, sub for fx w rout heal
		M48.41XG	Fatigue fx vert, occipt-atlan-ax rgn, sub for fx w delay heal
		M48.42XD	Fatigue fx vertebra, cerv region, subs for fx w routn heal
		M48.42XG	Fatigue fx vertebra, cerv region, subs for fx w delay heal
		M48.43XD	Fatigue fx vert, cervicothor rgn, subs for fx w routn heal
		M48.43XG	Fatigue fx vert, cervicothor rgn, subs for fx w delay heal
		M48.44XD	Fatigue fx vertebra, thor region, subs for fx w routn heal
		M48.44XG	Fatigue fx vertebra, thor region, subs for fx w delay heal
		M48.45XD	Fatigue fx vertebra, thrclm region, subs for fx w routn heal
		M48.45XG	Fatigue fx vertebra, thrclm region, subs for fx w delay heal
		M48.46XD	Fatigue fx vertebra, lumbar region, subs for fx w routn heal
		M48.46XG	Fatigue fx vertebra, lumbar region, subs for fx w delay heal
		M48.47XD	Fatigue fx vert, lumbosacr region, subs for fx w routn heal
		M48.47XG	Fatigue fx vert, lumbosacr region, subs for fx w delay heal
		M48.48XD	Fatigue fx vert, sacr/sacrocygl rgn, sub for fx w rout heal
	(Continued on next page)	**M48.48XG**	Fatigue fx vert, sacr/sacrocygl rgn, sub for fx w delay heal

ICD-9-CM		ICD-10-CM	
V54.27	AFTERCARE HEALING PATHOLOGIC FRACTURE VERTEBRAE **(Continued)**	**M48.5ØXD**	Collapsed vertebra, NEC, site unsp, subs for fx w routn heal
		M48.5ØXG	Collapsed vertebra, NEC, site unsp, subs for fx w delay heal
		M48.51XD	Collapsed vert, NEC, occipt-atlan-ax rgn, sub for fx w rout heal
		M48.51XG	Collapsed vert, NEC, occipt-atlan-ax rgn, sub for fx w delay heal
		M48.52XD	Collapsed vert, NEC, cerv region, subs for fx w routn heal
		M48.52XG	Collapsed vert, NEC, cerv region, subs for fx w delay heal
		M48.53XD	Collapsed vert, NEC, cervicothor rgn, sub for fx w rout heal
		M48.53XG	Collapsed vert, NEC, cervicothor rgn, sub for fx w delay heal
		M48.54XD	Collapsed vert, NEC, thor region, subs for fx w routn heal
		M48.54XG	Collapsed vert, NEC, thor region, subs for fx w delay heal
		M48.55XD	Collapsed vert, NEC, thrclm region, subs for fx w routn heal
		M48.55XG	Collapsed vert, NEC, thrclm region, subs for fx w delay heal
		M48.56XD	Collapsed vert, NEC, lumbar region, subs for fx w routn heal
		M48.56XG	Collapsed vert, NEC, lumbar region, subs for fx w delay heal
		M48.57XD	Collapsed vert, NEC, lumbosacr rgn, subs for fx w routn heal
		M48.57XG	Collapsed vert, NEC, lumbosacr rgn, subs for fx w delay heal
		M48.58XD	Collapsed vert, NEC, sacr/sacrocygl rgn, sub for fx w rout heal
		M48.58XG	Collapsed vert, NEC, sacr/sacrocygl rgn, sub for fx w delay heal
		M8Ø.Ø8XD	Age-rel osteopor w crnt path fx, verteb, sub for fx w rout heal
		M8Ø.Ø8XG	Age-rel osteopor w crnt path fx, verteb, sub for fx w delay heal
		M8Ø.88XD	Oth osteopor w crnt path fx, verteb, sub for fx w rout heal
		M8Ø.88XG	Oth osteopor w crnt path fx, verteb, sub for fx w delay heal
		M84.4ØXD	Pathological fracture, unsp site, subs for fx w routn heal
		M84.58XD	Path fx in neopltc disease, oth spec site, subs for fx w routn heal
		M84.58XG	Path fx in neopltc disease, oth spec site, subs for fx w delay heal
		M84.68XD	Path fx in oth disease, oth site, subs for fx w routn heal
V54.29	AFTERCARE HEALING PATHOLOGIC FRACTURE OTHER BONE	**M8Ø.ØØXD**	Age-rel osteopor w crnt path fx, unsp site, sub for fx w rout heal
		M8Ø.ØØXG	Age-rel osteopor w crnt path fx, unsp site, sub for fx w delay heal
		M8Ø.8ØXD	Oth osteopor w crnt path fx, unsp site, sub for fx w rout heal
		M8Ø.8ØXG	Oth osteopor w crnt path fx, unsp site, sub for fx w delay heal
		M84.3ØXD	Stress fracture, unsp site, subs for fx w routn heal
		M84.3ØXG	Stress fracture, unsp site, subs for fx w delay heal
		M84.35ØD	Stress fracture, pelvis, subs for fx w routn heal
		M84.35ØG	Stress fracture, pelvis, subs for fx w delay heal
		M84.38XD	Stress fracture, oth site, subs for fx w routn heal
		M84.38XG	Stress fracture, oth site, subs for fx w delay heal
		M84.4ØXD	Pathological fracture, unsp site, subs for fx w routn heal
		M84.4ØXG	Pathological fracture, unsp site, subs for fx w delay heal
		M84.454D	Pathological fracture, pelvis, subs for fx w routn heal
		M84.454G	Pathological fracture, pelvis, subs for fx w delay heal
		M84.48XD	Pathological fracture, oth site, subs for fx w routn heal
		M84.48XG	Pathological fracture, oth site, subs for fx w delay heal
		M84.5ØXD	Path fx in neopltc dis, unsp site, subs for fx w routn heal
		M84.5ØXG	Path fx in neopltc dis, unsp site, subs for fx w delay heal
		M84.55ØD	Path fx in neopltc disease, pelvis, subs for fx w routn heal
		M84.55ØG	Path fx in neopltc disease, pelvis, subs for fx w delay heal
		M84.6ØXD	Path fx in oth disease, unsp site, subs for fx w routn heal
		M84.6ØXG	Path fx in oth disease, unsp site, subs for fx w delay heal
		M84.65ØD	Path fx in oth disease, pelvis, subs for fx w routn heal
		M84.65ØG	Path fx in oth disease, pelvis, subs for fx w delay heal
		M84.68XD	Path fx in oth disease, oth site, subs for fx w routn heal
		M84.68XG	Path fx in oth disease, oth site, subs for fx w delay heal
		T84.Ø48D	Periprosth fracture around oth internal prosth joint, subs
		T84.Ø49D	Periprosth fracture around unsp internal prosth joint, subs
V54.81	AFTERCARE FOLLOWING JOINT REPLACEMENT	➡ **Z47.1**	Aftercare following joint replacement surgery
V54.82	AFTERCARE FOLLOW EXPLANTATION JOINT PROSTHESIS	**Z47.31**	Aftercare following explantation of shoulder jt prosthesis
		Z47.32	Aftercare following explantation of hip joint prosthesis
		Z47.33	Aftercare following explantation of knee joint prosthesis
V54.89	OTHER ORTHOPEDIC AFTERCARE	**Z47.81**	Encounter for orthopedic aftercare following surgical amp
		Z47.82	Encounter for orth aftercare following scoliosis surgery
		Z47.89	Encounter for other orthopedic aftercare
V54.9	UNSPECIFIED ORTHOPEDIC AFTERCARE	**Z51.89**	Encounter for other specified aftercare
V55.Ø	ATTENTION TO TRACHEOSTOMY	➡ **Z43.Ø**	Encounter for attention to tracheostomy
V55.1	ATTENTION TO GASTROSTOMY	➡ **Z43.1**	Encounter for attention to gastrostomy
V55.2	ATTENTION TO ILEOSTOMY	➡ **Z43.2**	Encounter for attention to ileostomy
V55.3	ATTENTION TO COLOSTOMY	➡ **Z43.3**	Encounter for attention to colostomy
V55.4	ATTN OTHER ARTIFICIAL OPENING DIGESTIVE TRACT	➡ **Z43.4**	Encounter for attn to oth artif openings of digestive tract
V55.5	ATTENTION TO CYSTOSTOMY	➡ **Z43.5**	Encounter for attention to cystostomy
V55.6	ATTENTION OTHER ARTIFICIAL OPENING URINARY TRACT	➡ **Z43.6**	Encounter for attn to oth artif openings of urinary tract
V55.7	ATTENTION TO ARTIFICIAL VAGINA	➡ **Z43.7**	Encounter for attention to artificial vagina
V55.8	ATTENTION TO OTHER SPECIFIED ARTIFICIAL OPENING	➡ **Z43.8**	Encounter for attention to other artificial openings
V55.9	ATTENTION TO UNSPECIFIED ARTIFICIAL OPENING	➡ **Z43.9**	Encounter for attention to unspecified artificial opening
V56.Ø	ENCOUNTER FOR EXTRACORPOREAL DIALYSIS	**Z49.31**	Encounter for adequacy testing for hemodialysis
V56.1	FITTING&ADJ EXTRACORPOREAL DIALYSIS CATHETER	➡ **Z49.Ø1**	Encounter for fit/adjst of extracorporeal dialysis catheter
V56.2	FITTING&ADJUSTMENT PERITONEAL DIALYSIS CATHETER	➡ **Z49.Ø2**	Encounter for fit/adjst of peritoneal dialysis catheter
V56.31	ENCOUNTER FOR ADEQUACY TESTING FOR HEMODIALYSIS	**Z49.31**	Encounter for adequacy testing for hemodialysis
V56.32	ENCOUNTER ADEQUACY TESTING PERITONEAL DIALYSIS	**Z49.32**	Encounter for adequacy testing for peritoneal dialysis
V56.8	ENCOUNTER OTHER DIALYSIS	**Z49.32**	Encounter for adequacy testing for peritoneal dialysis

ICD-9-CM			ICD-10-CM	
V57.Ø	CARE INVOLVING BREATHING EXERCISES		**Z51.89**	Encounter for other specified aftercare
V57.1	OTHER PHYSICAL THERAPY		**Z51.89**	Encounter for other specified aftercare
V57.21	ENCOUNTER FOR OCCUPATIONAL THERAPY		**Z51.89**	Encounter for other specified aftercare
V57.22	ENCOUNTER FOR VOCATIONAL THERAPY		**Z51.89**	Encounter for other specified aftercare
V57.3	CARE INVOLVING USE REHAB SPEECH-LANGUAGE TX		**Z51.89**	Encounter for other specified aftercare
V57.4	ORTHOPTIC TRAINING		**Z51.89**	Encounter for other specified aftercare
V57.81	ORTHOTIC TRAINING		**Z51.89**	Encounter for other specified aftercare
V57.89	OTHER SPECIFIED REHABILITATION PROCEDURE OTHER		**Z51.89**	Encounter for other specified aftercare
V57.9	UNSPECIFIED REHABILITATION PROCEDURE		**Z51.89**	Encounter for other specified aftercare
V58.Ø	RADIOTHERAPY	➡	**Z51.Ø**	Encounter for antineoplastic radiation therapy
V58.11	ENCOUNTER FOR ANTINEOPLASTIC CHEMOTHERAPY	➡	**Z51.11**	Encounter for antineoplastic chemotherapy
V58.12	ENCOUNTER FOR ANTINEOPLASTIC IMMUNOTHERAPY	➡	**Z51.12**	Encounter for antineoplastic immunotherapy
V58.2	BLOOD TRANSFUSION WITHOUT REPORTED DIAGNOSIS		**Z51.89**	Encounter for other specified aftercare
V58.3Ø	ENCOUNTER CHG/REMOVAL NONSURGICAL WOUND DRESSING	➡	**Z48.ØØ**	Encounter for change or removal of nonsurg wound dressing
V58.31	ENCOUNTER CHANGE/REMOVAL SURGICAL WOUND DRESSING	➡	**Z48.Ø1**	Encounter for change or removal of surgical wound dressing
V58.32	ENCOUNTER FOR REMOVAL OF SUTURES	➡	**Z48.Ø2**	Encounter for removal of sutures
V58.41	PLANNED POSTOPERATIVE WOUND CLOSURE	➡	**Z48.1**	Encounter for planned postprocedural wound closure
V58.42	AFTERCARE FOLLOWING SURGERY FOR NEOPLASM	➡	**Z48.3**	Aftercare following surgery for neoplasm
V58.43	AFTERCARE FOLLOWING SURGERY INJURY AND TRAUMA		**Z48.89**	Encounter for other specified surgical aftercare
V58.44	AFTERCARE FOLLOWING ORGAN TRANSPLANT	□ □ □ □ □ □ □ □	**Z48.21** **Z48.22** **Z48.23** **Z48.24** **Z48.28Ø** **Z48.288** **Z48.29Ø** **Z48.298**	Encounter for aftercare following heart transplant Encounter for aftercare following kidney transplant Encounter for aftercare following liver transplant Encounter for aftercare following lung transplant Encounter for aftercare following heart-lung transplant Encounter for aftercare following multiple organ transplant Encounter for aftercare following bone marrow transplant Encounter for aftercare following other organ transplant
V58.49	OTHER SPECIFIED AFTERCARE FOLLOWING SURGERY		**Z48.Ø3** **Z48.89**	Encounter for change or removal of drains Encounter for other specified surgical aftercare
V58.5	ORTHODONTICS AFTERCARE		**Z46.4**	Encounter for fitting and adjustment of orthodontic device
V58.61	LONG-TERM (CURRENT) USE OF ANTICOAGULANTS	➡	**Z79.Ø1**	Long term (current) use of anticoagulants
V58.62	LONG-TERM (CURRENT) USE OF ANTIBIOTICS	➡	**Z79.2**	Long term (current) use of antibiotics
V58.63	LONG-TERM USE OF ANTIPLATELET/ANTITHROMBOTIC	➡	**Z79.Ø2**	Long term (current) use of antithrombotics/antiplatelets
V58.64	LONG-TERM USE NON-STEROIDAL ANTI-INFLAMMATORIES	➡	**Z79.1**	Long term (current) use of non-steroidal non-inflam (NSAID)
V58.65	LONG-TERM USE OF STEROIDS		**Z79.51** **Z79.52**	Long term (current) use of inhaled steroids Long term (current) use of systemic steroids
V58.66	LONG-TERM USE OF ASPIRIN	➡	**Z79.82**	Long term (current) use of aspirin
V58.67	LONG-TERM USE OF INSULIN	➡	**Z79.4**	Long term (current) use of insulin
V58.68	LONG TERM CURRENT USE OF BISPHOSPHONATES	➡	**Z79.83**	Long term (current) use of bisphosphonates
V58.69	LONG-TERM (CURRENT) USE OF OTHER MEDICATIONS		**Z79.3** **Z79.891** **Z79.899**	Long term (current) use of hormonal contraceptives Long term (current) use of opiate analgesic Other long term (current) drug therapy
V58.71	AFTERCARE FOLLOWING SURGERY THE SENSE ORGANS NEC	➡	**Z48.81Ø**	Encntr for surgical aftcr fol surgery on the sense organs
V58.72	AFTERCARE FOLLOWING SURGERY NERVOUS SYSTEM NEC	➡	**Z48.811**	Encntr for surgical aftcr fol surgery on the nervous sys
V58.73	AFTERCARE FOLLOWING SURGERY CIRC SYSTEM NEC	➡	**Z48.812**	Encntr for surgical aftcr following surgery on the circ sys
V58.74	AFTERCARE FOLLOW SURGERY RESPIRATORY SYSTEM NEC	➡	**Z48.813**	Encntr for surgical aftcr following surgery on the resp sys
V58.75	AFTERCARE FLW SURG TEETH ORL CAV&DIGESTV SYS NEC		**Z48.814** **Z48.815**	Encntr for surg aftcr fol surg on the teeth or oral cavity Encntr for surgical aftcr following surgery on the dgstv sys
V58.76	AFTERCARE FOLLOW SURGERY GU SYSTEM NEC	➡	**Z48.816**	Encounter for surgical aftcr following surgery on the GU sys
V58.77	AFTERCARE FOLLOW SURGERY SKIN&SUBCUT TISSUE NEC	➡	**Z48.817**	Encntr for surgical aftcr fol surgery on the skin, subcu
V58.78	AFTERCARE FOLLOW SURGERY MUSCULOSKEL SYSTEM NEC		**Z48.89**	Encounter for other specified surgical aftercare
V58.81	FITTING AND ADJUSTMENT OF VASCULAR CATHETER	➡	**Z45.2**	Encounter for adjustment and management of VAD
V58.82	ENCOUNTER FITTING&ADJ NON-VASCULAR CATHETER NEC		**Z45.1** **Z46.82**	Encounter for adjustment and management of infusion pump Encounter for fit/adjst of non-vascular catheter
V58.83	ENCOUNTER FOR THERAPEUTIC DRUG MONITORING	➡	**Z51.81**	Encounter for therapeutic drug level monitoring
V58.89	ENCOUNTER FOR OTHER SPECIFIED AFTERCARE **(Continued on next page)**		**SØØ.ØØXD** **SØØ.Ø1XD** **SØØ.Ø2XD** **SØØ.Ø3XD** **SØØ.Ø4XD** **SØØ.Ø5XD** **SØØ.Ø6XD** **SØØ.Ø7XD** **SØØ.1ØXD** **SØØ.11XD** **SØØ.12XD** **SØØ.2Ø1D** **SØØ.2Ø2D** **SØØ.2Ø9D** **SØØ.211D** **SØØ.212D**	Unspecified superficial injury of scalp, subs encntr Abrasion of scalp, subsequent encounter Blister (nonthermal) of scalp, subsequent encounter Contusion of scalp, subsequent encounter External constriction of part of scalp, subsequent encounter Superficial foreign body of scalp, subsequent encounter Insect bite (nonvenomous) of scalp, subsequent encounter Other superficial bite of scalp, subsequent encounter Contusion of unsp eyelid and periocular area, subs encntr Contusion of right eyelid and periocular area, subs encntr Contusion of left eyelid and periocular area, subs encntr Unsp superfic inj right eyelid and periocułr area, subs Unsp superfic injury of left eyelid and periocułr area, subs Unsp superfic injury of unsp eyelid and periocułr area, subs Abrasion of right eyelid and periocular area, subs encntr Abrasion of left eyelid and periocular area, subs encntr

ICD-9-CM		ICD-10-CM	
V58.89	ENCOUNTER FOR OTHER SPECIFIED AFTERCARE **(Continued)**	**S00.219D**	Abrasion of unsp eyelid and periocular area, subs encntr
		S00.221D	Blister of right eyelid and periocular area, subs
		S00.222D	Blister of left eyelid and periocular area, subs
		S00.229D	Blister of unsp eyelid and periocular area, subs
		S00.241D	External constrict of right eyelid and periocular area, subs
		S00.242D	External constrict of left eyelid and periocular area, subs
		S00.249D	External constrict of unsp eyelid and periocular area, subs
		S00.251D	Superficial fb of right eyelid and periocular area, subs
		S00.252D	Superficial fb of left eyelid and periocular area, subs
		S00.259D	Superficial fb of unsp eyelid and periocular area, subs
		S00.261D	Insect bite of right eyelid and periocular area, subs
		S00.262D	Insect bite of left eyelid and periocular area, subs
		S00.269D	Insect bite of unsp eyelid and periocular area, subs
		S00.271D	Oth superfic bite of right eyelid and periocular area, subs
		S00.272D	Oth superfic bite of left eyelid and periocular area, subs
		S00.279D	Oth superfic bite of unsp eyelid and periocular area, subs
		S00.30XD	Unspecified superficial injury of nose, subsequent encounter
		S00.31XD	Abrasion of nose, subsequent encounter
		S00.32XD	Blister (nonthermal) of nose, subsequent encounter
		S00.33XD	Contusion of nose, subsequent encounter
		S00.34XD	External constriction of nose, subsequent encounter
		S00.35XD	Superficial foreign body of nose, subsequent encounter
		S00.36XD	Insect bite (nonvenomous) of nose, subsequent encounter
		S00.37XD	Other superficial bite of nose, subsequent encounter
		S00.401D	Unspecified superficial injury of right ear, subs encntr
		S00.402D	Unspecified superficial injury of left ear, subs encntr
		S00.409D	Unsp superficial injury of unspecified ear, subs encntr
		S00.411D	Abrasion of right ear, subsequent encounter
		S00.412D	Abrasion of left ear, subsequent encounter
		S00.419D	Abrasion of unspecified ear, subsequent encounter
		S00.421D	Blister (nonthermal) of right ear, subsequent encounter
		S00.422D	Blister (nonthermal) of left ear, subsequent encounter
		S00.429D	Blister (nonthermal) of unspecified ear, subs encntr
		S00.431D	Contusion of right ear, subsequent encounter
		S00.432D	Contusion of left ear, subsequent encounter
		S00.439D	Contusion of unspecified ear, subsequent encounter
		S00.441D	External constriction of right ear, subsequent encounter
		S00.442D	External constriction of left ear, subsequent encounter
		S00.449D	External constriction of unspecified ear, subs encntr
		S00.451D	Superficial foreign body of right ear, subsequent encounter
		S00.452D	Superficial foreign body of left ear, subsequent encounter
		S00.459D	Superficial foreign body of unspecified ear, subs encntr
		S00.461D	Insect bite (nonvenomous) of right ear, subsequent encounter
		S00.462D	Insect bite (nonvenomous) of left ear, subsequent encounter
		S00.469D	Insect bite (nonvenomous) of unspecified ear, subs encntr
		S00.471D	Other superficial bite of right ear, subsequent encounter
		S00.472D	Other superficial bite of left ear, subsequent encounter
		S00.479D	Other superficial bite of unspecified ear, subs encntr
		S00.501D	Unspecified superficial injury of lip, subsequent encounter
		S00.502D	Unspecified superficial injury of oral cavity, subs encntr
		S00.511D	Abrasion of lip, subsequent encounter
		S00.512D	Abrasion of oral cavity, subsequent encounter
		S00.521D	Blister (nonthermal) of lip, subsequent encounter
		S00.522D	Blister (nonthermal) of oral cavity, subsequent encounter
		S00.531D	Contusion of lip, subsequent encounter
		S00.532D	Contusion of oral cavity, subsequent encounter
		S00.541D	External constriction of lip, subsequent encounter
		S00.542D	External constriction of oral cavity, subsequent encounter
		S00.551D	Superficial foreign body of lip, subsequent encounter
		S00.552D	Superficial foreign body of oral cavity, subs encntr
		S00.561D	Insect bite (nonvenomous) of lip, subsequent encounter
		S00.562D	Insect bite (nonvenomous) of oral cavity, subs encntr
		S00.571D	Other superficial bite of lip, subsequent encounter
		S00.572D	Other superficial bite of oral cavity, subsequent encounter
		S00.80XD	Unsp superficial injury of other part of head, subs encntr
		S00.81XD	Abrasion of other part of head, subsequent encounter
		S00.82XD	Blister (nonthermal) of other part of head, subs encntr
		S00.83XD	Contusion of other part of head, subsequent encounter
		S00.84XD	External constriction of other part of head, subs encntr
		S00.85XD	Superficial foreign body of other part of head, subs encntr
		S00.86XD	Insect bite (nonvenomous) of other part of head, subs encntr
		S00.87XD	Other superficial bite of other part of head, subs encntr
		S00.90XD	Unsp superficial injury of unsp part of head, subs encntr
		S00.91XD	Abrasion of unspecified part of head, subsequent encounter
		S00.92XD	Blister (nonthermal) of unsp part of head, subs encntr
		S00.93XD	Contusion of unspecified part of head, subsequent encounter
		S00.94XD	External constriction of unsp part of head, subs encntr
		S00.95XD	Superficial foreign body of unsp part of head, subs encntr
		S00.96XD	Insect bite (nonvenomous) of unsp part of head, subs encntr
		S00.97XD	Other superficial bite of unsp part of head, subs encntr
		S01.00XD	Unspecified open wound of scalp, subsequent encounter
		S01.01XD	Laceration without foreign body of scalp, subs encntr
	(Continued on next page)	**S01.02XD**	Laceration with foreign body of scalp, subsequent encounter

ICD-9-CM		ICD-10-CM	
V58.89	ENCOUNTER FOR OTHER SPECIFIED AFTERCARE **(Continued)**	**S01.03XD**	Puncture wound without foreign body of scalp, subs encntr
		S01.04XD	Puncture wound with foreign body of scalp, subs encntr
		S01.05XD	Open bite of scalp, subsequent encounter
		S01.101D	Unsp open wound of right eyelid and periocular area, subs
		S01.102D	Unsp open wound of left eyelid and periocular area, subs
		S01.109D	Unsp open wound of unsp eyelid and periocular area, subs
		S01.111D	Laceration w/o fb of right eyelid and periocular area, subs
		S01.112D	Laceration w/o fb of left eyelid and periocular area, subs
		S01.119D	Laceration w/o fb of unsp eyelid and periocular area, subs
		S01.121D	Laceration w fb of right eyelid and periocular area, subs
		S01.122D	Laceration w fb of left eyelid and periocular area, subs
		S01.129D	Laceration w fb of unsp eyelid and periocular area, subs
		S01.131D	Pnctr w/o fb of right eyelid and periocular area, subs
		S01.132D	Pnctr w/o fb of left eyelid and periocular area, subs
		S01.139D	Pnctr w/o fb of unsp eyelid and periocular area, subs
		S01.141D	Pnctr w fb of right eyelid and periocular area, subs
		S01.142D	Pnctr w fb of left eyelid and periocular area, subs
		S01.149D	Pnctr w fb of unsp eyelid and periocular area, subs
		S01.151D	Open bite of right eyelid and periocular area, subs encntr
		S01.152D	Open bite of left eyelid and periocular area, subs encntr
		S01.159D	Open bite of unsp eyelid and periocular area, subs encntr
		S01.20XD	Unspecified open wound of nose, subsequent encounter
		S01.21XD	Laceration without foreign body of nose, subs encntr
		S01.22XD	Laceration with foreign body of nose, subsequent encounter
		S01.23XD	Puncture wound without foreign body of nose, subs encntr
		S01.24XD	Puncture wound with foreign body of nose, subs encntr
		S01.25XD	Open bite of nose, subsequent encounter
		S01.301D	Unspecified open wound of right ear, subsequent encounter
		S01.302D	Unspecified open wound of left ear, subsequent encounter
		S01.309D	Unspecified open wound of unspecified ear, subs encntr
		S01.311D	Laceration without foreign body of right ear, subs encntr
		S01.312D	Laceration without foreign body of left ear, subs encntr
		S01.319D	Laceration without foreign body of unsp ear, subs encntr
		S01.321D	Laceration with foreign body of right ear, subs encntr
		S01.322D	Laceration with foreign body of left ear, subs encntr
		S01.329D	Laceration with foreign body of unspecified ear, subs encntr
		S01.331D	Puncture wound w/o foreign body of right ear, subs encntr
		S01.332D	Puncture wound without foreign body of left ear, subs encntr
		S01.339D	Puncture wound without foreign body of unsp ear, subs encntr
		S01.341D	Puncture wound with foreign body of right ear, subs encntr
		S01.342D	Puncture wound with foreign body of left ear, subs encntr
		S01.349D	Puncture wound with foreign body of unsp ear, subs encntr
		S01.351D	Open bite of right ear, subsequent encounter
		S01.352D	Open bite of left ear, subsequent encounter
		S01.359D	Open bite of unspecified ear, subsequent encounter
		S01.401D	Unsp open wound of right cheek and TMJ area, subs
		S01.402D	Unsp open wound of left cheek and TMJ area, subs
		S01.409D	Unsp open wound of unsp cheek and TMJ area, subs
		S01.411D	Laceration w/o fb of right cheek and TMJ area, subs
		S01.412D	Laceration w/o foreign body of left cheek and TMJ area, subs
		S01.419D	Laceration w/o foreign body of unsp cheek and TMJ area, subs
		S01.421D	Laceration w foreign body of right cheek and TMJ area, subs
		S01.422D	Laceration w foreign body of left cheek and TMJ area, subs
		S01.429D	Laceration w foreign body of unsp cheek and TMJ area, subs
		S01.431D	Pnctr w/o foreign body of right cheek and TMJ area, subs
		S01.432D	Pnctr w/o foreign body of left cheek and TMJ area, subs
		S01.439D	Pnctr w/o foreign body of unsp cheek and TMJ area, subs
		S01.441D	Pnctr w foreign body of right cheek and TMJ area, subs
		S01.442D	Pnctr w foreign body of left cheek and TMJ area, subs
		S01.449D	Pnctr w foreign body of unsp cheek and TMJ area, subs
		S01.451D	Open bite of right cheek and temporomandibular area, subs
		S01.452D	Open bite of left cheek and temporomandibular area, subs
		S01.459D	Open bite of unsp cheek and temporomandibular area, subs
		S01.501D	Unspecified open wound of lip, subsequent encounter
		S01.502D	Unspecified open wound of oral cavity, subsequent encounter
		S01.511D	Laceration without foreign body of lip, subsequent encounter
		S01.512D	Laceration without foreign body of oral cavity, subs encntr
		S01.521D	Laceration with foreign body of lip, subsequent encounter
		S01.522D	Laceration with foreign body of oral cavity, subs encntr
		S01.531D	Puncture wound without foreign body of lip, subs encntr
		S01.532D	Puncture wound w/o foreign body of oral cavity, subs encntr
		S01.541D	Puncture wound with foreign body of lip, subs encntr
		S01.542D	Puncture wound with foreign body of oral cavity, subs encntr
		S01.551D	Open bite of lip, subsequent encounter
		S01.552D	Open bite of oral cavity, subsequent encounter
		S01.80XD	Unspecified open wound of other part of head, subs encntr
		S01.81XD	Laceration w/o foreign body of oth part of head, subs encntr
		S01.82XD	Laceration w foreign body of oth part of head, subs encntr
		S01.83XD	Puncture wound w/o foreign body oth prt head, subs encntr
		S01.84XD	Puncture wound w foreign body oth prt head, subs encntr
		S01.85XD	Open bite of other part of head, subsequent encounter
		S01.90XD	Unsp open wound of unspecified part of head, subs encntr
	(Continued on next page)	**S01.91XD**	Laceration w/o foreign body of unsp part of head, subs

ICD-9-CM		ICD-10-CM	
V58.89	ENCOUNTER FOR OTHER SPECIFIED AFTERCARE **(Continued)**	**S01.92XD**	Laceration w foreign body of unsp part of head, subs encntr
		S01.93XD	Puncture wound w/o foreign body of unsp part of head, subs
		S01.94XD	Puncture wound w foreign body of unsp part of head, subs
		S01.95XD	Open bite of unspecified part of head, subsequent encounter
		S03.0XXD	Dislocation of jaw, subsequent encounter
		S03.1XXD	Dislocation of septal cartilage of nose, subs encntr
		S03.2XXD	Dislocation of tooth, subsequent encounter
		S03.4XXD	Sprain of jaw, subsequent encounter
		S03.8XXD	Sprain of joints and ligaments of oth prt head, subs encntr
		S03.9XXD	Sprain of joints and ligaments of unsp parts of head, subs
		S04.011D	Injury of optic nerve, right eye, subsequent encounter
		S04.012D	Injury of optic nerve, left eye, subsequent encounter
		S04.019D	Injury of optic nerve, unspecified eye, subsequent encounter
		S04.02XD	Injury of optic chiasm, subsequent encounter
		S04.031D	Injury of optic tract and pathways, right eye, subs encntr
		S04.032D	Injury of optic tract and pathways, left eye, subs encntr
		S04.039D	Injury of optic tract and pathways, unsp eye, subs encntr
		S04.041D	Injury of visual cortex, right eye, subsequent encounter
		S04.042D	Injury of visual cortex, left eye, subsequent encounter
		S04.049D	Injury of visual cortex, unspecified eye, subs encntr
		S04.10XD	Injury of oculomotor nerve, unspecified side, subs encntr
		S04.11XD	Injury of oculomotor nerve, right side, subsequent encounter
		S04.12XD	Injury of oculomotor nerve, left side, subsequent encounter
		S04.20XD	Injury of trochlear nerve, unspecified side, subs encntr
		S04.21XD	Injury of trochlear nerve, right side, subsequent encounter
		S04.22XD	Injury of trochlear nerve, left side, subsequent encounter
		S04.30XD	Injury of trigeminal nerve, unspecified side, subs encntr
		S04.31XD	Injury of trigeminal nerve, right side, subsequent encounter
		S04.32XD	Injury of trigeminal nerve, left side, subsequent encounter
		S04.40XD	Injury of abducent nerve, unspecified side, subs encntr
		S04.41XD	Injury of abducent nerve, right side, subsequent encounter
		S04.42XD	Injury of abducent nerve, left side, subsequent encounter
		S04.50XD	Injury of facial nerve, unspecified side, subs encntr
		S04.51XD	Injury of facial nerve, right side, subsequent encounter
		S04.52XD	Injury of facial nerve, left side, subsequent encounter
		S04.60XD	Injury of acoustic nerve, unspecified side, subs encntr
		S04.61XD	Injury of acoustic nerve, right side, subsequent encounter
		S04.62XD	Injury of acoustic nerve, left side, subsequent encounter
		S04.70XD	Injury of accessory nerve, unspecified side, subs encntr
		S04.71XD	Injury of accessory nerve, right side, subsequent encounter
		S04.72XD	Injury of accessory nerve, left side, subsequent encounter
		S04.811D	Injury of olfactory nerve, right side, subsequent encounter
		S04.812D	Injury of olfactory nerve, left side, subsequent encounter
		S04.819D	Injury of olfactory nerve, unspecified side, subs encntr
		S04.891D	Injury of other cranial nerves, right side, subs encntr
		S04.892D	Injury of other cranial nerves, left side, subs encntr
		S04.899D	Injury of other cranial nerves, unsp side, subs encntr
		S04.9XXD	Injury of unspecified cranial nerve, subsequent encounter
		S05.00XD	Inj conjunctiva and corneal abrasion w/o fb, unsp eye, subs
		S05.01XD	Inj conjunctiva and corneal abrasion w/o fb, right eye, subs
		S05.02XD	Inj conjunctiva and corneal abrasion w/o fb, left eye, subs
		S05.10XD	Contusion of eyeball and orbital tissues, unsp eye, subs
		S05.11XD	Contusion of eyeball and orbital tissues, right eye, subs
		S05.12XD	Contusion of eyeball and orbital tissues, left eye, subs
		S05.20XD	Oclr lac/rupt w prolaps/loss of intraoc tiss, unsp eye, subs
		S05.21XD	Oclr lac/rupt w prolaps/loss of intraoc tissue, r eye, subs
		S05.22XD	Oclr lac/rupt w prolaps/loss of intraoc tissue, l eye, subs
		S05.30XD	Oclr lac w/o prolaps/loss of intraoc tissue, unsp eye, subs
		S05.31XD	Ocular lac w/o prolaps/loss of intraoc tissue, r eye, subs
		S05.32XD	Ocular lac w/o prolaps/loss of intraoc tissue, l eye, subs
		S05.40XD	Penetrating wound of orbit w or w/o fb, unsp eye, subs
		S05.41XD	Penetrating wound of orbit w or w/o fb, right eye, subs
		S05.42XD	Penetrating wound of orbit w or w/o fb, left eye, subs
		S05.50XD	Penetrating wound w foreign body of unsp eyeball, subs
		S05.51XD	Penetrating wound w foreign body of right eyeball, subs
		S05.52XD	Penetrating wound w foreign body of left eyeball, subs
		S05.60XD	Penetrating wound w/o foreign body of unsp eyeball, subs
		S05.61XD	Penetrating wound w/o foreign body of right eyeball, subs
		S05.62XD	Penetrating wound w/o foreign body of left eyeball, subs
		S05.70XD	Avulsion of unspecified eye, subsequent encounter
		S05.71XD	Avulsion of right eye, subsequent encounter
		S05.72XD	Avulsion of left eye, subsequent encounter
		S05.8X1D	Other injuries of right eye and orbit, subsequent encounter
		S05.8X2D	Other injuries of left eye and orbit, subsequent encounter
		S05.8X9D	Other injuries of unspecified eye and orbit, subs encntr
		S05.90XD	Unspecified injury of unspecified eye and orbit, subs encntr
		S05.91XD	Unspecified injury of right eye and orbit, subs encntr
		S05.92XD	Unspecified injury of left eye and orbit, subs encntr
		S06.0X0D	Concussion without loss of consciousness, subs encntr
		S06.0X1D	Concussion w LOC of 30 minutes or less, subs
		S06.0X2D	Concussion w loss of consciousness of 31-59 min, subs
		S06.0X3D	Concussion w loss of consciousness of 1-5 hrs 59 min, subs
	(Continued on next page)	**S06.0X4D**	Concussion w LOC of 6 hours to 24 hours, subs

ICD-9-CM		ICD-10-CM	
V58.89	ENCOUNTER FOR OTHER SPECIFIED AFTERCARE **(Continued)**	**SØ6.ØX5D**	Concussion w LOC >24 hr w ret consc lev, subs
		SØ6.ØX6D	Concussion w LOC >24 hr w/o ret consc w surv, subs
		SØ6.ØX7D	Concussion w LOC w death due to brain injury bf consc, subs
		SØ6.ØX8D	Concussion w LOC w death due to oth cause bf consc, subs
		SØ6.ØX9D	Concussion w loss of consciousness of unsp duration, subs
		SØ6.1XØD	Traumatic cerebral edema w/o loss of consciousness, subs
		SØ6.1X1D	Traumatic cerebral edema w LOC of 30 minutes or less, subs
		SØ6.1X2D	Traumatic cerebral edema w LOC of 31-59 min, subs
		SØ6.1X3D	Traumatic cerebral edema w LOC of 1-5 hrs 59 min, subs
		SØ6.1X4D	Traumatic cerebral edema w LOC of 6 hours to 24 hours, subs
		SØ6.1X5D	Traumatic cerebral edema w LOC >24 hr w ret consc lev, subs
		SØ6.1X6D	Traum cerebral edema w LOC >24 hr w/o ret consc w surv, subs
		SØ6.1X7D	Traum cereb edema w LOC w death d/t brain inj bf consc, subs
		SØ6.1X8D	Traum cereb edema w LOC w death d/t oth cause bf consc, subs
		SØ6.1X9D	Traumatic cerebral edema w LOC of unsp duration, subs
		SØ6.2XØD	Diffuse TBI w/o loss of consciousness, subs
		SØ6.2X1D	Diffuse TBI w LOC of 30 minutes or less, subs
		SØ6.2X2D	Diffuse TBI w loss of consciousness of 31-59 min, subs
		SØ6.2X3D	Diffuse TBI w loss of consciousness of 1-5 hrs 59 min, subs
		SØ6.2X4D	Diffuse TBI w LOC of 6 hours to 24 hours, subs
		SØ6.2X5D	Diffuse TBI w LOC >24 hr w return to conscious levels, subs
		SØ6.2X6D	Diffuse TBI w LOC >24 hr w/o ret consc w surv, subs
		SØ6.2X7D	Diffuse TBI w LOC w death due to brain injury bf consc, subs
		SØ6.2X8D	Diffuse TBI w LOC w death due to oth cause bf consc, subs
		SØ6.2X9D	Diffuse TBI w loss of consciousness of unsp duration, subs
		SØ6.3ØØD	Unsp focal TBI w/o loss of consciousness, subs
		SØ6.3Ø1D	Unsp focal TBI w LOC of 30 minutes or less, subs
		SØ6.3Ø2D	Unsp focal TBI w loss of consciousness of 31-59 min, subs
		SØ6.3Ø3D	Unsp focal TBI w LOC of 1-5 hrs 59 min, subs
		SØ6.3Ø4D	Unsp focal TBI w LOC of 6 hours to 24 hours, subs
		SØ6.3Ø5D	Unsp focal TBI w LOC >24 hr w ret consc lev, subs
		SØ6.3Ø6D	Unsp focal TBI w LOC >24 hr w/o ret consc w surv, subs
		SØ6.3Ø7D	Unsp focal TBI w LOC w death d/t brain injury bf consc, subs
		SØ6.3Ø8D	Unsp focal TBI w LOC w death due to oth cause bf consc, subs
		SØ6.3Ø9D	Unsp focal TBI w LOC of unsp duration, subs
		SØ6.31ØD	Contus/lac right cerebrum w/o loss of consciousness, subs
		SØ6.311D	Contus/lac right cerebrum w LOC of 30 minutes or less, subs
		SØ6.312D	Contus/lac right cerebrum w LOC of 31-59 min, subs
		SØ6.313D	Contus/lac right cerebrum w LOC of 1-5 hrs 59 min, subs
		SØ6.314D	Contus/lac right cerebrum w LOC of 6 hours to 24 hours, subs
		SØ6.315D	Contus/lac right cerebrum w LOC >24 hr w ret consc lev, subs
		SØ6.316D	Contus/lac r cereb w LOC >24 hr w/o ret consc w surv, subs
		SØ6.317D	Contus/lac r cereb w LOC w dth d/t brain inj bf consc, subs
		SØ6.318D	Contus/lac r cereb w LOC w dth d/t oth cause bf consc, subs
		SØ6.319D	Contus/lac right cerebrum w LOC of unsp duration, subs
		SØ6.32ØD	Contus/lac left cerebrum w/o loss of consciousness, subs
		SØ6.321D	Contus/lac left cerebrum w LOC of 30 minutes or less, subs
		SØ6.322D	Contus/lac left cerebrum w LOC of 31-59 min, subs
		SØ6.323D	Contus/lac left cerebrum w LOC of 1-5 hrs 59 min, subs
		SØ6.324D	Contus/lac left cerebrum w LOC of 6 hours to 24 hours, subs
		SØ6.325D	Contus/lac left cerebrum w LOC >24 hr w ret consc lev, subs
		SØ6.326D	Contus/lac l cereb w LOC >24 hr w/o ret consc w surv, subs
		SØ6.327D	Contus/lac l cereb w LOC w dth d/t brain inj bf consc, subs
		SØ6.328D	Contus/lac l cereb w LOC w dth d/t oth cause bf consc, subs
		SØ6.329D	Contus/lac left cerebrum w LOC of unsp duration, subs
		SØ6.33ØD	Contus/lac cereb, w/o loss of consciousness, subs
		SØ6.331D	Contus/lac cereb, w LOC of 30 minutes or less, subs
		SØ6.332D	Contus/lac cereb, w loss of consciousness of 31-59 min, subs
		SØ6.333D	Contus/lac cereb, w LOC of 1-5 hrs 59 min, subs
		SØ6.334D	Contus/lac cereb, w LOC of 6 hours to 24 hours, subs
		SØ6.335D	Contus/lac cereb, w LOC >24 hr w ret consc lev, subs
		SØ6.336D	Contus/lac cereb, w LOC >24 hr w/o ret consc w surv, subs
		SØ6.337D	Contus/lac cereb, w LOC w death d/t brain inj bf consc, subs
		SØ6.338D	Contus/lac cereb, w LOC w death d/t oth cause bf consc, subs
		SØ6.339D	Contus/lac cereb, w LOC of unsp duration, subs
		SØ6.34ØD	Traum hemor right cerebrum w/o loss of consciousness, subs
		SØ6.341D	Traum hemor right cerebrum w LOC of 30 minutes or less, subs
		SØ6.342D	Traum hemor right cerebrum w LOC of 31-59 min, subs
		SØ6.343D	Traum hemor right cerebrum w LOC of 1-5 hrs 59 minutes, subs
		SØ6.344D	Traum hemor right cerebrum w LOC of 6-24 hrs, subs
		SØ6.345D	Traum hemor r cereb w LOC >24 hr w ret consc lev, subs
		SØ6.346D	Traum hemor r cereb w LOC >24 hr w/o ret consc w surv, subs
		SØ6.347D	Traum hemor r cereb w LOC w dth d/t brain inj bf consc, subs
		SØ6.348D	Traum hemor r cereb w LOC w dth d/t oth cause bf consc, subs
		SØ6.349D	Traum hemor right cerebrum w LOC of unsp duration, subs
		SØ6.35ØD	Traum hemor left cerebrum w/o loss of consciousness, subs
		SØ6.351D	Traum hemor left cerebrum w LOC of 30 minutes or less, subs
		SØ6.352D	Traum hemor left cerebrum w LOC of 31-59 min, subs
		SØ6.353D	Traum hemor left cerebrum w LOC of 1-5 hrs 59 minutes, subs
		SØ6.354D	Traum hemor left cerebrum w LOC of 6 hours to 24 hours, subs
		SØ6.355D	Traum hemor left cerebrum w LOC >24 hr w ret consc lev, subs
		SØ6.356D	Traum hemor l cereb w LOC >24 hr w/o ret consc w surv, subs
	(Continued on next page)	**SØ6.357D**	Traum hemor l cereb w LOC w dth d/t brain inj bf consc, subs

ICD-9-CM		ICD-10-CM	
V58.89	ENCOUNTER FOR OTHER SPECIFIED AFTERCARE **(Continued)**	**S06.358D**	Traum hemor l cereb w LOC w dth d/t oth cause bf consc, subs
		S06.359D	Traum hemor left cerebrum w LOC of unsp duration, subs
		S06.360D	Traum hemor cereb, w/o loss of consciousness, subs
		S06.361D	Traum hemor cereb, w LOC of 30 minutes or less, subs
		S06.362D	Traum hemor cereb, w LOC of 31-59 min, subs
		S06.363D	Traum hemor cereb, w LOC of 1-5 hrs 59 minutes, subs
		S06.364D	Traum hemor cereb, w LOC of 6 hours to 24 hours, subs
		S06.365D	Traum hemor cereb, w LOC >24 hr w ret consc lev, subs
		S06.366D	Traum hemor cereb, w LOC >24 hr w/o ret consc w surv, subs
		S06.367D	Traum hemor cereb, w LOC w dth d/t brain inj bf consc, subs
		S06.368D	Traum hemor cereb, w LOC w dth d/t oth cause bf consc, subs
		S06.369D	Traum hemor cereb, w LOC of unsp duration, subs
		S06.370D	Contus/lac/hem crblm w/o loss of consciousness, subs
		S06.371D	Contus/lac/hem crblm w LOC of 30 minutes or less, subs
		S06.372D	Contus/lac/hem crblm w LOC of 31-59 min, subs
		S06.373D	Contus/lac/hem crblm w LOC of 1-5 hrs 59 min, subs
		S06.374D	Contus/lac/hem crblm w LOC of 6 hours to 24 hours, subs
		S06.375D	Contus/lac/hem crblm w LOC >24 hr w ret consc lev, subs
		S06.376D	Contus/lac/hem crblm w LOC >24 hr w/o ret consc w surv, subs
		S06.377D	Contus/lac/hem crblm w LOC w dth d/t brain inj bf consc,subs
		S06.378D	Contus/lac/hem crblm w LOC w dth d/t oth cause bf consc,subs
		S06.379D	Contus/lac/hem crblm w LOC of unsp duration, subs
		S06.380D	Contus/lac/hem brainstem w/o loss of consciousness, subs
		S06.381D	Contus/lac/hem brainstem w LOC of 30 minutes or less, subs
		S06.382D	Contus/lac/hem brainstem w LOC of 31-59 min, subs
		S06.383D	Contus/lac/hem brainstem w LOC of 1-5 hrs 59 min, subs
		S06.384D	Contus/lac/hem brainstem w LOC of 6 hours to 24 hours, subs
		S06.385D	Contus/lac/hem brainstem w LOC >24 hr w ret consc lev, subs
		S06.386D	Contus/lac/hem brnst w LOC >24 hr w/o ret consc w surv, subs
		S06.387D	Contus/lac/hem brnst w LOC w dth d/t brain inj bf consc,subs
		S06.388D	Contus/lac/hem brnst w LOC w dth d/t oth cause bf consc,subs
		S06.389D	Contus/lac/hem brainstem w LOC of unsp duration, subs
		S06.4X0D	Epidural hemorrhage w/o loss of consciousness, subs encntr
		S06.4X1D	Epidural hemorrhage w LOC of 30 minutes or less, subs
		S06.4X2D	Epidural hemorrhage w LOC of 31-59 min, subs
		S06.4X3D	Epidural hemorrhage w LOC of 1-5 hrs 59 min, subs
		S06.4X4D	Epidural hemorrhage w LOC of 6 hours to 24 hours, subs
		S06.4X5D	Epidural hemorrhage w LOC >24 hr w ret consc lev, subs
		S06.4X6D	Epidural hemorrhage w LOC >24 hr w/o ret consc w surv, subs
		S06.4X7D	Epidur hemor w LOC w death d/t brain injury bf consc, subs
		S06.4X8D	Epidur hemor w LOC w death due to oth causes bf consc, subs
		S06.4X9D	Epidural hemorrhage w LOC of unsp duration, subs
		S06.5X0D	Traum subdr hem w/o loss of consciousness, subs
		S06.5X1D	Traum subdr hem w LOC of 30 minutes or less, subs
		S06.5X2D	Traum subdr hem w loss of consciousness of 31-59 min, subs
		S06.5X3D	Traum subdr hem w LOC of 1-5 hrs 59 min, subs
		S06.5X4D	Traum subdr hem w LOC of 6 hours to 24 hours, subs
		S06.5X5D	Traum subdr hem w LOC >24 hr w ret consc lev, subs
		S06.5X6D	Traum subdr hem w LOC >24 hr w/o ret consc w surv, subs
		S06.5X7D	Traum subdr hem w LOC w dth d/t brain inj bef reg consc,subs
		S06.5X8D	Traum subdr hem w LOC w dth d/t oth cause bef reg consc,subs
		S06.5X9D	Traum subdr hem w LOC of unsp duration, subs
		S06.6X0D	Traum subrac hem w/o loss of consciousness, subs
		S06.6X1D	Traum subrac hem w LOC of 30 minutes or less, subs
		S06.6X2D	Traum subrac hem w loss of consciousness of 31-59 min, subs
		S06.6X3D	Traum subrac hem w LOC of 1-5 hrs 59 min, subs
		S06.6X4D	Traum subrac hem w LOC of 6 hours to 24 hours, subs
		S06.6X5D	Traum subrac hem w LOC >24 hr w ret consc lev, subs
		S06.6X6D	Traum subrac hem w LOC >24 hr w/o ret consc w surv, subs
		S06.6X7D	Traum subrac hem w LOC w death d/t brain inj bf consc, subs
		S06.6X8D	Traum subrac hem w LOC w death d/t oth cause bf consc, subs
		S06.6X9D	Traum subrac hem w LOC of unsp duration, subs
		S06.810D	Injury of r int carotid, intcr w/o LOC, subs
		S06.811D	Inj r int carotid, intcr w LOC of 30 minutes or less, subs
		S06.812D	Injury of r int carotid, intcr w LOC of 31-59 min, subs
		S06.813D	Injury of r int carotid, intcr w LOC of 1-5 hrs 59 min, subs
		S06.814D	Injury of r int carotid, intcr w LOC of 6-24 hrs, subs
		S06.815D	Inj r int carotid, intcr w LOC >24 hr w ret consc lev, subs
		S06.816D	Inj r int crtd,intcr w LOC >24 hr w/o ret consc w surv, subs
		S06.817D	Inj r int crtd,intcr w LOC w dth d/t brain inj bf consc,subs
		S06.818D	Inj r int crtd,intcr w LOC w dth d/t oth cause bf consc,subs
		S06.819D	Injury of r int carotid, intcr w LOC of unsp duration, subs
		S06.820D	Injury of l int carotid, intcr w/o LOC, subs
		S06.821D	Inj l int carotid, intcr w LOC of 30 minutes or less, subs
		S06.822D	Injury of l int carotid, intcr w LOC of 31-59 min, subs
		S06.823D	Injury of l int carotid, intcr w LOC of 1-5 hrs 59 min, subs
		S06.824D	Injury of l int carotid, intcr w LOC of 6-24 hrs, subs
		S06.825D	Inj l int carotid, intcr w LOC >24 hr w ret consc lev, subs
		S06.826D	Inj l int crtd,intcr w LOC >24 hr w/o ret consc w surv, subs
		S06.827D	Inj l int crtd,intcr w LOC w dth d/t brain inj bf consc,subs
		S06.828D	Inj l int crtd,intcr w LOC w dth d/t oth cause bf consc,subs
		S06.829D	Injury of l int carotid, intcr w LOC of unsp duration, subs
	(Continued on next page)	**S06.890D**	Intcran inj w/o loss of consciousness, subs encntr

ICD-9-CM		ICD-10-CM	
V58.89	ENCOUNTER FOR OTHER SPECIFIED AFTERCARE **(Continued)**	**S06.891D**	Intcran inj w LOC of 30 minutes or less, subs
		S06.892D	Intcran inj w loss of consciousness of 31-59 min, subs
		S06.893D	Intcran inj w loss of consciousness of 1-5 hrs 59 min, subs
		S06.894D	Intcran inj w LOC of 6 hours to 24 hours, subs
		S06.895D	Intcran inj w LOC >24 hr w ret consc lev, subs
		S06.896D	Intcran inj w LOC >24 hr w/o ret consc w surv, subs
		S06.897D	Intcran inj w LOC w death due to brain injury bf consc, subs
		S06.898D	Intcran inj w LOC w death due to oth cause bf consc, subs
		S06.899D	Intcran inj w loss of consciousness of unsp duration, subs
		S06.9X0D	Unsp intracranial injury w/o loss of consciousness, subs
		S06.9X1D	Unsp intracranial injury w LOC of 30 minutes or less, subs
		S06.9X2D	Unsp intracranial injury w LOC of 31-59 min, subs
		S06.9X3D	Unsp intracranial injury w LOC of 1-5 hrs 59 min, subs
		S06.9X4D	Unsp intracranial injury w LOC of 6 hours to 24 hours, subs
		S06.9X5D	Unsp intracranial injury w LOC >24 hr w ret consc lev, subs
		S06.9X6D	Unsp intcrn injury w LOC >24 hr w/o ret consc w surv, subs
		S06.9X7D	Unsp intcrn inj w LOC w death d/t brain inj bf consc, subs
		S06.9X8D	Unsp intcrn inj w LOC w death d/t oth cause bf consc, subs
		S06.9X9D	Unsp intracranial injury w LOC of unsp duration, subs
		S07.0XXD	Crushing injury of face, subsequent encounter
		S07.1XXD	Crushing injury of skull, subsequent encounter
		S07.8XXD	Crushing injury of other parts of head, subsequent encounter
		S07.9XXD	Crushing injury of head, part unspecified, subs encntr
		S08.0XXD	Avulsion of scalp, subsequent encounter
		S08.111D	Complete traumatic amputation of right ear, subs encntr
		S08.112D	Complete traumatic amputation of left ear, subs encntr
		S08.119D	Complete traumatic amputation of unsp ear, subs encntr
		S08.121D	Partial traumatic amputation of right ear, subs encntr
		S08.122D	Partial traumatic amputation of left ear, subs encntr
		S08.129D	Partial traumatic amputation of unspecified ear, subs encntr
		S08.811D	Complete traumatic amputation of nose, subsequent encounter
		S08.812D	Partial traumatic amputation of nose, subsequent encounter
		S08.89XD	Traumatic amputation of other parts of head, subs encntr
		S09.0XXD	Injury of blood vessels of head, NEC, subs
		S09.10XD	Unspecified injury of muscle and tendon of head, subs encntr
		S09.11XD	Strain of muscle and tendon of head, subsequent encounter
		S09.12XD	Laceration of muscle and tendon of head, subs encntr
		S09.19XD	Oth injury of muscle and tendon of head, subs encntr
		S09.20XD	Traumatic rupture of unspecified ear drum, subs encntr
		S09.21XD	Traumatic rupture of right ear drum, subsequent encounter
		S09.22XD	Traumatic rupture of left ear drum, subsequent encounter
		S09.301D	Unsp injury of right middle and inner ear, subs encntr
		S09.302D	Unspecified injury of left middle and inner ear, subs encntr
		S09.309D	Unsp injury of unspecified middle and inner ear, subs encntr
		S09.311D	Primary blast injury of right ear, subsequent encounter
		S09.312D	Primary blast injury of left ear, subsequent encounter
		S09.313D	Primary blast injury of ear, bilateral, subsequent encounter
		S09.319D	Primary blast injury of unspecified ear, subs encntr
		S09.391D	Oth injury of right middle and inner ear, subs encntr
		S09.392D	Oth injury of left middle and inner ear, subs encntr
		S09.399D	Oth injury of unspecified middle and inner ear, subs encntr
		S09.8XXD	Other specified injuries of head, subsequent encounter
		S09.90XD	Unspecified injury of head, subsequent encounter
		S09.91XD	Unspecified injury of ear, subsequent encounter
		S09.92XD	Unspecified injury of nose, subsequent encounter
		S09.93XD	Unspecified injury of face, subsequent encounter
		S10.0XXD	Contusion of throat, subsequent encounter
		S10.10XD	Unspecified superficial injuries of throat, subs encntr
		S10.11XD	Abrasion of throat, subsequent encounter
		S10.12XD	Blister (nonthermal) of throat, subsequent encounter
		S10.14XD	External constriction of part of throat, subs encntr
		S10.15XD	Superficial foreign body of throat, subsequent encounter
		S10.16XD	Insect bite (nonvenomous) of throat, subsequent encounter
		S10.17XD	Other superficial bite of throat, subsequent encounter
		S10.80XD	Unsp superficial injury of oth part of neck, subs encntr
		S10.81XD	Abrasion of other specified part of neck, subs encntr
		S10.82XD	Blister (nonthermal) of oth part of neck, subs encntr
		S10.83XD	Contusion of other specified part of neck, subs encntr
		S10.84XD	External constriction of oth part of neck, subs encntr
		S10.85XD	Superficial foreign body of oth part of neck, subs encntr
		S10.86XD	Insect bite of other specified part of neck, subs encntr
		S10.87XD	Other superficial bite of oth part of neck, subs encntr
		S10.90XD	Unsp superficial injury of unsp part of neck, subs encntr
		S10.91XD	Abrasion of unspecified part of neck, subsequent encounter
		S10.92XD	Blister (nonthermal) of unsp part of neck, subs encntr
		S10.93XD	Contusion of unspecified part of neck, subsequent encounter
		S10.94XD	External constriction of unsp part of neck, subs encntr
		S10.95XD	Superficial foreign body of unsp part of neck, subs encntr
		S10.96XD	Insect bite of unspecified part of neck, subs encntr
		S10.97XD	Other superficial bite of unsp part of neck, subs encntr
		S11.011D	Laceration without foreign body of larynx, subs encntr
		S11.012D	Laceration with foreign body of larynx, subsequent encounter
	(Continued on next page)	**S11.013D**	Puncture wound without foreign body of larynx, subs encntr

ICD-9-CM		ICD-10-CM	
V58.89	ENCOUNTER FOR OTHER SPECIFIED AFTERCARE **(Continued)**	**S11.014D**	Puncture wound with foreign body of larynx, subs encntr
		S11.015D	Open bite of larynx, subsequent encounter
		S11.019D	Unspecified open wound of larynx, subsequent encounter
		S11.021D	Laceration without foreign body of trachea, subs encntr
		S11.022D	Laceration with foreign body of trachea, subs encntr
		S11.023D	Puncture wound without foreign body of trachea, subs encntr
		S11.024D	Puncture wound with foreign body of trachea, subs encntr
		S11.025D	Open bite of trachea, subsequent encounter
		S11.029D	Unspecified open wound of trachea, subsequent encounter
		S11.031D	Laceration without foreign body of vocal cord, subs encntr
		S11.032D	Laceration with foreign body of vocal cord, subs encntr
		S11.033D	Puncture wound w/o foreign body of vocal cord, subs encntr
		S11.034D	Puncture wound with foreign body of vocal cord, subs encntr
		S11.035D	Open bite of vocal cord, subsequent encounter
		S11.039D	Unspecified open wound of vocal cord, subsequent encounter
		S11.10XD	Unspecified open wound of thyroid gland, subs encntr
		S11.11XD	Laceration w/o foreign body of thyroid gland, subs encntr
		S11.12XD	Laceration with foreign body of thyroid gland, subs encntr
		S11.13XD	Puncture wound w/o foreign body of thyroid gland, subs
		S11.14XD	Puncture wound w foreign body of thyroid gland, subs encntr
		S11.15XD	Open bite of thyroid gland, subsequent encounter
		S11.20XD	Unsp open wound of pharynx and cervical esophagus, subs
		S11.21XD	Laceration w/o fb of pharynx and cervical esophagus, subs
		S11.22XD	Laceration w fb of pharynx and cervical esophagus, subs
		S11.23XD	Pnctr w/o fb of pharynx and cervical esophagus, subs
		S11.24XD	Pnctr w foreign body of pharynx and cervical esophagus, subs
		S11.25XD	Open bite of pharynx and cervical esophagus, subs encntr
		S11.80XD	Unspecified open wound of oth part of neck, subs encntr
		S11.81XD	Laceration w/o foreign body of oth part of neck, subs encntr
		S11.82XD	Laceration w foreign body of oth part of neck, subs encntr
		S11.83XD	Puncture wound w/o foreign body oth prt neck, subs encntr
		S11.84XD	Puncture wound w foreign body oth prt neck, subs encntr
		S11.85XD	Open bite of other specified part of neck, subs encntr
		S11.89XD	Other open wound of oth part of neck, subs encntr
		S11.90XD	Unsp open wound of unspecified part of neck, subs encntr
		S11.91XD	Laceration w/o foreign body of unsp part of neck, subs
		S11.92XD	Laceration w foreign body of unsp part of neck, subs encntr
		S11.93XD	Puncture wound w/o foreign body of unsp part of neck, subs
		S11.94XD	Puncture wound w foreign body of unsp part of neck, subs
		S11.95XD	Open bite of unspecified part of neck, subsequent encounter
		S13.0XXD	Traumatic rupture of cervical intervertebral disc, subs
		S13.100D	Subluxation of unspecified cervical vertebrae, subs encntr
		S13.101D	Dislocation of unspecified cervical vertebrae, subs encntr
		S13.110D	Subluxation of C0/C1 cervical vertebrae, subs encntr
		S13.111D	Dislocation of C0/C1 cervical vertebrae, subs encntr
		S13.120D	Subluxation of C1/C2 cervical vertebrae, subs encntr
		S13.121D	Dislocation of C1/C2 cervical vertebrae, subs encntr
		S13.130D	Subluxation of C2/C3 cervical vertebrae, subs encntr
		S13.131D	Dislocation of C2/C3 cervical vertebrae, subs encntr
		S13.140D	Subluxation of C3/C4 cervical vertebrae, subs encntr
		S13.141D	Dislocation of C3/C4 cervical vertebrae, subs encntr
		S13.150D	Subluxation of C4/C5 cervical vertebrae, subs encntr
		S13.151D	Dislocation of C4/C5 cervical vertebrae, subs encntr
		S13.160D	Subluxation of C5/C6 cervical vertebrae, subs encntr
		S13.161D	Dislocation of C5/C6 cervical vertebrae, subs encntr
		S13.170D	Subluxation of C6/C7 cervical vertebrae, subs encntr
		S13.171D	Dislocation of C6/C7 cervical vertebrae, subs encntr
		S13.180D	Subluxation of C7/T1 cervical vertebrae, subs encntr
		S13.181D	Dislocation of C7/T1 cervical vertebrae, subs encntr
		S13.20XD	Dislocation of unspecified parts of neck, subs encntr
		S13.29XD	Dislocation of other parts of neck, subsequent encounter
		S13.4XXD	Sprain of ligaments of cervical spine, subsequent encounter
		S13.5XXD	Sprain of thyroid region, subsequent encounter
		S13.8XXD	Sprain of joints and ligaments of oth prt neck, subs encntr
		S13.9XXD	Sprain of joints and ligaments of unsp parts of neck, subs
		S14.0XXD	Concussion and edema of cervical spinal cord, subs encntr
		S14.101D	Unsp injury at C1 level of cervical spinal cord, subs encntr
		S14.102D	Unsp injury at C2 level of cervical spinal cord, subs encntr
		S14.103D	Unsp injury at C3 level of cervical spinal cord, subs encntr
		S14.104D	Unsp injury at C4 level of cervical spinal cord, subs encntr
		S14.105D	Unsp injury at C5 level of cervical spinal cord, subs encntr
		S14.106D	Unsp injury at C6 level of cervical spinal cord, subs encntr
		S14.107D	Unsp injury at C7 level of cervical spinal cord, subs encntr
		S14.108D	Unsp injury at C8 level of cervical spinal cord, subs encntr
		S14.109D	Unsp injury at unsp level of cervical spinal cord, subs
		S14.111D	Complete lesion at C1 level of cervical spinal cord, subs
		S14.112D	Complete lesion at C2 level of cervical spinal cord, subs
		S14.113D	Complete lesion at C3 level of cervical spinal cord, subs
		S14.114D	Complete lesion at C4 level of cervical spinal cord, subs
		S14.115D	Complete lesion at C5 level of cervical spinal cord, subs
		S14.116D	Complete lesion at C6 level of cervical spinal cord, subs
		S14.117D	Complete lesion at C7 level of cervical spinal cord, subs
		S14.118D	Complete lesion at C8 level of cervical spinal cord, subs

(Continued on next page)

ICD-9-CM		ICD-10-CM	
V58.89	ENCOUNTER FOR OTHER SPECIFIED AFTERCARE **(Continued)**	**S14.119D**	Complete lesion at unsp level of cervical spinal cord, subs
		S14.121D	Central cord syndrome at C1, subs
		S14.122D	Central cord syndrome at C2, subs
		S14.123D	Central cord syndrome at C3, subs
		S14.124D	Central cord syndrome at C4, subs
		S14.125D	Central cord syndrome at C5, subs
		S14.126D	Central cord syndrome at C6, subs
		S14.127D	Central cord syndrome at C7, subs
		S14.128D	Central cord syndrome at C8, subs
		S14.129D	Central cord synd at unsp level of cerv spinal cord, subs
		S14.131D	Anterior cord syndrome at C1, subs
		S14.132D	Anterior cord syndrome at C2, subs
		S14.133D	Anterior cord syndrome at C3, subs
		S14.134D	Anterior cord syndrome at C4, subs
		S14.135D	Anterior cord syndrome at C5, subs
		S14.136D	Anterior cord syndrome at C6, subs
		S14.137D	Anterior cord syndrome at C7, subs
		S14.138D	Anterior cord syndrome at C8, subs
		S14.139D	Ant cord syndrome at unsp level of cerv spinal cord, subs
		S14.141D	Brown-Sequard syndrome at C1, subs
		S14.142D	Brown-Sequard syndrome at C2, subs
		S14.143D	Brown-Sequard syndrome at C3, subs
		S14.144D	Brown-Sequard syndrome at C4, subs
		S14.145D	Brown-Sequard syndrome at C5, subs
		S14.146D	Brown-Sequard syndrome at C6, subs
		S14.147D	Brown-Sequard syndrome at C7, subs
		S14.148D	Brown-Sequard syndrome at C8, subs
		S14.149D	Brown-Sequard synd at unsp level of cerv spinal cord, subs
		S14.151D	Oth incomplete lesion at C1, subs
		S14.152D	Oth incomplete lesion at C2, subs
		S14.153D	Oth incomplete lesion at C3, subs
		S14.154D	Oth incomplete lesion at C4, subs
		S14.155D	Oth incomplete lesion at C5, subs
		S14.156D	Oth incomplete lesion at C6, subs
		S14.157D	Oth incomplete lesion at C7, subs
		S14.158D	Oth incomplete lesion at C8, subs
		S14.159D	Oth incmpl lesion at unsp level of cerv spinal cord, subs
		S14.2XXD	Injury of nerve root of cervical spine, subsequent encounter
		S14.3XXD	Injury of brachial plexus, subsequent encounter
		S14.4XXD	Injury of peripheral nerves of neck, subsequent encounter
		S14.5XXD	Injury of cervical sympathetic nerves, subsequent encounter
		S14.8XXD	Injury of other specified nerves of neck, subs encntr
		S14.9XXD	Injury of unspecified nerves of neck, subsequent encounter
		S15.ØØ1D	Unspecified injury of right carotid artery, subs encntr
		S15.ØØ2D	Unspecified injury of left carotid artery, subs encntr
		S15.ØØ9D	Unsp injury of unspecified carotid artery, subs encntr
		S15.Ø11D	Minor laceration of right carotid artery, subs encntr
		S15.Ø12D	Minor laceration of left carotid artery, subs encntr
		S15.Ø19D	Minor laceration of unspecified carotid artery, subs encntr
		S15.Ø21D	Major laceration of right carotid artery, subs encntr
		S15.Ø22D	Major laceration of left carotid artery, subs encntr
		S15.Ø29D	Major laceration of unspecified carotid artery, subs encntr
		S15.Ø91D	Other specified injury of right carotid artery, subs encntr
		S15.Ø92D	Other specified injury of left carotid artery, subs encntr
		S15.Ø99D	Oth injury of unspecified carotid artery, subs encntr
		S15.1Ø1D	Unspecified injury of right vertebral artery, subs encntr
		S15.1Ø2D	Unspecified injury of left vertebral artery, subs encntr
		S15.1Ø9D	Unsp injury of unspecified vertebral artery, subs encntr
		S15.111D	Minor laceration of right vertebral artery, subs encntr
		S15.112D	Minor laceration of left vertebral artery, subs encntr
		S15.119D	Minor laceration of unsp vertebral artery, subs encntr
		S15.121D	Major laceration of right vertebral artery, subs encntr
		S15.122D	Major laceration of left vertebral artery, subs encntr
		S15.129D	Major laceration of unsp vertebral artery, subs encntr
		S15.191D	Oth injury of right vertebral artery, subs encntr
		S15.192D	Other specified injury of left vertebral artery, subs encntr
		S15.199D	Oth injury of unspecified vertebral artery, subs encntr
		S15.2Ø1D	Unsp injury of right external jugular vein, subs encntr
		S15.2Ø2D	Unsp injury of left external jugular vein, subs encntr
		S15.2Ø9D	Unsp injury of unsp external jugular vein, subs encntr
		S15.211D	Minor laceration of right external jugular vein, subs encntr
		S15.212D	Minor laceration of left external jugular vein, subs encntr
		S15.219D	Minor laceration of unsp external jugular vein, subs encntr
		S15.221D	Major laceration of right external jugular vein, subs encntr
		S15.222D	Major laceration of left external jugular vein, subs encntr
		S15.229D	Major laceration of unsp external jugular vein, subs encntr
		S15.291D	Oth injury of right external jugular vein, subs encntr
		S15.292D	Oth injury of left external jugular vein, subs encntr
		S15.299D	Oth injury of unspecified external jugular vein, subs encntr
		S15.3Ø1D	Unsp injury of right internal jugular vein, subs encntr
		S15.3Ø2D	Unsp injury of left internal jugular vein, subs encntr
		S15.3Ø9D	Unsp injury of unsp internal jugular vein, subs encntr
	(Continued on next page)	**S15.311D**	Minor laceration of right internal jugular vein, subs encntr

ICD-9-CM		ICD-10-CM	
V58.89	ENCOUNTER FOR OTHER SPECIFIED AFTERCARE **(Continued)**	**S15.312D**	Minor laceration of left internal jugular vein, subs encntr
		S15.319D	Minor laceration of unsp internal jugular vein, subs encntr
		S15.321D	Major laceration of right internal jugular vein, subs encntr
		S15.322D	Major laceration of left internal jugular vein, subs encntr
		S15.329D	Major laceration of unsp internal jugular vein, subs encntr
		S15.391D	Oth injury of right internal jugular vein, subs encntr
		S15.392D	Oth injury of left internal jugular vein, subs encntr
		S15.399D	Oth injury of unspecified internal jugular vein, subs encntr
		S15.8XXD	Injury of oth blood vessels at neck level, subs encntr
		S15.9XXD	Injury of unsp blood vessel at neck level, subs encntr
		S16.1XXD	Strain of muscle, fascia and tendon at neck level, subs
		S16.2XXD	Laceration of muscle, fascia and tendon at neck level, subs
		S16.8XXD	Inj muscle, fascia and tendon at neck level, subs encntr
		S16.9XXD	Unsp injury of muscle, fascia and tendon at neck level, subs
		S17.ØXXD	Crushing injury of larynx and trachea, subsequent encounter
		S17.8XXD	Crushing injury of oth parts of neck, subs encntr
		S17.9XXD	Crushing injury of neck, part unspecified, subs encntr
		S19.8ØXD	Oth injuries of unspecified part of neck, subs encntr
		S19.81XD	Other specified injuries of larynx, subsequent encounter
		S19.82XD	Other specified injuries of cervical trachea, subs encntr
		S19.83XD	Other specified injuries of vocal cord, subsequent encounter
		S19.84XD	Other specified injuries of thyroid gland, subs encntr
		S19.85XD	Oth injuries of pharynx and cervical esophagus, subs encntr
		S19.89XD	Oth injuries of other specified part of neck, subs encntr
		S19.9XXD	Unspecified injury of neck, subsequent encounter
		S2Ø.ØØXD	Contusion of breast, unspecified breast, subs encntr
		S2Ø.Ø1XD	Contusion of right breast, subsequent encounter
		S2Ø.Ø2XD	Contusion of left breast, subsequent encounter
		S2Ø.1Ø1D	Unsp superficial injuries of breast, right breast, subs
		S2Ø.1Ø2D	Unsp superficial injuries of breast, left breast, subs
		S2Ø.1Ø9D	Unsp superficial injuries of breast, unsp breast, subs
		S2Ø.111D	Abrasion of breast, right breast, subsequent encounter
		S2Ø.112D	Abrasion of breast, left breast, subsequent encounter
		S2Ø.119D	Abrasion of breast, unspecified breast, subsequent encounter
		S2Ø.121D	Blister (nonthermal) of breast, right breast, subs encntr
		S2Ø.122D	Blister (nonthermal) of breast, left breast, subs encntr
		S2Ø.129D	Blister (nonthermal) of breast, unsp breast, subs encntr
		S2Ø.141D	External constriction of part of breast, right breast, subs
		S2Ø.142D	External constriction of part of breast, left breast, subs
		S2Ø.149D	External constriction of part of breast, unsp breast, subs
		S2Ø.151D	Superficial foreign body of breast, right breast, subs
		S2Ø.152D	Superficial foreign body of breast, left breast, subs encntr
		S2Ø.159D	Superficial foreign body of breast, unsp breast, subs encntr
		S2Ø.161D	Insect bite (nonvenomous) of breast, right breast, subs
		S2Ø.162D	Insect bite (nonvenomous) of breast, left breast, subs
		S2Ø.169D	Insect bite (nonvenomous) of breast, unsp breast, subs
		S2Ø.171D	Other superficial bite of breast, right breast, subs encntr
		S2Ø.172D	Other superficial bite of breast, left breast, subs encntr
		S2Ø.179D	Other superficial bite of breast, unsp breast, subs encntr
		S2Ø.2ØXD	Contusion of thorax, unspecified, subsequent encounter
		S2Ø.211D	Contusion of right front wall of thorax, subs encntr
		S2Ø.212D	Contusion of left front wall of thorax, subsequent encounter
		S2Ø.219D	Contusion of unspecified front wall of thorax, subs encntr
		S2Ø.221D	Contusion of right back wall of thorax, subsequent encounter
		S2Ø.222D	Contusion of left back wall of thorax, subsequent encounter
		S2Ø.229D	Contusion of unspecified back wall of thorax, subs encntr
		S2Ø.3Ø1D	Unsp superficial injuries of r frnt wl of thorax, subs
		S2Ø.3Ø2D	Unsp superficial injuries of left front wall of thorax, subs
		S2Ø.3Ø9D	Unsp superficial injuries of unsp front wall of thorax, subs
		S2Ø.311D	Abrasion of right front wall of thorax, subsequent encounter
		S2Ø.312D	Abrasion of left front wall of thorax, subsequent encounter
		S2Ø.319D	Abrasion of unspecified front wall of thorax, subs encntr
		S2Ø.321D	Blister (nonthermal) of right front wall of thorax, subs
		S2Ø.322D	Blister (nonthermal) of left front wall of thorax, subs
		S2Ø.329D	Blister (nonthermal) of unsp front wall of thorax, subs
		S2Ø.341D	External constriction of right front wall of thorax, subs
		S2Ø.342D	External constriction of left front wall of thorax, subs
		S2Ø.349D	External constriction of unsp front wall of thorax, subs
		S2Ø.351D	Superficial foreign body of right front wall of thorax, subs
		S2Ø.352D	Superficial foreign body of left front wall of thorax, subs
		S2Ø.359D	Superficial foreign body of unsp front wall of thorax, subs
		S2Ø.361D	Insect bite (nonvenomous) of r frnt wl of thorax, subs
		S2Ø.362D	Insect bite (nonvenomous) of left front wall of thorax, subs
		S2Ø.369D	Insect bite (nonvenomous) of unsp front wall of thorax, subs
		S2Ø.371D	Oth superficial bite of right front wall of thorax, subs
		S2Ø.372D	Oth superficial bite of left front wall of thorax, subs
		S2Ø.379D	Oth superficial bite of unsp front wall of thorax, subs
		S2Ø.4Ø1D	Unsp superficial injuries of right back wall of thorax, subs
		S2Ø.4Ø2D	Unsp superficial injuries of left back wall of thorax, subs
		S2Ø.4Ø9D	Unsp superficial injuries of unsp back wall of thorax, subs
		S2Ø.411D	Abrasion of right back wall of thorax, subsequent encounter
		S2Ø.412D	Abrasion of left back wall of thorax, subsequent encounter
	(Continued on next page)	**S2Ø.419D**	Abrasion of unspecified back wall of thorax, subs encntr

ICD-9-CM		ICD-10-CM	
V58.89	ENCOUNTER FOR OTHER SPECIFIED AFTERCARE **(Continued)**	**S2Ø.421D**	Blister (nonthermal) of right back wall of thorax, subs
		S2Ø.422D	Blister (nonthermal) of left back wall of thorax, subs
		S2Ø.429D	Blister (nonthermal) of unsp back wall of thorax, subs
		S2Ø.441D	External constriction of right back wall of thorax, subs
		S2Ø.442D	External constriction of left back wall of thorax, subs
		S2Ø.449D	External constriction of unsp back wall of thorax, subs
		S2Ø.451D	Superficial foreign body of right back wall of thorax, subs
		S2Ø.452D	Superficial foreign body of left back wall of thorax, subs
		S2Ø.459D	Superficial foreign body of unsp back wall of thorax, subs
		S2Ø.461D	Insect bite (nonvenomous) of right back wall of thorax, subs
		S2Ø.462D	Insect bite (nonvenomous) of left back wall of thorax, subs
		S2Ø.469D	Insect bite (nonvenomous) of unsp back wall of thorax, subs
		S2Ø.471D	Oth superficial bite of right back wall of thorax, subs
		S2Ø.472D	Oth superficial bite of left back wall of thorax, subs
		S2Ø.479D	Oth superficial bite of unsp back wall of thorax, subs
		S2Ø.9ØXD	Unsp superficial injury of unsp parts of thorax, subs encntr
		S2Ø.91XD	Abrasion of unspecified parts of thorax, subs encntr
		S2Ø.92XD	Blister (nonthermal) of unsp parts of thorax, subs encntr
		S2Ø.94XD	External constriction of unsp parts of thorax, subs encntr
		S2Ø.95XD	Superficial foreign body of unsp parts of thorax, subs
		S2Ø.96XD	Insect bite (nonvenomous) of unsp parts of thorax, subs
		S2Ø.97XD	Other superficial bite of unsp parts of thorax, subs encntr
		S21.ØØ1D	Unspecified open wound of right breast, subsequent encounter
		S21.ØØ2D	Unspecified open wound of left breast, subsequent encounter
		S21.ØØ9D	Unspecified open wound of unspecified breast, subs encntr
		S21.Ø11D	Laceration without foreign body of right breast, subs encntr
		S21.Ø12D	Laceration without foreign body of left breast, subs encntr
		S21.Ø19D	Laceration without foreign body of unsp breast, subs encntr
		S21.Ø21D	Laceration with foreign body of right breast, subs encntr
		S21.Ø22D	Laceration with foreign body of left breast, subs encntr
		S21.Ø29D	Laceration with foreign body of unsp breast, subs encntr
		S21.Ø31D	Puncture wound w/o foreign body of right breast, subs encntr
		S21.Ø32D	Puncture wound w/o foreign body of left breast, subs encntr
		S21.Ø39D	Puncture wound w/o foreign body of unsp breast, subs encntr
		S21.Ø41D	Puncture wound w foreign body of right breast, subs encntr
		S21.Ø42D	Puncture wound with foreign body of left breast, subs encntr
		S21.Ø49D	Puncture wound with foreign body of unsp breast, subs encntr
		S21.Ø51D	Open bite of right breast, subsequent encounter
		S21.Ø52D	Open bite of left breast, subsequent encounter
		S21.Ø59D	Open bite of unspecified breast, subsequent encounter
		S21.1Ø1D	Unsp opn wnd r frnt wl of thorax w/o penet thor cavity, subs
		S21.1Ø2D	Unsp opn wnd l frnt wl of thorax w/o penet thor cavity, subs
		S21.1Ø9D	Unsp opn wnd unsp frnt wall of thrx w/o penet thor cav, subs
		S21.111D	Lac w/o fb of r frnt wl of thorax w/o penet thor cav, subs
		S21.112D	Lac w/o fb of l frnt wl of thorax w/o penet thor cav, subs
		S21.119D	Lac w/o fb of unsp frnt wl of thrx w/o penet thor cav, subs
		S21.121D	Lac w fb of r frnt wl of thorax w/o penet thor cavity, subs
		S21.122D	Lac w fb of l frnt wl of thorax w/o penet thor cavity, subs
		S21.129D	Lac w fb of unsp front wall of thrx w/o penet thor cav, subs
		S21.131D	Pnctr w/o fb of r frnt wl of thorax w/o penet thor cav, subs
		S21.132D	Pnctr w/o fb of l frnt wl of thorax w/o penet thor cav, subs
		S21.139D	Pnctr w/o fb of unsp frnt wl of thrx w/o penet thor cav,subs
		S21.141D	Pnctr w fb of r frnt wl of thorax w/o penet thor cav, subs
		S21.142D	Pnctr w fb of l frnt wl of thorax w/o penet thor cav, subs
		S21.149D	Pnctr w fb of unsp frnt wl of thrx w/o penet thor cav, subs
		S21.151D	Open bite of r frnt wl of thorax w/o penet thor cavity, subs
		S21.152D	Open bite of l frnt wl of thorax w/o penet thor cavity, subs
		S21.159D	Open bite of unsp frnt wall of thrx w/o penet thor cav, subs
		S21.2Ø1D	Unsp opn wnd r bk wl of thorax w/o penet thor cavity, subs
		S21.2Ø2D	Unsp opn wnd l bk wl of thorax w/o penet thor cavity, subs
		S21.2Ø9D	Unsp opn wnd unsp bk wl of thorax w/o penet thor cav, subs
		S21.211D	Lac w/o fb of r bk wl of thorax w/o penet thor cavity, subs
		S21.212D	Lac w/o fb of l bk wl of thorax w/o penet thor cavity, subs
		S21.219D	Lac w/o fb of unsp bk wl of thorax w/o penet thor cav, subs
		S21.221D	Lac w fb of r bk wl of thorax w/o penet thor cavity, subs
		S21.222D	Lac w fb of l bk wl of thorax w/o penet thor cavity, subs
		S21.229D	Lac w fb of unsp bk wl of thorax w/o penet thor cavity, subs
		S21.231D	Pnctr w/o fb of r bk wl of thorax w/o penet thor cav, subs
		S21.232D	Pnctr w/o fb of l bk wl of thorax w/o penet thor cav, subs
		S21.239D	Pnctr w/o fb of unsp bk wl of thrx w/o penet thor cav, subs
		S21.241D	Pnctr w fb of r bk wl of thorax w/o penet thor cavity, subs
		S21.242D	Pnctr w fb of l bk wl of thorax w/o penet thor cavity, subs
		S21.249D	Pnctr w fb of unsp bk wl of thorax w/o penet thor cav, subs
		S21.251D	Open bite of r bk wl of thorax w/o penet thor cavity, subs
		S21.252D	Open bite of l bk wl of thorax w/o penet thor cavity, subs
		S21.259D	Open bite of unsp bk wl of thorax w/o penet thor cav, subs
		S21.3Ø1D	Unsp opn wnd r frnt wl of thorax w penet thor cavity, subs
		S21.3Ø2D	Unsp opn wnd l frnt wl of thorax w penet thor cavity, subs
		S21.3Ø9D	Unsp opn wnd unsp front wall of thrx w penet thor cav, subs
		S21.311D	Lac w/o fb of r frnt wl of thorax w penet thor cavity, subs
		S21.312D	Lac w/o fb of l frnt wl of thorax w penet thor cavity, subs
		S21.319D	Lac w/o fb of unsp front wall of thrx w penet thor cav, subs
		S21.321D	Lac w fb of r frnt wl of thorax w penet thor cavity, subs

(Continued on next page)

ICD-9-CM		ICD-10-CM	
V58.89	ENCOUNTER FOR OTHER SPECIFIED AFTERCARE **(Continued)**	**S21.322D**	Lac w fb of l frnt wl of thorax w penet thor cavity, subs
		S21.329D	Lac w fb of unsp front wall of thorax w penet thor cav, subs
		S21.331D	Pnctr w/o fb of r frnt wl of thorax w penet thor cav, subs
		S21.332D	Pnctr w/o fb of l frnt wl of thorax w penet thor cav, subs
		S21.339D	Pnctr w/o fb of unsp frnt wl of thrx w penet thor cav, subs
		S21.341D	Pnctr w fb of r frnt wl of thorax w penet thor cavity, subs
		S21.342D	Pnctr w fb of l frnt wl of thorax w penet thor cavity, subs
		S21.349D	Pnctr w fb of unsp front wall of thrx w penet thor cav, subs
		S21.351D	Open bite of r frnt wl of thorax w penet thor cavity, subs
		S21.352D	Open bite of l frnt wl of thorax w penet thor cavity, subs
		S21.359D	Open bite of unsp front wall of thrx w penet thor cav, subs
		S21.4Ø1D	Unsp opn wnd r bk wl of thorax w penet thoracic cavity, subs
		S21.4Ø2D	Unsp opn wnd l bk wl of thorax w penet thoracic cavity, subs
		S21.4Ø9D	Unsp opn wnd unsp bk wl of thorax w penet thor cavity, subs
		S21.411D	Lac w/o fb of r bk wl of thorax w penet thor cavity, subs
		S21.412D	Lac w/o fb of l bk wl of thorax w penet thor cavity, subs
		S21.419D	Lac w/o fb of unsp bk wl of thorax w penet thor cavity, subs
		S21.421D	Lac w fb of r bk wl of thorax w penet thoracic cavity, subs
		S21.422D	Lac w fb of l bk wl of thorax w penet thoracic cavity, subs
		S21.429D	Lac w fb of unsp bk wl of thorax w penet thor cavity, subs
		S21.431D	Pnctr w/o fb of r bk wl of thorax w penet thor cavity, subs
		S21.432D	Pnctr w/o fb of l bk wl of thorax w penet thor cavity, subs
		S21.439D	Pnctr w/o fb of unsp bk wl of thorax w penet thor cav, subs
		S21.441D	Pnctr w fb of r bk wl of thorax w penet thor cavity, subs
		S21.442D	Pnctr w fb of l bk wl of thorax w penet thor cavity, subs
		S21.449D	Pnctr w fb of unsp bk wl of thorax w penet thor cavity, subs
		S21.451D	Open bite of r bk wl of thorax w penet thoracic cavity, subs
		S21.452D	Open bite of l bk wl of thorax w penet thoracic cavity, subs
		S21.459D	Open bite of unsp bk wl of thorax w penet thor cavity, subs
		S21.9ØXD	Unsp open wound of unspecified part of thorax, subs encntr
		S21.91XD	Laceration w/o foreign body of unsp part of thorax, subs
		S21.92XD	Laceration w foreign body of unsp part of thorax, subs
		S21.93XD	Puncture wound w/o foreign body of unsp part of thorax, subs
		S21.94XD	Puncture wound w foreign body of unsp part of thorax, subs
		S21.95XD	Open bite of unspecified part of thorax, subs encntr
		S23.ØXXD	Traumatic rupture of thoracic intervertebral disc, subs
		S23.1ØØD	Subluxation of unspecified thoracic vertebra, subs encntr
		S23.1Ø1D	Dislocation of unspecified thoracic vertebra, subs encntr
		S23.11ØD	Subluxation of T1/T2 thoracic vertebra, subsequent encounter
		S23.111D	Dislocation of T1/T2 thoracic vertebra, subsequent encounter
		S23.12ØD	Subluxation of T2/T3 thoracic vertebra, subsequent encounter
		S23.121D	Dislocation of T2/T3 thoracic vertebra, subsequent encounter
		S23.122D	Subluxation of T3/T4 thoracic vertebra, subsequent encounter
		S23.123D	Dislocation of T3/T4 thoracic vertebra, subsequent encounter
		S23.13ØD	Subluxation of T4/T5 thoracic vertebra, subsequent encounter
		S23.131D	Dislocation of T4/T5 thoracic vertebra, subsequent encounter
		S23.132D	Subluxation of T5/T6 thoracic vertebra, subsequent encounter
		S23.133D	Dislocation of T5/T6 thoracic vertebra, subsequent encounter
		S23.14ØD	Subluxation of T6/T7 thoracic vertebra, subsequent encounter
		S23.141D	Dislocation of T6/T7 thoracic vertebra, subsequent encounter
		S23.142D	Subluxation of T7/T8 thoracic vertebra, subsequent encounter
		S23.143D	Dislocation of T7/T8 thoracic vertebra, subsequent encounter
		S23.15ØD	Subluxation of T8/T9 thoracic vertebra, subsequent encounter
		S23.151D	Dislocation of T8/T9 thoracic vertebra, subsequent encounter
		S23.152D	Subluxation of T9/T10 thoracic vertebra, subs encntr
		S23.153D	Dislocation of T9/T10 thoracic vertebra, subs encntr
		S23.16ØD	Subluxation of T10/T11 thoracic vertebra, subs encntr
		S23.161D	Dislocation of T10/T11 thoracic vertebra, subs encntr
		S23.162D	Subluxation of T11/T12 thoracic vertebra, subs encntr
		S23.163D	Dislocation of T11/T12 thoracic vertebra, subs encntr
		S23.17ØD	Subluxation of T12/L1 thoracic vertebra, subs encntr
		S23.171D	Dislocation of T12/L1 thoracic vertebra, subs encntr
		S23.2ØXD	Dislocation of unspecified part of thorax, subs encntr
		S23.29XD	Dislocation of other parts of thorax, subsequent encounter
		S23.3XXD	Sprain of ligaments of thoracic spine, subsequent encounter
		S23.41XD	Sprain of ribs, subsequent encounter
		S23.42ØD	Sprain of sternoclavicular (joint) (ligament), subs encntr
		S23.421D	Sprain of chondrosternal joint, subsequent encounter
		S23.428D	Other sprain of sternum, subsequent encounter
		S23.429D	Unspecified sprain of sternum, subsequent encounter
		S23.8XXD	Sprain of other specified parts of thorax, subs encntr
		S23.9XXD	Sprain of unspecified parts of thorax, subsequent encounter
		S24.ØXXD	Concussion and edema of thoracic spinal cord, subs encntr
		S24.1Ø1D	Unsp injury at T1 level of thoracic spinal cord, subs encntr
		S24.1Ø2D	Unsp injury at T2-T6 level of thoracic spinal cord, subs
		S24.1Ø3D	Unsp injury at T7-T10 level of thoracic spinal cord, subs
		S24.1Ø4D	Unsp injury at T11-T12 level of thoracic spinal cord, subs
		S24.1Ø9D	Unsp injury at unsp level of thoracic spinal cord, subs
		S24.111D	Complete lesion at T1 level of thoracic spinal cord, subs
		S24.112D	Complete lesion at T2-T6 level of thoracic spinal cord, subs
		S24.113D	Complete lesion at T7-T10, subs
		S24.114D	Complete lesion at T11-T12, subs
	(Continued on next page)	**S24.119D**	Complete lesion at unsp level of thoracic spinal cord, subs

ICD-9-CM		ICD-10-CM	
V58.89	ENCOUNTER FOR OTHER SPECIFIED AFTERCARE **(Continued)**	**S24.131D**	Anterior cord syndrome at T1, subs
		S24.132D	Anterior cord syndrome at T2-T6, subs
		S24.133D	Anterior cord syndrome at T7-T10, subs
		S24.134D	Anterior cord syndrome at T11-T12, subs
		S24.139D	Ant cord syndrome at unsp level of thor spinal cord, subs
		S24.141D	Brown-Sequard syndrome at T1, subs
		S24.142D	Brown-Sequard syndrome at T2-T6, subs
		S24.143D	Brown-Sequard syndrome at T7-T10, subs
		S24.144D	Brown-Sequard syndrome at T11-T12, subs
		S24.149D	Brown-Sequard synd at unsp level of thor spinal cord, subs
		S24.151D	Oth incomplete lesion at T1, subs
		S24.152D	Oth incomplete lesion at T2-T6, subs
		S24.153D	Oth incomplete lesion at T7-T10, subs
		S24.154D	Oth incomplete lesion at T11-T12, subs
		S24.159D	Oth incmpl lesion at unsp level of thor spinal cord, subs
		S24.2XXD	Injury of nerve root of thoracic spine, subsequent encounter
		S24.3XXD	Injury of peripheral nerves of thorax, subsequent encounter
		S24.4XXD	Injury of thoracic sympathetic nervous system, subs encntr
		S24.8XXD	Injury of other specified nerves of thorax, subs encntr
		S24.9XXD	Injury of unspecified nerve of thorax, subsequent encounter
		S25.00XD	Unspecified injury of thoracic aorta, subsequent encounter
		S25.01XD	Minor laceration of thoracic aorta, subsequent encounter
		S25.02XD	Major laceration of thoracic aorta, subsequent encounter
		S25.09XD	Other specified injury of thoracic aorta, subs encntr
		S25.101D	Unsp injury of right innominate or subclavian artery, subs
		S25.102D	Unsp injury of left innominate or subclavian artery, subs
		S25.109D	Unsp injury of unsp innominate or subclavian artery, subs
		S25.111D	Minor laceration of right innominate or subclav art, subs
		S25.112D	Minor laceration of left innominate or subclav art, subs
		S25.119D	Minor laceration of unsp innominate or subclav art, subs
		S25.121D	Major laceration of right innominate or subclav art, subs
		S25.122D	Major laceration of left innominate or subclav art, subs
		S25.129D	Major laceration of unsp innominate or subclav art, subs
		S25.191D	Inj right innominate or subclavian artery, subs encntr
		S25.192D	Inj left innominate or subclavian artery, subs encntr
		S25.199D	Inj unsp innominate or subclavian artery, subs encntr
		S25.20XD	Unspecified injury of superior vena cava, subs encntr
		S25.21XD	Minor laceration of superior vena cava, subsequent encounter
		S25.22XD	Major laceration of superior vena cava, subsequent encounter
		S25.29XD	Other specified injury of superior vena cava, subs encntr
		S25.301D	Unsp injury of right innominate or subclavian vein, subs
		S25.302D	Unsp injury of left innominate or subclavian vein, subs
		S25.309D	Unsp injury of unsp innominate or subclavian vein, subs
		S25.311D	Minor laceration of right innominate or subclav vein, subs
		S25.312D	Minor laceration of left innominate or subclavian vein, subs
		S25.319D	Minor laceration of unsp innominate or subclavian vein, subs
		S25.321D	Major laceration of right innominate or subclav vein, subs
		S25.322D	Major laceration of left innominate or subclavian vein, subs
		S25.329D	Major laceration of unsp innominate or subclavian vein, subs
		S25.391D	Inj right innominate or subclavian vein, subs encntr
		S25.392D	Inj left innominate or subclavian vein, subs encntr
		S25.399D	Inj unsp innominate or subclavian vein, subs encntr
		S25.401D	Unsp injury of right pulmonary blood vessels, subs encntr
		S25.402D	Unsp injury of left pulmonary blood vessels, subs encntr
		S25.409D	Unsp injury of unsp pulmonary blood vessels, subs encntr
		S25.411D	Minor laceration of right pulmonary blood vessels, subs
		S25.412D	Minor laceration of left pulmonary blood vessels, subs
		S25.419D	Minor laceration of unsp pulmonary blood vessels, subs
		S25.421D	Major laceration of right pulmonary blood vessels, subs
		S25.422D	Major laceration of left pulmonary blood vessels, subs
		S25.429D	Major laceration of unsp pulmonary blood vessels, subs
		S25.491D	Oth injury of right pulmonary blood vessels, subs encntr
		S25.492D	Oth injury of left pulmonary blood vessels, subs encntr
		S25.499D	Oth injury of unsp pulmonary blood vessels, subs encntr
		S25.501D	Unsp injury of intercostal blood vessels, right side, subs
		S25.502D	Unsp injury of intercostal blood vessels, left side, subs
		S25.509D	Unsp injury of intercostal blood vessels, unsp side, subs
		S25.511D	Laceration of intercostal blood vessels, right side, subs
		S25.512D	Laceration of intercostal blood vessels, left side, subs
		S25.519D	Laceration of intercostal blood vessels, unsp side, subs
		S25.591D	Inj intercostal blood vessels, right side, subs encntr
		S25.592D	Inj intercostal blood vessels, left side, subs encntr
		S25.599D	Inj intercostal blood vessels, unsp side, subs encntr
		S25.801D	Unsp injury of oth blood vessels of thorax, right side, subs
		S25.802D	Unsp injury of oth blood vessels of thorax, left side, subs
		S25.809D	Unsp injury of oth blood vessels of thorax, unsp side, subs
		S25.811D	Laceration of oth blood vessels of thorax, right side, subs
		S25.812D	Laceration of oth blood vessels of thorax, left side, subs
		S25.819D	Laceration of oth blood vessels of thorax, unsp side, subs
		S25.891D	Inj oth blood vessels of thorax, right side, subs encntr
		S25.892D	Inj oth blood vessels of thorax, left side, subs encntr
		S25.899D	Inj oth blood vessels of thorax, unsp side, subs encntr
	(Continued on next page)	**S25.90XD**	Unsp injury of unsp blood vessel of thorax, subs encntr

ICD-9-CM	ICD-10-CM	
V58.89 ENCOUNTER FOR OTHER SPECIFIED AFTERCARE **(Continued)**	**S25.91XD**	Laceration of unsp blood vessel of thorax, subs encntr
	S25.99XD	Oth injury of unsp blood vessel of thorax, subs encntr
	S26.00XD	Unsp injury of heart with hemopericardium, subs encntr
	S26.01XD	Contusion of heart with hemopericardium, subs encntr
	S26.020D	Mild laceration of heart with hemopericardium, subs encntr
	S26.021D	Moderate laceration of heart w hemopericardium, subs encntr
	S26.022D	Major laceration of heart with hemopericardium, subs encntr
	S26.09XD	Other injury of heart with hemopericardium, subs encntr
	S26.10XD	Unsp injury of heart without hemopericardium, subs encntr
	S26.11XD	Contusion of heart without hemopericardium, subs encntr
	S26.12XD	Laceration of heart without hemopericardium, subs encntr
	S26.19XD	Other injury of heart without hemopericardium, subs encntr
	S26.90XD	Unsp injury of heart, unsp w or w/o hemopericardium, subs
	S26.91XD	Contusion of heart, unsp w or w/o hemopericardium, subs
	S26.92XD	Laceration of heart, unsp w or w/o hemopericardium, subs
	S26.99XD	Inj heart, unsp w or w/o hemopericardium, subs encntr
	S27.0XXD	Traumatic pneumothorax, subsequent encounter
	S27.1XXD	Traumatic hemothorax, subsequent encounter
	S27.2XXD	Traumatic hemopneumothorax, subsequent encounter
	S27.301D	Unspecified injury of lung, unilateral, subsequent encounter
	S27.302D	Unspecified injury of lung, bilateral, subsequent encounter
	S27.309D	Unspecified injury of lung, unspecified, subs encntr
	S27.311D	Primary blast injury of lung, unilateral, subs encntr
	S27.312D	Primary blast injury of lung, bilateral, subs encntr
	S27.319D	Primary blast injury of lung, unspecified, subs encntr
	S27.321D	Contusion of lung, unilateral, subsequent encounter
	S27.322D	Contusion of lung, bilateral, subsequent encounter
	S27.329D	Contusion of lung, unspecified, subsequent encounter
	S27.331D	Laceration of lung, unilateral, subsequent encounter
	S27.332D	Laceration of lung, bilateral, subsequent encounter
	S27.339D	Laceration of lung, unspecified, subsequent encounter
	S27.391D	Other injuries of lung, unilateral, subsequent encounter
	S27.392D	Other injuries of lung, bilateral, subsequent encounter
	S27.399D	Other injuries of lung, unspecified, subsequent encounter
	S27.401D	Unspecified injury of bronchus, unilateral, subs encntr
	S27.402D	Unspecified injury of bronchus, bilateral, subs encntr
	S27.409D	Unspecified injury of bronchus, unspecified, subs encntr
	S27.411D	Primary blast injury of bronchus, unilateral, subs encntr
	S27.412D	Primary blast injury of bronchus, bilateral, subs encntr
	S27.419D	Primary blast injury of bronchus, unspecified, subs encntr
	S27.421D	Contusion of bronchus, unilateral, subsequent encounter
	S27.422D	Contusion of bronchus, bilateral, subsequent encounter
	S27.429D	Contusion of bronchus, unspecified, subsequent encounter
	S27.431D	Laceration of bronchus, unilateral, subsequent encounter
	S27.432D	Laceration of bronchus, bilateral, subsequent encounter
	S27.439D	Laceration of bronchus, unspecified, subsequent encounter
	S27.491D	Other injury of bronchus, unilateral, subsequent encounter
	S27.492D	Other injury of bronchus, bilateral, subsequent encounter
	S27.499D	Other injury of bronchus, unspecified, subsequent encounter
	S27.50XD	Unspecified injury of thoracic trachea, subsequent encounter
	S27.51XD	Primary blast injury of thoracic trachea, subs encntr
	S27.52XD	Contusion of thoracic trachea, subsequent encounter
	S27.53XD	Laceration of thoracic trachea, subsequent encounter
	S27.59XD	Other injury of thoracic trachea, subsequent encounter
	S27.60XD	Unspecified injury of pleura, subsequent encounter
	S27.63XD	Laceration of pleura, subsequent encounter
	S27.69XD	Other injury of pleura, subsequent encounter
	S27.802D	Contusion of diaphragm, subsequent encounter
	S27.803D	Laceration of diaphragm, subsequent encounter
	S27.808D	Other injury of diaphragm, subsequent encounter
	S27.809D	Unspecified injury of diaphragm, subsequent encounter
	S27.812D	Contusion of esophagus (thoracic part), subsequent encounter
	S27.813D	Laceration of esophagus (thoracic part), subs encntr
	S27.818D	Other injury of esophagus (thoracic part), subs encntr
	S27.819D	Unspecified injury of esophagus (thoracic part), subs encntr
	S27.892D	Contusion of oth intrathoracic organs, subs encntr
	S27.893D	Laceration of oth intrathoracic organs, subs encntr
	S27.898D	Other injury of oth intrathoracic organs, subs encntr
	S27.899D	Unspecified injury of oth intrathoracic organs, subs encntr
	S27.9XXD	Injury of unspecified intrathoracic organ, subs encntr
	S28.0XXD	Crushed chest, subsequent encounter
	S28.1XXD	Traumatic amp of part of thorax, except breast, subs
	S28.211D	Complete traumatic amputation of right breast, subs encntr
	S28.212D	Complete traumatic amputation of left breast, subs encntr
	S28.219D	Complete traumatic amputation of unsp breast, subs encntr
	S28.221D	Partial traumatic amputation of right breast, subs encntr
	S28.222D	Partial traumatic amputation of left breast, subs encntr
	S28.229D	Partial traumatic amputation of unsp breast, subs encntr
	S29.001D	Unsp injury of msl/tnd of front wall of thorax, subs
	S29.002D	Unsp injury of msl/tnd of back wall of thorax, subs
	S29.009D	Unsp injury of msl/tnd of unsp wall of thorax, subs
	S29.011D	Strain of muscle and tendon of front wall of thorax, subs
(Continued on next page)	**S29.012D**	Strain of muscle and tendon of back wall of thorax, subs

ICD-9-CM		ICD-10-CM	
V58.89	ENCOUNTER FOR OTHER SPECIFIED AFTERCARE **(Continued)**	**S29.Ø19D**	Strain of muscle and tendon of unsp wall of thorax, subs
		S29.Ø21D	Laceration of msl/tnd of front wall of thorax, subs
		S29.Ø22D	Laceration of muscle and tendon of back wall of thorax, subs
		S29.Ø29D	Laceration of muscle and tendon of unsp wall of thorax, subs
		S29.Ø91D	Inj muscle and tendon of front wall of thorax, subs encntr
		S29.Ø92D	Inj muscle and tendon of back wall of thorax, subs encntr
		S29.Ø99D	Inj muscle and tendon of unsp wall of thorax, subs encntr
		S29.8XXD	Other specified injuries of thorax, subsequent encounter
		S29.9XXD	Unspecified injury of thorax, subsequent encounter
		S3Ø.ØXXD	Contusion of lower back and pelvis, subsequent encounter
		S3Ø.1XXD	Contusion of abdominal wall, subsequent encounter
		S3Ø.2Ø1D	Contusion of unsp external genital organ, male, subs encntr
		S3Ø.2Ø2D	Contusion of unsp external genital organ, female, subs
		S3Ø.21XD	Contusion of penis, subsequent encounter
		S3Ø.22XD	Contusion of scrotum and testes, subsequent encounter
		S3Ø.23XD	Contusion of vagina and vulva, subsequent encounter
		S3Ø.3XXD	Contusion of anus, subsequent encounter
		S3Ø.81ØD	Abrasion of lower back and pelvis, subsequent encounter
		S3Ø.811D	Abrasion of abdominal wall, subsequent encounter
		S3Ø.812D	Abrasion of penis, subsequent encounter
		S3Ø.813D	Abrasion of scrotum and testes, subsequent encounter
		S3Ø.814D	Abrasion of vagina and vulva, subsequent encounter
		S3Ø.815D	Abrasion of unsp external genital organs, male, subs encntr
		S3Ø.816D	Abrasion of unsp external genital organs, female, subs
		S3Ø.817D	Abrasion of anus, subsequent encounter
		S3Ø.82ØD	Blister (nonthermal) of lower back and pelvis, subs encntr
		S3Ø.821D	Blister (nonthermal) of abdominal wall, subsequent encounter
		S3Ø.822D	Blister (nonthermal) of penis, subsequent encounter
		S3Ø.823D	Blister (nonthermal) of scrotum and testes, subs encntr
		S3Ø.824D	Blister (nonthermal) of vagina and vulva, subs encntr
		S3Ø.825D	Blister of unsp external genital organs, male, subs
		S3Ø.826D	Blister of unsp external genital organs, female, subs
		S3Ø.827D	Blister (nonthermal) of anus, subsequent encounter
		S3Ø.84ØD	External constriction of lower back and pelvis, subs encntr
		S3Ø.841D	External constriction of abdominal wall, subs encntr
		S3Ø.842D	External constriction of penis, subsequent encounter
		S3Ø.843D	External constriction of scrotum and testes, subs encntr
		S3Ø.844D	External constriction of vagina and vulva, subs encntr
		S3Ø.845D	Extrn constrict of unsp external genital organs, male, subs
		S3Ø.846D	Extrn constrict of unsp extrn genital organs, female, subs
		S3Ø.85ØD	Superficial foreign body of lower back and pelvis, subs
		S3Ø.851D	Superficial foreign body of abdominal wall, subs encntr
		S3Ø.852D	Superficial foreign body of penis, subsequent encounter
		S3Ø.853D	Superficial foreign body of scrotum and testes, subs encntr
		S3Ø.854D	Superficial foreign body of vagina and vulva, subs encntr
		S3Ø.855D	Superficial fb of unsp external genital organs, male, subs
		S3Ø.856D	Superficial fb of unsp external genital organs, female, subs
		S3Ø.857D	Superficial foreign body of anus, subsequent encounter
		S3Ø.86ØD	Insect bite (nonvenomous) of lower back and pelvis, subs
		S3Ø.861D	Insect bite (nonvenomous) of abdominal wall, subs encntr
		S3Ø.862D	Insect bite (nonvenomous) of penis, subsequent encounter
		S3Ø.863D	Insect bite (nonvenomous) of scrotum and testes, subs encntr
		S3Ø.864D	Insect bite (nonvenomous) of vagina and vulva, subs encntr
		S3Ø.865D	Insect bite of unsp external genital organs, male, subs
		S3Ø.866D	Insect bite of unsp external genital organs, female, subs
		S3Ø.867D	Insect bite (nonvenomous) of anus, subsequent encounter
		S3Ø.87ØD	Other superficial bite of lower back and pelvis, subs encntr
		S3Ø.871D	Other superficial bite of abdominal wall, subs encntr
		S3Ø.872D	Other superficial bite of penis, subsequent encounter
		S3Ø.873D	Other superficial bite of scrotum and testes, subs encntr
		S3Ø.874D	Other superficial bite of vagina and vulva, subs encntr
		S3Ø.875D	Oth superfic bite of unsp extrn genital organs, male, subs
		S3Ø.876D	Oth superfic bite of unsp extrn genital organs, female, subs
		S3Ø.877D	Other superficial bite of anus, subsequent encounter
		S3Ø.91XD	Unsp superficial injury of lower back and pelvis, subs
		S3Ø.92XD	Unsp superficial injury of abdominal wall, subs encntr
		S3Ø.93XD	Unspecified superficial injury of penis, subs encntr
		S3Ø.94XD	Unsp superficial injury of scrotum and testes, subs encntr
		S3Ø.95XD	Unsp superficial injury of vagina and vulva, subs encntr
		S3Ø.96XD	Unsp superfic inj unsp external genital organs, male, subs
		S3Ø.97XD	Unsp superfic inj unsp external genital organs, female, subs
		S3Ø.98XD	Unspecified superficial injury of anus, subsequent encounter
		S31.ØØØD	Unsp opn wnd low back and pelv w/o penet retroperiton, subs
		S31.ØØ1D	Unsp opn wnd low back and pelvis w penet retroperiton, subs
		S31.Ø1ØD	Lac w/o fb of low back and pelv w/o penet retroperiton, subs
		S31.Ø11D	Lac w/o fb of low back and pelvis w penet retroperiton, subs
		S31.Ø2ØD	Lac w fb of low back and pelvis w/o penet retroperiton, subs
		S31.Ø21D	Lac w fb of lower back and pelvis w penet retroperiton, subs
		S31.Ø3ØD	Pnctr w/o fb of low back & pelv w/o penet retroperiton, subs
		S31.Ø31D	Pnctr w/o fb of low back and pelv w penet retroperiton, subs
		S31.Ø4ØD	Pnctr w fb of low back and pelv w/o penet retroperiton, subs
		S31.Ø41D	Pnctr w fb of low back and pelvis w penet retroperiton, subs
	(Continued on next page)	**S31.Ø5ØD**	Open bite of low back and pelv w/o penet retroperiton, subs

ICD-9-CM		ICD-10-CM	
V58.89	ENCOUNTER FOR OTHER SPECIFIED AFTERCARE **(Continued)**	**S31.Ø51D**	Open bite of low back and pelvis w penet retroperiton, subs
		S31.1ØØD	Unsp opn wnd abd wall, r upper q w/o penet perit cav, subs
		S31.1Ø1D	Unsp opn wnd abd wall, l upr q w/o penet perit cav, subs
		S31.1Ø2D	Unsp opn wnd abd wall, epigst rgn w/o penet perit cav, subs
		S31.1Ø3D	Unsp opn wnd abd wall, right low q w/o penet perit cav, subs
		S31.1Ø4D	Unsp opn wnd abd wall, left low q w/o penet perit cav, subs
		S31.1Ø5D	Unsp opn wnd abd wall, periumb rgn w/o penet perit cav, subs
		S31.1Ø9D	Unsp opn wnd abd wall, unsp q w/o penet perit cav, subs
		S31.11ØD	Lac w/o fb of abd wall, r upper q w/o penet perit cav, subs
		S31.111D	Lac w/o fb of abd wall, l upr q w/o penet perit cav, subs
		S31.112D	Lac w/o fb of abd wall, epigst rgn w/o penet perit cav, subs
		S31.113D	Lac w/o fb of abd wall, r low q w/o penet perit cav, subs
		S31.114D	Lac w/o fb of abd wall, left low q w/o penet perit cav, subs
		S31.115D	Lac w/o fb of abd wl, periumb rgn w/o penet perit cav, subs
		S31.119D	Lac w/o fb of abd wall, unsp q w/o penet perit cav, subs
		S31.12ØD	Lacerat abd wall w fb, r upper q w/o penet perit cav, subs
		S31.121D	Lacerat abd wall w fb, l upr q w/o penet perit cav, subs
		S31.122D	Lacerat abd wall w fb, epigst rgn w/o penet perit cav, subs
		S31.123D	Lacerat abd wall w fb, right low q w/o penet perit cav, subs
		S31.124D	Lacerat abd wall w fb, left low q w/o penet perit cav, subs
		S31.125D	Lacerat abd wall w fb, periumb rgn w/o penet perit cav, subs
		S31.129D	Lacerat abd wall w fb, unsp q w/o penet perit cav, subs
		S31.13ØD	Pnctr of abd wall w/o fb, r upr q w/o penet perit cav, subs
		S31.131D	Pnctr of abd wall w/o fb, l upr q w/o penet perit cav, subs
		S31.132D	Pnctr of abd wl w/o fb, epigst rgn w/o penet perit cav, subs
		S31.133D	Pnctr of abd wall w/o fb, r low q w/o penet perit cav, subs
		S31.134D	Pnctr of abd wall w/o fb, l low q w/o penet perit cav, subs
		S31.135D	Pnctr of abd wl w/o fb,periumb rgn w/o penet perit cav, subs
		S31.139D	Pnctr of abd wall w/o fb, unsp q w/o penet perit cav, subs
		S31.14ØD	Pnctr of abd wall w fb, r upper q w/o penet perit cav, subs
		S31.141D	Pnctr of abd wall w fb, l upr q w/o penet perit cav, subs
		S31.142D	Pnctr of abd wall w fb, epigst rgn w/o penet perit cav, subs
		S31.143D	Pnctr of abd wall w fb, r low q w/o penet perit cav, subs
		S31.144D	Pnctr of abd wall w fb, left low q w/o penet perit cav, subs
		S31.145D	Pnctr of abd wl w fb, periumb rgn w/o penet perit cav, subs
		S31.149D	Pnctr of abd wall w fb, unsp q w/o penet perit cav, subs
		S31.15ØD	Open bite of abd wall, r upper q w/o penet perit cav, subs
		S31.151D	Open bite of abd wall, l upr q w/o penet perit cav, subs
		S31.152D	Open bite of abd wall, epigst rgn w/o penet perit cav, subs
		S31.153D	Open bite of abd wall, right low q w/o penet perit cav, subs
		S31.154D	Open bite of abd wall, left low q w/o penet perit cav, subs
		S31.155D	Open bite of abd wall, periumb rgn w/o penet perit cav, subs
		S31.159D	Open bite of abd wall, unsp q w/o penet perit cav, subs
		S31.2ØXD	Unspecified open wound of penis, subsequent encounter
		S31.21XD	Laceration without foreign body of penis, subs encntr
		S31.22XD	Laceration with foreign body of penis, subsequent encounter
		S31.23XD	Puncture wound without foreign body of penis, subs encntr
		S31.24XD	Puncture wound with foreign body of penis, subs encntr
		S31.25XD	Open bite of penis, subsequent encounter
		S31.3ØXD	Unspecified open wound of scrotum and testes, subs encntr
		S31.31XD	Laceration w/o foreign body of scrotum and testes, subs
		S31.32XD	Laceration w foreign body of scrotum and testes, subs encntr
		S31.33XD	Puncture wound w/o foreign body of scrotum and testes, subs
		S31.34XD	Puncture wound w foreign body of scrotum and testes, subs
		S31.35XD	Open bite of scrotum and testes, subsequent encounter
		S31.4ØXD	Unspecified open wound of vagina and vulva, subs encntr
		S31.41XD	Laceration w/o foreign body of vagina and vulva, subs encntr
		S31.42XD	Laceration w foreign body of vagina and vulva, subs encntr
		S31.43XD	Puncture wound w/o foreign body of vagina and vulva, subs
		S31.44XD	Puncture wound w foreign body of vagina and vulva, subs
		S31.45XD	Open bite of vagina and vulva, subsequent encounter
		S31.5Ø1D	Unsp open wound of unsp external genital organs, male, subs
		S31.5Ø2D	Unsp opn wnd unsp external genital organs, female, subs
		S31.511D	Lac w/o fb of unsp external genital organs, male, subs
		S31.512D	Lac w/o fb of unsp external genital organs, female, subs
		S31.521D	Laceration w fb of unsp external genital organs, male, subs
		S31.522D	Lac w fb of unsp external genital organs, female, subs
		S31.531D	Pnctr w/o fb of unsp external genital organs, male, subs
		S31.532D	Pnctr w/o fb of unsp external genital organs, female, subs
		S31.541D	Pnctr w fb of unsp external genital organs, male, subs
		S31.542D	Pnctr w fb of unsp external genital organs, female, subs
		S31.551D	Open bite of unsp external genital organs, male, subs encntr
		S31.552D	Open bite of unsp external genital organs, female, subs
		S31.6ØØD	Unsp opn wnd abd wall, right upper q w penet perit cav, subs
		S31.6Ø1D	Unsp open wound of abd wall, l upr q w penet perit cav, subs
		S31.6Ø2D	Unsp opn wnd abd wall, epigst rgn w penet perit cav, subs
		S31.6Ø3D	Unsp opn wnd abd wall, right lower q w penet perit cav, subs
		S31.6Ø4D	Unsp opn wnd abd wall, left lower q w penet perit cav, subs
		S31.6Ø5D	Unsp opn wnd abd wall, periumb rgn w penet perit cav, subs
		S31.6Ø9D	Unsp opn wnd abd wall, unsp quadrant w penet perit cav, subs
		S31.61ØD	Lac w/o fb of abd wall, r upper q w penet perit cav, subs
		S31.611D	Lac w/o fb of abd wall, l upr q w penet perit cav, subs
	(Continued on next page)	**S31.612D**	Lac w/o fb of abd wall, epigst rgn w penet perit cav, subs

ICD-9-CM		ICD-10-CM	
V58.89	ENCOUNTER FOR OTHER SPECIFIED AFTERCARE **(Continued)**	**S31.613D**	Lac w/o fb of abd wall, right low q w penet perit cav, subs
		S31.614D	Lac w/o fb of abd wall, left lower q w penet perit cav, subs
		S31.615D	Lac w/o fb of abd wall, periumb rgn w penet perit cav, subs
		S31.619D	Lac w/o fb of abd wall, unsp q w penet perit cav, subs
		S31.620D	Lac w fb of abd wall, right upper q w penet perit cav, subs
		S31.621D	Laceration w fb of abd wall, l upr q w penet perit cav, subs
		S31.622D	Lac w fb of abd wall, epigst rgn w penet perit cav, subs
		S31.623D	Lac w fb of abd wall, right lower q w penet perit cav, subs
		S31.624D	Lac w fb of abd wall, left lower q w penet perit cav, subs
		S31.625D	Lac w fb of abd wall, periumb rgn w penet perit cav, subs
		S31.629D	Lac w fb of abd wall, unsp quadrant w penet perit cav, subs
		S31.630D	Pnctr w/o fb of abd wall, r upper q w penet perit cav, subs
		S31.631D	Pnctr w/o fb of abd wall, l upr q w penet perit cav, subs
		S31.632D	Pnctr w/o fb of abd wall, epigst rgn w penet perit cav, subs
		S31.633D	Pnctr w/o fb of abd wall, r low q w penet perit cav, subs
		S31.634D	Pnctr w/o fb of abd wall, left low q w penet perit cav, subs
		S31.635D	Pnctr w/o fb of abd wl, periumb rgn w penet perit cav, subs
		S31.639D	Pnctr w/o fb of abd wall, unsp q w penet perit cav, subs
		S31.640D	Pnctr w fb of abd wall, r upper q w penet perit cav, subs
		S31.641D	Pnctr w fb of abd wall, l upr q w penet perit cav, subs
		S31.642D	Pnctr w fb of abd wall, epigst rgn w penet perit cav, subs
		S31.643D	Pnctr w fb of abd wall, right low q w penet perit cav, subs
		S31.644D	Pnctr w fb of abd wall, left lower q w penet perit cav, subs
		S31.645D	Pnctr w fb of abd wall, periumb rgn w penet perit cav, subs
		S31.649D	Pnctr w fb of abd wall, unsp q w penet perit cav, subs
		S31.650D	Open bite of abd wall, right upper q w penet perit cav, subs
		S31.651D	Open bite of abdominal wall, l upr q w penet perit cav, subs
		S31.652D	Open bite of abd wall, epigst rgn w penet perit cav, subs
		S31.653D	Open bite of abd wall, right lower q w penet perit cav, subs
		S31.654D	Open bite of abd wall, left lower q w penet perit cav, subs
		S31.655D	Open bite of abd wall, periumb rgn w penet perit cav, subs
		S31.659D	Open bite of abd wall, unsp quadrant w penet perit cav, subs
		S31.801D	Laceration without foreign body of unsp buttock, subs encntr
		S31.802D	Laceration with foreign body of unsp buttock, subs encntr
		S31.803D	Puncture wound w/o foreign body of unsp buttock, subs encntr
		S31.804D	Puncture wound w foreign body of unsp buttock, subs encntr
		S31.805D	Open bite of unspecified buttock, subsequent encounter
		S31.809D	Unspecified open wound of unspecified buttock, subs encntr
		S31.811D	Laceration w/o foreign body of right buttock, subs encntr
		S31.812D	Laceration with foreign body of right buttock, subs encntr
		S31.813D	Puncture wound w/o foreign body of right buttock, subs
		S31.814D	Puncture wound w foreign body of right buttock, subs encntr
		S31.815D	Open bite of right buttock, subsequent encounter
		S31.819D	Unspecified open wound of right buttock, subs encntr
		S31.821D	Laceration without foreign body of left buttock, subs encntr
		S31.822D	Laceration with foreign body of left buttock, subs encntr
		S31.823D	Puncture wound w/o foreign body of left buttock, subs encntr
		S31.824D	Puncture wound w foreign body of left buttock, subs encntr
		S31.825D	Open bite of left buttock, subsequent encounter
		S31.829D	Unspecified open wound of left buttock, subsequent encounter
		S31.831D	Laceration without foreign body of anus, subs encntr
		S31.832D	Laceration with foreign body of anus, subsequent encounter
		S31.833D	Puncture wound without foreign body of anus, subs encntr
		S31.834D	Puncture wound with foreign body of anus, subs encntr
		S31.835D	Open bite of anus, subsequent encounter
		S31.839D	Unspecified open wound of anus, subsequent encounter
		S33.0XXD	Traumatic rupture of lumbar intervertebral disc, subs encntr
		S33.100D	Subluxation of unspecified lumbar vertebra, subs encntr
		S33.101D	Dislocation of unspecified lumbar vertebra, subs encntr
		S33.110D	Subluxation of L1/L2 lumbar vertebra, subsequent encounter
		S33.111D	Dislocation of L1/L2 lumbar vertebra, subsequent encounter
		S33.120D	Subluxation of L2/L3 lumbar vertebra, subsequent encounter
		S33.121D	Dislocation of L2/L3 lumbar vertebra, subsequent encounter
		S33.130D	Subluxation of L3/L4 lumbar vertebra, subsequent encounter
		S33.131D	Dislocation of L3/L4 lumbar vertebra, subsequent encounter
		S33.140D	Subluxation of L4/L5 lumbar vertebra, subsequent encounter
		S33.141D	Dislocation of L4/L5 lumbar vertebra, subsequent encounter
		S33.2XXD	Dislocation of sacroiliac and sacrococcygeal joint, subs
		S33.30XD	Dislocation of unsp parts of lumbar spine and pelvis, subs
		S33.39XD	Dislocation of oth prt lumbar spine and pelvis, subs encntr
		S33.4XXD	Traumatic rupture of symphysis pubis, subsequent encounter
		S33.5XXD	Sprain of ligaments of lumbar spine, subsequent encounter
		S33.6XXD	Sprain of sacroiliac joint, subsequent encounter
		S33.8XXD	Sprain of oth parts of lumbar spine and pelvis, subs encntr
		S33.9XXD	Sprain of unsp parts of lumbar spine and pelvis, subs encntr
		S34.01XD	Concussion and edema of lumbar spinal cord, subs encntr
		S34.02XD	Concussion and edema of sacral spinal cord, subs encntr
		S34.101D	Unsp injury to L1 level of lumbar spinal cord, subs encntr
		S34.102D	Unsp injury to L2 level of lumbar spinal cord, subs encntr
		S34.103D	Unsp injury to L3 level of lumbar spinal cord, subs encntr
		S34.104D	Unsp injury to L4 level of lumbar spinal cord, subs encntr
		S34.105D	Unsp injury to L5 level of lumbar spinal cord, subs encntr
	(Continued on next page)	**S34.109D**	Unsp injury to unsp level of lumbar spinal cord, subs encntr

ICD-9-CM		ICD-10-CM	
V58.89	ENCOUNTER FOR OTHER SPECIFIED AFTERCARE **(Continued)**	**S34.111D**	Complete lesion of L1 level of lumbar spinal cord, subs
		S34.112D	Complete lesion of L2 level of lumbar spinal cord, subs
		S34.113D	Complete lesion of L3 level of lumbar spinal cord, subs
		S34.114D	Complete lesion of L4 level of lumbar spinal cord, subs
		S34.115D	Complete lesion of L5 level of lumbar spinal cord, subs
		S34.119D	Complete lesion of unsp level of lumbar spinal cord, subs
		S34.121D	Incomplete lesion of L1 level of lumbar spinal cord, subs
		S34.122D	Incomplete lesion of L2 level of lumbar spinal cord, subs
		S34.123D	Incomplete lesion of L3 level of lumbar spinal cord, subs
		S34.124D	Incomplete lesion of L4 level of lumbar spinal cord, subs
		S34.125D	Incomplete lesion of L5 level of lumbar spinal cord, subs
		S34.129D	Incomplete lesion of unsp level of lumbar spinal cord, subs
		S34.131D	Complete lesion of sacral spinal cord, subsequent encounter
		S34.132D	Incomplete lesion of sacral spinal cord, subs encntr
		S34.139D	Unspecified injury to sacral spinal cord, subs encntr
		S34.21XD	Injury of nerve root of lumbar spine, subsequent encounter
		S34.22XD	Injury of nerve root of sacral spine, subsequent encounter
		S34.3XXD	Injury of cauda equina, subsequent encounter
		S34.4XXD	Injury of lumbosacral plexus, subsequent encounter
		S34.5XXD	Injury of lumbar, sacral and pelvic sympathetic nerves, subs
		S34.6XXD	Inj prph nerve(s) at abd, low back and pelvis level, subs
		S34.8XXD	Injury of nerves at abdomen, low back and pelvis level, subs
		S34.9XXD	Inj unsp nerves at abdomen, low back and pelvis level, subs
		S35.00XD	Unspecified injury of abdominal aorta, subsequent encounter
		S35.01XD	Minor laceration of abdominal aorta, subsequent encounter
		S35.02XD	Major laceration of abdominal aorta, subsequent encounter
		S35.09XD	Other injury of abdominal aorta, subsequent encounter
		S35.10XD	Unspecified injury of inferior vena cava, subs encntr
		S35.11XD	Minor laceration of inferior vena cava, subsequent encounter
		S35.12XD	Major laceration of inferior vena cava, subsequent encounter
		S35.19XD	Other injury of inferior vena cava, subsequent encounter
		S35.211D	Minor laceration of celiac artery, subsequent encounter
		S35.212D	Major laceration of celiac artery, subsequent encounter
		S35.218D	Other injury of celiac artery, subsequent encounter
		S35.219D	Unspecified injury of celiac artery, subsequent encounter
		S35.221D	Minor laceration of superior mesenteric artery, subs encntr
		S35.222D	Major laceration of superior mesenteric artery, subs encntr
		S35.228D	Other injury of superior mesenteric artery, subs encntr
		S35.229D	Unsp injury of superior mesenteric artery, subs encntr
		S35.231D	Minor laceration of inferior mesenteric artery, subs encntr
		S35.232D	Major laceration of inferior mesenteric artery, subs encntr
		S35.238D	Other injury of inferior mesenteric artery, subs encntr
		S35.239D	Unsp injury of inferior mesenteric artery, subs encntr
		S35.291D	Minor laceration of branches of celiac and mesent art, subs
		S35.292D	Major laceration of branches of celiac and mesent art, subs
		S35.298D	Inj branches of celiac and mesenteric artery, subs encntr
		S35.299D	Unsp injury of branches of celiac and mesent art, subs
		S35.311D	Laceration of portal vein, subsequent encounter
		S35.318D	Other specified injury of portal vein, subsequent encounter
		S35.319D	Unspecified injury of portal vein, subsequent encounter
		S35.321D	Laceration of splenic vein, subsequent encounter
		S35.328D	Other specified injury of splenic vein, subsequent encounter
		S35.329D	Unspecified injury of splenic vein, subsequent encounter
		S35.331D	Laceration of superior mesenteric vein, subsequent encounter
		S35.338D	Oth injury of superior mesenteric vein, subs encntr
		S35.339D	Unspecified injury of superior mesenteric vein, subs encntr
		S35.341D	Laceration of inferior mesenteric vein, subsequent encounter
		S35.348D	Oth injury of inferior mesenteric vein, subs encntr
		S35.349D	Unspecified injury of inferior mesenteric vein, subs encntr
		S35.401D	Unspecified injury of right renal artery, subs encntr
		S35.402D	Unspecified injury of left renal artery, subs encntr
		S35.403D	Unspecified injury of unspecified renal artery, subs encntr
		S35.404D	Unspecified injury of right renal vein, subsequent encounter
		S35.405D	Unspecified injury of left renal vein, subsequent encounter
		S35.406D	Unspecified injury of unspecified renal vein, subs encntr
		S35.411D	Laceration of right renal artery, subsequent encounter
		S35.412D	Laceration of left renal artery, subsequent encounter
		S35.413D	Laceration of unspecified renal artery, subsequent encounter
		S35.414D	Laceration of right renal vein, subsequent encounter
		S35.415D	Laceration of left renal vein, subsequent encounter
		S35.416D	Laceration of unspecified renal vein, subsequent encounter
		S35.491D	Other specified injury of right renal artery, subs encntr
		S35.492D	Other specified injury of left renal artery, subs encntr
		S35.493D	Oth injury of unspecified renal artery, subs encntr
		S35.494D	Other specified injury of right renal vein, subs encntr
		S35.495D	Other specified injury of left renal vein, subs encntr
		S35.496D	Oth injury of unspecified renal vein, subs encntr
		S35.50XD	Injury of unspecified iliac blood vessel(s), subs encntr
		S35.511D	Injury of right iliac artery, subsequent encounter
		S35.512D	Injury of left iliac artery, subsequent encounter
		S35.513D	Injury of unspecified iliac artery, subsequent encounter
		S35.514D	Injury of right iliac vein, subsequent encounter
	(Continued on next page)	**S35.515D**	Injury of left iliac vein, subsequent encounter

ICD-9-CM		ICD-10-CM	
V58.89	ENCOUNTER FOR OTHER SPECIFIED AFTERCARE	**S35.516D**	Injury of unspecified iliac vein, subsequent encounter
	(Continued)	**S35.531D**	Injury of right uterine artery, subsequent encounter
		S35.532D	Injury of left uterine artery, subsequent encounter
		S35.533D	Injury of unspecified uterine artery, subsequent encounter
		S35.534D	Injury of right uterine vein, subsequent encounter
		S35.535D	Injury of left uterine vein, subsequent encounter
		S35.536D	Injury of unspecified uterine vein, subsequent encounter
		S35.59XD	Injury of other iliac blood vessels, subsequent encounter
		S35.8X1D	Lacerat blood vesls at abd, low back and pelvis level, subs
		S35.8X8D	Inj oth blood vesls at abd, low back and pelvis level, subs
		S35.8X9D	Unsp inj blood vesls at abd, low back and pelvis level, subs
		S35.90XD	Unsp inj unsp bld vess at abd, low back and pelv level, subs
		S35.91XD	Lacerat unsp bld vess at abd, low back and pelv level, subs
		S35.99XD	Inj unsp blood vess at abd, low back and pelvis level, subs
		S36.00XD	Unspecified injury of spleen, subsequent encounter
		S36.020D	Minor contusion of spleen, subsequent encounter
		S36.021D	Major contusion of spleen, subsequent encounter
		S36.029D	Unspecified contusion of spleen, subsequent encounter
		S36.030D	Superficial (capsular) laceration of spleen, subs encntr
		S36.031D	Moderate laceration of spleen, subsequent encounter
		S36.032D	Major laceration of spleen, subsequent encounter
		S36.039D	Unspecified laceration of spleen, subsequent encounter
		S36.09XD	Other injury of spleen, subsequent encounter
		S36.112D	Contusion of liver, subsequent encounter
		S36.113D	Laceration of liver, unspecified degree, subs encntr
		S36.114D	Minor laceration of liver, subsequent encounter
		S36.115D	Moderate laceration of liver, subsequent encounter
		S36.116D	Major laceration of liver, subsequent encounter
		S36.118D	Other injury of liver, subsequent encounter
		S36.119D	Unspecified injury of liver, subsequent encounter
		S36.122D	Contusion of gallbladder, subsequent encounter
		S36.123D	Laceration of gallbladder, subsequent encounter
		S36.128D	Other injury of gallbladder, subsequent encounter
		S36.129D	Unspecified injury of gallbladder, subsequent encounter
		S36.13XD	Injury of bile duct, subsequent encounter
		S36.200D	Unspecified injury of head of pancreas, subsequent encounter
		S36.201D	Unspecified injury of body of pancreas, subsequent encounter
		S36.202D	Unspecified injury of tail of pancreas, subsequent encounter
		S36.209D	Unsp injury of unspecified part of pancreas, subs encntr
		S36.220D	Contusion of head of pancreas, subsequent encounter
		S36.221D	Contusion of body of pancreas, subsequent encounter
		S36.222D	Contusion of tail of pancreas, subsequent encounter
		S36.229D	Contusion of unspecified part of pancreas, subs encntr
		S36.230D	Laceration of head of pancreas, unsp degree, subs encntr
		S36.231D	Laceration of body of pancreas, unsp degree, subs encntr
		S36.232D	Laceration of tail of pancreas, unsp degree, subs encntr
		S36.239D	Laceration of unsp part of pancreas, unsp degree, subs
		S36.240D	Minor laceration of head of pancreas, subsequent encounter
		S36.241D	Minor laceration of body of pancreas, subsequent encounter
		S36.242D	Minor laceration of tail of pancreas, subsequent encounter
		S36.249D	Minor laceration of unsp part of pancreas, subs encntr
		S36.250D	Moderate laceration of head of pancreas, subs encntr
		S36.251D	Moderate laceration of body of pancreas, subs encntr
		S36.252D	Moderate laceration of tail of pancreas, subs encntr
		S36.259D	Moderate laceration of unsp part of pancreas, subs encntr
		S36.260D	Major laceration of head of pancreas, subsequent encounter
		S36.261D	Major laceration of body of pancreas, subsequent encounter
		S36.262D	Major laceration of tail of pancreas, subsequent encounter
		S36.269D	Major laceration of unsp part of pancreas, subs encntr
		S36.290D	Other injury of head of pancreas, subsequent encounter
		S36.291D	Other injury of body of pancreas, subsequent encounter
		S36.292D	Other injury of tail of pancreas, subsequent encounter
		S36.299D	Other injury of unspecified part of pancreas, subs encntr
		S36.30XD	Unspecified injury of stomach, subsequent encounter
		S36.32XD	Contusion of stomach, subsequent encounter
		S36.33XD	Laceration of stomach, subsequent encounter
		S36.39XD	Other injury of stomach, subsequent encounter
		S36.400D	Unspecified injury of duodenum, subsequent encounter
		S36.408D	Unsp injury of other part of small intestine, subs encntr
		S36.409D	Unsp injury of unsp part of small intestine, subs encntr
		S36.410D	Primary blast injury of duodenum, subsequent encounter
		S36.418D	Primary blast injury oth prt small intestine, subs encntr
		S36.419D	Primary blast injury of unsp part of small intestine, subs
		S36.420D	Contusion of duodenum, subsequent encounter
		S36.428D	Contusion of other part of small intestine, subs encntr
		S36.429D	Contusion of unsp part of small intestine, subs encntr
		S36.430D	Laceration of duodenum, subsequent encounter
		S36.438D	Laceration of other part of small intestine, subs encntr
		S36.439D	Laceration of unsp part of small intestine, subs encntr
		S36.490D	Other injury of duodenum, subsequent encounter
		S36.498D	Other injury of other part of small intestine, subs encntr
		S36.499D	Other injury of unsp part of small intestine, subs encntr
	(Continued on next page)	**S36.500D**	Unspecified injury of ascending colon, subsequent encounter

[Brackets] indicate valid character values for each code. Character value meanings provided for each code grouping.

ICD-9-CM		ICD-10-CM	
V58.89	ENCOUNTER FOR OTHER SPECIFIED AFTERCARE **(Continued)**	**S36.5Ø1D**	Unspecified injury of transverse colon, subsequent encounter
		S36.5Ø2D	Unspecified injury of descending colon, subsequent encounter
		S36.5Ø3D	Unspecified injury of sigmoid colon, subsequent encounter
		S36.5Ø8D	Unspecified injury of other part of colon, subs encntr
		S36.5Ø9D	Unspecified injury of unspecified part of colon, subs encntr
		S36.51ØD	Primary blast injury of ascending colon, subs encntr
		S36.511D	Primary blast injury of transverse colon, subs encntr
		S36.512D	Primary blast injury of descending colon, subs encntr
		S36.513D	Primary blast injury of sigmoid colon, subsequent encounter
		S36.518D	Primary blast injury of other part of colon, subs encntr
		S36.519D	Primary blast injury of unsp part of colon, subs encntr
		S36.52ØD	Contusion of ascending [right] colon, subsequent encounter
		S36.521D	Contusion of transverse colon, subsequent encounter
		S36.522D	Contusion of descending [left] colon, subsequent encounter
		S36.523D	Contusion of sigmoid colon, subsequent encounter
		S36.528D	Contusion of other part of colon, subsequent encounter
		S36.529D	Contusion of unspecified part of colon, subsequent encounter
		S36.53ØD	Laceration of ascending [right] colon, subsequent encounter
		S36.531D	Laceration of transverse colon, subsequent encounter
		S36.532D	Laceration of descending [left] colon, subsequent encounter
		S36.533D	Laceration of sigmoid colon, subsequent encounter
		S36.538D	Laceration of other part of colon, subsequent encounter
		S36.539D	Laceration of unspecified part of colon, subs encntr
		S36.59ØD	Other injury of ascending colon, subsequent encounter
		S36.591D	Other injury of transverse colon, subsequent encounter
		S36.592D	Other injury of descending colon, subsequent encounter
		S36.593D	Other injury of sigmoid colon, subsequent encounter
		S36.598D	Other injury of other part of colon, subsequent encounter
		S36.599D	Other injury of unspecified part of colon, subs encntr
		S36.6ØXD	Unspecified injury of rectum, subsequent encounter
		S36.61XD	Primary blast injury of rectum, subsequent encounter
		S36.62XD	Contusion of rectum, subsequent encounter
		S36.63XD	Laceration of rectum, subsequent encounter
		S36.69XD	Other injury of rectum, subsequent encounter
		S36.81XD	Injury of peritoneum, subsequent encounter
		S36.892D	Contusion of other intra-abdominal organs, subs encntr
		S36.893D	Laceration of other intra-abdominal organs, subs encntr
		S36.898D	Other injury of other intra-abdominal organs, subs encntr
		S36.899D	Unsp injury of other intra-abdominal organs, subs encntr
		S36.9ØXD	Unsp injury of unsp intra-abdominal organ, subs encntr
		S36.92XD	Contusion of unspecified intra-abdominal organ, subs encntr
		S36.93XD	Laceration of unspecified intra-abdominal organ, subs encntr
		S36.99XD	Other injury of unsp intra-abdominal organ, subs encntr
		S37.ØØ1D	Unspecified injury of right kidney, subsequent encounter
		S37.ØØ2D	Unspecified injury of left kidney, subsequent encounter
		S37.ØØ9D	Unspecified injury of unspecified kidney, subs encntr
		S37.Ø11D	Minor contusion of right kidney, subsequent encounter
		S37.Ø12D	Minor contusion of left kidney, subsequent encounter
		S37.Ø19D	Minor contusion of unspecified kidney, subsequent encounter
		S37.Ø21D	Major contusion of right kidney, subsequent encounter
		S37.Ø22D	Major contusion of left kidney, subsequent encounter
		S37.Ø29D	Major contusion of unspecified kidney, subsequent encounter
		S37.Ø31D	Laceration of right kidney, unspecified degree, subs encntr
		S37.Ø32D	Laceration of left kidney, unspecified degree, subs encntr
		S37.Ø39D	Laceration of unsp kidney, unspecified degree, subs encntr
		S37.Ø41D	Minor laceration of right kidney, subsequent encounter
		S37.Ø42D	Minor laceration of left kidney, subsequent encounter
		S37.Ø49D	Minor laceration of unspecified kidney, subsequent encounter
		S37.Ø51D	Moderate laceration of right kidney, subsequent encounter
		S37.Ø52D	Moderate laceration of left kidney, subsequent encounter
		S37.Ø59D	Moderate laceration of unspecified kidney, subs encntr
		S37.Ø61D	Major laceration of right kidney, subsequent encounter
		S37.Ø62D	Major laceration of left kidney, subsequent encounter
		S37.Ø69D	Major laceration of unspecified kidney, subsequent encounter
		S37.Ø91D	Other injury of right kidney, subsequent encounter
		S37.Ø92D	Other injury of left kidney, subsequent encounter
		S37.Ø99D	Other injury of unspecified kidney, subsequent encounter
		S37.1ØXD	Unspecified injury of ureter, subsequent encounter
		S37.12XD	Contusion of ureter, subsequent encounter
		S37.13XD	Laceration of ureter, subsequent encounter
		S37.19XD	Other injury of ureter, subsequent encounter
		S37.2ØXD	Unspecified injury of bladder, subsequent encounter
		S37.22XD	Contusion of bladder, subsequent encounter
		S37.23XD	Laceration of bladder, subsequent encounter
		S37.29XD	Other injury of bladder, subsequent encounter
		S37.3ØXD	Unspecified injury of urethra, subsequent encounter
		S37.32XD	Contusion of urethra, subsequent encounter
		S37.33XD	Laceration of urethra, subsequent encounter
		S37.39XD	Other injury of urethra, subsequent encounter
		S37.4Ø1D	Unspecified injury of ovary, unilateral, subs encntr
		S37.4Ø2D	Unspecified injury of ovary, bilateral, subsequent encounter
		S37.4Ø9D	Unspecified injury of ovary, unspecified, subs encntr
	(Continued on next page)	**S37.421D**	Contusion of ovary, unilateral, subsequent encounter

V58.89–V58.89

ICD-9-CM		ICD-10-CM	
V58.89	ENCOUNTER FOR OTHER SPECIFIED AFTERCARE **(Continued)**	**S37.422D**	Contusion of ovary, bilateral, subsequent encounter
		S37.429D	Contusion of ovary, unspecified, subsequent encounter
		S37.431D	Laceration of ovary, unilateral, subsequent encounter
		S37.432D	Laceration of ovary, bilateral, subsequent encounter
		S37.439D	Laceration of ovary, unspecified, subsequent encounter
		S37.491D	Other injury of ovary, unilateral, subsequent encounter
		S37.492D	Other injury of ovary, bilateral, subsequent encounter
		S37.499D	Other injury of ovary, unspecified, subsequent encounter
		S37.5Ø1D	Unsp injury of fallopian tube, unilateral, subs encntr
		S37.5Ø2D	Unspecified injury of fallopian tube, bilateral, subs encntr
		S37.5Ø9D	Unsp injury of fallopian tube, unspecified, subs encntr
		S37.511D	Primary blast injury of fallopian tube, unilateral, subs
		S37.512D	Primary blast injury of fallopian tube, bilateral, subs
		S37.519D	Primary blast injury of fallopian tube, unsp, subs encntr
		S37.521D	Contusion of fallopian tube, unilateral, subs encntr
		S37.522D	Contusion of fallopian tube, bilateral, subsequent encounter
		S37.529D	Contusion of fallopian tube, unspecified, subs encntr
		S37.531D	Laceration of fallopian tube, unilateral, subs encntr
		S37.532D	Laceration of fallopian tube, bilateral, subs encntr
		S37.539D	Laceration of fallopian tube, unspecified, subs encntr
		S37.591D	Other injury of fallopian tube, unilateral, subs encntr
		S37.592D	Other injury of fallopian tube, bilateral, subs encntr
		S37.599D	Other injury of fallopian tube, unspecified, subs encntr
		S37.6ØXD	Unspecified injury of uterus, subsequent encounter
		S37.62XD	Contusion of uterus, subsequent encounter
		S37.63XD	Laceration of uterus, subsequent encounter
		S37.69XD	Other injury of uterus, subsequent encounter
		S37.812D	Contusion of adrenal gland, subsequent encounter
		S37.813D	Laceration of adrenal gland, subsequent encounter
		S37.818D	Other injury of adrenal gland, subsequent encounter
		S37.819D	Unspecified injury of adrenal gland, subsequent encounter
		S37.822D	Contusion of prostate, subsequent encounter
		S37.823D	Laceration of prostate, subsequent encounter
		S37.828D	Other injury of prostate, subsequent encounter
		S37.829D	Unspecified injury of prostate, subsequent encounter
		S37.892D	Contusion of other urinary and pelvic organ, subs encntr
		S37.893D	Laceration of other urinary and pelvic organ, subs encntr
		S37.898D	Other injury of other urinary and pelvic organ, subs encntr
		S37.899D	Unsp injury of other urinary and pelvic organ, subs encntr
		S37.9ØXD	Unsp injury of unsp urinary and pelvic organ, subs encntr
		S37.92XD	Contusion of unsp urinary and pelvic organ, subs encntr
		S37.93XD	Laceration of unsp urinary and pelvic organ, subs encntr
		S37.99XD	Other injury of unsp urinary and pelvic organ, subs encntr
		S38.ØØ1D	Crushing injury of unsp external genital organs, male, subs
		S38.ØØ2D	Crushing inj unsp external genital organs, female, subs
		S38.Ø1XD	Crushing injury of penis, subsequent encounter
		S38.Ø2XD	Crushing injury of scrotum and testis, subsequent encounter
		S38.Ø3XD	Crushing injury of vulva, subsequent encounter
		S38.1XXD	Crushing injury of abdomen, lower back, and pelvis, subs
		S38.211D	Complete traum amp of female external genital organs, subs
		S38.212D	Partial traum amp of female external genital organs, subs
		S38.221D	Complete traumatic amputation of penis, subsequent encounter
		S38.222D	Partial traumatic amputation of penis, subsequent encounter
		S38.231D	Complete traumatic amputation of scrotum and testis, subs
		S38.232D	Partial traumatic amputation of scrotum and testis, subs
		S38.3XXD	Transection (partial) of abdomen, subsequent encounter
		S39.ØØ1D	Unsp injury of muscle, fascia and tendon of abdomen, subs
		S39.ØØ2D	Unsp injury of muscle, fascia and tendon of lower back, subs
		S39.ØØ3D	Unsp injury of muscle, fascia and tendon of pelvis, subs
		S39.Ø11D	Strain of muscle, fascia and tendon of abdomen, subs encntr
		S39.Ø12D	Strain of muscle, fascia and tendon of lower back, subs
		S39.Ø13D	Strain of muscle, fascia and tendon of pelvis, subs encntr
		S39.Ø21D	Laceration of muscle, fascia and tendon of abdomen, subs
		S39.Ø22D	Laceration of muscle, fascia and tendon of lower back, subs
		S39.Ø23D	Laceration of muscle, fascia and tendon of pelvis, subs
		S39.Ø91D	Inj muscle, fascia and tendon of abdomen, subs encntr
		S39.Ø92D	Inj muscle, fascia and tendon of lower back, subs encntr
		S39.Ø93D	Inj muscle, fascia and tendon of pelvis, subs encntr
		S39.81XD	Other specified injuries of abdomen, subsequent encounter
		S39.82XD	Other specified injuries of lower back, subsequent encounter
		S39.83XD	Other specified injuries of pelvis, subsequent encounter
		S39.84ØD	Fracture of corpus cavernosum penis, subsequent encounter
		S39.848D	Other specified injuries of external genitals, subs encntr
		S39.91XD	Unspecified injury of abdomen, subsequent encounter
		S39.92XD	Unspecified injury of lower back, subsequent encounter
		S39.93XD	Unspecified injury of pelvis, subsequent encounter
		S39.94XD	Unspecified injury of external genitals, subs encntr
		S4Ø.Ø11D	Contusion of right shoulder, subsequent encounter
		S4Ø.Ø12D	Contusion of left shoulder, subsequent encounter
		S4Ø.Ø19D	Contusion of unspecified shoulder, subsequent encounter
		S4Ø.Ø21D	Contusion of right upper arm, subsequent encounter
		S4Ø.Ø22D	Contusion of left upper arm, subsequent encounter
	(Continued on next page)	**S4Ø.Ø29D**	Contusion of unspecified upper arm, subsequent encounter

ICD-9-CM		ICD-10-CM	
V58.89	ENCOUNTER FOR OTHER SPECIFIED AFTERCARE **(Continued)**	**S4Ø.211D**	Abrasion of right shoulder, subsequent encounter
		S4Ø.212D	Abrasion of left shoulder, subsequent encounter
		S4Ø.219D	Abrasion of unspecified shoulder, subsequent encounter
		S4Ø.221D	Blister (nonthermal) of right shoulder, subsequent encounter
		S4Ø.222D	Blister (nonthermal) of left shoulder, subsequent encounter
		S4Ø.229D	Blister (nonthermal) of unspecified shoulder, subs encntr
		S4Ø.241D	External constriction of right shoulder, subs encntr
		S4Ø.242D	External constriction of left shoulder, subsequent encounter
		S4Ø.249D	External constriction of unspecified shoulder, subs encntr
		S4Ø.251D	Superficial foreign body of right shoulder, subs encntr
		S4Ø.252D	Superficial foreign body of left shoulder, subs encntr
		S4Ø.259D	Superficial foreign body of unsp shoulder, subs encntr
		S4Ø.261D	Insect bite (nonvenomous) of right shoulder, subs encntr
		S4Ø.262D	Insect bite (nonvenomous) of left shoulder, subs encntr
		S4Ø.269D	Insect bite (nonvenomous) of unsp shoulder, subs encntr
		S4Ø.271D	Other superficial bite of right shoulder, subs encntr
		S4Ø.272D	Other superficial bite of left shoulder, subs encntr
		S4Ø.279D	Other superficial bite of unspecified shoulder, subs encntr
		S4Ø.811D	Abrasion of right upper arm, subsequent encounter
		S4Ø.812D	Abrasion of left upper arm, subsequent encounter
		S4Ø.819D	Abrasion of unspecified upper arm, subsequent encounter
		S4Ø.821D	Blister (nonthermal) of right upper arm, subs encntr
		S4Ø.822D	Blister (nonthermal) of left upper arm, subsequent encounter
		S4Ø.829D	Blister (nonthermal) of unspecified upper arm, subs encntr
		S4Ø.841D	External constriction of right upper arm, subs encntr
		S4Ø.842D	External constriction of left upper arm, subs encntr
		S4Ø.849D	External constriction of unspecified upper arm, subs encntr
		S4Ø.851D	Superficial foreign body of right upper arm, subs encntr
		S4Ø.852D	Superficial foreign body of left upper arm, subs encntr
		S4Ø.859D	Superficial foreign body of unsp upper arm, subs encntr
		S4Ø.861D	Insect bite (nonvenomous) of right upper arm, subs encntr
		S4Ø.862D	Insect bite (nonvenomous) of left upper arm, subs encntr
		S4Ø.869D	Insect bite (nonvenomous) of unsp upper arm, subs encntr
		S4Ø.871D	Other superficial bite of right upper arm, subs encntr
		S4Ø.872D	Other superficial bite of left upper arm, subs encntr
		S4Ø.879D	Other superficial bite of unspecified upper arm, subs encntr
		S4Ø.911D	Unsp superficial injury of right shoulder, subs encntr
		S4Ø.912D	Unspecified superficial injury of left shoulder, subs encntr
		S4Ø.919D	Unsp superficial injury of unspecified shoulder, subs encntr
		S4Ø.921D	Unsp superficial injury of right upper arm, subs encntr
		S4Ø.922D	Unsp superficial injury of left upper arm, subs encntr
		S4Ø.929D	Unsp superficial injury of unsp upper arm, subs encntr
		S41.ØØ1D	Unspecified open wound of right shoulder, subs encntr
		S41.ØØ2D	Unspecified open wound of left shoulder, subs encntr
		S41.ØØ9D	Unspecified open wound of unspecified shoulder, subs encntr
		S41.Ø11D	Laceration w/o foreign body of right shoulder, subs encntr
		S41.Ø12D	Laceration w/o foreign body of left shoulder, subs encntr
		S41.Ø19D	Laceration w/o foreign body of unsp shoulder, subs encntr
		S41.Ø21D	Laceration with foreign body of right shoulder, subs encntr
		S41.Ø22D	Laceration with foreign body of left shoulder, subs encntr
		S41.Ø29D	Laceration with foreign body of unsp shoulder, subs encntr
		S41.Ø31D	Puncture wound w/o foreign body of right shoulder, subs
		S41.Ø32D	Puncture wound w/o foreign body of left shoulder, subs
		S41.Ø39D	Puncture wound w/o foreign body of unsp shoulder, subs
		S41.Ø41D	Puncture wound w foreign body of right shoulder, subs encntr
		S41.Ø42D	Puncture wound w foreign body of left shoulder, subs encntr
		S41.Ø49D	Puncture wound w foreign body of unsp shoulder, subs encntr
		S41.Ø51D	Open bite of right shoulder, subsequent encounter
		S41.Ø52D	Open bite of left shoulder, subsequent encounter
		S41.Ø59D	Open bite of unspecified shoulder, subsequent encounter
		S41.1Ø1D	Unspecified open wound of right upper arm, subs encntr
		S41.1Ø2D	Unspecified open wound of left upper arm, subs encntr
		S41.1Ø9D	Unspecified open wound of unspecified upper arm, subs encntr
		S41.111D	Laceration w/o foreign body of right upper arm, subs encntr
		S41.112D	Laceration w/o foreign body of left upper arm, subs encntr
		S41.119D	Laceration w/o foreign body of unsp upper arm, subs encntr
		S41.121D	Laceration with foreign body of right upper arm, subs encntr
		S41.122D	Laceration with foreign body of left upper arm, subs encntr
		S41.129D	Laceration with foreign body of unsp upper arm, subs encntr
		S41.131D	Puncture wound w/o foreign body of right upper arm, subs
		S41.132D	Puncture wound w/o foreign body of left upper arm, subs
		S41.139D	Puncture wound w/o foreign body of unsp upper arm, subs
		S41.141D	Puncture wound w foreign body of right upper arm, subs
		S41.142D	Puncture wound w foreign body of left upper arm, subs encntr
		S41.149D	Puncture wound w foreign body of unsp upper arm, subs encntr
		S41.151D	Open bite of right upper arm, subsequent encounter
		S41.152D	Open bite of left upper arm, subsequent encounter
		S41.159D	Open bite of unspecified upper arm, subsequent encounter
		S43.ØØ1D	Unspecified subluxation of right shoulder joint, subs encntr
		S43.ØØ2D	Unspecified subluxation of left shoulder joint, subs encntr
		S43.ØØ3D	Unsp subluxation of unspecified shoulder joint, subs encntr
		S43.ØØ4D	Unspecified dislocation of right shoulder joint, subs encntr
	(Continued on next page)	**S43.ØØ5D**	Unspecified dislocation of left shoulder joint, subs encntr

ICD-9-CM	ICD-10-CM	
V58.89 ENCOUNTER FOR OTHER SPECIFIED AFTERCARE **(Continued)**	**S43.006D**	Unsp dislocation of unspecified shoulder joint, subs encntr
	S43.011D	Anterior subluxation of right humerus, subsequent encounter
	S43.012D	Anterior subluxation of left humerus, subsequent encounter
	S43.013D	Anterior subluxation of unspecified humerus, subs encntr
	S43.014D	Anterior dislocation of right humerus, subsequent encounter
	S43.015D	Anterior dislocation of left humerus, subsequent encounter
	S43.016D	Anterior dislocation of unspecified humerus, subs encntr
	S43.021D	Posterior subluxation of right humerus, subsequent encounter
	S43.022D	Posterior subluxation of left humerus, subsequent encounter
	S43.023D	Posterior subluxation of unspecified humerus, subs encntr
	S43.024D	Posterior dislocation of right humerus, subsequent encounter
	S43.025D	Posterior dislocation of left humerus, subsequent encounter
	S43.026D	Posterior dislocation of unspecified humerus, subs encntr
	S43.031D	Inferior subluxation of right humerus, subsequent encounter
	S43.032D	Inferior subluxation of left humerus, subsequent encounter
	S43.033D	Inferior subluxation of unspecified humerus, subs encntr
	S43.034D	Inferior dislocation of right humerus, subsequent encounter
	S43.035D	Inferior dislocation of left humerus, subsequent encounter
	S43.036D	Inferior dislocation of unspecified humerus, subs encntr
	S43.081D	Other subluxation of right shoulder joint, subs encntr
	S43.082D	Other subluxation of left shoulder joint, subs encntr
	S43.083D	Other subluxation of unspecified shoulder joint, subs encntr
	S43.084D	Other dislocation of right shoulder joint, subs encntr
	S43.085D	Other dislocation of left shoulder joint, subs encntr
	S43.086D	Other dislocation of unspecified shoulder joint, subs encntr
	S43.101D	Unsp dislocation of right acromioclavicular joint, subs
	S43.102D	Unsp dislocation of left acromioclavicular joint, subs
	S43.109D	Unsp dislocation of unsp acromioclavicular joint, subs
	S43.111D	Subluxation of right acromioclavicular joint, subs encntr
	S43.112D	Subluxation of left acromioclavicular joint, subs encntr
	S43.119D	Subluxation of unsp acromioclavicular joint, subs encntr
	S43.121D	Dislocation of r acromioclav jt, 100%-200% displacmnt, subs
	S43.122D	Dislocation of l acromioclav jt, 100%-200% displacmnt, subs
	S43.129D	Disloc of unsp acromioclav jt, 100%-200% displacmnt, subs
	S43.131D	Dislocation of r acromioclav jt, > 200% displacmnt, subs
	S43.132D	Dislocation of l acromioclav jt, > 200% displacmnt, subs
	S43.139D	Dislocation of unsp acromioclav jt, > 200% displacmnt, subs
	S43.141D	Inferior dislocation of right acromioclavicular joint, subs
	S43.142D	Inferior dislocation of left acromioclavicular joint, subs
	S43.149D	Inferior dislocation of unsp acromioclavicular joint, subs
	S43.151D	Posterior dislocation of right acromioclavicular joint, subs
	S43.152D	Posterior dislocation of left acromioclavicular joint, subs
	S43.159D	Posterior dislocation of unsp acromioclavicular joint, subs
	S43.201D	Unsp subluxation of right sternoclavicular joint, subs
	S43.202D	Unsp subluxation of left sternoclavicular joint, subs encntr
	S43.203D	Unsp subluxation of unsp sternoclavicular joint, subs encntr
	S43.204D	Unsp dislocation of right sternoclavicular joint, subs
	S43.205D	Unsp dislocation of left sternoclavicular joint, subs encntr
	S43.206D	Unsp dislocation of unsp sternoclavicular joint, subs encntr
	S43.211D	Anterior subluxation of right sternoclavicular joint, subs
	S43.212D	Anterior subluxation of left sternoclavicular joint, subs
	S43.213D	Anterior subluxation of unsp sternoclavicular joint, subs
	S43.214D	Anterior dislocation of right sternoclavicular joint, subs
	S43.215D	Anterior dislocation of left sternoclavicular joint, subs
	S43.216D	Anterior dislocation of unsp sternoclavicular joint, subs
	S43.221D	Posterior subluxation of right sternoclavicular joint, subs
	S43.222D	Posterior subluxation of left sternoclavicular joint, subs
	S43.223D	Posterior subluxation of unsp sternoclavicular joint, subs
	S43.224D	Posterior dislocation of right sternoclavicular joint, subs
	S43.225D	Posterior dislocation of left sternoclavicular joint, subs
	S43.226D	Posterior dislocation of unsp sternoclavicular joint, subs
	S43.301D	Subluxation of unsp parts of right shoulder girdle, subs
	S43.302D	Subluxation of unsp parts of left shoulder girdle, subs
	S43.303D	Subluxation of unsp parts of unsp shoulder girdle, subs
	S43.304D	Dislocation of unsp parts of right shoulder girdle, subs
	S43.305D	Dislocation of unsp parts of left shoulder girdle, subs
	S43.306D	Dislocation of unsp parts of unsp shoulder girdle, subs
	S43.311D	Subluxation of right scapula, subsequent encounter
	S43.312D	Subluxation of left scapula, subsequent encounter
	S43.313D	Subluxation of unspecified scapula, subsequent encounter
	S43.314D	Dislocation of right scapula, subsequent encounter
	S43.315D	Dislocation of left scapula, subsequent encounter
	S43.316D	Dislocation of unspecified scapula, subsequent encounter
	S43.391D	Subluxation of oth prt right shoulder girdle, subs encntr
	S43.392D	Subluxation of oth prt left shoulder girdle, subs encntr
	S43.393D	Subluxation of oth prt unsp shoulder girdle, subs encntr
	S43.394D	Dislocation of oth prt right shoulder girdle, subs encntr
	S43.395D	Dislocation of oth prt left shoulder girdle, subs encntr
	S43.396D	Dislocation of oth prt unsp shoulder girdle, subs encntr
	S43.401D	Unspecified sprain of right shoulder joint, subs encntr
	S43.402D	Unspecified sprain of left shoulder joint, subs encntr
	S43.409D	Unsp sprain of unspecified shoulder joint, subs encntr
(Continued on next page)	**S43.411D**	Sprain of right coracohumeral (ligament), subs encntr

[Brackets] indicate valid character values for each code. Character value meanings provided for each code grouping.

ICD-9-CM		ICD-10-CM	
V58.89	ENCOUNTER FOR OTHER SPECIFIED AFTERCARE **(Continued)**	**S43.412D**	Sprain of left coracohumeral (ligament), subs encntr
		S43.419D	Sprain of unspecified coracohumeral (ligament), subs encntr
		S43.421D	Sprain of right rotator cuff capsule, subsequent encounter
		S43.422D	Sprain of left rotator cuff capsule, subsequent encounter
		S43.429D	Sprain of unspecified rotator cuff capsule, subs encntr
		S43.431D	Superior glenoid labrum lesion of right shoulder, subs
		S43.432D	Superior glenoid labrum lesion of left shoulder, subs encntr
		S43.439D	Superior glenoid labrum lesion of unsp shoulder, subs encntr
		S43.491D	Other sprain of right shoulder joint, subsequent encounter
		S43.492D	Other sprain of left shoulder joint, subsequent encounter
		S43.499D	Other sprain of unspecified shoulder joint, subs encntr
		S43.5ØXD	Sprain of unspecified acromioclavicular joint, subs encntr
		S43.51XD	Sprain of right acromioclavicular joint, subs encntr
		S43.52XD	Sprain of left acromioclavicular joint, subsequent encounter
		S43.6ØXD	Sprain of unspecified sternoclavicular joint, subs encntr
		S43.61XD	Sprain of right sternoclavicular joint, subsequent encounter
		S43.62XD	Sprain of left sternoclavicular joint, subsequent encounter
		S43.8ØXD	Sprain of oth parts of unsp shoulder girdle, subs encntr
		S43.81XD	Sprain of oth parts of right shoulder girdle, subs encntr
		S43.82XD	Sprain of oth parts of left shoulder girdle, subs encntr
		S43.9ØXD	Sprain of unsp parts of unsp shoulder girdle, subs encntr
		S43.91XD	Sprain of unsp parts of right shoulder girdle, subs encntr
		S43.92XD	Sprain of unsp parts of left shoulder girdle, subs encntr
		S44.ØØXD	Injury of ulnar nerve at upper arm level, unsp arm, subs
		S44.Ø1XD	Injury of ulnar nerve at upper arm level, right arm, subs
		S44.Ø2XD	Injury of ulnar nerve at upper arm level, left arm, subs
		S44.1ØXD	Injury of median nerve at upper arm level, unsp arm, subs
		S44.11XD	Injury of median nerve at upper arm level, right arm, subs
		S44.12XD	Injury of median nerve at upper arm level, left arm, subs
		S44.2ØXD	Injury of radial nerve at upper arm level, unsp arm, subs
		S44.21XD	Injury of radial nerve at upper arm level, right arm, subs
		S44.22XD	Injury of radial nerve at upper arm level, left arm, subs
		S44.3ØXD	Injury of axillary nerve, unspecified arm, subs encntr
		S44.31XD	Injury of axillary nerve, right arm, subsequent encounter
		S44.32XD	Injury of axillary nerve, left arm, subsequent encounter
		S44.4ØXD	Injury of musculocutaneous nerve, unsp arm, subs encntr
		S44.41XD	Injury of musculocutaneous nerve, right arm, subs encntr
		S44.42XD	Injury of musculocutaneous nerve, left arm, subs encntr
		S44.5ØXD	Inj cutan sensory nerve at shldr/up arm, unsp arm, subs
		S44.51XD	Inj cutan sensory nerve at shldr/up arm, right arm, subs
		S44.52XD	Inj cutan sensory nerve at shldr/up arm, left arm, subs
		S44.8X1D	Injury of nerves at shldr/up arm, right arm, subs
		S44.8X2D	Injury of nerves at shldr/up arm, left arm, subs
		S44.8X9D	Injury of nerves at shldr/up arm, unsp arm, subs
		S44.9ØXD	Injury of unsp nerve at shldr/up arm, unsp arm, subs
		S44.91XD	Injury of unsp nerve at shldr/up arm, right arm, subs
		S44.92XD	Injury of unsp nerve at shldr/up arm, left arm, subs
		S45.ØØ1D	Unsp injury of axillary artery, right side, subs encntr
		S45.ØØ2D	Unsp injury of axillary artery, left side, subs encntr
		S45.ØØ9D	Unsp injury of axillary artery, unsp side, subs encntr
		S45.Ø11D	Laceration of axillary artery, right side, subs encntr
		S45.Ø12D	Laceration of axillary artery, left side, subs encntr
		S45.Ø19D	Laceration of axillary artery, unspecified side, subs encntr
		S45.Ø91D	Oth injury of axillary artery, right side, subs encntr
		S45.Ø92D	Oth injury of axillary artery, left side, subs encntr
		S45.Ø99D	Oth injury of axillary artery, unspecified side, subs encntr
		S45.1Ø1D	Unsp injury of brachial artery, right side, subs encntr
		S45.1Ø2D	Unsp injury of brachial artery, left side, subs encntr
		S45.1Ø9D	Unsp injury of brachial artery, unsp side, subs encntr
		S45.111D	Laceration of brachial artery, right side, subs encntr
		S45.112D	Laceration of brachial artery, left side, subs encntr
		S45.119D	Laceration of brachial artery, unspecified side, subs encntr
		S45.191D	Oth injury of brachial artery, right side, subs encntr
		S45.192D	Oth injury of brachial artery, left side, subs encntr
		S45.199D	Oth injury of brachial artery, unspecified side, subs encntr
		S45.2Ø1D	Unsp injury of axillary or brachial vein, right side, subs
		S45.2Ø2D	Unsp injury of axillary or brachial vein, left side, subs
		S45.2Ø9D	Unsp injury of axillary or brachial vein, unsp side, subs
		S45.211D	Laceration of axillary or brachial vein, right side, subs
		S45.212D	Laceration of axillary or brachial vein, left side, subs
		S45.219D	Laceration of axillary or brachial vein, unsp side, subs
		S45.291D	Inj axillary or brachial vein, right side, subs encntr
		S45.292D	Inj axillary or brachial vein, left side, subs encntr
		S45.299D	Inj axillary or brachial vein, unsp side, subs encntr
		S45.3Ø1D	Unsp injury of superfic vn at shldr/up arm, right arm, subs
		S45.3Ø2D	Unsp injury of superfic vn at shldr/up arm, left arm, subs
		S45.3Ø9D	Unsp injury of superfic vn at shldr/up arm, unsp arm, subs
		S45.311D	Laceration of superfic vn at shldr/up arm, right arm, subs
		S45.312D	Laceration of superfic vn at shldr/up arm, left arm, subs
		S45.319D	Laceration of superfic vn at shldr/up arm, unsp arm, subs
		S45.391D	Inj superficial vein at shldr/up arm, right arm, subs
		S45.392D	Inj superficial vein at shldr/up arm, left arm, subs
	(Continued on next page)	**S45.399D**	Inj superficial vein at shldr/up arm, unsp arm, subs

ICD-9-CM		ICD-10-CM	
V58.89	ENCOUNTER FOR OTHER SPECIFIED AFTERCARE **(Continued)**	**S45.801D**	Unsp inj blood vessels at shldr/up arm, right arm, subs
		S45.802D	Unsp injury of blood vessels at shldr/up arm, left arm, subs
		S45.809D	Unsp injury of blood vessels at shldr/up arm, unsp arm, subs
		S45.811D	Laceration of blood vessels at shldr/up arm, right arm, subs
		S45.812D	Laceration of blood vessels at shldr/up arm, left arm, subs
		S45.819D	Laceration of blood vessels at shldr/up arm, unsp arm, subs
		S45.891D	Inj oth blood vessels at shldr/up arm, right arm, subs
		S45.892D	Inj oth blood vessels at shldr/up arm, left arm, subs
		S45.899D	Inj oth blood vessels at shldr/up arm, unsp arm, subs
		S45.901D	Unsp inj unsp blood vess at shldr/up arm, right arm, subs
		S45.902D	Unsp inj unsp blood vess at shldr/up arm, left arm, subs
		S45.909D	Unsp inj unsp blood vess at shldr/up arm, unsp arm, subs
		S45.911D	Lacerat unsp blood vessel at shldr/up arm, right arm, subs
		S45.912D	Lacerat unsp blood vessel at shldr/up arm, left arm, subs
		S45.919D	Lacerat unsp blood vessel at shldr/up arm, unsp arm, subs
		S45.991D	Inj unsp blood vessel at shldr/up arm, right arm, subs
		S45.992D	Inj unsp blood vessel at shldr/up arm, left arm, subs
		S45.999D	Inj unsp blood vessel at shldr/up arm, unsp arm, subs
		S46.001D	Unsp inj musc/tend the rotator cuff of r shoulder, subs
		S46.002D	Unsp inj musc/tend the rotator cuff of l shoulder, subs
		S46.009D	Unsp inj musc/tend the rotator cuff of unsp shoulder, subs
		S46.011D	Strain of musc/tend the rotator cuff of right shoulder, subs
		S46.012D	Strain of musc/tend the rotator cuff of left shoulder, subs
		S46.019D	Strain of musc/tend the rotator cuff of unsp shoulder, subs
		S46.021D	Laceration of musc/tend the rotator cuff of r shoulder, subs
		S46.022D	Lacerat musc/tend the rotator cuff of left shoulder, subs
		S46.029D	Lacerat musc/tend the rotator cuff of unsp shoulder, subs
		S46.091D	Inj musc/tend the rotator cuff of right shoulder, subs
		S46.092D	Inj musc/tend the rotator cuff of left shoulder, subs
		S46.099D	Inj musc/tend the rotator cuff of unsp shoulder, subs
		S46.101D	Unsp injury of musc/fasc/tend long hd bicep, right arm, subs
		S46.102D	Unsp injury of musc/fasc/tend long hd bicep, left arm, subs
		S46.109D	Unsp injury of musc/fasc/tend long hd bicep, unsp arm, subs
		S46.111D	Strain of musc/fasc/tend long hd bicep, right arm, subs
		S46.112D	Strain of musc/fasc/tend long head of biceps, left arm, subs
		S46.119D	Strain of musc/fasc/tend long head of biceps, unsp arm, subs
		S46.121D	Laceration of musc/fasc/tend long hd bicep, right arm, subs
		S46.122D	Laceration of musc/fasc/tend long hd bicep, left arm, subs
		S46.129D	Laceration of musc/fasc/tend long hd bicep, unsp arm, subs
		S46.191D	Inj musc/fasc/tend long head of biceps, right arm, subs
		S46.192D	Inj musc/fasc/tend long head of biceps, left arm, subs
		S46.199D	Inj musc/fasc/tend long head of biceps, unsp arm, subs
		S46.201D	Unsp injury of musc/fasc/tend prt biceps, right arm, subs
		S46.202D	Unsp injury of musc/fasc/tend prt biceps, left arm, subs
		S46.209D	Unsp injury of musc/fasc/tend prt biceps, unsp arm, subs
		S46.211D	Strain of musc/fasc/tend prt biceps, right arm, subs
		S46.212D	Strain of musc/fasc/tend prt biceps, left arm, subs
		S46.219D	Strain of musc/fasc/tend prt biceps, unsp arm, subs
		S46.221D	Laceration of musc/fasc/tend prt biceps, right arm, subs
		S46.222D	Laceration of musc/fasc/tend prt biceps, left arm, subs
		S46.229D	Laceration of musc/fasc/tend prt biceps, unsp arm, subs
		S46.291D	Inj muscle, fascia and tendon of prt biceps, right arm, subs
		S46.292D	Inj muscle, fascia and tendon of prt biceps, left arm, subs
		S46.299D	Inj muscle, fascia and tendon of prt biceps, unsp arm, subs
		S46.301D	Unsp injury of musc/fasc/tend triceps, right arm, subs
		S46.302D	Unsp injury of musc/fasc/tend triceps, left arm, subs
		S46.309D	Unsp injury of musc/fasc/tend triceps, unsp arm, subs
		S46.311D	Strain of musc/fasc/tend triceps, right arm, subs
		S46.312D	Strain of musc/fasc/tend triceps, left arm, subs
		S46.319D	Strain of musc/fasc/tend triceps, unsp arm, subs
		S46.321D	Laceration of musc/fasc/tend triceps, right arm, subs
		S46.322D	Laceration of musc/fasc/tend triceps, left arm, subs
		S46.329D	Laceration of musc/fasc/tend triceps, unsp arm, subs
		S46.391D	Inj muscle, fascia and tendon of triceps, right arm, subs
		S46.392D	Inj muscle, fascia and tendon of triceps, left arm, subs
		S46.399D	Inj muscle, fascia and tendon of triceps, unsp arm, subs
		S46.801D	Unsp inj musc/fasc/tend at shldr/up arm, right arm, subs
		S46.802D	Unsp inj musc/fasc/tend at shldr/up arm, left arm, subs
		S46.809D	Unsp inj musc/fasc/tend at shldr/up arm, unsp arm, subs
		S46.811D	Strain of musc/fasc/tend at shldr/up arm, right arm, subs
		S46.812D	Strain of musc/fasc/tend at shldr/up arm, left arm, subs
		S46.819D	Strain of musc/fasc/tend at shldr/up arm, unsp arm, subs
		S46.821D	Lacerat musc/fasc/tend at shldr/up arm, right arm, subs
		S46.822D	Laceration of musc/fasc/tend at shldr/up arm, left arm, subs
		S46.829D	Laceration of musc/fasc/tend at shldr/up arm, unsp arm, subs
		S46.891D	Inj musc/fasc/tend at shldr/up arm, right arm, subs
		S46.892D	Inj musc/fasc/tend at shldr/up arm, left arm, subs
		S46.899D	Inj musc/fasc/tend at shldr/up arm, unsp arm, subs
		S46.901D	Unsp inj unsp musc/fasc/tend at shldr/up arm, r arm, subs
		S46.902D	Unsp inj unsp musc/fasc/tend at shldr/up arm, left arm, subs
		S46.909D	Unsp inj unsp musc/fasc/tend at shldr/up arm, unsp arm, subs
		S46.911D	Strain unsp musc/fasc/tend at shldr/up arm, right arm, subs
	(Continued on next page)	**S46.912D**	Strain unsp musc/fasc/tend at shldr/up arm, left arm, subs

ICD-9-CM		ICD-10-CM	
V58.89	ENCOUNTER FOR OTHER SPECIFIED AFTERCARE **(Continued)**	S46.919D	Strain unsp musc/fasc/tend at shldr/up arm, unsp arm, subs
		S46.921D	Lacerat unsp musc/fasc/tend at shldr/up arm, right arm, subs
		S46.922D	Lacerat unsp musc/fasc/tend at shldr/up arm, left arm, subs
		S46.929D	Lacerat unsp musc/fasc/tend at shldr/up arm, unsp arm, subs
		S46.991D	Inj unsp musc/fasc/tend at shldr/up arm, right arm, subs
		S46.992D	Inj unsp musc/fasc/tend at shldr/up arm, left arm, subs
		S46.999D	Inj unsp musc/fasc/tend at shldr/up arm, unsp arm, subs
		S47.1XXD	Crushing injury of right shoulder and upper arm, subs encntr
		S47.2XXD	Crushing injury of left shoulder and upper arm, subs encntr
		S47.9XXD	Crushing injury of shoulder and upper arm, unsp arm, subs
		S48.Ø11D	Complete traumatic amputation at right shoulder joint, subs
		S48.Ø12D	Complete traumatic amputation at left shoulder joint, subs
		S48.Ø19D	Complete traumatic amputation at unsp shoulder joint, subs
		S48.Ø21D	Partial traumatic amputation at right shoulder joint, subs
		S48.Ø22D	Partial traumatic amputation at left shoulder joint, subs
		S48.Ø29D	Partial traumatic amputation at unsp shoulder joint, subs
		S48.111D	Complete traum amp at level betw r shoulder and elbow, subs
		S48.112D	Complete traum amp at level betw l shoulder and elbow, subs
		S48.119D	Complete traum amp at level betw unsp shldr and elbow, subs
		S48.121D	Partial traum amp at level betw r shoulder and elbow, subs
		S48.122D	Partial traum amp at level betw l shoulder and elbow, subs
		S48.129D	Partial traum amp at level betw unsp shldr and elbow, subs
		S48.911D	Complete traum amp of right shldr/up arm, level unsp, subs
		S48.912D	Complete traum amp of left shldr/up arm, level unsp, subs
		S48.919D	Complete traum amp of unsp shldr/up arm, level unsp, subs
		S48.921D	Partial traum amp of right shldr/up arm, level unsp, subs
		S48.922D	Partial traumatic amp of left shldr/up arm, level unsp, subs
		S48.929D	Partial traumatic amp of unsp shldr/up arm, level unsp, subs
		S49.8ØXD	Oth injuries of shoulder and upper arm, unsp arm, subs
		S49.81XD	Oth injuries of right shoulder and upper arm, subs encntr
		S49.82XD	Oth injuries of left shoulder and upper arm, subs encntr
		S49.9ØXD	Unsp injury of shoulder and upper arm, unsp arm, subs encntr
		S49.91XD	Unsp injury of right shoulder and upper arm, subs encntr
		S49.92XD	Unsp injury of left shoulder and upper arm, subs encntr
		S5Ø.ØØXD	Contusion of unspecified elbow, subsequent encounter
		S5Ø.Ø1XD	Contusion of right elbow, subsequent encounter
		S5Ø.Ø2XD	Contusion of left elbow, subsequent encounter
		S5Ø.1ØXD	Contusion of unspecified forearm, subsequent encounter
		S5Ø.11XD	Contusion of right forearm, subsequent encounter
		S5Ø.12XD	Contusion of left forearm, subsequent encounter
		S5Ø.311D	Abrasion of right elbow, subsequent encounter
		S5Ø.312D	Abrasion of left elbow, subsequent encounter
		S5Ø.319D	Abrasion of unspecified elbow, subsequent encounter
		S5Ø.321D	Blister (nonthermal) of right elbow, subsequent encounter
		S5Ø.322D	Blister (nonthermal) of left elbow, subsequent encounter
		S5Ø.329D	Blister (nonthermal) of unspecified elbow, subs encntr
		S5Ø.341D	External constriction of right elbow, subsequent encounter
		S5Ø.342D	External constriction of left elbow, subsequent encounter
		S5Ø.349D	External constriction of unspecified elbow, subs encntr
		S5Ø.351D	Superficial foreign body of right elbow, subs encntr
		S5Ø.352D	Superficial foreign body of left elbow, subsequent encounter
		S5Ø.359D	Superficial foreign body of unspecified elbow, subs encntr
		S5Ø.361D	Insect bite (nonvenomous) of right elbow, subs encntr
		S5Ø.362D	Insect bite (nonvenomous) of left elbow, subs encntr
		S5Ø.369D	Insect bite (nonvenomous) of unspecified elbow, subs encntr
		S5Ø.371D	Other superficial bite of right elbow, subsequent encounter
		S5Ø.372D	Other superficial bite of left elbow, subsequent encounter
		S5Ø.379D	Other superficial bite of unspecified elbow, subs encntr
		S5Ø.811D	Abrasion of right forearm, subsequent encounter
		S5Ø.812D	Abrasion of left forearm, subsequent encounter
		S5Ø.819D	Abrasion of unspecified forearm, subsequent encounter
		S5Ø.821D	Blister (nonthermal) of right forearm, subsequent encounter
		S5Ø.822D	Blister (nonthermal) of left forearm, subsequent encounter
		S5Ø.829D	Blister (nonthermal) of unspecified forearm, subs encntr
		S5Ø.841D	External constriction of right forearm, subsequent encounter
		S5Ø.842D	External constriction of left forearm, subsequent encounter
		S5Ø.849D	External constriction of unspecified forearm, subs encntr
		S5Ø.851D	Superficial foreign body of right forearm, subs encntr
		S5Ø.852D	Superficial foreign body of left forearm, subs encntr
		S5Ø.859D	Superficial foreign body of unspecified forearm, subs encntr
		S5Ø.861D	Insect bite (nonvenomous) of right forearm, subs encntr
		S5Ø.862D	Insect bite (nonvenomous) of left forearm, subs encntr
		S5Ø.869D	Insect bite (nonvenomous) of unsp forearm, subs encntr
		S5Ø.871D	Other superficial bite of right forearm, subs encntr
		S5Ø.872D	Other superficial bite of left forearm, subsequent encounter
		S5Ø.879D	Other superficial bite of unspecified forearm, subs encntr
		S5Ø.9Ø1D	Unspecified superficial injury of right elbow, subs encntr
		S5Ø.9Ø2D	Unspecified superficial injury of left elbow, subs encntr
		S5Ø.9Ø9D	Unsp superficial injury of unspecified elbow, subs encntr
		S5Ø.911D	Unspecified superficial injury of right forearm, subs encntr
		S5Ø.912D	Unspecified superficial injury of left forearm, subs encntr
		S5Ø.919D	Unsp superficial injury of unspecified forearm, subs encntr
	(Continued on next page)	S51.ØØ1D	Unspecified open wound of right elbow, subsequent encounter

ICD-9-CM		ICD-10-CM	
V58.89	ENCOUNTER FOR OTHER SPECIFIED AFTERCARE **(Continued)**	**S51.ØØ2D**	Unspecified open wound of left elbow, subsequent encounter
		S51.ØØ9D	Unspecified open wound of unspecified elbow, subs encntr
		S51.Ø11D	Laceration without foreign body of right elbow, subs encntr
		S51.Ø12D	Laceration without foreign body of left elbow, subs encntr
		S51.Ø19D	Laceration without foreign body of unsp elbow, subs encntr
		S51.Ø21D	Laceration with foreign body of right elbow, subs encntr
		S51.Ø22D	Laceration with foreign body of left elbow, subs encntr
		S51.Ø29D	Laceration with foreign body of unsp elbow, subs encntr
		S51.Ø31D	Puncture wound w/o foreign body of right elbow, subs encntr
		S51.Ø32D	Puncture wound w/o foreign body of left elbow, subs encntr
		S51.Ø39D	Puncture wound w/o foreign body of unsp elbow, subs encntr
		S51.Ø41D	Puncture wound with foreign body of right elbow, subs encntr
		S51.Ø42D	Puncture wound with foreign body of left elbow, subs encntr
		S51.Ø49D	Puncture wound with foreign body of unsp elbow, subs encntr
		S51.Ø51D	Open bite, right elbow, subsequent encounter
		S51.Ø52D	Open bite, left elbow, subsequent encounter
		S51.Ø59D	Open bite, unspecified elbow, subsequent encounter
		S51.8Ø1D	Unspecified open wound of right forearm, subs encntr
		S51.8Ø2D	Unspecified open wound of left forearm, subsequent encounter
		S51.8Ø9D	Unspecified open wound of unspecified forearm, subs encntr
		S51.811D	Laceration w/o foreign body of right forearm, subs encntr
		S51.812D	Laceration without foreign body of left forearm, subs encntr
		S51.819D	Laceration without foreign body of unsp forearm, subs encntr
		S51.821D	Laceration with foreign body of right forearm, subs encntr
		S51.822D	Laceration with foreign body of left forearm, subs encntr
		S51.829D	Laceration with foreign body of unsp forearm, subs encntr
		S51.831D	Puncture wound w/o foreign body of right forearm, subs
		S51.832D	Puncture wound w/o foreign body of left forearm, subs encntr
		S51.839D	Puncture wound w/o foreign body of unsp forearm, subs encntr
		S51.841D	Puncture wound w foreign body of right forearm, subs encntr
		S51.842D	Puncture wound w foreign body of left forearm, subs encntr
		S51.849D	Puncture wound w foreign body of unsp forearm, subs encntr
		S51.851D	Open bite of right forearm, subsequent encounter
		S51.852D	Open bite of left forearm, subsequent encounter
		S51.859D	Open bite of unspecified forearm, subsequent encounter
		S53.ØØ1D	Unspecified subluxation of right radial head, subs encntr
		S53.ØØ2D	Unspecified subluxation of left radial head, subs encntr
		S53.ØØ3D	Unsp subluxation of unspecified radial head, subs encntr
		S53.ØØ4D	Unspecified dislocation of right radial head, subs encntr
		S53.ØØ5D	Unspecified dislocation of left radial head, subs encntr
		S53.ØØ6D	Unsp dislocation of unspecified radial head, subs encntr
		S53.Ø11D	Anterior subluxation of right radial head, subs encntr
		S53.Ø12D	Anterior subluxation of left radial head, subs encntr
		S53.Ø13D	Anterior subluxation of unspecified radial head, subs encntr
		S53.Ø14D	Anterior dislocation of right radial head, subs encntr
		S53.Ø15D	Anterior dislocation of left radial head, subs encntr
		S53.Ø16D	Anterior dislocation of unspecified radial head, subs encntr
		S53.Ø21D	Posterior subluxation of right radial head, subs encntr
		S53.Ø22D	Posterior subluxation of left radial head, subs encntr
		S53.Ø23D	Posterior subluxation of unsp radial head, subs encntr
		S53.Ø24D	Posterior dislocation of right radial head, subs encntr
		S53.Ø25D	Posterior dislocation of left radial head, subs encntr
		S53.Ø26D	Posterior dislocation of unsp radial head, subs encntr
		S53.Ø31D	Nursemaid's elbow, right elbow, subsequent encounter
		S53.Ø32D	Nursemaid's elbow, left elbow, subsequent encounter
		S53.Ø33D	Nursemaid's elbow, unspecified elbow, subsequent encounter
		S53.Ø91D	Other subluxation of right radial head, subsequent encounter
		S53.Ø92D	Other subluxation of left radial head, subsequent encounter
		S53.Ø93D	Other subluxation of unspecified radial head, subs encntr
		S53.Ø94D	Other dislocation of right radial head, subsequent encounter
		S53.Ø95D	Other dislocation of left radial head, subsequent encounter
		S53.Ø96D	Other dislocation of unspecified radial head, subs encntr
		S53.1Ø1D	Unsp subluxation of right ulnohumeral joint, subs encntr
		S53.1Ø2D	Unsp subluxation of left ulnohumeral joint, subs encntr
		S53.1Ø3D	Unsp subluxation of unsp ulnohumeral joint, subs encntr
		S53.1Ø4D	Unsp dislocation of right ulnohumeral joint, subs encntr
		S53.1Ø5D	Unsp dislocation of left ulnohumeral joint, subs encntr
		S53.1Ø6D	Unsp dislocation of unsp ulnohumeral joint, subs encntr
		S53.111D	Anterior subluxation of right ulnohumeral joint, subs encntr
		S53.112D	Anterior subluxation of left ulnohumeral joint, subs encntr
		S53.113D	Anterior subluxation of unsp ulnohumeral joint, subs encntr
		S53.114D	Anterior dislocation of right ulnohumeral joint, subs encntr
		S53.115D	Anterior dislocation of left ulnohumeral joint, subs encntr
		S53.116D	Anterior dislocation of unsp ulnohumeral joint, subs encntr
		S53.121D	Posterior subluxation of right ulnohumeral joint, subs
		S53.122D	Posterior subluxation of left ulnohumeral joint, subs encntr
		S53.123D	Posterior subluxation of unsp ulnohumeral joint, subs encntr
		S53.124D	Posterior dislocation of right ulnohumeral joint, subs
		S53.125D	Posterior dislocation of left ulnohumeral joint, subs encntr
		S53.126D	Posterior dislocation of unsp ulnohumeral joint, subs encntr
		S53.131D	Medial subluxation of right ulnohumeral joint, subs encntr
		S53.132D	Medial subluxation of left ulnohumeral joint, subs encntr
	(Continued on next page)	**S53.133D**	Medial subluxation of unsp ulnohumeral joint, subs encntr

ICD-9-CM		ICD-10-CM	
V58.89	ENCOUNTER FOR OTHER SPECIFIED AFTERCARE **(Continued)**	**S53.134D**	Medial dislocation of right ulnohumeral joint, subs encntr
		S53.135D	Medial dislocation of left ulnohumeral joint, subs encntr
		S53.136D	Medial dislocation of unsp ulnohumeral joint, subs encntr
		S53.141D	Lateral subluxation of right ulnohumeral joint, subs encntr
		S53.142D	Lateral subluxation of left ulnohumeral joint, subs encntr
		S53.143D	Lateral subluxation of unsp ulnohumeral joint, subs encntr
		S53.144D	Lateral dislocation of right ulnohumeral joint, subs encntr
		S53.145D	Lateral dislocation of left ulnohumeral joint, subs encntr
		S53.146D	Lateral dislocation of unsp ulnohumeral joint, subs encntr
		S53.191D	Other subluxation of right ulnohumeral joint, subs encntr
		S53.192D	Other subluxation of left ulnohumeral joint, subs encntr
		S53.193D	Other subluxation of unsp ulnohumeral joint, subs encntr
		S53.194D	Other dislocation of right ulnohumeral joint, subs encntr
		S53.195D	Other dislocation of left ulnohumeral joint, subs encntr
		S53.196D	Other dislocation of unsp ulnohumeral joint, subs encntr
		S53.2ØXD	Traumatic rupture of unsp radial collateral ligament, subs
		S53.21XD	Traumatic rupture of right radial collateral ligament, subs
		S53.22XD	Traumatic rupture of left radial collateral ligament, subs
		S53.3ØXD	Traumatic rupture of unsp ulnar collateral ligament, subs
		S53.31XD	Traumatic rupture of right ulnar collateral ligament, subs
		S53.32XD	Traumatic rupture of left ulnar collateral ligament, subs
		S53.4Ø1D	Unspecified sprain of right elbow, subsequent encounter
		S53.4Ø2D	Unspecified sprain of left elbow, subsequent encounter
		S53.4Ø9D	Unspecified sprain of unspecified elbow, subs encntr
		S53.411D	Radiohumeral (joint) sprain of right elbow, subs encntr
		S53.412D	Radiohumeral (joint) sprain of left elbow, subs encntr
		S53.419D	Radiohumeral (joint) sprain of unsp elbow, subs encntr
		S53.421D	Ulnohumeral (joint) sprain of right elbow, subs encntr
		S53.422D	Ulnohumeral (joint) sprain of left elbow, subs encntr
		S53.429D	Ulnohumeral (joint) sprain of unspecified elbow, subs encntr
		S53.431D	Radial collateral ligament sprain of right elbow, subs
		S53.432D	Radial collateral ligament sprain of left elbow, subs encntr
		S53.439D	Radial collateral ligament sprain of unsp elbow, subs encntr
		S53.441D	Ulnar collateral ligament sprain of right elbow, subs encntr
		S53.442D	Ulnar collateral ligament sprain of left elbow, subs encntr
		S53.449D	Ulnar collateral ligament sprain of unsp elbow, subs encntr
		S53.491D	Other sprain of right elbow, subsequent encounter
		S53.492D	Other sprain of left elbow, subsequent encounter
		S53.499D	Other sprain of unspecified elbow, subsequent encounter
		S54.ØØXD	Injury of ulnar nerve at forearm level, unsp arm, subs
		S54.Ø1XD	Injury of ulnar nerve at forearm level, right arm, subs
		S54.Ø2XD	Injury of ulnar nerve at forearm level, left arm, subs
		S54.1ØXD	Injury of median nerve at forearm level, unsp arm, subs
		S54.11XD	Injury of median nerve at forearm level, right arm, subs
		S54.12XD	Injury of median nerve at forearm level, left arm, subs
		S54.2ØXD	Injury of radial nerve at forearm level, unsp arm, subs
		S54.21XD	Injury of radial nerve at forearm level, right arm, subs
		S54.22XD	Injury of radial nerve at forearm level, left arm, subs
		S54.3ØXD	Injury of cutan sensory nerve at forarm lv, unsp arm, subs
		S54.31XD	Injury of cutan sensory nerve at forarm lv, right arm, subs
		S54.32XD	Injury of cutan sensory nerve at forarm lv, left arm, subs
		S54.8X1D	Unsp injury of oth nerves at forearm level, right arm, subs
		S54.8X2D	Unsp injury of oth nerves at forearm level, left arm, subs
		S54.8X9D	Unsp injury of oth nerves at forearm level, unsp arm, subs
		S54.9ØXD	Injury of unsp nerve at forearm level, unsp arm, subs encntr
		S54.91XD	Injury of unsp nerve at forearm level, right arm, subs
		S54.92XD	Injury of unsp nerve at forearm level, left arm, subs encntr
		S55.ØØ1D	Unsp injury of ulnar artery at forarm lv, right arm, subs
		S55.ØØ2D	Unsp injury of ulnar artery at forearm level, left arm, subs
		S55.ØØ9D	Unsp injury of ulnar artery at forearm level, unsp arm, subs
		S55.Ø11D	Laceration of ulnar artery at forearm level, right arm, subs
		S55.Ø12D	Laceration of ulnar artery at forearm level, left arm, subs
		S55.Ø19D	Laceration of ulnar artery at forearm level, unsp arm, subs
		S55.Ø91D	Inj ulnar artery at forearm level, right arm, subs encntr
		S55.Ø92D	Inj ulnar artery at forearm level, left arm, subs encntr
		S55.Ø99D	Inj ulnar artery at forearm level, unsp arm, subs encntr
		S55.1Ø1D	Unsp injury of radial artery at forarm lv, right arm, subs
		S55.1Ø2D	Unsp injury of radial artery at forarm lv, left arm, subs
		S55.1Ø9D	Unsp injury of radial artery at forarm lv, unsp arm, subs
		S55.111D	Laceration of radial artery at forarm lv, right arm, subs
		S55.112D	Laceration of radial artery at forearm level, left arm, subs
		S55.119D	Laceration of radial artery at forearm level, unsp arm, subs
		S55.191D	Inj radial artery at forearm level, right arm, subs encntr
		S55.192D	Inj radial artery at forearm level, left arm, subs encntr
		S55.199D	Inj radial artery at forearm level, unsp arm, subs encntr
		S55.2Ø1D	Unsp injury of vein at forearm level, right arm, subs encntr
		S55.2Ø2D	Unsp injury of vein at forearm level, left arm, subs encntr
		S55.2Ø9D	Unsp injury of vein at forearm level, unsp arm, subs encntr
		S55.211D	Laceration of vein at forearm level, right arm, subs encntr
		S55.212D	Laceration of vein at forearm level, left arm, subs encntr
		S55.219D	Laceration of vein at forearm level, unsp arm, subs encntr
		S55.291D	Oth injury of vein at forearm level, right arm, subs encntr
	(Continued on next page)	**S55.292D**	Oth injury of vein at forearm level, left arm, subs encntr

ICD-9-CM		ICD-10-CM	
V58.89	ENCOUNTER FOR OTHER SPECIFIED AFTERCARE **(Continued)**	**S55.299D**	Oth injury of vein at forearm level, unsp arm, subs encntr
		S55.801D	Unsp injury of blood vessels at forarm lv, right arm, subs
		S55.802D	Unsp injury of blood vessels at forarm lv, left arm, subs
		S55.809D	Unsp injury of blood vessels at forarm lv, unsp arm, subs
		S55.811D	Laceration of blood vessels at forarm lv, right arm, subs
		S55.812D	Laceration of blood vessels at forearm level, left arm, subs
		S55.819D	Laceration of blood vessels at forearm level, unsp arm, subs
		S55.891D	Inj oth blood vessels at forearm level, right arm, subs
		S55.892D	Inj oth blood vessels at forearm level, left arm, subs
		S55.899D	Inj oth blood vessels at forearm level, unsp arm, subs
		S55.901D	Unsp injury of unsp blood vess at forarm lv, right arm, subs
		S55.902D	Unsp injury of unsp blood vess at forarm lv, left arm, subs
		S55.909D	Unsp injury of unsp blood vess at forarm lv, unsp arm, subs
		S55.911D	Lacerat unsp blood vessel at forarm lv, right arm, subs
		S55.912D	Laceration of unsp blood vessel at forarm lv, left arm, subs
		S55.919D	Laceration of unsp blood vessel at forarm lv, unsp arm, subs
		S55.991D	Inj unsp blood vessel at forearm level, right arm, subs
		S55.992D	Inj unsp blood vessel at forearm level, left arm, subs
		S55.999D	Inj unsp blood vessel at forearm level, unsp arm, subs
		S56.001D	Unsp inj flexor musc/fasc/tend r thm at forarm lv, subs
		S56.002D	Unsp inj flexor musc/fasc/tend l thm at forarm lv, subs
		S56.009D	Unsp injury of flexor musc/fasc/tend thmb at forarm lv, subs
		S56.011D	Strain of flexor musc/fasc/tend r thm at forarm lv, subs
		S56.012D	Strain of flexor musc/fasc/tend l thm at forarm lv, subs
		S56.019D	Strain of flexor musc/fasc/tend thmb at forearm level, subs
		S56.021D	Lacerat flexor musc/fasc/tend right thumb at forarm lv, subs
		S56.022D	Lacerat flexor musc/fasc/tend left thumb at forarm lv, subs
		S56.029D	Laceration of flexor musc/fasc/tend thmb at forarm lv, subs
		S56.091D	Inj flexor musc/fasc/tend right thumb at forearm level, subs
		S56.092D	Inj flexor musc/fasc/tend left thumb at forearm level, subs
		S56.099D	Inj flexor musc/fasc/tend thmb at forearm level, subs
		S56.101D	Unsp inj flexor musc/fasc/tend r idx fngr at forarm lv, subs
		S56.102D	Unsp inj flexor musc/fasc/tend l idx fngr at forarm lv, subs
		S56.103D	Unsp inj flexor musc/fasc/tend r mid fngr at forarm lv, subs
		S56.104D	Unsp inj flexor musc/fasc/tend l mid fngr at forarm lv, subs
		S56.105D	Unsp inj flexor musc/fasc/tend r rng fngr at forarm lv, subs
		S56.106D	Unsp inj flexor musc/fasc/tend l rng fngr at forarm lv, subs
		S56.107D	Unsp inj flxr musc/fasc/tend r lit fngr at forarm lv, subs
		S56.108D	Unsp inj flxr musc/fasc/tend l lit fngr at forarm lv, subs
		S56.109D	Unsp inj flexor musc/fasc/tend unsp fngr at forarm lv, subs
		S56.111D	Strain flexor musc/fasc/tend r idx fngr at forarm lv, subs
		S56.112D	Strain flexor musc/fasc/tend l idx fngr at forarm lv, subs
		S56.113D	Strain flexor musc/fasc/tend r mid finger at forarm lv, subs
		S56.114D	Strain flexor musc/fasc/tend l mid finger at forarm lv, subs
		S56.115D	Strain flexor musc/fasc/tend r rng fngr at forarm lv, subs
		S56.116D	Strain flexor musc/fasc/tend l rng fngr at forarm lv, subs
		S56.117D	Strain flxr musc/fasc/tend r little fngr at forarm lv, subs
		S56.118D	Strain flxr musc/fasc/tend l little fngr at forarm lv, subs
		S56.119D	Strain flexor musc/fasc/tend of unsp fngr at forarm lv, subs
		S56.121D	Lacerat flexor musc/fasc/tend r idx fngr at forarm lv, subs
		S56.122D	Lacerat flexor musc/fasc/tend l idx fngr at forarm lv, subs
		S56.123D	Lacerat flexor musc/fasc/tend r mid fngr at forarm lv, subs
		S56.124D	Lacerat flexor musc/fasc/tend l mid fngr at forarm lv, subs
		S56.125D	Lacerat flexor musc/fasc/tend r rng fngr at forarm lv, subs
		S56.126D	Lacerat flexor musc/fasc/tend l rng fngr at forarm lv, subs
		S56.127D	Lacerat flxr musc/fasc/tend r little fngr at forarm lv, subs
		S56.128D	Lacerat flxr musc/fasc/tend l little fngr at forarm lv, subs
		S56.129D	Lacerat flexor musc/fasc/tend unsp finger at forarm lv, subs
		S56.191D	Inj flexor musc/fasc/tend r idx fngr at forearm level, subs
		S56.192D	Inj flexor musc/fasc/tend l idx fngr at forearm level, subs
		S56.193D	Inj flexor musc/fasc/tend r mid finger at forarm lv, subs
		S56.194D	Inj flexor musc/fasc/tend l mid finger at forarm lv, subs
		S56.195D	Inj flexor musc/fasc/tend r rng fngr at forearm level, subs
		S56.196D	Inj flexor musc/fasc/tend l rng fngr at forearm level, subs
		S56.197D	Inj flexor musc/fasc/tend r little finger at forarm lv, subs
		S56.198D	Inj flexor musc/fasc/tend l little finger at forarm lv, subs
		S56.199D	Inj flexor musc/fasc/tend unsp finger at forearm level, subs
		S56.201D	Unsp inj flexor musc/fasc/tend at forarm lv, right arm, subs
		S56.202D	Unsp inj flexor musc/fasc/tend at forarm lv, left arm, subs
		S56.209D	Unsp inj flexor musc/fasc/tend at forarm lv, unsp arm, subs
		S56.211D	Strain flexor musc/fasc/tend at forarm lv, right arm, subs
		S56.212D	Strain of flexor musc/fasc/tend at forarm lv, left arm, subs
		S56.219D	Strain of flexor musc/fasc/tend at forarm lv, unsp arm, subs
		S56.221D	Lacerat flexor musc/fasc/tend at forarm lv, right arm, subs
		S56.222D	Lacerat flexor musc/fasc/tend at forarm lv, left arm, subs
		S56.229D	Lacerat flexor musc/fasc/tend at forarm lv, unsp arm, subs
		S56.291D	Inj oth flexor musc/fasc/tend at forarm lv, right arm, subs
		S56.292D	Inj oth flexor musc/fasc/tend at forarm lv, left arm, subs
		S56.299D	Inj oth flexor musc/fasc/tend at forarm lv, unsp arm, subs
		S56.301D	Unsp inj extn/abdr musc/fasc/tend of r thm at forarm lv,subs
		S56.302D	Unsp inj extn/abdr musc/fasc/tend of l thm at forarm lv,subs
		S56.309D	Unsp inj extn/abdr musc/fasc/tend of thmb at forarm lv, subs
	(Continued on next page)	**S56.311D**	Strain extn/abdr musc/fasc/tend of r thm at forarm lv, subs

ICD-9-CM		ICD-10-CM	
V58.89	ENCOUNTER FOR OTHER SPECIFIED AFTERCARE **(Continued)**	**S56.312D**	Strain extn/abdr musc/fasc/tend of l thm at forarm lv, subs
		S56.319D	Strain extn/abdr musc/fasc/tend of thmb at forarm lv, subs
		S56.321D	Lacerat extn/abdr musc/fasc/tend of r thm at forarm lv, subs
		S56.322D	Lacerat extn/abdr musc/fasc/tend of l thm at forarm lv, subs
		S56.329D	Lacerat extn/abdr musc/fasc/tend of thmb at forarm lv, subs
		S56.391D	Inj extn/abdr musc/fasc/tend of r thm at forarm lv, subs
		S56.392D	Inj extn/abdr musc/fasc/tend of l thm at forarm lv, subs
		S56.399D	Inj extn/abdr musc/fasc/tend of thmb at forearm level, subs
		S56.401D	Unsp inj extn musc/fasc/tend r idx fngr at forarm lv, subs
		S56.402D	Unsp inj extn musc/fasc/tend l idx fngr at forarm lv, subs
		S56.403D	Unsp inj extn musc/fasc/tend r mid finger at forarm lv, subs
		S56.404D	Unsp inj extn musc/fasc/tend l mid finger at forarm lv, subs
		S56.405D	Unsp inj extn musc/fasc/tend r rng fngr at forarm lv, subs
		S56.406D	Unsp inj extn musc/fasc/tend l rng fngr at forarm lv, subs
		S56.407D	Unsp inj extn musc/fasc/tend r lit fngr at forarm lv, subs
		S56.408D	Unsp inj extn musc/fasc/tend l lit fngr at forarm lv, subs
		S56.409D	Unsp inj extn musc/fasc/tend unsp finger at forarm lv, subs
		S56.411D	Strain extensor musc/fasc/tend r idx fngr at forarm lv, subs
		S56.412D	Strain extensor musc/fasc/tend l idx fngr at forarm lv, subs
		S56.413D	Strain extn musc/fasc/tend r mid finger at forarm lv, subs
		S56.414D	Strain extn musc/fasc/tend l mid finger at forarm lv, subs
		S56.415D	Strain extensor musc/fasc/tend r rng fngr at forarm lv, subs
		S56.416D	Strain extensor musc/fasc/tend l rng fngr at forarm lv, subs
		S56.417D	Strain extn musc/fasc/tend r little fngr at forarm lv, subs
		S56.418D	Strain extn musc/fasc/tend l little fngr at forarm lv, subs
		S56.419D	Strain extn musc/fasc/tend fngr,unsp fngr at forarm lv, subs
		S56.421D	Lacerat extn musc/fasc/tend r idx fngr at forarm lv, subs
		S56.422D	Lacerat extn musc/fasc/tend l idx fngr at forarm lv, subs
		S56.423D	Lacerat extn musc/fasc/tend r mid finger at forarm lv, subs
		S56.424D	Lacerat extn musc/fasc/tend l mid finger at forarm lv, subs
		S56.425D	Lacerat extn musc/fasc/tend r rng fngr at forarm lv, subs
		S56.426D	Lacerat extn musc/fasc/tend l rng fngr at forarm lv, subs
		S56.427D	Lacerat extn musc/fasc/tend r little fngr at forarm lv, subs
		S56.428D	Lacerat extn musc/fasc/tend l little fngr at forarm lv, subs
		S56.429D	Lacerat extn musc/fasc/tend unsp finger at forarm lv, subs
		S56.491D	Inj extensor musc/fasc/tend r idx fngr at forarm lv, subs
		S56.492D	Inj extensor musc/fasc/tend l idx fngr at forarm lv, subs
		S56.493D	Inj extensor musc/fasc/tend r mid finger at forarm lv, subs
		S56.494D	Inj extensor musc/fasc/tend l mid finger at forarm lv, subs
		S56.495D	Inj extensor musc/fasc/tend r rng fngr at forarm lv, subs
		S56.496D	Inj extensor musc/fasc/tend l rng fngr at forarm lv, subs
		S56.497D	Inj extn musc/fasc/tend r little finger at forarm lv, subs
		S56.498D	Inj extn musc/fasc/tend l little finger at forarm lv, subs
		S56.499D	Inj extensor musc/fasc/tend unsp finger at forarm lv, subs
		S56.501D	Unsp inj extn musc/fasc/tend at forarm lv, right arm, subs
		S56.502D	Unsp inj extn musc/fasc/tend at forarm lv, left arm, subs
		S56.509D	Unsp inj extn musc/fasc/tend at forarm lv, unsp arm, subs
		S56.511D	Strain of extn musc/fasc/tend at forarm lv, right arm, subs
		S56.512D	Strain of extn musc/fasc/tend at forarm lv, left arm, subs
		S56.519D	Strain of extn musc/fasc/tend at forarm lv, unsp arm, subs
		S56.521D	Lacerat extn musc/fasc/tend at forarm lv, right arm, subs
		S56.522D	Lacerat extn musc/fasc/tend at forarm lv, left arm, subs
		S56.529D	Lacerat extn musc/fasc/tend at forarm lv, unsp arm, subs
		S56.591D	Inj extn musc/fasc/tend at forearm level, right arm, subs
		S56.592D	Inj extn musc/fasc/tend at forearm level, left arm, subs
		S56.599D	Inj extn musc/fasc/tend at forearm level, unsp arm, subs
		S56.801D	Unsp injury of musc/fasc/tend at forarm lv, right arm, subs
		S56.802D	Unsp injury of musc/fasc/tend at forarm lv, left arm, subs
		S56.809D	Unsp injury of musc/fasc/tend at forarm lv, unsp arm, subs
		S56.811D	Strain of musc/fasc/tend at forearm level, right arm, subs
		S56.812D	Strain of musc/fasc/tend at forearm level, left arm, subs
		S56.819D	Strain of musc/fasc/tend at forearm level, unsp arm, subs
		S56.821D	Laceration of musc/fasc/tend at forarm lv, right arm, subs
		S56.822D	Laceration of musc/fasc/tend at forarm lv, left arm, subs
		S56.829D	Laceration of musc/fasc/tend at forarm lv, unsp arm, subs
		S56.891D	Inj musc/fasc/tend at forearm level, right arm, subs encntr
		S56.892D	Inj musc/fasc/tend at forearm level, left arm, subs encntr
		S56.899D	Inj musc/fasc/tend at forearm level, unsp arm, subs encntr
		S56.901D	Unsp inj unsp musc/fasc/tend at forarm lv, right arm, subs
		S56.902D	Unsp inj unsp musc/fasc/tend at forarm lv, left arm, subs
		S56.909D	Unsp inj unsp musc/fasc/tend at forarm lv, unsp arm, subs
		S56.911D	Strain of unsp musc/fasc/tend at forarm lv, right arm, subs
		S56.912D	Strain of unsp musc/fasc/tend at forarm lv, left arm, subs
		S56.919D	Strain of unsp musc/fasc/tend at forarm lv, unsp arm, subs
		S56.921D	Lacerat unsp musc/fasc/tend at forarm lv, right arm, subs
		S56.922D	Lacerat unsp musc/fasc/tend at forarm lv, left arm, subs
		S56.929D	Lacerat unsp musc/fasc/tend at forarm lv, unsp arm, subs
		S56.991D	Inj unsp musc/fasc/tend at forearm level, right arm, subs
		S56.992D	Inj unsp musc/fasc/tend at forearm level, left arm, subs
		S56.999D	Inj unsp musc/fasc/tend at forearm level, unsp arm, subs
		S57.00XD	Crushing injury of unspecified elbow, subsequent encounter
		S57.01XD	Crushing injury of right elbow, subsequent encounter
	(Continued on next page)	**S57.02XD**	Crushing injury of left elbow, subsequent encounter

ICD-9-CM		ICD-10-CM	
V58.89	ENCOUNTER FOR OTHER SPECIFIED AFTERCARE **(Continued)**	**S57.8ØXD**	Crushing injury of unspecified forearm, subsequent encounter
		S57.81XD	Crushing injury of right forearm, subsequent encounter
		S57.82XD	Crushing injury of left forearm, subsequent encounter
		S58.Ø11D	Complete traumatic amp at elbow level, right arm, subs
		S58.Ø12D	Complete traumatic amputation at elbow level, left arm, subs
		S58.Ø19D	Complete traumatic amputation at elbow level, unsp arm, subs
		S58.Ø21D	Partial traumatic amputation at elbow level, right arm, subs
		S58.Ø22D	Partial traumatic amputation at elbow level, left arm, subs
		S58.Ø29D	Partial traumatic amputation at elbow level, unsp arm, subs
		S58.111D	Complete traum amp at lev betw elbow and wrist, r arm, subs
		S58.112D	Complete traum amp at lev betw elbow and wrs, left arm, subs
		S58.119D	Complete traum amp at lev betw elbow and wrs, unsp arm, subs
		S58.121D	Part traum amp at lev betw elbow and wrist, right arm, subs
		S58.122D	Part traum amp at level betw elbow and wrist, left arm, subs
		S58.129D	Part traum amp at level betw elbow and wrist, unsp arm, subs
		S58.911D	Complete traumatic amputation of r forearm, level unsp, subs
		S58.912D	Complete traumatic amputation of l forearm, level unsp, subs
		S58.919D	Complete traumatic amp of unsp forearm, level unsp, subs
		S58.921D	Partial traumatic amputation of r forearm, level unsp, subs
		S58.922D	Partial traumatic amputation of l forearm, level unsp, subs
		S58.929D	Partial traumatic amp of unsp forearm, level unsp, subs
		S59.8Ø1D	Other specified injuries of right elbow, subs encntr
		S59.8Ø2D	Other specified injuries of left elbow, subsequent encounter
		S59.8Ø9D	Other specified injuries of unspecified elbow, subs encntr
		S59.811D	Other specified injuries right forearm, subsequent encounter
		S59.812D	Other specified injuries left forearm, subsequent encounter
		S59.819D	Other specified injuries unspecified forearm, subs encntr
		S59.9Ø1D	Unspecified injury of right elbow, subsequent encounter
		S59.9Ø2D	Unspecified injury of left elbow, subsequent encounter
		S59.9Ø9D	Unspecified injury of unspecified elbow, subs encntr
		S59.911D	Unspecified injury of right forearm, subsequent encounter
		S59.912D	Unspecified injury of left forearm, subsequent encounter
		S59.919D	Unspecified injury of unspecified forearm, subs encntr
		S6Ø.ØØXD	Contusion of unsp finger without damage to nail, subs encntr
		S6Ø.Ø11D	Contusion of right thumb without damage to nail, subs encntr
		S6Ø.Ø12D	Contusion of left thumb without damage to nail, subs encntr
		S6Ø.Ø19D	Contusion of unsp thumb without damage to nail, subs encntr
		S6Ø.Ø21D	Contusion of right index finger w/o damage to nail, subs
		S6Ø.Ø22D	Contusion of left index finger w/o damage to nail, subs
		S6Ø.Ø29D	Contusion of unsp index finger w/o damage to nail, subs
		S6Ø.Ø31D	Contusion of right middle finger w/o damage to nail, subs
		S6Ø.Ø32D	Contusion of left middle finger w/o damage to nail, subs
		S6Ø.Ø39D	Contusion of unsp middle finger w/o damage to nail, subs
		S6Ø.Ø41D	Contusion of right ring finger w/o damage to nail, subs
		S6Ø.Ø42D	Contusion of left ring finger w/o damage to nail, subs
		S6Ø.Ø49D	Contusion of unsp ring finger w/o damage to nail, subs
		S6Ø.Ø51D	Contusion of right little finger w/o damage to nail, subs
		S6Ø.Ø52D	Contusion of left little finger w/o damage to nail, subs
		S6Ø.Ø59D	Contusion of unsp little finger w/o damage to nail, subs
		S6Ø.1ØXD	Contusion of unsp finger with damage to nail, subs encntr
		S6Ø.111D	Contusion of right thumb with damage to nail, subs encntr
		S6Ø.112D	Contusion of left thumb with damage to nail, subs encntr
		S6Ø.119D	Contusion of unsp thumb with damage to nail, subs encntr
		S6Ø.121D	Contusion of right index finger w damage to nail, subs
		S6Ø.122D	Contusion of left index finger w damage to nail, subs encntr
		S6Ø.129D	Contusion of unsp index finger w damage to nail, subs encntr
		S6Ø.131D	Contusion of right middle finger w damage to nail, subs
		S6Ø.132D	Contusion of left middle finger w damage to nail, subs
		S6Ø.139D	Contusion of unsp middle finger w damage to nail, subs
		S6Ø.141D	Contusion of right ring finger w damage to nail, subs encntr
		S6Ø.142D	Contusion of left ring finger w damage to nail, subs encntr
		S6Ø.149D	Contusion of unsp ring finger w damage to nail, subs encntr
		S6Ø.151D	Contusion of right little finger w damage to nail, subs
		S6Ø.152D	Contusion of left little finger w damage to nail, subs
		S6Ø.159D	Contusion of unsp little finger w damage to nail, subs
		S6Ø.211D	Contusion of right wrist, subsequent encounter
		S6Ø.212D	Contusion of left wrist, subsequent encounter
		S6Ø.219D	Contusion of unspecified wrist, subsequent encounter
		S6Ø.221D	Contusion of right hand, subsequent encounter
		S6Ø.222D	Contusion of left hand, subsequent encounter
		S6Ø.229D	Contusion of unspecified hand, subsequent encounter
		S6Ø.311D	Abrasion of right thumb, subsequent encounter
		S6Ø.312D	Abrasion of left thumb, subsequent encounter
		S6Ø.319D	Abrasion of unspecified thumb, subsequent encounter
		S6Ø.321D	Blister (nonthermal) of right thumb, subsequent encounter
		S6Ø.322D	Blister (nonthermal) of left thumb, subsequent encounter
		S6Ø.329D	Blister (nonthermal) of unspecified thumb, subs encntr
		S6Ø.341D	External constriction of right thumb, subsequent encounter
		S6Ø.342D	External constriction of left thumb, subsequent encounter
		S6Ø.349D	External constriction of unspecified thumb, subs encntr
		S6Ø.351D	Superficial foreign body of right thumb, subs encntr
		S6Ø.352D	Superficial foreign body of left thumb, subsequent encounter
	(Continued on next page)	**S6Ø.359D**	Superficial foreign body of unspecified thumb, subs encntr

ICD-9-CM		ICD-10-CM	
V58.89	ENCOUNTER FOR OTHER SPECIFIED AFTERCARE **(Continued)**	**S60.361D**	Insect bite (nonvenomous) of right thumb, subs encntr
		S60.362D	Insect bite (nonvenomous) of left thumb, subs encntr
		S60.369D	Insect bite (nonvenomous) of unspecified thumb, subs encntr
		S60.371D	Other superficial bite of right thumb, subsequent encounter
		S60.372D	Other superficial bite of left thumb, subsequent encounter
		S60.379D	Other superficial bite of unspecified thumb, subs encntr
		S60.391D	Other superficial injuries of right thumb, subs encntr
		S60.392D	Other superficial injuries of left thumb, subs encntr
		S60.399D	Other superficial injuries of unspecified thumb, subs encntr
		S60.410D	Abrasion of right index finger, subsequent encounter
		S60.411D	Abrasion of left index finger, subsequent encounter
		S60.412D	Abrasion of right middle finger, subsequent encounter
		S60.413D	Abrasion of left middle finger, subsequent encounter
		S60.414D	Abrasion of right ring finger, subsequent encounter
		S60.415D	Abrasion of left ring finger, subsequent encounter
		S60.416D	Abrasion of right little finger, subsequent encounter
		S60.417D	Abrasion of left little finger, subsequent encounter
		S60.418D	Abrasion of other finger, subsequent encounter
		S60.419D	Abrasion of unspecified finger, subsequent encounter
		S60.420D	Blister (nonthermal) of right index finger, subs encntr
		S60.421D	Blister (nonthermal) of left index finger, subs encntr
		S60.422D	Blister (nonthermal) of right middle finger, subs encntr
		S60.423D	Blister (nonthermal) of left middle finger, subs encntr
		S60.424D	Blister (nonthermal) of right ring finger, subs encntr
		S60.425D	Blister (nonthermal) of left ring finger, subs encntr
		S60.426D	Blister (nonthermal) of right little finger, subs encntr
		S60.427D	Blister (nonthermal) of left little finger, subs encntr
		S60.428D	Blister (nonthermal) of other finger, subsequent encounter
		S60.429D	Blister (nonthermal) of unspecified finger, subs encntr
		S60.440D	External constriction of right index finger, subs encntr
		S60.441D	External constriction of left index finger, subs encntr
		S60.442D	External constriction of right middle finger, subs encntr
		S60.443D	External constriction of left middle finger, subs encntr
		S60.444D	External constriction of right ring finger, subs encntr
		S60.445D	External constriction of left ring finger, subs encntr
		S60.446D	External constriction of right little finger, subs encntr
		S60.447D	External constriction of left little finger, subs encntr
		S60.448D	External constriction of other finger, subsequent encounter
		S60.449D	External constriction of unspecified finger, subs encntr
		S60.450D	Superficial foreign body of right index finger, subs encntr
		S60.451D	Superficial foreign body of left index finger, subs encntr
		S60.452D	Superficial foreign body of right middle finger, subs encntr
		S60.453D	Superficial foreign body of left middle finger, subs encntr
		S60.454D	Superficial foreign body of right ring finger, subs encntr
		S60.455D	Superficial foreign body of left ring finger, subs encntr
		S60.456D	Superficial foreign body of right little finger, subs encntr
		S60.457D	Superficial foreign body of left little finger, subs encntr
		S60.458D	Superficial foreign body of other finger, subs encntr
		S60.459D	Superficial foreign body of unspecified finger, subs encntr
		S60.460D	Insect bite (nonvenomous) of right index finger, subs encntr
		S60.461D	Insect bite (nonvenomous) of left index finger, subs encntr
		S60.462D	Insect bite (nonvenomous) of right middle finger, subs
		S60.463D	Insect bite (nonvenomous) of left middle finger, subs encntr
		S60.464D	Insect bite (nonvenomous) of right ring finger, subs encntr
		S60.465D	Insect bite (nonvenomous) of left ring finger, subs encntr
		S60.466D	Insect bite (nonvenomous) of right little finger, subs
		S60.467D	Insect bite (nonvenomous) of left little finger, subs encntr
		S60.468D	Insect bite (nonvenomous) of other finger, subs encntr
		S60.469D	Insect bite (nonvenomous) of unspecified finger, subs encntr
		S60.470D	Other superficial bite of right index finger, subs encntr
		S60.471D	Other superficial bite of left index finger, subs encntr
		S60.472D	Other superficial bite of right middle finger, subs encntr
		S60.473D	Other superficial bite of left middle finger, subs encntr
		S60.474D	Other superficial bite of right ring finger, subs encntr
		S60.475D	Other superficial bite of left ring finger, subs encntr
		S60.476D	Other superficial bite of right little finger, subs encntr
		S60.477D	Other superficial bite of left little finger, subs encntr
		S60.478D	Other superficial bite of other finger, subsequent encounter
		S60.479D	Other superficial bite of unspecified finger, subs encntr
		S60.511D	Abrasion of right hand, subsequent encounter
		S60.512D	Abrasion of left hand, subsequent encounter
		S60.519D	Abrasion of unspecified hand, subsequent encounter
		S60.521D	Blister (nonthermal) of right hand, subsequent encounter
		S60.522D	Blister (nonthermal) of left hand, subsequent encounter
		S60.529D	Blister (nonthermal) of unspecified hand, subs encntr
		S60.541D	External constriction of right hand, subsequent encounter
		S60.542D	External constriction of left hand, subsequent encounter
		S60.549D	External constriction of unspecified hand, subs encntr
		S60.551D	Superficial foreign body of right hand, subsequent encounter
		S60.552D	Superficial foreign body of left hand, subsequent encounter
		S60.559D	Superficial foreign body of unspecified hand, subs encntr
		S60.561D	Insect bite (nonvenomous) of right hand, subs encntr
	(Continued on next page)	**S60.562D**	Insect bite (nonvenomous) of left hand, subsequent encounter

ICD-9-CM		ICD-10-CM	
V58.89	ENCOUNTER FOR OTHER SPECIFIED AFTERCARE **(Continued)**	**S60.569D**	Insect bite (nonvenomous) of unspecified hand, subs encntr
		S60.571D	Other superficial bite of hand of right hand, subs encntr
		S60.572D	Other superficial bite of hand of left hand, subs encntr
		S60.579D	Other superficial bite of hand of unsp hand, subs encntr
		S60.811D	Abrasion of right wrist, subsequent encounter
		S60.812D	Abrasion of left wrist, subsequent encounter
		S60.819D	Abrasion of unspecified wrist, subsequent encounter
		S60.821D	Blister (nonthermal) of right wrist, subsequent encounter
		S60.822D	Blister (nonthermal) of left wrist, subsequent encounter
		S60.829D	Blister (nonthermal) of unspecified wrist, subs encntr
		S60.841D	External constriction of right wrist, subsequent encounter
		S60.842D	External constriction of left wrist, subsequent encounter
		S60.849D	External constriction of unspecified wrist, subs encntr
		S60.851D	Superficial foreign body of right wrist, subs encntr
		S60.852D	Superficial foreign body of left wrist, subsequent encounter
		S60.859D	Superficial foreign body of unspecified wrist, subs encntr
		S60.861D	Insect bite (nonvenomous) of right wrist, subs encntr
		S60.862D	Insect bite (nonvenomous) of left wrist, subs encntr
		S60.869D	Insect bite (nonvenomous) of unspecified wrist, subs encntr
		S60.871D	Other superficial bite of right wrist, subsequent encounter
		S60.872D	Other superficial bite of left wrist, subsequent encounter
		S60.879D	Other superficial bite of unspecified wrist, subs encntr
		S60.911D	Unspecified superficial injury of right wrist, subs encntr
		S60.912D	Unspecified superficial injury of left wrist, subs encntr
		S60.919D	Unsp superficial injury of unspecified wrist, subs encntr
		S60.921D	Unspecified superficial injury of right hand, subs encntr
		S60.922D	Unspecified superficial injury of left hand, subs encntr
		S60.929D	Unsp superficial injury of unspecified hand, subs encntr
		S60.931D	Unspecified superficial injury of right thumb, subs encntr
		S60.932D	Unspecified superficial injury of left thumb, subs encntr
		S60.939D	Unsp superficial injury of unspecified thumb, subs encntr
		S60.940D	Unsp superficial injury of right index finger, subs encntr
		S60.941D	Unsp superficial injury of left index finger, subs encntr
		S60.942D	Unsp superficial injury of right middle finger, subs encntr
		S60.943D	Unsp superficial injury of left middle finger, subs encntr
		S60.944D	Unsp superficial injury of right ring finger, subs encntr
		S60.945D	Unsp superficial injury of left ring finger, subs encntr
		S60.946D	Unsp superficial injury of right little finger, subs encntr
		S60.947D	Unsp superficial injury of left little finger, subs encntr
		S60.948D	Unspecified superficial injury of other finger, subs encntr
		S60.949D	Unsp superficial injury of unspecified finger, subs encntr
		S61.001D	Unsp open wound of right thumb w/o damage to nail, subs
		S61.002D	Unsp open wound of left thumb w/o damage to nail, subs
		S61.009D	Unsp open wound of unsp thumb w/o damage to nail, subs
		S61.011D	Laceration w/o fb of right thumb w/o damage to nail, subs
		S61.012D	Laceration w/o fb of left thumb w/o damage to nail, subs
		S61.019D	Laceration w/o foreign body of thmb w/o damage to nail, subs
		S61.021D	Laceration w fb of right thumb w/o damage to nail, subs
		S61.022D	Laceration w fb of left thumb w/o damage to nail, subs
		S61.029D	Laceration w foreign body of thmb w/o damage to nail, subs
		S61.031D	Pnctr w/o fb of right thumb w/o damage to nail, subs
		S61.032D	Pnctr w/o fb of left thumb w/o damage to nail, subs
		S61.039D	Pnctr w/o foreign body of thmb w/o damage to nail, subs
		S61.041D	Pnctr w foreign body of right thumb w/o damage to nail, subs
		S61.042D	Pnctr w foreign body of left thumb w/o damage to nail, subs
		S61.049D	Pnctr w foreign body of thmb w/o damage to nail, subs
		S61.051D	Open bite of right thumb without damage to nail, subs encntr
		S61.052D	Open bite of left thumb without damage to nail, subs encntr
		S61.059D	Open bite of unsp thumb without damage to nail, subs encntr
		S61.101D	Unsp open wound of right thumb w damage to nail, subs encntr
		S61.102D	Unsp open wound of left thumb w damage to nail, subs encntr
		S61.109D	Unsp open wound of unsp thumb w damage to nail, subs encntr
		S61.111D	Laceration w/o fb of right thumb w damage to nail, subs
		S61.112D	Laceration w/o fb of left thumb w damage to nail, subs
		S61.119D	Laceration w/o foreign body of thmb w damage to nail, subs
		S61.121D	Laceration w fb of right thumb w damage to nail, subs
		S61.122D	Laceration w fb of left thumb w damage to nail, subs
		S61.129D	Laceration w foreign body of thmb w damage to nail, subs
		S61.131D	Pnctr w/o foreign body of right thumb w damage to nail, subs
		S61.132D	Pnctr w/o foreign body of left thumb w damage to nail, subs
		S61.139D	Pnctr w/o foreign body of thmb w damage to nail, subs
		S61.141D	Pnctr w foreign body of right thumb w damage to nail, subs
		S61.142D	Pnctr w foreign body of left thumb w damage to nail, subs
		S61.149D	Puncture wound w foreign body of thmb w damage to nail, subs
		S61.151D	Open bite of right thumb with damage to nail, subs encntr
		S61.152D	Open bite of left thumb with damage to nail, subs encntr
		S61.159D	Open bite of unsp thumb with damage to nail, subs encntr
		S61.200D	Unsp open wound of r idx fngr w/o damage to nail, subs
		S61.201D	Unsp open wound of l idx fngr w/o damage to nail, subs
		S61.202D	Unsp open wound of r mid finger w/o damage to nail, subs
		S61.203D	Unsp open wound of l mid finger w/o damage to nail, subs
		S61.204D	Unsp open wound of r rng fngr w/o damage to nail, subs
	(Continued on next page)	**S61.205D**	Unsp open wound of left ring finger w/o damage to nail, subs

[Brackets] indicate valid character values for each code. Character value meanings provided for each code grouping.

ICD-9-CM		ICD-10-CM	
V58.89	ENCOUNTER FOR OTHER SPECIFIED AFTERCARE **(Continued)**	**S61.206D**	Unsp open wound of r little finger w/o damage to nail, subs
		S61.207D	Unsp open wound of l little finger w/o damage to nail, subs
		S61.208D	Unsp open wound of oth finger w/o damage to nail, subs
		S61.209D	Unsp open wound of unsp finger w/o damage to nail, subs
		S61.210D	Laceration w/o fb of r idx fngr w/o damage to nail, subs
		S61.211D	Laceration w/o fb of l idx fngr w/o damage to nail, subs
		S61.212D	Laceration w/o fb of r mid finger w/o damage to nail, subs
		S61.213D	Laceration w/o fb of l mid finger w/o damage to nail, subs
		S61.214D	Laceration w/o fb of r rng fngr w/o damage to nail, subs
		S61.215D	Laceration w/o fb of l rng fngr w/o damage to nail, subs
		S61.216D	Lac w/o fb of r little finger w/o damage to nail, subs
		S61.217D	Lac w/o fb of l little finger w/o damage to nail, subs
		S61.218D	Laceration w/o fb of finger w/o damage to nail, subs
		S61.219D	Laceration w/o fb of unsp finger w/o damage to nail, subs
		S61.220D	Laceration w fb of r idx fngr w/o damage to nail, subs
		S61.221D	Laceration w fb of l idx fngr w/o damage to nail, subs
		S61.222D	Laceration w fb of r mid finger w/o damage to nail, subs
		S61.223D	Laceration w fb of l mid finger w/o damage to nail, subs
		S61.224D	Laceration w fb of r rng fngr w/o damage to nail, subs
		S61.225D	Laceration w fb of l rng fngr w/o damage to nail, subs
		S61.226D	Laceration w fb of r little finger w/o damage to nail, subs
		S61.227D	Laceration w fb of l little finger w/o damage to nail, subs
		S61.228D	Laceration w foreign body of finger w/o damage to nail, subs
		S61.229D	Laceration w fb of unsp finger w/o damage to nail, subs
		S61.230D	Pnctr w/o fb of r idx fngr w/o damage to nail, subs
		S61.231D	Pnctr w/o fb of l idx fngr w/o damage to nail, subs
		S61.232D	Pnctr w/o fb of r mid finger w/o damage to nail, subs
		S61.233D	Pnctr w/o fb of l mid finger w/o damage to nail, subs
		S61.234D	Pnctr w/o fb of r rng fngr w/o damage to nail, subs
		S61.235D	Pnctr w/o fb of l rng fngr w/o damage to nail, subs
		S61.236D	Pnctr w/o fb of r little finger w/o damage to nail, subs
		S61.237D	Pnctr w/o fb of l little finger w/o damage to nail, subs
		S61.238D	Pnctr w/o foreign body of finger w/o damage to nail, subs
		S61.239D	Pnctr w/o fb of unsp finger w/o damage to nail, subs
		S61.240D	Pnctr w foreign body of r idx fngr w/o damage to nail, subs
		S61.241D	Pnctr w foreign body of l idx fngr w/o damage to nail, subs
		S61.242D	Pnctr w fb of r mid finger w/o damage to nail, subs
		S61.243D	Pnctr w fb of l mid finger w/o damage to nail, subs
		S61.244D	Pnctr w foreign body of r rng fngr w/o damage to nail, subs
		S61.245D	Pnctr w foreign body of l rng fngr w/o damage to nail, subs
		S61.246D	Pnctr w fb of r little finger w/o damage to nail, subs
		S61.247D	Pnctr w fb of l little finger w/o damage to nail, subs
		S61.248D	Pnctr w foreign body of finger w/o damage to nail, subs
		S61.249D	Pnctr w foreign body of unsp finger w/o damage to nail, subs
		S61.250D	Open bite of right index finger w/o damage to nail, subs
		S61.251D	Open bite of left index finger w/o damage to nail, subs
		S61.252D	Open bite of right middle finger w/o damage to nail, subs
		S61.253D	Open bite of left middle finger w/o damage to nail, subs
		S61.254D	Open bite of right ring finger w/o damage to nail, subs
		S61.255D	Open bite of left ring finger w/o damage to nail, subs
		S61.256D	Open bite of right little finger w/o damage to nail, subs
		S61.257D	Open bite of left little finger w/o damage to nail, subs
		S61.258D	Open bite of other finger w/o damage to nail, subs encntr
		S61.259D	Open bite of unsp finger without damage to nail, subs encntr
		S61.300D	Unsp open wound of right index finger w damage to nail, subs
		S61.301D	Unsp open wound of left index finger w damage to nail, subs
		S61.302D	Unsp open wound of r mid finger w damage to nail, subs
		S61.303D	Unsp open wound of left middle finger w damage to nail, subs
		S61.304D	Unsp open wound of right ring finger w damage to nail, subs
		S61.305D	Unsp open wound of left ring finger w damage to nail, subs
		S61.306D	Unsp open wound of r little finger w damage to nail, subs
		S61.307D	Unsp open wound of left little finger w damage to nail, subs
		S61.308D	Unsp open wound of oth finger w damage to nail, subs encntr
		S61.309D	Unsp open wound of unsp finger w damage to nail, subs encntr
		S61.310D	Laceration w/o fb of r idx fngr w damage to nail, subs
		S61.311D	Laceration w/o fb of l idx fngr w damage to nail, subs
		S61.312D	Laceration w/o fb of r mid finger w damage to nail, subs
		S61.313D	Laceration w/o fb of l mid finger w damage to nail, subs
		S61.314D	Laceration w/o fb of r rng fngr w damage to nail, subs
		S61.315D	Laceration w/o fb of l rng fngr w damage to nail, subs
		S61.316D	Laceration w/o fb of r little finger w damage to nail, subs
		S61.317D	Laceration w/o fb of l little finger w damage to nail, subs
		S61.318D	Laceration w/o foreign body of finger w damage to nail, subs
		S61.319D	Laceration w/o fb of unsp finger w damage to nail, subs
		S61.320D	Laceration w fb of r idx fngr w damage to nail, subs
		S61.321D	Laceration w fb of l idx fngr w damage to nail, subs
		S61.322D	Laceration w fb of r mid finger w damage to nail, subs
		S61.323D	Laceration w fb of l mid finger w damage to nail, subs
		S61.324D	Laceration w fb of r rng fngr w damage to nail, subs
		S61.325D	Laceration w fb of l rng fngr w damage to nail, subs
		S61.326D	Laceration w fb of r little finger w damage to nail, subs
		S61.327D	Laceration w fb of l little finger w damage to nail, subs
	(Continued on next page)	**S61.328D**	Laceration w foreign body of finger w damage to nail, subs

ICD-9-CM		ICD-10-CM	
V58.89	ENCOUNTER FOR OTHER SPECIFIED AFTERCARE **(Continued)**	**S61.329D**	Laceration w fb of unsp finger w damage to nail, subs
		S61.33ØD	Pnctr w/o foreign body of r idx fngr w damage to nail, subs
		S61.331D	Pnctr w/o foreign body of l idx fngr w damage to nail, subs
		S61.332D	Pnctr w/o fb of r mid finger w damage to nail, subs
		S61.333D	Pnctr w/o fb of l mid finger w damage to nail, subs
		S61.334D	Pnctr w/o foreign body of r rng fngr w damage to nail, subs
		S61.335D	Pnctr w/o foreign body of l rng fngr w damage to nail, subs
		S61.336D	Pnctr w/o fb of r little finger w damage to nail, subs
		S61.337D	Pnctr w/o fb of l little finger w damage to nail, subs
		S61.338D	Pnctr w/o foreign body of finger w damage to nail, subs
		S61.339D	Pnctr w/o foreign body of unsp finger w damage to nail, subs
		S61.34ØD	Pnctr w foreign body of r idx fngr w damage to nail, subs
		S61.341D	Pnctr w foreign body of l idx fngr w damage to nail, subs
		S61.342D	Pnctr w foreign body of r mid finger w damage to nail, subs
		S61.343D	Pnctr w foreign body of l mid finger w damage to nail, subs
		S61.344D	Pnctr w foreign body of r rng fngr w damage to nail, subs
		S61.345D	Pnctr w foreign body of l rng fngr w damage to nail, subs
		S61.346D	Pnctr w fb of r little finger w damage to nail, subs
		S61.347D	Pnctr w fb of l little finger w damage to nail, subs
		S61.348D	Pnctr w foreign body of finger w damage to nail, subs
		S61.349D	Pnctr w foreign body of unsp finger w damage to nail, subs
		S61.35ØD	Open bite of right index finger w damage to nail, subs
		S61.351D	Open bite of left index finger w damage to nail, subs encntr
		S61.352D	Open bite of right middle finger w damage to nail, subs
		S61.353D	Open bite of left middle finger w damage to nail, subs
		S61.354D	Open bite of right ring finger w damage to nail, subs encntr
		S61.355D	Open bite of left ring finger w damage to nail, subs encntr
		S61.356D	Open bite of right little finger w damage to nail, subs
		S61.357D	Open bite of left little finger w damage to nail, subs
		S61.358D	Open bite of other finger with damage to nail, subs encntr
		S61.359D	Open bite of unsp finger with damage to nail, subs encntr
		S61.4Ø1D	Unspecified open wound of right hand, subsequent encounter
		S61.4Ø2D	Unspecified open wound of left hand, subsequent encounter
		S61.4Ø9D	Unspecified open wound of unspecified hand, subs encntr
		S61.411D	Laceration without foreign body of right hand, subs encntr
		S61.412D	Laceration without foreign body of left hand, subs encntr
		S61.419D	Laceration without foreign body of unsp hand, subs encntr
		S61.421D	Laceration with foreign body of right hand, subs encntr
		S61.422D	Laceration with foreign body of left hand, subs encntr
		S61.429D	Laceration with foreign body of unsp hand, subs encntr
		S61.431D	Puncture wound w/o foreign body of right hand, subs encntr
		S61.432D	Puncture wound w/o foreign body of left hand, subs encntr
		S61.439D	Puncture wound w/o foreign body of unsp hand, subs encntr
		S61.441D	Puncture wound with foreign body of right hand, subs encntr
		S61.442D	Puncture wound with foreign body of left hand, subs encntr
		S61.449D	Puncture wound with foreign body of unsp hand, subs encntr
		S61.451D	Open bite of right hand, subsequent encounter
		S61.452D	Open bite of left hand, subsequent encounter
		S61.459D	Open bite of unspecified hand, subsequent encounter
		S61.5Ø1D	Unspecified open wound of right wrist, subsequent encounter
		S61.5Ø2D	Unspecified open wound of left wrist, subsequent encounter
		S61.5Ø9D	Unspecified open wound of unspecified wrist, subs encntr
		S61.511D	Laceration without foreign body of right wrist, subs encntr
		S61.512D	Laceration without foreign body of left wrist, subs encntr
		S61.519D	Laceration without foreign body of unsp wrist, subs encntr
		S61.521D	Laceration with foreign body of right wrist, subs encntr
		S61.522D	Laceration with foreign body of left wrist, subs encntr
		S61.529D	Laceration with foreign body of unsp wrist, subs encntr
		S61.531D	Puncture wound w/o foreign body of right wrist, subs encntr
		S61.532D	Puncture wound w/o foreign body of left wrist, subs encntr
		S61.539D	Puncture wound w/o foreign body of unsp wrist, subs encntr
		S61.541D	Puncture wound with foreign body of right wrist, subs encntr
		S61.542D	Puncture wound with foreign body of left wrist, subs encntr
		S61.549D	Puncture wound with foreign body of unsp wrist, subs encntr
		S61.551D	Open bite of right wrist, subsequent encounter
		S61.552D	Open bite of left wrist, subsequent encounter
		S61.559D	Open bite of unspecified wrist, subsequent encounter
		S63.ØØ1D	Unspecified subluxation of right wrist and hand, subs encntr
		S63.ØØ2D	Unspecified subluxation of left wrist and hand, subs encntr
		S63.ØØ3D	Unsp subluxation of unspecified wrist and hand, subs encntr
		S63.ØØ4D	Unspecified dislocation of right wrist and hand, subs encntr
		S63.ØØ5D	Unspecified dislocation of left wrist and hand, subs encntr
		S63.ØØ6D	Unsp dislocation of unspecified wrist and hand, subs encntr
		S63.Ø11D	Subluxation of distal radioulnar joint of right wrist, subs
		S63.Ø12D	Subluxation of distal radioulnar joint of left wrist, subs
		S63.Ø13D	Subluxation of distal radioulnar joint of unsp wrist, subs
		S63.Ø14D	Dislocation of distal radioulnar joint of right wrist, subs
		S63.Ø15D	Dislocation of distal radioulnar joint of left wrist, subs
		S63.Ø16D	Dislocation of distal radioulnar joint of unsp wrist, subs
		S63.Ø21D	Subluxation of radiocarpal joint of right wrist, subs encntr
		S63.Ø22D	Subluxation of radiocarpal joint of left wrist, subs encntr
		S63.Ø23D	Subluxation of radiocarpal joint of unsp wrist, subs encntr
	(Continued on next page)	**S63.Ø24D**	Dislocation of radiocarpal joint of right wrist, subs encntr

ICD-9-CM		ICD-10-CM	
V58.89	ENCOUNTER FOR OTHER SPECIFIED AFTERCARE **(Continued)**	**S63.Ø25D**	Dislocation of radiocarpal joint of left wrist, subs encntr
		S63.Ø26D	Dislocation of radiocarpal joint of unsp wrist, subs encntr
		S63.Ø31D	Subluxation of midcarpal joint of right wrist, subs encntr
		S63.Ø32D	Subluxation of midcarpal joint of left wrist, subs encntr
		S63.Ø33D	Subluxation of midcarpal joint of unsp wrist, subs encntr
		S63.Ø34D	Dislocation of midcarpal joint of right wrist, subs encntr
		S63.Ø35D	Dislocation of midcarpal joint of left wrist, subs encntr
		S63.Ø36D	Dislocation of midcarpal joint of unsp wrist, subs encntr
		S63.Ø41D	Subluxation of carpometacarpal joint of right thumb, subs
		S63.Ø42D	Subluxation of carpometacarpal joint of left thumb, subs
		S63.Ø43D	Subluxation of carpometacarpal joint of unsp thumb, subs
		S63.Ø44D	Dislocation of carpometacarpal joint of right thumb, subs
		S63.Ø45D	Dislocation of carpometacarpal joint of left thumb, subs
		S63.Ø46D	Dislocation of carpometacarpal joint of unsp thumb, subs
		S63.Ø51D	Subluxation of oth carpometacarpal joint of right hand, subs
		S63.Ø52D	Subluxation of oth carpometacarpal joint of left hand, subs
		S63.Ø53D	Subluxation of oth carpometacarpal joint of unsp hand, subs
		S63.Ø54D	Dislocation of oth carpometacarpal joint of right hand, subs
		S63.Ø55D	Dislocation of oth carpometacarpal joint of left hand, subs
		S63.Ø56D	Dislocation of oth carpometacarpal joint of unsp hand, subs
		S63.Ø61D	Sublux of MC (bone), proximal end of right hand, subs
		S63.Ø62D	Sublux of metacarpal (bone), proximal end of left hand, subs
		S63.Ø63D	Sublux of metacarpal (bone), proximal end of unsp hand, subs
		S63.Ø64D	Disloc of MC (bone), proximal end of right hand, subs
		S63.Ø65D	Disloc of metacarpal (bone), proximal end of left hand, subs
		S63.Ø66D	Disloc of metacarpal (bone), proximal end of unsp hand, subs
		S63.Ø71D	Subluxation of distal end of right ulna, subs encntr
		S63.Ø72D	Subluxation of distal end of left ulna, subsequent encounter
		S63.Ø73D	Subluxation of distal end of unspecified ulna, subs encntr
		S63.Ø74D	Dislocation of distal end of right ulna, subs encntr
		S63.Ø75D	Dislocation of distal end of left ulna, subsequent encounter
		S63.Ø76D	Dislocation of distal end of unspecified ulna, subs encntr
		S63.Ø91D	Other subluxation of right wrist and hand, subs encntr
		S63.Ø92D	Other subluxation of left wrist and hand, subs encntr
		S63.Ø93D	Other subluxation of unspecified wrist and hand, subs encntr
		S63.Ø94D	Other dislocation of right wrist and hand, subs encntr
		S63.Ø95D	Other dislocation of left wrist and hand, subs encntr
		S63.Ø96D	Other dislocation of unspecified wrist and hand, subs encntr
		S63.1Ø1D	Unspecified subluxation of right thumb, subsequent encounter
		S63.1Ø2D	Unspecified subluxation of left thumb, subsequent encounter
		S63.1Ø3D	Unspecified subluxation of unspecified thumb, subs encntr
		S63.1Ø4D	Unspecified dislocation of right thumb, subsequent encounter
		S63.1Ø5D	Unspecified dislocation of left thumb, subsequent encounter
		S63.1Ø6D	Unspecified dislocation of unspecified thumb, subs encntr
		S63.111D	Subluxation of MCP joint of right thumb, subs
		S63.112D	Subluxation of metacarpophalangeal joint of left thumb, subs
		S63.113D	Subluxation of metacarpophalangeal joint of unsp thumb, subs
		S63.114D	Dislocation of MCP joint of right thumb, subs
		S63.115D	Dislocation of metacarpophalangeal joint of left thumb, subs
		S63.116D	Dislocation of metacarpophalangeal joint of unsp thumb, subs
		S63.121D	Subluxation of unsp interphaln joint of right thumb, subs
		S63.122D	Subluxation of unsp interphaln joint of left thumb, subs
		S63.123D	Subluxation of unsp interphalangeal joint of thmb, subs
		S63.124D	Dislocation of unsp interphaln joint of right thumb, subs
		S63.125D	Dislocation of unsp interphaln joint of left thumb, subs
		S63.126D	Dislocation of unsp interphalangeal joint of thmb, subs
		S63.131D	Subluxation of proximal interphaln joint of r thm, subs
		S63.132D	Subluxation of proximal interphaln joint of left thumb, subs
		S63.133D	Subluxation of proximal interphalangeal joint of thmb, subs
		S63.134D	Disloc of proximal interphaln joint of right thumb, subs
		S63.135D	Dislocation of proximal interphaln joint of left thumb, subs
		S63.136D	Dislocation of proximal interphalangeal joint of thmb, subs
		S63.141D	Subluxation of distal interphaln joint of right thumb, subs
		S63.142D	Subluxation of distal interphaln joint of left thumb, subs
		S63.143D	Subluxation of distal interphalangeal joint of thmb, subs
		S63.144D	Dislocation of distal interphaln joint of right thumb, subs
		S63.145D	Dislocation of distal interphaln joint of left thumb, subs
		S63.146D	Dislocation of distal interphalangeal joint of thmb, subs
		S63.2ØØD	Unspecified subluxation of right index finger, subs encntr
		S63.2Ø1D	Unspecified subluxation of left index finger, subs encntr
		S63.2Ø2D	Unspecified subluxation of right middle finger, subs encntr
		S63.2Ø3D	Unspecified subluxation of left middle finger, subs encntr
		S63.2Ø4D	Unspecified subluxation of right ring finger, subs encntr
		S63.2Ø5D	Unspecified subluxation of left ring finger, subs encntr
		S63.2Ø6D	Unspecified subluxation of right little finger, subs encntr
		S63.2Ø7D	Unspecified subluxation of left little finger, subs encntr
		S63.2Ø8D	Unspecified subluxation of other finger, subs encntr
		S63.2Ø9D	Unspecified subluxation of unspecified finger, subs encntr
		S63.21ØD	Subluxation of MCP joint of right index finger, subs
		S63.211D	Subluxation of MCP joint of left index finger, subs
		S63.212D	Subluxation of MCP joint of right middle finger, subs
		S63.213D	Subluxation of MCP joint of left middle finger, subs
	(Continued on next page)	**S63.214D**	Subluxation of MCP joint of right ring finger, subs

ICD-9-CM		ICD-10-CM	
V58.89	ENCOUNTER FOR OTHER SPECIFIED AFTERCARE **(Continued)**	**S63.215D**	Subluxation of MCP joint of left ring finger, subs
		S63.216D	Subluxation of MCP joint of right little finger, subs
		S63.217D	Subluxation of MCP joint of left little finger, subs
		S63.218D	Subluxation of metacarpophalangeal joint of oth finger, subs
		S63.219D	Subluxation of MCP joint of unsp finger, subs
		S63.220D	Subluxation of unsp interphaln joint of r idx fngr, subs
		S63.221D	Subluxation of unsp interphaln joint of l idx fngr, subs
		S63.222D	Subluxation of unsp interphaln joint of r mid finger, subs
		S63.223D	Subluxation of unsp interphaln joint of l mid finger, subs
		S63.224D	Subluxation of unsp interphaln joint of r rng fngr, subs
		S63.225D	Subluxation of unsp interphaln joint of l rng fngr, subs
		S63.226D	Sublux of unsp interphaln joint of r little finger, subs
		S63.227D	Sublux of unsp interphaln joint of l little finger, subs
		S63.228D	Subluxation of unsp interphalangeal joint of finger, subs
		S63.229D	Subluxation of unsp interphaln joint of unsp finger, subs
		S63.230D	Subluxation of proximal interphaln joint of r idx fngr, subs
		S63.231D	Subluxation of proximal interphaln joint of l idx fngr, subs
		S63.232D	Sublux of proximal interphaln joint of r mid finger, subs
		S63.233D	Sublux of proximal interphaln joint of l mid finger, subs
		S63.234D	Subluxation of proximal interphaln joint of r rng fngr, subs
		S63.235D	Subluxation of proximal interphaln joint of l rng fngr, subs
		S63.236D	Sublux of proximal interphaln joint of r little finger, subs
		S63.237D	Sublux of proximal interphaln joint of l little finger, subs
		S63.238D	Subluxation of proximal interphaln joint of finger, subs
		S63.239D	Sublux of proximal interphaln joint of unsp finger, subs
		S63.240D	Subluxation of distal interphaln joint of r idx fngr, subs
		S63.241D	Subluxation of distal interphaln joint of l idx fngr, subs
		S63.242D	Subluxation of distal interphaln joint of r mid finger, subs
		S63.243D	Subluxation of distal interphaln joint of l mid finger, subs
		S63.244D	Subluxation of distal interphaln joint of r rng fngr, subs
		S63.245D	Subluxation of distal interphaln joint of l rng fngr, subs
		S63.246D	Sublux of distal interphaln joint of r little finger, subs
		S63.247D	Sublux of distal interphaln joint of l little finger, subs
		S63.248D	Subluxation of distal interphalangeal joint of finger, subs
		S63.249D	Subluxation of distal interphaln joint of unsp finger, subs
		S63.250D	Unspecified dislocation of right index finger, subs encntr
		S63.251D	Unspecified dislocation of left index finger, subs encntr
		S63.252D	Unspecified dislocation of right middle finger, subs encntr
		S63.253D	Unspecified dislocation of left middle finger, subs encntr
		S63.254D	Unspecified dislocation of right ring finger, subs encntr
		S63.255D	Unspecified dislocation of left ring finger, subs encntr
		S63.256D	Unspecified dislocation of right little finger, subs encntr
		S63.257D	Unspecified dislocation of left little finger, subs encntr
		S63.258D	Unspecified dislocation of other finger, subs encntr
		S63.259D	Unspecified dislocation of unspecified finger, subs encntr
		S63.260D	Dislocation of MCP joint of right index finger, subs
		S63.261D	Dislocation of MCP joint of left index finger, subs
		S63.262D	Dislocation of MCP joint of right middle finger, subs
		S63.263D	Dislocation of MCP joint of left middle finger, subs
		S63.264D	Dislocation of MCP joint of right ring finger, subs
		S63.265D	Dislocation of MCP joint of left ring finger, subs
		S63.266D	Dislocation of MCP joint of right little finger, subs
		S63.267D	Dislocation of MCP joint of left little finger, subs
		S63.268D	Dislocation of metacarpophalangeal joint of oth finger, subs
		S63.269D	Dislocation of MCP joint of unsp finger, subs
		S63.270D	Dislocation of unsp interphaln joint of r idx fngr, subs
		S63.271D	Dislocation of unsp interphaln joint of l idx fngr, subs
		S63.272D	Dislocation of unsp interphaln joint of r mid finger, subs
		S63.273D	Dislocation of unsp interphaln joint of l mid finger, subs
		S63.274D	Dislocation of unsp interphaln joint of r rng fngr, subs
		S63.275D	Dislocation of unsp interphaln joint of l rng fngr, subs
		S63.276D	Disloc of unsp interphaln joint of r little finger, subs
		S63.277D	Disloc of unsp interphaln joint of l little finger, subs
		S63.278D	Dislocation of unsp interphalangeal joint of finger, subs
		S63.279D	Dislocation of unsp interphaln joint of unsp finger, subs
		S63.280D	Dislocation of proximal interphaln joint of r idx fngr, subs
		S63.281D	Dislocation of proximal interphaln joint of l idx fngr, subs
		S63.282D	Disloc of proximal interphaln joint of r mid finger, subs
		S63.283D	Disloc of proximal interphaln joint of l mid finger, subs
		S63.284D	Dislocation of proximal interphaln joint of r rng fngr, subs
		S63.285D	Dislocation of proximal interphaln joint of l rng fngr, subs
		S63.286D	Disloc of proximal interphaln joint of r little finger, subs
		S63.287D	Disloc of proximal interphaln joint of l little finger, subs
		S63.288D	Dislocation of proximal interphaln joint of finger, subs
		S63.289D	Disloc of proximal interphaln joint of unsp finger, subs
		S63.290D	Dislocation of distal interphaln joint of r idx fngr, subs
		S63.291D	Dislocation of distal interphaln joint of l idx fngr, subs
		S63.292D	Dislocation of distal interphaln joint of r mid finger, subs
		S63.293D	Dislocation of distal interphaln joint of l mid finger, subs
		S63.294D	Dislocation of distal interphaln joint of r rng fngr, subs
		S63.295D	Dislocation of distal interphaln joint of l rng fngr, subs
		S63.296D	Disloc of distal interphaln joint of r little finger, subs
	(Continued on next page)	**S63.297D**	Disloc of distal interphaln joint of l little finger, subs

ICD-9-CM		ICD-10-CM	
V58.89	ENCOUNTER FOR OTHER SPECIFIED AFTERCARE **(Continued)**	**S63.298D**	Dislocation of distal interphalangeal joint of finger, subs
		S63.299D	Dislocation of distal interphaln joint of unsp finger, subs
		S63.301D	Traumatic rupture of unsp ligament of right wrist, subs
		S63.302D	Traumatic rupture of unsp ligament of left wrist, subs
		S63.309D	Traumatic rupture of unsp ligament of unsp wrist, subs
		S63.311D	Traumatic rupture of collateral ligament of r wrist, subs
		S63.312D	Traumatic rupture of collateral ligament of left wrist, subs
		S63.319D	Traumatic rupture of collateral ligament of unsp wrist, subs
		S63.321D	Traumatic rupture of right radiocarpal ligament, subs encntr
		S63.322D	Traumatic rupture of left radiocarpal ligament, subs encntr
		S63.329D	Traumatic rupture of unsp radiocarpal ligament, subs encntr
		S63.331D	Traum rupture of right ulnocarpal (palmar) ligament, subs
		S63.332D	Traumatic rupture of left ulnocarpal (palmar) ligament, subs
		S63.339D	Traumatic rupture of unsp ulnocarpal (palmar) ligament, subs
		S63.391D	Traumatic rupture of oth ligament of right wrist, subs
		S63.392D	Traumatic rupture of oth ligament of left wrist, subs encntr
		S63.399D	Traumatic rupture of oth ligament of unsp wrist, subs encntr
		S63.400D	Traum rupture of unsp ligmt of r idx fngr at MCP/IP jt, subs
		S63.401D	Traum rupture of unsp ligmt of l idx fngr at MCP/IP jt, subs
		S63.402D	Traum rupt of unsp ligmt of r mid finger at MCP/IP jt, subs
		S63.403D	Traum rupt of unsp ligmt of l mid finger at MCP/IP jt, subs
		S63.404D	Traum rupture of unsp ligmt of r rng fngr at MCP/IP jt, subs
		S63.405D	Traum rupture of unsp ligmt of l rng fngr at MCP/IP jt, subs
		S63.406D	Traum rupt of unsp ligmt of r little fngr at MCP/IP jt, subs
		S63.407D	Traum rupt of unsp ligmt of l little fngr at MCP/IP jt, subs
		S63.408D	Traum rupture of unsp ligament of finger at MCP/IP jt, subs
		S63.409D	Traum rupt of unsp ligmt of unsp finger at MCP/IP jt, subs
		S63.410D	Traum rupt of collat ligmt of r idx fngr at MCP/IP jt, subs
		S63.411D	Traum rupt of collat ligmt of l idx fngr at MCP/IP jt, subs
		S63.412D	Traum rupt of collat ligmt of r mid fngr at MCP/IP jt, subs
		S63.413D	Traum rupt of collat ligmt of l mid fngr at MCP/IP jt, subs
		S63.414D	Traum rupt of collat ligmt of r rng fngr at MCP/IP jt, subs
		S63.415D	Traum rupt of collat ligmt of l rng fngr at MCP/IP jt, subs
		S63.416D	Traum rupt of collat ligmt of r lit fngr at MCP/IP jt, subs
		S63.417D	Traum rupt of collat ligmt of l lit fngr at MCP/IP jt, subs
		S63.418D	Traum rupture of collat ligmt of finger at MCP/IP jt, subs
		S63.419D	Traum rupt of collat ligmt of unsp finger at MCP/IP jt, subs
		S63.420D	Traum rupt of palmar ligmt of r idx fngr at MCP/IP jt, subs
		S63.421D	Traum rupt of palmar ligmt of l idx fngr at MCP/IP jt, subs
		S63.422D	Traum rupt of palmar ligmt of r mid fngr at MCP/IP jt, subs
		S63.423D	Traum rupt of palmar ligmt of l mid fngr at MCP/IP jt, subs
		S63.424D	Traum rupt of palmar ligmt of r rng fngr at MCP/IP jt, subs
		S63.425D	Traum rupt of palmar ligmt of l rng fngr at MCP/IP jt, subs
		S63.426D	Traum rupt of palmar ligmt of r lit fngr at MCP/IP jt, subs
		S63.427D	Traum rupt of palmar ligmt of l lit fngr at MCP/IP jt, subs
		S63.428D	Traum rupture of palmar ligmt of finger at MCP/IP jt, subs
		S63.429D	Traum rupt of palmar ligmt of unsp finger at MCP/IP jt, subs
		S63.430D	Traum rupt of volar plate of r idx fngr at MCP/IP jt, subs
		S63.431D	Traum rupt of volar plate of l idx fngr at MCP/IP jt, subs
		S63.432D	Traum rupt of volar plate of r mid finger at MCP/IP jt, subs
		S63.433D	Traum rupt of volar plate of l mid finger at MCP/IP jt, subs
		S63.434D	Traum rupt of volar plate of r rng fngr at MCP/IP jt, subs
		S63.435D	Traum rupt of volar plate of l rng fngr at MCP/IP jt, subs
		S63.436D	Traum rupt of volar plate of r lit fngr at MCP/IP jt, subs
		S63.437D	Traum rupt of volar plate of l lit fngr at MCP/IP jt, subs
		S63.438D	Traum rupture of volar plate of finger at MCP/IP jt, subs
		S63.439D	Traum rupt of volar plate of unsp finger at MCP/IP jt, subs
		S63.490D	Traum rupture of ligament of r idx fngr at MCP/IP jt, subs
		S63.491D	Traum rupture of ligament of l idx fngr at MCP/IP jt, subs
		S63.492D	Traum rupture of ligament of r mid finger at MCP/IP jt, subs
		S63.493D	Traum rupture of ligament of l mid finger at MCP/IP jt, subs
		S63.494D	Traum rupture of ligament of r rng fngr at MCP/IP jt, subs
		S63.495D	Traum rupture of ligament of l rng fngr at MCP/IP jt, subs
		S63.496D	Traum rupture of ligmt of r little finger at MCP/IP jt, subs
		S63.497D	Traum rupture of ligmt of l little finger at MCP/IP jt, subs
		S63.498D	Traumatic rupture of ligament of finger at MCP/IP jt, subs
		S63.499D	Traum rupture of ligament of unsp finger at MCP/IP jt, subs
		S63.501D	Unspecified sprain of right wrist, subsequent encounter
		S63.502D	Unspecified sprain of left wrist, subsequent encounter
		S63.509D	Unspecified sprain of unspecified wrist, subs encntr
		S63.511D	Sprain of carpal joint of right wrist, subsequent encounter
		S63.512D	Sprain of carpal joint of left wrist, subsequent encounter
		S63.519D	Sprain of carpal joint of unspecified wrist, subs encntr
		S63.521D	Sprain of radiocarpal joint of right wrist, subs encntr
		S63.522D	Sprain of radiocarpal joint of left wrist, subs encntr
		S63.529D	Sprain of radiocarpal joint of unsp wrist, subs encntr
		S63.591D	Other specified sprain of right wrist, subsequent encounter
		S63.592D	Other specified sprain of left wrist, subsequent encounter
		S63.599D	Other specified sprain of unspecified wrist, subs encntr
		S63.601D	Unspecified sprain of right thumb, subsequent encounter
		S63.602D	Unspecified sprain of left thumb, subsequent encounter
		S63.609D	Unspecified sprain of unspecified thumb, subs encntr
	(Continued on next page)	**S63.610D**	Unspecified sprain of right index finger, subs encntr

ICD-9-CM		ICD-10-CM	
V58.89	ENCOUNTER FOR OTHER SPECIFIED AFTERCARE **(Continued)**	**S63.611D**	Unspecified sprain of left index finger, subs encntr
		S63.612D	Unspecified sprain of right middle finger, subs encntr
		S63.613D	Unspecified sprain of left middle finger, subs encntr
		S63.614D	Unspecified sprain of right ring finger, subs encntr
		S63.615D	Unspecified sprain of left ring finger, subsequent encounter
		S63.616D	Unspecified sprain of right little finger, subs encntr
		S63.617D	Unspecified sprain of left little finger, subs encntr
		S63.618D	Unspecified sprain of other finger, subsequent encounter
		S63.619D	Unspecified sprain of unspecified finger, subs encntr
		S63.621D	Sprain of interphalangeal joint of right thumb, subs encntr
		S63.622D	Sprain of interphalangeal joint of left thumb, subs encntr
		S63.629D	Sprain of interphalangeal joint of unsp thumb, subs encntr
		S63.630D	Sprain of interphalangeal joint of right index finger, subs
		S63.631D	Sprain of interphalangeal joint of left index finger, subs
		S63.632D	Sprain of interphalangeal joint of right middle finger, subs
		S63.633D	Sprain of interphalangeal joint of left middle finger, subs
		S63.634D	Sprain of interphalangeal joint of right ring finger, subs
		S63.635D	Sprain of interphalangeal joint of left ring finger, subs
		S63.636D	Sprain of interphalangeal joint of right little finger, subs
		S63.637D	Sprain of interphalangeal joint of left little finger, subs
		S63.638D	Sprain of interphalangeal joint of other finger, subs encntr
		S63.639D	Sprain of interphalangeal joint of unsp finger, subs encntr
		S63.641D	Sprain of metacarpophalangeal joint of right thumb, subs
		S63.642D	Sprain of metacarpophalangeal joint of left thumb, subs
		S63.649D	Sprain of metacarpophalangeal joint of unsp thumb, subs
		S63.650D	Sprain of MCP joint of right index finger, subs
		S63.651D	Sprain of MCP joint of left index finger, subs
		S63.652D	Sprain of MCP joint of right middle finger, subs
		S63.653D	Sprain of MCP joint of left middle finger, subs
		S63.654D	Sprain of MCP joint of right ring finger, subs
		S63.655D	Sprain of MCP joint of left ring finger, subs
		S63.656D	Sprain of MCP joint of right little finger, subs
		S63.657D	Sprain of MCP joint of left little finger, subs
		S63.658D	Sprain of metacarpophalangeal joint of oth finger, subs
		S63.659D	Sprain of metacarpophalangeal joint of unsp finger, subs
		S63.681D	Other sprain of right thumb, subsequent encounter
		S63.682D	Other sprain of left thumb, subsequent encounter
		S63.689D	Other sprain of unspecified thumb, subsequent encounter
		S63.690D	Other sprain of right index finger, subsequent encounter
		S63.691D	Other sprain of left index finger, subsequent encounter
		S63.692D	Other sprain of right middle finger, subsequent encounter
		S63.693D	Other sprain of left middle finger, subsequent encounter
		S63.694D	Other sprain of right ring finger, subsequent encounter
		S63.695D	Other sprain of left ring finger, subsequent encounter
		S63.696D	Other sprain of right little finger, subsequent encounter
		S63.697D	Other sprain of left little finger, subsequent encounter
		S63.698D	Other sprain of other finger, subsequent encounter
		S63.699D	Other sprain of unspecified finger, subsequent encounter
		S63.8X1D	Sprain of other part of right wrist and hand, subs encntr
		S63.8X2D	Sprain of other part of left wrist and hand, subs encntr
		S63.8X9D	Sprain of other part of unsp wrist and hand, subs encntr
		S63.90XD	Sprain of unsp part of unsp wrist and hand, subs encntr
		S63.91XD	Sprain of unsp part of right wrist and hand, subs encntr
		S63.92XD	Sprain of unsp part of left wrist and hand, subs encntr
		S64.00XD	Injury of ulnar nerve at wrs/hnd lv of unsp arm, subs
		S64.01XD	Injury of ulnar nerve at wrs/hnd lv of right arm, subs
		S64.02XD	Injury of ulnar nerve at wrs/hnd lv of left arm, subs
		S64.10XD	Injury of median nerve at wrs/hnd lv of unsp arm, subs
		S64.11XD	Injury of median nerve at wrs/hnd lv of right arm, subs
		S64.12XD	Injury of median nerve at wrs/hnd lv of left arm, subs
		S64.20XD	Injury of radial nerve at wrs/hnd lv of unsp arm, subs
		S64.21XD	Injury of radial nerve at wrs/hnd lv of right arm, subs
		S64.22XD	Injury of radial nerve at wrs/hnd lv of left arm, subs
		S64.30XD	Injury of digital nerve of unspecified thumb, subs encntr
		S64.31XD	Injury of digital nerve of right thumb, subsequent encounter
		S64.32XD	Injury of digital nerve of left thumb, subsequent encounter
		S64.40XD	Injury of digital nerve of unspecified finger, subs encntr
		S64.490D	Injury of digital nerve of right index finger, subs encntr
		S64.491D	Injury of digital nerve of left index finger, subs encntr
		S64.492D	Injury of digital nerve of right middle finger, subs encntr
		S64.493D	Injury of digital nerve of left middle finger, subs encntr
		S64.494D	Injury of digital nerve of right ring finger, subs encntr
		S64.495D	Injury of digital nerve of left ring finger, subs encntr
		S64.496D	Injury of digital nerve of right little finger, subs encntr
		S64.497D	Injury of digital nerve of left little finger, subs encntr
		S64.498D	Injury of digital nerve of other finger, subs encntr
		S64.8X1D	Injury of nerves at wrist and hand level of right arm, subs
		S64.8X2D	Injury of nerves at wrist and hand level of left arm, subs
		S64.8X9D	Injury of nerves at wrist and hand level of unsp arm, subs
		S64.90XD	Injury of unsp nerve at wrs/hnd lv of unsp arm, subs
		S64.91XD	Injury of unsp nerve at wrs/hnd lv of right arm, subs
		S64.92XD	Injury of unsp nerve at wrs/hnd lv of left arm, subs
		S65.001D	Unsp injury of ulnar artery at wrs/hnd lv of right arm, subs

(Continued on next page)

[Brackets] indicate valid character values for each code. Character value meanings provided for each code grouping.

ICD-9-CM		ICD-10-CM	
V58.89	ENCOUNTER FOR OTHER SPECIFIED AFTERCARE **(Continued)**	**S65.002D**	Unsp injury of ulnar artery at wrs/hnd lv of left arm, subs
		S65.009D	Unsp injury of ulnar artery at wrs/hnd lv of unsp arm, subs
		S65.011D	Laceration of ulnar artery at wrs/hnd lv of right arm, subs
		S65.012D	Laceration of ulnar artery at wrs/hnd lv of left arm, subs
		S65.019D	Laceration of ulnar artery at wrs/hnd lv of unsp arm, subs
		S65.091D	Inj ulnar artery at wrist and hand level of right arm, subs
		S65.092D	Inj ulnar artery at wrist and hand level of left arm, subs
		S65.099D	Inj ulnar artery at wrist and hand level of unsp arm, subs
		S65.101D	Unsp injury of radial art at wrs/hnd lv of right arm, subs
		S65.102D	Unsp injury of radial artery at wrs/hnd lv of left arm, subs
		S65.109D	Unsp injury of radial artery at wrs/hnd lv of unsp arm, subs
		S65.111D	Laceration of radial artery at wrs/hnd lv of right arm, subs
		S65.112D	Laceration of radial artery at wrs/hnd lv of left arm, subs
		S65.119D	Laceration of radial artery at wrs/hnd lv of unsp arm, subs
		S65.191D	Inj radial artery at wrist and hand level of right arm, subs
		S65.192D	Inj radial artery at wrist and hand level of left arm, subs
		S65.199D	Inj radial artery at wrist and hand level of unsp arm, subs
		S65.201D	Unsp injury of superficial palmar arch of right hand, subs
		S65.202D	Unsp injury of superficial palmar arch of left hand, subs
		S65.209D	Unsp injury of superficial palmar arch of unsp hand, subs
		S65.211D	Laceration of superficial palmar arch of right hand, subs
		S65.212D	Laceration of superficial palmar arch of left hand, subs
		S65.219D	Laceration of superficial palmar arch of unsp hand, subs
		S65.291D	Inj superficial palmar arch of right hand, subs encntr
		S65.292D	Inj superficial palmar arch of left hand, subs encntr
		S65.299D	Inj superficial palmar arch of unsp hand, subs encntr
		S65.301D	Unsp injury of deep palmar arch of right hand, subs encntr
		S65.302D	Unsp injury of deep palmar arch of left hand, subs encntr
		S65.309D	Unsp injury of deep palmar arch of unsp hand, subs encntr
		S65.311D	Laceration of deep palmar arch of right hand, subs encntr
		S65.312D	Laceration of deep palmar arch of left hand, subs encntr
		S65.319D	Laceration of deep palmar arch of unsp hand, subs encntr
		S65.391D	Oth injury of deep palmar arch of right hand, subs encntr
		S65.392D	Oth injury of deep palmar arch of left hand, subs encntr
		S65.399D	Oth injury of deep palmar arch of unsp hand, subs encntr
		S65.401D	Unsp injury of blood vessel of right thumb, subs encntr
		S65.402D	Unsp injury of blood vessel of left thumb, subs encntr
		S65.409D	Unsp injury of blood vessel of unsp thumb, subs encntr
		S65.411D	Laceration of blood vessel of right thumb, subs encntr
		S65.412D	Laceration of blood vessel of left thumb, subs encntr
		S65.419D	Laceration of blood vessel of unspecified thumb, subs encntr
		S65.491D	Oth injury of blood vessel of right thumb, subs encntr
		S65.492D	Oth injury of blood vessel of left thumb, subs encntr
		S65.499D	Oth injury of blood vessel of unspecified thumb, subs encntr
		S65.500D	Unsp injury of blood vessel of right index finger, subs
		S65.501D	Unsp injury of blood vessel of left index finger, subs
		S65.502D	Unsp injury of blood vessel of right middle finger, subs
		S65.503D	Unsp injury of blood vessel of left middle finger, subs
		S65.504D	Unsp injury of blood vessel of right ring finger, subs
		S65.505D	Unsp injury of blood vessel of left ring finger, subs encntr
		S65.506D	Unsp injury of blood vessel of right little finger, subs
		S65.507D	Unsp injury of blood vessel of left little finger, subs
		S65.508D	Unsp injury of blood vessel of other finger, subs encntr
		S65.509D	Unsp injury of blood vessel of unsp finger, subs encntr
		S65.510D	Laceration of blood vessel of right index finger, subs
		S65.511D	Laceration of blood vessel of left index finger, subs encntr
		S65.512D	Laceration of blood vessel of right middle finger, subs
		S65.513D	Laceration of blood vessel of left middle finger, subs
		S65.514D	Laceration of blood vessel of right ring finger, subs encntr
		S65.515D	Laceration of blood vessel of left ring finger, subs encntr
		S65.516D	Laceration of blood vessel of right little finger, subs
		S65.517D	Laceration of blood vessel of left little finger, subs
		S65.518D	Laceration of blood vessel of other finger, subs encntr
		S65.519D	Laceration of blood vessel of unsp finger, subs encntr
		S65.590D	Inj blood vessel of right index finger, subs encntr
		S65.591D	Oth injury of blood vessel of left index finger, subs encntr
		S65.592D	Inj blood vessel of right middle finger, subs encntr
		S65.593D	Inj blood vessel of left middle finger, subs encntr
		S65.594D	Oth injury of blood vessel of right ring finger, subs encntr
		S65.595D	Oth injury of blood vessel of left ring finger, subs encntr
		S65.596D	Inj blood vessel of right little finger, subs encntr
		S65.597D	Inj blood vessel of left little finger, subs encntr
		S65.598D	Oth injury of blood vessel of other finger, subs encntr
		S65.599D	Oth injury of blood vessel of unsp finger, subs encntr
		S65.801D	Unsp inj blood vessels at wrs/hnd lv of right arm, subs
		S65.802D	Unsp injury of blood vessels at wrs/hnd lv of left arm, subs
		S65.809D	Unsp injury of blood vessels at wrs/hnd lv of unsp arm, subs
		S65.811D	Laceration of blood vessels at wrs/hnd lv of right arm, subs
		S65.812D	Laceration of blood vessels at wrs/hnd lv of left arm, subs
		S65.819D	Laceration of blood vessels at wrs/hnd lv of unsp arm, subs
		S65.891D	Inj oth blood vessels at wrs/hnd lv of right arm, subs
		S65.892D	Inj oth blood vessels at wrs/hnd lv of left arm, subs
	(Continued on next page)	**S65.899D**	Inj oth blood vessels at wrs/hnd lv of unsp arm, subs

ICD-9-CM		ICD-10-CM	
V58.89	ENCOUNTER FOR OTHER SPECIFIED AFTERCARE **(Continued)**	**S65.901D**	Unsp inj unsp blood vess at wrs/hnd lv of right arm, subs
		S65.902D	Unsp inj unsp blood vess at wrs/hnd lv of left arm, subs
		S65.909D	Unsp inj unsp blood vess at wrs/hnd lv of unsp arm, subs
		S65.911D	Lacerat unsp blood vessel at wrs/hnd lv of right arm, subs
		S65.912D	Lacerat unsp blood vessel at wrs/hnd lv of left arm, subs
		S65.919D	Lacerat unsp blood vessel at wrs/hnd lv of unsp arm, subs
		S65.991D	Inj unsp blood vessel at wrist and hand of right arm, subs
		S65.992D	Inj unsp blood vessel at wrist and hand of left arm, subs
		S65.999D	Inj unsp blood vessel at wrist and hand of unsp arm, subs
		S66.001D	Unsp inj long flxr musc/fasc/tend r thm at wrs/hnd lv, subs
		S66.002D	Unsp inj long flxr musc/fasc/tend l thm at wrs/hnd lv, subs
		S66.009D	Unsp inj long flexor musc/fasc/tend thmb at wrs/hnd lv, subs
		S66.011D	Strain long flexor musc/fasc/tend r thm at wrs/hnd lv, subs
		S66.012D	Strain long flexor musc/fasc/tend l thm at wrs/hnd lv, subs
		S66.019D	Strain long flexor musc/fasc/tend thmb at wrs/hnd lv, subs
		S66.021D	Lacerat long flexor musc/fasc/tend r thm at wrs/hnd lv, subs
		S66.022D	Lacerat long flexor musc/fasc/tend l thm at wrs/hnd lv, subs
		S66.029D	Lacerat long flexor musc/fasc/tend thmb at wrs/hnd lv, subs
		S66.091D	Inj long flexor musc/fasc/tend r thm at wrs/hnd lv, subs
		S66.092D	Inj long flexor musc/fasc/tend l thm at wrs/hnd lv, subs
		S66.099D	Inj long flexor musc/fasc/tend thmb at wrs/hnd lv, subs
		S66.100D	Unsp inj flxr musc/fasc/tend r idx fngr at wrs/hnd lv, subs
		S66.101D	Unsp inj flxr musc/fasc/tend l idx fngr at wrs/hnd lv, subs
		S66.102D	Unsp inj flxr musc/fasc/tend r mid fngr at wrs/hnd lv, subs
		S66.103D	Unsp inj flxr musc/fasc/tend l mid fngr at wrs/hnd lv, subs
		S66.104D	Unsp inj flxr musc/fasc/tend r rng fngr at wrs/hnd lv, subs
		S66.105D	Unsp inj flxr musc/fasc/tend l rng fngr at wrs/hnd lv, subs
		S66.106D	Unsp inj flxr musc/fasc/tend r lit fngr at wrs/hnd lv, subs
		S66.107D	Unsp inj flxr musc/fasc/tend l lit fngr at wrs/hnd lv, subs
		S66.108D	Unsp inj flexor musc/fasc/tend finger at wrs/hnd lv, subs
		S66.109D	Unsp inj flexor musc/fasc/tend unsp fngr at wrs/hnd lv, subs
		S66.110D	Strain flexor musc/fasc/tend r idx fngr at wrs/hnd lv, subs
		S66.111D	Strain flexor musc/fasc/tend l idx fngr at wrs/hnd lv, subs
		S66.112D	Strain flexor musc/fasc/tend r mid fngr at wrs/hnd lv, subs
		S66.113D	Strain flexor musc/fasc/tend l mid fngr at wrs/hnd lv, subs
		S66.114D	Strain flexor musc/fasc/tend r rng fngr at wrs/hnd lv, subs
		S66.115D	Strain flexor musc/fasc/tend l rng fngr at wrs/hnd lv, subs
		S66.116D	Strain flxr musc/fasc/tend r little fngr at wrs/hnd lv, subs
		S66.117D	Strain flxr musc/fasc/tend l little fngr at wrs/hnd lv, subs
		S66.118D	Strain of flexor musc/fasc/tend finger at wrs/hnd lv, subs
		S66.119D	Strain flexor musc/fasc/tend unsp finger at wrs/hnd lv, subs
		S66.120D	Lacerat flexor musc/fasc/tend r idx fngr at wrs/hnd lv, subs
		S66.121D	Lacerat flexor musc/fasc/tend l idx fngr at wrs/hnd lv, subs
		S66.122D	Lacerat flexor musc/fasc/tend r mid fngr at wrs/hnd lv, subs
		S66.123D	Lacerat flexor musc/fasc/tend l mid fngr at wrs/hnd lv, subs
		S66.124D	Lacerat flexor musc/fasc/tend r rng fngr at wrs/hnd lv, subs
		S66.125D	Lacerat flexor musc/fasc/tend l rng fngr at wrs/hnd lv, subs
		S66.126D	Lacerat flxr musc/fasc/tend r lit fngr at wrs/hnd lv, subs
		S66.127D	Lacerat flxr musc/fasc/tend l lit fngr at wrs/hnd lv, subs
		S66.128D	Lacerat flexor musc/fasc/tend finger at wrs/hnd lv, subs
		S66.129D	Lacerat flexor musc/fasc/tend unsp fngr at wrs/hnd lv, subs
		S66.190D	Inj flexor musc/fasc/tend r idx fngr at wrs/hnd lv, subs
		S66.191D	Inj flexor musc/fasc/tend l idx fngr at wrs/hnd lv, subs
		S66.192D	Inj flexor musc/fasc/tend r mid finger at wrs/hnd lv, subs
		S66.193D	Inj flexor musc/fasc/tend l mid finger at wrs/hnd lv, subs
		S66.194D	Inj flexor musc/fasc/tend r rng fngr at wrs/hnd lv, subs
		S66.195D	Inj flexor musc/fasc/tend l rng fngr at wrs/hnd lv, subs
		S66.196D	Inj flexor musc/fasc/tend r little fngr at wrs/hnd lv, subs
		S66.197D	Inj flexor musc/fasc/tend l little fngr at wrs/hnd lv, subs
		S66.198D	Inj flexor musc/fasc/tend finger at wrs/hnd lv, subs
		S66.199D	Inj flexor musc/fasc/tend unsp finger at wrs/hnd lv, subs
		S66.201D	Unsp inj extensor musc/fasc/tend r thm at wrs/hnd lv, subs
		S66.202D	Unsp inj extensor musc/fasc/tend l thm at wrs/hnd lv, subs
		S66.209D	Unsp inj extensor musc/fasc/tend thmb at wrs/hnd lv, subs
		S66.211D	Strain of extensor musc/fasc/tend r thm at wrs/hnd lv, subs
		S66.212D	Strain of extensor musc/fasc/tend l thm at wrs/hnd lv, subs
		S66.219D	Strain of extensor musc/fasc/tend thmb at wrs/hnd lv, subs
		S66.221D	Lacerat extensor musc/fasc/tend r thm at wrs/hnd lv, subs
		S66.222D	Lacerat extensor musc/fasc/tend l thm at wrs/hnd lv, subs
		S66.229D	Lacerat extensor musc/fasc/tend thmb at wrs/hnd lv, subs
		S66.291D	Inj extensor musc/fasc/tend right thumb at wrs/hnd lv, subs
		S66.292D	Inj extensor musc/fasc/tend left thumb at wrs/hnd lv, subs
		S66.299D	Inj extensor musc/fasc/tend thmb at wrs/hnd lv, subs
		S66.300D	Unsp inj extn musc/fasc/tend r idx fngr at wrs/hnd lv, subs
		S66.301D	Unsp inj extn musc/fasc/tend l idx fngr at wrs/hnd lv, subs
		S66.302D	Unsp inj extn musc/fasc/tend r mid fngr at wrs/hnd lv, subs
		S66.303D	Unsp inj extn musc/fasc/tend l mid fngr at wrs/hnd lv, subs
		S66.304D	Unsp inj extn musc/fasc/tend r rng fngr at wrs/hnd lv, subs
		S66.305D	Unsp inj extn musc/fasc/tend l rng fngr at wrs/hnd lv, subs
		S66.306D	Unsp inj extn musc/fasc/tend r lit fngr at wrs/hnd lv, subs
		S66.307D	Unsp inj extn musc/fasc/tend l lit fngr at wrs/hnd lv, subs
		S66.308D	Unsp inj extensor musc/fasc/tend finger at wrs/hnd lv, subs
	(Continued on next page)	**S66.309D**	Unsp inj extn musc/fasc/tend unsp finger at wrs/hnd lv, subs

ICD-9-CM		ICD-10-CM	
V58.89	ENCOUNTER FOR OTHER SPECIFIED AFTERCARE **(Continued)**	**S66.310D**	Strain extn musc/fasc/tend r idx fngr at wrs/hnd lv, subs
		S66.311D	Strain extn musc/fasc/tend l idx fngr at wrs/hnd lv, subs
		S66.312D	Strain extn musc/fasc/tend r mid finger at wrs/hnd lv, subs
		S66.313D	Strain extn musc/fasc/tend l mid finger at wrs/hnd lv, subs
		S66.314D	Strain extn musc/fasc/tend r rng fngr at wrs/hnd lv, subs
		S66.315D	Strain extn musc/fasc/tend l rng fngr at wrs/hnd lv, subs
		S66.316D	Strain extn musc/fasc/tend r little fngr at wrs/hnd lv, subs
		S66.317D	Strain extn musc/fasc/tend l little fngr at wrs/hnd lv, subs
		S66.318D	Strain of extensor musc/fasc/tend finger at wrs/hnd lv, subs
		S66.319D	Strain extn musc/fasc/tend unsp finger at wrs/hnd lv, subs
		S66.320D	Lacerat extn musc/fasc/tend r idx fngr at wrs/hnd lv, subs
		S66.321D	Lacerat extn musc/fasc/tend l idx fngr at wrs/hnd lv, subs
		S66.322D	Lacerat extn musc/fasc/tend r mid finger at wrs/hnd lv, subs
		S66.323D	Lacerat extn musc/fasc/tend l mid finger at wrs/hnd lv, subs
		S66.324D	Lacerat extn musc/fasc/tend r rng fngr at wrs/hnd lv, subs
		S66.325D	Lacerat extn musc/fasc/tend l rng fngr at wrs/hnd lv, subs
		S66.326D	Lacerat extn musc/fasc/tend r lit fngr at wrs/hnd lv, subs
		S66.327D	Lacerat extn musc/fasc/tend l lit fngr at wrs/hnd lv, subs
		S66.328D	Lacerat extensor musc/fasc/tend finger at wrs/hnd lv, subs
		S66.329D	Lacerat extn musc/fasc/tend unsp finger at wrs/hnd lv, subs
		S66.390D	Inj extensor musc/fasc/tend r idx fngr at wrs/hnd lv, subs
		S66.391D	Inj extensor musc/fasc/tend l idx fngr at wrs/hnd lv, subs
		S66.392D	Inj extensor musc/fasc/tend r mid finger at wrs/hnd lv, subs
		S66.393D	Inj extensor musc/fasc/tend l mid finger at wrs/hnd lv, subs
		S66.394D	Inj extensor musc/fasc/tend r rng fngr at wrs/hnd lv, subs
		S66.395D	Inj extensor musc/fasc/tend l rng fngr at wrs/hnd lv, subs
		S66.396D	Inj extn musc/fasc/tend r little finger at wrs/hnd lv, subs
		S66.397D	Inj extn musc/fasc/tend l little finger at wrs/hnd lv, subs
		S66.398D	Inj extensor musc/fasc/tend finger at wrs/hnd lv, subs
		S66.399D	Inj extensor musc/fasc/tend unsp finger at wrs/hnd lv, subs
		S66.401D	Unsp inj intrinsic musc/fasc/tend r thm at wrs/hnd lv, subs
		S66.402D	Unsp inj intrinsic musc/fasc/tend l thm at wrs/hnd lv, subs
		S66.409D	Unsp inj intrinsic musc/fasc/tend thmb at wrs/hnd lv, subs
		S66.411D	Strain of intrinsic musc/fasc/tend r thm at wrs/hnd lv, subs
		S66.412D	Strain of intrinsic musc/fasc/tend l thm at wrs/hnd lv, subs
		S66.419D	Strain of intrinsic musc/fasc/tend thmb at wrs/hnd lv, subs
		S66.421D	Lacerat intrinsic musc/fasc/tend r thm at wrs/hnd lv, subs
		S66.422D	Lacerat intrinsic musc/fasc/tend l thm at wrs/hnd lv, subs
		S66.429D	Lacerat intrinsic musc/fasc/tend thmb at wrs/hnd lv, subs
		S66.491D	Inj intrinsic musc/fasc/tend right thumb at wrs/hnd lv, subs
		S66.492D	Inj intrinsic musc/fasc/tend left thumb at wrs/hnd lv, subs
		S66.499D	Inj intrinsic musc/fasc/tend thmb at wrs/hnd lv, subs
		S66.500D	Unsp inj intrns musc/fasc/tend r idx fngr at wrs/hnd lv,subs
		S66.501D	Unsp inj intrns musc/fasc/tend l idx fngr at wrs/hnd lv,subs
		S66.502D	Unsp inj intrns musc/fasc/tend r mid fngr at wrs/hnd lv,subs
		S66.503D	Unsp inj intrns musc/fasc/tend l mid fngr at wrs/hnd lv,subs
		S66.504D	Unsp inj intrns musc/fasc/tend r rng fngr at wrs/hnd lv,subs
		S66.505D	Unsp inj intrns musc/fasc/tend l rng fngr at wrs/hnd lv,subs
		S66.506D	Unsp inj intrns musc/fasc/tend r lit fngr at wrs/hnd lv,subs
		S66.507D	Unsp inj intrns musc/fasc/tend l lit fngr at wrs/hnd lv,subs
		S66.508D	Unsp inj intrinsic musc/fasc/tend finger at wrs/hnd lv, subs
		S66.509D	Unsp inj intrns musc/fasc/tend unsp fngr at wrs/hnd lv, subs
		S66.510D	Strain intrns musc/fasc/tend r idx fngr at wrs/hnd lv, subs
		S66.511D	Strain intrns musc/fasc/tend l idx fngr at wrs/hnd lv, subs
		S66.512D	Strain intrns musc/fasc/tend r mid fngr at wrs/hnd lv, subs
		S66.513D	Strain intrns musc/fasc/tend l mid fngr at wrs/hnd lv, subs
		S66.514D	Strain intrns musc/fasc/tend r rng fngr at wrs/hnd lv, subs
		S66.515D	Strain intrns musc/fasc/tend l rng fngr at wrs/hnd lv, subs
		S66.516D	Strain intrns musc/fasc/tend r lit fngr at wrs/hnd lv, subs
		S66.517D	Strain intrns musc/fasc/tend l lit fngr at wrs/hnd lv, subs
		S66.518D	Strain of intrns musc/fasc/tend finger at wrs/hnd lv, subs
		S66.519D	Strain intrns musc/fasc/tend unsp finger at wrs/hnd lv, subs
		S66.520D	Lacerat intrns musc/fasc/tend r idx fngr at wrs/hnd lv, subs
		S66.521D	Lacerat intrns musc/fasc/tend l idx fngr at wrs/hnd lv, subs
		S66.522D	Lacerat intrns musc/fasc/tend r mid fngr at wrs/hnd lv, subs
		S66.523D	Lacerat intrns musc/fasc/tend l mid fngr at wrs/hnd lv, subs
		S66.524D	Lacerat intrns musc/fasc/tend r rng fngr at wrs/hnd lv, subs
		S66.525D	Lacerat intrns musc/fasc/tend l rng fngr at wrs/hnd lv, subs
		S66.526D	Lacerat intrns musc/fasc/tend r lit fngr at wrs/hnd lv, subs
		S66.527D	Lacerat intrns musc/fasc/tend l lit fngr at wrs/hnd lv, subs
		S66.528D	Lacerat intrinsic musc/fasc/tend finger at wrs/hnd lv, subs
		S66.529D	Lacerat intrns musc/fasc/tend unsp fngr at wrs/hnd lv, subs
		S66.590D	Inj intrinsic musc/fasc/tend r idx fngr at wrs/hnd lv, subs
		S66.591D	Inj intrinsic musc/fasc/tend l idx fngr at wrs/hnd lv, subs
		S66.592D	Inj intrns musc/fasc/tend r mid finger at wrs/hnd lv, subs
		S66.593D	Inj intrns musc/fasc/tend l mid finger at wrs/hnd lv, subs
		S66.594D	Inj intrinsic musc/fasc/tend r rng fngr at wrs/hnd lv, subs
		S66.595D	Inj intrinsic musc/fasc/tend l rng fngr at wrs/hnd lv, subs
		S66.596D	Inj intrns musc/fasc/tend r little fngr at wrs/hnd lv, subs
		S66.597D	Inj intrns musc/fasc/tend l little fngr at wrs/hnd lv, subs
		S66.598D	Inj intrinsic musc/fasc/tend finger at wrs/hnd lv, subs
		S66.599D	Inj intrinsic musc/fasc/tend unsp finger at wrs/hnd lv, subs
	(Continued on next page)	**S66.801D**	Unsp injury of musc/fasc/tend at wrs/hnd lv, r hand, subs

ICD-9-CM		ICD-10-CM	
V58.89	ENCOUNTER FOR OTHER SPECIFIED AFTERCARE **(Continued)**	**S66.802D**	Unsp injury of musc/fasc/tend at wrs/hnd lv, left hand, subs
		S66.809D	Unsp injury of musc/fasc/tend at wrs/hnd lv, unsp hand, subs
		S66.811D	Strain of musc/fasc/tend at wrs/hnd lv, right hand, subs
		S66.812D	Strain of musc/fasc/tend at wrs/hnd lv, left hand, subs
		S66.819D	Strain of musc/fasc/tend at wrs/hnd lv, unsp hand, subs
		S66.821D	Laceration of musc/fasc/tend at wrs/hnd lv, right hand, subs
		S66.822D	Laceration of musc/fasc/tend at wrs/hnd lv, left hand, subs
		S66.829D	Laceration of musc/fasc/tend at wrs/hnd lv, unsp hand, subs
		S66.891D	Inj musc/fasc/tend at wrist and hand level, right hand, subs
		S66.892D	Inj musc/fasc/tend at wrist and hand level, left hand, subs
		S66.899D	Inj musc/fasc/tend at wrist and hand level, unsp hand, subs
		S66.901D	Unsp inj unsp musc/fasc/tend at wrs/hnd lv, r hand, subs
		S66.902D	Unsp inj unsp musc/fasc/tend at wrs/hnd lv, left hand, subs
		S66.909D	Unsp inj unsp musc/fasc/tend at wrs/hnd lv, unsp hand, subs
		S66.911D	Strain of unsp musc/fasc/tend at wrs/hnd lv, r hand, subs
		S66.912D	Strain of unsp musc/fasc/tend at wrs/hnd lv, left hand, subs
		S66.919D	Strain of unsp musc/fasc/tend at wrs/hnd lv, unsp hand, subs
		S66.921D	Lacerat unsp musc/fasc/tend at wrs/hnd lv, right hand, subs
		S66.922D	Lacerat unsp musc/fasc/tend at wrs/hnd lv, left hand, subs
		S66.929D	Lacerat unsp musc/fasc/tend at wrs/hnd lv, unsp hand, subs
		S66.991D	Inj unsp musc/fasc/tend at wrs/hnd lv, right hand, subs
		S66.992D	Inj unsp musc/fasc/tend at wrs/hnd lv, left hand, subs
		S66.999D	Inj unsp musc/fasc/tend at wrs/hnd lv, unsp hand, subs
		S67.00XD	Crushing injury of unspecified thumb, subsequent encounter
		S67.01XD	Crushing injury of right thumb, subsequent encounter
		S67.02XD	Crushing injury of left thumb, subsequent encounter
		S67.10XD	Crushing injury of unspecified finger(s), subs encntr
		S67.190D	Crushing injury of right index finger, subsequent encounter
		S67.191D	Crushing injury of left index finger, subsequent encounter
		S67.192D	Crushing injury of right middle finger, subsequent encounter
		S67.193D	Crushing injury of left middle finger, subsequent encounter
		S67.194D	Crushing injury of right ring finger, subsequent encounter
		S67.195D	Crushing injury of left ring finger, subsequent encounter
		S67.196D	Crushing injury of right little finger, subsequent encounter
		S67.197D	Crushing injury of left little finger, subsequent encounter
		S67.198D	Crushing injury of other finger, subsequent encounter
		S67.20XD	Crushing injury of unspecified hand, subsequent encounter
		S67.21XD	Crushing injury of right hand, subsequent encounter
		S67.22XD	Crushing injury of left hand, subsequent encounter
		S67.30XD	Crushing injury of unspecified wrist, subsequent encounter
		S67.31XD	Crushing injury of right wrist, subsequent encounter
		S67.32XD	Crushing injury of left wrist, subsequent encounter
		S67.40XD	Crushing injury of unspecified wrist and hand, subs encntr
		S67.41XD	Crushing injury of right wrist and hand, subs encntr
		S67.42XD	Crushing injury of left wrist and hand, subsequent encounter
		S67.90XD	Crush inj unsp part(s) of unsp wrist, hand and fingers, subs
		S67.91XD	Crushing inj unsp part(s) of r wrist, hand and fingers, subs
		S67.92XD	Crushing inj unsp part(s) of l wrist, hand and fingers, subs
		S68.011D	Complete traumatic MCP amputation of right thumb, subs
		S68.012D	Complete traumatic MCP amputation of left thumb, subs
		S68.019D	Complete traumatic MCP amputation of thmb, subs
		S68.021D	Partial traumatic MCP amputation of right thumb, subs
		S68.022D	Partial traumatic MCP amputation of left thumb, subs
		S68.029D	Partial traumatic MCP amputation of thmb, subs
		S68.110D	Complete traumatic MCP amputation of r idx fngr, subs
		S68.111D	Complete traumatic MCP amputation of left index finger, subs
		S68.112D	Complete traumatic MCP amputation of r mid finger, subs
		S68.113D	Complete traumatic MCP amputation of l mid finger, subs
		S68.114D	Complete traumatic MCP amputation of right ring finger, subs
		S68.115D	Complete traumatic MCP amputation of left ring finger, subs
		S68.116D	Complete traumatic MCP amputation of r little finger, subs
		S68.117D	Complete traumatic MCP amputation of l little finger, subs
		S68.118D	Complete traumatic MCP amputation of finger, subs
		S68.119D	Complete traumatic MCP amputation of unsp finger, subs
		S68.120D	Partial traumatic MCP amputation of right index finger, subs
		S68.121D	Partial traumatic MCP amputation of left index finger, subs
		S68.122D	Partial traumatic MCP amputation of r mid finger, subs
		S68.123D	Partial traumatic MCP amputation of left middle finger, subs
		S68.124D	Partial traumatic MCP amputation of right ring finger, subs
		S68.125D	Partial traumatic MCP amputation of left ring finger, subs
		S68.126D	Partial traumatic MCP amputation of r little finger, subs
		S68.127D	Partial traumatic MCP amputation of left little finger, subs
		S68.128D	Partial traumatic MCP amputation of finger, subs
		S68.129D	Partial traumatic MCP amputation of unsp finger, subs
		S68.411D	Complete traumatic amp of right hand at wrist level, subs
		S68.412D	Complete traumatic amp of left hand at wrist level, subs
		S68.419D	Complete traumatic amp of unsp hand at wrist level, subs
		S68.421D	Partial traumatic amp of right hand at wrist level, subs
		S68.422D	Partial traumatic amp of left hand at wrist level, subs
		S68.429D	Partial traumatic amp of unsp hand at wrist level, subs
		S68.511D	Complete traumatic trnsphal amputation of right thumb, subs
		S68.512D	Complete traumatic trnsphal amputation of left thumb, subs
	(Continued on next page)	**S68.519D**	Complete traumatic transphalangeal amputation of thmb, subs

ICD-9-CM		ICD-10-CM	
V58.89	ENCOUNTER FOR OTHER SPECIFIED AFTERCARE **(Continued)**	**S68.521D**	Partial traumatic trnsphal amputation of right thumb, subs
		S68.522D	Partial traumatic trnsphal amputation of left thumb, subs
		S68.529D	Partial traumatic transphalangeal amputation of thmb, subs
		S68.610D	Complete traumatic trnsphal amputation of r idx fngr, subs
		S68.611D	Complete traumatic trnsphal amputation of l idx fngr, subs
		S68.612D	Complete traumatic trnsphal amputation of r mid finger, subs
		S68.613D	Complete traumatic trnsphal amputation of l mid finger, subs
		S68.614D	Complete traumatic trnsphal amputation of r rng fngr, subs
		S68.615D	Complete traumatic trnsphal amputation of l rng fngr, subs
		S68.616D	Complete traumatic trnsphal amp of r little finger, subs
		S68.617D	Complete traumatic trnsphal amp of l little finger, subs
		S68.618D	Complete traumatic trnsphal amputation of finger, subs
		S68.619D	Complete traumatic trnsphal amputation of unsp finger, subs
		S68.620D	Partial traumatic trnsphal amputation of r idx fngr, subs
		S68.621D	Partial traumatic trnsphal amputation of l idx fngr, subs
		S68.622D	Partial traumatic trnsphal amputation of r mid finger, subs
		S68.623D	Partial traumatic trnsphal amputation of l mid finger, subs
		S68.624D	Partial traumatic trnsphal amputation of r rng fngr, subs
		S68.625D	Partial traumatic trnsphal amputation of l rng fngr, subs
		S68.626D	Partial traumatic trnsphal amp of r little finger, subs
		S68.627D	Partial traumatic trnsphal amp of l little finger, subs
		S68.628D	Partial traumatic transphalangeal amputation of finger, subs
		S68.629D	Partial traumatic trnsphal amputation of unsp finger, subs
		S68.711D	Complete traumatic transmetcrpl amp of right hand, subs
		S68.712D	Complete traumatic transmetcrpl amp of left hand, subs
		S68.719D	Complete traumatic transmetcrpl amp of unsp hand, subs
		S68.721D	Partial traumatic transmetcrpl amp of right hand, subs
		S68.722D	Partial traumatic transmetcrpl amputation of left hand, subs
		S68.729D	Partial traumatic transmetcrpl amputation of unsp hand, subs
		S69.80XD	Oth injuries of unsp wrist, hand and finger(s), subs encntr
		S69.81XD	Oth injuries of right wrist, hand and finger(s), subs encntr
		S69.82XD	Oth injuries of left wrist, hand and finger(s), subs encntr
		S69.90XD	Unsp injury of unsp wrist, hand and finger(s), subs encntr
		S69.91XD	Unsp injury of right wrist, hand and finger(s), subs encntr
		S69.92XD	Unsp injury of left wrist, hand and finger(s), subs encntr
		S70.00XD	Contusion of unspecified hip, subsequent encounter
		S70.01XD	Contusion of right hip, subsequent encounter
		S70.02XD	Contusion of left hip, subsequent encounter
		S70.10XD	Contusion of unspecified thigh, subsequent encounter
		S70.11XD	Contusion of right thigh, subsequent encounter
		S70.12XD	Contusion of left thigh, subsequent encounter
		S70.211D	Abrasion, right hip, subsequent encounter
		S70.212D	Abrasion, left hip, subsequent encounter
		S70.219D	Abrasion, unspecified hip, subsequent encounter
		S70.221D	Blister (nonthermal), right hip, subsequent encounter
		S70.222D	Blister (nonthermal), left hip, subsequent encounter
		S70.229D	Blister (nonthermal), unspecified hip, subsequent encounter
		S70.241D	External constriction, right hip, subsequent encounter
		S70.242D	External constriction, left hip, subsequent encounter
		S70.249D	External constriction, unspecified hip, subsequent encounter
		S70.251D	Superficial foreign body, right hip, subsequent encounter
		S70.252D	Superficial foreign body, left hip, subsequent encounter
		S70.259D	Superficial foreign body, unspecified hip, subs encntr
		S70.261D	Insect bite (nonvenomous), right hip, subsequent encounter
		S70.262D	Insect bite (nonvenomous), left hip, subsequent encounter
		S70.269D	Insect bite (nonvenomous), unspecified hip, subs encntr
		S70.271D	Other superficial bite of hip, right hip, subs encntr
		S70.272D	Other superficial bite of hip, left hip, subs encntr
		S70.279D	Other superficial bite of hip, unspecified hip, subs encntr
		S70.311D	Abrasion, right thigh, subsequent encounter
		S70.312D	Abrasion, left thigh, subsequent encounter
		S70.319D	Abrasion, unspecified thigh, subsequent encounter
		S70.321D	Blister (nonthermal), right thigh, subsequent encounter
		S70.322D	Blister (nonthermal), left thigh, subsequent encounter
		S70.329D	Blister (nonthermal), unspecified thigh, subs encntr
		S70.341D	External constriction, right thigh, subsequent encounter
		S70.342D	External constriction, left thigh, subsequent encounter
		S70.349D	External constriction, unspecified thigh, subs encntr
		S70.351D	Superficial foreign body, right thigh, subsequent encounter
		S70.352D	Superficial foreign body, left thigh, subsequent encounter
		S70.359D	Superficial foreign body, unspecified thigh, subs encntr
		S70.361D	Insect bite (nonvenomous), right thigh, subsequent encounter
		S70.362D	Insect bite (nonvenomous), left thigh, subsequent encounter
		S70.369D	Insect bite (nonvenomous), unspecified thigh, subs encntr
		S70.371D	Other superficial bite of right thigh, subsequent encounter
		S70.372D	Other superficial bite of left thigh, subsequent encounter
		S70.379D	Other superficial bite of unspecified thigh, subs encntr
		S70.911D	Unspecified superficial injury of right hip, subs encntr
		S70.912D	Unspecified superficial injury of left hip, subs encntr
		S70.919D	Unsp superficial injury of unspecified hip, subs encntr
		S70.921D	Unspecified superficial injury of right thigh, subs encntr
		S70.922D	Unspecified superficial injury of left thigh, subs encntr
	(Continued on next page)	**S70.929D**	Unsp superficial injury of unspecified thigh, subs encntr

ICD-9-CM		ICD-10-CM	
V58.89	ENCOUNTER FOR OTHER SPECIFIED AFTERCARE **(Continued)**	**S71.ØØ1D**	Unspecified open wound, right hip, subsequent encounter
		S71.ØØ2D	Unspecified open wound, left hip, subsequent encounter
		S71.ØØ9D	Unspecified open wound, unspecified hip, subs encntr
		S71.Ø11D	Laceration without foreign body, right hip, subs encntr
		S71.Ø12D	Laceration without foreign body, left hip, subs encntr
		S71.Ø19D	Laceration without foreign body, unsp hip, subs encntr
		S71.Ø21D	Laceration with foreign body, right hip, subs encntr
		S71.Ø22D	Laceration with foreign body, left hip, subsequent encounter
		S71.Ø29D	Laceration with foreign body, unspecified hip, subs encntr
		S71.Ø31D	Puncture wound without foreign body, right hip, subs encntr
		S71.Ø32D	Puncture wound without foreign body, left hip, subs encntr
		S71.Ø39D	Puncture wound without foreign body, unsp hip, subs encntr
		S71.Ø41D	Puncture wound with foreign body, right hip, subs encntr
		S71.Ø42D	Puncture wound with foreign body, left hip, subs encntr
		S71.Ø49D	Puncture wound with foreign body, unsp hip, subs encntr
		S71.Ø51D	Open bite, right hip, subsequent encounter
		S71.Ø52D	Open bite, left hip, subsequent encounter
		S71.Ø59D	Open bite, unspecified hip, subsequent encounter
		S71.1Ø1D	Unspecified open wound, right thigh, subsequent encounter
		S71.1Ø2D	Unspecified open wound, left thigh, subsequent encounter
		S71.1Ø9D	Unspecified open wound, unspecified thigh, subs encntr
		S71.111D	Laceration without foreign body, right thigh, subs encntr
		S71.112D	Laceration without foreign body, left thigh, subs encntr
		S71.119D	Laceration without foreign body, unsp thigh, subs encntr
		S71.121D	Laceration with foreign body, right thigh, subs encntr
		S71.122D	Laceration with foreign body, left thigh, subs encntr
		S71.129D	Laceration with foreign body, unspecified thigh, subs encntr
		S71.131D	Puncture wound w/o foreign body, right thigh, subs encntr
		S71.132D	Puncture wound without foreign body, left thigh, subs encntr
		S71.139D	Puncture wound without foreign body, unsp thigh, subs encntr
		S71.141D	Puncture wound with foreign body, right thigh, subs encntr
		S71.142D	Puncture wound with foreign body, left thigh, subs encntr
		S71.149D	Puncture wound with foreign body, unsp thigh, subs encntr
		S71.151D	Open bite, right thigh, subsequent encounter
		S71.152D	Open bite, left thigh, subsequent encounter
		S71.159D	Open bite, unspecified thigh, subsequent encounter
		S73.ØØ1D	Unspecified subluxation of right hip, subsequent encounter
		S73.ØØ2D	Unspecified subluxation of left hip, subsequent encounter
		S73.ØØ3D	Unspecified subluxation of unspecified hip, subs encntr
		S73.ØØ4D	Unspecified dislocation of right hip, subsequent encounter
		S73.ØØ5D	Unspecified dislocation of left hip, subsequent encounter
		S73.ØØ6D	Unspecified dislocation of unspecified hip, subs encntr
		S73.Ø11D	Posterior subluxation of right hip, subsequent encounter
		S73.Ø12D	Posterior subluxation of left hip, subsequent encounter
		S73.Ø13D	Posterior subluxation of unspecified hip, subs encntr
		S73.Ø14D	Posterior dislocation of right hip, subsequent encounter
		S73.Ø15D	Posterior dislocation of left hip, subsequent encounter
		S73.Ø16D	Posterior dislocation of unspecified hip, subs encntr
		S73.Ø21D	Obturator subluxation of right hip, subsequent encounter
		S73.Ø22D	Obturator subluxation of left hip, subsequent encounter
		S73.Ø23D	Obturator subluxation of unspecified hip, subs encntr
		S73.Ø24D	Obturator dislocation of right hip, subsequent encounter
		S73.Ø25D	Obturator dislocation of left hip, subsequent encounter
		S73.Ø26D	Obturator dislocation of unspecified hip, subs encntr
		S73.Ø31D	Other anterior subluxation of right hip, subs encntr
		S73.Ø32D	Other anterior subluxation of left hip, subsequent encounter
		S73.Ø33D	Other anterior subluxation of unspecified hip, subs encntr
		S73.Ø34D	Other anterior dislocation of right hip, subs encntr
		S73.Ø35D	Other anterior dislocation of left hip, subsequent encounter
		S73.Ø36D	Other anterior dislocation of unspecified hip, subs encntr
		S73.Ø41D	Central subluxation of right hip, subsequent encounter
		S73.Ø42D	Central subluxation of left hip, subsequent encounter
		S73.Ø43D	Central subluxation of unspecified hip, subsequent encounter
		S73.Ø44D	Central dislocation of right hip, subsequent encounter
		S73.Ø45D	Central dislocation of left hip, subsequent encounter
		S73.Ø46D	Central dislocation of unspecified hip, subsequent encounter
		S73.1Ø1D	Unspecified sprain of right hip, subsequent encounter
		S73.1Ø2D	Unspecified sprain of left hip, subsequent encounter
		S73.1Ø9D	Unspecified sprain of unspecified hip, subsequent encounter
		S73.111D	Iliofemoral ligament sprain of right hip, subs encntr
		S73.112D	Iliofemoral ligament sprain of left hip, subs encntr
		S73.119D	Iliofemoral ligament sprain of unspecified hip, subs encntr
		S73.121D	Ischiocapsular ligament sprain of right hip, subs encntr
		S73.122D	Ischiocapsular ligament sprain of left hip, subs encntr
		S73.129D	Ischiocapsular ligament sprain of unsp hip, subs encntr
		S73.191D	Other sprain of right hip, subsequent encounter
		S73.192D	Other sprain of left hip, subsequent encounter
		S73.199D	Other sprain of unspecified hip, subsequent encounter
		S74.ØØXD	Injury of sciatic nrv at hip and thigh level, unsp leg, subs
		S74.Ø1XD	Injury of sciatic nrv at hip and thi lev, right leg, subs
		S74.Ø2XD	Injury of sciatic nrv at hip and thigh level, left leg, subs
		S74.1ØXD	Injury of femoral nrv at hip and thigh level, unsp leg, subs
	(Continued on next page)	**S74.11XD**	Injury of femoral nrv at hip and thi lev, right leg, subs

ICD-9-CM		ICD-10-CM	
V58.89	ENCOUNTER FOR OTHER SPECIFIED AFTERCARE **(Continued)**	**S74.12XD**	Injury of femoral nrv at hip and thigh level, left leg, subs
		S74.20XD	Inj cutan sensory nerve at hip and thi lev, unsp leg, subs
		S74.21XD	Inj cutan sens nerve at hip and high level, right leg, subs
		S74.22XD	Inj cutan sensory nerve at hip and thi lev, left leg, subs
		S74.8X1D	Injury of oth nerves at hip and thigh level, right leg, subs
		S74.8X2D	Injury of oth nerves at hip and thigh level, left leg, subs
		S74.8X9D	Injury of oth nerves at hip and thigh level, unsp leg, subs
		S74.90XD	Injury of unsp nerve at hip and thigh level, unsp leg, subs
		S74.91XD	Injury of unsp nerve at hip and thigh level, right leg, subs
		S74.92XD	Injury of unsp nerve at hip and thigh level, left leg, subs
		S75.001D	Unspecified injury of femoral artery, right leg, subs encntr
		S75.002D	Unspecified injury of femoral artery, left leg, subs encntr
		S75.009D	Unsp injury of femoral artery, unspecified leg, subs encntr
		S75.011D	Minor laceration of femoral artery, right leg, subs encntr
		S75.012D	Minor laceration of femoral artery, left leg, subs encntr
		S75.019D	Minor laceration of femoral artery, unsp leg, subs encntr
		S75.021D	Major laceration of femoral artery, right leg, subs encntr
		S75.022D	Major laceration of femoral artery, left leg, subs encntr
		S75.029D	Major laceration of femoral artery, unsp leg, subs encntr
		S75.091D	Oth injury of femoral artery, right leg, subs encntr
		S75.092D	Oth injury of femoral artery, left leg, subs encntr
		S75.099D	Oth injury of femoral artery, unspecified leg, subs encntr
		S75.101D	Unsp inj femor vein at hip and thi lev, right leg, subs
		S75.102D	Unsp injury of femor vein at hip and thi lev, left leg, subs
		S75.109D	Unsp injury of femor vein at hip and thi lev, unsp leg, subs
		S75.111D	Minor lacerat femor vein at hip and thi lev, right leg, subs
		S75.112D	Minor lacerat femor vein at hip and thi lev, left leg, subs
		S75.119D	Minor lacerat femor vein at hip and thi lev, unsp leg, subs
		S75.121D	Major lacerat femor vein at hip and thi lev, right leg, subs
		S75.122D	Major lacerat femor vein at hip and thi lev, left leg, subs
		S75.129D	Major lacerat femor vein at hip and thi lev, unsp leg, subs
		S75.191D	Inj femoral vein at hip and thigh level, right leg, subs
		S75.192D	Inj femoral vein at hip and thigh level, left leg, subs
		S75.199D	Inj femoral vein at hip and thigh level, unsp leg, subs
		S75.201D	Unsp inj great saphenous at hip and thi lev, right leg, subs
		S75.202D	Unsp inj great saphenous at hip and thi lev, left leg, subs
		S75.209D	Unsp inj great saphenous at hip and thi lev, unsp leg, subs
		S75.211D	Minor lacerat great saph at hip and thi lev, right leg, subs
		S75.212D	Minor lacerat great saph at hip and thi lev, left leg, subs
		S75.219D	Minor lacerat great saph at hip and thi lev, unsp leg, subs
		S75.221D	Major lacerat great saph at hip and thi lev, right leg, subs
		S75.222D	Major lacerat great saph at hip and thi lev, left leg, subs
		S75.229D	Major lacerat great saph at hip and thi lev, unsp leg, subs
		S75.291D	Inj great saphenous at hip and thigh level, right leg, subs
		S75.292D	Inj great saphenous at hip and thigh level, left leg, subs
		S75.299D	Inj great saphenous at hip and thigh level, unsp leg, subs
		S75.801D	Unsp inj blood vessels at hip and thi lev, right leg, subs
		S75.802D	Unsp inj blood vessels at hip and thi lev, left leg, subs
		S75.809D	Unsp inj blood vessels at hip and thi lev, unsp leg, subs
		S75.811D	Lacerat blood vessels at hip and thi lev, right leg, subs
		S75.812D	Lacerat blood vessels at hip and thigh level, left leg, subs
		S75.819D	Lacerat blood vessels at hip and thigh level, unsp leg, subs
		S75.891D	Inj oth blood vessels at hip and thi lev, right leg, subs
		S75.892D	Inj oth blood vessels at hip and thigh level, left leg, subs
		S75.899D	Inj oth blood vessels at hip and thigh level, unsp leg, subs
		S75.901D	Unsp inj unsp blood vess at hip and thi lev, right leg, subs
		S75.902D	Unsp inj unsp blood vess at hip and thi lev, left leg, subs
		S75.909D	Unsp inj unsp blood vess at hip and thi lev, unsp leg, subs
		S75.911D	Lacerat unsp blood vess at hip and thi lev, right leg, subs
		S75.912D	Lacerat unsp blood vess at hip and thi lev, left leg, subs
		S75.919D	Lacerat unsp blood vess at hip and thi lev, unsp leg, subs
		S75.991D	Inj unsp blood vess at hip and thigh level, right leg, subs
		S75.992D	Inj unsp blood vessel at hip and thigh level, left leg, subs
		S75.999D	Inj unsp blood vessel at hip and thigh level, unsp leg, subs
		S76.001D	Unsp injury of muscle, fascia and tendon of right hip, subs
		S76.002D	Unsp injury of muscle, fascia and tendon of left hip, subs
		S76.009D	Unsp injury of muscle, fascia and tendon of unsp hip, subs
		S76.011D	Strain of muscle, fascia and tendon of right hip, subs
		S76.012D	Strain of muscle, fascia and tendon of left hip, subs encntr
		S76.019D	Strain of muscle, fascia and tendon of unsp hip, subs encntr
		S76.021D	Laceration of muscle, fascia and tendon of right hip, subs
		S76.022D	Laceration of muscle, fascia and tendon of left hip, subs
		S76.029D	Laceration of muscle, fascia and tendon of unsp hip, subs
		S76.091D	Inj muscle, fascia and tendon of right hip, subs encntr
		S76.092D	Inj muscle, fascia and tendon of left hip, subs encntr
		S76.099D	Inj muscle, fascia and tendon of unsp hip, subs encntr
		S76.101D	Unsp injury of right quadriceps musc/fasc/tend, subs
		S76.102D	Unsp injury of left quadriceps musc/fasc/tend, subs
		S76.109D	Unsp injury of unsp quadriceps musc/fasc/tend, subs
		S76.111D	Strain of right quadriceps muscle, fascia and tendon, subs
		S76.112D	Strain of left quadriceps muscle, fascia and tendon, subs
		S76.119D	Strain of unsp quadriceps muscle, fascia and tendon, subs
	(Continued on next page)	**S76.121D**	Laceration of right quadriceps musc/fasc/tend, subs

ICD-9-CM		ICD-10-CM	
V58.89	ENCOUNTER FOR OTHER SPECIFIED AFTERCARE **(Continued)**	**S76.122D**	Laceration of left quadriceps musc/fasc/tend, subs
		S76.129D	Laceration of unsp quadriceps musc/fasc/tend, subs
		S76.191D	Inj right quadriceps muscle, fascia and tendon, subs encntr
		S76.192D	Inj left quadriceps muscle, fascia and tendon, subs encntr
		S76.199D	Inj unsp quadriceps muscle, fascia and tendon, subs encntr
		S76.2Ø1D	Unsp injury of adductor musc/fasc/tend right thigh, subs
		S76.2Ø2D	Unsp injury of adductor musc/fasc/tend left thigh, subs
		S76.2Ø9D	Unsp injury of adductor musc/fasc/tend unsp thigh, subs
		S76.211D	Strain of adductor musc/fasc/tend right thigh, subs
		S76.212D	Strain of adductor musc/fasc/tend left thigh, subs
		S76.219D	Strain of adductor musc/fasc/tend unsp thigh, subs
		S76.221D	Laceration of adductor musc/fasc/tend right thigh, subs
		S76.222D	Laceration of adductor musc/fasc/tend left thigh, subs
		S76.229D	Laceration of adductor musc/fasc/tend unsp thigh, subs
		S76.291D	Inj adductor muscle, fascia and tendon of right thigh, subs
		S76.292D	Inj adductor muscle, fascia and tendon of left thigh, subs
		S76.299D	Inj adductor muscle, fascia and tendon of unsp thigh, subs
		S76.3Ø1D	Unsp inj msl/fasc/tnd post grp at thi lev, right thigh, subs
		S76.3Ø2D	Unsp inj msl/fasc/tnd post grp at thi lev, left thigh, subs
		S76.3Ø9D	Unsp inj msl/fasc/tnd post grp at thi lev, unsp thigh, subs
		S76.311D	Strain msl/fasc/tnd post grp at thi lev, right thigh, subs
		S76.312D	Strain of msl/fasc/tnd post grp at thi lev, left thigh, subs
		S76.319D	Strain of msl/fasc/tnd post grp at thi lev, unsp thigh, subs
		S76.321D	Lacerat msl/fasc/tnd post grp at thi lev, right thigh, subs
		S76.322D	Lacerat msl/fasc/tnd post grp at thi lev, left thigh, subs
		S76.329D	Lacerat msl/fasc/tnd post grp at thi lev, unsp thigh, subs
		S76.391D	Inj msl/fasc/tnd posterior grp at thi lev, right thigh, subs
		S76.392D	Inj msl/fasc/tnd posterior grp at thi lev, left thigh, subs
		S76.399D	Inj msl/fasc/tnd posterior grp at thi lev, unsp thigh, subs
		S76.8Ø1D	Unsp injury of musc/fasc/tend at thi lev, right thigh, subs
		S76.8Ø2D	Unsp injury of musc/fasc/tend at thi lev, left thigh, subs
		S76.8Ø9D	Unsp injury of musc/fasc/tend at thi lev, unsp thigh, subs
		S76.811D	Strain of musc/fasc/tend at thigh level, right thigh, subs
		S76.812D	Strain of musc/fasc/tend at thigh level, left thigh, subs
		S76.819D	Strain of musc/fasc/tend at thigh level, unsp thigh, subs
		S76.821D	Lacerat musc/fasc/tend at thigh level, right thigh, subs
		S76.822D	Lacerat musc/fasc/tend at thigh level, left thigh, subs
		S76.829D	Lacerat musc/fasc/tend at thigh level, unsp thigh, subs
		S76.891D	Inj musc/fasc/tend at thigh level, right thigh, subs encntr
		S76.892D	Inj musc/fasc/tend at thigh level, left thigh, subs encntr
		S76.899D	Inj musc/fasc/tend at thigh level, unsp thigh, subs encntr
		S76.9Ø1D	Unsp inj unsp musc/fasc/tend at thi lev, right thigh, subs
		S76.9Ø2D	Unsp inj unsp musc/fasc/tend at thi lev, left thigh, subs
		S76.9Ø9D	Unsp inj unsp musc/fasc/tend at thi lev, unsp thigh, subs
		S76.911D	Strain of unsp musc/fasc/tend at thi lev, right thigh, subs
		S76.912D	Strain of unsp musc/fasc/tend at thi lev, left thigh, subs
		S76.919D	Strain of unsp musc/fasc/tend at thi lev, unsp thigh, subs
		S76.921D	Lacerat unsp musc/fasc/tend at thi lev, right thigh, subs
		S76.922D	Lacerat unsp musc/fasc/tend at thigh level, left thigh, subs
		S76.929D	Lacerat unsp musc/fasc/tend at thigh level, unsp thigh, subs
		S76.991D	Inj unsp musc/fasc/tend at thigh level, right thigh, subs
		S76.992D	Inj unsp musc/fasc/tend at thigh level, left thigh, subs
		S76.999D	Inj unsp musc/fasc/tend at thigh level, unsp thigh, subs
		S77.ØØXD	Crushing injury of unspecified hip, subsequent encounter
		S77.Ø1XD	Crushing injury of right hip, subsequent encounter
		S77.Ø2XD	Crushing injury of left hip, subsequent encounter
		S77.1ØXD	Crushing injury of unspecified thigh, subsequent encounter
		S77.11XD	Crushing injury of right thigh, subsequent encounter
		S77.12XD	Crushing injury of left thigh, subsequent encounter
		S77.2ØXD	Crushing injury of unspecified hip with thigh, subs encntr
		S77.21XD	Crushing injury of right hip with thigh, subs encntr
		S77.22XD	Crushing injury of left hip with thigh, subsequent encounter
		S78.Ø11D	Complete traumatic amputation at right hip joint, subs
		S78.Ø12D	Complete traumatic amputation at left hip joint, subs encntr
		S78.Ø19D	Complete traumatic amputation at unsp hip joint, subs encntr
		S78.Ø21D	Partial traumatic amputation at right hip joint, subs encntr
		S78.Ø22D	Partial traumatic amputation at left hip joint, subs encntr
		S78.Ø29D	Partial traumatic amputation at unsp hip joint, subs encntr
		S78.111D	Complete traumatic amp at level betw r hip and knee, subs
		S78.112D	Complete traumatic amp at level betw left hip and knee, subs
		S78.119D	Complete traumatic amp at level betw unsp hip and knee, subs
		S78.121D	Partial traumatic amp at level betw right hip and knee, subs
		S78.122D	Partial traumatic amp at level betw left hip and knee, subs
		S78.129D	Partial traumatic amp at level betw unsp hip and knee, subs
		S78.911D	Complete traumatic amp of r hip and thigh, level unsp, subs
		S78.912D	Complete traum amp of left hip and thigh, level unsp, subs
		S78.919D	Complete traum amp of unsp hip and thigh, level unsp, subs
		S78.921D	Partial traumatic amp of r hip and thigh, level unsp, subs
		S78.922D	Partial traum amp of left hip and thigh, level unsp, subs
		S78.929D	Partial traum amp of unsp hip and thigh, level unsp, subs
		S79.811D	Other specified injuries of right hip, subsequent encounter
		S79.812D	Other specified injuries of left hip, subsequent encounter
	(Continued on next page)	**S79.819D**	Other specified injuries of unspecified hip, subs encntr

ICD-9-CM		ICD-10-CM	
V58.89	ENCOUNTER FOR OTHER SPECIFIED AFTERCARE **(Continued)**	**S79.821D**	Other specified injuries of right thigh, subs encntr
		S79.822D	Other specified injuries of left thigh, subsequent encounter
		S79.829D	Other specified injuries of unspecified thigh, subs encntr
		S79.911D	Unspecified injury of right hip, subsequent encounter
		S79.912D	Unspecified injury of left hip, subsequent encounter
		S79.919D	Unspecified injury of unspecified hip, subsequent encounter
		S79.921D	Unspecified injury of right thigh, subsequent encounter
		S79.922D	Unspecified injury of left thigh, subsequent encounter
		S79.929D	Unspecified injury of unspecified thigh, subs encntr
		S80.00XD	Contusion of unspecified knee, subsequent encounter
		S80.01XD	Contusion of right knee, subsequent encounter
		S80.02XD	Contusion of left knee, subsequent encounter
		S80.10XD	Contusion of unspecified lower leg, subsequent encounter
		S80.11XD	Contusion of right lower leg, subsequent encounter
		S80.12XD	Contusion of left lower leg, subsequent encounter
		S80.211D	Abrasion, right knee, subsequent encounter
		S80.212D	Abrasion, left knee, subsequent encounter
		S80.219D	Abrasion, unspecified knee, subsequent encounter
		S80.221D	Blister (nonthermal), right knee, subsequent encounter
		S80.222D	Blister (nonthermal), left knee, subsequent encounter
		S80.229D	Blister (nonthermal), unspecified knee, subsequent encounter
		S80.241D	External constriction, right knee, subsequent encounter
		S80.242D	External constriction, left knee, subsequent encounter
		S80.249D	External constriction, unspecified knee, subs encntr
		S80.251D	Superficial foreign body, right knee, subsequent encounter
		S80.252D	Superficial foreign body, left knee, subsequent encounter
		S80.259D	Superficial foreign body, unspecified knee, subs encntr
		S80.261D	Insect bite (nonvenomous), right knee, subsequent encounter
		S80.262D	Insect bite (nonvenomous), left knee, subsequent encounter
		S80.269D	Insect bite (nonvenomous), unspecified knee, subs encntr
		S80.271D	Other superficial bite of right knee, subsequent encounter
		S80.272D	Other superficial bite of left knee, subsequent encounter
		S80.279D	Other superficial bite of unspecified knee, subs encntr
		S80.811D	Abrasion, right lower leg, subsequent encounter
		S80.812D	Abrasion, left lower leg, subsequent encounter
		S80.819D	Abrasion, unspecified lower leg, subsequent encounter
		S80.821D	Blister (nonthermal), right lower leg, subsequent encounter
		S80.822D	Blister (nonthermal), left lower leg, subsequent encounter
		S80.829D	Blister (nonthermal), unspecified lower leg, subs encntr
		S80.841D	External constriction, right lower leg, subsequent encounter
		S80.842D	External constriction, left lower leg, subsequent encounter
		S80.849D	External constriction, unspecified lower leg, subs encntr
		S80.851D	Superficial foreign body, right lower leg, subs encntr
		S80.852D	Superficial foreign body, left lower leg, subs encntr
		S80.859D	Superficial foreign body, unspecified lower leg, subs encntr
		S80.861D	Insect bite (nonvenomous), right lower leg, subs encntr
		S80.862D	Insect bite (nonvenomous), left lower leg, subs encntr
		S80.869D	Insect bite (nonvenomous), unsp lower leg, subs encntr
		S80.871D	Other superficial bite, right lower leg, subs encntr
		S80.872D	Other superficial bite, left lower leg, subsequent encounter
		S80.879D	Other superficial bite, unspecified lower leg, subs encntr
		S80.911D	Unspecified superficial injury of right knee, subs encntr
		S80.912D	Unspecified superficial injury of left knee, subs encntr
		S80.919D	Unsp superficial injury of unspecified knee, subs encntr
		S80.921D	Unsp superficial injury of right lower leg, subs encntr
		S80.922D	Unsp superficial injury of left lower leg, subs encntr
		S80.929D	Unsp superficial injury of unsp lower leg, subs encntr
		S81.001D	Unspecified open wound, right knee, subsequent encounter
		S81.002D	Unspecified open wound, left knee, subsequent encounter
		S81.009D	Unspecified open wound, unspecified knee, subs encntr
		S81.011D	Laceration without foreign body, right knee, subs encntr
		S81.012D	Laceration without foreign body, left knee, subs encntr
		S81.019D	Laceration without foreign body, unsp knee, subs encntr
		S81.021D	Laceration with foreign body, right knee, subs encntr
		S81.022D	Laceration with foreign body, left knee, subs encntr
		S81.029D	Laceration with foreign body, unspecified knee, subs encntr
		S81.031D	Puncture wound without foreign body, right knee, subs encntr
		S81.032D	Puncture wound without foreign body, left knee, subs encntr
		S81.039D	Puncture wound without foreign body, unsp knee, subs encntr
		S81.041D	Puncture wound with foreign body, right knee, subs encntr
		S81.042D	Puncture wound with foreign body, left knee, subs encntr
		S81.049D	Puncture wound with foreign body, unsp knee, subs encntr
		S81.051D	Open bite, right knee, subsequent encounter
		S81.052D	Open bite, left knee, subsequent encounter
		S81.059D	Open bite, unspecified knee, subsequent encounter
		S81.801D	Unspecified open wound, right lower leg, subs encntr
		S81.802D	Unspecified open wound, left lower leg, subsequent encounter
		S81.809D	Unspecified open wound, unspecified lower leg, subs encntr
		S81.811D	Laceration w/o foreign body, right lower leg, subs encntr
		S81.812D	Laceration without foreign body, left lower leg, subs encntr
		S81.819D	Laceration without foreign body, unsp lower leg, subs encntr
		S81.821D	Laceration with foreign body, right lower leg, subs encntr
	(Continued on next page)	**S81.822D**	Laceration with foreign body, left lower leg, subs encntr

ICD-9-CM		ICD-10-CM	
V58.89	ENCOUNTER FOR OTHER SPECIFIED AFTERCARE **(Continued)**	**S81.829D**	Laceration with foreign body, unsp lower leg, subs encntr
		S81.831D	Puncture wound w/o foreign body, right lower leg, subs
		S81.832D	Puncture wound w/o foreign body, left lower leg, subs encntr
		S81.839D	Puncture wound w/o foreign body, unsp lower leg, subs encntr
		S81.841D	Puncture wound w foreign body, right lower leg, subs encntr
		S81.842D	Puncture wound w foreign body, left lower leg, subs encntr
		S81.849D	Puncture wound w foreign body, unsp lower leg, subs encntr
		S81.851D	Open bite, right lower leg, subsequent encounter
		S81.852D	Open bite, left lower leg, subsequent encounter
		S81.859D	Open bite, unspecified lower leg, subsequent encounter
		S83.ØØ1D	Unspecified subluxation of right patella, subs encntr
		S83.ØØ2D	Unspecified subluxation of left patella, subs encntr
		S83.ØØ3D	Unspecified subluxation of unspecified patella, subs encntr
		S83.ØØ4D	Unspecified dislocation of right patella, subs encntr
		S83.ØØ5D	Unspecified dislocation of left patella, subs encntr
		S83.ØØ6D	Unspecified dislocation of unspecified patella, subs encntr
		S83.Ø11D	Lateral subluxation of right patella, subsequent encounter
		S83.Ø12D	Lateral subluxation of left patella, subsequent encounter
		S83.Ø13D	Lateral subluxation of unspecified patella, subs encntr
		S83.Ø14D	Lateral dislocation of right patella, subsequent encounter
		S83.Ø15D	Lateral dislocation of left patella, subsequent encounter
		S83.Ø16D	Lateral dislocation of unspecified patella, subs encntr
		S83.Ø91D	Other subluxation of right patella, subsequent encounter
		S83.Ø92D	Other subluxation of left patella, subsequent encounter
		S83.Ø93D	Other subluxation of unspecified patella, subs encntr
		S83.Ø94D	Other dislocation of right patella, subsequent encounter
		S83.Ø95D	Other dislocation of left patella, subsequent encounter
		S83.Ø96D	Other dislocation of unspecified patella, subs encntr
		S83.1Ø1D	Unspecified subluxation of right knee, subsequent encounter
		S83.1Ø2D	Unspecified subluxation of left knee, subsequent encounter
		S83.1Ø3D	Unspecified subluxation of unspecified knee, subs encntr
		S83.1Ø4D	Unspecified dislocation of right knee, subsequent encounter
		S83.1Ø5D	Unspecified dislocation of left knee, subsequent encounter
		S83.1Ø6D	Unspecified dislocation of unspecified knee, subs encntr
		S83.111D	Anterior sublux of proximal end of tibia, right knee, subs
		S83.112D	Anterior sublux of proximal end of tibia, left knee, subs
		S83.113D	Anterior sublux of proximal end of tibia, unsp knee, subs
		S83.114D	Anterior disloc of proximal end of tibia, right knee, subs
		S83.115D	Anterior disloc of proximal end of tibia, left knee, subs
		S83.116D	Anterior disloc of proximal end of tibia, unsp knee, subs
		S83.121D	Posterior sublux of proximal end of tibia, right knee, subs
		S83.122D	Posterior sublux of proximal end of tibia, left knee, subs
		S83.123D	Posterior sublux of proximal end of tibia, unsp knee, subs
		S83.124D	Posterior disloc of proximal end of tibia, right knee, subs
		S83.125D	Posterior disloc of proximal end of tibia, left knee, subs
		S83.126D	Posterior disloc of proximal end of tibia, unsp knee, subs
		S83.131D	Medial sublux of proximal end of tibia, right knee, subs
		S83.132D	Medial subluxation of proximal end of tibia, left knee, subs
		S83.133D	Medial subluxation of proximal end of tibia, unsp knee, subs
		S83.134D	Medial disloc of proximal end of tibia, right knee, subs
		S83.135D	Medial dislocation of proximal end of tibia, left knee, subs
		S83.136D	Medial dislocation of proximal end of tibia, unsp knee, subs
		S83.141D	Lateral sublux of proximal end of tibia, right knee, subs
		S83.142D	Lateral sublux of proximal end of tibia, left knee, subs
		S83.143D	Lateral sublux of proximal end of tibia, unsp knee, subs
		S83.144D	Lateral disloc of proximal end of tibia, right knee, subs
		S83.145D	Lateral disloc of proximal end of tibia, left knee, subs
		S83.146D	Lateral disloc of proximal end of tibia, unsp knee, subs
		S83.191D	Other subluxation of right knee, subsequent encounter
		S83.192D	Other subluxation of left knee, subsequent encounter
		S83.193D	Other subluxation of unspecified knee, subsequent encounter
		S83.194D	Other dislocation of right knee, subsequent encounter
		S83.195D	Other dislocation of left knee, subsequent encounter
		S83.196D	Other dislocation of unspecified knee, subsequent encounter
		S83.2ØØD	Bucket-hndl tear of unsp mensc, current injury, r knee, subs
		S83.2Ø1D	Bucket-hndl tear of unsp mensc, current injury, l knee, subs
		S83.2Ø2D	Bucket-hndl tear of unsp mensc, crnt injury, unsp knee, subs
		S83.2Ø3D	Oth tear of unsp meniscus, current injury, right knee, subs
		S83.2Ø4D	Oth tear of unsp meniscus, current injury, left knee, subs
		S83.2Ø5D	Oth tear of unsp meniscus, current injury, unsp knee, subs
		S83.2Ø6D	Unsp tear of unsp meniscus, current injury, right knee, subs
		S83.2Ø7D	Unsp tear of unsp meniscus, current injury, left knee, subs
		S83.2Ø9D	Unsp tear of unsp meniscus, current injury, unsp knee, subs
		S83.211D	Bucket-hndl tear of medial mensc, crnt injury, r knee, subs
		S83.212D	Bucket-hndl tear of medial mensc, crnt injury, l knee, subs
		S83.219D	Bucket-hndl tear of medial mensc, crnt inj, unsp knee, subs
		S83.221D	Prph tear of medial meniscus, current injury, r knee, subs
		S83.222D	Prph tear of medial meniscus, current injury, l knee, subs
		S83.229D	Prph tear of medial mensc, current injury, unsp knee, subs
		S83.231D	Complex tear of medial mensc, current injury, r knee, subs
		S83.232D	Complex tear of medial mensc, current injury, l knee, subs
		S83.239D	Cmplx tear of medial mensc, current injury, unsp knee, subs
	(Continued on next page)	**S83.241D**	Oth tear of medial meniscus, current injury, r knee, subs

ICD-9-CM		ICD-10-CM	
V58.89	ENCOUNTER FOR OTHER SPECIFIED AFTERCARE **(Continued)**	**S83.242D**	Oth tear of medial meniscus, current injury, left knee, subs
		S83.249D	Oth tear of medial meniscus, current injury, unsp knee, subs
		S83.251D	Bucket-hndl tear of lat mensc, current injury, r knee, subs
		S83.252D	Bucket-hndl tear of lat mensc, current injury, l knee, subs
		S83.259D	Bucket-hndl tear of lat mensc, crnt injury, unsp knee, subs
		S83.261D	Prph tear of lat mensc, current injury, right knee, subs
		S83.262D	Prph tear of lat mensc, current injury, left knee, subs
		S83.269D	Prph tear of lat mensc, current injury, unsp knee, subs
		S83.271D	Complex tear of lat mensc, current injury, right knee, subs
		S83.272D	Complex tear of lat mensc, current injury, left knee, subs
		S83.279D	Complex tear of lat mensc, current injury, unsp knee, subs
		S83.281D	Oth tear of lat mensc, current injury, right knee, subs
		S83.282D	Oth tear of lat mensc, current injury, left knee, subs
		S83.289D	Oth tear of lat mensc, current injury, unsp knee, subs
		S83.30XD	Tear of articular cartilage of unsp knee, current, subs
		S83.31XD	Tear of articular cartilage of right knee, current, subs
		S83.32XD	Tear of articular cartilage of left knee, current, subs
		S83.401D	Sprain of unsp collateral ligament of right knee, subs
		S83.402D	Sprain of unsp collateral ligament of left knee, subs encntr
		S83.409D	Sprain of unsp collateral ligament of unsp knee, subs encntr
		S83.411D	Sprain of medial collateral ligament of right knee, subs
		S83.412D	Sprain of medial collateral ligament of left knee, subs
		S83.419D	Sprain of medial collateral ligament of unsp knee, subs
		S83.421D	Sprain of lateral collateral ligament of right knee, subs
		S83.422D	Sprain of lateral collateral ligament of left knee, subs
		S83.429D	Sprain of lateral collateral ligament of unsp knee, subs
		S83.501D	Sprain of unsp cruciate ligament of right knee, subs encntr
		S83.502D	Sprain of unsp cruciate ligament of left knee, subs encntr
		S83.509D	Sprain of unsp cruciate ligament of unsp knee, subs encntr
		S83.511D	Sprain of anterior cruciate ligament of right knee, subs
		S83.512D	Sprain of anterior cruciate ligament of left knee, subs
		S83.519D	Sprain of anterior cruciate ligament of unsp knee, subs
		S83.521D	Sprain of posterior cruciate ligament of right knee, subs
		S83.522D	Sprain of posterior cruciate ligament of left knee, subs
		S83.529D	Sprain of posterior cruciate ligament of unsp knee, subs
		S83.60XD	Sprain of super tibiofibul joint and ligmt, unsp knee, subs
		S83.61XD	Sprain of the super tibiofibul joint and ligmt, r knee, subs
		S83.62XD	Sprain of the super tibiofibul joint and ligmt, l knee, subs
		S83.8X1D	Sprain of other specified parts of right knee, subs encntr
		S83.8X2D	Sprain of other specified parts of left knee, subs encntr
		S83.8X9D	Sprain of oth parts of unspecified knee, subs encntr
		S83.90XD	Sprain of unspecified site of unspecified knee, subs encntr
		S83.91XD	Sprain of unspecified site of right knee, subs encntr
		S83.92XD	Sprain of unspecified site of left knee, subs encntr
		S84.00XD	Injury of tibial nerve at lower leg level, unsp leg, subs
		S84.01XD	Injury of tibial nerve at lower leg level, right leg, subs
		S84.02XD	Injury of tibial nerve at lower leg level, left leg, subs
		S84.10XD	Injury of peroneal nerve at lower leg level, unsp leg, subs
		S84.11XD	Injury of peroneal nerve at lower leg level, right leg, subs
		S84.12XD	Injury of peroneal nerve at lower leg level, left leg, subs
		S84.20XD	Inj cutan sensory nerve at lower leg level, unsp leg, subs
		S84.21XD	Inj cutan sensory nerve at lower leg level, right leg, subs
		S84.22XD	Inj cutan sensory nerve at lower leg level, left leg, subs
		S84.801D	Injury of oth nerves at lower leg level, right leg, subs
		S84.802D	Injury of oth nerves at lower leg level, left leg, subs
		S84.809D	Injury of oth nerves at lower leg level, unsp leg, subs
		S84.90XD	Injury of unsp nerve at lower leg level, unsp leg, subs
		S84.91XD	Injury of unsp nerve at lower leg level, right leg, subs
		S84.92XD	Injury of unsp nerve at lower leg level, left leg, subs
		S85.001D	Unsp injury of popliteal artery, right leg, subs encntr
		S85.002D	Unsp injury of popliteal artery, left leg, subs encntr
		S85.009D	Unsp injury of popliteal artery, unsp leg, subs encntr
		S85.011D	Laceration of popliteal artery, right leg, subs encntr
		S85.012D	Laceration of popliteal artery, left leg, subs encntr
		S85.019D	Laceration of popliteal artery, unspecified leg, subs encntr
		S85.091D	Oth injury of popliteal artery, right leg, subs encntr
		S85.092D	Oth injury of popliteal artery, left leg, subs encntr
		S85.099D	Oth injury of popliteal artery, unspecified leg, subs encntr
		S85.101D	Unsp injury of unsp tibial artery, right leg, subs encntr
		S85.102D	Unsp injury of unsp tibial artery, left leg, subs encntr
		S85.109D	Unsp injury of unsp tibial artery, unsp leg, subs encntr
		S85.111D	Laceration of unsp tibial artery, right leg, subs encntr
		S85.112D	Laceration of unsp tibial artery, left leg, subs encntr
		S85.119D	Laceration of unsp tibial artery, unsp leg, subs encntr
		S85.121D	Oth injury of unsp tibial artery, right leg, subs encntr
		S85.122D	Oth injury of unsp tibial artery, left leg, subs encntr
		S85.129D	Oth injury of unsp tibial artery, unsp leg, subs encntr
		S85.131D	Unsp injury of anterior tibial artery, right leg, subs
		S85.132D	Unsp injury of anterior tibial artery, left leg, subs encntr
		S85.139D	Unsp injury of anterior tibial artery, unsp leg, subs encntr
		S85.141D	Laceration of anterior tibial artery, right leg, subs encntr
		S85.142D	Laceration of anterior tibial artery, left leg, subs encntr
	(Continued on next page)	**S85.149D**	Laceration of anterior tibial artery, unsp leg, subs encntr

V58.89–V58.89

ICD-9-CM		ICD-10-CM	
V58.89	ENCOUNTER FOR OTHER SPECIFIED AFTERCARE **(Continued)**	**S85.151D**	Oth injury of anterior tibial artery, right leg, subs encntr
		S85.152D	Oth injury of anterior tibial artery, left leg, subs encntr
		S85.159D	Oth injury of anterior tibial artery, unsp leg, subs encntr
		S85.161D	Unsp injury of posterior tibial artery, right leg, subs
		S85.162D	Unsp injury of posterior tibial artery, left leg, subs
		S85.169D	Unsp injury of posterior tibial artery, unsp leg, subs
		S85.171D	Laceration of posterior tibial artery, right leg, subs
		S85.172D	Laceration of posterior tibial artery, left leg, subs encntr
		S85.179D	Laceration of posterior tibial artery, unsp leg, subs encntr
		S85.181D	Inj posterior tibial artery, right leg, subs encntr
		S85.182D	Oth injury of posterior tibial artery, left leg, subs encntr
		S85.189D	Oth injury of posterior tibial artery, unsp leg, subs encntr
		S85.201D	Unsp injury of peroneal artery, right leg, subs encntr
		S85.202D	Unspecified injury of peroneal artery, left leg, subs encntr
		S85.209D	Unsp injury of peroneal artery, unspecified leg, subs encntr
		S85.211D	Laceration of peroneal artery, right leg, subs encntr
		S85.212D	Laceration of peroneal artery, left leg, subs encntr
		S85.219D	Laceration of peroneal artery, unspecified leg, subs encntr
		S85.291D	Oth injury of peroneal artery, right leg, subs encntr
		S85.292D	Oth injury of peroneal artery, left leg, subs encntr
		S85.299D	Oth injury of peroneal artery, unspecified leg, subs encntr
		S85.301D	Unsp inj great saphenous at lower leg level, right leg, subs
		S85.302D	Unsp inj great saphenous at lower leg level, left leg, subs
		S85.309D	Unsp inj great saphenous at lower leg level, unsp leg, subs
		S85.311D	Lacerat great saphenous at lower leg level, right leg, subs
		S85.312D	Lacerat great saphenous at lower leg level, left leg, subs
		S85.319D	Lacerat great saphenous at lower leg level, unsp leg, subs
		S85.391D	Inj great saphenous at lower leg level, right leg, subs
		S85.392D	Inj great saphenous at lower leg level, left leg, subs
		S85.399D	Inj great saphenous at lower leg level, unsp leg, subs
		S85.401D	Unsp inj less saphenous at lower leg level, right leg, subs
		S85.402D	Unsp inj less saphenous at lower leg level, left leg, subs
		S85.409D	Unsp inj less saphenous at lower leg level, unsp leg, subs
		S85.411D	Lacerat less saphenous at lower leg level, right leg, subs
		S85.412D	Lacerat less saphenous at lower leg level, left leg, subs
		S85.419D	Lacerat less saphenous at lower leg level, unsp leg, subs
		S85.491D	Inj less saphenous at lower leg level, right leg, subs
		S85.492D	Inj lesser saphenous vein at lower leg level, left leg, subs
		S85.499D	Inj lesser saphenous vein at lower leg level, unsp leg, subs
		S85.501D	Unspecified injury of popliteal vein, right leg, subs encntr
		S85.502D	Unspecified injury of popliteal vein, left leg, subs encntr
		S85.509D	Unsp injury of popliteal vein, unspecified leg, subs encntr
		S85.511D	Laceration of popliteal vein, right leg, subs encntr
		S85.512D	Laceration of popliteal vein, left leg, subsequent encounter
		S85.519D	Laceration of popliteal vein, unspecified leg, subs encntr
		S85.591D	Oth injury of popliteal vein, right leg, subs encntr
		S85.592D	Oth injury of popliteal vein, left leg, subs encntr
		S85.599D	Oth injury of popliteal vein, unspecified leg, subs encntr
		S85.801D	Unsp inj blood vessels at lower leg level, right leg, subs
		S85.802D	Unsp inj blood vessels at lower leg level, left leg, subs
		S85.809D	Unsp inj blood vessels at lower leg level, unsp leg, subs
		S85.811D	Lacerat blood vessels at lower leg level, right leg, subs
		S85.812D	Lacerat blood vessels at lower leg level, left leg, subs
		S85.819D	Lacerat blood vessels at lower leg level, unsp leg, subs
		S85.891D	Inj oth blood vessels at lower leg level, right leg, subs
		S85.892D	Inj oth blood vessels at lower leg level, left leg, subs
		S85.899D	Inj oth blood vessels at lower leg level, unsp leg, subs
		S85.901D	Unsp inj unsp blood vess at lower leg level, right leg, subs
		S85.902D	Unsp inj unsp blood vess at lower leg level, left leg, subs
		S85.909D	Unsp inj unsp blood vess at lower leg level, unsp leg, subs
		S85.911D	Lacerat unsp blood vess at lower leg level, right leg, subs
		S85.912D	Lacerat unsp blood vessel at lower leg level, left leg, subs
		S85.919D	Lacerat unsp blood vessel at lower leg level, unsp leg, subs
		S85.991D	Inj unsp blood vessel at lower leg level, right leg, subs
		S85.992D	Inj unsp blood vessel at lower leg level, left leg, subs
		S85.999D	Inj unsp blood vessel at lower leg level, unsp leg, subs
		S86.001D	Unspecified injury of right Achilles tendon, subs encntr
		S86.002D	Unspecified injury of left Achilles tendon, subs encntr
		S86.009D	Unsp injury of unspecified Achilles tendon, subs encntr
		S86.011D	Strain of right Achilles tendon, subsequent encounter
		S86.012D	Strain of left Achilles tendon, subsequent encounter
		S86.019D	Strain of unspecified Achilles tendon, subsequent encounter
		S86.021D	Laceration of right Achilles tendon, subsequent encounter
		S86.022D	Laceration of left Achilles tendon, subsequent encounter
		S86.029D	Laceration of unspecified Achilles tendon, subs encntr
		S86.091D	Other specified injury of right Achilles tendon, subs encntr
		S86.092D	Other specified injury of left Achilles tendon, subs encntr
		S86.099D	Oth injury of unspecified Achilles tendon, subs encntr
		S86.101D	Unsp inj musc/tend post grp at low leg lev, right leg, subs
		S86.102D	Unsp inj musc/tend post grp at low leg level, left leg, subs
		S86.109D	Unsp inj musc/tend post grp at low leg level, unsp leg, subs
		S86.111D	Strain musc/tend post grp at low leg level, right leg, subs
	(Continued on next page)	**S86.112D**	Strain musc/tend post grp at low leg level, left leg, subs

ICD-9-CM		ICD-10-CM	
V58.89	ENCOUNTER FOR OTHER SPECIFIED AFTERCARE **(Continued)**	**S86.119D**	Strain musc/tend post grp at low leg level, unsp leg, subs
		S86.121D	Lacerat musc/tend post grp at low leg level, right leg, subs
		S86.122D	Lacerat musc/tend post grp at low leg level, left leg, subs
		S86.129D	Lacerat musc/tend post grp at low leg level, unsp leg, subs
		S86.191D	Inj oth musc/tend post grp at low leg level, right leg, subs
		S86.192D	Inj oth musc/tend post grp at low leg level, left leg, subs
		S86.199D	Inj oth musc/tend post grp at low leg level, unsp leg, subs
		S86.201D	Unsp inj musc/tend ant grp at low leg level, right leg, subs
		S86.202D	Unsp inj musc/tend ant grp at low leg level, left leg, subs
		S86.209D	Unsp inj musc/tend ant grp at low leg level, unsp leg, subs
		S86.211D	Strain musc/tend ant grp at low leg level, right leg, subs
		S86.212D	Strain musc/tend ant grp at low leg level, left leg, subs
		S86.219D	Strain musc/tend ant grp at low leg level, unsp leg, subs
		S86.221D	Lacerat musc/tend ant grp at low leg level, right leg, subs
		S86.222D	Lacerat musc/tend ant grp at low leg level, left leg, subs
		S86.229D	Lacerat musc/tend ant grp at low leg level, unsp leg, subs
		S86.291D	Inj musc/tend anterior grp at low leg level, right leg, subs
		S86.292D	Inj musc/tend anterior grp at low leg level, left leg, subs
		S86.299D	Inj musc/tend anterior grp at low leg level, unsp leg, subs
		S86.301D	Unsp inj musc/tend peroneal grp at low leg lev, r leg, subs
		S86.302D	Unsp inj musc/tend peroneal grp at low leg lev, l leg, subs
		S86.309D	Unsp inj musc/tend peroneal grp at low leg lev,unsp leg,subs
		S86.311D	Strain musc/tend peroneal grp at low leg lev, r leg, subs
		S86.312D	Strain musc/tend peroneal grp at low leg lev, left leg, subs
		S86.319D	Strain musc/tend peroneal grp at low leg lev, unsp leg, subs
		S86.321D	Lacerat musc/tend peroneal grp at low leg lev, r leg, subs
		S86.322D	Lacerat musc/tend peroneal grp at low leg lev, l leg, subs
		S86.329D	Lacerat musc/tend peroneal grp at low leg lev,unsp leg, subs
		S86.391D	Inj musc/tend peroneal grp at low leg level, right leg, subs
		S86.392D	Inj musc/tend peroneal grp at low leg level, left leg, subs
		S86.399D	Inj musc/tend peroneal grp at low leg level, unsp leg, subs
		S86.801D	Unsp injury of musc/tend at lower leg level, right leg, subs
		S86.802D	Unsp injury of musc/tend at lower leg level, left leg, subs
		S86.809D	Unsp injury of musc/tend at lower leg level, unsp leg, subs
		S86.811D	Strain of musc/tend at lower leg level, right leg, subs
		S86.812D	Strain of musc/tend at lower leg level, left leg, subs
		S86.819D	Strain of musc/tend at lower leg level, unsp leg, subs
		S86.821D	Laceration of musc/tend at lower leg level, right leg, subs
		S86.822D	Laceration of musc/tend at lower leg level, left leg, subs
		S86.829D	Laceration of musc/tend at lower leg level, unsp leg, subs
		S86.891D	Inj oth musc/tend at lower leg level, right leg, subs
		S86.892D	Inj oth musc/tend at lower leg level, left leg, subs
		S86.899D	Inj oth musc/tend at lower leg level, unsp leg, subs
		S86.901D	Unsp inj unsp musc/tend at lower leg level, right leg, subs
		S86.902D	Unsp inj unsp musc/tend at lower leg level, left leg, subs
		S86.909D	Unsp inj unsp musc/tend at lower leg level, unsp leg, subs
		S86.911D	Strain of unsp musc/tend at lower leg level, right leg, subs
		S86.912D	Strain of unsp musc/tend at lower leg level, left leg, subs
		S86.919D	Strain of unsp musc/tend at lower leg level, unsp leg, subs
		S86.921D	Lacerat unsp musc/tend at lower leg level, right leg, subs
		S86.922D	Lacerat unsp musc/tend at lower leg level, left leg, subs
		S86.929D	Lacerat unsp musc/tend at lower leg level, unsp leg, subs
		S86.991D	Inj unsp musc/tend at lower leg level, right leg, subs
		S86.992D	Inj unsp musc/tend at lower leg level, left leg, subs
		S86.999D	Inj unsp musc/tend at lower leg level, unsp leg, subs
		S87.00XD	Crushing injury of unspecified knee, subsequent encounter
		S87.01XD	Crushing injury of right knee, subsequent encounter
		S87.02XD	Crushing injury of left knee, subsequent encounter
		S87.80XD	Crushing injury of unspecified lower leg, subs encntr
		S87.81XD	Crushing injury of right lower leg, subsequent encounter
		S87.82XD	Crushing injury of left lower leg, subsequent encounter
		S88.011D	Complete traumatic amputation at knee level, r low leg, subs
		S88.012D	Complete traumatic amputation at knee level, l low leg, subs
		S88.019D	Complete traumatic amp at knee level, unsp lower leg, subs
		S88.021D	Partial traumatic amputation at knee level, r low leg, subs
		S88.022D	Partial traumatic amputation at knee level, l low leg, subs
		S88.029D	Partial traumatic amp at knee level, unsp lower leg, subs
		S88.111D	Complete traum amp at lev betw kn and ankl, r low leg, subs
		S88.112D	Complete traum amp at lev betw kn and ankl, l low leg, subs
		S88.119D	Complete traum amp at lev betw kn & ankl, unsp low leg, subs
		S88.121D	Part traum amp at level betw knee and ankle, r low leg, subs
		S88.122D	Part traum amp at level betw knee and ankle, l low leg, subs
		S88.129D	Part traum amp at lev betw knee and ankl, unsp low leg, subs
		S88.911D	Complete traumatic amputation of r low leg, level unsp, subs
		S88.912D	Complete traumatic amputation of l low leg, level unsp, subs
		S88.919D	Complete traumatic amp of unsp lower leg, level unsp, subs
		S88.921D	Partial traumatic amputation of r low leg, level unsp, subs
		S88.922D	Partial traumatic amputation of l low leg, level unsp, subs
		S88.929D	Partial traumatic amp of unsp lower leg, level unsp, subs
		S89.80XD	Oth injuries of unspecified lower leg, subs encntr
		S89.81XD	Other specified injuries of right lower leg, subs encntr
		S89.82XD	Other specified injuries of left lower leg, subs encntr
	(Continued on next page)	**S89.90XD**	Unspecified injury of unspecified lower leg, subs encntr

ICD-9-CM		ICD-10-CM	
V58.89	ENCOUNTER FOR OTHER SPECIFIED AFTERCARE **(Continued)**	**S89.91XD**	Unspecified injury of right lower leg, subsequent encounter
		S89.92XD	Unspecified injury of left lower leg, subsequent encounter
		S9Ø.ØØXD	Contusion of unspecified ankle, subsequent encounter
		S9Ø.Ø1XD	Contusion of right ankle, subsequent encounter
		S9Ø.Ø2XD	Contusion of left ankle, subsequent encounter
		S9Ø.111D	Contusion of right great toe w/o damage to nail, subs encntr
		S9Ø.112D	Contusion of left great toe w/o damage to nail, subs encntr
		S9Ø.119D	Contusion of unsp great toe w/o damage to nail, subs encntr
		S9Ø.121D	Contusion of right lesser toe(s) w/o damage to nail, subs
		S9Ø.122D	Contusion of left lesser toe(s) w/o damage to nail, subs
		S9Ø.129D	Contusion of unsp lesser toe(s) w/o damage to nail, subs
		S9Ø.211D	Contusion of right great toe w damage to nail, subs encntr
		S9Ø.212D	Contusion of left great toe with damage to nail, subs encntr
		S9Ø.219D	Contusion of unsp great toe with damage to nail, subs encntr
		S9Ø.221D	Contusion of right lesser toe(s) w damage to nail, subs
		S9Ø.222D	Contusion of left lesser toe(s) w damage to nail, subs
		S9Ø.229D	Contusion of unsp lesser toe(s) w damage to nail, subs
		S9Ø.3ØXD	Contusion of unspecified foot, subsequent encounter
		S9Ø.31XD	Contusion of right foot, subsequent encounter
		S9Ø.32XD	Contusion of left foot, subsequent encounter
		S9Ø.411D	Abrasion, right great toe, subsequent encounter
		S9Ø.412D	Abrasion, left great toe, subsequent encounter
		S9Ø.413D	Abrasion, unspecified great toe, subsequent encounter
		S9Ø.414D	Abrasion, right lesser toe(s), subsequent encounter
		S9Ø.415D	Abrasion, left lesser toe(s), subsequent encounter
		S9Ø.416D	Abrasion, unspecified lesser toe(s), subsequent encounter
		S9Ø.421D	Blister (nonthermal), right great toe, subsequent encounter
		S9Ø.422D	Blister (nonthermal), left great toe, subsequent encounter
		S9Ø.423D	Blister (nonthermal), unspecified great toe, subs encntr
		S9Ø.424D	Blister (nonthermal), right lesser toe(s), subs encntr
		S9Ø.425D	Blister (nonthermal), left lesser toe(s), subs encntr
		S9Ø.426D	Blister (nonthermal), unspecified lesser toe(s), subs encntr
		S9Ø.441D	External constriction, right great toe, subsequent encounter
		S9Ø.442D	External constriction, left great toe, subsequent encounter
		S9Ø.443D	External constriction, unspecified great toe, subs encntr
		S9Ø.444D	External constriction, right lesser toe(s), subs encntr
		S9Ø.445D	External constriction, left lesser toe(s), subs encntr
		S9Ø.446D	External constriction, unsp lesser toe(s), subs encntr
		S9Ø.451D	Superficial foreign body, right great toe, subs encntr
		S9Ø.452D	Superficial foreign body, left great toe, subs encntr
		S9Ø.453D	Superficial foreign body, unspecified great toe, subs encntr
		S9Ø.454D	Superficial foreign body, right lesser toe(s), subs encntr
		S9Ø.455D	Superficial foreign body, left lesser toe(s), subs encntr
		S9Ø.456D	Superficial foreign body, unsp lesser toe(s), subs encntr
		S9Ø.461D	Insect bite (nonvenomous), right great toe, subs encntr
		S9Ø.462D	Insect bite (nonvenomous), left great toe, subs encntr
		S9Ø.463D	Insect bite (nonvenomous), unsp great toe, subs encntr
		S9Ø.464D	Insect bite (nonvenomous), right lesser toe(s), subs encntr
		S9Ø.465D	Insect bite (nonvenomous), left lesser toe(s), subs encntr
		S9Ø.466D	Insect bite (nonvenomous), unsp lesser toe(s), subs encntr
		S9Ø.471D	Other superficial bite of right great toe, subs encntr
		S9Ø.472D	Other superficial bite of left great toe, subs encntr
		S9Ø.473D	Other superficial bite of unspecified great toe, subs encntr
		S9Ø.474D	Other superficial bite of right lesser toe(s), subs encntr
		S9Ø.475D	Other superficial bite of left lesser toe(s), subs encntr
		S9Ø.476D	Other superficial bite of unsp lesser toe(s), subs encntr
		S9Ø.511D	Abrasion, right ankle, subsequent encounter
		S9Ø.512D	Abrasion, left ankle, subsequent encounter
		S9Ø.519D	Abrasion, unspecified ankle, subsequent encounter
		S9Ø.521D	Blister (nonthermal), right ankle, subsequent encounter
		S9Ø.522D	Blister (nonthermal), left ankle, subsequent encounter
		S9Ø.529D	Blister (nonthermal), unspecified ankle, subs encntr
		S9Ø.541D	External constriction, right ankle, subsequent encounter
		S9Ø.542D	External constriction, left ankle, subsequent encounter
		S9Ø.549D	External constriction, unspecified ankle, subs encntr
		S9Ø.551D	Superficial foreign body, right ankle, subsequent encounter
		S9Ø.552D	Superficial foreign body, left ankle, subsequent encounter
		S9Ø.559D	Superficial foreign body, unspecified ankle, subs encntr
		S9Ø.561D	Insect bite (nonvenomous), right ankle, subsequent encounter
		S9Ø.562D	Insect bite (nonvenomous), left ankle, subsequent encounter
		S9Ø.569D	Insect bite (nonvenomous), unspecified ankle, subs encntr
		S9Ø.571D	Other superficial bite of ankle, right ankle, subs encntr
		S9Ø.572D	Other superficial bite of ankle, left ankle, subs encntr
		S9Ø.579D	Other superficial bite of ankle, unsp ankle, subs encntr
		S9Ø.811D	Abrasion, right foot, subsequent encounter
		S9Ø.812D	Abrasion, left foot, subsequent encounter
		S9Ø.819D	Abrasion, unspecified foot, subsequent encounter
		S9Ø.821D	Blister (nonthermal), right foot, subsequent encounter
		S9Ø.822D	Blister (nonthermal), left foot, subsequent encounter
		S9Ø.829D	Blister (nonthermal), unspecified foot, subsequent encounter
		S9Ø.841D	External constriction, right foot, subsequent encounter
		S9Ø.842D	External constriction, left foot, subsequent encounter
	(Continued on next page)	**S9Ø.849D**	External constriction, unspecified foot, subs encntr

ICD-9-CM		ICD-10-CM	
V58.89	ENCOUNTER FOR OTHER SPECIFIED AFTERCARE **(Continued)**	**S90.851D**	Superficial foreign body, right foot, subsequent encounter
		S90.852D	Superficial foreign body, left foot, subsequent encounter
		S90.859D	Superficial foreign body, unspecified foot, subs encntr
		S90.861D	Insect bite (nonvenomous), right foot, subsequent encounter
		S90.862D	Insect bite (nonvenomous), left foot, subsequent encounter
		S90.869D	Insect bite (nonvenomous), unspecified foot, subs encntr
		S90.871D	Other superficial bite of right foot, subsequent encounter
		S90.872D	Other superficial bite of left foot, subsequent encounter
		S90.879D	Other superficial bite of unspecified foot, subs encntr
		S90.911D	Unspecified superficial injury of right ankle, subs encntr
		S90.912D	Unspecified superficial injury of left ankle, subs encntr
		S90.919D	Unsp superficial injury of unspecified ankle, subs encntr
		S90.921D	Unspecified superficial injury of right foot, subs encntr
		S90.922D	Unspecified superficial injury of left foot, subs encntr
		S90.929D	Unsp superficial injury of unspecified foot, subs encntr
		S90.931D	Unsp superficial injury of right great toe, subs encntr
		S90.932D	Unsp superficial injury of left great toe, subs encntr
		S90.933D	Unsp superficial injury of unsp great toe, subs encntr
		S90.934D	Unsp superficial injury of right lesser toe(s), subs encntr
		S90.935D	Unsp superficial injury of left lesser toe(s), subs encntr
		S90.936D	Unsp superficial injury of unsp lesser toe(s), subs encntr
		S91.001D	Unspecified open wound, right ankle, subsequent encounter
		S91.002D	Unspecified open wound, left ankle, subsequent encounter
		S91.009D	Unspecified open wound, unspecified ankle, subs encntr
		S91.011D	Laceration without foreign body, right ankle, subs encntr
		S91.012D	Laceration without foreign body, left ankle, subs encntr
		S91.019D	Laceration without foreign body, unsp ankle, subs encntr
		S91.021D	Laceration with foreign body, right ankle, subs encntr
		S91.022D	Laceration with foreign body, left ankle, subs encntr
		S91.029D	Laceration with foreign body, unspecified ankle, subs encntr
		S91.031D	Puncture wound w/o foreign body, right ankle, subs encntr
		S91.032D	Puncture wound without foreign body, left ankle, subs encntr
		S91.039D	Puncture wound without foreign body, unsp ankle, subs encntr
		S91.041D	Puncture wound with foreign body, right ankle, subs encntr
		S91.042D	Puncture wound with foreign body, left ankle, subs encntr
		S91.049D	Puncture wound with foreign body, unsp ankle, subs encntr
		S91.051D	Open bite, right ankle, subsequent encounter
		S91.052D	Open bite, left ankle, subsequent encounter
		S91.059D	Open bite, unspecified ankle, subsequent encounter
		S91.101D	Unsp open wound of right great toe w/o damage to nail, subs
		S91.102D	Unsp open wound of left great toe w/o damage to nail, subs
		S91.103D	Unsp open wound of unsp great toe w/o damage to nail, subs
		S91.104D	Unsp opn wnd right lesser toe(s) w/o damage to nail, subs
		S91.105D	Unsp opn wnd left lesser toe(s) w/o damage to nail, subs
		S91.106D	Unsp opn wnd unsp lesser toe(s) w/o damage to nail, subs
		S91.109D	Unsp open wound of unsp toe(s) w/o damage to nail, subs
		S91.111D	Lac w/o fb of right great toe w/o damage to nail, subs
		S91.112D	Laceration w/o fb of left great toe w/o damage to nail, subs
		S91.113D	Laceration w/o fb of unsp great toe w/o damage to nail, subs
		S91.114D	Lac w/o fb of right lesser toe(s) w/o damage to nail, subs
		S91.115D	Lac w/o fb of left lesser toe(s) w/o damage to nail, subs
		S91.116D	Lac w/o fb of unsp lesser toe(s) w/o damage to nail, subs
		S91.119D	Laceration w/o fb of unsp toe w/o damage to nail, subs
		S91.121D	Laceration w fb of right great toe w/o damage to nail, subs
		S91.122D	Laceration w fb of left great toe w/o damage to nail, subs
		S91.123D	Laceration w fb of unsp great toe w/o damage to nail, subs
		S91.124D	Lac w fb of right lesser toe(s) w/o damage to nail, subs
		S91.125D	Lac w fb of left lesser toe(s) w/o damage to nail, subs
		S91.126D	Lac w fb of unsp lesser toe(s) w/o damage to nail, subs
		S91.129D	Laceration w fb of unsp toe(s) w/o damage to nail, subs
		S91.131D	Pnctr w/o fb of right great toe w/o damage to nail, subs
		S91.132D	Pnctr w/o fb of left great toe w/o damage to nail, subs
		S91.133D	Pnctr w/o fb of unsp great toe w/o damage to nail, subs
		S91.134D	Pnctr w/o fb of right lesser toe(s) w/o damage to nail, subs
		S91.135D	Pnctr w/o fb of left lesser toe(s) w/o damage to nail, subs
		S91.136D	Pnctr w/o fb of unsp lesser toe(s) w/o damage to nail, subs
		S91.139D	Pnctr w/o fb of unsp toe(s) w/o damage to nail, subs
		S91.141D	Pnctr w fb of right great toe w/o damage to nail, subs
		S91.142D	Pnctr w fb of left great toe w/o damage to nail, subs
		S91.143D	Pnctr w fb of unsp great toe w/o damage to nail, subs
		S91.144D	Pnctr w fb of right lesser toe(s) w/o damage to nail, subs
		S91.145D	Pnctr w fb of left lesser toe(s) w/o damage to nail, subs
		S91.146D	Pnctr w fb of unsp lesser toe(s) w/o damage to nail, subs
		S91.149D	Pnctr w foreign body of unsp toe(s) w/o damage to nail, subs
		S91.151D	Open bite of right great toe w/o damage to nail, subs encntr
		S91.152D	Open bite of left great toe w/o damage to nail, subs encntr
		S91.153D	Open bite of unsp great toe w/o damage to nail, subs encntr
		S91.154D	Open bite of right lesser toe(s) w/o damage to nail, subs
		S91.155D	Open bite of left lesser toe(s) w/o damage to nail, subs
		S91.156D	Open bite of unsp lesser toe(s) w/o damage to nail, subs
		S91.159D	Open bite of unsp toe(s) without damage to nail, subs encntr
		S91.201D	Unsp open wound of right great toe w damage to nail, subs
	(Continued on next page)	**S91.202D**	Unsp open wound of left great toe w damage to nail, subs

ICD-9-CM		ICD-10-CM	
V58.89	ENCOUNTER FOR OTHER SPECIFIED AFTERCARE **(Continued)**	**S91.203D**	Unsp open wound of unsp great toe w damage to nail, subs
		S91.204D	Unsp opn wnd right lesser toe(s) w damage to nail, subs
		S91.205D	Unsp open wound of left lesser toe(s) w damage to nail, subs
		S91.206D	Unsp open wound of unsp lesser toe(s) w damage to nail, subs
		S91.209D	Unsp open wound of unsp toe(s) w damage to nail, subs encntr
		S91.211D	Laceration w/o fb of right great toe w damage to nail, subs
		S91.212D	Laceration w/o fb of left great toe w damage to nail, subs
		S91.213D	Laceration w/o fb of unsp great toe w damage to nail, subs
		S91.214D	Lac w/o fb of right lesser toe(s) w damage to nail, subs
		S91.215D	Lac w/o fb of left lesser toe(s) w damage to nail, subs
		S91.216D	Lac w/o fb of unsp lesser toe(s) w damage to nail, subs
		S91.219D	Laceration w/o fb of unsp toe(s) w damage to nail, subs
		S91.221D	Laceration w fb of right great toe w damage to nail, subs
		S91.222D	Laceration w fb of left great toe w damage to nail, subs
		S91.223D	Laceration w fb of unsp great toe w damage to nail, subs
		S91.224D	Lac w fb of right lesser toe(s) w damage to nail, subs
		S91.225D	Laceration w fb of left lesser toe(s) w damage to nail, subs
		S91.226D	Laceration w fb of unsp lesser toe(s) w damage to nail, subs
		S91.229D	Laceration w fb of unsp toe(s) w damage to nail, subs
		S91.231D	Pnctr w/o fb of right great toe w damage to nail, subs
		S91.232D	Pnctr w/o fb of left great toe w damage to nail, subs
		S91.233D	Pnctr w/o fb of unsp great toe w damage to nail, subs
		S91.234D	Pnctr w/o fb of right lesser toe(s) w damage to nail, subs
		S91.235D	Pnctr w/o fb of left lesser toe(s) w damage to nail, subs
		S91.236D	Pnctr w/o fb of unsp lesser toe(s) w damage to nail, subs
		S91.239D	Pnctr w/o foreign body of unsp toe(s) w damage to nail, subs
		S91.241D	Pnctr w fb of right great toe w damage to nail, subs
		S91.242D	Pnctr w fb of left great toe w damage to nail, subs
		S91.243D	Pnctr w fb of unsp great toe w damage to nail, subs
		S91.244D	Pnctr w fb of right lesser toe(s) w damage to nail, subs
		S91.245D	Pnctr w fb of left lesser toe(s) w damage to nail, subs
		S91.246D	Pnctr w fb of unsp lesser toe(s) w damage to nail, subs
		S91.249D	Pnctr w foreign body of unsp toe(s) w damage to nail, subs
		S91.251D	Open bite of right great toe w damage to nail, subs encntr
		S91.252D	Open bite of left great toe with damage to nail, subs encntr
		S91.253D	Open bite of unsp great toe with damage to nail, subs encntr
		S91.254D	Open bite of right lesser toe(s) w damage to nail, subs
		S91.255D	Open bite of left lesser toe(s) w damage to nail, subs
		S91.256D	Open bite of unsp lesser toe(s) w damage to nail, subs
		S91.259D	Open bite of unsp toe(s) with damage to nail, subs encntr
		S91.301D	Unspecified open wound, right foot, subsequent encounter
		S91.302D	Unspecified open wound, left foot, subsequent encounter
		S91.309D	Unspecified open wound, unspecified foot, subs encntr
		S91.311D	Laceration without foreign body, right foot, subs encntr
		S91.312D	Laceration without foreign body, left foot, subs encntr
		S91.319D	Laceration without foreign body, unsp foot, subs encntr
		S91.321D	Laceration with foreign body, right foot, subs encntr
		S91.322D	Laceration with foreign body, left foot, subs encntr
		S91.329D	Laceration with foreign body, unspecified foot, subs encntr
		S91.331D	Puncture wound without foreign body, right foot, subs encntr
		S91.332D	Puncture wound without foreign body, left foot, subs encntr
		S91.339D	Puncture wound without foreign body, unsp foot, subs encntr
		S91.341D	Puncture wound with foreign body, right foot, subs encntr
		S91.342D	Puncture wound with foreign body, left foot, subs encntr
		S91.349D	Puncture wound with foreign body, unsp foot, subs encntr
		S91.351D	Open bite, right foot, subsequent encounter
		S91.352D	Open bite, left foot, subsequent encounter
		S91.359D	Open bite, unspecified foot, subsequent encounter
		S93.01XD	Subluxation of right ankle joint, subsequent encounter
		S93.02XD	Subluxation of left ankle joint, subsequent encounter
		S93.03XD	Subluxation of unspecified ankle joint, subsequent encounter
		S93.04XD	Dislocation of right ankle joint, subsequent encounter
		S93.05XD	Dislocation of left ankle joint, subsequent encounter
		S93.06XD	Dislocation of unspecified ankle joint, subsequent encounter
		S93.101D	Unspecified subluxation of right toe(s), subs encntr
		S93.102D	Unspecified subluxation of left toe(s), subsequent encounter
		S93.103D	Unspecified subluxation of unspecified toe(s), subs encntr
		S93.104D	Unspecified dislocation of right toe(s), subs encntr
		S93.105D	Unspecified dislocation of left toe(s), subsequent encounter
		S93.106D	Unspecified dislocation of unspecified toe(s), subs encntr
		S93.111D	Dislocation of interphaln joint of right great toe, subs
		S93.112D	Dislocation of interphalangeal joint of left great toe, subs
		S93.113D	Dislocation of interphalangeal joint of unsp great toe, subs
		S93.114D	Dislocation of interphaln joint of right lesser toe(s), subs
		S93.115D	Dislocation of interphaln joint of left lesser toe(s), subs
		S93.116D	Dislocation of interphaln joint of unsp lesser toe(s), subs
		S93.119D	Dislocation of interphalangeal joint of unsp toe(s), subs
		S93.121D	Dislocation of MTP joint of right great toe, subs
		S93.122D	Dislocation of MTP joint of left great toe, subs
		S93.123D	Dislocation of MTP joint of unsp great toe, subs
		S93.124D	Dislocation of MTP joint of right lesser toe(s), subs
		S93.125D	Dislocation of MTP joint of left lesser toe(s), subs
	(Continued on next page)	**S93.126D**	Dislocation of MTP joint of unsp lesser toe(s), subs

[Brackets] indicate valid character values for each code. Character value meanings provided for each code grouping.

ICD-9-CM		ICD-10-CM	
V58.89	ENCOUNTER FOR OTHER SPECIFIED AFTERCARE	**S93.129D**	Dislocation of MTP joint of unsp toe(s), subs
	(Continued)	**S93.131D**	Subluxation of interphaln joint of right great toe, subs
		S93.132D	Subluxation of interphalangeal joint of left great toe, subs
		S93.133D	Subluxation of interphalangeal joint of unsp great toe, subs
		S93.134D	Subluxation of interphaln joint of right lesser toe(s), subs
		S93.135D	Subluxation of interphaln joint of left lesser toe(s), subs
		S93.136D	Subluxation of interphaln joint of unsp lesser toe(s), subs
		S93.139D	Subluxation of interphalangeal joint of unsp toe(s), subs
		S93.141D	Subluxation of MTP joint of right great toe, subs
		S93.142D	Subluxation of MTP joint of left great toe, subs
		S93.143D	Subluxation of MTP joint of unsp great toe, subs
		S93.144D	Subluxation of MTP joint of right lesser toe(s), subs
		S93.145D	Subluxation of MTP joint of left lesser toe(s), subs
		S93.146D	Subluxation of MTP joint of unsp lesser toe(s), subs
		S93.149D	Subluxation of MTP joint of unsp toe(s), subs
		S93.301D	Unspecified subluxation of right foot, subsequent encounter
		S93.302D	Unspecified subluxation of left foot, subsequent encounter
		S93.303D	Unspecified subluxation of unspecified foot, subs encntr
		S93.304D	Unspecified dislocation of right foot, subsequent encounter
		S93.305D	Unspecified dislocation of left foot, subsequent encounter
		S93.306D	Unspecified dislocation of unspecified foot, subs encntr
		S93.311D	Subluxation of tarsal joint of right foot, subs encntr
		S93.312D	Subluxation of tarsal joint of left foot, subs encntr
		S93.313D	Subluxation of tarsal joint of unspecified foot, subs encntr
		S93.314D	Dislocation of tarsal joint of right foot, subs encntr
		S93.315D	Dislocation of tarsal joint of left foot, subs encntr
		S93.316D	Dislocation of tarsal joint of unspecified foot, subs encntr
		S93.321D	Subluxation of tarsometatarsal joint of right foot, subs
		S93.322D	Subluxation of tarsometatarsal joint of left foot, subs
		S93.323D	Subluxation of tarsometatarsal joint of unsp foot, subs
		S93.324D	Dislocation of tarsometatarsal joint of right foot, subs
		S93.325D	Dislocation of tarsometatarsal joint of left foot, subs
		S93.326D	Dislocation of tarsometatarsal joint of unsp foot, subs
		S93.331D	Other subluxation of right foot, subsequent encounter
		S93.332D	Other subluxation of left foot, subsequent encounter
		S93.333D	Other subluxation of unspecified foot, subsequent encounter
		S93.334D	Other dislocation of right foot, subsequent encounter
		S93.335D	Other dislocation of left foot, subsequent encounter
		S93.336D	Other dislocation of unspecified foot, subsequent encounter
		S93.401D	Sprain of unspecified ligament of right ankle, subs encntr
		S93.402D	Sprain of unspecified ligament of left ankle, subs encntr
		S93.409D	Sprain of unsp ligament of unspecified ankle, subs encntr
		S93.411D	Sprain of calcaneofibular ligament of right ankle, subs
		S93.412D	Sprain of calcaneofibular ligament of left ankle, subs
		S93.419D	Sprain of calcaneofibular ligament of unsp ankle, subs
		S93.421D	Sprain of deltoid ligament of right ankle, subs encntr
		S93.422D	Sprain of deltoid ligament of left ankle, subs encntr
		S93.429D	Sprain of deltoid ligament of unspecified ankle, subs encntr
		S93.431D	Sprain of tibiofibular ligament of right ankle, subs encntr
		S93.432D	Sprain of tibiofibular ligament of left ankle, subs encntr
		S93.439D	Sprain of tibiofibular ligament of unsp ankle, subs encntr
		S93.491D	Sprain of other ligament of right ankle, subs encntr
		S93.492D	Sprain of other ligament of left ankle, subsequent encounter
		S93.499D	Sprain of other ligament of unspecified ankle, subs encntr
		S93.501D	Unspecified sprain of right great toe, subsequent encounter
		S93.502D	Unspecified sprain of left great toe, subsequent encounter
		S93.503D	Unspecified sprain of unspecified great toe, subs encntr
		S93.504D	Unspecified sprain of right lesser toe(s), subs encntr
		S93.505D	Unspecified sprain of left lesser toe(s), subs encntr
		S93.506D	Unspecified sprain of unspecified lesser toe(s), subs encntr
		S93.509D	Unspecified sprain of unspecified toe(s), subs encntr
		S93.511D	Sprain of interphalangeal joint of right great toe, subs
		S93.512D	Sprain of interphalangeal joint of left great toe, subs
		S93.513D	Sprain of interphalangeal joint of unsp great toe, subs
		S93.514D	Sprain of interphalangeal joint of right lesser toe(s), subs
		S93.515D	Sprain of interphalangeal joint of left lesser toe(s), subs
		S93.516D	Sprain of interphalangeal joint of unsp lesser toe(s), subs
		S93.519D	Sprain of interphalangeal joint of unsp toe(s), subs encntr
		S93.521D	Sprain of metatarsophalangeal joint of right great toe, subs
		S93.522D	Sprain of metatarsophalangeal joint of left great toe, subs
		S93.523D	Sprain of metatarsophalangeal joint of unsp great toe, subs
		S93.524D	Sprain of MTP joint of right lesser toe(s), subs
		S93.525D	Sprain of MTP joint of left lesser toe(s), subs
		S93.526D	Sprain of MTP joint of unsp lesser toe(s), subs
		S93.529D	Sprain of metatarsophalangeal joint of unsp toe(s), subs
		S93.601D	Unspecified sprain of right foot, subsequent encounter
		S93.602D	Unspecified sprain of left foot, subsequent encounter
		S93.609D	Unspecified sprain of unspecified foot, subsequent encounter
		S93.611D	Sprain of tarsal ligament of right foot, subs encntr
		S93.612D	Sprain of tarsal ligament of left foot, subsequent encounter
		S93.619D	Sprain of tarsal ligament of unspecified foot, subs encntr
		S93.621D	Sprain of tarsometatarsal ligament of right foot, subs
	(Continued on next page)	**S93.622D**	Sprain of tarsometatarsal ligament of left foot, subs encntr

V58.89–V58.89

ICD-9-CM		ICD-10-CM	
V58.89	ENCOUNTER FOR OTHER SPECIFIED AFTERCARE **(Continued)**	**S93.629D**	Sprain of tarsometatarsal ligament of unsp foot, subs encntr
		S93.691D	Other sprain of right foot, subsequent encounter
		S93.692D	Other sprain of left foot, subsequent encounter
		S93.699D	Other sprain of unspecified foot, subsequent encounter
		S94.00XD	Injury of lateral plantar nerve, unsp leg, subs encntr
		S94.01XD	Injury of lateral plantar nerve, right leg, subs encntr
		S94.02XD	Injury of lateral plantar nerve, left leg, subs encntr
		S94.10XD	Injury of medial plantar nerve, unspecified leg, subs encntr
		S94.11XD	Injury of medial plantar nerve, right leg, subs encntr
		S94.12XD	Injury of medial plantar nerve, left leg, subs encntr
		S94.20XD	Injury of deep peroneal nrv at ank/ft level, unsp leg, subs
		S94.21XD	Injury of deep peroneal nrv at ank/ft level, right leg, subs
		S94.22XD	Injury of deep peroneal nrv at ank/ft level, left leg, subs
		S94.30XD	Inj cutan sensory nerve at ank/ft level, unsp leg, subs
		S94.31XD	Inj cutan sensory nerve at ank/ft level, right leg, subs
		S94.32XD	Inj cutan sensory nerve at ank/ft level, left leg, subs
		S94.8X1D	Injury of nerves at ankle and foot level, right leg, subs
		S94.8X2D	Injury of oth nerves at ankle and foot level, left leg, subs
		S94.8X9D	Injury of oth nerves at ankle and foot level, unsp leg, subs
		S94.90XD	Injury of unsp nerve at ankle and foot level, unsp leg, subs
		S94.91XD	Injury of unsp nerve at ank/ft level, right leg, subs
		S94.92XD	Injury of unsp nerve at ankle and foot level, left leg, subs
		S95.001D	Unsp injury of dorsal artery of right foot, subs encntr
		S95.002D	Unsp injury of dorsal artery of left foot, subs encntr
		S95.009D	Unsp injury of dorsal artery of unsp foot, subs encntr
		S95.011D	Laceration of dorsal artery of right foot, subs encntr
		S95.012D	Laceration of dorsal artery of left foot, subs encntr
		S95.019D	Laceration of dorsal artery of unspecified foot, subs encntr
		S95.091D	Oth injury of dorsal artery of right foot, subs encntr
		S95.092D	Oth injury of dorsal artery of left foot, subs encntr
		S95.099D	Oth injury of dorsal artery of unspecified foot, subs encntr
		S95.101D	Unsp injury of plantar artery of right foot, subs encntr
		S95.102D	Unsp injury of plantar artery of left foot, subs encntr
		S95.109D	Unsp injury of plantar artery of unsp foot, subs encntr
		S95.111D	Laceration of plantar artery of right foot, subs encntr
		S95.112D	Laceration of plantar artery of left foot, subs encntr
		S95.119D	Laceration of plantar artery of unsp foot, subs encntr
		S95.191D	Oth injury of plantar artery of right foot, subs encntr
		S95.192D	Oth injury of plantar artery of left foot, subs encntr
		S95.199D	Oth injury of plantar artery of unsp foot, subs encntr
		S95.201D	Unspecified injury of dorsal vein of right foot, subs encntr
		S95.202D	Unspecified injury of dorsal vein of left foot, subs encntr
		S95.209D	Unsp injury of dorsal vein of unspecified foot, subs encntr
		S95.211D	Laceration of dorsal vein of right foot, subs encntr
		S95.212D	Laceration of dorsal vein of left foot, subsequent encounter
		S95.219D	Laceration of dorsal vein of unspecified foot, subs encntr
		S95.291D	Oth injury of dorsal vein of right foot, subs encntr
		S95.292D	Oth injury of dorsal vein of left foot, subs encntr
		S95.299D	Oth injury of dorsal vein of unspecified foot, subs encntr
		S95.801D	Unsp inj blood vessels at ank/ft level, right leg, subs
		S95.802D	Unsp injury of blood vessels at ank/ft level, left leg, subs
		S95.809D	Unsp injury of blood vessels at ank/ft level, unsp leg, subs
		S95.811D	Laceration of blood vessels at ank/ft level, right leg, subs
		S95.812D	Laceration of blood vessels at ank/ft level, left leg, subs
		S95.819D	Laceration of blood vessels at ank/ft level, unsp leg, subs
		S95.891D	Inj oth blood vessels at ank/ft level, right leg, subs
		S95.892D	Inj oth blood vessels at ank/ft level, left leg, subs
		S95.899D	Inj oth blood vessels at ank/ft level, unsp leg, subs
		S95.901D	Unsp inj unsp blood vess at ank/ft level, right leg, subs
		S95.902D	Unsp inj unsp blood vess at ank/ft level, left leg, subs
		S95.909D	Unsp inj unsp blood vess at ank/ft level, unsp leg, subs
		S95.911D	Lacerat unsp blood vessel at ank/ft level, right leg, subs
		S95.912D	Lacerat unsp blood vessel at ank/ft level, left leg, subs
		S95.919D	Lacerat unsp blood vessel at ank/ft level, unsp leg, subs
		S95.991D	Inj unsp blood vessel at ank/ft level, right leg, subs
		S95.992D	Inj unsp blood vessel at ank/ft level, left leg, subs
		S95.999D	Inj unsp blood vessel at ank/ft level, unsp leg, subs
		S96.001D	Unsp inj msl/tnd lng flxr msl toe at ank/ft lev, r ft, subs
		S96.002D	Unsp inj msl/tnd lng flxr msl toe at ank/ft lev, l ft, subs
		S96.009D	Unsp inj msl/tnd lng flxr msl toe at ank/ft lev,unsp ft,subs
		S96.011D	Strain msl/tnd lng flxr msl toe at ank/ft lev, r foot, subs
		S96.012D	Strain msl/tnd lng flxr msl toe at ank/ft lev, l foot, subs
		S96.019D	Strain msl/tnd lng flxr msl toe at ank/ft lev, unsp ft, subs
		S96.021D	Lacerat msl/tnd lng flxr msl toe at ank/ft lev, r foot, subs
		S96.022D	Lacerat msl/tnd lng flxr msl toe at ank/ft lev, l foot, subs
		S96.029D	Lacerat msl/tnd lng flxr msl toe at ank/ft lev,unsp ft, subs
		S96.091D	Inj msl/tnd lng flxr msl toe at ank/ft level, r foot, subs
		S96.092D	Inj msl/tnd lng flxr msl toe at ank/ft level, l foot, subs
		S96.099D	Inj msl/tnd lng flxr msl toe at ank/ft lev, unsp foot, subs
		S96.101D	Unsp inj msl/tnd lng extn msl toe at ank/ft lev, r ft, subs
		S96.102D	Unsp inj msl/tnd lng extn msl toe at ank/ft lev, l ft, subs
		S96.109D	Unsp inj msl/tnd lng extn msl toe at ank/ft lev,unsp ft,subs
	(Continued on next page)	**S96.111D**	Strain msl/tnd lng extn msl toe at ank/ft lev, r foot, subs

ICD-9-CM		ICD-10-CM	
V58.89	ENCOUNTER FOR OTHER SPECIFIED AFTERCARE **(Continued)**	**S96.112D**	Strain msl/tnd lng extn msl toe at ank/ft lev, l foot, subs
		S96.119D	Strain msl/tnd lng extn msl toe at ank/ft lev, unsp ft, subs
		S96.121D	Lacerat msl/tnd lng extn msl toe at ank/ft lev, r foot, subs
		S96.122D	Lacerat msl/tnd lng extn msl toe at ank/ft lev, l foot, subs
		S96.129D	Lacerat msl/tnd lng extn msl toe at ank/ft lev,unsp ft, subs
		S96.191D	Inj msl/tnd lng extn msl toe at ank/ft level, r foot, subs
		S96.192D	Inj msl/tnd lng extn msl toe at ank/ft level, l foot, subs
		S96.199D	Inj msl/tnd lng extn msl toe at ank/ft lev, unsp foot, subs
		S96.201D	Unsp inj intrinsic msl/tnd at ank/ft level, r foot, subs
		S96.202D	Unsp inj intrinsic msl/tnd at ank/ft level, left foot, subs
		S96.209D	Unsp inj intrinsic msl/tnd at ank/ft level, unsp foot, subs
		S96.211D	Strain of intrinsic msl/tnd at ank/ft level, r foot, subs
		S96.212D	Strain of intrinsic msl/tnd at ank/ft level, left foot, subs
		S96.219D	Strain of intrinsic msl/tnd at ank/ft level, unsp foot, subs
		S96.221D	Lacerat intrinsic msl/tnd at ank/ft level, right foot, subs
		S96.222D	Lacerat intrinsic msl/tnd at ank/ft level, left foot, subs
		S96.229D	Lacerat intrinsic msl/tnd at ank/ft level, unsp foot, subs
		S96.291D	Inj intrinsic msl/tnd at ank/ft level, right foot, subs
		S96.292D	Inj intrinsic msl/tnd at ank/ft level, left foot, subs
		S96.299D	Inj intrinsic msl/tnd at ank/ft level, unsp foot, subs
		S96.801D	Unsp inj muscles and tendons at ank/ft level, r foot, subs
		S96.802D	Unsp inj muscles and tendons at ank/ft level, l foot, subs
		S96.809D	Unsp inj musc and tendons at ank/ft level, unsp foot, subs
		S96.811D	Strain of muscles and tendons at ank/ft level, r foot, subs
		S96.812D	Strain of muscles and tendons at ank/ft level, l foot, subs
		S96.819D	Strain muscles and tendons at ank/ft level, unsp foot, subs
		S96.821D	Lacerat muscles and tendons at ank/ft level, r foot, subs
		S96.822D	Lacerat muscles and tendons at ank/ft level, left foot, subs
		S96.829D	Lacerat muscles and tendons at ank/ft level, unsp foot, subs
		S96.891D	Inj oth muscles and tendons at ank/ft level, r foot, subs
		S96.892D	Inj oth muscles and tendons at ank/ft level, left foot, subs
		S96.899D	Inj oth muscles and tendons at ank/ft level, unsp foot, subs
		S96.901D	Unsp injury of unsp msl/tnd at ank/ft level, r foot, subs
		S96.902D	Unsp injury of unsp msl/tnd at ank/ft level, left foot, subs
		S96.909D	Unsp injury of unsp msl/tnd at ank/ft level, unsp foot, subs
		S96.911D	Strain of unsp msl/tnd at ank/ft level, right foot, subs
		S96.912D	Strain of unsp msl/tnd at ank/ft level, left foot, subs
		S96.919D	Strain of unsp msl/tnd at ank/ft level, unsp foot, subs
		S96.921D	Laceration of unsp msl/tnd at ank/ft level, right foot, subs
		S96.922D	Laceration of unsp msl/tnd at ank/ft level, left foot, subs
		S96.929D	Laceration of unsp msl/tnd at ank/ft level, unsp foot, subs
		S96.991D	Inj unsp msl/tnd at ankle and foot level, right foot, subs
		S96.992D	Inj unsp msl/tnd at ankle and foot level, left foot, subs
		S96.999D	Inj unsp msl/tnd at ankle and foot level, unsp foot, subs
		S97.00XD	Crushing injury of unspecified ankle, subsequent encounter
		S97.01XD	Crushing injury of right ankle, subsequent encounter
		S97.02XD	Crushing injury of left ankle, subsequent encounter
		S97.101D	Crushing injury of unspecified right toe(s), subs encntr
		S97.102D	Crushing injury of unspecified left toe(s), subs encntr
		S97.109D	Crushing injury of unspecified toe(s), subsequent encounter
		S97.111D	Crushing injury of right great toe, subsequent encounter
		S97.112D	Crushing injury of left great toe, subsequent encounter
		S97.119D	Crushing injury of unspecified great toe, subs encntr
		S97.121D	Crushing injury of right lesser toe(s), subsequent encounter
		S97.122D	Crushing injury of left lesser toe(s), subsequent encounter
		S97.129D	Crushing injury of unspecified lesser toe(s), subs encntr
		S97.80XD	Crushing injury of unspecified foot, subsequent encounter
		S97.81XD	Crushing injury of right foot, subsequent encounter
		S97.82XD	Crushing injury of left foot, subsequent encounter
		S98.011D	Complete traumatic amp of right foot at ankle level, subs
		S98.012D	Complete traumatic amp of left foot at ankle level, subs
		S98.019D	Complete traumatic amp of unsp foot at ankle level, subs
		S98.021D	Partial traumatic amp of right foot at ankle level, subs
		S98.022D	Partial traumatic amp of left foot at ankle level, subs
		S98.029D	Partial traumatic amp of unsp foot at ankle level, subs
		S98.111D	Complete traumatic amputation of right great toe, subs
		S98.112D	Complete traumatic amputation of left great toe, subs encntr
		S98.119D	Complete traumatic amputation of unsp great toe, subs encntr
		S98.121D	Partial traumatic amputation of right great toe, subs encntr
		S98.122D	Partial traumatic amputation of left great toe, subs encntr
		S98.129D	Partial traumatic amputation of unsp great toe, subs encntr
		S98.131D	Complete traumatic amputation of one right lesser toe, subs
		S98.132D	Complete traumatic amputation of one left lesser toe, subs
		S98.139D	Complete traumatic amputation of one unsp lesser toe, subs
		S98.141D	Partial traumatic amputation of one right lesser toe, subs
		S98.142D	Partial traumatic amputation of one left lesser toe, subs
		S98.149D	Partial traumatic amputation of one unsp lesser toe, subs
		S98.211D	Complete traum amp of two or more right lesser toes, subs
		S98.212D	Complete traumatic amp of two or more left lesser toes, subs
		S98.219D	Complete traumatic amp of two or more unsp lesser toes, subs
		S98.221D	Partial traumatic amp of two or more right lesser toes, subs
		S98.222D	Partial traumatic amp of two or more left lesser toes, subs
	(Continued on next page)	**S98.229D**	Partial traumatic amp of two or more unsp lesser toes, subs

ICD-9-CM		ICD-10-CM	
V58.89	ENCOUNTER FOR OTHER SPECIFIED AFTERCARE **(Continued)**	**S98.311D**	Complete traumatic amputation of right midfoot, subs encntr
		S98.312D	Complete traumatic amputation of left midfoot, subs encntr
		S98.319D	Complete traumatic amputation of unsp midfoot, subs encntr
		S98.321D	Partial traumatic amputation of right midfoot, subs encntr
		S98.322D	Partial traumatic amputation of left midfoot, subs encntr
		S98.329D	Partial traumatic amputation of unsp midfoot, subs encntr
		S98.911D	Complete traumatic amp of right foot, level unsp, subs
		S98.912D	Complete traumatic amputation of left foot, level unsp, subs
		S98.919D	Complete traumatic amputation of unsp foot, level unsp, subs
		S98.921D	Partial traumatic amputation of right foot, level unsp, subs
		S98.922D	Partial traumatic amputation of left foot, level unsp, subs
		S98.929D	Partial traumatic amputation of unsp foot, level unsp, subs
		S99.811D	Other specified injuries of right ankle, subs encntr
		S99.812D	Other specified injuries of left ankle, subsequent encounter
		S99.819D	Other specified injuries of unspecified ankle, subs encntr
		S99.821D	Other specified injuries of right foot, subsequent encounter
		S99.822D	Other specified injuries of left foot, subsequent encounter
		S99.829D	Other specified injuries of unspecified foot, subs encntr
		S99.911D	Unspecified injury of right ankle, subsequent encounter
		S99.912D	Unspecified injury of left ankle, subsequent encounter
		S99.919D	Unspecified injury of unspecified ankle, subs encntr
		S99.921D	Unspecified injury of right foot, subsequent encounter
		S99.922D	Unspecified injury of left foot, subsequent encounter
		S99.929D	Unspecified injury of unspecified foot, subsequent encounter
		T15.ØØXD	Foreign body in cornea, unspecified eye, subs encntr
		T15.Ø1XD	Foreign body in cornea, right eye, subsequent encounter
		T15.Ø2XD	Foreign body in cornea, left eye, subsequent encounter
		T15.1ØXD	Foreign body in conjunctival sac, unsp eye, subs encntr
		T15.11XD	Foreign body in conjunctival sac, right eye, subs encntr
		T15.12XD	Foreign body in conjunctival sac, left eye, subs encntr
		T15.8ØXD	Fb in oth and multiple parts of external eye, unsp eye, subs
		T15.81XD	Fb in oth and multiple parts of external eye, r eye, subs
		T15.82XD	Fb in oth and multiple parts of external eye, left eye, subs
		T15.9ØXD	Foreign body on external eye, part unsp, unsp eye, subs
		T15.91XD	Foreign body on external eye, part unsp, right eye, subs
		T15.92XD	Foreign body on external eye, part unsp, left eye, subs
		T16.1XXD	Foreign body in right ear, subsequent encounter
		T16.2XXD	Foreign body in left ear, subsequent encounter
		T16.9XXD	Foreign body in ear, unspecified ear, subsequent encounter
		T17.ØXXD	Foreign body in nasal sinus, subsequent encounter
		T17.1XXD	Foreign body in nostril, subsequent encounter
		T17.2ØØD	Unsp foreign body in pharynx causing asphyxiation, subs
		T17.2Ø8D	Unsp foreign body in pharynx causing oth injury, subs encntr
		T17.21ØD	Gastric contents in pharynx causing asphyxiation, subs
		T17.218D	Gastric contents in pharynx causing oth injury, subs encntr
		T17.22ØD	Food in pharynx causing asphyxiation, subsequent encounter
		T17.228D	Food in pharynx causing other injury, subsequent encounter
		T17.29ØD	Oth foreign object in pharynx causing asphyxiation, subs
		T17.298D	Oth foreign object in pharynx causing oth injury, subs
		T17.3ØØD	Unsp foreign body in larynx causing asphyxiation, subs
		T17.3Ø8D	Unsp foreign body in larynx causing oth injury, subs encntr
		T17.31ØD	Gastric contents in larynx causing asphyxiation, subs encntr
		T17.318D	Gastric contents in larynx causing other injury, subs encntr
		T17.32ØD	Food in larynx causing asphyxiation, subsequent encounter
		T17.328D	Food in larynx causing other injury, subsequent encounter
		T17.39ØD	Oth foreign object in larynx causing asphyxiation, subs
		T17.398D	Oth foreign object in larynx causing oth injury, subs encntr
		T17.4ØØD	Unsp foreign body in trachea causing asphyxiation, subs
		T17.4Ø8D	Unsp foreign body in trachea causing oth injury, subs encntr
		T17.41ØD	Gastric contents in trachea causing asphyxiation, subs
		T17.418D	Gastric contents in trachea causing oth injury, subs encntr
		T17.42ØD	Food in trachea causing asphyxiation, subsequent encounter
		T17.428D	Food in trachea causing other injury, subsequent encounter
		T17.49ØD	Oth foreign object in trachea causing asphyxiation, subs
		T17.498D	Oth foreign object in trachea causing oth injury, subs
		T17.5ØØD	Unsp foreign body in bronchus causing asphyxiation, subs
		T17.5Ø8D	Unsp foreign body in bronchus causing oth injury, subs
		T17.51ØD	Gastric contents in bronchus causing asphyxiation, subs
		T17.518D	Gastric contents in bronchus causing oth injury, subs encntr
		T17.52ØD	Food in bronchus causing asphyxiation, subsequent encounter
		T17.528D	Food in bronchus causing other injury, subsequent encounter
		T17.59ØD	Oth foreign object in bronchus causing asphyxiation, subs
		T17.598D	Oth foreign object in bronchus causing oth injury, subs
		T17.8ØØD	Unsp foreign body in oth prt resp tract causing asphyx, subs
		T17.8Ø8D	Unsp fb in oth prt resp tract causing oth injury, subs
		T17.81ØD	Gastric contents in oth prt resp tract causing asphyx, subs
		T17.818D	Gastr contents in oth prt resp tract cause oth injury, subs
		T17.82ØD	Food in oth prt respiratory tract causing asphyxiation, subs
		T17.828D	Food in oth prt respiratory tract causing oth injury, subs
		T17.89ØD	Oth foreign object in oth prt resp tract cause asphyx, subs
		T17.898D	Oth forn object in oth prt resp tract cause oth injury, subs
		T17.9ØØD	Unsp fb in resp tract, part unsp causing asphyx, subs
		T17.9Ø8D	Unsp fb in resp tract, part unsp causing oth injury, subs

(Continued on next page)

ICD-9-CM		ICD-10-CM	
V58.89	ENCOUNTER FOR OTHER SPECIFIED AFTERCARE **(Continued)**	**T17.910D**	Gastric contents in resp tract, part unsp cause asphyx, subs
		T17.918D	Gastr contents in resp tract, part unsp cause oth inj, subs
		T17.920D	Food in resp tract, part unsp causing asphyxiation, subs
		T17.928D	Food in resp tract, part unsp causing oth injury, subs
		T17.990D	Oth forn obj in resp tract, part unsp in cause asphyx, subs
		T17.998D	Oth forn object in resp tract, part unsp cause oth inj, subs
		T18.0XXD	Foreign body in mouth, subsequent encounter
		T18.100D	Unsp fb in esophagus causing compression of trachea, subs
		T18.108D	Unsp foreign body in esophagus causing oth injury, subs
		T18.110D	Gastric contents in esoph causing comprsn of trachea, subs
		T18.118D	Gastric contents in esophagus causing oth injury, subs
		T18.120D	Food in esophagus causing compression of trachea, subs
		T18.128D	Food in esophagus causing other injury, subsequent encounter
		T18.190D	Oth foreign object in esoph causing comprsn of trachea, subs
		T18.198D	Oth foreign object in esophagus causing oth injury, subs
		T18.2XXD	Foreign body in stomach, subsequent encounter
		T18.3XXD	Foreign body in small intestine, subsequent encounter
		T18.4XXD	Foreign body in colon, subsequent encounter
		T18.5XXD	Foreign body in anus and rectum, subsequent encounter
		T18.8XXD	Foreign body in other parts of alimentary tract, subs encntr
		T18.9XXD	Foreign body of alimentary tract, part unsp, subs encntr
		T19.0XXD	Foreign body in urethra, subsequent encounter
		T19.1XXD	Foreign body in bladder, subsequent encounter
		T19.2XXD	Foreign body in vulva and vagina, subsequent encounter
		T19.3XXD	Foreign body in uterus, subsequent encounter
		T19.4XXD	Foreign body in penis, subsequent encounter
		T19.8XXD	Foreign body in oth prt genitourinary tract, subs encntr
		T19.9XXD	Foreign body in genitourinary tract, part unsp, subs encntr
		T20.00XD	Burn of unsp degree of head, face, and neck, unsp site, subs
		T20.011D	Burn of unspecified degree of right ear, subs encntr
		T20.012D	Burn of unspecified degree of left ear, subsequent encounter
		T20.019D	Burn of unspecified degree of unspecified ear, subs encntr
		T20.02XD	Burn of unspecified degree of lip(s), subsequent encounter
		T20.03XD	Burn of unspecified degree of chin, subsequent encounter
		T20.04XD	Burn of unspecified degree of nose (septum), subs encntr
		T20.05XD	Burn of unspecified degree of scalp, subsequent encounter
		T20.06XD	Burn of unsp degree of forehead and cheek, subs encntr
		T20.07XD	Burn of unspecified degree of neck, subsequent encounter
		T20.09XD	Burn of unsp deg mult sites of head, face, and neck, subs
		T20.10XD	Burn first degree of head, face, and neck, unsp site, subs
		T20.111D	Burn of first degree of right ear, subsequent encounter
		T20.112D	Burn of first degree of left ear, subsequent encounter
		T20.119D	Burn of first degree of unspecified ear, subs encntr
		T20.12XD	Burn of first degree of lip(s), subsequent encounter
		T20.13XD	Burn of first degree of chin, subsequent encounter
		T20.14XD	Burn of first degree of nose (septum), subsequent encounter
		T20.15XD	Burn of first degree of scalp, subsequent encounter
		T20.16XD	Burn of first degree of forehead and cheek, subs encntr
		T20.17XD	Burn of first degree of neck, subsequent encounter
		T20.19XD	Burn of first deg mult sites of head, face, and neck, subs
		T20.20XD	Burn second degree of head, face, and neck, unsp site, subs
		T20.211D	Burn of second degree of right ear, subsequent encounter
		T20.212D	Burn of second degree of left ear, subsequent encounter
		T20.219D	Burn of second degree of unspecified ear, subs encntr
		T20.22XD	Burn of second degree of lip(s), subsequent encounter
		T20.23XD	Burn of second degree of chin, subsequent encounter
		T20.24XD	Burn of second degree of nose (septum), subsequent encounter
		T20.25XD	Burn of second degree of scalp, subsequent encounter
		T20.26XD	Burn of second degree of forehead and cheek, subs encntr
		T20.27XD	Burn of second degree of neck, subsequent encounter
		T20.29XD	Burn of 2nd deg mul sites of head, face, and neck, subs
		T20.30XD	Burn third degree of head, face, and neck, unsp site, subs
		T20.311D	Burn of third degree of right ear, subsequent encounter
		T20.312D	Burn of third degree of left ear, subsequent encounter
		T20.319D	Burn of third degree of unspecified ear, subs encntr
		T20.32XD	Burn of third degree of lip(s), subsequent encounter
		T20.33XD	Burn of third degree of chin, subsequent encounter
		T20.34XD	Burn of third degree of nose (septum), subsequent encounter
		T20.35XD	Burn of third degree of scalp, subsequent encounter
		T20.36XD	Burn of third degree of forehead and cheek, subs encntr
		T20.37XD	Burn of third degree of neck, subsequent encounter
		T20.39XD	Burn of 3rd deg mu sites of head, face, and neck, subs
		T20.40XD	Corros unsp degree of head, face, and neck, unsp site, subs
		T20.411D	Corrosion of unspecified degree of right ear, subs encntr
		T20.412D	Corrosion of unspecified degree of left ear, subs encntr
		T20.419D	Corrosion of unsp degree of unspecified ear, subs encntr
		T20.42XD	Corrosion of unspecified degree of lip(s), subs encntr
		T20.43XD	Corrosion of unspecified degree of chin, subs encntr
		T20.44XD	Corrosion of unsp degree of nose (septum), subs encntr
		T20.45XD	Corrosion of unspecified degree of scalp, subs encntr
		T20.46XD	Corrosion of unsp degree of forehead and cheek, subs encntr
		T20.47XD	Corrosion of unspecified degree of neck, subs encntr
	(Continued on next page)	**T20.49XD**	Corros unsp deg mult sites of head, face, and neck, subs

ICD-9-CM		ICD-10-CM	
V58.89	ENCOUNTER FOR OTHER SPECIFIED AFTERCARE **(Continued)**	**T20.50XD**	Corros first degree of head, face, and neck, unsp site, subs
		T20.511D	Corrosion of first degree of right ear, subsequent encounter
		T20.512D	Corrosion of first degree of left ear, subsequent encounter
		T20.519D	Corrosion of first degree of unspecified ear, subs encntr
		T20.52XD	Corrosion of first degree of lip(s), subsequent encounter
		T20.53XD	Corrosion of first degree of chin, subsequent encounter
		T20.54XD	Corrosion of first degree of nose (septum), subs encntr
		T20.55XD	Corrosion of first degree of scalp, subsequent encounter
		T20.56XD	Corrosion of first degree of forehead and cheek, subs encntr
		T20.57XD	Corrosion of first degree of neck, subsequent encounter
		T20.59XD	Corros first deg mult sites of head, face, and neck, subs
		T20.60XD	Corros second deg of head, face, and neck, unsp site, subs
		T20.611D	Corrosion of second degree of right ear, subs encntr
		T20.612D	Corrosion of second degree of left ear, subsequent encounter
		T20.619D	Corrosion of second degree of unspecified ear, subs encntr
		T20.62XD	Corrosion of second degree of lip(s), subsequent encounter
		T20.63XD	Corrosion of second degree of chin, subsequent encounter
		T20.64XD	Corrosion of second degree of nose (septum), subs encntr
		T20.65XD	Corrosion of second degree of scalp, subsequent encounter
		T20.66XD	Corrosion of second degree of forehead and cheek, subs
		T20.67XD	Corrosion of second degree of neck, subsequent encounter
		T20.69XD	Corrosion of 2nd deg mul sites of head, face, and neck, subs
		T20.70XD	Corros third degree of head, face, and neck, unsp site, subs
		T20.711D	Corrosion of third degree of right ear, subsequent encounter
		T20.712D	Corrosion of third degree of left ear, subsequent encounter
		T20.719D	Corrosion of third degree of unspecified ear, subs encntr
		T20.72XD	Corrosion of third degree of lip(s), subsequent encounter
		T20.73XD	Corrosion of third degree of chin, subsequent encounter
		T20.74XD	Corrosion of third degree of nose (septum), subs encntr
		T20.75XD	Corrosion of third degree of scalp, subsequent encounter
		T20.76XD	Corrosion of third degree of forehead and cheek, subs encntr
		T20.77XD	Corrosion of third degree of neck, subsequent encounter
		T20.79XD	Corrosion of 3rd deg mu sites of head, face, and neck, subs
		T21.00XD	Burn of unsp degree of trunk, unspecified site, subs encntr
		T21.01XD	Burn of unspecified degree of chest wall, subs encntr
		T21.02XD	Burn of unspecified degree of abdominal wall, subs encntr
		T21.03XD	Burn of unspecified degree of upper back, subs encntr
		T21.04XD	Burn of unspecified degree of lower back, subs encntr
		T21.05XD	Burn of unspecified degree of buttock, subsequent encounter
		T21.06XD	Burn of unsp degree of male genital region, subs encntr
		T21.07XD	Burn of unsp degree of female genital region, subs encntr
		T21.09XD	Burn of unsp degree of other site of trunk, subs encntr
		T21.10XD	Burn of first degree of trunk, unspecified site, subs encntr
		T21.11XD	Burn of first degree of chest wall, subsequent encounter
		T21.12XD	Burn of first degree of abdominal wall, subsequent encounter
		T21.13XD	Burn of first degree of upper back, subsequent encounter
		T21.14XD	Burn of first degree of lower back, subsequent encounter
		T21.15XD	Burn of first degree of buttock, subsequent encounter
		T21.16XD	Burn of first degree of male genital region, subs encntr
		T21.17XD	Burn of first degree of female genital region, subs encntr
		T21.19XD	Burn of first degree of other site of trunk, subs encntr
		T21.20XD	Burn of second degree of trunk, unsp site, subs encntr
		T21.21XD	Burn of second degree of chest wall, subsequent encounter
		T21.22XD	Burn of second degree of abdominal wall, subs encntr
		T21.23XD	Burn of second degree of upper back, subsequent encounter
		T21.24XD	Burn of second degree of lower back, subsequent encounter
		T21.25XD	Burn of second degree of buttock, subsequent encounter
		T21.26XD	Burn of second degree of male genital region, subs encntr
		T21.27XD	Burn of second degree of female genital region, subs encntr
		T21.29XD	Burn of second degree of other site of trunk, subs encntr
		T21.30XD	Burn of third degree of trunk, unspecified site, subs encntr
		T21.31XD	Burn of third degree of chest wall, subsequent encounter
		T21.32XD	Burn of third degree of abdominal wall, subsequent encounter
		T21.33XD	Burn of third degree of upper back, subsequent encounter
		T21.34XD	Burn of third degree of lower back, subsequent encounter
		T21.35XD	Burn of third degree of buttock, subsequent encounter
		T21.36XD	Burn of third degree of male genital region, subs encntr
		T21.37XD	Burn of third degree of female genital region, subs encntr
		T21.39XD	Burn of third degree of other site of trunk, subs encntr
		T21.40XD	Corrosion of unsp degree of trunk, unsp site, subs encntr
		T21.41XD	Corrosion of unspecified degree of chest wall, subs encntr
		T21.42XD	Corrosion of unsp degree of abdominal wall, subs encntr
		T21.43XD	Corrosion of unspecified degree of upper back, subs encntr
		T21.44XD	Corrosion of unspecified degree of lower back, subs encntr
		T21.45XD	Corrosion of unspecified degree of buttock, subs encntr
		T21.46XD	Corrosion of unsp degree of male genital region, subs encntr
		T21.47XD	Corrosion of unsp degree of female genital region, subs
		T21.49XD	Corrosion of unsp degree of other site of trunk, subs encntr
		T21.50XD	Corrosion of first degree of trunk, unsp site, subs encntr
		T21.51XD	Corrosion of first degree of chest wall, subs encntr
		T21.52XD	Corrosion of first degree of abdominal wall, subs encntr
		T21.53XD	Corrosion of first degree of upper back, subs encntr
	(Continued on next page)	**T21.54XD**	Corrosion of first degree of lower back, subs encntr

ICD-9-CM		ICD-10-CM	
V58.89	ENCOUNTER FOR OTHER SPECIFIED AFTERCARE **(Continued)**	**T21.55XD**	Corrosion of first degree of buttock, subsequent encounter
		T21.56XD	Corrosion of first degree of male genital region, subs
		T21.57XD	Corrosion of first degree of female genital region, subs
		T21.59XD	Corrosion of first degree of oth site of trunk, subs encntr
		T21.60XD	Corrosion of second degree of trunk, unsp site, subs encntr
		T21.61XD	Corrosion of second degree of chest wall, subs encntr
		T21.62XD	Corrosion of second degree of abdominal wall, subs encntr
		T21.63XD	Corrosion of second degree of upper back, subs encntr
		T21.64XD	Corrosion of second degree of lower back, subs encntr
		T21.65XD	Corrosion of second degree of buttock, subsequent encounter
		T21.66XD	Corrosion of second degree of male genital region, subs
		T21.67XD	Corrosion of second degree of female genital region, subs
		T21.69XD	Corrosion of second degree of oth site of trunk, subs encntr
		T21.70XD	Corrosion of third degree of trunk, unsp site, subs encntr
		T21.71XD	Corrosion of third degree of chest wall, subs encntr
		T21.72XD	Corrosion of third degree of abdominal wall, subs encntr
		T21.73XD	Corrosion of third degree of upper back, subs encntr
		T21.74XD	Corrosion of third degree of lower back, subs encntr
		T21.75XD	Corrosion of third degree of buttock, subsequent encounter
		T21.76XD	Corrosion of third degree of male genital region, subs
		T21.77XD	Corrosion of third degree of female genital region, subs
		T21.79XD	Corrosion of third degree of oth site of trunk, subs encntr
		T22.00XD	Burn unsp deg of shldr/up lmb, ex wrs/hnd, unsp site, subs
		T22.011D	Burn of unspecified degree of right forearm, subs encntr
		T22.012D	Burn of unspecified degree of left forearm, subs encntr
		T22.019D	Burn of unsp degree of unspecified forearm, subs encntr
		T22.021D	Burn of unspecified degree of right elbow, subs encntr
		T22.022D	Burn of unspecified degree of left elbow, subs encntr
		T22.029D	Burn of unspecified degree of unspecified elbow, subs encntr
		T22.031D	Burn of unspecified degree of right upper arm, subs encntr
		T22.032D	Burn of unspecified degree of left upper arm, subs encntr
		T22.039D	Burn of unsp degree of unspecified upper arm, subs encntr
		T22.041D	Burn of unspecified degree of right axilla, subs encntr
		T22.042D	Burn of unspecified degree of left axilla, subs encntr
		T22.049D	Burn of unsp degree of unspecified axilla, subs encntr
		T22.051D	Burn of unspecified degree of right shoulder, subs encntr
		T22.052D	Burn of unspecified degree of left shoulder, subs encntr
		T22.059D	Burn of unsp degree of unspecified shoulder, subs encntr
		T22.061D	Burn of unsp degree of right scapular region, subs encntr
		T22.062D	Burn of unsp degree of left scapular region, subs encntr
		T22.069D	Burn of unsp degree of unsp scapular region, subs encntr
		T22.091D	Burn unsp deg mult sites of r shldr/up lmb, ex wrs/hnd, subs
		T22.092D	Burn unsp deg mult site of l shldr/up lmb, ex wrs/hnd, subs
		T22.099D	Burn unsp deg mult sites of shldr/up lmb, ex wrs/hnd, subs
		T22.10XD	Burn first deg of shldr/up lmb, ex wrs/hnd, unsp site, subs
		T22.111D	Burn of first degree of right forearm, subsequent encounter
		T22.112D	Burn of first degree of left forearm, subsequent encounter
		T22.119D	Burn of first degree of unspecified forearm, subs encntr
		T22.121D	Burn of first degree of right elbow, subsequent encounter
		T22.122D	Burn of first degree of left elbow, subsequent encounter
		T22.129D	Burn of first degree of unspecified elbow, subs encntr
		T22.131D	Burn of first degree of right upper arm, subs encntr
		T22.132D	Burn of first degree of left upper arm, subsequent encounter
		T22.139D	Burn of first degree of unspecified upper arm, subs encntr
		T22.141D	Burn of first degree of right axilla, subsequent encounter
		T22.142D	Burn of first degree of left axilla, subsequent encounter
		T22.149D	Burn of first degree of unspecified axilla, subs encntr
		T22.151D	Burn of first degree of right shoulder, subsequent encounter
		T22.152D	Burn of first degree of left shoulder, subsequent encounter
		T22.159D	Burn of first degree of unspecified shoulder, subs encntr
		T22.161D	Burn of first degree of right scapular region, subs encntr
		T22.162D	Burn of first degree of left scapular region, subs encntr
		T22.169D	Burn of first degree of unsp scapular region, subs encntr
		T22.191D	Burn 1st deg mult sites of r shldr/up lmb, ex wrs/hnd, subs
		T22.192D	Burn 1st deg mult site of l shldr/up lmb, ex wrs/hnd, subs
		T22.199D	Burn first deg mult sites of shldr/up lmb, ex wrs/hnd, subs
		T22.20XD	Burn second deg of shldr/up lmb, ex wrs/hnd, unsp site, subs
		T22.211D	Burn of second degree of right forearm, subsequent encounter
		T22.212D	Burn of second degree of left forearm, subsequent encounter
		T22.219D	Burn of second degree of unspecified forearm, subs encntr
		T22.221D	Burn of second degree of right elbow, subsequent encounter
		T22.222D	Burn of second degree of left elbow, subsequent encounter
		T22.229D	Burn of second degree of unspecified elbow, subs encntr
		T22.231D	Burn of second degree of right upper arm, subs encntr
		T22.232D	Burn of second degree of left upper arm, subs encntr
		T22.239D	Burn of second degree of unspecified upper arm, subs encntr
		T22.241D	Burn of second degree of right axilla, subsequent encounter
		T22.242D	Burn of second degree of left axilla, subsequent encounter
		T22.249D	Burn of second degree of unspecified axilla, subs encntr
		T22.251D	Burn of second degree of right shoulder, subs encntr
		T22.252D	Burn of second degree of left shoulder, subsequent encounter
		T22.259D	Burn of second degree of unspecified shoulder, subs encntr
	(Continued on next page)	**T22.261D**	Burn of second degree of right scapular region, subs encntr

ICD-9-CM		ICD-10-CM	
V58.89	ENCOUNTER FOR OTHER SPECIFIED AFTERCARE **(Continued)**	**T22.262D**	Burn of second degree of left scapular region, subs encntr
		T22.269D	Burn of second degree of unsp scapular region, subs encntr
		T22.291D	Burn 2nd deg mul sites of r shldr/up lmb, ex wrs/hnd, subs
		T22.292D	Burn 2nd deg mul site of left shldr/up lmb, ex wrs/hnd, subs
		T22.299D	Burn 2nd deg mul sites of shldr/up lmb, except wrs/hnd, subs
		T22.30XD	Burn third deg of shldr/up lmb, ex wrs/hnd, unsp site, subs
		T22.311D	Burn of third degree of right forearm, subsequent encounter
		T22.312D	Burn of third degree of left forearm, subsequent encounter
		T22.319D	Burn of third degree of unspecified forearm, subs encntr
		T22.321D	Burn of third degree of right elbow, subsequent encounter
		T22.322D	Burn of third degree of left elbow, subsequent encounter
		T22.329D	Burn of third degree of unspecified elbow, subs encntr
		T22.331D	Burn of third degree of right upper arm, subs encntr
		T22.332D	Burn of third degree of left upper arm, subsequent encounter
		T22.339D	Burn of third degree of unspecified upper arm, subs encntr
		T22.341D	Burn of third degree of right axilla, subsequent encounter
		T22.342D	Burn of third degree of left axilla, subsequent encounter
		T22.349D	Burn of third degree of unspecified axilla, subs encntr
		T22.351D	Burn of third degree of right shoulder, subsequent encounter
		T22.352D	Burn of third degree of left shoulder, subsequent encounter
		T22.359D	Burn of third degree of unspecified shoulder, subs encntr
		T22.361D	Burn of third degree of right scapular region, subs encntr
		T22.362D	Burn of third degree of left scapular region, subs encntr
		T22.369D	Burn of third degree of unsp scapular region, subs encntr
		T22.391D	Burn 3rd deg mu sites of r shldr/up lmb, ex wrs/hnd, subs
		T22.392D	Burn 3rd deg mu sites of left shldr/up lmb, ex wrs/hnd, subs
		T22.399D	Burn 3rd deg mu sites of shldr/up lmb, except wrs/hnd, subs
		T22.40XD	Corros unsp deg of shldr/up lmb, ex wrs/hnd, unsp site, subs
		T22.411D	Corrosion of unsp degree of right forearm, subs encntr
		T22.412D	Corrosion of unspecified degree of left forearm, subs encntr
		T22.419D	Corrosion of unsp degree of unspecified forearm, subs encntr
		T22.421D	Corrosion of unspecified degree of right elbow, subs encntr
		T22.422D	Corrosion of unspecified degree of left elbow, subs encntr
		T22.429D	Corrosion of unsp degree of unspecified elbow, subs encntr
		T22.431D	Corrosion of unsp degree of right upper arm, subs encntr
		T22.432D	Corrosion of unsp degree of left upper arm, subs encntr
		T22.439D	Corrosion of unsp degree of unsp upper arm, subs encntr
		T22.441D	Corrosion of unspecified degree of right axilla, subs encntr
		T22.442D	Corrosion of unspecified degree of left axilla, subs encntr
		T22.449D	Corrosion of unsp degree of unspecified axilla, subs encntr
		T22.451D	Corrosion of unsp degree of right shoulder, subs encntr
		T22.452D	Corrosion of unsp degree of left shoulder, subs encntr
		T22.459D	Corrosion of unsp degree of unsp shoulder, subs encntr
		T22.461D	Corrosion of unsp degree of right scapular region, subs
		T22.462D	Corrosion of unsp degree of left scapular region, subs
		T22.469D	Corrosion of unsp degree of unsp scapular region, subs
		T22.491D	Corros unsp deg mult site of r shldr/up lmb,ex wrs/hnd, subs
		T22.492D	Corros unsp deg mult site of l shldr/up lmb,ex wrs/hnd, subs
		T22.499D	Corros unsp deg mult sites of shldr/up lmb, ex wrs/hnd, subs
		T22.50XD	Corros first deg of shldr/up lmb, ex wrs/hnd unsp site, subs
		T22.511D	Corrosion of first degree of right forearm, subs encntr
		T22.512D	Corrosion of first degree of left forearm, subs encntr
		T22.519D	Corrosion of first degree of unsp forearm, subs encntr
		T22.521D	Corrosion of first degree of right elbow, subs encntr
		T22.522D	Corrosion of first degree of left elbow, subs encntr
		T22.529D	Corrosion of first degree of unspecified elbow, subs encntr
		T22.531D	Corrosion of first degree of right upper arm, subs encntr
		T22.532D	Corrosion of first degree of left upper arm, subs encntr
		T22.539D	Corrosion of first degree of unsp upper arm, subs encntr
		T22.541D	Corrosion of first degree of right axilla, subs encntr
		T22.542D	Corrosion of first degree of left axilla, subs encntr
		T22.549D	Corrosion of first degree of unspecified axilla, subs encntr
		T22.551D	Corrosion of first degree of right shoulder, subs encntr
		T22.552D	Corrosion of first degree of left shoulder, subs encntr
		T22.559D	Corrosion of first degree of unsp shoulder, subs encntr
		T22.561D	Corrosion of first degree of right scapular region, subs
		T22.562D	Corrosion of first degree of left scapular region, subs
		T22.569D	Corrosion of first degree of unsp scapular region, subs
		T22.591D	Corros 1st deg mult site of r shldr/up lmb, ex wrs/hnd, subs
		T22.592D	Corros 1st deg mult site of l shldr/up lmb, ex wrs/hnd, subs
		T22.599D	Corros 1st deg mult sites of shldr/up lmb, ex wrs/hnd, subs
		T22.60XD	Corros 2nd deg of shldr/up lmb, ex wrs/hnd, unsp site, subs
		T22.611D	Corrosion of second degree of right forearm, subs encntr
		T22.612D	Corrosion of second degree of left forearm, subs encntr
		T22.619D	Corrosion of second degree of unsp forearm, subs encntr
		T22.621D	Corrosion of second degree of right elbow, subs encntr
		T22.622D	Corrosion of second degree of left elbow, subs encntr
		T22.629D	Corrosion of second degree of unspecified elbow, subs encntr
		T22.631D	Corrosion of second degree of right upper arm, subs encntr
		T22.632D	Corrosion of second degree of left upper arm, subs encntr
		T22.639D	Corrosion of second degree of unsp upper arm, subs encntr
		T22.641D	Corrosion of second degree of right axilla, subs encntr
	(Continued on next page)	**T22.642D**	Corrosion of second degree of left axilla, subs encntr

[Brackets] indicate valid character values for each code. Character value meanings provided for each code grouping.

ICD-9-CM		ICD-10-CM	
V58.89	ENCOUNTER FOR OTHER SPECIFIED AFTERCARE **(Continued)**	**T22.649D**	Corrosion of second degree of unsp axilla, subs encntr
		T22.651D	Corrosion of second degree of right shoulder, subs encntr
		T22.652D	Corrosion of second degree of left shoulder, subs encntr
		T22.659D	Corrosion of second degree of unsp shoulder, subs encntr
		T22.661D	Corrosion of second degree of right scapular region, subs
		T22.662D	Corrosion of second degree of left scapular region, subs
		T22.669D	Corrosion of second degree of unsp scapular region, subs
		T22.691D	Corros 2nd deg mul sites of r shldr/up lmb, ex wrs/hnd, subs
		T22.692D	Corros 2nd deg mul site of l shldr/up lmb, ex wrs/hnd, subs
		T22.699D	Corros 2nd deg mul sites of shldr/up lmb, ex wrs/hnd, subs
		T22.70XD	Corros 3rd deg of shldr/up lmb, ex wrs/hnd, unsp site, subs
		T22.711D	Corrosion of third degree of right forearm, subs encntr
		T22.712D	Corrosion of third degree of left forearm, subs encntr
		T22.719D	Corrosion of third degree of unsp forearm, subs encntr
		T22.721D	Corrosion of third degree of right elbow, subs encntr
		T22.722D	Corrosion of third degree of left elbow, subs encntr
		T22.729D	Corrosion of third degree of unspecified elbow, subs encntr
		T22.731D	Corrosion of third degree of right upper arm, subs encntr
		T22.732D	Corrosion of third degree of left upper arm, subs encntr
		T22.739D	Corrosion of third degree of unsp upper arm, subs encntr
		T22.741D	Corrosion of third degree of right axilla, subs encntr
		T22.742D	Corrosion of third degree of left axilla, subs encntr
		T22.749D	Corrosion of third degree of unspecified axilla, subs encntr
		T22.751D	Corrosion of third degree of right shoulder, subs encntr
		T22.752D	Corrosion of third degree of left shoulder, subs encntr
		T22.759D	Corrosion of third degree of unsp shoulder, subs encntr
		T22.761D	Corrosion of third degree of right scapular region, subs
		T22.762D	Corrosion of third degree of left scapular region, subs
		T22.769D	Corrosion of third degree of unsp scapular region, subs
		T22.791D	Corros 3rd deg mu sites of r shldr/up lmb, ex wrs/hnd, subs
		T22.792D	Corros 3rd deg mu site of l shldr/up lmb, ex wrs/hnd, subs
		T22.799D	Corros 3rd deg mu sites of shldr/up lmb, ex wrs/hnd, subs
		T23.001D	Burn of unsp degree of right hand, unsp site, subs encntr
		T23.002D	Burn of unsp degree of left hand, unsp site, subs encntr
		T23.009D	Burn of unsp degree of unsp hand, unsp site, subs encntr
		T23.011D	Burn of unsp degree of right thumb (nail), subs encntr
		T23.012D	Burn of unspecified degree of left thumb (nail), subs encntr
		T23.019D	Burn of unsp degree of unspecified thumb (nail), subs encntr
		T23.021D	Burn unsp degree of single r finger except thumb, subs
		T23.022D	Burn unsp degree of single l finger except thumb, subs
		T23.029D	Burn unsp degree of unsp single finger except thumb, subs
		T23.031D	Burn unsp deg mult right fingers (nail), not inc thumb, subs
		T23.032D	Burn unsp deg mult left fingers (nail), not inc thumb, subs
		T23.039D	Burn unsp degree of unsp mult fngr, not inc thumb, subs
		T23.041D	Burn of unsp deg mult right fingers (nail), inc thumb, subs
		T23.042D	Burn of unsp deg mult left fingers (nail), inc thumb, subs
		T23.049D	Burn unsp degree of unsp mult fngr (nail), inc thumb, subs
		T23.051D	Burn of unspecified degree of right palm, subs encntr
		T23.052D	Burn of unspecified degree of left palm, subs encntr
		T23.059D	Burn of unspecified degree of unspecified palm, subs encntr
		T23.061D	Burn of unsp degree of back of right hand, subs encntr
		T23.062D	Burn of unspecified degree of back of left hand, subs encntr
		T23.069D	Burn of unsp degree of back of unspecified hand, subs encntr
		T23.071D	Burn of unspecified degree of right wrist, subs encntr
		T23.072D	Burn of unspecified degree of left wrist, subs encntr
		T23.079D	Burn of unspecified degree of unspecified wrist, subs encntr
		T23.091D	Burn of unsp deg mult sites of right wrist and hand, subs
		T23.092D	Burn of unsp deg mult sites of left wrist and hand, subs
		T23.099D	Burn of unsp deg mult sites of unsp wrist and hand, subs
		T23.101D	Burn of first degree of right hand, unsp site, subs encntr
		T23.102D	Burn of first degree of left hand, unsp site, subs encntr
		T23.109D	Burn of first degree of unsp hand, unsp site, subs encntr
		T23.111D	Burn of first degree of right thumb (nail), subs encntr
		T23.112D	Burn of first degree of left thumb (nail), subs encntr
		T23.119D	Burn of first degree of unsp thumb (nail), subs encntr
		T23.121D	Burn first degree of single r finger except thumb, subs
		T23.122D	Burn first degree of single l finger except thumb, subs
		T23.129D	Burn first degree of unsp single finger except thumb, subs
		T23.131D	Burn first deg mult right fngr (nail), not inc thumb, subs
		T23.132D	Burn first deg mult left fingers (nail), not inc thumb, subs
		T23.139D	Burn first degree of unsp mult fngr, not inc thumb, subs
		T23.141D	Burn of first deg mult right fingers (nail), inc thumb, subs
		T23.142D	Burn of first deg mult left fingers (nail), inc thumb, subs
		T23.149D	Burn first degree of unsp mult fngr (nail), inc thumb, subs
		T23.151D	Burn of first degree of right palm, subsequent encounter
		T23.152D	Burn of first degree of left palm, subsequent encounter
		T23.159D	Burn of first degree of unspecified palm, subs encntr
		T23.161D	Burn of first degree of back of right hand, subs encntr
		T23.162D	Burn of first degree of back of left hand, subs encntr
		T23.169D	Burn of first degree of back of unsp hand, subs encntr
		T23.171D	Burn of first degree of right wrist, subsequent encounter
		T23.172D	Burn of first degree of left wrist, subsequent encounter
	(Continued on next page)	**T23.179D**	Burn of first degree of unspecified wrist, subs encntr

ICD-9-CM		ICD-10-CM	
V58.89	ENCOUNTER FOR OTHER SPECIFIED AFTERCARE **(Continued)**	**T23.191D**	Burn of first deg mult sites of right wrist and hand, subs
		T23.192D	Burn of first deg mult sites of left wrist and hand, subs
		T23.199D	Burn of first deg mult sites of unsp wrist and hand, subs
		T23.201D	Burn of second degree of right hand, unsp site, subs encntr
		T23.202D	Burn of second degree of left hand, unsp site, subs encntr
		T23.209D	Burn of second degree of unsp hand, unsp site, subs encntr
		T23.211D	Burn of second degree of right thumb (nail), subs encntr
		T23.212D	Burn of second degree of left thumb (nail), subs encntr
		T23.219D	Burn of second degree of unsp thumb (nail), subs encntr
		T23.221D	Burn second degree of single r finger except thumb, subs
		T23.222D	Burn second degree of single l finger except thumb, subs
		T23.229D	Burn second degree of unsp single finger except thumb, subs
		T23.231D	Burn 2nd deg mul right fingers (nail), not inc thumb, subs
		T23.232D	Burn of 2nd deg mul left fingers (nail), not inc thumb, subs
		T23.239D	Burn second degree of unsp mult fngr, not inc thumb, subs
		T23.241D	Burn of 2nd deg mul right fingers (nail), inc thumb, subs
		T23.242D	Burn of 2nd deg mul left fingers (nail), inc thumb, subs
		T23.249D	Burn second degree of unsp mult fngr (nail), inc thumb, subs
		T23.251D	Burn of second degree of right palm, subsequent encounter
		T23.252D	Burn of second degree of left palm, subsequent encounter
		T23.259D	Burn of second degree of unspecified palm, subs encntr
		T23.261D	Burn of second degree of back of right hand, subs encntr
		T23.262D	Burn of second degree of back of left hand, subs encntr
		T23.269D	Burn of second degree of back of unsp hand, subs encntr
		T23.271D	Burn of second degree of right wrist, subsequent encounter
		T23.272D	Burn of second degree of left wrist, subsequent encounter
		T23.279D	Burn of second degree of unspecified wrist, subs encntr
		T23.291D	Burn of 2nd deg mul sites of right wrist and hand, subs
		T23.292D	Burn of 2nd deg mul sites of left wrist and hand, subs
		T23.299D	Burn of 2nd deg mul sites of unsp wrist and hand, subs
		T23.301D	Burn of third degree of right hand, unsp site, subs encntr
		T23.302D	Burn of third degree of left hand, unsp site, subs encntr
		T23.309D	Burn of third degree of unsp hand, unsp site, subs encntr
		T23.311D	Burn of third degree of right thumb (nail), subs encntr
		T23.312D	Burn of third degree of left thumb (nail), subs encntr
		T23.319D	Burn of third degree of unsp thumb (nail), subs encntr
		T23.321D	Burn third degree of single r finger except thumb, subs
		T23.322D	Burn third degree of single l finger except thumb, subs
		T23.329D	Burn third degree of unsp single finger except thumb, subs
		T23.331D	Burn of 3rd deg mu right fingers (nail), not inc thumb, subs
		T23.332D	Burn of 3rd deg mu left fingers (nail), not inc thumb, subs
		T23.339D	Burn third degree of unsp mult fngr, not inc thumb, subs
		T23.341D	Burn of 3rd deg mu right fingers (nail), inc thumb, subs
		T23.342D	Burn of 3rd deg mu left fingers (nail), inc thumb, subs
		T23.349D	Burn third degree of unsp mult fngr (nail), inc thumb, subs
		T23.351D	Burn of third degree of right palm, subsequent encounter
		T23.352D	Burn of third degree of left palm, subsequent encounter
		T23.359D	Burn of third degree of unspecified palm, subs encntr
		T23.361D	Burn of third degree of back of right hand, subs encntr
		T23.362D	Burn of third degree of back of left hand, subs encntr
		T23.369D	Burn of third degree of back of unsp hand, subs encntr
		T23.371D	Burn of third degree of right wrist, subsequent encounter
		T23.372D	Burn of third degree of left wrist, subsequent encounter
		T23.379D	Burn of third degree of unspecified wrist, subs encntr
		T23.391D	Burn of 3rd deg mu sites of right wrist and hand, subs
		T23.392D	Burn of 3rd deg mu sites of left wrist and hand, subs
		T23.399D	Burn of 3rd deg mu sites of unsp wrist and hand, subs
		T23.401D	Corrosion of unsp degree of right hand, unsp site, subs
		T23.402D	Corrosion of unsp degree of left hand, unsp site, subs
		T23.409D	Corrosion of unsp degree of unsp hand, unsp site, subs
		T23.411D	Corrosion of unsp degree of right thumb (nail), subs encntr
		T23.412D	Corrosion of unsp degree of left thumb (nail), subs encntr
		T23.419D	Corrosion of unsp degree of unsp thumb (nail), subs encntr
		T23.421D	Corros unsp degree of single r finger except thumb, subs
		T23.422D	Corros unsp degree of single l finger except thumb, subs
		T23.429D	Corros unsp degree of unsp single finger except thumb, subs
		T23.431D	Corros unsp deg mult right fngr (nail), not inc thumb, subs
		T23.432D	Corros unsp deg mult left fngr (nail), not inc thumb, subs
		T23.439D	Corros unsp degree of unsp mult fngr, not inc thumb, subs
		T23.441D	Corros unsp deg mult right fingers (nail), inc thumb, subs
		T23.442D	Corros unsp deg mult left fingers (nail), inc thumb, subs
		T23.449D	Corros unsp degree of unsp mult fngr (nail), inc thumb, subs
		T23.451D	Corrosion of unspecified degree of right palm, subs encntr
		T23.452D	Corrosion of unspecified degree of left palm, subs encntr
		T23.459D	Corrosion of unsp degree of unspecified palm, subs encntr
		T23.461D	Corrosion of unsp degree of back of right hand, subs encntr
		T23.462D	Corrosion of unsp degree of back of left hand, subs encntr
		T23.469D	Corrosion of unsp degree of back of unsp hand, subs encntr
		T23.471D	Corrosion of unspecified degree of right wrist, subs encntr
		T23.472D	Corrosion of unspecified degree of left wrist, subs encntr
		T23.479D	Corrosion of unsp degree of unspecified wrist, subs encntr
		T23.491D	Corrosion of unsp deg mult sites of right wrs/hnd, subs
	(Continued on next page)	**T23.492D**	Corrosion of unsp deg mult sites of left wrs/hnd, subs

ICD-9-CM		ICD-10-CM	
V58.89	ENCOUNTER FOR OTHER SPECIFIED AFTERCARE **(Continued)**	**T23.499D**	Corrosion of unsp deg mult sites of unsp wrs/hnd, subs
		T23.501D	Corrosion of first degree of right hand, unsp site, subs
		T23.502D	Corrosion of first degree of left hand, unsp site, subs
		T23.509D	Corrosion of first degree of unsp hand, unsp site, subs
		T23.511D	Corrosion of first degree of right thumb (nail), subs encntr
		T23.512D	Corrosion of first degree of left thumb (nail), subs encntr
		T23.519D	Corrosion of first degree of unsp thumb (nail), subs encntr
		T23.521D	Corros first degree of single r finger except thumb, subs
		T23.522D	Corros first degree of single l finger except thumb, subs
		T23.529D	Corros first degree of unsp single finger except thumb, subs
		T23.531D	Corros first deg mult right fngr (nail), not inc thumb, subs
		T23.532D	Corros first deg mult left fngr (nail), not inc thumb, subs
		T23.539D	Corros first degree of unsp mult fngr, not inc thumb, subs
		T23.541D	Corros first deg mult right fingers (nail), inc thumb, subs
		T23.542D	Corros first deg mult left fingers (nail), inc thumb, subs
		T23.549D	Corros first degree of unsp mult fngr, inc thumb, subs
		T23.551D	Corrosion of first degree of right palm, subs encntr
		T23.552D	Corrosion of first degree of left palm, subsequent encounter
		T23.559D	Corrosion of first degree of unspecified palm, subs encntr
		T23.561D	Corrosion of first degree of back of right hand, subs encntr
		T23.562D	Corrosion of first degree of back of left hand, subs encntr
		T23.569D	Corrosion of first degree of back of unsp hand, subs encntr
		T23.571D	Corrosion of first degree of right wrist, subs encntr
		T23.572D	Corrosion of first degree of left wrist, subs encntr
		T23.579D	Corrosion of first degree of unspecified wrist, subs encntr
		T23.591D	Corrosion of first deg mult sites of right wrs/hnd, subs
		T23.592D	Corrosion of first deg mult sites of left wrs/hnd, subs
		T23.599D	Corrosion of first deg mult sites of unsp wrs/hnd, subs
		T23.601D	Corrosion of second degree of right hand, unsp site, subs
		T23.602D	Corrosion of second degree of left hand, unsp site, subs
		T23.609D	Corrosion of second degree of unsp hand, unsp site, subs
		T23.611D	Corrosion of second degree of right thumb (nail), subs
		T23.612D	Corrosion of second degree of left thumb (nail), subs encntr
		T23.619D	Corrosion of second degree of unsp thumb (nail), subs encntr
		T23.621D	Corros second degree of single r finger except thumb, subs
		T23.622D	Corros second degree of single l finger except thumb, subs
		T23.629D	Corros second deg of unsp single finger except thumb, subs
		T23.631D	Corros 2nd deg mul right fingers (nail), not inc thumb, subs
		T23.632D	Corros 2nd deg mul left fingers (nail), not inc thumb, subs
		T23.639D	Corros second degree of unsp mult fngr, not inc thumb, subs
		T23.641D	Corros 2nd deg mul right fingers (nail), inc thumb, subs
		T23.642D	Corros 2nd deg mul left fingers (nail), inc thumb, subs
		T23.649D	Corros second degree of unsp mult fngr, inc thumb, subs
		T23.651D	Corrosion of second degree of right palm, subs encntr
		T23.652D	Corrosion of second degree of left palm, subs encntr
		T23.659D	Corrosion of second degree of unspecified palm, subs encntr
		T23.661D	Corrosion of second degree back of right hand, subs encntr
		T23.662D	Corrosion of second degree back of left hand, subs encntr
		T23.669D	Corrosion of second degree back of unsp hand, subs encntr
		T23.671D	Corrosion of second degree of right wrist, subs encntr
		T23.672D	Corrosion of second degree of left wrist, subs encntr
		T23.679D	Corrosion of second degree of unspecified wrist, subs encntr
		T23.691D	Corrosion of 2nd deg mul sites of right wrist and hand, subs
		T23.692D	Corrosion of 2nd deg mul sites of left wrist and hand, subs
		T23.699D	Corrosion of 2nd deg mul sites of unsp wrist and hand, subs
		T23.701D	Corrosion of third degree of right hand, unsp site, subs
		T23.702D	Corrosion of third degree of left hand, unsp site, subs
		T23.709D	Corrosion of third degree of unsp hand, unsp site, subs
		T23.711D	Corrosion of third degree of right thumb (nail), subs encntr
		T23.712D	Corrosion of third degree of left thumb (nail), subs encntr
		T23.719D	Corrosion of third degree of unsp thumb (nail), subs encntr
		T23.721D	Corros third degree of single r finger except thumb, subs
		T23.722D	Corros third degree of single l finger except thumb, subs
		T23.729D	Corros third degree of unsp single finger except thumb, subs
		T23.731D	Corros 3rd deg mu right fingers (nail), not inc thumb, subs
		T23.732D	Corros 3rd deg mu left fingers (nail), not inc thumb, subs
		T23.739D	Corros third degree of unsp mult fngr, not inc thumb, subs
		T23.741D	Corros 3rd deg mu right fingers (nail), inc thumb, subs
		T23.742D	Corros 3rd deg mu left fingers (nail), including thumb, subs
		T23.749D	Corros third degree of unsp mult fngr, inc thumb, subs
		T23.751D	Corrosion of third degree of right palm, subs encntr
		T23.752D	Corrosion of third degree of left palm, subsequent encounter
		T23.759D	Corrosion of third degree of unspecified palm, subs encntr
		T23.761D	Corrosion of third degree of back of right hand, subs encntr
		T23.762D	Corrosion of third degree of back of left hand, subs encntr
		T23.769D	Corrosion of third degree back of unsp hand, subs encntr
		T23.771D	Corrosion of third degree of right wrist, subs encntr
		T23.772D	Corrosion of third degree of left wrist, subs encntr
		T23.779D	Corrosion of third degree of unspecified wrist, subs encntr
		T23.791D	Corrosion of 3rd deg mu sites of right wrist and hand, subs
		T23.792D	Corrosion of 3rd deg mu sites of left wrist and hand, subs
		T23.799D	Corrosion of 3rd deg mu sites of unsp wrist and hand, subs
	(Continued on next page)	**T24.001D**	Burn unsp deg of unsp site right lower limb, ex ank/ft, subs

ICD-9-CM		ICD-10-CM	
V58.89	ENCOUNTER FOR OTHER SPECIFIED AFTERCARE **(Continued)**	**T24.ØØ2D**	Burn unsp deg of unsp site left lower limb, ex ank/ft, subs
		T24.ØØ9D	Burn unsp deg of unsp site unsp lower limb, ex ank/ft, subs
		T24.Ø11D	Burn of unspecified degree of right thigh, subs encntr
		T24.Ø12D	Burn of unspecified degree of left thigh, subs encntr
		T24.Ø19D	Burn of unspecified degree of unspecified thigh, subs encntr
		T24.Ø21D	Burn of unspecified degree of right knee, subs encntr
		T24.Ø22D	Burn of unspecified degree of left knee, subs encntr
		T24.Ø29D	Burn of unspecified degree of unspecified knee, subs encntr
		T24.Ø31D	Burn of unspecified degree of right lower leg, subs encntr
		T24.Ø32D	Burn of unspecified degree of left lower leg, subs encntr
		T24.Ø39D	Burn of unsp degree of unspecified lower leg, subs encntr
		T24.Ø91D	Burn unsp deg mult sites of right low limb, ex ank/ft, subs
		T24.Ø92D	Burn unsp deg mult sites of left lower limb, ex ank/ft, subs
		T24.Ø99D	Burn unsp deg mult sites of unsp lower limb, ex ank/ft, subs
		T24.1Ø1D	Burn 1st deg of unsp site right lower limb, ex ank/ft, subs
		T24.1Ø2D	Burn first deg of unsp site left lower limb, ex ank/ft, subs
		T24.1Ø9D	Burn first deg of unsp site unsp lower limb, ex ank/ft, subs
		T24.111D	Burn of first degree of right thigh, subsequent encounter
		T24.112D	Burn of first degree of left thigh, subsequent encounter
		T24.119D	Burn of first degree of unspecified thigh, subs encntr
		T24.121D	Burn of first degree of right knee, subsequent encounter
		T24.122D	Burn of first degree of left knee, subsequent encounter
		T24.129D	Burn of first degree of unspecified knee, subs encntr
		T24.131D	Burn of first degree of right lower leg, subs encntr
		T24.132D	Burn of first degree of left lower leg, subsequent encounter
		T24.139D	Burn of first degree of unspecified lower leg, subs encntr
		T24.191D	Burn 1st deg mult sites of right lower limb, ex ank/ft, subs
		T24.192D	Burn 1st deg mult sites of left lower limb, ex ank/ft, subs
		T24.199D	Burn 1st deg mult sites of unsp lower limb, ex ank/ft, subs
		T24.2Ø1D	Burn 2nd deg of unsp site right lower limb, ex ank/ft, subs
		T24.2Ø2D	Burn 2nd deg of unsp site left lower limb, ex ank/ft, subs
		T24.2Ø9D	Burn 2nd deg of unsp site unsp lower limb, ex ank/ft, subs
		T24.211D	Burn of second degree of right thigh, subsequent encounter
		T24.212D	Burn of second degree of left thigh, subsequent encounter
		T24.219D	Burn of second degree of unspecified thigh, subs encntr
		T24.221D	Burn of second degree of right knee, subsequent encounter
		T24.222D	Burn of second degree of left knee, subsequent encounter
		T24.229D	Burn of second degree of unspecified knee, subs encntr
		T24.231D	Burn of second degree of right lower leg, subs encntr
		T24.232D	Burn of second degree of left lower leg, subs encntr
		T24.239D	Burn of second degree of unspecified lower leg, subs encntr
		T24.291D	Burn 2nd deg mul sites of right lower limb, ex ank/ft, subs
		T24.292D	Burn 2nd deg mul sites of left lower limb, ex ank/ft, subs
		T24.299D	Burn 2nd deg mul sites of unsp lower limb, ex ank/ft, subs
		T24.3Ø1D	Burn third deg of unsp site right low limb, ex ank/ft, subs
		T24.3Ø2D	Burn third deg of unsp site left lower limb, ex ank/ft, subs
		T24.3Ø9D	Burn third deg of unsp site unsp lower limb, ex ank/ft, subs
		T24.311D	Burn of third degree of right thigh, subsequent encounter
		T24.312D	Burn of third degree of left thigh, subsequent encounter
		T24.319D	Burn of third degree of unspecified thigh, subs encntr
		T24.321D	Burn of third degree of right knee, subsequent encounter
		T24.322D	Burn of third degree of left knee, subsequent encounter
		T24.329D	Burn of third degree of unspecified knee, subs encntr
		T24.331D	Burn of third degree of right lower leg, subs encntr
		T24.332D	Burn of third degree of left lower leg, subsequent encounter
		T24.339D	Burn of third degree of unspecified lower leg, subs encntr
		T24.391D	Burn 3rd deg mu sites of right lower limb, ex ank/ft, subs
		T24.392D	Burn 3rd deg mu sites of left lower limb, ex ank/ft, subs
		T24.399D	Burn 3rd deg mu sites of unsp lower limb, ex ank/ft, subs
		T24.4Ø1D	Corros unsp deg of unsp site right low limb, ex ank/ft, subs
		T24.4Ø2D	Corros unsp deg of unsp site left low limb, ex ank/ft, subs
		T24.4Ø9D	Corros unsp deg of unsp site unsp low limb, ex ank/ft, subs
		T24.411D	Corrosion of unspecified degree of right thigh, subs encntr
		T24.412D	Corrosion of unspecified degree of left thigh, subs encntr
		T24.419D	Corrosion of unsp degree of unspecified thigh, subs encntr
		T24.421D	Corrosion of unspecified degree of right knee, subs encntr
		T24.422D	Corrosion of unspecified degree of left knee, subs encntr
		T24.429D	Corrosion of unsp degree of unspecified knee, subs encntr
		T24.431D	Corrosion of unsp degree of right lower leg, subs encntr
		T24.432D	Corrosion of unsp degree of left lower leg, subs encntr
		T24.439D	Corrosion of unsp degree of unsp lower leg, subs encntr
		T24.491D	Corros unsp deg mult sites of r low limb, ex ank/ft, subs
		T24.492D	Corros unsp deg mult sites of left low limb, ex ank/ft, subs
		T24.499D	Corros unsp deg mult sites of unsp low limb, ex ank/ft, subs
		T24.5Ø1D	Corros 1st deg of unsp site right low limb, ex ank/ft, subs
		T24.5Ø2D	Corros 1st deg of unsp site left lower limb, ex ank/ft, subs
		T24.5Ø9D	Corros 1st deg of unsp site unsp lower limb, ex ank/ft, subs
		T24.511D	Corrosion of first degree of right thigh, subs encntr
		T24.512D	Corrosion of first degree of left thigh, subs encntr
		T24.519D	Corrosion of first degree of unspecified thigh, subs encntr
		T24.521D	Corrosion of first degree of right knee, subs encntr
		T24.522D	Corrosion of first degree of left knee, subsequent encounter
	(Continued on next page)	**T24.529D**	Corrosion of first degree of unspecified knee, subs encntr

ICD-9-CM		ICD-10-CM	
V58.89	ENCOUNTER FOR OTHER SPECIFIED AFTERCARE **(Continued)**	**T24.531D**	Corrosion of first degree of right lower leg, subs encntr
		T24.532D	Corrosion of first degree of left lower leg, subs encntr
		T24.539D	Corrosion of first degree of unsp lower leg, subs encntr
		T24.591D	Corros 1st deg mult sites of right low limb, ex ank/ft, subs
		T24.592D	Corros 1st deg mult sites of left low limb, ex ank/ft, subs
		T24.599D	Corros 1st deg mult sites of unsp low limb, ex ank/ft, subs
		T24.6Ø1D	Corros 2nd deg of unsp site right low limb, ex ank/ft, subs
		T24.6Ø2D	Corros 2nd deg of unsp site left lower limb, ex ank/ft, subs
		T24.6Ø9D	Corros 2nd deg of unsp site unsp lower limb, ex ank/ft, subs
		T24.611D	Corrosion of second degree of right thigh, subs encntr
		T24.612D	Corrosion of second degree of left thigh, subs encntr
		T24.619D	Corrosion of second degree of unspecified thigh, subs encntr
		T24.621D	Corrosion of second degree of right knee, subs encntr
		T24.622D	Corrosion of second degree of left knee, subs encntr
		T24.629D	Corrosion of second degree of unspecified knee, subs encntr
		T24.631D	Corrosion of second degree of right lower leg, subs encntr
		T24.632D	Corrosion of second degree of left lower leg, subs encntr
		T24.639D	Corrosion of second degree of unsp lower leg, subs encntr
		T24.691D	Corros 2nd deg mul sites of right low limb, ex ank/ft, subs
		T24.692D	Corros 2nd deg mul sites of left lower limb, ex ank/ft, subs
		T24.699D	Corros 2nd deg mul sites of unsp lower limb, ex ank/ft, subs
		T24.7Ø1D	Corros third deg of unsp site r low limb, ex ank/ft, subs
		T24.7Ø2D	Corros third deg of unsp site left low limb, ex ank/ft, subs
		T24.7Ø9D	Corros third deg of unsp site unsp low limb, ex ank/ft, subs
		T24.711D	Corrosion of third degree of right thigh, subs encntr
		T24.712D	Corrosion of third degree of left thigh, subs encntr
		T24.719D	Corrosion of third degree of unspecified thigh, subs encntr
		T24.721D	Corrosion of third degree of right knee, subs encntr
		T24.722D	Corrosion of third degree of left knee, subsequent encounter
		T24.729D	Corrosion of third degree of unspecified knee, subs encntr
		T24.731D	Corrosion of third degree of right lower leg, subs encntr
		T24.732D	Corrosion of third degree of left lower leg, subs encntr
		T24.739D	Corrosion of third degree of unsp lower leg, subs encntr
		T24.791D	Corros 3rd deg mu sites of right lower limb, ex ank/ft, subs
		T24.792D	Corros 3rd deg mu sites of left lower limb, ex ank/ft, subs
		T24.799D	Corros 3rd deg mu sites of unsp lower limb, ex ank/ft, subs
		T25.Ø11D	Burn of unspecified degree of right ankle, subs encntr
		T25.Ø12D	Burn of unspecified degree of left ankle, subs encntr
		T25.Ø19D	Burn of unspecified degree of unspecified ankle, subs encntr
		T25.Ø21D	Burn of unspecified degree of right foot, subs encntr
		T25.Ø22D	Burn of unspecified degree of left foot, subs encntr
		T25.Ø29D	Burn of unspecified degree of unspecified foot, subs encntr
		T25.Ø31D	Burn of unsp degree of right toe(s) (nail), subs encntr
		T25.Ø32D	Burn of unsp degree of left toe(s) (nail), subs encntr
		T25.Ø39D	Burn of unsp degree of unsp toe(s) (nail), subs encntr
		T25.Ø91D	Burn of unsp deg mult sites of right ankle and foot, subs
		T25.Ø92D	Burn of unsp deg mult sites of left ankle and foot, subs
		T25.Ø99D	Burn of unsp deg mult sites of unsp ankle and foot, subs
		T25.111D	Burn of first degree of right ankle, subsequent encounter
		T25.112D	Burn of first degree of left ankle, subsequent encounter
		T25.119D	Burn of first degree of unspecified ankle, subs encntr
		T25.121D	Burn of first degree of right foot, subsequent encounter
		T25.122D	Burn of first degree of left foot, subsequent encounter
		T25.129D	Burn of first degree of unspecified foot, subs encntr
		T25.131D	Burn of first degree of right toe(s) (nail), subs encntr
		T25.132D	Burn of first degree of left toe(s) (nail), subs encntr
		T25.139D	Burn of first degree of unsp toe(s) (nail), subs encntr
		T25.191D	Burn of first deg mult sites of right ankle and foot, subs
		T25.192D	Burn of first deg mult sites of left ankle and foot, subs
		T25.199D	Burn of first deg mult sites of unsp ankle and foot, subs
		T25.211D	Burn of second degree of right ankle, subsequent encounter
		T25.212D	Burn of second degree of left ankle, subsequent encounter
		T25.219D	Burn of second degree of unspecified ankle, subs encntr
		T25.221D	Burn of second degree of right foot, subsequent encounter
		T25.222D	Burn of second degree of left foot, subsequent encounter
		T25.229D	Burn of second degree of unspecified foot, subs encntr
		T25.231D	Burn of second degree of right toe(s) (nail), subs encntr
		T25.232D	Burn of second degree of left toe(s) (nail), subs encntr
		T25.239D	Burn of second degree of unsp toe(s) (nail), subs encntr
		T25.291D	Burn of 2nd deg mul sites of right ankle and foot, subs
		T25.292D	Burn of 2nd deg mul sites of left ankle and foot, subs
		T25.299D	Burn of 2nd deg mul sites of unsp ankle and foot, subs
		T25.311D	Burn of third degree of right ankle, subsequent encounter
		T25.312D	Burn of third degree of left ankle, subsequent encounter
		T25.319D	Burn of third degree of unspecified ankle, subs encntr
		T25.321D	Burn of third degree of right foot, subsequent encounter
		T25.322D	Burn of third degree of left foot, subsequent encounter
		T25.329D	Burn of third degree of unspecified foot, subs encntr
		T25.331D	Burn of third degree of right toe(s) (nail), subs encntr
		T25.332D	Burn of third degree of left toe(s) (nail), subs encntr
		T25.339D	Burn of third degree of unsp toe(s) (nail), subs encntr
		T25.391D	Burn of 3rd deg mu sites of right ankle and foot, subs
	(Continued on next page)	**T25.392D**	Burn of 3rd deg mu sites of left ankle and foot, subs

ICD-9-CM		ICD-10-CM	
V58.89	ENCOUNTER FOR OTHER SPECIFIED AFTERCARE **(Continued)**	**T25.399D**	Burn of 3rd deg mu sites of unsp ankle and foot, subs
		T25.411D	Corrosion of unspecified degree of right ankle, subs encntr
		T25.412D	Corrosion of unspecified degree of left ankle, subs encntr
		T25.419D	Corrosion of unsp degree of unspecified ankle, subs encntr
		T25.421D	Corrosion of unspecified degree of right foot, subs encntr
		T25.422D	Corrosion of unspecified degree of left foot, subs encntr
		T25.429D	Corrosion of unsp degree of unspecified foot, subs encntr
		T25.431D	Corrosion of unsp degree of right toe(s) (nail), subs encntr
		T25.432D	Corrosion of unsp degree of left toe(s) (nail), subs encntr
		T25.439D	Corrosion of unsp degree of unsp toe(s) (nail), subs encntr
		T25.491D	Corrosion of unsp deg mult sites of right ank/ft, subs
		T25.492D	Corrosion of unsp deg mult sites of left ank/ft, subs
		T25.499D	Corrosion of unsp deg mult sites of unsp ank/ft, subs
		T25.511D	Corrosion of first degree of right ankle, subs encntr
		T25.512D	Corrosion of first degree of left ankle, subs encntr
		T25.519D	Corrosion of first degree of unspecified ankle, subs encntr
		T25.521D	Corrosion of first degree of right foot, subs encntr
		T25.522D	Corrosion of first degree of left foot, subsequent encounter
		T25.529D	Corrosion of first degree of unspecified foot, subs encntr
		T25.531D	Corrosion of first degree of right toe(s) (nail), subs
		T25.532D	Corrosion of first degree of left toe(s) (nail), subs encntr
		T25.539D	Corrosion of first degree of unsp toe(s) (nail), subs encntr
		T25.591D	Corrosion of first deg mult sites of right ank/ft, subs
		T25.592D	Corrosion of first deg mult sites of left ank/ft, subs
		T25.599D	Corrosion of first deg mult sites of unsp ank/ft, subs
		T25.611D	Corrosion of second degree of right ankle, subs encntr
		T25.612D	Corrosion of second degree of left ankle, subs encntr
		T25.619D	Corrosion of second degree of unspecified ankle, subs encntr
		T25.621D	Corrosion of second degree of right foot, subs encntr
		T25.622D	Corrosion of second degree of left foot, subs encntr
		T25.629D	Corrosion of second degree of unspecified foot, subs encntr
		T25.631D	Corrosion of second degree of right toe(s) (nail), subs
		T25.632D	Corrosion of second degree of left toe(s) (nail), subs
		T25.639D	Corrosion of second degree of unsp toe(s) (nail), subs
		T25.691D	Corrosion of second degree of right ankle and foot, subs
		T25.692D	Corrosion of second degree of left ankle and foot, subs
		T25.699D	Corrosion of second degree of unsp ankle and foot, subs
		T25.711D	Corrosion of third degree of right ankle, subs encntr
		T25.712D	Corrosion of third degree of left ankle, subs encntr
		T25.719D	Corrosion of third degree of unspecified ankle, subs encntr
		T25.721D	Corrosion of third degree of right foot, subs encntr
		T25.722D	Corrosion of third degree of left foot, subsequent encounter
		T25.729D	Corrosion of third degree of unspecified foot, subs encntr
		T25.731D	Corrosion of third degree of right toe(s) (nail), subs
		T25.732D	Corrosion of third degree of left toe(s) (nail), subs encntr
		T25.739D	Corrosion of third degree of unsp toe(s) (nail), subs encntr
		T25.791D	Corrosion of 3rd deg mu sites of right ankle and foot, subs
		T25.792D	Corrosion of 3rd deg mu sites of left ankle and foot, subs
		T25.799D	Corrosion of 3rd deg mu sites of unsp ankle and foot, subs
		T26.00XD	Burn of unspecified eyelid and periocular area, subs encntr
		T26.01XD	Burn of right eyelid and periocular area, subs encntr
		T26.02XD	Burn of left eyelid and periocular area, subs encntr
		T26.10XD	Burn of cornea and conjunctival sac, unsp eye, subs encntr
		T26.11XD	Burn of cornea and conjunctival sac, right eye, subs encntr
		T26.12XD	Burn of cornea and conjunctival sac, left eye, subs encntr
		T26.20XD	Burn w resulting rupture and dest of unsp eyeball, subs
		T26.21XD	Burn w resulting rupture and dest of right eyeball, subs
		T26.22XD	Burn w resulting rupture and dest of left eyeball, subs
		T26.30XD	Burns of oth parts of unsp eye and adnexa, subs encntr
		T26.31XD	Burns of oth parts of right eye and adnexa, subs encntr
		T26.32XD	Burns of oth parts of left eye and adnexa, subs encntr
		T26.40XD	Burn of unsp eye and adnexa, part unspecified, subs encntr
		T26.41XD	Burn of right eye and adnexa, part unspecified, subs encntr
		T26.42XD	Burn of left eye and adnexa, part unspecified, subs encntr
		T26.50XD	Corrosion of unsp eyelid and periocular area, subs encntr
		T26.51XD	Corrosion of right eyelid and periocular area, subs encntr
		T26.52XD	Corrosion of left eyelid and periocular area, subs encntr
		T26.60XD	Corrosion of cornea and conjunctival sac, unsp eye, subs
		T26.61XD	Corrosion of cornea and conjunctival sac, right eye, subs
		T26.62XD	Corrosion of cornea and conjunctival sac, left eye, subs
		T26.70XD	Corrosion w resulting rupture and dest of unsp eyeball, subs
		T26.71XD	Corros w resulting rupture and dest of right eyeball, subs
		T26.72XD	Corrosion w resulting rupture and dest of left eyeball, subs
		T26.80XD	Corrosions of oth parts of unsp eye and adnexa, subs encntr
		T26.81XD	Corrosions of oth parts of right eye and adnexa, subs encntr
		T26.82XD	Corrosions of oth parts of left eye and adnexa, subs encntr
		T26.90XD	Corrosion of unsp eye and adnexa, part unsp, subs encntr
		T26.91XD	Corrosion of right eye and adnexa, part unsp, subs encntr
		T26.92XD	Corrosion of left eye and adnexa, part unsp, subs encntr
		T27.0XXD	Burn of larynx and trachea, subsequent encounter
		T27.1XXD	Burn involving larynx and trachea with lung, subs encntr
		T27.2XXD	Burn of other parts of respiratory tract, subs encntr
	(Continued on next page)	**T27.3XXD**	Burn of respiratory tract, part unspecified, subs encntr

ICD-9-CM		ICD-10-CM	
V58.89	ENCOUNTER FOR OTHER SPECIFIED AFTERCARE **(Continued)**	**T27.4XXD**	Corrosion of larynx and trachea, subsequent encounter
		T27.5XXD	Corrosion involving larynx and trachea w lung, subs encntr
		T27.6XXD	Corrosion of other parts of respiratory tract, subs encntr
		T27.7XXD	Corrosion of respiratory tract, part unsp, subs encntr
		T28.ØXXD	Burn of mouth and pharynx, subsequent encounter
		T28.1XXD	Burn of esophagus, subsequent encounter
		T28.2XXD	Burn of other parts of alimentary tract, subs encntr
		T28.3XXD	Burn of internal genitourinary organs, subsequent encounter
		T28.4ØXD	Burn of unspecified internal organ, subsequent encounter
		T28.411D	Burn of right ear drum, subsequent encounter
		T28.412D	Burn of left ear drum, subsequent encounter
		T28.419D	Burn of unspecified ear drum, subsequent encounter
		T28.49XD	Burn of other internal organ, subsequent encounter
		T28.5XXD	Corrosion of mouth and pharynx, subsequent encounter
		T28.6XXD	Corrosion of esophagus, subsequent encounter
		T28.7XXD	Corrosion of other parts of alimentary tract, subs encntr
		T28.8XXD	Corrosion of internal genitourinary organs, subs encntr
		T28.9ØXD	Corrosions of unspecified internal organs, subs encntr
		T28.911D	Corrosions of right ear drum, subsequent encounter
		T28.912D	Corrosions of left ear drum, subsequent encounter
		T28.919D	Corrosions of unspecified ear drum, subsequent encounter
		T28.99XD	Corrosions of other internal organs, subsequent encounter
		T33.Ø11D	Superficial frostbite of right ear, subsequent encounter
		T33.Ø12D	Superficial frostbite of left ear, subsequent encounter
		T33.Ø19D	Superficial frostbite of unspecified ear, subs encntr
		T33.Ø2XD	Superficial frostbite of nose, subsequent encounter
		T33.Ø9XD	Superficial frostbite of other part of head, subs encntr
		T33.1XXD	Superficial frostbite of neck, subsequent encounter
		T33.2XXD	Superficial frostbite of thorax, subsequent encounter
		T33.3XXD	Superfic frostbite of abd wall, lower back and pelvis, subs
		T33.4ØXD	Superficial frostbite of unspecified arm, subs encntr
		T33.41XD	Superficial frostbite of right arm, subsequent encounter
		T33.42XD	Superficial frostbite of left arm, subsequent encounter
		T33.511D	Superficial frostbite of right wrist, subsequent encounter
		T33.512D	Superficial frostbite of left wrist, subsequent encounter
		T33.519D	Superficial frostbite of unspecified wrist, subs encntr
		T33.521D	Superficial frostbite of right hand, subsequent encounter
		T33.522D	Superficial frostbite of left hand, subsequent encounter
		T33.529D	Superficial frostbite of unspecified hand, subs encntr
		T33.531D	Superficial frostbite of right finger(s), subs encntr
		T33.532D	Superficial frostbite of left finger(s), subs encntr
		T33.539D	Superficial frostbite of unspecified finger(s), subs encntr
		T33.6ØXD	Superficial frostbite of unsp hip and thigh, subs encntr
		T33.61XD	Superficial frostbite of right hip and thigh, subs encntr
		T33.62XD	Superficial frostbite of left hip and thigh, subs encntr
		T33.7ØXD	Superficial frostbite of unsp knee and lower leg, subs
		T33.71XD	Superficial frostbite of right knee and lower leg, subs
		T33.72XD	Superficial frostbite of left knee and lower leg, subs
		T33.811D	Superficial frostbite of right ankle, subsequent encounter
		T33.812D	Superficial frostbite of left ankle, subsequent encounter
		T33.819D	Superficial frostbite of unspecified ankle, subs encntr
		T33.821D	Superficial frostbite of right foot, subsequent encounter
		T33.822D	Superficial frostbite of left foot, subsequent encounter
		T33.829D	Superficial frostbite of unspecified foot, subs encntr
		T33.831D	Superficial frostbite of right toe(s), subsequent encounter
		T33.832D	Superficial frostbite of left toe(s), subsequent encounter
		T33.839D	Superficial frostbite of unspecified toe(s), subs encntr
		T33.9ØXD	Superficial frostbite of unspecified sites, subs encntr
		T33.99XD	Superficial frostbite of other sites, subsequent encounter
		T34.Ø11D	Frostbite with tissue necrosis of right ear, subs encntr
		T34.Ø12D	Frostbite with tissue necrosis of left ear, subs encntr
		T34.Ø19D	Frostbite with tissue necrosis of unsp ear, subs encntr
		T34.Ø2XD	Frostbite with tissue necrosis of nose, subsequent encounter
		T34.Ø9XD	Frostbite w tissue necrosis of oth part of head, subs encntr
		T34.1XXD	Frostbite with tissue necrosis of neck, subsequent encounter
		T34.2XXD	Frostbite with tissue necrosis of thorax, subs encntr
		T34.3XXD	Frstbte w tissue necros abd wall, low back and pelvis, subs
		T34.4ØXD	Frostbite with tissue necrosis of unsp arm, subs encntr
		T34.41XD	Frostbite with tissue necrosis of right arm, subs encntr
		T34.42XD	Frostbite with tissue necrosis of left arm, subs encntr
		T34.511D	Frostbite with tissue necrosis of right wrist, subs encntr
		T34.512D	Frostbite with tissue necrosis of left wrist, subs encntr
		T34.519D	Frostbite with tissue necrosis of unsp wrist, subs encntr
		T34.521D	Frostbite with tissue necrosis of right hand, subs encntr
		T34.522D	Frostbite with tissue necrosis of left hand, subs encntr
		T34.529D	Frostbite with tissue necrosis of unsp hand, subs encntr
		T34.531D	Frostbite w tissue necrosis of right finger(s), subs encntr
		T34.532D	Frostbite w tissue necrosis of left finger(s), subs encntr
		T34.539D	Frostbite w tissue necrosis of unsp finger(s), subs encntr
		T34.6ØXD	Frostbite w tissue necrosis of unsp hip and thigh, subs
		T34.61XD	Frostbite w tissue necrosis of right hip and thigh, subs
		T34.62XD	Frostbite w tissue necrosis of left hip and thigh, subs
	(Continued on next page)	**T34.7ØXD**	Frostbite w tissue necrosis of unsp knee and lower leg, subs

ICD-9-CM		ICD-10-CM	
V58.89	ENCOUNTER FOR OTHER SPECIFIED AFTERCARE **(Continued)**	**T34.71XD**	Frostbite w tissue necros right knee and lower leg, subs
		T34.72XD	Frostbite w tissue necrosis of left knee and lower leg, subs
		T34.811D	Frostbite with tissue necrosis of right ankle, subs encntr
		T34.812D	Frostbite with tissue necrosis of left ankle, subs encntr
		T34.819D	Frostbite with tissue necrosis of unsp ankle, subs encntr
		T34.821D	Frostbite with tissue necrosis of right foot, subs encntr
		T34.822D	Frostbite with tissue necrosis of left foot, subs encntr
		T34.829D	Frostbite with tissue necrosis of unsp foot, subs encntr
		T34.831D	Frostbite with tissue necrosis of right toe(s), subs encntr
		T34.832D	Frostbite with tissue necrosis of left toe(s), subs encntr
		T34.839D	Frostbite with tissue necrosis of unsp toe(s), subs encntr
		T34.9ØXD	Frostbite with tissue necrosis of unsp sites, subs encntr
		T34.99XD	Frostbite with tissue necrosis of other sites, subs encntr
		T36.ØX1D	Poisoning by penicillins, accidental (unintentional), subs
		T36.ØX2D	Poisoning by penicillins, intentional self-harm, subs encntr
		T36.ØX3D	Poisoning by penicillins, assault, subsequent encounter
		T36.ØX4D	Poisoning by penicillins, undetermined, subsequent encounter
		T36.ØX5D	Adverse effect of penicillins, subsequent encounter
		T36.1X1D	Poisoning by cephalospor/oth beta-lactm antibiot, acc, subs
		T36.1X2D	Poisn by cephalospor/oth beta-lactm antibiot, slf-hrm, subs
		T36.1X3D	Poisn by cephalospor/oth beta-lactm antibiot, assault, subs
		T36.1X4D	Poisn by cephalospor/oth beta-lactm antibiot, undet, subs
		T36.1X5D	Adverse effect of cephalospor/oth beta-lactm antibiot, subs
		T36.2X1D	Poisoning by chloramphenicol group, accidental, subs
		T36.2X2D	Poisoning by chloramphenicol group, self-harm, subs
		T36.2X3D	Poisoning by chloramphenicol group, assault, subs encntr
		T36.2X4D	Poisoning by chloramphenicol group, undetermined, subs
		T36.2X5D	Adverse effect of chloramphenicol group, subs encntr
		T36.3X1D	Poisoning by macrolides, accidental (unintentional), subs
		T36.3X2D	Poisoning by macrolides, intentional self-harm, subs encntr
		T36.3X3D	Poisoning by macrolides, assault, subsequent encounter
		T36.3X4D	Poisoning by macrolides, undetermined, subsequent encounter
		T36.3X5D	Adverse effect of macrolides, subsequent encounter
		T36.4X1D	Poisoning by tetracyclines, accidental (unintentional), subs
		T36.4X2D	Poisoning by tetracyclines, intentional self-harm, subs
		T36.4X3D	Poisoning by tetracyclines, assault, subsequent encounter
		T36.4X4D	Poisoning by tetracyclines, undetermined, subs encntr
		T36.4X5D	Adverse effect of tetracyclines, subsequent encounter
		T36.5X1D	Poisoning by aminoglycosides, accidental, subs
		T36.5X2D	Poisoning by aminoglycosides, intentional self-harm, subs
		T36.5X3D	Poisoning by aminoglycosides, assault, subsequent encounter
		T36.5X4D	Poisoning by aminoglycosides, undetermined, subs encntr
		T36.5X5D	Adverse effect of aminoglycosides, subsequent encounter
		T36.6X1D	Poisoning by rifampicins, accidental (unintentional), subs
		T36.6X2D	Poisoning by rifampicins, intentional self-harm, subs encntr
		T36.6X3D	Poisoning by rifampicins, assault, subsequent encounter
		T36.6X4D	Poisoning by rifampicins, undetermined, subsequent encounter
		T36.6X5D	Adverse effect of rifampicins, subsequent encounter
		T36.7X1D	Poisoning by antifungal antibiot, sys used, acc, subs
		T36.7X2D	Poisoning by antifungal antibiot, sys used, self-harm, subs
		T36.7X3D	Poisoning by antifungal antibiotics, sys used, assault, subs
		T36.7X4D	Poisoning by antifungal antibiotics, sys used, undet, subs
		T36.7X5D	Adverse effect of antifungal antibiotics, sys used, subs
		T36.8X1D	Poisoning by oth systemic antibiotics, accidental, subs
		T36.8X2D	Poisoning by oth systemic antibiotics, self-harm, subs
		T36.8X3D	Poisoning by oth systemic antibiotics, assault, subs encntr
		T36.8X4D	Poisoning by oth systemic antibiotics, undetermined, subs
		T36.8X5D	Adverse effect of other systemic antibiotics, subs encntr
		T36.91XD	Poisoning by unsp systemic antibiotic, accidental, subs
		T36.92XD	Poisoning by unsp systemic antibiotic, self-harm, subs
		T36.93XD	Poisoning by unsp systemic antibiotic, assault, subs encntr
		T36.94XD	Poisoning by unsp systemic antibiotic, undetermined, subs
		T36.95XD	Adverse effect of unsp systemic antibiotic, subs encntr
		T37.ØX1D	Poisoning by sulfonamides, accidental (unintentional), subs
		T37.ØX2D	Poisoning by sulfonamides, intentional self-harm, subs
		T37.ØX3D	Poisoning by sulfonamides, assault, subsequent encounter
		T37.ØX4D	Poisoning by sulfonamides, undetermined, subs encntr
		T37.ØX5D	Adverse effect of sulfonamides, subsequent encounter
		T37.1X1D	Poisoning by antimycobac drugs, accidental, subs
		T37.1X2D	Poisoning by antimycobacterial drugs, self-harm, subs
		T37.1X3D	Poisoning by antimycobacterial drugs, assault, subs encntr
		T37.1X4D	Poisoning by antimycobacterial drugs, undetermined, subs
		T37.1X5D	Adverse effect of antimycobacterial drugs, subs encntr
		T37.2X1D	Poisn by antimalari/drugs acting on bld protzoa, acc, subs
		T37.2X2D	Poisn by antimalari/drugs act on bld protzoa, slf-hrm, subs
		T37.2X3D	Poisn by antimalari/drugs acting on bld protzoa, asslt, subs
		T37.2X4D	Poisn by antimalari/drugs acting on bld protzoa, undet, subs
		T37.2X5D	Advrs effect of antimalari/drugs acting on bld protzoa, subs
		T37.3X1D	Poisoning by oth antiprotozoal drugs, accidental, subs
		T37.3X2D	Poisoning by oth antiprotozoal drugs, self-harm, subs
		T37.3X3D	Poisoning by other antiprotozoal drugs, assault, subs encntr
		T37.3X4D	Poisoning by oth antiprotozoal drugs, undetermined, subs
	(Continued on next page)	**T37.3X5D**	Adverse effect of other antiprotozoal drugs, subs encntr

ICD-9-CM		ICD-10-CM	
V58.89	ENCOUNTER FOR OTHER SPECIFIED AFTERCARE **(Continued)**	**T37.4X1D**	Poisoning by anthelminthics, accidental, subs
		T37.4X2D	Poisoning by anthelminthics, intentional self-harm, subs
		T37.4X3D	Poisoning by anthelminthics, assault, subsequent encounter
		T37.4X4D	Poisoning by anthelminthics, undetermined, subs encntr
		T37.4X5D	Adverse effect of anthelminthics, subsequent encounter
		T37.5X1D	Poisoning by antiviral drugs, accidental, subs
		T37.5X2D	Poisoning by antiviral drugs, intentional self-harm, subs
		T37.5X3D	Poisoning by antiviral drugs, assault, subsequent encounter
		T37.5X4D	Poisoning by antiviral drugs, undetermined, subs encntr
		T37.5X5D	Adverse effect of antiviral drugs, subsequent encounter
		T37.8X1D	Poisoning by oth systemic anti-infect/parasit, acc, subs
		T37.8X2D	Poisn by oth systemic anti-infect/parasit, self-harm, subs
		T37.8X3D	Poisoning by oth systemic anti-infect/parasit, assault, subs
		T37.8X4D	Poisoning by oth systemic anti-infect/parasit, undet, subs
		T37.8X5D	Adverse effect of systemic anti-infect/parasit, subs
		T37.91XD	Poisn by unsp sys anti-infect and antiparastc, acc, subs
		T37.92XD	Poisn by unsp sys anti-infect and antiparastc, slf-hrm, subs
		T37.93XD	Poisn by unsp sys anti-infect and antiparastc, assault, subs
		T37.94XD	Poisn by unsp sys anti-infect and antiparastc, undet, subs
		T37.95XD	Advrs effect of unsp sys anti-infect and antiparasitic, subs
		T38.ØX1D	Poisoning by glucocort/synth analog, accidental, subs
		T38.ØX2D	Poisoning by glucocort/synth analog, self-harm, subs
		T38.ØX3D	Poisoning by glucocort/synth analog, assault, subs
		T38.ØX4D	Poisoning by glucocort/synth analog, undetermined, subs
		T38.ØX5D	Adverse effect of glucocort/synth analog, subs
		T38.1X1D	Poisoning by thyroid hormones and sub, accidental, subs
		T38.1X2D	Poisoning by thyroid hormones and sub, self-harm, subs
		T38.1X3D	Poisoning by thyroid hormones and substitutes, assault, subs
		T38.1X4D	Poisoning by thyroid hormones and substitutes, undet, subs
		T38.1X5D	Adverse effect of thyroid hormones and substitutes, subs
		T38.2X1D	Poisoning by antithyroid drugs, accidental, subs
		T38.2X2D	Poisoning by antithyroid drugs, intentional self-harm, subs
		T38.2X3D	Poisoning by antithyroid drugs, assault, subs encntr
		T38.2X4D	Poisoning by antithyroid drugs, undetermined, subs encntr
		T38.2X5D	Adverse effect of antithyroid drugs, subsequent encounter
		T38.3X1D	Poisoning by insulin and oral hypoglycemic drugs, acc, subs
		T38.3X2D	Poisn by insulin and oral hypoglycemic drugs, slf-hrm, subs
		T38.3X3D	Poisn by insulin and oral hypoglycemic drugs, assault, subs
		T38.3X4D	Poisn by insulin and oral hypoglycemic drugs, undet, subs
		T38.3X5D	Adverse effect of insulin and oral hypoglycemic drugs, subs
		T38.4X1D	Poisoning by oral contraceptives, accidental, subs
		T38.4X2D	Poisoning by oral contraceptives, self-harm, subs
		T38.4X3D	Poisoning by oral contraceptives, assault, subs encntr
		T38.4X4D	Poisoning by oral contraceptives, undetermined, subs encntr
		T38.4X5D	Adverse effect of oral contraceptives, subsequent encounter
		T38.5X1D	Poisoning by oth estrogens and progstrn, accidental, subs
		T38.5X2D	Poisoning by oth estrogens and progestogens, self-harm, subs
		T38.5X3D	Poisoning by oth estrogens and progestogens, assault, subs
		T38.5X4D	Poisoning by oth estrogens and progstrn, undetermined, subs
		T38.5X5D	Adverse effect of oth estrogens and progestogens, subs
		T38.6X1D	Poisoning by antigonadtr/antiestr/antiandrg, NEC, acc, subs
		T38.6X2D	Poisn by antigonadtr/antiestr/antiandrg, NEC, slf-hrm, subs
		T38.6X3D	Poisn by antigonadtr/antiestr/antiandrg, NEC, assault, subs
		T38.6X4D	Poisn by antigonadtr/antiestr/antiandrg, NEC, undet, subs
		T38.6X5D	Adverse effect of antigonadtr/antiestr/antiandrg, NEC, subs
		T38.7X1D	Poisoning by androgens and anabolic congeners, acc, subs
		T38.7X2D	Poisn by androgens and anabolic congeners, self-harm, subs
		T38.7X3D	Poisoning by androgens and anabolic congeners, assault, subs
		T38.7X4D	Poisoning by androgens and anabolic congeners, undet, subs
		T38.7X5D	Adverse effect of androgens and anabolic congeners, subs
		T38.8Ø1D	Poisoning by unsp hormones and synthetic sub, acc, subs
		T38.8Ø2D	Poisn by unsp hormones and synthetic sub, self-harm, subs
		T38.8Ø3D	Poisoning by unsp hormones and synthetic sub, assault, subs
		T38.8Ø4D	Poisoning by unsp hormones and synthetic sub, undet, subs
		T38.8Ø5D	Adverse effect of unsp hormones and synthetic sub, subs
		T38.811D	Poisoning by anterior pituitary hormones, accidental, subs
		T38.812D	Poisoning by anterior pituitary hormones, self-harm, subs
		T38.813D	Poisoning by anterior pituitary hormones, assault, subs
		T38.814D	Poisoning by anterior pituitary hormones, undetermined, subs
		T38.815D	Adverse effect of anterior pituitary hormones, subs encntr
		T38.891D	Poisoning by oth hormones and synthetic sub, acc, subs
		T38.892D	Poisoning by oth hormones and synthetic sub, self-harm, subs
		T38.893D	Poisoning by oth hormones and synthetic sub, assault, subs
		T38.894D	Poisoning by oth hormones and synthetic sub, undet, subs
		T38.895D	Adverse effect of hormones and synthetic substitutes, subs
		T38.9Ø1D	Poisoning by unsp hormone antagonists, accidental, subs
		T38.9Ø2D	Poisoning by unsp hormone antagonists, self-harm, subs
		T38.9Ø3D	Poisoning by unsp hormone antagonists, assault, subs encntr
		T38.9Ø4D	Poisoning by unsp hormone antagonists, undetermined, subs
		T38.9Ø5D	Adverse effect of unsp hormone antagonists, subs encntr
		T38.991D	Poisoning by oth hormone antagonists, accidental, subs
		T38.992D	Poisoning by oth hormone antagonists, self-harm, subs
	(Continued on next page)	**T38.993D**	Poisoning by other hormone antagonists, assault, subs encntr

ICD-9-CM		ICD-10-CM	
V58.89	ENCOUNTER FOR OTHER SPECIFIED AFTERCARE **(Continued)**	**T38.994D**	Poisoning by oth hormone antagonists, undetermined, subs
		T38.995D	Adverse effect of other hormone antagonists, subs encntr
		T39.011D	Poisoning by aspirin, accidental (unintentional), subs
		T39.012D	Poisoning by aspirin, intentional self-harm, subs encntr
		T39.013D	Poisoning by aspirin, assault, subsequent encounter
		T39.014D	Poisoning by aspirin, undetermined, subsequent encounter
		T39.015D	Adverse effect of aspirin, subsequent encounter
		T39.091D	Poisoning by salicylates, accidental (unintentional), subs
		T39.092D	Poisoning by salicylates, intentional self-harm, subs encntr
		T39.093D	Poisoning by salicylates, assault, subsequent encounter
		T39.094D	Poisoning by salicylates, undetermined, subsequent encounter
		T39.095D	Adverse effect of salicylates, subsequent encounter
		T39.1X1D	Poisoning by 4-Aminophenol derivatives, accidental, subs
		T39.1X2D	Poisoning by 4-Aminophenol derivatives, self-harm, subs
		T39.1X3D	Poisoning by 4-Aminophenol derivatives, assault, subs encntr
		T39.1X4D	Poisoning by 4-Aminophenol derivatives, undetermined, subs
		T39.1X5D	Adverse effect of 4-Aminophenol derivatives, subs encntr
		T39.2X1D	Poisoning by pyrazolone derivatives, accidental, subs
		T39.2X2D	Poisoning by pyrazolone derivatives, self-harm, subs
		T39.2X3D	Poisoning by pyrazolone derivatives, assault, subs encntr
		T39.2X4D	Poisoning by pyrazolone derivatives, undetermined, subs
		T39.2X5D	Adverse effect of pyrazolone derivatives, subs encntr
		T39.311D	Poisoning by propionic acid derivatives, accidental, subs
		T39.312D	Poisoning by propionic acid derivatives, self-harm, subs
		T39.313D	Poisoning by propionic acid derivatives, assault, subs
		T39.314D	Poisoning by propionic acid derivatives, undetermined, subs
		T39.315D	Adverse effect of propionic acid derivatives, subs encntr
		T39.391D	Poisoning by oth nonsteroid anti-inflam drugs, acc, subs
		T39.392D	Poisn by oth nonsteroid anti-inflam drugs, self-harm, subs
		T39.393D	Poisoning by oth nonsteroid anti-inflam drugs, assault, subs
		T39.394D	Poisoning by oth nonsteroid anti-inflam drugs, undet, subs
		T39.395D	Adverse effect of nonsteroidal anti-inflammatory drugs, subs
		T39.4X1D	Poisoning by antirheumatics, NEC, accidental, subs
		T39.4X2D	Poisoning by antirheumatics, NEC, self-harm, subs
		T39.4X3D	Poisoning by antirheumatics, NEC, assault, subs
		T39.4X4D	Poisoning by antirheumatics, NEC, undetermined, subs
		T39.4X5D	Adverse effect of antirheumatics, NEC, subs
		T39.8X1D	Poisoning by oth nonopio analges/antipyret, NEC, acc, subs
		T39.8X2D	Poisn by oth nonopio analges/antipyret, NEC, self-harm, subs
		T39.8X3D	Poisn by oth nonopio analges/antipyret, NEC, assault, subs
		T39.8X4D	Poisoning by oth nonopio analges/antipyret, NEC, undet, subs
		T39.8X5D	Adverse effect of nonopioid analges/antipyret, NEC, subs
		T39.91XD	Poisoning by unsp nonopi analgs/antipyr/antirheu, acc, subs
		T39.92XD	Poisn by unsp nonopi analgs/antipyr/antirheu, slf-hrm, subs
		T39.93XD	Poisn by unsp nonopi analgs/antipyr/antirheu, assault, subs
		T39.94XD	Poisn by unsp nonopi analgs/antipyr/antirheu, undet, subs
		T39.95XD	Adverse effect of unsp nonopi analgs/antipyr/antirheu, subs
		T40.0X1D	Poisoning by opium, accidental (unintentional), subs encntr
		T40.0X2D	Poisoning by opium, intentional self-harm, subs encntr
		T40.0X3D	Poisoning by opium, assault, subsequent encounter
		T40.0X4D	Poisoning by opium, undetermined, subsequent encounter
		T40.0X5D	Adverse effect of opium, subsequent encounter
		T40.1X1D	Poisoning by heroin, accidental (unintentional), subs encntr
		T40.1X2D	Poisoning by heroin, intentional self-harm, subs encntr
		T40.1X3D	Poisoning by heroin, assault, subsequent encounter
		T40.1X4D	Poisoning by heroin, undetermined, subsequent encounter
		T40.2X1D	Poisoning by oth opioids, accidental (unintentional), subs
		T40.2X2D	Poisoning by oth opioids, intentional self-harm, subs encntr
		T40.2X3D	Poisoning by other opioids, assault, subsequent encounter
		T40.2X4D	Poisoning by other opioids, undetermined, subs encntr
		T40.2X5D	Adverse effect of other opioids, subsequent encounter
		T40.3X1D	Poisoning by methadone, accidental (unintentional), subs
		T40.3X2D	Poisoning by methadone, intentional self-harm, subs encntr
		T40.3X3D	Poisoning by methadone, assault, subsequent encounter
		T40.3X4D	Poisoning by methadone, undetermined, subsequent encounter
		T40.3X5D	Adverse effect of methadone, subsequent encounter
		T40.4X1D	Poisoning by oth synthetic narcotics, accidental, subs
		T40.4X2D	Poisoning by oth synthetic narcotics, self-harm, subs
		T40.4X3D	Poisoning by other synthetic narcotics, assault, subs encntr
		T40.4X4D	Poisoning by oth synthetic narcotics, undetermined, subs
		T40.4X5D	Adverse effect of other synthetic narcotics, subs encntr
		T40.5X1D	Poisoning by cocaine, accidental (unintentional), subs
		T40.5X2D	Poisoning by cocaine, intentional self-harm, subs encntr
		T40.5X3D	Poisoning by cocaine, assault, subsequent encounter
		T40.5X4D	Poisoning by cocaine, undetermined, subsequent encounter
		T40.5X5D	Adverse effect of cocaine, subsequent encounter
		T40.601D	Poisoning by unsp narcotics, accidental, subs
		T40.602D	Poisoning by unsp narcotics, intentional self-harm, subs
		T40.603D	Poisoning by unspecified narcotics, assault, subs encntr
		T40.604D	Poisoning by unsp narcotics, undetermined, subs encntr
		T40.605D	Adverse effect of unspecified narcotics, subs encntr
	(Continued on next page)	**T40.691D**	Poisoning by oth narcotics, accidental (unintentional), subs

ICD-9-CM		ICD-10-CM	
V58.89	ENCOUNTER FOR OTHER SPECIFIED AFTERCARE **(Continued)**	**T40.692D**	Poisoning by oth narcotics, intentional self-harm, subs
		T40.693D	Poisoning by other narcotics, assault, subsequent encounter
		T40.694D	Poisoning by other narcotics, undetermined, subs encntr
		T40.695D	Adverse effect of other narcotics, subsequent encounter
		T40.7X1D	Poisoning by cannabis (derivatives), accidental, subs
		T40.7X2D	Poisoning by cannabis (derivatives), self-harm, subs
		T40.7X3D	Poisoning by cannabis (derivatives), assault, subs encntr
		T40.7X4D	Poisoning by cannabis (derivatives), undetermined, subs
		T40.7X5D	Adverse effect of cannabis (derivatives), subs encntr
		T40.8X1D	Poisoning by lysergide, accidental (unintentional), subs
		T40.8X2D	Poisoning by lysergide, intentional self-harm, subs encntr
		T40.8X3D	Poisoning by lysergide [LSD], assault, subsequent encounter
		T40.8X4D	Poisoning by lysergide, undetermined, subsequent encounter
		T40.901D	Poisoning by unsp psychodyslept, accidental, subs
		T40.902D	Poisoning by unsp psychodysleptics, self-harm, subs
		T40.903D	Poisoning by unsp psychodysleptics, assault, subs encntr
		T40.904D	Poisoning by unsp psychodysleptics, undetermined, subs
		T40.905D	Adverse effect of unspecified psychodysleptics, subs encntr
		T40.991D	Poisoning by oth psychodyslept, accidental, subs
		T40.992D	Poisoning by oth psychodysleptics, self-harm, subs
		T40.993D	Poisoning by other psychodysleptics, assault, subs encntr
		T40.994D	Poisoning by oth psychodysleptics, undetermined, subs encntr
		T40.995D	Adverse effect of other psychodysleptics, subs encntr
		T41.0X1D	Poisoning by inhaled anesthetics, accidental, subs
		T41.0X2D	Poisoning by inhaled anesthetics, self-harm, subs
		T41.0X3D	Poisoning by inhaled anesthetics, assault, subs encntr
		T41.0X4D	Poisoning by inhaled anesthetics, undetermined, subs encntr
		T41.0X5D	Adverse effect of inhaled anesthetics, subsequent encounter
		T41.1X1D	Poisoning by intravenous anesthetics, accidental, subs
		T41.1X2D	Poisoning by intravenous anesthetics, self-harm, subs
		T41.1X3D	Poisoning by intravenous anesthetics, assault, subs encntr
		T41.1X4D	Poisoning by intravenous anesthetics, undetermined, subs
		T41.1X5D	Adverse effect of intravenous anesthetics, subs encntr
		T41.201D	Poisoning by unsp general anesthetics, accidental, subs
		T41.202D	Poisoning by unsp general anesthetics, self-harm, subs
		T41.203D	Poisoning by unsp general anesthetics, assault, subs encntr
		T41.204D	Poisoning by unsp general anesthetics, undetermined, subs
		T41.205D	Adverse effect of unsp general anesthetics, subs encntr
		T41.291D	Poisoning by oth general anesthetics, accidental, subs
		T41.292D	Poisoning by oth general anesthetics, self-harm, subs
		T41.293D	Poisoning by other general anesthetics, assault, subs encntr
		T41.294D	Poisoning by oth general anesthetics, undetermined, subs
		T41.295D	Adverse effect of other general anesthetics, subs encntr
		T41.3X1D	Poisoning by local anesthetics, accidental, subs
		T41.3X2D	Poisoning by local anesthetics, intentional self-harm, subs
		T41.3X3D	Poisoning by local anesthetics, assault, subs encntr
		T41.3X4D	Poisoning by local anesthetics, undetermined, subs encntr
		T41.3X5D	Adverse effect of local anesthetics, subsequent encounter
		T41.41XD	Poisoning by unsp anesthetic, accidental, subs
		T41.42XD	Poisoning by unsp anesthetic, intentional self-harm, subs
		T41.43XD	Poisoning by unspecified anesthetic, assault, subs encntr
		T41.44XD	Poisoning by unsp anesthetic, undetermined, subs encntr
		T41.45XD	Adverse effect of unspecified anesthetic, subs encntr
		T41.5X1D	Poisoning by therapeutic gases, accidental, subs
		T41.5X2D	Poisoning by therapeutic gases, intentional self-harm, subs
		T41.5X3D	Poisoning by therapeutic gases, assault, subs encntr
		T41.5X4D	Poisoning by therapeutic gases, undetermined, subs encntr
		T41.5X5D	Adverse effect of therapeutic gases, subsequent encounter
		T42.0X1D	Poisoning by hydantoin derivatives, accidental, subs
		T42.0X2D	Poisoning by hydantoin derivatives, self-harm, subs
		T42.0X3D	Poisoning by hydantoin derivatives, assault, subs encntr
		T42.0X4D	Poisoning by hydantoin derivatives, undetermined, subs
		T42.0X5D	Adverse effect of hydantoin derivatives, subs encntr
		T42.1X1D	Poisoning by iminostilbenes, accidental, subs
		T42.1X2D	Poisoning by iminostilbenes, intentional self-harm, subs
		T42.1X3D	Poisoning by iminostilbenes, assault, subsequent encounter
		T42.1X4D	Poisoning by iminostilbenes, undetermined, subs encntr
		T42.1X5D	Adverse effect of iminostilbenes, subsequent encounter
		T42.2X1D	Poisoning by succinimides and oxazolidinediones, acc, subs
		T42.2X2D	Poisn by succinimides and oxazolidinediones, self-harm, subs
		T42.2X3D	Poisn by succinimides and oxazolidinediones, assault, subs
		T42.2X4D	Poisoning by succinimides and oxazolidinediones, undet, subs
		T42.2X5D	Adverse effect of succinimides and oxazolidinediones, subs
		T42.3X1D	Poisoning by barbiturates, accidental (unintentional), subs
		T42.3X2D	Poisoning by barbiturates, intentional self-harm, subs
		T42.3X3D	Poisoning by barbiturates, assault, subsequent encounter
		T42.3X4D	Poisoning by barbiturates, undetermined, subs encntr
		T42.3X5D	Adverse effect of barbiturates, subsequent encounter
		T42.4X1D	Poisoning by benzodiazepines, accidental, subs
		T42.4X2D	Poisoning by benzodiazepines, intentional self-harm, subs
		T42.4X3D	Poisoning by benzodiazepines, assault, subsequent encounter
	(Continued on next page)	**T42.4X4D**	Poisoning by benzodiazepines, undetermined, subs encntr

ICD-9-CM		ICD-10-CM	
V58.89	ENCOUNTER FOR OTHER SPECIFIED AFTERCARE **(Continued)**	**T42.4X5D**	Adverse effect of benzodiazepines, subsequent encounter
		T42.5X1D	Poisoning by mixed antiepileptics, accidental, subs
		T42.5X2D	Poisoning by mixed antiepileptics, self-harm, subs
		T42.5X3D	Poisoning by mixed antiepileptics, assault, subs encntr
		T42.5X4D	Poisoning by mixed antiepileptics, undetermined, subs encntr
		T42.5X5D	Adverse effect of mixed antiepileptics, subsequent encounter
		T42.6X1D	Poisoning by oth antieplptc and sed-hypntc drugs, acc, subs
		T42.6X2D	Poisn by oth antieplptc and sed-hypntc drugs, slf-hrm, subs
		T42.6X3D	Poisn by oth antieplptc and sed-hypntc drugs, assault, subs
		T42.6X4D	Poisn by oth antieplptc and sed-hypntc drugs, undet, subs
		T42.6X5D	Adverse effect of antiepileptic and sed-hypntc drugs, subs
		T42.71XD	Poisn by unsp antieplptc and sed-hypntc drugs, acc, subs
		T42.72XD	Poisn by unsp antieplptc and sed-hypntc drugs, slf-hrm, subs
		T42.73XD	Poisn by unsp antieplptc and sed-hypntc drugs, assault, subs
		T42.74XD	Poisn by unsp antieplptc and sed-hypntc drugs, undet, subs
		T42.75XD	Adverse effect of unsp antieplptc and sed-hypntc drugs, subs
		T42.8X1D	Poisn by antiparkns drug/centr musc-tone depr, acc, subs
		T42.8X2D	Poisn by antiparkns drug/centr musc-tone depr, slf-hrm, subs
		T42.8X3D	Poisn by antiparkns drug/centr musc-tone depr, assault, subs
		T42.8X4D	Poisn by antiparkns drug/centr musc-tone depr, undet, subs
		T42.8X5D	Adverse effect of antiparkns drug/centr musc-tone depr, subs
		T43.011D	Poisoning by tricyclic antidepressants, accidental, subs
		T43.012D	Poisoning by tricyclic antidepressants, self-harm, subs
		T43.013D	Poisoning by tricyclic antidepressants, assault, subs encntr
		T43.014D	Poisoning by tricyclic antidepressants, undetermined, subs
		T43.015D	Adverse effect of tricyclic antidepressants, subs encntr
		T43.021D	Poisoning by tetracyclic antidepressants, accidental, subs
		T43.022D	Poisoning by tetracyclic antidepressants, self-harm, subs
		T43.023D	Poisoning by tetracyclic antidepressants, assault, subs
		T43.024D	Poisoning by tetracyclic antidepressants, undetermined, subs
		T43.025D	Adverse effect of tetracyclic antidepressants, subs encntr
		T43.1X1D	Poisoning by MAO inhib antidepressants, accidental, subs
		T43.1X2D	Poisoning by MAO inhib antidepressants, self-harm, subs
		T43.1X3D	Poisoning by MAO inhib antidepressants, assault, subs
		T43.1X4D	Poisoning by MAO inhib antidepressants, undetermined, subs
		T43.1X5D	Adverse effect of MAO inhib antidepressants, subs
		T43.201D	Poisoning by unsp antidepressants, accidental, subs
		T43.202D	Poisoning by unsp antidepressants, self-harm, subs
		T43.203D	Poisoning by unsp antidepressants, assault, subs encntr
		T43.204D	Poisoning by unsp antidepressants, undetermined, subs encntr
		T43.205D	Adverse effect of unspecified antidepressants, subs encntr
		T43.211D	Poisn by slctv seroton/norepineph reup inhibtr, acc, subs
		T43.212D	Poisn by slctv seroton/norepineph reup inhibtr,slf-hrm, subs
		T43.213D	Poisn by slctv seroton/norepineph reup inhibtr, asslt, subs
		T43.214D	Poisn by slctv seroton/norepineph reup inhibtr, undet, subs
		T43.215D	Advrs effect of slctv seroton/norepineph reup inhibtr, subs
		T43.221D	Poisn by selective serotonin reuptake inhibtr, acc, subs
		T43.222D	Poisn by slctv serotonin reuptake inhibtr, self-harm, subs
		T43.223D	Poisn by selective serotonin reuptake inhibtr, assault, subs
		T43.224D	Poisn by selective serotonin reuptake inhibtr, undet, subs
		T43.225D	Adverse effect of selective serotonin reuptake inhibtr, subs
		T43.291D	Poisoning by oth antidepressants, accidental, subs
		T43.292D	Poisoning by oth antidepressants, self-harm, subs
		T43.293D	Poisoning by other antidepressants, assault, subs encntr
		T43.294D	Poisoning by oth antidepressants, undetermined, subs encntr
		T43.295D	Adverse effect of other antidepressants, subs encntr
		T43.3X1D	Poisoning by phenothiaz antipsychot/neurolept, acc, subs
		T43.3X2D	Poisn by phenothiaz antipsychot/neurolept, self-harm, subs
		T43.3X3D	Poisoning by phenothiaz antipsychot/neurolept, assault, subs
		T43.3X4D	Poisoning by phenothiaz antipsychot/neurolept, undet, subs
		T43.3X5D	Adverse effect of phenothiazine antipsychot/neurolept, subs
		T43.4X1D	Poisoning by butyrophen/thiothixen neuroleptc, acc, subs
		T43.4X2D	Poisn by butyrophen/thiothixen neuroleptc, self-harm, subs
		T43.4X3D	Poisoning by butyrophen/thiothixen neuroleptc, assault, subs
		T43.4X4D	Poisoning by butyrophen/thiothixen neuroleptc, undet, subs
		T43.4X5D	Adverse effect of butyrophen/thiothixen neuroleptics, subs
		T43.501D	Poisoning by unsp antipsychot/neurolept, accidental, subs
		T43.502D	Poisoning by unsp antipsychot/neurolept, self-harm, subs
		T43.503D	Poisoning by unsp antipsychot/neurolept, assault, subs
		T43.504D	Poisoning by unsp antipsychot/neurolept, undetermined, subs
		T43.505D	Adverse effect of unsp antipsychotics and neuroleptics, subs
		T43.591D	Poisoning by oth antipsychot/neurolept, accidental, subs
		T43.592D	Poisoning by oth antipsychot/neurolept, self-harm, subs
		T43.593D	Poisoning by oth antipsychot/neurolept, assault, subs
		T43.594D	Poisoning by oth antipsychot/neurolept, undetermined, subs
		T43.595D	Adverse effect of oth antipsychotics and neuroleptics, subs
		T43.601D	Poisoning by unsp psychostim, accidental, subs
		T43.602D	Poisoning by unsp psychostimulants, self-harm, subs
		T43.603D	Poisoning by unsp psychostimulants, assault, subs encntr
		T43.604D	Poisoning by unsp psychostimulants, undetermined, subs
		T43.605D	Adverse effect of unspecified psychostimulants, subs encntr
		T43.611D	Poisoning by caffeine, accidental (unintentional), subs
	(Continued on next page)	**T43.612D**	Poisoning by caffeine, intentional self-harm, subs encntr

ICD-9-CM		ICD-10-CM	
V58.89	ENCOUNTER FOR OTHER SPECIFIED AFTERCARE **(Continued)**	**T43.613D**	Poisoning by caffeine, assault, subsequent encounter
		T43.614D	Poisoning by caffeine, undetermined, subsequent encounter
		T43.615D	Adverse effect of caffeine, subsequent encounter
		T43.621D	Poisoning by amphetamines, accidental (unintentional), subs
		T43.622D	Poisoning by amphetamines, intentional self-harm, subs
		T43.623D	Poisoning by amphetamines, assault, subsequent encounter
		T43.624D	Poisoning by amphetamines, undetermined, subs encntr
		T43.625D	Adverse effect of amphetamines, subsequent encounter
		T43.631D	Poisoning by methylphenidate, accidental, subs
		T43.632D	Poisoning by methylphenidate, intentional self-harm, subs
		T43.633D	Poisoning by methylphenidate, assault, subsequent encounter
		T43.634D	Poisoning by methylphenidate, undetermined, subs encntr
		T43.635D	Adverse effect of methylphenidate, subsequent encounter
		T43.691D	Poisoning by oth psychostim, accidental, subs
		T43.692D	Poisoning by oth psychostimulants, self-harm, subs
		T43.693D	Poisoning by other psychostimulants, assault, subs encntr
		T43.694D	Poisoning by oth psychostimulants, undetermined, subs encntr
		T43.695D	Adverse effect of other psychostimulants, subs encntr
		T43.8X1D	Poisoning by oth psychotropic drugs, accidental, subs
		T43.8X2D	Poisoning by oth psychotropic drugs, self-harm, subs
		T43.8X3D	Poisoning by other psychotropic drugs, assault, subs encntr
		T43.8X4D	Poisoning by oth psychotropic drugs, undetermined, subs
		T43.8X5D	Adverse effect of other psychotropic drugs, subs encntr
		T43.91XD	Poisoning by unsp psychotropic drug, accidental, subs
		T43.92XD	Poisoning by unsp psychotropic drug, self-harm, subs
		T43.93XD	Poisoning by unsp psychotropic drug, assault, subs encntr
		T43.94XD	Poisoning by unsp psychotropic drug, undetermined, subs
		T43.95XD	Adverse effect of unspecified psychotropic drug, subs encntr
		T44.ØX1D	Poisoning by anticholin agents, accidental, subs
		T44.ØX2D	Poisoning by anticholinesterase agents, self-harm, subs
		T44.ØX3D	Poisoning by anticholinesterase agents, assault, subs encntr
		T44.ØX4D	Poisoning by anticholinesterase agents, undetermined, subs
		T44.ØX5D	Adverse effect of anticholinesterase agents, subs encntr
		T44.1X1D	Poisoning by oth parasympath, accidental, subs
		T44.1X2D	Poisoning by oth parasympathomimetics, self-harm, subs
		T44.1X3D	Poisoning by oth parasympathomimetics, assault, subs encntr
		T44.1X4D	Poisoning by oth parasympathomimetics, undetermined, subs
		T44.1X5D	Adverse effect of other parasympathomimetics, subs encntr
		T44.2X1D	Poisoning by ganglionic blocking drugs, accidental, subs
		T44.2X2D	Poisoning by ganglionic blocking drugs, self-harm, subs
		T44.2X3D	Poisoning by ganglionic blocking drugs, assault, subs encntr
		T44.2X4D	Poisoning by ganglionic blocking drugs, undetermined, subs
		T44.2X5D	Adverse effect of ganglionic blocking drugs, subs encntr
		T44.3X1D	Poisoning by oth parasympath and spasmolytics, acc, subs
		T44.3X2D	Poisn by oth parasympath and spasmolytics, self-harm, subs
		T44.3X3D	Poisoning by oth parasympath and spasmolytics, assault, subs
		T44.3X4D	Poisoning by oth parasympath and spasmolytics, undet, subs
		T44.3X5D	Adverse effect of parasympatholytics and spasmolytics, subs
		T44.4X1D	Poisoning by predom alpha-adrenocpt agonists, acc, subs
		T44.4X2D	Poisn by predom alpha-adrenocpt agonists, self-harm, subs
		T44.4X3D	Poisoning by predom alpha-adrenocpt agonists, assault, subs
		T44.4X4D	Poisoning by predom alpha-adrenocpt agonists, undet, subs
		T44.4X5D	Adverse effect of predom alpha-adrenocpt agonists, subs
		T44.5X1D	Poisoning by predom beta-adrenocpt agonists, acc, subs
		T44.5X2D	Poisoning by predom beta-adrenocpt agonists, self-harm, subs
		T44.5X3D	Poisoning by predom beta-adrenocpt agonists, assault, subs
		T44.5X4D	Poisoning by predom beta-adrenocpt agonists, undet, subs
		T44.5X5D	Adverse effect of predom beta-adrenocpt agonists, subs
		T44.6X1D	Poisoning by alpha-adrenocpt antagonists, accidental, subs
		T44.6X2D	Poisoning by alpha-adrenocpt antagonists, self-harm, subs
		T44.6X3D	Poisoning by alpha-adrenoreceptor antagonists, assault, subs
		T44.6X4D	Poisoning by alpha-adrenocpt antagonists, undetermined, subs
		T44.6X5D	Adverse effect of alpha-adrenoreceptor antagonists, subs
		T44.7X1D	Poisoning by beta-adrenocpt antagonists, accidental, subs
		T44.7X2D	Poisoning by beta-adrenocpt antagonists, self-harm, subs
		T44.7X3D	Poisoning by beta-adrenoreceptor antagonists, assault, subs
		T44.7X4D	Poisoning by beta-adrenocpt antagonists, undetermined, subs
		T44.7X5D	Adverse effect of beta-adrenoreceptor antagonists, subs
		T44.8X1D	Poisoning by centr-acting/adren-neurn-block agnt, acc, subs
		T44.8X2D	Poisn by centr-acting/adren-neurn-block agnt, slf-hrm, subs
		T44.8X3D	Poisn by centr-acting/adren-neurn-block agnt, assault, subs
		T44.8X4D	Poisn by centr-acting/adren-neurn-block agnt, undet, subs
		T44.8X5D	Adverse effect of centr-acting/adren-neurn-block agnt, subs
		T44.9Ø1D	Poisn by unsp drugs aff the autonm nervous sys, acc, subs
		T44.9Ø2D	Poisn by unsp drugs aff the autonm nrv sys, slf-hrm, subs
		T44.9Ø3D	Poisn by unsp drugs aff the autonm nervous sys, asslt, subs
		T44.9Ø4D	Poisn by unsp drugs aff the autonm nervous sys, undet, subs
		T44.9Ø5D	Advrs effect of unsp drugs aff the autonm nervous sys, subs
		T44.991D	Poisoning by oth drug aff the autonm nervous sys, acc, subs
		T44.992D	Poisn by oth drug aff the autonm nervous sys, slf-hrm, subs
		T44.993D	Poisn by oth drug aff the autonm nervous sys, assault, subs
		T44.994D	Poisn by oth drug aff the autonm nervous sys, undet, subs
		T44.995D	Adverse effect of drug aff the autonomic nervous sys, subs

(Continued on next page)

ICD-9-CM		ICD-10-CM	
V58.89	ENCOUNTER FOR OTHER SPECIFIED AFTERCARE **(Continued)**	**T45.ØX1D**	Poisoning by antiallerg/antiemetic, accidental, subs
		T45.ØX2D	Poisoning by antiallerg/antiemetic, self-harm, subs
		T45.ØX3D	Poisoning by antiallerg/antiemetic, assault, subs
		T45.ØX4D	Poisoning by antiallerg/antiemetic, undetermined, subs
		T45.ØX5D	Adverse effect of antiallergic and antiemetic drugs, subs
		T45.1X1D	Poisoning by antineopl and immunosup drugs, acc, subs
		T45.1X2D	Poisoning by antineopl and immunosup drugs, self-harm, subs
		T45.1X3D	Poisoning by antineopl and immunosup drugs, assault, subs
		T45.1X4D	Poisoning by antineopl and immunosup drugs, undet, subs
		T45.1X5D	Adverse effect of antineoplastic and immunosup drugs, subs
		T45.2X1D	Poisoning by vitamins, accidental (unintentional), subs
		T45.2X2D	Poisoning by vitamins, intentional self-harm, subs encntr
		T45.2X3D	Poisoning by vitamins, assault, subsequent encounter
		T45.2X4D	Poisoning by vitamins, undetermined, subsequent encounter
		T45.2X5D	Adverse effect of vitamins, subsequent encounter
		T45.3X1D	Poisoning by enzymes, accidental (unintentional), subs
		T45.3X2D	Poisoning by enzymes, intentional self-harm, subs encntr
		T45.3X3D	Poisoning by enzymes, assault, subsequent encounter
		T45.3X4D	Poisoning by enzymes, undetermined, subsequent encounter
		T45.3X5D	Adverse effect of enzymes, subsequent encounter
		T45.4X1D	Poisoning by iron and its compounds, accidental, subs
		T45.4X2D	Poisoning by iron and its compounds, self-harm, subs
		T45.4X3D	Poisoning by iron and its compounds, assault, subs encntr
		T45.4X4D	Poisoning by iron and its compounds, undetermined, subs
		T45.4X5D	Adverse effect of iron and its compounds, subs encntr
		T45.511D	Poisoning by anticoagulants, accidental, subs
		T45.512D	Poisoning by anticoagulants, intentional self-harm, subs
		T45.513D	Poisoning by anticoagulants, assault, subsequent encounter
		T45.514D	Poisoning by anticoagulants, undetermined, subs encntr
		T45.515D	Adverse effect of anticoagulants, subsequent encounter
		T45.521D	Poisoning by antithrombotic drugs, accidental, subs
		T45.522D	Poisoning by antithrombotic drugs, self-harm, subs
		T45.523D	Poisoning by antithrombotic drugs, assault, subs encntr
		T45.524D	Poisoning by antithrombotic drugs, undetermined, subs encntr
		T45.525D	Adverse effect of antithrombotic drugs, subsequent encounter
		T45.6Ø1D	Poisoning by unsp fibrin-affct drugs, accidental, subs
		T45.6Ø2D	Poisoning by unsp fibrin-affct drugs, self-harm, subs
		T45.6Ø3D	Poisoning by unsp fibrin-affct drugs, assault, subs
		T45.6Ø4D	Poisoning by unsp fibrin-affct drugs, undetermined, subs
		T45.6Ø5D	Adverse effect of unsp fibrinolysis-affecting drugs, subs
		T45.611D	Poisoning by thrombolytic drug, accidental, subs
		T45.612D	Poisoning by thrombolytic drug, intentional self-harm, subs
		T45.613D	Poisoning by thrombolytic drug, assault, subs encntr
		T45.614D	Poisoning by thrombolytic drug, undetermined, subs encntr
		T45.615D	Adverse effect of thrombolytic drugs, subsequent encounter
		T45.621D	Poisoning by hemostatic drug, accidental, subs
		T45.622D	Poisoning by hemostatic drug, intentional self-harm, subs
		T45.623D	Poisoning by hemostatic drug, assault, subsequent encounter
		T45.624D	Poisoning by hemostatic drug, undetermined, subs encntr
		T45.625D	Adverse effect of hemostatic drug, subsequent encounter
		T45.691D	Poisoning by oth fibrin-affct drugs, accidental, subs
		T45.692D	Poisoning by oth fibrin-affct drugs, self-harm, subs
		T45.693D	Poisoning by oth fibrinolysis-affecting drugs, assault, subs
		T45.694D	Poisoning by oth fibrin-affct drugs, undetermined, subs
		T45.695D	Adverse effect of oth fibrinolysis-affecting drugs, subs
		T45.7X1D	Poisn by anticoag antag, vitamin K and oth coag, acc, subs
		T45.7X2D	Poisn by anticoag antag, vit K and oth coag, slf-hrm, subs
		T45.7X3D	Poisn by anticoag antag, vit K and oth coag, assault, subs
		T45.7X4D	Poisn by anticoag antag, vitamin K and oth coag, undet, subs
		T45.7X5D	Adverse effect of anticoag antag, vit K and oth coag, subs
		T45.8X1D	Poisn by oth prim systemic and hematolog agents, acc, subs
		T45.8X2D	Poisn by oth prim sys and hematolog agents, slf-hrm, subs
		T45.8X3D	Poisn by oth prim sys and hematolog agents, assault, subs
		T45.8X4D	Poisn by oth prim systemic and hematolog agents, undet, subs
		T45.8X5D	Adverse effect of prim systemic and hematolog agents, subs
		T45.91XD	Poisn by unsp prim systemic and hematolog agent, acc, subs
		T45.92XD	Poisn by unsp prim sys and hematolog agent, slf-hrm, subs
		T45.93XD	Poisn by unsp prim sys and hematolog agent, assault, subs
		T45.94XD	Poisn by unsp prim systemic and hematolog agent, undet, subs
		T45.95XD	Adverse effect of unsp prim sys and hematolog agent, subs
		T46.ØX1D	Poisoning by cardi-stim glycos/drug simlar act, acc, subs
		T46.ØX2D	Poisn by cardi-stim glycos/drug simlar act, self-harm, subs
		T46.ØX3D	Poisn by cardi-stim glycos/drug simlar act, assault, subs
		T46.ØX4D	Poisoning by cardi-stim glycos/drug simlar act, undet, subs
		T46.ØX5D	Adverse effect of cardi-stim glycos/drug simlar act, subs
		T46.1X1D	Poisoning by calcium-channel blockers, accidental, subs
		T46.1X2D	Poisoning by calcium-channel blockers, self-harm, subs
		T46.1X3D	Poisoning by calcium-channel blockers, assault, subs encntr
		T46.1X4D	Poisoning by calcium-channel blockers, undetermined, subs
		T46.1X5D	Adverse effect of calcium-channel blockers, subs encntr
		T46.2X1D	Poisoning by oth antidysrhythmic drugs, accidental, subs
		T46.2X2D	Poisoning by oth antidysrhythmic drugs, self-harm, subs
	(Continued on next page)	**T46.2X3D**	Poisoning by oth antidysrhythmic drugs, assault, subs encntr

ICD-9-CM		ICD-10-CM	
V58.89	ENCOUNTER FOR OTHER SPECIFIED AFTERCARE **(Continued)**	**T46.2X4D**	Poisoning by oth antidysrhythmic drugs, undetermined, subs
		T46.2X5D	Adverse effect of other antidysrhythmic drugs, subs encntr
		T46.3X1D	Poisoning by coronary vasodilators, accidental, subs
		T46.3X2D	Poisoning by coronary vasodilators, self-harm, subs
		T46.3X3D	Poisoning by coronary vasodilators, assault, subs encntr
		T46.3X4D	Poisoning by coronary vasodilators, undetermined, subs
		T46.3X5D	Adverse effect of coronary vasodilators, subs encntr
		T46.4X1D	Poisoning by angiotens-convert-enzyme inhibitors, acc, subs
		T46.4X2D	Poisn by angiotens-convert-enzyme inhibtr, self-harm, subs
		T46.4X3D	Poisoning by angiotens-convert-enzyme inhibtr, assault, subs
		T46.4X4D	Poisoning by angiotens-convert-enzyme inhibtr, undet, subs
		T46.4X5D	Adverse effect of angiotens-convert-enzyme inhibitors, subs
		T46.5X1D	Poisoning by oth antihypertn drugs, accidental, subs
		T46.5X2D	Poisoning by oth antihypertensive drugs, self-harm, subs
		T46.5X3D	Poisoning by oth antihypertensive drugs, assault, subs
		T46.5X4D	Poisoning by oth antihypertensive drugs, undetermined, subs
		T46.5X5D	Adverse effect of other antihypertensive drugs, subs encntr
		T46.6X1D	Poisoning by antihyperlip and antiarterio drugs, acc, subs
		T46.6X2D	Poisn by antihyperlip and antiarterio drugs, self-harm, subs
		T46.6X3D	Poisn by antihyperlip and antiarterio drugs, assault, subs
		T46.6X4D	Poisoning by antihyperlip and antiarterio drugs, undet, subs
		T46.6X5D	Adverse effect of antihyperlip and antiarterio drugs, subs
		T46.7X1D	Poisoning by peripheral vasodilators, accidental, subs
		T46.7X2D	Poisoning by peripheral vasodilators, self-harm, subs
		T46.7X3D	Poisoning by peripheral vasodilators, assault, subs encntr
		T46.7X4D	Poisoning by peripheral vasodilators, undetermined, subs
		T46.7X5D	Adverse effect of peripheral vasodilators, subs encntr
		T46.8X1D	Poisoning by antivaric drugs, inc scler agents, acc, subs
		T46.8X2D	Poisn by antivaric drugs, inc scler agents, self-harm, subs
		T46.8X3D	Poisn by antivaric drugs, inc scler agents, assault, subs
		T46.8X4D	Poisoning by antivaric drugs, inc scler agents, undet, subs
		T46.8X5D	Adverse effect of antivaric drugs, inc scler agents, subs
		T46.9Ø1D	Poisoning by unsp agents aff the cardiovasc sys, acc, subs
		T46.9Ø2D	Poisn by unsp agents aff the cardiovasc sys, self-harm, subs
		T46.9Ø3D	Poisn by unsp agents aff the cardiovasc sys, assault, subs
		T46.9Ø4D	Poisoning by unsp agents aff the cardiovasc sys, undet, subs
		T46.9Ø5D	Adverse effect of unsp agents aff the cardiovasc sys, subs
		T46.991D	Poisoning by oth agents aff the cardiovasc sys, acc, subs
		T46.992D	Poisn by oth agents aff the cardiovasc sys, self-harm, subs
		T46.993D	Poisn by oth agents aff the cardiovasc sys, assault, subs
		T46.994D	Poisoning by oth agents aff the cardiovasc sys, undet, subs
		T46.995D	Adverse effect of agents aff the cardiovascular sys, subs
		T47.ØX1D	Poisoning by histamine H2-receptor blockers, acc, subs
		T47.ØX2D	Poisoning by histamine H2-receptor blockers, self-harm, subs
		T47.ØX3D	Poisoning by histamine H2-receptor blockers, assault, subs
		T47.ØX4D	Poisoning by histamine H2-receptor blockers, undet, subs
		T47.ØX5D	Adverse effect of histamine H2-receptor blockers, subs
		T47.1X1D	Poisn by oth antacids and anti-gstrc-sec drugs, acc, subs
		T47.1X2D	Poisn by oth antacids & anti-gstrc-sec drugs, slf-hrm, subs
		T47.1X3D	Poisn by oth antacids and anti-gstrc-sec drugs, asslt, subs
		T47.1X4D	Poisn by oth antacids and anti-gstrc-sec drugs, undet, subs
		T47.1X5D	Adverse effect of antacids and anti-gstrc-sec drugs, subs
		T47.2X1D	Poisoning by stimulant laxatives, accidental, subs
		T47.2X2D	Poisoning by stimulant laxatives, self-harm, subs
		T47.2X3D	Poisoning by stimulant laxatives, assault, subs encntr
		T47.2X4D	Poisoning by stimulant laxatives, undetermined, subs encntr
		T47.2X5D	Adverse effect of stimulant laxatives, subsequent encounter
		T47.3X1D	Poisoning by saline and osmotic laxatives, accidental, subs
		T47.3X2D	Poisoning by saline and osmotic laxatives, self-harm, subs
		T47.3X3D	Poisoning by saline and osmotic laxatives, assault, subs
		T47.3X4D	Poisoning by saline and osmotic laxatives, undet, subs
		T47.3X5D	Adverse effect of saline and osmotic laxatives, subs encntr
		T47.4X1D	Poisoning by oth laxatives, accidental (unintentional), subs
		T47.4X2D	Poisoning by oth laxatives, intentional self-harm, subs
		T47.4X3D	Poisoning by other laxatives, assault, subsequent encounter
		T47.4X4D	Poisoning by other laxatives, undetermined, subs encntr
		T47.4X5D	Adverse effect of other laxatives, subsequent encounter
		T47.5X1D	Poisoning by digestants, accidental (unintentional), subs
		T47.5X2D	Poisoning by digestants, intentional self-harm, subs encntr
		T47.5X3D	Poisoning by digestants, assault, subsequent encounter
		T47.5X4D	Poisoning by digestants, undetermined, subsequent encounter
		T47.5X5D	Adverse effect of digestants, subsequent encounter
		T47.6X1D	Poisoning by antidiarrheal drugs, accidental, subs
		T47.6X2D	Poisoning by antidiarrheal drugs, self-harm, subs
		T47.6X3D	Poisoning by antidiarrheal drugs, assault, subs encntr
		T47.6X4D	Poisoning by antidiarrheal drugs, undetermined, subs encntr
		T47.6X5D	Adverse effect of antidiarrheal drugs, subsequent encounter
		T47.7X1D	Poisoning by emetics, accidental (unintentional), subs
		T47.7X2D	Poisoning by emetics, intentional self-harm, subs encntr
		T47.7X3D	Poisoning by emetics, assault, subsequent encounter
		T47.7X4D	Poisoning by emetics, undetermined, subsequent encounter
		T47.7X5D	Adverse effect of emetics, subsequent encounter
		T47.8X1D	Poisoning by oth agents aff GI sys, accidental, subs

(Continued on next page)

ICD-9-CM		ICD-10-CM	
V58.89	ENCOUNTER FOR OTHER SPECIFIED AFTERCARE **(Continued)**	**T47.8X2D**	Poisoning by oth agents aff GI sys, self-harm, subs
		T47.8X3D	Poisoning by oth agents aff GI sys, assault, subs
		T47.8X4D	Poisoning by oth agents aff GI sys, undetermined, subs
		T47.8X5D	Adverse effect of agents primarily affecting GI sys, subs
		T47.91XD	Poisoning by unsp agents aff the GI sys, accidental, subs
		T47.92XD	Poisoning by unsp agents aff the GI sys, self-harm, subs
		T47.93XD	Poisoning by unsp agents aff the GI sys, assault, subs
		T47.94XD	Poisoning by unsp agents aff the GI sys, undetermined, subs
		T47.95XD	Adverse effect of unsp agents aff the GI sys, subs
		T48.ØX1D	Poisoning by oxytocic drugs, accidental, subs
		T48.ØX2D	Poisoning by oxytocic drugs, intentional self-harm, subs
		T48.ØX3D	Poisoning by oxytocic drugs, assault, subsequent encounter
		T48.ØX4D	Poisoning by oxytocic drugs, undetermined, subs encntr
		T48.ØX5D	Adverse effect of oxytocic drugs, subsequent encounter
		T48.1X1D	Poisoning by skeletal muscle relaxants, accidental, subs
		T48.1X2D	Poisoning by skeletal muscle relaxants, self-harm, subs
		T48.1X3D	Poisoning by skeletal muscle relaxants, assault, subs encntr
		T48.1X4D	Poisoning by skeletal muscle relaxants, undetermined, subs
		T48.1X5D	Adverse effect of skeletal muscle relaxants, subs encntr
		T48.2Ø1D	Poisoning by unsp drugs acting on muscles, accidental, subs
		T48.2Ø2D	Poisoning by unsp drugs acting on muscles, self-harm, subs
		T48.2Ø3D	Poisoning by unsp drugs acting on muscles, assault, subs
		T48.2Ø4D	Poisoning by unsp drugs acting on muscles, undet, subs
		T48.2Ø5D	Adverse effect of unsp drugs acting on muscles, subs encntr
		T48.291D	Poisoning by oth drugs acting on muscles, accidental, subs
		T48.292D	Poisoning by oth drugs acting on muscles, self-harm, subs
		T48.293D	Poisoning by oth drugs acting on muscles, assault, subs
		T48.294D	Poisoning by oth drugs acting on muscles, undetermined, subs
		T48.295D	Adverse effect of other drugs acting on muscles, subs encntr
		T48.3X1D	Poisoning by antitussives, accidental (unintentional), subs
		T48.3X2D	Poisoning by antitussives, intentional self-harm, subs
		T48.3X3D	Poisoning by antitussives, assault, subsequent encounter
		T48.3X4D	Poisoning by antitussives, undetermined, subs encntr
		T48.3X5D	Adverse effect of antitussives, subsequent encounter
		T48.4X1D	Poisoning by expectorants, accidental (unintentional), subs
		T48.4X2D	Poisoning by expectorants, intentional self-harm, subs
		T48.4X3D	Poisoning by expectorants, assault, subsequent encounter
		T48.4X4D	Poisoning by expectorants, undetermined, subs encntr
		T48.4X5D	Adverse effect of expectorants, subsequent encounter
		T48.5X1D	Poisoning by oth anti-cmn-cold drugs, accidental, subs
		T48.5X2D	Poisoning by oth anti-common-cold drugs, self-harm, subs
		T48.5X3D	Poisoning by oth anti-common-cold drugs, assault, subs
		T48.5X4D	Poisoning by oth anti-common-cold drugs, undetermined, subs
		T48.5X5D	Adverse effect of other anti-common-cold drugs, subs encntr
		T48.6X1D	Poisoning by antiasthmatics, accidental, subs
		T48.6X2D	Poisoning by antiasthmatics, intentional self-harm, subs
		T48.6X3D	Poisoning by antiasthmatics, assault, subsequent encounter
		T48.6X4D	Poisoning by antiasthmatics, undetermined, subs encntr
		T48.6X5D	Adverse effect of antiasthmatics, subsequent encounter
		T48.9Ø1D	Poisn by unsp agents prim acting on the resp sys, acc, subs
		T48.9Ø2D	Poisn by unsp agents prim act on the resp sys, slf-hrm, subs
		T48.9Ø3D	Poisn by unsp agents prim act on the resp sys, asslt, subs
		T48.9Ø4D	Poisn by unsp agents prim act on the resp sys, undet, subs
		T48.9Ø5D	Advrs effect of unsp agents prim act on the resp sys, subs
		T48.991D	Poisn by oth agents prim acting on the resp sys, acc, subs
		T48.992D	Poisn by oth agents prim act on the resp sys, slf-hrm, subs
		T48.993D	Poisn by oth agents prim acting on the resp sys, asslt, subs
		T48.994D	Poisn by oth agents prim acting on the resp sys, undet, subs
		T48.995D	Adverse effect of agents prim acting on the resp sys, subs
		T49.ØX1D	Poisoning by local antifung/infect/inflamm drugs, acc, subs
		T49.ØX2D	Poisn by local antifung/infect/inflamm drugs, slf-hrm, subs
		T49.ØX3D	Poisn by local antifung/infect/inflamm drugs, assault, subs
		T49.ØX4D	Poisn by local antifung/infect/inflamm drugs, undet, subs
		T49.ØX5D	Adverse effect of local antifung/infect/inflamm drugs, subs
		T49.1X1D	Poisoning by antipruritics, accidental (unintentional), subs
		T49.1X2D	Poisoning by antipruritics, intentional self-harm, subs
		T49.1X3D	Poisoning by antipruritics, assault, subsequent encounter
		T49.1X4D	Poisoning by antipruritics, undetermined, subs encntr
		T49.1X5D	Adverse effect of antipruritics, subsequent encounter
		T49.2X1D	Poisoning by local astringents/detergents, accidental, subs
		T49.2X2D	Poisoning by local astringents/detergents, self-harm, subs
		T49.2X3D	Poisoning by local astringents/detergents, assault, subs
		T49.2X4D	Poisoning by local astringents/detergents, undet, subs
		T49.2X5D	Adverse effect of local astringents/detergents, subs
		T49.3X1D	Poisoning by emollients, demulcents and protect, acc, subs
		T49.3X2D	Poisn by emollients, demulcents and protect, self-harm, subs
		T49.3X3D	Poisn by emollients, demulcents and protect, assault, subs
		T49.3X4D	Poisoning by emollients, demulcents and protect, undet, subs
		T49.3X5D	Adverse effect of emollients, demulcents and protect, subs
		T49.4X1D	Poisoning by keratolyt/keratplst/hair trmt drug, acc, subs
		T49.4X2D	Poisn by keratolyt/keratplst/hair trmt drug, self-harm, subs
		T49.4X3D	Poisn by keratolyt/keratplst/hair trmt drug, assault, subs
	(Continued on next page)	**T49.4X4D**	Poisoning by keratolyt/keratplst/hair trmt drug, undet, subs

ICD-9-CM		ICD-10-CM	
V58.89	ENCOUNTER FOR OTHER SPECIFIED AFTERCARE **(Continued)**	**T49.4X5D**	Adverse effect of keratolyt/keratplst/hair trmt drug, subs
		T49.5X1D	Poisoning by opth drugs and preparations, accidental, subs
		T49.5X2D	Poisoning by opth drugs and preparations, self-harm, subs
		T49.5X3D	Poisoning by opth drugs and preparations, assault, subs
		T49.5X4D	Poisoning by opth drugs and preparations, undetermined, subs
		T49.5X5D	Adverse effect of opth drugs and preparations, subs
		T49.6X1D	Poisoning by otorhino drugs and prep, accidental, subs
		T49.6X2D	Poisoning by otorhino drugs and prep, self-harm, subs
		T49.6X3D	Poisoning by otorhino drugs and preparations, assault, subs
		T49.6X4D	Poisoning by otorhino drugs and prep, undetermined, subs
		T49.6X5D	Adverse effect of otorhino drugs and preparations, subs
		T49.7X1D	Poisoning by dental drugs, topically applied, acc, subs
		T49.7X2D	Poisn by dental drugs, topically applied, self-harm, subs
		T49.7X3D	Poisoning by dental drugs, topically applied, assault, subs
		T49.7X4D	Poisoning by dental drugs, topically applied, undet, subs
		T49.7X5D	Adverse effect of dental drugs, topically applied, subs
		T49.8X1D	Poisoning by oth topical agents, accidental, subs
		T49.8X2D	Poisoning by oth topical agents, intentional self-harm, subs
		T49.8X3D	Poisoning by other topical agents, assault, subs encntr
		T49.8X4D	Poisoning by other topical agents, undetermined, subs encntr
		T49.8X5D	Adverse effect of other topical agents, subsequent encounter
		T49.91XD	Poisoning by unsp topical agent, accidental, subs
		T49.92XD	Poisoning by unsp topical agent, intentional self-harm, subs
		T49.93XD	Poisoning by unspecified topical agent, assault, subs encntr
		T49.94XD	Poisoning by unsp topical agent, undetermined, subs encntr
		T49.95XD	Adverse effect of unspecified topical agent, subs encntr
		T5Ø.ØX1D	Poisoning by mineralocorticoids and their antag, acc, subs
		T5Ø.ØX2D	Poisoning by mineralocorticoids and antag, self-harm, subs
		T5Ø.ØX3D	Poisoning by mineralocorticoids and antag, assault, subs
		T5Ø.ØX4D	Poisoning by mineralocorticoids and their antag, undet, subs
		T5Ø.ØX5D	Adverse effect of mineralocorticoids and their antag, subs
		T5Ø.1X1D	Poisoning by loop diuretics, accidental, subs
		T5Ø.1X2D	Poisoning by loop diuretics, intentional self-harm, subs
		T5Ø.1X3D	Poisoning by loop diuretics, assault, subsequent encounter
		T5Ø.1X4D	Poisoning by loop diuretics, undetermined, subs encntr
		T5Ø.1X5D	Adverse effect of loop diuretics, subsequent encounter
		T5Ø.2X1D	Poisn by crbnc-anhydr inhibtr, benzo/oth diuretc, acc, subs
		T5Ø.2X2D	Poisn by crbnc-anhydr inhibtr,benzo/oth diuretc,slf-hrm,subs
		T5Ø.2X3D	Poisn by crbnc-anhydr inhibtr,benzo/oth diuretc, asslt, subs
		T5Ø.2X4D	Poisn by crbnc-anhydr inhibtr,benzo/oth diuretc, undet, subs
		T5Ø.2X5D	Advrs eff of crbnc-anhydr inhibtr, benzo/oth diuretc, subs
		T5Ø.3X1D	Poisoning by electrolytic/caloric/wtr-bal agnt, acc, subs
		T5Ø.3X2D	Poisn by electrolytic/caloric/wtr-bal agnt, self-harm, subs
		T5Ø.3X3D	Poisn by electrolytic/caloric/wtr-bal agnt, assault, subs
		T5Ø.3X4D	Poisoning by electrolytic/caloric/wtr-bal agnt, undet, subs
		T5Ø.3X5D	Adverse effect of electrolytic/caloric/wtr-bal agnt, subs
		T5Ø.4X1D	Poisoning by drugs affecting uric acid metab, acc, subs
		T5Ø.4X2D	Poisoning by drugs aff uric acid metab, self-harm, subs
		T5Ø.4X3D	Poisoning by drugs affecting uric acid metab, assault, subs
		T5Ø.4X4D	Poisoning by drugs affecting uric acid metab, undet, subs
		T5Ø.4X5D	Adverse effect of drugs affecting uric acid metabolism, subs
		T5Ø.5X1D	Poisoning by appetite depressants, accidental, subs
		T5Ø.5X2D	Poisoning by appetite depressants, self-harm, subs
		T5Ø.5X3D	Poisoning by appetite depressants, assault, subs encntr
		T5Ø.5X4D	Poisoning by appetite depressants, undetermined, subs encntr
		T5Ø.5X5D	Adverse effect of appetite depressants, subsequent encounter
		T5Ø.6X1D	Poisoning by antidotes and chelating agents, acc, subs
		T5Ø.6X2D	Poisoning by antidotes and chelating agents, self-harm, subs
		T5Ø.6X3D	Poisoning by antidotes and chelating agents, assault, subs
		T5Ø.6X4D	Poisoning by antidotes and chelating agents, undet, subs
		T5Ø.6X5D	Adverse effect of antidotes and chelating agents, subs
		T5Ø.7X1D	Poisn by analeptics and opioid receptor antag, acc, subs
		T5Ø.7X2D	Poisn by analeptics and opioid receptor antag, slf-hrm, subs
		T5Ø.7X3D	Poisn by analeptics and opioid receptor antag, assault, subs
		T5Ø.7X4D	Poisn by analeptics and opioid receptor antag, undet, subs
		T5Ø.7X5D	Adverse effect of analeptics and opioid receptor antag, subs
		T5Ø.8X1D	Poisoning by diagnostic agents, accidental, subs
		T5Ø.8X2D	Poisoning by diagnostic agents, intentional self-harm, subs
		T5Ø.8X3D	Poisoning by diagnostic agents, assault, subs encntr
		T5Ø.8X4D	Poisoning by diagnostic agents, undetermined, subs encntr
		T5Ø.8X5D	Adverse effect of diagnostic agents, subsequent encounter
		T5Ø.9Ø1D	Poisoning by unsp drug/meds/biol subst, accidental, subs
		T5Ø.9Ø2D	Poisoning by unsp drug/meds/biol subst, self-harm, subs
		T5Ø.9Ø3D	Poisoning by unsp drug/meds/biol subst, assault, subs
		T5Ø.9Ø4D	Poisoning by unsp drug/meds/biol subst, undetermined, subs
		T5Ø.9Ø5D	Adverse effect of unsp drug/meds/biol subst, subs
		T5Ø.991D	Poisoning by oth drug/meds/biol subst, accidental, subs
		T5Ø.992D	Poisoning by oth drug/meds/biol subst, self-harm, subs
		T5Ø.993D	Poisoning by oth drug/meds/biol subst, assault, subs
		T5Ø.994D	Poisoning by oth drug/meds/biol subst, undetermined, subs
		T5Ø.995D	Adverse effect of oth drug/meds/biol subst, subs
		T5Ø.A11D	Poisn by pertuss vaccine, inc combin w pertuss, acc, subs
	(Continued on next page)	**T5Ø.A12D**	Poisn by pertuss vaccn, inc combin w pertuss, slf-hrm, subs

See Appendix A ➡ Equivalent Mapping Scenario Scenario

ICD-9-CM		ICD-10-CM	
V58.89	ENCOUNTER FOR OTHER SPECIFIED AFTERCARE **(Continued)**	**T5Ø.A13D**	Poisn by pertuss vaccine, inc combin w pertuss, asslt, subs
		T5Ø.A14D	Poisn by pertuss vaccine, inc combin w pertuss, undet, subs
		T5Ø.A15D	Advrs effect of pertuss vaccine, inc combin w pertuss, subs
		T5Ø.A21D	Poisoning by mixed bact vaccines w/o a pertuss, acc, subs
		T5Ø.A22D	Poisn by mixed bact vaccines w/o a pertuss, self-harm, subs
		T5Ø.A23D	Poisn by mixed bact vaccines w/o a pertuss, assault, subs
		T5Ø.A24D	Poisoning by mixed bact vaccines w/o a pertuss, undet, subs
		T5Ø.A25D	Adverse effect of mixed bact vaccines w/o a pertuss, subs
		T5Ø.A91D	Poisoning by oth bacterial vaccines, accidental, subs
		T5Ø.A92D	Poisoning by oth bacterial vaccines, self-harm, subs
		T5Ø.A93D	Poisoning by other bacterial vaccines, assault, subs encntr
		T5Ø.A94D	Poisoning by oth bacterial vaccines, undetermined, subs
		T5Ø.A95D	Adverse effect of other bacterial vaccines, subs encntr
		T5Ø.B11D	Poisoning by smallpox vaccines, accidental, subs
		T5Ø.B12D	Poisoning by smallpox vaccines, intentional self-harm, subs
		T5Ø.B13D	Poisoning by smallpox vaccines, assault, subs encntr
		T5Ø.B14D	Poisoning by smallpox vaccines, undetermined, subs encntr
		T5Ø.B15D	Adverse effect of smallpox vaccines, subsequent encounter
		T5Ø.B91D	Poisoning by oth viral vaccines, accidental, subs
		T5Ø.B92D	Poisoning by oth viral vaccines, intentional self-harm, subs
		T5Ø.B93D	Poisoning by other viral vaccines, assault, subs encntr
		T5Ø.B94D	Poisoning by other viral vaccines, undetermined, subs encntr
		T5Ø.B95D	Adverse effect of other viral vaccines, subsequent encounter
		T5Ø.Z11D	Poisoning by immunoglobulin, accidental, subs
		T5Ø.Z12D	Poisoning by immunoglobulin, intentional self-harm, subs
		T5Ø.Z13D	Poisoning by immunoglobulin, assault, subsequent encounter
		T5Ø.Z14D	Poisoning by immunoglobulin, undetermined, subs encntr
		T5Ø.Z15D	Adverse effect of immunoglobulin, subsequent encounter
		T5Ø.Z91D	Poisoning by oth vaccines and biolg substances, acc, subs
		T5Ø.Z92D	Poisoning by oth vaccines and biolg substnc, self-harm, subs
		T5Ø.Z93D	Poisoning by oth vaccines and biolg substnc, assault, subs
		T5Ø.Z94D	Poisoning by oth vaccines and biolg substances, undet, subs
		T5Ø.Z95D	Adverse effect of vaccines and biological substances, subs
		T51.ØX1D	Toxic effect of ethanol, accidental (unintentional), subs
		T51.ØX2D	Toxic effect of ethanol, intentional self-harm, subs encntr
		T51.ØX3D	Toxic effect of ethanol, assault, subsequent encounter
		T51.ØX4D	Toxic effect of ethanol, undetermined, subsequent encounter
		T51.1X1D	Toxic effect of methanol, accidental (unintentional), subs
		T51.1X2D	Toxic effect of methanol, intentional self-harm, subs encntr
		T51.1X3D	Toxic effect of methanol, assault, subsequent encounter
		T51.1X4D	Toxic effect of methanol, undetermined, subsequent encounter
		T51.2X1D	Toxic effect of 2-Propanol, accidental (unintentional), subs
		T51.2X2D	Toxic effect of 2-Propanol, intentional self-harm, subs
		T51.2X3D	Toxic effect of 2-Propanol, assault, subsequent encounter
		T51.2X4D	Toxic effect of 2-Propanol, undetermined, subs encntr
		T51.3X1D	Toxic effect of fusel oil, accidental (unintentional), subs
		T51.3X2D	Toxic effect of fusel oil, intentional self-harm, subs
		T51.3X3D	Toxic effect of fusel oil, assault, subsequent encounter
		T51.3X4D	Toxic effect of fusel oil, undetermined, subs encntr
		T51.8X1D	Toxic effect of alcohols, accidental (unintentional), subs
		T51.8X2D	Toxic effect of oth alcohols, intentional self-harm, subs
		T51.8X3D	Toxic effect of other alcohols, assault, subs encntr
		T51.8X4D	Toxic effect of other alcohols, undetermined, subs encntr
		T51.91XD	Toxic effect of unsp alcohol, accidental, subs
		T51.92XD	Toxic effect of unsp alcohol, intentional self-harm, subs
		T51.93XD	Toxic effect of unspecified alcohol, assault, subs encntr
		T51.94XD	Toxic effect of unsp alcohol, undetermined, subs encntr
		T52.ØX1D	Toxic effect of petroleum products, accidental, subs
		T52.ØX2D	Toxic effect of petroleum products, self-harm, subs
		T52.ØX3D	Toxic effect of petroleum products, assault, subs encntr
		T52.ØX4D	Toxic effect of petroleum products, undetermined, subs
		T52.1X1D	Toxic effect of benzene, accidental (unintentional), subs
		T52.1X2D	Toxic effect of benzene, intentional self-harm, subs encntr
		T52.1X3D	Toxic effect of benzene, assault, subsequent encounter
		T52.1X4D	Toxic effect of benzene, undetermined, subsequent encounter
		T52.2X1D	Toxic effect of homologues of benzene, accidental, subs
		T52.2X2D	Toxic effect of homologues of benzene, self-harm, subs
		T52.2X3D	Toxic effect of homologues of benzene, assault, subs encntr
		T52.2X4D	Toxic effect of homologues of benzene, undetermined, subs
		T52.3X1D	Toxic effect of glycols, accidental (unintentional), subs
		T52.3X2D	Toxic effect of glycols, intentional self-harm, subs encntr
		T52.3X3D	Toxic effect of glycols, assault, subsequent encounter
		T52.3X4D	Toxic effect of glycols, undetermined, subsequent encounter
		T52.4X1D	Toxic effect of ketones, accidental (unintentional), subs
		T52.4X2D	Toxic effect of ketones, intentional self-harm, subs encntr
		T52.4X3D	Toxic effect of ketones, assault, subsequent encounter
		T52.4X4D	Toxic effect of ketones, undetermined, subsequent encounter
		T52.8X1D	Toxic effect of organic solvents, accidental, subs
		T52.8X2D	Toxic effect of organic solvents, self-harm, subs
		T52.8X3D	Toxic effect of other organic solvents, assault, subs encntr
		T52.8X4D	Toxic effect of oth organic solvents, undetermined, subs
		T52.91XD	Toxic effect of unsp organic solvent, accidental, subs
		T52.92XD	Toxic effect of unsp organic solvent, self-harm, subs

(Continued on next page)

[Brackets] indicate valid character values for each code. Character value meanings provided for each code grouping.

ICD-9-CM		ICD-10-CM	
V58.89	ENCOUNTER FOR OTHER SPECIFIED AFTERCARE **(Continued)**	**T52.93XD**	Toxic effect of unsp organic solvent, assault, subs encntr
		T52.94XD	Toxic effect of unsp organic solvent, undetermined, subs
		T53.ØX1D	Toxic effect of carbon tetrachloride, accidental, subs
		T53.ØX2D	Toxic effect of carbon tetrachloride, self-harm, subs
		T53.ØX3D	Toxic effect of carbon tetrachloride, assault, subs encntr
		T53.ØX4D	Toxic effect of carbon tetrachloride, undetermined, subs
		T53.1X1D	Toxic effect of chloroform, accidental (unintentional), subs
		T53.1X2D	Toxic effect of chloroform, intentional self-harm, subs
		T53.1X3D	Toxic effect of chloroform, assault, subsequent encounter
		T53.1X4D	Toxic effect of chloroform, undetermined, subs encntr
		T53.2X1D	Toxic effect of trichloroethylene, accidental, subs
		T53.2X2D	Toxic effect of trichloroethylene, self-harm, subs
		T53.2X3D	Toxic effect of trichloroethylene, assault, subs encntr
		T53.2X4D	Toxic effect of trichloroethylene, undetermined, subs encntr
		T53.3X1D	Toxic effect of tetrachloroethylene, accidental, subs
		T53.3X2D	Toxic effect of tetrachloroethylene, self-harm, subs
		T53.3X3D	Toxic effect of tetrachloroethylene, assault, subs encntr
		T53.3X4D	Toxic effect of tetrachloroethylene, undetermined, subs
		T53.4X1D	Toxic effect of dichloromethane, accidental, subs
		T53.4X2D	Toxic effect of dichloromethane, intentional self-harm, subs
		T53.4X3D	Toxic effect of dichloromethane, assault, subs encntr
		T53.4X4D	Toxic effect of dichloromethane, undetermined, subs encntr
		T53.5X1D	Toxic effect of chlorofluorocarbons, accidental, subs
		T53.5X2D	Toxic effect of chlorofluorocarbons, self-harm, subs
		T53.5X3D	Toxic effect of chlorofluorocarbons, assault, subs encntr
		T53.5X4D	Toxic effect of chlorofluorocarbons, undetermined, subs
		T53.6X1D	Toxic eff of halgn deriv of aliphatic hydrocrb, acc, subs
		T53.6X2D	Tox eff of halgn deriv of aliphatic hydrocrb, slf-hrm, subs
		T53.6X3D	Toxic eff of halgn deriv of aliphatic hydrocrb, asslt, subs
		T53.6X4D	Toxic eff of halgn deriv of aliphatic hydrocrb, undet, subs
		T53.7X1D	Toxic effect of halgn deriv of aromatic hydrocrb, acc, subs
		T53.7X2D	Toxic eff of halgn deriv of aromatic hydrocrb, slf-hrm, subs
		T53.7X3D	Toxic eff of halgn deriv of aromatic hydrocrb, asslt, subs
		T53.7X4D	Toxic eff of halgn deriv of aromatic hydrocrb, undet, subs
		T53.91XD	Toxic eff of unsp halgn deriv of aromat hydrocrb, acc, subs
		T53.92XD	Tox eff of unsp halgn deriv of aromat hydrocrb,slf-hrm, subs
		T53.93XD	Tox eff of unsp halgn deriv of aromat hydrocrb, asslt, subs
		T53.94XD	Tox eff of unsp halgn deriv of aromat hydrocrb, undet, subs
		T54.ØX1D	Toxic effect of phenol and phenol homologues, acc, subs
		T54.ØX2D	Toxic effect of phenol and phenol homolog, self-harm, subs
		T54.ØX3D	Toxic effect of phenol and phenol homologues, assault, subs
		T54.ØX4D	Toxic effect of phenol and phenol homologues, undet, subs
		T54.1X1D	Toxic effect of corrosive organic compounds, acc, subs
		T54.1X2D	Toxic effect of corrosive organic compounds, self-harm, subs
		T54.1X3D	Toxic effect of corrosive organic compounds, assault, subs
		T54.1X4D	Toxic effect of corrosive organic compounds, undet, subs
		T54.2X1D	Toxic eff of corrosv acids and acid-like substnc, acc, subs
		T54.2X2D	Tox eff of corrosv acids & acid-like substnc, slf-hrm, subs
		T54.2X3D	Tox eff of corrosv acids and acid-like substnc, asslt, subs
		T54.2X4D	Tox eff of corrosv acids and acid-like substnc, undet, subs
		T54.3X1D	Tox eff of corrosv alkalis and alk-like substnc, acc, subs
		T54.3X2D	Tox eff of corrosv alkalis & alk-like substnc, slf-hrm, subs
		T54.3X3D	Tox eff of corrosv alkalis and alk-like substnc, asslt, subs
		T54.3X4D	Tox eff of corrosv alkalis and alk-like substnc, undet, subs
		T54.91XD	Toxic effect of unsp corrosive substance, accidental, subs
		T54.92XD	Toxic effect of unsp corrosive substance, self-harm, subs
		T54.93XD	Toxic effect of unsp corrosive substance, assault, subs
		T54.94XD	Toxic effect of unsp corrosive substance, undetermined, subs
		T55.ØX1D	Toxic effect of soaps, accidental (unintentional), subs
		T55.ØX2D	Toxic effect of soaps, intentional self-harm, subs encntr
		T55.ØX3D	Toxic effect of soaps, assault, subsequent encounter
		T55.ØX4D	Toxic effect of soaps, undetermined, subsequent encounter
		T55.1X1D	Toxic effect of detergents, accidental (unintentional), subs
		T55.1X2D	Toxic effect of detergents, intentional self-harm, subs
		T55.1X3D	Toxic effect of detergents, assault, subsequent encounter
		T55.1X4D	Toxic effect of detergents, undetermined, subs encntr
		T56.ØX1D	Toxic effect of lead and its compounds, accidental, subs
		T56.ØX2D	Toxic effect of lead and its compounds, self-harm, subs
		T56.ØX3D	Toxic effect of lead and its compounds, assault, subs encntr
		T56.ØX4D	Toxic effect of lead and its compounds, undetermined, subs
		T56.1X1D	Toxic effect of mercury and its compounds, accidental, subs
		T56.1X2D	Toxic effect of mercury and its compounds, self-harm, subs
		T56.1X3D	Toxic effect of mercury and its compounds, assault, subs
		T56.1X4D	Toxic effect of mercury and its compounds, undet, subs
		T56.2X1D	Toxic effect of chromium and its compounds, acc, subs
		T56.2X2D	Toxic effect of chromium and its compounds, self-harm, subs
		T56.2X3D	Toxic effect of chromium and its compounds, assault, subs
		T56.2X4D	Toxic effect of chromium and its compounds, undet, subs
		T56.3X1D	Toxic effect of cadmium and its compounds, accidental, subs
		T56.3X2D	Toxic effect of cadmium and its compounds, self-harm, subs
		T56.3X3D	Toxic effect of cadmium and its compounds, assault, subs
		T56.3X4D	Toxic effect of cadmium and its compounds, undet, subs
	(Continued on next page)	**T56.4X1D**	Toxic effect of copper and its compounds, accidental, subs

ICD-9-CM		ICD-10-CM	
V58.89	ENCOUNTER FOR OTHER SPECIFIED AFTERCARE **(Continued)**	**T56.4X2D**	Toxic effect of copper and its compounds, self-harm, subs
		T56.4X3D	Toxic effect of copper and its compounds, assault, subs
		T56.4X4D	Toxic effect of copper and its compounds, undetermined, subs
		T56.5X1D	Toxic effect of zinc and its compounds, accidental, subs
		T56.5X2D	Toxic effect of zinc and its compounds, self-harm, subs
		T56.5X3D	Toxic effect of zinc and its compounds, assault, subs encntr
		T56.5X4D	Toxic effect of zinc and its compounds, undetermined, subs
		T56.6X1D	Toxic effect of tin and its compounds, accidental, subs
		T56.6X2D	Toxic effect of tin and its compounds, self-harm, subs
		T56.6X3D	Toxic effect of tin and its compounds, assault, subs encntr
		T56.6X4D	Toxic effect of tin and its compounds, undetermined, subs
		T56.7X1D	Toxic effect of beryllium and its compounds, acc, subs
		T56.7X2D	Toxic effect of beryllium and its compounds, self-harm, subs
		T56.7X3D	Toxic effect of beryllium and its compounds, assault, subs
		T56.7X4D	Toxic effect of beryllium and its compounds, undet, subs
		T56.811D	Toxic effect of thallium, accidental (unintentional), subs
		T56.812D	Toxic effect of thallium, intentional self-harm, subs encntr
		T56.813D	Toxic effect of thallium, assault, subsequent encounter
		T56.814D	Toxic effect of thallium, undetermined, subsequent encounter
		T56.891D	Toxic effect of oth metals, accidental (unintentional), subs
		T56.892D	Toxic effect of oth metals, intentional self-harm, subs
		T56.893D	Toxic effect of other metals, assault, subsequent encounter
		T56.894D	Toxic effect of other metals, undetermined, subs encntr
		T56.91XD	Toxic effect of unsp metal, accidental (unintentional), subs
		T56.92XD	Toxic effect of unsp metal, intentional self-harm, subs
		T56.93XD	Toxic effect of unspecified metal, assault, subs encntr
		T56.94XD	Toxic effect of unspecified metal, undetermined, subs encntr
		T57.ØX1D	Toxic effect of arsenic and its compounds, accidental, subs
		T57.ØX2D	Toxic effect of arsenic and its compounds, self-harm, subs
		T57.ØX3D	Toxic effect of arsenic and its compounds, assault, subs
		T57.ØX4D	Toxic effect of arsenic and its compounds, undet, subs
		T57.1X1D	Toxic effect of phosphorus and its compounds, acc, subs
		T57.1X2D	Toxic effect of phosphorus and its compnd, self-harm, subs
		T57.1X3D	Toxic effect of phosphorus and its compounds, assault, subs
		T57.1X4D	Toxic effect of phosphorus and its compounds, undet, subs
		T57.2X1D	Toxic effect of manganese and its compounds, acc, subs
		T57.2X2D	Toxic effect of manganese and its compounds, self-harm, subs
		T57.2X3D	Toxic effect of manganese and its compounds, assault, subs
		T57.2X4D	Toxic effect of manganese and its compounds, undet, subs
		T57.3X1D	Toxic effect of hydrogen cyanide, accidental, subs
		T57.3X2D	Toxic effect of hydrogen cyanide, self-harm, subs
		T57.3X3D	Toxic effect of hydrogen cyanide, assault, subs encntr
		T57.3X4D	Toxic effect of hydrogen cyanide, undetermined, subs encntr
		T57.8X1D	Toxic effect of inorganic substances, accidental, subs
		T57.8X2D	Toxic effect of inorganic substances, self-harm, subs
		T57.8X3D	Toxic effect of oth inorganic substances, assault, subs
		T57.8X4D	Toxic effect of oth inorganic substances, undetermined, subs
		T57.91XD	Toxic effect of unsp inorganic substance, accidental, subs
		T57.92XD	Toxic effect of unsp inorganic substance, self-harm, subs
		T57.93XD	Toxic effect of unsp inorganic substance, assault, subs
		T57.94XD	Toxic effect of unsp inorganic substance, undetermined, subs
		T58.Ø1XD	Toxic effect of carb monx from mtr veh exhaust, acc, subs
		T58.Ø2XD	Toxic eff of carb monx from mtr veh exhaust, slf-hrm, subs
		T58.Ø3XD	Toxic effect of carb monx from mtr veh exhaust, asslt, subs
		T58.Ø4XD	Toxic effect of carb monx from mtr veh exhaust, undet, subs
		T58.11XD	Toxic effect of carb monx from utility gas, acc, subs
		T58.12XD	Toxic effect of carb monx from utility gas, self-harm, subs
		T58.13XD	Toxic effect of carb monx from utility gas, assault, subs
		T58.14XD	Toxic effect of carb monx from utility gas, undet, subs
		T58.2X1D	Tox eff of carb monx fr incmpl combst dmst fuel, acc, subs
		T58.2X2D	Tox eff of carb monx fr incmpl combst dmst fuel,slf-hrm,subs
		T58.2X3D	Tox eff of carb monx fr incmpl combst dmst fuel, asslt, subs
		T58.2X4D	Tox eff of carb monx fr incmpl combst dmst fuel, undet, subs
		T58.8X1D	Toxic effect of carb monx from oth source, accidental, subs
		T58.8X2D	Toxic effect of carb monx from oth source, self-harm, subs
		T58.8X3D	Toxic effect of carb monx from oth source, assault, subs
		T58.8X4D	Toxic effect of carb monx from oth source, undet, subs
		T58.91XD	Toxic effect of carb monx from unsp source, acc, subs
		T58.92XD	Toxic effect of carb monx from unsp source, self-harm, subs
		T58.93XD	Toxic effect of carb monx from unsp source, assault, subs
		T58.94XD	Toxic effect of carb monx from unsp source, undet, subs
		T59.ØX1D	Toxic effect of nitrogen oxides, accidental, subs
		T59.ØX2D	Toxic effect of nitrogen oxides, intentional self-harm, subs
		T59.ØX3D	Toxic effect of nitrogen oxides, assault, subs encntr
		T59.ØX4D	Toxic effect of nitrogen oxides, undetermined, subs encntr
		T59.1X1D	Toxic effect of sulfur dioxide, accidental, subs
		T59.1X2D	Toxic effect of sulfur dioxide, intentional self-harm, subs
		T59.1X3D	Toxic effect of sulfur dioxide, assault, subs encntr
		T59.1X4D	Toxic effect of sulfur dioxide, undetermined, subs encntr
		T59.2X1D	Toxic effect of formaldehyde, accidental, subs
		T59.2X2D	Toxic effect of formaldehyde, intentional self-harm, subs
		T59.2X3D	Toxic effect of formaldehyde, assault, subsequent encounter
		T59.2X4D	Toxic effect of formaldehyde, undetermined, subs encntr

(Continued on next page)

ICD-9-CM		ICD-10-CM	
V58.89	ENCOUNTER FOR OTHER SPECIFIED AFTERCARE **(Continued)**	**T59.3X1D**	Toxic effect of lacrimogenic gas, accidental, subs
		T59.3X2D	Toxic effect of lacrimogenic gas, self-harm, subs
		T59.3X3D	Toxic effect of lacrimogenic gas, assault, subs encntr
		T59.3X4D	Toxic effect of lacrimogenic gas, undetermined, subs encntr
		T59.4X1D	Toxic effect of chlorine gas, accidental, subs
		T59.4X2D	Toxic effect of chlorine gas, intentional self-harm, subs
		T59.4X3D	Toxic effect of chlorine gas, assault, subsequent encounter
		T59.4X4D	Toxic effect of chlorine gas, undetermined, subs encntr
		T59.5X1D	Toxic eff of fluorine gas and hydrogen fluoride, acc, subs
		T59.5X2D	Tox eff of fluorine gas and hydrogen fluoride, slf-hrm, subs
		T59.5X3D	Toxic eff of fluorine gas and hydrogen fluoride, asslt, subs
		T59.5X4D	Toxic eff of fluorine gas and hydrogen fluoride, undet, subs
		T59.6X1D	Toxic effect of hydrogen sulfide, accidental, subs
		T59.6X2D	Toxic effect of hydrogen sulfide, self-harm, subs
		T59.6X3D	Toxic effect of hydrogen sulfide, assault, subs encntr
		T59.6X4D	Toxic effect of hydrogen sulfide, undetermined, subs encntr
		T59.7X1D	Toxic effect of carbon dioxide, accidental, subs
		T59.7X2D	Toxic effect of carbon dioxide, intentional self-harm, subs
		T59.7X3D	Toxic effect of carbon dioxide, assault, subs encntr
		T59.7X4D	Toxic effect of carbon dioxide, undetermined, subs encntr
		T59.811D	Toxic effect of smoke, accidental (unintentional), subs
		T59.812D	Toxic effect of smoke, intentional self-harm, subs encntr
		T59.813D	Toxic effect of smoke, assault, subsequent encounter
		T59.814D	Toxic effect of smoke, undetermined, subsequent encounter
		T59.891D	Toxic effect of gases, fumes and vapors, accidental, subs
		T59.892D	Toxic effect of gases, fumes and vapors, self-harm, subs
		T59.893D	Toxic effect of oth gases, fumes and vapors, assault, subs
		T59.894D	Toxic effect of gases, fumes and vapors, undetermined, subs
		T59.91XD	Toxic effect of unsp gases, fumes and vapors, acc, subs
		T59.92XD	Toxic effect of unsp gases, fumes and vapors, slf-hrm, subs
		T59.93XD	Toxic effect of unsp gases, fumes and vapors, assault, subs
		T59.94XD	Toxic effect of unsp gases, fumes and vapors, undet, subs
		T60.0X1D	Toxic effect of organophos and carbamate insect, acc, subs
		T60.0X2D	Toxic eff of organophos and carbamate insect, slf-hrm, subs
		T60.0X3D	Toxic effect of organophos and carbamate insect, asslt, subs
		T60.0X4D	Toxic effect of organophos and carbamate insect, undet, subs
		T60.1X1D	Toxic effect of halogenated insecticides, accidental, subs
		T60.1X2D	Toxic effect of halogenated insecticides, self-harm, subs
		T60.1X3D	Toxic effect of halogenated insecticides, assault, subs
		T60.1X4D	Toxic effect of halogenated insecticides, undetermined, subs
		T60.2X1D	Toxic effect of insecticides, accidental, subs
		T60.2X2D	Toxic effect of insecticides, intentional self-harm, subs
		T60.2X3D	Toxic effect of other insecticides, assault, subs encntr
		T60.2X4D	Toxic effect of oth insecticides, undetermined, subs encntr
		T60.3X1D	Toxic effect of herbicides and fungicides, accidental, subs
		T60.3X2D	Toxic effect of herbicides and fungicides, self-harm, subs
		T60.3X3D	Toxic effect of herbicides and fungicides, assault, subs
		T60.3X4D	Toxic effect of herbicides and fungicides, undet, subs
		T60.4X1D	Toxic effect of rodenticides, accidental, subs
		T60.4X2D	Toxic effect of rodenticides, intentional self-harm, subs
		T60.4X3D	Toxic effect of rodenticides, assault, subsequent encounter
		T60.4X4D	Toxic effect of rodenticides, undetermined, subs encntr
		T60.8X1D	Toxic effect of pesticides, accidental (unintentional), subs
		T60.8X2D	Toxic effect of oth pesticides, intentional self-harm, subs
		T60.8X3D	Toxic effect of other pesticides, assault, subs encntr
		T60.8X4D	Toxic effect of other pesticides, undetermined, subs encntr
		T60.91XD	Toxic effect of unsp pesticide, accidental, subs
		T60.92XD	Toxic effect of unsp pesticide, intentional self-harm, subs
		T60.93XD	Toxic effect of unspecified pesticide, assault, subs encntr
		T60.94XD	Toxic effect of unsp pesticide, undetermined, subs encntr
		T61.01XD	Ciguatera fish poisoning, accidental (unintentional), subs
		T61.02XD	Ciguatera fish poisoning, intentional self-harm, subs encntr
		T61.03XD	Ciguatera fish poisoning, assault, subsequent encounter
		T61.04XD	Ciguatera fish poisoning, undetermined, subsequent encounter
		T61.11XD	Scombroid fish poisoning, accidental (unintentional), subs
		T61.12XD	Scombroid fish poisoning, intentional self-harm, subs encntr
		T61.13XD	Scombroid fish poisoning, assault, subsequent encounter
		T61.14XD	Scombroid fish poisoning, undetermined, subsequent encounter
		T61.771D	Oth fish poisoning, accidental (unintentional), subs encntr
		T61.772D	Other fish poisoning, intentional self-harm, subs encntr
		T61.773D	Other fish poisoning, assault, subsequent encounter
		T61.774D	Other fish poisoning, undetermined, subsequent encounter
		T61.781D	Oth shellfish poisoning, accidental (unintentional), subs
		T61.782D	Oth shellfish poisoning, intentional self-harm, subs encntr
		T61.783D	Other shellfish poisoning, assault, subsequent encounter
		T61.784D	Other shellfish poisoning, undetermined, subs encntr
		T61.8X1D	Toxic effect of seafood, accidental (unintentional), subs
		T61.8X2D	Toxic effect of oth seafood, intentional self-harm, subs
		T61.8X3D	Toxic effect of other seafood, assault, subsequent encounter
		T61.8X4D	Toxic effect of other seafood, undetermined, subs encntr
		T61.91XD	Toxic effect of unsp seafood, accidental, subs
		T61.92XD	Toxic effect of unsp seafood, intentional self-harm, subs
	(Continued on next page)	**T61.93XD**	Toxic effect of unspecified seafood, assault, subs encntr

ICD-9-CM		ICD-10-CM	
V58.89	ENCOUNTER FOR OTHER SPECIFIED AFTERCARE **(Continued)**	**T61.94XD**	Toxic effect of unsp seafood, undetermined, subs encntr
		T62.ØX1D	Toxic effect of ingested mushrooms, accidental, subs
		T62.ØX2D	Toxic effect of ingested mushrooms, self-harm, subs
		T62.ØX3D	Toxic effect of ingested mushrooms, assault, subs encntr
		T62.ØX4D	Toxic effect of ingested mushrooms, undetermined, subs
		T62.1X1D	Toxic effect of ingested berries, accidental, subs
		T62.1X2D	Toxic effect of ingested berries, self-harm, subs
		T62.1X3D	Toxic effect of ingested berries, assault, subs encntr
		T62.1X4D	Toxic effect of ingested berries, undetermined, subs encntr
		T62.2X1D	Toxic effect of ingested (parts of) plant(s), acc, subs
		T62.2X2D	Toxic effect of ingested (parts of) plant(s), slf-hrm, subs
		T62.2X3D	Toxic effect of ingested (parts of) plant(s), assault, subs
		T62.2X4D	Toxic effect of ingested (parts of) plant(s), undet, subs
		T62.8X1D	Toxic effect of noxious substances eaten as food, acc, subs
		T62.8X2D	Toxic effect of noxious substnc eaten as food, slf-hrm, subs
		T62.8X3D	Toxic effect of noxious substnc eaten as food, assault, subs
		T62.8X4D	Toxic effect of noxious substnc eaten as food, undet, subs
		T62.91XD	Toxic effect of unsp noxious sub eaten as food, acc, subs
		T62.92XD	Toxic eff of unsp noxious sub eaten as food, slf-hrm, subs
		T62.93XD	Toxic effect of unsp noxious sub eaten as food, asslt, subs
		T62.94XD	Toxic effect of unsp noxious sub eaten as food, undet, subs
		T63.ØØ1D	Toxic effect of unsp snake venom, accidental, subs
		T63.ØØ2D	Toxic effect of unsp snake venom, self-harm, subs
		T63.ØØ3D	Toxic effect of unsp snake venom, assault, subs encntr
		T63.ØØ4D	Toxic effect of unsp snake venom, undetermined, subs encntr
		T63.Ø11D	Toxic effect of rattlesnake venom, accidental, subs
		T63.Ø12D	Toxic effect of rattlesnake venom, self-harm, subs
		T63.Ø13D	Toxic effect of rattlesnake venom, assault, subs encntr
		T63.Ø14D	Toxic effect of rattlesnake venom, undetermined, subs encntr
		T63.Ø21D	Toxic effect of coral snake venom, accidental, subs
		T63.Ø22D	Toxic effect of coral snake venom, self-harm, subs
		T63.Ø23D	Toxic effect of coral snake venom, assault, subs encntr
		T63.Ø24D	Toxic effect of coral snake venom, undetermined, subs encntr
		T63.Ø31D	Toxic effect of taipan venom, accidental, subs
		T63.Ø32D	Toxic effect of taipan venom, intentional self-harm, subs
		T63.Ø33D	Toxic effect of taipan venom, assault, subsequent encounter
		T63.Ø34D	Toxic effect of taipan venom, undetermined, subs encntr
		T63.Ø41D	Toxic effect of cobra venom, accidental, subs
		T63.Ø42D	Toxic effect of cobra venom, intentional self-harm, subs
		T63.Ø43D	Toxic effect of cobra venom, assault, subsequent encounter
		T63.Ø44D	Toxic effect of cobra venom, undetermined, subs encntr
		T63.Ø61D	Toxic effect of venom of N & S American snake, acc, subs
		T63.Ø62D	Toxic effect of venom of N & S American snake, slf-hrm, subs
		T63.Ø63D	Toxic effect of venom of N & S American snake, assault, subs
		T63.Ø64D	Toxic effect of venom of N & S American snake, undet, subs
		T63.Ø71D	Toxic effect of venom of Australian snake, accidental, subs
		T63.Ø72D	Toxic effect of venom of Australian snake, self-harm, subs
		T63.Ø73D	Toxic effect of venom of oth Australian snake, assault, subs
		T63.Ø74D	Toxic effect of venom of Australian snake, undet, subs
		T63.Ø81D	Toxic effect of venom of African and Asian snake, acc, subs
		T63.Ø82D	Toxic eff of venom of African and Asian snake, slf-hrm, subs
		T63.Ø83D	Toxic eff of venom of African and Asian snake, asslt, subs
		T63.Ø84D	Toxic eff of venom of African and Asian snake, undet, subs
		T63.Ø91D	Toxic effect of venom of snake, accidental, subs
		T63.Ø92D	Toxic effect of venom of snake, intentional self-harm, subs
		T63.Ø93D	Toxic effect of venom of other snake, assault, subs encntr
		T63.Ø94D	Toxic effect of venom of oth snake, undetermined, subs
		T63.111D	Toxic effect of venom of gila monster, accidental, subs
		T63.112D	Toxic effect of venom of gila monster, self-harm, subs
		T63.113D	Toxic effect of venom of gila monster, assault, subs encntr
		T63.114D	Toxic effect of venom of gila monster, undetermined, subs
		T63.121D	Toxic effect of venom of venomous lizard, accidental, subs
		T63.122D	Toxic effect of venom of venomous lizard, self-harm, subs
		T63.123D	Toxic effect of venom of oth venomous lizard, assault, subs
		T63.124D	Toxic effect of venom of venomous lizard, undetermined, subs
		T63.191D	Toxic effect of venom of reptiles, accidental, subs
		T63.192D	Toxic effect of venom of reptiles, self-harm, subs
		T63.193D	Toxic effect of venom of oth reptiles, assault, subs encntr
		T63.194D	Toxic effect of venom of oth reptiles, undetermined, subs
		T63.2X1D	Toxic effect of venom of scorpion, accidental, subs
		T63.2X2D	Toxic effect of venom of scorpion, self-harm, subs
		T63.2X3D	Toxic effect of venom of scorpion, assault, subs encntr
		T63.2X4D	Toxic effect of venom of scorpion, undetermined, subs encntr
		T63.3Ø1D	Toxic effect of unsp spider venom, accidental, subs
		T63.3Ø2D	Toxic effect of unsp spider venom, self-harm, subs
		T63.3Ø3D	Toxic effect of unsp spider venom, assault, subs encntr
		T63.3Ø4D	Toxic effect of unsp spider venom, undetermined, subs encntr
		T63.311D	Toxic effect of venom of black widow spider, acc, subs
		T63.312D	Toxic effect of venom of black widow spider, self-harm, subs
		T63.313D	Toxic effect of venom of black widow spider, assault, subs
		T63.314D	Toxic effect of venom of black widow spider, undet, subs
		T63.321D	Toxic effect of venom of tarantula, accidental, subs
		T63.322D	Toxic effect of venom of tarantula, self-harm, subs

(Continued on next page)

ICD-9-CM		ICD-10-CM	
V58.89	ENCOUNTER FOR OTHER SPECIFIED AFTERCARE **(Continued)**	**T63.323D**	Toxic effect of venom of tarantula, assault, subs encntr
		T63.324D	Toxic effect of venom of tarantula, undetermined, subs
		T63.331D	Toxic effect of venom of brown recluse spider, acc, subs
		T63.332D	Toxic effect of venom of brown recluse spider, slf-hrm, subs
		T63.333D	Toxic effect of venom of brown recluse spider, assault, subs
		T63.334D	Toxic effect of venom of brown recluse spider, undet, subs
		T63.391D	Toxic effect of venom of spider, accidental, subs
		T63.392D	Toxic effect of venom of spider, intentional self-harm, subs
		T63.393D	Toxic effect of venom of other spider, assault, subs encntr
		T63.394D	Toxic effect of venom of oth spider, undetermined, subs
		T63.411D	Toxic effect of venom of centipede/millipede, acc, subs
		T63.412D	Toxic effect of venom of centipede/millipede, slf-hrm, subs
		T63.413D	Toxic effect of venom of centipede/millipede, assault, subs
		T63.414D	Toxic effect of venom of centipede/millipede, undet, subs
		T63.421D	Toxic effect of venom of ants, accidental, subs
		T63.422D	Toxic effect of venom of ants, intentional self-harm, subs
		T63.423D	Toxic effect of venom of ants, assault, subsequent encounter
		T63.424D	Toxic effect of venom of ants, undetermined, subs encntr
		T63.431D	Toxic effect of venom of caterpillars, accidental, subs
		T63.432D	Toxic effect of venom of caterpillars, self-harm, subs
		T63.433D	Toxic effect of venom of caterpillars, assault, subs encntr
		T63.434D	Toxic effect of venom of caterpillars, undetermined, subs
		T63.441D	Toxic effect of venom of bees, accidental, subs
		T63.442D	Toxic effect of venom of bees, intentional self-harm, subs
		T63.443D	Toxic effect of venom of bees, assault, subsequent encounter
		T63.444D	Toxic effect of venom of bees, undetermined, subs encntr
		T63.451D	Toxic effect of venom of hornets, accidental, subs
		T63.452D	Toxic effect of venom of hornets, self-harm, subs
		T63.453D	Toxic effect of venom of hornets, assault, subs encntr
		T63.454D	Toxic effect of venom of hornets, undetermined, subs encntr
		T63.461D	Toxic effect of venom of wasps, accidental, subs
		T63.462D	Toxic effect of venom of wasps, intentional self-harm, subs
		T63.463D	Toxic effect of venom of wasps, assault, subs encntr
		T63.464D	Toxic effect of venom of wasps, undetermined, subs encntr
		T63.481D	Toxic effect of venom of arthropod, accidental, subs
		T63.482D	Toxic effect of venom of arthropod, self-harm, subs
		T63.483D	Toxic effect of venom of oth arthropod, assault, subs encntr
		T63.484D	Toxic effect of venom of oth arthropod, undetermined, subs
		T63.511D	Toxic effect of contact w stingray, accidental, subs
		T63.512D	Toxic effect of contact w stingray, self-harm, subs
		T63.513D	Toxic effect of contact with stingray, assault, subs encntr
		T63.514D	Toxic effect of contact w stingray, undetermined, subs
		T63.591D	Toxic effect of contact w oth venomous fish, acc, subs
		T63.592D	Toxic effect of contact w oth venomous fish, self-harm, subs
		T63.593D	Toxic effect of contact w oth venomous fish, assault, subs
		T63.594D	Toxic effect of contact w oth venomous fish, undet, subs
		T63.611D	Toxic effect of contact w Portugese Man-o-war, acc, subs
		T63.612D	Toxic effect of contact w Portugese Man-o-war, slf-hrm, subs
		T63.613D	Toxic effect of contact w Portugese Man-o-war, assault, subs
		T63.614D	Toxic effect of contact w Portugese Man-o-war, undet, subs
		T63.621D	Toxic effect of contact w oth jellyfish, accidental, subs
		T63.622D	Toxic effect of contact w oth jellyfish, self-harm, subs
		T63.623D	Toxic effect of contact w oth jellyfish, assault, subs
		T63.624D	Toxic effect of contact w oth jellyfish, undetermined, subs
		T63.631D	Toxic effect of contact w sea anemone, accidental, subs
		T63.632D	Toxic effect of contact w sea anemone, self-harm, subs
		T63.633D	Toxic effect of contact w sea anemone, assault, subs encntr
		T63.634D	Toxic effect of contact w sea anemone, undetermined, subs
		T63.691D	Toxic effect of cntct w oth venom marine animals, acc, subs
		T63.692D	Toxic eff of cntct w oth venom marine animals, slf-hrm, subs
		T63.693D	Toxic eff of cntct w oth venom marine animals, asslt, subs
		T63.694D	Toxic eff of cntct w oth venom marine animals, undet, subs
		T63.711D	Toxic effect of contact w venomous marine plant, acc, subs
		T63.712D	Toxic effect of contact w venom marine plant, slf-hrm, subs
		T63.713D	Toxic effect of contact w venom marine plant, assault, subs
		T63.714D	Toxic effect of contact w venomous marine plant, undet, subs
		T63.791D	Toxic effect of contact w oth venomous plant, acc, subs
		T63.792D	Toxic effect of contact w oth venomous plant, slf-hrm, subs
		T63.793D	Toxic effect of contact w oth venomous plant, assault, subs
		T63.794D	Toxic effect of contact w oth venomous plant, undet, subs
		T63.811D	Toxic effect of contact w venomous frog, accidental, subs
		T63.812D	Toxic effect of contact w venomous frog, self-harm, subs
		T63.813D	Toxic effect of contact w venomous frog, assault, subs
		T63.814D	Toxic effect of contact w venomous frog, undetermined, subs
		T63.821D	Toxic effect of contact w venomous toad, accidental, subs
		T63.822D	Toxic effect of contact w venomous toad, self-harm, subs
		T63.823D	Toxic effect of contact w venomous toad, assault, subs
		T63.824D	Toxic effect of contact w venomous toad, undetermined, subs
		T63.831D	Toxic effect of contact w oth venomous amphibian, acc, subs
		T63.832D	Toxic effect of contact w oth venomous amphib, slf-hrm, subs
		T63.833D	Toxic effect of contact w oth venomous amphib, assault, subs
		T63.834D	Toxic effect of contact w oth venomous amphib, undet, subs
	(Continued on next page)	**T63.891D**	Toxic effect of contact w oth venomous animals, acc, subs

ICD-9-CM		ICD-10-CM	
V58.89	ENCOUNTER FOR OTHER SPECIFIED AFTERCARE **(Continued)**	**T63.892D**	Toxic effect of contact w oth venom animals, slf-hrm, subs
		T63.893D	Toxic effect of contact w oth venom animals, assault, subs
		T63.894D	Toxic effect of contact w oth venomous animals, undet, subs
		T63.91XD	Toxic effect of contact w unsp venomous animal, acc, subs
		T63.92XD	Toxic effect of contact w unsp venom animal, slf-hrm, subs
		T63.93XD	Toxic effect of contact w unsp venom animal, assault, subs
		T63.94XD	Toxic effect of contact w unsp venomous animal, undet, subs
		T64.Ø1XD	Toxic effect of aflatoxin, accidental (unintentional), subs
		T64.Ø2XD	Toxic effect of aflatoxin, intentional self-harm, subs
		T64.Ø3XD	Toxic effect of aflatoxin, assault, subsequent encounter
		T64.Ø4XD	Toxic effect of aflatoxin, undetermined, subs encntr
		T64.81XD	Toxic effect of mycotoxin food contamnt, accidental, subs
		T64.82XD	Toxic effect of mycotoxin food contaminants, self-harm, subs
		T64.83XD	Toxic effect of mycotoxin food contaminants, assault, subs
		T64.84XD	Toxic effect of mycotoxin food contamnt, undetermined, subs
		T65.ØX1D	Toxic effect of cyanides, accidental (unintentional), subs
		T65.ØX2D	Toxic effect of cyanides, intentional self-harm, subs encntr
		T65.ØX3D	Toxic effect of cyanides, assault, subsequent encounter
		T65.ØX4D	Toxic effect of cyanides, undetermined, subsequent encounter
		T65.1X1D	Toxic effect of strychnine and its salts, accidental, subs
		T65.1X2D	Toxic effect of strychnine and its salts, self-harm, subs
		T65.1X3D	Toxic effect of strychnine and its salts, assault, subs
		T65.1X4D	Toxic effect of strychnine and its salts, undetermined, subs
		T65.211D	Toxic effect of chewing tobacco, accidental, subs
		T65.212D	Toxic effect of chewing tobacco, intentional self-harm, subs
		T65.213D	Toxic effect of chewing tobacco, assault, subs encntr
		T65.214D	Toxic effect of chewing tobacco, undetermined, subs encntr
		T65.221D	Toxic effect of tobacco cigarettes, accidental, subs
		T65.222D	Toxic effect of tobacco cigarettes, self-harm, subs
		T65.223D	Toxic effect of tobacco cigarettes, assault, subs encntr
		T65.224D	Toxic effect of tobacco cigarettes, undetermined, subs
		T65.291D	Toxic effect of tobacco and nicotine, accidental, subs
		T65.292D	Toxic effect of tobacco and nicotine, self-harm, subs
		T65.293D	Toxic effect of oth tobacco and nicotine, assault, subs
		T65.294D	Toxic effect of oth tobacco and nicotine, undetermined, subs
		T65.3X1D	Toxic eff of nitrodrv/aminodrv of benzn/homolog, acc, subs
		T65.3X2D	Tox eff of nitrodrv/aminodrv of benzn/homolog, slf-hrm, subs
		T65.3X3D	Toxic eff of nitrodrv/aminodrv of benzn/homolog, asslt, subs
		T65.3X4D	Toxic eff of nitrodrv/aminodrv of benzn/homolog, undet, subs
		T65.4X1D	Toxic effect of carbon disulfide, accidental, subs
		T65.4X2D	Toxic effect of carbon disulfide, self-harm, subs
		T65.4X3D	Toxic effect of carbon disulfide, assault, subs encntr
		T65.4X4D	Toxic effect of carbon disulfide, undetermined, subs encntr
		T65.5X1D	Tox eff of nitro and oth nitric acids and esters, acc, subs
		T65.5X2D	Tox eff of nitro & oth nitric acids & esters, slf-hrm, subs
		T65.5X3D	Tox eff of nitro & oth nitric acids and esters, asslt, subs
		T65.5X4D	Tox eff of nitro & oth nitric acids and esters, undet, subs
		T65.6X1D	Toxic effect of paints and dyes, NEC, accidental, subs
		T65.6X2D	Toxic effect of paints and dyes, NEC, self-harm, subs
		T65.6X3D	Toxic effect of paints and dyes, NEC, assault, subs
		T65.6X4D	Toxic effect of paints and dyes, NEC, undetermined, subs
		T65.811D	Toxic effect of latex, accidental (unintentional), subs
		T65.812D	Toxic effect of latex, intentional self-harm, subs encntr
		T65.813D	Toxic effect of latex, assault, subsequent encounter
		T65.814D	Toxic effect of latex, undetermined, subsequent encounter
		T65.821D	Toxic effect of harmful algae and algae toxins, acc, subs
		T65.822D	Toxic eff of harmful algae and algae toxins, slf-hrm, subs
		T65.823D	Toxic effect of harmful algae and algae toxins, asslt, subs
		T65.824D	Toxic effect of harmful algae and algae toxins, undet, subs
		T65.831D	Toxic effect of fiberglass, accidental (unintentional), subs
		T65.832D	Toxic effect of fiberglass, intentional self-harm, subs
		T65.833D	Toxic effect of fiberglass, assault, subsequent encounter
		T65.834D	Toxic effect of fiberglass, undetermined, subs encntr
		T65.891D	Toxic effect of substances, accidental (unintentional), subs
		T65.892D	Toxic effect of oth substances, intentional self-harm, subs
		T65.893D	Toxic effect of oth substances, assault, subs encntr
		T65.894D	Toxic effect of oth substances, undetermined, subs encntr
		T65.91XD	Toxic effect of unsp substance, accidental, subs
		T65.92XD	Toxic effect of unsp substance, intentional self-harm, subs
		T65.93XD	Toxic effect of unspecified substance, assault, subs encntr
		T65.94XD	Toxic effect of unsp substance, undetermined, subs encntr
		T66.XXXD	Radiation sickness, unspecified, subsequent encounter
		T67.ØXXD	Heatstroke and sunstroke, subsequent encounter
		T67.1XXD	Heat syncope, subsequent encounter
		T67.2XXD	Heat cramp, subsequent encounter
		T67.3XXD	Heat exhaustion, anhydrotic, subsequent encounter
		T67.4XXD	Heat exhaustion due to salt depletion, subsequent encounter
		T67.5XXD	Heat exhaustion, unspecified, subsequent encounter
		T67.6XXD	Heat fatigue, transient, subsequent encounter
		T67.7XXD	Heat edema, subsequent encounter
		T67.8XXD	Other effects of heat and light, subsequent encounter
		T67.9XXD	Effect of heat and light, unspecified, subsequent encounter
	(Continued on next page)	**T68.XXXD**	Hypothermia, subsequent encounter

[Brackets] indicate valid character values for each code. Character value meanings provided for each code grouping.

ICD-9-CM		ICD-10-CM	
V58.89	ENCOUNTER FOR OTHER SPECIFIED AFTERCARE **(Continued)**	**T69.Ø11D**	Immersion hand, right hand, subsequent encounter
		T69.Ø12D	Immersion hand, left hand, subsequent encounter
		T69.Ø19D	Immersion hand, unspecified hand, subsequent encounter
		T69.Ø21D	Immersion foot, right foot, subsequent encounter
		T69.Ø22D	Immersion foot, left foot, subsequent encounter
		T69.Ø29D	Immersion foot, unspecified foot, subsequent encounter
		T69.1XXD	Chilblains, subsequent encounter
		T69.8XXD	Other specified effects of reduced temperature, subs encntr
		T69.9XXD	Effect of reduced temperature, unspecified, subs encntr
		T7Ø.ØXXD	Otitic barotrauma, subsequent encounter
		T7Ø.1XXD	Sinus barotrauma, subsequent encounter
		T7Ø.2ØXD	Unspecified effects of high altitude, subsequent encounter
		T7Ø.29XD	Other effects of high altitude, subsequent encounter
		T7Ø.3XXD	Caisson disease, subsequent encounter
		T7Ø.4XXD	Effects of high-pressure fluids, subsequent encounter
		T7Ø.8XXD	Oth effects of air pressure and water pressure, subs encntr
		T7Ø.9XXD	Effect of air pressure and water pressure, unsp, subs encntr
		T71.111D	Asphyx due to smothering under pillow, accidental, subs
		T71.112D	Asphyxiation due to smothering under pillow, self-harm, subs
		T71.113D	Asphyxiation due to smothering under pillow, assault, subs
		T71.114D	Asphyx due to smothering under pillow, undetermined, subs
		T71.121D	Asphyxiation due to plastic bag, accidental, subs encntr
		T71.122D	Asphyxiation due to plastic bag, intentional self-harm, subs
		T71.123D	Asphyxiation due to plastic bag, assault, subs encntr
		T71.124D	Asphyxiation due to plastic bag, undetermined, subs encntr
		T71.131D	Asphyx due to being trapped in bed linens, accidental, subs
		T71.132D	Asphyx due to being trapped in bed linens, self-harm, subs
		T71.133D	Asphyx due to being trapped in bed linens, assault, subs
		T71.134D	Asphyx due to being trapped in bed linens, undet, subs
		T71.141D	Asphyx due to smothr under another person's body, acc, subs
		T71.143D	Asphyx d/t smothr under another person's body, asslt, subs
		T71.144D	Asphyx d/t smothr under another person's body, undet, subs
		T71.151D	Asphyx due to smothering in furniture, accidental, subs
		T71.152D	Asphyxiation due to smothering in furniture, self-harm, subs
		T71.153D	Asphyxiation due to smothering in furniture, assault, subs
		T71.154D	Asphyx due to smothering in furniture, undetermined, subs
		T71.161D	Asphyxiation due to hanging, accidental, subs encntr
		T71.162D	Asphyxiation due to hanging, intentional self-harm, subs
		T71.163D	Asphyxiation due to hanging, assault, subsequent encounter
		T71.164D	Asphyxiation due to hanging, undetermined, subs encntr
		T71.191D	Asphyx d/t mech threat to breathe d/t oth cause, acc, subs
		T71.192D	Asphyx d/t mech thrt to breathe d/t oth cause, slf-hrm, subs
		T71.193D	Asphyx d/t mech threat to breathe d/t oth cause, asslt, subs
		T71.194D	Asphyx d/t mech threat to breathe d/t oth cause, undet, subs
		T71.2ØXD	Asphyx d/t sys oxy defic d/t low oxy in air unsp cause, subs
		T71.21XD	Asphyxiation due to cave-in or falling earth, subs encntr
		T71.221D	Asphyx due to being trapped in a car trunk, accidental, subs
		T71.222D	Asphyx due to being trapped in a car trunk, self-harm, subs
		T71.223D	Asphyx due to being trapped in a car trunk, assault, subs
		T71.224D	Asphyx due to being trapped in a car trunk, undet, subs
		T71.231D	Asphyx due to being trap in a (discarded) refrig, acc, subs
		T71.232D	Asphyx d/t being trap in a (discarded) refrig, slf-hrm, subs
		T71.233D	Asphyx d/t being trap in a (discarded) refrig, asslt, subs
		T71.234D	Asphyx d/t being trap in a (discarded) refrig, undet, subs
		T71.29XD	Asphyx due to being trap in oth low oxygen environment, subs
		T71.9XXD	Asphyxiation due to unspecified cause, subsequent encounter
		T73.ØXXD	Starvation, subsequent encounter
		T73.1XXD	Deprivation of water, subsequent encounter
		T73.2XXD	Exhaustion due to exposure, subsequent encounter
		T73.3XXD	Exhaustion due to excessive exertion, subsequent encounter
		T73.8XXD	Other effects of deprivation, subsequent encounter
		T73.9XXD	Effect of deprivation, unspecified, subsequent encounter
		T74.Ø1XD	Adult neglect or abandonment, confirmed, subs encntr
		T74.Ø2XD	Child neglect or abandonment, confirmed, subs encntr
		T74.11XD	Adult physical abuse, confirmed, subsequent encounter
		T74.12XD	Child physical abuse, confirmed, subsequent encounter
		T74.21XD	Adult sexual abuse, confirmed, subsequent encounter
		T74.22XD	Child sexual abuse, confirmed, subsequent encounter
		T74.31XD	Adult psychological abuse, confirmed, subsequent encounter
		T74.32XD	Child psychological abuse, confirmed, subsequent encounter
		T74.4XXD	Shaken infant syndrome, subsequent encounter
		T74.91XD	Unspecified adult maltreatment, confirmed, subs encntr
		T74.92XD	Unspecified child maltreatment, confirmed, subs encntr
		T75.ØØXD	Unspecified effects of lightning, subsequent encounter
		T75.Ø1XD	Shock due to being struck by lightning, subsequent encounter
		T75.Ø9XD	Other effects of lightning, subsequent encounter
		T75.1XXD	Unsp effects of drowning and nonfatal submersion, subs
		T75.2ØXD	Unspecified effects of vibration, subsequent encounter
		T75.21XD	Pneumatic hammer syndrome, subsequent encounter
		T75.22XD	Traumatic vasospastic syndrome, subsequent encounter
		T75.23XD	Vertigo from infrasound, subsequent encounter
		T75.29XD	Other effects of vibration, subsequent encounter
	(Continued on next page)	**T75.3XXD**	Motion sickness, subsequent encounter

ICD-9-CM		ICD-10-CM	
V58.89	ENCOUNTER FOR OTHER SPECIFIED AFTERCARE **(Continued)**	**T75.4XXD**	Electrocution, subsequent encounter
		T75.81XD	Effects of abnormal gravitation forces, subsequent encounter
		T75.82XD	Effects of weightlessness, subsequent encounter
		T75.89XD	Other specified effects of external causes, subs encntr
		T76.Ø1XD	Adult neglect or abandonment, suspected, subs encntr
		T76.Ø2XD	Child neglect or abandonment, suspected, subs encntr
		T76.11XD	Adult physical abuse, suspected, subsequent encounter
		T76.12XD	Child physical abuse, suspected, subsequent encounter
		T76.21XD	Adult sexual abuse, suspected, subsequent encounter
		T76.22XD	Child sexual abuse, suspected, subsequent encounter
		T76.31XD	Adult psychological abuse, suspected, subsequent encounter
		T76.32XD	Child psychological abuse, suspected, subsequent encounter
		T76.91XD	Unspecified adult maltreatment, suspected, subs encntr
		T76.92XD	Unspecified child maltreatment, suspected, subs encntr
		T78.ØØXD	Anaphylactic reaction due to unspecified food, subs encntr
		T78.Ø1XD	Anaphylactic reaction due to peanuts, subsequent encounter
		T78.Ø2XD	Anaphylactic reaction due to shellfish (crustaceans), subs
		T78.Ø3XD	Anaphylactic reaction due to other fish, subs encntr
		T78.Ø4XD	Anaphylactic reaction due to fruits and vegetables, subs
		T78.Ø5XD	Anaphylactic reaction due to tree nuts and seeds, subs
		T78.Ø6XD	Anaphylactic reaction due to food additives, subs encntr
		T78.Ø7XD	Anaphylactic reaction due to milk and dairy products, subs
		T78.Ø8XD	Anaphylactic reaction due to eggs, subsequent encounter
		T78.Ø9XD	Anaphylactic reaction due to oth food products, subs encntr
		T78.1XXD	Oth adverse food reactions, not elsewhere classified, subs
		T78.2XXD	Anaphylactic shock, unspecified, subsequent encounter
		T78.3XXD	Angioneurotic edema, subsequent encounter
		T78.4ØXD	Allergy, unspecified, subsequent encounter
		T78.41XD	Arthus phenomenon, subsequent encounter
		T78.49XD	Other allergy, subsequent encounter
		T78.8XXD	Other adverse effects, not elsewhere classified, subs encntr
		T79.ØXXD	Air embolism (traumatic), subsequent encounter
		T79.1XXD	Fat embolism (traumatic), subsequent encounter
		T79.2XXD	Traumatic secondary and recurrent hemor and seroma, subs
		T79.4XXD	Traumatic shock, subsequent encounter
		T79.5XXD	Traumatic anuria, subsequent encounter
		T79.6XXD	Traumatic ischemia of muscle, subsequent encounter
		T79.7XXD	Traumatic subcutaneous emphysema, subsequent encounter
		T79.8XXD	Other early complications of trauma, subsequent encounter
		T79.9XXD	Unspecified early complication of trauma, subs encntr
		T79.AØXD	Compartment syndrome, unspecified, subsequent encounter
		T79.A11D	Traumatic compartment syndrome of r up extrem, subs
		T79.A12D	Traumatic compartment syndrome of left upper extremity, subs
		T79.A19D	Traumatic compartment syndrome of unsp upper extremity, subs
		T79.A21D	Traumatic compartment syndrome of r low extrem, subs
		T79.A22D	Traumatic compartment syndrome of left lower extremity, subs
		T79.A29D	Traumatic compartment syndrome of unsp lower extremity, subs
		T79.A3XD	Traumatic compartment syndrome of abdomen, subs encntr
		T79.A9XD	Traumatic compartment syndrome of other sites, subs encntr
		T8Ø.ØXXD	Air embolism fol infusion, tranfs and theraputc inject, subs
		T8Ø.1XXD	Vascular comp fol infusn, tranfs and theraputc inject, subs
		T8Ø.211D	Bloodstream infection due to central venous catheter, subs
		T8Ø.212D	Local infection due to central venous catheter, subs encntr
		T8Ø.218D	Other infection due to central venous catheter, subs encntr
		T8Ø.219D	Unsp infection due to central venous catheter, subs encntr
		T8Ø.22XD	Acute infct fol tranfs,infusn,inject blood/products, subs
		T8Ø.29XD	Infct fol oth infusion, transfuse and theraputc inject, subs
		T8Ø.3ØXD	ABO incompat react due to tranfs of bld/bld prod, unsp, subs
		T8Ø.31ØD	ABO incompatibility w acute hemolytic transfs react, subs
		T8Ø.311D	ABO incompatibility w delayed hemolytic transfs react, subs
		T8Ø.319D	ABO incompatibility w hemolytic transfs react, unsp, subs
		T8Ø.39XD	Oth ABO incompat react due to tranfs of bld/bld prod, subs
		T8Ø.4ØXD	Rh incompat react due to tranfs of bld/bld prod, unsp, subs
		T8Ø.41ØD	Rh incompatibility w acute hemolytic transfs react, subs
		T8Ø.411D	Rh incompatibility w delayed hemolytic transfs react, subs
		T8Ø.419D	Rh incompatibility w hemolytic transfs react, unsp, subs
		T8Ø.49XD	Oth Rh incompat reaction due to tranfs of bld/bld prod, subs
		T8Ø.51XD	Anaphylactic reaction due to admin blood/products, subs
		T8Ø.52XD	Anaphylactic reaction due to vaccination, subs encntr
		T8Ø.59XD	Anaphylactic reaction due to other serum, subs encntr
		T8Ø.61XD	Oth serum reaction due to admin blood/products, subs
		T8Ø.62XD	Other serum reaction due to vaccination, subs encntr
		T8Ø.69XD	Other serum reaction due to other serum, subs encntr
		T8Ø.81ØD	Extravasation of vesicant antineoplastic chemotherapy, subs
		T8Ø.818D	Extravasation of other vesicant agent, subsequent encounter
		T8Ø.89XD	Oth comp fol infusion, transfuse and theraputc inject, subs
		T8Ø.9ØXD	Unsp comp following infusion and therapeutic injection, subs
		T8Ø.91ØD	Acute hemolytic transfs react, unsp incompatibility, subs
		T8Ø.911D	Delayed hemolytic transfs react, unsp incompatibility, subs
		T8Ø.919D	Hemolytic transfs react, unsp incompat, unsp ac/delay, subs
		T8Ø.92XD	Unspecified transfusion reaction, subsequent encounter
		T8Ø.AØXD	Non-ABO incompat react d/t tranfs of bld/bld prod,unsp, subs
	(Continued on next page)	**T8Ø.A1ØD**	Non-ABO incompat w acute hemolytic transfs react, subs

ICD-9-CM		ICD-10-CM	
V58.89	ENCOUNTER FOR OTHER SPECIFIED AFTERCARE **(Continued)**	**T8Ø.A11D**	Non-ABO incompat w delayed hemolytic transfs react, subs
		T8Ø.A19D	Non-ABO incompat w hemolytic transfs react, unsp, subs
		T8Ø.A9XD	Oth non-ABO incompat react d/t tranfs of bld/bld prod, subs
		T81.1ØXD	Postprocedural shock unspecified, subsequent encounter
		T81.11XD	Postprocedural cardiogenic shock, subsequent encounter
		T81.12XD	Postprocedural septic shock, subsequent encounter
		T81.19XD	Other postprocedural shock, subsequent encounter
		T81.3ØXD	Disruption of wound, unspecified, subsequent encounter
		T81.31XD	Disruption of external operation (surgical) wound, NEC, subs
		T81.32XD	Disruption of internal operation (surgical) wound, NEC, subs
		T81.33XD	Disruption of traumatic injury wound repair, subs encntr
		T81.4XXD	Infection following a procedure, subsequent encounter
		T81.5ØØD	Unsp comp of fb acc left in body fol surgical op, subs
		T81.5Ø1D	Unsp comp of fb acc left in body fol infusn/transfusn, subs
		T81.5Ø2D	Unsp comp of fb acc left in body fol kidney dialysis, subs
		T81.5Ø3D	Unsp comp of fb acc left in body fol inject or immuniz, subs
		T81.5Ø4D	Unsp comp of fb acc left in body following endo exam, subs
		T81.5Ø5D	Unsp comp of fb acc left in body following heart cath, subs
		T81.5Ø6D	Unsp comp of fb acc left in body following punctr/cath, subs
		T81.5Ø7D	Unsp comp of fb acc left in body fol remov cath/pack, subs
		T81.5Ø8D	Unsp comp of fb acc left in body fol oth procedure, subs
		T81.5Ø9D	Unsp comp of fb acc left in body fol unsp procedure, subs
		T81.51ØD	Adhes due to fb acc left in body fol surgical op, subs
		T81.511D	Adhes due to fb acc left in body fol infusn/transfusn, subs
		T81.512D	Adhes due to fb acc left in body fol kidney dialysis, subs
		T81.513D	Adhes due to fb acc left in body fol inject or immuniz, subs
		T81.514D	Adhes due to fb acc left in body following endo exam, subs
		T81.515D	Adhes due to fb acc left in body following heart cath, subs
		T81.516D	Adhes due to fb acc left in body following punctr/cath, subs
		T81.517D	Adhes due to fb acc left in body fol remov cath/pack, subs
		T81.518D	Adhes due to fb acc left in body fol oth procedure, subs
		T81.519D	Adhes due to fb acc left in body fol unsp procedure, subs
		T81.52ØD	Obst due to fb acc left in body fol surgical operation, subs
		T81.521D	Obst due to fb acc left in body fol infusn/transfusn, subs
		T81.522D	Obst due to fb acc left in body fol kidney dialysis, subs
		T81.523D	Obst due to fb acc left in body fol inject or immuniz, subs
		T81.524D	Obst due to fb acc left in body following endo exam, subs
		T81.525D	Obst due to fb acc left in body following heart cath, subs
		T81.526D	Obst due to fb acc left in body following punctr/cath, subs
		T81.527D	Obst due to fb acc left in body fol remov cath/pack, subs
		T81.528D	Obst due to fb acc left in body fol oth procedure, subs
		T81.529D	Obst due to fb acc left in body fol unsp procedure, subs
		T81.53ØD	Perf due to fb acc left in body fol surgical operation, subs
		T81.531D	Perf due to fb acc left in body fol infusn/transfusn, subs
		T81.532D	Perf due to fb acc left in body fol kidney dialysis, subs
		T81.533D	Perf due to fb acc left in body fol inject or immuniz, subs
		T81.534D	Perf due to fb acc left in body following endo exam, subs
		T81.535D	Perf due to fb acc left in body following heart cath, subs
		T81.536D	Perf due to fb acc left in body following punctr/cath, subs
		T81.537D	Perf due to fb acc left in body fol remov cath/pack, subs
		T81.538D	Perf due to fb acc left in body fol oth procedure, subs
		T81.539D	Perf due to fb acc left in body fol unsp procedure, subs
		T81.59ØD	Oth comp of fb acc left in body fol surgical operation, subs
		T81.591D	Oth comp of fb acc left in body fol infusn/transfusn, subs
		T81.592D	Oth comp of fb acc left in body fol kidney dialysis, subs
		T81.593D	Oth comp of fb acc left in body fol inject or immuniz, subs
		T81.594D	Oth comp of fb acc left in body following endo exam, subs
		T81.595D	Oth comp of fb acc left in body following heart cath, subs
		T81.596D	Oth comp of fb acc left in body following punctr/cath, subs
		T81.597D	Oth comp of fb acc left in body fol remov cath/pack, subs
		T81.598D	Oth comp of fb acc left in body fol oth procedure, subs
		T81.599D	Oth comp of fb acc left in body fol unsp procedure, subs
		T81.6ØXD	Unsp acute reaction to foreign sub acc left dur proc, subs
		T81.61XD	Aseptic peritonitis due to forn sub acc left dur proc, subs
		T81.69XD	Oth acute reaction to foreign sub acc left dur proc, subs
		T81.71ØD	Complication of mesent art following a procedure, NEC, subs
		T81.711D	Comp of renal artery following a procedure, NEC, subs
		T81.718D	Complication of artery following a procedure, NEC, subs
		T81.719D	Complication of unsp artery following a procedure, NEC, subs
		T81.72XD	Complication of vein following a procedure, NEC, subs
		T81.81XD	Complication of inhalation therapy, subsequent encounter
		T81.82XD	Emphysema (subcutaneous) resulting from a procedure, subs
		T81.83XD	Persistent postprocedural fistula, subsequent encounter
		T81.89XD	Oth complications of procedures, NEC, subs
		T81.9XXD	Unspecified complication of procedure, subsequent encounter
		T82.Ø1XD	Breakdown (mechanical) of heart valve prosthesis, subs
		T82.Ø2XD	Displacement of heart valve prosthesis, subsequent encounter
		T82.Ø3XD	Leakage of heart valve prosthesis, subsequent encounter
		T82.Ø9XD	Mech compl of heart valve prosthesis, subsequent encounter
		T82.11ØD	Breakdown (mechanical) of cardiac electrode, subs encntr
		T82.111D	Breakdown of cardiac pulse generator (battery), subs
		T82.118D	Breakdown (mechanical) of cardiac electronic device, subs
	(Continued on next page)	**T82.119D**	Breakdown of unsp cardiac electronic device, subs

ICD-9-CM		ICD-10-CM	
V58.89	ENCOUNTER FOR OTHER SPECIFIED AFTERCARE **(Continued)**	**T82.120D**	Displacement of cardiac electrode, subsequent encounter
		T82.121D	Displacement of cardiac pulse generator (battery), subs
		T82.128D	Displacement of other cardiac electronic device, subs encntr
		T82.129D	Displacement of unsp cardiac electronic device, subs encntr
		T82.190D	Mech compl of cardiac electrode, subsequent encounter
		T82.191D	Mech compl of cardiac pulse generator (battery), subs encntr
		T82.198D	Mech compl of other cardiac electronic device, subs encntr
		T82.199D	Mech compl of unspecified cardiac device, subs encntr
		T82.211D	Breakdown (mechanical) of coronary artery bypass graft, subs
		T82.212D	Displacement of coronary artery bypass graft, subs encntr
		T82.213D	Leakage of coronary artery bypass graft, subs encntr
		T82.218D	Mech compl of coronary artery bypass graft, subs encntr
		T82.221D	Breakdown (mechanical) of biological heart valve graft, subs
		T82.222D	Displacement of biological heart valve graft, subs encntr
		T82.223D	Leakage of biological heart valve graft, subs encntr
		T82.228D	Mech compl of biological heart valve graft, subs encntr
		T82.310D	Breakdown (mechanical) of aortic (bifurcation) graft, subs
		T82.311D	Breakdown of carotid arterial graft (bypass), subs
		T82.312D	Breakdown of femoral arterial graft (bypass), subs
		T82.318D	Breakdown (mechanical) of other vascular grafts, subs encntr
		T82.319D	Breakdown (mechanical) of unsp vascular grafts, subs encntr
		T82.320D	Displacement of aortic (bifurcation) graft, subs
		T82.321D	Displacement of carotid arterial graft (bypass), subs encntr
		T82.322D	Displacement of femoral arterial graft (bypass), subs encntr
		T82.328D	Displacement of other vascular grafts, subsequent encounter
		T82.329D	Displacement of unspecified vascular grafts, subs encntr
		T82.330D	Leakage of aortic (bifurcation) graft (replacement), subs
		T82.331D	Leakage of carotid arterial graft (bypass), subs encntr
		T82.332D	Leakage of femoral arterial graft (bypass), subs encntr
		T82.338D	Leakage of other vascular grafts, subsequent encounter
		T82.339D	Leakage of unspecified vascular graft, subsequent encounter
		T82.390D	Mech compl of aortic (bifurcation) graft (replacement), subs
		T82.391D	Mech compl of carotid arterial graft (bypass), subs encntr
		T82.392D	Mech compl of femoral arterial graft (bypass), subs encntr
		T82.398D	Mech compl of other vascular grafts, subsequent encounter
		T82.399D	Mech compl of unspecified vascular grafts, subs encntr
		T82.41XD	Breakdown (mechanical) of vascular dialysis catheter, subs
		T82.42XD	Displacement of vascular dialysis catheter, subs encntr
		T82.43XD	Leakage of vascular dialysis catheter, subsequent encounter
		T82.49XD	Oth complication of vascular dialysis catheter, subs encntr
		T82.510D	Breakdown of surgically created AV fistula, subs
		T82.511D	Breakdown (mechanical) of surgically created AV shunt, subs
		T82.512D	Breakdown (mechanical) of artificial heart, subs encntr
		T82.513D	Breakdown of balloon (counterpulsation) device, subs
		T82.514D	Breakdown (mechanical) of infusion catheter, subs encntr
		T82.515D	Breakdown (mechanical) of umbrella device, subs encntr
		T82.518D	Breakdown of cardiac and vascular devices and implants, subs
		T82.519D	Brkdwn unsp cardiac and vascular devices and implants, subs
		T82.520D	Displacement of surgically created AV fistula, subs
		T82.521D	Displacement of surgically created arteriovenous shunt, subs
		T82.522D	Displacement of artificial heart, subsequent encounter
		T82.523D	Displacement of balloon (counterpulsation) device, subs
		T82.524D	Displacement of infusion catheter, subsequent encounter
		T82.525D	Displacement of umbrella device, subsequent encounter
		T82.528D	Displacmnt of cardiac and vascular devices and implnt, subs
		T82.529D	Displacmnt of unsp cardiac and vasc devices and implnt, subs
		T82.530D	Leakage of surgically created arteriovenous fistula, subs
		T82.531D	Leakage of surgically created arteriovenous shunt, subs
		T82.532D	Leakage of artificial heart, subsequent encounter
		T82.533D	Leakage of balloon (counterpulsation) device, subs encntr
		T82.534D	Leakage of infusion catheter, subsequent encounter
		T82.535D	Leakage of umbrella device, subsequent encounter
		T82.538D	Leakage of cardiac and vascular devices and implants, subs
		T82.539D	Leakage of unsp cardiac and vasc devices and implnt, subs
		T82.590D	Mech compl of surgically created arteriovenous fistula, subs
		T82.591D	Mech compl of surgically created arteriovenous shunt, subs
		T82.592D	Mech compl of artificial heart, subsequent encounter
		T82.593D	Mech compl of balloon (counterpulsation) device, subs encntr
		T82.594D	Mech compl of infusion catheter, subsequent encounter
		T82.595D	Mech compl of umbrella device, subsequent encounter
		T82.598D	Mech compl of cardiac and vascular devices and implnt, subs
		T82.599D	Mech compl of unsp cardiac and vasc devices and implnt, subs
		T82.6XXD	Infect/inflm reaction due to cardiac valve prosthesis, subs
		T82.7XXD	Infect/inflm react d/t oth cardi/vasc dev/implnt/grft, subs
		T82.817D	Embolism of cardiac prosth dev/grft, subs
		T82.818D	Embolism of vascular prosth dev/grft, subs
		T82.827D	Fibrosis of cardiac prosth dev/grft, subs
		T82.828D	Fibrosis of vascular prosth dev/grft, subs
		T82.837D	Hemorrhage of cardiac prosth dev/grft, subs
		T82.838D	Hemorrhage of vascular prosth dev/grft, subs
		T82.847D	Pain from cardiac prosth dev/grft, subs
		T82.848D	Pain from vascular prosth dev/grft, subs
	(Continued on next page)	**T82.857D**	Stenosis of cardiac prosth dev/grft, subs

ICD-9-CM		ICD-10-CM	
V58.89	ENCOUNTER FOR OTHER SPECIFIED AFTERCARE **(Continued)**	**T82.858D**	Stenosis of vascular prosth dev/grft, subs
		T82.867D	Thrombosis of cardiac prosth dev/grft, subs
		T82.868D	Thrombosis of vascular prosth dev/grft, subs
		T82.897D	Oth complication of cardiac prosth dev/grft, subs
		T82.898D	Oth complication of vascular prosth dev/grft, subs
		T82.9XXD	Unsp comp of cardiac and vascular prosth dev/grft, subs
		T83.010D	Breakdown (mechanical) of cystostomy catheter, subs encntr
		T83.018D	Breakdown (mechanical) of indwelling urethral catheter, subs
		T83.020D	Displacement of cystostomy catheter, subsequent encounter
		T83.028D	Displacement of oth indwelling urethral catheter, subs
		T83.030D	Leakage of cystostomy catheter, subsequent encounter
		T83.038D	Leakage of other indwelling urethral catheter, subs encntr
		T83.090D	Mech compl of cystostomy catheter, subsequent encounter
		T83.098D	Mech compl of oth indwelling urethral catheter, subs encntr
		T83.110D	Breakdown of urinary electronic stimulator device, subs
		T83.111D	Breakdown (mechanical) of urinary sphincter implant, subs
		T83.112D	Breakdown (mechanical) of urinary stent, subs encntr
		T83.118D	Breakdown (mechanical) of urinary devices and implants, subs
		T83.120D	Displacement of urinary electronic stimulator device, subs
		T83.121D	Displacement of urinary sphincter implant, subs encntr
		T83.122D	Displacement of urinary stent, subsequent encounter
		T83.128D	Displacement of oth urinary devices and implants, subs
		T83.190D	Mech compl of urinary electronic stimulator device, subs
		T83.191D	Mech compl of urinary sphincter implant, subs encntr
		T83.192D	Mech compl of urinary stent, subsequent encounter
		T83.198D	Mech compl of oth urinary devices and implants, subs encntr
		T83.21XD	Breakdown (mechanical) of graft of urinary organ, subs
		T83.22XD	Displacement of graft of urinary organ, subsequent encounter
		T83.23XD	Leakage of graft of urinary organ, subsequent encounter
		T83.29XD	Mech compl of graft of urinary organ, subsequent encounter
		T83.31XD	Breakdown (mechanical) of intrauterine contracep dev, subs
		T83.32XD	Displacement of intrauterine contraceptive device, subs
		T83.39XD	Mech compl of intrauterine contraceptive device, subs encntr
		T83.410D	Breakdown of penile (implanted) prosthesis, subs
		T83.418D	Breakdown of prosth dev/implnt/grft of genitl trct, subs
		T83.420D	Displacement of penile (implanted) prosthesis, subs encntr
		T83.428D	Displacement of prosth dev/implnt/grft of genitl trct, subs
		T83.490D	Mech compl of penile (implanted) prosthesis, subs encntr
		T83.498D	Mech compl of prosth dev/implnt/grft of genital tract, subs
		T83.51XD	Infect/inflm reaction due to indwell urinary catheter, subs
		T83.59XD	Infect/inflm react d/t prosth dev/grft in urinry sys, subs
		T83.6XXD	Infect/inflm react d/t prosth dev/grft in genitl trct, subs
		T83.711D	Erosion of implnt vag prstht mtrl to surrnd org/tiss, subs
		T83.718D	Erosion of implanted prstht mtrl to surrnd org/tiss, subs
		T83.721D	Exposure of implnt vag prstht mtrl into vagina, subs encntr
		T83.728D	Exposure of implanted prstht mtrl to surrnd org/tiss, subs
		T83.81XD	Embolism of genitourinary prosth dev/grft, subs
		T83.82XD	Fibrosis of genitourinary prosth dev/grft, subs
		T83.83XD	Hemorrhage of genitourinary prosth dev/grft, subs
		T83.84XD	Pain from genitourinary prosth dev/grft, subs
		T83.85XD	Stenosis of genitourinary prosth dev/grft, subs
		T83.86XD	Thrombosis of genitourinary prosth dev/grft, subs
		T83.89XD	Oth complication of genitourinary prosth dev/grft, subs
		T83.9XXD	Unsp complication of genitourinary prosth dev/grft, subs
		T84.010D	Broken internal right hip prosthesis, subsequent encounter
		T84.011D	Broken internal left hip prosthesis, subsequent encounter
		T84.012D	Broken internal right knee prosthesis, subsequent encounter
		T84.013D	Broken internal left knee prosthesis, subsequent encounter
		T84.018D	Broken internal joint prosthesis, other site, subs encntr
		T84.019D	Broken internal joint prosthesis, unsp site, subs encntr
		T84.020D	Dislocation of internal right hip prosthesis, subs encntr
		T84.021D	Dislocation of internal left hip prosthesis, subs encntr
		T84.022D	Instability of internal right knee prosthesis, subs encntr
		T84.023D	Instability of internal left knee prosthesis, subs encntr
		T84.028D	Dislocation of other internal joint prosthesis, subs encntr
		T84.029D	Dislocation of unsp internal joint prosthesis, subs encntr
		T84.030D	Mech loosening of internal right hip prosthetic joint, subs
		T84.031D	Mech loosening of internal left hip prosthetic joint, subs
		T84.032D	Mech loosening of internal right knee prosthetic joint, subs
		T84.033D	Mech loosening of internal left knee prosthetic joint, subs
		T84.038D	Mechanical loosening of oth internal prosthetic joint, subs
		T84.039D	Mechanical loosening of unsp internal prosthetic joint, subs
		T84.050D	Periprosth osteolysis of internal prosthetic r hip jt, subs
		T84.051D	Periprosth osteolysis of internal prosthetic l hip jt, subs
		T84.052D	Periprosth osteolysis of internal prosthetic r knee jt, subs
		T84.053D	Periprosth osteolysis of internal prosthetic l knee jt, subs
		T84.058D	Periprosthetic osteolysis of internal prosthetic joint, subs
		T84.059D	Periprosth osteolys of unsp internal prosthetic joint, subs
		T84.060D	Wear of artic bearing surface of int prosth r hip jt, subs
		T84.061D	Wear of artic bearing surface of int prosth l hip jt, subs
		T84.062D	Wear of artic bearing surface of int prosth r knee jt, subs
		T84.063D	Wear of artic bearing surface of int prosth l knee jt, subs
	(Continued on next page)	**T84.068D**	Wear of artic bearing surface of internal prosth joint, subs

ICD-9-CM		ICD-10-CM	
V58.89	ENCOUNTER FOR OTHER SPECIFIED AFTERCARE **(Continued)**	**T84.Ø69D**	Wear of artic bearing surface of unsp int prosth joint, subs
		T84.Ø9ØD	Mech compl of internal right hip prosthesis, subs encntr
		T84.Ø91D	Mech compl of internal left hip prosthesis, subs encntr
		T84.Ø92D	Mech compl of internal right knee prosthesis, subs encntr
		T84.Ø93D	Mech compl of internal left knee prosthesis, subs encntr
		T84.Ø98D	Mech compl of other internal joint prosthesis, subs encntr
		T84.Ø99D	Mech compl of unsp internal joint prosthesis, subs encntr
		T84.11ØD	Breakdown (mechanical) of int fix of right humerus, subs
		T84.111D	Breakdown (mechanical) of int fix of left humerus, subs
		T84.112D	Breakdown (mechanical) of int fix of bone of r forearm, subs
		T84.113D	Breakdown of int fix of bone of left forearm, subs
		T84.114D	Breakdown (mechanical) of int fix of right femur, subs
		T84.115D	Breakdown (mechanical) of int fix of left femur, subs
		T84.116D	Breakdown (mechanical) of int fix of bone of r low leg, subs
		T84.117D	Breakdown (mechanical) of int fix of bone of l low leg, subs
		T84.119D	Breakdown (mechanical) of int fix of unsp bone of limb, subs
		T84.12ØD	Displacement of int fix of right humerus, subs
		T84.121D	Displacement of int fix of left humerus, subs
		T84.122D	Displacement of int fix of bone of right forearm, subs
		T84.123D	Displacement of int fix of bone of left forearm, subs
		T84.124D	Displacement of int fix of right femur, subs
		T84.125D	Displacement of internal fixation device of left femur, subs
		T84.126D	Displacement of int fix of bone of right lower leg, subs
		T84.127D	Displacement of int fix of bone of left lower leg, subs
		T84.129D	Displacement of int fix of unsp bone of limb, subs
		T84.19ØD	Mech compl of int fix of right humerus, subs
		T84.191D	Mech compl of internal fixation device of left humerus, subs
		T84.192D	Mech compl of int fix of bone of right forearm, subs
		T84.193D	Mech compl of int fix of bone of left forearm, subs
		T84.194D	Mech compl of internal fixation device of right femur, subs
		T84.195D	Mech compl of internal fixation device of left femur, subs
		T84.196D	Mech compl of int fix of bone of right lower leg, subs
		T84.197D	Mech compl of int fix of bone of left lower leg, subs
		T84.199D	Mech compl of int fix of unsp bone of limb, subs
		T84.21ØD	Breakdown of int fix of bones of hand and fingers, subs
		T84.213D	Breakdown of int fix of bones of foot and toes, subs
		T84.216D	Breakdown (mechanical) of int fix of vertebrae, subs
		T84.218D	Breakdown (mechanical) of int fix of bones, subs
		T84.22ØD	Displacement of int fix of bones of hand and fingers, subs
		T84.223D	Displacement of int fix of bones of foot and toes, subs
		T84.226D	Displacement of internal fixation device of vertebrae, subs
		T84.228D	Displacement of internal fixation device of oth bones, subs
		T84.29ØD	Mech compl of int fix of bones of hand and fingers, subs
		T84.293D	Mech compl of int fix of bones of foot and toes, subs
		T84.296D	Mech compl of internal fixation device of vertebrae, subs
		T84.298D	Mech compl of internal fixation device of oth bones, subs
		T84.31ØD	Breakdown (mechanical) of electronic bone stimulator, subs
		T84.318D	Breakdown of bone devices, implants and grafts, subs
		T84.32ØD	Displacement of electronic bone stimulator, subs encntr
		T84.328D	Displacement of oth bone devices, implants and grafts, subs
		T84.39ØD	Mech compl of electronic bone stimulator, subs encntr
		T84.398D	Mech compl of oth bone devices, implants and grafts, subs
		T84.41ØD	Breakdown (mechanical) of muscle and tendon graft, subs
		T84.418D	Brkdwn internal orth devices, implants and grafts, subs
		T84.42ØD	Displacement of muscle and tendon graft, subs encntr
		T84.428D	Displacmnt of internal orth devices, implnt and grafts, subs
		T84.49ØD	Mech compl of muscle and tendon graft, subsequent encounter
		T84.498D	Mech compl of internal orth devices, implnt and grafts, subs
		T84.5ØXD	Infect/inflm reaction due to unsp int joint prosth, subs
		T84.51XD	Infect/inflm reaction due to internal right hip prosth, subs
		T84.52XD	Infect/inflm reaction due to internal left hip prosth, subs
		T84.53XD	Infect/inflm reaction due to internal r knee prosth, subs
		T84.54XD	Infect/inflm reaction due to internal left knee prosth, subs
		T84.59XD	Infect/inflm reaction due to oth internal joint prosth, subs
		T84.6ØXD	Infect/inflm reaction due to int fix of unsp site, subs
		T84.61ØD	Infect/inflm reaction due to int fix of right humerus, subs
		T84.611D	Infect/inflm reaction due to int fix of left humerus, subs
		T84.612D	Infect/inflm reaction due to int fix of right radius, subs
		T84.613D	Infect/inflm reaction due to int fix of left radius, subs
		T84.614D	Infect/inflm reaction due to int fix of right ulna, subs
		T84.615D	Infect/inflm reaction due to int fix of left ulna, subs
		T84.619D	Infect/inflm react due to int fix of unsp bone of arm, subs
		T84.62ØD	Infect/inflm reaction due to int fix of right femur, subs
		T84.621D	Infect/inflm reaction due to int fix of left femur, subs
		T84.622D	Infect/inflm reaction due to int fix of right tibia, subs
		T84.623D	Infect/inflm reaction due to int fix of left tibia, subs
		T84.624D	Infect/inflm reaction due to int fix of right fibula, subs
		T84.625D	Infect/inflm reaction due to int fix of left fibula, subs
		T84.629D	Infect/inflm react due to int fix of unsp bone of leg, subs
		T84.63XD	Infect/inflm reaction due to int fix of spine, subs
		T84.69XD	Infect/inflm reaction due to int fix of site, subs
		T84.7XXD	Infect/inflm react due to oth int orth prosth dev/grft, subs
	(Continued on next page)	**T84.81XD**	Embolism due to internal orthopedic prosth dev/grft, subs

ICD-9-CM		ICD-10-CM	
V58.89	ENCOUNTER FOR OTHER SPECIFIED AFTERCARE **(Continued)**	**T84.82XD**	Fibrosis due to internal orthopedic prosth dev/grft, subs
		T84.83XD	Hemorrhage due to internal orthopedic prosth dev/grft, subs
		T84.84XD	Pain due to internal orthopedic prosth dev/grft, subs
		T84.85XD	Stenosis due to internal orthopedic prosth dev/grft, subs
		T84.86XD	Thrombosis due to internal orthopedic prosth dev/grft, subs
		T84.89XD	Oth comp of internal orthopedic prosth dev/grft, subs
		T84.9XXD	Unsp comp of internal orthopedic prosth dev/grft, subs
		T85.Ø1XD	Breakdown of ventricular intracranial shunt, subs
		T85.Ø2XD	Displacement of ventricular intracranial shunt, subs
		T85.Ø3XD	Leakage of ventricular intracranial shunt, subs
		T85.Ø9XD	Mech compl of ventricular intracranial shunt, subs
		T85.11ØD	Brkdwn implanted electronic neurostim of brain, subs
		T85.111D	Brkdwn implanted electronic neurostim of periph nrv, subs
		T85.112D	Brkdwn implanted electronic neurostim of spinal cord, subs
		T85.118D	Brkdwn implanted electronic stimulator of nervous sys, subs
		T85.12ØD	Displacmnt of implanted electronic neurostim of brain, subs
		T85.121D	Displacmnt of implnt electrnc neurostim of periph nrv, subs
		T85.122D	Displacmnt of implnt electrnc neurostim of spinal cord, subs
		T85.128D	Displacmnt of implnt electrnc stimultr of nervous sys, subs
		T85.19ØD	Mech compl of implanted electronic neurostim of brain, subs
		T85.191D	Mech compl of implnt electrnc neurostim of periph nrv, subs
		T85.192D	Mech compl of implnt electrnc neurostim of spinal cord, subs
		T85.199D	Mech compl of implnt electrnc stimultr of nervous sys, subs
		T85.21XD	Breakdown (mechanical) of intraocular lens, subs encntr
		T85.22XD	Displacement of intraocular lens, subsequent encounter
		T85.29XD	Mech compl of intraocular lens, subsequent encounter
		T85.31ØD	Breakdown of prosthetic orbit of right eye, subs
		T85.311D	Breakdown (mechanical) of prosthetic orbit of left eye, subs
		T85.318D	Breakdown (mechanical) of ocular prosth dev/grft, subs
		T85.32ØD	Displacement of prosthetic orbit of right eye, subs encntr
		T85.321D	Displacement of prosthetic orbit of left eye, subs encntr
		T85.328D	Displacement of ocular prosth dev/grft, subs
		T85.39ØD	Mech compl of prosthetic orbit of right eye, subs encntr
		T85.391D	Mech compl of prosthetic orbit of left eye, subs encntr
		T85.398D	Mech compl of ocular prosth dev/grft, subs
		T85.41XD	Breakdown of breast prosthesis and implant, subs encntr
		T85.42XD	Displacement of breast prosthesis and implant, subs encntr
		T85.43XD	Leakage of breast prosthesis and implant, subs encntr
		T85.44XD	Capsular contracture of breast implant, subsequent encounter
		T85.49XD	Mech compl of breast prosthesis and implant, subs encntr
		T85.51ØD	Breakdown (mechanical) of bile duct prosthesis, subs encntr
		T85.511D	Breakdown of esophageal anti-reflux device, subs
		T85.518D	Breakdown (mechanical) of GI prosth dev/grft, subs
		T85.52ØD	Displacement of bile duct prosthesis, subsequent encounter
		T85.521D	Displacement of esophageal anti-reflux device, subs encntr
		T85.528D	Displacement of gastrointestinal prosth dev/grft, subs
		T85.59ØD	Mech compl of bile duct prosthesis, subsequent encounter
		T85.591D	Mech compl of esophageal anti-reflux device, subs encntr
		T85.598D	Mech compl of gastrointestinal prosth dev/grft, subs
		T85.61ØD	Breakdown of epidural and subdural infusion catheter, subs
		T85.611D	Breakdown of intraperitoneal dialysis catheter, subs
		T85.612D	Breakdown (mechanical) of permanent sutures, subs encntr
		T85.613D	Breakdown of artificial skin grft /decellular alloderm, subs
		T85.614D	Breakdown (mechanical) of insulin pump, subsequent encounter
		T85.618D	Breakdown (mechanical) of internal prosth dev/grft, subs
		T85.62ØD	Displacmnt of epidural and subdural infusion catheter, subs
		T85.621D	Displacement of intraperitoneal dialysis catheter, subs
		T85.622D	Displacement of permanent sutures, subsequent encounter
		T85.623D	Displacmnt of artif skin grft /decellular alloderm, subs
		T85.624D	Displacement of insulin pump, subsequent encounter
		T85.628D	Displacement of internal prosth dev/grft, subs
		T85.63ØD	Leakage of epidural and subdural infusion catheter, subs
		T85.631D	Leakage of intraperitoneal dialysis catheter, subs encntr
		T85.633D	Leakage of insulin pump, subsequent encounter
		T85.638D	Leakage of internal prosth dev/grft, subs
		T85.69ØD	Mech compl of epidural and subdural infusion catheter, subs
		T85.691D	Mech compl of intraperitoneal dialysis catheter, subs encntr
		T85.692D	Mech compl of permanent sutures, subsequent encounter
		T85.693D	Mech compl of artif skin grft /decellular alloderm, subs
		T85.694D	Mech compl of insulin pump, subsequent encounter
		T85.698D	Mech compl of internal prosth dev/grft, subs
		T85.71XD	Infect/inflm reaction due to periton dialysis catheter, subs
		T85.72XD	Infect/inflm reaction due to insulin pump, subs
		T85.79XD	Infect/inflm reaction due to oth int prosth dev/grft, subs
		T85.81XD	Embolism due to internal prosth dev/grft, NEC, subs
		T85.82XD	Fibrosis due to internal prosth dev/grft, NEC, subs
		T85.83XD	Hemorrhage due to internal prosth dev/grft, NEC, subs
		T85.84XD	Pain due to internal prosth dev/grft, NEC, subs
		T85.85XD	Stenosis due to internal prosth dev/grft, NEC, subs
		T85.86XD	Thrombosis due to internal prosth dev/grft, NEC, subs
		T85.89XD	Oth complication of internal prosth dev/grft, NEC, subs
		T85.9XXD	Unsp complication of internal prosth dev/grft, subs
	(Continued on next page)	**T88.ØXXD**	Infection following immunization, subsequent encounter

V58.89–V58.89

ICD-9-CM			ICD-10-CM	
V58.89	ENCOUNTER FOR OTHER SPECIFIED AFTERCARE **(Continued)**		**T88.1XXD**	Oth complications following immunization, NEC, subs
			T88.2XXD	Shock due to anesthesia, subsequent encounter
			T88.3XXD	Malignant hyperthermia due to anesthesia, subs encntr
			T88.4XXD	Failed or difficult intubation, subsequent encounter
			T88.51XD	Hypothermia following anesthesia, subsequent encounter
			T88.52XD	Failed moderate sedation during procedure, subs encntr
			T88.59XD	Other complications of anesthesia, subsequent encounter
			T88.6XXD	Anaphyl reaction due to advrs eff drug/med prop admin, subs
			T88.7XXD	Unsp adverse effect of drug or medicament, subs encntr
			T88.8XXD	Oth complications of surgical and medical care, NEC, subs
			T88.9XXD	Complication of surgical and medical care, unsp, subs encntr
			Z51.89	Encounter for other specified aftercare
V58.9	UNSPECIFIED AFTERCARE		**Z51.89**	Encounter for other specified aftercare
V59.Ø1	WHOLE BLOOD DONOR		**Z52.ØØØ**	Unspecified donor, whole blood
			Z52.Ø1Ø	Autologous donor, whole blood
			Z52.Ø9Ø	Other blood donor, whole blood
V59.Ø2	STEM CELL DONOR		**Z52.ØØ1**	Unspecified donor, stem cells
			Z52.Ø11	Autologous donor, stem cells
			Z52.Ø91	Other blood donor, stem cells
V59.Ø9	BLOOD DONOR, OTHER		**Z52.ØØ8**	Unspecified donor, other blood
			Z52.Ø18	Autologous donor, other blood
			Z52.Ø98	Other blood donor, other blood
V59.1	SKIN DONOR		**Z52.1Ø**	Skin donor, unspecified
			Z52.11	Skin donor, autologous
			Z52.19	Skin donor, other
V59.2	BONE DONOR		**Z52.2Ø**	Bone donor, unspecified
			Z52.21	Bone donor, autologous
			Z52.29	Bone donor, other
V59.3	BONE MARROW DONOR	➡	**Z52.3**	Bone marrow donor
V59.4	KIDNEY DONOR	➡	**Z52.4**	Kidney donor
V59.5	CORNEA DONOR	➡	**Z52.5**	Cornea donor
V59.6	LIVER DONOR	➡	**Z52.6**	Liver donor
V59.7Ø	EGG DONOR UNSPECIFIED	➡	**Z52.819**	Egg (Oocyte) donor, unspecified
V59.71	EGG DONOR UNDER AGE 35 ANONYMOUS RECIPIENT	➡	**Z52.81Ø**	Egg (Oocyte) donor under age 35, anonymous recipient
V59.72	EGG DONOR UNDER AGE 35 DESIGNATED RECIPIENT	➡	**Z52.811**	Egg (Oocyte) donor under age 35, designated recipient
V59.73	EGG DONOR AGE 35 & OVER ANONYMOUS RECIPIENT	➡	**Z52.812**	Egg (Oocyte) donor age 35 and over, anonymous recipient
V59.74	EGG DONOR AGE 35 & OVER DESIGNATED RECIPIENT	➡	**Z52.813**	Egg (Oocyte) donor age 35 and over, designated recipient
V59.8	DONOR OF OTHER SPECIFIED ORGAN OR TISSUE	➡	**Z52.89**	Donor of other specified organs or tissues
V59.9	DONOR OF UNSPECIFIED ORGAN OR TISSUE	➡	**Z52.9**	Donor of unspecified organ or tissue
V6Ø.Ø	LACK OF HOUSING		**Z59.Ø**	Homelessness
V6Ø.1	INADEQUATE HOUSING	➡	**Z59.1**	Inadequate housing
V6Ø.2	INADEQUATE MATERIAL RESOURCES		**Z59.4**	Lack of adequate food and safe drinking water
			Z59.5	Extreme poverty
			Z59.6	Low income
			Z59.7	Insufficient social insurance and welfare support
V6Ø.3	PERSON LIVING ALONE		**Z6Ø.2**	Problems related to living alone
V6Ø.4	NO OTHER HOUSEHOLD MEMBER ABLE TO RENDER CARE		**Z74.2**	Need for assist at home & no house memb able to render care
V6Ø.5	HOLIDAY RELIEF CARE	➡	**Z75.5**	Holiday relief care
V6Ø.6	PERSON LIVING IN RESIDENTIAL INSTITUTION	➡	**Z59.3**	Problems related to living in residential institution
V6Ø.81	FOSTER CARE STATUS		**Z62.21**	Child in welfare custody
V6Ø.89	OTHER SPECIFIED HOUSING/ECONOMIC CIRCUMSTANCES		**Z56.82**	Military deployment status
			Z59.2	Discord with neighbors, lodgers and landlord
			Z59.8	Other problems related to housing and economic circumstances
			Z74.1	Need for assistance with personal care
			Z74.3	Need for continuous supervision
			Z74.8	Other problems related to care provider dependency
V6Ø.9	UNSPECIFIED HOUSING OR ECONOMIC CIRCUMSTANCE		**Z59.9**	Problem related to housing and economic circumstances, unsp
			Z74.9	Problem related to care provider dependency, unspecified
V61.Ø1	FAM DISRUPT D/T FAM MEMBER MILITARY DEPLOYMENT		**Z63.32**	Other absence of family member
V61.Ø2	FAM DISRUPT D/T RETURN MEMBER MILITARY DEPLOYMNT		**Z63.8**	Other specified problems related to primary support group
V61.Ø3	FAMILY DISRUPTION D/T DIVORCE/LEGAL SEPARATION		**Z63.5**	Disruption of family by separation and divorce
V61.Ø4	FAMILY DISRUPTION D/T PARENT-CHILD ESTRANGEMENT		**Z63.8**	Other specified problems related to primary support group
V61.Ø5	FAMILY DISRUPTION D/T CHILD IN WELFARE CUSTODY		**Z63.32**	Other absence of family member
V61.Ø6	FAM DISRUPT CHILD IN FOSTER CARE/CARE NON-PARENT		**Z62.22**	Institutional upbringing
			Z62.29	Other upbringing away from parents
			Z63.32	Other absence of family member
V61.Ø7	FAMILY DISRUPTION DUE TO DEATH FAMILY MEMBER		**Z63.4**	Disappearance and death of family member
V61.Ø8	FAMILY DISRUPT DUE OTH EXT ABSENCE FAM MEMBER		**Z63.32**	Other absence of family member
V61.Ø9	OTHER FAMILY DISRUPTION		**Z63.8**	Other specified problems related to primary support group
V61.1Ø	COUNSELING MARITAL&PARTNER PROBLEMS UNSPECIFIED		**Z71.89**	Other specified counseling
V61.11	COUNSELING VICTIM OF SPOUSAL AND PARTNER ABUSE	➡	**Z69.11**	Encntr for mntl hlth serv for victim of spous or prtnr abuse
V61.12	COUNSELING PERPETRATOR OF SPOUSAL&PARTNER ABUSE	➡	**Z69.12**	Encntr for mental hlth serv for perp of spous or prtnr abuse
V61.2Ø	COUNSELING FOR PARENT-CHILD PROBLEM UNSPECIFIED		**Z71.89**	Other specified counseling

[Brackets] indicate valid character values for each code. Character value meanings provided for each code grouping.

ICD-9-CM		ICD-10-CM	
V61.21	COUNSELING FOR VICTIM OF CHILD ABUSE	**Z69.Ø1Ø** **Z69.Ø2Ø**	Encntr for mental hlth serv for victim of prntl child abuse Encntr for mntl hlth serv for vctm of non-prntl child abuse
V61.22	COUNSELING PERPETRATOR OF PARENT CHILD ABUSE	➡ **Z69.Ø11**	Encntr for mental health serv for perp of prntl child abuse
V61.23	COUNSELING FOR PARENT-BIOLOGICAL CHILD PROBLEM	**Z71.89**	Other specified counseling
V61.24	COUNSELING FOR PARENT-ADOPTED CHILD PROBLEM	**Z71.89**	Other specified counseling
V61.25	COUNSELING PARENT GUARDIAN-FOSTER CHILD PROBLEM	**Z71.89**	Other specified counseling
V61.29	OTHER PARENT-CHILD PROBLEMS	**Z62.Ø** **Z62.1** **Z62.3** **Z62.6** **Z62.81Ø** **Z62.811** **Z62.812** **Z62.819** **Z62.82Ø** **Z62.821** **Z62.822** **Z62.89Ø** **Z62.898** **Z62.9**	Inadequate parental supervision and control Parental overprotection Hostility towards and scapegoating of child Inappropriate (excessive) parental pressure Personal history of physical and sexual abuse in childhood Personal history of psychological abuse in childhood Personal history of neglect in childhood Personal history of unspecified abuse in childhood Parent-biological child conflict Parent-adopted child conflict Parent-foster child conflict Parent-child estrangement NEC Other specified problems related to upbringing Problem related to upbringing, unspecified
V61.3	PROBLEMS WITH AGED PARENTS OR IN-LAWS	**Z63.79**	Other stressful life events affecting family and household
V61.41	ALCOHOLISM IN FAMILY	**Z63.72**	Alcoholism and drug addiction in family
V61.42	SUBSTANCE ABUSE IN FAMILY	**Z63.79**	Other stressful life events affecting family and household
V61.49	OTHER HEALTH PROBLEM WITHIN THE FAMILY	**Z63.6** **Z63.79**	Dependent relative needing care at home Other stressful life events affecting family and household
V61.5	MULTIPARITY	**Z64.1**	Problems related to multiparity
V61.6	ILLEGITIMACY OR ILLEGITIMATE PREGNANCY	**Z64.Ø**	Problems related to unwanted pregnancy
V61.7	OTHER UNWANTED PREGNANCY	**Z64.Ø**	Problems related to unwanted pregnancy
V61.8	OTHER SPECIFIED FAMILY CIRCUMSTANCE	**Z62.22** **Z62.29** **Z62.891** **Z63.Ø** **Z63.1** **Z63.31** **Z63.32** **Z63.4** **Z63.71** **Z63.8**	Institutional upbringing Other upbringing away from parents Sibling rivalry Problems in relationship with spouse or partner Problems in relationship with in-laws Absence of family member due to military deployment Other absence of family member Disappearance and death of family member Stress on fam d/t return of family member from miltry deploy Other specified problems related to primary support group
V61.9	UNSPECIFIED FAMILY CIRCUMSTANCE	**Z63.9**	Problem related to primary support group, unspecified
V62.Ø	UNEMPLOYMENT	**Z56.Ø**	Unemployment, unspecified
V62.1	ADVERSE EFFECTS OF WORK ENVIRONMENT	**Z56.2** **Z56.3** **Z56.4** **Z56.5** **Z56.6** **Z56.81** **Z56.89** **Z56.9** **Z57.Ø** **Z57.1** **Z57.2** **Z57.31** **Z57.39** **Z57.4** **Z57.5** **Z57.6** **Z57.7** **Z57.8** **Z57.9**	Threat of job loss Stressful work schedule Discord with boss and workmates Uncongenial work environment Other physical and mental strain related to work Sexual harassment on the job Other problems related to employment Unspecified problems related to employment Occupational exposure to noise Occupational exposure to radiation Occupational exposure to dust Occupational exposure to environmental tobacco smoke Occupational exposure to other air contaminants Occupational exposure to toxic agents in agriculture Occupational exposure to toxic agents in other industries Occupational exposure to extreme temperature Occupational exposure to vibration Occupational exposure to other risk factors Occupational exposure to unspecified risk factor
V62.21	PERSONAL CURRENT MILITARY DEPLOYMENT STATUS	**Z65.8**	Oth problems related to psychosocial circumstances
V62.22	PERSONAL HX OF RETURN FROM MILITARY DEPLOYMENT	**Z65.5**	Exposure to disaster, war and other hostilities
V62.29	OTHER OCCUPATIONAL CIRCUMSTANCES/MALADJUSTMENT	**Z56.1** **Z65.8**	Change of job Oth problems related to psychosocial circumstances
V62.3	EDUCATIONAL CIRCUMSTANCE	**Z55.Ø** **Z55.1** **Z55.2** **Z55.3** **Z55.4** **Z55.8** **Z55.9**	Illiteracy and low-level literacy Schooling unavailable and unattainable Failed school examinations Underachievement in school Educational maladjustment & discord w teachers & classmates Other problems related to education and literacy Problems related to education and literacy, unspecified
V62.4	SOCIAL MALADJUSTMENT	**Z6Ø.3** **Z6Ø.4** **Z6Ø.5** **Z73.4** **Z73.5**	Acculturation difficulty Social exclusion and rejection Target of (perceived) adverse discrimination and persecution Inadequate social skills, not elsewhere classified Social role conflict, not elsewhere classified

ICD-9-CM		ICD-10-CM	
V62.5	LEGAL CIRCUMSTANCE	**Z65.Ø** **Z65.1** **Z65.2** **Z65.3**	Conviction in civil & criminal proceedings w/o imprisonment Imprisonment and other incarceration Problems related to release from prison Problems related to other legal circumstances
V62.6	REFUSAL TREATMENT REASONS RELIGION OR CONSCIENCE	**Z53.1**	Proc/trtmt not crd out bec pt belief and group pressure
V62.81	INTERPERSONAL PROBLEM NOT ELSEWHERE CLASSIFIED	**Z65.8**	Oth problems related to psychosocial circumstances
V62.82	BEREAVEMENT UNCOMPLICATED NEC	**Z63.4**	Disappearance and death of family member
V62.83	COUNSELING PERP OF PHYSICAL/SEXUAL ABUSE NEC	**Z69.Ø21** **Z69.82**	Encntr for mntl hlth serv for perp of non-prntl child abuse Encounter for mental health services for perp of abuse
V62.84	SUICIDAL IDEATION	➡ **R45.851**	Suicidal ideations
V62.85	HOMICIDAL IDEATION	➡ **R45.85Ø**	Homicidal ideations
V62.89	OTHER PSYCHOLOGICAL OR PHYSICAL STRESS NEC OTHER	**R41.83** **Z6Ø.Ø** **Z6Ø.8** **Z6Ø.9** **Z64.4** **Z65.4** **Z65.8** **Z73.6**	Borderline intellectual functioning Problems of adjustment to life-cycle transitions Other problems related to social environment Problem related to social environment, unspecified Discord with counselors Victim of crime and terrorism Oth problems related to psychosocial circumstances Limitation of activities due to disability
V62.9	UNSPECIFIED PSYCHOSOCIAL CIRCUMSTANCE NEC	**Z65.9**	Problem related to unspecified psychosocial circumstances
V63.Ø	RESIDENCE REMOTE FROM HOSP/OTH HLTH CARE FACL	**Z75.3**	Unavailability and inaccessibility of health-care facilities
V63.1	MEDICAL SERVICES IN HOME NOT AVAILABLE	➡ **Z75.Ø**	Medical services not available in home
V63.2	PERSON AWAITING ADMISSION ADEQUATE FACILITY ELSW	➡ **Z75.1**	Person awaiting admission to adequate facility elsewhere
V63.8	OTH SPEC REASON UNAVAILABILITY MED FACILITIES	**Z75.2** **Z75.4** **Z75.8**	Other waiting period for investigation and treatment Unavailability and inaccessibility of other helping agencies Oth prob related to medical facilities and oth health care
V63.9	UNSPEC REASON UNAVAILABILITY MEDICAL FACILITIES	**Z75.3** **Z75.9**	Unavailability and inaccessibility of health-care facilities Unsp problem related to med facilities and oth health care
V64.ØØ	VACCINATION NOT CARRIED OUT UNSPECIFIED REASON	➡ **Z28.9**	Immunization not carried out for unspecified reason
V64.Ø1	VACCINATION NOT CARRIED OUT ACUTE ILLNESS	➡ **Z28.Ø1**	Immunization not crd out because of acute illness of patient
V64.Ø2	VACCINATION NOT CARRIED OUT CHRONIC ILLNESS/COND	➡ **Z28.Ø2**	Immuniz not crd out bec chronic illness or cond of patient
V64.Ø3	VACCINATION NOT CARRIED OUT IMMUNE COMPROMISED	➡ **Z28.Ø3**	Immuniz not crd out bec immune compromised state of patient
V64.Ø4	VACCINATION NOT CARRIED OUT ALLERGY VACC/COMPONT	➡ **Z28.Ø4**	Immuniz not crd out bec patient allergy to vaccine or cmpnt
V64.Ø5	VACCINATION NOT CARRIED OUT CAREGIVER REFUSAL	➡ **Z28.82**	Immunization not carried out because of caregiver refusal
V64.Ø6	VACCINATION NOT CARRIED OUT PATIENT REFUSAL	**Z28.21** **Z53.1** **Z53.2Ø** **Z53.21** **Z53.29**	Immunization not carried out because of patient refusal Proc/trtmt not crd out bec pt belief and group pressure Proc/trtmt not crd out bec pt decision for unsp reasons Proc/trtmt not crd out d/t pt lv bef seen by hlth care prov Proc/trtmt not crd out bec pt decision for oth reasons
V64.Ø7	VACCINATION NOT CARRIED OUT RELIGIOUS REASONS	➡ **Z28.1**	Immuniz not crd out because of patient belief/grp pressr
V64.Ø8	VACC NOT CARRIED OUT PT HAD DZ BEING VACC AGNST	➡ **Z28.81**	Immuniz not crd out due to patient having had the disease
V64.Ø9	VACCINATION NOT CARRIED OUT FOR OTHER REASON	**Z28.Ø9** **Z28.2Ø** **Z28.29** **Z28.89**	Immunization not carried out because of oth contraindication Immuniz not crd out bec patient decision for unsp reason Immuniz not crd out bec patient decision for oth reason Immunization not carried out for other reason
V64.1	SURG/OTH PROC NOT DONE BECAUSE CONTRAINDICATION	**Z53.Ø1** **Z53.Ø9**	Proc/trtmt not carried out due to patient smoking Proc/trtmt not carried out because of contraindication
V64.2	SURG/OTH PROC NOT CARRIED OUT BECAUSE PTS DECN	**Z53.1** **Z53.2Ø** **Z53.21** **Z53.29**	Proc/trtmt not crd out bec pt belief and group pressure Proc/trtmt not crd out bec pt decision for unsp reasons Proc/trtmt not crd out d/t pt lv bef seen by hlth care prov Proc/trtmt not crd out bec pt decision for oth reasons
V64.3	PROCEDURE NOT CARRIED OUT FOR OTHER REASONS	**Z53.8** **Z53.9**	Procedure and treatment not carried out for other reasons Procedure and treatment not carried out, unspecified reason
V64.41	LAPAROSCOPIC SURGICAL PROC COVERTED OPEN PROC	NO DIAGNOSIS	
V64.42	THORACOSCOPIC SURGICAL PROC CONVRT OPEN PROC	NO DIAGNOSIS	
V64.43	ARTHROSCOPIC SURGICAL PROC CONVRT OPEN PROC	NO DIAGNOSIS	
V65.Ø	HEALTHY PERSON ACCOMPANYING SICK PERSON	**Z76.3** **Z76.4**	Healthy person accompanying sick person Other boarder to healthcare facility
V65.11	PEDIATRIC PRE-BIRTH VISIT FOR EXPECTANT PARENTS	➡ **Z76.81**	Expectant parent(s) prebirth pediatrician visit
V65.19	OTHER PERSON CONSULTING BEHALF OF ANOTHER PERSON	➡ **Z71.Ø**	Prsn encntr hlth serv to consult on behalf of another person
V65.2	PERSON FEIGNING ILLNESS	➡ **Z76.5**	Malingerer [conscious simulation]
V65.3	DIETARY SURVEILLANCE AND COUNSELING	➡ **Z71.3**	Dietary counseling and surveillance
V65.4Ø	COUNSELING NOS	**Z71.9**	Counseling, unspecified
V65.41	EXCERCISE COUNSELING	**Z71.89**	Other specified counseling
V65.42	COUNSELING ON SUBSTANCE USE AND ABUSE	**Z71.41** **Z71.42** **Z71.51** **Z71.52** **Z71.6**	Alcohol abuse counseling and surveillance of alcoholic Counseling for family member of alcoholic Drug abuse counseling and surveillance of drug abuser Counseling for family member of drug abuser Tobacco abuse counseling
V65.43	COUNSELING ON INJURY PREVENTION	**Z71.89**	Other specified counseling
V65.44	HUMAN IMMUNODEFICIENCY VIRUS COUNSELING	➡ **Z71.7**	Human immunodeficiency virus [HIV] counseling
V65.45	COUNSELING OTHER SEXUALLY TRANSMITTED DISEASES	**Z71.89**	Other specified counseling
V65.46	ENCOUNTER FOR INSULIN PUMP TRAINING	**Z46.81**	Encounter for fitting and adjustment of insulin pump

ICD-9-CM			ICD-10-CM	
V65.49	OTHER SPECIFIED COUNSELING		**Z32.2** **Z32.3** **Z69.81** **Z7Ø.Ø** **Z7Ø.1** **Z7Ø.2** **Z7Ø.3** **Z7Ø.8** **Z7Ø.9** **Z71.81** **Z71.89** **Z76.89**	Encounter for childbirth instruction Encounter for childcare instruction Encounter for mental health services for victim of oth abuse Counseling related to sexual attitude Counseling related to patient's sexual behavior and orientn Cnsl related to sexual behavior and orientn of third party Cnsl rel to comb concrn rgrd sex attitude, behav and orientn Other sex counseling Sex counseling, unspecified Spiritual or religious counseling Other specified counseling Persons encountering health services in oth circumstances
V65.5	PERSON W/FEARED COMPLAINT WHOM NO DX WAS MADE	➡	**Z71.1**	Person w feared hlth complaint in whom no diagnosis is made
V65.8	OTHER REASONS FOR SEEKING CONSULTATION		**Z71.2** **Z76.89**	Person consulting for explanation of exam or test findings Persons encountering health services in oth circumstances
V65.9	UNSPECIFIED REASON FOR CONSULTATION		**Z71.9**	Counseling, unspecified
V66.Ø	CONVALESCENCE FOLLOWING SURGERY		**Z51.89**	Encounter for other specified aftercare
V66.1	CONVALESCENCE FOLLOWING RADIOTHERAPY		**Z51.89**	Encounter for other specified aftercare
V66.2	CONVALESCENCE FOLLOWING CHEMOTHERAPY		**Z51.89**	Encounter for other specified aftercare
V66.3	CONVALESCENCE FLW PSYCHOTHAPY&OTH TX MENTL D/O		**Z51.89**	Encounter for other specified aftercare
V66.4	CONVALESCENCE FOLLOWING TREATMENT OF FRACTURE		**Z51.89**	Encounter for other specified aftercare
V66.5	CONVALESCENCE FOLLOWING OTHER TREATMENT		**Z51.89**	Encounter for other specified aftercare
V66.6	CONVALESCENCE FOLLOWING COMBINED TREATMENT		**Z51.89**	Encounter for other specified aftercare
V66.7	ENCOUNTER FOR PALLIATIVE CARE	➡	**Z51.5**	Encounter for palliative care
V66.9	UNSPECIFIED CONVALESCENCE		**Z51.89**	Encounter for other specified aftercare
V67.ØØ	FOLLOW-UP EXAMINATION FOLLOWING UNSPEC SURGERY		**ZØ9**	Encntr for f/u exam aft trtmt for cond oth than malig neoplm
V67.Ø1	FOLLOWING SURGERY FOLLOW-UP VAGINAL PAP SMEAR		**ZØ8**	Encntr for follow-up exam after trtmt for malignant neoplasm
V67.Ø9	FOLLOW-UP EXAMINATION FOLLOWING OTHER SURGERY		**ZØ9**	Encntr for f/u exam aft trtmt for cond oth than malig neoplm
V67.1	RADIOTHERAPY FOLLOW-UP EXAMINATION		**ZØ8** **ZØ9**	Encntr for follow-up exam after trtmt for malignant neoplasm Encntr for f/u exam aft trtmt for cond oth than malig neoplm
V67.2	CHEMOTHERAPY FOLLOW-UP EXAMINATION		**ZØ8** **ZØ9**	Encntr for follow-up exam after trtmt for malignant neoplasm Encntr for f/u exam aft trtmt for cond oth than malig neoplm
V67.3	PSYCHOTHAPY&OTH TX MENTAL DISORDER F/U EXAM		**ZØ9**	Encntr for f/u exam aft trtmt for cond oth than malig neoplm
V67.4	TREATMENT HEALED FRACTURE FOLLOW-UP EXAMINATION		**ZØ9**	Encntr for f/u exam aft trtmt for cond oth than malig neoplm
V67.51	F/U EXAM FOLLOW CMPL TX W/HIGH-RISK MED NEC		**ZØ9**	Encntr for f/u exam aft trtmt for cond oth than malig neoplm
V67.59	OTHER FOLLOW-UP EXAMINATION OTHER		**ZØ8** **ZØ9**	Encntr for follow-up exam after trtmt for malignant neoplasm Encntr for f/u exam aft trtmt for cond oth than malig neoplm
V67.6	COMBINED TREATMENT FOLLOW-UP EXAMINATION		**ZØ8** **ZØ9**	Encntr for follow-up exam after trtmt for malignant neoplasm Encntr for f/u exam aft trtmt for cond oth than malig neoplm
V67.9	UNSPECIFIED FOLLOW-UP EXAMINATION		**ZØ8** **ZØ9**	Encntr for follow-up exam after trtmt for malignant neoplasm Encntr for f/u exam aft trtmt for cond oth than malig neoplm
V68.Ø1	DISABILITY EXAMINATION	➡	**ZØ2.71**	Encounter for disability determination
V68.Ø9	OTHER ISSUE OF MEDICAL CERTIFICATES	➡	**ZØ2.79**	Encounter for issue of other medical certificate
V68.1	ISSUE OF REPEAT PRESCRIPTIONS	➡	**Z76.Ø**	Encounter for issue of repeat prescription
V68.2	REQUEST FOR EXPERT EVIDENCE		**ZØ4.8**	Encounter for examination and observation for oth reasons
V68.81	REFERRAL PATIENT WITHOUT EXAMINATION/TREATMENT		**ZØ4.9**	Encounter for examination and observation for unsp reason
V68.89	ENCOUNTERS OTHER SPEC ADMINISTRATIVE PURPOSE OTH		**ZØ2.89**	Encounter for other administrative examinations
V68.9	ENCOUNTERS UNSPECIFIED ADMINISTRATIVE PURPOSE		**ZØ2.9**	Encounter for administrative examinations, unspecified
V69.Ø	PROBLEMS RELATED TO LACK OF PHYSICAL EXCERCISE	➡	**Z72.3**	Lack of physical exercise
V69.1	PROBS RELATED INAPPROPRIATE DIET&EATING HABITS	➡	**Z72.4**	Inappropriate diet and eating habits
V69.2	PROBLEMS RELATED TO HIGH-RISK SEXUAL BEHAVIOR		**Z72.51** **Z72.52** **Z72.53**	High risk heterosexual behavior High risk homosexual behavior High risk bisexual behavior
V69.3	PROBLEMS RELATED TO GAMBLING AND BETTING	➡	**Z72.6**	Gambling and betting
V69.4	LACK OF ADEQUATE SLEEP	➡	**Z72.82Ø**	Sleep deprivation
V69.5	BEHAVIORAL INSOMNIA OF CHILDHOOD		**Z73.81Ø** **Z73.811** **Z73.812** **Z73.819** **Z73.89**	Behavioral insomnia of childhood, sleep-onset assoc type Behavioral insomnia of childhood, limit setting type Behavioral insomnia of childhood, combined type Behavioral insomnia of childhood, unspecified type Other problems related to life management difficulty
V69.8	OTHER PROBLEMS RELATED TO LIFESTYLE		**Z72.Ø** **Z72.821** **Z72.89** **Z73.Ø** **Z73.1** **Z73.2** **Z73.3**	Tobacco use Inadequate sleep hygiene Other problems related to lifestyle Burn-out Type A behavior pattern Lack of relaxation and leisure Stress, not elsewhere classified
V69.9	UNSPECIFIED PROBLEMS RELATED TO LIFESTYLE		**Z72.9** **Z73.9**	Problem related to lifestyle, unspecified Problem related to life management difficulty, unspecified
V7Ø.Ø	ROUTINE GENERAL MEDICAL EXAM@HEALTH CARE FACL		**ZØØ.ØØ** **ZØØ.Ø1**	Encntr for general adult medical exam w/o abnormal findings Encounter for general adult medical exam w abnormal findings
V7Ø.1	GENERAL PSYC EXAMINATION REQUESTED AUTHORITY	➡	**ZØ4.6**	Encntr for general psychiatric exam, requested by authority
V7Ø.2	OTHER&UNSPEC GENERAL PSYCHIATRIC EXAMINATION		**ZØØ.8**	Encounter for other general examination

ICD-9-CM			ICD-10-CM	
V7Ø.3	OTH GENERAL MEDICAL EXAMINATION ADMIN PURPOSES		**Z02.Ø**	Encounter for exam for admission to educational institution
			ZØ2.2	Encounter for exam for admission to residential institution
			ZØ2.4	Encounter for examination for driving license
			ZØ2.5	Encounter for examination for participation in sport
			ZØ2.6	Encounter for examination for insurance purposes
			ZØ2.82	Encounter for adoption services
			ZØ2.89	Encounter for other administrative examinations
V7Ø.4	EXAMINATION FOR MEDICOLEGAL REASON		**ZØ2.81**	Encounter for paternity testing
			ZØ2.83	Encounter for blood-alcohol and blood-drug test
V7Ø.5	HEALTH EXAMINATION OF DEFINED SUBPOPULATION		**ZØ2.1**	Encounter for pre-employment examination
			ZØ2.3	Encounter for examination for recruitment to armed forces
			ZØ2.89	Encounter for other administrative examinations
V7Ø.6	HEALTH EXAMINATION IN POPULATION SURVEY		**ZØØ.8**	Encounter for other general examination
V7Ø.7	EXAMINATION OF PARTICIPANT IN CLINICAL TRIAL	➡	**ZØØ.6**	Encntr for exam for nrml cmprsn and ctrl in clncl rsrch prog
V7Ø.8	OTHER SPECIFIED GENERAL MEDICAL EXAMINATION		**ZØØ.5**	Encounter for exam of potential donor of organ and tissue
			ZØØ.7Ø	Encntr for exam for delay growth in chldhd w/o abn findings
			ZØØ.71	Encntr for exam for delay growth in chldhd w abn findings
			ZØØ.8	Encounter for other general examination
V7Ø.9	UNSPECIFIED GENERAL MEDICAL EXAMINATION		**ZØØ.8**	Encounter for other general examination
V71.Ø1	OBSERVATION OF ADULT ANTISOCIAL BEHAVIOR		**ZØ3.89**	Encntr for obs for oth suspected diseases and cond ruled out
			Z72.811	Adult antisocial behavior
V71.Ø2	OBSERVATION CHILDHOOD/ADOLES ANTISOCIAL BEHAVIOR		**ZØ3.89**	Encntr for obs for oth suspected diseases and cond ruled out
			Z72.81Ø	Child and adolescent antisocial behavior
V71.Ø9	OBSERVATION OF OTHER SUSPECTED MENTAL CONDITION		**ZØ3.89**	Encntr for obs for oth suspected diseases and cond ruled out
V71.1	OBSERVATION FOR SUSPECTED MALIGNANT NEOPLASM		**ZØ3.89**	Encntr for obs for oth suspected diseases and cond ruled out
V71.2	OBSERVATION FOR SUSPECTED TUBERCULOSIS		**ZØ3.89**	Encntr for obs for oth suspected diseases and cond ruled out
V71.3	OBSERVATION FOLLOWING ACCIDENT AT WORK	➡	**ZØ4.2**	Encounter for exam and observation following work accident
V71.4	OBSERVATION FOLLOWING OTHER ACCIDENT		**ZØ4.1**	Encounter for exam and obs following transport accident
			ZØ4.3	Encounter for exam and observation following oth accident
V71.5	OBSERVATION FOLLOWING ALLEGED RAPE OR SEDUCTION		**ZØ4.41**	Encounter for exam and obs following alleged adult rape
			ZØ4.42	Encounter for exam and obs following alleged child rape
V71.6	OBSERVATION FOLLOWING OTHER INFLICTED INJURY		**ZØ4.8**	Encounter for examination and observation for oth reasons
V71.7	OBSERVATION FOR SUSPECTED CARDIOVASCULAR DISEASE		**ZØ3.89**	Encntr for obs for oth suspected diseases and cond ruled out
V71.81	OBSERVATION FOR SUSPECTED ABUSE AND NEGLECT		**ZØ4.71**	Encntr for exam and obs fol alleged adult physical abuse
			ZØ4.72	Encntr for exam and obs fol alleged child physical abuse
V71.82	OBSERVATION&EVALUATION SUSPECTED EXPOS ANTHRAX	➡	**ZØ3.81Ø**	Encntr for obs for suspected exposure to anthrax ruled out
V71.83	OBSERVATION&EVAL SPCT EXPOS OTH BIOLOGIC AGT	➡	**ZØ3.818**	Encntr for obs for susp expsr to oth biolg agents ruled out
V71.89	OBSERVATION OTHER SPECIFIED SUSPECTED CONDITIONS		**ZØ3.6**	Encntr for obs for susp toxic eff from ingest sub ruled out
			ZØ3.89	Encntr for obs for oth suspected diseases and cond ruled out
V71.9	OBSERVATION FOR UNSPECIFIED SUSPECTED CONDITION		**ZØ4.9**	Encounter for examination and observation for unsp reason
V72.Ø	EXAMINATION OF EYES AND VISION		**ZØ1.ØØ**	Encounter for exam of eyes and vision w/o abnormal findings
			ZØ1.Ø1	Encounter for exam of eyes and vision w abnormal findings
V72.11	ENCOUNTER HEARING EXAM FOLLOW FAILED HEARING SCR	➡	**ZØ1.11Ø**	Encounter for hearing exam following failed hear screening
V72.12	ENCOUNTER FOR HEARING CONSERVATION AND TREATMENT	➡	**ZØ1.12**	Encounter for hearing conservation and treatment
V72.19	OTHER EXAMINATION OF EARS AND HEARING		**ZØ1.1Ø**	Encounter for exam of ears and hearing w/o abnormal findings
			ZØ1.118	Encntr for exam of ears and hearing w oth abnormal findings
V72.2	DENTAL EXAMINATION		**ZØ1.2Ø**	Encounter for dental exam and cleaning w/o abnormal findings
			ZØ1.21	Encounter for dental exam and cleaning w abnormal findings
V72.31	ROUTINE GYNECOLOGICAL EXAMINATION		**ZØ1.411**	Encntr for gyn exam (general) (routine) w abnormal findings
			ZØ1.419	Encntr for gyn exam (general) (routine) w/o abn findings
V72.32	ENCOUNTER PAP CERV SMER CONFIRM NL SMER FLW ABN	➡	**ZØ1.42**	Encntr for cerv smear to cnfrm norm smr fol init abn smear
V72.4Ø	PREGNANCY EXAMINATION/TEST PREGNANCY UNCONFIRMED	➡	**Z32.ØØ**	Encounter for pregnancy test, result unknown
V72.41	PREGNANCY EXAMINATION OR TEST NEGATIVE RESULT	➡	**Z32.Ø2**	Encounter for pregnancy test, result negative
V72.42	PREGNANCY EXAMINATION OR TEST POSITIVE RESULT	➡	**Z32.Ø1**	Encounter for pregnancy test, result positive
V72.5	RADIOLOGICAL EXAMINATION NEC		**ZØ1.89**	Encounter for other specified special examinations
V72.6Ø	LABORATORY EXAMINATION UNSPECIFIED		**ZØØ.ØØ**	Encntr for general adult medical exam w/o abnormal findings
V72.61	ANTIBODY RESPONSE EXAMINATION	➡	**ZØ1.84**	Encounter for antibody response examination
V72.62	LABORATORY EXAM ORDER PART ROUTINE GEN MED EXAM		**ZØØ.ØØ**	Encntr for general adult medical exam w/o abnormal findings
V72.63	PRE-PROCEDURAL LABORATORY EXAMINATION	➡	**ZØ1.812**	Encounter for preprocedural laboratory examination
V72.69	OTHER LABORATORY EXAMINATION		**ZØ1.89**	Encounter for other specified special examinations
V72.7	DIAGNOSTIC SKIN AND SENSITIZATION TESTS		**ZØ1.82**	Encounter for allergy testing
			ZØ1.89	Encounter for other specified special examinations
V72.81	PRE-OPERATIVE CARDIOVASCULAR EXAMINATION	➡	**ZØ1.81Ø**	Encounter for preprocedural cardiovascular examination
V72.82	PRE-OPERATIVE RESPIRATORY EXAMINATION	➡	**ZØ1.811**	Encounter for preprocedural respiratory examination
V72.83	OTHER SPECIFIED PRE-OPERATIVE EXAMINATION		**ZØ1.818**	Encounter for other preprocedural examination
V72.84	UNSPECIFIED PRE-OPERATIVE EXAMINATION		**ZØ1.812**	Encounter for preprocedural laboratory examination
			ZØ1.818	Encounter for other preprocedural examination
V72.85	OTHER SPECIFIED EXAMINATION		**ZØ1.3Ø**	Encounter for exam of blood pressure w/o abnormal findings
			ZØ1.31	Encounter for exam of blood pressure w abnormal findings
			ZØ1.89	Encounter for other specified special examinations
V72.86	ENCOUNTER FOR BLOOD TYPING	➡	**ZØ1.83**	Encounter for blood typing
V72.9	UNSPECIFIED EXAMINATION		**ZØ1.89**	Encounter for other specified special examinations

ICD-9-CM			ICD-10-CM	
V73.Ø	SCREENING EXAMINATION FOR POLIOMYELITIS		**Z11.59**	Encounter for screening for other viral diseases
V73.1	SCREENING EXAMINATION FOR SMALLPOX		**Z11.59**	Encounter for screening for other viral diseases
V73.2	SCREENING EXAMINATION FOR MEASLES		**Z11.59**	Encounter for screening for other viral diseases
V73.3	SCREENING EXAMINATION FOR RUBELLA		**Z11.59**	Encounter for screening for other viral diseases
V73.4	SCREENING EXAMINATION FOR YELLOW FEVER		**Z11.59**	Encounter for screening for other viral diseases
V73.5	SCR EXAMINATION OTH ARTHROPOD-BORNE VIRAL DZ		**Z11.59**	Encounter for screening for other viral diseases
V73.6	SCREENING EXAMINATION FOR TRACHOMA		**Z11.59**	Encounter for screening for other viral diseases
V73.81	SPECIAL SCREENING EXAMINATION HUMAN PAPILVIRUS	➡	**Z11.51**	Encounter for screening for human papillomavirus (HPV)
V73.88	SPECIAL SCR EXAMINATION OTH SPEC CHLAMYDIAL DZ		**Z11.8**	Encounter for screening for oth infec/parastc diseases
V73.89	SPECIAL SCREENING EXAMINATION OTH SPEC VIRAL DZ		**Z11.4** **Z11.59**	Encounter for screening for human immunodeficiency virus Encounter for screening for other viral diseases
V73.98	SPECIAL SCR EXAM UNSPEC CHLAMYDIAL DISEASE		**Z11.8**	Encounter for screening for oth infec/parastc diseases
V73.99	SPECIAL SCR EXAMINATION UNSPEC VIRAL DISEASE		**Z11.59**	Encounter for screening for other viral diseases
V74.Ø	SCREENING EXAMINATION FOR CHOLERA		**Z11.Ø**	Encounter for screening for intestinal infectious diseases
V74.1	SCREENING EXAMINATION FOR PULMONARY TUBERCULOSIS	➡	**Z11.1**	Encounter for screening for respiratory tuberculosis
V74.2	SCREENING EXAMINATION FOR LEPROSY		**Z11.2**	Encounter for screening for other bacterial diseases
V74.3	SCREENING EXAMINATION FOR DIPHTHERIA		**Z11.2**	Encounter for screening for other bacterial diseases
V74.4	SCREENING EXAMINATION BACTERIAL CONJUNCTIVITIS		**Z11.2**	Encounter for screening for other bacterial diseases
V74.5	SCREENING EXAMINATION FOR VENEREAL DISEASE	➡	**Z11.3**	Encntr screen for infections w sexl mode of transmiss
V74.6	SCREENING EXAMINATION FOR YAWS		**Z11.8**	Encounter for screening for oth infec/parastc diseases
V74.8	SCR EXAMINATION OTH SPEC BACTERL&SPIROCHETAL DZ		**Z11.2** **Z11.8**	Encounter for screening for other bacterial diseases Encounter for screening for oth infec/parastc diseases
V74.9	SCR EXAMINATION UNSPEC BACTERL&SPIROCHETAL DZ		**Z11.2**	Encounter for screening for other bacterial diseases
V75.Ø	SCREENING EXAMINATION FOR RICKETTSIAL DISEASES		**Z11.8**	Encounter for screening for oth infec/parastc diseases
V75.1	SCREENING EXAMINATION FOR MALARIA		**Z11.6**	Encntr screen for oth protozoal diseases and helminthiases
V75.2	SCREENING EXAMINATION FOR LEISHMANIASIS		**Z11.6**	Encntr screen for oth protozoal diseases and helminthiases
V75.3	SCREENING EXAMINATION FOR TRYPANOSOMIASIS		**Z11.6**	Encntr screen for oth protozoal diseases and helminthiases
V75.4	SCREENING EXAMINATION FOR MYCOTIC INFECTIONS		**Z11.8**	Encounter for screening for oth infec/parastc diseases
V75.5	SCREENING EXAMINATION FOR SCHISTOSOMIASIS		**Z11.6**	Encntr screen for oth protozoal diseases and helminthiases
V75.6	SCREENING EXAMINATION FOR FILARIASIS		**Z11.6**	Encntr screen for oth protozoal diseases and helminthiases
V75.7	SCREENING EXAMINATION INTESTINAL HELMINTHIASIS		**Z11.6**	Encntr screen for oth protozoal diseases and helminthiases
V75.8	SCREENING EXAMINATION OTH SPEC PARASITIC INFS		**Z11.Ø** **Z11.8**	Encounter for screening for intestinal infectious diseases Encounter for screening for oth infec/parastc diseases
V75.9	SCREENING EXAMINATION UNSPEC INFECTIOUS DISEASE	➡	**Z11.9**	Encounter for screening for infec/parastc diseases, unsp
V76.Ø	SPECIAL SCREENING MALIG NEOPLASM RESP ORGN	➡	**Z12.2**	Encntr screen for malignant neoplasm of respiratory organs
V76.1Ø	UNSPECIFIED BREAST SCREENING		**Z12.39**	Encounter for oth screening for malignant neoplasm of breast
V76.11	SCREENING MAMMOGRAM FOR HIGH-RISK PATIENT		**Z12.31**	Encntr screen mammogram for malignant neoplasm of breast
V76.12	OTHER SCREENING MAMMOGRAM		**Z12.31**	Encntr screen mammogram for malignant neoplasm of breast
V76.19	OTHER SCREENING BREAST EXAMINATION		**Z12.39**	Encounter for oth screening for malignant neoplasm of breast
V76.2	SCREENING FOR MALIGNANT NEOPLASM OF THE CERVIX	➡	**Z12.4**	Encounter for screening for malignant neoplasm of cervix
V76.3	SCREENING FOR MALIGNANT NEOPLASM OF THE BLADDER	➡	**Z12.6**	Encounter for screening for malignant neoplasm of bladder
V76.41	SCREENING FOR MALIGNANT NEOPLASM OF THE RECTUM	➡	**Z12.12**	Encounter for screening for malignant neoplasm of rectum
V76.42	SCREENING MALIGNANT NEOPLASM OF THE ORAL CAVITY	➡	**Z12.81**	Encntr screen for malignant neoplasm of oral cavity
V76.43	SCREENING FOR MALIGNANT NEOPLASM OF THE SKIN	➡	**Z12.83**	Encounter for screening for malignant neoplasm of skin
V76.44	SPECIAL SCREENING MALIGNANT NEOPLASM OF PROSTATE	➡	**Z12.5**	Encounter for screening for malignant neoplasm of prostate
V76.45	SPECIAL SCREENING MALIGNANT NEOPLASM OF TESTIS	➡	**Z12.71**	Encounter for screening for malignant neoplasm of testis
V76.46	SPECIAL SCREENING FOR MALIGNANT NEOPLASMS OVARY	➡	**Z12.73**	Encounter for screening for malignant neoplasm of ovary
V76.47	SPECIAL SCREENING FOR MALIGNANT NEOPLASMS VAGINA		**Z12.72**	Encounter for screening for malignant neoplasm of vagina
V76.49	SPECIAL SCREENING MALIG NEOPLASMS OTHER SITES		**Z12.Ø** **Z12.79** **Z12.89**	Encounter for screening for malignant neoplasm of stomach Encntr screen for malignant neoplasm of genitourinary organs Encounter for screening for malignant neoplasm of oth sites
V76.5Ø	SPECIAL SCREENING MALIG NEOPLSM INTESTINE UNSPEC	➡	**Z12.1Ø**	Encntr screen for malignant neoplasm of intest tract, unsp
V76.51	SPECIAL SCREENING FOR MALIGNANT NEOPLASMS COLON	➡	**Z12.11**	Encounter for screening for malignant neoplasm of colon
V76.52	SPECIAL SCREENING MALIG NEOPLSM SMALL INTESTINE	➡	**Z12.13**	Encntr screen for malignant neoplasm of small intestine
V76.81	SPECIAL SCREENING MALIG NEOPLASMS NERVOUS SYSTEM	➡	**Z12.82**	Encntr screen for malignant neoplasm of nervous system
V76.89	SPECIAL SCREENING FOR OTHER MALIGNANT NEOPLASM		**Z12.89**	Encounter for screening for malignant neoplasm of oth sites
V76.9	SCREENING FOR UNSPECIFIED MALIGNANT NEOPLASM	➡	**Z12.9**	Encounter for screening for malignant neoplasm, site unsp
V77.Ø	SCREENING FOR THYROID DISORDER		**Z13.29**	Encounter for screening for oth suspected endocrine disorder
V77.1	SCREENING FOR DIABETES MELLITUS	➡	**Z13.1**	Encounter for screening for diabetes mellitus
V77.2	SCREENING FOR MALNUTRITION		**Z13.21**	Encounter for screening for nutritional disorder
V77.3	SCREENING FOR PHENYLKETONURIA		**Z13.228**	Encounter for screening for other metabolic disorders
V77.4	SCREENING FOR GALACTOSEMIA		**Z13.228**	Encounter for screening for other metabolic disorders
V77.5	SCREENING FOR GOUT		**Z13.89**	Encounter for screening for other disorder
V77.6	SCREENING FOR CYSTIC FIBROSIS		**Z13.228**	Encounter for screening for other metabolic disorders
V77.7	SCREENING FOR OTHER INBORN ERRORS OF METABOLISM		**Z13.228**	Encounter for screening for other metabolic disorders
V77.8	SCREENING FOR OBESITY		**Z13.89**	Encounter for screening for other disorder
V77.91	SCREENING FOR LIPOID DISORDERS	➡	**Z13.22Ø**	Encounter for screening for lipoid disorders

ICD-9-CM			ICD-10-CM	
V77.99	OTH&UNSPEC ENDOCRN NUTRIT METAB&IMMUNITY D/O		**Z13.21** **Z13.228** **Z13.29**	Encounter for screening for nutritional disorder Encounter for screening for other metabolic disorders Encounter for screening for oth suspected endocrine disorder
V78.Ø	SCREENING FOR IRON DEFICIENCY ANEMIA		**Z13.Ø**	Encntr screen for dis of the bld/bld-form org/immun mechnsm
V78.1	SCREENING OTHER&UNSPECIFIED DEFICIENCY ANEMIA		**Z13.Ø**	Encntr screen for dis of the bld/bld-form org/immun mechnsm
V78.2	SCREENING FOR SICKLE-CELL DISEASE OR TRAIT		**Z13.Ø**	Encntr screen for dis of the bld/bld-form org/immun mechnsm
V78.3	SCREENING FOR OTHER HEMOGLOBINOPATHIES		**Z13.Ø**	Encntr screen for dis of the bld/bld-form org/immun mechnsm
V78.8	SCREENING OTH DISORDERS BLD&BLD-FORMING ORGANS		**Z13.Ø**	Encntr screen for dis of the bld/bld-form org/immun mechnsm
V78.9	SCREENING UNSPEC DISORDER BLD&BLD-FORMING ORGANS		**Z13.Ø**	Encntr screen for dis of the bld/bld-form org/immun mechnsm
V79.Ø	SCREENING FOR DEPRESSION		**Z13.89**	Encounter for screening for other disorder
V79.1	SCREENING FOR ALCOHOLISM		**Z13.89**	Encounter for screening for other disorder
V79.2	SCREENING FOR INTELLECTUAL DISABILITIES		**Z13.4**	Encntr screen for certain developmental disorders in chldhd
V79.3	SCREENING DVLPMENTL HANDICAPS EARLY CHILDHOOD		**Z13.4**	Encntr screen for certain developmental disorders in chldhd
V79.8	SCR OTH SPEC MENTAL D/O&DVLPMENTL HANDICAPS		**Z13.4**	Encntr screen for certain developmental disorders in chldhd
V79.9	SCR UNSPEC MENTAL DISORDER&DVLPMENTL HANDICAP		**Z13.89**	Encounter for screening for other disorder
V8Ø.Ø1	SPECIAL SCREENING FOR TRAUMATIC BRAIN INJURY	➡	**Z13.85Ø**	Encounter for screening for traumatic brain injury
V8Ø.Ø9	SPECIAL SCREENING OTHER NEUROLOGICAL CONDITIONS	➡	**Z13.858**	Encounter for screening for other nervous system disorders
V8Ø.1	SCREENING FOR GLAUCOMA		**Z13.5**	Encounter for screening for eye and ear disorders
V8Ø.2	SCREENING FOR OTHER EYE CONDITIONS		**Z13.5**	Encounter for screening for eye and ear disorders
V8Ø.3	SCREENING FOR EAR DISEASES		**Z13.5**	Encounter for screening for eye and ear disorders
V81.Ø	SCREENING FOR ISCHEMIC HEART DISEASE		**Z13.6**	Encounter for screening for cardiovascular disorders
V81.1	SCREENING FOR HYPERTENSION		**Z13.6**	Encounter for screening for cardiovascular disorders
V81.2	SCREENING OTHER&UNSPEC CARDIOVASCULAR CONDITIONS		**Z13.6**	Encounter for screening for cardiovascular disorders
V81.3	SCREENING FOR CHRONIC BRONCHITIS AND EMPHYSEMA		**Z13.83**	Encounter for screening for respiratory disorder NEC
V81.4	SCREENING OTHER&UNSPEC RESPIRATORY CONDITION		**Z13.83**	Encounter for screening for respiratory disorder NEC
V81.5	SCREENING FOR NEPHROPATHY		**Z13.89**	Encounter for screening for other disorder
V81.6	SCREENING OTHER&UNSPEC GENITOURINARY CONDITION		**Z13.89**	Encounter for screening for other disorder
V82.Ø	SCREENING FOR SKIN CONDITION		**Z13.89**	Encounter for screening for other disorder
V82.1	SCREENING FOR RHEUMATOID ARTHRITIS		**Z13.828**	Encounter for screening for other musculoskeletal disorder
V82.2	SCREENING FOR OTHER RHEUMATIC DISORDER		**Z13.89**	Encounter for screening for other disorder
V82.3	SCREENING FOR CONGENITAL DISLOCATION OF HIP		**Z13.828**	Encounter for screening for other musculoskeletal disorder
V82.4	MATERNAL POSTNATAL SCREENING CHROMOSM ANOMALIES		**Z13.89**	Encounter for screening for other disorder
V82.5	SCREENING CHEMICAL POISONING&OTHER CONTAMINATION	➡	**Z13.88**	Encntr screen for disorder due to exposure to contaminants
V82.6	MULTIPHASIC SCREENING		**Z13.89**	Encounter for screening for other disorder
V82.71	SCREENING FOR GENETIC DISEASE CARRIER STATUS		**Z13.71**	Encntr for nonprocreat screen for genetic dis carrier status
V82.79	OTHER GENETIC SCREENING		**Z13.79** **Z13.89**	Encntr for oth screening for genetic and chromsoml anomalies Encounter for screening for other disorder
V82.81	SPECIAL SCREENING FOR OSTEOPOROSIS	➡	**Z13.82Ø**	Encounter for screening for osteoporosis
V82.89	SPECIAL SCREENING FOR OTHER SPECIFIED CONDITIONS		**Z13.81Ø** **Z13.811** **Z13.818** **Z13.828** **Z13.84** **Z13.89**	Encounter for screening for upper gastrointestinal disorder Encounter for screening for lower gastrointestinal disorder Encounter for screening for other digestive system disorders Encounter for screening for other musculoskeletal disorder Encounter for screening for dental disorders Encounter for screening for other disorder
V82.9	SCREENING FOR UNSPECIFIED CONDITION		**Z13.9**	Encounter for screening, unspecified
V83.Ø1	ASYMPTOMATIC HEMOPHILIA A CARRIER	➡	**Z14.Ø1**	Asymptomatic hemophilia A carrier
V83.Ø2	SYMPTOMATIC HEMOPHILIA A CARRIER	➡	**Z14.Ø2**	Symptomatic hemophilia A carrier
V83.81	CYSTIC FIBROSIS GENE CARRIER	➡	**Z14.1**	Cystic fibrosis carrier
V83.89	OTHER GENETIC CARRIER STATUS	➡	**Z14.8**	Genetic carrier of other disease
V84.Ø1	GENETIC SUSCEPTIBILITY MALIGNANT NEOPLASM BREAST	➡	**Z15.Ø1**	Genetic susceptibility to malignant neoplasm of breast
V84.Ø2	GENETIC SUSCEPTIBILITY MALIGNANT NEOPLASM OVARY	➡	**Z15.Ø2**	Genetic susceptibility to malignant neoplasm of ovary
V84.Ø3	GENETIC SUSCEPTIBILITY MALIG NEOPLASM PROSTATE	➡	**Z15.Ø3**	Genetic susceptibility to malignant neoplasm of prostate
V84.Ø4	GENETIC SUSECPT MALIG NEOPLASM ENDOMETRIUM	➡	**Z15.Ø4**	Genetic susceptibility to malignant neoplasm of endometrium
V84.Ø9	GENETIC SUSCEPTIBILITY OTHER MALIGNANT NEOPLASM	➡	**Z15.Ø9**	Genetic susceptibility to other malignant neoplasm
V84.81	GENETIC SUSCEPTIBILITY TO MX ENDOCRINE NEOPLASM	➡	**Z15.81**	Genetic susceptibility to multiple endocrine neoplasia [MEN]
V84.89	GENETIC SUSCEPTIBILITY TO OTHER DISEASE	➡	**Z15.89**	Genetic susceptibility to other disease
V85.Ø	BODY MASS INDEX LESS THAN 19 ADULT		**Z68.1**	Body mass index (BMI) 19 or less, adult
V85.1	BODY MASS INDEX BETWEEN 19-24 ADULT		**Z68.2Ø** **Z68.21** **Z68.22** **Z68.23** **Z68.24**	Body mass index (BMI) 20.0-20.9, adult Body mass index (BMI) 21.0-21.9, adult Body mass index (BMI) 22.0-22.9, adult Body mass index (BMI) 23.0-23.9, adult Body mass index (BMI) 24.0-24.9, adult
V85.21	BODY MASS INDEX 25.0-25.9 ADULT	➡	**Z68.25**	Body mass index (BMI) 25.0-25.9, adult
V85.22	BODY MASS INDEX 26.0-26.9 ADULT	➡	**Z68.26**	Body mass index (BMI) 26.0-26.9, adult
V85.23	BODY MASS INDEX 27.0-27.9 ADULT	➡	**Z68.27**	Body mass index (BMI) 27.0-27.9, adult
V85.24	BODY MASS INDEX 28.0-28.9 ADULT	➡	**Z68.28**	Body mass index (BMI) 28.0-28.9, adult
V85.25	BODY MASS INDEX 29.0-29.9 ADULT	➡	**Z68.29**	Body mass index (BMI) 29.0-29.9, adult
V85.3Ø	BODY MASS INDEX 30.0-30.9 ADULT	➡	**Z68.3Ø**	Body mass index (BMI) 30.0-30.9, adult
V85.31	BODY MASS INDEX 31.0-31.9 ADULT	➡	**Z68.31**	Body mass index (BMI) 31.0-31.9, adult

ICD-9-CM			ICD-10-CM	
V85.32	BODY MASS INDEX 32.0-32.9 ADULT	➡	**Z68.32**	Body mass index (BMI) 32.0-32.9, adult
V85.33	BODY MASS INDEX 33.0-33.9 ADULT	➡	**Z68.33**	Body mass index (BMI) 33.0-33.9, adult
V85.34	BODY MASS INDEX 34.0-34.9 ADULT	➡	**Z68.34**	Body mass index (BMI) 34.0-34.9, adult
V85.35	BODY MASS INDEX 35.0-35.9 ADULT	➡	**Z68.35**	Body mass index (BMI) 35.0-35.9, adult
V85.36	BODY MASS INDEX 36.0-36.9 ADULT	➡	**Z68.36**	Body mass index (BMI) 36.0-36.9, adult
V85.37	BODY MASS INDEX 37.0-37.9 ADULT	➡	**Z68.37**	Body mass index (BMI) 37.0-37.9, adult
V85.38	BODY MASS INDEX 38.0-38.9 ADULT	➡	**Z68.38**	Body mass index (BMI) 38.0-38.9, adult
V85.39	BODY MASS INDEX 39.0-39.9 ADULT	➡	**Z68.39**	Body mass index (BMI) 39.0-39.9, adult
V85.41	BODY MASS INDEX 40.0-44.9 ADULT	➡	**Z68.41**	Body mass index (BMI) 40.0-44.9, adult
V85.42	BODY MASS INDEX 45.0-49.9 ADULT	➡	**Z68.42**	Body mass index (BMI) 45.0-49.9, adult
V85.43	BODY MASS INDEX 50.0-59.9 ADULT	➡	**Z68.43**	Body mass index (BMI) 50-59.9 , adult
V85.44	BODY MASS INDEX 60.0-69.9 ADULT	➡	**Z68.44**	Body mass index (BMI) 60.0-69.9, adult
V85.45	BODY MASS INDEX 70 AND OVER ADULT	➡	**Z68.45**	Body mass index (BMI) 70 or greater, adult
V85.51	BODY MASS INDEX PEDIATRIC < 5TH PERCENTILE AGE	➡	**Z68.51**	BMI pediatric, less than 5th percentile for age
V85.52	BODY MASS INDEX PED 5TH % TO < 85TH % AGE	➡	**Z68.52**	BMI pediatric, 5th percentile to less than 85% for age
V85.53	BODY MASS INDEX PED 85TH % TO < 95TH % AGE	➡	**Z68.53**	BMI pediatric, 85% to less than 95th percentile for age
V85.54	BODY MASS INDEX PED >/EQUAL TO 95TH % AGE	➡	**Z68.54**	BMI pediatric, greater than or equal to 95% for age
V86.Ø	ESTROGEN RECEPTOR POSITIVE STATUS	➡	**Z17.Ø**	Estrogen receptor positive status [ER+]
V86.1	ESTROGEN RECEPTOR NEGATIVE STATUS	➡	**Z17.1**	Estrogen receptor negative status [ER-]
V87.Ø1	CONTACT WITH AND SUSPECTED EXPOSURE TO ARSENIC	➡	**Z77.Ø1Ø**	Contact with and (suspected) exposure to arsenic
V87.Ø2	CONTACT WITH AND SUSPECTED EXPOSURE TO URANIUM		**Z77.Ø12**	Contact with and (suspected) exposure to uranium
V87.Ø9	CONTACT & SUSPECTED EXPOSURE OTH HAZARDOUS METAL		**Z77.Ø18**	Contact w and (suspected) exposure to oth hazardous metals
V87.11	CONTACT & SUSPECTED EXPOSURE TO AROMATIC AMINES	➡	**Z77.Ø2Ø**	Contact with and (suspected) exposure to aromatic amines
V87.12	CONTACT WITH AND SUSPECTED EXPOSURE TO BENZENE	➡	**Z77.Ø21**	Contact with and (suspected) exposure to benzene
V87.19	CONTACT & SUSPECTED EXP OTH HAZ AROMATIC COMP		**Z77.Ø28**	Contact w and exposure to oth hazardous aromatic compounds
V87.2	CONTACT & SUSPECTED EXP OTH POTENTIAL HAZ CHEM		**Z77.Ø98**	Contact w and expsr to oth hazard, chiefly nonmed, chemicals
V87.31	CONTACT WITH AND SUSPECTED EXPOSURE TO MOLD	➡	**Z77.12Ø**	Contact with and (suspected) exposure to mold (toxic)
V87.32	CONTACT WITH AND EXPOSURE TO ALGAE BLOOM		**Z77.121**	Contact w and exposure to harmful algae and algae toxins
V87.39	CONTACT & SUSPECTED EXP OTH POTENTIAL HAZ SUBST		**Z77.29**	Contact w and (suspected) exposure to oth hazardous substnc
V87.41	PERSONAL HISTORY OF ANTINEOPLASTIC CHEMOTHERAPY	➡	**Z92.21**	Personal history of antineoplastic chemotherapy
V87.42	PERSONAL HISTORY OF MONOCLONAL DRUG THERAPY	➡	**Z92.22**	Personal history of monoclonal drug therapy
V87.43	PERSONAL HISTORY OF ESTROGEN THERAPY	➡	**Z92.23**	Personal history of estrogen therapy
V87.44	PERSONAL HISTORY OF INHALED STEROID THERAPY	➡	**Z92.24Ø**	Personal history of inhaled steroid therapy
V87.45	PERSONAL HISTORY OF SYSTEMIC STEROID THERAPY	➡	**Z92.241**	Personal history of systemic steroid therapy
V87.46	PERSONAL HISTORY OF IMMUNOSUPPRESSION THERAPY	➡	**Z92.25**	Personal history of immunosupression therapy
V87.49	PERSONAL HISTORY OF OTHER DRUG THERAPY	➡	**Z92.29**	Personal history of other drug therapy
V88.Ø1	ACQUIRED ABSENCE OF BOTH CERVIX AND UTERUS	➡	**Z9Ø.71Ø**	Acquired absence of both cervix and uterus
V88.Ø2	ACQUIRED ABSENCE OF UTERUS W/REMAIN CERVL STUMP	➡	**Z9Ø.711**	Acquired absence of uterus with remaining cervical stump
V88.Ø3	ACQUIRED ABSENCE OF CERVIX WITH REMAINING UTERUS	➡	**Z9Ø.712**	Acquired absence of cervix with remaining uterus
V88.11	ACQUIRED TOTAL ABSENCE OF PANCREAS	➡	**Z9Ø.41Ø**	Acquired total absence of pancreas
V88.12	ACQUIRED PARTIAL ABSENCE OF PANCREAS	➡	**Z9Ø.411**	Acquired partial absence of pancreas
V88.21	ACQUIRED ABSENCE OF HIP JOINT		**Z89.621**	Acquired absence of right hip joint
			Z89.622	Acquired absence of left hip joint
			Z89.629	Acquired absence of unspecified hip joint
V88.22	ACQUIRED ABSENCE OF KNEE JOINT		**Z89.521**	Acquired absence of right knee
			Z89.522	Acquired absence of left knee
			Z89.529	Acquired absence of unspecified knee
V88.29	ACQUIRED ABSENCE OF OTHER JOINT		**Z89.9**	Acquired absence of limb, unspecified
V89.Ø1	SPCT PROB W/AMNIOTIC CAVITY & MEMBRANE NOT FOUND	➡	**ZØ3.71**	Encntr for susp prob w amnio cavity and membrane ruled out
V89.Ø2	SUSPECTED PLACENTAL PROBLEM NOT FOUND	➡	**ZØ3.72**	Encounter for suspected placental problem ruled out
V89.Ø3	SUSPECTED FETAL ANOMALY NOT FOUND	➡	**ZØ3.73**	Encounter for suspected fetal anomaly ruled out
V89.Ø4	SUSPECTED PROBLEM WITH FETAL GROWTH NOT FOUND	➡	**ZØ3.74**	Encounter for suspected problem with fetal growth ruled out
V89.Ø5	SUSPECTED CERVICAL SHORTENING NOT FOUND	➡	**ZØ3.75**	Encounter for suspected cervical shortening ruled out
V89.Ø9	OTH SUSPECTED MATERNAL & FETAL COND NOT FOUND	➡	**ZØ3.79**	Encntr for oth suspected maternal and fetal cond ruled out
V9Ø.Ø1	RETAINED DEPLETED URANIUM FRAGMENTS	➡	**Z18.Ø1**	Retained depleted uranium fragments
V9Ø.Ø9	OTHER RETAINED RADIOACTIVE FRAGMENTS	➡	**Z18.Ø9**	Other retained radioactive fragments
V9Ø.1Ø	RETAINED METAL FRAGMENTS UNSPECIFIED	➡	**Z18.1Ø**	Retained metal fragments, unspecified
V9Ø.11	RETAINED MAGNETIC METAL FRAGMENTS	➡	**Z18.11**	Retained magnetic metal fragments
V9Ø.12	RETAINED NONMAGNETIC METAL FRAGMENTS	➡	**Z18.12**	Retained nonmagnetic metal fragments
V9Ø.2	RETAINED PLASTIC FRAGMENTS	➡	**Z18.2**	Retained plastic fragments
V9Ø.31	RETAINED ANIMAL QUILLS OR SPINES	➡	**Z18.31**	Retained animal quills or spines
V9Ø.32	RETAINED TOOTH	➡	**Z18.32**	Retained tooth
V9Ø.33	RETAINED WOOD FRAGMENTS	➡	**Z18.33**	Retained wood fragments
V9Ø.39	OTHER RETAINED ORGANIC FRAGMENTS	➡	**Z18.39**	Other retained organic fragments
V9Ø.81	RETAINED GLASS FRAGMENTS	➡	**Z18.81**	Retained glass fragments
V9Ø.83	RETAINED STONE OR CRYSTALLINE FRAGMENTS	➡	**Z18.83**	Retained stone or crystalline fragments
V9Ø.89	OTHER SPECIFIED RETAINED FOREIGN BODY	➡	**Z18.89**	Other specified retained foreign body fragments

ICD-9-CM		ICD-10-CM		
V90.9	RETAINED FOREIGN BODY UNSPECIFIED MATERIAL	➡	Z18.9	Retained foreign body fragments, unspecified material
V91.00	TWIN GESTATION UNS # PLACNTA UNS # AMNIOTIC SACS		O30.001	Twin preg, unsp num plcnta & amnio sacs, first trimester
			O30.002	Twin preg, unsp num plcnta & amnio sacs, second trimester
			O30.003	Twin preg, unsp num plcnta & amnio sacs, third trimester
			O30.009	Twin pregnancy, unsp num plcnta & amnio sacs, unsp trimester
V91.01	TWIN GEST MONOCHORIONIC/MONOAMNIOTC		O30.011	Twin pregnancy, monochorionic/monoamniotic, first trimester
			O30.012	Twin pregnancy, monochorionic/monoamniotic, second trimester
			O30.013	Twin pregnancy, monochorionic/monoamniotic, third trimester
			O30.019	Twin pregnancy, monochorionic/monoamniotic, unsp trimester
V91.02	TWIN GEST MONOCHORIONIC/DIAMNIOTIC		O30.031	Twin pregnancy, monochorionic/diamniotic, first trimester
			O30.032	Twin pregnancy, monochorionic/diamniotic, second trimester
			O30.033	Twin pregnancy, monochorionic/diamniotic, third trimester
			O30.039	Twin pregnancy, monochorionic/diamniotic, unsp trimester
V91.03	TWIN GEST DICHORIONIC/DIAMNIOTIC		O30.041	Twin pregnancy, dichorionic/diamniotic, first trimester
			O30.042	Twin pregnancy, dichorionic/diamniotic, second trimester
			O30.043	Twin pregnancy, dichorionic/diamniotic, third trimester
			O30.049	Twin pregnancy, dichorionic/diamniotic, unsp trimester
V91.09	TWIN GEST UNABLE DETRM # PLACNTA # AMNIOTIC SACS		O30.091	Twin preg, unable to dtrm num plcnta & amnio sacs, first tri
			O30.092	Twin preg, unable to dtrm num plcnta & amnio sacs, 2nd tri
			O30.093	Twin preg, unable to dtrm num plcnta & amnio sacs, third tri
			O30.099	Twin preg, unable to dtrm num plcnta & amnio sacs, unsp tri
V91.10	TRIPLT GEST UNS # PLACNTA UNS # AMNIOTIC SACS		O30.101	Triplet preg, unsp num plcnta & amnio sacs, first trimester
			O30.102	Triplet preg, unsp num plcnta & amnio sacs, second trimester
			O30.103	Triplet preg, unsp num plcnta & amnio sacs, third trimester
			O30.109	Triplet preg, unsp num plcnta & amnio sacs, unsp trimester
V91.11	TRIPLET GESTATION W/2/MORE MONOCHORIONIC FETUSES		O30.111	Triplet preg w two or more monochorionic fetuses, first tri
			O30.112	Triplet preg w two or more monochorionic fetuses, second tri
			O30.113	Triplet preg w two or more monochorionic fetuses, third tri
			O30.119	Triplet preg w two or more monochorionic fetuses, unsp tri
V91.12	TRIPLET GESTATION W/2/MORE MONOAMNIOTIC FETUSES		O30.121	Triplet preg w two or more monoamnio fetuses, first tri
			O30.122	Triplet preg w two or more monoamnio fetuses, second tri
			O30.123	Triplet preg w two or more monoamnio fetuses, third tri
			O30.129	Triplet preg w two or more monoamnio fetuses, unsp trimester
V91.19	TRIPLT GEST UNABL DETRM # PLACNTA # AMNIOTC SACS		O30.191	Trp preg, unable to dtrm num plcnta & amnio sacs, first tri
			O30.192	Trp preg, unable to dtrm num plcnta & amnio sacs, second tri
			O30.193	Trp preg, unable to dtrm num plcnta & amnio sacs, third tri
			O30.199	Trp preg, unable to dtrm num plcnta & amnio sacs, unsp tri
V91.20	QUADRUPLET GEST UNS # PLACNTA & # AMNIOTIC SACS		O30.201	Quad preg, unsp num plcnta & amnio sacs, first trimester
			O30.202	Quad preg, unsp num plcnta & amnio sacs, second trimester
			O30.203	Quad preg, unsp num plcnta & amnio sacs, third trimester
			O30.209	Quad pregnancy, unsp num plcnta & amnio sacs, unsp trimester
V91.21	QUADRUPLET GEST W/2/MORE MONOCHORIONIC FETUSES		O30.211	Quad preg w two or more monochorionic fetuses, first tri
			O30.212	Quad preg w two or more monochorionic fetuses, second tri
			O30.213	Quad preg w two or more monochorionic fetuses, third tri
			O30.219	Quad preg w two or more monochorionic fetuses, unsp tri
V91.22	QUADRUPLET GEST W/2/MORE MONOAMNIOTIC FETUSES		O30.221	Quad preg w two or more monoamnio fetuses, first trimester
			O30.222	Quad preg w two or more monoamnio fetuses, second trimester
			O30.223	Quad preg w two or more monoamnio fetuses, third trimester
			O30.229	Quad preg w two or more monoamnio fetuses, unsp trimester
V91.29	QUAD GEST UNABLE DETRM # PLACNTA # AMNIOTIC SACS		O30.291	Quad preg, unable to dtrm num plcnta & amnio sacs, first tri
			O30.292	Quad preg, unable to dtrm num plcnta & amnio sacs, 2nd tri
			O30.293	Quad preg, unable to dtrm num plcnta & amnio sacs, third tri
			O30.299	Quad preg, unable to dtrm num plcnta & amnio sacs, unsp tri
V91.90	OTH SPEC MX GEST UNS # PLACNTA & # AMNIOTIC SACS		O30.801	Oth multiple gest, unsp num plcnta & amnio sacs, first tri
			O30.802	Oth multiple gest, unsp num plcnta & amnio sacs, second tri
			O30.803	Oth multiple gest, unsp num plcnta & amnio sacs, third tri
			O30.809	Oth multiple gest, unsp num plcnta & amnio sacs, unsp tri
V91.91	MX GEST W/2/> MONOCHORIONIC FETUSES		O30.811	Oth mult gest w two or more monochorionic fetuses, first tri
			O30.812	Oth mult gest w two or more monochorionic fetuses, 2nd tri
			O30.813	Oth mult gest w two or more monochorionic fetuses, third tri
			O30.819	Oth mult gest w two or more monochorionic fetuses, unsp tri
V91.92	OTH MX GESTATION W/2/MORE MONOAMNIOTIC FETUSES		O30.821	Oth multiple gest w two or more monoamnio fetuses, first tri
			O30.822	Oth mult gest w two or more monoamnio fetuses, second tri
			O30.823	Oth multiple gest w two or more monoamnio fetuses, third tri
			O30.829	Oth multiple gest w two or more monoamnio fetuses, unsp tri
V91.99	OTH MX GEST UNABL DETRM # PLACNTA # AMNIOTC SACS		O30.891	Oth mult gest, unab to dtrm num plcnta & amnio sacs, 1st tri
			O30.892	Oth mult gest, unab to dtrm num plcnta & amnio sacs, 2nd tri
			O30.893	Oth mult gest, unab to dtrm num plcnta & amnio sacs, 3rd tri
			O30.899	Oth mult gest,unab to dtrm num plcnta & amnio sacs, unsp tri

[Brackets] indicate valid character values for each code. Character value meanings provided for each code grouping.

E Codes

ICD-9-CM			ICD-10-CM	
E000.0	CIVILIAN ACTIVITY DONE FOR INCOME OR PAY	➡	**Y99.0**	Civilian activity done for income or pay
E000.1	MILITARY ACTIVITY	➡	**Y99.1**	Military activity
E000.2	VOLUNTEER ACTIVITY	➡	**Y99.2**	Volunteer activity
E000.8	OTHER EXTERNAL CAUSE STATUS	➡	**Y99.8**	Other external cause status
E000.9	UNSPECIFIED EXTERNAL CAUSE STATUS	➡	**Y99.9**	Unspecified external cause status
E001.0	ACTIVITIES INVOLVING WALKING MARCHING & HIKING	➡	**Y93.01**	Activity, walking, marching and hiking
E001.1	ACTIVITIES INVOLVING RUNNING	➡	**Y93.02**	Activity, running
E002.0	ACTIVITIES INVOLVING SWIMMING	➡	**Y93.11**	Activity, swimming
E002.1	ACTIVITIES INVOLV SPRINGBOARD & PLATFORM DIVING	➡	**Y93.12**	Activity, springboard and platform diving
E002.2	ACTIVITIES INVOLVING WATER POLO	➡	**Y93.13**	Activity, water polo
E002.3	ACTIVITIES INVLV WATER AEROBICS & WATER EXERCISE	➡	**Y93.14**	Activity, water aerobics and water exercise
E002.4	ACTIVITIES INVOLV UNDERWATER DIVING & SNORKELING	➡	**Y93.15**	Activity, underwater diving and snorkeling
E002.5	ACT INVLV ROW CANOEING KAYAKING RAFTING & TUBING	➡	**Y93.16**	Activity, rowing, canoeing, kayaking, rafting and tubing
E002.6	ACTIVITIES INVOLV WATER SKIING AND WAKE BOARDING	➡	**Y93.17**	Activity, water skiing and wake boarding
E002.7	ACT INVLV SURFING WINDSURFING & BOOGIE BOARDING	➡	**Y93.18**	Activity, surfing, windsurfing and boogie boarding
E002.8	ACTIVITIES INVOLVING WATER SLIDING		**Y93.19**	Activity, other involving water and watercraft
E002.9	OTHER ACTIVITY INVOLVING WATER AND WATERCRAFT		**Y93.19**	Activity, other involving water and watercraft
E003.0	ACTIVITIES INVOLVING ICE SKATING	➡	**Y93.21**	Activity, ice skating
E003.1	ACTIVITIES INVOLVING ICE HOCKEY	➡	**Y93.22**	Activity, ice hockey
E003.2	ACT INVLV SNOW SKI BOARD SLED TOBOGGAN & TUBING	➡	**Y93.23**	Actvty,snow (alp/dwnhl) ski, snow brd, sled, tobogn & tubing
E003.3	ACTIVITIES INVOLVING CROSS COUNTRY SKIING	➡	**Y93.24**	Activity, cross country skiing
E003.9	OTHER ACTIVITY INVOLVING ICE AND SNOW	➡	**Y93.29**	Activity, other involving ice and snow
E004.0	ACT INVLV MOUNTAIN CLIMB ROCK CLIMB & WALL CLIMB	➡	**Y93.31**	Activity, mountain climbing, rock climbing and wall climbing
E004.1	ACTIVITIES INVOLVING RAPPELLING	➡	**Y93.32**	Activity, rappelling
E004.2	ACTIVITIES INVOLVING CLIMBING BASE JUMPING	➡	**Y93.33**	Activity, BASE jumping
E004.3	ACTIVITIES INVOLVING BUNGEE JUMPING	➡	**Y93.34**	Activity, bungee jumping
E004.4	ACTIVITIES INVOLVING HANG GLIDING	➡	**Y93.35**	Activity, hang gliding
E004.9	OTH ACT INVLV CLIMBING RAPPELLING & JUMPING OFF	➡	**Y93.39**	Activity, oth involving climbing, rappelling and jumping off
E005.0	ACTIVITIES INVOLVING DANCING	➡	**Y93.41**	Activity, dancing
E005.1	ACTIVITIES INVOLVING YOGA	➡	**Y93.42**	Activity, yoga
E005.2	ACTIVITIES INVOLVING GYMNASTICS	➡	**Y93.43**	Activity, gymnastics
E005.3	ACTIVITIES INVOLVING TRAMPOLINE	➡	**Y93.44**	Activity, trampolining
E005.4	ACTIVITIES INVOLVING CHEERLEADING	➡	**Y93.45**	Activity, cheerleading
E005.9	OTHER ACT INVLV DANCING & OTH RHYTHMIC MOVEMENTS	➡	**Y93.49**	Activity, oth involving dancing and other rhythmic movements
E006.0	ACTIVITIES INVLV ROLLER SKATING & SKATEBOARDING	➡	**Y93.51**	Activity, roller skating (inline) and skateboarding
E006.1	ACTIVITIES INVOLVING HORSEBACK RIDING	➡	**Y93.52**	Activity, horseback riding
E006.2	ACTIVITIES INVOLVING GOLF	➡	**Y93.53**	Activity, golf
E006.3	ACTIVITIES INVOLVING BOWLING	➡	**Y93.54**	Activity, bowling
E006.4	ACTIVITIES INVOLVING BIKE RIDING	➡	**Y93.55**	Activity, bike riding
E006.5	ACTIVITIES INVOLVING JUMP ROPE	➡	**Y93.56**	Activity, jumping rope
E006.6	ACTIVITIES INVLV NON-RUNNING TRACK & FIELD EVNTS	➡	**Y93.57**	Activity, non-running track and field events
E006.9	OTH ACT INVLV OTH SPORTS & ATHLETICS PLAYED IND	➡	**Y93.59**	Activity, oth w oth sports and athletics played individ
E007.0	ACTIVITIES INVOLVING AMERICAN TACKLE FOOTBALL	➡	**Y93.61**	Activity, american tackle football
E007.1	ACTIVITIES INVOLV AMERICAN FLAG/TOUCH FOOTBALL	➡	**Y93.62**	Activity, american flag or touch football
E007.2	ACTIVITIES INVOLVING RUGBY	➡	**Y93.63**	Activity, rugby
E007.3	ACTIVITIES INVOLVING BASEBALL	➡	**Y93.64**	Activity, baseball
E007.4	ACTIVITIES INVOLVING LACROSSE AND FIELD HOCKEY	➡	**Y93.65**	Activity, lacrosse and field hockey
E007.5	ACTIVITIES INVOLVING SOCCER	➡	**Y93.66**	Activity, soccer
E007.6	ACTIVITIES INVOLVING BASKETBALL	➡	**Y93.67**	Activity, basketball
E007.7	ACTIVITIES INVOLVING VOLLEYBALL BEACH COURT	➡	**Y93.68**	Activity, volleyball (beach) (court)
E007.8	ACT INVLV PHYS GAMES ASSOC W/RECESS CAMP & CHLD	➡	**Y93.6A**	Actvty,physcl games assoc w school recess, sumr camp & child
E007.9	OTH ACT INVLV OTHER SPORTS AND ATHLETCS TEAM/GRP	➡	**Y93.69**	Actvty, oth w oth sports & athletics played as a team or grp
E008.0	ACTIVITIES INVOLVING BOXING	➡	**Y93.71**	Activity, boxing
E008.1	ACTIVITIES INVOLVING WRESTLING	➡	**Y93.72**	Activity, wrestling
E008.2	ACTIVITIES INVOLVING RACQUET AND HAND SPORTS	➡	**Y93.73**	Activity, racquet and hand sports
E008.3	ACTIVITIES INVOLVING FRISBEE	➡	**Y93.74**	Activity, frisbee
E008.4	ACTIVITIES INVOLVING MARTIAL ARTS	➡	**Y93.75**	Activity, martial arts
E008.9	OTHER SPECIFIED SPORTS AND ATHLETICS ACTIVITIES	➡	**Y93.79**	Activity, other specified sports and athletics
E009.0	ACT INVLV EXER MACH PRIM CARDIORESPIRTRY COND	➡	**Y93.A1**	Activity, exercise machines prim for cardioresp conditioning
E009.1	ACTIVITY INVOLVING CALISTHENICS	➡	**Y93.A2**	Activity, calisthenics
E009.2	ACTIVITY INVOLVING AEROBIC AND STEP EXERCISE	➡	**Y93.A3**	Activity, aerobic and step exercise
E009.3	ACTIVITY INVOLVING CIRCUIT TRAINING	➡	**Y93.A4**	Activity, circuit training
E009.4	ACTIVITY INVOLVING OBSTACLE COURSE	➡	**Y93.A5**	Activity, obstacle course
E009.5	ACTIVITY INVOLVING GRASS DRILLS	➡	**Y93.A6**	Activity, grass drills
E009.9	OTHER ACTIVITY INVOLV CARDIORESPIRATORY EXERCISE	➡	**Y93.A9**	Activity, other involving cardiorespiratory exercise
E010.0	ACT INVLV EXER MACH PRIM MUSCLE STRENGTHENING	➡	**Y93.B1**	Activity, exercise machines prim for muscle strengthening
E010.1	ACTIVITY INVOLVING PUSH-UPS PULL-UPS SIT-UPS	➡	**Y93.B2**	Activity, push-ups, pull-ups, sit-ups

ICD-9-CM			ICD-10-CM	
EØ1Ø.2	ACTIVITY INVOLVING FREE WEIGHTS	➡	Y93.B3	Activity, free weights
EØ1Ø.3	ACTIVITY INVOLVING PILATES	➡	Y93.B4	Activity, pilates
EØ1Ø.9	OTH ACT INVLV OTH MUSCLE STRENGTHENING EXERCISES	➡	Y93.B9	Activity, other involving muscle strengthening exercises
EØ11.Ø	ACTIVITIES INVOLVING COMPUTER KEYBOARDING	➡	Y93.C1	Activity, computer keyboarding
EØ11.1	ACT INVLV HAND HELD INTERACTIVE ELECTRONIC DEVC	➡	Y93.C2	Activity, hand held interactive electronic device
EØ11.9	OTH ACT INVLV CMPT TECHNOLOGY & ELECTRONIC DEVC	➡	Y93.C9	Activity, oth involving computer tech and electrnc devices
EØ12.Ø	ACTIVITIES INVOLVING KNITTING AND CROCHETING	➡	Y93.D1	Activity, knitting and crocheting
EØ12.1	ACTIVITIES INVOLVING SEWING	➡	Y93.D2	Activity, sewing
EØ12.2	ACTIVITIES INVLV FURNITURE BUILDING & FINISHING	➡	Y93.D3	Activity, furniture building and finishing
EØ12.9	ACTIVITY INVOLVING OTHER ARTS AND HANDCRAFTS	➡	Y93.D9	Activity, other involving arts and handcrafts
EØ13.Ø	ACTIVITIES INVOLV PERSONAL BATHING AND SHOWERING	➡	Y93.E1	Activity, personal bathing and showering
EØ13.1	ACTIVITIES INVOLVING LAUNDRY	➡	Y93.E2	Activity, laundry
EØ13.2	ACTIVITIES INVOLVING VACUUMING	➡	Y93.E3	Activity, vacuuming
EØ13.3	ACTIVITIES INVOLVING IRONING	➡	Y93.E4	Activity, ironing
EØ13.4	ACTIVITIES INVOLVING FLOOR MOPPING AND CLEANING	➡	Y93.E5	Activity, floor mopping and cleaning
EØ13.5	ACTIVITIES INVOLVING RESIDENTIAL RELOCATION	➡	Y93.E6	Activity, residential relocation
EØ13.8	ACT INVLV OTHER PERSONAL HYGIENE	➡	Y93.E8	Activity, other personal hygiene
EØ13.9	ACT INVLV OTHER HOUSEHOLD MAINTENANCE	➡	Y93.E9	Activity, other interior property and clothing maintenance
EØ14.Ø	ACT INVLV CAREGIVING INVOLVING BATHING	➡	Y93.F1	Activity, caregiving, bathing
EØ14.1	ACT INVLV CAREGIVING INVOLVING LIFTING	➡	Y93.F2	Activity, caregiving, lifting
EØ14.9	OTH ACTIVITY INVOLV PERSON PROVIDING CAREGIVING	➡	Y93.F9	Activity, other caregiving
EØ15.Ø	ACTIVITIES INVOLVING FOOD PREPARATION & CLEAN UP	➡	Y93.G1	Activity, food preparation and clean up
EØ15.1	ACTIVITIES INVOLVING GRILLING AND SMOKING FOOD	➡	Y93.G2	Activity, grilling and smoking food
EØ15.2	ACTIVITIES INVOLVING COOKING AND BAKING	➡	Y93.G3	Activity, cooking and baking
EØ15.9	OTHER ACTIVITY INVOLVING COOKING AND GRILLING	➡	Y93.G9	Activity, other involving cooking and grilling
EØ16.Ø	ACTIVITIES INVOLVING DIGGING SHOVELING & RAKING	➡	Y93.H1	Activity, digging, shoveling and raking
EØ16.1	ACTIVITIES INVOLVING GARDENING AND LANDSCAPING	➡	Y93.H2	Activity, gardening and landscaping
EØ16.2	ACTIVITIES INVOLVING BUILDING AND CONSTRUCTION	➡	Y93.H3	Activity, building and construction
EØ16.9	OTH ACT INVOLV PROPERTY & LAND MAINT BLDG & CNST	➡	Y93.H9	Actvty,oth w exter property & land maint, bldg and construct
EØ17.Ø	ACTIVITIES INVOLVING ROLLER COASTER RIDING	➡	Y93.I1	Activity, roller coaster riding
EØ17.9	OTHER ACTIVITY INVOLVING EXTERNAL MOTION	➡	Y93.I9	Activity, other involving external motion
EØ18.Ø	ACTIVITIES INVOLVING PIANO PLAYING	➡	Y93.J1	Activity, piano playing
EØ18.1	ACT INVOLV DRUM & OTH PERCUSSION INSTRUMENT	➡	Y93.J2	Activity, drum and other percussion instrument playing
EØ18.2	ACTIVITIES INVOLVING STRING INSTRUMENT PLAYING	➡	Y93.J3	Activity, string instrument playing
EØ18.3	ACTIVITIES INVOLVING WIND & BRASS INSTRMNT PLYNG	➡	Y93.J4	Activity, winds and brass instrument playing
EØ19.Ø	ACTIVITIES INVOLVING WALKING AN ANIMAL	➡	Y93.K1	Activity, walking an animal
EØ19.1	ACTIVITIES INVOLVING MILKING AN ANIMAL	➡	Y93.K2	Activity, milking an animal
EØ19.2	ACTIVITIES INVOLVING GROOMING & SHEARING ANIMAL	➡	Y93.K3	Activity, grooming and shearing an animal
EØ19.9	OTHER ACTIVITY INVOLVING ANIMAL CARE	➡	Y93.K9	Activity, other involving animal care
EØ29.Ø	ACTIVITY INVOLVING REFEREEING A SPORTS ACTIVITY	➡	Y93.81	Activity, refereeing a sports activity
EØ29.1	ACTIVITY INVOLVING SPECTATOR AT AN EVENT	➡	Y93.82	Activity, spectator at an event
EØ29.2	ACTIVITY INVOLVING ROUGH HOUSING AND HORSEPLAY	➡	Y93.83	Activity, rough housing and horseplay
EØ29.9	OTHER ACTIVITY		Y93.84 Y93.89	Activity, sleeping Activity, other specified
EØ3Ø	UNSPECIFIED ACTIVITY	➡	Y93.9	Activity, unspecified
E8ØØ.Ø	RW ACC INVLV COLL W/ROLL STOCK INJR RW EMPLOYEE		V81.2XXA	Occ of rail trn/veh inj in collisn/hit by roll stok, init
E8ØØ.1	RW ACC INVLV COLL W/ROLLING STOCK INJR PSGR RW		V81.2XXA V81.2XXD	Occ of rail trn/veh inj in collisn/hit by roll stok, init Occ of rail trn/veh inj in collisn/hit by roll stok, subs
E8ØØ.2	RW ACC INVLV COLL W/ROLLING STOCK INJR PEDSTRN		V81.2XXA	Occ of rail trn/veh inj in collisn/hit by roll stok, init
E8ØØ.3	RW ACC INVLV COLL W/ROLL STOCK INJR PEDL CYCLS		V15.2XXA	Unsp pedl cyclst inj in clsn w rail trn/veh nontraf, init
E8ØØ.8	RW ACC INVLV COLL W/ROLL STOCK INJR OTH PERS		V81.2XXA	Occ of rail trn/veh inj in collisn/hit by roll stok, init
E8ØØ.9	RW ACC INVLV COLL W/ROLL STOCK INJR UNSPEC PERS		V81.2XXA	Occ of rail trn/veh inj in collisn/hit by roll stok, init
E8Ø1.Ø	RW ACC INVLV COLL W/OTH OBJ INJR RW EMPLOYEE		V81.3XXA	Occupant of rail trn/veh injured in clsn w oth object, init
E8Ø1.1	RW ACC INVLV COLL W/OTH OBJ INJR PSGR RW		V81.3XXA V81.3XXD	Occupant of rail trn/veh injured in clsn w oth object, init Occupant of rail trn/veh injured in clsn w oth object, subs
E8Ø1.2	RAILWAY ACC INVLV COLL W/OTH OBJ INJR PEDSTRN		V81.3XXA	Occupant of rail trn/veh injured in clsn w oth object, init
E8Ø1.3	RW ACC INVLV COLL W/OTH OBJ INJR PEDAL CYCLIST		V15.2XXA V15.2XXD V15.3XXA V15.3XXD V15.4XXA V15.4XXD V15.5XXA V15.5XXD V15.9XXA V15.9XXD	Unsp pedl cyclst inj in clsn w rail trn/veh nontraf, init Unsp pedl cyclst inj in clsn w rail trn/veh nontraf, subs Prsn brd/alit pedl cyc injured in clsn w rail trn/veh, init Prsn brd/alit pedl cyc injured in clsn w rail trn/veh, subs Pedl cyc driver injured in clsn w rail trn/veh in traf, init Pedl cyc driver injured in clsn w rail trn/veh in traf, subs Pedl cyc pasngr injured in clsn w rail trn/veh in traf, init Pedl cyc pasngr injured in clsn w rail trn/veh in traf, subs Unsp pedl cyclst inj in clsn w rail trn/veh in traf, init Unsp pedl cyclst inj in clsn w rail trn/veh in traf, subs

ICD-9-CM		ICD-10-CM	
E801.8	RW ACC INVLV COLL W/OTH OBJ INJR OTH SPEC PERS	**V80.61XA** **V80.61XD** **V80.62XA** **V80.62XD** **V82.2XXA**	Animal-rider injured in collision w rail trn/veh, init Animal-rider injured in collision w rail trn/veh, subs Occ of anml-drn vehicle injured in clsn w rail trn/veh, init Occ of anml-drn vehicle injured in clsn w rail trn/veh, subs Occupant of stcar injured in collisn/hit by roll stok, init
E801.9	RW ACC INVLV COLL W/OTH OBJ INJR UNSPEC PERS	**V82.2XXA** **V82.2XXD**	Occupant of stcar injured in collisn/hit by roll stok, init Occupant of stcar injured in collisn/hit by roll stok, subs
E802.0	RW ACC INVLV DERAIL WO COLL-INJUR RAIL PASSENGER	**V81.7XXA**	Occ of rail trn/veh inj in derail w/o antecedent clsn, init
E802.1	RW ACC INVLV DERAIL WO COLL-INJURING PEDESTRIAN	**V81.7XXA** **V81.7XXD**	Occ of rail trn/veh inj in derail w/o antecedent clsn, init Occ of rail trn/veh inj in derail w/o antecedent clsn, subs
E802.2	RW ACC INVLV DERAIL WO COLL-INJUR PEDAL CYCLIST	**V81.7XXA**	Occ of rail trn/veh inj in derail w/o antecedent clsn, init
E802.3	RW ACC INVLV DERAIL WO COLL-INJUR OTH SPEC PERSO	**V15.2XXA**	Unsp pedl cyclst inj in clsn w rail trn/veh nontraf, init
E802.8	RW ACC INVLV DERAIL WO COLL-INJURING UNS PERSON	**V81.7XXA**	Occ of rail trn/veh inj in derail w/o antecedent clsn, init
E802.9	RW-DERAILMENT WO COLLISION-INJURING UNS PERSON	**V81.7XXA**	Occ of rail trn/veh inj in derail w/o antecedent clsn, init
E803.0	RW ACC INVLV EXPLO FIRE/BURNING INJR RW EMPLOYEE	**V15.9XXA**	Unsp pedl cyclst inj in clsn w rail trn/veh in traf, init
E803.1	RW ACC INVLV EXPLO FIRE/BURNING INJR PSGR RW	**V81.81XA** **V81.81XD**	Occ of rail trn/veh inj d/t explosn or fire on train, init Occ of rail trn/veh inj d/t explosn or fire on train, subs
E803.2	RW ACC INVLV EXPLO FIRE/BURNING INJR PEDSTRN	**V81.81XA**	Occ of rail trn/veh inj d/t explosn or fire on train, init
E803.3	RW ACC INVLV EXPLO FIRE/BURNINJR PEDAL CYCLIST	**V15.2XXA**	Unsp pedl cyclst inj in clsn w rail trn/veh nontraf, init
E803.8	RW ACC INVLV EXPLO FIRE/BURNINJR OTH SPEC PERS	**V81.81XA**	Occ of rail trn/veh inj d/t explosn or fire on train, init
E803.9	RW ACC INVLV EXPLO FIRE/BURNING INJR UNSPEC PERS	**V81.81XA**	Occ of rail trn/veh inj d/t explosn or fire on train, init
E804.0	FALL IN ON/FROM RW TRAIN INJR RAILWAY EMPLOYEE	**V81.81XA**	Occ of rail trn/veh inj d/t explosn or fire on train, init
E804.1	FALL IN ON/FROM RW TRAIN INJR PASSENGER RAILWAY	**V81.4XXA** **V81.4XXD** **V81.5XXA** **V81.5XXD** **V81.6XXA** **V81.6XXD**	Person injured wh brd/alit from rail trn/veh, init Person injured wh brd/alit from rail trn/veh, subs Occ of rail trn/veh injured by fall in rail trn/veh, init Occ of rail trn/veh injured by fall in rail trn/veh, subs Occ of rail trn/veh injured by fall from rail trn/veh, init Occ of rail trn/veh injured by fall from rail trn/veh, subs
E804.2	FALL IN ON/FROM RW TRAIN INJURING PEDESTRIAN	**V81.5XXA**	Occ of rail trn/veh injured by fall in rail trn/veh, init
E804.3	FALL IN ON/FROM RW TRAIN INJURING PEDAL CYCLIST	**V15.2XXA**	Unsp pedl cyclst inj in clsn w rail trn/veh nontraf, init
E804.8	FALL IN ON/FROM RW TRAIN INJURING OTH SPEC PERSO	**V81.5XXA**	Occ of rail trn/veh injured by fall in rail trn/veh, init
E804.9	FALL IN ON/FROM RW TRAIN INJURING UNSPEC PERSON	**V81.5XXA**	Occ of rail trn/veh injured by fall in rail trn/veh, init
E805.0	RAILWAY EMPLOYEE HIT BY ROLLING STOCK	**V81.2XXA**	Occ of rail trn/veh inj in collisn/hit by roll stok, init
E805.1	PASSENGER ON RAILWAY HIT BY ROLLING STOCK	**V81.2XXA**	Occ of rail trn/veh inj in collisn/hit by roll stok, init
E805.2	PEDESTRIAN HIT BY ROLLING STOCK	**V05.00XA** **V05.00XD** **V05.01XA** **V05.01XD** **V05.02XA** **V05.02XD** **V05.09XA** **V05.09XD**	Ped on foot injured in clsn w rail trn/veh nontraf, init Ped on foot injured in clsn w rail trn/veh nontraf, subs Ped on rolr-skt injured in clsn w rail trn/veh nontraf, init Ped on rolr-skt injured in clsn w rail trn/veh nontraf, subs Ped on sktbrd injured in clsn w rail trn/veh nontraf, init Ped on sktbrd injured in clsn w rail trn/veh nontraf, subs Ped w convey injured in clsn w rail trn/veh nontraf, init Ped w convey injured in clsn w rail trn/veh nontraf, subs
E805.3	PEDAL CYCLIST HIT BY ROLLING STOCK	**V15.2XXA**	Unsp pedl cyclst inj in clsn w rail trn/veh nontraf, init
E805.8	OTHER SPECIFIED PERSON HIT BY ROLLING STOCK	**V81.2XXA**	Occ of rail trn/veh inj in collisn/hit by roll stok, init
E805.9	UNSPECIFIED PERSON HIT BY ROLLING STOCK	**V81.2XXA**	Occ of rail trn/veh inj in collisn/hit by roll stok, init
E806.0	OTH SPEC RAILWAY ACCIDENT INJR RAILWAY EMPLOYEE	**V81.89XA**	Occ of rail trn/veh injured due to oth railway acc, init
E806.1	OTH SPEC RAILWAY ACCIDENT INJR PASSENGER RAILWAY	**V81.82XA** **V81.82XD** **V81.83XA** **V81.83XD** **V81.89XA** **V81.89XD**	Occ of rail trn/veh inj due to object fall onto train, init Occ of rail trn/veh inj due to object fall onto train, subs Occ of rail trn/veh inj due to clsn w miltry vehicle, init Occ of rail trn/veh inj due to clsn w miltry vehicle, subs Occ of rail trn/veh injured due to oth railway acc, init Occ of rail trn/veh injured due to oth railway acc, subs
E806.2	OTHER SPEC RAILWAY ACCIDENT INJURING PEDESTRIAN	**V81.89XA**	Occ of rail trn/veh injured due to oth railway acc, init
E806.3	OTH SPEC RAILWAY ACCIDENT INJURING PEDAL CYCLIST	**V15.2XXA**	Unsp pedl cyclst inj in clsn w rail trn/veh nontraf, init
E806.8	OTH SPEC RAILWAY ACCIDENT INJR OTH SPEC PERSON	**V81.89XA**	Occ of rail trn/veh injured due to oth railway acc, init
E806.9	OTH SPEC RAILWAY ACCIDENT INJURING UNSPEC PERSON	**V81.89XA**	Occ of rail trn/veh injured due to oth railway acc, init
E807.0	RAILWAY ACC UNSPEC NATURE INJR RAILWAY EMPLOYEE	**V81.9XXA**	Occupant of rail trn/veh injured in unsp railway acc, init
E807.1	RAILWAY ACCIDENT UNSPEC NATURE INJR PSGR RAILWAY	**V81.9XXA** **V81.9XXD**	Occupant of rail trn/veh injured in unsp railway acc, init Occupant of rail trn/veh injured in unsp railway acc, subs
E807.2	RAILWAY ACCIDENT UNSPEC NATURE INJR PEDESTRIAN	**V05.90XA** **V05.90XD** **V05.91XA** **V05.91XD** **V05.92XA** **V05.92XD** **V05.99XA** **V05.99XD**	Ped on foot injured in collision w rail trn/veh, unsp, init Ped on foot injured in collision w rail trn/veh, unsp, subs Ped on rolr-skt injured in clsn w rail trn/veh, unsp, init Ped on rolr-skt injured in clsn w rail trn/veh, unsp, subs Ped on sktbrd injured in clsn w rail trn/veh, unsp, init Ped on sktbrd injured in clsn w rail trn/veh, unsp, subs Ped w convey injured in collision w rail trn/veh, unsp, init Ped w convey injured in collision w rail trn/veh, unsp, subs
E807.3	RAILWAY ACC UNSPEC NATURE INJR PEDAL CYCLIST	**V15.2XXA**	Unsp pedl cyclst inj in clsn w rail trn/veh nontraf, init
E807.8	RAILWAY ACC UNSPEC NATURE INJR OTH SPEC PERSON	**V81.9XXA**	Occupant of rail trn/veh injured in unsp railway acc, init
E807.9	RAILWAY ACC UNSPEC NATURE INJR UNSPEC PERSON	**V81.9XXA**	Occupant of rail trn/veh injured in unsp railway acc, init

ICD-9-CM		ICD-10-CM	
E810.0	MOTOR VEH COLLISION W/TRAIN-INJURING MV DRIVER	**V35.5XXA**	Driver of 3-whl mv inj in clsn w rail trn/veh in traf, init
		V35.5XXD	Driver of 3-whl mv inj in clsn w rail trn/veh in traf, subs
		V45.5XXA	Car driver injured in collision w rail trn/veh in traf, init
		V45.5XXD	Car driver injured in collision w rail trn/veh in traf, subs
		V55.5XXA	Driver of pk-up/van inj in clsn w rail trn/veh in traf, init
		V55.5XXD	Driver of pk-up/van inj in clsn w rail trn/veh in traf, subs
		V65.5XXA	Driver of hv veh inj in clsn w rail trn/veh in traf, init
		V65.5XXD	Driver of hv veh inj in clsn w rail trn/veh in traf, subs
		V75.5XXA	Driver of bus injured in clsn w rail trn/veh in traf, init
		V75.5XXD	Driver of bus injured in clsn w rail trn/veh in traf, subs
E810.1	MOTOR VEH COLLISION W/TRAIN-INJR MV PASSENGER	**V35.6XXA**	Pasngr in 3-whl mv inj in clsn w rail trn/veh in traf, init
		V35.6XXD	Pasngr in 3-whl mv inj in clsn w rail trn/veh in traf, subs
		V45.6XXA	Car passenger injured in clsn w rail trn/veh in traf, init
		V45.6XXD	Car passenger injured in clsn w rail trn/veh in traf, subs
		V55.6XXA	Pasngr in pk-up/van inj in clsn w rail trn/veh in traf, init
		V55.6XXD	Pasngr in pk-up/van inj in clsn w rail trn/veh in traf, subs
		V65.6XXA	Pasngr in hv veh inj in clsn w rail trn/veh in traf, init
		V65.6XXD	Pasngr in hv veh inj in clsn w rail trn/veh in traf, subs
		V75.6XXA	Pasngr on bus injured in clsn w rail trn/veh in traf, init
		V75.6XXD	Pasngr on bus injured in clsn w rail trn/veh in traf, subs
E810.2	MOTOR VEH COLLISION W/TRAIN INJR MOTORCYCLIST	**V25.4XXA**	Mtrcy driver injured in clsn w rail trn/veh in traf, init
		V25.4XXD	Mtrcy driver injured in clsn w rail trn/veh in traf, subs
E810.3	MOTOR VEH COLLISION W/TRAIN INJR PSGR MOTORCYCLE	**V25.5XXA**	Mtrcy passenger injured in clsn w rail trn/veh in traf, init
		V25.5XXD	Mtrcy passenger injured in clsn w rail trn/veh in traf, subs
E810.4	MOTOR VEH COLLISION W/TRAIN INJR OCC STREETCAR	**V82.8XXA**	Occupant of streetcar injured in oth transport acc, init
E810.5	MOTOR VEH COLLISION W/TRAIN-INJR ANIMAL RIDER	**V80.61XA**	Animal-rider injured in collision w rail trn/veh, init
		V80.62XA	Occ of anml-drn vehicle injured in clsn w rail trn/veh, init
E810.6	MOTOR VEH COLLISION W/TRAIN INJR PEDAL CYCLIST	**V15.9XXA**	Unsp pedl cyclst inj in clsn w rail trn/veh in traf, init
E810.7	MOTOR VEHICLE COLLISION W/TRAIN INJR PEDESTRIAN	**V05.10XA**	Ped on foot injured in clsn w rail trn/veh in traf, init
		V05.10XD	Ped on foot injured in clsn w rail trn/veh in traf, subs
		V05.11XA	Ped on rolr-skt injured in clsn w rail trn/veh in traf, init
		V05.11XD	Ped on rolr-skt injured in clsn w rail trn/veh in traf, subs
		V05.12XA	Ped on sktbrd injured in clsn w rail trn/veh in traf, init
		V05.12XD	Ped on sktbrd injured in clsn w rail trn/veh in traf, subs
		V05.19XA	Ped w convey injured in clsn w rail trn/veh in traf, init
		V05.19XD	Ped w convey injured in clsn w rail trn/veh in traf, subs
E810.8	MOTOR VEH COLLISION W/TRAIN INJR OTH SPEC PERSON	**V35.7XXA**	Prsn outsd 3-whl mv inj in clsn w rail trn/veh in traf, init
		V35.7XXD	Prsn outsd 3-whl mv inj in clsn w rail trn/veh in traf, subs
		V45.7XXA	Person outside car inj in clsn w rail trn/veh in traf, init
		V45.7XXD	Person outside car inj in clsn w rail trn/veh in traf, subs
		V55.7XXA	Prsn outsd pk-up/van inj in clsn w rail trn/veh in traf,init
		V55.7XXD	Prsn outsd pk-up/van inj in clsn w rail trn/veh in traf,subs
		V65.7XXA	Person outsd hv veh inj in clsn w rail trn/veh in traf, init
		V65.7XXD	Person outsd hv veh inj in clsn w rail trn/veh in traf, subs
		V75.7XXA	Person outside bus inj in clsn w rail trn/veh in traf, init
		V75.7XXD	Person outside bus inj in clsn w rail trn/veh in traf, subs
		V81.1XXA	Occ of rail trn/veh injured in clsn w mtr veh in traf, init
		V81.1XXD	Occ of rail trn/veh injured in clsn w mtr veh in traf, subs
E810.9	MOTOR VEH COLLISION W/TRAIN INJR UNSPEC PERSON	**V25.9XXA**	Unsp mtrcy rider inj in clsn w rail trn/veh in traf, init
		V25.9XXD	Unsp mtrcy rider inj in clsn w rail trn/veh in traf, subs
		V35.9XXA	Occup of 3-whl mv inj in clsn w rail trn/veh in traf, init
		V35.9XXD	Occup of 3-whl mv inj in clsn w rail trn/veh in traf, subs
		V45.9XXA	Unsp car occ injured in clsn w rail trn/veh in traf, init
		V45.9XXD	Unsp car occ injured in clsn w rail trn/veh in traf, subs
		V55.9XXA	Occup of pk-up/van inj in clsn w rail trn/veh in traf, init
		V55.9XXD	Occup of pk-up/van inj in clsn w rail trn/veh in traf, subs
		V65.9XXA	Occup of hv veh injured in clsn w rail trn/veh in traf, init
		V65.9XXD	Occup of hv veh injured in clsn w rail trn/veh in traf, subs
		V75.9XXA	Occup of bus injured in clsn w rail trn/veh in traf, init
		V75.9XXD	Occup of bus injured in clsn w rail trn/veh in traf, subs
		V87.6XXA	Person injured in collision betw rail trn/veh and car, init
		V87.6XXD	Person injured in collision betw rail trn/veh and car, subs
E811.0	MOTR VEH RE-ENTRANT COLL W/MV-INJR MV DRIVER	**V49.40XA**	Driver injured in collision w unsp mv in traf, init
E811.1	MOTR VEH RE-ENTRANT COLL W/MV-INJR MV PSGR	**V49.50XA**	Passenger injured in collision w unsp mv in traf, init
E811.2	MOTR VEH RE-ENTRANT COLL W/MV-INJR MOTRCYCLST	**V29.40XA**	Mtrcy driver injured in collision w unsp mv in traf, init
E811.3	MOTR VEH RE-ENTRANT COLL W/MV-INJR MC PSGR	**V29.50XA**	Mtrcy passenger injured in collision w unsp mv in traf, init
E811.4	MOTR VEH RE-ENTRANT COLL W/MV-INJR ST CAR RIDR	**V82.1XXA**	Occupant of stcar injured in clsn w mtr veh in traf, init
E811.5	MOTR VEH RE-ENTRANT COLL W/MV-INJR ANIMAL RIDR	**V80.41XA**	Animl-ridr inj pk-up truck, pick-up truck, van, hv veh, init
		V80.42XA	Occ animal-drwn veh injured collision hvy veh, init encntr
E811.6	MOTR VEH RE-ENTRANT COLL W/MV-INJURING CYCLIST	**V13.9XXA**	Unsp pedl cyclst inj pick-up truck, pk-up/van in traf, init
E811.7	MOTR VEH RE-ENTRANT COLL W/MV-INJR PEDESTRIAN	**V03.10XA**	Ped on foot injured pick-up truck, pk-up/van in traf, init
E811.8	MOTR VEH RE-ENTRANT COLL W/MV-INJR OTH PERSON	**V49.88XA**	Car occupant (driver) injured in oth transport acc, init
E811.9	MOTR VEH RE-ENTRANT COLL W/MV-INJR UNS PERSON	**V49.88XA**	Car occupant (driver) injured in oth transport acc, init

[Brackets] indicate valid character values for each code. Character value meanings provided for each code grouping.

ICD-9-CM		ICD-10-CM	
E812.Ø	OTH MOTR VEH COLL W/MOTR VEH-INJR MV DRIVER	**V32.5XXA**	Driver of 3-whl mv inj in clsn w 2/3-whl mv in traf, init
		V32.5XXD	Driver of 3-whl mv inj in clsn w 2/3-whl mv in traf, subs
		V33.5XXA	Driver of 3-whl mv inj pk-up truck, pk-up/van in traf, init
		V33.5XXD	Driver of 3-whl mv inj pk-up truck, pk-up/van in traf, subs
		V34.5XXA	Driver of 3-whl mv injured in clsn w hv veh in traf, init
		V34.5XXD	Driver of 3-whl mv injured in clsn w hv veh in traf, subs
		V39.4ØXA	Driver of 3-whl mv injured in clsn w unsp mv in traf, init
		V39.4ØXD	Driver of 3-whl mv injured in clsn w unsp mv in traf, subs
		V39.49XA	Driver of 3-whl mv injured in clsn w oth mv in traf, init
		V39.49XD	Driver of 3-whl mv injured in clsn w oth mv in traf, subs
		V39.81XA	Occ of 3-whl mv injured in trnsp acc w miltry vehicle, init
		V39.81XD	Occ of 3-whl mv injured in trnsp acc w miltry vehicle, subs
		V42.5XXA	Car driver injured in collision w 2/3-whl mv in traf, init
		V42.5XXD	Car driver injured in collision w 2/3-whl mv in traf, subs
		V43.51XA	Car driver injured in collision w SUV in traf, init
		V43.51XD	Car driver injured in collision w SUV in traf, subs
		V43.52XA	Car driver injured in collision w car in traf, init
		V43.52XD	Car driver injured in collision w car in traf, subs
		V43.53XA	Car driver injured in clsn w pick-up truck in traf, init
		V43.53XD	Car driver injured in clsn w pick-up truck in traf, subs
		V43.54XA	Car driver injured in collision w van in traf, init
		V43.54XD	Car driver injured in collision w van in traf, subs
		V44.5XXA	Car driver injured in collision w hv veh in traf, init
		V44.5XXD	Car driver injured in collision w hv veh in traf, subs
		V47.51XA	Driver of SUV injured in clsn w statnry object in traf, init
		V47.51XD	Driver of SUV injured in clsn w statnry object in traf, subs
		V47.52XA	Driver of car injured in clsn w statnry object in traf, init
		V47.52XD	Driver of car injured in clsn w statnry object in traf, subs
		V49.4ØXA	Driver injured in collision w unsp mv in traf, init
		V49.4ØXD	Driver injured in collision w unsp mv in traf, subs
		V49.49XA	Driver injured in collision w oth mv in traf, init
		V49.49XD	Driver injured in collision w oth mv in traf, subs
		V49.81XA	Car occupant injured in trnsp acc w military vehicle, init
		V49.81XD	Car occupant injured in trnsp acc w military vehicle, subs
		V49.88XA	Car occupant (driver) injured in oth transport acc, init
		V49.88XD	Car occupant (driver) injured in oth transport acc, subs
		V52.5XXA	Driver of pk-up/van inj in clsn w 2/3-whl mv in traf, init
		V52.5XXD	Driver of pk-up/van inj in clsn w 2/3-whl mv in traf, subs
		V53.5XXA	Driver of pk-up/van inj pk-up truck, pk-up/van in traf, init
		V53.5XXD	Driver of pk-up/van inj pk-up truck, pk-up/van in traf, subs
		V54.5XXA	Driver of pk-up/van injured in clsn w hv veh in traf, init
		V54.5XXD	Driver of pk-up/van injured in clsn w hv veh in traf, subs
		V59.4ØXA	Driver of pk-up/van injured in clsn w unsp mv in traf, init
		V59.4ØXD	Driver of pk-up/van injured in clsn w unsp mv in traf, subs
		V59.49XA	Driver of pk-up/van injured in clsn w oth mv in traf, init
		V59.49XD	Driver of pk-up/van injured in clsn w oth mv in traf, subs
		V62.5XXA	Driver of hv veh injured in clsn w 2/3-whl mv in traf, init
		V62.5XXD	Driver of hv veh injured in clsn w 2/3-whl mv in traf, subs
		V63.5XXA	Driver of hv veh inj pick-up truck, pk-up/van in traf, init
		V63.5XXD	Driver of hv veh inj pick-up truck, pk-up/van in traf, subs
		V64.5XXA	Driver of hv veh injured in collision w hv veh in traf, init
		V64.5XXD	Driver of hv veh injured in collision w hv veh in traf, subs
		V69.4ØXA	Driver of hv veh injured in clsn w unsp mv in traf, init
		V69.4ØXD	Driver of hv veh injured in clsn w unsp mv in traf, subs
		V69.49XA	Driver of hv veh injured in collision w oth mv in traf, init
		V69.49XD	Driver of hv veh injured in collision w oth mv in traf, subs
		V69.81XA	Occ of hv veh injured in trnsp acc w miltry vehicle, init
		V69.81XD	Occ of hv veh injured in trnsp acc w miltry vehicle, subs
		V69.88XA	Occupant (driver) of hv veh injured in oth trnsp acc, init
		V69.88XD	Occupant (driver) of hv veh injured in oth trnsp acc, subs
		V69.9XXA	Occupant (driver) of hv veh injured in unsp traf, init
		V69.9XXD	Occupant (driver) of hv veh injured in unsp traf, subs
		V72.5XXA	Driver of bus injured in clsn w 2/3-whl mv in traf, init
		V72.5XXD	Driver of bus injured in clsn w 2/3-whl mv in traf, subs
		V73.5XXA	Driver of bus injured pick-up truck, pk-up/van in traf, init
		V73.5XXD	Driver of bus injured pick-up truck, pk-up/van in traf, subs
		V74.5XXA	Driver of bus injured in collision w hv veh in traf, init
		V74.5XXD	Driver of bus injured in collision w hv veh in traf, subs
		V79.4ØXA	Driver of bus injured in collision w unsp mv in traf, init
		V79.4ØXD	Driver of bus injured in collision w unsp mv in traf, subs
		V79.49XA	Driver of bus injured in collision w oth mv in traf, init
		V79.49XD	Driver of bus injured in collision w oth mv in traf, subs
		V79.81XA	Bus occupant injured in trnsp acc w military vehicle, init
		V79.81XD	Bus occupant injured in trnsp acc w military vehicle, subs
		V79.88XA	Bus occupant (driver) injured in oth transport acc, init
		V79.88XD	Bus occupant (driver) injured in oth transport acc, subs
		V79.9XXA	Bus occupant (driver) (passenger) injured in unsp traf, init
		V79.9XXD	Bus occupant (driver) (passenger) injured in unsp traf, subs
		V84.ØXXA	Driver of special agricultural vehicle injured in traf, init
		V84.ØXXD	Driver of special agricultural vehicle injured in traf, subs
		V85.ØXXA	Driver of special construction vehicle injured in traf, init
		V85.ØXXD	Driver of special construction vehicle injured in traf, subs

ICD-9-CM		ICD-10-CM	
E812.1	OTH MOTR VEH COLL W/MOTR VEH-INJR MV PASSENGER	**V32.6XXA**	Pasngr in 3-whl mv inj in clsn w 2/3-whl mv in traf, init
		V32.6XXD	Pasngr in 3-whl mv inj in clsn w 2/3-whl mv in traf, subs
		V33.6XXA	Pasngr in 3-whl mv inj pk-up truck, pk-up/van in traf, init
		V33.6XXD	Pasngr in 3-whl mv inj pk-up truck, pk-up/van in traf, subs
		V34.6XXA	Passenger in 3-whl mv injured in clsn w hv veh in traf, init
		V34.6XXD	Passenger in 3-whl mv injured in clsn w hv veh in traf, subs
		V39.5ØXA	Pasngr in 3-whl mv injured in clsn w unsp mv in traf, init
		V39.5ØXD	Pasngr in 3-whl mv injured in clsn w unsp mv in traf, subs
		V39.59XA	Passenger in 3-whl mv injured in clsn w oth mv in traf, init
		V39.59XD	Passenger in 3-whl mv injured in clsn w oth mv in traf, subs
		V42.6XXA	Car passenger injured in clsn w 2/3-whl mv in traf, init
		V42.6XXD	Car passenger injured in clsn w 2/3-whl mv in traf, subs
		V43.61XA	Car passenger injured in collision w SUV in traf, init
		V43.61XD	Car passenger injured in collision w SUV in traf, subs
		V43.62XA	Car passenger injured in collision w car in traf, init
		V43.62XD	Car passenger injured in collision w car in traf, subs
		V43.63XA	Car passenger injured in clsn w pick-up truck in traf, init
		V43.63XD	Car passenger injured in clsn w pick-up truck in traf, subs
		V43.64XA	Car passenger injured in collision w van in traf, init
		V43.64XD	Car passenger injured in collision w van in traf, subs
		V44.6XXA	Car passenger injured in collision w hv veh in traf, init
		V44.6XXD	Car passenger injured in collision w hv veh in traf, subs
		V47.61XA	Pasngr of SUV injured in clsn w statnry object in traf, init
		V47.61XD	Pasngr of SUV injured in clsn w statnry object in traf, subs
		V47.62XA	Pasngr of car injured in clsn w statnry object in traf, init
		V47.62XD	Pasngr of car injured in clsn w statnry object in traf, subs
		V47.7XXA	Person outsd car inj in clsn w statnry object in traf, init
		V47.7XXD	Person outsd car inj in clsn w statnry object in traf, subs
		V49.5ØXA	Passenger injured in collision w unsp mv in traf, init
		V49.5ØXD	Passenger injured in collision w unsp mv in traf, subs
		V49.59XA	Passenger injured in collision w oth mv in traf, init
		V49.59XD	Passenger injured in collision w oth mv in traf, subs
		V52.6XXA	Pasngr in pk-up/van inj in clsn w 2/3-whl mv in traf, init
		V52.6XXD	Pasngr in pk-up/van inj in clsn w 2/3-whl mv in traf, subs
		V53.6XXA	Pasngr in pk-up/van inj pk-up truck, pk-up/van in traf, init
		V53.6XXD	Pasngr in pk-up/van inj pk-up truck, pk-up/van in traf, subs
		V54.6XXA	Pasngr in pk-up/van injured in clsn w hv veh in traf, init
		V54.6XXD	Pasngr in pk-up/van injured in clsn w hv veh in traf, subs
		V59.5ØXA	Pasngr in pk-up/van injured in clsn w unsp mv in traf, init
		V59.5ØXD	Pasngr in pk-up/van injured in clsn w unsp mv in traf, subs
		V59.59XA	Pasngr in pk-up/van injured in clsn w oth mv in traf, init
		V59.59XD	Pasngr in pk-up/van injured in clsn w oth mv in traf, subs
		V59.81XA	Occ of pk-up/van injured in trnsp acc w miltry vehicle, init
		V59.81XD	Occ of pk-up/van injured in trnsp acc w miltry vehicle, subs
		V59.88XA	Occupant of pk-up/van injured in oth trnsp acc, init
		V59.88XD	Occupant of pk-up/van injured in oth trnsp acc, subs
		V62.6XXA	Pasngr in hv veh injured in clsn w 2/3-whl mv in traf, init
		V62.6XXD	Pasngr in hv veh injured in clsn w 2/3-whl mv in traf, subs
		V63.6XXA	Pasngr in hv veh inj pick-up truck, pk-up/van in traf, init
		V63.6XXD	Pasngr in hv veh inj pick-up truck, pk-up/van in traf, subs
		V64.6XXA	Passenger in hv veh injured in clsn w hv veh in traf, init
		V64.6XXD	Passenger in hv veh injured in clsn w hv veh in traf, subs
		V69.5ØXA	Passenger in hv veh injured in clsn w unsp mv in traf, init
		V69.5ØXD	Passenger in hv veh injured in clsn w unsp mv in traf, subs
		V69.59XA	Passenger in hv veh injured in clsn w oth mv in traf, init
		V69.59XD	Passenger in hv veh injured in clsn w oth mv in traf, subs
		V72.6XXA	Passenger on bus injured in clsn w 2/3-whl mv in traf, init
		V72.6XXD	Passenger on bus injured in clsn w 2/3-whl mv in traf, subs
		V73.6XXA	Pasngr on bus injured pick-up truck, pk-up/van in traf, init
		V73.6XXD	Pasngr on bus injured pick-up truck, pk-up/van in traf, subs
		V74.6XXA	Passenger on bus injured in collision w hv veh in traf, init
		V74.6XXD	Passenger on bus injured in collision w hv veh in traf, subs
		V79.5ØXA	Passenger on bus injured in clsn w unsp mv in traf, init
		V79.5ØXD	Passenger on bus injured in clsn w unsp mv in traf, subs
		V79.59XA	Passenger on bus injured in collision w oth mv in traf, init
		V79.59XD	Passenger on bus injured in collision w oth mv in traf, subs
		V84.1XXA	Passenger of special agri vehicle injured in traf, init
		V84.1XXD	Passenger of special agri vehicle injured in traf, subs
		V85.1XXA	Passenger of special construct vehicle injured in traf, init
		V85.1XXD	Passenger of special construct vehicle injured in traf, subs
E812.2	OTH MOTR VEH COLL W/MOTR VEH-INJR MOTORCYCLIST	**V21.4XXA**	Mtrcy driver injured in collision w pedl cyc in traf, init
		V21.4XXD	Mtrcy driver injured in collision w pedl cyc in traf, subs
		V23.4XXA	Mtrcy driver injured pick-up truck, pk-up/van in traf, init
		V23.4XXD	Mtrcy driver injured pick-up truck, pk-up/van in traf, subs
		V24.4XXA	Mtrcy driver injured in collision w hv veh in traf, init
		V24.4XXD	Mtrcy driver injured in collision w hv veh in traf, subs
		V29.4ØXA	Mtrcy driver injured in collision w unsp mv in traf, init
		V29.4ØXD	Mtrcy driver injured in collision w unsp mv in traf, subs
		V29.49XA	Mtrcy driver injured in collision w oth mv in traf, init
		V29.49XD	Mtrcy driver injured in collision w oth mv in traf, subs

ICD-9-CM		ICD-10-CM	
E812.3	OTH MOTR VEH COLL W/MOTR VEH-INJR MC PASSENGER	**V23.5XXA**	Mtrcy pasngr injured pick-up truck, pk-up/van in traf, init
		V23.5XXD	Mtrcy pasngr injured pick-up truck, pk-up/van in traf, subs
		V24.5XXA	Mtrcy passenger injured in collision w hv veh in traf, init
		V24.5XXD	Mtrcy passenger injured in collision w hv veh in traf, subs
		V26.5XXA	Mtrcy pasngr injured in clsn w nonmtr vehicle in traf, init
		V26.5XXD	Mtrcy pasngr injured in clsn w nonmtr vehicle in traf, subs
		V29.5ØXA	Mtrcy passenger injured in collision w unsp mv in traf, init
		V29.5ØXD	Mtrcy passenger injured in collision w unsp mv in traf, subs
		V29.59XA	Mtrcy passenger injured in collision w oth mv in traf, init
		V29.59XD	Mtrcy passenger injured in collision w oth mv in traf, subs
E812.4	OTH MOTR VEH COLL W/MOTR VEH-INJR ST CAR RIDER	**V82.1XXA**	Occupant of stcar injured in clsn w mtr veh in traf, init
E812.5	OTH MOTR VEH COLL W/MOTR VEH-INJR ANIMAL RIDER	**V8Ø.41XA**	Animl-ridr inj pk-up truck, pick-up truck, van, hv veh, init
E812.6	OTH MOTR VEH COLL W/MOTR VEH-INJR PEDL CYCLS	**V13.9XXA**	Unsp pedl cyclst inj pick-up truck, pk-up/van in traf, init
E812.7	OTH MOTR VEH COLL W/MOTR VEH-INJR PEDESTRIAN	**VØ3.1ØXA**	Ped on foot injured pick-up truck, pk-up/van in traf, init
E812.8	OTH MOTR VEH COLL W/MOTR VEH-INJR OTH PERSON	**V32.7XXA**	Person outsd 3-whl mv inj in clsn w 2/3-whl mv in traf, init
		V32.7XXD	Person outsd 3-whl mv inj in clsn w 2/3-whl mv in traf, subs
		V33.7XXA	Prsn outsd 3-whl mv inj pk-up truck, pk-up/van in traf, init
		V33.7XXD	Prsn outsd 3-whl mv inj pk-up truck, pk-up/van in traf, subs
		V34.7XXA	Person outside 3-whl mv inj in clsn w hv veh in traf, init
		V34.7XXD	Person outside 3-whl mv inj in clsn w hv veh in traf, subs
		V41.7XXA	Person outside car injured in clsn w pedl cyc in traf, init
		V41.7XXD	Person outside car injured in clsn w pedl cyc in traf, subs
		V42.7XXA	Person outside car inj in clsn w 2/3-whl mv in traf, init
		V42.7XXD	Person outside car inj in clsn w 2/3-whl mv in traf, subs
		V43.71XA	Person outside car injured in collision w SUV in traf, init
		V43.71XD	Person outside car injured in collision w SUV in traf, subs
		V43.72XA	Person outside car injured in collision w car in traf, init
		V43.72XD	Person outside car injured in collision w car in traf, subs
		V43.73XA	Person outside car inj in clsn w pick-up truck in traf, init
		V43.73XD	Person outside car inj in clsn w pick-up truck in traf, subs
		V43.74XA	Person outside car injured in collision w van in traf, init
		V43.74XD	Person outside car injured in collision w van in traf, subs
		V44.7XXA	Person outside car injured in clsn w hv veh in traf, init
		V44.7XXD	Person outside car injured in clsn w hv veh in traf, subs
		V52.7XXA	Prsn outsd pk-up/van inj in clsn w 2/3-whl mv in traf, init
		V52.7XXD	Prsn outsd pk-up/van inj in clsn w 2/3-whl mv in traf, subs
		V53.7XXA	Prsn outsd pk-up/van inj pk-up truck,pk-up/van in traf, init
		V53.7XXD	Prsn outsd pk-up/van inj pk-up truck,pk-up/van in traf, subs
		V54.7XXA	Person outside pk-up/van inj in clsn w hv veh in traf, init
		V54.7XXD	Person outside pk-up/van inj in clsn w hv veh in traf, subs
		V62.7XXA	Person outside hv veh inj in clsn w 2/3-whl mv in traf, init
		V62.7XXD	Person outside hv veh inj in clsn w 2/3-whl mv in traf, subs
		V63.7XXA	Person outsd hv veh inj pk-up truck, pk-up/van in traf, init
		V63.7XXD	Person outsd hv veh inj pk-up truck, pk-up/van in traf, subs
		V64.7XXA	Person outside hv veh injured in clsn w hv veh in traf, init
		V64.7XXD	Person outside hv veh injured in clsn w hv veh in traf, subs
		V72.7XXA	Person outside bus inj in clsn w 2/3-whl mv in traf, init
		V72.7XXD	Person outside bus inj in clsn w 2/3-whl mv in traf, subs
		V73.7XXA	Person outsd bus inj pick-up truck, pk-up/van in traf, init
		V73.7XXD	Person outsd bus inj pick-up truck, pk-up/van in traf, subs
		V74.7XXA	Person outside bus injured in clsn w hv veh in traf, init
		V74.7XXD	Person outside bus injured in clsn w hv veh in traf, subs
		V84.2XXA	Person outside special agri vehicle injured in traf, init
		V84.2XXD	Person outside special agri vehicle injured in traf, subs
		V85.2XXA	Person outside special construct vehicle inj in traf, init
		V85.2XXD	Person outside special construct vehicle inj in traf, subs
E812.9	OTH MOTR VEH COLL W/MOTR VEH-INJR UNS PERSON	**V22.9XXA**	Unsp mtrcy rider injured in clsn w 2/3-whl mv in traf, init
		V22.9XXD	Unsp mtrcy rider injured in clsn w 2/3-whl mv in traf, subs
		V23.2XXA	Unsp mtrcy rider inj pick-up truck, pk-up/van nontraf, init
		V23.2XXD	Unsp mtrcy rider inj pick-up truck, pk-up/van nontraf, subs
		V23.9XXA	Unsp mtrcy rider inj pick-up truck, pk-up/van in traf, init
		V23.9XXD	Unsp mtrcy rider inj pick-up truck, pk-up/van in traf, subs
		V24.9XXA	Unsp mtrcy rider injured in collision w hv veh in traf, init
		V24.9XXD	Unsp mtrcy rider injured in collision w hv veh in traf, subs
		V29.6ØXA	Unsp mtrcy rider injured in clsn w unsp mv in traf, init
		V29.6ØXD	Unsp mtrcy rider injured in clsn w unsp mv in traf, subs
		V29.69XA	Unsp mtrcy rider injured in collision w oth mv in traf, init
		V29.69XD	Unsp mtrcy rider injured in collision w oth mv in traf, subs
		V32.9XXA	Occup of 3-whl mv injured in clsn w 2/3-whl mv in traf, init
		V32.9XXD	Occup of 3-whl mv injured in clsn w 2/3-whl mv in traf, subs
		V33.9XXA	Occup of 3-whl mv inj pick-up truck, pk-up/van in traf, init
		V33.9XXD	Occup of 3-whl mv inj pick-up truck, pk-up/van in traf, subs
		V34.9XXA	Occup of 3-whl mv injured in clsn w hv veh in traf, init
		V34.9XXD	Occup of 3-whl mv injured in clsn w hv veh in traf, subs
		V39.6ØXA	Occup of 3-whl mv injured in clsn w unsp mv in traf, init
		V39.6ØXD	Occup of 3-whl mv injured in clsn w unsp mv in traf, subs
		V39.69XA	Occup of 3-whl mv injured in clsn w oth mv in traf, init
		V39.69XD	Occup of 3-whl mv injured in clsn w oth mv in traf, subs
		V42.9XXA	Unsp car occupant injured in clsn w 2/3-whl mv in traf, init
		V42.9XXD	Unsp car occupant injured in clsn w 2/3-whl mv in traf, subs
		V43.91XA	Unsp car occupant injured in collision w SUV in traf, init

(Continued on next page)

ICD-9-CM		ICD-10-CM	
E812.9	OTH MOTR VEH COLL W/MOTR VEH-INJR UNS PERSON **(Continued)**	**V43.91XD**	Unsp car occupant injured in collision w SUV in traf, subs
		V43.92XA	Unsp car occupant injured in collision w car in traf, init
		V43.92XD	Unsp car occupant injured in collision w car in traf, subs
		V43.93XA	Unsp car occ injured in clsn w pick-up truck in traf, init
		V43.93XD	Unsp car occ injured in clsn w pick-up truck in traf, subs
		V43.94XA	Unsp car occupant injured in collision w van in traf, init
		V43.94XD	Unsp car occupant injured in collision w van in traf, subs
		V44.9XXA	Unsp car occupant injured in clsn w hv veh in traf, init
		V44.9XXD	Unsp car occupant injured in clsn w hv veh in traf, subs
		V47.91XA	Occup of SUV injured in clsn w statnry object in traf, init
		V47.91XD	Occup of SUV injured in clsn w statnry object in traf, subs
		V47.92XA	Occup of car injured in clsn w statnry object in traf, init
		V47.92XD	Occup of car injured in clsn w statnry object in traf, subs
		V49.6ØXA	Unsp car occupant injured in clsn w unsp mv in traf, init
		V49.6ØXD	Unsp car occupant injured in clsn w unsp mv in traf, subs
		V49.69XA	Unsp car occupant injured in clsn w oth mv in traf, init
		V49.69XD	Unsp car occupant injured in clsn w oth mv in traf, subs
		V52.9XXA	Occup of pk-up/van inj in clsn w 2/3-whl mv in traf, init
		V52.9XXD	Occup of pk-up/van inj in clsn w 2/3-whl mv in traf, subs
		V53.9XXA	Occup of pk-up/van inj pk-up truck, pk-up/van in traf, init
		V53.9XXD	Occup of pk-up/van inj pk-up truck, pk-up/van in traf, subs
		V54.9XXA	Occup of pk-up/van injured in clsn w hv veh in traf, init
		V54.9XXD	Occup of pk-up/van injured in clsn w hv veh in traf, subs
		V59.6ØXA	Occup of pk-up/van injured in clsn w unsp mv in traf, init
		V59.6ØXD	Occup of pk-up/van injured in clsn w unsp mv in traf, subs
		V59.69XA	Occup of pk-up/van injured in clsn w oth mv in traf, init
		V59.69XD	Occup of pk-up/van injured in clsn w oth mv in traf, subs
		V62.9XXA	Occup of hv veh injured in clsn w 2/3-whl mv in traf, init
		V62.9XXD	Occup of hv veh injured in clsn w 2/3-whl mv in traf, subs
		V63.9XXA	Occup of hv veh inj pick-up truck, pk-up/van in traf, init
		V63.9XXD	Occup of hv veh inj pick-up truck, pk-up/van in traf, subs
		V64.9XXA	Occup of hv veh injured in collision w hv veh in traf, init
		V64.9XXD	Occup of hv veh injured in collision w hv veh in traf, subs
		V69.6ØXA	Occup of hv veh injured in collision w unsp mv in traf, init
		V69.6ØXD	Occup of hv veh injured in collision w unsp mv in traf, subs
		V69.69XA	Occup of hv veh injured in collision w oth mv in traf, init
		V69.69XD	Occup of hv veh injured in collision w oth mv in traf, subs
		V72.9XXA	Occup of bus injured in collision w 2/3-whl mv in traf, init
		V72.9XXD	Occup of bus injured in collision w 2/3-whl mv in traf, subs
		V73.9XXA	Occup of bus injured pick-up truck, pk-up/van in traf, init
		V73.9XXD	Occup of bus injured pick-up truck, pk-up/van in traf, subs
		V74.9XXA	Occup of bus injured in collision w hv veh in traf, init
		V74.9XXD	Occup of bus injured in collision w hv veh in traf, subs
		V79.6ØXA	Unsp bus occupant injured in clsn w unsp mv in traf, init
		V79.6ØXD	Unsp bus occupant injured in clsn w unsp mv in traf, subs
		V79.69XA	Unsp bus occupant injured in clsn w oth mv in traf, init
		V79.69XD	Unsp bus occupant injured in clsn w oth mv in traf, subs
		V84.3XXA	Occup of special agricultural vehicle injured in traf, init
		V84.3XXD	Occup of special agricultural vehicle injured in traf, subs
		V85.3XXA	Occup of special construction vehicle injured in traf, init
		V85.3XXD	Occup of special construction vehicle injured in traf, subs
		V87.ØXXA	Person injured in clsn betw car and 2/3-whl pwr veh, init
		V87.ØXXD	Person injured in clsn betw car and 2/3-whl pwr veh, subs
		V87.1XXA	Person injured in clsn betw mtr veh and 2/3-whl mv, init
		V87.1XXD	Person injured in clsn betw mtr veh and 2/3-whl mv, subs
		V87.2XXA	Person injured in collision betw car and pk-up/van, init
		V87.2XXD	Person injured in collision betw car and pk-up/van, subs
		V87.3XXA	Person injured in collision betw car and bus (traffic), init
		V87.3XXD	Person injured in collision betw car and bus (traffic), subs
		V87.4XXA	Person injured in collision betw car and hv veh, init
		V87.4XXD	Person injured in collision betw car and hv veh, subs
		V87.5XXA	Person injured in collision betw hv veh and bus, init
		V87.5XXD	Person injured in collision betw hv veh and bus, subs
		V87.7XXA	Person injured in collision betw oth mtr veh (traffic), init
		V87.7XXD	Person injured in collision betw oth mtr veh (traffic), subs
E813.Ø	MOTR VEH COLLISION W/OTH VEH-INJR MV DRIVER	**V31.5XXA**	Driver of 3-whl mv injured in clsn w pedl cyc in traf, init
		V31.5XXD	Driver of 3-whl mv injured in clsn w pedl cyc in traf, subs
		V36.5XXA	Driver of 3-whl mv inj in clsn w nonmtr veh in traf, init
		V36.5XXD	Driver of 3-whl mv inj in clsn w nonmtr veh in traf, subs
		V39.89XA	Occupant (driver) of 3-whl mv injured in oth trnsp acc, init
		V39.89XD	Occupant (driver) of 3-whl mv injured in oth trnsp acc, subs
		V41.5XXA	Car driver injured in collision w pedal cycle in traf, init
		V41.5XXD	Car driver injured in collision w pedal cycle in traf, subs
		V46.5XXA	Car driver injured in clsn w nonmtr vehicle in traf, init
		V46.5XXD	Car driver injured in clsn w nonmtr vehicle in traf, subs
		V51.5XXA	Driver of pk-up/van injured in clsn w pedl cyc in traf, init
		V51.5XXD	Driver of pk-up/van injured in clsn w pedl cyc in traf, subs
		V56.5XXA	Driver of pk-up/van inj in clsn w nonmtr veh in traf, init
		V56.5XXD	Driver of pk-up/van inj in clsn w nonmtr veh in traf, subs
		V61.5XXA	Driver of hv veh injured in clsn w pedl cyc in traf, init
		V61.5XXD	Driver of hv veh injured in clsn w pedl cyc in traf, subs
	(Continued on next page)	**V66.5XXA**	Driver of hv veh inj in clsn w nonmtr vehicle in traf, init

ICD-9-CM		ICD-10-CM	
E813.Ø	MOTR VEH COLLISION W/OTH VEH-INJR MV DRIVER **(Continued)**	**V66.5XXD**	Driver of hv veh inj in clsn w nonmtr vehicle in traf, subs
		V71.5XXA	Driver of bus injured in collision w pedl cyc in traf, init
		V71.5XXD	Driver of bus injured in collision w pedl cyc in traf, subs
		V76.5XXA	Driver of bus injured in clsn w nonmtr vehicle in traf, init
		V76.5XXD	Driver of bus injured in clsn w nonmtr vehicle in traf, subs
E813.1	MOTR VEH COLLISION W/OTH VEH-INJR MV PASSENGER	**V36.6XXA**	Pasngr in 3-whl mv inj in clsn w nonmtr veh in traf, init
		V36.6XXD	Pasngr in 3-whl mv inj in clsn w nonmtr veh in traf, subs
		V41.6XXA	Car passenger injured in collision w pedl cyc in traf, init
		V41.6XXD	Car passenger injured in collision w pedl cyc in traf, subs
		V46.6XXA	Car passenger injured in clsn w nonmtr vehicle in traf, init
		V46.6XXD	Car passenger injured in clsn w nonmtr vehicle in traf, subs
		V51.6XXA	Pasngr in pk-up/van injured in clsn w pedl cyc in traf, init
		V51.6XXD	Pasngr in pk-up/van injured in clsn w pedl cyc in traf, subs
		V56.6XXA	Pasngr in pk-up/van inj in clsn w nonmtr veh in traf, init
		V56.6XXD	Pasngr in pk-up/van inj in clsn w nonmtr veh in traf, subs
		V61.6XXA	Passenger in hv veh injured in clsn w pedl cyc in traf, init
		V61.6XXD	Passenger in hv veh injured in clsn w pedl cyc in traf, subs
		V66.6XXA	Pasngr in hv veh inj in clsn w nonmtr vehicle in traf, init
		V66.6XXD	Pasngr in hv veh inj in clsn w nonmtr vehicle in traf, subs
		V71.6XXA	Passenger on bus injured in clsn w pedl cyc in traf, init
		V71.6XXD	Passenger on bus injured in clsn w pedl cyc in traf, subs
		V76.6XXA	Pasngr on bus injured in clsn w nonmtr vehicle in traf, init
		V76.6XXD	Pasngr on bus injured in clsn w nonmtr vehicle in traf, subs
E813.2	MOTR VEH COLLISION W/OTH VEH-INJR MOTORCYCLIST	**V21.3XXA**	Prsn brd/alit mtrcy injured in collision w pedal cycle, init
		V21.3XXD	Prsn brd/alit mtrcy injured in collision w pedal cycle, subs
		V26.4XXA	Mtrcy driver injured in clsn w nonmtr vehicle in traf, init
		V26.4XXD	Mtrcy driver injured in clsn w nonmtr vehicle in traf, subs
E813.3	MOTR VEH COLLISION W/OTH VEH-INJR MC PASSENGER	**V21.5XXA**	Mtrcy passenger injured in clsn w pedl cyc in traf, init
		V21.5XXD	Mtrcy passenger injured in clsn w pedl cyc in traf, subs
E813.4	MOTR VEH COLLISION W/OTH VEH-INJR ST CAR RIDER	**V82.1XXA**	Occupant of stcar injured in clsn w mtr veh in traf, init
		V82.1XXD	Occupant of stcar injured in clsn w mtr veh in traf, subs
E813.5	MOTR VEH COLLISION W/OTH VEH-INJR ANIMAL RIDER	**V8Ø.31XA**	Animal-rider injured in collision w 2/3-whl mv, init
		V8Ø.31XD	Animal-rider injured in collision w 2/3-whl mv, subs
		V8Ø.32XA	Occ of anml-drn vehicle injured in clsn w 2/3-whl mv, init
		V8Ø.32XD	Occ of anml-drn vehicle injured in clsn w 2/3-whl mv, subs
		V8Ø.41XA	Animl-ridr inj pk-up truck, pick-up truck, van, hv veh, init
		V8Ø.41XD	Animl-ridr inj pk-up truck, pick-up truck, van, hv veh, subs
		V8Ø.42XA	Occ animal-drwn veh injured collision hvy veh, init encntr
		V8Ø.42XD	Occ animal-drwn veh injured collision hvy veh, subs encntr
		V8Ø.51XA	Animal-rider injured in collision w mtr veh, init encntr
		V8Ø.51XD	Animal-rider injured in collision w mtr veh, subs encntr
		V8Ø.52XA	Occupant of anml-drn vehicle injured in clsn w mtr veh, init
		V8Ø.52XD	Occupant of anml-drn vehicle injured in clsn w mtr veh, subs
E813.6	MOTR VEH COLLISION W/OTH VEH-INJR PEDAL CYCLIST	**V12.4XXA**	Pedl cyc driver injured in clsn w 2/3-whl mv in traf, init
		V12.4XXD	Pedl cyc driver injured in clsn w 2/3-whl mv in traf, subs
		V12.5XXA	Pedl cyc pasngr injured in clsn w 2/3-whl mv in traf, init
		V12.5XXD	Pedl cyc pasngr injured in clsn w 2/3-whl mv in traf, subs
		V12.9XXA	Unsp pedl cyclst injured in clsn w 2/3-whl mv in traf, init
		V12.9XXD	Unsp pedl cyclst injured in clsn w 2/3-whl mv in traf, subs
		V13.4XXA	Pedl cyc driver inj pick-up truck, pk-up/van in traf, init
		V13.4XXD	Pedl cyc driver inj pick-up truck, pk-up/van in traf, subs
		V13.5XXA	Pedl cyc pasngr inj pick-up truck, pk-up/van in traf, init
		V13.5XXD	Pedl cyc pasngr inj pick-up truck, pk-up/van in traf, subs
		V13.9XXA	Unsp pedl cyclst inj pick-up truck, pk-up/van in traf, init
		V13.9XXD	Unsp pedl cyclst inj pick-up truck, pk-up/van in traf, subs
		V14.4XXA	Pedl cyc driver injured in collision w hv veh in traf, init
		V14.4XXD	Pedl cyc driver injured in collision w hv veh in traf, subs
		V14.5XXA	Pedl cyc passenger injured in clsn w hv veh in traf, init
		V14.5XXD	Pedl cyc passenger injured in clsn w hv veh in traf, subs
		V14.9XXA	Unsp pedl cyclst injured in collision w hv veh in traf, init
		V14.9XXD	Unsp pedl cyclst injured in collision w hv veh in traf, subs
		V19.4ØXA	Pedl cyc driver injured in collision w unsp mv in traf, init
		V19.4ØXD	Pedl cyc driver injured in collision w unsp mv in traf, subs
		V19.49XA	Pedl cyc driver injured in collision w oth mv in traf, init
		V19.49XD	Pedl cyc driver injured in collision w oth mv in traf, subs
		V19.5ØXA	Pedl cyc passenger injured in clsn w unsp mv in traf, init
		V19.5ØXD	Pedl cyc passenger injured in clsn w unsp mv in traf, subs
		V19.59XA	Pedl cyc passenger injured in clsn w oth mv in traf, init
		V19.59XD	Pedl cyc passenger injured in clsn w oth mv in traf, subs
		V19.6ØXA	Unsp pedl cyclst injured in clsn w unsp mv in traf, init
		V19.6ØXD	Unsp pedl cyclst injured in clsn w unsp mv in traf, subs
		V19.69XA	Unsp pedl cyclst injured in collision w oth mv in traf, init
		V19.69XD	Unsp pedl cyclst injured in collision w oth mv in traf, subs
E813.7	MOTR VEH COLLISION W/OTH VEH-INJR PEDESTRIAN	**VØ3.1ØXA**	Ped on foot injured pick-up truck, pk-up/van in traf, init

ICD-9-CM		ICD-10-CM	
E813.8	MOTR VEH COLLISION W/OTH VEH-INJR OTH PERSON	**V31.6XXA**	Pasngr in 3-whl mv injured in clsn w pedl cyc in traf, init
		V31.6XXD	Pasngr in 3-whl mv injured in clsn w pedl cyc in traf, subs
		V31.7XXA	Person outside 3-whl mv inj in clsn w pedl cyc in traf, init
		V31.7XXD	Person outside 3-whl mv inj in clsn w pedl cyc in traf, subs
		V36.7XXA	Person outsd 3-whl mv inj in clsn w nonmtr veh in traf, init
		V36.7XXD	Person outsd 3-whl mv inj in clsn w nonmtr veh in traf, subs
		V46.7XXA	Person outsd car inj in clsn w nonmtr vehicle in traf, init
		V46.7XXD	Person outsd car inj in clsn w nonmtr vehicle in traf, subs
		V51.7XXA	Person outsd pk-up/van inj in clsn w pedl cyc in traf, init
		V51.7XXD	Person outsd pk-up/van inj in clsn w pedl cyc in traf, subs
		V56.7XXA	Prsn outsd pk-up/van inj in clsn w nonmtr veh in traf, init
		V56.7XXD	Prsn outsd pk-up/van inj in clsn w nonmtr veh in traf, subs
		V61.7XXA	Person outside hv veh inj in clsn w pedl cyc in traf, init
		V61.7XXD	Person outside hv veh inj in clsn w pedl cyc in traf, subs
		V66.7XXA	Person outsd hv veh inj in clsn w nonmtr veh in traf, init
		V66.7XXD	Person outsd hv veh inj in clsn w nonmtr veh in traf, subs
		V71.7XXA	Person outside bus injured in clsn w pedl cyc in traf, init
		V71.7XXD	Person outside bus injured in clsn w pedl cyc in traf, subs
		V76.7XXA	Person outsd bus inj in clsn w nonmtr vehicle in traf, init
		V76.7XXD	Person outsd bus inj in clsn w nonmtr vehicle in traf, subs
E813.9	MOTR VEH COLLISION W/OTH VEH-INJR UNS PERSON	**V21.9XXA**	Unsp mtrcy rider injured in clsn w pedl cyc in traf, init
		V21.9XXD	Unsp mtrcy rider injured in clsn w pedl cyc in traf, subs
		V26.9XXA	Unsp mtrcy rider inj in clsn w nonmtr vehicle in traf, init
		V26.9XXD	Unsp mtrcy rider inj in clsn w nonmtr vehicle in traf, subs
		V31.9XXA	Occup of 3-whl mv injured in clsn w pedl cyc in traf, init
		V31.9XXD	Occup of 3-whl mv injured in clsn w pedl cyc in traf, subs
		V36.9XXA	Occup of 3-whl mv inj in clsn w nonmtr vehicle in traf, init
		V36.9XXD	Occup of 3-whl mv inj in clsn w nonmtr vehicle in traf, subs
		V41.9XXA	Unsp car occupant injured in clsn w pedl cyc in traf, init
		V41.9XXD	Unsp car occupant injured in clsn w pedl cyc in traf, subs
		V46.9XXA	Unsp car occ injured in clsn w nonmtr vehicle in traf, init
		V46.9XXD	Unsp car occ injured in clsn w nonmtr vehicle in traf, subs
		V51.9XXA	Occup of pk-up/van injured in clsn w pedl cyc in traf, init
		V51.9XXD	Occup of pk-up/van injured in clsn w pedl cyc in traf, subs
		V56.9XXA	Occup of pk-up/van inj in clsn w nonmtr veh in traf, init
		V56.9XXD	Occup of pk-up/van inj in clsn w nonmtr veh in traf, subs
		V61.9XXA	Occup of hv veh injured in clsn w pedl cyc in traf, init
		V61.9XXD	Occup of hv veh injured in clsn w pedl cyc in traf, subs
		V66.9XXA	Occup of hv veh inj in clsn w nonmtr vehicle in traf, init
		V66.9XXD	Occup of hv veh inj in clsn w nonmtr vehicle in traf, subs
		V71.9XXA	Occup of bus injured in collision w pedl cyc in traf, init
		V71.9XXD	Occup of bus injured in collision w pedl cyc in traf, subs
		V76.9XXA	Occup of bus injured in clsn w nonmtr vehicle in traf, init
		V76.9XXD	Occup of bus injured in clsn w nonmtr vehicle in traf, subs
		V87.9XXA	Person injured in oth transport acc involving non-mv, init
		V87.9XXD	Person injured in oth transport acc involving non-mv, subs
E814.Ø	MOTOR VEH COLLISION W/PEDSTRN-INJR MV DRIVER	**V3Ø.5XXA**	Driver of 3-whl mv injured in clsn w ped/anml in traf, init
		V3Ø.5XXD	Driver of 3-whl mv injured in clsn w ped/anml in traf, subs
		V4Ø.5XXA	Car driver injured in collision w ped/anml in traf, init
		V4Ø.5XXD	Car driver injured in collision w ped/anml in traf, subs
		V5Ø.5XXA	Driver of pk-up/van injured in clsn w ped/anml in traf, init
		V5Ø.5XXD	Driver of pk-up/van injured in clsn w ped/anml in traf, subs
		V6Ø.5XXA	Driver of hv veh injured in clsn w ped/anml in traf, init
		V6Ø.5XXD	Driver of hv veh injured in clsn w ped/anml in traf, subs
		V7Ø.5XXA	Driver of bus injured in collision w ped/anml in traf, init
		V7Ø.5XXD	Driver of bus injured in collision w ped/anml in traf, subs
E814.1	MOTOR VEH COLLISION W/PEDSTRN-INJR MV PASSENGER	**V3Ø.6XXA**	Pasngr in 3-whl mv injured in clsn w ped/anml in traf, init
		V3Ø.6XXD	Pasngr in 3-whl mv injured in clsn w ped/anml in traf, subs
		V4Ø.6XXA	Car passenger injured in collision w ped/anml in traf, init
		V4Ø.6XXD	Car passenger injured in collision w ped/anml in traf, subs
		V5Ø.6XXA	Pasngr in pk-up/van injured in clsn w ped/anml in traf, init
		V5Ø.6XXD	Pasngr in pk-up/van injured in clsn w ped/anml in traf, subs
		V6Ø.6XXA	Passenger in hv veh injured in clsn w ped/anml in traf, init
		V6Ø.6XXD	Passenger in hv veh injured in clsn w ped/anml in traf, subs
		V7Ø.6XXA	Passenger on bus injured in clsn w ped/anml in traf, init
		V7Ø.6XXD	Passenger on bus injured in clsn w ped/anml in traf, subs
E814.2	MOTOR VEH COLLISION W/PEDSTRN-INJR MOTORCYCLIST	**V2Ø.4XXA**	Mtrcy driver injured in collision w ped/anml in traf, init
		V2Ø.4XXD	Mtrcy driver injured in collision w ped/anml in traf, subs
E814.3	MOTOR VEH COLL W/PEDSTRN-INJR PSNGR MOTRCYCLE	**V2Ø.5XXA**	Mtrcy passenger injured in clsn w ped/anml in traf, init
		V2Ø.5XXD	Mtrcy passenger injured in clsn w ped/anml in traf, subs
E814.4	MOTOR VEH COLL W/PEDSTRN-INJR OCC STREETCAR	**V82.1XXA**	Occupant of stcar injured in clsn w mtr veh in traf, init
E814.5	MOTOR VEH COLL W/PEDSTRN-INJR ANIMAL RIDER	**V8Ø.41XA**	Animl-ridr inj pk-up truck, pick-up truck, van, hv veh, init
E814.6	MOTOR VEH COLLISION W/PEDSTRN-INJR PEDAL CYCLIST	**V13.9XXA**	Unsp pedl cyclst inj pick-up truck, pk-up/van in traf, init
E814.7	MOTOR VEH COLLISION W/PEDSTRN-INJR PEDSTRN	**VØ2.1ØXA**	Ped on foot injured in collision w 2/3-whl mv in traf, init
		VØ2.1ØXD	Ped on foot injured in collision w 2/3-whl mv in traf, subs
		VØ2.11XA	Ped on rolr-skt injured in clsn w 2/3-whl mv in traf, init
		VØ2.11XD	Ped on rolr-skt injured in clsn w 2/3-whl mv in traf, subs
		VØ2.12XA	Ped on sktbrd injured in clsn w 2/3-whl mv in traf, init
		VØ2.12XD	Ped on sktbrd injured in clsn w 2/3-whl mv in traf, subs
		VØ2.19XA	Ped w convey injured in collision w 2/3-whl mv in traf, init
	(Continued on next page)	**VØ2.19XD**	Ped w convey injured in collision w 2/3-whl mv in traf, subs

ICD-9-CM		ICD-10-CM	
E814.7	MOTOR VEH COLLISION W/PEDSTRN-INJR PEDSTRN **(Continued)**	**VØ2.9ØXA**	Ped on foot injured in collision w 2/3-whl mv, unsp, init
		VØ2.9ØXD	Ped on foot injured in collision w 2/3-whl mv, unsp, subs
		VØ2.91XA	Ped on rolr-skt injured in clsn w 2/3-whl mv, unsp, init
		VØ2.91XD	Ped on rolr-skt injured in clsn w 2/3-whl mv, unsp, subs
		VØ2.92XA	Ped on sktbrd injured in collision w 2/3-whl mv, unsp, init
		VØ2.92XD	Ped on sktbrd injured in collision w 2/3-whl mv, unsp, subs
		VØ2.99XA	Ped w convey injured in collision w 2/3-whl mv, unsp, init
		VØ2.99XD	Ped w convey injured in collision w 2/3-whl mv, unsp, subs
		VØ3.1ØXA	Ped on foot injured pick-up truck, pk-up/van in traf, init
		VØ3.1ØXD	Ped on foot injured pick-up truck, pk-up/van in traf, subs
		VØ3.11XA	Ped on rolr-skt inj pick-up truck, pk-up/van in traf, init
		VØ3.11XD	Ped on rolr-skt inj pick-up truck, pk-up/van in traf, subs
		VØ3.12XA	Ped on sktbrd injured pick-up truck, pk-up/van in traf, init
		VØ3.12XD	Ped on sktbrd injured pick-up truck, pk-up/van in traf, subs
		VØ3.19XA	Ped w convey injured pick-up truck, pk-up/van in traf, init
		VØ3.19XD	Ped w convey injured pick-up truck, pk-up/van in traf, subs
		VØ3.9ØXA	Ped on foot injured pick-up truck, pk-up/van, unsp, init
		VØ3.9ØXD	Ped on foot injured pick-up truck, pk-up/van, unsp, subs
		VØ3.91XA	Ped on rolr-skt injured pick-up truck, pk-up/van, unsp, init
		VØ3.91XD	Ped on rolr-skt injured pick-up truck, pk-up/van, unsp, subs
		VØ3.92XA	Ped on sktbrd injured pick-up truck, pk-up/van, unsp, init
		VØ3.92XD	Ped on sktbrd injured pick-up truck, pk-up/van, unsp, subs
		VØ3.99XA	Ped w convey injured pick-up truck, pk-up/van, unsp, init
		VØ3.99XD	Ped w convey injured pick-up truck, pk-up/van, unsp, subs
		VØ4.1ØXA	Ped on foot injured in collision w hv veh in traf, init
		VØ4.1ØXD	Ped on foot injured in collision w hv veh in traf, subs
		VØ4.11XA	Ped on rolr-skt injured in collision w hv veh in traf, init
		VØ4.11XD	Ped on rolr-skt injured in collision w hv veh in traf, subs
		VØ4.12XA	Ped on sktbrd injured in collision w hv veh in traf, init
		VØ4.12XD	Ped on sktbrd injured in collision w hv veh in traf, subs
		VØ4.19XA	Ped w convey injured in collision w hv veh in traf, init
		VØ4.19XD	Ped w convey injured in collision w hv veh in traf, subs
		VØ4.9ØXA	Pedestrian on foot injured in collision w hv veh, unsp, init
		VØ4.9ØXD	Pedestrian on foot injured in collision w hv veh, unsp, subs
		VØ4.91XA	Ped on rolr-skt injured in collision w hv veh, unsp, init
		VØ4.91XD	Ped on rolr-skt injured in collision w hv veh, unsp, subs
		VØ4.92XA	Ped on skateboard injured in collision w hv veh, unsp, init
		VØ4.92XD	Ped on skateboard injured in collision w hv veh, unsp, subs
		VØ4.99XA	Ped w convey injured in collision w hv veh, unsp, init
		VØ4.99XD	Ped w convey injured in collision w hv veh, unsp, subs
		VØ9.2ØXA	Pedestrian injured in traf involving unsp mv, init
		VØ9.2ØXD	Pedestrian injured in traf involving unsp mv, subs
		VØ9.21XA	Pedestrian injured in traf involving military vehicle, init
		VØ9.21XD	Pedestrian injured in traf involving military vehicle, subs
		VØ9.29XA	Pedestrian injured in traf involving oth mv, init
		VØ9.29XD	Pedestrian injured in traf involving oth mv, subs
E814.8	MOTOR VEH COLL W/PEDSTRN-INJR OTH SPEC PERSON	**V3Ø.7XXA**	Person outside 3-whl mv inj in clsn w ped/anml in traf, init
		V3Ø.7XXD	Person outside 3-whl mv inj in clsn w ped/anml in traf, subs
		V4Ø.7XXA	Person outside car injured in clsn w ped/anml in traf, init
		V4Ø.7XXD	Person outside car injured in clsn w ped/anml in traf, subs
		V5Ø.7XXA	Person outsd pk-up/van inj in clsn w ped/anml in traf, init
		V5Ø.7XXD	Person outsd pk-up/van inj in clsn w ped/anml in traf, subs
		V6Ø.7XXA	Person outside hv veh inj in clsn w ped/anml in traf, init
		V6Ø.7XXD	Person outside hv veh inj in clsn w ped/anml in traf, subs
		V7Ø.7XXA	Person outside bus injured in clsn w ped/anml in traf, init
		V7Ø.7XXD	Person outside bus injured in clsn w ped/anml in traf, subs
E814.9	MOTOR VEH COLLISION W/PEDSTRN-INJR UNS PERSON	**V2Ø.9XXA**	Unsp mtrcy rider injured in clsn w ped/anml in traf, init
		V2Ø.9XXD	Unsp mtrcy rider injured in clsn w ped/anml in traf, subs
		V3Ø.9XXA	Occup of 3-whl mv injured in clsn w ped/anml in traf, init
		V3Ø.9XXD	Occup of 3-whl mv injured in clsn w ped/anml in traf, subs
		V4Ø.9XXA	Unsp car occupant injured in clsn w ped/anml in traf, init
		V4Ø.9XXD	Unsp car occupant injured in clsn w ped/anml in traf, subs
		V5Ø.9XXA	Occup of pk-up/van injured in clsn w ped/anml in traf, init
		V5Ø.9XXD	Occup of pk-up/van injured in clsn w ped/anml in traf, subs
		V6Ø.9XXA	Occup of hv veh injured in clsn w ped/anml in traf, init
		V6Ø.9XXD	Occup of hv veh injured in clsn w ped/anml in traf, subs
		V7Ø.9XXA	Occup of bus injured in collision w ped/anml in traf, init
		V7Ø.9XXD	Occup of bus injured in collision w ped/anml in traf, subs
E815.Ø	OTH MOTR VEH COLL W/OBJ HIWAY-INJURING DRIVER	**V37.5XXA**	Drvr of 3-whl mv inj in clsn w statnry object in traf, init
		V37.5XXD	Drvr of 3-whl mv inj in clsn w statnry object in traf, subs
		V39.9XXA	Occupant (driver) of 3-whl mv injured in unsp traf, init
		V39.9XXD	Occupant (driver) of 3-whl mv injured in unsp traf, subs
		V57.5XXA	Drvr of pk-up/van inj in clsn w statnry object in traf, init
		V57.5XXD	Drvr of pk-up/van inj in clsn w statnry object in traf, subs
		V67.5XXA	Driver of hv veh inj in clsn w statnry object in traf, init
		V67.5XXD	Driver of hv veh inj in clsn w statnry object in traf, subs
		V77.5XXA	Driver of bus injured in clsn w statnry object in traf, init
		V77.5XXD	Driver of bus injured in clsn w statnry object in traf, subs
		V86.Ø1XA	Driver of amblnc/fire eng injured in traffic accident, init
		V86.Ø1XD	Driver of amblnc/fire eng injured in traffic accident, subs
		V86.Ø2XA	Driver of snowmobile injured in traffic accident, init
	(Continued on next page)	**V86.Ø2XD**	Driver of snowmobile injured in traffic accident, subs

ICD-9-CM		ICD-10-CM	
E815.Ø	OTH MOTR VEH COLL W/OBJ HIWAY-INJURING DRIVER **(Continued)**	**V86.Ø3XA**	Driver of dune buggy injured in traffic accident, init
		V86.Ø3XD	Driver of dune buggy injured in traffic accident, subs
		V86.Ø4XA	Driver of military vehicle injured in traffic accident, init
		V86.Ø4XD	Driver of military vehicle injured in traffic accident, subs
		V86.Ø9XA	Driver of oth sp off-rd mv injured in traffic accident, init
		V86.Ø9XD	Driver of oth sp off-rd mv injured in traffic accident, subs
E815.1	OTH MOTR VEH COLL W/OBJ HIWAY-INJR PASSENGER	**V37.6XXA**	Pasngr in 3-whl mv inj in clsn w statnry obj in traf, init
		V37.6XXD	Pasngr in 3-whl mv inj in clsn w statnry obj in traf, subs
		V57.6XXA	Pasngr in pk-up/van inj in clsn w statnry obj in traf, init
		V57.6XXD	Pasngr in pk-up/van inj in clsn w statnry obj in traf, subs
		V67.6XXA	Pasngr in hv veh inj in clsn w statnry object in traf, init
		V67.6XXD	Pasngr in hv veh inj in clsn w statnry object in traf, subs
		V77.6XXA	Pasngr on bus injured in clsn w statnry object in traf, init
		V77.6XXD	Pasngr on bus injured in clsn w statnry object in traf, subs
		V86.11XA	Passenger of amblnc/fire eng injured in traf, init
		V86.11XD	Passenger of amblnc/fire eng injured in traf, subs
		V86.12XA	Passenger of snowmobile injured in traffic accident, init
		V86.12XD	Passenger of snowmobile injured in traffic accident, subs
		V86.13XA	Passenger of dune buggy injured in traffic accident, init
		V86.13XD	Passenger of dune buggy injured in traffic accident, subs
		V86.14XA	Passenger of military vehicle injured in traf, init
		V86.14XD	Passenger of military vehicle injured in traf, subs
		V86.19XA	Passenger of sp off-rd mv injured in traffic accident, init
		V86.19XD	Passenger of sp off-rd mv injured in traffic accident, subs
E815.2	OTH MOTR VEH COLL W/OBJ HIWAY-INJR MOTORCYCLIST	**V27.4XXA**	Mtrcy driver injured in clsn w statnry object in traf, init
		V27.4XXD	Mtrcy driver injured in clsn w statnry object in traf, subs
		V29.81XA	Mtrcy rider injured in trnsp acc w military vehicle, init
		V29.81XD	Mtrcy rider injured in trnsp acc w military vehicle, subs
		V29.88XA	Mtrcy rider (driver) injured in oth transport acc, init
		V29.88XD	Mtrcy rider (driver) injured in oth transport acc, subs
E815.3	OTH MOTR VEH COLL W/OBJ HIWAY-INJR MC PSNGR	**V27.5XXA**	Mtrcy pasngr injured in clsn w statnry object in traf, init
		V27.5XXD	Mtrcy pasngr injured in clsn w statnry object in traf, subs
E815.4	OTH MOTR VEH COLL W/OBJ HIWAY INJR OCC STREETCAR	**V82.1XXA**	Occupant of stcar injured in clsn w mtr veh in traf, init
E815.5	OTH MOTR VEH COLL W/OBJ HIWAY-INJR ANIMAL RIDER	**V8Ø.41XA**	Animl-ridr inj pk-up truck, pick-up truck, van, hv veh, init
E815.6	OTH MOTR VEH COLL W/OBJ HIWAY-INJR PEDAL CYCLIST	**V13.9XXA**	Unsp pedl cyclst inj pick-up truck, pk-up/van in traf, init
E815.7	OTH MOTR VEH COLL W/OBJ HIWAY-INJR PEDESTRIAN	**VØ3.1ØXA**	Ped on foot injured pick-up truck, pk-up/van in traf, init
E815.8	OTH MOTR VEH COLL W/OBJ HIWAY-INJR OTH PERSON	**V37.7XXA**	Prsn outsd 3-whl mv inj in clsn w statnry obj in traf, init
		V37.7XXD	Prsn outsd 3-whl mv inj in clsn w statnry obj in traf, subs
		V57.7XXA	Prsn outsd pk-up/van inj in clsn w statnry obj in traf, init
		V57.7XXD	Prsn outsd pk-up/van inj in clsn w statnry obj in traf, subs
		V67.7XXA	Person outsd hv veh inj in clsn w statnry obj in traf, init
		V67.7XXD	Person outsd hv veh inj in clsn w statnry obj in traf, subs
		V77.7XXA	Person outsd bus inj in clsn w statnry object in traf, init
		V77.7XXD	Person outsd bus inj in clsn w statnry object in traf, subs
		V86.21XA	Person on outside of amblnc/fire eng injured in traf, init
		V86.21XD	Person on outside of amblnc/fire eng injured in traf, subs
		V86.22XA	Person on outside of snowmobile injured in traf, init
		V86.22XD	Person on outside of snowmobile injured in traf, subs
		V86.23XA	Person on outside of dune buggy injured in traf, init
		V86.23XD	Person on outside of dune buggy injured in traf, subs
		V86.24XA	Person on outside of military vehicle injured in traf, init
		V86.24XD	Person on outside of military vehicle injured in traf, subs
		V86.29XA	Person on outside of sp off-rd mv injured in traf, init
		V86.29XD	Person on outside of sp off-rd mv injured in traf, subs
E815.9	OTH MOTR VEH COLL W/OBJ HIWAY-INJR UNS PERSON	**V27.9XXA**	Unsp mtrcy rider inj in clsn w statnry object in traf, init
		V27.9XXD	Unsp mtrcy rider inj in clsn w statnry object in traf, subs
		V37.9XXA	Occup of 3-whl mv inj in clsn w statnry object in traf, init
		V37.9XXD	Occup of 3-whl mv inj in clsn w statnry object in traf, subs
		V57.9XXA	Occup of pk-up/van inj in clsn w statnry obj in traf, init
		V57.9XXD	Occup of pk-up/van inj in clsn w statnry obj in traf, subs
		V67.9XXA	Occup of hv veh inj in clsn w statnry object in traf, init
		V67.9XXD	Occup of hv veh inj in clsn w statnry object in traf, subs
		V77.9XXA	Occup of bus injured in clsn w statnry object in traf, init
		V77.9XXD	Occup of bus injured in clsn w statnry object in traf, subs
		V86.31XA	Occup of amblnc/fire eng injured in traffic accident, init
		V86.31XD	Occup of amblnc/fire eng injured in traffic accident, subs
		V86.32XA	Occup of snowmobile injured in traffic accident, init encntr
		V86.32XD	Occup of snowmobile injured in traffic accident, subs encntr
		V86.33XA	Occup of dune buggy injured in traffic accident, init encntr
		V86.33XD	Occup of dune buggy injured in traffic accident, subs encntr
		V86.34XA	Occup of military vehicle injured in traffic accident, init
		V86.34XD	Occup of military vehicle injured in traffic accident, subs
		V86.39XA	Occup of oth sp off-rd mv injured in traffic accident, init
		V86.39XD	Occup of oth sp off-rd mv injured in traffic accident, subs

ICD-9-CM		ICD-10-CM	
E816.Ø	MOTR VEH LOSS CNTRL W/O COLL HIWAY-INJR DRIVER	**V38.5XXA**	Driver of 3-whl mv inj in nonclsn trnsp acc in traf, init
		V38.5XXD	Driver of 3-whl mv inj in nonclsn trnsp acc in traf, subs
		V48.5XXA	Car driver injured in nonclsn trnsp accident in traf, init
		V48.5XXD	Car driver injured in nonclsn trnsp accident in traf, subs
		V58.5XXA	Driver of pk-up/van inj in nonclsn trnsp acc in traf, init
		V58.5XXD	Driver of pk-up/van inj in nonclsn trnsp acc in traf, subs
		V68.5XXA	Driver of hv veh injured in nonclsn trnsp acc in traf, init
		V68.5XXD	Driver of hv veh injured in nonclsn trnsp acc in traf, subs
		V78.5XXA	Driver of bus injured in nonclsn trnsp acc in traf, init
		V78.5XXD	Driver of bus injured in nonclsn trnsp acc in traf, subs
E816.1	MOTR VEH LOSS CNTRL W/O COLL HIWAY-INJR PSNGR	**V38.6XXA**	Pasngr in 3-whl mv inj in nonclsn trnsp acc in traf, init
		V38.6XXD	Pasngr in 3-whl mv inj in nonclsn trnsp acc in traf, subs
		V48.6XXA	Car pasngr injured in nonclsn trnsp accident in traf, init
		V48.6XXD	Car pasngr injured in nonclsn trnsp accident in traf, subs
		V58.6XXA	Pasngr in pk-up/van inj in nonclsn trnsp acc in traf, init
		V58.6XXD	Pasngr in pk-up/van inj in nonclsn trnsp acc in traf, subs
		V68.6XXA	Pasngr in hv veh injured in nonclsn trnsp acc in traf, init
		V68.6XXD	Pasngr in hv veh injured in nonclsn trnsp acc in traf, subs
		V78.6XXA	Pasngr on bus injured in nonclsn trnsp acc in traf, init
		V78.6XXD	Pasngr on bus injured in nonclsn trnsp acc in traf, subs
E816.2	MOTR VEH LOSS CNTRL W/O COLL HIWAY-MOTORCYCLIST	**V28.4XXA**	Mtrcy driver injured in nonclsn trnsp accident in traf, init
		V28.4XXD	Mtrcy driver injured in nonclsn trnsp accident in traf, subs
E816.3	MOTR VEH LOSS CNTRL W/O COLL HIWAY-INJR MC PSNGR	**V28.5XXA**	Mtrcy pasngr injured in nonclsn trnsp accident in traf, init
		V28.5XXD	Mtrcy pasngr injured in nonclsn trnsp accident in traf, subs
E816.4	MOTR VEH LOSS CNTRL W/O COLL HIWAY-ST CAR RIDER	**V82.9XXA**	Occupant of streetcar injured in unsp traffic accident, init
E816.5	MOTR VEH LOSS CNTRL W/O COLL HIWAY-ANIMAL RIDER	**V8Ø.929A**	Occupant of anml-drn vehicle injured in unsp trnsp acc, init
E816.6	MOTR VEH LOSS CNTRL W/O COLL HIWAY-PEDAL CYCLIST	**V19.3XXA**	Pedl cyclst (driver) injured in unsp nontraf, init
E816.7	MOTR VEH LOSS CNTRL W/O COLL HIWAY-INJR PEDSTRN	**VØ9.1XXA**	Pedestrian injured in unsp nontraffic accident, init encntr
E816.8	MOTR VEH LOSS CNTRL W/O COLL HIWAY-INJR OTH PERS	**V38.7XXA**	Person outsd 3-whl mv inj in nonclsn trnsp acc in traf, init
		V38.7XXD	Person outsd 3-whl mv inj in nonclsn trnsp acc in traf, subs
		V48.7XXA	Person outside car inj in nonclsn trnsp acc in traf, init
		V48.7XXD	Person outside car inj in nonclsn trnsp acc in traf, subs
		V58.7XXA	Prsn outsd pk-up/van inj in nonclsn trnsp acc in traf, init
		V58.7XXD	Prsn outsd pk-up/van inj in nonclsn trnsp acc in traf, subs
		V68.7XXA	Person outside hv veh inj in nonclsn trnsp acc in traf, init
		V68.7XXD	Person outside hv veh inj in nonclsn trnsp acc in traf, subs
E816.9	MOTR VEH LOSS CNTRL W/O COLL HIWAY-INJR UNS PERS	**V28.9XXA**	Unsp mtrcy rider injured in nonclsn trnsp acc in traf, init
		V28.9XXD	Unsp mtrcy rider injured in nonclsn trnsp acc in traf, subs
		V38.9XXA	Occup of 3-whl mv injured in nonclsn trnsp acc in traf, init
		V38.9XXD	Occup of 3-whl mv injured in nonclsn trnsp acc in traf, subs
		V48.9XXA	Unsp car occupant injured in nonclsn trnsp acc in traf, init
		V48.9XXD	Unsp car occupant injured in nonclsn trnsp acc in traf, subs
		V58.9XXA	Occup of pk-up/van inj in nonclsn trnsp acc in traf, init
		V58.9XXD	Occup of pk-up/van inj in nonclsn trnsp acc in traf, subs
		V68.9XXA	Occup of hv veh injured in nonclsn trnsp acc in traf, init
		V68.9XXD	Occup of hv veh injured in nonclsn trnsp acc in traf, subs
		V78.9XXA	Occup of bus injured in nonclsn trnsp accident in traf, init
		V78.9XXD	Occup of bus injured in nonclsn trnsp accident in traf, subs
E817.Ø	NONCOLL MOTR VEH ACC BOARD/ALIGHT-INJR DRIVER	**V48.4XXA**	Prsn brd/alit a car injured in nonclsn trnsp accident, init
E817.1	NONCOLL MOTR VEH ACC BOARD/ALIGHT-INJR PASNGR	**V48.4XXA**	Prsn brd/alit a car injured in nonclsn trnsp accident, init
E817.2	NONCOLL MOTR VEH ACC BOARD/ALIGHT-INJR MTRCYCLST	**V28.3XXA**	Prsn brd/alit mtrcy injured in nonclsn trnsp accident, init
E817.3	NONCOLL MOTR VEH ACC BOARD/ALIGHT-INJR MC PSNGR	**V28.3XXA**	Prsn brd/alit mtrcy injured in nonclsn trnsp accident, init
E817.4	NONCOLL MOTR VEH ACC BOARD/ALIGHT-ST CAR RIDER	**V82.4XXA**	Person injured wh brd/alit from streetcar, init
E817.5	NONCOLL MOTR VEH ACC BOARD/ALIGHT-ANIMAL RIDER	**V8Ø.918A**	Animal-rider injured in oth transport accident, init encntr
E817.6	NONCOLL MOTR VEH ACC BOARD/ALIGHT-PEDAL CYCLST	**V18.3XXA**	Prsn brd/alit pedl cyc injured in nonclsn trnsp acc, init
E817.7	NONCOLL MOTR VEH ACC BOARD/ALIGHT-INJR PEDSTRN	**VØ9.2ØXA**	Pedestrian injured in traf involving unsp mv, init
E817.8	NONCOLL MOTR VEH ACC BOARD/ALIGHT-INJR OTH PERS	**V48.4XXA**	Prsn brd/alit a car injured in nonclsn trnsp accident, init
		V48.4XXD	Prsn brd/alit a car injured in nonclsn trnsp accident, subs
E817.9	NONCOLL MOTR VEH ACC BOARD/ALIGHT-INJR UNS PERS	**V87.8XXA**	Person injured in oth nonclsn transport acc w mtr veh, init
E818.Ø	OTH NONCOLL MOTOR VEH ACC-INJURING MV DRIVER	**V48.5XXA**	Car driver injured in nonclsn trnsp accident in traf, init
E818.1	OTH NONCOLL MOTOR VEH ACC-INJR MV PASSENGER	**V48.6XXA**	Car pasngr injured in nonclsn trnsp accident in traf, init
E818.2	OTH NONCOLL MOTOR VEH ACC-INJR MOTORCYCLIST	**V28.4XXA**	Mtrcy driver injured in nonclsn trnsp accident in traf, init
E818.3	OTH NONCOLL MOTOR VEH ACC-INJR MC PASSENGER	**V28.5XXA**	Mtrcy pasngr injured in nonclsn trnsp accident in traf, init
E818.4	OTH NONCOLL MOTOR VEH ACC-INJR STREETCAR RIDER	**V82.8XXA**	Occupant of streetcar injured in oth transport acc, init
E818.5	OTH NONCOLL MOTOR VEH ACC-INJR ANIMAL RIDER	**V8Ø.918A**	Animal-rider injured in oth transport accident, init encntr
E818.6	OTH NONCOLL MOTOR VEH ACC-INJR PEDAL CYCLIST	**V18.9XXA**	Unsp pedl cyclst injured in nonclsn trnsp acc in traf, init
E818.7	OTH NONCOLL MOTOR VEH ACC-INJR PEDESTRIAN	**VØ9.3XXA**	Pedestrian injured in unsp traffic accident, init encntr
E818.8	OTH NONCOLL MOTOR VEH ACC-INJR OTH SPEC PERS	**V78.7XXA**	Person outside bus inj in nonclsn trnsp acc in traf, init
		V78.7XXD	Person outside bus inj in nonclsn trnsp acc in traf, subs
E818.9	OTH NONCOLL MOTOR VEH ACC-INJR UNS PERSON	**V87.8XXA**	Person injured in oth nonclsn transport acc w mtr veh, init
		V87.8XXD	Person injured in oth nonclsn transport acc w mtr veh, subs
E819.Ø	MOTOR VEH ACC UNS NATURE-INJR MOTOR VEH DRIVER	**V49.9XXA**	Car occupant (driver) (passenger) injured in unsp traf, init
		V49.9XXD	Car occupant (driver) (passenger) injured in unsp traf, subs
		V59.9XXA	Occupant (driver) of pk-up/van injured in unsp traf, init
		V59.9XXD	Occupant (driver) of pk-up/van injured in unsp traf, subs
		V69.9XXA	Occupant (driver) of hv veh injured in unsp traf, init

ICD-9-CM		ICD-10-CM	
E819.1	MOTOR VEH ACC UNS NATURE-INJR MOTOR VEH PSNGR	**V49.9XXA**	Car occupant (driver) (passenger) injured in unsp traf, init
		V59.9XXA	Occupant (driver) of pk-up/van injured in unsp traf, init
		V69.9XXA	Occupant (driver) of hv veh injured in unsp traf, init
E819.2	MOTOR VEH ACC UNS NATURE-INJURING MOTRCYCLIST	**V29.9XXA**	Motorcycle rider (driver) injured in unsp traf, init
		V29.9XXD	Motorcycle rider (driver) injured in unsp traf, subs
E819.3	MOTOR VEH ACC UNS NATURE-INJR PSNGR MOTRCYCLE	**V29.9XXA**	Motorcycle rider (driver) injured in unsp traf, init
E819.4	MOTR VEH TRAFFIC ACC UNS NATR INJR OCC STREETCAR	**V82.9XXA**	Occupant of streetcar injured in unsp traffic accident, init
E819.5	MOTOR VEH ACC UNS NATURE-INJURING ANIMAL RIDER	**V8Ø.919A**	Animal-rider injured in unsp transport accident, init encntr
E819.6	MOTOR VEH ACC UNS NATURE-INJURING PEDAL CYCLIST	**V19.9XXA**	Pedl cyclst (driver) (passenger) injured in unsp traf, init
E819.7	MOTOR VEH ACC UNS NATURE-INJURING PEDESTRIAN	**VØ9.3XXA**	Pedestrian injured in unsp traffic accident, init encntr
E819.8	MOTOR VEH ACC UNS NATURE-INJURING OTH PERSON	**V89.2XXA**	Person injured in unsp motor-vehicle accident, traffic, init
E819.9	MOTOR VEH ACC UNS NATURE-INJURING UNS PERSON	**V89.2XXA**	Person injured in unsp motor-vehicle accident, traffic, init
		V89.2XXD	Person injured in unsp motor-vehicle accident, traffic, subs
		V89.3XXA	Person injured in unsp nonmotor-vehicle acc, traffic, init
		V89.3XXD	Person injured in unsp nonmotor-vehicle acc, traffic, subs
		V89.9XXA	Person injured in unspecified vehicle accident, init encntr
		V89.9XXD	Person injured in unspecified vehicle accident, subs encntr
E82Ø.Ø	NONTRFF ACC MOTOR SNOW VEH-INJR MV DRIVER	**V86.52XA**	Driver of snowmobile injured in nontraffic accident, init
		V86.52XD	Driver of snowmobile injured in nontraffic accident, subs
E82Ø.1	NONTRFF ACC MOTOR SNOW VEH-INJR MV PASSENGER	**V86.62XA**	Passenger of snowmobile injured in nontraffic accident, init
		V86.62XD	Passenger of snowmobile injured in nontraffic accident, subs
E82Ø.2	NONTRFF ACC MOTOR SNOW VEH-INJR MOTORCYCLIST	**V88.8XXA**	Person inj in oth nonclsn trnsp acc w mtr veh, nontraf, init
E82Ø.3	NONTRFF ACC MOTOR SNOW VEH-INJR MC PASSENGER	**V88.8XXA**	Person inj in oth nonclsn trnsp acc w mtr veh, nontraf, init
E82Ø.4	NONTRFF ACC MOTOR SNOW VEH-INJR ST CAR RIDER	**V88.8XXA**	Person inj in oth nonclsn trnsp acc w mtr veh, nontraf, init
E82Ø.5	NONTRFF ACC MOTOR SNOW VEH-INJR ANIMAL RIDER	**V88.8XXA**	Person inj in oth nonclsn trnsp acc w mtr veh, nontraf, init
E82Ø.6	NONTRFF ACC MOTOR SNOW VEH-INJR PEDAL CYCLIST	**V88.8XXA**	Person inj in oth nonclsn trnsp acc w mtr veh, nontraf, init
E82Ø.7	NONTRFF ACC MOTOR SNOW VEH-INJURING PEDESTRIAN	**V88.8XXA**	Person inj in oth nonclsn trnsp acc w mtr veh, nontraf, init
E82Ø.8	NONTRFF ACC MOTOR SNOW VEH-INJURING OTH PERSON	**V86.42XA**	Person injured wh brd/alit from snowmobile, init
		V86.42XD	Person injured wh brd/alit from snowmobile, subs
		V86.72XA	Person on outside of snowmobile injured nontraf, init
		V86.72XD	Person on outside of snowmobile injured nontraf, subs
E82Ø.9	NONTRFF ACC MOTOR SNOW VEH-INJURING UNS PERSON	**V86.92XA**	Occup of snowmobile injured in nontraffic accident, init
		V86.92XD	Occup of snowmobile injured in nontraffic accident, subs
E821.Ø	NONTRFF ACC OTH OFF-ROAD MOTR VEH-INJR DRIVER	**V86.53XA**	Driver of dune buggy injured in nontraffic accident, init
		V86.53XD	Driver of dune buggy injured in nontraffic accident, subs
		V86.59XA	Driver of sp off-rd mv injured in nontraffic accident, init
		V86.59XD	Driver of sp off-rd mv injured in nontraffic accident, subs
E821.1	NONTRFF ACC OTH OFF-ROAD MOTR VEH-INJR MV PSNGR	**V86.63XA**	Passenger of dune buggy injured in nontraffic accident, init
		V86.63XD	Passenger of dune buggy injured in nontraffic accident, subs
		V86.69XA	Passenger of sp off-rd mv injured nontraf, init
		V86.69XD	Passenger of sp off-rd mv injured nontraf, subs
E821.2	NONTRFF ACC OTH OFF-ROAD MOTR VEH-INJR MTRCYCL	**V88.8XXA**	Person inj in oth nonclsn trnsp acc w mtr veh, nontraf, init
E821.3	NONTRFF ACC OTH OFF-ROAD MOTR VEH-INJR MC PSNGR	**V88.8XXA**	Person inj in oth nonclsn trnsp acc w mtr veh, nontraf, init
E821.4	NONTRFF ACC OTH OFF-ROAD MOTR VEH-ST CAR RIDER	**V88.8XXA**	Person inj in oth nonclsn trnsp acc w mtr veh, nontraf, init
E821.5	NONTRFF ACC OTH OFF-ROAD MOTR VEH-ANIMAL RIDER	**V88.8XXA**	Person inj in oth nonclsn trnsp acc w mtr veh, nontraf, init
E821.6	NONTRFF ACC OTH OFF-ROAD MOTR VEH-PEDAL CYCLIST	**V88.8XXA**	Person inj in oth nonclsn trnsp acc w mtr veh, nontraf, init
E821.7	NONTRFF ACC OTH OFF-ROAD MOTR VEH-INJR PEDSTRN	**V88.8XXA**	Person inj in oth nonclsn trnsp acc w mtr veh, nontraf, init
E821.8	NONTRFF ACC OTH OFF-ROAD MOTR VEH-INJR OTH PERS	**V86.43XA**	Person injured wh brd/alit from dune buggy, init
		V86.43XD	Person injured wh brd/alit from dune buggy, subs
		V86.49XA	Person injured wh brd/alit from oth sp off-rd mv, init
		V86.49XD	Person injured wh brd/alit from oth sp off-rd mv, subs
		V86.73XA	Person on outside of dune buggy injured nontraf, init
		V86.73XD	Person on outside of dune buggy injured nontraf, subs
		V86.79XA	Person on outside of sp off-rd mv injured nontraf, init
		V86.79XD	Person on outside of sp off-rd mv injured nontraf, subs
E821.9	NONTRFF ACC OTH OFF-ROAD MOTR VEH-INJR UNS PERS	**V86.93XA**	Occup of dune buggy injured in nontraffic accident, init
		V86.93XD	Occup of dune buggy injured in nontraffic accident, subs
		V86.99XA	Occup of sp off-rd mv injured in nontraffic accident, init
		V86.99XD	Occup of sp off-rd mv injured in nontraffic accident, subs
E822.Ø	OTH MOTR VEH NONTRFF COLL W/MOV OBJ-INJR DRIVER	**V3Ø.ØXXA**	Driver of 3-whl mv injured in clsn w ped/anml nontraf, init
		V3Ø.ØXXD	Driver of 3-whl mv injured in clsn w ped/anml nontraf, subs
		V31.ØXXA	Driver of 3-whl mv injured in clsn w pedl cyc nontraf, init
		V31.ØXXD	Driver of 3-whl mv injured in clsn w pedl cyc nontraf, subs
		V32.ØXXA	Driver of 3-whl mv inj in clsn w 2/3-whl mv nontraf, init
		V32.ØXXD	Driver of 3-whl mv inj in clsn w 2/3-whl mv nontraf, subs
		V33.ØXXA	Driver of 3-whl mv inj pk-up truck, pk-up/van nontraf, init
		V33.ØXXD	Driver of 3-whl mv inj pk-up truck, pk-up/van nontraf, subs
		V34.ØXXA	Driver of 3-whl mv injured in clsn w hv veh nontraf, init
		V34.ØXXD	Driver of 3-whl mv injured in clsn w hv veh nontraf, subs
		V35.ØXXA	Driver of 3-whl mv inj in clsn w rail trn/veh nontraf, init
		V35.ØXXD	Driver of 3-whl mv inj in clsn w rail trn/veh nontraf, subs
		V36.ØXXA	Driver of 3-whl mv inj in clsn w nonmtr veh nontraf, init
		V36.ØXXD	Driver of 3-whl mv inj in clsn w nonmtr veh nontraf, subs
		V39.ØØXA	Driver of 3-whl mv injured in clsn w unsp mv nontraf, init
		V39.ØØXD	Driver of 3-whl mv injured in clsn w unsp mv nontraf, subs
	(Continued on next page)	**V39.Ø9XA**	Driver of 3-whl mv injured in clsn w oth mv nontraf, init

[Brackets] indicate valid character values for each code. Character value meanings provided for each code grouping.

ICD-9-CM		ICD-10-CM	
E822.Ø	OTH MOTR VEH NONTRFF COLL W/MOV OBJ-INJR DRIVER **(Continued)**	**V39.Ø9XD**	Driver of 3-whl mv injured in clsn w oth mv nontraf, subs
		V4Ø.ØXXA	Car driver injured in collision w ped/anml nontraf, init
		V4Ø.ØXXD	Car driver injured in collision w ped/anml nontraf, subs
		V41.ØXXA	Car driver injured in collision w pedal cycle nontraf, init
		V41.ØXXD	Car driver injured in collision w pedal cycle nontraf, subs
		V42.ØXXA	Car driver injured in collision w 2/3-whl mv nontraf, init
		V42.ØXXD	Car driver injured in collision w 2/3-whl mv nontraf, subs
		V43.Ø1XA	Car driver injured in collision w SUV nontraf, init
		V43.Ø1XD	Car driver injured in collision w SUV nontraf, subs
		V43.Ø2XA	Car driver injured in collision w car nontraf, init
		V43.Ø2XD	Car driver injured in collision w car nontraf, subs
		V43.Ø3XA	Car driver injured in clsn w pick-up truck nontraf, init
		V43.Ø3XD	Car driver injured in clsn w pick-up truck nontraf, subs
		V43.Ø4XA	Car driver injured in collision w van nontraf, init
		V43.Ø4XD	Car driver injured in collision w van nontraf, subs
		V44.ØXXA	Car driver injured in collision w hv veh nontraf, init
		V44.ØXXD	Car driver injured in collision w hv veh nontraf, subs
		V45.ØXXA	Car driver injured in collision w rail trn/veh nontraf, init
		V45.ØXXD	Car driver injured in collision w rail trn/veh nontraf, subs
		V46.ØXXA	Car driver injured in clsn w nonmtr vehicle nontraf, init
		V46.ØXXD	Car driver injured in clsn w nonmtr vehicle nontraf, subs
		V48.ØXXA	Car driver injured in nonclsn trnsp accident nontraf, init
		V48.ØXXD	Car driver injured in nonclsn trnsp accident nontraf, subs
		V49.ØØXA	Driver injured in collision w unsp mv nontraf, init
		V49.ØØXD	Driver injured in collision w unsp mv nontraf, subs
		V49.Ø9XA	Driver injured in collision w oth mv nontraf, init
		V49.Ø9XD	Driver injured in collision w oth mv nontraf, subs
		V5Ø.ØXXA	Driver of pk-up/van injured in clsn w ped/anml nontraf, init
		V5Ø.ØXXD	Driver of pk-up/van injured in clsn w ped/anml nontraf, subs
		V51.ØXXA	Driver of pk-up/van injured in clsn w pedl cyc nontraf, init
		V51.ØXXD	Driver of pk-up/van injured in clsn w pedl cyc nontraf, subs
		V52.ØXXA	Driver of pk-up/van inj in clsn w 2/3-whl mv nontraf, init
		V52.ØXXD	Driver of pk-up/van inj in clsn w 2/3-whl mv nontraf, subs
		V53.ØXXA	Driver of pk-up/van inj pk-up truck, pk-up/van nontraf, init
		V53.ØXXD	Driver of pk-up/van inj pk-up truck, pk-up/van nontraf, subs
		V54.ØXXA	Driver of pk-up/van injured in clsn w hv veh nontraf, init
		V54.ØXXD	Driver of pk-up/van injured in clsn w hv veh nontraf, subs
		V55.ØXXA	Driver of pk-up/van inj in clsn w rail trn/veh nontraf, init
		V55.ØXXD	Driver of pk-up/van inj in clsn w rail trn/veh nontraf, subs
		V56.ØXXA	Driver of pk-up/van inj in clsn w nonmtr veh nontraf, init
		V56.ØXXD	Driver of pk-up/van inj in clsn w nonmtr veh nontraf, subs
		V59.ØØXA	Driver of pk-up/van injured in clsn w unsp mv nontraf, init
		V59.ØØXD	Driver of pk-up/van injured in clsn w unsp mv nontraf, subs
		V59.Ø9XA	Driver of pk-up/van injured in clsn w oth mv nontraf, init
		V59.Ø9XD	Driver of pk-up/van injured in clsn w oth mv nontraf, subs
		V6Ø.ØXXA	Driver of hv veh injured in clsn w ped/anml nontraf, init
		V6Ø.ØXXD	Driver of hv veh injured in clsn w ped/anml nontraf, subs
		V61.ØXXA	Driver of hv veh injured in clsn w pedl cyc nontraf, init
		V61.ØXXD	Driver of hv veh injured in clsn w pedl cyc nontraf, subs
		V62.ØXXA	Driver of hv veh injured in clsn w 2/3-whl mv nontraf, init
		V62.ØXXD	Driver of hv veh injured in clsn w 2/3-whl mv nontraf, subs
		V63.ØXXA	Driver of hv veh inj pick-up truck, pk-up/van nontraf, init
		V63.ØXXD	Driver of hv veh inj pick-up truck, pk-up/van nontraf, subs
		V64.ØXXA	Driver of hv veh injured in collision w hv veh nontraf, init
		V64.ØXXD	Driver of hv veh injured in collision w hv veh nontraf, subs
		V65.ØXXA	Driver of hv veh inj in clsn w rail trn/veh nontraf, init
		V65.ØXXD	Driver of hv veh inj in clsn w rail trn/veh nontraf, subs
		V66.ØXXA	Driver of hv veh inj in clsn w nonmtr vehicle nontraf, init
		V66.ØXXD	Driver of hv veh inj in clsn w nonmtr vehicle nontraf, subs
		V69.ØØXA	Driver of hv veh injured in clsn w unsp mv nontraf, init
		V69.ØØXD	Driver of hv veh injured in clsn w unsp mv nontraf, subs
		V69.Ø9XA	Driver of hv veh injured in collision w oth mv nontraf, init
		V69.Ø9XD	Driver of hv veh injured in collision w oth mv nontraf, subs
		V7Ø.ØXXA	Driver of bus injured in collision w ped/anml nontraf, init
		V7Ø.ØXXD	Driver of bus injured in collision w ped/anml nontraf, subs
		V71.ØXXA	Driver of bus injured in collision w pedl cyc nontraf, init
		V71.ØXXD	Driver of bus injured in collision w pedl cyc nontraf, subs
		V72.ØXXA	Driver of bus injured in clsn w 2/3-whl mv nontraf, init
		V72.ØXXD	Driver of bus injured in clsn w 2/3-whl mv nontraf, subs
		V73.ØXXA	Driver of bus injured pick-up truck, pk-up/van nontraf, init
		V73.ØXXD	Driver of bus injured pick-up truck, pk-up/van nontraf, subs
		V74.ØXXA	Driver of bus injured in collision w hv veh nontraf, init
		V74.ØXXD	Driver of bus injured in collision w hv veh nontraf, subs
		V75.ØXXA	Driver of bus injured in clsn w rail trn/veh nontraf, init
		V75.ØXXD	Driver of bus injured in clsn w rail trn/veh nontraf, subs
		V76.ØXXA	Driver of bus injured in clsn w nonmtr vehicle nontraf, init
		V76.ØXXD	Driver of bus injured in clsn w nonmtr vehicle nontraf, subs
		V79.ØØXA	Driver of bus injured in collision w unsp mv nontraf, init
		V79.ØØXD	Driver of bus injured in collision w unsp mv nontraf, subs
		V79.Ø9XA	Driver of bus injured in collision w oth mv nontraf, init
		V79.Ø9XD	Driver of bus injured in collision w oth mv nontraf, subs
	(Continued on next page)	**V84.5XXA**	Driver of special agricultural vehicle injured nontraf, init

ICD-9-CM		ICD-10-CM	
E822.Ø	OTH MOTR VEH NONTRFF COLL W/MOV OBJ-INJR DRIVER **(Continued)**	**V84.5XXD**	Driver of special agricultural vehicle injured nontraf, subs
		V85.5XXA	Driver of special construction vehicle injured nontraf, init
		V85.5XXD	Driver of special construction vehicle injured nontraf, subs
		V86.51XA	Driver of amblnc/fire eng injured nontraf, init
		V86.51XD	Driver of amblnc/fire eng injured nontraf, subs
		V86.54XA	Driver of military vehicle injured nontraf, init
		V86.54XD	Driver of military vehicle injured nontraf, subs
E822.1	OTH MOTR VEH NONTRFF COLL W/MOV OBJ-INJR PSNGR	**V3Ø.1XXA**	Pasngr in 3-whl mv injured in clsn w ped/anml nontraf, init
		V3Ø.1XXD	Pasngr in 3-whl mv injured in clsn w ped/anml nontraf, subs
		V31.1XXA	Pasngr in 3-whl mv injured in clsn w pedl cyc nontraf, init
		V31.1XXD	Pasngr in 3-whl mv injured in clsn w pedl cyc nontraf, subs
		V32.1XXA	Pasngr in 3-whl mv inj in clsn w 2/3-whl mv nontraf, init
		V32.1XXD	Pasngr in 3-whl mv inj in clsn w 2/3-whl mv nontraf, subs
		V33.1XXA	Pasngr in 3-whl mv inj pk-up truck, pk-up/van nontraf, init
		V33.1XXD	Pasngr in 3-whl mv inj pk-up truck, pk-up/van nontraf, subs
		V34.1XXA	Passenger in 3-whl mv injured in clsn w hv veh nontraf, init
		V34.1XXD	Passenger in 3-whl mv injured in clsn w hv veh nontraf, subs
		V35.1XXA	Pasngr in 3-whl mv inj in clsn w rail trn/veh nontraf, init
		V35.1XXD	Pasngr in 3-whl mv inj in clsn w rail trn/veh nontraf, subs
		V36.1XXA	Pasngr in 3-whl mv inj in clsn w nonmtr veh nontraf, init
		V36.1XXD	Pasngr in 3-whl mv inj in clsn w nonmtr veh nontraf, subs
		V39.1ØXA	Pasngr in 3-whl mv injured in clsn w unsp mv nontraf, init
		V39.1ØXD	Pasngr in 3-whl mv injured in clsn w unsp mv nontraf, subs
		V39.19XA	Passenger in 3-whl mv injured in clsn w oth mv nontraf, init
		V39.19XD	Passenger in 3-whl mv injured in clsn w oth mv nontraf, subs
		V4Ø.1XXA	Car passenger injured in collision w ped/anml nontraf, init
		V4Ø.1XXD	Car passenger injured in collision w ped/anml nontraf, subs
		V41.1XXA	Car passenger injured in collision w pedl cyc nontraf, init
		V41.1XXD	Car passenger injured in collision w pedl cyc nontraf, subs
		V42.1XXA	Car passenger injured in clsn w 2/3-whl mv nontraf, init
		V42.1XXD	Car passenger injured in clsn w 2/3-whl mv nontraf, subs
		V43.11XA	Car passenger injured in collision w SUV nontraf, init
		V43.11XD	Car passenger injured in collision w SUV nontraf, subs
		V43.12XA	Car passenger injured in collision w car nontraf, init
		V43.12XD	Car passenger injured in collision w car nontraf, subs
		V43.13XA	Car passenger injured in collision w pick-up nontraf, init
		V43.13XD	Car passenger injured in collision w pick-up nontraf, subs
		V43.14XA	Car passenger injured in collision w van nontraf, init
		V43.14XD	Car passenger injured in collision w van nontraf, subs
		V44.1XXA	Car passenger injured in collision w hv veh nontraf, init
		V44.1XXD	Car passenger injured in collision w hv veh nontraf, subs
		V45.1XXA	Car passenger injured in clsn w rail trn/veh nontraf, init
		V45.1XXD	Car passenger injured in clsn w rail trn/veh nontraf, subs
		V46.1XXA	Car passenger injured in clsn w nonmtr vehicle nontraf, init
		V46.1XXD	Car passenger injured in clsn w nonmtr vehicle nontraf, subs
		V48.1XXA	Car pasngr injured in nonclsn trnsp accident nontraf, init
		V48.1XXD	Car pasngr injured in nonclsn trnsp accident nontraf, subs
		V49.1ØXA	Passenger injured in collision w unsp mv nontraf, init
		V49.1ØXD	Passenger injured in collision w unsp mv nontraf, subs
		V49.19XA	Passenger injured in collision w oth mv nontraf, init
		V49.19XD	Passenger injured in collision w oth mv nontraf, subs
		V5Ø.1XXA	Pasngr in pk-up/van injured in clsn w ped/anml nontraf, init
		V5Ø.1XXD	Pasngr in pk-up/van injured in clsn w ped/anml nontraf, subs
		V51.1XXA	Pasngr in pk-up/van injured in clsn w pedl cyc nontraf, init
		V51.1XXD	Pasngr in pk-up/van injured in clsn w pedl cyc nontraf, subs
		V52.1XXA	Pasngr in pk-up/van inj in clsn w 2/3-whl mv nontraf, init
		V52.1XXD	Pasngr in pk-up/van inj in clsn w 2/3-whl mv nontraf, subs
		V53.1XXA	Pasngr in pk-up/van inj pk-up truck, pk-up/van nontraf, init
		V53.1XXD	Pasngr in pk-up/van inj pk-up truck, pk-up/van nontraf, subs
		V54.1XXA	Pasngr in pk-up/van injured in clsn w hv veh nontraf, init
		V54.1XXD	Pasngr in pk-up/van injured in clsn w hv veh nontraf, subs
		V55.1XXA	Pasngr in pk-up/van inj in clsn w rail trn/veh nontraf, init
		V55.1XXD	Pasngr in pk-up/van inj in clsn w rail trn/veh nontraf, subs
		V56.1XXA	Pasngr in pk-up/van inj in clsn w nonmtr veh nontraf, init
		V56.1XXD	Pasngr in pk-up/van inj in clsn w nonmtr veh nontraf, subs
		V59.1ØXA	Pasngr in pk-up/van injured in clsn w unsp mv nontraf, init
		V59.1ØXD	Pasngr in pk-up/van injured in clsn w unsp mv nontraf, subs
		V59.19XA	Pasngr in pk-up/van injured in clsn w oth mv nontraf, init
		V59.19XD	Pasngr in pk-up/van injured in clsn w oth mv nontraf, subs
		V6Ø.1XXA	Passenger in hv veh injured in clsn w ped/anml nontraf, init
		V6Ø.1XXD	Passenger in hv veh injured in clsn w ped/anml nontraf, subs
		V61.1XXA	Passenger in hv veh injured in clsn w pedl cyc nontraf, init
		V61.1XXD	Passenger in hv veh injured in clsn w pedl cyc nontraf, subs
		V62.1XXA	Pasngr in hv veh injured in clsn w 2/3-whl mv nontraf, init
		V62.1XXD	Pasngr in hv veh injured in clsn w 2/3-whl mv nontraf, subs
		V63.1XXA	Pasngr in hv veh inj pick-up truck, pk-up/van nontraf, init
		V63.1XXD	Pasngr in hv veh inj pick-up truck, pk-up/van nontraf, subs
		V64.1XXA	Passenger in hv veh injured in clsn w hv veh nontraf, init
		V64.1XXD	Passenger in hv veh injured in clsn w hv veh nontraf, subs
		V65.1XXA	Pasngr in hv veh inj in clsn w rail trn/veh nontraf, init
		V65.1XXD	Pasngr in hv veh inj in clsn w rail trn/veh nontraf, subs
	(Continued on next page)	**V66.1XXA**	Pasngr in hv veh inj in clsn w nonmtr vehicle nontraf, init

 [Brackets] indicate valid character values for each code. Character value meanings provided for each code grouping.

ICD-9-CM		ICD-10-CM	
E822.1	OTH MOTR VEH NONTRFF COLL W/MOV OBJ-INJR PSNGR **(Continued)**	**V66.1XXD**	Pasngr in hv veh inj in clsn w nonmtr vehicle nontraf, subs
		V69.1ØXA	Passenger in hv veh injured in clsn w unsp mv nontraf, init
		V69.1ØXD	Passenger in hv veh injured in clsn w unsp mv nontraf, subs
		V69.19XA	Passenger in hv veh injured in clsn w oth mv nontraf, init
		V69.19XD	Passenger in hv veh injured in clsn w oth mv nontraf, subs
		V7Ø.1XXA	Passenger on bus injured in clsn w ped/anml nontraf, init
		V7Ø.1XXD	Passenger on bus injured in clsn w ped/anml nontraf, subs
		V71.1XXA	Passenger on bus injured in clsn w pedl cyc nontraf, init
		V71.1XXD	Passenger on bus injured in clsn w pedl cyc nontraf, subs
		V72.1XXA	Passenger on bus injured in clsn w 2/3-whl mv nontraf, init
		V72.1XXD	Passenger on bus injured in clsn w 2/3-whl mv nontraf, subs
		V73.1XXA	Pasngr on bus injured pick-up truck, pk-up/van nontraf, init
		V73.1XXD	Pasngr on bus injured pick-up truck, pk-up/van nontraf, subs
		V74.1XXA	Passenger on bus injured in collision w hv veh nontraf, init
		V74.1XXD	Passenger on bus injured in collision w hv veh nontraf, subs
		V75.1XXA	Pasngr on bus injured in clsn w rail trn/veh nontraf, init
		V75.1XXD	Pasngr on bus injured in clsn w rail trn/veh nontraf, subs
		V76.1XXA	Pasngr on bus injured in clsn w nonmtr vehicle nontraf, init
		V76.1XXD	Pasngr on bus injured in clsn w nonmtr vehicle nontraf, subs
		V79.1ØXA	Passenger on bus injured in clsn w unsp mv nontraf, init
		V79.1ØXD	Passenger on bus injured in clsn w unsp mv nontraf, subs
		V79.19XA	Passenger on bus injured in collision w oth mv nontraf, init
		V79.19XD	Passenger on bus injured in collision w oth mv nontraf, subs
		V84.6XXA	Passenger of special agri vehicle injured nontraf, init
		V84.6XXD	Passenger of special agri vehicle injured nontraf, subs
		V85.6XXA	Passenger of special construct vehicle injured nontraf, init
		V85.6XXD	Passenger of special construct vehicle injured nontraf, subs
		V86.61XA	Passenger of amblnc/fire eng injured nontraf, init
		V86.61XD	Passenger of amblnc/fire eng injured nontraf, subs
		V86.64XA	Passenger of military vehicle injured nontraf, init
		V86.64XD	Passenger of military vehicle injured nontraf, subs
E822.2	OTH MOTR VEH NONTRFF COLL W/MOV OBJ-MTRCYCLST	**V2Ø.ØXXA**	Mtrcy driver injured in collision w ped/anml nontraf, init
		V2Ø.ØXXD	Mtrcy driver injured in collision w ped/anml nontraf, subs
		V21.ØXXA	Mtrcy driver injured in collision w pedl cyc nontraf, init
		V21.ØXXD	Mtrcy driver injured in collision w pedl cyc nontraf, subs
		V22.ØXXA	Mtrcy driver injured in collision w 2/3-whl mv nontraf, init
		V22.ØXXD	Mtrcy driver injured in collision w 2/3-whl mv nontraf, subs
		V22.4XXA	Mtrcy driver injured in collision w 2/3-whl mv in traf, init
		V22.4XXD	Mtrcy driver injured in collision w 2/3-whl mv in traf, subs
		V23.ØXXA	Mtrcy driver injured pick-up truck, pk-up/van nontraf, init
		V23.ØXXD	Mtrcy driver injured pick-up truck, pk-up/van nontraf, subs
		V24.ØXXA	Mtrcy driver injured in collision w hv veh nontraf, init
		V24.ØXXD	Mtrcy driver injured in collision w hv veh nontraf, subs
		V25.ØXXA	Mtrcy driver injured in clsn w rail trn/veh nontraf, init
		V25.ØXXD	Mtrcy driver injured in clsn w rail trn/veh nontraf, subs
		V26.ØXXA	Mtrcy driver injured in clsn w nonmtr vehicle nontraf, init
		V26.ØXXD	Mtrcy driver injured in clsn w nonmtr vehicle nontraf, subs
		V29.ØØXA	Mtrcy driver injured in collision w unsp mv nontraf, init
		V29.ØØXD	Mtrcy driver injured in collision w unsp mv nontraf, subs
		V29.Ø9XA	Mtrcy driver injured in collision w oth mv nontraf, init
		V29.Ø9XD	Mtrcy driver injured in collision w oth mv nontraf, subs
E822.3	OTH MOTR VEH NONTRFF COLL W/MOV OBJ-MC PSNGR	**V2Ø.1XXA**	Mtrcy passenger injured in clsn w ped/anml nontraf, init
		V2Ø.1XXD	Mtrcy passenger injured in clsn w ped/anml nontraf, subs
		V21.1XXA	Mtrcy passenger injured in clsn w pedl cyc nontraf, init
		V21.1XXD	Mtrcy passenger injured in clsn w pedl cyc nontraf, subs
		V22.1XXA	Mtrcy passenger injured in clsn w 2/3-whl mv nontraf, init
		V22.1XXD	Mtrcy passenger injured in clsn w 2/3-whl mv nontraf, subs
		V22.5XXA	Mtrcy passenger injured in clsn w 2/3-whl mv in traf, init
		V22.5XXD	Mtrcy passenger injured in clsn w 2/3-whl mv in traf, subs
		V23.1XXA	Mtrcy pasngr injured pick-up truck, pk-up/van nontraf, init
		V23.1XXD	Mtrcy pasngr injured pick-up truck, pk-up/van nontraf, subs
		V24.1XXA	Mtrcy passenger injured in collision w hv veh nontraf, init
		V24.1XXD	Mtrcy passenger injured in collision w hv veh nontraf, subs
		V25.1XXA	Mtrcy passenger injured in clsn w rail trn/veh nontraf, init
		V25.1XXD	Mtrcy passenger injured in clsn w rail trn/veh nontraf, subs
		V26.1XXA	Mtrcy pasngr injured in clsn w nonmtr vehicle nontraf, init
		V26.1XXD	Mtrcy pasngr injured in clsn w nonmtr vehicle nontraf, subs
		V29.1ØXA	Mtrcy passenger injured in collision w unsp mv nontraf, init
		V29.1ØXD	Mtrcy passenger injured in collision w unsp mv nontraf, subs
E822.4	OTH MOTR VEH NONTRFF COLL W/MOV OBJ-ST CAR RIDR	**V82.ØXXA**	Occupant of stcar injured in clsn w mtr veh nontraf, init
		V82.ØXXD	Occupant of stcar injured in clsn w mtr veh nontraf, subs
E822.5	OTH MOTR VEH NONTRFF COLL W/MOV OBJ-ANIM RIDER	**V8Ø.918A**	Animal-rider injured in oth transport accident, init encntr
E822.6	OTH MOTR VEH NONTRFF COLL W/MOV OBJ-PED CYCLST	**V12.ØXXA**	Pedl cyc driver injured in clsn w 2/3-whl mv nontraf, init
		V12.ØXXD	Pedl cyc driver injured in clsn w 2/3-whl mv nontraf, subs
		V12.1XXA	Pedl cyc pasngr injured in clsn w 2/3-whl mv nontraf, init
		V12.1XXD	Pedl cyc pasngr injured in clsn w 2/3-whl mv nontraf, subs
		V12.2XXA	Unsp pedl cyclst injured in clsn w 2/3-whl mv nontraf, init
		V12.2XXD	Unsp pedl cyclst injured in clsn w 2/3-whl mv nontraf, subs
		V13.ØXXA	Pedl cyc driver inj pick-up truck, pk-up/van nontraf, init
		V13.ØXXD	Pedl cyc driver inj pick-up truck, pk-up/van nontraf, subs
		V13.1XXA	Pedl cyc pasngr inj pick-up truck, pk-up/van nontraf, init
	(Continued on next page)	**V13.1XXD**	Pedl cyc pasngr inj pick-up truck, pk-up/van nontraf, subs

ICD-9-CM		ICD-10-CM	
E822.6	OTH MOTR VEH NONTRFF COLL W/MOV OBJ-PED CYCLST **(Continued)**	**V13.2XXA**	Unsp pedl cyclst inj pick-up truck, pk-up/van nontraf, init
		V13.2XXD	Unsp pedl cyclst inj pick-up truck, pk-up/van nontraf, subs
		V14.0XXA	Pedl cyc driver injured in collision w hv veh nontraf, init
		V14.0XXD	Pedl cyc driver injured in collision w hv veh nontraf, subs
		V14.1XXA	Pedl cyc passenger injured in clsn w hv veh nontraf, init
		V14.1XXD	Pedl cyc passenger injured in clsn w hv veh nontraf, subs
		V14.2XXA	Unsp pedl cyclst injured in collision w hv veh nontraf, init
		V14.2XXD	Unsp pedl cyclst injured in collision w hv veh nontraf, subs
		V15.0XXA	Pedl cyc driver injured in clsn w rail trn/veh nontraf, init
		V15.0XXD	Pedl cyc driver injured in clsn w rail trn/veh nontraf, subs
		V15.1XXA	Pedl cyc pasngr injured in clsn w rail trn/veh nontraf, init
		V15.1XXD	Pedl cyc pasngr injured in clsn w rail trn/veh nontraf, subs
		V19.00XA	Pedl cyc driver injured in collision w unsp mv nontraf, init
		V19.00XD	Pedl cyc driver injured in collision w unsp mv nontraf, subs
		V19.09XA	Pedl cyc driver injured in collision w oth mv nontraf, init
		V19.09XD	Pedl cyc driver injured in collision w oth mv nontraf, subs
		V19.10XA	Pedl cyc passenger injured in clsn w unsp mv nontraf, init
		V19.10XD	Pedl cyc passenger injured in clsn w unsp mv nontraf, subs
		V19.19XA	Pedl cyc passenger injured in clsn w oth mv nontraf, init
		V19.19XD	Pedl cyc passenger injured in clsn w oth mv nontraf, subs
		V19.20XA	Unsp pedl cyclst injured in clsn w unsp mv nontraf, init
		V19.20XD	Unsp pedl cyclst injured in clsn w unsp mv nontraf, subs
		V19.29XA	Unsp pedl cyclst injured in collision w oth mv nontraf, init
		V19.29XD	Unsp pedl cyclst injured in collision w oth mv nontraf, subs
		V19.81XA	Pedl cyclst injured in trnsp acc w military vehicle, init
		V19.81XD	Pedl cyclst injured in trnsp acc w military vehicle, subs
E822.7	OTH MOTR VEH NONTRFF COLL W/MOV OBJ-PEDSTRN	**V02.00XA**	Ped on foot injured in collision w 2/3-whl mv nontraf, init
		V02.00XD	Ped on foot injured in collision w 2/3-whl mv nontraf, subs
		V02.01XA	Ped on rolr-skt injured in clsn w 2/3-whl mv nontraf, init
		V02.01XD	Ped on rolr-skt injured in clsn w 2/3-whl mv nontraf, subs
		V02.02XA	Ped on sktbrd injured in clsn w 2/3-whl mv nontraf, init
		V02.02XD	Ped on sktbrd injured in clsn w 2/3-whl mv nontraf, subs
		V02.09XA	Ped w convey injured in collision w 2/3-whl mv nontraf, init
		V02.09XD	Ped w convey injured in collision w 2/3-whl mv nontraf, subs
		V03.00XA	Ped on foot injured pick-up truck, pk-up/van nontraf, init
		V03.00XD	Ped on foot injured pick-up truck, pk-up/van nontraf, subs
		V03.01XA	Ped on rolr-skt inj pick-up truck, pk-up/van nontraf, init
		V03.01XD	Ped on rolr-skt inj pick-up truck, pk-up/van nontraf, subs
		V03.02XA	Ped on sktbrd injured pick-up truck, pk-up/van nontraf, init
		V03.02XD	Ped on sktbrd injured pick-up truck, pk-up/van nontraf, subs
		V03.09XA	Ped w convey injured pick-up truck, pk-up/van nontraf, init
		V03.09XD	Ped w convey injured pick-up truck, pk-up/van nontraf, subs
		V04.00XA	Ped on foot injured in collision w hv veh nontraf, init
		V04.00XD	Ped on foot injured in collision w hv veh nontraf, subs
		V04.01XA	Ped on rolr-skt injured in collision w hv veh nontraf, init
		V04.01XD	Ped on rolr-skt injured in collision w hv veh nontraf, subs
		V04.02XA	Ped on sktbrd injured in collision w hv veh nontraf, init
		V04.02XD	Ped on sktbrd injured in collision w hv veh nontraf, subs
		V04.09XA	Ped w convey injured in collision w hv veh nontraf, init
		V04.09XD	Ped w convey injured in collision w hv veh nontraf, subs
		V09.00XA	Pedestrian injured nontraf involving unsp mv, init
		V09.00XD	Pedestrian injured nontraf involving unsp mv, subs
		V09.01XA	Pedestrian injured nontraf involving military vehicle, init
		V09.01XD	Pedestrian injured nontraf involving military vehicle, subs
		V09.09XA	Pedestrian injured nontraf involving oth mv, init
		V09.09XD	Pedestrian injured nontraf involving oth mv, subs
E822.8	OTH MOTR VEH NONTRFF COLL W/MOV OBJ-OTH PERSON	**V30.2XXA**	Person outside 3-whl mv inj in clsn w ped/anml nontraf, init
		V30.2XXD	Person outside 3-whl mv inj in clsn w ped/anml nontraf, subs
		V31.2XXA	Person outside 3-whl mv inj in clsn w pedl cyc nontraf, init
		V31.2XXD	Person outside 3-whl mv inj in clsn w pedl cyc nontraf, subs
		V32.2XXA	Person outsd 3-whl mv inj in clsn w 2/3-whl mv nontraf, init
		V32.2XXD	Person outsd 3-whl mv inj in clsn w 2/3-whl mv nontraf, subs
		V33.2XXA	Prsn outsd 3-whl mv inj pk-up truck, pk-up/van nontraf, init
		V33.2XXD	Prsn outsd 3-whl mv inj pk-up truck, pk-up/van nontraf, subs
		V34.2XXA	Person outside 3-whl mv inj in clsn w hv veh nontraf, init
		V34.2XXD	Person outside 3-whl mv inj in clsn w hv veh nontraf, subs
		V35.2XXA	Prsn outsd 3-whl mv inj in clsn w rail trn/veh nontraf, init
		V35.2XXD	Prsn outsd 3-whl mv inj in clsn w rail trn/veh nontraf, subs
		V36.2XXA	Person outsd 3-whl mv inj in clsn w nonmtr veh nontraf, init
		V36.2XXD	Person outsd 3-whl mv inj in clsn w nonmtr veh nontraf, subs
		V40.2XXA	Person outside car injured in clsn w ped/anml nontraf, init
		V40.2XXD	Person outside car injured in clsn w ped/anml nontraf, subs
		V41.2XXA	Person outside car injured in clsn w pedl cyc nontraf, init
		V41.2XXD	Person outside car injured in clsn w pedl cyc nontraf, subs
		V42.2XXA	Person outside car inj in clsn w 2/3-whl mv nontraf, init
		V42.2XXD	Person outside car inj in clsn w 2/3-whl mv nontraf, subs
		V43.21XA	Person outside car injured in collision w SUV nontraf, init
		V43.21XD	Person outside car injured in collision w SUV nontraf, subs
		V43.22XA	Person outside car injured in collision w car nontraf, init
		V43.22XD	Person outside car injured in collision w car nontraf, subs
		V43.23XA	Person outside car inj in clsn w pick-up truck nontraf, init
		V43.23XD	Person outside car inj in clsn w pick-up truck nontraf, subs
	(Continued on next page)	**V43.24XA**	Person outside car injured in collision w van nontraf, init

ICD-9-CM		ICD-10-CM	
E822.8	OTH MOTR VEH NONTRFF COLL W/MOV OBJ-OTH PERSON **(Continued)**	**V43.24XD**	Person outside car injured in collision w van nontraf, subs
		V44.2XXA	Person outside car injured in clsn w hv veh nontraf, init
		V44.2XXD	Person outside car injured in clsn w hv veh nontraf, subs
		V45.2XXA	Person outside car inj in clsn w rail trn/veh nontraf, init
		V45.2XXD	Person outside car inj in clsn w rail trn/veh nontraf, subs
		V46.2XXA	Person outsd car inj in clsn w nonmtr vehicle nontraf, init
		V46.2XXD	Person outsd car inj in clsn w nonmtr vehicle nontraf, subs
		V48.2XXA	Person outside car inj in nonclsn trnsp acc nontraf, init
		V48.2XXD	Person outside car inj in nonclsn trnsp acc nontraf, subs
		V5Ø.2XXA	Person outsd pk-up/van inj in clsn w ped/anml nontraf, init
		V5Ø.2XXD	Person outsd pk-up/van inj in clsn w ped/anml nontraf, subs
		V51.2XXA	Person outsd pk-up/van inj in clsn w pedl cyc nontraf, init
		V51.2XXD	Person outsd pk-up/van inj in clsn w pedl cyc nontraf, subs
		V52.2XXA	Prsn outsd pk-up/van inj in clsn w 2/3-whl mv nontraf, init
		V52.2XXD	Prsn outsd pk-up/van inj in clsn w 2/3-whl mv nontraf, subs
		V53.2XXA	Prsn outsd pk-up/van inj pk-up truck,pk-up/van nontraf, init
		V53.2XXD	Prsn outsd pk-up/van inj pk-up truck,pk-up/van nontraf, subs
		V54.2XXA	Person outside pk-up/van inj in clsn w hv veh nontraf, init
		V54.2XXD	Person outside pk-up/van inj in clsn w hv veh nontraf, subs
		V55.2XXA	Prsn outsd pk-up/van inj in clsn w rail trn/veh nontraf,init
		V55.2XXD	Prsn outsd pk-up/van inj in clsn w rail trn/veh nontraf,subs
		V56.2XXA	Prsn outsd pk-up/van inj in clsn w nonmtr veh nontraf, init
		V56.2XXD	Prsn outsd pk-up/van inj in clsn w nonmtr veh nontraf, subs
		V6Ø.2XXA	Person outside hv veh inj in clsn w ped/anml nontraf, init
		V6Ø.2XXD	Person outside hv veh inj in clsn w ped/anml nontraf, subs
		V61.2XXA	Person outside hv veh inj in clsn w pedl cyc nontraf, init
		V61.2XXD	Person outside hv veh inj in clsn w pedl cyc nontraf, subs
		V62.2XXA	Person outside hv veh inj in clsn w 2/3-whl mv nontraf, init
		V62.2XXD	Person outside hv veh inj in clsn w 2/3-whl mv nontraf, subs
		V63.2XXA	Person outsd hv veh inj pk-up truck, pk-up/van nontraf, init
		V63.2XXD	Person outsd hv veh inj pk-up truck, pk-up/van nontraf, subs
		V64.2XXA	Person outside hv veh injured in clsn w hv veh nontraf, init
		V64.2XXD	Person outside hv veh injured in clsn w hv veh nontraf, subs
		V65.2XXA	Person outsd hv veh inj in clsn w rail trn/veh nontraf, init
		V65.2XXD	Person outsd hv veh inj in clsn w rail trn/veh nontraf, subs
		V66.2XXA	Person outsd hv veh inj in clsn w nonmtr veh nontraf, init
		V66.2XXD	Person outsd hv veh inj in clsn w nonmtr veh nontraf, subs
		V7Ø.2XXA	Person outside bus injured in clsn w ped/anml nontraf, init
		V7Ø.2XXD	Person outside bus injured in clsn w ped/anml nontraf, subs
		V71.2XXA	Person outside bus injured in clsn w pedl cyc nontraf, init
		V71.2XXD	Person outside bus injured in clsn w pedl cyc nontraf, subs
		V72.2XXA	Person outside bus inj in clsn w 2/3-whl mv nontraf, init
		V72.2XXD	Person outside bus inj in clsn w 2/3-whl mv nontraf, subs
		V73.2XXA	Person outsd bus inj pick-up truck, pk-up/van nontraf, init
		V73.2XXD	Person outsd bus inj pick-up truck, pk-up/van nontraf, subs
		V74.2XXA	Person outside bus injured in clsn w hv veh nontraf, init
		V74.2XXD	Person outside bus injured in clsn w hv veh nontraf, subs
		V75.2XXA	Person outside bus inj in clsn w rail trn/veh nontraf, init
		V75.2XXD	Person outside bus inj in clsn w rail trn/veh nontraf, subs
		V76.2XXA	Person outsd bus inj in clsn w nonmtr vehicle nontraf, init
		V76.2XXD	Person outsd bus inj in clsn w nonmtr vehicle nontraf, subs
		V81.ØXXA	Occ of rail trn/veh injured in clsn w mtr veh nontraf, init
		V81.ØXXD	Occ of rail trn/veh injured in clsn w mtr veh nontraf, subs
		V84.7XXA	Person outside special agri vehicle injured nontraf, init
		V84.7XXD	Person outside special agri vehicle injured nontraf, subs
		V85.7XXA	Person outside special construct vehicle inj nontraf, init
		V85.7XXD	Person outside special construct vehicle inj nontraf, subs
		V86.71XA	Person on outside of amblnc/fire eng injured nontraf, init
		V86.71XD	Person on outside of amblnc/fire eng injured nontraf, subs
		V88.ØXXA	Person inj in clsn betw car and 2/3-whl mv, nontraf, init
		V88.ØXXD	Person inj in clsn betw car and 2/3-whl mv, nontraf, subs
		V88.1XXA	Prsn inj in clsn betw mtr veh and 2/3-whl mv, nontraf, init
		V88.1XXD	Prsn inj in clsn betw mtr veh and 2/3-whl mv, nontraf, subs
		V88.2XXA	Person injured in clsn betw car and pk-up/van, nontraf, init
		V88.2XXD	Person injured in clsn betw car and pk-up/van, nontraf, subs
		V88.3XXA	Person injured in collision betw car and bus, nontraf, init
		V88.3XXD	Person injured in collision betw car and bus, nontraf, subs
		V88.4XXA	Person injured in clsn betw car and hv veh, nontraf, init
		V88.4XXD	Person injured in clsn betw car and hv veh, nontraf, subs
		V88.5XXA	Person injured in clsn betw hv veh and bus, nontraf, init
		V88.5XXD	Person injured in clsn betw hv veh and bus, nontraf, subs
		V88.6XXA	Person inj in clsn betw rail trn/veh and car, nontraf, init
		V88.6XXD	Person inj in clsn betw rail trn/veh and car, nontraf, subs
		V88.7XXA	Person injured in collision betw mtr veh, nontraffic, init
		V88.7XXD	Person injured in collision betw mtr veh, nontraffic, subs
		V88.8XXA	Person inj in oth nonclsn trnsp acc w mtr veh, nontraf, init
		V88.8XXD	Person inj in oth nonclsn trnsp acc w mtr veh, nontraf, subs
		V88.9XXA	Person injured in oth transport acc w non-mv, nontraf, init
		V88.9XXD	Person injured in oth transport acc w non-mv, nontraf, subs

ICD-9-CM		ICD-10-CM	
E822.9	OTH MOTR VEH NONTRFF COLL W/MOV OBJ-UNS PERSON	**V20.2XXA**	Unsp mtrcy rider injured in clsn w ped/anml nontraf, init
		V20.2XXD	Unsp mtrcy rider injured in clsn w ped/anml nontraf, subs
		V21.2XXA	Unsp mtrcy rider injured in clsn w pedl cyc nontraf, init
		V21.2XXD	Unsp mtrcy rider injured in clsn w pedl cyc nontraf, subs
		V22.2XXA	Unsp mtrcy rider injured in clsn w 2/3-whl mv nontraf, init
		V22.2XXD	Unsp mtrcy rider injured in clsn w 2/3-whl mv nontraf, subs
		V24.2XXA	Unsp mtrcy rider injured in collision w hv veh nontraf, init
		V24.2XXD	Unsp mtrcy rider injured in collision w hv veh nontraf, subs
		V25.2XXA	Unsp mtrcy rider inj in clsn w rail trn/veh nontraf, init
		V25.2XXD	Unsp mtrcy rider inj in clsn w rail trn/veh nontraf, subs
		V26.2XXA	Unsp mtrcy rider inj in clsn w nonmtr vehicle nontraf, init
		V26.2XXD	Unsp mtrcy rider inj in clsn w nonmtr vehicle nontraf, subs
		V29.19XA	Mtrcy passenger injured in collision w oth mv nontraf, init
		V29.19XD	Mtrcy passenger injured in collision w oth mv nontraf, subs
		V29.20XA	Unsp mtrcy rider injured in clsn w unsp mv nontraf, init
		V29.20XD	Unsp mtrcy rider injured in clsn w unsp mv nontraf, subs
		V29.29XA	Unsp mtrcy rider injured in collision w oth mv nontraf, init
		V29.29XD	Unsp mtrcy rider injured in collision w oth mv nontraf, subs
		V30.3XXA	Occup of 3-whl mv injured in clsn w ped/anml nontraf, init
		V30.3XXD	Occup of 3-whl mv injured in clsn w ped/anml nontraf, subs
		V31.3XXA	Occup of 3-whl mv injured in clsn w pedl cyc nontraf, init
		V31.3XXD	Occup of 3-whl mv injured in clsn w pedl cyc nontraf, subs
		V32.3XXA	Occup of 3-whl mv injured in clsn w 2/3-whl mv nontraf, init
		V32.3XXD	Occup of 3-whl mv injured in clsn w 2/3-whl mv nontraf, subs
		V33.3XXA	Occup of 3-whl mv inj pick-up truck, pk-up/van nontraf, init
		V33.3XXD	Occup of 3-whl mv inj pick-up truck, pk-up/van nontraf, subs
		V34.3XXA	Occup of 3-whl mv injured in clsn w hv veh nontraf, init
		V34.3XXD	Occup of 3-whl mv injured in clsn w hv veh nontraf, subs
		V35.3XXA	Occup of 3-whl mv inj in clsn w rail trn/veh nontraf, init
		V35.3XXD	Occup of 3-whl mv inj in clsn w rail trn/veh nontraf, subs
		V36.3XXA	Occup of 3-whl mv inj in clsn w nonmtr vehicle nontraf, init
		V36.3XXD	Occup of 3-whl mv inj in clsn w nonmtr vehicle nontraf, subs
		V39.20XA	Occup of 3-whl mv injured in clsn w unsp mv nontraf, init
		V39.20XD	Occup of 3-whl mv injured in clsn w unsp mv nontraf, subs
		V39.29XA	Occup of 3-whl mv injured in clsn w oth mv nontraf, init
		V39.29XD	Occup of 3-whl mv injured in clsn w oth mv nontraf, subs
		V40.3XXA	Unsp car occupant injured in clsn w ped/anml nontraf, init
		V40.3XXD	Unsp car occupant injured in clsn w ped/anml nontraf, subs
		V41.3XXA	Unsp car occupant injured in clsn w pedl cyc nontraf, init
		V41.3XXD	Unsp car occupant injured in clsn w pedl cyc nontraf, subs
		V42.3XXA	Unsp car occupant injured in clsn w 2/3-whl mv nontraf, init
		V42.3XXD	Unsp car occupant injured in clsn w 2/3-whl mv nontraf, subs
		V43.31XA	Unsp car occupant injured in collision w SUV nontraf, init
		V43.31XD	Unsp car occupant injured in collision w SUV nontraf, subs
		V43.32XA	Unsp car occupant injured in collision w car nontraf, init
		V43.32XD	Unsp car occupant injured in collision w car nontraf, subs
		V43.33XA	Unsp car occ injured in clsn w pick-up truck nontraf, init
		V43.33XD	Unsp car occ injured in clsn w pick-up truck nontraf, subs
		V43.34XA	Unsp car occupant injured in collision w van nontraf, init
		V43.34XD	Unsp car occupant injured in collision w van nontraf, subs
		V44.3XXA	Unsp car occupant injured in clsn w hv veh nontraf, init
		V44.3XXD	Unsp car occupant injured in clsn w hv veh nontraf, subs
		V45.3XXA	Unsp car occ injured in clsn w rail trn/veh nontraf, init
		V45.3XXD	Unsp car occ injured in clsn w rail trn/veh nontraf, subs
		V46.3XXA	Unsp car occ injured in clsn w nonmtr vehicle nontraf, init
		V46.3XXD	Unsp car occ injured in clsn w nonmtr vehicle nontraf, subs
		V48.3XXA	Unsp car occupant injured in nonclsn trnsp acc nontraf, init
		V48.3XXD	Unsp car occupant injured in nonclsn trnsp acc nontraf, subs
		V49.20XA	Unsp car occupant injured in clsn w unsp mv nontraf, init
		V49.20XD	Unsp car occupant injured in clsn w unsp mv nontraf, subs
		V49.29XA	Unsp car occupant injured in clsn w oth mv nontraf, init
		V49.29XD	Unsp car occupant injured in clsn w oth mv nontraf, subs
		V50.3XXA	Occup of pk-up/van injured in clsn w ped/anml nontraf, init
		V50.3XXD	Occup of pk-up/van injured in clsn w ped/anml nontraf, subs
		V51.3XXA	Occup of pk-up/van injured in clsn w pedl cyc nontraf, init
		V51.3XXD	Occup of pk-up/van injured in clsn w pedl cyc nontraf, subs
		V52.3XXA	Occup of pk-up/van inj in clsn w 2/3-whl mv nontraf, init
		V52.3XXD	Occup of pk-up/van inj in clsn w 2/3-whl mv nontraf, subs
		V53.3XXA	Occup of pk-up/van inj pk-up truck, pk-up/van nontraf, init
		V53.3XXD	Occup of pk-up/van inj pk-up truck, pk-up/van nontraf, subs
		V54.3XXA	Occup of pk-up/van injured in clsn w hv veh nontraf, init
		V54.3XXD	Occup of pk-up/van injured in clsn w hv veh nontraf, subs
		V55.3XXA	Occup of pk-up/van inj in clsn w rail trn/veh nontraf, init
		V55.3XXD	Occup of pk-up/van inj in clsn w rail trn/veh nontraf, subs
		V56.3XXA	Occup of pk-up/van inj in clsn w nonmtr veh nontraf, init
		V56.3XXD	Occup of pk-up/van inj in clsn w nonmtr veh nontraf, subs
		V59.20XA	Occup of pk-up/van injured in clsn w unsp mv nontraf, init
		V59.20XD	Occup of pk-up/van injured in clsn w unsp mv nontraf, subs
		V59.29XA	Occup of pk-up/van injured in clsn w oth mv nontraf, init
		V59.29XD	Occup of pk-up/van injured in clsn w oth mv nontraf, subs
		V60.3XXA	Occup of hv veh injured in clsn w ped/anml nontraf, init
		V60.3XXD	Occup of hv veh injured in clsn w ped/anml nontraf, subs
		V61.3XXA	Occup of hv veh injured in clsn w pedl cyc nontraf, init

(Continued on next page)

ICD-9-CM		ICD-10-CM	
E822.9	OTH MOTR VEH NONTRFF COLL W/MOV OBJ-UNS PERSON **(Continued)**	**V61.3XXD**	Occup of hv veh injured in clsn w pedl cyc nontraf, subs
		V62.3XXA	Occup of hv veh injured in clsn w 2/3-whl mv nontraf, init
		V62.3XXD	Occup of hv veh injured in clsn w 2/3-whl mv nontraf, subs
		V63.3XXA	Occup of hv veh inj pick-up truck, pk-up/van nontraf, init
		V63.3XXD	Occup of hv veh inj pick-up truck, pk-up/van nontraf, subs
		V64.3XXA	Occup of hv veh injured in collision w hv veh nontraf, init
		V64.3XXD	Occup of hv veh injured in collision w hv veh nontraf, subs
		V65.3XXA	Occup of hv veh injured in clsn w rail trn/veh nontraf, init
		V65.3XXD	Occup of hv veh injured in clsn w rail trn/veh nontraf, subs
		V66.3XXA	Occup of hv veh inj in clsn w nonmtr vehicle nontraf, init
		V66.3XXD	Occup of hv veh inj in clsn w nonmtr vehicle nontraf, subs
		V69.2ØXA	Occup of hv veh injured in collision w unsp mv nontraf, init
		V69.2ØXD	Occup of hv veh injured in collision w unsp mv nontraf, subs
		V69.29XA	Occup of hv veh injured in collision w oth mv nontraf, init
		V69.29XD	Occup of hv veh injured in collision w oth mv nontraf, subs
		V7Ø.3XXA	Occup of bus injured in collision w ped/anml nontraf, init
		V7Ø.3XXD	Occup of bus injured in collision w ped/anml nontraf, subs
		V71.3XXA	Occup of bus injured in collision w pedl cyc nontraf, init
		V71.3XXD	Occup of bus injured in collision w pedl cyc nontraf, subs
		V72.3XXA	Occup of bus injured in collision w 2/3-whl mv nontraf, init
		V72.3XXD	Occup of bus injured in collision w 2/3-whl mv nontraf, subs
		V73.3XXA	Occup of bus injured pick-up truck, pk-up/van nontraf, init
		V73.3XXD	Occup of bus injured pick-up truck, pk-up/van nontraf, subs
		V74.3XXA	Occup of bus injured in collision w hv veh nontraf, init
		V74.3XXD	Occup of bus injured in collision w hv veh nontraf, subs
		V75.3XXA	Occup of bus injured in clsn w rail trn/veh nontraf, init
		V75.3XXD	Occup of bus injured in clsn w rail trn/veh nontraf, subs
		V76.3XXA	Occup of bus injured in clsn w nonmtr vehicle nontraf, init
		V76.3XXD	Occup of bus injured in clsn w nonmtr vehicle nontraf, subs
		V79.2ØXA	Unsp bus occupant injured in clsn w unsp mv nontraf, init
		V79.2ØXD	Unsp bus occupant injured in clsn w unsp mv nontraf, subs
		V79.29XA	Unsp bus occupant injured in clsn w oth mv nontraf, init
		V79.29XD	Unsp bus occupant injured in clsn w oth mv nontraf, subs
		V84.9XXA	Occup of special agricultural vehicle injured nontraf, init
		V84.9XXD	Occup of special agricultural vehicle injured nontraf, subs
		V85.9XXA	Occup of special construction vehicle injured nontraf, init
		V85.9XXD	Occup of special construction vehicle injured nontraf, subs
E823.Ø	OTH MOTR VEH NONTRFF COLL W/STATION OBJ-DRIVER	**V37.ØXXA**	Drvr of 3-whl mv inj in clsn w statnry object nontraf, init
		V37.ØXXD	Drvr of 3-whl mv inj in clsn w statnry object nontraf, subs
		V47.Ø1XA	Driver of SUV injured in clsn w statnry object nontraf, init
		V47.Ø1XD	Driver of SUV injured in clsn w statnry object nontraf, subs
		V47.Ø2XA	Driver of car injured in clsn w statnry object nontraf, init
		V47.Ø2XD	Driver of car injured in clsn w statnry object nontraf, subs
		V57.ØXXA	Drvr of pk-up/van inj in clsn w statnry object nontraf, init
		V57.ØXXD	Drvr of pk-up/van inj in clsn w statnry object nontraf, subs
		V67.ØXXA	Driver of hv veh inj in clsn w statnry object nontraf, init
		V67.ØXXD	Driver of hv veh inj in clsn w statnry object nontraf, subs
		V77.ØXXA	Driver of bus injured in clsn w statnry object nontraf, init
		V77.ØXXD	Driver of bus injured in clsn w statnry object nontraf, subs
E823.1	OTH MOTR VEH NONTRFF COLL W/STATION OBJ-PSNGR	**V37.1XXA**	Pasngr in 3-whl mv inj in clsn w statnry obj nontraf, init
		V37.1XXD	Pasngr in 3-whl mv inj in clsn w statnry obj nontraf, subs
		V47.11XA	Pasngr of SUV injured in clsn w statnry object nontraf, init
		V47.11XD	Pasngr of SUV injured in clsn w statnry object nontraf, subs
		V47.12XA	Pasngr of car injured in clsn w statnry object nontraf, init
		V47.12XD	Pasngr of car injured in clsn w statnry object nontraf, subs
		V47.2XXA	Person outsd car inj in clsn w statnry object nontraf, init
		V47.2XXD	Person outsd car inj in clsn w statnry object nontraf, subs
		V57.1XXA	Pasngr in pk-up/van inj in clsn w statnry obj nontraf, init
		V57.1XXD	Pasngr in pk-up/van inj in clsn w statnry obj nontraf, subs
		V67.1XXA	Pasngr in hv veh inj in clsn w statnry object nontraf, init
		V67.1XXD	Pasngr in hv veh inj in clsn w statnry object nontraf, subs
		V77.1XXA	Pasngr on bus injured in clsn w statnry object nontraf, init
		V77.1XXD	Pasngr on bus injured in clsn w statnry object nontraf, subs
E823.2	OTH MOTR VEH NONTRFF COLL W/STATION OBJ-MTRCYLST	**V27.ØXXA**	Mtrcy driver injured in clsn w statnry object nontraf, init
		V27.ØXXD	Mtrcy driver injured in clsn w statnry object nontraf, subs
E823.3	OTH MOTR VEH NONTRFF COLL W/STATION OBJ-MC PSNGR	**V27.1XXA**	Mtrcy pasngr injured in clsn w statnry object nontraf, init
		V27.1XXD	Mtrcy pasngr injured in clsn w statnry object nontraf, subs
E823.4	OTH MOTR VEH NONTRFF COLL W/STATION OBJ-ST CAR	**V82.3XXA**	Occupant of streetcar injured in clsn w oth object, init
E823.5	OTH MOTR VEH NONTRFF COLL W/STATION OBJ-ANM RIDR	**V8Ø.81XA**	Animal-rider injured in collision w statnry object, init
E823.6	OTH MOTR VEH NONTRFF COLL W/STATION OBJ-CYCLIST	**V17.2XXA**	Unsp pedl cyclst inj in clsn w statnry object nontraf, init
E823.7	OTH MOTR VEH NONTRFF COLL W/STATION OBJ-PEDSTRN	**VØ9.9XXA**	Pedestrian injured in unsp transport accident, init encntr
E823.8	OTH MOTR VEH NONTRFF COLL W/STATION OBJ-OTH PERS	**V37.2XXA**	Prsn outsd 3-whl mv inj in clsn w statnry obj nontraf, init
		V37.2XXD	Prsn outsd 3-whl mv inj in clsn w statnry obj nontraf, subs
		V57.2XXA	Prsn outsd pk-up/van inj in clsn w statnry obj nontraf, init
		V57.2XXD	Prsn outsd pk-up/van inj in clsn w statnry obj nontraf, subs
		V67.2XXA	Person outsd hv veh inj in clsn w statnry obj nontraf, init
		V67.2XXD	Person outsd hv veh inj in clsn w statnry obj nontraf, subs
		V77.2XXA	Person outsd bus inj in clsn w statnry object nontraf, init
		V77.2XXD	Person outsd bus inj in clsn w statnry object nontraf, subs

ICD-9-CM		ICD-10-CM	
E823.9	OTH MOTR VEH NONTRFF COLL W/STATION OBJ-UNS PERS	**V27.2XXA**	Unsp mtrcy rider inj in clsn w statnry object nontraf, init
		V27.2XXD	Unsp mtrcy rider inj in clsn w statnry object nontraf, subs
		V37.3XXA	Occup of 3-whl mv inj in clsn w statnry object nontraf, init
		V37.3XXD	Occup of 3-whl mv inj in clsn w statnry object nontraf, subs
		V47.31XA	Occup of SUV injured in clsn w statnry object nontraf, init
		V47.31XD	Occup of SUV injured in clsn w statnry object nontraf, subs
		V47.32XA	Occup of car injured in clsn w statnry object nontraf, init
		V47.32XD	Occup of car injured in clsn w statnry object nontraf, subs
		V47.4XXA	Prsn brd/alit a car injured in clsn w statnry object, init
		V47.4XXD	Prsn brd/alit a car injured in clsn w statnry object, subs
		V57.3XXA	Occup of pk-up/van inj in clsn w statnry obj nontraf, init
		V57.3XXD	Occup of pk-up/van inj in clsn w statnry obj nontraf, subs
		V67.3XXA	Occup of hv veh inj in clsn w statnry object nontraf, init
		V67.3XXD	Occup of hv veh inj in clsn w statnry object nontraf, subs
		V77.3XXA	Occup of bus injured in clsn w statnry object nontraf, init
		V77.3XXD	Occup of bus injured in clsn w statnry object nontraf, subs
E824.Ø	OTH MOTR VEH NONTRFF ACC BOARD&ALIGHT-INJR DRIVE	**V43.42XA**	Prsn brd/alit a car injured in collision w car, init
E824.1	OTH MOTR VEH NONTRFF ACC BOARD&ALIGHT-INJR PSNGR	**V43.42XA**	Prsn brd/alit a car injured in collision w car, init
E824.2	OTH MOTR VEH NONTRFF ACC BOARD&ALIGHT-MTRCYCLST	**V2Ø.3XXA**	Prsn brd/alit mtrcy injured in collision w ped/anml, init
		V2Ø.3XXD	Prsn brd/alit mtrcy injured in collision w ped/anml, subs
		V22.3XXA	Prsn brd/alit mtrcy injured in collision w 2/3-whl mv, init
		V22.3XXD	Prsn brd/alit mtrcy injured in collision w 2/3-whl mv, subs
		V23.3XXA	Prsn brd/alit mtrcy injured pick-up truck, pk-up/van, init
		V23.3XXD	Prsn brd/alit mtrcy injured pick-up truck, pk-up/van, subs
		V24.3XXA	Prsn brd/alit mtrcy injured in collision w hv veh, init
		V24.3XXD	Prsn brd/alit mtrcy injured in collision w hv veh, subs
		V25.3XXA	Prsn brd/alit mtrcy injured in clsn w rail trn/veh, init
		V25.3XXD	Prsn brd/alit mtrcy injured in clsn w rail trn/veh, subs
		V26.3XXA	Prsn brd/alit mtrcy injured in clsn w nonmtr vehicle, init
		V26.3XXD	Prsn brd/alit mtrcy injured in clsn w nonmtr vehicle, subs
		V27.3XXA	Prsn brd/alit mtrcy injured in clsn w statnry object, init
		V27.3XXD	Prsn brd/alit mtrcy injured in clsn w statnry object, subs
		V28.3XXA	Prsn brd/alit mtrcy injured in nonclsn trnsp accident, init
		V28.3XXD	Prsn brd/alit mtrcy injured in nonclsn trnsp accident, subs
E824.3	OTH MOTR VEH NONTRFF ACC BOARD&ALIGHT-MC PSNGR	**V23.3XXA**	Prsn brd/alit mtrcy injured pick-up truck, pk-up/van, init
E824.4	OTH MOTR VEH NONTRFF ACC BOARD&ALIGHT-ST CAR	**V82.4XXA**	Person injured wh brd/alit from streetcar, init
E824.5	OTH MOTR VEH NONTRFF ACC BOARD&ALIGHT-ANIM RIDER	**V8Ø.918A**	Animal-rider injured in oth transport accident, init encntr
E824.6	OTH MOTR VEH NONTRFF ACC BOARD&ALIGHT-PED CYCLST	**V12.3XXA**	Prsn brd/alit pedl cyc injured in clsn w 2/3-whl mv, init
		V12.3XXD	Prsn brd/alit pedl cyc injured in clsn w 2/3-whl mv, subs
		V13.3XXA	Prsn brd/alit pedl cyc inj pick-up truck, pk-up/van, init
		V13.3XXD	Prsn brd/alit pedl cyc inj pick-up truck, pk-up/van, subs
		V14.3XXA	Prsn brd/alit pedl cyc injured in collision w hv veh, init
		V14.3XXD	Prsn brd/alit pedl cyc injured in collision w hv veh, subs
		V18.3XXA	Prsn brd/alit pedl cyc injured in nonclsn trnsp acc, init
E824.7	OTH MOTOR VEH NONTRFF ACC INJR PEDSTRN BD&ALIGHT	**VØ9.9XXA**	Pedestrian injured in unsp transport accident, init encntr
E824.8	OTH MOTR VEH NONTRFF ACC INJR OTH PERS BD&ALGHT	**V3Ø.4XXA**	Prsn brd/alit a 3-whl mv injured in clsn w ped/anml, init
		V3Ø.4XXD	Prsn brd/alit a 3-whl mv injured in clsn w ped/anml, subs
		V31.4XXA	Prsn brd/alit a 3-whl mv injured in clsn w pedl cyc, init
		V31.4XXD	Prsn brd/alit a 3-whl mv injured in clsn w pedl cyc, subs
		V32.4XXA	Prsn brd/alit a 3-whl mv injured in clsn w 2/3-whl mv, init
		V32.4XXD	Prsn brd/alit a 3-whl mv injured in clsn w 2/3-whl mv, subs
		V33.4XXA	Prsn brd/alit a 3-whl mv inj pick-up truck, pk-up/van, init
		V33.4XXD	Prsn brd/alit a 3-whl mv inj pick-up truck, pk-up/van, subs
		V34.4XXA	Prsn brd/alit a 3-whl mv injured in collision w hv veh, init
		V34.4XXD	Prsn brd/alit a 3-whl mv injured in collision w hv veh, subs
		V35.4XXA	Prsn brd/alit a 3-whl mv inj in clsn w rail trn/veh, init
		V35.4XXD	Prsn brd/alit a 3-whl mv inj in clsn w rail trn/veh, subs
		V36.4XXA	Prsn brd/alit a 3-whl mv inj in clsn w nonmtr vehicle, init
		V36.4XXD	Prsn brd/alit a 3-whl mv inj in clsn w nonmtr vehicle, subs
		V37.4XXA	Prsn brd/alit a 3-whl mv inj in clsn w statnry object, init
		V37.4XXD	Prsn brd/alit a 3-whl mv inj in clsn w statnry object, subs
		V38.4XXA	Prsn brd/alit a 3-whl mv injured in nonclsn trnsp acc, init
		V38.4XXD	Prsn brd/alit a 3-whl mv injured in nonclsn trnsp acc, subs
		V4Ø.4XXA	Prsn brd/alit a car injured in collision w ped/anml, init
		V4Ø.4XXD	Prsn brd/alit a car injured in collision w ped/anml, subs
		V41.4XXA	Prsn brd/alit a car injured in collision w pedal cycle, init
		V41.4XXD	Prsn brd/alit a car injured in collision w pedal cycle, subs
		V42.4XXA	Prsn brd/alit a car injured in collision w 2/3-whl mv, init
		V42.4XXD	Prsn brd/alit a car injured in collision w 2/3-whl mv, subs
		V43.41XA	Prsn brd/alit a car injured in collision w SUV, init
		V43.41XD	Prsn brd/alit a car injured in collision w SUV, subs
		V43.42XA	Prsn brd/alit a car injured in collision w car, init
		V43.42XD	Prsn brd/alit a car injured in collision w car, subs
		V43.43XA	Prsn brd/alit a car injured in clsn w pick-up truck, init
		V43.43XD	Prsn brd/alit a car injured in clsn w pick-up truck, subs
		V43.44XA	Prsn brd/alit a car injured in collision w van, init
		V43.44XD	Prsn brd/alit a car injured in collision w van, subs
		V44.4XXA	Prsn brd/alit a car injured in collision w hv veh, init
		V44.4XXD	Prsn brd/alit a car injured in collision w hv veh, subs
		V45.4XXA	Prsn brd/alit a car injured in clsn w rail trn/veh, init
	(Continued on next page)	**V45.4XXD**	Prsn brd/alit a car injured in clsn w rail trn/veh, subs

ICD-9-CM		ICD-10-CM	
E824.8	OTH MOTR VEH NONTRFF ACC INJR OTH PERS BD&ALGHT **(Continued)**	**V46.4XXA**	Prsn brd/alit a car injured in clsn w nonmtr vehicle, init
		V46.4XXD	Prsn brd/alit a car injured in clsn w nonmtr vehicle, subs
		V5Ø.4XXA	Prsn brd/alit pk-up/van injured in clsn w ped/anml, init
		V5Ø.4XXD	Prsn brd/alit pk-up/van injured in clsn w ped/anml, subs
		V51.4XXA	Prsn brd/alit pk-up/van injured in clsn w pedl cyc, init
		V51.4XXD	Prsn brd/alit pk-up/van injured in clsn w pedl cyc, subs
		V52.4XXA	Prsn brd/alit pk-up/van injured in clsn w 2/3-whl mv, init
		V52.4XXD	Prsn brd/alit pk-up/van injured in clsn w 2/3-whl mv, subs
		V53.4XXA	Prsn brd/alit pk-up/van inj pick-up truck, pk-up/van, init
		V53.4XXD	Prsn brd/alit pk-up/van inj pick-up truck, pk-up/van, subs
		V54.4XXA	Prsn brd/alit pk-up/van injured in collision w hv veh, init
		V54.4XXD	Prsn brd/alit pk-up/van injured in collision w hv veh, subs
		V55.4XXA	Prsn brd/alit pk-up/van injured in clsn w rail trn/veh, init
		V55.4XXD	Prsn brd/alit pk-up/van injured in clsn w rail trn/veh, subs
		V56.4XXA	Prsn brd/alit pk-up/van inj in clsn w nonmtr vehicle, init
		V56.4XXD	Prsn brd/alit pk-up/van inj in clsn w nonmtr vehicle, subs
		V57.4XXA	Prsn brd/alit pk-up/van inj in clsn w statnry object, init
		V57.4XXD	Prsn brd/alit pk-up/van inj in clsn w statnry object, subs
		V58.4XXA	Prsn brd/alit pk-up/van injured in nonclsn trnsp acc, init
		V58.4XXD	Prsn brd/alit pk-up/van injured in nonclsn trnsp acc, subs
		V6Ø.4XXA	Prsn brd/alit hv veh injured in collision w ped/anml, init
		V6Ø.4XXD	Prsn brd/alit hv veh injured in collision w ped/anml, subs
		V61.4XXA	Prsn brd/alit hv veh inj in clsn w pedl cyc wh brd/alit,init
		V61.4XXD	Prsn brd/alit hv veh inj in clsn w pedl cyc wh brd/alit,subs
		V62.4XXA	Prsn brd/alit hv veh injured in collision w 2/3-whl mv, init
		V62.4XXD	Prsn brd/alit hv veh injured in collision w 2/3-whl mv, subs
		V63.4XXA	Prsn brd/alit hv veh injured pick-up truck, pk-up/van, init
		V63.4XXD	Prsn brd/alit hv veh injured pick-up truck, pk-up/van, subs
		V64.4XXA	Prsn brd/alit hv veh inj in clsn w hv veh wh brd/alit, init
		V64.4XXD	Prsn brd/alit hv veh inj in clsn w hv veh wh brd/alit, subs
		V65.4XXA	Prsn brd/alit hv veh injured in clsn w rail trn/veh, init
		V65.4XXD	Prsn brd/alit hv veh injured in clsn w rail trn/veh, subs
		V66.4XXA	Prsn brd/alit hv veh injured in clsn w nonmtr vehicle, init
		V66.4XXD	Prsn brd/alit hv veh injured in clsn w nonmtr vehicle, subs
		V67.4XXA	Prsn brd/alit hv veh injured in clsn w statnry object, init
		V67.4XXD	Prsn brd/alit hv veh injured in clsn w statnry object, subs
		V68.4XXA	Prsn brd/alit hv veh injured in nonclsn trnsp accident, init
		V68.4XXD	Prsn brd/alit hv veh injured in nonclsn trnsp accident, subs
		V7Ø.4XXA	Prsn brd/alit from bus injured in collision w ped/anml, init
		V7Ø.4XXD	Prsn brd/alit from bus injured in collision w ped/anml, subs
		V71.4XXA	Prsn brd/alit from bus injured in collision w pedl cyc, init
		V71.4XXD	Prsn brd/alit from bus injured in collision w pedl cyc, subs
		V72.4XXA	Prsn brd/alit from bus injured in clsn w 2/3-whl mv, init
		V72.4XXD	Prsn brd/alit from bus injured in clsn w 2/3-whl mv, subs
		V73.4XXA	Prsn brd/alit from bus inj pick-up truck, pk-up/van, init
		V73.4XXD	Prsn brd/alit from bus inj pick-up truck, pk-up/van, subs
		V74.4XXA	Prsn brd/alit from bus injured in collision w hv veh, init
		V74.4XXD	Prsn brd/alit from bus injured in collision w hv veh, subs
		V75.4XXA	Prsn brd/alit from bus injured in clsn w rail trn/veh, init
		V75.4XXD	Prsn brd/alit from bus injured in clsn w rail trn/veh, subs
		V76.4XXA	Prsn brd/alit from bus inj in clsn w nonmtr vehicle, init
		V76.4XXD	Prsn brd/alit from bus inj in clsn w nonmtr vehicle, subs
		V77.4XXA	Prsn brd/alit from bus inj in clsn w statnry object, init
		V77.4XXD	Prsn brd/alit from bus inj in clsn w statnry object, subs
		V78.4XXA	Prsn brd/alit from bus injured in nonclsn trnsp acc, init
		V78.4XXD	Prsn brd/alit from bus injured in nonclsn trnsp acc, subs
		V84.4XXA	Person injured wh brd/alit from special agri vehicle, init
		V84.4XXD	Person injured wh brd/alit from special agri vehicle, subs
		V85.4XXA	Person inj wh brd/alit from special construct vehicle, init
		V85.4XXD	Person inj wh brd/alit from special construct vehicle, subs
		V86.41XA	Person injured wh brd/alit from amblnc/fire eng, init
		V86.41XD	Person injured wh brd/alit from amblnc/fire eng, subs
		V86.44XA	Person injured wh brd/alit from military vehicle, init
		V86.44XD	Person injured wh brd/alit from military vehicle, subs
E824.9	OTH MOTR VEH NONTRFF ACC INJR UNS PERS BD&ALGHT	**V88.8XXA**	Person inj in oth nonclsn trnsp acc w mtr veh, nontraf, init
E825.Ø	OTH MOTR VEH NONTRFF OTH&UNS NATR-INJR DRIVER	**V38.ØXXA**	Driver of 3-whl mv inj in nonclsn trnsp acc nontraf, init
		V38.ØXXD	Driver of 3-whl mv inj in nonclsn trnsp acc nontraf, subs
		V39.3XXA	Occupant (driver) of 3-whl mv injured in unsp nontraf, init
		V39.3XXD	Occupant (driver) of 3-whl mv injured in unsp nontraf, subs
		V58.ØXXA	Driver of pk-up/van inj in nonclsn trnsp acc nontraf, init
		V58.ØXXD	Driver of pk-up/van inj in nonclsn trnsp acc nontraf, subs
		V59.3XXA	Occupant (driver) of pk-up/van injured in unsp nontraf, init
		V59.3XXD	Occupant (driver) of pk-up/van injured in unsp nontraf, subs
		V68.ØXXA	Driver of hv veh injured in nonclsn trnsp acc nontraf, init
		V68.ØXXD	Driver of hv veh injured in nonclsn trnsp acc nontraf, subs
		V69.3XXA	Occupant (driver) of hv veh injured in unsp nontraf, init
		V69.3XXD	Occupant (driver) of hv veh injured in unsp nontraf, subs
		V78.ØXXA	Driver of bus injured in nonclsn trnsp acc nontraf, init
		V78.ØXXD	Driver of bus injured in nonclsn trnsp acc nontraf, subs
		V79.3XXA	Bus occupant (driver) injured in unsp nontraf, init
		V79.3XXD	Bus occupant (driver) injured in unsp nontraf, subs

ICD-9-CM		ICD-10-CM	
E825.1	OTH MOTR VEH NONTRFF OTH&UNS NATR-INJR PSNGR	**V38.1XXA**	Pasngr in 3-whl mv inj in nonclsn trnsp acc nontraf, init
		V38.1XXD	Pasngr in 3-whl mv inj in nonclsn trnsp acc nontraf, subs
		V49.3XXA	Car occupant (driver) injured in unsp nontraf, init
		V49.3XXD	Car occupant (driver) injured in unsp nontraf, subs
		V58.1XXA	Pasngr in pk-up/van inj in nonclsn trnsp acc nontraf, init
		V58.1XXD	Pasngr in pk-up/van inj in nonclsn trnsp acc nontraf, subs
		V68.1XXA	Pasngr in hv veh injured in nonclsn trnsp acc nontraf, init
		V68.1XXD	Pasngr in hv veh injured in nonclsn trnsp acc nontraf, subs
		V78.1XXA	Pasngr on bus injured in nonclsn trnsp acc nontraf, init
		V78.1XXD	Pasngr on bus injured in nonclsn trnsp acc nontraf, subs
E825.2	OTH MOTR VEH NONTRFF OTH&UNS NATR-INJR MTRCYCLST	**V28.ØXXA**	Mtrcy driver injured in nonclsn trnsp accident nontraf, init
		V28.ØXXD	Mtrcy driver injured in nonclsn trnsp accident nontraf, subs
		V29.3XXA	Motorcycle rider (driver) injured in unsp nontraf, init
		V29.3XXD	Motorcycle rider (driver) injured in unsp nontraf, subs
E825.3	OTH MOTR VEH NONTRFF OTH&UNS NATR-INJR MC PSNGR	**V28.1XXA**	Mtrcy pasngr injured in nonclsn trnsp accident nontraf, init
		V28.1XXD	Mtrcy pasngr injured in nonclsn trnsp accident nontraf, subs
E825.4	OTH MOTR VEH NONTRFF OTH&UNS NATR-ST CAR RIDER	**V82.8XXA**	Occupant of streetcar injured in oth transport acc, init
E825.5	OTH MOTR VEH NONTRFF OTH&UNS NATR-INJR ANIM RIDR	**V8Ø.918A**	Animal-rider injured in oth transport accident, init encntr
E825.6	OTH MOTR VEH NONTRFF OTH&UNS NATR-INJR PED CYCL	**V19.88XA**	Pedl cyclst (driver) injured in oth transport acc, init
E825.7	OTH MOTR VEH NONTRFF OTH&UNS NATR-INJR PEDSTRN	**VØ9.ØØXA**	Pedestrian injured nontraf involving unsp mv, init
E825.8	OTH MOTR VEH NONTRFF OTH&UNS NATR-INJR OTH PERS	**V38.2XXA**	Person outsd 3-whl mv inj in nonclsn trnsp acc nontraf, init
		V38.2XXD	Person outsd 3-whl mv inj in nonclsn trnsp acc nontraf, subs
		V58.2XXA	Prsn outsd pk-up/van inj in nonclsn trnsp acc nontraf, init
		V58.2XXD	Prsn outsd pk-up/van inj in nonclsn trnsp acc nontraf, subs
		V68.2XXA	Person outside hv veh inj in nonclsn trnsp acc nontraf, init
		V68.2XXD	Person outside hv veh inj in nonclsn trnsp acc nontraf, subs
		V78.2XXA	Person outside bus inj in nonclsn trnsp acc nontraf, init
		V78.2XXD	Person outside bus inj in nonclsn trnsp acc nontraf, subs
		V86.74XA	Person on outside of military vehicle injured nontraf, init
		V86.74XD	Person on outside of military vehicle injured nontraf, subs
E825.9	OTH MOTR VEH NONTRFF OTH&UNS NATR-INJR UNS PERS	**V28.2XXA**	Unsp mtrcy rider injured in nonclsn trnsp acc nontraf, init
		V28.2XXD	Unsp mtrcy rider injured in nonclsn trnsp acc nontraf, subs
		V38.3XXA	Occup of 3-whl mv injured in nonclsn trnsp acc nontraf, init
		V38.3XXD	Occup of 3-whl mv injured in nonclsn trnsp acc nontraf, subs
		V58.3XXA	Occup of pk-up/van inj in nonclsn trnsp acc nontraf, init
		V58.3XXD	Occup of pk-up/van inj in nonclsn trnsp acc nontraf, subs
		V68.3XXA	Occup of hv veh injured in nonclsn trnsp acc nontraf, init
		V68.3XXD	Occup of hv veh injured in nonclsn trnsp acc nontraf, subs
		V78.3XXA	Occup of bus injured in nonclsn trnsp accident nontraf, init
		V78.3XXD	Occup of bus injured in nonclsn trnsp accident nontraf, subs
		V86.91XA	Occup of amblnc/fire eng injured nontraf, init
		V86.91XD	Occup of amblnc/fire eng injured nontraf, subs
		V86.94XA	Occup of military vehicle injured nontraf, init
		V86.94XD	Occup of military vehicle injured nontraf, subs
		V89.ØXXA	Person injured in unsp motor-vehicle accident, nontraf, init
		V89.ØXXD	Person injured in unsp motor-vehicle accident, nontraf, subs
E826.Ø	PEDAL CYCLE ACCIDENT INJURING PEDESTRIAN	**VØ1.ØØXA**	Ped on foot injured in collision w pedl cyc nontraf, init
		VØ1.ØØXD	Ped on foot injured in collision w pedl cyc nontraf, subs
		VØ1.Ø1XA	Ped on rolr-skt injured in clsn w pedl cyc nontraf, init
		VØ1.Ø1XD	Ped on rolr-skt injured in clsn w pedl cyc nontraf, subs
		VØ1.Ø2XA	Ped on sktbrd injured in collision w pedl cyc nontraf, init
		VØ1.Ø2XD	Ped on sktbrd injured in collision w pedl cyc nontraf, subs
		VØ1.Ø9XA	Ped w convey injured in collision w pedl cyc nontraf, init
		VØ1.Ø9XD	Ped w convey injured in collision w pedl cyc nontraf, subs
		VØ1.1ØXA	Ped on foot injured in collision w pedl cyc in traf, init
		VØ1.1ØXD	Ped on foot injured in collision w pedl cyc in traf, subs
		VØ1.11XA	Ped on rolr-skt injured in clsn w pedl cyc in traf, init
		VØ1.11XD	Ped on rolr-skt injured in clsn w pedl cyc in traf, subs
		VØ1.12XA	Ped on sktbrd injured in collision w pedl cyc in traf, init
		VØ1.12XD	Ped on sktbrd injured in collision w pedl cyc in traf, subs
		VØ1.19XA	Ped w convey injured in collision w pedl cyc in traf, init
		VØ1.19XD	Ped w convey injured in collision w pedl cyc in traf, subs
		VØ1.9ØXA	Ped on foot injured in collision w pedl cyc, unsp, init
		VØ1.9ØXD	Ped on foot injured in collision w pedl cyc, unsp, subs
		VØ1.91XA	Ped on rolr-skt injured in collision w pedl cyc, unsp, init
		VØ1.91XD	Ped on rolr-skt injured in collision w pedl cyc, unsp, subs
		VØ1.92XA	Ped on sktbrd injured in collision w pedl cyc, unsp, init
		VØ1.92XD	Ped on sktbrd injured in collision w pedl cyc, unsp, subs
		VØ1.99XA	Ped w convey injured in collision w pedl cyc, unsp, init
		VØ1.99XD	Ped w convey injured in collision w pedl cyc, unsp, subs
E826.1	PEDAL CYCLE ACCIDENT INJURING PEDAL CYCLIST	**V1Ø.ØXXA**	Pedl cyc driver injured in clsn w ped/anml nontraf, init
		V1Ø.ØXXD	Pedl cyc driver injured in clsn w ped/anml nontraf, subs
		V1Ø.1XXA	Pedl cyc passenger injured in clsn w ped/anml nontraf, init
		V1Ø.1XXD	Pedl cyc passenger injured in clsn w ped/anml nontraf, subs
		V1Ø.3XXA	Prsn brd/alit pedl cyc injured in collision w ped/anml, init
		V1Ø.3XXD	Prsn brd/alit pedl cyc injured in collision w ped/anml, subs
		V1Ø.4XXA	Pedl cyc driver injured in clsn w ped/anml in traf, init
		V1Ø.4XXD	Pedl cyc driver injured in clsn w ped/anml in traf, subs
		V1Ø.5XXA	Pedl cyc passenger injured in clsn w ped/anml in traf, init
		V1Ø.5XXD	Pedl cyc passenger injured in clsn w ped/anml in traf, subs
	(Continued on next page)	**V11.ØXXA**	Pedl cyc driver injured in clsn w oth pedl cyc nontraf, init

ICD-9-CM		ICD-10-CM	
E826.1	PEDAL CYCLE ACCIDENT INJURING PEDAL CYCLIST **(Continued)**	**V11.ØXXD**	Pedl cyc driver injured in clsn w oth pedl cyc nontraf, subs
		V11.1XXA	Pedl cyc pasngr injured in clsn w oth pedl cyc nontraf, init
		V11.1XXD	Pedl cyc pasngr injured in clsn w oth pedl cyc nontraf, subs
		V11.3XXA	Prsn brd/alit pedl cyc injured in clsn w oth pedl cyc, init
		V11.3XXD	Prsn brd/alit pedl cyc injured in clsn w oth pedl cyc, subs
		V11.4XXA	Pedl cyc driver injured in clsn w oth pedl cyc in traf, init
		V11.4XXD	Pedl cyc driver injured in clsn w oth pedl cyc in traf, subs
		V11.5XXA	Pedl cyc pasngr injured in clsn w oth pedl cyc in traf, init
		V11.5XXD	Pedl cyc pasngr injured in clsn w oth pedl cyc in traf, subs
		V16.ØXXA	Pedl cyc driver inj in clsn w nonmtr vehicle nontraf, init
		V16.ØXXD	Pedl cyc driver inj in clsn w nonmtr vehicle nontraf, subs
		V16.1XXA	Pedl cyc pasngr inj in clsn w nonmtr vehicle nontraf, init
		V16.1XXD	Pedl cyc pasngr inj in clsn w nonmtr vehicle nontraf, subs
		V16.3XXA	Prsn brd/alit pedl cyc inj in clsn w nonmtr veh nontraf,init
		V16.3XXD	Prsn brd/alit pedl cyc inj in clsn w nonmtr veh nontraf,subs
		V16.4XXA	Pedl cyc driver inj in clsn w nonmtr vehicle in traf, init
		V16.4XXD	Pedl cyc driver inj in clsn w nonmtr vehicle in traf, subs
		V16.5XXA	Pedl cyc pasngr inj in clsn w nonmtr vehicle in traf, init
		V16.5XXD	Pedl cyc pasngr inj in clsn w nonmtr vehicle in traf, subs
		V17.ØXXA	Pedl cyc driver inj in clsn w statnry object nontraf, init
		V17.ØXXD	Pedl cyc driver inj in clsn w statnry object nontraf, subs
		V17.1XXA	Pedl cyc pasngr inj in clsn w statnry object nontraf, init
		V17.1XXD	Pedl cyc pasngr inj in clsn w statnry object nontraf, subs
		V17.3XXA	Prsn brd/alit pedl cyc inj in clsn w statnry object, init
		V17.3XXD	Prsn brd/alit pedl cyc inj in clsn w statnry object, subs
		V17.4XXA	Pedl cyc driver inj in clsn w statnry object in traf, init
		V17.4XXD	Pedl cyc driver inj in clsn w statnry object in traf, subs
		V17.5XXA	Pedl cyc pasngr inj in clsn w statnry object in traf, init
		V17.5XXD	Pedl cyc pasngr inj in clsn w statnry object in traf, subs
		V18.ØXXA	Pedl cyc driver injured in nonclsn trnsp acc nontraf, init
		V18.ØXXD	Pedl cyc driver injured in nonclsn trnsp acc nontraf, subs
		V18.1XXA	Pedl cyc pasngr injured in nonclsn trnsp acc nontraf, init
		V18.1XXD	Pedl cyc pasngr injured in nonclsn trnsp acc nontraf, subs
		V18.3XXA	Prsn brd/alit pedl cyc injured in nonclsn trnsp acc, init
		V18.3XXD	Prsn brd/alit pedl cyc injured in nonclsn trnsp acc, subs
		V18.4XXA	Pedl cyc driver injured in nonclsn trnsp acc in traf, init
		V18.4XXD	Pedl cyc driver injured in nonclsn trnsp acc in traf, subs
		V18.5XXA	Pedl cyc pasngr injured in nonclsn trnsp acc in traf, init
		V18.5XXD	Pedl cyc pasngr injured in nonclsn trnsp acc in traf, subs
		V19.3XXA	Pedl cyclst (driver) injured in unsp nontraf, init
		V19.3XXD	Pedl cyclst (driver) injured in unsp nontraf, subs
		V19.88XA	Pedl cyclst (driver) injured in oth transport acc, init
		V19.88XD	Pedl cyclst (driver) injured in oth transport acc, subs
		V19.9XXA	Pedl cyclst (driver) (passenger) injured in unsp traf, init
		V19.9XXD	Pedl cyclst (driver) (passenger) injured in unsp traf, subs
E826.2	PEDAL CYCLE ACCIDENT INJURING RIDER OF ANIMAL	**V8Ø.21XA**	Animal-rider injured in collision w pedal cycle, init encntr
		V8Ø.21XD	Animal-rider injured in collision w pedal cycle, subs encntr
E826.3	PEDAL CYCLE ACCIDENT INJR OCC ANIMAL-DRAWN VEH	**V8Ø.22XA**	Occ of anml-drn vehicle injured in clsn w pedl cyc, init
		V8Ø.22XD	Occ of anml-drn vehicle injured in clsn w pedl cyc, subs
E826.4	PEDAL CYCLE ACCIDENT INJURING OCCUPANT STREETCAR	**V82.8XXA**	Occupant of streetcar injured in oth transport acc, init
E826.8	PEDAL CYCLE ACCIDENT INJURING OTHER SPEC PERSON	**V18.2XXA**	Unsp pedl cyclst injured in nonclsn trnsp acc nontraf, init
E826.9	PEDAL CYCLE ACCIDENT INJURING UNSPECIFIED PERSON	**V1Ø.2XXA**	Unsp pedl cyclst injured in clsn w ped/anml nontraf, init
		V1Ø.2XXD	Unsp pedl cyclst injured in clsn w ped/anml nontraf, subs
		V1Ø.9XXA	Unsp pedl cyclst injured in clsn w ped/anml in traf, init
		V1Ø.9XXD	Unsp pedl cyclst injured in clsn w ped/anml in traf, subs
		V11.2XXA	Unsp pedl cyclst inj in clsn w oth pedl cyc nontraf, init
		V11.2XXD	Unsp pedl cyclst inj in clsn w oth pedl cyc nontraf, subs
		V11.9XXA	Unsp pedl cyclst inj in clsn w oth pedl cyc in traf, init
		V11.9XXD	Unsp pedl cyclst inj in clsn w oth pedl cyc in traf, subs
		V16.2XXA	Unsp pedl cyclst inj in clsn w nonmtr vehicle nontraf, init
		V16.2XXD	Unsp pedl cyclst inj in clsn w nonmtr vehicle nontraf, subs
		V16.9XXA	Unsp pedl cyclst inj in clsn w nonmtr vehicle in traf, init
		V16.9XXD	Unsp pedl cyclst inj in clsn w nonmtr vehicle in traf, subs
		V17.2XXA	Unsp pedl cyclst inj in clsn w statnry object nontraf, init
		V17.2XXD	Unsp pedl cyclst inj in clsn w statnry object nontraf, subs
		V17.9XXA	Unsp pedl cyclst inj in clsn w statnry object in traf, init
		V17.9XXD	Unsp pedl cyclst inj in clsn w statnry object in traf, subs
		V18.2XXA	Unsp pedl cyclst injured in nonclsn trnsp acc nontraf, init
		V18.2XXD	Unsp pedl cyclst injured in nonclsn trnsp acc nontraf, subs
		V18.9XXA	Unsp pedl cyclst injured in nonclsn trnsp acc in traf, init
		V18.9XXD	Unsp pedl cyclst injured in nonclsn trnsp acc in traf, subs
E827.Ø	ANIMAL-DRAWN VEHICLE ACCIDENT INJR PEDESTRIAN	**VØ9.1XXA**	Pedestrian injured in unsp nontraffic accident, init encntr
E827.2	ANIMAL-DRAWN VEHICLE ACCIDENT INJR RIDER ANIMAL	**V8Ø.71ØA**	Animal-rider injured in collision w animl being ridden, init
		V8Ø.71ØD	Animal-rider injured in collision w animl being ridden, subs
		V8Ø.72ØA	Animal-rider injured in collision w anml-drn vehicle, init
		V8Ø.72ØD	Animal-rider injured in collision w anml-drn vehicle, subs

ICD-9-CM		ICD-10-CM	
E827.3	ANIMAL-DRAWN VEH ACC INJR OCC ANIMAL-DRAWN VEH	**V8Ø.Ø2XA**	Occ of anml-drn veh inj by fall fr veh in nonclsn acc, init
		V8Ø.Ø2XD	Occ of anml-drn veh inj by fall fr veh in nonclsn acc, subs
		V8Ø.12XA	Occ of anml-drn vehicle injured in clsn w ped/anml, init
		V8Ø.12XD	Occ of anml-drn vehicle injured in clsn w ped/anml, subs
		V8Ø.711A	Occ of anml-drn veh inj in clsn w animal being ridden, init
		V8Ø.711D	Occ of anml-drn veh inj in clsn w animal being ridden, subs
		V8Ø.721A	Occ of anml-drn vehicle injured in collisn with same, init
		V8Ø.721D	Occ of anml-drn vehicle injured in collisn with same, subs
		V8Ø.731A	Occupant of anml-drn vehicle injured in clsn w stcar, init
		V8Ø.731D	Occupant of anml-drn vehicle injured in clsn w stcar, subs
		V8Ø.791A	Occ of anml-drn vehicle injured in clsn w nonmtr veh, init
		V8Ø.791D	Occ of anml-drn vehicle injured in clsn w nonmtr veh, subs
		V8Ø.82XA	Occ of anml-drn vehicle inj in clsn w statnry object, init
		V8Ø.82XD	Occ of anml-drn vehicle inj in clsn w statnry object, subs
		V8Ø.92ØA	Occ of anml-drn veh inj in trnsp acc w miltry vehicle, init
		V8Ø.92ØD	Occ of anml-drn veh inj in trnsp acc w miltry vehicle, subs
		V8Ø.928A	Occupant of anml-drn vehicle injured in oth trnsp acc, init
		V8Ø.928D	Occupant of anml-drn vehicle injured in oth trnsp acc, subs
		V8Ø.929A	Occupant of anml-drn vehicle injured in unsp trnsp acc, init
		V8Ø.929D	Occupant of anml-drn vehicle injured in unsp trnsp acc, subs
E827.4	ANIMAL-DRAWN VEHICLE ACCIDENT INJR OCC STREETCAR	**V82.8XXA**	Occupant of streetcar injured in oth transport acc, init
E827.8	ANIMAL-DRAWN VEH ACCIDENT INJR OTH SPEC PERSON	**V88.9XXA**	Person injured in oth transport acc w non-mv, nontraf, init
E827.9	ANIMAL-DRAWN VEHICLE ACCIDENT INJR UNSPEC PERSON	**V88.9XXA**	Person injured in oth transport acc w non-mv, nontraf, init
E828.Ø	ACCIDENT INVLV ANIMAL BEING RIDDEN INJR PEDSTRN	**VØ9.1XXA**	Pedestrian injured in unsp nontraffic accident, init encntr
E828.2	ACC INVLV ANIMAL BEING RIDDEN INJR RIDER ANIMAL	**V8Ø.Ø1ØA**	Animl-ridr injured by fall fr horse in nonclsn acc, init
		V8Ø.Ø1ØD	Animl-ridr injured by fall fr horse in nonclsn acc, subs
		V8Ø.Ø18A	Animl-ridr injured by fall fr animl in nonclsn acc, init
		V8Ø.Ø18D	Animl-ridr injured by fall fr animl in nonclsn acc, subs
		V8Ø.11XA	Animal-rider injured in collision w ped/anml, init
		V8Ø.11XD	Animal-rider injured in collision w ped/anml, subs
		V8Ø.73ØA	Animal-rider injured in collision w streetcar, init encntr
		V8Ø.73ØD	Animal-rider injured in collision w streetcar, subs encntr
		V8Ø.79ØA	Animal-rider injured in collision w nonmtr vehicles, init
		V8Ø.79ØD	Animal-rider injured in collision w nonmtr vehicles, subs
		V8Ø.81XA	Animal-rider injured in collision w statnry object, init
		V8Ø.81XD	Animal-rider injured in collision w statnry object, subs
		V8Ø.91ØA	Animl-ridr injured in trnsp acc w military vehicle, init
		V8Ø.91ØD	Animl-ridr injured in trnsp acc w military vehicle, subs
		V8Ø.918A	Animal-rider injured in oth transport accident, init encntr
		V8Ø.918D	Animal-rider injured in oth transport accident, subs encntr
		V8Ø.919A	Animal-rider injured in unsp transport accident, init encntr
		V8Ø.919D	Animal-rider injured in unsp transport accident, subs encntr
E828.4	ACC INVLV ANIMAL BEING RIDDEN INJR OCC STREETCAR	**V82.8XXA**	Occupant of streetcar injured in oth transport acc, init
E828.8	ACC INVLV ANIMAL BEING RIDDEN INJR OTH SPEC PERS	**V88.9XXA**	Person injured in oth transport acc w non-mv, nontraf, init
E828.9	ACC INVLV ANIMAL BEING RIDDEN INJR UNSPEC PERSON	**V88.9XXA**	Person injured in oth transport acc w non-mv, nontraf, init
E829.Ø	OTHER ROAD VEHICLE ACCIDENTS INJURING PEDESTRIAN	**VØ6.ØØXA**	Ped on foot injured in clsn w nonmtr vehicle nontraf, init
		VØ6.ØØXD	Ped on foot injured in clsn w nonmtr vehicle nontraf, subs
		VØ6.Ø1XA	Ped on rolr-skt inj in clsn w nonmtr vehicle nontraf, init
		VØ6.Ø1XD	Ped on rolr-skt inj in clsn w nonmtr vehicle nontraf, subs
		VØ6.Ø2XA	Ped on sktbrd injured in clsn w nonmtr vehicle nontraf, init
		VØ6.Ø2XD	Ped on sktbrd injured in clsn w nonmtr vehicle nontraf, subs
		VØ6.Ø9XA	Ped w convey injured in clsn w nonmtr vehicle nontraf, init
		VØ6.Ø9XD	Ped w convey injured in clsn w nonmtr vehicle nontraf, subs
		VØ6.1ØXA	Ped on foot injured in clsn w nonmtr vehicle in traf, init
		VØ6.1ØXD	Ped on foot injured in clsn w nonmtr vehicle in traf, subs
		VØ6.11XA	Ped on rolr-skt inj in clsn w nonmtr vehicle in traf, init
		VØ6.11XD	Ped on rolr-skt inj in clsn w nonmtr vehicle in traf, subs
		VØ6.12XA	Ped on sktbrd injured in clsn w nonmtr vehicle in traf, init
		VØ6.12XD	Ped on sktbrd injured in clsn w nonmtr vehicle in traf, subs
		VØ6.19XA	Ped w convey injured in clsn w nonmtr vehicle in traf, init
		VØ6.19XD	Ped w convey injured in clsn w nonmtr vehicle in traf, subs
		VØ6.9ØXA	Ped on foot injured in clsn w nonmtr vehicle, unsp, init
		VØ6.9ØXD	Ped on foot injured in clsn w nonmtr vehicle, unsp, subs
		VØ6.91XA	Ped on rolr-skt injured in clsn w nonmtr vehicle, unsp, init
		VØ6.91XD	Ped on rolr-skt injured in clsn w nonmtr vehicle, unsp, subs
		VØ6.92XA	Ped on sktbrd injured in clsn w nonmtr vehicle, unsp, init
		VØ6.92XD	Ped on sktbrd injured in clsn w nonmtr vehicle, unsp, subs
		VØ6.99XA	Ped w convey injured in clsn w nonmtr vehicle, unsp, init
		VØ6.99XD	Ped w convey injured in clsn w nonmtr vehicle, unsp, subs
		VØ9.1XXA	Pedestrian injured in unsp nontraffic accident, init encntr
		VØ9.1XXD	Pedestrian injured in unsp nontraffic accident, subs encntr
		VØ9.3XXA	Pedestrian injured in unsp traffic accident, init encntr
		VØ9.3XXD	Pedestrian injured in unsp traffic accident, subs encntr
		VØ9.9XXA	Pedestrian injured in unsp transport accident, init encntr
		VØ9.9XXD	Pedestrian injured in unsp transport accident, subs encntr

ICD-9-CM		ICD-10-CM	
E829.4	OTH ROAD VEHICLE ACC INJURING OCCUPANT STREETCAR	**V82.3XXA**	Occupant of streetcar injured in clsn w oth object, init
		V82.3XXD	Occupant of streetcar injured in clsn w oth object, subs
		V82.4XXA	Person injured wh brd/alit from streetcar, init
		V82.4XXD	Person injured wh brd/alit from streetcar, subs
		V82.5XXA	Occupant of streetcar injured by fall in streetcar, init
		V82.5XXD	Occupant of streetcar injured by fall in streetcar, subs
		V82.6XXA	Occupant of streetcar injured by fall from streetcar, init
		V82.6XXD	Occupant of streetcar injured by fall from streetcar, subs
		V82.7XXA	Occ of stcar injured in derail w/o antecedent clsn, init
		V82.7XXD	Occ of stcar injured in derail w/o antecedent clsn, subs
		V82.8XXA	Occupant of streetcar injured in oth transport acc, init
		V82.8XXD	Occupant of streetcar injured in oth transport acc, subs
		V82.9XXA	Occupant of streetcar injured in unsp traffic accident, init
		V82.9XXD	Occupant of streetcar injured in unsp traffic accident, subs
E829.8	OTH ROAD VEHICLE ACC INJURING OTH SPEC PERSON	**V88.9XXA**	Person injured in oth transport acc w non-mv, nontraf, init
E829.9	OTH ROAD VEHICLE ACC INJURING UNSPEC PERSON	**V89.1XXA**	Person injured in unsp nonmotor-vehicle acc, nontraf, init
		V89.1XXD	Person injured in unsp nonmotor-vehicle acc, nontraf, subs
E83Ø.Ø	ACC WATRCRFT CAUS SUBMERS-OCC SM UNPOWR BOAT	**V9Ø.89XA**	Drown due to oth accident to unsp watercraft, init
E83Ø.1	ACC WATRCRFT CAUS SUBMERS-OCC SM POWR BOAT	**V9Ø.89XA**	Drown due to oth accident to unsp watercraft, init
E83Ø.2	ACC WATERCRAFT CAUS SUBMERSION-CREW	**V9Ø.89XA**	Drown due to oth accident to unsp watercraft, init
E83Ø.3	ACC WATERCRAFT CAUS SUBMERSION-OCC NOT CREW	**V9Ø.89XA**	Drown due to oth accident to unsp watercraft, init
E83Ø.4	ACC WATERCRAFT CAUS SUBMERSION-WATER SKIER	**V9Ø.89XA**	Drown due to oth accident to unsp watercraft, init
E83Ø.5	ACC WATERCRAFT CAUS SUBMERSION-INJR SWIMMER	**V9Ø.89XA**	Drown due to oth accident to unsp watercraft, init
E83Ø.6	ACC WATERCRAFT CAUS SUBMERSION-DOCKERS-WORKRS	**V9Ø.89XA**	Drown due to oth accident to unsp watercraft, init
E83Ø.7	ACC WATERCRAFT SUBMERSION OCC MILITARY WATERCRFT	**V9Ø.89XA**	Drown due to oth accident to unsp watercraft, init
E83Ø.8	ACC WATERCRAFT CAUS SUBMERSION-INJR OTH PERS	**V9Ø.89XA**	Drown due to oth accident to unsp watercraft, init
E83Ø.9	ACC WATERCRAFT CAUS SUBMERSION-INJR UNSPEC PERS	**V9Ø.ØØXA**	Drown due to merchant ship overturning, init
		V9Ø.ØØXD	Drown due to merchant ship overturning, subs
		V9Ø.Ø1XA	Drown due to passenger ship overturning, init
		V9Ø.Ø1XD	Drown due to passenger ship overturning, subs
		V9Ø.Ø2XA	Drown due to fishing boat overturning, init
		V9Ø.Ø2XD	Drown due to fishing boat overturning, subs
		V9Ø.Ø3XA	Drown due to oth powered watercraft overturning, init
		V9Ø.Ø3XD	Drown due to oth powered watercraft overturning, subs
		V9Ø.Ø4XA	Drowning and submersion due to sailboat overturning, init
		V9Ø.Ø4XD	Drowning and submersion due to sailboat overturning, subs
		V9Ø.Ø5XA	Drown due to canoe or kayak overturning, init
		V9Ø.Ø5XD	Drown due to canoe or kayak overturning, subs
		V9Ø.Ø6XA	Drown due to (nonpowered) inflatable craft overturning, init
		V9Ø.Ø6XD	Drown due to (nonpowered) inflatable craft overturning, subs
		V9Ø.Ø8XA	Drown due to unpowr wtrcrft overturning, init
		V9Ø.Ø8XD	Drown due to unpowr wtrcrft overturning, subs
		V9Ø.Ø9XA	Drown due to unsp watercraft overturning, init
		V9Ø.Ø9XD	Drown due to unsp watercraft overturning, subs
		V9Ø.1ØXA	Drowning and submersion due to merchant ship sinking, init
		V9Ø.1ØXD	Drowning and submersion due to merchant ship sinking, subs
		V9Ø.11XA	Drowning and submersion due to passenger ship sinking, init
		V9Ø.11XD	Drowning and submersion due to passenger ship sinking, subs
		V9Ø.12XA	Drowning and submersion due to fishing boat sinking, init
		V9Ø.12XD	Drowning and submersion due to fishing boat sinking, subs
		V9Ø.13XA	Drown due to oth powered watercraft sinking, init
		V9Ø.13XD	Drown due to oth powered watercraft sinking, subs
		V9Ø.14XA	Drowning and submersion due to sailboat sinking, init encntr
		V9Ø.14XD	Drowning and submersion due to sailboat sinking, subs encntr
		V9Ø.15XA	Drowning and submersion due to canoe or kayak sinking, init
		V9Ø.15XD	Drowning and submersion due to canoe or kayak sinking, subs
		V9Ø.16XA	Drown due to (nonpowered) inflatable craft sinking, init
		V9Ø.16XD	Drown due to (nonpowered) inflatable craft sinking, subs
		V9Ø.18XA	Drowning and submersion due to unpowr wtrcrft sinking, init
		V9Ø.18XD	Drowning and submersion due to unpowr wtrcrft sinking, subs
		V9Ø.19XA	Drowning and submersion due to unsp watercraft sinking, init
		V9Ø.19XD	Drowning and submersion due to unsp watercraft sinking, subs
		V9Ø.2ØXA	Drown due to fall/jump fr burning merchant ship, init
		V9Ø.2ØXD	Drown due to fall/jump fr burning merchant ship, subs
		V9Ø.21XA	Drown due to fall/jump fr burning passenger ship, init
		V9Ø.21XD	Drown due to fall/jump fr burning passenger ship, subs
		V9Ø.22XA	Drown due to fall/jump fr burning fishing boat, init
		V9Ø.22XD	Drown due to fall/jump fr burning fishing boat, subs
		V9Ø.23XA	Drown due to fall/jump fr oth burning powered wtrcrft, init
		V9Ø.23XD	Drown due to fall/jump fr oth burning powered wtrcrft, subs
		V9Ø.24XA	Drown due to falling or jumping from burning sailboat, init
		V9Ø.24XD	Drown due to falling or jumping from burning sailboat, subs
		V9Ø.25XA	Drown due to fall/jump fr burning canoe or kayak, init
		V9Ø.25XD	Drown due to fall/jump fr burning canoe or kayak, subs
		V9Ø.26XA	Drown due to fall/jump fr burning inflatbl crft, init
		V9Ø.26XD	Drown due to fall/jump fr burning inflatbl crft, subs
		V9Ø.27XA	Drown due to fall/jump fr burning water-skis, init
		V9Ø.27XD	Drown due to fall/jump fr burning water-skis, subs
		V9Ø.28XA	Drown due to fall/jump fr oth burning unpowr wtrcrft, init
		V9Ø.28XD	Drown due to fall/jump fr oth burning unpowr wtrcrft, subs

(Continued on next page)

ICD-9-CM		ICD-10-CM	
E83Ø.9	ACC WATERCRAFT CAUS SUBMERSION-INJR UNSPEC PERS **(Continued)**	**V9Ø.29XA**	Drown due to fall/jump fr unsp burning watercraft, init
		V9Ø.29XD	Drown due to fall/jump fr unsp burning watercraft, subs
		V9Ø.3ØXA	Drown due to fall/jump fr crushed merchant ship, init
		V9Ø.3ØXD	Drown due to fall/jump fr crushed merchant ship, subs
		V9Ø.31XA	Drown due to fall/jump fr crushed passenger ship, init
		V9Ø.31XD	Drown due to fall/jump fr crushed passenger ship, subs
		V9Ø.32XA	Drown due to fall/jump fr crushed fishing boat, init
		V9Ø.32XD	Drown due to fall/jump fr crushed fishing boat, subs
		V9Ø.33XA	Drown due to fall/jump fr oth crushed powered wtrcrft, init
		V9Ø.33XD	Drown due to fall/jump fr oth crushed powered wtrcrft, subs
		V9Ø.34XA	Drown due to falling or jumping from crushed sailboat, init
		V9Ø.34XD	Drown due to falling or jumping from crushed sailboat, subs
		V9Ø.35XA	Drown due to fall/jump fr crushed canoe or kayak, init
		V9Ø.35XD	Drown due to fall/jump fr crushed canoe or kayak, subs
		V9Ø.36XA	Drown due to fall/jump fr crushed inflatbl crft, init
		V9Ø.36XD	Drown due to fall/jump fr crushed inflatbl crft, subs
		V9Ø.37XA	Drown due to fall/jump fr crushed water-skis, init
		V9Ø.37XD	Drown due to fall/jump fr crushed water-skis, subs
		V9Ø.38XA	Drown due to fall/jump fr oth crushed unpowr wtrcrft, init
		V9Ø.38XD	Drown due to fall/jump fr oth crushed unpowr wtrcrft, subs
		V9Ø.39XA	Drown due to fall/jump fr crushed unsp watercraft, init
		V9Ø.39XD	Drown due to fall/jump fr crushed unsp watercraft, subs
		V9Ø.8ØXA	Drown due to oth accident to merchant ship, init
		V9Ø.8ØXD	Drown due to oth accident to merchant ship, subs
		V9Ø.81XA	Drown due to oth accident to passenger ship, init
		V9Ø.81XD	Drown due to oth accident to passenger ship, subs
		V9Ø.82XA	Drown due to oth accident to fishing boat, init
		V9Ø.82XD	Drown due to oth accident to fishing boat, subs
		V9Ø.83XA	Drown due to oth accident to oth powered watercraft, init
		V9Ø.83XD	Drown due to oth accident to oth powered watercraft, subs
		V9Ø.84XA	Drown due to oth accident to sailboat, init
		V9Ø.84XD	Drown due to oth accident to sailboat, subs
		V9Ø.85XA	Drown due to oth accident to canoe or kayak, init
		V9Ø.85XD	Drown due to oth accident to canoe or kayak, subs
		V9Ø.86XA	Drown due to oth accident to inflatbl crft, init
		V9Ø.86XD	Drown due to oth accident to inflatbl crft, subs
		V9Ø.87XA	Drown due to oth accident to water-skis, init
		V9Ø.87XD	Drown due to oth accident to water-skis, subs
		V9Ø.88XA	Drown due to oth accident to unpowr wtrcrft, init
		V9Ø.88XD	Drown due to oth accident to unpowr wtrcrft, subs
		V9Ø.89XA	Drown due to oth accident to unsp watercraft, init
		V9Ø.89XD	Drown due to oth accident to unsp watercraft, subs
E831.Ø	ACC WATRCRFT CAUS OTH INJURY OCC-SM UNPOWER BOAT	**V91.89XA**	Oth injury due to oth accident to unsp watercraft, init
E831.1	ACC WATERCRAFT CAUS OTH INJURY OCC-SM POWER BOAT	**V91.89XA**	Oth injury due to oth accident to unsp watercraft, init
E831.2	ACC WATERCRAFT CAUSING OTHER INJURY-CREW	**V91.89XA**	Oth injury due to oth accident to unsp watercraft, init
E831.3	ACC WATERCRAFT CAUSING OTH INJURY-NOT CREW	**V91.89XA**	Oth injury due to oth accident to unsp watercraft, init
E831.4	ACC WATERCRAFT CAUSING OTH INJURY-WATER SKIER	**V91.89XA**	Oth injury due to oth accident to unsp watercraft, init
E831.5	ACC WATERCRAFT CAUSING OTHER INJURY-SWIMMER	**V91.89XA**	Oth injury due to oth accident to unsp watercraft, init
E831.6	ACC WATRCRFT CAUS OTH INJR-DOCKERS STEVEDORES	**V91.89XA**	Oth injury due to oth accident to unsp watercraft, init
E831.7	ACC WATERCRFT CAUS OTH INJ OCC MILITARY WATRCRFT	**V91.89XA**	Oth injury due to oth accident to unsp watercraft, init
E831.8	ACC WATERCRAFT CAUS OTH INJURY-OTH SPEC PERSON	**V91.89XA**	Oth injury due to oth accident to unsp watercraft, init
E831.9	ACC WATERCRAFT CAUS OTH INJURY-UNSPEC PERSON	**V91.ØØXA**	Burn due to merchant ship on fire, initial encounter
		V91.ØØXD	Burn due to merchant ship on fire, subsequent encounter
		V91.Ø1XA	Burn due to passenger ship on fire, initial encounter
		V91.Ø1XD	Burn due to passenger ship on fire, subsequent encounter
		V91.Ø2XA	Burn due to fishing boat on fire, initial encounter
		V91.Ø2XD	Burn due to fishing boat on fire, subsequent encounter
		V91.Ø3XA	Burn due to other powered watercraft on fire, init encntr
		V91.Ø3XD	Burn due to other powered watercraft on fire, subs encntr
		V91.Ø4XA	Burn due to sailboat on fire, initial encounter
		V91.Ø4XD	Burn due to sailboat on fire, subsequent encounter
		V91.Ø5XA	Burn due to canoe or kayak on fire, initial encounter
		V91.Ø5XD	Burn due to canoe or kayak on fire, subsequent encounter
		V91.Ø6XA	Burn due to (nonpowered) inflatable craft on fire, init
		V91.Ø6XD	Burn due to (nonpowered) inflatable craft on fire, subs
		V91.Ø7XA	Burn due to water-skis on fire, initial encounter
		V91.Ø7XD	Burn due to water-skis on fire, subsequent encounter
		V91.Ø8XA	Burn due to other unpowered watercraft on fire, init encntr
		V91.Ø8XD	Burn due to other unpowered watercraft on fire, subs encntr
		V91.Ø9XA	Burn due to unspecified watercraft on fire, init encntr
		V91.Ø9XD	Burn due to unspecified watercraft on fire, subs encntr
		V91.1ØXA	Crush betw merch ship and oth wtrcrft/obj due to clsn, init
		V91.1ØXD	Crush betw merch ship and oth wtrcrft/obj due to clsn, subs
		V91.11XA	Crush betw pasngr ship and oth wtrcrft/obj due to clsn, init
		V91.11XD	Crush betw pasngr ship and oth wtrcrft/obj due to clsn, subs
		V91.12XA	Crush betw fish boat and oth wtrcrft/obj due to clsn, init
		V91.12XD	Crush betw fish boat and oth wtrcrft/obj due to clsn, subs
		V91.13XA	Crush betw oth pwr wtrcrft & oth wtrcrft/obj d/t clsn, init
		V91.13XD	Crush betw oth pwr wtrcrft & oth wtrcrft/obj d/t clsn, subs
	(Continued on next page)	**V91.14XA**	Crushed betw sailboat and oth wtrcrft/obj due to clsn, init

ICD-9-CM		ICD-10-CM	
E831.9	ACC WATERCRAFT CAUS OTH INJURY-UNSPEC PERSON **(Continued)**	**V91.14XD**	Crushed betw sailboat and oth wtrcrft/obj due to clsn, subs
		V91.15XA	Crush betw canoe/kayk and oth wtrcrft/obj due to clsn, init
		V91.15XD	Crush betw canoe/kayk and oth wtrcrft/obj due to clsn, subs
		V91.16XA	Crush betw inflatbl crft and oth wtrcrft/obj d/t clsn, init
		V91.16XD	Crush betw inflatbl crft and oth wtrcrft/obj d/t clsn, subs
		V91.18XA	Crush betw unpowr wtrcrft and oth wtrcrft/obj d/t clsn, init
		V91.18XD	Crush betw unpowr wtrcrft and oth wtrcrft/obj d/t clsn, subs
		V91.19XA	Crush betw unsp wtrcrft and oth wtrcrft/obj d/t clsn, init
		V91.19XD	Crush betw unsp wtrcrft and oth wtrcrft/obj d/t clsn, subs
		V91.2ØXA	Fall due to clsn betw merch ship and oth wtrcrft/obj, init
		V91.2ØXD	Fall due to clsn betw merch ship and oth wtrcrft/obj, subs
		V91.21XA	Fall due to clsn betw pasngr ship and oth wtrcrft/obj, init
		V91.21XD	Fall due to clsn betw pasngr ship and oth wtrcrft/obj, subs
		V91.22XA	Fall due to clsn betw fishing boat and oth wtrcrft/obj, init
		V91.22XD	Fall due to clsn betw fishing boat and oth wtrcrft/obj, subs
		V91.23XA	Fall d/t clsn betw oth pwr wtrcrft and oth wtrcrft/obj, init
		V91.23XD	Fall d/t clsn betw oth pwr wtrcrft and oth wtrcrft/obj, subs
		V91.24XA	Fall due to clsn betw sailboat and oth wtrcrft/obj, init
		V91.24XD	Fall due to clsn betw sailboat and oth wtrcrft/obj, subs
		V91.25XA	Fall due to clsn betw canoe/kayk and oth wtrcrft/obj, init
		V91.25XD	Fall due to clsn betw canoe/kayk and oth wtrcrft/obj, subs
		V91.26XA	Fall d/t clsn betw inflatbl crft and oth wtrcrft/obj, init
		V91.26XD	Fall d/t clsn betw inflatbl crft and oth wtrcrft/obj, subs
		V91.29XA	Fall due to clsn betw unsp wtrcrft and oth wtrcrft/obj, init
		V91.29XD	Fall due to clsn betw unsp wtrcrft and oth wtrcrft/obj, subs
		V91.3ØXA	Hit by falling object due to accident to merchant ship, init
		V91.3ØXD	Hit by falling object due to accident to merchant ship, subs
		V91.31XA	Hit by falling object due to accident to pasngr ship, init
		V91.31XD	Hit by falling object due to accident to pasngr ship, subs
		V91.32XA	Hit by falling object due to accident to fishing boat, init
		V91.32XD	Hit by falling object due to accident to fishing boat, subs
		V91.33XA	Hit by fall object due to acc to oth powered wtrcrft, init
		V91.33XD	Hit by fall object due to acc to oth powered wtrcrft, subs
		V91.34XA	Hit by falling object due to accident to sailboat, init
		V91.34XD	Hit by falling object due to accident to sailboat, subs
		V91.35XA	Hit by falling object due to accident to canoe/kayk, init
		V91.35XD	Hit by falling object due to accident to canoe/kayk, subs
		V91.36XA	Hit by falling object due to accident to inflatbl crft, init
		V91.36XD	Hit by falling object due to accident to inflatbl crft, subs
		V91.37XA	Hit by falling object due to accident to water-skis, init
		V91.37XD	Hit by falling object due to accident to water-skis, subs
		V91.38XA	Hit by falling object due to acc to unpowr wtrcrft, init
		V91.38XD	Hit by falling object due to acc to unpowr wtrcrft, subs
		V91.39XA	Hit by falling object due to accident to unsp wtrcrft, init
		V91.39XD	Hit by falling object due to accident to unsp wtrcrft, subs
		V91.8ØXA	Oth injury due to oth accident to merchant ship, init encntr
		V91.8ØXD	Oth injury due to oth accident to merchant ship, subs encntr
		V91.81XA	Oth injury due to oth accident to passenger ship, init
		V91.81XD	Oth injury due to oth accident to passenger ship, subs
		V91.82XA	Oth injury due to oth accident to fishing boat, init encntr
		V91.82XD	Oth injury due to oth accident to fishing boat, subs encntr
		V91.83XA	Oth injury due to oth accident to oth powered wtrcrft, init
		V91.83XD	Oth injury due to oth accident to oth powered wtrcrft, subs
		V91.84XA	Other injury due to other accident to sailboat, init encntr
		V91.84XD	Other injury due to other accident to sailboat, subs encntr
		V91.85XA	Oth injury due to oth accident to canoe or kayak, init
		V91.85XD	Oth injury due to oth accident to canoe or kayak, subs
		V91.86XA	Oth injury due to oth accident to inflatbl crft, init
		V91.86XD	Oth injury due to oth accident to inflatbl crft, subs
		V91.87XA	Oth injury due to other accident to water-skis, init encntr
		V91.87XD	Oth injury due to other accident to water-skis, subs encntr
		V91.88XA	Oth injury due to oth accident to unpowr wtrcrft, init
		V91.88XD	Oth injury due to oth accident to unpowr wtrcrft, subs
		V91.89XA	Oth injury due to oth accident to unsp watercraft, init
		V91.89XD	Oth injury due to oth accident to unsp watercraft, subs
E832.Ø	OTH ACC SUBMERS/DROWN WATER TRNSPRT-UNPWR BOAT	**V92.Ø9XA**	Drown due to fall off unsp watercraft, init
E832.1	OTH ACC SUBMERS/DROWN WATER TRNSPRT-POWER BOAT	**V92.Ø9XA**	Drown due to fall off unsp watercraft, init
E832.2	OTH ACC SUBMERS/DROWN WATER TRANSPORT-CREW	**V92.Ø9XA**	Drown due to fall off unsp watercraft, init
E832.3	OTH ACC SUBMERS/DROWN WATER TRANSPORT-NOT CREW	**V92.Ø9XA**	Drown due to fall off unsp watercraft, init
E832.4	OTH ACC SUBMERS/DROWN WATER TRNSPRT-WATER SKIER	**V92.Ø9XA**	Drown due to fall off unsp watercraft, init
E832.5	OTH ACC SUBMERS/DROWN H2O TRNSPRT ACC INJR SWMR	**V92.Ø9XA**	Drown due to fall off unsp watercraft, init
E832.6	OTH ACC SUBMERS/DROWN WATER TRNSPRT-DOCKERS	**V92.Ø9XA**	Drown due to fall off unsp watercraft, init
E832.7	OTH ACC SUBMERS/DROWN WATER TRNSPRT OCC MILITARY	**V92.Ø9XA**	Drown due to fall off unsp watercraft, init
E832.8	OTH ACC SUBMERS/DROWN WATER TRNSPRT-OTH PERSON	**V92.Ø9XA**	Drown due to fall off unsp watercraft, init
E832.9	OTH ACC SUBMERS/DROWN WATER TRNSPRT-UNS PERSON	**V92.ØØXA**	Drowning and submersion due to fall off merchant ship, init
		V92.ØØXD	Drowning and submersion due to fall off merchant ship, subs
		V92.Ø1XA	Drowning and submersion due to fall off passenger ship, init
		V92.Ø1XD	Drowning and submersion due to fall off passenger ship, subs
		V92.Ø2XA	Drowning and submersion due to fall off fishing boat, init
	(Continued on next page)	**V92.Ø2XD**	Drowning and submersion due to fall off fishing boat, subs

ICD-9-CM		ICD-10-CM	
E832.9	OTH ACC SUBMERS/DROWN WATER TRNSPRT-UNS PERSON **(Continued)**	**V92.Ø3XA**	Drown due to fall off oth powered watercraft, init
		V92.Ø3XD	Drown due to fall off oth powered watercraft, subs
		V92.Ø4XA	Drowning and submersion due to fall off sailboat, init
		V92.Ø4XD	Drowning and submersion due to fall off sailboat, subs
		V92.Ø5XA	Drowning and submersion due to fall off canoe or kayak, init
		V92.Ø5XD	Drowning and submersion due to fall off canoe or kayak, subs
		V92.Ø6XA	Drown due to fall off (nonpowered) inflatable craft, init
		V92.Ø6XD	Drown due to fall off (nonpowered) inflatable craft, subs
		V92.Ø7XA	Drowning and submersion due to fall off water-skis, init
		V92.Ø7XD	Drowning and submersion due to fall off water-skis, subs
		V92.Ø8XA	Drowning and submersion due to fall off unpowr wtrcrft, init
		V92.Ø8XD	Drowning and submersion due to fall off unpowr wtrcrft, subs
		V92.Ø9XA	Drown due to fall off unsp watercraft, init
		V92.Ø9XD	Drown due to fall off unsp watercraft, subs
		V92.1ØXA	Drown d/t being thrown ovrbrd by motion of merch ship, init
		V92.1ØXD	Drown d/t being thrown ovrbrd by motion of merch ship, subs
		V92.11XA	Drown d/t being thrown ovrbrd by motion of pasngr ship, init
		V92.11XD	Drown d/t being thrown ovrbrd by motion of pasngr ship, subs
		V92.12XA	Drown d/t being thrown ovrbrd by motion of fish boat, init
		V92.12XD	Drown d/t being thrown ovrbrd by motion of fish boat, subs
		V92.13XA	Drown d/t thrown ovrbrd by motion of power wtrcrft, init
		V92.13XD	Drown d/t thrown ovrbrd by motion of power wtrcrft, subs
		V92.14XA	Drown due to being thrown ovrbrd by motion of sailboat, init
		V92.14XD	Drown due to being thrown ovrbrd by motion of sailboat, subs
		V92.15XA	Drown d/t being thrown ovrbrd by motion of canoe/kayk, init
		V92.15XD	Drown d/t being thrown ovrbrd by motion of canoe/kayk, subs
		V92.16XA	Drown d/t thrown ovrbrd by motion of inflatbl crft, init
		V92.16XD	Drown d/t thrown ovrbrd by motion of inflatbl crft, subs
		V92.19XA	Drown d/t thrown ovrbrd by motion of unsp wtrcrft, init
		V92.19XD	Drown d/t thrown ovrbrd by motion of unsp wtrcrft, subs
		V92.2ØXA	Drown due to being washed overboard from merchant ship, init
		V92.2ØXD	Drown due to being washed overboard from merchant ship, subs
		V92.21XA	Drown due to being washed ovrbrd from passenger ship, init
		V92.21XD	Drown due to being washed ovrbrd from passenger ship, subs
		V92.22XA	Drown due to being washed overboard from fishing boat, init
		V92.22XD	Drown due to being washed overboard from fishing boat, subs
		V92.23XA	Drown d/t being washed ovrbrd from oth power wtrcrft, init
		V92.23XD	Drown d/t being washed ovrbrd from oth power wtrcrft, subs
		V92.24XA	Drown due to being washed overboard from sailboat, init
		V92.24XD	Drown due to being washed overboard from sailboat, subs
		V92.25XA	Drown due to being washed overboard from canoe/kayk, init
		V92.25XD	Drown due to being washed overboard from canoe/kayk, subs
		V92.26XA	Drown due to being washed overboard from inflatbl crft, init
		V92.26XD	Drown due to being washed overboard from inflatbl crft, subs
		V92.27XA	Drown due to being washed overboard from water-skis, init
		V92.27XD	Drown due to being washed overboard from water-skis, subs
		V92.28XA	Drown due to being washed ovrbrd from unpowr wtrcrft, init
		V92.28XD	Drown due to being washed ovrbrd from unpowr wtrcrft, subs
		V92.29XA	Drown due to being washed overboard from unsp wtrcrft, init
		V92.29XD	Drown due to being washed overboard from unsp wtrcrft, subs
E833.Ø	FALL STAIRS/LADDERS WATR TRNSPRT-UNPOWR BOAT	**V93.38XA**	Fall on board other unpowered watercraft, initial encounter
E833.1	FALL STAIRS/LADDERS WATR TRNSPRT-POWR BOAT	**V93.33XA**	Fall on board other powered watercraft, initial encounter
E833.2	FALL STAIRS/LADDERS WATR TRNSPRT-INJR CREW	**V93.39XA**	Fall on board unspecified watercraft, initial encounter
E833.3	FALL STAIRS/LADDERS WATR TRNSPRT-INJR NOT CREW	**V93.39XA**	Fall on board unspecified watercraft, initial encounter
E833.4	FALL STAIRS/LADDERS WATR TRNSPRT-INJR WATR SKIER	**V93.39XA**	Fall on board unspecified watercraft, initial encounter
E833.5	FALL STAIRS/LADDERS WATR TRNSPRT-INJR SWIMMER	**V93.39XA**	Fall on board unspecified watercraft, initial encounter
E833.6	FALL STAIRS/LADDERS WATR TRNSPRT-INJR DOCKERS	**V93.39XA**	Fall on board unspecified watercraft, initial encounter
E833.7	FALL STAIRS/LADDER WATER TRANSPORT OCC MILITARY	**V93.39XA**	Fall on board unspecified watercraft, initial encounter
E833.8	FALL STAIRS/LADDERS WATR TRNSPRT-INJR OTH PERS	**V93.39XA**	Fall on board unspecified watercraft, initial encounter
E833.9	FALL STAIRS/LADDERS WATR TRNSPRT-INJR UNS PERS	**V93.39XA**	Fall on board unspecified watercraft, initial encounter
E834.Ø	OTH FALL 1 LEVEL TO OTH WATR TRNSPRT-UNPOWR BOAT	**V93.38XA**	Fall on board other unpowered watercraft, initial encounter
E834.1	OTH FALL 1 LEVEL TO OTH WATR TRNSPRT-POWR BOAT	**V93.33XA**	Fall on board other powered watercraft, initial encounter
E834.2	OTH FALL 1 LEVEL TO OTH WATER TRANSPORT-CREW	**V93.39XA**	Fall on board unspecified watercraft, initial encounter
E834.3	OTH FALL 1 LEVEL TO OTH WATR TRNSPRT-NOT CREW	**V93.39XA**	Fall on board unspecified watercraft, initial encounter
E834.4	OTH FALL 1 LEVL TO OTH WATER TRNSPRT INJR SKIER	**V93.39XA**	Fall on board unspecified watercraft, initial encounter
E834.5	OTH FALL 1 LEVL TO OTH WATER TRNSPRT INJR SWIMR	**V93.39XA**	Fall on board unspecified watercraft, initial encounter
E834.6	OTH FALL 1 LEVEL TO OTH WATER TRANSPORT-DOCKERS	**V93.39XA**	Fall on board unspecified watercraft, initial encounter
E834.7	OTH FALL 1 LEVL TO OTH WATR TRNSPRT OCC MILITARY	**V93.39XA**	Fall on board unspecified watercraft, initial encounter
E834.8	OTH FALL 1 LEVL TO OTH WTR TRNSPRT INJR OTH PERS	**V93.39XA**	Fall on board unspecified watercraft, initial encounter
E834.9	OTH FALL 1 LEVL TO OTH WTR TRNSPRT INJR UNS PERS	**V93.39XA**	Fall on board unspecified watercraft, initial encounter
E835.Ø	OTH&UNS FALL WATR TRNSPRT-INJR OCC UNPOWR BOAT	**V93.38XA**	Fall on board other unpowered watercraft, initial encounter
E835.1	OTH&UNS FALL WATER TRNSPRT-INJR OCC POWER BOAT	**V93.33XA**	Fall on board other powered watercraft, initial encounter
E835.2	OTH&UNS FALL WATR TRNSPRT-INJR WATRCRFT CREW	**V93.39XA**	Fall on board unspecified watercraft, initial encounter
E835.3	OTH&UNS FALL WATER TRANSPORT-INJURING NOT CREW	**V93.39XA**	Fall on board unspecified watercraft, initial encounter
E835.4	OTH&UNS FALL WATER TRANSPORT-INJR WATER SKIER	**V93.39XA**	Fall on board unspecified watercraft, initial encounter
E835.5	OTH&UNS FALL WATER TRANSPORT-INJURING SWIMMER	**V93.39XA**	Fall on board unspecified watercraft, initial encounter

[Brackets] indicate valid character values for each code. Character value meanings provided for each code grouping.

ICD-9-CM		ICD-10-CM	
E835.6	OTH&UNS FALL WATER TRANSPORT-INJR DOCKERS	**V93.39XA**	Fall on board unspecified watercraft, initial encounter
E835.7	OTH&UNS FALL WATER TRANSPORT OCCUPANT MILITARY	**V93.39XA**	Fall on board unspecified watercraft, initial encounter
E835.8	OTH&UNS FALL WATER TRANSPORT-INJR OTH SPEC PERS	**V93.39XA**	Fall on board unspecified watercraft, initial encounter
E835.9	OTH&UNS FALL WATER TRANSPORT-INJR UNS PERSON	**V93.30XA**	Fall on board merchant ship, initial encounter
		V93.30XD	Fall on board merchant ship, subsequent encounter
		V93.31XA	Fall on board passenger ship, initial encounter
		V93.31XD	Fall on board passenger ship, subsequent encounter
		V93.32XA	Fall on board fishing boat, initial encounter
		V93.32XD	Fall on board fishing boat, subsequent encounter
		V93.33XA	Fall on board other powered watercraft, initial encounter
		V93.33XD	Fall on board other powered watercraft, subsequent encounter
		V93.34XA	Fall on board sailboat, initial encounter
		V93.34XD	Fall on board sailboat, subsequent encounter
		V93.35XA	Fall on board canoe or kayak, initial encounter
		V93.35XD	Fall on board canoe or kayak, subsequent encounter
		V93.36XA	Fall on board (nonpowered) inflatable craft, init encntr
		V93.36XD	Fall on board (nonpowered) inflatable craft, subs encntr
		V93.38XA	Fall on board other unpowered watercraft, initial encounter
		V93.38XD	Fall on board other unpowered watercraft, subs encntr
		V93.39XA	Fall on board unspecified watercraft, initial encounter
		V93.39XD	Fall on board unspecified watercraft, subsequent encounter
E836.0	MACHINERY ACC WATR TRNSPRT-OCC UNPOWR BOAT	**V93.64XA**	Machinery accident on board sailboat, initial encounter
E836.1	MACHINERY ACC WATR TRNSPRT-OCC POWER BOAT	**V93.63XA**	Machinery accident on board oth powered watercraft, init
E836.2	MACHINERY ACC WATER TRANSPORT-INJURING CREW	**V93.69XA**	Machinery accident on board unsp watercraft, init encntr
E836.3	MACHINERY ACC WATER TRANSPORT-INJURING NOT CREW	**V93.69XA**	Machinery accident on board unsp watercraft, init encntr
E836.4	MACHINERY ACC WATER TRANSPORT-INJR WATER SKIER	**V93.69XA**	Machinery accident on board unsp watercraft, init encntr
E836.5	MACHINERY ACC WATER TRANSPORT-INJURING SWIMMER	**V93.69XA**	Machinery accident on board unsp watercraft, init encntr
E836.6	MACHINERY ACC WATER TRNSPRT-INJR DOCKERS	**V93.69XA**	Machinery accident on board unsp watercraft, init encntr
E836.7	MACHINERY ACC WATER TRANSPORT OCCUPANT MILITARY	**V93.69XA**	Machinery accident on board unsp watercraft, init encntr
E836.8	MACHINERY ACC WATER TRANSPORT-INJR OTH PERSON	**V93.69XA**	Machinery accident on board unsp watercraft, init encntr
E836.9	MACHINERY ACC WATER TRANSPORT-INJR UNS PERSON	**V93.60XA**	Machinery accident on board merchant ship, initial encounter
		V93.60XD	Machinery accident on board merchant ship, subs encntr
		V93.61XA	Machinery accident on board passenger ship, init encntr
		V93.61XD	Machinery accident on board passenger ship, subs encntr
		V93.62XA	Machinery accident on board fishing boat, initial encounter
		V93.62XD	Machinery accident on board fishing boat, subs encntr
		V93.63XA	Machinery accident on board oth powered watercraft, init
		V93.63XD	Machinery accident on board oth powered watercraft, subs
		V93.64XA	Machinery accident on board sailboat, initial encounter
		V93.64XD	Machinery accident on board sailboat, subsequent encounter
		V93.69XA	Machinery accident on board unsp watercraft, init encntr
		V93.69XD	Machinery accident on board unsp watercraft, subs encntr
E837.0	EXPLO FIRE/BURNWATRCRAFT INJR OCC SM UNPWR BOAT	**V93.14XA**	Other burn on board sailboat, initial encounter
E837.1	EXPLO FIRE/BURNWATRCRAFT INJR OCC SM PWR BOAT	**V93.53XA**	Explosion on board other powered watercraft, init encntr
E837.2	EXPLOSION FIRE/BURN WATERCRAFT-INJURING CREW	**V93.09XA**	Burn due to localized fire on board unsp watercraft, init
E837.3	EXPLOSION FIRE/BURN WATERCRAFT-INJR NOT CREW	**V93.09XA**	Burn due to localized fire on board unsp watercraft, init
E837.4	EXPLOSION FIRE/BURN WATERCRAFT-INJR WATR SKIER	**V93.09XA**	Burn due to localized fire on board unsp watercraft, init
E837.5	EXPLOSION FIRE/BURN WATERCRAFT-INJURING SWIMMER	**V93.09XA**	Burn due to localized fire on board unsp watercraft, init
E837.6	EXPLOSION FIRE/BURN WATERCRAFT-INJURING DOCKERS	**V93.09XA**	Burn due to localized fire on board unsp watercraft, init
E837.7	EXPLOSION FIRE/BURN WATRCRAFT INJ OCC MILITARY	**V93.19XA**	Other burn on board unspecified watercraft, init encntr
E837.8	EXPLOSION FIRE/BURN WATERCRAFT-INJR OTH PERSON	**V93.09XA**	Burn due to localized fire on board unsp watercraft, init
E837.9	EXPLOSION FIRE/BURN WATERCRAFT-INJR UNS PERSON	**V93.00XA**	Burn due to localized fire on board merchant vessel, init
		V93.00XD	Burn due to localized fire on board merchant vessel, subs
		V93.01XA	Burn due to localized fire on board passenger vessel, init
		V93.01XD	Burn due to localized fire on board passenger vessel, subs
		V93.02XA	Burn due to localized fire on board fishing boat, init
		V93.02XD	Burn due to localized fire on board fishing boat, subs
		V93.03XA	Burn due to loc fire on board oth powered wtrcrft, init
		V93.03XD	Burn due to loc fire on board oth powered wtrcrft, subs
		V93.04XA	Burn due to localized fire on board sailboat, init encntr
		V93.04XD	Burn due to localized fire on board sailboat, subs encntr
		V93.09XA	Burn due to localized fire on board unsp watercraft, init
		V93.09XD	Burn due to localized fire on board unsp watercraft, subs
		V93.10XA	Other burn on board merchant vessel, initial encounter
		V93.10XD	Other burn on board merchant vessel, subsequent encounter
		V93.11XA	Other burn on board passenger vessel, initial encounter
		V93.11XD	Other burn on board passenger vessel, subsequent encounter
		V93.12XA	Other burn on board fishing boat, initial encounter
		V93.12XD	Other burn on board fishing boat, subsequent encounter
		V93.13XA	Other burn on board other powered watercraft, init encntr
		V93.13XD	Other burn on board other powered watercraft, subs encntr
		V93.14XA	Other burn on board sailboat, initial encounter
		V93.14XD	Other burn on board sailboat, subsequent encounter
		V93.19XA	Other burn on board unspecified watercraft, init encntr
		V93.19XD	Other burn on board unspecified watercraft, subs encntr
		V93.50XA	Explosion on board merchant ship, initial encounter
	(Continued on next page)	**V93.50XD**	Explosion on board merchant ship, subsequent encounter

ICD-9-CM		ICD-10-CM	
E837.9	EXPLOSION FIRE/BURN WATERCRAFT-INJR UNS PERSON **(Continued)**	**V93.51XA**	Explosion on board passenger ship, initial encounter
		V93.51XD	Explosion on board passenger ship, subsequent encounter
		V93.52XA	Explosion on board fishing boat, initial encounter
		V93.52XD	Explosion on board fishing boat, subsequent encounter
		V93.53XA	Explosion on board other powered watercraft, init encntr
		V93.53XD	Explosion on board other powered watercraft, subs encntr
		V93.54XA	Explosion on board sailboat, initial encounter
		V93.54XD	Explosion on board sailboat, subsequent encounter
		V93.59XA	Explosion on board unspecified watercraft, initial encounter
		V93.59XD	Explosion on board unspecified watercraft, subs encntr
E838.Ø	OTH&UNS WATER TRANSPORT ACC-OCC UNPOWR BOAT	**V94.21XA**	Rider of nonpowr wtrcrft struck by oth nonpowr wtrcrft, init
		V94.21XD	Rider of nonpowr wtrcrft struck by oth nonpowr wtrcrft, subs
		V94.31XA	Inj to rider of recreatl wtrcrft puld beh oth wtrcrft, init
		V94.31XD	Inj to rider of recreatl wtrcrft puld beh oth wtrcrft, subs
		V94.32XA	Inj to rider of nonrecr wtrcrft puld beh oth wtrcrft, init
		V94.32XD	Inj to rider of nonrecr wtrcrft puld beh oth wtrcrft, subs
E838.1	OTH&UNS WATER TRANSPORT ACC-OCC POWER BOAT	**V94.22XA**	Rider of nonpowr wtrcrft struck by powered watercraft, init
		V94.22XD	Rider of nonpowr wtrcrft struck by powered watercraft, subs
E838.2	OTH&UNS WATER TRNSPRT ACC-INJURING CREW	**V94.89XA**	Other water transport accident, initial encounter
E838.3	OTH&UNS WATER TRANSPORT ACC-INJURING NOT CREW	**V94.89XA**	Other water transport accident, initial encounter
E838.4	OTH&UNS WATER TRANSPORT ACC-INJR WATER SKIER	**V94.4XXA**	Injury to barefoot water-skier, initial encounter
		V94.4XXD	Injury to barefoot water-skier, subsequent encounter
E838.5	OTH&UNS WATER TRANSPORT ACC-INJR SWIMMER	**V94.11XA**	Bather struck by powered watercraft, initial encounter
		V94.11XD	Bather struck by powered watercraft, subsequent encounter
		V94.12XA	Bather struck by nonpowered watercraft, initial encounter
		V94.12XD	Bather struck by nonpowered watercraft, subsequent encounter
		V94.811A	Civilian in water injured by military watercraft, init
		V94.811D	Civilian in water injured by military watercraft, subs
E838.6	OTH&UNS WATER TRANSPORT ACC-INJR DOCKERS	**V94.89XA**	Other water transport accident, initial encounter
E838.7	OTH&UNS WATER TRANSPORT ACC OCCUPANT MILITARY	**V94.89XA**	Other water transport accident, initial encounter
E838.8	OTH&UNS WATER TRANSPORT ACC-INJR OTH PERSON	**V94.89XA**	Other water transport accident, initial encounter
E838.9	OTH&UNS WATER TRANSPORT ACC-INJR UNS PERSON	**V93.2ØXA**	Heat exposure on board merchant ship, initial encounter
		V93.2ØXD	Heat exposure on board merchant ship, subsequent encounter
		V93.21XA	Heat exposure on board passenger ship, initial encounter
		V93.21XD	Heat exposure on board passenger ship, subsequent encounter
		V93.22XA	Heat exposure on board fishing boat, initial encounter
		V93.22XD	Heat exposure on board fishing boat, subsequent encounter
		V93.23XA	Heat exposure on board other powered watercraft, init encntr
		V93.23XD	Heat exposure on board other powered watercraft, subs encntr
		V93.24XA	Heat exposure on board sailboat, initial encounter
		V93.24XD	Heat exposure on board sailboat, subsequent encounter
		V93.29XA	Heat exposure on board unspecified watercraft, init encntr
		V93.29XD	Heat exposure on board unspecified watercraft, subs encntr
		V93.4ØXA	Struck by falling object on merchant ship, initial encounter
		V93.4ØXD	Struck by falling object on merchant ship, subs encntr
		V93.41XA	Struck by falling object on passenger ship, init encntr
		V93.41XD	Struck by falling object on passenger ship, subs encntr
		V93.42XA	Struck by falling object on fishing boat, initial encounter
		V93.42XD	Struck by falling object on fishing boat, subs encntr
		V93.43XA	Struck by falling object on oth powered watercraft, init
		V93.43XD	Struck by falling object on oth powered watercraft, subs
		V93.44XA	Struck by falling object on sailboat, initial encounter
		V93.44XD	Struck by falling object on sailboat, subsequent encounter
		V93.48XA	Struck by falling object on unpowr wtrcrft, init encntr
		V93.48XD	Struck by falling object on unpowr wtrcrft, subs encntr
		V93.49XA	Struck by falling object on unsp watercraft, init encntr
		V93.49XD	Struck by falling object on unsp watercraft, subs encntr
		V93.8ØXA	Oth injury due to oth accident on board merchant ship, init
		V93.8ØXD	Oth injury due to oth accident on board merchant ship, subs
		V93.81XA	Oth injury due to oth accident on board passenger ship, init
		V93.81XD	Oth injury due to oth accident on board passenger ship, subs
		V93.82XA	Oth injury due to oth accident on board fishing boat, init
		V93.82XD	Oth injury due to oth accident on board fishing boat, subs
		V93.83XA	Oth injury due to oth acc on board oth powered wtrcrft, init
		V93.83XD	Oth injury due to oth acc on board oth powered wtrcrft, subs
		V93.84XA	Oth injury due to oth accident on board sailboat, init
		V93.84XD	Oth injury due to oth accident on board sailboat, subs
		V93.85XA	Oth injury due to oth accident on board canoe or kayak, init
		V93.85XD	Oth injury due to oth accident on board canoe or kayak, subs
		V93.86XA	Oth injury due to oth accident on board inflatbl crft, init
		V93.86XD	Oth injury due to oth accident on board inflatbl crft, subs
		V93.87XA	Oth injury due to oth accident on board water-skis, init
		V93.87XD	Oth injury due to oth accident on board water-skis, subs
		V93.88XA	Oth injury due to oth accident on board unpowr wtrcrft, init
		V93.88XD	Oth injury due to oth accident on board unpowr wtrcrft, subs
		V93.89XA	Oth injury due to oth accident on board unsp wtrcrft, init
		V93.89XD	Oth injury due to oth accident on board unsp wtrcrft, subs
		V94.ØXXA	Hitting obj/botm of body of wtr d/t fall from wtrcrft, init
	(Continued on next page)	**V94.ØXXD**	Hitting obj/botm of body of wtr d/t fall from wtrcrft, subs

ICD-9-CM		ICD-10-CM	
E838.9	OTH&UNS WATER TRANSPORT ACC-INJR UNS PERSON **(Continued)**	**V94.810A**	Civilian wtrcrft in water trnsp acc w military wtrcrft, init
		V94.810D	Civilian wtrcrft in water trnsp acc w military wtrcrft, subs
		V94.818A	Oth water transport accident w military wtrcrft, init
		V94.818D	Oth water transport accident w military wtrcrft, subs
		V94.89XA	Other water transport accident, initial encounter
		V94.89XD	Other water transport accident, subsequent encounter
		V94.9XXA	Unspecified water transport accident, initial encounter
		V94.9XXD	Unspecified water transport accident, subsequent encounter
E840.0	ACC PWR AIRCRFT@TAKEOFF/LAND INJR OCC SPACECRFT	**V95.42XA**	Forced landing of spacecraft injuring occupant, init encntr
E840.1	ACC POWR AIRCRFT TAKEOFF/LAND-OCC MILTRY AIRCRFT	**V97.818A**	Oth air transport accident involving military aircraft, init
E840.2	ACC POWR AIRCRFT TAKEOFF/LAND-CREW COMMERCIAL	**V95.32XA**	Forced landing of commrcl fix-wing arcrft inj occupant, init
E840.3	ACC POWR AIRCRFT TAKEOFF/LAND-OTH OCC COMMERCIAL	**V95.01XA**	Helicopter crash injuring occupant, initial encounter
		V95.01XD	Helicopter crash injuring occupant, subsequent encounter
		V95.02XA	Forced landing of helicopter injuring occupant, init encntr
		V95.02XD	Forced landing of helicopter injuring occupant, subs encntr
		V95.03XA	Helicopter collision injuring occupant, initial encounter
		V95.03XD	Helicopter collision injuring occupant, subsequent encounter
		V95.04XA	Helicopter fire injuring occupant, initial encounter
		V95.04XD	Helicopter fire injuring occupant, subsequent encounter
		V95.05XA	Helicopter explosion injuring occupant, initial encounter
		V95.05XD	Helicopter explosion injuring occupant, subsequent encounter
		V95.21XA	Oth private fix-wing aircraft crash injuring occupant, init
		V95.21XD	Oth private fix-wing aircraft crash injuring occupant, subs
		V95.22XA	Forced landing of private fix-wing arcrft inj occupant, init
		V95.22XD	Forced landing of private fix-wing arcrft inj occupant, subs
		V95.23XA	Oth private fix-wing aircraft clsn injuring occupant, init
		V95.23XD	Oth private fix-wing aircraft clsn injuring occupant, subs
		V95.24XA	Oth private fixed-wing aircraft fire injuring occupant, init
		V95.24XD	Oth private fixed-wing aircraft fire injuring occupant, subs
		V95.25XA	Oth private fix-wing arcrft explosn injuring occupant, init
		V95.25XD	Oth private fix-wing arcrft explosn injuring occupant, subs
		V95.29XA	Oth acc to oth private fix-wing arcrft inj occupant, init
		V95.29XD	Oth acc to oth private fix-wing arcrft inj occupant, subs
		V95.31XA	Commercial fixed-wing aircraft crash injuring occupant, init
		V95.31XD	Commercial fixed-wing aircraft crash injuring occupant, subs
		V95.32XA	Forced landing of commrcl fix-wing arcrft inj occupant, init
		V95.32XD	Forced landing of commrcl fix-wing arcrft inj occupant, subs
		V95.33XA	Commrcl fix-wing aircraft collision injuring occupant, init
		V95.33XD	Commrcl fix-wing aircraft collision injuring occupant, subs
		V95.34XA	Commercial fixed-wing aircraft fire injuring occupant, init
		V95.34XD	Commercial fixed-wing aircraft fire injuring occupant, subs
		V95.35XA	Commrcl fix-wing aircraft explosion injuring occupant, init
		V95.35XD	Commrcl fix-wing aircraft explosion injuring occupant, subs
E840.4	ACC POWR AIRCRFT TAKEOFF/LAND-OCC COMMERCIAL	**V95.31XA**	Commercial fixed-wing aircraft crash injuring occupant, init
E840.5	ACC POWR AIRCRFT TAKEOFF/LAND-OTH POWR AIRCRFT	**V95.29XA**	Oth acc to oth private fix-wing arcrft inj occupant, init
E840.6	ACC POWR AIRCRFT TAKEOFF/LAND-OTH UNPOWR AIRCRFT	**V95.11XA**	Ultralt/microlt/pwr-glider crash injuring occupant, init
		V95.11XD	Ultralt/microlt/pwr-glider crash injuring occupant, subs
		V95.12XA	Forced landing of ultralt/microlt/pwr-glider inj occ, init
		V95.12XD	Forced landing of ultralt/microlt/pwr-glider inj occ, subs
		V95.13XA	Ultralt/microlt/pwr-glider collision injuring occupant, init
		V95.13XD	Ultralt/microlt/pwr-glider collision injuring occupant, subs
		V95.14XA	Ultralt/microlt/pwr-glider fire injuring occupant, init
		V95.14XD	Ultralt/microlt/pwr-glider fire injuring occupant, subs
		V95.15XA	Ultralt/microlt/pwr-glider explosion injuring occupant, init
		V95.15XD	Ultralt/microlt/pwr-glider explosion injuring occupant, subs
		V95.19XA	Oth ultralt/microlt/pwr-glider acc injuring occupant, init
		V95.19XD	Oth ultralt/microlt/pwr-glider acc injuring occupant, subs
E840.7	ACC POWR AIRCRFT TAKEOFF/LAND-PARACHUTIST	**V97.22XA**	Parachutist injured on landing, initial encounter
E840.8	ACC POWR AIRCRFT TAKEOFF/LAND-GROUND CREW EMPLOY	**V97.39XA**	Oth injury to person on ground due to air trnsp acc, init
E840.9	ACC POWR AIRCRFT TAKEOFF/LAND-OTHER PERSON	**V97.39XA**	Oth injury to person on ground due to air trnsp acc, init
E841.0	ACC POWR AIRC OTH&UNSPEC INJR OCCUPANT SPACECRFT	**V95.43XA**	Spacecraft collision injuring occupant, initial encounter
E841.1	ACC POWR AIRC OTH&UNS INJR OCC MILITARY AIRC	**V97.818A**	Oth air transport accident involving military aircraft, init
		V97.818D	Oth air transport accident involving military aircraft, subs
E841.2	ACC POWR AIRC OTH&UNS-INJR CREW COMMER AIRC	**V95.33XA**	Commrcl fix-wing aircraft collision injuring occupant, init
E841.3	ACC POWR AIRC OTH&UNS-INJR OTH OCC COMMER AIRC	**V95.00XA**	Unsp helicopter accident injuring occupant, init encntr
		V95.00XD	Unsp helicopter accident injuring occupant, subs encntr
		V95.09XA	Other helicopter accident injuring occupant, init encntr
		V95.09XD	Other helicopter accident injuring occupant, subs encntr
		V95.10XA	Unsp ultralt/microlt/pwr-glider acc injuring occupant, init
		V95.10XD	Unsp ultralt/microlt/pwr-glider acc injuring occupant, subs
		V95.20XA	Unsp acc to oth private fix-wing arcrft, inj occupant, init
		V95.20XD	Unsp acc to oth private fix-wing arcrft, inj occupant, subs
		V95.30XA	Unsp acc to commrcl fix-wing arcrft injuring occupant, init
		V95.30XD	Unsp acc to commrcl fix-wing arcrft injuring occupant, subs
		V95.39XA	Oth acc to commrcl fix-wing aircraft injuring occupant, init
		V95.39XD	Oth acc to commrcl fix-wing aircraft injuring occupant, subs
		V95.8XXA	Oth powered aircraft accidents injuring occupant, init
		V95.8XXD	Oth powered aircraft accidents injuring occupant, subs
		V95.9XXA	Unspecified aircraft accident injuring occupant, init encntr
		V95.9XXD	Unspecified aircraft accident injuring occupant, subs encntr

ICD-9-CM		ICD-10-CM	
E841.4	ACC POWR AIRC OTH&UNS-INJR OCC-COMMERCIAL AIRC	V95.33XA	Commrcl fix-wing aircraft collision injuring occupant, init
E841.5	ACC POWR AIRC OTH&UNS-INJR OCC OTH POWR AIRC	V95.23XA	Oth private fix-wing aircraft clsn injuring occupant, init
E841.6	ACC POWR AIRC OTH&UNS-INJR OCC-UNPOWR AIRC	V95.13XA	Ultralt/microlt/pwr-glider collision injuring occupant, init
E841.7	ACCIDENT POWR AIRCRAFT OTH&UNSPEC INJR PRACHUTST	V97.29XA	Other parachutist accident, initial encounter
E841.8	ACC POWR AIRC OTH&UNS-INJR GRND CREW-EMPLOYEE	V97.39XA	Oth injury to person on ground due to air trnsp acc, init
E841.9	ACCIDENT POWR AIRC OTH&UNSPEC INJR OTH PERSON	V97.39XA	Oth injury to person on ground due to air trnsp acc, init
E842.6	ACC UNPOWR AIRCRAFT-INJR OCC UNPOWR AIRCRAFT	V96.ØØXA	Unspecified balloon accident injuring occupant, init encntr
		V96.ØØXD	Unspecified balloon accident injuring occupant, subs encntr
		V96.Ø1XA	Balloon crash injuring occupant, initial encounter
		V96.Ø1XD	Balloon crash injuring occupant, subsequent encounter
		V96.Ø2XA	Forced landing of balloon injuring occupant, init encntr
		V96.Ø2XD	Forced landing of balloon injuring occupant, subs encntr
		V96.Ø3XA	Balloon collision injuring occupant, initial encounter
		V96.Ø3XD	Balloon collision injuring occupant, subsequent encounter
		V96.Ø4XA	Balloon fire injuring occupant, initial encounter
		V96.Ø4XD	Balloon fire injuring occupant, subsequent encounter
		V96.Ø5XA	Balloon explosion injuring occupant, initial encounter
		V96.Ø5XD	Balloon explosion injuring occupant, subsequent encounter
		V96.Ø9XA	Other balloon accident injuring occupant, initial encounter
		V96.Ø9XD	Other balloon accident injuring occupant, subs encntr
		V96.1ØXA	Unsp hang-glider accident injuring occupant, init encntr
		V96.1ØXD	Unsp hang-glider accident injuring occupant, subs encntr
		V96.11XA	Hang-glider crash injuring occupant, initial encounter
		V96.11XD	Hang-glider crash injuring occupant, subsequent encounter
		V96.12XA	Forced landing of hang-glider injuring occupant, init encntr
		V96.12XD	Forced landing of hang-glider injuring occupant, subs encntr
		V96.13XA	Hang-glider collision injuring occupant, initial encounter
		V96.13XD	Hang-glider collision injuring occupant, subs encntr
		V96.14XA	Hang-glider fire injuring occupant, initial encounter
		V96.14XD	Hang-glider fire injuring occupant, subsequent encounter
		V96.15XA	Hang-glider explosion injuring occupant, initial encounter
		V96.15XD	Hang-glider explosion injuring occupant, subs encntr
		V96.19XA	Other hang-glider accident injuring occupant, init encntr
		V96.19XD	Other hang-glider accident injuring occupant, subs encntr
		V96.2ØXA	Unsp glider (nonpowered) accident injuring occupant, init
		V96.2ØXD	Unsp glider (nonpowered) accident injuring occupant, subs
		V96.21XA	Glider (nonpowered) crash injuring occupant, init encntr
		V96.21XD	Glider (nonpowered) crash injuring occupant, subs encntr
		V96.22XA	Forced landing of glider injuring occupant, init
		V96.22XD	Forced landing of glider injuring occupant, subs
		V96.23XA	Glider (nonpowered) collision injuring occupant, init encntr
		V96.23XD	Glider (nonpowered) collision injuring occupant, subs encntr
		V96.24XA	Glider (nonpowered) fire injuring occupant, init encntr
		V96.24XD	Glider (nonpowered) fire injuring occupant, subs encntr
		V96.25XA	Glider (nonpowered) explosion injuring occupant, init encntr
		V96.25XD	Glider (nonpowered) explosion injuring occupant, subs encntr
		V96.29XA	Oth glider (nonpowered) accident injuring occupant, init
		V96.29XD	Oth glider (nonpowered) accident injuring occupant, subs
		V96.8XXA	Oth nonpowered-aircraft accidents injuring occupant, init
		V96.8XXD	Oth nonpowered-aircraft accidents injuring occupant, subs
		V96.9XXA	Unsp nonpowered-aircraft accident injuring occupant, init
		V96.9XXD	Unsp nonpowered-aircraft accident injuring occupant, subs
E842.7	ACCIDENT UNPOWERED AIRCRAFT INJURING PARACHUTIST	V97.29XA	Other parachutist accident, initial encounter
E842.8	ACC UNPOWR AIRCRAFT-INJR GRND CREW-EMPLOYEE	V97.39XA	Oth injury to person on ground due to air trnsp acc, init
E842.9	ACCIDENT UNPOWERED AIRCRAFT INJURING OTH PERSON	V97.39XA	Oth injury to person on ground due to air trnsp acc, init
E843.Ø	FALL IN ON/FROM AIRCRAFT INJR OCC SPACECRAFT	V97.ØXXA	Occupant of aircraft injured in oth air transport acc, init
E843.1	FALL IN ON/FROM AIRCRAFT INJR OCC MILITARY AIRC	V97.818A	Oth air transport accident involving military aircraft, init
E843.2	FALL IN-ON/FROM AIRC-INJR CREW-COMMER AIRC	V97.ØXXA	Occupant of aircraft injured in oth air transport acc, init
E843.3	FALL IN-ON/FROM AIRC-INJR OTH OCC COMMER AIRC	V97.ØXXA	Occupant of aircraft injured in oth air transport acc, init
		V97.ØXXD	Occupant of aircraft injured in oth air transport acc, subs
E843.4	FALL IN-ON/FROM AIRC-INJR OCC-COMMERCIAL AIRC	V97.ØXXA	Occupant of aircraft injured in oth air transport acc, init
E843.5	FALL IN ON/FROM AIRC INJR OCC OTH POWR AIRC	V97.ØXXA	Occupant of aircraft injured in oth air transport acc, init
E843.6	FALL IN ON/FROM AIRCRFT INJR OCC UNPWR AIRCRFT	V97.ØXXA	Occupant of aircraft injured in oth air transport acc, init
E843.7	FALL IN ON/FROM AIRCRAFT INJURING PARACHUTIST	V97.21XA	Parachutist entangled in object, initial encounter
		V97.21XD	Parachutist entangled in object, subsequent encounter
		V97.22XA	Parachutist injured on landing, initial encounter
		V97.22XD	Parachutist injured on landing, subsequent encounter
		V97.29XA	Other parachutist accident, initial encounter
E843.8	FALL IN ON/FROM AIRC INJR GRND CREW EMPLOYEE	V97.39XA	Oth injury to person on ground due to air trnsp acc, init
E843.9	FALL IN ON/FROM AIRCRAFT INJURING OTHER PERSON	V97.1XXA	Person injured wh brd/alit from aircraft, init
		V97.1XXD	Person injured wh brd/alit from aircraft, subs
E844.Ø	OTH AIR TRNSPRT ACCS INJR OCCUPANT SPACECRFT	V97.ØXXA	Occupant of aircraft injured in oth air transport acc, init
E844.1	OTH AIR TRNSPRT ACCS INJR OCCUPANT MILITARY AIRC	V97.ØXXA	Occupant of aircraft injured in oth air transport acc, init
		V97.811A	Civilian injured by military aircraft, initial encounter
		V97.811D	Civilian injured by military aircraft, subsequent encounter
E844.2	OTH AIR TRNSPRT ACC-INJR CREW COMMER AIRCRFT	V97.ØXXA	Occupant of aircraft injured in oth air transport acc, init

ICD-9-CM		ICD-10-CM	
E844.3	OTH AIR TRNSPRT ACC-INJR OTH OCC COMMER AIRCRFT	**V97.ØXXA**	Occupant of aircraft injured in oth air transport acc, init
		V97.ØXXD	Occupant of aircraft injured in oth air transport acc, subs
E844.4	OTH AIR TRNSPRT ACC-INJR OCC-COMMERCIAL AIRCRFT	**V97.ØXXA**	Occupant of aircraft injured in oth air transport acc, init
E844.5	OTH AIR TRNSPRT ACCS INJR OCCUPANT OTH POWR AIRC	**V97.ØXXA**	Occupant of aircraft injured in oth air transport acc, init
E844.6	OTH AIR TRNSPRT ACC-INJR OCC-UNPOWERED AIRCRFT	**V97.ØXXA**	Occupant of aircraft injured in oth air transport acc, init
E844.7	OTH AIR TRANSPORT ACCIDENTS INJR PARACHUTIST	**V97.29XA**	Other parachutist accident, initial encounter
		V97.29XD	Other parachutist accident, subsequent encounter
E844.8	OTH AIR TRNSPRT ACC-INJR GROUND CREW-EMPLOYEE	**V97.39XA**	Oth injury to person on ground due to air trnsp acc, init
E844.9	OTH AIR TRANSPORT ACCIDENTS INJR OTH PERSON	**V97.31XA**	Hit by object falling from aircraft, initial encounter
		V97.31XD	Hit by object falling from aircraft, subsequent encounter
		V97.32XA	Injured by rotating propeller, initial encounter
		V97.32XD	Injured by rotating propeller, subsequent encounter
		V97.33XA	Sucked into jet engine, initial encounter
		V97.33XD	Sucked into jet engine, subsequent encounter
		V97.39XA	Oth injury to person on ground due to air trnsp acc, init
		V97.39XD	Oth injury to person on ground due to air trnsp acc, subs
		V97.81ØA	Civilian aircraft in air trnsp acc w military aircraft, init
		V97.81ØD	Civilian aircraft in air trnsp acc w military aircraft, subs
		V97.89XA	Oth air transport accidents, not elsewhere classified, init
		V97.89XD	Oth air transport accidents, not elsewhere classified, subs
E845.Ø	ACCIDENT INVLV SPACECRAFT INJR OCC SPACECRAFT	**V95.4ØXA**	Unsp spacecraft accident injuring occupant, init encntr
		V95.4ØXD	Unsp spacecraft accident injuring occupant, subs encntr
		V95.41XA	Spacecraft crash injuring occupant, initial encounter
		V95.41XD	Spacecraft crash injuring occupant, subsequent encounter
		V95.42XA	Forced landing of spacecraft injuring occupant, init encntr
		V95.42XD	Forced landing of spacecraft injuring occupant, subs encntr
		V95.43XA	Spacecraft collision injuring occupant, initial encounter
		V95.43XD	Spacecraft collision injuring occupant, subsequent encounter
		V95.44XA	Spacecraft fire injuring occupant, initial encounter
		V95.44XD	Spacecraft fire injuring occupant, subsequent encounter
		V95.45XA	Spacecraft explosion injuring occupant, initial encounter
		V95.45XD	Spacecraft explosion injuring occupant, subsequent encounter
		V95.49XA	Other spacecraft accident injuring occupant, init encntr
		V95.49XD	Other spacecraft accident injuring occupant, subs encntr
E845.8	ACC INVLV SPACECRAFT-INJR GROUND CREW-EMPLOYEE	**V97.39XA**	Oth injury to person on ground due to air trnsp acc, init
E845.9	ACCIDENT INVOLVING SPACECRAFT INJR OTH PERSON	**V95.49XA**	Other spacecraft accident injuring occupant, init encntr
E846	ACC-POWER VEHICLE USED ONLY IN INDUST/COMMERCE	**V83.ØXXA**	Driver of special industrial vehicle injured in traf, init
		V83.ØXXD	Driver of special industrial vehicle injured in traf, subs
		V83.1XXA	Passenger of special industr vehicle injured in traf, init
		V83.1XXD	Passenger of special industr vehicle injured in traf, subs
		V83.2XXA	Person outside special industr vehicle injured in traf, init
		V83.2XXD	Person outside special industr vehicle injured in traf, subs
		V83.3XXA	Occup of special industrial vehicle injured in traf, init
		V83.3XXD	Occup of special industrial vehicle injured in traf, subs
		V83.4XXA	Person inj wh brd/alit from special industr vehicle, init
		V83.4XXD	Person inj wh brd/alit from special industr vehicle, subs
		V83.5XXA	Driver of special industrial vehicle injured nontraf, init
		V83.5XXD	Driver of special industrial vehicle injured nontraf, subs
		V83.6XXA	Passenger of special industr vehicle injured nontraf, init
		V83.6XXD	Passenger of special industr vehicle injured nontraf, subs
		V83.7XXA	Person outside special industr vehicle injured nontraf, init
		V83.7XXD	Person outside special industr vehicle injured nontraf, subs
		V83.9XXA	Occup of special industrial vehicle injured nontraf, init
		V83.9XXD	Occup of special industrial vehicle injured nontraf, subs
E847	ACCIDENTS INVOLVING CABLE CARS NOT RUNNING RAILS	**V98.ØXXA**	Accident to, on or involving cable-car, not on rails, init
		V98.ØXXD	Accident to, on or involving cable-car, not on rails, subs
		V98.3XXA	Accident to, on or involving ski lift, initial encounter
		V98.3XXD	Accident to, on or involving ski lift, subsequent encounter
E848	ACC INVOLVING OTH VEHICLES NOT ELSW CLASSIFIABLE	**V98.1XXA**	Accident to, on or involving land-yacht, initial encounter
		V98.1XXD	Accident to, on or involving land-yacht, subs encntr
		V98.2XXA	Accident to, on or involving ice yacht, initial encounter
		V98.2XXD	Accident to, on or involving ice yacht, subsequent encounter
		V98.8XXA	Other specified transport accidents, initial encounter
		V98.8XXD	Other specified transport accidents, subsequent encounter
		V99.XXXA	Unspecified transport accident, initial encounter
		V99.XXXD	Unspecified transport accident, subsequent encounter
E849.Ø	PLACE OF OCCURRENCE, HOME	**Y92.ØØØ**	Kitchen of unsp non-institut (private) residence as place
		Y92.ØØ1	Dining room of unsp non-institut residence as place
		Y92.ØØ2	Bathroom of unsp non-inst (private) resdnce sngl-fmly house as place
		Y92.ØØ3	Bedroom of unsp non-institut (private) residence as place
		Y92.ØØ7	Garden or yard of unsp non-institut residence as place
		Y92.ØØ8	Oth place in unsp non-institut (private) residence as place
		Y92.ØØ9	Unsp place in unsp non-institut (private) residence as place
		Y92.Ø1Ø	Kitchen of single-family (private) house as place
		Y92.Ø11	Dining room of single-family (private) house as place
		Y92.Ø12	Bathroom of single-family (private) house as place
		Y92.Ø13	Bedroom of single-family (private) house as place
		Y92.Ø14	Private driveway to single-family (private) house as place
		Y92.Ø15	Private garage of single-family (private) house as place
		Y92.Ø16	Swm-pool in sngl-fmly (private) house or garden as place

(Continued on next page)

ICD-9-CM		ICD-10-CM	
E849.Ø	PLACE OF OCCURRENCE, HOME **(Continued)**	**Y92.Ø17**	Garden or yard in single-family (private) house as place
		Y92.Ø18	Oth place in single-family (private) house as place
		Y92.Ø19	Unsp place in single-family (private) house as place
		Y92.Ø2Ø	Kitchen in mobile home as place
		Y92.Ø21	Dining room in mobile home as place
		Y92.Ø22	Bathroom in mobile home as place
		Y92.Ø23	Bedroom in mobile home as place
		Y92.Ø24	Driveway of mobile home as place
		Y92.Ø25	Garage of mobile home as place
		Y92.Ø26	Swimming-pool of mobile home as place
		Y92.Ø27	Garden or yard of mobile home as place
		Y92.Ø28	Oth place in mobile home as place
		Y92.Ø29	Unsp place in mobile home as place
		Y92.Ø3Ø	Kitchen in apartment as place
		Y92.Ø31	Bathroom in apartment as place
		Y92.Ø32	Bedroom in apartment as place
		Y92.Ø38	Oth place in apartment as place
		Y92.Ø39	Unsp place in apartment as place
		Y92.Ø4Ø	Kitchen in boarding-house as place
		Y92.Ø41	Bathroom in boarding-house as place
		Y92.Ø42	Bedroom in boarding-house as place
		Y92.Ø43	Driveway of boarding-house as place
		Y92.Ø44	Garage of boarding-house as place
		Y92.Ø45	Swimming-pool of boarding-house as place
		Y92.Ø46	Garden or yard of boarding-house as place
		Y92.Ø48	Oth place in boarding-house as place
		Y92.Ø49	Unsp place in boarding-house as place
		Y92.Ø9Ø	Kitchen in oth non-institutional residence as place
		Y92.Ø91	Bathroom in oth non-institutional residence as place
		Y92.Ø92	Bedroom in oth non-institutional residence as place
		Y92.Ø93	Driveway of non-institutional residence as place
		Y92.Ø94	Garage of non-institutional residence as place
		Y92.Ø95	Swimming-pool of non-institutional residence as place
		Y92.Ø96	Garden or yard of non-institutional residence as place
		Y92.Ø98	Oth place in oth non-institutional residence as place
		Y92.Ø99	Unsp place in oth non-institutional residence as place
		Y92.1Ø	Unsp residential institution as place
E849.1	PLACE OF OCCURRENCE, FARM	**Y92.71**	Barn as the place of occurrence of the external cause
		Y92.72	Chicken coop as place
		Y92.73	Farm field as the place of occurrence of the external cause
		Y92.74	Orchard as the place of occurrence of the external cause
		Y92.79	Oth farm location as place
E849.2	PLACE OF OCCURRENCE MINE AND QUARRY	**Y92.64**	Mine or pit as the place of occurrence of the external cause
E849.3	PLACE OF OCCURRENCE INDUSTRIAL PLACES&PREMISES	**Y92.61**	Building under construction as place
		Y92.62	Dock or shipyard as place
		Y92.63	Factory as the place of occurrence of the external cause
		Y92.65	Oil rig as the place of occurrence of the external cause
		Y92.69	Oth industrial and construction area as place
E849.4	PLACE OF OCCURRENCE PLACE RECREATION AND SPORT	**Y92.31Ø**	Basketball court as place
		Y92.311	Squash court as place
		Y92.312	Tennis court as place
		Y92.318	Oth athletic court as place
		Y92.32Ø	Baseball field as place
		Y92.321	Football field as place
		Y92.322	Soccer field as place
		Y92.328	Oth athletic field as place
		Y92.33Ø	Ice skating rink (indoor) (outdoor) as place
		Y92.331	Roller skating rink as place
		Y92.34	Swimming pool (public) as place
		Y92.39	Oth sports and athletic area as place
		Y92.83Ø	Public park as the place of occurrence of the external cause
		Y92.831	Amusement park as place
		Y92.832	Beach as the place of occurrence of the external cause
		Y92.833	Campsite as the place of occurrence of the external cause
		Y92.834	Zoological garden (Zoo) as place
		Y92.838	Oth recreation area as place
E849.5	PLACE OF OCCURRENCE STREET AND HIGHWAY	**Y92.41Ø**	Unsp street and highway as place
		Y92.411	Interstate highway as place
		Y92.412	Parkway as the place of occurrence of the external cause
		Y92.413	State road as the place of occurrence of the external cause
		Y92.414	Local residential or business street as place
		Y92.415	Exit ramp or entrance ramp of street or highway as place
		Y92.48Ø	Sidewalk as the place of occurrence of the external cause
		Y92.481	Parking lot as the place of occurrence of the external cause
		Y92.482	Bike path as the place of occurrence of the external cause
		Y92.488	Oth paved roadways as place

ICD-9-CM		ICD-10-CM	
E849.6	PLACE OF OCCURRENCE PUBLIC BUILDING	**Y92.210**	Daycare center as place
		Y92.211	Elementary school as place
		Y92.212	Middle school as place
		Y92.213	High school as the place of occurrence of the external cause
		Y92.214	College as the place of occurrence of the external cause
		Y92.215	Trade school as place
		Y92.218	Oth school as the place of occurrence of the external cause
		Y92.219	Unsp school as the place of occurrence of the external cause
		Y92.22	Religious institution as place
		Y92.240	Courthouse as the place of occurrence of the external cause
		Y92.241	Library as the place of occurrence of the external cause
		Y92.242	Post office as the place of occurrence of the external cause
		Y92.243	City hall as the place of occurrence of the external cause
		Y92.248	Oth public administrative building as place
		Y92.250	Art Gallery as the place of occurrence of the external cause
		Y92.251	Museum as the place of occurrence of the external cause
		Y92.252	Music hall as the place of occurrence of the external cause
		Y92.253	Opera house as the place of occurrence of the external cause
		Y92.254	Theater (live) as place
		Y92.258	Oth cultural public building as place
		Y92.26	Movie house or cinema as place
		Y92.29	Oth public building as place
		Y92.510	Bank as the place of occurrence of the external cause
		Y92.511	Restaurant or cafe as place
		Y92.512	Supermarket, store or market as place
		Y92.513	Shop (commercial) as place
		Y92.520	Airport as the place of occurrence of the external cause
		Y92.521	Bus station as the place of occurrence of the external cause
		Y92.522	Railway station as place
		Y92.523	Highway rest stop as place
		Y92.524	Gas station as the place of occurrence of the external cause
		Y92.530	Ambulatory surgery center as place
		Y92.531	Health care provider office as place
		Y92.532	Urgent care center as place
		Y92.538	Oth ambulatory health services establishments as place
		Y92.59	Oth trade areas as place
E849.7	PLACE OF OCCURRENCE RESIDENTIAL INSTITUTION	**Y92.110**	Kitchen in children's home and orphanage as place
		Y92.111	Bathroom in children's home and orphanage as place
		Y92.112	Bedroom in children's home and orphanage as place
		Y92.113	Driveway of children's home and orphanage as place
		Y92.114	Garage of children's home and orphanage as place
		Y92.115	Swimming-pool of children's home and orphanage as place
		Y92.116	Garden or yard of children's home and orphanage as place
		Y92.118	Oth place in children's home and orphanage as place
		Y92.119	Unsp place in children's home and orphanage as place
		Y92.120	Kitchen in nursing home as place
		Y92.121	Bathroom in nursing home as place
		Y92.122	Bedroom in nursing home as place
		Y92.123	Driveway of nursing home as place
		Y92.124	Garage of nursing home as place
		Y92.125	Swimming-pool of nursing home as place
		Y92.126	Garden or yard of nursing home as place
		Y92.128	Oth place in nursing home as place
		Y92.129	Unsp place in nursing home as place
		Y92.140	Kitchen in prison as place
		Y92.141	Dining room in prison as place
		Y92.142	Bathroom in prison as place
		Y92.143	Cell of prison as place
		Y92.146	Swimming-pool of prison as place
		Y92.147	Courtyard of prison as place
		Y92.148	Oth place in prison as place
		Y92.149	Unsp place in prison as place
		Y92.150	Kitchen in reform school as place
		Y92.151	Dining room in reform school as place
		Y92.152	Bathroom in reform school as place
		Y92.153	Bedroom in reform school as place
		Y92.154	Driveway of reform school as place
		Y92.155	Garage of reform school as place
		Y92.156	Swimming-pool of reform school as place
		Y92.157	Garden or yard of reform school as place
		Y92.158	Oth place in reform school as place
		Y92.159	Unsp place in reform school as place
		Y92.160	Kitchen in school dormitory as place
		Y92.161	Dining room in school dormitory as place
		Y92.162	Bathroom in school dormitory as place
		Y92.163	Bedroom in school dormitory as place
		Y92.168	Oth place in school dormitory as place
		Y92.169	Unsp place in school dormitory as place
		Y92.190	Kitchen in oth residential institution as place
		Y92.191	Dining room in oth residential institution as place
		Y92.192	Bathroom in oth residential institution as place
		Y92.193	Bedroom in oth residential institution as place

(Continued on next page)

ICD-9-CM		ICD-10-CM	
E849.7	PLACE OF OCCURRENCE RESIDENTIAL INSTITUTION **(Continued)**	**Y92.194**	Driveway of residential institution as place
		Y92.195	Garage of residential institution as place
		Y92.196	Pool of residential institution as place
		Y92.197	Garden or yard of residential institution as place
		Y92.198	Oth place in oth residential institution as place
		Y92.199	Unsp place in oth residential institution as place
		Y92.230	Patient room in hospital as place
		Y92.231	Patient bathroom in hospital as place
		Y92.232	Corridor of hospital as place
		Y92.233	Cafeteria of hospital as place
		Y92.234	Operating room of hospital as place
		Y92.238	Oth place in hospital as place
		Y92.239	Unsp place in hospital as place
E849.8	OTHER SPECIFIED PLACE OF OCCURRENCE	**Y92.130**	Kitchen on military base as place
		Y92.131	Mess hall on military base as place
		Y92.133	Barracks on military base as place
		Y92.135	Garage on military base as place
		Y92.136	Swimming-pool on military base as place
		Y92.137	Garden or yard on military base as place
		Y92.138	Oth place on military base as place
		Y92.139	Unsp place military base as place
		Y92.810	Car as the place of occurrence of the external cause
		Y92.811	Bus as the place of occurrence of the external cause
		Y92.812	Truck as the place of occurrence of the external cause
		Y92.813	Airplane as the place of occurrence of the external cause
		Y92.814	Boat as the place of occurrence of the external cause
		Y92.815	Train as the place of occurrence of the external cause
		Y92.816	Subway car as the place of occurrence of the external cause
		Y92.818	Oth transport vehicle as place
		Y92.820	Desert as the place of occurrence of the external cause
		Y92.821	Forest as the place of occurrence of the external cause
		Y92.828	Oth wilderness area as place
		Y92.84	Military training ground as place
		Y92.85	Railroad track as place
		Y92.86	Slaughter house as place
		Y92.89	Oth places as the place of occurrence of the external cause
E849.9	UNSPECIFIED PLACE OF OCCURRENCE	**Y92.9**	Unspecified place or not applicable
E850.0	ACCIDENTAL POISONING BY HEROIN	**T40.1X1A**	Poisoning by heroin, accidental (unintentional), init encntr
E850.1	ACCIDENTAL POISONING BY METHADONE	**T40.3X1A**	Poisoning by methadone, accidental (unintentional), init
E850.2	ACCIDENTAL POISN OTH OPIATES&RELATED NARCOTICS	**T40.0X1A**	Poisoning by opium, accidental (unintentional), init encntr
		T40.2X1A	Poisoning by oth opioids, accidental (unintentional), init
		T40.4X1A	Poisoning by oth synthetic narcotics, accidental, init
		T40.601A	Poisoning by unsp narcotics, accidental, init
		T40.691A	Poisoning by oth narcotics, accidental (unintentional), init
E850.3	ACCIDENTAL POISONING BY SALICYLATES	**T39.011A**	Poisoning by aspirin, accidental (unintentional), init
		T39.091A	Poisoning by salicylates, accidental (unintentional), init
E850.4	ACCIDENTAL POISONING BY AROMATIC ANALGESICS NEC	**T39.1X1A**	Poisoning by 4-Aminophenol derivatives, accidental, init
E850.5	ACCIDENTAL POISONING BY PYRAZOLE DERIVATIVES	**T39.2X1A**	Poisoning by pyrazolone derivatives, accidental, init
E850.6	ACCIDENTAL POISONING BY ANTIRHEUMATICS	**T39.391A**	Poisoning by oth nonsteroid anti-inflam drugs, acc, init
		T39.4X1A	Poisoning by antirheumatics, NEC, accidental, init
E850.7	ACCIDENTAL POISONING OTH NON-NARCOTIC ANALGESICS	**T39.311A**	Poisoning by propionic acid derivatives, accidental, init
		T39.8X1A	Poisoning by oth nonopio analges/antipyret, NEC, acc, init
		T39.91XA	Poisoning by unsp nonopi analgs/antipyr/antirheu, acc, init
E850.8	ACCIDENTAL POISN OTH SPEC ANALGES&ANTIPYRETICS	NO DIAGNOSIS	
E850.9	ACCIDENTAL POISN UNSPEC ANALGESIC/ANTIPYRETIC	NO DIAGNOSIS	
E851	ACCIDENTAL POISONING BY BARBITURATES	**T42.3X1A**	Poisoning by barbiturates, accidental (unintentional), init
E852.0	ACCIDENTAL POISONING BY CHLORAL HYDRATE GROUP	NO DIAGNOSIS	
E852.1	ACCIDENTAL POISONING BY PARALDEHYDE	NO DIAGNOSIS	
E852.2	ACCIDENTAL POISONING BY BROMINE COMPOUNDS	NO DIAGNOSIS	
E852.3	ACCIDENTAL POISONING BY METHAQUALONE COMPOUNDS	NO DIAGNOSIS	
E852.4	ACCIDENTAL POISONING BY GLUTETHIMIDE GROUP	NO DIAGNOSIS	
E852.5	ACCIDENTAL POISONING BY MIXED SEDATIVES NEC	NO DIAGNOSIS	
E852.8	ACCIDENTAL POISONING OTH SPEC SEDATIVE&HYPNOTIC	**T42.6X1A**	Poisoning by oth antieplptc and sed-hypntc drugs, acc, init
		T42.71XA	Poisn by unsp antieplptc and sed-hypntc drugs, acc, init
E852.9	ACCIDENTAL POISONING UNSPEC SEDATIVE/HYPNOTIC	NO DIAGNOSIS	
E853.0	ACCIDENTAL POISN PHENOTHIAZINE-BASED TRANQ	**T43.3X1A**	Poisoning by phenothiaz antipsychot/neurolept, acc, init
E853.1	ACCIDENTAL POISN BUTYROPHENONE-BASED TRANQ	**T43.4X1A**	Poisoning by butyrophen/thiothixen neuroleptc, acc, init
E853.2	ACCIDENTAL POISN BENZODIAZEPINE-BASED TRANQ	**T42.4X1A**	Poisoning by benzodiazepines, accidental, init
E853.8	ACCIDENTAL POISONING OTHER SPEC TRANQUILIZERS	NO DIAGNOSIS	
E853.9	ACCIDENTAL POISONING BY UNSPECIFIED TRANQUILIZER	NO DIAGNOSIS	

[Brackets] indicate valid character values for each code. Character value meanings provided for each code grouping.

ICD-9-CM		ICD-10-CM	
E854.Ø	ACCIDENTAL POISONING BY ANTIDEPRESSANTS	**T43.Ø11A**	Poisoning by tricyclic antidepressants, accidental, init
		T43.Ø21A	Poisoning by tetracyclic antidepressants, accidental, init
		T43.1X1A	Poisoning by MAO inhib antidepressants, accidental, init
		T43.2Ø1A	Poisoning by unsp antidepressants, accidental, init
		T43.211A	Poisn by slctv seroton/norepineph reup inhibtr, acc, init
		T43.221A	Poisn by selective serotonin reuptake inhibtr, acc, init
		T43.291A	Poisoning by oth antidepressants, accidental, init
E854.1	ACCIDENTAL POISONING BY PSYCHODYSLEPTICS	**T4Ø.7X1A**	Poisoning by cannabis (derivatives), accidental, init
		T4Ø.8X1A	Poisoning by lysergide, accidental (unintentional), init
		T4Ø.9Ø1A	Poisoning by unsp psychodyslept, accidental, init
		T4Ø.991A	Poisoning by oth psychodyslept, accidental, init
E854.2	ACCIDENTAL POISONING BY PSYCHOSTIMULANTS	**T4Ø.5X1A**	Poisoning by cocaine, accidental (unintentional), init
		T43.6Ø1A	Poisoning by unsp psychostim, accidental, init
		T43.611A	Poisoning by caffeine, accidental (unintentional), init
		T43.621A	Poisoning by amphetamines, accidental (unintentional), init
		T43.631A	Poisoning by methylphenidate, accidental, init
		T43.691A	Poisoning by oth psychostim, accidental, init
E854.3	ACCIDENTAL POISONING CNTRL NERV SYS STIMULANTS	**T5Ø.7X1A**	Poisn by analeptics and opioid receptor antag, acc, init
E854.8	ACCIDENTAL POISONING OTHER PSYCHOTROPIC AGENTS	**T43.5Ø1A**	Poisoning by unsp antipsychot/neurolept, accidental, init
		T43.591A	Poisoning by oth antipsychot/neurolept, accidental, init
		T43.8X1A	Poisoning by oth psychotropic drugs, accidental, init
		T43.91XA	Poisoning by unsp psychotropic drug, accidental, init
E855.Ø	ACC POISN ANTICONVULSANT&ANTI-PARKINSONISM RX	**T42.ØX1A**	Poisoning by hydantoin derivatives, accidental, init
		T42.8X1A	Poisn by antiparkns drug/centr musc-tone depr, acc, init
E855.1	ACCIDENTAL POISONING OTH CNTRL NERV SYS DEPTSSNT	**T41.ØX1A**	Poisoning by inhaled anesthetics, accidental, init
		T41.1X1A	Poisoning by intravenous anesthetics, accidental, init
		T41.2Ø1A	Poisoning by unsp general anesthetics, accidental, init
		T41.291A	Poisoning by oth general anesthetics, accidental, init
		T41.41XA	Poisoning by unsp anesthetic, accidental, init
E855.2	ACCIDENTAL POISONING BY LOCAL ANESTHETICS	**T41.3X1A**	Poisoning by local anesthetics, accidental, init
E855.3	ACCIDENTAL POISONING BY PARASYMPATHOMIMETICS	**T44.ØX1A**	Poisoning by anticholin agents, accidental, init
		T44.1X1A	Poisoning by oth parasympath, accidental, init
E855.4	ACCIDENTAL POISN PARASYMPATHOLYTICS&SPASMOLYTICS	**T44.3X1A**	Poisoning by oth parasympath and spasmolytics, acc, init
E855.5	ACCIDENTAL POISONING BY SYMPATHOMIMETICS	**T44.4X1A**	Poisoning by predom alpha-adrenocpt agonists, acc, init
		T44.5X1A	Poisoning by predom beta-adrenocpt agonists, acc, init
E855.6	ACCIDENTAL POISONING BY SYMPATHOLYTICS	**T44.6X1A**	Poisoning by alpha-adrenocpt antagonists, accidental, init
		T44.7X1A	Poisoning by beta-adrenocpt antagonists, accidental, init
		T44.8X1A	Poisoning by centr-acting/adren-neurn-block agnt, acc, init
E855.8	ACC POISN OTH SPEC RX ACT CNTRL&AUTONOM NERV SYS	**T42.1X1A**	Poisoning by iminostilbenes, accidental, init
		T42.2X1A	Poisoning by succinimides and oxazolidinediones, acc, init
		T42.5X1A	Poisoning by mixed antiepileptics, accidental, init
		T44.2X1A	Poisoning by ganglionic blocking drugs, accidental, init
		T44.9Ø1A	Poisn by unsp drugs aff the autonm nervous sys, acc, init
		T44.991A	Poisoning by oth drug aff the autonm nervous sys, acc, init
E855.9	ACC POISN UNS RX ACTING CNTRL&AUTONOM NERV SYS	NO DIAGNOSIS	
E856	ACCIDENTAL POISONING BY ANTIBIOTICS	**T36.ØX1A**	Poisoning by penicillins, accidental (unintentional), init
		T36.1X1A	Poisoning by cephalospor/oth beta-lactm antibiot, acc, init
		T36.2X1A	Poisoning by chloramphenicol group, accidental, init
		T36.3X1A	Poisoning by macrolides, accidental (unintentional), init
		T36.4X1A	Poisoning by tetracyclines, accidental (unintentional), init
		T36.5X1A	Poisoning by aminoglycosides, accidental, init
		T36.6X1A	Poisoning by rifampicins, accidental (unintentional), init
		T36.7X1A	Poisoning by antifungal antibiot, sys used, acc, init
		T36.8X1A	Poisoning by oth systemic antibiotics, accidental, init
		T36.91XA	Poisoning by unsp systemic antibiotic, accidental, init
E857	ACCIDENTAL POISONING BY OTHER ANTI-INFECTIVES	**T37.ØX1A**	Poisoning by sulfonamides, accidental (unintentional), init
		T37.1X1A	Poisoning by antimycobac drugs, accidental, init
		T37.2X1A	Poisn by antimalari/drugs acting on bld protzoa, acc, init
		T37.3X1A	Poisoning by oth antiprotozoal drugs, accidental, init
		T37.4X1A	Poisoning by anthelminthics, accidental, init
		T37.5X1A	Poisoning by antiviral drugs, accidental, init
		T37.8X1A	Poisoning by oth systemic anti-infect/parasit, acc, init
		T37.91XA	Poisn by unsp sys anti-infect and antiparastc, acc, init

ICD-9-CM		ICD-10-CM	
E858.Ø	ACCIDENTAL POISN HORMONES&SYNTHETIC SUBSTITUTES	**T38.ØX1A**	Poisoning by glucocort/synth analog, accidental, init
		T38.1X1A	Poisoning by thyroid hormones and sub, accidental, init
		T38.2X1A	Poisoning by antithyroid drugs, accidental, init
		T38.4X1A	Poisoning by oral contraceptives, accidental, init
		T38.5X1A	Poisoning by oth estrogens and progstrn, accidental, init
		T38.6X1A	Poisoning by antigonadtr/antiestr/antiandrg, NEC, acc, init
		T38.7X1A	Poisoning by androgens and anabolic congeners, acc, init
		T38.8Ø1A	Poisoning by unsp hormones and synthetic sub, acc, init
		T38.811A	Poisoning by anterior pituitary hormones, accidental, init
		T38.891A	Poisoning by oth hormones and synthetic sub, acc, init
		T38.9Ø1A	Poisoning by unsp hormone antagonists, accidental, init
		T38.991A	Poisoning by oth hormone antagonists, accidental, init
		T48.ØX1A	Poisoning by oxytocic drugs, accidental, init
		T5Ø.ØX1A	Poisoning by mineralocorticoids and their antag, acc, init
E858.1	ACCIDENTAL POISONING PRIMARILY SYSTEMIC AGENTS	**T45.1X1A**	Poisoning by antineopl and immunosup drugs, acc, init
		T45.8X1A	Poisn by oth prim systemic and hematolog agents, acc, init
		T45.91XA	Poisn by unsp prim systemic and hematolog agent, acc, init
		T5Ø.A11A	Poisn by pertuss vaccine, inc combin w pertuss, acc, init
		T5Ø.A21A	Poisoning by mixed bact vaccines w/o a pertuss, acc, init
		T5Ø.A91A	Poisoning by oth bacterial vaccines, accidental, init
		T5Ø.B11A	Poisoning by smallpox vaccines, accidental, init
		T5Ø.B91A	Poisoning by oth viral vaccines, accidental, init
		T5Ø.Z11A	Poisoning by immunoglobulin, accidental, init
		T5Ø.Z91A	Poisoning by oth vaccines and biolg substances, acc, init
E858.2	ACC POISN AGTS PRIM AFFECT BLD CONSTITUENTS	**T45.4X1A**	Poisoning by iron and its compounds, accidental, init
		T45.511A	Poisoning by anticoagulants, accidental, init
		T45.521A	Poisoning by antithrombotic drugs, accidental, init
		T45.6Ø1A	Poisoning by unsp fibrin-affct drugs, accidental, init
		T45.611A	Poisoning by thrombolytic drug, accidental, init
		T45.621A	Poisoning by hemostatic drug, accidental, init
		T45.691A	Poisoning by oth fibrin-affct drugs, accidental, init
		T45.7X1A	Poisn by anticoag antag, vitamin K and oth coag, acc, init
		T45.8X1A	Poisn by oth prim systemic and hematolog agents, acc, init
		T45.91XA	Poisn by unsp prim systemic and hematolog agent, acc, init
E858.3	ACCIDENTAL POISN AGTS PRIMARILY AFFECT CV SYSTEM	**T46.ØX1A**	Poisoning by cardi-stim glycos/drug simlar act, acc, init
		T46.1X1A	Poisoning by calcium-channel blockers, accidental, init
		T46.2X1A	Poisoning by oth antidysrhythmic drugs, accidental, init
		T46.3X1A	Poisoning by coronary vasodilators, accidental, init
		T46.4X1A	Poisoning by angiotens-convert-enzyme inhibitors, acc, init
		T46.5X1A	Poisoning by oth antihypertn drugs, accidental, init
		T46.6X1A	Poisoning by antihyperlip and antiarterio drugs, acc, init
		T46.7X1A	Poisoning by peripheral vasodilators, accidental, init
		T46.8X1A	Poisoning by antivaric drugs, inc scler agents, acc, init
		T46.9Ø1A	Poisoning by unsp agents aff the cardiovasc sys, acc, init
		T46.991A	Poisoning by oth agents aff the cardiovasc sys, acc, init
E858.4	ACCIDENTAL POISN AGTS PRIMARILY AFFECT GI SYSTEM	**T47.ØX1A**	Poisoning by histamine H2-receptor blockers, acc, init
		T47.1X1A	Poisn by oth antacids and anti-gstrc-sec drugs, acc, init
		T47.2X1A	Poisoning by stimulant laxatives, accidental, init
		T47.3X1A	Poisoning by saline and osmotic laxatives, accidental, init
		T47.4X1A	Poisoning by oth laxatives, accidental (unintentional), init
		T47.5X1A	Poisoning by digestants, accidental (unintentional), init
		T47.6X1A	Poisoning by antidiarrheal drugs, accidental, init
		T47.7X1A	Poisoning by emetics, accidental (unintentional), init
		T47.8X1A	Poisoning by oth agents aff GI sys, accidental, init
		T47.91XA	Poisoning by unsp agents aff the GI sys, accidental, init
E858.5	ACC POISN BY WATR MINERAL&URIC ACID METAB RX	**T5Ø.1X1A**	Poisoning by loop diuretics, accidental, init
		T5Ø.1X4A	Poisoning by loop diuretics, undetermined, initial encounter
		T5Ø.2X1A	Poisn by crbnc-anhydr inhibtr, benzo/oth diuretc, acc, init
		T5Ø.3X1A	Poisoning by electrolytic/caloric/wtr-bal agnt, acc, init
		T5Ø.4X1A	Poisoning by drugs affecting uric acid metab, acc, init
E858.6	ACC POISN AGT PRIM ACT SMOOTH&SKEL MUSC&RESP SYS	**T41.5X1A**	Poisoning by therapeutic gases, accidental, init
		T48.1X1A	Poisoning by skeletal muscle relaxants, accidental, init
		T48.2Ø1A	Poisoning by unsp drugs acting on muscles, accidental, init
		T48.291A	Poisoning by oth drugs acting on muscles, accidental, init
		T48.3X1A	Poisoning by antitussives, accidental (unintentional), init
		T48.4X1A	Poisoning by expectorants, accidental (unintentional), init
		T48.5X1A	Poisoning by oth anti-cmn-cold drugs, accidental, init
		T48.6X1A	Poisoning by antiasthmatics, accidental, init
		T48.9Ø1A	Poisn by unsp agents prim acting on the resp sys, acc, init
		T48.991A	Poisn by oth agents prim acting on the resp sys, acc, init

ICD-9-CM		ICD-10-CM	
E858.7	ACCIDENTAL POISONING BY SKIN-MUCOUS MEMB AGENTS	**T49.ØX1A**	Poisoning by local antifung/infect/inflamm drugs, acc, init
		T49.1X1A	Poisoning by antipruritics, accidental (unintentional), init
		T49.2X1A	Poisoning by local astringents/detergents, accidental, init
		T49.3X1A	Poisoning by emollients, demulcents and protect, acc, init
		T49.4X1A	Poisoning by keratolyt/keratplst/hair trmt drug, acc, init
		T49.5X1A	Poisoning by opth drugs and preparations, accidental, init
		T49.6X1A	Poisoning by otorhino drugs and prep, accidental, init
		T49.7X1A	Poisoning by dental drugs, topically applied, acc, init
		T49.8X1A	Poisoning by oth topical agents, accidental, init
		T49.91XA	Poisoning by unsp topical agent, accidental, init
E858.8	ACCIDENTAL POISONING BY OTHER SPECIFIED DRUGS	**T38.3X1A**	Poisoning by insulin and oral hypoglycemic drugs, acc, init
		T42.6X1A	Poisoning by oth antieplptc and sed-hypntc drugs, acc, init
		T42.71XA	Poisn by unsp antieplptc and sed-hypntc drugs, acc, init
		T45.ØX1A	Poisoning by antiallerg/antiemetic, accidental, init
		T45.2X1A	Poisoning by vitamins, accidental (unintentional), init
		T45.3X1A	Poisoning by enzymes, accidental (unintentional), init
		T5Ø.5X1A	Poisoning by appetite depressants, accidental, init
		T5Ø.6X1A	Poisoning by antidotes and chelating agents, acc, init
		T5Ø.8X1A	Poisoning by diagnostic agents, accidental, init
		T5Ø.9Ø1A	Poisoning by unsp drug/meds/biol subst, accidental, init
		T5Ø.991A	Poisoning by oth drug/meds/biol subst, accidental, init
E858.9	ACCIDENTAL POISONING BY UNSPECIFIED DRUG		NO DIAGNOSIS
E86Ø.Ø	ACCIDENTAL POISONING BY ALCOHOLIC BEVERAGES		NO DIAGNOSIS
E86Ø.1	ACC POISN OTH&UNSPEC ETHYL ALCOHOL&ITS PRODUCTS	**T51.ØX1A**	Toxic effect of ethanol, accidental (unintentional), init
E86Ø.2	ACCIDENTAL POISONING BY METHYL ALCOHOL	**T51.1X1A**	Toxic effect of methanol, accidental (unintentional), init
E86Ø.3	ACCIDENTAL POISONING BY ISOPROPYL ALCOHOL	**T51.2X1A**	Toxic effect of 2-Propanol, accidental (unintentional), init
E86Ø.4	ACCIDENTAL POISONING BY FUSEL OIL	**T51.3X1A**	Toxic effect of fusel oil, accidental (unintentional), init
E86Ø.8	ACCIDENTAL POISONING BY OTHER SPECIFIED ALCOHOLS	**T51.8X1A**	Toxic effect of alcohols, accidental (unintentional), init
E86Ø.9	ACCIDENTAL POISONING BY UNSPECIFIED ALCOHOL	**T51.91XA**	Toxic effect of unsp alcohol, accidental, init
E861.Ø	ACCIDENTAL POISONING SYNTHETIC DETRGNTS&SHAMPOOS	**T55.1X1A**	Toxic effect of detergents, accidental (unintentional), init
E861.1	ACCIDENTAL POISONING BY SOAP PRODUCTS	**T55.ØX1A**	Toxic effect of soaps, accidental (unintentional), init
E861.2	ACCIDENTAL POISONING BY POLISHES		NO DIAGNOSIS
E861.3	ACCIDENTAL POISN OTH CLEANSING&POLISHING AGTS		NO DIAGNOSIS
E861.4	ACCIDENTAL POISONING BY DISINFECTANTS		NO DIAGNOSIS
E861.5	ACCIDENTAL POISONING BY LEAD PAINTS		NO DIAGNOSIS
E861.6	ACCIDENTAL POISONING OTHER PAINTS AND VARNISHES	**T65.6X1A**	Toxic effect of paints and dyes, NEC, accidental, init
E861.9	ACC POISON-UNS CLEAN-POLISH-DISINFECTANT-PAINT		NO DIAGNOSIS
E862.Ø	ACCIDENTAL POISONING BY PETROLEUM SOLVENTS		NO DIAGNOSIS
E862.1	ACCIDENTAL POISONING BY PETROLEUM FUELS&CLEANERS	**T52.ØX1A**	Toxic effect of petroleum products, accidental, init
E862.2	ACCIDENTAL POISONING BY LUBRICATING OILS		NO DIAGNOSIS
E862.3	ACCIDENTAL POISONING BY PETROLEUM SOLIDS		NO DIAGNOSIS
E862.4	ACCIDENTAL POISONING BY OTHER SPECIFIED SOLVENTS	**T52.1X1A**	Toxic effect of benzene, accidental (unintentional), init
		T52.2X1A	Toxic effect of homologues of benzene, accidental, init
		T52.3X1A	Toxic effect of glycols, accidental (unintentional), init
		T52.4X1A	Toxic effect of ketones, accidental (unintentional), init
		T52.8X1A	Toxic effect of organic solvents, accidental, init
		T52.91XA	Toxic effect of unsp organic solvent, accidental, init
E862.9	ACCIDENTAL POISONING BY UNSPECIFIED SOLVENT		NO DIAGNOSIS
E863.Ø	ACC POISN INSECTICIDES ORGANOCHLORINE COMPND		NO DIAGNOSIS
E863.1	ACC POISN INSECTICIDES ORGANOPHOSPHORUS COMPND	**T6Ø.ØX1A**	Toxic effect of organophos and carbamate insect, acc, init
E863.2	ACCIDENTAL POISONING BY CARBAMATES		NO DIAGNOSIS
E863.3	ACCIDENTAL POISONING BY MIXTURES OF INSECTICIDES		NO DIAGNOSIS
E863.4	ACCIDENTAL POISONING OTHER&UNSPEC INSECTICIDES	**T6Ø.1X1A**	Toxic effect of halogenated insecticides, accidental, init
		T6Ø.2X1A	Toxic effect of insecticides, accidental, init
		T6Ø.8X1A	Toxic effect of pesticides, accidental (unintentional), init
		T6Ø.91XA	Toxic effect of unsp pesticide, accidental, init
E863.5	ACCIDENTAL POISONING BY HERBICIDES	**T6Ø.3X1A**	Toxic effect of herbicides and fungicides, accidental, init
E863.6	ACCIDENTAL POISONING BY FUNGICIDES		NO DIAGNOSIS
E863.7	ACCIDENTAL POISONING BY RODENTICIDES	**T6Ø.4X1A**	Toxic effect of rodenticides, accidental, init
E863.8	ACCIDENTAL POISONING BY FUMIGANTS		NO DIAGNOSIS
E863.9	ACCID POISON-OTH AGRICULT-HORTICULT CHEM-RX PREP		NO DIAGNOSIS
E864.Ø	ACCIDENTAL POISONING BY CORROSIVE AROMATICS NEC	**T54.ØX1A**	Toxic effect of phenol and phenol homologues, acc, init
E864.1	ACCIDENTAL POISONING BY ACIDS NEC	**T65.5X1A**	Tox eff of nitro and oth nitric acids and esters, acc, init
E864.2	ACCIDENTAL POISONING BY CAUSTIC ALKALIS NEC		NO DIAGNOSIS
E864.3	ACC POISN OTH SPEC CORROSIVES&CAUSTICS NEC	**T57.1X1A**	Toxic effect of phosphorus and its compounds, acc, init
E864.4	ACCIDENTAL POISN UNSPEC CORROSIVES&CAUSTICS NEC	**T56.4X1A**	Toxic effect of copper and its compounds, accidental, init
E865.Ø	ACCIDENTAL POISONING BY MEAT		NO DIAGNOSIS
E865.1	ACCIDENTAL POISONING BY SHELLFISH	**T61.781A**	Oth shellfish poisoning, accidental (unintentional), init

ICD-9-CM		ICD-10-CM	
E865.2	ACCIDENTAL POISONING FROM OTHER FISH	**T61.Ø1XA**	Ciguatera fish poisoning, accidental (unintentional), init
		T61.11XA	Scombroid fish poisoning, accidental (unintentional), init
		T61.771A	Oth fish poisoning, accidental (unintentional), init encntr
		T61.8X1A	Toxic effect of seafood, accidental (unintentional), init
		T61.91XA	Toxic effect of unsp seafood, accidental, init
E865.3	ACCIDENTAL POISONING FROM BERRIES AND SEEDS	**T62.1X1A**	Toxic effect of ingested berries, accidental, init
E865.4	ACCIDENTAL POISONING FROM OTHER SPECIFIED PLANTS	**T62.2X1A**	Toxic effect of ingested (parts of) plant(s), acc, init
E865.5	ACCIDENTAL POISONING FROM MUSHROOMS&OTHER FUNGI	**T62.ØX1A**	Toxic effect of ingested mushrooms, accidental, init
E865.8	ACCIDENTAL POISONING FROM OTHER SPECIFIED FOODS	**T62.8X1A**	Toxic effect of noxious substances eaten as food, acc, init
E865.9	ACC POISN FROM UNSPEC FOODSTUFF/POISONOUS PLANT	**T62.91XA**	Toxic effect of unsp noxious sub eaten as food, acc, init
E866.Ø	ACCIDENTAL POISONING LEAD&ITS COMPOUNDS&FUMES	**T56.ØX1A**	Toxic effect of lead and its compounds, accidental, init
E866.1	ACCIDENTAL POISONING MERCURY&ITS COMPOUNDS&FUMES	**T56.1X1A**	Toxic effect of mercury and its compounds, accidental, init
E866.2	ACCIDENTAL POISONING ANTIMONY&ITS COMPND&FUMES	NO DIAGNOSIS	
E866.3	ACCIDENTAL POISONING ARSENIC&ITS COMPOUNDS&FUMES	**T57.ØX1A**	Toxic effect of arsenic and its compounds, accidental, init
E866.4	ACCIDENTAL POISN OTH METALS&THEIR COMPND&FUMES	**T56.2X1A**	Toxic effect of chromium and its compounds, acc, init
		T56.3X1A	Toxic effect of cadmium and its compounds, accidental, init
		T56.5X1A	Toxic effect of zinc and its compounds, accidental, init
		T56.6X1A	Toxic effect of tin and its compounds, accidental, init
		T56.7X1A	Toxic effect of beryllium and its compounds, acc, init
		T56.811A	Toxic effect of thallium, accidental (unintentional), init
		T56.891A	Toxic effect of oth metals, accidental (unintentional), init
		T56.91XA	Toxic effect of unsp metal, accidental (unintentional), init
		T57.2X1A	Toxic effect of manganese and its compounds, acc, init
E866.5	ACCIDENTAL POISONING PLANT FOODS AND FERTILIZERS	NO DIAGNOSIS	
E866.6	ACCIDENTAL POISONING BY GLUES AND ADHESIVES	NO DIAGNOSIS	
E866.7	ACCIDENTAL POISONING BY COSMETICS	NO DIAGNOSIS	
E866.8	ACCIDENTAL POISN OTH SPEC SOLID/LIQUID SBSTNC	**T57.8X1A**	Toxic effect of inorganic substances, accidental, init
		T57.91XA	Toxic effect of unsp inorganic substance, accidental, init
		T64.Ø1XA	Toxic effect of aflatoxin, accidental (unintentional), init
		T64.81XA	Toxic effect of mycotoxin food contamnt, accidental, init
		T65.ØX1A	Toxic effect of cyanides, accidental (unintentional), init
		T65.1X1A	Toxic effect of strychnine and its salts, accidental, init
		T65.211A	Toxic effect of chewing tobacco, accidental, init
		T65.221A	Toxic effect of tobacco cigarettes, accidental, init
		T65.291A	Toxic effect of tobacco and nicotine, accidental, init
		T65.3X1A	Toxic eff of nitrodrv/aminodrv of benzn/homolog, acc, init
		T65.4X1A	Toxic effect of carbon disulfide, accidental, init
		T65.811A	Toxic effect of latex, accidental (unintentional), init
		T65.831A	Toxic effect of fiberglass, accidental (unintentional), init
		T65.891A	Toxic effect of substances, accidental (unintentional), init
		T65.91XA	Toxic effect of unsp substance, accidental, init
E866.9	ACCIDENTAL POISN UNSPEC SOLID/LIQUID SUBSTANCE	NO DIAGNOSIS	
E867	ACCIDENTAL POISONING GAS DISTRIBUTED PIPELINE	NO DIAGNOSIS	
E868.Ø	ACCID POISON-LIQUEF PETRO GAS IN MOBILE CONTAINR	NO DIAGNOSIS	
E868.1	ACCIDENTAL POISONING OTHER&UNSPEC UTILITY GAS	**T58.11XA**	Toxic effect of carb monx from utility gas, acc, init
E868.2	ACCIDENTAL POISONING MOTOR VEHICLE EXHAUST GAS	**T58.Ø1XA**	Toxic effect of carb monx from mtr veh exhaust, acc, init
E868.3	ACCID POISON-INCOMPLETE CARBON MONOXIDE COMBUST	**T58.2X1A**	Tox eff of carb monx fr incmpl combst dmst fuel, acc, init
E868.8	ACCIDENTAL POISN CARB MONOXIDE FROM OTH SOURCES	**T58.8X1A**	Toxic effect of carb monx from oth source, accidental, init
E868.9	ACCIDENTAL POISONING UNSPECIFIED CARBON MONOXIDE	**T58.91XA**	Toxic effect of carb monx from unsp source, acc, init
E869.Ø	ACCIDENTAL POISONING BY NITROGEN OXIDES	**T59.ØX1A**	Toxic effect of nitrogen oxides, accidental, init
E869.1	ACCIDENTAL POISONING BY SULFUR DIOXIDE	**T59.1X1A**	Toxic effect of sulfur dioxide, accidental, init
E869.2	ACCIDENTAL POISONING BY FREON	**T53.5X1A**	Toxic effect of chlorofluorocarbons, accidental, init
E869.3	ACCIDENTAL POISONING BY LACRIMOGENIC GAS	**T59.3X1A**	Toxic effect of lacrimogenic gas, accidental, init
E869.4	ACCIDENTAL POISONING SECOND-HAND TOBACCO SMOKE	NO DIAGNOSIS	
E869.8	ACCIDENTAL POISONING OTHER SPEC GASES&VAPORS	**T53.ØX1A**	Toxic effect of carbon tetrachloride, accidental, init
		T53.1X1A	Toxic effect of chloroform, accidental (unintentional), init
		T53.2X1A	Toxic effect of trichloroethylene, accidental, init
		T53.3X1A	Toxic effect of tetrachloroethylene, accidental, init
		T53.4X1A	Toxic effect of dichloromethane, accidental, init
		T53.6X1A	Toxic eff of halgn deriv of aliphatic hydrocrb, acc, init
		T53.7X1A	Toxic effect of halgn deriv of aromatic hydrocrb, acc, init
		T53.91XA	Toxic eff of unsp halgn deriv of aromat hydrocrb, acc, init
		T57.3X1A	Toxic effect of hydrogen cyanide, accidental, init
		T59.2X1A	Toxic effect of formaldehyde, accidental, init
		T59.4X1A	Toxic effect of chlorine gas, accidental, init
		T59.5X1A	Toxic eff of fluorine gas and hydrogen fluoride, acc, init
		T59.6X1A	Toxic effect of hydrogen sulfide, accidental, init
		T59.7X1A	Toxic effect of carbon dioxide, accidental, init
		T59.811A	Toxic effect of smoke, accidental (unintentional), init
		T59.891A	Toxic effect of gases, fumes and vapors, accidental, init
		T59.894A	Toxic effect of gases, fumes and vapors, undetermined, init
		T59.91XA	Toxic effect of unsp gases, fumes and vapors, acc, init
E869.9	ACCIDENTAL POISONING UNSPECIFIED GASES&VAPORS	NO DIAGNOSIS	

[Brackets] indicate valid character values for each code. Character value meanings provided for each code grouping.

ICD-9-CM			ICD-10-CM	
E870.Ø	ACC CUT PUNCT PERF/HEMORR DURING SURG OPERATION		NO DIAGNOSIS	
E870.1	ACC CUT PUNCT PERF/HEMORR DURING INFUS/TRANSFUS		NO DIAGNOSIS	
E870.2	ACC CUT PUNCT PERF/HEMORR DUR DIALYSIS/PERFUSION		NO DIAGNOSIS	
E870.3	ACC CUT PUNCT PERF/HEMORR DURING INJECTION/VACC		NO DIAGNOSIS	
E870.4	ACC CUT PUNCT PERF/HEMORR DURING ENDO EXAM		NO DIAGNOSIS	
E870.5	ACC CUT/HEMMOR DUR FLUID ASPIRAT-PUNCT-CATH		NO DIAGNOSIS	
E870.6	ACCIDENTAL CUT PUNCT PERF/HEMORR DURING HRT CATH		NO DIAGNOSIS	
E870.7	ACC CUT PUNCT PERF/HEMORR DURING ADMIN ENEMA		NO DIAGNOSIS	
E870.8	ACC CUT PUNCT PERF/HEMORR DUR OTH SPEC MED CARE		NO DIAGNOSIS	
E870.9	ACC CUT PUNCT PERF/HEMORR DUR UNSPEC MED CARE		NO DIAGNOSIS	
E871.Ø	FOREIGN OBJECT LEFT BODY DURING SURG OPERATION		NO DIAGNOSIS	
E871.1	FOREIGN OBJECT LEFT BODY DURING INFUS/TRANSFUS		NO DIAGNOSIS	
E871.2	FOREIGN OBJ LEFT IN BODY DUR DIALYSIS/PERFUSION		NO DIAGNOSIS	
E871.3	FOREIGN OBJECT LEFT BODY DURING INJECTION/VACC		NO DIAGNOSIS	
E871.4	FOREIGN OBJECT LEFT BODY DURING ENDO EXAMINATION		NO DIAGNOSIS	
E871.5	FOREIGN OBJ LT BDY DUR ASPIR FL/TISS PUNCT&CATH		NO DIAGNOSIS	
E871.6	FOREIGN OBJECT LEFT BODY DURING HEART CATH		NO DIAGNOSIS	
E871.7	FOREIGN OBJ LT BDY DURING REMOVAL CATH/PACKING		NO DIAGNOSIS	
E871.8	FOREIGN OBJECT LEFT BODY DURING OTH SPEC PROC		NO DIAGNOSIS	
E871.9	FOREIGN OBJECT LEFT BODY DURING UNSPEC PROCEDURE		NO DIAGNOSIS	
E872.Ø	FAIL STERL PRECAUTION DURING SURGICAL OPERATION	➡	Y62.Ø	Failure of sterile precautions during surgical operation
E872.1	FAIL STERILE PRECAUTIONS DURING INFUS/TRANSFUS	➡	Y62.1	Failure of sterile precautions during infusn/transfusn
E872.2	FAILED STERILE PRECAUTIONS DUR DIALYSIS/PERFUS	➡	Y62.2	Fail of steril precaut dur kidney dialysis and oth perfusion
E872.3	FAIL STERL PRECAUTION DURING INJECTION/VACC	➡	Y62.3	Failure of steril precaut during injection or immunization
E872.4	FAIL STERILE PRECAUTIONS DURING ENDO EXAMINATION	➡	Y62.4	Failure of sterile precautions during endoscopic examination
E872.5	FAILED STERILE PRECAUT DURING ASPIRAT-PUNCT-CATH	➡	Y62.6	Failure of steril precaut during aspirat, pnctr and oth cath
E872.6	FAILURE STERILE PRECAUTIONS DURING HEART CATH	➡	Y62.5	Failure of sterile precautions during heart catheterization
E872.8	FAILURE STERILE PRECAUTIONS DURING OTH SPEC PROC	➡	Y62.8	Failure of steril precaut during oth surg and medical care
E872.9	FAILURE STERILE PRECAUTIONS DURING UNSPEC PROC	➡	Y62.9	Failure of steril precaut during unsp surg and medical care
E873.Ø	EXCESS AMOUNT BLD/OTH FL DURING TRANSFUS/INFUS	➡	Y63.Ø	Excess amount of bld or oth fluid given dur tranfs or infusn
E873.1	INCORRECT DILUTION OF FLUID DURING INFUSION	➡	Y63.1	Incorrect dilution of fluid used during infusion
E873.2	OVERDOSE OF RADIATION IN THERAPY	➡	Y63.2	Overdose of radiation given during therapy
E873.3	INADVERTENT EXPOS PT RAD DURING MEDICAL CARE	➡	Y63.3	Inadvertent expsr of patient to radiation during med care
E873.4	FAILURE DOSE ELECTROSHOCK/INSULIN-SHOCK THERAPY	➡	Y63.4	Failure in dosage in electroshock or insulin-shock therapy
E873.5	INAPPROPRIATE TEMP LOCAL APPLICATION&PACKING	➡	Y63.5	Inappropriate temperature in local application and packing
E873.6	NONADMIN NECESSARY DRUG/MEDICINAL SUBSTANCE		Y63.6	Undrdose & nonadmin of necess drug, medicament or biolg sub
E873.8	OTHER SPECIFIED FAILURE IN DOSAGE		Y63.6 Y63.8	Undrdose & nonadmin of necess drug, medicament or biolg sub Failure in dosage during other surgical and medical care
E873.9	UNSPECIFIED FAILURE IN DOSAGE	➡	Y63.9	Failure in dosage during unsp surgical and medical care
E874.Ø	MECH FAIL INSTRUMENT/APPARAT DUR SURG OPERATION		NO DIAGNOSIS	
E874.1	MECH FAIL INSTRUMENT/APPARAT DUR INFUS&TRANSFUS		NO DIAGNOSIS	
E874.2	MECH FAIL-INSTRUMNT/APPARATUS DUR DIALYS-PERFUS		NO DIAGNOSIS	
E874.3	MECH FAIL INSTRUMENT/APPARAT DURING ENDO EXAM		NO DIAGNOSIS	
E874.4	MECH FAIL-INSTRUMENT DUR ASPIRATION-PUNCT-CATH		NO DIAGNOSIS	
E874.5	MECH FAIL INSTRUMENT/APPARAT DURING HEART CATH		NO DIAGNOSIS	
E874.8	MECH FAIL INSTRUMENT/APPARAT DUR OTH SPEC PROC		NO DIAGNOSIS	
E874.9	MECH FAIL INSTRUMENT/APPARAT DURING UNSPEC PROC		NO DIAGNOSIS	
E875.Ø	CONTAMINATED SUBSTANCE TRANSFUSED OR INFUSED	➡	Y64.Ø	Contaminated med/biolog sub, transfused or infused
E875.1	CONTAMINATED SUBSTANCE INJECTED/USED VACCINATION	➡	Y64.1	Contaminated med/biolog sub, injected or used for immuniz
E875.2	CONTAMINAT RX/BIOLOGICAL SBSTNC ADMIN OTH MEANS	➡	Y64.8	Contaminated med/biolog sub administered by oth means
E875.8	OTHER CONTAMINATION PATIENT DURING MEDICAL CARE		Y64.8	Contaminated med/biolog sub administered by oth means
E875.9	UNSPEC CONTAMINATION PATIENT DURING MEDICAL CARE	➡	Y64.9	Contaminated med/biolog sub administered by unsp means
E876.Ø	MISMATCHED BLOOD IN TRANSFUSION	➡	Y65.Ø	Mismatched blood in transfusion
E876.1	WRONG FLUID IN INFUSION	➡	Y65.1	Wrong fluid used in infusion
E876.2	FAIL SUTURE&LIGATURE DURING SURGICAL OPERATION	➡	Y65.2	Failure in suture or ligature during surgical operation
E876.3	ET WRONGLY PLACED DURING ANESTHETIC PROC	➡	Y65.3	Endotracheal tube wrongly placed during anesthetic procedure
E876.4	FAILURE INTRODUCE/TO REMOVE OTH TUBE/INSTRUMENT	➡	Y65.4	Failure to introduce or to remove other tube or instrument
E876.5	PERFORMANCE OF WRNG OPERATION ON CORRECT PT	➡	Y65.51	Performance of wrong procedure (op) on correct patient
E876.6	PERFORM OPERATION ON PT NOT SCHEDULED SURGERY	➡	Y65.52	Perform of proc (op) on patient not scheduled for surgery
E876.7	PERFORM CORRECT OPERATION ON WRONG SIDE/BDY PART	➡	Y65.53	Perform of correct procedure (op) on wrong side or body part
E876.8	OTHER SPECIFIED MISADVENTURE DURING MEDICAL CARE		Y65.8 Y66	Oth misadventures during surgical and medical care Nonadministration of surgical and medical care
E876.9	UNSPECIFIED MISADVENTURE DURING MEDICAL CARE	➡	Y69	Unspecified misadventure during surgical and medical care
E878.Ø	ABNORM REACT/COMPLI D/T WHOLE ORGAN TRANSPLNT SX	➡	Y83.Ø	Txplt of whole organ cause abn react/compl, w/o misadvnt
E878.1	ABNORM REACT D/T ARTIFICIAL INTERN DEVICE IMPLNT	➡	Y83.1	Implnt of artif int dev cause abn react/compl, w/o misadvnt
E878.2	ABNORM REACT D/T ANASTOMOSIS-BYPASS/GRAFT SURG	➡	Y83.2	Anastomos,bypass or grft cause abn react/compl, w/o misadvnt
E878.3	ABNORM REACT D/T EXTERNAL STOMA FORMATION SURG	➡	Y83.3	Form of external stoma cause abn react/compl, w/o misadvnt

ICD-9-CM			ICD-10-CM	
E878.4	ABNORM REACT/COMPLI D/T OTH RESTORATIVE SURGERY	➡	**Y83.4**	Oth recnst surgery cause abn react/compl, w/o misadvnt
E878.5	ABNORMAL REACT/COMPLI D/T AMPUTATION OF LIMB(S)	➡	**Y83.5**	Amputation of limb(s) cause abn react/compl, w/o misadvnt
E878.6	ABNORM REACT D/T REMOVE-OTH ORGAN (PARTIAL/TOTAL	➡	**Y83.6**	Remov org (total) cause abn react/compl, w/o misadvnt
E878.8	ABNORMAL REACTION/COMPLICAT D/T OTH SPEC SURGERY	➡	**Y83.8**	Oth surgical procedures cause abn react/compl, w/o misadvnt
E878.9	ABNORM REACT/COMPLI D/T SURGICAL OP & PROCEDURES		**Y83.9** **Y84.9**	Surgical proc, unsp cause abn react/compl, w/o misadvnt Medical procedure, unsp cause abn react/compl, w/o misadvnt
E879.Ø	ABNORMAL REACTION/COMPLICATION D/T CARDIAC CATH	➡	**Y84.Ø**	Cardiac catheterization cause abn react/compl, w/o misadvnt
E879.1	ABNORMAL REACTION/COMPLICAT D/T KIDNEY DIALYSIS	➡	**Y84.1**	Kidney dialysis cause abn react/compl, w/o misadvnt
E879.2	ABNORM REACT/COMPLI D/T RADIOLOGY-RADIOTHERAPY	➡	**Y84.2**	Radiolog proc/radiothrpy cause abn react/compl, w/o misadvnt
E879.3	ABNORMAL REACTION/COMPLICATION D/T SHOCK THERAPY	➡	**Y84.3**	Shock therapy cause abn react/compl, w/o misadvnt
E879.4	ABNORMAL REACTION/COMPLICAT D/T ASPIRATION-FLUID	➡	**Y84.4**	Aspiration of fluid cause abn react/compl, w/o misadvnt
E879.5	ABNORM REACT D/T INSERT-GASTRIC/DUODENAL SOUND	➡	**Y84.5**	Insrt gastr/duodnl sound cause abn react/compl, w/o misadvnt
E879.6	ABNORMAL REACTION/COMPLICATION D/T URINARY CATH	➡	**Y84.6**	Urinary catheterization cause abn react/compl, w/o misadvnt
E879.7	ABNORMAL REACTION/COMPLICAT D/T BLOOD SAMPLING	➡	**Y84.7**	Blood-sampling cause abn react/compl, w/o misadvnt
E879.8	ABNORMAL REACTION/COMPLICAT D/T OTH SPEC PROCED		**Y84.8**	Oth medical procedures cause abn react/compl, w/o misadvnt
E879.9	ABNORMAL REACTION/COMPLICAT D/T UNS PROCEDURE		**Y84.8**	Oth medical procedures cause abn react/compl, w/o misadvnt
E88Ø.Ø	ACCIDENTAL FALL ON OR FROM ESCALATOR		**W1Ø.ØXXA** **W1Ø.ØXXD**	Fall (on)(from) escalator, initial encounter Fall (on)(from) escalator, subsequent encounter
E88Ø.1	ACCIDENTAL FALL ON OR FROM SIDEWALK CURB		**W1Ø.1XXA** **W1Ø.1XXD**	Fall (on)(from) sidewalk curb, initial encounter Fall (on)(from) sidewalk curb, subsequent encounter
E88Ø.9	ACCIDENTAL FALL ON OR FROM OTHER STAIRS OR STEPS		**W1Ø.2XXA** **W1Ø.2XXD** **W1Ø.8XXA** **W1Ø.8XXD** **W1Ø.9XXA** **W1Ø.9XXD**	Fall (on)(from) incline, initial encounter Fall (on)(from) incline, subsequent encounter Fall (on) (from) other stairs and steps, initial encounter Fall (on) (from) other stairs and steps, subs encntr Fall (on) (from) unspecified stairs and steps, init encntr Fall (on) (from) unspecified stairs and steps, subs encntr
E881.Ø	ACCIDENTAL FALL FROM LADDER		**W11.XXXA** **W11.XXXD**	Fall on and from ladder, initial encounter Fall on and from ladder, subsequent encounter
E881.1	ACCIDENTAL FALL FROM SCAFFOLDING		**W12.XXXA** **W12.XXXD**	Fall on and from scaffolding, initial encounter Fall on and from scaffolding, subsequent encounter
E882	ACCIDENTAL FALL FROM/OUT BUILDING/OTH STRUCTURE		**W13.ØXXA** **W13.ØXXD** **W13.1XXA** **W13.1XXD** **W13.2XXA** **W13.2XXD** **W13.3XXA** **W13.3XXD** **W13.4XXA** **W13.4XXD** **W13.8XXA** **W13.8XXD** **W13.9XXA** **W13.9XXD**	Fall from, out of or through balcony, initial encounter Fall from, out of or through balcony, subsequent encounter Fall from, out of or through bridge, initial encounter Fall from, out of or through bridge, subsequent encounter Fall from, out of or through roof, initial encounter Fall from, out of or through roof, subsequent encounter Fall through floor, initial encounter Fall through floor, subsequent encounter Fall from, out of or through window, initial encounter Fall from, out of or through window, subsequent encounter Fall from, out of or through oth building or structure, init Fall from, out of or through oth building or structure, subs Fall from, out of or through bldg, not otherwise spcf, init Fall from, out of or through bldg, not otherwise spcf, subs
E883.Ø	ACCIDENT FROM DIVING OR JUMPING INTO WATER		**W16.Ø11A** **W16.Ø11D** **W16.Ø12A** **W16.Ø12D** **W16.Ø21A** **W16.Ø21D** **W16.Ø22A** **W16.Ø22D** **W16.Ø31A** **W16.Ø31D** **W16.Ø32A** **W16.Ø32D** **W16.111A** **W16.111D** **W16.112A** **W16.112D** **W16.121A** **W16.121D** **W16.122A** **W16.122D** **W16.131A** **W16.131D** **W16.132A** **W16.132D** **W16.211A** **W16.211D** **W16.212A** **W16.212D** **W16.221A** **W16.221D** **W16.222A** **W16.222D** **W16.311A**	Fall into swimming pool striking surfc causing drown, init Fall into swimming pool striking surfc causing drown, subs Fall into swimming pool strk surfc causing oth injury, init Fall into swimming pool strk surfc causing oth injury, subs Fall into swimming pool striking bottom causing drown, init Fall into swimming pool striking bottom causing drown, subs Fall into swimming pool strk bottom causing oth injury, init Fall into swimming pool strk bottom causing oth injury, subs Fall into swimming pool striking wall causing drown, init Fall into swimming pool striking wall causing drown, subs Fall into swimming pool strk wall causing oth injury, init Fall into swimming pool strk wall causing oth injury, subs Fall into natural body of water strk surfc cause drown, init Fall into natural body of water strk surfc cause drown, subs Fall into natrl body of water strk surfc cause oth inj, init Fall into natrl body of water strk surfc cause oth inj, subs Fall into natrl body of water strk bottom cause drown, init Fall into natrl body of water strk bottom cause drown, subs Fall into natrl body of water strk botm cause oth inj, init Fall into natrl body of water strk botm cause oth inj, subs Fall into natural body of water strk side cause drown, init Fall into natural body of water strk side cause drown, subs Fall into natrl body of water strk side cause oth inj, init Fall into natrl body of water strk side cause oth inj, subs Fall in (into) filled bathtub causing drown, init Fall in (into) filled bathtub causing drown, subs Fall in (into) filled bathtub causing oth injury, init Fall in (into) filled bathtub causing oth injury, subs Fall in (into) bucket of water causing drown, init Fall in (into) bucket of water causing drown, subs Fall in (into) bucket of water causing oth injury, init Fall in (into) bucket of water causing oth injury, subs Fall into oth water striking surfc causing drown, init

(Continued on next page)

ICD-9-CM		ICD-10-CM	
E883.Ø	ACCIDENT FROM DIVING OR JUMPING INTO WATER **(Continued)**	**W16.311D**	Fall into oth water striking surfc causing drown, subs
		W16.312A	Fall into oth water striking surfc causing oth injury, init
		W16.312D	Fall into oth water striking surfc causing oth injury, subs
		W16.321A	Fall into oth water striking bottom causing drown, init
		W16.321D	Fall into oth water striking bottom causing drown, subs
		W16.322A	Fall into oth water striking bottom causing oth injury, init
		W16.322D	Fall into oth water striking bottom causing oth injury, subs
		W16.331A	Fall into oth water striking wall causing drown, init
		W16.331D	Fall into oth water striking wall causing drown, subs
		W16.332A	Fall into oth water striking wall causing oth injury, init
		W16.332D	Fall into oth water striking wall causing oth injury, subs
		W16.41XA	Fall into unsp water causing drowning and submersion, init
		W16.41XD	Fall into unsp water causing drowning and submersion, subs
		W16.42XA	Fall into unsp water causing other injury, init encntr
		W16.42XD	Fall into unsp water causing other injury, subs encntr
		W16.511A	Jump/div into swimming pool strk surfc causing drown, init
		W16.511D	Jump/div into swimming pool strk surfc causing drown, subs
		W16.512A	Jump/div into swim pool strk surfc causing oth injury, init
		W16.512D	Jump/div into swim pool strk surfc causing oth injury, subs
		W16.521A	Jump/div into swimming pool strk bottom causing drown, init
		W16.521D	Jump/div into swimming pool strk bottom causing drown, subs
		W16.522A	Jump/div into swim pool strk bottom causing oth injury, init
		W16.522D	Jump/div into swim pool strk bottom causing oth injury, subs
		W16.531A	Jump/div into swimming pool strk wall causing drown, init
		W16.531D	Jump/div into swimming pool strk wall causing drown, subs
		W16.532A	Jump/div into swim pool strk wall causing oth injury, init
		W16.532D	Jump/div into swim pool strk wall causing oth injury, subs
		W16.611A	Jump/div into natrl body of wtr strk surfc cause drown, init
		W16.611D	Jump/div into natrl body of wtr strk surfc cause drown, subs
		W16.612A	Jump/div in natrl body of wtr strk surfc cause oth inj, init
		W16.612D	Jump/div in natrl body of wtr strk surfc cause oth inj, subs
		W16.621A	Jump/div into natrl body of wtr strk botm cause drown, init
		W16.621D	Jump/div into natrl body of wtr strk botm cause drown, subs
		W16.622A	Jump/div in natrl body of wtr strk botm cause oth inj, init
		W16.622D	Jump/div in natrl body of wtr strk botm cause oth inj, subs
		W16.711A	Jump/div from boat striking surfc causing drown, init
		W16.711D	Jump/div from boat striking surfc causing drown, subs
		W16.712A	Jump/div from boat striking surfc causing oth injury, init
		W16.712D	Jump/div from boat striking surfc causing oth injury, subs
		W16.721A	Jump/div from boat striking bottom causing drown, init
		W16.721D	Jump/div from boat striking bottom causing drown, subs
		W16.722A	Jump/div from boat striking bottom causing oth injury, init
		W16.722D	Jump/div from boat striking bottom causing oth injury, subs
		W16.811A	Jump/div into oth water striking surfc causing drown, init
		W16.811D	Jump/div into oth water striking surfc causing drown, subs
		W16.812A	Jump/div into oth water strk surfc causing oth injury, init
		W16.812D	Jump/div into oth water strk surfc causing oth injury, subs
		W16.821A	Jump/div into oth water striking bottom causing drown, init
		W16.821D	Jump/div into oth water striking bottom causing drown, subs
		W16.822A	Jump/div into oth water strk bottom causing oth injury, init
		W16.822D	Jump/div into oth water strk bottom causing oth injury, subs
		W16.831A	Jump/div into oth water striking wall causing drown, init
		W16.831D	Jump/div into oth water striking wall causing drown, subs
		W16.832A	Jump/div into oth water strk wall causing oth injury, init
		W16.832D	Jump/div into oth water strk wall causing oth injury, subs
		W16.91XA	Jumping or diving into unsp water causing drown, init
		W16.91XD	Jumping or diving into unsp water causing drown, subs
		W16.92XA	Jumping or diving into unsp water causing oth injury, init
		W16.92XD	Jumping or diving into unsp water causing oth injury, subs
E883.1	ACCIDENTAL FALL INTO WELL	**W17.ØXXA**	Fall into well, initial encounter
		W17.ØXXD	Fall into well, subsequent encounter
E883.2	ACCIDENTAL FALL INTO STORM DRAIN OR MANHOLE	**W17.1XXA**	Fall into storm drain or manhole, initial encounter
		W17.1XXD	Fall into storm drain or manhole, subsequent encounter
E883.9	ACCIDENTAL FALL INTO OTH HOLE/OTH OPENING SURFCE	**W17.2XXA**	Fall into hole, initial encounter
		W17.2XXD	Fall into hole, subsequent encounter
		W17.3XXA	Fall into empty swimming pool, initial encounter
		W17.3XXD	Fall into empty swimming pool, subsequent encounter
		W17.4XXA	Fall from dock, initial encounter
		W17.4XXD	Fall from dock, subsequent encounter
E884.Ø	ACCIDENTAL FALL FROM PLAYGROUND EQUIPMENT	**WØ9.ØXXA**	Fall on or from playground slide, initial encounter
		WØ9.ØXXD	Fall on or from playground slide, subsequent encounter
		WØ9.1XXA	Fall from playground swing, initial encounter
		WØ9.1XXD	Fall from playground swing, subsequent encounter
		WØ9.2XXA	Fall on or from jungle gym, initial encounter
		WØ9.2XXD	Fall on or from jungle gym, subsequent encounter
		WØ9.8XXA	Fall on or from other playground equipment, init encntr
		WØ9.8XXD	Fall on or from other playground equipment, subs encntr
E884.1	ACCIDENTAL FALL FROM CLIFF	**W15.XXXA**	Fall from cliff, initial encounter
		W15.XXXD	Fall from cliff, subsequent encounter
E884.2	ACCIDENTAL FALL FROM CHAIR	**WØ7.XXXA**	Fall from chair, initial encounter
		WØ7.XXXD	Fall from chair, subsequent encounter

ICD-9-CM		ICD-10-CM	
E884.3	ACCIDENTAL FALL FROM WHEELCHAIR	**V00.811A**	Fall from moving wheelchair (powered), initial encounter
		V00.811D	Fall from moving wheelchair (powered), subsequent encounter
		V00.812A	Wheelchair (powered) colliding w stationary object, init
		V00.812D	Wheelchair (powered) colliding w stationary object, subs
		V00.818A	Other accident with wheelchair (powered), initial encounter
		V00.818D	Other accident with wheelchair (powered), subs encntr
		V00.831A	Fall from motorized mobility scooter, initial encounter
		V00.831D	Fall from motorized mobility scooter, subsequent encounter
		V00.832A	Motorized mobility scooter colliding w statnry obj, init
		V00.832D	Motorized mobility scooter colliding w statnry obj, subs
		V00.838A	Other accident with motorized mobility scooter, init encntr
		V00.838D	Other accident with motorized mobility scooter, subs encntr
		W05.0XXA	Fall from non-moving wheelchair, initial encounter
		W05.0XXD	Fall from non-moving wheelchair, subsequent encounter
		W05.1XXA	Fall from non-moving nonmotorized scooter, initial encounter
		W05.1XXD	Fall from non-moving nonmotorized scooter, subs encntr
		W05.2XXA	Fall from non-moving motorized mobility scooter, init encntr
		W05.2XXD	Fall from non-moving motorized mobility scooter, subs encntr
E884.4	ACCIDENTAL FALL FROM BED	**W06.XXXA**	Fall from bed, initial encounter
		W06.XXXD	Fall from bed, subsequent encounter
E884.5	ACCIDENTAL FALL FROM OTHER FURNITURE	**V00.821A**	Fall from babystroller, initial encounter
		V00.821D	Fall from babystroller, subsequent encounter
		V00.822A	Babystroller colliding with stationary object, init encntr
		V00.822D	Babystroller colliding with stationary object, subs encntr
		V00.828A	Other accident with babystroller, initial encounter
		V00.828D	Other accident with babystroller, subsequent encounter
		W08.XXXA	Fall from other furniture, initial encounter
		W08.XXXD	Fall from other furniture, subsequent encounter
E884.6	ACCIDENTAL FALL FROM COMMODE	**W18.11XA**	Fall from or off toilet w/o strike against object, init
		W18.11XD	Fall from or off toilet w/o strike against object, subs
		W18.12XA	Fall from or off toilet w strike against object, init
		W18.12XD	Fall from or off toilet w strike against object, subs
E884.9	OTHER ACCIDENTAL FALL FROM ONE LEVEL TO ANOTHER	**V00.891A**	Fall from other pedestrian conveyance, initial encounter
		V00.891D	Fall from other pedestrian conveyance, subsequent encounter
		V00.892A	Ped on oth pedestrian convey colliding w statnry obj, init
		V00.892D	Ped on oth pedestrian convey colliding w statnry obj, subs
		V00.898A	Other accident on other pedestrian conveyance, init encntr
		V00.898D	Other accident on other pedestrian conveyance, subs encntr
		W00.1XXA	Fall from stairs and steps due to ice and snow, init encntr
		W00.1XXD	Fall from stairs and steps due to ice and snow, subs encntr
		W00.2XXA	Oth fall from one level to another due to ice and snow, init
		W00.2XXD	Oth fall from one level to another due to ice and snow, subs
		W14.XXXA	Fall from tree, initial encounter
		W14.XXXD	Fall from tree, subsequent encounter
		W17.81XA	Fall down embankment (hill), initial encounter
		W17.81XD	Fall down embankment (hill), subsequent encounter
		W17.82XA	Fall from (out of) grocery cart, initial encounter
		W17.82XD	Fall from (out of) grocery cart, subsequent encounter
		W17.89XA	Other fall from one level to another, initial encounter
		W17.89XD	Other fall from one level to another, subsequent encounter
E885.0	FALL ON SAME LEVEL FROM SCOOTER	**V00.141A**	Fall from scooter (nonmotorized), initial encounter
		V00.141D	Fall from scooter (nonmotorized), subsequent encounter
		V00.142A	Scooter (nonmotorized) colliding w stationary object, init
		V00.142D	Scooter (nonmotorized) colliding w stationary object, subs
		V00.148A	Other scooter (nonmotorized) accident, initial encounter
		V00.148D	Other scooter (nonmotorized) accident, subsequent encounter
E885.1	FALL FROM ROLLER SKATES	**V00.111A**	Fall from in-line roller-skates, initial encounter
		V00.111D	Fall from in-line roller-skates, subsequent encounter
		V00.112A	In-line roller-skater colliding w stationary object, init
		V00.112D	In-line roller-skater colliding w stationary object, subs
		V00.118A	Other in-line roller-skate accident, initial encounter
		V00.118D	Other in-line roller-skate accident, subsequent encounter
		V00.121A	Fall from non-in-line roller-skates, initial encounter
		V00.121D	Fall from non-in-line roller-skates, subsequent encounter
		V00.122A	Non-in-line roller-skater colliding w statnry obj, init
		V00.122D	Non-in-line roller-skater colliding w statnry obj, subs
		V00.128A	Other non-in-line roller-skating accident, initial encounter
		V00.128D	Other non-in-line roller-skating accident, subs encntr
		V00.151A	Fall from heelies, initial encounter
		V00.151D	Fall from heelies, subsequent encounter
		V00.152A	Heelies colliding with stationary object, initial encounter
		V00.152D	Heelies colliding with stationary object, subs encntr
		V00.158A	Other heelies accident, initial encounter
		V00.158D	Other heelies accident, subsequent encounter
E885.2	FALL FROM SKATEBOARD	**V00.131A**	Fall from skateboard, initial encounter
		V00.131D	Fall from skateboard, subsequent encounter
		V00.132A	Skateboarder colliding with stationary object, init encntr
		V00.132D	Skateboarder colliding with stationary object, subs encntr
		V00.138A	Other skateboard accident, initial encounter
		V00.138D	Other skateboard accident, subsequent encounter

ICD-9-CM		ICD-10-CM	
E885.3	FALL FROM SKIS	**VØØ.321A**	Fall from snow-skis, initial encounter
		VØØ.321D	Fall from snow-skis, subsequent encounter
		VØØ.322A	Snow-skier colliding with stationary object, init encntr
		VØØ.322D	Snow-skier colliding with stationary object, subs encntr
		VØØ.328A	Other snow-ski accident, initial encounter
		VØØ.328D	Other snow-ski accident, subsequent encounter
E885.4	FALL FROM SNOWBOARD	**VØØ.311A**	Fall from snowboard, initial encounter
		VØØ.311D	Fall from snowboard, subsequent encounter
		VØØ.312A	Snowboarder colliding with stationary object, init encntr
		VØØ.312D	Snowboarder colliding with stationary object, subs encntr
		VØØ.318A	Other snowboard accident, initial encounter
		VØØ.318D	Other snowboard accident, subsequent encounter
E885.9	FALL FROM OTHER SLIPPING TRIPPING OR STUMBLING	**VØØ.181A**	Fall from oth rolling-type pedestrian conveyance, init
		VØØ.181D	Fall from oth rolling-type pedestrian conveyance, subs
		VØØ.182A	Ped on oth roll-type ped convey collid w statnry obj, init
		VØØ.182D	Ped on oth roll-type ped convey collid w statnry obj, subs
		VØØ.211A	Fall from ice-skates, initial encounter
		VØØ.211D	Fall from ice-skates, subsequent encounter
		VØØ.212A	Ice-skater colliding with stationary object, init encntr
		VØØ.212D	Ice-skater colliding with stationary object, subs encntr
		VØØ.221A	Fall from sled, initial encounter
		VØØ.221D	Fall from sled, subsequent encounter
		VØØ.222A	Sledder colliding with stationary object, initial encounter
		VØØ.222D	Sledder colliding with stationary object, subs encntr
		VØØ.281A	Fall from gliding-type pedestrian conveyance, init encntr
		VØØ.281D	Fall from gliding-type pedestrian conveyance, subs encntr
		VØØ.282A	Ped on gliding-type ped convey colliding w statnry obj, init
		VØØ.282D	Ped on gliding-type ped convey colliding w statnry obj, subs
		VØØ.381A	Fall from flat-bottomed pedestrian conveyance, init encntr
		VØØ.381D	Fall from flat-bottomed pedestrian conveyance, subs encntr
		VØØ.382A	Ped on flat-bottomed ped convey collid w statnry obj, init
		VØØ.382D	Ped on flat-bottomed ped convey collid w statnry obj, subs
		WØØ.ØXXA	Fall on same level due to ice and snow, initial encounter
		WØØ.ØXXD	Fall on same level due to ice and snow, subsequent encounter
		WØØ.9XXA	Unspecified fall due to ice and snow, initial encounter
		WØØ.9XXD	Unspecified fall due to ice and snow, subsequent encounter
		WØ1.ØXXA	Fall same lev from slip/trip w/o strike against object, init
		WØ1.ØXXD	Fall same lev from slip/trip w/o strike against object, subs
		W18.2XXA	Fall in (into) shower or empty bathtub, initial encounter
		W18.2XXD	Fall in (into) shower or empty bathtub, subsequent encounter
		W18.4ØXA	Slipping, tripping and stumbling w/o falling, unsp, init
		W18.4ØXD	Slipping, tripping and stumbling w/o falling, unsp, subs
		W18.41XA	Slip/trip w/o falling due to stepping on object, init
		W18.41XD	Slip/trip w/o falling due to stepping on object, subs
		W18.42XA	Slip/trip w/o falling due to step into hole or opening, init
		W18.42XD	Slip/trip w/o falling due to step into hole or opening, subs
		W18.43XA	Slip/trip w/o fall d/t step from one level to another, init
		W18.43XD	Slip/trip w/o fall d/t step from one level to another, subs
		W18.49XA	Oth slipping, tripping and stumbling w/o falling, init
		W18.49XD	Oth slipping, tripping and stumbling w/o falling, subs
E886.Ø	FALL-SAME LEVEL-COLLIS-PUSH/SHOVE IN SPORTS	**WØ3.XXXA**	Oth fall same lev due to collision w another person, init
		WØ3.XXXD	Oth fall same lev due to collision w another person, subs
E886.9	OTH & UNS ACCIDENTAL FALL ON SAME LEVEL	**VØØ.188A**	Oth accident on oth rolling-type pedestrian conveyance, init
		VØØ.188D	Oth accident on oth rolling-type pedestrian conveyance, subs
		VØØ.218A	Other ice-skates accident, initial encounter
		VØØ.218D	Other ice-skates accident, subsequent encounter
		VØØ.228A	Other sled accident, initial encounter
		VØØ.228D	Other sled accident, subsequent encounter
		VØØ.288A	Oth accident on gliding-type pedestrian conveyance, init
		VØØ.288D	Oth accident on gliding-type pedestrian conveyance, subs
		VØØ.388A	Oth accident on flat-bottomed pedestrian conveyance, init
		VØØ.388D	Oth accident on flat-bottomed pedestrian conveyance, subs
E887	FRACTURE IN ACCIDENTAL FALL CAUSE UNSPECIFIED	**W19.XXXA**	Unspecified fall, initial encounter
E888.Ø	FALL RESULTING IN STRIKING AGAINST SHARP OBJECT	**WØ1.1ØXA**	Fall same lev from slip/trip w strike agnst unsp obj, init
		WØ1.1ØXD	Fall same lev from slip/trip w strike agnst unsp obj, subs
		WØ1.11ØA	Fall same lev from slip/trip w strk agnst sharp glass, init
		WØ1.11ØD	Fall same lev from slip/trip w strk agnst sharp glass, subs
		WØ1.111A	Fall same lev from slip/trip w strk agnst pwr tl/machn, init
		WØ1.111D	Fall same lev from slip/trip w strk agnst pwr tl/machn, subs
		WØ1.118A	Fall same lev fr slip/trip w strk agnst oth sharp obj, init
		WØ1.118D	Fall same lev fr slip/trip w strk agnst oth sharp obj, subs
		WØ1.119A	Fall same lev fr slip/trip w strk agnst unsp sharp obj, init
		WØ1.119D	Fall same lev fr slip/trip w strk agnst unsp sharp obj, subs
		W18.Ø2XA	Striking against glass with subsequent fall, init encntr
		W18.Ø2XD	Striking against glass with subsequent fall, subs encntr

ICD-9-CM		ICD-10-CM	
E888.1	FALL RESULTING IN STRIKING AGAINST OTHER OBJECT	**WØ1.19ØA**	Fall same lev from slip/trip w strike agnst furniture, init
		WØ1.19ØD	Fall same lev from slip/trip w strike agnst furniture, subs
		WØ1.198A	Fall same lev from slip/trip w strike agnst oth object, init
		WØ1.198D	Fall same lev from slip/trip w strike agnst oth object, subs
		W18.ØØXA	Striking against unsp object w subsequent fall, init encntr
		W18.ØØXD	Striking against unsp object w subsequent fall, subs encntr
		W18.Ø1XA	Striking against sports equipment w subsequent fall, init
		W18.Ø1XD	Striking against sports equipment w subsequent fall, subs
		W18.Ø9XD	Striking against oth object w subsequent fall, subs encntr
E888.8	OTHER FALL	**WØ4.XXXA**	Fall while being carried or supported by oth persons, init
		WØ4.XXXD	Fall while being carried or supported by oth persons, subs
		W18.3ØXA	Fall on same level, unspecified, initial encounter
		W18.3ØXD	Fall on same level, unspecified, subsequent encounter
		W18.31XA	Fall on same level due to stepping on an object, init encntr
		W18.31XD	Fall on same level due to stepping on an object, subs encntr
		W18.39XA	Other fall on same level, initial encounter
		W18.39XD	Other fall on same level, subsequent encounter
E888.9	UNSPECIFIED FALL	**W19.XXXA**	Unspecified fall, initial encounter
		W19.XXXD	Unspecified fall, subsequent encounter
E89Ø.Ø	EXPLOSION CAUSED CONFLAGRATION PRIVATE DWELLING	**XØØ.8XXA**	Oth exposure to uncontrolled fire in bldg, init
E89Ø.1	PVC FUMES-COMBUST-CONFLAGRAT IN PRIVATE DWELLING	**XØ8.8XXA**	Exposure to oth smoke, fire and flames, init encntr
E89Ø.2	OTH SMOKE&FUMES FROM CONFLAGRAT PRIVATE DWELLING	**XØØ.1XXA**	Exposure to smoke in uncontrolled fire in bldg, init
		XØØ.1XXD	Exposure to smoke in uncontrolled fire in bldg, subs
		XØ2.1XXA	Exposure to smoke in controlled fire in bldg, init
		XØ2.1XXD	Exposure to smoke in controlled fire in bldg, subs
E89Ø.3	BURNING CAUSED CONFLAGRATION IN PRIVATE DWELLING	**XØØ.ØXXA**	Exposure to flames in uncontrolled fire in bldg, init
		XØØ.ØXXD	Exposure to flames in uncontrolled fire in bldg, subs
		XØ2.ØXXA	Exposure to flames in controlled fire in bldg, init
		XØ2.ØXXD	Exposure to flames in controlled fire in bldg, subs
E89Ø.8	OTH ACC RESULT FROM CONFLAGRAT PRIVATE DWELLING	**XØØ.2XXA**	Injury due to collapse of burn bldg in uncntrld fire, init
		XØØ.2XXD	Injury due to collapse of burn bldg in uncntrld fire, subs
		XØØ.3XXA	Fall from burning bldg in uncontrolled fire, init
		XØØ.3XXD	Fall from burning bldg in uncontrolled fire, subs
		XØØ.4XXA	Hit by object from burning bldg in uncontrolled fire, init
		XØØ.4XXD	Hit by object from burning bldg in uncontrolled fire, subs
		XØØ.5XXA	Jump from burning bldg in uncontrolled fire, init
		XØØ.5XXD	Jump from burning bldg in uncontrolled fire, subs
		XØØ.8XXA	Oth exposure to uncontrolled fire in bldg, init
		XØØ.8XXD	Oth exposure to uncontrolled fire in bldg, subs
		XØ2.2XXA	Injury due to collapse of burning bldg in ctrl fire, init
		XØ2.2XXD	Injury due to collapse of burning bldg in ctrl fire, subs
		XØ2.3XXA	Fall from burning bldg in controlled fire, init
		XØ2.3XXD	Fall from burning bldg in controlled fire, subs
		XØ2.4XXA	Hit by object from burning bldg in controlled fire, init
		XØ2.4XXD	Hit by object from burning bldg in controlled fire, subs
		XØ2.5XXA	Jump from burning bldg in controlled fire, init
		XØ2.5XXD	Jump from burning bldg in controlled fire, subs
		XØ2.8XXD	Oth exposure to controlled fire in bldg, subs
E89Ø.9	UNSPEC ACC RESULT FROM CONFLAGRAT PRIVATE DWELL	**XØØ.8XXA**	Oth exposure to uncontrolled fire in bldg, init
E891.Ø	EXPLO CAUS CONFLAGRAT OTH&UNSPEC BLDG/STRUCTURE	**XØØ.8XXA**	Oth exposure to uncontrolled fire in bldg, init
E891.1	PVC FUMES-COMBUSTION-CONFLAGRAT IN OTH-UNS BUILD	**XØ8.8XXA**	Exposure to oth smoke, fire and flames, init encntr
E891.2	OTH SMOKE&FUMES CONFLAGRAT OTH&UNS BLDG/STRCT	**XØØ.1XXA**	Exposure to smoke in uncontrolled fire in bldg, init
E891.3	BURNING CAUS CONFLAGRAT OTH&UNSPEC BLDG/STRCT	**XØØ.ØXXA**	Exposure to flames in uncontrolled fire in bldg, init
E891.8	OTH ACC RSLT FROM CONFLAGRAT OTH&UNS BLDG/STRCT	**XØØ.8XXA**	Oth exposure to uncontrolled fire in bldg, init
E891.9	UNS ACC RSLT FROM CONFLAGRAT OTH&UNS BLDG/STRCT	**XØØ.8XXA**	Oth exposure to uncontrolled fire in bldg, init
E892	CONFLAGRATION NOT IN BUILDING OR STRUCTURE	**XØ1.ØXXA**	Exposure to flames in uncontrolled fire, not in bldg, init
		XØ1.ØXXD	Exposure to flames in uncontrolled fire, not in bldg, subs
		XØ1.1XXA	Exposure to smoke in uncontrolled fire, not in bldg, init
		XØ1.1XXD	Exposure to smoke in uncontrolled fire, not in bldg, subs
		XØ1.3XXA	Fall due to uncontrolled fire, not in bldg, init
		XØ1.3XXD	Fall due to uncontrolled fire, not in bldg, subs
		XØ1.4XXA	Hit by object due to uncontrolled fire, not in bldg, init
		XØ1.4XXD	Hit by object due to uncontrolled fire, not in bldg, subs
		XØ1.8XXA	Oth exposure to uncontrolled fire, not in bldg, init
		XØ1.8XXD	Oth exposure to uncontrolled fire, not in bldg, subs
E893.Ø	ACC CAUS IGNITION CLOTHING CNTRL FIRE PRIV DWELL	**XØ5.XXXA**	Exposure to ignition or melting of nightwear, init encntr
		XØ5.XXXD	Exposure to ignition or melting of nightwear, subs encntr
E893.1	ACC CAUS IGNITION CLOTHES-CNTRL FIRE OTH BUILD	**XØ2.ØXXA**	Exposure to flames in controlled fire in bldg, init
E893.2	ACC CAUS IGNITION CLOTHES-CNTRL FIRE-NOT IN BLDG	**XØ3.ØXXA**	Exposure to flames in controlled fire, not in bldg, init
E893.8	ACC CAUSED IGNITION CLOTHING FROM OTH SPEC SRC	**XØ6.ØXXA**	Exposure to ignition of plastic jewelry, initial encounter
		XØ6.ØXXD	Exposure to ignition of plastic jewelry, subs encntr
		XØ6.1XXA	Exposure to melting of plastic jewelry, initial encounter
		XØ6.1XXD	Exposure to melting of plastic jewelry, subsequent encounter
		XØ6.2XXA	Exposure to ignition of oth clothing and apparel, init
		XØ6.2XXD	Exposure to ignition of oth clothing and apparel, subs
		XØ6.3XXA	Exposure to melting of oth clothing and apparel, init encntr
		XØ6.3XXD	Exposure to melting of oth clothing and apparel, subs encntr
E893.9	ACCIDENT CAUSED IGNITION CLOTHING UNSPEC SOURCE	**XØ8.8XXA**	Exposure to oth smoke, fire and flames, init encntr

ICD-9-CM		ICD-10-CM	
E894	IGNITION OF HIGHLY INFLAMMABLE MATERIAL	**X04.XXXA**	Exposure to ignition of highly flammable material, init
		X04.XXXD	Exposure to ignition of highly flammable material, subs
E895	ACCIDENT CAUSED CONTROLLED FIRE PRIVATE DWELLING	**X02.8XXA**	Oth exposure to controlled fire in bldg, init
E896	ACC CAUSED CNTRL FIRE OTH&UNSPEC BLDG/STRUCTURE	**X02.8XXA**	Oth exposure to controlled fire in bldg, init
E897	ACCIDENT CAUSED CNTRL FIRE NOT BLDG/STRUCTURE	**X03.0XXA**	Exposure to flames in controlled fire, not in bldg, init
		X03.0XXD	Exposure to flames in controlled fire, not in bldg, subs
		X03.1XXA	Exposure to smoke in controlled fire, not in bldg, init
		X03.1XXD	Exposure to smoke in controlled fire, not in bldg, subs
		X03.3XXA	Fall due to controlled fire, not in bldg, init
		X03.3XXD	Fall due to controlled fire, not in bldg, subs
		X03.4XXA	Hit by object due to controlled fire, not in bldg, init
		X03.4XXD	Hit by object due to controlled fire, not in bldg, subs
		X03.8XXA	Oth exposure to controlled fire, not in bldg, init
		X03.8XXD	Oth exposure to controlled fire, not in bldg, subs
E898.0	ACCIDENT CAUSED BY BURNING BEDCLOTHES	**X08.09XA**	Exposure to bed fire due to oth burning material, init
		X08.09XD	Exposure to bed fire due to oth burning material, subs
E898.1	ACCIDENT CAUSED BY OTHER BURNING MATERIALS	**X08.00XA**	Exposure to bed fire due to unsp burning material, init
		X08.00XD	Exposure to bed fire due to unsp burning material, subs
		X08.01XA	Exposure to bed fire due to burning cigarette, init encntr
		X08.01XD	Exposure to bed fire due to burning cigarette, subs encntr
		X08.10XA	Exposure to sofa fire due to unsp burning material, init
		X08.10XD	Exposure to sofa fire due to unsp burning material, subs
		X08.11XA	Exposure to sofa fire due to burning cigarette, init encntr
		X08.11XD	Exposure to sofa fire due to burning cigarette, subs encntr
		X08.19XA	Exposure to sofa fire due to oth burning material, init
		X08.19XD	Exposure to sofa fire due to oth burning material, subs
		X08.20XA	Expsr to oth furniture fire due to unsp burn material, init
		X08.20XD	Expsr to oth furniture fire due to unsp burn material, subs
		X08.21XA	Expsr to oth furniture fire due to burning cigarette, init
		X08.21XD	Expsr to oth furniture fire due to burning cigarette, subs
		X08.29XA	Expsr to oth furniture fire due to oth burn material, init
		X08.29XD	Expsr to oth furniture fire due to oth burn material, subs
		X08.8XXA	Exposure to oth smoke, fire and flames, init encntr
		X08.8XXD	Exposure to oth smoke, fire and flames, subs encntr
E899	ACCIDENT CAUSED BY UNSPECIFIED FIRE	**X08.8XXA**	Exposure to oth smoke, fire and flames, init encntr
E900.0	ACCIDENT DUE EXCESSIVE HEAT WEATHER CONDITIONS	**X30.XXXA**	Exposure to excessive natural heat, initial encounter
		X30.XXXD	Exposure to excessive natural heat, subsequent encounter
		X32.XXXA	Exposure to sunlight, initial encounter
		X32.XXXD	Exposure to sunlight, subsequent encounter
E900.1	ACCIDENT DUE TO EXCESSIVE HEAT MAN-MADE ORIGIN	**W92.XXXA**	Exposure to excessive heat of man-made origin, init encntr
		W92.XXXD	Exposure to excessive heat of man-made origin, subs encntr
E900.9	ACCIDENT DUE EXCESSIVE HEAT UNSPECIFIED ORIGIN	**X30.XXXA**	Exposure to excessive natural heat, initial encounter
E901.0	ACCIDENT DUE EXCESSIVE COLD WEATHER CONDITIONS	**X31.XXXA**	Exposure to excessive natural cold, initial encounter
		X31.XXXD	Exposure to excessive natural cold, subsequent encounter
E901.1	ACCIDENT DUE TO EXCESSIVE COLD MAN-MADE ORIGIN	**W93.01XA**	Contact with dry ice, initial encounter
		W93.01XD	Contact with dry ice, subsequent encounter
		W93.02XA	Inhalation of dry ice, initial encounter
		W93.02XD	Inhalation of dry ice, subsequent encounter
		W93.11XA	Contact with liquid air, initial encounter
		W93.11XD	Contact with liquid air, subsequent encounter
		W93.12XA	Inhalation of liquid air, initial encounter
		W93.12XD	Inhalation of liquid air, subsequent encounter
		W93.2XXA	Prolonged exposure in deep freeze unit or refrigerator, init
		W93.2XXD	Prolonged exposure in deep freeze unit or refrigerator, subs
E901.8	ACCIDENT DUE EXCESSIVE COLD OTHER SPEC ORIGIN	**W93.8XXA**	Exposure to oth excessive cold of man-made origin, init
		W93.8XXD	Exposure to oth excessive cold of man-made origin, subs
E901.9	ACCIDENT DUE EXCESSIVE COLD UNSPECIFIED ORIGIN	**X31.XXXA**	Exposure to excessive natural cold, initial encounter
E902.0	ACC DUE RESIDENCE/PROLONG VISIT@HIGH ALTITUDE	**W94.0XXA**	Exposure to prolonged high air pressure, initial encounter
		W94.0XXD	Exposure to prolonged high air pressure, subs encntr
		W94.11XA	Expsr to resdnce or prolonged visit at high altitude, init
		W94.11XD	Expsr to resdnce or prolonged visit at high altitude, subs
E902.1	ACCIDENT DUE TO CHANGES AIRPRESSURE AIRCRAFT	**W94.23XA**	Expsr to chng in air pressure in arcrft during ascent, init
		W94.23XD	Expsr to chng in air pressure in arcrft during ascent, subs
		W94.29XA	Expsr to oth rapid changes in air pressr during ascent, init
		W94.29XD	Expsr to oth rapid changes in air pressr during ascent, subs
		W94.31XA	Expsr to chng in air pressr in arcrft dur desc, init
		W94.31XD	Expsr to chng in air pressr in arcrft dur desc, subs
E902.2	ACCIDENT DUE CHANGES AIR PRESSURE DUE DIVING	**W94.21XA**	Expsr to rdct in atmos pressr wh surfc fr dp-watr div, init
		W94.21XD	Expsr to rdct in atmos pressr wh surfc fr dp-watr div, subs
		W94.32XA	Expsr to high air pressure from rapid descent in water, init
		W94.32XD	Expsr to high air pressure from rapid descent in water, subs
		W94.39XA	Expsr to oth rapid changes in air pressr dur descent, init
		W94.39XD	Expsr to oth rapid changes in air pressr dur descent, subs
E902.8	ACCIDENT DUE CHGS AIR PRESS DUE OTH SPEC CAUSE	**W94.12XA**	Exposure to other prolonged low air pressure, init encntr
		W94.12XD	Exposure to other prolonged low air pressure, subs encntr
		W94.22XA	Expsr to rdct in atmos pressr wh surfc fr underground, init
		W94.22XD	Expsr to rdct in atmos pressr wh surfc fr underground, subs
		W99.XXXA	Exposure to oth man-made environmental factors, init encntr
		W99.XXXD	Exposure to oth man-made environmental factors, subs encntr

ICD-9-CM		ICD-10-CM	
E902.9	ACCIDENT DUE CHGS AIR PRESSURE FROM UNSPEC CAUSE	**W99.XXXA**	Exposure to oth man-made environmental factors, init encntr
E903	ACCIDENT DUE TO TRAVEL AND MOTION	**T75.3XXA**	Motion sickness, initial encounter
E904.0	ACC DUE ABANDONMENT/NEGLECT INFNT&HELPLESS PERS	**T74.01XA**	Adult neglect or abandonment, confirmed, initial encounter
		T74.02XA	Child neglect or abandonment, confirmed, initial encounter
E904.1	ACCIDENT DUE TO LACK OF FOOD	**T73.0XXA**	Starvation, initial encounter
E904.2	ACCIDENT DUE TO LACK OF WATER	**T73.1XXA**	Deprivation of water, initial encounter
E904.3	ACCIDENT DUE EXPOSURE NOT ELSEWHERE CLASSIFIABLE	**T73.2XXA**	Exhaustion due to exposure, initial encounter
E904.9	ACCIDENT DUE TO UNQUALIFIED PRIVATION	**T73.8XXA**	Other effects of deprivation, initial encounter
		T73.9XXA	Effect of deprivation, unspecified, initial encounter
E905.0	VENOMOUS SNAKES&LIZARDS AS CAUSE POISN&TOX REACT	**T63.001A**	Toxic effect of unsp snake venom, accidental, init
		T63.011A	Toxic effect of rattlesnake venom, accidental, init
		T63.021A	Toxic effect of coral snake venom, accidental, init
		T63.031A	Toxic effect of taipan venom, accidental, init
		T63.041A	Toxic effect of cobra venom, accidental, init
		T63.061A	Toxic effect of venom of N & S American snake, acc, init
		T63.071A	Toxic effect of venom of Australian snake, accidental, init
		T63.081A	Toxic effect of venom of African and Asian snake, acc, init
		T63.091A	Toxic effect of venom of snake, accidental, init
		T63.111A	Toxic effect of venom of gila monster, accidental, init
		T63.121A	Toxic effect of venom of venomous lizard, accidental, init
		T63.191A	Toxic effect of venom of reptiles, accidental, init
E905.1	VENOMOUS SPIDERS AS CAUSE POISN&TOXIC REACTIONS	**T63.301A**	Toxic effect of unsp spider venom, accidental, init
		T63.311A	Toxic effect of venom of black widow spider, acc, init
		T63.321A	Toxic effect of venom of tarantula, accidental, init
		T63.331A	Toxic effect of venom of brown recluse spider, acc, init
		T63.391A	Toxic effect of venom of spider, accidental, init
E905.2	SCORPION STING AS CAUSE POISN&TOXIC REACTIONS	**T63.2X1A**	Toxic effect of venom of scorpion, accidental, init
E905.3	STING HORNETS WASPS&BEES CAUSE POISN&TOX REACT	**T63.441A**	Toxic effect of venom of bees, accidental, init
		T63.451A	Toxic effect of venom of hornets, accidental, init
		T63.461A	Toxic effect of venom of wasps, accidental, init
E905.4	POISION-TOXIC REACT D/T CENTIPEDE-VENOM MILLPEDE	**T63.411A**	Toxic effect of venom of centipede/millipede, acc, init
E905.5	OTH VENOMOUS ARTHROPODS AS CAUSE POISN&TOX REACT	**T63.421A**	Toxic effect of venom of ants, accidental, init
		T63.431A	Toxic effect of venom of caterpillars, accidental, init
		T63.481A	Toxic effect of venom of arthropod, accidental, init
E905.6	VNOM MARINE ANIMALS&PLANTS CAUSE POISN&TOX REACT	**T63.511A**	Toxic effect of contact w stingray, accidental, init
		T63.591A	Toxic effect of contact w oth venomous fish, acc, init
		T63.611A	Toxic effect of contact w Portugese Man-o-war, acc, init
		T63.621A	Toxic effect of contact w oth jellyfish, accidental, init
		T63.631A	Toxic effect of contact w sea anemone, accidental, init
		T63.691A	Toxic effect of cntct w oth venom marine animals, acc, init
		T63.711A	Toxic effect of contact w venomous marine plant, acc, init
		T63.791A	Toxic effect of contact w oth venomous plant, acc, init
		T63.811A	Toxic effect of contact w venomous frog, accidental, init
		T63.821A	Toxic effect of contact w venomous toad, accidental, init
		T63.831A	Toxic effect of contact w oth venomous amphibian, acc, init
		T63.891A	Toxic effect of contact w oth venomous animals, acc, init
		T63.91XA	Toxic effect of contact w unsp venomous animal, acc, init
E905.7	POISONING&TOXIC REACTIONS CAUSED OTHER PLANTS		NO DIAGNOSIS
E905.8	POISN&TOXIC REACT CAUSED OTH SPEC ANIMALS&PLANTS		NO DIAGNOSIS
E905.9	POISN&TOXIC REACTS CAUSED UNSPEC ANIMALS&PLANTS		NO DIAGNOSIS
E906.0	DOG BITE	**W54.0XXA**	Bitten by dog, initial encounter
		W54.0XXD	Bitten by dog, subsequent encounter
E906.1	RAT BITE	**W53.01XA**	Bitten by mouse, initial encounter
		W53.01XD	Bitten by mouse, subsequent encounter
		W53.09XA	Other contact with mouse, initial encounter
		W53.09XD	Other contact with mouse, subsequent encounter
		W53.11XA	Bitten by rat, initial encounter
		W53.11XD	Bitten by rat, subsequent encounter
		W53.19XA	Other contact with rat, initial encounter
		W53.19XD	Other contact with rat, subsequent encounter
E906.2	BITE OF NONVENOMOUS SNAKES AND LIZARDS	**W59.01XA**	Bitten by nonvenomous lizards, initial encounter
		W59.01XD	Bitten by nonvenomous lizards, subsequent encounter
		W59.11XA	Bitten by nonvenomous snake, initial encounter
		W59.11XD	Bitten by nonvenomous snake, subsequent encounter
		W59.81XA	Bitten by other nonvenomous reptiles, initial encounter
		W59.81XD	Bitten by other nonvenomous reptiles, subsequent encounter
E906.3	BITE OF OTHER ANIMAL EXCEPT ARTHROPOD	**W53.21XA**	Bitten by squirrel, initial encounter
		W53.21XD	Bitten by squirrel, subsequent encounter
		W53.81XA	Bitten by other rodent, initial encounter
		W53.81XD	Bitten by other rodent, subsequent encounter
		W55.01XA	Bitten by cat, initial encounter
		W55.01XD	Bitten by cat, subsequent encounter
		W55.11XA	Bitten by horse, initial encounter
		W55.11XD	Bitten by horse, subsequent encounter
		W55.21XA	Bitten by cow, initial encounter
		W55.21XD	Bitten by cow, subsequent encounter

(Continued on next page)

ICD-9-CM		ICD-10-CM	
E906.3	BITE OF OTHER ANIMAL EXCEPT ARTHROPOD **(Continued)**	**W55.31XA**	Bitten by other hoof stock, initial encounter
		W55.31XD	Bitten by other hoof stock, subsequent encounter
		W55.41XA	Bitten by pig, initial encounter
		W55.41XD	Bitten by pig, subsequent encounter
		W55.51XA	Bitten by raccoon, initial encounter
		W55.51XD	Bitten by raccoon, subsequent encounter
		W55.81XA	Bitten by other mammals, initial encounter
		W55.81XD	Bitten by other mammals, subsequent encounter
		W56.01XA	Bitten by dolphin, initial encounter
		W56.01XD	Bitten by dolphin, subsequent encounter
		W56.11XA	Bitten by sea lion, initial encounter
		W56.11XD	Bitten by sea lion, subsequent encounter
		W56.21XA	Bitten by orca, initial encounter
		W56.21XD	Bitten by orca, subsequent encounter
		W56.31XA	Bitten by other marine mammals, initial encounter
		W56.31XD	Bitten by other marine mammals, subsequent encounter
		W56.41XA	Bitten by shark, initial encounter
		W56.41XD	Bitten by shark, subsequent encounter
		W56.51XA	Bitten by other fish, initial encounter
		W56.51XD	Bitten by other fish, subsequent encounter
		W56.81XA	Bitten by other nonvenomous marine animals, init encntr
		W56.81XD	Bitten by other nonvenomous marine animals, subs encntr
		W58.01XA	Bitten by alligator, initial encounter
		W58.01XD	Bitten by alligator, subsequent encounter
		W58.09XA	Other contact with alligator, initial encounter
		W58.09XD	Other contact with alligator, subsequent encounter
		W58.11XA	Bitten by crocodile, initial encounter
		W58.11XD	Bitten by crocodile, subsequent encounter
		W58.19XA	Other contact with crocodile, initial encounter
		W58.19XD	Other contact with crocodile, subsequent encounter
		W59.21XA	Bitten by turtle, initial encounter
		W59.21XD	Bitten by turtle, subsequent encounter
		W61.01XA	Bitten by parrot, initial encounter
		W61.01XD	Bitten by parrot, subsequent encounter
		W61.11XA	Bitten by macaw, initial encounter
		W61.11XD	Bitten by macaw, subsequent encounter
		W61.21XA	Bitten by other psittacines, initial encounter
		W61.21XD	Bitten by other psittacines, subsequent encounter
		W61.51XA	Bitten by goose, initial encounter
		W61.51XD	Bitten by goose, subsequent encounter
		W61.61XA	Bitten by duck, initial encounter
		W61.61XD	Bitten by duck, subsequent encounter
		W61.91XA	Bitten by other birds, initial encounter
		W61.91XD	Bitten by other birds, subsequent encounter
E906.4	BITE OF NONVENOMOUS ARTHROPOD	**W57.XXXA**	Bit/stung by nonvenom insect & oth nonvenom arthropods, init
		W57.XXXD	Bit/stung by nonvenom insect & oth nonvenom arthropods, subs
E906.5	BITE BY UNSPECIFIED ANIMAL	**W55.81XA**	Bitten by other mammals, initial encounter
E906.8	OTHER SPECIFIED INJURY CAUSED BY ANIMAL	**W53.29XA**	Other contact with squirrel, initial encounter
		W53.29XD	Other contact with squirrel, subsequent encounter
		W53.89XA	Other contact with other rodent, initial encounter
		W53.89XD	Other contact with other rodent, subsequent encounter
		W54.1XXA	Struck by dog, initial encounter
		W54.1XXD	Struck by dog, subsequent encounter
		W54.8XXA	Other contact with dog, initial encounter
		W54.8XXD	Other contact with dog, subsequent encounter
		W55.03XA	Scratched by cat, initial encounter
		W55.03XD	Scratched by cat, subsequent encounter
		W55.09XA	Other contact with cat, initial encounter
		W55.09XD	Other contact with cat, subsequent encounter
		W55.12XA	Struck by horse, initial encounter
		W55.12XD	Struck by horse, subsequent encounter
		W55.19XA	Other contact with horse, initial encounter
		W55.19XD	Other contact with horse, subsequent encounter
		W55.22XA	Struck by cow, initial encounter
		W55.22XD	Struck by cow, subsequent encounter
		W55.29XA	Other contact with cow, initial encounter
		W55.29XD	Other contact with cow, subsequent encounter
		W55.32XA	Struck by other hoof stock, initial encounter
		W55.32XD	Struck by other hoof stock, subsequent encounter
		W55.39XA	Other contact with other hoof stock, initial encounter
		W55.39XD	Other contact with other hoof stock, subsequent encounter
		W55.42XA	Struck by pig, initial encounter
		W55.42XD	Struck by pig, subsequent encounter
		W55.49XA	Other contact with pig, initial encounter
		W55.49XD	Other contact with pig, subsequent encounter
		W55.52XA	Struck by raccoon, initial encounter
		W55.52XD	Struck by raccoon, subsequent encounter
		W55.59XA	Other contact with raccoon, initial encounter
		W55.59XD	Other contact with raccoon, subsequent encounter
		W55.82XA	Struck by other mammals, initial encounter
		W55.82XD	Struck by other mammals, subsequent encounter
	(Continued on next page)	**W55.89XA**	Other contact with other mammals, initial encounter

ICD-9-CM		ICD-10-CM	
E9Ø6.8	OTHER SPECIFIED INJURY CAUSED BY ANIMAL **(Continued)**	**W55.89XD**	Other contact with other mammals, subsequent encounter
		W56.Ø2XA	Struck by dolphin, initial encounter
		W56.Ø2XD	Struck by dolphin, subsequent encounter
		W56.Ø9XA	Other contact with dolphin, initial encounter
		W56.Ø9XD	Other contact with dolphin, subsequent encounter
		W56.12XA	Struck by sea lion, initial encounter
		W56.12XD	Struck by sea lion, subsequent encounter
		W56.19XA	Other contact with sea lion, initial encounter
		W56.19XD	Other contact with sea lion, subsequent encounter
		W56.22XA	Struck by orca, initial encounter
		W56.22XD	Struck by orca, subsequent encounter
		W56.29XA	Other contact with orca, initial encounter
		W56.29XD	Other contact with orca, subsequent encounter
		W56.32XA	Struck by other marine mammals, initial encounter
		W56.32XD	Struck by other marine mammals, subsequent encounter
		W56.39XA	Other contact with other marine mammals, initial encounter
		W56.39XD	Other contact with other marine mammals, subs encntr
		W56.42XA	Struck by shark, initial encounter
		W56.42XD	Struck by shark, subsequent encounter
		W56.49XA	Other contact with shark, initial encounter
		W56.49XD	Other contact with shark, subsequent encounter
		W56.52XA	Struck by other fish, initial encounter
		W56.52XD	Struck by other fish, subsequent encounter
		W56.59XA	Other contact with other fish, initial encounter
		W56.59XD	Other contact with other fish, subsequent encounter
		W56.82XA	Struck by other nonvenomous marine animals, init encntr
		W56.82XD	Struck by other nonvenomous marine animals, subs encntr
		W56.89XA	Oth contact with oth nonvenomous marine animals, init encntr
		W56.89XD	Oth contact with oth nonvenomous marine animals, subs encntr
		W58.Ø2XA	Struck by alligator, initial encounter
		W58.Ø2XD	Struck by alligator, subsequent encounter
		W58.Ø3XA	Crushed by alligator, initial encounter
		W58.Ø3XD	Crushed by alligator, subsequent encounter
		W58.12XA	Struck by crocodile, initial encounter
		W58.12XD	Struck by crocodile, subsequent encounter
		W58.13XA	Crushed by crocodile, initial encounter
		W58.13XD	Crushed by crocodile, subsequent encounter
		W59.Ø2XA	Struck by nonvenomous lizards, initial encounter
		W59.Ø2XD	Struck by nonvenomous lizards, subsequent encounter
		W59.Ø9XA	Other contact with nonvenomous lizards, initial encounter
		W59.Ø9XD	Other contact with nonvenomous lizards, subsequent encounter
		W59.12XA	Struck by nonvenomous snake, initial encounter
		W59.12XD	Struck by nonvenomous snake, subsequent encounter
		W59.13XA	Crushed by nonvenomous snake, initial encounter
		W59.13XD	Crushed by nonvenomous snake, subsequent encounter
		W59.19XA	Other contact with nonvenomous snake, initial encounter
		W59.19XD	Other contact with nonvenomous snake, subsequent encounter
		W59.22XA	Struck by turtle, initial encounter
		W59.22XD	Struck by turtle, subsequent encounter
		W59.29XA	Other contact with turtle, initial encounter
		W59.29XD	Other contact with turtle, subsequent encounter
		W59.82XA	Struck by other nonvenomous reptiles, initial encounter
		W59.82XD	Struck by other nonvenomous reptiles, subsequent encounter
		W59.83XA	Crushed by other nonvenomous reptiles, initial encounter
		W59.83XD	Crushed by other nonvenomous reptiles, subsequent encounter
		W59.89XA	Other contact with other nonvenomous reptiles, init encntr
		W59.89XD	Other contact with other nonvenomous reptiles, subs encntr
		W61.Ø2XA	Struck by parrot, initial encounter
		W61.Ø2XD	Struck by parrot, subsequent encounter
		W61.Ø9XA	Other contact with parrot, initial encounter
		W61.Ø9XD	Other contact with parrot, subsequent encounter
		W61.12XA	Struck by macaw, initial encounter
		W61.12XD	Struck by macaw, subsequent encounter
		W61.19XA	Other contact with macaw, initial encounter
		W61.19XD	Other contact with macaw, subsequent encounter
		W61.22XA	Struck by other psittacines, initial encounter
		W61.22XD	Struck by other psittacines, subsequent encounter
		W61.29XA	Other contact with other psittacines, initial encounter
		W61.29XD	Other contact with other psittacines, subsequent encounter
		W61.32XA	Struck by chicken, initial encounter
		W61.32XD	Struck by chicken, subsequent encounter
		W61.33XA	Pecked by chicken, initial encounter
		W61.33XD	Pecked by chicken, subsequent encounter
		W61.39XA	Other contact with chicken, initial encounter
		W61.39XD	Other contact with chicken, subsequent encounter
		W61.42XA	Struck by turkey, initial encounter
		W61.42XD	Struck by turkey, subsequent encounter
		W61.43XA	Pecked by turkey, initial encounter
		W61.43XD	Pecked by turkey, subsequent encounter
		W61.49XA	Other contact with turkey, initial encounter
		W61.49XD	Other contact with turkey, subsequent encounter
E9Ø6.8	**(Continued on next page)**	**W61.52XA**	Struck by goose, initial encounter

 [Brackets] indicate valid character values for each code. Character value meanings provided for each code grouping.

ICD-9-CM		ICD-10-CM	
E9Ø6.8	OTHER SPECIFIED INJURY CAUSED BY ANIMAL **(Continued)**	**W61.52XD**	Struck by goose, subsequent encounter
		W61.59XA	Other contact with goose, initial encounter
		W61.59XD	Other contact with goose, subsequent encounter
		W61.62XA	Struck by duck, initial encounter
		W61.62XD	Struck by duck, subsequent encounter
		W61.69XA	Other contact with duck, initial encounter
		W61.69XD	Other contact with duck, subsequent encounter
		W61.92XA	Struck by other birds, initial encounter
		W61.92XD	Struck by other birds, subsequent encounter
		W61.99XA	Other contact with other birds, initial encounter
		W61.99XD	Other contact with other birds, subsequent encounter
		W62.ØXXA	Contact with nonvenomous frogs, initial encounter
		W62.ØXXD	Contact with nonvenomous frogs, subsequent encounter
		W62.1XXA	Contact with nonvenomous toads, initial encounter
		W62.1XXD	Contact with nonvenomous toads, subsequent encounter
		W62.9XXA	Contact with other nonvenomous amphibians, initial encounter
		W62.9XXD	Contact with other nonvenomous amphibians, subs encntr
E9Ø6.9	UNSPECIFIED INJURY CAUSED BY ANIMAL	**W64.XXXA**	Exposure to other animate mechanical forces, init encntr
		W64.XXXD	Exposure to other animate mechanical forces, subs encntr
E9Ø7	ACCIDENT DUE TO LIGHTNING	**X39.8XXA**	Other exposure to forces of nature, initial encounter
E9Ø8.Ø	ACCIDENT DUE TO HURRICANE	**X37.ØXXA**	Hurricane, initial encounter
		X37.ØXXD	Hurricane, subsequent encounter
		X37.42XA	Tidal wave due to storm, initial encounter
		X37.42XD	Tidal wave due to storm, subsequent encounter
E9Ø8.1	ACCIDENT DUE TO TORNADO	**X37.1XXA**	Tornado, initial encounter
		X37.1XXD	Tornado, subsequent encounter
E9Ø8.2	ACCIDENT DUE TO FLOODS	**X38.XXXA**	Flood, initial encounter
		X38.XXXD	Flood, subsequent encounter
E9Ø8.3	ACCIDENT DUE TO BLIZZARD	**X37.2XXA**	Blizzard (snow)(ice), initial encounter
		X37.2XXD	Blizzard (snow)(ice), subsequent encounter
E9Ø8.4	ACCIDENT DUE TO DUST STORM	**X37.3XXA**	Dust storm, initial encounter
		X37.3XXD	Dust storm, subsequent encounter
E9Ø8.8	ACCIDENT DUE TO OTHER CATACLYSMIC STORMS	**X37.8XXA**	Other cataclysmic storms, initial encounter
		X37.8XXD	Other cataclysmic storms, subsequent encounter
E9Ø8.9	ACC DUE UNS CATACLYS STORMS&FLOODS RSLT STORMS	**X37.9XXA**	Unspecified cataclysmic storm, initial encounter
		X37.9XXD	Unspecified cataclysmic storm, subsequent encounter
E9Ø9.Ø	EARTHQUAKES	**X34.XXXA**	Earthquake, initial encounter
		X34.XXXD	Earthquake, subsequent encounter
E9Ø9.1	VOLCANIC ERUPTIONS	**X35.XXXA**	Volcanic eruption, initial encounter
		X35.XXXD	Volcanic eruption, subsequent encounter
E9Ø9.2	AVALANCHE, LANDSLIDE, OR MUDSLIDE	**X36.1XXA**	Avalanche, landslide, or mudslide, initial encounter
		X36.1XXD	Avalanche, landslide, or mudslide, subsequent encounter
E9Ø9.3	COLLAPSE OF DAM OR MAN-MADE STRUCTURE	**X36.ØXXA**	Collapse of dam or man-made struct cause earth movmnt, init
		X36.ØXXD	Collapse of dam or man-made struct cause earth movmnt, subs
E9Ø9.4	TIDALWAVE CAUSED BY EARTHQUAKE	**X37.41XA**	Tidal wave due to earthquake or volcanic eruption, init
		X37.41XD	Tidal wave due to earthquake or volcanic eruption, subs
E9Ø9.8	OTH CATACLYS EARTH SURFACE MOVEMENTS&ERUPTIONS	**X37.43XA**	Tidal wave due to landslide, initial encounter
		X37.43XD	Tidal wave due to landslide, subsequent encounter
		X39.8XXA	Other exposure to forces of nature, initial encounter
E9Ø9.9	UNSPEC CATACLYS ERTH SURFACE MOVEMENTS&ERUPTIONS	**X39.8XXA**	Other exposure to forces of nature, initial encounter
E91Ø.Ø	ACCIDENTAL DROWNING AND SUBMERSION WATER-SKIING	**W69.XXXA**	Accidental drown while in natural water, init
E91Ø.1	ACCID DROWN-SUBMERS W DIVING EQUIP-SPORT/RECREAT	**W69.XXXA**	Accidental drown while in natural water, init
E91Ø.2	ACCID DROWN-SUBMERS-NO DIVE EQUIP-SPORT/RECREAT	**W69.XXXA**	Accidental drown while in natural water, init
		W69.XXXD	Accidental drown while in natural water, subs
E91Ø.3	ACCID DROWN-SUBMERS-SWIM/DIVE-NON RECREAT/SPORT	**W69.XXXA**	Accidental drown while in natural water, init
E91Ø.4	ACCIDENTAL DROWNING AND SUBMERSION IN BATHTUB	**W65.XXXA**	Accidental drowning and submersion while in bath-tub, init
		W65.XXXD	Accidental drowning and submersion while in bath-tub, subs
		Y21.ØXXA	Drown while in bathtub, undetermined intent, init
		Y21.ØXXD	Drown while in bathtub, undetermined intent, subs
		Y21.1XXA	Drown after fall into bathtub, undetermined intent, init
		Y21.1XXD	Drown after fall into bathtub, undetermined intent, subs
E91Ø.8	OTHER ACCIDENTAL DROWNING OR SUBMERSION	**W67.XXXA**	Accidental drown while in swimming-pool, init
		W67.XXXD	Accidental drown while in swimming-pool, subs
		W73.XXXA	Oth cause of accidental non-transport drown, init
		W73.XXXD	Oth cause of accidental non-transport drown, subs
		Y21.2XXA	Drown while in swimming pool, undetermined intent, init
		Y21.2XXD	Drown while in swimming pool, undetermined intent, subs
		Y21.3XXA	Drown after fall into swimming pool, undet intent, init
		Y21.3XXD	Drown after fall into swimming pool, undet intent, subs
		Y21.4XXA	Drown in natural water, undetermined intent, init
		Y21.4XXD	Drown in natural water, undetermined intent, subs
		Y21.8XXA	Oth drowning and submersion, undetermined intent, init
		Y21.8XXD	Oth drowning and submersion, undetermined intent, subs
E91Ø.9	UNSPECIFIED ACCIDENTAL DROWNING OR SUBMERSION	**W74.XXXA**	Unsp cause of accidental drowning and submersion, init
		W74.XXXD	Unsp cause of accidental drowning and submersion, subs

ICD-9-CM		ICD-10-CM	
E911	INHAL&INGESTION FOOD CAUS OBST RESP TRACT/SUFFOC	**T17.21ØA**	Gastric contents in pharynx causing asphyxiation, init
		T17.218A	Gastric contents in pharynx causing oth injury, init encntr
		T17.22ØA	Food in pharynx causing asphyxiation, initial encounter
		T17.228A	Food in pharynx causing other injury, initial encounter
		T17.31ØA	Gastric contents in larynx causing asphyxiation, init encntr
		T17.318A	Gastric contents in larynx causing other injury, init encntr
		T17.32ØA	Food in larynx causing asphyxiation, initial encounter
		T17.328A	Food in larynx causing other injury, initial encounter
		T17.41ØA	Gastric contents in trachea causing asphyxiation, init
		T17.418A	Gastric contents in trachea causing oth injury, init encntr
		T17.42ØA	Food in trachea causing asphyxiation, initial encounter
		T17.428A	Food in trachea causing other injury, initial encounter
		T17.51ØA	Gastric contents in bronchus causing asphyxiation, init
		T17.518A	Gastric contents in bronchus causing oth injury, init encntr
		T17.52ØA	Food in bronchus causing asphyxiation, initial encounter
		T17.528A	Food in bronchus causing other injury, initial encounter
		T17.81ØA	Gastric contents in oth prt resp tract causing asphyx, init
		T17.818A	Gastr contents in oth prt resp tract cause oth injury, init
		T17.82ØA	Food in oth prt respiratory tract causing asphyxiation, init
		T17.828A	Food in oth prt respiratory tract causing oth injury, init
		T17.91ØA	Gastric contents in resp tract, part unsp cause asphyx, init
		T17.918A	Gastr contents in resp tract, part unsp cause oth inj, init
		T17.92ØA	Food in resp tract, part unsp causing asphyxiation, init
		T17.928A	Food in resp tract, part unsp causing oth injury, init
		T18.11ØA	Gastric contents in esoph causing comprsn of trachea, init
		T18.12ØA	Food in esophagus causing compression of trachea, init
E912	OBST/SUFFOCAT D/T INHALING-INGESTING OTH OBJECT	**T17.2ØØA**	Unsp foreign body in pharynx causing asphyxiation, init
		T17.29ØA	Oth foreign object in pharynx causing asphyxiation, init
		T17.3ØØA	Unsp foreign body in larynx causing asphyxiation, init
		T17.39ØA	Oth foreign object in larynx causing asphyxiation, init
		T17.4ØØA	Unsp foreign body in trachea causing asphyxiation, init
		T17.49ØA	Oth foreign object in trachea causing asphyxiation, init
		T17.5ØØA	Unsp foreign body in bronchus causing asphyxiation, init
		T17.59ØA	Oth foreign object in bronchus causing asphyxiation, init
		T17.8ØØA	Unsp foreign body in oth prt resp tract causing asphyx, init
		T17.89ØA	Oth foreign object in oth prt resp tract cause asphyx, init
		T17.898A	Oth forn object in oth prt resp tract cause oth injury, init
		T17.9ØØA	Unsp fb in resp tract, part unsp causing asphyx, init
		T17.99ØA	Oth forn obj in resp tract, part unsp in cause asphyx, init
		T18.1ØØA	Unsp fb in esophagus causing compression of trachea, init
		T18.19ØA	Oth foreign object in esoph causing comprsn of trachea, init
E913.Ø	ACCIDENTAL MECHANICAL SUFFOCATION BED OR CRADLE	**T71.111A**	Asphyx due to smothering under pillow, accidental, init
		T71.131A	Asphyx due to being trapped in bed linens, accidental, init
		T71.141A	Asphyx due to smothr under another person's body, acc, init
E913.1	ACCIDENTAL MECHANICAL SUFFOCATION BY PLASTIC BAG	**T71.121A**	Asphyxiation due to plastic bag, accidental, init encntr
E913.2	ACCIDENTAL MECHANICAL SUFFOCATION DUE LACK AIR	**T71.2ØXA**	Asphyx d/t sys oxy defic d/t low oxy in air unsp cause, init
		T71.221A	Asphyx due to being trapped in a car trunk, accidental, init
		T71.231A	Asphyx due to being trap in a (discarded) refrig, acc, init
		T71.29XA	Asphyx due to being trap in oth low oxygen environment, init
E913.3	ACC MECH SUFFOCAT FALLING ERTH/OTH SUBSTANCE	**T71.21XA**	Asphyxiation due to cave-in or falling earth, init encntr
E913.8	ACCIDENTAL MECH SUFFOCATION OTHER SPEC MEANS	**T71.151A**	Asphyx due to smothering in furniture, accidental, init
		T71.161A	Asphyxiation due to hanging, accidental, initial encounter
		T71.191A	Asphyx d/t mech threat to breathe d/t oth cause, acc, init
E913.9	ACCIDENTAL MECHANICAL SUFFOCATION UNSPEC MEANS	**T71.9XXA**	Asphyxiation due to unspecified cause, initial encounter
E914	FOREIGN BODY ACCIDENTALLY ENTERING EYE&ADNEXA	**T15.ØØXA**	Foreign body in cornea, unspecified eye, initial encounter
		T15.Ø1XA	Foreign body in cornea, right eye, initial encounter
		T15.Ø2XA	Foreign body in cornea, left eye, initial encounter
		T15.1ØXA	Foreign body in conjunctival sac, unsp eye, init encntr
		T15.11XA	Foreign body in conjunctival sac, right eye, init encntr
		T15.12XA	Foreign body in conjunctival sac, left eye, init encntr
		T15.8ØXA	Fb in oth and multiple parts of external eye, unsp eye, init
		T15.81XA	Fb in oth and multiple parts of external eye, r eye, init
		T15.82XA	Fb in oth and multiple parts of external eye, left eye, init
		T15.9ØXA	Foreign body on external eye, part unsp, unsp eye, init
		T15.91XA	Foreign body on external eye, part unsp, right eye, init
		T15.92XA	Foreign body on external eye, part unsp, left eye, init
E915	FOREIGN BODY ACCIDENTALLY ENTERING OTHER ORIFICE	**T16.1XXA**	Foreign body in right ear, initial encounter
		T16.2XXA	Foreign body in left ear, initial encounter
		T16.9XXA	Foreign body in ear, unspecified ear, initial encounter
		T17.ØXXA	Foreign body in nasal sinus, initial encounter
		T17.1XXA	Foreign body in nostril, initial encounter
		T17.2Ø8A	Unsp foreign body in pharynx causing oth injury, init encntr
		T17.298A	Oth foreign object in pharynx causing oth injury, init
		T17.3Ø8A	Unsp foreign body in larynx causing oth injury, init encntr
		T17.398A	Oth foreign object in larynx causing oth injury, init encntr
		T17.4Ø8A	Unsp foreign body in trachea causing oth injury, init encntr
	(Continued on next page)	**T17.498A**	Oth foreign object in trachea causing oth injury, init
		T17.5Ø8A	Unsp foreign body in bronchus causing oth injury, init

ICD-9-CM		ICD-10-CM	
E915	FOREIGN BODY ACCIDENTALLY ENTERING OTHER ORIFICE **(Continued)**	**T17.598A**	Oth foreign object in bronchus causing oth injury, init
		T17.8Ø8A	Unsp fb in oth prt resp tract causing oth injury, init
		T17.9Ø8A	Unsp fb in resp tract, part unsp causing oth injury, init
		T17.998A	Oth forn object in resp tract, part unsp cause oth inj, init
		T18.ØXXA	Foreign body in mouth, initial encounter
		T18.1Ø8A	Unsp foreign body in esophagus causing oth injury, init
		T18.118A	Gastric contents in esophagus causing oth injury, init
		T18.128A	Food in esophagus causing other injury, initial encounter
		T18.198A	Oth foreign object in esophagus causing oth injury, init
		T18.2XXA	Foreign body in stomach, initial encounter
		T18.3XXA	Foreign body in small intestine, initial encounter
		T18.4XXA	Foreign body in colon, initial encounter
		T18.5XXA	Foreign body in anus and rectum, initial encounter
		T18.8XXA	Foreign body in other parts of alimentary tract, init encntr
		T18.9XXA	Foreign body of alimentary tract, part unsp, init encntr
		T19.ØXXA	Foreign body in urethra, initial encounter
		T19.1XXA	Foreign body in bladder, initial encounter
		T19.2XXA	Foreign body in vulva and vagina, initial encounter
		T19.3XXA	Foreign body in uterus, initial encounter
		T19.4XXA	Foreign body in penis, initial encounter
		T19.8XXA	Foreign body in oth prt genitourinary tract, init encntr
		T19.9XXA	Foreign body in genitourinary tract, part unsp, init encntr
E916	STRUCK ACCIDENTALLY BY FALLING OBJECT	**W2Ø.ØXXA**	Struck by falling object in cave-in, initial encounter
		W2Ø.ØXXD	Struck by falling object in cave-in, subsequent encounter
		W2Ø.1XXA	Struck by object due to collapse of building, init encntr
		W2Ø.1XXD	Struck by object due to collapse of building, subs encntr
		W2Ø.8XXA	Oth cause of strike by thrown, projected or fall obj, init
		W2Ø.8XXD	Oth cause of strike by thrown, projected or fall obj, subs
E917.Ø	STRIKE AGNST/STRUCK ACC SPORTS W/O SUBSQT FALL	**W21.ØØXA**	Struck by hit or thrown ball, unspecified type, init encntr
		W21.ØØXD	Struck by hit or thrown ball, unspecified type, subs encntr
		W21.Ø1XA	Struck by football, initial encounter
		W21.Ø1XD	Struck by football, subsequent encounter
		W21.Ø2XA	Struck by soccer ball, initial encounter
		W21.Ø2XD	Struck by soccer ball, subsequent encounter
		W21.Ø3XA	Struck by baseball, initial encounter
		W21.Ø3XD	Struck by baseball, subsequent encounter
		W21.Ø4XA	Struck by golf ball, initial encounter
		W21.Ø4XD	Struck by golf ball, subsequent encounter
		W21.Ø5XA	Struck by basketball, initial encounter
		W21.Ø5XD	Struck by basketball, subsequent encounter
		W21.Ø6XA	Struck by volleyball, initial encounter
		W21.Ø6XD	Struck by volleyball, subsequent encounter
		W21.Ø7XA	Struck by softball, initial encounter
		W21.Ø7XD	Struck by softball, subsequent encounter
		W21.Ø9XA	Struck by other hit or thrown ball, initial encounter
		W21.Ø9XD	Struck by other hit or thrown ball, subsequent encounter
		W21.11XA	Struck by baseball bat, initial encounter
		W21.11XD	Struck by baseball bat, subsequent encounter
		W21.12XA	Struck by tennis racquet, initial encounter
		W21.12XD	Struck by tennis racquet, subsequent encounter
		W21.13XA	Struck by golf club, initial encounter
		W21.13XD	Struck by golf club, subsequent encounter
		W21.19XA	Struck by other bat, racquet or club, initial encounter
		W21.19XD	Struck by other bat, racquet or club, subsequent encounter
		W21.21ØA	Struck by ice hockey stick, initial encounter
		W21.21ØD	Struck by ice hockey stick, subsequent encounter
		W21.211A	Struck by field hockey stick, initial encounter
		W21.211D	Struck by field hockey stick, subsequent encounter
		W21.22ØA	Struck by ice hockey puck, initial encounter
		W21.22ØD	Struck by ice hockey puck, subsequent encounter
		W21.221A	Struck by field hockey puck, initial encounter
		W21.221D	Struck by field hockey puck, subsequent encounter
		W21.31XA	Struck by shoe cleats, initial encounter
		W21.31XD	Struck by shoe cleats, subsequent encounter
		W21.32XA	Struck by skate blades, initial encounter
		W21.32XD	Struck by skate blades, subsequent encounter
		W21.39XA	Struck by other sports foot wear, initial encounter
		W21.39XD	Struck by other sports foot wear, subsequent encounter
		W21.4XXA	Striking against diving board, initial encounter
		W21.4XXD	Striking against diving board, subsequent encounter
		W21.81XA	Striking against or struck by football helmet, init encntr
		W21.81XD	Striking against or struck by football helmet, subs encntr
		W21.89XA	Striking against or struck by oth sports equipment, init
		W21.89XD	Striking against or struck by oth sports equipment, subs
		W21.9XXA	Striking against or struck by unsp sports equipment, init
		W21.9XXD	Striking against or struck by unsp sports equipment, subs
E917.1	STRIKE AGNST/STRUCK ACC CROWD W/O SUBSQT FALL	**W52.XXXA**	Crushd/pushd/stepd on by crowd or human stampede, init
		W52.XXXD	Crushd/pushd/stepd on by crowd or human stampede, subs
E917.2	STRIKE AGNST/STRUCK ACC RUN WTR W/O SUBSQT FALL	**W2Ø.8XXA**	Oth cause of strike by thrown, projected or fall obj, init
E917.3	STRIKE AGNST/STRUCK ACC FURN W/O SUBSEQUENT FALL	**W22.Ø3XA**	Walked into furniture, initial encounter
		W22.Ø3XD	Walked into furniture, subsequent encounter

ICD-9-CM		ICD-10-CM	
E917.4	STRIKE AGNST/STRUCK ACC OTH STATNRY OBJ W/O FALL	**W22.01XA**	Walked into wall, initial encounter
		W22.01XD	Walked into wall, subsequent encounter
		W22.02XA	Walked into lamppost, initial encounter
		W22.02XD	Walked into lamppost, subsequent encounter
		W22.041A	Striking against wall of swimming pool causing drown, init
		W22.041D	Striking against wall of swimming pool causing drown, subs
		W22.042A	Strike wall of swimming pool causing oth injury, init
		W22.042D	Strike wall of swimming pool causing oth injury, subs
		W22.09XA	Striking against other stationary object, initial encounter
		W22.09XD	Striking against other stationary object, subs encntr
		W22.10XA	Striking against or struck by unsp automobile airbag, init
		W22.10XD	Striking against or struck by unsp automobile airbag, subs
		W22.11XA	Strike/struck by driver side automobile airbag, init
		W22.11XD	Strike/struck by driver side automobile airbag, subs
		W22.12XA	Strike/struck by front passenger side auto airbag, init
		W22.12XD	Strike/struck by front passenger side auto airbag, subs
		W22.19XA	Striking against or struck by oth automobile airbag, init
		W22.19XD	Striking against or struck by oth automobile airbag, subs
		W22.8XXA	Striking against or struck by other objects, init encntr
		W22.8XXD	Striking against or struck by other objects, subs encntr
E917.5	STRIKE AGNST/STRUCK ACC OTH OBJ SPORTS W/FALL	**W50.0XXA**	Accidental hit or strike by another person, init encntr
E917.6	STRIKE AGNST/STRUCK ACC CROWD FEAR/PANIC W/FALL	**W52.XXXA**	Crushd/pushd/stepd on by crowd or human stampede, init
E917.7	STRIKE AGAINST/STRUCK ACC FURN W/SUBSEQUENT FALL	**W18.09XA**	Striking against oth object w subsequent fall, init encntr
E917.8	STRIKE AGNST/STRUCK ACC OTH STATNRY OBJ W/FALL	**W18.09XA**	Striking against oth object w subsequent fall, init encntr
E917.9	OTHER STRIKING AGAINST W/WO SUBSEQUENT FALL	**V00.01XA**	Ped on foot injured in collision w roller-skater, init
		V00.01XD	Ped on foot injured in collision w roller-skater, subs
		V00.02XA	Pedestrian on foot injured in collision w skateboarder, init
		V00.02XD	Pedestrian on foot injured in collision w skateboarder, subs
		V00.09XA	Ped on foot injured in collision w oth ped convey, init
		V00.09XD	Ped on foot injured in collision w oth ped convey, subs
		W50.0XXA	Accidental hit or strike by another person, init encntr
		W50.0XXD	Accidental hit or strike by another person, subs encntr
		W50.1XXA	Accidental kick by another person, initial encounter
		W50.1XXD	Accidental kick by another person, subsequent encounter
		W50.2XXA	Accidental twist by another person, initial encounter
		W50.2XXD	Accidental twist by another person, subsequent encounter
		W50.4XXA	Accidental scratch by another person, initial encounter
		W50.4XXD	Accidental scratch by another person, subsequent encounter
		W51.XXXA	Accidental strike or bumped into by another person, init
		W51.XXXD	Accidental strike or bumped into by another person, subs
E918	CAUGHT ACCIDENTALLY IN OR BETWEEN OBJECTS	**W23.0XXA**	Caught, crush, jammed, or pinched betw moving objects, init
		W23.0XXD	Caught, crush, jammed, or pinched betw moving objects, subs
		W23.1XXA	Caught, crush, jammed, or pinched betw stationry obj, init
		W23.1XXD	Caught, crush, jammed, or pinched betw stationry obj, subs
E919.0	ACCIDENT CAUSED BY AGRICULTURAL MACHINES	**W30.0XXA**	Contact with combine harvester, initial encounter
		W30.0XXD	Contact with combine harvester, subsequent encounter
		W30.1XXA	Contact with power take-off devices (PTO), initial encounter
		W30.1XXD	Contact with power take-off devices (PTO), subs encntr
		W30.2XXA	Contact with hay derrick, initial encounter
		W30.2XXD	Contact with hay derrick, subsequent encounter
		W30.3XXA	Contact with grain storage elevator, initial encounter
		W30.3XXD	Contact with grain storage elevator, subsequent encounter
		W30.81XA	Contact w agri transport vehicle in stationary use, init
		W30.81XD	Contact w agri transport vehicle in stationary use, subs
		W30.89XA	Contact with oth agricultural machinery, init encntr
		W30.89XD	Contact with oth agricultural machinery, subs encntr
		W30.9XXA	Contact with unspecified agricultural machinery, init encntr
		W30.9XXD	Contact with unspecified agricultural machinery, subs encntr
E919.1	ACCIDENT CAUSED MINING&EARTH-DRILLING MACHINERY	**W31.0XXA**	Contact w mining and earth-drilling machinery, init encntr
		W31.0XXD	Contact w mining and earth-drilling machinery, subs encntr
E919.2	ACCIDENT CAUSED LIFTING MACHINES AND APPLIANCES	**W24.0XXA**	Contact w lifting devices, not elsewhere classified, init
		W24.0XXD	Contact w lifting devices, not elsewhere classified, subs
E919.3	ACCIDENT CAUSED BY METALWORKING MACHINES	**W31.1XXA**	Contact with metalworking machines, initial encounter
		W31.1XXD	Contact with metalworking machines, subsequent encounter
E919.4	ACCIDENT CAUSED WOODWORKING AND FORMING MACHINES	**W31.2XXA**	Contact w powered woodworking and forming machines, init
		W31.2XXD	Contact w powered woodworking and forming machines, subs
E919.5	ACCIDENT CAUSED PRIME MOVERS EXCEPT ELEC MOTORS	**W31.3XXA**	Contact with prime movers, initial encounter
		W31.3XXD	Contact with prime movers, subsequent encounter
E919.6	ACCIDENT CAUSED BY TRANSMISSION MACHINERY	**W24.1XXA**	Contact w transmission devices, NEC, init
		W24.1XXD	Contact w transmission devices, NEC, subs
E919.7	ACC CAUS ERTH MOV SCRAPING&OTH EXCAVATING MACHS	**W31.83XA**	Contact w special construct vehicle in stationary use, init
		W31.83XD	Contact w special construct vehicle in stationary use, subs
E919.8	ACCIDENT CAUSED BY OTHER SPECIFIED MACHINERY	**W31.81XA**	Contact with recreational machinery, initial encounter
		W31.81XD	Contact with recreational machinery, subsequent encounter
		W31.82XA	Contact with other commercial machinery, initial encounter
		W31.82XD	Contact with other commercial machinery, subs encntr
		W31.89XA	Contact with other specified machinery, initial encounter
		W31.89XD	Contact with other specified machinery, subsequent encounter

 [Brackets] indicate valid character values for each code. Character value meanings provided for each code grouping.

ICD-9-CM		ICD-10-CM	
E919.9	ACCIDENT CAUSED BY UNSPECIFIED MACHINERY	**W31.9XXA**	Contact with unspecified machinery, initial encounter
		W31.9XXD	Contact with unspecified machinery, subsequent encounter
E920.0	ACCIDENT CAUSED BY POWERED LAWN MOWER	**W28.XXXA**	Contact with powered lawn mower, initial encounter
		W28.XXXD	Contact with powered lawn mower, subsequent encounter
E920.1	ACCIDENT CAUSED BY OTHER POWERED HAND TOOLS	**W29.3XXA**	Cntct w powered garden and outdoor hand tools and mach, init
		W29.3XXD	Cntct w powered garden and outdoor hand tools and mach, subs
		W29.4XXA	Contact with nail gun, initial encounter
		W29.4XXD	Contact with nail gun, subsequent encounter
		W29.8XXA	Cntct w oth power power hand tools and household mach, init
		W29.8XXD	Cntct w oth power power hand tools and household mach, subs
E920.2	ACC CAUSED POWER HOUSEHOLD APPLINCS&IMPLEMENTS	**W29.0XXA**	Contact with powered kitchen appliance, initial encounter
		W29.0XXD	Contact with powered kitchen appliance, subsequent encounter
		W29.1XXA	Contact with electric knife, initial encounter
		W29.1XXD	Contact with electric knife, subsequent encounter
		W29.2XXA	Contact with other powered household machinery, init encntr
		W29.2XXD	Contact with other powered household machinery, subs encntr
E920.3	ACCIDENT CAUSED BY KNIVES SWORDS AND DAGGERS	**W26.0XXA**	Contact with knife, initial encounter
		W26.0XXD	Contact with knife, subsequent encounter
		W26.1XXA	Contact with sword or dagger, initial encounter
		W26.1XXD	Contact with sword or dagger, subsequent encounter
E920.4	ACCIDENT CAUSED OTHER HAND TOOLS AND IMPLEMENTS	**W27.0XXA**	Contact with workbench tool, initial encounter
		W27.0XXD	Contact with workbench tool, subsequent encounter
		W27.1XXA	Contact with garden tool, initial encounter
		W27.1XXD	Contact with garden tool, subsequent encounter
		W27.2XXA	Contact with scissors, initial encounter
		W27.2XXD	Contact with scissors, subsequent encounter
		W27.3XXA	Contact with needle (sewing), initial encounter
		W27.3XXD	Contact with needle (sewing), subsequent encounter
		W27.4XXA	Contact with kitchen utensil, initial encounter
		W27.4XXD	Contact with kitchen utensil, subsequent encounter
		W27.5XXA	Contact with paper-cutter, initial encounter
		W27.5XXD	Contact with paper-cutter, subsequent encounter
		W27.8XXA	Contact with other nonpowered hand tool, initial encounter
		W27.8XXD	Contact with other nonpowered hand tool, subs encntr
E920.5	ACCIDENT CAUSED BY HYPODERMIC NEEDLE	**W46.0XXA**	Contact with hypodermic needle, initial encounter
		W46.0XXD	Contact with hypodermic needle, subsequent encounter
		W46.1XXA	Contact with contaminated hypodermic needle, init encntr
		W46.1XXD	Contact with contaminated hypodermic needle, subs encntr
E920.8	ACC CAUSED OTH SPEC CUT&PIERCING INSTRUM/OBJS	**W25.XXXA**	Contact with sharp glass, initial encounter
		W25.XXXD	Contact with sharp glass, subsequent encounter
		W45.0XXA	Nail entering through skin, initial encounter
		W45.0XXD	Nail entering through skin, subsequent encounter
		W45.1XXA	Paper entering through skin, initial encounter
		W45.1XXD	Paper entering through skin, subsequent encounter
		W45.2XXA	Lid of can entering through skin, initial encounter
		W45.2XXD	Lid of can entering through skin, subsequent encounter
		W45.8XXA	Oth foreign body or object entering through skin, init
		W45.8XXD	Oth foreign body or object entering through skin, subs
		W60.XXXA	Cntct w nonvenom plant thorns & spines & sharp leaves, init
		W60.XXXD	Cntct w nonvenom plant thorns & spines & sharp leaves, subs
E920.9	ACC CAUSED UNSPEC CUT&PIERCING INSTRUMENT/OBJ	**W45.8XXA**	Oth foreign body or object entering through skin, init
E921.0	ACCIDENT CAUSED BY EXPLOSION OF BOILERS	**W35.XXXA**	Explosion and rupture of boiler, initial encounter
		W35.XXXD	Explosion and rupture of boiler, subsequent encounter
E921.1	ACCIDENT CAUSED BY EXPLOSION OF GAS CYLINDERS	**W36.2XXA**	Explosion and rupture of air tank, initial encounter
		W36.2XXD	Explosion and rupture of air tank, subsequent encounter
		W36.3XXA	Explosion and rupture of pressurized-gas tank, init encntr
		W36.3XXD	Explosion and rupture of pressurized-gas tank, subs encntr
		W36.8XXA	Explosion and rupture of other gas cylinder, init encntr
		W36.8XXD	Explosion and rupture of other gas cylinder, subs encntr
		W36.9XXA	Explosion and rupture of unsp gas cylinder, init encntr
		W36.9XXD	Explosion and rupture of unsp gas cylinder, subs encntr
E921.8	ACCIDENT CAUSED EXPLO OTH SPEC PRESSURE VESSELS	**W36.1XXA**	Explosion and rupture of aerosol can, initial encounter
		W36.1XXD	Explosion and rupture of aerosol can, subsequent encounter
		W37.0XXA	Explosion of bicycle tire, initial encounter
		W37.0XXD	Explosion of bicycle tire, subsequent encounter
		W37.8XXA	Explosn and rupture of pressurized tire, pipe or hose, init
		W37.8XXD	Explosn and rupture of pressurized tire, pipe or hose, subs
		W38.XXXA	Explosion and rupture of oth pressurized devices, init
		W38.XXXD	Explosion and rupture of oth pressurized devices, subs
E921.9	ACCIDENT CAUSED EXPLOSION UNSPEC PRESSURE VESSEL	**W38.XXXA**	Explosion and rupture of oth pressurized devices, init
E922.0	ACCIDENT CAUSED BY HANDGUN	**W32.0XXA**	Accidental handgun discharge, initial encounter
		W32.0XXD	Accidental handgun discharge, subsequent encounter
		W32.1XXA	Accidental handgun malfunction, initial encounter
		W32.1XXD	Accidental handgun malfunction, subsequent encounter
E922.1	ACCIDENT CAUSED BY SHOTGUN	**W33.01XA**	Accidental discharge of shotgun, initial encounter
		W33.01XD	Accidental discharge of shotgun, subsequent encounter
		W33.11XA	Accidental malfunction of shotgun, initial encounter
		W33.11XD	Accidental malfunction of shotgun, subsequent encounter

ICD-9-CM		ICD-10-CM	
E922.2	ACCIDENT CAUSED BY HUNTING RIFLE	**W33.02XA**	Accidental discharge of hunting rifle, initial encounter
		W33.02XD	Accidental discharge of hunting rifle, subsequent encounter
		W33.12XA	Accidental malfunction of hunting rifle, initial encounter
		W33.12XD	Accidental malfunction of hunting rifle, subs encntr
E922.3	ACCIDENT CAUSED BY MILITARY FIREARMS	**W33.03XA**	Accidental discharge of machine gun, initial encounter
		W33.03XD	Accidental discharge of machine gun, subsequent encounter
		W33.13XA	Accidental malfunction of machine gun, initial encounter
		W33.13XD	Accidental malfunction of machine gun, subsequent encounter
E922.4	ACCIDENT CAUSED BY AIR GUN	**W34.010A**	Accidental discharge of airgun, initial encounter
		W34.010D	Accidental discharge of airgun, subsequent encounter
		W34.110A	Accidental malfunction of airgun, initial encounter
		W34.110D	Accidental malfunction of airgun, subsequent encounter
E922.5	ACCIDENT CAUSED BY PAINTBALL GUN	**W34.011A**	Accidental discharge of paintball gun, initial encounter
		W34.011D	Accidental discharge of paintball gun, subsequent encounter
		W34.111A	Accidental malfunction of paintball gun, initial encounter
		W34.111D	Accidental malfunction of paintball gun, subs encntr
E922.8	ACCIDENT CAUSED OTHER SPECIFIED FIREARM MISSILE	**W33.09XA**	Accidental discharge of other larger firearm, init encntr
		W33.09XD	Accidental discharge of other larger firearm, subs encntr
		W33.19XA	Accidental malfunction of other larger firearm, init encntr
		W33.19XD	Accidental malfunction of other larger firearm, subs encntr
		W34.018A	Accidental discharge of gas, air or sprng-op gun, init
		W34.018D	Accidental discharge of gas, air or sprng-op gun, subs
		W34.09XA	Accidental discharge from oth firearms, init encntr
		W34.09XD	Accidental discharge from oth firearms, subs encntr
		W34.118A	Accidental malfunction of gas, air or sprng-op gun, init
		W34.118D	Accidental malfunction of gas, air or sprng-op gun, subs
		W34.19XA	Accidental malfunction from oth firearms, init encntr
		W34.19XD	Accidental malfunction from oth firearms, subs encntr
E922.9	ACCIDENT CAUSED BY UNSPECIFIED FIREARM MISSILE	**W33.00XA**	Accidental discharge of unsp larger firearm, init encntr
		W33.00XD	Accidental discharge of unsp larger firearm, subs encntr
		W33.10XA	Accidental malfunction of unsp larger firearm, init encntr
		W33.10XD	Accidental malfunction of unsp larger firearm, subs encntr
		W34.00XA	Accidental discharge from unsp firearms or gun, init encntr
		W34.00XD	Accidental discharge from unsp firearms or gun, subs encntr
		W34.10XA	Accidental malfunction from unsp firearms or gun, init
		W34.10XD	Accidental malfunction from unsp firearms or gun, subs
E923.0	ACCIDENT CAUSED BY FIREWORKS	**W39.XXXA**	Discharge of firework, initial encounter
		W39.XXXD	Discharge of firework, subsequent encounter
E923.1	ACCIDENT CAUSED BY BLASTING MATERIALS	**W40.0XXA**	Explosion of blasting material, initial encounter
		W40.0XXD	Explosion of blasting material, subsequent encounter
E923.2	ACCIDENT CAUSED BY EXPLOSIVE GASES	**W40.1XXA**	Explosion of explosive gases, initial encounter
		W40.1XXD	Explosion of explosive gases, subsequent encounter
E923.8	ACCIDENT CAUSED BY OTHER EXPLOSIVE MATERIALS	**W40.8XXA**	Explosion of oth explosive materials, init encntr
		W40.8XXD	Explosion of oth explosive materials, subs encntr
E923.9	ACCIDENT CAUSED UNSPECIFIED EXPLOSIVE MATERIAL	**W40.9XXA**	Explosion of unspecified explosive materials, init encntr
		W40.9XXD	Explosion of unspecified explosive materials, subs encntr
E924.0	ACCIDENT CAUSED HOT LIQUIDS&VAPORS INCL STEAM	**X10.0XXA**	Contact with hot drinks, initial encounter
		X10.0XXD	Contact with hot drinks, subsequent encounter
		X10.1XXA	Contact with hot food, initial encounter
		X10.1XXD	Contact with hot food, subsequent encounter
		X10.2XXA	Contact with fats and cooking oils, initial encounter
		X10.2XXD	Contact with fats and cooking oils, subsequent encounter
		X12.XXXA	Contact with other hot fluids, initial encounter
		X12.XXXD	Contact with other hot fluids, subsequent encounter
		X13.0XXA	Inhalation of steam and other hot vapors, initial encounter
		X13.0XXD	Inhalation of steam and other hot vapors, subs encntr
		X13.1XXA	Other contact with steam and other hot vapors, init encntr
		X13.1XXD	Other contact with steam and other hot vapors, subs encntr
		X14.0XXA	Inhalation of hot air and gases, initial encounter
		X14.0XXD	Inhalation of hot air and gases, subsequent encounter
		X14.1XXA	Other contact with hot air and other hot gases, init encntr
		X14.1XXD	Other contact with hot air and other hot gases, subs encntr
		X18.XXXA	Contact with other hot metals, initial encounter
		X18.XXXD	Contact with other hot metals, subsequent encounter
E924.1	ACCIDENT CAUSED CAUSTIC AND CORROSIVE SUBSTANCES	**T54.1X1A**	Toxic effect of corrosive organic compounds, acc, init
		T54.1X4A	Toxic effect of corrosive organic compounds, undet, init
		T54.2X1A	Toxic eff of corrosv acids and acid-like substnc, acc, init
		T54.2X4A	Tox eff of corrosv acids and acid-like substnc, undet, init
		T54.3X1A	Tox eff of corrosv alkalis and alk-like substnc, acc, init
		T54.3X4A	Tox eff of corrosv alkalis and alk-like substnc, undet, init
		T54.91XA	Toxic effect of unsp corrosive substance, accidental, init
E924.2	ACCIDENT CAUSED BY HOT TAP WATER	**X11.0XXA**	Contact with hot water in bath or tub, initial encounter
		X11.0XXD	Contact with hot water in bath or tub, subsequent encounter
		X11.1XXA	Contact with running hot water, initial encounter
		X11.1XXD	Contact with running hot water, subsequent encounter
		X11.8XXA	Contact with other hot tap-water, initial encounter
		X11.8XXD	Contact with other hot tap-water, subsequent encounter

ICD-9-CM		ICD-10-CM	
E924.8	ACCIDENT CAUSED BY OTHER HOT SUBSTANCE OR OBJECT	X15.ØXXA	Contact with hot stove (kitchen), initial encounter
		X15.ØXXD	Contact with hot stove (kitchen), subsequent encounter
		X15.1XXA	Contact with hot toaster, initial encounter
		X15.1XXD	Contact with hot toaster, subsequent encounter
		X15.2XXA	Contact with hotplate, initial encounter
		X15.2XXD	Contact with hotplate, subsequent encounter
		X15.3XXA	Contact with hot saucepan or skillet, initial encounter
		X15.3XXD	Contact with hot saucepan or skillet, subsequent encounter
		X15.8XXA	Contact with other hot household appliances, init encntr
		X15.8XXD	Contact with other hot household appliances, subs encntr
		X16.XXXA	Contact w hot heating appliances, radiators and pipes, init
		X16.XXXD	Contact w hot heating appliances, radiators and pipes, subs
		X17.XXXA	Contact with hot engines, machinery and tools, init encntr
		X17.XXXD	Contact with hot engines, machinery and tools, subs encntr
		X19.XXXA	Contact with other heat and hot substances, init encntr
		X19.XXXD	Contact with other heat and hot substances, subs encntr
E924.9	ACCIDENT CAUSED UNSPECIFIED HOT SUBSTANCE/OBJECT	X19.XXXA	Contact with other heat and hot substances, init encntr
E925.Ø	ELEC ACCIDENT CAUSED BY DOMESTIC WIRING&APPLINCS	W86.ØXXA	Exposure to domestic wiring and appliances, init encntr
		W86.ØXXD	Exposure to domestic wiring and appliances, subs encntr
E925.1	ELEC ACC CAUSED BY POWER PLANTS-STATION-LINES	W85.XXXA	Exposure to electric transmission lines, initial encounter
		W85.XXXD	Exposure to electric transmission lines, subs encntr
E925.2	ELEC ACC CAUS INDUST WIRING APPLINCS&ELEC MACHRY	W86.1XXA	Expsr to industr wiring, appliances & electrical mach, init
		W86.1XXD	Expsr to industr wiring, appliances & electrical mach, subs
E925.8	ACCIDENT CAUSED BY OTHER ELECTRIC CURRENT	W86.8XXA	Exposure to other electric current, initial encounter
		W86.8XXD	Exposure to other electric current, subsequent encounter
E925.9	ACCIDENT CAUSED BY UNSPECIFIED ELECTRIC CURRENT	W86.8XXA	Exposure to other electric current, initial encounter
E926.Ø	EXPOSURE TO RADIOFREQUENCY RADIATION	W9Ø.ØXXA	Exposure to radiofrequency, initial encounter
		W9Ø.ØXXD	Exposure to radiofrequency, subsequent encounter
E926.1	EXPOSURE INFRARED RADIATION FROM HEATERS&LAMPS	W9Ø.1XXA	Exposure to infrared radiation, initial encounter
		W9Ø.1XXD	Exposure to infrared radiation, subsequent encounter
E926.2	EXPOSURE TO VISIBLE&ULTRAVIOLET LIGHT SOURCES	W89.ØXXA	Exposure to welding light (arc), initial encounter
		W89.ØXXD	Exposure to welding light (arc), subsequent encounter
		W89.1XXA	Exposure to tanning bed, initial encounter
		W89.1XXD	Exposure to tanning bed, subsequent encounter
		W89.8XXA	Exposure to oth man-made visible and ultraviolet light, init
		W89.8XXD	Exposure to oth man-made visible and ultraviolet light, subs
		W89.9XXA	Expsr to unsp man-made visible and ultraviolet light, init
		W89.9XXD	Expsr to unsp man-made visible and ultraviolet light, subs
E926.3	EXPOS X-RAYS&OTH ELECTROMAGNETIC IONIZING RAD	W88.ØXXA	Exposure to X-rays, initial encounter
		W88.ØXXD	Exposure to X-rays, subsequent encounter
		W88.8XXA	Exposure to other ionizing radiation, initial encounter
		W88.8XXD	Exposure to other ionizing radiation, subsequent encounter
E926.4	EXPOSURE TO LASERS	W9Ø.2XXA	Exposure to laser radiation, initial encounter
		W9Ø.2XXD	Exposure to laser radiation, subsequent encounter
E926.5	EXPOSURE TO RADIOACTIVE ISOTOPES	W88.1XXA	Exposure to radioactive isotopes, initial encounter
		W88.1XXD	Exposure to radioactive isotopes, subsequent encounter
E926.8	EXPOSURE TO OTHER SPECIFIED RADIATION	W88.1XXA	Exposure to radioactive isotopes, initial encounter
		W9Ø.8XXA	Exposure to other nonionizing radiation, initial encounter
		W9Ø.8XXD	Exposure to other nonionizing radiation, subs encntr
		X39.Ø1XA	Exposure to radon, initial encounter
		X39.Ø1XD	Exposure to radon, subsequent encounter
		X39.Ø8XA	Exposure to other natural radiation, initial encounter
		X39.Ø8XD	Exposure to other natural radiation, subsequent encounter
E926.9	EXPOSURE TO UNSPECIFIED RADIATION	W9Ø.8XXA	Exposure to other nonionizing radiation, initial encounter
E927.Ø	OVEREXERTION FROM SUDDEN STRENUOUS MOVEMENT	NO DIAGNOSIS	
E927.1	OVEREXERTION FROM PROLONGED STATIC POSITION	NO DIAGNOSIS	
E927.2	EXCESSIVE PHYS EXERTION FROM PROLONGED ACTIVITY	T73.3XXA	Exhaustion due to excessive exertion, initial encounter
E927.3	CUMULATIVE TRAUMA FROM REPETITIVE MOTION	NO DIAGNOSIS	
E927.4	CUMULATIVE TRAUMA FROM REPETITIVE IMPACT	NO DIAGNOSIS	
E927.8	OTH OVEREXERT&STRENUOUS&REPETITIVE MVMNTS/LOADS	NO DIAGNOSIS	
E927.9	UNS OVEREXERT& STRENUOUS&REPETITIVE MVMNTS/LOADS	NO DIAGNOSIS	
E928.Ø	PROLONGED STAY IN WEIGHTLESS ENVIRONMENT	X52.XXXA	Prolonged stay in weightless environment, initial encounter
		X52.XXXD	Prolonged stay in weightless environment, subs encntr
E928.1	EXPOSURE TO NOISE	W42.ØXXA	Exposure to supersonic waves, initial encounter
		W42.ØXXD	Exposure to supersonic waves, subsequent encounter
		W42.9XXA	Exposure to other noise, initial encounter
		W42.9XXD	Exposure to other noise, subsequent encounter
E928.2	ACCIDENT CAUSED BY VIBRATION	X58.XXXA	Exposure to other specified factors, initial encounter
E928.3	ACCIDENTAL HUMAN BITE	W5Ø.3XXA	Accidental bite by another person, initial encounter
		W5Ø.3XXD	Accidental bite by another person, subsequent encounter
E928.4	EXTERNAL CONSTRICTION CAUSED BY HAIR	W49.Ø1XA	Hair causing external constriction, initial encounter
		W49.Ø1XD	Hair causing external constriction, subsequent encounter

ICD-9-CM		ICD-10-CM	
E928.5	EXTERNAL CONSTRICTION CAUSED BY OTHER OBJECT	**W49.Ø2XA**	String or thread causing external constriction, init encntr
		W49.Ø2XD	String or thread causing external constriction, subs encntr
		W49.Ø3XA	Rubber band causing external constriction, initial encounter
		W49.Ø3XD	Rubber band causing external constriction, subs encntr
		W49.Ø4XA	Ring or oth jewelry causing external constriction, init
		W49.Ø4XD	Ring or oth jewelry causing external constriction, subs
		W49.Ø9XA	Oth item causing external constriction, init encntr
		W49.Ø9XD	Oth item causing external constriction, subs encntr
E928.6	ENVIRONMENTAL EXPOSURE HARMFUL ALGAE&TOXINS	**T65.821A**	Toxic effect of harmful algae and algae toxins, acc, init
		T65.824A	Toxic effect of harmful algae and algae toxins, undet, init
E928.7	ENVIRO & ACC CAUSE MECH/COMPNT FIREARM & AIR GUN	**X58.XXXA**	Exposure to other specified factors, initial encounter
E928.8	OTHER ACCIDENT	**W49.9XXA**	Exposure to other inanimate mechanical forces, init encntr
		W49.9XXD	Exposure to other inanimate mechanical forces, subs encntr
		X39.8XXA	Other exposure to forces of nature, initial encounter
		X39.8XXD	Other exposure to forces of nature, subsequent encounter
		X58.XXXA	Exposure to other specified factors, initial encounter
		X58.XXXD	Exposure to other specified factors, subsequent encounter
E928.9	UNSPECIFIED ACCIDENT	**X58.XXXA**	Exposure to other specified factors, initial encounter
E929.Ø	LATE EFFECTS OF MOTOR VEHICLE ACCIDENT	**VØ2.ØØXS**	Ped on foot injured in clsn w 2/3-whl mv nontraf, sequela
		VØ2.Ø1XS	Ped on rolr-skt inj in clsn w 2/3-whl mv nontraf, sequela
		VØ2.Ø2XS	Ped on sktbrd injured in clsn w 2/3-whl mv nontraf, sequela
		VØ2.Ø9XS	Ped w convey injured in clsn w 2/3-whl mv nontraf, sequela
		VØ2.1ØXS	Ped on foot injured in clsn w 2/3-whl mv in traf, sequela
		VØ2.11XS	Ped on rolr-skt inj in clsn w 2/3-whl mv in traf, sequela
		VØ2.12XS	Ped on sktbrd injured in clsn w 2/3-whl mv in traf, sequela
		VØ2.19XS	Ped w convey injured in clsn w 2/3-whl mv in traf, sequela
		VØ2.9ØXS	Ped on foot injured in collision w 2/3-whl mv, unsp, sequela
		VØ2.91XS	Ped on rolr-skt injured in clsn w 2/3-whl mv, unsp, sequela
		VØ2.92XS	Ped on sktbrd injured in clsn w 2/3-whl mv, unsp, sequela
		VØ2.99XS	Ped w convey injured in clsn w 2/3-whl mv, unsp, sequela
		VØ3.ØØXS	Ped on foot inj pick-up truck, pk-up/van nontraf, sequela
		VØ3.Ø1XS	Ped on rolr-skt inj pk-up truck, pk-up/van nontraf, sequela
		VØ3.Ø2XS	Ped on sktbrd inj pick-up truck, pk-up/van nontraf, sequela
		VØ3.Ø9XS	Ped w convey inj pick-up truck, pk-up/van nontraf, sequela
		VØ3.1ØXS	Ped on foot inj pick-up truck, pk-up/van in traf, sequela
		VØ3.11XS	Ped on rolr-skt inj pk-up truck, pk-up/van in traf, sequela
		VØ3.12XS	Ped on sktbrd inj pick-up truck, pk-up/van in traf, sequela
		VØ3.19XS	Ped w convey inj pick-up truck, pk-up/van in traf, sequela
		VØ3.9ØXS	Ped on foot injured pick-up truck, pk-up/van, unsp, sequela
		VØ3.91XS	Ped on rolr-skt inj pick-up truck, pk-up/van, unsp, sequela
		VØ3.92XS	Ped on sktbrd inj pick-up truck, pk-up/van, unsp, sequela
		VØ3.99XS	Ped w convey injured pick-up truck, pk-up/van, unsp, sequela
		VØ4.ØØXS	Ped on foot injured in collision w hv veh nontraf, sequela
		VØ4.Ø1XS	Ped on rolr-skt injured in clsn w hv veh nontraf, sequela
		VØ4.Ø2XS	Ped on sktbrd injured in collision w hv veh nontraf, sequela
		VØ4.Ø9XS	Ped w convey injured in collision w hv veh nontraf, sequela
		VØ4.1ØXS	Ped on foot injured in collision w hv veh in traf, sequela
		VØ4.11XS	Ped on rolr-skt injured in clsn w hv veh in traf, sequela
		VØ4.12XS	Ped on sktbrd injured in collision w hv veh in traf, sequela
		VØ4.19XS	Ped w convey injured in collision w hv veh in traf, sequela
		VØ4.9ØXS	Ped on foot injured in collision w hv veh, unsp, sequela
		VØ4.91XS	Ped on rolr-skt injured in collision w hv veh, unsp, sequela
		VØ4.92XS	Ped on sktbrd injured in collision w hv veh, unsp, sequela
		VØ4.99XS	Ped w convey injured in collision w hv veh, unsp, sequela
		VØ5.1ØXS	Ped on foot injured in clsn w rail trn/veh in traf, sequela
		VØ5.11XS	Ped on rolr-skt inj in clsn w rail trn/veh in traf, sequela
		VØ5.12XS	Ped on sktbrd inj in clsn w rail trn/veh in traf, sequela
		VØ5.19XS	Ped w convey injured in clsn w rail trn/veh in traf, sequela
		VØ9.ØØXS	Pedestrian injured nontraf involving unsp mv, sequela
		VØ9.Ø1XS	Ped injured nontraf involving military vehicle, sequela
		VØ9.Ø9XS	Pedestrian injured nontraf involving oth mv, sequela
		VØ9.2ØXS	Pedestrian injured in traf involving unsp mv, sequela
		VØ9.21XS	Ped injured in traf involving military vehicle, sequela
		VØ9.29XS	Pedestrian injured in traf involving oth mv, sequela
		V12.ØXXS	Pedl cyc driver inj in clsn w 2/3-whl mv nontraf, sequela
		V12.1XXS	Pedl cyc pasngr inj in clsn w 2/3-whl mv nontraf, sequela
		V12.2XXS	Unsp pedl cyclst inj in clsn w 2/3-whl mv nontraf, sequela
		V12.3XXS	Prsn brd/alit pedl cyc injured in clsn w 2/3-whl mv, sequela
		V12.4XXS	Pedl cyc driver inj in clsn w 2/3-whl mv in traf, sequela
		V12.5XXS	Pedl cyc pasngr inj in clsn w 2/3-whl mv in traf, sequela
		V12.9XXS	Unsp pedl cyclst inj in clsn w 2/3-whl mv in traf, sequela
		V13.ØXXS	Pedl cyc driver inj pk-up truck, pk-up/van nontraf, sequela
		V13.1XXS	Pedl cyc pasngr inj pk-up truck, pk-up/van nontraf, sequela
		V13.2XXS	Unsp pedl cyclst inj pk-up truck, pk-up/van nontraf, sequela
		V13.3XXS	Prsn brd/alit pedl cyc inj pick-up truck, pk-up/van, sequela
		V13.4XXS	Pedl cyc driver inj pk-up truck, pk-up/van in traf, sequela
		V13.5XXS	Pedl cyc pasngr inj pk-up truck, pk-up/van in traf, sequela
		V13.9XXS	Unsp pedl cyclst inj pk-up truck, pk-up/van in traf, sequela
		V14.ØXXS	Pedl cyc driver injured in clsn w hv veh nontraf, sequela
		V14.1XXS	Pedl cyc passenger injured in clsn w hv veh nontraf, sequela
	(Continued on next page)	**V14.2XXS**	Unsp pedl cyclst injured in clsn w hv veh nontraf, sequela

[Brackets] indicate valid character values for each code. Character value meanings provided for each code grouping.

ICD-9-CM		ICD-10-CM	
E929.Ø	LATE EFFECTS OF MOTOR VEHICLE ACCIDENT **(Continued)**	**V14.3XXS**	Prsn brd/alit pedl cyc injured in clsn w hv veh, sequela
		V14.4XXS	Pedl cyc driver injured in clsn w hv veh in traf, sequela
		V14.5XXS	Pedl cyc passenger injured in clsn w hv veh in traf, sequela
		V14.9XXS	Unsp pedl cyclst injured in clsn w hv veh in traf, sequela
		V15.ØXXS	Pedl cyc driver inj in clsn w rail trn/veh nontraf, sequela
		V15.1XXS	Pedl cyc pasngr inj in clsn w rail trn/veh nontraf, sequela
		V19.ØØXS	Pedl cyc driver injured in clsn w unsp mv nontraf, sequela
		V19.Ø9XS	Pedl cyc driver injured in clsn w oth mv nontraf, sequela
		V19.1ØXS	Pedl cyc pasngr injured in clsn w unsp mv nontraf, sequela
		V19.19XS	Pedl cyc passenger injured in clsn w oth mv nontraf, sequela
		V19.2ØXS	Unsp pedl cyclst injured in clsn w unsp mv nontraf, sequela
		V19.29XS	Unsp pedl cyclst injured in clsn w oth mv nontraf, sequela
		V19.4ØXS	Pedl cyc driver injured in clsn w unsp mv in traf, sequela
		V19.49XS	Pedl cyc driver injured in clsn w oth mv in traf, sequela
		V19.5ØXS	Pedl cyc pasngr injured in clsn w unsp mv in traf, sequela
		V19.59XS	Pedl cyc passenger injured in clsn w oth mv in traf, sequela
		V19.6ØXS	Unsp pedl cyclst injured in clsn w unsp mv in traf, sequela
		V19.69XS	Unsp pedl cyclst injured in clsn w oth mv in traf, sequela
		V19.81XS	Pedl cyclst injured in trnsp acc w military vehicle, sequela
		V2Ø.ØXXS	Mtrcy driver injured in clsn w ped/anml nontraf, sequela
		V2Ø.1XXS	Mtrcy passenger injured in clsn w ped/anml nontraf, sequela
		V2Ø.2XXS	Unsp mtrcy rider injured in clsn w ped/anml nontraf, sequela
		V2Ø.3XXS	Prsn brd/alit mtrcy injured in collision w ped/anml, sequela
		V2Ø.4XXS	Mtrcy driver injured in clsn w ped/anml in traf, sequela
		V2Ø.5XXS	Mtrcy passenger injured in clsn w ped/anml in traf, sequela
		V2Ø.9XXS	Unsp mtrcy rider injured in clsn w ped/anml in traf, sequela
		V21.ØXXS	Mtrcy driver injured in clsn w pedl cyc nontraf, sequela
		V21.1XXS	Mtrcy passenger injured in clsn w pedl cyc nontraf, sequela
		V21.2XXS	Unsp mtrcy rider injured in clsn w pedl cyc nontraf, sequela
		V21.3XXS	Prsn brd/alit mtrcy injured in collision w pedl cyc, sequela
		V21.4XXS	Mtrcy driver injured in clsn w pedl cyc in traf, sequela
		V21.5XXS	Mtrcy passenger injured in clsn w pedl cyc in traf, sequela
		V21.9XXS	Unsp mtrcy rider injured in clsn w pedl cyc in traf, sequela
		V22.ØXXS	Mtrcy driver injured in clsn w 2/3-whl mv nontraf, sequela
		V22.1XXS	Mtrcy pasngr injured in clsn w 2/3-whl mv nontraf, sequela
		V22.2XXS	Unsp mtrcy rider inj in clsn w 2/3-whl mv nontraf, sequela
		V22.3XXS	Prsn brd/alit mtrcy injured in clsn w 2/3-whl mv, sequela
		V22.4XXS	Mtrcy driver injured in clsn w 2/3-whl mv in traf, sequela
		V22.5XXS	Mtrcy pasngr injured in clsn w 2/3-whl mv in traf, sequela
		V22.9XXS	Unsp mtrcy rider inj in clsn w 2/3-whl mv in traf, sequela
		V23.ØXXS	Mtrcy driver inj pick-up truck, pk-up/van nontraf, sequela
		V23.1XXS	Mtrcy pasngr inj pick-up truck, pk-up/van nontraf, sequela
		V23.2XXS	Unsp mtrcy rider inj pk-up truck, pk-up/van nontraf, sequela
		V23.3XXS	Prsn brd/alit mtrcy inj pick-up truck, pk-up/van, sequela
		V23.4XXS	Mtrcy driver inj pick-up truck, pk-up/van in traf, sequela
		V23.5XXS	Mtrcy pasngr inj pick-up truck, pk-up/van in traf, sequela
		V23.9XXS	Unsp mtrcy rider inj pk-up truck, pk-up/van in traf, sequela
		V24.ØXXS	Mtrcy driver injured in collision w hv veh nontraf, sequela
		V24.1XXS	Mtrcy passenger injured in clsn w hv veh nontraf, sequela
		V24.2XXS	Unsp mtrcy rider injured in clsn w hv veh nontraf, sequela
		V24.3XXS	Prsn brd/alit mtrcy injured in collision w hv veh, sequela
		V24.4XXS	Mtrcy driver injured in collision w hv veh in traf, sequela
		V24.5XXS	Mtrcy passenger injured in clsn w hv veh in traf, sequela
		V24.9XXS	Unsp mtrcy rider injured in clsn w hv veh in traf, sequela
		V25.ØXXS	Mtrcy driver injured in clsn w rail trn/veh nontraf, sequela
		V25.1XXS	Mtrcy pasngr injured in clsn w rail trn/veh nontraf, sequela
		V25.2XXS	Unsp mtrcy rider inj in clsn w rail trn/veh nontraf, sequela
		V25.3XXS	Prsn brd/alit mtrcy injured in clsn w rail trn/veh, sequela
		V25.4XXS	Mtrcy driver injured in clsn w rail trn/veh in traf, sequela
		V25.5XXS	Mtrcy pasngr injured in clsn w rail trn/veh in traf, sequela
		V25.9XXS	Unsp mtrcy rider inj in clsn w rail trn/veh in traf, sequela
		V26.ØXXS	Mtrcy driver inj in clsn w nonmtr vehicle nontraf, sequela
		V26.1XXS	Mtrcy pasngr inj in clsn w nonmtr vehicle nontraf, sequela
		V26.2XXS	Unsp mtrcy rider inj in clsn w nonmtr vehicle nontraf, sqla
		V26.3XXS	Prsn brd/alit mtrcy inj in clsn w nonmtr vehicle, sequela
		V26.4XXS	Mtrcy driver inj in clsn w nonmtr vehicle in traf, sequela
		V26.5XXS	Mtrcy pasngr inj in clsn w nonmtr vehicle in traf, sequela
		V26.9XXS	Unsp mtrcy rider inj in clsn w nonmtr vehicle in traf, sqla
		V27.ØXXS	Mtrcy driver inj in clsn w statnry object nontraf, sequela
		V27.1XXS	Mtrcy pasngr inj in clsn w statnry object nontraf, sequela
		V27.2XXS	Unsp mtrcy rider inj in clsn w statnry object nontraf, sqla
		V27.3XXS	Prsn brd/alit mtrcy inj in clsn w statnry object, sequela
		V27.4XXS	Mtrcy driver inj in clsn w statnry object in traf, sequela
		V27.5XXS	Mtrcy pasngr inj in clsn w statnry object in traf, sequela
		V27.9XXS	Unsp mtrcy rider inj in clsn w statnry object in traf, sqla
		V28.ØXXS	Mtrcy driver injured in nonclsn trnsp acc nontraf, sequela
		V28.1XXS	Mtrcy pasngr injured in nonclsn trnsp acc nontraf, sequela
		V28.2XXS	Unsp mtrcy rider inj in nonclsn trnsp acc nontraf, sequela
		V28.3XXS	Prsn brd/alit mtrcy injured in nonclsn trnsp acc, sequela
		V28.4XXS	Mtrcy driver injured in nonclsn trnsp acc in traf, sequela
		V28.5XXS	Mtrcy pasngr injured in nonclsn trnsp acc in traf, sequela
	(Continued on next page)	**V28.9XXS**	Unsp mtrcy rider inj in nonclsn trnsp acc in traf, sequela

ICD-9-CM		ICD-10-CM	
E929.Ø	LATE EFFECTS OF MOTOR VEHICLE ACCIDENT **(Continued)**	**V29.ØØXS**	Mtrcy driver injured in collision w unsp mv nontraf, sequela
		V29.Ø9XS	Mtrcy driver injured in collision w oth mv nontraf, sequela
		V29.1ØXS	Mtrcy passenger injured in clsn w unsp mv nontraf, sequela
		V29.19XS	Mtrcy passenger injured in clsn w oth mv nontraf, sequela
		V29.2ØXS	Unsp mtrcy rider injured in clsn w unsp mv nontraf, sequela
		V29.29XS	Unsp mtrcy rider injured in clsn w oth mv nontraf, sequela
		V29.3XXS	Motorcycle rider (driver) injured in unsp nontraf, sequela
		V29.4ØXS	Mtrcy driver injured in collision w unsp mv in traf, sequela
		V29.49XS	Mtrcy driver injured in collision w oth mv in traf, sequela
		V29.5ØXS	Mtrcy passenger injured in clsn w unsp mv in traf, sequela
		V29.59XS	Mtrcy passenger injured in clsn w oth mv in traf, sequela
		V29.6ØXS	Unsp mtrcy rider injured in clsn w unsp mv in traf, sequela
		V29.69XS	Unsp mtrcy rider injured in clsn w oth mv in traf, sequela
		V29.81XS	Mtrcy rider injured in trnsp acc w military vehicle, sequela
		V29.88XS	Mtrcy rider (driver) injured in oth transport acc, sequela
		V29.9XXS	Motorcycle rider (driver) injured in unsp traf, sequela
		V3Ø.ØXXS	Driver of 3-whl mv inj in clsn w ped/anml nontraf, sequela
		V3Ø.1XXS	Pasngr in 3-whl mv inj in clsn w ped/anml nontraf, sequela
		V3Ø.2XXS	Person outsd 3-whl mv inj in clsn w ped/anml nontraf, sqla
		V3Ø.3XXS	Occup of 3-whl mv inj in clsn w ped/anml nontraf, sequela
		V3Ø.4XXS	Prsn brd/alit a 3-whl mv injured in clsn w ped/anml, sequela
		V3Ø.5XXS	Driver of 3-whl mv inj in clsn w ped/anml in traf, sequela
		V3Ø.6XXS	Pasngr in 3-whl mv inj in clsn w ped/anml in traf, sequela
		V3Ø.7XXS	Person outsd 3-whl mv inj in clsn w ped/anml in traf, sqla
		V3Ø.9XXS	Occup of 3-whl mv inj in clsn w ped/anml in traf, sequela
		V31.ØXXS	Driver of 3-whl mv inj in clsn w pedl cyc nontraf, sequela
		V31.1XXS	Pasngr in 3-whl mv inj in clsn w pedl cyc nontraf, sequela
		V31.2XXS	Person outsd 3-whl mv inj in clsn w pedl cyc nontraf, sqla
		V31.3XXS	Occup of 3-whl mv inj in clsn w pedl cyc nontraf, sequela
		V31.4XXS	Prsn brd/alit a 3-whl mv injured in clsn w pedl cyc, sequela
		V31.5XXS	Driver of 3-whl mv inj in clsn w pedl cyc in traf, sequela
		V31.6XXS	Pasngr in 3-whl mv inj in clsn w pedl cyc in traf, sequela
		V31.7XXS	Person outsd 3-whl mv inj in clsn w pedl cyc in traf, sqla
		V31.9XXS	Occup of 3-whl mv inj in clsn w pedl cyc in traf, sequela
		V32.ØXXS	Driver of 3-whl mv inj in clsn w 2/3-whl mv nontraf, sequela
		V32.1XXS	Pasngr in 3-whl mv inj in clsn w 2/3-whl mv nontraf, sequela
		V32.2XXS	Person outsd 3-whl mv inj in clsn w 2/3-whl mv nontraf, sqla
		V32.3XXS	Occup of 3-whl mv inj in clsn w 2/3-whl mv nontraf, sequela
		V32.4XXS	Prsn brd/alit a 3-whl mv inj in clsn w 2/3-whl mv, sequela
		V32.5XXS	Driver of 3-whl mv inj in clsn w 2/3-whl mv in traf, sequela
		V32.6XXS	Pasngr in 3-whl mv inj in clsn w 2/3-whl mv in traf, sequela
		V32.7XXS	Person outsd 3-whl mv inj in clsn w 2/3-whl mv in traf, sqla
		V32.9XXS	Occup of 3-whl mv inj in clsn w 2/3-whl mv in traf, sequela
		V33.ØXXS	Driver of 3-whl mv inj pk-up truck, pk-up/van nontraf, sqla
		V33.1XXS	Pasngr in 3-whl mv inj pk-up truck, pk-up/van nontraf, sqla
		V33.2XXS	Prsn outsd 3-whl mv inj pk-up truck, pk-up/van nontraf, sqla
		V33.3XXS	Occup of 3-whl mv inj pk-up truck, pk-up/van nontraf, sqla
		V33.4XXS	Prsn brd/alit a 3-whl mv inj pk-up truck, pk-up/van, sequela
		V33.5XXS	Driver of 3-whl mv inj pk-up truck, pk-up/van in traf, sqla
		V33.6XXS	Pasngr in 3-whl mv inj pk-up truck, pk-up/van in traf, sqla
		V33.7XXS	Prsn outsd 3-whl mv inj pk-up truck, pk-up/van in traf, sqla
		V33.9XXS	Occup of 3-whl mv inj pk-up truck, pk-up/van in traf, sqla
		V34.ØXXS	Driver of 3-whl mv injured in clsn w hv veh nontraf, sequela
		V34.1XXS	Pasngr in 3-whl mv injured in clsn w hv veh nontraf, sequela
		V34.2XXS	Person outsd 3-whl mv inj in clsn w hv veh nontraf, sequela
		V34.3XXS	Occup of 3-whl mv injured in clsn w hv veh nontraf, sequela
		V34.4XXS	Prsn brd/alit a 3-whl mv injured in clsn w hv veh, sequela
		V34.5XXS	Driver of 3-whl mv injured in clsn w hv veh in traf, sequela
		V34.6XXS	Pasngr in 3-whl mv injured in clsn w hv veh in traf, sequela
		V34.7XXS	Person outsd 3-whl mv inj in clsn w hv veh in traf, sequela
		V34.9XXS	Occup of 3-whl mv injured in clsn w hv veh in traf, sequela
		V35.ØXXS	Driver of 3-whl mv inj in clsn w rail trn/veh nontraf, sqla
		V35.1XXS	Pasngr in 3-whl mv inj in clsn w rail trn/veh nontraf, sqla
		V35.2XXS	Prsn outsd 3-whl mv inj in clsn w rail trn/veh nontraf, sqla
		V35.3XXS	Occup of 3-whl mv inj in clsn w rail trn/veh nontraf, sqla
		V35.4XXS	Prsn brd/alit a 3-whl mv inj in clsn w rail trn/veh, sequela
		V35.5XXS	Driver of 3-whl mv inj in clsn w rail trn/veh in traf, sqla
		V35.6XXS	Pasngr in 3-whl mv inj in clsn w rail trn/veh in traf, sqla
		V35.7XXS	Prsn outsd 3-whl mv inj in clsn w rail trn/veh in traf, sqla
		V35.9XXS	Occup of 3-whl mv inj in clsn w rail trn/veh in traf, sqla
		V36.ØXXS	Driver of 3-whl mv inj in clsn w nonmtr veh nontraf, sqla
		V36.1XXS	Pasngr in 3-whl mv inj in clsn w nonmtr veh nontraf, sqla
		V36.2XXS	Person outsd 3-whl mv inj in clsn w nonmtr veh nontraf, sqla
		V36.3XXS	Occup of 3-whl mv inj in clsn w nonmtr vehicle nontraf, sqla
		V36.4XXS	Prsn brd/alit a 3-whl mv inj in clsn w nonmtr vehicle, sqla
		V36.5XXS	Driver of 3-whl mv inj in clsn w nonmtr veh in traf, sqla
		V36.6XXS	Pasngr in 3-whl mv inj in clsn w nonmtr veh in traf, sqla
		V36.7XXS	Person outsd 3-whl mv inj in clsn w nonmtr veh in traf, sqla
		V36.9XXS	Occup of 3-whl mv inj in clsn w nonmtr vehicle in traf, sqla
		V37.ØXXS	Drvr of 3-whl mv inj in clsn w statnry object nontraf, sqla
		V37.1XXS	Pasngr in 3-whl mv inj in clsn w statnry obj nontraf, sqla
	(Continued on next page)	**V37.2XXS**	Prsn outsd 3-whl mv inj in clsn w statnry obj nontraf, sqla

[Brackets] indicate valid character values for each code. Character value meanings provided for each code grouping.

ICD-9-CM		ICD-10-CM	
E929.Ø	LATE EFFECTS OF MOTOR VEHICLE ACCIDENT **(Continued)**	**V37.3XXS**	Occup of 3-whl mv inj in clsn w statnry object nontraf, sqla
		V37.4XXS	Prsn brd/alit a 3-whl mv inj in clsn w statnry object, sqla
		V37.5XXS	Drvr of 3-whl mv inj in clsn w statnry object in traf, sqla
		V37.6XXS	Pasngr in 3-whl mv inj in clsn w statnry obj in traf, sqla
		V37.7XXS	Prsn outsd 3-whl mv inj in clsn w statnry obj in traf, sqla
		V37.9XXS	Occup of 3-whl mv inj in clsn w statnry object in traf, sqla
		V38.ØXXS	Driver of 3-whl mv inj in nonclsn trnsp acc nontraf, sequela
		V38.1XXS	Pasngr in 3-whl mv inj in nonclsn trnsp acc nontraf, sequela
		V38.2XXS	Person outsd 3-whl mv inj in nonclsn trnsp acc nontraf, sqla
		V38.3XXS	Occup of 3-whl mv inj in nonclsn trnsp acc nontraf, sequela
		V38.4XXS	Prsn brd/alit a 3-whl mv inj in nonclsn trnsp acc, sequela
		V38.5XXS	Driver of 3-whl mv inj in nonclsn trnsp acc in traf, sequela
		V38.6XXS	Pasngr in 3-whl mv inj in nonclsn trnsp acc in traf, sequela
		V38.7XXS	Person outsd 3-whl mv inj in nonclsn trnsp acc in traf, sqla
		V38.9XXS	Occup of 3-whl mv inj in nonclsn trnsp acc in traf, sequela
		V39.ØØXS	Driver of 3-whl mv inj in clsn w unsp mv nontraf, sequela
		V39.Ø9XS	Driver of 3-whl mv injured in clsn w oth mv nontraf, sequela
		V39.1ØXS	Pasngr in 3-whl mv inj in clsn w unsp mv nontraf, sequela
		V39.19XS	Pasngr in 3-whl mv injured in clsn w oth mv nontraf, sequela
		V39.2ØXS	Occup of 3-whl mv injured in clsn w unsp mv nontraf, sequela
		V39.29XS	Occup of 3-whl mv injured in clsn w oth mv nontraf, sequela
		V39.3XXS	Occupant of 3-whl mv injured in unsp nontraf, sequela
		V39.4ØXS	Driver of 3-whl mv inj in clsn w unsp mv in traf, sequela
		V39.49XS	Driver of 3-whl mv injured in clsn w oth mv in traf, sequela
		V39.5ØXS	Pasngr in 3-whl mv inj in clsn w unsp mv in traf, sequela
		V39.59XS	Pasngr in 3-whl mv injured in clsn w oth mv in traf, sequela
		V39.6ØXS	Occup of 3-whl mv injured in clsn w unsp mv in traf, sequela
		V39.69XS	Occup of 3-whl mv injured in clsn w oth mv in traf, sequela
		V39.81XS	Occ of 3-whl mv inj in trnsp acc w miltry vehicle, sequela
		V39.89XS	Occupant of 3-whl mv injured in oth trnsp acc, sequela
		V39.9XXS	Occupant (driver) of 3-whl mv injured in unsp traf, sequela
		V4Ø.ØXXS	Car driver injured in collision w ped/anml nontraf, sequela
		V4Ø.1XXS	Car passenger injured in clsn w ped/anml nontraf, sequela
		V4Ø.2XXS	Person outside car inj in clsn w ped/anml nontraf, sequela
		V4Ø.3XXS	Unsp car occ injured in clsn w ped/anml nontraf, sequela
		V4Ø.4XXS	Prsn brd/alit a car injured in collision w ped/anml, sequela
		V4Ø.5XXS	Car driver injured in collision w ped/anml in traf, sequela
		V4Ø.6XXS	Car passenger injured in clsn w ped/anml in traf, sequela
		V4Ø.7XXS	Person outside car inj in clsn w ped/anml in traf, sequela
		V4Ø.9XXS	Unsp car occ injured in clsn w ped/anml in traf, sequela
		V41.ØXXS	Car driver injured in collision w pedl cyc nontraf, sequela
		V41.1XXS	Car passenger injured in clsn w pedl cyc nontraf, sequela
		V41.2XXS	Person outside car inj in clsn w pedl cyc nontraf, sequela
		V41.3XXS	Unsp car occ injured in clsn w pedl cyc nontraf, sequela
		V41.4XXS	Prsn brd/alit a car injured in collision w pedl cyc, sequela
		V41.5XXS	Car driver injured in collision w pedl cyc in traf, sequela
		V41.6XXS	Car passenger injured in clsn w pedl cyc in traf, sequela
		V41.7XXS	Person outside car inj in clsn w pedl cyc in traf, sequela
		V41.9XXS	Unsp car occ injured in clsn w pedl cyc in traf, sequela
		V42.ØXXS	Car driver injured in clsn w 2/3-whl mv nontraf, sequela
		V42.1XXS	Car passenger injured in clsn w 2/3-whl mv nontraf, sequela
		V42.2XXS	Person outside car inj in clsn w 2/3-whl mv nontraf, sequela
		V42.3XXS	Unsp car occ injured in clsn w 2/3-whl mv nontraf, sequela
		V42.4XXS	Prsn brd/alit a car injured in clsn w 2/3-whl mv, sequela
		V42.5XXS	Car driver injured in clsn w 2/3-whl mv in traf, sequela
		V42.6XXS	Car passenger injured in clsn w 2/3-whl mv in traf, sequela
		V42.7XXS	Person outside car inj in clsn w 2/3-whl mv in traf, sequela
		V42.9XXS	Unsp car occ injured in clsn w 2/3-whl mv in traf, sequela
		V43.Ø1XS	Car driver injured in collision w SUV nontraf, sequela
		V43.Ø2XS	Car driver injured in collision w car nontraf, sequela
		V43.Ø3XS	Car driver injured in clsn w pick-up truck nontraf, sequela
		V43.Ø4XS	Car driver injured in collision w van nontraf, sequela
		V43.11XS	Car passenger injured in collision w SUV nontraf, sequela
		V43.12XS	Car passenger injured in collision w car nontraf, sequela
		V43.13XS	Car passenger injured in clsn w pick-up nontraf, sequela
		V43.14XS	Car passenger injured in collision w van nontraf, sequela
		V43.21XS	Person outside car injured in clsn w SUV nontraf, sequela
		V43.22XS	Person outside car injured in clsn w car nontraf, sequela
		V43.23XS	Person outsd car inj in clsn w pk-up truck nontraf, sequela
		V43.24XS	Person outside car injured in clsn w van nontraf, sequela
		V43.31XS	Unsp car occupant injured in clsn w SUV nontraf, sequela
		V43.32XS	Unsp car occupant injured in clsn w car nontraf, sequela
		V43.33XS	Unsp car occ inj in clsn w pick-up truck nontraf, sequela
		V43.34XS	Unsp car occupant injured in clsn w van nontraf, sequela
		V43.41XS	Prsn brd/alit a car injured in collision w SUV, sequela
		V43.42XS	Prsn brd/alit a car injured in collision w car, sequela
		V43.43XS	Prsn brd/alit a car injured in clsn w pick-up truck, sequela
		V43.44XS	Prsn brd/alit a car injured in collision w van, sequela
		V43.51XS	Car driver injured in collision w SUV in traf, sequela
		V43.52XS	Car driver injured in collision w car in traf, sequela
		V43.53XS	Car driver injured in clsn w pick-up truck in traf, sequela
		V43.54XS	Car driver injured in collision w van in traf, sequela
	(Continued on next page)	**V43.61XS**	Car passenger injured in collision w SUV in traf, sequela

ICD-9-CM		ICD-10-CM	
E929.Ø	LATE EFFECTS OF MOTOR VEHICLE ACCIDENT **(Continued)**	**V43.62XS**	Car passenger injured in collision w car in traf, sequela
		V43.63XS	Car pasngr injured in clsn w pick-up truck in traf, sequela
		V43.64XS	Car passenger injured in collision w van in traf, sequela
		V43.71XS	Person outside car injured in clsn w SUV in traf, sequela
		V43.72XS	Person outside car injured in clsn w car in traf, sequela
		V43.73XS	Person outsd car inj in clsn w pk-up truck in traf, sequela
		V43.74XS	Person outside car injured in clsn w van in traf, sequela
		V43.91XS	Unsp car occupant injured in clsn w SUV in traf, sequela
		V43.92XS	Unsp car occupant injured in clsn w car in traf, sequela
		V43.93XS	Unsp car occ inj in clsn w pick-up truck in traf, sequela
		V43.94XS	Unsp car occupant injured in clsn w van in traf, sequela
		V44.ØXXS	Car driver injured in collision w hv veh nontraf, sequela
		V44.1XXS	Car passenger injured in collision w hv veh nontraf, sequela
		V44.2XXS	Person outside car injured in clsn w hv veh nontraf, sequela
		V44.3XXS	Unsp car occupant injured in clsn w hv veh nontraf, sequela
		V44.4XXS	Prsn brd/alit a car injured in collision w hv veh, sequela
		V44.5XXS	Car driver injured in collision w hv veh in traf, sequela
		V44.6XXS	Car passenger injured in collision w hv veh in traf, sequela
		V44.7XXS	Person outside car injured in clsn w hv veh in traf, sequela
		V44.9XXS	Unsp car occupant injured in clsn w hv veh in traf, sequela
		V45.ØXXS	Car driver injured in clsn w rail trn/veh nontraf, sequela
		V45.1XXS	Car pasngr injured in clsn w rail trn/veh nontraf, sequela
		V45.2XXS	Person outsd car inj in clsn w rail trn/veh nontraf, sequela
		V45.3XXS	Unsp car occ injured in clsn w rail trn/veh nontraf, sequela
		V45.4XXS	Prsn brd/alit a car injured in clsn w rail trn/veh, sequela
		V45.5XXS	Car driver injured in clsn w rail trn/veh in traf, sequela
		V45.6XXS	Car pasngr injured in clsn w rail trn/veh in traf, sequela
		V45.7XXS	Person outsd car inj in clsn w rail trn/veh in traf, sequela
		V45.9XXS	Unsp car occ injured in clsn w rail trn/veh in traf, sequela
		V46.ØXXS	Car driver injured in clsn w nonmtr vehicle nontraf, sequela
		V46.1XXS	Car pasngr injured in clsn w nonmtr vehicle nontraf, sequela
		V46.2XXS	Person outsd car inj in clsn w nonmtr vehicle nontraf, sqla
		V46.3XXS	Unsp car occ inj in clsn w nonmtr vehicle nontraf, sequela
		V46.4XXS	Prsn brd/alit a car inj in clsn w nonmtr vehicle, sequela
		V46.5XXS	Car driver injured in clsn w nonmtr vehicle in traf, sequela
		V46.6XXS	Car pasngr injured in clsn w nonmtr vehicle in traf, sequela
		V46.7XXS	Person outsd car inj in clsn w nonmtr vehicle in traf, sqla
		V46.9XXS	Unsp car occ inj in clsn w nonmtr vehicle in traf, sequela
		V47.Ø1XS	Driver of SUV inj in clsn w statnry object nontraf, sequela
		V47.Ø2XS	Driver of car inj in clsn w statnry object nontraf, sequela
		V47.11XS	Pasngr of SUV inj in clsn w statnry object nontraf, sequela
		V47.12XS	Pasngr of car inj in clsn w statnry object nontraf, sequela
		V47.2XXS	Person outsd car inj in clsn w statnry object nontraf, sqla
		V47.31XS	Occup of SUV inj in clsn w statnry object nontraf, sequela
		V47.32XS	Occup of car inj in clsn w statnry object nontraf, sequela
		V47.4XXS	Prsn brd/alit a car inj in clsn w statnry object, sequela
		V47.51XS	Driver of SUV inj in clsn w statnry object in traf, sequela
		V47.52XS	Driver of car inj in clsn w statnry object in traf, sequela
		V47.61XS	Pasngr of SUV inj in clsn w statnry object in traf, sequela
		V47.62XS	Pasngr of car inj in clsn w statnry object in traf, sequela
		V47.7XXS	Person outsd car inj in clsn w statnry object in traf, sqla
		V47.91XS	Occup of SUV inj in clsn w statnry object in traf, sequela
		V47.92XS	Occup of car inj in clsn w statnry object in traf, sequela
		V48.ØXXS	Car driver injured in nonclsn trnsp acc nontraf, sequela
		V48.1XXS	Car pasngr injured in nonclsn trnsp acc nontraf, sequela
		V48.2XXS	Person outside car inj in nonclsn trnsp acc nontraf, sequela
		V48.3XXS	Unsp car occ injured in nonclsn trnsp acc nontraf, sequela
		V48.4XXS	Prsn brd/alit a car injured in nonclsn trnsp acc, sequela
		V48.5XXS	Car driver injured in nonclsn trnsp acc in traf, sequela
		V48.6XXS	Car pasngr injured in nonclsn trnsp acc in traf, sequela
		V48.7XXS	Person outside car inj in nonclsn trnsp acc in traf, sequela
		V48.9XXS	Unsp car occ injured in nonclsn trnsp acc in traf, sequela
		V49.ØØXS	Driver injured in collision w unsp mv nontraf, sequela
		V49.Ø9XS	Driver injured in collision w oth mv nontraf, sequela
		V49.1ØXS	Passenger injured in collision w unsp mv nontraf, sequela
		V49.19XS	Passenger injured in collision w oth mv nontraf, sequela
		V49.2ØXS	Unsp car occupant injured in clsn w unsp mv nontraf, sequela
		V49.29XS	Unsp car occupant injured in clsn w oth mv nontraf, sequela
		V49.3XXS	Car occupant (driver) injured in unsp nontraf, sequela
		V49.4ØXS	Driver injured in collision w unsp mv in traf, sequela
		V49.49XS	Driver injured in collision w oth mv in traf, sequela
		V49.5ØXS	Passenger injured in collision w unsp mv in traf, sequela
		V49.59XS	Passenger injured in collision w oth mv in traf, sequela
		V49.6ØXS	Unsp car occupant injured in clsn w unsp mv in traf, sequela
		V49.69XS	Unsp car occupant injured in clsn w oth mv in traf, sequela
		V49.81XS	Car occupant injured in trnsp acc w miltry vehicle, sequela
		V49.88XS	Car occupant (driver) injured in oth transport acc, sequela
		V49.9XXS	Car occupant (driver) injured in unsp traf, sequela
		V5Ø.ØXXS	Driver of pk-up/van inj in clsn w ped/anml nontraf, sequela
		V5Ø.1XXS	Pasngr in pk-up/van inj in clsn w ped/anml nontraf, sequela
		V5Ø.2XXS	Person outsd pk-up/van inj in clsn w ped/anml nontraf, sqla
		V5Ø.3XXS	Occup of pk-up/van inj in clsn w ped/anml nontraf, sequela
	(Continued on next page)	**V5Ø.4XXS**	Prsn brd/alit pk-up/van injured in clsn w ped/anml, sequela

ICD-9-CM		ICD-10-CM	
E929.Ø	LATE EFFECTS OF MOTOR VEHICLE ACCIDENT **(Continued)**	**V5Ø.5XXS**	Driver of pk-up/van inj in clsn w ped/anml in traf, sequela
		V5Ø.6XXS	Pasngr in pk-up/van inj in clsn w ped/anml in traf, sequela
		V5Ø.7XXS	Person outsd pk-up/van inj in clsn w ped/anml in traf, sqla
		V5Ø.9XXS	Occup of pk-up/van inj in clsn w ped/anml in traf, sequela
		V51.ØXXS	Driver of pk-up/van inj in clsn w pedl cyc nontraf, sequela
		V51.1XXS	Pasngr in pk-up/van inj in clsn w pedl cyc nontraf, sequela
		V51.2XXS	Person outsd pk-up/van inj in clsn w pedl cyc nontraf, sqla
		V51.3XXS	Occup of pk-up/van inj in clsn w pedl cyc nontraf, sequela
		V51.4XXS	Prsn brd/alit pk-up/van injured in clsn w pedl cyc, sequela
		V51.5XXS	Driver of pk-up/van inj in clsn w pedl cyc in traf, sequela
		V51.6XXS	Pasngr in pk-up/van inj in clsn w pedl cyc in traf, sequela
		V51.7XXS	Person outsd pk-up/van inj in clsn w pedl cyc in traf, sqla
		V51.9XXS	Occup of pk-up/van inj in clsn w pedl cyc in traf, sequela
		V52.ØXXS	Driver of pk-up/van inj in clsn w 2/3-whl mv nontraf, sqla
		V52.1XXS	Pasngr in pk-up/van inj in clsn w 2/3-whl mv nontraf, sqla
		V52.2XXS	Prsn outsd pk-up/van inj in clsn w 2/3-whl mv nontraf, sqla
		V52.3XXS	Occup of pk-up/van inj in clsn w 2/3-whl mv nontraf, sequela
		V52.4XXS	Prsn brd/alit pk-up/van inj in clsn w 2/3-whl mv, sequela
		V52.5XXS	Driver of pk-up/van inj in clsn w 2/3-whl mv in traf, sqla
		V52.6XXS	Pasngr in pk-up/van inj in clsn w 2/3-whl mv in traf, sqla
		V52.7XXS	Prsn outsd pk-up/van inj in clsn w 2/3-whl mv in traf, sqla
		V52.9XXS	Occup of pk-up/van inj in clsn w 2/3-whl mv in traf, sequela
		V53.ØXXS	Driver of pk-up/van inj pk-up truck, pk-up/van nontraf, sqla
		V53.1XXS	Pasngr in pk-up/van inj pk-up truck, pk-up/van nontraf, sqla
		V53.2XXS	Prsn outsd pk-up/van inj pk-up truck,pk-up/van nontraf, sqla
		V53.3XXS	Occup of pk-up/van inj pk-up truck, pk-up/van nontraf, sqla
		V53.4XXS	Prsn brd/alit pk-up/van inj pk-up truck, pk-up/van, sequela
		V53.5XXS	Driver of pk-up/van inj pk-up truck, pk-up/van in traf, sqla
		V53.6XXS	Pasngr in pk-up/van inj pk-up truck, pk-up/van in traf, sqla
		V53.7XXS	Prsn outsd pk-up/van inj pk-up truck,pk-up/van in traf, sqla
		V53.9XXS	Occup of pk-up/van inj pk-up truck, pk-up/van in traf, sqla
		V54.ØXXS	Driver of pk-up/van inj in clsn w hv veh nontraf, sequela
		V54.1XXS	Pasngr in pk-up/van inj in clsn w hv veh nontraf, sequela
		V54.2XXS	Person outsd pk-up/van inj in clsn w hv veh nontraf, sequela
		V54.3XXS	Occup of pk-up/van injured in clsn w hv veh nontraf, sequela
		V54.4XXS	Prsn brd/alit pk-up/van injured in clsn w hv veh, sequela
		V54.5XXS	Driver of pk-up/van inj in clsn w hv veh in traf, sequela
		V54.6XXS	Pasngr in pk-up/van inj in clsn w hv veh in traf, sequela
		V54.7XXS	Person outsd pk-up/van inj in clsn w hv veh in traf, sequela
		V54.9XXS	Occup of pk-up/van injured in clsn w hv veh in traf, sequela
		V55.ØXXS	Driver of pk-up/van inj in clsn w rail trn/veh nontraf, sqla
		V55.1XXS	Pasngr in pk-up/van inj in clsn w rail trn/veh nontraf, sqla
		V55.2XXS	Prsn outsd pk-up/van inj in clsn w rail trn/veh nontraf,sqla
		V55.3XXS	Occup of pk-up/van inj in clsn w rail trn/veh nontraf, sqla
		V55.4XXS	Prsn brd/alit pk-up/van inj in clsn w rail trn/veh, sequela
		V55.5XXS	Driver of pk-up/van inj in clsn w rail trn/veh in traf, sqla
		V55.6XXS	Pasngr in pk-up/van inj in clsn w rail trn/veh in traf, sqla
		V55.7XXS	Prsn outsd pk-up/van inj in clsn w rail trn/veh in traf,sqla
		V55.9XXS	Occup of pk-up/van inj in clsn w rail trn/veh in traf, sqla
		V56.ØXXS	Driver of pk-up/van inj in clsn w nonmtr veh nontraf, sqla
		V56.1XXS	Pasngr in pk-up/van inj in clsn w nonmtr veh nontraf, sqla
		V56.2XXS	Prsn outsd pk-up/van inj in clsn w nonmtr veh nontraf, sqla
		V56.3XXS	Occup of pk-up/van inj in clsn w nonmtr veh nontraf, sqla
		V56.4XXS	Prsn brd/alit pk-up/van inj in clsn w nonmtr vehicle, sqla
		V56.5XXS	Driver of pk-up/van inj in clsn w nonmtr veh in traf, sqla
		V56.6XXS	Pasngr in pk-up/van inj in clsn w nonmtr veh in traf, sqla
		V56.7XXS	Prsn outsd pk-up/van inj in clsn w nonmtr veh in traf, sqla
		V56.9XXS	Occup of pk-up/van inj in clsn w nonmtr veh in traf, sqla
		V57.ØXXS	Drvr of pk-up/van inj in clsn w statnry object nontraf, sqla
		V57.1XXS	Pasngr in pk-up/van inj in clsn w statnry obj nontraf, sqla
		V57.2XXS	Prsn outsd pk-up/van inj in clsn w statnry obj nontraf, sqla
		V57.3XXS	Occup of pk-up/van inj in clsn w statnry obj nontraf, sqla
		V57.4XXS	Prsn brd/alit pk-up/van inj in clsn w statnry object, sqla
		V57.5XXS	Drvr of pk-up/van inj in clsn w statnry object in traf, sqla
		V57.6XXS	Pasngr in pk-up/van inj in clsn w statnry obj in traf, sqla
		V57.7XXS	Prsn outsd pk-up/van inj in clsn w statnry obj in traf, sqla
		V57.9XXS	Occup of pk-up/van inj in clsn w statnry obj in traf, sqla
		V58.ØXXS	Driver of pk-up/van inj in nonclsn trnsp acc nontraf, sqla
		V58.1XXS	Pasngr in pk-up/van inj in nonclsn trnsp acc nontraf, sqla
		V58.2XXS	Prsn outsd pk-up/van inj in nonclsn trnsp acc nontraf, sqla
		V58.3XXS	Occup of pk-up/van inj in nonclsn trnsp acc nontraf, sequela
		V58.4XXS	Prsn brd/alit pk-up/van inj in nonclsn trnsp acc, sequela
		V58.5XXS	Driver of pk-up/van inj in nonclsn trnsp acc in traf, sqla
		V58.6XXS	Pasngr in pk-up/van inj in nonclsn trnsp acc in traf, sqla
		V58.7XXS	Prsn outsd pk-up/van inj in nonclsn trnsp acc in traf, sqla
		V58.9XXS	Occup of pk-up/van inj in nonclsn trnsp acc in traf, sequela
		V59.ØØXS	Driver of pk-up/van inj in clsn w unsp mv nontraf, sequela
		V59.Ø9XS	Driver of pk-up/van inj in clsn w oth mv nontraf, sequela
		V59.1ØXS	Pasngr in pk-up/van inj in clsn w unsp mv nontraf, sequela
		V59.19XS	Pasngr in pk-up/van inj in clsn w oth mv nontraf, sequela
		V59.2ØXS	Occup of pk-up/van inj in clsn w unsp mv nontraf, sequela
		V59.29XS	Occup of pk-up/van injured in clsn w oth mv nontraf, sequela
	(Continued on next page)	**V59.3XXS**	Occupant of pk-up/van injured in unsp nontraf, sequela

ICD-9-CM		ICD-10-CM	
E929.Ø	LATE EFFECTS OF MOTOR VEHICLE ACCIDENT **(Continued)**	**V59.4ØXS**	Driver of pk-up/van inj in clsn w unsp mv in traf, sequela
		V59.49XS	Driver of pk-up/van inj in clsn w oth mv in traf, sequela
		V59.5ØXS	Pasngr in pk-up/van inj in clsn w unsp mv in traf, sequela
		V59.59XS	Pasngr in pk-up/van inj in clsn w oth mv in traf, sequela
		V59.6ØXS	Occup of pk-up/van inj in clsn w unsp mv in traf, sequela
		V59.69XS	Occup of pk-up/van injured in clsn w oth mv in traf, sequela
		V59.81XS	Occ of pk-up/van inj in trnsp acc w miltry vehicle, sequela
		V59.88XS	Occupant of pk-up/van injured in oth trnsp acc, sequela
		V59.9XXS	Occupant (driver) of pk-up/van injured in unsp traf, sequela
		V6Ø.ØXXS	Driver of hv veh injured in clsn w ped/anml nontraf, sequela
		V6Ø.1XXS	Pasngr in hv veh injured in clsn w ped/anml nontraf, sequela
		V6Ø.2XXS	Person outsd hv veh inj in clsn w ped/anml nontraf, sequela
		V6Ø.3XXS	Occup of hv veh injured in clsn w ped/anml nontraf, sequela
		V6Ø.4XXS	Prsn brd/alit hv veh injured in clsn w ped/anml, sequela
		V6Ø.5XXS	Driver of hv veh injured in clsn w ped/anml in traf, sequela
		V6Ø.6XXS	Pasngr in hv veh injured in clsn w ped/anml in traf, sequela
		V6Ø.7XXS	Person outsd hv veh inj in clsn w ped/anml in traf, sequela
		V6Ø.9XXS	Occup of hv veh injured in clsn w ped/anml in traf, sequela
		V61.ØXXS	Driver of hv veh injured in clsn w pedl cyc nontraf, sequela
		V61.1XXS	Pasngr in hv veh injured in clsn w pedl cyc nontraf, sequela
		V61.2XXS	Person outsd hv veh inj in clsn w pedl cyc nontraf, sequela
		V61.3XXS	Occup of hv veh injured in clsn w pedl cyc nontraf, sequela
		V61.4XXS	Prsn brd/alit hv veh inj in clsn w pedl cyc wh brd/alit,sqla
		V61.5XXS	Driver of hv veh injured in clsn w pedl cyc in traf, sequela
		V61.6XXS	Pasngr in hv veh injured in clsn w pedl cyc in traf, sequela
		V61.7XXS	Person outsd hv veh inj in clsn w pedl cyc in traf, sequela
		V61.9XXS	Occup of hv veh injured in clsn w pedl cyc in traf, sequela
		V62.ØXXS	Driver of hv veh inj in clsn w 2/3-whl mv nontraf, sequela
		V62.1XXS	Pasngr in hv veh inj in clsn w 2/3-whl mv nontraf, sequela
		V62.2XXS	Person outsd hv veh inj in clsn w 2/3-whl mv nontraf, sqla
		V62.3XXS	Occup of hv veh inj in clsn w 2/3-whl mv nontraf, sequela
		V62.4XXS	Prsn brd/alit hv veh injured in clsn w 2/3-whl mv, sequela
		V62.5XXS	Driver of hv veh inj in clsn w 2/3-whl mv in traf, sequela
		V62.6XXS	Pasngr in hv veh inj in clsn w 2/3-whl mv in traf, sequela
		V62.7XXS	Person outsd hv veh inj in clsn w 2/3-whl mv in traf, sqla
		V62.9XXS	Occup of hv veh inj in clsn w 2/3-whl mv in traf, sequela
		V63.ØXXS	Driver of hv veh inj pk-up truck, pk-up/van nontraf, sequela
		V63.1XXS	Pasngr in hv veh inj pk-up truck, pk-up/van nontraf, sequela
		V63.2XXS	Person outsd hv veh inj pk-up truck, pk-up/van nontraf, sqla
		V63.3XXS	Occup of hv veh inj pk-up truck, pk-up/van nontraf, sequela
		V63.4XXS	Prsn brd/alit hv veh inj pick-up truck, pk-up/van, sequela
		V63.5XXS	Driver of hv veh inj pk-up truck, pk-up/van in traf, sequela
		V63.6XXS	Pasngr in hv veh inj pk-up truck, pk-up/van in traf, sequela
		V63.7XXS	Person outsd hv veh inj pk-up truck, pk-up/van in traf, sqla
		V63.9XXS	Occup of hv veh inj pk-up truck, pk-up/van in traf, sequela
		V64.ØXXS	Driver of hv veh injured in clsn w hv veh nontraf, sequela
		V64.1XXS	Pasngr in hv veh injured in clsn w hv veh nontraf, sequela
		V64.2XXS	Person outside hv veh inj in clsn w hv veh nontraf, sequela
		V64.3XXS	Occup of hv veh injured in clsn w hv veh nontraf, sequela
		V64.4XXS	Prsn brd/alit hv veh inj in clsn w hv veh wh brd/alit, sqla
		V64.5XXS	Driver of hv veh injured in clsn w hv veh in traf, sequela
		V64.6XXS	Pasngr in hv veh injured in clsn w hv veh in traf, sequela
		V64.7XXS	Person outside hv veh inj in clsn w hv veh in traf, sequela
		V64.9XXS	Occup of hv veh injured in clsn w hv veh in traf, sequela
		V65.ØXXS	Driver of hv veh inj in clsn w rail trn/veh nontraf, sequela
		V65.1XXS	Pasngr in hv veh inj in clsn w rail trn/veh nontraf, sequela
		V65.2XXS	Person outsd hv veh inj in clsn w rail trn/veh nontraf, sqla
		V65.3XXS	Occup of hv veh inj in clsn w rail trn/veh nontraf, sequela
		V65.4XXS	Prsn brd/alit hv veh injured in clsn w rail trn/veh, sequela
		V65.5XXS	Driver of hv veh inj in clsn w rail trn/veh in traf, sequela
		V65.6XXS	Pasngr in hv veh inj in clsn w rail trn/veh in traf, sequela
		V65.7XXS	Person outsd hv veh inj in clsn w rail trn/veh in traf, sqla
		V65.9XXS	Occup of hv veh inj in clsn w rail trn/veh in traf, sequela
		V66.ØXXS	Driver of hv veh inj in clsn w nonmtr vehicle nontraf, sqla
		V66.1XXS	Pasngr in hv veh inj in clsn w nonmtr vehicle nontraf, sqla
		V66.2XXS	Person outsd hv veh inj in clsn w nonmtr veh nontraf, sqla
		V66.3XXS	Occup of hv veh inj in clsn w nonmtr vehicle nontraf, sqla
		V66.4XXS	Prsn brd/alit hv veh inj in clsn w nonmtr vehicle, sequela
		V66.5XXS	Driver of hv veh inj in clsn w nonmtr vehicle in traf, sqla
		V66.6XXS	Pasngr in hv veh inj in clsn w nonmtr vehicle in traf, sqla
		V66.7XXS	Person outsd hv veh inj in clsn w nonmtr veh in traf, sqla
		V66.9XXS	Occup of hv veh inj in clsn w nonmtr vehicle in traf, sqla
		V67.ØXXS	Driver of hv veh inj in clsn w statnry object nontraf, sqla
		V67.1XXS	Pasngr in hv veh inj in clsn w statnry object nontraf, sqla
		V67.2XXS	Person outsd hv veh inj in clsn w statnry obj nontraf, sqla
		V67.3XXS	Occup of hv veh inj in clsn w statnry object nontraf, sqla
		V67.4XXS	Prsn brd/alit hv veh inj in clsn w statnry object, sequela
		V67.5XXS	Driver of hv veh inj in clsn w statnry object in traf, sqla
		V67.6XXS	Pasngr in hv veh inj in clsn w statnry object in traf, sqla
		V67.7XXS	Person outsd hv veh inj in clsn w statnry obj in traf, sqla
		V67.9XXS	Occup of hv veh inj in clsn w statnry object in traf, sqla
		V68.ØXXS	Driver of hv veh inj in nonclsn trnsp acc nontraf, sequela
	(Continued on next page)	**V68.1XXS**	Pasngr in hv veh inj in nonclsn trnsp acc nontraf, sequela

ICD-9-CM		ICD-10-CM	
E929.Ø	LATE EFFECTS OF MOTOR VEHICLE ACCIDENT **(Continued)**	**V68.2XXS**	Person outsd hv veh inj in nonclsn trnsp acc nontraf, sqla
		V68.3XXS	Occup of hv veh inj in nonclsn trnsp acc nontraf, sequela
		V68.4XXS	Prsn brd/alit hv veh injured in nonclsn trnsp acc, sequela
		V68.5XXS	Driver of hv veh inj in nonclsn trnsp acc in traf, sequela
		V68.6XXS	Pasngr in hv veh inj in nonclsn trnsp acc in traf, sequela
		V68.7XXS	Person outsd hv veh inj in nonclsn trnsp acc in traf, sqla
		V68.9XXS	Occup of hv veh inj in nonclsn trnsp acc in traf, sequela
		V69.ØØXS	Driver of hv veh injured in clsn w unsp mv nontraf, sequela
		V69.Ø9XS	Driver of hv veh injured in clsn w oth mv nontraf, sequela
		V69.1ØXS	Pasngr in hv veh injured in clsn w unsp mv nontraf, sequela
		V69.19XS	Pasngr in hv veh injured in clsn w oth mv nontraf, sequela
		V69.2ØXS	Occup of hv veh injured in clsn w unsp mv nontraf, sequela
		V69.29XS	Occup of hv veh injured in clsn w oth mv nontraf, sequela
		V69.3XXS	Occupant (driver) of hv veh injured in unsp nontraf, sequela
		V69.4ØXS	Driver of hv veh injured in clsn w unsp mv in traf, sequela
		V69.49XS	Driver of hv veh injured in clsn w oth mv in traf, sequela
		V69.5ØXS	Pasngr in hv veh injured in clsn w unsp mv in traf, sequela
		V69.59XS	Pasngr in hv veh injured in clsn w oth mv in traf, sequela
		V69.6ØXS	Occup of hv veh injured in clsn w unsp mv in traf, sequela
		V69.69XS	Occup of hv veh injured in clsn w oth mv in traf, sequela
		V69.81XS	Occ of hv veh injured in trnsp acc w miltry vehicle, sequela
		V69.88XS	Occupant of hv veh injured in oth trnsp acc, sequela
		V69.9XXS	Occupant (driver) of hv veh injured in unsp traf, sequela
		V7Ø.ØXXS	Driver of bus injured in clsn w ped/anml nontraf, sequela
		V7Ø.1XXS	Passenger on bus injured in clsn w ped/anml nontraf, sequela
		V7Ø.2XXS	Person outside bus inj in clsn w ped/anml nontraf, sequela
		V7Ø.3XXS	Occup of bus injured in clsn w ped/anml nontraf, sequela
		V7Ø.4XXS	Prsn brd/alit from bus injured in clsn w ped/anml, sequela
		V7Ø.5XXS	Driver of bus injured in clsn w ped/anml in traf, sequela
		V7Ø.6XXS	Passenger on bus injured in clsn w ped/anml in traf, sequela
		V7Ø.7XXS	Person outside bus inj in clsn w ped/anml in traf, sequela
		V7Ø.9XXS	Occup of bus injured in clsn w ped/anml in traf, sequela
		V71.ØXXS	Driver of bus injured in clsn w pedl cyc nontraf, sequela
		V71.1XXS	Passenger on bus injured in clsn w pedl cyc nontraf, sequela
		V71.2XXS	Person outside bus inj in clsn w pedl cyc nontraf, sequela
		V71.3XXS	Occup of bus injured in clsn w pedl cyc nontraf, sequela
		V71.4XXS	Prsn brd/alit from bus injured in clsn w pedl cyc, sequela
		V71.5XXS	Driver of bus injured in clsn w pedl cyc in traf, sequela
		V71.6XXS	Passenger on bus injured in clsn w pedl cyc in traf, sequela
		V71.7XXS	Person outside bus inj in clsn w pedl cyc in traf, sequela
		V71.9XXS	Occup of bus injured in clsn w pedl cyc in traf, sequela
		V72.ØXXS	Driver of bus injured in clsn w 2/3-whl mv nontraf, sequela
		V72.1XXS	Pasngr on bus injured in clsn w 2/3-whl mv nontraf, sequela
		V72.2XXS	Person outside bus inj in clsn w 2/3-whl mv nontraf, sequela
		V72.3XXS	Occup of bus injured in clsn w 2/3-whl mv nontraf, sequela
		V72.4XXS	Prsn brd/alit from bus injured in clsn w 2/3-whl mv, sequela
		V72.5XXS	Driver of bus injured in clsn w 2/3-whl mv in traf, sequela
		V72.6XXS	Pasngr on bus injured in clsn w 2/3-whl mv in traf, sequela
		V72.7XXS	Person outside bus inj in clsn w 2/3-whl mv in traf, sequela
		V72.9XXS	Occup of bus injured in clsn w 2/3-whl mv in traf, sequela
		V73.ØXXS	Driver of bus inj pick-up truck, pk-up/van nontraf, sequela
		V73.1XXS	Pasngr on bus inj pick-up truck, pk-up/van nontraf, sequela
		V73.2XXS	Person outsd bus inj pk-up truck, pk-up/van nontraf, sequela
		V73.3XXS	Occup of bus inj pick-up truck, pk-up/van nontraf, sequela
		V73.4XXS	Prsn brd/alit from bus inj pick-up truck, pk-up/van, sequela
		V73.5XXS	Driver of bus inj pick-up truck, pk-up/van in traf, sequela
		V73.6XXS	Pasngr on bus inj pick-up truck, pk-up/van in traf, sequela
		V73.7XXS	Person outsd bus inj pk-up truck, pk-up/van in traf, sequela
		V73.9XXS	Occup of bus inj pick-up truck, pk-up/van in traf, sequela
		V74.ØXXS	Driver of bus injured in collision w hv veh nontraf, sequela
		V74.1XXS	Passenger on bus injured in clsn w hv veh nontraf, sequela
		V74.2XXS	Person outside bus injured in clsn w hv veh nontraf, sequela
		V74.3XXS	Occup of bus injured in collision w hv veh nontraf, sequela
		V74.4XXS	Prsn brd/alit from bus injured in clsn w hv veh, sequela
		V74.5XXS	Driver of bus injured in collision w hv veh in traf, sequela
		V74.6XXS	Passenger on bus injured in clsn w hv veh in traf, sequela
		V74.7XXS	Person outside bus injured in clsn w hv veh in traf, sequela
		V74.9XXS	Occup of bus injured in collision w hv veh in traf, sequela
		V75.ØXXS	Driver of bus inj in clsn w rail trn/veh nontraf, sequela
		V75.1XXS	Pasngr on bus inj in clsn w rail trn/veh nontraf, sequela
		V75.2XXS	Person outsd bus inj in clsn w rail trn/veh nontraf, sequela
		V75.3XXS	Occup of bus injured in clsn w rail trn/veh nontraf, sequela
		V75.4XXS	Prsn brd/alit from bus inj in clsn w rail trn/veh, sequela
		V75.5XXS	Driver of bus inj in clsn w rail trn/veh in traf, sequela
		V75.6XXS	Pasngr on bus inj in clsn w rail trn/veh in traf, sequela
		V75.7XXS	Person outsd bus inj in clsn w rail trn/veh in traf, sequela
		V75.9XXS	Occup of bus injured in clsn w rail trn/veh in traf, sequela
		V76.ØXXS	Driver of bus inj in clsn w nonmtr vehicle nontraf, sequela
		V76.1XXS	Pasngr on bus inj in clsn w nonmtr vehicle nontraf, sequela
		V76.2XXS	Person outsd bus inj in clsn w nonmtr vehicle nontraf, sqla
		V76.3XXS	Occup of bus inj in clsn w nonmtr vehicle nontraf, sequela
		V76.4XXS	Prsn brd/alit from bus inj in clsn w nonmtr vehicle, sequela
	(Continued on next page)	**V76.5XXS**	Driver of bus inj in clsn w nonmtr vehicle in traf, sequela

ICD-9-CM		ICD-10-CM	
E929.Ø	LATE EFFECTS OF MOTOR VEHICLE ACCIDENT **(Continued)**	**V76.6XXS**	Pasngr on bus inj in clsn w nonmtr vehicle in traf, sequela
		V76.7XXS	Person outsd bus inj in clsn w nonmtr vehicle in traf, sqla
		V76.9XXS	Occup of bus inj in clsn w nonmtr vehicle in traf, sequela
		V77.ØXXS	Driver of bus inj in clsn w statnry object nontraf, sequela
		V77.1XXS	Pasngr on bus inj in clsn w statnry object nontraf, sequela
		V77.2XXS	Person outsd bus inj in clsn w statnry object nontraf, sqla
		V77.3XXS	Occup of bus inj in clsn w statnry object nontraf, sequela
		V77.4XXS	Prsn brd/alit from bus inj in clsn w statnry object, sequela
		V77.5XXS	Driver of bus inj in clsn w statnry object in traf, sequela
		V77.6XXS	Pasngr on bus inj in clsn w statnry object in traf, sequela
		V77.7XXS	Person outsd bus inj in clsn w statnry object in traf, sqla
		V77.9XXS	Occup of bus inj in clsn w statnry object in traf, sequela
		V78.ØXXS	Driver of bus injured in nonclsn trnsp acc nontraf, sequela
		V78.1XXS	Pasngr on bus injured in nonclsn trnsp acc nontraf, sequela
		V78.2XXS	Person outside bus inj in nonclsn trnsp acc nontraf, sequela
		V78.3XXS	Occup of bus injured in nonclsn trnsp acc nontraf, sequela
		V78.4XXS	Prsn brd/alit from bus injured in nonclsn trnsp acc, sequela
		V78.5XXS	Driver of bus injured in nonclsn trnsp acc in traf, sequela
		V78.6XXS	Pasngr on bus injured in nonclsn trnsp acc in traf, sequela
		V78.7XXS	Person outside bus inj in nonclsn trnsp acc in traf, sequela
		V78.9XXS	Occup of bus injured in nonclsn trnsp acc in traf, sequela
		V79.ØØXS	Driver of bus injured in clsn w unsp mv nontraf, sequela
		V79.Ø9XS	Driver of bus injured in collision w oth mv nontraf, sequela
		V79.1ØXS	Passenger on bus injured in clsn w unsp mv nontraf, sequela
		V79.19XS	Passenger on bus injured in clsn w oth mv nontraf, sequela
		V79.2ØXS	Unsp bus occupant injured in clsn w unsp mv nontraf, sequela
		V79.29XS	Unsp bus occupant injured in clsn w oth mv nontraf, sequela
		V79.3XXS	Bus occupant (driver) injured in unsp nontraf, sequela
		V79.4ØXS	Driver of bus injured in clsn w unsp mv in traf, sequela
		V79.49XS	Driver of bus injured in collision w oth mv in traf, sequela
		V79.5ØXS	Passenger on bus injured in clsn w unsp mv in traf, sequela
		V79.59XS	Passenger on bus injured in clsn w oth mv in traf, sequela
		V79.6ØXS	Unsp bus occupant injured in clsn w unsp mv in traf, sequela
		V79.69XS	Unsp bus occupant injured in clsn w oth mv in traf, sequela
		V79.81XS	Bus occupant injured in trnsp acc w miltry vehicle, sequela
		V79.88XS	Bus occupant (driver) injured in oth transport acc, sequela
		V79.9XXS	Bus occupant (driver) injured in unsp traf, sequela
		V8Ø.31XS	Animal-rider injured in collision w 2/3-whl mv, sequela
		V8Ø.32XS	Occ of anml-drn vehicle inj in clsn w 2/3-whl mv, sequela
		V8Ø.41XS	Animl-ridr inj pk-up truck, pk-up truck, van, hv veh, sqla
		V8Ø.42XS	Occ animal-drwn veh injured collision hvy veh, sequela
		V8Ø.51XS	Animal-rider injured in collision w mtr veh, sequela
		V8Ø.52XS	Occ of anml-drn vehicle injured in clsn w mtr veh, sequela
		V81.ØXXS	Occ of rail trn/veh inj in clsn w mtr veh nontraf, sequela
		V81.1XXS	Occ of rail trn/veh inj in clsn w mtr veh in traf, sequela
		V82.ØXXS	Occupant of stcar injured in clsn w mtr veh nontraf, sequela
		V82.1XXS	Occupant of stcar injured in clsn w mtr veh in traf, sequela
		V84.ØXXS	Driver of special agri vehicle injured in traf, sequela
		V84.1XXS	Passenger of special agri vehicle injured in traf, sequela
		V84.2XXS	Person outside special agri vehicle injured in traf, sequela
		V84.3XXS	Occup of special agri vehicle injured in traf, sequela
		V84.4XXS	Person inj wh brd/alit from special agri vehicle, sequela
		V84.5XXS	Driver of special agri vehicle injured nontraf, sequela
		V84.6XXS	Passenger of special agri vehicle injured nontraf, sequela
		V84.7XXS	Person outside special agri vehicle injured nontraf, sequela
		V84.9XXS	Occup of special agri vehicle injured nontraf, sequela
		V85.ØXXS	Driver of special construct vehicle injured in traf, sequela
		V85.1XXS	Pasngr of special construct vehicle injured in traf, sequela
		V85.2XXS	Person outsd special construct vehicle inj in traf, sequela
		V85.3XXS	Occup of special construct vehicle injured in traf, sequela
		V85.4XXS	Person inj wh brd/alit from special construct vehicle, sqla
		V85.5XXS	Driver of special construct vehicle injured nontraf, sequela
		V85.6XXS	Pasngr of special construct vehicle injured nontraf, sequela
		V85.7XXS	Person outsd special construct vehicle inj nontraf, sequela
		V85.9XXS	Occup of special construct vehicle injured nontraf, sequela
		V86.Ø1XS	Driver of amblnc/fire eng injured in traf, sequela
		V86.Ø2XS	Driver of snowmobile injured in traffic accident, sequela
		V86.Ø3XS	Driver of dune buggy injured in traffic accident, sequela
		V86.Ø4XS	Driver of military vehicle injured in traf, sequela
		V86.Ø9XS	Driver of sp off-rd mv injured in traffic accident, sequela
		V86.11XS	Passenger of amblnc/fire eng injured in traf, sequela
		V86.12XS	Passenger of snowmobile injured in traffic accident, sequela
		V86.13XS	Passenger of dune buggy injured in traffic accident, sequela
		V86.14XS	Passenger of military vehicle injured in traf, sequela
		V86.19XS	Passenger of sp off-rd mv injured in traf, sequela
		V86.21XS	Person outside amblnc/fire eng injured in traf, sequela
		V86.22XS	Person on outside of snowmobile injured in traf, sequela
		V86.23XS	Person on outside of dune buggy injured in traf, sequela
		V86.24XS	Person outside military vehicle injured in traf, sequela
		V86.29XS	Person on outside of sp off-rd mv injured in traf, sequela
		V86.31XS	Occup of amblnc/fire eng injured in traf, sequela
		V86.32XS	Occup of snowmobile injured in traffic accident, sequela
	(Continued on next page)	**V86.33XS**	Occup of dune buggy injured in traffic accident, sequela

ICD-9-CM		ICD-10-CM	
E929.Ø	LATE EFFECTS OF MOTOR VEHICLE ACCIDENT **(Continued)**	**V86.34XS**	Occup of military vehicle injured in traf, sequela
		V86.39XS	Occup of sp off-rd mv injured in traffic accident, sequela
		V86.41XS	Person injured wh brd/alit from amblnc/fire eng, sequela
		V86.42XS	Person injured wh brd/alit from snowmobile, sequela
		V86.43XS	Person injured wh brd/alit from dune buggy, sequela
		V86.44XS	Person injured wh brd/alit from military vehicle, sequela
		V86.49XS	Person injured wh brd/alit from oth sp off-rd mv, sequela
		V86.51XS	Driver of amblnc/fire eng injured nontraf, sequela
		V86.52XS	Driver of snowmobile injured in nontraffic accident, sequela
		V86.53XS	Driver of dune buggy injured in nontraffic accident, sequela
		V86.54XS	Driver of military vehicle injured nontraf, sequela
		V86.59XS	Driver of sp off-rd mv injured nontraf, sequela
		V86.61XS	Passenger of amblnc/fire eng injured nontraf, sequela
		V86.62XS	Passenger of snowmobile injured nontraf, sequela
		V86.63XS	Passenger of dune buggy injured nontraf, sequela
		V86.64XS	Passenger of military vehicle injured nontraf, sequela
		V86.69XS	Passenger of sp off-rd mv injured nontraf, sequela
		V86.71XS	Person outside amblnc/fire eng injured nontraf, sequela
		V86.72XS	Person on outside of snowmobile injured nontraf, sequela
		V86.73XS	Person on outside of dune buggy injured nontraf, sequela
		V86.74XS	Person outside military vehicle injured nontraf, sequela
		V86.79XS	Person on outside of sp off-rd mv injured nontraf, sequela
		V86.91XS	Occup of amblnc/fire eng injured nontraf, sequela
		V86.92XS	Occup of snowmobile injured in nontraffic accident, sequela
		V86.93XS	Occup of dune buggy injured in nontraffic accident, sequela
		V86.94XS	Occup of military vehicle injured nontraf, sequela
		V86.99XS	Occup of sp off-rd mv injured nontraf, sequela
		V87.ØXXS	Person inj in clsn betw car and 2/3-whl pwr veh, sequela
		V87.1XXS	Person injured in clsn betw mtr veh and 2/3-whl mv, sequela
		V87.2XXS	Person injured in collision betw car and pk-up/van, sequela
		V87.3XXS	Person injured in collision betw car and bus, sequela
		V87.4XXS	Person injured in collision betw car and hv veh, sequela
		V87.5XXS	Person injured in collision betw hv veh and bus, sequela
		V87.6XXS	Person injured in clsn betw rail trn/veh and car, sequela
		V87.7XXS	Person injured in collision betw oth mtr veh, sequela
		V87.8XXS	Person injured in oth nonclsn trnsp acc w mtr veh, sequela
		V87.9XXS	Person injured in oth transport acc w non-mv, sequela
		V88.ØXXS	Person inj in clsn betw car and 2/3-whl mv, nontraf, sequela
		V88.1XXS	Prsn inj in clsn betw mtr veh and 2/3-whl mv, nontraf, sqla
		V88.2XXS	Person inj in clsn betw car and pk-up/van, nontraf, sequela
		V88.3XXS	Person injured in clsn betw car and bus, nontraf, sequela
		V88.4XXS	Person injured in clsn betw car and hv veh, nontraf, sequela
		V88.5XXS	Person injured in clsn betw hv veh and bus, nontraf, sequela
		V88.6XXS	Person inj in clsn betw rail trn/veh and car, nontraf, sqla
		V88.7XXS	Person injured in collision betw mtr veh, nontraf, sequela
		V88.8XXS	Person inj in oth nonclsn trnsp acc w mtr veh, nontraf, sqla
		V89.ØXXS	Person injured in unsp motor-vehicle acc, nontraf, sequela
		V89.2XXS	Person injured in unsp motor-vehicle acc, traffic, sequela
		V89.3XXS	Person inj in unsp nonmotor-vehicle acc, traffic, sequela
		V89.9XXS	Person injured in unspecified vehicle accident, sequela
E929.1	LATE EFFECTS OF OTHER TRANSPORT ACCIDENT	**VØ1.ØØXS**	Ped on foot injured in collision w pedl cyc nontraf, sequela
		VØ1.Ø1XS	Ped on rolr-skt injured in clsn w pedl cyc nontraf, sequela
		VØ1.Ø2XS	Ped on sktbrd injured in clsn w pedl cyc nontraf, sequela
		VØ1.Ø9XS	Ped w convey injured in clsn w pedl cyc nontraf, sequela
		VØ1.1ØXS	Ped on foot injured in collision w pedl cyc in traf, sequela
		VØ1.11XS	Ped on rolr-skt injured in clsn w pedl cyc in traf, sequela
		VØ1.12XS	Ped on sktbrd injured in clsn w pedl cyc in traf, sequela
		VØ1.19XS	Ped w convey injured in clsn w pedl cyc in traf, sequela
		VØ1.9ØXS	Ped on foot injured in collision w pedl cyc, unsp, sequela
		VØ1.91XS	Ped on rolr-skt injured in clsn w pedl cyc, unsp, sequela
		VØ1.92XS	Ped on sktbrd injured in collision w pedl cyc, unsp, sequela
		VØ1.99XS	Ped w convey injured in collision w pedl cyc, unsp, sequela
		VØ5.ØØXS	Ped on foot injured in clsn w rail trn/veh nontraf, sequela
		VØ5.Ø1XS	Ped on rolr-skt inj in clsn w rail trn/veh nontraf, sequela
		VØ5.Ø2XS	Ped on sktbrd inj in clsn w rail trn/veh nontraf, sequela
		VØ5.Ø9XS	Ped w convey injured in clsn w rail trn/veh nontraf, sequela
		VØ5.9ØXS	Ped on foot injured in clsn w rail trn/veh, unsp, sequela
		VØ5.91XS	Ped on rolr-skt inj in clsn w rail trn/veh, unsp, sequela
		VØ5.92XS	Ped on sktbrd injured in clsn w rail trn/veh, unsp, sequela
		VØ5.99XS	Ped w convey injured in clsn w rail trn/veh, unsp, sequela
		VØ6.ØØXS	Ped on foot inj in clsn w nonmtr vehicle nontraf, sequela
		VØ6.Ø1XS	Ped on rolr-skt inj in clsn w nonmtr vehicle nontraf, sqla
		VØ6.Ø2XS	Ped on sktbrd inj in clsn w nonmtr vehicle nontraf, sequela
		VØ6.Ø9XS	Ped w convey inj in clsn w nonmtr vehicle nontraf, sequela
		VØ6.1ØXS	Ped on foot inj in clsn w nonmtr vehicle in traf, sequela
		VØ6.11XS	Ped on rolr-skt inj in clsn w nonmtr vehicle in traf, sqla
		VØ6.12XS	Ped on sktbrd inj in clsn w nonmtr vehicle in traf, sequela
		VØ6.19XS	Ped w convey inj in clsn w nonmtr vehicle in traf, sequela
		VØ6.9ØXS	Ped on foot injured in clsn w nonmtr vehicle, unsp, sequela
		VØ6.91XS	Ped on rolr-skt inj in clsn w nonmtr vehicle, unsp, sequela
		VØ6.92XS	Ped on sktbrd inj in clsn w nonmtr vehicle, unsp, sequela
		VØ6.99XS	Ped w convey injured in clsn w nonmtr vehicle, unsp, sequela
	(Continued on next page)	**VØ9.1XXS**	Pedestrian injured in unsp nontraffic accident, sequela

ICD-9-CM		ICD-10-CM	
E929.1	LATE EFFECTS OF OTHER TRANSPORT ACCIDENT **(Continued)**	**V09.3XXS**	Pedestrian injured in unspecified traffic accident, sequela
		V09.9XXS	Pedestrian injured in unsp transport accident, sequela
		V10.0XXS	Pedl cyc driver injured in clsn w ped/anml nontraf, sequela
		V10.1XXS	Pedl cyc pasngr injured in clsn w ped/anml nontraf, sequela
		V10.2XXS	Unsp pedl cyclst injured in clsn w ped/anml nontraf, sequela
		V10.3XXS	Prsn brd/alit pedl cyc injured in clsn w ped/anml, sequela
		V10.4XXS	Pedl cyc driver injured in clsn w ped/anml in traf, sequela
		V10.5XXS	Pedl cyc pasngr injured in clsn w ped/anml in traf, sequela
		V10.9XXS	Unsp pedl cyclst injured in clsn w ped/anml in traf, sequela
		V11.0XXS	Pedl cyc driver inj in clsn w oth pedl cyc nontraf, sequela
		V11.1XXS	Pedl cyc pasngr inj in clsn w oth pedl cyc nontraf, sequela
		V11.2XXS	Unsp pedl cyclst inj in clsn w oth pedl cyc nontraf, sequela
		V11.3XXS	Prsn brd/alit pedl cyc inj in clsn w oth pedl cyc, sequela
		V11.4XXS	Pedl cyc driver inj in clsn w oth pedl cyc in traf, sequela
		V11.5XXS	Pedl cyc pasngr inj in clsn w oth pedl cyc in traf, sequela
		V11.9XXS	Unsp pedl cyclst inj in clsn w oth pedl cyc in traf, sequela
		V15.2XXS	Unsp pedl cyclst inj in clsn w rail trn/veh nontraf, sequela
		V15.3XXS	Prsn brd/alit pedl cyc inj in clsn w rail trn/veh, sequela
		V15.4XXS	Pedl cyc driver inj in clsn w rail trn/veh in traf, sequela
		V15.5XXS	Pedl cyc pasngr inj in clsn w rail trn/veh in traf, sequela
		V15.9XXS	Unsp pedl cyclst inj in clsn w rail trn/veh in traf, sequela
		V16.0XXS	Pedl cyc driver inj in clsn w nonmtr vehicle nontraf, sqla
		V16.1XXS	Pedl cyc pasngr inj in clsn w nonmtr vehicle nontraf, sqla
		V16.2XXS	Unsp pedl cyclst inj in clsn w nonmtr vehicle nontraf, sqla
		V16.3XXS	Prsn brd/alit pedl cyc inj in clsn w nonmtr veh nontraf,sqla
		V16.4XXS	Pedl cyc driver inj in clsn w nonmtr vehicle in traf, sqla
		V16.5XXS	Pedl cyc pasngr inj in clsn w nonmtr vehicle in traf, sqla
		V16.9XXS	Unsp pedl cyclst inj in clsn w nonmtr vehicle in traf, sqla
		V17.0XXS	Pedl cyc driver inj in clsn w statnry object nontraf, sqla
		V17.1XXS	Pedl cyc pasngr inj in clsn w statnry object nontraf, sqla
		V17.2XXS	Unsp pedl cyclst inj in clsn w statnry object nontraf, sqla
		V17.3XXS	Prsn brd/alit pedl cyc inj in clsn w statnry object, sequela
		V17.4XXS	Pedl cyc driver inj in clsn w statnry object in traf, sqla
		V17.5XXS	Pedl cyc pasngr inj in clsn w statnry object in traf, sqla
		V17.9XXS	Unsp pedl cyclst inj in clsn w statnry object in traf, sqla
		V18.0XXS	Pedl cyc driver inj in nonclsn trnsp acc nontraf, sequela
		V18.1XXS	Pedl cyc pasngr inj in nonclsn trnsp acc nontraf, sequela
		V18.2XXS	Unsp pedl cyclst inj in nonclsn trnsp acc nontraf, sequela
		V18.3XXS	Prsn brd/alit pedl cyc injured in nonclsn trnsp acc, sequela
		V18.4XXS	Pedl cyc driver inj in nonclsn trnsp acc in traf, sequela
		V18.5XXS	Pedl cyc pasngr inj in nonclsn trnsp acc in traf, sequela
		V18.9XXS	Unsp pedl cyclst inj in nonclsn trnsp acc in traf, sequela
		V19.3XXS	Pedl cyclst (driver) injured in unsp nontraf, sequela
		V19.88XS	Pedl cyclst (driver) injured in oth transport acc, sequela
		V19.9XXS	Pedl cyclst (driver) injured in unsp traf, sequela
		V80.010S	Animl-ridr injured by fall fr horse in nonclsn acc, sequela
		V80.018S	Animl-ridr injured by fall fr animl in nonclsn acc, sequela
		V80.02XS	Occ of anml-drn veh inj by fall fr veh in nonclsn acc, sqla
		V80.11XS	Animal-rider injured in collision w ped/anml, sequela
		V80.12XS	Occ of anml-drn vehicle injured in clsn w ped/anml, sequela
		V80.21XS	Animal-rider injured in collision with pedal cycle, sequela
		V80.22XS	Occ of anml-drn vehicle injured in clsn w pedl cyc, sequela
		V80.61XS	Animal-rider injured in collision w rail trn/veh, sequela
		V80.62XS	Occ of anml-drn vehicle inj in clsn w rail trn/veh, sequela
		V80.710S	Animl-ridr injured in clsn w animl being ridden, sequela
		V80.711S	Occ of anml-drn veh inj in clsn w animal being ridden, sqla
		V80.720S	Animl-ridr injured in collision w anml-drn vehicle, sequela
		V80.721S	Occ of anml-drn vehicle inj in collisn with same, sequela
		V80.730S	Animal-rider injured in collision with streetcar, sequela
		V80.731S	Occ of anml-drn vehicle injured in clsn w stcar, sequela
		V80.790S	Animal-rider injured in collision w nonmtr vehicles, sequela
		V80.791S	Occ of anml-drn vehicle inj in clsn w nonmtr veh, sequela
		V80.81XS	Animal-rider injured in collision w statnry object, sequela
		V80.82XS	Occ of anml-drn vehicle inj in clsn w statnry object, sqla
		V80.910S	Animl-ridr injured in trnsp acc w military vehicle, sequela
		V80.918S	Animal-rider injured in other transport accident, sequela
		V80.919S	Animal-rider injured in unsp transport accident, sequela
		V80.920S	Occ of anml-drn veh inj in trnsp acc w miltry vehicle, sqla
		V80.928S	Occ of anml-drn vehicle injured in oth trnsp acc, sequela
		V80.929S	Occ of anml-drn vehicle injured in unsp trnsp acc, sequela
		V81.2XXS	Occ of rail trn/veh inj in collisn/hit by roll stok, sequela
		V81.3XXS	Occ of rail trn/veh injured in clsn w oth object, sequela
		V81.4XXS	Person injured wh brd/alit from rail trn/veh, sequela
		V81.5XXS	Occ of rail trn/veh injured by fall in rail trn/veh, sequela
		V81.6XXS	Occ of rail trn/veh inj by fall from rail trn/veh, sequela
		V81.7XXS	Occ of rail trn/veh inj in derail w/o antecedent clsn, sqla
		V81.81XS	Occ of rail trn/veh inj d/t explosn or fire on train, sqla
		V81.82XS	Occ of rail trn/veh inj due to object fall onto train, sqla
		V81.83XS	Occ of rail trn/veh inj due to clsn w miltry vehicle, sqla
		V81.89XS	Occ of rail trn/veh injured due to oth railway acc, sequela
		V81.9XXS	Occ of rail trn/veh injured in unsp railway acc, sequela
	(Continued on next page)	**V82.2XXS**	Occ of stcar injured in collisn/hit by roll stok, sequela

ICD-9-CM		ICD-10-CM	
E929.1	LATE EFFECTS OF OTHER TRANSPORT ACCIDENT **(Continued)**	**V82.3XXS**	Occupant of streetcar injured in clsn w oth object, sequela
		V82.4XXS	Person injured wh brd/alit from streetcar, sequela
		V82.5XXS	Occupant of streetcar injured by fall in streetcar, sequela
		V82.6XXS	Occupant of stcar injured by fall from streetcar, sequela
		V82.7XXS	Occ of stcar injured in derail w/o antecedent clsn, sequela
		V82.8XXS	Occupant of streetcar injured in oth transport acc, sequela
		V82.9XXS	Occupant of streetcar injured in unsp traf, sequela
		V83.0XXS	Driver of special industr vehicle injured in traf, sequela
		V83.1XXS	Pasngr of special industr vehicle injured in traf, sequela
		V83.2XXS	Person outside special industr vehicle inj in traf, sequela
		V83.3XXS	Occup of special industrial vehicle injured in traf, sequela
		V83.4XXS	Person inj wh brd/alit from special industr vehicle, sequela
		V83.5XXS	Driver of special industr vehicle injured nontraf, sequela
		V83.6XXS	Pasngr of special industr vehicle injured nontraf, sequela
		V83.7XXS	Person outside special industr vehicle inj nontraf, sequela
		V83.9XXS	Occup of special industrial vehicle injured nontraf, sequela
		V88.9XXS	Person injured in oth trnsp acc w non-mv, nontraf, sequela
		V89.1XXS	Person inj in unsp nonmotor-vehicle acc, nontraf, sequela
		V90.00XS	Drown due to merchant ship overturning, sequela
		V90.01XS	Drown due to passenger ship overturning, sequela
		V90.02XS	Drown due to fishing boat overturning, sequela
		V90.03XS	Drown due to oth powered watercraft overturning, sequela
		V90.04XS	Drowning and submersion due to sailboat overturning, sequela
		V90.05XS	Drown due to canoe or kayak overturning, sequela
		V90.06XS	Drown due to (nonpowered) inflatbl crft overturning, sequela
		V90.08XS	Drown due to unpowr wtrcrft overturning, sequela
		V90.09XS	Drown due to unsp watercraft overturning, sequela
		V90.10XS	Drown due to merchant ship sinking, sequela
		V90.11XS	Drown due to passenger ship sinking, sequela
		V90.12XS	Drowning and submersion due to fishing boat sinking, sequela
		V90.13XS	Drown due to oth powered watercraft sinking, sequela
		V90.14XS	Drowning and submersion due to sailboat sinking, sequela
		V90.15XS	Drown due to canoe or kayak sinking, sequela
		V90.16XS	Drown due to (nonpowered) inflatable craft sinking, sequela
		V90.18XS	Drown due to unpowr wtrcrft sinking, sequela
		V90.19XS	Drown due to unsp watercraft sinking, sequela
		V90.20XS	Drown due to fall/jump fr burning merchant ship, sequela
		V90.21XS	Drown due to fall/jump fr burning passenger ship, sequela
		V90.22XS	Drown due to fall/jump fr burning fishing boat, sequela
		V90.23XS	Drown due to fall/jump fr oth burn powered wtrcrft, sequela
		V90.24XS	Drown due to fall/jump fr burning sailboat, sequela
		V90.25XS	Drown due to fall/jump fr burning canoe or kayak, sequela
		V90.26XS	Drown due to fall/jump fr burning inflatbl crft, sequela
		V90.27XS	Drown due to fall/jump fr burning water-skis, sequela
		V90.28XS	Drown due to fall/jump fr oth burn unpowr wtrcrft, sequela
		V90.29XS	Drown due to fall/jump fr unsp burning watercraft, sequela
		V90.30XS	Drown due to fall/jump fr crushed merchant ship, sequela
		V90.31XS	Drown due to fall/jump fr crushed passenger ship, sequela
		V90.32XS	Drown due to fall/jump fr crushed fishing boat, sequela
		V90.33XS	Drown due to fall/jump fr oth crush powered wtrcrft, sequela
		V90.34XS	Drown due to fall/jump fr crushed sailboat, sequela
		V90.35XS	Drown due to fall/jump fr crushed canoe or kayak, sequela
		V90.36XS	Drown due to fall/jump fr crushed inflatbl crft, sequela
		V90.37XS	Drown due to fall/jump fr crushed water-skis, sequela
		V90.38XS	Drown due to fall/jump fr oth crush unpowr wtrcrft, sequela
		V90.39XS	Drown due to fall/jump fr crushed unsp watercraft, sequela
		V90.80XS	Drown due to oth accident to merchant ship, sequela
		V90.81XS	Drown due to oth accident to passenger ship, sequela
		V90.82XS	Drown due to oth accident to fishing boat, sequela
		V90.83XS	Drown due to oth accident to oth powered watercraft, sequela
		V90.84XS	Drown due to oth accident to sailboat, sequela
		V90.85XS	Drown due to oth accident to canoe or kayak, sequela
		V90.86XS	Drown due to oth accident to inflatbl crft, sequela
		V90.87XS	Drown due to oth accident to water-skis, sequela
		V90.88XS	Drown due to oth accident to unpowr wtrcrft, sequela
		V90.89XS	Drown due to oth accident to unsp watercraft, sequela
		V91.00XS	Burn due to merchant ship on fire, sequela
		V91.01XS	Burn due to passenger ship on fire, sequela
		V91.02XS	Burn due to fishing boat on fire, sequela
		V91.03XS	Burn due to other powered watercraft on fire, sequela
		V91.04XS	Burn due to sailboat on fire, sequela
		V91.05XS	Burn due to canoe or kayak on fire, sequela
		V91.06XS	Burn due to (nonpowered) inflatable craft on fire, sequela
		V91.07XS	Burn due to water-skis on fire, sequela
		V91.08XS	Burn due to other unpowered watercraft on fire, sequela
		V91.09XS	Burn due to unspecified watercraft on fire, sequela
		V91.10XS	Crush betw merch ship and oth wtrcrft/obj due to clsn, sqla
		V91.11XS	Crush betw pasngr ship and oth wtrcrft/obj due to clsn, sqla
		V91.12XS	Crush betw fish boat and oth wtrcrft/obj due to clsn, sqla
		V91.13XS	Crush betw oth pwr wtrcrft & oth wtrcrft/obj d/t clsn, sqla
		V91.14XS	Crushed betw sailbt and oth wtrcrft/obj due to clsn, sequela
	(Continued on next page)	**V91.15XS**	Crush betw canoe/kayk and oth wtrcrft/obj due to clsn, sqla

ICD-9-CM		ICD-10-CM	
E929.1	LATE EFFECTS OF OTHER TRANSPORT ACCIDENT **(Continued)**	**V91.16XS**	Crush betw inflatbl crft and oth wtrcrft/obj d/t clsn, sqla
		V91.18XS	Crush betw unpowr wtrcrft and oth wtrcrft/obj d/t clsn, sqla
		V91.19XS	Crush betw unsp wtrcrft and oth wtrcrft/obj d/t clsn, sqla
		V91.20XS	Fall due to clsn betw merch ship and oth wtrcrft/obj, sqla
		V91.21XS	Fall due to clsn betw pasngr ship and oth wtrcrft/obj, sqla
		V91.22XS	Fall due to clsn betw fish boat and oth wtrcrft/obj, sequela
		V91.23XS	Fall d/t clsn betw oth pwr wtrcrft and oth wtrcrft/obj, sqla
		V91.24XS	Fall due to clsn betw sailboat and oth wtrcrft/obj, sequela
		V91.25XS	Fall due to clsn betw canoe/kayk and oth wtrcrft/obj, sqla
		V91.26XS	Fall d/t clsn betw inflatbl crft and oth wtrcrft/obj, sqla
		V91.29XS	Fall due to clsn betw unsp wtrcrft and oth wtrcrft/obj, sqla
		V91.30XS	Hit by falling object due to accident to merch ship, sequela
		V91.31XS	Hit by falling object due to acc to pasngr ship, sequela
		V91.32XS	Hit by falling object due to acc to fishing boat, sequela
		V91.33XS	Hit by fall object due to acc to oth power wtrcrft, sequela
		V91.34XS	Hit by falling object due to accident to sailboat, sequela
		V91.35XS	Hit by falling object due to accident to canoe/kayk, sequela
		V91.36XS	Hit by falling object due to acc to inflatbl crft, sequela
		V91.37XS	Hit by falling object due to accident to water-skis, sequela
		V91.38XS	Hit by falling object due to acc to unpowr wtrcrft, sequela
		V91.39XS	Hit by falling object due to acc to unsp wtrcrft, sequela
		V91.80XS	Other injury due to other accident to merchant ship, sequela
		V91.81XS	Oth injury due to other accident to passenger ship, sequela
		V91.82XS	Other injury due to other accident to fishing boat, sequela
		V91.83XS	Oth injury due to oth acc to oth powered wtrcrft, sequela
		V91.84XS	Other injury due to other accident to sailboat, sequela
		V91.85XS	Oth injury due to other accident to canoe or kayak, sequela
		V91.86XS	Oth injury due to oth accident to inflatbl crft, sequela
		V91.87XS	Other injury due to other accident to water-skis, sequela
		V91.88XS	Oth injury due to oth accident to unpowr wtrcrft, sequela
		V91.89XS	Oth injury due to other accident to unsp watercraft, sequela
		V92.00XS	Drown due to fall off merchant ship, sequela
		V92.01XS	Drown due to fall off passenger ship, sequela
		V92.02XS	Drown due to fall off fishing boat, sequela
		V92.03XS	Drown due to fall off oth powered watercraft, sequela
		V92.04XS	Drowning and submersion due to fall off sailboat, sequela
		V92.05XS	Drown due to fall off canoe or kayak, sequela
		V92.06XS	Drown due to fall off (nonpowered) inflatable craft, sequela
		V92.07XS	Drowning and submersion due to fall off water-skis, sequela
		V92.08XS	Drown due to fall off unpowr wtrcrft, sequela
		V92.09XS	Drown due to fall off unsp watercraft, sequela
		V92.10XS	Drown d/t being thrown ovrbrd by motion of merch ship, sqla
		V92.11XS	Drown d/t being thrown ovrbrd by motion of pasngr ship, sqla
		V92.12XS	Drown d/t being thrown ovrbrd by motion of fish boat, sqla
		V92.13XS	Drown d/t thrown ovrbrd by motion of power wtrcrft, sqla
		V92.14XS	Drown due to being thrown ovrbrd by motion of sailbt, sqla
		V92.15XS	Drown d/t being thrown ovrbrd by motion of canoe/kayk, sqla
		V92.16XS	Drown d/t thrown ovrbrd by motion of inflatbl crft, sqla
		V92.19XS	Drown d/t thrown ovrbrd by motion of unsp wtrcrft, sqla
		V92.20XS	Drown due to being washed overboard from merch ship, sequela
		V92.21XS	Drown due to being washed ovrbrd from pasngr ship, sequela
		V92.22XS	Drown due to being washed ovrbrd from fishing boat, sequela
		V92.23XS	Drown d/t being washed ovrbrd from oth power wtrcrft, sqla
		V92.24XS	Drown due to being washed overboard from sailboat, sequela
		V92.25XS	Drown due to being washed overboard from canoe/kayk, sequela
		V92.26XS	Drown due to being washed ovrbrd from inflatbl crft, sequela
		V92.27XS	Drown due to being washed overboard from water-skis, sequela
		V92.28XS	Drown due to being washed ovrbrd from unpowr wtrcrft, sqla
		V92.29XS	Drown due to being washed ovrbrd from unsp wtrcrft, sequela
		V93.00XS	Burn due to localized fire on board merchant vessel, sequela
		V93.01XS	Burn due to loc fire on board passenger vessel, sequela
		V93.02XS	Burn due to localized fire on board fishing boat, sequela
		V93.03XS	Burn due to loc fire on board oth powered wtrcrft, sequela
		V93.04XS	Burn due to localized fire on board sailboat, sequela
		V93.09XS	Burn due to localized fire on board unsp watercraft, sequela
		V93.10XS	Other burn on board merchant vessel, sequela
		V93.11XS	Other burn on board passenger vessel, sequela
		V93.12XS	Other burn on board fishing boat, sequela
		V93.13XS	Other burn on board other powered watercraft, sequela
		V93.14XS	Other burn on board sailboat, sequela
		V93.19XS	Other burn on board unspecified watercraft, sequela
		V93.20XS	Heat exposure on board merchant ship, sequela
		V93.21XS	Heat exposure on board passenger ship, sequela
		V93.22XS	Heat exposure on board fishing boat, sequela
		V93.23XS	Heat exposure on board other powered watercraft, sequela
		V93.24XS	Heat exposure on board sailboat, sequela
		V93.29XS	Heat exposure on board unspecified watercraft, sequela
		V93.30XS	Fall on board merchant ship, sequela
		V93.31XS	Fall on board passenger ship, sequela
		V93.32XS	Fall on board fishing boat, sequela
		V93.33XS	Fall on board other powered watercraft, sequela
	(Continued on next page)	**V93.34XS**	Fall on board sailboat, sequela

[Brackets] indicate valid character values for each code. Character value meanings provided for each code grouping.

ICD-9-CM		ICD-10-CM	
E929.1	LATE EFFECTS OF OTHER TRANSPORT ACCIDENT **(Continued)**	**V93.35XS**	Fall on board canoe or kayak, sequela
		V93.36XS	Fall on board (nonpowered) inflatable craft, sequela
		V93.38XS	Fall on board other unpowered watercraft, sequela
		V93.39XS	Fall on board unspecified watercraft, sequela
		V93.40XS	Struck by falling object on merchant ship, sequela
		V93.41XS	Struck by falling object on passenger ship, sequela
		V93.42XS	Struck by falling object on fishing boat, sequela
		V93.43XS	Struck by falling object on oth powered watercraft, sequela
		V93.44XS	Struck by falling object on sailboat, sequela
		V93.48XS	Struck by falling object on unpowr wtrcrft, sequela
		V93.49XS	Struck by falling object on unspecified watercraft, sequela
		V93.50XS	Explosion on board merchant ship, sequela
		V93.51XS	Explosion on board passenger ship, sequela
		V93.52XS	Explosion on board fishing boat, sequela
		V93.53XS	Explosion on board other powered watercraft, sequela
		V93.54XS	Explosion on board sailboat, sequela
		V93.59XS	Explosion on board unspecified watercraft, sequela
		V93.60XS	Machinery accident on board merchant ship, sequela
		V93.61XS	Machinery accident on board passenger ship, sequela
		V93.62XS	Machinery accident on board fishing boat, sequela
		V93.63XS	Machinery accident on board oth powered watercraft, sequela
		V93.64XS	Machinery accident on board sailboat, sequela
		V93.69XS	Machinery accident on board unspecified watercraft, sequela
		V93.80XS	Oth injury due to oth accident on board merch ship, sequela
		V93.81XS	Oth injury due to oth accident on board pasngr ship, sequela
		V93.82XS	Oth injury due to oth acc on board fishing boat, sequela
		V93.83XS	Oth injury due to oth acc on board oth power wtrcrft, sqla
		V93.84XS	Oth injury due to other accident on board sailboat, sequela
		V93.85XS	Oth injury due to oth accident on board canoe/kayk, sequela
		V93.86XS	Oth injury due to oth acc on board inflatbl crft, sequela
		V93.87XS	Oth injury due to oth accident on board water-skis, sequela
		V93.88XS	Oth injury due to oth acc on board unpowr wtrcrft, sequela
		V93.89XS	Oth injury due to oth acc on board unsp wtrcrft, sequela
		V94.0XXS	Hitting obj/botm of body of wtr d/t fall from wtrcrft, sqla
		V94.11XS	Bather struck by powered watercraft, sequela
		V94.12XS	Bather struck by nonpowered watercraft, sequela
		V94.21XS	Rider of nonpowr wtrcrft struck by oth nonpowr wtrcrft, sqla
		V94.22XS	Rider of nonpowr wtrcrft struck by powered wtrcrft, sequela
		V94.31XS	Inj to rider of recreatl wtrcrft puld beh oth wtrcrft, sqla
		V94.32XS	Inj to rider of nonrecr wtrcrft puld beh oth wtrcrft, sqla
		V94.4XXS	Injury to barefoot water-skier, sequela
		V94.810S	Civ wtrcrft in water trnsp acc w military wtrcrft, sequela
		V94.811S	Civilian in water injured by military watercraft, sequela
		V94.818S	Oth water transport accident w military wtrcrft, sequela
		V94.89XS	Other water transport accident, sequela
		V94.9XXS	Unspecified water transport accident, sequela
		V95.00XS	Unspecified helicopter accident injuring occupant, sequela
		V95.01XS	Helicopter crash injuring occupant, sequela
		V95.02XS	Forced landing of helicopter injuring occupant, sequela
		V95.03XS	Helicopter collision injuring occupant, sequela
		V95.04XS	Helicopter fire injuring occupant, sequela
		V95.05XS	Helicopter explosion injuring occupant, sequela
		V95.09XS	Other helicopter accident injuring occupant, sequela
		V95.10XS	Unsp ultralt/microlt/pwr-glider acc inj occupant, sequela
		V95.11XS	Ultralt/microlt/pwr-glider crash injuring occupant, sequela
		V95.12XS	Forced land of ultralt/microlt/pwr-glider inj occ, sequela
		V95.13XS	Ultralt/microlt/pwr-glider clsn injuring occupant, sequela
		V95.14XS	Ultralt/microlt/pwr-glider fire injuring occupant, sequela
		V95.15XS	Ultralt/microlt/pwr-glider explosn inj occupant, sequela
		V95.19XS	Oth ultralt/microlt/pwr-glider acc inj occupant, sequela
		V95.20XS	Unsp acc to oth private fix-wing arcrft, inj occ, sequela
		V95.21XS	Oth private fix-wing arcrft crash injuring occupant, sequela
		V95.22XS	Forced landing of private fix-wing arcrft inj occ, sequela
		V95.23XS	Oth private fix-wing arcrft clsn injuring occupant, sequela
		V95.24XS	Oth private fix-wing arcrft fire injuring occupant, sequela
		V95.25XS	Oth private fix-wing arcrft explosn inj occupant, sequela
		V95.29XS	Oth acc to oth private fix-wing arcrft inj occupant, sequela
		V95.30XS	Unsp acc to commrcl fix-wing arcrft inj occupant, sequela
		V95.31XS	Commrcl fixed-wing aircraft crash injuring occupant, sequela
		V95.32XS	Forced landing of commrcl fix-wing arcrft inj occ, sequela
		V95.33XS	Commrcl fix-wing aircraft clsn injuring occupant, sequela
		V95.34XS	Commrcl fixed-wing aircraft fire injuring occupant, sequela
		V95.35XS	Commrcl fix-wing aircraft explosn injuring occupant, sequela
		V95.39XS	Oth acc to commrcl fix-wing arcrft inj occupant, sequela
		V95.40XS	Unspecified spacecraft accident injuring occupant, sequela
		V95.41XS	Spacecraft crash injuring occupant, sequela
		V95.42XS	Forced landing of spacecraft injuring occupant, sequela
		V95.43XS	Spacecraft collision injuring occupant, sequela
		V95.44XS	Spacecraft fire injuring occupant, sequela
		V95.45XS	Spacecraft explosion injuring occupant, sequela
		V95.49XS	Other spacecraft accident injuring occupant, sequela
	(Continued on next page)	**V95.8XXS**	Other powered aircraft accidents injuring occupant, sequela

ICD-9-CM		ICD-10-CM	
E929.1	LATE EFFECTS OF OTHER TRANSPORT ACCIDENT **(Continued)**	**V95.9XXS**	Unspecified aircraft accident injuring occupant, sequela
		V96.00XS	Unspecified balloon accident injuring occupant, sequela
		V96.01XS	Balloon crash injuring occupant, sequela
		V96.02XS	Forced landing of balloon injuring occupant, sequela
		V96.03XS	Balloon collision injuring occupant, sequela
		V96.04XS	Balloon fire injuring occupant, sequela
		V96.05XS	Balloon explosion injuring occupant, sequela
		V96.09XS	Other balloon accident injuring occupant, sequela
		V96.10XS	Unspecified hang-glider accident injuring occupant, sequela
		V96.11XS	Hang-glider crash injuring occupant, sequela
		V96.12XS	Forced landing of hang-glider injuring occupant, sequela
		V96.13XS	Hang-glider collision injuring occupant, sequela
		V96.14XS	Hang-glider fire injuring occupant, sequela
		V96.15XS	Hang-glider explosion injuring occupant, sequela
		V96.19XS	Other hang-glider accident injuring occupant, sequela
		V96.20XS	Unsp glider (nonpowered) accident injuring occupant, sequela
		V96.21XS	Glider (nonpowered) crash injuring occupant, sequela
		V96.22XS	Forced landing of glider injuring occupant, sequela
		V96.23XS	Glider (nonpowered) collision injuring occupant, sequela
		V96.24XS	Glider (nonpowered) fire injuring occupant, sequela
		V96.25XS	Glider (nonpowered) explosion injuring occupant, sequela
		V96.29XS	Oth glider (nonpowered) accident injuring occupant, sequela
		V96.8XXS	Oth nonpowered-aircraft accidents injuring occupant, sequela
		V96.9XXS	Unsp nonpowered-aircraft accident injuring occupant, sequela
		V97.0XXS	Occupant of aircraft injured in oth air trnsp acc, sequela
		V97.1XXS	Person injured wh brd/alit from aircraft, sequela
		V97.21XS	Parachutist entangled in object, sequela
		V97.22XS	Parachutist injured on landing, sequela
		V97.29XS	Other parachutist accident, sequela
		V97.31XS	Hit by object falling from aircraft, sequela
		V97.32XS	Injured by rotating propeller, sequela
		V97.33XS	Sucked into jet engine, sequela
		V97.39XS	Oth injury to person on ground due to air trnsp acc, sequela
		V97.810S	Civilian arcrft in air trnsp acc w military arcrft, sequela
		V97.811S	Civilian injured by military aircraft, sequela
		V97.818S	Oth air transport accident w military aircraft, sequela
		V97.89XS	Oth air transport accidents, NEC, sequela
		V98.0XXS	Accident to, on or w cable-car, not on rails, sequela
		V98.1XXS	Accident to, on or involving land-yacht, sequela
		V98.2XXS	Accident to, on or involving ice yacht, sequela
		V98.3XXS	Accident to, on or involving ski lift, sequela
		V98.8XXS	Other specified transport accidents, sequela
		V99.XXXS	Unspecified transport accident, sequela
E929.2	LATE EFFECTS OF ACCIDENTAL POISONING	**T36.0X1S**	Poisoning by penicillins, accidental, sequela
		T36.1X1S	Poisn by cephalospor/oth beta-lactm antibiot, acc, sequela
		T36.2X1S	Poisoning by chloramphenicol group, accidental, sequela
		T36.3X1S	Poisoning by macrolides, accidental (unintentional), sequela
		T36.4X1S	Poisoning by tetracyclines, accidental, sequela
		T36.5X1S	Poisoning by aminoglycosides, accidental, sequela
		T36.6X1S	Poisoning by rifampicins, accidental, sequela
		T36.7X1S	Poisoning by antifungal antibiot, sys used, acc, sequela
		T36.8X1S	Poisoning by oth systemic antibiotics, accidental, sequela
		T36.91XS	Poisoning by unsp systemic antibiotic, accidental, sequela
		T37.0X1S	Poisoning by sulfonamides, accidental, sequela
		T37.1X1S	Poisoning by antimycobac drugs, accidental, sequela
		T37.2X1S	Poisn by antimalari/drugs acting on bld protzoa, acc, sqla
		T37.3X1S	Poisoning by oth antiprotozoal drugs, accidental, sequela
		T37.4X1S	Poisoning by anthelminthics, accidental, sequela
		T37.5X1S	Poisoning by antiviral drugs, accidental, sequela
		T37.8X1S	Poisoning by oth systemic anti-infect/parasit, acc, sequela
		T37.91XS	Poisn by unsp sys anti-infect and antiparastc, acc, sequela
		T38.0X1S	Poisoning by glucocort/synth analog, accidental, sequela
		T38.1X1S	Poisoning by thyroid hormones and sub, accidental, sequela
		T38.2X1S	Poisoning by antithyroid drugs, accidental, sequela
		T38.3X1S	Poisn by insulin and oral hypoglycemic drugs, acc, sequela
		T38.4X1S	Poisoning by oral contraceptives, accidental, sequela
		T38.5X1S	Poisoning by oth estrogens and progstrn, acc, sequela
		T38.6X1S	Poisn by antigonadtr/antiestr/antiandrg, NEC, acc, sequela
		T38.7X1S	Poisoning by androgens and anabolic congeners, acc, sequela
		T38.801S	Poisoning by unsp hormones and synthetic sub, acc, sequela
		T38.811S	Poisoning by anterior pituitary hormones, acc, sequela
		T38.891S	Poisoning by oth hormones and synthetic sub, acc, sequela
		T38.901S	Poisoning by unsp hormone antagonists, accidental, sequela
		T38.991S	Poisoning by oth hormone antagonists, accidental, sequela
		T39.011S	Poisoning by aspirin, accidental (unintentional), sequela
		T39.091S	Poisoning by salicylates, accidental, sequela
		T39.1X1S	Poisoning by 4-Aminophenol derivatives, accidental, sequela
		T39.2X1S	Poisoning by pyrazolone derivatives, accidental, sequela
		T39.311S	Poisoning by propionic acid deriv, accidental, sequela
		T39.391S	Poisoning by oth nonsteroid anti-inflam drugs, acc, sequela
	(Continued on next page)	**T39.4X1S**	Poisoning by antirheumatics, NEC, accidental, sequela

ICD-9-CM		ICD-10-CM	
E929.2	LATE EFFECTS OF ACCIDENTAL POISONING (Continued)	T39.8X1S	Poisn by oth nonopio analges/antipyret, NEC, acc, sequela
		T39.91XS	Poisn by unsp nonopi analgs/antipyr/antirheu, acc, sequela
		T40.0X1S	Poisoning by opium, accidental (unintentional), sequela
		T40.1X1S	Poisoning by heroin, accidental (unintentional), sequela
		T40.2X1S	Poisoning by oth opioids, accidental, sequela
		T40.3X1S	Poisoning by methadone, accidental (unintentional), sequela
		T40.4X1S	Poisoning by oth synthetic narcotics, accidental, sequela
		T40.5X1S	Poisoning by cocaine, accidental (unintentional), sequela
		T40.601S	Poisoning by unsp narcotics, accidental, sequela
		T40.691S	Poisoning by oth narcotics, accidental, sequela
		T40.7X1S	Poisoning by cannabis (derivatives), accidental, sequela
		T40.8X1S	Poisoning by lysergide, accidental (unintentional), sequela
		T40.901S	Poisoning by unsp psychodyslept, accidental, sequela
		T40.991S	Poisoning by oth psychodyslept, accidental, sequela
		T41.0X1S	Poisoning by inhaled anesthetics, accidental, sequela
		T41.1X1S	Poisoning by intravenous anesthetics, accidental, sequela
		T41.201S	Poisoning by unsp general anesthetics, accidental, sequela
		T41.291S	Poisoning by oth general anesthetics, accidental, sequela
		T41.3X1S	Poisoning by local anesthetics, accidental, sequela
		T41.41XS	Poisoning by unsp anesthetic, accidental, sequela
		T41.5X1S	Poisoning by therapeutic gases, accidental, sequela
		T42.0X1S	Poisoning by hydantoin derivatives, accidental, sequela
		T42.1X1S	Poisoning by iminostilbenes, accidental, sequela
		T42.2X1S	Poisn by succinimides and oxazolidinediones, acc, sequela
		T42.3X1S	Poisoning by barbiturates, accidental, sequela
		T42.4X1S	Poisoning by benzodiazepines, accidental, sequela
		T42.5X1S	Poisoning by mixed antiepileptics, accidental, sequela
		T42.6X1S	Poisn by oth antieplptc and sed-hypntc drugs, acc, sequela
		T42.71XS	Poisn by unsp antieplptc and sed-hypntc drugs, acc, sequela
		T42.8X1S	Poisn by antiparkns drug/centr musc-tone depr, acc, sequela
		T43.011S	Poisoning by tricyclic antidepressants, accidental, sequela
		T43.021S	Poisoning by tetracyclic antidepress, accidental, sequela
		T43.1X1S	Poisoning by MAO inhib antidepressants, accidental, sequela
		T43.201S	Poisoning by unsp antidepressants, accidental, sequela
		T43.211S	Poisn by slctv seroton/norepineph reup inhibtr, acc, sqla
		T43.221S	Poisn by selective serotonin reuptake inhibtr, acc, sequela
		T43.291S	Poisoning by oth antidepressants, accidental, sequela
		T43.3X1S	Poisoning by phenothiaz antipsychot/neurolept, acc, sequela
		T43.4X1S	Poisoning by butyrophen/thiothixen neuroleptc, acc, sequela
		T43.501S	Poisoning by unsp antipsychot/neurolept, acc, sequela
		T43.591S	Poisoning by oth antipsychot/neurolept, accidental, sequela
		T43.601S	Poisoning by unsp psychostim, accidental, sequela
		T43.611S	Poisoning by caffeine, accidental (unintentional), sequela
		T43.621S	Poisoning by amphetamines, accidental, sequela
		T43.631S	Poisoning by methylphenidate, accidental, sequela
		T43.691S	Poisoning by oth psychostim, accidental, sequela
		T43.8X1S	Poisoning by oth psychotropic drugs, accidental, sequela
		T43.91XS	Poisoning by unsp psychotropic drug, accidental, sequela
		T44.0X1S	Poisoning by anticholin agents, accidental, sequela
		T44.1X1S	Poisoning by oth parasympath, accidental, sequela
		T44.2X1S	Poisoning by ganglionic blocking drugs, accidental, sequela
		T44.3X1S	Poisoning by oth parasympath and spasmolytics, acc, sequela
		T44.4X1S	Poisoning by predom alpha-adrenocpt agonists, acc, sequela
		T44.5X1S	Poisoning by predom beta-adrenocpt agonists, acc, sequela
		T44.6X1S	Poisoning by alpha-adrenocpt antag, accidental, sequela
		T44.7X1S	Poisoning by beta-adrenocpt antag, accidental, sequela
		T44.8X1S	Poisn by centr-acting/adren-neurn-block agnt, acc, sequela
		T44.901S	Poisn by unsp drugs aff the autonm nrv sys, acc, sequela
		T44.991S	Poisn by oth drug aff the autonm nervous sys, acc, sequela
		T45.0X1S	Poisoning by antiallerg/antiemetic, accidental, sequela
		T45.1X1S	Poisoning by antineopl and immunosup drugs, acc, sequela
		T45.2X1S	Poisoning by vitamins, accidental (unintentional), sequela
		T45.3X1S	Poisoning by enzymes, accidental (unintentional), sequela
		T45.4X1S	Poisoning by iron and its compounds, accidental, sequela
		T45.511S	Poisoning by anticoagulants, accidental, sequela
		T45.521S	Poisoning by antithrombotic drugs, accidental, sequela
		T45.601S	Poisoning by unsp fibrin-affct drugs, accidental, sequela
		T45.611S	Poisoning by thrombolytic drug, accidental, sequela
		T45.621S	Poisoning by hemostatic drug, accidental, sequela
		T45.691S	Poisoning by oth fibrin-affct drugs, accidental, sequela
		T45.7X1S	Poisn by anticoag antag, vit K and oth coag, acc, sequela
		T45.8X1S	Poisn by oth prim sys and hematolog agents, acc, sequela
		T45.91XS	Poisn by unsp prim sys and hematolog agent, acc, sequela
		T46.0X1S	Poisn by cardi-stim glycos/drug simlar act, acc, sequela
		T46.1X1S	Poisoning by calcium-channel blockers, accidental, sequela
		T46.2X1S	Poisoning by oth antidysrhythmic drugs, accidental, sequela
		T46.3X1S	Poisoning by coronary vasodilators, accidental, sequela
		T46.4X1S	Poisoning by angiotens-convert-enzyme inhibtr, acc, sequela
	(Continued on next page)	T46.5X1S	Poisoning by oth antihypertn drugs, accidental, sequela

ICD-9-CM		ICD-10-CM	
E929.2	LATE EFFECTS OF ACCIDENTAL POISONING **(Continued)**	**T46.6X1S**	Poisn by antihyperlip and antiarterio drugs, acc, sequela
		T46.7X1S	Poisoning by peripheral vasodilators, accidental, sequela
		T46.8X1S	Poisn by antivaric drugs, inc scler agents, acc, sequela
		T46.9Ø1S	Poisn by unsp agents aff the cardiovasc sys, acc, sequela
		T46.991S	Poisn by oth agents aff the cardiovasc sys, acc, sequela
		T47.ØX1S	Poisoning by histamine H2-receptor blockers, acc, sequela
		T47.1X1S	Poisn by oth antacids and anti-gstrc-sec drugs, acc, sqla
		T47.2X1S	Poisoning by stimulant laxatives, accidental, sequela
		T47.3X1S	Poisoning by saline and osmotic laxatives, acc, sequela
		T47.4X1S	Poisoning by oth laxatives, accidental, sequela
		T47.5X1S	Poisoning by digestants, accidental (unintentional), sequela
		T47.6X1S	Poisoning by antidiarrheal drugs, accidental, sequela
		T47.7X1S	Poisoning by emetics, accidental (unintentional), sequela
		T47.8X1S	Poisoning by oth agents aff GI sys, accidental, sequela
		T47.91XS	Poisoning by unsp agents aff the GI sys, acc, sequela
		T48.ØX1S	Poisoning by oxytocic drugs, accidental, sequela
		T48.1X1S	Poisoning by skeletal muscle relaxants, accidental, sequela
		T48.2Ø1S	Poisoning by unsp drugs acting on muscles, acc, sequela
		T48.291S	Poisoning by oth drugs acting on muscles, acc, sequela
		T48.3X1S	Poisoning by antitussives, accidental, sequela
		T48.4X1S	Poisoning by expectorants, accidental, sequela
		T48.5X1S	Poisoning by oth anti-cmn-cold drugs, accidental, sequela
		T48.6X1S	Poisoning by antiasthmatics, accidental, sequela
		T48.9Ø1S	Poisn by unsp agents prim acting on the resp sys, acc, sqla
		T48.991S	Poisn by oth agents prim acting on the resp sys, acc, sqla
		T49.ØX1S	Poisn by local antifung/infect/inflamm drugs, acc, sequela
		T49.1X1S	Poisoning by antipruritics, accidental, sequela
		T49.2X1S	Poisoning by local astringents/detergents, acc, sequela
		T49.3X1S	Poisn by emollients, demulcents and protect, acc, sequela
		T49.4X1S	Poisn by keratolyt/keratplst/hair trmt drug, acc, sequela
		T49.5X1S	Poisoning by opth drugs and prep, accidental, sequela
		T49.6X1S	Poisoning by otorhino drugs and prep, accidental, sequela
		T49.7X1S	Poisoning by dental drugs, topically applied, acc, sequela
		T49.8X1S	Poisoning by oth topical agents, accidental, sequela
		T49.91XS	Poisoning by unsp topical agent, accidental, sequela
		T5Ø.ØX1S	Poisoning by mineralocorticoids and antag, acc, sequela
		T5Ø.1X1S	Poisoning by loop diuretics, accidental, sequela
		T5Ø.2X1S	Poisn by crbnc-anhydr inhibtr, benzo/oth diuretc, acc, sqla
		T5Ø.3X1S	Poisn by electrolytic/caloric/wtr-bal agnt, acc, sequela
		T5Ø.4X1S	Poisoning by drugs affecting uric acid metab, acc, sequela
		T5Ø.5X1S	Poisoning by appetite depressants, accidental, sequela
		T5Ø.6X1S	Poisoning by antidotes and chelating agents, acc, sequela
		T5Ø.7X1S	Poisn by analeptics and opioid receptor antag, acc, sequela
		T5Ø.8X1S	Poisoning by diagnostic agents, accidental, sequela
		T5Ø.9Ø1S	Poisoning by unsp drug/meds/biol subst, accidental, sequela
		T5Ø.991S	Poisoning by oth drug/meds/biol subst, accidental, sequela
		T5Ø.A11S	Poisn by pertuss vaccine, inc combin w pertuss, acc, sqla
		T5Ø.A21S	Poisn by mixed bact vaccines w/o a pertuss, acc, sequela
		T5Ø.A91S	Poisoning by oth bacterial vaccines, accidental, sequela
		T5Ø.B11S	Poisoning by smallpox vaccines, accidental, sequela
		T5Ø.B91S	Poisoning by oth viral vaccines, accidental, sequela
		T5Ø.Z11S	Poisoning by immunoglobulin, accidental, sequela
		T5Ø.Z91S	Poisoning by oth vaccines and biolg substnc, acc, sequela
		T6Ø.ØX1S	Toxic effect of organophos and carbamate insect, acc, sqla
		T6Ø.1X1S	Toxic effect of halogenated insect, accidental, sequela
		T6Ø.2X1S	Toxic effect of insecticides, accidental, sequela
		T6Ø.3X1S	Toxic effect of herbicides and fungicides, acc, sequela
		T6Ø.4X1S	Toxic effect of rodenticides, accidental, sequela
		T6Ø.8X1S	Toxic effect of pesticides, accidental, sequela
		T6Ø.91XS	Toxic effect of unsp pesticide, accidental, sequela
		T61.Ø1XS	Ciguatera fish poisoning, accidental, sequela
		T61.11XS	Scombroid fish poisoning, accidental, sequela
		T61.771S	Other fish poisoning, accidental (unintentional), sequela
		T61.781S	Oth shellfish poisoning, accidental (unintentional), sequela
		T61.8X1S	Toxic effect of seafood, accidental (unintentional), sequela
		T61.91XS	Toxic effect of unsp seafood, accidental, sequela
		T62.ØX1S	Toxic effect of ingested mushrooms, accidental, sequela
		T62.1X1S	Toxic effect of ingested berries, accidental, sequela
		T62.2X1S	Toxic effect of ingested (parts of) plant(s), acc, sequela
		T62.8X1S	Toxic effect of noxious substnc eaten as food, acc, sequela
		T62.91XS	Toxic effect of unsp noxious sub eaten as food, acc, sqla
		T63.ØØ2S	Toxic effect of unsp snake venom, self-harm, sequela
		T63.Ø11S	Toxic effect of rattlesnake venom, accidental, sequela
		T63.Ø21S	Toxic effect of coral snake venom, accidental, sequela
		T63.Ø31S	Toxic effect of taipan venom, accidental, sequela
		T63.Ø41S	Toxic effect of cobra venom, accidental, sequela
		T63.Ø61S	Toxic effect of venom of N & S American snake, acc, sequela
		T63.Ø71S	Toxic effect of venom of Australian snake, acc, sequela
	(Continued on next page)	**T63.Ø81S**	Toxic effect of venom of African and Asian snake, acc, sqla

ICD-9-CM		ICD-10-CM	
E929.2	LATE EFFECTS OF ACCIDENTAL POISONING **(Continued)**	**T63.Ø91S**	Toxic effect of venom of snake, accidental, sequela
		T63.111S	Toxic effect of venom of gila monster, accidental, sequela
		T63.121S	Toxic effect of venom of venomous lizard, acc, sequela
		T63.191S	Toxic effect of venom of reptiles, accidental, sequela
		T63.2X1S	Toxic effect of venom of scorpion, accidental, sequela
		T63.3Ø1S	Toxic effect of unsp spider venom, accidental, sequela
		T63.311S	Toxic effect of venom of black widow spider, acc, sequela
		T63.321S	Toxic effect of venom of tarantula, accidental, sequela
		T63.331S	Toxic effect of venom of brown recluse spider, acc, sequela
		T63.391S	Toxic effect of venom of spider, accidental, sequela
		T63.411S	Toxic effect of venom of centipede/millipede, acc, sequela
		T63.421S	Toxic effect of venom of ants, accidental, sequela
		T63.431S	Toxic effect of venom of caterpillars, accidental, sequela
		T63.441S	Toxic effect of venom of bees, accidental, sequela
		T63.451S	Toxic effect of venom of hornets, accidental, sequela
		T63.461S	Toxic effect of venom of wasps, accidental, sequela
		T63.481S	Toxic effect of venom of arthropod, accidental, sequela
		T63.511S	Toxic effect of contact w stingray, accidental, sequela
		T63.591S	Toxic effect of contact w oth venomous fish, acc, sequela
		T63.611S	Toxic effect of contact w Portugese Man-o-war, acc, sequela
		T63.621S	Toxic effect of contact w oth jellyfish, acc, sequela
		T63.631S	Toxic effect of contact w sea anemone, accidental, sequela
		T63.691S	Toxic effect of cntct w oth venom marine animals, acc, sqla
		T63.711S	Toxic effect of contact w venom marine plant, acc, sequela
		T63.791S	Toxic effect of contact w oth venomous plant, acc, sequela
		T63.811S	Toxic effect of contact w venomous frog, acc, sequela
		T63.821S	Toxic effect of contact w venomous toad, acc, sequela
		T63.831S	Toxic effect of contact w oth venomous amphib, acc, sequela
		T63.891S	Toxic effect of contact w oth venom animals, acc, sequela
		T63.91XS	Toxic effect of contact w unsp venom animal, acc, sequela
		T64.Ø1XS	Toxic effect of aflatoxin, accidental, sequela
		T64.81XS	Toxic effect of mycotoxin food contamnt, acc, sequela
		T65.ØX1S	Toxic effect of cyanides, accidental, sequela
		T65.1X1S	Toxic effect of strychnine and its salts, acc, sequela
		T65.211S	Toxic effect of chewing tobacco, accidental, sequela
		T65.221S	Toxic effect of tobacco cigarettes, accidental, sequela
		T65.291S	Toxic effect of tobacco and nicotine, accidental, sequela
		T65.3X1S	Toxic eff of nitrodrv/aminodrv of benzn/homolog, acc, sqla
		T65.4X1S	Toxic effect of carbon disulfide, accidental, sequela
		T65.5X1S	Tox eff of nitro and oth nitric acids and esters, acc, sqla
		T65.6X1S	Toxic effect of paints and dyes, NEC, accidental, sequela
		T65.811S	Toxic effect of latex, accidental (unintentional), sequela
		T65.821S	Toxic effect of harmful algae and algae toxins, acc, sqla
		T65.831S	Toxic effect of fiberglass, accidental, sequela
		T65.891S	Toxic effect of substances, accidental, sequela
		T65.91XS	Toxic effect of unsp substance, accidental, sequela
E929.3	LATE EFFECTS OF ACCIDENTAL FALL	**VØØ.111S**	Fall from in-line roller-skates, sequela
		VØØ.112S	In-line roller-skater colliding w stationary object, sequela
		VØØ.118S	Other in-line roller-skate accident, sequela
		VØØ.121S	Fall from non-in-line roller-skates, sequela
		VØØ.122S	Non-in-line roller-skater colliding w statnry obj, sequela
		VØØ.128S	Other non-in-line roller-skating accident, sequela
		VØØ.131S	Fall from skateboard, sequela
		VØØ.132S	Skateboarder colliding with stationary object, sequela
		VØØ.138S	Other skateboard accident, sequela
		VØØ.141S	Fall from scooter (nonmotorized), sequela
		VØØ.142S	Scooter (nonmotorized) colliding w statnry obj, sequela
		VØØ.148S	Other scooter (nonmotorized) accident, sequela
		VØØ.151S	Fall from heelies, sequela
		VØØ.152S	Heelies colliding with stationary object, sequela
		VØØ.158S	Other heelies accident, sequela
		VØØ.181S	Fall from other rolling-type pedestrian conveyance, sequela
		VØØ.182S	Ped on oth roll-type ped convey collid w statnry obj, sqla
		VØØ.188S	Oth accident on oth roll-type pedestrian conveyance, sequela
		VØØ.211S	Fall from ice-skates, sequela
		VØØ.212S	Ice-skater colliding with stationary object, sequela
		VØØ.218S	Other ice-skates accident, sequela
		VØØ.221S	Fall from sled, sequela
		VØØ.222S	Sledder colliding with stationary object, sequela
		VØØ.228S	Other sled accident, sequela
		VØØ.281S	Fall from other gliding-type pedestrian conveyance, sequela
		VØØ.282S	Ped on gliding-type ped convey collid w statnry obj, sequela
		VØØ.288S	Oth accident on gliding-type pedestrian conveyance, sequela
		VØØ.311S	Fall from snowboard, sequela
		VØØ.312S	Snowboarder colliding with stationary object, sequela
		VØØ.318S	Other snowboard accident, sequela
		VØØ.321S	Fall from snow-skis, sequela
		VØØ.322S	Snow-skier colliding with stationary object, sequela
		VØØ.328S	Other snow-ski accident, sequela
		VØØ.381S	Fall from other flat-bottomed pedestrian conveyance, sequela
	(Continued on next page)	**VØØ.382S**	Ped on flat-bottomed ped convey collid w statnry obj, sqla

ICD-9-CM		ICD-10-CM	
E929.3	LATE EFFECTS OF ACCIDENTAL FALL **(Continued)**	**V00.388S**	Oth accident on flat-bottomed pedestrian conveyance, sequela
		V00.811S	Fall from moving wheelchair (powered), sequela
		V00.812S	Wheelchair (powered) colliding w stationary object, sequela
		V00.818S	Other accident with wheelchair (powered), sequela
		V00.821S	Fall from babystroller, sequela
		V00.822S	Babystroller colliding with stationary object, sequela
		V00.828S	Other accident with babystroller, sequela
		V00.831S	Fall from motorized mobility scooter, sequela
		V00.832S	Motorized mobility scooter colliding w statnry obj, sequela
		V00.838S	Other accident with motorized mobility scooter, sequela
		V00.891S	Fall from other pedestrian conveyance, sequela
		V00.892S	Ped on oth ped convey colliding w statnry obj, sequela
		V00.898S	Other accident on other pedestrian conveyance, sequela
		W00.0XXS	Fall on same level due to ice and snow, sequela
		W00.1XXS	Fall from stairs and steps due to ice and snow, sequela
		W00.2XXS	Oth fall from one level to another due to ice and snow, sqla
		W00.9XXS	Unspecified fall due to ice and snow, sequela
		W01.0XXS	Fall same lev from slip/trip w/o strike agnst object, sqla
		W01.10XS	Fall same lev from slip/trip w strike agnst unsp obj, sqla
		W01.110S	Fall same lev from slip/trip w strk agnst sharp glass, sqla
		W01.111S	Fall same lev from slip/trip w strk agnst pwr tl/machn, sqla
		W01.118S	Fall same lev fr slip/trip w strk agnst oth sharp obj, sqla
		W01.119S	Fall same lev fr slip/trip w strk agnst unsp sharp obj, sqla
		W01.190S	Fall same lev from slip/trip w strike agnst furniture, sqla
		W01.198S	Fall same lev from slip/trip w strike agnst oth object, sqla
		W03.XXXS	Oth fall same lev due to collision w another person, sequela
		W04.XXXS	Fall while being carried or supported by oth persons, sqla
		W05.0XXS	Fall from non-moving wheelchair, sequela
		W05.1XXS	Fall from non-moving nonmotorized scooter, sequela
		W05.2XXS	Fall from non-moving motorized mobility scooter, sequela
		W06.XXXS	Fall from bed, sequela
		W07.XXXS	Fall from chair, sequela
		W08.XXXS	Fall from other furniture, sequela
		W09.0XXS	Fall on or from playground slide, sequela
		W09.1XXS	Fall from playground swing, sequela
		W09.2XXS	Fall on or from jungle gym, sequela
		W09.8XXS	Fall on or from other playground equipment, sequela
		W10.0XXS	Fall (on)(from) escalator, sequela
		W10.1XXS	Fall (on)(from) sidewalk curb, sequela
		W10.2XXS	Fall (on)(from) incline, sequela
		W10.8XXS	Fall (on) (from) other stairs and steps, sequela
		W10.9XXS	Fall (on) (from) unspecified stairs and steps, sequela
		W11.XXXS	Fall on and from ladder, sequela
		W12.XXXS	Fall on and from scaffolding, sequela
		W13.0XXS	Fall from, out of or through balcony, sequela
		W13.1XXS	Fall from, out of or through bridge, sequela
		W13.2XXS	Fall from, out of or through roof, sequela
		W13.3XXS	Fall through floor, sequela
		W13.4XXS	Fall from, out of or through window, sequela
		W13.8XXS	Fall from, out of or through oth bldg, sequela
		W13.9XXS	Fall from, out of or through bldg, not otherwise spcf, sqla
		W14.XXXS	Fall from tree, sequela
		W15.XXXS	Fall from cliff, sequela
		W16.011S	Fall into swimming pool strk surfc causing drown, sequela
		W16.012S	Fall into swim pool strk surfc causing oth injury, sequela
		W16.021S	Fall into swimming pool strk bottom causing drown, sequela
		W16.022S	Fall into swim pool strk bottom causing oth injury, sequela
		W16.031S	Fall into swimming pool striking wall causing drown, sequela
		W16.032S	Fall into swim pool strk wall causing oth injury, sequela
		W16.111S	Fall into natrl body of water strk surfc cause drown, sqla
		W16.112S	Fall into natrl body of water strk surfc cause oth inj, sqla
		W16.121S	Fall into natrl body of water strk bottom cause drown, sqla
		W16.122S	Fall into natrl body of water strk botm cause oth inj, sqla
		W16.131S	Fall into natrl body of water strk side cause drown, sequela
		W16.132S	Fall into natrl body of water strk side cause oth inj, sqla
		W16.211S	Fall in (into) filled bathtub causing drown, sequela
		W16.212S	Fall in (into) filled bathtub causing other injury, sequela
		W16.221S	Fall in (into) bucket of water causing drown, sequela
		W16.222S	Fall in (into) bucket of water causing other injury, sequela
		W16.311S	Fall into oth water striking surfc causing drown, sequela
		W16.312S	Fall into oth water strk surfc causing oth injury, sequela
		W16.321S	Fall into oth water striking bottom causing drown, sequela
		W16.322S	Fall into oth water strk bottom causing oth injury, sequela
		W16.331S	Fall into oth water striking wall causing drown, sequela
		W16.332S	Fall into oth water strk wall causing oth injury, sequela
		W16.41XS	Fall into unsp water causing drown, sequela
		W16.42XS	Fall into unspecified water causing other injury, sequela
		W16.511S	Jump/div into swim pool strk surfc causing drown, sequela
		W16.512S	Jump/div into swim pool strk surfc cause oth injury, sequela
		W16.521S	Jump/div into swim pool strk bottom causing drown, sequela
		W16.522S	Jump/div into swim pool strk bottom cause oth injury, sqla
	(Continued on next page)	**W16.531S**	Jump/div into swimming pool strk wall causing drown, sequela

ICD-9-CM		ICD-10-CM	
E929.3	LATE EFFECTS OF ACCIDENTAL FALL **(Continued)**	**W16.532S**	Jump/div into swim pool strk wall cause oth injury, sequela
		W16.611S	Jump/div into natrl body of wtr strk surfc cause drown, sqla
		W16.612S	Jump/div in natrl body of wtr strk surfc cause oth inj, sqla
		W16.621S	Jump/div into natrl body of wtr strk botm cause drown, sqla
		W16.622S	Jump/div in natrl body of wtr strk botm cause oth inj, sqla
		W16.711S	Jump/div from boat striking surfc causing drown, sequela
		W16.712S	Jump/div from boat strk surfc causing oth injury, sequela
		W16.721S	Jump/div from boat striking bottom causing drown, sequela
		W16.722S	Jump/div from boat strk bottom causing oth injury, sequela
		W16.811S	Jump/div into oth water strk surfc causing drown, sequela
		W16.812S	Jump/div into oth water strk surfc cause oth injury, sequela
		W16.821S	Jump/div into oth water strk bottom causing drown, sequela
		W16.822S	Jump/div into oth water strk bottom cause oth injury, sqla
		W16.831S	Jump/div into oth water striking wall causing drown, sequela
		W16.832S	Jump/div into oth water strk wall cause oth injury, sequela
		W16.91XS	Jumping or diving into unsp water causing drown, sequela
		W16.92XS	Jump/div into unsp water causing oth injury, sequela
		W17.ØXXS	Fall into well, sequela
		W17.1XXS	Fall into storm drain or manhole, sequela
		W17.2XXS	Fall into hole, sequela
		W17.3XXS	Fall into empty swimming pool, sequela
		W17.4XXS	Fall from dock, sequela
		W17.81XS	Fall down embankment (hill), sequela
		W17.82XS	Fall from (out of) grocery cart, sequela
		W17.89XS	Other fall from one level to another, sequela
		W18.ØØXS	Striking against unsp object with subsequent fall, sequela
		W18.Ø1XS	Striking against sports equipment w subsequent fall, sequela
		W18.Ø2XS	Striking against glass with subsequent fall, sequela
		W18.Ø9XS	Striking against other object with subsequent fall, sequela
		W18.11XS	Fall from or off toilet w/o strike against object, sequela
		W18.12XS	Fall from or off toilet w strike against object, sequela
		W18.2XXS	Fall in (into) shower or empty bathtub, sequela
		W18.3ØXS	Fall on same level, unspecified, sequela
		W18.31XS	Fall on same level due to stepping on an object, sequela
		W18.39XS	Other fall on same level, sequela
		W18.4ØXS	Slipping, tripping and stumbling w/o falling, unsp, sequela
		W18.41XS	Slip/trip w/o falling due to stepping on object, sequela
		W18.42XS	Slip/trip w/o fall due to step into hole or opening, sequela
		W18.43XS	Slip/trip w/o fall d/t step from one level to another, sqla
		W18.49XS	Other slipping, tripping and stumbling w/o falling, sequela
		W19.XXXS	Unspecified fall, sequela
E929.4	LATE EFFECTS OF ACCIDENT CAUSED BY FIRE	**XØØ.ØXXS**	Exposure to flames in uncontrolled fire in bldg, sequela
		XØØ.1XXS	Exposure to smoke in uncontrolled fire in bldg, sequela
		XØØ.2XXS	Injury due to collapse of burn bldg in uncntrld fire, sqla
		XØØ.3XXS	Fall from burning bldg in uncontrolled fire, sequela
		XØØ.4XXS	Hit by object from burning bldg in uncntrld fire, sequela
		XØØ.5XXS	Jump from burning bldg in uncontrolled fire, sequela
		XØØ.8XXS	Oth exposure to uncontrolled fire in bldg, sequela
		XØ1.ØXXS	Exposure to flames in uncntrld fire, not in bldg, sequela
		XØ1.1XXS	Exposure to smoke in uncontrolled fire, not in bldg, sequela
		XØ1.3XXS	Fall due to uncontrolled fire, not in bldg, sequela
		XØ1.4XXS	Hit by object due to uncontrolled fire, not in bldg, sequela
		XØ1.8XXS	Oth exposure to uncontrolled fire, not in bldg, sequela
		XØ2.ØXXS	Exposure to flames in controlled fire in bldg, sequela
		XØ2.1XXS	Exposure to smoke in controlled fire in bldg, sequela
		XØ2.2XXS	Injury due to collapse of burning bldg in ctrl fire, sequela
		XØ2.3XXS	Fall from burning bldg in controlled fire, sequela
		XØ2.4XXS	Hit by object from burning bldg in controlled fire, sequela
		XØ2.5XXS	Jump from burning bldg in controlled fire, sequela
		XØ2.8XXS	Oth exposure to controlled fire in bldg, sequela
		XØ3.ØXXS	Exposure to flames in controlled fire, not in bldg, sequela
		XØ3.1XXS	Exposure to smoke in controlled fire, not in bldg, sequela
		XØ3.3XXS	Fall due to controlled fire, not in bldg, sequela
		XØ3.4XXS	Hit by object due to controlled fire, not in bldg, sequela
		XØ3.8XXS	Oth exposure to controlled fire, not in bldg, sequela
		XØ4.XXXS	Exposure to ignition of highly flammable material, sequela
		XØ5.XXXS	Exposure to ignition or melting of nightwear, sequela
		XØ6.ØXXS	Exposure to ignition of plastic jewelry, sequela
		XØ6.1XXS	Exposure to melting of plastic jewelry, sequela
		XØ6.2XXS	Exposure to ignition of other clothing and apparel, sequela
		XØ6.3XXS	Exposure to melting of other clothing and apparel, sequela
		XØ8.ØØXS	Exposure to bed fire due to unsp burning material, sequela
		XØ8.Ø1XS	Exposure to bed fire due to burning cigarette, sequela
		XØ8.Ø9XS	Exposure to bed fire due to other burning material, sequela
		XØ8.1ØXS	Exposure to sofa fire due to unsp burning material, sequela
		XØ8.11XS	Exposure to sofa fire due to burning cigarette, sequela
		XØ8.19XS	Exposure to sofa fire due to other burning material, sequela
		XØ8.2ØXS	Expsr to oth furniture fire due to unsp burn material, sqla
		XØ8.21XS	Expsr to oth furniture fire due to burn cigarette, sequela
		XØ8.29XS	Expsr to oth furniture fire due to oth burn material, sqla
		XØ8.8XXS	Exposure to other specified smoke, fire and flames, sequela

ICD-9-CM		ICD-10-CM	
E929.5	LATE EFF ACCIDENT DUE NATURAL&ENVIR FACTORS	**W53.Ø1XS**	Bitten by mouse, sequela
		W53.Ø9XS	Other contact with mouse, sequela
		W53.11XS	Bitten by rat, sequela
		W53.19XS	Other contact with rat, sequela
		W53.21XS	Bitten by squirrel, sequela
		W53.29XS	Other contact with squirrel, sequela
		W53.81XS	Bitten by other rodent, sequela
		W53.89XS	Other contact with other rodent, sequela
		W54.ØXXS	Bitten by dog, sequela
		W54.1XXS	Struck by dog, sequela
		W54.8XXS	Other contact with dog, sequela
		W55.Ø1XS	Bitten by cat, sequela
		W55.Ø3XS	Scratched by cat, sequela
		W55.Ø9XS	Other contact with cat, sequela
		W55.11XS	Bitten by horse, sequela
		W55.12XS	Struck by horse, sequela
		W55.19XS	Other contact with horse, sequela
		W55.21XS	Bitten by cow, sequela
		W55.22XS	Struck by cow, sequela
		W55.29XS	Other contact with cow, sequela
		W55.31XS	Bitten by other hoof stock, sequela
		W55.32XS	Struck by other hoof stock, sequela
		W55.39XS	Other contact with other hoof stock, sequela
		W55.41XS	Bitten by pig, sequela
		W55.42XS	Struck by pig, sequela
		W55.49XS	Other contact with pig, sequela
		W55.51XS	Bitten by raccoon, sequela
		W55.52XS	Struck by raccoon, sequela
		W55.59XS	Other contact with raccoon, sequela
		W55.81XS	Bitten by other mammals, sequela
		W55.82XS	Struck by other mammals, sequela
		W55.89XS	Other contact with other mammals, sequela
		W56.Ø1XS	Bitten by dolphin, sequela
		W56.Ø2XS	Struck by dolphin, sequela
		W56.Ø9XS	Other contact with dolphin, sequela
		W56.11XS	Bitten by sea lion, sequela
		W56.12XS	Struck by sea lion, sequela
		W56.19XS	Other contact with sea lion, sequela
		W56.21XS	Bitten by orca, sequela
		W56.22XS	Struck by orca, sequela
		W56.29XS	Other contact with orca, sequela
		W56.31XS	Bitten by other marine mammals, sequela
		W56.32XS	Struck by other marine mammals, sequela
		W56.39XS	Other contact with other marine mammals, sequela
		W56.41XS	Bitten by shark, sequela
		W56.42XS	Struck by shark, sequela
		W56.49XS	Other contact with shark, sequela
		W56.51XS	Bitten by other fish, sequela
		W56.52XS	Struck by other fish, sequela
		W56.59XS	Other contact with other fish, sequela
		W56.81XS	Bitten by other nonvenomous marine animals, sequela
		W56.82XS	Struck by other nonvenomous marine animals, sequela
		W56.89XS	Other contact with other nonvenomous marine animals, sequela
		W57.XXXS	Bit/stung by nonvenom insect & oth nonvenom arthropods, sqla
		W58.Ø1XS	Bitten by alligator, sequela
		W58.Ø2XS	Struck by alligator, sequela
		W58.Ø3XS	Crushed by alligator, sequela
		W58.Ø9XS	Other contact with alligator, sequela
		W58.11XS	Bitten by crocodile, sequela
		W58.12XS	Struck by crocodile, sequela
		W58.13XS	Crushed by crocodile, sequela
		W58.19XS	Other contact with crocodile, sequela
		W59.Ø1XS	Bitten by nonvenomous lizards, sequela
		W59.Ø2XS	Struck by nonvenomous lizards, sequela
		W59.Ø9XS	Other contact with nonvenomous lizards, sequela
		W59.11XS	Bitten by nonvenomous snake, sequela
		W59.12XS	Struck by nonvenomous snake, sequela
		W59.13XS	Crushed by nonvenomous snake, sequela
		W59.19XS	Other contact with nonvenomous snake, sequela
		W59.21XS	Bitten by turtle, sequela
		W59.22XS	Struck by turtle, sequela
		W59.29XS	Other contact with turtle, sequela
		W59.81XS	Bitten by other nonvenomous reptiles, sequela
		W59.82XS	Struck by other nonvenomous reptiles, sequela
		W59.83XS	Crushed by other nonvenomous reptiles, sequela
		W59.89XS	Other contact with other nonvenomous reptiles, sequela
		W61.Ø1XS	Bitten by parrot, sequela
		W61.Ø2XS	Struck by parrot, sequela
		W61.Ø9XS	Other contact with parrot, sequela
		W61.11XS	Bitten by macaw, sequela
		W61.12XS	Struck by macaw, sequela
		W61.19XS	Other contact with macaw, sequela
	(Continued on next page)	**W61.21XS**	Bitten by other psittacines, sequela

ICD-9-CM		ICD-10-CM		
E929.5	LATE EFF ACCIDENT DUE NATURAL&ENVIR FACTORS **(Continued)**		**W61.22XS**	Struck by other psittacines, sequela
			W61.29XS	Other contact with other psittacines, sequela
			W61.32XS	Struck by chicken, sequela
			W61.33XS	Pecked by chicken, sequela
			W61.39XS	Other contact with chicken, sequela
			W61.42XS	Struck by turkey, sequela
			W61.43XS	Pecked by turkey, sequela
			W61.49XS	Other contact with turkey, sequela
			W61.51XS	Bitten by goose, sequela
			W61.52XS	Struck by goose, sequela
			W61.59XS	Other contact with goose, sequela
			W61.61XS	Bitten by duck, sequela
			W61.62XS	Struck by duck, sequela
			W61.69XS	Other contact with duck, sequela
			W61.91XS	Bitten by other birds, sequela
			W61.92XS	Struck by other birds, sequela
			W61.99XS	Other contact with other birds, sequela
			W62.ØXXS	Contact with nonvenomous frogs, sequela
			W62.1XXS	Contact with nonvenomous toads, sequela
			W62.9XXS	Contact with other nonvenomous amphibians, sequela
			W64.XXXS	Exposure to other animate mechanical forces, sequela
			W92.XXXS	Exposure to excessive heat of man-made origin, sequela
			W93.Ø1XS	Contact with dry ice, sequela
			W93.Ø2XS	Inhalation of dry ice, sequela
			W93.11XS	Contact with liquid air, sequela
			W93.12XS	Inhalation of liquid air, sequela
			W93.2XXS	Prolonged exposure in deep freeze unit or refrig, sequela
			W93.8XXS	Exposure to other excessive cold of man-made origin, sequela
			W94.ØXXS	Exposure to prolonged high air pressure, sequela
			W94.11XS	Expsr to resdnce or prolonged visit at high altitude, sqla
			W94.12XS	Exposure to other prolonged low air pressure, sequela
			W94.21XS	Expsr to rdct in atmos pressr wh surfc fr dp-watr div, sqla
			W94.22XS	Expsr to rdct in atmos pressr wh surfc fr underground, sqla
			W94.23XS	Expsr to chng in air pressr in arcrft during ascent, sequela
			W94.29XS	Expsr to oth rapid changes in air pressr during ascent, sqla
			W94.31XS	Expsr to chng in air pressr in arcrft dur desc, sqla
			W94.32XS	Expsr to high air pressr from rapid descent in water, sqla
			W94.39XS	Expsr to oth rapid changes in air pressr dur descent, sqla
			W99.XXXS	Exposure to other man-made environmental factors, sequela
			X3Ø.XXXS	Exposure to excessive natural heat, sequela
			X31.XXXS	Exposure to excessive natural cold, sequela
			X32.XXXS	Exposure to sunlight, sequela
			X34.XXXS	Earthquake, sequela
			X35.XXXS	Volcanic eruption, sequela
			X36.ØXXS	Collapse of dam or man-made struct cause earth movmnt, sqla
			X36.1XXS	Avalanche, landslide, or mudslide, sequela
			X37.ØXXS	Hurricane, sequela
			X37.1XXS	Tornado, sequela
			X37.2XXS	Blizzard (snow)(ice), sequela
			X37.3XXS	Dust storm, sequela
			X37.41XS	Tidal wave due to earthquake or volcanic eruption, sequela
			X37.42XS	Tidal wave due to storm, sequela
			X37.43XS	Tidal wave due to landslide, sequela
			X37.8XXS	Other cataclysmic storms, sequela
			X37.9XXS	Unspecified cataclysmic storm, sequela
			X38.XXXS	Flood, sequela
			X39.8XXS	Other exposure to forces of nature, sequela
E929.8	LATE EFFECTS OF OTHER ACCIDENTS	◘	**T71.161S**	Asphyxiation due to hanging, accidental, sequela
			VØØ.Ø1XS	Ped on foot injured in collision w roller-skater, sequela
			VØØ.Ø2XS	Ped on foot injured in collision w skateboarder, sequela
			VØØ.Ø9XS	Ped on foot injured in collision w oth ped convey, sequela
			W2Ø.ØXXS	Struck by falling object in cave-in, sequela
			W2Ø.1XXS	Struck by object due to collapse of building, sequela
			W2Ø.8XXS	Oth cause of strike by thrown, projected or fall obj, sqla
			W21.ØØXS	Struck by hit or thrown ball, unspecified type, sequela
			W21.Ø1XS	Struck by football, sequela
			W21.Ø2XS	Struck by soccer ball, sequela
			W21.Ø3XS	Struck by baseball, sequela
			W21.Ø4XS	Struck by golf ball, sequela
			W21.Ø5XS	Struck by basketball, sequela
			W21.Ø6XS	Struck by volleyball, sequela
			W21.Ø7XS	Struck by softball, sequela
			W21.Ø9XS	Struck by other hit or thrown ball, sequela
			W21.11XS	Struck by baseball bat, sequela
			W21.12XS	Struck by tennis racquet, sequela
			W21.13XS	Struck by golf club, sequela
			W21.19XS	Struck by other bat, racquet or club, sequela
			W21.21ØS	Struck by ice hockey stick, sequela
			W21.211S	Struck by field hockey stick, sequela
			W21.22ØS	Struck by ice hockey puck, sequela
			W21.221S	Struck by field hockey puck, sequela
			W21.31XS	Struck by shoe cleats, sequela
	(Continued on next page)		**W21.32XS**	Struck by skate blades, sequela

ICD-9-CM		ICD-10-CM	
E929.8	LATE EFFECTS OF OTHER ACCIDENTS **(Continued)**	**W21.39XS**	Struck by other sports foot wear, sequela
		W21.4XXS	Striking against diving board, sequela
		W21.81XS	Striking against or struck by football helmet, sequela
		W21.89XS	Striking against or struck by oth sports equipment, sequela
		W21.9XXS	Striking against or struck by unsp sports equipment, sequela
		W22.01XS	Walked into wall, sequela
		W22.02XS	Walked into lamppost, sequela
		W22.03XS	Walked into furniture, sequela
		W22.041S	Strike wall of swimming pool causing drown, sequela
		W22.042S	Strike wall of swimming pool causing oth injury, sequela
		W22.09XS	Striking against other stationary object, sequela
		W22.10XS	Strike/struck by unsp automobile airbag, sequela
		W22.11XS	Strike/struck by driver side automobile airbag, sequela
		W22.12XS	Strike/struck by front passenger side auto airbag, sequela
		W22.19XS	Striking against or struck by oth automobile airbag, sequela
		W22.8XXS	Striking against or struck by other objects, sequela
		W23.0XXS	Caught, crush, jammed, or pinched betw moving obj, sequela
		W23.1XXS	Caught, crush, jammed, or pinched betw stationry obj, sqla
		W24.0XXS	Contact w lifting devices, not elsewhere classified, sequela
		W24.1XXS	Contact w transmission devices, NEC, sequela
		W25.XXXS	Contact with sharp glass, sequela
		W26.0XXS	Contact with knife, sequela
		W26.1XXS	Contact with sword or dagger, sequela
		W27.0XXS	Contact with workbench tool, sequela
		W27.1XXS	Contact with garden tool, sequela
		W27.2XXS	Contact with scissors, sequela
		W27.3XXS	Contact with needle (sewing), sequela
		W27.4XXS	Contact with kitchen utensil, sequela
		W27.5XXS	Contact with paper-cutter, sequela
		W27.8XXS	Contact with other nonpowered hand tool, sequela
		W28.XXXS	Contact with powered lawn mower, sequela
		W29.0XXS	Contact with powered kitchen appliance, sequela
		W29.1XXS	Contact with electric knife, sequela
		W29.2XXS	Contact with other powered household machinery, sequela
		W29.3XXS	Cntct w power garden and outdoor hand tools and mach, sqla
		W29.4XXS	Contact with nail gun, sequela
		W29.8XXS	Cntct w oth power power hand tools and household mach, sqla
		W30.0XXS	Contact with combine harvester, sequela
		W30.1XXS	Contact with power take-off devices (PTO), sequela
		W30.2XXS	Contact with hay derrick, sequela
		W30.3XXS	Contact with grain storage elevator, sequela
		W30.81XS	Contact w agri transport vehicle in stationary use, sequela
		W30.89XS	Contact with other specified agricultural machinery, sequela
		W30.9XXS	Contact with unspecified agricultural machinery, sequela
		W31.0XXS	Contact with mining and earth-drilling machinery, sequela
		W31.1XXS	Contact with metalworking machines, sequela
		W31.2XXS	Contact w powered woodworking and forming machines, sequela
		W31.3XXS	Contact with prime movers, sequela
		W31.81XS	Contact with recreational machinery, sequela
		W31.82XS	Contact with other commercial machinery, sequela
		W31.83XS	Cntct w special construct vehicle in stationry use, sequela
		W31.89XS	Contact with other specified machinery, sequela
		W31.9XXS	Contact with unspecified machinery, sequela
		W32.0XXS	Accidental handgun discharge, sequela
		W32.1XXS	Accidental handgun malfunction, sequela
		W33.00XS	Accidental discharge of unspecified larger firearm, sequela
		W33.01XS	Accidental discharge of shotgun, sequela
		W33.02XS	Accidental discharge of hunting rifle, sequela
		W33.03XS	Accidental discharge of machine gun, sequela
		W33.09XS	Accidental discharge of other larger firearm, sequela
		W33.10XS	Accidental malfunction of unsp larger firearm, sequela
		W33.11XS	Accidental malfunction of shotgun, sequela
		W33.12XS	Accidental malfunction of hunting rifle, sequela
		W33.13XS	Accidental malfunction of machine gun, sequela
		W33.19XS	Accidental malfunction of other larger firearm, sequela
		W34.00XS	Accidental discharge from unsp firearms or gun, sequela
		W34.010S	Accidental discharge of airgun, sequela
		W34.011S	Accidental discharge of paintball gun, sequela
		W34.018S	Accidental discharge of gas, air or sprng-op gun, sequela
		W34.09XS	Accidental discharge from other specified firearms, sequela
		W34.10XS	Accidental malfunction from unsp firearms or gun, sequela
		W34.110S	Accidental malfunction of airgun, sequela
		W34.111S	Accidental malfunction of paintball gun, sequela
		W34.118S	Accidental malfunction of gas, air or sprng-op gun, sequela
		W34.19XS	Accidental malfunction from oth firearms, sequela
		W35.XXXS	Explosion and rupture of boiler, sequela
		W36.1XXS	Explosion and rupture of aerosol can, sequela
		W36.2XXS	Explosion and rupture of air tank, sequela
		W36.3XXS	Explosion and rupture of pressurized-gas tank, sequela
		W36.8XXS	Explosion and rupture of other gas cylinder, sequela
		W36.9XXS	Explosion and rupture of unspecified gas cylinder, sequela
	(Continued on next page)	**W37.0XXS**	Explosion of bicycle tire, sequela

ICD-9-CM		ICD-10-CM	
E929.8	LATE EFFECTS OF OTHER ACCIDENTS **(Continued)**	**W37.8XXS**	Explosn and rupt of pressurized tire, pipe or hose, sequela
		W38.XXXS	Explosion and rupture of oth pressurized devices, sequela
		W39.XXXS	Discharge of firework, sequela
		W40.0XXS	Explosion of blasting material, sequela
		W40.1XXS	Explosion of explosive gases, sequela
		W40.8XXS	Explosion of other specified explosive materials, sequela
		W40.9XXS	Explosion of unspecified explosive materials, sequela
		W42.0XXS	Exposure to supersonic waves, sequela
		W42.9XXS	Exposure to other noise, sequela
		W45.0XXS	Nail entering through skin, sequela
		W45.1XXS	Paper entering through skin, sequela
		W45.2XXS	Lid of can entering through skin, sequela
		W45.8XXS	Other foreign body or object entering through skin, sequela
		W46.0XXS	Contact with hypodermic needle, sequela
		W46.1XXS	Contact with contaminated hypodermic needle, sequela
		W49.01XS	Hair causing external constriction, sequela
		W49.02XS	String or thread causing external constriction, sequela
		W49.03XS	Rubber band causing external constriction, sequela
		W49.04XS	Ring or other jewelry causing external constriction, sequela
		W49.09XS	Other specified item causing external constriction, sequela
		W49.9XXS	Exposure to other inanimate mechanical forces, sequela
		W50.0XXS	Accidental hit or strike by another person, sequela
		W50.1XXS	Accidental kick by another person, sequela
		W50.2XXS	Accidental twist by another person, sequela
		W50.3XXS	Accidental bite by another person, sequela
		W50.4XXS	Accidental scratch by another person, sequela
		W51.XXXS	Accidental strike or bumped into by another person, sequela
		W52.XXXS	Crushd/pushd/stepd on by crowd or human stampede, sequela
		W60.XXXS	Cntct w nonvenom plant thorns & spines & sharp leaves, sqla
		W65.XXXS	Accidental drown while in bath-tub, sequela
		W67.XXXS	Accidental drown while in swimming-pool, sequela
		W69.XXXS	Accidental drown while in natural water, sequela
		W73.XXXS	Oth cause of accidental non-transport drown, sequela
		W74.XXXS	Unsp cause of accidental drowning and submersion, sequela
		W85.XXXS	Exposure to electric transmission lines, sequela
		W86.0XXS	Exposure to domestic wiring and appliances, sequela
		W86.1XXS	Expsr to industr wiring, appliances & electrical mach, sqla
		W86.8XXS	Exposure to other electric current, sequela
		W88.0XXS	Exposure to X-rays, sequela
		W88.1XXS	Exposure to radioactive isotopes, sequela
		W88.8XXS	Exposure to other ionizing radiation, sequela
		W89.0XXS	Exposure to welding light (arc), sequela
		W89.1XXS	Exposure to tanning bed, sequela
		W89.8XXS	Expsr to oth man-made visible and ultraviolet light, sequela
		W89.9XXS	Expsr to unsp man-made visible and ultraviolet light, sqla
		W90.0XXS	Exposure to radiofrequency, sequela
		W90.1XXS	Exposure to infrared radiation, sequela
		W90.2XXS	Exposure to laser radiation, sequela
		W90.8XXS	Exposure to other nonionizing radiation, sequela
		X10.0XXS	Contact with hot drinks, sequela
		X10.1XXS	Contact with hot food, sequela
		X10.2XXS	Contact with fats and cooking oils, sequela
		X11.0XXS	Contact with hot water in bath or tub, sequela
		X11.1XXS	Contact with running hot water, sequela
		X11.8XXS	Contact with other hot tap-water, sequela
		X12.XXXS	Contact with other hot fluids, sequela
		X13.0XXS	Inhalation of steam and other hot vapors, sequela
		X13.1XXS	Other contact with steam and other hot vapors, sequela
		X14.0XXS	Inhalation of hot air and gases, sequela
		X14.1XXS	Other contact with hot air and other hot gases, sequela
		X15.0XXS	Contact with hot stove (kitchen), sequela
		X15.1XXS	Contact with hot toaster, sequela
		X15.2XXS	Contact with hotplate, sequela
		X15.3XXS	Contact with hot saucepan or skillet, sequela
		X15.8XXS	Contact with other hot household appliances, sequela
		X16.XXXS	Cntct w hot heating appliances, radiators and pipes, sequela
		X17.XXXS	Contact with hot engines, machinery and tools, sequela
		X18.XXXS	Contact with other hot metals, sequela
		X19.XXXS	Contact with other heat and hot substances, sequela
		X39.01XS	Exposure to radon, sequela
		X39.08XS	Exposure to other natural radiation, sequela
		X52.XXXS	Prolonged stay in weightless environment, sequela
		X58.XXXS	Exposure to other specified factors, sequela
		Y21.0XXS	Drown while in bathtub, undetermined intent, sequela
		Y21.1XXS	Drown after fall into bathtub, undetermined intent, sequela
		Y21.2XXS	Drown while in swimming pool, undetermined intent, sequela
		Y21.3XXS	Drown after fall into swimming pool, undet intent, sequela
		Y21.4XXS	Drown in natural water, undetermined intent, sequela
		Y21.8XXS	Other drowning and submersion, undetermined intent, sequela
		Y21.9XXS	Unsp drowning and submersion, undetermined intent, sequela
		Y22.XXXS	Handgun discharge, undetermined intent, sequela
	(Continued on next page)	**Y23.0XXS**	Shotgun discharge, undetermined intent, sequela

ICD-9-CM		ICD-10-CM	
E929.8	LATE EFFECTS OF OTHER ACCIDENTS **(Continued)**	**Y23.1XXS**	Hunting rifle discharge, undetermined intent, sequela
		Y23.2XXS	Military firearm discharge, undetermined intent, sequela
		Y23.3XXS	Machine gun discharge, undetermined intent, sequela
		Y23.8XXS	Other larger firearm discharge, undetermined intent, sequela
		Y23.9XXS	Unsp larger firearm discharge, undetermined intent, sequela
		Y24.ØXXS	Airgun discharge, undetermined intent, sequela
		Y24.8XXS	Other firearm discharge, undetermined intent, sequela
		Y24.9XXS	Unspecified firearm discharge, undetermined intent, sequela
		Y25.XXXS	Contact w explosive material, undetermined intent, sequela
		Y26.XXXS	Exposure to smoke, fire and flames, undet intent, sequela
		Y27.ØXXS	Contact w steam and hot vapors, undetermined intent, sequela
		Y27.1XXS	Contact with hot tap water, undetermined intent, sequela
		Y27.2XXS	Contact with hot fluids, undetermined intent, sequela
		Y27.3XXS	Contact w hot household appliance, undet intent, sequela
		Y27.8XXS	Contact with other hot objects, undetermined intent, sequela
		Y27.9XXS	Contact with unsp hot objects, undetermined intent, sequela
		Y28.ØXXS	Contact with sharp glass, undetermined intent, sequela
		Y28.1XXS	Contact with knife, undetermined intent, sequela
		Y28.2XXS	Contact with sword or dagger, undetermined intent, sequela
		Y28.8XXS	Contact with oth sharp object, undetermined intent, sequela
		Y28.9XXS	Contact with unsp sharp object, undetermined intent, sequela
		Y29.XXXS	Contact with blunt object, undetermined intent, sequela
		Y3Ø.XXXS	Fall, jump or pushed from a high place, undet intent, sqla
		Y31.XXXS	Fall/lying/running bef/into moving obj, undet intent, sqla
		Y32.XXXS	Crashing of motor vehicle, undetermined intent, sequela
		Y33.XXXS	Other specified events, undetermined intent, sequela
E929.9	LATE EFFECTS OF UNSPECIFIED ACCIDENT	**X58.XXXS**	Exposure to other specified factors, sequela
E93Ø.Ø	PENICILLINS CAUS ADVERSE EFFECT THERAPEUTIC USE	**T36.ØX5A**	Adverse effect of penicillins, initial encounter
		T36.ØX5S	Adverse effect of penicillins, sequela
E93Ø.1	ANTIFUNGAL ABXS CAUS ADVRS EFF THERAPEUTIC USE	**T36.7X5A**	Adverse effect of antifungal antibiotics, sys used, init
		T36.7X5S	Adverse effect of antifungal antibiotics, sys used, sequela
E93Ø.2	CHLORAMPHENICOL GRP CAUS ADVRS EFF TX USE	**T36.2X5A**	Adverse effect of chloramphenicol group, initial encounter
		T36.2X5S	Adverse effect of chloramphenicol group, sequela
E93Ø.3	ERYTH&OTH MACROLIDES CAUS ADVRS EFF TX USE	**T36.3X5A**	Adverse effect of macrolides, initial encounter
		T36.3X5S	Adverse effect of macrolides, sequela
E93Ø.4	TETRACYCLINE GRP CAUS ADVRS EFF THERAPEUTIC USE	**T36.4X5A**	Adverse effect of tetracyclines, initial encounter
		T36.4X5S	Adverse effect of tetracyclines, sequela
E93Ø.5	CEPHALOSPORIN GRP CAUS ADVRS EFF THERAPEUTIC USE	**T36.1X5A**	Adverse effect of cephalospor/oth beta-lactm antibiot, init
		T36.1X5S	Advrs effect of cephalospor/oth beta-lactm antibiot, sequela
E93Ø.6	ANTIMYCOBACTERL ABXS CAUS ADVRS EFF TX USE	**T36.6X5A**	Adverse effect of rifampicins, initial encounter
		T36.6X5S	Adverse effect of rifampicins, sequela
		T37.1X5A	Adverse effect of antimycobacterial drugs, initial encounter
		T37.1X5S	Adverse effect of antimycobacterial drugs, sequela
E93Ø.7	ANTINEOPLSTC ABXS CAUS ADVRS EFF THERAPEUTIC USE		NO DIAGNOSIS
E93Ø.8	OTH SPEC ABXS CAUS ADVRS EFFECT THERAPEUTIC USE	**T36.5X5A**	Adverse effect of aminoglycosides, initial encounter
		T36.5X5S	Adverse effect of aminoglycosides, sequela
		T36.8X5A	Adverse effect of other systemic antibiotics, init encntr
		T36.8X5S	Adverse effect of other systemic antibiotics, sequela
		T36.95XA	Adverse effect of unsp systemic antibiotic, init encntr
		T36.95XS	Adverse effect of unspecified systemic antibiotic, sequela
E93Ø.9	UNSPEC ABX CAUS ADVERSE EFFECT THERAPEUTIC USE		NO DIAGNOSIS
E931.Ø	SULFONAMIDES CAUS ADVERSE EFFECT THERAPEUTIC USE	**T37.ØX5A**	Adverse effect of sulfonamides, initial encounter
		T37.ØX5S	Adverse effect of sulfonamides, sequela
E931.1	ARSENICAL ANTI-INFECTVS CAUS ADVRS EFF TX USE		NO DIAGNOSIS
E931.2	HEAVY METAL ANTI-INFECTVS CAUS ADVRS EFF TX USE		NO DIAGNOSIS
E931.3	QUINOLINE-HYDROXYQUINOLIN CAUS ADVRSE EFF TX USE		NO DIAGNOSIS
E931.4	ANTIMALARIALS OTH PROTZOA CAUS ADVRSE EFF TX USE	**T37.2X5A**	Advrs effect of antimalari/drugs acting on bld protzoa, init
		T37.2X5S	Advrs effect of antimalari/drugs acting on bld protzoa, sqla
E931.5	OTH ANTIPROTOZOAL RX CAUS ADVRS EFF TX USE	**T37.3X5A**	Adverse effect of other antiprotozoal drugs, init encntr
		T37.3X5S	Adverse effect of other antiprotozoal drugs, sequela
E931.6	ANTHELMINTICS CAUS ADVRS EFFECT THERAPEUTIC USE	**T37.4X5A**	Adverse effect of anthelminthics, initial encounter
		T37.4X5S	Adverse effect of anthelminthics, sequela
E931.7	ANTIVIRAL RX CAUS ADVERSE EFFECT THERAPEUTIC USE	**T37.5X5A**	Adverse effect of antiviral drugs, initial encounter
		T37.5X5S	Adverse effect of antiviral drugs, sequela
E931.8	OTH ANTIMYCOBACTERL RX CAUS ADVRS EFF TX USE		NO DIAGNOSIS
E931.9	OTH&UNSPEC ANTI-INFECTVS CAUS ADVRS EFF TX USE	**T37.8X5A**	Adverse effect of systemic anti-infect/parasit, init
		T37.8X5S	Adverse effect of systemic anti-infect/parasit, sequela
		T37.95XA	Advrs effect of unsp sys anti-infect and antiparasitic, init
		T37.95XS	Advrs effect of unsp sys anti-infect and antiparasitic, sqla
E932.Ø	ADRENL CORTICAL STEROIDS CAUS ADVRS EFF TX USE	**T38.ØX5A**	Adverse effect of glucocort/synth analog, init
		T38.ØX5S	Adverse effect of glucocort/synth analog, sequela
		T5Ø.ØX5A	Adverse effect of mineralocorticoids and their antag, init
		T5Ø.ØX5S	Adverse effect of mineralocorticoids and antag, sequela
E932.1	ANDROGEN&ANABOL CONGENER CAUS ADVRSE EFF TX USE	**T38.7X5A**	Adverse effect of androgens and anabolic congeners, init
		T38.7X5S	Adverse effect of androgens and anabolic congeners, sequela

ICD-9-CM		ICD-10-CM	
E932.2	OVARY HORMONE-SYNTH SUBST CAUS ADVRSE EFF TX USE	T38.4X5A	Adverse effect of oral contraceptives, initial encounter
		T38.4X5S	Adverse effect of oral contraceptives, sequela
		T38.5X5A	Adverse effect of oth estrogens and progestogens, init
		T38.5X5S	Adverse effect of other estrogens and progestogens, sequela
E932.3	INSULINS&ANTIDIAB AGTS CAUS ADVRS EFF TX USE	T38.3X5A	Adverse effect of insulin and oral hypoglycemic drugs, init
		T38.3X5S	Advrs effect of insulin and oral hypoglycemic drugs, sequela
E932.4	ANT PITUITARY HORMONES CAUS ADVRS EFF TX USE	T38.815A	Adverse effect of anterior pituitary hormones, init encntr
		T38.815S	Adverse effect of anterior pituitary hormones, sequela
E932.5	POST PITUITARY HORMONES CAUS ADVRS EFF TX USE		NO DIAGNOSIS
E932.6	PARATHYROID & DERIVATIVES CAUS ADVRSE EFF TX USE		NO DIAGNOSIS
E932.7	THYROID & DERIVATIVES CAUS ADVRSE EFF TX USE	T38.1X5A	Adverse effect of thyroid hormones and substitutes, init
		T38.1X5S	Adverse effect of thyroid hormones and substitutes, sequela
E932.8	ANTITHYROID AGTS CAUS ADVRS EFF THERAPEUTIC USE	T38.2X5A	Adverse effect of antithyroid drugs, initial encounter
		T38.2X5S	Adverse effect of antithyroid drugs, sequela
E932.9	UNS HORMONES&SYNTH SUBSTS CAUS ADVRS EFF TX USE	T38.6X5A	Adverse effect of antigonadtr/antiestr/antiandrg, NEC, init
		T38.6X5S	Advrs effect of antigonadtr/antiestr/antiandrg, NEC, sequela
		T38.8Ø5A	Adverse effect of unsp hormones and synthetic sub, init
		T38.8Ø5S	Adverse effect of unsp hormones and synthetic sub, sequela
		T38.895A	Adverse effect of hormones and synthetic substitutes, init
		T38.895S	Adverse effect of hormones and synthetic sub, sequela
		T38.9Ø5A	Adverse effect of unsp hormone antagonists, init encntr
		T38.9Ø5S	Adverse effect of unspecified hormone antagonists, sequela
		T38.995A	Adverse effect of other hormone antagonists, init encntr
		T38.995S	Adverse effect of other hormone antagonists, sequela
E933.Ø	ANTIALLERG&ANTIEMETIC RX CAUS ADVRS EFF TX USE	T45.ØX5A	Adverse effect of antiallergic and antiemetic drugs, init
		T45.ØX5S	Adverse effect of antiallergic and antiemetic drugs, sequela
E933.1	ANTINEOPLASTIC-IMMUNOSUPP CAUS ADVRSE EFF TX USE	T45.1X5A	Adverse effect of antineoplastic and immunosup drugs, init
		T45.1X5S	Adverse effect of antineopl and immunosup drugs, sequela
E933.2	ACIDIFYING AGTS CAUS ADVRS EFF THERAPEUTIC USE		NO DIAGNOSIS
E933.3	ALKALIZING AGTS CAUS ADVRS EFF THERAPEUTIC USE		NO DIAGNOSIS
E933.4	ENZYMES NEC CAUS ADVERSE EFFECT THERAPEUTIC USE	T45.3X5A	Adverse effect of enzymes, initial encounter
		T45.3X5S	Adverse effect of enzymes, sequela
E933.5	VITAMINS NEC CAUS ADVERSE EFFECT THERAPEUTIC USE	T45.2X5A	Adverse effect of vitamins, initial encounter
		T45.2X5S	Adverse effect of vitamins, sequela
E933.6	DRUG ADV EFFECT, ORAL BISPHOSPHONATES	T45.8X5A	Adverse effect of prim systemic and hematolog agents, init
		T45.8X5S	Adverse effect of prim sys and hematolog agents, sequela
E933.7	DRUG ADVRSE EFFCT, INTRAVENOUS BISPHOSPHONATES	T45.8X5A	Adverse effect of prim systemic and hematolog agents, init
		T45.8X5S	Adverse effect of prim sys and hematolog agents, sequela
E933.8	OTH SYS AGTS NEC CAUS ADVRS EFF THERAPEUTIC USE	T45.8X5A	Adverse effect of prim systemic and hematolog agents, init
		T45.8X5S	Adverse effect of prim sys and hematolog agents, sequela
E933.9	UNSPEC SYS AGT CAUS ADVRS EFFECT THERAPEUTIC USE	T45.95XA	Adverse effect of unsp prim sys and hematolog agent, init
E934.Ø	IRON&ITS COMPND CAUS ADVRS EFF THERAPEUTIC USE	T45.4X5A	Adverse effect of iron and its compounds, initial encounter
		T45.4X5S	Adverse effect of iron and its compounds, sequela
E934.1	LIVER-OTH ANTIANEMIC AGT CAUS ADVRSE EFF TX USE		NO DIAGNOSIS
E934.2	ANTICOAG CAUSING ADVERSE EFFECT THERAPEUTIC USE	T45.515A	Adverse effect of anticoagulants, initial encounter
		T45.515S	Adverse effect of anticoagulants, sequela
		T45.525A	Adverse effect of antithrombotic drugs, initial encounter
		T45.525S	Adverse effect of antithrombotic drugs, sequela
E934.3	VITAMIN K CAUSING ADVERSE EFFECT THERAPEUTIC USE		NO DIAGNOSIS
E934.4	FIBRINOLYSIS-AFFCT RX CAUS ADVRS EFF TX USE	T45.6Ø5A	Adverse effect of unsp fibrinolysis-affecting drugs, init
		T45.6Ø5S	Adverse effect of unsp fibrinolysis-affecting drugs, sequela
		T45.615A	Adverse effect of thrombolytic drugs, initial encounter
		T45.615S	Adverse effect of thrombolytic drugs, sequela
		T45.695A	Adverse effect of oth fibrinolysis-affecting drugs, init
		T45.695S	Adverse effect of oth fibrinolysis-affecting drugs, sequela
E934.5	ANTICOAG ANTAGONISTS CAUS ADVRSE EFF TX USE	T45.7X5A	Adverse effect of anticoag antag, vit K and oth coag, init
		T45.7X5S	Advrs effect of anticoag antag, vit K and oth coag, sequela
E934.6	GAMMA GLOB CAUS ADVERSE EFFECT THERAPEUTIC USE	T5Ø.Z15A	Adverse effect of immunoglobulin, initial encounter
		T5Ø.Z15S	Adverse effect of immunoglobulin, sequela
E934.7	NATURAL BLD&BLD PRODUCTS CAUS ADVRS EFF TX USE		NO DIAGNOSIS
E934.8	OTH AGT BLD CONSTITUNTS CAUS ADVRSE EFF TX USE	T45.625A	Adverse effect of hemostatic drug, initial encounter
		T45.625S	Adverse effect of hemostatic drug, sequela
		T45.8X5A	Adverse effect of prim systemic and hematolog agents, init
		T45.8X5S	Adverse effect of prim sys and hematolog agents, sequela
E934.9	UNS AGT BLD CONSTITUNTS CAUS ADVRSE EFF TX USE	T45.95XA	Adverse effect of unsp prim sys and hematolog agent, init
		T45.95XS	Adverse effect of unsp prim sys and hematolog agent, sequela
E935.Ø	HEROIN CAUSING ADVERSE EFFECT IN THERAPEUTIC USE	T4Ø.ØX5A	Adverse effect of opium, initial encounter
		T4Ø.ØX5S	Adverse effect of opium, sequela
E935.1	METHADONE CAUSING AVERSE EFFECT THERAPEUTIC USE	T4Ø.3X5A	Adverse effect of methadone, initial encounter
		T4Ø.3X5S	Adverse effect of methadone, sequela

ICD-9-CM		ICD-10-CM	
E935.2	OTH OPIATES&REL NARCOTICS CAUS ADVRS EFF TX USE	**T40.ØX5A**	Adverse effect of opium, initial encounter
		T40.ØX5S	Adverse effect of opium, sequela
		T40.2X5A	Adverse effect of other opioids, initial encounter
		T40.2X5S	Adverse effect of other opioids, sequela
		T40.4X5A	Adverse effect of other synthetic narcotics, init encntr
		T40.4X5S	Adverse effect of other synthetic narcotics, sequela
		T40.6Ø5A	Adverse effect of unspecified narcotics, initial encounter
		T40.6Ø5S	Adverse effect of unspecified narcotics, sequela
		T40.695A	Adverse effect of other narcotics, initial encounter
		T40.695S	Adverse effect of other narcotics, sequela
E935.3	SALICYLATES CAUS ADVERSE EFFECT THERAPEUTIC USE	**T39.Ø15A**	Adverse effect of aspirin, initial encounter
		T39.Ø15S	Adverse effect of aspirin, sequela
		T39.Ø95A	Adverse effect of salicylates, initial encounter
		T39.Ø95S	Adverse effect of salicylates, sequela
		T39.1X5A	Adverse effect of 4-Aminophenol derivatives, init encntr
		T39.1X5S	Adverse effect of 4-Aminophenol derivatives, sequela
E935.4	AROMATIC ANALGES NEC CAUS ADVRS EFF TX USE	NO DIAGNOSIS	
E935.5	PYRAZOLE DERIVATIVES CAUS ADVRS EFF TX USE	**T39.2X5A**	Adverse effect of pyrazolone derivatives, initial encounter
		T39.2X5S	Adverse effect of pyrazolone derivatives, sequela
E935.6	ANTIRHEUMATICS CAUS ADVRS EFFECT THERAPEUTIC USE	**T39.4X5A**	Adverse effect of antirheumatics, NEC, init
		T39.4X5S	Adverse effect of antirheumatics, NEC, sequela
E935.7	OTH NON-NARCOTIC ANALGES CAUS ADVRS EFF TX USE	**T39.315A**	Adverse effect of propionic acid derivatives, init encntr
		T39.315S	Adverse effect of propionic acid derivatives, sequela
		T39.395A	Adverse effect of nonsteroidal anti-inflammatory drugs, init
		T39.395S	Adverse effect of nonsteroidal anti-inflam drugs, sequela
		T39.8X5A	Adverse effect of nonopioid analges/antipyret, NEC, init
		T39.8X5S	Adverse effect of nonopioid analges/antipyret, NEC, sequela
		T39.95XA	Adverse effect of unsp nonopi analgs/antipyr/antirheu, init
		T39.95XS	Advrs effect of unsp nonopi analgs/antipyr/antirheu, sequela
E935.8	OTH ANALGES&ANTIPYRETICS CAUS ADVRS EFF TX USE	NO DIAGNOSIS	
E935.9	UNS ANALGESIC&ANTIPYRETIC CAUS ADVRS EFF TX USE	NO DIAGNOSIS	
E936.Ø	OXAZOLIDINE DERIVATIVES CAUS ADVRS EFF TX USE	**T42.2X5A**	Adverse effect of succinimides and oxazolidinediones, init
		T42.2X5S	Advrs effect of succinimides and oxazolidinediones, sequela
E936.1	HYDANTOIN DERIVATIVES CAUS ADVRS EFF TX USE	**T42.ØX5A**	Adverse effect of hydantoin derivatives, initial encounter
		T42.ØX5S	Adverse effect of hydantoin derivatives, sequela
E936.2	SUCCINIMIDES CAUS ADVERSE EFFECT THERAPEUTIC USE	**T42.2X5A**	Adverse effect of succinimides and oxazolidinediones, init
		T42.2X5S	Advrs effect of succinimides and oxazolidinediones, sequela
E936.3	OTH&UNSPEC ANTICONVUL CAUS ADVRS EFF TX USE	**T42.1X5A**	Adverse effect of iminostilbenes, initial encounter
		T42.1X5S	Adverse effect of iminostilbenes, sequela
		T42.5X5A	Adverse effect of mixed antiepileptics, initial encounter
		T42.5X5S	Adverse effect of mixed antiepileptics, sequela
		T42.6X5A	Adverse effect of antiepileptic and sed-hypntc drugs, init
		T42.6X5S	Adverse effect of antieplptc and sed-hypntc drugs, sequela
		T42.75XA	Adverse effect of unsp antieplptc and sed-hypntc drugs, init
		T42.75XS	Advrs effect of unsp antieplptc and sed-hypntc drugs, sqla
E936.4	ANTI-PARKINSONISM RX CAUS ADVRS EFF TX USE	**T42.8X5A**	Adverse effect of antiparkns drug/centr musc-tone depr, init
		T42.8X5S	Advrs effect of antiparkns drug/centr musc-tone depr, sqla
E937.Ø	BARBITURATES CAUS ADVERSE EFFECT THERAPEUTIC USE	**T42.3X5A**	Adverse effect of barbiturates, initial encounter
		T42.3X5S	Adverse effect of barbiturates, sequela
E937.1	CHLORL HYDRATE GRP CAUS ADVRS EFF TX USE	NO DIAGNOSIS	
E937.2	PARALDEHYDE CAUS ADVERSE EFFECT THERAPEUTIC USE	NO DIAGNOSIS	
E937.3	BROMINE COMPND CAUS ADVRS EFFECT THERAPEUTIC USE	NO DIAGNOSIS	
E937.4	METHAQUALONE COMPND CAUS ADVRS EFF TX USE	NO DIAGNOSIS	
E937.5	GLUTETHIMIDE GRP CAUS ADVRS EFF THERAPEUTIC USE	NO DIAGNOSIS	
E937.6	MIX SEDAT NEC CAUS ADVRS EFFECT THERAPEUTIC USE	NO DIAGNOSIS	
E937.8	OTH SEDAT&HYPNOT CAUS ADVRS EFF THERAPEUTIC USE	**T42.6X5A**	Adverse effect of antiepileptic and sed-hypntc drugs, init
		T42.6X5S	Adverse effect of antieplptc and sed-hypntc drugs, sequela
E937.9	UNSPEC SEDAT&HYPNOT CAUS ADVRS EFF TX USE	**T42.75XA**	Adverse effect of unsp antieplptc and sed-hypntc drugs, init
		T42.75XS	Advrs effect of unsp antieplptc and sed-hypntc drugs, sqla
E938.Ø	CNS MUSC-TONE DEPRSSNT CAUS ADVRSE EFF TX USE	NO DIAGNOSIS	
E938.1	HALOTHANE CAUSING ADVERSE EFFECT THERAPEUTIC USE	NO DIAGNOSIS	
E938.2	OTH GASEOUS ANES CAUS ADVRS EFF THERAPEUTIC USE	**T41.ØX5A**	Adverse effect of inhaled anesthetics, initial encounter
		T41.ØX5S	Adverse effect of inhaled anesthetics, sequela
E938.3	IV ANES CAUS ADVERSE EFFECT THERAPEUTIC USE	**T41.1X5A**	Adverse effect of intravenous anesthetics, initial encounter
		T41.1X5S	Adverse effect of intravenous anesthetics, sequela
E938.4	OTH&UNSPEC GEN ANES CAUS ADVRS EFF TX USE	**T41.2Ø5A**	Adverse effect of unsp general anesthetics, init encntr
		T41.2Ø5S	Adverse effect of unspecified general anesthetics, sequela
		T41.295A	Adverse effect of other general anesthetics, init encntr
		T41.295S	Adverse effect of other general anesthetics, sequela
E938.5	SURFCE&INFILTRATION ANES CAUS ADVRS EFF TX USE	NO DIAGNOSIS	
E938.6	PERIPH NRV-PLEXS-BLK ANES CAUS ADVRSE EFF TX USE	NO DIAGNOSIS	
E938.7	SPINAL ANES CAUS ADVERSE EFFECT THERAPEUTIC USE	NO DIAGNOSIS	

[Brackets] indicate valid character values for each code. Character value meanings provided for each code grouping.

ICD-9-CM		ICD-10-CM	
E938.9	OTH&UNSPEC LOC ANES CAUS ADVRS EFF TX USE	**T41.3X5A**	Adverse effect of local anesthetics, initial encounter
		T41.3X5S	Adverse effect of local anesthetics, sequela
		T41.45XA	Adverse effect of unspecified anesthetic, initial encounter
		T41.45XS	Adverse effect of unspecified anesthetic, sequela
E939.Ø	ANTIDEPTSSNT CAUS ADVERSE EFFECT THERAPEUTIC USE	**T43.Ø15A**	Adverse effect of tricyclic antidepressants, init encntr
		T43.Ø15S	Adverse effect of tricyclic antidepressants, sequela
		T43.Ø25A	Adverse effect of tetracyclic antidepressants, init encntr
		T43.Ø25S	Adverse effect of tetracyclic antidepressants, sequela
		T43.1X5A	Adverse effect of MAO inhib antidepressants, init
		T43.1X5S	Adverse effect of MAO inhib antidepressants, sequela
		T43.2Ø5A	Adverse effect of unspecified antidepressants, init encntr
		T43.2Ø5S	Adverse effect of unspecified antidepressants, sequela
		T43.215A	Advrs effect of slctv seroton/norepineph reup inhibtr, init
		T43.215S	Advrs effect of slctv seroton/norepineph reup inhibtr, sqla
		T43.225A	Adverse effect of selective serotonin reuptake inhibtr, init
		T43.225S	Adverse effect of slctv serotonin reuptake inhibtr, sequela
		T43.295A	Adverse effect of other antidepressants, initial encounter
		T43.295S	Adverse effect of other antidepressants, sequela
E939.1	PHENOTHIAZINE-BASED TRANQ CAUS ADVRS EFF TX USE	**T43.3X5A**	Adverse effect of phenothiazine antipsychot/neurolept, init
		T43.3X5S	Adverse effect of phenothiaz antipsychot/neurolept, sequela
E939.2	BUTYROPHENONE-BASED TRANQ CAUS ADVRS EFF TX USE	**T43.4X5A**	Adverse effect of butyrophen/thiothixen neuroleptics, init
		T43.4X5S	Adverse effect of butyrophen/thiothixen neuroleptc, sequela
E939.3	OTH ANTIPSYCHOT-NEUROLEPT CAUS ADVRSE EFF TX USE	**T43.5Ø5A**	Adverse effect of unsp antipsychotics and neuroleptics, init
		T43.5Ø5S	Adverse effect of unsp antipsychot/neurolept, sequela
		T43.595A	Adverse effect of oth antipsychotics and neuroleptics, init
		T43.595S	Adverse effect of antipsychotics and neuroleptics, sequela
E939.4	BENZODIAZEPINE-BASED TRANQ CAUS ADVRS EFF TX USE	**T42.4X5A**	Adverse effect of benzodiazepines, initial encounter
		T42.4X5S	Adverse effect of benzodiazepines, sequela
E939.5	OTH TRANQ CAUS ADVERSE EFFECT THERAPEUTIC USE	NO DIAGNOSIS	
E939.6	PSYCHODYSLEPTICS CAUS ADVRS EFF THERAPEUTIC USE	**T4Ø.7X5A**	Adverse effect of cannabis (derivatives), initial encounter
		T4Ø.7X5S	Adverse effect of cannabis (derivatives), sequela
		T4Ø.9Ø5A	Adverse effect of unspecified psychodysleptics, init encntr
		T4Ø.9Ø5S	Adverse effect of unspecified psychodysleptics, sequela
		T4Ø.995A	Adverse effect of other psychodysleptics, initial encounter
		T4Ø.995S	Adverse effect of other psychodysleptics, sequela
E939.7	PSYCHOSTIMS CAUS ADVERSE EFFECT THERAPEUTIC USE	**T4Ø.5X5A**	Adverse effect of cocaine, initial encounter
		T4Ø.5X5S	Adverse effect of cocaine, sequela
		T43.6Ø5A	Adverse effect of unspecified psychostimulants, init encntr
		T43.6Ø5S	Adverse effect of unspecified psychostimulants, sequela
		T43.615A	Adverse effect of caffeine, initial encounter
		T43.615S	Adverse effect of caffeine, sequela
		T43.625A	Adverse effect of amphetamines, initial encounter
		T43.625S	Adverse effect of amphetamines, sequela
		T43.635A	Adverse effect of methylphenidate, initial encounter
		T43.635S	Adverse effect of methylphenidate, sequela
		T43.695A	Adverse effect of other psychostimulants, initial encounter
		T43.695S	Adverse effect of other psychostimulants, sequela
E939.8	OTH PSYCHOTRP AGTS CAUS ADVRS EFF TX USE	**T43.8X5A**	Adverse effect of other psychotropic drugs, init encntr
		T43.8X5S	Adverse effect of other psychotropic drugs, sequela
E939.9	UNSPEC PSYCHOTRP AGT CAUS ADVRS EFF TX USE	**T43.95XA**	Adverse effect of unspecified psychotropic drug, init encntr
		T43.95XS	Adverse effect of unspecified psychotropic drug, sequela
E94Ø.Ø	ANALEPTICS CAUS ADVERSE EFFECT THERAPEUTIC USE	**T5Ø.7X5A**	Adverse effect of analeptics and opioid receptor antag, init
		T5Ø.7X5S	Advrs effect of analeptics and opioid receptor antag, sqla
E94Ø.1	OPIATE ANTAGONISTS CAUS ADVRS EFF TX USE	**T5Ø.7X5A**	Adverse effect of analeptics and opioid receptor antag, init
		T5Ø.7X5S	Advrs effect of analeptics and opioid receptor antag, sqla
E94Ø.8	OTH CNTRL NRV SYS STIMS CAUS ADVRS EFF TX USE	NO DIAGNOSIS	
E94Ø.9	UNSPEC CNTRL NERV SYS STIM CAUS ADVRS EFF TX USE	NO DIAGNOSIS	
E941.Ø	PRASYMPTHOMIMET CAUS ADVRS EFF THERAPEUTIC USE	**T44.ØX5A**	Adverse effect of anticholinesterase agents, init encntr
		T44.ØX5S	Adverse effect of anticholinesterase agents, sequela
		T44.1X5A	Adverse effect of other parasympathomimetics, init encntr
		T44.1X5S	Adverse effect of other parasympathomimetics, sequela
E941.1	PARASYMPATHOLYTICS CAUS ADVRSE EFF IN TX USE	**T44.3X5A**	Adverse effect of parasympatholytics and spasmolytics, init
		T44.3X5S	Adverse effect of parasympath and spasmolytics, sequela
E941.2	SYMPATHOMIMETS CAUS ADVRS EFFECT THERAPEUTIC USE	**T44.4X5A**	Adverse effect of predom alpha-adrenocpt agonists, init
		T44.4X5S	Adverse effect of predom alpha-adrenocpt agonists, sequela
		T44.5X5A	Adverse effect of predom beta-adrenocpt agonists, init
		T44.5X5S	Adverse effect of predom beta-adrenocpt agonists, sequela
E941.3	SYMPATHOLYTICS CAUS ADVRS EFFECT THERAPEUTIC USE	**T44.6X5A**	Adverse effect of alpha-adrenoreceptor antagonists, init
		T44.6X5S	Adverse effect of alpha-adrenoreceptor antagonists, sequela
		T44.7X5A	Adverse effect of beta-adrenoreceptor antagonists, init
		T44.7X5S	Adverse effect of beta-adrenoreceptor antagonists, sequela
		T44.8X5A	Adverse effect of centr-acting/adren-neurn-block agnt, init
		T44.8X5S	Advrs effect of centr-acting/adren-neurn-block agnt, sequela

ICD-9-CM		ICD-10-CM	
E941.9	UNS RX AUTONOM NERV SYS CAUS ADVRSE EFF TX USE	**T44.2X5A**	Adverse effect of ganglionic blocking drugs, init encntr
		T44.2X5S	Adverse effect of ganglionic blocking drugs, sequela
		T44.905A	Advrs effect of unsp drugs aff the autonm nervous sys, init
		T44.905S	Advrs effect of unsp drugs aff the autonm nrv sys, sequela
		T44.995A	Adverse effect of drug aff the autonomic nervous sys, init
		T44.995S	Adverse effect of drug aff the autonm nervous sys, sequela
E942.0	CARD RHYTHM REGULATORS CAUS ADVRS EFF TX USE	**T46.1X5A**	Adverse effect of calcium-channel blockers, init encntr
		T46.1X5S	Adverse effect of calcium-channel blockers, sequela
		T46.2X5A	Adverse effect of other antidysrhythmic drugs, init encntr
		T46.2X5S	Adverse effect of other antidysrhythmic drugs, sequela
E942.1	CARDIOTONIC GLYCOSIDES CAUS ADVRSE EFF TX USE	**T46.0X5A**	Adverse effect of cardi-stim glycos/drug simlar act, init
		T46.0X5S	Adverse effect of cardi-stim glycos/drug simlar act, sequela
E942.2	ANTIARTERIOSCLEROTIC RX CAUS ADVRSE EFF TX USE	**T46.6X5A**	Adverse effect of antihyperlip and antiarterio drugs, init
		T46.6X5S	Advrs effect of antihyperlip and antiarterio drugs, sequela
E942.3	GANG-BLK AGTS CAUS ADVRS EFFECT THERAPEUTIC USE		NO DIAGNOSIS
E942.4	COR VASODILATS CAUS ADVRS EFFECT THERAPEUTIC USE	**T46.3X5A**	Adverse effect of coronary vasodilators, initial encounter
		T46.3X5S	Adverse effect of coronary vasodilators, sequela
E942.5	OTH VASODILATS CAUS ADVRS EFFECT THERAPEUTIC USE	**T46.7X5A**	Adverse effect of peripheral vasodilators, initial encounter
		T46.7X5S	Adverse effect of peripheral vasodilators, sequela
E942.6	OTH ANTIHTN AGTS CAUS ADVRS EFF THERAPEUTIC USE	**T46.4X5A**	Adverse effect of angiotens-convert-enzyme inhibitors, init
		T46.4X5S	Adverse effect of angiotens-convert-enzyme inhibtr, sequela
		T46.5X5A	Adverse effect of other antihypertensive drugs, init encntr
		T46.5X5S	Adverse effect of other antihypertensive drugs, sequela
E942.7	ANTIVARICOS RX SCLROS AGT CAUS ADVRSE EFF TX USE	**T46.8X5A**	Adverse effect of antivaric drugs, inc scler agents, init
		T46.8X5S	Adverse effect of antivaric drugs, inc scler agents, sequela
E942.8	CAPILLARY-ACTV RX CAUS ADVRS EFF THERAPEUTIC USE		NO DIAGNOSIS
E942.9	UNS AGT PRIM AFFCT CV SYS CAUS ADVRS EFF TX USE	**T46.905A**	Adverse effect of unsp agents aff the cardiovasc sys, init
		T46.905S	Advrs effect of unsp agents aff the cardiovasc sys, sequela
		T46.995A	Adverse effect of agents aff the cardiovascular sys, init
		T46.995S	Adverse effect of agents aff the cardiovascular sys, sequela
E943.0	ANTACID&ANTIGASTRIC RX CAUS ADVRSE EFF TX USE	**T47.0X5A**	Adverse effect of histamine H2-receptor blockers, init
		T47.0X5S	Adverse effect of histamine H2-receptor blockers, sequela
		T47.1X5A	Adverse effect of antacids and anti-gstrc-sec drugs, init
		T47.1X5S	Adverse effect of antacids and anti-gstrc-sec drugs, sequela
E943.1	IRRITANT CATHRT CAUS ADVRS EFF THERAPEUTIC USE	**T47.2X5A**	Adverse effect of stimulant laxatives, initial encounter
		T47.2X5S	Adverse effect of stimulant laxatives, sequela
E943.2	EMOLLIENT CATHRT CAUS ADVRS EFF THERAPEUTIC USE	**T47.3X5A**	Adverse effect of saline and osmotic laxatives, init encntr
		T47.3X5S	Adverse effect of saline and osmotic laxatives, sequela
E943.3	OTH CATHARTICS RX CAUS ADVRSE EFF TX USE	**T47.4X5A**	Adverse effect of other laxatives, initial encounter
		T47.4X5S	Adverse effect of other laxatives, sequela
E943.4	DIGESTANTS CAUS ADVERSE EFFECT THERAPEUTIC USE	**T47.5X5A**	Adverse effect of digestants, initial encounter
		T47.5X5S	Adverse effect of digestants, sequela
E943.5	ANTIDIARRHEAL RX CAUS ADVRS EFF THERAPEUTIC USE	**T47.6X5A**	Adverse effect of antidiarrheal drugs, initial encounter
		T47.6X5S	Adverse effect of antidiarrheal drugs, sequela
E943.6	EMETICS CAUSING ADVERSE EFFECT THERAPEUTIC USE	**T47.7X5A**	Adverse effect of emetics, initial encounter
		T47.7X5S	Adverse effect of emetics, sequela
E943.8	OTH AGT PRIM AFFCT GI SYS CAUS ADVRS EFF TX USE	**T47.8X5A**	Adverse effect of agents primarily affecting GI sys, init
		T47.8X5S	Adverse effect of agents primarily affecting GI sys, sequela
E943.9	UNS AGT PRIM AFFCT GI SYS CAUS ADVRS EFF TX USE	**T47.95XA**	Adverse effect of unsp agents aff the GI sys, init
		T47.95XS	Adverse effect of unsp agents aff the GI sys, sequela
E944.0	MERCURIAL DIURETICS CAUS ADVRS EFF TX USE		NO DIAGNOSIS
E944.1	PURIN DERIVATIVE DIURETICS CAUS ADVRS EFF TX USE		NO DIAGNOSIS
E944.2	CRBNC ACID ANHYDRAS INHIB CAUS ADVRSE EFF TX USE	**T50.2X5A**	Advrs eff of crbnc-anhydr inhibtr, benzo/oth diuretc, init
		T50.2X5S	Advrs eff of crbnc-anhydr inhibtr, benzo/oth diuretc, sqla
E944.3	SALURETICS CAUS ADVERSE EFFECT THERAPEUTIC USE		NO DIAGNOSIS
E944.4	OTH DIURETICS CAUS ADVRS EFFECT THERAPEUTIC USE	**T50.1X5A**	Adverse effect of loop diuretics, initial encounter
		T50.1X5S	Adverse effect of loop [high-ceiling] diuretics, sequela
E944.5	ELECTOLYT-CALOR-WATR-BAL CAUS ADVRSE EFF TX USE	**T50.3X5A**	Adverse effect of electrolytic/caloric/wtr-bal agnt, init
		T50.3X5S	Adverse effect of electrolytic/caloric/wtr-bal agnt, sequela
E944.6	OTH MINERL SALTS NEC CAUS ADVRS EFF TX USE		NO DIAGNOSIS
E944.7	URIC ACID METAB RX CAUS ADVRS EFF TX USE	**T50.4X5A**	Adverse effect of drugs affecting uric acid metabolism, init
		T50.4X5S	Adverse effect of drugs affecting uric acid metab, sequela
E945.0	OXYTOCIC AGTS CAUS ADVRS EFFECT THERAPEUTIC USE	**T48.0X5A**	Adverse effect of oxytocic drugs, initial encounter
		T48.0X5S	Adverse effect of oxytocic drugs, sequela
E945.1	SMOOTH MUSC RELAXANTS CAUS ADVRS EFF TX USE		NO DIAGNOSIS
E945.2	SKEL MUSC RELAXANTS CAUS ADVRS EFF TX USE	**T48.1X5A**	Adverse effect of skeletal muscle relaxants, init encntr
		T48.1X5S	Adverse effect of skeletal muscle relaxants, sequela
E945.3	OTH&UNSPEC RX ACTING MUSC CAUS ADVRS EFF TX USE	**T48.205A**	Adverse effect of unsp drugs acting on muscles, init encntr
		T48.205S	Adverse effect of unsp drugs acting on muscles, sequela
		T48.295A	Adverse effect of other drugs acting on muscles, init encntr
		T48.295S	Adverse effect of other drugs acting on muscles, sequela

[Brackets] indicate valid character values for each code. Character value meanings provided for each code grouping.

ICD-9-CM		ICD-10-CM	
E945.4	ANTITUSSIVES CAUS ADVERSE EFFECT THERAPEUTIC USE	T48.3X5A	Adverse effect of antitussives, initial encounter
		T48.3X5S	Adverse effect of antitussives, sequela
E945.5	EXPECTORANTS CAUS ADVERSE EFFECT THERAPEUTIC USE	T48.4X5A	Adverse effect of expectorants, initial encounter
		T48.4X5S	Adverse effect of expectorants, sequela
E945.6	ANTI-COMMON COLD RX CAUS ADVRS EFF TX USE	T48.5X5A	Adverse effect of other anti-common-cold drugs, init encntr
		T48.5X5S	Adverse effect of other anti-common-cold drugs, sequela
E945.7	ANTIASTHMATICS CAUS ADVRS EFFECT THERAPEUTIC USE	T48.6X5A	Adverse effect of antiasthmatics, initial encounter
		T48.6X5S	Adverse effect of antiasthmatics, sequela
E945.8	OTH&UNSPEC RESP RX CAUS ADVRS EFF TX USE	T41.5X5A	Adverse effect of therapeutic gases, initial encounter
		T41.5X5S	Adverse effect of therapeutic gases, sequela
		T48.905A	Advrs effect of unsp agents prim act on the resp sys, init
		T48.905S	Advrs effect of unsp agents prim act on the resp sys, sqla
		T48.995A	Adverse effect of agents prim acting on the resp sys, init
		T48.995S	Advrs effect of agents prim acting on the resp sys, sequela
E946.0	LOC ANTI-INFECT-INFLAM RX CAUS ADVRSE EFF TX USE	T49.0X5A	Adverse effect of local antifung/infect/inflamm drugs, init
		T49.0X5S	Advrs effect of local antifung/infect/inflamm drugs, sequela
E946.1	ANTIPRURITICS CAUS ADVRS EFFECT THERAPEUTIC USE	T49.1X5A	Adverse effect of antipruritics, initial encounter
		T49.1X5S	Adverse effect of antipruritics, sequela
E946.2	LOC ASTRINGENTS&DETRGNT CAUS ADVRSE EFF TX USE	T49.2X5A	Adverse effect of local astringents/detergents, init
		T49.2X5S	Adverse effect of local astringents/detergents, sequela
E946.3	EMOLLIENTS & PROTECTANTS CAUS ADVRSE EFF TX USE	T49.3X5A	Adverse effect of emollients, demulcents and protect, init
		T49.3X5S	Advrs effect of emollients, demulcents and protect, sequela
E946.4	KERATOLYTIC-KERATOPLSTIC CAUS ADVRSE EFF TX USE	T49.4X5A	Adverse effect of keratolyt/keratplst/hair trmt drug, init
		T49.4X5S	Advrs effect of keratolyt/keratplst/hair trmt drug, sequela
E946.5	EYE ANTI-INFECTIVES&OTH RX CAUS ADVRSE EFF TX US	T49.5X5A	Adverse effect of opth drugs and preparations, init
		T49.5X5S	Adverse effect of opth drugs and preparations, sequela
E946.6	ANTI-INFECT & OTH ENT RX CAUS ADVRSE EFF TX USE	T49.6X5A	Adverse effect of otorhino drugs and preparations, init
		T49.6X5S	Adverse effect of otorhino drugs and preparations, sequela
E946.7	DENTAL RX TOPIC APPLIC CAUS ADVRS EFF TX USE	T49.7X5A	Adverse effect of dental drugs, topically applied, init
		T49.7X5S	Adverse effect of dental drugs, topically applied, sequela
E946.8	OTH AGT SKIN-MUCOS MEMB CAUS ADVRSE EFF TX USE	T49.8X5A	Adverse effect of other topical agents, initial encounter
		T49.8X5S	Adverse effect of other topical agents, sequela
E946.9	UNS AGT SKIN-MUCOS MEMB CAUS ADVRSE EFF TX USE	T49.95XA	Adverse effect of unspecified topical agent, init encntr
		T49.95XS	Adverse effect of unspecified topical agent, sequela
E947.0	DIETETICS CAUSING ADVERSE EFFECT THERAPEUTIC USE	T50.5X5A	Adverse effect of appetite depressants, initial encounter
		T50.5X5S	Adverse effect of appetite depressants, sequela
E947.1	LIPOTROPIC RX CAUS ADVRS EFFECT THERAPEUTIC USE		NO DIAGNOSIS
E947.2	ANTIDOTES&CHELAT AGT-NEC CAUS ADVRSE EFF TX USE	T50.6X5A	Adverse effect of antidotes and chelating agents, init
		T50.6X5S	Adverse effect of antidotes and chelating agents, sequela
E947.3	ALCOHL DETERRENTS CAUS ADVRS EFF THERAPEUTIC USE		NO DIAGNOSIS
E947.4	PHARMACEUTICAL EXCIPIENTS CAUS ADVRS EFF TX USE		NO DIAGNOSIS
E947.8	OTH RX&MEDICINAL SBSTNC CAUS ADVRS EFF TX USE	T50.8X5A	Adverse effect of diagnostic agents, initial encounter
		T50.8X5S	Adverse effect of diagnostic agents, sequela
		T50.995A	Adverse effect of drug/meds/biol subst, init
		T50.995S	Adverse effect of drug/meds/biol subst, sequela
E947.9	UNSPEC RX/MEDICINAL SBSTNC CAUS ADVRS EFF TX USE	R50.2	Drug induced fever
		T50.905A	Adverse effect of unsp drug/meds/biol subst, init
		T50.905S	Adverse effect of unsp drug/meds/biol subst, sequela
E948.0	BCG VACCINE CAUS ADVERSE EFFECT THERAPEUTIC USE		NO DIAGNOSIS
E948.1	TYPHOID&PARATYPHOID VACCS CAUS ADVRS EFF TX USE		NO DIAGNOSIS
E948.2	CHOLERA VACC CAUS ADVERSE EFFECT THERAPEUTIC USE		NO DIAGNOSIS
E948.3	PLAGUE VACC CAUS ADVERSE EFFECT THERAPEUTIC USE		NO DIAGNOSIS
E948.4	TETANUS VACC CAUS ADVERSE EFFECT THERAPEUTIC USE		NO DIAGNOSIS
E948.5	DIPHTH VACC CAUS ADVERSE EFFECT THERAPEUTIC USE		NO DIAGNOSIS
E948.6	PERTUSSIS VACC INCL COMBO CAUS ADVRSE EFF TX USE	T50.A15A	Advrs effect of pertuss vaccine, inc combin w pertuss, init
		T50.A15S	Advrs effect of pertuss vaccine, inc combin w pertuss, sqla
E948.8	OTH&UNSPEC BACTERL VACCS CAUS ADVRS EFF TX USE	T50.A95A	Adverse effect of other bacterial vaccines, init encntr
		T50.A95S	Adverse effect of other bacterial vaccines, sequela
E948.9	MIXED VACC W/O PERTUSS CAUS ADVRSE EFF TX USE	T50.A25A	Adverse effect of mixed bact vaccines w/o a pertuss, init
		T50.A25S	Adverse effect of mixed bact vaccines w/o a pertuss, sequela
E949.0	SMPOX VACC CAUS ADVERSE EFFECT THERAPEUTIC USE	T50.B15A	Adverse effect of smallpox vaccines, initial encounter
		T50.B15S	Adverse effect of smallpox vaccines, sequela
E949.1	RABIES VACC CAUS ADVERSE EFFECT THERAPEUTIC USE		NO DIAGNOSIS
E949.2	TYPHUS VACC CAUS ADVERSE EFFECT THERAPEUTIC USE		NO DIAGNOSIS
E949.3	YELLOW FEVER VACC CAUS ADVRS EFF THERAPEUTIC USE		NO DIAGNOSIS
E949.4	MEASLES VACC CAUS ADVERSE EFFECT THERAPEUTIC USE		NO DIAGNOSIS
E949.5	POLIOMYEL VACC CAUS ADVRS EFFECT THERAPEUTIC USE		NO DIAGNOSIS
E949.6	UNS VIRL&RICKETTS VACCS CAUS ADVRS EFF TX USE	T50.B95A	Adverse effect of other viral vaccines, initial encounter
		T50.B95S	Adverse effect of other viral vaccines, sequela
E949.7	MIX VACC WO PERTUSS CAUS ADVRSE EFF TX USE		NO DIAGNOSIS

ICD-9-CM		ICD-10-CM	
E949.9	OTH&UNS VACC&BIOLOG SBSTNC CAUS ADVRS EFF TX USE	**T50.Z95A**	Adverse effect of vaccines and biological substances, init
		T50.Z95S	Adverse effect of vaccines and biolg substances, sequela
E950.0	SUI&SLF-INFLCT PSN-ANALGES-ANTIPYRET-ANTIRHEUMAT	**T39.012A**	Poisoning by aspirin, intentional self-harm, init encntr
		T39.092A	Poisoning by salicylates, intentional self-harm, init encntr
		T39.1X2A	Poisoning by 4-Aminophenol derivatives, self-harm, init
		T39.2X2A	Poisoning by pyrazolone derivatives, self-harm, init
		T39.312A	Poisoning by propionic acid derivatives, self-harm, init
		T39.392A	Poisn by oth nonsteroid anti-inflam drugs, self-harm, init
		T39.4X2A	Poisoning by antirheumatics, NEC, self-harm, init
		T39.8X2A	Poisn by oth nonopio analges/antipyret, NEC, self-harm, init
		T39.92XA	Poisn by unsp nonopi analgs/antipyr/antirheu, slf-hrm, init
		T40.0X2A	Poisoning by opium, intentional self-harm, initial encounter
		T40.1X2A	Poisoning by heroin, intentional self-harm, init encntr
		T40.2X2A	Poisoning by oth opioids, intentional self-harm, init encntr
		T40.3X2A	Poisoning by methadone, intentional self-harm, init encntr
		T40.4X2A	Poisoning by oth synthetic narcotics, self-harm, init
		T41.1X2A	Poisoning by intravenous anesthetics, self-harm, init
		T41.202A	Poisoning by unsp general anesthetics, self-harm, init
		T41.292A	Poisoning by oth general anesthetics, self-harm, init
		T41.3X2A	Poisoning by local anesthetics, intentional self-harm, init
		T41.42XA	Poisoning by unsp anesthetic, intentional self-harm, init
E950.1	SUICIDE&SELF-INFLICTED POISONING BARBITURATES	**T42.3X2A**	Poisoning by barbiturates, intentional self-harm, init
E950.2	SUICIDE&SELF-INFLICTED POISN OTH SEDAT&HYPNOT	**T40.7X2A**	Poisoning by cannabis (derivatives), self-harm, init
		T42.4X2A	Poisoning by benzodiazepines, intentional self-harm, init
		T42.6X2A	Poisn by oth antieplptc and sed-hypntc drugs, slf-hrm, init
		T42.6X4A	Poisn by oth antieplptc and sed-hypntc drugs, undet, init
E950.3	SUI&SLF-INFLICT POISN TRANQ&OTH PSYCHOTRP AGT	**T40.8X2A**	Poisoning by lysergide, intentional self-harm, init encntr
		T40.902A	Poisoning by unsp psychodysleptics, self-harm, init
		T40.992A	Poisoning by oth psychodysleptics, self-harm, init
		T42.72XA	Poisn by unsp antieplptc and sed-hypntc drugs, slf-hrm, init
		T43.012A	Poisoning by tricyclic antidepressants, self-harm, init
		T43.022A	Poisoning by tetracyclic antidepressants, self-harm, init
		T43.1X2A	Poisoning by MAO inhib antidepressants, self-harm, init
		T43.202A	Poisoning by unsp antidepressants, self-harm, init
		T43.212A	Poisn by slctv seroton/norepineph reup inhibtr,slf-hrm, init
		T43.222A	Poisn by slctv serotonin reuptake inhibtr, self-harm, init
		T43.292A	Poisoning by oth antidepressants, self-harm, init
		T43.3X2A	Poisn by phenothiaz antipsychot/neurolept, self-harm, init
		T43.4X2A	Poisn by butyrophen/thiothixen neuroleptc, self-harm, init
		T43.502A	Poisoning by unsp antipsychot/neurolept, self-harm, init
		T43.592A	Poisoning by oth antipsychot/neurolept, self-harm, init
		T43.602A	Poisoning by unsp psychostimulants, self-harm, init
		T43.612A	Poisoning by caffeine, intentional self-harm, init encntr
		T43.622A	Poisoning by amphetamines, intentional self-harm, init
		T43.632A	Poisoning by methylphenidate, intentional self-harm, init
		T43.692A	Poisoning by oth psychostimulants, self-harm, init
		T43.8X2A	Poisoning by oth psychotropic drugs, self-harm, init
		T43.92XA	Poisoning by unsp psychotropic drug, self-harm, init
E950.4	SUI&SLF-INFLICT POISN OTH RX&MEDICINAL SBSTNC	**T36.0X2A**	Poisoning by penicillins, intentional self-harm, init encntr
		T36.1X2A	Poisn by cephalospor/oth beta-lactm antibiot, slf-hrm, init
		T36.2X2A	Poisoning by chloramphenicol group, self-harm, init
		T36.3X2A	Poisoning by macrolides, intentional self-harm, init encntr
		T36.4X2A	Poisoning by tetracyclines, intentional self-harm, init
		T36.5X2A	Poisoning by aminoglycosides, intentional self-harm, init
		T36.6X2A	Poisoning by rifampicins, intentional self-harm, init encntr
		T36.7X2A	Poisoning by antifungal antibiot, sys used, self-harm, init
		T36.8X2A	Poisoning by oth systemic antibiotics, self-harm, init
		T36.92XA	Poisoning by unsp systemic antibiotic, self-harm, init
		T37.0X2A	Poisoning by sulfonamides, intentional self-harm, init
		T37.1X2A	Poisoning by antimycobacterial drugs, self-harm, init
		T37.2X2A	Poisn by antimalari/drugs act on bld protzoa, slf-hrm, init
		T37.3X2A	Poisoning by oth antiprotozoal drugs, self-harm, init
		T37.4X2A	Poisoning by anthelminthics, intentional self-harm, init
		T37.5X2A	Poisoning by antiviral drugs, intentional self-harm, init
		T37.8X2A	Poisn by oth systemic anti-infect/parasit, self-harm, init
		T37.92XA	Poisn by unsp sys anti-infect and antiparastc, slf-hrm, init
		T38.0X2A	Poisoning by glucocort/synth analog, self-harm, init
		T38.1X2A	Poisoning by thyroid hormones and sub, self-harm, init
		T38.2X2A	Poisoning by antithyroid drugs, intentional self-harm, init
		T38.3X2A	Poisn by insulin and oral hypoglycemic drugs, slf-hrm, init
		T38.4X2A	Poisoning by oral contraceptives, self-harm, init
		T38.5X2A	Poisoning by oth estrogens and progestogens, self-harm, init
		T38.6X2A	Poisn by antigonadtr/antiestr/antiandrg, NEC, slf-hrm, init
		T38.7X2A	Poisn by androgens and anabolic congeners, self-harm, init
		T38.802A	Poisn by unsp hormones and synthetic sub, self-harm, init
		T38.812A	Poisoning by anterior pituitary hormones, self-harm, init
		T38.892A	Poisoning by oth hormones and synthetic sub, self-harm, init

(Continued on next page)

ICD-9-CM		ICD-10-CM	
E95Ø.4	SUI&SLF-INFLICT POISN OTH RX&MEDICINAL SBSTNC **(Continued)**	**T38.9Ø2A**	Poisoning by unsp hormone antagonists, self-harm, init
		T38.992A	Poisoning by oth hormone antagonists, self-harm, init
		T4Ø.5X2A	Poisoning by cocaine, intentional self-harm, init encntr
		T4Ø.6Ø2A	Poisoning by unsp narcotics, intentional self-harm, init
		T4Ø.692A	Poisoning by oth narcotics, intentional self-harm, init
		T42.ØX2A	Poisoning by hydantoin derivatives, self-harm, init
		T42.1X2A	Poisoning by iminostilbenes, intentional self-harm, init
		T42.2X2A	Poisn by succinimides and oxazolidinediones, self-harm, init
		T42.5X2A	Poisoning by mixed antiepileptics, self-harm, init
		T42.6X2A	Poisn by oth antieplptc and sed-hypntc drugs, slf-hrm, init
		T42.72XA	Poisn by unsp antieplptc and sed-hypntc drugs, slf-hrm, init
		T42.8X2A	Poisn by antiparkns drug/centr musc-tone depr, slf-hrm, init
		T44.ØX2A	Poisoning by anticholinesterase agents, self-harm, init
		T44.1X2A	Poisoning by oth parasympathomimetics, self-harm, init
		T44.2X2A	Poisoning by ganglionic blocking drugs, self-harm, init
		T44.3X2A	Poisn by oth parasympath and spasmolytics, self-harm, init
		T44.4X2A	Poisn by predom alpha-adrenocpt agonists, self-harm, init
		T44.5X2A	Poisoning by predom beta-adrenocpt agonists, self-harm, init
		T44.6X2A	Poisoning by alpha-adrenocpt antagonists, self-harm, init
		T44.7X2A	Poisoning by beta-adrenocpt antagonists, self-harm, init
		T44.8X2A	Poisn by centr-acting/adren-neurn-block agnt, slf-hrm, init
		T44.9Ø2A	Poisn by unsp drugs aff the autonm nrv sys, slf-hrm, init
		T44.992A	Poisn by oth drug aff the autonm nervous sys, slf-hrm, init
		T45.ØX2A	Poisoning by antiallerg/antiemetic, self-harm, init
		T45.1X2A	Poisoning by antineopl and immunosup drugs, self-harm, init
		T45.2X2A	Poisoning by vitamins, intentional self-harm, init encntr
		T45.3X2A	Poisoning by enzymes, intentional self-harm, init encntr
		T45.4X2A	Poisoning by iron and its compounds, self-harm, init
		T45.512A	Poisoning by anticoagulants, intentional self-harm, init
		T45.522A	Poisoning by antithrombotic drugs, self-harm, init
		T45.6Ø2A	Poisoning by unsp fibrin-affct drugs, self-harm, init
		T45.612A	Poisoning by thrombolytic drug, intentional self-harm, init
		T45.622A	Poisoning by hemostatic drug, intentional self-harm, init
		T45.692A	Poisoning by oth fibrin-affct drugs, self-harm, init
		T45.7X2A	Poisn by anticoag antag, vit K and oth coag, slf-hrm, init
		T45.8X2A	Poisn by oth prim sys and hematolog agents, slf-hrm, init
		T45.92XA	Poisn by unsp prim sys and hematolog agent, slf-hrm, init
		T46.ØX2A	Poisn by cardi-stim glycos/drug simlar act, self-harm, init
		T46.1X2A	Poisoning by calcium-channel blockers, self-harm, init
		T46.2X2A	Poisoning by oth antidysrhythmic drugs, self-harm, init
		T46.3X2A	Poisoning by coronary vasodilators, self-harm, init
		T46.4X2A	Poisn by angiotens-convert-enzyme inhibtr, self-harm, init
		T46.5X2A	Poisoning by oth antihypertensive drugs, self-harm, init
		T46.6X2A	Poisn by antihyperlip and antiarterio drugs, self-harm, init
		T46.7X2A	Poisoning by peripheral vasodilators, self-harm, init
		T46.8X2A	Poisn by antivaric drugs, inc scler agents, self-harm, init
		T46.9Ø2A	Poisn by unsp agents aff the cardiovasc sys, self-harm, init
		T46.992A	Poisn by oth agents aff the cardiovasc sys, self-harm, init
		T47.ØX2A	Poisoning by histamine H2-receptor blockers, self-harm, init
		T47.1X2A	Poisn by oth antacids & anti-gstrc-sec drugs, slf-hrm, init
		T47.2X2A	Poisoning by stimulant laxatives, self-harm, init
		T47.3X2A	Poisoning by saline and osmotic laxatives, self-harm, init
		T47.4X2A	Poisoning by oth laxatives, intentional self-harm, init
		T47.5X2A	Poisoning by digestants, intentional self-harm, init encntr
		T47.6X2A	Poisoning by antidiarrheal drugs, self-harm, init
		T47.7X2A	Poisoning by emetics, intentional self-harm, init encntr
		T47.8X2A	Poisoning by oth agents aff GI sys, self-harm, init
		T47.92XA	Poisoning by unsp agents aff the GI sys, self-harm, init
		T48.ØX2A	Poisoning by oxytocic drugs, intentional self-harm, init
		T48.1X2A	Poisoning by skeletal muscle relaxants, self-harm, init
		T48.2Ø2A	Poisoning by unsp drugs acting on muscles, self-harm, init
		T48.292A	Poisoning by oth drugs acting on muscles, self-harm, init
		T48.3X2A	Poisoning by antitussives, intentional self-harm, init
		T48.4X2A	Poisoning by expectorants, intentional self-harm, init
		T48.5X2A	Poisoning by oth anti-common-cold drugs, self-harm, init
		T48.6X2A	Poisoning by antiasthmatics, intentional self-harm, init
		T48.9Ø2A	Poisn by unsp agents prim act on the resp sys, slf-hrm, init
		T48.992A	Poisn by oth agents prim act on the resp sys, slf-hrm, init
		T49.ØX2A	Poisn by local antifung/infect/inflamm drugs, slf-hrm, init
		T49.1X2A	Poisoning by antipruritics, intentional self-harm, init
		T49.2X2A	Poisoning by local astringents/detergents, self-harm, init
		T49.3X2A	Poisn by emollients, demulcents and protect, self-harm, init
		T49.4X2A	Poisn by keratolyt/keratplst/hair trmt drug, self-harm, init
		T49.5X2A	Poisoning by opth drugs and preparations, self-harm, init
		T49.6X2A	Poisoning by otorhino drugs and prep, self-harm, init
		T49.7X2A	Poisn by dental drugs, topically applied, self-harm, init
		T49.8X2A	Poisoning by oth topical agents, intentional self-harm, init
		T49.92XA	Poisoning by unsp topical agent, intentional self-harm, init
		T5Ø.ØX2A	Poisoning by mineralocorticoids and antag, self-harm, init

(Continued on next page)

ICD-9-CM		ICD-10-CM	
E95Ø.4	SUI&SLF-INFLICT POISN OTH RX&MEDICINAL SBSTNC **(Continued)**	**T5Ø.1X2A**	Poisoning by loop diuretics, intentional self-harm, init
		T5Ø.2X2A	Poisn by crbnc-anhydr inhibtr,benzo/oth diuretc,slf-hrm,init
		T5Ø.3X2A	Poisn by electrolytic/caloric/wtr-bal agnt, self-harm, init
		T5Ø.4X2A	Poisoning by drugs aff uric acid metab, self-harm, init
		T5Ø.5X2A	Poisoning by appetite depressants, self-harm, init
		T5Ø.6X2A	Poisoning by antidotes and chelating agents, self-harm, init
		T5Ø.7X2A	Poisn by analeptics and opioid receptor antag, slf-hrm, init
		T5Ø.8X2A	Poisoning by diagnostic agents, intentional self-harm, init
		T5Ø.9Ø2A	Poisoning by unsp drug/meds/biol subst, self-harm, init
		T5Ø.992A	Poisoning by oth drug/meds/biol subst, self-harm, init
		T5Ø.A12A	Poisn by pertuss vaccn, inc combin w pertuss, slf-hrm, init
		T5Ø.A22A	Poisn by mixed bact vaccines w/o a pertuss, self-harm, init
		T5Ø.A92A	Poisoning by oth bacterial vaccines, self-harm, init
		T5Ø.B12A	Poisoning by smallpox vaccines, intentional self-harm, init
		T5Ø.B92A	Poisoning by oth viral vaccines, intentional self-harm, init
		T5Ø.Z12A	Poisoning by immunoglobulin, intentional self-harm, init
		T5Ø.Z92A	Poisoning by oth vaccines and biolg substnc, self-harm, init
E95Ø.5	SUI&SLF-INFLICT POISN UNS RX/MEDICINAL SBSTNC	NO DIAGNOSIS	
E95Ø.6	SUI&SLF-INFLCT POISN-AGRICUL-HORTICUL CHEM PREP	**T6Ø.ØX2A**	Toxic eff of organophos and carbamate insect, slf-hrm, init
		T6Ø.1X2A	Toxic effect of halogenated insecticides, self-harm, init
		T6Ø.2X2A	Toxic effect of insecticides, intentional self-harm, init
		T6Ø.3X2A	Toxic effect of herbicides and fungicides, self-harm, init
		T6Ø.4X2A	Toxic effect of rodenticides, intentional self-harm, init
		T6Ø.8X2A	Toxic effect of oth pesticides, intentional self-harm, init
		T6Ø.92XA	Toxic effect of unsp pesticide, intentional self-harm, init
E95Ø.7	SUI&SLF-INFLICT POISN CORROSIVE&CAUSTIC SBSTNC	**T54.ØX2A**	Toxic effect of phenol and phenol homolog, self-harm, init
		T54.1X2A	Toxic effect of corrosive organic compounds, self-harm, init
		T54.2X2A	Tox eff of corrosv acids & acid-like substnc, slf-hrm, init
		T54.3X2A	Tox eff of corrosv alkalis & alk-like substnc, slf-hrm, init
		T54.92XA	Toxic effect of unsp corrosive substance, self-harm, init
		T55.ØX2A	Toxic effect of soaps, intentional self-harm, init encntr
		T55.1X2A	Toxic effect of detergents, intentional self-harm, init
		T57.1X2A	Toxic effect of phosphorus and its compnd, self-harm, init
		T57.2X2A	Toxic effect of manganese and its compounds, self-harm, init
E95Ø.8	SUICIDE&SELF-INFLICTED POISN ARSENIC&ITS COMPND	**T57.ØX2A**	Toxic effect of arsenic and its compounds, self-harm, init
E95Ø.9	SUICIDE&SELF-INFLICT POISN UNS SOLID&LQD SBSTNC	**T51.ØX2A**	Toxic effect of ethanol, intentional self-harm, init encntr
		T51.1X2A	Toxic effect of methanol, intentional self-harm, init encntr
		T51.2X2A	Toxic effect of 2-Propanol, intentional self-harm, init
		T51.3X2A	Toxic effect of fusel oil, intentional self-harm, init
		T51.8X2A	Toxic effect of oth alcohols, intentional self-harm, init
		T51.92XA	Toxic effect of unsp alcohol, intentional self-harm, init
		T52.ØX2A	Toxic effect of petroleum products, self-harm, init
		T52.1X2A	Toxic effect of benzene, intentional self-harm, init encntr
		T52.2X2A	Toxic effect of homologues of benzene, self-harm, init
		T52.3X2A	Toxic effect of glycols, intentional self-harm, init encntr
		T52.4X2A	Toxic effect of ketones, intentional self-harm, init encntr
		T52.8X2A	Toxic effect of organic solvents, self-harm, init
		T52.92XA	Toxic effect of unsp organic solvent, self-harm, init
		T53.ØX2A	Toxic effect of carbon tetrachloride, self-harm, init
		T53.1X2A	Toxic effect of chloroform, intentional self-harm, init
		T53.2X2A	Toxic effect of trichloroethylene, self-harm, init
		T53.3X2A	Toxic effect of tetrachloroethylene, self-harm, init
		T53.4X2A	Toxic effect of dichloromethane, intentional self-harm, init
		T53.6X2A	Tox eff of halgn deriv of aliphatic hydrocrb, slf-hrm, init
		T53.7X2A	Toxic eff of halgn deriv of aromatic hydrocrb, slf-hrm, init
		T53.92XA	Tox eff of unsp halgn deriv of aromat hydrocrb,slf-hrm, init
		T56.ØX2A	Toxic effect of lead and its compounds, self-harm, init
		T56.1X2A	Toxic effect of mercury and its compounds, self-harm, init
		T56.2X2A	Toxic effect of chromium and its compounds, self-harm, init
		T56.3X2A	Toxic effect of cadmium and its compounds, self-harm, init
		T56.4X2A	Toxic effect of copper and its compounds, self-harm, init
		T56.5X2A	Toxic effect of zinc and its compounds, self-harm, init
		T56.6X2A	Toxic effect of tin and its compounds, self-harm, init
		T56.7X2A	Toxic effect of beryllium and its compounds, self-harm, init
		T56.812A	Toxic effect of thallium, intentional self-harm, init encntr
		T56.892A	Toxic effect of oth metals, intentional self-harm, init
		T56.92XA	Toxic effect of unsp metal, intentional self-harm, init
		T57.8X2A	Toxic effect of inorganic substances, self-harm, init
		T57.92XA	Toxic effect of unsp inorganic substance, self-harm, init
		T61.Ø2XA	Ciguatera fish poisoning, intentional self-harm, init encntr
		T61.12XA	Scombroid fish poisoning, intentional self-harm, init encntr
		T61.772A	Other fish poisoning, intentional self-harm, init encntr
		T61.782A	Oth shellfish poisoning, intentional self-harm, init encntr
		T61.8X2A	Toxic effect of oth seafood, intentional self-harm, init
		T61.92XA	Toxic effect of unsp seafood, intentional self-harm, init
		T62.ØX2A	Toxic effect of ingested mushrooms, self-harm, init
		T62.1X2A	Toxic effect of ingested berries, self-harm, init
	(Continued on next page)	**T62.2X2A**	Toxic effect of ingested (parts of) plant(s), slf-hrm, init

ICD-9-CM		ICD-10-CM	
E95Ø.9	SUICIDE&SELF-INFLICT POISN UNS SOLID&LQD SBSTNC **(Continued)**	**T62.8X2A**	Toxic effect of noxious substnc eaten as food, slf-hrm, init
		T62.92XA	Toxic eff of unsp noxious sub eaten as food, slf-hrm, init
		T63.ØØ2A	Toxic effect of unsp snake venom, self-harm, init
		T63.Ø12A	Toxic effect of rattlesnake venom, self-harm, init
		T63.Ø22A	Toxic effect of coral snake venom, self-harm, init
		T63.Ø32A	Toxic effect of taipan venom, intentional self-harm, init
		T63.Ø42A	Toxic effect of cobra venom, intentional self-harm, init
		T63.Ø62A	Toxic effect of venom of N & S American snake, slf-hrm, init
		T63.Ø72A	Toxic effect of venom of Australian snake, self-harm, init
		T63.Ø82A	Toxic eff of venom of African and Asian snake, slf-hrm, init
		T63.Ø92A	Toxic effect of venom of snake, intentional self-harm, init
		T63.112A	Toxic effect of venom of gila monster, self-harm, init
		T63.122A	Toxic effect of venom of venomous lizard, self-harm, init
		T63.192A	Toxic effect of venom of reptiles, self-harm, init
		T63.2X2A	Toxic effect of venom of scorpion, self-harm, init
		T63.3Ø2A	Toxic effect of unsp spider venom, self-harm, init
		T63.312A	Toxic effect of venom of black widow spider, self-harm, init
		T63.322A	Toxic effect of venom of tarantula, self-harm, init
		T63.332A	Toxic effect of venom of brown recluse spider, slf-hrm, init
		T63.392A	Toxic effect of venom of spider, intentional self-harm, init
		T63.412A	Toxic effect of venom of centipede/millipede, slf-hrm, init
		T63.422A	Toxic effect of venom of ants, intentional self-harm, init
		T63.432A	Toxic effect of venom of caterpillars, self-harm, init
		T63.442A	Toxic effect of venom of bees, intentional self-harm, init
		T63.452A	Toxic effect of venom of hornets, self-harm, init
		T63.462A	Toxic effect of venom of wasps, intentional self-harm, init
		T63.482A	Toxic effect of venom of arthropod, self-harm, init
		T63.512A	Toxic effect of contact w stingray, self-harm, init
		T63.592A	Toxic effect of contact w oth venomous fish, self-harm, init
		T63.612A	Toxic effect of contact w Portugese Man-o-war, slf-hrm, init
		T63.622A	Toxic effect of contact w oth jellyfish, self-harm, init
		T63.632A	Toxic effect of contact w sea anemone, self-harm, init
		T63.692A	Toxic eff of cntct w oth venom marine animals, slf-hrm, init
		T63.712A	Toxic effect of contact w venom marine plant, slf-hrm, init
		T63.792A	Toxic effect of contact w oth venomous plant, slf-hrm, init
		T63.812A	Toxic effect of contact w venomous frog, self-harm, init
		T63.822A	Toxic effect of contact w venomous toad, self-harm, init
		T63.832A	Toxic effect of contact w oth venomous amphib, slf-hrm, init
		T63.892A	Toxic effect of contact w oth venom animals, slf-hrm, init
		T63.92XA	Toxic effect of contact w unsp venom animal, slf-hrm, init
		T64.Ø2XA	Toxic effect of aflatoxin, intentional self-harm, init
		T64.82XA	Toxic effect of mycotoxin food contaminants, self-harm, init
		T65.ØX2A	Toxic effect of cyanides, intentional self-harm, init encntr
		T65.1X2A	Toxic effect of strychnine and its salts, self-harm, init
		T65.212A	Toxic effect of chewing tobacco, intentional self-harm, init
		T65.222A	Toxic effect of tobacco cigarettes, self-harm, init
		T65.292A	Toxic effect of tobacco and nicotine, self-harm, init
		T65.3X2A	Tox eff of nitrodrv/aminodrv of benzn/homolog, slf-hrm, init
		T65.4X2A	Toxic effect of carbon disulfide, self-harm, init
		T65.5X2A	Tox eff of nitro & oth nitric acids & esters, slf-hrm, init
		T65.6X2A	Toxic effect of paints and dyes, NEC, self-harm, init
		T65.812A	Toxic effect of latex, intentional self-harm, init encntr
		T65.822A	Toxic eff of harmful algae and algae toxins, slf-hrm, init
		T65.832A	Toxic effect of fiberglass, intentional self-harm, init
		T65.892A	Toxic effect of oth substances, intentional self-harm, init
		T65.92XA	Toxic effect of unsp substance, intentional self-harm, init
E951.Ø	SUICIDE&SELF-INFLICTED POISN GAS DSTRBD PIPELINE	NO DIAGNOSIS	
E951.1	SUI&SLF-INFLCT POISN-LIQ PETRO GAS-MOBIL CONTANR	NO DIAGNOSIS	
E951.8	SUICIDE&SELF-INFLICTED POISONING OTH UTILITY GAS	NO DIAGNOSIS	
E952.Ø	SUICIDE&SELF-INFLICT POISN MOTOR VEH EXHAUST GAS	**T58.Ø2XA**	Toxic eff of carb monx from mtr veh exhaust, slf-hrm, init
E952.1	SUICIDE&SELF-INFLICTED POISN OTH CARB MONOXIDE	**T58.12XA**	Toxic effect of carb monx from utility gas, self-harm, init
		T58.2X2A	Tox eff of carb monx fr incmpl combst dmst fuel,slf-hrm,init
		T58.8X2A	Toxic effect of carb monx from oth source, self-harm, init
		T58.92XA	Toxic effect of carb monx from unsp source, self-harm, init
E952.8	SUICIDE&SELF-INFLICT POISN OTH SPEC GASES&VAPORS	**T41.ØX2A**	Poisoning by inhaled anesthetics, self-harm, init
		T41.5X2A	Poisoning by therapeutic gases, intentional self-harm, init
		T53.5X2A	Toxic effect of chlorofluorocarbons, self-harm, init
		T57.3X2A	Toxic effect of hydrogen cyanide, self-harm, init
		T59.ØX2A	Toxic effect of nitrogen oxides, intentional self-harm, init
		T59.1X2A	Toxic effect of sulfur dioxide, intentional self-harm, init
		T59.2X2A	Toxic effect of formaldehyde, intentional self-harm, init
		T59.3X2A	Toxic effect of lacrimogenic gas, self-harm, init
		T59.4X2A	Toxic effect of chlorine gas, intentional self-harm, init
		T59.5X2A	Tox eff of fluorine gas and hydrogen fluoride, slf-hrm, init
		T59.6X2A	Toxic effect of hydrogen sulfide, self-harm, init
		T59.7X2A	Toxic effect of carbon dioxide, intentional self-harm, init
		T59.812A	Toxic effect of smoke, intentional self-harm, init encntr
		T59.892A	Toxic effect of gases, fumes and vapors, self-harm, init

ICD-9-CM		ICD-10-CM		
E952.9	SUICIDE&SELF-INFLICTED POISN UNSPEC GASES&VAPORS	**T59.92XA**	Toxic effect of unsp gases, fumes and vapors, slf-hrm, init	
E953.Ø	SUICIDE AND SELF-INFLICTED INJURY BY HANGING	**T71.162A**	Asphyxiation due to hanging, intentional self-harm, init	
E953.1	SUICIDE&SELF-INFLICTED INJURY SUFFOCAT PLSTC BAG	**T71.122A**	Asphyxiation due to plastic bag, intentional self-harm, init	
		T71.152A	Asphyxiation due to smothering in furniture, self-harm, init	
E953.8	SUI&SLF INJR HANG STRANG&SUFFOCAT OTH SPEC	**T71.112A**	Asphyxiation due to smothering under pillow, self-harm, init	
		T71.132A	Asphyx due to being trapped in bed linens, self-harm, init	
		T71.192A	Asphyx d/t mech thrt to breathe d/t oth cause, slf-hrm, init	
		T71.222A	Asphyx due to being trapped in a car trunk, self-harm, init	
		T71.232A	Asphyx d/t being trap in a (discarded) refrig, slf-hrm, init	
E953.9	SUI&SELF INJURY HANG STRANG&SUFFOCAT UNS MEANS	NO DIAGNOSIS		
E954	SUICIDE AND SELF-INFLICTED INJURY BY SUBMERSION	**X71.ØXXA**	Intentional self-harm by drown while in bathtub, init	
		X71.ØXXD	Intentional self-harm by drown while in bathtub, subs	
		X71.1XXA	Intentional self-harm by drown while in swimming pool, init	
		X71.1XXD	Intentional self-harm by drown while in swimming pool, subs	
		X71.2XXA	Self-harm by drown after jump into swimming pool, init	
		X71.2XXD	Self-harm by drown after jump into swimming pool, subs	
		X71.3XXA	Intentional self-harm by drown in natural water, init	
		X71.3XXD	Intentional self-harm by drown in natural water, subs	
		X71.8XXA	Oth intentional self-harm by drowning and submersion, init	
		X71.8XXD	Oth intentional self-harm by drowning and submersion, subs	
		X71.9XXA	Intentional self-harm by drowning and submersion, unsp, init	
		X71.9XXD	Intentional self-harm by drowning and submersion, unsp, subs	
E955.Ø	SUICIDE AND SELF-INFLICTED INJURY BY HANDGUN	**X72.XXXA**	Intentional self-harm by handgun discharge, init encntr	
		X72.XXXD	Intentional self-harm by handgun discharge, subs encntr	
E955.1	SUICIDE AND SELF-INFLICTED INJURY BY SHOTGUN	**X73.ØXXA**	Intentional self-harm by shotgun discharge, init encntr	
		X73.ØXXD	Intentional self-harm by shotgun discharge, subs encntr	
E955.2	SUICIDE AND SELF-INFLICTED INJURY HUNTING RIFLE	**X73.1XXA**	Intentional self-harm by hunting rifle discharge, init	
		X73.1XXD	Intentional self-harm by hunting rifle discharge, subs	
E955.3	SUICIDE&SELF-INFLICTED INJURY MILITARY FIREARMS	**X73.2XXA**	Intentional self-harm by machine gun discharge, init encntr	
		X73.2XXD	Intentional self-harm by machine gun discharge, subs encntr	
E955.4	SUICIDE&SELF-INFLICTED INJURY OTH&UNSPEC FIREARM	**X73.8XXA**	Intentional self-harm by oth larger firearm discharge, init	
		X73.8XXD	Intentional self-harm by oth larger firearm discharge, subs	
		X73.9XXA	Intentional self-harm by unsp larger firearm discharge, init	
		X73.9XXD	Intentional self-harm by unsp larger firearm discharge, subs	
		X74.8XXA	Intentional self-harm by oth firearm discharge, init encntr	
		X74.8XXD	Intentional self-harm by oth firearm discharge, subs encntr	
E955.5	SUICIDE AND SELF-INFLICTED INJURY BY EXPLOSIVES	**X75.XXXA**	Intentional self-harm by explosive material, init encntr	
		X75.XXXD	Intentional self-harm by explosive material, subs encntr	
E955.6	SUICIDE AND SELF-INFLICTED INJURY BY AIR GUN	**X74.Ø1XA**	Intentional self-harm by airgun, initial encounter	
		X74.Ø1XD	Intentional self-harm by airgun, subsequent encounter	
		X74.Ø9XA	Self-harm by oth gas, air or spring-operated gun, init	
		X74.Ø9XD	Self-harm by oth gas, air or spring-operated gun, subs	
E955.7	SUICIDE AND SELF-INFLICTED INJURY PAINTBALL GUN	**X74.Ø2XA**	Intentional self-harm by paintball gun, initial encounter	
		X74.Ø2XD	Intentional self-harm by paintball gun, subsequent encounter	
E955.9	SUI&SLF-INFLICT INJR BY FIRARMS&EXPLOSIVES UNS	**X74.9XXA**	Intentional self-harm by unsp firearm discharge, init encntr	
		X74.9XXD	Intentional self-harm by unsp firearm discharge, subs encntr	
E956	SUICIDE&SELF-INFLICT INJURY CUT&PIERCING INSTRUM	**X78.ØXXA**	Intentional self-harm by sharp glass, initial encounter	
		X78.ØXXD	Intentional self-harm by sharp glass, subsequent encounter	
		X78.1XXA	Intentional self-harm by knife, initial encounter	
		X78.1XXD	Intentional self-harm by knife, subsequent encounter	
		X78.2XXA	Intentional self-harm by sword or dagger, initial encounter	
		X78.2XXD	Intentional self-harm by sword or dagger, subs encntr	
		X78.8XXA	Intentional self-harm by other sharp object, init encntr	
		X78.8XXD	Intentional self-harm by other sharp object, subs encntr	
		X78.9XXA	Intentional self-harm by unsp sharp object, init encntr	
		X78.9XXD	Intentional self-harm by unsp sharp object, subs encntr	
E957.Ø	SUI&SLF-INFLICT INJR BY JUMP FRM RES PREMISES	**X8Ø.XXXA**	Intentional self-harm by jumping from a high place, init	*and*
		Y92.ØØ9	Unsp place in unsp non-institut (private) residence as place	
E957.1	SUICIDE&SLF-INFLICT INJR JUMP OTH MAN-MADE STRCT	**X8Ø.XXXA**	Intentional self-harm by jumping from a high place, init	*and*
		Y92.89	Oth places as the place of occurrence of the external cause	
E957.2	SUI&SLF-INFLICT INJR BY JUMP FROM NATURAL SITE	**X8Ø.XXXA**	Intentional self-harm by jumping from a high place, init	*and*
		Y92.828	Oth wilderness area as place	*or*
		Y92.838	Oth recreation area as place	
E957.9	SUICIDE&SLF-INFLICT INJURIES JUMP FROM UNS SITE	**X8Ø.XXXD**	Intentional self-harm by jumping from a high place, subs	
		X8Ø.XXXA	Intentional self-harm by jumping from a high place, init	*and*
		Y92.9	Unspecified place or not applicable	
E958.Ø	SUI&SLF-INFLICT INJR JUMP/LYING BEFORE MOV OBJ	**X81.ØXXA**	Self-harm by jumping or lying in front of mtr veh, init	
		X81.ØXXD	Self-harm by jumping or lying in front of mtr veh, subs	
		X81.1XXA	Slf-hrm by jumping or lying in front of (subway) train, init	
		X81.1XXD	Slf-hrm by jumping or lying in front of (subway) train, subs	
		X81.8XXA	Slf-hrm by jumping or lying in front of moving object, init	
		X81.8XXD	Slf-hrm by jumping or lying in front of moving object, subs	

ICD-9-CM		ICD-10-CM	
E958.1	SUICIDE AND SELF-INFLICTED INJURY BY BURNS FIRE	**X76.XXXA**	Intentional self-harm by smoke, fire and flames, init encntr
		X76.XXXD	Intentional self-harm by smoke, fire and flames, subs encntr
		X77.3XXA	Intentional self-harm by hot household appliances, init
		X77.3XXD	Intentional self-harm by hot household appliances, subs
		X77.8XXA	Intentional self-harm by other hot objects, init encntr
		X77.8XXD	Intentional self-harm by other hot objects, subs encntr
		X77.9XXA	Intentional self-harm by unsp hot objects, init encntr
		X77.9XXD	Intentional self-harm by unsp hot objects, subs encntr
E958.2	SUICIDE AND SELF-INFLICTED INJURY BY SCALD	**X77.ØXXA**	Intentional self-harm by steam or hot vapors, init encntr
		X77.ØXXD	Intentional self-harm by steam or hot vapors, subs encntr
		X77.1XXA	Intentional self-harm by hot tap water, initial encounter
		X77.1XXD	Intentional self-harm by hot tap water, subsequent encounter
		X77.2XXA	Intentional self-harm by other hot fluids, initial encounter
		X77.2XXD	Intentional self-harm by other hot fluids, subs encntr
E958.3	SUICIDE&SELF-INFLICTED INJURY EXTREMES OF COLD	**X83.2XXA**	Intentional self-harm by exposure to extremes of cold, init
		X83.2XXD	Intentional self-harm by exposure to extremes of cold, subs
E958.4	SUICIDE AND SELF-INFLICTED INJURY ELECTROCUTION	**X83.1XXA**	Intentional self-harm by electrocution, initial encounter
		X83.1XXD	Intentional self-harm by electrocution, subsequent encounter
E958.5	SUICIDE&SELF-INFLICTED INJURY CRASHING MOTOR VEH	**X82.ØXXA**	Intentional collision of motor vehicle w mtr veh, init
		X82.ØXXD	Intentional collision of motor vehicle w mtr veh, subs
		X82.1XXA	Intentional collision of motor vehicle w train, init encntr
		X82.1XXD	Intentional collision of motor vehicle w train, subs encntr
		X82.2XXA	Intentional collision of motor vehicle w tree, init encntr
		X82.2XXD	Intentional collision of motor vehicle w tree, subs encntr
		X82.8XXA	Oth intentional self-harm by crashing of motor vehicle, init
		X82.8XXD	Oth intentional self-harm by crashing of motor vehicle, subs
E958.6	SUICIDE&SELF-INFLICTED INJURY CRASHING AIRCRAFT	**X83.ØXXA**	Intentional self-harm by crashing of aircraft, init encntr
		X83.ØXXD	Intentional self-harm by crashing of aircraft, subs encntr
E958.7	SUICIDE&SLF-INFLICT INJR CAUSTIC SBSTNC NO POISN	**X83.8XXA**	Intentional self-harm by other specified means, init encntr
		X83.8XXD	Intentional self-harm by other specified means, subs encntr
E958.8	SUICIDE&SELF-INFLICTED INJURY OTHER SPEC MEANS	**X79.XXXA**	Intentional self-harm by blunt object, initial encounter
		X79.XXXD	Intentional self-harm by blunt object, subsequent encounter
		X83.8XXA	Intentional self-harm by other specified means, init encntr
		X83.8XXD	Intentional self-harm by other specified means, subs encntr
E958.9	SUICIDE&SELF-INFLICTED INJURY UNSPECIFIED MEANS	**T14.91**	Suicide attempt
		X83.8XXA	Intentional self-harm by other specified means, init encntr
E959	LATE EFFECTS OF SELF-INFLICTED INJURY	**T36.ØX2S**	Poisoning by penicillins, intentional self-harm, sequela
		T36.1X2S	Poisn by cephalospor/oth beta-lactm antibiot, slf-hrm, sqla
		T36.2X2S	Poisoning by chloramphenicol group, self-harm, sequela
		T36.3X2S	Poisoning by macrolides, intentional self-harm, sequela
		T36.4X2S	Poisoning by tetracyclines, intentional self-harm, sequela
		T36.5X2S	Poisoning by aminoglycosides, intentional self-harm, sequela
		T36.6X2S	Poisoning by rifampicins, intentional self-harm, sequela
		T36.7X2S	Poisoning by antifung antibiot, sys used, self-harm, sequela
		T36.8X2S	Poisoning by oth systemic antibiotics, self-harm, sequela
		T36.92XS	Poisoning by unsp systemic antibiotic, self-harm, sequela
		T37.ØX2S	Poisoning by sulfonamides, intentional self-harm, sequela
		T37.1X2S	Poisoning by antimycobacterial drugs, self-harm, sequela
		T37.2X2S	Poisn by antimalari/drugs act on bld protzoa, slf-hrm, sqla
		T37.3X2S	Poisoning by oth antiprotozoal drugs, self-harm, sequela
		T37.4X2S	Poisoning by anthelminthics, intentional self-harm, sequela
		T37.5X2S	Poisoning by antiviral drugs, intentional self-harm, sequela
		T37.8X2S	Poisn by oth systemic anti-infect/parasit, slf-hrm, sequela
		T37.92XS	Poisn by unsp sys anti-infect and antiparastc, slf-hrm, sqla
		T38.ØX2S	Poisoning by glucocort/synth analog, self-harm, sequela
		T38.1X2S	Poisoning by thyroid hormones and sub, self-harm, sequela
		T38.2X2S	Poisoning by antithyroid drugs, self-harm, sequela
		T38.3X2S	Poisn by insulin and oral hypoglycemic drugs, slf-hrm, sqla
		T38.4X2S	Poisoning by oral contraceptives, self-harm, sequela
		T38.5X2S	Poisoning by oth estrogens and progstrn, self-harm, sequela
		T38.6X2S	Poisn by antigonadtr/antiestr/antiandrg, NEC, slf-hrm, sqla
		T38.7X2S	Poisn by androgens and anabolic congeners, slf-hrm, sequela
		T38.8Ø2S	Poisn by unsp hormones and synthetic sub, self-harm, sequela
		T38.812S	Poisoning by anterior pituitary hormones, self-harm, sequela
		T38.892S	Poisn by oth hormones and synthetic sub, self-harm, sequela
		T38.9Ø2S	Poisoning by unsp hormone antagonists, self-harm, sequela
		T38.992S	Poisoning by oth hormone antagonists, self-harm, sequela
		T39.Ø12S	Poisoning by aspirin, intentional self-harm, sequela
		T39.Ø92S	Poisoning by salicylates, intentional self-harm, sequela
		T39.1X2S	Poisoning by 4-Aminophenol derivatives, self-harm, sequela
		T39.2X2S	Poisoning by pyrazolone derivatives, self-harm, sequela
		T39.312S	Poisoning by propionic acid derivatives, self-harm, sequela
		T39.392S	Poisn by oth nonsteroid anti-inflam drugs, slf-hrm, sequela
		T39.4X2S	Poisoning by antirheumatics, NEC, self-harm, sequela
		T39.8X2S	Poisn by oth nonopio analges/antipyret, NEC, slf-hrm, sqla
		T39.92XS	Poisn by unsp nonopi analgs/antipyr/antirheu, slf-hrm, sqla
		T4Ø.ØX2S	Poisoning by opium, intentional self-harm, sequela
	(Continued on next page)	**T4Ø.1X2S**	Poisoning by heroin, intentional self-harm, sequela

ICD-9-CM		ICD-10-CM	
E959	LATE EFFECTS OF SELF-INFLICTED INJURY **(Continued)**	**T4Ø.2X2S**	Poisoning by other opioids, intentional self-harm, sequela
		T4Ø.3X2S	Poisoning by methadone, intentional self-harm, sequela
		T4Ø.4X2S	Poisoning by oth synthetic narcotics, self-harm, sequela
		T4Ø.5X2S	Poisoning by cocaine, intentional self-harm, sequela
		T4Ø.6Ø2S	Poisoning by unsp narcotics, intentional self-harm, sequela
		T4Ø.692S	Poisoning by other narcotics, intentional self-harm, sequela
		T4Ø.7X2S	Poisoning by cannabis (derivatives), self-harm, sequela
		T4Ø.8X2S	Poisoning by lysergide [LSD], intentional self-harm, sequela
		T4Ø.9Ø2S	Poisoning by unsp psychodysleptics, self-harm, sequela
		T4Ø.992S	Poisoning by oth psychodysleptics, self-harm, sequela
		T41.ØX2S	Poisoning by inhaled anesthetics, self-harm, sequela
		T41.1X2S	Poisoning by intravenous anesthetics, self-harm, sequela
		T41.2Ø2S	Poisoning by unsp general anesthetics, self-harm, sequela
		T41.292S	Poisoning by oth general anesthetics, self-harm, sequela
		T41.3X2S	Poisoning by local anesthetics, self-harm, sequela
		T41.42XS	Poisoning by unsp anesthetic, intentional self-harm, sequela
		T41.5X2S	Poisoning by therapeutic gases, self-harm, sequela
		T42.ØX2S	Poisoning by hydantoin derivatives, self-harm, sequela
		T42.1X2S	Poisoning by iminostilbenes, intentional self-harm, sequela
		T42.2X2S	Poisn by succinimides and oxazolidinediones, slf-hrm, sqla
		T42.3X2S	Poisoning by barbiturates, intentional self-harm, sequela
		T42.4X2S	Poisoning by benzodiazepines, intentional self-harm, sequela
		T42.5X2S	Poisoning by mixed antiepileptics, self-harm, sequela
		T42.6X2S	Poisn by oth antieplptc and sed-hypntc drugs, slf-hrm, sqla
		T42.72XS	Poisn by unsp antieplptc and sed-hypntc drugs, slf-hrm, sqla
		T42.8X2S	Poisn by antiparkns drug/centr musc-tone depr, slf-hrm, sqla
		T43.Ø12S	Poisoning by tricyclic antidepressants, self-harm, sequela
		T43.Ø22S	Poisoning by tetracyclic antidepressants, self-harm, sequela
		T43.1X2S	Poisoning by MAO inhib antidepressants, self-harm, sequela
		T43.2Ø2S	Poisoning by unsp antidepressants, self-harm, sequela
		T43.212S	Poisn by slctv seroton/norepineph reup inhibtr,slf-hrm, sqla
		T43.222S	Poisn by slctv serotonin reuptake inhibtr, slf-hrm, sequela
		T43.292S	Poisoning by oth antidepressants, self-harm, sequela
		T43.3X2S	Poisn by phenothiaz antipsychot/neurolept, slf-hrm, sequela
		T43.4X2S	Poisn by butyrophen/thiothixen neuroleptc, slf-hrm, sequela
		T43.5Ø2S	Poisoning by unsp antipsychot/neurolept, self-harm, sequela
		T43.592S	Poisoning by oth antipsychot/neurolept, self-harm, sequela
		T43.6Ø2S	Poisoning by unsp psychostimulants, self-harm, sequela
		T43.612S	Poisoning by caffeine, intentional self-harm, sequela
		T43.622S	Poisoning by amphetamines, intentional self-harm, sequela
		T43.632S	Poisoning by methylphenidate, intentional self-harm, sequela
		T43.692S	Poisoning by oth psychostimulants, self-harm, sequela
		T43.8X2S	Poisoning by oth psychotropic drugs, self-harm, sequela
		T43.92XS	Poisoning by unsp psychotropic drug, self-harm, sequela
		T44.ØX2S	Poisoning by anticholinesterase agents, self-harm, sequela
		T44.1X2S	Poisoning by oth parasympathomimetics, self-harm, sequela
		T44.2X2S	Poisoning by ganglionic blocking drugs, self-harm, sequela
		T44.3X2S	Poisn by oth parasympath and spasmolytics, slf-hrm, sequela
		T44.4X2S	Poisn by predom alpha-adrenocpt agonists, self-harm, sequela
		T44.5X2S	Poisn by predom beta-adrenocpt agonists, self-harm, sequela
		T44.6X2S	Poisoning by alpha-adrenocpt antagonists, self-harm, sequela
		T44.7X2S	Poisoning by beta-adrenocpt antagonists, self-harm, sequela
		T44.8X2S	Poisn by centr-acting/adren-neurn-block agnt, slf-hrm, sqla
		T44.9Ø2S	Poisn by unsp drugs aff the autonm nrv sys, slf-hrm, sequela
		T44.992S	Poisn by oth drug aff the autonm nrv sys, slf-hrm, sequela
		T45.ØX2S	Poisoning by antiallerg/antiemetic, self-harm, sequela
		T45.1X2S	Poisn by antineopl and immunosup drugs, self-harm, sequela
		T45.2X2S	Poisoning by vitamins, intentional self-harm, sequela
		T45.3X2S	Poisoning by enzymes, intentional self-harm, sequela
		T45.4X2S	Poisoning by iron and its compounds, self-harm, sequela
		T45.512S	Poisoning by anticoagulants, intentional self-harm, sequela
		T45.522S	Poisoning by antithrombotic drugs, self-harm, sequela
		T45.6Ø2S	Poisoning by unsp fibrin-affct drugs, self-harm, sequela
		T45.612S	Poisoning by thrombolytic drug, self-harm, sequela
		T45.622S	Poisoning by hemostatic drug, intentional self-harm, sequela
		T45.692S	Poisoning by oth fibrin-affct drugs, self-harm, sequela
		T45.7X2S	Poisn by anticoag antag, vit K and oth coag, slf-hrm, sqla
		T45.8X2S	Poisn by oth prim sys and hematolog agents, slf-hrm, sequela
		T45.92XS	Poisn by unsp prim sys and hematolog agent, slf-hrm, sequela
		T46.ØX2S	Poisn by cardi-stim glycos/drug simlar act, slf-hrm, sequela
		T46.1X2S	Poisoning by calcium-channel blockers, self-harm, sequela
		T46.2X2S	Poisoning by oth antidysrhythmic drugs, self-harm, sequela
		T46.3X2S	Poisoning by coronary vasodilators, self-harm, sequela
		T46.4X2S	Poisn by angiotens-convert-enzyme inhibtr, slf-hrm, sequela
		T46.5X2S	Poisoning by oth antihypertensive drugs, self-harm, sequela
		T46.6X2S	Poisn by antihyperlip and antiarterio drugs, slf-hrm, sqla
		T46.7X2S	Poisoning by peripheral vasodilators, self-harm, sequela
		T46.8X2S	Poisn by antivaric drugs, inc scler agents, slf-hrm, sequela
	(Continued on next page)	**T46.9Ø2S**	Poisn by unsp agents aff the cardiovasc sys, slf-hrm, sqla

ICD-9-CM		ICD-10-CM	
E959	LATE EFFECTS OF SELF-INFLICTED INJURY **(Continued)**	**T46.992S**	Poisn by oth agents aff the cardiovasc sys, slf-hrm, sequela
		T47.0X2S	Poisn by histamine H2-receptor blockers, self-harm, sequela
		T47.1X2S	Poisn by oth antacids & anti-gstrc-sec drugs, slf-hrm, sqla
		T47.2X2S	Poisoning by stimulant laxatives, self-harm, sequela
		T47.3X2S	Poisoning by saline and osmotic laxtv, self-harm, sequela
		T47.4X2S	Poisoning by other laxatives, intentional self-harm, sequela
		T47.5X2S	Poisoning by digestants, intentional self-harm, sequela
		T47.6X2S	Poisoning by antidiarrheal drugs, self-harm, sequela
		T47.7X2S	Poisoning by emetics, intentional self-harm, sequela
		T47.8X2S	Poisoning by oth agents aff GI sys, self-harm, sequela
		T47.92XS	Poisoning by unsp agents aff the GI sys, self-harm, sequela
		T48.0X2S	Poisoning by oxytocic drugs, intentional self-harm, sequela
		T48.1X2S	Poisoning by skeletal muscle relaxants, self-harm, sequela
		T48.202S	Poisn by unsp drugs acting on muscles, self-harm, sequela
		T48.292S	Poisoning by oth drugs acting on muscles, self-harm, sequela
		T48.3X2S	Poisoning by antitussives, intentional self-harm, sequela
		T48.4X2S	Poisoning by expectorants, intentional self-harm, sequela
		T48.5X2S	Poisoning by oth anti-common-cold drugs, self-harm, sequela
		T48.6X2S	Poisoning by antiasthmatics, intentional self-harm, sequela
		T48.902S	Poisn by unsp agents prim act on the resp sys, slf-hrm, sqla
		T48.992S	Poisn by oth agents prim act on the resp sys, slf-hrm, sqla
		T49.0X2S	Poisn by local antifung/infect/inflamm drugs, slf-hrm, sqla
		T49.1X2S	Poisoning by antipruritics, intentional self-harm, sequela
		T49.2X2S	Poisn by local astringents/detergents, self-harm, sequela
		T49.3X2S	Poisn by emollients, demulcents and protect, slf-hrm, sqla
		T49.4X2S	Poisn by keratolyt/keratplst/hair trmt drug, slf-hrm, sqla
		T49.5X2S	Poisoning by opth drugs and preparations, self-harm, sequela
		T49.6X2S	Poisoning by otorhino drugs and prep, self-harm, sequela
		T49.7X2S	Poisn by dental drugs, topically applied, self-harm, sequela
		T49.8X2S	Poisoning by oth topical agents, self-harm, sequela
		T49.92XS	Poisoning by unsp topical agent, self-harm, sequela
		T50.0X2S	Poisn by mineralocorticoids and antag, self-harm, sequela
		T50.1X2S	Poisoning by loop diuretics, intentional self-harm, sequela
		T50.2X2S	Poisn by crbnc-anhydr inhibtr,benzo/oth diuretc,slf-hrm,sqla
		T50.3X2S	Poisn by electrolytic/caloric/wtr-bal agnt, slf-hrm, sequela
		T50.4X2S	Poisoning by drugs aff uric acid metab, self-harm, sequela
		T50.5X2S	Poisoning by appetite depressants, self-harm, sequela
		T50.6X2S	Poisn by antidotes and chelating agents, self-harm, sequela
		T50.7X2S	Poisn by analeptics and opioid receptor antag, slf-hrm, sqla
		T50.8X2S	Poisoning by diagnostic agents, self-harm, sequela
		T50.902S	Poisoning by unsp drug/meds/biol subst, self-harm, sequela
		T50.992S	Poisoning by oth drug/meds/biol subst, self-harm, sequela
		T50.A12S	Poisn by pertuss vaccn, inc combin w pertuss, slf-hrm, sqla
		T50.A22S	Poisn by mixed bact vaccines w/o a pertuss, slf-hrm, sequela
		T50.A92S	Poisoning by oth bacterial vaccines, self-harm, sequela
		T50.B12S	Poisoning by smallpox vaccines, self-harm, sequela
		T50.B92S	Poisoning by oth viral vaccines, self-harm, sequela
		T50.Z12S	Poisoning by immunoglobulin, intentional self-harm, sequela
		T50.Z92S	Poisn by oth vaccines and biolg substnc, self-harm, sequela
		T60.0X2S	Toxic eff of organophos and carbamate insect, slf-hrm, sqla
		T60.1X2S	Toxic effect of halogenated insecticides, self-harm, sequela
		T60.2X2S	Toxic effect of insecticides, intentional self-harm, sequela
		T60.3X2S	Toxic effect of herbicides and fungicides, slf-hrm, sequela
		T60.4X2S	Toxic effect of rodenticides, intentional self-harm, sequela
		T60.8X2S	Toxic effect of pesticides, intentional self-harm, sequela
		T60.92XS	Toxic effect of unsp pesticide, self-harm, sequela
		T61.02XS	Ciguatera fish poisoning, intentional self-harm, sequela
		T61.12XS	Scombroid fish poisoning, intentional self-harm, sequela
		T61.772S	Other fish poisoning, intentional self-harm, sequela
		T61.782S	Other shellfish poisoning, intentional self-harm, sequela
		T61.8X2S	Toxic effect of oth seafood, intentional self-harm, sequela
		T61.92XS	Toxic effect of unsp seafood, intentional self-harm, sequela
		T62.0X2S	Toxic effect of ingested mushrooms, self-harm, sequela
		T62.1X2S	Toxic effect of ingested berries, self-harm, sequela
		T62.2X2S	Toxic effect of ingest (parts of) plant(s), slf-hrm, sequela
		T62.8X2S	Toxic effect of noxious substnc eaten as food, slf-hrm, sqla
		T62.92XS	Toxic eff of unsp noxious sub eaten as food, slf-hrm, sqla
		T63.003S	Toxic effect of unspecified snake venom, assault, sequela
		T63.012S	Toxic effect of rattlesnake venom, self-harm, sequela
		T63.022S	Toxic effect of coral snake venom, self-harm, sequela
		T63.032S	Toxic effect of taipan venom, intentional self-harm, sequela
		T63.042S	Toxic effect of cobra venom, intentional self-harm, sequela
		T63.062S	Toxic effect of venom of N & S American snake, slf-hrm, sqla
		T63.072S	Toxic effect of venom of Australian snake, slf-hrm, sequela
		T63.082S	Toxic eff of venom of African and Asian snake, slf-hrm, sqla
		T63.092S	Toxic effect of venom of snake, self-harm, sequela
		T63.112S	Toxic effect of venom of gila monster, self-harm, sequela
		T63.122S	Toxic effect of venom of venomous lizard, self-harm, sequela
	(Continued on next page)	**T63.192S**	Toxic effect of venom of reptiles, self-harm, sequela

ICD-9-CM		ICD-10-CM	
E959	LATE EFFECTS OF SELF-INFLICTED INJURY **(Continued)**	**T63.2X2S**	Toxic effect of venom of scorpion, self-harm, sequela
		T63.302S	Toxic effect of unsp spider venom, self-harm, sequela
		T63.312S	Toxic effect of venom of black widow spider, slf-hrm, sqla
		T63.322S	Toxic effect of venom of tarantula, self-harm, sequela
		T63.332S	Toxic effect of venom of brown recluse spider, slf-hrm, sqla
		T63.392S	Toxic effect of venom of spider, self-harm, sequela
		T63.412S	Toxic effect of venom of centipede/millipede, slf-hrm, sqla
		T63.422S	Toxic effect of venom of ants, self-harm, sequela
		T63.432S	Toxic effect of venom of caterpillars, self-harm, sequela
		T63.442S	Toxic effect of venom of bees, self-harm, sequela
		T63.452S	Toxic effect of venom of hornets, self-harm, sequela
		T63.462S	Toxic effect of venom of wasps, self-harm, sequela
		T63.482S	Toxic effect of venom of arthropod, self-harm, sequela
		T63.512S	Toxic effect of contact w stingray, self-harm, sequela
		T63.592S	Toxic effect of contact w oth venom fish, slf-hrm, sequela
		T63.612S	Toxic effect of cntct w Portugese Man-o-war, slf-hrm, sqla
		T63.622S	Toxic effect of contact w oth jellyfish, self-harm, sequela
		T63.632S	Toxic effect of contact w sea anemone, self-harm, sequela
		T63.692S	Toxic eff of cntct w oth venom marine animals, slf-hrm, sqla
		T63.712S	Toxic effect of cntct w venom marine plant, slf-hrm, sequela
		T63.792S	Toxic effect of contact w oth venom plant, slf-hrm, sequela
		T63.812S	Toxic effect of contact w venomous frog, self-harm, sequela
		T63.822S	Toxic effect of contact w venomous toad, self-harm, sequela
		T63.832S	Toxic effect of contact w oth venom amphib, slf-hrm, sequela
		T63.892S	Toxic effect of cntct w oth venom animals, slf-hrm, sequela
		T63.92XS	Toxic effect of cntct w unsp venom animal, slf-hrm, sequela
		T64.02XS	Toxic effect of aflatoxin, intentional self-harm, sequela
		T64.82XS	Toxic effect of mycotoxin food contamnt, self-harm, sequela
		T65.0X2S	Toxic effect of cyanides, intentional self-harm, sequela
		T65.1X2S	Toxic effect of strychnine and its salts, self-harm, sequela
		T65.212S	Toxic effect of chewing tobacco, self-harm, sequela
		T65.222S	Toxic effect of tobacco cigarettes, self-harm, sequela
		T65.292S	Toxic effect of tobacco and nicotine, self-harm, sequela
		T65.3X2S	Tox eff of nitrodrv/aminodrv of benzn/homolog, slf-hrm, sqla
		T65.4X2S	Toxic effect of carbon disulfide, self-harm, sequela
		T65.5X2S	Tox eff of nitro & oth nitric acids & esters, slf-hrm, sqla
		T65.6X2S	Toxic effect of paints and dyes, NEC, self-harm, sequela
		T65.812S	Toxic effect of latex, intentional self-harm, sequela
		T65.822S	Toxic eff of harmful algae and algae toxins, slf-hrm, sqla
		T65.832S	Toxic effect of fiberglass, intentional self-harm, sequela
		T65.892S	Toxic effect of substances, intentional self-harm, sequela
		T65.92XS	Toxic effect of unsp substance, self-harm, sequela
		T71.162S	Asphyxiation due to hanging, intentional self-harm, sequela
		X71.0XXS	Intentional self-harm by drown while in bathtub, sequela
		X71.1XXS	Self-harm by drown while in swimming pool, sequela
		X71.2XXS	Self-harm by drown after jump into swimming pool, sequela
		X71.3XXS	Intentional self-harm by drown in natural water, sequela
		X71.8XXS	Oth intentional self-harm by drown, sequela
		X71.9XXS	Intentional self-harm by drown, unsp, sequela
		X72.XXXS	Intentional self-harm by handgun discharge, sequela
		X73.0XXS	Intentional self-harm by shotgun discharge, sequela
		X73.1XXS	Intentional self-harm by hunting rifle discharge, sequela
		X73.2XXS	Intentional self-harm by machine gun discharge, sequela
		X73.8XXS	Self-harm by oth larger firearm discharge, sequela
		X73.9XXS	Self-harm by unsp larger firearm discharge, sequela
		X74.01XS	Intentional self-harm by airgun, sequela
		X74.02XS	Intentional self-harm by paintball gun, sequela
		X74.09XS	Self-harm by oth gas, air or spring-operated gun, sequela
		X74.8XXS	Intentional self-harm by other firearm discharge, sequela
		X74.9XXS	Intentional self-harm by unsp firearm discharge, sequela
		X75.XXXS	Intentional self-harm by explosive material, sequela
		X76.XXXS	Intentional self-harm by smoke, fire and flames, sequela
		X77.0XXS	Intentional self-harm by steam or hot vapors, sequela
		X77.1XXS	Intentional self-harm by hot tap water, sequela
		X77.2XXS	Intentional self-harm by other hot fluids, sequela
		X77.3XXS	Intentional self-harm by hot household appliances, sequela
		X77.8XXS	Intentional self-harm by other hot objects, sequela
		X77.9XXS	Intentional self-harm by unspecified hot objects, sequela
		X78.0XXS	Intentional self-harm by sharp glass, sequela
		X78.1XXS	Intentional self-harm by knife, sequela
		X78.2XXS	Intentional self-harm by sword or dagger, sequela
		X78.8XXS	Intentional self-harm by other sharp object, sequela
		X78.9XXS	Intentional self-harm by unspecified sharp object, sequela
		X79.XXXS	Intentional self-harm by blunt object, sequela
		X80.XXXS	Intentional self-harm by jumping from a high place, sequela
		X81.0XXS	Self-harm by jumping or lying in front of mtr veh, sequela
		X81.1XXS	Slf-hrm by jumping or lying in front of train, sequela
		X81.8XXS	Slf-hrm by jump or lying in front of moving object, sequela
		X82.0XXS	Intentional collision of motor vehicle w mtr veh, sequela
	(Continued on next page)	**X82.1XXS**	Intentional collision of motor vehicle with train, sequela
		X82.2XXS	Intentional collision of motor vehicle with tree, sequela

ICD-9-CM			ICD-10-CM	
E959	LATE EFFECTS OF SELF-INFLICTED INJURY **(Continued)**		**X82.8XXS**	Oth self-harm by crashing of motor vehicle, sequela
			X83.ØXXS	Intentional self-harm by crashing of aircraft, sequela
			X83.1XXS	Intentional self-harm by electrocution, sequela
			X83.2XXS	Self-harm by exposure to extremes of cold, sequela
			X83.8XXS	Intentional self-harm by other specified means, sequela
E96Ø.Ø	UNARMED FIGHT OR BRAWL		**YØ4.ØXXA**	Assault by unarmed brawl or fight, initial encounter
			YØ4.ØXXD	Assault by unarmed brawl or fight, subsequent encounter
			YØ4.2XXA	Asslt by strike agnst or bumped into by another person, init
			YØ4.2XXD	Asslt by strike agnst or bumped into by another person, subs
			YØ4.8XXA	Assault by other bodily force, initial encounter
			YØ4.8XXD	Assault by other bodily force, subsequent encounter
E96Ø.1	RAPE		**YØ4.8XXA**	Assault by other bodily force, initial encounter
E961	ASSAULT CORROSIVE/CAUSTIC SUBSTANCE NO POISONING	◘	**T54.ØX3A**	Toxic effect of phenol and phenol homologues, assault, init
		◘	**T54.1X3A**	Toxic effect of corrosive organic compounds, assault, init
		◘	**T54.2X3A**	Tox eff of corrosv acids and acid-like substnc, asslt, init
		◘	**T54.3X3A**	Tox eff of corrosv alkalis and alk-like substnc, asslt, init
		◘	**T54.93XA**	Toxic effect of unsp corrosive substance, assault, init
E962.Ø	ASSAULT BY DRUGS AND MEDICINAL SUBSTANCES	◘	**T36.ØX3A**	Poisoning by penicillins, assault, initial encounter
		◘	**T36.1X3A**	Poisn by cephalospor/oth beta-lactm antibiot, assault, init
		◘	**T36.2X3A**	Poisoning by chloramphenicol group, assault, init encntr
		◘	**T36.3X3A**	Poisoning by macrolides, assault, initial encounter
		◘	**T36.4X3A**	Poisoning by tetracyclines, assault, initial encounter
		◘	**T36.5X3A**	Poisoning by aminoglycosides, assault, initial encounter
		◘	**T36.6X3A**	Poisoning by rifampicins, assault, initial encounter
		◘	**T36.7X3A**	Poisoning by antifungal antibiotics, sys used, assault, init
		◘	**T36.8X3A**	Poisoning by oth systemic antibiotics, assault, init encntr
		◘	**T36.93XA**	Poisoning by unsp systemic antibiotic, assault, init encntr
		◘	**T37.ØX3A**	Poisoning by sulfonamides, assault, initial encounter
		◘	**T37.1X3A**	Poisoning by antimycobacterial drugs, assault, init encntr
		◘	**T37.2X3A**	Poisn by antimalari/drugs acting on bld protzoa, asslt, init
		◘	**T37.3X3A**	Poisoning by other antiprotozoal drugs, assault, init encntr
		◘	**T37.4X3A**	Poisoning by anthelminthics, assault, initial encounter
		◘	**T37.5X3A**	Poisoning by antiviral drugs, assault, initial encounter
		◘	**T37.8X3A**	Poisoning by oth systemic anti-infect/parasit, assault, init
		◘	**T37.93XA**	Poisn by unsp sys anti-infect and antiparastc, assault, init
		◘	**T38.ØX3A**	Poisoning by glucocort/synth analog, assault, init
		◘	**T38.1X3A**	Poisoning by thyroid hormones and substitutes, assault, init
		◘	**T38.2X3A**	Poisoning by antithyroid drugs, assault, initial encounter
		◘	**T38.3X3A**	Poisn by insulin and oral hypoglycemic drugs, assault, init
		◘	**T38.4X3A**	Poisoning by oral contraceptives, assault, initial encounter
		◘	**T38.5X3A**	Poisoning by oth estrogens and progestogens, assault, init
		◘	**T38.6X3A**	Poisn by antigonadtr/antiestr/antiandrg, NEC, assault, init
		◘	**T38.7X3A**	Poisoning by androgens and anabolic congeners, assault, init
		◘	**T38.8Ø3A**	Poisoning by unsp hormones and synthetic sub, assault, init
		◘	**T38.813A**	Poisoning by anterior pituitary hormones, assault, init
		◘	**T38.893A**	Poisoning by oth hormones and synthetic sub, assault, init
		◘	**T38.9Ø3A**	Poisoning by unsp hormone antagonists, assault, init encntr
		◘	**T38.993A**	Poisoning by other hormone antagonists, assault, init encntr
		◘	**T39.Ø13A**	Poisoning by aspirin, assault, initial encounter
		◘	**T39.Ø93A**	Poisoning by salicylates, assault, initial encounter
		◘	**T39.1X3A**	Poisoning by 4-Aminophenol derivatives, assault, init encntr
		◘	**T39.2X3A**	Poisoning by pyrazolone derivatives, assault, init encntr
		◘	**T39.313A**	Poisoning by propionic acid derivatives, assault, init
		◘	**T39.393A**	Poisoning by oth nonsteroid anti-inflam drugs, assault, init
		◘	**T39.4X3A**	Poisoning by antirheumatics, NEC, assault, init
		◘	**T39.8X3A**	Poisn by oth nonopio analges/antipyret, NEC, assault, init
		◘	**T39.93XA**	Poisn by unsp nonopi analgs/antipyr/antirheu, assault, init
		◘	**T4Ø.ØX3A**	Poisoning by opium, assault, initial encounter
		◘	**T4Ø.1X3A**	Poisoning by heroin, assault, initial encounter
		◘	**T4Ø.2X3A**	Poisoning by other opioids, assault, initial encounter
		◘	**T4Ø.3X3A**	Poisoning by methadone, assault, initial encounter
		◘	**T4Ø.4X3A**	Poisoning by other synthetic narcotics, assault, init encntr
		◘	**T4Ø.5X3A**	Poisoning by cocaine, assault, initial encounter
		◘	**T4Ø.6Ø3A**	Poisoning by unspecified narcotics, assault, init encntr
		◘	**T4Ø.693A**	Poisoning by other narcotics, assault, initial encounter
		◘	**T4Ø.7X3A**	Poisoning by cannabis (derivatives), assault, init encntr
		◘	**T4Ø.8X3A**	Poisoning by lysergide [LSD], assault, initial encounter
		◘	**T4Ø.9Ø3A**	Poisoning by unsp psychodysleptics, assault, init encntr
		◘	**T4Ø.993A**	Poisoning by other psychodysleptics, assault, init encntr
		◘	**T41.ØX3A**	Poisoning by inhaled anesthetics, assault, initial encounter
		◘	**T41.1X3A**	Poisoning by intravenous anesthetics, assault, init encntr
		◘	**T41.2Ø3A**	Poisoning by unsp general anesthetics, assault, init encntr
		◘	**T41.293A**	Poisoning by other general anesthetics, assault, init encntr
		◘	**T41.3X3A**	Poisoning by local anesthetics, assault, initial encounter
		◘	**T41.43XA**	Poisoning by unspecified anesthetic, assault, init encntr
		◘	**T41.5X3A**	Poisoning by therapeutic gases, assault, initial encounter
		◘	**T42.ØX3A**	Poisoning by hydantoin derivatives, assault, init encntr
		◘	**T42.1X3A**	Poisoning by iminostilbenes, assault, initial encounter
	(Continued on next page)			

ICD-9-CM		ICD-10-CM	
E962.Ø	ASSAULT BY DRUGS AND MEDICINAL SUBSTANCES **(Continued)**	**T42.2X3A**	Poisn by succinimides and oxazolidinediones, assault, init
		T42.3X3A	Poisoning by barbiturates, assault, initial encounter
		T42.4X3A	Poisoning by benzodiazepines, assault, initial encounter
		T42.5X3A	Poisoning by mixed antiepileptics, assault, init encntr
		T42.6X3A	Poisn by oth antieplptc and sed-hypntc drugs, assault, init
		T42.73XA	Poisn by unsp antieplptc and sed-hypntc drugs, assault, init
		T42.8X3A	Poisn by antiparkns drug/centr musc-tone depr, assault, init
		T43.Ø13A	Poisoning by tricyclic antidepressants, assault, init encntr
		T43.Ø23A	Poisoning by tetracyclic antidepressants, assault, init
		T43.1X3A	Poisoning by MAO inhib antidepressants, assault, init
		T43.2Ø3A	Poisoning by unsp antidepressants, assault, init encntr
		T43.213A	Poisn by slctv seroton/norepineph reup inhibtr, asslt, init
		T43.223A	Poisn by selective serotonin reuptake inhibtr, assault, init
		T43.293A	Poisoning by other antidepressants, assault, init encntr
		T43.3X3A	Poisoning by phenothiaz antipsychot/neurolept, assault, init
		T43.4X3A	Poisoning by butyrophen/thiothixen neuroleptc, assault, init
		T43.5Ø3A	Poisoning by unsp antipsychot/neurolept, assault, init
		T43.593A	Poisoning by oth antipsychot/neurolept, assault, init
		T43.6Ø3A	Poisoning by unsp psychostimulants, assault, init encntr
		T43.613A	Poisoning by caffeine, assault, initial encounter
		T43.623A	Poisoning by amphetamines, assault, initial encounter
		T43.633A	Poisoning by methylphenidate, assault, initial encounter
		T43.693A	Poisoning by other psychostimulants, assault, init encntr
		T43.8X3A	Poisoning by other psychotropic drugs, assault, init encntr
		T43.93XA	Poisoning by unsp psychotropic drug, assault, init encntr
		T44.ØX3A	Poisoning by anticholinesterase agents, assault, init encntr
		T44.1X3A	Poisoning by oth parasympathomimetics, assault, init encntr
		T44.2X3A	Poisoning by ganglionic blocking drugs, assault, init encntr
		T44.3X3A	Poisoning by oth parasympath and spasmolytics, assault, init
		T44.4X3A	Poisoning by predom alpha-adrenocpt agonists, assault, init
		T44.5X3A	Poisoning by predom beta-adrenocpt agonists, assault, init
		T44.6X3A	Poisoning by alpha-adrenoreceptor antagonists, assault, init
		T44.7X3A	Poisoning by beta-adrenoreceptor antagonists, assault, init
		T44.8X3A	Poisn by centr-acting/adren-neurn-block agnt, assault, init
		T44.9Ø3A	Poisn by unsp drugs aff the autonm nervous sys, asslt, init
		T44.993A	Poisn by oth drug aff the autonm nervous sys, assault, init
		T45.ØX3A	Poisoning by antiallerg/antiemetic, assault, init
		T45.1X3A	Poisoning by antineopl and immunosup drugs, assault, init
		T45.2X3A	Poisoning by vitamins, assault, initial encounter
		T45.3X3A	Poisoning by enzymes, assault, initial encounter
		T45.4X3A	Poisoning by iron and its compounds, assault, init encntr
		T45.513A	Poisoning by anticoagulants, assault, initial encounter
		T45.523A	Poisoning by antithrombotic drugs, assault, init encntr
		T45.6Ø3A	Poisoning by unsp fibrin-affct drugs, assault, init
		T45.613A	Poisoning by thrombolytic drug, assault, initial encounter
		T45.623A	Poisoning by hemostatic drug, assault, initial encounter
		T45.693A	Poisoning by oth fibrinolysis-affecting drugs, assault, init
		T45.7X3A	Poisn by anticoag antag, vit K and oth coag, assault, init
		T45.8X3A	Poisn by oth prim sys and hematolog agents, assault, init
		T45.93XA	Poisn by unsp prim sys and hematolog agent, assault, init
		T46.ØX3A	Poisn by cardi-stim glycos/drug simlar act, assault, init
		T46.1X3A	Poisoning by calcium-channel blockers, assault, init encntr
		T46.2X3A	Poisoning by oth antidysrhythmic drugs, assault, init encntr
		T46.3X3A	Poisoning by coronary vasodilators, assault, init encntr
		T46.4X3A	Poisoning by angiotens-convert-enzyme inhibtr, assault, init
		T46.5X3A	Poisoning by oth antihypertensive drugs, assault, init
		T46.6X3A	Poisn by antihyperlip and antiarterio drugs, assault, init
		T46.7X3A	Poisoning by peripheral vasodilators, assault, init encntr
		T46.8X3A	Poisn by antivaric drugs, inc scler agents, assault, init
		T46.9Ø3A	Poisn by unsp agents aff the cardiovasc sys, assault, init
		T46.993A	Poisn by oth agents aff the cardiovasc sys, assault, init
		T47.ØX3A	Poisoning by histamine H2-receptor blockers, assault, init
		T47.1X3A	Poisn by oth antacids and anti-gstrc-sec drugs, asslt, init
		T47.2X3A	Poisoning by stimulant laxatives, assault, initial encounter
		T47.3X3A	Poisoning by saline and osmotic laxatives, assault, init
		T47.4X3A	Poisoning by other laxatives, assault, initial encounter
		T47.5X3A	Poisoning by digestants, assault, initial encounter
		T47.6X3A	Poisoning by antidiarrheal drugs, assault, initial encounter
		T47.7X3A	Poisoning by emetics, assault, initial encounter
		T47.8X3A	Poisoning by oth agents aff GI sys, assault, init
		T47.93XA	Poisoning by unsp agents aff the GI sys, assault, init
		T48.ØX3A	Poisoning by oxytocic drugs, assault, initial encounter
		T48.1X3A	Poisoning by skeletal muscle relaxants, assault, init encntr
		T48.2Ø3A	Poisoning by unsp drugs acting on muscles, assault, init
		T48.293A	Poisoning by oth drugs acting on muscles, assault, init
		T48.3X3A	Poisoning by antitussives, assault, initial encounter
		T48.4X3A	Poisoning by expectorants, assault, initial encounter
		T48.5X3A	Poisoning by oth anti-common-cold drugs, assault, init
	(Continued on next page)	**T48.6X3A**	Poisoning by antiasthmatics, assault, initial encounter

ICD-9-CM		ICD-10-CM	
E962.Ø	ASSAULT BY DRUGS AND MEDICINAL SUBSTANCES **(Continued)**	**T48.9Ø3A**	Poisn by unsp agents prim act on the resp sys, asslt, init
		T48.993A	Poisn by oth agents prim acting on the resp sys, asslt, init
		T49.ØX3A	Poisn by local antifung/infect/inflamm drugs, assault, init
		T49.1X3A	Poisoning by antipruritics, assault, initial encounter
		T49.2X3A	Poisoning by local astringents/detergents, assault, init
		T49.3X3A	Poisn by emollients, demulcents and protect, assault, init
		T49.4X3A	Poisn by keratolyt/keratplst/hair trmt drug, assault, init
		T49.5X3A	Poisoning by opth drugs and preparations, assault, init
		T49.6X3A	Poisoning by otorhino drugs and preparations, assault, init
		T49.7X3A	Poisoning by dental drugs, topically applied, assault, init
		T49.8X3A	Poisoning by other topical agents, assault, init encntr
		T49.93XA	Poisoning by unspecified topical agent, assault, init encntr
		T5Ø.ØX3A	Poisoning by mineralocorticoids and antag, assault, init
		T5Ø.1X3A	Poisoning by loop diuretics, assault, initial encounter
		T5Ø.2X3A	Poisn by crbnc-anhydr inhibtr,benzo/oth diuretc, asslt, init
		T5Ø.3X3A	Poisn by electrolytic/caloric/wtr-bal agnt, assault, init
		T5Ø.4X3A	Poisoning by drugs affecting uric acid metab, assault, init
		T5Ø.5X3A	Poisoning by appetite depressants, assault, init encntr
		T5Ø.6X3A	Poisoning by antidotes and chelating agents, assault, init
		T5Ø.7X3A	Poisn by analeptics and opioid receptor antag, assault, init
		T5Ø.8X3A	Poisoning by diagnostic agents, assault, initial encounter
		T5Ø.9Ø3A	Poisoning by unsp drug/meds/biol subst, assault, init
		T5Ø.993A	Poisoning by oth drug/meds/biol subst, assault, init
		T5Ø.A13A	Poisn by pertuss vaccine, inc combin w pertuss, asslt, init
		T5Ø.A23A	Poisn by mixed bact vaccines w/o a pertuss, assault, init
		T5Ø.A93A	Poisoning by other bacterial vaccines, assault, init encntr
		T5Ø.B13A	Poisoning by smallpox vaccines, assault, initial encounter
		T5Ø.B93A	Poisoning by other viral vaccines, assault, init encntr
		T5Ø.Z13A	Poisoning by immunoglobulin, assault, initial encounter
		T5Ø.Z93A	Poisoning by oth vaccines and biolg substnc, assault, init
E962.1	ASSAULT BY OTHER SOLID AND LIQUID SUBSTANCES	**T51.ØX3A**	Toxic effect of ethanol, assault, initial encounter
		T51.1X3A	Toxic effect of methanol, assault, initial encounter
		T51.2X3A	Toxic effect of 2-Propanol, assault, initial encounter
		T51.3X3A	Toxic effect of fusel oil, assault, initial encounter
		T51.8X3A	Toxic effect of other alcohols, assault, initial encounter
		T51.93XA	Toxic effect of unspecified alcohol, assault, init encntr
		T52.ØX3A	Toxic effect of petroleum products, assault, init encntr
		T52.1X3A	Toxic effect of benzene, assault, initial encounter
		T52.2X3A	Toxic effect of homologues of benzene, assault, init encntr
		T52.3X3A	Toxic effect of glycols, assault, initial encounter
		T52.4X3A	Toxic effect of ketones, assault, initial encounter
		T52.8X3A	Toxic effect of other organic solvents, assault, init encntr
		T52.93XA	Toxic effect of unsp organic solvent, assault, init encntr
		T55.ØX3A	Toxic effect of soaps, assault, initial encounter
		T55.1X3A	Toxic effect of detergents, assault, initial encounter
		T56.ØX3A	Toxic effect of lead and its compounds, assault, init encntr
		T56.1X3A	Toxic effect of mercury and its compounds, assault, init
		T56.2X3A	Toxic effect of chromium and its compounds, assault, init
		T56.3X3A	Toxic effect of cadmium and its compounds, assault, init
		T56.4X3A	Toxic effect of copper and its compounds, assault, init
		T56.5X3A	Toxic effect of zinc and its compounds, assault, init encntr
		T56.6X3A	Toxic effect of tin and its compounds, assault, init encntr
		T56.7X3A	Toxic effect of beryllium and its compounds, assault, init
		T56.813A	Toxic effect of thallium, assault, initial encounter
		T56.893A	Toxic effect of other metals, assault, initial encounter
		T56.93XA	Toxic effect of unspecified metal, assault, init encntr
		T57.ØX3A	Toxic effect of arsenic and its compounds, assault, init
		T57.1X3A	Toxic effect of phosphorus and its compounds, assault, init
		T57.2X3A	Toxic effect of manganese and its compounds, assault, init
		T57.3X3A	Toxic effect of hydrogen cyanide, assault, initial encounter
		T57.8X3A	Toxic effect of oth inorganic substances, assault, init
		T6Ø.ØX3A	Toxic effect of organophos and carbamate insect, asslt, init
		T6Ø.1X3A	Toxic effect of halogenated insecticides, assault, init
		T6Ø.2X3A	Toxic effect of other insecticides, assault, init encntr
		T6Ø.3X3A	Toxic effect of herbicides and fungicides, assault, init
		T6Ø.4X3A	Toxic effect of rodenticides, assault, initial encounter
		T6Ø.8X3A	Toxic effect of other pesticides, assault, initial encounter
		T6Ø.93XA	Toxic effect of unspecified pesticide, assault, init encntr
		T61.Ø3XA	Ciguatera fish poisoning, assault, initial encounter
		T61.13XA	Scombroid fish poisoning, assault, initial encounter
		T61.773A	Other fish poisoning, assault, initial encounter
		T61.783A	Other shellfish poisoning, assault, initial encounter
		T61.8X3A	Toxic effect of other seafood, assault, initial encounter
		T61.93XA	Toxic effect of unspecified seafood, assault, init encntr
		T62.ØX3A	Toxic effect of ingested mushrooms, assault, init encntr
		T62.1X3A	Toxic effect of ingested berries, assault, initial encounter
		T62.2X3A	Toxic effect of ingested (parts of) plant(s), assault, init
		T62.8X3A	Toxic effect of noxious substnc eaten as food, assault, init
	(Continued on next page)	**T62.93XA**	Toxic effect of unsp noxious sub eaten as food, asslt, init

ICD-9-CM		ICD-10-CM	
E962.1	ASSAULT BY OTHER SOLID AND LIQUID SUBSTANCES **(Continued)**	**T63.ØØ3A**	Toxic effect of unsp snake venom, assault, init encntr
		T63.Ø13A	Toxic effect of rattlesnake venom, assault, init encntr
		T63.Ø23A	Toxic effect of coral snake venom, assault, init encntr
		T63.Ø33A	Toxic effect of taipan venom, assault, initial encounter
		T63.Ø43A	Toxic effect of cobra venom, assault, initial encounter
		T63.Ø63A	Toxic effect of venom of N & S American snake, assault, init
		T63.Ø73A	Toxic effect of venom of oth Australian snake, assault, init
		T63.Ø83A	Toxic eff of venom of African and Asian snake, asslt, init
		T63.Ø93A	Toxic effect of venom of other snake, assault, init encntr
		T63.113A	Toxic effect of venom of gila monster, assault, init encntr
		T63.123A	Toxic effect of venom of oth venomous lizard, assault, init
		T63.193A	Toxic effect of venom of oth reptiles, assault, init encntr
		T63.2X3A	Toxic effect of venom of scorpion, assault, init encntr
		T63.3Ø3A	Toxic effect of unsp spider venom, assault, init encntr
		T63.313A	Toxic effect of venom of black widow spider, assault, init
		T63.323A	Toxic effect of venom of tarantula, assault, init encntr
		T63.333A	Toxic effect of venom of brown recluse spider, assault, init
		T63.393A	Toxic effect of venom of other spider, assault, init encntr
		T63.413A	Toxic effect of venom of centipede/millipede, assault, init
		T63.423A	Toxic effect of venom of ants, assault, initial encounter
		T63.433A	Toxic effect of venom of caterpillars, assault, init encntr
		T63.443A	Toxic effect of venom of bees, assault, initial encounter
		T63.453A	Toxic effect of venom of hornets, assault, initial encounter
		T63.463A	Toxic effect of venom of wasps, assault, initial encounter
		T63.483A	Toxic effect of venom of oth arthropod, assault, init encntr
		T63.513A	Toxic effect of contact with stingray, assault, init encntr
		T63.593A	Toxic effect of contact w oth venomous fish, assault, init
		T63.613A	Toxic effect of contact w Portugese Man-o-war, assault, init
		T63.623A	Toxic effect of contact w oth jellyfish, assault, init
		T63.633A	Toxic effect of contact w sea anemone, assault, init encntr
		T63.693A	Toxic eff of cntct w oth venom marine animals, asslt, init
		T63.713A	Toxic effect of contact w venom marine plant, assault, init
		T63.793A	Toxic effect of contact w oth venomous plant, assault, init
		T63.813A	Toxic effect of contact w venomous frog, assault, init
		T63.823A	Toxic effect of contact w venomous toad, assault, init
		T63.833A	Toxic effect of contact w oth venomous amphib, assault, init
		T63.893A	Toxic effect of contact w oth venom animals, assault, init
		T63.93XA	Toxic effect of contact w unsp venom animal, assault, init
		T64.Ø3XA	Toxic effect of aflatoxin, assault, initial encounter
		T64.83XA	Toxic effect of mycotoxin food contaminants, assault, init
		T65.ØX3A	Toxic effect of cyanides, assault, initial encounter
		T65.1X3A	Toxic effect of strychnine and its salts, assault, init
		T65.213A	Toxic effect of chewing tobacco, assault, initial encounter
		T65.223A	Toxic effect of tobacco cigarettes, assault, init encntr
		T65.293A	Toxic effect of oth tobacco and nicotine, assault, init
		T65.3X3A	Toxic eff of nitrodrv/aminodrv of benzn/homolog, asslt, init
		T65.4X3A	Toxic effect of carbon disulfide, assault, initial encounter
		T65.5X3A	Tox eff of nitro & oth nitric acids and esters, asslt, init
		T65.6X3A	Toxic effect of paints and dyes, NEC, assault, init
		T65.813A	Toxic effect of latex, assault, initial encounter
		T65.823A	Toxic effect of harmful algae and algae toxins, asslt, init
		T65.833A	Toxic effect of fiberglass, assault, initial encounter
		T65.893A	Toxic effect of oth substances, assault, init encntr
E962.2	ASSAULT BY OTHER GASES AND VAPORS	**T53.ØX3A**	Toxic effect of carbon tetrachloride, assault, init encntr
		T53.1X3A	Toxic effect of chloroform, assault, initial encounter
		T53.2X3A	Toxic effect of trichloroethylene, assault, init encntr
		T53.3X3A	Toxic effect of tetrachloroethylene, assault, init encntr
		T53.4X3A	Toxic effect of dichloromethane, assault, initial encounter
		T53.5X3A	Toxic effect of chlorofluorocarbons, assault, init encntr
		T53.6X3A	Toxic eff of halgn deriv of aliphatic hydrocrb, asslt, init
		T53.7X3A	Toxic eff of halgn deriv of aromatic hydrocrb, asslt, init
		T53.93XA	Tox eff of unsp halgn deriv of aromat hydrocrb, asslt, init
		T58.Ø3XA	Toxic effect of carb monx from mtr veh exhaust, asslt, init
		T58.13XA	Toxic effect of carb monx from utility gas, assault, init
		T58.2X3A	Tox eff of carb monx fr incmpl combst dmst fuel, asslt, init
		T58.8X3A	Toxic effect of carb monx from oth source, assault, init
		T58.93XA	Toxic effect of carb monx from unsp source, assault, init
		T59.ØX3A	Toxic effect of nitrogen oxides, assault, initial encounter
		T59.1X3A	Toxic effect of sulfur dioxide, assault, initial encounter
		T59.2X3A	Toxic effect of formaldehyde, assault, initial encounter
		T59.3X3A	Toxic effect of lacrimogenic gas, assault, initial encounter
		T59.4X3A	Toxic effect of chlorine gas, assault, initial encounter
		T59.5X3A	Toxic eff of fluorine gas and hydrogen fluoride, asslt, init
		T59.6X3A	Toxic effect of hydrogen sulfide, assault, initial encounter
		T59.7X3A	Toxic effect of carbon dioxide, assault, initial encounter
		T59.813A	Toxic effect of smoke, assault, initial encounter
		T59.893A	Toxic effect of oth gases, fumes and vapors, assault, init
		T59.93XA	Toxic effect of unsp gases, fumes and vapors, assault, init

ICD-9-CM		ICD-10-CM	
E962.9	ASSAULT BY UNSPECIFIED POISONING	**T57.93XA**	Toxic effect of unsp inorganic substance, assault, init
		T65.93XA	Toxic effect of unspecified substance, assault, init encntr
E963	ASSAULT BY HANGING AND STRANGULATION	**T71.113A**	Asphyxiation due to smothering under pillow, assault, init
		T71.123A	Asphyxiation due to plastic bag, assault, initial encounter
		T71.133A	Asphyx due to being trapped in bed linens, assault, init
		T71.143A	Asphyx d/t smothr under another person's body, asslt, init
		T71.153A	Asphyxiation due to smothering in furniture, assault, init
		T71.163A	Asphyxiation due to hanging, assault, initial encounter
		T71.193A	Asphyx d/t mech threat to breathe d/t oth cause, asslt, init
		T71.223A	Asphyx due to being trapped in a car trunk, assault, init
		T71.233A	Asphyx d/t being trap in a (discarded) refrig, asslt, init
E964	ASSAULT BY SUBMERSION	**X92.ØXXA**	Assault by drowning and submersion while in bathtub, init
		X92.ØXXD	Assault by drowning and submersion while in bathtub, subs
		X92.1XXA	Assault by drown while in swimming pool, init
		X92.1XXD	Assault by drown while in swimming pool, subs
		X92.2XXA	Assault by drown after push into swimming pool, init
		X92.2XXD	Assault by drown after push into swimming pool, subs
		X92.3XXA	Assault by drowning and submersion in natural water, init
		X92.3XXD	Assault by drowning and submersion in natural water, subs
		X92.8XXA	Other assault by drowning and submersion, initial encounter
		X92.8XXD	Other assault by drowning and submersion, subs encntr
		X92.9XXA	Assault by drowning and submersion, unspecified, init encntr
		X92.9XXD	Assault by drowning and submersion, unspecified, subs encntr
E965.Ø	ASSAULT BY HANDGUN	**X93.XXXA**	Assault by handgun discharge, initial encounter
		X93.XXXD	Assault by handgun discharge, subsequent encounter
E965.1	ASSAULT BY SHOTGUN	**X94.ØXXA**	Assault by shotgun, initial encounter
		X94.ØXXD	Assault by shotgun, subsequent encounter
E965.2	ASSAULT BY HUNTING RIFLE	**X94.1XXA**	Assault by hunting rifle, initial encounter
		X94.1XXD	Assault by hunting rifle, subsequent encounter
E965.3	ASSAULT BY MILITARY FIREARMS	**X94.2XXA**	Assault by machine gun, initial encounter
		X94.2XXD	Assault by machine gun, subsequent encounter
E965.4	ASSAULT BY OTHER AND UNSPECIFIED FIREARM	**X94.8XXA**	Assault by other larger firearm discharge, initial encounter
		X94.8XXD	Assault by other larger firearm discharge, subs encntr
		X94.9XXA	Assault by unspecified larger firearm discharge, init encntr
		X94.9XXD	Assault by unspecified larger firearm discharge, subs encntr
		X95.Ø2XA	Assault by paintball gun discharge, initial encounter
		X95.Ø2XD	Assault by paintball gun discharge, subsequent encounter
		X95.Ø9XA	Assault by oth gas, air or spring-operated gun, init encntr
		X95.Ø9XD	Assault by oth gas, air or spring-operated gun, subs encntr
		X95.8XXA	Assault by other firearm discharge, initial encounter
		X95.8XXD	Assault by other firearm discharge, subsequent encounter
		X95.9XXA	Assault by unspecified firearm discharge, initial encounter
		X95.9XXD	Assault by unspecified firearm discharge, subs encntr
E965.5	ASSAULT BY ANTIPERSONNEL BOMB	**X96.ØXXA**	Assault by antipersonnel bomb, initial encounter
		X96.ØXXD	Assault by antipersonnel bomb, subsequent encounter
E965.6	ASSAULT BY GASOLINE BOMB	**X96.1XXA**	Assault by gasoline bomb, initial encounter
		X96.1XXD	Assault by gasoline bomb, subsequent encounter
E965.7	ASSAULT BY LETTER BOMB	**X96.2XXA**	Assault by letter bomb, initial encounter
		X96.2XXD	Assault by letter bomb, subsequent encounter
E965.8	ASSAULT BY OTHER SPECIFIED EXPLOSIVE	**X96.3XXA**	Assault by fertilizer bomb, initial encounter
		X96.3XXD	Assault by fertilizer bomb, subsequent encounter
		X96.4XXA	Assault by pipe bomb, initial encounter
		X96.4XXD	Assault by pipe bomb, subsequent encounter
		X96.8XXA	Assault by other specified explosive, initial encounter
		X96.8XXD	Assault by other specified explosive, subsequent encounter
E965.9	ASSAULT BY UNSPECIFIED EXPLOSIVE	**X96.9XXA**	Assault by unspecified explosive, initial encounter
		X96.9XXD	Assault by unspecified explosive, subsequent encounter
E966	ASSAULT BY CUTTING AND PIERCING INSTRUMENT	**X99.ØXXA**	Assault by sharp glass, initial encounter
		X99.ØXXD	Assault by sharp glass, subsequent encounter
		X99.1XXA	Assault by knife, initial encounter
		X99.1XXD	Assault by knife, subsequent encounter
		X99.2XXA	Assault by sword or dagger, initial encounter
		X99.2XXD	Assault by sword or dagger, subsequent encounter
		X99.8XXA	Assault by other sharp object, initial encounter
		X99.8XXD	Assault by other sharp object, subsequent encounter
		X99.9XXA	Assault by unspecified sharp object, initial encounter
		X99.9XXD	Assault by unspecified sharp object, subsequent encounter
E967.Ø	CHILD&ADLT BATTERING&OTH MALTX FATHER/STEPFATHER	**YØ7.11**	Biological father, perpetrator of maltreatment and neglect
		YØ7.13	Adoptive father, perpetrator of maltreatment and neglect
		YØ7.43Ø	Stepfather, perpetrator of maltreatment and neglect
		YØ7.432	Male friend of parent, perpetrator of maltreat and neglect
E967.1	CHILD&ADULT BATTERING&OTH MALTX OTH SPEC PERSON	**YØ7.499**	Other family member, perpetrator of maltreatment and neglect
E967.2	CHILD&ADULT BATTERING&OTH MALTX MOTH/STEPMOTH	**YØ7.12**	Biological mother, perpetrator of maltreatment and neglect
		YØ7.14	Adoptive mother, perpetrator of maltreatment and neglect
		YØ7.433	Stepmother, perpetrator of maltreatment and neglect
		YØ7.434	Female friend of parent, perp of maltreat and neglect

ICD-9-CM		ICD-10-CM	
E967.3	CHILD&ADULT BATTERING&OTH MALTX SPOUSE/PARTNER	**Y07.01**	Husband, perpetrator of maltreatment and neglect
		Y07.02	Wife, perpetrator of maltreatment and neglect
		Y07.03	Male partner, perpetrator of maltreatment and neglect
		Y07.04	Female partner, perpetrator of maltreatment and neglect
E967.4	CHILD&ADULT BATTERING&OTHER MALTREATMENT CHILD	**Y07.50**	Unsp non-family member, perpetrator of maltreat and neglect
E967.5	CHILD&ADULT BATTERING&OTHER MALTREATMENT SIBLING	**Y07.410**	Brother, perpetrator of maltreatment and neglect
		Y07.411	Sister, perpetrator of maltreatment and neglect
		Y07.435	Stepbrother, perpetrator or maltreatment and neglect
		Y07.436	Stepsister, perpetrator of maltreatment and neglect
E967.6	CHILD&ADULT BATTERING&OTH MALTX GRANDPARENT	**Y07.499**	Other family member, perpetrator of maltreatment and neglect
E967.7	CHILD&ADULT BATTERING&OTH MALTX OTH RELATIVE	**Y07.490**	Male cousin, perpetrator of maltreatment and neglect
		Y07.491	Female cousin, perpetrator of maltreatment and neglect
		Y07.499	Other family member, perpetrator of maltreatment and neglect
E967.8	CHLD&ADLT BATTER&OTH MALTX NON-RELATED CAREGIVER	**Y07.420**	Foster father, perpetrator of maltreatment and neglect
		Y07.421	Foster mother, perpetrator of maltreatment and neglect
		Y07.50	Unsp non-family member, perpetrator of maltreat and neglect
		Y07.510	At-home childcare provider, perp of maltreat and neglect
		Y07.511	Daycare center childcare prov, perp of maltreat and neglect
		Y07.512	At-home adultcare provider, perp of maltreat and neglect
		Y07.513	Adultcare center provider, perp of maltreat and neglect
		Y07.519	Unsp daycare provider, perpetrator of maltreat and neglect
		Y07.521	Mental health provider, perpetrator of maltreat and neglect
		Y07.528	Oth therapist or healthcare prov, perp of maltreat & neglect
		Y07.529	Unsp healthcare provider, perp of maltreat and neglect
		Y07.53	Teacher or instructor, perpetrator of maltreat and neglect
		Y07.59	Oth non-family member, perpetrator of maltreat and neglect
E967.9	CHILD&ADULT BATTERING&OTH MALTX UNSPEC PERSON	**Y07.9**	Unspecified perpetrator of maltreatment and neglect
E968.0	ASSAULT BY FIRE	**X97.XXXA**	Assault by smoke, fire and flames, initial encounter
		X97.XXXD	Assault by smoke, fire and flames, subsequent encounter
E968.1	ASSAULT BY PUSHING FROM HIGH PLACE	**Y01.XXXA**	Assault by pushing from high place, initial encounter
		Y01.XXXD	Assault by pushing from high place, subsequent encounter
E968.2	ASSAULT BY STRIKING BY BLUNT OR THROWN OBJECT	**Y00.XXXA**	Assault by blunt object, initial encounter
		Y00.XXXD	Assault by blunt object, subsequent encounter
		Y08.01XA	Assault by strike by hockey stick, initial encounter
		Y08.01XD	Assault by strike by hockey stick, subsequent encounter
		Y08.02XA	Assault by strike by baseball bat, initial encounter
		Y08.02XD	Assault by strike by baseball bat, subsequent encounter
		Y08.09XA	Assault by strike by oth type of sport equipment, init
		Y08.09XD	Assault by strike by oth type of sport equipment, subs
E968.3	ASSAULT BY HOT LIQUID	**X98.1XXA**	Assault by hot tap water, initial encounter
		X98.1XXD	Assault by hot tap water, subsequent encounter
		X98.2XXA	Assault by hot fluids, initial encounter
		X98.2XXD	Assault by hot fluids, subsequent encounter
E968.4	CRIMINAL NEGLECT	**Y07.01**	Husband, perpetrator of maltreatment and neglect
		Y07.02	Wife, perpetrator of maltreatment and neglect
		Y07.03	Male partner, perpetrator of maltreatment and neglect
		Y07.04	Female partner, perpetrator of maltreatment and neglect
		Y07.11	Biological father, perpetrator of maltreatment and neglect
		Y07.12	Biological mother, perpetrator of maltreatment and neglect
		Y07.13	Adoptive father, perpetrator of maltreatment and neglect
		Y07.14	Adoptive mother, perpetrator of maltreatment and neglect
		Y07.410	Brother, perpetrator of maltreatment and neglect
		Y07.411	Sister, perpetrator of maltreatment and neglect
		Y07.420	Foster father, perpetrator of maltreatment and neglect
		Y07.421	Foster mother, perpetrator of maltreatment and neglect
		Y07.430	Stepfather, perpetrator of maltreatment and neglect
		Y07.432	Male friend of parent, perpetrator of maltreat and neglect
		Y07.433	Stepmother, perpetrator of maltreatment and neglect
		Y07.434	Female friend of parent, perp of maltreat and neglect
		Y07.435	Stepbrother, perpetrator or maltreatment and neglect
		Y07.436	Stepsister, perpetrator of maltreatment and neglect
		Y07.490	Male cousin, perpetrator of maltreatment and neglect
		Y07.491	Female cousin, perpetrator of maltreatment and neglect
		Y07.499	Other family member, perpetrator of maltreatment and neglect
		Y07.50	Unsp non-family member, perpetrator of maltreat and neglect
		Y07.510	At-home childcare provider, perp of maltreat and neglect
		Y07.511	Daycare center childcare prov, perp of maltreat and neglect
		Y07.512	At-home adultcare provider, perp of maltreat and neglect
		Y07.513	Adultcare center provider, perp of maltreat and neglect
		Y07.519	Unsp daycare provider, perpetrator of maltreat and neglect
		Y07.521	Mental health provider, perpetrator of maltreat and neglect
		Y07.528	Oth therapist or healthcare prov, perp of maltreat & neglect
		Y07.529	Unsp healthcare provider, perp of maltreat and neglect
		Y07.53	Teacher or instructor, perpetrator of maltreat and neglect
		Y07.59	Oth non-family member, perpetrator of maltreat and neglect

ICD-9-CM		ICD-10-CM	
E968.5	ASSAULT BY TRANSPORT VEHICLE	**YØ2.ØXXA**	Assault by push/place victim in front of motor vehicle, init
		YØ2.ØXXD	Assault by push/place victim in front of motor vehicle, subs
		YØ2.1XXA	Assault by push/place victim in front of train, init
		YØ2.1XXD	Assault by push/place victim in front of train, subs
		YØ2.8XXA	Assault by push/place victim in front of moving object, init
		YØ2.8XXD	Assault by push/place victim in front of moving object, subs
		YØ3.ØXXA	Assault by being hit or run over by motor vehicle, init
		YØ3.ØXXD	Assault by being hit or run over by motor vehicle, subs
		YØ3.8XXA	Other assault by crashing of motor vehicle, init encntr
		YØ3.8XXD	Other assault by crashing of motor vehicle, subs encntr
		YØ8.81XA	Assault by crashing of aircraft, initial encounter
		YØ8.81XD	Assault by crashing of aircraft, subsequent encounter
E968.6	ASSAULT BY AIR GUN	**X95.Ø1XA**	Assault by airgun discharge, initial encounter
		X95.Ø1XD	Assault by airgun discharge, subsequent encounter
E968.7	ASSAULT BY HUMAN BITE	**YØ4.1XXA**	Assault by human bite, initial encounter
		YØ4.1XXD	Assault by human bite, subsequent encounter
E968.8	ASSAULT BY OTHER SPECIFIED MEANS	**X98.ØXXA**	Assault by steam or hot vapors, initial encounter
		X98.ØXXD	Assault by steam or hot vapors, subsequent encounter
		X98.3XXA	Assault by hot household appliances, initial encounter
		X98.3XXD	Assault by hot household appliances, subsequent encounter
		X98.8XXA	Assault by other hot objects, initial encounter
		X98.8XXD	Assault by other hot objects, subsequent encounter
		X98.9XXA	Assault by unspecified hot objects, initial encounter
		X98.9XXD	Assault by unspecified hot objects, subsequent encounter
		YØ8.89XA	Assault by other specified means, initial encounter
		YØ8.89XD	Assault by other specified means, subsequent encounter
E968.9	ASSAULT BY UNSPECIFIED MEANS	➡ **YØ9**	Assault by unspecified means
E969	LATE EFF INJURY PURPOSELY INFLICTED OTH PERSON	**T36.ØX3S**	Poisoning by penicillins, assault, sequela
		T36.1X3S	Poisn by cephalospor/oth beta-lactm antibiot, asslt, sequela
		T36.2X3S	Poisoning by chloramphenicol group, assault, sequela
		T36.3X3S	Poisoning by macrolides, assault, sequela
		T36.4X3S	Poisoning by tetracyclines, assault, sequela
		T36.5X3S	Poisoning by aminoglycosides, assault, sequela
		T36.6X3S	Poisoning by rifampicins, assault, sequela
		T36.7X3S	Poisoning by antifungal antibiot, sys used, assault, sequela
		T36.8X3S	Poisoning by other systemic antibiotics, assault, sequela
		T36.93XS	Poisoning by unsp systemic antibiotic, assault, sequela
		T37.ØX3S	Poisoning by sulfonamides, assault, sequela
		T37.1X3S	Poisoning by antimycobacterial drugs, assault, sequela
		T37.2X3S	Poisn by antimalari/drugs acting on bld protzoa, asslt, sqla
		T37.3X3S	Poisoning by other antiprotozoal drugs, assault, sequela
		T37.4X3S	Poisoning by anthelminthics, assault, sequela
		T37.5X3S	Poisoning by antiviral drugs, assault, sequela
		T37.8X3S	Poisn by oth systemic anti-infect/parasit, assault, sequela
		T37.93XS	Poisn by unsp sys anti-infect and antiparastc, asslt, sqla
		T38.ØX3S	Poisoning by glucocort/synth analog, assault, sequela
		T38.1X3S	Poisoning by thyroid hormones and sub, assault, sequela
		T38.2X3S	Poisoning by antithyroid drugs, assault, sequela
		T38.3X3S	Poisn by insulin and oral hypoglycemic drugs, asslt, sequela
		T38.4X3S	Poisoning by oral contraceptives, assault, sequela
		T38.5X3S	Poisoning by oth estrogens and progstrn, assault, sequela
		T38.6X3S	Poisn by antigonadtr/antiestr/antiandrg, NEC, asslt, sequela
		T38.7X3S	Poisn by androgens and anabolic congeners, assault, sequela
		T38.8Ø3S	Poisn by unsp hormones and synthetic sub, assault, sequela
		T38.813S	Poisoning by anterior pituitary hormones, assault, sequela
		T38.893S	Poisn by oth hormones and synthetic sub, assault, sequela
		T38.9Ø3S	Poisoning by unsp hormone antagonists, assault, sequela
		T38.993S	Poisoning by other hormone antagonists, assault, sequela
		T39.Ø13S	Poisoning by aspirin, assault, sequela
		T39.Ø93S	Poisoning by salicylates, assault, sequela
		T39.1X3S	Poisoning by 4-Aminophenol derivatives, assault, sequela
		T39.2X3S	Poisoning by pyrazolone derivatives, assault, sequela
		T39.313S	Poisoning by propionic acid derivatives, assault, sequela
		T39.393S	Poisn by oth nonsteroid anti-inflam drugs, assault, sequela
		T39.4X3S	Poisoning by antirheumatics, NEC, assault, sequela
		T39.8X3S	Poisn by oth nonopio analges/antipyret, NEC, asslt, sequela
		T39.93XS	Poisn by unsp nonopi analgs/antipyr/antirheu, asslt, sequela
		T4Ø.ØX3S	Poisoning by opium, assault, sequela
		T4Ø.1X3S	Poisoning by heroin, assault, sequela
		T4Ø.2X3S	Poisoning by other opioids, assault, sequela
		T4Ø.3X3S	Poisoning by methadone, assault, sequela
		T4Ø.4X3S	Poisoning by other synthetic narcotics, assault, sequela
		T4Ø.5X3S	Poisoning by cocaine, assault, sequela
		T4Ø.6Ø3S	Poisoning by unspecified narcotics, assault, sequela
		T4Ø.693S	Poisoning by other narcotics, assault, sequela
		T4Ø.7X3S	Poisoning by cannabis (derivatives), assault, sequela
		T4Ø.8X3S	Poisoning by lysergide [LSD], assault, sequela
		T4Ø.9Ø3S	Poisoning by unspecified psychodysleptics, assault, sequela
	(Continued on next page)	**T4Ø.993S**	Poisoning by other psychodysleptics, assault, sequela

ICD-9-CM		ICD-10-CM	
E969	LATE EFF INJURY PURPOSELY INFLICTED OTH PERSON **(Continued)**	**T41.ØX3S**	Poisoning by inhaled anesthetics, assault, sequela
		T41.1X3S	Poisoning by intravenous anesthetics, assault, sequela
		T41.2Ø3S	Poisoning by unsp general anesthetics, assault, sequela
		T41.293S	Poisoning by other general anesthetics, assault, sequela
		T41.3X3S	Poisoning by local anesthetics, assault, sequela
		T41.43XS	Poisoning by unspecified anesthetic, assault, sequela
		T41.5X3S	Poisoning by therapeutic gases, assault, sequela
		T42.ØX3S	Poisoning by hydantoin derivatives, assault, sequela
		T42.1X3S	Poisoning by iminostilbenes, assault, sequela
		T42.2X3S	Poisn by succinimides and oxazolidinediones, asslt, sequela
		T42.3X3S	Poisoning by barbiturates, assault, sequela
		T42.4X3S	Poisoning by benzodiazepines, assault, sequela
		T42.5X3S	Poisoning by mixed antiepileptics, assault, sequela
		T42.6X3S	Poisn by oth antieplptc and sed-hypntc drugs, asslt, sequela
		T42.73XS	Poisn by unsp antieplptc and sed-hypntc drugs, asslt, sqla
		T42.8X3S	Poisn by antiparkns drug/centr musc-tone depr, asslt, sqla
		T43.Ø13S	Poisoning by tricyclic antidepressants, assault, sequela
		T43.Ø23S	Poisoning by tetracyclic antidepressants, assault, sequela
		T43.1X3S	Poisoning by MAO inhib antidepressants, assault, sequela
		T43.2Ø3S	Poisoning by unspecified antidepressants, assault, sequela
		T43.213S	Poisn by slctv seroton/norepineph reup inhibtr, asslt, sqla
		T43.223S	Poisn by slctv serotonin reuptake inhibtr, assault, sequela
		T43.293S	Poisoning by other antidepressants, assault, sequela
		T43.3X3S	Poisn by phenothiaz antipsychot/neurolept, assault, sequela
		T43.4X3S	Poisn by butyrophen/thiothixen neuroleptc, assault, sequela
		T43.5Ø3S	Poisoning by unsp antipsychot/neurolept, assault, sequela
		T43.593S	Poisoning by oth antipsychot/neurolept, assault, sequela
		T43.6Ø3S	Poisoning by unspecified psychostimulants, assault, sequela
		T43.613S	Poisoning by caffeine, assault, sequela
		T43.623S	Poisoning by amphetamines, assault, sequela
		T43.633S	Poisoning by methylphenidate, assault, sequela
		T43.693S	Poisoning by other psychostimulants, assault, sequela
		T43.8X3S	Poisoning by other psychotropic drugs, assault, sequela
		T43.93XS	Poisoning by unspecified psychotropic drug, assault, sequela
		T44.ØX3S	Poisoning by anticholinesterase agents, assault, sequela
		T44.1X3S	Poisoning by other parasympathomimetics, assault, sequela
		T44.2X3S	Poisoning by ganglionic blocking drugs, assault, sequela
		T44.3X3S	Poisn by oth parasympath and spasmolytics, assault, sequela
		T44.4X3S	Poisn by predom alpha-adrenocpt agonists, assault, sequela
		T44.5X3S	Poisn by predom beta-adrenocpt agonists, assault, sequela
		T44.6X3S	Poisoning by alpha-adrenocpt antagonists, assault, sequela
		T44.7X3S	Poisoning by beta-adrenocpt antagonists, assault, sequela
		T44.8X3S	Poisn by centr-acting/adren-neurn-block agnt, asslt, sequela
		T44.9Ø3S	Poisn by unsp drugs aff the autonm nrv sys, asslt, sequela
		T44.993S	Poisn by oth drug aff the autonm nervous sys, asslt, sequela
		T45.ØX3S	Poisoning by antiallerg/antiemetic, assault, sequela
		T45.1X3S	Poisoning by antineopl and immunosup drugs, assault, sequela
		T45.2X3S	Poisoning by vitamins, assault, sequela
		T45.3X3S	Poisoning by enzymes, assault, sequela
		T45.4X3S	Poisoning by iron and its compounds, assault, sequela
		T45.513S	Poisoning by anticoagulants, assault, sequela
		T45.523S	Poisoning by antithrombotic drugs, assault, sequela
		T45.6Ø3S	Poisoning by unsp fibrin-affct drugs, assault, sequela
		T45.613S	Poisoning by thrombolytic drug, assault, sequela
		T45.623S	Poisoning by hemostatic drug, assault, sequela
		T45.693S	Poisoning by oth fibrin-affct drugs, assault, sequela
		T45.7X3S	Poisn by anticoag antag, vit K and oth coag, asslt, sequela
		T45.8X3S	Poisn by oth prim sys and hematolog agents, assault, sequela
		T45.93XS	Poisn by unsp prim sys and hematolog agent, assault, sequela
		T46.ØX3S	Poisn by cardi-stim glycos/drug simlar act, assault, sequela
		T46.1X3S	Poisoning by calcium-channel blockers, assault, sequela
		T46.2X3S	Poisoning by other antidysrhythmic drugs, assault, sequela
		T46.3X3S	Poisoning by coronary vasodilators, assault, sequela
		T46.4X3S	Poisn by angiotens-convert-enzyme inhibtr, assault, sequela
		T46.5X3S	Poisoning by other antihypertensive drugs, assault, sequela
		T46.6X3S	Poisn by antihyperlip and antiarterio drugs, asslt, sequela
		T46.7X3S	Poisoning by peripheral vasodilators, assault, sequela
		T46.8X3S	Poisn by antivaric drugs, inc scler agents, assault, sequela
		T46.9Ø3S	Poisn by unsp agents aff the cardiovasc sys, asslt, sequela
		T46.993S	Poisn by oth agents aff the cardiovasc sys, assault, sequela
		T47.ØX3S	Poisn by histamine H2-receptor blockers, assault, sequela
		T47.1X3S	Poisn by oth antacids and anti-gstrc-sec drugs, asslt, sqla
		T47.2X3S	Poisoning by stimulant laxatives, assault, sequela
		T47.3X3S	Poisoning by saline and osmotic laxatives, assault, sequela
		T47.4X3S	Poisoning by other laxatives, assault, sequela
		T47.5X3S	Poisoning by digestants, assault, sequela
		T47.6X3S	Poisoning by antidiarrheal drugs, assault, sequela
		T47.7X3S	Poisoning by emetics, assault, sequela
	(Continued on next page)	**T47.8X3S**	Poisoning by oth agents aff GI sys, assault, sequela

ICD-9-CM		ICD-10-CM	
E969	LATE EFF INJURY PURPOSELY INFLICTED OTH PERSON **(Continued)**	**T47.93XS**	Poisoning by unsp agents aff the GI sys, assault, sequela
		T48.ØX3S	Poisoning by oxytocic drugs, assault, sequela
		T48.1X3S	Poisoning by skeletal muscle relaxants, assault, sequela
		T48.2Ø3S	Poisoning by unsp drugs acting on muscles, assault, sequela
		T48.293S	Poisoning by other drugs acting on muscles, assault, sequela
		T48.3X3S	Poisoning by antitussives, assault, sequela
		T48.4X3S	Poisoning by expectorants, assault, sequela
		T48.5X3S	Poisoning by other anti-common-cold drugs, assault, sequela
		T48.6X3S	Poisoning by antiasthmatics, assault, sequela
		T48.9Ø3S	Poisn by unsp agents prim act on the resp sys, asslt, sqla
		T48.993S	Poisn by oth agents prim acting on the resp sys, asslt, sqla
		T49.ØX3S	Poisn by local antifung/infect/inflamm drugs, asslt, sequela
		T49.1X3S	Poisoning by antipruritics, assault, sequela
		T49.2X3S	Poisoning by local astringents/detergents, assault, sequela
		T49.3X3S	Poisn by emollients, demulcents and protect, asslt, sequela
		T49.4X3S	Poisn by keratolyt/keratplst/hair trmt drug, asslt, sequela
		T49.5X3S	Poisoning by opth drugs and preparations, assault, sequela
		T49.6X3S	Poisoning by otorhino drugs and prep, assault, sequela
		T49.7X3S	Poisn by dental drugs, topically applied, assault, sequela
		T49.8X3S	Poisoning by other topical agents, assault, sequela
		T49.93XS	Poisoning by unspecified topical agent, assault, sequela
		T5Ø.ØX3S	Poisoning by mineralocorticoids and antag, assault, sequela
		T5Ø.1X3S	Poisoning by loop [high-ceiling] diuretics, assault, sequela
		T5Ø.2X3S	Poisn by crbnc-anhydr inhibtr,benzo/oth diuretc, asslt, sqla
		T5Ø.3X3S	Poisn by electrolytic/caloric/wtr-bal agnt, assault, sequela
		T5Ø.4X3S	Poisoning by drugs aff uric acid metab, assault, sequela
		T5Ø.5X3S	Poisoning by appetite depressants, assault, sequela
		T5Ø.6X3S	Poisn by antidotes and chelating agents, assault, sequela
		T5Ø.7X3S	Poisn by analeptics and opioid receptor antag, asslt, sqla
		T5Ø.8X3S	Poisoning by diagnostic agents, assault, sequela
		T5Ø.9Ø3S	Poisoning by unsp drug/meds/biol subst, assault, sequela
		T5Ø.993S	Poisoning by oth drug/meds/biol subst, assault, sequela
		T5Ø.A13S	Poisn by pertuss vaccine, inc combin w pertuss, asslt, sqla
		T5Ø.A23S	Poisn by mixed bact vaccines w/o a pertuss, assault, sequela
		T5Ø.A93S	Poisoning by other bacterial vaccines, assault, sequela
		T5Ø.B13S	Poisoning by smallpox vaccines, assault, sequela
		T5Ø.B93S	Poisoning by other viral vaccines, assault, sequela
		T5Ø.Z13S	Poisoning by immunoglobulin, assault, sequela
		T5Ø.Z93S	Poisn by oth vaccines and biolg substnc, assault, sequela
		T6Ø.ØX3S	Toxic effect of organophos and carbamate insect, asslt, sqla
		T6Ø.1X3S	Toxic effect of halogenated insecticides, assault, sequela
		T6Ø.2X3S	Toxic effect of other insecticides, assault, sequela
		T6Ø.3X3S	Toxic effect of herbicides and fungicides, assault, sequela
		T6Ø.4X3S	Toxic effect of rodenticides, assault, sequela
		T6Ø.8X3S	Toxic effect of other pesticides, assault, sequela
		T6Ø.93XS	Toxic effect of unspecified pesticide, assault, sequela
		T61.Ø3XS	Ciguatera fish poisoning, assault, sequela
		T61.13XS	Scombroid fish poisoning, assault, sequela
		T61.773S	Other fish poisoning, assault, sequela
		T61.783S	Other shellfish poisoning, assault, sequela
		T61.8X3S	Toxic effect of other seafood, assault, sequela
		T61.93XS	Toxic effect of unspecified seafood, assault, sequela
		T62.ØX3S	Toxic effect of ingested mushrooms, assault, sequela
		T62.1X3S	Toxic effect of ingested berries, assault, sequela
		T62.2X3S	Toxic effect of ingest (parts of) plant(s), assault, sequela
		T62.8X3S	Toxic effect of noxious substnc eaten as food, asslt, sqla
		T62.93XS	Toxic effect of unsp noxious sub eaten as food, asslt, sqla
		T63.ØØ4S	Toxic effect of unsp snake venom, undetermined, sequela
		T63.Ø13S	Toxic effect of rattlesnake venom, assault, sequela
		T63.Ø23S	Toxic effect of coral snake venom, assault, sequela
		T63.Ø33S	Toxic effect of taipan venom, assault, sequela
		T63.Ø43S	Toxic effect of cobra venom, assault, sequela
		T63.Ø63S	Toxic effect of venom of N & S American snake, asslt, sqla
		T63.Ø73S	Toxic effect of venom of Australian snake, assault, sequela
		T63.Ø83S	Toxic eff of venom of African and Asian snake, asslt, sqla
		T63.Ø93S	Toxic effect of venom of other snake, assault, sequela
		T63.113S	Toxic effect of venom of gila monster, assault, sequela
		T63.123S	Toxic effect of venom of venomous lizard, assault, sequela
		T63.193S	Toxic effect of venom of other reptiles, assault, sequela
		T63.2X3S	Toxic effect of venom of scorpion, assault, sequela
		T63.3Ø3S	Toxic effect of unspecified spider venom, assault, sequela
		T63.313S	Toxic effect of venom of black widow spider, asslt, sequela
		T63.323S	Toxic effect of venom of tarantula, assault, sequela
		T63.333S	Toxic effect of venom of brown recluse spider, asslt, sqla
		T63.393S	Toxic effect of venom of other spider, assault, sequela
		T63.413S	Toxic effect of venom of centipede/millipede, asslt, sequela
		T63.423S	Toxic effect of venom of ants, assault, sequela
		T63.433S	Toxic effect of venom of caterpillars, assault, sequela
	(Continued on next page)	**T63.443S**	Toxic effect of venom of bees, assault, sequela

ICD-9-CM		ICD-10-CM	
E969	LATE EFF INJURY PURPOSELY INFLICTED OTH PERSON **(Continued)**	**T63.453S**	Toxic effect of venom of hornets, assault, sequela
		T63.463S	Toxic effect of venom of wasps, assault, sequela
		T63.483S	Toxic effect of venom of other arthropod, assault, sequela
		T63.513S	Toxic effect of contact with stingray, assault, sequela
		T63.593S	Toxic effect of contact w oth venom fish, assault, sequela
		T63.613S	Toxic effect of cntct w Portugese Man-o-war, asslt, sequela
		T63.623S	Toxic effect of contact with oth jellyfish, assault, sequela
		T63.633S	Toxic effect of contact with sea anemone, assault, sequela
		T63.693S	Toxic eff of cntct w oth venom marine animals, asslt, sqla
		T63.713S	Toxic effect of contact w venom marine plant, asslt, sequela
		T63.793S	Toxic effect of contact w oth venom plant, assault, sequela
		T63.813S	Toxic effect of contact with venomous frog, assault, sequela
		T63.823S	Toxic effect of contact with venomous toad, assault, sequela
		T63.833S	Toxic effect of contact w oth venom amphib, assault, sequela
		T63.893S	Toxic effect of contact w oth venom animals, asslt, sequela
		T63.93XS	Toxic effect of contact w unsp venom animal, asslt, sequela
		T64.03XS	Toxic effect of aflatoxin, assault, sequela
		T64.83XS	Toxic effect of mycotoxin food contamnt, assault, sequela
		T65.0X3S	Toxic effect of cyanides, assault, sequela
		T65.1X3S	Toxic effect of strychnine and its salts, assault, sequela
		T65.213S	Toxic effect of chewing tobacco, assault, sequela
		T65.223S	Toxic effect of tobacco cigarettes, assault, sequela
		T65.293S	Toxic effect of other tobacco and nicotine, assault, sequela
		T65.3X3S	Toxic eff of nitrodrv/aminodrv of benzn/homolog, asslt, sqla
		T65.4X3S	Toxic effect of carbon disulfide, assault, sequela
		T65.5X3S	Tox eff of nitro & oth nitric acids and esters, asslt, sqla
		T65.6X3S	Toxic effect of paints and dyes, NEC, assault, sequela
		T65.813S	Toxic effect of latex, assault, sequela
		T65.823S	Toxic effect of harmful algae and algae toxins, asslt, sqla
		T65.833S	Toxic effect of fiberglass, assault, sequela
		T65.893S	Toxic effect of other specified substances, assault, sequela
		T65.93XS	Toxic effect of unspecified substance, assault, sequela
		T71.163S	Asphyxiation due to hanging, assault, sequela
		X92.0XXS	Assault by drowning and submersion while in bathtub, sequela
		X92.1XXS	Assault by drown while in swimming pool, sequela
		X92.2XXS	Assault by drown after push into swimming pool, sequela
		X92.3XXS	Assault by drowning and submersion in natural water, sequela
		X92.8XXS	Other assault by drowning and submersion, sequela
		X92.9XXS	Assault by drowning and submersion, unspecified, sequela
		X93.XXXS	Assault by handgun discharge, sequela
		X94.0XXS	Assault by shotgun, sequela
		X94.1XXS	Assault by hunting rifle, sequela
		X94.2XXS	Assault by machine gun, sequela
		X94.8XXS	Assault by other larger firearm discharge, sequela
		X94.9XXS	Assault by unspecified larger firearm discharge, sequela
		X95.01XS	Assault by airgun discharge, sequela
		X95.02XS	Assault by paintball gun discharge, sequela
		X95.09XS	Assault by other gas, air or spring-operated gun, sequela
		X95.8XXS	Assault by other firearm discharge, sequela
		X95.9XXS	Assault by unspecified firearm discharge, sequela
		X96.0XXS	Assault by antipersonnel bomb, sequela
		X96.1XXS	Assault by gasoline bomb, sequela
		X96.2XXS	Assault by letter bomb, sequela
		X96.3XXS	Assault by fertilizer bomb, sequela
		X96.4XXS	Assault by pipe bomb, sequela
		X96.8XXS	Assault by other specified explosive, sequela
		X96.9XXS	Assault by unspecified explosive, sequela
		X97.XXXS	Assault by smoke, fire and flames, sequela
		X98.0XXS	Assault by steam or hot vapors, sequela
		X98.1XXS	Assault by hot tap water, sequela
		X98.2XXS	Assault by hot fluids, sequela
		X98.3XXS	Assault by hot household appliances, sequela
		X98.8XXS	Assault by other hot objects, sequela
		X98.9XXS	Assault by unspecified hot objects, sequela
		X99.0XXS	Assault by sharp glass, sequela
		X99.1XXS	Assault by knife, sequela
		X99.2XXS	Assault by sword or dagger, sequela
		X99.8XXS	Assault by other sharp object, sequela
		X99.9XXS	Assault by unspecified sharp object, sequela
		Y00.XXXS	Assault by blunt object, sequela
		Y01.XXXS	Assault by pushing from high place, sequela
		Y02.0XXS	Assault by push/place victim in front of mtr veh, sequela
		Y02.1XXS	Assault by push/place victim in front of train, sequela
		Y02.8XXS	Asslt by push/place victim in front of moving object, sqla
		Y03.0XXS	Assault by being hit or run over by motor vehicle, sequela
		Y03.8XXS	Other assault by crashing of motor vehicle, sequela
		Y04.0XXS	Assault by unarmed brawl or fight, sequela
		Y04.1XXS	Assault by human bite, sequela
		Y04.2XXS	Asslt by strike agnst or bumped into by another person, sqla
		Y04.8XXS	Assault by other bodily force, sequela

(Continued on next page)

[Brackets] indicate valid character values for each code. Character value meanings provided for each code grouping.

ICD-9-CM		ICD-10-CM	
E969	LATE EFF INJURY PURPOSELY INFLICTED OTH PERSON **(Continued)**	**Y08.01XS**	Assault by strike by hockey stick, sequela
		Y08.02XS	Assault by strike by baseball bat, sequela
		Y08.09XS	Assault by strike by oth type of sport equipment, sequela
		Y08.81XS	Assault by crashing of aircraft, sequela
		Y08.89XS	Assault by other specified means, sequela
E970	INJURY DUE TO LEGAL INTERVENTION BY FIREARMS	**Y35.001A**	Lgl intervnt w unsp firearm disch, law enforc offl inj, init
		Y35.001D	Lgl intervnt w unsp firearm disch, law enforc offl inj, subs
		Y35.002A	Legal intervnt w unsp firearm disch, bystand injured, init
		Y35.002D	Legal intervnt w unsp firearm disch, bystand injured, subs
		Y35.003A	Legal intervnt w unsp firearm disch, suspect injured, init
		Y35.003D	Legal intervnt w unsp firearm disch, suspect injured, subs
		Y35.011A	Legal intervnt w inj by mch gun, law enforc offl inj, init
		Y35.011D	Legal intervnt w inj by mch gun, law enforc offl inj, subs
		Y35.012A	Legal intervnt w injury by mch gun, bystand injured, init
		Y35.012D	Legal intervnt w injury by mch gun, bystand injured, subs
		Y35.013A	Legal intervnt w injury by mch gun, suspect injured, init
		Y35.013D	Legal intervnt w injury by mch gun, suspect injured, subs
		Y35.021A	Legal intervnt w inj by handgun, law enforc offl inj, init
		Y35.021D	Legal intervnt w inj by handgun, law enforc offl inj, subs
		Y35.022A	Legal intervnt w injury by handgun, bystand injured, init
		Y35.022D	Legal intervnt w injury by handgun, bystand injured, subs
		Y35.023A	Legal intervnt w injury by handgun, suspect injured, init
		Y35.023D	Legal intervnt w injury by handgun, suspect injured, subs
		Y35.031A	Lgl intervnt w inj by rifl pelet, law enforc offl inj, init
		Y35.031D	Lgl intervnt w inj by rifl pelet, law enforc offl inj, subs
		Y35.032A	Legal intervnt w injury by rifl pelet, bystand injured, init
		Y35.032D	Legal intervnt w injury by rifl pelet, bystand injured, subs
		Y35.033A	Legal intervnt w injury by rifl pelet, suspect injured, init
		Y35.033D	Legal intervnt w injury by rifl pelet, suspect injured, subs
		Y35.041A	Lgl intervnt w inj by rubr bulet, law enforc offl inj, init
		Y35.041D	Lgl intervnt w inj by rubr bulet, law enforc offl inj, subs
		Y35.042A	Legal intervnt w injury by rubr bulet, bystand injured, init
		Y35.042D	Legal intervnt w injury by rubr bulet, bystand injured, subs
		Y35.043A	Legal intervnt w injury by rubr bulet, suspect injured, init
		Y35.043D	Legal intervnt w injury by rubr bulet, suspect injured, subs
		Y35.091A	Legal intervnt w firearm disch, law enforc offl inj, init
		Y35.091D	Legal intervnt w firearm disch, law enforc offl inj, subs
		Y35.092A	Legal intervnt w firearm disch, bystand injured, init
		Y35.092D	Legal intervnt w firearm disch, bystand injured, subs
		Y35.093A	Legal intervnt w firearm disch, suspect injured, init
		Y35.093D	Legal intervnt w firearm disch, suspect injured, subs
E971	INJURY DUE TO LEGAL INTERVENTION BY EXPLOSIVES	**Y35.101A**	Legal intervnt w unsp explosv, law enforc offl injured, init
		Y35.101D	Legal intervnt w unsp explosv, law enforc offl injured, subs
		Y35.102A	Legal intervnt involving unsp explosv, bystand injured, init
		Y35.102D	Legal intervnt involving unsp explosv, bystand injured, subs
		Y35.103A	Legal intervnt involving unsp explosv, suspect injured, init
		Y35.103D	Legal intervnt involving unsp explosv, suspect injured, subs
		Y35.111A	Legal intervnt w inj by dynamite, law enforc offl inj, init
		Y35.111D	Legal intervnt w inj by dynamite, law enforc offl inj, subs
		Y35.112A	Legal intervnt w injury by dynamite, bystand injured, init
		Y35.112D	Legal intervnt w injury by dynamite, bystand injured, subs
		Y35.113A	Legal intervnt w injury by dynamite, suspect injured, init
		Y35.113D	Legal intervnt w injury by dynamite, suspect injured, subs
		Y35.121A	Lgl intervnt w inj by explosv shl, law enforc offl inj, init
		Y35.121D	Lgl intervnt w inj by explosv shl, law enforc offl inj, subs
		Y35.122A	Legal intervnt w injury by explosv shell, bystand inj, init
		Y35.122D	Legal intervnt w injury by explosv shell, bystand inj, subs
		Y35.123A	Legal intervnt w injury by explosv shell, suspect inj, init
		Y35.123D	Legal intervnt w injury by explosv shell, suspect inj, subs
		Y35.191A	Legal intervnt w oth explosv, law enforc offl injured, init
		Y35.191D	Legal intervnt w oth explosv, law enforc offl injured, subs
		Y35.192A	Legal intervnt involving oth explosv, bystand injured, init
		Y35.192D	Legal intervnt involving oth explosv, bystand injured, subs
		Y35.193A	Legal intervnt involving oth explosv, suspect injured, init
		Y35.193D	Legal intervnt involving oth explosv, suspect injured, subs

ICD-9-CM		ICD-10-CM	
E972	INJURY DUE TO LEGAL INTERVENTION BY GAS	**Y35.201A**	Legal intervnt w unsp gas, law enforc offl injured, init
		Y35.201D	Legal intervnt w unsp gas, law enforc offl injured, subs
		Y35.202A	Legal intervnt involving unsp gas, bystander injured, init
		Y35.202D	Legal intervnt involving unsp gas, bystander injured, subs
		Y35.203A	Legal intervention involving unsp gas, suspect injured, init
		Y35.203D	Legal intervention involving unsp gas, suspect injured, subs
		Y35.211A	Legal intervnt w inj by tear gas, law enforc offl inj, init
		Y35.211D	Legal intervnt w inj by tear gas, law enforc offl inj, subs
		Y35.212A	Legal intervnt w injury by tear gas, bystand injured, init
		Y35.212D	Legal intervnt w injury by tear gas, bystand injured, subs
		Y35.213A	Legal intervnt w injury by tear gas, suspect injured, init
		Y35.213D	Legal intervnt w injury by tear gas, suspect injured, subs
		Y35.291A	Legal intervnt w oth gas, law enforc offl injured, init
		Y35.291D	Legal intervnt w oth gas, law enforc offl injured, subs
		Y35.292A	Legal intervnt involving oth gas, bystander injured, init
		Y35.292D	Legal intervnt involving oth gas, bystander injured, subs
		Y35.293A	Legal intervention involving oth gas, suspect injured, init
		Y35.293D	Legal intervention involving oth gas, suspect injured, subs
		Y35.291D	Legal intervnt w oth gas, law enforc offl injured, subs
		Y35.292A	Legal intervnt involving oth gas, bystander injured, init
		Y35.292D	Legal intervnt involving oth gas, bystander injured, subs
		Y35.293A	Legal intervention involving oth gas, suspect injured, init
		Y35.293D	Legal intervention involving oth gas, suspect injured, subs
E973	INJURY DUE TO LEGAL INTERVENTION BY BLUNT OBJECT	**Y35.301A**	Legal intervnt w unsp blunt obj, law enforc offl inj, init
		Y35.301D	Legal intervnt w unsp blunt obj, law enforc offl inj, subs
		Y35.302A	Legal intervnt w unsp blunt objects, bystand injured, init
		Y35.302D	Legal intervnt w unsp blunt objects, bystand injured, subs
		Y35.303A	Legal intervnt w unsp blunt objects, suspect injured, init
		Y35.303D	Legal intervnt w unsp blunt objects, suspect injured, subs
		Y35.311A	Legal intervnt w baton, law enforc offl injured, init
		Y35.311D	Legal intervnt w baton, law enforc offl injured, subs
		Y35.312A	Legal intervention involving baton, bystander injured, init
		Y35.312D	Legal intervention involving baton, bystander injured, subs
		Y35.313A	Legal intervention involving baton, suspect injured, init
		Y35.313D	Legal intervention involving baton, suspect injured, subs
		Y35.391A	Legal intervnt w oth blunt obj, law enforc offl inj, init
		Y35.391D	Legal intervnt w oth blunt obj, law enforc offl inj, subs
		Y35.392A	Legal intervnt w oth blunt objects, bystand injured, init
		Y35.392D	Legal intervnt w oth blunt objects, bystand injured, subs
		Y35.393A	Legal intervnt w oth blunt objects, suspect injured, init
		Y35.393D	Legal intervnt w oth blunt objects, suspect injured, subs
E974	INJURY DUE LEGAL INTERVEN CUT&PIERCING INSTRUM	**Y35.401A**	Legal intervnt w unsp sharp obj, law enforc offl inj, init
		Y35.401D	Legal intervnt w unsp sharp obj, law enforc offl inj, subs
		Y35.402A	Legal intervnt w unsp sharp objects, bystand injured, init
		Y35.402D	Legal intervnt w unsp sharp objects, bystand injured, subs
		Y35.403A	Legal intervnt w unsp sharp objects, suspect injured, init
		Y35.403D	Legal intervnt w unsp sharp objects, suspect injured, subs
		Y35.411A	Legal intervnt w bayonet, law enforc offl injured, init
		Y35.411D	Legal intervnt w bayonet, law enforc offl injured, subs
		Y35.412A	Legal intervnt involving bayonet, bystander injured, init
		Y35.412D	Legal intervnt involving bayonet, bystander injured, subs
		Y35.413A	Legal intervention involving bayonet, suspect injured, init
		Y35.413D	Legal intervention involving bayonet, suspect injured, subs
		Y35.491A	Legal intervnt w oth sharp obj, law enforc offl inj, init
		Y35.491D	Legal intervnt w oth sharp obj, law enforc offl inj, subs
		Y35.492A	Legal intervnt w oth sharp objects, bystand injured, init
		Y35.492D	Legal intervnt w oth sharp objects, bystand injured, subs
		Y35.493A	Legal intervnt w oth sharp objects, suspect injured, init
		Y35.493D	Legal intervnt w oth sharp objects, suspect injured, subs
E975	INJURY DUE LEGAL INTERVENTION OTHER SPEC MEANS	**Y35.811A**	Legal intervnt w manhandling, law enforc offl injured, init
		Y35.811D	Legal intervnt w manhandling, law enforc offl injured, subs
		Y35.812A	Legal intervnt involving manhandling, bystand injured, init
		Y35.812D	Legal intervnt involving manhandling, bystand injured, subs
		Y35.813A	Legal intervnt involving manhandling, suspect injured, init
		Y35.813D	Legal intervnt involving manhandling, suspect injured, subs
		Y35.891A	Legal intervnt w oth means, law enforc offl injured, init
		Y35.891D	Legal intervnt w oth means, law enforc offl injured, subs
		Y35.892A	Legal intervnt involving oth means, bystander injured, init
		Y35.892D	Legal intervnt involving oth means, bystander injured, subs
		Y35.893A	Legal intervnt involving oth means, suspect injured, init
		Y35.893D	Legal intervnt involving oth means, suspect injured, subs
E976	INJURY DUE LEGAL INTERVENTION UNSPECIFIED MEANS	**Y35.91XA**	Legal intervnt, means unsp, law enforc offl injured, init
		Y35.91XD	Legal intervnt, means unsp, law enforc offl injured, subs
		Y35.92XA	Legal intervention, means unsp, bystander injured, init
		Y35.92XD	Legal intervention, means unsp, bystander injured, subs
		Y35.93XA	Legal intervention, means unsp, suspect injured, init encntr
		Y35.93XD	Legal intervention, means unsp, suspect injured, subs encntr

ICD-9-CM		ICD-10-CM	
E977	LATE EFFECTS INJURIES DUE TO LEGAL INTERVENTION	**Y35.001S**	Lgl intervnt w unsp firearm disch, law enforc offl inj, sqla
		Y35.002S	Legal intervnt w unsp firearm disch, bystand inj, sequela
		Y35.003S	Legal intervnt w unsp firearm disch, suspect inj, sequela
		Y35.011S	Legal intervnt w inj by mch gun, law enforc offl inj, sqla
		Y35.012S	Legal intervnt w injury by mch gun, bystand injured, sequela
		Y35.013S	Legal intervnt w injury by mch gun, suspect injured, sequela
		Y35.021S	Legal intervnt w inj by handgun, law enforc offl inj, sqla
		Y35.022S	Legal intervnt w injury by handgun, bystand injured, sequela
		Y35.023S	Legal intervnt w injury by handgun, suspect injured, sequela
		Y35.031S	Lgl intervnt w inj by rifl pelet, law enforc offl inj, sqla
		Y35.032S	Legal intervnt w injury by rifl pelet, bystand inj, sequela
		Y35.033S	Legal intervnt w injury by rifl pelet, suspect inj, sequela
		Y35.041S	Lgl intervnt w inj by rubr bulet, law enforc offl inj, sqla
		Y35.042S	Legal intervnt w injury by rubr bulet, bystand inj, sequela
		Y35.043S	Legal intervnt w injury by rubr bulet, suspect inj, sequela
		Y35.091S	Legal intervnt w firearm disch, law enforc offl inj, sequela
		Y35.092S	Legal intervnt w firearm disch, bystand injured, sequela
		Y35.093S	Legal intervnt w firearm disch, suspect injured, sequela
		Y35.101S	Legal intervnt w unsp explosv, law enforc offl inj, sequela
		Y35.102S	Legal intervnt w unsp explosv, bystand injured, sequela
		Y35.103S	Legal intervnt w unsp explosv, suspect injured, sequela
		Y35.111S	Legal intervnt w inj by dynamite, law enforc offl inj, sqla
		Y35.112S	Legal intervnt w injury by dynamite, bystand inj, sequela
		Y35.113S	Legal intervnt w injury by dynamite, suspect inj, sequela
		Y35.121S	Lgl intervnt w inj by explosv shl, law enforc offl inj, sqla
		Y35.122S	Legal intervnt w injury by explosv shell, bystand inj, sqla
		Y35.123S	Legal intervnt w injury by explosv shell, suspect inj, sqla
		Y35.191S	Legal intervnt w oth explosv, law enforc offl inj, sequela
		Y35.192S	Legal intervnt w oth explosv, bystand injured, sequela
		Y35.193S	Legal intervnt w oth explosv, suspect injured, sequela
		Y35.201S	Legal intervnt w unsp gas, law enforc offl injured, sequela
		Y35.202S	Legal intervnt involving unsp gas, bystand injured, sequela
		Y35.203S	Legal intervnt involving unsp gas, suspect injured, sequela
		Y35.211S	Legal intervnt w inj by tear gas, law enforc offl inj, sqla
		Y35.212S	Legal intervnt w injury by tear gas, bystand inj, sequela
		Y35.213S	Legal intervnt w injury by tear gas, suspect inj, sequela
		Y35.291S	Legal intervnt w oth gas, law enforc offl injured, sequela
		Y35.292S	Legal intervnt involving oth gas, bystander injured, sequela
		Y35.293S	Legal intervnt involving oth gas, suspect injured, sequela
		Y35.301S	Legal intervnt w unsp blunt obj, law enforc offl inj, sqla
		Y35.302S	Legal intervnt w unsp blunt objects, bystand inj, sequela
		Y35.303S	Legal intervnt w unsp blunt objects, suspect inj, sequela
		Y35.311S	Legal intervnt w baton, law enforc offl injured, sequela
		Y35.312S	Legal intervnt involving baton, bystander injured, sequela
		Y35.313S	Legal intervention involving baton, suspect injured, sequela
		Y35.391S	Legal intervnt w oth blunt obj, law enforc offl inj, sequela
		Y35.392S	Legal intervnt w oth blunt objects, bystand injured, sequela
		Y35.393S	Legal intervnt w oth blunt objects, suspect injured, sequela
		Y35.401S	Legal intervnt w unsp sharp obj, law enforc offl inj, sqla
		Y35.402S	Legal intervnt w unsp sharp objects, bystand inj, sequela
		Y35.403S	Legal intervnt w unsp sharp objects, suspect inj, sequela
		Y35.411S	Legal intervnt w bayonet, law enforc offl injured, sequela
		Y35.412S	Legal intervnt involving bayonet, bystander injured, sequela
		Y35.413S	Legal intervnt involving bayonet, suspect injured, sequela
		Y35.491S	Legal intervnt w oth sharp obj, law enforc offl inj, sequela
		Y35.492S	Legal intervnt w oth sharp objects, bystand injured, sequela
		Y35.493S	Legal intervnt w oth sharp objects, suspect injured, sequela
		Y35.811S	Legal intervnt w manhandling, law enforc offl inj, sequela
		Y35.812S	Legal intervnt w manhandling, bystand injured, sequela
		Y35.813S	Legal intervnt w manhandling, suspect injured, sequela
		Y35.891S	Legal intervnt w oth means, law enforc offl injured, sequela
		Y35.892S	Legal intervnt involving oth means, bystand injured, sequela
		Y35.893S	Legal intervnt involving oth means, suspect injured, sequela
		Y35.91XS	Legal intervnt, means unsp, law enforc offl injured, sequela
		Y35.92XS	Legal intervention, means unsp, bystander injured, sequela
		Y35.93XS	Legal intervention, means unsp, suspect injured, sequela
E978	LEGAL EXECUTION	NO DIAGNOSIS	
E979.0	TERRORISM INVOLVING EXPLOSION OF MARINE WEAPONS	**Y38.0X1A**	Terorsm w explosn of marine weap, publ sfty offcl inj, init
		Y38.0X1D	Terorsm w explosn of marine weap, publ sfty offcl inj, subs
		Y38.0X2A	Terorsm w explosn of marine weapons, civilian injured, init
		Y38.0X2D	Terorsm w explosn of marine weapons, civilian injured, subs
		Y38.0X3A	Terorsm w explosn of marine weapons, terrorist injured, init
		Y38.0X3D	Terorsm w explosn of marine weapons, terrorist injured, subs
E979.1	TERRORISM INVOLVING DESTRUCTION OF AIRCRAFT	**Y38.1X1A**	Terrorism w dest arcrft, publ sfty offcl injured, init
		Y38.1X1D	Terrorism w dest arcrft, publ sfty offcl injured, subs
		Y38.1X2A	Terrorism involving dest arcrft, civilian injured, init
		Y38.1X2D	Terrorism involving dest arcrft, civilian injured, subs
		Y38.1X3A	Terrorism involving dest arcrft, terrorist injured, init
		Y38.1X3D	Terrorism involving dest arcrft, terrorist injured, subs

ICD-9-CM		ICD-10-CM	
E979.2	TERRORISM INVOLVING OTHER EXPLOSIONS&FRAGMENTS	**Y38.2X1A**	Terorsm w oth explosn and fragmt, publ sfty offcl inj, init
		Y38.2X1D	Terorsm w oth explosn and fragmt, publ sfty offcl inj, subs
		Y38.2X2A	Terrorism w oth explosn and fragmt, civilian injured, init
		Y38.2X2D	Terrorism w oth explosn and fragmt, civilian injured, subs
		Y38.2X3A	Terrorism w oth explosn and fragmt, terrorist injured, init
		Y38.2X3D	Terrorism w oth explosn and fragmt, terrorist injured, subs
E979.3	TERRORISM INVLV FIRES CONFLAGRAT&HOT SUBSTANCES	**Y38.3X1A**	Terrorism w fire/hot subst, publ sfty offcl injured, init
		Y38.3X1D	Terrorism w fire/hot subst, publ sfty offcl injured, subs
		Y38.3X2A	Terrorism involving fire/hot subst, civilian injured, init
		Y38.3X2D	Terrorism involving fire/hot subst, civilian injured, subs
		Y38.3X3A	Terrorism involving fire/hot subst, terrorist injured, init
		Y38.3X3D	Terrorism involving fire/hot subst, terrorist injured, subs
E979.4	TERRORISM INVOLVING FIREARMS	**Y38.4X1A**	Terrorism involving firearms, publ sfty offcl injured, init
		Y38.4X1D	Terrorism involving firearms, publ sfty offcl injured, subs
		Y38.4X2A	Terrorism involving firearms, civilian injured, init encntr
		Y38.4X2D	Terrorism involving firearms, civilian injured, subs encntr
		Y38.4X3A	Terrorism involving firearms, terrorist injured, init encntr
		Y38.4X3D	Terrorism involving firearms, terrorist injured, subs encntr
E979.5	TERRORISM INVOLVING NUCLEAR WEAPONS	**Y38.5X1A**	Terrorism w nuclear weapons, publ sfty offcl injured, init
		Y38.5X1D	Terrorism w nuclear weapons, publ sfty offcl injured, subs
		Y38.5X2A	Terrorism involving nuclear weapons, civilian injured, init
		Y38.5X2D	Terrorism involving nuclear weapons, civilian injured, subs
		Y38.5X3A	Terrorism involving nuclear weapons, terrorist injured, init
		Y38.5X3D	Terrorism involving nuclear weapons, terrorist injured, subs
E979.6	TERRORISM INVOLVING BIOLOGICAL WEAPONS	**Y38.6X1A**	Terrorism w biolg weapons, publ sfty offcl injured, init
		Y38.6X1D	Terrorism w biolg weapons, publ sfty offcl injured, subs
		Y38.6X2A	Terrorism involving biolg weapons, civilian injured, init
		Y38.6X2D	Terrorism involving biolg weapons, civilian injured, subs
		Y38.6X3A	Terrorism involving biolg weapons, terrorist injured, init
		Y38.6X3D	Terrorism involving biolg weapons, terrorist injured, subs
E979.7	TERRORISM INVOLVING CHEMICAL WEAPONS	**Y38.7X1A**	Terrorism w chemical weapons, publ sfty offcl injured, init
		Y38.7X1D	Terrorism w chemical weapons, publ sfty offcl injured, subs
		Y38.7X2A	Terrorism involving chemical weapons, civilian injured, init
		Y38.7X2D	Terrorism involving chemical weapons, civilian injured, subs
		Y38.7X3A	Terrorism w chemical weapons, terrorist injured, init
		Y38.7X3D	Terrorism w chemical weapons, terrorist injured, subs
E979.8	TERRORISM INVOLVING OTHER MEANS	**Y38.8ØXA**	Terrorism involving unspecified means, initial encounter
		Y38.8ØXD	Terrorism involving unspecified means, subsequent encounter
		Y38.811A	Terrorism w suicide bomber, publ sfty offcl injured, init
		Y38.811D	Terrorism w suicide bomber, publ sfty offcl injured, subs
		Y38.812A	Terrorism involving suicide bomber, civilian injured, init
		Y38.812D	Terrorism involving suicide bomber, civilian injured, subs
		Y38.891A	Terrorism involving oth means, publ sfty offcl injured, init
		Y38.891D	Terrorism involving oth means, publ sfty offcl injured, subs
		Y38.892A	Terrorism involving oth means, civilian injured, init encntr
		Y38.892D	Terrorism involving oth means, civilian injured, subs encntr
		Y38.893A	Terrorism involving oth means, terrorist injured, init
		Y38.893D	Terrorism involving oth means, terrorist injured, subs
E979.9	TERRORISM SECONDARY EFFECTS	**Y38.9X1A**	Terrorism, secondary effects, publ sfty offcl injured, init
		Y38.9X1D	Terrorism, secondary effects, publ sfty offcl injured, subs
		Y38.9X2A	Terrorism, secondary effects, civilian injured, init encntr
		Y38.9X2D	Terrorism, secondary effects, civilian injured, subs encntr
E98Ø.Ø	POISN-ANALGES-ANTIPYRET-ANTIRHEUM-UNDETERM CAUSE	**T39.Ø14A**	Poisoning by aspirin, undetermined, initial encounter
		T39.Ø94A	Poisoning by salicylates, undetermined, initial encounter
		T39.1X4A	Poisoning by 4-Aminophenol derivatives, undetermined, init
		T39.2X4A	Poisoning by pyrazolone derivatives, undetermined, init
		T39.314A	Poisoning by propionic acid derivatives, undetermined, init
		T39.394A	Poisoning by oth nonsteroid anti-inflam drugs, undet, init
		T39.4X4A	Poisoning by antirheumatics, NEC, undetermined, init
		T39.8X4A	Poisoning by oth nonopio analges/antipyret, NEC, undet, init
		T39.94XA	Poisn by unsp nonopi analgs/antipyr/antirheu, undet, init
		T4Ø.ØX4A	Poisoning by opium, undetermined, initial encounter
		T4Ø.1X4A	Poisoning by heroin, undetermined, initial encounter
		T4Ø.2X4A	Poisoning by other opioids, undetermined, initial encounter
		T4Ø.3X4A	Poisoning by methadone, undetermined, initial encounter
		T4Ø.4X4A	Poisoning by oth synthetic narcotics, undetermined, init
E98Ø.1	POISN BARBITURATES UNDETERM ACC/PURPOSE INFLICT	**T42.3X4A**	Poisoning by barbiturates, undetermined, initial encounter
E98Ø.2	POISN OTH SEDAT&HYPNOT UNDET ACC/PRPOSLY INFLICT	**T4Ø.7X4A**	Poisoning by cannabis (derivatives), undetermined, init
		T4Ø.8X4A	Poisoning by lysergide, undetermined, initial encounter
		T4Ø.9Ø4A	Poisoning by unsp psychodysleptics, undetermined, init
		T4Ø.994A	Poisoning by oth psychodysleptics, undetermined, init encntr
		T42.4X4A	Poisoning by benzodiazepines, undetermined, init encntr

ICD-9-CM		ICD-10-CM	
E98Ø.3	POISON-TRANQUILIZER-PSYCHOTROPIC-UNDETERM CAUSE	**T43.Ø14A**	Poisoning by tricyclic antidepressants, undetermined, init
		T43.Ø24A	Poisoning by tetracyclic antidepressants, undetermined, init
		T43.1X4A	Poisoning by MAO inhib antidepressants, undetermined, init
		T43.2Ø4A	Poisoning by unsp antidepressants, undetermined, init encntr
		T43.214A	Poisn by slctv seroton/norepineph reup inhibtr, undet, init
		T43.224A	Poisn by selective serotonin reuptake inhibtr, undet, init
		T43.294A	Poisoning by oth antidepressants, undetermined, init encntr
		T43.3X4A	Poisoning by phenothiaz antipsychot/neurolept, undet, init
		T43.4X4A	Poisoning by butyrophen/thiothixen neuroleptc, undet, init
		T43.5Ø4A	Poisoning by unsp antipsychot/neurolept, undetermined, init
		T43.594A	Poisoning by oth antipsychot/neurolept, undetermined, init
		T43.6Ø4A	Poisoning by unsp psychostimulants, undetermined, init
		T43.614A	Poisoning by caffeine, undetermined, initial encounter
		T43.624A	Poisoning by amphetamines, undetermined, initial encounter
		T43.634A	Poisoning by methylphenidate, undetermined, init encntr
		T43.694A	Poisoning by oth psychostimulants, undetermined, init encntr
		T43.8X4A	Poisoning by oth psychotropic drugs, undetermined, init
		T43.94XA	Poisoning by unsp psychotropic drug, undetermined, init
E98Ø.4	POISONING BY OTH DRUG & MEDICINE-UNDETERM CAUSE	**T36.ØX4A**	Poisoning by penicillins, undetermined, initial encounter
		T36.1X4A	Poisn by cephalospor/oth beta-lactm antibiot, undet, init
		T36.2X4A	Poisoning by chloramphenicol group, undetermined, init
		T36.3X4A	Poisoning by macrolides, undetermined, initial encounter
		T36.4X4A	Poisoning by tetracyclines, undetermined, initial encounter
		T36.5X4A	Poisoning by aminoglycosides, undetermined, init encntr
		T36.6X4A	Poisoning by rifampicins, undetermined, initial encounter
		T36.7X4A	Poisoning by antifungal antibiotics, sys used, undet, init
		T36.8X4A	Poisoning by oth systemic antibiotics, undetermined, init
		T36.94XA	Poisoning by unsp systemic antibiotic, undetermined, init
		T37.ØX4A	Poisoning by sulfonamides, undetermined, initial encounter
		T37.1X4A	Poisoning by antimycobacterial drugs, undetermined, init
		T37.2X4A	Poisn by antimalari/drugs acting on bld protzoa, undet, init
		T37.3X4A	Poisoning by oth antiprotozoal drugs, undetermined, init
		T37.4X4A	Poisoning by anthelminthics, undetermined, initial encounter
		T37.5X4A	Poisoning by antiviral drugs, undetermined, init encntr
		T37.8X4A	Poisoning by oth systemic anti-infect/parasit, undet, init
		T37.94XA	Poisn by unsp sys anti-infect and antiparastc, undet, init
		T38.ØX4A	Poisoning by glucocort/synth analog, undetermined, init
		T38.1X4A	Poisoning by thyroid hormones and substitutes, undet, init
		T38.2X4A	Poisoning by antithyroid drugs, undetermined, init encntr
		T38.3X4A	Poisn by insulin and oral hypoglycemic drugs, undet, init
		T38.4X4A	Poisoning by oral contraceptives, undetermined, init encntr
		T38.5X4A	Poisoning by oth estrogens and progstrn, undetermined, init
		T38.6X4A	Poisn by antigonadtr/antiestr/antiandrg, NEC, undet, init
		T38.7X4A	Poisoning by androgens and anabolic congeners, undet, init
		T38.8Ø4A	Poisoning by unsp hormones and synthetic sub, undet, init
		T38.814A	Poisoning by anterior pituitary hormones, undetermined, init
		T38.894A	Poisoning by oth hormones and synthetic sub, undet, init
		T38.9Ø4A	Poisoning by unsp hormone antagonists, undetermined, init
		T38.994A	Poisoning by oth hormone antagonists, undetermined, init
		T4Ø.5X4A	Poisoning by cocaine, undetermined, initial encounter
		T4Ø.6Ø4A	Poisoning by unsp narcotics, undetermined, init encntr
		T4Ø.694A	Poisoning by other narcotics, undetermined, init encntr
		T41.ØX4A	Poisoning by inhaled anesthetics, undetermined, init encntr
		T41.1X4A	Poisoning by intravenous anesthetics, undetermined, init
		T41.2Ø4A	Poisoning by unsp general anesthetics, undetermined, init
		T41.294A	Poisoning by oth general anesthetics, undetermined, init
		T41.3X4A	Poisoning by local anesthetics, undetermined, init encntr
		T41.44XA	Poisoning by unsp anesthetic, undetermined, init encntr
		T41.5X4A	Poisoning by therapeutic gases, undetermined, init encntr
		T42.ØX4A	Poisoning by hydantoin derivatives, undetermined, init
		T42.1X4A	Poisoning by iminostilbenes, undetermined, initial encounter
		T42.2X4A	Poisoning by succinimides and oxazolidinediones, undet, init
		T42.5X4A	Poisoning by mixed antiepileptics, undetermined, init encntr
		T42.6X4A	Poisn by oth antieplptc and sed-hypntc drugs, undet, init
		T42.74XA	Poisn by unsp antieplptc and sed-hypntc drugs, undet, init
		T42.8X4A	Poisn by antiparkns drug/centr musc-tone depr, undet, init
		T44.ØX4A	Poisoning by anticholinesterase agents, undetermined, init
		T44.1X4A	Poisoning by oth parasympathomimetics, undetermined, init
		T44.2X4A	Poisoning by ganglionic blocking drugs, undetermined, init
		T44.3X4A	Poisoning by oth parasympath and spasmolytics, undet, init
		T44.4X4A	Poisoning by predom alpha-adrenocpt agonists, undet, init
		T44.5X4A	Poisoning by predom beta-adrenocpt agonists, undet, init
		T44.6X4A	Poisoning by alpha-adrenocpt antagonists, undetermined, init
		T44.7X4A	Poisoning by beta-adrenocpt antagonists, undetermined, init
		T44.8X4A	Poisn by centr-acting/adren-neurn-block agnt, undet, init
		T44.9Ø4A	Poisn by unsp drugs aff the autonm nervous sys, undet, init
		T44.994A	Poisn by oth drug aff the autonm nervous sys, undet, init
		T45.ØX4A	Poisoning by antiallerg/antiemetic, undetermined, init
		T45.1X4A	Poisoning by antineopl and immunosup drugs, undet, init

(Continued on next page)

ICD-9-CM		ICD-10-CM	
E980.4	POISONING BY OTH DRUG & MEDICINE-UNDETERM CAUSE **(Continued)**	**T45.2X4A**	Poisoning by vitamins, undetermined, initial encounter
		T45.3X4A	Poisoning by enzymes, undetermined, initial encounter
		T45.4X4A	Poisoning by iron and its compounds, undetermined, init
		T45.514A	Poisoning by anticoagulants, undetermined, initial encounter
		T45.524A	Poisoning by antithrombotic drugs, undetermined, init encntr
		T45.604A	Poisoning by unsp fibrin-affct drugs, undetermined, init
		T45.614A	Poisoning by thrombolytic drug, undetermined, init encntr
		T45.624A	Poisoning by hemostatic drug, undetermined, init encntr
		T45.694A	Poisoning by oth fibrin-affct drugs, undetermined, init
		T45.7X4A	Poisn by anticoag antag, vitamin K and oth coag, undet, init
		T45.8X4A	Poisn by oth prim systemic and hematolog agents, undet, init
		T45.94XA	Poisn by unsp prim systemic and hematolog agent, undet, init
		T46.0X4A	Poisoning by cardi-stim glycos/drug simlar act, undet, init
		T46.1X4A	Poisoning by calcium-channel blockers, undetermined, init
		T46.2X4A	Poisoning by oth antidysrhythmic drugs, undetermined, init
		T46.3X4A	Poisoning by coronary vasodilators, undetermined, init
		T46.4X4A	Poisoning by angiotens-convert-enzyme inhibtr, undet, init
		T46.5X4A	Poisoning by oth antihypertensive drugs, undetermined, init
		T46.6X4A	Poisoning by antihyperlip and antiarterio drugs, undet, init
		T46.7X4A	Poisoning by peripheral vasodilators, undetermined, init
		T46.8X4A	Poisoning by antivaric drugs, inc scler agents, undet, init
		T46.904A	Poisoning by unsp agents aff the cardiovasc sys, undet, init
		T46.994A	Poisoning by oth agents aff the cardiovasc sys, undet, init
		T47.0X4A	Poisoning by histamine H2-receptor blockers, undet, init
		T47.1X4A	Poisn by oth antacids and anti-gstrc-sec drugs, undet, init
		T47.2X4A	Poisoning by stimulant laxatives, undetermined, init encntr
		T47.3X4A	Poisoning by saline and osmotic laxatives, undet, init
		T47.4X4A	Poisoning by other laxatives, undetermined, init encntr
		T47.5X4A	Poisoning by digestants, undetermined, initial encounter
		T47.6X4A	Poisoning by antidiarrheal drugs, undetermined, init encntr
		T47.7X4A	Poisoning by emetics, undetermined, initial encounter
		T47.8X4A	Poisoning by oth agents aff GI sys, undetermined, init
		T47.94XA	Poisoning by unsp agents aff the GI sys, undetermined, init
		T48.0X4A	Poisoning by oxytocic drugs, undetermined, initial encounter
		T48.1X4A	Poisoning by skeletal muscle relaxants, undetermined, init
		T48.204A	Poisoning by unsp drugs acting on muscles, undet, init
		T48.294A	Poisoning by oth drugs acting on muscles, undetermined, init
		T48.3X4A	Poisoning by antitussives, undetermined, initial encounter
		T48.4X4A	Poisoning by expectorants, undetermined, initial encounter
		T48.5X4A	Poisoning by oth anti-common-cold drugs, undetermined, init
		T48.6X4A	Poisoning by antiasthmatics, undetermined, initial encounter
		T48.904A	Poisn by unsp agents prim act on the resp sys, undet, init
		T48.994A	Poisn by oth agents prim acting on the resp sys, undet, init
		T49.0X4A	Poisn by local antifung/infect/inflamm drugs, undet, init
		T49.1X4A	Poisoning by antipruritics, undetermined, initial encounter
		T49.2X4A	Poisoning by local astringents/detergents, undet, init
		T49.3X4A	Poisoning by emollients, demulcents and protect, undet, init
		T49.4X4A	Poisoning by keratolyt/keratplst/hair trmt drug, undet, init
		T49.5X4A	Poisoning by opth drugs and preparations, undetermined, init
		T49.6X4A	Poisoning by otorhino drugs and prep, undetermined, init
		T49.7X4A	Poisoning by dental drugs, topically applied, undet, init
		T49.8X4A	Poisoning by other topical agents, undetermined, init encntr
		T49.94XA	Poisoning by unsp topical agent, undetermined, init encntr
		T50.0X4A	Poisoning by mineralocorticoids and their antag, undet, init
		T50.2X4A	Poisn by crbnc-anhydr inhibtr,benzo/oth diuretc, undet, init
		T50.3X4A	Poisoning by electrolytic/caloric/wtr-bal agnt, undet, init
		T50.4X4A	Poisoning by drugs affecting uric acid metab, undet, init
		T50.5X4A	Poisoning by appetite depressants, undetermined, init encntr
		T50.6X4A	Poisoning by antidotes and chelating agents, undet, init
		T50.7X4A	Poisn by analeptics and opioid receptor antag, undet, init
		T50.8X4A	Poisoning by diagnostic agents, undetermined, init encntr
		T50.994A	Poisoning by oth drug/meds/biol subst, undetermined, init
		T50.A14A	Poisn by pertuss vaccine, inc combin w pertuss, undet, init
		T50.A24A	Poisoning by mixed bact vaccines w/o a pertuss, undet, init
		T50.A94A	Poisoning by oth bacterial vaccines, undetermined, init
		T50.B14A	Poisoning by smallpox vaccines, undetermined, init encntr
		T50.B94A	Poisoning by other viral vaccines, undetermined, init encntr
		T50.Z14A	Poisoning by immunoglobulin, undetermined, initial encounter
		T50.Z94A	Poisoning by oth vaccines and biolg substances, undet, init
E980.5	POISONING BY UNS DRUG OR MEDICINE-UNDETERM CAUSE	**T50.904A**	Poisoning by unsp drug/meds/biol subst, undetermined, init
E980.6	POISON-CORROSIVE-CAUSTIC SUBSTNCE-UNDETERM CAUSE	**T54.0X4A**	Toxic effect of phenol and phenol homologues, undet, init
		T54.94XA	Toxic effect of unsp corrosive substance, undetermined, init
		T55.0X4A	Toxic effect of soaps, undetermined, initial encounter
		T55.1X4A	Toxic effect of detergents, undetermined, initial encounter
		T57.1X4A	Toxic effect of phosphorus and its compounds, undet, init
		T57.2X4A	Toxic effect of manganese and its compounds, undet, init

ICD-9-CM		ICD-10-CM	
E980.7	POISON-AGRICULT-HORTICULT CHEM-UNDETERM CAUSE	**T60.0X4A**	Toxic effect of organophos and carbamate insect, undet, init
		T60.1X4A	Toxic effect of halogenated insecticides, undetermined, init
		T60.2X4A	Toxic effect of oth insecticides, undetermined, init encntr
		T60.3X4A	Toxic effect of herbicides and fungicides, undet, init
		T60.4X4A	Toxic effect of rodenticides, undetermined, init encntr
		T60.8X4A	Toxic effect of other pesticides, undetermined, init encntr
		T60.94XA	Toxic effect of unsp pesticide, undetermined, init encntr
E980.8	PSN ARSENIC&ITS COMPND UNDET ACC/PRPSLY INFLICT	**T57.0X4A**	Toxic effect of arsenic and its compounds, undet, init
E980.9	POISN-OTH&UNS SOLID&LIQUID SUBSTANCE-UNDET CAUSE	**T51.0X4A**	Toxic effect of ethanol, undetermined, initial encounter
		T51.1X4A	Toxic effect of methanol, undetermined, initial encounter
		T51.2X4A	Toxic effect of 2-Propanol, undetermined, initial encounter
		T51.3X4A	Toxic effect of fusel oil, undetermined, initial encounter
		T51.8X4A	Toxic effect of other alcohols, undetermined, init encntr
		T51.94XA	Toxic effect of unsp alcohol, undetermined, init encntr
		T52.0X4A	Toxic effect of petroleum products, undetermined, init
		T52.1X4A	Toxic effect of benzene, undetermined, initial encounter
		T52.2X4A	Toxic effect of homologues of benzene, undetermined, init
		T52.3X4A	Toxic effect of glycols, undetermined, initial encounter
		T52.4X4A	Toxic effect of ketones, undetermined, initial encounter
		T52.8X4A	Toxic effect of oth organic solvents, undetermined, init
		T52.94XA	Toxic effect of unsp organic solvent, undetermined, init
		T53.0X4A	Toxic effect of carbon tetrachloride, undetermined, init
		T53.1X4A	Toxic effect of chloroform, undetermined, initial encounter
		T53.2X4A	Toxic effect of trichloroethylene, undetermined, init encntr
		T53.3X4A	Toxic effect of tetrachloroethylene, undetermined, init
		T53.4X4A	Toxic effect of dichloromethane, undetermined, init encntr
		T53.6X4A	Toxic eff of halgn deriv of aliphatic hydrocrb, undet, init
		T53.7X4A	Toxic eff of halgn deriv of aromatic hydrocrb, undet, init
		T53.94XA	Tox eff of unsp halgn deriv of aromat hydrocrb, undet, init
		T56.0X4A	Toxic effect of lead and its compounds, undetermined, init
		T56.1X4A	Toxic effect of mercury and its compounds, undet, init
		T56.2X4A	Toxic effect of chromium and its compounds, undet, init
		T56.3X4A	Toxic effect of cadmium and its compounds, undet, init
		T56.4X4A	Toxic effect of copper and its compounds, undetermined, init
		T56.5X4A	Toxic effect of zinc and its compounds, undetermined, init
		T56.6X4A	Toxic effect of tin and its compounds, undetermined, init
		T56.7X4A	Toxic effect of beryllium and its compounds, undet, init
		T56.814A	Toxic effect of thallium, undetermined, initial encounter
		T56.894A	Toxic effect of other metals, undetermined, init encntr
		T56.94XA	Toxic effect of unspecified metal, undetermined, init encntr
		T57.8X4A	Toxic effect of oth inorganic substances, undetermined, init
		T57.94XA	Toxic effect of unsp inorganic substance, undetermined, init
		T61.04XA	Ciguatera fish poisoning, undetermined, initial encounter
		T61.14XA	Scombroid fish poisoning, undetermined, initial encounter
		T61.774A	Other fish poisoning, undetermined, initial encounter
		T61.784A	Other shellfish poisoning, undetermined, initial encounter
		T61.8X4A	Toxic effect of other seafood, undetermined, init encntr
		T61.94XA	Toxic effect of unsp seafood, undetermined, init encntr
		T62.0X4A	Toxic effect of ingested mushrooms, undetermined, init
		T62.1X4A	Toxic effect of ingested berries, undetermined, init encntr
		T62.2X4A	Toxic effect of ingested (parts of) plant(s), undet, init
		T62.8X4A	Toxic effect of noxious substnc eaten as food, undet, init
		T62.94XA	Toxic effect of unsp noxious sub eaten as food, undet, init
		T63.004A	Toxic effect of unsp snake venom, undetermined, init encntr
		T63.014A	Toxic effect of rattlesnake venom, undetermined, init encntr
		T63.024A	Toxic effect of coral snake venom, undetermined, init encntr
		T63.034A	Toxic effect of taipan venom, undetermined, init encntr
		T63.044A	Toxic effect of cobra venom, undetermined, initial encounter
		T63.064A	Toxic effect of venom of N & S American snake, undet, init
		T63.074A	Toxic effect of venom of Australian snake, undet, init
		T63.084A	Toxic eff of venom of African and Asian snake, undet, init
		T63.094A	Toxic effect of venom of oth snake, undetermined, init
		T63.114A	Toxic effect of venom of gila monster, undetermined, init
		T63.124A	Toxic effect of venom of venomous lizard, undetermined, init
		T63.194A	Toxic effect of venom of oth reptiles, undetermined, init
		T63.2X4A	Toxic effect of venom of scorpion, undetermined, init encntr
		T63.304A	Toxic effect of unsp spider venom, undetermined, init encntr
		T63.314A	Toxic effect of venom of black widow spider, undet, init
		T63.324A	Toxic effect of venom of tarantula, undetermined, init
		T63.334A	Toxic effect of venom of brown recluse spider, undet, init
		T63.394A	Toxic effect of venom of oth spider, undetermined, init
		T63.414A	Toxic effect of venom of centipede/millipede, undet, init
		T63.424A	Toxic effect of venom of ants, undetermined, init encntr
		T63.434A	Toxic effect of venom of caterpillars, undetermined, init
		T63.444A	Toxic effect of venom of bees, undetermined, init encntr
		T63.454A	Toxic effect of venom of hornets, undetermined, init encntr
		T63.464A	Toxic effect of venom of wasps, undetermined, init encntr
		T63.484A	Toxic effect of venom of oth arthropod, undetermined, init
	(Continued on next page)	**T63.514A**	Toxic effect of contact w stingray, undetermined, init

ICD-9-CM		ICD-10-CM	
E980.9	POISN-OTH&UNS SOLID&LIQUID SUBSTANCE-UNDET CAUSE **(Continued)**	**T63.594A**	Toxic effect of contact w oth venomous fish, undet, init
		T63.614A	Toxic effect of contact w Portugese Man-o-war, undet, init
		T63.624A	Toxic effect of contact w oth jellyfish, undetermined, init
		T63.634A	Toxic effect of contact w sea anemone, undetermined, init
		T63.694A	Toxic eff of cntct w oth venom marine animals, undet, init
		T63.714A	Toxic effect of contact w venomous marine plant, undet, init
		T63.794A	Toxic effect of contact w oth venomous plant, undet, init
		T63.814A	Toxic effect of contact w venomous frog, undetermined, init
		T63.824A	Toxic effect of contact w venomous toad, undetermined, init
		T63.834A	Toxic effect of contact w oth venomous amphib, undet, init
		T63.894A	Toxic effect of contact w oth venomous animals, undet, init
		T63.94XA	Toxic effect of contact w unsp venomous animal, undet, init
		T64.04XA	Toxic effect of aflatoxin, undetermined, initial encounter
		T64.84XA	Toxic effect of mycotoxin food contamnt, undetermined, init
		T65.0X4A	Toxic effect of cyanides, undetermined, initial encounter
		T65.1X4A	Toxic effect of strychnine and its salts, undetermined, init
		T65.214A	Toxic effect of chewing tobacco, undetermined, init encntr
		T65.224A	Toxic effect of tobacco cigarettes, undetermined, init
		T65.294A	Toxic effect of oth tobacco and nicotine, undetermined, init
		T65.3X4A	Toxic eff of nitrodrv/aminodrv of benzn/homolog, undet, init
		T65.4X4A	Toxic effect of carbon disulfide, undetermined, init encntr
		T65.5X4A	Tox eff of nitro & oth nitric acids and esters, undet, init
		T65.6X4A	Toxic effect of paints and dyes, NEC, undetermined, init
		T65.814A	Toxic effect of latex, undetermined, initial encounter
		T65.834A	Toxic effect of fiberglass, undetermined, initial encounter
		T65.894A	Toxic effect of oth substances, undetermined, init encntr
		T65.94XA	Toxic effect of unsp substance, undetermined, init encntr
E981.0	PSN GAS DSTRBD PIPELINE UNDET ACC/PRPSLY INFLICT	NO DIAGNOSIS	
E981.1	POISON-LIQ GAS IN MOBILE CONTAINR-UNDETERM CAUSE	NO DIAGNOSIS	
E981.8	POISN OTH UTILITY GAS UNDET ACC/PRPSLY INFLICT	NO DIAGNOSIS	
E982.0	POISON-MOTOR VEHICLE EXHAUST GAS-UNDETERM CAUSE	**T58.04XA**	Toxic effect of carb monx from mtr veh exhaust, undet, init
E982.1	POISN OTH CARB MONOXIDE UNDET ACC/PRPSLY INFLICT	**T58.14XA**	Toxic effect of carb monx from utility gas, undet, init
		T58.2X4A	Tox eff of carb monx fr incmpl combst dmst fuel, undet, init
		T58.8X4A	Toxic effect of carb monx from oth source, undet, init
		T58.94XA	Toxic effect of carb monx from unsp source, undet, init
E982.8	POISN OTH GASES&VAPORS UNDET ACC/PRPSLY INFLICT	**T53.5X4A**	Toxic effect of chlorofluorocarbons, undetermined, init
		T57.3X4A	Toxic effect of hydrogen cyanide, undetermined, init encntr
		T59.0X4A	Toxic effect of nitrogen oxides, undetermined, init encntr
		T59.1X4A	Toxic effect of sulfur dioxide, undetermined, init encntr
		T59.2X4A	Toxic effect of formaldehyde, undetermined, init encntr
		T59.3X4A	Toxic effect of lacrimogenic gas, undetermined, init encntr
		T59.4X4A	Toxic effect of chlorine gas, undetermined, init encntr
		T59.5X4A	Toxic eff of fluorine gas and hydrogen fluoride, undet, init
		T59.6X4A	Toxic effect of hydrogen sulfide, undetermined, init encntr
		T59.7X4A	Toxic effect of carbon dioxide, undetermined, init encntr
		T59.814A	Toxic effect of smoke, undetermined, initial encounter
		T59.94XA	Toxic effect of unsp gases, fumes and vapors, undet, init
E982.9	POISN UNS GASES&VAPORS UNDET ACC/PRPSLY INFLICT	NO DIAGNOSIS	
E983.0	HANGING UNDET WHETHER ACC/PURPOSELY INFLICTED	**T71.164A**	Asphyxiation due to hanging, undetermined, initial encounter
E983.1	SUFFOC-PASTIC BAG UNDET ACC/PURPOSELY INFLICTED	**T71.124A**	Asphyxiation due to plastic bag, undetermined, init encntr
E983.8	STRANGULAT/SUFFOCAT BY OTH MEANS-UNDETERM CAUSE	**T71.114A**	Asphyx due to smothering under pillow, undetermined, init
		T71.134A	Asphyx due to being trapped in bed linens, undet, init
		T71.144A	Asphyx d/t smothr under another person's body, undet, init
		T71.154A	Asphyx due to smothering in furniture, undetermined, init
		T71.194A	Asphyx d/t mech threat to breathe d/t oth cause, undet, init
		T71.224A	Asphyx due to being trapped in a car trunk, undet, init
		T71.234A	Asphyx d/t being trap in a (discarded) refrig, undet, init
E983.9	STRANGULAT/SUFFOCAT BY UNS MEANS-UNDETERM CAUSE	NO DIAGNOSIS	
E984	SUBMERSION UNDET WHETHER ACC/PURPOSELY INFLICTED	**Y21.9XXA**	Unsp drowning and submersion, undetermined intent, init
		Y21.9XXD	Unsp drowning and submersion, undetermined intent, subs
E985.0	INJURY BY HANDGUN UNDETERM ACC/PURPOSELY INFLICT	**Y22.XXXA**	Handgun discharge, undetermined intent, initial encounter
		Y22.XXXD	Handgun discharge, undetermined intent, subsequent encounter
E985.1	INJURY SHOTGUN UNDET ACC/PRPOSLY INFLICTED	**Y23.0XXA**	Shotgun discharge, undetermined intent, initial encounter
		Y23.0XXD	Shotgun discharge, undetermined intent, subsequent encounter
E985.2	INJURY HUNTING RIFLE UNDET ACC/PRPOSLY INFLICTED	**Y23.1XXA**	Hunting rifle discharge, undetermined intent, init encntr
		Y23.1XXD	Hunting rifle discharge, undetermined intent, subs encntr
E985.3	INJURY MILITARY FIRARMS UNDET ACC/PRPSLY INFLICT	**Y23.2XXA**	Military firearm discharge, undetermined intent, init encntr
		Y23.2XXD	Military firearm discharge, undetermined intent, subs encntr
		Y23.3XXA	Machine gun discharge, undetermined intent, init encntr
		Y23.3XXD	Machine gun discharge, undetermined intent, subs encntr
E985.4	INJURY AIR GUN UNDETERM ACC/PURPOSEFULLY INFLICT	**Y23.8XXA**	Oth larger firearm discharge, undetermined intent, init
		Y23.8XXD	Oth larger firearm discharge, undetermined intent, subs
		Y23.9XXA	Unsp larger firearm discharge, undetermined intent, init
		Y23.9XXD	Unsp larger firearm discharge, undetermined intent, subs
		Y24.9XXA	Unsp firearm discharge, undetermined intent, init encntr
		Y24.9XXD	Unsp firearm discharge, undetermined intent, subs encntr

ICD-9-CM		ICD-10-CM	
E985.5	INJURY EXPLOSIVES UNDET ACC/PRPOSLY INFLICTED	**Y25.XXXA**	Contact w explosive material, undetermined intent, init
		Y25.XXXD	Contact w explosive material, undetermined intent, subs
E985.6	INJURY AIR GUN UNDET ACCOR PRPOSFULLY INFLICTED	**Y24.ØXXA**	Airgun discharge, undetermined intent, initial encounter
		Y24.ØXXD	Airgun discharge, undetermined intent, subsequent encounter
E985.7	INJURY PAINTBALL GUN UNDET ACC/PRPOSFULL INFLICT	**Y24.8XXA**	Other firearm discharge, undetermined intent, init encntr
		Y24.8XXD	Other firearm discharge, undetermined intent, subs encntr
E986	INJR CUT&PIERC INSTRUM UNDET ACC/PRPSLY INFLICT	**Y28.ØXXA**	Contact with sharp glass, undetermined intent, init encntr
		Y28.ØXXD	Contact with sharp glass, undetermined intent, subs encntr
		Y28.1XXA	Contact with knife, undetermined intent, initial encounter
		Y28.1XXD	Contact with knife, undetermined intent, subs encntr
		Y28.2XXA	Contact w sword or dagger, undetermined intent, init encntr
		Y28.2XXD	Contact w sword or dagger, undetermined intent, subs encntr
		Y28.8XXA	Contact w oth sharp object, undetermined intent, init encntr
		Y28.8XXD	Contact w oth sharp object, undetermined intent, subs encntr
		Y28.9XXA	Contact w unsp sharp object, undetermined intent, init
		Y28.9XXD	Contact w unsp sharp object, undetermined intent, subs
E987.Ø	FALL-HIGH PLACE-RESIDENT PREMISES-UNDETERM CAUSE	**Y3Ø.XXXA**	Fall, jump or pushed from a high place, undet intent, init
E987.1	FALL-HIGH PLACE-MAN-MADE STRUCT-UNDETERM CAUSE	**Y3Ø.XXXA**	Fall, jump or pushed from a high place, undet intent, init
E987.2	FALL FROM HIGH PLACE-NATURAL SITE-UNDETERM CAUSE	**Y3Ø.XXXA**	Fall, jump or pushed from a high place, undet intent, init
E987.9	FALLING UNS HI PLACE UNDET ACC/PRPSLY INFLICT	**Y3Ø.XXXA**	Fall, jump or pushed from a high place, undet intent, init
		Y3Ø.XXXD	Fall, jump or pushed from a high place, undet intent, subs
E988.Ø	INJURY-JUMP/LYING BEFORE MOVE OBJ-UNDETERM CAUSE	**Y31.XXXA**	Fall/lying/running bef/into moving obj, undet intent, init
		Y31.XXXD	Fall/lying/running bef/into moving obj, undet intent, subs
E988.1	INJURY BURNS/FIRE UNDET ACC/PRPOSLY INFLICTED	**Y26.XXXA**	Exposure to smoke, fire and flames, undet intent, init
		Y26.XXXD	Exposure to smoke, fire and flames, undet intent, subs
		Y27.3XXA	Contact w hot household appliance, undetermined intent, init
		Y27.3XXD	Contact w hot household appliance, undetermined intent, subs
		Y27.8XXA	Contact w oth hot objects, undetermined intent, init encntr
		Y27.8XXD	Contact w oth hot objects, undetermined intent, subs encntr
		Y27.9XXA	Contact w unsp hot objects, undetermined intent, init encntr
		Y27.9XXD	Contact w unsp hot objects, undetermined intent, subs encntr
E988.2	INJURY SCALD UNDET WHETHER ACC/PRPOSLY INFLICTED	**Y27.ØXXA**	Contact w steam and hot vapors, undetermined intent, init
		Y27.ØXXD	Contact w steam and hot vapors, undetermined intent, subs
		Y27.1XXA	Contact with hot tap water, undetermined intent, init encntr
		Y27.1XXD	Contact with hot tap water, undetermined intent, subs encntr
		Y27.2XXA	Contact with hot fluids, undetermined intent, init encntr
		Y27.2XXD	Contact with hot fluids, undetermined intent, subs encntr
E988.3	INJURY EXTREMS COLD UNDET ACC/PRPOSLY INFLICTED	**Y33.XXXA**	Other specified events, undetermined intent, init encntr
E988.4	INJR BY ELECTROCUTE UNDETRM ACC/PURPOSELY INFLCT	**Y33.XXXA**	Other specified events, undetermined intent, init encntr
E988.5	INJR CRASHING MOTR VEH UNDET ACC/PRPSLY INFLICT	**Y32.XXXA**	Crashing of motor vehicle, undetermined intent, init encntr
		Y32.XXXD	Crashing of motor vehicle, undetermined intent, subs encntr
E988.6	INJURY CRASHING AIRCRFT UNDET ACC/PRPSLY INFLICT	**Y33.XXXA**	Other specified events, undetermined intent, init encntr
E988.7	INJ-CAUSTIC SUBSTANCE-NOT POISON-UNDETERM CAUSE	**Y33.XXXA**	Other specified events, undetermined intent, init encntr
E988.8	INJURY OTH SPEC MEANS UNDET ACC/PRPOSLY INFLICT	**Y29.XXXA**	Contact with blunt object, undetermined intent, init encntr
		Y29.XXXD	Contact with blunt object, undetermined intent, subs encntr
		Y33.XXXA	Other specified events, undetermined intent, init encntr
		Y33.XXXD	Other specified events, undetermined intent, subs encntr
E988.9	INJURY UNSPEC MEANS UNDET ACC/PRPOSLY INFLICTED	**Y33.XXXA**	Other specified events, undetermined intent, init encntr
E989	LATE EFF INJURY UNDET ACC/PRPOSLY INFLICTED	**T36.ØX4S**	Poisoning by penicillins, undetermined, sequela
		T36.1X4S	Poisn by cephalospor/oth beta-lactm antibiot, undet, sequela
		T36.2X4S	Poisoning by chloramphenicol group, undetermined, sequela
		T36.3X4S	Poisoning by macrolides, undetermined, sequela
		T36.4X4S	Poisoning by tetracyclines, undetermined, sequela
		T36.5X4S	Poisoning by aminoglycosides, undetermined, sequela
		T36.6X4S	Poisoning by rifampicins, undetermined, sequela
		T36.7X4S	Poisoning by antifungal antibiot, sys used, undet, sequela
		T36.8X4S	Poisoning by oth systemic antibiotics, undetermined, sequela
		T36.94XS	Poisoning by unsp systemic antibiotic, undetermined, sequela
		T37.ØX4S	Poisoning by sulfonamides, undetermined, sequela
		T37.1X4S	Poisoning by antimycobacterial drugs, undetermined, sequela
		T37.2X4S	Poisn by antimalari/drugs acting on bld protzoa, undet, sqla
		T37.3X4S	Poisoning by oth antiprotozoal drugs, undetermined, sequela
		T37.4X4S	Poisoning by anthelminthics, undetermined, sequela
		T37.5X4S	Poisoning by antiviral drugs, undetermined, sequela
		T37.8X4S	Poisn by oth systemic anti-infect/parasit, undet, sequela
		T37.94XS	Poisn by unsp sys anti-infect and antiparastc, undet, sqla
		T38.ØX4S	Poisoning by glucocort/synth analog, undetermined, sequela
		T38.1X4S	Poisoning by thyroid hormones and sub, undet, sequela
		T38.2X4S	Poisoning by antithyroid drugs, undetermined, sequela
		T38.3X4S	Poisn by insulin and oral hypoglycemic drugs, undet, sequela
		T38.4X4S	Poisoning by oral contraceptives, undetermined, sequela
		T38.5X4S	Poisoning by oth estrogens and progstrn, undet, sequela
		T38.6X4S	Poisn by antigonadtr/antiestr/antiandrg, NEC, undet, sequela
		T38.7X4S	Poisn by androgens and anabolic congeners, undet, sequela
		T38.8Ø4S	Poisoning by unsp hormones and synthetic sub, undet, sequela
		T38.814S	Poisoning by anterior pituitary hormones, undet, sequela
		T38.894S	Poisoning by oth hormones and synthetic sub, undet, sequela

(Continued on next page)

ICD-9-CM		ICD-10-CM	
E989	LATE EFF INJURY UNDET ACC/PRPOSLY INFLICTED (Continued)	T38.9Ø4S	Poisoning by unsp hormone antagonists, undetermined, sequela
		T38.994S	Poisoning by oth hormone antagonists, undetermined, sequela
		T39.Ø14S	Poisoning by aspirin, undetermined, sequela
		T39.Ø94S	Poisoning by salicylates, undetermined, sequela
		T39.1X4S	Poisoning by 4-Aminophenol derivatives, undet, sequela
		T39.2X4S	Poisoning by pyrazolone derivatives, undetermined, sequela
		T39.314S	Poisoning by propionic acid derivatives, undet, sequela
		T39.394S	Poisn by oth nonsteroid anti-inflam drugs, undet, sequela
		T39.4X4S	Poisoning by antirheumatics, NEC, undetermined, sequela
		T39.8X4S	Poisn by oth nonopio analges/antipyret, NEC, undet, sequela
		T39.94XS	Poisn by unsp nonopi analgs/antipyr/antirheu, undet, sequela
		T4Ø.ØX4S	Poisoning by opium, undetermined, sequela
		T4Ø.1X4S	Poisoning by heroin, undetermined, sequela
		T4Ø.2X4S	Poisoning by other opioids, undetermined, sequela
		T4Ø.3X4S	Poisoning by methadone, undetermined, sequela
		T4Ø.4X4S	Poisoning by oth synthetic narcotics, undetermined, sequela
		T4Ø.5X4S	Poisoning by cocaine, undetermined, sequela
		T4Ø.6Ø4S	Poisoning by unspecified narcotics, undetermined, sequela
		T4Ø.694S	Poisoning by other narcotics, undetermined, sequela
		T4Ø.7X4S	Poisoning by cannabis (derivatives), undetermined, sequela
		T4Ø.8X4S	Poisoning by lysergide [LSD], undetermined, sequela
		T4Ø.9Ø4S	Poisoning by unsp psychodysleptics, undetermined, sequela
		T4Ø.994S	Poisoning by other psychodysleptics, undetermined, sequela
		T41.ØX4S	Poisoning by inhaled anesthetics, undetermined, sequela
		T41.1X4S	Poisoning by intravenous anesthetics, undetermined, sequela
		T41.2Ø4S	Poisoning by unsp general anesthetics, undetermined, sequela
		T41.294S	Poisoning by oth general anesthetics, undetermined, sequela
		T41.3X4S	Poisoning by local anesthetics, undetermined, sequela
		T41.44XS	Poisoning by unspecified anesthetic, undetermined, sequela
		T41.5X4S	Poisoning by therapeutic gases, undetermined, sequela
		T42.ØX4S	Poisoning by hydantoin derivatives, undetermined, sequela
		T42.1X4S	Poisoning by iminostilbenes, undetermined, sequela
		T42.2X4S	Poisn by succinimides and oxazolidinediones, undet, sequela
		T42.3X4S	Poisoning by barbiturates, undetermined, sequela
		T42.4X4S	Poisoning by benzodiazepines, undetermined, sequela
		T42.5X4S	Poisoning by mixed antiepileptics, undetermined, sequela
		T42.6X4S	Poisn by oth antieplptc and sed-hypntc drugs, undet, sequela
		T42.74XS	Poisn by unsp antieplptc and sed-hypntc drugs, undet, sqla
		T42.8X4S	Poisn by antiparkns drug/centr musc-tone depr, undet, sqla
		T43.Ø14S	Poisoning by tricyclic antidepress, undetermined, sequela
		T43.Ø24S	Poisoning by tetracyclic antidepress, undetermined, sequela
		T43.1X4S	Poisoning by MAO inhib antidepress, undetermined, sequela
		T43.2Ø4S	Poisoning by unsp antidepressants, undetermined, sequela
		T43.214S	Poisn by slctv seroton/norepineph reup inhibtr, undet, sqla
		T43.224S	Poisn by slctv serotonin reuptake inhibtr, undet, sequela
		T43.294S	Poisoning by other antidepressants, undetermined, sequela
		T43.3X4S	Poisn by phenothiaz antipsychot/neurolept, undet, sequela
		T43.4X4S	Poisn by butyrophen/thiothixen neuroleptc, undet, sequela
		T43.5Ø4S	Poisoning by unsp antipsychot/neurolept, undet, sequela
		T43.594S	Poisoning by oth antipsychot/neurolept, undet, sequela
		T43.6Ø4S	Poisoning by unsp psychostimulants, undetermined, sequela
		T43.614S	Poisoning by caffeine, undetermined, sequela
		T43.624S	Poisoning by amphetamines, undetermined, sequela
		T43.634S	Poisoning by methylphenidate, undetermined, sequela
		T43.694S	Poisoning by other psychostimulants, undetermined, sequela
		T43.8X4S	Poisoning by other psychotropic drugs, undetermined, sequela
		T43.94XS	Poisoning by unsp psychotropic drug, undetermined, sequela
		T44.ØX4S	Poisoning by anticholin agents, undetermined, sequela
		T44.1X4S	Poisoning by oth parasympathomimetics, undetermined, sequela
		T44.2X4S	Poisoning by ganglionic blocking drugs, undet, sequela
		T44.3X4S	Poisn by oth parasympath and spasmolytics, undet, sequela
		T44.4X4S	Poisoning by predom alpha-adrenocpt agonists, undet, sequela
		T44.5X4S	Poisoning by predom beta-adrenocpt agonists, undet, sequela
		T44.6X4S	Poisoning by alpha-adrenocpt antagonists, undet, sequela
		T44.7X4S	Poisoning by beta-adrenocpt antagonists, undet, sequela
		T44.8X4S	Poisn by centr-acting/adren-neurn-block agnt, undet, sequela
		T44.9Ø4S	Poisn by unsp drugs aff the autonm nrv sys, undet, sequela
		T44.994S	Poisn by oth drug aff the autonm nervous sys, undet, sequela
		T45.ØX4S	Poisoning by antiallerg/antiemetic, undetermined, sequela
		T45.1X4S	Poisoning by antineopl and immunosup drugs, undet, sequela
		T45.2X4S	Poisoning by vitamins, undetermined, sequela
		T45.3X4S	Poisoning by enzymes, undetermined, sequela
		T45.4X4S	Poisoning by iron and its compounds, undetermined, sequela
		T45.514S	Poisoning by anticoagulants, undetermined, sequela
		T45.524S	Poisoning by antithrombotic drugs, undetermined, sequela
		T45.6Ø4S	Poisoning by unsp fibrin-affct drugs, undetermined, sequela
		T45.614S	Poisoning by thrombolytic drug, undetermined, sequela
		T45.624S	Poisoning by hemostatic drug, undetermined, sequela
	(Continued on next page)	T45.694S	Poisoning by oth fibrin-affct drugs, undetermined, sequela

ICD-9-CM		ICD-10-CM	
E989	LATE EFF INJURY UNDET ACC/PRPOSLY INFLICTED **(Continued)**	**T45.7X4S**	Poisn by anticoag antag, vit K and oth coag, undet, sequela
		T45.8X4S	Poisn by oth prim sys and hematolog agents, undet, sequela
		T45.94XS	Poisn by unsp prim sys and hematolog agent, undet, sequela
		T46.ØX4S	Poisn by cardi-stim glycos/drug simlar act, undet, sequela
		T46.1X4S	Poisoning by calcium-channel blockers, undetermined, sequela
		T46.2X4S	Poisoning by oth antidysrhy drugs, undetermined, sequela
		T46.3X4S	Poisoning by coronary vasodilators, undetermined, sequela
		T46.4X4S	Poisn by angiotens-convert-enzyme inhibtr, undet, sequela
		T46.5X4S	Poisoning by oth antihypertn drugs, undetermined, sequela
		T46.6X4S	Poisn by antihyperlip and antiarterio drugs, undet, sequela
		T46.7X4S	Poisoning by peripheral vasodilators, undetermined, sequela
		T46.8X4S	Poisn by antivaric drugs, inc scler agents, undet, sequela
		T46.9Ø4S	Poisn by unsp agents aff the cardiovasc sys, undet, sequela
		T46.994S	Poisn by oth agents aff the cardiovasc sys, undet, sequela
		T47.ØX4S	Poisoning by histamine H2-receptor blockers, undet, sequela
		T47.1X4S	Poisn by oth antacids and anti-gstrc-sec drugs, undet, sqla
		T47.2X4S	Poisoning by stimulant laxatives, undetermined, sequela
		T47.3X4S	Poisoning by saline and osmotic laxatives, undet, sequela
		T47.4X4S	Poisoning by other laxatives, undetermined, sequela
		T47.5X4S	Poisoning by digestants, undetermined, sequela
		T47.6X4S	Poisoning by antidiarrheal drugs, undetermined, sequela
		T47.7X4S	Poisoning by emetics, undetermined, sequela
		T47.8X4S	Poisoning by oth agents aff GI sys, undetermined, sequela
		T47.94XS	Poisoning by unsp agents aff the GI sys, undet, sequela
		T48.ØX4S	Poisoning by oxytocic drugs, undetermined, sequela
		T48.1X4S	Poisoning by skeletal muscle relaxants, undet, sequela
		T48.2Ø4S	Poisoning by unsp drugs acting on muscles, undet, sequela
		T48.294S	Poisoning by oth drugs acting on muscles, undet, sequela
		T48.3X4S	Poisoning by antitussives, undetermined, sequela
		T48.4X4S	Poisoning by expectorants, undetermined, sequela
		T48.5X4S	Poisoning by oth anti-cmn-cold drugs, undetermined, sequela
		T48.6X4S	Poisoning by antiasthmatics, undetermined, sequela
		T48.9Ø4S	Poisn by unsp agents prim act on the resp sys, undet, sqla
		T48.994S	Poisn by oth agents prim acting on the resp sys, undet, sqla
		T49.ØX4S	Poisn by local antifung/infect/inflamm drugs, undet, sequela
		T49.1X4S	Poisoning by antipruritics, undetermined, sequela
		T49.2X4S	Poisoning by local astringents/detergents, undet, sequela
		T49.3X4S	Poisn by emollients, demulcents and protect, undet, sequela
		T49.4X4S	Poisn by keratolyt/keratplst/hair trmt drug, undet, sequela
		T49.5X4S	Poisoning by opth drugs and prep, undetermined, sequela
		T49.6X4S	Poisoning by otorhino drugs and prep, undetermined, sequela
		T49.7X4S	Poisoning by dental drugs, topically applied, undet, sequela
		T49.8X4S	Poisoning by other topical agents, undetermined, sequela
		T49.94XS	Poisoning by unsp topical agent, undetermined, sequela
		T5Ø.ØX4S	Poisoning by mineralocorticoids and antag, undet, sequela
		T5Ø.1X4S	Poisoning by loop diuretics, undetermined, sequela
		T5Ø.2X4S	Poisn by crbnc-anhydr inhibtr,benzo/oth diuretc, undet, sqla
		T5Ø.3X4S	Poisn by electrolytic/caloric/wtr-bal agnt, undet, sequela
		T5Ø.4X4S	Poisoning by drugs affecting uric acid metab, undet, sequela
		T5Ø.5X4S	Poisoning by appetite depressants, undetermined, sequela
		T5Ø.6X4S	Poisoning by antidotes and chelating agents, undet, sequela
		T5Ø.7X4S	Poisn by analeptics and opioid receptor antag, undet, sqla
		T5Ø.8X4S	Poisoning by diagnostic agents, undetermined, sequela
		T5Ø.9Ø4S	Poisoning by unsp drug/meds/biol subst, undet, sequela
		T5Ø.994S	Poisoning by oth drug/meds/biol subst, undetermined, sequela
		T5Ø.A14S	Poisn by pertuss vaccine, inc combin w pertuss, undet, sqla
		T5Ø.A24S	Poisn by mixed bact vaccines w/o a pertuss, undet, sequela
		T5Ø.A94S	Poisoning by other bacterial vaccines, undetermined, sequela
		T5Ø.B14S	Poisoning by smallpox vaccines, undetermined, sequela
		T5Ø.B94S	Poisoning by other viral vaccines, undetermined, sequela
		T5Ø.Z14S	Poisoning by immunoglobulin, undetermined, sequela
		T5Ø.Z94S	Poisoning by oth vaccines and biolg substnc, undet, sequela
		T6Ø.ØX4S	Toxic effect of organophos and carbamate insect, undet, sqla
		T6Ø.1X4S	Toxic effect of halogenated insect, undetermined, sequela
		T6Ø.2X4S	Toxic effect of other insecticides, undetermined, sequela
		T6Ø.3X4S	Toxic effect of herbicides and fungicides, undet, sequela
		T6Ø.4X4S	Toxic effect of rodenticides, undetermined, sequela
		T6Ø.8X4S	Toxic effect of other pesticides, undetermined, sequela
		T6Ø.94XS	Toxic effect of unspecified pesticide, undetermined, sequela
		T61.Ø4XS	Ciguatera fish poisoning, undetermined, sequela
		T61.14XS	Scombroid fish poisoning, undetermined, sequela
		T61.774S	Other fish poisoning, undetermined, sequela
		T61.784S	Other shellfish poisoning, undetermined, sequela
		T61.8X4S	Toxic effect of other seafood, undetermined, sequela
		T61.94XS	Toxic effect of unspecified seafood, undetermined, sequela
		T62.ØX4S	Toxic effect of ingested mushrooms, undetermined, sequela
		T62.1X4S	Toxic effect of ingested berries, undetermined, sequela
		T62.2X4S	Toxic effect of ingested (parts of) plant(s), undet, sequela
	(Continued on next page)	**T62.8X4S**	Toxic effect of noxious substnc eaten as food, undet, sqla

ICD-9-CM		ICD-10-CM	
E989	LATE EFF INJURY UNDET ACC/PRPOSLY INFLICTED **(Continued)**	**T62.94XS**	Toxic effect of unsp noxious sub eaten as food, undet, sqla
		T63.001S	Toxic effect of unsp snake venom, accidental, sequela
		T63.014S	Toxic effect of rattlesnake venom, undetermined, sequela
		T63.024S	Toxic effect of coral snake venom, undetermined, sequela
		T63.034S	Toxic effect of taipan venom, undetermined, sequela
		T63.044S	Toxic effect of cobra venom, undetermined, sequela
		T63.064S	Toxic effect of venom of N & S American snake, undet, sqla
		T63.074S	Toxic effect of venom of Australian snake, undet, sequela
		T63.084S	Toxic eff of venom of African and Asian snake, undet, sqla
		T63.094S	Toxic effect of venom of other snake, undetermined, sequela
		T63.114S	Toxic effect of venom of gila monster, undetermined, sequela
		T63.124S	Toxic effect of venom of venomous lizard, undet, sequela
		T63.194S	Toxic effect of venom of oth reptiles, undetermined, sequela
		T63.2X4S	Toxic effect of venom of scorpion, undetermined, sequela
		T63.304S	Toxic effect of unsp spider venom, undetermined, sequela
		T63.314S	Toxic effect of venom of black widow spider, undet, sequela
		T63.324S	Toxic effect of venom of tarantula, undetermined, sequela
		T63.334S	Toxic effect of venom of brown recluse spider, undet, sqla
		T63.394S	Toxic effect of venom of other spider, undetermined, sequela
		T63.414S	Toxic effect of venom of centipede/millipede, undet, sequela
		T63.424S	Toxic effect of venom of ants, undetermined, sequela
		T63.434S	Toxic effect of venom of caterpillars, undetermined, sequela
		T63.444S	Toxic effect of venom of bees, undetermined, sequela
		T63.454S	Toxic effect of venom of hornets, undetermined, sequela
		T63.464S	Toxic effect of venom of wasps, undetermined, sequela
		T63.484S	Toxic effect of venom of arthropod, undetermined, sequela
		T63.514S	Toxic effect of contact with stingray, undetermined, sequela
		T63.594S	Toxic effect of contact w oth venomous fish, undet, sequela
		T63.614S	Toxic effect of cntct w Portugese Man-o-war, undet, sequela
		T63.624S	Toxic effect of contact w oth jellyfish, undet, sequela
		T63.634S	Toxic effect of contact w sea anemone, undetermined, sequela
		T63.694S	Toxic eff of cntct w oth venom marine animals, undet, sqla
		T63.714S	Toxic effect of contact w venom marine plant, undet, sequela
		T63.794S	Toxic effect of contact w oth venomous plant, undet, sequela
		T63.814S	Toxic effect of contact w venomous frog, undet, sequela
		T63.824S	Toxic effect of contact w venomous toad, undet, sequela
		T63.834S	Toxic effect of contact w oth venom amphib, undet, sequela
		T63.894S	Toxic effect of contact w oth venom animals, undet, sequela
		T63.94XS	Toxic effect of contact w unsp venom animal, undet, sequela
		T64.04XS	Toxic effect of aflatoxin, undetermined, sequela
		T64.84XS	Toxic effect of mycotoxin food contamnt, undet, sequela
		T65.0X4S	Toxic effect of cyanides, undetermined, sequela
		T65.1X4S	Toxic effect of strychnine and its salts, undet, sequela
		T65.214S	Toxic effect of chewing tobacco, undetermined, sequela
		T65.224S	Toxic effect of tobacco cigarettes, undetermined, sequela
		T65.294S	Toxic effect of tobacco and nicotine, undetermined, sequela
		T65.3X4S	Toxic eff of nitrodrv/aminodrv of benzn/homolog, undet, sqla
		T65.4X4S	Toxic effect of carbon disulfide, undetermined, sequela
		T65.5X4S	Tox eff of nitro & oth nitric acids and esters, undet, sqla
		T65.6X4S	Toxic effect of paints and dyes, NEC, undetermined, sequela
		T65.814S	Toxic effect of latex, undetermined, sequela
		T65.824S	Toxic effect of harmful algae and algae toxins, undet, sqla
		T65.834S	Toxic effect of fiberglass, undetermined, sequela
		T65.894S	Toxic effect of oth substances, undetermined, sequela
		T65.94XS	Toxic effect of unspecified substance, undetermined, sequela
		T71.164S	Asphyxiation due to hanging, undetermined, sequela
E990.0	INJURY DUE TO WAR OPERATIONS FROM GASOLINE BOMB	**Y36.310A**	War operations involving gasoline bomb, milt, init
		Y36.310D	War operations involving gasoline bomb, milt, subs
		Y36.311A	War operations involving gasoline bomb, civilian, init
		Y36.311D	War operations involving gasoline bomb, civilian, subs
		Y37.310A	Milt op involving gasoline bomb, military personnel, init
		Y37.310D	Milt op involving gasoline bomb, military personnel, subs
		Y37.311A	Military operations involving gasoline bomb, civilian, init
		Y37.311D	Military operations involving gasoline bomb, civilian, subs
E990.1	INJURY DUE TO WAR OPERATIONS FROM FLAMETHROWER	**Y36.330A**	War operations involving flamethrower, milt, init
		Y36.330D	War operations involving flamethrower, milt, subs
		Y36.331A	War operations involving flamethrower, civilian, init encntr
		Y36.331D	War operations involving flamethrower, civilian, subs encntr
		Y37.330A	Milt op involving flamethrower, military personnel, init
		Y37.330D	Milt op involving flamethrower, military personnel, subs
		Y37.331A	Military operations involving flamethrower, civilian, init
		Y37.331D	Military operations involving flamethrower, civilian, subs
E990.2	INJURY DUE WAR OPERATIONS FROM INCENDIARY BULLET	**Y36.320A**	War operations involving incendiary bullet, milt, init
		Y36.320D	War operations involving incendiary bullet, milt, subs
		Y36.321A	War operations involving incendiary bullet, civilian, init
		Y36.321D	War operations involving incendiary bullet, civilian, subs
		Y37.320A	Milt op involving incendiary bullet, milt, init
		Y37.320D	Milt op involving incendiary bullet, milt, subs
		Y37.321A	Milt op involving incendiary bullet, civilian, init
		Y37.321D	Milt op involving incendiary bullet, civilian, subs

ICD-9-CM		ICD-10-CM	
E99Ø.3	INJ DUE WAR OP FIRE INDIRCTLY CONVENTIONL WEAPON	**Y36.39ØA**	War operations involving oth fire/hot subst, milt, init
		Y36.39ØD	War operations involving oth fire/hot subst, milt, subs
		Y36.391A	War operations involving oth fire/hot subst, civilian, init
		Y36.391D	War operations involving oth fire/hot subst, civilian, subs
		Y37.39ØA	Milt op involving oth fire/hot subst, milt, init
		Y37.39ØD	Milt op involving oth fire/hot subst, milt, subs
		Y37.391A	Milt op involving oth fire/hot subst, civilian, init
		Y37.391D	Milt op involving oth fire/hot subst, civilian, subs
E99Ø.9	INJURY DUE WAR OPERATIONS FROM OTH&UNSPEC SOURCE	**Y36.3ØØA**	War op involving unsp fire/conflagr/hot subst, milt, init
		Y36.3ØØD	War op involving unsp fire/conflagr/hot subst, milt, subs
		Y36.3Ø1A	War op w unsp fire/conflagr/hot subst, civilian, init
		Y36.3Ø1D	War op w unsp fire/conflagr/hot subst, civilian, subs
		Y36.9ØXA	War operations, unspecified, initial encounter
		Y36.9ØXD	War operations, unspecified, subsequent encounter
		Y36.92XA	War operations involving friendly fire, initial encounter
		Y36.92XD	War operations involving friendly fire, subsequent encounter
		Y37.3ØØA	Milt op involving unsp fire/conflagr/hot subst, milt, init
		Y37.3ØØD	Milt op involving unsp fire/conflagr/hot subst, milt, subs
		Y37.3Ø1A	Milt op w unsp fire/conflagr/hot subst, civilian, init
		Y37.3Ø1D	Milt op w unsp fire/conflagr/hot subst, civilian, subs
		Y37.9ØXA	Military operations, unspecified, initial encounter
		Y37.9ØXD	Military operations, unspecified, subsequent encounter
		Y37.92XA	Military operations involving friendly fire, init encntr
		Y37.92XD	Military operations involving friendly fire, subs encntr
E991.Ø	INJURY DUE TO WAR OPERATIONS FROM RUBBER BULLETS	**Y36.41ØA**	War operations involving rubber bullets, milt, init
		Y36.41ØD	War operations involving rubber bullets, milt, subs
		Y36.411A	War operations involving rubber bullets, civilian, init
		Y36.411D	War operations involving rubber bullets, civilian, subs
		Y37.41ØA	Milt op involving rubber bullets, military personnel, init
		Y37.41ØD	Milt op involving rubber bullets, military personnel, subs
		Y37.411A	Military operations involving rubber bullets, civilian, init
		Y37.411D	Military operations involving rubber bullets, civilian, subs
E991.1	INJURY DUE TO WAR OPERATIONS FROM PELLETS	**Y36.42ØA**	War operations involving firearms pellets, milt, init
		Y36.42ØD	War operations involving firearms pellets, milt, subs
		Y36.421A	War operations involving firearms pellets, civilian, init
		Y36.421D	War operations involving firearms pellets, civilian, subs
		Y37.42ØA	Milt op involving firearms pellets, military personnel, init
		Y37.42ØD	Milt op involving firearms pellets, military personnel, subs
		Y37.421A	Milt op involving firearms pellets, civilian, init
		Y37.421D	Milt op involving firearms pellets, civilian, subs
E991.2	INJURY DUE TO WAR OPERATIONS FROM OTHER BULLETS	**Y36.43ØA**	War operations involving oth firearms discharge, milt, init
		Y36.43ØD	War operations involving oth firearms discharge, milt, subs
		Y36.431A	War op involving oth firearms discharge, civilian, init
		Y36.431D	War op involving oth firearms discharge, civilian, subs
		Y37.43ØA	Milt op involving oth firearms discharge, milt, init
		Y37.43ØD	Milt op involving oth firearms discharge, milt, subs
		Y37.431A	Milt op involving oth firearms discharge, civilian, init
		Y37.431D	Milt op involving oth firearms discharge, civilian, subs
E991.3	INJURY DUE WAR OP FROM ANTIPERSONNEL BOMB	**Y36.29ØA**	War op involving oth explosn and fragments, milt, init
		Y36.29ØD	War op involving oth explosn and fragments, milt, subs
		Y36.291A	War op involving oth explosn and fragments, civilian, init
		Y36.291D	War op involving oth explosn and fragments, civilian, subs
E991.4	INJURY DUE TO WAR OP BY FRAGMENTS FROM MUNITIONS	**Y36.25ØA**	War op involving fragments from munitions, milt, init
		Y36.25ØD	War op involving fragments from munitions, milt, subs
		Y36.251A	War op involving fragments from munitions, civilian, init
		Y36.251D	War op involving fragments from munitions, civilian, subs
		Y37.25ØA	Milt op involving fragments from munitions, milt, init
		Y37.25ØD	Milt op involving fragments from munitions, milt, subs
		Y37.251A	Milt op involving fragments from munitions, civilian, init
		Y37.251D	Milt op involving fragments from munitions, civilian, subs
E991.5	INJ DUE WAR OP FRAGMENTS FROM PERSON-BORNE IED	**Y36.26ØA**	War op involving fragmt of improv explosv device, milt, init
		Y36.26ØD	War op involving fragmt of improv explosv device, milt, subs
		Y36.261A	War op w fragmt of improv explosv device, civilian, init
		Y36.261D	War op w fragmt of improv explosv device, civilian, subs
		Y37.26ØA	Milt op w fragmt of improv explosv device, milt, init
		Y37.26ØD	Milt op w fragmt of improv explosv device, milt, subs
		Y37.261A	Milt op w fragmt of improv explosv device, civilian, init
		Y37.261D	Milt op w fragmt of improv explosv device, civilian, subs
E991.6	INJ DUE WAR OP FRAGMENTS FROM VEHICLE-BORNE IED	**Y36.26ØA**	War op involving fragmt of improv explosv device, milt, init
		Y36.26ØD	War op involving fragmt of improv explosv device, milt, subs
		Y36.261A	War op w fragmt of improv explosv device, civilian, init
		Y36.261D	War op w fragmt of improv explosv device, civilian, subs
		Y37.26ØA	Milt op w fragmt of improv explosv device, milt, init
		Y37.26ØD	Milt op w fragmt of improv explosv device, milt, subs
		Y37.261A	Milt op w fragmt of improv explosv device, civilian, init
		Y37.261D	Milt op w fragmt of improv explosv device, civilian, subs

ICD-9-CM		ICD-10-CM	
E991.7	INJURY DUE WAR OP FRAGMENTS FROM OTHER IED	**Y36.26ØA**	War op involving fragmt of improv explosv device, milt, init
		Y36.26ØD	War op involving fragmt of improv explosv device, milt, subs
		Y36.261A	War op w fragmt of improv explosv device, civilian, init
		Y36.261D	War op w fragmt of improv explosv device, civilian, subs
		Y37.26ØA	Milt op w fragmt of improv explosv device, milt, init
		Y37.26ØD	Milt op w fragmt of improv explosv device, milt, subs
		Y37.261A	Milt op w fragmt of improv explosv device, civilian, init
		Y37.261D	Milt op w fragmt of improv explosv device, civilian, subs
E991.8	INJURY DUE WAR OPERATIONS FRAGMENTS FROM WEAPONS	**Y36.27ØA**	War operations involving fragments from weapons, milt, init
		Y36.27ØD	War operations involving fragments from weapons, milt, subs
		Y36.271A	War op involving fragments from weapons, civilian, init
		Y36.271D	War op involving fragments from weapons, civilian, subs
		Y37.27ØA	Milt op involving fragments from weapons, milt, init
		Y37.27ØD	Milt op involving fragments from weapons, milt, subs
		Y37.271A	Milt op involving fragments from weapons, civilian, init
		Y37.271D	Milt op involving fragments from weapons, civilian, subs
E991.9	INJURY DUE WAR OPERATIONS FROM OTH&UNSPEC FRAGS	**Y36.2ØØA**	War op involving unsp explosion and fragments, milt, init
		Y36.2ØØD	War op involving unsp explosion and fragments, milt, subs
		Y36.2Ø1A	War op involving unsp explosn and fragments, civilian, init
		Y36.2Ø1D	War op involving unsp explosn and fragments, civilian, subs
E992.Ø	INJURY WAR OP EXPL DUE TO TORPEDO	**Y36.Ø4ØA**	War operations involving explosion of torpedo, milt, init
		Y36.Ø4ØD	War operations involving explosion of torpedo, milt, subs
		Y36.Ø41A	War op involving explosion of torpedo, civilian, init
		Y36.Ø41D	War op involving explosion of torpedo, civilian, subs
		Y37.Ø4ØA	Milt op involving explosion of torpedo, milt, init
		Y37.Ø4ØD	Milt op involving explosion of torpedo, milt, subs
		Y37.Ø41A	Milt op involving explosion of torpedo, civilian, init
		Y37.Ø41D	Milt op involving explosion of torpedo, civilian, subs
E992.1	INJURY WAR OPER DUE TO DEPTH CHARGE	**Y36.Ø1ØA**	War operations involving explosion of depth-chg, milt, init
		Y36.Ø1ØD	War operations involving explosion of depth-chg, milt, subs
		Y36.Ø11A	War op involving explosion of depth-chg, civilian, init
		Y36.Ø11D	War op involving explosion of depth-chg, civilian, subs
		Y37.Ø1ØA	Milt op involving explosion of depth-charge, milt, init
		Y37.Ø1ØD	Milt op involving explosion of depth-charge, milt, subs
		Y37.Ø11A	Milt op involving explosion of depth-charge, civilian, init
		Y37.Ø11D	Milt op involving explosion of depth-charge, civilian, subs
E992.2	INJURY DUE TO WAR OPERATIONS - MARINE MINES	**Y36.Ø2ØA**	War op involving explosion of marine mine, milt, init
		Y36.Ø2ØD	War op involving explosion of marine mine, milt, subs
		Y36.Ø21A	War op involving explosion of marine mine, civilian, init
		Y36.Ø21D	War op involving explosion of marine mine, civilian, subs
		Y37.Ø2ØA	Milt op involving explosion of marine mine, milt, init
		Y37.Ø2ØD	Milt op involving explosion of marine mine, milt, subs
		Y37.Ø21A	Milt op involving explosion of marine mine, civilian, init
		Y37.Ø21D	Milt op involving explosion of marine mine, civilian, subs
E992.3	INJURY DUE TO WAR OPS SEA-BASED ARTILLERY SHELL	**Y36.Ø3ØA**	War op w explosn of sea-based artlry shell, milt, init
		Y36.Ø3ØD	War op w explosn of sea-based artlry shell, milt, subs
		Y36.Ø31A	War op w explosn of sea-based artlry shell, civilian, init
		Y36.Ø31D	War op w explosn of sea-based artlry shell, civilian, subs
		Y37.Ø3ØA	Milt op w explosn of sea-based artlry shell, milt, init
		Y37.Ø3ØD	Milt op w explosn of sea-based artlry shell, milt, subs
		Y37.Ø31A	Milt op w explosn of sea-based artlry shell, civilian, init
		Y37.Ø31D	Milt op w explosn of sea-based artlry shell, civilian, subs
E992.8	INJURY DUE TO WAR OPERATION OTHER MARINE WEAPONS	**Y36.Ø9ØA**	War op involving explosion of marine weapons, milt, init
		Y36.Ø9ØD	War op involving explosion of marine weapons, milt, subs
		Y36.Ø91A	War op involving explosion of marine weapons, civilian, init
		Y36.Ø91D	War op involving explosion of marine weapons, civilian, subs
		Y37.Ø9ØA	Milt op involving explosion of marine weapons, milt, init
		Y37.Ø9ØD	Milt op involving explosion of marine weapons, milt, subs
		Y37.Ø91A	Milt op involving explosn of marine weapons, civilian, init
		Y37.Ø91D	Milt op involving explosn of marine weapons, civilian, subs
E992.9	INJURY DUE TO WAR OPERATIONS UNS MARINE WEAPON	**Y36.ØØØA**	War op involving explosion of unsp marine weapon, milt, init
		Y36.ØØØD	War op involving explosion of unsp marine weapon, milt, subs
		Y36.ØØ1A	War op w explosn of unsp marine weapon, civilian, init
		Y36.ØØ1D	War op w explosn of unsp marine weapon, civilian, subs
		Y36.Ø5ØA	War op w acc deton onboard marine weapons, milt, init
		Y36.Ø5ØD	War op w acc deton onboard marine weapons, milt, subs
		Y36.Ø51A	War op w acc deton onboard marine weapons, civilian, init
		Y36.Ø51D	War op w acc deton onboard marine weapons, civilian, subs
		Y37.ØØØA	Milt op involving explosn of unsp marine weapon, milt, init
		Y37.ØØØD	Milt op involving explosn of unsp marine weapon, milt, subs
		Y37.ØØ1A	Milt op w explosn of unsp marine weapon, civilian, init
		Y37.ØØ1D	Milt op w explosn of unsp marine weapon, civilian, subs
		Y37.Ø5ØA	Milt op w acc deton onboard marine weapons, milt, init
		Y37.Ø5ØD	Milt op w acc deton onboard marine weapons, milt, subs
		Y37.Ø51A	Milt op w acc deton onboard marine weapons, civilian, init
		Y37.Ø51D	Milt op w acc deton onboard marine weapons, civilian, subs

ICD-9-CM		ICD-10-CM	
E993.Ø	INJURY DUE TO WAR OPERATIONS BY AERIAL BOMB	**Y36.21ØA**	War op involving explosion of aerial bomb, milt, init
		Y36.21ØD	War op involving explosion of aerial bomb, milt, subs
		Y36.211A	War op involving explosion of aerial bomb, civilian, init
		Y36.211D	War op involving explosion of aerial bomb, civilian, subs
		Y37.21ØA	Milt op involving explosion of aerial bomb, milt, init
		Y37.21ØD	Milt op involving explosion of aerial bomb, milt, subs
		Y37.211A	Milt op involving explosion of aerial bomb, civilian, init
		Y37.211D	Milt op involving explosion of aerial bomb, civilian, subs
E993.1	INJURY DUE TO WAR OPERATIONS BY GUIDED MISSILE	**Y36.22ØA**	War op involving explosion of guided missile, milt, init
		Y36.22ØD	War op involving explosion of guided missile, milt, subs
		Y36.221A	War op involving explosion of guided missile, civilian, init
		Y36.221D	War op involving explosion of guided missile, civilian, subs
		Y37.22ØA	Milt op involving explosion of guided missile, milt, init
		Y37.22ØD	Milt op involving explosion of guided missile, milt, subs
		Y37.221A	Milt op involving explosn of guided missile, civilian, init
		Y37.221D	Milt op involving explosn of guided missile, civilian, subs
E993.2	INJURY DUE TO WAR OPERATIONS BY MORTAR	**Y36.29ØA**	War op involving oth explosn and fragments, milt, init
		Y36.29ØD	War op involving oth explosn and fragments, milt, subs
		Y36.291A	War op involving oth explosn and fragments, civilian, init
		Y36.291D	War op involving oth explosn and fragments, civilian, subs
		Y37.29ØA	Milt op involving oth explosions and fragments, milt, init
		Y37.29ØD	Milt op involving oth explosions and fragments, milt, subs
		Y37.291A	Milt op involving oth explosn and fragments, civilian, init
		Y37.291D	Milt op involving oth explosn and fragments, civilian, subs
E993.3	INJURY DUE TO WAR OPERATIONS BY PERSON BORNE IED	**Y36.23ØA**	War op w explosn of improv explosv device, milt, init
		Y36.23ØD	War op w explosn of improv explosv device, milt, subs
		Y36.231A	War op w explosn of improv explosv device, civilian, init
		Y36.231D	War op w explosn of improv explosv device, civilian, subs
		Y37.23ØA	Milt op w explosn of improv explosv device, milt, init
		Y37.23ØD	Milt op w explosn of improv explosv device, milt, subs
		Y37.231A	Milt op w explosn of improv explosv device, civilian, init
		Y37.231D	Milt op w explosn of improv explosv device, civilian, subs
E993.4	INJURY DUE TO WAR OPERATION BY VEHICLE BORNE IED	**Y36.23ØA**	War op w explosn of improv explosv device, milt, init
		Y36.23ØD	War op w explosn of improv explosv device, milt, subs
		Y36.231A	War op w explosn of improv explosv device, civilian, init
		Y36.231D	War op w explosn of improv explosv device, civilian, subs
		Y37.23ØA	Milt op w explosn of improv explosv device, milt, init
		Y37.23ØD	Milt op w explosn of improv explosv device, milt, subs
		Y37.231A	Milt op w explosn of improv explosv device, civilian, init
		Y37.231D	Milt op w explosn of improv explosv device, civilian, subs
E993.5	INJURY DUE TO WAR OPERATIONS BY OTHER IED	**Y36.23ØA**	War op w explosn of improv explosv device, milt, init
		Y36.23ØD	War op w explosn of improv explosv device, milt, subs
		Y36.231A	War op w explosn of improv explosv device, civilian, init
		Y36.231D	War op w explosn of improv explosv device, civilian, subs
		Y37.23ØA	Milt op w explosn of improv explosv device, milt, init
		Y37.23ØD	Milt op w explosn of improv explosv device, milt, subs
		Y37.231A	Milt op w explosn of improv explosv device, civilian, init
		Y37.231D	Milt op w explosn of improv explosv device, civilian, subs
E993.6	INJ DUE WAR OP UNINTENTIONAL DET OWN MUNITIONS	**Y36.24ØA**	War op w explosn due to acc disch of own munit, milt, init
		Y36.24ØD	War op w explosn due to acc disch of own munit, milt, subs
		Y36.241A	War op w explosn due to acc disch of own munit, civ, init
		Y36.241D	War op w explosn due to acc disch of own munit, civ, subs
		Y37.24ØA	Milt op w explosn due to acc disch of own munit, milt, init
		Y37.24ØD	Milt op w explosn due to acc disch of own munit, milt, subs
		Y37.241A	Milt op w explosn due to acc disch of own munit, civ, init
		Y37.241D	Milt op w explosn due to acc disch of own munit, civ, subs
E993.7	INJ WAR OP UNINTENTIONL DISCHRG OWN LAUNCH DEVIC	**Y36.24ØA**	War op w explosn due to acc disch of own munit, milt, init
		Y36.24ØD	War op w explosn due to acc disch of own munit, milt, subs
		Y36.241A	War op w explosn due to acc disch of own munit, civ, init
		Y36.241D	War op w explosn due to acc disch of own munit, civ, subs
		Y37.24ØA	Milt op w explosn due to acc disch of own munit, milt, init
		Y37.24ØD	Milt op w explosn due to acc disch of own munit, milt, subs
		Y37.241A	Milt op w explosn due to acc disch of own munit, civ, init
		Y37.241D	Milt op w explosn due to acc disch of own munit, civ, subs
E993.8	INJURY DUE WAR OPERATIONS OTHER SPEC EXPLOSION	**Y36.29ØA**	War op involving oth explosn and fragments, milt, init
		Y36.29ØD	War op involving oth explosn and fragments, milt, subs
		Y36.291A	War op involving oth explosn and fragments, civilian, init
		Y36.291D	War op involving oth explosn and fragments, civilian, subs
		Y37.29ØA	Milt op involving oth explosions and fragments, milt, init
		Y37.29ØD	Milt op involving oth explosions and fragments, milt, subs
		Y37.291A	Milt op involving oth explosn and fragments, civilian, init
		Y37.291D	Milt op involving oth explosn and fragments, civilian, subs
E993.9	INJURY DUE WAR OPERATIONS UNSPECIFIED EXPLOSION	**Y36.2ØØA**	War op involving unsp explosion and fragments, milt, init
		Y36.2ØØD	War op involving unsp explosion and fragments, milt, subs
		Y36.2Ø1A	War op involving unsp explosn and fragments, civilian, init
		Y36.2Ø1D	War op involving unsp explosn and fragments, civilian, subs
		Y37.2ØØA	Milt op involving unsp explosion and fragments, milt, init
		Y37.2ØØD	Milt op involving unsp explosion and fragments, milt, subs
		Y37.2Ø1A	Milt op involving unsp explosn and fragments, civilian, init
		Y37.2Ø1D	Milt op involving unsp explosn and fragments, civilian, subs

ICD-9-CM		ICD-10-CM	
E994.Ø	INJ DUE WAR OP DESTRUCTN AIRCRAFT DUE ENEMY FIRE	**Y36.11ØA**	War op w dest arcrft due to enmy fire/expls, milt, init
		Y36.11ØD	War op w dest arcrft due to enmy fire/expls, milt, subs
		Y36.111A	War op w dest arcrft due to enmy fire/expls, civilian, init
		Y36.111D	War op w dest arcrft due to enmy fire/expls, civilian, subs
		Y37.11ØA	Milt op w dest arcrft due to enmy fire/expls, milt, init
		Y37.11ØD	Milt op w dest arcrft due to enmy fire/expls, milt, subs
		Y37.111A	Milt op w dest arcrft due to enmy fire/expls, civilian, init
		Y37.111D	Milt op w dest arcrft due to enmy fire/expls, civilian, subs
E994.1	INJ WAR OP DESTRUCTN AIRCRAFT ONBOARD EXPLOSION	**Y36.14ØA**	War op w dest arcrft d/t acc deton onbrd munit, milt, init
		Y36.14ØD	War op w dest arcrft d/t acc deton onbrd munit, milt, subs
		Y36.141A	War op w dest arcrft due to acc deton onbrd munit, civ, init
		Y36.141D	War op w dest arcrft due to acc deton onbrd munit, civ, subs
		Y37.14ØA	Milt op w dest arcrft d/t acc deton onbrd munit, milt, init
		Y37.14ØD	Milt op w dest arcrft d/t acc deton onbrd munit, milt, subs
		Y37.141A	Milt op w dest arcrft d/t acc deton onbrd munit, civ, init
		Y37.141D	Milt op w dest arcrft d/t acc deton onbrd munit, civ, subs
E994.2	INJ WAR DESTRUCT AIRCRAFT COLLISION OTH AIRCRAFT	**Y36.12ØA**	War op w dest arcrft due to clsn w oth aircraft, milt, init
		Y36.12ØD	War op w dest arcrft due to clsn w oth aircraft, milt, subs
		Y36.121A	War op w dest arcrft due to clsn w oth arcrft, civ, init
		Y36.121D	War op w dest arcrft due to clsn w oth arcrft, civ, subs
		Y37.12ØA	Milt op w dest arcrft due to clsn w oth aircraft, milt, init
		Y37.12ØD	Milt op w dest arcrft due to clsn w oth aircraft, milt, subs
		Y37.121A	Milt op w dest arcrft due to clsn w oth arcrft, civ, init
		Y37.121D	Milt op w dest arcrft due to clsn w oth arcrft, civ, subs
E994.3	INJURY WAR OP DESTRUCT AIRCRAFT DUE ONBOARD FIRE	**Y36.13ØA**	War op involving dest arcrft due to onboard fire, milt, init
		Y36.13ØD	War op involving dest arcrft due to onboard fire, milt, subs
		Y36.131A	War op w dest arcrft due to onboard fire, civilian, init
		Y36.131D	War op w dest arcrft due to onboard fire, civilian, subs
		Y37.13ØA	Milt op w dest arcrft due to onboard fire, milt, init
		Y37.13ØD	Milt op w dest arcrft due to onboard fire, milt, subs
		Y37.131A	Milt op w dest arcrft due to onboard fire, civilian, init
		Y37.131D	Milt op w dest arcrft due to onboard fire, civilian, subs
E994.8	INJURY DUE TO WAR OP OTHER DESTRUCTION AIRCRAFT	**Y36.19ØA**	War operations involving oth dest arcrft, milt, init
		Y36.19ØD	War operations involving oth dest arcrft, milt, subs
		Y36.191A	War operations involving oth dest arcrft, civilian, init
		Y36.191D	War operations involving oth dest arcrft, civilian, subs
		Y37.19ØA	Milt op involving oth dest arcrft, military personnel, init
		Y37.19ØD	Milt op involving oth dest arcrft, military personnel, subs
		Y37.191A	Milt op involving oth dest arcrft, civilian, init
		Y37.191D	Milt op involving oth dest arcrft, civilian, subs
E994.9	INJURY DUE TO WAR OP UNS DESTRUCTION AIRCRAFT	**Y36.1ØØA**	War operations involving unsp dest arcrft, milt, init
		Y36.1ØØD	War operations involving unsp dest arcrft, milt, subs
		Y36.1Ø1A	War operations involving unsp dest arcrft, civilian, init
		Y36.1Ø1D	War operations involving unsp dest arcrft, civilian, subs
		Y37.1ØØA	Milt op involving unsp dest arcrft, military personnel, init
		Y37.1ØØD	Milt op involving unsp dest arcrft, military personnel, subs
		Y37.1Ø1A	Milt op involving unsp dest arcrft, civilian, init
		Y37.1Ø1D	Milt op involving unsp dest arcrft, civilian, subs
E995.Ø	INJURY DUE TO WAR OP UNARMED HAND-TO-HAND COMBAT	**Y36.44ØA**	War op involving unarmed hand to hand combat, milt, init
		Y36.44ØD	War op involving unarmed hand to hand combat, milt, subs
		Y36.441A	War op involving unarmed hand to hand combat, civilian, init
		Y36.441D	War op involving unarmed hand to hand combat, civilian, subs
		Y37.44ØA	Milt op involving unarmed hand to hand combat, milt, init
		Y37.44ØD	Milt op involving unarmed hand to hand combat, milt, subs
		Y37.441A	Milt op w unarmed hand to hand combat, civilian, init
		Y37.441D	Milt op w unarmed hand to hand combat, civilian, subs
E995.1	INJURY DUE WAR OPERATIONS STRUCK BLUNT OBJECT	**Y36.45ØA**	War op involving combat using blunt/pierc object, milt, init
		Y36.45ØD	War op involving combat using blunt/pierc object, milt, subs
		Y36.451A	War op w combat using blunt/pierc object, civilian, init
		Y36.451D	War op w combat using blunt/pierc object, civilian, subs
		Y37.45ØA	Milt op w combat using blunt/pierc object, milt, init
		Y37.45ØD	Milt op w combat using blunt/pierc object, milt, subs
		Y37.451A	Milt op w combat using blunt/pierc object, civilian, init
		Y37.451D	Milt op w combat using blunt/pierc object, civilian, subs
E995.2	INJURY DUE TO WAR OPERATIONS BY PIERCING OBJECT	**Y36.45ØA**	War op involving combat using blunt/pierc object, milt, init
		Y36.45ØD	War op involving combat using blunt/pierc object, milt, subs
		Y36.451A	War op w combat using blunt/pierc object, civilian, init
		Y36.451D	War op w combat using blunt/pierc object, civilian, subs
		Y37.45ØA	Milt op w combat using blunt/pierc object, milt, init
		Y37.45ØD	Milt op w combat using blunt/pierc object, milt, subs
		Y37.451A	Milt op w combat using blunt/pierc object, civilian, init
		Y37.451D	Milt op w combat using blunt/pierc object, civilian, subs
E995.3	INJ DUE WAR OP INTENTIONAL RESTRICT AIR & AIRWAY	**Y36.46ØA**	War op involving intentl restrict of air/airwy, milt, init
		Y36.46ØD	War op involving intentl restrict of air/airwy, milt, subs
		Y36.461A	War op w intentl restrict of air/airwy, civilian, init
		Y36.461D	War op w intentl restrict of air/airwy, civilian, subs
		Y37.46ØA	Milt op involving intentl restrict of air/airwy, milt, init
		Y37.46ØD	Milt op involving intentl restrict of air/airwy, milt, subs
		Y37.461A	Milt op w intentl restrict of air/airwy, civilian, init
		Y37.461D	Milt op w intentl restrict of air/airwy, civilian, subs

ICD-9-CM		ICD-10-CM	
E995.4	INJ WAR OP UNINTENTIONAL DROWN INABILITY SURFACE	**Y36.47ØA**	War op involving unintent restrict of air/airwy, milt, init
		Y36.47ØD	War op involving unintent restrict of air/airwy, milt, subs
		Y36.471A	War op w unintent restrict of air/airwy, civilian, init
		Y36.471D	War op w unintent restrict of air/airwy, civilian, subs
		Y37.47ØA	Milt op involving unintent restrict of air/airwy, milt, init
		Y37.47ØD	Milt op involving unintent restrict of air/airwy, milt, subs
		Y37.471A	Milt op w unintent restrict of air/airwy, civilian, init
		Y37.471D	Milt op w unintent restrict of air/airwy, civilian, subs
E995.8	INJURY DUE WAR OP OTH FORM CONVENTIONAL WARFARE	**Y36.49ØA**	War operations involving oth conventl warfare, milt, init
		Y36.49ØD	War operations involving oth conventl warfare, milt, subs
		Y36.491A	War op involving oth conventl warfare, civilian, init
		Y36.491D	War op involving oth conventl warfare, civilian, subs
		Y37.49ØA	Milt op involving oth conventional warfare, milt, init
		Y37.49ØD	Milt op involving oth conventional warfare, milt, subs
		Y37.491A	Milt op involving oth conventional warfare, civilian, init
E995.9	INJURY DUE WAR OP UNS FORM CONVENTIONAL WARFARE	**Y36.49ØA**	War operations involving oth conventl warfare, milt, init
		Y36.49ØD	War operations involving oth conventl warfare, milt, subs
		Y36.491A	War op involving oth conventl warfare, civilian, init
		Y36.491D	War op involving oth conventl warfare, civilian, subs
		Y37.49ØA	Milt op involving oth conventional warfare, milt, init
		Y37.49ØD	Milt op involving oth conventional warfare, milt, subs
		Y37.491D	Milt op involving oth conventional warfare, civilian, subs
E996.Ø	INJ DUE WAR OP DIRCT BLAST EFFECT NUCLEAR WEAPON	**Y36.51ØA**	War op w direct blast effect of nuclear weapon, milt, init
		Y36.51ØD	War op w direct blast effect of nuclear weapon, milt, subs
		Y36.511A	War op w direct blast effect of nuclear weapon, civ, init
		Y36.511D	War op w direct blast effect of nuclear weapon, civ, subs
		Y37.51ØA	Milt op w direct blast effect of nuclear weapon, milt, init
		Y37.51ØD	Milt op w direct blast effect of nuclear weapon, milt, subs
		Y37.511A	Milt op w direct blast effect of nuclear weapon, civ, init
		Y37.511D	Milt op w direct blast effect of nuclear weapon, civ, subs
E996.1	INJ WAR OP INDIRECT BLAST EFFECT NUCLEAR WEAPON	**Y36.52ØA**	War op w indirect blast effect of nuclear weapon, milt, init
		Y36.52ØD	War op w indirect blast effect of nuclear weapon, milt, subs
		Y36.521A	War op w indirect blast effect of nuclear weapon, civ, init
		Y36.521D	War op w indirect blast effect of nuclear weapon, civ, subs
		Y37.52ØA	Milt op w indir blast effect of nuclear weapon, milt, init
		Y37.52ØD	Milt op w indir blast effect of nuclear weapon, milt, subs
		Y37.521A	Milt op w indirect blast effect of nuclear weapon, civ, init
		Y37.521D	Milt op w indirect blast effect of nuclear weapon, civ, subs
E996.2	INJ DUE WAR OP THERMAL RAD EFFECT NUCLEAR WEAPON	**Y36.53ØA**	War op w thermal radn effect of nuclear weapon, milt, init
		Y36.53ØD	War op w thermal radn effect of nuclear weapon, milt, subs
		Y36.531A	War op w thermal radn effect of nuclear weapon, civ, init
		Y36.531D	War op w thermal radn effect of nuclear weapon, civ, subs
		Y37.53ØA	Milt op w thermal radn effect of nuclear weapon, milt, init
		Y37.53ØD	Milt op w thermal radn effect of nuclear weapon, milt, subs
		Y37.531A	Milt op w thermal radn effect of nuclear weapon, civ, init
		Y37.531D	Milt op w thermal radn effect of nuclear weapon, civ, subs
E996.3	INJURY DUE WAR OP NUCLEAR RADIATION EFFECTS	**Y36.54ØA**	War op w nuclear radiation eff of nuclear weapon, milt, init
		Y36.54ØD	War op w nuclear radiation eff of nuclear weapon, milt, subs
		Y36.541A	War op w nuclear radiation eff of nuclear weapon, civ, init
		Y36.541D	War op w nuclear radiation eff of nuclear weapon, civ, subs
		Y37.54ØA	Miltry op w nuclr radiation eff of nuclr weapon, milt, init
		Y37.54ØD	Miltry op w nuclr radiation eff of nuclr weapon, milt, subs
		Y37.541A	Miltry op w nuclr radiation eff of nuclear weapon, civ, init
		Y37.541D	Miltry op w nuclr radiation eff of nuclear weapon, civ, subs
E996.8	INJURY DUE WAR OP OTHER EFFECTS NUCLEAR WEAPONS	**Y36.59ØA**	War operation w oth effects of nuclear weapons, milt, init
		Y36.59ØD	War operation w oth effects of nuclear weapons, milt, subs
		Y36.591A	War op w oth effects of nuclear weapons, civilian, init
		Y36.591D	War op w oth effects of nuclear weapons, civilian, subs
		Y37.59ØA	Military op w oth effects of nuclear weapons, milt, init
		Y37.59ØD	Military op w oth effects of nuclear weapons, milt, subs
		Y37.591A	Military op w oth effects of nuclear weapons, civilian, init
		Y37.591D	Military op w oth effects of nuclear weapons, civilian, subs
E996.9	INJURY DUE TO WAR OP UNS EFFECT NUCLEAR WEAPON	**Y36.5ØØA**	War op involving unsp effect of nuclear weapon, milt, init
		Y36.5ØØD	War op involving unsp effect of nuclear weapon, milt, subs
		Y36.5Ø1A	War op w unsp effect of nuclear weapon, civilian, init
		Y36.5Ø1D	War op w unsp effect of nuclear weapon, civilian, subs
		Y37.5ØØA	Milt op involving unsp effect of nuclear weapon, milt, init
		Y37.5ØØD	Milt op involving unsp effect of nuclear weapon, milt, subs
		Y37.5Ø1A	Milt op w unsp effect of nuclear weapon, civilian, init
		Y37.5Ø1D	Milt op w unsp effect of nuclear weapon, civilian, subs
E997.Ø	INJURY DUE TO WAR OPERATIONS BY LASERS	**Y36.7XØA**	War op w chem weapons and oth unconvtl warfare, milt, init
		Y36.7XØD	War op w chem weapons and oth unconvtl warfare, milt, subs
		Y36.7X1A	War op w chem weapons and oth unconvtl warfare, civ, init
		Y36.7X1D	War op w chem weapons and oth unconvtl warfare, civ, subs

ICD-9-CM		ICD-10-CM	
E997.1	INJURY DUE TO WAR OPERATIONS BIOLOGICAL WARFARE	**Y36.6XØA**	War operations involving biological weapons, milt, init
		Y36.6XØD	War operations involving biological weapons, milt, subs
		Y36.6X1A	War operations involving biological weapons, civilian, init
		Y36.6X1D	War operations involving biological weapons, civilian, subs
		Y37.6XØA	Milt op involving biological weapons, milt, init
		Y37.6XØD	Milt op involving biological weapons, milt, subs
		Y37.6X1A	Milt op involving biological weapons, civilian, init
		Y37.6X1D	Milt op involving biological weapons, civilian, subs
E997.2	INJURY DUE WAR OPERATIONS GASES FUMES&CHEMICALS	**Y36.7XØA**	War op w chem weapons and oth unconvtl warfare, milt, init
		Y36.7XØD	War op w chem weapons and oth unconvtl warfare, milt, subs
		Y36.7X1A	War op w chem weapons and oth unconvtl warfare, civ, init
		Y36.7X1D	War op w chem weapons and oth unconvtl warfare, civ, subs
		Y37.7XØA	Milt op w chem weapons and oth unconvtl warfare, milt, init
		Y37.7XØD	Milt op w chem weapons and oth unconvtl warfare, milt, subs
		Y37.7X1A	Milt op w chem weapons and oth unconvtl warfare, civ, init
		Y37.7X1D	Milt op w chem weapons and oth unconvtl warfare, civ, subs
E997.3	INJURY DUE TO WAR OPERATIONS BY WMD UNSPECIFIED	**Y36.91XA**	War operations involving unsp weapon of mass dest, init
		Y36.91XD	War operations involving unsp weapon of mass dest, subs
		Y37.91XA	Milt op involving unsp weapon of mass destruction, init
		Y37.91XD	Milt op involving unsp weapon of mass destruction, subs
E997.8	INJURY DUE OTH SPEC FORMS UNCONVENTIONAL WARFARE	**Y36.7XØA**	War op w chem weapons and oth unconvtl warfare, milt, init
		Y36.7XØD	War op w chem weapons and oth unconvtl warfare, milt, subs
E997.9	INJURY DUE UNSPEC FORM UNCONVENTIONAL WARFARE	**Y36.7X1A**	War op w chem weapons and oth unconvtl warfare, civ, init
		Y36.7X1D	War op w chem weapons and oth unconvtl warfare, civ, subs
E998.Ø	INJ WAR AFTER CESSATION HOSTILITIES EXPLOS MINES	**Y36.81ØA**	Explosn of mine place dur war op but expld aft, milt, init
		Y36.81ØD	Explosn of mine place dur war op but expld aft, milt, subs
		Y36.811A	Explosn of mine place dur war op but expld after, civ, init
		Y36.811D	Explosn of mine place dur war op but expld after, civ, subs
E998.1	INJ WAR AFTER CESSATION HOSTILITIES EXPLOS BOMBS	**Y36.82ØA**	Explosn of bomb place dur war op but expld aft, milt, init
		Y36.82ØD	Explosn of bomb place dur war op but expld aft, milt, subs
		Y36.821A	Explosn of bomb place dur war op but expld after, civ, init
		Y36.821D	Explosn of bomb place dur war op but expld after, civ, subs
E998.8	INJ OTH WAR OP OCCUR AFTER CESSATION HOSTILIES	**Y36.88ØA**	Oth war operations occurring after, milt, init
		Y36.88ØD	Oth war operations occurring after, milt, subs
		Y36.881A	Oth war operations occurring after, civilian, init
		Y36.881D	Oth war operations occurring after, civilian, subs
E998.9	INJ UNS WAR OP OCCUR AFTER CESSATION HOSTILITIES	**Y36.89ØA**	Unsp war operations occurring after, milt, init
		Y36.89ØD	Unsp war operations occurring after, milt, subs
		Y36.891A	Unsp war operations occurring after, civilian, init
		Y36.891D	Unsp war operations occurring after, civilian, subs
E999.Ø	LATE EFFECT OF INJURY DUE TO WAR OPERATIONS	**Y36.ØØØS**	War op w explosn of unsp marine weapon, milt, sequela
		Y36.ØØ1S	War op w explosn of unsp marine weapon, civilian, sequela
		Y36.Ø1ØS	War op involving explosion of depth-chg, milt, sequela
		Y36.Ø11S	War op involving explosion of depth-chg, civilian, sequela
		Y36.Ø2ØS	War op involving explosion of marine mine, milt, sequela
		Y36.Ø21S	War op involving explosion of marine mine, civilian, sequela
		Y36.Ø3ØS	War op w explosn of sea-based artlry shell, milt, sequela
		Y36.Ø31S	War op w explosn of sea-based artlry shell, civ, sequela
		Y36.Ø4ØS	War operations involving explosion of torpedo, milt, sequela
		Y36.Ø41S	War op involving explosion of torpedo, civilian, sequela
		Y36.Ø5ØS	War op w acc deton onboard marine weapons, milt, sequela
		Y36.Ø51S	War op w acc deton onboard marine weapons, civilian, sequela
		Y36.Ø9ØS	War op involving explosion of marine weapons, milt, sequela
		Y36.Ø91S	War op w explosn of marine weapons, civilian, sequela
		Y36.1ØØS	War operations involving unsp dest arcrft, milt, sequela
		Y36.1Ø1S	War operations involving unsp dest arcrft, civilian, sequela
		Y36.11ØS	War op w dest arcrft due to enmy fire/expls, milt, sequela
		Y36.111S	War op w dest arcrft due to enmy fire/expls, civ, sequela
		Y36.12ØS	War op w dest arcrft due to clsn w oth arcrft, milt, sequela
		Y36.121S	War op w dest arcrft due to clsn w oth arcrft, civ, sequela
		Y36.13ØS	War op w dest arcrft due to onboard fire, milt, sequela
		Y36.131S	War op w dest arcrft due to onboard fire, civilian, sequela
		Y36.14ØS	War op w dest arcrft d/t acc deton onbrd munit, milt, sqla
		Y36.141S	War op w dest arcrft due to acc deton onbrd munit, civ, sqla
		Y36.19ØS	War operations involving oth dest arcrft, milt, sequela
		Y36.191S	War operations involving oth dest arcrft, civilian, sequela
		Y36.2ØØS	War op involving unsp explosion and fragments, milt, sequela
		Y36.2Ø1S	War op involving unsp explosn and fragmt, civilian, sequela
		Y36.21ØS	War op involving explosion of aerial bomb, milt, sequela
		Y36.211S	War op involving explosion of aerial bomb, civilian, sequela
		Y36.22ØS	War op involving explosion of guided missile, milt, sequela
		Y36.221S	War op w explosn of guided missile, civilian, sequela
		Y36.23ØS	War op w explosn of improv explosv device, milt, sequela
		Y36.231S	War op w explosn of improv explosv device, civilian, sequela
		Y36.24ØS	War op w explosn due to acc disch of own munit, milt, sqla
		Y36.241S	War op w explosn due to acc disch of own munit, civ, sequela
		Y36.25ØS	War op involving fragments from munitions, milt, sequela
		Y36.251S	War op involving fragments from munitions, civilian, sequela
		Y36.26ØS	War op w fragmt of improv explosv device, milt, sequela
		Y36.261S	War op w fragmt of improv explosv device, civilian, sequela

(Continued on next page)

ICD-9-CM		ICD-10-CM	
E999.Ø	LATE EFFECT OF INJURY DUE TO WAR OPERATIONS **(Continued)**	**Y36.27ØS**	War op involving fragments from weapons, milt, sequela
		Y36.271S	War op involving fragments from weapons, civilian, sequela
		Y36.29ØS	War op involving oth explosn and fragments, milt, sequela
		Y36.291S	War op involving oth explosn and fragmt, civilian, sequela
		Y36.3ØØS	War op involving unsp fire/conflagr/hot subst, milt, sequela
		Y36.3Ø1S	War op w unsp fire/conflagr/hot subst, civilian, sequela
		Y36.31ØS	War operations involving gasoline bomb, milt, sequela
		Y36.311S	War operations involving gasoline bomb, civilian, sequela
		Y36.32ØS	War operations involving incendiary bullet, milt, sequela
		Y36.321S	War op involving incendiary bullet, civilian, sequela
		Y36.33ØS	War operations involving flamethrower, milt, sequela
		Y36.331S	War operations involving flamethrower, civilian, sequela
		Y36.39ØS	War operations involving oth fire/hot subst, milt, sequela
		Y36.391S	War op involving oth fire/hot subst, civilian, sequela
		Y36.41ØS	War operations involving rubber bullets, milt, sequela
		Y36.411S	War operations involving rubber bullets, civilian, sequela
		Y36.42ØS	War operations involving firearms pellets, milt, sequela
		Y36.421S	War operations involving firearms pellets, civilian, sequela
		Y36.43ØS	War op involving oth firearms discharge, milt, sequela
		Y36.431S	War op involving oth firearms discharge, civilian, sequela
		Y36.44ØS	War op involving unarmed hand to hand combat, milt, sequela
		Y36.441S	War op w unarmed hand to hand combat, civilian, sequela
		Y36.45ØS	War op w combat using blunt/pierc object, milt, sequela
		Y36.451S	War op w combat using blunt/pierc object, civilian, sequela
		Y36.46ØS	War op w intentl restrict of air/airwy, milt, sequela
		Y36.461S	War op w intentl restrict of air/airwy, civilian, sequela
		Y36.47ØS	War op w unintent restrict of air/airwy, milt, sequela
		Y36.471S	War op w unintent restrict of air/airwy, civilian, sequela
		Y36.49ØS	War operations involving oth conventl warfare, milt, sequela
		Y36.491S	War op involving oth conventl warfare, civilian, sequela
		Y36.5ØØS	War op w unsp effect of nuclear weapon, milt, sequela
		Y36.5Ø1S	War op w unsp effect of nuclear weapon, civilian, sequela
		Y36.51ØS	War op w direct blast effect of nuclr weapon, milt, sequela
		Y36.511S	War op w direct blast effect of nuclear weapon, civ, sequela
		Y36.52ØS	War op w indir blast effect of nuclear weapon, milt, sequela
		Y36.521S	War op w indir blast effect of nuclear weapon, civ, sequela
		Y36.53ØS	War op w thermal radn effect of nuclr weapon, milt, sequela
		Y36.531S	War op w thermal radn effect of nuclear weapon, civ, sequela
		Y36.54ØS	War op w nuclr radiation eff of nuclr weapon, milt, sequela
		Y36.541S	War op w nuclr radiation eff of nuclear weapon, civ, sequela
		Y36.59ØS	War op w oth effects of nuclear weapons, milt, sequela
		Y36.591S	War op w oth effects of nuclear weapons, civilian, sequela
		Y36.6XØS	War operations involving biological weapons, milt, sequela
		Y36.6X1S	War operations involving biolg weapons, civilian, sequela
		Y36.7XØS	War op w chem weapons and oth unconvtl warfare, milt, sqla
		Y36.7X1S	War op w chem weapons and oth unconvtl warfare, civ, sequela
		Y36.81ØS	Explosn of mine place dur war op but expld aft, milt, sqla
		Y36.811S	Explosn of mine place dur war op but expld after, civ, sqla
		Y36.82ØS	Explosn of bomb place dur war op but expld aft, milt, sqla
		Y36.821S	Explosn of bomb place dur war op but expld after, civ, sqla
		Y36.88ØS	Oth war operations occurring after, milt, sequela
		Y36.881S	Oth war operations occurring after, civilian, sequela
		Y36.89ØS	Unsp war operations occurring after, milt, sequela
		Y36.891S	Unsp war operations occurring after, civilian, sequela
		Y36.9ØXS	War operations, unspecified, sequela
		Y36.91XS	War operations involving unsp weapon of mass dest, sequela
		Y36.92XS	War operations involving friendly fire, sequela
		Y37.ØØØS	Milt op w explosn of unsp marine weapon, milt, sequela
		Y37.ØØ1S	Milt op w explosn of unsp marine weapon, civilian, sequela
		Y37.Ø1ØS	Milt op involving explosion of depth-charge, milt, sequela
		Y37.Ø11S	Milt op involving explosion of depth-chg, civilian, sequela
		Y37.Ø2ØS	Milt op involving explosion of marine mine, milt, sequela
		Y37.Ø21S	Milt op involving explosn of marine mine, civilian, sequela
		Y37.Ø3ØS	Milt op w explosn of sea-based artlry shell, milt, sequela
		Y37.Ø31S	Milt op w explosn of sea-based artlry shell, civ, sequela
		Y37.Ø4ØS	Milt op involving explosion of torpedo, milt, sequela
		Y37.Ø41S	Milt op involving explosion of torpedo, civilian, sequela
		Y37.Ø5ØS	Milt op w acc deton onboard marine weapons, milt, sequela
		Y37.Ø51S	Milt op w acc deton onboard marine weapons, civ, sequela
		Y37.Ø9ØS	Milt op involving explosion of marine weapons, milt, sequela
		Y37.Ø91S	Milt op w explosn of marine weapons, civilian, sequela
		Y37.1ØØS	Milt op involving unsp dest arcrft, milt, sequela
		Y37.1Ø1S	Milt op involving unsp dest arcrft, civilian, sequela
		Y37.11ØS	Milt op w dest arcrft due to enmy fire/expls, milt, sequela
		Y37.111S	Milt op w dest arcrft due to enmy fire/expls, civ, sequela
		Y37.12ØS	Milt op w dest arcrft due to clsn w oth arcrft, milt, sqla
		Y37.121S	Milt op w dest arcrft due to clsn w oth arcrft, civ, sequela
		Y37.13ØS	Milt op w dest arcrft due to onboard fire, milt, sequela
		Y37.131S	Milt op w dest arcrft due to onboard fire, civilian, sequela
		Y37.14ØS	Milt op w dest arcrft d/t acc deton onbrd munit, milt, sqla
		Y37.141S	Milt op w dest arcrft d/t acc deton onbrd munit, civ, sqla
	(Continued on next page)	**Y37.19ØS**	Milt op involving oth dest arcrft, milt, sequela

ICD-9-CM		ICD-10-CM	
E999.Ø	LATE EFFECT OF INJURY DUE TO WAR OPERATIONS **(Continued)**	**Y37.191S**	Milt op involving oth dest arcrft, civilian, sequela
		Y37.2ØØS	Milt op involving unsp explosn and fragments, milt, sequela
		Y37.2Ø1S	Milt op involving unsp explosn and fragmt, civilian, sequela
		Y37.21ØS	Milt op involving explosion of aerial bomb, milt, sequela
		Y37.211S	Milt op involving explosn of aerial bomb, civilian, sequela
		Y37.22ØS	Milt op involving explosion of guided missile, milt, sequela
		Y37.221S	Milt op w explosn of guided missile, civilian, sequela
		Y37.23ØS	Milt op w explosn of improv explosv device, milt, sequela
		Y37.231S	Milt op w explosn of improv explosv device, civ, sequela
		Y37.24ØS	Milt op w explosn due to acc disch of own munit, milt, sqla
		Y37.241S	Milt op w explosn due to acc disch of own munit, civ, sqla
		Y37.25ØS	Milt op involving fragments from munitions, milt, sequela
		Y37.251S	Milt op involving fragmt from munitions, civilian, sequela
		Y37.26ØS	Milt op w fragmt of improv explosv device, milt, sequela
		Y37.261S	Milt op w fragmt of improv explosv device, civilian, sequela
		Y37.27ØS	Milt op involving fragments from weapons, milt, sequela
		Y37.271S	Milt op involving fragments from weapons, civilian, sequela
		Y37.29ØS	Milt op involving oth explosn and fragments, milt, sequela
		Y37.291S	Milt op involving oth explosn and fragmt, civilian, sequela
		Y37.3ØØS	Milt op w unsp fire/conflagr/hot subst, milt, sequela
		Y37.3Ø1S	Milt op w unsp fire/conflagr/hot subst, civilian, sequela
		Y37.31ØS	Milt op involving gasoline bomb, military personnel, sequela
		Y37.311S	Milt op involving gasoline bomb, civilian, sequela
		Y37.32ØS	Milt op involving incendiary bullet, milt, sequela
		Y37.321S	Milt op involving incendiary bullet, civilian, sequela
		Y37.33ØS	Milt op involving flamethrower, military personnel, sequela
		Y37.331S	Milt op involving flamethrower, civilian, sequela
		Y37.39ØS	Milt op involving oth fire/hot subst, milt, sequela
		Y37.391S	Milt op involving oth fire/hot subst, civilian, sequela
		Y37.41ØS	Milt op involving rubber bullets, milt, sequela
		Y37.411S	Milt op involving rubber bullets, civilian, sequela
		Y37.42ØS	Milt op involving firearms pellets, milt, sequela
		Y37.421S	Milt op involving firearms pellets, civilian, sequela
		Y37.43ØS	Milt op involving oth firearms discharge, milt, sequela
		Y37.431S	Milt op involving oth firearms discharge, civilian, sequela
		Y37.44ØS	Milt op involving unarmed hand to hand combat, milt, sequela
		Y37.441S	Milt op w unarmed hand to hand combat, civilian, sequela
		Y37.45ØS	Milt op w combat using blunt/pierc object, milt, sequela
		Y37.451S	Milt op w combat using blunt/pierc object, civilian, sequela
		Y37.46ØS	Milt op w intentl restrict of air/airwy, milt, sequela
		Y37.461S	Milt op w intentl restrict of air/airwy, civilian, sequela
		Y37.47ØS	Milt op w unintent restrict of air/airwy, milt, sequela
		Y37.471S	Milt op w unintent restrict of air/airwy, civilian, sequela
		Y37.49ØS	Milt op involving oth conventional warfare, milt, sequela
		Y37.491S	Milt op involving oth conventl warfare, civilian, sequela
		Y37.5ØØS	Milt op w unsp effect of nuclear weapon, milt, sequela
		Y37.5Ø1S	Milt op w unsp effect of nuclear weapon, civilian, sequela
		Y37.51ØS	Milt op w direct blast effect of nuclr weapon, milt, sequela
		Y37.511S	Milt op w direct blast effect of nuclr weapon, civ, sequela
		Y37.52ØS	Milt op w indir blast effect of nuclr weapon, milt, sequela
		Y37.521S	Milt op w indir blast effect of nuclear weapon, civ, sequela
		Y37.53ØS	Milt op w thermal radn effect of nuclr weapon, milt, sequela
		Y37.531S	Milt op w thermal radn effect of nuclr weapon, civ, sequela
		Y37.54ØS	Miltry op w nuclr radiation eff of nuclr weapon, milt, sqla
		Y37.541S	Miltry op w nuclr radiation eff of nuclr weapon, civ, sqla
		Y37.59ØS	Military op w oth effects of nuclear weapons, milt, sequela
		Y37.591S	Military op w oth effects of nuclear weapons, civ, sequela
		Y37.6XØS	Milt op involving biological weapons, milt, sequela
		Y37.6X1S	Milt op involving biological weapons, civilian, sequela
		Y37.7XØS	Milt op w chem weapons and oth unconvtl warfare, milt, sqla
		Y37.7X1S	Milt op w chem weapons and oth unconvtl warfare, civ, sqla
		Y37.9ØXS	Military operations, unspecified, sequela
		Y37.91XS	Milt op involving unsp weapon of mass destruction, sequela
		Y37.92XS	Military operations involving friendly fire, sequela
E999.1	LATE EFFECT OF INJURY DUE TO TERRORISM	**Y38.ØX1S**	Terorsm w explosn of marine weap, publ sfty offcl inj, sqla
		Y38.ØX2S	Terorsm w explosn of marine weapons, civ injured, sequela
		Y38.ØX3S	Terorsm w explosn of marine weapons, terrorist inj, sequela
		Y38.1X1S	Terrorism w dest arcrft, publ sfty offcl injured, sequela
		Y38.1X2S	Terrorism involving dest arcrft, civilian injured, sequela
		Y38.1X3S	Terrorism involving dest arcrft, terrorist injured, sequela
		Y38.2X1S	Terorsm w oth explosn and fragmt, publ sfty offcl inj, sqla
		Y38.2X2S	Terorsm w oth explosn and fragmt, civilian injured, sequela
		Y38.2X3S	Terorsm w oth explosn and fragmt, terrorist injured, sequela
		Y38.3X1S	Terrorism w fire/hot subst, publ sfty offcl injured, sequela
		Y38.3X2S	Terrorism w fire/hot subst, civilian injured, sequela
		Y38.3X3S	Terrorism w fire/hot subst, terrorist injured, sequela
		Y38.4X1S	Terrorism w firearms, publ sfty offcl injured, sequela
		Y38.4X2S	Terrorism involving firearms, civilian injured, sequela
		Y38.4X3S	Terrorism involving firearms, terrorist injured, sequela
		Y38.5X1S	Terorsm w nuclear weapons, publ sfty offcl injured, sequela
		Y38.5X2S	Terrorism w nuclear weapons, civilian injured, sequela
	(Continued on next page)	**Y38.5X3S**	Terrorism w nuclear weapons, terrorist injured, sequela

ICD-9-CM		ICD-10-CM	
E999.1	LATE EFFECT OF INJURY DUE TO TERRORISM **(Continued)**	**Y38.6X1S**	Terrorism w biolg weapons, publ sfty offcl injured, sequela
		Y38.6X2S	Terrorism involving biolg weapons, civilian injured, sequela
		Y38.6X3S	Terrorism w biolg weapons, terrorist injured, sequela
		Y38.7X1S	Terorsm w chemical weapons, publ sfty offcl injured, sequela
		Y38.7X2S	Terrorism w chemical weapons, civilian injured, sequela
		Y38.7X3S	Terrorism w chemical weapons, terrorist injured, sequela
		Y38.8ØXS	Terrorism involving unspecified means, sequela
		Y38.811S	Terrorism w suicide bomber, publ sfty offcl injured, sequela
		Y38.812S	Terrorism w suicide bomber, civilian injured, sequela
		Y38.891S	Terrorism w oth means, publ sfty offcl injured, sequela
		Y38.892S	Terrorism involving other means, civilian injured, sequela
		Y38.893S	Terrorism involving other means, terrorist injured, sequela
		Y38.9X1S	Terrorism, sec effects, publ sfty offcl injured, sequela
		Y38.9X2S	Terrorism, secondary effects, civilian injured, sequela

Appendix A. ICD-10-CM Combination Mappings

In the ICD-10-CM to ICD-9-CM mappings (backward mapping) there are cases in which the ICD-9-CM code contains more clinical detail than exists in ICD-10-CM. This occurs especially when the clinical concept or axis classification in ICD-9-CM is considered no longer essential. For these cases a single ICD-10-CM code maps to multiple ICD-9-CM codes. Due to the format of this manual, the presentation of the multiple coding scenarios for the ICD-10-CM to ICD-9-CM mapping was not possible. The ICD-10-CM codes that map to combinations of ICD-9-CM codes are flagged in the tabular listing of this book. This appendix provides the complete combination coding for these cases. The listing is by ICD-10-CM codes, and the multiple ICD-9-CM codes that satisfy the mapping are listed.

AØ2.1	ØØ3.1 and 995.91
A18.Ø1	Ø15.ØØ and 711.48; Ø15.ØØ and 72Ø.81; Ø15.ØØ and 73Ø.88; Ø15.ØØ and 737.4Ø
A18.Ø2	Ø15.1Ø and 711.45; Ø15.2Ø and 711.46; Ø15.8Ø and 711.48
A18.Ø3	Ø15.7Ø and 73Ø.88
A18.14	Ø16.5Ø and 6Ø1.4
A18.51	Ø17.3Ø and 379.Ø9
A18.52	Ø17.3Ø and 37Ø.31; Ø17.3Ø and 37Ø.59
A18.53	Ø17.3Ø and 363.13
A18.54	Ø17.3Ø and 364.11
A18.84	Ø17.9Ø and 42Ø.Ø; Ø17.9Ø and 422.Ø; Ø17.9Ø and 424.91; Ø17.9Ø and 425.8
A22.1	Ø22.1 and 484.5
A22.7	Ø22.3 and 995.91
A26.7	Ø27.1 and 995.91
A32.7	Ø27.Ø and 995.91
A37.Ø1	Ø33.Ø and 484.3
A37.11	Ø33.1 and 484.3
A37.81	Ø33.8 and 484.3
A37.91	Ø33.9 and 484.3
A4Ø.Ø	Ø38.Ø and 995.91
A4Ø.1	Ø38.Ø and 995.91
A4Ø.3	Ø38.Ø and 995.91; Ø38.2 and 995.91
A4Ø.8	Ø38.Ø and 995.91
A4Ø.9	Ø38.Ø and 995.91
A41.Ø1	Ø38.11 and 995.91
A41.Ø2	Ø38.12 and 995.91
A41.1	Ø38.19 and 995.91
A41.2	Ø38.1Ø and 995.91
A41.3	Ø38.41 and 995.91
A41.4	Ø38.3 and 995.91
A41.5Ø	Ø38.4Ø and 995.91
A41.51	Ø38.42 and 995.91
A41.52	Ø38.43 and 995.91
A41.53	Ø38.44 and 995.91
A41.59	Ø38.49 and 995.91
A41.81	Ø38.8 and 995.91
A41.89	Ø38.8 and 995.91
A41.9	Ø38.9 and 995.91
A42.7	Ø38.8 and 995.91
A52.15	Ø94.89 and 357.4
A52.16	Ø94.Ø and 713.5
A54.86	Ø98.89 and 995.91
A56.Ø1	Ø99.53 and 595.4
A56.Ø2	Ø99.53 and 616.11
A56.11	Ø99.54 and 614.9
B25.Ø	Ø78.5 and 484.1
B25.1	Ø78.5 and 573.1
B25.2	Ø78.5 and 577.Ø
B37.7	112.5 and 995.91
B44.Ø	117.3 and 484.6
B45.1	117.5 and 321.Ø
B52.Ø	Ø84.9 and 581.81
B6Ø.12	136.21 and 372.15
B6Ø.13	136.21 and 37Ø.8
B77.81	127.Ø and 484.8
D57.Ø1	282.62 and 517.3
D57.Ø2	282.62 and 289.52
D57.211	282.64 and 517.3
D57.212	282.64 and 289.52
D57.411	282.42 and 517.3
D57.412	282.42 and 289.52
D57.811	282.69 and 517.3
D57.812	282.69 and 289.52
EØ8.21	249.4Ø and 581.81
EØ8.22	249.4Ø and 581.81
EØ8.29	249.4Ø and 581.81
EØ8.311	249.5Ø and 362.Ø1 and 362.Ø7
EØ8.319	249.5Ø and 362.Ø1
EØ8.321	249.5Ø and 362.Ø4 and 362.Ø7
EØ8.329	249.5Ø and 362.Ø4
EØ8.331	249.5Ø and 362.Ø1 and 362.Ø7
EØ8.339	249.5Ø and 362.Ø1
EØ8.341	249.5Ø and 362.Ø1 and 362.Ø7
EØ8.349	249.5Ø and 362.Ø1
EØ8.351	249.5Ø and 362.Ø2 and 362.Ø7
EØ8.359	249.5Ø and 362.Ø2
EØ8.36	249.5Ø and 366.41
EØ8.4Ø	249.6Ø and 357.2
EØ8.41	249.6Ø and 355.9
EØ8.42	249.6Ø and 357.2
EØ8.43	249.6Ø and 536.3
EØ8.44	249.6Ø and 353.5
EØ8.49	249.6Ø and 349.89
EØ8.51	249.7Ø and 443.81
EØ8.52	249.7Ø and 443.81 and 785.4
EØ8.61Ø	249.6Ø and 713.5
EØ8.618	249.8Ø and 716.8Ø
EØ8.628	249.8Ø and 7Ø9.8
EØ8.63Ø	249.8Ø and 523.8
EØ8.638	249.8Ø and 528.9
EØ8.649	249.8Ø and 251.1
EØ9.21	249.4Ø and 581.81; 249.4Ø and 583.81
EØ9.22	249.4Ø and 581.81; 249.4Ø and 583.81
EØ9.29	249.4Ø and 581.81; 249.4Ø and 583.81
EØ9.311	249.5Ø and 362.Ø1 and 362.Ø7
EØ9.319	249.5Ø and 362.Ø1
EØ9.321	249.5Ø and 362.Ø4 and 362.Ø7
EØ9.329	249.5Ø and 362.Ø4
EØ9.331	249.5Ø and 362.Ø1 and 362.Ø7
EØ9.339	249.5Ø and 362.Ø1
EØ9.341	249.5Ø and 362.Ø1 and 362.Ø7
EØ9.349	249.5Ø and 362.Ø1
EØ9.351	249.5Ø and 362.Ø2 and 362.Ø7
EØ9.359	249.5Ø and 362.Ø2
EØ9.36	249.5Ø and 366.41
EØ9.4Ø	249.6Ø and 357.2
EØ9.41	249.6Ø and 355.9
EØ9.42	249.6Ø and 357.2
EØ9.43	249.6Ø and 536.3
EØ9.44	249.6Ø and 353.5
EØ9.49	249.6Ø and 349.89
EØ9.51	249.7Ø and 443.81
EØ9.52	249.7Ø and 443.81 and 785.4
EØ9.61Ø	249.6Ø and 713.5
EØ9.618	249.8Ø and 716.8Ø
EØ9.628	249.8Ø and 7Ø9.8
EØ9.63Ø	249.8Ø and 523.8
EØ9.638	249.8Ø and 528.9
E1Ø.311	25Ø.51 and 362.Ø1 and 362.Ø7
E1Ø.319	25Ø.51 and 362.Ø1
E1Ø.321	25Ø.51 and 362.Ø4 and 362.Ø7
E1Ø.329	25Ø.51 and 362.Ø4
E1Ø.331	25Ø.51 and 362.Ø5 and 362.Ø7
E1Ø.339	25Ø.51 and 362.Ø5
E1Ø.341	25Ø.51 and 362.Ø6 and 362.Ø7
E1Ø.349	25Ø.51 and 362.Ø6
E1Ø.351	25Ø.51 and 362.Ø2 and 362.Ø7
E1Ø.359	25Ø.51 and 362.Ø2
E1Ø.36	25Ø.51 and 366.41
E1Ø.4Ø	25Ø.61 and 357.2
E1Ø.41	25Ø.61 and 355.9
E1Ø.42	25Ø.61 and 357.2
E1Ø.43	25Ø.61 and 536.3
E1Ø.44	25Ø.61 and 353.5
E1Ø.49	25Ø.61 and 349.89
E1Ø.51	25Ø.71 and 443.81
E1Ø.52	25Ø.71 and 443.81 and 785.4
E1Ø.61Ø	25Ø.61 and 713.5
E1Ø.618	25Ø.81 and 716.8Ø
E1Ø.63Ø	25Ø.81 and 523.8
E11.311	25Ø.5Ø and 362.Ø1 and 362.Ø7
E11.319	25Ø.5Ø and 362.Ø1
E11.321	25Ø.5Ø and 362.Ø4 and 362.Ø7
E11.329	25Ø.5Ø and 362.Ø4
E11.331	25Ø.5Ø and 362.Ø5 and 362.Ø7
E11.339	25Ø.5Ø and 362.Ø5
E11.341	25Ø.5Ø and 362.Ø6 and 362.Ø7
E11.349	25Ø.5Ø and 362.Ø6
E11.351	25Ø.5Ø and 362.Ø2 and 362.Ø7
E11.359	25Ø.5Ø and 362.Ø2
E11.36	25Ø.5Ø and 366.41
E11.4Ø	25Ø.6Ø and 357.2
E11.41	25Ø.6Ø and 355.9
E11.42	25Ø.6Ø and 357.2
E11.43	25Ø.6Ø and 536.3
E11.44	25Ø.6Ø and 353.5
E11.49	25Ø.6Ø and 349.89
E11.51	25Ø.7Ø and 443.81
E11.52	25Ø.7Ø and 443.81 and 785.4

ICD-10-CM	ICD-9-CM
E11.610	250.60 and 713.5
E11.618	250.80 and 716.80
E11.630	250.80 and 523.8
E13.311	249.50 and 362.01 and 362.07; 250.50 and 362.01 and 362.07
E13.319	249.50 and 362.01; 250.50 and 362.01
E13.321	249.50 and 362.04 and 362.07; 250.50 and 362.04 and 362.07
E13.329	249.50 and 362.04; 250.50 and 362.04
E13.331	249.50 and 362.05 and 362.07; 250.50 and 362.05 and 362.07
E13.339	249.50 and 362.05; 250.50 and 362.05
E13.341	249.50 and 362.06 and 362.07; 250.50 and 362.06 and 362.07
E13.349	249.50 and 362.06; 250.50 and 362.06
E13.351	249.50 and 362.02 and 362.07; 250.50 and 362.02 and 362.07
E13.359	249.50 and 362.02; 250.50 and 362.02
E13.36	249.50 and 366.41; 250.50 and 366.41
E13.40	249.60 and 357.2; 250.60 and 357.2
E13.41	249.60 and 355.9; 250.60 and 355.9
E13.42	249.60 and 357.2; 250.60 and 357.2
E13.43	249.60 and 536.3; 250.60 and 536.3
E13.44	249.60 and 353.5; 250.60 and 353.5
E13.49	249.60 and 349.89; 250.60 and 349.89
E13.51	249.70 and 443.81; 250.70 and 443.81
E13.52	249.70 and 443.81 and 785.4; 250.70 and 443.81 and 785.4
E13.610	249.60 and 713.5; 250.60 and 713.5
E13.618	249.80 and 716.80; 250.80 and 716.80
E13.630	249.80 and 523.8; 250.80 and 523.8
F11.220	292.2 and 304.00
F11.221	292.81 and 304.00
F11.222	292.89 and 304.00
F11.229	292.2 and 304.00
F11.23	292.0 and 304.00
F11.24	292.84 and 304.00
F11.250	292.11 and 304.00
F11.251	292.12 and 304.00
F11.259	292.89 and 304.00
F11.281	292.89 and 304.00
F11.282	292.85 and 304.00
F11.288	292.89 and 304.00
F11.29	292.9 and 304.00
F12.220	292.2 and 304.30
F12.221	292.81 and 304.30
F12.222	292.89 and 304.30
F12.229	292.2 and 304.30
F12.250	292.11 and 304.30
F12.251	292.12 and 304.30
F12.259	292.89 and 304.30
F12.280	292.89 and 304.30
F12.288	292.89 and 304.30
F12.29	292.9 and 304.30
F13.220	292.2 and 304.10
F13.221	292.81 and 304.10
F13.229	292.2 and 304.10
F13.230	292.0 and 304.10
F13.231	292.0 and 304.10
F13.232	292.0 and 304.10
F13.239	292.0 and 304.10
F13.24	292.84 and 304.10
F13.250	292.11 and 304.10
F13.251	292.12 and 304.10
F13.259	292.89 and 304.10
F13.26	292.83 and 304.10
F13.27	292.82 and 304.10
F13.280	292.89 and 304.10
F13.281	292.89 and 304.10
F13.282	292.85 and 304.10
F13.288	292.89 and 304.10
F13.29	292.9 and 304.10
F14.220	292.2 and 304.20
F14.221	292.81 and 304.20
F14.222	292.89 and 304.20
F14.229	292.2 and 304.20
F14.23	292.0 and 304.20
F14.24	292.84 and 304.20
F14.250	292.11 and 304.20
F14.251	292.12 and 304.20
F14.259	292.89 and 304.20
F14.280	292.89 and 304.20
F14.281	292.89 and 304.20
F14.282	292.85 and 304.20
F14.288	292.89 and 304.20
F14.29	292.9 and 304.20
F15.220	292.2 and 304.40
F15.221	292.81 and 304.40
F15.222	292.89 and 304.40
F15.229	292.2 and 304.40
F15.23	292.0 and 304.40
F15.24	292.84 and 304.40
F15.250	292.11 and 304.40
F15.251	292.12 and 304.40
F15.259	292.89 and 304.40
F15.280	292.89 and 304.40
F15.281	292.89 and 304.40
F15.282	292.85 and 304.40
F15.288	292.89 and 304.40
F15.29	292.9 and 304.40
F16.220	292.2 and 304.50
F16.221	292.81 and 304.50
F16.229	292.2 and 304.50
F16.24	292.84 and 304.50
F16.250	292.11 and 304.50
F16.251	292.12 and 304.50
F16.259	292.89 and 304.50
F16.280	292.89 and 304.50
F16.283	292.89 and 304.50
F16.288	292.89 and 304.50
F16.29	292.9 and 304.50
F18.220	292.2 and 304.60
F18.221	292.81 and 304.60
F18.229	292.2 and 304.60
F18.24	292.84 and 304.60
F18.250	292.11 and 304.60
F18.251	292.12 and 304.60
F18.259	292.89 and 304.60
F18.27	292.82 and 304.60
F18.280	292.89 and 304.60
F18.288	292.89 and 304.60
F18.29	292.9 and 304.60
F19.220	292.2 and 304.60
F19.221	292.81 and 304.60
F19.222	292.89 and 304.60
F19.229	292.2 and 304.60
F19.230	292.0 and 304.60
F19.231	292.0 and 304.60
F19.232	292.0 and 304.60
F19.239	292.0 and 304.60
F19.24	292.84 and 304.60
F19.250	292.11 and 304.60
F19.251	292.12 and 304.60
F19.259	292.89 and 304.60
F19.26	292.83 and 304.60
F19.27	292.82 and 304.60
F19.280	292.89 and 304.60
F19.281	292.89 and 304.60
F19.282	292.85 and 304.60
F19.288	292.89 and 304.60
F19.29	292.9 and 304.60
F68.13	300.16 and 301.51
H16.261	370.32 and 372.13
H16.262	370.32 and 372.13
H16.263	370.32 and 372.13
H16.269	370.32 and 372.13
H40.10X0	365.10 and 365.70
H40.10X1	365.10 and 365.71
H40.10X2	365.10 and 365.72
H40.10X3	365.10 and 365.73
H40.10X4	365.10 and 365.74
H40.11X0	365.11 and 365.70
H40.11X1	365.11 and 365.71
H40.11X2	365.11 and 365.72
H40.11X3	365.11 and 365.73
H40.11X4	365.11 and 365.74
H40.1210	365.12 and 365.70
H40.1211	365.12 and 365.71
H40.1212	365.12 and 365.72
H40.1213	365.12 and 365.73
H40.1214	365.12 and 365.74
H40.1220	365.12 and 365.70
H40.1221	365.12 and 365.71
H40.1222	365.12 and 365.72
H40.1223	365.12 and 365.73
H40.1224	365.12 and 365.74
H40.1230	365.12 and 365.70
H40.1231	365.12 and 365.71
H40.1232	365.12 and 365.72
H40.1233	365.12 and 365.73
H40.1234	365.12 and 365.74
H40.1290	365.12 and 365.70
H40.1291	365.12 and 365.71
H40.1292	365.12 and 365.72
H40.1293	365.12 and 365.73
H40.1294	365.12 and 365.74
H40.1310	365.13 and 365.70
H40.1311	365.13 and 365.71
H40.1312	365.13 and 365.72
H40.1313	365.13 and 365.73
H40.1314	365.13 and 365.74
H40.1320	365.13 and 365.70
H40.1321	365.13 and 365.71
H40.1322	365.13 and 365.72
H40.1323	365.13 and 365.73
H40.1324	365.13 and 365.74
H40.1330	365.13 and 365.70
H40.1331	365.13 and 365.71
H40.1332	365.13 and 365.72
H40.1333	365.13 and 365.73
H40.1334	365.13 and 365.74
H40.1390	365.13 and 365.70
H40.1391	365.13 and 365.71
H40.1392	365.13 and 365.72
H40.1393	365.13 and 365.73
H40.1394	365.13 and 365.74
H40.1410	365.52 and 365.70
H40.1411	365.52 and 365.71
H40.1412	365.52 and 365.72
H40.1413	365.52 and 365.73

ICD-10-CM	ICD-9-CM
H40.1414	365.52 and 365.74
H40.1420	365.52 and 365.70
H40.1421	365.52 and 365.71
H40.1422	365.52 and 365.72
H40.1423	365.52 and 365.73
H40.1424	365.52 and 365.74
H40.1430	365.52 and 365.70
H40.1431	365.52 and 365.71
H40.1432	365.52 and 365.72
H40.1433	365.52 and 365.73
H40.1434	365.52 and 365.74
H40.1490	365.52 and 365.70
H40.1491	365.52 and 365.71
H40.1492	365.52 and 365.72
H40.1493	365.52 and 365.73
H40.1494	365.52 and 365.74
H40.20X0	365.20 and 365.70
H40.20X1	365.20 and 365.71
H40.20X2	365.20 and 365.72
H40.20X3	365.20 and 365.73
H40.20X4	365.20 and 365.74
H40.2210	365.23 and 365.70
H40.2211	365.23 and 365.71
H40.2212	365.23 and 365.72
H40.2213	365.23 and 365.73
H40.2214	365.23 and 365.74
H40.2220	365.23 and 365.70
H40.2221	365.23 and 365.71
H40.2222	365.23 and 365.72
H40.2223	365.23 and 365.73
H40.2224	365.23 and 365.74
H40.2230	365.23 and 365.70
H40.2231	365.23 and 365.71
H40.2232	365.23 and 365.72
H40.2233	365.23 and 365.73
H40.2234	365.23 and 365.74
H40.2290	365.23 and 365.70
H40.2291	365.23 and 365.71
H40.2292	365.23 and 365.72
H40.2293	365.23 and 365.73
H40.2294	365.23 and 365.74
H40.30X0	365.65 and 365.70
H40.30X1	365.65 and 365.71
H40.30X2	365.65 and 365.72
H40.30X3	365.65 and 365.73
H40.30X4	365.65 and 365.74
H40.31X0	365.65 and 365.70
H40.31X1	365.65 and 365.71
H40.31X2	365.65 and 365.72
H40.31X3	365.65 and 365.73
H40.31X4	365.65 and 365.74
H40.32X0	365.65 and 365.70
H40.32X1	365.65 and 365.71
H40.32X2	365.65 and 365.72
H40.32X3	365.65 and 365.73
H40.32X4	365.65 and 365.74
H40.33X0	365.65 and 365.70
H40.33X1	365.65 and 365.71
H40.33X2	365.65 and 365.72
H40.33X3	365.65 and 365.73
H40.33X4	365.65 and 365.74
H40.40X0	365.62 and 365.70
H40.40X1	365.62 and 365.71
H40.40X2	365.62 and 365.72
H40.40X3	365.62 and 365.73
H40.40X4	365.62 and 365.74
H40.41X0	365.62 and 365.70
H40.41X1	365.62 and 365.71
H40.41X2	365.62 and 365.72
H40.41X3	365.62 and 365.73
H40.41X4	365.62 and 365.74
H40.42X0	365.62 and 365.70
H40.42X1	365.62 and 365.71
H40.42X2	365.62 and 365.72
H40.42X3	365.62 and 365.73
H40.42X4	365.62 and 365.74
H40.43X0	365.62 and 365.70
H40.43X1	365.62 and 365.71
H40.43X2	365.62 and 365.72
H40.43X3	365.62 and 365.73
H40.43X4	365.62 and 365.74
H40.50X0	365.59 or 365.60 or 365.61 or 365.64 and 365.70
H40.50X1	365.59 or 365.60 or 365.61 or 365.64 and 365.71
H40.50X2	365.59 or 365.60 or 365.61 or 365.64 and 365.72
H40.50X3	365.59 or 365.60 or 365.61 or 365.64 and 365.73
H40.50X4	365.59 or 365.60 or 365.61 or 365.64 and 365.74
H40.51X0	365.59 or 365.60 or 365.61 or 365.64 and 365.70
H40.51X1	365.59 or 365.60 or 365.61 or 365.64 and 365.71
H40.51X2	365.59 or 365.60 or 365.61 or 365.64 and 365.72
H40.51X3	365.59 or 365.60 or 365.61 or 365.64 and 365.73
H40.51X4	365.59 or 365.60 or 365.61 or 365.64 and 365.74
H40.52X0	365.59 or 365.60 or 365.61 or 365.64 and 365.70
H40.52X1	365.59 or 365.60 or 365.61 or 365.64 and 365.71
H40.52X2	365.59 or 365.60 or 365.61 or 365.64 and 365.72
H40.52X3	365.59 or 365.60 or 365.61 or 365.64 and 365.73
H40.52X4	365.59 or 365.60 or 365.61 or 365.64 and 365.74
H40.53X0	365.59 or 365.60 or 365.61 or 365.64 and 365.70
H40.53X1	365.59 or 365.60 or 365.61 or 365.64 and 365.71
H40.53X2	365.59 or 365.60 or 365.61 or 365.64 and 365.72
H40.53X3	365.59 or 365.60 or 365.61 or 365.64 and 365.73
H40.53X4	365.59 or 365.60 or 365.61 or 365.64 and 365.74
H40.60X0	365.31 or 365.32 and 365.70
H40.60X1	365.31 or 365.32 and 365.71
H40.60X2	365.31 or 365.32 and 365.72
H40.60X3	365.31 or 365.32 and 365.73
H40.60X4	365.31 or 365.32 and 365.74
H40.61X0	365.31 or 365.32 and 365.70
H40.61X1	365.31 or 365.32 and 365.71
H40.61X2	365.31 or 365.32 and 365.72
H40.61X3	365.31 or 365.32 and 365.73
H40.61X4	365.31 or 365.32 and 365.74
H40.62X0	365.31 or 365.32 and 365.70
H40.62X1	365.31 or 365.32 and 365.71
H40.62X2	365.31 or 365.32 and 365.72
H40.62X3	365.31 or 365.32 and 365.73
H40.62X4	365.31 or 365.32 and 365.74
H40.63X0	365.31 or 365.32 and 365.70
H40.63X1	365.31 or 365.32 and 365.71
H40.63X2	365.31 or 365.32 and 365.72
H40.63X3	365.31 or 365.32 and 365.73
H40.63X4	365.31 or 365.32 and 365.74
I25.110	411.1 and 414.01
I25.111	413.9 and 414.01
I25.118	413.9 and 414.01
I25.119	413.9 and 414.01
I25.700	411.1 and 414.05
I25.701	413.9 and 414.05
I25.708	413.9 and 414.05
I25.709	413.9 and 414.05
I25.710	411.1 and 414.02
I25.711	413.9 and 414.02
I25.718	413.9 and 414.02
I25.719	413.9 and 414.02
I25.720	411.1 and 414.04
I25.721	413.9 and 414.04
I25.728	413.9 and 414.04
I25.729	413.9 and 414.04
I25.730	411.1 and 414.03
I25.731	413.9 and 414.03
I25.738	413.9 and 414.03
I25.739	413.9 and 414.03
I25.750	411.1 and 414.06
I25.751	413.9 and 414.06
I25.758	413.9 and 414.06
I25.759	413.9 and 414.06
I25.760	411.1 and 414.07
I25.761	413.9 and 414.07
I25.768	413.9 and 414.07
I25.769	413.9 and 414.07
I25.790	411.1 and 414.04; 411.1 and 414.05
I25.791	413.9 and 414.04; 413.9 and 414.05
I25.798	413.9 and 414.04; 413.9 and 414.05
I25.799	413.9 and 414.04; 413.9 and 414.05
I26.01	415.0 and 415.12
I26.02	415.0 and 415.13
I26.09	415.0 and 415.19
I50.20	428.0 and 428.20
I50.21	428.0 and 428.21
I50.22	428.0 and 428.22
I50.23	428.0 and 428.23
I50.30	428.0 and 428.30
I50.31	428.0 and 428.31
I50.32	428.0 and 428.32
I50.33	428.0 and 428.33
I50.40	428.0 and 428.40
I50.41	428.0 and 428.41
I50.42	428.0 and 428.42
I50.43	428.0 and 428.43
I70.231	440.23 and 707.11
I70.232	440.23 and 707.12
I70.233	440.23 and 707.13
I70.234	440.23 and 707.14
I70.235	440.23 and 707.15
I70.238	440.23 and 707.19
I70.239	440.23 and 707.19
I70.241	440.23 and 707.11
I70.242	440.23 and 707.12
I70.243	440.23 and 707.13
I70.244	440.23 and 707.14
I70.245	440.23 and 707.15
I70.248	440.23 and 707.19
I70.249	440.23 and 707.19
I70.25	440.23 and 707.9
I70.331	440.30 and 707.11
I70.332	440.30 and 707.12
I70.333	440.30 and 707.13
I70.334	440.30 and 707.14
I70.335	440.30 and 707.15
I70.338	440.30 and 707.19
I70.339	440.30 and 707.19
I70.341	440.30 and 707.11
I70.342	440.30 and 707.12

I7Ø.343	44Ø.3Ø and 7Ø7.13
I7Ø.344	44Ø.3Ø and 7Ø7.14
I7Ø.345	44Ø.3Ø and 7Ø7.15
I7Ø.348	44Ø.3Ø and 7Ø7.19
I7Ø.349	44Ø.3Ø and 7Ø7.19
I7Ø.35	44Ø.3Ø and 7Ø7.9
I7Ø.361	44Ø.3Ø and 785.4
I7Ø.362	44Ø.3Ø and 785.4
I7Ø.363	44Ø.3Ø and 785.4
I7Ø.368	44Ø.3Ø and 785.4
I7Ø.369	44Ø.3Ø and 785.4
I7Ø.431	44Ø.31 and 7Ø7.11
I7Ø.432	44Ø.31 and 7Ø7.12
I7Ø.433	44Ø.31 and 7Ø7.13
I7Ø.434	44Ø.31 and 7Ø7.14
I7Ø.435	44Ø.31 and 7Ø7.15
I7Ø.438	44Ø.31 and 7Ø7.19
I7Ø.439	44Ø.31 and 7Ø7.19
I7Ø.441	44Ø.31 and 7Ø7.11
I7Ø.442	44Ø.31 and 7Ø7.12
I7Ø.443	44Ø.31 and 7Ø7.13
I7Ø.444	44Ø.31 and 7Ø7.14
I7Ø.445	44Ø.31 and 7Ø7.15
I7Ø.448	44Ø.31 and 7Ø7.19
I7Ø.449	44Ø.31 and 7Ø7.19
I7Ø.45	44Ø.31 and 7Ø7.9
I7Ø.461	44Ø.31 and 785.4
I7Ø.462	44Ø.31 and 785.4
I7Ø.463	44Ø.31 and 785.4
I7Ø.468	44Ø.31 and 785.4
I7Ø.469	44Ø.31 and 785.4
I7Ø.531	44Ø.32 and 7Ø7.11
I7Ø.532	44Ø.32 and 7Ø7.12
I7Ø.533	44Ø.32 and 7Ø7.13
I7Ø.534	44Ø.32 and 7Ø7.14
I7Ø.535	44Ø.32 and 7Ø7.15
I7Ø.538	44Ø.32 and 7Ø7.19
I7Ø.539	44Ø.32 and 7Ø7.19
I7Ø.541	44Ø.32 and 7Ø7.11
I7Ø.542	44Ø.32 and 7Ø7.12
I7Ø.543	44Ø.32 and 7Ø7.13
I7Ø.544	44Ø.32 and 7Ø7.14
I7Ø.545	44Ø.32 and 7Ø7.15
I7Ø.548	44Ø.32 and 7Ø7.19
I7Ø.549	44Ø.32 and 7Ø7.19
I7Ø.55	44Ø.32 and 7Ø7.9
I7Ø.561	44Ø.32 and 785.4
I7Ø.562	44Ø.32 and 785.4
I7Ø.563	44Ø.32 and 785.4
I7Ø.568	44Ø.32 and 785.4
I7Ø.569	44Ø.32 and 785.4
I7Ø.631	44Ø.3Ø and 7Ø7.11
I7Ø.632	44Ø.3Ø and 7Ø7.12
I7Ø.633	44Ø.3Ø and 7Ø7.13
I7Ø.634	44Ø.3Ø and 7Ø7.14
I7Ø.635	44Ø.3Ø and 7Ø7.15
I7Ø.638	44Ø.3Ø and 7Ø7.19
I7Ø.639	44Ø.3Ø and 7Ø7.19
I7Ø.641	44Ø.3Ø and 7Ø7.11
I7Ø.642	44Ø.3Ø and 7Ø7.12
I7Ø.643	44Ø.3Ø and 7Ø7.13
I7Ø.644	44Ø.3Ø and 7Ø7.14
I7Ø.645	44Ø.3Ø and 7Ø7.15
I7Ø.648	44Ø.3Ø and 7Ø7.19
I7Ø.649	44Ø.3Ø and 7Ø7.19
I7Ø.65	44Ø.3Ø and 7Ø7.9
I7Ø.661	44Ø.3Ø and 785.4
I7Ø.662	44Ø.3Ø and 785.4
I7Ø.663	44Ø.3Ø and 785.4
I7Ø.668	44Ø.3Ø and 785.4
I7Ø.669	44Ø.3Ø and 785.4
I7Ø.731	44Ø.3Ø and 7Ø7.11
I7Ø.732	44Ø.3Ø and 7Ø7.12
I7Ø.733	44Ø.3Ø and 7Ø7.13
I7Ø.734	44Ø.3Ø and 7Ø7.14
I7Ø.735	44Ø.3Ø and 7Ø7.15
I7Ø.738	44Ø.3Ø and 7Ø7.19
I7Ø.739	44Ø.3Ø and 7Ø7.19
I7Ø.741	44Ø.3Ø and 7Ø7.11
I7Ø.742	44Ø.3Ø and 7Ø7.12
I7Ø.743	44Ø.3Ø and 7Ø7.13
I7Ø.744	44Ø.3Ø and 7Ø7.14
I7Ø.745	44Ø.3Ø and 7Ø7.15
I7Ø.748	44Ø.3Ø and 7Ø7.19
I7Ø.749	44Ø.3Ø and 7Ø7.19
I7Ø.75	44Ø.3Ø and 7Ø7.9
I7Ø.761	44Ø.3Ø and 785.4
I7Ø.762	44Ø.3Ø and 785.4
I7Ø.763	44Ø.3Ø and 785.4
I7Ø.768	44Ø.3Ø and 785.4
I7Ø.769	44Ø.3Ø and 785.4
I73.Ø1	443.Ø and 785.4
I97.11Ø	429.4 and 997.1
I97.111	429.4 and 997.1
I97.12Ø	429.4 and 997.1
I97.121	429.4 and 997.1
I97.13Ø	429.4 and 997.1
I97.131	429.4 and 997.1
I97.19Ø	429.4 and 997.1
I97.191	429.4 and 997.1
J2Ø.Ø	Ø41.81 and 466.Ø
J2Ø.1	Ø41.5 and 466.Ø
J2Ø.2	Ø41.ØØ and 466.Ø
J2Ø.3	Ø79.2 and 466.Ø
J2Ø.4	Ø79.89 and 466.Ø
J2Ø.5	Ø79.6 and 466.Ø
J2Ø.6	Ø79.3 and 466.Ø
J2Ø.7	Ø79.1 and 466.Ø
KØ2.51	521.Ø1 and 521.Ø6
KØ2.52	521.Ø2 and 521.Ø6
KØ2.53	521.Ø3 and 521.Ø6
KØ2.61	521.Ø1 and 521.Ø7
KØ2.62	521.Ø2 and 521.Ø7
KØ2.63	521.Ø3 and 521.Ø7
KØ8.1Ø1	525.1Ø and 525.41
KØ8.1Ø2	525.1Ø and 525.42
KØ8.1Ø3	525.1Ø and 525.43
KØ8.1Ø4	525.1Ø and 525.44
KØ8.1Ø9	525.1Ø and 525.4Ø
KØ8.111	525.11 and 525.41
KØ8.112	525.11 and 525.42
KØ8.113	525.11 and 525.43
KØ8.114	525.11 and 525.44
KØ8.119	525.11 and 525.4Ø
KØ8.121	525.12 and 525.41
KØ8.122	525.12 and 525.42
KØ8.123	525.12 and 525.43
KØ8.124	525.12 and 525.44
KØ8.129	525.12 and 525.4Ø
KØ8.131	525.13 and 525.41
KØ8.132	525.13 and 525.42
KØ8.133	525.13 and 525.43
KØ8.134	525.13 and 525.44
KØ8.139	525.13 and 525.4Ø
KØ8.191	525.19 and 525.41
KØ8.192	525.19 and 525.42
KØ8.193	525.19 and 525.43
KØ8.194	525.19 and 525.44
KØ8.199	525.19 and 525.4Ø
KØ8.4Ø1	525.1Ø and 525.51
KØ8.4Ø2	525.1Ø and 525.52
KØ8.4Ø3	525.1Ø and 525.53
KØ8.4Ø4	525.1Ø and 525.54
KØ8.4Ø9	525.1Ø and 525.5Ø
KØ8.411	525.11 and 525.51
KØ8.412	525.11 and 525.52
KØ8.413	525.11 and 525.53
KØ8.414	525.11 and 525.54
KØ8.419	525.11 and 525.5Ø
KØ8.421	525.12 and 525.51
KØ8.422	525.12 and 525.52
KØ8.423	525.12 and 525.53
KØ8.424	525.12 and 525.54
KØ8.429	525.12 and 525.5Ø
KØ8.431	525.13 and 525.51
KØ8.432	525.13 and 525.52
KØ8.433	525.13 and 525.53
KØ8.434	525.13 and 525.54
KØ8.439	525.13 and 525.5Ø
KØ8.491	525.19 and 525.51
KØ8.492	525.19 and 525.52
KØ8.493	525.19 and 525.53
KØ8.494	525.19 and 525.54
KØ8.499	525.19 and 525.5Ø
K5Ø.Ø12	555.Ø and 56Ø.9
K5Ø.Ø13	555.Ø and 569.81
K5Ø.Ø14	555.Ø and 569.5
K5Ø.112	555.1 and 56Ø.9
K5Ø.113	555.1 and 569.81
K5Ø.114	555.1 and 569.5
K5Ø.812	555.2 and 56Ø.9
K5Ø.813	555.2 and 569.81
K5Ø.814	555.2 and 569.5
K5Ø.912	555.9 and 56Ø.9
K5Ø.913	555.9 and 569.81
K5Ø.914	555.9 and 569.5
K51.Ø12	556.6 and 56Ø.89
K51.Ø13	556.6 and 569.81
K51.Ø14	556.6 and 569.5
K51.212	556.2 and 56Ø.89
K51.213	556.2 and 569.81
K51.214	556.2 and 569.5
K51.312	556.3 and 56Ø.89
K51.313	556.3 and 569.81
K51.314	556.3 and 569.5
K51.412	556.4 and 56Ø.89
K51.413	556.4 and 569.81
K51.414	556.4 and 569.5
K51.512	556.5 and 56Ø.89
K51.513	556.5 and 569.81
K51.514	556.5 and 569.5
K51.812	556.8 and 56Ø.89
K51.813	556.8 and 569.81
K51.814	556.8 and 569.5
K51.912	556.9 and 56Ø.89
K51.913	556.9 and 569.81
K51.914	556.9 and 569.5
K57.ØØ	562.Ø1 and 569.5
K57.Ø1	562.Ø3 and 569.5
K57.2Ø	562.11 and 569.5
K57.21	562.13 and 569.5
K57.4Ø	562.Ø1 and 562.11 and 569.5
K57.41	562.Ø3 and 562.13 and 569.5
K57.5Ø	562.ØØ and 562.1Ø
K57.51	562.Ø2 and 562.12
K57.52	562.Ø1 and 562.11
K57.53	562.Ø3 and 562.13
K57.8Ø	562.11 and 569.5
K57.81	562.13 and 569.5
K7Ø.41	571.3 and 572.2
K71.11	572.2 and 573.3
K72.Ø1	57Ø and 572.2
K72.11	572.2 and 572.8
K72.91	572.2 and 572.8
K8Ø.12	574.ØØ and 574.1Ø
K8Ø.13	574.Ø1 and 574.11

K80.30	574.50 and 576.1
K80.31	574.51 and 576.1
K80.32	574.50 and 576.1
K80.33	574.51 and 576.1
K80.34	574.50 and 576.1
K80.35	574.51 and 576.1
K80.36	574.50 and 576.1
K80.37	574.51 and 576.1
K80.46	574.30 and 574.40
K80.47	574.31 and 574.41
L89.000	707.01 and 707.25
L89.001	707.01 and 707.21
L89.002	707.01 and 707.22
L89.003	707.01 and 707.23
L89.004	707.01 and 707.24
L89.009	707.01 and 707.20
L89.010	707.01 and 707.25
L89.011	707.01 and 707.21
L89.012	707.01 and 707.22
L89.013	707.01 and 707.23
L89.014	707.01 and 707.24
L89.019	707.01 and 707.20
L89.020	707.01 and 707.25
L89.021	707.01 and 707.21
L89.022	707.01 and 707.22
L89.023	707.01 and 707.23
L89.024	707.01 and 707.24
L89.029	707.01 and 707.20
L89.100	707.02 and 707.25
L89.101	707.02 and 707.21
L89.102	707.02 and 707.22
L89.103	707.02 and 707.23
L89.104	707.02 and 707.24
L89.109	707.02 and 707.20
L89.110	707.02 and 707.25
L89.111	707.02 and 707.21
L89.112	707.02 and 707.22
L89.113	707.02 and 707.23
L89.114	707.02 and 707.24
L89.119	707.02 and 707.20
L89.120	707.02 and 707.25
L89.121	707.02 and 707.21
L89.122	707.02 and 707.22
L89.123	707.02 and 707.23
L89.124	707.02 and 707.24
L89.129	707.02 and 707.20
L89.130	707.03 and 707.25
L89.131	707.03 and 707.21
L89.132	707.03 and 707.22
L89.133	707.03 and 707.23
L89.134	707.03 and 707.24
L89.139	707.03 and 707.20
L89.140	707.03 and 707.25
L89.141	707.03 and 707.21
L89.142	707.03 and 707.22
L89.143	707.03 and 707.23
L89.144	707.03 and 707.24
L89.149	707.03 and 707.20
L89.150	707.03 and 707.25
L89.151	707.03 and 707.21
L89.152	707.03 and 707.22
L89.153	707.03 and 707.23
L89.154	707.03 and 707.24
L89.159	707.03 and 707.20
L89.200	707.04 and 707.25
L89.201	707.04 and 707.21
L89.202	707.04 and 707.22
L89.203	707.04 and 707.23
L89.204	707.04 and 707.24
L89.209	707.04 and 707.20
L89.210	707.04 and 707.25
L89.211	707.04 and 707.21
L89.212	707.04 and 707.22
L89.213	707.04 and 707.23
L89.214	707.04 and 707.24
L89.219	707.04 and 707.20
L89.220	707.04 and 707.25
L89.221	707.04 and 707.21
L89.222	707.04 and 707.22
L89.223	707.04 and 707.23
L89.224	707.04 and 707.24
L89.229	707.04 and 707.20
L89.300	707.05 and 707.25
L89.301	707.05 and 707.21
L89.302	707.05 and 707.22
L89.303	707.05 and 707.23
L89.304	707.05 and 707.24
L89.309	707.05 and 707.20
L89.310	707.05 and 707.25
L89.311	707.05 and 707.21
L89.312	707.05 and 707.22
L89.313	707.05 and 707.23
L89.314	707.05 and 707.24
L89.319	707.05 and 707.20
L89.320	707.05 and 707.25
L89.321	707.05 and 707.21
L89.322	707.05 and 707.22
L89.323	707.05 and 707.23
L89.324	707.05 and 707.24
L89.329	707.05 and 707.20
L89.40	707.03 and 707.04 and 707.05 and 707.20
L89.41	707.03 and 707.04 and 707.05 and 707.21
L89.42	707.03 and 707.04 and 707.05 and 707.22
L89.43	707.03 and 707.04 and 707.05 and 707.23
L89.44	707.03 and 707.04 and 707.05 and 707.24
L89.45	707.03 and 707.04 and 707.05 and 707.25
L89.500	707.06 and 707.25
L89.501	707.06 and 707.21
L89.502	707.06 and 707.22
L89.503	707.06 and 707.23
L89.504	707.06 and 707.24
L89.509	707.06 and 707.20
L89.510	707.06 and 707.25
L89.511	707.06 and 707.21
L89.512	707.06 and 707.22
L89.513	707.06 and 707.23
L89.514	707.06 and 707.24
L89.519	707.06 and 707.20
L89.520	707.06 and 707.25
L89.521	707.06 and 707.21
L89.522	707.06 and 707.22
L89.523	707.06 and 707.23
L89.524	707.06 and 707.24
L89.529	707.06 and 707.20
L89.600	707.07 and 707.25
L89.601	707.07 and 707.21
L89.602	707.07 and 707.22
L89.603	707.07 and 707.23
L89.604	707.07 and 707.24
L89.609	707.07 and 707.20
L89.610	707.07 and 707.25
L89.611	707.07 and 707.21
L89.612	707.07 and 707.22
L89.613	707.07 and 707.23
L89.614	707.07 and 707.24
L89.619	707.07 and 707.20
L89.620	707.07 and 707.25
L89.621	707.07 and 707.21
L89.622	707.07 and 707.22
L89.623	707.07 and 707.23
L89.624	707.07 and 707.24
L89.629	707.07 and 707.20
L89.810	707.09 and 707.25
L89.811	707.09 and 707.21
L89.812	707.09 and 707.22
L89.813	707.09 and 707.23
L89.814	707.09 and 707.24
L89.819	707.09 and 707.20
L89.890	707.09 and 707.25
L89.891	707.09 and 707.21
L89.892	707.09 and 707.22
L89.893	707.09 and 707.23
L89.894	707.09 and 707.24
L89.899	707.09 and 707.20
L89.90	707.00 and 707.20
L89.91	707.00 and 707.21
L89.92	707.00 and 707.22
L89.93	707.00 and 707.23
L89.94	707.00 and 707.24
L89.95	707.00 and 707.25
M00.00	041.10 and 711.00
M00.011	041.10 and 711.01
M00.012	041.10 and 711.01
M00.019	041.10 and 711.01
M00.021	041.10 and 711.02
M00.022	041.10 and 711.02
M00.029	041.10 and 711.02
M00.031	041.10 and 711.03
M00.032	041.10 and 711.03
M00.039	041.10 and 711.03
M00.041	041.10 and 711.04
M00.042	041.10 and 711.04
M00.049	041.10 and 711.04
M00.051	041.10 and 711.05
M00.052	041.10 and 711.05
M00.059	041.10 and 711.05
M00.061	041.10 and 711.06
M00.062	041.10 and 711.06
M00.069	041.10 and 711.06
M00.071	041.10 and 711.07
M00.072	041.10 and 711.07
M00.079	041.10 and 711.07
M00.08	041.10 and 711.08
M00.09	041.10 and 711.08
M00.10	041.2 and 711.00
M00.111	041.2 and 711.01
M00.112	041.2 and 711.01
M00.119	041.2 and 711.01
M00.121	041.2 and 711.02
M00.122	041.2 and 711.02
M00.129	041.2 and 711.02
M00.131	041.2 and 711.03
M00.132	041.2 and 711.03
M00.139	041.2 and 711.03
M00.141	041.2 and 711.04
M00.142	041.2 and 711.04
M00.149	041.2 and 711.04
M00.151	041.2 and 711.05
M00.152	041.2 and 711.05
M00.159	041.2 and 711.05
M00.161	041.2 and 711.06
M00.162	041.2 and 711.06
M00.169	041.2 and 711.06
M00.171	041.2 and 711.07
M00.172	041.2 and 711.07
M00.179	041.2 and 711.07
M00.18	041.2 and 711.08
M00.19	041.2 and 711.09
M00.20	041.09 and 711.00
M00.211	041.09 and 711.01

MØØ.212 Ø41.Ø9 and 711.Ø1
MØØ.219 Ø41.Ø9 and 711.Ø1
MØØ.221 Ø41.Ø9 and 711.Ø2
MØØ.222 Ø41.Ø9 and 711.Ø2
MØØ.229 Ø41.Ø9 and 711.Ø2
MØØ.231 Ø41.Ø9 and 711.Ø3
MØØ.232 Ø41.Ø9 and 711.Ø3
MØØ.239 Ø41.Ø9 and 711.Ø3
MØØ.241 Ø41.Ø9 and 711.Ø4
MØØ.242 Ø41.Ø9 and 711.Ø4
MØØ.249 Ø41.Ø9 and 711.Ø4
MØØ.251 Ø41.Ø9 and 711.Ø5
MØØ.252 Ø41.Ø9 and 711.Ø5
MØØ.259 Ø41.Ø9 and 711.Ø5
MØØ.261 Ø41.Ø9 and 711.Ø6
MØØ.262 Ø41.Ø9 and 711.Ø6
MØØ.269 Ø41.Ø9 and 711.Ø6
MØØ.271 Ø41.Ø9 and 711.Ø7
MØØ.272 Ø41.Ø9 and 711.Ø7
MØØ.279 Ø41.Ø9 and 711.Ø7
MØØ.28 Ø41.Ø9 and 711.Ø8
MØØ.29 Ø41.Ø9 and 711.Ø9
MØØ.8Ø Ø41.89 and 711.ØØ
MØØ.811 Ø41.89 and 711.Ø1
MØØ.812 Ø41.89 and 711.Ø1
MØØ.819 Ø41.89 and 711.Ø1
MØØ.821 Ø41.89 and 711.Ø2
MØØ.822 Ø41.89 and 711.Ø2
MØØ.829 Ø41.89 and 711.Ø2
MØØ.831 Ø41.89 and 711.Ø3
MØØ.832 Ø41.89 and 711.Ø3
MØØ.839 Ø41.89 and 711.Ø3
MØØ.841 Ø41.89 and 711.Ø4
MØØ.842 Ø41.89 and 711.Ø4
MØØ.849 Ø41.89 and 711.Ø4
MØØ.851 Ø41.89 and 711.Ø5
MØØ.852 Ø41.89 and 711.Ø5
MØØ.859 Ø41.89 and 711.Ø5
MØØ.861 Ø41.89 and 711.Ø6
MØØ.862 Ø41.89 and 711.Ø6
MØØ.869 Ø41.89 and 711.Ø6
MØØ.871 Ø41.89 and 711.Ø7
MØØ.872 Ø41.89 and 711.Ø7
MØØ.879 Ø41.89 and 711.Ø7
MØØ.88 Ø41.89 and 711.Ø8
MØØ.89 Ø41.89 and 711.Ø9
MØ2.211 713.6 and 999.52
MØ2.212 713.6 and 999.52
MØ2.219 713.6 and 999.52
MØ2.221 713.6 and 999.52
MØ2.222 713.6 and 999.52
MØ2.229 713.6 and 999.52
MØ2.231 713.6 and 999.52
MØ2.232 713.6 and 999.52
MØ2.239 713.6 and 999.52
MØ2.241 713.6 and 999.52
MØ2.242 713.6 and 999.52
MØ2.249 713.6 and 999.52
MØ2.251 713.6 and 999.52
MØ2.252 713.6 and 999.52
MØ2.259 713.6 and 999.52
MØ2.261 713.6 and 999.52
MØ2.262 713.6 and 999.52
MØ2.269 713.6 and 999.52
MØ2.271 713.6 and 999.52
MØ2.272 713.6 and 999.52
MØ2.279 713.6 and 999.52
MØ2.28 713.6 and 999.52
MØ2.29 713.6 and 999.52
MØ2.3Ø Ø99.3 and 711.1Ø
MØ2.311 Ø99.3 and 711.11
MØ2.312 Ø99.3 and 711.11
MØ2.319 Ø99.3 and 711.11
MØ2.321 Ø99.3 and 711.12
MØ2.322 Ø99.3 and 711.12
MØ2.329 Ø99.3 and 711.12
MØ2.331 Ø99.3 and 711.13
MØ2.332 Ø99.3 and 711.13
MØ2.339 Ø99.3 and 711.13
MØ2.341 Ø99.3 and 711.14
MØ2.342 Ø99.3 and 711.14
MØ2.349 Ø99.3 and 711.14
MØ2.351 Ø99.3 and 711.15
MØ2.352 Ø99.3 and 711.15
MØ2.359 Ø99.3 and 711.15
MØ2.361 Ø99.3 and 711.16
MØ2.362 Ø99.3 and 711.16
MØ2.369 Ø99.3 and 711.16
MØ2.371 Ø99.3 and 711.17
MØ2.372 Ø99.3 and 711.17
MØ2.379 Ø99.3 and 711.17
MØ2.38 Ø99.3 and 711.18
MØ2.39 Ø99.3 and 711.19
MØ5.4Ø 359.6 and 714.Ø
MØ5.411 359.6 and 714.Ø
MØ5.412 359.6 and 714.Ø
MØ5.419 359.6 and 714.Ø
MØ5.421 359.6 and 714.Ø
MØ5.422 359.6 and 714.Ø
MØ5.429 359.6 and 714.Ø
MØ5.431 359.6 and 714.Ø
MØ5.432 359.6 and 714.Ø
MØ5.439 359.6 and 714.Ø
MØ5.441 359.6 and 714.Ø
MØ5.442 359.6 and 714.Ø
MØ5.449 359.6 and 714.Ø
MØ5.451 359.6 and 714.Ø
MØ5.452 359.6 and 714.Ø
MØ5.459 359.6 and 714.Ø
MØ5.461 359.6 and 714.Ø
MØ5.462 359.6 and 714.Ø
MØ5.469 359.6 and 714.Ø
MØ5.471 359.6 and 714.Ø
MØ5.472 359.6 and 714.Ø
MØ5.479 359.6 and 714.Ø
MØ5.49 359.6 and 714.Ø
MØ5.5Ø 357.1 and 714.Ø
MØ5.511 357.1 and 714.Ø
MØ5.512 357.1 and 714.Ø
MØ5.519 357.1 and 714.Ø
MØ5.521 357.1 and 714.Ø
MØ5.522 357.1 and 714.Ø
MØ5.529 357.1 and 714.Ø
MØ5.531 357.1 and 714.Ø
MØ5.532 357.1 and 714.Ø
MØ5.539 357.1 and 714.Ø
MØ5.541 357.1 and 714.Ø
MØ5.542 357.1 and 714.Ø
MØ5.549 357.1 and 714.Ø
MØ5.551 357.1 and 714.Ø
MØ5.552 357.1 and 714.Ø
MØ5.559 357.1 and 714.Ø
MØ5.561 357.1 and 714.Ø
MØ5.562 357.1 and 714.Ø
MØ5.569 357.1 and 714.Ø
MØ5.571 357.1 and 714.Ø
MØ5.572 357.1 and 714.Ø
MØ5.579 357.1 and 714.Ø
MØ5.59 357.1 and 714.Ø
MØ7.6Ø 713.1 and 716.8Ø
MØ7.611 713.1 and 716.81
MØ7.612 713.1 and 716.81
MØ7.619 713.1 and 716.81
MØ7.621 713.1 and 716.82
MØ7.622 713.1 and 716.82
MØ7.629 713.1 and 716.82
MØ7.631 713.1 and 716.83
MØ7.632 713.1 and 716.83
MØ7.639 713.1 and 716.83
MØ7.641 713.1 and 716.84
MØ7.642 713.1 and 716.84
MØ7.649 713.1 and 716.84
MØ7.651 713.1 and 716.85
MØ7.652 713.1 and 716.85
MØ7.659 713.1 and 716.85
MØ7.661 713.1 and 716.86
MØ7.662 713.1 and 716.86
MØ7.669 713.1 and 716.86
MØ7.671 713.1 and 716.87
MØ7.672 713.1 and 716.87
MØ7.679 713.1 and 716.87
MØ7.68 713.1 and 716.88
MØ7.69 713.1 and 716.89
M32.11 424.91 and 71Ø.Ø
M32.12 42Ø.Ø and 71Ø.Ø
M32.13 517.8 and 71Ø.Ø
M32.14 583.81 and 71Ø.Ø
M32.15 583.81 and 71Ø.Ø
M33.Ø1 517.8 and 71Ø.3
M33.Ø2 359.6 and 71Ø.3
M33.11 517.8 and 71Ø.3
M33.12 359.6 and 71Ø.3
M33.21 517.8 and 71Ø.4
M33.22 359.6 and 71Ø.4
M33.91 517.8 and 71Ø.3
M33.92 359.6 and 71Ø.3
M34.81 517.2 and 71Ø.1
M34.82 359.6 and 71Ø.1
M34.83 357.4 and 71Ø.1
M35.Ø2 517.8 and 71Ø.2
M35.Ø3 359.6 and 71Ø.2
M35.Ø4 583.81 and 71Ø.2
M35.2 136.1 and 711.2Ø
M9Ø.5Ø 731.8 and 733.4Ø
M9Ø.511 731.8 and 733.41
M9Ø.512 731.8 and 733.41
M9Ø.519 731.8 and 733.41
M9Ø.521 731.8 and 733.49
M9Ø.522 731.8 and 733.49
M9Ø.529 731.8 and 733.49
M9Ø.531 731.8 and 733.49
M9Ø.532 731.8 and 733.49
M9Ø.539 731.8 and 733.49
M9Ø.541 731.8 and 733.49
M9Ø.542 731.8 and 733.49
M9Ø.549 731.8 and 733.49
M9Ø.551 731.8 and 733.42
M9Ø.552 731.8 and 733.42
M9Ø.559 731.8 and 733.42
M9Ø.561 731.8 and 733.49
M9Ø.562 731.8 and 733.49
M9Ø.569 731.8 and 733.49
M9Ø.571 731.8 and 733.49
M9Ø.572 731.8 and 733.49
M9Ø.579 731.8 and 733.49
M9Ø.58 731.8 and 733.49
M9Ø.59 731.8 and 733.49

ICD-10-CM	ICD-9-CM
N11.1	590.01 and 593.3; 590.01 and 593.4
N13.1[1]	591 and 593.3
N13.2[1]	591 and 592.0; 591 and 592.1
N13.9[2]	592.9
N36.43	599.81 and 599.82
O12.20	646.10 and 646.20
O12.21	646.11 and 646.21; 646.13 and 646.23
O12.22	646.11 and 646.21; 646.13 and 646.23
O12.23	646.11 and 646.21; 646.13 and 646.23
O30.001	651.01 and V91.00; 651.03 and V91.00
O30.002	651.01 and V91.00; 651.03 and V91.00
O30.003	651.01 and V91.00; 651.03 and V91.00
O30.009	651.00 and V91.00
O30.011	651.01 and V91.01; 651.03 and V91.01
O30.012	651.01 and V91.01; 651.03 and V91.01
O30.013	651.01 and V91.01; 651.03 and V91.01
O30.019	651.00 and V91.01
O30.031	651.01 and V91.02; 651.03 and V91.02
O30.032	651.01 and V91.02; 651.03 and V91.02
O30.033	651.01 and V91.02; 651.03 and V91.02
O30.039	651.00 and V91.02
O30.041	651.01 and V91.03; 651.03 and V91.03
O30.042	651.01 and V91.03; 651.03 and V91.03
O30.043	651.01 and V91.03; 651.03 and V91.03
O30.049	651.00 and V91.03
O30.091	651.01 and V91.09; 651.03 and V91.09
O30.092	651.01 and V91.09; 651.03 and V91.09
O30.093	651.01 and V91.09; 651.03 and V91.09
O30.099	651.00 and V91.09
O30.101	651.11 and V91.10; 651.13 and V91.10
O30.102	651.11 and V91.10; 651.13 and V91.10
O30.103	651.11 and V91.10; 651.13 and V91.10
O30.109	651.10 and V91.10
O30.111	651.11 and V91.11; 651.13 and V91.11
O30.112	651.11 and V91.11; 651.13 and V91.11
O30.113	651.11 and V91.11; 651.13 and V91.11
O30.119	651.10 and V91.11
O30.121	651.11 and V91.12; 651.13 and V91.12
O30.122	651.11 and V91.12; 651.13 and V91.12
O30.123	651.11 and V91.12; 651.13 and V91.12
O30.129	651.10 and V91.12
O30.191	651.11 and V91.19; 651.13 and V91.19
O30.192	651.11 and V91.19; 651.13 and V91.19
O30.193	651.11 and V91.19; 651.13 and V91.19
O30.199	651.10 and V91.19
O30.201	651.21 and V91.20; 651.23 and V91.20
O30.202	651.21 and V91.20; 651.23 and V91.20
O30.203	651.21 and V91.20; 651.23 and V91.20
O30.209	651.20 and V91.20
O30.211	651.21 and V91.21; 651.23 and V91.21
O30.212	651.21 and V91.21; 651.23 and V91.21
O30.213	651.21 and V91.21; 651.23 and V91.21
O30.219	651.20 and V91.21
O30.221	651.21 and V91.22; 651.23 and V91.22
O30.222	651.21 and V91.22; 651.23 and V91.22
O30.223	651.21 and V91.22; 651.23 and V91.22
O30.229	651.20 and V91.22
O30.291	651.21 and V91.29; 651.23 and V91.29
O30.292	651.21 and V91.29; 651.23 and V91.29
O30.293	651.21 and V91.29; 651.23 and V91.29
O30.299	651.20 and V91.29
O30.801	651.81 and V91.90; 651.83 and V91.90
O30.802	651.81 and V91.90; 651.83 and V91.90
O30.803	651.81 and V91.90; 651.83 and V91.90
O30.809	651.80 and V91.90
O30.811	651.81 and V91.91; 651.83 and V91.91
O30.812	651.81 and V91.91; 651.83 and V91.91
O30.813	651.81 and V91.91; 651.83 and V91.91
O30.819	651.80 and V91.91
O30.821	651.81 and V91.92; 651.83 and V91.92
O30.822	651.81 and V91.92; 651.83 and V91.92
O30.823	651.81 and V91.92; 651.83 and V91.92
O30.829	651.80 and V91.92
O30.891	651.81 and V91.99; 651.83 and V91.99
O30.892	651.81 and V91.99; 651.83 and V91.99
O30.893	651.81 and V91.99; 651.83 and V91.99
O30.899	651.80 and V91.99
O64.1XX0	652.21 and 660.01
O64.1XX1	652.21 and 660.01
O64.1XX2	652.21 and 660.01
O64.1XX3	652.21 and 660.01
O64.1XX4	652.21 and 660.01
O64.1XX5	652.21 and 660.01
O64.1XX9	652.21 and 660.01
O64.2XX0	652.41 and 660.01
O64.2XX1	652.41 and 660.01
O64.2XX2	652.41 and 660.01
O64.2XX3	652.41 and 660.01
O64.2XX4	652.41 and 660.01
O64.2XX5	652.41 and 660.01
O64.2XX9	652.41 and 660.01
O64.3XX0	652.41 and 660.01
O64.3XX1	652.41 and 660.01
O64.3XX2	652.41 and 660.01
O64.3XX3	652.41 and 660.01
O64.3XX4	652.41 and 660.01
O64.3XX5	652.41 and 660.01
O64.3XX9	652.41 and 660.01
O64.4XX0	652.81 and 660.01
O64.4XX1	652.81 and 660.01
O64.4XX2	652.81 and 660.01
O64.4XX3	652.81 and 660.01
O64.4XX4	652.81 and 660.01
O64.4XX5	652.81 and 660.01
O64.4XX9	652.81 and 660.01
O64.5XX0	652.81 and 660.01
O64.5XX1	652.81 and 660.01
O64.5XX2	652.81 and 660.01
O64.5XX3	652.81 and 660.01
O64.5XX4	652.81 and 660.01
O64.5XX5	652.81 and 660.01
O64.5XX9	652.81 and 660.01
O64.8XX0	652.81 and 660.01
O64.8XX1	652.81 and 660.01
O64.8XX2	652.81 and 660.01
O64.8XX3	652.81 and 660.01
O64.8XX4	652.81 and 660.01
O64.8XX5	652.81 and 660.01
O64.8XX9	652.81 and 660.01
O64.9XX0	652.91 and 660.01
O64.9XX1	652.91 and 660.01
O64.9XX2	652.91 and 660.01
O64.9XX3	652.91 and 660.01
O64.9XX4	652.91 and 660.01
O64.9XX5	652.91 and 660.01
O64.9XX9	652.91 and 660.01
O65.0	653.01 and 660.11
O65.1	653.11 and 660.11
O65.2	653.21 and 660.11
O65.3	653.31 and 660.11
O65.4	653.41 and 660.11
O65.8	654.91 and 660.21
O65.9	654.91 and 660.21
O66.2	653.51 and 660.81
O66.6	652.61 and 660.81
O99.820	648.93 and V02.51
O99.824	648.91 and V02.51
O99.825	648.94 and V02.51
R16.2	789.1 and 789.2
R50.2	780.60 and E947.9
R65.21	785.52 and 995.92
S06.1X0A	348.5 and 854.01
S06.1X1A	348.5 and 854.02
S06.1X2A	348.5 and 854.02
S06.1X3A	348.5 and 854.03

1. Official ICD-10-CM GEM update summary indicates ICD-9-CM code 592.9 should be included in Choice List 2 with GEM flag 10112 for the cluster/combination map for ICD-10-CM code N13.2, but this is not included in the Official ICD-10-CM GEM file as of date of publication.
2. Official ICD-10-CM GEM files show ICD-10-CM code N13.9 mapped to ICD-9-CM code 592.9 as a cluster/combination Choice List 2 GEM flag 10112 without an option for a Choice List 1 GEM flag 10111 as of date of publication.

S06.1X4A	348.5 and 854.03
S06.1X5A	348.5 and 854.04
S06.1X6A	348.5 and 854.05
S06.1X7A	348.5 and 854.05
S06.1X8A	348.5 and 854.05
S06.1X9A	348.5 and 854.06
T14.91	959.9 and E958.9
T15.00XA	930.0 and E914
T15.01XA	930.0 and E914
T15.02XA	930.0 and E914
T15.10XA	930.1 and E914
T15.11XA	930.1 and E914
T15.12XA	930.1 and E914
T15.80XA	930.2 and E914; 930.8 and E914
T15.81XA	930.2 and E914; 930.8 and E914
T15.82XA	930.2 and E914; 930.8 and E914
T15.90XA	930.9 and E914
T15.91XA	930.9 and E914
T15.92XA	930.9 and E914
T16.1XXA	931 and E915
T16.2XXA	931 and E915
T16.9XXA	931 and E915
T17.0XXA	932 and E915
T17.1XXA	932 and E915
T17.200A	933.0 and E912
T17.208A	933.0 and E915
T17.210A	933.0 and E911
T17.218A	933.0 and E911
T17.220A	933.0 and E911
T17.228A	933.0 and E911
T17.290A	933.0 and E912
T17.298A	933.0 and E915
T17.300A	933.1 and E912
T17.308A	933.1 and E915
T17.310A	933.1 and E911
T17.318A	933.1 and E911
T17.320A	933.1 and E911
T17.328A	933.1 and E911
T17.390A	933.1 and E912
T17.398A	933.1 and E915
T17.400A	934.0 and E912
T17.408A	934.0 and E915
T17.410A	934.0 and E911
T17.418A	934.0 and E911
T17.420A	934.0 and E911
T17.428A	934.0 and E911
T17.490A	934.0 and E912
T17.498A	934.0 and E915
T17.500A	934.1 and E912
T17.508A	934.1 and E915
T17.510A	934.1 and E911
T17.518A	934.1 and E911
T17.520A	934.1 and E911
T17.528A	934.1 and E911
T17.590A	934.1 and E912
T17.598A	934.1 and E915
T17.800A	934.8 and E912
T17.808A	934.8 and E915
T17.810A	934.8 and E911
T17.818A	934.8 and E911
T17.820A	934.8 and E911
T17.828A	934.8 and E911
T17.890A	934.8 and E912
T17.898A	934.8 and E912
T17.900A	934.9 and E912
T17.908A	934.9 and E915
T17.910A	934.9 and E911
T17.918A	934.9 and E911
T17.920A	934.9 and E911
T17.928A	934.9 and E911
T17.990A	934.9 and E912
T17.998A	934.9 and E915
T18.0XXA	935.0 and E915
T18.100A	935.1 and E912
T18.108A	935.1 and E915
T18.110A	935.1 and E911
T18.118A	935.1 and E915
T18.120A	935.1 and E911
T18.128A	935.1 and E915
T18.190A	935.1 and E912
T18.198A	935.1 and E915
T18.2XXA	935.2 and E915
T18.3XXA	936 and E915
T18.4XXA	936 and E915
T18.5XXA	937 and E915
T18.8XXA	938 and E915
T18.9XXA	938 and E915
T19.0XXA	939.0 and E915
T19.1XXA	939.0 and E915
T19.2XXA	939.2 and E915
T19.3XXA	939.1 and E915
T19.4XXA	939.3 and E915
T19.8XXA	939.9 and E915
T19.9XXA	939.9 and E915
T36.0X1A	960.0 and E856
T36.0X1S	909.0 and E929.2
T36.0X2A	960.0 and E950.4
T36.0X2S	909.0 and E959
T36.0X3A	960.0 and E962.0
T36.0X3S	909.0 and E969
T36.0X4A	960.0 and E980.4
T36.0X4S	909.0 and E989
T36.0X5A	995.29 and E930.0
T36.0X5S	909.5 and E930.0
T36.1X1A	960.5 and E856
T36.1X1S	909.0 and E929.2
T36.1X2A	960.5 and E950.4
T36.1X2S	909.0 and E959
T36.1X3A	960.5 and E962.0
T36.1X3S	909.0 and E969
T36.1X4A	960.5 and E980.4
T36.1X4S	909.0 and E989
T36.1X5A	995.29 and E930.5
T36.1X5S	909.5 and E930.5
T36.2X1A	960.2 and E856
T36.2X1S	909.0 and E929.2
T36.2X2A	960.2 and E950.4
T36.2X2S	909.0 and E959
T36.2X3A	960.2 and E962.0
T36.2X3S	909.0 and E969
T36.2X4A	960.2 and E980.4
T36.2X4S	909.0 and E989
T36.2X5A	995.29 and E930.2
T36.2X5S	909.5 and E930.2
T36.3X1A	960.3 and E856
T36.3X1S	909.0 and E929.2
T36.3X2A	960.3 and E950.4
T36.3X2S	909.0 and E959
T36.3X3A	960.3 and E962.0
T36.3X3S	909.0 and E969
T36.3X4A	960.3 and E980.4
T36.3X4S	909.0 and E989
T36.3X5A	995.29 and E930.3
T36.3X5S	909.5 and E930.3
T36.4X1A	960.4 and E856
T36.4X1S	909.0 and E929.2
T36.4X2A	960.4 and E950.4
T36.4X2S	909.0 and E959
T36.4X3A	960.4 and E962.0
T36.4X3S	909.0 and E969
T36.4X4A	960.4 and E980.4
T36.4X4S	909.0 and E989
T36.4X5A	995.29 and E930.4
T36.4X5S	909.5 and E930.4
T36.5X1A	960.8 and E856
T36.5X1S	909.0 and E929.2
T36.5X2A	960.8 and E950.4
T36.5X2S	909.0 and E959
T36.5X3A	960.8 and E962.0
T36.5X3S	909.0 and E969
T36.5X4A	960.8 and E950.4
T36.5X4S	909.0 and E989
T36.5X5A	995.29 and E930.8
T36.5X5S	909.5 and E930.8
T36.6X1A	960.6 and E856
T36.6X1S	909.0 and E929.2
T36.6X2A	960.6 and E950.4
T36.6X2S	909.0 and E959
T36.6X3A	960.6 and E962.0
T36.6X3S	909.0 and E969
T36.6X4A	960.6 and E980.4
T36.6X4S	909.0 and E989
T36.6X5A	995.29 and E930.6
T36.6X5S	909.5 and E930.6
T36.7X1A	960.1 and E856
T36.7X1S	909.0 and E929.2
T36.7X2A	960.1 and E950.4
T36.7X2S	909.0 and E959
T36.7X3A	960.1 and E962.0
T36.7X3S	909.0 and E969
T36.7X4A	960.1 and E980.4
T36.7X4S	909.0 and E989
T36.7X5A	995.29 and E930.1
T36.7X5S	909.5 and E930.1
T36.8X1A	960.8 and E856
T36.8X1S	909.0 and E929.2
T36.8X2A	960.8 and E950.4
T36.8X2S	909.0 and E959
T36.8X3A	960.8 and E962.0
T36.8X3S	909.0 and E969
T36.8X4A	960.8 and E980.4
T36.8X4S	909.0 and E989
T36.8X5A	995.29 and E930.8
T36.8X5S	909.5 and E930.8
T36.91XA	960.9 and E856
T36.91XS	909.0 and E929.2
T36.92XA	960.9 and E950.4
T36.92XS	909.0 and E959
T36.93XA	960.9 and E962.0
T36.93XS	909.0 and E969
T36.94XA	960.9 and E980.4
T36.94XS	909.0 and E989
T36.95XA	995.29 and E930.8
T36.95XS	909.5 and E930.8
T37.0X1A	961.0 and E857
T37.0X1S	909.0 and E929.2
T37.0X2A	961.0 and E950.4
T37.0X2S	909.0 and E959
T37.0X3A	961.0 and E962.0
T37.0X3S	909.0 and E969
T37.0X4A	961.0 and E980.4
T37.0X4S	909.0 and E989
T37.0X5A	995.29 and E931.0
T37.0X5S	909.5 and E931.0
T37.1X1A	961.8 and E857
T37.1X1S	909.0 and E929.2
T37.1X2A	961.8 and E950.4
T37.1X2S	909.0 and E959
T37.1X3A	961.8 and E962.0
T37.1X3S	909.0 and E969
T37.1X4A	961.8 and E980.4
T37.1X4S	909.0 and E989
T37.1X5A	995.29 and E930.6

T37.1X5S	909.5 and E930.6
T37.2X1A	961.4 and E857
T37.2X1S	909.0 and E929.2
T37.2X2A	961.4 and E950.4
T37.2X2S	909.0 and E959
T37.2X3A	961.4 and E962.0
T37.2X3S	909.0 and E969
T37.2X4A	961.4 and E980.4
T37.2X4S	909.0 and E989
T37.2X5A	995.29 and E931.4
T37.2X5S	909.5 and E931.4
T37.3X1A	961.5 and E857
T37.3X1S	909.0 and E929.2
T37.3X2A	961.5 and E950.4
T37.3X2S	909.0 and E959
T37.3X3A	961.5 and E962.0
T37.3X3S	909.0 and E969
T37.3X4A	961.5 and E980.4
T37.3X4S	909.0 and E989
T37.3X5A	995.29 and E931.5
T37.3X5S	909.5 and E931.5
T37.4X1A	961.6 and E857
T37.4X1S	909.0 and E929.2
T37.4X2A	961.6 and E950.4
T37.4X2S	909.0 and E959
T37.4X3A	961.6 and E962.0
T37.4X3S	909.0 and E969
T37.4X4A	961.6 and E980.4
T37.4X4S	909.0 and E989
T37.4X5A	995.29 and E931.6
T37.4X5S	909.5 and E931.6
T37.5X1A	961.7 and E857
T37.5X1S	909.0 and E929.2
T37.5X2A	961.7 and E950.4
T37.5X2S	909.0 and E959
T37.5X3A	961.7 and E962.0
T37.5X3S	909.0 and E969
T37.5X4A	961.7 and E980.4
T37.5X4S	909.0 and E989
T37.5X5A	995.29 and E931.7
T37.5X5S	909.5 and E931.7
T37.8X1A	961.9 and E857
T37.8X1S	909.0 and E929.2
T37.8X2A	961.9 and E950.4
T37.8X2S	909.0 and E959
T37.8X3A	961.9 and E962.0
T37.8X3S	909.0 and E969
T37.8X4A	961.9 and E980.4
T37.8X4S	909.0 and E989
T37.8X5A	995.29 and E931.9
T37.8X5S	909.5 and E931.9
T37.91XA	961.9 and E857
T37.91XS	909.0 and E929.2
T37.92XA	961.9 and E950.4
T37.92XS	909.0 and E959
T37.93XA	961.9 and E962.0
T37.93XS	909.0 and E969
T37.94XA	961.9 and E980.4
T37.94XS	909.0 and E989
T37.95XA	995.29 and E931.9
T37.95XS	909.5 and E931.9
T38.0X1A	962.0 and E858.0
T38.0X1S	909.0 and E929.2
T38.0X2A	962.0 and E950.4
T38.0X2S	909.0 and E959
T38.0X3A	962.0 and E962.0
T38.0X3S	909.0 and E969
T38.0X4A	962.0 and E980.4
T38.0X4S	909.0 and E989
T38.0X5A	995.29 and E932.0
T38.0X5S	909.5 and E932.0
T38.1X1A	962.7 and E858.0
T38.1X1S	909.0 and E929.2
T38.1X2A	962.7 and E950.4
T38.1X2S	909.0 and E959
T38.1X3A	962.7 and E962.0
T38.1X3S	909.0 and E969
T38.1X4A	962.7 and E980.4
T38.1X4S	909.0 and E989
T38.1X5A	995.29 and E932.7
T38.1X5S	909.5 and E932.7
T38.2X1A	962.8 and E858.0
T38.2X1S	909.0 and E929.2
T38.2X2A	962.8 and E950.4
T38.2X2S	909.0 and E959
T38.2X3A	962.8 and E962.0
T38.2X3S	909.0 and E969
T38.2X4A	962.8 and E980.4
T38.2X4S	909.0 and E989
T38.2X5A	995.29 and E932.8
T38.2X5S	909.5 and E932.8
T38.3X1A	962.3 and E858.8
T38.3X1S	909.0 and E929.2
T38.3X2A	962.3 and E950.4
T38.3X2S	909.0 and E959
T38.3X3A	962.3 and E962.0
T38.3X3S	909.0 and E969
T38.3X4A	962.3 and E980.4
T38.3X4S	909.0 and E989
T38.3X5A	995.23 and E932.3
T38.3X5S	909.5 and E932.3
T38.4X1A	962.2 and E858.0
T38.4X1S	909.0 and E929.2
T38.4X2A	962.2 and E950.4
T38.4X2S	909.0 and E959
T38.4X3A	962.2 and E962.0
T38.4X3S	909.0 and E969
T38.4X4A	962.2 and E980.4
T38.4X4S	909.0 and E989
T38.4X5A	995.29 and E932.2
T38.4X5S	909.5 and E932.2
T38.5X1A	962.2 and E858.0
T38.5X1S	909.0 and E929.2
T38.5X2A	962.2 and E950.4
T38.5X2S	909.0 and E959
T38.5X3A	962.2 and E962.0
T38.5X3S	909.0 and E969
T38.5X4A	962.2 and E980.4
T38.5X4S	909.0 and E989
T38.5X5A	995.29 and E932.2
T38.5X5S	909.5 and E932.2
T38.6X1A	962.1 and E858.0
T38.6X1S	909.0 and E929.2
T38.6X2A	962.1 and E950.4
T38.6X2S	909.0 and E959
T38.6X3A	962.1 and E962.0
T38.6X3S	909.0 and E969
T38.6X4A	962.1 and E980.4
T38.6X4S	909.0 and E989
T38.6X5A	995.29 and E932.9
T38.6X5S	909.5 and E932.9
T38.7X1A	962.1 and E858.0
T38.7X1S	909.0 and E929.2
T38.7X2A	962.1 and E950.4
T38.7X2S	909.0 and E959
T38.7X3A	962.1 and E962.0
T38.7X3S	909.0 and E969
T38.7X4A	962.1 and E980.4
T38.7X4S	909.0 and E989
T38.7X5A	995.29 and E932.1
T38.7X5S	909.5 and E932.1
T38.801A	962.9 and E858.0
T38.801S	909.0 and E929.2
T38.802A	962.9 and E950.4
T38.802S	909.0 and E959
T38.803A	962.9 and E962.0
T38.803S	909.0 and E969
T38.804A	962.9 and E980.4
T38.804S	909.0 and E989
T38.805A	995.29 and E932.9
T38.805S	909.5 and E932.9
T38.811A	962.4 and E858.0
T38.811S	909.0 and E929.2
T38.812A	962.4 and E950.4
T38.812S	909.0 and E959
T38.813A	962.4 and E962.0
T38.813S	909.0 and E969
T38.814A	962.4 and E980.4
T38.814S	909.0 and E989
T38.815A	995.29 and E932.4
T38.815S	909.5 and E932.4
T38.891A	962.9 and E858.0
T38.891S	909.0 and E929.2
T38.892A	962.9 and E950.4
T38.892S	909.0 and E959
T38.893A	962.9 and E962.0
T38.893S	909.0 and E969
T38.894A	962.9 and E980.4
T38.894S	909.0 and E989
T38.895A	995.29 and E932.9
T38.895S	909.5 and E932.9
T38.901A	962.9 and E858.0
T38.901S	909.0 and E929.2
T38.902A	962.9 and E950.4
T38.902S	909.0 and E959
T38.903A	962.9 and E962.0
T38.903S	909.0 and E969
T38.904A	962.9 and E980.4
T38.904S	909.0 and E989
T38.905A	995.29 and E932.9
T38.905S	909.5 and E932.9
T38.991A	962.9 and E858.0
T38.991S	909.0 and E929.2
T38.992A	962.9 and E950.4
T38.992S	909.0 and E959
T38.993A	962.9 and E962.0
T38.993S	909.0 and E969
T38.994A	962.9 and E980.4
T38.994S	909.0 and E989
T38.995A	995.29 and E932.9
T38.995S	909.5 and E932.9
T39.011A	965.1 and E850.3
T39.011S	909.0 and E929.2
T39.012A	965.1 and E950.0
T39.012S	909.0 and E959
T39.013A	965.1 and E962.0
T39.013S	909.0 and E969
T39.014A	965.1 and E980.0
T39.014S	909.0 and E989
T39.015A	995.29 and E935.3
T39.015S	909.5 and E935.3
T39.091A	965.1 and E850.3
T39.091S	909.0 and E929.2
T39.092A	965.1 and E950.0
T39.092S	909.0 and E959
T39.093A	965.1 and E962.0
T39.093S	909.0 and E969
T39.094A	965.1 and E980.0
T39.094S	909.0 and E989
T39.095A	995.29 and E935.3
T39.095S	909.5 and E935.3
T39.1X1A	965.4 and E850.4
T39.1X1S	909.0 and E929.2
T39.1X2A	965.4 and E950.0
T39.1X2S	909.0 and E959
T39.1X3A	965.4 and E962.0

ICD-10-CM	ICD-9-CM
T39.1X3S	9Ø9.Ø and E969
T39.1X4A	965.4 and E98Ø.Ø
T39.1X4S	9Ø9.Ø and E989
T39.1X5A	995.29 and E935.3
T39.1X5S	9Ø9.5 and E935.3
T39.2X1A	965.5 and E85Ø.5
T39.2X1S	9Ø9.Ø and E929.2
T39.2X2A	965.5 and E95Ø.Ø
T39.2X2S	9Ø9.Ø and E959
T39.2X3A	965.5 and E962.Ø
T39.2X3S	9Ø9.Ø and E969
T39.2X4A	965.5 and E98Ø.Ø
T39.2X4S	9Ø9.Ø and E989
T39.2X5A	995.29 and E935.5
T39.2X5S	9Ø9.5 and E935.5
T39.311A	965.61 and E85Ø.7
T39.311S	9Ø9.Ø and E929.2
T39.312A	965.61 and E95Ø.Ø
T39.312S	9Ø9.Ø and E959
T39.313A	965.61 and E962.Ø
T39.313S	9Ø9.Ø and E969
T39.314A	965.1 and E98Ø.Ø
T39.314S	9Ø9.Ø and E989
T39.315A	995.29 and E935.7
T39.315S	9Ø9.5 and E935.7
T39.391A	965.61 and E85Ø.6
T39.391S	9Ø9.Ø and E929.2
T39.392A	965.61 and E95Ø.Ø
T39.392S	9Ø9.Ø and E959
T39.393A	965.61 and E962.Ø
T39.393S	9Ø9.Ø and E969
T39.394A	965.61 and E98Ø.Ø
T39.394S	9Ø9.Ø and E989
T39.395A	995.29 and E935.7
T39.395S	9Ø9.5 and E935.7
T39.4X1A	965.69 and E85Ø.6
T39.4X1S	9Ø9.Ø and E929.2
T39.4X2A	965.69 and E95Ø.Ø
T39.4X2S	9Ø9.Ø and E959
T39.4X3A	965.69 and E962.Ø
T39.4X3S	9Ø9.Ø and E969
T39.4X4A	965.69 and E98Ø.Ø
T39.4X4S	9Ø9.Ø and E989
T39.4X5A	995.29 and E935.6
T39.4X5S	9Ø9.5 and E935.6
T39.8X1A	965.7 and E85Ø.7
T39.8X1S	9Ø9.Ø and E929.2
T39.8X2A	965.7 and E95Ø.Ø
T39.8X2S	9Ø9.Ø and E959
T39.8X3A	965.7 and E962.Ø
T39.8X3S	9Ø9.Ø and E969
T39.8X4A	965.7 and E98Ø.Ø
T39.8X4S	9Ø9.Ø and E989
T39.8X5A	995.29 and E935.7
T39.8X5S	9Ø9.5 and E935.7
T39.91XA	965.9 and E85Ø.7
T39.91XS	9Ø9.Ø and E929.2
T39.92XA	965.9 and E95Ø.Ø
T39.92XS	9Ø9.Ø and E959
T39.93XA	965.9 and E962.Ø
T39.93XS	9Ø9.Ø and E969
T39.94XA	965.9 and E98Ø.Ø
T39.94XS	9Ø9.Ø and E989
T39.95XA	995.29 and E935.7
T39.95XS	9Ø9.5 and E935.7
T4Ø.ØX1A	965.ØØ and E85Ø.2
T4Ø.ØX1S	9Ø9.Ø and E929.2
T4Ø.ØX2A	965.ØØ and E95Ø.Ø
T4Ø.ØX2S	9Ø9.Ø and E959
T4Ø.ØX3A	965.ØØ and E962.Ø
T4Ø.ØX3S	9Ø9.Ø and E969
T4Ø.ØX4A	965.ØØ and E98Ø.Ø
T4Ø.ØX4S	9Ø9.Ø and E989
T4Ø.ØX5A	995.29 and E935.2; 995.29 and E935.Ø
T4Ø.ØX5S	9Ø9.5 and E935.2; 9Ø9.5 and E935.Ø
T4Ø.1X1A	965.Ø1 and E85Ø.Ø
T4Ø.1X1S	9Ø9.Ø and E929.2
T4Ø.1X2A	965.Ø1 and E95Ø.Ø
T4Ø.1X2S	9Ø9.Ø and E959
T4Ø.1X3A	965.Ø1 and E962.Ø
T4Ø.1X3S	9Ø9.Ø and E969
T4Ø.1X4A	965.Ø1 and E98Ø.Ø
T4Ø.1X4S	9Ø9.Ø and E989
T4Ø.2X1A	965.Ø9 and E85Ø.2
T4Ø.2X1S	9Ø9.Ø and E929.2
T4Ø.2X2A	965.Ø9 and E95Ø.Ø
T4Ø.2X2S	9Ø9.Ø and E959
T4Ø.2X3A	965.Ø9 and E962.Ø
T4Ø.2X3S	9Ø9.Ø and E969
T4Ø.2X4A	965.Ø9 and E98Ø.Ø
T4Ø.2X4S	9Ø9.Ø and E989
T4Ø.2X5A	995.29 and E935.2
T4Ø.2X5S	9Ø9.5 and E935.2
T4Ø.3X1A	965.Ø2 and E85Ø.1
T4Ø.3X1S	9Ø9.Ø and E929.2
T4Ø.3X2A	965.Ø2 and E95Ø.Ø
T4Ø.3X2S	9Ø9.Ø and E959
T4Ø.3X3A	965.Ø2 and E962.Ø
T4Ø.3X3S	9Ø9.Ø and E969
T4Ø.3X4A	965.Ø2 and E98Ø.Ø
T4Ø.3X4S	9Ø9.Ø and E989
T4Ø.3X5A	995.29 and E935.1
T4Ø.3X5S	9Ø9.5 and E935.1
T4Ø.4X1A	965.Ø9 and E85Ø.2
T4Ø.4X1S	9Ø9.Ø and E929.2
T4Ø.4X2A	965.Ø9 and E95Ø.Ø
T4Ø.4X2S	9Ø9.Ø and E959
T4Ø.4X3A	965.Ø9 and E962.Ø
T4Ø.4X3S	9Ø9.Ø and E969
T4Ø.4X4A	965.Ø9 and E98Ø.Ø
T4Ø.4X4S	9Ø9.Ø and E989
T4Ø.4X5A	995.29 and E935.2
T4Ø.4X5S	9Ø9.5 and E935.2
T4Ø.5X1A	97Ø.81 and E854.2
T4Ø.5X1S	9Ø9.Ø and E929.2
T4Ø.5X2A	97Ø.81 and E95Ø.4
T4Ø.5X2S	9Ø9.Ø and E959
T4Ø.5X3A	97Ø.81 and E962.Ø
T4Ø.5X3S	9Ø9.Ø and E969
T4Ø.5X4A	97Ø.81 and E98Ø.4
T4Ø.5X4S	9Ø9.Ø and E989
T4Ø.5X5A	995.29 and E939.7
T4Ø.5X5S	9Ø9.5 and E939.7
T4Ø.6Ø1A	965.Ø9 and E85Ø.2
T4Ø.6Ø1S	9Ø9.Ø and E929.2
T4Ø.6Ø2A	965.Ø9 and E95Ø.4
T4Ø.6Ø2S	9Ø9.Ø and E959
T4Ø.6Ø3A	965.Ø9 and E962.Ø
T4Ø.6Ø3S	9Ø9.Ø and E969
T4Ø.6Ø4A	965.Ø9 and E98Ø.4
T4Ø.6Ø4S	9Ø9.Ø and E989
T4Ø.6Ø5A	995.29 and E935.2
T4Ø.6Ø5S	9Ø9.5 and E935.2
T4Ø.691A	965.Ø9 and E85Ø.2
T4Ø.691S	9Ø9.Ø and E929.2
T4Ø.692A	965.Ø9 and E95Ø.4
T4Ø.692S	9Ø9.Ø and E959
T4Ø.693A	965.Ø9 and E962.Ø
T4Ø.693S	9Ø9.Ø and E969
T4Ø.694A	965.Ø9 and E98Ø.4
T4Ø.694S	9Ø9.Ø and E989
T4Ø.695A	995.29 and E935.2
T4Ø.695S	9Ø9.5 and E935.2
T4Ø.7X1A	969.6 and E854.1
T4Ø.7X1S	9Ø9.Ø and E929.2
T4Ø.7X2A	969.6 and E95Ø.2
T4Ø.7X2S	9Ø9.Ø and E959
T4Ø.7X3A	969.6 and E962.Ø
T4Ø.7X3S	9Ø9.Ø and E969
T4Ø.7X4A	969.6 and E98Ø.2
T4Ø.7X4S	9Ø9.Ø and E989
T4Ø.7X5A	995.29 and E939.6
T4Ø.7X5S	9Ø9.5 and E939.6
T4Ø.8X1A	969.6 and E854.1
T4Ø.8X1S	9Ø9.Ø and E929.2
T4Ø.8X2A	969.6 and E95Ø.3
T4Ø.8X2S	9Ø9.Ø and E959
T4Ø.8X3A	969.6 and E962.Ø
T4Ø.8X3S	9Ø9.Ø and E969
T4Ø.8X4A	969.6 and E98Ø.2
T4Ø.8X4S	9Ø9.Ø and E989
T4Ø.8X5A	995.29 and E939.6
T4Ø.8X5S	9Ø9.5 and E939.6
T4Ø.9Ø1A	969.6 and E854.1
T4Ø.9Ø1S	9Ø9.Ø and E929.2
T4Ø.9Ø2A	969.6 and E95Ø.3
T4Ø.9Ø2S	9Ø9.Ø and E959
T4Ø.9Ø3A	969.6 and E962.Ø
T4Ø.9Ø3S	9Ø9.Ø and E969
T4Ø.9Ø4A	969.6 and E98Ø.2
T4Ø.9Ø4S	9Ø9.Ø and E989
T4Ø.9Ø5A	995.29 and E939.6
T4Ø.9Ø5S	9Ø9.5 and E939.6
T4Ø.991A	969.6 and E854.1
T4Ø.991S	9Ø9.Ø and E929.2
T4Ø.992A	969.6 and E95Ø.3
T4Ø.992S	9Ø9.Ø and E959
T4Ø.993A	969.6 and E962.Ø
T4Ø.993S	9Ø9.Ø and E969
T4Ø.994A	969.6 and E98Ø.2
T4Ø.994S	9Ø9.Ø and E989
T4Ø.995A	995.29 and E939.6
T4Ø.995S	9Ø9.5 and E939.6
T41.ØX1A	968.1 and E855.1; 968.2 and E855.1
T41.ØX1S	9Ø9.Ø and E929.2
T41.ØX2A	968.1 and E952.8; 968.2 and E952.8
T41.ØX2S	9Ø9.Ø and E959
T41.ØX3A	968.1 and E962.Ø; 968.2 and E962.Ø
T41.ØX3S	9Ø9.Ø and E969
T41.ØX4A	968.1 and E98Ø.4; 968.2 and E98Ø.4
T41.ØX4S	9Ø9.Ø and E989
T41.ØX5A	995.22 and E938.2
T41.ØX5S	9Ø9.5 and E938.2
T41.1X1A	968.3 and E855.1
T41.1X1S	9Ø9.Ø and E929.2
T41.1X2A	968.3 and E95Ø.Ø
T41.1X2S	9Ø9.Ø and E959
T41.1X3A	968.3 and E962.Ø
T41.1X3S	9Ø9.Ø and E969
T41.1X4A	968.3 and E98Ø.4
T41.1X4S	9Ø9.Ø and E989
T41.1X5A	995.22 and E938.3
T41.1X5S	9Ø9.5 and E938.3
T41.2Ø1A	968.4 and E855.1
T41.2Ø1S	9Ø9.Ø and E929.2
T41.2Ø2A	968.4 and E95Ø.Ø
T41.2Ø2S	9Ø9.Ø and E959
T41.2Ø3A	968.4 and E962.Ø
T41.2Ø3S	9Ø9.Ø and E969
T41.2Ø4A	968.4 and E98Ø.4

T41.204S	909.0 and E989
T41.205A	995.22 and E938.4
T41.205S	909.5 and E938.4
T41.291A	968.4 and E855.1
T41.291S	909.0 and E929.2
T41.292A	968.4 and E950.0
T41.292S	909.0 and E959
T41.293A	968.4 and E962.0
T41.293S	909.0 and E969
T41.294A	968.4 and E980.4
T41.294S	909.0 and E989
T41.295A	995.22 and E938.4
T41.295S	909.5 and E938.4
T41.3X1A	968.5 and E855.2; 968.9 and E855.2
T41.3X1S	909.0 and E929.2
T41.3X2A	968.5 and E950.0; 968.9 and E950.0
T41.3X2S	909.0 and E959
T41.3X3A	968.5 and E962.0; 968.9 and E962.0
T41.3X3S	909.0 and E969
T41.3X4A	968.5 and E980.4; 968.9 and E980.4
T41.3X4S	909.0 and E989
T41.3X5A	995.22 and E938.9
T41.3X5S	909.5 and E938.9
T41.41XA	968.9 and E855.1
T41.41XS	909.0 and E929.2
T41.42XA	968.9 and E950.0
T41.42XS	909.0 and E959
T41.43XA	968.9 and E962.0
T41.43XS	909.0 and E969
T41.44XA	968.9 and E980.4
T41.44XS	909.0 and E989
T41.45XA	995.22 and E938.9
T41.45XS	909.5 and E938.9
T41.5X1A	975.8 and E858.6
T41.5X1S	909.0 and E929.2
T41.5X2A	975.8 and E952.8
T41.5X2S	909.0 and E959
T41.5X3A	975.8 and E962.0
T41.5X3S	909.0 and E969
T41.5X4A	975.8 and E980.4
T41.5X4S	909.0 and E989
T41.5X5A	995.29 and E945.8
T41.5X5S	909.5 and E945.8
T42.0X1A	966.1 and E855.0
T42.0X1S	909.0 and E929.2
T42.0X2A	966.1 and E950.4
T42.0X2S	909.0 and E959
T42.0X3A	966.1 and E962.0
T42.0X3S	909.0 and E969
T42.0X4A	966.1 and E980.4
T42.0X4S	909.0 and E989
T42.0X5A	995.29 and E936.1
T42.0X5S	909.5 and E936.1
T42.1X1A	966.3 and E855.8
T42.1X1S	909.0 and E929.2
T42.1X2A	966.3 and E950.4
T42.1X2S	909.0 and E959
T42.1X3A	966.3 and E962.0
T42.1X3S	909.0 and E969
T42.1X4A	966.3 and E980.4
T42.1X4S	909.0 and E989
T42.1X5A	995.29 and E936.3
T42.1X5S	909.5 and E936.3
T42.2X1A	966.0 and E855.8; 966.2 and E855.8
T42.2X1S	909.0 and E929.2
T42.2X2A	966.0 and E950.4; 966.2 and E950.4
T42.2X2S	909.0 and E959
T42.2X3A	966.0 and E962.0; 966.2 and E962.0
T42.2X3S	909.0 and E969
T42.2X4A	966.0 and E980.4; 966.2 and E980.4
T42.2X4S	909.0 and E989
T42.2X5A	995.29 and E936.0; 995.29 and E936.2
T42.2X5S	909.5 and E936.0; 909.5 and E936.2
T42.3X1A	967.0 and E851
T42.3X1S	909.0 and E929.2
T42.3X2A	967.0 and E950.1
T42.3X2S	909.0 and E959
T42.3X3A	967.0 and E962.0
T42.3X3S	909.0 and E969
T42.3X4A	967.0 and E980.1
T42.3X4S	909.0 and E989
T42.3X5A	995.29 and E937.0
T42.3X5S	909.5 and E937.0
T42.4X1A	969.4 and E853.2
T42.4X1S	909.0 and E929.2
T42.4X2A	969.4 and E950.2
T42.4X2S	909.0 and E959
T42.4X3A	969.4 and E962.0
T42.4X3S	909.0 and E969
T42.4X4A	969.4 and E980.2
T42.4X4S	909.0 and E989
T42.4X5A	995.29 and E939.4
T42.4X5S	909.5 and E939.4
T42.5X1A	966.3 and E855.8
T42.5X1S	909.0 and E929.2
T42.5X2A	966.3 and E950.4
T42.5X2S	909.0 and E959
T42.5X3A	966.3 and E962.0
T42.5X3S	909.0 and E969
T42.5X4A	966.3 and E980.4
T42.5X4S	909.0 and E989
T42.5X5A	995.29 and E936.3
T42.5X5S	909.5 and E936.3
T42.6X1A	966.3 and E858.8; 967.1 and E858.8; 967.2 and E858.8; 967.3 and E858.8; 967.4 and E858.8; 967.5 and E858.8; 967.6 and E858.8; 967.8 and E852.8
T42.6X1S	909.0 and E929.2
T42.6X2A	966.3 and E950.4; 967.1 and E950.4; 967.2 and E950.4; 967.3 and E950.4; 967.4 and E950.4; 967.5 and E950.4; 967.6 and E950.4; 967.8 and E950.2
T42.6X2S	909.0 and E959
T42.6X3A	966.3 and E962.0; 967.1 and E962.0; 967.2 and E962.0; 967.3 and E962.0; 967.4 and E962.0; 967.5 and E962.0; 967.6 and E962.0;967.8 and E962.0
T42.6X3S	909.0 and E969
T42.6X4A	966.3 and E980.4; 967.1 and E980.4; 967.2 and E980.4; 967.3 and E980.4; 967.4 and E980.4; 967.5 and E980.4; 967.6 and E980.4;967.8 and E950.2
T42.6X4S	909.0 and E989
T42.6X5A	995.29 and E936.3; 995.29 and E937.8
T42.6X5S	909.5 and E936.3; 909.5 and E937.8
T42.71XA	966.3 and E858.8; 967.9 and E852.8
T42.71XS	909.0 and E929.2
T42.72XA	966.3 and E950.4; 967.9 and E950.3
T42.72XS	909.0 and E959
T42.73XA	966.3 and E962.0; 967.9 and E962.0
T42.73XS	909.0 and E969
T42.74XA	966.3 and E980.4; 967.9 and E980.4
T42.74XS	909.0 and E989
T42.75XA	995.29 and E936.3; 995.29 and E937.9
T42.75XS	909.5 and E936.3; 909.5 and E937.9
T42.8X1A	966.4 and E855.0; 968.0 and E855.0
T42.8X1S	909.0 and E929.2
T42.8X2A	966.4 and E950.4; 968.0 and E950.4
T42.8X2S	909.0 and E959
T42.8X3A	966.4 and E962.0; 968.0 and E962.0
T42.8X3S	909.0 and E969
T42.8X4A	966.4 and E980.4; 968.0 and E980.4
T42.8X4S	909.0 and E989
T42.8X5A	995.29 and E936.4
T42.8X5S	909.5 and E936.4
T43.011A	969.05 and E854.0
T43.011S	909.0 and E929.2
T43.012A	969.05 and E950.3
T43.012S	909.0 and E959
T43.013A	969.05 and E962.0
T43.013S	909.0 and E969
T43.014A	969.05 and E980.3
T43.014S	909.0 and E989
T43.015A	995.29 and E939.0
T43.015S	909.5 and E939.0
T43.021A	969.04 and E854.0
T43.021S	909.0 and E929.2
T43.022A	969.04 and E950.3
T43.022S	909.0 and E959
T43.023A	969.04 and E962.0
T43.023S	909.0 and E969
T43.024A	969.04 and E980.3
T43.024S	909.0 and E989
T43.025A	995.29 and E939.0
T43.025S	909.5 and E939.0
T43.1X1A	969.01 and E854.0
T43.1X1S	909.0 and E929.2
T43.1X2A	969.01 and E950.3
T43.1X2S	909.0 and E959
T43.1X3A	969.01 and E962.0
T43.1X3S	909.0 and E969
T43.1X4A	969.01 and E980.3
T43.1X4S	909.0 and E989
T43.1X5A	995.29 and E939.0
T43.1X5S	909.5 and E939.0
T43.201A	969.00 and E854.0
T43.201S	909.0 and E929.2
T43.202A	969.00 and E950.3
T43.202S	909.0 and E959
T43.203A	969.00 and E962.0
T43.203S	909.0 and E969
T43.204A	969.00 and E980.3
T43.204S	909.0 and E989
T43.205A	995.29 and E939.0
T43.205S	909.5 and E939.0

T43.211A	969.02 and E854.0
T43.211S	909.0 and E929.2
T43.212A	969.02 and E950.3
T43.212S	909.0 and E959
T43.213A	969.02 and E962.0
T43.213S	909.0 and E969
T43.214A	969.02 and E980.3
T43.214S	909.0 and E989
T43.215A	995.29 and E939.0
T43.215S	909.5 and E939.0
T43.221A	969.03 and E854.0
T43.221S	909.0 and E929.2
T43.222A	969.03 and E950.3
T43.222S	909.0 and E959
T43.223A	969.03 and E962.0
T43.223S	909.0 and E969
T43.224A	969.03 and E980.3
T43.224S	909.0 and E989
T43.225A	995.29 and E939.0
T43.225S	909.5 and E939.0
T43.291A	969.09 and E854.0
T43.291S	909.0 and E929.2
T43.292A	969.09 and E950.3
T43.292S	909.0 and E959
T43.293A	969.09 and E962.0
T43.293S	909.0 and E969
T43.294A	969.09 and E980.3
T43.294S	909.0 and E989
T43.295A	995.29 and E939.0
T43.295S	909.5 and E939.0
T43.3X1A	969.1 and E853.0
T43.3X1S	909.0 and E929.2
T43.3X2A	969.1 and E950.3
T43.3X2S	909.0 and E959
T43.3X3A	969.1 and E962.0
T43.3X3S	909.0 and E969
T43.3X4A	969.1 and E980.3
T43.3X4S	909.0 and E989
T43.3X5A	995.29 and E939.1
T43.3X5S	909.5 and E939.1
T43.4X1A	969.2 and E853.1
T43.4X1S	909.0 and E929.2
T43.4X2A	969.2 and E950.3
T43.4X2S	909.0 and E959
T43.4X3A	969.2 and E962.0
T43.4X3S	909.0 and E969
T43.4X4A	969.2 and E980.3
T43.4X4S	909.0 and E989
T43.4X5A	995.29 and E939.2
T43.4X5S	909.5 and E939.2
T43.501A	969.3 and E854.8
T43.501S	909.0 and E929.2
T43.502A	969.3 and E950.3
T43.502S	909.0 and E959
T43.503A	969.3 and E962.0
T43.503S	909.0 and E969
T43.504A	969.3 and E980.3
T43.504S	909.0 and E989
T43.505A	995.29 and E939.3
T43.505S	909.5 and E939.3
T43.591A	969.3 and E854.8
T43.591S	909.0 and E929.2
T43.592A	969.3 and E950.3
T43.592S	909.0 and E959
T43.593A	969.3 and E962.0
T43.593S	909.0 and E969
T43.594A	969.3 and E980.3
T43.594S	909.0 and E989
T43.595A	995.29 and E939.3
T43.595S	909.5 and E939.3
T43.601A	969.70 and E854.2
T43.601S	909.0 and E929.2
T43.602A	969.70 and E950.3
T43.602S	909.0 and E959
T43.603A	969.70 and E962.0
T43.603S	909.0 and E969
T43.604A	969.70 and E980.3
T43.604S	909.0 and E989
T43.605A	995.29 and E939.7
T43.605S	909.5 and E939.7
T43.611A	969.71 and E854.2
T43.611S	909.0 and E929.2
T43.612A	969.71 and E950.3
T43.612S	909.0 and E959
T43.613A	969.71 and E962.0
T43.613S	909.0 and E969
T43.614A	969.71 and E980.3
T43.614S	909.0 and E989
T43.615A	995.29 and E939.7
T43.615S	909.5 and E939.7
T43.621A	969.72 and E854.2
T43.621S	909.0 and E929.2
T43.622A	969.72 and E950.3
T43.622S	909.0 and E959
T43.623A	969.72 and E962.0
T43.623S	909.0 and E969
T43.624A	969.72 and E980.3
T43.624S	909.0 and E989
T43.625A	995.29 and E939.7
T43.625S	909.5 and E939.7
T43.631A	969.73 and E854.2
T43.631S	909.0 and E929.2
T43.632A	969.73 and E950.3
T43.632S	909.0 and E959
T43.633A	969.73 and E962.0
T43.633S	909.0 and E969
T43.634A	969.73 and E980.3
T43.634S	909.0 and E989
T43.635A	995.29 and E939.7
T43.635S	909.5 and E939.7
T43.691A	969.79 and E854.2
T43.691S	909.0 and E929.2
T43.692A	969.79 and E950.3
T43.692S	909.0 and E959
T43.693A	969.79 and E962.0
T43.693S	909.0 and E969
T43.694A	969.79 and E980.3
T43.694S	909.0 and E989
T43.695A	995.29 and E939.7
T43.695S	909.5 and E939.7
T43.8X1A	969.8 and E854.8
T43.8X1S	909.0 and E929.2
T43.8X2A	969.8 and E950.3
T43.8X2S	909.0 and E959
T43.8X3A	969.8 and E962.0
T43.8X3S	909.0 and E969
T43.8X4A	969.8 and E980.3
T43.8X4S	909.0 and E989
T43.8X5A	995.29 and E939.8
T43.8X5S	909.5 and E939.8
T43.91XA	969.9 and E854.8
T43.91XS	909.0 and E929.2
T43.92XA	969.9 and E950.3
T43.92XS	909.0 and E959
T43.93XA	969.9 and E962.0
T43.93XS	909.0 and E969
T43.94XA	969.9 and E980.3
T43.94XS	909.0 and E989
T43.95XA	995.29 and E939.9
T43.95XS	909.5 and E939.9
T44.0X1A	971.0 and E855.3
T44.0X1S	909.0 and E929.2
T44.0X2A	971.0 and E950.4
T44.0X2S	909.0 and E959
T44.0X3A	971.0 and E962.0
T44.0X3S	909.0 and E969
T44.0X4A	971.0 and E980.4
T44.0X4S	909.0 and E989
T44.0X5A	995.29 and E941.0
T44.0X5S	909.5 and E941.0
T44.1X1A	971.0 and E855.3
T44.1X1S	909.0 and E929.2
T44.1X2A	971.0 and E950.4
T44.1X2S	909.0 and E959
T44.1X3A	971.0 and E962.0
T44.1X3S	909.0 and E969
T44.1X4A	971.0 and E980.4
T44.1X4S	909.0 and E989
T44.1X5A	995.29 and E941.0
T44.1X5S	909.5 and E941.0
T44.2X1A	972.3 and E855.8
T44.2X1S	909.0 and E929.2
T44.2X2A	972.3 and E950.4
T44.2X2S	909.0 and E959
T44.2X3A	972.3 and E962.0
T44.2X3S	909.0 and E969
T44.2X4A	972.3 and E980.4
T44.2X4S	909.0 and E989
T44.2X5A	995.29 and E941.9
T44.2X5S	909.5 and E941.9
T44.3X1A	971.1 and E855.4
T44.3X1S	909.0 and E929.2
T44.3X2A	971.1 and E950.4
T44.3X2S	909.0 and E959
T44.3X3A	971.1 and E962.0
T44.3X3S	909.0 and E969
T44.3X4A	971.1 and E980.4
T44.3X4S	909.0 and E989
T44.3X5A	995.29 and E941.1
T44.3X5S	909.5 and E941.1
T44.4X1A	971.2 and E855.5
T44.4X1S	909.0 and E929.2
T44.4X2A	971.2 and E950.4
T44.4X2S	909.0 and E959
T44.4X3A	971.2 and E962.0
T44.4X3S	909.0 and E969
T44.4X4A	971.2 and E980.4
T44.4X4S	909.0 and E989
T44.4X5A	995.29 and E941.2
T44.4X5S	909.5 and E941.2
T44.5X1A	971.2 and E855.5
T44.5X1S	909.0 and E929.2
T44.5X2A	971.2 and E950.4
T44.5X2S	909.0 and E959
T44.5X3A	971.2 and E962.0
T44.5X3S	909.0 and E969
T44.5X4A	971.2 and E980.4
T44.5X4S	909.0 and E989
T44.5X5A	995.29 and E941.2
T44.5X5S	909.5 and E941.2
T44.6X1A	971.3 and E855.6
T44.6X1S	909.0 and E929.2
T44.6X2A	971.3 and E950.4
T44.6X2S	909.0 and E959
T44.6X3A	971.3 and E962.0
T44.6X3S	909.0 and E969
T44.6X4A	971.3 and E980.4
T44.6X4S	909.0 and E989
T44.6X5A	995.29 and E941.3
T44.6X5S	909.5 and E941.3
T44.7X1A	971.3 and E855.6
T44.7X1S	909.0 and E929.2
T44.7X2A	971.3 and E950.4
T44.7X2S	909.0 and E959
T44.7X3A	971.3 and E962.0
T44.7X3S	909.0 and E969

T44.7X4A	971.3 and E980.4
T44.7X4S	909.0 and E989
T44.7X5A	995.29 and E941.3
T44.7X5S	909.5 and E941.3
T44.8X1A	971.3 and E855.6
T44.8X1S	909.0 and E929.2
T44.8X2A	971.3 and E950.4
T44.8X2S	909.0 and E959
T44.8X3A	971.3 and E962.0
T44.8X3S	909.0 and E969
T44.8X4A	971.3 and E980.4
T44.8X4S	909.0 and E989
T44.8X5A	995.29 and E941.3
T44.8X5S	909.5 and E941.3
T44.901A	971.9 and E855.8
T44.901S	909.0 and E929.2
T44.902A	971.9 and E950.4
T44.902S	909.0 and E959
T44.903A	971.9 and E962.0
T44.903S	909.0 and E969
T44.904A	971.9 and E980.4
T44.904S	909.0 and E989
T44.905A	995.29 and E941.9
T44.905S	909.5 and E941.9
T44.991A	971.9 and E855.8
T44.991S	909.0 and E929.2
T44.992A	971.9 and E950.4
T44.992S	909.0 and E959
T44.993A	971.9 and E962.0
T44.993S	909.0 and E969
T44.994A	971.9 and E980.4
T44.994S	909.0 and E989
T44.995A	995.29 and E941.9
T44.995S	909.5 and E941.9
T45.0X1A	963.0 and E858.8
T45.0X1S	909.0 and E929.2
T45.0X2A	963.0 and E950.4
T45.0X2S	909.0 and E959
T45.0X3A	963.0 and E962.0
T45.0X3S	909.0 and E969
T45.0X4A	963.0 and E980.4
T45.0X4S	909.0 and E989
T45.0X5A	995.29 and E933.0
T45.0X5S	909.5 and E933.0
T45.1X1A	963.1 and E858.1
T45.1X1S	909.0 and E929.2
T45.1X2A	963.1 and E950.4
T45.1X2S	909.0 and E959
T45.1X3A	963.1 and E962.0
T45.1X3S	909.0 and E969
T45.1X4A	963.1 and E980.4
T45.1X4S	909.0 and E989
T45.1X5A	995.29 and E933.1
T45.1X5S	909.5 and E933.1
T45.2X1A	963.5 and E858.8
T45.2X1S	909.0 and E929.2
T45.2X2A	963.5 and E950.4
T45.2X2S	909.0 and E959
T45.2X3A	963.5 and E962.0
T45.2X3S	909.0 and E969
T45.2X4A	963.5 and E980.4
T45.2X4S	909.0 and E989
T45.2X5A	995.29 and E933.5
T45.2X5S	909.5 and E933.5
T45.3X1A	963.4 and E858.8
T45.3X1S	909.0 and E929.2
T45.3X2A	963.4 and E950.4
T45.3X2S	909.0 and E959
T45.3X3A	963.4 and E962.0
T45.3X3S	909.0 and E969
T45.3X4A	963.4 and E980.4
T45.3X4S	909.0 and E989
T45.3X5A	995.29 and E933.4
T45.3X5S	909.5 and E933.4
T45.4X1A	964.0 and E858.2
T45.4X1S	909.0 and E929.2
T45.4X2A	964.0 and E950.4
T45.4X2S	909.0 and E959
T45.4X3A	964.0 and E962.0
T45.4X3S	909.0 and E969
T45.4X4A	964.0 and E980.4
T45.4X4S	909.0 and E989
T45.4X5A	995.29 and E934.0
T45.4X5S	909.5 and E934.0
T45.511A	964.2 and E858.2
T45.511S	909.0 and E929.2
T45.512A	964.2 and E950.4
T45.512S	909.0 and E959
T45.513A	964.2 and E962.0
T45.513S	909.0 and E969
T45.514A	964.2 and E980.4
T45.514S	909.0 and E989
T45.515A	995.29 and E934.2
T45.515S	909.5 and E934.2
T45.521A	964.2 and E858.2
T45.521S	909.0 and E929.2
T45.522A	964.2 and E950.4
T45.522S	909.0 and E959
T45.523A	964.2 and E962.0
T45.523S	909.0 and E969
T45.524A	964.2 and E980.4
T45.524S	909.0 and E989
T45.525A	995.29 and E934.2
T45.525S	909.5 and E934.2
T45.601A	964.4 and E858.2
T45.601S	909.0 and E929.2
T45.602A	964.4 and E950.4
T45.602S	909.0 and E959
T45.603A	964.4 and E962.0
T45.603S	909.0 and E969
T45.604A	964.4 and E980.4
T45.604S	909.0 and E989
T45.605A	995.29 and E934.4
T45.605S	909.5 and E934.4
T45.611A	964.4 and E858.2
T45.611S	909.0 and E929.2
T45.612A	964.4 and E950.4
T45.612S	909.0 and E959
T45.613A	964.4 and E962.0
T45.613S	909.0 and E969
T45.614A	964.4 and E980.4
T45.614S	909.0 and E989
T45.615A	995.29 and E934.4
T45.615S	909.5 and E934.4
T45.621A	964.8 and E858.2
T45.621S	909.0 and E929.2
T45.622A	964.8 and E950.4
T45.622S	909.0 and E959
T45.623A	964.8 and E962.0
T45.623S	909.0 and E969
T45.624A	964.8 and E980.4
T45.624S	909.0 and E989
T45.625A	995.29 and E934.8
T45.625S	909.5 and E934.8
T45.691A	964.4 and E858.2
T45.691S	909.0 and E929.2
T45.692A	964.4 and E950.4
T45.692S	909.0 and E959
T45.693A	964.4 and E962.0
T45.693S	909.0 and E969
T45.694A	964.4 and E980.4
T45.694S	909.0 and E989
T45.695A	995.29 and E934.4
T45.695S	909.5 and E934.4
T45.7X1A	964.5 and E858.2
T45.7X1S	909.0 and E929.2
T45.7X2A	964.3 and E950.4; 964.5 and E950.4
T45.7X2S	909.0 and E959
T45.7X3A	964.3 and E962.0; 964.5 and E962.0
T45.7X3S	909.0 and E969
T45.7X4A	964.5 and E980.4
T45.7X4S	909.0 and E989
T45.7X5A	995.29 and E934.5
T45.7X5S	909.5 and E934.5
T45.8X1A	963.8 and E858.1; 964.8 and E858.2
T45.8X1S	909.0 and E929.2
T45.8X2A	963.8 and E950.4; 964.8 and E950.4
T45.8X2S	909.0 and E959
T45.8X3A	963.8 and E962.0; 964.8 and E962.0
T45.8X3S	909.0 and E969
T45.8X4A	963.8 and E980.4; 964.8 and E980.4
T45.8X4S	909.0 and E989
T45.8X5A	995.29 and E933.6; 995.29 and E933.7; 995.29 and E933.8; 995.29 and E934.8
T45.8X5S	909.5 and E933.6; 909.5 and E933.7; 909.5 and E933.8; 909.5 and E934.8
T45.91XA	963.9 and E858.1; 964.9 and E858.2
T45.91XS	909.0 and E929.2
T45.92XA	963.9 and E950.4; 964.9 and E950.4
T45.92XS	909.0 and E959
T45.93XA	963.9 and E962.0; 964.9 and E962.0
T45.93XS	909.0 and E969
T45.94XA	963.9 and E980.4; 964.9 and E980.4
T45.94XS	909.0 and E989
T45.95XA	995.29 and E933.9; 995.29 and E934.9
T45.95XS	909.5 and E934.9
T46.0X1A	972.1 and E858.3
T46.0X1S	909.0 and E929.2
T46.0X2A	972.1 and E950.4
T46.0X2S	909.0 and E959
T46.0X3A	972.1 and E962.0
T46.0X3S	909.0 and E969
T46.0X4A	972.1 and E980.4
T46.0X4S	909.0 and E989
T46.0X5A	995.29 and E942.1
T46.0X5S	909.5 and E942.1
T46.1X1A	972.9 and E858.3
T46.1X1S	909.0 and E929.2
T46.1X2A	972.9 and E950.4
T46.1X2S	909.0 and E959
T46.1X3A	972.9 and E962.0
T46.1X3S	909.0 and E969
T46.1X4A	972.9 and E980.4
T46.1X4S	909.0 and E989
T46.1X5A	995.29 and E942.0
T46.1X5S	909.5 and E942.0
T46.2X1A	972.0 and E858.3
T46.2X1S	909.0 and E929.2
T46.2X2A	972.0 and E950.4
T46.2X2S	909.0 and E959
T46.2X3A	972.0 and E962.0
T46.2X3S	909.0 and E969
T46.2X4A	972.0 and E980.4

T46.2X4S	9Ø9.Ø and E989
T46.2X5A	995.29 and E942.Ø
T46.2X5S	9Ø9.5 and E942.Ø
T46.3X1A	972.4 and E858.3
T46.3X1S	9Ø9.Ø and E929.2
T46.3X2A	972.4 and E95Ø.4
T46.3X2S	9Ø9.Ø and E959
T46.3X3A	972.4 and E962.Ø
T46.3X3S	9Ø9.Ø and E969
T46.3X4A	972.4 and E98Ø.4
T46.3X4S	9Ø9.Ø and E989
T46.3X5A	995.29 and E942.4
T46.3X5S	9Ø9.5 and E942.4
T46.4X1A	972.6 and E858.3
T46.4X1S	9Ø9.Ø and E929.2
T46.4X2A	972.6 and E95Ø.4
T46.4X2S	9Ø9.Ø and E959
T46.4X3A	972.6 and E962.Ø
T46.4X3S	9Ø9.Ø and E969
T46.4X4A	972.6 and E98Ø.4
T46.4X4S	9Ø9.Ø and E989
T46.4X5A	995.29 and E942.6
T46.4X5S	9Ø9.5 and E942.6
T46.5X1A	972.6 and E858.3
T46.5X1S	9Ø9.Ø and E929.2
T46.5X2A	972.6 and E95Ø.4
T46.5X2S	9Ø9.Ø and E959
T46.5X3A	972.6 and E962.Ø
T46.5X3S	9Ø9.Ø and E969
T46.5X4A	972.6 and E98Ø.4
T46.5X4S	9Ø9.Ø and E989
T46.5X5A	995.29 and E942.6
T46.5X5S	9Ø9.5 and E942.6
T46.6X1A	972.2 and E858.3
T46.6X1S	9Ø9.Ø and E929.2
T46.6X2A	972.2 and E95Ø.4
T46.6X2S	9Ø9.Ø and E959
T46.6X3A	972.2 and E962.Ø
T46.6X3S	9Ø9.Ø and E969
T46.6X4A	972.2 and E98Ø.4
T46.6X4S	9Ø9.Ø and E989
T46.6X5A	995.29 and E942.2
T46.6X5S	9Ø9.5 and E942.2
T46.7X1A	972.5 and E858.3
T46.7X1S	9Ø9.Ø and E929.2
T46.7X2A	972.5 and E95Ø.4
T46.7X2S	9Ø9.Ø and E959
T46.7X3A	972.5 and E962.Ø
T46.7X3S	9Ø9.Ø and E969
T46.7X4A	972.5 and E98Ø.4
T46.7X4S	9Ø9.Ø and E989
T46.7X5A	995.29 and E942.5
T46.7X5S	9Ø9.5 and E942.5
T46.8X1A	972.7 and E858.3
T46.8X1S	9Ø9.Ø and E929.2
T46.8X2A	972.7 and E95Ø.4
T46.8X2S	9Ø9.Ø and E959
T46.8X3A	972.7 and E962.Ø
T46.8X3S	9Ø9.Ø and E969
T46.8X4A	972.7 and E98Ø.4
T46.8X4S	9Ø9.Ø and E989
T46.8X5A	995.29 and E942.7
T46.8X5S	9Ø9.5 and E942.7
T46.9Ø1A	972.9 and E858.3
T46.9Ø1S	9Ø9.Ø and E929.2
T46.9Ø2A	972.9 and E95Ø.4
T46.9Ø2S	9Ø9.Ø and E959
T46.9Ø3A	972.9 and E962.Ø
T46.9Ø3S	9Ø9.Ø and E969
T46.9Ø4A	972.9 and E98Ø.4
T46.9Ø4S	9Ø9.Ø and E989
T46.9Ø5A	995.29 and E942.9
T46.9Ø5S	9Ø9.5 and E942.9
T46.991A	972.9 and E858.3
T46.991S	9Ø9.Ø and E929.2
T46.992A	972.9 and E95Ø.4
T46.992S	9Ø9.Ø and E959
T46.993A	972.9 and E962.Ø
T46.993S	9Ø9.Ø and E969
T46.994A	972.9 and E98Ø.4
T46.994S	9Ø9.Ø and E989
T46.995A	995.29 and E942.9
T46.995S	9Ø9.5 and E942.9
T47.ØX1A	973.Ø and E858.4
T47.ØX1S	9Ø9.Ø and E929.2
T47.ØX2A	973.Ø and E95Ø.4
T47.ØX2S	9Ø9.Ø and E959
T47.ØX3A	973.Ø and E962.Ø
T47.ØX3S	9Ø9.Ø and E969
T47.ØX4A	973.Ø and E98Ø.4
T47.ØX4S	9Ø9.Ø and E989
T47.ØX5A	995.29 and E943.Ø
T47.ØX5S	9Ø9.5 and E943.Ø
T47.1X1A	973.Ø and E858.4
T47.1X1S	9Ø9.Ø and E929.2
T47.1X2A	973.Ø and E95Ø.4
T47.1X2S	9Ø9.Ø and E959
T47.1X3A	973.Ø and E962.Ø
T47.1X3S	9Ø9.Ø and E969
T47.1X4A	973.Ø and E98Ø.4
T47.1X4S	9Ø9.Ø and E989
T47.1X5A	995.29 and E943.Ø
T47.1X5S	9Ø9.5 and E943.Ø
T47.2X1A	973.1 and E858.4
T47.2X1S	9Ø9.Ø and E929.2
T47.2X2A	973.1 and E95Ø.4
T47.2X2S	9Ø9.Ø and E959
T47.2X3A	973.1 and E962.Ø
T47.2X3S	9Ø9.Ø and E969
T47.2X4A	973.1 and E98Ø.4
T47.2X4S	9Ø9.Ø and E989
T47.2X5A	995.29 and E943.1
T47.2X5S	9Ø9.5 and E943.1
T47.3X1A	973.2 and E858.4
T47.3X1S	9Ø9.Ø and E929.2
T47.3X2A	973.2 and E95Ø.4
T47.3X2S	9Ø9.Ø and E959
T47.3X3A	973.2 and E962.Ø
T47.3X3S	9Ø9.Ø and E969
T47.3X4A	973.2 and E98Ø.4
T47.3X4S	9Ø9.Ø and E989
T47.3X5A	995.29 and E943.2
T47.3X5S	9Ø9.5 and E943.2
T47.4X1A	973.3 and E858.4
T47.4X1S	9Ø9.Ø and E929.2
T47.4X2A	973.3 and E95Ø.4
T47.4X2S	9Ø9.Ø and E959
T47.4X3A	973.3 and E962.Ø
T47.4X3S	9Ø9.Ø and E969
T47.4X4A	973.3 and E98Ø.4
T47.4X4S	9Ø9.Ø and E989
T47.4X5A	995.29 and E943.3
T47.4X5S	9Ø9.5 and E943.3
T47.5X1A	973.4 and E858.4
T47.5X1S	9Ø9.Ø and E929.2
T47.5X2A	973.4 and E95Ø.4
T47.5X2S	9Ø9.Ø and E959
T47.5X3A	973.4 and E962.Ø
T47.5X3S	9Ø9.Ø and E969
T47.5X4A	973.4 and E98Ø.4
T47.5X4S	9Ø9.Ø and E989
T47.5X5A	995.29 and E943.4
T47.5X5S	9Ø9.5 and E943.4
T47.6X1A	973.5 and E858.4
T47.6X1S	9Ø9.Ø and E929.2
T47.6X2A	973.5 and E95Ø.4
T47.6X2S	9Ø9.Ø and E959
T47.6X3A	973.5 and E962.Ø
T47.6X3S	9Ø9.Ø and E969
T47.6X4A	973.5 and E98Ø.4
T47.6X4S	9Ø9.Ø and E989
T47.6X5A	995.29 and E943.5
T47.6X5S	9Ø9.5 and E943.5
T47.7X1A	973.6 and E858.4
T47.7X1S	9Ø9.Ø and E929.2
T47.7X2A	973.6 and E95Ø.4
T47.7X2S	9Ø9.Ø and E959
T47.7X3A	973.6 and E962.Ø
T47.7X3S	9Ø9.Ø and E969
T47.7X4A	973.6 and E98Ø.4
T47.7X4S	9Ø9.Ø and E989
T47.7X5A	995.29 and E943.6
T47.7X5S	9Ø9.5 and E943.6
T47.8X1A	973.8 and E858.4
T47.8X1S	9Ø9.Ø and E929.2
T47.8X2A	973.8 and E95Ø.4
T47.8X2S	9Ø9.Ø and E959
T47.8X3A	973.8 and E962.Ø
T47.8X3S	9Ø9.Ø and E969
T47.8X4A	973.8 and E98Ø.4
T47.8X4S	9Ø9.Ø and E989
T47.8X5A	995.29 and E943.8
T47.8X5S	9Ø9.5 and E943.8
T47.91XA	973.9 and E858.4
T47.91XS	9Ø9.Ø and E929.2
T47.92XA	973.9 and E95Ø.4
T47.92XS	9Ø9.Ø and E959
T47.93XA	973.9 and E962.Ø
T47.93XS	9Ø9.Ø and E969
T47.94XA	973.9 and E98Ø.4
T47.94XS	9Ø9.Ø and E989
T47.95XA	995.29 and E943.9
T47.95XS	9Ø9.5 and E943.9
T48.ØX1A	975.Ø and E858.Ø
T48.ØX1S	9Ø9.Ø and E929.2
T48.ØX2A	975.Ø and E95Ø.4
T48.ØX2S	9Ø9.Ø and E959
T48.ØX3A	975.Ø and E962.Ø
T48.ØX3S	9Ø9.Ø and E969
T48.ØX4A	975.Ø and E98Ø.4
T48.ØX4S	9Ø9.Ø and E989
T48.ØX5A	995.29 and E945.Ø
T48.ØX5S	9Ø9.5 and E945.Ø
T48.1X1A	975.2 and E858.6
T48.1X1S	9Ø9.Ø and E929.2
T48.1X2A	975.2 and E95Ø.4
T48.1X2S	9Ø9.Ø and E959
T48.1X3A	975.2 and E962.Ø
T48.1X3S	9Ø9.Ø and E969
T48.1X4A	975.2 and E98Ø.4
T48.1X4S	9Ø9.Ø and E989
T48.1X5A	995.29 and E945.2
T48.1X5S	9Ø9.5 and E945.2
T48.2Ø1A	975.1 and E858.6; 975.3 and E858.6
T48.2Ø1S	9Ø9.Ø and E929.2
T48.2Ø2A	975.3 and E95Ø.4
T48.2Ø2S	9Ø9.Ø and E959
T48.2Ø3A	975.3 and E962.Ø
T48.2Ø3S	9Ø9.Ø and E969
T48.2Ø4A	975.3 and E98Ø.4
T48.2Ø4S	9Ø9.Ø and E989
T48.2Ø5A	995.29 and E945.3
T48.2Ø5S	9Ø9.5 and E945.3
T48.291A	975.1 and E858.6; 975.3 and E858.6

T48.291S	9Ø9.Ø and E929.2
T48.292A	975.3 and E95Ø.4
T48.292S	9Ø9.Ø and E959
T48.293A	975.3 and E962.Ø
T48.293S	9Ø9.Ø and E969
T48.294A	975.3 and E98Ø.4
T48.294S	9Ø9.Ø and E989
T48.295A	995.29 and E945.3
T48.295S	9Ø9.5 and E945.3
T48.3X1A	975.4 and E858.6
T48.3X1S	9Ø9.Ø and E929.2
T48.3X2A	975.4 and E95Ø.4
T48.3X2S	9Ø9.Ø and E959
T48.3X3A	975.4 and E962.Ø
T48.3X3S	9Ø9.Ø and E969
T48.3X4A	975.4 and E98Ø.4
T48.3X4S	9Ø9.Ø and E989
T48.3X5A	995.29 and E945.4
T48.3X5S	9Ø9.5 and E945.4
T48.4X1A	975.5 and E858.6
T48.4X1S	9Ø9.Ø and E929.2
T48.4X2A	975.5 and E95Ø.4
T48.4X2S	9Ø9.Ø and E959
T48.4X3A	975.5 and E962.Ø
T48.4X3S	9Ø9.Ø and E969
T48.4X4A	975.5 and E98Ø.4
T48.4X4S	9Ø9.Ø and E989
T48.4X5A	995.29 and E945.5
T48.4X5S	9Ø9.5 and E945.5
T48.5X1A	975.6 and E858.6
T48.5X1S	9Ø9.Ø and E929.2
T48.5X2A	975.6 and E95Ø.4
T48.5X2S	9Ø9.Ø and E959
T48.5X3A	975.6 and E962.Ø
T48.5X3S	9Ø9.Ø and E969
T48.5X4A	975.6 and E98Ø.4
T48.5X4S	9Ø9.Ø and E989
T48.5X5A	995.29 and E945.6
T48.5X5S	9Ø9.5 and E945.6
T48.6X1A	975.7 and E858.6
T48.6X1S	9Ø9.Ø and E929.2
T48.6X2A	975.7 and E95Ø.4
T48.6X2S	9Ø9.Ø and E959
T48.6X3A	975.7 and E962.Ø
T48.6X3S	9Ø9.Ø and E969
T48.6X4A	975.7 and E98Ø.4
T48.6X4S	9Ø9.Ø and E989
T48.6X5A	995.29 and E945.7
T48.6X5S	9Ø9.5 and E945.7
T48.9Ø1A	975.8 and E858.6
T48.9Ø1S	9Ø9.Ø and E929.2
T48.9Ø2A	975.8 and E95Ø.4
T48.9Ø2S	9Ø9.Ø and E959
T48.9Ø3A	975.8 and E962.Ø
T48.9Ø3S	9Ø9.Ø and E969
T48.9Ø4A	975.8 and E98Ø.4
T48.9Ø4S	9Ø9.Ø and E989
T48.9Ø5A	995.29 and E945.8
T48.9Ø5S	9Ø9.5 and E945.8
T48.991A	975.8 and E858.6
T48.991S	9Ø9.Ø and E929.2
T48.992A	975.8 and E95Ø.4
T48.992S	9Ø9.Ø and E959
T48.993A	975.8 and E962.Ø
T48.993S	9Ø9.Ø and E969
T48.994A	975.8 and E98Ø.4
T48.994S	9Ø9.Ø and E989
T48.995A	995.29 and E945.8
T48.995S	9Ø9.5 and E945.8
T49.ØX1A	976.Ø and E858.7
T49.ØX1S	9Ø9.Ø and E929.2
T49.ØX2A	976.Ø and E95Ø.4
T49.ØX2S	9Ø9.Ø and E959
T49.ØX3A	976.Ø and E962.Ø
T49.ØX3S	9Ø9.Ø and E969
T49.ØX4A	976.Ø and E98Ø.4
T49.ØX4S	9Ø9.Ø and E989
T49.ØX5A	995.29 and E946.Ø
T49.ØX5S	9Ø9.5 and E946.Ø
T49.1X1A	976.1 and E858.7
T49.1X1S	9Ø9.Ø and E929.2
T49.1X2A	976.1 and E95Ø.4
T49.1X2S	9Ø9.Ø and E959
T49.1X3A	976.1 and E962.Ø
T49.1X3S	9Ø9.Ø and E969
T49.1X4A	976.1 and E98Ø.4
T49.1X4S	9Ø9.Ø and E989
T49.1X5A	995.29 and E946.1
T49.1X5S	9Ø9.5 and E946.1
T49.2X1A	976.2 and E858.7
T49.2X1S	9Ø9.Ø and E929.2
T49.2X2A	976.2 and E95Ø.4
T49.2X2S	9Ø9.Ø and E959
T49.2X3A	976.2 and E962.Ø
T49.2X3S	9Ø9.Ø and E969
T49.2X4A	976.2 and E98Ø.4
T49.2X4S	9Ø9.Ø and E989
T49.2X5A	995.29 and E946.2
T49.2X5S	9Ø9.5 and E946.2
T49.3X1A	976.3 and E858.7
T49.3X1S	9Ø9.Ø and E929.2
T49.3X2A	976.3 and E95Ø.4
T49.3X2S	9Ø9.Ø and E959
T49.3X3A	976.3 and E962.Ø
T49.3X3S	9Ø9.Ø and E969
T49.3X4A	976.3 and E98Ø.4
T49.3X4S	9Ø9.Ø and E989
T49.3X5A	995.29 and E946.3
T49.3X5S	9Ø9.5 and E946.3
T49.4X1A	976.4 and E858.7
T49.4X1S	9Ø9.Ø and E929.2
T49.4X2A	976.4 and E95Ø.4
T49.4X2S	9Ø9.Ø and E959
T49.4X3A	976.4 and E962.Ø
T49.4X3S	9Ø9.Ø and E969
T49.4X4A	976.4 and E98Ø.4
T49.4X4S	9Ø9.Ø and E989
T49.4X5A	995.29 and E946.4
T49.4X5S	9Ø9.5 and E946.4
T49.5X1A	976.5 and E858.7
T49.5X1S	9Ø9.Ø and E929.2
T49.5X2A	976.5 and E95Ø.4
T49.5X2S	9Ø9.Ø and E959
T49.5X3A	976.5 and E962.Ø
T49.5X3S	9Ø9.Ø and E969
T49.5X4A	976.5 and E98Ø.4
T49.5X4S	9Ø9.Ø and E989
T49.5X5A	995.29 and E946.5
T49.5X5S	9Ø9.5 and E946.5
T49.6X1A	976.6 and E858.7
T49.6X1S	9Ø9.Ø and E929.2
T49.6X2A	976.6 and E95Ø.4
T49.6X2S	9Ø9.Ø and E959
T49.6X3A	976.6 and E962.Ø
T49.6X3S	9Ø9.Ø and E969
T49.6X4A	976.6 and E98Ø.4
T49.6X4S	9Ø9.Ø and E989
T49.6X5A	995.29 and E946.6
T49.6X5S	9Ø9.5 and E946.6
T49.7X1A	976.7 and E858.7
T49.7X1S	9Ø9.Ø and E929.2
T49.7X2A	976.7 and E95Ø.4
T49.7X2S	9Ø9.Ø and E959
T49.7X3A	976.7 and E962.Ø
T49.7X3S	9Ø9.Ø and E969
T49.7X4A	976.7 and E98Ø.4
T49.7X4S	9Ø9.Ø and E989
T49.7X5A	995.29 and E946.7
T49.7X5S	9Ø9.5 and E946.7
T49.8X1A	976.8 and E858.7
T49.8X1S	9Ø9.Ø and E929.2
T49.8X2A	976.8 and E95Ø.4
T49.8X2S	9Ø9.Ø and E959
T49.8X3A	976.8 and E962.Ø
T49.8X3S	9Ø9.Ø and E969
T49.8X4A	976.8 and E98Ø.4
T49.8X4S	9Ø9.Ø and E989
T49.8X5A	995.29 and E946.8
T49.8X5S	9Ø9.5 and E946.8
T49.91XA	976.9 and E858.7
T49.91XS	9Ø9.Ø and E929.2
T49.92XA	976.9 and E95Ø.4
T49.92XS	9Ø9.Ø and E959
T49.93XA	976.9 and E962.Ø
T49.93XS	9Ø9.Ø and E969
T49.94XA	976.9 and E98Ø.4
T49.94XS	9Ø9.Ø and E989
T49.95XA	995.29 and E946.9
T49.95XS	9Ø9.5 and E946.9
T5Ø.ØX1A	962.Ø and E858.Ø
T5Ø.ØX1S	9Ø9.Ø and E929.2
T5Ø.ØX2A	962.Ø and E95Ø.4
T5Ø.ØX2S	9Ø9.Ø and E959
T5Ø.ØX3A	962.Ø and E962.Ø
T5Ø.ØX3S	9Ø9.Ø and E969
T5Ø.ØX4A	962.Ø and E98Ø.4
T5Ø.ØX4S	9Ø9.Ø and E989
T5Ø.ØX5A	995.29 and E932.Ø
T5Ø.ØX5S	9Ø9.5 and E932.Ø
T5Ø.1X1A	974.4 and E858.5
T5Ø.1X1S	9Ø9.Ø and E929.2
T5Ø.1X2A	974.4 and E95Ø.4
T5Ø.1X2S	9Ø9.Ø and E959
T5Ø.1X3A	974.4 and E962.Ø
T5Ø.1X3S	9Ø9.Ø and E969
T5Ø.1X4A	974.4 and E858.5
T5Ø.1X4S	9Ø9.Ø and E989
T5Ø.1X5A	995.29 and E944.4
T5Ø.1X5S	9Ø9.5 and E944.4
T5Ø.2X1A	974.2 and E858.5; 974.4 and E858.5
T5Ø.2X1S	9Ø9.Ø and E929.2
T5Ø.2X2A	974.2 and E95Ø.4; 974.4 and E95Ø.4
T5Ø.2X2S	9Ø9.Ø and E959
T5Ø.2X3A	974.2 and E962.Ø; 974.4 and E962.Ø
T5Ø.2X3S	9Ø9.Ø and E969
T5Ø.2X4A	974.2 and E98Ø.4; 974.4 and E98Ø.4
T5Ø.2X4S	9Ø9.Ø and E989
T5Ø.2X5A	995.29 and E944.2
T5Ø.2X5S	9Ø9.5 and E944.2
T5Ø.3X1A	974.5 and E858.5
T5Ø.3X1S	9Ø9.Ø and E929.2
T5Ø.3X2A	974.5 and E95Ø.4
T5Ø.3X2S	9Ø9.Ø and E959
T5Ø.3X3A	974.5 and E962.Ø
T5Ø.3X3S	9Ø9.Ø and E969
T5Ø.3X4A	974.5 and E98Ø.4
T5Ø.3X4S	9Ø9.Ø and E989
T5Ø.3X5A	995.29 and E944.5
T5Ø.3X5S	9Ø9.5 and E944.5
T5Ø.4X1A	974.7 and E858.5
T5Ø.4X1S	9Ø9.Ø and E929.2
T5Ø.4X2A	974.7 and E95Ø.4

T50.4X2S	909.0 and E959
T50.4X3A	974.7 and E962.0
T50.4X3S	909.0 and E969
T50.4X4A	974.7 and E980.4
T50.4X4S	909.0 and E989
T50.4X5A	995.29 and E944.7
T50.4X5S	909.5 and E944.7
T50.5X1A	977.0 and E858.8
T50.5X1S	909.0 and E929.2
T50.5X2A	977.0 and E950.4
T50.5X2S	909.0 and E959
T50.5X3A	977.0 and E962.0
T50.5X3S	909.0 and E969
T50.5X4A	977.0 and E980.4
T50.5X4S	909.0 and E989
T50.5X5A	995.29 and E947.0
T50.5X5S	909.5 and E947.0
T50.6X1A	977.2 and E858.8
T50.6X1S	909.0 and E929.2
T50.6X2A	977.2 and E950.4
T50.6X2S	909.0 and E959
T50.6X3A	977.2 and E962.0
T50.6X3S	909.0 and E969
T50.6X4A	977.2 and E980.4
T50.6X4S	909.0 and E989
T50.6X5A	995.29 and E947.2
T50.6X5S	909.5 and E947.2
T50.7X1A	970.0 and E854.3; 970.1 and E854.3
T50.7X1S	909.0 and E929.2
T50.7X2A	970.0 and E950.4; 970.1 and E950.4
T50.7X2S	909.0 and E959
T50.7X3A	970.0 and E962.0; 970.1 and E962.0
T50.7X3S	909.0 and E969
T50.7X4A	970.0 and E980.4; 970.1 and E980.4
T50.7X4S	909.0 and E989
T50.7X5A	995.29 and E940.0; 995.29 and E940.1
T50.7X5S	909.5 and E940.0; 909.5 and E940.1
T50.8X1A	977.8 and E858.8
T50.8X1S	909.0 and E929.2
T50.8X2A	977.8 and E950.4
T50.8X2S	909.0 and E959
T50.8X3A	977.8 and E962.0
T50.8X3S	909.0 and E969
T50.8X4A	977.8 and E980.4
T50.8X4S	909.0 and E989
T50.8X5A	995.29 and E947.8
T50.8X5S	909.5 and E947.8
T50.901A	977.9 and E858.8
T50.901S	909.0 and E929.2
T50.902A	977.9 and E950.4
T50.902S	909.0 and E959
T50.903A	977.9 and E962.0
T50.903S	909.0 and E969
T50.904A	977.9 and E980.5
T50.904S	909.0 and E989
T50.905A	995.20 and E947.9
T50.905S	909.5 and E947.9
T50.991A	979.9 and E858.8
T50.991S	909.0 and E929.2
T50.992A	979.9 and E950.4
T50.992S	909.0 and E959
T50.993A	979.9 and E962.0
T50.993S	909.0 and E969
T50.994A	979.9 and E980.4
T50.994S	909.0 and E989
T50.995A	995.29 and E947.8
T50.995S	909.5 and E947.8
T50.A11A	978.6 and E858.1
T50.A11S	909.0 and E929.2
T50.A12A	978.6 and E950.4
T50.A12S	909.0 and E959
T50.A13A	978.6 and E962.0
T50.A13S	909.0 and E969
T50.A14A	978.6 and E980.4
T50.A14S	909.0 and E989
T50.A15A	995.29 and E948.6
T50.A15S	909.5 and E948.6
T50.A21A	978.9 and E858.1
T50.A21S	909.0 and E929.2
T50.A22A	978.9 and E950.4
T50.A22S	909.0 and E959
T50.A23A	978.9 and E962.0
T50.A23S	909.0 and E969
T50.A24A	978.9 and E980.4
T50.A24S	909.0 and E989
T50.A25A	995.29 and E948.9
T50.A25S	909.5 and E948.9
T50.A91A	978.8 and E858.1
T50.A91S	909.0 and E929.2
T50.A92A	978.8 and E950.4
T50.A92S	909.0 and E959
T50.A93A	978.8 and E962.0
T50.A93S	909.0 and E969
T50.A94A	978.8 and E980.4
T50.A94S	909.0 and E989
T50.A95A	995.29 and E948.8
T50.A95S	909.5 and E948.8
T50.B11A	979.0 and E858.1
T50.B11S	909.0 and E929.2
T50.B12A	979.0 and E950.4
T50.B12S	909.0 and E959
T50.B13A	979.0 and E962.0
T50.B13S	909.0 and E969
T50.B14A	979.0 and E980.4
T50.B14S	909.0 and E989
T50.B15A	995.29 and E949.0
T50.B15S	909.5 and E949.0
T50.B91A	979.6 and E858.1
T50.B91S	909.0 and E929.2
T50.B92A	979.6 and E950.4
T50.B92S	909.0 and E959
T50.B93A	979.6 and E962.0
T50.B93S	909.0 and E969
T50.B94A	979.6 and E980.4
T50.B94S	909.0 and E989
T50.B95A	995.29 and E949.6
T50.B95S	909.5 and E949.6
T50.Z11A	964.6 and E858.1
T50.Z11S	909.0 and E929.2
T50.Z12A	964.6 and E950.4
T50.Z12S	909.0 and E959
T50.Z13A	964.6 and E962.0
T50.Z13S	909.0 and E969
T50.Z14A	964.6 and E980.4
T50.Z14S	909.0 and E989
T50.Z15A	995.29 and E934.6
T50.Z15S	909.5 and E934.6
T50.Z91A	979.9 and E858.1
T50.Z91S	909.0 and E929.2
T50.Z92A	979.9 and E950.4
T50.Z92S	909.0 and E959
T50.Z93A	979.9 and E962.0
T50.Z93S	909.0 and E969
T50.Z94A	979.9 and E980.4
T50.Z94S	909.0 and E989
T50.Z95A	995.29 and E949.9
T50.Z95S	909.5 and E949.9
T51.0X1A	980.0 and E860.1
T51.0X2A	980.0 and E950.9
T51.0X3A	980.0 and E962.1
T51.0X4A	980.0 and E980.9
T51.1X1A	980.1 and E860.2
T51.1X2A	980.1 and E950.9
T51.1X3A	980.1 and E962.1
T51.1X4A	980.1 and E980.9
T51.2X1A	980.2 and E860.3
T51.2X2A	980.2 and E950.9
T51.2X3A	980.2 and E962.1
T51.2X4A	980.2 and E980.9
T51.3X1A	980.3 and E860.4
T51.3X2A	980.3 and E950.9
T51.3X3A	980.3 and E962.1
T51.3X4A	980.3 and E980.9
T51.8X1A	980.8 and E860.8
T51.8X2A	980.8 and E950.9
T51.8X3A	980.8 and E962.1
T51.8X4A	980.8 and E980.9
T51.91XA	980.9 and E860.9
T51.92XA	980.9 and E950.9
T51.93XA	980.9 and E962.1
T51.94XA	980.9 and E980.9
T52.0X1A	981 and E862.1
T52.0X2A	981 and E950.9
T52.0X3A	981 and E962.1
T52.0X4A	981 and E980.9
T52.1X1A	982.0 and E862.4
T52.1X2A	982.0 and E950.9
T52.1X3A	982.0 and E962.1
T52.1X4A	982.0 and E980.9
T52.2X1A	982.0 and E862.4
T52.2X2A	982.0 and E950.9
T52.2X3A	982.0 and E962.1
T52.2X4A	982.0 and E980.9
T52.3X1A	982.4 and E862.4
T52.3X2A	982.4 and E950.9
T52.3X3A	982.4 and E962.1
T52.3X4A	982.4 and E980.9
T52.4X1A	982.8 and E862.4
T52.4X2A	982.8 and E950.9
T52.4X3A	982.8 and E962.1
T52.4X4A	982.8 and E980.9
T52.8X1A	982.8 and E862.4
T52.8X2A	982.8 and E950.9
T52.8X3A	982.8 and E962.1
T52.8X4A	982.8 and E980.9
T52.91XA	982.8 and E862.4
T52.92XA	982.8 and E950.9
T52.93XA	982.8 and E962.1
T52.94XA	982.8 and E980.9
T53.0X1A	982.1 and E869.8
T53.0X2A	982.1 and E950.9
T53.0X3A	982.1 and E962.2
T53.0X4A	982.1 and E980.9
T53.1X1A	982.3 and E869.8
T53.1X2A	982.3 and E950.9
T53.1X3A	982.3 and E962.2
T53.1X4A	982.3 and E980.9
T53.2X1A	982.3 and E869.8
T53.2X2A	982.3 and E950.9
T53.2X3A	982.3 and E962.2
T53.2X4A	982.3 and E980.9
T53.3X1A	982.3 and E869.8
T53.3X2A	982.3 and E950.9
T53.3X3A	982.3 and E962.2
T53.3X4A	982.3 and E980.9
T53.4X1A	982.3 and E869.8
T53.4X2A	982.3 and E950.9
T53.4X3A	982.3 and E962.2
T53.4X4A	982.3 and E980.9
T53.5X1A	987.4 and E869.2

ICD-10-CM	ICD-9-CM
T53.5X2A	987.4 and E952.8
T53.5X3A	987.4 and E962.2
T53.5X4A	987.4 and E982.8
T53.6X1A	982.3 and E869.8
T53.6X2A	982.3 and E950.9
T53.6X3A	982.3 and E962.2
T53.6X4A	982.3 and E980.9
T53.7X1A	982.3 and E869.8
T53.7X2A	982.3 and E950.9
T53.7X3A	982.3 and E962.2
T53.7X4A	982.3 and E980.9
T53.91XA	982.3 and E869.8; 989.2 and E869.8
T53.92XA	982.3 and E950.9; 989.2 and E950.9
T53.93XA	982.3 and E962.2; 989.2 and E962.2
T53.94XA	982.3 and E980.9; 989.2 and E980.9
T54.0X1A	983.0 and E864.0
T54.0X2A	983.0 and E950.7
T54.0X3A	983.0 and E961
T54.0X4A	983.0 and E980.6
T54.1X1A	983.9 and E924.1
T54.1X2A	983.9 and E950.7
T54.1X3A	983.9 and E961
T54.1X4A	983.9 and E924.1
T54.2X1A	983.1 and E924.1
T54.2X2A	983.1 and E950.7
T54.2X3A	983.1 and E961
T54.2X4A	983.1 and E924.1
T54.3X1A	983.2 and E924.1
T54.3X2A	983.2 and E950.7
T54.3X3A	983.2 and E961
T54.3X4A	983.2 and E924.1
T54.91XA	983.9 and E924.1
T54.92XA	983.9 and E950.7
T54.93XA	983.9 and E961
T54.94XA	983.9 and E980.6
T55.0X1A	989.6 and E861.1
T55.0X2A	989.6 and E950.7
T55.0X3A	989.6 and E962.1
T55.0X4A	989.6 and E980.6
T55.1X1A	989.6 and E861.0
T55.1X2A	989.6 and E950.7
T55.1X3A	989.6 and E962.1
T55.1X4A	989.6 and E980.6
T56.0X1A	984.9 and E866.0
T56.0X2A	984.9 and E950.9
T56.0X3A	984.9 and E962.1
T56.0X4A	980.9 and 984.9
T56.1X1A	985.0 and E866.1
T56.1X2A	985.0 and E950.9
T56.1X3A	985.0 and E962.1
T56.1X4A	985.0 and E980.9
T56.2X1A	985.6 and E866.4
T56.2X2A	985.6 and E950.9
T56.2X3A	985.6 and E962.1
T56.2X4A	985.6 and E980.9
T56.3X1A	985.5 and E866.4
T56.3X2A	985.5 and E950.9
T56.3X3A	985.5 and E962.1
T56.3X4A	985.5 and E980.9
T56.4X1A	985.8 and E864.4
T56.4X2A	985.8 and E950.9
T56.4X3A	985.8 and E962.1
T56.4X4A	985.8 and E980.9
T56.5X1A	985.8 and E866.4
T56.5X2A	985.8 and E950.9
T56.5X3A	985.8 and E962.1
T56.5X4A	985.8 and E980.9
T56.6X1A	985.8 and E866.4
T56.6X2A	985.8 and E950.9
T56.6X3A	985.8 and E962.1
T56.6X4A	985.8 and E980.9
T56.7X1A	985.3 and E866.4
T56.7X2A	985.3 and E950.9
T56.7X3A	985.3 and E962.1
T56.7X4A	985.3 and E980.9
T56.811A	985.8 and E866.4
T56.812A	985.8 and E950.9
T56.813A	985.8 and E962.1
T56.814A	985.8 and E980.9
T56.891A	985.8 and E866.4
T56.892A	985.8 and E950.9
T56.893A	985.8 and E962.1
T56.894A	985.8 and E980.9
T56.91XA	985.9 and E866.4
T56.92XA	985.9 and E950.9
T56.93XA	985.9 and E962.1
T56.94XA	985.9 and E980.9
T57.0X1A	985.1 and E866.3
T57.0X2A	985.1 and E950.8
T57.0X3A	985.1 and E962.1
T57.0X4A	985.1 and E980.8
T57.1X1A	983.9 and E864.3
T57.1X2A	983.9 and E950.7
T57.1X3A	983.9 and E962.1
T57.1X4A	983.9 and E980.6
T57.2X1A	985.2 and E866.4
T57.2X2A	985.2 and E950.7
T57.2X3A	985.2 and E962.1
T57.2X4A	985.2 and E980.6
T57.3X1A	987.7 and E869.8
T57.3X2A	987.7 and E952.8
T57.3X3A	987.7 and E962.1
T57.3X4A	987.7 and E982.8
T57.8X1A	989.89 and E866.8
T57.8X2A	989.89 and E950.9
T57.8X3A	989.89 and E962.1
T57.8X4A	989.89 and E980.9
T57.91XA	989.9 and E866.8
T57.92XA	989.9 and E950.9
T57.93XA	989.9 and E962.9
T57.94XA	989.9 and E980.9
T58.01XA	986 and E868.2
T58.02XA	986 and E952.0
T58.03XA	986 and E962.2
T58.04XA	986 and E982.0
T58.11XA	986 and E868.1
T58.12XA	986 and E952.1
T58.13XA	986 and E962.2
T58.14XA	986 and E982.1
T58.2X1A	986 and E868.3
T58.2X2A	986 and E952.1
T58.2X3A	986 and E962.2
T58.2X4A	986 and E982.1
T58.8X1A	986 and E868.8
T58.8X2A	986 and E952.1
T58.8X3A	986 and E962.2
T58.8X4A	986 and E982.1
T58.91XA	986 and E868.9
T58.92XA	986 and E952.1
T58.93XA	986 and E962.2
T58.94XA	986 and E982.1
T59.0X1A	987.2 and E869.0
T59.0X2A	987.2 and E952.8
T59.0X3A	987.2 and E962.2
T59.0X4A	987.2 and E982.8
T59.1X1A	987.3 and E869.1
T59.1X2A	987.3 and E952.8
T59.1X3A	987.3 and E962.2
T59.1X4A	987.3 and E982.8
T59.2X1A	987.1 and E869.8
T59.2X2A	987.1 and E952.8
T59.2X3A	987.1 and E962.2
T59.2X4A	987.1 and E982.8
T59.3X1A	987.5 and E869.3
T59.3X2A	987.5 and E952.8
T59.3X3A	987.5 and E962.2
T59.3X4A	987.5 and E982.8
T59.4X1A	987.6 and E869.8
T59.4X2A	987.6 and E952.8
T59.4X3A	987.6 and E962.2
T59.4X4A	987.6 and E982.8
T59.5X1A	987.8 and E869.8
T59.5X2A	987.8 and E952.8
T59.5X3A	987.8 and E962.2
T59.5X4A	987.8 and E982.8
T59.6X1A	987.8 and E869.8
T59.6X2A	987.8 and E952.8
T59.6X3A	987.8 and E962.2
T59.6X4A	987.8 and E982.8
T59.7X1A	987.8 and E869.8
T59.7X2A	987.8 and E952.8
T59.7X3A	987.8 and E962.2
T59.7X4A	987.8 and E982.8
T59.811A	987.9 and E869.8
T59.812A	987.9 and E952.8
T59.813A	987.9 and E962.2
T59.814A	987.9 and E982.8
T59.891A	987.9 and E869.8
T59.892A	987.9 and E952.8
T59.893A	987.9 and E962.2
T59.894A	987.9 and E869.8
T59.91XA	987.9 and E869.8
T59.92XA	987.9 and E952.9
T59.93XA	987.9 and E962.2
T59.94XA	987.9 and E982.8
T60.0X1A	989.3 and E863.1
T60.0X1S	909.1 and E929.2
T60.0X2A	989.3 and E950.6
T60.0X2S	909.1 and E959
T60.0X3A	989.3 and E962.1
T60.0X3S	909.1 and E969
T60.0X4A	989.3 and E980.7
T60.0X4S	909.1 and E989
T60.1X1A	989.4 and E863.4
T60.1X1S	909.1 and E929.2
T60.1X2A	989.4 and E950.6
T60.1X2S	909.1 and E959
T60.1X3A	989.4 and E962.1
T60.1X3S	909.1 and E969
T60.1X4A	989.4 and E980.7
T60.1X4S	909.1 and E989
T60.2X1A	989.4 and E863.4
T60.2X1S	909.1 and E929.2
T60.2X2A	989.4 and E950.6
T60.2X2S	909.1 and E959
T60.2X3A	989.4 and E962.1
T60.2X3S	909.1 and E969
T60.2X4A	989.4 and E980.7
T60.2X4S	909.1 and E989
T60.3X1A	989.89 and E863.5
T60.3X1S	909.1 and E929.2
T60.3X2A	989.89 and E950.6
T60.3X2S	909.1 and E959
T60.3X3A	989.89 and E962.1
T60.3X3S	909.1 and E969
T60.3X4A	989.89 and E980.7
T60.3X4S	909.1 and E989
T60.4X1A	989.4 and E863.7
T60.4X1S	909.1 and E929.2
T60.4X2A	989.4 and E950.6
T60.4X2S	909.1 and E959
T60.4X3A	989.4 and E962.1

T60.4X3S 909.1 and E969
T60.4X4A 989.4 and E980.7
T60.4X4S 909.1 and E989
T60.8X1A 989.4 and E863.4
T60.8X1S 909.1 and E929.2
T60.8X2A 989.4 and E950.6
T60.8X2S 909.1 and E959
T60.8X3A 989.4 and E962.1
T60.8X3S 909.1 and E969
T60.8X4A 989.4 and E980.7
T60.8X4S 909.1 and E989
T60.91XA 989.4 and E863.4
T60.91XS 909.1 and E929.2
T60.92XA 989.4 and E950.6
T60.92XS 909.1 and E959
T60.93XA 989.4 and E962.1
T60.93XS 909.1 and E969
T60.94XA 989.4 and E980.7
T60.94XS 909.1 and E989
T61.01XA 988.0 and E865.2
T61.01XS 909.1 and E929.2
T61.02XA 988.0 and E950.9
T61.02XS 909.1 and E959
T61.03XA 988.0 and E962.1
T61.03XS 909.1 and E969
T61.04XA 988.0 and E980.9
T61.04XS 909.1 and E989
T61.11XA 988.0 and E865.2
T61.11XS 909.1 and E929.2
T61.12XA 988.0 and E950.9
T61.12XS 909.1 and E959
T61.13XA 988.0 and E962.1
T61.13XS 909.1 and E969
T61.14XA 988.0 and E980.9
T61.14XS 909.1 and E989
T61.771A 988.0 and E865.2
T61.771S 909.1 and E929.2
T61.772A 988.0 and E950.9
T61.772S 909.1 and E959
T61.773A 988.0 and E962.1
T61.773S 909.1 and E969
T61.774A 988.0 and E980.9
T61.774S 909.1 and E989
T61.781A 988.0 and E865.1
T61.781S 909.1 and E929.2
T61.782A 988.0 and E950.9
T61.782S 909.1 and E959
T61.783A 988.0 and E962.1
T61.783S 909.1 and E969
T61.784A 988.0 and E980.9
T61.784S 909.1 and E989
T61.8X1A 988.0 and E865.2
T61.8X1S 909.1 and E929.2
T61.8X2A 988.0 and E950.9
T61.8X2S 909.1 and E959
T61.8X3A 988.0 and E962.1
T61.8X3S 909.1 and E969
T61.8X4A 988.0 and E980.9
T61.8X4S 909.1 and E989
T61.91XA 988.0 and E865.2
T61.91XS 909.1 and E929.2
T61.92XA 988.0 and E950.9
T61.92XS 909.1 and E959
T61.93XA 988.0 and E962.1
T61.93XS 909.1 and E969
T61.94XA 988.0 and E980.9
T61.94XS 909.1 and E989
T62.0X1A 988.1 and E865.5
T62.0X1S 909.1 and E929.2
T62.0X2A 988.1 and E950.9
T62.0X2S 909.1 and E959
T62.0X3A 988.1 and E962.1
T62.0X3S 909.1 and E969
T62.0X4A 988.1 and E980.9
T62.0X4S 909.1 and E989
T62.1X1A 988.2 and E865.3
T62.1X1S 909.1 and E929.2
T62.1X2A 988.2 and E950.9
T62.1X2S 909.1 and E959
T62.1X3A 988.2 and E962.1
T62.1X3S 909.1 and E969
T62.1X4A 988.2 and E980.9
T62.1X4S 909.1 and E989
T62.2X1A 988.2 and E865.4
T62.2X1S 909.1 and E929.2
T62.2X2A 988.2 and E950.9
T62.2X2S 909.1 and E959
T62.2X3A 988.2 and E962.1
T62.2X3S 909.1 and E969
T62.2X4A 988.2 and E980.9
T62.2X4S 909.1 and E989
T62.8X1A 988.8 and E865.8
T62.8X1S 909.1 and E929.2
T62.8X2A 988.8 and E950.9
T62.8X2S 909.1 and E959
T62.8X3A 988.8 and E962.1
T62.8X3S 909.1 and E969
T62.8X4A 988.8 and E980.9
T62.8X4S 909.1 and E989
T62.91XA 988.9 and E865.9
T62.91XS 909.1 and E929.2
T62.92XA 988.9 and E950.9
T62.92XS 909.1 and E959
T62.93XA 988.9 and E962.1
T62.93XS 909.1 and E969
T62.94XA 988.9 and E980.9
T62.94XS 909.1 and E989
T63.001A 989.5 and E905.0
T63.001S 909.1 and E989
T63.002A 989.5 and E950.9
T63.002S 909.1 and E929.2
T63.003A 989.5 and E962.1
T63.003S 909.1 and E959
T63.004A 989.5 and E980.9
T63.004S 909.1 and E969
T63.011A 989.5 and E905.0
T63.011S 909.1 and E929.2
T63.012A 989.5 and E950.9
T63.012S 909.1 and E959
T63.013A 989.5 and E962.1
T63.013S 909.1 and E969
T63.014A 989.5 and E980.9
T63.014S 909.1 and E989
T63.021A 989.5 and E905.0
T63.021S 909.1 and E929.2
T63.022A 989.5 and E950.9
T63.022S 909.1 and E959
T63.023A 989.5 and E962.1
T63.023S 909.1 and E969
T63.024A 989.5 and E980.9
T63.024S 909.1 and E989
T63.031A 989.5 and E905.0
T63.031S 909.1 and E929.2
T63.032A 989.5 and E950.9
T63.032S 909.1 and E959
T63.033A 989.5 and E962.1
T63.033S 909.1 and E969
T63.034A 989.5 and E980.9
T63.034S 909.1 and E989
T63.041A 989.5 and E905.0
T63.041S 909.1 and E929.2
T63.042A 989.5 and E950.9
T63.042S 909.1 and E959
T63.043A 989.5 and E962.1
T63.043S 909.1 and E969
T63.044A 989.5 and E980.9
T63.044S 909.1 and E989
T63.061A 989.5 and E905.0
T63.061S 909.1 and E929.2
T63.062A 989.5 and E950.9
T63.062S 909.1 and E959
T63.063A 989.5 and E962.1
T63.063S 909.1 and E969
T63.064A 989.5 and E980.9
T63.064S 909.1 and E989
T63.071A 989.5 and E905.0
T63.071S 909.1 and E929.2
T63.072A 989.5 and E950.9
T63.072S 909.1 and E959
T63.073A 989.5 and E962.1
T63.073S 909.1 and E969
T63.074A 989.5 and E980.9
T63.074S 909.1 and E989
T63.081A 989.5 and E905.0
T63.081S 909.1 and E929.2
T63.082A 989.5 and E950.9
T63.082S 909.1 and E959
T63.083A 989.5 and E962.1
T63.083S 909.1 and E969
T63.084A 989.5 and E980.9
T63.084S 909.1 and E989
T63.091A 989.5 and E905.0
T63.091S 909.1 and E929.2
T63.092A 989.5 and E950.9
T63.092S 909.1 and E959
T63.093A 989.5 and E962.1
T63.093S 909.1 and E969
T63.094A 989.5 and E980.9
T63.094S 909.1 and E989
T63.111A 989.5 and E905.0
T63.111S 909.1 and E929.2
T63.112A 989.5 and E950.9
T63.112S 909.1 and E959
T63.113A 989.5 and E962.1
T63.113S 909.1 and E969
T63.114A 989.5 and E980.9
T63.114S 909.1 and E989
T63.121A 989.5 and E905.0
T63.121S 909.1 and E929.2
T63.122A 989.5 and E950.9
T63.122S 909.1 and E959
T63.123A 989.5 and E962.1
T63.123S 909.1 and E969
T63.124A 989.5 and E980.9
T63.124S 909.1 and E989
T63.191A 989.5 and E905.0
T63.191S 909.1 and E929.2
T63.192A 989.5 and E950.9
T63.192S 909.1 and E959
T63.193A 989.5 and E962.1
T63.193S 909.1 and E969
T63.194A 989.5 and E980.9
T63.194S 909.1 and E989
T63.2X1A 989.5 and E905.2
T63.2X1S 909.1 and E929.2
T63.2X2A 989.5 and E950.9
T63.2X2S 909.1 and E959
T63.2X3A 989.5 and E962.1
T63.2X3S 909.1 and E969
T63.2X4A 989.5 and E980.9
T63.2X4S 909.1 and E989
T63.301A 989.5 and E905.1
T63.301S 909.1 and E929.2
T63.302A 989.5 and E950.9
T63.302S 909.1 and E959
T63.303A 989.5 and E962.1

ICD-10-CM	ICD-9-CM
T63.3Ø3S	9Ø9.1 and E969
T63.3Ø4A	989.5 and E98Ø.9
T63.3Ø4S	9Ø9.1 and E989
T63.311A	989.5 and E9Ø5.1
T63.311S	9Ø9.1 and E929.2
T63.312A	989.5 and E95Ø.9
T63.312S	9Ø9.1 and E959
T63.313A	989.5 and E962.1
T63.313S	9Ø9.1 and E969
T63.314A	989.5 and E98Ø.9
T63.314S	9Ø9.1 and E989
T63.321A	989.5 and E9Ø5.1
T63.321S	9Ø9.1 and E929.2
T63.322A	989.5 and E95Ø.9
T63.322S	9Ø9.1 and E959
T63.323A	989.5 and E962.1
T63.323S	9Ø9.1 and E969
T63.324A	989.5 and E98Ø.9
T63.324S	9Ø9.1 and E989
T63.331A	989.5 and E9Ø5.1
T63.331S	9Ø9.1 and E929.2
T63.332A	989.5 and E95Ø.9
T63.332S	9Ø9.1 and E959
T63.333A	989.5 and E962.1
T63.333S	9Ø9.1 and E969
T63.334A	989.5 and E98Ø.9
T63.334S	9Ø9.1 and E989
T63.391A	989.5 and E9Ø5.1
T63.391S	9Ø9.1 and E929.2
T63.392A	989.5 and E95Ø.9
T63.392S	9Ø9.1 and E959
T63.393A	989.5 and E962.1
T63.393S	9Ø9.1 and E969
T63.394A	989.5 and E98Ø.9
T63.394S	9Ø9.1 and E989
T63.411A	989.5 and E9Ø5.4
T63.411S	9Ø9.1 and E929.2
T63.412A	989.5 and E95Ø.9
T63.412S	9Ø9.1 and E959
T63.413A	989.5 and E962.1
T63.413S	9Ø9.1 and E969
T63.414A	989.5 and E98Ø.9
T63.414S	9Ø9.1 and E989
T63.421A	989.5 and E9Ø5.5
T63.421S	9Ø9.1 and E929.2
T63.422A	989.5 and E95Ø.9
T63.422S	9Ø9.1 and E959
T63.423A	989.5 and E962.1
T63.423S	9Ø9.1 and E969
T63.424A	989.5 and E98Ø.9
T63.424S	9Ø9.1 and E989
T63.431A	989.5 and E9Ø5.5
T63.431S	9Ø9.1 and E929.2
T63.432A	989.5 and E95Ø.9
T63.432S	9Ø9.1 and E959
T63.433A	989.5 and E962.1
T63.433S	9Ø9.1 and E969
T63.434A	989.5 and E98Ø.9
T63.434S	9Ø9.1 and E989
T63.441A	989.5 and E9Ø5.3
T63.441S	9Ø9.1 and E929.2
T63.442A	989.5 and E95Ø.9
T63.442S	9Ø9.1 and E959
T63.443A	989.5 and E962.1
T63.443S	9Ø9.1 and E969
T63.444A	989.5 and E98Ø.9
T63.444S	9Ø9.1 and E989
T63.451A	989.5 and E9Ø5.3
T63.451S	9Ø9.1 and E929.2
T63.452A	989.5 and E95Ø.9
T63.452S	9Ø9.1 and E959
T63.453A	989.5 and E962.1
T63.453S	9Ø9.1 and E969
T63.454A	989.5 and E98Ø.9
T63.454S	9Ø9.1 and E989
T63.461A	989.5 and E9Ø5.3
T63.461S	9Ø9.1 and E929.2
T63.462A	989.5 and E95Ø.9
T63.462S	9Ø9.1 and E959
T63.463A	989.5 and E962.1
T63.463S	9Ø9.1 and E969
T63.464A	989.5 and E98Ø.9
T63.464S	9Ø9.1 and E989
T63.481A	989.5 and E9Ø5.5
T63.481S	9Ø9.1 and E929.2
T63.482A	989.5 and E95Ø.9
T63.482S	9Ø9.1 and E959
T63.483A	989.5 and E962.1
T63.483S	9Ø9.1 and E969
T63.484A	989.5 and E98Ø.9
T63.484S	9Ø9.1 and E989
T63.511A	989.5 and E9Ø5.6
T63.511S	9Ø9.1 and E929.2
T63.512A	989.5 and E95Ø.9
T63.512S	9Ø9.1 and E959
T63.513A	989.5 and E962.1
T63.513S	9Ø9.1 and E969
T63.514A	989.5 and E98Ø.9
T63.514S	9Ø9.1 and E989
T63.591A	989.5 and E9Ø5.6
T63.591S	9Ø9.1 and E929.2
T63.592A	989.5 and E95Ø.9
T63.592S	9Ø9.1 and E959
T63.593A	989.5 and E962.1
T63.593S	9Ø9.1 and E969
T63.594A	989.5 and E98Ø.9
T63.594S	9Ø9.1 and E989
T63.611A	989.5 and E9Ø5.6
T63.611S	9Ø9.1 and E929.2
T63.612A	989.5 and E95Ø.9
T63.612S	9Ø9.1 and E959
T63.613A	989.5 and E962.1
T63.613S	9Ø9.1 and E969
T63.614A	989.5 and E98Ø.9
T63.614S	9Ø9.1 and E989
T63.621A	989.5 and E9Ø5.6
T63.621S	9Ø9.1 and E929.2
T63.622A	989.5 and E95Ø.9
T63.622S	9Ø9.1 and E959
T63.623A	989.5 and E962.1
T63.623S	9Ø9.1 and E969
T63.624A	989.5 and E98Ø.9
T63.624S	9Ø9.1 and E989
T63.631A	989.5 and E9Ø5.6
T63.631S	9Ø9.1 and E929.2
T63.632A	989.5 and E95Ø.9
T63.632S	9Ø9.1 and E959
T63.633A	989.5 and E962.1
T63.633S	9Ø9.1 and E969
T63.634A	989.5 and E98Ø.9
T63.634S	9Ø9.1 and E989
T63.691A	989.5 and E9Ø5.6
T63.691S	9Ø9.1 and E929.2
T63.692A	989.5 and E95Ø.9
T63.692S	9Ø9.1 and E959
T63.693A	989.5 and E962.1
T63.693S	9Ø9.1 and E969
T63.694A	989.5 and E98Ø.9
T63.694S	9Ø9.1 and E989
T63.711A	989.5 and E9Ø5.6
T63.711S	9Ø9.1 and E929.2
T63.712A	989.5 and E95Ø.9
T63.712S	9Ø9.1 and E959
T63.713A	989.5 and E962.1
T63.713S	9Ø9.1 and E969
T63.714A	989.5 and E98Ø.9
T63.714S	9Ø9.1 and E989
T63.791A	989.5 and E9Ø5.6
T63.791S	9Ø9.1 and E929.2
T63.792A	989.5 and E95Ø.9
T63.792S	9Ø9.1 and E959
T63.793A	989.5 and E962.1
T63.793S	9Ø9.1 and E969
T63.794A	989.5 and E98Ø.9
T63.794S	9Ø9.1 and E989
T63.811A	989.5 and E9Ø5.6
T63.811S	9Ø9.1 and E929.2
T63.812A	989.5 and E95Ø.9
T63.812S	9Ø9.1 and E959
T63.813A	989.5 and E962.1
T63.813S	9Ø9.1 and E969
T63.814A	989.5 and E98Ø.9
T63.814S	9Ø9.1 and E989
T63.821A	989.5 and E9Ø5.6
T63.821S	9Ø9.1 and E929.2
T63.822A	989.5 and E95Ø.9
T63.822S	9Ø9.1 and E959
T63.823A	989.5 and E962.1
T63.823S	9Ø9.1 and E969
T63.824A	989.5 and E98Ø.9
T63.824S	9Ø9.1 and E989
T63.831A	989.5 and E9Ø5.6
T63.831S	9Ø9.1 and E929.2
T63.832A	989.5 and E95Ø.9
T63.832S	9Ø9.1 and E959
T63.833A	989.5 and E962.1
T63.833S	9Ø9.1 and E969
T63.834A	989.5 and E98Ø.9
T63.834S	9Ø9.1 and E989
T63.891A	989.5 and E9Ø5.6
T63.891S	9Ø9.1 and E929.2
T63.892A	989.5 and E95Ø.9
T63.892S	9Ø9.1 and E959
T63.893A	989.5 and E962.1
T63.893S	9Ø9.1 and E969
T63.894A	989.5 and E98Ø.9
T63.894S	9Ø9.1 and E989
T63.91XA	989.5 and E9Ø5.6
T63.91XS	9Ø9.1 and E929.2
T63.92XA	989.5 and E95Ø.9
T63.92XS	9Ø9.1 and E959
T63.93XA	989.5 and E962.1
T63.93XS	9Ø9.1 and E969
T63.94XA	989.5 and E98Ø.9
T63.94XS	9Ø9.1 and E989
T64.Ø1XA	989.7 and E866.8
T64.Ø1XS	9Ø9.1 and E929.2
T64.Ø2XA	989.7 and E95Ø.9
T64.Ø2XS	9Ø9.1 and E959
T64.Ø3XA	989.7 and E962.1
T64.Ø3XS	9Ø9.1 and E969
T64.Ø4XA	989.7 and E98Ø.9
T64.Ø4XS	9Ø9.1 and E989
T64.81XA	989.7 and E866.8
T64.81XS	9Ø9.1 and E929.2
T64.82XA	989.7 and E95Ø.9
T64.82XS	9Ø9.1 and E959
T64.83XA	989.7 and E962.1
T64.83XS	9Ø9.1 and E969
T64.84XA	989.7 and E98Ø.9
T64.84XS	9Ø9.1 and E989
T65.ØX1A	989.Ø and E866.8
T65.ØX1S	9Ø9.1 and E929.2
T65.ØX2A	989.Ø and E95Ø.9
T65.ØX2S	9Ø9.1 and E959
T65.ØX3A	989.Ø and E962.1

T65.ØX3S 9Ø9.1 and E969
T65.ØX4A 989.Ø and E98Ø.9
T65.ØX4S 9Ø9.1 and E989
T65.1X1A 989.1 and E866.8
T65.1X1S 9Ø9.1 and E929.2
T65.1X2A 989.1 and E95Ø.9
T65.1X2S 9Ø9.1 and E959
T65.1X3A 989.1 and E962.1
T65.1X3S 9Ø9.1 and E969
T65.1X4A 989.1 and E98Ø.9
T65.1X4S 9Ø9.1 and E989
T65.211A 989.84 and E866.8
T65.211S 9Ø9.1 and E929.2
T65.212A 989.84 and E95Ø.9
T65.212S 9Ø9.1 and E959
T65.213A 989.84 and E962.1
T65.213S 9Ø9.1 and E969
T65.214A 989.84 and E98Ø.9
T65.214S 9Ø9.1 and E989
T65.221A 989.84 and E866.8
T65.221S 9Ø9.1 and E929.2
T65.222A 989.84 and E95Ø.9
T65.222S 9Ø9.1 and E959
T65.223A 989.84 and E962.1
T65.223S 9Ø9.1 and E969
T65.224A 989.84 and E98Ø.9
T65.224S 9Ø9.1 and E989
T65.291A 989.84 and E866.8
T65.291S 9Ø9.1 and E929.2
T65.292A 989.84 and E95Ø.9
T65.292S 9Ø9.1 and E959
T65.293A 989.84 and E962.1
T65.293S 9Ø9.1 and E969
T65.294A 989.84 and E98Ø.9
T65.294S 9Ø9.1 and E989
T65.3X1A 982.Ø and E866.8
T65.3X1S 9Ø9.1 and E929.2
T65.3X2A 982.Ø and E95Ø.9
T65.3X2S 9Ø9.1 and E959
T65.3X3A 982.Ø and E962.1
T65.3X3S 9Ø9.1 and E969
T65.3X4A 982.Ø and E98Ø.9
T65.3X4S 9Ø9.1 and E989
T65.4X1A 982.2 and E866.8
T65.4X1S 9Ø9.1 and E929.2
T65.4X2A 982.2 and E95Ø.9
T65.4X2S 9Ø9.1 and E959
T65.4X3A 982.2 and E962.1
T65.4X3S 9Ø9.1 and E969
T65.4X4A 982.2 and E98Ø.9
T65.4X4S 9Ø9.1 and E989
T65.5X1A 989.89 and E864.1
T65.5X1S 9Ø9.1 and E929.2
T65.5X2A 989.89 and E95Ø.9
T65.5X2S 9Ø9.1 and E959
T65.5X3A 989.89 and E962.1
T65.5X3S 9Ø9.1 and E969
T65.5X4A 989.89 and E98Ø.9
T65.5X4S 9Ø9.1 and E989
T65.6X1A 989.89 and E861.6
T65.6X1S 9Ø9.1 and E929.2
T65.6X2A 989.89 and E95Ø.9
T65.6X2S 9Ø9.1 and E959
T65.6X3A 989.89 and E962.1
T65.6X3S 9Ø9.1 and E969
T65.6X4A 989.89 and E98Ø.9
T65.6X4S 9Ø9.1 and E989
T65.811A 989.82 and E866.8
T65.811S 9Ø9.1 and E929.2
T65.812A 989.82 and E95Ø.9
T65.812S 9Ø9.1 and E959
T65.813A 989.82 and E962.1
T65.813S 9Ø9.1 and E969
T65.814A 989.82 and E98Ø.9
T65.814S 9Ø9.1 and E989
T65.821A 989.89 and E928.6
T65.821S 9Ø9.1 and E929.2
T65.822A 989.89 and E95Ø.9
T65.822S 9Ø9.1 and E959
T65.823A 989.89 and E962.1
T65.823S 9Ø9.1 and E969
T65.824A 989.89 and E928.6
T65.824S 9Ø9.1 and E989
T65.831A 989.89 and E866.8
T65.831S 9Ø9.1 and E929.2
T65.832A 989.89 and E95Ø.9
T65.832S 9Ø9.1 and E959
T65.833A 989.89 and E962.1
T65.833S 9Ø9.1 and E969
T65.834A 989.89 and E98Ø.9
T65.834S 9Ø9.1 and E989
T65.891A 989.89 and E866.8
T65.891S 9Ø9.1 and E929.2
T65.892A 989.89 and E95Ø.9
T65.892S 9Ø9.1 and E959
T65.893A 989.89 and E962.1
T65.893S 9Ø9.1 and E969
T65.894A 989.89 and E98Ø.9
T65.894S 9Ø9.1 and E989
T65.91XA 989.9 and E866.8
T65.91XS 9Ø9.1 and E929.2
T65.92XA 989.9 and E95Ø.9
T65.92XS 9Ø9.1 and E959
T65.93XA 989.9 and E962.9
T65.93XS 9Ø9.1 and E969
T65.94XA 989.9 and E98Ø.9
T65.94XS 9Ø9.1 and E989
T71.111A 994.7 and E913.Ø
T71.112A 994.7 and E953.8
T71.113A 994.7 and E963
T71.114A 994.7 and E983.8
T71.121A 994.7 and E913.1
T71.122A 994.7 and E953.1
T71.123A 994.7 and E963
T71.124A 994.7 and E983.1
T71.131A 994.7 and E913.Ø
T71.132A 994.7 and E953.8
T71.133A 994.7 and E963
T71.134A 994.7 and E983.8
T71.141A 994.7 and E913.Ø
T71.143A 994.7 and E963
T71.144A 994.7 and E983.8
T71.151A 994.7 and E913.8
T71.152A 994.7 and E953.1
T71.153A 994.7 and E963
T71.154A 994.7 and E983.8
T71.161A 994.7 and E913.8
T71.161S 9Ø9.4 and E929.8
T71.162A 994.7 and E953.Ø
T71.162S 9Ø9.4 and E959
T71.163A 994.7 and E963
T71.163S 9Ø9.4 and E969
T71.164A 994.7 and E983.Ø
T71.164S 9Ø9.4 and E989
T71.191A 994.7 and E913.8
T71.192A 994.7 and E953.8
T71.193A 994.7 and E963
T71.194A 994.7 and E983.8
T71.2ØXA 994.7 and E913.2
T71.21XA 994.7 and E913.3
T71.221A 994.7 and E913.2
T71.222A 994.7 and E953.8
T71.223A 994.7 and E963
T71.224A 994.7 and E983.8
T71.231A 994.7 and E913.2
T71.232A 994.7 and E953.8
T71.233A 994.7 and E963
T71.234A 994.7 and E983.8
T71.29XA 994.7 and E913.2
T71.9XXA 994.7 and E913.9
T73.ØXXA 994.2 and E9Ø4.1
T73.1XXA 994.3 and E9Ø4.2
T73.2XXA 994.4 and E9Ø4.3
T73.3XXA 994.5 and E927.2
T73.8XXA 994.9 and E9Ø4.9
T73.9XXA 994.9 and E9Ø4.9
T74.Ø1XA 995.84 and E9Ø4.Ø
T74.Ø2XA 995.52 and E9Ø4.Ø
T75.3XXA 994.6 and E9Ø3
T86.3Ø 996.83 and 996.84
T86.31 996.83 and 996.84
T86.32 996.83 and 996.84
T86.33 996.83 and 996.84
T86.39 996.83 and 996.84
Z48.21 V42.1 and V58.44
Z48.22 V42.Ø and V58.44
Z48.23 V42.7 and V58.44
Z48.24 V42.6 and V58.44
Z48.28Ø V42.1 and V42.6 and V58.44
Z48.288 V42.9 and V58.44
Z48.29Ø V42.81 and V58.44
Z48.298 V42.89 and V58.44
Z94.3 V42.1 and V42.6

Appendix B. Abbreviations

A&D	ADMISSION AND DISCHARGE
AA	ABDOMINAL AORTA, AMINO ACID
AAA	ABDOMINAL AORTIC ANEURYSM(ECTOMY), ACUTE ANXIETY ATTACK
AB	ABDO(MEN)(MINAL), ABORT(ER)(ION), ANTIBODY
AB-	AB NEGATIVE BLOOD TYPE
AB+	AB POSITIVE BLOOD TYPE
ABD	ABDO(MEN)(MINAL)(MINO)
ABDUC(T)	ABDUCENT, ABDUCTION, ABDUCTOR
ABER	ABERRANT
ABG	AORTOILLIAC BYPASS GRAFT, ARTERIAL BLOOD GAS(ES)
ABL(AT)	ABLAT(ION)(IVE)
ABMT	AUTOLOGOUS BONE MARROW TRANSPLANTATION
ABN	ABNORMAL(ITY)(ITIES), ADVANCE BENEFICIARY NOTICE
ABNORM	ABNORMAL(ITY)(ITIES)
ABRAS	ABRASION
ABS	ABUSE
ABSC	ABSCESS
ABSN(T)	ABSENT
ABSORB	ABSORBABLE
ABSORP	ABSORPTION, ABSORPTIVE
ABUT	ABUTMENT
ABV	ARTHROPOD-BORNE VIRUS
ABVE	ABOVE
ABX	ANTIBIOTIC(S)
AC	ACROMIOCLAVICULAR, ACUTE
ACC	ACCIDENT(ALLY)(AL)(S)
ACCEL	ACCELERATOR
ACCESS	ACCESSION, ACCESSORY(IES)
ACCOM	ACCOMMODATION
ACEI	ANGIOTENSIN-CONVERTING-ENZYME INHIBITORS
ACETAB	ACETAB(ULAR)(UM)
ACFT	AIRCRAFT
ACH(LL)	ADRENAL CORTICAL HORMONE, ACHILLES
ACL	ANTERIOR CRUCIATE LIGAMENT
ACOUS	ACOUSTIC
ACQ	ACQUIRED
ACQN	ACQUISITION
ACRM(CL)	ACROMIAL, ACROMIOCLAVICULAR
ACROMNECT	ACROMIONECTOMY
ACROMPLSTY	ACROMIOPLASTY
ACRYLC	ACRYLIC
ACSS	ACCESS
ACT	ACTING
ACTAT	ACETATE
ACTB	ACETABUL(UM)(I)
ACTV	ACTIVE, ACTIVITY(IES)
AD	ADNEXA, ADRENAL, ANTIDEPRESSANT
ADAPT	ADAPT(ATION)(ER)(OR)
ADD	ADD(ED)(ING)(ITION)(ITIONAL)(S), ATTENTION DEFICIT DISORDER
ADDUC(T)	ADDUCTION, ADDUCTOR
ADEM	ACUTE DISSEMINATED ENCEPHALITIS
ADHES	ADHESION(S), ADHESIVE
ADJ	ADJACENT, ADJUST(ABLE)(MENT)
ADJST(BL)	ADJUST(ABLE)(ED)
ADLT	ADULT
ADM	ADMISSION
ADM(I)N	ADMINI(STER)(STERED)(STRATED) (STRATION) (STRATIVE)
ADMIS	ADMISSION
ADOLES	ADOLESCENT
ADPT	ADAPT(ATION)
ADRENALECT	ADRENALECTOMY
ADSORPT	ADSORPTION
ADV	ADVANCE(MENT)
ADVRS	ADVERSE
AER(S)	AEROBIC, AEROSOL
AF	ANTIFUNGAL
AFF(CT)	AFFECT(ING)(IVE)
AFTR	AFTER
AG	ARTERIAL GRAFT
AGCY	AGENCY(IES)
AGNST	AGAINST
AGNT, AGT	AGENT(S)
AGRAN	AGRANULOCYTOSIS
AGRIC	AGRICULTUR(E)(AL)
AGT	AGENT
AIDS	ACQUIRED IMMUNODEFICIENCY SYNDROME
AIF	ANTI-INFLAMMATORY
AIRCRFT	AIRCRAFT
AIRPLNE	AIRPLANE
AK	ABOVE KNEE
ALB	ALBINISM
ALC	ALCOHOL(IC)(ISM)
ALDOST	ALDOSTERONISM
ALGN	ALIGN(MENT)
ALGT	ALIGHTING
A-LINE	ARTERIAL CATHETER
ALK	ALKAL(IS)(OSIS)
ALLOGFT	ALLOGRAFT
ALLOPLAS	ALLOPLASTIC
ALLOW	ALLOWANCE
ALLRG	ALLER(GEN)(GENIC)(GIC)(Y)
ALS	ADVANCED LIFE SUPPORT
ALT(ER)	ALTER(ATION)(ED), ALTERNAT(E)(IVE)
ALV(EOL)	ALVEO(LAR)(LITIS)(LUS)
ALZ	ALZHEIMER'S (DISEASE)
AMB	AMBULANCE, AMBULATORY
AMINODER	AMINODERIVATIVES
AMNIO	AMNIOCENTESIS, AMNIO(N)(TIC)
AMP	AMPUTAT(E)(ED)(ION), AMPUTEE, AMPULA
AMPCLLN	AMPICILLIN
AMPHET	AMPHETAMINE
AMT	AMOUNT
ANAER	ANAEROBE
ANALG(ES)	ANALGES(IA)(IC)(ICS)
ANALY	ANALYS(ES)(IS), ANALYZE®
ANAPHYLACT	ANAPHYLACTIC
ANAST(OM)	ANASTOMOSIS
ANAT	ANATOMIC(AL)
ANCHR	ANCHORING
ANCILLRY	ANCILLARY
ANDR	ANDROGEN(IC)(S)
ANEM	ANEMIA(S), ANEMIC
ANES	ANESTHESIA, ANESTHETIC(S)
ANEUR	ANEURYSM(S)
ANG	ANGINA, ANGLE
ANGIO	ANGIO(GRAM)(GRAPHY)(SCOPE) (SCOPY)
ANGPLSTY	ANGIOPLASTY
ANK	ANKLE
ANML	ANIMAL
ANOM(AL)	ANOMALY(IES)
ANORECTVAGPLSTY	ANORECTOVAGINOPLASTY
ANRYSM	ANEURYSM(S)
ANSCPY	ANOSCOPY

ANT	ANTERIOR
ANTAG	ANTAGONISTS
ANTCP(Y)	ANTICIPATE, ANTICIPATORY
ANTIBIO	ANTIBIOTIC(S)
ANTICOAG	ANTICOAGULANT(S)
ANTICONVUL	ANTICONVULSANT(S)
ANTIDIAB	ANTIDIABETIC
ANTIDIARR	ANTIDIARRHEAL
ANTIDIUR	ANTIDIURETIC
ANTIDPRSNT	ANTIDEPRESSANT(S)
ANTIEMET	ANTIEMETIC(S)
ANTIEPI	ANTIEPILEPTIC
ANTIER	ANTIESTROGENS
ANTIFUNG	ANTIFUNGAL
ANTIG	ANTIGEN(IC)(S)
ANTIGN	ANTIGONADOTROPHINS
ANTIHTN	ANTIHYPERTENSIVE
ANTI-INFEC	ANTI-INFECTIVE(S)
ANTIPARASIT	ANTIPARASITICS
ANTIPRKNSN	ANTIPARKINSONISM
ANTIPSYCH(OT)	ANTIPSYCHOTIC(S)
ANTIPYRET	ANTIPYRETIC(S)
ANTIREFLX	ANTIREFLUX
ANTIRH(EUM)	ANTIRHEUMATIC
ANTISEP	ANTISEPTIC
ANTITHYMCYT	ANTITHYMOCYTE
ANTPRT(M)	ANTEPARTUM
ANTR	ANTR(AL)(UM)
ANTROST	ANTROSTOMY
ANTROT	ANTROTOMY
ANX	ANXIETY
AO(RTC)	AORTA, AORTIC
AORTGRPH	AORTOGRAPHY
AP	ANTEPARTUM, ANTEROPOSTERIOR
APC/C	ANTEPARTUM CONDITION/ COMPLICATION
APEXIFICAT	APEXIFICATION
APGAR	APPEARANCE PULSE GRIMACE ACTIVITY AND RESPIRATION
APHAK	APHAKIA
APHAS	APHASIA
APHERES	APHERESIS
APK	ANTIPARKINSONISM
APNECT	APPENDECTOMY
APOPHYSL	APOPHYSEAL
APPARAT	APPARATUS
APPDX	APPENDIX
APPEAR	APPEARANCE
APPL(IC)	APPLIANCE, APPLICA(BLE)(TION)(TOR), APPLIED
APPNDICULR	APPENDICULAR
APPR, APPRCH	APPROACH
APPROP	APPROPRIATE(LY)(NESS)
APPROX	APPROXIMATELY
APPRVD	APPROVED
APPT	APPOINTMENT
AQ	AQUEOUS
ARISE	ARISING
ARNG(MT)	ARRANGE(MENT)
AROSL	AEROSOL
ARRHY(TH)	ARRHYTHMIA(S), ARRHYTHMOGENIC
ART(IF)(FICL)	ARTER(IAL)(IES)(Y), ARTIFICIAL
ARTC(LR)	ARTICULAR, ARTICULATING
ARTENOIDECT	ARTENOIDECTOMY
ARTERGM	ARTERIOGRAM(S)
ARTHPLSTY	ARTHROPLASTY
ARTHRDSIS	ARTHRODESIS
ARTHRIT	ARTHRITIS
ARTHROCEN	ARTHROCENTESIS
ARTHROGM	ARTHROGRAM
ARTHROGRPH	ARTHROGRAPHY
ARTHROP	ARTHROPATHY
ARTHROT	ARTHROTOMY
ARTHSCPY	ARTHROSCOP(Y)(ICALLY)
ARTIC(LR)	ARTICULAR, ARTICULAT(E)(ED)(ING)(TION)
ARTRGRPH	ARTERIOGRAPHY
ARTRIOSCLROT	ARTERIOSCLEROTIC
ARWAY	AIRWAY
AS	ATHEROSCLERO(SIS)(TIC)
ASA	AMERICAN SOCIETY OF ANESTHESIOLOGISTS
ASBEST	ASBESTOS
ASC	ASCENDING
ASEP	ASEPTIC
ASLT	ASSAULT
ASP(IR)	ASPIRAT(E)(ION)(IONAL)
ASPHRCITY	ASPHERICITY
ASPHYX	ASPHYXIATION
ASSESS	ASSESSMENT
ASSIST	ASSISTING
ASSLT	ASSAULT
ASSMBL	ASSEMBLY
ASSOC	ASSOCIATED, ASSOCIATION
ASST(D)	ASSIST(ANT)(ED)
ASTH(MATC)	ASTHMA(TICUS)
ASTIG(MA)	ASTIGMATISM
ASYM(PT)	ASYMMETRIC(AL), ASYMPTOMATIC
AT	ATRI(AL)(UM)
ATD	ATTEND
ATHERECT	ATHERECTOMY
ATHEROSCLER	ATHEROSCLEROSIS
ATMPT	ATTEMPT(ED)
ATR	ATRI(AL)(UM)
ATROPH	ATROPH(IC)(Y)
ATROPIN	ATROPINE
ATTCH	ATTACH(ED)(MENT)(MENTS)
ATTEMP	ATTEMPTED
ATTEND	ATTEND(ANCE)(ED)
ATTN	ATTENTION
ATV	ALL-TERRAIN VEHICLE
ATYP	ATYPICAL
AUD(ITRY)	AUDI(OMETRY)(TORY)
AUG	AUGMENT(ATION)(ATIVE)
AUTHNTC	AUTHENTIC
AUTO	AUTO(LOGOUS)(MATED)(MATIC)(MATION)
AUTOCLVBL	AUTOCLAVABLE
AUTOGEN	AUTOGENOUS
AUTOGFT	AUTOGRAFT(S)
AUTONOM	AUTONOMIC
AV	AORTIC VALVE, ARTERIOVENOUS
AVL, AVUL	AVULSION
AW	ABDOMINAL WALL, AIRWAY
AX	AXILLA(RY)
BA	BARIUM, BIOACTIVE, BRACHIAL ARTERY
BACT	BACTERIA(L)
BAL	BALANCE(D)
BALLN	BALLOON
BALLST	BALLAST
BANDGE	BANDAGE
BARB	BARBITUATE
BART	BARTON'S
BARTH	BARTHOLIN'S
BASL	BASILAR
BATT	BATTERY(IES)
BATTER	BATTERING
BCUG	BILATERAL CYSTOURETHROGRAM
BD	BILE DUCT, BOARD
BDY	BODY
BEAR	BEARING
BEDSID	BEDSIDE
BEHAV	BEHAVIOR(AL)
BELW	BELOW

BEN	BENIGN
BENDR	BENDER
BENZ	BENZATHINE
BENZDIAZ	BENZODIAZEPINE
BERKLY	BERKELEY
BETA-ADRN	BETA-ADRENORECEPTOR
BETR	BETTER
BETWN	BETWEEN
BFO	BLOOD-FORMING ORGAN(S)
BGS	BONE GROWTH STIMULATOR
BHT	BUCKET-HANDLE TEAR
BHV	BEHAVIOR
BICARB	BICARBONATE
BICNDYL	BICONDYLAR
BICORON	BICORONAL
BICPS	BICEPS
BICUSP	BICUSPID
BIF(URCAT)(N)	BIFURCAT(ED)(ION)
BIFOCL	BIFOCAL
BIFRNT	BIFRONTAL
BIL	BILATERAL
BILAMIN	BILAMINATE
BILI	BILIARY, BILIRUBIN
BIMAL	BIMALLEOLAR
BIO(LOG)	BIOLOG(IC)(ICAL)
BIPLR	BIPOLAR
BIVALV	BIVALVING
BK	BACK, BELOW KNEE
BL	BETA-LACTAM
BLAD	BLADDER
BLAZR	BLAZER
BLD	BLOOD, BUILD
BLDG	BUILDING
BLEED	BLEEDING
BLEPH(PLSTY)	BLEPHAROPLASTY
BLEPHAROPT	BLEPHAROPTOSIS
BLISTR	BLISTER(S)
BLK	BLOCK(ING)
BLND	BLIND(NESS)
BLNT	BLUNT
BLS	BASIC LIFE SUPPORT
BLST(R)	BLAST, BLISTER
BLZZ	BLIZZARD
BMR	BASAL METABOLIC RATE
BN(S)	BONE(S)
BNT	BENT
BOARD	BOARDING
BOND	BONDED
BORD	BORDER
BORN	BORNE
BP	BIPOLAR, BLOOD PRESSURE, BRACHIAL PLEXUS, BYPASS
BR	BRANCH, BY REPORT
BRACH	BRACHIAL
BRACHCEPH	BRACHIOCEPHALIC
BREAK	BREAKING
BRF	BRIEF
BRKDWN	BREAKDOWN
BRN	BURN, BRAIN
BRNCH	BRANCH(ES)
BRNCHSCPY	BRONCHOSCOPY
BRNSTM	BRAINSTEM
BRON(CH)	BRONCH(IAL)(US)
BRONCHIECT	BRONCHIECT(ASIS)(OMY)
BRONCHIOL	BRONCHIOLITIS
BRONCHIT	BRONCHITIS
BRONCHOGRPH	BRONCHOGRAPHY
BRSH	BRUSH
BRST	BREAST
BRTH	BIRTH, BREATH
BSA	BODY SURFACE AREA
BSKT	BASKET
BT	BOAT
BTTM	BOTTOM
BTWN	BETWEEN
BUCC	BUCCAL
BULBR	BULBAR
BUN	BUNNION
BURS(IT)	BURS(AE)(ITIS)
BUTYROPHEN	BUTYROPHENONE
BV	BLOOD VESSEL(S)
BWT	BIRTHWEIGHT
BX	BIOPSY(IES)
BYPS	BYPASS
C	CELL
C/S	C-SECTION
C1-C7	CERVICAL VERTEBRA 1 THROUGH 7
C9	GLOSSOPHARYNGEAL NERVE
CA	CANCER, CARCINOMA, CELIAC ARTERY, CORONARY ARTERY
CABG	CORONARY ARTERY BYPASS GRAFT
CADVR	CADAVER
CAG	CORONARY ARTERY GRAFT
CAI	CARBONIC-ANHYDRASE INHIBITORS
CAL	CALCIUM, CALORIES
CALCAN	CALCANE(AL)(US)
CALCIF	CALCIFICATION
CALCM	CALCIUM
CALCU	CALCUL(I)(US)
CALIBRTD	CALIBRATED
CALIPR	CALIPER
CANB	CANNABIS
CANCL	CANCELED
CANCR	CANCER
CANNSTR	CANNISTER
CANNUL(AT)	CANNULATION
CANTHORR	CANTHORRHAPHY
CAP	CAPITATE, CAPSULE
CAPABL	CAPABLE
CAPACTY	CAPACITY
CAPSLDSIS	CAPSULODESIS
CAPSULOT	CAPSULOTOMY
CAPSUR	CAPSURE
CARB(S)	CARBOHYDRATE(S), CARBON
CARBCL	CARBUNCLE
CARBMAZ	CARBAMAZEPINE
CARBMTE	CARBAMATE
CARD	CARDIAC
CARDIECT	CARDIECTOMY
CARDIOVERT	CARDIOVERTER
CARDPULM	CARDIOPULMONARY
CARDRESP	CARDIORESPIRATORY
CARDTHOR	CARDIOTHORACIC
CARDVRT	CARDIOVERTER
CARDVSC	CARDIOVASCULAR
CARR	CARRIER
CART	CARTILAGE
CARTD	CAROTID
CARTLG	CARTILAGE(NOUS)
CASTR	CASTER
CAT	CATEGORY, COMPUTERIZED AXIAL TOMOGRAPHY
CATACLYS	CATACLYSMIC
CATAR	CATARACT
CATGY	CATEGORY
CATH	CATHETER(S)(IZATION)
CATHRT	CATHARTICS
CAUD	CAUDAL
CAUS	CAUS(E)(ED)(ES)(ING)
CAUT	CAUTER(IZATION)(Y)
CAV	CAVITY
CB	CHILDBIRTH
CCA	COMMON CAROTID ARTERY
CD	CESAREAN DELIVERY

CECOST	CECOSTOMY
CEL	CELIAC
CELL(R)	CELLULAR(ITY)
CENT	CENTRAL
CEPH	CEPHALIC
CERAM	CERAMIC
CERBLLR	CEREBELLAR
CERBRL	CEREBRAL
CERBRVSC	CEREBROVASCULAR
CERC	CERCLAGE
CERT	CERTIFICATION, CERTIFIED
CERV	CERV(ICAL)(IX)
CERVICECT	CERVICECTOMY
CESS	CESSATION
CF	CYSTIC FIBROSIS
CFA	COMMON FEMORAL ARTERY
CHAMB	CHAMBER
CHAR	CHARACTER(ISTICS)
CHEILECT	CHEILECTOMY
CHEL	CHELAT(ABLE)(ION)
CHEM	CHEMICAL, CHEMISTRY
CHEMO	CHEMOTHERAP(Y)(EUTIC)
CHF	CONGESTIVE HEART FAILURE
CHG	CHANGE
CHKR	CHECKER
CHL(ORID)	CHLORIDE
CHLAMYD	CHLAMYDIA
CHLD	CHILD(REN)(HOOD)
CHMBR	CHAMBER
CHOL(EST)	CHOLESTEROL
CHOL(E)CYST(GRPH)(OST)(TOT)	CHOLECYST(ECTOMY)(ITIS)(OGRAPHY)(OSTOMY)(OTOMY)
CHOLEDOCH(OST)(OT)	CHOLEDOCHO(STOMY)(TOMY)
CHONDRCALC	CHONDROCALCINOSIS
CHONDRCYT	CHONDROCYTE
CHONDROCALCINOS	CHONDROCALCINOSIS
CHORD	CHORDAE, CHOROID(AL)
CHORIRET	CHORIORETINAL
CHR(O)(N)	CHRONIC
CHRG	CHARGE
CHROM	CHROMOSOM(AL)(E)
CHROMATGRPH	CHROMATOGRAPHY
CHROMOSM	CHROMOSOM(E)(AL)
CHST	CHEST
CIA	COMMON ILIAC ARTERY
CILRY	CILIARY
CINERADIGRPH	CINERADIOGRAPHY
CIRC	CIRCULA(R)(TING)(TION)(TORY), CIRCUMCISION, CIRCUMFEREN(CE)(TIAL), CIRCLE
CIRR	CIRRHOSIS
CIS-DDP	CISPLATIN
CIV	CIVILIAN
CK	CREATINE KINASE
CK	CHECK
CKD	CHRONIC KIDNEY DISEASE
CL	CLOS(ED)(URE)
CLASS	CLASSIFIED
CLAUD(ICAT)	CLAUDICATION
CLAV	CLAVIC(LE)(ULAR)
CLCT	COLLECT(ED)(ION)(IONS)
CLFT	CLEFT
CLIN	CLINICAL
CLNR	CLEANER
CLO(S)	CLOS(E)(ED)(ING)(URE)
CLOST	CLOSTRIDIUM
CLOT	CLOTTING
CLR	CLEAR(ED)
CLV	CLAVIC(LE)(ULAR)
CM	CENTIMETER
CMC	CARPOMETACARPAL
CMINTD, CMMINT	COMMINUTED
CMN	COMMON
CMNCT	COMMUNICAT(E)(ING)(IVE)(ION)(IONS)
CMNUT	COMMINUTED
CMPCT	COMPACT
CMPL	COMPLET(E)(ED)(ELY)(ION), COMPLICAT(ED)(ION)
CMPLX	COMPLEX(ITY)
CMPND	COMPOUND
CMPNT	COMPONENT
CMPRTMT	COMPARTMENT(S)
CMPT	COMPUTE(D)(R)
CMRCL	COMMERCIAL
CMTY	COMMUNITY
CMV	CYTOMEGALOVIR(AL)(US)
CN	CERVICAL PLEXUS
CN 4	TROCHLEAR NERVE
CN 5	TRIGEMINAL NERVE
CN 6	ABDUCENS NERVE
CN 7	FACIAL NERVE
CN 9	GLOSSOPHARYNGEAL NERVE
CN 10	VAGUS NERVE
CN 11	ACCESSORY NERVE
CN 12	HYPOGLOSSAL NERVE
CNCT(R)(V)	CONNECT(OR)(IVE)
CNDYL	CONDYL(AR)(E)
CNJCT	CONJUNCTIV(A)(ITIS)
CNS	CENTRAL NERVOUS SYSTEM
CNSC	CONSCIOUS(NESS)
CNSL	COUNSEL(ING)
CNSLT	CONSULT(ATION)(ATIVE)(ING)
CNSTR	CONSTRUCT
CNT	COUNT
CNTAM	CONTAMINANT, CONTAMINATED
CNTC	CONTACT
CNTN	CONTENT(S)
CNTRL	CENTRAL, CONTROL(LED)(LING)
CNTRL NERV SYS	CENTRAL NERVOUS SYSTEM
CNTRLAT	CONTRALATERAL
CNTRLY	CENTRALLY
CNTRST	CONTRAST
CNTUS	CONTUSION
CNVLS	CONVULS(ION)(IVE)
CNVRT	CONVER(SION)(T)
CO	CARBON MONOXIDE
COAD	CHRONIC OBSTRUCTIVE AIRWAY DISEASE
COAG(ULAT)	COAGULA(NT)(TING)(TION)
COARCT	COARCTATION
COAT	COATING
COC	COCCY(X)(GEAL)
COC	COCAINE
COCCX	COCCYX
COCCY	COCCYGEAL
COCHL	COCHLEAR
COCHLEOVEST	COCHLEOVESTIBULAR
COINCDENC	COINCIDENCE
COL	COLONOSCOPY
COLECT	COLECTOMY
COLL	COLL(AGEN)(IDING)(ISION)
COLLAB(ORAT)	COLLABORATION
COLLAT	COLLATERAL
COLLR	COLLAR
COLM	COLUMN
COLN	COLON(IC)
COLNSCPY	COLONOSCOPY
COLOREC	COLORECTAL
COLOST	COLOSTOMY
COLOT	COLOTOMY
COLP(ECT)(ORR)(OT)(OURETHRCYSTPXY)	COLPORRHAPHY, COLPECTOMY, COLPORRHAPHY, COLPOTOMY, COLPO-URETHROCYSTOPEXY

COLR	COLOR
COLUM	COLUMN(S)
COMB	COMBI(NATION)(NATIONS)(NE)(NED)(NING), COMBO(S)
COMBUST	COMBUSTION
COMM	COMMERCIAL, COMMINUTED
COMMISSUROT	COMMISSUROTOMY
COMMUN	COMMUNICA(BLE)(TION), COMMUNITY
COMN	COMMON
COMP(L)	COMPLICA(TED)(TING)(TION), COMPREHENSIVE, COMPENSAT(E)(OR)
COMPAN	COMPANION
COMPAR	COMPARISON
COMPAT	COMPATIB(ILITY)(LE)
COMPET	COMPETEN(CE)(T)
COMPND	COMPOUND(S)
COMPON	COMPONENT
COMPOS	COMPOSITE
COMPRS	COMPRESS(ED)(ION)(OR)
COMPRT	COMPARTMENT
CON	CONSCIOUS
CONC	CONCENTRAT(E)(ED)(ION)(OR)
CONCN	CONCENTRA(TED)(TION)
CONCNTRC	CONCENTRIC
CONCUS(S)	CONCUSSION
COND(CTR)(UCT)	CONDITION(S), CONDUCT(ION)(OR)
CONDYLECT	CONDYLECTOMY
CONDYLR	CONDYLAR
CONF	CONFERENCE, CONFIRMA(TION)(TORY)
CONFIG	CONFIGURATION
CONFLAG(RAT)	CONFLAGRATION
CONG(E)N	CONGENITAL
CONGST	CONGEST(ION)(IVE)
CONIZ	CONIZATION
CONJ(UGAT)	CONJUGATION
CONJ(UNCT)	CONJUNCTIV(A)(AL)(ITIS)(O)
CONJN	CONJOINED
CONJUNCTPLSTY	CONJUNCTIVOPLASTY
CONNECT	CONNECTION
CONSC	CONSCIOUS(NESS)
CONSLT	CONSULTATION
CONSTIT(UNTS)	CONSTITUENTS
CONSTR(UCT)	CONSTRUCTION
CONT	CONTINENT, CONTINU(ATION)(E)(ED)(ING)(ITY)(OUS)
CONTAG	CONTAGIOSUM
CONTAINMNT	CONTAINMENT
CONTAMIN(AT)	CONTAMINAT(E)(ED)
CONTOUR	CONTOURING
CONTR	CONTRACTION
CONTRA	CONTRAINDICATION
CONTRACEPT	CONTRACEPTIVE
CONTRALAT	CONTRALATERAL
CONTRST	CONTRAST
CONTUS	CONTUSION
CONVNTION	CONVENTIONAL
CONVRT	CONVERT(ED)
CONVUL	CONVUL(SIVE)(TION)
CONVXITY	CONVEXITY
COORD	COORDINATE(D), COORDINATING
COPD	CHRONIC OBSTRUCTIVE PULMONARY DISEASE
COR	CORONARY, CORROSIVE
CORAC	CORACOID
CORDECT	CORDECTOMY
CORDOT	CORDOTOMY
CORN	CORNEA
CORPECT	CORPECTOMY
CORR(ECT)	CORRECT(ION)
CORROS	CORROS(ION)(IVE)
CORT(X)	CORTEX, CORTICAL
CORUGATD	CORRUGATED

COUNSL	COUNSELING
COVR	COVER(ED)
CP	CARDIOPULMONARY, CERVICAL PLEXUS
CPA	CEREBELLOPONTINE ANGLE
CPAP	CONTINUOUS POSITIVE AIRWAY PRESSURE
CPR	CARDIOPULMONARY RESUSCITATION
CPSLORR	CAPSULORRHAPHY
CR	CARDIAC RHYTHM
CRACD	CORACOID
CRANI(ECT)	CRANIAL, CRANIECTOMY
CRANIOPHARYNG	CRANIOPHAYNGEAL
CRANIOT	CRANIOTOMY
CRBL(M)	CEREBELLUM
CRBRL	CEREBRAL
CRBRUM	CEREBRUM
CRD	CORD
CREAT	CREATION
CRIS	CRISIS
CRIT	CRITICAL
CRPL	CARPAL
CRSH	CRUSH(ED)(ING)
CRTCH	CRUTCH
CRTL	CRITICAL
CRUC	CRUCIATE
CRV	CERVICAL
CRYGLB	CRYOGLOBULINEMIA
CRYO	CRYOSURGERY
CRYPTSPOR	CRYPTOSPORIDIUM
CRYST(ALNE)	CRYSTAL(LINE)
CS	CESAREAN SECTION
C-SECT	CESAREAN SECTION
C-SPINE	CERVICAL SPINE
CSTM	CUSTOM
CT	CHORDAE TENDINEAE, COMPUTERIZED TOMOGRAPHY
CTRL	CONTROL(LED)
CUB	CUBIC, CUBOID
CULT	CULTURE
CUNE	CUNEIFORM
CUR(ET)	CURETTAGE
CURR(NT)	CURRNT
CURV	CURVATURE
CUSHN	CUSHION
CUST	CUSTOM
CUT	CUTANEOUS, CUTTING
CUTDN	CUTDOWN
CV	CARDIOVASCULAR, CERVICAL VERTEBRAE
CVC	CENTRAL VENOUS CATHETER
CVS	CARDIOVASCULAR SYSTEM
CX	CERVIX
CYBR(O)NIC	CYBERONIC(S)
CYCL	CYCLE
CYCLECT	CYCLECTOMY
CYCLOSPOR	CYCLOSPORIASIS
CYL	CYLINDER
CYND	CYANIDE
CYSTECT	CYSTECTOMY
CYSTOHISTOLGC	CYSTOHISTOLOGIC
CYSTORR	CYSTORRHAPHY
CYSTOST	CYSTOSTOMY
CYSTOT	CYSTOTOMY
CYSTPLSTY	CYSTOPLASTY
CYSTSCPY	CYSTOSCOPY
CYSTURETHRPLSTY	CYSTOURETHROPLASTY
CYSTURETHRSCPY	CYSTOURETHROSCOPY
CYTOL	CYTOLOGIC
CYTOMTY	CYTOMETRY
CYTRABIN	CYTARABINE
D	DAY(S)
D&C	DILATION & CURETTAGE

D&E	DILATION AND EVACUATION
D&I	DEBRIDEMENT AND IRRIGATION
D&T	DIAGNOSIS AND TREATMENT
D/C	DISCHARGE
D/O	DISORDER(S)
D/T	DUE TO
DA	DAY(S), DUCTUS ARTERIOSUS
DAMGE	DAMAGE
DBL	DOUBLE
DCE	DISEASE CLASSIFIED ELSEWHERE
DCID	DECIDUOUS
DCRS	DECREASE(D)
DCUB	DECUBIT(AL)(US)
DEBRID	DEBRIDEMENT
DECLOT	DECLOTTING
DECN	DECISION
DECOMP	DECOMPRESS(ION)(IVE)
DECORTIC	DECORTICATION
DECR	DECREASE(D)
DEF(EC)	DEFECT(IVE)(S)
DEFIB	DEFIBRILLA(TION)(TOR)
DEFIC	DEFICIENCY(IES)
DEFLCTBLE	DEFLECTABLE
DEFN(ITV)	DEFINITIVE
DEFNDR	DEFENDER
DEFORM	DEFORM(ED)(ITY)(ITIES)
DEG	DEGREE
DEGEN	DEGENERATION
DEHIS	DEHISCENCE
DEL	DELETE(D), DELIVERED, DELUSIONAL
DELAY	DELAYED
DELIRM	DELIRIUM
DELV	DELIVER(ED)(IES)(Y)
DEM(ENT)	DEMENTIA, DEMONSTRAT(E)(ED)(ION)
DENERVAT	DENERVATION
DENS	DENSITY
DENT	DENT(AL)(ITION)(URE)
DENTITN	DENTITION
DEP(END)	DEPOSIT, DEPENDEN(CE)(T)
DEPLET	DEPLETION
DEPT	DEPARTMENT
DER(IV)	DERIVATIVE(S)
DERAIL	DERAILMENT
DERM	DERM(ABRASION)(AL)(ATOLOGIC)
DESC	DESCENDING, DESCRIBE(D), DESCRIP(TION)(TIONS)(TIVE)(TOR)
DESENZT	DESENSITIZ(ATION)(IZING)
DESN	DESIGN
DESR	DESIRE
DESTR(UC)	DESTRUC(TION)(TIVE)
DET	DETAIL(ED)
DET(E)RM	DETERMIN(ATION)(ATIVE)(E)(ED)
DETACH(BLE)(MNT)	DETACH(ABLE)(MENT)
DETECT	DETECTION
DETON	DETONATION
DETRGNT	DETERGENT(S)
DEV	DEVELOP(ING)(MENT)(MENTAL), DEVICE(S)
DEVITALIZ	DEVITALIZE(D)
DEXA	DUAL ENERGY X-RAY ABSORPTIOMETRY
DFFCLT	DIFFICULT
DFIB	DEFIBRILLA(TION)(TOR)
DFORM	DEFORMANS, DEFORMITY(IES)
DG	DEGREE
DGEN	DEGENERAT(ION)(IVE)
DGR	DEGREE
DGT	DIGIT(AL)
DHISC	DEHISCENCE
DIAB	DIABET(ES)(IC)
DIAL	DIALYSIS
DIAM	DIAMETER
DIAMND	DIAMOND
DIAPH	DIAPHRAGM(ATIC)
DIAS	DIASTOLIC
DIAZ	DIAZEPAM
DIET	DIETARY
DIFF	DIFFERENT(IAL)(IATION)
DIFFUS	DIFFUS(IBLE)(ING)(ION)
DIGESTV	DIGESTIVE
DIGT(S)	DIGIT(S)
DIGTIZD	DIGITIZED
DIGTL	DIGITAL
DIL(AT)	DILAT(ATION)(E)(ED)(ION)(OR)
DILUT	DILUTION
DIMEN	DIMENSION
DIOX	DIOXIDE
DIPHTH	DIPHTHERIA
DIPSTIC	DIPSTICK
DIR	DIRECT(OR)
DIRECT	DIRECTION
DIS	DISEASE
DISABL	DISABILITY
DISAPP	DISAPPEARANCE
DISART	DISARTICULAT(E)(ION)
DISCH	DISCHARGE
DISCON	DISCONNECT
DISKECT	DISKECTOMY
DISL(OC)	DISLOCAT(E)(ED)(ING)(ION)
DISNTGRATV	DISINTEGRATIVE
DISOD	DISODIUM
DISORG	DISORGANIZE(D)
DISP	DISPENS(E)(ER)(ING)
DISP(BL)	DISPOS(E)(ABLE)
DISRUPT	DISRUPTION
DISSECT	DISSECTION
DISSEM	DISSEMINAT(E)(ED)(ION)
DIST	DISTAL, DISTANCE, DISTILL(ED), DISTRIBUT(E)(ION), DISTURB(ANCE)
DISULF	DISULFIDE
DIV	DIVISION
DIVERTIC(LECT)	DIVERTICUL(A)(ECTOMY)(UM)
DJD	DEGENERATED JOINT DISEASE
DLA	DELAY(ED)
DLAY	DELAY
DM	DIABETES MELLITUS
DME	DURABLE MEDICAL EQUIPMENT
DMND	DIAMOND
DMNSN(L)	DIMENSION(AL)(S)
DMYEL	DEMYELINATING
DNSITY	DENSITY
DOA	DEAD ON ARRIVAL
DOB	DATE OF BIRTH
DOC	DOCUMENT(ATION)(ED)
DOM	DOMINANT
DOMEST	DOMESTIC
DONR	DONOR
DOPPLR	DOPPLER
DORS	DORSAL
DOSE	DOSAGE
DOZ	DOZEN
DP	DEEP
DPH(GM)	DIAPHRAGM(ATIC)
DPND	DEPEND
DPRSD	DEPRESSED
DPRSNT	DEPRESSANT(S)
DPRSV	DEPRESSIVE
DR(AI)N	DRAINAGE
DRANG	DERANGEMENT
DROWN	DROWNING
DRSG	DRESSING(S)
DRV	DRIV(ER)(ING)
DRVWY	DRIVEWAY
DSBL	DISAB(LE)(ILITY)
DSG	DRESSING(S)

DSP(L)(LCD)	DISPLACE(D)
DSRPT	DISRUPT
DSTRB	DISTURBANCE(S)
DSTRUC	DESTRUCT(ION)(IVE)
DT	DELIRIUM TREMENS
DTACH(BLE)	DETACH(ABLE)
DTAP	DIPHTERIA AND TETANUS TOXOIDS WITH ACELLULAR PERTUSSIS VACCINE
DTH	DEATH
DTL	DETAIL(ED)(ING)
DTP	DIPTHERIA AND TETANUS TOXOIDS WITH PERTUSSIS VACCINE
DTPA	DIPTHERIA AND TETANUS TOXOIDS WITH ACELLULAR PERTUSSIS VACCINE
DTX	DETOXIFICATION
DUI	DRIVING UNDER THE INFLUENCE
DUL	DUAL
DULMESH	DUALMESH
DUOD(NM)	DUODEN(AL)(UM)
DUODENECT	DUODENECTOMY
DUP	DUPLICATE(D)
DUR	DURAT(E)(ION)
DVLP	DEVELOPMENT(AL)
DVRTC	DIVERTICUL(A)(AR)(OSIS)(UM)
DWELL	DWELLING
DX	DIAGNOS(ED)(IS)(TIC)
DXT	DEXTROSE
DYN	DYNAMIC
DYSF	DYSFUNCTION
DYSPL	DYSPLASIA
DYSTR	DYSTROPHY
DZ	DISEASE(S)
E COLI	ESCHERICHIA COLI
E&M	EVALUATION AND MANAGEMENT (SERVICES)
EA	EACH
EAC	EXTERNAL AUDITORY CANAL
EB	ENDOBRONCHIAL
EB	EPSTEIN-BARR
ECA	EXTERNAL CAROTID ARTERY
ECCE	EXTRACAPSULAR CATARACT EXTRACTION
ECCNTRIC	ECCENTRIC
ECG	ELECTROCARDIO(GRAM)(GRAPHIC) (GRAPHY)
ECHO	ECHOCARDIO(GRAM)(GRAPHIC) (GRAPHY), ECHOENCEPHALOGRAPHY, ECHOGRAPHY
ECLMP	ECLAMPSIA
ECTOP	ECTOPIC
ECTPAR	ECTPARASITE
ECTROP	ECTROPIC, ECTROPION
ECZM	ECZEMA(TOUS)
ED	EDUCATION
EDMA	EDEMA
EDNTULS	EDENTULOUS
EEG	ELECTROENCEPHALO(GRAM)(GRAPHIC) (GRAPHY)
EF(D)	ENEMY FIRE, EXTERNAL FIXATION (DEVICE)
EFF	EFFECT(S)(IVE)
EFFUS	EFFUSION
EG	FOR EXAMPLE
EGD	ESOPHAGOGASTRODUODENOSCOPY
EGG	ELECTROGASTROGRAPHY
EIA	EXTERNAL ILIAC ARTERY
EJ	EJECTION
EJAC(ULAT)	EJACULATION
ELAST	ELASTIC
ELB	ELBOW
ELDER	ELDERLY
ELEC	ELECT(IVE)(RIC)(RO)(RONIC)(ROCUTION)
ELEC-COAG	ELECTROCOAGULATION
ELEC-CONV	ELECTROCONVULSIVE
ELEC-DX	ELECTRODIAGNOSTIC
ELECGM	ELECTROGRAM(S)
ELEC-PHORE	ELECTROPHORE(SIS)(TIC)
ELECPHYSIOL	ELECTROPHYSIOLOGY
ELEC-SURG	ELECTROSURG(ERY)(ICAL)
ELECTLYT	ELECTROLYTE(S)
ELECTRD	ELECTRODE(S)
ELEM	ELEMENT
ELEV	ELEVAT(E)(ING)(ION)
ELIG(BLITY)	ELIGIBILITY
ELIX	ELIXIR
ELSW	ELSEWHERE
ELUT	ELUTING
EMBO(LIZ)	EMBOL(ECTOMY)(ISM)(IZATION)
EMERG	EMERGENCY(IES)
EMG	ELECTROMYO(GRAM)(GRAPH) (GRAPHIC) (GRAPHY)
E-MICRO	ELECTRON MICROSCOPY
EMOL	EMOLLIENT
EMOT	EMOTION
EMP	EXTRAMEDULLARY PLASMACYTOMA
EMPHYS	EMPHYSEMA(TOUS)
EMPLOY	EMPLOY(ED)(EE)(MENT)
EMT	EMERGENCY MEDICAL TECHNICIAN
EN	ENCOUNTER
ENC(NTR)	ENCOUNTER
ENCEPHALGRPH	ENCEPHALOGRAPHY
ENCEPHALIT	ENCEPHALITIS
END	END(ED)(ING)
ENDARTERECT	ENDARTERECTOMY
ENDO	ENDODONTIC, ENDOSCOP(E)(IC)(Y)
ENDOBRONCH	ENDOBRONCHIAL
ENDOCARDIT	ENDOCARDITIS
ENDOCERV	ENDOCERVICAL
ENDOCRN	ENDOCRINE
ENDOLUMINL	ENDOLUMINAL
ENDOMET	ENDOMETRIAL
ENDOMYCARD	ENDOMYOCARDIAL
ENDOSC	ENDOSCOP(IC)(Y)
ENDOSONC	ENDOSONICS
ENDOTRACH	ENDOTRACHEAL
ENE FIRE	ENEMY FIRE
ENHNCD	ENHANCED
ENL	ENLARGED
ENMY	ENEMY
ENT	EARS NOSE THROAT
ENTANGL	ENTANGLEMENT
ENTERECT	ENTERECTOMY
ENTERIT	ENTERITIS
ENTEROENTEROST	ENTEROENTEROSTOMY
ENTERSCPY	ENTEROSCOPY
ENTR	ENTERING
ENTRAL	ENTERAL
ENTRCL	ENTEROCELE
ENTROP	ENTROPION
ENTROST	ENTEROSTOMY
ENTROT	ENTEROTOMY
ENTRSTML	ENTEROSTOMAL
ENTRVRUS	ENTEROVIRUS
ENUC(LEAT)	ENUCLEATION
ENVIR	ENVIRONMENT(AL)
ENZYM	ENZYME
EOC	EPISODE OF CARE
EOG	ELECTRO-OCULOGRAM
EP	ELECTROPHYSIOLOGIC(AL)
EPCNDL	EPICONDYLE
EPI	EPILEP(SY)(TIC), EPIGLOTTIS
EPICARD	EPICARDIAL
EPICOND	EPICONDYLAR
EPID	EPIDERMAL, EPIDURAL

EPIDIDYMGRPH	EPIDIDYMOGRAPHY
EPIDIDYMIT	EPIDIDYMITIS
EPIDIDYMOVASOST	EPIDIDYMOVASOSTOMY
EPIG(STRC)	EPIGASTRIC
EPIGL	EPIGLOTTIS
EPIL	EPILEP(SY)(TIC)
EPILAT	EPILATION
EPIPHYSDSIS	EPIPHYSIODESIS
EPIPHYSL	EPIPHYSEAL
EPIS	EPISODE
EPISCL	EPISCLERA
EPISPAD	EPISPADIUS
EPISTX	EPISTAXIS
EPITH(EL)	EPITHEL(IAL)(IUM)
EPITHLIPATH	EPITHELIOPATHY
EQ	EQUIN(A)(E)
EQP	EQUIPMENT
EQUILIB	EQUILIBRIUM
EQUL	EQUAL
EQUVALNT	EQUIVALENT
ER	EMERGENCY ROOM
ERCP	ENDOSCOPIC RETROGRADE CHOLANGIOPANCREATOGRAPHY
ERLY	EARLY
EROS	EROSION
ERR	ERROR(S)
ERS	EARS
ERTH	EARTH
ERUCT	ERUCTATION
ERUPT	ERUPTIONS
ERYTH	ERYTHROMYCIN
ERYTHMA	ERYTHEMA
ES	EPILEPTIC SYNDROMES
ESOPH	ESOPHAG(EAL)(US)
ESOPHAGECT	ESOPHAGECTOMY
ESOPHAGOGASTROST	ESOPHAGOGASTROSTOMY
ESOPHAGOST	ESOPHAGOSTOMY
ESOPHGPLSTY	ESOPHAGOPLASTY
ESOPHGSCPY	ESOPHAGOSCOPY
ESRD	END STAGE RENAL DISEASE
EST(AB)	ESTABLISH(ED)(ING)(MENT), ESTIMATION
E-STIM	ELECTRICAL STIMULATION
ET	ENDOTRACHEAL
ET AL	AND OTHERS
ETH(MO)	ETHMOID(AL)
ETHMOECT	ETHMOIDECTOMY
ETHOL	ETHANOL
ETT	ENDOTRACHEAL TUBE
EUST(ACH)	EUSTACHIAN
EVAC	EVACUATION
EVAL	EVALUAT(E)(ION)(IVE)
EVISC	EVISCERAT(E)(ION)
EX	EXAM, EXAMPLE, EXCEPT, EXCISE, EXCISION
EXAC(E)RBAT	EXACERBATION
EXAM	EXAMIN(ATION)(E)(ED)(ING)
EXC	EXCIS(E)(ED)(ION)(IONAL)
EXCESS	EXCESSIVE
EXCHG	EXCHANGE(R)(S)
EXCLD	EXCLUD(E)(ED)(ES)(ING)
EXCLU(S)	EXCLUS(ION)(IVE)(IVELY)
EXCRANI	EXTRACRANIAL
EXCURSN	EXCURSION
EXER	EXERCISE(S)
EXOPHTH	EXOPHTHALM(IC)(OS)
EXOSKL	EXOSKELETAL
EXOTROP	EXOTROPIA
EXP	EXPOS(ED)(URE)
EXP LAP	EXPLORATORY LAPARTOMY
EXPAN	EXPANSION
EXPCT	EXPECTORANTS
EXPL	EXPLORAT(ION)(ORY)
EXPLO	EXPLOSION
EXPNDR	EXPANDER
EXP(O)S	EXPOSURE
EXT	EXTEND(ED)(ING), EXTENS(ION)(IVE)(OR), EXTERNAL(LY), EXTREMITY, EXTRACTION
EXTIRPAT	EXTIRPATION
EXTRAARTIC	EXTRAARTICULAR
EXTRACT	EXTRACTION
EXTRALUM	EXTRALUMINAL
EXTRAV	EXTRAVASATION
EXTRCORP	EXTRACORPOREAL
EXTRDUR	EXTRADURAL
EXTREM	EXTREME, EXTREMITY(IES)
EXTRHEP	EXTRAHEPATIC
EXTRIN	EXTRINSIC
EXTRMED	EXTRAMEDULLARY
EXTRN	EXTERNAL
EXTRNOD	EXTRANODAL
EXTRNSL	EXTRANASAL
EXTROC	EXTRAOCULAR
EXTROR	EXTRAORAL
EXTRPELV	EXTRAPELVIC
EXTRPERIOST	EXTRAPERIOSTEAL
EXTRPERIT	EXTRAPERITONEAL
EXTRPLEUR	EXTRAPLEURAL
EXUD	EXUDATIVE
EYBLL	EYEBALL
EYELD	EYELID(S)
F	FASCIA, FEMALE
F/U	FOLLOW-UP
FA	FEMORAL ARTERY
FAB	FABRICAT(E)(ED)(ION)
FACL	FACIAL, FACILITATE, FACILITY
FACT	FACTOR
FAIL	FAIL(ED)(URE)
FALLOP	FALLOPIAN
FAM	FAMILY(IES)
FARM	FOREARM
FASC(ECT)(IT)(OT)	FASC(IA)(IECTOMY)(IITIS)(IOTOMY)
FB	FOREIGN BODY(IES)
FBG	FASTING BLOOD GLUCOSE
FCE	FAC(E)(IAL)
FCT	FACTOR(S)
FD	FOOD, FEEDING
FDA	FOOD AND DRUG ADMINISTRATION
FDBRN	FOODBORNE
FE	FEMALE
FEATUR	FEATURE(S)
FEB	FEBRILE
FEED	FEEDING
FEM	FEMUR, FEMORAL
FEMFEM	FEMORAL FEMORAL
FEMPOP	FEMORAL POPLITEAL
FEMTIB	FEMORAL TIBIAL
FERT	FERTILIZATION
FET(L)	FET(AL)(US)
FEV(R)	FEVER
FF	FRIENDLY FIRE
F-GLSS	FIBERGLASS
FHEAD	FOREHEAD
FIB	FIBRILLATION, FIBULA
FIBRD	FIBROID
FIBRGLS	FIBERGLASS
FIBRNLYS	FIBRINOLYSIS
FIBRO	FIBRO(SIS)(US)
FIBROADNO	FIBROADENOMA
FIL	FILL(ED)(ER)(ING)
FILTR	FILTER(ED)
FIND	FINDING(S)
FIRARM	FIREARM

FISH	FISHING
FISS	FISSURE
FISSURECT	FISSURECTOMY
FIST	FISTULA
FISTULECT	FISTULECTOMY
FISTULIZ	FISTULIZATION
FISTULOT	FISTULOTOMY
FIT	FIT(TED)(TING)
FIX	FIX(ATION)(ATIVE)(ED)
FL	FLUID
FLAC	FLACCID
FLAT	FLATULANCE
FLD	FIELD
FLEX	FLEX(IBLE)(ION)(OR)
FLEXSIG	FLEXIBLE SIGMOIDOSCOPY
FLNGE	FLANGE
FLP	FLAP
FLR	FLOOR
FLTR	FILTER
FLU	INFLUENZA
FLUO	FLUOTHANE
FLUORO	FLUOROSCOP(IC)(IES)(Y)
FLUT	FLUTTER
FLW	FOLLOW(ING)
FLX	FLEX(IBLE)(ION)(OR)
FM	FAMIL(IAL)(Y)
FNCT	FUNCTION(AL)(S)
FND	FINDING(S)
FNG(R)	FINGER(S)
FOC	FOCUS
FOCL	FOCAL
FOCUS	FOCUSED
FOLD	FOLDING
FOLLIC	FOLLICLE, FOLLICULAR
FOLW	FOLLOWING
FOLY	FOLEY
FOOTRST	FOOTRESTS
FORAMINOT	FORAMINOTOMY
FORARM	FOREARM
FORM	FORMATION
FORMLATION	FORMULATION(S)
FORMUL	FORMULAE
FOX	FOCAL
FRAC	FRACTION(AL)
FRAG(MENT)	FRAGMENT(ATION)
FRAGL	FRAGILE, FRAGILIS
FRARM	FOREARM
FREQ	FREQUENCY, FREQUENT(LY)
FRGN	FOREIGN
FRIC	FRICTION
FRM	FORM(S), FORMATION
FRME	FRAME
FRND	FRIEND(LY)
FRNT(L)	FRONT(AL)
FRZN	FROZEN
FSC	FASCIA
FSG	FASTING SERUM GLUCOSE
FSH	FOLLICLE-STIMULATING HORMONE
FT	FEET, FOOT, FULL TERM
FTB	FOOTBALL
FTG	FULL THICKNESS GRAFT
FTIG	FATIGUE
FTL	FETAL
FTSG	FULL THINCKNESS SKIN GRAFT
FU(D)	FOLLOW-UP (DAYS)
FULG	FULGURATION
FULL	FULLY
FUNC(T)	FUNCTION(AL)(S)
FURN	FURNITURE
FURNC	FURUNCLE
FUS	FUSION
FUSD	FUSED
FX	FRACTURE(D)(S)
G	GRADE
GANG	GANGLION
GANGREN	GANGRENE
GARMNT	GARMENT
GASTR	GASTRIC
GASTRECT	GASTRECTOMY
GASTROC	GASTOCNEMIUS
GASTRODUOD	GASTRODUODENAL
GASTROJEJ(UN)	GASTROJEJUNAL
GASTRORR	GASTRORRHAPHY
GASTROST	GASTROSTOMY
GASTROT	GASTROTOMY
GASTRPLSTY	GASTROPLASTY
GAUNTLT	GAUNTLET
GB	GALLBLADDER
GC	GONOCOCCAL, GONORRHEA
GE	GASTROESOPHAGEAL
GEN(IT)	GENERAL(IZED), GENERAT(E)(ED)(ING)(ION)(OR), GENITAL(ALIA)(S)
GENE	GENETIC
GENT	GENTAMICIN
GENTL	GENITAL(IA)(S)
GEST	GESTATION
GFT	GRAFT(ING)(S)
GI	GASTROINTESTINAL
GIFT	GAMETE INTRAFALLOPION TRANSFER
GING	GINGIV(A)(ECTOMY)
GIRDL	GIRDLE
GITT	GLUCOSE INSULIN TOLERANCE TEST
GJ	GASTROJEJUNOSTOMY
GL	GLAND
GLAUC	GLAUCOMA
GLC	GLAUCOMA
GLEN	GLENOID
GLID(R)	GLID(ER)(ING)
GLND	GLAND(S), GLENOID
GLOB	GLOBULIN
GLOM	GLOMERULAR
GLOSSECT	GLOSSECTOMY
GLOV	GLOVE
GLU	GLUCOSE
GLUC	GLUCAGON
GLUT(L)	GLUTEAL
GLYCEROPHOSHATE	GLYCEROPHOSPHATE
GLYCPROT	GLYCOPROTEIN
GM	GRAM
GN	GLOMERULONEPHRITIS
GNA	GALANTHUS NIVALIS AGGLUTININ
GOIT	GOITER
GONOCCL	GONOCOCCAL
GONORHEA	GONORRHEA
GONSCPY	GONIOSCOPY
GOR-TX	GORE-TEX
GR	GROSS
GR(T)	GREAT(ER)
GRAD(E)(I)NT	GRADIENT
GRANL	GRANUL(ATION)(OMA)
GRAV(D)	GRAVID
GRND	GROUND
GRNSTCK	GREENSTICK
GRP	GROUP(ING)(S)
GRVITY	GRAVITY
GRWTH	GROWTH
GT	GREATER
G-TUBE	GASTROSTOMY TUBE
GU(I)	GENITOURINARY (INFECTION)
GUID	GUID(ANCE)(E)(ED)(ING)
GY	GRAY
GYN	GYNECOLOG(IC)(ICAL)(Y)
GYNECOMAS	GYNECOMASTIA
H PYLORI	HELICOBACTER PYLORI

H&D	HEAD AND NECK
HA	HEADACHE, HEPATIC ARTERY
HAB	HABITUAL
HALGN	HALOGEN
HALLUC	HALLUCIN(ATION)(OGEN)
HALX	HALLUX
HARV(EST)	HARVEST(ING)
HAZ	HAZARD(OUS)
HB	HOMEBOUND, HOUSEBOUND
HBP	HIGH BLOOD PRESSURE
HC	HYDROCARBONS
HCFA	HEALTH CARE FINANCING ADMINISTRATION
HCG	HUMAN CHORIONIC GONADOTROPIN
HCI	HYDROCHLORIC ACID
HCL	HYDROCHLORIDE
HCPCS	HCFA COMMON PROCEDURAL CODING SYSTEM
HCT	HEMATOCRIT
HCV	HEPATITIS C VIRUS
HD	HEAD, HEMODIALYSIS
HDL	HIGH-DENSITY LIPOPROTEIN
HEAL	HEALING
HEAR	HEARING
HEAT	HEATED
HEENT	HEAD EYES EARS NOSE AND THROAT
HELMNTH	HELMINTHIASIS
HEM	HEMORRHAGE
HEMARTH	HEMARTHROSIS
HEMAT	HEMATOMA
HEMATOLOG	HEMATOLOGICAL
HEMDIAL	HEMODIALYSIS
HEMI	HEMISPHERE
HEMIPHALANGECT	HEMIPHALANGECTOMY
HEMIPL	HEMIPLEGIA
HEMISPHERECT	HEMISPHERECTOMY
HEMODIAL	HEMODIALYSIS
HEMOLYS	HEMOLYSIS
HEMOLYT	HEMOLYTIC
HEMOR(R)	HEMORRHAGE
HEMORRHOIDECT	HEMORRHOIDECTOMY
HEMPHIL	HEMOPHILI(A)(C)
HEMRD	HEMORRHOID(S)
HEMTM	HEMATOMA
HEMTOG	HEMATOGENOUS
HEMTUR	HEMATURIA
HEP(AT)	HEPAT(IC)(ITIS)
HEPARN	HEPARIN
HEPATECT	HEPATECTOMY
HEPBIL	HEPATOBILIARY
HERED	HEREDITARY
HERED(IT)	HEREDITARY
HERN	HERNIA(TED)
HERNIORR	HERNIORRHAPHY
HERNIOT	HERNIOTOMY
HERNIPLSTY	HERNIOPLASTY
HEVY	HEAVY
HF	HYDROGEN FLUORIDE
HFC	HYDROFLUOROCARBON
HGB	HEMOGLOBIN
HGT	HEIGHT
HHC	HOME HEALTH CARE
HI	HIGH(ER)(EST)
HIB	HAEMOPHILUS INFLUENZAE TYPE B
HIDRAD(EN)	HIDRADENITIS
HIE	HYPOXI-ISCHEMIC-ENCEPHALOPATHY
HISTAM	HISTAMINE
HISTCYT	HISTIOCYTIC
HIT	HOME INFUSION THERAPY
HIV	HUMAN IMMUNODEFICIENCY VIRUS
HIWY	HIGHWAY
HK	HOOK
HL	HEALING, HEARING LOSS
HLDR	HOLDER
HLNG	HEALING
HLP(R)	HELP(ER)
HLTH	HEALTH
HMO	HEALTH MAINTENANCE ORGANIZATION
HMSTRG	HAMSTRING
HND(S)	HAND(S)
HNDQTR	HINDQUARTER
HNGS	HINGES
HODG(KINS)	HODGKIN'S DISEASE
HOM	HOME
HOMOGFT	HOMOGRAFT
HOMOLOG	HOMOLOG(OUS)(UES)
HORM	HORMONE(S)
HOSP	HOSPITAL(IZED)(IZATION)
HOUS	HOUSING
HP	HARD PALATE
HPB	HEPATOBILIARY
HR	HOUR(S)
HRNSS	HARNESS
HRT	HEART
HSG	HYSEROSALPINGOGRAPHY
HSHLD	HOUSEHOLD
HT	HEIGHT
HTN	HYPERTENS(ION)(IVE)
HTV	HEAVY TRANSPORTATION VEHICLE
HUM	HUMER(AL)(US)
HUMDIFIR	HUMIDIFIER
HUMIDFICATN	HUMIDIFICATION
HUMN	HUMAN
HVY	HEAVY
HX	HISTORY
HYD	HYDRATION
HYDRCARB	HYDROCARBONS
HYDRCEPHAL	HYDROCEPHALIC
HYDRGN	HYDROGEN
HYDROCELECT	HYDROCELECTOMY
HYDROPHIL	HYDROPHILIC
HYPERTON	HYPERTONIC
HYPERTROPH	HYPERTROPHIC
HYPNOT	HYPNOTIC(S)
HYPOCALC	HYPOCALCEMIA
HYPOFNCT	HYPOFUNCTION
HYPOPHYSECT	HYPOPHYSECTOMY
HYPOSASTR	HYPOGASTRIC
HYPOSPAD	HYPOSPADIAS
HYPOTEN(S)	HYPOTENSION
HYPOTHERM	HYPOTHERMIA
HYPRACT	HYPERACTIV(E)(ITY)
HYPRAL	HYPERALIMENTATION
HYPRBR	HYPERBARIC
HYPRCOAG	HYPERCOAGULABLE
HYPREXT	HYPEREXTENSION
HYPRPLAS	HYPERPLAS(IA)(TIC)
HYPRSENS	HYPERSENSITIV(E)(ITY)
HYPRSOMN	HYPERSOMNIA
HYPRTHYR	HYPERTHYROIDISM
HYPRTROP	HYPERTROPH(IC)(Y)
HYPRVENT	HYPERVENTILATION
HYPTHALM	HYPOTHALAMUS
HYST	HYSTERECTOMY
HYSTEROSALPINGGRPHY	HYSTEROSALPINGOGRAPHY
HYSTEROSC	HYSTEROSCOPY
HYSTERSONOGRPHY	HYSTEROSONOGRAPHY
I&A	IRRIGATION AND ASPIRATION
I&D	INCISION AND DRAINAGE
I&R	INSERTION AND REMOVAL
IA	INTRA-ARTICULAR, INNOMINATE ARTERY
IATRO(GEN)	IATROGENIC
IC	INTRACONDYLAR

IC	INTRACRANIAL
ICA	INTERNAL CAROTID ARTERY
ICD 9 CM	INTERNATIONAL CLASSIFICATION OF DISEASES 9TH REVISION CLINICAL MODIFICATION
ICH	INTRACRANIAL HEMORRHAGE
ICI	INTRACRANIAL INJURY
ICU	INTENSIVE CARE UNIT
ICW	INTRACRANIAL WOUND
ID	IDENTIF(IABLE)(ICATION)(IED)(IFY)(IFYING), THE SAME
IDD	INSULIN-DEPENDENT DIABETES
IDDM	INSULIN-DEPENDENT DIABETES MELLITUS
IDIO(PATH)	IDIOPATHIC
IE	IDIOPATHIC EPILEPSY, THAT IS
IF(D)	INDEX FINGER, INTERNAL FIXATION (DEVICE)
IG	IMMUNE GLOBULIN
IGA	IMMUNOGLOBULIN A
IGD	IMMUNOGLOBULIN D
IGE	IMMUNOGLOBULIN E
IGG	IMMUNOGLOBULIN G
IGM	IMMUNOGLOBULIN M
IIA	INTERNAL ILIAC ARTERY
III	IIIA B/C
IIIA B/C	IIIA IIIB/IIIC
IL	ILIUM
ILEOPROCTOST	ILEOPROCTOSTOMY
ILEOST	ILEOSTOMY
ILESCPY	ILEOSCOPY
ILL-DEFIND	ILL-DEFINED
ILLEG	ILLEGAL(LY)
ILPBC	ILIOPUBIC
ILPUB	ILIOPUBIC
ILSCHIAL	ILIOISCHIAL
IM	INTRAMUSCULAR
IMA	INFERIOR MESENTERIC ARTERY, INTERNAL MAMMARY ARTERY
IMAG	IMAG(E)(ING)
IMF	INTRAMEDULLARY FIXATION
IMM	IMMUN(E)(OLOGICAL)
IMMATUR	IMMATURITY
IMMDEFIC	IMMUNODEFICIEN(CY)(T)
IMMED	IMMEDIATE(LY)
IMMGLOB	IMMUNOGLOBULIN(S)
IMMIZ	IMMUNIZATION(S)
IMMOB	IMMOBILITY
IMMOBLIZR	IMMOBILIZER
IMMSUPP	IMMUNOSUPPRESS(ED)(IVE)
IMMU(N)(NLGIC)	IMMUN(ITY)(IZATION)(OLOGICAL)
IMMUNOFLUORES	IMMUNOFLUORESCEN(CE)(T)
IMMUNOTX	IMMUNOTHERAPY
IMP(ACT)	IMPACT(ED)
IMPAIR	IMPAIRMENT
IMPERF	IMPERORATE
IMPERM	IMPERMEABLE
IMPL	IMPLANT(ABLE)(ATION)(ED)(ING)(S)
IMPLEMENT	IMPLEMENTATION
IMPR	IMPAIR(ED)
IMPREGNTD	IMPREGNATED
IMPRESS	IMPRESSION
IMPRV	IMPROVE
IMPS	IMPOSE(D)(ING)
IMS	IMMUNOSUPPRESSED
IN	INCH(ES), INITIAL
IN VIT	IN VITRO
INAPP	INAPPROPRIATE
INC	INCORPORATE(D), INCLUDE
INCAR(CERAT)	INCARCERATED
INCD	INCIDENTS
INCI	INCISION(AL)(S)
INCL	INCLUDE(E)(ED)(ING), INCLUSIONAL
INCOMP(AT)(ETNCE)(REHENS)	INCOMPREHENSIBLE, INCOMPATIBLE, INCOMPETENCE
INCONT	INCONTINEN(CE)(T)
INCPL	INCOMPLETE
INCR	INCREAS(E)(ED)(ING)
IND	INDICAT(E)(OR), INDIVIDUAL(LY), INDUCED
INDEP	INDEPENDENT(LY)
INDICAT	INDICATION
INDIR	INDIRECT
INDUCD	INDUCE(D)
INDUCT	INDUCTION
INDUST	INDUSTRIAL
INDV	INDIVIDUAL(S)
INDW(E)LL	INDWELLING
INDX	INDEX
INF	INFECT(ED)(ION)(IOUS), INFERIOR
INFARCT	INFARCTION
INFEC(TV)	INFECTIVE
INFER	INFERIOR
INFERT	INFERTILITY
INFEST	INFESTATION
INFILTRAT	INFILTRATIVE
INFLAM	INFLAMMAT(ION)(ORY)
INFLAT	INFLATABLE
INFLICT	INFLICTED
INFNT	INFANT
INFO	INFORM(ANTS)(ATION)(ED)
INFRARD	INFRARED
INFRATENTOR	INFRATENTORIAL
INFRCT	INFARCTION
INFST	INFESTATION
INFT	INFANT
INFUNDIB	INFUNDIBULAR
INFUS	INFUSION
ING	INGUINAL
INGN	INGROWN
INGST	INGESTED
INHAL	INHAL(ATION)(ER)
INHIB	INHIBIT(ED)(ION)(OR)(ORY)
INIT	INITIA(L)(TE)(TIAL)(TING)
INJ	INJECT(ABLE)(ED)(ION)(ORS), INJUR(ED)(IES)(ING)(Y)
INNOM(IN)	INNOMINATE
INNR	INNER
INOC(ULAT)	INOCULATION
INOP	INOPERABLE
INORG	INORGANIC
INPT	INPATIENT
INS	INSERT, INSURANCE
INS(E)RT	INSERT(ED)(ING)(ION)
INSCT	INSECT
INSCTCID	INSECTICIDE
INSEM	INSEMINATION
INSIP	INSIPIDUS
INSLN	INSULIN
INSPECT	INSPECTION
INST	INSTITUTION(AL)
INSTAB	INSTABILITY
INSTILL	INSTILLATION
INSTL	INSTALLATION, INSTILLATION
INSTR	INSTRUCTION(S), INSTRUMENT
INSTRUM	INSTRUMENT(AL)(ATION)(S)
INSUF(F)	INSUFFICIEN(CY)(T)
INT	INTEREST(ED), INTERMEDIATE, INTERNAL
INTDERM	INTRADERMAL
INTEG	INTEGUMENT(ARY)
INTEGR	INTEGRITY
INTENS	INTENSITY
INTEPR	INTERPRET(ATION)(IVE)(S)

INTERCNDYL	INTERCONDYLAR
INTERMED	INTERMEDIATE
INTERMIT	INTERMITTENT
INTEROP	INTEROPERATIVE
INTERST	INTERSTITIAL
INTERVEN	INTERVENTION(AL)
INTEST	INTESTIN(AL)(E)(ES)
INTF	INTERFACE
INTGR	INTEGRAT(E)(ED)(ION)
INTGRL	INTEGRAL
INTL	INITIAL
INTNT	INTENT
INTOL	INTOLERANCE
INTOX(ICAT)	INTOXICATION
INTRABD	INTRA-ABDOMINAL
INTRACT	INTRACTABLE
INTRARTIC	INTRA-ARTICULAR
INTRBDY	INTERBODY
INTRCAP	INTRACAPSULAR
INTRCARD	INTRACARDIAL
INTRCAV	INTRACAVITARY
INTRCEREB	INTRACEREBRAL
INTRCOND	INTERCONDYLAR
INTRCOR	INTRACORONARY
INTRCORP	INTRACORPOREAL
INTRCOST	INTERCOSTAL
INTRCPTV	INTERCEPTIVE
INTRCRN	INTRACRANIAL
INTRCUT	INTRACUTANEOUS
INTRDNTL	INTERDENTAL
INTRDUCR	INTRODUCER
INTRDUR	INTRADURAL
INTRFALLOP	INTRAFALLOPIAN
INTRFER	INTERFERON
INTRHEP	INTRAHEPATIC
INTRIN	INTRINSIC
INTRL	INTERNAL
INTRLES	INTRALESIONAL
INTRLUM	INTRALUMINAL
INTRM	INTERIM
INTRMED	INTERMEDIATE
INTRMEDLLRY	INTRAMEDULLARY
INTRMITT	INTERMITTENT
INTRMUR	INTRAMURAL
INTRNAS	INTRANASAL
INTRNS	INTRINSIC
INTRNUCL	INTERNUCLEAR
INTRO	INTRODUC(E)(ED)(TION)(TORY)
INTROC(ULR)	INTRAOCULAR
INTROP	INTRAOPERATIVE
INTRORL	INTRAORAL
INTROSS	INTRAOSSEOUS
INTRP	INTERRUPT(ION)
INTRPELV	INTRAPELVIC
INTRPER(IT)	INTRAPERITONEAL
INTRPLM	INTRAPULMONARY
INTRSP	INTERSPACE
INTRSPINAL	INTRASPINAL
INTRSTIT	INTERSTITIAL
INTRTHEC	INTRATHECAL
INTRTHOR	INTRATHORACIC
INTRU	INTRUSION
INTRV	INTERVERTEBRAL
INTRVASC	INTRAVASCULAR
INTRVENT	INTRAVENTRICULAR
INTRVESC	INTRAVESICAL
INTRVL	INTERVAL
INTRVN	INTERVENTION(AL)
INTUB(AT)	INTUBAT(E)(ION)
INTUSS	INTUSSUSCEPTION
INVASV	INVASIVE
INVESTIGAT	INVESTIGATION

INVLV	INVOLV(E)(ED)(EMENT)(ES)(ING)
INVOL	INVOLUNTARY
IOL	INTRAOCULAR LENS
IP	INPATIENT(S), INTERPHALANGEAL
IPPB	INTERMITTENT POSITIVE PRESSURE BREATHING
IQ	INTELLIGENCE QUOTIENT
IRIDCYC	IRIDOCYCLITIS
IRIDECT	IRIDECTOMY
IRIDOT	IRIDOTOMY
IRRADATD	IRRADIATED
IRREG	IRREGULAR
IRRIG	IRRIGATION(S)
IRRIT	IRRITAB(ILITY)(LE), IRRITANT
IS	IMMUNOSUPPRESSIVE
ISCH	ISCHEMIA
ISCH(M)	ISCHI(AL)(UM)
ISOIMM	ISOIMMUNIZATION
ISOL(AT)	ISOLAT(ES)(ION)
ISTH(MUSECT)	ISTHMUS(ECTOMY)
IT	INTERTROCHANTERIC, IT IS
IU(D)	INTRAUTERINE (DEVICE)
IV	INTRAVENOUS, INTERVERTEBRAL
IVASC	INTRAVASCULAR
IVF	IN VITRO FERTILIZATION
JACKT	JACKET
JAUND	JAUNDICE
JDGMT	JUDGMENT
J(E)JUN	JEJUNUM
J(E)JUNOST	JEJUNOSTOMY
JMML	JUVENILE MYELOMONOCYTIC LEUKEMIA
JNCT	JUNCTION
J(N)T	JOINT(S)
JP	JACKSON-PRATT
JR	JUNIOR
J-TUBE	JEJUNOSTOMY TUBE
JUG	JUGULAR
J(U)MP	JUMPING
JUNC	JUNCTION(AL)
JUV	JUVENILE
K+	POTASSIUM
KAP	KAPOSI'S
KERIT	KERATITIS
KETN	KETONE
KETOACID	KETOACIDOSIS
KG	KILOGRAM
KID	KIDNEY
KN	KNEE, KNOWN
KNUCKL	KNUCKLE
KNWN	KNOWN
L	LOW
L&D	LABOR AND DELIVERY
L&R	LEFT AND RIGHT
L1-L5	LUMBAR VERTEBRAE 1 THROUGH 5
L5-S1	LUMBAR FIFTH VERTEBRA TO SACRAL FIRST VERTEBRA
LAB	LABORATORY(IES)
LABR	LABOR
LABYRINTHIN	LABYRINTHINE
LABYRINTHOT	LABYRINTHOTOMY
LAC	LACERAT(E)(ION)
LACR	LACRIMAL
LACT	LACTATE
LAD	LEFT ANTERIOR DESCENDING CORONARY ARTERY
LAMINECT	LAMINECTOMY
LAND	LANDING
LANG	LANGUAGE
LAP(AROT)	LAPARO(SCOPIC)(SCOPY)(TOMY)
LAR	LARYNX
LARYNG	LARYNGEAL

LARYNGECT	LARYNGECTOMY
LARYNGOT	LARYNGOTOMY
LARYNGPLSTY	LARYNGOPLASTY
LARYNGRPH	LARYNGOGRAPHY
LARYNGSCPY	LARYNGOSCOPY
LASR	LASER
LAT	LATER(AL)(O)
LATISS	LATISSIMUS
LATX	LATEX
LAVH	LAPROSCOPICALLY ASSISTED VAGINAL HYSTERECTOMY
LAX	LAXATIVE
LAY	LAYER(ED)
LB	LIVEBORN
LBR	LABOR
LCA	LEFT CORONARY ARTERY
LCH	LANGERHANS-CELL HISTIOCYTOSIS
LD	LEAD
LE	LEG, LOWER EXTREMITY
LEATHR	LEATHER
LEEP	LOOP ELECTROSURGICAL EXCISION PROCEDURE
LEGL	LEGAL(ITY)(LY)
LEGRST	LEGREST(S)
LEISHMAN	LEISHMANIASIS
LEN	LENGTH(ENING)(Y)
LEP	LEPROSY
LES	LESION(S)
LESR	LESSER
LEUK(EM)	LEUKEMI(A)(C)
LEVL	LEVEL
LF	LITTLE FINGER
L-F-D	LIGHT-FOR-DATES
LG	LARGE
LGHT	LIGHT
LGHTWT	LIGHTWEIGHT
LGTH	LENGTH
LGTNG	LIGHTNING
LIC	LICENSE(D)
LIDO	LIDOCAINE
LIG	LIGAMENT(OUS), LIGATION, LIGATURE
LING	LINGULA
LINR	LINEAR
LIP	LIPID
LIQD	LIQUID
LIST	LISTED
LITH	LITHOLAPAXY, LITHOTOMY, LITHOTRIPSY
LITL	LITTLE
LIV(R)	LIVER
LIVEB(RN)	LIVEBORN
LK	LEAK(AGE)
LL	LOWER (LIMB) (LOBE)
LLQ	LEFT LOWER QUADRANT
LMCA	LEFT MAIN CORONARY ARTERY
LN	LINED
LNDSLD	LANDSLIDE
LNG(S)	LONG, LUNG(S)
LOAD	LOADING
LOBECT	LOBECTOMY
LOBP	LOSS OF BODY PART
LOC	LOCAL(IZATION)(IZED)(IZING), LOSS OF CONSCIOUSNESS
LOCK	LOCKING
LOCM	LOW-OSMOLALITY CONTRAST MEDIA
LODGNG	LODGING
LONG(I)T(UDNL)	LONGITUDINAL
LOW	LOWER
LP(S)	LIP(S)
LPN	LICENSED PRACTICAL NURSE
LQD	LIQUID
LRYN	LARYN(GEAL)(X)

LS	LUMBAR SPINAL, LUMBOSACRAL
LT	LEFT, LIGHT
LTD	LIMITED
LTL	LITTLE
LTR	LATER
LU	LUNG(S)
LUBRICNT	LUBRICANT
LUMB	LUMBAR
LUMBOSUBARACH	LUMBOSUBARACHNOID
LUNA	LAPAROSCOPIC UTEROSACRAL NERVE ABLATION
LUQ	LEFT UPPER QUADRANT
LV	LUMBAR VERTEBRA
LV ANGIO	LEFT VENTRICULAR ANGIOGRAM
LVAD	LEFT VENTRICULAR ASSIST DEVICE
LVL	LEVEL
LW(R)	LOW(ER)
LYM DZ	LYME DISEASE
LYMPH	LYMPHADENECTOMY, LYMPHATIC
LYMPHCYT	LYMPHOCYT(E)(IC)
LYMPHECT	LYMPHADENECTOMY
LYMPHOM	LYMPHOMA
LYR	LAYER
LYTES	ELECTROLYTES
M	MEDIAL, MUSCLE
M&F	MALE AND FEMALE
M&T	MUSCLE (FASCIA) & TENDON
M/F	MALE OR FEMALE
MA (TUBE)	MILLER ABBOT TUBE
MAC	MACULA(R)
MACER	MACERATED
MACH	MACHINE(RY)
MAG(NET)	MAGNETIC
MAGN	MAGNUM
MAINT	MAINTENANCE
MAISN	MAISONNEUVES
MAISONV	MAISONNEUVES
MAJ	MAJOR
MAL	MALIG(NANCY)(NANT)
MALAB(SORP)	MALABSORPTION
MALADJ	MALADJUSTMENT
MALF(NCT)	MALFORMATION(S), MALFUNCTION
MALIG	MALIGNAN(T)(CIES)(CY)
MALL	MALLEOLUS
MALNUT	MALNUTRITION
MALPOS	MALPRESENTATION
MALR	MALAR
MALROTAT	MALROTATION
MALTREAT	MALTREATMENT
MALUN	MALUNION
MAMM	MAMMARY
MAMMO	MAMMO(GRAM)(GRAPHIC)(GRAPHY)(PLASTY)
MAN	MANS
MAN(I)FST	MANIFESTATION(S)
MAND	MANDIB(LE)(ULAR)
MANIP	MANIPULA(TION)(TIVE)
MAN-MD	MAN-MADE
MAOI	MONOAMINE-OXIDASE-INHIBITOR
MAP	MAPPING
MARG	MARGIN(AL)(S)
MARKR	MARKER
MARSUP	MARSUPIALIZATION
MARTHON	MARATHON
MASTECT	MASTECTOMY
MASTOIDOT	MASTOIDOTOMY
MASTOIECT	MASTOIDECTOMY
MAT	MATERIAL(S), MATUR(ATION)(ITY)
MATCHD	MATCHED
MATL	MATERIAL(S)
MATNL	MATERNAL
MATTRSS	MATTRESS

MAVRCK	MAVERICK
MAX	MAXI(L)(MAL)
MAXIL	MAXILLA(RY)
MC	METACARPAL
MCI	MILLICURIE
MCL	MEDIAL COLLATERAL LIGAMENT
MCP	METACARPOPHALANGEAL
MCR	MEDICARE
MCYCL	MOTORCYCL(E)(IST)
MD	MEDICAL DOCTOR
MDL	MODEL
MDRXYPRGESTRON	MEDROXYPROGESTERONE
ME	MACULAR EDEMA
MEATOT	MEATOTOMY
MEC	MECONIUM
MECH	MECHAN(ICAL)(ISM)(IZED)
MED	MED(IA)(IAL)(IAN)(IUM), MEDICA(LLY)(TED)(TION), MEDICINE
MED OBL	MEDULLA OBLONGATA
MEDC	MEDIC(AL)(AMENT)(ATION)(INE)
MEDIAST	MEDIAST(INAL)(INUM)
MEDIASTINOT	MEDIASTINOTOMY
MEDIASTINSCPY	MEDIASTINSCOPY
MEDM	MEDIUM
MEDS	MEDICAMENTS
MEDTRON	MEDTRONIC
MEDUL(RY)	MEDULLA(RY)
MEET	MEETING
MEGASONC	MEGASONICS
MELL	MELLITUS
MELNOM	MELANOMA
MEM	MEMORY
MEMB	MEMBRANE(S), MEMBRANOUS
MEN(G)	MENING(EAL)(ES)
MENGCOC	MININGOCOCCUS
MENGENCEPH	MENINGOCENCEPHALITIS
MENGIT	MENINGITIS
MENISC	MENISC(AL)(US)
MENO	MENOPAUSE
MENST(RUAT)	MENS(TRUAL)(TRUATION)
MENT(L)	MENTAL
MERC	MERCURY
MERCH	MERCHANT
MES(NTR)	MESEN(TERIC)(TERY), MESIAL
METAB	METABOL(IC)(ISM)(ITES)
METAS	METASTATIC
METH	METHOD(S), METHODOLOGY(IES)
METL	METAL
METRD	METERED
METS	METASTAS(ES)(IS)
MF	MIDDLE FINGER
MFD	MAXIMUM FRACTIONS PER DAY
MG	MAGNESIUM, MILLIGRAM
MGMT	MANAGEMENT
MI	MYOCARDIAL INFARCTION
MIC	MICROSCOP(E)(IC)(Y)
MIC-LGT	MICRO-LIGHT
MICROCALC	MICROCALCIFICATION
MICROLIT	MICROLIGHT
MICROPHTH	MICROPHTHALMAS
MICROPIGM	MICROPIGMENTATION
MICRPROCSS	MICROPROCESSOR
MICRSC	MICROSCOPIC
MICRVASC	MICROVASCULAR
MICSURG	MICROSURGICAL
MICVASC	MICROVASCULAR
MID	MIDDLE
MIDCRV	MIDCERVICAL
MIDFT	MIDFOOT
MIDLN	MIDLINE
MIL(IT)	MILITARY
MIN	MINIM(ALLY)(UM), MINOR, MINUTE(S)
MINERL	MINERAL
MINI	MINIATURIZED, MINIM(AL)(UM)
MISAD(V)	MISADVENTURE
MISC	MISCELLANEOUS
MITRL	MITRAL
MIX	MIX(ED)(TURES)
ML	MILLILITER, MID LOBE
MLDSTRB	MALDISTRIBUTION
MLNUTRIT	MALNUTRITION
MLTANG	MULTIANGULAR
MLWAKEE	MILWAUKEE
MM	MILLIMETERS OF MERCURY
MMC	METHYLMETHACRYLATE
MMR	MEASLES MUMPS & RUBELLA
MN	MEDIAN NERVE
MNG	MANAGE
MNIC	MANIC
MNINGOCOCCL	MENINGOCOCCAL
MNL	MANUAL
MOBL(IZ)	MOBIL(E)(ITY)(IZATION)
MOD	MOD(ERATE)(IFICATIONS)(IFIED)(IFIERS)(IFYING)(ULAR)
MODAL	MODALITY(IES)
MODULATD	MODULATED
MOIST(R)	MOISTURE
MOISTURZR	MOISTURIZERS
MOLD	MOLD(ED)(ING)
MOLECLR	MOLECULAR
MOLLUSC	MOLLUSCUM
MOM	MOTHER
MON	MONITOR(ING)
MONCYT	MONOCYTIC
MONO	INFECTIOUS MONONUCLEOSIS
MONOC	MONOCULAR
MONOCLON	MONOCLONAL
MONOPLEG	MONOPLEGIA
MONOX	MONOXIDE
MONTG	MONTEGGIA'S
MORBD(TY)	MORBID(ITY)
MORPH	MORPHINE
MOSQT	MOSQUITO-BORNE
MOT	MOTION
MOTR(IZD)	MOTOR(IZED)
MOV(MNT)	MOVE(MENT)(MENTS)(RS)
MPJ	METACARPAL PHALANGEAL JOINT
MR(A)	MAGNETIC RESONANCE (ANGIOGRAPHY)
MRCELLATR	MORCELLATOR
MRE	MOST RECENT EPISODE
MRI	MAGNETIC RESONANCE IMAGING
MRINE	MARINE
MRTALTY	MORTALITY
MRTHON	MARTHON
MS	MULTIPLE SCLEROSIS
MSC	MUSCLE(S)
MSG	MONOSODIUM GLUTAMATE, MESSAGE(S)
MSK(L)	MUSCULOSKELETAL
MSR	MEASURE(D)(MENT)(MENTS), MEASURING
MSTD(IT)	MASTOID(ITIS)
MT	METATARSAL, MUSCLE TONE
MTH	MOUTH
MTN	MOTION, MOUNTAIN
MTP	METATARSOPHALANGEAL
MTR	MOTOR
MTRCYCLST	MOTORCYCLIST
MTRN	MATERN(AL)(ITY)
MU	MALUNION
MUC	MUCOSA(L)
MUCOCUT	MUCOCUTANEOUS
MUCOPUR	MUCOPURULENT

MUCOS	MUCOSAL, MUCOUS, MUCOSA
MUCOSECT	MUCOSECTOMY
MUDSLD	MUDSLIDE
MULT	MULTIPLE
MULTFOC	MULTIFOCAL
MULTGRAV	MULTIGRAVIDA
MULTP(AR)	MULTIPARITY
MUSC	MUSCLE(S), MUSCUL(AR)(ATURE)
MUSCUTAN	MUSCULOCUTANEOUS
MUSH	MUSHROOMS
MUTAT	MUTATION
MV	MITRAL VALVE, MOVE, MOTOR VEHICLE(S)
MX	MULTIPLE(S)
MXAXL	MULTIAXIAL
MYALG	MYALGIA
MYCOPLAS	MYCOPLASMA
MYCOTOX	MYCOTOXIN
MYELEC	MYOELECTRONICALLY
MYELOP	MYELOPATHY
MYELPROLIF	MYELOPROLIFERATIVE
MYOCARD	MYOCARDIAL
MYOCUT	MYOCUTANEOUS
MYOELECTRNICALY	MYOELECTRONICALLY
MYOMECT	MYOMECTOMY
MYOP	MYOPATHY
MYOSIT	MYOSITIS
MYOT	MYOTOMY
MYRINGOT	MYRINGOTOMY
NA	NOT APPLICABLE
NARC	NARCOTIC(S)
NAS	NASAL
NASL	NASAL
NASOLAC	NASOPHARYNGITIS
NASOMAXIL	NASOMAXILLARY
NASOPHAR(YNG)	NASOPHARYNG(EAL)(ITIS)
NAT(RL)	NATURAL
NATV	NATIVE
NAVIC	NAVICULAR
NB	NEONATE, NEWBORN
N(C)K	NECK
NDLE	NEEDLE
NDSPLC	NONDISPLACED
NEB	NEBULIZER
NEC	NECESS(ARILY)(ARY)(ITATING)(ITY), NOT ELSEWHERE CLASSIFIED
NECR(OS)	NECROSIS, NECROTIZING
NEG	NEGATIVE
NEGL	NEGLECT
NEO	NEOPLSM
NEODERM	NEODERMIS
NEONAT	NEONATAL, NEONATE
NEOPL	NEO(PLASM)(PLASTIC)
NEOPLSM	NEOPLASM(S)
NEOVASC	NEOVASCULARIZATION
NEPHR	NEPH(RITIC)(ROPATHY)
NEPHRECT	NEPHRECTOMY
NEPHRIT	NEPHRITIS
NEPHRO	NEPHROGRAM
NEPHROST	NEPHROSTOMY
NEPHROTOMGRPH	NEPHROTOMOGRAPHY
NEPHRPXY	NEPHROPEXY
NERV	NERVE(S), NERVOUS
NES	NOT ELSEWHERE SPECIFIED
NEURAX	NEURAXIAL
NEURIT	NEURITIS
NEURL	NEURAL
NEURLYT	NEUROLYTIC
NEURMUSC	NEUROMUSCULAR
NEURO	NEUROLOG(ICAL)(Y)
NEUROCYBRNTIC	NEUROCYBERNETIC
NEUROGEN	NEUROGENIC
NEUROL	NEURO(LOGIC)(LOGICAL)
NEUROLEP(T)	NEUROLEPTIC(S)
NEUROP	NEURO(PATHIC)(PATHY)
NEUROVASC	NEUROVASCULAR
NEURPLSTY	NEUROPLASTY
NEURSTIM	NEUROSTIMU(LATOR)(LATION)
NEURSYPH	NEUROSYPHILIS
NEURTROPH	NEUROTROPHIC
NEV	NEV(I)(US)
NFS	NOT FURTHER SPECIFIED
NG	NASOGASTRIC, NITROGLYCERIN
NG TUBE	NASOGASTRIC TUBE
NGHBR	NEIGHBOR(ING)
NGT	NIGHT
NIC	NICOTINE
NICKL	NICKEL
NICU	NEONATAL INTENSIVE CARE UNIT
NIP	NIPPLE
NITR	NITRIC
NITRO(DER)	NITRO(DERIVITIVES)(GEN)(GLYCERINE)
NL	NAIL, NASOLACRIMAL, NORMAL
NLD	NASOLACRIMAL DUCT
NMV	NONMOTOR VEHICLE
NO	EXCEPT, NORTH, NUMBERS, WITHOUT
NOA	NONOPIOID ANALGESIC
NOC	NOCTURNAL, NOT OTHERWISE CLASSIFIED
NOD	NOD(ES)(ULAR)(ULE)
NODES	LYMPH NODES
NODUL	NODULE
NODULR	NODULAR
NOM	NONSUPPURATIVE OTITIS MEDIA
NON/MALUNION	NONUNION/MALUNION
NONADJ	NONADJUSTABLE
NONADM	NONADMINISTRATION
NONARTHR	NONARTHROPOD
NONASPH	NONASPHERIC
NONAUTO(G)(L)	NONAUTOLOGOUS
NONBAC	NONBACTERIAL
NONBIO	NONBIOLOGICAL
NONCHEMO	NONCHEMOTHERAPEUTIC
NONCOLL	NONCOLLISION
NON-DECB	NON-DECUBITUS
NONDISP	NONDISPOSABLE
NONDISPL	NONDISPLACED
NONDISSOLV	NONDISSOLVABLE
NONDOM	NONDOMINANT
NONDSPLC(D)	NONDISPLACED
NONDYSENT	NONDYSENTERIC
NONELECTR	NONELECTRIC
NONER	NONEMERGENCY
NONEXC	NONEXCISIONAL
NONEXT	NONEXTENSIVE
NONEXUD	NONEXUDATIVE
NON-HODG	NON-HODGKIN'S
NONINF	NONINFECTIOUS
NONINFLAM	NONINFLAMMATORY
NON-INST	NON-INSTITUTIONAL
NONINV	NONINVASIVE
NONMAG	NONMAGNETIC
NONMECH	NONMECHANICAL
NONMED	NONMEDICINAL
NONMTR	NONMOTOR
NONOB	NONOBSTETRICAL
NONOBLIT	NONOBLITERATIVE
NONODONT	NONODONTOGENIC
NONOP	NONOPIOID
NONORG	NONORGANIC
NONPARAL	NONPARALYTIC
NONPERF	NONPERFORATING
NONPETROL	NONPETROLEUM
NONPWR	NONPOWERED

NONPYO	NONPYOGENIC
NONRECOMB	NONRECOMBINANT
NONRMV	NONREMOVABLE
NONSTEREOTAC	NONSTEREOTACTIC
NONTHRM	NONTHERMAL
NONTRAU	NONTRAUMATIC
NONTRFF	NONTRAFFIC
NONTRNSPT	NONTRANSPORT
NONUN	NONUNION
NONVEN	NONVENOMOUS
NON-WK	NONWORK
NORM	NORMAL(IZED)(LY)
NOS	NOT OTHERWISE SPECIFIED, UNSPECIFIED
NOX	NOXIOUS
NP(HX)	NASOPHARYNX
NPPL	NIPPLE
NR	NEAR
NRI	NOREPINEPHRINE REUPTAKE INHIBITORS
NRS	NURS(E)(ING)
NRV	NERVE(S), NERVOUS
NS	NERVOUS SYSTEM
NSE	NOSE
NST	NONSTRESS TEST
NTV	NATIVE
NU	NONUNION
NUC(L)	NUCLEAR
NUT	NUTRITION
NUTR(IT)	NUTRITION(AL)
NVICLR	NAVICULAR
NYSTAG	NYSTAGMUS
O2	OXYGEN
O-A-AX	OCCIPITO-ATLANTO-AXIAL
OA	OSTEOARTHROSIS
OB	OBSTETRIC(AL)
OBES	OBESITY
OBJ	OBJECT(S)
OBL	OBLIQUE(S)
OBLIQ	OBLIQUE(S)
OBLIT	OBLITER(ATE)(ATION)(ATIVE)
OBS	OBSERVATION(S)
OBSC	OBSCURE
OBSERV	OBSERVATION(S)
OBST(R)	OBSTRUCT(ING)(ION)(IVE)
OBTUR	OBTURATOR
OC	OCULAR, OSTEOCHONDRAL
OCC(IP)	OCCIPITAL, OCCUPANT
OCCL	OCCLUD(ED)(ING), OCCLUS(AL)(ION)(IONAL)(IVE)
OCCUP	OCCUPANT, OCCUPATIONAL
OCCUR	OCCURRENCE
OCULOMTR	OCULOMOTOR
OCULR	OCULAR
ODONT	ODONTOGENIC
ODONTOGN	ODONTOGENIC
OFC	OFFICE(S)
OFFC	OFFICIAL
OFF-RD	OFF-ROAD
OINTMNT	OINTMENTS
OL(E)CRN	OLECRANON
OLF	OLFACTORY
OM	OTITIS MEDIA
OM1	FIRST OBTUSE MARGINAL BRANCH
OM2	SECOND OBTUSE MARGINAL BRANCH
OMENTECT	OMENTECTOMY
OMN	OCULOMOTOR NERVE
OMPHAL	OMPHALOCELE
OMT	OSTEOPATHIC MANIPULATIVE TECHNIQUE
ON	OPTIC NERVE
OOPHORECT	OOPHORECTOMY

OP	OPEN, OPERAT(ED)(S)(ING)(ION)(IONS)(IVE), OPIOID, ORGANOPHOSPHATE, OSTEOPOROSIS, OUTPATIENT, OUTPUT
OPAC	OPAC(IFICATION)(ITY)
OPHTH	OPHTHALM(IA)(IC)(OLOGIC)(OLOGICAL)(OLOGY)(OPATHY)(OSCOPIC)(OSCOPY)
OPHTHPLEG	OPHTHALMOPLEGIA
OPN(G)	OPEN(ING)
OPQ	OPAQUE
OPT(C)	OPTIC(AL)
OPTOKIN	OPTOKINETIC
OR IMPL	ORTHOPEDIC IMPLANT
ORB	ORBIT(AL)
ORBITOT	ORBITOTOMY
ORCHECT	ORCHIECTOMY
ORCHIT	ORCHITIS
ORD	ORDER
ORDR	ORDER(ING)
ORG	ORGAN(IC)(ISM)(S)
ORGN	ORGAN(S)
ORGNSM	ORGANISM, ORGASM
ORGPHOS	ORGANOPHOSPHATE
ORIF	OPEN REDUCTION INTERNAL FIXATION
ORIG	ORIGIN(AL)(ATING)
ORL	ORAL, OTORHINOLARYNGOLOGICAL
OROMAX	OROMAXILLARY
OROPHRYN	OROPHARYNGEAL
ORR	ORRHAPHY
ORTH(OPED)	ORTHOPEDIC
ORTHDNT	ORTHODONTIC
ORTHOS	ORTHOPEDICS
ORTHOT	ORTHOTIC
OSCILLAT	OSCILLATING
OSM	OSMOLAR
OSS	OSSEOUS
OSSF	OSSFI(CANS)(CATION)
OSSIC	OSSICLES
OSSIF	OSSIFICATION
OST	OSTEITIS, OSTOMY
OSTCHOND	OSTEOCHON(DRAL)(DROPATHIES)(DROPATHY)(DROSIS)
OSTEC	OSTECTOMY
OSTEOARTHROS	OSTEOARTHROSIS
OSTEOCHNDRL	OSTEOCHONDRAL
OSTEOCHNDRTIS	OSTEOCHONDRITIS
OSTEOMYEL	OSTEOMYELITIS
OSTEOPATH	OSTEOPATHIC
OSTEOPHYTECT	OSTEOPHYTECTOMY
OSTEOQ	OSTEOCUTANEOUS
OSTEOT	OSTEOTOM(IES)(Y)
OSTEPLSTY	OSTEOPLASTY
OSTGEN	OSTEOGEN(ESIS)(IC)
OSTMYL	OSTEOMYELITIS
OSTNCR	OSTEONECROSIS
OSTOGNS	OSTEOGENESIS
OSTPATH	OSTEOPATHY
OSTPHYT	OSTEOPHYTE
OSTPOR	OSTEOPOROSIS
OT	OTOM(IES)(Y)
OTH	OTHER
OTIT	OTITIS
OTOAC	OTOACOUSTIC
OTOSCLER	OTOSCLEROSIS
OUTRIG	OUTRIGGER
OUTSD	OUTSIDE
OV	OFFICE VISIT, OVARY
OVERTURN	OVERTURNING
OVL	OVAL
OVR	OVER
OVRACT	OVERACTIVITY
OVRBRD	OVERBOARD
OVRCORR	OVERCORRECTION

OVRLAP	OVERLAP(PING)
OVRLAY	OVERLAY
OVRTRN	OVERTURNING
OVRUSE	OVERUSE
OVRY	OVARY
OWND	OWNED
OXAZOL	OXAZOLIDINEDIONES
OXFRD	OXFORD
OXI	OXIDES
OXYGNTR	OXYGENATOR
OZ	OUNCE
P/S	POLYUNSATURATED TO SATURATED FATTY ACIDS RATIO
PA	POSTEROANTERIOR, PULMONARY ARTERY
PACE	PACING
PACEMKR	PACEMAKER
PAL	PALATE
PALAT	PALATINE
PALATL	PALATAL
PALATPLSTY	PALATOPLASTY
PALL	PALLIATIVE
PALLADM	PALLADIUM
PALND	PALINDROMIC
PALS	PALSY
PANC	PANCREAS, PANCREATIC
PANCRATGRPH	PANCREATOGRAPHY
PANCREATECT	PANCREATECTOMY
PANENCEPH	PANENCEPHALITIS
PANL	PANEL
PANN	PANNICULITIS
PAP	PAPANICOLAOUM, PAPILLARY
PAP SMEAR	PAPANICOLAOU'S SMEAR
PAPIL	PAPILLOMA
PAPILLED	PAPILLEDEMA
PAR	PARING
PARACERV	PARACERVICAL
PARAGANG	PARAGANGLION
PARAGRN(ULOM)	PARAGRANULOMA
PARAINFLU	PARAINFLUENZA
PARAL(YT)	PARALYTIC
PARANAS	PARANASAL
PARAPHARYNG	PARAPHARYNGEAL
PARASIT	PARASITIC
PARATHYROIDECT	PARATHYROIDECTOMY
PARENCHY	PARENCHYMA
PARENT	PARENTERAL
PARIET	PARIETAL
PARK	PARKING
PARKSM	PARKINSONISM
PARM	PARAMETER
PARNTRAL	PARENTERAL
PARSIT	PARA(SITE)(SITIC)(SITOLOGY)
PARSYMP	PARASYMPATHOLYTIC
PART	PART(IAL)(LY)(S)
PARTHY	PARATHYROID
PARTYPH	PARATYPHOID
PASSG	PASSAGE(S)
PASSV	PASSIVE
PAT	PATELLA(R)
PATEL	PATELLA
PATH	OPATHY, PATHAL, PATHO(GENIC)(LOGIC) (LOGICAL)(LOGIST) (LOGY)
PATHWY	PATHWAYS
PAY	PAYMENT
PC	PIECE
PC/P	PREGRNANCY, CHILDBIRTH & PUERPERIUM
PCK	PACKING
PCKET	PACKET
PCN	PENICILLIN(S)
PCP	PNEUMOOCYSTIS CARINII PNEMONIA
PCTA	PERCUTANEOUS TRANSLUMINAL ANGIOPLASTY
PDA	PATENT DUCTUS ARTERIOSUS
PDR	PHYSICIANS DESK REFERENCE
PEC	PECTOR(AL)(IS)
PECE	PIECE
PED	PEDESTRIAN, PEDIATRIC(S)
PEDCL	PEDICLE
PEDL	PEDAL
PEDST	PEDESTRIAN
PELL	PELLETS
PELV	PELVIC, PELVIS
PEN	PENETRAT(E) (ING), PENILE, PENIS
PEND	PENDULOUS
PENDUNCULOT	PENDUNCULOTOMY
PENETR(AT)	PENETRAT(ING)(ION)
PENTR	PENETRATION
PEPTC	PEPTIC
PER	PERSON
PERC	PERCUTANEOUS
PERCEP	PERCEPTION
PERF	PERFORA(TING)(TION)(TIONS)(TORS)
PERFRM	PERFORMANCE
PERFUS	PERFUSION
PERIACETAB	PERIACETABULAR
PERIAN	PERIANAL
PERIART	PERIARTERIAL
PERIARTIC	PERIARTICULAR
PERICARD	PERICARD(IAL)(ITIS)(IUM)
PERICARDIECT	PERICARDIECTOMY
PERICARDIT	PERICARDIUM
PERIN	PERIN(EAL)(EUM)
PERINAT	PERINATAL
PERINL	PERINEAL
PERINTL	PERINATAL
PERIOC	PERIOCULAR
PERIODNT	PERIODONTAL
PERIORB	PERIORBITAL
PERIPANC	PERIPANCREATIC
PERIPH	PERIPHERAL
PERIREC	PERIRECTAL
PERISTOM	PERISTOMAL
PERIT	PERITON(EAL)(EUM)
PERITN	PERITONEAL
PERITON	PERITON(EAL)(EUM)
PERIUMB	PERIUMBILIC(AL)
PERIVENT	PERIVENTRICULAR
PERM	PERMANENT
PERMBL	PERMEABLE
PERON(L)	PERONEAL
PERP	PERPETRATOR
PERQ	PERCUTANEOUS
PERS	PERSON(AL)(NEL)
PERSIS(T)	PERSISTENT
PERTUSS	PERTUSSIS
PEST	PESTICIDE(S)
PET	POSITRON-EMISSION TOMOGRAPHY
PETR	PETROUS
PETROL	PETROLEUM
PFND	PROFOUND
PG	PAROTID GLAND, PREGNANT(CY)(CIES)
PHAL(ANG)(X)	PHALAN(GEAL)(GES)(X)
PHAR	PHARYNX
PHARM	PHARMA(CEUTICAL)(COLOGIC)
PHARYNGOGASTROST	PHARYNGOGASTROSTOMY
PHARYNGOLARYNGECT	PHARYNGOLARYNGECTOMY
PHELPLSTY	PHELOPLASTY
PHENL	PHENEL
PHENO	PHENOTYPE
PHENOTHIAZ	PHENOTHIAZINE
PHENPROP	PHENPROPIONATE
PHENTOLAM	PHENTOLAMINE

PHENTZ	PHENOTHIAZINE
PHEOCHROM	PHEOCHROMOCYTOMA
PHER(ES)	PHERESIS
PHLBIT	PHLEBITIS
PHLBTHRMB	PHLEBOTHROMBOSIS
PHLEB	PHLEBERRHAPHY
PHLYCT	PHLYCTENULAR
PHN	PHRENIC NERVE
PHOS	PHOS(PHATASE)(PHATE)(PHORUS)
PHOTOCOAG	PHOTOCOAGULATE
PHREN	PHRENIC
PHRM	PHARMACY
PHRM(CL)	PHARMAC(OLOGIC)(Y)
PHRMSEED	PHARMASEED
PHRYN	PHARYN(GEAL)(X)
PHRYNIT	PHARYNGITIS
PHSL	PHYSEAL
PHYS	PHYSICAL, PHYSICIAN(S)
PHYS PT	PHYSICAL THERAPY
PHYSIO(LOG)	PHYSIOLOGICAL
PHYSL	PHYSEAL
PIG(M)	PIGMENT(ATION)(S)
PIN	PINNING
PISFRM	PISIFORM
PIT(UIT)	PITUITARY
PKD	POLYCYSTIC KIDNEY DISEASE
PKG	PACKAGE
PKP	PENETRATING KERATOPLASTY
PKU	PHENYLKETONURIA
PK-UP	PICK-UP
PLAC	PLACENTA(L), PLANING
PLACENTL	PLACENTAL
PLACNTA	PLACENTA(E)
PLACNTL	PLACENTAL
PLAN	PLANING
PLANTR	PLANTAR
PLAS(M)	PLASMA
PLAST(R)	PLASTER
PLAT	PLATE, PLATEAU
PLATLT	PLATELET
PLAYGRN	PLAYGROUND
PLC(D)(MT)	PLACE(D)(MENT)
PLERSY	PLUERISY
PLETHYSMGRPH	PLETHYSMOGRAPHY
PLEU(R)	PLEUR(AL)(ISY)
PLEURECT	PLEURECTOMY
PLEX	PLEXUS
PLM	PALM(AR)
PLN	PLAN
PLNT	PLANT
PLNTR	PLANTAR
PLSMA	PLASMA
PLST(C)	PLASTIC
PLT	PLATELET
PLUMB	PLUMBING
PLX	PLEXUS
PM	PACEMAKER, POSTMENOPAUSAL
PMH	PAST MEDICAL HISTORY
PN	PERIPHERAL NERVE, PNEUMONIA(E)
PNCT	PUNCTURE
PNEUM(AT)	PNEUMATIC
PNEUMCOC(CL)	PNEUMOCOCCAL
PNEUMCON	PNEUMOCONIOSIS
PNEUMHEM	PNEUMOHEMOTHORAX
PNEUMNIT	PNEUMONITIS
PNEUMO	PNEUMOTHORAX
PNEUMOCONIOS	PNEUMOCONIOSIS
PNEUMON	PNEUMONIA(E)
PNEUMONECT	PNEUMONECTOMY
PNEUMOPERIT	PNEUMOPERITONIUM
PNEUMTHOR	PNEUMOTHORAX
PNL	PANEL
PNS	PERIPHERAL NERVOUS SYSTEM
PNTS	POINTS
PO4	PHOSPHATE
POIS(N)	POISON(ING), POISON BY
POL(ARIZ)	POLAR(IZING)
POLCENT	POLYCENTRIC
POLIO(MYEL)	POLIOMYELITIS
POLYART	POLYARTERITIS
POLYARTC	POLYARTICULAR
POLYARTH	POLYARTHROPATHY
POLYCNTRC	POLYCENTRIC
POLYDACT	POLYDACTYL(OUS)(Y)
POLYGLND	POLYGLANDULAR
POLYNEUR	POLYNEUROPATHY
POLYNEURIT	POLYNEURITIS
POLYPECT	POLYPECTOMY
POLYSACC	POLYSACCHARIDE
POLYSOMNGRPH	POLYSOMNOGRAPHY
POOL	POOLED
POP(L)	POPLITEAL, POPULATION
PORCELN	PORCELAIN
PORT	PORTAL
PORTGRPH	PORTOGRAPHY
PORTN	PORTION
POS(IT)	POSITION
POSS	POSSIBL(E)(LY)
POST	POSTERIOR
POSTDYSNT	POSTDYSENTERIC
POSTERUP	POSTERUPTIVE
POSTHEM	POSTHEMORRHAGIC
POSTINFARCT	POSTINFARCTION
POSTINFLAM	POSTINFLAMMATORY
POSTLAMI	POSTLAMINECTOMY
POSTMAST	POSTMASTECTOMY
POSTMASTOID	POSTMASTOIDECTOMY
POSTMENO	POSTMENOPAUSE
POSTNAT	POSTNATAL
POSTOP	POSTOPERATIVE
POSTPHLEB	POSTPHLEBITIC
POSTP(ROC)(X)	POSTPROCEDUR(E)(AL)
POSTRHEUM	POSTRHEUMATIC
POST-TRAUM	POST-TRAUMATIC
POT	POTENTIAL
POWER	POWERED
POX	PULSE OXIMETRY
PP	POSTPARTUM
PPC	POSTPARTUM COMPLICATION
PPROM	PRETERM, PREMATURE RUPTURE OF MEMBRANES
PR	POOR, PRIOR
PRACHUTST	PARACHUTIST
PRASYMPTHOMIMET	PARASYMPATHOMIMETICS
PRC	PROCESS
PRCISN	PRECISION
PRD	PERIODIC
PRDONTIT	PERIDONTITIS
PRECAUT	PRECAUTION(S)
PRECEREB	PRECEREBRAL
PRECIP	PRECIPITA(TION)(TORS)
PRED	PREDNISOLONE
PREDICT	PREDICTION
PREDOM	PREDOMI(NANCE)(NANT)(NANTLY)(NATELY)
PRE-ECLAM(P)	PRE-ECLAMPSIA
PRE-EXIST	PRE-EXISTING
PREFAB	PREFABRICAT(ED)(ION)
PREG	PREGNANC(IES)(Y)
PREG-REL	PREGNANCY-RELATED
PREM	PREMATURE
PRENAT	PRENATAL
PREOP	PREOPERATIVE

PREP	PREPAR(ATORY)(ED)(ING), PREPARE FOR SURGERY, PREPERATION(S)
PREREC	PRERECORDED
PRES	PRESERVA(TION)(TIVE), PRESERV(ED)(ING)
PRES(E)NC	PRESENCE
PRESENIL	PRESENILE
PRESNT	PRESENTATION
PRESRV	PRESERVATION
PRESS	PRESSURE(S)
PRESUM(P)	PRESUM(ED)(PTIVE)
PRETIB	PRETIBIAL
PRETX	PRETREATMENT
PREV(NT)	PREVENT(ION)(IVE), PREVIA, PREVIOUS(LY)
PREVOC	PREVOCATIONAL
PREX	PRE-EXISTING
PRFAB	PREFABRICAT(ED)(ION)
PRFND	PROFUNDA
PRFRM	PERFORM(ANCE)(ED)
PRIM	PRIMAR(ILY)(Y)
PRIMIGRAV	PRIMIGRAVIDA
PRIO	PRIOR
PRIV	PRIVATE
PRLIM	PRELIMINARY
PRMOUNTD	PREMOUNTED
PROB	PROBLEM(S)
PROC	PROCEDURE(S), PROCESSOR
PROCESS	PROCESSING
PROCID	PROCIDENTIA
PROCREAT	PROCREATIVE
PROCTECT	PROCTECTOMY
PROCTOT	PROCTOTOMY
PROCTSIGIT	PROCTOSIGMOIDITIS
PROCTSIGMOIDSCPY	PROCTOSIGMOIDOSCOPY
PROD	PRODUCT
PROF	PROFESSIONAL(S)
PROFND	PROFOUND
PROFUND	PROFUNDUS
PROG	PROGRAM(MABLE)(MED)(MING)(S), PROGRESS(IVA)(IVE)
PROGEN	PROGENITOR
PROGS	PROGRESSIVE
PROGST	PROGESTOGENS
PROJ	PROJECT(ED)(ILE)(ION)(IVE)(S)
PROLAP(S)	PROLAPSE
PROLIF(ERAT)	PROLIFERATIVE
PROLNG	PROLONG(ED)
PRON(ATR)	PRONAT(ION)(OR)
PROP	PROPION(ATE)(IC)
PROPH(YL)	PROPHY(LACTIC)(LAXIS)
PROS	PROSTHE(SIS)(TIC), PROSTATE
PROST	PROSTAT(E)(IC)
PROSTATOT	PROSTATOTOMY
PROSTH	PROSTHES(ES)(IS), PROSTHETIC(S)
PROSTIT	PROSTATITIS
PROT	PROTEIN
PROTNT	PROTECTANTS
PROTVE	PROTECTIVE
PROV	PROVIDE(D)(R)(S), PROVIDING, PROVISION(AL)
PROVOC	PROVOCATION
PROX	PROXIMAL
PRPS	PURPOSE
PRS	PRESENT(ING)
PRSC	PRESCRIBE(D)(ING), PRESCRIPTION
PRSS	PRESS
PRT	PART, PORTION
PRTBLE	PORTABLE
PRTCP	PARTICIPANT
PRTECT	PROTECT(IVE)(OR)
PRTERM	PRETERM

PRTIC	PARTICULATE
PRTL	PARTIAL(LY)
PRTN	PORTION, PROTEIN(ASE)
PRTNUR	PROTEINURIA
PRTUSS	PERTUSSIS
PR-TX	PRETREATMENT
PRVS	PROVISION(AL)
PRX	PRE-EXISTING
PRXT	PRE-EXISTING
PSA	PROSTATE-SPECIFIC ANTIGEN
PSEUDAARTH	PSEUDOARTHROSIS
PSEUDANRYSM	PSEUDOANEURYSM
PSEUDCYST	PSEUDOCYST
PSEUDEXFOL	PSEUDOEXFOLIATIVE
PSEUDMEMB	PSEUDOMEMBRANOUS
PSGR	PASSENGER
PSN	POISON(ING)
PSNGR	PASSENGER
PSTN	POSITION(AL)(ING)(S)
PSV	PASSIVE
PSX	POSTSYMPTOM
PSYC(H)	PSYCHIA(TRIC)(TRY), PSYCHO(LOGIC)(LOGICAL)(SIS)(TIC)
PSYCHACTV	PSYCHOACTIVE
PSYCHDYS	PSYCHODYSLEPTICS
PSYCHED	PSYCHOEDUCATIONAL
PSYCHGEN	PSYCHOGENIC
PSYCHMOTR	PSYCHOMOTOR
PSYCHODYSLEPTICS	PSYCHODYSLEPTICS HALLUCINOGENS
PSYCHOS	PSYCHOSES
PSYCHOSEX	PSYCHOSEXUAL
PSYCHOT	PSYCHOTIC
PSYCHPHYS	PSYCHOPHYSIOLOGICAL
PSYCHSEX	PSYCHOSEXUAL
PSYCHSOC	PSYCHOSOCIAL
PSYCHTROP	PSYCHOTROPIC
PSYCHTX	PSYCHOTHERAPY
PT	PATIENT, PRETERM, PROTHROMBIN, PULMONARY TRUNK
PTERYG	PTERYGIUM
PTERYGMAX	PTERYGOMAXILLARY
PTL	PRETERM LABOR
PTNTL	POTENTIAL
PUB	PUB(IC)(IS), PUBLIC
PUD(EN)	PUDENDAL
PULM	PULMONARY
PULP	PULP(AL)(OTOMY)
PULS	PULSED
PUNC(T)	PUNCTURE
PURCH	PURCHASES
PURG	PURGING
PURIF(ICAT)	PURI(FICATION)(FIED)
PURS	PURSUIT
PUSH	PUSHED
PV	PULMONARY (VALVE) (VEIN)
PVT	PRIVATE
PWR	POWER(ED)
PX	PROCEDURE
PYELGRPH	PYELOGRAPHY
PYELNEPHR(IT)	PYELONEPHRITIS
PYELOST	PYELOSTOMY
PYELSCPY	PYELOSCOPY
PYEM	PYEMIC
PYLN	PYLON
PYLOR	PYLORUS
PYLORPLST	PYLOROPLASTY
PYOGEN	PYOGENIC
QUAD	QUAD(RANT)(RICEPS)(RIPLEGIC)(RUPLET)
QUADLAT	QUADRILATERAL
QUADPOL	QUADRAPOLAR
QUAL	QUALI(FIED)(FIES)(FYING)(TATIVE)(TY)

QUAN	QUANTI(FICATION)(TATION)(TATIVE)
R/R	RECESSION OR RESECTION
RA	RADIOACTIVE, RADIAL ARTERY, RHEUMATOID ARTHRITIS, RENAL ARTERY
RACC	RACCOON
RAD	RADI(ATION)(OLOGIC)(OLOGICAL)(OLOGIST)(OLOGY), RADIAL, RADICAL, RADIUS
RADIACT	RADIOACTIVE
RADIC	RADICULOPATHY
RADICRPL	RADIOCARPAL
RADIHUM	RADIOHUMERAL
RADIOL	RADIOLOGY
RADIOTX	RADIOTHERAPY
RADL	RADICAL
RADOPHRM	RADIOPHARMACEUTICAL
RADOPHRMACEUTCL	RADIOPHARMACEUTICAL
RADULN	RADIOULNAR
RADUS	RADIUS
RAIL	RAILS
RATLSNK	RATTLESNAKE
RBC	RED BLOOD CELL
RC	ROOT CANAL
RCA	RIGHT CORONARY ARTERY
RD	ROAD
RDR	RIDER
RDS	RESPIRATORY DISTRESS SYNDROME
RDUC	REDUCE(D), REDUCIBLE, REDUCING, REDUCTION
REACT	REACT(ION)(S)
REALIGN	REALIGNMENT
REATT	REATTACH(ED)(MENT)
REATTACH	REATTACHMENT
REC	RECORD(ING), RECREATION(AL)
RECALCIFICAT	RECALCIFICATION
RECEPT	RECEPTOR
RECERT	RECERTIFICATION
RECESS	RECESSION
RECIP	RECIPIENT
RECIPROCAT	RECIPROCATING
RECLIN	RECLINING
RECOM	RECOMMEND(ED)
RECOMB	RECOMBINANT
RECON	RECONSTRUCT(ED)(ION)(IVE)
RECONST	RECONSTRUCTIVE
RECR	RECRUITMENT
RECT	REC(TAL)(TUM)(TUS)
RECTSIG	RECTOSIGMOID
RECTURETH	RECTOURETHRAL
RECTVAG	RECTOVAGINAL
RECTVESC	RECTOVESICAL
RECUMBNT	RECUMBENT
RECUR	RECURRENCE, RECURRENT
RECV	RECEIVE(R)
RED	REDUC(ED)(TION)
REF	REFERENCE(S), REFERR(AL)(ED)(ING)
REFL	REFLUX
REFRIG	REFRIGERATOR
REFRM	REFORM
REG	RADIOENCEPHALOGRAM, REGU(LAR)(LATING)(LATION)(LATOR)
REGAIN	REGAINING
REGEN	REGENERATION
REGN	REGION(AL)
REGNING	REGAINING
REGURG	REGURGITATION
REHAB	REHABILITATION, REHABILITATIVE
REINS	REINSERT(ION)
REIT	REITER'S
REL	RELATE(D), RELATION
RELAPS	RELAPSING
RELAX	RELAXANTS
RELS	RELEASE
REM(AIN)	REMAINING, REMISSION
REMISS	REMISSION
REMV	REMOV(ABLE)(AL)(ALS)(ER)
REN(L)	RENAL
REP	REPAIR, REPRESENTATIVES
REPET	REPETITIVE
REPL	REPLACE(ABLE)(MENTS)
REPLACE	REPLACEMENT
REPLANT	REPLANTATION
REPOL	REPOLARIZATION
REPOS(IT)	REPOSITION(ING)
REPR	REPAIR(S)
REPRO(D)	REPRODUCTIVE
REPT	REPEAT, REPTILES
REQ	REQUESTED, REQUIR(ED)(ING)
RES	RESECTIONS, RESIDENCE, RESIDENT(IAL)
RESC	RESUSCITATION
RESECT	RESECTION
RESID	RESIDUAL
RESIN COMPOS	RESIN-BASED COMPOSITE
RESIST	RESIST(ANCE)(ANT)
RESL	RESULT(ING)(S)
RESLV	RESOL(UTION)(VED)(VING)
RESORB	RESORBABLE
RESORP	RESORPTION
RESP	RESPIRATION(S), RESPIRATORY
RESPON	RESPONS(E)(IVENESS)
RESPOND	RESPONDERS
RESRVOR	RESERVOIR
REST	RESTORATION
RESTRICT	RESTRICT(IVE)(ION)
RESULT	RESULTING
RET	RETAIN(ED)(ER), RETENTION, RETINAL
RET DETACH	RETINAL DETACHMENT
RETAIN	RETAINE(D)(R)
RETARD	RETARDATION
RETIC	RETICULOCYTE
RETICLD	RETICULOID
RETICSARC	RETICULOSARCOMA
RETICULOENDOTHELIOS	RETICULOENDOTHELIOSIS
RETICULR	RETICULAR
RETN	RETAIN, RETENTION, RETINA(L)
RETNIT	RETINITIS
RETNOP	RETINOPATHY
RETRACT	RETRACTILE
RETRBULB	RETROBULBAR
RETREAT	RETREATMENT
RETR(O)(GR)	RETROGRADE
RETROPERITON	RETROPERITONEAL
RETROPHARYNG	RETROPHARYNGEAL
RETROVERT	RETROVERTED
RETRPERIT	RETROPERITONE(AL)(UM)
RETRPHRYN	RETROPHARYNGEAL
RETRPUB	RETROPUBIC
RETRV	RETRIEVAL
RETRVERT	RETROVERTED
RETRX	RETRACTIONS
REUSBL	REUSABLE
REV	REVERS(AL)(E), RE(VIEW)(VISED)(VISION)
REVASC	REVASCULARIZATION
RF	RING FINGER
RGN	REGION(AL)
RGN BLK	REGIONAL BLOCK ANESTHESIA
RGNING	REGAINING
RHD	RHEUMATIC HEART DISEASE
RHEOLYT	RHEOLYTIC
RHES	RHESUS
RHEUM	RHEUMA(TISM)(TOID)(TIC)
RHINO	RHINOPLASTY

RHINOT	RHINOTOMY
RHLYT	RHEOLYTIC
RHOGAM	RHO IMMUNE GLOBULIN
RHYTH	RHYTHM
RHYTIDECT	RHYTIDECTOMY
RICK(ETTS)	RICKETTSIAL
RIFL	RIFLE
RIG(D)	RIGID
RIGD/FOLD TYPE	RIGID/FOLD TYPE
RK	RADIAL KERATOTOMY
RLND	ROLANDO'S
RLQ	RIGHT LOWER QUADRANT
RLSE	RELEASE
RMINGTN	REMINGTON
RMV	REMOV(ABLE)(AL)(E)
RN	REGISTERED NURSE, REFLUX NEPHROPATHY
RNEW	RENEW
RNG	RANGE, RING
ROCKR	ROCKER
ROLL	ROLLING
ROLL-CSTR	ROLLERCOASTER
ROLL-SKT	ROLLER-SKAT(E)(ER)(ES)(ING)
ROLL-TYP	ROLLING-TYPE
ROT(AT)	ROTA(TING)(TION)(TOR)
RP	RETROPERITONEUM
RPG	RETROGRADE PYELOGRAM
RPT	REPORT
RQR	REQUIRE(S), REQUIRING
RR	RAILWAY
RS	RESPIRATORY SYSTEM
RSIST	RESIST(ANCE)(ANT)
RSK	RISK
RSLT	RESULT(ING) (FROM)
RSN	REASON(S), RESIN
RSPN	RESPOND, RESPONSE(S)
RSRV	RESERVE(D)
RSTRC	RESTRICT
RSV	RESPIRATORY SYNCYTIAL VIRUS
RT	RIGHT
RTN	RETURN, ROUTINE
RTX	RADIATION THERAPY
RUBR	RUBBER
RUN	RUNNING
RUP(T)	RUPTURE(D)
RUQ	RIGHT UPPER QUADRANT
RVRS	REVERSE
RW	RAILWAY
RX	DRUG(S), PRESCRI(BED)(PTION)
RXN	REACTION(S)
RXTV	REACTIVE
SA	SUBARACHNOID, SUBCLAVIAN ARTERY, SPLENIC ARTERY
SA NODE	SINOATRIAL NODE
SAC	SACRAL
SACR	SACR(AL)(UM)
SACR(O)IL	SACROILIAC
SAG(IT)	SAGITTAL
SAILBT	SAILBOAT
SALIV	SALIVARY
SAL(M)	SALMONELLA
SALPGIT	SALPINGITIS
SALPINGECT	SALPINGECTOMY
SAMP	SAMPLE(S), SAMPLING(S)
SANG	SANGUINOUS
SAPH	SAPHENOUS
SAT	SATURATION, SUBACUTE THYROIDITIS
SB	STILLBORN
SBDRL	SUBDURAL
SBSTNC	SUBSTANCE(S)
SC	SCOP(E)(IC), STERNCLAVICULAR
SC JNT	STERNOCLAVICULAR JOINT
SCAN	SCANNING
SCAP	SCAPULA(E)(R)
SCAPH(D)	SCAPHOID
SCHED	SCHEDULE
SCHIZ	SCHIZOPHREN(IA)(IC)
SCHIZAFF	SCHIZOAFFECTIVE
SCHIZO	SCHIZOPHREN(IA)(IC)
SCIAT	SCIATIC
SCKT	SOCKET
SCLER	SCLERA
SCLEROS	SCLEROS(ING)(IS)
SCLP	SCALP
SCLS	SCALES
SCM	STERNOCLEIDOMASTOID
SCN	SCIATIC NERVE
SCNNR	SCANNERS
SCOL	SCOLIOSIS
SCOR	SCORING
SCRCOCC	SACROCOCCYGEAL
SCR(N)	SCREENING
SCROT	SCROT(AL)(UM)
SD	SEED(ING), SUBDURAL
SDL	SADDLE
SE	STATUS EPILEPTICUS
SEAFD	SEAFOOD
SEAL(NT)	SEALANT(S)
SEB	SEBACEOUS
SEBORR	SEBORRHEIC
SEC	SECONDARY, SECRETION, SECTION
SECT	SECTION(ING)(S)
SECTL	SECTIONAL
SED	SEDIMENTATION
SEDAT	SEDATION, SEDATIVE(S)
SEDTV	SEDATIVE
SEG	SEGMENT(S)(AL)
SEIZ(UR)	SEIZURE(S)
SEL	SELECT(ABILITY)(ED)(ION)(IVE)
SELF-HRM	SELF-HARM
SEM	SEM(EN)(INAL)
SEMILUN	SEMILUNAR
SEMINL	SEMINAL
SEMIPNUMAT	SEMIPNEUMATIC
SEN	SENIL(E)(ITY)
SENIL	SENILE
SENS	SENSITIVITY, SENSOR(Y)
SENSNEUR	SENSORINEURAL
SEP	SEPARA(TED)(TION), SEPERATELY
SEP PROC	SEPARATE PROCEDURE
SEPS	SEPSIS
SEPT	SEPT(AL)(UM)
SEPTECT	SEPTECTOMY
SEPTM	SEPTUM
SEPTOST	SEPTOSTOMY
SEPTPLSTY	SEPTOPLASTY
SEQ	SEQUELA(E), SEQUENCE(S), SEQUEN(CING)(TIAL), SEQUESTRATION
SEQECT	SEQUESTRECTOMY
SER	SEROUS
SERIALGRPH	SERIALOGRAPHY
SERO-SANG	SEROSANGUINEOUS
SESAMOIDECT	SESAMOIDECTOMY
SESS	SESSION
SET	SETTING
SEV(R)	SEVER(E)(ITY)
SEX	SEXUAL(ISM)(LY)
SEXL	SEXUAL
SFT	SOFT
SFTY	SAFETY
SG	SALIVARY GLAND, SEGMENT(S)(AL)
SGN	SIGNS
SGOT	SERUM GLUTAMIC OXALOACETIC TRANSAMINASE

SGPT	SERUM GLUTAMATE PYRUVATE TRANSAMINASE
SHAP	SHAPE(D), SHAPING
SHAV	SHAVING
SHFT	SHAFT
SHIG	SHIGELLA
SHL	SENSORINEURAL HEARING LOSS
SHLD(R)	SHOULDER
SHNK	SHANK
SHNT	SHUNT
SHOVE	SHOVED
SHRP	SHARP
SHRT	SHORT(ENING)
SHTH	SHEATH
SHX	SOCIAL HISTORY
SI	SACROILIAC
SIBS	SIBLINGS
SIDS	SUDDEN INFANT DEATH SYNDROME
SIG	SIGMOID, SIGNIFICANT
SIGNIF	SIGNIFI(CANCE)(CANT)
SILCON	SILICONE
SIM	SIMILAR
SIMUL	SIMULATION, SIMULTANEOUS
SIN	SINUS
SINK	SINKING
SINUSOT	SINUSOTOMY
SIS	SISTER
SITE	SITES
SK	SKULL
SKBRD	SKATEBOARD(ER)
SK(E)L	SKELET(AL)(ON)
SKILL	SKILLED
SKL	SKELET(AL)(ON), SKILL(S)
SKN	SKIN
SKUL	SKULL
SLAT-HAR	SLATER-HARRIS
SLD	SLID(E)(ING)
SLF	SELF
SLF-ALIGN	SELF-ALIGNING
SLF-CONTAIND	SELF-CONTAINED
SL(I)P	SLIPPED, SLIPPING
SLT-HRS	SALTER HARRIS
SM	SMALL(ER), STATUS MIGRAINOSUS
SMA	SUPERIOR MESENTERIC ARTERY
SMER	SMEAR
SMK	SMOKE
SMPL	SIMPLE
SMPX	SMALLPOX
SMR	SKELETAL MUSCLE RELAXANTS
SMTH	SMITH'S
SMTHR	SMOTHERING
SMX	SUBMAXILLARY
SN	SYMPATHETIC NERVE
SNF	SKILLED NURSING FACILITY
SNK	SNAKE
SNSRY	SENSORY
SNW	SNOW
SNWBRD	SNOWBOARD(ER)
SNWICE	SNOWICE
SNWMOB	SNOWMOBILE
SNW-SKI	SNOW-SKI(ER)(S)
S-O	SALPINGO-OOPHORECTOMY
SO AMER	SOUTH AMERICAN
SO4	SULFATE
SOB	SHORTNESS OF BREATH
SOC	SOCIAL, STATE OF CONSCIOUSNESS
SOCKT	SOCKET
SOCL	SOCIAL
SODIM	SODIUM
SOL	SOLUTION
SOLD	SOLID
SOLV	SOLVENT(S)
SOLVNT	SOLVENT
SOM	SUPPURATIVE OTITIS MEDIA
SOMAT	SOMATIC
SONO	SONOGRAM
SP	SPIN(AL)(E), SEPARATE PROCEDURE, SOFT PALATE
SP FL	SPINAL FLUID
SP TAP	SPINAL TAP
SP TUBE	SUPRAPUBIC TUBE
SPACECRFT	SPACECRAFT
SPACR	SPACER
SPAS	SPASTIC
SPC	SPACE
SPCH	SPEECH
SPCL	SPECIAL
SPCL ED	SPECIAL EDUCATION
SPCRFT	SPACECRAFT
SPCT	SUSPECT(ED)
SPEC	SPECIAL(IZED), SPECIFI(CALLY) (CATIONS), SPECI(FIED)(FY)(MEN) (MENS)
SPECM	SPECIMEN(S)
SPECT	SINGLE-PHOTON EMISSION COMPUTED TOMOGRAPHY, SPECTACLE
SPECTRMTRY	SPECTROMETRY
SPECTRNET	SPECTRANETICS
SPECTRNT	SPECTRANETICS
SPHEN	SPHENOID(AL)
SPHENOIDECT	SPHENOIDECTOMY
SPHENOIDOT	SPHENOIDOTOMY
SPHER	SPHERE
SPHINCTROT	SPHINCTEROTOMY
SPHINCTRPLSTY	SPHINCTEROPLASTY
SPHNCT(R)	SPHINCTER
SPID	SPIDER
SPIROMT(RY)	SPIROMETR(IC)(Y)
SPL	SUPPLIES, SUPPLY
SPLEN	SPLEEN, SPLENIC
SPLENECT	SPLENECTOMY
SPLNT	SPLINT(ING)
SPN	SPINE
SPNDLTHSIS	SPONDYLOLISTHESIS
SPOKE	SPOKES
SPONDYL	SPONDYLO(PATHIES)(PATHY)(SIS)
SPONDYLITH	SPONDYLOLISTHESIS
SPONG	SPONGIOSUM
SPONT	SPONTANEOUS
SPRCOND	SUPRACONDYLAR
SPRL	SPIRAL
SPRN	SPRAIN
SPRNG	SPRING
SPS	SIMPLE PARTIAL SEIZURES
SPUT	SPUTUM
SQ	SQUAMOUS, SQUARE
SR	SUSTAINED RELEASE
SRC	SOURCE(S)
SRCOM	SARCOMA
SRG	SURGERY, SURGICAL(LY)
SRI	SEROTONIN REUPTAKE INHIBITORS
SRVC	SERVICE(S)
SSN	SOCIAL SECURITY NUMBER
ST	SUBTROCHANTERIC
STAIR	STAIRS
STAPEDECT	STADPEDECTOMY
STAPEDOT	STAPEDOTOMY
STAPH	STAPHYLO(COCCAL)(COCCUS)(MA)
STARY	SOLITARY
STAT	STAT(IC)(US)
STATN	STATIONARY
STATUT	STATUTORILY
STBL	STABILIZATION, STABLE

STD	SEXUALLY TRANSMITTED DISEASE(S), STANDARD(S)
STDNT	STUDENT
STDY	STUDIES, STUDY
STEEPR	STEEPER
STEERABL	STEERABLE
STEN(OS)	STENOS(ING)(IS)
STENT	STENTING
STEREO	STEROPSIS
STEREOT(AC)(X)	STEREO(TACTIC)(TAXIS)
STERL(IZ)	STERIL(E)(IZATION)
STERN	STERN(AL)(UM)
STERNCLAV	STERNOCLAVICULAR
STETH	STETHOSCOPE
STG	STAGE
STIFF	STIFFNESS
STILLB	STILLBORN
STIM	STIMU(LANT)(LATING)(LATION)(LATOR)
STIRUP	STIRRUP
STK	STOCKING
STMBL	STUMBLING
STND	STANDARDIZED
STNLESS	STAINLESS
STNT	STENT
STOM	STOMACH
STOR	STORAGE, STORE
STR	STRAIN
STRAB	STRABISMUS
STRAIT	STRAIGHT
STRANG	STRANGULA(TE)(TED)(TION)
STRANGULAT	STRANGULATED
STRAP	STRAPPING
STRBOSC	STROBOSCOPY
STRCAR	STREETCAR
STRCT	STRUCTURAL, STRUCTURE(S)
STREP	STREPTOCOCCAL, STREPTOCOCCUS
STRGTH	STRENGTH
STRICT	STRICTURE(S)
STRICTURPLSTY	STRICTUROPLASTY
STRIK	STRIKING
STRIP	STRIPPING
STRK	STRIKING, STRUCK
STRN	STRAIN
STRNG	STRANGULATED
STRNL	STERNAL
STRNM	STERNUM
STRNOCLEIDOMSTOID	STERNOCLEIDOMASTOID
STROBOSCPY	STROBOSCOPY
STRSS	STRESS
STRTR	STARTER
STRUCT	STRUCTUR(AL)(E)
STS	STATUS
STSG	SPLIT THICKNESS SKIN GRAFT
STYL	STYLE, STYLOID
SUB	SUBSEQUENT(LY), SUBSTITUTES
SUBAC	SUBACUTE
SUBACROM	SUBACROMIAL
SUBARACH	SUBARACHNOID
SUBAROT	SUBAROTIC
SUBCAPS	SUBCAPSULAR
SUBCHR	SUBCHRONIC
SUBCLV	SUBCLAVIAN
SUBCONJUNCT	SUBCONJUNCTIVAL
SUBCORT	SUBCORTICAL
SUBDELT	SUBDELTOID
SUBDRM	SUBDERMAL
SUBDUR	SUBDURAL
SUBEND	SUBENDOCARDIAL
SUBEPITH	SUBEPITHELIAL
SUBFASC	SUBFASCIAL
SUBJ	SUBJECTIVE
SUBL(NG)	SUBLINGUAL
SUBLUX	SUBLUXATION
SUBMAND	SUBMANDIBULAR
SUBMAX	SUBMAXILLARY
SUBMER(S)	SUBMERSION
SUBMNTL	SUBMENTAL
SUBMUC	SUBMU(COSAL)(COUS)
SUBMUSC	SUBMUSCULAR
SUBPERIOST	SUBPERIOSTEAL
SUBQ	SUBCUTANEOUS
SUBS	SUBSTANCE(S)
SUBSEG	SUBSEGMENTAL
SUBSQT	SUBSEQUENT(LY)
SUBST	SUBSTANCE(S), SUBSTI(TUTE)(TUTION)
SUBSTERN	SUBSTERNAL
SUBSTRN	SUBSTERNAL
SUBTOT	SUBTOTAL
SUBTRACT	SUBTRACTION
SUBTROCH	SUBTROCHANTERIC
SUBVALV	SUBVALVULAR
SUC	SUCCESS(FUL)
SUCC	SUCCINIMIDES
SUCCNAT	SUCCINATE
SUCTN	SUCTION
SUDD	SUDDEN
SUFF(OCAT)	SUFFOCATION
SUGG	SUGGESTIVE
SUGR	SUGAR
SUI(C)	SUICIDE
SULF	SULFUR
SULFAT	SULFATE
SUN	SUNDAYS
SUP	SUPERFICIAL(IS), SUPERIOR, SUPERVIS(ED)(ING)(ION), SUPINATION
SUPCONDYL	SUPRACONDYLAR
SUPINATR	SUPINATOR
SUPL(MNTL)	SUPPLEMENT(AL)(S), SUPPL(IES)(Y)
SUPP	SUPPERATIVE, SUPPORT(D)(TIVE), SUPPOSITORY
SUPPOS	SUPPOSITORY
SUPPR	SUPPRESSION
SUPPUR	SUPPURATIVE
SUPRAGLOT	SUPRAGLOTTIC
SUPRATENTOR	SUPRATENTORIAL
SUPRGLOTT	SUPRAGLOTTIC
SUPRORB	SUPRAORBITAL
SUPRPUB	SUPRAPUBIC
SUPRV	SUPERVISION
SUPSCAP	SUPRASCAPULAR
SUPTENT	SUPRATENTORIAL
SUR	SURGEON(S)
SURF	SURFACE(S)
SURG	SURGERY, SURGICAL
SURV	SURVEILLANCE
SURVL	SURVIVAL
SUSECPT	SUSCEPTIBILITY
SUSP	SUSPECT(ED), SUS(PEND)(PENSION)(PENSORY)
SUT	SUTURE, SUTURING
SUV	SPORT UTILITY VEHICLE
SV	SAPHENOUS VEIN, SUPTRAVENTRICULAR
SVC	SERVICE(S)
SWALL	SWALLOWING
SWELL	SWELLING
SWG	SWING
SWIM	SWIM(MER)(MING)
SWMR	SWIMMER
SWTCH	SWITCH
SX	SYMPTOM(S), SYMPTOMATIC
SYMBLEPH	SYMBLEPHARON
SYMM	SYMMETRICAL
SYMP(ATHECT)	SYMPATHECTOMY, SYMPATHETIC

SYMPATHET	SYMPATHETIC
SYMPATHOMIMET	SYMPATHOMIMETIC
SYMPH	SYMPHYSIS
SYMPHYSIOT	SYMPHYSIOTOMY
SYN	SYNOVIAL
SYNCH	SYNCHRONOUS
SYNCHRMD	SYNCHROMED
SYND	SYNDROME(S)
SYNDACT	SYNDACTYLY
SYNOST	SYNOSTOSIS
SYNOV	SYNOVI(AL)(UM)
SYNOVECT	SYNOVECTOMY
SYNOVIT	SYNOVITIS
SYNRGY	SYNERGY
SYNTH	SYNTHETIC
SYPH	SYPHI(LIS)(LITIC)
SYPHLIT	SYPHILITIC
SYR	SYRINGE
SYRP	SYRUP
SYS(T)	SYSTEM(IC)(S)
SYST BP	SYSTOLIC BLOOD PRESSURE
SYST(OL)	SYSTOLIC
SZ	SEIZURE, SIZE
T CELL	SMALL LYMPHOCYTE
T&A	TONSILLECTOMY AND ADENOIDECTOMY, TONSILS AND ADENOIDS
T&H	TYPE AND HOLD
T&S	TYPE AND SCREEN
T&X	TYPE AND CROSS MATCH
T1-T12	THORACIC VERTEBRAE 1 THROUGH 12
T4	THYROXINE
TA	TEMPORAL ARTERY
TAB	TABLET
TAH	TOTAL ABDOMINAL HYSTERECTOMY
TAHBSO	TOTAL ABDOMINAL HYSTERECTOMY BILATERAL SALPINGO-OOPHORECTOMY
TAL	TALUS
TALNT	TALENT
TAPR	TAPERING
TARS	TARSAL
TARSCNJCT	TARSOCONJUNCTIVAL
TARSORR	TARSORRHAPHY
TART	TARTRATE
TATT	TATTOO(ING)
TB	TUBERCULOSIS
TBA	TO BE ANNOUNCED, TO BE ARRANGED, TO BE ASSESSED, TOTAL BODY AREA
TBD	TO BE DETERMINED
TBE	TO BE EVALUATED
TBL	TABLESPOON
TBOMA	TUBERCULOMA
TBSA	TOTAL BODY SURFACE AREA
TBT	TRACHEOBRONCHIAL TREE
TCP	THROMBOCYTOPENIA
TE	TRACHEOESOPHAGEAL
TEAR/INJ	TEAR OR INJURY
TECH	TECH(NICAL)(NICIAN)(NIQUE)(NIQUES)(NOLOGIST)(NOLOGY)
TECHTUM	TECHNETIUM
TEDS	THROMBOEMBOLIC DISEASE STOCKINGS
TEL	TELEMETRIC, TELEMETRY, TELEPHONE, TELEPHONIC
TELANG	TELANGIECTAS(IA)(IS)
TEMP	TEMPERATURE, TEMPORAL(LY), TEMPORARY
TEND	TENDON(S)
TENODSIS	TENODESIS
TENOSYN	TENOSYNOVITIS
TENOT	TENOTOMY
TENPLSTY	TENOPLASTY
TENS	TENSION, TRANSCUTANEOUS ELECTRICAL NERVE STIMULATION
TERM	TERMINAL, TERMINATION, TERMINOLOGY
TERR	TERROR(ISM)(IST)
TERT	TERTIARY
TEST	TEST(ES)(ICLE)(ICULAR)(IS)
TESTO(ST)	TESTOSTERONE
TET	TETENANUS, TETRACHLORIDE
TETH	TETHERED
TH	THORACIC, THORAX, THROAT
TH CULT	THROAT CULTURE
THAL	THALA(MUS)(SSEMIA)
THCK	THICKENING
THEOPH	THEOPHYLLINE
THI	THIGH
THICK	THICKNESS
THMB	THUMB
THOR	THORACIC, THORAX
THORACOT	THORACOTOMY
THORACPLSTY	THORACOPLASTY
THORACSCPY	THORACOSCOPY
THORC	THORA(CIC)(X)
THORCABD	THORACOABDOMINAL
THORCLUMB	THORACOLUMBAR
THR	THYROID
THREAT	THREATENING
THRESH	THRESHOLD
THRMB	THROM(BOSED)(BOSIS)(BOTIC)
THRMBANGIIT	THROMBOANGIITIS
THRMBCT	THROMBECTOMY
THRMBOLYT	THROMBOLYTIC
THRMBPHLEB	THROMBOPHLEBITIS
THRML	THERMAL
THROMB	THROMBOSIS, THROMBUS
THROMBECT	THROMBECTOMY
THROMBENDART	THROMBOENDARTERECTOMY
THROMBOPHLEB	THROMBOPHLEBITIS
THRT	THROAT
THRU	THROUGH
THRWN	THROWN
THYMECT	THYMECTOMY
THYR(D)	THYROID
THYRGLOSS	THYROGLOSSAL
THYRIT	THYROIDITIS
THYROIDECT	THYROIDECTOMY
THYRTOX	THYROTOXICOSIS
TIA	TRANSIENT ISCHEMIC ATTACK
TIB	THYROTOXIC, TIBIA(L)(LIS)
TIBFIB	TIBIOFIBULAR
TIBPERON	TIBIOPERONEAL
TILLR	TILLER
TINCT	TINCTURE
TIP	TIPPED
TISS	TISSUE(S)
TM	TEAM, TIME
TMJ	TEMPOROMANDIBULAR JOINT
TMT	TARSOMETATARSOL
T-NAIL	TOENAIL
TND	TENDON(S)
TNDNIT	TENDINITIS
TOBAC	TOBACCO
TOL(ERNC)	TOLERANCE
TOLL	TOLLS
TOMOGRPH	TOMOGRAPH(IC)(Y)
TONG	TONGUE
TOP	TOPICAL
TORQ	TORQUE
TORS	TORSION
TOT	TOTAL
TOX	TOX(EMIA)(IC)(IN)(OIDS)
TOXPLAS(MOS)	TOXOPLASMOSIS

TP	THROMBOPHLEBITIS
TPLNT	TRANSPLANT(ATIONS)(ED)(S)
TPN	TOTAL PARENTERAL NUTRITION
TR	TRACHEA(L)
TRABECULECT	TRABECULECTOMY
TRAC	TRACTION
TRACH	TRACHEA(L), TRACHEOSTOMY
TRACHBRONCH	TRACHEOBRONCHIAL
TRACHELECT	TRACHELECTOMY
TRACHEOPHARYNG	TRACHEOPHARYNGEAL
TRACHEORR	TRACHEORRHAPHY
TRACHEOST	TRACHEOSTOMY
TRACHEOT	TRACHEOTOMY
TRACHEPLSTY	TRACHEOPLASTY
TRACHESCPY	TRACHEOSCOPY
TRACHOMAT	TRACHOMATIS
TRACHPHRYN	TRACHEOPHARYNGEAL
TRACK	TRACKING
TRACTOT	TRACTOTOMY
TRAFF	TRAFFIC
TRAM	TRANSVERSE RECTUS ABDOMINOUS MYOCUTANEOUS FLAP
TRANQ	TRANQUILIZER(S)
TRANSPHLNG	TRANSPHALANGEAL
TRANSPL	TRANSPLANTATION
TRAP	TRAPPED
TRAPEZ	TRAPEZE
TRAPZ	TRAPEZ(IUM)(OID)
TRAUM	TRAUMA(TIC)
TRAUMAT	TRAUMATIC
TRCK	TRUCK
TRCT	TRACT
TREATD	TREATED
TREN	TRENDELENBURG
TREPHINAT	TREPHINATION
TRF	TRAFFIC
TRI	TRIMESTER
TRIAN	TRIANGULAR
TRICH	TRICH(IASIS)(OMONAS)
TRICP	TRICEPS
TRICSP(D)	TRICUSPID
TRIFASC	TRIFASCICULAR
TRIFOC(L)	TRIFOCAL
TRIG	TRIGGER
TRIGEM	TRIGEMINAL
TRIMAL	TRIMALLEOLAR
TRIMSTR	TRIMESTER
TRIP(L)(LT)	TRIPLET
TRIQ	TRIQUETRUM
TRK	TRACK(ING)
TRN	TRAIN(ING)
TRNK	TRUNK
TRNS	TRANSVENOUS, TRANSVERSE
TRNSCATH	TRANSCATHETER
TRNSCNDYL	TRANSCONDYLAR
TRNSDUODEN	TRANSDUODENAL
TRNSECT	TRANSECTION
TRNSF	TRANSFER(RED)(S), TRANSFUSION
TRNSFORM	TRANSFORMATION
TRNSIT	TRANSI(TION)(TORY)
TRNSITIONL	TRANSITIONAL
TRNSITRY	TRANSITORY
TRNSLOC(AT)	TRANSLOCATION
TRNSLUM	TRANSLUMINAL
TRNSLUMB	TRANSLUMBAR
TRNSMC	TRANSMETACARPAL
TRNSMIT	TRANSMITTED
TRNSMRL	TRANSMURAL
TRNSMS	TRANSMISSION
TRNSMT	TRANSMIT(TER)
TRNSMYOCARD	TRANSMYOCARDIAL
TRNSPERITON	TRANSPERITONEAL
TRNSPL	TRANSPLANT(ATION)(ED)
TRNSPOS	TRANSPOSITION
TRNSPRT	TRANSPARENT, TRANSPORT(ATION)
TRNSPSTN	TRANSPOSITION
TRNSPT	TRANSPORT
TRNSPUPLLRY	TRANSPUPILLARY
TRNSQ	TRANSCUTANEOUS
TRNST	TRANSFERRED, TRANSIENT
TRNSTEMPRL	TRANSTEMPORAL
TRNSURETEROURETEROST	TRANSURETEROURETEROSTOMY
TRNSURETH	TRANSURETHRAL
TRNSV	TRANSVERSE
TRNSVEN	TRANSVENOUS
TRNSV-POST	TRANSVERSE-POSTERIOR
TROCH	TROCHANTER(IC)
TROPHBLAS	TROPHOBLASTIC
TRPST	THERAPIST(S)
TRVL	TRAVEL
TRYPANOS	TRYPANOSOMIASIS
TSH	THYROID STIMULATING HORMONE
TSN	THORACIC SYMPATHETIC NERVE
TSP	TEASPOON
T-SPINE	THORACIC SPINE
TST	TEST(ING)
TU	TRANSURETHRAL
TUBERCL	TUBERCLE
TUBEROS	TUBEROSITY
TUBULARIZ	TUBULARIZATION
TUM(R)	TUMOR
TUN(NLD)	TUNNELED
TUNA	TRANURETHRAL NEEDLE ABLATION
TUR BLDR	TRANSURETHRAL RESECTION OF THE BLADDER
TURB(IN)	TURBINATE
TURP	TRANSURETHRAL RESECTION OF PROSTATE
TV	THORACIC VERTEBRAE, TRICUSPID VALVE
TVH	TOTAL VAGINAL HYSTERECTOMY
T-WAVE	VENTRICULAR REPOLARIZATION
TX	TREATMENT(S), THERAP(EUTIC)(Y), TRACTION
TX EX	THERAPEUTIC EXERCISE
TYMP	TYMPANIC, TYMPANO(GRAM)(PLASTY)(STOMY)
TYMPSCLER(OS)	TYMPANOSCLEROSIS
TYP	TYPE
TYPANOT	TYMPANOTOMY
TYPE	TYPING
TYPH	TYPHOID
U	UNIT
UA	URINALYSIS
UE	UPPER EXTREMITY
UGI	UPPER GASTROINTESTINAL SERIES
UI	UPPER-INNER
UL	UPPER LOBE, UPPER LIMB
ULC	ULCER(ATION)(ATIVE)
ULCGLND	ULCEROGLANDULAR
ULCR	ULCER
ULN	ULNA(R)
ULNHUM	ULNOHUMERAL
ULTRLGT	ULTRALIGHT
ULTSENS	ULTRASENSITIVE
UMB	UMBILICAL
UNAGGRESS	UNAGGRESSIVE
UNCERT	UNCERTAIN
UNCMPL	UNCOMPLICATED
UNCNTRL	UNCONTROLLED
UNCNVN(TIONL)	UNCONVENTIONAL
UNCOMP	UNCOMPLICATED
UNCRTN	UNCERTAIN
UNCTRL	UNCONTROLLED

UND UNDER
UNDERLY UNDERLYING
UNDESC UNDESCENDED
UNDET(RM) UNDETERMINE(D)
UNDIFF UNDIFFERENTIATED
UNDRACHV UNDERACHIEVEMENT
UNDRDOS UNDERDOSING
UNDRLY UNDERLYING
UNDRSOC UNDERSOCIALIZED
UNERUPTD UNERUPTED
UNEXPL UNEXPLAINED
UNI UNILATERAL
UNICOND UNICONDYLAR
UNINTN UNINTENTIONAL
UNINTRPED UNINTERRUPTED
UNKN UNKNOWN
UNL UNLESS, UNLISTED
UNPWR UNPOWER(ED)
UNREL UNRELATED
UNS UNSPECIFIED
UNSAT UNSATURATED
UNSCH UNSCHEDULED
UNSTB(L) UNSTABLE
UNSUC UNSUCCESSFUL
UNUSUAL UNUSUALLY
UO UPPER-OUTER
UP UPPER
UPGRD UPGRADE
UPHLSTR UPHOLSTERY
UR URINARY
URETER URETHERAL
URETERECT URETERECTOMY
URETERGRAPH URETEROGRAPHY
URETERNEOCYSTOST URETERONEOCYSTOSTOMY
URETEROPYELGRPH URETEROPYELOGRAPHY
URETEROST URETEROSTOMY
URETERSCPY URETEROSCOPY
URETERSIGMOIDOST URETEROSIGMOIDOSTOMY
URETH(RAL) URETHERAL
URETHRPLSTY URETHROPLASTY
URETR URETER(AL)
URETRL URETERAL
URG URGENT
URI UPPER RESPIRATORY INFECTION
URIN URIN(ARY)(E)
UROGEN UROGENITAL
UROGRPH UROGRAPHY
US ULTRASONIC, ULTRASOUND
UTER(N) UTER(INE)(US)
UTI URINARY TRACT INFECTION
UTIL UTIL(ITY)(IZATION)(IZE)(IZING)
UTRUS UTERUS
UV ULTRAVIOLET
UW UNCONVENTIONAL WARFARE
V VERBAL, VOLT
VA VERTEBRAL ARTERY
VAC(C) VACCINATION, VACCINE(S), VACUUM,
VAD VASCULAR ACCESS DEVICE
VAG VAGINA(L)(LIS)
VAGINECT VAGNIECTOMY
VAGNIT VAGINITIS
VAGOT VAGOTOMY
VALT VAULT
VALV VALVE
VALVOT VALVOTOMY
VALVULPLSTY VALVULOPLASTY
VANGRD VANGUARD
VAP VAPOR(IZATION)(S)
VAPORIZ VAPORIZATION
VAR VARIABLE
VARIBL VARIABLE
VARIC VARICES
VARICOS VARICOSE
VASC(IT) VASCUL(AR)(ITIS)
VASDIL VASODILATORS
VASGRPH VASOGRAPHY
VASOT VASOTOMY
VBAC VAGINAL BIRTH AFTER CESAREAN
VC VARICOSE, VENA CAVA, VOCAL CORD
VCL VOCAL
VEG VEGETABLES
VEH VEHICLE(S)
VEL VELOCITY
VEN(M) VENOM(OUS)
VENT VENTILATION, VENTILATOR, VENTRICLE, VENTRICULAR
VENTRICGRM VENTRICULOGRAM
VENTRICGRPH VENTRICULOGRAPHY
VENTRICULOMYOT VENTRICULOMYOTOMY
VENTRL VENTRAL
VERBL VERBAL
VERFICATN VERIFICATION
VERT VERTEBRA(L)
VERT-BAS VERTEBRO-BASILAR
VERTICL VERTICAL
VERTPLSTY VERTEBROPLASTY
VES VESSEL(S)
VESCL VESICLE(S)
VESCURTR-RFLX VESICOURETERAL-REFLUX
VESCUTER VESICOUTERINE
VESCVAG VESICOVAGINAL
VESICOURTRL VESICOURETERAL
VESICULGRPH VESICULOGRAPHY
VESS VESSEL(S)
VEST VESTIBU(LAR)(LE)
VG VENUS GRAFT
VIAB VIABILITY
VIB VIBRATION
VICT VICTIM
VID VIDEO
VILL VILLAGE
VILLNOD VILLONODULAR
VIR VIRUS
VIRL VIRAL
VIS VIS(IBLE)(ION)(UAL)
VISC VISCERAL
VISL VISUAL
VISN VISION
VIT VITAMIN
VITR VITREOUS
VITRECT VITRECTOMY
VLOCTY VELOCITY
VLR VOLAR
VLV VALVE(S)
VN VEIN(S), VENOUS
VNEREL VENEREAL
VNOM VENOM(OUS)
VNRL VENEREAL
VNS VEINS
VOCAB VOCABULARY
VOID VOIDING
VOL(M) VOLUME(TRIC), VOLUNTEER
VOLUN VOLUNTEER
VOLV VOLVULUS
VP VENTRICULO-PERITONEAL
VRC VARICELLA
VRITY VARIETY
VRL VIRAL
VRNL VERNAL
VRT VERTICLE
VRTC VERTICAL
VRTGO VERTIGO
VS VENTRICULAR SEPTUM
VST VISIT

VTACH	VENTRICULAR TACHYCARDIA
VULVECT	VULVECTOMY
W/	WITH
W/I(N)	WITHIN
W/O	WITHOUT
W/WO	WITH OR WITHOUT
WAIV	WAIVER
WALK	WALKER, WALKING
WAR(FAR)	WARFARE
WASH	WASHINGS
WATR	WATER
WATRCRFT	WATERCRAFT
WBC	WHITE BLOOD COUNT
WC	WHEELCHAIR
WDG	WEDGE
WDRL	WITHDRAWAL
WDTH	WIDTH
WDW	WIDOW
WEBSTR	WEBSTER
WGTLESS	WEIGHT(LESS)(LESSNESS)
WHCH	WHICH
WHETH	WHETHER
WHL	WHEEL(ED)
WHLCHAIR	WHEELCHAIR
WHLS	WHEELS
WHOOP	WHOOPING
WK	WEEK(LY)(S)
WKNS	WEAKNESS
WND(S)	WOUND(S)
WNDW	WINDOW
WOMAN	WOMANS
WPN(S)	WEAPON(S)
WRK	WORK(ING)
WRST	WRIST
WSH	WASHED
WT	WEIGHT(ED)(ING)
WTR	WATER
WTR-BAL	WATER-BALANCE
WTRCRFT	WATERCRAFT
WTR-SKI	WATER-SKI(ER)(S)
WV	WAVE(S)
XACRBAT	EXACERBATE
XAN	XANTHELASMA
XARTIC	EXTRAARTIC
XCESS	EXCESS
XCITMNT	EXCITEMENT
XER	XEROSIS
XERO	XERODERMA
XIPH	XIPHOID
X-MATCH	CROSSMATCH
XPND	EXPAND(ED)
X-RAY	RADIOGRAPHIC IMAGES
XST	EXIST(ING)
XTRA	EXTRA
XTRACAPSLR	EXTRACAPSULAR
XTRACORP	EXTRACORPOREAL
XTRACRAN	EXTRACRANIAL
XTRADURL	EXTRADURAL
XTRAMEDLLRY	EXTRAMEDULLARY
XTRANOD	EXTRANODAL
XTRAOCULR	EXTRAOCULAR
XTRAORL	EXTRAORAL
XTRAPER	EXTRAPERITONEAL
XTRCT	EXTRACT
YAG	YTTRIUM ALUMINUM GARNET (LASER)
YD	YARD
YNG	YOUNG
YR	YEAR(S)
ZN	ZINC
ZOOPLSTC	ZOOPLASTIC
ZSTR	ZOSTER
ZYG(O)	ZYGOMA(TIC)